ICD~10~CM
Complete Draft Code Set
2015

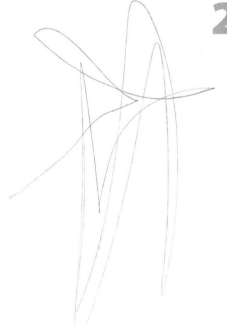

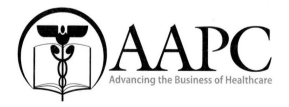

AAPC
Advancing the Business of Healthcare

PUBLISHER'S NOTICE

Coding, billing, and reimbursement decisions should not be made based solely upon information within this ICD-10-CM code book. Application of the information in this book does not imply or guarantee claims payment. Make inquiries of your local carriers' bulletins, policy announcements, etc., to resolve local billing requirements. Finally, the law, applicable regulations, payers' instructions, interpretations, enforcement, etc., of ICD-10-CM codes may change at any time in any particular area. Information in this book is solely based on ICD-10-CM rules and regulations.

This ICD-10-CM is designed to be an accurate and authoritative source regarding coding, and every reasonable effort has been made to ensure accuracy and completeness of content. However, this publisher makes no guarantee, warrantee, or representation that this publication is complete, accurate, or without errors. It is understood that this publisher is not rendering any legal or professional services or advice in this code book and bears no liability for any results or consequences arising from use of this ICD-10-CM book.

AAPC'S COMMITMENT TO ACCURACY

This publisher is committed to providing our members accurate and reliable materials. However, codes and the guidelines by which they are applied change or are reinterpreted through the year. Check www.aapc.com periodically for updates. To report corrections and updates, please contact AAPC Customer Service via 1-800-626-2633 or via email to code.books@aapc.com.

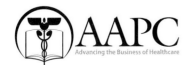
AAPC
Advancing the Business of Healthcare

Copyright 2014 © AAPC
ISBN: 978-1-626881-662

ACKNOWLEDGEMENTS PAGE

Reviewers:

We wish to acknowledge the following AAPC members for helping with the development of the 2015 ICD-10-CM Draft code book. We are extremely grateful to them for sharing their expertise and experience.

Alysia Martinez, CPC-A

Angela Teasley

Anita Robinson, CPC, CPC-H, CPC-P, CPMA, CPC-I

Anja Aplan, CPC

Belinda Shaw, RHIT, CCS, CPC

Betty Hovey, CPC, CPC-H, CPB, CPMA, CPC-I, CPCD

Beverly Abernathy, CPC

Brenda Edwards, CPC, CPB, CPMA, CPC-I, CEMC

Brooke Bierman, CPC

Camille Y. Betters, CPC, CMC, CMOM

Cathy Jennings, BS, CPC, CEDC, CHONC

Chandra Stephenson, CPC, CPC-H, CPCO, CPMA, CPC-I CANPC, CEMC, CFPC, CGSC, CIMC, COSC

Chastity Radcliff, CPC, CPMA

Danielle Wombough CPC-P

Darlene Britton, CPC, CPC-I, CEDC, RHIT

Darrelyn Rodman, CPC-A

Deborah Frizzle CPC, CIMC

Deborah Santos, CPC, CPMA

Diana Vincent, CPC

Elaine Griffel, CPC

Ellen Ontko, CPC

Geanetta Johnson Agbona, CPC, CPC-I, CBCS

Gerry Pape, BA, CPC

Hope Dendy, CPC, CPC-P

Ila Callagan, CPC

Irene Castillo Leon, CPC, CEMC

Irene Quast-Beck, CPC, CPCO, CPMA, CPPM, CEMC

Jackie Stack, CPC, CPB, CPC-I, CEMC, CFPC, CIMC, CPEDC

Jacqueline Baer, RN, MSN, CPC-H

Jennifer Bartunek, CPC, CPB

Jerri Freeman, CPC, CPC-P, CPC-I

Joyce McCoy, CPC

Judy Wilson

Julie Lytle, CPC-A

Karen K. Tritz, CPC

Karen Leonard, CPC, CPMA

Katalin Kerekes, CPC, CMCO

Kathleen Galioto, CPC-A

Katrina R. Tweedy, CPC, CPMA

Kent Williston BA, MS, CPC

Kim Pasienza, CPC

Kim Pichon, CPC

Kimberly Kiper-Mills, CPC

Kristy Urban, CPC

Lena Staniscia,CPC

Leonta Julien-Williams, CPC

Lillian J. Galindo-Bryson, CPC

Linda Bovis, RN, CPC

Linda Gilbreath, CPC, CPC-I, CPC-H, CEMC, AHFI, CHCA

Linda Vargas, CPC, CPC-I, CEMC

Lisa A. Oakes CPC

Loretta Gaither, CPC, COBGC

Lynn Rawlings, CPC, CPMA, CPC-I, CCVTC, CEMC, CCVTC

Marcie Barker, CPC, CPMA

Maria Puerto, CPC-H, CPMA

Marie Guido, CPC-A

Martha B (Martie) Gaskin

Martha Sims-Green, BS, CPC

Mary E. Wilds, CPC, CEMC

Mary Homer, CPC, CPC-H, CIRCC, CPC-I

Melody Irvine, CPC, CPMA, CPC-I, CEMC, CFPC

Melody Whilden, CPC

Michael Ann Fowler, CPC, CPMA, CPC-I

Michelle Lane, CPC-A

N. Carol Mitchell, CPC

Nancy Clark, CPC, CPB, CPMA, CPC-I

Patricia Henry, CPC, CCA

Paula M Wright, CPC, CIRCC, CPMA, CEMC, CPC-I

Pearl Evelyn Parker-Hartfield, CPC-A

Peggy Stilley, CPC, CPB, CPMA, CPC-I, COBGC

Rhonda Buckholtz, CPC, CPMA, CPC-I, CENTC, CGSC, COBGC, CPEDC

Ronda Seubert, BSBM, CPC

Rose Gibbs, CPC

Rose Mukkadan, CPC

Ruby Woodward, BSN, CPC, COSC,

Sandra Pedersen, CPC, CEMC, CPMA

Sarah Mros, RHIT, CPC, CPMA

Shelia G. Hickman, RHIT, CPC

Shelly Noll, CPC, CHONC

Shirley Holtz, CCS-P, CPC-H, CPC, ACS-AN

Stacey L. Murphy, MPA, RHIA, CPC

Staci Foster, CPC

Susan O'Loughlin

Susan Ward, CPC, CPC-H, CPC-I, CEMC, CPCD, CPRC

Susie Kottkamp, CPC

Suzanne L. Haile, CPC

Suzette Long, CPC, CPC-H

Thomas Penta, CPC, CCS, CHDA, PMP

Valerie Jones, CPC

Valerie McClanahan, CPC

Vanessa Coles, RHIT, CPC, CPMA, CEMC

Yvonne Dailey, CPC, CPB, CPC-I

Table of Contents ICD-10-CM

ICD-10-CM Official Preface

This 2015 update of the International Classification of Diseases and, 10th revision, Clinical Modification (ICD-10-CM) is being published by the United States Government in recognition of its responsibility to promulgate this classification throughout the United States for morbidity coding. The International Classification of Diseases and Related Health Problems, 10th Revision (ICD-10), published by the World Health Organization (WHO), is the foundation of ICD-10-CM. ICD-10 continues to be the classification used in cause-of-death coding in the United States. The ICD-10-CM is comparable with the ICD-10. The WHO Collaborating Center for the Family of International Classifications in North America, housed at the Centers for Disease Control and Prevention's National Center for Health Statistics (NCHS), has responsibility for the implementation of ICD and other WHO-FIC classifications and serves as a liaison with the WHO, fulfilling international obligations for comparable classifications and the national health data needs of the United States. The historical background of ICD and ICD-10 can be found in the Introduction to the International Classification of Diseases and Related Health Problems (ICD-10), 2008, World Health Organization, Geneva, Switzerland.

ICD-10-CM is the United States' clinical modification of the World Health Organization's ICD-10. The term "clinical" is used to emphasize the modification's intent: to serve as a useful tool in the area of classification of morbidity data for indexing of health records, medical care review, and ambulatory and other health care programs, as well as for basic health statistics. To describe the clinical picture of the patient the codes must be more precise than those needed only for statistical groupings and trend analysis.

Characteristics of ICD-10-CM

ICD-10-CM far exceeds its predecessors in the number of concepts and codes provided. The disease classification has been expanded to include health-related conditions and to provide greater specificity at the sixth and seventh character level. The sixth and seventh characters are not optional and are intended for use in recording the information documented in the clinical record.

ICD-10-CM: The Complete Draft Code Set

This *ICD-10-CM: The Complete Draft Code Set* edition includes the following features, designed in consultation with coding consultants and ICD-10 trainers, to provide a comprehensive and easy-to-use reference manual:

- A table of contents page
- The complete 2015 ICD-10-CM code set
- Full code descriptions
- Special color coding throughout to highlight instructional notes, bilateral indicators, and other features.
- Color coding for Medicare code edits to highlight age, sex, manifestation, other specified and unspecified codes
- Illustrations
- ICD-10-CM conventions
- ICD-10-CM official coding guidelines
- Official index to the tabular section
- Official index to external causes
- Table of drugs and chemicals
- Neoplasm table
- Extention "X" alert symbol to alert readers to the new ICD-10-CM placeholder "x" convention
- Anatomy and physiology drawings interspersed throughout and used to explain particular categories
- Trimester icon for O30 and O31 categories

List of Features

ICD-10-CM is essential to documenting medical necessity for services rendered, and accurate codes mean better outcomes for the patient, your claims, and your practice or facility.

Count on this manual to help you choose and report the right ICD-10-CM code. Unique features, intuitive design, and expert features that coders developed assure this manual will keep your coding on target.

This manual includes ICD-10-CM Volume 2 (Alphabetic Index) and ICD-10-CM Volume 1 (Tabular List), effective for 2015.

To help you make the most of ICD-10-CM Volumes 1 and 2, this manual also includes the following features:

- ICD-10-CM Official Guidelines for Coding and Reporting for 2015; the Health Insurance Portability and Accountability Act (HIPAA) requires all entities assigning ICD-10-CM codes to follow these guidelines

- ICD-9-CM to ICD-10-CM Crosswalks covering the top codes by specialty

- ICD-10-CM implementation checklist to help ensure that you are ready for the rollover to the new code set

- Chapter-specific guidelines before each Tabular List chapter containing codes pertaining to the guidelines to help you get a quick sense of the guidelines to review

- Anatomy descriptions before Tabular List chapters containing codes pertaining to specific body anatomy

- Full illustrations of body systems at the front of the book so you don't have to search the manual for these large color images of body systems

- Illustrations of anatomy and conditions throughout the Tabular List to help you to better understand how to assign specific codes

- ICD-9-CM history and legacy, revealing the advances and changes that have affected coders

- Symbols indicating "Additional digit required" so you know when a code requires an additional digit for code specificity and validity (provided in both the Alphabetic Index and Tabular List)

- Age and sex edits showing which codes have restrictions on use based on age or sex of the patient

- Highlighted coding instructional and informational notes help you recognize important code usage guidance for specific sections

- Intuitive color-coded symbols and alerts identify critical coding and reimbursement issues quickly, such as "Other Specified" and "Unspecified" diagnosis alerts

- Manifestation code alerts so you properly use codes that represent manifestations of an underlying disease and know when you must use two codes

- A user-friendly page design, including dictionary-style headers, color bleed tabs, and legend keys

- Key word - Green font is used to differentiate key words that appear in similar code descriptions in a given category.

Practical Steps for Using the ICD-10-CM Manual

This manual includes the diagnosis code set from the International Classification of Diseases, Tenth Revision, Clinical Modification (ICD-10-CM).

Understand Code Structure to Choose the Most Specific Code

ICD-10-CM codes are made up of a minimum of three characters and a maximum of seven characters:

- Character 1 – capital letter A-Z, except the letter U, which is not used
- Character 2 – number
- Character 3 – number
- Character 4 – number or letter – capital or lowercase
- Character 5 – number or letter – capital or lowercase
- Character 6 – number or letter – capital or lowercase
- Character 7 – number or letter – capital or lowercase; character 7 is only used in specific chapters, including pregnancy, musculoskeletal, injuries, and external causes of morbidity

Each Tabular List chapter is divided into subchapters, which are also called blocks. Subchapters are divided into groups of categories (3 characters).

Each chapter starts with a summary of the blocks within the chapter.

Subchapters are divided into:

Categories (3 characters) – Represents one disease or a group of diseases or related conditions. If a category does not have a further subdivision, it is called a code.

Categories are divided into:

Subcategories (4-6 characters) – Represents greater specificity of one disease or a group of diseases.

Subcategories are divided into:

Codes (4-7 characters) – Codes are the final level which cannot be subdivided further. Codes that are 7 characters are always called "codes" because 7 is the maximum number of characters in a code.

Review the ICD-10-CM Volumes Included in This Manual

This manual includes:

- Volume 1, Tabular List, includes diagnosis codes in numerical order and their official descriptors in 21 chapters
- Volume 2, Alphabetic Index, includes three sections:
  - o Index to Diseases, which you'll use to search for the vast majority of codes
  - o Two tables you'll find at the end of the Index to Diseases:
    - Neoplasm Table
    - Table of Drugs and Chemicals
  - o Alphabetic Index to External Causes of Injury and Poisoning

This manual follows the industry standard of placing Volume 2 (Alphabetic Index) before Volume 1 (Tabular List) because when you search for a code, you should always check the Index first to make a preliminary code choice and then check the Tabular List for confirmation.

Code Diagnoses With Confidence Following This Approach

- ➤ The first step in choosing the proper ICD-10-CM code is reading the medical documentation to identify the diagnosis the provider documents and confirms. If there is no confirmed diagnosis, look for the sign or symptom that brought the patient in or other reason for the encounter.
  - Be sure to check online or hard copy references, such as medical dictionaries and anatomy resources to look up unfamiliar terms.
- ➤ Next, decide which main term you will search in the Index based on the patient's specific case. ICD-10-CM doesn't use body sites as main terms. Instead, look for the disease, sign, symptom, etc. You can find the body site as a subterm. For neoplasm diagnoses, review the Neoplasm Table for the appropriate diagnosis.
- ➤ Once you find the term in the Index, note the recommended code. Start with the main term and review any available subterms. Also note whether the Index offers any other clues to proper coding, such as the need for additional characters or the need for an additional code.
- ➤ Turn to that code in the Tabular List, and read the full code descriptor. Keep in mind that you may need to read the subcategory and category titles as well as the code descriptor to get the full meaning of the code.
- ➤ Check to see whether ICD-10-CM requires additional characters for that code. If so, review the code definitions of any available categories and subcategories.
  - Remember, if a code has seven characters available, you must report all seven characters, both to comply with coding rules and to prevent insurers from denying your claim. Similarly, if a code has four characters, with no fifth character available, you must report all four characters rather than a

three-character code. This manual will alert you to the need for an additional character using easily identifiable symbols.

➤ If the Index points you to a code that includes the terms other, unspecified, NOS (not otherwise specified), or NEC (not elsewhere classified), double check that a more specific code isn't available. Always report the most specific code the medical record supports.

➤ Before making your final code decision, review all applicable notes and instructions to be sure they don't affect your choice. You'll find these notes and instructions on every level, from the chapter to the code itself. Also review the surrounding codes to be sure there isn't a more appropriate code available.

➤ Finally, take a moment to confirm that your code choice complies with the philosophy of ethical coding. Never report an ICD-10-CM code simply because it will support reimbursement from a payer. Report only those codes the documentation supports.

Factor In the Other Resources in This Manual

In addition to Volumes 1 and 2, you'll find the following materials in this manual.

Conventions Specific to This ICD-10-CM Manual: To be sure you make the most of all of the resources and instructional symbols this manual includes, read this section.

Test Yourself: ICD-10-CM Challenge: Assess the strengths and weaknesses in your ICD-10-CM preparations with this quiz, featuring carefully explained solutions.

ICD-10-CM Official Guidelines for Coding and Reporting: No coder should let a year go by without reviewing the Official Guidelines. These authoritative rules provide many instructions not available in the Tabular List.

Additional Content in Tabular List Chapters: At the beginning of specific Tabular List chapters, you'll find anatomy descriptions and Official Guidelines pertinent to that chapter to help you to better understand and assign codes.

ICD-10-CM Draft Official Conventions

The conventions for the ICD-10-CM are the general rules for use of the classification independent of the guidelines. These conventions are incorporated within the Alphabetic Index and Tabular List of the ICD-10-CM as instructional notes.

Format and Structure

The ICD-10-CM Tabular List contains categories, subcategories and codes. Characters for categories, subcategories and codes may be either a letter or a number. All categories are 3 characters. A three-character category that has no further subdivision is equivalent to a code. Subcategories are either 4 or 5 characters. Codes may be 3, 4, 5, 6 or 7 characters. That is, each level of subdivision after a category is a subcategory. The final level of subdivision is a code. Codes that have applicable 7th characters are still referred to as codes, not subcategories. A code that has an applicable 7th character is considered invalid without the 7th character.

The ICD-10-CM uses an indented format for ease in reference.

Codes for reporting purposes

For reporting purposes only codes, are permissible, not categories or subcategories, and any applicable 7th character is required.

Placeholder Character

The ICD-10-CM utilizes a placeholder character "X". The "X" is used as a placeholder at certain codes to allow for future expansion. An example of this is at the poisoning, adverse effect and underdosing codes, categories T36-T50.

Where a placeholder exists, the X must be used in order for the code to be considered a valid code.

7th Characters

Certain ICD-10-CM categories have applicable 7th characters. The applicable 7th character is required for all codes within the category, or as the notes in the Tabular List instruct. The 7th character must always be the 7th character in the data field. If a code that requires a 7th character is not 6 characters, a placeholder X must be used to fill in the empty characters.

Abbreviations

a. Alphabetic Index abbreviations

NEC   "Not elsewhere classifiable"

This abbreviation in the Alphabetic Index represents "other specified". When a specific code is not available for a condition, the Alphabetic Index directs the coder to the "other specified" code in the Tabular List.

NOS   "Not otherwise specified"

This abbreviation is the equivalent of unspecified.

b. Tabular List abbreviations

NEC   "Not elsewhere classifiable"

This abbreviation in the Tabular List represents "other specified". When a specific code is not available for a condition the Tabular List includes an NEC entry under a code to identify the code as the "other specified" code.

NOS   "Not otherwise specified"

This abbreviation is the equivalent of unspecified.

Punctuation

[ ] Brackets are used in the Tabular List to enclose synonyms, alternative wording or explanatory phrases. Brackets are used in the Alphabetic Index to identify manifestation codes.

( ) Parentheses are used in both the Alphabetic Index and Tabular List to enclose supplementary words that may be present or absent in the statement of a disease or procedure without affecting the code number to which it is assigned. The terms within the parentheses are referred to as nonessential modifiers.

: Colons are used in the Tabular List after an incomplete term which needs one or more of the modifiers following the colon to make it assignable to a given category.

Notes

Other and Unspecified codes

a. "Other" codes

Codes titled "other" or "other specified" are for use when the information in the medical record provides detail for which a specific code does not exist. Alphabetic Index entries with NEC in the line designate "other" codes in the Tabular List. These Alphabetic Index entries represent specific disease entities for which no specific code exists so the term is included within an "other" code.

b. "Unspecified" codes

Codes titled "unspecified" are for use when the information in the medical record is insufficient to assign a more specific code. For those categories for which an unspecified code is not provided, the "other specified" code may represent both other and unspecified.

Includes Notes

This note appears immediately under a three character code title to further define, or give examples of, the content of the category.

Inclusion Terms

A list of terms is included under some codes. These terms are the conditions for which that code is to be used. The terms may be synonyms of the code title, or, in the case of "other specified" codes, the terms are a list of the various conditions assigned to that code. The inclusion terms are not necessarily exhaustive. Additional terms found only in the Alphabetic Index may also be assigned to a code.

Excludes Notes

The ICD-10-CM has two types of excludes notes. Each type of note has a different definition for use but they are all similar in that they indicate that codes excluded from each other are independent of each other.

   a. Excludes 1

   A type 1 Excludes note is a pure excludes note. It means "NOT CODED HERE!" An Excludes1 note indicates that the code excluded should never be used at the same time as the code above the Excludes1 note. An Excludes1 is used when two conditions cannot occur together, such as a congenital form versus an acquired form of the same condition.

   b. Excludes 2

   A type 2 Excludes note represents "Not included here". An Excludes2 note indicates that the condition excluded is not part of the condition represented by the code, but a patient may have both conditions at the same time. When an Excludes2 note appears under a code, it is acceptable to use both the code and the excluded code together, when appropriate.

Etiology/Manifestation Codes

Etiology/manifestation convention ("code first", "use additional code" and "in diseases classified elsewhere" notes)

Certain conditions have both an underlying etiology and multiple body system manifestations due to the underlying etiology. For such conditions, the ICD-10-CM has a coding convention that requires the underlying condition be sequenced first followed by the manifestation. Wherever such a combination exists, there is a "use additional code" note at the etiology code, and a "code first" note at the manifestation code. These instructional notes indicate the proper sequencing order of the codes, etiology followed by manifestation.

In most cases the manifestation codes will have in the code title, "in diseases classified elsewhere." Codes with this title are a component of the etiology/ manifestation convention. The code title indicates that it is a manifestation code. "In diseases classified elsewhere" codes are never permitted to be used as first-listed or principal diagnosis codes. They must be used in conjunction with an underlying condition code and they must be listed following the underlying condition.

There are manifestation codes that do not have "in diseases classified elsewhere" in the title. For such codes, there is a "use additional code" note at the etiology code and a "code first" note at the manifestation code and the rules for sequencing apply.

In addition to the notes in the Tabular List, these conditions also have a specific Alphabetic Index entry structure. In the Alphabetic Index both conditions are listed together with the etiology code first followed by the manifestation codes in brackets. The code in brackets is always to be sequenced second.

An example of the etiology/manifestation convention is dementia in Parkinson's disease. In the Alphabetic Index, code G20 is listed first, followed by code F02.80 or F02.81 in brackets. Code G20 represents the underlying etiology, Parkinson's disease, and must be sequenced first, whereas codes F02.80 and F02.81 represent the manifestation of dementia in diseases classified elsewhere, with or without behavioral disturbance.

"Code first" and "Use additional code" notes are also used as sequencing rules in the classification for certain codes that are not part of an etiology/ manifestation combination.

And/With/See Also

   a. "And"

   The word "and" should be interpreted to mean either "and" or "or" when it appears in a title.

   For example, cases of "tuberculosis of bones", "tuberculosis of joints" and "tuberculosis of bones and joints" are classified to subcategory A18.0, Tuberculosis of bones and joints.

   b. "With"

   The word "with" should be interpreted to mean "associated with" or "due to" when it appears in a code title, the Alphabetic Index, or an instructional note in the Tabular List.

   The word "with" in the Alphabetic Index is sequenced immediately following the main term, not in alphabetical order.

   c. "See" and "See Also"

   The "see" instruction following a main term in the Alphabetic Index indicates that another term should be referenced. It is necessary to go to the main term referenced with the "see" note to locate the correct code.

   A "see also" instruction following a main term in the Alphabetic Index instructs that there is another main term that may also be referenced that may provide additional Alphabetic Index entries that may be useful. It is not necessary to follow the "see also" note when the original main term provides the necessary code.

Code Also

A "code also" note instructs that two codes may be required to fully describe a condition, but this note does not provide sequencing direction.

Default Codes

A code listed next to a main term in the ICD-10-CM Alphabetic Index is referred to as a default code. The default code represents that condition that is most commonly associated with the main term, or is the unspecified code for the condition. If a condition is documented in a medical record (for example, appendicitis) without any additional information, such as acute or chronic, the default code should be assigned.

Symbols and Conventions

Additional Characters Required

- [4th] This red symbol cautions that the code requires an additional fourth character.
- [5th] This red symbol cautions that the code requires an additional fifth character.
- [6th] This red symbol cautions that the code requires an additional sixth character.
- [7th] This red symbol cautions that the code requires an additional seventh character.

Extension "X" Alert

- [7th] This blue symbol cautions that the code requires an additional seventh character following the placeholder X.

Medicare Code Edits Symbols and Colors

The Medicare Code Editor (MCE) Version-V31R detects and reports errors in the coding claims data. The coding edit information in this manual is effective from 10/01/2013 to 09/30/2014. However, it is not intended to be used to process claims as the ICD-10 code set will not be mandated for use until the implementation of ICD-10.

Age Conflict

The Medicare Code Editor detects inconsistencies between a patient's age and any diagnosis on the patient's record. For example, a five-year-old patient with benign prostatic hypertrophy or a 78-year-old patient coded with a delivery.

- [N] Age of 0 years; a subset of diagnoses intended only for newborns and neonates (e.g., fetal distress, perinatal jaundice).
- [P] Age range is 0–17 years inclusive (e.g., Reye's syndrome, routine child health exam).
- [M] Age range is 12–55 years inclusive (e.g., diabetes in pregnancy, antepartum pulmonary complication).
- [A] Age range is 15–124 years inclusive (e.g., senile delirium, mature cataract).

Sex Conflict

Medicare Code Editor detects inconsistencies between a patient's sex and any diagnosis or procedure on the patient's record. For example, a male patient with cervical cancer (diagnosis) or a female patient with a prostatectomy (procedure).

In both instances, the indicated diagnosis or the procedure conflicts with the stated sex of the patient. Therefore, either the patient's diagnosis, procedure or sex is presumed to be incorrect.

- ♂ This symbol indicates diagnoses for male only
- ♀ This symbol indicates diagnoses for females only

Manifestation Codes

Code description is highlighted with light blue color. Manifestation codes describe the manifestation of an underlying disease, not the disease itself, and therefore should not be used as a principal diagnosis.

Other Symbols and Color Coding

Key Terms

Bold green font is used in code descriptions throughout the Tabular List of Diseases to quickly identify key terms in a given category.

Other Specified Codes

Code description is highlighted with gray color. These codes are assigned when the documentation indicates a specified diagnosis, but the ICD-10-CM system does not have a specific code that describes the condition

Unspecified Codes

Code description is highlighted with yellow color. These codes are assigned when neither the diagnostic statement nor the documentation provides enough information to assign a more specific code.

PDx Principal Diagnosis Only

Certain Z codes may only be reported as the principal/first-listed diagnosis, except when there are multiple encounters on the same day and the medical records for the encounters are combined. A list of these codes can be found in ICD-10-CM official guidelines.

Checklist for ICD-10-CM Preparation

Preparing for the implementation of ICD-10-CM and ICD-10-PCS is essential, especially as colleagues in your practice, group, or facility look to coders for answers. Most providers have started preparing, but take advantage the new Oct. 1, 2015 date. Here are some tips that will help you be ready:

- Make sure your place of employment has an implementation plan. Share the checklist below with your supervisor or administrator.

- Refresh and broaden your knowledge of anatomy and pathophysiology (A&P). The new codes require a better understanding for accurate reporting. Buy an anatomy and pathophysiology book, attend classes, or use AAPC's online course.

- Get an ICD-10-CM book, and become familiar with its conventions. Some are similar to ICD-9-CM, and some are new.

- Attend chapter meetings, especially those where A&P and ICD-10-CM are being discussed. Talk to your colleagues about ICD-10.

- Take advantage of AAPC's inexpensive in-person and online trainings. Become conversant on ICD-10-CM and the A&P needed to understand documentation.

- Demonstrate ICD-10-CMpProficiency.

- Look at your documentation. Does it have what you will need to code ICD-10-CM? Share what you learn about ICD-10 with your providers.

- Participate in preparations at your workplace.

Follow These 9 Steps for Successful ICD-10 Implementation:

1 – Inform	5 – Prepare	9 - Evaluate
2 – Assign	6 - Train	
3 – Assess	7 - Test	
4 – Plan	8 - Implement	

Step 1: Inform

Give practice decision makers a high-level overview of ICD-10 and get buy-in to begin implementation preparation:

- Prepare briefing materials for providers and staff to review related to the scope of work needed for the implementation of ICD-10 and HIPAA 5010.

- Meet with practice decision makers to explain what ICD-10 is and why ICD-9-CM is being phased out.

- Resources for this step: High Level Overview of ICD-10 (webinar series)

- Meet with practice decision makers for a high-level review of the Department of Health and Human Services (HHS) final rule and CMS memorandums.

- Perform a 360° degree high-level assessment of how a diagnosis code is impacted from the time a patient makes an appointment to when payment has been received for a service:

  o Follow each process through the office looking for potential impacts, and note all systems impacted by ICD-10 including front desk, clinical areas, documentation, coding systems, etc.

  o Show practice decision makers this assessment to help them understand the changes needed. Be sure to list potential benefits of changes and how the practice can implement them such as improved disease management and tracking, possible changes in policies, etc.

- Obtain buy-in from practice decision makers on the urgency of ICD-10, the need to begin preparing now, and to steps and tasks outlined in this tracker.

Step 2: Assign

Assign teams to oversee the implementation effort:

- Assign a PROJECT MANAGER the ownership of the ICD-10 implementation project. This role should be filled by a key staff member such as an office manager, administrator, or lead physician. Make sure this individual understands the full scope of this project and can effectively manage it.

- Establish a COMMUNICATION COMMITTEE or COMMUNICATION LIAISON with responsibility for updates to the PROJECT MANAGER, STEERING COMMITTEE, STAFF, VENDORS, and HEALTH PLANS. Communication methods can include e-mail, newsletters, webinars, staff briefings, etc.

- Once teams/individuals are selected, outline the ICD-10 Implementation scope of work and the steps in this tracker, and make assignments for each.

- Establish a regular meeting schedule with activity and result reporting.

Step 3: Assess

Assess all areas of practice and determine what has to change:

- Complete a review of regulatory requirements of ICD-10 to identify impacts to your practice.

- Evaluate clinical documentation to determine if current specificity allows an ICD-10 code to be assigned. Assess by disease process, by provider, by specialty, or by group, and run a report to indicate the most frequently used diagnosis codes within the practice. Share results of the assessment with providers to educate them on new specificity requirements of ICD-10.

- Complete an in-depth systems review to list the impact that ICD-10 will have, and determine compatibility if upgrades will be necessary:

  o Evaluate all systems, coding applications, and software to ensure compatibility with 5010 and ICD-10. **Note**: Systems must support both ICD-9-CM and ICD-10 code sets for a period of time.

- Have a STEERING COMMITTEE create flow charts of current procedures and processes for their respective departments to determine changes needed for ICD-10 and the affect on how things are currently done.

- Evaluate health plan contract changes to determine the impact on reimbursement, and determine if the practice will continue to participate with the health plan. **Note:** This step may need to be postponed until health plans have completed their ICD-10 changes.

- Determine ICD-10 requirements and expectations for/from all affected departments, system users, and internal and external system vendors to determine product timelines for upgrades, testing, and changes for each system.

- Based on the results from your assessments above, complete a detailed report of existing systems, processes, procedures, policies, and technology that ICD-10 will impact:

  o Account for all areas of the practice where an ICD-9-CM code currently exists.

  o Share the report with the PROJECT MANAGER and STEERING COMMITTEE.

Step 4: Plan

Plan the Implementation of ICD-10:

- Create a budget based on the areas identified in the practice as being impacted (IT systems, software, hardware, implementation/code deployment, cross-walking, staff training and education, documentation readiness audits, overtime during the transition, etc.).

- Work with vendors to schedule timeframes for practice management/EMR/coding systems upgrades, testing, and integration.

- List the policies identified with change requirements, and make assignments to rewrite and implement.

- Plan staff training schedules on implementation, documentation, code set, systems, policies, and procedures.

- Plan steps to measure learning and proficiency after the training has been provided.

- Have a COMMUNICATION COMMITTEE OR LIAISON plan a schedule for communication throughout the implementation process.

- Acquire resources needed to execute plans.

Step 5: Prepare

Prepare the changes for ICD-10:

- Create staff training materials:

  o Identify the best training methods based on each staff member's learning style: on-line, in person, self-study, etc.

  o Consider training on implementation, clinical documentation (based on documentation assessments), anatomy & pathophysiology (for non-clinical staff), general and specialty code sets, and ICD 10 PCS (if required).

- Update internal policies such as the use of ABNs, referrals, pharmacy, lab orders, new LCDs and NCDs, etc.

- Create flow charts for new procedures and processes for ICD-10. Modify them as needed until ICD-10 is supported in all processes and flows. Although a goal of compliance is sufficient, we recommend you take the opportunity to develop improved operations, performance, quality, etc.

Step 6: Train

Train staff on the changes made for ICD-10:

- If needed, re-train providers on specificity requirements of ICD-10 by utilizing existing documentation from patient encounters. Repeat the cycle of assessing documentation and training until providers reach 90 percent accuracy.

- Train coders and staff on medical terminology as it relates to ICD-10-PCS (if being utilized).

- Train coders with limited clinical knowledge on anatomy & pathophysiology for ICD-10

- Train coders on ICD-10 general code set

- Train coders on ICD-10-PCS (if being utilized).

- Train staff on policy and procedure changes. Utilize newly created flow charts and policy revisions.

- Train users on system and software upgrades.

- Resources for this step: Anatomy & Pathophysiology for ICD-10

Step 7: Test

Test all changes for ICD-10 prior to implementation:

- Perform internal and external testing of software and hardware to verify compatibility with upgrades and existing systems:

- o Ensure integrated changes into production systems have been accomplished via internal testing and external testing.
- o Be sure to run complete testing of systems with clearinghouses, payers, etc. (60-90 days)
- Test updated policies and procedures to ensure both compliance and improved efficiencies.
- If needed, re-evaluate clinical documentation for ICD-10 readiness. Again, at least 90 percent accuracy is recommended.
- Test knowledge of staff to validate preparedness for ICD-10.
- Resources for this step: ICD-10 Proficiency Assessment

Step 8: Implement

Implement ICD-10:

- Push upgrades to systems live, and turn on production mode in systems.
- Begin using ICD-10 and ICD-9-CM code sets in tandem.
- Make all new policies and procedures effective.

Step 9: Evaluate

Evaluate the implementation results:

- Re-evaluate medical record documentation for compliance through readiness assessments. Re-train providers as necessary.
- Analyze any claim denials, and make appropriate adjustments to reduce them.
- Assess whether staff is following new policies, and determine the effectiveness of each. Compare expectations to actual results.
- Monitor and measure coding and billing productivity. Set goals, and plan for ongoing training to improve productivity.
- Monitor and measure productivity outcomes of all staff on a regular basis.
- Audit systems and software for accuracy.
- Analyze all changes, and look for gaps between expectations and actual results to determine areas that need additional adjustments.
- Provide additional training as needed in the areas where you identify deficiencies.

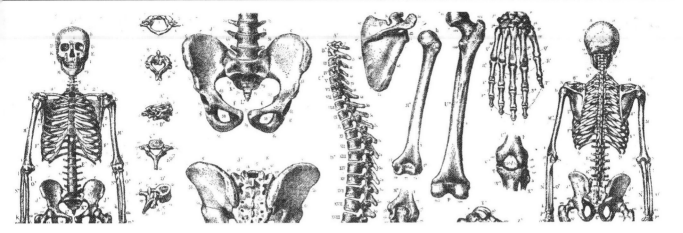

S ince 1979, the U.S. has used the International Classification of Diseases, Ninth Revision, Clinical Modifications (ICD-9-CM) to identify diagnoses related to morbidity and mortality. Twenty five years later, we will transition from ICD-9-CM to ICD-10-CM, on Oct, 2015.

We have become very familiar with ICD-9-CM; and, it is all many providers and coders have ever known for diagnosis coding. As we transition from this long used code set, let's take a quick look back to see what has brought us to where we are today.

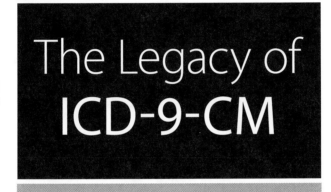

The Legacy of ICD-9-CM

A LONG-TIME GOAL

Efforts to catalogue and classify disease reach back at least 400 years and burgeoned during the 18th Century. Responding to an 1853 request of the newly formed International Statistical Congress, English medical statistician William Farr and Swiss physician Marc d'Espine each prepared a uniform classification of causes of death to present to the International Statistical Congress in Paris. The resulting hybrid system of classification was never internationally adopted but we derive the principle of categorizing diseases by anatomical site from these attempts.

The prototype International Classification of Disease (ICD) was adopted in 1893 by the International Statistical Institute. By 1938, the classification system would undergo five revisions. International interest led to a sixth revision by the newly created World Health Organization (WHO) in 1948. The seventh and eighth revisions followed in 1955 and 1965. The ninth revision, released in 1975, forms the basis of our current codes.

The National Center for Health Statistics applied clinical modifications (CM) to ICD-9 in 1977. The code set provided for a wide variety of signs, symptoms, abnormal findings, complaints, social circumstances, and procedures. ICD-9-CM was adopted nationally in 1979.

ADVENT OF ICD-10

WHO member states began adopting the tenth revision of the ICD in 1994. Compared to ICD-9-CM, ICD-10 provides for greater specificity, promising to enhance the clarity of shared patient data. AAPC provides the following crosswalk of the most reported ICD-9-CM diagnoses to ICD-10-CM codes for a number of specialties.

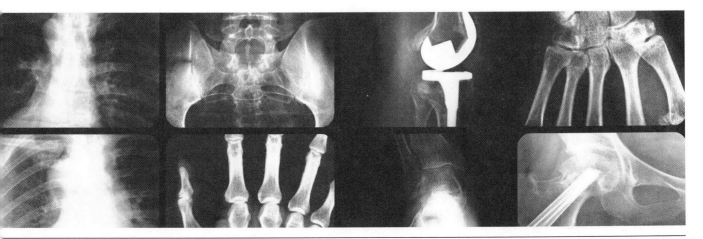

1982

ICD-9-CM became the driver of the new Diagnosis Related Group (DRG) reimbursement system. This facility inpatient payment system relies largely on the diagnoses and procedures documented for a patient by using ICD-9-CM codes.

1991

The nomenclature for Human Immuno-deficiency Virus (HIV) was clarified, adding the 042-V044 series of categories.

1996

The Health Insurance Portability and Accountability Act's (HIPAA) Title II administration simplifications clause make ICD-9-CM one of the official codesets to be used in all healthcare transactions.

2001

The September 11 terror attacks resulted in a new set of U codes to describe mortality and morbidity related to terror attacks. And E999, which was used previously to denote the late effects of war operations, was modified to include late effects of terrorism in 2001.

2006

Present on Admissions rules were added to the ICD-9-CM Guidelines Oct. 1, 2006.

2009

The prevalence of traumatic brain injury (TBI) suffered by solders falling victim to improvised explosive devices in the Iraq War motivated the U.S. Department of Defense to request new codes for sequela related to TBI (799.21-799.29), as well as codes for TBI screening (V80.01) and personal history of traumatic brain injury (V15.52). The new codes joined ICD-9-CM in October 2009.

2013

With conversion to ICD-10-CM and ICD-10-PCS near, 2013 brings no changes to the diagnostic codes and one new code in Vol. 3.

1986

An interim classification characterizing the causative agent of AIDS was added.

1988

The Catastrophic Coverage Act of made the use of the ICD-9-CM system on all Medicare claims mandatory.

1994

042 becomes the single code for HIV disease and V08 is added for *Asymptomatic HIV infection*. HIV-specific guidelines are added to assist coders in selection and sequencing of HIV-related illness.

2000

Worries about a computer-crushing "Millennium Bug" prompted the federal government to freeze ICD-9-CM for the 2000 code year. No new codes were implemented in October 1999 but updates resumed the following year when fears passed.

2003

Severe Acute Respiratory Syndrome (SARS) virus in 2003 prompted the addition of both 480.31 *Pneumonia due to SARS-associated coronavirus* and V01.82 *Exposure to SARS-associated coronavirus*s

2009

The emergence of "swine flu" (2009 H1N1) led to the creation of a new diagnosis code in 2009. Several years later, the influenza codes were once again overhauled to allow reporting of novel influenza A virus.

2009

E codes reflecting new exercise and sporting activities such as boogie boarding and windsurfing (E002.7); bungee jumping (E004.3); and Pilates (E010.3) were added in 2009. Other activity E codes for knitting and crocheting (E012.0); laundry (E013.1); vacuuming (E013.2); ironing (E013.3); and floor mopping and cleaning (E013.4) also made their ICD-9-CM debut in 2009.

The following crosswalks were developed by AAPC based on the ICD-10 Fast Forward crosswalking quick reference tools. If you'd like to purchase a laminated Fast Forward for your specialty, please go to www.aapc.com.

Anesthesia

D-9 722.32
ICD-10 **M51.37** Other intervertebral disc degeneration, lumbosacral region
721.3
ICD-10 **M47.817** Spondylosis without myelopathy or radiculopathy, lumbosacral region
D-9 724.2
ICD-10 **M54.5** Low back pain
D-9 724.4
ICD-10 **M54.14** Radiculopathy, thoracic region
M54.17 Radiculopathy, lumbosacral region
D-9 724.02
ICD-10 **M48.06** Spinal stenosis, lumbar region
D-9 720.2
ICD-10 **M46.1** Sacroiliitis, not elsewhere classified
724.8
ICD-10 **R29.898** Other symptoms and signs involving the musculoskeletal system
D-9 721.42
ICD-10 **M47.16** Other spondylosis with myelopathy, lumbar region
D-9 723.1
ICD-10 **M54.2** Cervicalgia
D-9 729.1
ICD-10 **M79.1** Myalgia
M79.7 Fibromyalgia
M60.9 Myositis, unspecified
** There are more specific code choice selections available in ICD-10-CM. These include:
M60.811 Other myositis, right shoulder
M60.822 Other myositis, left shoulder
M60.819 Other myositiis, unspecified shoulder
M60.821 Other myositis, right upper arm
M60.822 Other myositis, left upper arm
M60.829 Other myositis, unspecified upper arm
M60.831 Other myositis, right forearm
M60.832 Other myositis, left forearm
M60.839 Other myositis, unspecified forearm
M60.841 Other myositis, right hand
M60.842 Other myositis, left hand
M60.849 Other myositis, unspecified hand
M60.851 Other myositis, right thigh
M60.852 Other myositis, left thigh
M60.859 Other myositis, unspecified thigh
M60.861 Other myositis, right lower leg
M60.862 Other myositis, left lower leg
M60.869 Other myositis, unspecified lower leg
M60.871 Other myositis, right ankle and foot
M60.872 Other myositis, left ankle and foot
M60.879 Other myositis, unspecified ankle and foot
D-9 722.6
ICD-10 **M51.34** Other intervertebral disc degeneration, thoracic region
M51.35 Other intervertebral disc degeneration, thoracolumbar region
M51.36 Other intervertebral disc degeneration, lumbar region
M51.37 Other intervertebral disc degeneration, lumbosacral region
D-9 715.00
ICD-10 **M15.0** Primary generalized (osteo)arthritis
M15.4 Erosive (osteo)arthritis
M15.8 Other polyosteoarthritis
M15.9 Polyosteoarthritis, unspecified
D-9 726.5
ICD-10 **M70.60** Trochanteric bursitis, unspecified hip
M70.61 Trochanteric bursitis, right hip
M70.62 Trochanteric bursitis, left hip
M70.70 Other bursitis, unspecified hip
M70.71 Other bursitis, right hip
M70.72 Other bursitis, left hip
* Use additional external cause code to identify activity causing disorder (Y93-)
M76.10 Psoas tendinitis, unspecified hip
M76.11 Psoas tendinitis, right hip
M76.12 Psoas tendinitis, left hip
M76.20 Iliac crest spur, unspecified hip
M76.21 Iliac crest spur, right hip
M76.22 Iliac crest spur, left hip
D-9 726.19
ICD-10 **M75.80** Other shoulder lesions, unspecified shoulder
M75.81 Other shoulder lesions, right shoulder
M75.82 Other shoulder lesions, left shoulder

ICD-9 719.41
ICD-10 **M25.511** Pain in right shoulder
M25.512 Pain in left shoulder
M25.519 Pain in unspecified shoulder
ICD-9 719.45
ICD-10 **M25.551** Pain in right hip
M25.552 Pain in left hip
M25.559 Pain in unspecified hip
ICD-9 722.4
ICD-10 **M50.30** Other cervical disc degeneration, unspecified cervical region
M50.31 Other cervical disc degeneration, occipito-atlanto-axial region
M50.32 Other cervical disc degeneration, mid-cervical region
M50.33 Other cervical disc degeneration, cervicothoracic region
ICD-9 719.40
ICD-10 **M25.50** Pain in unspecified joint
** There are more specific code choice selections available in ICD-10-CM. These include:
M25.511 Pain in right shoulder
M25.512 Pain in left shoulder
M25.519 Pain in unspecified shoulder
M25.521 Pain in right elbow
M25.522 Pain in left elbow
M25.529 Pain in unspecified elbow
M25.531 Pain in right wrist
M25.532 Pain in left wrist
M25.539 Pain in unspecified wrist
M25.551 Pain in right hip
M25.552 Pain in left hip
M25.559 Pain in unspecified hip
M25.561 Pain in right knee
M25.562 Pain in left knee
M25.569 Pain in unspecified knee
M25.571 Pain in right ankle and joints of the right foot
M25.572 Pain in left ankle and joints of the left foot
M25.579 Pain in unspecified ankle
ICD-9 162.9
ICD-10 **C34.90** Malignant neoplasm of unspecified part of unspecified bronchus or lung
** There are more specific code choice selections available in ICD-10-CM. These include:
C34.00 Malignant neoplasm of unspecified main bronchus
C34.01 Malignant neoplasm of right main bronchus
C34.02 Malignant neoplasm of left main bronchus
C34.10 Malignant neoplasm of upper lobe, unspecified bronchus or lung
C34.11 Malignant neoplasm of upper lobe, right bronchus or lung
C34.12 Malignant neoplasm of upper lobe, left bronchus or lung
C34.2 Malignant neoplasm of middle lobe, bronchus or lung
C34.30 Malignant neoplasm of lower lobe, unspecified bronchus or lung
C34.31 Malignant neoplasm of lower lobe, right bronchus or lung
C34.32 Malignant neoplasm of lower lobe, left bronchus or lung
C34.80 Malignant neoplasm of overlapping sites of unspecified bronchus or lung
C34.81 Malignant neoplasm of overlapping sites of right bronchus or lung
C34.82 Malignant neoplasm of overlapping sites of left bronchus or lung
C34.91 Malignant neoplasm of unspecified part of right bronchus or lung
C34.92 Malignant neoplasm of unspecified part of left bronchus or lung
ICD-9 721.0
ICD-10 **M47.812** Spondylosis without myelopathy or radiculopathy, cervical region
ICD-9 337.22
ICD-10 **G90.529** Complex regional pain syndrome I of unspecified lower limb
** There are more specific code choice selections available in ICD-10-CM. These include:
G90.521 Complex regional pain syndrome I of right lower limb
G90.522 Complex regional pain syndrome I of left lower limb
G90.523 Complex regional pain syndrome I of lower limb, bilateral
ICD-9 722.10
ICD-10 **M51.26** Other intervertebral disc displacement, lumbar region
ICD-9 338.4
ICD-10 **G89.4** Chronic pain syndrome
* Code also related psychological factors associated with pain (G54.42-)
ICD-9 724.6
ICD-10 **M53.3** Sacrococcygeal disorders, not elsewhere classified
M43.28 Fusion of spine, sacral and sacrococcygeal region

M53.2x8 Spinal instabilities, sacral and sacrococcygeal region
ICD-9 355.8
ICD-10 **G57.90** Unspecified mononeuropathy of unspecified lower limb
** There are more specific code choice selections available in ICD-10-CM. These include:
G57.91 Unspecified mononeuropathy of right lower limb
G57.92 Unspecified mononeuropathy of left lower limb
G57.80 Other specified mononeuropathies of unspecified lower limb
G57.81 Other specified mononeuropathies of right lower limb
G57.82 Other specified mononeuropathies of left lower limb
ICD-9 337.29
ICD-10 **G90.59** Complex regional pain syndrome I of other specified site
ICD-9 789.03
ICD-10 **R10.31** Right lower quadrant pain
ICD-9 738.4
ICD-10 **M43.10** Spondylolisthesis, site unspecified
M43.11 Spondylolisthesis, occipito-atlanto-axial region
M43.12 Spondylolisthesis, cervical region
M43.13 Spondylolisthesis, cervicothoracic region
M43.14 Spondylolisthesis, thoracic region
M43.15 Spondylolisthesis, thoracolumbar region
M43.16 Spondylolisthesis, lumbar region
M43.17 Spondylolisthesis, lumbosacral region
M43.18 Spondylolisthesis, sacral and sacrococcygeal region
M43.19 Spondylolisthesis, multiple sites in spine
ICD-9 723.4
ICD-10 **M54.12** Radiculopathy, cervical region
M54.13 Radiculopathy, cervicothoracic region
ICD-9 354.2
ICD-10 **G56.20** Lesion of ulnar nerve, unspecified upper limb
G56.21 Lesion of ulnar nerve, right upper limb
G56.22 Lesion of ulnar nerve, left upper limb
ICD-9 722.51
ICD-10 **M51.34** Other intervertebral disc degeneration, thoracic region
M51.35 Other intervertebral disc degeneration, thoracolumbar region
M51.36 Other intervertebral disc degeneration, lumbar region
M51.37 Other intervertebral disc degeneration, lumbosacral region
ICD-9 346.00
ICD-10 **G43.109** Migraine with aura, not intractable, without status migrainosus
** Code also any associated seizure (G40-, R56.9)
ICD-9 726.60
ICD-10 **M70.50** Other bursitis of knee, unspecified knee
M70.51 Other bursitis of knee, right knee
M70.52 Other bursitis of knee, left knee
** Use additional external cause code to identify activity causing disorder (Y93-)
M76.50 Patellar tendinitis, unspecified knee
M76.51 Patellar tendinitis, right knee
M76.52 Patellar tendinitis, left knee
ICD-9 322.9
ICD-10 **G03.9** Meningitis, unspecified
** There are more specific code choice selections available in ICD-10-CM. These include:
G00.0 Hemophilus meningitis
G00.1 Pneumococcal meningitis
G00.2 Streptococcal meningitis
G00.3 Staphylococcal meningitis
Use additional code to further identify organism (B96.61-B95.8)
G00.8 Other bacterial meningitis
Use additional code to further identify organism (B96-)
G00.9 Bacterial meningitis, unspecified
G01 Meningitis in bacterial diseases classified elsewhere
** Code first underlying disease
G02 Meningitis in other infectious and parasitic diseases classified elsewhere
** Code first underlying disease, such as: poliovirus infection (A80-)
G03.0 Nonpyogenic meningitis
G03.1 Chronic meningitis
G03.2 Benign recurrent meningitis (Mollaret)
G03.8 Meningitis due to other specified causes
ICD-9 170.9
ICD-10 **C41.9** Malignant neoplasm of bone and articular cartilage, unspecified
** There are more specific code choice selections available in ICD-10-CM. These include:
C41.0 Malignant neoplasm of bones of skull and face
C41.1 Malignant neoplasm of mandible
C41.2 Malignant neoplasm of vertebral column
C41.3 Malignant neoplasm of ribs, sternum and clavicle
C41.4 Malignant neoplasm of pelvic bones, sacrum and coccyx
ICD-9 722.80
ICD-10 **M96.1** Postlaminectomy syndrome, not elsewhere classified

ICD-9 338.21
ICD-10 G89.21 Chronic pain due to trauma
** Code also related psychological factors associated with pain (F45.42)

ICD-9 789.00
ICD-10 R10.9 Unspecified abdominal pain
** There are more specific code choice selections available in ICD-10-CM. These include:
  R10.0 Acute abdomen
  R10.10 Upper abdominal pain, unspecified
  R10.11 Right upper quadrant pain
  R10.12 Left upper quadrant pain
  R10.13 Epigastric pain
  R10.2 Pelvic and perineal pain
  R10.30 Lower abdominal pain, unspecified
  R10.31 Right lower quadrant pain
  R10.32 Left lower quadrant pain
  R10.33 Periumbilical pain
  R10.84 Generalized abdominal pain

ICD-9 786.59
ICD-10 R07.82 Intercostal pain
  R07.89 Other chest pain

ICD-9 724.1
ICD-10 M54.6 Pain in thoracic spine

ICD-9 724.3
ICD-10 M54.30 Sciatica, unspecified site
  M54.31 Sciatica, right side
  M54.32 Sciatica, left side

ICD-9 356.9
ICD-10 G60.9 Hereditary and idiopathic neuropathy, unspecified
** There are more specific code choice selections available in ICD-10-CM. These include:
  G60.0 Hereditary motor and sensory neuropathy
  G60.3 Idiopathic progressive neuropathy
  G60.8 Other hereditary and idiopathic neuropathies

ICD-9 789.05
ICD-10 R10.33 Periumbilic pain

ICD-9 724.00
ICD-10 M48.00 Spinal stenosis, site unspecified
** There are more specific code choice selections available in ICD-10-CM. These include:
  M48.01 Spinal stenosis, occipito-atlanto-axial region
  M48.02 Spinal stenosis, cervical region
  M48.03 Spinal stenosis, cervicothoracic region
  M48.04 Spinal stenosis, thoracic region
  M48.05 Spinal stenosis, thoracolumbar region
  M48.06 Spinal stenosis, lumbar region
  M48.07 Spinal stenosis, lumbosacral region
  M48.08 Spinal stenosis, sacral and sacrococcygeal region

ICD-9 726.0
ICD-10 M75.00 Adhesive capsulitis of unspecified shoulder
  M75.01 Adhesive capsulitis of right shoulder
  M75.02 Adhesive capsulitis of left shoulder

ICD-9 569.42
ICD-10 K62.89 Other specified diseases of anus and rectum
Use additional code for any associated fecal incontinence (R15-)

ICD-9 723.8
ICD-10 M53.1 Cervicobrachial syndrome
  Q76.1 Klippel-Feil syndrome
  M53.82 Other specified dorsopathies, cervical region
  M53.83 Other specified dorsopathies, cervicothoracic region

ICD-9 337.21
ICD-10 G90.519 Complex regional pain syndrome I of unspecified upper limb
** There are more specific code choice selections available in ICD-10-CM. These include:
  G90.511 Complex regional pain syndrome I of right upper limb
  G90.512 Complex regional pain syndrome I of left upper limb
  G90.513 Complex regional pain syndrome I of upper limb, bilateral

ICD-9 338.28
ICD-10 G89.28 Other chronic postprocedural pain
** Code also related psychological factors associated with pain (F45.42)

ICD-9 354.9
ICD-10 G56.90 Unspecified mononeuropathy of unspecified upper limb
  G56.91 Unspecified mononeuropathy of right upper limb
  G56.92 Unspecified mononeuropathy of left upper limb

ICD-9 349.0
ICD-10 G97.1 Other reaction to spinal and lumbar puncture

Behavioral Health

ICD-9 309.9
ICD-10 F43.20 Adjustment disorder, unspecified
** There are more specific code choice selections available in ICD-10-CM. These include:
  F43.21 Adjustment disorder with depressed mood
  F43.22 Adjustment disorder with anxiety

  F43.23 Adjustment disorder with mixed anxiety and depressed mood
  F43.24 Adjustment disorder with disturbance of conduct
  F43.25 Adjustment disorder with mixed disturbance of emotions and conduct
  F43.29 Adjustment disorder with other symptoms

ICD-9 296.36
ICD-10 F33.42 Major depressive disorder, recurrent, in full remission

ICD-9 300.00
ICD-10 F41.9 Anxiety disorder, unspecified
** There are more specific code choice selections available in ICD-10-CM. These include:
  F41.1 Generalized anxiety disorder
  F41.8 Other specified anxiety disorders

ICD-9 296.32
ICD-10 F33.1 Major depressive disorder, recurrent, moderate

ICD-9 311
ICD-10 F32.9 Major depressive disorder, single episode, unspecified
** There are more specific code choice selections available in ICD-10-CM. These include:
  F32.0 Major depressive disorder, single episode, mild
  F32.1 Major depressive disorder, single episode, moderate
  F32.2 Major depressive disorder, single episode, severe without psychotic features
  F32.3 Major depressive disorder, single episode, severe with psychotic features
  F32.4 Major depressive disorder, single episode, in partial remission
  F32.5 Major depressive disorder, single episode, in full remission
  F32.8 Other depressive episodes

ICD-9 314.9
ICD-10 F90.0 Attention-deficit hyperactivity disorder, predominantly inattentive type
  F90.1 Attention-deficit hyperactivity disorder, predominantly hyperactive type
  F90.2 Attention-deficit hyperactivity disorder, combined type
  F90.8 Attention-deficit hyperactivity disorder, other type
  F90.9 Attention-deficit hyperactivity disorder, unspecified type

ICD-9 296.31
ICD-10 F33.0 Major depressive disorder, recurrent, mild

ICD-9 296.7
ICD-10 F31.9 Bipolar disorder, unspecified
** There are more specific code choice selections available in ICD-10-CM. These include:
  F31.0 Bipolar disorder, current episode hypomanic
  F31.10 Bipolar disorder, current episode manic without psychotic features, unspecified
  F31.11 Bipolar disorder, current episode manic without psychotic features, mild
  F31.12 Bipolar disorder, current episode manic without psychotic features, moderate
  F31.13 Bipolar disorder, current episode manic without psychotic features, severe
  F31.30 Bipolar disorder, current episode depressed, mild or moderate severity, unspecified
  F31.31 Bipolar disorder, current episode depressed, mild
  F31.32 Bipolar disorder, current episode depressed, moderate
  F31.4 Bipolar disorder, current episode depressed, severe, without psychotic features
  F31.5 Bipolar disorder, current episode depressed, severe, with psychotic features
  F31.60 Bipolar disorder, current episode mixed, unspecified
  F31.61 Bipolar disorder, current episode mixed, mild
  F31.62 Bipolar disorder, current episode mixed, moderate
  F31.63 Bipolar disorder, current episode mixed, severe, without psychotic features
  F31.64 Bipolar disorder, current episode mixed, severe, with psychotic features
  F31.70 Bipolar disorder, currently in remission most recent episode unspecified
  F31.71 Bipolar disorder, currently in partial remission, most recent episode hypomanic
  F31.72 Bipolar disorder, currently in full remission, most recent episode hypomanic
  F31.73 Bipolar disorder, currently in partial remission, most recent episode manic
  F31.74 Bipolar disorder, currently in full remission, most recent episode manic
  F31.75 Bipolar disorder, currently in partial remission, most recent episode depressed
  F31.76 Bipolar disorder, currently in full remission, most recent episode depressed
  F31.77 Bipolar disorder, currently in partial remission, most recent episode mixed

  F31.78 Bipolar disorder, currently in full remission, most recent episode mixed

ICD-9 300.4
ICD-10 F34.1 Dysthymic disorder

ICD-9 300.3
ICD-10 F42 Obsessive-compulsive disorder

ICD-9 296.90
ICD-10 F39 Unspecified mood [affective] disorder

ICD-9 295.70
ICD-10 F25.9 Schizoaffective disorder, unspecified
** There are more specific code choice selections available in ICD-10-CM. These include:
  F25.0 Schizoaffective disorder, bipolar type
  F25.1 Schizoaffective disorder, depressive type
  F25.8 Other schizoaffective disorders

ICD-9 294.8
ICD-10 F06.8 Other specified mental disorders due to known physiological condition

ICD-9 296.35
ICD-10 F33.41 Major depressive disorder, recurrent, in partial remission

ICD-9 309.28
ICD-10 F43.23 Adjustment disorder with mixed anxiety and depressed mood

ICD-9 298.9
ICD-10 F29 Unspecified psychosis not due to a substance or known physiological condition

ICD-9 294.9
ICD-10 F06.8 Other specified mental disorders due to known physiological condition

ICD-9 309.24
ICD-10 F43.22 Adjustment disorder with anxiety

ICD-9 296.89
ICD-10 F31.81 Bipolar II disorder
  F31.89 Other bipolar disorder

ICD-9 296.33
ICD-10 F33.2 Major depressive disorder, recurrent severe without psychotic features

ICD-9 296.66
ICD-10 F31.78 Bipolar disorder, in full remission, most recent episode mixed

ICD-9 302.6
ICD-10 F64.2 Gender identity disorder of childhood

ICD-9 296.80
ICD-10 F31.9 Bipolar disorder, unspecified
** There are more specific code choice selections available in ICD-10-CM. These include:
  F31.0 Bipolar disorder, current episode hypomanic
  F31.10 Bipolar disorder, current episode manic without psychotic features, unspecified
  F31.11 Bipolar disorder, current episode manic without psychotic features, mild
  F31.12 Bipolar disorder, current episode manic without psychotic features, moderate
  F31.13 Bipolar disorder, current episode manic without psychotic features, severe
  F31.30 Bipolar disorder, current episode depressed, mild or moderate severity, unspecified
  F31.31 Bipolar disorder, current episode depressed, mild
  F31.4 Bipolar disorder, current episode depressed, severe, without psychotic features
  F31.5 Bipolar disorder, current episode depressed, severe, with psychotic features
  F31.60 Bipolar disorder, current episode mixed, unspecified
  F31.61 Bipolar disorder, current episode mixed, mild
  F31.62 Bipolar disorder, current episode mixed, moderate
  F31.63 Bipolar disorder, current episode mixed, severe, without psychotic features
  F31.64 Bipolar disorder, current episode mixed, severe, with psychotic features
  F31.70 Bipolar disorder, currently in remission most recent episode unspecified
  F31.71 Bipolar disorder, currently in partial remission, most recent episode hypomanic
  F31.72 Bipolar disorder, currently in full remission, most recent episode hypomanic
  F31.73 Bipolar disorder, currently in partial remission, most recent episode manic
  F31.74 Bipolar disorder, currently in full remission, most recent episode manic
  F31.75 Bipolar disorder, currently in partial remission, most recent episode depressed

F31.76 Bipolar disorder, currently in full remission, most recent episode depressed

F31.77 Bipolar disorder, currently in partial remission, most recent episode mixed

F31.78 Bipolar disorder, currently in full remission, most recent episode mixed

ICD-9 300.02
ICD-10 F41.1 Generalized anxiety disorder

ICD-9 309.81
ICD-10 F43.10 Posttraumatic stress disorder, unspecified
F43.11 Posttraumatic stress disorder, acute
F43.12 Posttraumatic stress disorder, chronic

ICD-9 300.01
ICD-10 F41.0 Panic disorder [episodic paroxysmal anxiety] without agoraphobia

ICD-9 296.34
ICD-10 F33.3 Major depressive disorder, recurrent, severe with psychotic symptoms

ICD-9 331.0
ICD-10 G30.0 Alzheimer's disease with early onset
G30.1 Alzheimer's disease with late onset
G30.8 Other Alzheimer's disease
G30.9 Alzheimer's disease, unspecified

ICD-9 301.83
ICD-10 F60.3 Borderline personality disorder

ICD-9 296.52
ICD-10 F31.32 Bipolar disorder, current episode depressed, moderate

ICD-9 309.89
ICD-10 F34.8 Other reactions to severe stress

314.01
ICD-10 F90.0 Attention-deficit hyperactivity disorder, predominantly inattentive type
F90.1 Attention-deficit hyperactivity disorder, predominantly hyperactive type
F90.2 Attention-deficit hyperactivity disorder, combined type
F90.8 Attention-deficit hyperactivity disorder, other type
F90.9 Attention-deficit hyperactivity disorder, unspecified type

ICD-9 304.03
ICD-10 F11.21 Opioid dependence, in remission

ICD-9 296.62
ICD-10 F31.62 Bipolar disorder, current episode mixed, moderate

ICD-9 296.60
ICD-10 F31.60 Bipolar disorder, current episode mixed, unspecified
*There are more specific code choice selections available in ICD-10-CM. These include:
F31.61 Bipolar disorder, current episode mixed, mild
F31.62 Bipolar disorder, current episode mixed, moderate
F31.63 Bipolar disorder, current episode mixed, severe, without psychotic features
F31.64 Bipolar disorder, current episode mixed, severe, with psychotic features

ICD-9 293.83
ICD-10 F06.30 Mood disorder due to known physiological condition, unspecified
F06.31 Mood disorder due to known physiological condition with depressive features
F06.32 Mood disorder due to known physiological condition with major depressive-like episode
F06.33 Mood disorder due to known physiological condition with manic features
F06.34 Mood disorder due to known physiological condition with mixed features

ICD-9 314.8
ICD-10 F90.8 Attention-deficit hyperactivity disorder, other type

ICD-9 309.0
ICD-10 F43.21 Adjustment disorder with depressed mood

ICD-9 304.00
ICD-10 F11.20 Opioid dependence, uncomplicated
*There are more specific code choice selections available in ICD-10-CM. These include:
F11.21 Opioid dependence, in remission
F11.220 Opioid dependence with intoxication, uncomplicated
F11.221 Opioid dependence with intoxication delirium
F11.222 Opioid dependence with intoxication with perceptual disturbance
F11.229 Opioid dependence with intoxication, unspecified
F11.23 Opioid dependence with withdrawal
F11.24 Opioid dependence with opioid-induced mood disorder
F11.250 Opioid dependence with opioid-induced psychotic disorder with delusions
F11.251 Opioid dependence with opioid-induced psychotic disorder with hallucinations

F11.259 Opioid dependence with opioid-induced psychotic disorder, unspecified
F11.281 Opioid dependence with opioid-induced sexual dysfunction
F11.282 Opioid dependence with opioid-induced sleep disorder
F11.288 Opioid dependence with other opioid-induced disorder
F11.29 Opioid dependence with unspecified opioid-induced disorder

ICD-9 307.42
ICD-10 F51.01 Primary insomnia
F51.02 Adjustment insomnia
F51.03 Paradoxical insomnia
F51.04 Psychophysiologic insomnia
F51.05 Insomnia due to other mental disorder
**Code also associated mental disorder
F51.09 Other insomnia not due to a substance of known physiological condition

ICD-9 296.54
ICD-10 F31.5 Bipolar disorder, current episode depressed, severe, with psychotic features

ICD-9 300.23
ICD-10 F40.10 Social phobia, unspecified
F40.11 Social phobia, generalized

ICD-9 296.30
ICD-10 F33.9 Major depressive disorder, recurrent, unspecified
**There are more specific code choice selections available in ICD-10-CM. These include:
F33.0 Major depressive disorder, recurrent, mild
F33.1 Major depressive disorder, recurrent, moderate
F33.2 Major depressive disorder, recurrent severe without psychotic features
F33.3 Major depressive disorder, recurrent, severe with psychotic features
F33.40 Major depressive disorder, recurrent, in remission, unspecified
F33.41 Major depressive disorder, recurrent, in partial remission
F33.42 Major depressive disorder, recurrent, in full remission
F33.8 Other recurrent depressive disorders

ICD-9 309.3
ICD-10 F43.24 Adjustment disorder with disturbance of conduct

ICD-9 296.22
ICD-10 F32.1 Major depressive disorder, single episode, moderate

ICD-9 300.21
ICD-10 F40.01 Agoraphobia with panic disorder

ICD-9 296.53
ICD-10 F31.4 Bipolar disorder, current episode depressed, severe without psychotic features

ICD-9 293.0
ICD-10 F05 Delirium due to known physiological condition
**Code first the underlying physiological condition
301.3 Explosive personality disorder
F60.3 Borderline personality disorder

ICD-9 300.11
ICD-10 F44.4 Conversion disorder with motor symptom or deficit
F44.5 Conversion disorder with seizures or convulsions
F44.6 Conversion disorder with sensory symptom or deficit
F44.7 Conversion disorder with mixed symptom presentation
F44.89 Other dissociative and conversion disorders
F44.9 Dissociative and conversion disorder, unspecified

Cardiology

ICD-9 786.50
ICD-10 R07.9 Chest pain, unspecified
**There are more specific code choice selections available in ICD-10-CM. These include:
R07.89 Other chest pain
R07.2 Precordial pain
R07.1 Chest pain on breathing
R07.81 Pleurodynia

ICD-9 414.00
ICD-10 No map (No ICD-10 code exists for unspecified vessel; native or bypass graft must be indicated)

ICD-9 427.31
ICD-10 I48.0 Paroxysmal atrial fibrillation
I48.1 Persistent atrial fibrillation
I48.2 Chronic atrial fibrillation
I48.91 Unspecified atrial fibrillation

ICD-9 427.89
ICD-10 I49.8 Other specified cardiac arrhythmias

ICD-9 414.01
ICD-10 I25.10 Atherosclerotic heart disease of native coronary artery without angina pectoris

ICD-9 794.31
ICD-10 R94.31 Abnormal electrocardiogram

ICD-9 424.1
ICD-10 I35.9 Nonrheumatic aortic valve disorder, unspecified
I35.0 Nonrheumatic aortic (valve) stenosis
I35.1 Nonrheumatic aortic (valve) insufficiency
I35.2 Nonrheumatic aortic (valve) stenosis with insuffisiciency
I35.8 Other nonrheumatic aortic valve disorders

ICD-9 786.05
ICD-10 R06.02 Shortness of breath

ICD-9 427.69
ICD-10 I49.40 Unspecified premature depolarization
I49.1 Atrial premature depolarization
I49.2 Junctional premature depolarization
I49.3 Ventricular premature depolarization
I49.8 Other specified cardiac arrhythmias
I49.49 Other premature depolarization

ICD-9 427.1
ICD-10 I47.2 Ventricular tachycardia

ICD-9 425.4
ICD-10 I42.2 Other hypertrophic cardiomyopathy
I42.5 Other restrictive cardiomyopathy
I42.8 Other cardiomyopathies
I42.9 Cardiomyopathy, unspecified (familial)(idiopathic)

ICD-9 780.2
ICD-10 R55 Syncope and collapse

ICD-9 427.81
ICD-10 I49.5 Sick sinus syndrome

ICD-9 786.09
ICD-10 R06.89 Other abnormalities of breathing

ICD-9 424.0
ICD-10 I34.9 Nonrheumatic mitral valve disorder, unspecified
I34.0 Nonrheumatic mitral (valve) insufficiency
I34.1 Nonrheumatic mitral (valve) prolapse
I34.2 Nonrheumatic mitral (valve) stenosis
I34.8 Other nonrheumatic mitral valve disorders

ICD-9 794.30
ICD-10 R94.30 Abnormal result of cardiovascular function study, unspecified
R94.39 Abnormal result of other cardiovascular function study

ICD-9 427.9
ICD-10 I49.9 Cardiac arrhythmia, unspecified
** Code first cardiac arrhythmia complicating:
Abortion or ectopic or molar pregnancy (000-007, 008.8)
Obstetric surgery and procedures (075.4)
** There are more specific code choice selections available in ICD-10-CM. These include:
I47.0 Re-entry ventricular arrhythmia
I47.1 Supraventricular tachycardia
I47.2 Ventricular tachycardia
I47.9 Paroxysmal tachycardia, unspecified
** For I47.0–I47.9 Code first cardiac arrhythmia complicating:
Abortion or ectopic or molar pregnancy (000-007, 008.8)
Obstetric surgery and procedures (075.4)
I48.0 Atrial fibrillation
I48.1 Atrial flutter
I49.01 Ventricular fibrillation
I49.02 Ventricular flutter
I49.1 Atrial premature depolarization
I49.2 Junctional premature depolarization
I49.3 Ventricular premature depolarization
I49.40 Unspecified premature depolarization
I49.49 Other premature depolarization
I49.5 Sick sinus syndrome
I49.8 Other specified cardiac arrhythmias
** For I49.0–I49.9 Code first cardiac arrhythmia complicating:
Abortion or ectopic or molar pregnancy (000-007, 008.8)
Obstetric surgery and procedures (075.4)

ICD-9 785.1
ICD-10 R00.2 Palpitations
F45.8

ICD-9 429.3
ICD-10 I51.7 Cardiomegaly

ICD-9 428.22
ICD-10 I50.22 Chronic systolic (congestive) heart failure

ICD-9 427.61
ICD-10 I49.1 Atrial premature depolarization

ICD-9 427.0
ICD-10 I47.1 Supraventricular tachycardia

ICD-9 786.59
ICD-10 R07.89 Other chest pain NOS
R07.82 Intercostal pain

ICD-9 401.9
ICD-10 I10 Essential (primary) hypertension
ICD-9 426.0
ICD-10 I44.2 Atrioventricular block, complete
ICD-9 426.11
ICD-10 I44.0 Atrioventricular block, first degree
ICD-9 401.1
ICD-10 I10 Essential (primary) hypertension
ICD-9 272.4
ICD-10 E78.4 Other hyperlipidemia
    E78.5 Hyperlipidemia, unspecified
**There are more specific code choice selections available in ICD-10-CM. These include:
    E78.0 Pure hypercholesterolemia
    E78.1 Pure hyperglyceridemia
    E78.2 Mixed hyperlipidemia
    E78.3 Hyperchylomicronemia
    E78.6 Lipoprotein deficiency
ICD-9 V72.81
ICD-10 Z01.810 Encounter for preprocedural cardiovascular examination
ICD-9 785.2
ICD-10 R01.1 Cardiac murmur, unspecified
ICD-9 428.0
ICD-10 I50.9 Heart failure, unspecified
    I50.1 Left ventricular failure
    I50.20 Unspecified systolic (congestive) heart failure
    I50.21 Acute systolic (congestive) heart failure
    I50.22 Chronic systolic (congestive) heart failure
    I50.23 Acute on chronic systolic (congestive) heart failure
    I50.30 Unspecified diastolic (congestive) heart failure
    I50.31 Acute diastolic (congestive) heart failure
    I50.32 Chronic diastolic (congestive) heart failure
    I50.33 Acute on chronic diastolic (congestive) heart failure
    I50.40 Unspecified combined systolic (congestive) and diastolic (congestive) heart failure
    I50.41 Acute combined systolic (congestive) and diastolic (congestive) heart failure
    I50.42 Chronic combined systolic (congestive) and diastolic (congestive) heart failure
    I50.43 Acute on chronic combined systolic (congestive) and diastolic (congestive) heart failure
ICD-9 414.8
ICD-10 I25.89 Other forms of chronic ischemic heart disease
    I25.9 Ischemic heart disease; unspecified
ICD-9 427.32
ICD-10 I48.3 Typical atrial flutter
    I48.4 Atypical atrial flutter
    I48.92 Unspecified atrial flutter
ICD-9 426.4
ICD-10 I45.10 Unspecified right bundle-branch block
    I45.19 Other right bundle-branch block
    I45.2 Bifasicular block
ICD-9 780.79
ICD-10 R53.81 Other malaise
    R53.1 Weakness
    R53.83 Other fatigue
    G93.3 Postviral fatigue syndrome
ICD-9 413.9
ICD-10 I20.8 Other forms of angina pectoris
    I20.9 Angina pectoris, unspecified
    I20.0 Unstable angina
    I20.1 Angina pectoris with documented spasm
ICD-9 780.4
ICD-10 R42 Dizziness and giddiness
ICD-9 428.42
ICD-10 I50.42 Chronic combined systolic (congestive) and diastolic (congestive) heart failure
ICD-9 411.1
ICD-10 I20.0 Unstable angina
ICD-9 412
ICD-10 I25.2 Old myocardial infarction
ICD-9 426.3
ICD-10 I44.7 Left bundle-branch block, unspecified
    I45.2 Bifasicular block
    I44.60 Unspecified bifascicular block
    I44.4 Left anterior bifascicular block
    I44.5 Left posterior bifascicular block
ICD-9 426.50
ICD-10 I45.4 Nonspecific intraventricular block
    I44.30 Unspecified atrioventricular block

    I44.39 Other atrioventricular block
ICD-9 425.11
ICD-10 I42.1 Obstructive hypertrophic cardiomyopathy
ICD-9 424.2
ICD-10 I36.0 Nonrheumatic tricuspid (valve) stenosis
    I36.1 Nonrheumatic tricuspid (valve) insufficiency
    I36.2 Nonrheumatic tricuspid (valve) stenosis with insufficiency
    I36.8 Other nonrheumatic tricuspid valve disorders
    I36.9 Nonrheumatic tricuspid valve disorder, unspecified
ICD-9 410.40
ICD-10 I21.19 ST elevation (STEMI) myocardial infarction involving other coronary artery of inferior wall
    I22.1 Subsequent ST elevation (STEMI) myocardial infarction of inferior wall
ICD-9 785.0
ICD-10 R00.0 Tachycardia, unspecified
ICD-9 416.8
ICD-10 I27.2 Other secondary pulmonary hypertension
    I27.89 Other specified pulmonary heart disease
    I27.9 Pulmonary heart disease, unspecified
ICD-9 426.13
ICD-10 I44.1 Atrioventricular block, second degree
ICD-9 782.3
ICD-10 R60.0 Localized edema
    R60.1 Generalized edema
    R60.9 Edema, unspecified
ICD-9 427.41
ICD-10 I49.01 Ventricular fibrillation
ICD-9 416.0
ICD-10 I27.0 Primary pulmonary hypertension

Cardiothoracic and Vascular

ICD-9 433.10
ICD-10 I65.21 Occlusion and stenosis of right carotid artery
    I65.22 Occlusion and stenosis of left carotid artery
    I65.23 Occlusion and stenosis of bilateral carotid arteries
    I65.29 Occlusion and stenosis of unspecified carotid artery
ICD-9 440.21
ICD-10 I70.211 Atherosclerosis of native arteries of extremities with intermittent claudication, right leg
    I70.212 Atherosclerosis of native arteries of extremities with intermittent claudication, left leg
    I70.213 Atherosclerosis of native arteries of extremities with intermittent claudication, bilateral legs
    I70.218 Atherosclerosis of native arteries of extremities with intermittent claudication, other extremity
    I70.219 Atherosclerosis of native arteries of extremities with intermittent claudication, unspecified extremity
ICD-9 441.4
ICD-10 I71.4 Abdominal aortic aneurysm, without rupture
ICD-9 443.9
ICD-10 I73.9 Peripheral vascular disease, unspecified
** There are more specific code choice selections available. These include:
    I73.00 Raynaud's syndrome without gangrene
    I73.01 Raynaud's syndrome with gangrene
    I73.1 Thromboangiitis obliterans (Buerger's disease)
    I73.81 Erythromelalgia
    I73.89 Other specified peripheral vascular diseases
ICD-9 459.81
ICD-10 I87.2 Venous insufficiency (chronic) (peripheral)
ICD-9 585.6
ICD-10 N18.6 End stage renal disease
** Use additional code to identify dialysis status (Z99.2)
Code first any associated:
Diabetic chronic kidney disease (E08.22, E09.22, E10.22, E11.22, E13.22)
Hypertensive chronic kidney disease (I12.-, I13.-)
Use additional code to identify kidney transplant status, if applicable (Z94.0)
ICD-9 729.5
ICD-10 M79.609 Pain in unspecified limb
** There are more specific code choice selections available in ICD-10-CM. These include:
    M79.601 Pain in right arm
    M79.602 Pain in left arm
    M79.603 Pain in arm, unspecified
    M79.604 Pain in right leg
    M79.605 Pain in left leg
    M79.606 Pain in leg, unspecified
    M79.621 Pain in right upper arm
    M79.622 Pain in left upper arm
    M79.629 Pain in unspecified upper arm
    M79.631 Pain in right forearm

    M79.632 Pain in left forearm
    M79.639 Pain in unspecified forearm
    M79.641 Pain in right hand
    M79.642 Pain in left hand
    M79.643 Pain in unspecified hand
    M79.644 Pain in right finger(s)
    M79.645 Pain in left finger(s)
    M79.646 Pain in unspecified finger(s)
    M79.651 Pain in right thigh
    M79.652 Pain in left thigh
    M79.659 Pain in unspecified thigh
    M79.661 Pain in right lower leg
    M79.662 Pain in left lower leg
    M79.669 Pain in unspecified leg
    M79.671 Pain in right foot
    M79.672 Pain in left foot
    M79.673 Pain in unspecified foot
    M79.674 Pain in right toe(s)
    M79.675 Pain in left toe(s)
    M79.676 Pain in unspecified toe(s)
ICD-9 440.23
ICD-10 I70.25 Atherosclerosis of native arteries of other extremities with ulceration
** Use additional code to identify the severity of the ulcer (L98.49-)
* There are more specific code choice selections available in ICD-10-CM. These include:
    I70.231 Atherosclerosis of native arteries of right leg with ulceration of thigh
    I70.232 Atherosclerosis of native arteries of right leg with ulceration of calf
    I70.233 Atherosclerosis of native arteries of right leg with ulceration of ankle
    I70.234 Atherosclerosis of native arteries of right leg with ulceration of heel and midfoot
    I70.235 Atherosclerosis of native arteries of right leg with ulceration of other part of foot
    I70.238 Atherosclerosis of native arteries of right leg with ulceration of other part of lower right leg
    I70.239 Atherosclerosis of native arteries of right leg with ulceration of unspecified site
    I70.241 Atherosclerosis of native arteries of left leg with ulceration of thigh
    I70.242 Atherosclerosis of native arteries of left leg with ulceration of calf
    I70.243 Atherosclerosis of native arteries of left leg with ulceration of ankle
    I70.244 Atherosclerosis of native arteries of left leg with ulceration of heel and midfoot
    I70.245 Atherosclerosis of native arteries of left leg with ulceration of other part of foot
    I70.248 Atherosclerosis of native arteries of left leg with ulceration of other part of lower left leg
    I70.249 Atherosclerosis of native arteries of left leg with ulceration of unspecified site
ICD-9 454.0
ICD-10
** Use additional code to identify severity of ulcer (L97.0)
** There are more specific code choice selections available in ICD-10-CM. These include:
    I83.001 Varicose veins of unspecified lower extremity with ulcer of thigh
    I83.002 Varicose veins of unspecified lower extremity with ulcer of calf
    I83.003 Varicose veins of unspecified lower extremity with ulcer of ankle
    I83.004 Varicose veins of unspecified lower extremity with ulcer of heel and midfoot
    I83.005 Varicose veins of unspecified lower extremity with ulcer other part of foot
    I83.008 Varicose veins of unspecified lower extremity with ulcer other part of lower leg I83.009 Varicose veins of unspecified lower extremity with ulcer other part of lower leg
    I83.009 Varicose veins of unspecified lower extremity with ulcer of unspecified site
    I83.011 Varicose veins of right lower extremity with ulcer of thigh
    I83.012 Varicose veins of right lower extremity with ulcer of calf
    I83.013 Varicose veins of right lower extremity with ulcer of ankle
    I83.014 Varicose veins of right lower extremity with ulcer of heel and midfoot
    I83.015 Varicose veins of right lower extremity with ulcer other part of foot

I83.018 Varicose veins of right lower extremity with ulcer other part of lower leg

I03.019 Varicose veins of right lower extremity with ulcer of unspecified site

I83.021 Varicose veins of left lower extremity with ulcer of thigh

I83.022 Varicose veins of left lower extremity with ulcer of calf

I83.023 Varicose veins of left lower extremity with ulcer of ankle

I83.024 Varicose veins of left lower extremity with ulcer of heel and midfoot

I83.025 Varicose veins of left lower extremity with ulcer other part of foot

I83.028 Varicose veins of left lower extremity with ulcer other part of lower leg

I83.029 Varicose veins of left lower extremity with ulcer of unspecified site

D-9 440.20
ICD-10 **I70.209** Unspecified atherosclerosis of native arteries of extremities, unspecified extremity

Use additional code, if applicable, to identify chronic total occlusion of artery of extremity (I70.92)
There are more specific code choice selections available in ICD-10-CM. These include:

I70.201 Unspecified atherosclerosis of native arteries of extremities, right leg

I70.202 Unspecified atherosclerosis of native arteries of extremities, left leg

I70.203 Unspecified atherosclerosis of native arteries of extremities, bilateral legs

I70.208 Unspecified atherosclerosis of native arteries of extremities, other extremity

D-9 707.13
ICD-10 **L97.309** Non-pressure chronic ulcer of unspecified ankle with unspecified severity

Code first any associated underlying condition:
Atherosclerosis of the lower extremities (I70.23-, I70.24-, I70.33-, I70.34-, I70.43-, I70.44-, I70.53-, I70.54-, I70.63-, I70.64-, I70.73-, I70.74-)
Chronic venous hypertension (I87.31-, I87.33-)
Diabetic ulcers (E08.621, E08.622, E09.621, E09.622, E10.621, E10.622, E11.621, E11.622, E13.621, E13.622)
Postphlebetic syndrome (I87.01-, I87.03-)
Postthrombotic syndrome (I87.01-, I87.03-)
Varicose ulcer (I83.0-, I83.2-)
Code first any associated gangrene (I96)
There are more specific code choice selections available in ICD-10-CM. These include:

L97.301 Non-pressure chronic ulcer of unspecified ankle limited to breakdown of skin

L97.302 Non-pressure chronic ulcer of unspecified ankle with fat layer exposed

L97.303 Non-pressure chronic ulcer of unspecified ankle with necrosis of muscle

L97.304 Non-pressure chronic ulcer of unspecified ankle with necrosis of bone

L97.309 Non-pressure chronic uler of unspecified ankle with unspecified severity

L97.311 Non-pressure chronic ulcer of right ankle limited to breakdown of skin

L97.312 Non-pressure chronic ulcer of right ankle with fat layer exposed

L97.313 Non-pressure chronic ulcer of right ankle with necrosis of muscle

L97.314 Non-pressure chronic ulcer of right ankle with necrosis of bone

L97.319 Non-pressure chronic ulcer of right ankle with unspecified severity

L97.319 Non-pressure chronic ulcer of right ankle with unspecified severity

L97.321 Non-pressure chronic ulcer of left ankle limited to breakdown of skin

L97.322 Non-pressure chronic ulcer of left ankle with fat layer exposed

L97.323 Non-pressure chronic ulcer of left ankle with necrosis of muscle

L97.324 Non-pressure chronic ulcer of left ankle with necrosis of bone

L97.329 Non-pressure chronic ulcer of left ankle with unspecified severity

D-9 440.22
CD-10 **I70.229** Atherosclerosis of native arteries of extremities with rest pain, unspecified extremity

Use additional code to identify:
There are more specific code choice selections available in ICD-10-CM. These include:

I70.221 Atherosclerosis of native arteries of extremities with rest pain, right leg

I70.222 Atherosclerosis of native arteries of extremities with rest pain, left leg

I70.223 Atherosclerosis of native arteries of extremities with rest pain, bilateral legs

I70.228 Atherosclerosis of native arteries of extremities with rest pain, other extremity

*Use additional code, if applicable, to identify chronic total occlusion of artery of extremity (I70.92)

ICD-9 440.24
ICD-10 **I70.269** Atherosclerosis of native arteries of extremities with gangrene, unspecified extremity

** Use additional code to identify:
Use additional code to identify the severity of any ulcer (L98.49-) if applicable
** There are more specific code choice selections available in ICD-10-CM. These include:

I70.261 Atherosclerosis of native arteries of extremities with gangrene, right leg

I70.262 Atherosclerosis of native arteries of extremities with gangrene, left leg

I70.263 Atherosclerosis of native arteries of extremities with gangrene, bilateral legs

I70.268 Atherosclerosis of native arteries of extremities with gangrene, other extremity

*Use additional code, if applicable, to identify chronic total occlusion of artery of extremity (I70.92)

ICD-9 707.12
ICD-10 **L97.209** Non-pressure chronic ulcer of unspecified ankle with unspecified severity

** Code first any associated underlying condition:
Atherosclerosis of the lower extremities (I70.23-, I70.24-, I70.33-, I70.34-, I70.43-, I70.44-, I70.53-, I70.54-, I70.63-, I70.64-, I70.73-, I70.74-)
Chronic venous hypertension (I87.31-, I87.33-)
Diabetic ulcers (E08.621, E08.622, E09.621, E09.622, E10.621, E10.622, E11.621, E11.622, E13.621, E13.622)
Postphlebetic syndrome (I87.01-, I87.03-)
Postthrombotic syndrome (I87.01-, I87.03-)
Varicose ulcer (I83.0-, I83.2-)
Code first any associated gangrene (I96)
** There are more specific code choice selections available in ICD-10-CM. These include:

L97.201 Non-pressure chronic ulcer of unspecified calf limited to breakdown of skin

L97.202 Non-pressure chronic ulcer of unspecified calf with fat layer exposed

L97.203 Non-pressure chronic ulcer of unspecified calf with necrosis of muscle

L97.204 Non-pressure chronic ulcer of unspecified calf with necrosis of bone

L97.211 Non-pressure chronic ulcer of right calf limited to breakdown of skin

L97.212 Non-pressure chronic ulcer of right calf with fat layer exposed

L97.213 Non-pressure chronic ulcer of right calf with necrosis of muscle

L97.214 Non-pressure chronic ulcer of right calf with necrosis of bone

L97.219 Non-pressure chronic ulcer of right calf with unspecified severity

L97.221 Non-pressure chronic ulcer of left calf limited to breakdown of skin

L97.222 Non-pressure chronic ulcer of left calf with fat layer exposed

L97.223 Non-pressure chronic ulcer of left calf with necrosis of muscle

L97.224 Non-pressure chronic ulcer of left calf with necrosis of bone

L97.229 Non-pressure chronic ulcer of left calf with unspecified severity

ICD-9 V67.00
ICD-10 **Z09** Encounter for follow-up examination after completed treatment for conditions other than malignant neoplasm

** Use additional code to identify any applicable history of disease code (Z86.-, Z87.-)

ICD-9 414.01
ICD-10 **I25.10** Atherosclerotic heart disease of native coronary artery without angina pectoris

** Use additional code, if applicable, to identify coronary atherosclerosis due to lipid rich plaque (I25.83)

ICD-9 729.81
ICD-10 **M79.89** Other specified soft tissue disorders

ICD-9 424.1
ICD-10 **I35.0** Nonrheumatic aortic (valve) stenosis

I35.1 Nonrheumatic aortic (valve) insufficiency

I35.2 Nonrheumatic aortic (valve) stenosis with insufficiency

I35.8 Other nonrheumatic aortic valve disorders

I35.9 Nonrheumatic aortic valve disorder, unspecified

ICD-9 454.8
ICD-10 **I83.811** Varicose veins of right lower extremities with pain

I83.812 Varicose veins of left lower extremities with pain

I83.813 Varicose veins of bilateral lower extremities with pain

I83.819 Varicose veins of unspecified lower extremities with pain

I83.891 Varicose veins of right lower extremities with other complications

I83.892 Varicose veins of left lower extremities with other complications

I83.893 Varicose veins of bilateral lower extremities with other complications

I83.899 Varicose veins of unspecified lower extremities with other complications

ICD-9 996.73
ICD-10

The appropriate 7th character is to be added to each code from category T82:
A initial encounter
D subsequent encounter
S sequela
** These codes require a 7th character extender.

T82.818- Embolism of vascular prosthetic devices, implants and grafts

T82.828- Fibrosis of vascular prosthetic devices, implants and graft

T82.838- Hemorrhage of vascular prosthetic devices, implants and grafts

T82.848- Pain from vascular prosthetic devices, implants and grafts

T82.7XX- Infection and inflammatory reaction due to other cardiac and vascular devices, implants and grafts

** Use additional code to identify infection

T82.41X- Breakdown (mechanical) of vascular dialysis catheter

T82.42X- Displacement of vascular dialysis catheter

T82.43X- Leakage of vascular dialysis catheter

T82.49X- Other complication of vascular dialysis catheter

T82.858- Stenosis of vascular prosthetic devices, implants and grafts

T82.868- Thrombosis of vascular prosthetic devices, implants and grafts

T82.898- Other specified complication of vascular prosthetic devices, implants and grafts

ICD-9 707.14
ICD-10 **L97.409** Non-pressure chronic ulcer of unspecified heel and midfoot with unspecified severity

** Code first any associated underlying condition:
Atherosclerosis of the lower extremities (I70.23-, I70.24-, I70.33-, I70.34-, I70.43-, I70.44-, I70.53-, I70.54-, I70.63-, I70.64-, I70.73-, I70.74-)
Chronic venous hypertension (I87.31-, I87.33-)
Diabetic ulcers (E08.621, E08.622, E09.621, E09.622, E10.621, E10.622, E11.621, E11.622, E13.621, E13.622)
Postphlebetic syndrome (I87.01-, I87.03-)
Postthrombotic syndrome (I87.01-, I87.03-)
Varicose ulcer (I83.0-, I83.2-)
Code first any associated gangrene (I96)
** There are more specific code choice selections available in ICD-10-CM. These include:

L97.401 Non-pressure chronic ulcer of unspecified heel and midfoot limited to breakdown of skin

L97.402 Non-pressure chronic ulcer of unspecified heel and midfoot with fat layer exposed

L97.403 Non-pressure chronic ulcer of unspecified heel and midfoot with necrosis of muscle

L97.404 Non-pressure chronic ulcer of unspecified heel and midfoot with necrosis of bone

L97.411 Non-pressure chronic ulcer of right heel and midfoot limited to breakdown of skin

L97.412 Non-pressure chronic ulcer of right heel and midfoot with fat layer exposed

L97.413 Non-pressure chronic ulcer of right heel and midfoot with necrosis of muscle

L97.414 Non-pressure chronic ulcer of right heel and midfoot with necrosis of bone

L97.419 Non-pressure chronic ulcer of right heel and midfoot with unspecified severity

L97.421 Non-pressure chronic ulcer of left heel and midfoot limited to breakdown of skin

L97.422 Non-pressure chronic ulcer of left heel and midfoot with fat layer exposed

L97.423 Non-pressure chronic ulcer of left heel and midfoot with necrosis of muscle

L97.424 Non-pressure chronic ulcer of left heel and midfoot with necrosis of bone

L97.429 Non-pressure chronic ulcer of left heel and midfoot with unspecified severity

ICD-9 593.9
ICD-10 **N28.9** Disorder of kidney and ureter, unspecified
ICD-9 707.15
ICD-10 **L97.509** Non-pressure chronic ulcer of other part of unspecified foot with unspecified severity
** Code first any associated underlying condition:
Atherosclerosis of the lower extremities (I70.23-, I70.24-, I70.33-, I70.34-, I70.43-, I70.44-, I70.53-, I70.54-, I70.63-, I70.64-, I70.73-, I70.74-)
Chronic venous hypertension (I87.31-, I87.33-)
Diabetic ulcers (E08.621, E08.622, E09.621, E09.622, E10.621, E10.622, E11.621, E11.622, E13.621, E13.622)
Postphlebetic syndrome (I87.01-, I87.03-)
Postthrombotic syndrome (I87.01-, I87.03-)
Varicose ulcer (I83.0-, I83.2-)
Code first any associated gangrene
** There are more specific code choice selections available in ICD-10-CM. These include:

L97.501 Non-pressure chronic ulcer of other part of unspecified foot limited to breakdown of skin
L97.502 Non-pressure chronic ulcer of other part of unspecified foot with fat layer exposed
L97.503 Non-pressure chronic ulcer of other part of unspecified foot with necrosis of muscle
L97.504 Non-pressure chronic ulcer of other part of unspecified foot with necrosis of bone
L97.511 Non-pressure chronic ulcer of other part of right foot limited to breakdown of skin
L97.512 Non-pressure chronic ulcer of other part of right foot with fat layer exposed
L97.513 Non-pressure chronic ulcer of other part of right foot with necrosis of muscle
L97.514 Non-pressure chronic ulcer of other part of right foot with necrosis of bone
L97.519 Non-pressure chronic ulcer of other part of right foot with unspecified severity
L97.521 Non-pressure chronic ulcer of other part of left foot limited to breakdown of skin
L97.522 Non-pressure chronic ulcer of other part of left foot with fat layer exposed
L97.523 Non-pressure chronic ulcer of other part of left foot with necrosis of muscle
L97.524 Non-pressure chronic ulcer of other part of left foot with necrosis of bone
L97.529 Non-pressure chronic ulcer of other part of left foot with unspecified severity

ICD-9 162.9
ICD-10 **C34.90** Malignant neoplasm of unspecified part of unspecified bronchus or lung
** There are more specific code choice selections available. These include:
C34.00 Malignant neoplasm of unspecified main bronchus
C34.01 Malignant neoplasm of right main bronchus
C34.02 Malignant neoplasm of left main bronchus
C34.10 Malignant neoplasm of upper lobe, unspecified bronchus or lung
C34.11 Malignant neoplasm of upper lobe, right bronchus or lung
C34.12 Malignant neoplasm of upper lobe, left bronchus or lung
C34.2 Malignant neoplasm of middle lobe, bronchus or lung
C34.30 Malignant neoplasm of lower lobe, unspecified bronchus or lung
C34.31 Malignant neoplasm of lower lobe, right bronchus or lung
C34.32 Malignant neoplasm of lower lobe, left bronchus or lung
C34.80 Malignant neoplasm of overlapping sites of unspecified bronchus or lung
C34.81 Malignant neoplasm of overlapping sites of right bronchus or lung
C34.82 Malignant neoplasm of overlapping sites of left bronchus or lung
C34.91 Malignant neoplasm of unspecified part of right bronchus or lung
C34.92 Malignant neoplasm of unspecified part of left bronchus or lung

ICD-9 785.9
ICD-10 **R09.89** Other specified symptoms and signs involving the circulatory and respiratory systems
ICD-9 585.9
ICD-10 **N18.9** Chronic kidney disease, unspecified
** Code first any associated:
Diabetic chronic kidney disease (E08.22, E09.22, E10.22, E11.22, E13.22)
Hypertensive chronic kidney disease (I12-, I13-)
Use additional code to identify kidney transplant status, if applicable (Z94.0)
** There are more specific code choice selections available. These include:
N18.1 Chronic kidney disease, stage 1
N18.2 Chronic kidney disease, stage 2 (mild)

N18.3 Chronic kidney disease, stage 3 (moderate)
N18.4 Chronic kidney disease, stage 4 (severe)
N18.5 Chronic kidney disease, stage 5
N18.6 End stage renal disease
** Use additional code to identify dialysis status (Z99.2)
ICD-9 433.11
ICD-10 **I63.231** Cerebral infarction due to unspecified occlusion or stenosis of right carotid arteries
I63.232 Cerebral infarction due to unspecified occlusion or stenosis of left carotid arteries
I62.239 Cerebral infarction due to unspecified occlusion or stenosis of unspecified arteries
I63.131 Cerebral infarction due to embolism of right carotid artery
I63.132 Cerebral infarction due to embolism of left carotid artery
I63.139 Cerebral infarction due to embolism of unspecified carotid artery
ICD-9 441.2
ICD-10 **I71.2** Thoracic aortic aneurysm, without rupture
ICD-9 443.89
ICD-10 **I73.00** Raynaud's syndrome without gangrene
I73.01 Raynaud's syndrome with gangrene
I73.1 Thromboangiitis obliterans (Buerger's disease)
I73.81 Erythromelalgia
I73.89 Other specified peripheral vascular diseases
ICD-9 996.74
ICD-10
The appropriate 7th character is to be added to each code from category T82:
A initial encounter
D subsequent encounter
S sequela
** These codes require a 7th character extender.
T82.818- Embolism of vascular prosthetic devices, implants and grafts
T82.828- Fibrosis of vascular prosthetic devices, implants and graft
T82.838- Hemorrhage of vascular prosthetic devices, implants and grafts
T82.848- Pain from vascular prosthetic devices, implants and grafts
T82.7XX- Infection and inflammatory reaction due to other cardiac and vascular devices, implants and grafts
** Use additional code to identify infection
T82.858- Stenosis of vascular prosthetic devices, implants and grafts
T82.868- Thrombosis of vascular prosthetic devices, implants and grafts
T82.898- Other specified complication of vascular prosthetic devices, implants and grafts
ICD-9 585.5
ICD-10 **N18.5** Chronic kidney disease, stage 5
** Code first any associated:
Diabetic chronic kidney disease (E08.22, E09.22, E10.22, E11.22, E13.22)
Hypertensive chronic kidney disease (I12-, I13-)
Use additional code to identify kidney transplant status, if applicable (Z94.0)
ICD-9 440.0
ICD-10 **I70.0** Atherosclerosis of aorta
** Use additional code to identify:
Exposure to environmental tobacco smoke (Z77.22)
History of tobacco use (Z87.891)
Occupational exposure to environmental tobacco smoke (Z57.31)
Tobacco dependence (F17-)
Tobacco use (Z72.0)
ICD-9 442.3
ICD-10 **I72.4** Aneurysm of artery of lower extremity
ICD-9 998.83
ICD-10
The appropriate 7th character is to be added to each code from category T81:
A initial encounter
D subsequent encounter
S sequela
** This code requires a 7th character extender.
T81.89X- Other complications of procedures, not elsewhere classified
** Use additional code to specify complication, such as:
Postprocedural delirium (F05)
ICD-9 557.1
ICD-10 **K55.1** Chronic vascular disorders of intestine
K55.8 Other vascular disorders of intestine
K55.9 Vascular disorder of intestine, unspecified
ICD-9 424.0
ICD-10 **I05.0** Rheumatic mitral stenosis
I05.1 Rheumatic mitral insufficiency
I05.2 Rheumatic mitral stenosis with insufficiency
I05.8 Other rheumatic mitral valve diseases
I05.9 Rheumatic mitral valve disease, unspecified

ICD-9 454.1
ICD-10 **I83.10** Varicose veins of unspecified lower extremity with inflammation
I83.11 Varicose veins of right lower extremity with inflammatic
I83.12 Varicose veins of left lower extremity with inflammatior
ICD-9 250.70
ICD-10 **E11.59** Type 2 diabetes mellitus with other circulatory complications
** Use additional code to identify any insulin use (Z79.4)
ICD-9 996.1
ICD-10
The appropriate 7th character is to be added to each code from category T82:
A initial encounter
D subsequent encounter
S sequela
** These codes require a 7th character extender.
T82.390- Other mechanical complication of aortic (bifurcation) graft (replacement)
T82.391- Other mechanical complication of carotid arterial graft (bypass)
T82.392- Other mechanical complication of femoral arterial graft (bypass)
T82.398- Other mechanical complication of other vascular graft
T82.399- Other mechanical complication of unspecified vascular grafts
T82.49X- Other complication of vascular dialysis catheter
T82.590- Other mechanical complication of surgically created arteriovenous fistula
T82.591- Other mechanical complication of surgically created arteriovenous shunt
T82.593- Other mechanical complication of balloon (counterpulsation) device
T82.595- Other mechanical complication of umbrella device
T82.598- Other mechanical complication of other cardiac and vascular devices and implants
ICD-9 V67.09
ICD-10 **Z09** Encounter for follow-up examination after completed treatment for conditions other than malignant neoplasm
** Use additional code to identify any applicable history of disease code (Z86.-, Z87-)
ICD-9 405.91
ICD-10 **I15.0** Renovascular hypertension
** Code also underlying condition
ICD-9 998.89
ICD-10
The appropriate 7th character is to be added to each code from category T81:
A initial encounter
D subsequent encounter
S sequela
** This code requires a 7th character extender.
T81.89X- Other complications of procedures, not elsewhere classified
** Use additional code to specify complication, such as:
Postprocedural delirium (F05)
ICD-9 442.2
ICD-10 **I72.3** Aneurysm of iliac artery
ICD-9 585.4
ICD-10 **N18.4** Chronic kidney disease, stage 4 (severe)
** Code first any associated:
Diabetic chronic kidney disease (E08.22, E09.22, E10.22, E11.22, E13.22)
Hypertensive chronic kidney disease (I12-, I13-)
Use additional code to identify kidney transplant status, if applicable (Z94.0)
ICD-9 401.1
ICD-10 **I10** Essential (primary) hypertension
ICD-9 435.9
ICD-10 **G45.9** Transient cerebral ischemic attack, unspecified
ICD-9 440.1
ICD-10 **I70.1** Atherosclerosis of renal artery
** Use additional code to identify:
Exposure to environmental tobacco smoke (Z77.22)
History of tobacco use (Z87.891)
Occupational exposure to environmental tobacco smoke (Z57.31)
Tobacco dependence (F17-)
Tobacco use (Z72.0)
ICD-9 451.19
ICD-10 **I80.209** Phlebitis and thrombophlebitis of unspecified deep vessels of unspecified lower extremity
** Code first phlebitis and thrombophlebitis complicating abortion, ectopic or molar pregnancy (O00-O07, O08.7)
Pregnancy, childbirth and the puerperium (O22-, O87-)
** There are more specific code choice selections available in ICD-10-CM. These include
I80.201 Phlebitis and thrombophlebitis of unspecified deep vessels of right lower extremity
I80.202 Phlebitis and thrombophlebitis of unspecified deep vessels of left lower extremity

I80.203 Phlebitis and thrombophlebitis of unspecified deep vessels of lower extremities, bilateral
I80.211 Phlebitis and thrombophlebitis of right iliac vein
I80.212 Phlebitis and thrombophlebitis of left iliac vein
I80.213 Phlebitis and thrombophlebitis of iliac vein, bilateral
I80.219 Phlebitis and thrombophlebitis of unspecified iliac vein
I80.221 Phlebitis and thrombophlebitis of right popliteal vein
I80.222 Phlebitis and thrombophlebitis of left popliteal vein
I80.223 Phlebitis and thrombophlebitis of popliteal vein, bilateral
I80.229 Phlebitis and thrombophlebitis of unspecified popliteal vein
I80.231 Phlebitis and thrombophlebitis of right tibial vein
I80.232 Phlebitis and thrombophlebitis of left tibial vein
I80.233 Phlebitis and thrombophlebitis of tibial vein, bilateral
I80.239 Phlebitis and thrombophlebitis of unspecified tibial vein
I80.291 Phlebitis and thrombophlebitis of other deep vessels of right lower extremity
I80.292 Phlebitis and thrombophlebitis of other deep vessels of left lower extremity
I80.293 Phlebitis and thrombophlebitis of other deep vessels of lower extremity, bilateral
I80.299 Phlebitis and thrombophlebitis of other deep vessels of unspecified lower extremity

D-9 **457.1**
ICD-10 **I89.0** Lymphedema, not elsewhere classified
D-9 **681.10**
ICD-10 **L03.039** Cellulitis of unspecified toe
L03.049 Acute lymphangitis of unspecified toe
There are more specific code choice selections available in ICD-10-CM. These include:
L03.031 Cellulitis of right toe
L03.032 Cellulitis of left toe
L03.041 Acute lymphangitis of right toe
L03.042 Acute lymphangitis of left toe

Dermatology

702.0
ICD-10 **L57.0** Actinic keratosis
Use additional code to identify the source of the ultraviolet radiation (W89, X32)
D-9 **173.30**
ICD-10 **C44.300** Unspecified malignant neoplasm of skin of unspecified part of face
C44.301 Unspecified malignant neoplasm of skin of nose
C44.309 Unspecified malignant neoplasm of skin of other parts of face
C44.310 Basal cell carcinoma of skin of unspecified part of face
C44.311 Basal cell carcinoma of skin of nose
C44.319 Basal cell carcinoma of skin of other parts of face
C44.320 Squamous cell carcinoma of skin of unspecified parts of face
C44.321 Squamous cell carcinoma of skin of nose
C44.329 Squamous cell carcinoma of other parts of face
C44.390 Other specified malignant neoplasm of skin of unspecified parts of face
C44.391 Other specified malignant neoplasm of skin of nose
C44.399 Other specified malignant neoplasm of other parts of face

239.2
ICD-10 **D49.2** Neoplasm of unspecified behavior of bone, soft tissue, and skin
D-9 **V10.83**
ICD-10 **Z85.828** Personal history of other malignant neoplasm of skin
There are more specific code choice selections available in ICD-10-CM. These include:
Z85.820 Personal history of malignant melanoma of skin
Z85.821 Personal history of Merkel cell carcinoma
D-9 **238.2**
ICD-10 **D48.5** Neoplasm of uncertain behavior of skin
D-9 **692.9**
ICD-10 **L25.9** Unspecified contact dermatitis, unspecified nature
Code first (T36-T65) to identify drug or substance
L30.9 Dermatitis, unspecified
There are more specific code choice selections available in ICD-10-CM. These include:
L25.0 Unspecified contact dermatitis due to cosmetics
L25.1 Unspecified contact dermatitis due to drugs in contact with skin
L25.2 Unspecified contact dermatitis due to dyes
L25.3 Unspecified contact dermatitis due to other chemical products
L25.4 Unspecified contact dermatitis due to food in contact with skin

L25.5 Unspecified contact dermatitis due to plants, except food
L25.8 Unspecified contact dermatitis due to other agents
**Use additional code for adverse effect, if applicable, to identify drug (T36-T50 with fifth or sixth character 5)
ICD-9 **696.1**
ICD-10 **L40.8** Other psoriasis
** There are more specific code choice selections available in ICD-10-CM. These include:
L40.0 Psoriasis vulgaris
L40.1 Generalized pustular psoriasis
L40.2 Acrodermatitis continua
L40.3 Pustulosis Palmaris et plantaris
L40.4 Guttate psoriasis
L40.50 Arthropathic psoriasis, unspecified
L40.51 Distal interphalangeal psoriatic arthropathy
L40.52 Psoriatic arthritis mutilans
L40.53 Psoriatic spondylitis
L40.54 Psoriatic juvenile arthropathy
L40.59 Other psoriatic arthropathy
ICD-9 **702.19**
ICD-10 **L82.1** Other seborrheic keratosis
ICD-9 **173.40**
ICD-10 **C44.40** Unspecified malignant neoplasm of skin of scalp and neck
C44.41 Basal cell carcinoma of skin of scalp and neck
C44.42 Squamous cell carcinoma of skin of scalp and neck
C44.49 Other specified malignant neoplasm of skin of scalp and neck
ICD-9 **702.11**
ICD-10 **L82.0** Inflamed seborrheic keratosis
ICD-9 **173.20**
ICD-10 **C44.201** Unspecified malignant neoplasm of skin of unspecified ear and external auricular canal
C44.202 Unspecified malignant neoplasm of skin of right ear and external auricular canal
C44.209 Unspecified malignant neoplasm of skin of left ear and external auricular canal
C44.211 Basal cell carcinoma of skin of unspecified ear and external auricular canal
C44.212 Basal cell carcinoma of skin of right ear and external auricular canal
C44.219 Basal cell carcinoma of skin of left ear and external auricular canal
C44.221 Squamous cell carcinoma of skin of unspecified ear and external auricular canal
C44.222 Squamous cell carcinoma of skin of right ear and external auricular canal
C44.229 Squamous cell carcinoma of skin of left ear and external auricular canal
C44.291 Other specified malignant neoplasm of unspecified ear and external auricular canal
C44.292 Other specified malignant neoplasm of skin of right ear and external auricular canal
C44.299 Other specified malignant neoplasm of skin of left ear and external auricular canal
ICD-9 **173.60**
ICD-10 **C44.601** Unspecified malignant neoplasm of skin of unspecified upper limb, including shoulder
C44.602 Unspecified malignant neoplasm of skin of right upper limb, including shoulder
C44.609 Unspecified malignant neoplasm of skin of left upper limb, including shoulder
C44.611 Basal cell carcinoma of skin of unspecified upper limb, including shoulder
C44.612 Basal cell carcinoma of skin of right upper limb, including shoulder
C44.619 Basal cell carcinoma of skin of left upper limb, including shoulder
C44.621 Squamous cell carcinoma of skin of unspecified upper limb, including shoulder
C44.622 Squamous cell carcinoma of skin of right upper limb, including shoulder
C44.629 Squamous cell carcinoma of skin of left upper limb, including shoulder
C44.691 Other specified malignant neoplasm of skin of unspecified upper limb, including shoulder
C44.692 Other specified malignant neoplasm of skin of right upper limb, including shoulder
C44.699 Other specified malignant neoplasm of skin of left upper limb, including shoulder
ICD-9 **V10.82**
ICD-10 **Z85.820** Personal history of malignant melanoma of skin

ICD-9 **173.70**
ICD-10 **C44.701** Unspecified malignant neoplasm of skin of unspecified lower limb, including hip
C44.702 Unspecified malignant neoplasm of skin of right lower limb, including hip
C44.709 Unspecified malignant neoplasm of skin of left lower limb, including hip
C44.711 Basal cell carcinoma of skin of unspecified lower limb, including hip
C44.712 Basal cell carcinoma of skin of right lower limb, including hip
C44.719 Basal cell carcinoma of skin of left lower limb, including hip
C44.721 Squamous cell carcinoma of skin of unspecified lower limb, including hip
C44.722 Squamous cell carcinoma of skin of right lower limb, including hip
C44.729 Squamous cell carcinoma of skin of left lower limb, including hip
C44.791 Other specified malignant neoplasm of skin of unspecified lower limb, including hip
C44.792 Other specified malignant neoplasm of skin of right lower limb, including hip
C44.799 Other specified malignant neoplasm of skin of left lower limb, including hip
ICD-9 **173.50**
ICD-10 **C44.500** Unspecified malignant neoplasm of anal skin
C44.501 Unspecified malignant neoplasm of skin of breast
C44.509 Unspecified malignant neoplasm of skin of other part of trunk
C44.510 Basal cell carcinoma of anal skin
C44.511 Basal cell carcinoma of skin of breast
C44.519 Basal cell carcinoma of skin of other part of trunk
C44.520 Squamous cell carcinoma of anal skin
C44.521 Squamous cell carcinoma of skin of breast
C44.529 Squamous cell carcinoma of skin of other part of trunk
C44.590 Other specified malignant neoplasm of anal skin
C44.591 Other specified malignant neoplasm of skin of breast
C44.599 Other specified malignant neoplasm of skin of other part of trunk
ICD-9 **454.1**
ICD-10 **I83.10** Varicose veins of unspecified lower extremity with inflammation
I83.11 Varicose veins of right lower extremity with inflammation
I83.12 Varicose veins of left lower extremity with inflammation
I87.2 Venous insufficiency (chronic)(peripheral)
ICD-9 **173.00**
ICD-10 **C44.00** Unspecified malignant neoplasm of skin of lip
C44.01 Basal cell carcinoma of skin of lip
C44.02 Squamous cell carcinoma of skin of lip
C44.09 Other specified malignant neoplasm of skin of lip
ICD-9 **706.2**
ICD-10 **L72.3** Sebaceous cyst
ICD-9 **173.10**
ICD-10 **C44.101** Unspecified malignant neoplasm of skin of unspecified eyelid, including canthus
C44.102 Unspecified malignant neoplasm of skin of right eyelid, including canthus
C44.109 Unspecified malignant neoplasm of skin of left eyelid, including canthus
C44.111 Basal cell carcinoma of skin of unspecified eyelid, including canthus
C44.112 Basal cell carcinoma of skin of right eyelid, including canthus
C44.119 Basal cell carcinoma of skin of left eyelid, including canthus
C44.121 Squamous cell carcinoma of skin of unspecified eyelid, including canthus
C44.122 Squamous cell carcinoma of skin of right eyelid, including canthus
C44.129 Squamous cell carcinoma of skin of left eyelid, including canthus
C44.191 Other specified malignant neoplasm of skin of unspecified eyelid, including canthus
C44.192 Other specified malignant neoplasm of skin of right eyelid, including canthus
C44.199 Other specified malignant neoplasm of skin of left eyelid, including canthus

ICD-9 172.3
ICD-10 **C43.30** Malignant melanoma of unspecified part of face
C43.31 Malignant melanoma of nose
C43.39 Malignant melanoma of other parts of face
D03.30 Melanoma in situ of unspecified part of face
D03.39 Melanoma in situ of other parts of face
ICD-9 216.5
ICD-10 **D23.5** Other benign neoplasm of skin of trunk
D22.5 Melanocytic nevi of trunk
ICD-9 692.79
ICD-10 **L56.4** Polymorphous light eruption
L56.8 Other specified acute skin changes due to ultraviolet radiation
L57.8 Other skin changes due to chronic exposure to nonionizing radiation
**Use additional code to identify the source of the ultraviolet radiation (W89, X32)
ICD-9 078.10
ICD-10 **B07.9** Viral wart, unspecified
** There are more specific code choice selections available in ICD-10-CM. These include:
B07.0 Plantar wart
B07.8 Other viral warts
ICD-9 695.3
ICD-10 **L71.0** Perioral dermatitis
L71.1 Rhinophyma
L71.8 Other rosacea
L71.9 Rosacea, unspecified
**Use additional code for adverse effect, if applicable, to identify drug (T36-T50 with fifth or sixth character 5)
ICD-9 698.3
ICD-10 **L28.0** Lichen simplex chronicus
L28.1 Prurigo nodularis
ICD-9 690.10
ICD-10 **L21.9** Seborrheic dermatitis, unspecified
* There are more specific code choice selections available in ICD-10-CM. These include:
L21.0 Seborrhea capitis
L21.1 Seborrheic infantile dermatitis
L21.8 Other seborrheic dermatitis
ICD-9 706.8
ICD-10 **L85.3** Xerosis cutis
L73.8 Other specified follicular disorders
ICD-9 709.09
ICD-10 **L81.9** Disorder of pigmentation, unspecified
* There are more specific code choice selections available in ICD-10-CM. These include:
L81.0 Postinflammatory hyperpigmentation
L81.1 Chloasma
L81.2 Freckles
L81.3 Café au lait spots
L81.4 Other melanin hyperpigmentation
L81.5 Leukoderma, NEC
L81.6 Other disorders of diminished melanin formation
L81.7 Pigmented purpuric dermatosis
L81.8 Other specified disorders of pigmentation
ICD-9 697.0
ICD-10 **L66.1** Lichen planopilaris
L43.0 Hypertrophic lichen planus
L43.1 Bullous lichen planus
L43.2 Lichenoid drug reaction
*Use additional code for adverse effect, if applicable, to identify drug (T36-T50 with fifth or sixth character 5)
L43.3 Subacute (active) lichen planus
L43.8 Other lichen planus
L43.9 Lichen planus, unspecified
ICD-9 704.8
ICD-10 **L01.02** Bockhart's impetigo
L66.3 Perifolliculitis capitis abscedens
L73.8 Other specified follicular disorders
ICD-9 691.8
ICD-10 **L20.0** Besnier's prurigo
L20.81 Atopic neurodermatitis
L20.82 Flexural eczema
L20.83 Infantile (acute) (chronic) eczema
L20.84 Intrinsic (allergic) eczema
L20.89 Other atopic dermatitis
L20.9 Atopic dermatitis, unspecified
ICD-9 701.9
ICD-10 **L90.9** Atrophic disorder of skin, unspecified
L91.9 Hypertrophic disorder of the skin, unspecified
*There are mores specific code choice selections available in ICD-10-CM. These include:
L90.0 Lichen sclerosus et atrophicus
L90.1 Anetoderma of Schweninger-Buzzi
L90.2 Anetoderma of Jadassohn-Pellizzari
L90.3 Atrophoderma of Pasini and Pierini

L90.4 Acrodermatitis chronica atrophicans
L90.5 Scar conditions and fibrosis of skin
L90.6 Striae atrophicae
L90.8 Other atrophic disorders of skin
L91.0 Hypertrophic scar
L91.8 Other hypertrophic disorders of the skin
ICD-9 706.1
ICD-10 **L70.0** Acne vulgaris
L70.1 Acne conglobata
L70.2 Acne varioliformis
L70.3 Acne tropica
L70.4 Infantile acne
L70.5 Acne excoriee des jeunes filles
L70.8 Other acne
L70.9 Acne, unspecified
L73.0 Acne keloid
ICD-9 695.89
ICD-10 **L26** Exfoliative dermatitis
L30.4 Erythema intertrigo
L44.0 Pityriasis rubra pilaris
L53.8 Other specified erythematous conditions
L92.0 Granuloma annulare
L95.1 Erythema elevatum diutinum
L98.2 Febrile neutrophilic dermatosis (Sweet)
ICD-9 707.9
ICD-10 **L98.499** Non-pressure chronic ulcer of skin of other sites with unspecified severity
*There are more specific code choice selections available in ICD-10-CM. These include:
L98.411 Non-pressure chronic ulcer of buttock limited to breakdown of skin
L98.412 Non-pressure chronic ulcer of buttock with fat layer exposed
L98.413 Non-pressure chronic ulcer of buttock with necrosis of muscle
L98.414 Non-pressure chronic ulcer of buttock with necrosis of bone
L98.419 Non-pressure chronic ulcer of buttock with unspecified severity
L98.421 Non-pressure chronic ulcer of back limited to breakdown of skin
L98.422 Non-pressure chronic ulcer of back with fat layer exposed
L98.423 Non-pressure chronic ulcer of back with necrosis of muscle
L98.424 Non-pressure chronic ulcer of back with necrosis of bone
L98.429 Non-pressure chronic ulcer of back with unspecified severity
L98.491 Non-pressure chronic ulcer of skin of other sites limited to breakdown of skin
L98.492 Non-pressure chronic ulcer of skin of other sites with fat layer exposed
L98.493 Non-pressure chronic ulcer of skin of other sites with necrosis of muscle
L98.494 Non-pressure chronic ulcer of skin of other sites with necrosis of bone
ICD-9 692.74
ICD-10 **L57.8** Other skin changes due to chronic exposure to nonionizing radiation
L57.9 Skin changes due to chronic exposure to nonionizing radiation, unspecified
**Use additional code to identify the source of the ultraviolet radiation (W89, X32)
ICD-9 701.4
ICD-10 **L91.0** Hypertrophic scar
ICD-9 782.1
ICD-10 **R21** Rash and other nonspecific skin eruption
ICD-9 694.5
ICD-10 **L12.0** Bullous pemphigoid
L12.1 Cicatricial pemphigoid
L12.2 Chronic bullous disease of childhood
L12.8 Other pemphigoid
L12.9 Pemphigoid, unspecified
L13.0 Dermatitis herpetiformis
ICD-9 701.0
ICD-10 **L94.0** Localized scleroderma (morphea)
L90.0 Lichen sclerosus et atrophicus
L94.1 Linear scleroderma
L94.3 Sclerodactyly
ICD-9 698.9
ICD-10 **L29.9** Pruritis, unspecified
** There are more specific code choice selections available in ICD-10-CM. These include:

L29.0 Pruritis ani
L29.1 Pruritis scroti
L29.2 Pruritis vulvae
L29.3 Anogenital pruritis, unspecified
L29.8 Other pruritis
ICD-9 172.5
ICD-10 **C43.51** Malignant melanoma of anal skin
C43.52 Malignant melanoma of skin of breast
C43.59 Malignant melanoma of other part of trunk
D03.51 Melanoma in situ of anal skin
D03.52 Melanoma in situ of breast (skin) (soft tissue)
D03.59 Melanoma in situ of other part of trunk
ICD-9 V58.32
ICD-10 **Z48.02** Encounter for removal of sutures
ICD-9 202.11
ICD-10 **C84.01** Mycosis fungoides, lymph nodes of head, face, and neck
ICD-9 704.00
ICD-10 **L65.9** Nonscarring hair loss, unspecified
**Use additional code for adverse effect, if applicable, to identify drug (T36-T50 with fifth or sixth character 5)
** There are more specific code choice selections available in ICD-10-CM. These includ
L63.0 Alopecia (capitis) totalis
L63.1 Alopecia universalis
L63.2 Ophiasis
L63.8 Other alopecia areata
L63.9 Alopecia areata, unspecified
L64.0 Drug-induced androgenic alopecia
**Use additional code for adverse effect, if applicable, to identify drug (T36-T50 with fifth or sixth character 5)
L64.8 Other androgenic alopecia
L64.9 Androgenic alopecia, unspecified
L65.0 Telogen effluvium
L65.1 Anagen effluvium
L65.2 Alopecia mucinosa
L65.8 Other specified nonscarring hair loss
ICD-9 693.0
ICD-10 **L27.0** Generalized skin eruption due to drugs and medicaments taken internally
L27.1 Localized skin eruption due to drugs and medicaments taken internally
**Use additional code for adverse effect, if applicable, to identify drug (T36-T50 with fifth or sixth character 5)
ICD-9 110.5
ICD-10 **B35.4** Tinea corporis
B35.5 Tinea imbricata
ICD-9 172.6
ICD-10 **C43.60** Malignant melanoma of unspecified upper limb, including shoulder
C43.61 Malignant melanoma of right upper limb, including shoulder
C43.62 Malignant melanoma of left upper limb, including should
D03.60 Melanoma in situ of unspecified upper limb, including shoulder
D03.61 Melanoma in situ of right upper limb, including shoulder
D03.62 Melanoma in situ of left upper limb, including shoulde
ICD-9 V16.8
ICD-10 **Z80.8** Family history of malignant neoplasm of other organs or systems
ICD-9 228.01
ICD-10 **D18.01** Hemangioma of skin and subcutaneous tissue
ICD-9 110.4
ICD-10 **B35.3** Tinea pedis

Emergency Department

ICD-9 786.50
ICD-10 **R07.9** Chest pain, unspecified
** There are more specific code choice selections available in ICD-10-CM. These inclu
R07.1 Chest pain on breathing
R07.2 Precordial pain
R07.81 Pleurodynia
R07.89 Other chest pain
ICD-9 789.09
ICD-10 **R10.10** Upper abdominal pain, unspecified
R10.2 Pelvic and perineal pain
R10.30 Lower abdominal pain, unspecified
ICD-9 959.01
** These codes require a 7th character extender.
ICD-10 **S09.90X-** Unspecified injury of head
** There are more specific code choice selections available in ICD-10-CM. These inclu
S09.8XX- Other specified injuries of head

S06.9X0- Unspecified intracranial injury without loss of consciousness

S06.9X1- Unspecified intracranial injury with loss of consciousness of 30 minutes or less

S06.9X2- Unspecified intracranial injury with loss of consciousness of 31 minutes to 59 minutes

S06.9X3- Unspecified intracranial injury with loss of consciousness of 1 hour to 5 hours 59 minutes

S06.9X4- Unspecified intracranial injury with loss of consciousness of 6 hours to 24 hours

S06.9X5- Unspecified intracranial injury with loss of consciousness of greater than 24 hours with return to pre-existing conscious level

S06.9X6- Unspecified intracranial injury with loss of consciousness of greater than 24 hours without return to pre-existing conscious level with patient surviving

S06.9X7- Unspecified intracranial injury with loss of consciousness of any duration with death due to brain injury prior to regaining consciousness

S06.9X8- Unspecified intracranial injury with loss of consciousness of any duration with death due to other cause prior to regaining consciousness

S06.9X9- Unspecified intracranial injury with loss of consciousness of unspecified duration

CD-9 784.0
ICD-10 R51 Headache
CD-9 780.2
ICD-10 R55 Syncope and collapse
CD-9 883

The appropriate 7th character is to be added to each code from category, S61

ICD-10 **S61.209-** Unspecified open wound of unspecified finger without damage to nail

* There are more specific code choice selections available in ICD-10-CM. These include:

S61.001- Unspecified open wound of right thumb without damage to nail

S61.002- Unspecified open wound of left thumb without damage to nail

S61.009- Unspecified open wound of unspecified thumb without damage to nail

S61.011- Laceration without foreign body of right thumb without damage to nail

S61.012- Laceration without foreign body of left thumb without damage to nail

S61.019- Laceration without foreign body of unspecified thumb without damage to nail

S61.021- Laceration with foreign body of right thumb without damage to nail

S61.022- Laceration with foreign body of left thumb without damage to nail

S61.029- Laceration with foreign body of unspecified thumb without damage to nail

S61.031- Puncture wound without foreign body of right thumb without damage to nail

S61.032- Puncture wound without foreign body of left thumb without damage to nail

S61.039- Puncture wound without foreign body of unspecified thumb without damage to nail

S61.041- Puncture wound with foreign body of right thumb without damage to nail

S61.042- Puncture wound with foreign body of left thumb without damage to nail

S61.049- Puncture wound with foreign body of unspecified thumb without damage to nail

S61.051- Open bite of right thumb without damage to nail
S61.052- Open bite of left thumb without damage to nail
S61.059- Open bite of unspecified thumb without damage to nail

S61.101- Unspecified open wound of right thumb with damage to nail

S61.102- Unspecified open wound of left thumb with damage to nail

S61.109- Unspecified open wound of unspecified thumb with damage to nail

S61.111- Laceration without foreign body of right thumb with damage to nail

S61.112- Laceration without foreign body of left thumb with damage to nail

S61.119- Laceration without foreign body of unspecified thumb with damage to nail

S61.121- Laceration with foreign body of right thumb with damage to nail

S61.122- Laceration with foreign body of left thumb with damage to nail

S61.129- Laceration with foreign body of unspecified thumb with damage to nail

** These codes require a 7th character extender.

S61.131- Puncture wound without foreign body of right thumb with damage to nail

S61.132- Puncture wound without foreign body of left thumb with damage to nail

S61.139- Puncture wound without foreign body of unspecified thumb with damage to nail

S61.141- Puncture wound with foreign body of right thumb with damage to nail

S61.142- Puncture wound with foreign body of left thumb with damage to nail

S61.149- Puncture wound with foreign body of unspecified thumb with damage to nail

S61.151- Open bite of right thumb with damage to nail
S61.152- Open bite of left thumb with damage to nail
S61.159- Open bite of unspecified thumb with damage to nail

S61.200- Unspecified open wound of right index finger without damage to nail

S61.201- Unspecified open wound of left index finger without damage to nail

S61.202- Unspecified open wound of right middle finger without damage to nail

S61.203- Unspecified open wound of left middle finger without damage to nail

S61.204- Unspecified open wound of right ring finger without damage to nail

S61.205- Unspecified open wound of left ring finger without damage to nail

S61.206- Unspecified open wound of right little finger without damage to nail

S61.207- Unspecified open wound of left little finger without damage to nail

S61.208- Unspecified open wound of other finger without damage to nail

S61.209- Unspecified open wound of unspecified finger without damage to nail

S61.210- Laceration without foreign body of right index finger without damage to nail

S61.211- Laceration without foreign body of left index finger without damage to nail

S61.212- Laceration without foreign body of right middle finger without damage to nail

S61.213- Laceration without foreign body of left middle finger without damage to nail

S61.214- Laceration without foreign body of right ring finger without damage to nail

S61.215- Laceration without foreign body of left ring finger without damage to nail

S61.216- Laceration without foreign body of right little finger without damage to nail

S61.217- Laceration without foreign body of left little finger without damage to nail

S61.218- Laceration without foreign body of other finger without damage to nail

S61.219- Laceration without foreign body of unspecified finger without damage to nail

S61.220- Laceration with foreign body of right index finger without damage to nail

S61.221- Laceration with foreign body of left index finger without damage to nail

S61.222- Laceration with foreign body of right middle finger without damage to nail

S61.223- Laceration with foreign body of left middle finger without damage to nail

S61.224- Laceration with foreign body of right ring finger without damage to nail

S61.225- Laceration with foreign body of left ring finger without damage to nail

S61.226- Laceration with foreign body of right little finger without damage to nail

S61.227- Laceration with foreign body of left little finger without damage to nail

S61.228- Laceration with foreign body of other finger without damage to nail

S61.229- Laceration with foreign body of unspecified finger without damage to nail

S61.230- Puncture wound without foreign body of right index finger without damage to nail

S61.231- Puncture wound without foreign body of left index finger without damage to nail

S61.232- Puncture wound without foreign body of right middle finger without damage to nail

S61.233- Puncture wound without foreign body of left middle finger without damage to nail

S61.234- Puncture wound without foreign body of right ring finger without damage to nail

S61.235- Puncture wound without foreign body of left ring finger without damage to nail

S61.236- Puncture wound without foreign body of right little finger without damage to nail

S61.237- Puncture wound without foreign body of left little finger without damage to nail

S61.238- Puncture wound without foreign body of other finger without damage to nail

S61.239- Puncture wound without foreign body of unspecified finger without damage to nail

S61.240- Puncture wound with foreign body of right index finger without damage to nail

S61.241- Puncture wound with foreign body of left index finger without damage to nail

S61.242- Puncture wound with foreign body of right middle finger without damage to nail

S61.243- Puncture wound with foreign body of left middle finger without damage to nail

S61.244- Puncture wound with foreign body of right ring finger without damage to nail

S61.245- Puncture wound with foreign body of left ring finger without damage to nail

S61.246- Puncture wound with foreign body of right little finger without damage to nail

S61.247- Puncture wound with foreign body of left little finger without damage to nail

S61.248- Puncture wound with foreign body of other finger without damage to nail

S61.249- Puncture wound with foreign body of unspecified finger without damage to nail

S61.250- Open bite of right index finger without damage to nail
S61.251- Open bite of left index finger without damage to nail
S61.252- Open bite of right middle finger without damage to nail
S61.253- Open bite of left middle finger without damage to nail
S61.254- Open bite of right ring finger without damage to nail
S61.255- Open bite of left ring finger without damage to nail
S61.256- Open bite of right little finger without damage to nail
S61.257- Open bite of left little finger without damage to nail
S61.258- Open bite of other finger without damage to nail
S61.259- Open bite of unspecified finger without damage to nail

S61.300- Unspecified open wound of right index finger with damage to nail

S61.301- Unspecified open wound of left index finger with damage to nail

S61.302- Unspecified open wound of right middle finger with damage to nail

S61.303- Unspecified open wound of left middle finger with damage to nail

S61.304- Unspecified open wound of right ring finger with damage to nail

S61.305- Unspecified open wound of left ring finger with damage to nail

S61.306- Unspecified open wound of right little finger with damage to nail

S61.307- Unspecified open wound of left little finger with damage to nail

S61.308- Unspecified open wound of other finger with damage to nail

S61.309- Unspecified open wound of unspecified finger with damage to nail

S61.310- Laceration without foreign body of right index finger with damage to nail

S61.311- Laceration without foreign body of left index finger with damage to nail

S61.312- Laceration without foreign body of right middle finger with damage to nail

S61.313- Laceration without foreign body of left middle finger with damage to nail

S61.314- Laceration without foreign body of right ring finger with damage to nail

S61.315- Laceration without foreign body of left ring finger with damage to nail

S61.316- Laceration without foreign body of right little finger with damage to nail

S61.317- Laceration without foreign body of left little finger with damage to nail

S61.318- Laceration without foreign body of other finger with damage to nail

S61.319- Laceration without foreign body of unspecified finger with damage to nail

S61.320- Laceration with foreign body of right index finger with damage to nail

S61.321- Laceration with foreign body of left index finger with damage to nail

S61.322- Laceration with foreign body of right middle finger with damage to nail

S61.323- Laceration with foreign body of left middle finger with damage to nail

S61.324- Laceration with foreign body of right ring finger with damage to nail

S61.325- Laceration with foreign body of left ring finger with damage to nail

S61.326- Laceration with foreign body of right little finger with damage to nail

S61.327- Laceration with foreign body of left little finger with damage to nail

S61.328- Laceration with foreign body of other finger with damage to nail

S61.329- Laceration with foreign body of unspecified finger with damage to nail

S61.330- Puncture wound without foreign body of right index finger with damage to nail

S61.331- Puncture wound without foreign body of left index finger with damage to nail

S61.332- Puncture wound without foreign body of right middle finger with damage to nail

S61.333- Puncture wound without foreign body of left middle finger with damage to nail

S61.334- Puncture wound without foreign body of right ring finger with damage to nail

S61.335- Puncture wound without foreign body of left ring finger with damage to nail

S61.336- Puncture wound without foreign body of right little finger with damage to nail

S61.337- Puncture wound without foreign body of left little finger with damage to nail

S61.338- Puncture wound without foreign body of other finger with damage to nail

S61.339- Puncture wound without foreign body of unspecified finger with damage to nail

S61.340- Puncture wound with foreign body of right index finger with damage to nail

S61.341- Puncture wound with foreign body of left index finger with damage to nail

S61.342- Puncture wound with foreign body of right middle finger with damage to nail

S61.343- Puncture wound with foreign body of left middle finger with damage to nail

S61.344- Puncture wound with foreign body of right ring finger with damage to nail

S61.345- Puncture wound with foreign body of left ring finger with damage to nail

S61.346- Puncture wound with foreign body of right little finger with damage to nail

S61.347- Puncture wound with foreign body of left little finger with damage to nail

S61.348- Puncture wound with foreign body of other finger with damage to nail

S61.349- Puncture wound with foreign body of unspecified finger with damage to nail

S61.350- Open bite of right index finger with damage to nail
S61.351- Open bite of left index finger with damage to nail
S61.352- Open bite of right middle finger with damage to nail
S61.353- Open bite of left middle finger with damage to nail
S61.354- Open bite of right ring finger with damage to nail
S61.355- Open bite of left ring finger with damage to nail
S61.356- Open bite of right little finger with damage to nail
S61.357- Open bite of left little finger with damage to nail
S61.358- Open bite of other finger with damage to nail

S61.359- Open bite of unspecified finger with damage to nail

ICD-9 845.00
The appropriate 7th character is to be added to each code from category S93 and S96
ICD-10 **S93.409-** Sprain of unspecified ligament of unspecified ankle
** There are more specific code choice selections available in ICD-10-CM. These include:
S93.401- Sprain of unspecified ligament of right ankle
S93.402- Sprain of unspecified ligament of left ankle
S93.411- Sprain of calcaneofibular ligament of right ankle
S93.412- Sprain of calcaneofibular ligament of left ankle
S93.419- Sprain of calcaneofibular ligament of unspecified ankle
S93.421- Sprain of deltoid ligament of right ankle
S93.422- Sprain of deltoid ligament of left ankle
S93.429- Sprain of deltoid ligament of unspecified ankle
S93.431- Sprain of tibiofibular ligament of right ankle
S93.432- Sprain of tibiofibular ligament of left ankle
S93.439- Sprain of tibiofibular ligament of unspecified ankle
S93.491- Sprain of other ligament of right ankle
S93.492- Sprain of other ligament of left ankle
S93.499- Sprain of other ligament of unspecified ankle
S96.011- Strain of muscle and tendon of long flexor muscle of toe at ankle and foot level, right foot
S96.012- Strain of muscle and tendon of long flexor muscle of toe at ankle and foot level, left foot
S96.019- Strain of muscle and tendon of long flexor muscle of toe at ankle and foot level, unspecified foot
S96.111- Strain of muscle and tendon of long extensor muscle of toe at ankle and foot level, right foot
S96.112- Strain of muscle and tendon of long extensor muscle of toe at ankle and foot level, left foot
S96.119- Strain of muscle and tendon of long extensor muscle of toe at ankle and foot, unspecified foot
S96.211- Strain of intrinsic muscle and tendon at ankle and foot level, right foot
S96.212- Strain of intrinsic muscle and tendon at ankle and foot level, left foot
S96.219- Strain of intrinsic muscle and tendon at ankle and foot level, unspecified foot
S96.811- Strain of other specified muscles and tendons at ankle and foot level, right foot
S96.812- Strain of other specified muscles and tendons at ankle and foot level, left foot
S96.819- Strain of other specified muscles and tendons at ankle and foot level, unspecified foot
S96.911- Strain of unspecified muscle and tendon at ankle and foot level, right foot
S96.912- Strain of unspecified muscle and tendon at ankle and foot level, left foot
S96.919- Strain of unspecified muscle and tendon at ankle and foot level, unspecified foot

ICD-9 486
ICD-10 **J18.9** Pneumonia, unspecified organism
J18.8 Other pneumonia, unspecified organism
** Code first associated influenza, if applicable (J09.X1, J10.0-, J11.0-)
ICD-9 780.60
ICD-10 **R50.9** Fever, unspecified
** There are more specific code choice selections available in ICD-10-CM. These include:
R50.2 Drug induced fever
**Use additional code for adverse effect, if applicable to identify drug (T36-T50 with fifth or sixth character 5)
R50.81 Fever presenting with conditions classified elsewhere
R50.82 Postprocedural fever
R50.83 Postvaccination fever
R50.84 Febrile nonhemolytic transfusion reaction
ICD-9 724.5
ICD-10 **M54.9** Dorsalgia, unspecified
** There are more specific code choice selections available for back pain. These include:
M54.89 Other dorsalgia
M54.6 Pain in thoracic spine
M54.5 Low back pain
M53.3 Sacrococcygeal disorders, not elsewhere classified
ICD-9 305.00
ICD-10 **F10.10** Alcohol abuse, uncomplicated
** Use additional code for blood alcohol level, if applicable (Y90-)
** There are more specific code choice selections available in ICD-10-CM. These include:
F10.120 Alcohol abuse with intoxication, uncomplicated
F10.121 Alcohol abuse with intoxication delirium
F10.129 Alcohol abuse with intoxication, unspecified
F10.14 Alcohol abuse with alcohol-induced mood disorder
F10.150 Alcohol abuse with alcohol-induced psychotic disorder with delusions

F10.151 Alcohol abuse with alcohol-induced psychotic disorde with hallucinations
F10.519 Alcohol abuse with alcohol-induced psychotic disorde unspecified
F10.159 Alcohol abuse with alcohol-induced anxiety disorder
F10.181 Alcohol abuse with alcohol-induced sexual dysfunction
F10.182 Alcohol abuse with alcohol-induced sleep disorder
F10.188 Alcohol abuse with other alcohol-induced disorder
ICD-9 729.5
ICD-10 **M79.609** Pain in unspecified limb
** There are more specific code choice selections available in ICD-10-CM. These includ
M79.601 Pain in right arm
M79.602 Pain in left arm
M79.603 Pain in arm, unspecified
M79.604 Pain in right leg
M79.605 Pain in left leg
M79.606 Pain in leg, unspecified
M79.621 Pain in right upper arm
M79.622 Pain in left upper arm
M79.629 Pain in unspecified upper arm
M79.631 Pain in right forearm
M79.632 Pain in left forearm
M79.639 Pain in unspecified forearm
M79.641 Pain in right hand
M79.642 Pain in left hand
M79.643 Pain in unspecified hand
M79.644 Pain in right finger(s)
M79.645 Pain in left finger(s)
M79.646 Pain in unspecified finger(s)
M79.651 Pain in right thigh
M79.652 Pain in left thigh
M79.659 Pain in unspecified thigh
M79.661 Pain in right lower leg
M79.662 Pain in left lower leg
M79.669 Pain in unspecified lower leg
M79.671 Pain in right foot
M79.672 Pain in left foot
M79.673 Pain in unspecified foot
M79.674 Pain in right toe(s)
M79.675 Pain in left toe(s)
M79.676 Pain in unspecified toes(s)
ICD-9 787.03
ICD-10 **R11.11** Vomiting without nausea
ICD-9 465.9
ICD-10 **J06.9** Acute upper respiratory infection, unspecified
J39.8 Other specified diseases of upper respiratory tract
ICD-9 724.2
ICD-10 **M54.5** Low back pain
ICD-9 789.00
ICD-10 **R10.9** Unspecified abdominal pain
** There are more specific code choice selections available in ICD-10-CM. These incluc
R10.0 Acute abdomen
R10.10 Upper abdominal pain, unspecified
R10.11 Right upper quadrant pain
R10.12 Left upper quadrant pain
R10.13 Epigastric pain
R10.2 Pelvic pain
R10.30 Lower abdominal pain, unspecified
R10.31 Right lower quadrant pain
R10.32 Left lower quadrant pain
R10.33 Periumbilical pain
R10.84 Generalized abdominal pain
ICD-9 780.99
ICD-10 **R68.89** Other general symptoms and signs
R45.84 Anhedonia
ICD-9 462
ICD-10 **J02.8** Acute pharyngitis due to other specified organisms
** Use additional code (B95-B97) to identify infectious agent
J02.0 Streptococcal pharyngitis
J02.9 Acute pharyngitis, unspecified
ICD-9 786.59
ICD-10 **R07.82** Intercostal pain
R07.89 Chest pain, other
ICD-9 599.0
ICD-10 **N39.0** Urinary tract infection, site not specified
** Use additional code (B95-B97) to identify infectious agent
** There are more specific code choice selections available in ICD-10-CM. These incluc
N30.00 Acute cystitis without hematuria
N30.01 Acute cystitis with hematuria
N30.10 Interstitial cystitis (chronic) without hematuria

N30.11 Interstitial cystitis (chronic) with hematuria
N30.20 Other chronic cystitis without hematuria
N30.21 Other chronic cystitis with hematuria
N30.30 Trigonitis without hematuria
N30.31 Trigonitis with hematuria
N30.40 Irradiation cystitis without hematuria
N30.41 Irradiation cystitis with hematuria
N30.80 Other cystitis without hematuria
N30.81 Other cystitis with hematuria
N30.90 Cystitis, unspecified without hematuria
N30.91 Cystitis, unspecified with hematuria
N15.9 Renal tubulo-interstitial disease, unspecified

ICD-9 **847.0**
e appropriate 7th character is to be added to each code from category **S13 and S16**
ICD-10 **S13.4XX-** Sprain of ligaments of cervical spine
S13.8XX- Sprain of joints and ligaments of other parts of neck
S16.1XX- Strain of muscle, fascia and tendon at neck level

311
ICD-10 **F32.9** Major depressive disorder, single episode, unspecified
There are more specific code choice selections available in ICD-10-CM. These include:
F32.0 Major depressive disorder, single episode, mild
F32.1 Major depressive disorder, single episode, moderate
F32.2 Major depressive disorder, single episode, severe without psychotic features
F32.3 Major depressive disorder, single episode, severe with psychotic features
F32.4 Major depressive disorder, single episode, in partial remission
F32.5 Major depressive disorder, single episode, in full remission
F32.8 Other depressive episodes

ICD-9 **300.00**
ICD-10 **F41.1** Generalized anxiety disorder
F41.8 Other specified anxiety disorders
F41.9 Anxiety disorder, unspecified

ICD-9 **525.9**
ICD-10 **K08.9** Disorder of teeth and supporting structures, unspecified
There are more specific code choice selections available in ICD-10-CM. These include:
K08.51 Open restoration margins of tooth
K08.530 Fractured dental restorative material without loss of material
K08.531 Fractured dental restorative material with loss of material
K08.539 Fractured dental restorative material, unspecified

786.09
ICD-10 **R06.83** Snoring
R06.3 Periodic breathing
R06.4 Hyperventilation
R06.00 Dyspnea, unspecified
R06.89 Other abnormalities of breathing

ICD-9 **787.01**
ICD-10 **R11.2** Nausea with vomiting, unspecified

ICD-9 **844.9**
e appropriate 7th character is to be added to each code from category **S83**
ICD-10 **S83.90X-** Sprain of unspecified site of unspecified knee
There are more specific code choice selections available in ICD-10-CM. These include:
S83.401- Sprain of unspecified collateral ligament of right knee
S83.402- Sprain of unspecified collateral ligament of left knee
S83.409- Sprain of unspecified collateral ligament of unspecified knee
S83.411- Sprain of medial collateral ligament of right knee
S83.412- Sprain of medial collateral ligament of left knee
S83.419- Sprain of medial collateral ligament of unspecified knee
S83.421- Sprain of lateral collateral ligament of right knee
S83.422- Sprain of lateral collateral ligament of left knee
S83.429- Sprain of lateral collateral ligament of unspecified knee
S83.501- Sprain of unspecified cruciate ligament of right knee
S83.502- Sprain of unspecified cruciate ligament of left knee
S83.509- Sprain of unspecified cruciate ligament of unspecified knee
S83.511- Sprain of anterior cruciate ligament of right knee
S83.512- Sprain of anterior cruciate ligament of left knee
S83.519- Sprain of anterior cruciate ligament of unspecified knee
S83.521- Sprain of posterior cruciate ligament of right knee
S83.522- Sprain of posterior cruciate ligament of left knee
S83.8X1- Sprain of other specified parts of right knee
S83.8X2- Sprain of other specified parts of left knee
S83.8X9- Sprain of other specified parts of unspecified knee
S83.91X- Sprain of unspecified site of right knee
S83.92X- Sprain of unspecified site of left knee

ICD-9 **789.03**
ICD-10 **R10.31** Right lower quadrant pain
ICD-9 **700.39**
ICD-10 **R56.9** Unspecified convulsions
** There are more specific code choice selections available in ICD-10-CM. These include:
R56.00 Simple febrile convulsions
R56.01 Complex febrile convulsions
R56.1 Post traumatic seizures
ICD-9 **780.4**
ICD-10 **R42** Dizziness and giddiness
ICD-9 **346.90**
ICD-10 **G43.909** Migraine, unspecified, not intractable, without status migrainosus
** There are more specific code choice selections available in ICD-10-CM. These include:
G43.009 Migraine without aura, not intractable, without status migrainosus
G43.109 Migraine with aura, not intractable, without status migrainosus
G43.409 Hemiplegic migraine, not intractable, without status migrainosus
G43.509 Persistent migraine aura without cerebral infarction, not intractable, without status migrainosus
G43.609 Persistent migraine aura with cerebral infarction, not intractable, without status migrainosus
G43.709 Chronic migraine without aura, not intractable, without status migrainosus
G43.B0 Ophthalmoplegic migraine, not intractable
G43.D0 Abdominal migraine, not intractable
G43.809 Other migraine, not intractable, without status migrainosus
ICD-9 **521.00**
ICD-10 **K02.9** Dental carries, unspecified
** There are more specific code choice selections available in ICD-10-CM. These include:
K02.51 Dental carries on pit and fissure surface limited to enamel
K02.52 Dental carries on pit and fissure surface penetrating into dentin
K02.53 Dental carries on pit and fissure surface penetrating into pulp
K02.61 Dental carries on smooth surface limited to enamel
K02.62 Dental carries on smooth surface penetrating into dentin
K02.63 Dental carries on smooth surface penetrating into pulp
K02.7 Dental root carries
ICD-9 **079.99**
ICD-10 **B34.9** Viral infection, unspecified
ICD-10 **490**
ICD-10 **J40** Bronchitis, not specified as acute or chronic
** There are more specific code choice selections available in ICD-10-CM. These include:
J20.0 Acute bronchitis due to Mycoplasma pneumoiae
J20.1 Acute bronchitis due to Hemophilus influenzae
J20.2 Acute bronchitis due to streptococcus
J20.3 Acute bronchitis due to coxsackievirus
J20.4 Acute bronchitis due to parainfluenza virus
J20.5 Acute bronchitis due to respiratory syncytial virus
J20.6 Acute bronchitis due to rhinovirus
J20.7 Acute bronchitis due to echovirus
J20.8 Acute bronchitis due to other specified organisms
J20.9 Acute bronchitis, unspecified
J41.0 Simple chronic bronchitis
J41.1 Mucopurulent chronic bronchitis
J41.8 Mixed simple and mucopurulent chronic bronchitis
J42 Unspecified chronic bronchitis
ICD-9 **789.06**
ICD-10 **R10.13** Epigastric pain
ICD-9 **682.6**
ICD-10 **L03.115** Cellulitis of right lower limb
L03.116 Cellulitis of left lower limb
L03.119 Cellulitis of unspecified part of limb
L03.125 Acute lymphangitis of right lower limb
L03.126 Acute lymphangitis of left lower limb
L03.129 Acute lymphangitis of unspecified part of limb
ICD-9 **719.46**
ICD-10 **M25.561** Pain in right knee
M25.562 Pain in left knee
M25.569 Pain in unspecified knee
ICD-9 **780.97**
ICD-10 **R41.82** Altered mental status, unspecified
** There are more specific code choice selections available in ICD-10-CM. These include:
R41.0 Disorientation, unspecified
R41.81 Age-related cognitive decline
R41.840 Attention and concentration deficit

R41.89 Other symptoms and signs involving cognitive functions and awareness
ICD-9 **427.31**
ICD-10 **I48.0** Paroxysmal atrial fibrillation
I48.1 Persistent atrial fibrillation
I48.2 Chronic atrial fibrillation
I48.91 Unspecified atrial fibrillation
ICD-9 **920**
The appropriate 7th character is to be added to each code from category **S00 and S10**
ICD-10 **S00.93X-** Contusion of unspecified part of head
S10.93X- Contusion of unspecified part of neck
** There are more specific code choice selections available in ICD-10-CM. These include:
S10.83X- Contusion of other specified part of neck
S00.83X- Contusion of other part of head
S00.03X- Contusion of scalp
S00.33X- Contusion of nose
S00.431- Contusion of right ear
S00.432- Contusion of left ear
S00.439- Contusion of unspecified ear
S00.531- Contusion of lip
ICD-9 **786.2**
ICD-10 **R05** Cough
ICD-9 **780.79**
ICD-10 **R53.81** Other malaise
R53.83 Other fatigue
R53.0 Neoplastic (malignant) related fatigue
R53.1 Weakness
G93.3 Postviral fatigue syndrome
ICD-9 **789.07**
ICD-10 **R10.84** Generalized abdominal pain
ICD-9 **882.0**
The appropriate 7th character is to be added to each code from category, **S61**
ICD-10 **S61.409-** Unspecified open wound of unspecified hand
** There are more specific code choice selections available in ICD-10-CM. These include:
S61.401- Unspecified open wound of right hand
S61.402- Unspecified open wound of left hand
S61.411- Laceration without foreign body of right hand
S61.412- Laceration without foreign body of left hand
S61.419- Laceration without foreign body of unspecified hand
S61.421- Laceration with foreign body of right hand
S61.422- Laceration with foreign body of left hand
S61.429- Laceration with foreign body of unspecified hand
S61.431- Puncture wound without foreign body of right hand
S61.432- Puncture wound without foreign body of left hand
S61.439- Puncture wound without foreign body of unspecified hand
S61.441- Puncture wound with foreign body of right hand
S61.442- Puncture wound with foreign body of left hand
S61.449- Puncture wound with foreign body of unspecified hand
S61.451- Open bite of right hand
S61.452- Open bite of left hand
S61.459- Open bite of unspecified hand
ICD-9 **592.0**
ICD-10 **N20.0** Calculus of kidney
ICD-9 **276.51**
ICD-10 **E86.0** Dehydration
ICD-9 **564.00**
ICD-10 **K59.00** Constipation, unspecified
** There are more specific code choice selections available in ICD-10-CM. These include:
K59.01 Slow transit constipation
K59.02 Outlet dysfunction constipation
K59.09 Other constipation
ICD-9 **786.52**
ICD-10 **R07.1** Chest pain on breathing
R07.81 Pleurodynia
R07.89 Other chest pain
ICD-9 **382.9**
ICD-10 **H66.90** Otitis media, unspecified, unspecified ear
** There are more specific code choice selections available in ICD-10-CM. These include:
H66.91 Otitis media, unspecified, right ear
H66.92 Otitis media, unspecified, let ear
H66.93 Otitis media, unspecified, bilateral
H65.00 Acute serous otitis media, unspecified ear
H65.01 Acute serous otitis media, right ear
H65.02 Acute serous otitis media, left ear
H65.03 Acute serous otitis media, bilateral
H65.04 Acute serous otitis media, recurrent, right ear
H65.05 Acute serous otitis media, recurrent, left ear
H65.06 Acute serous otitis media, recurrent, bilateral
H65.07 Acute serous otitis media, recurrent, unspecified ear

H65.111 Acute and subacute allergic otitis media (mucoid) (sanguinous) (serous), right ear

H65.112 Acute and subacute allergic otitis media (mucoid) (sanguinous) (serous), left ear

H65.113 Acute and subacute allergic otitis media (mucoid) (sanguinous) (serous), bilateral

H65.114 Acute and subacute allergic otitis media (mucoid) (sanguinous) (serous), recurrent, right ear

H65.115 Acute and subacute allergic otitis media (mucoid) (sanguinous) (serous), recurrent, left ear

H65.116 Acute and subacute allergic otitis media (mucoid) (sanguinous) (serous), recurrent, bilateral

H65.117 Acute and subacute allergic otitis media (mucoid) (sanguinous) (serous), recurrent, unspecified ear

H65.119 Acute and subacute allergic otitis media (mucoid) (sanguinous) (serous), unspecified ear

H65.191 Other acute nonsuppurative otitis media, right ear

H65.192 Other acute nonsuppurative otitis media, left ear

H65.193 Other acute nonsuppurative otitis media, bilateral

H65.194 Other acute nonsuppurative otitis media, recurrent, right ear

H65.195 Other acute nonsuppurative otitis media, recurrent, left ear

H65.196 Other acute nonsuppurative otitis media, recurrent, bilateral

H65.197 Other acute nonsuppurative otitis media, recurrent, unspecified ear

H65.199 Other acute nonsuppurative otitis media, unspecified ear

H65.20 Chronic serous otitis media, unspecified ear

H65.21 Chronic serous otitis media, right ear

H65.22 Chronic serous otitis media, left ear

H65.23 Chronic serous otitis media, bilateral

H65.30 Chronic mucoid otitis media, unspecified ear

H65.31 Chronic mucoid otitis media, right ear

H65.32 Chronic mucoid otitis media, left ear

H65.33 Chronic mucoid otitis media, bilateral

H65.411 Chronic allergic otitis media, right ear

H65.412 Chronic allergic otitis media, left ear

H65.413 Chronic allergic otitis media, bilateral

H65.419 Chronic allergic otitis media, unspecified ear

H65.491 Other chronic nonsuppurative otitis media, right ear

H65.492 Other chronic nonsuppurative otitis media, left ear

H65.493 Other chronic nonsuppurative otitis media, bilateral

H65.499 Other chronic nonsuppurative otitis media, unspecified ear

H65.90 Unspecified nonsuppurative otitis media, unspecified ear

H65.91 Unspecified nonsuppurative otitis media, right ear

H65.92 Unspecified nonsuppurative otitis media, left ear

H66.001 Acute suppurative otitis media without spontaneous rupture of ear drum, right ear

H66.002 Acute suppurative otitis media without spontaneous rupture of ear drum, left ear

H66.003 Acute suppurative otitis media without spontaneous rupture of ear drum, bilateral

H66.004 Acute suppurative otitis media without spontaneous rupture of ear drum, recurrent, right ear

H66.005 Acute suppurative otitis media without spontaneous rupture of ear drum, recurrent, left ear

H66.006 Acute suppurative otitis media without spontaneous rupture of ear drum, recurrent, bilateral

H66.007 Acute suppurative otitis media without spontaneous rupture of ear drum, recurrent, unspecified ear

H66.009 Acute suppurative otitis media without spontaneous rupture of ear drum, unspecified ear

H66.011 Acute suppurative otitis media with spontaneous rupture of ear drum, right ear

H66.012 Acute suppurative otitis media with spontaneous rupture of ear drum, left ear

H66.013 Acute suppurative otitis media with spontaneous rupture of ear drum, bilateral

H66.014 Acute suppurative otitis media with spontaneous rupture of ear drum, recurrent, right ear

H66.015 Acute suppurative otitis media with spontaneous rupture of ear drum, recurrent, left ear

H66.016 Acute suppurative otitis media with spontaneous rupture of ear drum, recurrent, bilateral

H66.017 Acute suppurative otitis media with spontaneous rupture of ear drum, recurrent, unspecified ear

H66.019 Acute suppurative otitis media with spontaneous rupture of ear drum, unspecified ear

H66.10 Chronic tubotympanic suppurative otitis media, unspecified

H66.11 Chronic tubotympanic suppurative otitis media, right ear

H66.12 Chronic tubotympanic suppurative otitis media, left ear

H66.13 Chronic tubotympanic suppurative otitis media, bilateral

H66.20 Chronic atticoantral suppurative otitis media, unspecified ear

H66.21 Chronic atticoantral suppurative otitis media, right ear

H66.22 Chronic atticoantral suppurative otitis media, left ear

H66.23 Chronic atticoantral suppurative otitis media, bilateral

H66.3X1 Other chronic suppurative otitis media, right ear

H66.3X2 Other chronic suppurative otitis media, left ear

H66.3X3 Other chronic suppurative otitis media, bilateral

H66.3X9 Other chronic suppurative otitis media, unspecified ear

H66.40 Suppurative otitis media, unspecified, unspecified ear

H66.41 Suppurative otitis media, unspecified, right ear

H66.42 Suppurative otitis media, unspecified, left ear

H66.43 Suppurative otitis media, unspecified, bilateral

H66.91 Unspecified otitis media, right ear

H66.92 Unspecified otitis media, left ear

H66.93 Unspecified otitis media, bilateral

ICD-9 787.91
ICD-10 R19.7 Diarrhea, unspecified

Family Practice

ICD-9 250.00
ICD-10 E11.9 Type 2 diabetes mellitus without complications

ICD-9 401.9
ICD-10 I10 Essential (primary) hypertension

ICD-9 272.4
ICD-10 E78.4 Other hyperlipidemia
E78.5 Hyperlipidemia, unspecified
*There are more specific code choice selections available in ICD-10-CM. These include:
E78.0 Pure hypercholesterolemia
E78.1 Pure hyperglyceridemia
E78.2 Mixed hyperlipidemia
E78.3 Hyperchylomicronemia
E78.6 Lipoprotein deficiency

ICD-9 724.5
ICD-10 M54.9 Dorsalgia, unspecified
*There are more specific code choice selections available in ICD-10-CM. These include:
M54.89 Other dorsalgia
M54.6 Pain in thoracic spine
M54.5 Low back pain
M53.3 Sacrococcygeal disorders, not elsewhere classified

ICD-9 V70.0
ICD-10 Z00.00 Encounter for general adult medical examination without abnormal findings
Z00.01 Encounter for general adult medical examination with abnormal findings
** Use additional code to identify abnormal findings

ICD-9 496
ICD-10 J44.9 Chronic obstructive pulmonary disease, unspecified
* There are more specific code choice selections available in ICD-10-CM. These include:
J44.0 Chronic obstructive pulmonary disease with acute lower respiratory infection
J44.1 Chronic obstructive pulmonary disease with (acute) exacerbation

ICD-9 V72.83
ICD-10 Z01.818 Encounter for other preprocedural examination

ICD-9 427.31
ICD-10 I48.0 Paroxysmal atrial fibrillation
I48.1 Persistent atrial fibrillation
I48.2 Chronic atrial fibrillation
I48.91 Unspecified atrial fibrillation

ICD-9 789.00
ICD-10 R10.9 Unspecified abdominal pain
*There are more specific code choice selections available in ICD-10-CM. These include:
R10.0 Acute abdomen
R10.10 Upper abdominal pain, unspecified
R10.11 Right upper quadrant pain
R10.12 Left upper quadrant pain
R10.13 Epigastric pain
R10.2 Pelvic and perineal pain
R10.30 Lower abdominal pain, unspecified
R10.31 Right lower quadrant pain
R10.32 Left lower quadrant pain
R10.33 Periumbilical pain
R10.84 Generalized abdominal pain

ICD-9 786.2
ICD-10 R05 Cough

ICD-9 414.00
ICD-10 No map (No ICD-10 code exists for unspecified vessel; native or bypass graft must be indicated)

ICD-9 338.4
ICD-10 G89.4 Chronic pain syndrome
* Code also related psychological factors associated with pain (F54.42-)

ICD-9 V04.81
ICD-10 Z23 Encounter for immunization
**Code first any routine childhood examination

ICD-9 599.0
ICD-10 N39.0 Urinary tract infection, site not specified
** Use additional code (B95-B97)to identify infectious agent
*There are more specific code choice selections available in ICD-10-CM. These include:
N30.00 Acute cystitis without hematuria
N30.01 Acute cystitis with hematuria
N30.10 Interstitial cystitis chronic without hematuria
N30.11 Interstitial cystitis chronic with hematuria
N30.20 Other chronic cystitis without hematuria
N30.21 Other chronic cystitis with hematuria
N30.30 Trigonitis without hematuria
N30.31 Trigonitis with hematuria
N30.40 Irradiation cystitis without hematuria
N30.41 Irradiation cystitis with hematuria
N30.80 Other cystitis without hematuria
N30.81 Other cystitis with hematuria
N30.90 Cystitis, unspecified without hematuria
N30.91 Cystitis, unspecified with hematuria
N15.9 Renal tubulo-interstitial disease, unspecified
N34.1 Nonspecific urethritis
N34.2 Other urethritis

ICD-9 300.00
ICD-10 F41.9 Anxiety disorder, unspecified
*There are more specific code choice selections available in ICD-10-CM. These include:
F41.1 Generalized anxiety disorder
F41.8 Other specified anxiety disorders

ICD-9 311
ICD-10 F32.9 Major depressive disorder, single episode, unspecified
*There are more specific code choice selections available in ICD-10-CM. These include:
F32.0 Major depressive disorder, single episode, mild
F32.1 Major depressive disorder, single episode, moderate
F32.2 Major depressive disorder, single episode, severe without psychotic features
F32.3 Major depressive disorder, single episode, severe with psychotic features
F32.4 Major depressive disorder, single episode, in partial remission
F32.5 Major depressive disorder, single episode, in full remission
F32.8 Other depressive episodes

ICD-9 530.81
ICD-10 K21.9 Gastro-esophageal reflux disease without esophagitis
K21.0 Gastro-esophageal reflux disease with esophagitis

ICD-9 729.5
ICD-10 M79.609 Pain in unspecified limb
** There are more specific code choice selections available in ICD-10-CM. These inclu
M79.601 Pain in right arm
M79.602 Pain in left arm
M79.603 Pain in arm, unspecified
M79.604 Pain in right leg
M79.605 Pain in left leg
M79.606 Pain in leg, unspecified
M79.621 Pain in right upper arm
M79.622 Pain in left upper arm
M79.629 Pain in unspecified upper arm
M79.631 Pain in right forearm
M79.632 Pain in left forearm
M79.639 Pain in unspecified forearm
M79.641 Pain in right hand
M79.642 Pain in left hand
M79.643 Pain in unspecified hand
M79.644 Pain in right finger(s)
M79.645 Pain in left finger(s)
M79.646 Pain in unspecified finger(s)
M79.651 Pain in right thigh
M79.652 Pain in left thigh
M79.659 Pain in unspecified thigh
M79.661 Pain in right lower leg
M79.662 Pain in left lower leg
M79.669 Pain in unspecified lower leg
M79.671 Pain in right foot
M79.672 Pain in left foot
M79.673 Pain in unspecified foot

M79.674 Pain in right toe(s)
M79.675 Pain in left toe(s)
M79.676 Pain in unspecified toe(s)

[ICD-9] 786.50
[ICD-10] R07.9 Chest pain, unspecified
There are more specific code choice selections available in ICD-10-CM. These include:
R07.1 Chest pain on breathing
R07.2 Precordial pain
R07.81 Pleurodynia
R07.89 Other chest pain

780.79
[ICD-10] R53.0 Neoplasm (malignant) related fatigue
R53.1 Weakness
R53.81 Other malaise
R53.83 Other fatigue
G93.3 Postviral fatigue syndrome

[ICD-9] 465.9
[ICD-10] J06.9 Acute upper respiratory infection, unspecified
J39.8 Other specified diseases of upper respiratory tract

[ICD-9] 486
[ICD-10] J18.9 Pneumonia, unspecified organism
Code first associated influenza, if applicable (J09.X1, J10.0- –J11.0-)

[ICD-9] 466.0
[ICD-10] J20.9 Acute bronchitis, unspecified
There are more specific code choice selections available in ICD-10-CM. These include:
J20.0 Acute bronchitis due to Mycoplasma pneumoniae
J20.1 Acute bronchitis due to Hemophilus influenzae
J20.2 Acute bronchitis due to streptococcus
J20.3 Acute bronchitis due to coxsackievirus
J20.4 Acute bronchitis due to parainfluenza virus
J20.5 Acute bronchitis due to respiratory syncytial virus
J20.6 Acute bronchitis due to rhinovirus
J20.7 Acute bronchitis due to echovirus
J20.8 Acute bronchitis due to other specified organisms

[ICD-9] 719.46
[ICD-10] M25.561 Pain in right knee
M25.562 Pain in left knee
M25.569 Pain in unspecified knee

[ICD-9] 428.0
[ICD-10] I50.9 Heart failure, unspecified
here are more specific code choice selections available in ICD-10-CM. These include:
I50.1 Left ventricular failure
I50.21 Acute systolic (congestive) heart failure
I50.22 Chronic systolic (congestive) heart failure
I50.23 Acute on chronic systolic (congestive) heart failure
I50.30 Unspecified diastolic (congestive) heart failure
I50.31 Acute diastolic (congestive) heart failure
I50.32 Chronic diastolic (congestive) heart failure
I50.33 Acute on chronic diastolic (congestive) heart failure
I50.40 Unspecified combined systolic (congestive) and diastolic (congestive) heart failure
I50.41 Acute combined systolic (congestive) and diastolic (congestive) heart failure
I50.42 Chronic combined systolic (congestive) and diastolic (congestive) heart failure
I50.43 Acute on chronic combined systolic (congestive) and diastolic (congestive) heart failure

[ICD-9] 780.4
[ICD-10] R42 Dizziness and giddiness

[ICD-9] 461.9
[ICD-10] J01.90 Acute sinusitis, unspecified
here are more specific code choice selections available in ICD-10-CM. These include:
J01.00 Acute maxillary sinusitis, unspecified
J01.10 Acute frontal sinusitis, unspecified
J01.20 Acute ethmoidal sinusitis, unspecified
J01.30 Acute sphenoidal sinusitis, unspecified
J01.40 Acute pansinusitis, unspecified
J01.80 Other acute sinusitis

[ICD-9] 782.3
[ICD-10] R60.0 Localized edema
R60.1 Generalized edema
R60.9 Edema, unspecified

[ICD-9] 477.9
[ICD-10] J30.9 Allergic rhinitis, unspecified
here are more specific code choice selections available in ICD-10-CM. These include:
J30.0 Vasomotor rhinitis
J30.1 Allergic rhinitis due to pollen
J30.2 Other seasonal allergic rhinitis
J30.5 Allergic rhinitis due to food
J30.81 Allergic rhinitis due to animal (cat) (dog) hair and dander

J30.89 Other allergic rhinitis

[ICD-9] 719.41
[ICD-10] M25.511 Pain in right shoulder
M25.512 Pain in left shoulder
M25.519 Pain in unspecified shoulder

[ICD-10] 784.0
[ICD-10] R51 Headache

[ICD-10] 380.4
[ICD-10] H61.21 Impacted cerumen, right ear
H61.22 Impacted cerumen, left ear
H61.23 Impacted cerumen, bilateral
H61.20 Impacted cerumen, unspecified ear

[ICD-10] 462
[ICD-10] J02.8 Acute pharyngitis due to other specified organisms
** Use additional code (B95-B97) to identify infectious agent
J02.0 Streptococcal pharyngitis
J02.9 Acute pharyngitis, unspecified

[ICD-10] 723.1
[ICD-10] M54.2 Cervicalgia

[ICD-10] 285.9
[ICD-10] D64.9 Anemia, unspecified
* There are more specific code choice selections available in ICD-10-CM. These include:
D64.0 Hereditary sideroblastic anemia
D64.1 Secondary sideroblastic anemia due to disease
D64.2 Secondary sideroblastic anemia due to drugs and toxins
Use additional code for adverse effect, if applicable, to identify drug (T36-T50 with fifth or sixth character 5)
D64.3 Other sideroblastic anemias (anemia is plural in code descriptor)
D64.81 Anemia due to antineoplastic chemotherapy
D64.89 Other specified anemias

[ICD-10] 782.1
[ICD-10] R21 Rash and other nonspecific skin eruption

[ICD-10] 787.91
[ICD-10] R19.7 Diarrhea, unspecified

[ICD-10] 493.90
[ICD-10] J45.909 Unspecified asthma, uncomplicated
** There are more specific code choice selections available in ICD-10-CM. These include:
J45.20 Mild intermittent asthma, uncomplicated
J45.21 Mild intermittent asthma with (acute) exacerbation
J45.22 Mild intermittent asthma with status asthmaticus
J45.30 Mild persistent asthma, uncomplicated
J45.31 Mild persistent asthma with (acute) exacerbation
J45.32 Mild persistent asthma with status asthmaticus
J45.40 Moderate persistent asthma, uncomplicated
J45.41 Moderate persistent asthma with (acute) exacerbation
J45.42 Moderate persistent asthma with status asthmaticus
J45.50 Severe persistent asthma, uncomplicated
J45.51 Severe persistent asthma with (acute) exacerbation
J45.52 Severe persistent asthma with status asthmaticus
J45.901 Unspecified asthma with (acute) exacerbation
J45.902 Unspecified asthma with status asthmaticus
J45.990 Exercise induced bronchospasm
J45.991 Cough variant asthma
J45.998 Other asthma

[ICD-10] 490
[ICD-10] J40 Bronchitis, not specified as acute or chronic
** There are more specific code choice selections available in ICD-10-CM. These include:
J20.0 Acute bronchitis due to Mycoplasma pneumoniae
J20.1 Acute bronchitis due to Hemophilus influenzae
J20.2 Acute bronchitis due to streptococcus
J20.3 Acute bronchitis due to coxsackievirus
J20.4 Acute bronchitis due to parainfluenza virus
J20.5 Acute bronchitis due to respiratory syncytial virus
J20.6 Acute bronchitis due to rhinovirus
J20.7 Acute bronchitis due to echovirus
J20.8 Acute bronchitis due to other specified organisms
J20.9 Acute bronchitis, unspecified
J41.0 Simple chronic bronchitis
J41.1 Mucopurulent chronic bronchitis
J41.8 Mixed simple and mucopurulent chronic bronchitis
J42 Unspecified chronic bronchitis

[ICD-9] 493.00
[ICD-10] J45.901 Unspecified asthma with (acute) exacerbation
J45.902 Unspecified asthma with status asthmaticus
J45.909 Unspecified asthma, uncomplicated

[ICD-9] 244.9
[ICD-10] E03.9 Hypothyroidism, unspecified
* There are more specific code choice selections available ICD-10-CM. These include:
E03.0 Congenital hypothyroidism with diffuse goiter

E03.1 Congenital hypothyroidism without goiter
E03.2 Hypothyroidism due to medicaments and other exogenous substances
Use additional code for adverse effect, if applicable, to identify drug (T36-T50 with fifth or sixth character 5)
E03.3 Postinfectious hypothyroidism
E03.4 Atrophy of thyroid (acquired)
E03.5 Myxedema coma
E03.8 Other specified hypothyroidism

[ICD-9] 788.1
[ICD-10] R30.0 Dysuria

[ICD-9] 786.05
[ICD-10] R06.02 Shortness of breath

[ICD-9] 309.9
[ICD-10] F43.20 Adjustment disorder, unspecified
* There are more specific code choice selections available ICD-10-CM. These include:
F43.21 Adjustment disorder with depressed mood
F43.22 Adjustment disorder with anxiety
F43.23 Adjustment disorder with mixed anxiety and depressed mood
F43.24 Adjustment disorder with disturbance of conduct
F43.25 Adjustment disorder with mixed disturbance of emotions and conduct
F43.29 Adjustment disorder with other symptoms

[ICD-9] 719.45
[ICD-10] M25.551 Pain in right hip
M25.552 Pain in left hip
M25.559 Pain in unspecified hip

[ICD-9] 786.09
[ICD-10] R06.83 Snoring
R06.00 Dyspnea, unspecified
R06.3 Periodic breathing
R06.4 Hyperventilation
R06.89 Other abnormalities of breathing

[ICD-9] 692.9
[ICD-10] L25.9 Unspecified contact dermatitis, unspecified nature
** Use additional code for adverse effect, if applicable, to identify drug (T36-T50 with fifth or sixth character 5)
L30.9 Dermatitis, unspecified
* There are more specific code choice selections available ICD-10-CM. These include:
L25.0 Unspecified contact dermatitis due to cosmetics
L25.1 Unspecified contact dermatitis due to drugs in contact with skin
L25.2 Unspecified contact dermatitis due to dyes
L25.3 Unspecified contact dermatitis due to other chemical products
L25.4 Unspecified contact dermatitis due to food in contact with skin
L25.5 Unspecified contact dermatitis due to plants, except food
L25.8 Unspecified contact dermatitis due to other agents
** Use additional code for adverse effect, if applicable, to identify drug (T36-T50 with fifth or sixth character 5)

[ICD-9] 724.2
[ICD-10] M54.5 Low back pain

[ICD-9] 682.6
[ICD-10] L03.115 Cellulitis of right lower limb
L03.116 Cellulitis of left lower limb
L03.119 Cellulitis of unspecified part of limb
L03.125 Acute lymphangitis of right lower limb
L03.126 Acute lymphangitis of left lower limb
L03.129 Acute lymphangitis of unspecified part of limb

[ICD-9] 455.5
[ICD-10] K64.4 Residual hemorrhoidal skin tags
K64.5 Perianal venous thrombosis

Gastroenterology

[ICD-9] V76.51
[ICD-10] Z12.11 Encounter for screening for malignant neoplasm of colon

[ICD-9] 211.3
[ICD-10] D12.6 Benign neoplasm of colon, unspecified
* There are more specific code choice selections available in ICD-10-CM. These include:
D12.0 Benign neoplasm of cecum
D12.1 Benign neoplasm of appendix
D12.2 Benign neoplasm of ascending colon
D12.3 Benign neoplasm of transverse colon
D12.4 Benign neoplasm of descending colon
D12.5 Benign neoplasm of sigmoid colon

[ICD-9] 789.00
[ICD-10] R10.9 Unspecified abdominal pain
* There are more specific code choice selections available in ICD-10-CM. These include:
R10.0 Acute abdomen

R10.10 Upper abdominal pain, unspecified
R10.11 Right upper quadrant pain
R10.12 Left upper quadrant pain
R10.13 Epigastric pain
R10.2 Pelvic and perineal pain
R10.30 Lower abdominal pain, unspecified
R10.31 Right lower quadrant pain
R10.32 Left lower quadrant pain
R10.33 Periumbilical pain
R10.84 Generalized abdominal pain

`ICD-9` **V12.72**
`ICD-10` **Z86.010** Personal history of colonic polyps

`ICD-9` **787.20**
`ICD-10` **R13.0** Aphagia
R13.10 Dysphagia
** Code first, if applicable, dysphagia following cerebrovascular disease (I69. with final characters -91)

`ICD-9` **V16.0**
`ICD-10` **Z80.0** Family history of primary malignant neoplasm of digestive organs

`ICD-9` **562.10**
`ICD-10` **K57.30** Diverticulosis of large intestine without perforation or abscess without bleeding

`ICD-9` **530.81**
`ICD-10` **K21.9** Gastro-esophageal reflux without esophagitis
K21.0 Gastro-esophageal reflux with esophagitis

`ICD-9` **787.91**
`ICD-10` **R19.7** Diarrhea, unspecified

`ICD-9` **530.85**
`ICD-10` **K22.70** Barrett's esophagus without dysplasia
K22.710 Barrett's esophagus with low grade dysplasia
K22.711 Barrett's esophagus with high grade dysplasia
K22.719 Barrett's esophagus with dysplasia, unspecified

`ICD-9` **578.9**
`ICD-10` **K92.2** Gastrointestinal hemorrhage, unspecified

`ICD-9` **793.4**
`ICD-10` **R93.3** Abnormal findings on diagnostic imaging of other parts of digestive tract

`ICD-9` **211.4**
`ICD-10` **D12.7** Benign neoplasm of rectosigmoid junction
D12.8 Benign neoplasm of rectum
D12.9 Benign neoplasm of anus and anal canal

`ICD-9` **574.50**
`ICD-10` **K80.50** Calculus of bile duct without cholangitis or cholecystitis without obstruction

`ICD-9` **535.10**
`ICD-10` **K29.40** Chronic atrophic gastritis without bleeding

`ICD-9` **555.9**
`ICD-10` **K50.90** Crohn's disease, unspecified, without complications
** Use additional code to identify manifestations, such as: pyoderma gangrenosum (L88)
* There are more specific code choice selections available in ICD-10-CM. These include:
K50.00 Crohn's disease of small intestine without complications
K50.011 Crohn's disease of small intestine with rectal bleeding
K50.012 Crohn's disease of small intestine with intestinal obstruction
K50.013 Crohn's disease of small intestine with fistula
K50.014 Crohn's disease of small intestine with abscess
K50.018 Crohn's disease of small intestine with other complication
K50.019 Crohn's disease of small intestine with unspecified complications
K50.10 Crohn's disease of large intestine without complications
K50.111 Crohn's disease of large intestine with rectal bleeding
K50.112 Crohn's disease of large intestine with intestinal obstruction
K50.113 Crohn's disease of large intestine with fistula
K50.114 Crohn's disease of large intestine with abscess
K50.118 Crohn's disease of large intestine with other complication
K50.119 Crohn's disease of large intestine with unspecified complications
K50.80 Crohn's disease of both small and large intestine without complications
K50.811 Crohn's disease of both small and large intestine with rectal bleeding
K50.812 Crohn's disease of both small and large intestine with intestinal obstruction
K50.813 Crohn's disease of both small and large intestine with fistula
K50.814 Crohn's disease of both small and large intestine with abscess

K50.818 Crohn's disease of both small and large intestine with other complication
K50.819 Crohn's disease of both small and large intestine with unspecified complications
K50.911 Crohn's disease, unspecified, with rectal bleeding
K50.912 Crohn's disease, unspecified, with intestinal obstruction
K50.913 Crohn's disease, unspecified, with fistula
K50.914 Crohn's disease, unspecified, with abscess
K50.918 Crohn's disease, unspecified, with other complication
K50.919 Crohn's disease, unspecified, with unspecified complications

`ICD-9` **569.3**
`ICD-10` **K62.5** Hemorrhage of anus and rectum

`ICD-9` **455.6**
`ICD-10` **K64.0** Hemorrhoids, 1st degree (grade/stage I)
K64.1 Hemorrhoids 2nd degree (grade/stage II)
K64.2 Hemorrhoids 3rd degree (grade/stage III)
K64.3 Hemorrhoids 4th degree (grade/stage IV)
K64.8 Hemorrhoids, other (without mention of degree)
K64.9 Hemorrhoids, unspecified (without mention of degree)

`ICD-9` **558.9**
`ICD-10` **K52.89** Other specified noninfective gastroenteritis and colitis
K52.9 Noninfective gastroenteritis and colitis, unspecified

`ICD-9` **571.5**
`ICD-10` **K74.60** Unspecified cirrhosis of liver
K74.69 Other cirrhosis of liver
** Code also, if applicable, viral hepatitis (acute) (chronic) (B15-B19)

`ICD-9` **530.3**
`ICD-10` **K22.2** Esophageal obstruction

`ICD-9` **553.3**
`ICD-10` **K44.9** Diaphragmatic hernia without obstruction or gangrene

`ICD-9` **787.99**
`ICD-10` **R19.8** Other specified symptoms and signs involving the digestive system and abdomen

`ICD-9` **564.00**
`ICD-10` **K59.00** Constipation, unspecified
* There are more specific code choice selections available in ICD-10-CM. These include:
K59.01 Slow transit constipation
K59.02 Outlet dysfunction constipation
K59.09 Other constipation

`ICD-9` **456.1**
`ICD-10` **I85.00** Esophageal varices without bleeding

`ICD-9` **285.9**
`ICD-10` **D64.9** Anemia, unspecified
* There are more specific code choice selections available in ICD-10-CM. These include:
D64.81 Anemia due to antineoplastic chemotherapy
D64.89 Other specified anemias

`ICD-9` **790.4**
`ICD-10` **R74.0** Nonspecific elevation of levels of transaminase and lactic acid dehydrogenase (LDH)

`ICD-9` **556.8**
`ICD-10` **K51.80** Other ulcerative colitis without complications
K51.811 Other ulcerative colitis with rectal bleeding
K51.812 Other ulcerative colitis with intestinal obstruction
K51.813 Other ulcerative colitis with fistula
K51.814 Other ulcerative colitis with abscess
K51.818 Other ulcerative colitis with other complication
K51.819 Other ulcerative colitis with unspecified complications
** Use additional code to identify manifestations, such as: pyoderma gangrenosum (L88)

`ICD-9` **530.10**
`ICD-10` **K20.9** Esophagitis, unspecified
* There are more specific code choice selections available in ICD-10-CM. These include:
K20.0 Eosinophilic esophagitis
K20.8 Other esophagitis
** Use additional code to identify: Alcohol abuse and dependence (F10-)

`ICD-9` **280.9**
`ICD-10` **D50.9** Iron deficiency anemia, unspecified
* There are more specific code choice selections available in ICD-10-CM. These include:
D50.0 Iron deficiency anemia secondary to blood loss (chronic)
D50.1 Sideropenic dysphagia
D50.8 Other iron deficiency anemias

`ICD-9` **536.8**
`ICD-10` **R10.13** Epigastric pain (dyspepsia)
K30 Functional dyspepsia
K31.0 Acute dilatation of stomach
K31.1 Adult hypertrophic pyloric stenosis
K31.2 Hourglass stricture and stenosis of stomach
K31.3 Pylorospasm, not elsewhere classified
K31.4 Gastric diverticulum
K31.5 Obstruction of duodenum
K31.6 Fistula of stomach and duodenum
K31.7 Polyp of stomach and duodenum

K31.811 Angiodysplasia of stomach and duodenum with bleeding
K31.819 Angiodysplasia of stomach and duodenum without bleeding
K31.82 Dieulafoy lesion (hemorrhagic) of stomach and duodenum
K31.83 Achlorhydria
K31.84 Gastroparesis
K31.89 Other disorders of stomach and duodenum

`ICD-9` **070.54**
`ICD-10` **B18.2** Chronic viral hepatitis C

`ICD-9` **789.06**
`ICD-10` **R10.13** Epigastric pain

`ICD-9` **211.1**
`ICD-10` **D13.1** Benign neoplasm of stomach

`ICD-9` **556.9**
`ICD-10` **K51.90** Ulcerative colitis, unspecified, without complications
* There are more specific code choice selections available in ICD-10-CM. These include:
K51.00 Ulcerative (chronic) pancolitis without complications
K51.011 Ulcerative (chronic) pancolitis with rectal bleeding
K51.012 Ulcerative (chronic) pancolitis with intestinal obstruction
K51.013 Ulcerative (chronic) pancolitis with fistula
K51.014 Ulcerative (chronic) pancolitis with abscess
K51.018 Ulcerative (chronic) pancolitis with other complication
K51.019 Ulcerative (chronic) pancolitis with unspecified complications
K51.20 Ulcerative (chronic) proctitis without complications
K51.211 Ulcerative (chronic) proctitis with rectal bleeding
K51.212 Ulcerative (chronic) proctitis with intestinal obstruction
K51.213 Ulcerative (chronic) proctitis with fistula
K51.214 Ulcerative (chronic) proctitis with abscess
K51.218 Ulcerative (chronic) proctitis with other complication
K51.219 Ulcerative (chronic) proctitis with unspecified complications
K51.30 Ulcerative (chronic) rectosigmoiditis without complication
K51.311 Ulcerative (chronic) rectosigmoiditis with rectal bleeding
K51.312 Ulcerative (chronic) rectosigmoiditis with intestinal obstruction
K51.313 Ulcerative (chronic) rectosigmoiditis with fistula
K51.314 Ulcerative (chronic) rectosigmoiditis with abscess
K51.318 Ulcerative (chronic) rectosigmoiditis with other complication
K51.319 Ulcerative (chronic) rectosigmoiditis with unspecified complications
K51.40 Inflammatory polyps of colon without complications
K51.411 Inflammatory polyps of colon with rectal bleeding
K51.412 Inflammatory polyps of colon with intestinal obstruction
K51.413 Inflammatory polyps of colon with fistula
K51.414 Inflammatory polyps of colon with abscess
K51.418 Inflammatory polyps of colon with other complication
K51.419 Inflammatory polyps of colon with unspecified complications
K51.50 Left sided colitis without complications
K51.511 Left sided colitis with rectal bleeding
K51.512 Left sided colitis with intestinal obstruction
K51.513 Left sided colitis with fistula
K51.514 Left sided colitis with abscess
K51.518 Left sided colitis with other complication
K51.519 Left sided colitis with unspecified complications
K51.80 Other ulcerative colitis without complications
K51.811 Other ulcerative colitis with rectal bleeding
K51.812 Other ulcerative colitis with intestinal obstruction
K51.813 Other ulcerative colitis with fistula
K51.814 Other ulcerative colitis with abscess
K51.818 Other ulcerative colitis with other complication
K51.819 Other ulcerative colitis with unspecified complication
K51.911 Ulcerative colitis, unspecified with rectal bleeding
K51.912 Ulcerative colitis, unspecified with intestinal obstruction
K51.913 Ulcerative colitis, unspecified with fistula
K51.914 Ulcerative colitis, unspecified with abscess
K51.918 Ulcerative colitis, unspecified with other complication
K51.919 Ulcerative colitis, unspecified with unspecified complications
** Use additional code to identify manifestations, such as: Pyoderma gangrenosum (L88)

`ICD-9` **571.2**
`ICD-10` **K70.30** Alcoholic cirrhosis of liver without ascites
K70.31 Alcoholic cirrhosis of liver with ascites
** Use additional code to identify: alcohol abuse and dependence (F10-)

`ICD-9` **578.1**
`ICD-10` **K92.1** Melena
R19.5 Other fecal abnormalities

`ICD-9` **150.9**
`ICD-10` **C15.9** Malignant neoplasm of esophagus, unspecified
* There are more specific code choice selections available in ICD-10-CM. These include:
C15.3 Malignant neoplasm of upper third of esophagus
C15.4 Malignant neoplasm of middle third of esophagus
C15.5 Malignant neoplasm of lower third of esophagus

C15.8 Malignant neoplasm of overlapping sites of esophagus
* Use additional code to identify: alcohol abuse and dependence (F10-)

ICD-9 V12.79
ICD-10 **Z87.19** Personal history of other diseases of the digestive system
* Code first any follow-up examination after treatment (Z09)

ICD-9 786.50
ICD-10 **R07.9** Chest pain, unspecified
There are more specific code choice selections available in ICD-10-CM. These include:
  R07.1 Chest pain on breathing
  R07.81 Pleurodynia
  R07.89 Other chest pain

ICD-9 577.2
ICD-10 **K86.2** Cyst of pancreas
  K86.3 Pseudocyst of pancreas

ICD-9 531.90
ICD-10 **K25.9** Gastric ulcer, unspecified as acute or chronic, without hemorrhage or perforation

ICD-9 V18.51
ICD-10 **Z83.71** Family history of colonic polyps

ICD-9 569.89
ICD-10 **K63.89** Other specified diseases of intestine
  K63.0 Abscess of intestine
  K63.1 Perforation of intestine (nontraumatic)
  K63.2 Fistula of intestine
  K63.3 Ulcer of intestine
  K63.4 Enteroptosis
  K63.5 Polyp of colon
  K63.81 Dieulafoy lesion of intestine

ICD-9 564.1
ICD-10 **K58.0** Irritable bowel syndrome with diarrhea
  K58.9 Irritable bowel syndrome without diarrhea

ICD-9 935.1
ICD-10
e appropriate 7th character is to be added to each code from category T18:
initial
subsequent
sequela
These codes require a 7th character extender.
  T18.100- Unspecified foreign body in esophagus causing compression of trachea
There are more specific code choice selections available in ICD-10-CM. These include:
  T18.108- Unspecified foreign body in esophagus causing other injury
  T18.110- Gastric contents in esophagus causing compression of trachea
  T18.118- Gastric contents in esophagus causing other injury
  T18.120- Food in esophagus causing compression of trachea
  T18.128- Food in esophagus causing other injury
  T18.190- Other foreign body in esophagus causing compression of trachea
  T18.198- Other foreign body in esophagus causing other injury

ICD-9 576.2
ICD-10 **K83.1** Obstruction of bile duct

ICD-9 530.11
ICD-10 **K21.0** Gastro-esophageal reflux disease with esophagitis
  K21.9 Gastro-esophageal reflux disease without esophagitis

ICD-9 794.8
ICD-10 **R94.5** Abnormal results of function studies of other organs and systems

ICD-9 V10.05
ICD-10 **Z85.030** Personal history of malignant carcinoid tumor of large intestine
  Z85.038 Personal history of other malignant neoplasm of large intestine

General Surgery

ICD-9 550.90
ICD-10 **K40.90** Unilateral inguinal hernia, without obstruction or gangrene, not specified as recurrent

ICD-9 278.01
ICD-10 **E66.01** Morbid (severe) obesity due to excess calories
* additional code to identify body mass index (BMI), if known (Z68-)

ICD-9 574.20
ICD-10 **K80.20** Calculus of gallbladder without cholecystitis without obstruction

ICD-9 211.3
ICD-10 **D12.0** Benign neoplasm of cecum
  D12.1 Benign neoplasm of appendix
  D12.2 Benign neoplasm of ascending colon
  D12.3 Benign neoplasm of transverse colon
  D12.4 Benign neoplasm of descending colon

  D12.5 Benign neoplasm of sigmoid colon
  D12.6 Benign neoplasm of colon, unspecified
  D12.7 Benign neoplasm of rectosigmoid junction
  K63.5 Polyp of colon

ICD-9 V10.05
ICD-10 **Z85.038** Personal history of other malignant neoplasm of large intestine
  Z85.030 Personal history of malignant carcinoid tumor of large intestine

ICD-9 530.81
ICD-10 **K21.0** Gastro-esophageal reflux disease with esophagitis
  K21.9 Gastro-esophageal reflux disease without esophagitis

ICD-9 553.21
ICD-10 **K43.0** Incisional hernia with obstruction, without gangrene
  K43.1 Incisional hernia with gangrene
  K43.2 Incisional hernia without obstruction or gangrene

ICD-9 154.1
ICD-10 **C20** Malignant neoplasm of rectum

ICD-9 V12.72
ICD-10 **Z86.010** Personal history of colonic polyps

ICD-9 V76.51
ICD-10 **Z12.11** Encounter for screening for malignant neoplasm of colon

ICD-9 455.2
ICD-10 **K64.0** First degree hemorrhoids
  K64.1 Second degree hemorrhoids
  K64.2 Third degree hemorrhoids
  K64.3 Fourth degree hemorrhoids
  K64.8 Other hemorrhoids
  K64.9 Unspecified hemorrhoids

ICD-9 789.00
ICD-10 **R10.0** Acute abdomen
  R10.10 Upper abdominal pain, unspecified
  R10.11 Right upper quadrant pain
  R10.12 Left upper quadrant pain
  R10.13 Epigastric pain
  R10.2 Pelvic and perineal pain
  R10.30 Lower abdominal pain, unspecified
  R10.31 Right lower quadrant pain
  R10.32 Left lower quadrant pain
  R10.33 Periumbilical pain
  R10.84 Generalized abdominal pain
  R10.9 Unspecified abdominal pain

ICD-9 553.3
ICD-10 **K44.9** Diaphragmatic hernia without obstruction or gangrene
  K44.0 Diaphragmatic hernia with obstruction, without gangrene
  K44.1 Diaphragmatic hernia with gangrene
  Q79.0 Congenital diaphragmatic hernia

ICD-9 540.9
ICD-10 **K35.80** Unspecified acute appendicitis
  K35.89 Other acute appendicitis

ICD-9 564.00
ICD-10 **K59.00** Constipation, unspecified
** There are more specific code choice selections available in ICD-10-CM. These include:
  K59.01 Slow transit constipation
  K59.02 Outlet dysfunction constipation
  K59.09 Other constipation

ICD-9 562.10
ICD-10 **K57.30** Diverticulosis of large intestine without perforation or abscess without bleeding

ICD-9 562.11
ICD-10 **K57.32** Diverticulitis of large intestine without perforation or abscess without bleeding
  K57.20 Diverticulitis of large intestine with perforation and abscess without bleeding

ICD-9 553.1
ICD-10 **K42.9** Umbilical hernia without obstruction or gangrene
  K42.0 Umbilical hernia with obstruction, without gangrene
  K42.1 Umbilical hernia with gangrene

ICD-9 565.0
ICD-10 **K60.0** Acute anal fissure
  K60.1 Chronic anal fissure
  K60.2 Anal fissure, unspecified

ICD-9 V16.0
ICD-10 **Z80.0** Family history of malignant neoplasm of digestive organs

ICD-9 552.1
ICD-10 **K42.0** Umbilical hernia with obstruction, without gangrene

ICD-9 553.20
ICD-10 **K43.6** Other and unspecified ventral hernia with obstruction, without gangrene

  K43.7 Other and unspecified ventral hernia with gangrene
  K43.9 Ventral hernia without obstruction or gangrene

ICD-9 575.10
ICD-10 **K81.9** Cholecystitis, unspecified
  K81.0 Acute cholecystitis
  K81.1 Chronic cholecystitis
  K81.2 Acute cholecystitis with chronic cholecystitis

ICD-9 565.1
ICD-10 **K60.3** Anal fistula

ICD-9 455.5
ICD-10 **K64.4** Residual hemorrhoid skin tags
  K64.5 Perianal venous thrombosis
  K64.8 Hemorrhoids, other
  K64.9 Hemorrhoids, unspecified

ICD-9 555.9
ICD-10 **K50.90** Crohn's disease, unspecified, without complications
** There are more specific code choice selections available in ICD-10-CM. These include:
  K50.00 Crohn's disease of small intestine without complications
  K50.011 Crohn's disease of small intestine with rectal bleeding
  K50.012 Crohn's disease of small intestine with intestinal obstruction
  K50.013 Crohn's disease of small intestine with fistula
  K50.014 Crohn's disease of small intestine with abscess
  K50.018 Crohn's disease of small intestine with other complication
  K50.019 Crohn's disease of small intestine with unspecified complications
  K50.10 Crohn's disease of large intestine without complications
  K50.111 Crohn's disease of large intestine with rectal bleeding
  K50.112 Crohn's disease of large intestine with intestinal obstruction
  K50.113 Crohn's disease of large intestine with fistula
  K50.114 Crohn's disease of large intestine with abscess
  K50.118 Crohn's disease of large intestine with other complication
  K50.119 Crohn's disease of large intestine with unspecified complications
  K50.80 Crohn's disease of both small and large intestine without complications
  K50.811 Crohn's disease of both small and large intestine with rectal bleeding
  K50.812 Crohn's disease of both small and large intestine with intestinal obstruction
  K50.813 Crohn's disease of both small and large intestine with fistula
  K50.814 Crohn's disease of both small and large intestine with abscess
  K50.818 Crohn's disease of both small and large intestine with other complication
  K50.819 Crohn's disease of both small and large intestine with unspecified complications
  K50.911 Crohn's disease, unspecified, with rectal bleeding
  K50.912 Crohn's disease, unspecified, with intestinal obstruction
  K50.913 Crohn's disease, unspecified, with fistula
  K50.914 Crohn's disease, unspecified, with abscess
  K50.918 Crohn's disease, unspecified, with other complication
  K50.919 Crohn's disease, unspecified, with unspecified complications

ICD-9 569.3
ICD-10 **K62.5** Hemorrhage of anus and rectum

ICD-9 574.10
ICD-10 **K80.00** Calculus of gallbladder with acute cholecystitis without obstruction

ICD-9 550.91
ICD-10 **K40.91** Unilateral inguinal hernia, without obstruction or gangrene, recurrent

ICD-9 783.1
ICD-10 **R63.5** Abnormal weight gain

ICD-9 787.60
ICD-10 **R15.9** Full incontinence of feces

ICD-9 250.00
ICD-10 **E11.9** Type 2 diabetes mellitus without complication

ICD-9 556.8
ICD-10 **K51.80** Other ulcerative colitis without complications
  K51.811 Other ulcerative colitis with rectal bleeding
  K51.812 Other ulcerative colitis with intestinal obstruction
  K51.813 Other ulcerative colitis with fistula
  K51.814 Other ulcerative colitis with abscess
  K51.818 Other ulcerative colitis with other complication
  K51.819 Other ulcerative colitis with unspecified complications

ICD-9 685.1
ICD-10 **L05.91** Pilonidal cyst without abscess
  L05.92 Pilonidal sinus without abscess

ICD-9 239.0

D49.0 Neoplasm of unspecified behavior of digestive system

ICD-9 **278.00**

E66.9 Obesity, unspecified
* Use additional code to identify body mass index (BMI), if known (Z68-)
** There are more specific code choice selections available in ICD-10-CM. These include:
- **E66.3** Overweight
- **E66.8** Other obesity
- **E66.1** Drug-induced obesity
* Use additional code for adverse effect, if applicable, to identify drug (T36-T50 with fifth or sixth character 5)

ICD-9 **560.9**

K56.60 Unspecified intestinal obstruction
** There are more specific code choice selections available in ICD-10-CM. These include:
- **K56.5** Intestinal adhesions (bands) with obstruction (postprocedural) (postinfection)
- **K56.0** Paralytic ileus
- **K56.3** Gallstone ileus
- **K56.2** Volvulus
- **K56.69** Other intestinal obstruction
- **K91.3** Postprocedural intestinal obstruction

ICD-9 **787.99**

R19.4 Change in bowel habit
- **R19.8** Other specified symptoms and signs involving the digestive system and abdomen

ICD-9 **157.9**

C25.9 Malignant neoplasm of pancreas, unspecified
* Use additional code to identify alcohol abuse and dependence (F10-)
** There are more specific code choice selections available in ICD-10-CM. These include:
- **C25.0** Malignant neoplasm of head of pancreas
- **C25.1** Malignant neoplasm of body of pancreas
- **C25.2** Malignant neoplasm of tail of pancreas
- **C25.3** Malignant neoplasm of pancreatic duct
- **C25.4** Malignant neoplasm of endocrine pancreas
* Use additional code to identify any functional activity
- **C25.7** Malignant neoplasm of other parts of pancreas
- **C25.8** Malignant neoplasm of overlapping sites of pancreas

ICD-9 **789.03**

R10.31 Right lower quadrant pain

ICD-9 **211.4**

D12.7 Benign neoplasm of rectosigmoid junction
- **D12.8** Benign neoplasm of rectum
- **D12.9** Benign neoplasm of anus and anal canal

ICD-9 **578.9**

K92.2 Gastrointestinal hemorrhage, unspecified

ICD-9 **250.02**

E11.65 Diabetes mellitus Type 2 with hyperglycemia

ICD-9 **569.49**

K62.89 Other specified diseases of anus and rectum

ICD-9 **569.1**

K62.2 Anal prolapse
- **K62.3** Rectal prolapse

ICD-9 **706.2**

L72.3 Sebaceous cyst

ICD-9 **575.8**

K82.8 Other specified diseases of the gallbladder
- **K82.0** Obstruction of gallbladder
- **K82.1** Hydrops of gallbladder
- **K82.2** Perforation of the gallbladder
- **K82.3** Fistula of gallbladder
- **K82.4** Cholesterolosis of gallbladder
- **K82.9** Diseases of gallbladder, unspecified

ICD-9 **078.11**

A63.0 Anogenital (venereal) warts

ICD-9 **153.0**

C18.3 Malignant neoplasm of hepatic flexure

Ob/Gyn

ICD-9 **V72.31**

Z01.411 Encounter for gynecological examination (general) (routine) with abnormal findings
* Use additional code to identify abnormal findings
- **Z01.419** Encounter for gynecological examination (general) (routine) without abnormal findings

ICD-9 **701.0**

L94.0 Localized scleroderma [morphea]
- **L90.0** Lichen sclerosus et atrophicus
- **L94.1** Linear scleroderma
- **L94.3** Sclerodactyly

ICD-9 **624.9**

N90.9 Noninflammatory disorder of vulva and perineum, unspecified

*There are more specific code choice selections available in ICD-10-CM. These include:
- **N90.0** Mild vulvar dysplasia
- **N90.1** Moderate vulvar dysplasia
- **N90.3** Dysplasia of vulva, unspecified
- **N90.4** Leukoplakia of vulva
- **N90.5** Atrophy of vulva
- **N90.6** Hypertrophy of vulva
- **N90.7** Vulvar cyst
- **N90.810** Female genital mutilation status, unspecified
- **N90.811** Female genital mutilation status, Type I status
- **N90.812** Female genital mutilation status, Type II status
- **N90.813** Female genital mutilation status, Type III status
- **N90.818** Other female genital mutilation status
- **N90.89** Other specified noninflammatory disorders of vulva and perineum

ICD-9 **627.1**

N95.0 Postmenopausal bleeding

ICD-9 **625.9**

N94.89 Other specified conditions associated with female genital organs and menstrual cycle
- **N94.9** Unspecified condition associated with female genital organs and menstrual cycle
- **R10.2** Pelvic and perineal pain
- **R19.8** Other specified symptoms and signs involving the digestive system and abdomen
- **R39.9** Unspecified symptoms and signs involving the genitourinary system

ICD-9 **644.03**

O47.00 False labor before 37 weeks of completed gestation, unspecified trimester
- **O47.02** False labor before 37 completed weeks of gestation, second trimester
- **O47.03** False labor before 37 completed weeks of gestation, third trimester
- **O47.1** False labor at or after 37 completed weeks of gestation
- **O47.9** False labor, unspecified
** An additional code from category Z3A is needed to specify the weeks of gestation of the pregnancy.

ICD-9 **618.01**

N81.11 Cystocele, midline

ICD-9 **626.2**

N92.0 Excessive and frequent menstruation with regular cycle
- **N92.1** Excessive and frequent menstruation with irregular cycle
- **N92.2** Excessive menstruation at puberty
- **N92.4** Excessive bleeding in the premenopausal period

ICD-9 **648.33**

O99.320 Drug use complicating pregnancy, unspecified trimester
- **O99.321** Drug use complicating pregnancy, first trimester
- **O99.322** Drug use complicating pregnancy, second trimester
- **O99.323** Drug use complicating pregnancy, third trimester
** The codes from this subcategory require an additional code from F11-F16 and F18-F19 to identify manifestations of the drug use.
** An additional code from category Z3A is needed to specify the weeks of gestation of the pregnancy.

ICD-9 **627.3**

N95.2 Postmenopausal atrophic vaginitis

ICD-9 **646.83**

O26.891 Other specified pregnancy related conditions, first trimester
- **O26.892** Other specified pregnancy related conditions, second trimester
- **O26.893** Other specified pregnancy related conditions, third trimester
- **O26.899** Other specified pregnancy related conditions, unspecified trimester
* There are other code selections avialable for codes previously coded to 646.83:
- **O26.10** Low weight gain in pregnancy, unspecified trimester
- **O26.11** Low weight gain in pregnancy, first trimester
- **O26.12** Low weight gain in pregnancy, second trimester
- **O26.13** Low weight gain in pregnancy, third trimester
- **O26.40** Herpes gestationis, unspecified trimester
- **O26.41** Herpes gestationis, first trimester
- **O26.42** Herpes gestationis, second trimester
- **O26.43** Herpes gestationis, third trimester
- **O26.811** Pregnancy related exhaustion and fatigue, first trimester
- **O26.812** Pregnancy related exhaustion and fatigue, second trimester
- **O26.813** Pregnancy related exhaustion and fatigue, third trimester
- **O26.819** Pregnancy related exhaustion and fatigue, unspecified trimester

** An additional code from category Z3A is needed to specify the weeks of gestation of the pregnancy.

ICD-9 **632**

O02.1 Missed abortion
** Use additional code from category O08 to identify any associated complication
** An additional code from category Z3A is needed to specify the weeks of gestation of the pregnancy.

ICD-9 **616.10**

N76.0 Acute vaginitis
**Use additional code (B95-B97), to identify infectious agent
There are other codes from this subcategory to describe vaginitis:
- **N76.1** Subacute and chronic vaginitis
- **N76.2** Acute vulvitis
- **N76.3** Subacute and chronic vulvitis
- **N76.89** Other specified inflammation of vagina and vulva

ICD-9 **618.00**

N81.9 Female genital prolapse, unspecified
*There are more specific code choice selections available in ICD-10-CM. These include:
- **N81.0** Urethrocele
- **N81.10** Cystocele, unspecified
- **N81.11** Cystocele, midline
- **N81.12** Cystocele, lateral
- **N81.2** Incomplete uterovaginal prolapse
- **N81.3** Complete uterovaginal prolapsed
- **N81.4** Uterovaginal prolapsed, unspecified
- **N81.5** Vaginal enterocele
- **N81.6** Rectocele
- **N81.81** Perineocele
- **N81.82** Incompetence or weakening of pubocervical tissue
- **N81.83** Incompetence or weakening of rectovaginal tissue
- **N81.84** Pelvic muscle wasting
- **N81.85** Cervical stump prolapsed
- **N81.89** Other female genital prolapsed

ICD-9 **620.2**

N83.20 Unspecified ovarian cysts
- **N83.29** Other ovarian cysts
* There are more specific code choice selections available in ICD-10-CM. These include:
- **N83.1** Corpus luteum cyst
- **N83.0** Follicular cyst of ovary
- **D27.9** Benign neoplasm of unspecified ovary
- **Q50.1** Developmental ovarian cyst
- **O34.80** Maternal care for other abnormalities of pelvic organs, unspecified trimester
- **O34.81** Maternal care for other abnormalities of pelvic organs, first trimester
- **O34.82** Maternal care for other abnormalities of pelvic organs, second trimester
- **O34.83** Maternal care for other abnormalities of pelvic organs, third trimester
- **O65.5** Obstructed labor due to abnormality of maternal pelvic organs
** An additional code from category Z3A is needed to specify the weeks of gestation of the pregnancy.

ICD-9 **623.9**

N89.8 Other specified noninflammatory disorders of vagina
* There are more specific code choice selections available in ICD-10-CM. These includ
- **N89.0** Mild vaginal dysplasia
- **N89.1** Moderate vaginal dysplasia
- **N89.3** Dysplasia of vagina, unspecified
- **N89.4** Leukoplakia of vagina
- **N89.5** Stricture and atresia of vagina
- **N89.6** Tight hymenal ring
- **N89.7** Hematocolpos
- **N89.9** Noninflammatory disorder of vagina, unspecified

ICD-9 **V25.2**

Z30.2 Encounter for sterilization

ICD-9 **618.1**

N81.2 Incomplete uterovaginal prolapse
- **N81.3** Complete uterovaginal prolapse
- **N81.4** Uterovaginal prolapse, unspecified

ICD-9 **788.20**

R33.9 Retention of urine, unspecified
* There are more specific code choice selections available in ICD-10-CM. These includ
- **R33.8** Other retention of urine
- **R33.0** Drug induced retention of urine
** Use additional code for adverse effect, if applicable, to identify drug (T36-T50 with fifth or sixth character 5)
- **F45.8** Other somatoform disorders

ICD-9 **788.31**

N39.41 Urge incontinence
** Code also any associated overactive bladder (N32.81)

ICD-9 788.33
ICD-10 N39.46 Mixed incontinence
Code also any associated overactive bladder symptoms (N32.81)

ICD-9 789.03
ICD-10 R10.31 Right lower quadrant pain

ICD-9 625.6
ICD-10 N39.3 Stress incontinence (female) (male)
Code also any associated overactive bladder symptoms (N32.81)

ICD-9 V22.1
ICD-10 Z34.80 Encounter for supervision of other normal pregnancy, unspecified trimester
Z34.81 Encounter for supervision of other normal pregnancy, first trimester
Z34.82 Encounter for supervision of other normal pregnancy, second trimester
Z34.83 Encounter for supervision of other normal pregnancy, third trimester

ICD-9 611.72
ICD-10 N63 Unspecified lump in breast

ICD-9 599.0
ICD-10 N39.0 Urinary tract infection, site not specified
Use additional code (B95-B97), to identify infectious agent
here are more specific code choice selections available in ICD-10-CM. These include:
N30.00 Acute cystitis without hematuria
N30.01 Acute cystitis with hematuria
N30.10 Interstitial cystitis (chronic) without hematuria
N30.11 Interstitial cystitis (chronic) with hematuria
N30.20 Other chronic cystitis without hematuria
N30.21 Other chronic cystitis with hematuria
N30.30 Trigonitis without hematuria
N30.31 Trigonitis with hematuria
N30.40 Irradiation cystitis without hematuria
N30.41 Irradiation cystitis with hematuria
N30.80 Other cystitis without hematuria
N30.81 Other cystitis with hematuria
N30.90 Cystitis, unspecified without hematuria
N30.91 Cystitis, unspecified with hematuria
N15.9 Renal tubule-interstitial disease, unspecified
N34.1 Nonspecific urethritis
N34.2 Other urethritis

ICD-9 627.9
ICD-10 N95.9 Unspecified menopausal and perimenopausal disorder
ere are more specific code choice selections available in ICD-10-CM. These include:
N95.0 Postmenopausal bleeding
N95.1 Menopausal and female climacteric states
N95.2 Postmenopausal atrophic vaginitis
N95.8 Other specified menopausal and perimenopausal disorders

ICD-9 788.34
ICD-10 N39.42 Incontinence without sensory awareness
Code also any associated overactive bladder (N32.81)

ICD-9 642.43
ICD-10 O14.00 Mild to moderate pre-eclampsia, unspecified trimester
O14.02 Mild to moderate pre-eclampsia, second trimester
O14.03 Mild to moderate pre-eclampsia, third trimester
O14.90 Unspecified pre-eclampsia, unspecified trimester
O14.92 Unspecified pre-eclampsia, second trimester
O14.93 Unspecified pre-eclampsia, third trimester
n additional code from category Z3A is needed to specify the weeks of gestation
f the pregnancy.

ICD-9 795.01
ICD-10 R87.610 Atypical squamous cells of undetermined significance on cytologic smear of cervix (ASC-US)
ere are more specific code choice selections available in ICD-10-CM. These include:
R87.611 Atypical squamous cells cannot exclude high grade squamous intraepithelial lesion on cytologic smear of cervix (ASC-H)
R87.612 Low grade squamous intraepithelial lesion on cytologic smear of cervix (LGSIL)
R87.613 High grade squamous intraepithelial lesion on cytologic smear of cervix (HGSIL)
R87.614 Cytologic evidence of malignancy on smear of cervix
R87.615 Unsatisfactory cytologic smear of cervix
R87.616 Satisfactory cervical smear but lacking transformation zone
R87.618 Other abnormal cytological findings on specimens from cervix uteri
R87.619 Unspecified abnormal cytological findings in specimens from cervix uteri

ICD-9 626.4
ICD-10 N92.5 Other specified irregular menstruation
N92.6 Irregular menstruation, unspecified

---

* There are more specific code choice selections available in ICD-10-CM. These include:
N92.0 Excessive and frequent menstruation with regular cycle
N92.1 Excessive and frequent menstruation with irregular cycle
N92.2 Excessive menstruation at puberty
N92.4 Excessive bleeding in the premenopausal period

ICD-9 651.03
ICD-10 O30.001 Twin pregnancy, unspecified number of placenta and unspecified number of amniotic sacs, first trimester
O30.002 Twin pregnancy, unspecified number of placenta and unspecified number of amniotic sacs, second trimester
O30.003 Twin pregnancy, unspecified number of placenta and unspecified number of amniotic sacs, third trimester
O30.009 Twin pregnancy, unspecified number of placenta and unspecified number of amniotic sacs, unspecified trimester
O30.011 Twin pregnancy, monochorionic/monoamniotic, first trimester
O30.012 Twin pregnancy, monochorionic/monoamniotic, second trimester
O30.013 Twin pregnancy, monochorionic/monoamniotic, third trimester
O30.019 Twin pregnancy, monochorionic/monoamniotic, unspecified trimester
O30.031 Twin pregnancy, monochorionic/diamniotic, first trimester
O30.032 Twin pregnancy, monochorionic/diamniotic, second trimester
O30.033 Twin pregnancy, monochorionic/diamniotic, third trimester
O30.039 Twin pregnancy, monochorionic/diamniotic, unspecified trimester
O30.041 Twin pregnancy, dichorionic/diamniotic, first trimester
O30.042 Twin pregnancy, dichorionic/diamniotic, second trimester
O30.043 Twin pregnancy, dichorionic/diamniotic, third trimester
O30.049 Twin pregnancy, dichorionic/diamniotic, unspecified trimester
O30.091 Twin pregnancy, unable to determine number of placenta and number of amniotic sacs, first trimester
O30.092 Twin pregnancy, unable to determine number of placenta and number of amniotic sacs, second trimester
O30.093 Twin pregnancy, unable to determine number of placenta and number of amniotic sacs, third trimester
O30.099 Twin pregnancy, unable to determine number of placenta and number of amniotic sacs, unspecified trimester
** An additional code from category Z3A is needed to specify the weeks of gestation of the pregnancy.

ICD-9 795.03
ICD-10 R87.612 Low grade squamous intraepithelial lesion on cytologic smear of cervix (LGSIL)

ICD-9 623.5
ICD-10 N89.8 Other specified noninflammatory disorders of vagina

ICD-9 V25.11
ICD-10 Z30.430 Encounter for insertion of intrauterine contraceptive device

ICD-9 658.23
ICD-10 O42.111 Preterm premature rupture of membranes, onset of labor more than 24 hours following rupture, first trimester
O42.112 Preterm premature rupture of membranes, onset of labor more than 24 hours following rupture, second trimester
O42.113 Preterm premature rupture of membranes, onset of labor more than 24 hours following rupture, third trimester
O42.119 Preterm premature rupture of membranes, onset of labor more than 24 hours following rupture, unspecified trimester
** An additional code from category Z3A is needed to specify the weeks of gestation of the pregnancy.

ICD-9 789.00
ICD-10 R10.9 Unspecified abdominal pain
* There are more specific code choice selections available in ICD-10-CM. These include:
R10.0 Acute abdomen
R10.10 Upper abdominal pain, unspecified
R10.11 Right upper quadrant pain
R10.12 Left upper quadrant pain
R10.13 Epigastric pain
R10.2 Pelvic and perineal pain

R10.30 Lower abdominal pain, unspecified
R10.31 Right lower quadrant pain
R10.32 Left lower quadrant pain
R10.33 Periumbilical pain
R10.84 Generalized abdominal pain

ICD-9 V28.3
ICD-10 Z36 Encounter for antenatal screening of mother

ICD-9 V76.2
ICD-10 Z12.4 Encounter for screening for malignant neoplasm of cervix

ICD-9 655.13
ICD-10

* A 7th character extender must be assigned to code under category O35.
O35.1XX0 Maternal care for (suspected) chromosomal abnormality in fetus, not applicable or unspecified
O35.1XX1 Maternal care for (suspected) chromosomal abnormality in fetus, fetus 1
O35.1XX2 Maternal care for (suspected) chromosomal abnormality in fetus, fetus 2
O35.1XX3 Maternal care for (suspected) chromosomal abnormality in fetus, fetus 3
O35.1XX4 Maternal care for (suspected) chromosomal abnormality in fetus, fetus 4
O35.1XX5 Maternal care for (suspected) chromosomal abnormality in fetus, fetus 5
O35.1XX9 Maternal care for (suspected) chromosomal abnormality in fetus, other fetus

One of the following 7th characters is to be assigned to each code under category O35. 7th character 0 is for single gestations and multiple gestations where the fetus is unspecified. 7th character 1 through 9 are for cases of multiple gestations to identify the fetus for which the code applies. The appropriate code from category O30, multiple gestation, must also be assigned when assigning a code from category O35 that has a 7th character of 1 through 9.
7th Character extenders for subcategory O35-
0 Not Applicable or unspecified
1 Fetus 1
2 Fetus 2
3 Fetus 3
4 Fetus 4
5 Fetus 5
9 Other fetus
** An additional code from category Z3A is needed to specify the weeks of gestation of the pregnancy.

ICD-9 789.04
ICD-10 R10.32 Left lower quadrant pain

ICD-9 789.07
ICD-10 R10.84 Generalized abdominal pain

ICD-9 595.1
ICD-10 N30.10 Interstitial cystitis (chronic) without hematuria
N30.11 Interstitial cystitis (chronic) with hematuria

ICD-9 595.9
ICD-10 N30.90 Cystitis, unspecified without hematuria
N30.91 Cystitis, unspecified with hematuria
** Use additional code to identify infectious agent (B95-B97)
* There are more specific code choice selections available in ICD-10-CM. These include:
N30.00 Acute cystitis without hematuria
N30.01 Acute cystitis with hematuria
N30.10 Interstitial cystitis (chronic) without hematuria
N30.11 Interstitial cystitis (chronic) with hematuria
N30.20 Other chronic cystitis without hematuria
N30.21 Other chronic cystitis with hematuria
N30.30 Trigonitis without hematuria
N30.31 Trigonitis with hematuria
N30.40 Irradiation cystitis without hematuria
N30.41 Irradiation cystitis with hematuria
N30.80 Other cystitis without hematuria
N30.81 Other cystitis with hematuria

ICD-9 788.43
ICD-10 R35.1 Nocturia

ICD-9 112.1
ICD-10 B37.3 Candidiasis of vulva and vagina

ICD-9 616.2
ICD-10 N75.0 Cyst of Bartholin's gland

ICD-9 616.4
ICD-10 N76.4 Abscess of vulva

ICD-9 V25.09
ICD-10 Z30.09 Encounter for other general counseling and advice on contraception
Z30.8 Encounter for other contraceptive management

ICD-9 659.73
ICD-10 O76 Abnormality in fetal heart rate and rhythm complicating labor and delivery

---

ICD-10 **Z3A.00** Weeks of gestation of pregnancy not specified
Z3A.01 Less than 8 weeks gestation of pregnancy
Z3A.08 8 weeks gestation of pregnancy
Z3A.09 9 weeks gestation of pregnancy
Z3A.10 10 weeks gestation of pregnancy
Z3A.11 11 weeks gestation of pregnancy
Z3A.12 12 weeks gestation of pregnancy
Z3A.13 13 weeks gestation of pregnancy
Z3A.14 14 weeks gestation of pregnancy
Z3A.15 15 weeks gestation of pregnancy
Z3A.16 16 weeks gestation of pregnancy
Z3A.17 17 weeks gestation of pregnancy
Z3A.18 18 weeks gestation of pregnancy
Z3A.19 19 weeks gestation of pregnancy
Z3A.20 20 weeks gestation of pregnancy
Z3A.21 21 weeks gestation of pregnancy
Z3A.22 22 weeks gestation of pregnancy
Z3A.23 23 weeks gestation of pregnancy
Z3A.24 24 weeks gestation of pregnancy
Z3A.25 25 weeks gestation of pregnancy
Z3A.26 26 weeks gestation of pregnancy
Z3A.27 27 weeks gestation of pregnancy
Z3A.28 28 weeks gestation of pregnancy
Z3A.29 29 weeks gestation of pregnancy
Z3A.30 30 weeks gestation of pregnancy
Z3A.31 31 weeks gestation of pregnancy
Z3A.32 32 weeks gestation of pregnancy
Z3A.33 33 weeks gestation of pregnancy
Z3A.34 34 weeks gestation of pregnancy
Z3A.35 35 weeks gestation of pregnancy
Z3A.36 36 weeks gestation of pregnancy
Z3A.37 37 weeks gestation of pregnancy
Z3A.38 38 weeks gestation of pregnancy
Z3A.39 39 weeks gestation of pregnancy
Z3A.40 40 weeks gestation of pregnancy
Z3A.41 41 weeks gestation of pregnancy
Z3A.42 42 weeks gestation of pregnancy
Z3A.49 Greater than 42 weeks gestation of pregnancy

Internal Medicine

ICD-9 **401.9**
ICD-10 **I10** Essential (primary) hypertension
ICD-9 **250.00**
ICD-10 **E11.9** Type 2 diabetes mellitus without complications
ICD-9 **272.4**
ICD-10 **E78.4** Other hyperlipidemia
E78.5 Hyperlipidemia, unspecified
** There are more specific code choice selections available in ICD-10-CM. These include:
E78.0 Pure hypercholesterolemia
E78.1 Pure hyperglyceridemia
E78.2 Mixed hyperlipidemia
E78.3 Hyperchylomicronemia
E78.6 Lipoprotein deficiency
ICD-9 **V70.0**
ICD-10 **Z00.00** Encounter for general adult medical examination without abnormal findings
Z00.01 Encounter for general adult medical examination with abnormal findings
** Use additional code to identify abnormal findings
ICD-9 **724.5**
ICD-10 **M54.9** Dorsalgia, unspecified
** There are more specific code choice selections available for back pain. These include:
M54.89 Other dorsalgia
M54.6 Pain in thoracic spine
M54.5 Low back pain
M53.3 Sacrococcygeal disorders, not elsewhere classified
ICD-9 **414.00**
ICD-10 **I25.10** Atherosclerotic heart disease of native coronary artery without angina pectoris
ICD-9 **V72.81**
ICD-10 **Z01.810** Encounter for preprocedural cardiovascular examination
ICD-9 **780.79**
ICD-10 **R53.1** Weakness
R53.81 Other malaise

R53.83 Other fatigue
G93.3 Postviral fatigue syndrome
R53.0 Neoplastic (malignant) related fatigue
* Code first associated neoplasm
ICD-9 **496**
ICD-10 **J44.9** Chronic obstructive pulmonary disease, unspecified
** There are more specific code choice selections available in ICD-10-CM. These include:
J44.0 Chronic obstructive pulmonary disease with acute lower respiratory infection
J44.1 Chronic obstructive pulmonary disease with (acute) exacerbation
** Code also type of asthma, if applicable (J45.-)
** Use additional code to identify:
Exposure to environmental tobacco smoke (Z77.22)
History of tobacco use (Z87.891)
Occupational exposure to environmental tobacco smoke (Z57.31)
Tobacco dependence (F17.-)
Tobacco use (Z72.0)
ICD-9 **427.31**
ICD-10 **I48.0** Paroxysmal atrial fibrillation
I48.1 Persistent atrial fibrillation
I48.2 Chronic atrial fibrillation
I48.91 Unspecified atrial fibrillation
ICD-9 **V04.81**
ICD-10 **Z23** Encounter for immunization
ICD-9 **786.2**
ICD-10 **R05** Cough
ICD-9 **311**
ICD-10 **F32.9** Major depressive disorder, single episode, unspecified
** There are more specific code choice selections available for depression. These include:
F32.0 Major depressive disorder, single episode, mild
F32.1 Major depressive disorder, single episode, moderate
F32.2 Major depressive disorder, single episode, severe without psychotic features
F32.3 Major depressive disorder, single episode, severe with psychotic features
F32.4 Major depressive disorder, single episode, in partial remission
F32.5 Major depressive disorder, single episode, in full remission
F32.8 Other depressive episodes
ICD-9 **250.02**
ICD-10 **E11.65** Type 2 diabetes mellitus with hyperglycemia
ICD-9 **729.5**
ICD-10 **M79.609** Pain in unspecified limb
** There are more specific code choice selections available in ICD-10-CM. These include:
M79.601 Pain in right arm
M79.602 Pain in left arm
M79.603 Pain in arm, unspecified
M79.604 Pain in right leg
M79.605 Pain in left leg
M79.606 Pain in leg, unspecified
M79.621 Pain in right upper arm
M79.622 Pain in left upper arm
M79.629 Pain in unspecified upper arm
M79.631 Pain in right forearm
M79.632 Pain in left forearm
M79.639 Pain in unspecified forearm
M79.641 Pain in right hand
M79.642 Pain in left hand
M79.643 Pain in unspecified hand
M79.644 Pain in right finger(s)
M79.645 Pain in left finger(s)
M79.646 Pain in unspecified finger(s)
M79.671 Pain in right foot
M79.672 Pain in left foot
M79.673 Pain in unspecified foot
M79.674 Pain in right toe(s)
M79.675 Pain in left toe(s)
M79.676 Pain in unspecified toe(s)
M79.651 Pain in right thigh
M79.652 Pain in left thigh
M79.659 Pain in unspecified thigh
M79.661 Pain in right lower leg
M79.662 Pain in left lower leg
M79.669 Pain in unspecified lower leg
ICD-9 **428.0**
ICD-10 **I50.9** Heart failure, unspecified
** There are more specific code choice selections available in ICD-10-CM. These include:
I50.1 Left ventricular failure
I50.21 Acute systolic (congestive) heart failure
I50.22 Chronic systolic (congestive) heart failure

I50.23 Acute on chronic systolic (congestive) heart failure
I50.31 Acute diastolic (congestive) heart failure
I50.32 Chronic diastolic (congestive) heart failure
I50.33 Acute on chronic diastolic (congestive) heart failure
I50.41 Acute combined systolic (congestive) and diastolic (congestive) heart failure
I50.42 Chronic combined systolic (congestive) and diastolic (congestive) heart failure
I50.43 Acute on chronic combined systolic (congestive) and diastolic (congestive) heart failure
ICD-9 **782.1**
ICD-10 **R21** Rash and other nonspecific skin changes
ICD-9 **786.50**
ICD-10 **R07.9** Chest pain, unspecified
** There are more specific code choice selections available in ICD-10-CM. These include:
R07.1 Chest pain on breathing
R07.81 Pleurodynia
R07.89 Other chest pain
ICD-9 **789.00**
ICD-10 **R10.9** Unspecified abdominal pain
** There are more specific code choice selections available for abdominal pain. These include:
R10.0 Acute abdomen
R10.10 Upper abdominal pain, unspecified
R10.11 Right upper quadrant pain
R10.12 Left upper quadrant pain
R10.13 Epigastric pain
R10.2 Pelvic and perineal pain
R10.30 Lower abdominal pain, unspecified
R10.31 Right lower quadrant pain
R10.32 Left lower quadrant pain
R10.33 Periumbilical pain
R10.84 Generalized abdominal pain
ICD-9 **719.46**
ICD-10 **M25.561** Pain in right knee
M25.562 Pain in left knee
M25.569 Pain in unspecified knee
ICD-9 **782.3**
ICD-10 **R60.0** Localized edema
R60.1 Generalized edema
R60.9 Edema, unspecified
ICD-9 **300.00**
ICD-10 **F41.1** Generalized anxiety disorder
F41.8 Other specified anxiety disorders
F41.9 Anxiety disorder, unspecified
ICD-9 **V72.83**
ICD-10 **Z01.818** Encounter for other preprocedural examination
ICD-9 **780.4**
ICD-10 **R42** Dizziness and giddiness
ICD-9 **466.0**
ICD-10 **J20.9** Acute bronchitis, unspecified
** There are more specific code choice selections available in ICD-10-CM. These include:
J20.0 Acute bronchitis due to Mycoplasma pneumoniae
J20.1 Acute bronchitis due to Hemophilus influenzae
J20.2 Acute bronchitis due to streptococcus
J20.3 Acute bronchitis due to coxsackievirus
J20.4 Acute bronchitis due to parainfluenza virus
J20.5 Acute bronchitis due to respiratory syncytial virus
J20.6 Acute bronchitis due to rhinovirus
J20.7 Acute bronchitis due to echovirus
J20.8 Acute bronchitis due to other specified organisms
ICD-9 **786.05**
ICD-10 **R06.02** Shortness of breath
ICD-9 **465.9**
ICD-10 **J06.9** Acute upper respiratory infection, unspecified
J39.8 Other specified diseases of upper respiratory tract
ICD-9 **530.81**
ICD-10 **K21.9** Gastro-esophageal reflux disease without esophagitis
K21.0 Gastro-esophageal reflux disease with esophagitis
ICD-9 **599.0**
ICD-10 **N39.0** Urinary tract infection, site not specified
** Use additional code (B95-B97)to identify infectious agent
** There are more specific code choice selections available in ICD-10-CM. These include:
N30.00 Acute cystitis without hematuria
N30.01 Acute cystitis with hematuria
N30.10 Interstitial cystitis (chronic) without hematuria
N30.11 Interstitial cystitis (chronic) with hematuria
N30.20 Other chronic cystitis without hematuria
N30.21 Other chronic cystitis with hematuria
N30.30 Trigonitis without hematuria

N30.31 Trigonitis with hematuria
N30.40 Irradiation cystitis without hematuria
N30.41 Irradiation cystitis with hematuria
N30.80 Other cystitis without hematuria
N30.81 Other cystitis with hematuria
N30.80 Other cystitis without hematuria
N30.81 Other cystitis with hematuria
N30.90 Cystitis, unspecified without hematuria
N30.91 Cystitis, unspecified with hematuria
N15.9 Renal tubule-interstitial disease, unspecified
N34.1 Nonspecific urethritis
N34.2 Other urethritis

ICD-9 724.4
ICD-10 M54.14 Radiculopathy, thoracic region
M54.15 Radiculopathy, thoracolumbar region
M54.16 Radiculopathy, lumbar region
M54.17 Radiculopathy, lumbosacral region

ICD-9 244.9
ICD-10 E03.9 Hypothyroidism, unspecified
* There are more specific code choice selections available for hypothyroidism. These include:
E03.0 Congenital hypothyroidism with diffuse goiter
E03.1 Congenital hypothyroidism without goiter
E03.2 Hypothyroidism due to medicaments and other exogenous substances
* Code first poisoning due to drug or toxin, if applicable (T36–T65 with fifth or sixth character 1–4 or 6)
* Use additional code for adverse effect, if applicable, to identify drug (T36–T50 with fifth or sixth character 5)
E03.3 Postinfectious hypothyroidism
E03.4 Atrophy of thyroid (acquired)
E03.5 Myxedema coma
E03.8 Other specified hypothyroidism

ICD-9 380.4
ICD-10 H61.21 Impacted cerumen, right ear
H61.22 Impacted cerumen, left ear
H61.23 Impacted cerumen, bilateral
H61.20 Impacted cerumen, unspecified ear

ICD-9 719.41
ICD-10 M25.511 Pain in right shoulder
M25.512 Pain in left shoulder
M25.519 Pain in unspecified shoulder

ICD-9 290.0
ICD-10 F03.9 Unspecified dementia

ICD-9 723.1
ICD-10 M54.2 Cervicalgia

ICD-9 787.91
ICD-10 R19.7 Diarrhea, unspecified

ICD-9 285.9
ICD-10 D64.9 Anemia, unspecified
There are more specific code choice selections available for use. These include:
D64.0 Hereditary sideroblastic anemia
D64.1 Secondary sideroblastic anemia due to disease
Code first underlying disease
D64.2 Secondary sideroblastic anemia due to drugs and toxins
Code first (T36-T65) to identify drug or toxin
Code first poisoning due to drug or toxin, if applicable (T36–T65 with fifth or sixth character 1–4 or 6)
Use additional code for adverse effect, if applicable, to identify drug (T36–T50 with fifth or sixth character 5)
D64.3 Other sideroblastic anemia
D64.81 Anemia due to antineoplastic chemotherapy
D64.89 Other specified anemias

ICD-9 461.9
ICD-10 J01.90 Acute sinusitis, unspecified
There are more specific code choice selections available in ICD-10-CM. These include:
J01.00 Acute maxillary sinusitis, unspecified
J01.01 Acute recurrent maxillary sinusitis
J01.10 Acute frontal sinusitis, unspecified
J01.11 Acute recurrent frontal sinusitis
J01.20 Acute ethmoidal sinusitis, unspecified
J01.21 Acute recurrent ethmoidal sinusitis
J01.30 Acute sphenoidal sinusitis
J01.31 Acute recurrent sphenoidal sinusitis
J01.40 Acute pansinusitis, unspecified
J01.41 Acute recurrent pansinusitis
J01.80 Other acute sinusitis
J01.81 Other acute recurrent sinusitis, unspecified
J01.91 Acute recurrent sinusitis, unspecified

ICD-9 719.45
ICD-10 M25.551 Pain in right hip
M25.552 Pain in left hip
M25.559 Pain in unspecified hip

ICD-9 477.9
ICD-10 J30.9 Allergic rhinitis, unspecified
** There are more specific code choice selections available for allergic rhinitis. These include:
J30.0 Vasomotor rhinitis
J30.1 Allergic rhinitis due to pollen
J30.2 Other seasonal allergic rhinitis
J30.5 Allergic rhinitis due to food
J30.81 Allergic rhinitis due to animal (cat) (dog) hair and dander
J30.89 Other allergic rhinitis

ICD-9 784.0
ICD-10 R51 Headache

ICD-9 564.00
ICD-10 K59.00 Constipation, unspecified
** There are more specific code choice selections available for constipation. These include:
K59.01 Slow transit constipation
K59.02 Outlet dysfunction constipation
K59.09 Other constipation

ICD-9 486
ICD-10 J18.9 Pneumonia, unspecified organism
J18.8 Other pneumonia, unspecified organism
** Code first associated influenza, if applicable (J09.X1, J10.0- to J11.0-)

ICD-9 338.4
ICD-10 G89.4 Chronic pain syndrome

ICD-9 796.2
ICD-10 R03.0 Elevated blood-pressure reading, without diagnosis of hypertension

ICD-9 780.2
ICD-10 R55 Syncope and collapse

ICD-9 493.90
ICD-10 J45.909 Unspecified asthma, uncomplicated
** There are more specific code choice selections available for asthma. These include:
J45.20 Mild intermittent asthma, uncomplicated
J45.21 Mild intermittent asthma with (acute) exacerbation
J45.22 Mild intermittent asthma with status asthmaticus
J45.30 Mild persistent asthma, uncomplicated
J45.31 Mild persistent asthma with (acute) exacerbation
J45.32 Mild persistent asthma with status asthmaticus
J45.40 Moderate persistent asthma, uncomplicated
J45.41 Moderate persistent asthma with (acute) exacerbation
J45.42 Moderate persistent asthma with status asthmaticus
J45.50 Severe persistent asthma, uncomplicated
J45.51 Severe persistent asthma with (acute) exacerbation
J45.52 Severe persistent asthma with status asthmaticus
J45.901 Unspecified asthma with (acute) exacerbation
J45.902 Unspecified asthma with status asthmaticus
J45.990 Exercise induced bronchospasm
J45.991 Cough variant asthma
J45.998 Other asthma
* Use additional code to identify:
exposure to environmental tobacco smoke (Z77.22)
exposure to tobacco smoke in the perinatal period (P96.81)
history of tobacco use (Z87.891)
occupational exposure to environmental tobacco smoke (Z57.31)
tobacco dependence (F17-)
tobacco use (Z72.0)

ICD-9 724.2
ICD-10 M54.5 Low back pain

ICD-9 682.6
ICD-10 L03.115 Cellulitis of right lower limb
L03.116 Cellulitis of left lower limb
L03.119 Cellulitis of unspecified part of limb
L03.125 Acute lymphangitis of right lower limb
L03.126 Acute lymphangitis of left lower limb
L03.129 Acute lymphangitis of unspecified part of limb

ICD-9 462
ICD-10 J02.8 Acute pharyngitis due to other specified organisms
** Use additional code (B95–B97) to identify infectious agent
J02.0 Streptococcal pharyngitis
J02.9 Acute pharyngitis, unspecified

Orthopedics — Lower

ICD-9 715.36
ICD-10 M16.0 Bilateral primary osteoarthritis of hip
M16.10 Unilateral primary osteoarthritis, unspecified hip
M16.11 Unilateral primary osteoarthritis, right hip
M16.12 Unilateral primary osteoarthritis, left hip
M16.6 Other bilateral secondary osteoarthritis of hip
M16.7 Other unilateral secondary osteoarthritis of hip
M16.9 Osteoarthritis of hip, unspecified
M17.0 Bilateral primary osteoarthritis of knee

M17.10 Unilateral primary osteoarthritis, unspecified knee
M17.11 Unilateral primary osteoarthritis, right knee
M17.12 Unilateral primary osteoarthritis, left knee
M19.271 Secondary osteoarthritis, right ankle and foot
M19.272 Secondary osteoarthritis, left ankle and foot
M19.279 Secondary osteoarthritis, unspecified ankle and foot

ICD-9 715.35
ICD-10 M16.0 Bilateral primary osteoarthritis of hip
M16.10 Unilateral primary osteoarthritis, unspecified hip
M16.11 Unilateral primary osteoarthritis, right hip
M16.12 Unilateral primary osteoarthritis, left hip
M16.6 Other bilateral secondary osteoarthritis of hip
M16.7 Other unilateral secondary osteoarthritis of hip
M16.9 Osteoarthritis of hip, unspecified

ICD-9 719.46
ICD-10 M25.551 Pain in right hip
M25.552 Pain in left hip
M25.559 Pain in unspecified hip
M25.561 Pain in right knee
M25.562 Pain in left knee
M25.569 Pain in unspecified knee

ICD-9 719.45
ICD-10 M25.551 Pain in right hip
M25.552 Pain in left hip
M25.559 Pain in unspecified hip

ICD-9 836.0
The appropriate 7th character is to be added to each code from category S83
ICD-10 S83.211 Bucket-handle tear of medial meniscus, current injury, right knee
S83.212 Bucket-handle tear of medial meniscus, current injury, left knee
S83.219 Bucket-handle tear of medial meniscus, current injury, unspecified knee
S83.221 Peripheral tear of medial meniscus, current injury,
S83.222 Peripheral tear of medial meniscus, current injury, left knee
S83.229 Peripheral tear of medial meniscus, current injury, unspecified knee
S83.231 Complex tear of medial meniscus, current injury, right knee
S83.232 Complex tear of medial meniscus, current injury, left knee
S83.239 Complex tear of medial meniscus, current injury, unspecified knee
S83.241 Other tear of medial meniscus, current injury, right knee
S83.242 Other tear of medial meniscus, current injury, left knee
S83.249 Other tear of medical meniscus, current injury, unspecified knee

ICD-9 824.6
The appropriate 7th character is to be added to each code from category S82.85
ICD-10 S82.851 Displaced trimalleolar fracture of right lower leg
S82.852 Displaced trimalleolar fracture of left lower leg
S82.853 Displaced trimalleolar fracture of unspecified lower leg
S82.854 Nondisplaced trimalleolar fracture of right lower leg
S82.855 Nondisplaced trimalleolar fracture of left lower leg
S82.856 Nondisplaced trimalleolar fracture of unspecified lower leg

ICD-9 996.78
The appropriate 7th character is to be added to each code from category T84
ICD-10 T84.81X Embolism due to internal orthopedic prosthetic devices, implants and grafts
T84.82X Fibrosis due to internal orthopedic prosthetic devices, implants and grafts
T84.83X Hemorrhage due to internal orthopedic prosthetic devices, implants and grafts
T84.84X Pain due to internal orthopedic prosthetic devices, implants and grafts
T84.85X Stenosis due to internal orthopedic prosthetic devices, implants and grafts
T84.86X Thrombosis due to internal orthopedic prosthetic devices, implants and grafts
T84.89X Other specified complication of internal orthopedic prosthetic devices, implants and grafts

ICD-9 715.89
ICD-10 M15.3 Secondary multiple arthritis
M15.8 Other polyosteoarthritis
844.2 Sprain and strain of cruciate ligament of knee
The appropriate 7th character is to be added to each code from category S83
S83.501 Sprain of unspecified cruciate ligament of right knee
S83.502 Sprain of unspecified cruciate ligament of left knee

S83.509 Sprain of unspecified cruciate ligament of unspecified knee

** There are more specific code choice selections available in ICD-10-CM. These include:

S83.511 Sprain of anterior cruciate ligament of right knee
S83.512 Sprain of anterior cruciate ligament of left knee
S83.519 Sprain of anterior cruciate ligament of unspecified knee
S83.521 Sprain of posterior cruciate ligament of right knee
S83.522 Sprain of posterior cruciate ligament of left knee
S83.529 Sprain of posterior cruciate ligament of unspecified knee

`ICD-9` **726.5**
`ICD-10` **M76.891** Other specified enthesopathies of right lower limb, excluding foot
M76.892 Other specified enthesopathies of left lower limb, excluding foot
M76.899 Other specified enthesopathies of unspecified lower limb, excluding foot
M76.9 Unspecified enthesopathy, lower limb, excluding foot

`ICD-9` **825.25**
The appropriate 7th character is to be added to each code from category S92
`ICD-10` **S92.301** Fracture of unspecified metatarsal bone(s), right foot
S92.302 Fracture of unspecified metatarsal bone(s), left foot
S92.309 Fracture of unspecified metatarsal bone(s), unspecified foot
S92.311 Displaced fracture of first metatarsal bone, right foot
S92.312 Displaced fracture of first metatarsal bone, left foot
S92.319 Displaced fracture of first metatarsal bone, unspecified foot
S92.314 Nondisplaced fracture of first metatarsal bone, right foot
S92.315 Nondisplaced fracture of first metatarsal bone, left foot
S92.316 Nondisplaced fracture of first metatarsal bone, unspecified foot
S92.321 Displaced fracture of second metatarsal bone, right foot
S92.322 Displaced fracture of second metatarsal bone, left foot
S92.323 Displaced fracture of second metatarsal bone, unspecified foot
S92.324 Nondisplaced fracture of second metatarsal bone, right foot
S92.325 Nondisplaced fracture of second metatarsal bone, left foot
S92.326 Nondisplaced fracture of second metatarsal bone, unspecified foot
S92.331 Displaced fracture of third metatarsal bone, right foot
S92.332 Displaced fracture of third metatarsal bone, left foot
S92.333 Displaced fracture of third metatarsal bone, unspecified foot
S92.334 Nondisplaced fracture of third metatarsal bone, right foot
S92.335 Nondisplaced fracture of third metatarsal bone, left foot
S92.336 Nondisplaced fracture of third metatarsal bone, unspecified foot
S92.341 Displaced fracture of fourth metatarsal, right foot
S92.342 Displaced fracture of fourth metatarsal, left foot
S92.343 Displaced fracture of fourth metatarsal, unspecified foot
S92.344 Nondisplaced fracture of fourth metatarsal, right foot
S92.345 Nondisplaced fracture of fourth metatarsal, left foot
S92.346 Nondisplaced fracture of fourth metatarsal, unspecified foot
S92.351 Displaced fracture of fifth metatarsal bone, right foot
S92.352 Displaced fracture of fifth metatarsal bone, left foot
S92.353 Displaced fracture of fifth metatarsal bone, unspecified foot
S92.354 Nondisplaced fracture of fifth metatarsal bone, right foot
S92.355 Nondisplaced fracture of fifth metatarsal bone, left foot
S92.356 Nondisplaced fracture of fifth metatarsal bone, unspecified foot

`ICD-9` **820.8**
The appropriate 7th character is to be added to each code from category S72
`ICD-10` **S72.001** Fracture of unspecified part of neck of right femur
S72.002 Fracture of unspecified part of neck of left femur
S72.009 Fracture of unspecified part of neck of unspecified femur

`ICD-9` **820.21**
The appropriate 7th character is to be added to each code from category S72
`ICD-10` **S72.141** Displaced intertrochanteric fracture of right femur
S72.142 Displaced intertrochanteric fracture of left femur
S72.143 Displaced intertrochanteric fracture of unspecified femur
S72.144 Nondisplaced intertrochanteric fracture of right femur
S72.145 Nondisplaced intertrochanteric fracture of left femur
S72.146 Nondisplaced intertrochanteric fracture of unspecified femur

`ICD-9` **719.47**
`ICD-10` **M25.571** Pain in right ankle

M25.572 Pain in left ankle
M25.573 Pain in unspecified ankle

`ICD-9` **717.2**
`ICD-10` **M23.321** Other meniscus derangements, posterior horn of medial meniscus, right knee
M23.322 Other meniscus derangements, posterior horn of medial meniscus, left knee
M23.329 Other meniscus derangements, posterior horn of medial meniscus, unspecified knee

`ICD-9` **735.0**
`ICD-10` **M20.10** Hallux valgus (acquired), unspecified foot
M20.11 Hallux valgus (acquired), right foot
M20.12 Hallux valgus (acquired), left foot

`ICD-9` **733.82**
`ICD-10`
In ICD-10-CM, a nonunion is coded by site and represented by the appropriate 7th character extension.*

`ICD-9` **735.4**
`ICD-10` **M20.40** Other hammer toe(s) (acquired), unspecified foot
M20.41 Other hammer toe(s) (acquired), right foot
M20.42 Other hammer toe(s) (acquired), left foot

`ICD-9` **735.2**
`ICD-10` **M20.20** Hallux rigidus, unspecified foot
M20.21 Hallux rigidus, right foot
M20.22 Hallux rigidus, left foot

`ICD-9` **836.2**
The appropriate 7th character is to be added to each code from category S83
`ICD-10` **S83.203** Other tear of unspecified meniscus, current injury, right knee
S83.204 Other tear of unspecified meniscus, current injury, left knee
S83.205 Other tear of unspecified meniscus, current injury, unspecified knee

`ICD-9` **250.00**
`ICD-10` **E11.9** Type 2 diabetes mellitus without complications
`ICD-9` **729.5**
`ICD-10` **M79.609** Pain in unspecified limb
M79.601 Pain in right arm
M79.602 Pain in left arm
M79.603 Pain in arm, unspecified
M79.604 Pain in right leg
M79.605 Pain in left leg
M79.606 Pain in leg, unspecified
M79.621 Pain in right upper arm
M79.622 Pain in left upper arm
M79.629 Pain in unspecified upper arm
M79.631 Pain in right forearm
M79.632 Pain in left forearm
M79.639 Pain in unspecified forearm
M79.641 Pain in right hand
M79.642 Pain in left hand
M79.643 Pain in unspecified hand
M79.644 Pain in right finger(s)
M79.645 Pain in left finger(s)
M79.646 Pain in unspecified finger(s)
M79.651 Pain in right thigh
M79.652 Pain in left thigh
M79.659 Pain in unspecified thigh
M79.661 Pain in right lower leg
M79.662 Pain in left lower leg
M79.669 Pain in unspecified lower leg
M79.671 Pain in right foot
M79.672 Pain in left foot
M79.673 Pain in unspecified foot
M79.674 Pain in right toe(s)
M79.675 Pain in left toe(s)
M79.676 Pain in unspecified toe(s)

`ICD-9` **823.0**
The appropriate 7th character is to be added to each code from category S82.1
`ICD-10` **S82.101** Unspecified fracture of upper end of right tibia
S82.102 Unspecified fracture of upper end of left tibia
S82.109 Unspecified fracture of upper end of unspecified tibia
S82.111 Displaced fracture of right tibial spine
S82.112 Displaced fracture of left tibial spine
S82.113 Displaced fracture of unspecified tibial spine
S82.114 Nondisplaced fracture of right tibial spine
S82.115 Nondisplaced fracture of left tibial spine
S82.116 Nondisplaced fracture of unspecified tibial spine
S82.121 Displaced fracture of lateral condyle of right tibia
S82.122 Displaced fracture of lateral condyle of left tibia

S82.123 Displaced fracture of lateral condyle of unspecified tibia
S82.124 Nondisplaced fracture of lateral condyle of right tibia
S82.125 Nondisplaced fracture of lateral condyle of left tibia
S82.126 Nondisplaced fracture of lateral condyle of unspecified tibia
S82.131 Displaced fracture of medial condyle of right tibia
S82.132 Displaced fracture of medial condyle of left tibia
S82.133 Displaced fracture of medial condyle of unspecified tibia
S82.134 Nondisplaced fracture of medial condyle of right tibia
S82.135 Nondisplaced fracture of medial condyle of left tibia
S82.136 Nondisplaced fracture of medial condyle of unspecified tibia
S82.141 Displaced bicondylar fracture of right tibia
S82.142 Displaced bicondylar fracture of left tibia
S82.143 Displaced bicondylar fracture of unspecified tibia
S82.144 Nondisplaced bicondylar fracture of right tibia
S82.145 Nondisplaced bicondylar fracture of left tibia
S82.146 Nondisplaced bicondylar fracture of unspecified tibia
S82.151 Displaced fracture of right tibial tuberosity
S82.152 Displaced fracture of left tibial tuberosity
S82.153 Displaced fracture of unspecified tibial tuberosity
S82.154 Nondisplaced fracture of right tibial tuberosity
S82.155 Nondisplaced fracture of left tibial tuberosity
S82.156 Nondisplaced fracture of unspecified tibial tuberosity

`ICD-9` **717.3**
`ICD-10` **M23.231** Derangement of other medial meniscus due to old tear or injury, right knee
M23.232 Derangement of other medial meniscus due to old tear or injury, left knee
M23.239 Derangement of other medial meniscus due to old tear or injury, unspecified knee
M23.303 Other meniscus derangements, unspecified medial meniscus, right knee
M23.304 Other meniscus derangements, unspecified medial meniscus, left knee
M23.305 Other meniscus derangements, unspecified medial meniscus, unspecified knee
M23.331 Other meniscus derangements, other medial meniscus, right knee
M23.332 Other meniscus derangements, other medial meniscus, left knee
M23.339 Other meniscus derangements, other medial meniscus, unspecified knee

`ICD-9` **726.1**
`ICD-10` **M76.60** Achilles tendinitis, unspecified leg
M76.61 Achilles tendinitis, right leg
M76.62 Achilles tendinitis, left leg

`ICD-9` **845.09**
The appropriate 7th character is to be added to each code from category S93
`ICD-10` **S93.401** Sprain of unspecified ligament of right ankle
S93.402 Sprain of unspecified ligament of left ankle
S93.409 Sprain of unspecified ligament of unspecified ankle
S93.411 Sprain of calcaneofibular ligament of right ankle
S93.412 Sprain of calcaneofibular ligament of left ankle
S93.419 Sprain of calcaneofibular ligament of unspecified ankle
S93.421 Sprain of deltoid ligament of right ankle
S93.422 Sprain of deltoid ligament of left ankle
S93.429 Sprain of deltoid ligament of unspecified ankle
S93.431 Sprain of tibiofibular ligament of right ankle
S93.432 Sprain of tibiofibular ligament of left ankle
S93.439 Sprain of tibiofibular ligament of unspecified ankle
S93.491 Sprain of other ligament of right ankle
S93.492 Sprain of other ligament of left ankle
S93.499 Sprain of other ligament of unspecified ankle
S93.601 Unspecified sprain of right foot
S93.602 Unspecified sprain of left foot
S93.609 Unspecified sprain of unspecified foot
S93.611 Sprain of tarsal ligament of right foot
S93.612 Sprain of tarsal ligament of left foot
S93.619 Sprain of tarsal ligament of unspecified foot
S93.621 Sprain of tarsometatarsal ligament of right foot
S93.622 Sprain of tarsometatarsal ligament of left foot
S93.629 Sprain of tarsometatarsal ligament of unspecified foot
S93.691 Other sprain of right foot
S93.692 Other sprain of left foot
S93.699 Other sprain of unspecified foot

`ICD-9` **715.17**
`ICD-10` **M19.071** Primary osteoarthritis, right ankle and foot
M19.072 Primary osteoarthritis, left ankle and foot
M19.079 Primary osteoarthritis, unspecified ankle and foot

M23.611 Other spontaneous disruption of anterior cruciate ligament of right knee
M23.612 Other spontaneous disruption of anterior cruciate ligament of left knee
M23.619 Other spontaneous disruption of anterior cruciate ligament of unspecified knee

ICD-9 727.06

M65.171 Other infective (teno)synovitis, right ankle and foot
M65.172 Other infective (teno)synovitis, left ankle and foot
M65.179 Other infective (teno)synovitis, unspecified ankle and foot
M65.871 Other synovitis and tenosynovitis, right ankle and foot
M65.872 Other synovitis and tenosynovitis, left ankle and foot
M65.879 Other synovitis and tenosynovitis, unspecified ankle and foot

ICD-9 822.0
The appropriate 7th character is to be added to each code from category S82.0

S82.001 Unspecified fracture of right patella
S82.002 Unspecified fracture of left patella
S82.009 Unspecified fracture of unspecified patella
S82.011 Displaced osteochondral fracture of right patella
S82.012 Displaced osteochondral fracture of left patella
S82.013 Displaced osteochondral fracture of unspecified patella
S82.014 Nondisplaced osteochondral fracture of right patella
S82.015 Nondisplaced osteochondral fracture of left patella
S82.016 Nondisplaced osteochondral fracture of unspecified patella
S82.021 Displaced longitudinal fracture of right patella
S82.022 Displaced longitudinal fracture of left patella
S82.023 Displaced longitudinal fracture of unspecified patella
S82.024 Nondisplaced longitudinal fracture of right patella
S82.025 Nondisplaced longitudinal fracture of left patella
S82.026 Nondisplaced longitudinal fracture of unspecified patella
S82.031 Displaced transverse facture of right patella
S82.032 Displaced transverse facture of left patella
S82.033 Displaced transverse facture of unspecified patella
S82.034 Nondisplaced transverse fracture of right patella
S82.035 Nondisplaced transverse fracture of left patella
S82.036 Nondisplaced transverse fracture of unspecified patella
S82.041 Displaced comminuted fracture of right patella
S82.042 Displaced comminuted fracture of left patella
S82.043 Displaced comminuted fracture of unspecified patella
S82.044 Nondisplaced comminuted fracture of right patella
S82.045 Nondisplaced comminuted fracture of left patella
S82.046 Nondisplaced comminuted fracture of unspecified patella
S82.091 Other fracture of right patella
S82.092 Other fracture of left patella
S82.099 Other fracture of unspecified patella

ICD-9 733.42

M87.051 Idiopathic aseptic necrosis of right femur
M87.052 Idiopathic aseptic necrosis of left femur
M87.059 Idiopathic aseptic necrosis of unspecified femur

ICD-9 736.79

M21.6x1 Other acquired deformities of right foot
M21.6x2 Other acquired deformities of left foot
M21.6x9 Other acquired deformities of unspecified foot
M21.961 Unspecified acquired deformity of right lower leg
M21.962 Unspecified acquired deformity of left lower leg
M21.969 Unspecified acquired deformity of unspecified lower leg

ICD-9 715.96

M16.0 Bilateral primary osteoarthritis of hip
M16.10 Unilateral primary osteoarthritis, unspecified hip
M16.11 Unilateral primary osteoarthritis, right hip
M16.12 Unilateral primary osteoarthritis, left hip
M16.6 Other bilateral secondary osteoarthritis of hip
M16.7 Other unilateral secondary osteoarthritis of hip
M16.9 Osteoarthritis of hip, unspecified
M17.0 Bilateral primary osteoarthritis of knee
M17.10 Unilateral primary osteoarthritis, unspecified knee
M17.11 Unilateral primary osteoarthritis, right knee
M17.12 Unilateral primary osteoarthritis, left knee
M19.271 Secondary osteoarthritis, right ankle and foot
M19.272 Secondary osteoarthritis, left ankle and foot
M19.279 Secondary osteoarthritis, unspecified ankle and foot

ICD-9 821.20
appropriate 7th character is to be added to each code from category S72

S72.401 Unspecified fracture of lower end of right femur
S72.402 Unspecified fracture of lower end of left femur

S72.409 Unspecified fracture of lower end of unspecified femur

ICD-9 996.49
The appropriate 7th character is to be added to each code from category T84
* The characters listed below are subcategories, further detail is necessary.

T84.03 Mechanical loosening of internal prosthetic joint
T84.09 Other mechanical complication of internal joint prosthesis
T84.11 Breakdown (mechanical) of internal fixation device of bones of limbs
T84.19 Other mechanical complication of internal fixation device of bones of limb
T84.21 Breakdown (mechanical) of internal fixation device of other bones
T84.29 Other mechanical complication of internal fixation device of other bones
T84.31 Breakdown (mechanical) of other bone devices, implants and grafts
T84.39 Other mechanical complication of other bone devices, implants and grafts
T84.41 Breakdown (mechanical) of other internal orthopedic devices, implants and grafts
T84.49 Other mechanical complication of other internal orthopedic devices, implants and grafts

ICD-9 836.1
The appropriate 7th character is to be added to each code from category S83

S83.251 Bucket-handle tear of lateral meniscus, current injury, right knee
S83.252 Bucket-handle tear of lateral meniscus, current injury, left knee
S83.259 Bucket-handle tear of lateral meniscus, current injury, unspecified knee
S83.261 Peripheral tear of lateral meniscus, current injury, right knee
S83.262 Peripheral tear of lateral meniscus, current injury, left knee
S83.269 Peripheral tear of lateral meniscus, current injury, unspecified knee
S83.271 Complex tear of lateral meniscus, current injury, right knee
S83.272 Complex tear of lateral meniscus, current injury, left knee
S83.279 Complex tear of lateral meniscus, current injury, unspecified knee
S83.281 Other tear of lateral meniscus, current injury, right knee
S83.282 Other tear of lateral meniscus, current injury, left knee
S83.289 Other tear of lateral meniscus, current injury, unspecified knee

ICD-9 726.72

M76.821 Posterior tibial tendinitis, right leg
M76.822 Posterior tibial tendinitis, left leg
M76.829 Posterior tibial tendinitis, unspecified leg

ICD-9 215.3

D21.20 Benign neoplasm of connective and other soft tissue of unspecified lower limb, including hip
D21.21 Benign neoplasm of connective and other soft tissue of right lower limb, including hip
D21.22 Benign neoplasm of connective and other soft tissue of left lower limb, including hip

ICD-9 250.61

E10.40 Type 1 diabetes mellitus with diabetic neuropathy, unspecified
E10.41 Type 1 diabetes mellitus with diabetic mononeuropathy
E10.42 Type 1 diabetes mellitus with diabetic polyneuropathy
E10.43 Type 1 diabetes mellitus with diabetic autonomic (poly) neuropathy
E10.44 Type 1 diabetes mellitus with diabetic amyotrophy
E10.49 Type 1 diabetes mellitus with other diabetic neurological complication

ICD-9 726.91

M89.9 Disorder of bone, unspecified

ICD-9 824.2
The appropriate 7th character is to be added to each code from category S82

S82.61x Displaced fracture of lateral malleolus of right fibula
S82.62x Displaced fracture of lateral malleolus of left fibula
S82.63x Displaced fracture of lateral malleolus of unspecified fibula
S82.64x Nondisplaced fracture of lateral malleolus of right fibula
S82.65x Nondisplaced fracture of lateral malleolus of left fibula
S82.66x Nondisplaced fracture of lateral malleolus of unspecified fibula

ICD-9 821.00
The appropriate 7th character is to be added to each code from category S42

S42.201 Unspecified fracture of upper end of right humerus
S42.202 Unspecified fracture of upper end of left humerus
S42.209 Unspecified fracture of upper end of unspecified humerus
S42.271 Torus fracture of upper end of right humerus
S42.272 Torus fracture of upper end of left humerus
S42.279 Torus fracture of upper end of unspecified humerus
S42.291 Other displaced fracture of upper end of right humerus
S42.292 Other displaced fracture of upper end of left humerus
S42.293 Other displaced fracture of upper end of unspecified humerus
S42.294 Other nondisplaced fracture of upper end of right humerus
S42.295 Other nondisplaced fracture of upper end of left humerus
S42.296 Other nondisplaced fracture of upper end of unspecified humerus

ICD-9 727.68

M66.871 Spontaneous rupture of other tendons, right ankle and foot
M66.872 Spontaneous rupture of other tendons, left ankle and foot
M66.879 Spontaneous rupture of other tendons, unspecified ankle and foot

ICD-9 738.4

M43.10 Spondylolisthesis, site unspecified
M43.11 Spondylolisthesis, occipito-atlanto-axial region
M43.12 Spondylolisthesis, cervical region
M43.13 Spondylolisthesis, cervicothoracic region
M43.14 Spondylolisthesis, thoracic region
M43.15 Spondylolisthesis, thoracolumbar region
M43.16 Spondylolisthesis, lumbar region
M43.17 Spondylolisthesis, lumbosacral region
M43.18 Spondylolisthesis, sacral and sacrococcygeal region
M43.19 Spondylolisthesis, multiple sites in spine

ICD-9 730.17

M86.671 Other chronic osteomyelitis, right ankle and foot
M86.672 Other chronic osteomyelitis, left ankle and foot
M86.679 Other chronic osteomyelitis, unspecified ankle and foot

ICD-9 728.71

M72.2 Plantar fascial fibromatosis

ICD-9 821.00
The appropriate 7th character is to be added to each code from category S72

S72.90x Unspecified fracture of unspecified femur
S72.91x Unspecified fracture of right femur
S72.92x Unspecified fracture of left femur
S72.8x1 Other fracture of right femur
S72.8x2 Other fracture of left femur
S72.8x9 Other fracture of unspecified femur

ICD-9 824.7
The appropriate 7th character is to be added to each code from subcategory S82.8

S82.851 Displaced trimalleolar fracture of right lower leg
S82.852 Displaced trimalleolar fracture of left lower leg
S82.853 Displaced trimalleolar fracture of unspecified lower leg
S82.854 Nondisplaced trimalleolar fracture of right lower leg
S82.855 Nondisplaced trimalleolar fracture of left lower leg
S82.856 Nondisplaced trimalleolar fracture of unspecified lower leg

ICD-9 718.56

M24.651 Ankylosis, right hip
M24.652 Ankylosis, left hip
M24.659 Ankylosis, unspecified hip
M24.661 Ankylosis, right knee
M24.662 Ankylosis, left knee
M24.669 Ankylosis, unspecified knee
M24.671 Ankylosis, right ankle
M24.672 Ankylosis, left ankle
M24.673 Ankylosis, unspecified ankle
M24.674 Ankylosis, right foot
M24.675 Ankylosis, left foot
M24.676 Ankylosis, unspecified foot

ICD-9 716.17

M12.571 Traumatic arthropathy, right ankle and foot
M12.572 Traumatic arthropathy, left ankle and foot
M12.579 Traumatic arthropathy, unspecified ankle and foot

For any category that requires a 7th character extender that does not include 6 characters, a dummy placeholder must be used to fill in the missing characters. In ICD-10-CM this is identified by the letter x.
In ICD-10-CM a fracture not indicated as nondisplaced or displaced should be classified to displaced. A fracture not indicated as open or closed should be coded to closed.

Orthopedics — Upper

ICD-9 724.2
ICD-10 M54.5 Low back pain (Lumbago, NOS)
M54.40 Lumbago with sciatica, unspecified site
M54.41 Lumbago with sciatica, right side
M54.42 Lumbago with sciatica, left side

ICD-9 724.02
ICD-10 M48.06 Spinal stenosis, lumbar region
M48.07 Spinal stenosis, lumbosacral region

ICD-9 722.52
ICD-10 M51.36 Other intervertebral disc degeneration, lumbar region
M51.37 Other intervertebral disc degeneration, lumbosacral region

ICD-9 723.1
ICD-10 M54.2 Cervicalgia

ICD-9 724.3
ICD-10 M54.30 Sciatica, unspecified site
M54.31 Sciatica, right side
M54.32 Sciatica, left side
M54.40 Lumbago with sciatica, unspecified site
M54.41 Lumbago with sciatica, right side
M54.42 Lumbago with sciatica, left side

ICD-9 722.10
ICD-10 M51.26 Other intervertebral disc displacement, lumbar region
M51.27 Other intervertebral disc displacement, lumbosacral region

ICD-9 722.4
ICD-10 M50.30 Other cervical disc degeneration, unspecified cervical region
M50.31 Other cervical disc degeneration, occipito-atlanto-axial region
M50.32 Other cervical disc degeneration, mid-cervical region
M50.33 Other cervical disc degeneration, cervicothoracic region

ICD-9 737.30
ICD-10 M41.112 Juvenile idiopathic scoliosis, cervical region
M41.113 Juvenile idiopathic scoliosis, cervicothoracic region
M41.114 Juvenile idiopathic scoliosis, thoracic region
M41.115 Juvenile idiopathic scoliosis, thoracolumbar region
M41.116 Juvenile idiopathic scoliosis, lumbar region
M41.117 Juvenile idiopathic scoliosis, lumbosacral region
M41.119 Juvenile idiopathic scoliosis, site unspecified
M41.122 Adolescent idiopathic scoliosis, cervical region
M41.123 Adolescent idiopathic scoliosis, cervicothoracic region
M41.124 Adolescent idiopathic scoliosis, thoracic region
M41.125 Adolescent idiopathic scoliosis, thoracolumbar region
M41.126 Adolescent idiopathic scoliosis, lumbar region
M41.127 Adolescent idiopathic scoliosis, lumbosacral region
M41.129 Adolescent idiopathic scoliosis, site unspecified
M41.20 Other idiopathic scoliosis, site unspecified
M41.22 Other idiopathic scoliosis, cervical region
M41.23 Other idiopathic scoliosis, cervicothoracic region
M41.24 Other idiopathic scoliosis, thoracic region
M41.25 Other idiopathic scoliosis, thoracolumbar region
M41.26 Other idiopathic scoliosis, lumbar region
M41.27 Other idiopathic scoliosis, lumbosacral region

ICD-9 719.41
ICD-10 M25.511 Pain in right shoulder
M25.512 Pain in left shoulder
M25.519 Pain in unspecified shoulder

ICD-9 840.4
The appropriate 7th character is to be added to each code from category S43.
ICD-10 S43.421 Sprain of right rotator cuff capsule
S43.422 Sprain of left rotator cuff capsule
S43.429 Sprain of unspecified rotator cuff capsule

ICD-9 729.5
ICD-10 M79.609 Pain in unspecified limb
** There are more specific code choice selections available in ICD-10-CM. These include:
M79.601 Pain in right arm'
M79.602 Pain in left arm
M79.603 Pain in arm, unspecified
M79.604 Pain in right leg
M79.605 Pain in left leg
M79.606 Pain in leg, unspecified
M79.631 Pain in right upper arm
M79.622 Pain in left upper arm
M79.629 Pain in unspecified upper arm
M79.631 Pain in right forearm
M79.632 Pain in left forearm
M79.639 Pain in unspecified forearm
M79.651 Pain in right thigh

M79.652 Pain in left thigh
M79.659 Pain in unspecified thigh
M79.661 Pain in right lower leg
M79.662 Pain in left lower leg
M79.669 Pain in unspecified lower leg

ICD-9 715.91
ICD-10 M19.011 Primary osteoarthritis, right shoulder
M19.012 Primary osteoarthritis, left shoulder
M19.019 Primary osteoarthritis, unspecified shoulder

ICD-9 727.61
ICD-10 M75.100 Unspecified rotator cuff tear or rupture of unspecified shoulder, not specified as traumatic
M75.101 Unspecified rotator cuff tear or rupture of right shoulder, not specified as traumatic
M75.102 Unspecified rotator cuff tear or rupture of unspecified shoulder, not specified as traumatic
M75.110 Incomplete rotator cuff tear or rupture of unspecified shoulder, not specified as traumatic
M75.111 Incomplete rotator cuff tear or rupture of right shoulder, not specified as traumatic
M75.112 Incomplete rotator cuff tear or rupture of left shoulder, not specified as traumatic
M75.120 Complete rotator cuff tear or rupture of unspecified shoulder, not specified as traumatic
M75.121 Complete rotator cuff tear or rupture of right shoulder, not specified as traumatic
M75.122 Complete rotator cuff tear or rupture of left shoulder, not specified as traumatic

ICD-9 756.12
ICD-10 Q76.2 Congenital spondylolisthesis

ICD-9 812.00
The appropriate 7th character is to be added to each code from category S42.
ICD-10 S42.201 Unspecified fracture of upper end of right humerus
S42.202 Unspecified fracture of upper end of left humerus
S42.209 Unspecified fracture of upper end of unspecified humerus
** There are more specific code choice selections available in ICD-10-CM. These include:
S42.211 Unspecified displaced fracture of surgical neck of right humerus
S42.212 Unspecified displaced fracture of surgical neck of left humerus
S42.214 Unspecified nondisplaced fracture of surgical neck of right humerus
S42.215 Unspecified nondisplaced fracture of surgical neck of left humerus
S42.216 Unspecified nondisplaced fracture of surgical neck of unspecified humerus
S42.219 Unspecified displaced fracture of surgical neck of unspecified humerus
S42.221 2-part displaced fracture of surgical neck of right humerus
S42.222 2-part displaced fracture of surgical neck of left humerus
S42.223 2-part displaced fracture of surgical neck of unspecified humerus
S42.224 2-part nondisplaced fracture of surgical neck of right humerus
S42.225 2-part nondisplaced fracture of surgical neck of left humerus
S42.226 2-part nondisplaced fracture of surgical neck of unspecified humerus
S42.231 3-part fracture of surgical neck of right humerus
S42.232 3-part fracture of surgical neck of left humerus
S42.239 3-part fracture of surgical neck of unspecified humerus
S42.241 4-part fracture of surgical neck of right humerus
S42.242 4-part fracture of surgical neck of left humerus
S42.249 4-part fracture of surgical neck of unspecified humerus
S42.251 Displaced fracture of greater tuberosity of right humerus
S42.252 Displaced fracture of greater tuberosity of left humerus
S42.253 Displaced fracture of greater tuberosity of unspecified humerus
S42.254 Nondisplaced fracture of greater tuberosity of right humerus
S42.255 Nondisplaced fracture of greater tuberosity of left humerus
S42.256 Nondisplaced fracture of greater tuberosity of unspecified humerus
S42.261 Displaced fracture of lesser tuberosity of right humerus
S42.262 Displaced fracture of lesser tuberosity of left humerus
S42.263 Displaced fracture of lesser tuberosity of unspecified humerus
S42.264 Nondisplaced fracture of lesser tuberosity of right humerus

S42.265 Nondisplaced fracture of lesser tuberosity of left humerus
S42.266 Nondisplaced fracture of lesser tuberosity of unspecified humerus
S42.271 Torus fracture of upper end of right humerus
S42.272 Torus fracture of upper end of left humerus
S42.279 Torus fracture of upper end of unspecified humerus
S42.291 Other displaced fracture of upper end of right humerus
S42.292 Other displaced fracture of upper end of left humerus
S42.293 Other displaced fracture of upper end of unspecified humerus
S42.294 Other nondisplaced fracture of upper end of right humerus
S42.295 Other nondisplaced fracture of upper end of left humerus
S42.296 Other nondisplaced fracture of upper end of unspecified humerus

ICD-9 738.4
ICD-10 M43.10 Spondylolisthesis, site unspecified
M43.11 Spondylolisthesis, occipito-atlanto-axial region
M43.12 Spondylolisthesis, cervical region
M43.13 Spondylolisthesis, cervicothoracic region
M43.14 Spondylolisthesis, thoracic region
M43.15 Spondylolisthesis, thoracolumbar region
M43.16 Spondylolisthesis, lumbar region
M43.17 Spondylolithesis, lumbosacral region
M43.18 Spondylolisthesis, sacral and sacrococcygeal region
M43.19 Spondylolisthesis, multiple sites in spine

ICD-9 722.2
ICD-10 M50.20 Other cervical disc displacement, unspecified cervical region
M50.21 Other cervical disc displacement, occipito-atlanto-axial region
M50.22 Other cervical disc displacement, mid-cervical region
M50.23 Other cervical disc displacement, cervicothoracic region

ICD-9 724.00
ICD-10 M48.00 Spinal stenosis, site unspecified
** There are more specific code choice selections available in ICD-10-CM. These inclu
M48.01 Spinal stenosis, occipito-atlanto-axial region
M48.02 Spinal stenosis, cervical region
M48.03 Spinal stenosis, cervicothoracic region
M48.04 Spinal stenosis, thoracic region
M48.05 Spinal stenosis, thoracolumbar region
M48.06 Spinal stenosis, lumbar region
M48.07 Spinal stenosis, lumbosacral region
M48.08 Spinal stenosis, sacral and sacrococcygeal region

ICD-9 840.6
The appropriate 7th character is to be added to each code from category S43.
ICD-10 S43.50 Sprain of unspecified acromioclavicular joint
S43.51 Sprain of right acromioclavicular joint
S43.52 Sprain of left acromioclavicular joint
S43.60 Sprain of unspecified sternoclavicular joint
S43.61 Sprain of right sternoclavicular joint
S43.62 Sprain of left sternoclavicular joint
S43.8 Sprain of other specified parts of unspecified shoulder girdle
S43.81 Sprain of other specified parts of right shoulder girdle
S43.82 Sprain of other specified parts of left shoulder girdle
S43.90 Sprain of unspecified parts of unspecified shoulder gir
S43.91 Sprain of unspecified parts of right shoulder girdle
S43.92 Sprain of unspecified parts of the left shoulder girdle
S43.491 Other sprain of right shoulder joint
S43.492 Other sprain of left shoulder joint
S43.499 Other sprain of unspecified shoulder joint

ICD-9 805.02
The appropriate 7th character is to be added to each code from category S12.0–S12.6
ICD-10 S12.100 Unspecified displaced fracture of second cervical vertebra
S12.101 Unspecified nondisplaced fracture of second cervical vertebra
** There are more specific code choice selections available in ICD-10-CM. These inclu
S12.01 Stable burst fracture of the first cervical vertebra
S12.02 Unstable burst fracture of first cervical vertebra
S12.030 Displaced posterior arch fracture of first cervical vertebra
S12.031 Nondisplaces posterior arch fracture of first cervical vertebra
S12.040 Displaced lateral mass fracture of first cervical vertek
S12.041 Nondisplaced lateral mass fracture of first cervical vertebra
S12.090 Other displaced fracture of first cervical vertebra
S12.091 Other nondisplaced fracture of first cervical vertebra
S12.110 Anterior displaced Type II dens fracture

S12.111 Posterior displaced Type II dens fracture
S12.112 Nondisplaced Type II dens fracture
S12.120 Other displaced dens fracture
S12.121 Other nondisplaced dens fracture
S12.190 Other displaced fracture of second cervical vertebra
S12.191 Other nondisplaced fracture of second cervical vertebra.

de also any associated cervical spinal cord injury (S14.0, S14.1-)

[CD-9] 721.1
[CD-10] M47.12 Other spondylosis with myelopathy, cervical region

[CD-9] 805.4
e appropriate 7ᵗʰ character is to be added to each code from category S32.
There are more specific code choice selections available in ICD-10-CM. These include:
[CD-10] S32.000- Wedge compression fracture of unspecified lumbar vertebra
S32.001- Stable burst fracture of unspecified lumbar vertebra
S32.008- Other fracture of unspecified lumbar vertebra
S32.009- Unspecified fracture of unspecified lumbar vertebra
S32.010- Wedge compression fracture of first lumbar vertebra
S32.011- Stable burst fracture of first lumbar vertebra
S32.012- Unstable burst fracture of first lumbar vertebra
S32.019- Unspecified fracture of first lumbar vertebra
S32.020- Wedge compression fracture of second lumbar vertebra
S32.021- Stable burst fracture of second lumbar vertebra
S32.022- Unstable burst fracture of second lumbar vertebra
S32.028- Other fracture of second lumbar vertebra
S32.029- Unspecified fracture of second lumbar vertebra
S32.030- Wedge compression fracture of third lumbar vertebra
S32.031- Stable burst fracture of third lumbar vertebra
S32.032- Unstable burst fracture of third lumbar vertebra
S32.038- Other fracture of third lumbar vertebra
S32.039- Unspecified fracture of third lumbar vertebra
S32.040- Wedge compression fracture of fourth lumbar vertebra
S32.041- Stable burst fracture of fourth lumbar vertebra
S32.042- Unstable burst fracture of fourth lumbar vertebra
S32.048- Other fracture of fourth lumbar vertebra
S32.049- Unspecified fracture of fourth lumbar vertebra
S32.050- Wedge compression fracture of fifth lumbar vertebra
S32.051- Stable burst fracture of fifth lumbar vertebra
S32.052- Unstable burst fracture of fifth lumbar vertebra
S32.058- Other fracture of fifth lumbar vertebra
S32.059- Unspecified fracture of fifth lumbar vertebra

[CD-9] 810.00
e appropriate 7ᵗʰ character is to be added to each code from category S42.
[CD-10] S42.009 Fracture of unspecified part of unspecified clavicle
There are more specific code choice selections available in ICD-10-CM. These include:
S42.001 Fracture of unspecified part of right clavicle
S42.002 Fracture of unspecified part of left clavicle
S42.011 Anterior displaced fracture of sternal end of right clavicle
S42.012 Anterior displaced fracture of sternal end of left clavicle
S42.013 Anterior displaced fracture of sternal end of unspecified clavicle
S42.014 Posterior displaced fracture of sternal end of right clavicle
S42.015 Posterior displaced fracture of sternal end of left clavicle
S42.016 Posterior displaced fracture of sternal end of unspecified clavicle
S42.017 Nondisplaced fracture of sternal end of right clavicle
S42.018 Nondisplaced fracture of sternal end of left clavicle
S42.019 Nondisplaced fracture of sternal end of unspecified clavicle
S42.021 Displaced fracture of shaft of right clavicle
S42.022 Displaced fracture of shaft of left clavicle
S42.023 Displaced fracture of shaft of unspecified clavicle
S42.024 Nondisplaced fracture of shaft of right clavicle
S42.025 Nondisplaced fracture of shaft of left clavicle
S42.026 Nondisplaced fracture of shaft of unspecified clavicle
S42.031 Displaced fracture of lateral end of right clavicle
S42.032 Displaced fracture of lateral end of left clavicle
S42.033 Displaced fracture of lateral end of unspecified clavicle
S42.034 Nondisplaced fracture of lateral end of right clavicle
S42.035 Nondisplaced fracture of lateral end of left clavicle
S42.036 Nondisplaced fracture of lateral end of unspecified clavicle

[CD-9] 805.2
e appropriate 7ᵗʰ character is to be added to each code from category S22.
[CD-10] S22.078 Other fracture of T9-T10 vertebra
S22.079 Unspecified fracture of T9-T10 vertebra
S22.080 Wedge compression fracture of T11-T12 vertebra
S22.081 Stable burst fracture of T11-T12 vertebra
S22.082 Unstable burst fracture of T11-T12 vertebra

S22.088 Other fracture of T11-T12 vertebra
S22.089 Unspecified fracture of T11-T12 vertebra
* Code first any associated: injury of intrathoracic organ (S27-), spinal cord injury (S24.0-, S24.1-).
[CD-9] 721.90
[CD-10] M47.819 Spondylosis without myelopathy or radiculopathy, site unspecified
** There are more specific code choice selections available in ICD-10-CM. These include:
M47.811 Spondylosis without myelopathy or radiculopathy, occipito-atlanto-axial region
M47.812 Spondylosis without myelopathy or radiculopathy, cervical region
M47.813 Spondylosis without myelopathy or radiculopathy, cervicothoracic region
M47.814 Spondylosis without myelopathy or radiculopathy, thoracic region
M47.815 Spondylosis without myelopathy or radiculopathy, thoracolumbar region
M47.816 Spondylosis without myelopathy or radiculopathy, lumbar region
M47.817 Spondylosis without myelopathy or radiculopathy, lumbosacral region
M47.818 Spondylosis without myelopathy or radiculopathy, sacral and sacrococcygeal region
M47.20 Other spondylosis with radiculopathy, site unspecified
M47.899 Other spondylosis, site unspecified
M47.9 Spondylosis, unspecified

[CD-9] 726.2
[CD-10] M75.00 Adhesive capsulitis of unspecified shoulder
M75.01 Adhesive capsulitis of right shoulder
M75.02 Adhesive capsulitis of left shoulder
M75.30 Calcific tendinitis of unspecified shoulder
M75.31 Calcific tendinitis of right shoulder
M75.32 Calcific tendinitis of left shoulder
M75.40 Impingement syndrome of unspecified shoulder
M75.41 Impingement syndrome of right shoulder
M75.42 Impingement syndrome of left shoulder
M75.50 Bursitis of unspecified shoulder
M75.51 Bursitis of right shoulder
M75.52 Bursitis of left shoulder
M75.80 Other shoulder lesions, unspecified shoulder
M75.81 Other shoulder lesions, right shoulder
M75.82 Other shoulder lesions, left shoulder
M75.90 Shoulder lesion, unspecified, unspecified shoulder
M75.91 Shoulder lesion, unspecified, right shoulder
M75.92 Shoulder lesion, unspecified, left shoulder
M25.711 Osteophyte, right shoulder
M25.712 Osteophyte, left shoulder
M25.719 Osteophyte, unspecified shoulder

[CD-9] 718.81
[CD-10] M24.811 Other specific joint derangements of right shoulder, not elsewhere classified
M24.812 Other specific joint derangements of left shoulder, not elsewhere classified
M24.819 Other specific joint derangements of unspecified shoulder, not elsewhere classified
M25.211 Flail joint, right shoulder
M25.212 Flail joint, left shoulder
M25.219 Flail joint, unspecified shoulder
M25.311 Other instability, right shoulder
M25.312 Other instability, left shoulder
M25.319 Other instability, unspecified shoulder

[CD-9] 724.1
[CD-10] M54.6 Pain in thoracic spine
[CD-9] 812.21
The appropriate 7ᵗʰ character is to be added to each code from category S42.
[CD-10] S42.301 Unspecified fracture of shaft of humerus, right arm
S42.302 Unspecified fracture of shaft of humerus, left arm
S42.309 Unspecified fracture of shaft of humerus, unspecified arm
S42.311 Greenstick fracture of shaft of humerus, right arm
S42.312 Greenstick fracture of shaft of humerus, left arm
S42.319 Greenstick fracture of shaft of humerus, unspecified arm
S42.321 Displaced transverse fracture of shaft of humerus, right arm
S42.322 Displaced transverse fracture of shaft of humerus, left arm
S42.323 Displaced transverse fracture of shaft of humerus, unspecified arm

---

S42.324 Nondisplaced transverse fracture of shaft of humerus, right arm
S42.325 Nondisplaced transverse fracture of shaft of humerus, left arm
S42.326 Nondisplaced transverse fracture of shaft of humerus, unspecified arm
S42.331 Displaced oblique fracture of shaft of humerus, right arm
S42.332 Displaced oblique fracture of shaft of humerus, left arm
S42.333 Displaced oblique fracture of shaft of humerus, unspecified arm
S42.334 Nondisplaced oblique fracture of shaft of humerus, right arm
S42.335 Nondisplaced oblique fracture of shaft of humerus, left arm
S42.336 Nondisplaced oblique fracture of shaft of humerus, unspecified arm
S42.411 Displaced simple supracondylar fracture without intercondylar fracture of right humerus
S42.412 Displaced simple supracondylar fracture without intercondylar fracture of left humerus
S42.413 Displaced simple supracondylar fracture without intercondylar fracture of unspecified humerus
S42.414 Nondisplaced simple supracondylar fracture without intercondylar fracture of right humerus
S42.415 Nondisplaced simple supracondylar fracture without intercondylar fracture of left humerus
S42.416 Nondisplaced simple supracondylar fracture without intercondylar fracture of unspecified humerus
S42.421 Displaced comminuted supracondylar fracture without intercondylar fracture of right humerus
S42.422 Displaced comminuted supracondylar fracture without intercondylar fracture of left humerus
S42.423 Displaced comminuted supracondylar fracture without intercondylar fracture of unspecified humerus
S42.424 Nondisplaced comminuted supracondylar fracture without intercondylar fracture of right humerus
S42.425 Nondisplaced comminuted supracondylar fracture without intercondylar fracture of left humerus
S42.426 Nondisplaced comminuted supracondylar fracture without intercondylar fracture of unspecified humerus
S42.431 Displaced spiral fracture of shaft of humerus, right arm
S42.432 Displaced spiral fracture of shaft of humerus, left arm
S42.433 Displaced spiral fracture of shaft of humerus, unspecified arm
S42.434 Nondisplaced spiral fracture of shaft of humerus, right arm
S42.435 Nondisplaced spiral fracture of shaft of humerus, left arm
S42.436 Nondisplaced spiral fracture of shaft of humerus, unspecified arm
S42.351 Displaced comminuted fracture of shaft of humerus, right arm
S42.352 Displaced comminuted fracture of shaft of humerus, left arm
S42.353 Displaced comminuted fracture of shaft of humerus, unspecified arm
S42.354 Nondisplaced comminuted fracture of shaft of humerus, right arm
S42.355 Nondisplaced comminuted fracture of shaft of humerus, left arm
S42.356 Nondisplaced comminuted fracture of shaft of humerus, unspecified arm
S42.361 Displaced segmental fracture of shaft of humerus, right arm
S42.362 Displaced segmental fracture of shaft of humerus, left arm
S42.363 Displaced segmental fracture of shaft of humerus, unspecified arm
S42.364 Nondisplaced segmental fracture of shaft of humerus, right arm
S42.365 Nondisplaced segmental fracture of shaft of humerus, left arm
S42.366 Nondisplaced segmental fracture of shaft of humerus, unspecified arm
S42.391 Other fracture of shaft of right humerus
S42.392 Other fracture of shaft of left humerus
S42.399 Other fracture of shaft of unspecified humerus

ICD-9 737.10
ICD-10 **M40.00** Postural kyphosis, site unspecified
M40.03 Postural kyphosis, cervicothoracic region
M40.04 Postural kyphosis, thoracic region
M40.05 Postural kyposis, thoracolumbar region
M40.10 Other secondary kyphosis, site unspecified
M40.12 Other secondary kyphosis, cervical region
M40.13 Other secondary kyphosis, cervicothoracic region
M40.14 Other secondary kyphosis, thoracic region
M40.15 Other secondary kyphosis, thoracolumbar region
M40.202 Unspecified kyphosis, cervical region
M40.203 Unspecified kyphosis, cervicothoracic region
M40.204 Unspecified kyphosis, thoracic region
M40.205 Unspecified kyphosis, thoracolumbar region
M40.209 Unspecified kyphosis, site unspecified
M40.292 Other kyphosis, cervical region
M40.293 Other kyphosis, cervicothoracic region
M40.294 Other kyphosis, thoracic region
M40.295 Other kyphosis, thoracolumbar region
M40.299 Other kyphosis, site unspecified

ICD-9 813.42
The appropriate 7th character is to be added to each code from category S52.
ICD-10 **S52.501** Unspecified fracture of the lower end of right radius
S52.502 Unspecified fracture of the lower end of left radius
S52.509 Unspecified fracture of the lower end of unspecified radius
S52.511 Displaced fracture of right radial styloid process
S52.512 Displaced fracture of left radial styloid process
S52.513 Displaced fracture of unspecified radial styloid process
S52.514 Nondisplaced fracture of right radial styloid process
S52.515 Nondisplaced fracture of left radial styloid process
S52.516 Nondisplaced fracture of unspecified radial styloid process
S52.551 Other extraarticular fracture of lower end of right radius
S52.552 Other extraarticular fracture of lower end of left radius
S52.559 Other extraarticular fracture of lower end of unspecified radius
S52.561 Barton's fracture of right radius
S52.562 Barton's fracture of left radius
S52.569 Barton's fracture of unspecified radius
S52.571 Other intraarticular fracture of lower end of right radius
S52.572 Other intraarticular fracture of lower end of left radius
S52.579 Other intraarticular fracture of lower end of unspecified radius
S52.591 Other fracture of lower end of right radius
S52.592 Other fracture of lower end of left radius
S52.599 Other fracture of lower end of unspecified radius

ICD-9 718.31
ICD-10 **M24.411** Recurrent dislocation, right shoulder
M24.412 Recurrent dislocation, left shoulder
M24.419 Recurrent dislocation, unspecified shoulder

ICD-9 810.02
ICD-10 **S42.021** Displaced fracture of shaft of right clavicle
S42.022 Displaced fracture of shaft of left clavicle
S42.023 Displaced fracture of shaft of unspecified clavicle
S42.024 Nondisplaced fracture of shaft of right clavicle
S42.025 Nondisplaced fracture of shaft of left clavicle
S42.026 Nondisplaced fracture of shaft of unspecified clavicle

ICD-9 354.2
ICD-10 **G56.20** Lesion of ulnar nerve, unspecified upper limb
G56.21 Lesion of ulnar nerve, right upper limb
G56.22 Lesion of ulnar nerve, left upper limb

ICD-9 727.00
ICD-10 **M65.89** Other synovitis and tenosynovitis, other site
There are additional code choice options in ICD-10-CM:
M65.80 Other synovitis and tenosynovitis, unspecified site
M65.811 Other synovitis and tenosynovitis, right shoulder
M65.812 Other synovitis and tenosynovitis, left shoulder
M65.819 Other synovitis and tenosynovitis, unspecified shoulder
M65.821 Other synovitis and tenosynovitis, right upper arm
M65.822 Other synovitis and tenosynovitis, left upper arm
M65.829 Other synovitis and tenosynovitis, unspecified upper arm
M65.831 Other synovitis and tenosynovitis, right forearm
M65.832 Other synovitis and tenosynovitis, left forearm
M65.839 Other synovitis and tenosynovitis, unspecified forearm
M65.841 Other synovitis and tenosynovitis, right hand
M65.842 Other synovitis and tenosynovitis, left hand
M65.849 Other synovitis and tenosynovitis, unspecified hand
M65.851 Other synovitis and tenosynovitis, right thigh

M65.852 Other synovitis and tenosynovitis, left thigh
M65.859 Other synovitis and tenosynovitis, unspecified thigh
M65.861 Other synovitis and tenosynovitis, right lower leg
M65.862 Other synovitis and tenosynovitis, left lower leg
M65.863 Other synovitis and tenosynovitis, unspecified lower leg
M65.871 Other synovitis and tenosynovitis, right ankle and foot
M65.872 Other synovitis and tenosynovitis, left ankle and foot
M65.879 Other synovitis and tenosynovitis, unspecified ankle and foot

ICD-9 723.0
ICD-10 **M48.02** Spinal stenosis, cervical region

ICD-9 726.10
ICD-10 **M75.50** Bursitis of unspecified shoulder
M75.51 Bursitis of right shoulder
M75.52 Bursitis of left shoulder

ICD-9 840.8
The appropriate 7th character is to be added to each code from category S43 and S46.
ICD-10 **S43.90** Sprain of unspecified parts of unspecified shoulder girdle
S43.91 Sprain of unspecified parts of right shoulder
S43.92 Sprain of unspecified parts of left shoulder
S46.011 Strain of muscle(s) and tendon(s) of the rotator cuff of the right shoulder
S46.012 Strain of the muscle(s) and tendon(s) of the rotator cuff of the left shoulder
S46.019 Strain of the muscle(s) and tendon(s) of the rotator cuff of the left shoulder
S46.811 Strain of other muscles, fascia and tendons at shoulder and upper arm level, right arm
S46.812 Strain of other muscles, fascia and tendons at shoulder and upper arm level, left arm
S46.819 Strain of other muscles, fascia and tendons at shoulder and upper arm level, unspecified arm
* Code also any associated open wound (S41-).

ICD-9 805.06
The appropriate 7th character is to be added to each code from category S12.
ICD-10 **S12.500** Unspecified displaced fracture of sixth cervical vertebra
S12.501 Unspecified nondisplaced fracture of sixth vertebra

ICD-9 840.7
The appropriate 7th character is to be added to each code from category S43.
ICD-10 **S43.431** Superior glenoid labrum lesion of right shoulder
S43.432 Superior glenoid labrum lesion of left shoulder
S43.439 Superior glenoid labrum lesion of unspecified shoulder

ICD-9 726.0
ICD-10 **M75.00** Adhesive capsulitis of unspecified shoulder
M75.01 Adhesive capsulitis of right shoulder
M75.02 Adhesive capsulitis of left shoulder

ICD-9 733.13
ICD-10 **M84.48** Pathological fracture, other site, initial encounter for fracture

ICD-9 805.01
The appropriate 7th character is to be added to each code from category M80.
* These codes require a 7th character extender and consist of dummy placeholders.
ICD-10 **M80.08** Age-related osteoporosis with current pathological fracture, vertebra(e)
M84.48 Pathological fracture, other site, initial encounter for fracture
M80.08 Age-related osteoporosis with current pathological fracture, vertebra(e)
M84.58- Pathological fracture in neoplastic disease, vertebrae, initial encounter for fracture
M84.68 Pathological fracture in other disease, other site, initial encounter for fracture

ICD-9 812.41
ICD-10 **M84.68** Pathological fracture in other disease, other site, initial encounter for fracture

ICD-9 718.01
ICD-10 **M24.119** Other articular cartilage disorders, unspecified shoulder

ICD-9 726.11
ICD-10 **M75.30** Calcific tendinitis of unspecified shoulder
M75.31 Calcific tendinitis of right shoulder
M75.32 Calcific tendinitis of left shoulder

ICD-9 812.01
The appropriate 7th character is to be added to each code from category S42.
ICD-10 **S42.211** Unspecified displaced fracture of surgical neck of right humerus
S42.212 Unspecified displaced fracture of surgical neck, left humerus
S42.213 Unspecified displaced fracture of surgical neck of unspecified humerus
S42.214 Unspecified nondisplaced fracture of surgical neck of right humerus

S42.215 Unspecified nondisplaced fracture of surgical neck of left humerus
S42.216 Unspecified nondisplaced fracture of surgical neck of unspecified humerus

ICD-9 727.62
ICD-10 **M66.221** Spontaneous rupture of extensor tendons, right upper arm
M66.222 Spontaneous rupture of extensor tendons, left upper arm
M66.229 Spontaneous rupture of extensor tendons, unspecified upper arm
M66.30 Spontaneous rupture of flexor tendons, unspecified site
M66.311 Spontaneous rupture of flexor tendons, right shoulder
M66.312 Spontaneous rupture of flexor tendons, left shoulder
M66.319 Spontaneous rupture of flexor tendons, unspecified shoulder
M66.321 Spontaneous rupture of flexor tendons, right upper arm
M66.322 Spontaneous rupture of flexor tendons, left upper arm
M66.329 Spontaneous rupture of flexor tendons, unspecified upper arm
M66.821 Spontaneous rupture of other tendons, right upper arm
M66.822 Spontaneous rupture of other tendons, left upper arm
M66.829 Spontaneous rupture of other tendons, unspecified upper arm shoulder

ICD-9 810.01
The appropriate 7th character is to be added to each code from category S42.
ICD-10 **S42.011** Anterior displaced fracture of sternal end of right clavicle
S42.012 Anterior displaced fracture of sternal end of left clavicle
S42.013 Anterior displaced fracture of sternal end of unspecified clavicle
S42.014 Posterior displaced fracture of sternal end of right clavicle
S42.015 Posterior displaced fracture of sternal end of left clavicle
S42.016 Posterior displaced fracture of sternal end of unspecified clavicle
S42.017 Nondisplaced fracture of sternal end of right clavicle
S42.018 Nondisplaced fracture of sternal end of left clavicle
S42.019 Nondisplaced fracture of sternal end of unspecified clavicle

ICD-9 724.5
ICD-10 **M54.9** Dorsalgia, unspecified
M53.3 Sacroliliac (Sacrococcygeal disorders, NEC)
M54.89 Other dorsalgia

ICD-9 811.00
The appropriate 7th character is to be added to each code from category S42.
ICD-10 **S42.101** Fracture of unspecified part of scapula, right shoulder initial encounter for closed fracture
S42.102 Fracture of unspecified part of scapula, left shoulder, initial encounter for closed fracture
S42.109 Fracture of unspecified part of scapula, unspecified shoulder, initial encounter for closed fracture

ICD-9 812.20
The appropriate 7th character is to be added to each code from category S42.
ICD-10 **S42.301** Unspecified fracture of shaft of humerus, right arm, initial encounter for closed fracture
S42.302 Unspecified fracture of shaft of humerus, left arm, initial encounter for closed fracture
S42.309 Unspecified fracture of shaft of humerus, unspecified arm, initial encounter for closed fracture
S42.90 Fracture of unspecified shoulder girdle, part unspecified initial encounter for closed fracture
S42.91 Fracture of right shoulder girdle, part unspecified, initial encounter for closed fracture
S42.92 Fracture of left shoulder girdle, part unspecified, initial encounter for closed fracture

Otolaryngology

ICD-9 474.00
ICD-10 **J35.01** Chronic tonsillitis
* Use additional code to identify:
Exposure to environmental tobacco smoke (Z77.22)
Exposure to tobacco smoke in the perinatal period (P96.81)
History of tobacco use (Z87.891)
Occupational exposure to environmental tobacco smoke (Z57.31)
Tobacco dependence (F17-)
Tobacco use (Z72.0)

ICD-9 382.3
ICD-10 **H66.3x1** Other chronic suppurative otitis media, right ear
H66.3x2 Other chronic suppurative otitis media, left ear
H66.3x3 Other chronic suppurative otitis media, bilateral
H66.3x9 Other chronic suppurative otitis media, unspecified

Use additional code for any associated perforated tympanic membrane (H72-)
Use additional code to identify:
Exposure to environmental tobacco smoke (Z77.22)
Exposure to tobacco smoke in the perinatal period (P96.81)
History of tobacco use (Z87.891)
Occupational exposure to environmental tobacco smoke (Z57.31)
Tobacco dependence (F17-)
Tobacco use (Z72.0)

D-9 474.10
ICD-10 J35.3 Hypertrophy of tonsils with hypertrophy of adenoids
Use additional code to identify:
Exposure to environmental tobacco smoke (Z77.22)
Exposure to tobacco smoke in the perinatal period (P96.81)
History of tobacco use (Z87.891)
Occupational exposure to environmental tobacco smoke (Z57.31)
Tobacco dependence (F17-)
Tobacco use (Z72.0)

D-9 381.10
ICD-10 H65.20 Chronic serous otitis media, unspecified ear
H65.21 Chronic serous otitis media, right ear
H65.22 Chronic serous otitis media, left ear
H65.23 Chronic serous otitis media, bilateral
Use additional code for any associated perforated tympanic membrane (H72-)
Use additional code to identify:
Exposure to environmental tobacco smoke (Z77.22)
Exposure to tobacco smoke in the perinatal period (P96.81)
History of tobacco use (Z87.891)
Occupational exposure to environmental tobacco smoke (Z57.31)
Tobacco dependence (F17-)
Tobacco use (Z72.0)

D-9 470
ICD-10 J34.2 Deviated nasal septum

D-9 327.23
ICD-10 G47.33 Obstructive sleep apnea (adult)(pediatric)
Code also any associated underlying condition

D-9 384.20
ICD-10 H72.90 Unspecified perforation of tympanic membrane, unspecified ear
Code first any associated otitis media (H65-, H66.1-, H66.2-, H66.3-, H66.4-, H66.9-, H67-)
H72.91 Unspecified perforation of tympanic membrane, right ear
H72.92 Unspecified perforation of tympanic membrane, left ear
H72.93 Unspecified perforation of tympanic membrane, bilateral
There are more specific code choice selections available in ICD-10-CM. These include:
H72.00 Central perforation of tympanic membrane, unspecified ear
H72.01 Central perforation of tympanic membrane, right ear
H72.02 Central perforation of tympanic membrane, left ear
H72.03 Central perforation of tympanic membrane, bilateral
H72.10 Attic perforation of tympanic membrane, unspecified ear
H72.11 Attic perforation of tympanic membrane, right ear
H72.12 Attic perforation of tympanic membrane, left ear
H72.13 Attic perforation of tympanic membrane, bilateral
H72.2x1 Other marginal perforations of tympanic membrane, right ear
H72.2x2 Other marginal perforations of tympanic membrane, left ear
H72.2x3 Other marginal perforations of tympanic membrane, bilateral
H72.2x9 Other marginal perforations of tympanic membrane, unspecified ear
H72.811 Multiple perforations of tympanic membrane, right ear
H72.812 Multiple perforations of tympanic membrane, left ear
H72.813 Multiple perforations of tympanic membrane, bilateral
H72.819 Multiple perforations of tympanic membrane, unspecified ear
H72.821 Total perforations of tympanic membrane, right ear
H72.822 Total perforations of tympanic membrane, left ear
H72.823 Total perforations of tympanic membrane, bilateral
H72.829 Total perforations of tympanic membrane, unspecified ear

D-9 382.9
ICD-10 H66.90 Otitis media, unspecified, unspecified ear
Use additional code for any associated perforated tympanic membrane (H72-)
Use additional code to identify:
Exposure to environmental tobacco smoke (Z77.22)
Exposure to tobacco smoke in the perinatal period (P96.81)
History of tobacco use (Z87.891)
Occupational exposure to environmental tobacco smoke (Z57.31)
Tobacco dependence (F17-)
Tobacco use (Z72.0)
There are more specific code choice selections available in ICD-10-CM. These include:
H66.91 Otitis media, unspecified, right ear
H66.92 Otitis media, unspecified, let ear
H66.93 Otitis media, unspecified, bilateral
There are more specific codes available for otis media. These include:
H65.00 Acute serous otitis media, unspecified ear

H65.01 Acute serous otitis media, right ear
H65.02 Acute serous otitis media, left ear
H65.03 Acute serous otitis media, bilateral
H65.04 Acute serous otitis media, recurrent, right ear
H65.05 Acute serous otitis media, recurrent, left ear
H65.06 Acute serous otitis media, recurrent, bilateral
H65.07 Acute serous otitis media, recurrent, unspecified ear
H65.111 Acute and subacute allergic otitis media (mucoid) (sanguinous) (serous), right ear
H65.112 Acute and subacute allergic otitis media (mucoid) (sanguinous) (serous), left ear
H65.113 Acute and subacute allergic otitis media (mucoid) (sanguinous) (serous), bilateral
H65.114 Acute and subacute allergic otitis media (mucoid) (sanguinous) (serous), recurrent, right ear
H65.115 Acute and subacute allergic otitis media (mucoid) (sanguinous) (serous), recurrent, left ear
H65.116 Acute and subacute allergic otitis media (mucoid) (sanguinous) (serous), recurrent, bilateral
H65.117 Acute and subacute allergic otitis media (mucoid) (sanguinous) (serous), recurrent, unspecified ear
H65.119 Acute and subacute allergic otitis media (mucoid) (sanguinous) (serous), unspecified ear
H65.191 Other acute nonsuppurative otitis media, right ear
H65.192 Other acute nonsuppurative otitis media, left ear
H65.193 Other acute nonsuppurative otitis media, bilateral
H65.194 Other acute nonsuppurative otitis media, recurrent, right ear
H65.195 Other acute nonsuppurative otitis media, recurrent, left ear
H65.196 Other acute nonsuppurative otitis media, recurrent, bilateral
H65.197 Other acute nonsuppurative otitis media, recurrent, unspecified ear
H65.199 Other acute nonsuppurative otitis media, unspecified ear
H65.20 Chronic serous otitis media, unspecified ear
H65.21 Chronic serous otitis media, right ear
H65.22 Chronic serous otitis media, left ear
H65.23 Chronic serous otitis media, bilateral
H65.30 Chronic mucoid otitis media, unspecified ear
H65.31 Chronic mucoid otitis media, right ear
H65.32 Chronic mucoid otitis media, left ear
H65.33 Chronic mucoid otitis media, bilateral
H65.411 Chronic allergic otitis media, right ear
H65.412 Chronic allergic otitis media, left ear
H65.413 Chronic allergic otitis media, bilateral
H65.419 Chronic allergic otitis media, unspecified ear
H65.491 Other chronic nonsuppurative otitis media, right ear
H65.492 Other chronic nonsuppurative otitis media, left ear
H65.493 Other chronic nonsuppurative otitis media, bilateral
H65.499 Other chronic nonsuppurative otitis media, unspecified ear
H65.90 Unspecified nonsuppurative otitis media, unspecified ear
H65.91 Unspecified nonsuppurative otitis media, right ear
H65.92 Unspecified nonsuppurative otitis media, left ear
H65.93 Unspecified nonsuppurative otitis media, bilateral
H66.001 Acute suppurative otitis media without spontaneous rupture of ear drum, right ear
H66.002 Acute suppurative otitis media without spontaneous rupture of ear drum, left ear
H66.003 Acute suppurative otitis media without spontaneous rupture of ear drum, bilateral
H66.004 Acute suppurative otitis media without spontaneous rupture of ear drum, recurrent, right ear
H66.005 Acute suppurative otitis media without spontaneous rupture of ear drum, recurrent, left ear
H66.006 Acute suppurative otitis media without spontaneous rupture of ear drum, recurrent, bilateral
H66.007 Acute suppurative otitis media without spontaneous rupture of ear drum, recurrent, unspecified ear
H66.009 Acute suppurative otitis media without spontaneous rupture of ear drum, unspecified ear
H66.011 Acute suppurative otitis media with spontaneous rupture of ear drum, right ear
H66.012 Acute suppurative otitis media with spontaneous rupture of ear drum, left ear
H66.013 Acute suppurative otitis media with spontaneous rupture of ear drum, bilateral

H66.014 Acute suppurative otitis media with spontaneous rupture of ear drum, recurrent, right ear
H66.015 Acute suppurative otitis media with spontaneous rupture of ear drum, recurrent, left ear
H66.016 Acute suppurative otitis media with spontaneous rupture of ear drum, recurrent, bilateral
H66.017 Acute suppurative otitis media with spontaneous rupture of ear drum, recurrent, unspecified ear
H66.019 Acute suppurative otitis media with spontaneous rupture of ear drum, unspecified ear
H66.10 Chronic tubotympanic suppurative otitis media, unspecified
H66.11 Chronic tubotympanic suppurative otitis media, right ear
H66.12 Chronic tubotympanic suppurative otitis media, left ear
H66.13 Chronic tubotympanic suppurative otitis media, bilateral
H66.20 Chronic atticoantral suppurative otitis media, unspecified
H66.21 Chronic atticoantral suppurative otitis media, right ear
H66.22 Chronic atticoantral suppurative otitis media, left ear
H66.23 Chronic atticoantral suppurative otitis media, bilateral
H66.3X1 Other chronic suppurative otitis media, right ear
H66.3X2 Other chronic suppurative otitis media, left ear
H66.3X3 Other chronic suppurative otitis media, bilateral
H66.3X9 Other chronic suppurative otitis media, unspecified ear
H66.40 Suppurative otitis media, unspecified, unspecified ear
H66.41 Suppurative otitis media, unspecified, right ear
H66.42 Suppurative otitis media, unspecified, left ear
H66.43 Suppurative otitis media, unspecified, bilateral
H66.91 Unspecified otitis media, right ear
H66.92 Unspecified otitis media, left ear
H66.93 Unspecified otitis media, bilateral

ICD-9 474.01
ICD-10 J35.02 Chronic adenoiditis

ICD-9 381.20
ICD-10 H65.30 Chronic mucoid otitis media, unspecified ear
H65.31 Chronic mucoid otitis media, right ear
H65.32 Chronic mucoid otitis media, left ear
H65.33 Chronic mucoid otitis media, bilateral

ICD-9 473.9
ICD-10 J32.9 Chronic sinusitis, unspecified
* Use additional code to identify:
Exposure to environmental tobacco smoke (Z77.22)
Exposure to tobacco smoke in the perinatal period (P96.81)
History of tobacco use (Z87.891)
Occupational exposure to environmental tobacco smoke (Z57.31)
Tobacco dependence (F17-)
Tobacco use (Z72.0)
** There are more specific code choice selections available in ICD-10-CM. These include:
J32.0 Chronic maxillary sinusitis
J32.1 Chronic frontal sinusitis
J32.2 Chronic ethmoidal sinusitis
J32.3 Chronic sphenoidal sinusitis
J32.4 Chronic pansinusitis
J32.8 Other chronic sinusitis

Pediatrics

ICD-9 V20.2
ICD-10 Z00.121 Encounter for routine child health examination with abnormal findings
** Use additional code to identify abnormal findings
Z00.129 Encounter for routine child health examination without abnormal findings

ICD-9 V72.19
ICD-10 Z01.10 Encounter for examination of ears and hearing without abnormal findings
Z01.110 Encounter for hearing examination following failed hearing screening
Z01.118 Encounter for examination of ears and hearing with other abnormal findings
** Use additional code to identify abnormal findings

ICD-9 V72.0
ICD-10 Z01.00 Encounter for examination of eyes and vision without abnormal findings
Z01.01 Encounter for examination of eyes and vision with abnormal findings
** Use additional code to identify abnormal findings

ICD-9 493.00
ICD-10 J45.901 Unspecified asthma with (acute) exacerbation
J45.902 Unspecified asthma with status asthmaticus
J45.909 Unspecified asthma, uncomplicated

ICD-9 465.9
ICD-10 J06.9 Acute upper respiratory infection, unspecified
J39.8 Other specified diseases of upper respiratory tract
ICD-9 382.9
ICD-10 H66.90 Otitis media, unspecified, unspecified ear
** There are more specific code choice selections available in ICD-10-CM. These include:

H66.91 Otitis media, unspecified, right ear
H66.92 Otitis media, unspecified, let ear
H66.93 Otitis media, unspecified, bilateral
There are more specific codes available for otis media. These include:

H65.00 Acute serous otitis media, unspecified ear
H65.01 Acute serous otitis media, right ear
H65.02 Acute serous otitis media, left ear
H65.03 Acute serous otitis media, bilateral
H65.04 Acute serous otitis media, recurrent, right ear
H65.05 Acute serous otitis media, recurrent, left ear
H65.06 Acute serous otitis media, recurrent, bilateral
H65.07 Acute serous otitis media, recurrent, unspecified ear
H65.111 Acute and subacute allergic otitis media (mucoid) (sanguinous) (serous), right ear
H65.112 Acute and subacute allergic otitis media (mucoid) (sanguinous) (serous), left ear
H65.113 Acute and subacute allergic otitis media (mucoid) (sanguinous) (serous), bilateral
H65.114 Acute and subacute allergic otitis media (mucoid) (sanguinous) (serous), recurrent, right ear
H65.115 Acute and subacute allergic otitis media (mucoid) (sanguinous) (serous), recurrent, left ear
H65.116 Acute and subacute allergic otitis media (mucoid) (sanguinous) (serous), recurrent, bilateral
H65.117 Acute and subacute allergic otitis media (mucoid) (sanguinous) (serous), recurrent, unspecified ear
H65.119 Acute and subacute allergic otitis media (mucoid) (sanguinous) (serous), unspecified ear
H65.191 Other acute nonsuppurative otitis media, right ear
H65.192 Other acute nonsuppurative otitis media, left ear
H65.193 Other acute nonsuppurative otitis media, bilateral
H65.194 Other acute nonsuppurative otitis media, recurrent, right ear
H65.195 Other acute nonsuppurative otitis media, recurrent, left ear
H65.196 Other acute nonsuppurative otitis media, recurrent, bilateral
H65.197 Other acute nonsuppurative otitis media, recurrent, unspecified ear
H65.199 Other acute nonsuppurative otitis media, unspecified ear
H65.20 Chronic serous otitis media, unspecified ear
H65.21 Chronic serous otitis media, right ear
H65.22 Chronic serous otitis media, left ear
H65.23 Chronic serous otitis media, bilateral
H65.30 Chronic mucoid otitis media, unspecified ear
H65.31 Chronic mucoid otitis media, right ear
H65.32 Chronic mucoid otitis media, left ear
H65.33 Chronic mucoid otitis media, bilateral
H65.411 Chronic allergic otitis media, right ear
H65.412 Chronic allergic otitis media, left ear
H65.413 Chronic allergic otitis media, bilateral
H65.419 Chronic allergic otitis media, unspecified ear
H65.491 Other chronic nonsuppurative otitis media, right ear
H65.492 Other chronic nonsuppurative otitis media, left ear
H65.493 Other chronic nonsuppurative otitis media, bilateral
H65.499 Other chronic nonsuppurative otitis media, unspecified ear
H65.90 Unspecified nonsuppurative otitis media, unspecified ear
H65.91 Unspecified nonsuppurative otitis media, right ear
H65.92 Unspecified nonsuppurative otitis media, left ear
H65.93 Unspecified nonsuppurative otitis media, bilateral
H66.001 Acute suppurative otitis media without spontaneous rupture of ear drum, right ear
H66.002 Acute suppurative otitis media without spontaneous rupture of ear drum, left ear
H66.003 Acute suppurative otitis media without spontaneous rupture of ear drum, bilateral
H66.004 Acute suppurative otitis media without spontaneous rupture of ear drum, recurrent, right ear
H66.005 Acute suppurative otitis media without spontaneous rupture of ear drum, recurrent, left ear
H66.006 Acute suppurative otitis media without spontaneous rupture of ear drum, recurrent, bilateral

H66.007 Acute suppurative otitis media without spontaneous rupture of ear drum, recurrent, unspecified ear
H66.009 Acute suppurative otitis media without spontaneous rupture of ear drum, unspecified ear
H66.011 Acute suppurative otitis media with spontaneous rupture of ear drum, right ear
H66.012 Acute suppurative otitis media with spontaneous rupture of ear drum, left ear
H66.013 Acute suppurative otitis media with spontaneous rupture of ear drum, bilateral
H66.014 Acute suppurative otitis media with spontaneous rupture of ear drum, recurrent, right ear
H66.015 Acute suppurative otitis media with spontaneous rupture of ear drum, recurrent, left ear
H66.016 Acute suppurative otitis media with spontaneous rupture of ear drum, recurrent, bilateral
H66.017 Acute suppurative otitis media with spontaneous rupture of ear drum, recurrent, unspecified ear
H66.019 Acute suppurative otitis media with spontaneous rupture of ear drum, unspecified ear
H66.10 Chronic tubotympanic suppurative otitis media, unspecified
H66.11 Chronic tubotympanic suppurative otitis media, right ear
H66.12 Chronic tubotympanic suppurative otitis media, left ear
H66.13 Chronic tubotympanic suppurative otitis media, bilateral
H66.20 Chronic atticoantral suppurative otitis media, unspecified ear
H66.21 Chronic atticoantral suppurative otitis media, right ear
H66.22 Chronic atticoantral suppurative otitis media, left ear
H66.23 Chronic atticoantral suppurative otitis media, bilateral
H66.3X1 Other chronic suppurative otitis media, right ear
H66.3X2 Other chronic suppurative otitis media, left ear
H66.3X3 Other chronic suppurative otitis media, bilateral
H66.3X9 Other chronic suppurative otitis media, unspecified ear
H66.40 Suppurative otitis media, unspecified, unspecified ear
H66.41 Suppurative otitis media, unspecified, right ear
H66.42 Suppurative otitis media, unspecified, left ear
H66.43 Suppurative otitis media, unspecified, bilateral
H67.1 Otitis media in diseases classified elsewhere, right ear
H67.2 Otitis media in diseases classified elsewhere, left ear
H67.3 Otitis media in diseases classified elsewhere, bilateral
H67.9 Otitis media in diseases classified elsewhere, unspecified ear

ICD-9 785.2
ICD-10 R01.1 Cardiac murmur, unspecified
ICD-9 462
ICD-10 J02.8 Acute pharyngitis due to other specified organisms
** Use additional code (B95-B97) to identify infectious agent
J02.0 Streptococcal pharyngitis
J02.9 Acute pharyngitis, unspecified
ICD-9 277.00
ICD-10 E84.9 Cystic fibrosis, unspecified
** There are more specific code choice selections available in ICD-10-CM. These include:
E84.0 Cystic fibrosis with pulmonary manifestations
** Use additional code to identify any infectious organism present, such as: Pseudomonas (B96.5)
E84.11 Meconium ileus in cystic fibrosis
E84.19 Cystic fibrosis with other intestinal manifestations
E84.8 Cystic fibrosis with other manifestations
ICD-9 204.00
ICD-10 C91.90 Lymphoid leukemia, unspecified not having achieved remission
** There are more specific code choice selections available in ICD-10-CM. These include:
C91.00 Acute lymphoblastic leukemia not having achieved remission
C91.10 Chronic lymphocytic leukemia of B-cell type not having achieved remission
C91.30 Prolymphocytic leukemia of B-cell type not having achieved remission
C91.40 Hairy cell leukemia not having achieved remission
C91.50 Adult T-cell lymphoma/leukemia (HTLV-1-associated) not having achieved remission
C91.60 Prolymphocytic leukemia of T-cell type not having achieved remission
C91.A0 Mature B-cell leukemia Burkitt-type not having achieved remission
C91.Z0 Other lymphoid leukemia not having achieved remission
ICD-9 250.01
ICD-10 E10.9 Type 1 diabetes mellitus without complications
ICD-9 194.0
ICD-10 C74.90 Malignant neoplasm of unspecified part of unspecified adrenal gland
** There are more specific code choice selections available in ICD-10-CM. These include:

C74.00 Malignant neoplasm of cortex of unspecified adrenal gland
C74.01 Malignant neoplasm of cortex of right adrenal gland
C74.02 Malignant neoplasm of cortex of left adrenal gland
C74.10 Malignant neoplasm of medulla of unspecified adrenal gland
C74.11 Malignant neoplasm of medulla of right adrenal gland
C74.12 Malignant neoplasm of medulla of left adrenal gland
C74.91 Malignant neoplasm of unspecified part of right adrenal gland
C74.92 Malignant neoplasm of unspecified part of left adrenal gland
ICD-9 V74.1
ICD-10 Z11.1 Encounter for screening for respiratory tuberculosis
ICD-9 786.2
ICD-10 R05 Cough
ICD-9 V01.1
ICD-10 Z20.1 Contact with and (suspected) exposure to tuberculosis
ICD-9 779.5
ICD-10 P96.1 Neonatal withdrawal symptoms from maternal use of drugs of addiction
P96.2 Withdrawal symptoms from therapeutic use of drugs in newborn
ICD-9 250.03
ICD-10 E10.65 Type 1 diabetes mellitus with hyperglycemia
ICD-9 530.81
ICD-10 K21.9 Gastro-esophageal reflux without esophagitis
K21.0 Gastro-esophageal reflux with esophagitis
ICD-9 564.00 *
ICD-10 K59.00 Constipation, unspecified
** There are more specific code choice selections available in ICD-10-CM. These includ
K59.01 Slow transit constipation
K59.02 Outlet dysfunction constipation
K59.09 Other constipation
ICD-9 493.90
ICD-10 J45.909 Unspecified asthma, uncomplicated
** There are more specific code choice selections available in ICD-10-CM. These includ
J45.20 Mild intermittent asthma, uncomplicated
J45.21 Mild intermittent asthma with (acute) exacerbation
J45.22 Mild intermittent asthma with status asthmaticus
J45.30 Mild persistent asthma, uncomplicated
J45.31 Mild persistent asthma with (acute) exacerbation
J45.32 Mild persistent asthma with status asthmaticus
J45.40 Moderate persistent asthma, uncomplicated
J45.41 Moderate persistent asthma with (acute) exacerbation
J45.42 Moderate persistent asthma with status asthmaticus
J45.50 Severe persistent asthma, uncomplicated
J45.51 Severe persistent asthma with (acute) exacerbation
J45.52 Severe persistent asthma with status asthmaticus
J45.901 Unspecified asthma with (acute) exacerbation
J45.902 Unspecified asthma with status asthmaticus
J45.990 Exercise induced bronchospasm
J45.991 Cough variant asthma
J45.998 Other asthma

ICD-9 745.4
ICD-10 Q21.0 Ventricular septal defect
ICD-9 745.5
ICD-10 Q21.1 Atrial septal defect
ICD-9 034.0
ICD-10 J02.0 Streptococcal pharyngitis
ICD-9 789.00
ICD-10 R10.9 Unspecified abdominal pain
** There are more specific code choice selections available for use. These include:
R10.0 Acute abdomen
R10.10 Upper abdominal pain, unspecified
R10.11 Right upper quadrant pain
R10.12 Left upper quadrant pain
R10.13 Epigastric pain
R10.2 Pelvic and perineal pain
R10.30 Lower abdominal pain, unspecified
R10.31 Right lower quadrant pain
R10.32 Left lower quadrant pain
R10.33 Periumbilical pain
R10.84 Generalized abdominal pain
ICD-9 555.2
ICD-10 K50.80 Crohn's disease of both small and large intestine withou complication
** There are more specific code choice selections available in ICD-10-CM. These includ
K50.811 Crohn's disease of both small and large intestine with rectal bleeding
K50.812 Crohn's disease of both small and large intestine with intestinal obstruction

K50.813 Crohn's disease of both small and large intestine with fistula

K50.814 Crohn's disease of both small and large intestine with abscess

K50.818 Crohn's disease of both small and large intestine with other complication

K50.819 Crohn's disease of both small and large intestine with unspecified complications

Use additional code to identify manifestations, such as: psyoderma gangrenosum (88)

D-9 079.99

ICD-10 B34.9 Viral infection, unspecified

D-9 314.01

ICD-10 F90.0 Attention-deficit hyperactivity disorder, predominantly inattentive type

F90.1 Attention-deficit hyperactivity disorder, predominantly hyperactive type

F90.2 Attention-deficit hyperactivity disorder, combined type

F90.8 Attention-deficit hyperactivity disorder, other type

F90.9 Attention-deficit hyperactivity disorder, unspecified type

D-9 V65.49

ICD-10 Z71.89 Other specified counseling

D-9 V70.0

ICD-10 Z00.00 Encounter for general adult medical examination without abnormal findings

Z00.01 Encounter for general adult medical examination with abnormal findings

Use additional code to identify abnormal findings

D-9 789.07

ICD-10 R10.84 Generalized abdominal pain

D-9 427.89

ICD-10 I49.8 Other specified cardiac arrhythmias

D-9 486

ICD-10 J18.9 Pneumonia, unspecified organism

Code first associated influenza, if applicable (J09.X1, J10.0-,-J11.0-)

D-9 780.60

ICD-10 R50.9 Fever, unspecified

There are more specific code choice selections available in ICD-10-CM. These include:

R50.2 Drug induced fever

R50.81 Fever presenting with conditions classified elsewhere

R50.82 Postprocedural fever

R50.83 Postvaccination fever

R50.84 Febrile nonhemolytic transfusion reaction

D-9 786.50

ICD-10 R07.9 Chest pain, unspecified

There are more specific code choice selections available in ICD-10-CM. These include:

R07.1 Chest pain on breathing

R07.81 Pleurodynia

R07.89 Other chest pain

D-9 714.30

ICD-10 M08.3 Juvenile rheumatoid polyarthritis (seronegative)

M08.00 Unspecified juvenile rheumatoid arthritis of unspecified site

Code also any associated underlying condition, such as: Regional enteritis (Crohn's ease) (K50-), Ulcerative colitis (K51-)

D-9 427.9

ICD-10 I49.9 Cardiac arrhythmia, unspecified

Code first cardiac arrhythmia complicating:
ortion or ectopic or molar pregnancy (000-007, 008.8)
stetric surgery and procedures (075.4)

There are more specific code choice selections available in ICD-10-CM. These include:

I47.0 Re-entry ventricular arrhythmia

I47.1 Supraventricular tachycardia

I47.2 Ventricular tachycardia

I47.9 Paroxysmal tachycardia, unspecified

For I47.0 – I47.9 Code first cardiac arrhythmia complicating:
ortion or ectopic or molar pregnancy (000-007, 008.8)
stetric surgery and procedures (075.4)

I48.0 Paroxysmal atrial fibrillation

I48.1 Persistent atrial fibrillation

I48.2 Chronic atrial fibrillation

I48.91 Unspecified atrial fibrillation

I49.01 Ventricular fibrillation

I49.02 Ventricular flutter

I49.1 Atrial premature depolarization

I49.2 Junctional premature depolarization

I49.3 Ventricular premature depolarization

I49.40 Unspecified premature depolarization

I49.49 Other premature depolarization

I49.5 Sick sinus syndrome

I49.8 Other specified cardiac arrhythmias

For I49.0-I49.9 Code first cardiac arrhythmia complicating:
ortion or ectopic or molar pregnancy (000-007, 008.8)
stetric surgery and procedures (075.4)

ICD-9 692.9

ICD-10 L25.9 Unspecified contact dermatitis, unspecified nature

** Code first (T36-T65) to identify drug or substance

L30.9 Dermatitis, unspecified

** There are more specific unspecified codes in ICD-10-CM. These include:

L25.0 Unspecified contact dermatitis due to cosmetics

L25.1 Unspecified contact dermatitis due to drugs in contact with skin

L25.2 Unspecified contact dermatitis due to dyes

L25.3 Unspecified contact dermatitis due to other chemical products

L25.4 Unspecified contact dermatitis due to food in contact with skin

L25.5 Unspecified contact dermatitis due to plants, except food

L25.8 Unspecified contact dermatitis due to other agents

** Use additional code for adverse effect, if applicable, to identify drug (T36-T50 with fifth or sixth character 5)

ICD-9 388.70

ICD-10 H92.09 Otalgia, unspecified ear

** There are more specific code choice selections available in ICD-10-CM. These include:

H92.01 Otalgia, right ear

H92.02 Otalgia, left ear

H92.03 Otalgia, bilateral

ICD-9 V04.81

ICD-10 Z23 Encounter for immunization

** Code first any routine childhood examination

** Note: Procedure codes are required to identify the types of immunizations given. In ICD-10-CM there is only one diagnostic code available for immunizations

ICD-9 783.43

ICD-10 E34.3 Short stature due to endocrine disorder

R62.52 Short stature (child)

ICD-9 204.01

ICD-10 C91.01 Acute lymphoblastic leukemia, in remission

ICD-9 277.02

ICD-10 E84.0 Cystic fibrosis with pulmonary manifestations

**Use additional code to identify any infectious organism present, such as: Pseudomonas (B96.5)

ICD-9 461.9

ICD-10 J01.90 Acute sinusitis, unspecified

** There are more specific code choice selections available in ICD-10-CM. These include:

J01.00 Acute maxillary sinusitis, unspecified

J01.01 Acute recurrent maxillary sinusitis

J01.10 Acute frontal sinusitis, unspecfied

J01.11 Acute recurrent frontal sinusitis

J01.20 Acute ethmoidal sinusitis, unspecified

J01.21 Acute recurrent ethmoidal sinusitis

J01.30 Acute sphenoidal sinusitis

J01.31 Acute recurrent sphenoidal sinusitis

J01.40 Acute pansinusitits, unspecified

J01.41 Acute recurrent pansinusitis

J01.80 Other acute sinusitis

J01.81 Other acute recurrent sinusitis, unspecified

J01.91 Acute recurrent sinusitis, unspecified

ICD-9 780.2

ICD-10 R55 Syncope and collapse

ICD-9 795.5

ICD-10 R76.1 Abnormal reaction to tuberculin test

R76.11 Nonspecific reaction to tuberculin skin test without active tuberculosis

R76.12 Nonspecific reaction to cell mediated immunity measurement of gamma interferon antigen response without active tuberculosis

ICD-9 787.91

ICD-10 R19.7 Diarrhea, unspecified

K59.1 Functional diarrhea

**There are many combination codes in ICD-10-CM that include diarrhea as a manifestation

ICD-9 493.92

ICD-10 J45.901 Unspecified asthma with (acute) exacerbation

** There are more specific code choice selections available in ICD-10-CM. These include:

J45.21 Mild intermittent asthma with (acute) exacerbation

J45.31 Mild persistent asthma with (acute) exacerbation

J45.41 Moderate persistent asthma with (acute) excerbatoin

J45.51 Severe persistent asthma with (acute) exacerbation

ICD-9 Multiple

ICD-10 Z23 Encounter for immunization

** Code first any routine childhood examination

** Note: Procedure codes are required to identify the types of immunizations given. In ICD-10-CM there is only one diagnostic code available for immunizations

---

Urology

ICD-9 185

ICD-10 C61 Malignant neoplasm of prostate

ICD-9 600.01

Two codes are required in ICD-10-CM:

ICD-10 N40.1 Enlarged prostate with lower urinary tract symptoms (LUTS); AND

N13.8 Other obstructive and reflux uropathy

** Note under N40.1 states – Use additional code for associated symptoms, when specified:
Incomplete bladder emptying (R39.14)
Nocturia (R35.1)
Straining on urination (R39.16)
Urinary frequency (R35.0)
Urinary hesitancy (R39.11)
Urinary incontinence (N39.4-)
Urinary obstruction (N13.8)
Urinary retention (R33.8)
Urinary urgency (R39.15)
Weak urinary stream (R39.12)

ICD-9 788.20

ICD-10 R33.9 Retention of urine, unspecified

** There are more specific code choice selections available in ICD-10-CM. These include:

R33.0 Drug induced retention of urine

** Use additional code for adverse effect, if applicable, to identify drug (T36-T50 with fifth or sixth character 5)

R33.8 Other retention of urine

** Code first, if applicable, any causal condition, such as: enlarged prostate (N40.1)

ICD-9 188.9

ICD-10 C67.9 Malignant neoplasm of bladder, unspecified

** There are more specific code choice selections available in ICD-10-CM. These include:

C67.0 Malignant neoplasm of trigone of bladder

C67.1 Malignant neoplasm of dome of bladder

C67.2 Malignant neoplasm of lateral wall of bladder

C67.3 Malignant neoplasm of anterior wall of bladder

C67.4 Malignant neoplasm of posterior wall of bladder

C67.5 Malignant neoplasm of bladder neck

C67.6 Malignant neoplasm of ureteric orifice

C67.7 Malignant neoplasm of urachus

C67.8 Malignant neoplasm of overlapping sites of bladder

ICD-9 607.84

ICD-10 N52.9 Male erectile dysfunction, unspecified

** There are more specific code choice selections available in ICD-10-CM. These include:

N52.01 Erectile dysfunction due to arterial insufficiency

N52.02 Corporo-venous occlusive erectile dysfunction

N52.03 Combined arterial insufficiency and corporo-venous occlusive erectile dysfunction

N52.1 Erectile dysfunction due to diseases classified elsewhere

** Code first underlying disease

N52.2 Drug-induced erectile dysfunction

N52.31 Erectile dysfunction following radical prostatectomy

N52.32 Erectile dysfunction following radical cystectomy

N52.33 Erectile dysfunction following urethral surgery

N52.34 Erectile dysfunction following simple prostatectomy

N52.39 Other post-surgical erectile dysfunction

N52.8 Other male erectile dysfunction

ICD-9 592.0

ICD-10 N20.0 Calculus of kidney

N20.9 Urinary calculus; unspecified

N20.2 Calculus of kidney and ureter

ICD-9 790.93

ICD-10 R97.2 Elevated prostate specific antigen (PSA)

ICD-9 788.21

ICD-10 N20.2 Calculus of kidney with calculus of ureter

ICD-9 788.31

ICD-10 N39.41 Urge incontinence

ICD-9 592.1

ICD-10 N20.1 Calculus of ureter

N20.2 Calculus of kidney with calculus of ureter

ICD-9 596.54

ICD-10 N31.9 Neuromuscular dysfunction of bladder, unspecified

** There are more specific code choice selections available in ICD-10-CM. These include:

N31.0 Uninhibited neuropathic bladder, not elsewhere classified

N31.1 Reflex neuropathic bladder, not elsewhere classified

N31.2 Flaccid neuropathic bladder, not elsewhere classified

N31.8 Other neuromuscular dysfunction of bladder

** Use additional code to identify any associated urinary incontinence (N39.3-N39.4-)

ICD-9 189.0

ICD-10 C64.1 Malignant neoplasm of right kidney, except renal pelvis

C64.2 Malignant neoplasm of left kidney, except renal pelvis

C64.9 Malignant neoplasm of unspecified kidney, except renal pelvis

ICD-9 788.41
ICD-10 R35.0 Frequency of micturition
** Code first, if applicable, any causal condition, such as enlarged prostate
ICD-9 599.0
ICD-10 N39.0 Urinary tract infection, site not specified
** Use additional code (B95-B97) to identify infectious agent
** There are more specific code choice selections available in ICD-10-CM. These include:
    N30.00 Acute cystitis without hematuria
    N30.01 Acute cystitis with hematuria
    N30.10 Interstitial cystitis (chronic) without hematuria
    N30.11 Interstitial cystitis (chronic) with hematuria
    N30.20 Other chronic cystitis without hematuria
    N30.21 Other chronic cystitis with hematuria
    N30.30 Trigonitis without hematuria
    N30.31 Trigonitis with hematuria
    N30.40 Irradiation cystitis without hematuria
    N30.41 Irradiation cystitis with hematuria
    N30.80 Other cystitis without hematuria
    N30.81 Other cystitis with hematuria
    N30.90 Cystitis, unspecified without hematuria
    N30.91 Cystitis, unspecified with hematuria
    N15.9 Renal tubule-interstitial disease, unspecified
    N34.1 Nonspecific urethritis
    N34.2 Other urethritis
ICD-9 625.6
ICD-10 N39.3 Stress incontinence (female) (male)
** Code also any associated overactive bladder (N32.81).
ICD-9 599.71
ICD-10 R31.0 Gross hematuria
    R31.1 Benign essential microscopic hematuria
    R31.2 Other microscopic hematuria
    R31.9 Unspecified hematuria
ICD-9 788.32
ICD-10 N39.3 Stress incontinence (female) (male)
** Code also any associated overactive bladder (N32.81).
ICD-9 239.5
ICD-10 D49.5 Neoplasm of unspecified behavior of other genitourinary organs
ICD-9 598.9
ICD-10 N35.9 Urethral stricture, unspecified
** There are more specific code choice selections available in ICD-10-CM. These include:
    N35.010 Post-traumatic urethral stricture, male, meatal
    N35.011 Post-traumatic bulbous urethral stricture
    N35.012 Post-traumatic membranous urethral stricture
    N35.013 Post-traumatic anterior urethral stricture
    N35.014 Post-traumatic urethral stricture, male, unspecified
    N35.021 Urethral stricture due to childbirth
    N35.028 Other post-traumatic urethral stricture, female
    N35.111 Postinfective urethral stricture, not elsewhere classified, male, meatal
    N35.112 Postinfective bulbous urethral stricture, not elsewhere classified
    N35.113 Postinfective membranous urethral stricture, not elsewhere classified
    N35.114 Postinfective anterior urethral stricture, not elsewhere classified
    N35.119 Postinfective urethral stricture, not elsewhere classified, male, unspecified
    N35.12 Postinfective urethral stricture, not elsewhere classified, female
    N35.8 Other urethral stricture, unspecified
ICD-9 605
ICD-10 N47.0 Adherent prepuce, newborn
    N47.1 Phimosis
    N47.2 Paraphimosis
    N47.8 Other disorders of prepuce
ICD-9 591
ICD-10 N13.30 Unspecified hydronephrosis
** There are more specific code choice selections available in ICD-10-CM. These include:
    N13.1 Hydronephrosis with ureteral stricture, not elsewhere classified
    N13.2 Hydronephrosis with renal and ureteral calculus obstruction
    N13.39 Other hydronephrosis
ICD-9 603.9
ICD-10 N43.3 Hydrocele, unspecified
** There are more specific code choice selections available in ICD-10-CM. These include:
    N43.0 Encysted hydrocele
    N43.1 Infected hydrocele
** Use additional code (B95-B97) to identify infectious agent
    N43.2 Other hydrocele

ICD-9 239.4
ICD-10 D49.4 Neoplasm of unspecified behavior of bladder
ICD-9 788.43
ICD-10 R35.1 Nocturia
ICD-9 257.2
ICD-10 E29.1 Testicular hypofunction
** Use additional code for adverse effect, if applicable, to identify drug (T36-T50 with fifth or sixth character 5)
ICD-9 600.91
Two codes are required in ICD-10-CM:
ICD-10 N40.1 Enlarged prostate with lower urinary tract symptoms (LUTS); AND
       N13.8 Other obstructive and reflux uropathy ***
** Note under N40.1 states – Use additional code for associated symptoms, when specified:
Incomplete bladder emptying (R39.14)
Nocturia (R35.1)
Straining on urination (R39.16)
Urinary frequency (R35.0)
Urinary hesitancy (R39.11)
Urinary incontinence (N39.4-)
Urinary obstruction (N13.8)
Urinary retention (R33.8)
Urinary urgency (R39.15)
Weak urinary stream (R39.12)
ICD-9 594.1
ICD-10 N21.0 Calculus in bladder
ICD-9 595.2
ICD-10 N30.20 Other chronic cystitis without hematuria
    N30.21 Other chronic cystitis with hematuria
** Use additional code to identify infectious agent (B95-B97).
ICD-9 601.1
ICD-10 N41.1 Chronic prostatitis
ICD-9 600.00
ICD-10 N40.0 Enlarged prostate without lower urinary tract symptoms (LUTS)
ICD-9 752.51
ICD-10 Q53.10 Unspecified undescended testicle, unilateral
    Q53.11 Abdominal testicle, unilateral
    Q53.12 Ectopic perineal testis, unilateral
    Q53.20 Undescended testicle, unspecified, bilateral
    Q53.21 Abdominal testis, bilateral
    Q53.22 Ectopic perineal testis, bilateral
    Q53.9 Hypospadias, unspecified
ICD-9 788.30
ICD-10 R32 Unspecified urinary incontinence
    R39.81 Functional urinary incontinence
    F98.0 Non-organic origin
** There are more specific code choice selections available in ICD-10-CM. These include:
    N39.3 Stress incontinence (female) (male)
** Code also associated overactive bladder (N32.81)
    N39.41 Urge incontinence
    N39.42 Incontinence without sensory awareness
    N39.43 Post-void dribbling
    N39.44 Nocturnal enuresis
    N39.45 Continuous leakage
    N39.46 Mixed incontinence
    N39.490 Overflow incontinence
    N39.498 Other specified urinary incontinence
ICD-9 595.1
ICD-10 N30.10 Interstitial cystitis (chronic) without hematuria **
    N30.11 Interstitial cystitis (chronic) with hematuria **
** Use additional code to identify infectious agent (B95-B97).
ICD-9 593.4
ICD-10 N13.8 Other obstructive and reflux uropathy
** Code first, if applicable, any causal condition, such as: enlarged prostate (N40.1).
ICD-9 585.9
ICD-10 N18.9 Chronic kidney disease, unspecified
** Code first any associated:
Diabetic chronic kidney disease (E08.22, E09.22, E10.22, E11.22, E13.22)
Hypertensive chronic kidney disease (I12-, I13-)
Use additional code to identify kidney transplant status, if applicable (Z94.0)
** There are more specific code choice selections available in ICD-10-CM. These include:
    N18.1 Chronic kidney disease, stage 1
    N18.2 Chronic kidney disease, stage 2 (mild)
    N18.3 Chronic kidney disease, stage 3 (moderate)
    N18.4 Chronic kidney disease, stage 4 (severe)
    N18.5 Chronic kidney disease, stage 5
    N18.6 End stage renal disease
** Use additional code to identify dialysis status (Z99.2)
ICD-9 788.63
ICD-10 R39.15 Urgency of urination
** Code first, if applicable, any causal condition, such as enlarged prostate (N40.1).
ICD-9 788.1
ICD-10 R30.0 Dysuria

ICD-9 599.70
ICD-10 R31.9 Hematuria, unspecified
** There are more specific code choice selections available in ICD-10-CM. These includ[e]
    R31.0 Gross hematuria
    R31.1 Benign essential microscopic hematuria
    R31.2 Other microscopic hematuria
    N02.0 Recurrent and persistent hematuria with minor glomerular abnormality
    N02.1 Recurrent and persistent hematuria with focal and segmental glomerular lesions
    N02.2 Recurrent and persistent hematuria with diffuse membranous glomerulonephritis
    N02.3 Recurrent and persistent hematuria with diffuse mesangial proliferative glomerulonephritis
    N02.4 Recurrent and persistent hematuria with diffuse endocapillary proliferative glomerulonephritis
    N02.5 Recurrent and persistent hematuria with diffuse mesangiocapillary glomerulonephritis
    N02.6 Recurrent and persistent hematuria with dense deposit disease
    N02.7 Recurrent and persistent hematuria with diffuse crescentic glomerulonephritis
    N02.8 Recurrent and persistent hematuria with other morphologic changes
    N02.9 Recurrent and persistent hematuria with unspecified morphologic changes
ICD-9 593.2
ICD-10 N28.1 Cyst of kidney, acquired
ICD-9 599.72
ICD-10 R31.1 Benign essential microscopic hematuria
    R31.2 Other microscopic hematuria
ICD-9 607.1
ICD-10 N47.6 Balanoposthitis
    N48.1 Balanitis
** Use additional code (B95-B97) to identify infectious agent.
ICD-9 789.0
ICD-10 R10.9 Unspecified abdominal pain
** There are more specific code choice selections available in ICD-10-CM. These includ[e]
    R10.0 Acute abdomen
    R10.10 Upper abdominal pain, unspecified
    R10.11 Right upper quadrant pain
    R10.12 Left upper quadrant pain
    R10.13 Epigastric pain
    R10.2 Pelvic and perineal pain
    R10.30 Lower abdominal pain, unspecified
    R10.31 Right lower quadrant pain
    R10.32 Left lower quadrant pain
    R10.33 Periumbilical pain
    R10.84 Generalized abdominal pain
ICD-9 752.61
ICD-10 Q54.9 Hypospadias, unspecified
** There are more specific code choice selections available in ICD-10-CM. These includ[e]
    Q54.0 Hypospadias, balanic
    Q54.1 Hypospadias, penile
    Q54.2 Hypospadias, penoscrotal
    Q54.3 Hypospadias, perineal
    Q54.8 Other hypospadias
ICD-9 596.9
ICD-10 N32.9 Bladder disorder, unspecified
** There are more specific code choice selections available in ICD-10-CM. These includ[e]
    N32.0 Bladder neck obstruction
    N32.3 Diverticulum of bladder
ICD-9 788.36
ICD-10 N39.44 Nocturnal enuresis
ICD-9 600.10
ICD-10 N40.0 Enlarged prostate without lower urinary tract symptom[s] (LUTS)
ICD-9 608.9
ICD-10 N50.9 Disorder of male genital organs, unspecified
ICD-9 604.90
ICD-10 N45.1 Epididymitis
    N45.2 Orchitis
    N45.3 Epididymo-orchitis
** Use additional code (B95-B97) to identify infectious agent
ICD-9 608.1
ICD-10 N43.40 Spermatocele of epididymis, unspecified
    N43.41 Spermatocele of epididymis, single
    N43.42 Spermatocele of epididymis, multiple
ICD-9 607.85
ICD-10 N48.6 Peyronie's disease

ICD-9 598.2

ICD-10 **N99.110** Postprocedural urethral stricture, male, meatal
N99.111 Postprocedural bulbous urethral stricture
N99.112 Postprocedural membranous urethral stricture
N99.113 Postprocedural anterior urethral stricture
N99.114 Postprocedural urethral stricture, male, unspecified
N99.12 Postprocedural urethral stricture, female

7th character extenders	
A	**initial encounter**
D	**subsequent**
S	**sequela**

7th character extenders for the Orthopedic catagories	
A	initial encounter for closed fracture
B	initial encounter for open fracture type I, or II initial encounter for open fracture NOS
C	initial encounter for open fracture type IIIA, IIB, or IIIC
D	subsequent encounter for closed fracture with routine healing
E	subsequent encounter for open fracture of type I or II with routine healing
F	subsequent encounter for open fracture type IIIA, IIIB, or IIIC with routine healing
G	subsequent encounter for closed fracture with delayed healing
H	subsequent encounter for open fracture type I or II with delayed healing
J	subsequent encounter for open fracture type IIIA, IIIB, or IIIC with delayed healing
K	subsequent encounter for closed fracture with nonunion
M	subsequent encounter for open fracture type I or II with nonunion
N	subsequent encounter for open fracture type IIIA, IIIB, or IIIC with nonunion
P	subsequent encounter for closed fracture with malunion
Q	subsequent encounter for open fracture type I or II with malunion
R	subsequent encounter for open fracture type IIIA, IIIB, or IIIC with malunion
S	sequela

Test Yourself: ICD-10-CM Challenge

The quiz below features questions related to ICD-10-CM, the diagnosis code set expected to replace ICD-9-CM in the near future. Use the quiz to test your familiarity with unique structural features of ICD-10-CM, transition tools, official guidelines, and proper coding for top diagnoses in several different specialties.

Directions: Answer the following questions using the 2015 ICD-10-CM code set, the 2015 General Equivalence Mappings, and the 2014 ICD-10-CM Official Guidelines for Coding and Reporting. Then flip to Test Yourself: ICD-10-CM Challenge (Answers) to check your responses.

Questions

1. **Which of the following is/are true for the use of "X" in an ICD-10-CM code?**

    A. The "X" serves as a placeholder for future expansion.
    B. The "X" serves as a placeholder to allow a code to meet the requirement of coding to the highest level of specificity when a code has fewer than six characters and requires a seventh character extension.
    C. Both A and B are correct.
    D. The "X" is a signal that the code is incomplete.

2. **The General Equivalence Mappings (GEMs) show ICD-9-CM code 649.53 (*Spotting complicating pregnancy, antepartum condition or complication*) does not have a specific one-to-one correlation to an ICD-10-CM code. Why?**

    A. You have to know the trimester to choose the proper ICD-10-CM code.
    B. Complication codes always translate into combination codes in ICD-10-CM.
    C. You won't find any complication codes in ICD-10-CM.
    D. None of the above apply.

3. **ICD-10-CM guidelines state, "An _____ note indicates that the code excluded should never be used at the same time as the code above the _____ note." Which term applies to both blanks?**

    A. Excludes
    B. Excludes1
    C. Excludes2
    D. Includes

4. **The physician documents mitral valve regurgitation, caused by a prior heart attack. The patient has no history of rheumatic fever. The most appropriate code to describe the valve disorder is:**

    A. Q23.3
    B. I05.1
    C. I34.1
    D. I34.0

5. **A patient presents to the emergency department via ambulance from a motorcycle accident. The exam reveals a few lacerations on the patient's scalp. Additionally, the patient experiences neck pain and has restricted neck movement. The physician documents "facial trauma." What is the ICD-10-CM code equivalent of 959.09 that pertains to injury of the face?**

    A. S09.93XA
    B. S19.9XXA
    C. S19.93XX
    D. S19.93XA

6. **Under ICD-10-CM, how do you report an adult checkup encounter when the provider documents abnormal findings?**

    A. Z00.00
    B. Z00.01
    C. Z00.121
    D. Z00.129

7. **What is the best possible choice of code(s) for the condition "lesion of plantar nerve, right and left lower limb"?**

    A. G57.61, G57.62
    B. G57.41, G57.42
    C. G57.31, G57.32
    D. G57.20

8. **A 35-year-old woman presents for an annual exam. She has not had a Pap smear in four years, and Pap results return ASC-US. The physician asks her to come back in three months for a repeat Pap to follow any abnormal cell progress. When the patient returns, you should support the appropriate E/M office visit with what code in ICD-10-CM?**

    A. R87.613
    B. R87.612
    C. R87.611
    D. R87.610

9. **In the eye clinic, an ophthalmologist diagnoses a 29-year-old male with myopia of both eyes. The coder assigned ICD-9-CM code 367.1. The most appropriate ICD-10-CM code to describe this clinical diagnosis is:**

    A. H52.03
    B. H52.11, H52.12
    C. H52.02
    D. H52.13

10. **According to ICD-10-CM guidelines, if your physician does not classify a fracture as "open" or "closed," you should code the fracture as "closed." If your physician does not classify a fracture as "displaced" or "nondisplaced," you should consider this _____.**

    A. Nondisplaced
    B. Displaced
    C. Unspecified
    D. Other

11. **Under ICD-10-CM, your acute cystitis diagnosis code choice will depend on what factor?**

   A. Whether the patient has hematuria
   B. Whether the patient is older or younger than age 9
   C. How long the patient has had the infection
   D. The patient's frequency of urination

Test Yourself: ICD-10-CM Challenge (Answers)

1. The answer is C: Both A and B.

ICD-10-CM uses the placeholder "X" to:

A) Provide room for future expansion while keeping the code's required structure (such as T65.0X2S, *Toxic effect of cyanides, intentional self-harm, sequela*).

AND

B) Meet the requirement of coding to the highest level of specificity when a code has fewer than six characters and the code requires a seventh character extension (such as S17.0XXA, *Crushing injury of larynx and trachea, initial encounter*).

Source: 2014 ICD-10-CM Official Guidelines for Coding and Reporting, Sections I.A.4 and I.A.5

2. The answer is A: You have to know the trimester to choose the proper ICD-10-CM code.

GEMs stand for General Equivalence Mappings. The GEMs are the raw material from which providers, health information vendors, and payers can derive specific applied code mappings to meet their needs. You can use GEMs to study the differences between ICD-9-CM and ICD-10-CM.

The important term to remember for GEMs is "General." Some codes won't match because one code set is more specific than the other. For instance, 649.53 (*Spotting complicating pregnancy, antepartum condition or complication*) does not cross neatly to one ICD-10-CM code because to arrive at the correct code in ICD-10-CM you have to know the trimester. The GEMs map 649.53 to the following codes:

- O26.851, *Spotting complicating pregnancy, first trimester*
- O26.852, *Spotting complicating pregnancy, second trimester*
- O26.853, *Spotting complicating pregnancy, third trimester*.

Note that the GEMs don't include all possible codes you may use in place of 649.53. For instance, the ICD-9-CM to ICD-10-CM GEMs do not map 649.53 to O26.859 (*Spotting complicating pregnancy, unspecified trimester*).

Source: 2015 GEMs and ICD-10-CM 2015

3. The answer is B: Excludes1.

ICD-9-CM uses Excludes notes, but ICD-10-CM uses both Excludes1 and Excludes2 notes. Before ICD-10-CM implementation, be sure you understand how these two notes differ. The following is a quote from the 2014 ICD-10-CM Official Guidelines, Section I.a.12:

a. Excludes1

A type 1 Excludes note is a pure excludes note. It means "NOT CODED HERE!" An Excludes1 note indicates that the code excluded should never be used at the same time as the code above the Excludes1 note. An Excludes1 is used when two conditions cannot occur together, such as a congenital form versus an acquired form of the same condition.

b. Excludes2

A type 2 Excludes note represents "Not included here." An excludes2 note indicates that the condition excluded is not part of the condition represented by the code, but a patient may have both conditions at the same time. When an Excludes2 note appears under a code, it is acceptable to use both the code and the excluded code together, when appropriate.

Source: 2014 ICD-10-CM Official Guidelines for Coding and Reporting, Section I.a.12

4. The answer is D: I34.0.

ICD-10-CM notes with I34.0 (*Nonrheumatic mitral [valve] insufficiency*) tell you that it is the proper code for mitral valve regurgitation (as well as insufficiency or incompetence). You should choose the nonrheumatic code because documentation shows the patient has no history of rheumatic fever and a prior heart attack caused the disorder.

Source: ICD-10-CM 2015

5. The answer is A: S09.93XA

ICD-10-CM expands 959.09 into two codes with different options for unspecified injuries to the face and neck: S09.93XA (*Unspecified injury of face, initial encounter*) and S19.9XXA (*Unspecified injury of neck, initial encounter*).

For facial trauma, the provider should check the patient's facial skeleton, which is divided into three sections: the forehead, the middle face, and the mandible or jaw. Code S09.93XA is the ICD-10-CM code you would use to describe injury to the face.

Code S19.9XXA pertains to injury to the neck. Codes S19.93XX and S19.93XA are not valid ICD-10-CM codes.

Source: ICD-10-CM 2015

6. The answer is B: Z00.01.

ICD-10-CM includes wellness check codes based on the patient's age and whether the provider documents any abnormal findings. Code Z00.01 (*Encounter for general adult medical examination with abnormal findings*) is specific to adult exams with abnormal findings.

The other answers represent the following:

- A standard exam of an adult where the provider does not discover abnormal findings (Z00.00)

- A pediatric well visit with abnormal findings (Z00.121)

- A pediatric well visit without abnormal findings (Z00.129).

Source: ICD-10-CM 2015

7. The answer is A: G57.61, G57.62.

Although in many cases ICD-10-CM offers a code specific to a condition found on both sides of the body, for plantar nerve lesions, you need to report individual codes for the left side and the right side: G57.61 (*Lesion of plantar nerve, right lower limb*) and G57.62 (*Lesion of plantar nerve, left lower limb*).

Source: ICD-10-CM 2015

8. The answer is D: R87.610.

You should report R87.610 (*Atypical squamous cells of undetermined significance on cytologic smear of cervix [ASC-US]*) because the physician repeats the Pap due to abnormal cells. Notice the question included the Pap results as returning ASC-US, and this term is included in the descriptor for R87.610.

Source: ICD-10-CM 2015

9. The answer is D: H52.13.

As the descriptor of H52.13 (*Myopia, bilateral*) indicates, it represents myopia of both eyes (or bilateral myopia).

You should not report separate codes for the left and right eyes because ICD-10-CM offers the more specific bilateral combination code.

Source: ICD-10-CM 2015

10. The answer is B: Displaced

You should consider an unclassified fracture to be "displaced." The precise wording from the 2014 ICD-10-CM Official Guidelines for Coding and Reporting is, "A fracture not indicated whether displaced or not displaced should be coded to displaced."

Displaced indicates a fracture in which the two ends of the broken bone are separated from one another. Nondisplaced indicates the bone breaks either partially or all the way through but still maintains its proper alignment.

Source: 2014 ICD-10-CM Official Guidelines for Coding and Reporting, Section I.C.19.c

11. The answer is A: Whether the patient has hematuria.

ICD-10-CM includes these options for acute cystitis:

- N30.00, *Acute cystitis without hematuria*

- N30.01, *Acute cystitis with hematuria*.

As you can see, the options differ based on documentation of with or without hematuria, which is blood in the urine.

Source: ICD-10-CM 2015

ICD-10-CM Official Guidelines for Coding and Reporting 2015

Narrative changes appear in **bold** text.

Items <u>underlined</u> have been moved within the guidelines since the 2013 version.

Italics are used to indicate revisions to heading changes.

The Centers for Medicare and Medicaid Services (CMS) and the National Center for Health Statistics (NCHS), two departments within the U.S. Federal Government's Department of Health and Human Services (DHHS), provide the following guidelines for coding and reporting using the International Classification of Diseases, 10th Revision, Clinical Modification (ICD-10-CM). These guidelines should be used as a companion document to the official version of the ICD-10-CM as published on the NCHS website. The ICD-10-CM is a morbidity classification published by the United States for classifying diagnoses and reason for visits in all health care settings. The ICD-10-CM is based on the ICD-10, the statistical classification of disease published by the World Health Organization (WHO).

These guidelines have been approved by the four organizations that make up the Cooperating Parties for the ICD-10-CM: the American Hospital Association (AHA), the American Health Information Management Association (AHIMA), CMS, and NCHS.

These guidelines are a set of rules that have been developed to accompany and complement the official conventions and instructions provided within the ICD-10-CM itself. The instructions and conventions of the classification take precedence over guidelines. These guidelines are based on the coding and sequencing instructions in the Tabular List and Alphabetic Index of ICD-10-CM, but provide additional instruction. Adherence to these guidelines when assigning ICD-10-CM diagnosis codes is required under the Health Insurance Portability and Accountability Act (HIPAA). The diagnosis codes (Tabular List and Alphabetic Index) have been adopted under HIPAA for all healthcare settings. A joint effort between the healthcare provider and the coder is essential to achieve complete and accurate documentation, code assignment, and reporting of diagnoses and procedures. These guidelines have been developed to assist both the healthcare provider and the coder in identifying those diagnoses that are to be reported. The importance of consistent, complete documentation in the medical record cannot be overemphasized. Without such documentation accurate coding cannot be achieved. The entire record should be reviewed to determine the specific reason for the encounter and the conditions treated.

The term encounter is used for all settings, including hospital admissions. In the context of these guidelines, the term provider is used throughout the guidelines to mean physician or any qualified health care practitioner who is legally accountable for establishing the patient's diagnosis. Only this set of guidelines, approved by the Cooperating Parties, is official.

The guidelines are organized into sections. Section I includes the structure and conventions of the classification and general guidelines that apply to the entire classification, and chapter-specific guidelines that correspond to the chapters as they are arranged in the classification. Section II includes guidelines for selection of principal diagnosis for non-outpatient settings. Section III includes guidelines for reporting additional diagnoses in non-outpatient settings. Section IV is for outpatient coding and reporting. It is necessary to review all sections of the guidelines to fully understand all of the rules and instructions needed to code properly.

Section I. Conventions, General Coding Guidelines and Chapter Specific Guidelines

The conventions, general guidelines and chapter-specific guidelines are applicable to all health care settings unless otherwise indicated. The conventions and instructions of the classification take precedence over guidelines.

A. Conventions for the ICD-10-CM

The conventions for the ICD-10-CM are the general rules for use of the classification independent of the guidelines. These conventions are incorporated within the Alphabetic Index and Tabular List of the ICD-10-CM as instructional notes.

1. **The Alphabetic Index and Tabular List**
   The ICD-10-CM is divided into the Alphabetic Index, an alphabetical list of terms and their corresponding code, and the Tabular List, a structured list of codes divided into chapters based on body system or condition. The Alphabetic Index consists of the following parts: the Index of Diseases and Injury, the Index of External Causes of Injury, the Table of Neoplasms and the Table of Drugs and Chemicals.

   See Section I.C2. General guidelines

   See Section I.C.19. Adverse Effects, Poisoning, Underdosing and Toxic Effects

2. **Format and Structure:**
   The ICD-10-CM Tabular List contains categories, subcategories and codes. Characters for categories, subcategories and codes may be either a letter or a number. All categories are 3 characters. A three-character category that has no further subdivision is equivalent to a code. Subcategories are either 4 or 5 characters. Codes may be 3, 4, 5, 6 or 7 characters. That is, each level of subdivision after a category is a subcategory. The final level of subdivision is a code. Codes that have applicable 7th characters are still referred to as codes, not subcategories. A code that has an applicable 7th character is considered invalid without the 7th character.

   The ICD-10-CM uses an indented format for ease in reference.

3. **Use of codes for reporting purposes**
   For reporting purposes only codes are permissible, not categories or subcategories, and any applicable 7th character is required.

4. **Placeholder character**
   The ICD-10-CM utilizes a placeholder character "X". The "X" is used as a placeholder at certain codes to allow for future expansion. An example of this is at the poisoning, adverse effect and underdosing codes, categories T36-T50.

   Where a placeholder exists, the X must be used in order for the code to be considered a valid code.

5. **7th Characters**
   Certain ICD-10-CM categories have applicable 7th characters. The applicable 7th character is required for all codes within the category, or as the notes in the Tabular List instruct. The 7th character must always be the 7th character in the data field. If a code that requires a 7th character is not 6 characters, a placeholder X must be used to fill in the empty characters.

6. **Abbreviations**
   a. **Alphabetic Index abbreviations**
      NEC   "Not elsewhere classifiable"

      This abbreviation in the Alphabetic Index represents "other specified". When a specific code is not available for a condition, the Alphabetic Index directs the coder to the "other specified" code in the Tabular List.

      NOS   "Not otherwise specified"

      This abbreviation is the equivalent of unspecified.

   b. **Tabular List Abbreviations**
      NEC   "Not elsewhere classifiable"

      This abbreviation in the Tabular List represents "other specified". When a specific code is not available for a condition the Tabular List includes an NEC entry under a code to identify the code as the "other specified" code.

      NOS   "Not otherwise specified"

      This abbreviation is the equivalent of unspecified.

7. **Punctuation**
   [ ]   Brackets are used in the Tabular List to enclose synonyms, alternative wording or explanatory phrases. Brackets are used in the Alphabetic Index to identify manifestation codes.

   ( )   Parentheses are used in both the Alphabetic Index and Tabular List to enclose supplementary words that may be present or absent in the statement of a disease or procedure without affecting the code number to which it is assigned. The terms within the parentheses are referred to as nonessential modifiers. **The nonessential modifiers in the Alphabetic Index to Diseases apply to subterms following a main term except when a nonessential modifier and a subentry are mutually exclusive, the subentry takes precedence. For example, in the ICD-10-CM Alphabetic Index under the main term Enteritis, "acute" is a nonessential modifier and "chronic" is a subentry. In this case, the nonessential modifier "acute" does not apply to the subentry "chronic".**

   :   Colons are used in the Tabular List after an incomplete term which needs one or more of the modifiers following the colon to make it assignable to a given category.

8. **Use of "And".**
   See Section I.A.14. Use of the term "And"

9. **Other and Unspecified codes**
   a. **"Other" codes**
      Codes titled "other" or "other specified" are for use when the information in the medical record provides detail for which a specific code does not exist. Alphabetic Index entries with NEC in the line designate "other" codes in the Tabular List. These Alphabetic Index entries represent specific disease entities for which no *specific* code exists so the term is included within an "other" code.

   b. **"Unspecified" codes**
      Codes titled "unspecified" are for use when the information in the medical record is insufficient to assign a more specific code. For those categories for which an unspecified code is not provided, the "other specified" code may represent both other and unspecified.

      See Section I.B.18 Use of Signs/Symptom/Unspecified Codes

10. **Includes Notes**
    This note appears immediately under a three character code title to further define, or give examples of, the content of the category.

11. **Inclusion terms**
    List of terms is included under some codes. These terms are the conditions for which that code is to be used. The terms may be synonyms of the code title, or, in the case of "other specified" codes, the terms are a list of the various conditions assigned to that code. The inclusion terms are not necessarily exhaustive. Additional terms found only in the Alphabetic Index may also be assigned to a code.

12. **Excludes Notes**
    The ICD-10-CM has two types of excludes notes. Each type of note has a different definition for use but they are all similar in that they indicate that codes excluded from each other are independent of each other.

    a. **Excludes1**
       A type 1 Excludes note is a pure excludes note. It means "NOT CODED HERE!" An Excludes1 note indicates that the code excluded should never be used at the same time as the code above the Excludes1 note. An Excludes1 is used when two conditions cannot occur together, such as a congenital form versus an acquired form of the same condition.

    b. **Excludes2**
       A type 2 Excludes note represents "Not included here". An Excludes2 note indicates that the condition excluded is not part of the condition represented by the code, but a patient may have both conditions at the same time. When an Excludes2 note appears under a code, it is acceptable to use both the code and the excluded code together, when appropriate.

13. **Etiology/Manifestation Convention ("code first", "use additional code" and "in diseases classified elsewhere" notes)**
    Certain conditions have both an underlying etiology and multiple body system manifestations due to the underlying etiology. For such conditions, the ICD-10-CM has a coding convention that requires the underlying condition be sequenced first followed by the manifestation. Wherever such a combination exists, there is a "use additional code" note at the etiology code, and a "code first" note at the manifestation

code. These instructional notes indicate the proper sequencing order of the codes, etiology followed by manifestation.

In most cases the manifestation codes will have in the code title, "in diseases classified elsewhere." Codes with this title are a component of the etiology/ manifestation convention. The code title indicates that it is a manifestation code. "In diseases classified elsewhere" codes are never permitted to be used as first-listed or principal diagnosis codes. They must be used in conjunction with an underlying condition code and they must be listed following the underlying condition. See category F02, Dementia in other diseases classified elsewhere, for an example of this convention.

There are manifestation codes that do not have "in diseases classified elsewhere" in the title. For such codes, there is a "use additional code" note at the etiology code and a "code first" note at the manifestation code and the rules for sequencing apply.

In addition to the notes in the Tabular List, these conditions also have a specific Alphabetic Index entry structure. In the Alphabetic Index both conditions are listed together with the etiology code first followed by the manifestation codes in brackets. The code in brackets is always to be sequenced second.

An example of the etiology/manifestation convention is dementia in Parkinson's disease. In the Alphabetic Index, code G20 is listed first, followed by code F02.80 or F02.81 in brackets. Code G20 represents the underlying etiology, Parkinson's disease, and must be sequenced first, whereas codes F02.80 and F02.81 represent the manifestation of dementia in diseases classified elsewhere, with or without behavioral disturbance.

"Code first" and "Use additional code" notes are also used as sequencing rules in the classification for certain codes that are not part of an etiology/ manifestation combination.

See Section I.B.7. Multiple Coding for a Single Condition.

14. "And"
The word "and" should be interpreted to mean either "and" or "or" when it appears in a title.

For example, cases of "tuberculosis of bones", "tuberculosis of joints" and "tuberculosis of bones and joints" are classified to subcategory A18.0, Tuberculosis of bones and joints.

15. "With"
The word "with" should be interpreted to mean "associated with" or "due to" when it appears in a code title, the Alphabetic Index, or an instructional note in the Tabular List.

The word "with" in the Alphabetic Index is sequenced immediately following the main term, not in alphabetical order.

16. "See" and "See Also"
The "see" instruction following a main term in the Alphabetic Index indicates that another term should be referenced. It is necessary to go to the main term referenced with the "see" note to locate the correct code.

A "see also" instruction following a main term in the Alphabetic Index instructs that there is another main term that may also be referenced that may provide additional Alphabetic Index entries that may be useful. It is not necessary to follow the "see also" note when the original main term provides the necessary code.

17. "Code Also" Note
A "code also" note instructs that two codes may be required to fully describe a condition, but this note does not provide sequencing direction.

18. Default codes
A code listed next to a main term in the ICD-10-CM Alphabetic Index is referred to as a default code. The default code represents that condition that is most commonly associated with the main term, or is the unspecified code for the condition. If a condition is documented in a medical record (for example, appendicitis) without any additional information, such as acute or chronic, the default code should be assigned.

B. General Coding Guidelines

1. Locating a code in the ICD-10-CM
To select a code in the classification that corresponds to a diagnosis or reason for visit documented in a medical record, first locate the term in the Alphabetic Index, and then verify the code in the Tabular List. Read and be guided by instructional notations that appear in both the Alphabetic Index and the Tabular List.

It is essential to use both the Alphabetic Index and Tabular List when locating and assigning a code. The Alphabetic Index does not always provide the full code. Selection of the full code, including laterality and any applicable 7th character can only be done in the Tabular List. A dash (-) at the end of an Alphabetic Index entry indicates that additional characters are required. Even if a dash is not included at the Alphabetic Index entry, it is necessary to refer to the Tabular List to verify that no 7th character is required.

2. Level of Detail in Coding
Diagnosis codes are to be used and reported at their highest number of characters available.

ICD-10-CM diagnosis codes are composed of codes with 3, 4, 5, 6 or 7 characters. Codes with three characters are included in ICD-10-CM as the heading of a category of codes that may be further subdivided by the use of fourth and/or fifth characters and/or sixth characters, which provide greater detail.

A three-character code is to be used only if it is not further subdivided. A code is invalid if it has not been coded to the full number of characters required for that code, including the 7th character, if applicable.

3. Code or codes from A00.0 through T88.9, Z00-Z99.8
The appropriate code or codes from A00.0 through T88.9, Z00-Z99.8 must be used to identify diagnoses, symptoms, conditions, problems, complaints or other reason(s) for the encounter/visit.

4. Signs and symptoms
Codes that describe symptoms and signs, as opposed to diagnoses, are acceptable for reporting purposes when a related definitive diagnosis has not been established (confirmed) by the provider. Chapter 18 of ICD-10-CM, Symptoms, Signs, and Abnormal Clinical and Laboratory Findings, Not Elsewhere Classified (codes R00.0 - R99) contains many, but not all codes for symptoms.

See Section I.B.18 Use of Signs/Symptom/Unspecified Codes

5. Conditions that are an integral part of a disease process
Signs and symptoms that are associated routinely with a disease process should not be assigned as additional codes, unless otherwise instructed by the classification.

6. Conditions that are not an integral part of a disease process
Additional signs and symptoms that may not be associated routinely with a disease process should be coded when present.

7. Multiple coding for a single condition
In addition to the etiology/manifestation convention that requires two codes to fully describe a single condition that affects multiple body systems, there are other single conditions that also require more than one code. "Use additional code" notes are found in the Tabular List at codes that are not part of an etiology/manifestation pair where a secondary code is useful to fully describe a condition. The sequencing rule is the same as the etiology/manifestation pair, "use additional code" indicates that a secondary code should be added.

For example, for bacterial infections that are not included in chapter 1, a secondary code from category B95, Streptococcus, Staphylococcus, and Enterococcus, as the cause of diseases classified elsewhere, or B96, Other bacterial agents as the cause of diseases classified elsewhere, may be required to identify the bacterial organism causing the infection. A "use additional code" note will normally be found at the infectious disease code, indicating a need for the organism code to be added as a secondary code.

"Code first" notes are also under certain codes that are not specifically manifestation codes but may be due to an underlying cause. When there is a "code first" note and an underlying condition is present, the underlying condition should be sequenced first.

"Code, if applicable, any causal condition first", notes indicate that this code may be assigned as a principal diagnosis when the causal condition is unknown or not applicable. If a causal condition is known, then the code for that condition should be sequenced as the principal or first-listed diagnosis.

Multiple codes may be needed for sequela, complication codes and obstetric codes to more fully describe a condition. See the specific guidelines for these conditions for further instruction.

8. Acute and Chronic Conditions
If the same condition is described as both acute (subacute) and chronic, and separate subentries exist in the Alphabetic Index at the same indentation level, code both and sequence the acute (subacute) code first.

9. Combination Code

A combination code is a single code used to classify:

Two diagnoses, or

A diagnosis with an associated secondary process (manifestation);

A diagnosis with an associated complication.

Combination codes are identified by referring to subterm entries in the Alphabetic Index and by reading the inclusion and exclusion notes in the Tabular List.

Assign only the combination code when that code fully identifies the diagnostic conditions involved or when the Alphabetic Index so directs. Multiple coding should not be used when the classification provides a combination code that clearly identifies all of the elements documented in the diagnosis. When the combination code lacks necessary specificity in describing the manifestation or complication, an additional code should be used as a secondary code.

10. Sequela (Late Effects)

A sequela is the residual effect (condition produced) after the acute phase of an illness or injury has terminated. There is no time limit on when a sequela code can be used. The residual may be apparent early, such as in cerebral infarction, or it may occur months or years later, such as that due to a previous injury. Coding of sequela generally requires two codes sequenced in the following order: The condition or nature of the sequela is sequenced first. The sequela code is sequenced second.

An exception to the above guidelines are those instances where the code for the sequela is followed by a manifestation code identified in the Tabular List and title, or the sequela code has been expanded (at the fourth, fifth or sixth character levels) to include the manifestation(s). The code for the acute phase of an illness or injury that led to the sequela is never used with a code for the late effect.

See Section I.C.9. Sequelae of Cerebrovascular Disease

See Section I.C.15. Sequelae of Complication of Pregnancy, Childbirth and the Puerperium

See Section I.C.19. Application of 7th characters for Chapter 19

11. Impending or Threatened Condition

Code any condition described at the time of discharge as "impending" or "threatened" as follows:

If it did occur, code as confirmed diagnosis.

If it did not occur, reference the Alphabetic Index to determine if the condition has a subentry term for "impending" or "threatened" and also reference main term entries for "Impending" and for "Threatened."

If the subterms are listed, assign the given code.

If the subterms are not listed, code the existing underlying condition(s) and not the condition described as impending or threatened.

12. Reporting Same Diagnosis Code More than Once

Each unique ICD-10-CM diagnosis code may be reported only once for an encounter. This applies to bilateral conditions when there are no distinct codes identifying laterality or two different conditions classified to the same ICD-10-CM diagnosis code.

13. Laterality

Some ICD-10-CM codes indicate laterality, specifying whether the condition occurs on the left, right or is bilateral. If no bilateral code is provided and the condition is bilateral, assign separate codes for both the left and right side. If the side is not identified in the medical record, assign the code for the unspecified side.

14. Documentation for BMI, Non-pressure Ulcers and Pressure Ulcer Stages

For the Body Mass Index (BMI), depth of non-pressure chronic ulcers and pressure ulcer stage codes, code assignment may be based on medical record documentation from clinicians who are not the patient's provider (i.e., physician or other qualified healthcare practitioner legally accountable for establishing the patient's diagnosis), since this information is typically documented by other clinicians involved in the care of the patient (e.g., a dietitian often documents the BMI and nurses often documents the pressure ulcer stages). However, the associated diagnosis (such as overweight, obesity, or pressure ulcer) must be documented by the patient's provider. If there is conflicting medical record documentation, either from the same clinician or different clinicians, the patient's attending provider should be queried for clarification.

The BMI codes should only be reported as secondary diagnoses. As with all other secondary diagnosis codes, the BMI codes should only be assigned when they meet the definition of a reportable additional diagnosis (see Section III, Reporting Additional Diagnoses).

15. Syndromes

Follow the Alphabetic Index guidance when coding syndromes. In the absence of Alphabetic Index guidance, assign codes for the documented manifestations of the syndrome. Additional codes for manifestations that are not an integral part of the disease process may also be assigned when the condition does not have a unique code.

16. Documentation of Complications of Care

Code assignment is based on the provider's documentation of the relationship between the condition and the care or procedure. The guideline extends to any complications of care, regardless of the chapter the code is located in. It is important to note that not all conditions that occur during or following medical care or surgery are classified as complications. There must be a cause-and-effect relationship between the care provided and the condition, and an indication in the documentation that it is a complication. Query the provider for clarification, if the complication is not clearly documented.

17. Borderline Diagnosis

If the provider documents a "borderline" diagnosis at the time of discharge, the diagnosis is coded as confirmed, unless the classification provides a specific entry (e.g., borderline diabetes). If a borderline condition has a specific index entry in ICD-10-CM, it should be coded as such. Since borderline conditions are not uncertain diagnoses, no distinction is made between the care setting (inpatient versus outpatient). Whenever the documentation is unclear regarding a borderline condition, coders are encouraged to query for clarification.

18. Use of Sign/Symptom/Unspecified Codes

Sign/symptom and "unspecified" codes have acceptable, even necessary, uses. While specific diagnosis codes should be reported when they are supported by the available medical record documentation and clinical knowledge of the patient's health condition, there are instances when signs/symptoms or unspecified codes are the best choices for accurately reflecting the healthcare encounter. Each healthcare encounter should be coded to the level of certainty known for that encounter.

If a definitive diagnosis has not been established by the end of the encounter, it is appropriate to report codes for sign(s) and/or symptom(s) in lieu of a definitive diagnosis. When sufficient clinical information isn't known or available about a particular health condition to assign a more specific code, it is acceptable to report the appropriate "unspecified" code (e.g., a diagnosis of pneumonia has been determined, but not the specific type). Unspecified codes should be reported when they are the codes that most accurately reflects what is known about the patient's condition at the time of that particular encounter. It would be inappropriate to select a specific code that is not supported by the medical record documentation or conduct medically unnecessary diagnostic testing in order to determine a more specific code.

C. Chapter-Specific Coding Guidelines

In addition to general coding guidelines, there are guidelines for specific diagnoses and/or conditions in the classification. Unless otherwise indicated, these guidelines apply to all health care settings. Please refer to Section II for guidelines on the selection of principal diagnosis.

1. Chapter 1: Certain Infectious and Parasitic Diseases (A00-B99)

a. Human Immunodeficiency Virus (HIV) Infections

1) Code only confirmed cases

Code only confirmed cases of HIV infection/illness. This is an exception to the hospital inpatient guideline Section II, H.

In this context, "confirmation" does not require documentation of positive serology or culture for HIV; the provider's diagnostic statement that the patient is HIV positive, or has an HIV-related illness is sufficient.

2) Selection and sequencing of HIV codes

(a) Patient admitted for HIV-related condition

If a patient is admitted for an HIV-related condition, the principal diagnosis should be B20, Human immunodeficiency virus [HIV] disease followed by additional diagnosis codes for all reported HIV-related conditions.

(b) **Patient with HIV disease admitted for unrelated condition**

If a patient with HIV disease is admitted for an unrelated condition (such as a traumatic injury), the code for the unrelated condition (e.g., the nature of injury code) should be the principal diagnosis. Other diagnoses would be B20 followed by additional diagnosis codes for all reported HIV-related conditions.

(c) **Whether the patient is newly diagnosed**

Whether the patient is newly diagnosed or has had previous admissions/encounters for HIV conditions is irrelevant to the sequencing decision.

(d) **Asymptomatic human immunodeficiency virus**

Z21, Asymptomatic human immunodeficiency virus [HIV] infection status, is to be applied when the patient without any documentation of symptoms is listed as being "HIV positive," "known HIV," "HIV test positive," or similar terminology. Do not use this code if the term "AIDS" is used or if the patient is treated for any HIV-related illness or is described as having any condition(s) resulting from his/her HIV positive status; use B20 in these cases.

(e) **Patients with inconclusive HIV serology**

Patients with inconclusive HIV serology, but no definitive diagnosis or manifestations of the illness, may be assigned code R75, Inconclusive laboratory evidence of human immunodeficiency virus [HIV].

(f) **Previously diagnosed HIV-related illness**

Patients with any known prior diagnosis of an HIV-related illness should be coded to B20. Once a patient has developed an HIV-related illness, the patient should always be assigned code B20 on every subsequent admission/encounter. Patients previously diagnosed with any HIV illness (B20) should never be assigned to R75 or Z21, Asymptomatic human immunodeficiency virus [HIV] infection status.

(g) **HIV Infection in pregnancy, childbirth and the puerperium**

During pregnancy, childbirth or the puerperium, a patient admitted (or presenting for a health care encounter) because of an HIV-related illness should receive a principal diagnosis code of O98.7-, Human immunodeficiency [HIV] disease complicating pregnancy, childbirth and the puerperium, followed by B20 and the code(s) for the HIV-related illness(es). Codes from Chapter 15 always take sequencing priority.

Patients with asymptomatic HIV infection status admitted (or presenting for a health care encounter) during pregnancy, childbirth, or the puerperium should receive codes of O98.7- and Z21.

(h) **Encounters for testing for HIV**

If a patient is being seen to determine his/her HIV status, use code Z11.4, Encounter for screening for human immunodeficiency virus [HIV]. Use additional codes for any associated high risk behavior.

If a patient with signs or symptoms is being seen for HIV testing, code the signs and symptoms. An additional counseling code Z71.7, Human immunodeficiency virus [HIV] counseling, may be used if counseling is provided during the encounter for the test.

When a patient returns to be informed of his/her HIV test results and the test result is negative, use code Z71.7, Human immunodeficiency virus [HIV] counseling.

If the results are positive, see previous guidelines and assign codes as appropriate.

b. **Infectious Agents as the Cause of Diseases Classified to Other Chapters**

Certain infections are classified in chapters other than Chapter 1 and no organism is identified as part of the infection code. In these instances, it is necessary to use an additional code from Chapter 1 to identify the organism. A code from category B95, Streptococcus, Staphylococcus, and Enterococcus as the cause of diseases classified to other chapters, B96, Other bacterial agents as the cause of diseases classified to other chapters, or B97, Viral agents as the cause of diseases classified to other chapters, is to be used as an additional code to identify the organism. An instructional note will be found at the infection code advising that an additional organism code is required.

c. **Infections Resistant to Antibiotics**

Many bacterial infections are resistant to current antibiotics. It is necessary to identify all infections documented as antibiotic resistant. Assign a code from category Z16, Resistance to antimicrobial drugs, following the infection code only if the infection code does not identify drug resistance.

d. **Sepsis, Severe Sepsis, and Septic Shock**

1) **Coding of Sepsis and Severe Sepsis**

   (a) **Sepsis**

   For a diagnosis of sepsis, assign the appropriate code for the underlying systemic infection. If the type of infection or causal organism is not further specified, assign code A41.9, Sepsis, unspecified organism.

   A code from subcategory R65.2, Severe sepsis, should not be assigned unless severe sepsis or an associated acute organ dysfunction is documented.

   (i) Negative or inconclusive blood cultures and sepsis

   Negative or inconclusive blood cultures do not preclude a diagnosis of sepsis in patients with clinical evidence of the condition, however, the provider should be queried.

   (ii) Urosepsis

   The term urosepsis is a nonspecific term. It is not to be considered synonymous with sepsis. It has no default code in the Alphabetic Index. Should a provider use this term, he/she must be queried for clarification.

   (iii) Sepsis with organ dysfunction

   If a patient has sepsis and associated acute organ dysfunction or multiple organ dysfunction (MOD), follow the instructions for coding severe sepsis.

   (iv) Acute organ dysfunction that is not clearly associated with the sepsis

   If a patient has sepsis and an acute organ dysfunction, but the medical record documentation indicates that the acute organ dysfunction is related to a medical condition other than the sepsis, do not assign a code from subcategory R65.2, Severe sepsis. An acute organ dysfunction must be associated with the sepsis in order to assign the severe sepsis code. If the documentation is not clear as to whether an acute organ dysfunction is related to the sepsis or another medical condition, query the provider.

   (b) **Severe sepsis**

   The coding of severe sepsis requires a minimum of 2 codes: first a code for the underlying systemic infection, followed by a code from subcategory R65.2, Severe sepsis. If the causal organism is not documented, assign code A41.9, Sepsis, unspecified organism, for the infection. Additional code(s) for the associated acute organ dysfunction are also required.

   Due to the complex nature of severe sepsis, some cases may require querying the provider prior to assignment of the codes.

2) **Septic Shock**

   (a) Septic shock generally refers to circulatory failure associated with severe sepsis, and therefore, it represents a type of acute organ dysfunction.

   For cases of septic shock, the code for the systemic infection should be sequenced first, followed by code R65.21, Severe sepsis with septic shock or code T81.12, Postprocedural septic shock. Any additional codes for the other acute organ dysfunctions should also be assigned. As noted in the sequencing instructions in the Tabular List, the code for septic shock cannot be assigned as a principal diagnosis.

3) **Sequencing of Severe Sepsis**

   If severe sepsis is present on admission, and meets the definition of principal diagnosis, the underlying systemic infection should be assigned as principal diagnosis followed by the appropriate code from subcategory R65.2 as required by the sequencing rules in the Tabular List. A code from subcategory R65.2 can never be assigned as a principal diagnosis.

When severe sepsis develops during an encounter (it was not present on admission) the underlying systemic infection and the appropriate code from subcategory R65.2 should be assigned as secondary diagnoses.

Severe sepsis may be present on admission but the diagnosis may not be confirmed until sometime after admission. If the documentation is not clear whether severe sepsis was present on admission, the provider should be queried.

4) Sepsis and Severe Sepsis with a Localized Infection

If the reason for admission is both sepsis or severe sepsis and a localized infection, such as pneumonia or cellulitis, a code(s) for the underlying systemic infection should be assigned first and the code for the localized infection should be assigned as a secondary diagnosis. If the patient has severe sepsis, a code from subcategory R65.2 should also be assigned as a secondary diagnosis. If the patient is admitted with a localized infection, such as pneumonia, and sepsis/severe sepsis doesn't develop until after admission, the localized infection should be assigned first, followed by the appropriate sepsis/severe sepsis codes.

5) Sepsis Due to a Postprocedural Infection

(a) Documentation of causal relationship

As with all postprocedural complications, code assignment is based on the provider's documentation of the relationship between the infection and the procedure.

(b) Sepsis due to a postprocedural infection

For such cases, the postprocedural infection code, such as, T80.2, Infections following infusion, transfusion, and therapeutic injection, T81.4, Infection following a procedure, T88.0, Infection following immunization, or O86.0, Infection of obstetric surgical wound, should be coded first, followed by the code for the specific infection. If the patient has severe sepsis the appropriate code from subcategory R65.2 should also be assigned with the additional code(s) for any acute organ dysfunction.

(c) Postprocedural infection and postprocedural septic shock

In cases where a postprocedural infection has occurred and has resulted in severe sepsis and postprocedural septic shock, the code for the precipitating complication such as code T81.4, Infection following a procedure, or O86.0, Infection of obstetrical surgical wound should be coded first followed by code R65.21, Severe sepsis with septic shock and a code for the systemic infection.

6) Sepsis and severe sepsis associated with a noninfectious process (condition)

In some cases a noninfectious process (condition), such as trauma, may lead to an infection which can result in sepsis or severe sepsis. If sepsis or severe sepsis is documented as associated with a noninfectious condition, such as a burn or serious injury, and this condition meets the definition for principal diagnosis, the code for the noninfectious condition should be sequenced first, followed by the code for the resulting infection. If severe sepsis, is present a code from subcategory R65.2 should also be assigned with any associated organ dysfunction(s) codes. It is not necessary to assign a code from subcategory R65.1, Systemic inflammatory response syndrome (SIRS) of non-infectious origin, for these cases.

If the infection meets the definition of principal diagnosis it should be sequenced before the non-infectious condition. When both the associated non-infectious condition and the infection meet the definition of principal diagnosis either may be assigned as principal diagnosis.

Only one code from category R65, Symptoms and signs specifically associated with systemic inflammation and infection, should be assigned. Therefore, when a non-infectious condition leads to an infection resulting in severe sepsis, assign the appropriate code from subcategory R65.2, Severe sepsis. Do not additionally assign a code from subcategory R65.1, Systemic inflammatory response syndrome (SIRS) of non-infectious origin.

See Section I.C.18. SIRS due to non-infectious process

7) Sepsis and septic shock complicating abortion, pregnancy, childbirth, and the puerperium

See Section I.C.15. Sepsis and septic shock complicating abortion, pregnancy, childbirth and the puerperium

8) Newborn sepsis

See Section I.C.16. f. Bacterial sepsis of Newborn

e. Methicillin Resistant Staphylococcus aureus (MRSA) Conditions

1) Selection and sequencing of MRSA codes

(a) Combination codes for MRSA infection

When a patient is diagnosed with an infection that is due to methicillin resistant *Staphylococcus aureus* (MRSA), and that infection has a combination code that includes the causal organism (e.g., sepsis, pneumonia) assign the appropriate combination code for the condition (e.g., code A41.02, Sepsis due to Methicillin resistant Staphylococcus aureus or code J15.212, Pneumonia due to Methicillin resistant Staphylococcus aureus). Do not assign code B95.62, Methicillin resistant Staphylococcus aureus infection as the cause of diseases classified elsewhere, as an additional code because the combination code includes the type of infection and the MRSA organism. Do not assign a code from subcategory Z16.11, Resistance to penicillins, as an additional diagnosis.

See Section C.1. for instructions on coding and sequencing of sepsis and severe sepsis.

(b) Other codes for MRSA infection

When there is documentation of a current infection (e.g., wound infection, stitch abscess, urinary tract infection) due to MRSA, and that infection does not have a combination code that includes the causal organism, assign the appropriate code to identify the condition along with code B95.62, Methicillin resistant Staphylococcus aureus infection as the cause of diseases classified elsewhere for the MRSA infection. Do not assign a code from subcategory Z16.11, Resistance to penicillins.

(c) Methicillin susceptible Staphylococcus aureus (MSSA) and MRSA colonization

The condition or state of being colonized or carrying MSSA or MRSA is called colonization or carriage, while an individual person is described as being colonized or being a carrier. Colonization means that MSSA or MSRA is present on or in the body without necessarily causing illness. A positive MRSA colonization test might be documented by the provider as "MRSA screen positive" or "MRSA nasal swab positive".

Assign code Z22.322, Carrier or suspected carrier of Methicillin resistant Staphylococcus aureus, for patients documented as having MRSA colonization. Assign code Z22.321, Carrier or suspected carrier of Methicillin susceptible Staphylococcus aureus, for patient documented as having MSSA colonization. Colonization is not necessarily indicative of a disease process or as the cause of a specific condition the patient may have unless documented as such by the provider.

(d) MRSA colonization and infection

If a patient is documented as having both MRSA colonization and infection during a hospital admission, code Z22.322, Carrier or suspected carrier of Methicillin resistant Staphylococcus aureus, and a code for the MRSA infection may both be assigned.

2. Chapter 2: Neoplasms (C00-D49)
General Guidelines

Chapter 2 of the ICD-10-CM contains the codes for most benign and all malignant neoplasms. Certain benign neoplasms, such as prostatic adenomas, may be found in the specific body system chapters. To properly code a neoplasm it is necessary to determine from the record if the neoplasm is benign, in-situ, malignant, or of uncertain histologic behavior. If malignant, any secondary (metastatic) sites should also be determined.

Primary malignant neoplasms overlapping site boundaries

A primary malignant neoplasm that overlaps two or more contiguous (next to each other) sites should be classified to the subcategory/code .8 ('overlapping lesion'), unless the combination is specifically indexed elsewhere. For multiple neoplasms of the same site that are not contiguous such as tumors in different quadrants of the same breast, codes for each site should be assigned.

Malignant neoplasm of ectopic tissue

Malignant neoplasms of ectopic tissue are to be coded to the site of origin mentioned, e.g., ectopic pancreatic malignant neoplasms involving the stomach are coded to pancreas, unspecified (C25.9).

The neoplasm table in the Alphabetic Index should be referenced first. However, if the histological term is documented, that term should be referenced first, rather than going immediately to the Neoplasm Table, in order to determine which column in the Neoplasm Table is appropriate. For example, if the documentation indicates "adenoma," refer to the term in the Alphabetic Index to review the entries under this term and the instructional note to "see also neoplasm, by site, benign." The table provides the proper code based on the type of neoplasm and the site. It is important to select the proper column in the table that corresponds to the type of neoplasm. The Tabular List should then be referenced to verify that the correct code has been selected from the table and that a more specific site code does not exist.

See Section I.C.21. Factors influencing health status and contact with health services, Status, for information regarding Z15.0, codes for genetic susceptibility to cancer.

a. Treatment directed at the malignancy

If the treatment is directed at the malignancy, designate the malignancy as the principal diagnosis.

The only exception to this guideline is if a patient admission/encounter is solely for the administration of chemotherapy, immunotherapy or radiation therapy, assign the appropriate Z51.-- code as the first-listed or principal diagnosis, and the diagnosis or problem for which the service is being performed as a secondary diagnosis.

b. Treatment of secondary site

When a patient is admitted because of a primary neoplasm with metastasis and treatment is directed toward the secondary site only, the secondary neoplasm is designated as the principal diagnosis even though the primary malignancy is still present.

c. Coding and sequencing of complications

Coding and sequencing of complications associated with the malignancies or with the therapy thereof are subject to the following guidelines:

1) Anemia associated with malignancy

When admission/encounter is for management of an anemia associated with the malignancy, and the treatment is only for anemia, the appropriate code for the malignancy is sequenced as the principal or first-listed diagnosis followed by the appropriate code for the anemia (such as code D63.0, Anemia in neoplastic disease).

2) Anemia associated with chemotherapy, immunotherapy and radiation therapy

When the admission/encounter is for management of an anemia associated with an adverse effect of the administration of chemotherapy or immunotherapy and the only treatment is for the anemia, the anemia code is sequenced first followed by the appropriate codes for the neoplasm and the adverse effect (T45.1X5, Adverse effect of antineoplastic and immunosuppressive drugs).

When the admission/encounter is for management of an anemia associated with an adverse effect of radiotherapy, the anemia code should be sequenced first, followed by the appropriate neoplasm code and code Y84.2, Radiological procedure and radiotherapy as the cause of abnormal reaction of the patient, or of later complication, without mention of misadventure at the time of the procedure.

3) Management of dehydration due to the malignancy

When the admission/encounter is for management of dehydration due to the malignancy and only the dehydration is being treated (intravenous rehydration), the dehydration is sequenced first, followed by the code(s) for the malignancy.

4) Treatment of a complication resulting from a surgical procedure

When the admission/encounter is for treatment of a complication resulting from a surgical procedure, designate the complication as the principal or first-listed diagnosis if treatment is directed at resolving the complication.

d. Primary malignancy previously excised

When a primary malignancy has been previously excised or eradicated from its site and there is no further treatment directed to that site and there is no evidence of any existing primary malignancy, a code from category Z85, Personal history of malignant neoplasm, should be used to indicate the former site of the malignancy. Any mention of extension, invasion, or metastasis to another site is coded as a secondary malignant neoplasm to that site. The secondary site may be the principal or first-listed with the Z85 code used as a secondary code.

e. Admissions/Encounters involving chemotherapy, immunotherapy and radiation therapy

1) Episode of care involves surgical removal of neoplasm

When an episode of care involves the surgical removal of a neoplasm, primary or secondary site, followed by adjunct chemotherapy or radiation treatment during the same episode of care, the code for the neoplasm should be assigned as principal or first-listed diagnosis.

2) Patient admission/encounter solely for administration of chemotherapy, immunotherapy and radiation therapy

If a patient admission/encounter is solely for the administration of chemotherapy, immunotherapy or radiation therapy assign code Z51.0, Encounter for antineoplastic radiation therapy, or Z51.11, Encounter for antineoplastic chemotherapy, or Z51.12, Encounter for antineoplastic immunotherapy as the first-listed or principal diagnosis. If a patient receives more than one of these therapies during the same admission more than one of these codes may be assigned, in any sequence.

The malignancy for which the therapy is being administered should be assigned as a secondary diagnosis.

3) Patient admitted for radiation therapy, chemotherapy or immunotherapy and develops complications

When a patient is admitted for the purpose of radiotherapy, immunotherapy or chemotherapy and develops complications such as uncontrolled nausea and vomiting or dehydration, the principal or first-listed diagnosis is Z51.0, Encounter for antineoplastic radiation therapy, or Z51.11, Encounter for antineoplastic chemotherapy, or Z51.12, Encounter for antineoplastic immunotherapy followed by any codes for the complications.

f. Admission/encounter to determine extent of malignancy

When the reason for admission/encounter is to determine the extent of the malignancy, or for a procedure such as paracentesis or thoracentesis, the primary malignancy or appropriate metastatic site is designated as the principal or first-listed diagnosis, even though chemotherapy or radiotherapy is administered.

g. Symptoms, signs, and abnormal findings listed in Chapter 18 associated with neoplasms

Symptoms, signs, and ill-defined conditions listed in Chapter 18 characteristic of, or associated with, an existing primary or secondary site malignancy cannot be used to replace the malignancy as principal or first-listed diagnosis, regardless of the number of admissions or encounters for treatment and care of the neoplasm.

See section I.C.21. Factors Influencing Health Status and Contact with Health Services, Encounter for Prophylactic Organ Removal.

h. Admission/encounter for pain control/management

See Section I.C.6. for information on coding admission/encounter for pain control/management.

i. Malignancy in two or more noncontiguous sites

A patient may have more than one malignant tumor in the same organ. These tumors may represent different primaries or metastatic disease, depending on the site. Should the documentation be unclear, the provider should be queried as to the status of each tumor so that the correct codes can be assigned.

j. Disseminated malignant neoplasm, unspecified

Code C80.0, Disseminated malignant neoplasm, unspecified, is for use only in those cases where the patient has advanced metastatic disease and no known primary or secondary sites are specified. It should not be used in place of assigning codes for the primary site and all known secondary sites.

k. Malignant neoplasm without specification of site
Code C80.1, Malignant (primary) neoplasm, unspecified, equates to Cancer, unspecified. This code should only be used when no determination can be made as to the primary site of a malignancy. This code should rarely be used in the inpatient setting.

l. Sequencing of neoplasm codes

1) Encounter for treatment of primary malignancy
If the reason for the encounter is for treatment of a primary malignancy, assign the malignancy as the principal/first-listed diagnosis. The primary site is to be sequenced first, followed by any metastatic sites.

2) Encounter for treatment of secondary malignancy
When an encounter is for a primary malignancy with metastasis and treatment is directed toward the metastatic (secondary) site(s) only, the metastatic site(s) is designated as the principal/first-listed diagnosis. The primary malignancy is coded as an additional code.

3) Malignant neoplasm in a pregnant patient
When a pregnant woman has a malignant neoplasm, a code from subcategory O9A.1-, Malignant neoplasm complicating pregnancy, childbirth, and the puerperium, should be sequenced first, followed by the appropriate code from Chapter 2 to indicate the type of neoplasm.

4) Encounter for complication associated with a neoplasm
When an encounter is for management of a complication associated with a neoplasm, such as dehydration, and the treatment is only for the complication, the complication is coded first, followed by the appropriate code(s) for the neoplasm.

The exception to this guideline is anemia. When the admission/encounter is for management of an anemia associated with the malignancy, and the treatment is only for anemia, the appropriate code for the malignancy is sequenced as the principal or first-listed diagnosis followed by code D63.0, Anemia in neoplastic disease.

5) Complication from surgical procedure for treatment of a neoplasm
When an encounter is for treatment of a complication resulting from a surgical procedure performed for the treatment of the neoplasm, designate the complication as the principal/first-listed diagnosis. See guideline regarding the coding of a current malignancy versus personal history to determine if the code for the neoplasm should also be assigned.

6) Pathologic fracture due to a neoplasm
When an encounter is for a pathological fracture due to a neoplasm, and the focus of treatment is the fracture, a code from subcategory M84.5, Pathological fracture in neoplastic disease, should be sequenced first, followed by the code for the neoplasm.

If the focus of treatment is the neoplasm with an associated pathological fracture, the neoplasm code should be sequenced first, followed by a code from M84.5 for the pathological fracture.

m. Current malignancy versus personal history of malignancy
When a primary malignancy has been excised but further treatment, such as an additional surgery for the malignancy, radiation therapy or chemotherapy is directed to that site, the primary malignancy code should be used until treatment is completed.

When a primary malignancy has been previously excised or eradicated from its site, there is no further treatment (of the malignancy) directed to that site, and there is no evidence of any existing primary malignancy, a code from category Z85, Personal history of malignant neoplasm, should be used to indicate the former site of the malignancy.

See Section I.C.21. Factors influencing health status and contact with health services, History (of)

n. Leukemia, Multiple Myeloma, and Malignant Plasma Cell Neoplasms in remission versus personal history
The categories for leukemia, and category C90, Multiple myeloma and malignant plasma cell neoplasms, have codes indicating whether or not the leukemia has achieved remission. There are also codes Z85.6, Personal history of leukemia, and Z85.79, Personal history of other malignant neoplasms of lymphoid, hematopoietic and related tissues. If the documentation is unclear, as to whether the leukemia has achieved remission, the provider should be queried.

See Section I.C.21. Factors influencing health status and contact with health services, History (of)

o. Aftercare following surgery for neoplasm
See Section I.C.21. Factors influencing health status and contact with health services, Aftercare

p. Follow-up care for completed treatment of a malignancy
See Section I.C.21. Factors influencing health status and contact with health services, Follow-up

q. Prophylactic organ removal for prevention of malignancy
See Section I.C. 21, Factors influencing health status and contact with health services, Prophylactic organ removal

r. Malignant neoplasm associated with transplanted organ
A malignant neoplasm of a transplanted organ should be coded as a transplant complication. Assign first the appropriate code from category T86.-, Complications of transplanted organs and tissue, followed by code C80.2, Malignant neoplasm associated with transplanted organ. Use an additional code for the specific malignancy.

3. Chapter 3: Disease of the blood and blood-forming organs and certain disorders involving the immune mechanism (D50-D89)
Reserved for future guideline expansion

4. Chapter 4: Endocrine, Nutritional, and Metabolic Diseases (E00-E89)

a. Diabetes mellitus
The diabetes mellitus codes are combination codes that include the type of diabetes mellitus, the body system affected, and the complications affecting that body system. As many codes within a particular category as are necessary to describe all of the complications of the disease may be used. They should be sequenced based on the reason for a particular encounter. Assign as many codes from categories E08 – E13 as needed to identify all of the associated conditions that the patient has.

1) Type of diabetes
The age of a patient is not the sole determining factor, though most type 1 diabetics develop the condition before reaching puberty. For this reason type 1 diabetes mellitus is also referred to as juvenile diabetes.

2) Type of diabetes mellitus not documented
If the type of diabetes mellitus is not documented in the medical record the default is E11.-, Type 2 diabetes mellitus.

3) Diabetes mellitus and the use of insulin
If the documentation in a medical record does not indicate the type of diabetes but does indicate that the patient uses insulin, code E11, Type 2 diabetes mellitus, should be assigned. Code Z79.4, Long-term (current) use of insulin, should also be assigned to indicate that the patient uses insulin. Code Z79.4 should not be assigned if insulin is given temporarily to bring a type 2 patient's blood sugar under control during an encounter.

4) Diabetes mellitus in pregnancy and gestational diabetes
See Section I.C.15. Diabetes mellitus in pregnancy.

See Section I.C.15. Gestational (pregnancy induced) diabetes

5) Complications due to insulin pump malfunction
(a) Underdose of insulin due to insulin pump failure

An underdose of insulin due to an insulin pump failure should be assigned to a code from subcategory T85.6, Mechanical complication of other specified internal and external prosthetic devices, implants and grafts, that specifies the type of pump malfunction, as the principal or first-listed code, followed by code T38.3x6-, Underdosing of insulin and oral hypoglycemic [antidiabetic] drugs. Additional codes for the type of diabetes mellitus and any associated complications due to the underdosing should also be assigned.

(b) Overdose of insulin due to insulin pump failure

The principal or first-listed code for an encounter due to an insulin pump malfunction resulting in an overdose of insulin, should also be T85.6-, Mechanical complication of other specified internal and external prosthetic devices, implants and grafts, followed by code T38.3x1-, Poisoning by insulin and oral hypoglycemic [antidiabetic] drugs, accidental (unintentional).

6) Secondary diabetes mellitus
Codes under categories E08, Diabetes mellitus due to underlying condition, E09, Drug or chemical induced diabetes mellitus, and

E13, Other specified diabetes mellitus, identify complications/ manifestations associated with secondary diabetes mellitus. Secondary diabetes is always caused by another condition or event (e.g., cystic fibrosis, malignant neoplasm of pancreas, pancreatectomy, adverse effect of drug, or poisoning).

(a) Secondary diabetes mellitus and the use of insulin

For patients who routinely use insulin, code Z79.4, Long-term (current) use of insulin, should also be assigned. Code Z79.4 should not be assigned if insulin is given temporarily to bring a patient's blood sugar under control during an encounter.

(b) Assigning and sequencing secondary diabetes codes and its causes

The sequencing of the secondary diabetes codes in relationship to codes for the cause of the diabetes is based on the Tabular List instructions for categories E08, E09 and E13.

(i) Secondary diabetes mellitus due to pancreatectomy

For postpancreatectomy diabetes mellitus (lack of insulin due to the surgical removal of all or part of the pancreas), assign code E89.1, Postprocedural hypoinsulinemia. Assign a code from category E13 and a code from subcategory Z90.41-, Acquired absence of pancreas, as additional codes.

(ii) Secondary diabetes due to drugs

Secondary diabetes may be caused by an adverse effect of correctly administered medications, poisoning or sequela of poisoning.

See section I.C.19.e for coding of adverse effects and poisoning, and section I.C.20 for external cause code reporting.

5. **Chapter 5: Mental, Behavioral and Neurodevelopmental Disorders (F01 – F99)**

a. **Pain disorders related to psychological factors**

Assign code F45.41, for pain that is exclusively related to psychological disorders. As indicated by the Excludes 1 note under category G89, a code from category G89 should not be assigned with code F45.41

Code F45.42, Pain disorders with related psychological factors, should be used with a code from category G89, Pain, not elsewhere classified, if there is documentation of a psychological component for a patient with acute or chronic pain.

See Section I.C.6. Pain

b. **Mental and behavioral disorders due to psychoactive substance use**

1) **In Remission**

Selection of codes for "in remission" for categories F10-F19, Mental and behavioral disorders due to psychoactive substance use (categories F10-F19 with -.21) requires the provider's clinical judgment. The appropriate codes for "in remission" are assigned only on the basis of provider documentation (as defined in the Official Guidelines for Coding and Reporting).

2) **Psychoactive Substance Use, Abuse And Dependence**

When the provider documentation refers to use, abuse and dependence of the same substance (e.g. alcohol, opioid, cannabis, etc.), only one code should be assigned to identify the pattern of use based on the following hierarchy:

- If both use and abuse are documented, assign only the code for abuse
- If both abuse and dependence are documented, assign only the code for dependence
- If use, abuse and dependence are all documented, assign only the code for dependence
- If both use and dependence are documented, assign only the code for dependence.

3) **Psychoactive Substance Use**

As with all other diagnoses, the codes for psychoactive substance use (F10.9-, F11.9-, F12.9-, F13.9-, F14.9-, F15.9-, F16.9-) should only be assigned based on provider documentation and when they meet the definition of a reportable diagnosis (see Section III, Reporting Additional Diagnoses). The codes are to be used only when the psychoactive substance use is associated with a mental or behavioral disorder, and such a relationship is documented by the provider.

6. **Chapter 6: Diseases of the Nervous System (G00-G99)**

a. **Dominant/nondominant side**

Codes from category G81, Hemiplegia and hemiparesis, and subcategories, G83.1, Monoplegia of lower limb, G83.2, Monoplegia of upper limb, and G83.3, Monoplegia, unspecified, identify whether the dominant or nondominant side is affected. Should the affected side be documented, but not specified as dominant or nondominant, and the classification system does not indicate a default, code selection is as follows:

- For ambidextrous patients, the default should be dominant.
- If the left side is affected, the default is non-dominant.
- If the right side is affected, the default is dominant.

b. **Pain - Category G89**

1) **General coding information**

Codes in category G89, Pain, not elsewhere classified, may be used in conjunction with codes from other categories and chapters to provide more detail about acute or chronic pain and neoplasm-related pain, unless otherwise indicated below.

If the pain is not specified as acute or chronic, post-thoracotomy, postprocedural, or neoplasm-related, do not assign codes from category G89.

A code from category G89 should not be assigned if the underlying (definitive) diagnosis is known, unless the reason for the encounter is pain control/ management and not management of the underlying condition.

When an admission or encounter is for a procedure aimed at treating the underlying condition (e.g., spinal fusion, kyphoplasty), a code for the underlying condition (e.g., vertebral fracture, spinal stenosis) should be assigned as the principal diagnosis. No code from category G89 should be assigned.

(a) **Category G89 codes as principal or first-listed diagnosis**

Category G89 codes are acceptable as principal diagnosis or the first-listed code:

- When pain control or pain management is the reason for the admission/encounter (e.g., a patient with displaced intervertebral disc, nerve impingement and severe back pain presents for injection of steroid into the spinal canal). The underlying cause of the pain should be reported as an additional diagnosis, if known.
- When a patient is admitted for the insertion of a neurostimulator for pain control, assign the appropriate pain code as the principal or first-listed diagnosis. When an admission or encounter is for a procedure aimed at treating the underlying condition and a neurostimulator is inserted for pain control during the same admission/ encounter, a code for the underlying condition should be assigned as the principal diagnosis and the appropriate pain code should be assigned as a secondary diagnosis.

(b) **Use of category G89 codes in conjunction with site specific pain codes**

(i) **Assigning category G89 and site-specific pain codes**

Codes from category G89 may be used in conjunction with codes that identify the site of pain (including codes from chapter 18) if the category G89 code provides additional information. For example, if the code describes the site of the pain, but does not fully describe whether the pain is acute or chronic, then both codes should be assigned.

(ii) **Sequencing of category G89 codes with site-specific pain codes**

The sequencing of category G89 codes with site-specific pain codes (including chapter 18 codes), is dependent on the circumstances of the encounter/admission as follows:

- If the encounter is for pain control or pain management, assign the code from category G89 followed by the code identifying the specific site of pain (e.g., encounter for pain management for acute neck pain from trauma is assigned code G89.11,

Acute pain due to trauma, followed by code M54.2, Cervicalgia, to identify the site of pain).

- If the encounter is for any other reason except pain control or pain management, and a related definitive diagnosis has not been established (confirmed) by the provider, assign the code for the specific site of pain first, followed by the appropriate code from category G89.

2) Pain due to devices, implants and grafts
See Section I.C.19. Pain due to medical devices

3) Postoperative Pain
The provider's documentation should be used to guide the coding of postoperative pain, as well as *Section III. Reporting Additional Diagnoses* and *Section IV. Diagnostic Coding and Reporting in the Outpatient Setting.*

The default for post-thoracotomy and other postoperative pain not specified as acute or chronic is the code for the acute form.

Routine or expected postoperative pain immediately after surgery should not be coded.

(a) Postoperative pain not associated with specific postoperative complication
Postoperative pain not associated with a specific postoperative complication is assigned to the appropriate postoperative pain code in category G89.

(b) Postoperative pain associated with specific postoperative complication
Postoperative pain associated with a specific postoperative complication (such as painful wire sutures) is assigned to the appropriate code(s) found in Chapter 19, Injury, poisoning, and certain other consequences of external causes. If appropriate, use additional code(s) from category G89 to identify acute or chronic pain (G89.18 or G89.28).

4) Chronic pain
Chronic pain is classified to subcategory G89.2. There is no time frame defining when pain becomes chronic pain. The provider's documentation should be used to guide use of these codes.

5) Neoplasm Related Pain
Code G89.3 is assigned to pain documented as being related, associated or due to cancer, primary or secondary malignancy, or tumor. This code is assigned regardless of whether the pain is acute or chronic.

This code may be assigned as the principal or first-listed code when the stated reason for the admission/encounter is documented as pain control/pain management. The underlying neoplasm should be reported as an additional diagnosis.

When the reason for the admission/encounter is management of the neoplasm and the pain associated with the neoplasm is also documented, code G89.3 may be assigned as an additional diagnosis. It is not necessary to assign an additional code for the site of the pain.

See Section I.C.2 for instructions on the sequencing of neoplasms for all other stated reasons for the admission/encounter (except for pain control/pain management).

6) Chronic pain syndrome
Central pain syndrome (G89.0) and chronic pain syndrome (G89.4) are different than the term "chronic pain," and therefore codes should only be used when the provider has specifically documented this condition.

See Section I.C.5. Pain disorders related to psychological factors

7. Chapter 7: Diseases of the Eye and Adnexa (H00-H59)
a. Glaucoma
1) Assigning Glaucoma Codes
Assign as many codes from category H40, Glaucoma, as needed to identify the type of glaucoma, the affected eye, and the glaucoma stage.

2) Bilateral glaucoma with same type and stage
When a patient has bilateral glaucoma and both eyes are documented as being the same type and stage, and there is a code for bilateral glaucoma, report only the code for the type of glaucoma, bilateral, with the seventh character for the stage.

When a patient has bilateral glaucoma and both eyes are documented as being the same type and stage, and the classification does not provide a code for bilateral glaucoma (i.e. subcategories H40.10, H40.11 and H40.20) report only one code for the type of glaucoma with the appropriate seventh character for the stage.

3) Bilateral glaucoma stage with different types or stages
When a patient has bilateral glaucoma and each eye is documented as having a different type or stage, and the classification distinguishes laterality, assign the appropriate code for each eye rather than the code for bilateral glaucoma.

When a patient has bilateral glaucoma and each eye is documented as having a different type, and the classification does not distinguish laterality (i.e. subcategories H40.10, H40.11 and H40.20), assign one code for each type of glaucoma with the appropriate seventh character for the stage.

When a patient has bilateral glaucoma and each eye is documented as having the same type, but different stage, and the classification does not distinguish laterality (i.e. subcategories H40.10, H40.11 and H40.20), assign a code for the type of glaucoma for each eye with the seventh character for the specific glaucoma stage documented for each eye.

4) Patient admitted with glaucoma and stage evolves during the admission
If a patient is admitted with glaucoma and the stage progresses during the admission, assign the code for highest stage documented.

5) Indeterminate stage glaucoma
Assignment of the seventh character "4" for "indeterminate stage" should be based on the clinical documentation. The seventh character "4" is used for glaucomas whose stage cannot be clinically determined. This seventh character should not be confused with the seventh character "0", unspecified, which should be assigned when there is no documentation regarding the stage of the glaucoma.

8. Chapter 8: Diseases of the Ear and Mastoid Process (H60-H95)
Reserved for future guideline expansion

9. Chapter 9: Diseases of the Circulatory System (I00-I99)
a. Hypertension
1) Hypertension with Heart Disease
Heart conditions classified to I50.- or I51.4-I51.9, are assigned to, a code from category I11, Hypertensive heart disease, when a causal relationship is stated (due to hypertension) or implied (hypertensive). Use an additional code from category I50, Heart failure, to identify the type of heart failure in those patients with heart failure.

The same heart conditions (I50.-, I51.4-I51.9) with hypertension, but without a stated causal relationship, are coded separately. Sequence according to the circumstances of the admission/encounter.

2) Hypertensive Chronic Kidney Disease
Assign codes from category I12, Hypertensive chronic kidney disease, when both hypertension and a condition classifiable to category N18, Chronic kidney disease (CKD), are present. Unlike hypertension with heart disease, ICD-10-CM presumes a cause-and-effect relationship and classifies chronic kidney disease with hypertension as hypertensive chronic kidney disease.

The appropriate code from category N18 should be used as a secondary code with a code from category I12 to identify the stage of chronic kidney disease.

See Section I.C.14. Chronic kidney disease.

If a patient has hypertensive chronic kidney disease and acute renal failure, an additional code for the acute renal failure is required.

3) Hypertensive Heart and Chronic Kidney Disease
Assign codes from combination category I13, Hypertensive heart and chronic kidney disease, when both hypertensive kidney disease and hypertensive heart disease are stated in the diagnosis. Assume a relationship between the hypertension and the chronic kidney disease, whether or not the condition is so designated. If heart failure is present, assign an additional code from category I50 to identify the type of heart failure.

The appropriate code from category N18, Chronic kidney disease, should be used as a secondary code with a code from category I13 to identify the stage of chronic kidney disease.

See Section I.C.14. Chronic kidney disease.

The codes in category I13, Hypertensive heart and chronic kidney disease, are combination codes that include hypertension, heart disease and chronic kidney disease. The Includes note at I13 specifies that the conditions included at I11 and I12 are included together in I13. If a patient has hypertension, heart disease and chronic kidney disease then a code from I13 should be used, not individual codes for hypertension, heart disease and chronic kidney disease, or codes from I11 or I12.

For patients with both acute renal failure and chronic kidney disease an additional code for acute renal failure is required.

4) **Hypertensive Cerebrovascular Disease**
For hypertensive cerebrovascular disease, first assign the appropriate code from categories I60-I69, followed by the appropriate hypertension code.

5) **Hypertensive Retinopathy**
Subcategory H35.0, Background retinopathy and retinal vascular changes, should be used with a code from category I10 – I15, Hypertensive disease to include the systemic hypertension. The sequencing is based on the reason for the encounter.

6) **Hypertension, Secondary**
Secondary hypertension is due to an underlying condition. Two codes are required: one to identify the underlying etiology and one from category I15 to identify the hypertension. Sequencing of codes is determined by the reason for admission/encounter.

7) **Hypertension, Transient**
Assign code R03.0, Elevated blood pressure reading without diagnosis of hypertension, unless patient has an established diagnosis of hypertension. Assign code O13.-, Gestational [pregnancy-induced] hypertension without significant proteinuria, or O14.-, Pre-eclampsia, for transient hypertension of pregnancy.

8) **Hypertension, Controlled**
This diagnostic statement usually refers to an existing state of hypertension under control by therapy. Assign the appropriate code from categories I10-I15, Hypertensive diseases.

9) **Hypertension, Uncontrolled**
Uncontrolled hypertension may refer to untreated hypertension or hypertension not responding to current therapeutic regimen. In either case, assign the appropriate code from categories I10-I15, Hypertensive diseases.

b. **Atherosclerotic Coronary Artery Disease and Angina**
ICD-10-CM has combination codes for atherosclerotic heart disease with angina pectoris. The subcategories for these codes are I25.11, Atherosclerotic heart disease of native coronary artery with angina pectoris and I25.7, Atherosclerosis of coronary artery bypass graft(s) and coronary artery of transplanted heart with angina pectoris.

When using one of these combination codes it is not necessary to use an additional code for angina pectoris. A causal relationship can be assumed in a patient with both atherosclerosis and angina pectoris, unless the documentation indicates the angina is due to something other than the atherosclerosis.

If a patient with coronary artery disease is admitted due to an acute myocardial infarction (AMI), the AMI should be sequenced before the coronary artery disease.

See Section I.C.9. Acute myocardial infarction (AMI)

c. **Intraoperative and Postprocedural Cerebrovascular Accident**

Medical record documentation should clearly specify the cause-and-effect relationship between the medical intervention and the cerebrovascular accident in order to assign a code for intraoperative or postprocedural cerebrovascular accident.

Proper code assignment depends on whether it was an infarction or hemorrhage and whether it occurred intraoperatively or postoperatively. If it was a cerebral hemorrhage, code assignment depends on the type of procedure performed.

d. **Sequelae of Cerebrovascular Disease**
1) **Category I69, Sequelae of Cerebrovascular disease**
Category I69 is used to indicate conditions classifiable to categories I60-I67 as the causes of sequela (neurologic deficits), themselves classified elsewhere. These "late effects" include neurologic deficits that persist after initial onset of conditions classifiable to categories I60-I67. The neurologic deficits caused by cerebrovascular disease may be present from the onset or may arise at any time after the onset of the condition classifiable to categories I60-I67.

Codes from category I69, Sequelae of cerebrovascular disease, that specify hemiplegia, hemiparesis and monoplegia identify whether the dominant or nondominant side is affected. Should the affected side be documented, but not specified as dominant or nondominant, and the classification system does not indicate a default, code selection is as follows:

- For ambidextrous patients, the default should be dominant.
- If the left side is affected, the default is non-dominant.
- If the right side is affected, the default is dominant.

2) **Codes from category I69 with codes from I60-I67**
Codes from category I69 may be assigned on a health care record with codes from I60-I67, if the patient has a current cerebrovascular disease and deficits from an old cerebrovascular disease.

3) **Codes from category I69 and Personal history of transient ischemic attack (TIA) and cerebral infarction (Z86.73)**
Codes from category I69 should not be assigned if the patient does not have neurologic deficits.

See Section I.C.21. 4. History (of) for use of personal history codes

e. **Acute myocardial infarction (AMI)**
1) **ST elevation myocardial infarction (STEMI) and non ST elevation myocardial infarction (NSTEMI)**
The ICD-10-CM codes for acute myocardial infarction (AMI) identify the site, such as anterolateral wall or true posterior wall. Subcategories I21.0-I21.2 and code I21.3 are used for ST elevation myocardial infarction (STEMI). Code I21.4, Non-ST elevation (NSTEMI) myocardial infarction, is used for non ST elevation myocardial infarction (NSTEMI) and nontransmural MIs.

If NSTEMI evolves to STEMI, assign the STEMI code. If STEMI converts to NSTEMI due to thrombolytic therapy, it is still coded as STEMI.

For encounters occurring while the myocardial infarction is equal to, or less than, four weeks old, including transfers to another acute setting or a postacute setting, and the patient requires continued care for the myocardial infarction, codes from category I21 may continue to be reported. For encounters after the 4 week time frame and the patient is still receiving care related to the myocardial infarction, the appropriate aftercare code should be assigned, rather than a code from category I21. For old or healed myocardial infarctions not requiring further care, code I25.2, Old myocardial infarction, may be assigned.

2) **Acute myocardial infarction, unspecified**
Code I21.3, ST elevation (STEMI) myocardial infarction of unspecified site, is the default for unspecified acute myocardial infarction. If only STEMI or transmural MI without the site is documented, assign code I21.3.

3) **AMI documented as nontransmural or subendocardial but site provided**
If an AMI is documented as nontransmural or subendocardial, but the site is provided, it is still coded as a subendocardial AMI.

See Section I.C.21.3 for information on coding status post administration of tPA in a different facility within the last 24 hours.

4) **Subsequent acute myocardial infarction**
A code from category I22, Subsequent ST elevation (STEMI) and non ST elevation (NSTEMI) myocardial infarction, is to be used when a patient who has suffered an AMI has a new AMI within the 4 week time frame of the initial AMI. A code from category I22 must be used in conjunction with a code from category I21. The sequencing of the I22 and I21 codes depends on the circumstances of the encounter.

10. **Chapter 10: Diseases of the Respiratory System (J00-J99)**
   a. **Chronic Obstructive Pulmonary Disease [COPD] and Asthma**
      1) **Acute exacerbation of chronic obstructive bronchitis and asthma**
      The codes in categories J44 and J45 distinguish between uncomplicated cases and those in acute exacerbation. An acute exacerbation is a worsening or a decompensation of a chronic condition. An acute exacerbation is not equivalent to an infection superimposed on a chronic condition, though an exacerbation may be triggered by an infection.

   b. **Acute Respiratory Failure**
      1) **Acute respiratory failure as principal diagnosis**
      A code from subcategory J96.0, Acute respiratory failure, or subcategory J96.2, Acute and chronic respiratory failure, may be assigned as a principal diagnosis when it is the condition established after study to be chiefly responsible for occasioning the admission to the hospital, and the selection is supported by the Alphabetic Index and Tabular List. However, chapter-specific coding guidelines (such as obstetrics, poisoning, HIV, newborn) that provide sequencing direction take precedence.

      2) **Acute respiratory failure as secondary diagnosis**
      Respiratory failure may be listed as a secondary diagnosis if it occurs after admission, or if it is present on admission, but does not meet the definition of principal diagnosis.

      3) **Sequencing of acute respiratory failure and another acute condition**
      When a patient is admitted with respiratory failure and another acute condition, (e.g., myocardial infarction, cerebrovascular accident, aspiration pneumonia), the principal diagnosis will not be the same in every situation. This applies whether the other acute condition is a respiratory or nonrespiratory condition. Selection of the principal diagnosis will be dependent on the circumstances of admission. If both the respiratory failure and the other acute condition are equally responsible for occasioning the admission to the hospital, and there are no chapter-specific sequencing rules, the guideline regarding two or more diagnoses that equally meet the definition for principal diagnosis (Section II, C.) may be applied in these situations.

      If the documentation is not clear as to whether acute respiratory failure and another condition are equally responsible for occasioning the admission, query the provider for clarification.

   c. **Influenza due to certain identified influenza viruses**
   Code only confirmed cases of influenza due to certain identified influenza viruses (category J09), and due to other identified influenza virus (category J10). This is an exception to the hospital inpatient guideline Section II, H. (Uncertain Diagnosis).

   In this context, "confirmation" does not require documentation of positive laboratory testing specific for avian or other novel influenza A or other identified influenza virus. However, coding should be based on the provider's diagnostic statement that the patient has avian influenza, or other novel influenza A, for category J09, or has another particular identified strain of influenza, such as H1N1 or H3N2, but not identified as novel or variant, for category J10.

   If the provider records "suspected" or "possible" or "probable" avian influenza, or novel influenza, or other identified influenza, then the appropriate influenza code from category J11, Influenza due to unidentified influenza virus, should be assigned. A code from category J09, Influenza due to certain identified influenza viruses, should not be assigned nor should a code from category J10, Influenza due to other identified influenza virus.

   d. **Ventilator associated Pneumonia**
      1) **Documentation of Ventilator associated Pneumonia**
      As with all procedural or postprocedural complications, code assignment is based on the provider's documentation of the relationship between the condition and the procedure.

      Code J95.851, Ventilator associated pneumonia, should be assigned only when the provider has documented ventilator associated pneumonia (VAP). An additional code to identify the organism (e.g., Pseudomonas aeruginosa, code B96.5) should also be assigned. Do not assign an additional code from categories J12-J18 to identify the type of pneumonia.

      Code J95.851 should not be assigned for cases where the patient has pneumonia and is on a mechanical ventilator and the provider has not specifically stated that the pneumonia is ventilator-associated pneumonia. If the documentation is unclear as to whether the patient has a pneumonia that is a complication attributable to the mechanical ventilator, query the provider.

      2) **Ventilator associated Pneumonia Develops after Admission**
      A patient may be admitted with one type of pneumonia (e.g., code J13, Pneumonia due to Streptococcus pneumonia) and subsequently develop VAP. In this instance, the principal diagnosis would be the appropriate code from categories J12-J18 for the pneumonia diagnosed at the time of admission. Code J95.851, Ventilator associated pneumonia, would be assigned as an additional diagnosis when the provider has also documented the presence of ventilator associated pneumonia.

11. **Chapter 11: Diseases of the Digestive System (K00-K95)**
   Reserved for future guideline expansion

12. **Chapter 12: Diseases of the Skin and Subcutaneous Tissue (L00-L99)**
   a. **Pressure ulcer stage codes**
      1) **Pressure ulcer stages**
      Codes from category L89, Pressure ulcer, are combination codes that identify the site of the pressure ulcer as well as the stage of the ulcer.

      The ICD-10-CM classifies pressure ulcer stages based on severity, which is designated by stages 1-4, unspecified stage and unstageable.

      Assign as many codes from category L89 as needed to identify all the pressure ulcers the patient has, if applicable.

      2) **Unstageable pressure ulcers**
      Assignment of the code for unstageable pressure ulcer (L89.--0) should be based on the clinical documentation. These codes are used for pressure ulcers whose stage cannot be clinically determined (e.g., the ulcer is covered by eschar or has been treated with a skin or muscle graft) and pressure ulcers that are documented as deep tissue injury but not documented as due to trauma. This code should not be confused with the codes for unspecified stage (L89.--9). When there is no documentation regarding the stage of the pressure ulcer, assign the appropriate code for unspecified stage (L89.--9).

      3) **Documented pressure ulcer stage**
      Assignment of the pressure ulcer stage code should be guided by clinical documentation of the stage or documentation of the terms found in the Alphabetic Index. For clinical terms describing the stage that are not found in the Alphabetic Index, and there is no documentation of the stage, the provider should be queried.

      4) **Patients admitted with pressure ulcers documented as healed**
      No code is assigned if the documentation states that the pressure ulcer is completely healed.

      5) **Patients admitted with pressure ulcers documented as healing**
      Pressure ulcers described as healing should be assigned the appropriate pressure ulcer stage code based on the documentation in the medical record. If the documentation does not provide information about the stage of the healing pressure ulcer, assign the appropriate code for unspecified stage.

      If the documentation is unclear as to whether the patient has a current (new) pressure ulcer or if the patient is being treated for a healing pressure ulcer, query the provider.

      6) **Patient admitted with pressure ulcer evolving into another stage during the admission**
      If a patient is admitted with a pressure ulcer at one stage and it progresses to a higher stage, assign the code for the highest stage reported for that site.

13. **Chapter 13: Diseases of the Musculoskeletal System and Connective Tissue (M00-M99)**
   a. **Site and laterality**
   Most of the codes within Chapter 13 have site and laterality designations. The site represents the bone, joint or the muscle involved. For some conditions where more than one bone, joint or muscle is usually involved, such as osteoarthritis, there is a "multiple sites" code available. For categories where no multiple site code is provided and more than one bone, joint or muscle is involved, multiple codes should be used to indicate the different sites involved.

1) Bone versus joint
For certain conditions, the bone may be affected at the upper or lower end, (e.g., avascular necrosis of bone, M87, Osteoporosis, M80, M81). Though the portion of the bone affected may be at the joint, the site designation will be the bone, not the joint.

b. Acute traumatic versus chronic or recurrent musculoskeletal conditions
Many musculoskeletal conditions are a result of previous injury or trauma to a site, or are recurrent conditions. Bone, joint or muscle conditions that are the result of a healed injury are usually found in chapter 13. Recurrent bone, joint or muscle conditions are also usually found in chapter 13. Any current, acute injury should be coded to the appropriate injury code from chapter 19. Chronic or recurrent conditions should generally be coded with a code from chapter 13. If it is difficult to determine from the documentation in the record which code is best to describe a condition, query the provider.

c. Coding of Pathologic Fractures
7th character A is for use as long as the patient is receiving active treatment for the fracture. Examples of active treatment are: surgical treatment, emergency department encounter, evaluation and treatment by a new physician. 7th character, D is to be used for encounters after the patient has completed active treatment. The other 7th characters, listed under each subcategory in the Tabular List, are to be used for subsequent encounters for treatment of problems associated with the healing, such as malunions, nonunions, and sequelae.

Care for complications of surgical treatment for fracture repairs during the healing or recovery phase should be coded with the appropriate complication codes.

See Section I.C.19. Coding of traumatic fractures.

d. Osteoporosis
Osteoporosis is a systemic condition, meaning that all bones of the musculoskeletal system are affected. Therefore, site is not a component of the codes under category M81, Osteoporosis without current pathological fracture. The site codes under category M80, Osteoporosis with current pathological fracture, identify the site of the fracture, not the osteoporosis.

1) Osteoporosis without pathological fracture
Category M81, Osteoporosis without current pathological fracture, is for use for patients with osteoporosis who do not currently have a pathologic fracture due to the osteoporosis, even if they have had a fracture in the past. For patients with a history of osteoporosis fractures, status code Z87.310, Personal history of (healed) osteoporosis fracture, should follow the code from M81.

2) Osteoporosis with current pathological fracture
Category M80, Osteoporosis with current pathological fracture, is for patients who have a current pathologic fracture at the time of an encounter. The codes under M80 identify the site of the fracture. A code from category M80, not a traumatic fracture code, should be used for any patient with known osteoporosis who suffers a fracture, even if the patient had a minor fall or trauma, if that fall or trauma would not usually break a normal, healthy bone.

14. Chapter 14: Diseases of Genitourinary System (N00-N99)
a. Chronic kidney disease
1) Stages of chronic kidney disease (CKD)
The ICD-10-CM classifies CKD based on severity. The severity of CKD is designated by stages 1-5. Stage 2, code N18.2, equates to mild CKD; stage 3, code N18.3, equates to moderate CKD; and stage 4, code N18.4, equates to severe CKD. Code N18.6, End stage renal disease (ESRD), is assigned when the provider has documented end-stage-renal disease (ESRD).

If both a stage of CKD and ESRD are documented, assign code N18.6 only.

2) Chronic kidney disease and kidney transplant status
Patients who have undergone kidney transplant may still have some form of chronic kidney disease (CKD) because the kidney transplant may not fully restore kidney function. Therefore, the presence of CKD alone does not constitute a transplant complication. Assign the appropriate N18 code for the patient's stage of CKD and code Z94.0, Kidney transplant status. If a transplant complication such as failure or rejection or other transplant complication is documented, see section I.C.19.g for information on coding complications of a kidney transplant. If the documentation is unclear as to whether the patient has a complication of the transplant, query the provider.

3) Chronic kidney disease with other conditions
Patients with CKD may also suffer from other serious conditions, most commonly diabetes mellitus and hypertension. The sequencing of the CKD code in relationship to codes for other contributing conditions is based on the conventions in the Tabular List.

See I.C.9. Hypertensive chronic kidney disease.

See I.C.19. Chronic kidney disease and kidney transplant complications.

15. Chapter 15: Pregnancy, Childbirth, and the Puerperium (O00-O9A)
a. General Rules for Obstetric Cases
1) Codes from chapter 15 and sequencing priority
Obstetric cases require codes from chapter 15, codes in the range O00-O9A, Pregnancy, Childbirth, and the Puerperium. Chapter 15 codes have sequencing priority over codes from other chapters. Additional codes from other chapters may be used in conjunction with chapter 15 codes to further specify conditions. Should the provider document that the pregnancy is incidental to the encounter, then code Z33.1, Pregnant state, incidental, should be used in place of any chapter 15 codes. It is the provider's responsibility to state that the condition being treated is not affecting the pregnancy.

2) Chapter 15 codes used only on the maternal record
Chapter 15 codes are to be used only on the maternal record, never on the record of the newborn.

3) Final character for trimester
The majority of codes in Chapter 15 have a final character indicating the trimester of pregnancy. The timeframes for the trimesters are indicated at the beginning of the chapter. If trimester is not a component of a code it is because the condition always occurs in a specific trimester, or the concept of trimester of pregnancy is not applicable. Certain codes have characters for only certain trimesters because the condition does not occur in all trimesters, but it may occur in more than just one.

Assignment of the final character for trimester should be based on the provider's documentation of the trimester (or number of weeks) for the current admission/encounter. This applies to the assignment of trimester for pre-existing conditions as well as those that develop during or are due to the pregnancy. The provider's documentation of the number of weeks may be used to assign the appropriate code identifying the trimester.

Whenever delivery occurs during the current admission, and there is an "in childbirth" option for the obstetric complication being coded, the "in childbirth" code should be assigned.

4) Selection of trimester for inpatient admissions that encompass more than one trimester
In instances when a patient is admitted to a hospital for complications of pregnancy during one trimester and remains in the hospital into a subsequent trimester, the trimester character for the antepartum complication code should be assigned on the basis of the trimester when the complication developed, not the trimester of the discharge. If the condition developed prior to the current admission/encounter or represents a pre-existing condition, the trimester character for the trimester at the time of the admission/encounter should be assigned.

5) Unspecified trimester
Each category that includes codes for trimester has a code for "unspecified trimester." The "unspecified trimester" code should rarely be used, such as when the documentation in the record is insufficient to determine the trimester and it is not possible to obtain clarification.

6) 7th character for Fetus Identification
Where applicable, a 7th character is to be assigned for certain categories (O31, O32, O33.3 - O33.6, O35, O36, O40, O41, O60.1, O60.2, O64, and O69) to identify the fetus for which the complication code applies.

Assign 7th character "0":

- For single gestations
- When the documentation in the record is insufficient to determine the fetus affected and it is not possible to obtain clarification.
- When it is not possible to clinically determine which fetus is affected.

b. Selection of OB Principal or First-listed Diagnosis

1) Routine outpatient prenatal visits

For routine outpatient prenatal visits when no complications are present, a code from category Z34, Encounter for supervision of normal pregnancy, should be used as the first-listed diagnosis. These codes should not be used in conjunction with chapter 15 codes.

2) Prenatal outpatient visits for high-risk patients

For routine prenatal outpatient visits for patients with high-risk pregnancies, a code from category O09, Supervision of high-risk pregnancy, should be used as the first-listed diagnosis. Secondary chapter 15 codes may be used in conjunction with these codes if appropriate.

3) Episodes when no delivery occurs

In episodes when no delivery occurs, the principal diagnosis should correspond to the principal complication of the pregnancy which necessitated the encounter. Should more than one complication exist, all of which are treated or monitored, any of the complications codes may be sequenced first.

4) When a delivery occurs

When a delivery occurs, the principal diagnosis should correspond to the main circumstances or complication of the delivery. In cases of cesarean delivery, the selection of the principal diagnosis should be the condition established after study that was responsible for the patient's admission. If the patient was admitted with a condition that resulted in the performance of a cesarean procedure, that condition should be selected as the principal diagnosis. If the reason for the admission/encounter was unrelated to the condition resulting in the cesarean delivery, the condition related to the reason for the admission/encounter should be selected as the principal diagnosis.

5) Outcome of delivery

A code from category Z37, Outcome of delivery, should be included on every maternal record when a delivery has occurred. These codes are not to be used on subsequent records or on the newborn record.

c. Pre-existing conditions versus conditions due to the pregnancy

Certain categories in Chapter 15 distinguish between conditions of the mother that existed prior to pregnancy (pre-existing) and those that are a direct result of pregnancy. When assigning codes from Chapter 15, it is important to assess if a condition was pre-existing prior to pregnancy or developed during or due to the pregnancy in order to assign the correct code.

Categories that do not distinguish between pre-existing and pregnancy-related conditions may be used for either. It is acceptable to use codes specifically for the puerperium with codes complicating pregnancy and childbirth if a condition arises postpartum during the delivery encounter.

d. Pre-existing hypertension in pregnancy

Category O10, Pre-existing hypertension complicating pregnancy, childbirth and the puerperium, includes codes for hypertensive heart and hypertensive chronic kidney disease. When assigning one of the O10 codes that includes hypertensive heart disease or hypertensive chronic kidney disease, it is necessary to add a secondary code from the appropriate hypertension category to specify the type of heart failure or chronic kidney disease.

See Section I.C.9. Hypertension.

e. Fetal Conditions Affecting the Management of the Mother

1) Codes from categories O35 and O36

Codes from categories O35, Maternal care for known or suspected fetal abnormality and damage, and O36, Maternal care for other fetal problems, are assigned only when the fetal condition is actually responsible for modifying the management of the mother, i.e., by requiring diagnostic studies, additional observation, special care, or termination of pregnancy. The fact that the fetal condition exists does not justify assigning a code from this series to the mother's record.

2) In utero surgery

In cases when surgery is performed on the fetus, a diagnosis code from category O35, Maternal care for known or suspected fetal abnormality and damage, should be assigned identifying the fetal condition. Assign the appropriate procedure code for the procedure performed.

No code from Chapter 16, the perinatal codes, should be used on the mother's record to identify fetal conditions. Surgery performed in utero on a fetus is still to be coded as an obstetric encounter.

f. HIV Infection in Pregnancy, Childbirth and the Puerperium

During pregnancy, childbirth or the puerperium, a patient admitted because of an HIV-related illness should receive a principal diagnosis from subcategory O98.7-, Human immunodeficiency [HIV] disease complicating pregnancy, childbirth and the puerperium, followed by the code(s) for the HIV-related illness(es).

Patients with asymptomatic HIV infection status admitted during pregnancy, childbirth, or the puerperium should receive codes of O98.7- and Z21, Asymptomatic human immunodeficiency virus [HIV] infection status.

g. Diabetes mellitus in pregnancy

Diabetes mellitus is a significant complicating factor in pregnancy. Pregnant women who are diabetic should be assigned a code from category O24, Diabetes mellitus in pregnancy, childbirth, and the puerperium, first, followed by the appropriate diabetes code(s) (E08-E13) from Chapter 4.

h. Long term use of insulin

Code Z79.4, Long-term (current) use of insulin, should also be assigned if the diabetes mellitus is being treated with insulin.

i. Gestational (pregnancy induced) diabetes

Gestational (pregnancy induced) diabetes can occur during the second and third trimester of pregnancy in women who were not diabetic prior to pregnancy. Gestational diabetes can cause complications in the pregnancy similar to those of pre-existing diabetes mellitus. It also puts the woman at greater risk of developing diabetes after the pregnancy. Codes for gestational diabetes are in subcategory O24.4, Gestational diabetes mellitus. No other code from category O24,

Diabetes mellitus in pregnancy, childbirth, and the puerperium, should be used with a code from O24.4

The codes under subcategory O24.4 include diet controlled and insulin controlled. If a patient with gestational diabetes is treated with both diet and insulin, only the code for insulin-controlled is required.

Code Z79.4, Long-term (current) use of insulin, should not be assigned with codes from subcategory O24.4.

An abnormal glucose tolerance in pregnancy is assigned a code from subcategory O99.81, Abnormal glucose complicating pregnancy, childbirth, and the puerperium.

j. Sepsis and septic shock complicating abortion, pregnancy, childbirth and the puerperium

When assigning a chapter 15 code for sepsis complicating abortion, pregnancy, childbirth, and the puerperium, a code for the specific type of infection should be assigned as an additional diagnosis. If severe sepsis is present, a code from subcategory R65.2, Severe sepsis, and code(s) for associated organ dysfunction(s) should also be assigned as additional diagnoses.

k. Puerperal sepsis

Code O85, Puerperal sepsis, should be assigned with a secondary code to identify the causal organism (e.g., for a bacterial infection, assign a code from category B95-B96, Bacterial infections in conditions classified elsewhere). A code from category A40, Streptococcal sepsis, or A41, Other sepsis, should not be used for puerperal sepsis. If applicable, use additional codes to identify severe sepsis (R65.2-) and any associated acute organ dysfunction.

l. Alcohol and tobacco use during pregnancy, childbirth and the puerperium

1) Alcohol use during pregnancy, childbirth and the puerperium

Codes under subcategory O99.31, Alcohol use complicating pregnancy, childbirth, and the puerperium, should be assigned for any pregnancy case when a mother uses alcohol during the pregnancy or postpartum. A secondary code from category F10, Alcohol related disorders, should also be assigned to identify manifestations of the alcohol use.

2) **Tobacco use during pregnancy, childbirth and the puerperium**
Codes under subcategory O99.33, Smoking (tobacco) complicating pregnancy, childbirth, and the puerperium, should be assigned for any pregnancy case when a mother uses any type of tobacco product during the pregnancy or postpartum. A secondary code from category F17, Nicotine dependence, should also be assigned to identify the type of nicotine dependence.

m. **Poisoning, toxic effects, adverse effects and underdosing in a pregnant patient**
A code from subcategory O9A.2, Injury, poisoning and certain other consequences of external causes complicating pregnancy, childbirth, and the puerperium, should be sequenced first, followed by the appropriate injury, poisoning, toxic effect, adverse effect or underdosing code, and then the additional code(s) that specifies the condition caused by the poisoning, toxic effect, adverse effect or underdosing.

See Section I.C.19. Adverse effects, poisoning, underdosing and toxic effects.

n. **Normal Delivery, Code O80**
1) **Encounter for full term uncomplicated delivery**
Code O80 should be assigned when a woman is admitted for a full-term normal delivery and delivers a single, healthy infant without any complications antepartum, during the delivery, or postpartum during the delivery episode. Code O80 is always a principal diagnosis. It is not to be used if any other code from chapter 15 is needed to describe a current complication of the antenatal, delivery, or perinatal period. Additional codes from other chapters may be used with code O80 if they are not related to or are in any way complicating the pregnancy.

2) **Uncomplicated delivery with resolved antepartum complication**
Code O80 may be used if the patient had a complication at some point during the pregnancy, but the complication is not present at the time of the admission for delivery.

3) **Outcome of delivery for O80**
Z37.0, Single live birth, is the only outcome of delivery code appropriate for use with O80.

o. **The Peripartum and Postpartum Periods**
1) **Peripartum and Postpartum periods**
The postpartum period begins immediately after delivery and continues for six weeks following delivery. The peripartum period is defined as the last month of pregnancy to five months postpartum.

2) **Peripartum and postpartum complication**
A postpartum complication is any complication occurring within the six-week period.

3) **Pregnancy-related complications after 6 week period**
Chapter 15 codes may also be used to describe pregnancy-related complications after the peripartum or postpartum period if the provider documents that a condition is pregnancy related.

4) **Admission for routine postpartum care following delivery outside hospital**
When the mother delivers outside the hospital prior to admission and is admitted for routine postpartum care and no complications are noted, code Z39.0, Encounter for care and examination of mother immediately after delivery, should be assigned as the principal diagnosis.

5) **Pregnancy associated cardiomyopathy**
Pregnancy associated cardiomyopathy, code O90.3, is unique in that it may be diagnosed in the third trimester of pregnancy but may continue to progress months after delivery. For this reason, it is referred to as peripartum cardiomyopathy. Code O90.3 is only for use when the cardiomyopathy develops as a result of pregnancy in a woman who did not have pre-existing heart disease.

p. **Code O94, Sequelae of complication of pregnancy, childbirth, and the puerperium**
1) **Code O94**
Code O94, Sequelae of complication of pregnancy, childbirth, and the puerperium, is for use in those cases when an initial complication of a pregnancy develops a sequelae requiring care or treatment at a future date.

2) **After the initial postpartum period**
This code may be used at any time after the initial postpartum period.

3) **Sequencing of Code O94**
This code, like all sequela codes, is to be sequenced following the code describing the sequelae of the complication.

q. **Termination of Pregnancy and Spontaneous abortions**
1) **Abortion with Liveborn Fetus**
When an attempted termination of pregnancy results in a liveborn fetus, assign code Z33.2, Encounter for elective termination of pregnancy and a code from category Z37, Outcome of Delivery.

2) **Retained Products of Conception following an abortion**
Subsequent encounters for retained products of conception following a spontaneous abortion or elective termination of pregnancy are assigned the appropriate code from category O03, Spontaneous abortion, or codes O07.4, Failed attempted termination of pregnancy without complication and Z33.2, Encounter for elective termination of pregnancy. This advice is appropriate even when the patient was discharged previously with a discharge diagnosis of complete abortion.

3) **Complications leading to abortion**
Codes from Chapter 15 may be used as additional codes to identify any documented complications of the pregnancy in conjunction with codes in categories in O07 and O08.

r. **Abuse in a pregnant patient**
For suspected or confirmed cases of abuse of a pregnant patient, a code(s) from subcategories O9A.3, Physical abuse complicating pregnancy, childbirth, and the puerperium, O9A.4, Sexual abuse complicating pregnancy, childbirth, and the puerperium, and O9A.5, Psychological abuse complicating pregnancy, childbirth, and the puerperium, should be sequenced first, followed by the appropriate codes (if applicable) to identify any associated current injury due to physical abuse, sexual abuse, and the perpetrator of abuse.

See Section I.C.19. Adult and child abuse, neglect and other maltreatment.

16. **Chapter 16: Certain Conditions Originating in the Perinatal Period (P00-P96)**
For coding and reporting purposes the perinatal period is defined as before birth through the 28th day following birth. The following guidelines are provided for reporting purposes

a. **General Perinatal Rules**
1) **Use of Chapter 16 Codes**
Codes in this chapter are never for use on the maternal record. Codes from Chapter 15, the obstetric chapter, are never permitted on the newborn record. Chapter 16 codes may be used throughout the life of the patient if the condition is still present.

2) **Principal Diagnosis for Birth Record**
When coding the birth episode in a newborn record, assign a code from category Z38, Liveborn infants according to place of birth and type of delivery, as the principal diagnosis. A code from category Z38 is assigned only once, to a newborn at the time of birth. If a newborn is transferred to another institution, a code from category Z38 should not be used at the receiving hospital.

A code from category Z38 is used only on the newborn record, not on the mother's record.

3) **Use of Codes from other Chapters with Codes from Chapter 16**
Codes from other chapters may be used with codes from chapter 16 if the codes from the other chapters provide more specific detail. Codes for signs and symptoms may be assigned when a definitive diagnosis has not been established. If the reason for the encounter is a perinatal condition, the code from chapter 16 should be sequenced first.

4) **Use of Chapter 16 Codes after the Perinatal Period**

Should a condition originate in the perinatal period, and continue throughout the life of the patient, the perinatal code should continue to be used regardless of the patient's age.

5) Birth process or community acquired conditions

If a newborn has a condition that may be either due to the birth process or community acquired and the documentation does not indicate which it is, the default is due to the birth process and the code from Chapter 16 should be used. If the condition is community-acquired, a code from Chapter 16 should not be assigned.

6) Code all clinically significant conditions

All clinically significant conditions noted on routine newborn examination should be coded. A condition is clinically significant if it requires:

- clinical evaluation; or
- therapeutic treatment; or
- diagnostic procedures; or
- extended length of hospital stay; or
- increased nursing care and/or monitoring; or
- has implications for future health care needs

   Note: The perinatal guidelines listed above are the same as the general coding guidelines for "additional diagnoses", except for the final point regarding implications for future health care needs. Codes should be assigned for conditions that have been specified by the provider as having implications for future health care needs.

b. Observation and Evaluation of Newborns for Suspected Conditions not Found

Reserved for future expansion

c. Coding Additional Perinatal Diagnoses

1) Assigning codes for conditions that require treatment

Assign codes for conditions that require treatment or further investigation, prolong the length of stay, or require resource utilization.

2) Codes for conditions specified as having implications for future health care needs

Assign codes for conditions that have been specified by the provider as having implications for future health care needs.

Note: This guideline should not be used for adult patients.

d. Prematurity and Fetal Growth Retardation

Providers utilize different criteria in determining prematurity. A code for prematurity should not be assigned unless it is documented. Assignment of codes in categories P05, Disorders of newborn related to slow fetal growth and fetal malnutrition, and P07, Disorders of newborn related to short gestation and low birth weight, not elsewhere classified, should be based on the recorded birth weight and estimated gestational age. Codes from category P05 should not be assigned with codes from category P07.

When both birth weight and gestational age are available, two codes from category P07 should be assigned, with the code for birth weight sequenced before the code for gestational age.

e. Low birth weight and immaturity status

Codes from category P07, Disorders of newborn related to short gestation and low birth weight, not elsewhere classified, are for use for a child or adult who was premature or had a low birth weight as a newborn and this is affecting the patient's current health status.

See Section I.C.21. Factors influencing health status and contact with health services, Status.

f. Bacterial Sepsis of Newborn

Category P36, Bacterial sepsis of newborn, includes congenital sepsis. If a perinate is documented as having sepsis without documentation of congenital or community acquired, the default is congenital and a code from category P36 should be assigned. If the P36 code includes the causal organism, an additional code from category B95, Streptococcus, Staphylococcus, and Enterococcus as the cause of diseases classified elsewhere, or B96, Other bacterial agents as the cause of diseases classified elsewhere, should not be assigned. If the P36 code does not include the causal organism, assign an additional code from category B96. If applicable, use additional codes to identify severe sepsis (R65.2-) and any associated acute organ dysfunction.

g. Stillbirth

Code P95, Stillbirth, is only for use in institutions that maintain separate records for stillbirths. No other code should be used with P95. Code P95 should not be used on the mother's record.

17. Chapter 17: Congenital malformations, deformations, and chromosomal abnormalities (Q00-Q99)

Assign an appropriate code(s) from categories Q00-Q99, Congenital malformations, deformations, and chromosomal abnormalities when a malformation/deformation or chromosomal abnormality is documented. A malformation/deformation/or chromosomal abnormality may be the principal/first-listed diagnosis on a record or a secondary diagnosis.

When a malformation/deformation/or chromosomal abnormality does not have a unique code assignment, assign additional code(s) for any manifestations that may be present.

When the code assignment specifically identifies the malformation/ deformation/or chromosomal abnormality, manifestations that are an inherent component of the anomaly should not be coded separately. Additional codes should be assigned for manifestations that are not an inherent component.

Codes from Chapter 17 may be used throughout the life of the patient. If a congenital malformation or deformity has been corrected, a personal history code should be used to identify the history of the malformation or deformity. Although present at birth, malformation/deformation/or chromosomal abnormality may not be identified until later in life. Whenever the condition is diagnosed by the physician, it is appropriate to assign a code from codes Q00-Q99.For the birth admission, the appropriate code from category Z38, Liveborn infants, according to place of birth and type of delivery, should be sequenced as the principal diagnosis, followed by any congenital anomaly codes, Q00- Q99.

18. Chapter 18: Symptoms, signs, and abnormal clinical and laboratory findings, not elsewhere classified (R00-R99)

Chapter 18 includes symptoms, signs, abnormal results of clinical or other investigative procedures, and ill-defined conditions regarding which no diagnosis classifiable elsewhere is recorded. Signs and symptoms that point to a specific diagnosis have been assigned to a category in other chapters of the classification.

a. Use of symptom codes

Codes that describe symptoms and signs are acceptable for reporting purposes when a related definitive diagnosis has not been established (confirmed) by the provider.

b. Use of a symptom code with a definitive diagnosis code

Codes for signs and symptoms may be reported in addition to a related definitive diagnosis when the sign or symptom is not routinely associated with that diagnosis, such as the various signs and symptoms associated with complex syndromes. The definitive diagnosis code should be sequenced before the symptom code.

Signs or symptoms that are associated routinely with a disease process should not be assigned as additional codes, unless otherwise instructed by the classification.

c. Combination codes that include symptoms

ICD-10-CM contains a number of combination codes that identify both the definitive diagnosis and common symptoms of that diagnosis. When using one of these combination codes, an additional code should not be assigned for the symptom.

d. Repeated falls

Code R29.6, Repeated falls, is for use for encounters when a patient has recently fallen and the reason for the fall is being investigated.

Code Z91.81, History of falling, is for use when a patient has fallen in the past and is at risk for future falls. When appropriate, both codes R29.6 and Z91.81 may be assigned together.

e. Coma scale

The coma scale codes (R40.2-) can be used in conjunction with traumatic brain injury codes, acute cerebrovascular disease or sequelae of cerebrovascular disease codes. These codes are primarily for use by trauma registries, but they may be used in any setting where this information is collected. The coma scale codes should be sequenced after the diagnosis code(s).

These codes, one from each subcategory, are needed to complete the scale. The 7th character indicates when the scale was recorded. The 7th character should match for all three codes.

At a minimum, report the initial score documented on presentation at your facility. This may be a score from the emergency medicine technician (EMT) or in the emergency department. If desired, a facility may choose to capture multiple coma scale scores.

Assign code R40.24, Glasgow coma scale, total score, when only the total score is documented in the medical record and not the individual score(s).

f. Functional quadriplegia
Functional quadriplegia (code R53.2) is the lack of ability to use one's limbs or to ambulate due to extreme debility. It is not associated with neurologic deficit or injury, and code R53.2 should not be used for cases of neurologic quadriplegia. It should only be assigned if functional quadriplegia is specifically documented in the medical record.

g. SIRS due to Non-Infectious Process
The systemic inflammatory response syndrome (SIRS) can develop as a result of certain non-infectious disease processes, such as trauma, malignant neoplasm, or pancreatitis. When SIRS is documented with a noninfectious condition, and no subsequent infection is documented, the code for the underlying condition, such as an injury, should be assigned, followed by code R65.10, Systemic inflammatory response syndrome (SIRS) of non-infectious origin without acute organ dysfunction, or code R65.11, Systemic inflammatory response syndrome (SIRS) of non-infectious origin with acute organ dysfunction. If an associated acute organ dysfunction is documented, the appropriate code(s) for the specific type of organ dysfunction(s) should be assigned in addition to code R65.11. If acute organ dysfunction is documented, but it cannot be determined if the acute organ dysfunction is associated with SIRS or due to another condition (e.g., directly due to the trauma), the provider should be queried.

h. Death NOS
Code R99, Ill-defined and unknown cause of mortality, is only for use in the very limited circumstance when a patient who has already died is brought into an emergency department or other healthcare facility and is pronounced dead upon arrival. It does not represent the discharge disposition of death.

19. Chapter 19: Injury, Poisoning, and Certain Other Consequences of External Causes (S00-T88)

a. Application of 7th Characters in Chapter 19
Most categories in chapter 19 have a 7th character requirement for each applicable code. Most categories in this chapter have three 7th character values (with the exception of fractures): A, initial encounter, D, subsequent encounter and S, sequela. Categories for traumatic fractures have additional 7th character values.

7th character "A", initial encounter is used while the patient is receiving active treatment for the condition. Examples of active treatment are: surgical treatment, emergency department encounter, and evaluation and treatment by a new physician.

7th character "D" subsequent encounter is used for encounters after the patient has received active treatment of the condition and is receiving routine care for the condition during the healing or recovery phase. Examples of subsequent care are: cast change or removal, removal of external or internal fixation device, medication adjustment, other aftercare and follow up visits following treatment of the injury or condition.

The aftercare Z codes should not be used for aftercare for conditions such as injuries or poisonings, where 7th characters are provided to identify subsequent care. For example, for aftercare of an injury, assign the acute injury code with the 7th character "D" (subsequent encounter).

7th character "S", sequela, is for use for complications or conditions that arise as a direct result of a condition, such as scar formation after a burn. The scars are sequelae of the burn. When using 7th character "S", it is necessary to use both the injury code that precipitated the sequela and the code for the sequela itself. The "S" is added only to the injury code, not the sequela code. The 7th character "S" identifies the injury responsible for the sequela. The specific type of sequela (e.g. scar) is sequenced first, followed by the injury code.

b. Coding of Injuries
When coding injuries, assign separate codes for each injury unless a combination code is provided, in which case the combination code is assigned. Code T07, Unspecified multiple injuries should not be assigned in the inpatient setting unless information for a more specific code is not available. Traumatic injury codes (S00-T14.9) are not to be used for normal, healing surgical wounds or to identify complications of surgical wounds.

The code for the most serious injury, as determined by the provider and the focus of treatment, is sequenced first.

1) Superficial injuries
Superficial injuries such as abrasions or contusions are not coded when associated with more severe injuries of the same site.

2) Primary injury with damage to nerves/blood vessels
When a primary injury results in minor damage to peripheral nerves or blood vessels, the primary injury is sequenced first with additional code(s) for injuries to nerves and spinal cord (such as category S04), and/or injury to blood vessels (such as category S15). When the primary injury is to the blood vessels or nerves, that injury should be sequenced first.

c. Coding of Traumatic Fractures
The principles of multiple coding of injuries should be followed in coding fractures. Fractures of specified sites are coded individually by site in accordance with both the provisions within categories S02, S12, S22, S32, S42, S49, S52, S59, S62, S72, S79, S82, S89, S92 and the level of detail furnished by medical record content.

A fracture not indicated as open or closed should be coded to closed. A fracture not indicated whether displaced or not displaced should be coded to displaced.

More specific guidelines are as follows:

1) Initial vs. Subsequent Encounter for Fractures
Traumatic fractures are coded using the appropriate 7th character for initial encounter (A, B, C) while the patient is receiving active treatment for the fracture. Examples of active treatment are: surgical treatment, emergency department encounter, and evaluation and treatment by a new physician. The appropriate 7th character for initial encounter should also be assigned for a patient who delayed seeking treatment for the fracture or nonunion.

Fractures are coded using the appropriate 7th character for subsequent care for encounters after the patient has completed active treatment of the fracture and is receiving routine care for the fracture during the healing or recovery phase. Examples of fracture aftercare are: cast change or removal, removal of external or internal fixation device, medication adjustment, and follow-up visits following fracture treatment.

Care for complications of surgical treatment for fracture repairs during the healing or recovery phase should be coded with the appropriate complication codes.

Care of complications of fractures, such as malunion and nonunion, should be reported with the appropriate 7th character for subsequent care with nonunion (K, M, N,) or subsequent care with malunion (P, Q, R).

A code from category M80, not a traumatic fracture code, should be used for any patient with known osteoporosis who suffers a fracture, even if the patient had a minor fall or trauma, if that fall or trauma would not usually break a normal, healthy bone.

See Section I.C.13. Osteoporosis.

The aftercare Z codes should not be used for aftercare for traumatic fractures. For aftercare of a traumatic fracture, assign the acute fracture code with the appropriate 7th character.

2) Multiple fractures sequencing
Multiple fractures are sequenced in accordance with the severity of the fracture.

d. Coding of Burns and Corrosions
The ICD-10-CM makes a distinction between burns and corrosions. The burn codes are for thermal burns, except sunburns, that come from a heat source, such as a fire or hot appliance. The burn codes are also for burns resulting from electricity and radiation. Corrosions are burns due to chemicals. The guidelines are the same for burns and corrosions.

Current burns (T20-T25) are classified by depth, extent and by agent (X code). Burns are classified by depth as first degree (erythema), second degree (blistering), and third degree (full-thickness involvement). Burns of the eye and internal organs (T26-T28) are classified by site, but not by degree.

1) **Sequencing of burn and related condition codes**
Sequence first the code that reflects the highest degree of burn when more than one burn is present.

   a. When the reason for the admission or encounter is for treatment of external multiple burns, sequence first the code that reflects the burn of the highest degree.

   b. When a patient has both internal and external burns, the circumstances of admission govern the selection of the principal diagnosis or first-listed diagnosis.

   c. When a patient is admitted for burn injuries and other related conditions such as smoke inhalation and/or respiratory failure, the circumstances of admission govern the selection of the principal or first-listed diagnosis.

2) **Burns of the same local site**
Classify burns of the same local site (three-character category level, T20-T28) but of different degrees to the subcategory identifying the highest degree recorded in the diagnosis.

3) **Non-healing burns**
Non-healing burns are coded as acute burns.

   Necrosis of burned skin should be coded as a non-healed burn.

4) **Infected Burn**
For any documented infected burn site, use an additional code for the infection.

5) **Assign separate codes for each burn site**
When coding burns, assign separate codes for each burn site. Category T30, Burn and corrosion, body region unspecified is extremely vague and should rarely be used.

6) **Burns and Corrosions Classified According to Extent of Body Surface Involved**
Assign codes from category T31, Burns classified according to extent of body surface involved, or T32, Corrosions classified according to extent of body surface involved, when the site of the burn is not specified or when there is a need for additional data. It is advisable to use category T31 as additional coding when needed to provide data for evaluating burn mortality, such as that needed by burn units. It is also advisable to use category T31 as an additional code for reporting purposes when there is mention of a third-degree burn involving 20 percent or more of the body surface.

Categories T31 and T32 are based on the classic "rule of nines" in estimating body surface involved: head and neck are assigned nine percent, each arm nine percent, each leg 18 percent, the anterior trunk 18 percent, posterior trunk 18 percent, and genitalia one percent. Providers may change these percentage assignments where necessary to accommodate infants and children who have proportionately larger heads than adults, and patients who have large buttocks, thighs, or abdomen that involve burns.

7) **Encounters for treatment of sequela of burns**
Encounters for the treatment of the late effects of burns or corrosions (i.e., scars or joint contractures) should be coded with a burn or corrosion code with the 7th character "S" for sequela.

8) **Sequelae with a late effect code and current burn**
When appropriate, both a code for a current burn or corrosion with 7th character "A" or "D" and a burn or corrosion code with 7th character "S" may be assigned on the same record (when both a current burn and sequelae of an old burn exist). Burns and corrosions do not heal at the same rate and a current healing wound may still exist with sequela of a healed burn or corrosion.

9) **Use of an external cause code with burns and corrosions**
An external cause code should be used with burns and corrosions to identify the source and intent of the burn, as well as the place where it occurred.

e. **Adverse Effects, Poisoning, Underdosing and Toxic Effects**
Codes in categories T36-T65 are combination codes that include the substance that was taken as well as the intent. No additional external cause code is required for poisonings, toxic effects, adverse effects and underdosing codes.

1) **Do not code directly from the Table of Drugs**
Do not code directly from the Table of Drugs and Chemicals. Always refer back to the Tabular List.

2) **Use as many codes as necessary to describe**
Use as many codes as necessary to describe completely all drugs, medicinal or biological substances.

3) **If the same code would describe the causative agent**
If the same code would describe the causative agent for more than one adverse reaction, poisoning, toxic effect or underdosing, assign the code only once.

4) **If two or more drugs, medicinal or biological substances**
If two or more drugs, medicinal or biological substances are reported, code each individually unless **a** combination code is listed in the Table of Drugs and Chemicals.

5) **The occurrence of drug toxicity is classified in ICD-10-CM as follows:**
   (a) **Adverse effect**
   When coding an adverse effect of a drug that has been correctly prescribed and properly administered, assign the appropriate code for the nature of the adverse effect followed by the appropriate code for the adverse effect of the drug (T36-T50). The code for the drug should have a 5th or 6th character "5" (for example T36.0X5-) Examples of the nature of an adverse effect are tachycardia, delirium, gastrointestinal hemorrhaging, vomiting, hypokalemia, hepatitis, renal failure, or respiratory failure.

   (b) **Poisoning**
   When coding a poisoning or reaction to the improper use of a medication (e.g., overdose, wrong substance given or taken in error, wrong route of administration), first assign the appropriate code from categories T36-T50. The poisoning codes have an associated intent as their 5th or 6th character (accidental, intentional self-harm, assault and undetermined. Use additional code(s) for all manifestations of poisonings.

   If there is also a diagnosis of abuse or dependence of the substance, the abuse or dependence is assigned as an additional code.

   Examples of poisoning include:

   (i) Error was made in drug prescription

   Errors made in drug prescription or in the administration of the drug by provider, nurse, patient, or other person.

   (ii) Overdose of a drug intentionally taken

   If an overdose of a drug was intentionally taken or administered and resulted in drug toxicity, it would be coded as a poisoning.

   (iii) Nonprescribed drug taken with correctly prescribed and properly administered drug

   If a nonprescribed drug or medicinal agent was taken in combination with a correctly prescribed and properly administered drug, any drug toxicity or other reaction resulting from the interaction of the two drugs would be classified as a poisoning.

   (iv) Interaction of drug(s) and alcohol

   When a reaction results from the interaction of a drug(s) and alcohol, this would be classified as poisoning.

   See Section I.C.4. if poisoning is the result of insulin pump malfunctions.

   (c) **Underdosing**
   Underdosing refers to taking less of a medication than is prescribed by a provider or a manufacturer's instruction. For underdosing, assign the code from categories T36-T50 (fifth or sixth character "6").

   Codes for underdosing should never be assigned as principal or first-listed codes. If a patient has a relapse or exacerbation of the medical condition for which the drug is prescribed because of the reduction in dose, then the medical condition itself should be coded.

Noncompliance (Z91.12-, Z91.13-) or complication of care (Y63.6-Y63.9) codes are to be used with an underdosing code to indicate intent, if known.

(d) Toxic Effects

When a harmful substance is ingested or comes in contact with a person, this is classified as a toxic effect. The toxic effect codes are in categories T51-T65.

Toxic effect codes have an associated intent: accidental, intentional self-harm, assault and undetermined.

f. Adult and child abuse, neglect and other maltreatment
Sequence first the appropriate code from categories T74.- (Adult and child abuse, neglect and other maltreatment, confirmed) or T76.- (Adult and child abuse, neglect and other maltreatment, suspected) for abuse, neglect and other maltreatment, followed by any accompanying mental health or injury code(s).

If the documentation in the medical record states abuse or neglect it is coded as confirmed (T74.-). It is coded as suspected if it is documented as suspected (T76.-).

For cases of confirmed abuse or neglect an external cause code from the assault section (X92-Y08) should be added to identify the cause of any physical injuries. A perpetrator code (Y07) should be added when the perpetrator of the abuse is known. For suspected cases of abuse or neglect, do not report external cause or perpetrator code.

If a suspected case of abuse, neglect or mistreatment is ruled out during an encounter code Z04.71, Encounter for examination and observation following alleged physical adult abuse, ruled out, or code Z04.72, Encounter for examination and observation following alleged child physical abuse, ruled out, should be used, not a code from T76.

If a suspected case of alleged rape or sexual abuse is ruled out during an encounter code Z04.41, Encounter for examination and observation following alleged physical abuse, ruled out, or code Z04.42, Encounter for examination and observation following alleged rape or sexual abuse, ruled out, should be used, not a code from T76.

See Section I.C.15. Abuse in a pregnant patient.

g. Complications of care
  1) General guidelines for complications of care
     (a) Documentation of complications of care

See Section I.B.16. for information on documentation of complications of care.

  2) Pain due to medical devices
Pain associated with devices, implants or grafts left in a surgical site (for example painful hip prosthesis) is assigned to the appropriate code(s) found in Chapter 19, Injury, poisoning, and certain other consequences of external causes. Specific codes for pain due to medical devices are found in the T code section of the ICD-10-CM. Use additional code(s) from category G89 to identify acute or chronic pain due to presence of the device, implant or graft (G89.18 or G89.28).

  3) Transplant complications
     (a) Transplant complications other than kidney

Codes under category T86, Complications of transplanted organs and tissues, are for use for both complications and rejection of transplanted organs. A transplant complication code is only assigned if the complication affects the function of the transplanted organ. Two codes are required to fully describe a transplant complication: the appropriate code from category T86 and a secondary code that identifies the complication.

Pre-existing conditions or conditions that develop after the transplant are not coded as complications unless they affect the function of the transplanted organs.

See I.C.21. for transplant organ removal status

See I.C.2. for malignant neoplasm associated with transplanted organ.

     (b) Kidney transplant complications

Patients who have undergone kidney transplant may still have some form of chronic kidney disease (CKD) because the kidney transplant may not fully restore kidney function. Code

T86.1- should be assigned for documented complications of a kidney transplant, such as transplant failure or rejection or other transplant complication. Code T86.1- should not be assigned for post kidney transplant patients who have chronic kidney (CKD) unless a transplant complication such as transplant failure or rejection is documented. If the documentation is unclear as to whether the patient has a complication of the transplant, query the provider.

Conditions that affect the function of the transplanted kidney, other than CKD, should be assigned a code from subcategory T86.1, Complications of transplanted organ, Kidney, and a secondary code that identifies the complication.

For patients with CKD following a kidney transplant, but who do not have a complication such as failure or rejection, *see section I.C.14. Chronic kidney disease and kidney transplant status.*

  4) Complication codes that include the external cause
As with certain other T codes, some of the complications of care codes have the external cause included in the code. The code includes the nature of the complication as well as the type of procedure that caused the complication. No external cause code indicating the type of procedure is necessary for these codes.

  5) Complications of care codes within the body system chapters
Intraoperative and postprocedural complication codes are found within the body system chapters with codes specific to the organs and structures of that body system. These codes should be sequenced first, followed by a code(s) for the specific complication, if applicable.

20. Chapter 20: External Causes of Morbidity (V00-Y99)
The external causes of morbidity codes should never be sequenced as the first-listed or principal diagnosis.

External cause codes are intended to provide data for injury research and evaluation of injury prevention strategies. These codes capture how the injury or health condition happened (cause), the intent (unintentional or accidental; or intentional, such as suicide or assault), the place where the event occurred the activity of the patient at the time of the event, and the person's status (e.g., civilian, military).

There is no national requirement for mandatory ICD-10-CM external cause code reporting. Unless a provider is subject to a state-based external cause code reporting mandate or these codes are required by a particular payer, reporting of ICD-10-CM codes in Chapter 20, External Causes of Morbidity, is not required. In the absence of a mandatory reporting requirement, providers are encouraged to voluntarily report external cause codes, as they provide valuable data for injury research and evaluation of injury prevention strategies.

a. General External Cause Coding Guidelines
  1) Used with any code in the range of A00.0-T88.9, Z00-Z99
An external cause code may be used with any code in the range of A00.0-T88.9, Z00-Z99, classification that is a health condition due to an external cause. Though they are most applicable to injuries, they are also valid for use with such things as infections or diseases due to an external source, and other health conditions, such as a heart attack that occurs during strenuous physical activity.

  2) External cause code used for length of treatment
Assign the external cause code, with the appropriate 7th character (initial encounter, subsequent encounter or sequela) for each encounter for which the injury or condition is being treated.

  3) Use the full range of external cause codes
Use the full range of external cause codes to completely describe the cause, the intent, the place of occurrence, and if applicable, the activity of the patient at the time of the event, and the patient's status, for all injuries, and other health conditions due to an external cause.

  4) Assign as many external cause codes as necessary
Assign as many external cause codes as necessary to fully explain each cause. If only one external code can be recorded, assign the code most related to the principal diagnosis.

  5) The selection of the appropriate external cause code

The selection of the appropriate external cause code is guided by the Alphabetic Index of External Causes and by Inclusion and Exclusion notes in the Tabular List.

6) **External cause code can never be a principal diagnosis**
An external cause code can never be a principal (first-listed) diagnosis.

7) **Combination external cause codes**
Certain of the external cause codes are combination codes that identify sequential events that result in an injury, such as a fall which results in striking against an object. The injury may be due to either event or both. The combination external cause code used should correspond to the sequence of events regardless of which caused the most serious injury.

8) **No external cause code needed in certain circumstances**
No external cause code from Chapter 20 is needed if the external cause and intent are included in a code from another chapter (e.g. T36.0X1- Poisoning by penicillins, accidental (unintentional)).

b. **Place of Occurrence Guideline**
Codes from category Y92, Place of occurrence of the external cause, are secondary codes for use after other external cause codes to identify the location of the patient at the time of injury or other condition.

A place of occurrence code is used only once, at the initial encounter for treatment. No 7th characters are used for Y92. Only one code from Y92 should be recorded on a medical record.

Do not use place of occurrence code Y92.9 if the place is not stated or is not applicable.

c. **Activity Code**
Assign a code from category Y93, Activity code, to describe the activity of the patient at the time the injury or other health condition occurred.

An activity code is used only once, at the initial encounter for treatment. Only one code from Y93 should be recorded on a medical record.

The activity codes are not applicable to poisonings, adverse effects, misadventures or sequela .

Do not assign Y93.9, Unspecified activity, if the activity is not stated.

A code from category Y93 is appropriate for use with external cause and intent codes if identifying the activity provides additional information about the event.

d. **Place of Occurrence, Activity, and Status Codes Used with other External Cause Code**
When applicable, place of occurrence, activity, and external cause status codes are sequenced after the main external cause code(s). Regardless of the number of external cause codes assigned, there should be only one place of occurrence code, one activity code, and one external cause status code assigned to an encounter.

e. **If the Reporting Format Limits the Number of External Cause Codes**
If the reporting format limits the number of external cause codes that can be used in reporting clinical data, report the code for the cause/intent most related to the principal diagnosis. If the format permits capture of additional external cause codes, the cause/intent, including medical misadventures, of the additional events should be reported rather than the codes for place, activity, or external status.

f. **Multiple External Cause Coding Guidelines**
More than one external cause code is required to fully describe the external cause of an illness or injury. The assignment of external cause codes should be sequenced in the following priority:

If two or more events cause separate injuries, an external cause code should be assigned for each cause. The first-listed external cause code will be selected in the following order:

External codes for child and adult abuse take priority over all other external cause codes.

See Section I.C.19., Child and Adult abuse guidelines.

External cause codes for terrorism events take priority over all other external cause codes except child and adult abuse.

External cause codes for cataclysmic events take priority over all other external cause codes except child and adult abuse and terrorism.

External cause codes for transport accidents take priority over all other external cause codes except cataclysmic events, child and adult abuse and terrorism.

Activity and external cause status codes are assigned following all causal (intent) external cause codes.

The first-listed external cause code should correspond to the cause of the most serious diagnosis due to an assault, accident, or self-harm, following the order of hierarchy listed above.

g. **Child and Adult Abuse Guideline**
Adult and child abuse, neglect and maltreatment are classified as assault. Any of the assault codes may be used to indicate the external cause of any injury resulting from the confirmed abuse.

For confirmed cases of abuse, neglect and maltreatment, when the perpetrator is known, a code from Y07, Perpetrator of maltreatment and neglect, should accompany any other assault codes.

See Section I.C.19. Adult and child abuse, neglect and other maltreatment

h. **Unknown or Undetermined Intent Guideline**
If the intent (accident, self-harm, assault) of the cause of an injury or other condition is unknown or unspecified, code the intent as accidental intent. All transport accident categories assume accidental intent.

1) **Use of undetermined intent**
External cause codes for events of undetermined intent are only for use if the documentation in the record specifies that the intent cannot be determined.

i. **Sequelae (Late Effects) of External Cause Guidelines**
1) **Sequelae external cause codes**
Sequela are reported using the external cause code with the 7th character "S" for sequela. These codes should be used with any report of a late effect or sequela resulting from a previous injury.

2) **Sequela external cause code with a related current injury**
A sequela external cause code should never be used with a related current nature of injury code.

3) **Use of sequela external cause codes for subsequent visits**
Use a late effect external cause code for subsequent visits when a late effect of the initial injury is being treated. Do not use a late effect external cause code for subsequent visits for follow-up care (e.g., to assess healing, to receive rehabilitative therapy) of the injury when no late effect of the injury has been documented.

j. **Terrorism Guidelines**
1) **Cause of injury identified by the Federal Government (FBI) as terrorism**
When the cause of an injury is identified by the Federal Government (FBI) as terrorism, the first-listed external cause code should be a code from category Y38, Terrorism. The definition of terrorism employed by the FBI is found at the inclusion note at the beginning of category Y38. Use additional code for place of occurrence (Y92.-). More than one Y38 code may be assigned if the injury is the result of more than one mechanism of terrorism.

2) **Cause of an injury is suspected to be the result of terrorism**
When the cause of an injury is suspected to be the result of terrorism a code from category Y38 should not be assigned. Suspected cases should be classified as assault.

3) **Code Y38.9, Terrorism, secondary effects**
Assign code Y38.9, Terrorism, secondary effects, for conditions occurring subsequent to the terrorist event. This code should not be assigned for conditions that are due to the initial terrorist act.

It is acceptable to assign code Y38.9 with another code from Y38 if there is an injury due to the initial terrorist event and an injury that is a subsequent result of the terrorist event.

k. **External cause status**
A code from category Y99, External cause status, should be assigned whenever any other external cause code is assigned for an encounter, including an Activity code, except for the events noted below. Assign a code from category Y99, External cause status,

to indicate the work status of the person at the time the event occurred. The status code indicates whether the event occurred during military activity, whether a non-military person was at work, whether an individual including a student or volunteer was involved in a non-work activity at the time of the causal event.

A code from Y99, External cause status, should be assigned, when applicable, with other external cause codes, such as transport accidents and falls. The external cause status codes are not applicable to poisonings, adverse effects, misadventures or late effects.

Do not assign a code from category Y99 if no other external cause codes (cause, activity) are applicable for the encounter.

An external cause status code is used only once, at the initial encounter for treatment. Only one code from Y99 should be recorded on a medical record.

Do not assign code Y99.9, Unspecified external cause status, if the status is not stated.

21. **Chapter 21: Factors Influencing Health Status and Contact with Health Services (Z00-Z99)**
Note: The chapter specific guidelines provide additional information about the use of Z codes for specified encounters.

a. **Use of Z codes in any healthcare setting**
Z codes are for use in any healthcare setting. Z codes may be used as either a first-listed (principal diagnosis code in the inpatient setting) or secondary code, depending on the circumstances of the encounter. Certain Z codes may only be used as first-listed or principal diagnosis.

b. **Z Codes indicate a reason for an encounter**
Z codes are not procedure codes. A corresponding procedure code must accompany a Z code to describe any procedure performed.

c. **Categories of Z Codes**
1) **Contact/Exposure**
Category Z20 indicates contact with, and suspected exposure to, communicable diseases. These codes are for patients who do not show any sign or symptom of a disease but are suspected to have been exposed to it by close personal contact with an infected individual or are in an area where a disease is epidemic.

Category Z77, indicates contact with and suspected exposures hazardous to health.

Contact/exposure codes may be used as a first-listed code to explain an encounter for testing, or, more commonly, as a secondary code to identify a potential risk.

2) **Inoculations and vaccinations**
Code Z23 is for encounters for inoculations and vaccinations. It indicates that a patient is being seen to receive a prophylactic inoculation against a disease. Procedure codes are required to identify the actual administration of the injection and the type(s) of immunizations given. Code Z23 may be used as a secondary code if the inoculation is given as a routine part of preventive health care, such as a well-baby visit.

3) **Status**
Status codes indicate that a patient is either a carrier of a disease or has the sequelae or residual of a past disease or condition. This includes such things as the presence of prosthetic or mechanical devices resulting from past treatment. A status code is informative, because the status may affect the course of treatment and its outcome. A status code is distinct from a history code. The history code indicates that the patient no longer has the condition.

A status code should not be used with a diagnosis code from one of the body system chapters, if the diagnosis code includes the information provided by the status code. For example, code Z94.1, Heart transplant status, should not be used with a code from subcategory T86.2, Complications of heart transplant. The status code does not provide additional information. The complication code indicates that the patient is a heart transplant patient.

For encounters for weaning from a mechanical ventilator, assign a code from subcategory J96.1, Chronic respiratory failure, followed by code Z99.11, Dependence on respirator [ventilator] status.

The status Z codes/categories are:

Z14 Genetic carrier

Genetic carrier status indicates that a person carries a gene, associated with a particular disease, which may be passed to offspring who may develop that disease. The person does not have the disease and is not at risk of developing the disease.

Z15 Genetic susceptibility to disease

Genetic susceptibility indicates that a person has a gene that increases the risk of that person developing the disease.

Codes from category Z15 should not be used as principal or first-listed codes. If the patient has the condition to which he/she is susceptible, and that condition is the reason for the encounter, the code for the current condition should be sequenced first. If the patient is being seen for follow-up after completed treatment for this condition, and the condition no longer exists, a follow-up code should be sequenced first, followed by the appropriate personal history and genetic susceptibility codes. If the purpose of the encounter is genetic counseling associated with procreative management, code Z31.5, Encounter for genetic counseling, should be assigned as the first-listed code, followed by a code from category Z15. Additional codes should be assigned for any applicable family or personal history.

Z16 Resistance to antimicrobial drugs

This code indicates that a patient has a condition that is resistant to antimicrobial drug treatment. Sequence the infection code first.

Z17 Estrogen receptor status

Z18 Retained foreign body fragments

Z21 Asymptomatic HIV infection status

This code indicates that a patient has tested positive for HIV but has manifested no signs or symptoms of the disease.

Z22 Carrier of infectious disease

Carrier status indicates that a person harbors the specific organisms of a disease without manifest symptoms and is capable of transmitting the infection.

Z28.3 Underimmunization status

Z33.1 Pregnant state, incidental

This code is a secondary code only for use when the pregnancy is in no way complicating the reason for visit. Otherwise, a code from the obstetric chapter is required.

Z66 Do not resuscitate

This code may be used when it is documented by the provider that a patient is on do not resuscitate status at any time during the stay.

Z67 Blood type

Z68 Body mass index (BMI)

Z74.01 Bed confinement status

Z76.82 Awaiting organ transplant status

Z78 Other specified health status

Code Z78.1, Physical restraint status, may be used when it is documented by the provider that a patient has been put in restraints during the current encounter. Please note that this code should not be reported when it is documented by the provider that a patient is temporarily restrained during a procedure.

Z79 Long-term (current) drug therapy

Codes from this category indicate a patient's continuous use of a prescribed drug (including such things as aspirin therapy) for the long-term treatment of a condition or for prophylactic use. It is not for use for patients who have addictions to drugs. This subcategory is not for use of medications for detoxification or maintenance programs to prevent withdrawal symptoms in patients with drug dependence (e.g., methadone maintenance for opiate dependence). Assign the appropriate code for the drug dependence instead.

Assign a code from Z79 if the patient is receiving a medication for an extended period as a prophylactic measure (such as for the prevention of deep vein thrombosis) or as treatment of a chronic condition (such as arthritis) or a disease requiring a lengthy course of treatment (such as cancer). Do not assign a code from category Z79 for medication being administered for a brief period of time to treat an acute illness or injury (such as a course of antibiotics to treat acute bronchitis).

Z88 Allergy status to drugs, medicaments and biological substances

Except: Z88.9, Allergy status to unspecified drugs, medicaments and biological substances status

Z89 Acquired absence of limb

Z90 Acquired absence of organs, not elsewhere classified

Z91.0- Allergy status, other than to drugs and biological substances

Z92.82 Status post administration of tPA (rtPA) in a different facility within the last 24 hours prior to admission to a current facility

Assign code Z92.82, Status post administration of tPA (rtPA) in a different facility within the last 24 hours prior to admission to current facility, as a secondary diagnosis when a patient is received by transfer into a facility and documentation indicates they were administered tissue plasminogen activator (tPA) within the last 24 hours prior to admission to the current facility.

This guideline applies even if the patient is still receiving the tPA at the time they are received into the current facility.

The appropriate code for the condition for which the tPA was administered (such as cerebrovascular disease or myocardial infarction) should be assigned first.

Code Z92.82 is only applicable to the receiving facility record and not to the transferring facility record.

Z93 Artificial opening status

Z94 Transplanted organ and tissue status

Z95 Presence of cardiac and vascular implants and grafts

Z96 Presence of other functional implants

Z97 Presence of other devices

Z98 Other postprocedural states

Assign code Z98.85, Transplanted organ removal status, to indicate that a transplanted organ has been previously removed. This code should not be assigned for the encounter in which the transplanted organ is removed. The complication necessitating removal of the transplant organ should be assigned for that encounter.

See section I.C19. for information on the coding of organ transplant complications.

Z99 Dependence on enabling machines and devices, not elsewhere classified

Note: Categories Z89-Z90 and Z93-Z99 are for use only if there are no complications or malfunctions of the organ or tissue replaced, the amputation site or the equipment on which the patient is dependent.

4) **History (of)**
There are two types of history Z codes, personal and family. Personal history codes explain a patient's past medical condition that no longer exists and is not receiving any treatment, but that has the potential for recurrence, and therefore may require continued monitoring.

Family history codes are for use when a patient has a family member(s) who has had a particular disease that causes the patient to be at higher risk of also contracting the disease.

Personal history codes may be used in conjunction with follow-up codes and family history codes may be used in conjunction with screening codes to explain the need for a test or procedure. History codes are also acceptable on any medical record regardless of the reason for visit. A history of an illness, even if no longer present, is important information that may alter the type of treatment ordered.

The history Z code categories are:

Z80 Family history of primary malignant neoplasm

Z81 Family history of mental and behavioral disorders

Z82 Family history of certain disabilities and chronic diseases (leading to disablement)

Z83 Family history of other specific disorders

Z84 Family history of other conditions

Z85 Personal history of malignant neoplasm

Z86 Personal history of certain other diseases

Z87 Personal history of other diseases and conditions

Z91.4- Personal history of psychological trauma, not elsewhere classified

Z91.5 Personal history of self-harm

Z91.8- Other specified personal risk factors, not elsewhere classified

Exception: Z91.83, Wandering in diseases classified elsewhere

Z92 Personal history of medical treatment

Except: Z92.0, Personal history of contraception

Except: Z92.82, Status post administration of tPA (rtPA) in a different facility within the last 24 hours prior to admission to a current facility

5) **Screening**
Screening is the testing for disease or disease precursors in seemingly well individuals so that early detection and treatment can be provided for those who test positive for the disease (e.g., screening mammogram).

The testing of a person to rule out or confirm a suspected diagnosis because the patient has some sign or symptom is a diagnostic examination, not a screening. In these cases, the sign or symptom is used to explain the reason for the test.

A screening code may be a first-listed code if the reason for the visit is specifically the screening exam. It may also be used as an additional code if the screening is done during an office visit for other health problems. A screening code is not necessary if the screening is inherent to a routine examination, such as a pap smear done during a routine pelvic examination.

Should a condition be discovered during the screening then the code for the condition may be assigned as an additional diagnosis.

The Z code indicates that a screening exam is planned. A procedure code is required to confirm that the screening was performed.

The screening Z codes/categories:

Z11 Encounter for screening for infectious and parasitic diseases

Z12 Encounter for screening for malignant neoplasms

Z13 Encounter for screening for other diseases and disorders

Except: Z13.9, Encounter for screening, unspecified

Z36 Encounter for antenatal screening for mother

6) **Observation**
There are two observation Z code categories. They are for use in very limited circumstances when a person is being observed for a suspected condition that is ruled out. The observation codes are not for use if an injury or illness or any signs or symptoms related to the suspected condition are present. In such cases the diagnosis/symptom code is used with the corresponding external cause code.

The observation codes are to be used as principal diagnosis only. Additional codes may be used in addition to the observation code but only if they are unrelated to the suspected condition being observed.

Codes from subcategory Z03.7, Encounter for suspected maternal and fetal conditions ruled out, may either be used as a first-listed or as an additional code assignment depending on the case. They are for use in very limited circumstances on a maternal record when an encounter is for a suspected maternal or fetal condition that is ruled out during that encounter (for example, a maternal or fetal condition may be suspected due to an abnormal test result). These codes should not be used when the condition is confirmed. In those cases, the confirmed condition should be coded. In addition, these codes are not for use if an illness or any signs or symptoms related to the suspected condition or problem are present. In such cases the diagnosis/symptom code is used.

Additional codes may be used in addition to the code from subcategory Z03.7, but only if they are unrelated to the suspected condition being evaluated.

Codes from subcategory Z03.7 may not be used for encounters for antenatal screening of mother. *See Section I.C.21. Screening.*

For encounters for suspected fetal condition that are inconclusive following testing and evaluation, assign the appropriate code from category O35, O36, O40 or O41.

The observation Z code categories:

Z03   Encounter for medical observation for suspected diseases and conditions ruled out

Z04   Encounter for examination and observation for other reasons

     Except: Z04.9, Encounter for examination and observation for unspecified reason

7) Aftercare

Aftercare visit codes cover situations when the initial treatment of a disease has been performed and the patient requires continued care during the healing or recovery phase, or for the long-term consequences of the disease. The aftercare Z code should not be used if treatment is directed at a current, acute disease. The diagnosis code is to be used in these cases. Exceptions to this rule are codes Z51.0, Encounter for antineoplastic radiation therapy, and codes from subcategory Z51.1, Encounter for antineoplastic chemotherapy and immunotherapy. These codes are to be first-listed, followed by the diagnosis code when a patient's encounter is solely to receive radiation therapy, chemotherapy, or immunotherapy for the treatment of a neoplasm. If the reason for the encounter is more than one type of antineoplastic therapy, code Z51.0 and a code from subcategory Z51.1 may be assigned together, in which case one of these codes would be reported as a secondary diagnosis.

The aftercare Z codes should also not be used for aftercare for injuries. For aftercare of an injury, assign the acute injury code with the appropriate 7th character (for subsequent encounter).

The aftercare codes are generally first-listed to explain the specific reason for the encounter. An aftercare code may be used as an additional code when some type of aftercare is provided in addition to the reason for admission and no diagnosis code is applicable. An example of this would be the closure of a colostomy during an encounter for treatment of another condition.

Aftercare codes should be used in conjunction with other aftercare codes or diagnosis codes to provide better detail on the specifics of an aftercare encounter visit, unless otherwise directed by the classification. Should a patient receive multiple types of antineoplastic therapy during the same encounter, code Z51.0, Encounter for antineoplastic radiation therapy, and codes from subcategory Z51.1, Encounter for antineoplastic chemotherapy and immunotherapy, may be used together on a record. The sequencing of multiple aftercare codes depends on the circumstances of the encounter.

Certain aftercare Z code categories need a secondary diagnosis code to describe the resolving condition or sequelae. For others, the condition is included in the code title.

Additional Z code aftercare category terms include fitting and adjustment, and attention to artificial openings.

Status Z codes may be used with aftercare Z codes to indicate the nature of the aftercare. For example code Z95.1, Presence of aortocoronary bypass graft, may be used with code Z48.812,

Encounter for surgical aftercare following surgery on the circulatory system, to indicate the surgery for which the aftercare is being performed. A status code should not be used when the aftercare code indicates the type of status, such as using Z43.0, Encounter for attention to tracheostomy, with Z93.0, Tracheostomy status.

The aftercare Z category/codes:

Z42   Encounter for plastic and reconstructive surgery following medical procedure or healed injury

Z43   Encounter for attention to artificial openings

Z44   Encounter for fitting and adjustment of external prosthetic device

Z45   Encounter for adjustment and management of implanted device

Z46   Encounter for fitting and adjustment of other devices

Z47   Orthopedic aftercare

Z48   Encounter for other postprocedural aftercare

Z49   Encounter for care involving renal dialysis

Z51   Encounter for other aftercare

8) Follow-up

The follow-up codes are used to explain continuing surveillance following completed treatment of a disease, condition, or injury. They imply that the condition has been fully treated and no longer exists. They should not be confused with aftercare codes, or injury codes with a 7th character for subsequent encounter, that explain ongoing care of a healing condition or its sequelae. Follow-up codes may be used in conjunction with history codes to provide the full picture of the healed condition and its treatment. The follow-up code is sequenced first, followed by the history code.

A follow-up code may be used to explain multiple visits. Should a condition be found to have recurred on the follow-up visit, then the diagnosis code for the condition should be assigned in place of the follow-up code.

The follow-up Z code categories:

Z08   Encounter for follow-up examination after completed treatment for malignant neoplasm

Z09   Encounter for follow-up examination after completed treatment for conditions other than malignant neoplasm

Z39   Encounter for maternal postpartum care and examination

9) Donor

Codes in category Z52, Donors of organs and tissues, are used for living individuals who are donating blood or other body tissue. These codes are only for individuals donating for others, not for self-donations. They are not used to identify cadaveric donations.

10) Counseling

Counseling Z codes are used when a patient or family member receives assistance in the aftermath of an illness or injury, or when support is required in coping with family or social problems. They are not used in conjunction with a diagnosis code when the counseling component of care is considered integral to standard treatment.

The counseling Z codes/categories:

Z30.0-   Encounter for general counseling and advice on contraception

Z31.5   Encounter for genetic counseling

Z31.6-   Encounter for general counseling and advice on procreation

Z32.2   Encounter for childbirth instruction

Z32.3   Encounter for childcare instruction

Z69   Encounter for mental health services for victim and perpetrator of abuse

Z70   Counseling related to sexual attitude, behavior and orientation

Z71   Persons encountering health services for other counseling and medical advice, not elsewhere classified

Z76.81 Expectant mother prebirth pediatrician visit

11) Encounters for Obstetrical and Reproductive Services
See Section I.C.15. Pregnancy, Childbirth, and the Puerperium, for further instruction on the use of these codes.

Z codes for pregnancy are for use in those circumstances when none of the problems or complications included in the codes from the Obstetrics chapter exist (a routine prenatal visit or postpartum care). Codes in category Z34, Encounter for supervision of normal pregnancy, are always first-listed and are not to be used with any other code from the OB chapter.

Codes in category Z3A, Weeks of gestation, may be assigned to provide additional information about the pregnancy. **The date of the admission should be used to determine weeks of gestation for inpatient admissions that encompass more than one gestational week.**

The outcome of delivery, category Z37, should be included on all maternal delivery records. It is always a secondary code. Codes in category Z37 should not be used on the newborn record.

Z codes for family planning (contraceptive) or procreative management and counseling should be included on an obstetric record either during the pregnancy or the postpartum stage, if applicable.

Z codes/categories for obstetrical and reproductive services:

Z30   Encounter for contraceptive management

Z31   Encounter for procreative management

Z32.2 Encounter for childbirth instruction

Z32.3 Encounter for childcare instruction

Z33   Pregnant state

Z34   Encounter for supervision of normal pregnancy

Z36   Encounter for antenatal screening of mother

Z3A   Weeks of gestation

Z37   Outcome of delivery

Z39   Encounter for maternal postpartum care and examination

Z76.81 Expectant mother prebirth pediatrician visit

12) Newborns and Infants
See Section I.C.16. Newborn (Perinatal) Guidelines, for further instruction on the use of these codes.

Newborn Z codes/categories:

Z76.1 Encounter for health supervision and care of foundling

Z00.1- Encounter for routine child health examination

Z38   Liveborn infants according to place of birth and type of delivery

13) Routine and Administrative Examinations
The Z codes allow for the description of encounters for routine examinations, such as, a general check-up, or, examinations for administrative purposes, such as, a pre-employment physical. The codes are not to be used if the examination is for diagnosis of a suspected condition or for treatment purposes. In such cases the diagnosis code is used. During a routine exam, should a diagnosis or condition be discovered, it should be coded as an additional code. Pre-existing and chronic conditions and history codes may also be included as additional codes as long as the examination is for administrative purposes and not focused on any particular condition.

Some of the codes for routine health examinations distinguish between "with" and "without" abnormal findings. Code assignment depends on the information that is known at the time the encounter is being coded. For example, if no abnormal findings were found during the examination, but the encounter is being coded before test results are back, it is acceptable to assign the code for "without abnormal findings." When assigning a code for "with abnormal findings," additional code(s) should be assigned to identify the specific abnormal finding(s).

Pre-operative examination and pre-procedural laboratory examination Z codes are for use only in those situations when a patient is being cleared for a procedure or surgery and no treatment is given.

The Z codes/categories for routine and administrative examinations:

Z00   Encounter for general examination without complaint, suspected or reported diagnosis

Z01   Encounter for other special examination without complaint, suspected or reported diagnosis

Z02   Encounter for administrative examination

     Except: Z02.9, Encounter for administrative examinations, unspecified

Z32.0- Encounter for pregnancy test

14) Miscellaneous Z Codes
The miscellaneous Z codes capture a number of other health care encounters that do not fall into one of the other categories. Certain of these codes identify the reason for the encounter; others are for use as additional codes that provide useful information on circumstances that may affect a patient's care and treatment.

Prophylactic Organ Removal

For encounters specifically for prophylactic removal of an organ (such as prophylactic removal of breasts due to a genetic susceptibility to cancer or a family history of cancer), the principal or first-listed code should be a code from category Z40, Encounter for prophylactic surgery, followed by the appropriate codes to identify the associated risk factor (such as genetic susceptibility or family history).

If the patient has a malignancy of one site and is having prophylactic removal at another site to prevent either a new primary malignancy or metastatic disease, a code for the malignancy should also be assigned in addition to a code from subcategory Z40.0, Encounter for prophylactic surgery for risk factors related to malignant neoplasms. A Z40.0 code should not be assigned if the patient is having organ removal for treatment of a malignancy, such as the removal of the testes for the treatment of prostate cancer.

Miscellaneous Z codes/categories:

Z28   Immunization not carried out

     Except: Z28.3, Underimmunization status

Z40   Encounter for prophylactic surgery

Z41   Encounter for procedures for purposes other than remedying health state

     Except: Z41.9, Encounter for procedure for purposes other than remedying health state, unspecified

Z53   Persons encountering health services for specific procedures and treatment, not carried out

Z55   Problems related to education and literacy

Z56   Problems related to employment and unemployment

Z57   Occupational exposure to risk factors

Z58   Problems related to physical environment

Z59   Problems related to housing and economic circumstances

Z60   Problems related to social environment

Z62   Problems related to upbringing

Z63   Other problems related to primary support group, including family circumstances

Z64   Problems related to certain psychosocial circumstances

Z65   Problems related to other psychosocial circumstances

Z72   Problems related to lifestyle

Z73   Problems related to life management difficulty

Z74   Problems related to care provider dependency

     Except: Z74.01, Bed confinement status

Z75   Problems related to medical facilities and other health care

Z76.0 Encounter for issue of repeat prescription

Z76.3 Healthy person accompanying sick person

Z76.4 Other boarder to healthcare facility

Z76.5 Malingerer [conscious simulation]

Z91.1- Patient's noncompliance with medical treatment and regimen

Z91.83 Wandering in diseases classified elsewhere

Z91.89 Other specified personal risk factors, not elsewhere classified

15) Nonspecific Z codes

Certain Z codes are so non-specific, or potentially redundant with other codes in the classification, that there can be little justification for their use in the inpatient setting. Their use in the outpatient setting should be limited to those instances when there is no further documentation to permit more precise coding. Otherwise, any sign or symptom or any other reason for visit that is captured in another code should be used.

Nonspecific Z codes/categories:

Z02.9 Encounter for administrative examinations, unspecified

Z04.9 Encounter for examination and observation for unspecified reason

Z13.9 Encounter for screening, unspecified

Z41.9 Encounter for procedure for purposes other than remedying health state, unspecified

Z52.9 Donor of unspecified organ or tissue

Z86.59 Personal history of other mental and behavioral disorders

Z88.9 Allergy status to unspecified drugs, medicaments and biological substances status

Z92.0 Personal history of contraception

16) Z Codes That May Only be Principal/First-Listed Diagnosis

The following Z codes/categories may only be reported as the principal/first-listed diagnosis, except when there are multiple encounters on the same day and the medical records for the encounters are combined:

Z00 Encounter for general examination without complaint, suspected or reported diagnosis

Z01 Encounter for other special examination without complaint, suspected or reported diagnosis

Z02 Encounter for administrative examination

Z03 Encounter for medical observation for suspected diseases and conditions ruled out

Z04 Encounter for examination and observation for other reasons

Z33.2 Encounter for elective termination of pregnancy

Z31.81 Encounter for male factor infertility in female patient

Z31.82 Encounter for Rh incompatibility status

Z31.83 Encounter for assisted reproductive fertility procedure cycle

Z31.84 Encounter for fertility preservation procedure

Z34 Encounter for supervision of normal pregnancy

Z39 Encounter for maternal postpartum care and examination

Z38 Liveborn infants according to place of birth and type of delivery

Z42 Encounter for plastic and reconstructive surgery following medical procedure or healed injury

Z51.0 Encounter for antineoplastic radiation therapy

Z51.1- Encounter for antineoplastic chemotherapy and immunotherapy

Z52 Donors of organs and tissues

Except: Z52.9, Donor of unspecified organ or tissue

Z76.1 Encounter for health supervision and care of foundling

Z76.2 Encounter for health supervision and care of other healthy infant and child

Z99.12 Encounter for respirator [ventilator] dependence during power failure

Section II. Selection of Principal Diagnosis

The circumstances of inpatient admission always govern the selection of principal diagnosis. The principal diagnosis is defined in the Uniform Hospital Discharge Data Set (UHDDS) as "that condition established after study to be chiefly responsible for occasioning the admission of the patient to the hospital for care."

The UHDDS definitions are used by hospitals to report inpatient data elements in a standardized manner. These data elements and their definitions can be found in the July 31, 1985, Federal Register (Vol. 50, No, 147), pp. 31038-40.

Since that time the application of the UHDDS definitions has been expanded to include all non-outpatient settings (acute care, short term, long term care and psychiatric hospitals; home health agencies; rehab facilities; nursing homes, etc).

In determining principal diagnosis, coding conventions in the ICD-10-CM, the Tabular List and Alphabetic Index take precedence over these official coding guidelines.

(See Section I.A., Conventions for the ICD-10-CM)

The importance of consistent, complete documentation in the medical record cannot be overemphasized. Without such documentation the application of all coding guidelines is a difficult, if not impossible, task.

A. Codes for symptoms, signs, and ill-defined conditions

Codes for symptoms, signs, and ill-defined conditions from Chapter 18 are not to be used as principal diagnosis when a related definitive diagnosis has been established.

B. Two or more interrelated conditions, each potentially meeting the definition for principal diagnosis.

When there are two or more interrelated conditions (such as diseases in the same ICD-10-CM chapter or manifestations characteristically associated with a certain disease) potentially meeting the definition of principal diagnosis, either condition may be sequenced first, unless the circumstances of the admission, the therapy provided, the Tabular List, or the Alphabetic Index indicate otherwise.

C. Two or more diagnoses that equally meet the definition for principal diagnosis

In the unusual instance when two or more diagnoses equally meet the criteria for principal diagnosis as determined by the circumstances of admission, diagnostic workup and/or therapy provided, and the Alphabetic Index, Tabular List, or another coding guidelines does not provide sequencing direction, any one of the diagnoses may be sequenced first.

D. Two or more comparative or contrasting conditions

In those rare instances when two or more contrasting or comparative diagnoses are documented as "either/or" (or similar terminology), they are coded as if the diagnoses were confirmed and the diagnoses are sequenced according to the circumstances of the admission. If no further determination can be made as to which diagnosis should be principal, either diagnosis may be sequenced first.

E. A symptom(s) followed by contrasting/comparative diagnoses

When a symptom(s) is followed by contrasting/comparative diagnoses, the symptom code is sequenced first. **However, if the symptom code is integral to the conditions listed, no code for the symptom is reported.** All the contrasting/comparative diagnoses should be coded as additional diagnoses.

F. Original treatment plan not carried out

Sequence as the principal diagnosis the condition, which after study occasioned the admission to the hospital, even though treatment may not have been carried out due to unforeseen circumstances.

G. Complications of surgery and other medical care

When the admission is for treatment of a complication resulting from surgery or other medical care, the complication code is sequenced as the principal diagnosis. If the complication is classified to the T80-T88 series and the code lacks the necessary specificity in describing the complication, an additional code for the specific complication should be assigned.

H. Uncertain Diagnosis

If the diagnosis documented at the time of discharge is qualified as "probable", "suspected", "likely", "questionable", "possible", or "still to be ruled out", or other similar terms indicating uncertainty, code the condition as if it existed or was established. The bases for these guidelines are the diagnostic workup, arrangements for further workup or observation, and initial therapeutic approach that correspond most closely with the established diagnosis.

Note: This guideline is applicable only to inpatient admissions to short-term, acute, long-term care and psychiatric hospitals.

I. Admission from Observation Unit

1. Admission Following Medical Observation

When a patient is admitted to an observation unit for a medical condition, which either worsens or does not improve, and is subsequently admitted as an inpatient of the same hospital for this same medical condition, the principal diagnosis would be the medical condition which led to the hospital admission.

2. Admission Following Post-Operative Observation

When a patient is admitted to an observation unit to monitor a condition (or complication) that develops following outpatient surgery, and then is subsequently admitted as an inpatient of the same hospital, hospitals should apply the Uniform Hospital Discharge Data Set (UHDDS) definition of principal diagnosis as "that condition established after study to be chiefly responsible for occasioning the admission of the patient to the hospital for care."

J. Admission from Outpatient Surgery

When a patient receives surgery in the hospital's outpatient surgery department and is subsequently admitted for continuing inpatient care at the same hospital, the following guidelines should be followed in selecting the principal diagnosis for the inpatient admission:

- If the reason for the inpatient admission is a complication, assign the complication as the principal diagnosis.
- If no complication, or other condition, is documented as the reason for the inpatient admission, assign the reason for the outpatient surgery as the principal diagnosis.
- If the reason for the inpatient admission is another condition unrelated to the surgery, assign the unrelated condition as the principal diagnosis.

K. Admissions/Encounters for Rehabilitation

When the purpose for the admission/encounter is rehabilitation, sequence first the code for the condition for which the service is being performed. For example, for an admission/encounter for rehabilitation for right-sided dominant hemiplegia following a cerebrovascular infarction, report code I69.351, Hemiplegia and hemiparesis following cerebral infarction affecting right dominant side, as the first-listed or principal diagnosis.

If the condition for which the rehabilitation service is no longer present, report the appropriate aftercare code as the first-listed or principal diagnosis. For example, if a patient with severe degenerative osteoarthritis of the hip, underwent hip replacement and the current encounter/admission is for rehabilitation, report code Z47.1, Aftercare following joint replacement surgery, as the first-listed or principal diagnosis.

See Section I.C.21.c.7, Factors influencing health states and contact with health services, Aftercare.

Section III. Reporting Additional Diagnoses

GENERAL RULES FOR OTHER (ADDITIONAL) DIAGNOSES

For reporting purposes the definition for "other diagnoses" is interpreted as additional conditions that affect patient care in terms of requiring:

clinical evaluation; or

therapeutic treatment; or

diagnostic procedures; or

extended length of hospital stay; or

increased nursing care and/or monitoring.

The UHDDS item #11-b defines Other Diagnoses as "all conditions that coexist at the time of admission, that develop subsequently, or that affect the treatment received and/or the length of stay. Diagnoses that relate to an earlier episode which have no bearing on the current hospital stay are to be excluded." UHDDS definitions apply to inpatients in acute care, short-term, long term care and psychiatric hospital setting. The UHDDS definitions are used by acute care short-term hospitals to report inpatient data elements in a standardized manner. These data elements and their definitions can be found in the July 31, 1985, Federal Register (Vol. 50, No, 147), pp. 31038-40.

Since that time the application of the UHDDS definitions has been expanded to include all non-outpatient settings (acute care, short term, long term care and psychiatric hospitals; home health agencies; rehab facilities; nursing homes, etc).

The following guidelines are to be applied in designating "other diagnoses" when neither the Alphabetic Index nor the Tabular List in ICD-10-CM provide direction. The listing of the diagnoses in the patient record is the responsibility of the attending provider.

A. Previous conditions

If the provider has included a diagnosis in the final diagnostic statement, such as the discharge summary or the face sheet, it should ordinarily be coded. Some providers include in the diagnostic statement resolved conditions or diagnoses and status-post procedures from previous admission that have no bearing on the current stay. Such conditions are not to be reported and are coded only if required by hospital policy.

However, history codes (categories Z80-Z87) may be used as secondary codes if the historical condition or family history has an impact on current care or influences treatment.

B. Abnormal findings

Abnormal findings (laboratory, x-ray, pathologic, and other diagnostic results) are not coded and reported unless the provider indicates their clinical significance. If the findings are outside the normal range and the attending provider has ordered other tests to evaluate the condition or prescribed treatment, it is appropriate to ask the provider whether the abnormal finding should be added.

Please note: This differs from the coding practices in the outpatient setting for coding encounters for diagnostic tests that have been interpreted by a provider.

C. Uncertain Diagnosis

If the diagnosis documented at the time of discharge is qualified as "probable", "suspected", "likely", "questionable", "possible", or "still to be ruled out" or other similar terms indicating uncertainty, code the condition as if it existed or was established. The bases for these guidelines are the diagnostic workup, arrangements for further workup or observation, and initial therapeutic approach that correspond most closely with the established diagnosis.

Note: This guideline is applicable only to inpatient admissions to short-term, acute, long-term care and psychiatric hospitals.

Section IV. Diagnostic Coding and Reporting Guidelines for Outpatient Services

These coding guidelines for outpatient diagnoses have been approved for use by hospitals/ providers in coding and reporting hospital-based outpatient services and provider-based office visits.

Information about the use of certain abbreviations, punctuation, symbols, and other conventions used in the ICD-10-CM Tabular List (code numbers and titles), can be found in Section IA of these guidelines, under "Conventions Used in the Tabular List." **Section I.B. contains general guidelines that apply to the entire classification. Section I.C. contains chapter-specific guidelines that correspond to the chapters as they are arranged in the classification.** Information about the correct sequence to use in finding a code is also described in Section I.

The terms encounter and visit are often used interchangeably in describing outpatient service contacts and, therefore, appear together in these guidelines without distinguishing one from the other.

Though the conventions and general guidelines apply to all settings, coding guidelines for outpatient and provider reporting of diagnoses will vary in a number of instances from those for inpatient diagnoses, recognizing that:

The Uniform Hospital Discharge Data Set (UHDDS) definition of principal diagnosis applies only to inpatients in acute, short-term, long-term care and psychiatric hospitals.

Coding guidelines for inconclusive diagnoses (probable, suspected, rule out, etc.) were developed for inpatient reporting and do not apply to outpatients.

A. Selection of first-listed condition

In the outpatient setting, the term first-listed diagnosis is used in lieu of principal diagnosis.

In determining the first-listed diagnosis the coding conventions of ICD-10-CM, as well as the general and disease specific guidelines take precedence over the outpatient guidelines.

Diagnoses often are not established at the time of the initial encounter/visit. It may take two or more visits before the diagnosis is confirmed.

The most critical rule involves beginning the search for the correct code assignment through the Alphabetic Index. Never begin searching initially in the Tabular List as this will lead to coding errors.

1. **Outpatient Surgery**
   When a patient presents for outpatient surgery (same day surgery), code the reason for the surgery as the first-listed diagnosis (reason for the encounter), even if the surgery is not performed due to a contraindication.

2. **Observation Stay**
   When a patient is admitted for observation for a medical condition, assign a code for the medical condition as the first-listed diagnosis.

   When a patient presents for outpatient surgery and develops complications requiring admission to observation, code the reason for the surgery as the first reported diagnosis (reason for the encounter), followed by codes for the complications as secondary diagnoses.

B. Codes from A00.0 through T88.9, Z00-Z99

The appropriate code(s) from A00.0 through T88.9, Z00-Z99 must be used to identify diagnoses, symptoms, conditions, problems, complaints, or other reason(s) for the encounter/visit.

C. Accurate reporting of ICD-10-CM diagnosis codes

For accurate reporting of ICD-10-CM diagnosis codes, the documentation should describe the patient's condition, using terminology which includes specific diagnoses as well as symptoms, problems, or reasons for the encounter. There are ICD-10-CM codes to describe all of these.

D. Codes that describe symptoms and signs

Codes that describe symptoms and signs, as opposed to diagnoses, are acceptable for reporting purposes when a diagnosis has not been established (confirmed) by the provider. Chapter 18 of ICD-10-CM, Symptoms, Signs, and Abnormal Clinical and Laboratory Findings Not Elsewhere Classified (codes R00-R99) contain many, but not all codes for symptoms.

E. Encounters for circumstances other than a disease or injury

ICD-10-CM provides codes to deal with encounters for circumstances other than a disease or injury. The Factors Influencing Health Status and Contact with Health Services codes (Z00-Z99) are provided to deal with occasions when circumstances other than a disease or injury are recorded as diagnosis or problems.

See Section I.C.21. Factors influencing health status and contact with health services.

F. Level of Detail in Coding

1. **ICD-10-CM codes with 3, 4, 5, 6 or 7 characters**
   ICD-10-CM is composed of codes with 3, 4, 5, 6 or 7 characters. Codes with three characters are included in ICD-10-CM as the heading of a category of codes that may be further subdivided by the use of fourth, fifth, sixth or seventh characters to provide greater specificity.

2. **Use of full number of characters required for a code**
   A three-character code is to be used only if it is not further subdivided. A code is invalid if it has not been coded to the full number of characters required for that code, including the 7th character, if applicable.

G. ICD-10-CM code for the diagnosis, condition, problem, or other reason for encounter/visit

List first the ICD-10-CM code for the diagnosis, condition, problem, or other reason for encounter/visit shown in the medical record to be chiefly responsible for the services provided. List additional codes that describe any coexisting conditions. In some cases the first-listed diagnosis may be a symptom when a diagnosis has not been established (confirmed) by the physician.

H. Uncertain diagnosis

Do not code diagnoses documented as "probable," "suspected," "questionable," "rule out," or "working diagnosis" or other similar terms indicating uncertainty. Rather, code the condition(s) to the highest degree of certainty for that encounter/visit, such as symptoms, signs, abnormal test results, or other reason for the visit.

Please note: This differs from the coding practices used by short-term, acute care, long-term care and psychiatric hospitals.

I. Chronic diseases

Chronic diseases treated on an ongoing basis may be coded and reported as many times as the patient receives treatment and care for the condition(s)

J. Code all documented conditions that coexist

Code all documented conditions that coexist at the time of the encounter/visit, and require or affect patient care treatment or management. Do not code conditions that were previously treated and no longer exist. However, history codes (categories Z80-Z87) may be used as secondary codes if the historical condition or family history has an impact on current care or influences treatment.

K. Patients receiving diagnostic services only

For patients receiving diagnostic services only during an encounter/visit, sequence first the diagnosis, condition, problem, or other reason for encounter/visit shown in the medical record to be chiefly responsible for the outpatient services provided during the encounter/visit. Codes for other diagnoses (e.g., chronic conditions) may be sequenced as additional diagnoses.

For encounters for routine laboratory/radiology testing in the absence of any signs, symptoms, or associated diagnosis, assign Z01.89, Encounter for other specified special examinations. If routine testing is performed during the same encounter as a test to evaluate a sign, symptom, or diagnosis, it is appropriate to assign both the Z code and the code describing the reason for the non-routine test.

For outpatient encounters for diagnostic tests that have been interpreted by a physician, and the final report is available at the time of coding, code any confirmed or definitive diagnosis(es) documented in the interpretation. Do not code related signs and symptoms as additional diagnoses.

Please note: This differs from the coding practice in the hospital inpatient setting regarding abnormal findings on test results.

L. Patients receiving therapeutic services only

For patients receiving therapeutic services only during an encounter/visit, sequence first the diagnosis, condition, problem, or other reason for encounter/visit shown in the medical record to be chiefly responsible for the outpatient services provided during the encounter/visit. Codes for other diagnoses (e.g., chronic conditions) may be sequenced as additional diagnoses.

The only exception to this rule is that when the primary reason for the admission/encounter is chemotherapy or radiation therapy, the appropriate Z code for the service is listed first, and the diagnosis or problem for which the service is being performed listed second.

M. Patients receiving preoperative evaluations only

For patients receiving preoperative evaluations only, sequence first a code from subcategory Z01.81, Encounter for pre-procedural examinations, to describe the pre-op consultations. Assign a code for the condition to describe the reason for the surgery as an additional diagnosis. Code also any findings related to the pre-op evaluation.

N. Ambulatory surgery

For ambulatory surgery, code the diagnosis for which the surgery was performed. If the postoperative diagnosis is known to be different from the preoperative diagnosis at the time the diagnosis is confirmed, select the postoperative diagnosis for coding, since it is the most definitive.

O. Routine outpatient prenatal visits

See Section I.C.15. Routine outpatient prenatal visits.

P. **Encounters for general medical examinations with abnormal findings**

The subcategories for encounters for general medical examinations, Z00.0-, provide codes for with and without abnormal findings. Should a general medical examination result in an abnormal finding, the code for general medical examination with abnormal finding should be assigned as the first-listed diagnosis. A secondary code for the abnormal finding should also be coded.

Q. **Encounters for routine health screenings**

See Section I.C.21. Factors influencing health status and contact with health services, Screening

Appendix I. Present on Admission Reporting Guidelines

Introduction

These guidelines are to be used as a supplement to the *ICD-10-CM Official Guidelines for Coding and Reporting* to facilitate the assignment of the Present on Admission (POA) indicator for each diagnosis and external cause of injury code reported on claim forms (UB-04 and 837 Institutional).

These guidelines are not intended to replace any guidelines in the main body of the *ICD-10-CM Official Guidelines for Coding and Reporting*. The POA guidelines are not intended to provide guidance on when a condition should be coded, but rather, how to apply the POA indicator to the final set of diagnosis codes that have been assigned in accordance with Sections I, II, and III of the official coding guidelines. Subsequent to the assignment of the ICD-10-CM codes, the POA indicator should then be assigned to those conditions that have been coded.

As stated in the Introduction to the ICD-10-CM Official Guidelines for Coding and Reporting, a joint effort between the healthcare provider and the coder is essential to achieve complete and accurate documentation, code assignment, and reporting of diagnoses and procedures. The importance of consistent, complete documentation in the medical record cannot be overemphasized. Medical record documentation from any provider involved in the care and treatment of the patient may be used to support the determination of whether a condition was present on admission or not. In the context of the official coding guidelines, the term "provider" means a physician or any qualified healthcare practitioner who is legally accountable for establishing the patient's diagnosis.

These guidelines are not a substitute for the provider's clinical judgment as to the determination of whether a condition was/was not present on admission. The provider should be queried regarding issues related to the linking of signs/symptoms, timing of test results, and the timing of findings.

General Reporting Requirements

All claims involving inpatient admissions to general acute care hospitals or other facilities that are subject to a law or regulation mandating collection of present on admission information.

Present on admission is defined as present at the time the order for inpatient admission occurs -- conditions that develop during an outpatient encounter, including emergency department, observation, or outpatient surgery, are considered as present on admission.

POA indicator is assigned to principal and secondary diagnoses (as defined in Section II of the Official Guidelines for Coding and Reporting) and the external cause of injury codes.

Issues related to inconsistent, missing, conflicting or unclear documentation must still be resolved by the provider.

If a condition would not be coded and reported based on UHDDS definitions and current official coding guidelines, then the POA indicator would not be reported.

Reporting Options

Y - Yes

N - No

U - Unknown

W – Clinically undetermined

Unreported/Not used – (Exempt from POA reporting)

Reporting Definitions

Y = present at the time of inpatient admission

N – not present at the time of inpatient admission

U = documentation is insufficient to determine if condition is present on admission

W = provider is unable to clinically determine whether condition was present on admission or not

Timeframe for POA Identification and Documentation

There is no required timeframe as to when a provider (per the definition of "provider" used in these guidelines) must identify or document a condition to be present on admission. In some clinical situations, it may not be possible for a provider to make a definitive diagnosis (or a condition may not be recognized or reported by the patient) for a period of time after admission. In some cases it may be several days before the provider arrives at a definitive diagnosis. This does not mean that the condition was not present on admission. Determination of whether the condition was present on admission or not will be based on the applicable POA guideline as identified in this document, or on the provider's best clinical judgment.

If at the time of code assignment the documentation is unclear as to whether a condition was present on admission or not, it is appropriate to query the provider for clarification.

Assigning the POA Indicator

Condition is on the "Exempt from Reporting" list

Leave the "present on admission" field blank if the condition is on the list of ICD-10-CM codes for which this field is not applicable. This is the only circumstance in which the field may be left blank.

POA Explicitly Documented

Assign Y for any condition the provider explicitly documents as being present on admission.

Assign N for any condition the provider explicitly documents as not present at the time of admission.

Conditions diagnosed prior to inpatient admission

Assign "Y" for conditions that were diagnosed prior to admission (example: hypertension, diabetes mellitus, asthma)

Conditions diagnosed during the admission but clearly present before admission

Assign "Y" for conditions diagnosed during the admission that were clearly present but not diagnosed until after admission occurred.

Diagnoses subsequently confirmed after admission are considered present on admission if at the time of admission they are documented as suspected, possible, rule out, differential diagnosis, or constitute an underlying cause of a symptom that is present at the time of admission.

Condition develops during outpatient encounter prior to inpatient admission

Assign Y for any condition that develops during an outpatient encounter prior to a written order for inpatient admission.

Documentation does not indicate whether condition was present on admission

Assign "U" when the medical record documentation is unclear as to whether the condition was present on admission. "U" should not be routinely assigned and used only in very limited circumstances. Coders are encouraged to query the providers when the documentation is unclear.

Documentation states that it cannot be determined whether the condition was or was not present on admission

Assign "W" when the medical record documentation indicates that it cannot be clinically determined whether or not the condition was present on admission.

Chronic condition with acute exacerbation during the admission

If a single code identifies both the chronic condition and the acute exacerbation, see POA guidelines pertaining to combination codes.

If a single code only identifies the chronic condition and not the acute exacerbation (e.g., acute exacerbation of chronic leukemia), assign "Y."

Conditions documented as possible, probable, suspected, or rule out at the time of discharge

If the final diagnosis contains a possible, probable, suspected, or rule out diagnosis, and this diagnosis was based on signs, symptoms or clinical findings suspected at the time of inpatient admission, assign "Y."

If the final diagnosis contains a possible, probable, suspected, or rule out diagnosis, and this diagnosis was based on signs, symptoms or clinical findings that were not present on admission, assign "N".

Conditions documented as impending or threatened at the time of discharge

If the final diagnosis contains an impending or threatened diagnosis, and this diagnosis is based on symptoms or clinical findings that were present on admission, assign "Y".

If the final diagnosis contains an impending or threatened diagnosis, and this diagnosis is based on symptoms or clinical findings that were not present on admission, assign "N".

Acute and Chronic Conditions

Assign "Y" for acute conditions that are present at time of admission and N for acute conditions that are not present at time of admission.

Assign "Y" for chronic conditions, even though the condition may not be diagnosed until after admission.

If a single code identifies both an acute and chronic condition, see the POA guidelines for combination codes.

Combination Codes

Assign "N" if any part of the combination code was not present on admission (e.g., COPD with acute exacerbation and the exacerbation was not present on admission; gastric ulcer that does not start bleeding until after admission; asthma patient develops status asthmaticus after admission)

Assign "Y" if all parts of the combination code were present on admission (e.g., patient with acute prostatitis admitted with hematuria)

If the final diagnosis includes comparative or contrasting diagnoses, and both were present, or suspected, at the time of admission, assign "Y".

For infection codes that include the causal organism, assign "Y" if the infection (or signs of the infection) was present on admission, even though the culture results may not be known until after admission (e.g., patient is admitted with pneumonia and the provider documents pseudomonas as the causal organism a few days later).

Same Diagnosis Code for Two or More Conditions

When the same ICD-10-CM diagnosis code applies to two or more conditions during the same encounter (e.g. two separate conditions classified to the same ICD-10-CM diagnosis code):

Assign "Y" if all conditions represented by the single ICD-10-CM code were present on admission (e.g. bilateral unspecified age-related cataracts).

Assign "N" if any of the conditions represented by the single ICD-10-CM code was not present on admission (e.g. traumatic secondary and recurrent hemorrhage and seroma is assigned to a single code T79.2, but only one of the conditions was present on admission).

Obstetrical conditions

Whether or not the patient delivers during the current hospitalization does not affect assignment of the POA indicator. The determining factor for POA assignment is whether the pregnancy complication or obstetrical condition described by the code was present at the time of admission or not.

If the pregnancy complication or obstetrical condition was present on admission (e.g., patient admitted in preterm labor), assign "Y".

If the pregnancy complication or obstetrical condition was not present on admission (e.g., 2nd degree laceration during delivery, postpartum hemorrhage that occurred during current hospitalization, fetal distress develops after admission), assign "N".

If the obstetrical code includes more than one diagnosis and any of the diagnoses identified by the code were not present on admission assign "N". (e.g., Category O11, Pre-existing hypertension with pre-eclampsia)

Perinatal conditions

Newborns are not considered to be admitted until after birth. Therefore, any condition present at birth or that developed in utero is considered present at admission and should be assigned "Y". This includes conditions that occur during delivery (e.g., injury during delivery, meconium aspiration, exposure to streptococcus B in the vaginal canal).

Congenital conditions and anomalies

Assign "Y" for congenital conditions and anomalies except for categories Q00-Q99, Congenital anomalies, which are on the exempt list. Congenital conditions are always considered present on admission.

External cause of injury codes

Assign "Y" for any external cause code representing an external cause of morbidity that occurred prior to inpatient admission (e.g., patient fell out of bed at home, patient fell out of bed in emergency room prior to admission)

Assign "N" for any external cause code representing an external cause of morbidity that occurred during inpatient hospitalization (e.g., patient fell out of hospital bed during hospital stay, patient experienced an adverse reaction to a medication administered after inpatient admission)

Categories and Codes Exempt from Diagnosis Present on Admission Requirement

Note: "Diagnosis present on admission" for these code categories are exempt because they represent circumstances regarding the healthcare encounter or factors influencing health status that do not represent a current disease or injury or are always present on admission

B90–B94	Sequelae of infectious and parasitic diseases
E64	Sequelae of malnutrition and other nutritional deficiencies
I25.2	Old myocardial infarction
I69	Sequelae of cerebrovascular disease
O09	Supervision of high risk pregnancy
O66.5	Attempted application of vacuum extractor and forceps
O80	Encounter for full-term uncomplicated delivery
O94	Sequelae of complication of pregnancy, childbirth, and the puerperium
P00	Newborn (suspected to be) affected by maternal conditions that may be unrelated to present pregnancy
Q00 – Q99	Congenital malformations, deformations and chromosomal abnormalities
S00-T88.9	Injury, poisoning and certain other consequences of external causes with 7th character representing subsequent encounter or sequela
V00- V09	Pedestrian injured in transport accident
	Except V00.81-, Accident with wheelchair (powered) V00.83-, Accident with motorized mobility scooter
V10-V19	Pedal cycle rider injured in transport accident
V20-V29	Motorcycle rider injured in transport accident
V30-V39	Occupant of three-wheeled motor vehicle injured in transport accident
V40-V49	Car occupant injured in transport accident
V50-V59	Occupant of pick-up truck or van injured in transport accident
V60-V69	Occupant of heavy transport vehicle injured in transport accident
V70-V79	Bus occupant injured in transport accident
V80-V89	Other land transport accidents
V90-V94	Water transport accidents
V95-V97	Air and space transport accidents
V98-V99	Other and unspecified transport accidents
W09	Fall on and from playground equipment
W14	Fall from tree
W15	Fall from cliff
W17.0	Fall into well
W17.1	Fall into storm drain or manhole
W18.01	Striking against sports equipment with subsequent fall
W21	Striking against or struck by sports equipment
W30	Contact with agricultural machinery
W31	Contact with other and unspecified machinery
W32-W34	Accidental handgun discharge and malfunction
W35- W40	Exposure to inanimate mechanical forces
W52	Crushed, pushed or stepped on by crowd or human stampede
W56	Contact with nonvenomous marine animal
W58	Contact with crocodile or alligator
W61	Contact with birds (domestic) (wild)
W62	Contact with nonvenomous amphibians
W89	Exposure to man-made visible and ultraviolet light
X02	Exposure to controlled fire in building or structure
X03	Exposure to controlled fire, not in building or structure

X04	Exposure to ignition of highly flammable material
X52	Prolonged stay in weightless environment
X71	Intentional self-harm by drowning and submersion
	Except X71.0-, Intentional self-harm by drowning and submersion while in bath tub
X72	Intentional self-harm by handgun discharge
X73	Intentional self-harm by rifle, shotgun and larger firearm discharge
X74	Intentional self-harm by other and unspecified firearm and gun discharge
X75	Intentional self-harm by explosive material
X76	Intentional self-harm by smoke, fire and flames
X77	Intentional self-harm by steam hot vapors and hot objects
X81	Intentional self-harm by jumping or lying in front of moving object
X82	Intentional self-harm by crashing of motor vehicle
X83	Intentional self-harm by other specified means
Y03	**Assault by crashing of motor vehicle**
Y07	**Perpetrator of assault, maltreatment and neglect**
Y08.8	**Assault by strike by sports equipment**
Y21	Drowning and submersion, undetermined intent
Y22	Handgun discharge, undetermined intent
Y23	Rifle, shotgun and larger firearm discharge, undetermined intent
Y24	Other and unspecified firearm discharge, undetermined intent
Y30	Falling, jumping or pushed from a high place, undetermined intent
Y32	**Assault by crashing of motor vehicle, undetermined intent**
Y37	Military operations
Y36	Operations of war
Y92	Place of occurrence of the external cause
Y93	Activity code
Y99	External cause status
Z00	Encounter for general examination without complaint, suspected or reported diagnosis
Z01	Encounter for other special examination without complaint, suspected or reported diagnosis
Z02	Encounter for administrative examination
Z03	Encounter for medical observation for suspected diseases and conditions ruled out
Z08	Encounter for follow-up examination following completed treatment for malignant neoplasm
Z09	Encounter for follow-up examination after completed treatment for conditions other than malignant neoplasm
Z11	Encounter for screening for infectious and parasitic diseases
Z11.8	Encounter for screening for other infectious and parasitic diseases
Z12	Encounter for screening for malignant neoplasms
Z13	Encounter for screening for other diseases and disorders
Z13.4	Encounter for screening for certain developmental disorders in childhood
Z13.5	Encounter for screening for eye and ear disorders
Z13.6	Encounter for screening for cardiovascular disorders
Z13.83	Encounter for screening for respiratory disorder NEC
Z13.89	Encounter for screening for other disorder
Z13.89	Encounter for screening for other disorder
Z14	Genetic carrier
Z15	Genetic susceptibility to disease
Z17	Estrogen receptor status
Z18	Retained foreign body fragments
Z22	Carrier of infectious disease
Z23	Encounter for immunization
Z28	Immunization not carried out and underimmunization status
Z28.3	Underimmunization status
Z30	Encounter for contraceptive management
Z31	Encounter for procreative management
Z34	Encounter for supervision of normal pregnancy
Z36	Encounter for antenatal screening of mother
Z37	Outcome of delivery

Z38	Liveborn infants according to place of birth and type of delivery
Z39	Encounter for maternal postpartum care and examination
Z41	Encounter for procedures for purposes other than remedying health state
Z42	Encounter for plastic and reconstructive surgery following medical procedure or healed injury
Z43	Encounter for attention to artificial openings
Z44	Encounter for fitting and adjustment of external prosthetic device
Z45	Encounter for adjustment and management of implanted device
Z46	Encounter for fitting and adjustment of other devices
Z47.8	Encounter for other orthopedic aftercare
Z49	Encounter for care involving renal dialysis
Z51	Encounter for other aftercare
Z51.5	Encounter for palliative care
Z51.8	Encounter for other specified aftercare
Z52	Donors of organs and tissues
Z59	Problems related to housing and economic circumstances
Z63	Other problems related to primary support group, including family circumstances
Z65	Problems related to other psychosocial circumstances
Z65.8	Other specified problems related to psychosocial circumstances
Z67.1 – Z67.9	Blood type
Z68	Body mass index (BMI)
Z72	Problems related to lifestyle
Z74.01	Bed confinement status
Z76	Persons encountering health services in other circumstances
Z77.110-Z77.128	Environmental pollution and hazards in the physical environment
Z78	Other specified health status
Z79	Long term (current) drug therapy
Z80	Family history of primary malignant neoplasm
Z81	Family history of mental and behavioral disorders
Z82	Family history of certain disabilities and chronic diseases (leading to disablement)
Z83	Family history of other specific disorders
Z84	Family history of other conditions
Z85	Personal history of primary malignant neoplasm
Z86	Personal history of certain other diseases
Z87	Personal history of other diseases and conditions
Z87.828	Personal history of other (healed) physical injury and trauma
Z87.891	Personal history of nicotine dependence
Z88	Allergy status to drugs, medicaments and biological substances
Z89	Acquired absence of limb
Z90.710	Acquired absence of both cervix and uterus
Z91.0	Allergy status, other than to drugs and biological substances
Z91.4	Personal history of psychological trauma, not elsewhere classified
Z91.5	Personal history of self-harm
Z91.8	Other specified risk factors, not elsewhere classified
Z92	Personal history of medical treatment
Z93	Artificial opening status
Z94	Transplanted organ and tissue status
Z95	Presence of cardiac and vascular implants and grafts
Z97	Presence of other devices
Z98	Other postprocedural states
Z99	Dependence on enabling machines and devices, not elsewhere classified

BRAIN FUNCTION

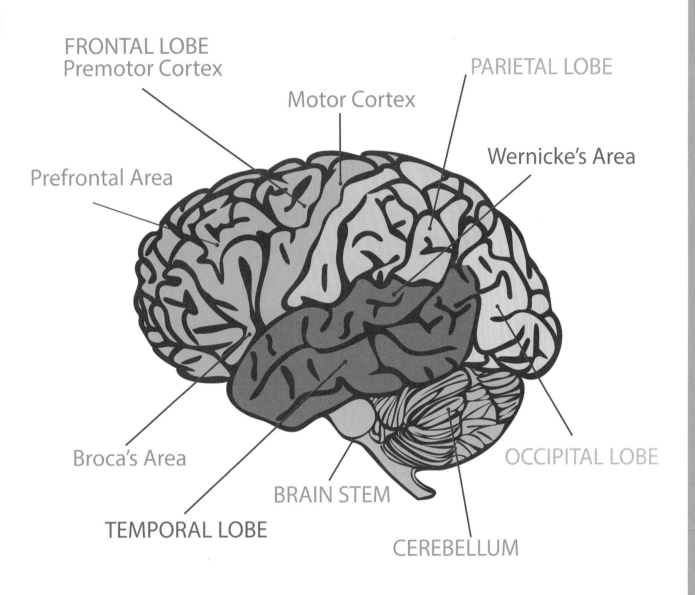

FRONTAL LOBE
Premotor Cortex

PARIETAL LOBE

Motor Cortex

Wernicke's Area

Prefrontal Area

Broca's Area

OCCIPITAL LOBE

TEMPORAL LOBE

BRAIN STEM

CEREBELLUM

BREAST ANATOMY

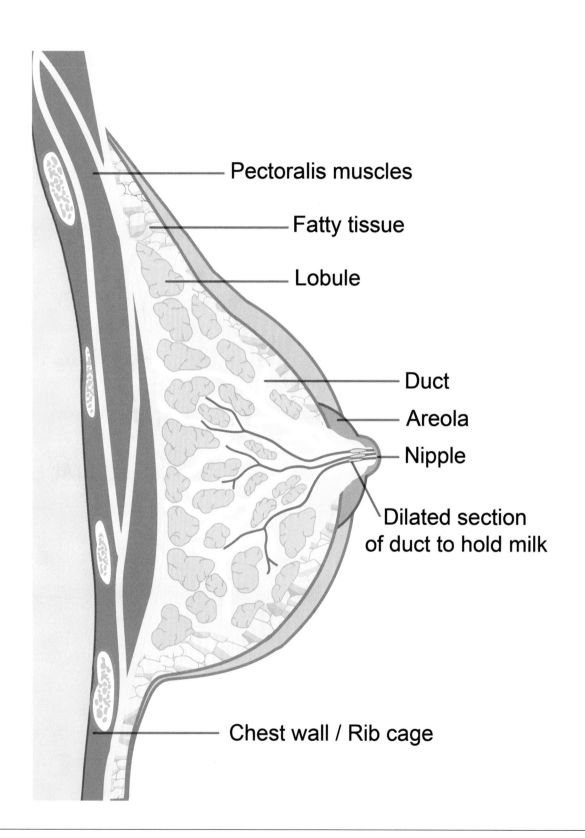

Pectoralis muscles

Fatty tissue

Lobule

Duct

Areola

Nipple

Dilated section
of duct to hold milk

Chest wall / Rib cage

CARDIAC CYCLE

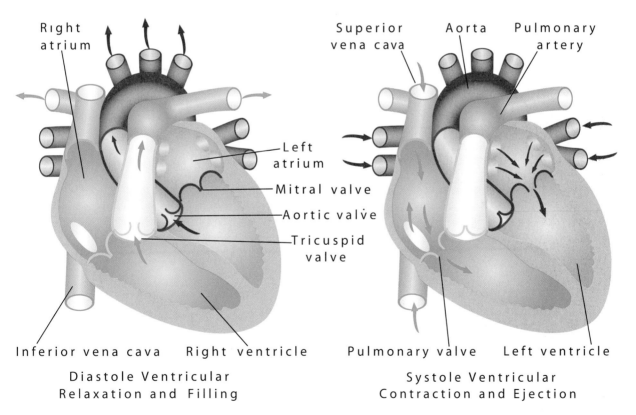

Brachiocephalic trunk

Ascending aorta

Right pulmonary artery

Superior vena cava

Pulmonary trung

Right pulmonary vens

Right atrium

Right coronary artery

Right ventricle

Inferior vena cava

Left common carotid artery

Left subclavian artery

Aortic arch

Ligamentum arteriosum

Left pulmonary artery

Left pulmonary vens

Left atrium

Circumflex artery

Left coronary artery

Left ventricle

Anterior interventricular artery

Apex

ANATOMY OF THE HEART

Right atrium

Left atrium

Mitral valve

Aortic valve

Tricuspid valve

Inferior vena cava   Right ventricle

Diastole Ventricular
Relaxation and Filling

Superior vena cava   Aorta   Pulmonary artery

Pulmonary valve   Left ventricle

Systole Ventricular
Contraction and Ejection

CIRCULARY SYSTEM

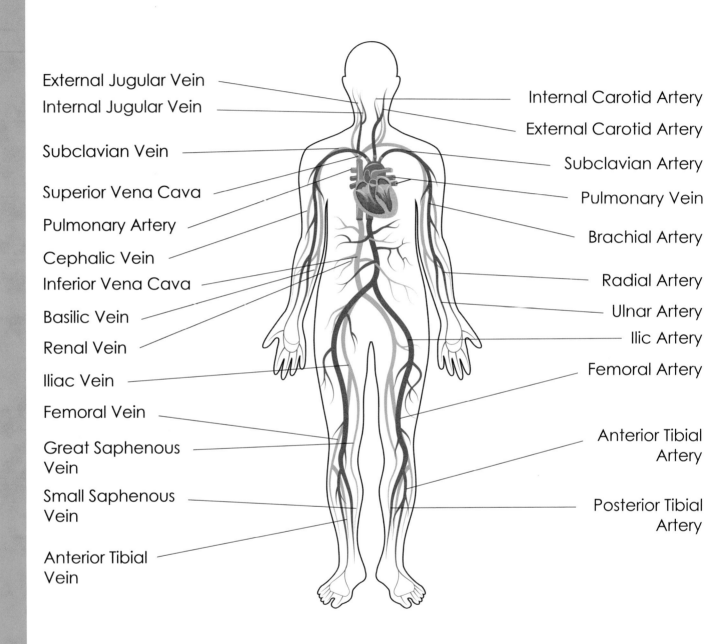

External Jugular Vein

Internal Jugular Vein

Subclavian Vein

Superior Vena Cava

Pulmonary Artery

Cephalic Vein

Inferior Vena Cava

Basilic Vein

Renal Vein

Iliac Vein

Femoral Vein

Great Saphenous Vein

Small Saphenous Vein

Anterior Tibial Vein

Internal Carotid Artery

External Carotid Artery

Subclavian Artery

Pulmonary Vein

Brachial Artery

Radial Artery

Ulnar Artery

Ilic Artery

Femoral Artery

Anterior Tibial Artery

Posterior Tibial Artery

DIGESTIVE SYSTEM

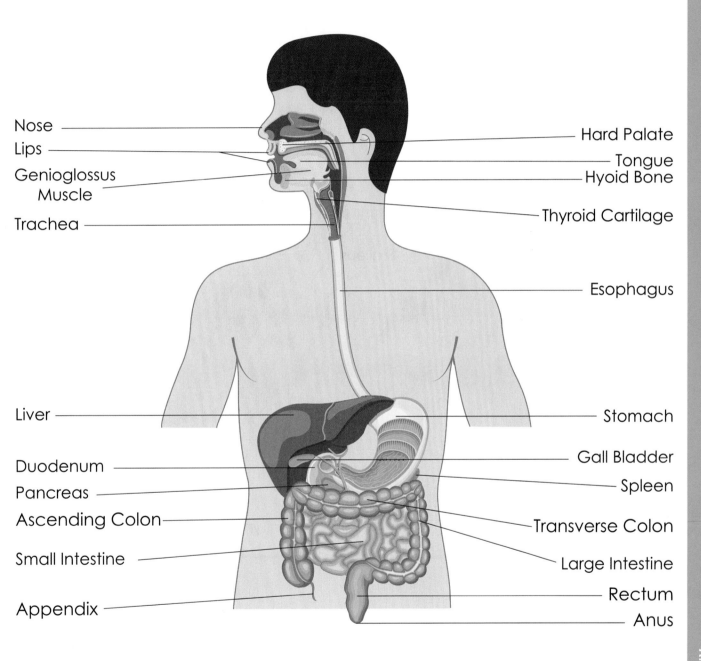

Nose

Lips

Genioglossus
Muscle

Trachea

Hard Palate

Tongue

Hyoid Bone

Thyroid Cartilage

Esophagus

Liver

Stomach

Gall Bladder

Duodenum

Pancreas

Spleen

Ascending Colon

Transverse Colon

Small Intestine

Large Intestine

Appendix

Rectum

Anus

EAR ANATOMY

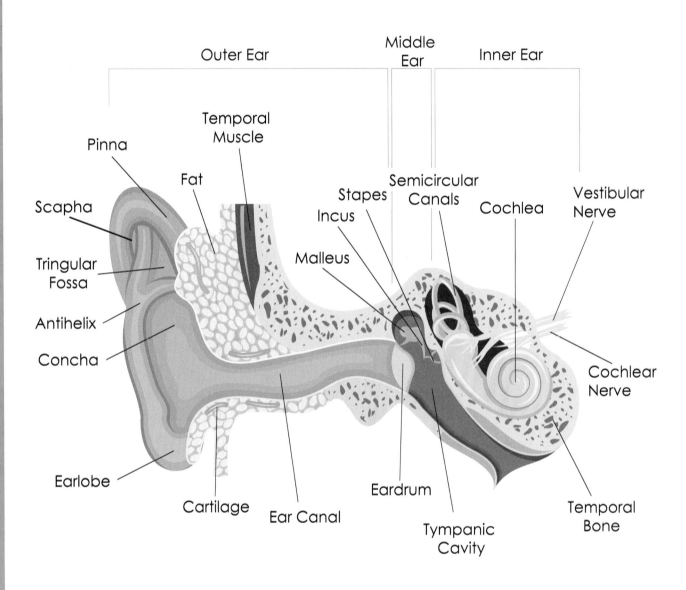

ENDOCRINE SYSTEM

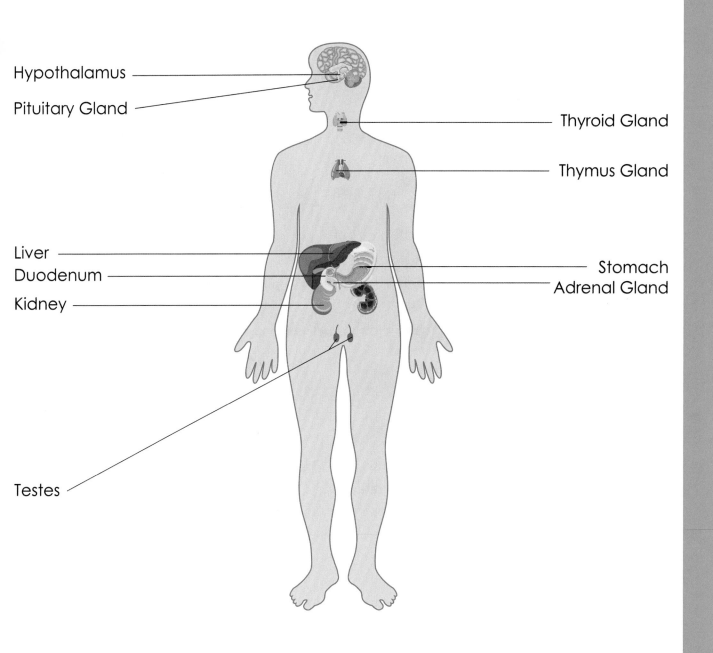

Hypothalamus

Pituitary Gland

Thyroid Gland

Thymus Gland

Liver

Duodenum

Kidney

Stomach

Adrenal Gland

Testes

EYE ANATOMY

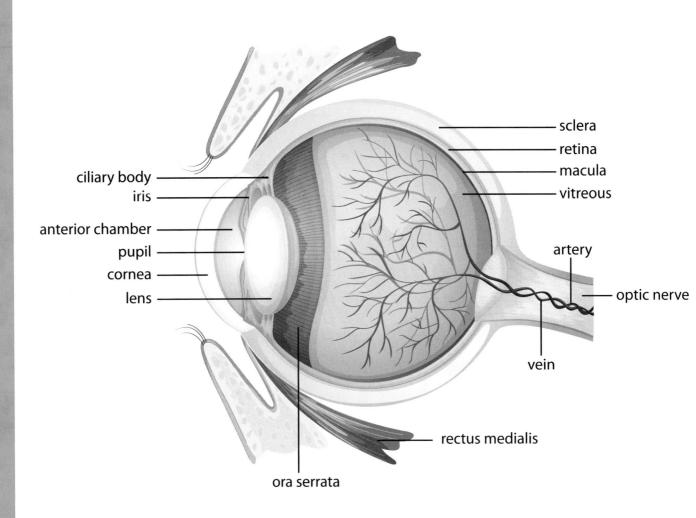

ciliary body
iris
anterior chamber
pupil
cornea
lens

sclera
retina
macula
vitreous

artery

optic nerve

vein

rectus medialis

ora serrata

FEMALE REPRODUCTIVE SYSTEM

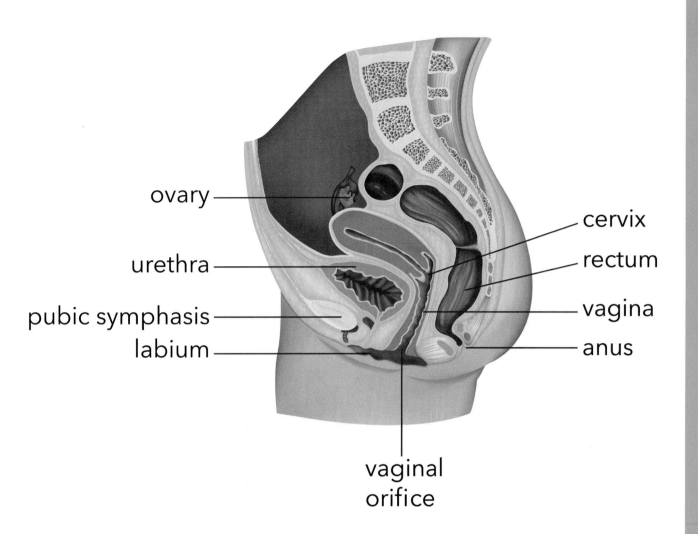

ovary

urethra

pubic symphasis

labium

cervix

rectum

vagina

anus

vaginal
orifice

FOOT BONES (right foot, lateral view)

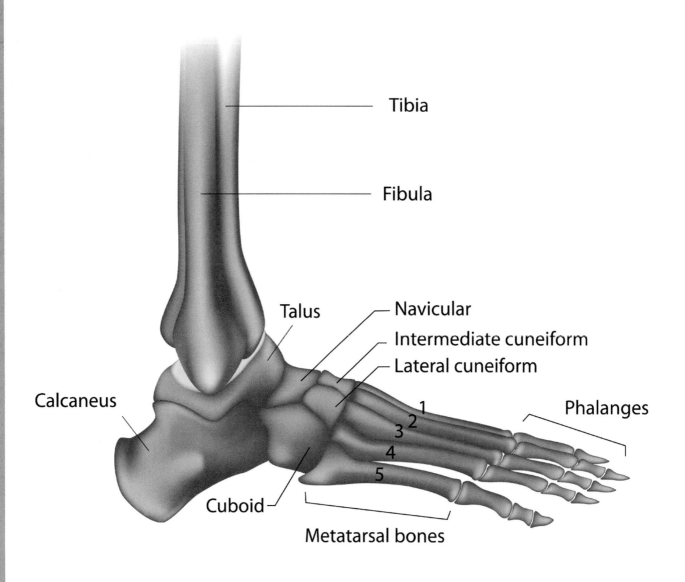

Tibia

Fibula

Talus

Navicular

Intermediate cuneiform

Lateral cuneiform

Calcaneus

1
2
3
4
5

Phalanges

Cuboid

Metatarsal bones

FOREARM MUSCLES
(right arm, posterior compartment)

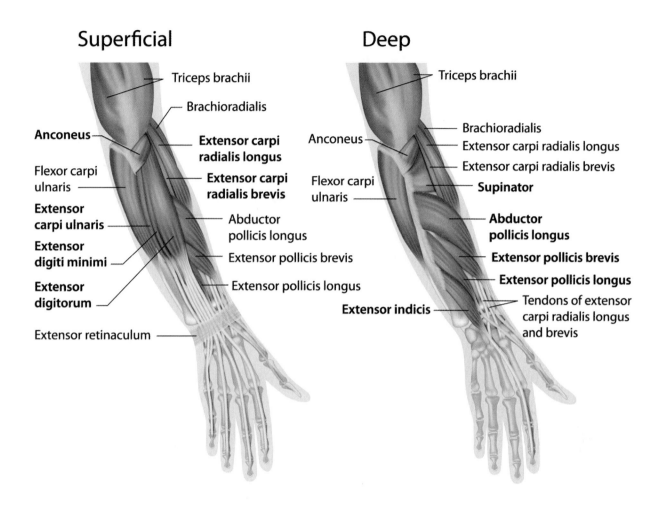

Superficial

Triceps brachii

Brachioradialis

Anconeus

Extensor carpi radialis longus

Flexor carpi ulnaris

Extensor carpi radialis brevis

Extensor carpi ulnaris

Abductor pollicis longus

Extensor digiti minimi

Extensor pollicis brevis

Extensor digitorum

Extensor pollicis longus

Extensor retinaculum

Deep

Triceps brachii

Anconeus

Brachioradialis

Extensor carpi radialis longus

Extensor carpi radialis brevis

Flexor carpi ulnaris

Supinator

Abductor pollicis longus

Extensor pollicis brevis

Extensor pollicis longus

Extensor indicis

Tendons of extensor carpi radialis longus and brevis

HAND BONES

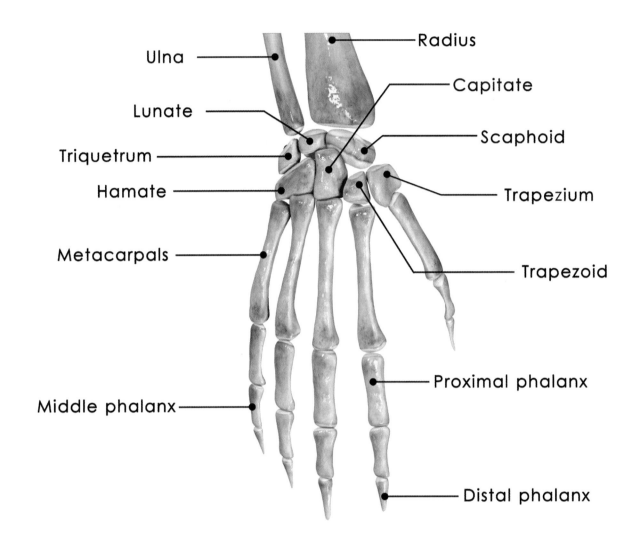

Ulna

Radius

Lunate

Capitate

Triquetrum

Scaphoid

Hamate

Trapezium

Metacarpals

Trapezoid

Proximal phalanx

Middle phalanx

Distal phalanx

KIDNEY ANATOMY

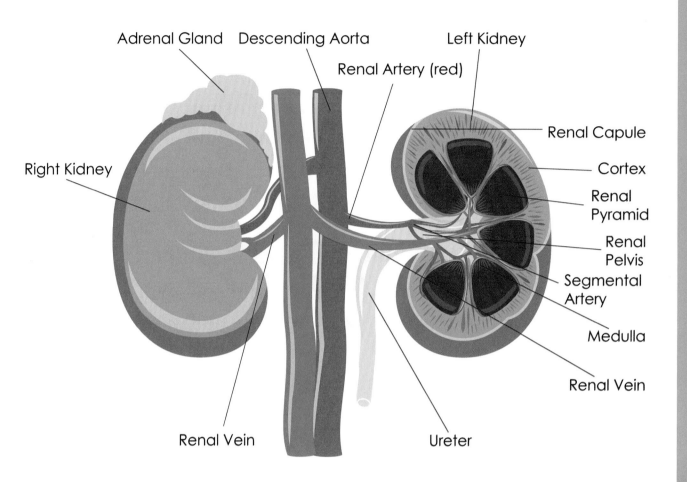

LARGE INTESTINE ANATOMY

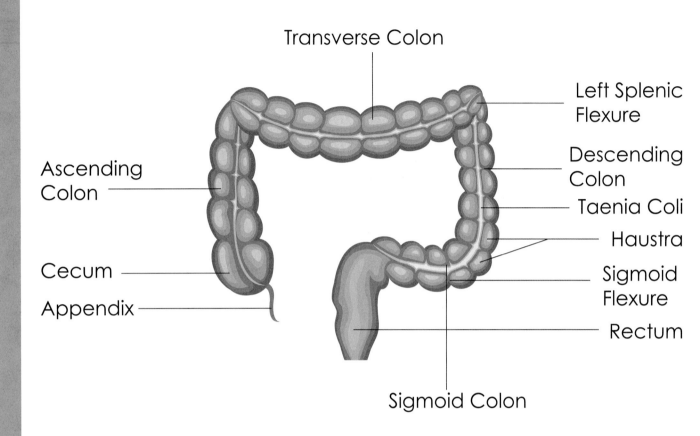

Transverse Colon

Left Splenic Flexure

Ascending Colon

Descending Colon

Taenia Coli

Haustra

Cecum

Sigmoid Flexure

Appendix

Rectum

Sigmoid Colon

LIVER ANATOMY

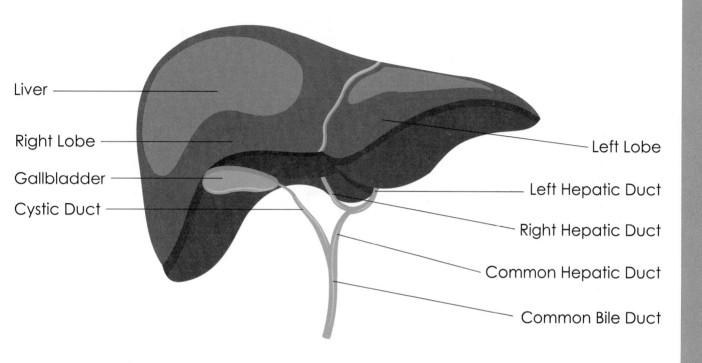

Liver

Right Lobe

Gallbladder

Cystic Duct

Left Lobe

Left Hepatic Duct

Right Hepatic Duct

Common Hepatic Duct

Common Bile Duct

LYMPHATIC SYSTEM

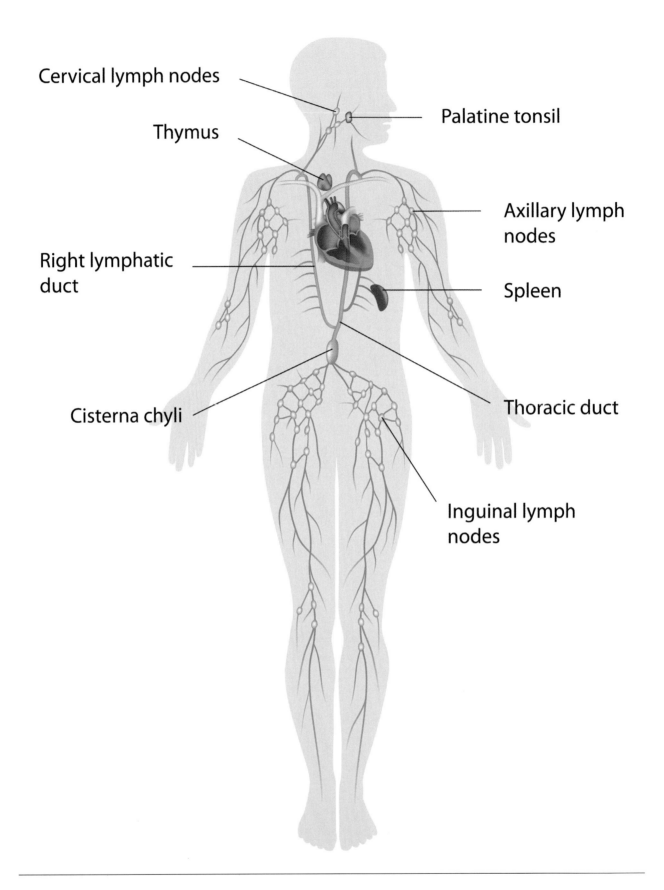

Cervical lymph nodes

Palatine tonsil

Thymus

Axillary lymph nodes

Right lymphatic duct

Spleen

Cisterna chyli

Thoracic duct

Inguinal lymph nodes

MALE REPRODUCTIVE SYSTEM

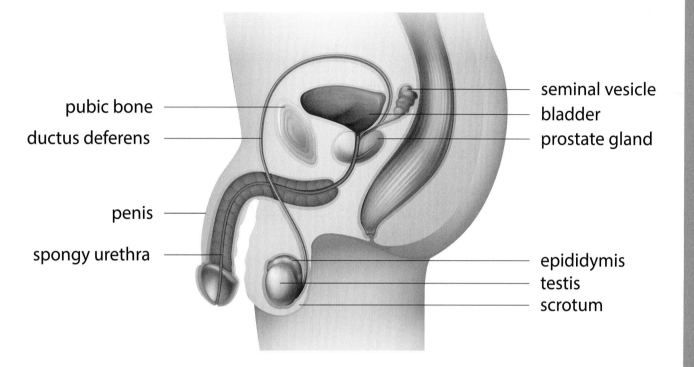

pubic bone

ductus deferens

penis

spongy urethra

seminal vesicle

bladder

prostate gland

epididymis

testis

scrotum

MOUTH ANATOMY

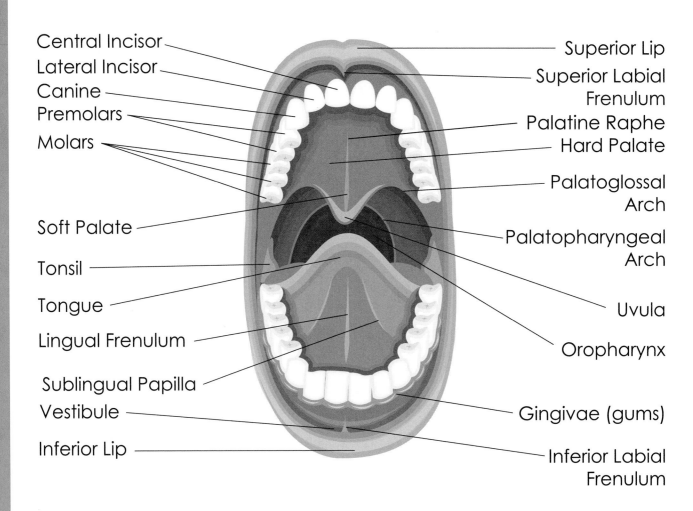

Central Incisor

Lateral Incisor

Canine

Premolars

Molars

Soft Palate

Tonsil

Tongue

Lingual Frenulum

Sublingual Papilla

Vestibule

Inferior Lip

Superior Lip

Superior Labial Frenulum

Palatine Raphe

Hard Palate

Palatoglossal Arch

Palatopharyngeal Arch

Uvula

Oropharynx

Gingivae (gums)

Inferior Labial Frenulum

MUSCLE SYSTEM

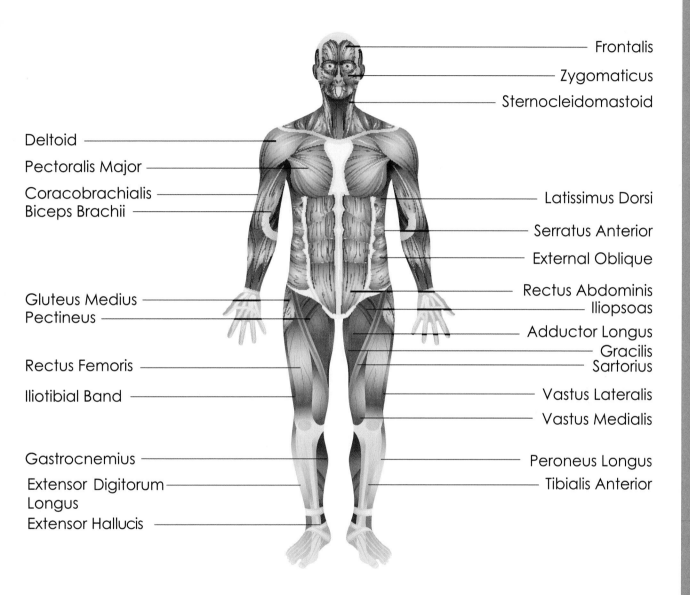

Frontalis

Zygomaticus

Sternocleidomastoid

Deltoid

Pectoralis Major

Coracobrachialis
Biceps Brachii

Latissimus Dorsi

Serratus Anterior

External Oblique

Gluteus Medius
Pectineus

Rectus Abdominis
Iliopsoas

Adductor Longus

Gracilis
Sartorius

Rectus Femoris

Iliotibial Band

Vastus Lateralis

Vastus Medialis

Gastrocnemius

Extensor Digitorum
Longus
Extensor Hallucis

Peroneus Longus

Tibialis Anterior

NERVOUS SYSTEM

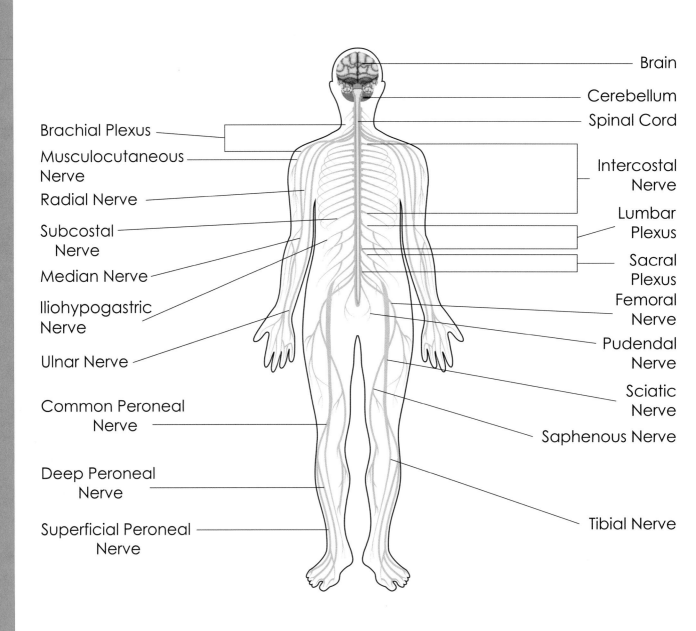

Brachial Plexus

Musculocutaneous Nerve

Radial Nerve

Subcostal Nerve

Median Nerve

Iliohypogastric Nerve

Ulnar Nerve

Common Peroneal Nerve

Deep Peroneal Nerve

Superficial Peroneal Nerve

Brain

Cerebellum

Spinal Cord

Intercostal Nerve

Lumbar Plexus

Sacral Plexus

Femoral Nerve

Pudendal Nerve

Sciatic Nerve

Saphenous Nerve

Tibial Nerve

NOSE ANATOMY

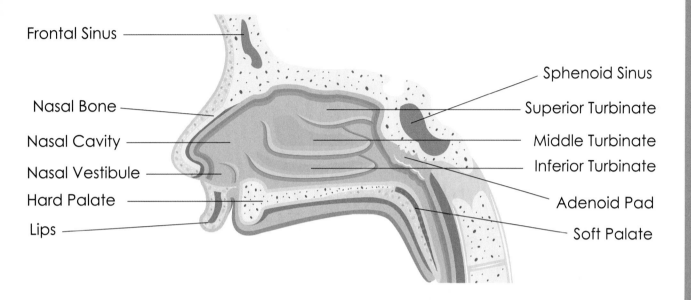

Frontal Sinus

Nasal Bone

Nasal Cavity

Nasal Vestibule

Hard Palate

Lips

Sphenoid Sinus

Superior Turbinate

Middle Turbinate

Inferior Turbinate

Adenoid Pad

Soft Palate

PANCREAS ANATOMY

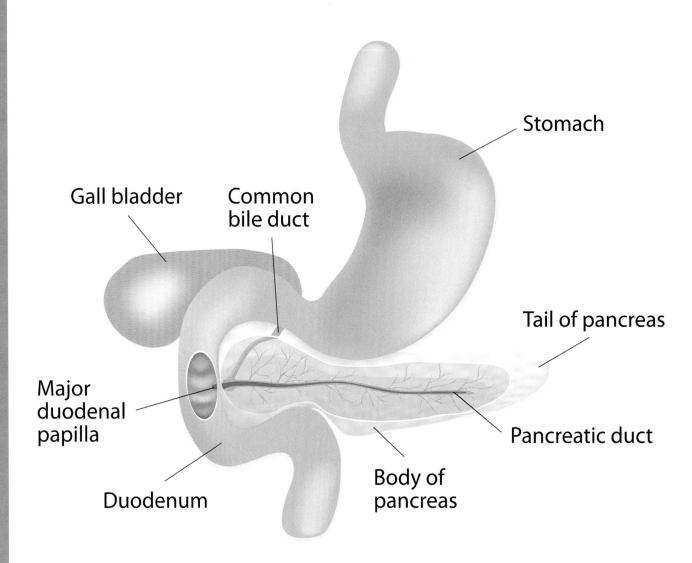

Stomach

Gall bladder

Common bile duct

Tail of pancreas

Major duodenal papilla

Pancreatic duct

Duodenum

Body of pancreas

PARASYMPATHETIC SYSTEM

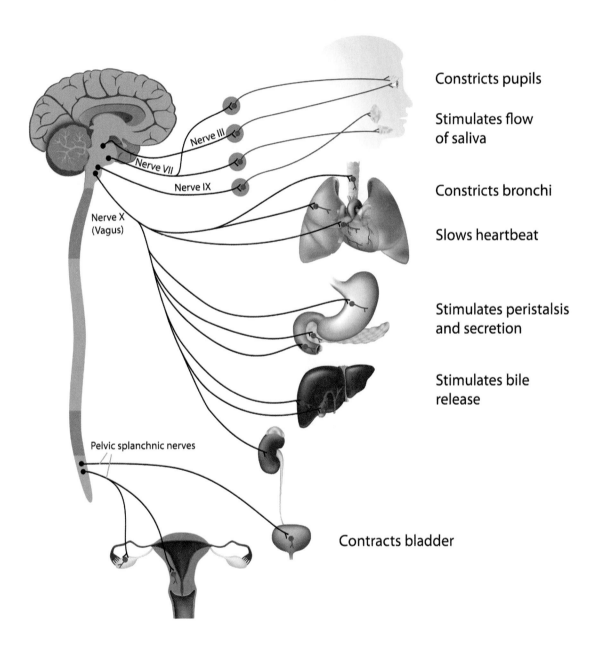

Constricts pupils

Stimulates flow of saliva

Nerve III

Nerve VII

Nerve IX

Nerve X (Vagus)

Constricts bronchi

Slows heartbeat

Stimulates peristalsis and secretion

Stimulates bile release

Pelvic splanchnic nerves

Contracts bladder

RESPIRATORY SYSTEM

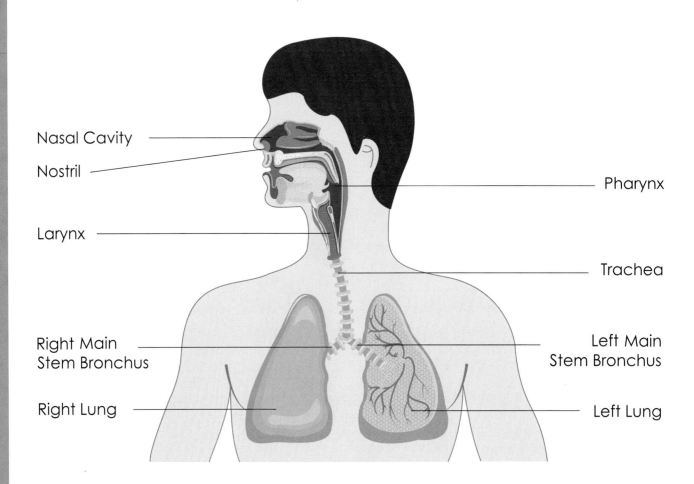

Nasal Cavity

Nostril

Larynx

Pharynx

Trachea

Right Main
Stem Bronchus

Right Lung

Left Main
Stem Bronchus

Left Lung

ROTATOR CUFF MUSCLES

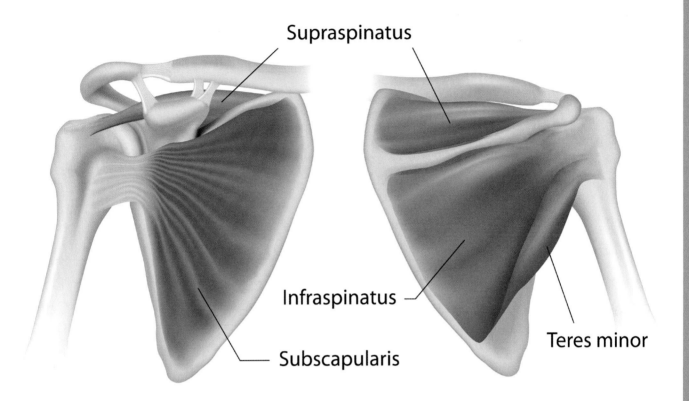

Supraspinatus

Infraspinatus

Subscapularis

Teres minor

Anterior view   Posterior view

SKELETAL SYSTEM

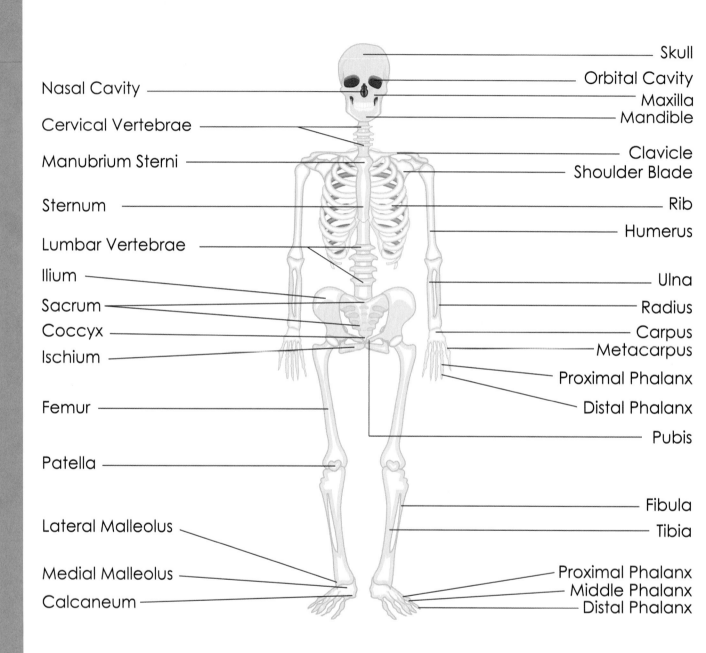

Skull

Orbital Cavity

Nasal Cavity

Maxilla

Mandible

Cervical Vertebrae

Clavicle

Manubrium Sterni

Shoulder Blade

Sternum

Rib

Lumbar Vertebrae

Humerus

Ilium

Ulna

Sacrum

Radius

Coccyx

Carpus

Ischium

Metacarpus

Proximal Phalanx

Femur

Distal Phalanx

Pubis

Patella

Fibula

Tibia

Lateral Malleolus

Proximal Phalanx

Medial Malleolus

Middle Phalanx

Calcaneum

Distal Phalanx

SKULL ANATOMY

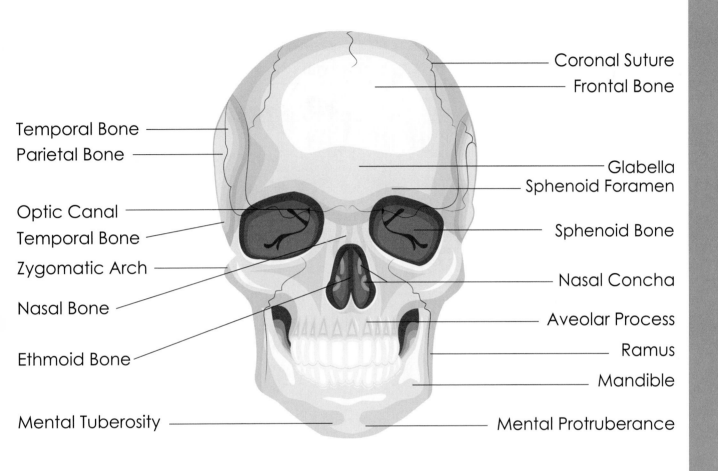

Coronal Suture

Frontal Bone

Temporal Bone

Parietal Bone

Glabella

Sphenoid Foramen

Optic Canal

Temporal Bone

Sphenoid Bone

Zygomatic Arch

Nasal Concha

Nasal Bone

Aveolar Process

Ramus

Ethmoid Bone

Mandible

Mental Tuberosity

Mental Protruberance

SMALL INTESTINE ANATOMY

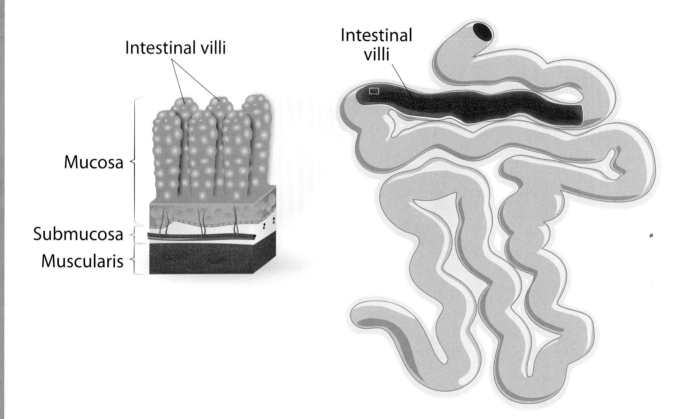

Intestinal villi

Mucosa

Submucosa

Muscularis

Intestinal villi

STOMACH ANATOMY

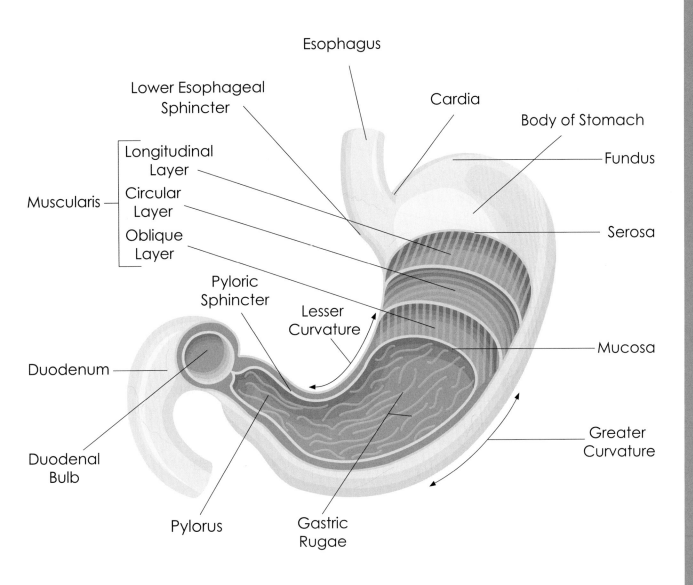

Esophagus

Lower Esophageal Sphincter

Cardia

Body of Stomach

Fundus

Muscularis

Longitudinal Layer

Circular Layer

Oblique Layer

Serosa

Pyloric Sphincter

Lesser Curvature

Duodenum

Mucosa

Duodenal Bulb

Greater Curvature

Pylorus

Gastric Rugae

SYMPATHETIC SYSTEM

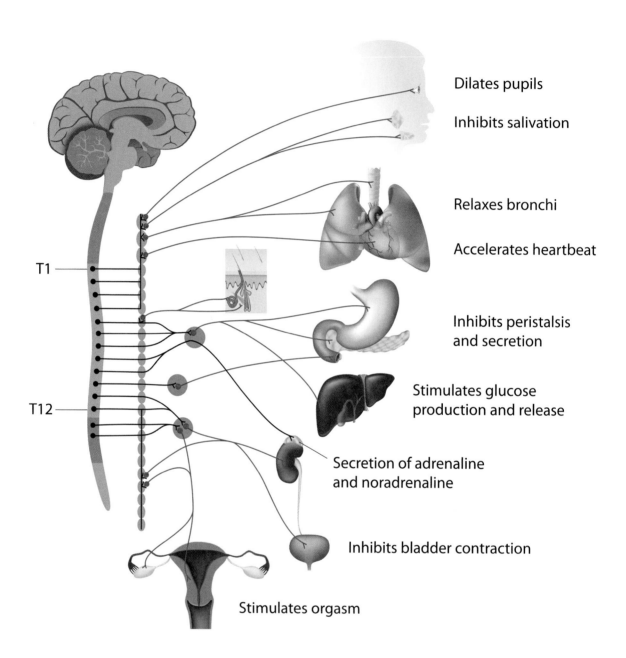

Dilates pupils

Inhibits salivation

Relaxes bronchi

Accelerates heartbeat

Inhibits peristalsis and secretion

Stimulates glucose production and release

Secretion of adrenaline and noradrenaline

Inhibits bladder contraction

Stimulates orgasm

T1

T12

THROAT ANATOMY

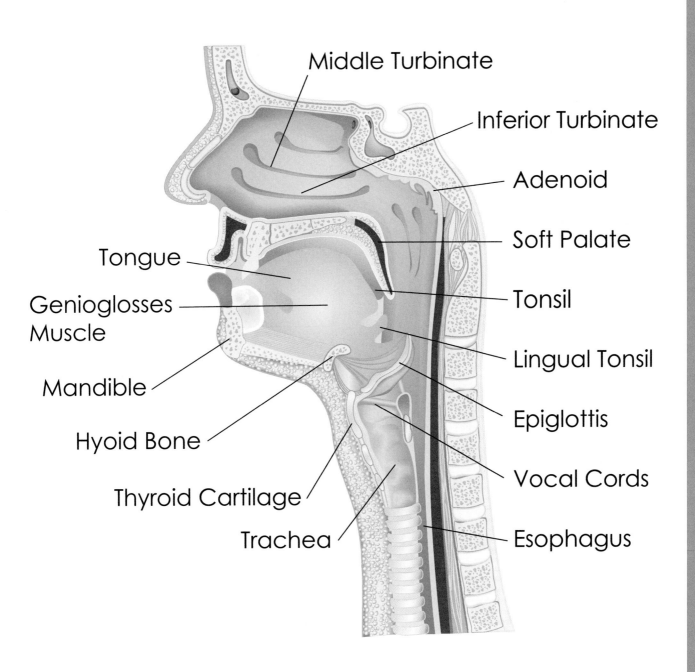

Middle Turbinate

Inferior Turbinate

Adenoid

Soft Palate

Tongue

Tonsil

Genioglosses Muscle

Lingual Tonsil

Mandible

Epiglottis

Hyoid Bone

Vocal Cords

Thyroid Cartilage

Trachea

Esophagus

URINARY SYSTEM

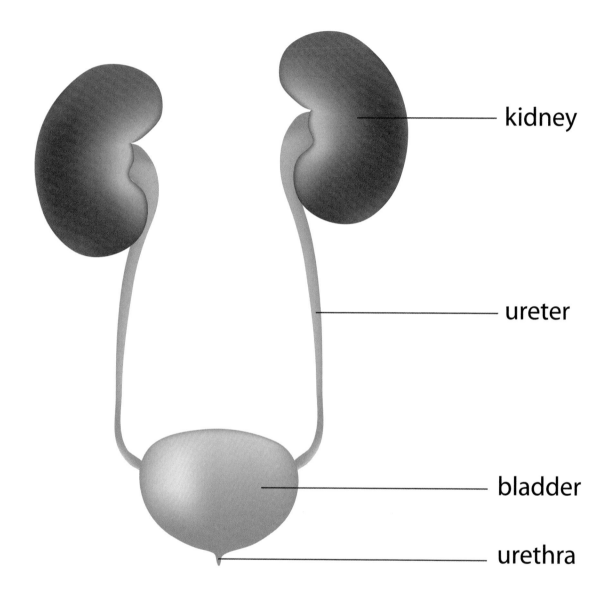

kidney

ureter

bladder

urethra

A

Aarskog's syndrome Q87.1
Abandonment — *see* Maltreatment
Abasia (-astasia) (hysterical) F44.4
Abderhalden-Kaufmann-Lignac syndrome
(cystinosis) E72.04
Abdomen, abdominal (*see also* condition)
  acute R10.0
  angina K55.1
  muscle deficiency syndrome Q79.4
Abdominalgia — *see* Pain, abdominal
Abduction contracture, hip or other joint — *see*
  Contraction, joint
Aberrant (congenital) (*see also* Malposition,
  congenital)
  adrenal gland Q89.1
  artery (peripheral) Q27.8
    basilar NEC Q28.1
    cerebral Q28.3
    coronary Q24.5
    digestive system Q27.8
    eye Q15.8
    lower limb Q27.8
    precerebral Q28.1
    pulmonary Q25.79
    renal Q27.2
    retina Q14.1
    specified site NEC Q27.8
    subclavian Q27.8
    upper limb Q27.8
    vertebral Q28.1
  breast Q83.8
  endocrine gland NEC Q89.2
  hepatic duct Q44.5
  pancreas Q45.3
  parathyroid gland Q89.2
  pituitary gland Q89.2
  sebaceous glands, mucous membrane, mouth,
    congenital Q38.6
  spleen Q89.09
  subclavian artery Q27.8
  thymus (gland) Q89.2
  thyroid gland Q89.2
  vein (peripheral) NEC Q27.8
    cerebral Q28.3
    digestive system Q27.8
    lower limb Q27.8
    precerebral Q28.1
    specified site NEC Q27.8
    upper limb Q27.8
Aberration
  distantial — *see* Disturbance, visual
  mental F99
Abetalipoproteinemia E78.6
Abiotrophy R68.89
Ablatio, ablation
  retinae — *see* Detachment, retina
Ablepharia, ablepharon Q10.3
Abnormal, abnormality, abnormalities (*see also*
  Anomaly)
  acid-base balance (mixed) E87.4
  albumin R77.0
  alphafetoprotein R77.2
  alveolar ridge K08.9
  anatomical relationship Q89.9
  apertures, congenital, diaphragm Q79.1
  auditory perception H93.29- ☑
    diplacusis — *see* Diplacusis
    hyperacusis — *see* Hyperacusis
    recruitment — *see* Recruitment, auditory
    threshold shift — *see* Shift, auditory threshold
  autosomes Q99.9
    fragile site Q95.5
  basal metabolic rate R94.8
  biosynthesis, testicular androgen E29.1
  bleeding time R79.1
  blood-gas level R79.81
  blood level (of)
    cobalt R79.0
    copper R79.0
    iron R79.0
    lithium R78.89
    magnesium R79.0
    mineral NEC R79.0
    zinc R79.0
  blood pressure
    elevated R03.0
    low reading (nonspecific) R03.1
  blood sugar R73.09
  bowel sounds R19.15

Abnormal — *continued*
  absent R19.11
  hyperactive R19.12
  brain scan R94.02
  breathing R06.9
  caloric test R94.138
  cerebrospinal fluid R83.9
    cytology R83.6
    drug level R83.2
    enzyme level R83.0
    hormones R83.1
    immunology R83.4
    microbiology R83.5
    nonmedicinal level R83.3
    specified type NEC R83.8
  chemistry, blood R79.9
    C-reactive protein R79.82
    drugs — *see* Findings, abnormal, in blood
    gas level R79.81
    minerals R79.0
    pancytopenia D61.818
    PTT R79.1
    specified NEC R79.89
    toxins — *see* Findings, abnormal, in blood
  chest sounds (friction) (rales) R09.89
  chromosome, chromosomal Q99.9
    with more than three X chromosomes, female
      Q97.1
    analysis result R89.8
      bronchial washings R84.8
      cerebrospinal fluid R83.8
      cervix uteri NEC R87.89
      nasal secretions R84.8
      nipple discharge R89.8
      peritoneal fluid R85.89
      pleural fluid R84.8
      prostatic secretions R86.8
      saliva R85.89
      seminal fluid R86.8
      sputum R84.8
      synovial fluid R89.8
      throat scrapings R84.8
      vagina R87.89
      vulva R87.89
      wound secretions R89.8
    dicentric replacement Q93.2
    ring replacement Q93.2
    sex Q99.8
      female phenotype Q97.9
        specified NEC Q97.8
      male phenotype Q98.9
        specified NEC Q98.8
      structural male Q98.6
    specified NEC Q99.8
  clinical findings NEC R68.89
  coagulation D68.9
    newborn, transient P61.6
    profile R79.1
    time R79.1
  communication — *see* Fistula
  conjunctiva, vascular H11.41- ☑
  coronary artery Q24.5
  cortisol-binding globulin E27.8
  course, eustachian tube Q17.8
  creatinine clearance R94.4
  cytology
    anus R85.619
      atypical squamous cells cannot exclude high
        grade squamous intraepithelial lesion
        (ASC-H) R85.611
      atypical squamous cells of undetermined
        significance (ASC-US) R85.610
      cytologic evidence of malignancy R85.614
      high grade squamous intraepithelial lesion
        (HGSIL) R85.613
      human papillomavirus (HPV) DNA test
        high risk positive R85.81
        low risk postive R85.82
      inadequate smear R85.615
      low grade squamous intraepithelial lesion
        (LGSIL) R85.612
      satisfactory anal smear but lacking
        transformation zone R85.616
      specified NEC R85.618
      unsatisfactory smear R85.615
    female genital organs — *see* Abnormal,
      Papanicolaou (smear)
  dark adaptation curve H53.61
  dentofacial NEC — *see* Anomaly, dentofacial
  development, developmental Q89.9
    central nervous system Q07.9
  diagnostic imaging

Abnormal — *continued*
  abdomen, abdominal region NEC R93.5
  biliary tract R93.2
  breast R92.8
  central nervous system NEC R90.89
  cerebrovascular NEC R90.89
  coronary circulation R93.1
  digestive tract NEC R93.3
  gastrointestinal (tract) R93.3
  genitourinary organs R93.8
  head R93.0
  heart R93.1
  intrathoracic organ NEC R93.8
  limbs R93.6
  liver R93.2
  lung (field) R91.8
  musculoskeletal system NEC R93.7
  retroperitoneum R93.5
  site specified NEC R93.8
  skin and subcutaneous tissue R93.8
  skull R93.0
  urinary organs R93.4
  direction, teeth, fully erupted M26.30
  ear ossicles, acquired NEC H74.39- ☑
    ankylosis — *see* Ankylosis, ear ossicles
    discontinuity — *see* Discontinuity, ossicles, ear
    partial loss — *see* Loss, ossicles, ear (partial)
  Ebstein Q22.5
  echocardiogram R93.1
  echoencephalogram R90.81
  echogram — *see* Abnormal, diagnostic imaging
  electrocardiogram [ECG] [EKG] R94.31
  electroencephalogram [EEG] R94.01
  electrolyte — *see* Imbalance, electrolyte
  electromyogram [EMG] R94.131
  electro-oculogram [EOG] R94.110
  electrophysiological intracardiac studies R94.39
  electroretinogram [ERG] R94.111
  erythrocytes
    congenital, with perinatal jaundice D58.9
  feces (color) (contents) (mucus) R19.5
  finding — *see* Findings, abnormal, without
    diagnosis
  fluid
    amniotic — *see* Abnormal, specimen, specified
    cerebrospinal — *see* Abnormal, cerebrospinal
      fluid
    peritoneal — *see* Abnormal, specimen,
      digestive organs
    pleural — *see* Abnormal, specimen, respiratory
      organs
    synovial — *see* Abnormal, specimen, specified
    thorax (bronchial washings) (pleural fluid)
      — *see* Abnormal, specimen, respiratory
      organs
    vaginal — *see* Abnormal, specimen, female
      genital organs
  form
    teeth K00.2
    uterus — *see* Anomaly, uterus
  function studies
    auditory R94.120
    bladder R94.8
    brain R94.09
    cardiovascular R94.30
    ear R94.128
    endocrine NEC R94.7
    eye NEC R94.118
    kidney R94.4
    liver R94.5
    nervous system
      central NEC R94.09
      peripheral NEC R94.138
    pancreas R94.8
    placenta R94.8
    pulmonary R94.2
    special senses NEC R94.128
    spleen R94.8
    thyroid R94.6
    vestibular R94.121
  gait — *see* Gait
    hysterical F44.4
  gastrin secretion E16.4
  globulin R77.1
    cortisol-binding E27.8
    thyroid-binding E07.89
  glomerular, minor (*see also* N00-N07 with fourth
    character .0) N05.0
  glucagon secretion E16.3
  glucose tolerance (test) (non-fasting) R73.09
  gravitational (G) forces or states (effect of)
    T75.81 ☑

Abnormal — *continued*
    hair (color) (shaft) L67.9
        specified NEC L67.8
    hard tissue formation in pulp (dental) K04.3
    head movement R25.0
    heart
        rate R00.9
            specified NEC R00.8
        shadow R93.1
        sounds NEC R01.2
    hemoglobin (disease) (*see also* Disease,
        hemoglobin) D58.2
        trait — *see* Trait, hemoglobin, abnormal
    histology NEC R89.7
    immunological findings R89.4
        in serum R76.9
            specified NEC R76.8
    increase in appetite R63.2
    involuntary movement — *see* Abnormal,
        movement, involuntary
    jaw closure M26.51
    karyotype R89.8
    kidney function test R94.4
    knee jerk R29.2
    leukocyte (cell) (differential) NEC D72.9
    liver
    loss of
        height R29.890
        weight R63.4
    mammogram NEC R92.8
        calcification (calculus) R92.1
        microcalcification R92.0
    Mantoux test R76.11
    movement (disorder) (*see also* Disorder,
        movement)
        head R25.0
        involuntary R25.9
            fasciculation R25.3
            of head R25.0
            spasm R25.2
            specified type NEC R25.8
            tremor R25.1
    myoglobin (Aberdeen) (Annapolis) R89.7
    neonatal screening P09
    oculomotor study R94.113
    palmar creases Q82.8
    Papanicolaou (smear)
        anus R85.619
            atypical squamous cells cannot exclude high
                grade squamous intraepithelial lesion
                (ASC-H) R85.611
            atypical squamous cells of undetermined
                significance (ASC-US) R85.610
            cytologic evidence of malignancy R85.614
            high grade squamous intraepithelial lesion
                (HGSIL) R85.613
            human papillomavirus (HPV) DNA test
                high risk positive R85.81
                low risk postive R85.82
            inadequate smear R85.615
            low grade squamous intraepithelial lesion
                (LGSIL) R85.612
            satisfactory anal smear but lacking
                transformation zone R85.616
            specified NEC R85.618
            unsatisfactory smear R85.615
        bronchial washings R84.6
        cerebrospinal fluid R83.6
        cervix R87.619
            atypical squamous cells cannot exclude high
                grade squamous intraepithelial lesion
                (ASC-H) R87.611
            atypical squamous cells of undetermined
                significance (ASC-US) R87.610
            cytologic evidence of malignancy R87.614
            high grade squamous intraepithelial lesion
                (HGSIL) R87.613
            inadequate smear R87.615
            low grade squamous intraepithelial lesion
                (LGSIL) R87.612
            non-atypical endometrial cells R87.618
            satisfactory cervical smear but lacking
                transformation zone R87.616
            specified NEC R87.618
            thin preparaton R87.619
            unsatisfactory smear R87.615
        nasal secretions R84.6
        nipple discharge R89.6
        peritoneal fluid R85.69
        pleural fluid R84.6
        prostatic secretions R86.6
        saliva R85.69

Abnormal — *continued*
    seminal fluid R86.6
    sites NEC R89.6
    sputum R84.6
    synovial fluid R89.6
    throat scrapings R84.6
    vagina R87.629
        atypical squamous cells cannot exclude high
            grade squamous intraepithelial lesion
            (ASC-H) R87.621
        atypical squamous cells of undetermined
            significance (ASC-US) R87.620
        cytologic evidence of malignancy R87.624
        high grade squamous intraepithelial lesion
            (HGSIL) R87.623
        inadequate smear R87.625
        low grade squamous intraepithelial lesion
            (LGSIL) R87.622
        specified NEC R87.628
        thin preparation R87.629
        unsatisfactory smear R87.625
    vulva R87.69
    wound secretions R89.6
    partial thromboplastin time (PTT) R79.1
    pelvis (bony) — *see* Deformity, pelvis
    percussion, chest (tympany) R09.89
    periods (grossly) — *see* Menstruation
    phonocardiogram R94.39
    plantar reflex R29.2
    plasma
        protein R77.9
            specified NEC R77.8
        viscosity R70.1
    pleural (folds) Q34.0
    posture R29.3
    product of conception O02.9
        specified type NEC O02.89
    prothrombin time (PT) R79.1
    pulmonary
        artery, congenital Q25.79
        function, newborn P28.89
        test results R94.2
    pulsations in neck R00.2
    pupillary H21.56- ☑
        function (reaction) (reflex) — *see* Anomaly,
            pupil, function
    radiological examination — *see* Abnormal,
        diagnostic imaging
    red blood cell (s) (morphology) (volume) R71.8
    reflex — *see* Reflex
    renal function test R94.4
    response to nerve stimulation R94.130
    retinal correspondence H53.31
    retinal function study R94.111
    rhythm, heart (*see also* Arrhythmia)
    saliva — *see* Abnormal, specimen, digestive
        organs
    scan
        kidney R94.4
        liver R93.2
        thyroid R94.6
    secretion
        gastrin E16.4
        glucagon E16.3
    semen, seminal fluid — *see* Abnormal, specimen,
        male genital organs
    serum level (of)
        acid phosphatase R74.8
        alkaline phosphatase R74.8
        amylase R74.8
        enzymes R74.9
            specified NEC R74.8
        lipase R74.8
        triacylglycerol lipase R74.8
    shape
        gravid uterus — *see* Anomaly, uterus
    sinus venosus Q21.1
    size, tooth, teeth K00.2
    spacing, tooth, teeth, fully erupted M26.30
    specimen
        digestive organs (peritoneal fluid) (saliva)
            R85.9
            cytology R85.69
            drug level R85.2
            enzyme level R85.0
            histology R85.7
            hormones R85.1
            immunology R85.4
            microbiology R85.5
            nonmedicinal level R85.3
            specified type NEC R85.89

Abnormal — *continued*
    female genital organs (secretions) (smears)
        R87.9
        cytology R87.69
            cervix R87.619
                human papillomavirus (HPV) DNA test
                    high risk positive R87.810
                    low risk positive R87.820
                inadequate (unsatisfactory) smear
                    R87.615
                non-atypical endometrial cells R87.618
                specified NEC R87.618
            vagina R87.629
                human papillomavirus (HPV) DNA test
                    high risk positive R87.811
                    low risk positive R87.821
                inadequate (unsatisfactory) smear
                    R87.625
            vulva R87.69
        drug level R87.2
        enzyme level R87.0
        histological R87.7
        hormones R87.1
        immunology R87.4
        microbiology R87.5
        nonmedicinal level R87.3
        specified type NEC R87.89
    male genital organs (prostatic secretions)
        (semen) R86.9
        cytology R86.6
        drug level R86.2
        enzyme level R86.0
        histological R86.7
        hormones R86.1
        immunology R86.4
        microbiology R86.5
        nonmedicinal level R86.3
        specified type NEC R86.8
    nipple discharge — *see* Abnormal, specimen,
        specified
    respiratory organs (bronchial washings) (nasal
        secretions) (pleural fluid) (sputum) R84.9
        cytology R84.6
        drug level R84.2
        enzyme level R84.0
        histology R84.7
        hormones R84.1
        immunology R84.4
        microbiology R84.5
        nonmedicinal level R84.3
        specified type NEC R84.8
    specified organ, system and tissue NOS R89.9
        cytology R89.6
        drug level R89.2
        enzyme level R89.0
        histology R89.7
        hormones R89.1
        immunology R89.4
        microbiology R89.5
        nonmedicinal level R89.3
        specified type NEC R89.8
    synovial fluid — *see* Abnormal, specimen,
        specified
    thorax (bronchial washings) (pleural fluids)
        — *see* Abnormal, specimen, respiratory
        organs
    vagina (secretion) (smear) R87.629
    vulva (secretion) (smear) R87.69
    wound secretion — *see* Abnormal, specimen,
        specified
    spermatozoa — *see* Abnormal, specimen, male
        genital organs
    sputum (amount) (color) (odor) R09.3
    stool (color) (contents) (mucus) R19.5
        bloody K92.1
        guaiac positive R19.5
    synchondrosis Q78.8
    thermography (*see also* Abnormal, diagnostic
        imaging) R93.8
    thyroid-binding globulin E07.89
    tooth, teeth (form) (size) K00.2
    toxicology (findings) R78.9
    transport protein E88.09
    tumor marker NEC R97.8
    ultrasound results — *see* Abnormal, diagnostic
        imaging
    umbilical cord complicating delivery O69.9 ☑
    urination NEC R39.19
    urine (constituents) R82.90
        bile R82.2
        cytological examination R82.8
        drugs R82.5

☑ **Additional character required**

Abnormal — *continued*
fat R82.0
glucose R81
heavy metals R82.6
hemoglobin R82.3
histological examination R82.8
ketones R82.4
microbiological examination (culture) R82.7
myoglobin R82.1
positive culture R82.7
protein — *see* Proteinuria
specified substance NEC R82.99
chromoabnormality NEC R82.91
substances nonmedical R82.6
uterine hemorrhage — *see* Hemorrhage, uterus
vectorcardiogram R94.39
visually evoked potential (VEP) R94.112
white blood cells D72.9
specified NEC D72.89
X-ray examination — *see* Abnormal, diagnostic imaging
Abnormity (any organ or part) — *see* Anomaly
Abocclusion M26.29
hemolytic disease (newborn) P55.1
incompatibility reaction ABO — *see* Complication(s), transfusion, incompatibility reaction, ABO
Abolition, language R48.8
Aborter, habitual or recurrent — *see* Loss (of), pregnancy, recurrent
Abortion (complete) (spontaneous) O03.9
with
retained products of conception — *see* Abortion, incomplete
attempted (elective) (failed) O07.4
complicated by O07.30
afibrinogenemia O07.1
cardiac arrest O07.36
chemical damage of pelvic organ (s) O07.34
circulatory collapse O07.31
cystitis O07.38
defibrination syndrome O07.1
electrolyte imbalance O07.33
embolism (air) (amniotic fluid) (blood clot) (fat) (pulmonary) (septic) (soap) O07.2
endometritis O07.0
genital tract and pelvic infection O07.0
hemolysis O07.1
hemorrhage (delayed) (excessive) O07.1
infection
genital tract or pelvic O07.0
urinary tract tract O07.38
intravascular coagulation O07.1
laceration of pelvic organ (s) O07.34
metabolic disorder O07.33
oliguria O07.32
oophoritis O07.0
parametritis O07.0
pelvic peritonitis O07.0
perforation of pelvic organ (s) O07.34
renal failure or shutdown O07.32
salpingitis or salpingo-oophoritis O07.0
sepsis O07.37
shock O07.31
specified condition NEC O07.39
tubular necrosis (renal) O07.32
uremia O07.32
urinary tract infection O07.38
venous complication NEC O07.35
embolism (air) (amniotic fluid) (blood clot) (fat) (pulmonary) (septic) (soap) O07.2
complicated (by) (following) O03.80
afibrinogenemia O03.6
cardiac arrest O03.86
chemical damage of pelvic organ (s) O03.84
circulatory collapse O03.81
cystitis O03.88
defibrination syndrome O03.6
electrolyte imbalance O03.83
embolism (air) (amniotic fluid) (blood clot) (fat) (pulmonary) (septic) (soap) O03.7
endometritis O03.5
genital tract and pelvic infection O03.5
hemolysis O03.6
hemorrhage (delayed) (excessive) O03.6
infection
genital tract or pelvic O03.5
urinary tract O03.88
intravascular coagulation O03.6
laceration of pelvic organ (s) O03.84
metabolic disorder O03.03
oliguria O03.82

Abortion — *continued*
oophoritis O03.5
parametritis O03.5
pelvic peritonitis O03.5
perforation of pelvic organ (s) O03.84
renal failure or shutdown O03.82
salpingitis or salpingo-oophoritis O03.5
sepsis O03.87
shock O03.81
specified condition NEC O03.89
tubular necrosis (renal) O03.82
uremia O03.82
urinary tract infection O03.88
venous complication NEC O03.85
embolism (air) (amniotic fluid) (blood clot) (fat) (pulmonary) (septic) (soap) O03.7
failed — *see* Abortion, attempted
habitual or recurrent N96
with current abortion — *see* categories O03-O06
without current pregnancy N96
care in current pregnancy O26.2- ☑
incomplete (spontaneous) O03.4
complicated (by) (following) O03.30
afibrinogenemia O03.1
cardiac arrest O03.36
chemical damage of pelvic organ (s) O03.34
circulatory collapse O03.31
cystitis O03.38
defibrination syndrome O03.1
electrolyte imbalance O03.33
embolism (air) (amniotic fluid) (blood clot) (fat) (pulmonary) (septic) (soap) O03.2
endometritis O03.0
genital tract and pelvic infection O03.0
hemolysis O03.1
hemorrhage (delayed) (excessive) O03.1
infection
genital tract or pelvic O03.0
urinary tract O03.38
intravascular coagulation O03.1
laceration of pelvic organ (s) O03.34
metabolic disorder O03.33
oliguria O03.32
oophoritis O03.0
parametritis O03.0
pelvic peritonitis O03.0
perforation of pelvic organ (s) O03.34
renal failure or shutdown O03.32
salpingitis or salpingo-oophoritis O03.0
sepsis O03.37
shock O03.31
specified condition NEC O03.39
tubular necrosis (renal) O03.32
uremia O03.32
urinary infection O03.38
venous complication NEC O03.35
embolism (air) (amniotic fluid) (blood clot) (fat) (pulmonary) (septic) (soap) O03.2
induced (encounter for) Z33.2
complicated by O04.80
afibrinogenemia O04.6
cardiac arrest O04.86
chemical damage of pelvic organ (s) O04.84
circulatory collapse O04.81
cystitis O04.88
defibrination syndrome O04.6
electrolyte imbalance O04.83
embolism (air) (amniotic fluid) (blood clot) (fat) (pulmonary) (septic) (soap) O04.7
endometritis O04.5
genital tract and pelvic infection O04.5
hemolysis O04.6
hemorrhage (delayed) (excessive) O04.6
infection
genital tract or pelvic O04.5
urinary tract O04.88
intravascular coagulation O04.6
laceration of pelvic organ (s) O04.84
metabolic disorder O04.83
oliguria O04.82
oophoritis O04.5
parametritis O04.5
pelvic peritonitis O04.5
perforation of pelvic organ (s) O04.84
renal failure or shutdown O04.82
salpingitis or salpingo-oophoritis O04.5
sepsis O04.87
shock O04.81
specified condition NEC O04.89
tubular necrosis (renal) O04.02
uremia O04.82

Abortion — *continued*
urinary tract infection O04.88
venous complication NEC O04.85
embolism (air) (amniotic fluid) (blood clot) (fat) (pulmonary) (septic) (soap) O04.7
missed O02.1
spontaneous — *see* Abortion (complete) (spontaneous)
threatened O20.0
threatened (spontaneous) O20.0
tubal O00.1
Abortus fever A23.1
Aboulomania F60.7
Abrami's disease D59.8
Abramov-Fiedler myocarditis (acute isolated myocarditis) I40.1
Abrasion T14.8
abdomen, abdominal (wall) S30.811 ☑
alveolar process S00.512 ☑
ankle S90.51- ☑
antecubital space — *see* Abrasion, elbow
anus S30.817 ☑
arm (upper) S40.81- ☑
auditory canal — *see* Abrasion, ear
auricle — *see* Abrasion, ear
axilla — *see* Abrasion, arm
back, lower S30.810 ☑
breast S20.11- ☑
brow S00.81 ☑
buttock S30.810 ☑
calf — *see* Abrasion, leg
canthus — *see* Abrasion, eyelid
cheek S00.81 ☑
internal S00.512 ☑
chest wall — *see* Abrasion, thorax
chin S00.81 ☑
clitoris S30.814 ☑
cornea S05.0- ☑
costal region — *see* Abrasion, thorax
dental K03.1
digit (s)
foot — *see* Abrasion, toe
hand — *see* Abrasion, finger
ear S00.41- ☑
elbow S50.31- ☑
epididymis S30.813 ☑
epigastric region S30.811 ☑
epiglottis S10.11 ☑
esophagus (thoracic) S27.818 ☑
cervical S10.11 ☑
eyebrow — *see* Abrasion, eyelid
eyelid S00.21- ☑
face S00.81 ☑
finger (s) S60.41- ☑
index S60.41- ☑
little S60.41- ☑
middle S60.41- ☑
ring S60.41- ☑
flank S30.811 ☑
foot (except toe(s) alone) S90.81- ☑
toe — *see* Abrasion, toe
forearm S50.81- ☑
elbow only — *see* Abrasion, elbow
forehead S00.81 ☑
genital organs, external
female S30.816 ☑
male S30.815 ☑
groin S30.811 ☑
gum S00.512 ☑
hand S60.51- ☑
head S00.91 ☑
ear — *see* Abrasion, ear
eyelid — *see* Abrasion, eyelid
lip S00.511 ☑
nose S00.31 ☑
oral cavity S00.512 ☑
scalp S00.01 ☑
specified site NEC S00.81 ☑
heel — *see* Abrasion, foot
hip S70.21- ☑
inguinal region S30.811 ☑
interscapular region S20.419 ☑
jaw S00.81 ☑
knee S80.21- ☑
labium (majus) (minus) S30.814 ☑
larynx S10.11 ☑
leg (lower) S80.81- ☑
knee — *see* Abrasion, knee
upper — *see* Abrasion, thigh
lip S00.511 ☑
lower back S30.810 ☑
lumbar region S30.810 ☑

Abrasion — *continued*
  malar region S00.81 ☑
  mammary — *see* Abrasion, breast
  mastoid region S00.81 ☑
  mouth S00.512 ☑
  nail
    finger — *see* Abrasion, finger
    toe — *see* Abrasion, toe
  nape S10.81 ☑
  nasal S00.31 ☑
  neck S10.91 ☑
    specified site NEC S10.81 ☑
    throat S10.11 ☑
  nose S00.31 ☑
  occipital region S00.01 ☑
  oral cavity S00.512 ☑
  orbital region — *see* Abrasion, eyelid
  palate S00.512 ☑
  palm — *see* Abrasion, hand
  parietal region S00.01 ☑
  pelvis S30.810 ☑
  penis S30.812 ☑
  perineum
    female S30.814 ☑
    male S30.810 ☑
  periocular area — *see* Abrasion, eyelid
  phalanges
    finger — *see* Abrasion, finger
    toe — *see* Abrasion, toe
  pharynx S10.11 ☑
  pinna — *see* Abrasion, ear
  popliteal space — *see* Abrasion, knee
  prepuce S30.812 ☑
  pubic region S30.810 ☑
  pudendum
    female S30.816 ☑
    male S30.815 ☑
  sacral region S30.810 ☑
  scalp S00.01 ☑
  scapular region — *see* Abrasion, shoulder
  scrotum S30.813 ☑
  shin — *see* Abrasion, leg
  shoulder S40.21- ☑
  skin NEC T14.8
  sternal region S20.319 ☑
  submaxillary region S00.81 ☑
  submental region S00.81 ☑
  subungual
    finger (s) — *see* Abrasion, finger
    toe (s) — *see* Abrasion, toe
  supraclavicular fossa S10.81 ☑
  supraorbital S00.81 ☑
  temple S00.81 ☑
  temporal region S00.81 ☑
  testis S30.813 ☑
  thigh S70.31- ☑
  thorax, thoracic (wall) S20.91 ☑
    back S20.41- ☑
    front S20.31- ☑
  throat S10.11 ☑
  thumb S60.31- ☑
  toe (s) (lesser) S90.416 ☑
    great S90.41- ☑
  tongue S00.512 ☑
  tooth, teeth (dentifrice) (habitual) (hard tissues) (occupational) (ritual) (traditional) K03.1
  trachea S10.11 ☑
  tunica vaginalis S30.813 ☑
  tympanum, tympanic membrane — *see* Abrasion, ear
  uvula S00.512 ☑
  vagina S30.814 ☑
  vocal cords S10.11 ☑
  vulva S30.814 ☑
  wrist S60.81- ☑
Abrism — *see* Poisoning, food, noxious, plant
Abruptio placentae O45.9- ☑
  with
    afibrinogenemia O45.01- ☑
    coagulation defect O45.00- ☑
      specified NEC O45.09- ☑
    disseminated intravascular coagulation O45.02- ☑
    hypofibrinogenemia O45.01- ☑
    specified NEC O45.8- ☑
Abruption, placenta — *see* Abruptio placentae
Abscess (connective tissue) (embolic) (fistulous) (infective) (metastatic) (multiple) (pernicious) (pyogenic) (septic) L02.91
  with
    diverticular disease (intestine) K57.80
      with bleeding K57.81
      large intestine K57.20

Abscess — *continued*
  with
    bleeding K57.21
    small intestine K57.40
      with bleeding K57.41
    small intestine K57.00
  with
    bleeding K57.01
    large intestine K57.40
      with bleeding K57.41
  lymphangitis - code by site under Abscess
  abdomen, abdominal
    cavity K65.1
    wall L02.211
  abdominopelvic K65.1
  accessory sinus — *see* Sinusitis
  adrenal (capsule) (gland) E27.8
  alveolar K04.7
    with sinus K04.6
  ambic A06.4
    brain (and liver or lung abscess) A06.6
    genitourinary tract A06.82
    liver (without mention of brain or lung abscess) A06.4
    lung (and liver) (without mention of brain abscess) A06.5
    specified site NEC A06.89
    spleen A06.89
  anerobic A48.0
  ankle — *see* Abscess, lower limb
  anorectal K61.2
  antecubital space — *see* Abscess, upper limb
  antrum (chronic) (Highmore) — *see* Sinusitis, maxillary
  anus K61.0
  apical (tooth) K04.7
    with sinus (alveolar) K04.6
  appendix K35.3
  areola (acute) (chronic) (nonpuerperal) N61
    puerperal, postpartum or gestational — *see* Infection, nipple
  arm (any part) — *see* Abscess, upper limb
  artery (wall) I77.89
  atheromatous I77.2
  auricle, ear — *see* Abscess, ear, external
  axilla (region) L02.41- ☑
    lymph gland or node L04.2
  back (any part, except buttock) L02.212
  Bartholin's gland N75.1
    with
      abortion — *see* Abortion, by type complicated by, sepsis
      ectopic or molar pregnancy O08.0
    following ectopic or molar pregnancy O08.0
  Bezold's — *see* Mastoiditis, acute
  bilharziasis B65.1
  bladder (wall) — *see* Cystitis, specified type NEC
  bone (subperiosteal) (*see also* Osteomyelitis, specified type NEC)
    accessory sinus (chronic) — *see* Sinusitis
    chronic or old — *see* Osteomyelitis, chronic
    jaw (lower) (upper) M27.2
    mastoid — *see* Mastoiditis, acute, subperiosteal
    petrous — *see* Petrositis
    spinal (tuberculous) A18.01
      nontuberculous — *see* Osteomyelitis, vertebra
  bowel K63.0
  brain (any part) (cystic) (otogenic) G06.0
    amebic (with abscess of any other site) A06.6
    gonococcal A54.82
    pheomycotic (chromomycotic) B43.1
    tuberculous A17.81
  breast (acute) (chronic) (nonpuerperal) N61
    newborn P39.0
    puerperal, postpartum, gestational — *see* Mastitis, obstetric, purulent
  broad ligament N73.2
    acute N73.0
    chronic N73.1
  Brodie's (localized) (chronic) M86.8X- ☑
  bronchi J98.09
  buccal cavity K12.2
  bulbourethral gland N34.0
  bursa M71.00
    ankle M71.07- ☑
    elbow M71.02- ☑
    foot M71.07- ☑
    hand M71.04- ☑
    hip M71.05- ☑
    knee M71.06- ☑
    multiple sites M71.09

Abscess — *continued*
  pharyngeal J39.1
    shoulder M71.01- ☑
    specified site NEC M71.08
    wrist M71.03- ☑
  buttock L02.31
  canthus — *see* Blepharoconjunctivitis
  cartilage — *see* Disorder, cartilage, specified type NEC
  cecum K35.3
  cerebellum, cerebellar G06.0
    sequelae G09
  cerebral (embolic) G06.0
    sequelae G09
  cervical (meaning neck) L02.11
    lymph gland or node L04.0
  cervix (stump) (uteri) — *see* Cervicitis
  cheek (external) L02.01
    inner K12.2
  chest J86.9
    with fistula J86.0
    wall L02.213
  chin L02.01
  choroid — *see* Inflammation, chorioretinal
  circumtonsillar J36
  cold (lung) (tuberculous) (*see also* Tuberculosis, abscess, lung)
    articular — *see* Tuberculosis, joint
  colon (wall) K63.0
  colostomy K94.02
  conjunctiva — *see* Conjunctivitis, acute
  cornea H16.31- ☑
  corpus
    cavernosum N48.21
    luteum — *see* Oophoritis
  Cowper's gland N34.0
  cranium G06.0
  cul-de-sac (Douglas') (posterior) — *see* Peritonitis, pelvic, female
  cutaneous — *see* Abscess, by site
  dental K04.7
    with sinus (alveolar) K04.6
  dentoalveolar K04.7
    with sinus K04.6
  diaphragm, diaphragmatic K65.1
  Douglas' cul-de-sac or pouch — *see* Peritonitis, pelvic, female
  Dubois A50.59
  ear (middle) (*see also* Otitis, media, suppurative)
    acute — *see* Otitis, media, suppurative, acute
    external H60.0- ☑
  entamebic — *see* Abscess, amebic
  enterostomy K94.12
  epididymis N45.4
  epidural G06.2
    brain G06.0
    spinal cord G06.1
  epiglottis J38.7
  epiploon, epiploic K65.1
  erysipelatous — *see* Erysipelas
  esophagus K20.8
  ethmoid (bone) (chronic) (sinus) J32.2
  external auditory canal — *see* Abscess, ear, external
  extradural G06.2
    brain G06.0
      sequelae G09
    spinal cord G06.1
  extraperitoneal K68.19
  eye — *see* Endophthalmitis, purulent
  eyelid H00.03- ☑
  face (any part, except ear, eye and nose) L02.01
  fallopian tube — *see* Salpingitis
  fascia M72.8
  fauces J39.1
  fecal K63.0
  femoral (region) — *see* Abscess, lower limb
  filaria, filarial — *see* Infestation, filarial
  finger (any) (*see also* Abscess, hand)
    nail — *see* Cellulitis, finger
  foot L02.61- ☑
  forehead L02.01
  frontal sinus (chronic) J32.1
  gallbladder K81.0
  genital organ or tract
    female (external) N76.4
    male N49.9
      multiple sites N49.8
      specified NEC N49.8
  gestational mammary O91.11- ☑
  gestational subareolar O91.11- ☑
  gingival K05.21

☑ **Additional character required**

Abscess — *continued*

gland, glandular (lymph) (acute) — *see*
  Lymphadenitis, acute
gluteal (region) L02.31
gonorrheal — *see* Gonococcus
groin L02.214
gum K05.21
hand L02.51- ☑
head NEC L02.811
  face (any part, except ear, eye and nose) L02.01
heart — *see* Carditis
heel — *see* Abscess, foot
helminthic — *see* Infestation, helminth
hepatic (cholangitic) (hematogenic)
  (lymphogenic) (pylephlebitic) K75.0
  amebic A06.4
hip (region) — *see* Abscess, lower limb
ileocecal K35.3
ileostomy (bud) K94.12
iliac (region) L02.214
  fossa K35.3
infraclavicular (fossa) — *see* Abscess, upper limb
inguinal (region) L02.214
  lymph gland or node L04.1
intestine, intestinal NEC K63.0
  rectal K61.1
intra-abdominal (*see also* Abscess, peritoneum)
  K65.1
  postoperative T81.4 ☑
  retroperitoneal K68.11
intracranial G06.0
intramammary — *see* Abscess, breast
intraorbital — *see* Abscess, orbit
intraperitoneal K65.1
intrasphincteric (anus) K61.4
intraspinal G06.1
intratonsillar J36
ischiorectal (fossa) K61.3
jaw (bone) (lower) (upper) M27.2
joint — *see* Arthritis, pyogenic or pyemic
  spine (tuberculous) A18.01
    nontuberculous — *see* Spondylopathy,
    infective
kidney N15.1
  with calculus N20.0
    with hydronephrosis N13.6
  puerperal (postpartum) O86.21
knee (*see also* Abscess, lower limb)
  joint M00.9
labium (majus) (minus) N76.4
lacrimal
  caruncle — *see* Inflammation, lacrimal,
    passages, acute
  gland — *see* Dacryoadenitis
  passages (duct) (sac) — *see* Inflammation,
    lacrimal, passages, acute
lacunar N34.0
larynx J38.7
lateral (alveolar) K04.7
  with sinus K04.6
leg (any part) — *see* Abscess, lower limb
lens H27.8
lingual K14.0
  tonsil J36
lip K13.0
Littre's gland N34.0
liver (cholangitic) (hematogenic) (lymphogenic)
  (pylephlebitic) (pyogenic) K75.0
  amebic (due to Entamoeba histolytica)
    (dysenteric) (tropical) A06.4
    with
      brain abscess (and liver or lung abscess)
      A06.6
      lung abscess A06.5
loin (region) L02.211
lower limb L02.41- ☑
lumbar (tuberculous) A18.01
  nontuberculous L02.212
lung (miliary) (putrid) J85.2
  with pneumonia J85.1
    due to specified organism (see Pneumonia,
      in (due to))
  amebic (with liver abscess) A06.5
    with
      brain abscess A06.6
      pneumonia A06.5
lymph, lymphatic, gland or node (acute) (*see also*
  Lymphadenitis, acute)
  mesentery I88.0
malar M27.2
mammary gland — *see* Abscess, breast
marginal, anus K61.0

Abscess — *continued*

mastoid — *see* Mastoiditis, acute
maxilla, maxillary M27.2
  molar (tooth) K04.7
    with sinus K04.6
  premolar K04.7
  sinus (chronic) J32.0
mediastinum J85.3
meibomian gland — *see* Hordeolum
meninges G06.2
mesentery, mesenteric K65.1
mesosalpinx — *see* Salpingitis
mons pubis L02.215
mouth (floor) K12.2
muscle — *see* Myositis, infective
myocardium I40.0
nabothian (follicle) — *see* Cervicitis
nasal J32.9
nasopharyngeal J39.1
navel L02.216
  newborn P38.9
    with mild hemorrhage P38.1
    without hemorrhage P38.9
neck (region) L02.11
  lymph gland or node L04.0
nephritic — *see* Abscess, kidney
nipple N61
  associated with
    lactation — *see* Pregnancy, complicated by,
    pregnancy — *see* Pregnancy, complicated by
nose (external) (fossa) (septum) J34.0
  sinus (chronic) — *see* Sinusitis
omentum K65.1
operative wound T81.4 ☑
orbit, orbital — *see* Cellulitis, orbit
otogenic G06.0
ovary, ovarian (corpus luteum) — *see* Oophoritis
oviduct — *see* Oophoritis
palate (soft) K12.2
  hard M27.2
palmar (space) — *see* Abscess, hand
pancreas (duct) — *see* Pancreatitis, acute
parafrenal N48.21
parametric, parametrium N73.2
  acute N73.0
  chronic N73.1
paranephric N15.1
parapancreatic — *see* Pancreatitis, acute
parapharyngeal J39.0
pararectal K61.1
parasinus — *see* Sinusitis
parauterine (*see also* Disease, pelvis,
  inflammatory) N73.2
paravaginal — *see* Vaginitis
parietal region (scalp) L02.811
parodontal K05.21
parotid (duct) (gland) K11.3
  region K12.2
pectoral (region) L02.213
pelvis, pelvic
  female — *see* Disease, pelvis, inflammatory
  male, peritoneal K65.1
penis N48.21
  gonococcal (accessory gland) (periurethral)
    A54.1
perianal K61.0
periapical K04.7
  with sinus (alveolar) K04.6
periappendicular K35.3
pericardial I30.1
pericecal K35.3
pericemental K05.21
pericholecystic — *see* Cholecystitis, acute
pericoronal K05.21
peridental K05.21
perimetric (*see also* Disease, pelvis,
  inflammatory) N73.2
perinephric, perinephritic — *see* Abscess, kidney
perineum, perineal (superficial) L02.215
  urethra N34.0
periodontal (parietal) K05.21
  apical K04.7
periosteum, periosteal (*see also* Osteomyelitis,
  specified type NEC)
  with osteomyelitis (*see also* Osteomyelitis,
    specified type NEC)
    acute — *see* Osteomyelitis, acute
    chronic — *see* Osteomyelitis, chronic
peripharyngeal J39.0
peripleuritic J86.9
  with fistula J86.0
periprostatic N41.2

Abscess — *continued*

perirectal K61.1
perirenal (tissue) — *see* Abscess, kidney
perisinuous (nose) — *see* Sinusitis
peritoneum, peritoneal (perforated) (ruptured)
  K65.1
  with appendicitis K35.3
  pelvic
    female — *see* Peritonitis, pelvic, female
    male K65.1
  postoperative T81.4 ☑
  puerperal, postpartum, childbirth O85
  tuberculous A18.31
peritonsillar J36
perityphlic K35.3
periureteral N28.89
periurethral N34.0
  gonococcal (accessory gland) (periurethral)
    A54.1
periuterine (*see also* Disease, pelvis,
  inflammatory) N73.2
perivesical — *see* Cystitis, specified type NEC
petrous bone — *see* Petrositis
phagedenic NOS L02.91
  chancroid A57
pharynx, pharyngeal (lateral) J39.1
pilonidal L05.01
pituitary (gland) E23.6
pleura J86.9
  with fistula J86.0
popliteal — *see* Abscess, lower limb
postcecal K35.3
postlaryngeal J38.7
postnasal J34.0
postoperative (any site) T81.4 ☑
  retroperitoneal K68.11
postpharyngeal J39.0
posttonsillar J36
post-typhoid A01.09
pouch of Douglas — *see* Peritonitis, pelvic, female
premammary — *see* Abscess, breast
prepatellar — *see* Abscess, lower limb
prostate N41.2
  gonococcal (acute) (chronic) A54.22
psoas muscle K68.12
puerperal - code by site under Puerperal, abscess
pulmonary — *see* Abscess, lung
pulp, pulpal (dental) K04.0
rectovaginal septum K63.0
rectovesical — *see* Cystitis, specified type NEC
rectum K61.1
renal — *see* Abscess, kidney
retina — *see* Inflammation, chorioretinal
retrobulbar — *see* Abscess, orbit
retrocecal K65.1
retrolaryngeal J38.7
retromammary — *see* Abscess, breast
retroperitoneal NEC K68.19
  postprocedural K68.11
retropharyngeal J39.0
retrouterine — *see* Peritonitis, pelvic, female
retrovesical — *see* Cystitis, specified type NEC
root, tooth K04.7
  with sinus (alveolar) K04.6
round ligament (*see also* Disease, pelvis,
  inflammatory) N73.2
rupture (spontaneous) NOS L02.91
sacrum (tuberculous) A18.01
  nontuberculous M46.28
salivary (duct) (gland) K11.3
scalp (any part) L02.811
scapular — *see* Osteomyelitis, specified type NEC
sclera — *see* Scleritis
scrofulous (tuberculous) A18.2
scrotum N49.2
seminal vesicle N49.0
septal, dental K04.7
  with sinus (alveolar) K04.6
serous — *see* Periostitis
shoulder (region) — *see* Abscess, upper limb
sigmoid K63.0
sinus (accessory) (chronic) (nasal) (*see also*
  Sinusitis)
  intracranial venous (any) G06.0
Skene's duct or gland N34.0
skin — *see* Abscess, by site
specified site NEC L02.818
spermatic cord N49.1
sphenoidal (sinus) (chronic) J32.3
spinal cord (any part) (staphylococcal) G06.1
  tuberculous A17.81
spine (column) (tuberculous) A18.01

Abscess — *continued*
  epidural G06.1
    nontuberculous — *see* Osteomyelitis, vertebra
  spleen D73.3
    amebic A06.89
  stitch T81.4 ☑
  subarachnoid G06.2
    brain G06.0
    spinal cord G06.1
  subareolar — *see* Abscess, breast
  subcecal K35.3
  subcutaneous (*see also* Abscess, by site)
    pheomycotic (chromomycotic) B43.2
  subdiaphragmatic K65.1
  subdural G06.2
    brain G06.0
      sequelae G09
    spinal cord G06.1
  subgaleal L02.811
  subhepatic K65.1
  sublingual K12.2
    gland K11.3
  submammary — *see* Abscess, breast
  submandibular (region) (space) (triangle) K12.2
    gland K11.3
  submaxillary (region) L02.01
    gland K11.3
  submental L02.01
    gland K11.3
  subperiosteal — *see* Osteomyelitis, specified type NEC
  subphrenic K65.1
    postoperative T81.4 ☑
  suburethral N34.0
  sudoriparous L75.8
  supraclavicular (fossa) — *see* Abscess, upper limb
  suprapelvic, acute N73.0
  suprarenal (capsule) (gland) E27.8
  sweat gland L74.8
  tear duct — *see* Inflammation, lacrimal, passages, acute
  temple L02.01
  temporal region L02.01
  temporosphenoidal G06.0
  tendon (sheath) M65.00
    ankle M65.07- ☑
    foot M65.07- ☑
    forearm M65.03- ☑
    hand M65.04- ☑
    lower leg M65.06- ☑
    pelvic region M65.05- ☑
    shoulder region M65.01- ☑
    specified site NEC M65.08
    thigh M65.05- ☑
    upper arm M65.02- ☑
  testis N45.4
  thigh — *see* Abscess, lower limb
  thorax J86.9
    with fistula J86.0
  throat J39.1
  thumb (*see also* Abscess, hand)
    nail — *see* Cellulitis, finger
  thymus (gland) E32.1
  thyroid (gland) E06.0
  toe (any) (*see also* Abscess, foot)
    nail — *see* Cellulitis, toe
  tongue (staphylococcal) K14.0
  tonsil (s) (lingual) J36
  tonsillopharyngeal J36
  tooth, teeth (root) K04.7
    with sinus (alveolar) K04.6
    supporting structures NEC K05.21
  trachea J39.8
  trunk L02.219
    abdominal wall L02.211
    back L02.212
    chest wall L02.213
    groin L02.214
    perineum L02.215
    umbilicus L02.216
  tubal — *see* Salpingitis
  tuberculous — *see* Tuberculosis, abscess
  tubo-ovarian — *see* Salpingo-oophoritis
  tunica vaginalis N49.1
  umbilicus L02.216
  upper
    limb L02.41- ☑
    respiratory J39.8
  urethral (gland) N34.0
  urinary N34.0
  uterus, uterine (wall) (*see also* Endometritis)

Abscess — *continued*
  ligament (*see also* Disease, pelvis, inflammatory) N73.2
  neck — *see* Cervicitis
  uvula K12.2
  vagina (wall) — *see* Vaginitis
  vaginorectal — *see* Vaginitis
  vas deferens N49.1
  vermiform appendix K35.3
  vertebra (column) (tuberculous) A18.01
    nontuberculous — *see* Osteomyelitis, vertebra
  vesical — *see* Cystitis, specified type NEC
  vesico-uterine pouch — *see* Peritonitis, pelvic, female
  vitreous (humor) — *see* Endophthalmitis, purulent
  vocal cord J38.3
  von Bezold's — *see* Mastoiditis, acute
  vulva N76.4
  vulvovaginal gland N75.1
  web space — *see* Abscess, hand
  wound T81.4 ☑
  wrist — *see* Abscess, upper limb
Absence (of) (organ or part) (complete or partial)
  adrenal (gland) (congenital) Q89.1
    acquired E89.6
  albumin in blood E88.09
  alimentary tract (congenital) Q45.8
    upper Q40.8
  alveolar process (acquired) — *see* Anomaly, alveolar
  ankle (acquired) Z89.44- ☑
  anus (congenital) Q42.3
    with fistula Q42.2
  aorta (congenital) Q25.4
  appendix, congenital Q42.8
  arm (acquired) Z89.20- ☑
    above elbow Z89.22- ☑
      congenital (with hand present) — *see* Agenesis, arm, with hand present
      and hand — *see* Agenesis, forearm, and hand
    below elbow Z89.21- ☑
      congenital (with hand present) — *see* Agenesis, arm, with hand present
      and hand — *see* Agenesis, forearm, and hand
    congenital — *see* Defect, reduction, upper limb
    shoulder (following explantation of shoulder joint prosthesis) (joint) (with or without presence of antibiotic-impregnated cement spacer) Z89.23- ☑
      congenital (with hand present) — *see* Agenesis, arm, with hand present
  artery (congenital) (peripheral) Q27.8
    brain Q28.3
    coronary Q24.5
    pulmonary Q25.79
    specified NEC Q27.8
    umbilical Q27.0
  atrial septum (congenital) Q21.1
  auditory canal (congenital) (external) Q16.1
  auricle (ear), congenital Q16.0
  bile, biliary duct, congenital Q44.5
  bladder (acquired) Z90.6
    congenital Q64.5
  bowel sounds R19.11
  brain Q00.0
    part of Q04.3
  breast (s) (and nipple(s)) (acquired) Z90.1- ☑
    congenital Q83.8
  broad ligament Q50.6
  bronchus (congenital) Q32.4
  canaliculus lacrimalis, congenital Q10.4
  cerebellum (vermis) Q04.3
  cervix (acquired) (with uterus) Z90.710
    with remaining uterus Z90.712
    congenital Q51.5
  chin, congenital Q18.8
  cilia (congenital) Q10.3
    acquired — *see* Madarosis
  clitoris (congenital) Q52.6
  coccyx, congenital Q76.49
  cold sense R20.8
  congenital
    lumen — *see* Atresia
    organ or site NEC — *see* Agenesis
    septum — *see* Imperfect, closure
  corpus callosum Q04.0
  cricoid cartilage, congenital Q31.8
  diaphragm (with hernia), congenital Q79.1
  digestive organ (s) or tract, congenital Q45.8

Absence — *continued*
  acquired NEC Z90.49
    upper Q40.8
  ductus arteriosus Q28.8
  duodenum (acquired) Z90.49
    congenital Q41.0
  ear, congenital Q16.9
    acquired H93.8- ☑
    auricle Q16.0
    external Q16.0
    inner Q16.5
    lobe, lobule Q17.8
    middle, except ossicles Q16.4
      ossicles Q16.3
    ossicles Q16.3
  ejaculatory duct (congenital) Q55.4
  endocrine gland (congenital) NEC Q89.2
    acquired E89.89
  epididymis (congenital) Q55.4
    acquired Z90.79
  epiglottis, congenital Q31.8
  esophagus (congenital) Q39.8
    acquired (partial) Z90.49
  eustachian tube (congenital) Q16.2
  extremity (acquired) Z89.9
    congenital Q73.0
    knee (following explantation of knee joint prosthesis) (joint) (with or without presence of antibiotic-impregnated cement spacer) Z89.52- ☑
    lower (above knee) Z89.619
      below knee Z89.51- ☑
    upper — *see* Absence, arm
  eye (acquired) Z90.01
    congenital Q11.1
    muscle (congenital) Q10.3
  eyeball (acquired) Z90.01
  eyelid (fold) (congenital) Q10.3
    acquired Z90.01
  face, specified part NEC Q18.8
  fallopian tube (s) (acquired) Z90.79
    congenital Q50.6
  family member (causing problem in home) NEC (*see also* Disruption, family) Z63.32
  femur, congenital — *see* Defect, reduction, lower limb, longitudinal, femur
  fibrinogen (congenital) D68.2
    acquired D65
  finger (s) (acquired) Z89.02- ☑
    congenital — *see* Agenesis, hand
  foot (acquired) Z89.43- ☑
    congenital — *see* Agenesis, foot
  forearm (acquired) — *see* Absence, arm, below elbow
  gallbladder (acquired) Z90.49
    congenital Q44.0
  gamma globulin in blood D80.1
    hereditary D80.0
  genital organs
    acquired (female) (male) Z90.79
    female, congenital Q52.8
      external Q52.71
      internal NEC Q52.8
    male, congenital Q55.8
  genitourinary organs, congenital NEC
    female Q52.8
    male Q55.8
  globe (acquired) Z90.01
    congenital Q11.1
  glottis, congenital Q31.8
  hand and wrist (acquired) Z89.11- ☑
    congenital — *see* Agenesis, hand
  head, part (acquired) NEC Z90.09
  heat sense R20.8
  hip (following explantation of hip joint prosthesis) (joint) (with or without presence of antibiotic-impregnated cement spacer) Z89.62- ☑
  hymen (congenital) Q52.4
  ileum (acquired) Z90.49
    congenital Q41.2
  immunoglobulin, isolated NEC D80.3
    IgA D80.2
    IgG D80.3
    IgM D80.4
  incus (acquired) — *see* Loss, ossicles, ear
    congenital Q16.3
  inner ear, congenital Q16.5
  intestine (acquired) (small) Z90.49
    congenital Q41.9
      specified NEC Q41.8
    large Z90.49

Absence — *continued*
    congenital Q42.9
        specified NEC Q42.8
    iris, congenital Q13.1
    jejunum (acquired) Z90.49
        congenital Q41.1
    joint
        acquired
            hip (following explantation of hip joint
                prosthesis) (with or without presence of
                antibiotic-impregnated cement spacer)
                Z89.62- ☑
            knee (following explantation of knee joint
                prosthesis) (with or without presence of
                antibiotic-impregnated cement spacer)
                Z89.52- ☑
            shoulder (following explantation of shoulder
                joint prosthesis) (with or without
                presence of antibiotic-impregnated
                cement spacer) Z89.23- ☑
        congenital NEC Q74.8
    kidney (s) (acquired) Z90.5
        congenital Q60.2
            bilateral Q60.1
            unilateral Q60.0
    knee (following explantation of knee joint
        prosthesis) (joint) (with or without presence
        of antibiotic-impregnated cement spacer)
        Z89.52- ☑
    labyrinth, membranous Q16.5
    larynx (congenital) Q31.8
        acquired Z90.02
    leg (acquired) (above knee) Z89.61- ☑
        below knee Z89.51- ☑
        congenital — *see* Defect, reduction, lower limb
    lens (acquired) (*see also* Aphakia)
        congenital Q12.3
        post cataract extraction Z98.4- ☑
    limb (acquired) — *see* Absence, extremity
    lip Q38.6
    liver (congenital) Q44.7
    lung (fissure) (lobe) (bilateral) (unilateral)
        (congenital) Q33.3
        acquired (any part) Z90.2
    menstruation — *see* Amenorrhea
    muscle (congenital) (pectoral) Q79.8
        ocular Q10.3
    neck, part Q18.8
    neutrophil — *see* Agranulocytosis
    nipple (s) (with breast(s)) (acquired) Z90.1- ☑
        congenital Q83.2
    nose (congenital) Q30.1
        acquired Z90.09
    organ
        of Corti, congenital Q16.5
        or site, congenital NEC Q89.8
            acquired NEC Z90.89
    osseous meatus (ear) Q16.4
    ovary (acquired)
        bilateral Z90.722
        congenital
            bilateral Q50.02
            unilateral Q50.01
        unilateral Z90.721
    oviduct (acquired)
        bilateral Z90.722
        congenital Q50.6
        unilateral Z90.721
    pancreas (congenital) Q45.0
        acquired Z90.410
            complete Z90.410
            partial Z90.411
            total Z90.410
    parathyroid gland (acquired) E89.2
        congenital Q89.2
    patella, congenital Q74.1
    penis (congenital) Q55.5
        acquired Z90.79
    pericardium (congenital) Q24.8
    pituitary gland (congenital) Q89.2
        acquired E89.3
    prostate (acquired) Z90.79
        congenital Q55.4
    pulmonary valve Q22.0
    punctum lacrimale (congenital) Q10.4
    radius, congenital — *see* Defect, reduction, upper
        limb, longitudinal, radius
    rectum (congenital) Q42.1
        with fistula Q42.0
        acquired Z90.49
    respiratory organ NOS Q34.9
    rib (acquired) Z90.89

Absence — *continued*
    congenital Q76.6
    sacrum, congenital Q76.49
    salivary gland (s), congenital Q38.4
    scrotum, congenital Q55.29
    seminal vesicles (congenital) Q55.4
        acquired Z90.79
    septum
        atrial (congenital) Q21.1
        between aorta and pulmonary artery Q21.4
        ventricular (congenital) Q20.4
    sex chromosome
        female phenotype Q97.8
        male phenotype Q98.8
    skull bone (congenital) Q75.8
        with
            anencephaly Q00.0
            encephalocele — *see* Encephalocele
            hydrocephalus Q03.9
                with spina bifida — *see* Spina bifida, by site,
                    with hydrocephalus
            microcephaly Q02
    spermatic cord, congenital Q55.4
    spine, congenital Q76.49
    spleen (congenital) Q89.01
        acquired Z90.81
    sternum, congenital Q76.7
    stomach (acquired) (partial) Z90.3
        congenital Q40.2
    superior vena cava, congenital Q26.8
    teeth, tooth (congenital) K00.0
        acquired (complete) K08.109
            class I K08.101
            class II K08.102
            class III K08.103
            class IV K08.104
            due to
                caries K08.139
                    class I K08.131
                    class II K08.132
                    class III K08.133
                    class IV K08.134
                periodontal disease K08.129
                    class I K08.121
                    class II K08.122
                    class III K08.123
                    class IV K08.124
                specified NEC K08.199
                    class I K08.191
                    class II K08.192
                    class III K08.193
                    class IV K08.194
                trauma K08.119
                    class I K08.111
                    class II K08.112
                    class III K08.113
                    class IV K08.114
            partial K08.409
                class I K08.401
                class II K08.402
                class III K08.403
                class IV K08.404
                due to
                    caries K08.439
                        class I K08.431
                        class II K08.432
                        class III K08.433
                        class IV K08.434
                    periodontal disease K08.429
                        class I K08.421
                        class II K08.422
                        class III K08.423
                        class IV K08.424
                    specified NEC K08.499
                        class I K08.491
                        class II K08.492
                        class III K08.493
                        class IV K08.494
                    trauma K08.419
                        class I K08.411
                        class II K08.412
                        class III K08.413
                        class IV K08.414
    tendon (congenital) Q79.8
    testis (congenital) Q55.0
        acquired Z90.79
    thumb (acquired) Z89.01- ☑
        congenital — *see* Agenesis, hand
    thymus gland Q89.2
    thyroid (gland) (acquired) E89.0
        cartilage, congenital Q31.8
        congenital E03.1

Absence — *continued*
    toe (s) (acquired) Z89.42- ☑
        with foot — *see* Absence, foot and ankle
        congenital — *see* Agenesis, foot
        great Z89.41- ☑
    tongue, congenital Q38.3
    trachea (cartilage), congenital Q32.1
    transverse aortic arch, congenital Q25.4
    tricuspid valve Q22.4
    umbilical artery, congenital Q27.0
    upper arm and forearm with hand present,
        congenital — *see* Agenesis, arm, with hand
        present
    ureter (congenital) Q62.4
        acquired Z90.6
    urethra, congenital Q64.5
    uterus (acquired) Z90.710
        with cervix Z90.710
        with remaining cervical stump Z90.711
        congenital Q51.0
    uvula, congenital Q38.5
    vagina, congenital Q52.0
    vas deferens (congenital) Q55.4
        acquired Z90.79
    vein (peripheral) congenital NEC Q27.8
        cerebral Q28.3
        digestive system Q27.8
        great Q26.8
        lower limb Q27.8
        portal Q26.5
        precerebral Q28.1
        specified site NEC Q27.8
        upper limb Q27.8
    vena cava (inferior) (superior), congenital Q26.8
    ventricular septum Q20.4
    vertebra, congenital Q76.49
    vulva, congenital Q52.71
    wrist (acquired) Z89.12- ☑
Absorbent system disease I87.8
Absorption
    carbohydrate, disturbance K90.4
    chemical — *see* Table of Drugs and Chemicals
        through placenta (newborn) P04.9
            environmental substance P04.6
            nutritional substance P04.5
            obstetric anesthetic or analgesic drug P04.0
    drug NEC — *see* Table of Drugs and Chemicals
        addictive
            through placenta (newborn) P04.49
                cocaine P04.41
        medicinal
            through placenta (newborn) P04.1
            through placenta (newborn) P04.1
                obstetric anesthetic or analgesic drug P04.0
    fat, disturbance K90.4
        pancreatic K90.3
    noxious substance — *see* Table of Drugs and
        Chemicals
    protein, disturbance K90.4
    starch, disturbance K90.4
    toxic substance — *see* Table of Drugs and
        Chemicals
    uremic — *see* Uremia
Abstinence symptoms, syndrome
    alcohol F10.239
        with delirium F10.231
    cocaine F14.23
    neonatal P96.1
    nicotine — *see* Dependence, drug, nicotine, with,
        withdrawal
    opioid F11.93
        with dependence F11.23
    psychoactive NEC F19.939
        with
            delirium F19.931
            dependence F19.239
                with
                    delirium F19.231
                    perceptual disturbance F19.232
                uncomplicated F19.230
            perceptual disturbance F19.932
        uncomplicated F19.930
    sedative F13.939
        with
            delirium F13.931
            dependence F13.239
                with
                    delirium F13.231
                    perceptual disturbance F13.232
                uncomplicated F13.230
            perceptual disturbance F13.932
        uncomplicated F13.930

Abstinence — *continued*
  stimulant NEC F15.93
    with dependence F15.23
Abulia R68.89
Abulomania F60.7
Abuse
  adult — *see* Maltreatment, adult
    as reason for
      couple seeking advice (including offender)
        Z63.0
  alcohol (non-dependent) F10.10
    with
      anxiety disorder F10.180
      intoxication F10.129
        with delirium F10.121
        uncomplicated F10.120
      mood disorder F10.14
      other specified disorder F10.188
      psychosis F10.159
        delusions F10.150
        hallucinations F10.151
      sexual dysfunction F10.181
      sleep disorder F10.182
      unspecified disorder F10.19
    counseling and surveillance Z71.41
  amphetamine (or related substance) — *see*
    Abuse, drug, stimulant NEC
  analgesics (non-prescribed) (over the counter)
    F55.8
  antacids F55.0
  antidepressants — *see* Abuse, drug, psychoactive
    NEC
  anxiolytic — *see* Abuse, drug, sedative
  barbiturates — *see* Abuse, drug, sedative
  caffeine — *see* Abuse, drug, stimulant NEC
  cannabis, cannabinoids — *see* Abuse, drug,
    cannabis
  child — *see* Maltreatment, child
  cocaine — *see* Abuse, drug, cocaine
  drug NEC (non-dependent) F19.10
    with sleep disorder F19.182
    amphetamine type — *see* Abuse, drug,
      stimulant NEC
    analgesics (non-prescribed) (over the counter)
      F55.8
    antacids F55.0
    antidepressants — *see* Abuse, drug,
      psychoactive NEC
    anxiolytics — *see* Abuse, drug, sedative
    barbiturates — *see* Abuse, drug, sedative
    caffeine — *see* Abuse, drug, stimulant NEC
    cannabis F12.10
      with
        anxiety disorder F12.180
        intoxication F12.129
          with
            delirium F12.121
            perceptual disturbance F12.122
          uncomplicated F12.120
        other specified disorder F12.188
        psychosis F12.159
          delusions F12.150
          hallucinations F12.151
        unspecified disorder F12.19
    cocaine F14.10
      with
        anxiety disorder F14.180
        intoxication F14.129
          with
            delirium F14.121
            perceptual disturbance F14.122
          uncomplicated F14.120
        mood disorder F14.14
        other specified disorder F14.188
        psychosis F14.159
          delusions F14.150
          hallucinations F14.151
        sexual dysfunction F14.181
        sleep disorder F14.182
        unspecified disorder F14.19
    counseling and surveillance Z71.51
    hallucinogen F16.10
      with
        anxiety disorder F16.180
        flashbacks F16.183
        intoxication F16.129
          with
            delirium F16.121
            perceptual disturbance F16.122
          uncomplicated F16.120
        mood disorder F16.14
        other specified disorder F16.188

Abuse — *continued*
      perception disorder, persisting F16.183
      psychosis F16.159
        delusions F16.150
        hallucinations F16.151
      unspecified disorder F16.19
  hashish — *see* Abuse, drug, cannabis
  herbal or folk remedies F55.1
  hormones F55.3
  hypnotics — *see* Abuse, drug, sedative
  inhalant F18.10
    with
      anxiety disorder F18.180
      dementia, persisting F18.17
      intoxication F18.129
        with delirium F18.121
        uncomplicated F18.120
      mood disorder F18.14
      other specified disorder F18.188
      psychosis F18.159
        delusions F18.150
        hallucinations F18.151
      unspecified disorder F18.19
  laxatives F55.2
  LSD — *see* Abuse, drug, hallucinogen
  marihuana — *see* Abuse, drug, cannabis
  morphine type (opioids) — *see* Abuse, drug,
    opioid
  opioid F11.10
    with
      intoxication F11.129
        with
          delirium F11.121
          perceptual disturbance F11.122
        uncomplicated F11.120
      mood disorder F11.14
      other specified disorder F11.188
      psychosis F11.159
        delusions F11.150
        hallucinations F11.151
      sexual dysfunction F11.181
      sleep disorder F11.182
      unspecified disorder F11.19
  PCP (phencyclidine) (or related substance) —
    see Abuse, drug, hallucinogen
  psychoactive NEC F19.10
    with
      amnestic disorder F19.16
      anxiety disorder F19.180
      dementia F19.17
      intoxication F19.129
        with
          delirium F19.121
          perceptual disturbance F19.122
        uncomplicated F19.120
      mood disorder F19.14
      other specified disorder F19.188
      psychosis F19.159
        delusions F19.150
        hallucinations F19.151
      sexual dysfunction F19.181
      sleep disorder F19.182
      unspecified disorder F19.19
  sedative, hypnotic or anxiolytic F13.10
    with
      anxiety disorder F13.180
      intoxication F13.129
        with delirium F13.121
        uncomplicated F13.120
      mood disorder F13.14
      other specified disorder F13.188
      psychosis F13.159
        delusions F13.150
        hallucinations F13.151
      sexual dysfunction F13.181
      sleep disorder F13.182
      unspecified disorder F13.19
  solvent — *see* Abuse, drug, inhalant
  steroids F55.3
  stimulant NEC F15.10
    with
      anxiety disorder F15.180
      intoxication F15.129
        with
          delirium F15.121
          perceptual disturbance F15.122
        uncomplicated F15.120
      mood disorder F15.14
      other specified disorder F15.188
      psychosis F15.159
        delusions F15.150
        hallucinations F15.151

Abuse — *continued*
      sexual dysfunction F15.181
      sleep disorder F15.182
      unspecified disorder F15.19
    tranquilizers — *see* Abuse, drug, sedative
    vitamins F55.4
  hallucinogens — *see* Abuse, drug, hallucinogen
  hashish — *see* Abuse, drug, cannabis
  herbal or folk remedies F55.1
  hormones F55.3
  hypnotic — *see* Abuse, drug, sedative
  inhalant — *see* Abuse, drug, inhalant
  laxatives F55.2
  LSD — *see* Abuse, drug, hallucinogen
  marihuana — *see* Abuse, drug, cannabis
  morphine type (opioids) — *see* Abuse, drug,
    opioid
  non-psychoactive substance NEC F55.8
    antacids F55.0
    folk remedies F55.1
    herbal remedies F55.1
    hormones F55.3
    laxatives F55.2
    steroids F55.3
    vitamins F55.4
  opioids — *see* Abuse, drug, opioid
  PCP (phencyclidine) (or related substance) — *see*
    Abuse, drug, hallucinogen
  physical (adult) (child) — *see* Maltreatment
  psychoactive substance — *see* Abuse, drug,
    psychoactive NEC
  psychological (adult) (child) — *see* Maltreatment
  sedative — *see* Abuse, drug, sedative
  sexual — *see* Maltreatment
  solvent — *see* Abuse, drug, inhalant
  steroids F55.3
  vitamins F55.4
Acalculia R48.8
  developmental F81.2
Acanthamebiasis (with) B60.10
  conjunctiva B60.12
  keratoconjunctivitis B60.13
  meningoencephalitis B60.11
  other specified B60.19
Acanthocephaliasis B83.8
Acanthocheilonemiasis B74.4
Acanthocytosis E78.6
Acantholysis L11.9
Acanthosis (acquired) (nigricans) L83
  benign Q82.8
  congenital Q82.8
  seborrheic L82.1
    inflamed L82.0
  tongue K14.3
Acapnia E87.3
Acarbia E87.2
Acardia, acardius Q89.8
Acardiacus amorphus Q89.8
Acardiotrophia I51.4
Acariasis B88.0
  scabies B86
Acarodermatitis (urticarioides) B88.0
Acarophobia F40.218
Acatalasemia, acatalasia E80.3
Acathisia (drug induced) G25.71
Accelerated atrioventricular conduction I45.6
Accentuation of personality traits (type A) Z73.1
Accessory (congenital)
  adrenal gland Q89.1
  anus Q43.4
  appendix Q43.4
  atrioventricular conduction I45.6
  auditory ossicles Q16.3
  auricle (ear) Q17.0
  biliary duct or passage Q44.5
  bladder Q64.79
  blood vessels NEC Q27.9
    coronary Q24.5
  bone NEC Q79.8
  breast tissue, axilla Q83.1
  carpal bones Q74.0
  cecum Q43.4
  chromosome (s) NEC (nonsex) Q92.9
    with complex rearrangements NEC Q92.5
      seen only at prometaphase Q92.8
    partial Q92.9
    sex
      female phenotype Q97.8
      13 — *see* Trisomy, 13
      18 — *see* Trisomy, 18
      21 — *see* Trisomy, 21
  coronary artery Q24.5

☑ **Additional character required**

Accessory — *continued*
  cusp (s), heart valve NEC Q24.8
    pulmonary Q22.3
  cystic duct Q44.5
  digit (s) Q69.9
  ear (auricle) (lobe) Q17.0
  endocrine gland NEC Q89.2
  eye muscle Q10.3
  eyelid Q10.3
  face bone (s) Q75.8
  fallopian tube (fimbria) (ostium) Q50.6
  finger (s) Q69.0
  foreskin N47.8
  frontonasal process Q75.8
  gallbladder Q44.1
  genital organ (s)
    female Q52.8
      external Q52.79
      internal NEC Q52.8
    male Q55.8
  genitourinary organs NEC Q89.8
    female Q52.8
    male Q55.8
  hallux Q69.2
  heart Q24.8
    valve NEC Q24.8
      pulmonary Q22.3
  hepatic ducts Q44.5
  hymen Q52.4
  intestine (large) (small) Q43.4
  kidney Q63.0
  lacrimal canal Q10.6
  leaflet, heart valve NEC Q24.8
  ligament, broad Q50.6
  liver Q44.7
    duct Q44.5
  lobule (ear) Q17.0
  lung (lobe) Q33.1
  muscle Q79.8
  navicular of carpus Q74.0
  nervous system, part NEC Q07.8
  nipple Q83.3
  nose Q30.8
  organ or site not listed — *see* Anomaly, by site
  ovary Q50.31
  oviduct Q50.6
  pancreas Q45.3
  parathyroid gland Q89.2
  parotid gland (and duct) Q38.4
  pituitary gland Q89.2
  preauricular appendage Q17.0
  prepuce N47.8
  renal arteries (multiple) Q27.2
  rib Q76.6
    cervical Q76.5
  roots (teeth) K00.2
  salivary gland Q38.4
  sesamoid bones Q74.8
    foot Q74.2
    hand Q74.0
  skin tags Q82.8
  spleen Q89.09
  sternum Q76.7
  submaxillary gland Q38.4
  tarsal bones Q74.2
  teeth, tooth K00.1
  tendon Q79.8
  thumb Q69.1
  thymus gland Q89.2
  thyroid gland Q89.2
  toes Q69.2
  tongue Q38.3
  tooth, teeth K00.1
  tragus Q17.0
  ureter Q62.5
  urethra Q64.79
  urinary organ or tract NEC Q64.8
  uterus Q51.2
  vagina Q52.10
  valve, heart NEC Q24.8
    pulmonary Q22.3
  vertebra Q76.49
  vocal cords Q31.8
  vulva Q52.79
Accident
  birth — *see* Birth, injury
  cardiac — *see* Infarct, myocardium
  cerebral I63.9
  cerebrovascular (embolic) (ischemic)
    (thrombotic) I63.9
    aborted I63.9

Accident — *continued*
  hemorrhagic — *see* Hemorrhage, intracranial,
    intracerebral
    old (without sequelae) Z86.73
      with sequelae (of) — *see* Sequelae, infarction,
        cerebral
  coronary — *see* Infarct, myocardium
  craniovascular I63.9
  vascular, brain I63.9
Accidental — *see* condition
Accommodation (disorder) (*see also* condition)
  hysterical paralysis of F44.89
  insufficiency of H52.4
  paresis — *see* Paresis, of accommodation
  spasm — *see* Spasm, of accommodation
Accouchement — *see* Delivery
Accreta placenta O43.21- ☑
Accretio cordis (nonrheumatic) I31.0
Accretions, tooth, teeth K03.6
Acculturation difficulty Z60.3
Accumulation secretion, prostate N42.89
Acephalia, acephalism, acephalus, acephaly Q00.0
Acephalobrachia monster Q89.8
Acephalochirus monster Q89.8
Acephalogaster Q89.8
Acephalostomus monster Q89.8
Acephalothorax Q89.8
Acerophobia F40.298
Acetonemia R79.89
  in Type 1 diabetes E10.10
    with coma E10.11
Acetonuria R82.4
Achalasia (cardia) (esophagus) K22.0
  congenital Q39.5
  pylorus Q40.0
  sphincteral NEC K59.8
Ache (s) — *see* Pain
Acheilia Q38.6
Achilloburitis — *see* Tendinitis, Achilles
Achillodynia — *see* Tendinitis, Achilles
Achlorhydria, achlorhydric (neurogenic) K31.83
  anemia D50.8
  diarrhea K31.83
  psychogenic F45.8
  secondary to vagotomy K91.1
Achluophobia F40.228
Acholia K82.8
Acholuric jaundice (familial) (splenomegalic) (*see
  also* Spherocytosis)
  acquired D59.8
Achondrogenesis Q77.0
Achondroplasia (osteosclerosis congenita) Q77.4
Achroma, cutis L80
Achromat (ism), achromatopsia (acquired)
  (congenital) H53.51
Achromia, congenital — *see* Albinism
Achromia parasitica B36.0
Achylia gastrica K31.89
  psychogenic F45.8
Acid
  burn — *see* Corrosion
  deficiency
    amide nicotinic E52
    ascorbic E54
    folic E53.8
    nicotinic E52
    pantothenic E53.8
  intoxication E87.2
  peptic disease K30
  phosphatase deficiency E83.39
  stomach K30
    psychogenic F45.8
Acidemia E87.2
  argininosuccinic E72.22
  isovaleric E71.110
  metabolic (newborn) P19.9
    first noted before onset of labor P19.0
    first noted during labor P19.1
    noted at birth P19.2
  methylmalonic E71.120
  pipecolic E72.3
  propionic E71.121
Acidity, gastric (high) K30
  psychogenic F45.8
Acidocytopenia — *see* Agranulocytosis
Acidocytosis D72.1
Acidopenia — *see* Agranulocytosis
Acidosis (lactic) (respiratory) E87.2
  in Type 1 diabetes E10.10
    with coma E10.11
  kidney, tubular N25.89
  lactic E87.2

Acidosis — *continued*
  metabolic NEC E87.2
    with respiratory acidosis E87.4
    late, of newborn P74.0
  mixed metabolic and respiratory, newborn P84
  newborn P84
  renal (hyperchloremic) (tubular) N25.89
  respiratory E87.2
    complicated by
      metabolic
        acidosis E87.4
        alkalosis E87.4
Aciduria
  argininosuccinic E72.22
  glutaric (type I) E72.3
    type II E71.313
    type III E71.5- ☑
  orotic (congenital) (hereditary) (pyrimidine
    deficiency) E79.8
    anemia D53.0
Acladiosis (skin) B36.0
Aclasis, diaphyseal Q78.6
Acleistocardia Q21.1
Aclusion — *see* Anomaly, dentofacial, malocclusion
Acne L70.9
  artificialis L70.8
  atrophica L70.2
  cachecticorum (Hebra) L70.8
  conglobata L70.1
  cystic L70.0
  decalvans L66.2
  excoriée des jeunes filles L70.5
  frontalis L70.2
  indurata L70.0
  infantile L70.4
  keloid L73.0
  lupoid L70.2
  necrotic, necrotica (miliaris) L70.2
  neonatal L70.4
  nodular L70.0
  occupational L70.8
  picker's L70.5
  pustular L70.0
  rodens L70.2
  rosacea L71.9
  specified NEC L70.8
  tropica L70.3
  varioliformis L70.2
  vulgaris L70.0
Acnitis (primary) A18.4
Acosta's disease T70.29 ☑
Acoustic — *see* condition
Acousticophobia F40.298
Acquired (*see also* condition)
  immunodeficiency syndrome (AIDS) B20
Acrania Q00.0
Acroangiodermatitis I78.9
Acroasphyxia, chronic I73.89
Acrobystitis N47.7
Acrocephalopolysyndactyly Q87.0
Acrocephalosyndactyly Q87.0
Acrocephaly Q75.0
Acrochondrohyperplasia — *see* Syndrome,
  Marfan's
Acrocyanosis I73.8 ☑
  newborn P28.2
    meaning transient blue hands and feet - omit
      code
Acrodermatitis L30.8
  atrophicans (chronica) L90.4
  continua (Hallopeau) L40.2
  enteropathica (hereditary) E83.2
  Hallopeau's L40.2
  infantile papular L44.4
  perstans L40.2
  pustulosa continua L40.2
  recalcitrant pustular L40.2
Acrodynia — *see* Poisoning, mercury
Acromegaly, acromegalia E22.0
Acromelalgia I73.81
Acromicria, acromikria Q79.8
Acronyx L60.0
Acropachy, thyroid — *see* Thyrotoxicosis
Acroparesthesia (simple) (vasomotor) I73.89
Acropathy, thyroid — *see* Thyrotoxicosis
Acrophobia F40.241
Acroposthitis N47.7
Acroscleriasis, acroscleroderma, acrosclerosis — *see*
  Sclerosis, systemic
Acrosphacelus I96
Acrospiroma, eccrine — *see* Neoplasm, skin, benign
Acrostealgia — *see* Osteochondropathy

Acrotrophodynia — *see* Immersion
ACTH ectopic syndrome E24.3
Actinic — *see* condition
Actinobacillosis, actinobacillus A28.8
　　mallei A24.0
　　muris A25.1
Actinomyces israelii (infection) — *see* Actinomycosis
Actinomycetoma (foot) B47.1
Actinomycosis, actinomycotic A42.9
　　with pneumonia A42.0
　　abdominal A42.1
　　cervicofacial A42.2
　　cutaneous A42.89
　　gastrointestinal A42.1
　　pulmonary A42.0
　　sepsis A42.7
　　specified site NEC A42.89
Actinoneuritis G62.82
Action, heart
　　disorder I49.9
　　irregular I49.9
　　　　psychogenic F45.8
Activated protein C resistance D68.51
Active — *see* condition
Acute (*see also* condition)
　　abdomen R10.0
　　gallbladder — *see* Cholecystitis, acute
Acyanotic heart disease (congenital) Q24.9
Acystia Q64.5
Adair-Dighton syndrome (brittle bones and blue sclera, deafness) Q78.0
Adamantinoblastoma — *see* Ameloblastoma
Adamantinoma (*see also* Cyst, calcifying odontogenic)
　　long bones C40.90
　　　　lower limb C40.2- ☑
　　　　upper limb C40.0- ☑
　　malignant C41.1
　　　　jaw (bone) (lower) C41.1
　　　　　　upper C41.0
　　tibial C40.2- ☑
Adamantoblastoma — *see* Ameloblastoma
Adams-Stokes (-Morgagni) disease or syndrome I45.9
Adaption reaction — *see* Disorder, adjustment
Addiction (*see also* Dependence) F19.20
　　alcohol, alcoholic (ethyl) (methyl) (wood) (without remission) F10.20
　　　　with remission F10.21
　　drug — *see* Dependence, drug
　　ethyl alcohol (without remission) F10.20
　　　　with remission F10.21
　　heroin — *see* Dependence, drug, opioid
　　methyl alcohol (without remission) F10.20
　　　　with remission F10.21
　　methylated spirit (without remission) F10.20
　　　　with remission F10.21
　　morphine (-like substances) — *see* Dependence, drug, opioid
　　nicotine — *see* Dependence, drug, nicotine
　　opium and opioids — *see* Dependence, drug, opioid
　　tobacco — *see* Dependence, drug, nicotine
Addisonian crisis E27.2
Addison's
　　anemia (pernicious) D51.0
　　disease (bronze) or syndrome E27.1
　　　　tuberculous A18.7
　　keloid L94.0
Addison-Biermer anemia (pernicious) D51.0
Addison-Schilder complex E71.528
Additional (*see also* Accessory)
　　chromosome (s) Q99.8
　　　　sex — *see* Abnormal, chromosome, sex
　　　　21 — *see* Trisomy, 21
Adduction contracture, hip or other joint — *see* Contraction, joint
Adenitis (*see also* Lymphadenitis)
　　acute, unspecified site L04.9
　　axillary I88.9
　　　　acute L04.2
　　　　chronic or subacute I88.1
　　Bartholin's gland N75.8
　　bulbourethral gland — *see* Urethritis
　　cervical I88.9
　　　　acute L04.0
　　　　chronic or subacute I88.1
　　chancroid (Hemophilus ducreyi) A57
　　chronic, unspecified site I88.1
　　Cowper's gland — *see* Urethritis
　　due to Pasteurella multocida (p. septica) A28.0
　　epidemic, acute B27.09

Adenitis — *continued*
　　gangrenous L04.9
　　gonorrheal NEC A54.89
　　groin I88.9
　　　　acute L04.1
　　　　chronic or subacute I88.1
　　infectious (acute) (epidemic) B27.09
　　inguinal I88.9
　　　　acute L04.1
　　　　chronic or subacute I88.1
　　lymph gland or node, except mesenteric I88.9
　　　　acute — *see* Lymphadenitis, acute
　　　　chronic or subacute I88.1
　　mesenteric (acute) (chronic) (nonspecific) (subacute) I88.0
　　parotid gland (suppurative) — *see* Sialoadenitis
　　salivary gland (any) (suppurative) — *see* Sialoadenitis
　　scrofulous (tuberculous) A18.2
　　Skene's duct or gland — *see* Urethritis
　　strumous, tuberculous A18.2
　　subacute, unspecified site I88.1
　　sublingual gland (suppurative) — *see* Sialoadenitis
　　submandibular gland (suppurative) — *see* Sialoadenitis
　　submaxillary gland (suppurative) — *see* Sialoadenitis
　　tuberculous — *see* Tuberculosis, lymph gland
　　urethral gland — *see* Urethritis
　　Wharton's duct (suppurative) — *see* Sialoadenitis
Adenoacanthoma — *see* Neoplasm, malignant, by site
Adenoameloblastoma — *see* Cyst, calcifying odontogenic
Adenocarcinoid (tumor) — *see* Neoplasm, malignant, by site
Adenocarcinoma (*see also* Neoplasm, malignant, by site)
　　acidophil
　　　　specified site — *see* Neoplasm, malignant, by site
　　　　unspecified site C75.1
　　adrenal cortical C74.0- ☑
　　alveolar — *see* Neoplasm, lung, malignant
　　apocrine
　　　　breast — *see* Neoplasm, breast, malignant
　　　　in situ
　　　　　　breast D05.8- ☑
　　　　　　specified site NEC — *see* Neoplasm, skin, in situ
　　　　　　unspecified site D04.9
　　　　specified site NEC — *see* Neoplasm, skin, malignant
　　　　unspecified site C44.99
　　basal cell
　　　　specified site — *see* Neoplasm, skin, malignant
　　　　unspecified site C08.9
　　basophil
　　　　specified site — *see* Neoplasm, malignant, by site
　　　　unspecified site C75.1
　　bile duct type C22.1
　　　　liver C22.1
　　　　specified site NEC — *see* Neoplasm, malignant, by site
　　　　unspecified site C22.1
　　bronchiolar — *see* Neoplasm, lung, malignant
　　bronchioloalveolar — *see* Neoplasm, lung, malignant
　　ceruminous C44.29- ☑
　　cervix, in situ (*see also* Carcinoma, cervix uteri, in situ) D06.9
　　chromophobe
　　　　specified site — *see* Neoplasm, malignant, by site
　　　　unspecified site C75.1
　　diffuse type
　　　　specified site — *see* Neoplasm, malignant, by site
　　　　unspecified site C16.9
　　duct
　　　　infiltrating
　　　　　　with Paget's disease — *see* Neoplasm, breast, malignant
　　　　　　specified site — *see* Neoplasm, malignant, by site
　　　　　　unspecified site (female) C50.91- ☑
　　　　　　　　male C50.92- ☑
　　　　specified site — *see* Neoplasm, malignant, by site
　　　　unspecified site

Adenocarcinoma — *continued*
　　female C56.9
　　male C61
　　eosinophil
　　　　specified site — *see* Neoplasm, malignant, by site
　　　　unspecified site C75.1
　　follicular
　　　　with papillary C73
　　　　moderately differentiated C73
　　　　specified site — *see* Neoplasm, malignant, by site
　　　　trabecular C73
　　　　unspecified site C73
　　　　well differentiated C73
　　Hurthle cell C73
　　in
　　　　adenomatous
　　　　　　polyposis coli C18.9
　　infiltrating duct
　　　　with Paget's disease — *see* Neoplasm, breast, malignant
　　　　specified site — *see* Neoplasm, by site, malignant
　　　　unspecified site (female) C50.91- ☑
　　　　　　male C50.92- ☑
　　inflammatory
　　　　specified site — *see* Neoplasm, by site, malignant
　　　　unspecified site (female) C50.91- ☑
　　　　　　male C50.92- ☑
　　intestinal type
　　　　specified site — *see* Neoplasm, by site, malignant
　　　　unspecified site C16.9
　　intracystic papillary
　　intraductal
　　　　breast D05.1- ☑
　　　　noninfiltrating
　　　　　　breast D05.1- ☑
　　　　papillary
　　　　　　with invasion
　　　　　　　　specified site — *see* Neoplasm, by site, malignant
　　　　　　　　unspecified site (female) C50.91- ☑
　　　　　　　　　　male C50.92- ☑
　　　　　　breast D05.1- ☑
　　　　　　specified site NEC — *see* Neoplasm, in situ, by site
　　　　　　unspecified site D05.1- ☑
　　　　specified site NEC — *see* Neoplasm, in situ, by site
　　　　unspecified site D05.1- ☑
　　papillary
　　　　with invasion
　　　　　　specified site — *see* Neoplasm, malignant, by site
　　　　　　unspecified site (female) C50.91- ☑
　　　　　　　　male C50.92- ☑
　　　　breast D05.1- ☑
　　　　specified site — *see* Neoplasm, in situ, by site
　　　　unspecified site D05.1- ☑
　　　　specified site NEC — *see* Neoplasm, in situ, by site
　　　　unspecified site D05.1- ☑
　　islet cell
　　　　with exocrine, mixed
　　　　　　specified site — *see* Neoplasm, malignant, by site
　　　　　　unspecified site C25.9
　　　　pancreas C25.4
　　　　specified site NEC — *see* Neoplasm, malignant, by site
　　　　unspecified site C25.4
　　lobular
　　　　in situ
　　　　　　breast D05.0- ☑
　　　　　　specified site NEC — *see* Neoplasm, in situ, by site
　　　　　　unspecified site D05.0- ☑
　　　　specified site — *see* Neoplasm, malignant, by site
　　　　unspecified site (female) C50.91- ☑
　　　　　　male C50.92- ☑
　　mucoid (*see also* Neoplasm, malignant, by site)
　　　　cell
　　　　　　specified site — *see* Neoplasm, malignant, by site
　　　　　　unspecified site C75.1
　　nonencapsulated sclerosing C73
　　papillary
　　　　with follicular C73

　　　　　☑ **Additional character required**

Adenocarcinoma — *continued*
  follicular variant C73
  intraductal (noninfiltrating)
    with invasion
      specified site — *see* Neoplasm, malignant, by site
      unspecified site (female) C50.91- ☑
        male C50.92- ☑
    breast D05.1- ☑
    specified site NEC — *see* Neoplasm, in situ, by site
    unspecified site D05.1- ☑
  serous
    specified site — *see* Neoplasm, malignant, by site
    unspecified site C56.9
  papillocystic
    specified site — *see* Neoplasm, malignant, by site
    unspecified site C56.9
  pseudomucinous
    specified site — *see* Neoplasm, malignant, by site
    unspecified site C56.9
  renal cell C64- ☑
  sebaceous — *see* Neoplasm, skin, malignant
  serous (*see also* Neoplasm, malignant, by site)
    papillary
      specified site — *see* Neoplasm, malignant, by site
      unspecified site C56.9
  sweat gland — *see* Neoplasm, skin, malignant
  water-clear cell C75.0
Adenocarcinoma-in-situ (*see also* Neoplasm, in situ, by site)
  breast D05.9- ☑
Adenofibroma
  clear cell — *see* Neoplasm, benign, by site
  endometrioid D27.9
    borderline malignancy D39.10
    malignant C56- ☑
  mucinous
    specified site — *see* Neoplasm, benign, by site
    unspecified site D27.9
  papillary
    specified site — *see* Neoplasm, benign, by site
    unspecified site D27.9
  prostate — *see* Enlargement, enlarged, prostate
  serous
    specified site — *see* Neoplasm, benign, by site
    unspecified site D27.9
  specified site — *see* Neoplasm, benign, by site
  unspecified site D27.9
Adenofibrosis
  breast — *see* Fibroadenosis, breast
  endometrioid N80.0
Adenoiditis (chronic) J35.02
  with tonsillitis J35.03
  acute J03.90
    recurrent J03.91
    specified organism NEC J03.80
      recurrent J03.81
    staphylococcal J03.80
      recurrent J03.81
    streptococcal J03.00
      recurrent J03.01
Adenoids — *see* condition
Adenolipoma — *see* Neoplasm, benign, by site
Adenolipomatosis, Launois-Bensaude E88.89
Adenolymphoma
  specified site — *see* Neoplasm, benign, by site
  unspecified site D11.9
Adenoma (*see also* Neoplasm, benign, by site)
  acidophil
    specified site — *see* Neoplasm, benign, by site
    unspecified site D35.2
  acidophil-basophil, mixed
    specified site — *see* Neoplasm, benign, by site
    unspecified site D35.2
  adrenal (cortical) D35.00
    clear cell D35.00
    compact cell D35.00
    glomerulosa cell D35.00
    heavily pigmented variant D35.00
    mixed cell D35.00
  alpha-cell
    pancreas D13.7
    specified site NEC — *see* Neoplasm, benign, by site
    unspecified site D13.7
  alveolar D14.30
  apocrine

Adenoma — *continued*
  breast D24- ☑
  specified site NEC — *see* Neoplasm, skin, benign, by site
  unspecified site D23.9
  basal cell D11.9
  basophil
    specified site — *see* Neoplasm, benign, by site
    unspecified site D35.2
  basophil-acidophil, mixed
    specified site — *see* Neoplasm, benign, by site
    unspecified site D35.2
  beta-cell
    pancreas D13.7
    specified site NEC — *see* Neoplasm, benign, by site
    unspecified site D13.7
  bile duct D13.4
    common D13.5
    extrahepatic D13.5
    intrahepatic D13.4
    specified site NEC — *see* Neoplasm, benign, by site
    unspecified site D13.4
  black D35.00
  bronchial D38.1
    cylindroid type — *see* Neoplasm, lung, malignant
  ceruminous D23.2- ☑
  chief cell D35.1
  chromophobe
    specified site — *see* Neoplasm, benign, by site
    unspecified site D35.2
  colloid
    specified site — *see* Neoplasm, benign, by site
    unspecified site D34
  duct
  eccrine, papillary — *see* Neoplasm, skin, benign
  endocrine, multiple
    single specified site — *see* Neoplasm, uncertain behavior, by site
    two or more specified sites D44- ☑
    unspecified site D44.9
  endometrioid (*see also* Neoplasm, benign)
    borderline malignancy — *see* Neoplasm, uncertain behavior, by site
  eosinophil
    specified site — *see* Neoplasm, benign, by site
    unspecified site D35.2
  fetal
    specified site — *see* Neoplasm, benign, by site
    unspecified site D34
  follicular
    specified site — *see* Neoplasm, benign, by site
    unspecified site D34
  hepatocellular D13.4
  Hurthle cell D34
  islet cell
    pancreas D13.7
    specified site NEC — *see* Neoplasm, benign, by site
    unspecified site D13.7
  liver cell D13.4
  macrofollicular
    specified site — *see* Neoplasm, benign, by site
    unspecified site D34
  malignant, malignum — *see* Neoplasm, malignant, by site
  microcystic
    pancreas D13.7
    specified site NEC — *see* Neoplasm, benign, by site
    unspecified site D13.7
  microfollicular
    specified site — *see* Neoplasm, benign, by site
    unspecified site D34
  mucoid cell
    specified site — *see* Neoplasm, benign, by site
    unspecified site D35.2
  multiple endocrine
    single specified site — *see* Neoplasm, uncertain behavior, by site
    two or more specified sites D44- ☑
    unspecified site D44.9
  nipple D24- ☑
  papillary (*see also* Neoplasm, benign, by site)
    eccrine — *see* Neoplasm, skin, benign, by site
  Pick's tubular
    specified site — *see* Neoplasm, benign, by site
    unspecified site
      female D27.9
      male D29.20

Adenoma — *continued*
  pleomorphic
    carcinoma in — *see* Neoplasm, salivary gland, malignant
      specified site — *see* Neoplasm, malignant, by site
      unspecified site C08.9
  polypoid (*see also* Neoplasm, benign)
    adenocarcinoma in — *see* Neoplasm, malignant, by site
    adenocarcinoma in situ — *see* Neoplasm, in situ, by site
  prostate — *see* Neoplasm, benign, prostate
  rete cell D29.20
  sebaceous — *see* Neoplasm, skin, benign
  Sertoli cell
    specified site — *see* Neoplasm, benign, by site
    unspecified site
      female D27.9
      male D29.20
  skin appendage — *see* Neoplasm, skin, benign
  sudoriferous gland — *see* Neoplasm, skin, benign
  sweat gland — *see* Neoplasm, skin, benign
  testicular
    specified site — *see* Neoplasm, benign, by site
    unspecified site
      female D27.9
      male D29.20
  tubular (*see also* Neoplasm, benign, by site)
    adenocarcinoma in — *see* Neoplasm, malignant, by site
    adenocarcinoma in situ — *see* Neoplasm, in situ, by site
    Pick's
      specified site — *see* Neoplasm, benign, by site
      unspecified site
        female D27.9
        male D29.20
  tubulovillous (*see also* Neoplasm, benign, by site)
    adenocarcinoma in — *see* Neoplasm, malignant, by site
    adenocarcinoma in situ — *see* Neoplasm, in situ, by site
  villous — *see* Neoplasm, uncertain behavior, by site
    adenocarcinoma in — *see* Neoplasm, malignant, by site
    adenocarcinoma in situ — *see* Neoplasm, in situ, by site
  water-clear cell D35.1
Adenomatosis
  endocrine (multiple) E31.20
    single specified site — *see* Neoplasm, uncertain behavior, by site
  erosive of nipple D24- ☑
  pluriendocrine — *see* Adenomatosis, endocrine
  pulmonary D38.1
    malignant — *see* Neoplasm, lung, malignant
  specified site — *see* Neoplasm, benign, by site
  unspecified site D12.6
Adenomatous
  goiter (nontoxic) E04.9
    with hyperthyroidism — *see* Hyperthyroidism, with, goiter, nodular
    toxic — *see* Hyperthyroidism, with, goiter, nodular
Adenomyoma (*see also* Neoplasm, benign, by site)
  prostate — *see* Enlarged, prostate
Adenomyometritis N80.0
Adenomyosis N80.0
Adenopathy (lymph gland) R59.9
  generalized R59.1
  inguinal R59.0
  localized R59.0
  mediastinal R59.0
  mesentery R59.0
  syphilitic (secondary) A51.49
  tracheobronchial R59.0
    tuberculous A15.4
      primary (progressive) A15.7
  tuberculous (*see also* Tuberculosis, lymph gland)
    tracheobronchial A15.4
      primary (progressive) A15.7
Adenosalpingitis — *see* Salpingitis
Adenosarcoma — *see* Neoplasm, malignant, by site
Adenosclerosis I88.8
Adenosis (sclerosing) breast — *see* Fibroadenosis, breast
Adenovirus, as cause of disease classified elsewhere B97.0
Adentia (complete) (partial) — *see* Absence, teeth

Adherent - Admission

Adherent (*see also* Adhesions)
labia (minora) N90.89
pericardium (nonrheumatic) I31.0
rheumatic I09.2
placenta (with hemorrhage) O72.0
without hemorrhage O73.0
prepuce, newborn N47.0
scar (skin) L90.5
tendon in scar L90.5
Adhesions, adhesive (postinfective) K66.0
with intestinal obstruction K56.5
abdominal (wall) — *see* Adhesions, peritoneum
appendix K38.8
bile duct (common) (hepatic) K83.8
bladder (sphincter) N32.89
bowel — *see* Adhesions, peritoneum
cardiac I31.0
rheumatic I09.2
cecum — *see* Adhesions, peritoneum
cervicovaginal N88.1
congenital Q52.8
postpartal O90.89
old N88.1
cervix N88.1
ciliary body NEC — *see* Adhesions, iris
clitoris N90.89
colon — *see* Adhesions, peritoneum
common duct K83.8
congenital (*see also* Anomaly, by site)
fingers — *see* Syndactylism, complex, fingers
omental, anomalous Q43.3
peritoneal Q43.3
tongue (to gum or roof of mouth) Q38.3
conjunctiva (acquired) H11.21- ☑
congenital Q15.8
cystic duct K82.8
diaphragm — *see* Adhesions, peritoneum
due to foreign body — *see* Foreign body
duodenum — *see* Adhesions, peritoneum
ear
middle H74.1- ☑
epididymis N50.8
epidural — *see* Adhesions, meninges
epiglottis J38.7
eyelid H02.59
female pelvis N73.6
gallbladder K82.8
globe H44.89
heart I31.0
rheumatic I09.2
ileocecal (coil) — *see* Adhesions, peritoneum
ileum — *see* Adhesions, peritoneum
intestine (*see also* Adhesions, peritoneum)
with obstruction K56.5
intra-abdominal — *see* Adhesions, peritoneum
iris H21.50- ☑
anterior H21.51- ☑
goniosynechiae H21.52- ☑
posterior H21.54- ☑
to corneal graft T85.89 ☑
joint — *see* Ankylosis
knee M23.8X ☑
temporomandibular M26.61
labium (majus) (minus), congenital Q52.5
liver — *see* Adhesions, peritoneum
lung J98.4
mediastinum J98.5
meninges (cerebral) (spinal) G96.12
congenital Q07.8
tuberculous (cerebral) (spinal) A17.0
mesenteric — *see* Adhesions, peritoneum
nasal (septum) (to turbinates) J34.89
ocular muscle — *see* Strabismus, mechanical
omentum — *see* Adhesions, peritoneum
ovary N73.6
congenital (to cecum, kidney or omentum) Q50.39
paraovarian N73.6
pelvic (peritoneal)
female N73.6
postprocedural N99.4
male — *see* Adhesions, peritoneum
postpartal (old) N73.6
tuberculous A18.17
penis to scrotum (congenital) Q55.8
periappendiceal (*see also* Adhesions, peritoneum)
pericardium (nonrheumatic) I31.0
focal I31.8
rheumatic I09.2
tuberculous A18.84
pericholecystic K82.8
perigastric — *see* Adhesions, peritoneum

Adhesions — *continued*
periovarian N73.6
periprostatic N42.89
perirectal — *see* Adhesions, peritoneum
perirenal N28.89
peritoneum, peritoneal (postinfective) (postprocedural) K66.0
with obstruction (intestinal) K56.5
congenital Q43.3
pelvic, female N73.6
postprocedural N99.4
postpartal, pelvic N73.6
to uterus N73.6
peritubal N73.6
periureteral N28.89
periuterine N73.6
perivesical N32.89
perivesicular (seminal vesicle) N50.8
pleura, pleuritic J94.8
tuberculous NEC A15.6
pleuropericardial J94.8
postoperative (gastrointestinal tract) K66.0
with obstruction K91.3
due to foreign body accidentally left in wound — *see* Foreign body, accidentally left during a procedure
pelvic peritoneal N99.4
urethra — *see* Stricture, urethra, postprocedural
vagina N99.2
postpartal, old (vulva or perineum) N90.89
preputial, prepuce N47.5
pulmonary J98.4
pylorus — *see* Adhesions, peritoneum
sciatic nerve — *see* Lesion, nerve, sciatic
seminal vesicle N50.8
shoulder (joint) — *see* Capsulitis, adhesive
sigmoid flexure — *see* Adhesions, peritoneum
spermatic cord (acquired) N50.8
congenital Q55.4
spinal canal G96.12
stomach — *see* Adhesions, peritoneum
subscapular — *see* Capsulitis, adhesive
temporomandibular M26.61
tendinitis (*see also* Tenosynovitis, specified type NEC)
shoulder — *see* Capsulitis, adhesive
testis N44.8
tongue, congenital (to gum or roof of mouth) Q38.3
acquired K14.8
trachea J39.8
tubo-ovarian N73.6
tunica vaginalis N44.8
uterus N73.6
internal N85.6
to abdominal wall N73.6
vagina (chronic) N89.5
postoperative N99.2
vitreomacular H43.82- ☑
vitreous H43.89
vulva N90.89
Adiaspiromycosis B48.8
Adie (-Holmes) pupil or syndrome — *see* Anomaly, pupil, function, tonic pupil
Adiponecrosis neonatorum P83.8
Adiposis (*see also* Obesity)
cerebralis E23.6
dolorosa E88.2
Adiposity (*see also* Obesity)
heart — *see* Degeneration, myocardial
localized E65
Adiposogenital dystrophy E23.6
Adjustment
disorder — *see* Disorder, adjustment
implanted device — *see* Encounter (for), adjustment (of)
prosthesis, external — *see* Fitting
reaction — *see* Disorder, adjustment
Administration of tPA (rtPA) in a different facility within the last 24 hours prior to admission to current facility Z92.82
Admission (for) (*see also* Encounter (for))
adjustment (of)
artificial
arm Z44.00- ☑
complete Z44.01- ☑
partial Z44.02- ☑
eye Z44.2 ☑
leg Z44.10- ☑
complete Z44.11- ☑
partial Z44.12- ☑
brain neuropacemaker Z46.2

Admission — *continued*
implanted Z45.42
breast
implant Z45.81 ☑
prosthesis (external) Z44.3 ☑
colostomy belt Z46.89
contact lenses Z46.0
cystostomy device Z46.6
dental prosthesis Z46.3
device NEC
abdominal Z46.89
implanted Z45.89
cardiac Z45.09
defibrillator (with synchronous cardiac pacemaker) Z45.02
pacemaker Z45.018
pulse generator Z45.010
hearing device Z45.328
bone conduction Z45.320
cochlear Z45.321
infusion pump Z45.1
nervous system Z45.49
CSF drainage Z45.41
hearing device — *see* Admission, adjustment, device, implanted, hearing device
neuropacemaker Z45.42
visual substitution Z45.31
specified NEC Z45.89
vascular access Z45.2
visual substitution Z45.31
nervous system Z46.2
implanted — *see* Admission, adjustment, device, implanted, nervous system
orthodontic Z46.4
prosthetic Z44.9
arm — *see* Admission, adjustment, artificial, arm
breast Z44.3 ☑
dental Z46.3
eye Z44.2 ☑
leg — *see* Admission, adjustment, artificial, leg
specified type NEC Z44.8
substitution
auditory Z46.2
implanted — *see* Admission, adjustment, device, implanted, hearing device
nervous system Z46.2
implanted — *see* Admission, adjustment, device, implanted, nervous system
visual Z46.2
implanted Z45.31
urinary Z46.6
hearing aid Z46.1
implanted — *see* Admission, adjustment, device, implanted, hearing device
ileostomy device Z46.89
intestinal appliance or device NEC Z46.89
neuropacemaker (brain) (peripheral nerve) (spinal cord) Z46.2
implanted Z45.42
orthodontic device Z46.4
orthopedic (brace) (cast) (device) (shoes) Z46.89
pacemaker
cardiac Z45.018
pulse generator Z45.010
nervous system Z46.2
implanted Z45.42
portacath (port-a-cath) Z45.2
prosthesis Z44.9
arm — *see* Admission, adjustment, artificial, arm
breast Z44.3 ☑
dental Z46.3
eye Z44.2 ☑
leg — *see* Admission, adjustment, artificial, leg
specified NEC Z44.8
spectacles Z46.0
aftercare (*see also* Aftercare) Z51.89
postpartum
immediately after delivery Z39.0
routine follow-up Z39.2
radiation therapy (antineoplastic) Z51.0
attention to artificial opening (of) Z43.9
artificial vagina Z43.7
colostomy Z43.3
cystostomy Z43.5
enterostomy Z43.4
gastrostomy Z43.1

☑ **Additional character required**

Admission — *continued*
ileostomy Z43.2
jejunostomy Z43.4
nephrostomy Z43.6
specified site NEC Z43.8
  intestinal tract Z43.4
  urinary tract Z43.6
tracheostomy Z43.0
ureterostomy Z43.6
urethrostomy Z43.6
breast augmentation or reduction Z41.1
breast reconstruction following mastectomy Z42.1
change of
  dressing (nonsurgical) Z48.00
  neuropacemaker device (brain) (peripheral nerve) (spinal cord) Z46.2
    implanted Z45.42
  surgical dressing Z48.01
circumcision, ritual or routine (in absence of diagnosis) Z41.2
clinical research investigation (control) (normal comparison) (participant) Z00.6
contraceptive management Z30.9
cosmetic surgery NEC Z41.1
counseling (*see also* Counseling)
  dietary Z71.3
  HIV Z71.7
  human immunodeficiency virus Z71.7
  nonattending third party Z71.0
  procreative management NEC Z31.69
delivery, full-term, uncomplicated O80
  cesarean, without indication O82
dietary surveillance and counseling Z71.3
ear piercing Z41.3
examination at health care facility (adult) (*see also* Examination) Z00.00
  with abnormal findings Z00.01
  clinical research investigation (control) (normal comparison) (participant) Z00.6
  dental Z01.20
    with abnormal findings Z01.21
  donor (potential) Z00.5
  ear Z01.10
    with abnormal findings NEC Z01.118
  eye Z01.00
    with abnormal findings Z01.01
  general, specified reason NEC Z00.8
  hearing Z01.10
    with abnormal findings NEC Z01.118
  postpartum checkup Z39.2
  psychiatric (general) Z00.8
    requested by authority Z04.6
  vision Z01.00
    with abnormal findings Z01.01
fitting (of)
  artificial
    arm — *see* Admission, adjustment, artificial, arm
    eye Z44.2 ☑
    leg — *see* Admission, adjustment, artificial, leg
  brain neuropacemaker Z46.2
    implanted Z45.42
  breast prosthesis (external) Z44.3 ☑
  colostomy belt Z46.89
  contact lenses Z46.0
  cystostomy device Z46.6
  dental prosthesis Z46.3
  dentures Z46.3
  device NEC
    abdominal Z46.89
    nervous system Z46.2
      implanted — *see* Admission, adjustment, device, implanted, nervous system
    orthodontic Z46.4
    prosthetic Z44.9
     breast Z44.3 ☑
     dental Z46.3
     eye Z44.2 ☑
    substitution
     auditory Z46.2
      implanted — *see* Admission, adjustment, device, implanted, hearing device
     nervous system Z46.2
      implanted — *see* Admission, adjustment, device, implanted, nervous system
     visual Z46.2
      implanted Z45.31
  hearing aid Z46.1
  ileostomy device Z46.89
  intestinal appliance or device NEC Z46.89

Admission — *continued*
  neuropacemaker (brain) (peripheral nerve) (spinal cord) Z46.2
    implanted Z45.42
  orthodontic device Z46.4
  orthopedic device (brace) (cast) (shoes) Z46.89
  prosthesis Z44.9
    arm — *see* Admission, adjustment, artificial, arm
    breast Z44.3 ☑
    dental Z46.3
    eye Z44.2 ☑
    leg — *see* Admission, adjustment, artificial, leg
    specified type NEC Z44.8
  spectacles Z46.0
follow-up examination Z09
intrauterine device management Z30.431
  initial prescription Z30.014
mental health evaluation Z00.8
  requested by authority Z04.6
observation — *see* Observation
Papanicolaou smear, cervix Z12.4
  for suspected malignant neoplasm Z12.4
plastic and reconstructive surgery following medical procedure or healed injury NEC Z42.8
plastic surgery, cosmetic NEC Z41.1
postpartum observation
  immediately after delivery Z39.0
  routine follow-up Z39.2
poststerilization (for restoration) Z31.0
  aftercare Z31.42
procreative management Z31.9
prophylactic (measure)
  organ removal Z40.00
    breast Z40.01
    ovary Z40.02
    specified organ NEC Z40.09
    testes Z40.09
  vaccination Z23
psychiatric examination (general) Z00.8
  requested by authority Z04.6
radiation therapy (antineoplastic) Z51.0
reconstructive surgery following medical procedure or healed injury NEC Z42.8
removal of
  cystostomy catheter Z43.5
  drains Z48.03
  dressing (nonsurgical) Z48.00
  intrauterine contraceptive device Z30.432
  neuropacemaker (brain) (peripheral nerve) (spinal cord) Z46.2
    implanted Z45.42
  staples Z48.02
  surgical dressing Z48.01
  sutures Z48.02
  ureteral stent Z46.6
respirator [ventilator] use during power failure Z99.12
restoration of organ continuity (poststerilization) Z31.0
  aftercare Z31.42
sensitivity test (*see also* Test, skin)
  allergy NEC Z01.82
  Mantoux Z11.1
tuboplasty following previous sterilization Z31.0
  aftercare Z31.42
vasoplasty following previous sterilization Z31.0
  aftercare Z31.42
vision examination Z01.00
  with abnormal findings Z01.01
waiting period for admission to other facility Z75.1

Adnexitis (suppurative) — *see* Salpingo-oophoritis
Adolescent X-linked adrenoleukodystrophy E71.521
Adrenal (gland) — *see* condition
Adrenalism, tuberculous A18.7
Adrenalitis, adrenitis E27.8
  autoimmune E27.1
  meningococcal, hemorrhagic A39.1
Adrenarche, premature E27.0
Adrenocortical syndrome — *see* Cushing's, syndrome
Adrenogenital syndrome E25.9
  acquired E25.8
  congenital E25.0
  salt loss E25.0
Adrenogenitalism, congenital E25.0
Adrenoleukodystrophy E71.529
  neonatal E71.511
  X-linked E71.529

Adrenoleukodystrophy — *continued*
  Addison only phenotype E71.528
  Addison-Schilder E71.528
  adolescent E71.521
  adrenomyeloneuropathy E71.522
  childhood cerebral E71.520
  other specified E71.528
Adrenomyeloneuropathy E71.522
Adventitious bursa — *see* Bursopathy, specified type NEC
Adverse effect — *see* Table of Drugs and Chemicals, categories T36-T50, with 6th character 5
Advice — *see* Counseling
Adynamia (episodica) (hereditary) (periodic) G72.3
Aeration lung imperfect, newborn — *see* Atelectasis
Aerobullosis T70.3 ☑
Aerocele — *see* Embolism, air
Aerodermectasia
  subcutaneous (traumatic) T79.7 ☑
Aerodontalgia T70.29 ☑
Aeroembolism T70.3 ☑
Aerogenes capsulatus infection A48.0
Aero-otitis media T70.0 ☑
Aerophagy, aerophagia (psychogenic) F45.8
Aerophobia F40.228
Aerosinusitis T70.1 ☑
Aerotitis T70.0 ☑
Affection — *see* Disease
Afibrinogenemia (*see also* Defect, coagulation) D68.8
  acquired D65
  congenital D68.2
  following ectopic or molar pregnancy O08.1
  in abortion — *see* Abortion, by type, complicated by, afibrinogenemia
  puerperal O72.3
African
  sleeping sickness B56.9
  tick fever A68.1
  trypanosomiasis B56.9
    gambian B56.0
    rhodesian B56.1
Aftercare (*see also* Care) Z51.89
  following surgery (for) (on)
    amputation Z47.81
    attention to
     drains Z48.03
     dressings (nonsurgical) Z48.00
      surgical Z48.01
     sutures Z48.02
    circulatory system Z48.812
    delayed (planned) wound closure Z48.1
    digestive system Z48.815
    explantation of joint prosthesis (staged procedure)
     hip Z47.32
     knee Z47.33
     shoulder Z47.31
    genitourinary system Z48.816
    joint replacement Z47.1
    neoplasm Z48.3
    nervous system Z48.811
    oral cavity Z48.814
    organ transplant
     bone marrow Z48.290
     heart Z48.21
     heart-lung Z48.280
     kidney Z48.22
     liver Z48.23
     lung Z48.24
     multiple organs NEC Z48.288
     specified NEC Z48.298
    orthopedic NEC Z47.89
    planned wound closure Z48.1
    removal of internal fixation device Z47.2
    respiratory system Z48.813
    scoliosis Z47.82
    sense organs Z48.810
    skin and subcutaneous tissue Z48.817
    specified body system
     circulatory Z48.812
     digestive Z48.815
     genitourinary Z48.816
     nervous Z48.811
     oral cavity Z48.814
     respiratory Z48.813
     sense organs Z48.810
     skin and subcutaneous tissue Z48.817
     teeth Z48.814
    specified NEC Z48.89
    spinal Z48.89
    teeth Z48.814

Aftercare — *continued*
  fracture - code to fracture with seventh character D
  involving
    removal of
      drains Z48.03
      dressings (nonsurgical) Z48.00
      staples Z48.02
      surgical dressings Z48.01
      sutures Z48.02
    neuropacemaker (brain) (peripheral nerve) (spinal cord) Z46.2
    implanted Z45.42
  orthopedic NEC Z47.89
  postprocedural — *see* Aftercare, following surgery
After-cataract — *see* Cataract, secondary
Agalactia (primary) O92.3
  elective, secondary or therapeutic O92.5
Agammaglobulinemia (acquired (secondary)) (nonfamilial) D80.1
  with
    immunoglobulin-bearing B-lymphocytes D80.1
    lymphopenia D81.9
  autosomal recessive (Swiss type) D80.0
  Bruton's X-linked D80.0
  common variable (CVAgamma) D80.1
  congenital sex-linked D80.0
  hereditary D80.0
  lymphopenic D81.9
  Swiss type (autosomal recessive) D80.0
  X-linked (with growth hormone deficiency) (Bruton) D80.0
Aganglionosis (bowel) (colon) Q43.1
Age (old) — *see* Senility
Agenesis
  adrenal (gland) Q89.1
  alimentary tract (complete) (partial) NEC Q45.8
    upper Q40.8
  anus, anal (canal) Q42.3
    with fistula Q42.2
  aorta Q25.4
  appendix Q42.8
  arm (complete) Q71.0- ☑
    with hand present Q71.1- ☑
  artery (peripheral) Q27.9
    brain Q28.3
    coronary Q24.5
    pulmonary Q25.79
    specified NEC Q27.8
    umbilical Q27.0
  auditory (canal) (external) Q16.1
  auricle (ear) Q16.0
  bile duct or passage Q44.5
  bladder Q64.5
  bone Q79.9
  brain Q00.0
    part of Q04.3
  breast (with nipple present) Q83.8
    with absent nipple Q83.0
  bronchus Q32.4
  canaliculus lacrimalis Q10.4
  carpus — *see* Agenesis, hand
  cartilage Q79.9
  cecum Q42.8
  cerebellum Q04.3
  cervix Q51.5
  chin Q18.8
  cilia Q10.3
  circulatory system, part NOS Q28.9
  clavicle Q74.0
  clitoris Q52.6
  coccyx Q76.49
  colon Q42.9
    specified NEC Q42.8
  corpus callosum Q04.0
  cricoid cartilage Q31.8
  diaphragm (with hernia) Q79.1
  digestive organ (s) or tract (complete) (partial) NEC Q45.8
    upper Q40.8
  ductus arteriosus Q28.8
  duodenum Q41.0
  ear Q16.9
    auricle Q16.0
    lobe Q17.8
  ejaculatory duct Q55.4
  endocrine (gland) NEC Q89.2
  epiglottis Q31.8
  esophagus Q39.8
  eustachian tube Q16.2
  eye Q11.1

Agenesis — *continued*
  adnexa Q15.8
  eyelid (fold) Q10.3
  face
    bones NEC Q75.8
    specified part NEC Q18.8
  fallopian tube Q50.6
  femur — *see* Defect, reduction, lower limb, longitudinal, femur
  fibula — *see* Defect, reduction, lower limb, longitudinal, fibula
  finger (complete) (partial) — *see* Agenesis, hand
  foot (and toes) (complete) (partial) Q72.3- ☑
  forearm (with hand present) — *see* Agenesis, arm, with hand present
    and hand Q71.2- ☑
  gallbladder Q44.0
  gastric Q40.2
  genitalia, genital (organ(s))
    female Q52.8
      external Q52.71
      internal NEC Q52.8
    male Q55.8
  glottis Q31.8
  hair Q84.0
  hand (and fingers) (complete) (partial) Q71.3- ☑
  heart Q24.8
    valve NEC Q24.8
      pulmonary Q22.0
  hepatic Q44.7
  humerus — *see* Defect, reduction, upper limb
  hymen Q52.4
  ileum Q41.2
  incus Q16.3
  intestine (small) Q41.9
    large Q42.9
      specified NEC Q42.8
  iris (dilator fibers) Q13.1
  jaw M26.09
  jejunum Q41.1
  kidney (s) (partial) Q60.2
    bilateral Q60.1
    unilateral Q60.0
  labium (majus) (minus) Q52.71
  labyrinth, membranous Q16.5
  lacrimal apparatus Q10.4
  larynx Q31.8
  leg (complete) Q72.0- ☑
    with foot present Q72.1- ☑
    lower leg (with foot present) — *see* Agenesis, leg, with foot present
      and foot Q72.2- ☑
  lens Q12.3
  limb (complete) Q73.0
    lower — *see* Agenesis, leg
    upper — *see* Agenesis, arm
  lip Q38.0
  liver Q44.7
  lung (fissure) (lobe) (bilateral) (unilateral) Q33.3
  mandible, maxilla M26.09
  metacarpus — *see* Agenesis, hand
  metatarsus — *see* Agenesis, foot
  muscle Q79.8
    eyelid Q10.3
    ocular Q15.8
  musculoskeletal system NEC Q79.8
  nail (s) Q84.3
  neck, part Q18.8
  nerve Q07.8
  nervous system, part NEC Q07.8
  nipple Q83.2
  nose Q30.1
  nuclear Q07.8
  organ
    of Corti Q16.5
    or site not listed — *see* Anomaly, by site
  osseous meatus (ear) Q16.1
  ovary
    bilateral Q50.02
    unilateral Q50.01
  oviduct Q50.6
  pancreas Q45.0
  parathyroid (gland) Q89.2
  parotid gland (s) Q38.4
  patella Q74.1
  pelvic girdle (complete) (partial) Q74.2
  penis Q55.5
  pericardium Q24.8
  pituitary (gland) Q89.2
  prostate Q55.4
  punctum lacrimale Q10.4
  radioulnar — *see* Defect, reduction, upper limb

Agenesis — *continued*
  radius — *see* Defect, reduction, upper limb, longitudinal, radius
  rectum Q42.1
    with fistula Q42.0
  renal Q60.2
    bilateral Q60.1
    unilateral Q60.0
  respiratory organ NEC Q34.8
  rib Q76.6
  roof of orbit Q75.8
  round ligament Q52.8
  sacrum Q76.49
  salivary gland Q38.4
  scapula Q74.0
  scrotum Q55.29
  seminal vesicles Q55.4
  septum
    atrial Q21.1
    between aorta and pulmonary artery Q21.4
    ventricular Q20.4
  shoulder girdle (complete) (partial) Q74.0
  skull (bone) Q75.8
    with
      anencephaly Q00.0
      encephalocele — *see* Encephalocele
      hydrocephalus Q03.9
        with spina bifida — *see* Spina bifida, by site, with hydrocephalus
      microcephaly Q02
  spermatic cord Q55.4
  spinal cord Q06.0
  spine Q76.49
  spleen Q89.01
  sternum Q76.7
  stomach Q40.2
  submaxillary gland (s) (congenital) Q38.4
  tarsus — *see* Agenesis, foot
  tendon Q79.8
  testicle Q55.0
  thymus (gland) Q89.2
  thyroid (gland) E03.1
    cartilage Q31.8
  tibia — *see* Defect, reduction, lower limb, longitudinal, tibia
  tibiofibular — *see* Defect, reduction, lower limb, specified type NEC
  toe (and foot) (complete) (partial) — *see* Agenesis, foot
  tongue Q38.3
  trachea (cartilage) Q32.1
  ulna — *see* Defect, reduction, upper limb, longitudinal, ulna
  upper limb — *see* Agenesis, arm
  ureter Q62.4
  urethra Q64.5
  urinary tract NEC Q64.8
  uterus Q51.0
  uvula Q38.5
  vagina Q52.0
  vas deferens Q55.4
  vein (s) (peripheral) Q27.9
    brain Q28.3
    great NEC Q26.8
    portal Q26.5
  vena cava (inferior) (superior) Q26.8
  vermis of cerebellum Q04.3
  vertebra Q76.49
  vulva Q52.71
Ageusia R43.2
Agitated — *see* condition
Agitation R45.1
Aglossia (congenital) Q38.3
Aglossia-adactylia syndrome Q87.0
Aglycogenosis E74.00
Agnosia (body image) (other senses) (tactile) R48.1
  developmental F88
  verbal R48.1
    auditory R48.1
      developmental F80.2
    developmental F80.2
  visual (object) R48.3
Agoraphobia F40.00
  with panic disorder F40.01
  without panic disorder F40.02
Agrammatism R48.8
Agranulocytopenia — *see* Agranulocytosis
Agranulocytosis (chronic) (cyclical) (genetic) (infantile) (periodic) (pernicious) (*see also* Neutropenia) D70.9
  congenital D70.0

☑ **Additional character required**

Agranulocytosis — continued
  cytoreductive cancer chemotherapy sequela D70.1
  drug-induced D70.2
    due to cytoreductive cancer chemotherapy D70.1
  due to infection D70.3
  secondary D70.4
    drug-induced D70.2
      due to cytoreductive cancer chemotherapy D70.1
Agraphia (absolute) R48.8
  with alexia R48.0
  developmental F81.81
Ague (dumb) — see Malaria
Agyria Q04.3
Ahumada-del Castillo syndrome E23.0
Aichomophobia F40.298
AIDS (related complex) B20
Ailment heart — see Disease, heart
Ailurophobia F40.218
Ainhum (disease) L94.6
AIPHI (acute idiopathic pulmonary hemorrhage in infants (over 28 days old)) R04.81
Air
  anterior mediastinum J98.2
  compressed, disease T70.3 ☑
  conditioner lung or pneumonitis J67.7
  embolism (artery) (cerebral) (any site) T79.0 ☑
    with ectopic or molar pregnancy O08.2
    due to implanted device NEC — see Complications, by site and type, specified NEC
    following
      abortion — see Abortion by type, complicated by, embolism
      ectopic or molar pregnancy O08.2
    infusion, therapeutic injection or transfusion T80.0 ☑
    in pregnancy, childbirth or puerperium — see Embolism, obstetric
    traumatic T79.0 ☑
  hunger, psychogenic F45.8
  rarefied, effects of — see Effect, adverse, high altitude
  sickness T75.3 ☑
Airplane sickness T75.3 ☑
Akathisia (drug-induced) (treatment-induced) G25.71
  neuroleptic induced (acute) G25.71
Akinesia R29.898
Akinetic mutism R41.89
Akureyri's disease G93.3
Alactasia, congenital E73.0
Alagille's syndrome Q44.7
Alastrim B03
Albers-Schönberg syndrome Q78.2
Albert's syndrome — see Tendinitis, Achilles
Albinism, albino E70.30
  with hematologic abnormality E70.339
    Chédiak-Higashi syndrome E70.330
    Hermansky-Pudlak syndrome E70.331
    other specified E70.338
    I E70.320
    II E70.321
  ocular E70.319
    autosomal recessive E70.311
    other specified E70.318
    X-linked E70.310
  oculocutaneous E70.329
    other specified E70.328
    tyrosinase (ty) negative E70.320
    tyrosinase (ty) positive E70.321
  other specified E70.39
Albinismus E70.30
Albright (-McCune)(-Sternberg) syndrome Q78.1
Albuminous — see condition
Albuminuria, albuminuric (acute) (chronic) (subacute) (see also Proteinuria) R80.9
  complicating pregnancy — see Proteinuria, gestational
    with
      gestational hypertension — see Pre-eclampsia
      pre-existing hypertension — see Hypertension, complicating pregnancy, pre-existing, with, pre-eclampsia
  gestational — see Proteinuria, gestational
    with
      gestational hypertension — see Pre-eclampsia

Albuminuria — continued
    pre-existing hypertension — see Hypertension, complicating pregnancy, pre-existing, with, pre-eclampsia
  orthostatic R80.2
  postural R80.2
  pre-eclamptic — see Pre-eclampsia
  scarlatinal A38.8
Albuminurophobia F40.298
Alcaptonuria E70.29
Alcohol, alcoholic, alcohol-induced
  addiction (without remission) F10.20
    with remission F10.21
  amnestic disorder, persisting F10.96
    with dependence F10.26
  brain syndrome, chronic F10.97
    with dependence F10.27
  cardiopathy I42.6
  counseling and surveillance Z71.41
    family member Z71.42
  delirium (acute) (tremens) (withdrawal) F10.231
    with intoxication F10.921
      in
        abuse F10.121
        dependence F10.221
  dementia F10.97
    with dependence F10.27
  deterioration F10.97
    with dependence F10.27
  hallucinosis (acute) F10.951
    in
      abuse F10.151
      dependence F10.251
  insanity F10.959
  intoxication (acute) (without dependence) F10.129
    with
      delirium F10.121
      dependence F10.229
        with delirium F10.221
        uncomplicated F10.220
    uncomplicated F10.120
  jealousy F10.988
  Korsakoff's, Korsakov's, Korsakow's F10.26
  liver K70.9
    acute — see Disease, liver, alcoholic, hepatitis
  mania (acute) (chronic) F10.959
  paranoia, paranoid (type) psychosis F10.950
  pellagra E52
  poisoning, accidental (acute) NEC — see Table of Drugs and Chemicals, alcohol, poisoning
  psychosis — see Psychosis, alcoholic
  withdrawal (without convulsions) F10.239
    with delirium F10.231
Alcoholism (chronic) (without remission) F10.20
  with
    psychosis — see Psychosis, alcoholic
    remission F10.21
  Korsakov's F10.96
    with dependence F10.26
Alder (-Reilly) anomaly or syndrome (leukocyte granulation) D72.0
Aldosteronism E26.9
  familial (type I) E26.02
  glucocorticoid-remediable E26.02
  primary (due to (bilateral) adrenal hyperplasia) E26.09
  primary NEC E26.09
  secondary E26.1
  specified NEC E26.89
Aldosteronoma D44.10
Aldrich (-Wiskott) syndrome (eczema-thrombocytopenia) D82.0
Alektorophobia F40.218
Aleppo boil B55.1
Aleukemic — see condition
Aleukia
  congenital D70.0
  hemorrhagica D61.9
    congenital D61.09
  splenica D73.1
Alexia R48.0
  developmental F81.0
  secondary to organic lesion R48.0
Algoneurodystrophy M89.00
  ankle M89.07- ☑
  foot M89.07- ☑
  forearm M89.03- ☑
  hand M89.04- ☑
  lower leg M89.06- ☑
  multiple sites M89.0- ☑
  shoulder M89.01- ☑

Algoneurodystrophy — continued
  specified site NEC M89.08
  thigh M89.05- ☑
  upper arm M89.02- ☑
Algophobia F40.298
Alienation, mental — see Psychosis
Alkalemia E87.3
Alkalosis E87.3
  metabolic E87.3
    with respiratory acidosis E87.4
  respiratory E87.3
Alkaptonuria E70.29
Allen-Masters syndrome N83.8
Allergy, allergic (reaction) (to) T78.40 ☑
  air-borne substance NEC (rhinitis) J30.89
  alveolitis (extrinsic) J67.9
    due to
      Aspergillus clavatus J67.4
      Cryptostroma corticale J67.6
      organisms (fungal, thermophilic actinomycete) growing in ventilation (air conditioning) systems J67.7
    specified type NEC J67.8
  anaphylactic reaction or shock T78.2 ☑
  angioneurotic edema T78.3 ☑
  animal (dander) (epidermal) (hair) (rhinitis) J30.81
  bee sting (anaphylactic shock) — see Toxicity, venom, arthropod, bee
  biological — see Allergy, drug
  colitis K52.2
  dander (animal) (rhinitis) J30.81
  dandruff (rhinitis) J30.81
  dental restorative material (existing) K08.55
  dermatitis — see Dermatitis, contact, allergic
  diathesis — see History, allergy
  drug, medicament & biological (any) (external) (internal) T78.40 ☑
    correct substance properly administered — see Table of Drugs and Chemicals, by drug, adverse effect
    wrong substance given or taken NEC (by accident) — see Table of Drugs and Chemicals, by drug, poisoning
  due to pollen J30.1
  dust (house) (stock) (rhinitis) J30.89
    with asthma — see Asthma, allergic extrinsic
  eczema — see Dermatitis, contact, allergic
  epidermal (animal) (rhinitis) J30.81
  feathers (rhinitis) J30.89
  food (any) (ingested) NEC T78.1 ☑
    anaphylactic shock — see Shock, anaphylactic, due to food
    dermatitis — see Dermatitis, due to, food
    dietary counseling and surveillance Z71.3
    in contact with skin L23.6
    rhinitis J30.5
    status (without reaction) Z91.018
      eggs Z91.012
      milk products Z91.011
      peanuts Z91.010
      seafood Z91.013
      specified NEC Z91.018
  gastrointestinal K52.2
  grain J30.1
  grass (hay fever) (pollen) J30.1
    asthma — see Asthma, allergic extrinsic
  hair (animal) (rhinitis) J30.81
  history (of) — see History, allergy
  horse serum — see Allergy, serum
  inhalant (rhinitis) J30.89
    pollen J30.1
  kapok (rhinitis) J30.89
  medicine — see Allergy, drug
  milk protein K52.2
  nasal, seasonal due to pollen J30.1
  pneumonia J82
  pollen (any) (hay fever) J30.1
    asthma — see Asthma, allergic extrinsic
  primrose J30.1
  primula J30.1
  purpura D69.0
  ragweed (hay fever) (pollen) J30.1
    asthma — see Asthma, allergic extrinsic
  rose (pollen) J30.1
  seasonal NEC J30.2
  Senecio jacobae (pollen) J30.1
  serum (see also Reaction, serum) T80.69 ☑
    anaphylactic shock T80.59 ☑
  shock (anaphylactic) T78.2 ☑
    due to
      administration of blood and blood products T80.51 ☑

Allergy — *continued*
    adverse effect of correct medicinal substance properly administered T88.6 ☑
      immunization T80.52 ☑
      serum NEC T80.59 ☑
      vaccination T80.52 ☑
    specific NEC T78.49 ☑
    tree (any) (hay fever) (pollen) J30.1
      asthma — *see* Asthma, allergic extrinsic
    upper respiratory J30.9
    urticaria L50.0
    vaccine — *see* Allergy, serum
    wheat — *see* Allergy, food
Allescheriasis B48.2
Alligator skin disease Q80.9
Allocheiria, allochiria R20.8
Almeida's disease — *see* Paracoccidioidomycosis
Alopecia (hereditaria) (seborrheica) L65.9
    androgenic L64.9
      drug-induced L64.0
      specified NEC L64.8
    areata L63.9
      ophiasis L63.2
      specified NEC L63.8
      totalis L63.0
      universalis L63.1
    cicatricial L66.9
      specified NEC L66.8
    circumscripta L63.9
    congenital, congenitalis Q84.0
    due to cytotoxic drugs NEC L65.8
    mucinosa L65.2
    postinfective NEC L65.8
    postpartum L65.0
    premature L64.8
    specific (syphilitic) A51.32
    specified NEC L65.8
    syphilitic (secondary) A51.32
    totalis (capitis) L63.0
    universalis (entire body) L63.1
    X-ray L58.1
Alpers' disease G31.81
Alpine sickness T70.29 ☑
Alport syndrome Q87.81
ALTE (apparent life threatening event) in newborn and infant R68.13
Alteration (of), Altered
    awareness, transient R40.4
    mental status R41.82
    pattern of family relationships affecting child Z62.898
    sensation
      following
        cerebrovascular disease I69.998
          cerebral infarction I69.398
          intracerebral hemorrhage I69.198
          nontraumatic intracranial hemorrhage NEC I69.298
          specified disease NEC I69.898
          subarachnoid hemorrhage I69.098
Alternating — *see* condition
Altitude, high (effects) — *see* Effect, adverse, high altitude
Aluminosis (of lung) J63.0
Alveolitis
    allergic (extrinsic) — *see* Pneumonitis, hypersensitivity
    due to
      Aspergillus clavatus J67.4
      Cryptostroma corticale J67.6
    fibrosing (cryptogenic) (idiopathic) J84.112
    jaw M27.3
    sicca dolorosa M27.3
Alveolus, alveolar — *see* condition
Alymphocytosis D72.810
    thymic (with immunodeficiency) D82.1
Alymphoplasia, thymic D82.1
Alzheimer's disease or sclerosis — *see* Disease, Alzheimer's
Amastia (with nipple present) Q83.8
    with absent nipple Q83.0
Amathophobia F40.228
Amaurosis (acquired) (congenital) (*see also* Blindness)
    fugax G45.3
    hysterical F44.6
    Leber's congenital H35.50
    uremic — *see* Uremia
Amaurotic idiocy (infantile) (juvenile) (late) E75.4
Amaxophobia F40.248
Ambiguous genitalia Q56.4

Amblyopia (congenital) (ex anopsia) (partial) (suppression) H53.00- ☑
    anisometropic — *see* Amblyopia, refractive
    deprivation H53.01- ☑
    hysterical F44.6
    nocturnal (*see also* Blindness, night)
      vitamin A deficiency E50.5
    refractive H53.02- ☑
    strabismic H53.03- ☑
    tobacco H53.8
    toxic NEC H53.8
    uremic — *see* Uremia
Ameba, amebic (histolytica) (*see also* Amebiasis)
    abscess (liver) A06.4
Amebiasis A06.9
    with abscess — *see* Abscess, amebic
    acute A06.0
    chronic (intestine) A06.1
      with abscess — *see* Abscess, amebic
    cutaneous A06.7
    cutis A06.7
    cystitis A06.81
    genitourinary tract NEC A06.82
    hepatic — *see* Abscess, liver, amebic
    intestine A06.0
    nondysenteric colitis A06.2
    skin A06.7
    specified site NEC A06.89
Ameboma (of intestine) A06.3
Amelia Q73.0
    lower limb — *see* Agenesis, leg
    upper limb — *see* Agenesis, arm
Ameloblastoma (*see also* Cyst, calcifying odontogenic)
    long bones C40.9- ☑
      lower limb C40.2- ☑
      upper limb C40.0- ☑
    malignant C41.1
      jaw (bone) (lower) C41.1
        upper C41.0
    tibial C40.2- ☑
Amelogenesis imperfecta K00.5
    nonhereditaria (segmentalis) K00.4
Amenorrhea N91.2
    hyperhormonal E28.8
    primary N91.0
    secondary N91.1
Amentia — *see* Disability, intellectual
    Meynert's (nonalcoholic) F04
American
    leishmaniasis B55.2
    mountain tick fever A93.2
Ametropia — *see* Disorder, refraction
Amianthosis J61
Amimia R48.8
Amino-acid disorder E72.9
    anemia D53.0
Aminoacidopathy E72.9
Aminoaciduria E72.9
Amnes (t)ic syndrome (post-traumatic) F04
    induced by
      alcohol F10.96
        with dependence F10.26
      psychoactive NEC F19.96
        with
          abuse F19.16
          dependence F19.26
      sedative F13.96
        with dependence F13.26
Amnesia R41.3
    anterograde R41.1
    auditory R48.8
    dissociative F44.0
    hysterical F44.0
    postictal in epilepsy — *see* Epilepsy
    psychogenic F44.0
    retrograde R41.2
    transient global G45.4
Amnion, amniotic — *see* condition
Amnionitis — *see* Pregnancy, complicated by
Amok F68.8
Amoral traits F60.89
Ampulla
    lower esophagus K22.8
    phrenic K22.8
Amputation (*see also* Absence, by site, acquired)
    neuroma (postoperative) (traumatic) — *see* Complications, amputation stump, neuroma
    stump (surgical)
      abnormal, painful, or with complication (late) — *see* Complications, amputation stump
      healed or old NOS Z89.9

Amputation — *continued*
    traumatic (complete) (partial)
      arm (upper) (complete) S48.91- ☑
        at
          elbow S58.01- ☑
            partial S58.02- ☑
          shoulder joint (complete) S48.01- ☑
            partial S48.02- ☑
        between
          elbow and wrist (complete) S58.11- ☑
            partial S58.12- ☑
          shoulder and elbow (complete) S48.11- ☑
            partial S48.12- ☑
        partial S48.92- ☑
      breast (complete) S28.21- ☑
        partial S28.22- ☑
      clitoris (complete) S38.211 ☑
        partial S38.212 ☑
      ear (complete) S08.11- ☑
        partial S08.12- ☑
      finger (complete) (metacarpophalangeal) S68.11- ☑
        index S68.11- ☑
        little S68.11- ☑
        middle S68.11- ☑
        partial S68.12- ☑
          index S68.12- ☑
          little S68.12- ☑
          middle S68.12- ☑
          ring S68.12- ☑
        ring S68.11- ☑
        thumb — *see* Amputation, traumatic, thumb
        transphalangeal (complete) S68.61- ☑
          index S68.61- ☑
          little S68.61- ☑
          middle S68.61- ☑
          partial S68.62- ☑
            index S68.62- ☑
            little S68.62- ☑
            middle S68.62- ☑
            ring S68.62- ☑
          ring S68.61- ☑
      foot (complete) S98.91- ☑
        at ankle level S98.01- ☑
          partial S98.02- ☑
        midfoot S98.31- ☑
          partial S98.32- ☑
        partial S98.92- ☑
      forearm (complete) S58.91- ☑
        at elbow level (complete) S58.01- ☑
          partial S58.02- ☑
        between elbow and wrist (complete) S58.11- ☑
          partial S58.12- ☑
        partial S58.92- ☑
      genital organ (s) (external)
        female (complete) S38.211 ☑
          partial S38.212 ☑
        male
          penis (complete) S38.221 ☑
            partial S38.222 ☑
          scrotum (complete) S38.231 ☑
            partial S38.232 ☑
          testes (complete) S38.231 ☑
            partial S38.232 ☑
      hand (complete) (wrist level) S68.41- ☑
        finger (s) alone — *see* Amputation, traumatic, finger
        partial S68.42- ☑
        thumb alone — *see* Amputation, traumatic, thumb
        transmetacarpal (complete) S68.71- ☑
          partial S68.72- ☑
      head
        ear — *see* Amputation, traumatic, ear
        nose (partial) S08.812 ☑
          complete S08.811 ☑
        part S08.89 ☑
        scalp S08.0 ☑
      hip (and thigh) (complete) S78.91- ☑
        at hip joint (complete) S78.01- ☑
          partial S78.02- ☑
        between hip and knee (complete) S78.11- ☑
          partial S78.12- ☑
        partial S78.92- ☑
      labium (majus) (minus) (complete) S38.21- ☑
        partial S38.21- ☑
      leg (lower) S88.91- ☑
        at knee level S88.01- ☑
          partial S88.02- ☑
        between knee and ankle S88.11- ☑
          partial S88.12- ☑
        partial S88.92- ☑

☑ **Additional character required**

Amputation — *continued*
  nose (partial) S08.812 ☑
    complete S08.811 ☑
  penis (complete) S38.221 ☑
    partial S38.222 ☑
  scrotum (complete) S38.231 ☑
    partial S38.232 ☑
  shoulder — *see* Amputation, traumatic, arm
    at shoulder joint — *see* Amputation,
      traumatic, arm, at shoulder joint
  testes (complete) S38.231 ☑
    partial S38.232 ☑
  thigh — *see* Amputation, traumatic, hip
  thorax, part of S28.1 ☑
    breast — *see* Amputation, traumatic, breast
  thumb (complete) (metacarpophalangeal)
    S68.01- ☑
    partial S68.02- ☑
    transphalangeal (complete) S68.51- ☑
      partial S68.52- ☑
  toe (lesser) S98.13- ☑
    great S98.11- ☑
      partial S98.12- ☑
    more than one S98.21- ☑
      partial S98.22- ☑
    partial S98.14- ☑
  vulva (complete) S38.211 ☑
    partial S38.212 ☑
Amputee (bilateral) (old) Z89.9
Amsterdam dwarfism Q87.1
Amusia R48.8
  developmental F80.89
Amyelencephalus, amyelencephaly Q00.0
Amyelia Q06.0
Amygdalitis — *see* Tonsillitis
Amygdalolith J35.8
Amyloid heart (disease) E85.4 [I43]
Amyloidosis (generalized) (primary) E85.9
  with lung involvement E85.4 [J99]
  familial E85.2
  genetic E85.2
  heart E85.4 [I43]
  hemodialysis-associated E85.3
  liver E85.4 [K77]
  localized E85.4
  neuropathic heredofamilial E85.1
  non-neuropathic heredofamilial E85.0
  organ limited E85.4
  Portuguese E85.1
  pulmonary E85.4 [J99]
  secondary systemic E85.3
  skin (lichen) (macular) E85.4 [L99]
  specified NEC E85.8
  subglottic E85.4 [J99]
Amylopectinosis (brancher enzyme deficiency)
    E74.03
Amylophagia — *see* Pica
Amyoplasia congenita Q79.8
Amyotonia M62.89
  congenita G70.2
Amyotrophia, amyotrophy, amyotrophic G71.8
  congenita Q79.8
  diabetic — *see* Diabetes, amyotrophy
  lateral sclerosis G12.21
  neuralgic G54.5
  spinal progressive G12.21
Anacidity, gastric K31.83
  psychogenic F45.8
Anaerosis of newborn P28.89
Analbuminemia E88.09
Analgesia — *see* Anesthesia
Analphalipoproteinemia E78.6
Anaphylactic
  purpura D69.0
  shock or reaction — *see* Shock, anaphylactic
Anaphylactoid shock or reaction — *see* Shock,
    anaphylactic
Anaphylactoid syndrome of pregnancy O88.01- ☑
Anaphylaxis — *see* Shock, anaphylactic
Anaplasia cervix (*see also* Dysplasia, cervix) N87.9
Anaplasmosis, human A77.49
Anarthria R47.1
Anasarca R60.1
  cardiac — *see* Failure, heart, congestive
  lung J18.2
  newborn P83.2
  nutritional E43
  pulmonary J18.2
  renal N04.9
Anastomosis
  aneurysmal — *see* Aneurysm
  arteriovenous ruptured brain I60.8

Anastomosis — *continued*
  intestinal K63.89
    complicated NEC K91.89
      involving urinary tract N99.89
  retinal and choroidal vessels (congenital) Q14.8
Anatomical narrow angle H40.03- ☑
Ancylostoma, ancylostomiasis (braziliense)
    (caninum) (ceylanicum) (duodenale) B76.0
    Necator americanus B76.1
Andersen's disease (glycogen storage) E74.09
Anderson-Fabry disease E75.21
Andes disease T70.29 ☑
Andrews' disease (bacterid) L08.89
Androblastoma
  benign
    specified site — *see* Neoplasm, benign, by site
    unspecified site
      female D27.9
      male D29.20
  malignant
    specified site — *see* Neoplasm, malignant, by
      site
    unspecified site
      female C56.9
      male C62.90
  specified site — *see* Neoplasm, uncertain
      behavior, by site
  tubular
    with lipid storage
      specified site — *see* Neoplasm, benign, by
        site
      unspecified site
        female D27.9
        male D29.20
    specified site — *see* Neoplasm, benign, by site
    unspecified site
      female D27.9
      male D29.20
  unspecified site
    female D39.10
    male D40.10
Androgen insensitivity syndrome (*see also*
    Syndrome, androgen insensitivity) E34.50
Androgen resistance syndrome (*see also* Syndrome,
    androgen insensitivity) E34.50
Android pelvis Q74.2
  with disproportion (fetopelvic) O33.3 ☑
    causing obstructed labor O65.3
Androphobia F40.290
Anectasis, pulmonary (newborn) — *see* Atelectasis
Anemia (essential) (general) (hemoglobin
    deficiency) (infantile) (primary) (profound) D64.9
  with (due to) (in)
    disorder of
      anaerobic glycolysis D55.2
      pentose phosphate pathway D55.1
    koilonychia D50.9
  achlorhydric D50.8
  achrestic D53.1
  Addison (-Biermer) (pernicious) D51.0
  agranulocytic — *see* Agranulocytosis
  amino-acid-deficiency D53.0
  aplastic D61.9
    congenital D61.09
    drug-induced D61.1
    due to
      drugs D61.1
      external agents NEC D61.2
      infection D61.2
      radiation D61.2
    idiopathic D61.3
    red cell (pure) D60.9
      chronic D60.0
      congenital D61.01
      specified type NEC D60.8
      transient D60.1
    specified type NEC D61.89
    toxic D61.2
  aregenerative
    congenital D61.09
  asiderotic D50.9
  atypical (primary) D64.9
  Baghdad spring D55.0
  Balantidium coli A07.0
  Biermer's (pernicious) D51.0
  blood loss (chronic) D50.0
    acute D62
  bothriocephalus B70.0 [D63.8]
  brickmaker's B76.9 [D63.8]
  cerebral I67.89
  childhood D58.9
  chlorotic D50.8

Anemia — *continued*
  chronic
    blood loss D50.0
    hemolytic D58.9
      idiopathic D59.9
    simple D53.9
  chronica congenita aregenerativa D61.09
  combined system disease NEC D51.0 [G32.0]
    due to dietary vitamin B12 deficiency D51.3
      [G32.0]
  complicating pregnancy, childbirth or
    puerperium — *see* Pregnancy, complicated
    by (management affected by), anemia
  congenital P61.4
    aplastic D61.09
    due to isoimmunization NOS P55.9
    dyserythropoietic, dyshematopoietic D64.4
    following fetal blood loss P61.3
    Heinz body D58.2
    hereditary hemolytic NOS D58.9
    pernicious D51.0
    spherocytic D58.0
  Cooley's (erythroblastic) D56.1
  cytogenic D51.0
  deficiency D53.9
    2, 3 diphosphoglycurate mutase D55.2
    2, 3 PG D55.2
    6 phosphogluconate dehydrogenase D55.1
    6-PGD D55.1
    amino-acid D53.0
    combined B12 and folate D53.1
    enzyme D55.9
      drug-induced (hemolytic) D59.2
      glucose-6-phosphate dehydrogenase (G6PD)
        D55.0
      glycolytic D55.2
      nucleotide metabolism D55.3
      related to hexose monophosphate (HMP)
        shunt pathway NEC D55.1
      specified type NEC D55.8
    erythrocytic glutathione D55.1
    folate D52.9
      dietary D52.0
      drug-induced D52.1
    folic acid D52.9
      dietary D52.0
      drug-induced D52.1
    G SH D55.1
    GGS-R D55.1
    glucose-6-phosphate dehydrogenase D55.0
    glutathione reductase D55.1
    glyceraldehyde phosphate dehydrogenase
      D55.2
    G6PD D55.0
    hexokinase D55.2
    iron D50.9
      secondary to blood loss (chronic) D50.0
    nutritional D53.9
      with
        poor iron absorption D50.8
        specified deficiency NEC D53.8
    phosphofructo-aldolase D55.2
    phosphoglycerate kinase D55.2
    PK D55.2
    protein D53.0
    pyruvate kinase D55.2
    transcobalamin II D51.2
    triose-phosphate isomerase D55.2
    vitamin B12 NOS D51.9
      dietary D51.3
      due to
        intrinsic factor deficiency D51.0
        selective vitamin B12 malabsorption with
          proteinuria D51.1
      pernicious D51.0
      specified type NEC D51.8
  Diamond-Blackfan (congenital hypoplastic)
    D61.01
  dibothriocephalus B70.0 [D63.8]
  dimorphic D53.1
  diphasic D53.1
  Diphyllobothrium (Dibothriocephalus) B70.0
    [D63.8]
  due to (in) (with)
    antineoplastic chemotherapy D64.81
    blood loss (chronic) D50.0
      acute D62
    chemotherapy, antineoplastic D64.81
    chronic disease classified elsewhere NEC D63.8
    chronic kidney disease D63.1
    deficiency
      amino-acid D53.0

Anemia

Anemia — *continued*
   copper D53.8
   folate (folic acid) D52.9
     dietary D52.0
     drug-induced D52.1
   molybdenum D53.8
   protein D53.0
   zinc D53.8
   dietary vitamin B12 deficiency D51.3
   disorder of
     glutathione metabolism D55.1
     nucleotide metabolism D55.3
   drug — *see* Anemia, by type (*see also* Table of Drugs and Chemicals)
   end stage renal disease D63.1
   enzyme disorder D55.9
   fetal blood loss P61.3
   fish tapeworm (D.latum) infestation B70.0 [D63.8]
   hemorrhage (chronic) D50.0
     acute D62
   impaired absorption D50.9
   loss of blood (chronic) D50.0
     acute D62
   myxedema E03.9 [D63.8]
   Necator americanus B76.1 [D63.8]
   prematurity P61.2
   selective vitamin B12 malabsorption with proteinuria D51.1
   transcobalamin II deficiency D51.2
  Dyke-Young type (secondary) (symptomatic) D59.1
  dyserythropoietic (congenital) D64.4
  dyshematopoietic (congenital) D64.4
  Egyptian B76.9 [D63.8]
  elliptocytosis — *see* Elliptocytosis
  enzyme-deficiency, drug-induced D59.2
  epidemic (*see also* Ancylostomiasis) B76.9 [D63.8]
  erythroblastic
   familial D56.1
     newborn (*see also* Disease, hemolytic) P55.9
   of childhood D56.1
  erythrocytic glutathione deficiency D55.1
  erythropoietin-resistant anemia (EPO resistant anemia) D63.1
  Faber's (achlorhydric anemia) D50.9
  factitious (self-induced blood letting) D50.0
  familial erythroblastic D56.1
  Fanconi's (congenital pancytopenia) D61.09
  favism D55.0
  fish tapeworm (D. latum) infestation B70.0 [D63.8]
  folate (folic acid) deficiency D52.9
  glucose-6-phosphate dehydrogenase (G6PD) deficiency D55.0
  glutathione-reductase deficiency D55.1
  goat's milk D52.0
  granulocytic — *see* Agranulocytosis
  Heinz body, congenital D58.2
  hemolytic D58.9
   acquired D59.9
     with hemoglobinuria NEC D59.6
     autoimmune NEC D59.1
     infectious D59.4
     specified type NEC D59.8
     toxic D59.4
   acute D59.9
     due to enzyme deficiency specified type NEC D55.8
     Lederer's D59.1
   autoimmune D59.1
     drug-induced D59.0
   chronic D58.9
     idiopathic D59.9
   cold type (secondary) (symptomatic) D59.1
   congenital (spherocytic) — *see* Spherocytosis
   due to
     cardiac conditions D59.4
     drugs (nonautoimmune) D59.2
       autoimmune D59.0
     enzyme disorder D55.9
       drug-induced D59.2
     presence of shunt or other internal prosthetic device D59.4
   familial D58.9
   hereditary D58.9
     due to enzyme disorder D55.9
       specified type NEC D55.8
     specified type NEC D58.8
   idiopathic (chronic) D59.9
   mechanical D59.4
   microangiopathic D59.4
   nonautoimmune D59.4
     drug-induced D59.2

Anemia — *continued*
  nonspherocytic
   congenital or hereditary NEC D55.8
     glucose-6-phosphate dehydrogenase deficiency D55.0
     pyruvate kinase deficiency D55.2
     type
       I D55.1
       II D55.2
   type
     I D55.1
     II D55.2
   secondary D59.4
     autoimmune D59.1
   specified (hereditary) type NEC D58.8
   Stransky-Regala type (*see also* Hemoglobinopathy) D58.8
   symptomatic D59.4
     autoimmune D59.1
   toxic D59.4
   warm type (secondary) (symptomatic) D59.1
  hemorrhagic (chronic) D50.0
   acute D62
  Herrick's D57.1
  hexokinase deficiency D55.2
  hookworm B76.9 [D63.8]
  hypochromic (idiopathic) (microcytic) (normoblastic) D50.9
   due to blood loss (chronic) D50.0
     acute D62
   familial sex-linked D64.0
   pyridoxine-responsive D64.3
   sideroblastic, sex-linked D64.0
  hypoplasia, red blood cells D61.9
   congenital or familial D61.01
  hypoplastic (idiopathic) D61.9
   congenital or familial (of childhood) D61.01
  hypoproliferative (refractive) D61.9
  idiopathic D64.9
   aplastic D61.3
   hemolytic, chronic D59.9
  in (due to) (with)
   chronic kidney disease D63.1
   end stage renal disease D63.1
   failure, kidney (renal) D63.1
   neoplastic disease (*see also* Neoplasm) D63.0
  intertropical (*see also* Ancylostomiasis) D63.8
  iron deficiency D50.9
   secondary to blood loss (chronic) D50.0
     acute D62
   specified type NEC D50.8
  Joseph-Diamond-Blackfan (congenital hypoplastic) D61.01
  Lederer's (hemolytic) D59.1
  leukoerythroblastic D61.82
  macrocytic D53.9
   nutritional D52.0
   tropical D52.8
  malarial (*see also* Malaria) B54 [D63.8]
  malignant (progressive) D51.0
  malnutrition D53.9
  marsh (*see also* Malaria) B54 [D63.8]
  Mediterranean (with other hemoglobinopathy) D56.9
  megaloblastic D53.1
   combined B12 and folate deficiency D53.1
   hereditary D51.1
   nutritional D52.0
   orotic aciduria D53.0
   refractory D53.1
   specified type NEC D53.1
  megalocytic D53.1
  microcytic (hypochromic) D50.9
   due to blood loss (chronic) D50.0
     acute D62
   familial D56.8
  microdrepanocytosis D57.40
  microelliptopoikilocytic (Rietti-Greppi- Micheli) D56.9
  miner's B76.9 [D63.8]
  myelodysplastic D46.9
  myelofibrosis D75.81
  myelogenous D64.89
  myelopathic D64.89
  myelophthisic D61.82
  myeloproliferative D47.Z9
  newborn P61.4
   due to
     ABO (antibodies, isoimmunization, maternal/fetal incompatibility) P55.1
     Rh (antibodies, isoimmunization, maternal/fetal incompatibility) P55.0

Anemia — *continued*
  following fetal blood loss P61.3
  posthemorrhagic (fetal) P61.3
  nonspherocytic hemolytic — *see* Anemia, hemolytic, nonspherocytic
  normocytic (infectional) D64.9
   due to blood loss (chronic) D50.0
     acute D62
   myelophthisic D61.82
  nutritional (deficiency) D53.9
   with
     poor iron absorption D50.8
     specified deficiency NEC D53.8
   megaloblastic D52.0
  of prematurity P61.2
  orotaciduric (congenital) (hereditary) D53.0
  osteosclerotic D64.89
  ovalocytosis (hereditary) — *see* Elliptocytosis
  paludal (*see also* Malaria) B54 [D63.8]
  pernicious (congenital) (malignant) (progressive) D51.0
  pleochromic D64.89
  of sprue D52.8
  posthemorrhagic (chronic) D50.0
   acute D62
   newborn P61.3
  postoperative (postprocedural)
   due to (acute) blood loss D62
     chronic blood loss D50.0
   specified NEC D64.9
  postpartum O90.81
  pressure D64.89
  progressive D64.9
   malignant D51.0
   pernicious D51.0
  protein-deficiency D53.0
  pseudoleukemica infantum D64.89
  pure red cell D60.9
   congenital D61.01
  pyridoxine-responsive D64.3
  pyruvate kinase deficiency D55.2
  refractory D46.4
   with
     excess of blasts D46.20
       1 (RAEB 1) D46.21
       2 (RAEB 2) D46.22
       in transformation (RAEB T) — *see* Leukemia, acute myeloblastic
     hemochromatosis D46.1
     sideroblasts (ring) (RARS) D46.1
   megaloblastic D53.1
   sideroblastic D46.1
   sideropenic D50.9
   without ring sideroblasts, so stated D46.0
   without sideroblasts without excess of blasts D46.0
  Rietti-Greppi-Micheli D56.9
  scorbutic D53.2
  secondary to
   blood loss (chronic) D50.0
     acute D62
   hemorrhage (chronic) D50.0
     acute D62
  semiplastic D61.89
  sickle-cell — *see* Disease, sickle-cell
  sideroblastic D64.3
   hereditary D64.0
   hypochromic, sex-linked D64.0
   pyridoxine-responsive NEC D64.3
   refractory D46.1
   secondary (due to)
     disease D64.1
     drugs and toxins D64.2
   specified type NEC D64.3
  sideropenic (refractory) D50.9
   due to blood loss (chronic) D50.0
     acute D62
  simple chronic D53.9
  specified type NEC D64.89
  spherocytic (hereditary) — *see* Spherocytosis
  splenic D64.89
  splenomegalic D64.89
  stomatocytosis D58.8
  syphilitic (acquired) (late) A52.79 [D63.8]
  target cell D64.89
  thalassemia D56.9
  thrombocytopenic — *see* Thrombocytopenia
  toxic D61.2
  tropical B76.9 [D63.8]
   macrocytic D52.8
  tuberculous A18.89 [D63.8]
  vegan D51.3

☑ **Additional character required**

Anemia — *continued*
  vitamin
    B6-responsive D64.3
    B12 deficiency (dietary) pernicious D51.0
    von Jaksch's D64.89
    Witts' (achlorhydric anemia) D50.8
Anemophobia F40.228
Anencephalus, anencephaly Q00.0
Anergasia — *see* Psychosis, organic
Anesthesia, anesthetic R20.0
  complication or reaction NEC (*see also*
      Complications, anesthesia) T88.59 ☑
    due to
      correct substance properly administered
          — *see* Table of Drugs and Chemicals, by
          drug, adverse effect
      overdose or wrong substance given — *see*
          Table of Drugs and Chemicals, by drug,
          poisoning
  cornea H18.81- ☑
  dissociative F44.6
  functional (hysterical) F44.6
  hyperesthetic, thalamic G89.0
  hysterical F44.6
  local skin lesion R20.0
  sexual (psychogenic) F52.1
  shock (due to) T88.2 ☑
  skin R20.0
  testicular N50.9
Anetoderma (maculosum) (of) L90.8
  Jadassohn-Pellizzari L90.2
  Schweniger-Buzzi L90.1
Aneurin deficiency E51.9
Aneurysm (anastomotic) (artery) (cirsoid) (diffuse)
    (false) (fusiform) (multiple) (saccular) I72.9
  abdominal (aorta) I71.4
    ruptured I71.3
    syphilitic A52.01
  aorta, aortic (nonsyphilitic) I71.9
    abdominal I71.4
      ruptured I71.3
    arch I71.2
      ruptured I71.1
    arteriosclerotic I71.9
      ruptured I71.8
    ascending I71.2
      ruptured I71.1
    congenital Q25.4
    descending I71.9
      abdominal I71.4
        ruptured I71.3
      ruptured I71.8
      thoracic I71.2
        ruptured I71.1
    ruptured I71.8
    sinus, congenital Q25.4
    syphilitic A52.01
    thoracic I71.2
      ruptured I71.1
    thoracoabdominal I71.6
      ruptured I71.5
    thorax, thoracic (arch) I71.2
      ruptured I71.1
    transverse I71.2
      ruptured I71.1
    valve (heart) (*see also* Endocarditis, aortic) I35.8
  arteriosclerotic I72.9
    cerebral I67.1
      ruptured — *see* Hemorrhage, intracranial,
          subarachnoid
  arteriovenous (congenital) (*see also*
      Malformation, arteriovenous)
    acquired I77.0
      brain I67.1
      coronary I25.41
      pulmonary I28.0
    brain Q28.2
      ruptured I60.8
    peripheral — *see* Malformation, arteriovenous,
        peripheral
    precerebral vessels Q28.0
    specified site NEC (*see also* Malformation,
        arteriovenous)
      acquired I77.0
  basal — *see* Aneurysm, brain
  berry (congenital) (nonruptured) I67.1
    ruptured I60.7
  brain I67.1
    arteriosclerotic I67.1
      ruptured — *see* Hemorrhage, intracranial,
          subarachnoid

Aneurysm — *continued*
  arteriovenous (congenital) (nonruptured)
      Q28.2
    acquired I67.1
      ruptured I60.8
    ruptured I60.8
  berry (congenital) (nonruptured) I67.1
    ruptured (*see also* Hemorrhage, intracranial,
        subarachnoid) I60.7
  congenital Q28.3
    ruptured I60.7
  meninges I67.1
    ruptured I60.8
  miliary (congenital) (nonruptured) I67.1
    ruptured (*see also* Hemorrhage, intracranial,
        subarachnoid) I60.7
  mycotic I33.0
  ruptured — *see* Hemorrhage, intracranial,
      subarachnoid
  syphilitic (hemorrhage) A52.05
  cardiac (false) (*see also* Aneurysm, heart) I25.3
  carotid artery (common) (external) I72.0
    internal (intracranial) I67.1
      extracranial portion I72.0
    ruptured into brain I60.0- ☑
    syphilitic A52.09
      intracranial A52.05
  cavernous sinus I67.1
    arteriovenous (congenital) (nonruptured)
        Q28.3
      ruptured I60.8
  celiac I72.8
  central nervous system, syphilitic A52.05
  cerebral — *see* Aneurysm, brain
  chest — *see* Aneurysm, thorax
  circle of Willis I67.1
    congenital Q28.3
      ruptured I60.6
    ruptured I60.6
  common iliac artery I72.3
  congenital (peripheral) Q27.8
    brain Q28.3
      ruptured I60.7
    coronary Q24.5
    digestive system Q27.8
    lower limb Q27.8
    pulmonary Q25.79
    retina Q14.1
    specified site NEC Q27.8
    upper limb Q27.8
  conjunctiva — *see* Abnormality, conjunctiva,
      vascular
  conus arteriosus — *see* Aneurysm, heart
  coronary (arteriosclerotic) (artery) I25.41
    arteriovenous, congenital Q24.5
    congenital Q24.5
    ruptured — *see* Infarct, myocardium
    syphilitic A52.06
    vein I25.89
  cylindroid (aorta) I71.9
    ruptured I71.8
    syphilitic A52.01
  ductus arteriosus Q25.0
  endocardial, infective (any valve) I33.0
  femoral (artery) (ruptured) I72.4
  gastroduodenal I72.8
  gastroepiploic I72.8
  heart (wall) (chronic or with a stated duration of
      over 4 weeks) I25.3
    valve — *see* Endocarditis
  hepatic I72.8
  iliac (common) (artery) (ruptured) I72.3
  infective I72.9
    endocardial (any valve) I33.0
  innominate (nonsyphilitic) I72.8
    syphilitic A52.09
  interauricular septum — *see* Aneurysm, heart
  interventricular septum — *see* Aneurysm, heart
  intrathoracic (nonsyphilitic) I71.2
    ruptured I71.1
    syphilitic A52.01
  lower limb I72.4
  lung (pulmonary artery) I28.1
  mediastinal (nonsyphilitic) I72.8
    syphilitic A52.09
  miliary (congenital) I67.1
    ruptured — *see* Hemorrhage, intracerebral,
        subarachnoid, intracranial
  mitral (heart) (valve) I34.8
  mural — *see* Aneurysm, heart
  mycotic I72.9
    endocardial (any valve) I33.0

Aneurysm — *continued*
  ruptured, brain — *see* Hemorrhage,
      intracerebral, subarachnoid
  myocardium — *see* Aneurysm, heart
  neck I72.0
  pancreaticoduodenal I72.8
  patent ductus arteriosus Q25.0
  peripheral NEC I72.8
    congenital Q27.8
      digestive system Q27.8
      lower limb Q27.8
      specified site NEC Q27.8
      upper limb Q27.8
  popliteal (artery) (ruptured) I72.4
  precerebral, congenital (nonruptured) Q28.1
  pulmonary I28.1
    arteriovenous Q25.72
      acquired I28.0
    syphilitic A52.09
    valve (heart) — *see* Endocarditis, pulmonary
  racemose (peripheral) I72.9
    congenital — *see* Aneurysm, congenital
  radial I72.1
  Rasmussen NEC A15.0
  renal (artery) I72.2
  retina (*see also* Disorder, retina, microaneurysms)
    congenital Q14.1
    diabetic — *see* Diabetes, microaneurysms,
        retinal
  sinus of Valsalva Q25.4
  specified NEC I72.8
  spinal (cord) I72.8
    syphilitic (hemorrhage) A52.09
  splenic I72.8
  subclavian (artery) (ruptured) I72.8
    syphilitic A52.09
  superior mesenteric I72.8
  syphilitic (aorta) A52.01
    central nervous system A52.05
    congenital (late) A50.54 [I79.0]
    spine, spinal A52.09
  thoracoabdominal (aorta) I71.6
    ruptured I71.5
    syphilitic A52.01
  thorax, thoracic (aorta) (arch) (nonsyphilitic) I71.2
    ruptured I71.1
    syphilitic A52.01
  traumatic (complication) (early), specified site —
      see Injury, blood vessel
  tricuspid (heart) (valve) I07.8
  ulnar I72.1
  upper limb (ruptured) I72.1
  valve, valvular — *see* Endocarditis
  venous (*see also* Varix) I86.8
    congenital Q27.8
      digestive system Q27.8
      lower limb Q27.8
      specified site NEC Q27.8
      upper limb Q27.8
  ventricle — *see* Aneurysm, heart
  visceral NEC I72.8
Angelman syndrome Q93.5
Anger R45.4
Angiectasis, angiectopia I99.8
Angiitis I77.6
  allergic granulomatous M30.1
  hypersensitivity M31.0
  necrotizing M31.9
    specified NEC M31.8
  nervous system, granulomatous I67.7
Angina (attack) (cardiac) (chest) (heart) (pectoris)
    (syndrome) (vasomotor) I20.9
  with
    atherosclerotic heart disease — *see*
        Arteriosclerosis, coronary (artery),
        documented spasm I20.1
  abdominal K55.1
  accelerated — *see* Angina, unstable
  agranulocytic — *see* Agranulocytosis
  angiospastic — *see* Angina, with documented
      spasm
  aphthous B08.5
  crescendo — *see* Angina, unstable
  croupous J05.0
  cruris I73.9
  de novo effort — *see* Angina, unstable
  diphtheritic, membranous A36.0
  equivalent I20.8
  exudative, chronic J37.0
  following acute myocardial infarction I23.7
  gangrenous diphtheritic A36.0
  intestinal K55.1

Angina — *continued*
Ludovici K12.2
Ludwig's K12.2
malignant diphtheritic A36.0
membranous J05.0
diphtheritic A36.0
Vincent's A69.1
mesenteric K55.1
monocytic — *see* Mononucleosis, infectious
of effort — *see* Angina, specified NEC
phlegmonous J36
diphtheritic A36.0
post-infarctional I23.7
pre-infarctional — *see* Angina, unstable
Prinzmetal — *see* Angina, with documented
spasm
progressive — *see* Angina, unstable
pseudomembranous A69.1
pultaceous, diphtheritic A36.0
spasm-induced — *see* Angina, with documented
spasm
specified NEC I20.8
stable I20.9
stenocardia — *see* Angina, specified NEC
stridulous, diphtheritic A36.2
tonsil J36
trachealis J05.0
unstable I20.0
variant — *see* Angina, with documented spasm
Vincent's A69.1
worsening effort — *see* Angina, unstable
Angioblastoma — *see* Neoplasm, connective tissue,
uncertain behavior
Angiocholecystitis — *see* Cholecystitis, acute
Angiocholitis (*see also* Cholecystitis, acute) K83.0
Angiodysgenesis spinalis G95.19
Angiodysplasia (cecum) (colon) K55.20
with bleeding K55.21
duodenum (and stomach) K31.819
with bleeding K31.811
stomach (and duodenum) K31.819
with bleeding K31.811
Angioedema (allergic) (any site) (with urticaria)
T78.3 ☑
hereditary D84.1
Angioendothelioma — *see* Neoplasm, uncertain
behavior, by site
benign D18.00
intra-abdominal D18.03
intracranial D18.02
skin D18.01
specified site NEC D18.09
bone — *see* Neoplasm, bone, malignant
Ewing's — *see* Neoplasm, bone, malignant
Angioendotheliomatosis C85.8- ☑
Angiofibroma (*see also* Neoplasm, benign, by site)
juvenile
specified site — *see* Neoplasm, benign, by site
unspecified site D10.6
Angiohemophilia (A) (B) D68.0
Angioid streaks (choroid) (macula) (retina) H35.33
Angiokeratoma — *see* Neoplasm, skin, benign
corporis diffusum E75.21
Angioleiomyoma — *see* Neoplasm, connective
tissue, benign
Angiolipoma (*see also* Lipoma)
infiltrating — *see* Lipoma
Angioma (*see also* Hemangioma, by site)
capillary I78.1
hemorrhagicum hereditaria I78.0
intra-abdominal D18.03
intracranial D18.02
malignant — *see* Neoplasm, connective tissue,
malignant
plexiform D18.00
intra-abdominal D18.03
intracranial D18.02
skin D18.01
specified site NEC D18.09
senile I78.1
serpiginosum L81.7
skin D18.01
specified site NEC D18.09
spider I78.1
stellate I78.1
venous Q28.3
Angiomatosis Q82.8
bacillary A79.89
encephalotrigeminal Q85.8
hemorrhagic familial I78.0
hereditary familial I78.0
liver K76.4

Angiomyolipoma — *see* Lipoma
Angiomyoliposarcoma — *see* Neoplasm,
connective tissue, malignant
Angiomyoma — *see* Neoplasm, connective tissue,
benign
Angiomyosarcoma — *see* Neoplasm, connective
tissue, malignant
Angiomyxoma — *see* Neoplasm, connective tissue,
uncertain behavior
Angioneurosis F45.8
Angioneurotic edema (allergic) (any site) (with
urticaria) T78.3 ☑
hereditary D84.1
Angiopathia, angiopathy I99.9
cerebral I67.9
amyloid E85.4 [I68.0]
diabetic (peripheral) — *see* Diabetes, angiopathy
peripheral I73.9
diabetic — *see* Diabetes, angiopathy
specified type NEC I73.89
retinae syphilitica A52.05
retinalis (juvenilis)
diabetic — *see* Diabetes, retinopathy
proliferative — *see* Retinopathy, proliferative
Angiosarcoma (*see also* Neoplasm, connective
tissue, malignant)
liver C22.3
Angiosclerosis — *see* Arteriosclerosis
Angiospasm (peripheral) (traumatic) (vessel) I73.9
brachial plexus G54.0
cerebral G45.9
cervical plexus G54.2
nerve
arm — *see* Mononeuropathy, upper limb
axillary G54.0
median — *see* Lesion, nerve, median
ulnar — *see* Lesion, nerve, ulnar
axillary G54.0
leg — *see* Mononeuropathy, lower limb
median — *see* Lesion, nerve, median
plantar — *see* Lesion, nerve, plantar
ulnar — *see* Lesion, nerve, ulnar
Angiospastic disease or edema I73.9
Angiostrongyliasis
due to
Parastrongylus
cantonensis B83.2
costaricensis B81.3
intestinal B81.3
Anguillulosis — *see* Strongyloidiasis
Angulation
cecum — *see* Obstruction, intestine
coccyx (acquired) (*see also* subcategory) M43.8 ☑
congenital NEC Q76.49
femur (acquired) (*see also* Deformity, limb,
specified type NEC, thigh)
congenital Q74.2
intestine (large) (small) — *see* Obstruction,
intestine
sacrum (acquired) (*see also* subcategory) M43.8 ☑
congenital NEC Q76.49
sigmoid (flexure) — *see* Obstruction, intestine
spine — *see* Dorsopathy, deforming, specified
NEC
tibia (acquired) (*see also* Deformity, limb,
specified type NEC, lower leg)
congenital Q74.2
ureter N13.5
with infection N13.6
wrist (acquired) (*see also* Deformity, limb,
specified type NEC, forearm)
congenital Q74.0
Angulus infectiosus (lips) K13.0
Anhedonia R45.84
Anhidrosis L74.4
Anhydration, anhydremia E86.0
with
hypernatremia E87.0
hyponatremia E87.1
Anhydremia E86.0
with
hypernatremia E87.0
hyponatremia E87.1
Anidrosis L74.4
Aniridia (congenital) Q13.1
Anisakiasis (infection) (infestation) B81.0
Anisakis larvae infestation B81.0
Aniseikonia H52.32
Anisocoria (pupil) H57.02
congenital Q13.2
Anisocytosis R71.8
Anisometropia (congenital) H52.31

Ankle — *see* condition
Ankyloblepharon (eyelid) (acquired) (*see also*
Blepharophimosis)
filiforme (adnatum) (congenital) Q10.3
total Q10.3
Ankyloglossia Q38.1
Ankylosis (fibrous) (osseous) (joint) M24.60
ankle M24.67- ☑
arthrodesis status Z98.1
cricoarytenoid (cartilage) (joint) (larynx) J38.7
dental K03.5
ear ossicles H74.31- ☑
elbow M24.62- ☑
foot M24.67- ☑
hand M24.64- ☑
hip M24.65- ☑
incostapedial joint (infectional) — *see* Ankylosis,
ear ossicles
jaw (temporomandibular) M26.61
knee M24.66- ☑
lumbosacral (joint) M43.27
postoperative (status) Z98.1
produced by surgical fusion, status Z98.1
sacro-iliac (joint) M43.28
shoulder M24.61- ☑
spine (joint) (*see also* Fusion, spine)
spondylitic — *see* Spondylitis, ankylosing
surgical Z98.1
temporomandibular M26.61
tooth, teeth (hard tissues) K03.5
wrist M24.63- ☑
Ankylostoma — *see* Ancylostoma
Ankylostomiasis — *see* Ancylostomiasis
Ankylurethria — *see* Stricture, urethra
Annular (*see also* condition)
detachment, cervix N88.8
organ or site, congenital NEC — *see* Distortion
pancreas (congenital) Q45.1
Anodontia (complete) (partial) (vera) K00.0
acquired K08.10 ☑
Anomaly, anomalous (congenital) (unspecified type)
Q89.9
abdominal wall NEC Q79.59
acoustic nerve Q07.8
adrenal (gland) Q89.1
Alder (-Reilly) (leukocyte granulation) D72.0
alimentary tract Q45.9
upper Q40.9
alveolar M26.70
hyperplasia M26.79
mandibular M26.72
maxillary M26.71
hypoplasia M26.79
mandibular M26.74
maxillary M26.73
ridge (process) M26.79
specified NEC M26.79
ankle (joint) Q74.2
anus Q43.9
aorta (arch) NEC Q25.4
coarctation (preductal) (postductal) Q25.1
aortic cusp or valve Q23.9
appendix Q43.8
apple peel syndrome Q41.1
aqueduct of Sylvius Q03.0
with spina bifida — *see* Spina bifida, with
hydrocephalus
arm Q74.0
arteriovenous NEC
coronary Q24.5
gastrointestinal Q27.33
acquired — *see* Angiodysplasia
artery (peripheral) Q27.9
basilar NEC Q28.1
cerebral Q28.3
coronary Q24.5
digestive system Q27.8
eye Q15.8
great Q25.9
specified NEC Q25.8
lower limb Q27.8
peripheral Q27.9
specified NEC Q27.8
pulmonary NEC Q25.79
renal Q27.2
retina Q14.1
specified site NEC Q27.8
subclavian Q27.8
umbilical Q27.0
upper limb Q27.8
vertebral NEC Q28.1
aryteno-epiglottic folds Q31.8

☑ **Additional character required**

Anomaly

Anomaly — *continued*
  atrial
    bands or folds Q20.8
    septa Q21.1
  atrioventricular
    excitation I45.6
    septum Q21.0
  auditory canal Q17.8
  auricle
    ear Q17.8
      causing impairment of hearing Q16.9
    heart Q20.8
  Axenfeld's Q15.0
  back Q89.9
  band
    atrial Q20.8
    heart Q24.8
    ventricular Q24.8
  Bartholin's duct Q38.4
  biliary duct or passage Q44.5
  bladder Q64.70
    absence Q64.5
    diverticulum Q64.6
    exstrophy Q64.10
      cloacal Q64.12
      extroversion Q64.19
      specified type NEC Q64.19
      supravesical fissure Q64.11
    neck obstruction Q64.31
    specified type NEC Q64.79
  bone Q79.9
    arm Q74.0
    face Q75.9
    leg Q74.2
    pelvic girdle Q74.2
    shoulder girdle Q74.0
    skull Q75.9
      with
        anencephaly Q00.0
        encephalocele — *see* Encephalocele
        hydrocephalus Q03.9
          with spina bifida — *see* Spina bifida, by
            site, with hydrocephalus
        microcephaly Q02
  brain (multiple) Q04.9
    vessel Q28.3
  breast Q83.9
  broad ligament Q50.6
  bronchus Q32.4
  bulbus cordis Q21.9
  bursa Q79.9
  canal of Nuck Q52.4
  canthus Q10.3
  capillary Q27.9
  cardiac Q24.9
    chambers Q20.9
      specified NEC Q20.8
    septal closure Q21.9
      specified NEC Q21.8
    valve NEC Q24.8
      pulmonary Q22.3
  cardiovascular system Q28.8
  carpus Q74.0
  caruncle, lacrimal Q10.6
  cascade stomach Q40.2
  cauda equina Q06.3
  cecum Q43.9
  cerebral Q04.9
    vessels Q28.3
  cervix Q51.9
  Chédiak-Higashi (-Steinbrinck) (congenital
    gigantism of peroxidase granules) E70.330
  cheek Q18.9
  chest wall Q67.8
    bones Q76.9
  chin Q18.9
  chordae tendineae Q24.8
  choroid Q14.3
    plexus Q07.8
  chromosomes, chromosomal Q99.9
    D (1) — *see* condition, chromosome 13
    E (3) — *see* condition, chromosome 18
    G — *see* condition, chromosome 21
    sex
      female phenotype Q97.8
      gonadal dysgenesis (pure) Q99.1
      Klinefelter's Q98.4
      male phenotype Q98.9
      Turner's Q96.9
    specified NEC Q99.8
  cilia Q10.3
  circulatory system Q28.9

Anomaly — *continued*
  clavicle Q74.0
  clitoris Q52.6
  coccyx Q76.49
  colon Q43.9
  common duct Q44.5
  communication
    coronary artery Q24.5
    left ventricle with right atrium Q21.0
  concha (ear) Q17.3
  connection
    portal vein Q26.5
    pulmonary venous Q26.4
      partial Q26.3
      total Q26.2
    renal artery with kidney Q27.2
  cornea (shape) Q13.4
  coronary artery or vein Q24.5
  cranium — *see* Anomaly, skull
  cricoid cartilage Q31.8
  cystic duct Q44.5
  dental
    alveolar — *see* Anomaly, alveolar
    arch relationship M26.20
      specified NEC M26.29
  dentofacial M26.9
    alveolar — *see* Anomaly, alveolar
    dental arch relationship M26.20
      specified NEC M26.29
    functional M26.50
      specified NEC M26.59
    jaw-cranial base relationship M26.10
      asymmetry M26.12
        maxillary M26.11
      specified type NEC M26.19
    jaw size M26.00
      macrogenia M26.05
      mandibular
        hyperplasia M26.03
        hypoplasia M26.04
      maxillary
        hyperplasia M26.01
        hypoplasia M26.02
      microgenia M26.06
      specified type NEC M26.09
    malocclusion M26.4
      dental arch relationship NEC M26.29
      jaw-cranial base relationship — *see* Anomaly,
        dentofacial, jaw-cranial base relationship
      jaw size — *see* Anomaly, dentofacial, jaw size
    specified type NEC M26.89
    temporomandibular joint M26.60
      adhesions M26.61
      ankylosis M26.61
      arthralgia M26.62
      articular disc M26.63
      specified type NEC M26.69
    tooth position, fully erupted M26.30
      specified NEC M26.39
  dermatoglyphic Q82.8
  diaphragm (apertures) NEC Q79.1
  digestive organ (s) or tract Q45.9
    lower Q43.9
    upper Q40.9
  distance, interarch (excessive) (inadequate)
    M26.25
  distribution, coronary artery Q24.5
  ductus
    arteriosus Q25.0
    botalli Q25.0
  duodenum Q43.9
  dura (brain) Q04.9
    spinal cord Q06.9
  ear (external) Q17.9
    causing impairment of hearing Q16.9
    inner Q16.5
    middle (causing impairment of hearing) Q16.4
    ossicles Q16.3
  Ebstein's (heart) (tricuspid valve) Q22.5
  ectodermal Q82.9
  Eisenmenger's (ventricular septal defect) Q21.8
  ejaculatory duct Q55.4
  elbow Q74.0
  endocrine gland NEC Q89.2
  epididymis Q55.4
  epiglottis Q31.8
  esophagus Q39.9
  eustachian tube Q17.8
  eye Q15.9
    anterior segment Q13.9
      specified NEC Q13.89
    posterior segment Q14.9

Anomaly — *continued*
    specified NEC Q14.8
    ptosis (eyelid) Q10.0
    specified NEC Q15.8
  eyebrow Q18.8
  eyelid Q10.3
    ptosis Q10.0
  face Q18.9
    bone (s) Q75.9
  fallopian tube Q50.6
  fascia Q79.9
  femur NEC Q74.2
  fibula NEC Q74.2
  finger Q74.0
  fixation, intestine Q43.3
  flexion (joint) NOS Q74.9
    hip or thigh Q65.89
  foot NEC Q74.2
    varus (congenital) Q66.3
  foramen
    Botalli Q21.1
    ovale Q21.1
  forearm Q74.0
  forehead Q75.8
  form, teeth K00.2
  fovea centralis Q14.1
  frontal bone — *see* Anomaly, skull
  gallbladder (position) (shape) (size) Q44.1
  Gartner's duct Q52.4
  gastrointestinal tract Q45.9
  genitalia, genital organ (s) or system
    female Q52.9
      external Q52.70
      internal NOS Q52.9
    male Q55.9
      hydrocele P83.5
      specified NEC Q55.8
  genitourinary NEC
    female Q52.9
    male Q55.9
  Gerbode Q21.0
  glottis Q31.8
  granulation or granulocyte, genetic
    (constitutional) (leukocyte) D72.0
  gum Q38.6
  gyri Q07.9
  hair Q84.2
  hand Q74.0
  hard tissue formation in pulp K04.3
  head — *see* Anomaly, skull
  heart Q24.9
    auricle Q20.8
    bands or folds Q24.8
    fibroelastosis cordis I42.4
    obstructive NEC Q22.6
    patent ductus arteriosus (Botalli) Q25.0
    septum Q21.9
      auricular Q21.1
      interatrial Q21.1
      interventricular Q21.0
        with pulmonary stenosis or atresia,
          dextraposition of aorta and
          hypertrophy of right ventricle Q21.3
      specified NEC Q21.8
      ventricular Q21.0
        with pulmonary stenosis or atresia,
          dextraposition of aorta and
          hypertrophy of right ventricle Q21.3
    tetralogy of Fallot Q21.3
    valve NEC Q24.8
      aortic
        bicuspid valve Q23.1
        insufficiency Q23.1
        stenosis Q23.0
          subaortic Q24.4
      mitral
        insufficiency Q23.3
        stenosis Q23.2
      pulmonary Q22.3
        atresia Q22.0
        insufficiency Q22.2
        stenosis Q22.1
          infundibular Q24.3
          subvalvular Q24.3
      tricuspid
        atresia Q22.4
        stenosis Q22.4
    ventricle Q20.8
  heel NEC Q74.2
  Hegglin's D72.0
  hemianencephaly Q00.0
  hemicephaly Q00.0

Anomaly — *continued*
  hemicrania Q00.0
  hepatic duct Q44.5
  hip NEC Q74.2
  hourglass stomach Q40.2
  humerus Q74.0
  hydatid of Morgagni
    female Q50.5
    male (epididymal) Q55.4
      testicular Q55.29
  hymen Q52.4
  hypersegmentation of neutrophils, hereditary
    D72.0
  hypophyseal Q89.2
  ileocecal (coil) (valve) Q43.9
  ileum Q43.9
  ilium NEC Q74.2
  integument Q84.9
    specified NEC Q84.8
  interarch distance (excessive) (inadequate)
    M26.25
  intervertebral cartilage or disc Q76.49
  intestine (large) (small) Q43.9
    with anomalous adhesions, fixation or
      malrotation Q43.3
  iris Q13.2
  ischium NEC Q74.2
  jaw — *see* Anomaly, dentofacial
    alveolar — *see* Anomaly, alveolar
  jaw-cranial base relationship — *see* Anomaly,
    dentofacial, jaw-cranial base relationship
  jejunum Q43.8
  joint Q74.9
    specified NEC Q74.8
  Jordan's D72.0
  kidney (s) (calyx) (pelvis) Q63.9
    artery Q27.2
    specified NEC Q63.8
  Klippel-Feil (brevicollis) Q76.1
  knee Q74.1
  labium (majus) (minus) Q52.70
  labyrinth, membranous Q16.5
  lacrimal apparatus or duct Q10.6
  larynx, laryngeal (muscle) Q31.9
    web (bed) Q31.0
  lens Q12.9
  leukocytes, genetic D72.0
    granulation (constitutional) D72.0
  lid (fold) Q10.3
  ligament Q79.9
    broad Q50.6
    round Q52.8
  limb Q74.9
    lower NEC Q74.2
      reduction deformity — *see* Defect, reduction,
        lower limb
    upper Q74.0
  lip Q38.0
  liver Q44.7
    duct Q44.5
  lower limb NEC Q74.2
  lumbosacral (joint) (region) Q76.49
    kyphosis — *see* Kyphosis, congenital
    lordosis — *see* Lordosis, congenital
  lung (fissure) (lobe) Q33.9
  mandible — *see* Anomaly, dentofacial
  maxilla — *see* Anomaly, dentofacial
  May (-Hegglin) D72.0
  meatus urinarius NEC Q64.79
  meningeal bands or folds Q07.9
    constriction of Q07.8
    spinal Q06.9
  meninges Q07.9
    cerebral Q04.8
    spinal Q06.9
  meningocele Q05.9
  mesentery Q45.9
  metacarpus Q74.0
  metatarsus NEC Q74.2
  middle ear Q16.4
    ossicles Q16.3
  mitral (leaflets) (valve) Q23.9
    insufficiency Q23.3
    specified NEC Q23.8
    stenosis Q23.2
  mouth Q38.6
  Müllerian (*see also* Anomaly, by site)
    uterus NEC Q51.818
  multiple NEC Q89.7
  muscle Q79.9
    eyelid Q10.3
  musculoskeletal system, except limbs Q79.9

Anomaly — *continued*
  myocardium Q24.8
  nail Q84.6
  narrowness, eyelid Q10.3
  nasal sinus (wall) Q30.8
  neck (any part) Q18.9
  nerve Q07.9
    acoustic Q07.8
    optic Q07.8
  nervous system (central) Q07.9
  nipple Q83.9
  nose, nasal (bones) (cartilage) (septum) (sinus)
    Q30.9
    specified NEC Q30.8
  ocular muscle Q15.8
  omphalomesenteric duct Q43.0
  opening, pulmonary veins Q26.4
  optic
    disc Q14.2
    nerve Q07.8
  opticociliary vessels Q13.2
  orbit (eye) Q10.7
  organ Q89.9
    of Corti Q16.5
  origin
    artery
      innominate Q25.8
      pulmonary Q25.79
      renal Q27.2
      subclavian Q25.8
  osseous meatus (ear) Q16.1
  ovary Q50.39
  oviduct Q50.6
  palate (hard) (soft) NEC Q38.5
  pancreas or pancreatic duct Q45.3
  papillary muscles Q24.8
  parathyroid gland Q89.2
  paraurethral ducts Q64.79
  parotid (gland) Q38.4
  patella Q74.1
  Pelger-Huët (hereditary hyposegmentation)
    D72.0
  pelvic girdle NEC Q74.2
  pelvis (bony) NEC Q74.2
    rachitic E64.3
  penis (glans) Q55.69
  pericardium Q24.8
  peripheral vascular system Q27.9
  Peter's Q13.4
  pharynx Q38.8
  pigmentation L81.9
    congenital Q82.8
  pituitary (gland) Q89.2
  pleural (folds) Q34.0
  portal vein Q26.5
    connection Q26.5
  position, tooth, teeth, fully erupted M26.30
    specified NEC M26.39
  precerebral vessel Q28.1
  prepuce Q55.69
  prostate Q55.4
  pulmonary Q33.9
    artery NEC Q25.79
    valve Q22.3
      atresia Q22.0
      insufficiency Q22.2
      specified type NEC Q22.3
      stenosis Q22.1
        infundibular Q24.3
        subvalvular Q24.3
    venous connection Q26.4
      partial Q26.3
      total Q26.2
  pupil Q13.2
    function H57.00
      anisocoria H57.02
      Argyll Robertson pupil H57.01
      miosis H57.03
      mydriasis H57.04
      specified type NEC H57.09
      tonic pupil H57.05- ☑
  pylorus Q40.3
  radius Q74.0
  rectum Q43.9
  reduction (extremity) (limb)
    femur (longitudinal) — *see* Defect, reduction,
      lower limb, longitudinal, femur
    fibula (longitudinal) — *see* Defect, reduction,
      lower limb, longitudinal, fibula
    lower limb — *see* Defect, reduction, lower limb
    radius (longitudinal) — *see* Defect, reduction,
      upper limb, longitudinal, radius

Anomaly — *continued*
  tibia (longitudinal) — *see* Defect, reduction,
    lower limb, longitudinal, tibia
  ulna (longitudinal) — *see* Defect, reduction,
    upper limb, longitudinal, ulna
  upper limb — *see* Defect, reduction, upper limb
  refraction — *see* Disorder, refraction
  renal Q63.9
    artery Q27.2
    pelvis Q63.9
      specified NEC Q63.8
  respiratory system Q34.9
    specified NEC Q34.8
  retina Q14.1
  rib Q76.6
    cervical Q76.5
  Rieger's Q13.81
  rotation — *see* Malrotation
    hip or thigh Q65.89
  round ligament Q52.8
  sacroiliac (joint) NEC Q74.2
  sacrum NEC Q76.49
    kyphosis — *see* Kyphosis, congenital
    lordosis — *see* Lordosis, congenital
  saddle nose, syphilitic A50.57
  salivary duct or gland Q38.4
  scapula Q74.0
  scrotum — *see* Malformation, testis and scrotum
  sebaceous gland Q82.9
  seminal vesicles Q55.4
  sense organs NEC Q07.8
  sex chromosomes NEC (*see also* Anomaly,
    chromosomes)
    female phenotype Q97.8
    male phenotype Q98.9
  shoulder (girdle) (joint) Q74.0
  sigmoid (flexure) Q43.9
  simian crease Q82.8
  sinus of Valsalva Q25.4
  skeleton generalized Q78.9
  skin (appendage) Q82.9
  skull Q75.9
    with
      anencephaly Q00.0
      encephalocele — *see* Encephalocele
      hydrocephalus Q03.9
        with spina bifida — *see* Spina bifida, by site,
          with hydrocephalus
      microcephaly Q02
  specified organ or site NEC Q89.8
  spermatic cord Q55.4
  spine, spinal NEC Q76.49
    column NEC Q76.49
      kyphosis — *see* Kyphosis, congenital
      lordosis — *see* Lordosis, congenital
    cord Q06.9
    nerve root Q07.8
  spleen Q89.09
    agenesis Q89.01
  stenonian duct Q38.4
  sternum NEC Q76.7
  stomach Q40.3
  submaxillary gland Q38.4
  tarsus NEC Q74.2
  tendon Q79.9
  testis — *see* Malformation, testis and scrotum
  thigh NEC Q74.2
  thorax (wall) Q67.8
    bony Q76.9
  throat Q38.8
  thumb Q74.0
  thymus gland Q89.2
  thyroid (gland) Q89.2
    cartilage Q31.8
  tibia NEC Q74.2
    saber A50.56
  toe Q74.2
  tongue Q38.3
  tooth, teeth K00.9
    eruption K00.6
    position, fully erupted M26.30
    spacing, fully erupted M26.30
  trachea (cartilage) Q32.1
  tragus Q17.9
  tricuspid (leaflet) (valve) Q22.9
    atresia or stenosis Q22.4
    Ebstein's Q22.5
  Uhl's (hypoplasia of myocardium, right ventricle)
    Q24.8
  ulna Q74.0
  umbilical artery Q27.0
  union

☑ **Additional character required**

Anomaly — continued
  cricoid cartilage and thyroid cartilage Q31.8
  thyroid cartilage and hyoid bone Q31.8
  trachea with larynx Q31.8
  upper limb Q74.0
  urachus Q64.4
  ureter Q62.8
    obstructive NEC Q62.39
      cecoureterocele Q62.32
      orthotopic ureterocele Q62.31
  urethra Q64.70
    absence Q64.5
    double Q64.74
    fistula to rectum Q64.73
    obstructive Q64.39
      stricture Q64.32
    prolapse Q64.71
    specified type NEC Q64.79
  urinary tract Q64.9
  uterus Q51.9
    with only one functioning horn Q51.4
  uvula Q38.5
  vagina Q52.4
  valleculae Q31.8
  valve (heart) NEC Q24.8
    coronary sinus Q24.5
    inferior vena cava Q24.8
    pulmonary Q22.3
    sinus coronario Q24.5
    venae cavae inferioris Q24.8
  vas deferens Q55.4
  vascular Q27.9
    brain Q28.3
    ring Q25.4
  vein (s) (peripheral) Q27.9
    brain Q28.3
    cerebral Q28.3
    coronary Q24.5
    developmental Q28.3
    great Q26.9
      specified NEC Q26.8
  vena cava (inferior) (superior) Q26.9
  venous — see Anomaly, vein(s)
  venous return Q26.8
  ventricular
    bands or folds Q24.8
    septa Q21.0
  vertebra Q76.49
    kyphosis — see Kyphosis, congenital
    lordosis — see Lordosis, congenital
  vesicourethral orifice Q64.79
  vessel (s) Q27.9
    optic papilla Q14.2
    precerebral Q28.1
  vitelline duct Q43.0
  vitreous body or humor Q14.0
  vulva Q52.70
  wrist (joint) Q74.0
Anomia R48.8
Anonychia (congenital) Q84.3
  acquired L60.8
Anophthalmos, anophthalmus (congenital) (globe)
  Q11.1
  acquired Z90.01
Anopia, anopsia H53.46- ☑
  quadrant H53.46- ☑
Anorchia, anorchism, anorchidism Q55.0
Anorexia R63.0
  hysterical F44.89
  nervosa F50.00
    atypical F50.9
    binge-eating type F50.2
      with purging F50.02
    restricting type F50.01
Anorgasmy, psychogenic (female) F52.31
  male F52.32
Anosmia R43.0
  hysterical F44.6
  postinfectional J39.8
Anosognosia R41.89
Anosteoplasia Q78.9
Anovulatory cycle N97.0
Anoxemia R09.02
  newborn P84
Anoxia (pathological) R09.02
  altitude T70.29 ☑
  cerebral G93.1
    complicating
      anesthesia (general) (local) or other sedation
        T88.59 ☑
      in labor and delivery O74.3
      in pregnancy O29.21- ☑

Anoxia — continued
  postpartum, puerperal O89.2
  delivery (cesarean) (instrumental) O75.4
  during a procedure G97.81
  newborn P84
  resulting from a procedure G97.82
  due to
    drowning T75.1 ☑
    high altitude T70.29 ☑
  heart — see Insufficiency, coronary
  intrauterine P84
  myocardial — see Insufficiency, coronary
  newborn P84
  spinal cord G95.11
  systemic (by suffocation) (low content in
    atmosphere) — see Asphyxia, traumatic
Anteflexion — see Anteversion
Antenatal
  care (normal pregnancy) Z34.90
  screening (encounter for) of mother Z36
Antepartum — see condition
Anterior — see condition
Antero-occlusion M26.220
Anteversion
  cervix — see Anteversion, uterus
  femur (neck), congenital Q65.89
  uterus, uterine (cervix) (postinfectional)
    (postpartal, old) N85.4
    congenital Q51.818
    in pregnancy or childbirth — see Pregnancy,
      complicated by
Anthophobia F40.228
Anthracosilicosis J60
Anthracosis (lung) (occupational) J60
  lingua K14.3
Anthrax A22.9
  with pneumonia A22.1
  cerebral A22.8
  colitis A22.2
  cutaneous A22.0
  gastrointestinal A22.2
  inhalation A22.1
  intestinal A22.2
  meningitis A22.8
  pulmonary A22.1
  respiratory A22.1
  sepsis A22.7
  specified manifestation NEC A22.8
Anthropoid pelvis Q74.2
  with disproportion (fetopelvic) O33.0
Anthropophobia F40.10
  generalized F40.11
Antibodies, maternal (blood group) — see
  Isoimmunization, affecting management of
  pregnancy
  anti-D — see Isoimmunization, affecting
    management of pregnancy, Rh
  newborn P55.0
Antibody
  anticardiolipin R76.0
    with
      hemorrhagic disorder D68.312
      hypercoagulable state D68.61
  antiphosphatidylglycerol R76.0
    with
      hemorrhagic disorder D68.312
      hypercoagulable state D68.61
  antiphosphatidylinositol R76.0
    with
      hemorrhagic disorder D68.312
      hypercoagulable state D68.61
  antiphosphatidylserine R76.0
    with
      hemorrhagic disorder D68.312
      hypercoagulable state D68.61
  antiphospholipid R76.0
    with
      hemorrhagic disorder D68.312
      hypercoagulable state D68.61
Anticardiolipin syndrome D68.61
Anticoagulant, circulating (intrinsic) (see also -
  Disorder, hemorrhagic) D68.318
  drug-induced (extrinsic) (see also - Disorder,
    hemorrhagic) D68.32
Antidiuretic hormone syndrome E22.2
Antimonial cholera — see Poisoning, antimony
Antiphospholipid
  antibody
    with hemorrhagic disorder D68.312
    syndrome D68.61
Antisocial personality F60.2

Antithrombinemia — see Circulating
  anticoagulants
Antithromboplastinemia D68.318
Antithromboplastinogenemia D68.318
Antitoxin complication or reaction — see
  Complications, vaccination
Antlophobia F40.228
Antritis J32.0
  maxilla J32.0
    acute J01.00
      recurrent J01.01
  stomach K29.60
    with bleeding K29.61
Antrum, antral — see condition
Anuria R34
  calculus (impacted) (recurrent) (see also
    Calculus, urinary) N20.9
  following
    abortion — see Abortion by type complicated
      by, renal failure
    ectopic or molar pregnancy O08.4
  newborn P96.0
  postprocedural N99.0
  postrenal N13.8
  traumatic (following crushing) T79.5 ☑
Anus, anal — see condition
Anusitis K62.89
Anxiety F41.9
  depression F41.8
  episodic paroxysmal F41.0
  generalized F41.1
  hysteria F41.8
  neurosis F41.1
  panic type F41.0
  reaction F41.1
  separation, abnormal (of childhood) F93.0
  specified NEC F41.8
  state F41.1
Aorta, aortic — see condition
Aortectasia — see Ectasia, aorta
  with aneurysm — see Aneurysm, aorta
Aortitis (nonsyphilitic) (calcific) I77.6
  arteriosclerotic I70.0
  Doehle-Heller A52.02
  luetic A52.02
  rheumatic — see Endocarditis, acute, rheumatic
  specific (syphilitic) A52.02
  syphilitic A52.02
    congenital A50.54 [I79.1]
Apathetic thyroid storm — see Thyrotoxicosis
Apathy R45.3
Apeirophobia F40.228
Apepsia K30
  psychogenic F45.8
Aperistalsis, esophagus K22.0
Apertognathia M26.29
Apert's syndrome Q87.0
Aphagia R13.0
  psychogenic F50.9
Aphakia (acquired) (postoperative) H27.0- ☑
  congenital Q12.3
Aphasia (amnestic) (global) (nominal) (semantic)
  (syntactic) R47.01
  acquired, with epilepsy (Landau-Kleffner
    syndrome) — see Epilepsy, specified NEC
  auditory (developmental) F80.2
  developmental (receptive type) F80.2
    expressive type F80.1
    Wernicke's F80.2
  following
    cerebrovascular disease I69.920
      cerebral infarction I69.320
      intracerebral hemorrhage I69.120
      nontraumatic intracranial hemorrhage NEC
        I69.220
      specified disease NEC I69.820
      subarachnoid hemorrhage I69.020
  primary progressive G31.01 [F02.80]
    with behavioral disturbance G31.01 [F02.81]
  progressive isolated G31.01 [F02.80]
    with behavioral disturbance G31.01 [F02.81]
  sensory F80.2
  syphilis, tertiary A52.19
  Wernicke's (developmental) F80.2
Aphonia (organic) R49.1
  hysterical F44.4
  psychogenic F44.4
Aphthae, aphthous (see also condition)
  Bednar's K12.0
  cachectic K14.0
  epizootic B08.8
  fever B08.8

Aphthae — *continued*
  oral (recurrent) K12.0
  stomatitis (major) (minor) K12.0
  thrush B37.0
  ulcer (oral) (recurrent) K12.0
    genital organ (s) NEC
      female N76.6
      male N50.8
    larynx J38.7
Apical — *see* condition
Apiphobia F40.218
Aplasia (*see also* Agenesis)
  abdominal muscle syndrome Q79.4
  alveolar process (acquired) — *see* Anomaly, alveolar
  congenital Q38.6
  aorta (congenital) Q25.4
  axialis extracorticalis (congenita) E75.29
  bone marrow (myeloid) D61.9
    congenital D61.01
  brain Q00.0
    part of Q04.3
  bronchus Q32.4
  cementum K00.4
  cerebellum Q04.3
  cervix (congenital) Q51.5
  congenital pure red cell D61.01
  corpus callosum Q04.0
  cutis congenita Q84.8
  erythrocyte congenital D61.01
  extracortical axial E75.29
  eye Q11.1
  fovea centralis (congenital) Q14.1
  gallbladder, congenital Q44.0
  iris Q13.1
  labyrinth, membranous Q16.5
  limb (congenital) Q73.8
    lower — *see* Defect, reduction, lower limb
    upper — *see* Agenesis, arm
  lung, congenital (bilateral) (unilateral) Q33.3
  pancreas Q45.0
  parathyroid-thymic D82.1
  Pelizaeus-Merzbacher E75.29
  penis Q55.5
  prostate Q55.4
  red cell (with thymoma) D60.9
    acquired D60.9
      due to drugs D60.9
    adult D60.9
    chronic D60.0
    congenital D61.01
    constitutional D61.01
    due to drugs D60.9
    hereditary D61.01
    of infants D61.01
    primary D61.01
    pure D61.01
      due to drugs D60.9
    specified type NEC D60.8
    transient D60.1
  round ligament Q52.8
  skin Q84.8
  spermatic cord Q55.4
  spleen Q89.01
  testicle Q55.0
  thymic, with immunodeficiency D82.1
  thyroid (congenital) (with myxedema) E03.1
  uterus Q51.0
  ventral horn cell Q06.1
Apnea, apneic (of) (spells) R06.81
  newborn NEC P28.4
    obstructive P28.4
    sleep (central) (obstructive) (primary) P28.3
  prematurity P28.4
  sleep G47.30
    central (primary) G47.31
      in conditions classified elsewhere G47.37
    obstructive (adult) (pediatric) G47.33
    primary central G47.31
    specified NEC G47.39
Apneumatosis, newborn P28.0
Apocrine metaplasia (breast) — *see* Dysplasia, mammary, specified type NEC
Apophysitis (bone) (*see also* Osteochondropathy)
  calcaneus M92.8
  juvenile M92.9
Apoplectiform convulsions (cerebral ischemia) I67.82
Apoplexia, apoplexy, apoplectic
  adrenal A39.1
  heart (auricle) (ventricle) — *see* Infarct, myocardium

Apoplexia — *continued*
  heat T67.0 ☑
  hemorrhagic (stroke) — *see* Hemorrhage, intracranial
  meninges, hemorrhagic — *see* Hemorrhage, intracranial, subarachnoid
  uremic N18.9 [I68.8]
Appearance
  bizarre R46.1
  specified NEC R46.89
  very low level of personal hygiene R46.0
Appendage
  epididymal (organ of Morgagni) Q55.4
  intestine (epiploic) Q43.8
  preauricular Q17.0
  testicular (organ of Morgagni) Q55.29
Appendicitis (pneumococcal) (retrocecal) K37
  with
    perforation or rupture K35.2
    peritoneal abscess K35.3
    peritonitis NEC K35.3
      generalized (with perforation or rupture) K35.2
      localized (with perforation or rupture) K35.3
  acute (catarrhal) (fulminating) (gangrenous) (obstructive) (retrocecal) (suppurative) K35.80
    with
      peritoneal abscess K35.3
      peritonitis NEC K35.3
        generalized (with perforation or rupture) K35.2
        localized (with perforation or rupture) K35.3
      specified NEC K35.89
  amebic A06.89
  chronic (recurrent) K36
  exacerbation — *see* Appendicitis, acute
  gangrenous — *see* Appendicitis, acute
  healed (obliterative) K36
  interval K36
  neurogenic K36
  obstructive K36
  recurrent K36
  relapsing K36
  subacute (adhesive) K36
  subsiding K36
  suppurative — *see* Appendicitis, acute
  tuberculous A18.32
Appendicopathia oxyurica B80
Appendix, appendicular (*see also* condition)
  epididymis Q55.4
  Morgagni
    female Q50.5
    male (epididymal) Q55.4
      testicular Q55.29
  testis Q55.29
Appetite
  depraved — *see* Pica
  excessive R63.2
  lack or loss (*see also* Anorexia) R63.0
    nonorganic origin F50.8
    psychogenic F50.8
  perverted (hysterical) — *see* Pica
Apple peel syndrome Q41.1
Apprehension state F41.1
Apprehensiveness, abnormal F41.9
Approximal wear K03.0
Apraxia (classic) (ideational) (ideokinetic) (ideomotor) (motor) (verbal) R48.2
  following
    cerebrovascular disease I69.990
      cerebral infarction I69.390
      intracerebral hemorrhage I69.190
      nontraumatic intracranial hemorrhage NEC I69.290
      specified disease NEC I69.890
      subarachnoid hemorrhage I69.090
  oculomotor, congenital H51.8
Aptyalism K11.7
Apudoma — *see* Neoplasm, uncertain behavior, by site
Aqueous misdirection H40.83- ☑
Arabicum elephantiasis — *see* Infestation, filarial
Arachnitis — *see* Meningitis
Arachnodactyly — *see* Syndrome, Marfan's
Arachnoiditis (acute) (adhesive) (basal) (brain) (cerebrospinal) — *see* Meningitis
Arachnophobia F40.210
Arboencephalitis, Australian A83.4
Arborization block (heart) I45.5
ARC (AIDS-related complex) B20

Arches — *see* condition
Arcuate uterus Q51.810
Arcuatus uterus Q51.810
Arcus (cornea) senilis — *see* Degeneration, cornea, senile
Arc-welder's lung J63.4
Areflexia R29.2
Areola — *see* condition
Argentaffinoma (*see also* Neoplasm, uncertain behavior, by site)
  malignant — *see* Neoplasm, malignant, by site
  syndrome E34.0
Argininemia E72.21
Arginosuccinic aciduria E72.22
Argyll Robertson phenomenon, pupil or syndrome (syphilitic) A52.19
  atypical H57.09
  nonsyphilitic H57.09
Argyria, argyriasis
  conjunctival H11.13- ☑
  from drug or medicament — *see* Table of Drugs and Chemicals, by substance
Argyrosis, conjunctival H11.13- ☑
Arhinencephaly Q04.1
Ariboflavinosis E53.0
Arm — *see* condition
Arnold-Chiari disease, obstruction or syndrome (type II) Q07.00
  with
    hydrocephalus Q07.02
      with spina bifida Q07.03
    spina bifida Q07.01
      with hydrocephalus Q07.03
  type III — *see* Encephalocele
  type IV Q04.8
Aromatic amino-acid metabolism disorder E70.9
  specified NEC E70.8
Arousals, confusional G47.51
Arrest, arrested
  cardiac I46.9
    complicating
      abortion — *see* Abortion, by type, complicated by, cardiac arrest
      anesthesia (general) (local) or other sedation — *see* Table of Drugs and Chemicals, by drug,
      in labor and delivery O74.2
      in pregnancy O29.11- ☑
      postpartum, puerperal O89.1
    delivery (cesarean) (instrumental) O75.4
    due to
      cardiac condition I46.2
      specified condition NEC I46.8
    intraoperative I97.71- ☑
    newborn P29.81
    postprocedural I97.12- ☑
      obstetric procedure O75.4
  cardiorespiratory — *see* Arrest, cardiac
  circulatory — *see* Arrest, cardiac
  deep transverse O64.0 ☑
  development or growth
    bone — *see* Disorder, bone, development or growth
    child R62.50
    tracheal rings Q32.1
  epiphyseal
    complete
      femur M89.15- ☑
      humerus M89.12- ☑
      tibia M89.16- ☑
      ulna M89.13- ☑
    forearm M89.13- ☑
      specified NEC M89.13- ☑
      ulna — *see* Arrest, epiphyseal, by type, ulna
    lower leg M89.16- ☑
      specified NEC M89.168
      tibia — *see* Arrest, epiphyseal, by type, tibia
    partial
      femur M89.15- ☑
      humerus M89.12- ☑
      tibia M89.16- ☑
      ulna M89.13- ☑
    specified NEC M89.18
  granulopoiesis — *see* Agranulocytosis
  growth plate — *see* Arrest, epiphyseal
  heart — *see* Arrest, cardiac
  legal, anxiety concerning Z65.3
  physeal — *see* Arrest, epiphyseal
  respiratory R09.2
    newborn P28.81
  sinus I45.5
  spermatogenesis (complete) — *see* Azoospermia

☑ **Additional character required**

Arrest — *continued*
  incomplete — *see* Oligospermia
  transverse (deep) O64.0 ☑
Arrhenoblastoma
  benign
    specified site — *see* Neoplasm, benign, by site
    unspecified site
      female D27.9
      male D29.20
  malignant
    specified site — *see* Neoplasm, malignant, by site
    unspecified site
      female C56.9
      male C62.90
  specified site — *see* Neoplasm, uncertain behavior, by site
  unspecified site
    female D39.10
    male D40.10
Arrhythmia (auricle)(cardiac)(juvenile)(nodal)(reflex)(sinus)(supraventricular)(transitory)(ventricle) I49.9
  block I45.9
  extrasystolic I49.49
  newborn
    bradycardia P29.12
    occurring before birth P03.819
      before onset of labor P03.810
      during labor P03.811
    tachycardia P29.11
  psychogenic F45.8
  specified NEC I49.8
  vagal R55
  ventricular re-entry I47.0
Arrillaga-Ayerza syndrome (pulmonary sclerosis with pulmonary hypertension) I27.0
Arsenical pigmentation L81.8
  from drug or medicament — *see* Table of Drugs and Chemicals
Arsenism — *see* Poisoning, arsenic
Arterial — *see* condition
Arteriofibrosis — *see* Arteriosclerosis
Arteriolar sclerosis — *see* Arteriosclerosis
Arteriolith — *see* Arteriosclerosis
Arteriolitis I77.6
  necrotizing, kidney I77.5
  renal — *see* Hypertension, kidney
Arteriolosclerosis — *see* Arteriosclerosis
Arterionephrosclerosis — *see* Hypertension, kidney
Arteriopathy I77.9
Arteriosclerosis, arteriosclerotic (diffuse)(obliterans) (of) (senile) (with calcification) I70.90
  aorta I70.0
  arteries of extremities — *see* Arteriosclerosis, extremities
  brain I67.2
  bypass graft
    coronary — *see* Arteriosclerosis, coronary, bypass graft
    extremities — *see* Arteriosclerosis, extremities, bypass graft
  cardiac — *see* Disease, heart, ischemic, atherosclerotic
  cardiopathy — *see* Disease, heart, ischemic, atherosclerotic
  cardiorenal — *see* Hypertension, cardiorenal
  cardiovascular — *see* Disease, heart, ischemic, atherosclerotic
  carotid (*see also* Occlusion, artery, carotid) I65.2- ☑
  central nervous system I67.2
  cerebral I67.2
  cerebrovascular I67.2
  coronary (artery) I25.10
    due to
      calcified coronary lesion (severely) I25.84
      lipid rich plaque I25.83
    bypass graft I25.810
      with
        angina pectoris I25.709
          with documented spasm I25.701
          specified type NEC I25.708
          unstable I25.700
        ischemic chest pain I25.709
      autologous artery I25.810
        with
          angina pectoris I25.729
            with documented spasm I25.721
            specified type I25.728
            unstable I25.720
          ischemic chest pain I25.729
      autologous vein I25.810

Arteriosclerosis — *continued*
  with
    angina pectoris I25.719
      with documented spasm I25.711
      specified type I25.718
      unstable I25.710
    ischemic chest pain I25.719
    nonautologous biological I25.810
      with
        angina pectoris I25.739
          with documented spasm I25.731
          specified type I25.738
          unstable I25.730
        ischemic chest pain I25.739
    specified type NEC I25.810
      with
        angina pectoris I25.799
          with documented spasm I25.791
          specified type I25.798
          unstable I25.790
        ischemic chest pain I25.799
  native vessel
    with
      angina pectoris I25.119
        with documented spasm I25.111
        specified type NEC I25.118
        unstable I25.110
      ischemic chest pain I25.119
  transplanted heart I25.811
    bypass graft I25.812
      with
        angina pectoris I25.769
          with documented spasm I25.761
          specified type I25.768
          unstable I25.760
        ischemic chest pain I25.769
    native coronary artery I25.811
      with
        angina pectoris I25.759
          with documented spasm I25.751
          specified type I25.758
          unstable I25.750
        ischemic chest pain I25.759
  extremities (native arteries) I70.209
    bypass graft I70.309
      autologous vein graft I70.409
        leg I70.409
          with
            gangrene (and intermittent claudication, rest pain and ulcer) I70.469
            intermittent claudication I70.419
            rest pain (and intermittent claudication) I70.429
          bilateral I70.403
            with
              gangrene (and intermittent claudication, rest pain and ulcer) I70.463
              intermittent claudication I70.413
              rest pain (and intermittent claudication) I70.423
              specified type NEC I70.493
          left I70.402
            with
              gangrene (and intermittent claudication, rest pain and ulcer) I70.462
              intermittent claudication I70.412
              rest pain (and intermittent claudication) I70.422
              ulceration (and intermittent claudication and rest pain) I70.449
                ankle I70.443
                calf I70.442
                foot site NEC I70.445
                heel I70.444
                lower leg NEC I70.448
                midfoot I70.444
                thigh I70.441
              specified type NEC I70.492
          right I70.401
            with
              gangrene (and intermittent claudication, rest pain and ulcer) I70.461
              intermittent claudication I70.411
              rest pain (and intermittent claudication) I70.421
              ulceration (and intermittent claudication and rest pain) I70.439

Arteriosclerosis — *continued*
                ankle I70.433
                calf I70.432
                foot site NEC I70.435
                heel I70.434
                lower leg NEC I70.438
                midfoot I70.434
                thigh I70.431
              specified type NEC I70.491
            specified type NEC I70.499
      specified NEC I70.408
        with
          gangrene (and intermittent claudication, rest pain and ulcer) I70.468
          intermittent claudication I70.418
          rest pain (and intermittent claudication) I70.428
          ulceration (and intermittent claudication and rest pain) I70.45
        specified type NEC I70.498
    leg I70.309
      with
        gangrene (and intermittent claudication, rest pain and ulcer) I70.369
        intermittent claudication I70.319
        rest pain (and intermittent claudication) I70.329
      bilateral I70.303
        with
          gangrene (and intermittent claudication, rest pain and ulcer) I70.363
          intermittent claudication I70.313
          rest pain (and intermittent claudication) I70.323
          specified type NEC I70.393
      left I70.302
        with
          gangrene (and intermittent claudication, rest pain and ulcer) I70.362
          intermittent claudication I70.312
          rest pain (and intermittent claudication) I70.322
          ulceration (and intermittent claudication and rest pain) I70.349
            ankle I70.343
            calf I70.342
            foot site NEC I70.345
            heel I70.344
            lower leg NEC I70.348
            midfoot I70.344
            thigh I70.341
         specified type NEC I70.392
      right I70.301
        with
          gangrene (and intermittent claudication, rest pain and ulcer) I70.361
          intermittent claudication I70.311
          rest pain (and intermittent claudication) I70.321
          ulceration (and intermittent claudication and rest pain) I70.339
            ankle I70.333
            calf I70.332
            foot site NEC I70.335
            heel I70.334
            lower leg NEC I70.338
            midfoot I70.334
            thigh I70.331
        specified type NEC I70.391
      specified type NEC I70.399
    nonautologous biological graft I70.509
      leg I70.509
        with
          gangrene (and intermittent claudication, rest pain and ulcer) I70.569
          intermittent claudication I70.519
          rest pain (and intermittent claudication) I70.529
      bilateral I70.503
        with
          gangrene (and intermittent claudication, rest pain and ulcer) I70.563
          intermittent claudication I70.513
          rest pain (and intermittent claudication) I70.523
          specified type NEC I70.593

Arteriosclerosis — *continued*

 left I70.502
  with
   gangrene (and intermittent
     claudication, rest pain and ulcer)
     I70.562
   intermittent claudication I70.512
   rest pain (and intermittent
     claudication) I70.522
   ulceration (and intermittent
     claudication and rest pain)
     I70.549
    ankle I70.543
    calf I70.542
    foot site NEC I70.545
    heel I70.544
    lower leg NEC I70.548
    midfoot I70.544
    thigh I70.541
   specified type NEC I70.592
 right I70.501
  with
   gangrene (and intermittent
     claudication, rest pain and ulcer)
     I70.561
   intermittent claudication I70.511
   rest pain (and intermittent
     claudication) I70.521
   ulceration (and intermittent
     claudication and rest pain)
     I70.539
    ankle I70.533
    calf I70.532
    foot site NEC I70.535
    heel I70.534
    lower leg NEC I70.538
    midfoot I70.534
    thigh I70.531
   specified type NEC I70.591
  specified type NEC I70.599
 specified NEC I70.508
  with
   gangrene (and intermittent
     claudication, rest pain and ulcer)
     I70.568
   intermittent claudication I70.518
   rest pain (and intermittent
     claudication) I70.528
   ulceration (and intermittent
     claudication and rest pain) I70.55
   specified type NEC I70.598
 nonbiological graft I70.609
  leg I70.609
   with
    gangrene (and intermittent
      claudication, rest pain and ulcer)
      I70.669
    intermittent claudication I70.619
    rest pain (and intermittent
      claudication) I70.629
   bilateral I70.603
    with
     gangrene (and intermittent
       claudication, rest pain and ulcer)
       I70.663
     intermittent claudication I70.613
     rest pain (and intermittent
       claudication) I70.623
    specified type NEC I70.693
   left I70.602
    with
     gangrene (and intermittent
       claudication, rest pain and ulcer)
       I70.662
     intermittent claudication I70.612
     rest pain (and intermittent
       claudication) I70.622
     ulceration (and intermittent
       claudication and rest pain) I70.649
      ankle I70.643
      calf I70.642
      foot site NEC I70.645
      heel I70.644
      lower leg NEC I70.648
      midfoot I70.644
      thigh I70.641
     specified type NEC I70.692
   right I70.601
    with
     gangrene (and intermittent
       claudication, rest pain and ulcer)
       I70.661

Arteriosclerosis — *continued*

     intermittent claudication I70.611
     rest pain (and intermittent
       claudication) I70.621
     ulceration (and intermittent
       claudication and rest pain)
       I70.639
      ankle I70.633
      calf I70.632
      foot site NEC I70.635
      heel I70.634
      lower leg NEC I70.638
      midfoot I70.634
      thigh I70.631
     specified type NEC I70.691
    specified type NEC I70.699
   specified NEC I70.608
    with
     gangrene (and intermittent
       claudication, rest pain and ulcer)
       I70.668
     intermittent claudication I70.618
     rest pain (and intermittent
       claudication) I70.628
     ulceration (and intermittent
       claudication and rest pain) I70.65
    specified type NEC I70.698
 specified graft NEC I70.709
  leg I70.709
   with
    gangrene (and intermittent
      claudication, rest pain and ulcer)
      I70.769
    intermittent claudication I70.719
    rest pain (and intermittent
      claudication) I70.729
   bilateral I70.703
    with
     gangrene (and intermittent
       claudication, rest pain and ulcer)
       I70.763
     intermittent claudication I70.713
     rest pain (and intermittent
       claudication) I70.723
    specified type NEC I70.793
   left I70.702
    with
     gangrene (and intermittent
       claudication, rest pain and ulcer)
       I70.762
     intermittent claudication I70.712
     rest pain (and intermittent
       claudication) I70.722
     ulceration (and intermittent
       claudication and rest pain)
       I70.749
      ankle I70.743
      calf I70.742
      foot site NEC I70.745
      heel I70.744
      lower leg NEC I70.748
      midfoot I70.744
      thigh I70.741
     specified type NEC I70.792
   right I70.701
    with
     gangrene (and intermittent
       claudication, rest pain and ulcer)
       I70.761
     intermittent claudication I70.711
     rest pain (and intermittent
       claudication) I70.721
     ulceration (and intermittent
       claudication and rest pain)
       I70.739
      ankle I70.733
      calf I70.732
      foot site NEC I70.735
      heel I70.734
      lower leg NEC I70.738
      midfoot I70.734
      thigh I70.731
     specified type NEC I70.791
    specified type NEC I70.799
   specified NEC I70.708
    with
     gangrene (and intermittent
       claudication, rest pain and ulcer)
       I70.768
     intermittent claudication I70.718
     rest pain (and intermittent
       claudication) I70.728

Arteriosclerosis — *continued*

     ulceration (and intermittent
       claudication and rest pain) I70.75
    specified type NEC I70.798
   specified NEC I70.308
    with
     gangrene (and intermittent claudication,
       rest pain and ulcer) I70.368
     intermittent claudication I70.318
     rest pain (and intermittent claudication)
       I70.328
     ulceration (and intermittent claudication
       and rest pain) I70.35
    specified type NEC I70.398
  leg I70.209
   with
    gangrene (and intermittent claudication,
      rest pain and ulcer) I70.269
    intermittent claudication I70.219
    rest pain (and intermittent claudication)
      I70.229
   bilateral I70.203
    with
     gangrene (and intermittent claudication,
       rest pain and ulcer) I70.263
     intermittent claudication I70.213
     rest pain (and intermittent claudication)
       I70.223
    specified type NEC I70.293
   left I70.202
    with
     gangrene (and intermittent claudication,
       rest pain and ulcer) I70.262
     intermittent claudication I70.212
     rest pain (and intermittent claudication)
       I70.222
     ulceration (and intermittent claudication
       and rest pain) I70.249
      ankle I70.243
      calf I70.242
      foot site NEC I70.245
      heel I70.244
      lower leg NEC I70.248
      midfoot I70.244
      thigh I70.241
     specified type NEC I70.292
   right I70.201
    with
     gangrene (and intermittent claudication,
       rest pain and ulcer) I70.261
     intermittent claudication I70.211
     rest pain (and intermittent claudication)
       I70.221
     ulceration (and intermittent claudication
       and rest pain) I70.239
      ankle I70.233
      calf I70.232
      foot site NEC I70.235
      heel I70.234
      lower leg NEC I70.238
      midfoot I70.234
      thigh I70.231
     specified type NEC I70.291
    specified type NEC I70.299
   specified site NEC I70.208
    with
     gangrene (and intermittent claudication,
       rest pain and ulcer) I70.268
     intermittent claudication I70.218
     rest pain (and intermittent claudication)
       I70.228
     ulceration (and intermittent claudication
       and rest pain) I70.25
    specified type NEC I70.298
 generalized I70.91
 heart (disease) — *see* Arteriosclerosis, coronary
   (artery),
 kidney — *see* Hypertension, kidney
 medial — *see* Arteriosclerosis, extremities
 mesenteric (artery) K55.1
 Mönckeberg's — *see* Arteriosclerosis, extremities
 myocarditis I51.4
 peripheral (of extremities) — *see* Arteriosclerosis,
   extremities
 pulmonary (idiopathic) I27.0
 renal (arterioles) (*see also* Hypertension, kidney)
   artery I70.1
 retina (vascular) I70.8 [H35.0- ☑]
 specified artery NEC I70.8
 spinal (cord) G95.19
 vertebral (artery) I67.2

☑ **Additional character required**

Arteriospasm I73.9
Arteriovenous — *see* condition
Arteritis I77.6
  allergic M31.0
  aorta (nonsyphilitic) I77.6
    syphilitic A52.02
  aortic arch M31.4
  brachiocephalic M31.4
  brain I67.7
    syphilitic A52.04
  cerebral I67.7
    in
      diseases classified elsewhere I68.2
      systemic lupus erythematosus M32.19
    listerial A32.89
    syphilitic A52.04
    tuberculous A18.89
  coronary (artery) I25.89
    rheumatic I01.8
      chronic I09.89
    syphilitic A52.06
  cranial (left) (right), giant cell M31.6
  deformans — *see* Arteriosclerosis
  giant cell NEC M31.6
    with polymyalgia rheumatica M31.5
  necrosing or necrotizing M31.9
    specified NEC M31.8
  nodosa M30.0
  obliterans — *see* Arteriosclerosis
  pulmonary I28.8
  rheumatic — *see* Fever, rheumatic
  senile — *see* Arteriosclerosis
  suppurative I77.2
  syphilitic (general) A52.09
    brain A52.04
    coronary A52.06
    spinal A52.09
  temporal, giant cell M31.6
  young female aortic arch syndrome M31.4
Artery, arterial (*see also* condition)
  abscess I77.89
  single umbilical Q27.0
Arthralgia (allergic) (*see also* Pain, joint)
  in caisson disease T70.3 ☑
  temporomandibular M26.62
Arthritis, arthritic (acute) (chronic) (nonpyogenic)
  (subacute) M19.90
  allergic — *see* Arthritis, specified form NEC
  ankylosing (crippling) (spine) (*see also*
    Spondylitis, ankylosing)
    sites other than spine — *see* Arthritis, specified
      form NEC
  atrophic — *see* Osteoarthritis
    spine — *see* Spondylitis, ankylosing
  back — *see* Spondylopathy, inflammatory
  blennorrhagic (gonococcal) A54.42
  Charcot's — *see* Arthropathy, neuropathic
    diabetic — *see* Diabetes, arthropathy,
      neuropathic
    syringomyelic G95.0
  chylous (filarial) (*see also* category M01) B74.9
  climacteric (any site) NEC — *see* Arthritis,
    specified form NEC
  crystal (-induced) — *see* Arthritis, in, crystals
  deformans — *see* Osteoarthritis
  degenerative — *see* Osteoarthritis
  due to or associated with
    acromegaly E22.0
    brucellosis — *see* Brucellosis
    caisson disease T70.3 ☑
    diabetes — *see* Diabetes, arthropathy
    dracontiasis (*see also* category M01) B72
    enteritis NEC
      regional — *see* Enteritis, regional
    erysipelas (*see also* category M01) A46
    erythema
      epidemic A25.1
      nodosum L52
    filariasis NOS B74.9
    glanders A24.0
    helminthiasis (*see also* category M01) B83.9
    hemophilia D66 [M36.2]
    Henoch- (Schönlein) purpura D69.0 [M36.4]
    human parvovirus (*see also* category M01)
      B97.6
    infectious disease NEC M01
    leprosy (see also category M01) (*see also*
      Leprosy) A30.9
    Lyme disease A69.23
    mycobacteria (*see also* category M01) A31.8
    parasitic disease NEC (*see also* category M01)
      B89

Arthritis — *continued*
  paratyphoid fever (see also category M01) (*see
    also* Fever, paratyphoid) A01.4
  rat bite fever (*see also* category M01) A25.1
  regional enteritis — *see* Enteritis, regional
  respiratory disorder NOS J98.9
  serum sickness (*see also* Reaction, serum)
    T80.69 ☑
  syringomyelia G95.0
  typhoid fever A01.04
  epidemic erythema A25.1
  febrile — *see* Fever, rheumatic
  gonococcal A54.42
  gouty (acute) — *see* Gout, idiopathic
  in (due to)
    acromegaly (*see also* subcategory M14.8-) E22.0
    amyloidosis (*see also* subcategory M14.8-) E85.4
    bacterial disease (*see also* subcategory M01)
      A49.9
    Behçet's syndrome M35.2
    caisson disease (*see also* subcategory M14.8-)
      T70.3 ☑
    coliform bacilli (Escherichia coli) — *see* Arthritis,
      in, pyogenic organism NEC
    crystals M11.9
      dicalcium phosphate — *see* Arthritis, in,
        crystals, specified type NEC
      hydroxyapatite M11.0- ☑
      pyrophosphate — *see* Arthritis, in, crystals,
        specified type NEC
      specified type NEC M11.80
        ankle M11.87- ☑
        elbow M11.82- ☑
        foot joint M11.87- ☑
        hand joint M11.84- ☑
        hip M11.85- ☑
        knee M11.86- ☑
        multiple sites M11.8- ☑
        shoulder M11.81- ☑
        vertebrae M11.88
        wrist M11.83- ☑
    dermatoarthritis, lipoid E78.81
    dracontiasis (dracunculiasis) (*see also* category
      M01) B72
    endocrine disorder NEC (*see also* subcategory
      M14.8-) E34.9
    enteritis, infectious NEC (*see also* category
      M01) A09
      specified organism NEC (*see also* category
        M01) A08.8
    erythema
      multiforme (*see also* subcategory M14.8-)
        L51.9
      nodosum (*see also* subcategory M14.8-) L52
    gout — *see* Gout, idiopathic
    helminthiasis NEC (*see also* category M01)
      B83.9
    hemochromatosis (*see also* subcategory M14.8-
) E83.118
    hemoglobinopathy NEC D58.2 [M36.3]
    hemophilia NEC D66 [M36.2]
    Hemophilus influenzae M00.8- ☑ [B96.3]
    Henoch (-Schönlein) purpura D69.0 [M36.4]
    hyperparathyroidism NEC (*see also* subcategory
      M14.8-) E21.3
    hypersensitivity reaction NEC T78.49 ☑ [M36.4]
    hypogammaglobulinemia (*see also*
      subcategory M14.8-) D80.1
    hypothyroidism NEC (*see also* subcategory
      M14.8-) E03.9
    infection — *see* Arthritis, pyogenic or pyemic
      spine — *see* Spondylopathy, infective
    infectious disease NEC M01
    leprosy (*see also* category M01) A30.9
    leukemia NEC C95.9- ☑ [M36.1]
    lipoid dermatoarthritis E78.81
    Lyme disease A69.23
    Mediterranean fever, familial (*see also*
      subcategory M14.8-) E85.0
    Meningococcus A39.83
    metabolic disorder NEC (*see also* subcategory
      M14.8-) E88.9
    multiple myelomatosis C90.0- ☑ [M36.1]
    mumps B26.85
    mycosis NEC (*see also* category M01) B49
    myelomatosis (multiple) C90.0- ☑ [M36.1]
    neurological disorder NEC G98.0
    ochronosis (*see also* subcategory M14.8-)
      E70.29
    O'nyong-nyong (*see also* category M01) A92.1
    parasitic disease NEC (*see also* category M01)
      B89

Arthritis — *continued*
  paratyphoid fever (*see also* category M01)
    A01.4
  Pseudomonas — *see* Arthritis, pyogenic,
    bacterial NEC
  psoriasis L40.50
  pyogenic organism NEC — *see* Arthritis,
    pyogenic, bacterial NEC
  Reiter's disease — *see* Reiter's disease
  respiratory disorder NEC (*see also* subcategory
    M14.8-) J98.9
  reticulosis, malignant (*see also* subcategory
    M14.8-) C86.0
  rubella B06.82
  Salmonella (arizonae) (cholerae-suis)
    (enteritidis) (typhimurium) A02.23
  sarcoidosis D86.86
  specified bacteria NEC — *see* Arthritis,
    pyogenic, bacterial NEC
  sporotrichosis B42.82
  syringomyelia G95.0
  thalassemia NEC D56.9 [M36.3]
  tuberculosis — *see* Tuberculosis, arthritis
  typhoid fever A01.04
  urethritis, Reiter's — *see* Reiter's disease
  viral disease NEC (*see also* category M01) B34.9
  infectious or infective (*see also* Arthritis, pyogenic
    or pyemic)
    spine — *see* Spondylopathy, infective
  juvenile M08.90
    with systemic onset — *see* Still's disease
    ankle M08.97- ☑
    elbow M08.92- ☑
    foot joint M08.97- ☑
    hand joint M08.94- ☑
    hip M08.95- ☑
    knee M08.96- ☑
    multiple site M08.99
    pauciarticular M08.40
      ankle M08.47- ☑
      elbow M08.42- ☑
      foot joint M08.47- ☑
      hand joint M08.44- ☑
      hip M08.45- ☑
      knee M08.46- ☑
      shoulder M08.41- ☑
      vertebrae M08.48
      wrist M08.43- ☑
    psoriatic L40.54
    rheumatoid — *see* Arthritis, rheumatoid,
      juvenile
    shoulder M08.91- ☑
    vertebra M08.98
    specified type NEC M08.80
      ankle M08.87- ☑
      elbow M08.82- ☑
      foot joint M08.87- ☑
      hand joint M08.84- ☑
      hip M08.85- ☑
      knee M08.86- ☑
      multiple site M08.89
      shoulder M08.81- ☑
      specified joint NEC M08.88
      vertebrae M08.88
      wrist M08.83- ☑
    wrist M08.93- ☑
  meaning osteoarthritis — *see* Osteoarthritis
  meningococcal A39.83
  menopausal (any site) NEC — *see* Arthritis,
    specified form NEC
  mutilans (psoriatic) L40.52
  mycotic NEC (*see also* category M01) B49
  neuropathic (Charcot) — *see* Arthropathy,
    neuropathic
    diabetic — *see* Diabetes, arthropathy,
      neuropathic
    nonsyphilitic NEC G98.0
    syringomyelic G95.0
  ochronotic (*see also* subcategory M14.8-) E70.29
  palindromic (any site) — *see* Rheumatism,
    palindromic
  pneumococcal M00.10
    ankle M00.17- ☑
    elbow M00.12- ☑
    foot joint — *see* Arthritis, pneumococcal, ankle
    hand joint M00.14- ☑
    hip M00.15- ☑
    knee M00.16- ☑
    multiple site M00.19
    shoulder M00.11- ☑
    vertebra M00.10
    wrist M00.13- ☑

Arthritis - Arthropathy

Arthritis — *continued*
  postdysenteric — *see* Arthropathy, postdysenteric
  postmeningococcal A39.84
  postrheumatic, chronic — *see* Arthropathy, postrheumatic, chronic
  primary progressive (*see also* Arthritis, specified form NEC)
    spine — *see* Spondylitis, ankylosing
  psoriatic L40.50
  purulent (any site except spine) — *see* Arthritis, pyogenic or pyemic
    spine — *see* Spondylopathy, infective
  pyogenic or pyemic (any site except spine) M00.9
    bacterial NEC M00.80
      ankle M00.87- ☑
      elbow M00.82- ☑
      foot joint — *see* Arthritis, pyogenic, bacterial NEC, ankle
      hand joint M00.84- ☑
      hip M00.85- ☑
      knee M00.86- ☑
      multiple site M00.89
      shoulder M00.81- ☑
      vertebra M00.88
      wrist M00.83- ☑
    pneumococcal — *see* Arthritis, pneumococcal
    spine — *see* Spondylopathy, infective
    staphylococcal — *see* Arthritis, staphylococcal
    streptococcal — *see* Arthritis, streptococcal NEC
      pneumococcal — *see* Arthritis, pneumococcal
  reactive — *see* Reiter's disease
  rheumatic (*see also* Arthritis, rheumatoid)
    acute or subacute — *see* Fever, rheumatic
  rheumatoid M06.9
    with
      carditis — *see* Rheumatoid, carditis
      endocarditis — *see* Rheumatoid, carditis
      heart involvement NEC — *see* Rheumatoid, carditis
      lung involvement — *see* Rheumatoid, lung
      myocarditis — *see* Rheumatoid, carditis
      myopathy — *see* Rheumatoid, myopathy
      pericarditis — *see* Rheumatoid, carditis
      polyneuropathy — *see* Rheumatoid, polyneuropathy
      rheumatoid factor — *see* Arthritis, rheumatoid, seropositive
      splenoadenomegaly and leukopenia — *see* Felty's syndrome
      vasculitis — *see* Rheumatoid, vasculitis
      visceral involvement NEC — *see* Rheumatoid, arthritis, with involvement of organs NEC
    juvenile (with or without rheumatoid factor) M08.00
      ankle M08.07- ☑
      elbow M08.02- ☑
      foot joint M08.07- ☑
      hand joint M08.04- ☑
      hip M08.05- ☑
      knee M08.06- ☑
      multiple site M08.09
      shoulder M08.01- ☑
      vertebra M08.08
      wrist M08.03- ☑
    seronegative M06.00
      ankle M06.07- ☑
      elbow M06.02- ☑
      foot joint M06.07- ☑
      hand joint M06.04- ☑
      hip M06.05- ☑
      knee M06.06- ☑
      multiple site M06.09
      shoulder M06.01- ☑
      vertebra M06.08
      wrist M06.03- ☑
    seropositive M05.9
      specified NEC M05.80
        ankle M05.87- ☑
        elbow M05.82- ☑
        foot joint M05.87- ☑
        hand joint M05.84- ☑
        hip M05.85- ☑
        knee M05.86- ☑
        multiple sites M05.89
        shoulder M05.81- ☑
        vertebra — *see* Spondylitis, ankylosing
        wrist M05.83- ☑
      without organ involvement M05.70
        ankle M05.77- ☑
        elbow M05.72- ☑
        foot joint M05.77- ☑

Arthritis — *continued*
        hand joint M05.74- ☑
        hip M05.75- ☑
        knee M05.76- ☑
        multiple sites M05.79
        shoulder M05.71- ☑
        vertebra — *see* Spondylitis, ankylosing
        wrist M05.73- ☑
    specified type NEC M06.80
      ankle M06.87- ☑
      elbow M06.82- ☑
      foot joint M06.87- ☑
      hand joint M06.84- ☑
      hip M06.85- ☑
      knee M06.86- ☑
      multiple site M06.89
      shoulder M06.81- ☑
      vertebra M06.88
      wrist M06.83- ☑
    spine — *see* Spondylitis, ankylosing
  rubella B06.82
  scorbutic (*see also* subcategory M14.8-) E54
  senile or senescent — *see* Osteoarthritis
  septic (any site except spine) — *see* Arthritis, pyogenic or pyemic
    spine — *see* Spondylopathy, infective
  serum (nontherapeutic) (therapeutic) — *see* Arthropathy, postimmunization
  specified form NEC M13.80
    ankle M13.87- ☑
    elbow M13.82- ☑
    foot joint M13.87- ☑
    hand joint M13.84- ☑
    hip M13.85- ☑
    knee M13.86- ☑
    multiple site M13.89
    shoulder M13.81- ☑
    specified joint NEC M13.88
    wrist M13.83- ☑
  spine (*see also* Spondylopathy, inflammatory)
    infectious or infective NEC — *see* Spondylopathy, infective
    Marie-Strümpell — *see* Spondylitis, ankylosing
    pyogenic — *see* Spondylopathy, infective
    rheumatoid — *see* Spondylitis, ankylosing
    traumatic (old) — *see* Spondylopathy, traumatic
    tuberculous A18.01
  staphylococcal M00.00
    ankle M00.07- ☑
    elbow M00.02- ☑
    foot joint — *see* Arthritis, staphylococcal, ankle
    hand joint M00.04- ☑
    hip M00.05- ☑
    knee M00.06- ☑
    multiple site M00.09
    shoulder M00.01- ☑
    vertebra M00.08
    wrist M00.03- ☑
  streptococcal NEC M00.20
    ankle M00.27- ☑
    elbow M00.22- ☑
    foot joint — *see* Arthritis, streptococcal, ankle
    hand joint M00.24- ☑
    hip M00.25- ☑
    knee M00.26- ☑
    multiple site M00.29
    shoulder M00.21- ☑
    vertebra M00.28
    wrist M00.23- ☑
  suppurative — *see* Arthritis, pyogenic or pyemic
  syphilitic (late) A52.16
    congenital A50.55 [M12.80]
  syphilitica deformans (Charcot) A52.16
  temporomandibular M26.69
  toxic of menopause (any site) — *see* Arthritis, specified form NEC
  transient — *see* Arthropathy, specified form NEC
  traumatic (chronic) — *see* Arthropathy, traumatic
  tuberculous A18.02
    spine A18.01
  uratic — *see* Gout, idiopathic
  urethritica (Reiter's) — *see* Reiter's disease
  vertebral — *see* Spondylopathy, inflammatory
  villous (any site) — *see* Arthropathy, specified form NEC
Arthrocele — *see* Effusion, joint
Arthrodesis status Z98.1
Arthrodynia (*see also* Pain, joint)
Arthrodysplasia Q74.9
Arthrofibrosis, joint — *see* Ankylosis
Arthrogryposis (congenital) Q68.8

Arthrokatadysis — *continued*
  multiplex congenita Q74.3
Arthrokatadysis M24.7
Arthropathy (*see also* Arthritis) M12.9
  Charcot's — *see* Arthropathy, neuropathic
    diabetic — *see* Diabetes, arthropathy, neuropathic
    syringomyelic G95.0
  cricoarytenoid J38.7
  crystal (-induced) — *see* Arthritis, in, crystals
  diabetic NEC — *see* Diabetes, arthropathy
  distal interphalangeal, psoriatic L40.51
  enteropathic M07.60
    ankle M07.67- ☑
    elbow M07.62- ☑
    foot joint M07.67- ☑
    hand joint M07.64- ☑
    hip M07.65- ☑
    knee M07.66- ☑
    multiple site M07.69
    shoulder M07.61- ☑
    vertebra M07.68
    wrist M07.63- ☑
  following intestinal bypass M02.00
    ankle M02.07- ☑
    elbow M02.02- ☑
    foot joint M02.07- ☑
    hand joint M02.04- ☑
    hip M02.05- ☑
    knee M02.06- ☑
    multiple site M02.09
    shoulder M02.01- ☑
    vertebra M02.08
    wrist M02.03- ☑
  gouty (*see also* Gout, idiopathic)
    in (due to)
      Lesch-Nyhan syndrome E79.1 [M14.8- ☑]
      sickle-cell disorders D57- ☑ [M14.8- ☑]
  hemophilic NEC D66 [M36.2]
    in (due to)
      hyperparathyroidism NEC E21.3 [M14.8- ☑]
      metabolic disease NOS E88.9 [M14.8- ☑]
  in (due to)
    acromegaly E22.0 [M14.8- ☑]
    amyloidosis E85.4 [M14.8- ☑]
    blood disorder NOS D75.9 [M36.3]
    diabetes — *see* Diabetes, arthropathy
    endocrine disease NOS E34.9 [M14.8- ☑]
    erythema
      multiforme L51.9 [M14.8- ☑]
      nodosum L52 [M14.8- ☑]
    hemochromatosis E83.118 [M14.8- ☑]
    hemoglobinopathy NEC D58.2 [M36.3]
    hemophilia NEC D66 [M36.2]
    Henoch-Schönlein purpura D69.0 [M36.4]
    hyperthyroidism E05.90 [M14.8- ☑]
    hypothyroidism E03.9 [M14.8- ☑]
    infective endocarditis I33.0 [M12.80]
    leukemia NEC C95.9- ☑ [M36.1]
    malignant histiocytosis C96.A [M36.1]
    metabolic disease NOS E88.9 [M14.8- ☑]
    multiple myeloma C90.0- ☑ [M36.1]
    neoplastic disease NOS (*see also* Neoplasm) D49.9 [M36.1]
    nutritional deficiency (*see also* subcategory M14.8-) E63.9
    psoriasis NOS L40.50
    sarcoidosis D86.86
    syphilis (late) A52.77
      congenital A50.55 [M12.80]
    thyrotoxicosis (*see also* subcategory M14.8-) E05.90
    ulcerative colitis K51.90 [M07.60]
    viral hepatitis (postinfectious) NEC B19.9 [M12.80]
    Whipple's disease (*see also* subcategory M14.8-) K90.81
  Jaccoud — *see* Arthropathy, postrheumatic, chronic
  juvenile — *see* Arthritis, juvenile
    psoriatic L40.54
  mutilans (psoriatic) L40.52
  neuropathic (Charcot) M14.60
    ankle M14.67- ☑
    diabetic — *see* Diabetes, arthropathy, neuropathic
    elbow M14.62- ☑
    foot joint M14.67- ☑
    hand joint M14.64- ☑
    hip M14.65- ☑
    knee M14.66- ☑
    multiple site M14.69

    ☑ **Additional character required**

Arthropathy — *continued*
  nonsyphilitic NEC G98.0
    shoulder M14.61- ☑
    syringomyelic G95.0
    vertebra M14.68
    wrist M14.63- ☑
  osteopulmonary — *see* Osteoarthropathy,
    hypertrophic, specified NEC
  postdysenteric M02.10
    ankle M02.17- ☑
    elbow M02.12- ☑
    foot joint M02.17- ☑
    hand joint M02.14- ☑
    hip M02.15- ☑
    knee M02.16- ☑
    multiple site M02.19
    shoulder M02.11- ☑
    vertebra M02.18
    wrist M02.13- ☑
  postimmunization M02.20
    ankle M02.27- ☑
    elbow M02.22- ☑
    foot joint M02.27- ☑
    hand joint M02.24- ☑
    hip M02.25- ☑
    knee M02.26- ☑
    multiple site M02.29
    shoulder M02.21- ☑
    vertebra M02.28
    wrist M02.23- ☑
  postinfectious NEC B99 ☑ [M12.80]
    in (due to)
      enteritis due to Yersinia enterocolitica A04.6
        [M12.80]
      syphilis A52.77
      viral hepatitis NEC B19.9 [M12.80]
  postrheumatic, chronic (Jaccoud) M12.00
    ankle M12.07- ☑
    elbow M12.02- ☑
    foot joint M12.07- ☑
    hand joint M12.04- ☑
    hip M12.05- ☑
    knee M12.06- ☑
    multiple site M12.09
    shoulder M12.01- ☑
    specified joint NEC M12.08
    vertebrae M12.08
    wrist M12.03- ☑
  psoriatic NEC L40.59
    interphalangeal, distal L40.51
  reactive M02.9
    in (due to)
      infective endocarditis I33.0 [M02.9]
    specified type NEC M02.80
      ankle M02.87- ☑
      elbow M02.82- ☑
      foot joint M02.87- ☑
      hand joint M02.84- ☑
      hip M02.85- ☑
      knee M02.86- ☑
      multiple site M02.89
      shoulder M02.81- ☑
      vertebra M02.88
      wrist M02.83- ☑
  specified form NEC M12.80
    ankle M12.87- ☑
    elbow M12.82- ☑
    foot joint M12.87- ☑
    hand joint M12.84- ☑
    hip M12.85- ☑
    knee M12.86- ☑
    multiple site M12.89
    shoulder M12.81- ☑
    specified joint NEC M12.88
    vertebrae M12.88
    wrist M12.83- ☑
  syringomyelic G95.0
  tabes dorsalis A52.16
  tabetic A52.16
  transient — *see* Arthropathy, specified form NEC
  traumatic M12.50
    ankle M12.57- ☑
    elbow M12.52- ☑
    foot joint M12.57- ☑
    hand joint M12.54- ☑
    hip M12.55- ☑
    knee M12.56- ☑
    multiple site M12.59
    shoulder M12.51- ☑
    specified joint NEC M12.58
    vertebrae M12.58
    wrist M12.53- ☑

Arthropyosis — *see* Arthritis, pyogenic or pyemic
Arthrosis (deformans) (degenerative) (localized) (*see also* Osteoarthritis) M19.90
  spine — *see* Spondylosis
Arthus' phenomenon or reaction T78.41 ☑
  due to
    drug — *see* Table of Drugs and Chemicals, by
      drug
Articular — *see* condition
Articulation, reverse (teeth) M26.24
Artificial
  insemination complication — *see* Complications,
    artificial, fertilization
  opening status (functioning) (without
    complication) Z93.9
    anus (colostomy) Z93.3
    colostomy Z93.3
    cystostomy Z93.50
      appendico-vesicostomy Z93.52
      cutaneous Z93.51
      specified NEC Z93.59
    enterostomy Z93.4
    gastrostomy Z93.1
    ileostomy Z93.2
    intestinal tract NEC Z93.4
    jejunostomy Z93.4
    nephrostomy Z93.6
    specified site NEC Z93.8
    tracheostomy Z93.0
    ureterostomy Z93.6
    urethrostomy Z93.6
    urinary tract NEC Z93.6
    vagina Z93.8
    vagina status Z93.8
Arytenoid — *see* condition
Asbestosis (occupational) J61
ASC-H (atypical squamous cells cannot exclude high
  grade squamous intraepithelial lesion on cytologic
  smear)
  anus R85.611
  cervix R87.611
  vagina R87.621
ASC-US (atypical squamous cells of undetermined
  significance on cytologic smear)
  anus R85.610
  cervix R87.610
  vagina R87.620
Ascariasis B77.9
  with
    complications NEC B77.89
    intestinal complications B77.0
    pneumonia, pneumonitis B77.81
Ascaridosis, ascaridiasis — *see* Ascariasis
Ascaris (infection) (infestation) (lumbricoides) — *see*
  Ascariasis
Ascending — *see* condition
Aschoff's bodies — *see* Myocarditis, rheumatic
Ascites (abdominal) R18.8
  cardiac I50.9
  chylous (nonfilarial) I89.8
    filarial — *see* Infestation, filarial
  due to
    cirrhosis, alcoholic K70.31
    hepatitis
      alcoholic K70.11
      chronic active K71.51
    S. japonicum B65.2
  heart I50.9
  malignant R18.0
  pseudochylous R18.8
  syphilitic A52.74
  tuberculous A18.31
Aseptic — *see* condition
Asherman's syndrome N85.6
Asialia K11.7
Asiatic cholera — *see* Cholera
Asimultagnosia (simultanagnosia) R48.3
Askin's tumor — *see* Neoplasm, connective tissue,
  malignant
Asocial personality F60.2
Asomatognosia R41.4
Aspartylglucosaminuria E77.1
Asperger's disease or syndrome F84.5
Aspergilloma — *see* Aspergillosis
Aspergillosis (with pneumonia) B44.9
  bronchopulmonary, allergic B44.81
  disseminated B44.7
  generalized B44.7
  pulmonary NEC B44.1
    allergic B44.81
    invasive B44.0
  specified NEC B44.89

Aspergillosis — *continued*
  tonsillar B44.2
Aspergillus (flavus) (fumigatus) (infection) (terreus)
  — *see* Aspergillosis
Aspermatogenesis — *see* Azoospermia
Aspermia (testis) — *see* Azoospermia
Asphyxia, asphyxiation (by) R09.01
  antenatal P84
  birth P84
  bunny bag — *see* Asphyxia, due to, mechanical
    threat to breathing, trapped in bed clothes
  crushing S28.0
  drowning T75.1 ☑
  gas, fumes, or vapor — *see* Table of Drugs and
    Chemicals
  inhalation — *see* Inhalation
  intrauterine P84
  local I73.00
    with gangrene I73.01
  mucus (*see also* Foreign body, respiratory tract,
    causing asphyxia)
  newborn P84
  pathological R09.01
  postnatal P84
    mechanical — *see* Asphyxia, due to, mechanical
      threat to breathing
  prenatal P84
  reticularis R23.1
  strangulation — *see* Asphyxia, due to, mechanical
    threat to breathing
  submersion T75.1 ☑
  traumatic T71.9 ☑
    due to
      crushed chest S28.0 ☑
      foreign body (in) — *see* Foreign body,
        respiratory tract, causing asphyxia
      low oxygen content of ambient air T71.20 ☑
        due to
          being trapped in
            low oxygen environment T71.29 ☑
              in car trunk T71.221 ☑
                circumstances undetermined
                  T71.224 ☑
                done with intent to harm by
                  another person T71.223 ☑
                  self T71.222 ☑
              in refrigerator T71.231 ☑
                circumstances undetermined
                  T71.234 ☑
                done with intent to harm by
                  another person T71.233 ☑
                  self T71.232 ☑
        cave-in T71.21 ☑
      mechanical threat to breathing (accidental)
        T71.191 ☑
        circumstances undetermined T71.194 ☑
        done with intent to harm by
          another person T71.193 ☑
          self T71.192 ☑
        hanging T71.161 ☑
        circumstances undetermined T71.164 ☑
        done with intent to harm by
          another person T71.163 ☑
          self T71.162 ☑
        plastic bag T71.121 ☑
        circumstances undetermined T71.124 ☑
        done with intent to harm by
          another person T71.123 ☑
          self T71.122 ☑
        smothering
          in furniture T71.151 ☑
            circumstances undetermined T71.154
              ☑
            done with intent to harm by
              another person T71.153 ☑
              self T71.152 ☑
          under
            another person's body T71.141 ☑
              circumstances undetermined
                T71.144 ☑
              done with intent to harm T71.143 ☑
            pillow T71.111 ☑
              circumstances undetermined
                T71.114 ☑
              done with intent to harm by
                another person T71.113 ☑
              self T71.112 ☑
        trapped in bed clothes T71.131 ☑
        circumstances undetermined T71.134 ☑
        done with intent to harm by
          another person T71.133 ☑
          self T71.132 ☑

Asphyxia — *continued*
  vomiting, vomitus — *see* Foreign body,
    respiratory tract, causing asphyxia
Aspiration
  amniotic (clear) fluid (newborn) P24.10
    with
      pneumonia (pneumonitis) P24.11
      respiratory symptoms P24.11
  blood
    newborn (without respiratory symptoms)
      P24.20
      with
        pneumonia (pneumonitis) P24.21
        respiratory symptoms P24.21
      specified age NEC — *see* Foreign body,
        respiratory tract
  bronchitis J69.0
  food or foreign body (with asphyxiation) — *see*
    Asphyxia, food
  liquor (amnii) (newborn) P24.10
    with
      pneumonia (pneumonitis) P24.11
      respiratory symptoms P24.11
  meconium (newborn) (without respiratory
    symptoms) P24.00
    with
      pneumonitis (pneumonitis) P24.01
      respiratory symptoms P24.01
  milk (newborn) (without respiratory symptoms)
    P24.30
    with
      pneumonia (pneumonitis) P24.31
      respiratory symptoms P24.31
    specified age NEC — *see* Foreign body,
      respiratory tract
  mucus (*see also* Foreign body, by site, causing
    asphyxia)
    newborn P24.10
      with
        pneumonia (pneumonitis) P24.11
        respiratory symptoms P24.11
  neonatal P24.9
    specific NEC (without respiratory symptoms)
      P24.80
      with
        pneumonia (pneumonitis) P24.81
        respiratory symptoms P24.81
  newborn P24.9
    specific NEC (without respiratory symptoms)
      P24.80
      with
        pneumonia (pneumonitis) P24.81
        respiratory symptoms P24.81
  pneumonia J69.0
  pneumonitis J69.0
  syndrome of newborn — *see* Aspiration, by
    substance, with pneumonia
  vernix caseosa (newborn) P24.80
    with
      pneumonia (pneumonitis) P24.81
      respiratory symptoms P24.81
  vomitus (*see also* Foreign body, respiratory tract)
    newborn (without respiratory symptoms)
      P24.30
      with
        pneumonia (pneumonitis) P24.31
        respiratory symptoms P24.31
Asplenia (congenital) Q89.01
  postsurgical Z90.81
Assam fever B55.0
Assault, sexual — *see* Maltreatment
Assmann's focus NEC A15.0
Astasia (-abasia) (hysterical) F44.4
Asteatosis cutis L85.3
Astereognosia, astereognosis R48.1
Asterixis R27.8
  in liver disease K71.3
Asteroid hyalitis — *see* Deposit, crystalline
Asthenia, asthenic R53.1
  cardiac (*see also* Failure, heart) I50.9
    psychogenic F45.8
  cardiovascular (*see also* Failure, heart) I50.9
    psychogenic F45.8
  heart (*see also* Failure, heart) I50.9
    psychogenic F45.8
  hysterical F44.4
  myocardial (*see also* Failure, heart) I50.9
    psychogenic F45.8
  nervous F48.8
  neurocirculatory F45.8
  neurotic F48.8
  psychogenic F48.8

Asthenia — *continued*
  psychoneurotic F48.8
  psychophysiologic F48.8
  reaction (psychophysiologic) F48.8
  senile R54
Asthenopia (*see also* Discomfort, visual)
  hysterical F44.6
  psychogenic F44.6
Asthenospermia — *see* Abnormal, specimen, male
  genital organs
Asthma, asthmatic (bronchial) (catarrh) (spasmodic)
  J45.909
  with
    chronic obstructive bronchitis J44.9
      with
        acute lower respiratory infection J44.0
        exacerbation (acute) J44.1
    chronic obstructive pulmonary disease J44.9
      with
        acute lower respiratory infection J44.0
        exacerbation (acute) J44.1
    exacerbation (acute) J45.901
    hay fever — *see* Asthma, allergic extrinsic
    rhinitis, allergic — *see* Asthma, allergic extrinsic
    status asthmaticus J45.902
  allergic extrinsic J45.909
    with
      exacerbation (acute) J45.901
      status asthmaticus J45.902
  atopic — *see* Asthma, allergic extrinsic
  cardiac — *see* Failure, ventricular, left
  cardiobronchial I50.1
  childhood J45.909
    with
      exacerbation (acute) J45.901
      status asthmaticus J45.902
  chronic obstructive J44.9
    with
      acute lower respiratory infection J44.0
      exacerbation (acute) J44.1
  collier's J60
  cough variant J45.991
  detergent J69.8
  due to
    detergent J69.8
    inhalation of fumes J68.3
  eosinophilic J82
  extrinsic, allergic — *see* Asthma, allergic extrinsic
  grinder's J62.8
  hay — *see* Asthma, allergic extrinsic
  heart I50.1
  idiosyncratic — *see* Asthma, nonallergic
  intermittent (mild) J45.20
    with
      exacerbation (acute) J45.21
      status asthmaticus J45.22
  intrinsic, nonallergic — *see* Asthma, nonallergic
  Kopp's E32.8
  late-onset J45.909
    with
      exacerbation (acute) J45.901
      status asthmaticus J45.902
  mild intermittent J45.20
    with
      exacerbation (acute) J45.21
      status asthmaticus J45.22
  mild persistent J45.30
    with
      exacerbation (acute) J45.31
      status asthmaticus J45.32
  Millar's (laryngismus stridulus) J38.5
  miner's J60
  mixed J45.909
    with
      exacerbation (acute) J45.901
      status asthmaticus J45.902
  moderate persistent J45.40
    with
      exacerbation (acute) J45.41
      status asthmaticus J45.42
  nervous — *see* Asthma, nonallergic
  nonallergic (intrinsic) J45.909
    with
      exacerbation (acute) J45.901
      status asthmaticus J45.902
  persistent
    mild J45.30
      with
        exacerbation (acute) J45.31
        status asthmaticus J45.32
    moderate J45.40
      with

Asthma — *continued*
    exacerbation (acute) J45.41
    status asthmaticus J45.42
  severe J45.50
    with
      exacerbation (acute) J45.51
      status asthmaticus J45.52
  platinum J45.998
  pneumoconiotic NEC J64
  potter's J62.8
  predominantly allergic J45.909
  psychogenic F54
  pulmonary eosinophilic J82
  red cedar J67.8
  Rostan's I50.1
  sandblaster's J62.8
  sequoiosis J67.8
  severe persistent J45.50
    with
      exacerbation (acute) J45.51
      status asthmaticus J45.52
  specified NEC J45.998
  stonemason's J62.8
  thymic E32.8
  tuberculous — *see* Tuberculosis, pulmonary
  Wichmann's (laryngismus stridulus) J38.5
  wood J67.8
Astigmatism (compound) (congenital) H52.20- ☑
  irregular H52.21- ☑
  regular H52.22- ☑
Astraphobia F40.220
Astroblastoma
  specified site — *see* Neoplasm, malignant, by site
  unspecified site C71.9
Astrocytoma (cystic)
  anaplastic
    specified site — *see* Neoplasm, malignant, by
      site
    unspecified site C71.9
  fibrillary
    specified site — *see* Neoplasm, malignant, by
      site
    unspecified site C71.9
  fibrous
    specified site — *see* Neoplasm, malignant, by
      site
    unspecified site C71.9
  gemistocytic
    specified site — *see* Neoplasm, malignant, by
      site
    unspecified site C71.9
  juvenile
    specified site — *see* Neoplasm, malignant, by
      site
    unspecified site C71.9
  pilocytic
    specified site — *see* Neoplasm, malignant, by
      site
    unspecified site C71.9
  piloid
    specified site — *see* Neoplasm, malignant, by
      site
    unspecified site C71.9
  protoplasmic
    specified site — *see* Neoplasm, malignant, by
      site
    unspecified site C71.9
  specified site NEC — *see* Neoplasm, malignant,
    by site
  subependymal D43.2
    giant cell
      specified site — *see* Neoplasm, uncertain
        behavior, by site
      unspecified site D43.2
    specified site — *see* Neoplasm, uncertain
      behavior, by site
    unspecified site D43.2
  unspecified site C71.9
Astroglioma
  specified site — *see* Neoplasm, malignant, by site
  unspecified site C71.9
Asymbolia R48.8
Asymmetry (*see also* Distortion)
  between native and reconstructed breast N65.1
  face Q67.0
  jaw (lower) — *see* Anomaly, dentofacial, jaw-
    cranial base relationship, asymmetry
Asynergia, asynergy R27.8
  ventricular I51.89
Asystole (heart) — *see* Arrest, cardiac
At risk
  for falling Z91.81

☑ **Additional character required**

Ataxia, ataxy, ataxic R27.0
  acute R27.8
  brain (hereditary) G11.9
  cerebellar (hereditary) G11.9
    with defective DNA repair G11.3
    alcoholic G31.2
    early-onset G11.1
    in
      alcoholism G31.2
      myxedema E03.9 [G13.2]
      neoplastic disease (see also Neoplasm) D49.9
        [G13.1]
      specified disease NEC G32.81
    late-onset (Marie's) G11.2
  cerebral (hereditary) G11.9
  congenital nonprogressive G11.0
  family, familial — see Ataxia, hereditary
  following
    cerebrovascular disease I69.993
      cerebral infarction I69.393
      intracerebral hemorrhage I69.193
      nontraumatic intracranial hemorrhage NEC
        I69.293
      specified disease NEC I69.893
      subarachnoid hemorrhage I69.093
  Friedreich's (heredofamilial) (cerebellar) (spinal)
    G11.1
  gait R26.0
    hysterical F44.4
  general R27.8
  gluten M35.9 [G32.81]
    with celiac disease K90.0 [G32.81]
  hereditary G11.9
    with neuropathy G60.2
    cerebellar — see Ataxia, cerebellar
    spastic G11.4
    specified NEC G11.8
    spinal (Friedreich's) G11.1
  heredofamilial — see Ataxia, hereditary
  Hunt's G11.1
  hysterical F44.4
  locomotor (progressive) (syphilitic) (partial)
    (spastic) A52.11
    diabetic — see Diabetes, ataxia
  Marie's (cerebellar) (heredofamilial) (late- onset)
    G11.2
  nonorganic origin F44.4
  nonprogressive, congenital G11.0
  psychogenic F44.4
  Roussy-Lévy G60.0
  Sanger-Brown's (hereditary) G11.2
  spastic hereditary G11.4
  spinal
    hereditary (Friedreich's) G11.1
    progressive (syphilitic) A52.11
  spinocerebellar, X-linked recessive G11.1
  telangiectasia (Louis-Bar) G11.3
Ataxia-telangiectasia (Louis-Bar) G11.3
Atelectasis (massive) (partial) (pressure)
    (pulmonary) J98.11
  newborn P28.10
    due to resorption P28.11
    partial P28.19
    primary P28.0
    secondary P28.19
  primary (newborn) P28.0
  tuberculous — see Tuberculosis, pulmonary
Atelocardia Q24.9
Atelomyelia Q06.1
Atheroembolism
  of
    extremities
      lower I75.02- ☑
      upper I75.01- ☑
    kidney I75.81
    specified NEC I75.89
Atheroma, atheromatous (see also Arteriosclerosis)
    I70.90
  aorta, aortic I70.0
    valve (see also Endocarditis, aortic) I35.8
  aorto-iliac I70.0
  artery — see Arteriosclerosis
  basilar (artery) I67.2
  carotid (artery) (common) (internal) I67.2
  cerebral (arteries) I67.2
  coronary (artery) I25.10
    with angina pectoris — see Arteriosclerosis,
      coronary (artery),
  degeneration — see Arteriosclerosis
  heart, cardiac — see Disease, heart, ischemic,
    atherosclerotic
  mitral (valve) I34.8

Atheroma — continued
  myocardium, myocardial — see Disease, heart,
    ischemic, atherosclerotic
  pulmonary valve (heart) (see also Endocarditis,
    pulmonary) I37.8
  tricuspid (heart) (valve) I36.8
  valve, valvular — see Endocarditis
  vertebral (artery) I67.2
Atheromatosis — see Arteriosclerosis
Atherosclerosis (see also Arteriosclerosis)
  coronary
    artery I25.10
      with angina pectoris — see Arteriosclerosis,
        coronary (artery),
      due to
        calcified coronary lesion (severely) I25.84
        lipid rich plaque I25.83
    transplanted heart I25.811
      bypass graft I25.812
        with angina pectoris — see Arteriosclerosis,
          coronary (artery),
      native coronary artery I25.811
        with angina pectoris — see Arteriosclerosis,
          coronary (artery),
Athetosis (acquired) R25.8
  bilateral (congenital) G80.3
  congenital (bilateral) (double) G80.3
  double (congenital) G80.3
  unilateral R25.8
Athlete's
  foot B35.3
  heart I51.7
Athrepsia E41
Athyrea (acquired) (see also Hypothyroidism)
  congenital E03.1
Atonia, atony, atonic
  bladder (sphincter) (neurogenic) N31.2
  capillary I78.8
  cecum K59.8
    psychogenic F45.8
  colon — see Atony, intestine
  congenital P94.2
  esophagus K22.8
  intestine K59.8
    psychogenic F45.8
  stomach K31.89
    neurotic or psychogenic F45.8
  uterus (during labor) O62.2
    with hemorrhage (postpartum) O72.1
    postpartum (with hemorrhage) O72.1
      without hemorrhage O75.89
Atopy — see History, allergy
Atransferrinemia, congenital E88.09
Atresia, atretic
  alimentary organ or tract NEC Q45.8
    upper Q40.8
  ani, anus, anal (canal) Q42.3
    with fistula Q42.2
  aorta (arch) (ring) Q25.2
  aortic (orifice) (valve) Q23.0
    arch Q25.2
    congenital with hypoplasia of ascending aorta
      and defective development of left ventricle
      (with mitral stenosis) Q23.4
    in hypoplastic left heart syndrome Q23.4
  aqueduct of Sylvius Q03.0
    with spina bifida — see Spina bifida, with
      hydrocephalus
  artery NEC Q27.8
    cerebral Q28.3
    coronary Q24.5
    digestive system Q27.8
    eye Q15.8
    lower limb Q27.8
    pulmonary Q25.5
    specified site NEC Q27.8
    umbilical Q27.0
    upper limb Q27.8
  auditory canal (external) Q16.1
  bile duct (common) (congenital) (hepatic) Q44.2
    acquired — see Obstruction, bile duct
  bladder (neck) Q64.39
    obstruction Q64.31
  bronchus Q32.4
  cecum Q42.8
  cervix (acquired) N88.2
    congenital Q51.828
    in pregnancy or childbirth — see Anomaly,
      cervix, in pregnancy or childbirth
      causing obstructed labor O65.5
  choana Q30.0
  colon Q42.9

Atresia — continued
  specified NEC Q42.8
  common duct Q44.2
  cricoid cartilage Q31.8
  cystic duct Q44.2
    acquired K82.8
      with obstruction K82.0
  digestive organs NEC Q45.8
  duodenum Q41.0
  ear canal Q16.1
  ejaculatory duct Q55.4
  epiglottis Q31.8
  esophagus Q39.0
    with tracheoesophageal fistula Q39.1
  eustachian tube Q17.8
  fallopian tube (congenital) Q50.6
    acquired N97.1
  follicular cyst N83.0
  foramen of
    Luschka Q03.1
      with spina bifida — see Spina bifida, with
        hydrocephalus
    Magendie Q03.1
      with spina bifida — see Spina bifida, with
        hydrocephalus
  gallbladder Q44.1
  genital organ
    external
      female Q52.79
      male Q55.8
    internal
      female Q52.8
      male Q55.8
  glottis Q31.8
  gullet Q39.0
    with tracheoesophageal fistula Q39.1
  heart valve NEC Q24.8
    pulmonary Q22.0
    tricuspid Q22.4
  hymen Q52.3
    acquired (postinfective) N89.6
  ileum Q41.2
  intestine (small) Q41.9
    large Q42.9
      specified NEC Q42.8
  iris, filtration angle Q15.0
  jejunum Q41.1
  lacrimal apparatus Q10.4
  larynx Q31.8
  meatus urinarius Q64.33
  mitral valve Q23.2
    in hypoplastic left heart syndrome Q23.4
  nares (anterior) (posterior) Q30.0
  nasopharynx Q34.8
  nose, nostril Q30.0
    acquired J34.89
  organ or site NEC Q89.8
  osseous meatus (ear) Q16.1
  oviduct (congenital) Q50.6
    acquired N97.1
  parotid duct Q38.4
    acquired K11.8
  pulmonary (artery) Q25.5
    valve Q22.0
  pulmonic Q22.0
  pupil Q13.2
  rectum Q42.1
    with fistula Q42.0
  salivary duct Q38.4
    acquired K11.8
  sublingual duct Q38.4
    acquired K11.8
  submandibular duct Q38.4
    acquired K11.8
  submaxillary duct Q38.4
    acquired K11.8
  thyroid cartilage Q31.8
  trachea Q32.1
  tricuspid valve Q22.4
  ureter Q62.10
    pelvic junction Q62.11
    vesical orifice Q62.12
  ureteropelvic junction Q62.11
  ureterovesical orifice Q62.12
  urethra (valvular) Q64.39
    stricture Q64.32
  urinary tract NEC Q64.8
  uterus Q51.818
    acquired N85.8
  vagina (congenital) Q52.4
    acquired (postinfectional) (senile) N89.5
  vas deferens Q55.3

Atresia — *continued*
  vascular NEC Q27.8
    cerebral Q28.3
    digestive system Q27.8
    lower limb Q27.8
    specified site NEC Q27.8
    upper limb Q27.8
  vein NEC Q27.8
    digestive system Q27.8
    great Q26.8
    lower limb Q27.8
    portal Q26.5
    pulmonary Q26.3
    specified site NEC Q27.8
    upper limb Q27.8
  vena cava (inferior) (superior) Q26.8
  vesicourethral orifice Q64.31
  vulva Q52.79
    acquired N90.5
Atrichia, atrichosis — *see* Alopecia
Atrophia (*see also* Atrophy)
  cutis senilis L90.8
    due to radiation L57.8
  gyrata of choroid and retina H31.23
  senilis R54
    dermatological L90.8
      due to radiation (nonionizing) (solar) L57.8
  unguium L60.3
    congenita Q84.6
Atrophie blanche (en plaque) (de Milian) L95.0
Atrophoderma, atrophodermia (of) L90.9
  diffusum (idiopathic) L90.4
  maculatum L90.8
    et striatum L90.8
      due to syphilis A52.79
    syphilitic A51.39
  neuriticum L90.8
  Pasini and Pierini L90.3
  pigmentosum Q82.1
  reticulatum symmetricum faciei L66.4
  senile L90.8
    due to radiation (nonionizing) (solar) L57.8
  vermiculata (cheeks) L66.4
Atrophy, atrophic (of)
  adrenal (capsule) (gland) E27.49
    primary (autoimmune) E27.1
  alveolar process or ridge (edentulous) K08.20
  anal sphincter (disuse) N81.84
  appendix K38.8
  arteriosclerotic — *see* Arteriosclerosis
  bile duct (common) (hepatic) K83.8
  bladder N32.89
    neurogenic N31.8
  blanche (en plaque) (of Milian) L95.0
  bone (senile) NEC (*see also* Disorder, bone, specified type NEC)
    due to
      tabes dorsalis (neurogenic) A52.11
  brain (cortex) (progressive) G31.9
    frontotemporal circumscribed G31.01 [F02.80]
      with behavioral disturbance G31.01 [F02.81]
    senile NEC G31.1
  breast N64.2
    obstetric — *see* Disorder, breast, specified type NEC
  buccal cavity K13.79
  cardiac — *see* Degeneration, myocardial
  cartilage (infectional) (joint) — *see* Disorder, cartilage, specified NEC
  cerebellar — *see* Atrophy, brain
  cerebral — *see* Atrophy, brain
  cervix (mucosa) (senile) (uteri) N88.8
    menopausal N95.8
  Charcot-Marie-Tooth G60.0
  choroid (central) (macular) (myopic) (retina) H31.10- ☑
    diffuse secondary H31.12- ☑
    gyrate H31.23
    senile H31.11- ☑
  ciliary body — *see* Atrophy, iris
  conjunctiva (senile) H11.89
  corpus cavernosum N48.89
  cortical — *see* Atrophy, brain
  cystic duct K82.8
  Déjérine-Thomas G23.8
  disuse NEC — *see* Atrophy, muscle
  Duchenne-Aran G12.21
  ear H93.8- ☑
  edentulous alveolar ridge K08.20
  endometrium (senile) N85.8
    cervix N88.8
  enteric K63.89

Atrophy — *continued*
  epididymis N50.8
  eyeball — *see* Disorder, globe, degenerated condition, atrophy
  eyelid (senile) — *see* Disorder, eyelid, degenerative
  facial (skin) L90.9
  fallopian tube (senile) N83.32
    with ovary N83.33
  fascioscapulohumeral (Landouzy- Déjérine) G71.0
  fatty, thymus (gland) E32.8
  gallbladder K82.8
  gastric K29.40
    with bleeding K29.41
  gastrointestinal K63.89
  glandular I89.8
  globe H44.52- ☑
  gum K06.0
  hair L67.8
  heart (brown) — *see* Degeneration, myocardial
  hemifacial Q67.4
    Romberg G51.8
  infantile E41
    paralysis, acute — *see* Poliomyelitis, paralytic
  intestine K63.89
  iris (essential) (progressive) H21.26- ☑
    specified NEC H21.29
  kidney (senile) (terminal) (*see also* Sclerosis, renal) N26.1
    congenital or infantile Q60.5
      bilateral Q60.4
      unilateral Q60.3
    hydronephrotic — *see* Hydronephrosis
  lacrimal gland (primary) H04.14- ☑
    secondary H04.15- ☑
  Landouzy-Déjérine G71.0
  laryngitis, infective J37.0
  larynx J38.7
  Leber's optic (hereditary) H47.22
  lip K13.0
  liver (yellow) K72.90
    with coma K72.91
    acute, subacute K72.00
      with coma K72.01
    chronic K72.10
      with coma K72.11
  lung (senile) J98.4
  macular (dermatological) L90.8
    syphilitic, skin A51.39
      striated A52.79
  mandible (edentulous) K08.20
    minimal K08.21
    moderate K08.22
    severe K08.23
  maxilla K08.20
    minimal K08.24
    moderate K08.25
    severe K08.26
  muscle, muscular (diffuse) (general) (idiopathic) (primary) M62.50
    ankle M62.57- ☑
    Duchenne-Aran G12.21
    foot M62.57- ☑
    forearm M62.53- ☑
    hand M62.54- ☑
    infantile spinal G12.0
    lower leg M62.56- ☑
    multiple sites M62.59
    myelopathic — *see* Atrophy, muscle, spinal
    myotonic G71.11
    neuritic G58.9
    neuropathic (peroneal) (progressive) G60.0
    pelvic (disuse) N81.84
    peroneal G60.0
    progressive (bulbar) G12.21
      adult G12.1
      infantile (spinal) G12.0
      spinal G12.9
        adult G12.1
        infantile G12.0
    pseudohypertrophic G71.0
    shoulder region M62.51- ☑
    specified site NEC M62.58
    spinal G12.9
      adult form G12.1
      Aran-Duchenne G12.21
      childhood form, type II G12.1
      distal G12.1
      hereditary NEC G12.1
      infantile, type I (Werdnig-Hoffmann) G12.0

Atrophy — *continued*
    juvenile form, type III (Kugelberg- Welander) G12.1
    progressive G12.21
    scapuloperoneal form G12.1
    specified NEC G12.8
  syphilitic A52.78
  thigh M62.55- ☑
  upper arm M62.52- ☑
  myocardium — *see* Degeneration, myocardial
  myometrium (senile) N85.8
    cervix N88.8
  myopathic NEC — *see* Atrophy, muscle
  myotonia G71.11
  nail L60.3
  nasopharynx J31.1
  nerve (*see also* Disorder, nerve)
    abducens — *see* Strabismus, paralytic, sixth nerve
    accessory G52.8
    acoustic or auditory H93.3
    cranial G52.9
      eighth (auditory) H93.3
      eleventh (accessory) G52.8
      fifth (trigeminal) G50.8
      first (olfactory) G52.0
      fourth (trochlear) — *see* Strabismus, paralytic, fourth nerve
      second (optic) H47.20
      sixth (abducens) — *see* Strabismus, paralytic, sixth nerve
      tenth (pneumogastric) (vagus) G52.2
      third (oculomotor) — *see* Strabismus, paralytic, third nerve
      twelfth (hypoglossal) G52.3
    hypoglossal G52.3
    oculomotor — *see* Strabismus, paralytic, third nerve
    olfactory G52.0
    optic (papillomacular bundle)
      syphilitic (late) A52.15
        congenital A50.44
    pneumogastric G52.2
    trigeminal G50.8
    trochlear — *see* Strabismus, paralytic, fourth nerve
    vagus (pneumogastric) G52.2
  neurogenic, bone, tabetic A52.11
  nutritional E41
  old age R54
  olivopontocerebellar G23.8
  optic (nerve) H47.20
    glaucomatous H47.23- ☑
    hereditary H47.22
    primary H47.21- ☑
    specified type NEC H47.29- ☑
    syphilitic (late) A52.15
      congenital A50.44
  orbit H05.31- ☑
  ovary (senile) N83.31
    with fallopian tube N83.33
  oviduct (senile) — *see* Atrophy, fallopian tube
  palsy, diffuse (progressive) G12.22
  pancreas (duct) (senile) K86.8
  parotid gland K11.0
  pelvic muscle N81.84
  penis N48.89
  pharynx J39.2
  pluriglandular E31.8
    autoimmune E31.0
  polyarthritis M15.9
  prostate N42.89
  pseudohypertrophic (muscle) G71.0
  renal (*see also* Sclerosis, renal) N26.1
  retina, retinal (postinfectional) H35.89
  rhinitis J31.0
  salivary gland K11.0
  scar L90.5
  sclerosis, lobar (of brain) G31.09 [F02.80]
    with behavioral disturbance G31.09 [F02.81]
  scrotum N50.8
  seminal vesicle N50.8
  senile R54
    due to radiation (nonionizing) (solar) L57.8
  skin (patches) (spots) L90.9
    degenerative (senile) L90.8
    due to radiation (nonionizing) (solar) L57.8
    senile L90.8
  spermatic cord N50.8
  spinal (acute) (cord) G95.89
    muscular — *see* Atrophy, muscle, spinal
    paralysis G12.20

☑ **Additional character required**

Atrophy — *continued*
  acute — *see* Poliomyelitis, paralytic
    meaning progressive muscular atrophy
    G12.21
  spine (column) — *see* Spondylopathy, specified
    NEC
  spleen (senile) D73.0
  stomach K29.40
    with bleeding K29.41
  striate (skin) L90.6
    syphilitic A52.79
  subcutaneous L90.9
  sublingual gland K11.0
  submandibular gland K11.0
  submaxillary gland K11.0
  Sudeck's — *see* Algoneurodystrophy
  suprarenal (capsule) (gland) E27.49
    primary E27.1
  systemic affecting central nervous system
    in
      myxedema E03.9 [G13.2]
      neoplastic disease (*see also* Neoplasm) D49.9
      [G13.1]
      specified disease NEC G13.8
  tarso-orbital fascia, congenital Q10.3
  testis N50.0
  thenar, partial — *see* Syndrome, carpal tunnel
  thymus (fatty) E32.8
  thyroid (gland) (acquired) E03.4
    with cretinism E03.1
    congenital (with myxedema) E03.1
  tongue (senile) K14.8
    papillae K14.4
  trachea J39.8
  tunica vaginalis N50.8
  turbinate J34.89
  tympanic membrane (nonflaccid) H73.82- ☑
    flaccid H73.81- ☑
  upper respiratory tract J39.8
  uterus, uterine (senile) N85.8
    cervix N88.8
    due to radiation (intended effect) N85.8
      adverse effect or misadventure N99.89
  vagina (senile) N95.2
  vas deferens N50.8
  vascular I99.8
  vertebra (senile) — *see* Spondylopathy, specified
    NEC
  vulva (senile) N90.5
  Werdnig-Hoffmann G12.0
  yellow — *see* Failure, hepatic
Attack, attacks
  with alteration of consciousness (with
    automatisms) — *see* Epilepsy, localization-
    related, symptomatic, with complex partial
    seizures
  Adams-Stokes I45.9
  akinetic — *see* Epilepsy, generalized, specified
    NEC
  angina — *see* Angina
  atonic — *see* Epilepsy, generalized, specified NEC
  benign shuddering G25.83
  cataleptic — *see* Catalepsy
  coronary — *see* Infarct, myocardium
  cyanotic, newborn P28.2
  drop NEC R55
  epileptic — *see* Epilepsy
  heart — *see* infarct, myocardium
  hysterical F44.9
  jacksonian — *see* Epilepsy, localization-related,
    symptomatic, with simple partial seizures
  myocardium, myocardial — *see* Infarct,
    myocardium
  myoclonic — *see* Epilepsy, generalized, specified
    NEC
  panic F41.0
  psychomotor — *see* Epilepsy, localization-related,
    symptomatic, with complex partial seizures
  salaam — *see* Epilepsy, spasms
  schizophreniform, brief F23
  shuddering, benign G25.83
  Stokes-Adams I45.9
  syncope R55
  transient ischemic (TIA) G45.9
    specified NEC G45.8
  unconsciousness R55
    hysterical F44.89
  vasomotor R55
  vasovagal (paroxysmal) (idiopathic) R55
  without alteration of consciousness — *see*
    Epilepsy, localization-related, symptomatic,
    with simple partial seizures

Attention (to)
  artificial
    opening (of) Z43.9
      digestive tract NEC Z43.4
        colon Z43.3
        ilium Z43.2
        stomach Z43.1
      specified NEC Z43.8
      trachea Z43.0
      urinary tract NEC Z43.6
        cystostomy Z43.5
        nephrostomy Z43.6
        ureterostomy Z43.6
        urethrostomy Z43.6
      vagina Z43.7
  colostomy Z43.3
  cystostomy Z43.5
  deficit disorder or syndrome F98.8
    with hyperactivity — *see* Disorder, attention-
      deficit hyperactivity
  gastrostomy Z43.1
  ileostomy Z43.2
  jejunostomy Z43.4
  nephrostomy Z43.6
  surgical dressings Z48.01
  sutures Z48.02
  tracheostomy Z43.0
  ureterostomy Z43.6
  urethrostomy Z43.6
Attrition
  gum K06.0
  tooth, teeth (excessive) (hard tissues) K03.0
Atypical, atypism (*see also* condition)
  cells (on cytolgocial smear) (endocervical)
    (endometrial) (glandular)
    cervix R87.619
    vagina R87.629
  cervical N87.9
  endometrium N85.9
    hyperplasia N85.00
  parenting situation Z62.9
Auditory — *see* condition
Aujeszky's disease B33.8
Aurantiasis, cutis E67.1
Auricle, auricular (*see also* condition)
  cervical Q18.2
Auriculotemporal syndrome G50.8
Austin Flint murmur (aortic insufficiency) I35.1
Australian
  Q fever A78
  X disease A83.4
Autism, autistic (childhood) (infantile) F84.0
  atypical F84.9
Autodigestion R68.89
Autoerythrocyte sensitization (syndrome) D69.2
Autographism L50.3
Autoimmune
  disease (systemic) M35.9
  inhibitors to clotting factors D68.311
  lymphoproliferative syndrome [ALPS] D89.82
  thyroiditis E06.3
Autointoxication R68.89
Automatism G93.89
  with temporal sclerosis G93.81
  epileptic — *see* Epilepsy, localization-related,
    symptomatic, with complex partial seizures
  paroxysmal, idiopathic — *see* Epilepsy,
    localization-related, symptomatic, with
    complex partial seizures
Autonomic, autonomous
  bladder (neurogenic) N31.2
  hysteria seizure F44.5
Autosensitivity, erythrocyte D69.2
Autosensitization, cutaneous L30.2
Autosome — *see* condition by chromosome
  involved
Autotopagnosia R48.1
Autotoxemia R68.89
Autumn — *see* condition
Avellis' syndrome G46.8
Aversion
  oral R63.3
    newborn P92.- ☑
    nonorganic origin F98.2 ☑
  sexual F52.1
Aviator's
  disease or sickness — *see* Effect, adverse, high
    altitude
  ear T70.0 ☑
Avitaminosis (multiple) (*see also* Deficiency,
  vitamin) E56.9
  B E53.9

Avitaminosis — *continued*
  with
    beriberi E51.11
    pellagra E52
  B2 E53.0
  B6 E53.1
  B12 E53.8
  D E55.9
    with rickets E55.0
  G E53.0
  K E56.1
  nicotinic acid E52
AVNRT (atrioventricular nodal re-entrant
tachycardia) I47.1
AVRT (atrioventricular nodal re-entrant tachycardia)
I47.1
Avulsion (traumatic)
  blood vessel — *see* Injury, blood vessel
  bone — *see* Fracture, by site
  cartilage (*see also* Dislocation, by site)
    symphyseal (inner), complicating delivery
    O71.6
  external site other than limb — *see* Wound,
    open, by site
  eye S05.7-
  head (intracranial)
    external site NEC S08.89 ☑
    scalp S08.0 ☑
  internal organ or site — *see* Injury, by site
  joint (*see also* Dislocation, by site)
    capsule — *see* Sprain, by site
  kidney S37.06-
  ligament — *see* Sprain, by site
  limb (*see also* Amputation, traumatic, by site)
    skin and subcutaneous tissue — *see* Wound,
    open, by site
  muscle — *see* Injury, muscle
  nerve (root) — *see* Injury, nerve
  scalp S08.0 ☑
  skin and subcutaneous tissue — *see* Wound,
    open, by site
  spleen S36.032 ☑
  symphyseal cartilage (inner), complicating
    delivery O71.6
  tendon — *see* Injury, muscle
  tooth S03.2 ☑
Awareness of heart beat R00.2
Axenfeld's
  anomaly or syndrome Q15.0
  degeneration (calcareous) Q13.4
Axilla, axillary (*see also* condition)
  breast Q83.1
Axonotmesis — *see* Injury, nerve
Ayerza's disease or syndrome (pulmonary artery
sclerosis with pulmonary hypertension) I27.0
Azoospermia (organic) N46.01
  due to
    drug therapy N46.021
    efferent duct obstruction N46.023
    infection N46.022
    radiation N46.024
    specified cause NEC N46.029
    systemic disease N46.025
Azotemia R79.89
  meaning uremia N19
Aztec ear Q17.3
Azygos
  continuation inferior vena cava Q26.8
  lobe (lung) Q33.1

B

Baastrup's disease — *see* Kissing spine
Babesiosis B60.0
Babington's disease (familial hemorrhagic telangiectasia) I78.0
Babinski's syndrome A52.79
Baby
  crying constantly R68.11
  floppy (syndrome) P94.2
Bacillary — *see* condition
Bacilluria N39.0
Bacillus (*see also* Infection, bacillus)
  abortus infection A23.1
  anthracis infection A22.9
  coli infection (*see also* Escherichia coli) B96.20
  Flexner's A03.1
  mallei infection A24.0
  Shiga's A03.0
  suipestifer infection — *see* Infection, salmonella
Back — *see* condition
Backache (postural) M54.9
  sacroiliac M53.3
  specified NEC M54.89
Backflow — *see* Reflux
Backward reading (dyslexia) F81.0
Bacteremia R78.81
  with sepsis — *see* Sepsis
Bactericholia — *see* Cholecystitis, acute
Bacterid, bacteride (pustular) L40.3
Bacterium, bacteria, bacterial
  agent NEC, as cause of disease classified elsewhere B96.89
  in blood — *see* Bacteremia
  in urine — *see* Bacteriuria
Bacteriuria, bacteruria N39.0
  asymptomatic N39.0
Bacteroides
  fragilis, as cause of disease classified elsewhere B96.6
Bad
  heart — *see* Disease, heart
  trip
    due to drug abuse — *see* Abuse, drug, hallucinogen
    due to drug dependence — *see* Dependence, drug, hallucinogen
Baelz's disease (cheilitis glandularis apostematosa) K13.0
Baerensprung's disease (eczema marginatum) B35.6
Bagasse disease or pneumonitis J67.1
Bagassosis J67.1
Baker's cyst — *see* Cyst, Baker's
Bakwin-Krida syndrome (craniometaphyseal dysplasia) Q78.5
Balancing side interference M26.56
Balanitis (circinata) (erosiva) (gangrenosa) (phagedenic) (vulgaris) N48.1
  amebic A06.82
  candidal B37.42
  due to Haemophilus ducreyi A57
  gonococcal (acute) (chronic) A54.09
  xerotica obliterans N48.0
Balanoposthitis N47.6
  gonococcal (acute) (chronic) A54.09
  ulcerative (specific) A63.8
Balanorrhagia — *see* Balanitis
Balantidiasis, balantidiosis A07.0
Bald tongue K14.4
Baldness (*see also* Alopecia)
  male-pattern — *see* Alopecia, androgenic
Balkan grippe A78
Balloon disease — *see* Effect, adverse, high altitude
Balo's disease (concentric sclerosis) G37.5
Bamberger-Marie disease — *see* Osteoarthropathy, hypertrophic, specified type NEC
Bancroft's filariasis B74.0
Band (s)
  adhesive — *see* Adhesions, peritoneum
  anomalous or congenital (*see also* Anomaly, by site)
    heart (atrial) (ventricular) Q24.8
    intestine Q43.3
    omentum Q43.3
  cervix N88.1
  constricting, congenital Q79.8
  gallbladder (congenital) Q44.1
  intestinal (adhesive) — *see* Adhesions, peritoneum
  obstructive

Band — *continued*
    intestine K56.5
    peritoneum K56.5
  periappendiceal, congenital Q43.3
  peritoneal (adhesive) — *see* Adhesions, peritoneum
  uterus N73.6
    internal N85.6
  vagina N89.5
Bandemia D72.825
Bandl's ring (contraction), complicating delivery O62.4
Bangkok hemorrhagic fever A91
Bang's disease (brucella abortus) A23.1
Bankruptcy, anxiety concerning Z59.8
Bannister's disease T78.3 ☑
  hereditary D84.1
Banti's disease or syndrome (with cirrhosis) (with portal hypertension) K76.6
Bar, median, prostate — *see* Enlargement, enlarged, prostate
Barcoo disease or rot — *see* Ulcer, skin
Barlow's disease E54
Barodontalgia T70.29 ☑
Baron Münchausen syndrome — *see* Disorder, factitious
Barosinusitis T70.1 ☑
Barotitis T70.0 ☑
Barotrauma T70.29 ☑
  odontalgia T70.29 ☑
  otitic T70.0 ☑
  sinus T70.1 ☑
Barraquer (-Simons) disease or syndrome (progressive lipodystrophy) E88.1
Barré-Guillain disease or syndrome G61.0
Barré-Liéou syndrome (posterior cervical sympathetic) M53.0
Barrel chest M95.4
Barrett's
  disease — *see* Barrett's, esophagus
  esophagus K22.70
    with dysplasia K22.719
      high grade K22.711
      low grade K22.710
    without dysplasia K22.70
  syndrome — *see* Barrett's, esophagus
  ulcer K22.10
    with bleeding K22.11
    without bleeding K22.10
Bársony (-Polgár) (-Teschendorf) syndrome (corkscrew esophagus) K22.4
Bartholinitis (suppurating) N75.8
  gonococcal (acute) (chronic) (with abscess) A54.1
Barth syndrome E78.71
Bartonellosis A44.9
  cutaneous A44.1
  mucocutaneous A44.1
  specified NEC A44.8
  systemic A44.0
Barton's fracture S52.56- ☑
Bartter's syndrome E26.81
Basal — *see* condition
Basan's (hidrotic) ectodermal dysplasia Q82.4
Baseball finger — *see* Dislocation, finger
Basedow's disease (exophthalmic goiter) — *see* Hyperthyroidism, with, goiter
Basic — *see* condition
Basilar — *see* condition
Bason's (hidrotic) ectodermal dysplasia Q82.4
Basopenia — *see* Agranulocytosis
Basophilia D72.824
Basophilism (cortico-adrenal) (Cushing's) (pituitary) E24.0
Bassen-Kornzweig disease or syndrome E78.6
Bat ear Q17.5
Bateman's
  disease B08.1
  purpura (senile) D69.2
Bathing cramp T75.1 ☑
Bathophobia F40.248
Batten (-Mayou) disease E75.4
  retina E75.4 [H36]
Batten-Steinert syndrome G71.11
Battered — *see* Maltreatment
Battey Mycobacterium infection A31.0
Battle exhaustion F43.0
Battledore placenta O43.19- ☑
Baumgarten-Cruveilhier cirrhosis, disease or syndrome K74.69
Bauxite fibrosis (of lung) J63.1
Bayle's disease (general paresis) A52.17
Bazin's disease (primary) (tuberculous) A18.4

Beach ear — *see* Swimmer's, ear
Beaded hair (congenital) Q84.1
Béal conjunctivitis or syndrome B30.2
Beard's disease (neurasthenia) F48.8
Beat (s)
  atrial, premature I49.1
  ectopic I49.49
  elbow — *see* Bursitis, elbow
  escaped, heart I49.49
  hand — *see* Bursitis, hand
  knee — *see* Bursitis, knee
  premature I49.40
    atrial I49.1
    auricular I49.1
    supraventricular I49.1
Beau's
  disease or syndrome — *see* Degeneration, myocardial
  lines (transverse furrows on fingernails) L60.4
Bechterev's syndrome — *see* Spondylitis, ankylosing
Beck's syndrome (anterior spinal artery occlusion) I65.8
Becker's
  cardiomyopathy I42.8
  disease
    idiopathic mural endomyocardial disease I42.3
    myotonia congenita, recessive form G71.12
  dystrophy G71.0
  pigmented hairy nevus D22.5
Beckwith-Wiedemann syndrome Q87.3
Bed confinement status Z74.01
Bed sore — *see* Ulcer, pressure, by site
Bedbug bite (s) — *see* Bite(s), by site, superficial, insect
Bedclothes, asphyxiation or suffocation by — *see* Asphyxia, traumatic, due to, mechanical, trapped
Bednar's
  aphthae K12.0
  tumor — *see* Neoplasm, malignant, by site
Bedridden Z74.01
Bedsore — *see* Ulcer, pressure, by site
Bedwetting — *see* Enuresis
Bee sting (with allergic or anaphylactic shock) — *see* Toxicity, venom, arthropod, bee
Beer drinker's heart (disease) I42.6
Begbie's disease (exophthalmic goiter) — *see* Hyperthyroidism, with, goiter
Behavior
  antisocial
    adult Z72.811
    child or adolescent Z72.810
  disorder, disturbance — *see* Disorder, conduct
  disruptive — *see* Disorder, conduct
  drug seeking Z72.89
  inexplicable R46.2
  marked evasiveness R46.5
  obsessive-compulsive R46.81
  overactivity R46.3
  poor responsiveness R46.4
  self-damaging (life-style) Z72.89
  sleep-incompatible Z72.821
  slowness R46.4
  specified NEC R46.89
  strange (and inexplicable) R46.2
  suspiciousness R46.5
  type A pattern Z73.1
  undue concern or preoccupation with stressful events R46.6
  verbosity and circumstantial detail obscuring reason for contact R46.7
Behçet's disease or syndrome M35.2
Behr's disease — *see* Degeneration, macula
Beigel's disease or morbus (white piedra) B36.2
Bejel A65
Bekhterev's syndrome — *see* Spondylitis, ankylosing
Belching — *see* Eructation
Bell's
  mania F30.8
  palsy, paralysis G51.0
    infant or newborn P11.3
  spasm G51.3
Bence Jones albuminuria or proteinuria NEC R80.3
Bends T70.3 ☑
Benedikt's paralysis or syndrome G46.3
Benign (*see also* condition)
  prostatic hyperplasia — *see* Hyperplasia, prostate
Bennett's fracture (displaced) S62.21- ☑
Benson's disease — *see* Deposit, crystalline
Bent
  back (hysterical) F44.4
  nose M95.0

☑ **Additional character required**

Bent — *continued*
　　congenital Q67.4
Bereavement (uncomplicated) Z63.4
Bergeron's disease (hysterical chorea) F44.4
Berger's disease — *see* Nephropathy, IgA
Beriberi (dry) E51.11
　　heart (disease) E51.12
　　polyneuropathy E51.11
　　wet E51.12
　　　　involving circulatory system E51.11
Berlin's disease or edema (traumatic) S05.8X- ☑
Berlock (berloque) dermatitis L56.2
Bernard-Horner syndrome G90.2
Bernard-Soulier disease or thrombopathia D69.1
Bernhardt (-Roth) disease — *see* Mononeuropathy, lower limb, meralgia paresthetica
Bernheim's syndrome — *see* Failure, heart, congestive
Bertielliasis B71.8
Berylliosis (lung) J63.2
Besnier-Boeck (-Schaumann) disease — *see* Sarcoidosis
Besnier's
　　lupus pernio D86.3
　　prurigo L20.0
Bestiality F65.89
Best's disease H35.50
Beta-mercaptolactate-cysteine disulfiduria E72.09
Betalipoproteinemia, broad or floating E78.2
Betting and gambling Z72.6
　　pathological (compulsive) F63.0
Bezoar T18.9 ☑
　　intestine T18.3 ☑
　　stomach T18.2 ☑
Bezold's abscess — *see* Mastoiditis, acute
Bianchi's syndrome R48.8
Bicornate or bicornis uterus Q51.3
　　in pregnancy or childbirth O34.59- ☑
　　　　causing obstructed labor O65.5
Bicuspid aortic valve Q23.1
Biedl-Bardet syndrome Q87.89
Bielschowsky (-Jansky) disease E75.4
Biermer's (pernicious) anemia or disease D51.0
Biett's disease L93.0
Bifid (congenital)
　　apex, heart Q24.8
　　clitoris Q52.6
　　kidney Q63.8
　　nose Q30.2
　　patella Q74.1
　　scrotum Q55.29
　　toe NEC Q74.2
　　tongue Q38.3
　　ureter Q62.8
　　uterus Q51.3
　　uvula Q35.7
Biforis uterus (suprasimplex) Q51.3
Bifurcation (congenital)
　　gallbladder Q44.1
　　kidney pelvis Q63.8
　　renal pelvis Q63.8
　　rib Q76.6
　　tongue, congenital Q38.3
　　trachea Q32.1
　　ureter Q62.8
　　urethra Q64.74
　　vertebra Q76.49
Big spleen syndrome D73.1
Bigeminal pulse R00.8
Bilateral — *see* condition
Bile
　　duct — *see* condition
　　pigments in urine R82.2
Bilharziasis (*see also* Schistosomiasis)
　　chyluria B65.0
　　cutaneous B65.3
　　galacturia B65.0
　　hematochyluria B65.0
　　intestinal B65.1
　　lipemia B65.9
　　lipuria B65.0
　　oriental B65.2
　　piarhemia B65.9
　　pulmonary NOS B65.9 [J99]
　　　　pneumonia B65.9 [J17]
　　tropical hematuria B65.0
　　vesical B65.0
Biliary — *see* condition
Bilirubin metabolism disorder E80.7
　　specified NEC E80.6
Bilirubinemia, familial nonhemolytic E80.4
Bilirubinuria R82.2

Biliuria R82.2
Bilocular stomach K31.2
Binswanger's disease I67.3
Biparta, bipartite
　　carpal scaphoid Q74.0
　　patella Q74.1
　　vagina Q52.10
Bird
　　face Q75.8
　　fancier's disease or lung J67.2
Birt-Hogg-Dube syndrome Q87.89
Birth
　　complications in mother — *see* Delivery, complicated
　　compression during NOS P15.9
　　defect — *see* Anomaly
　　immature (less than 37 completed weeks) — *see* Preterm, newborn
　　　　extremely (less than 28 completed weeks) — *see* Immaturity, extreme
　　inattention, at or after — *see* Maltreatment, child, neglect
　　injury NOS P15.9
　　　　basal ganglia P11.1
　　　　brachial plexus NEC P14.3
　　　　brain (compression) (pressure) P11.2
　　　　central nervous system NOS P11.9
　　　　cerebellum P11.1
　　　　cerebral hemorrhage P10.1
　　　　external genitalia P15.5
　　　　eye P15.3
　　　　face P15.4
　　　　fracture
　　　　　　bone P13.9
　　　　　　　　specified NEC P13.8
　　　　　　clavicle P13.4
　　　　　　femur P13.2
　　　　　　humerus P13.3
　　　　　　long bone, except femur P13.3
　　　　　　radius and ulna P13.3
　　　　　　skull P13.0
　　　　　　spine P11.5
　　　　　　tibia and fibula P13.3
　　　　intracranial P11.2
　　　　　　laceration or hemorrhage P10.9
　　　　　　　　specified NEC P10.8
　　　　　　intraventricular hemorrhage P10.2
　　　　laceration
　　　　　　brain P10.1
　　　　　　by scalpel P15.8
　　　　　　peripheral nerve P14.9
　　　　liver P15.0
　　　　meninges
　　　　　　brain P11.1
　　　　　　spinal cord P11.5
　　　　nerve
　　　　　　brachial plexus P14.3
　　　　　　cranial NEC (except facial) P11.4
　　　　　　facial P11.3
　　　　　　peripheral P14.9
　　　　　　phrenic (paralysis) P14.2
　　　　paralysis
　　　　　　facial nerve P11.3
　　　　　　spinal P11.5
　　　　penis P15.5
　　　　rupture
　　　　　　spinal cord P11.5
　　　　scalp P12.9
　　　　scalpel wound P15.8
　　　　scrotum P15.5
　　　　skull NEC P13.1
　　　　　　fracture P13.0
　　　　specified type NEC P15.8
　　　　spinal cord P11.5
　　　　spine P11.5
　　　　spleen P15.1
　　　　sternomastoid (hematoma) P15.2
　　　　subarachnoid hemorrhage P10.3
　　　　subcutaneous fat necrosis P15.6
　　　　subdural hemorrhage P10.0
　　　　tentorial tear P10.4
　　　　testes P15.5
　　　　vulva P15.5
　　lack of care, at or after — *see* Maltreatment, child, neglect
　　neglect, at or after — *see* Maltreatment, child, neglect
　　palsy or paralysis, newborn, NOS (birth injury) P14.9
　　premature (infant) — *see* Preterm, newborn
　　shock, newborn P96.89
　　trauma — *see* Birth, injury

Birth — *continued*
　　weight
　　　　low (2499 grams or less) — *see* Low, birthweight
　　　　　　extremely (999 grams or less) — *see* Low, birthweight, extreme
　　　　4000 grams to 4499 grams P08.1
　　　　4500 grams or more P08.0
Birthmark Q82.5
Bisalbuminemia E88.09
Biskra's button B55.1
Bite (s) (animal) (human)
　　abdomen, abdominal
　　　　wall S31.159 ☑
　　　　　　with penetration into peritoneal cavity S31.659 ☑
　　　　　　epigastric region S31.152 ☑
　　　　　　　　with penetration into peritoneal cavity S31.652 ☑
　　　　　　left
　　　　　　　　lower quadrant S31.154 ☑
　　　　　　　　　　with penetration into peritoneal cavity S31.654 ☑
　　　　　　　　upper quadrant S31.151 ☑
　　　　　　　　　　with penetration into peritoneal cavity S31.651 ☑
　　　　　　periumbilic region S31.155 ☑
　　　　　　　　with penetration into peritoneal cavity S31.655 ☑
　　　　　　right
　　　　　　　　lower quadrant S31.153 ☑
　　　　　　　　　　with penetration into peritoneal cavity S31.653 ☑
　　　　　　　　upper quadrant S31.150 ☑
　　　　　　　　　　with penetration into peritoneal cavity S31.650 ☑
　　　　　　superficial NEC S30.871 ☑
　　　　　　　　insect S30.861 ☑
　　alveolar (process) — *see* Bite, oral cavity
　　amphibian (venomous) — *see* Venom, bite, amphibian
　　animal (*see also* Bite, by site)
　　　　venomous — *see* Venom
　　ankle S91.05- ☑
　　　　superficial NEC S90.57- ☑
　　　　　　insect S90.56- ☑
　　antecubital space — *see* Bite, elbow
　　anus S31.835 ☑
　　　　superficial NEC S30.877 ☑
　　　　　　insect S30.867 ☑
　　arm (upper) S41.15- ☑
　　　　lower — *see* Bite, forearm
　　　　superficial NEC S40.87- ☑
　　　　　　insect S40.86- ☑
　　arthropod NEC — *see* Venom, bite, arthropod
　　auditory canal (external) (meatus) — *see* Bite, ear
　　auricle, ear — *see* Bite, ear
　　axilla — *see* Bite, arm
　　back (*see also* Bite, thorax, back)
　　　　lower S31.050 ☑
　　　　　　with penetration into retroperitoneal space S31.051 ☑
　　　　　　superficial NEC S30.870 ☑
　　　　　　　　insect S30.860 ☑
　　bedbug — *see* Bite(s), by site, superficial, insect
　　breast S21.05- ☑
　　　　superficial NEC S20.17- ☑
　　　　　　insect S20.16- ☑
　　brow — *see* Bite, head, specified site NEC
　　buttock S31.805 ☑
　　　　left S31.825 ☑
　　　　right S31.815 ☑
　　　　superficial NEC S30.870 ☑
　　　　　　insect S30.860 ☑
　　calf — *see* Bite, leg
　　canaliculus lacrimalis — *see* Bite, eyelid
　　canthus, eye — *see* Bite, eyelid
　　centipede — *see* Toxicity, venom, arthropod, centipede
　　cheek (external) S01.45- ☑
　　　　superficial NEC S00.87 ☑
　　　　　　insect S00.86 ☑
　　　　internal — *see* Bite, oral cavity
　　chest wall — *see* Bite, thorax
　　chigger B88.0
　　chin — *see* Bite, head, specified site NEC
　　clitoris — *see* Bite, vulva
　　costal region — *see* Bite, thorax
　　digit (s)
　　　　hand — *see* Bite, finger
　　　　toe — *see* Bite, toe
　　ear (canal) (external) S01.35- ☑

Bite — continued
superficial NEC S00.47- ☑
insect S00.46- ☑
elbow S51.05- ☑
superficial NEC S50.37- ☑
insect S50.36- ☑
epididymis — see Bite, testis
epigastric region — see Bite, abdomen
epiglottis — see Bite, neck, specified site NEC
esophagus, cervical S11.25 ☑
superficial NEC S10.17 ☑
insect S10.16 ☑
eyebrow — see Bite, eyelid
eyelid S01.15- ☑
superficial NEC S00.27- ☑
insect S00.26- ☑
face NEC — see Bite, head, specified site NEC
finger (s) S61.259 ☑
with
damage to nail S61.359 ☑
index S61.258 ☑
with
damage to nail S61.358 ☑
left S61.251 ☑
with
damage to nail S61.351 ☑
right S61.250 ☑
with
damage to nail S61.350 ☑
superficial NEC S60.478 ☑
insect S60.46- ☑
little S61.25- ☑
with
damage to nail S61.35- ☑
superficial NEC S60.47- ☑
insect S60.46- ☑
middle S61.25- ☑
with
damage to nail S61.35- ☑
superficial NEC S60.47- ☑
insect S60.46- ☑
ring S61.25- ☑
with
damage to nail S61.35- ☑
superficial NEC S60.47- ☑
insect S60.46- ☑
superficial NEC S60.479 ☑
insect S60.469 ☑
thumb — see Bite, thumb
flank — see Bite, abdomen, wall
flea — see Bite, by site, superficial, insect
foot (except toe(s) alone) S91.35- ☑
superficial NEC S90.87- ☑
insect S90.86- ☑
toe — see Bite, toe
forearm S51.85- ☑
elbow only — see Bite, elbow
superficial NEC S50.87- ☑
insect S50.86- ☑
forehead — see Bite, head, specified site NEC
genital organs, external
female S31.552 ☑
superficial NEC S30.876 ☑
insect S30.866 ☑
vagina and vulva — see Bite, vulva
male S31.551 ☑
penis — see Bite, penis
scrotum — see Bite, scrotum
superficial NEC S30.875 ☑
insect S30.865 ☑
testes — see Bite, testis
groin — see Bite, abdomen, wall
gum — see Bite, oral cavity
hand S61.45- ☑
finger — see Bite, finger
superficial NEC S60.57- ☑
insect S60.56- ☑
thumb — see Bite, thumb
head S01.95 ☑
cheek — see Bite, cheek
ear — see Bite, ear
eyelid — see Bite, eyelid
lip — see Bite, lip
nose — see Bite, nose
oral cavity — see Bite, oral cavity
scalp — see Bite, scalp
specified site NEC S01.85 ☑
superficial NEC S00.87 ☑
insect S00.86 ☑
superficial NEC S00.97 ☑
insect S00.96 ☑
temporomandibular area — see Bite, cheek

Bite — continued
heel — see Bite, foot
hip S71.05- ☑
superficial NEC S70.27- ☑
insect S70.26- ☑
hymen S31.45 ☑
hypochondrium — see Bite, abdomen, wall
hypogastric region — see Bite, abdomen, wall
inguinal region — see Bite, abdomen, wall
insect — see Bite, by site, superficial, insect
instep — see Bite, foot
interscapular region — see Bite, thorax, back
jaw — see Bite, head, specified site NEC
knee S81.05- ☑
superficial NEC S80.27- ☑
insect S80.26- ☑
labium (majus) (minus) — see Bite, vulva
lacrimal duct — see Bite, eyelid
larynx S11.015 ☑
superficial NEC S10.17 ☑
insect S10.16 ☑
leg (lower) S81.85- ☑
ankle — see Bite, ankle
foot — see Bite, foot
knee — see Bite, knee
superficial NEC S80.87- ☑
insect S80.86- ☑
toe — see Bite, toe
upper — see Bite, thigh
lip S01.551 ☑
superficial NEC S00.571 ☑
insect S00.561 ☑
lizard (venomous) — see Venom, bite, reptile
loin — see Bite, abdomen, wall
lower back — see Bite, back, lower
lumbar region — see Bite, back, lower
malar region — see Bite, head, specified site NEC
mammary — see Bite, breast
marine animals (venomous) — see Toxicity,
venom, marine animal
mastoid region — see Bite, head, specified site
NEC
mouth — see Bite, oral cavity
nail
finger — see Bite, finger
toe — see Bite, toe
nape — see Bite, neck, specified site NEC
nasal (septum) (sinus) — see Bite, nose
nasopharynx — see Bite, head, specified site NEC
neck S11.95 ☑
involving
cervical esophagus — see Bite, esophagus,
cervical
larynx — see Bite, larynx
pharynx — see Bite, pharynx
thyroid gland S11.15 ☑
trachea — see Bite, trachea
specified site NEC S11.85 ☑
superficial NEC S10.87 ☑
insect S10.86 ☑
superficial NEC S10.97 ☑
insect S10.96 ☑
throat S11.85 ☑
superficial NEC S10.17 ☑
insect S10.16 ☑
nose (septum) (sinus) S01.25 ☑
superficial NEC S00.37 ☑
insect S00.36 ☑
occipital region — see Bite, scalp
oral cavity S01.552 ☑
superficial NEC S00.572 ☑
insect S00.562 ☑
orbital region — see Bite, eyelid
palate — see Bite, oral cavity
palm — see Bite, hand
parietal region — see Bite, scalp
pelvis S31.050 ☑
with penetration into retroperitoneal space
S31.051 ☑
superficial NEC S30.870 ☑
insect S30.860 ☑
penis S31.25 ☑
superficial NEC S30.872 ☑
insect S30.862 ☑
perineum
female — see Bite, vulva
male — see Bite, pelvis
periocular area (with or without lacrimal
passages) — see Bite, eyelid
phalanges
finger — see Bite, finger
toe — see Bite, toe

Bite — continued
pharynx S11.25 ☑
superficial NEC S10.17 ☑
insect S10.16 ☑
pinna — see Bite, ear
poisonous — see Venom
popliteal space — see Bite, knee
prepuce — see Bite, penis
pubic region — see Bite, abdomen, wall
rectovaginal septum — see Bite, vulva
red bug B88.0
reptile NEC (see also Venom, bite, reptile)
nonvenomous — see Bite, by site
snake — see Venom, bite, snake
sacral region — see Bite, back, lower
sacroiliac region — see Bite, back, lower
salivary gland — see Bite, oral cavity
scalp S01.05 ☑
superficial NEC S00.07 ☑
insect S00.06 ☑
scapular region — see Bite, shoulder
scrotum S31.35 ☑
superficial NEC S30.873 ☑
insect S30.863 ☑
sea-snake (venomous) — see Toxicity, venom,
snake, sea snake
shin — see Bite, leg
shoulder S41.05- ☑
superficial NEC S40.27- ☑
insect S40.26- ☑
snake (see also Venom, bite, snake)
nonvenomous — see Bite, by site
spermatic cord — see Bite, testis
spider (venomous) — see Toxicity, venom, spider
nonvenomous — see Bite, by site, superficial,
insect
sternal region — see Bite, thorax, front
submaxillary region — see Bite, head, specified
site NEC
submental region — see Bite, head, specified
site NEC
subungual
finger (s) — see Bite, finger
toe — see Bite, toe
superficial — see Bite, by site, superficial
supraclavicular fossa S11.85 ☑
supraorbital — see Bite, head, specified site NEC
temple, temporal region — see Bite, head,
specified site NEC
temporomandibular area — see Bite, cheek
testis S31.35 ☑
superficial NEC S30.873 ☑
insect S30.863 ☑
thigh S71.15- ☑
superficial NEC S70.37- ☑
insect S70.36- ☑
thorax, thoracic (wall) S21.95 ☑
back S21.25- ☑
with penetration into thoracic cavity S21.45- ☑
breast — see Bite, breast
front S21.15- ☑
with penetration into thoracic cavity S21.35- ☑
superficial NEC S20.97 ☑
back S20.47- ☑
front S20.37- ☑
insect S20.96 ☑
back S20.46- ☑
front S20.36- ☑
throat — see Bite, neck, throat
thumb S61.05- ☑
with
damage to nail S61.15- ☑
superficial NEC S60.37- ☑
insect S60.36- ☑
thyroid S11.15 ☑
superficial NEC S10.87 ☑
insect S10.86 ☑
toe (s) S91.15- ☑
with
damage to nail S91.25- ☑
great S91.15- ☑
with
damage to nail S91.25- ☑
lesser S91.15- ☑
with
damage to nail S91.25- ☑
superficial NEC S90.47- ☑
great S90.47- ☑
insect S90.46- ☑
great S90.46- ☑
tongue S01.552 ☑
trachea S11.025 ☑

Bite — *continued*
　superficial NEC S10.17 ☑
　　insect S10.16 ☑
　tunica vaginalis — *see* Bite, testis
　tympanum, tympanic membrane — *see* Bite, ear
　umbilical region S31.155 ☑
　uvula — *see* Bite, oral cavity
　vagina — *see* Bite, vulva
　venomous — *see* Venom
　vocal cords S11.035 ☑
　　superficial NEC S10.17 ☑
　　　insect S10.16 ☑
　vulva S31.45 ☑
　　superficial NEC S30.874 ☑
　　　insect S30.864 ☑
　wrist S61.55- ☑
　　superficial NEC S60.87- ☑
　　　insect S60.86- ☑
Biting, cheek or lip K13.1
Biventricular failure (heart) I50.9
Björck (-Thorson) syndrome (malignant carcinoid) E34.0
Black
　death A20.9
　eye S00.1- ☑
　hairy tongue K14.3
　heel (foot) S90.3- ☑
　lung (disease) J60
　palm (hand) S60.22- ☑
Blackfan-Diamond anemia or syndrome (congenital hypoplastic anemia) D61.01
Blackhead L70.0
Blackout R55
Bladder — *see* condition
Blast (air) (hydraulic) (immersion) (underwater)
　blindness S05.8X- ☑
　injury
　　abdomen or thorax — *see* Injury, by site
　　ear (acoustic nerve trauma) — *see* Injury, nerve, acoustic, specified type NEC
　　syndrome NEC T70.8 ☑
Blastoma — *see* Neoplasm, malignant, by site
　pulmonary — *see* Neoplasm, lung, malignant
Blastomycosis, blastomycotic B40.9
　Brazilian — *see* Paracoccidioidomycosis
　cutaneous B40.3
　disseminated B40.7
　European — *see* Cryptococcosis
　generalized B40.7
　keloidal B48.0
　North American B40.9
　primary pulmonary B40.0
　pulmonary B40.2
　　acute B40.0
　　chronic B40.1
　skin B40.3
　South American — *see* Paracoccidioidomycosis
　specified NEC B40.89
Bleb (s) R23.8
　emphysematous (lung) (solitary) J43.9
　endophthalmitis H59.43
　filtering (vitreous), after glaucoma surgery Z98.83
　inflamed (infected), postprocedural H59.40
　　stage 1 H59.41
　　stage 2 H59.42
　　stage 3 H59.43
　lung (ruptured) J43.9
　　congenital — *see* Atelectasis
　　newborn P25.8
　subpleural (emphysematous) J43.9
Blebitis, postprocedural H59.40
　stage 1 H59.41
　stage 2 H59.42
　stage 3 H59.43
Bleeder (familial) (hereditary) — *see* Hemophilia
Bleeding (*see also* Hemorrhage)
　anal K62.5
　anovulatory N97.0
　atonic, following delivery O72.1
　capillary I78.8
　　puerperal O72.2
　contact (postcoital) N93.0
　due to uterine subinvolution N85.3
　ear — *see* Otorrhagia
　excessive, associated with menopausal onset N92.4
　familial — *see* Defect, coagulation
　following intercourse N93.0
　gastrointestinal K92.2
　hemorrhoids — *see* Hemorrhoids
　intermenstrual (regular) N92.3
　　irregular N92.1

Bleeding — *continued*
　intraoperative — *see* Complication, intraoperative, hemorrhage
　irregular N92.6
　menopausal N92.4
　newborn, intraventricular — *see* Newborn, affected by, hemorrhage, intraventricular
　nipple N64.59
　nose R04.0
　ovulation N92.3
　postclimacteric N95.0
　postcoital N93.0
　postmenopausal N95.0
　postoperative — *see* Complication, postprocedural, hemorrhage
　preclimacteric N92.4
　puberty (excessive, with onset of menstrual periods) N92.2
　rectum, rectal K62.5
　　newborn P54.2
　tendencies — *see* Defect, coagulation
　throat R04.1
　tooth socket (post-extraction) K91.840
　umbilical stump P51.9
　uterus, uterine NEC N93.9
　　climacteric N92.4
　　dysfunctional of functional N93.8
　　menopausal N92.4
　　preclimacteric or premenopausal N92.4
　　unrelated to menstrual cycle N93.9
　vagina, vaginal (abnormal) N93.9
　　dysfunctional or functional N93.8
　　newborn P54.6
　vicarious N94.89
Blennorrhagia, blennorrhagic — *see* Gonorrhea
Blennorrhea (acute) (chronic) (*see also* Gonorrhea)
　inclusion (neonatal) (newborn) P39.1
　lower genitourinary tract (gonococcal) A54.00
　neonatorum (gonococcal ophthalmia) A54.31
Blepharelosis — *see* Entropion
Blepharitis (angularis) (ciliaris) (eyelid) (marginal) (nonulcerative) H01.009
　herpes zoster B02.39
　left H01.006
　　lower H01.005
　　upper H01.004
　right H01.003
　　lower H01.002
　　upper H01.001
　squamous H01.029
　　left H01.026
　　　lower H01.025
　　　upper H01.024
　　right H01.023
　　　lower H01.022
　　　upper H01.021
　ulcerative H01.019
　　left H01.016
　　　lower H01.015
　　　upper H01.014
　　right H01.013
　　　lower H01.012
　　　upper H01.011
Blepharochalasis H02.30
　congenital Q10.0
　left H02.36
　　lower H02.35
　　upper H02.34
　right H02.33
　　lower H02.32
　　upper H02.31
Blepharoclonus H02.59
Blepharoconjunctivitis H10.50- ☑
　angular H10.52- ☑
　contact H10.53- ☑
　ligneous H10.51- ☑
Blepharophimosis (eyelid) H02.529
　congenital Q10.3
　left H02.526
　　lower H02.525
　　upper H02.524
　right H02.523
　　lower H02.522
　　upper H02.521
Blepharoptosis H02.40- ☑
　congenital Q10.0
　mechanical H02.41- ☑
　myogenic H02.42- ☑
　neurogenic H02.43- ☑
　paralytic H02.43- ☑
Blepharopyorrhea, gonococcal A54.39
Blepharospasm G24.5

Blepharospasm — *continued*
　drug induced G24.01
Blighted ovum O02.0
Blind (*see also* Blindness)
　bronchus (congenital) Q32.4
　loop syndrome K90.2
　　congenital Q43.8
　sac, fallopian tube (congenital) Q50.6
　spot, enlarged — *see* Defect, visual field, localized, scotoma, blind spot area
　tract or tube, congenital NEC — *see* Atresia, by site
Blindness (acquired) (congenital) (both eyes) H54.0
　blast S05.8X- ☑
　color — *see* Deficiency, color vision
　concussion S05.8X- ☑
　cortical H47.619
　　left brain H47.612
　　right brain H47.611
　day H53.11
　due to injury (current episode) S05.9- ☑
　　sequelae -- code to injury with seventh character S
　eclipse (total) — *see* Retinopathy, solar
　emotional (hysterical) F44.6
　face H53.16
　hysterical F44.6
　legal (both eyes) (USA definition) H54.8
　mind R48.8
　night H53.60
　　abnormal dark adaptation curve H53.61
　　acquired H53.62
　　congenital H53.63
　　specified type NEC H53.69
　　vitamin A deficiency E50.5
　one eye (other eye normal) H54.40
　　left (normal vision on right) H54.42
　　　low vision on right H54.12
　　low vision, other eye H54.10
　　right (normal vision on left) H54.41
　　　low vision on left H54.11
　psychic R48.8
　river B73.01
　snow — *see* Photokeratitis
　sun, solar — *see* Retinopathy, solar
　transient — *see* Disturbance, vision, subjective, loss, transient
　traumatic (current episode) S05.9- ☑
　word (developmental) F81.0
　　acquired R48.0
　　secondary to organic lesion R48.0
Blister (nonthermal)
　abdominal wall S30.821 ☑
　alveolar process S00.522 ☑
　ankle S90.52- ☑
　antecubital space — *see* Blister, elbow
　anus S30.827 ☑
　arm (upper) S40.82- ☑
　auditory canal — *see* Blister, ear
　auricle — *see* Blister, ear
　axilla — *see* Blister, arm
　back, lower S30.820 ☑
　beetle dermatitis L24.89
　breast S20.12- ☑
　brow S00.82 ☑
　calf — *see* Blister, leg
　canthus — *see* Blister, eyelid
　cheek S00.82 ☑
　　internal S00.522 ☑
　chest wall — *see* Blister, thorax
　chin S00.82 ☑
　costal region — *see* Blister, thorax
　digit (s)
　　foot — *see* Blister, toe
　　hand — *see* Blister, finger
　due to burn — *see* Burn, by site, second degree
　ear S00.42- ☑
　elbow S50.32- ☑
　epiglottis S10.12 ☑
　esophagus, cervical S10.12 ☑
　eyebrow — *see* Blister, eyelid
　eyelid S00.22- ☑
　face S00.82 ☑
　fever B00.1
　finger (s) S60.429 ☑
　　index S60.42- ☑
　　little S60.42- ☑
　　middle S60.42- ☑
　　ring S60.42- ☑
　foot (except toe(s) alone) S90.82- ☑
　　toe — *see* Blister, toe
　forearm S50.82- ☑

Blister — continued
elbow only — see Blister, elbow
forehead S00.82 ☑
fracture - omit code
genital organ
female S30.826 ☑
male S30.825 ☑
gum S00.522 ☑
hand S60.52- ☑
head S00.92 ☑
ear — see Blister, ear
eyelid — see Blister, eyelid
lip S00.521 ☑
nose S00.32 ☑
oral cavity S00.522 ☑
scalp S00.02 ☑
specified site NEC S00.82 ☑
heel — see Blister, foot
hip S70.22- ☑
interscapular region S20.429 ☑
jaw S00.82 ☑
knee S80.22- ☑
larynx S10.12 ☑
leg (lower) S80.82- ☑
knee — see Blister, knee
upper — see Blister, thigh
lip S00.521 ☑
malar region S00.82 ☑
mammary — see Blister, breast
mastoid region S00.82 ☑
mouth S00.522 ☑
multiple, skin, nontraumatic R23.8
nail
finger — see Blister, finger
toe — see Blister, toe
nasal S00.32 ☑
neck S10.92 ☑
specified site NEC S10.82 ☑
throat S10.12 ☑
nose S00.32 ☑
occipital region S00.02 ☑
oral cavity S00.522 ☑
orbital region — see Blister, eyelid
palate S00.522 ☑
palm — see Blister, hand
parietal region S00.02 ☑
pelvis S30.820 ☑
penis S30.822 ☑
periocular area — see Blister, eyelid
phalanges
finger — see Blister, finger
toe — see Blister, toe
pharynx S10.12 ☑
pinna — see Blister, ear
popliteal space — see Blister, knee
scalp S00.02 ☑
scapular region — see Blister, shoulder
scrotum S30.823 ☑
shin — see Blister, leg
shoulder S40.22- ☑
sternal region S20.329 ☑
submaxillary region S00.82 ☑
submental region S00.82 ☑
subungual
finger (s) — see Blister, finger
toe (s) — see Blister, toe
supraclavicular fossa S10.82 ☑
supraorbital S00.82 ☑
temple S00.82 ☑
temporal region S00.82 ☑
testis S30.823 ☑
thermal — see Burn, second degree, by site
thigh S70.32- ☑
thorax, thoracic (wall) S20.92 ☑
back S20.42- ☑
front S20.32- ☑
throat S10.12 ☑
thumb S60.32- ☑
toe (s) S90.42- ☑
great S90.42- ☑
tongue S00.522 ☑
trachea S10.12 ☑
tympanum, tympanic membrane — see Blister, ear
upper arm — see Blister, arm (upper)
uvula S00.522 ☑
vagina S30.824 ☑
vocal cords S10.12 ☑
vulva S30.824 ☑
wrist S60.82- ☑
Bloating R14.0
Bloch-Sulzberger disease or syndrome Q82.3

Block, blocked
alveolocapillary J84.10
arborization (heart) I45.5
arrhythmic I45.9
atrioventricular (incomplete) (partial) I44.30
with atrioventricular dissociation I44.2
complete I44.2
congenital Q24.6
congenital Q24.6
first degree I44.0
second degree (types I and II) I44.1
specified NEC I44.39
third degree I44.2
types I and II I44.1
auriculoventricular — see Block, atrioventricular
bifascicular (cardiac) I45.2
bundle-branch (complete) (false) (incomplete) I45.4
bilateral I45.2
left I44.7
with right bundle branch block I45.2
hemiblock I44.60
anterior I44.4
posterior I44.5
incomplete I44.7
with right bundle branch block I45.2
right I45.10
with
left bundle branch block I45.2
left fascicular block I45.2
specified NEC I45.19
Wilson's type I45.19
cardiac I45.9
conduction I45.9
complete I44.2
fascicular (left) I44.60
anterior I44.4
posterior I44.5
right I45.0
specified NEC I44.69
foramen Magendie (acquired) G91.1
congenital Q03.1
with spina bifida — see Spina bifida, by site, with hydrocephalus
heart I45.9
bundle branch I45.4
bilateral I45.2
complete (atrioventricular) I44.2
congenital Q24.6
first degree (atrioventricular) I44.0
second degree (atrioventricular) I44.1
specified type NEC I45.5
third degree (atrioventricular) I44.2
hepatic vein I82.0
intraventricular (nonspecific) I45.4
bundle branch
bilateral I45.2
kidney N28.9
postcystoscopic or postprocedural N99.0
Mobitz (types I and II) I44.1
myocardial — see Block, heart
nodal I45.5
organ or site, congenital NEC — see Atresia, by site
portal (vein) I81
second degree (types I and II) I44.1
sinoatrial I45.5
sinoauricular I45.5
third degree I44.2
trifascicular I45.3
tubal N97.1
vein NOS I82.90
Wenckebach (types I and II) I44.1
Blockage — see Obstruction
Blocq's disease F44.4
Blood
constituents, abnormal R78.9
disease D75.9
donor — see Donor, blood
dyscrasia D75.9
with
abortion — see Abortion, by type, complicated by, hemorrhage
ectopic pregnancy O08.1
molar pregnancy O08.1
following ectopic or molar pregnancy O08.1
newborn P61.9
puerperal, postpartum O72.3
flukes NEC — see Schistosomiasis
in
feces K92.1
occult R19.5

Blood — continued
urine — see Hematuria
mole O02.0
occult in feces R19.5
pressure
decreased, due to shock following injury T79.4 ☑
examination only Z01.30
fluctuating I99.8
high — see Hypertension
borderline R03.0
incidental reading, without diagnosis of hypertension R03.0
low (see also Hypotension)
incidental reading, without diagnosis of hypotension R03.1
spitting — see Hemoptysis
staining cornea — see Pigmentation, cornea, stromal
transfusion
reaction or complication — see Complications, transfusion
type
A (Rh positive) Z67.10
Rh negative Z67.11
AB (Rh positive) Z67.30
Rh negative Z67.31
B (Rh positive) Z67.20
Rh negative Z67.21
O (Rh positive) Z67.40
Rh negative Z67.41
Rh (positive) Z67.90
negative Z67.91
vessel rupture — see Hemorrhage
vomiting — see Hematemesis
Blood-forming organs, disease D75.9
Bloodgood's disease — see Mastopathy, cystic
Bloom (-Machacek)(-Torre) syndrome Q82.8
Blount's disease or osteochondrosis — see Osteochondrosis, juvenile, tibia
Blue
baby Q24.9
diaper syndrome E72.09
dome cyst (breast) — see Cyst, breast
dot cataract Q12.0
nevus D22.9
sclera Q13.5
with fragility of bone and deafness Q78.0
toe syndrome I75.02- ☑
Blueness — see Cyanosis
Blues, postpartal O90.6
baby O90.6
Blurring, visual H53.8
Blushing (abnormal) (excessive) R23.2
BMI — see Body, mass index
Boarder, hospital NEC Z76.4
accompanying sick person Z76.3
healthy infant or child Z76.2
foundling Z76.1
Bockhart's impetigo L01.02
Bodechtel-Guttman disease (subacute sclerosing panencephalitis) A81.1
Boder-Sedgwick syndrome (ataxia-telangiectasia) G11.3
Body, bodies
Aschoff's — see Myocarditis, rheumatic
asteroid, vitreous — see Deposit, crystalline
cytoid (retina) — see Occlusion, artery, retina
drusen (degenerative) (macula) (retinal) (see also Degeneration, macula, drusen)
optic disc — see Drusen, optic disc
foreign — see Foreign body
loose
joint, except knee — see Loose, body, joint
knee M23.4- ☑
sheath, tendon — see Disorder, tendon, specified type NEC
mass index (BMI)
adult
19 or less Z68.1
20.0-20.9 Z68.20
21.0-21.9 Z68.21
22.0-22.9 Z68.22
23.0-23.9 Z68.23
24.0-24.9 Z68.24
25.0-25.9 Z68.25
26.0-26.9 Z68.26
27.0-27.9 Z68.27
28.0-28.9 Z68.28
29.0-29.9 Z68.29
30.0-30.9 Z68.30
31.0-31.9 Z68.31

Body — continued
  32.0-32.9 Z68.32
  33.0-33.9 Z68.33
  34.0-34.9 Z68.34
  35.0-35.9 Z68.35
  36.0-36.9 Z68.36
  37.0-37.9 Z68.37
  38.0-38.9 Z68.38
  39.0-39.9 Z68.39
  40.0-44.9 Z68.41
  45.0-49.9 Z68.42
  50.0-59.9 Z68.43
  60.0-69.9 Z68.44
  70 and over Z68.45
  pediatric
    5th percentile to less than 85th percentile for age Z68.52
    85th percentile to less than 95th percentile for age Z68.53
    greater than or equal to ninety-fifth percentile for age Z68.54
    less than fifth percentile for age Z68.51
  Mooser's A75.2
  rice (see also Loose, body, joint)
    knee M23.4- ☑
  rocking F98.4
Boeck's
  disease or sarcoid — see Sarcoidosis
  lupoid (miliary) D86.3
Boerhaave's syndrome (spontaneous esophageal rupture) K22.3
Boggy
  cervix N88.8
  uterus N85.8
Boil (see also Furuncle, by site)
  Aleppo B55.1
  Baghdad B55.1
  Delhi B55.1
  lacrimal
    gland — see Dacryoadenitis
    passages (duct) (sac) — see Inflammation, lacrimal, passages, acute
  Natal B55.1
  orbit, orbital — see Abscess, orbit
  tropical B55.1
Bold hives — see Urticaria
Bombé, iris — see Membrane, pupillary
Bone — see condition
Bonnevie-Ullrich syndrome Q87.1
Bonnier's syndromeH81.8
Bonvale dam fever T73.3 ☑
Bony block of joint — see Ankylosis
BOOP (bronchiolitis obliterans organized pneumonia) J84.89
Borderline
  diabetes mellitus R73.09
  hypertension R03.0
  osteopenia M85.8- ☑
  pelvis, with obstruction during labor O65.1
  personality F60.3
Borna disease A83.9
Bornholm disease B33.0
Boston exanthem A88.0
Botalli, ductus (patent) (persistent) Q25.0
Bothriocephalus latus infestation B70.0
Botulism (foodborne intoxication) A05.1
  infant A48.51
  non-foodborne A48.52
  wound A48.52
Bouba — see Yaws
Bouchard's nodes (with arthropathy) M15.2
Bouffée délirante F23
Bouillaud's disease or syndrome (rheumatic heart disease) I01.9
Bourneville's disease Q85.1
Boutonniere deformity (finger) — see Deformity, finger, boutonniere
Bouveret (-Hoffmann) syndrome (paroxysmal tachycardia) I47.9
Bovine heart — see Hypertrophy, cardiac
Bowel — see condition
Bowen's
  dermatosis (precancerous) — see Neoplasm, skin, in situ
  disease — see Neoplasm, skin, in situ
  epithelioma — see Neoplasm, skin, in situ
  type
    epidermoid carcinoma-in-situ — see Neoplasm, skin, in situ
    intraepidermal squamous cell carcinoma — see Neoplasm, skin, in situ

Bowing
  femur (see also Deformity, limb, specified type NEC, thigh)
    congenital Q68.3
  fibula (see also Deformity, limb, specified type NEC, lower leg)
    congenital Q68.4
  forearm — see Deformity, limb, specified type NEC, forearm
  leg (s), long bones, congenital Q68.5
  radius — see Deformity, limb, specified type NEC, forearm
  tibia (see also Deformity, limb, specified type NEC, lower leg)
    congenital Q68.4
Bowleg (s) (acquired) M21.16- ☑
  congenital Q68.5
  rachitic E64.3
Boyd's dysentery A03.2
Brachial — see condition
Brachycardia R00.1
Brachycephaly Q75.0
Bradley's disease A08.19
Bradyarrhythmia, cardiac I49.8
Bradycardia (sinoatrial) (sinus) (vagal) R00.1
  neonatal P29.12
  reflex G90.09
  tachycardia syndrome I49.5
Bradykinesia R25.8
Bradypnea R06.89
Bradytachycardia I49.5
Brailsford's disease or osteochondrosis — see Osteochondrosis, juvenile, radius
Brain (see also condition)
  death G93.82
  syndrome — see Syndrome, brain
Branched-chain amino-acid disorder E71.2
Branchial — see condition
  cartilage, congenital Q18.2
Branchiogenic remnant (in neck) Q18.0
Brandt's syndrome (acrodermatitis enteropathica) E83.2
Brash (water) R12
Bravais-jacksonian epilepsy — see Epilepsy, localization-related, symptomatic, with simple partial seizures
Braxton Hicks contractions — see False, labor
Brazilian leishmaniasis B55.2
BRBPR K62.5
Break, retina (without detachment) H33.30- ☑
  with retinal detachment — see Detachment, retina
  horseshoe tear H33.31- ☑
  multiple H33.33- ☑
  round hole H33.32- ☑
Breakdown
  device, graft or implant (see also Complications, by site and type, mechanical) T85.618 ☑
    arterial graft NEC — see Complication, cardiovascular device, mechanical, vascular
    breast (implant) T85.41 ☑
    catheter NEC T85.618 ☑
      cystostomy T83.010 ☑
      dialysis (renal) T82.41 ☑
        intraperitoneal T85.611 ☑
      infusion NEC T82.514 ☑
        spinal (epidural) (subdural) T85.610 ☑
      urinary (indwelling) T83.018 ☑
    electronic (electrode) (pulse generator) (stimulator)
      bone T84.310 ☑
      cardiac T82.119 ☑
        electrode T82.110 ☑
        pulse generator T82.111 ☑
        specified type NEC T82.118 ☑
      nervous system — see Complication, prosthetic device, mechanical, electronic nervous system stimulator
      urinary — see Complication, genitourinary, device, urinary, mechanical
    fixation, internal (orthopedic) NEC — see Complication, fixation device, mechanical
    gastrointestinal — see Complications, prosthetic device, mechanical, gastrointestinal device
    genital NEC T83.418 ☑
      intrauterine contraceptive device T83.31 ☑
      penile prosthesis T83.410 ☑
    heart NEC — see Complication, cardiovascular device, mechanical
    joint prosthesis — see Complications..., joint prosthesis,internal, mechanical, by site

Breakdown — continued
    ocular NEC — see Complications, prosthetic device, mechanical, ocular device
    orthopedic NEC — see Complication, orthopedic, device, mechanical
    specified NEC T85.618 ☑
    sutures, permanent T85.612 ☑
      used in bone repair — see Complications, fixation device, internal (orthopedic), mechanical
    urinary NEC (see also Complication, genitourinary, device, urinary, mechanical)
      graft T83.21 ☑
    vascular NEC — see Complication, cardiovascular device, mechanical
    ventricular intracranial shunt T85.01 ☑
  nervous F48.8
  perineum O90.1
  respirator J95.850
    specified NEC J95.859
  ventilator J95.850
    specified NEC J95.859
Breast (see also condition)
  buds E30.1
    in newborn P96.89
  dense R92.2
  nodule N63
Breath
  foul R19.6
  holder, child R06.89
  holding spell R06.89
  shortness R06.02
Breathing
  labored — see Hyperventilation
  mouth R06.5
    causing malocclusion M26.5 ☑
  periodic R06.3
    high altitude G47.32
Breathlessness R06.81
Breda's disease — see Yaws
Breech presentation (mother) O32.1 ☑
  causing obstructed labor O64.1 ☑
  footling O32.8 ☑
    causing obstructed labor O64.8 ☑
  incomplete O32.8 ☑
    causing obstructed labor O64.8 ☑
Breisky's disease N90.4
Brennemann's syndrome I88.0
Brenner
  tumor (benign) D27.9
    borderline malignancy D39.1- ☑
    malignant C56 ☑
    proliferating D39.1- ☑
Bretonneau's disease or angina A36.0
Breus' mole O02.0
Brevicollis Q76.49
Brickmakers' anemia B76.9 [D63.8]
Bridge, myocardial Q24.5
Bright red blood per rectum (BRBPR) K62.5
Bright's disease (see also Nephritis)
  arteriosclerotic — see Hypertension, kidney
Brill (-Zinsser) disease (recrudescent typhus) A75.1
  flea-borne A75.2
  louse-borne A75.1
Brill-Symmers' disease C82.90
Brion-Kayser disease — see Fever, parathyroid
Briquet's disorder or syndrome F45.0
Brissaud's
  infantilism or dwarfism E23.0
  motor-verbal tic F95.2
Brittle
  bones disease Q78.0
  nails L60.3
    congenital Q84.6
Broad (see also condition)
  beta disease E78.2
  ligament laceration syndrome N83.8
Broad- or floating-betalipoproteinemia E78.2
Brock's syndrome (atelectasis due to enlarged lymph nodes) J98.19
Brocq-Duhring disease (dermatitis herpetiformis) L13.0
Brodie's abscess or disease M86.8X- ☑
Broken
  arches (see also Deformity, limb, flat foot)
  arm (meaning upper limb) — see Fracture, arm
  back — see Fracture, vertebra
  bone — see Fracture
  implant or internal device — see Complications, by site and type, mechanical
  leg (meaning lower limb) — see Fracture, leg
  nose S02.2 ☑

Broken — *continued*
  tooth, teeth — *see* Fracture, tooth
Bromhidrosis, bromidrosis L75.0
Bromidism, bromism G92
  due to
    correct substance properly administered — *see* Table of Drugs and Chemicals, by drug, adverse effect
    overdose or wrong substance given or taken — *see* Table of Drugs and Chemicals, by drug, poisoning
  chronic (dependence) F13.20
Bromidrosiphobia F40.298
Bronchi, bronchial — *see* condition
Bronchiectasis (cylindrical) (diffuse) (fusiform) (localized) (saccular) J47.9
  with
    acute
      bronchitis J47.0
      lower respiratory infection J47.0
    exacerbation (acute) J47.1
  congenital Q33.4
  tuberculous NEC — *see* Tuberculosis, pulmonary
Bronchiolectasis — *see* Bronchiectasis
Bronchiolitis (acute) (infective) (subacute) J21.9
  with
    bronchospasm or obstruction J21.9
    influenza, flu or grippe — *see* Influenza, with, respiratory manifestations NEC
  chemical (chronic) J68.4
    acute J68.0
  chronic (fibrosing) (obliterative) J44.9
  due to
    external agent — *see* Bronchitis, acute, due to
    human metapneumovirus J21.1
    respiratory syncytial virus J21.0
    specified organism NEC J21.8
  fibrosa obliterans J44.9
  influenzal — *see* Influenza, with, respiratory manifestations NEC
  obliterans J42
    with organizing pneumonia (BOOP) J84.89
  obliterative (chronic) (subacute) J44.9
    due to fumes or vapors J68.4
    due to chemicals, gases, fumes or vapors (inhalation) J68.4
  respiratory, interstitial lung disease J84.115
Bronchitis (diffuse) (fibrinous) (hypostatic) (infective) (membranous) J40
  with
    influenza, flu or grippe — *see* Influenza, with, respiratory manifestations NEC
    obstruction (airway) (lung) J44.9
    tracheitis (I5 years of age and above) J40
      acute or subacute J20.9
      chronic J42
      under I5 years of age J20.9
    acute or subacute (with bronchospasm or obstruction) J20.9
      with
        bronchiectasis J47.0
        chronic obstructive pulmonary disease J44.0
      chemical (due to gases, fumes or vapors) J68.0
      due to
        fumes or vapors J68.0
        Haemophilus influenzae J20.1
        Mycoplasma pneumoniae J20.0
        radiation J70.0
        specified organism NEC J20.8
        Streptococcus J20.2
        virus
          coxsackie J20.3
          echovirus J20.7
          parainfluenzae J20.4
          respiratory syncytial J20.5
          rhinovirus J20.6
        viral NEC J20.8
    allergic (acute) J45.909
      with
        exacerbation (acute) J45.901
        status asthmaticus J45.902
    arachidic T17.528 ☑
    aspiration (due to fumes or vapors) J68.0
    asthmatic J45.9 ☑
      chronic J44.9
        with
          acute lower respiratory infection J44.0
          exacerbation (acute) J44.1
    capillary — *see* Pneumonia, broncho
    caseous (tuberculous) A15.5
    Castellani's A69.8
    catarrhal (I5 years of age and above) J40

Bronchitis — *continued*
  acute — *see* Bronchitis, acute
  chronic J41.0
    under I5 years of age J20.9
  chemical (acute) (subacute) J68.0
    chronic J68.4
    due to fumes or vapors J68.0
      chronic J68.4
  chronic J42
    with
      airways obstruction J44.9
      tracheitis (chronic) J42
      asthmatic (obstructive) J44.9
    catarrhal J41.0
    chemical (due to fumes or vapors) J68.4
    due to
      chemicals, gases, fumes or vapors (inhalation) J68.4
      radiation J70.1
      tobacco smoking J41.0
    emphysematous J44.9
    mucopurulent J41.1
    non-obstructive J41.0
    obliterans J44.9
    obstructive J44.9
    purulent J41.1
    simple J41.0
  croupous — *see* Bronchitis, acute
  due to gases, fumes or vapors (chemical) J68.0
  emphysematous (obstructive) J44.9
  exudative — *see* Bronchitis, acute
  fetid J41.1
  grippal — *see* Influenza, with, respiratory manifestations NEC
  in those under I5 years age — *see* Bronchitis, acute
    chronic — *see* Bronchitis, chronic
  influenzal — *see* Influenza, with, respiratory manifestations NEC
  mixed simple and mucopurulent J41.8
  moulder's J62.8
  mucopurulent (chronic) (recurrent) J41.1
    acute or subacute J20.9
    simple (mixed) J41.8
  obliterans (chronic) J44.9
  obstructive (chronic) (diffuse) J44.9
  pituitous J41.1
  pneumococcal, acute or subacute J20.2
  pseudomembranous, acute or subacute — *see* Bronchitis, acute
  purulent (chronic) (recurrent) J41.1
    acute or subacute — *see* Bronchitis, acute
  putrid J41.1
  senile (chronic) J42
  simple and mucopurulent (mixed) J41.8
  smokers' J41.0
  spirochetal NEC A69.8
  subacute — *see* Bronchitis, acute
  suppurative (chronic) J41.1
    acute or subacute — *see* Bronchitis, acute
  tuberculous A15.5
    under I5 years of age — *see* Bronchitis, acute
    chronic — *see* Bronchitis, chronic
  viral NEC, acute or subacute (*see also* Bronchitis, acute) J20.8
Bronchoalveolitis J18.0
Bronchoaspergillosis B44.1
Bronchocele meaning goiter E04.0
Broncholithiasis J98.09
  tuberculous NEC A15.5
Bronchomalacia J98.09
  congenital Q32.2
Bronchomycosis NOS B49 [J99]
  candidal B37.1
Bronchopleuropneumonia — *see* Pneumonia, broncho
Bronchopneumonia — *see* Pneumonia, broncho
Bronchopneumonitis — *see* Pneumonia, broncho
Bronchopulmonary — *see* condition
Bronchopulmonitis — *see* Pneumonia, broncho
Bronchorrhagia (see Hemoptysis)
Bronchorrhea J98.09
  acute J20.9
  chronic (infective) (purulent) J42
Bronchospasm (acute) J98.01
  with
    bronchiolitis, acute J21.9
    bronchitis, acute (conditions in J20) — *see* Bronchitis, acute
  due to external agent — *see* condition, respiratory, acute, due to
  exercise induced J45.990

Bronchospirochetosis A69.8
  Castellani A69.8
Bronchostenosis J98.09
Bronchus — *see* condition
Brontophobia F40.220
Bronze baby syndrome P83.8
Brooke's tumor — *see* Neoplasm, skin, benign
Brown enamel of teeth (hereditary) K00.5
Brown's sheath syndrome H50.61- ☑
Brown-Séquard disease, paralysis or syndrome G83.81
Bruce sepsis A23.0
Brucellosis (infection) A23.9
  abortus A23.1
  canis A23.3
  dermatitis A23.9
  melitensis A23.0
  mixed A23.8
  sepsis A23.9
    melitensis A23.0
    specified NEC A23.8
  suis A23.2
Bruck-de Lange disease Q87.1
Bruck's disease — *see* Deformity, limb
Brugsch's syndrome Q82.8
Bruise (skin surface intact) (*see also* Contusion)
  with
    open wound — *see* Wound, open
    internal organ — *see* Injury, by site
  newborn P54.5
  scalp, due to birth injury, newborn P12.3
  umbilical cord O69.5 ☑
Bruit (arterial) R09.89
  cardiac R01.1
Brush burn — *see* Abrasion, by site
Bruton's X-linked agammaglobulinemia D80.0
Bruxism
  psychogenic F45.8
  sleep related G47.63
Bubbly lung syndrome P27.0
Bubo I88.8
  blennorrhagic (gonococcal) A54.89
  chancroidal A57
  climatic A55
  due to Haemophilus ducreyi A57
  gonococcal A54.89
  indolent (nonspecific) I88.8
  inguinal (nonspecific) I88.8
    chancroidal A57
    climatic A55
    due to H. ducreyi A57
    infective I88.8
  scrofulous (tuberculous) A18.2
  soft chancre A57
  suppurating — *see* Lymphadenitis, acute
  syphilitic (primary) A51.0
    congenital A50.07
  tropical A55
  virulent (chancroidal) A57
Bubonic plague A20.0
Bubonocele — *see* Hernia, inguinal
Buccal — *see* condition
Buchanan's disease or osteochondrosis M91.0
Buchem's syndrome (hyperostosis corticalis) M85.2
Bucket-handle fracture or tear (semilunar cartilage) — *see* Tear, meniscus
Budd-Chiari syndrome (hepatic vein thrombosis) I82.0
Budgerigar fancier's disease or lung J67.2
Buds
  breast E30.1
    in newborn P96.89
Buerger's disease (thromboangiitis obliterans) I73.1
Bulbar — *see* condition
Bulbus cordis (left ventricle) (persistent) Q21.8
Bulimia (nervosa) F50.2
  atypical F50.9
  normal weight F50.9
Bulky
  stools R19.5
  uterus N85.2
Bulla (e) R23.8
  lung (emphysematous) (solitary) J43.9
    newborn P25.8
Bullet wound (*see also* Wound, open)
  fracture - code as Fracture, by site
  internal organ — *see* Injury, by site
Bundle
  branch block (complete) (false) (incomplete) — *see* Block, bundle-branch
  of His — *see* condition
Bunion — *see* Deformity, toe, hallux valgus

☑ **Additional character required**

Buphthalmia, buphthalmos (congenital) Q15.0
Burdwan fever B55.0
Bürger-Grütz disease or syndrome E78.3
Buried
  penis (congenital) Q55.64
    acquired N48.83
  roots K08.3
Burke's syndrome K86.8
Burkitt
  cell leukemia C91.0- ☑
  lymphoma (malignant) C83.7- ☑
    small noncleaved, diffuse C83.7- ☑
    spleen C83.77
    undifferentiated C83.7- ☑
  tumor C83.7- ☑
  type
    acute lymphoblastic leukemia C91.0- ☑
    undifferentiated C83.7- ☑
Burn (electricity) (flame) (hot gas, liquid or hot object) (radiation) (steam) (thermal) T30.0
  abdomen, abdominal (muscle) (wall) T21.02 ☑
    first degree T21.12 ☑
    second degree T21.22 ☑
    third degree T21.32 ☑
  above elbow T22.039 ☑
    first degree T22.139 ☑
    left T22.032 ☑
      first degree T22.132 ☑
      second degree T22.232 ☑
      third degree T22.332 ☑
    right T22.031 ☑
      first degree T22.131 ☑
      second degree T22.231 ☑
      third degree T22.331 ☑
    second degree T22.239 ☑
    third degree T22.339 ☑
  acid (caustic) (external) (internal) — *see* Corrosion, by site
  alimentary tract NEC T28.2 ☑
    esophagus T28.1 ☑
    mouth T28.0 ☑
    pharynx T28.0 ☑
  alkaline (caustic) (external) (internal) — *see* Corrosion, by site
  ankle T25.019 ☑
    first degree T25.119 ☑
    left T25.012 ☑
      first degree T25.112 ☑
      second degree T25.212 ☑
      third degree T25.312 ☑
    multiple with foot — *see* Burn, lower, limb, multiple, ankle and foot
    right T25.011 ☑
      first degree T25.111 ☑
      second degree T25.211 ☑
      third degree T25.311 ☑
    second degree T25.219 ☑
    third degree T25.319 ☑
  anus — *see* Burn, buttock
  arm (lower) (upper) — *see* Burn, upper, limb
  axilla T22.049 ☑
    first degree T22.149 ☑
    left T22.042 ☑
      first degree T22.142 ☑
      second degree T22.242 ☑
      third degree T22.342 ☑
    right T22.041 ☑
      first degree T22.141 ☑
      second degree T22.241 ☑
      third degree T22.341 ☑
    second degree T22.249 ☑
    third degree T22.349 ☑
  back (lower) T21.04 ☑
    first degree T21.14 ☑
    second degree T21.24 ☑
    third degree T21.34 ☑
    upper T21.03 ☑
      first degree T21.13 ☑
      second degree T21.23 ☑
      third degree T21.33 ☑
  blisters - code as Burn, second degree, by site
  breast (s) — *see* Burn, chest wall
  buttock (s) T21.05 ☑
    first degree T21.15 ☑
    second degree T21.25 ☑
    third degree T21.35 ☑
  calf T24.039 ☑
    first degree T24.139 ☑
    left T24.032 ☑
      first degree T24.132 ☑
      second degree T24.232 ☑
      third degree T24.332 ☑

Burn — *continued*
  right T24.031 ☑
    first degree T24.131 ☑
    second degree T24.231 ☑
    third degree T24.331 ☑
  second degree T24.239 ☑
  third degree T24.339 ☑
  canthus (eye) — *see* Burn, eyelid
  caustic acid or alkaline — *see* Corrosion, by site
  cervix T28.3 ☑
  cheek T20.06 ☑
    first degree T20.16 ☑
    second degree T20.26 ☑
    third degree T20.36 ☑
  chemical (acids) (alkalines) (caustics) (external) (internal) — *see* Corrosion, by site
  chest wall T21.01 ☑
    first degree T21.11 ☑
    second degree T21.21 ☑
    third degree T21.31 ☑
  chin T20.03 ☑
    first degree T20.13 ☑
    second degree T20.23 ☑
    third degree T20.33 ☑
  colon T28.2 ☑
  conjunctiva (and cornea) — *see* Burn, cornea
  cornea (and conjunctiva) T26.1- ☑
    chemical — *see* Corrosion, cornea
  corrosion (external) (internal) — *see* Corrosion, by site
  deep necrosis of underlying tissue - code as Burn, third degree, by site
  dorsum of hand T23.069 ☑
    first degree T23.169 ☑
    left T23.062 ☑
      first degree T23.162 ☑
      second degree T23.262 ☑
      third degree T23.362 ☑
    right T23.061 ☑
      first degree T23.161 ☑
      second degree T23.261 ☑
      third degree T23.361 ☑
    second degree T23.269 ☑
    third degree T23.369 ☑
  due to ingested chemical agent — *see* Corrosion, by site
  ear (auricle) (external) (canal) T20.01 ☑
    first degree T20.11 ☑
    second degree T20.21 ☑
    third degree T20.31 ☑
  elbow T22.029 ☑
    first degree T22.129 ☑
    left T22.022 ☑
      first degree T22.122 ☑
      second degree T22.222 ☑
      third degree T22.322 ☑
    right T22.021 ☑
      first degree T22.121 ☑
      second degree T22.221 ☑
      third degree T22.321 ☑
    second degree T22.229 ☑
    third degree T22.329 ☑
  epidermal loss - code as Burn, second degree, by site
  erythema, erythematous - code as Burn, first degree, by site
  esophagus T28.1 ☑
  extent (percentage of body surface)
    less than 10 percent T31.0
    10-19 percent T31.10
      with 0-9 percent third degree burns T31.10
      with 10-19 percent third degree burns T31.11
    20-29 percent T31.20
      with 0-9 percent third degree burns T31.20
      with 10-19 percent third degree burns T31.21
      with 20-29 percent third degree burns T31.22
    30-39 percent T31.30
      with 0-9 percent third degree burns T31.30
      with 10-19 percent third degree burns T31.31
      with 20-29 percent third degree burns T31.32
      with 30-39 percent third degree burns T31.33
    40-49 percent T31.40
      with 0-9 percent third degree burns T31.40
      with 10-19 percent third degree burns T31.41
      with 20-29 percent third degree burns T31.42
      with 30-39 percent third degree burns T31.43
      with 40-49 percent third degree burns T31.44
    50-59 percent T31.50
      with 0-9 percent third degree burns T31.50
      with 10-19 percent third degree burns T31.51
      with 20-29 percent third degree burns T31.52
      with 30-39 percent third degree burns T31.53

Burn — *continued*
      with 40-49 percent third degree burns T31.54
      with 50-59 percent third degree burns T31.55
    60-69 percent T31.60
      with 0-9 percent third degree burns T31.60
      with 10-19 percent third degree burns T31.61
      with 20-29 percent third degree burns T31.62
      with 30-39 percent third degree burns T31.63
      with 40-49 percent third degree burns T31.64
      with 50-59 percent third degree burns T31.65
      with 60-69 percent third degree burns T31.66
    70-79 percent T31.70
      with 0-9 percent third degree burns T31.70
      with 10-19 percent third degree burns T31.71
      with 20-29 percent third degree burns T31.72
      with 30-39 percent third degree burns T31.73
      with 40-49 percent third degree burns T31.74
      with 50-59 percent third degree burns T31.75
      with 60-69 percent third degree burns T31.76
      with 70-79 percent third degree burns T31.77
    80-89 percent T31.80
      with 0-9 percent third degree burns T31.80
      with 10-19 percent third degree burns T31.81
      with 20-29 percent third degree burns T31.82
      with 30-39 percent third degree burns T31.83
      with 40-49 percent third degree burns T31.84
      with 50-59 percent third degree burns T31.85
      with 60-69 percent third degree burns T31.86
      with 70-79 percent third degree burns T31.87
      with 80-89 percent third degree burns T31.88
    90 percent or more T31.90
      with 0-9 percent third degree burns T31.90
      with 10-19 percent third degree burns T31.91
      with 20-29 percent third degree burns T31.92
      with 30-39 percent third degree burns T31.93
      with 40-49 percent third degree burns T31.94
      with 50-59 percent third degree burns T31.95
      with 60-69 percent third degree burns T31.96
      with 70-79 percent third degree burns T31.97
      with 80-89 percent third degree burns T31.98
      with 90 percent or more third degree burns T31.99
  extremity — *see* Burn, limb
  eye (s) and adnexa T26.4- ☑
    with resulting rupture and destruction of eyeball T26.2- ☑
    conjunctival sac — *see* Burn, cornea
    cornea — *see* Burn, cornea
    lid — *see* Burn, eyelid
    periocular area — *see* Burn, eyelid
    specified site NEC T26.3- ☑
  eyeball — *see* Burn, eye
  eyelid (s) T26.0- ☑
    chemical — *see* Corrosion, eyelid
  face — *see* Burn, head
  finger T23.029 ☑
    first degree T23.129 ☑
    left T23.022 ☑
      first degree T23.122 ☑
      second degree T23.222 ☑
      third degree T23.322 ☑
    multiple sites (without thumb) T23.039 ☑
      with thumb T23.049 ☑
        first degree T23.149 ☑
        left T23.042 ☑
          first degree T23.142 ☑
          second degree T23.242 ☑
          third degree T23.342 ☑
        right T23.041 ☑
          first degree T23.141 ☑
          second degree T23.241 ☑
          third degree T23.341 ☑
        second degree T23.249 ☑
        third degree T23.349 ☑
    first degree T23.139 ☑
    left T23.032 ☑
      first degree T23.132 ☑
      second degree T23.232 ☑
      third degree T23.332 ☑
    right T23.031 ☑
      first degree T23.131 ☑
      second degree T23.231 ☑
      third degree T23.331 ☑
    second degree T23.239 ☑
    third degree T23.339 ☑
    right T23.021 ☑
      first degree T23.121 ☑
      second degree T23.221 ☑
      third degree T23.321 ☑
    second degree T23.229 ☑
    third degree T23.329 ☑
  flank — *see* Burn, abdominal wall

Burn

Burn — continued
 foot T25.029 ☑
  first degree T25.129 ☑
  left T25.022 ☑
   first degree T25.122 ☑
   second degree T25.222 ☑
   third degree T25.322 ☑
  multiple with ankle — see Burn, lower, limb,
   multiple, ankle and foot
  right T25.021 ☑
   first degree T25.121 ☑
   second degree T25.221 ☑
   third degree T25.321 ☑
  second degree T25.229 ☑
  third degree T25.329 ☑
 forearm T22.019 ☑
  first degree T22.119 ☑
  left T22.012 ☑
   first degree T22.112 ☑
   second degree T22.212 ☑
   third degree T22.312 ☑
  right T22.011 ☑
   first degree T22.111 ☑
   second degree T22.211 ☑
   third degree T22.311 ☑
  second degree T22.219 ☑
  third degree T22.319 ☑
 forehead T20.06 ☑
  first degree T20.16 ☑
  second degree T20.26 ☑
  third degree T20.36 ☑
 fourth degree - code as Burn, third degree, by
  site
 friction — see Burn, by site
 from swallowing caustic or corrosive substance
  NEC — see Corrosion, by site
 full thickness skin loss - code as Burn, third
  degree, by site
 gastrointestinal tract NEC T28.2 ☑
  from swallowing caustic or corrosive substance
   T28.7 ☑
 genital organs
  external
   female T21.07 ☑
    first degree T21.17 ☑
    second degree T21.27 ☑
    third degree T21.37 ☑
   male T21.06 ☑
    first degree T21.16 ☑
    second degree T21.26 ☑
    third degree T21.36 ☑
  internal T28.3 ☑
   from caustic or corrosive substance T28.8 ☑
 groin — see Burn, abdominal wall
 hand (s) T23.009 ☑
  back — see Burn, dorsum of hand
  finger — see Burn, finger
  first degree T23.109 ☑
  left T23.002 ☑
   first degree T23.102 ☑
   second degree T23.202 ☑
   third degree T23.302 ☑
  multiple sites with wrist T23.099 ☑
   first degree T23.199 ☑
   left T23.092 ☑
    first degree T23.192 ☑
    second degree T23.292 ☑
    third degree T23.392 ☑
   right T23.091 ☑
    first degree T23.191 ☑
    second degree T23.291 ☑
    third degree T23.391 ☑
   second degree T23.299 ☑
   third degree T23.399 ☑
  palm — see Burn, palm
  right T23.001 ☑
   first degree T23.101 ☑
   second degree T23.201 ☑
   third degree T23.301 ☑
  second degree T23.209 ☑
  third degree T23.309 ☑
  thumb — see Burn, thumb
 head (and face) (and neck) T20.00 ☑
  cheek — see Burn, cheek
  chin — see Burn, chin
  ear — see Burn, ear
  eye (s) only — see Burn, eye
  first degree T20.10 ☑
  forehead — see Burn, forehead
  lip — see Burn, lip
  multiple sites T20.09 ☑
   first degree T20.19 ☑

Burn — continued
   second degree T20.29 ☑
   third degree T20.39 ☑
  neck — see Burn, neck
  nose — see Burn, nose
  scalp — see Burn, scalp
  second degree T20.20 ☑
  third degree T20.30 ☑
 hip (s) — see Burn, lower, limb
 inhalation — see Burn, respiratory tract
  caustic or corrosive substance (fumes) — see
   Corrosion, respiratory tract
 internal organ (s) T28.40 ☑
  alimentary tract T28.2 ☑
   esophagus T28.1 ☑
  eardrum T28.41 ☑
  esophagus T28.1 ☑
  from caustic or corrosive substance
   (swallowing) NEC — see Corrosion, by site
  genitourinary T28.3 ☑
  mouth T28.0 ☑
  pharynx T28.0 ☑
  respiratory tract — see Burn, respiratory tract
  specified organ NEC T28.49 ☑
 interscapular region — see Burn, back, upper
 intestine (large) (small) T28.2 ☑
 knee T24.029 ☑
  first degree T24.129 ☑
  left T24.022 ☑
   first degree T24.122 ☑
   second degree T24.222 ☑
   third degree T24.322 ☑
  right T24.021 ☑
   first degree T24.121 ☑
   second degree T24.221 ☑
   third degree T24.321 ☑
  second degree T24.229 ☑
  third degree T24.329 ☑
 labium (majus) (minus) — see Burn, genital
  organs, external, female
 lacrimal apparatus, duct, gland or sac — see Burn,
  eye, specified site NEC
 larynx T27.0 ☑
  with lung T27.1 ☑
 leg (s) (lower) (upper) — see Burn, lower, limb
 lightning — see Burn, by site
 limb (s)
  lower (except ankle or foot alone) — see Burn,
   lower, limb
  upper — see Burn, upper limb
 lip (s) T20.02 ☑
  first degree T20.12 ☑
  second degree T20.22 ☑
  third degree T20.32 ☑
 lower
  back — see Burn, back
  limb T24.009 ☑
   ankle — see Burn, ankle
   calf — see Burn, calf
   first degree T24.109 ☑
   foot — see Burn, foot
   hip — see Burn, thigh
   knee — see Burn, knee
   left T24.002 ☑
    first degree T24.102 ☑
    second degree T24.202 ☑
    third degree T24.302 ☑
   multiple sites, except ankle and foot T24.099
    ☑
   ankle and foot T25.099 ☑
    first degree T25.199 ☑
    left T25.092 ☑
     first degree T25.192 ☑
     second degree T25.292 ☑
     third degree T25.392 ☑
    right T25.091 ☑
     first degree T25.191 ☑
     second degree T25.291 ☑
     third degree T25.391 ☑
    second degree T25.299 ☑
    third degree T25.399 ☑
   first degree T24.199 ☑
   left T24.092 ☑
    first degree T24.192 ☑
    second degree T24.292 ☑
    third degree T24.392 ☑
   right T24.091 ☑
    first degree T24.191 ☑
    second degree T24.291 ☑
    third degree T24.391 ☑
   second degree T24.299 ☑
   third degree T24.399 ☑

Burn — continued
  right T24.001 ☑
   first degree T24.101 ☑
   second degree T24.201 ☑
   third degree T24.301 ☑
  second degree T24.209 ☑
  thigh — see Burn, thigh
  third degree T24.309 ☑
  toe — see Burn, toe
 lung (with larynx and trachea) T27.1 ☑
 mouth T28.0 ☑
 neck T20.07 ☑
  first degree T20.17 ☑
  second degree T20.27 ☑
  third degree T20.37 ☑
 nose (septum) T20.04 ☑
  first degree T20.14 ☑
  second degree T20.24 ☑
  third degree T20.34 ☑
 ocular adnexa — see Burn, eye
 orbit region — see Burn, eyelid
 palm T23.059 ☑
  first degree T23.159 ☑
  left T23.052 ☑
   first degree T23.152 ☑
   second degree T23.252 ☑
   third degree T23.352 ☑
  right T23.051 ☑
   first degree T23.151 ☑
   second degree T23.251 ☑
   third degree T23.351 ☑
  second degree T23.259 ☑
  third degree T23.359 ☑
 partial thickness - code as Burn, unspecified
  degree, by site
 pelvis — see Burn, trunk
 penis — see Burn, genital organs, external, male
 perineum
  female — see Burn, genital organs, external,
   female
  male — see Burn, genital organs, external, male
 periocular area — see Burn, eyelid
 pharynx T28.0 ☑
 rectum T28.2 ☑
 respiratory tract T27.3 ☑
  larynx — see Burn, larynx
  specified part NEC T27.2 ☑
  trachea — see Burn, trachea
 sac, lacrimal — see Burn, eye, specified site NEC
 scalp T20.05 ☑
  first degree T20.15 ☑
  second degree T20.25 ☑
  third degree T20.35 ☑
 scapular region T22.069 ☑
  first degree T22.169 ☑
  left T22.062 ☑
   first degree T22.162 ☑
   second degree T22.262 ☑
   third degree T22.362 ☑
  right T22.061 ☑
   first degree T22.161 ☑
   second degree T22.261 ☑
   third degree T22.361 ☑
  second degree T22.269 ☑
  third degree T22.369 ☑
 sclera — see Burn, eye, specified site NEC
 scrotum — see Burn, genital organs, external,
  male
 shoulder T22.059 ☑
  first degree T22.159 ☑
  left T22.052 ☑
   first degree T22.152 ☑
   second degree T22.252 ☑
   third degree T22.352 ☑
  right T22.051 ☑
   first degree T22.151 ☑
   second degree T22.251 ☑
   third degree T22.351 ☑
  second degree T22.259 ☑
  third degree T22.359 ☑
 stomach T28.2 ☑
 temple — see Burn, head
 testis — see Burn, genital organs, external, male
 thigh T24.019 ☑
  first degree T24.119 ☑
  left T24.012 ☑
   first degree T24.112 ☑
   second degree T24.212 ☑
   third degree T24.312 ☑
  right T24.011 ☑
   first degree T24.111 ☑
   second degree T24.211 ☑

☑ **Additional character required**

Burn — continued
    third degree T24.311 ☑
    second degree T24.219 ☑
    third degree T24.319 ☑
  thorax (external) — see Burn, trunk
  throat (meaning pharynx) T28.0 ☑
  thumb (s) T23.019 ☑
    first degree T23.119 ☑
    left T23.012 ☑
      first degree T23.112 ☑
      second degree T23.212 ☑
      third degree T23.312 ☑
    multiple sites with fingers T23.049 ☑
      first degree T23.149 ☑
      left T23.042 ☑
        first degree T23.142 ☑
        second degree T23.242 ☑
        third degree T23.342 ☑
      right T23.041 ☑
        first degree T23.141 ☑
        second degree T23.241 ☑
        third degree T23.341 ☑
      second degree T23.249 ☑
      third degree T23.349 ☑
    right T23.011 ☑
      first degree T23.111 ☑
      second degree T23.211 ☑
      third degree T23.311 ☑
    second degree T23.219 ☑
    third degree T23.319 ☑
  toe T25.039 ☑
    first degree T25.139 ☑
    left T25.032 ☑
      first degree T25.132 ☑
      second degree T25.232 ☑
      third degree T25.332 ☑
    right T25.031 ☑
      first degree T25.131 ☑
      second degree T25.231 ☑
      third degree T25.331 ☑
    second degree T25.239 ☑
    third degree T25.339 ☑
  tongue T28.0 ☑
  tonsil (s) T28.0 ☑
  trachea T27.0 ☑
    with lung T27.1 ☑
  trunk T21.00 ☑
    abdominal wall — see Burn, abdominal wall
    anus — see Burn, buttock
    axilla — see Burn, upper limb
    back — see Burn, back
    breast — see Burn, chest wall
    buttock — see Burn, buttock
    chest wall — see Burn, chest wall
    first degree T21.10 ☑
    flank — see Burn, abdominal wall
    genital
      female — see Burn, genital organs, external, female
      male — see Burn, genital organs, external, male
    groin — see Burn, abdominal wall
    interscapular region — see Burn, back, upper
    labia — see Burn, genital organs, external, female
    lower back — see Burn, back
    penis — see Burn, genital organs, external, male
    perineum
      female — see Burn, genital organs, external, female
      male — see Burn, genital organs, external, male
    scapula region — see Burn, scapular region
    scrotum — see Burn, genital organs, external, male
    second degree T21.20 ☑
    specified site NEC T21.09 ☑
      first degree T21.19 ☑
      second degree T21.29 ☑
      third degree T21.39 ☑
    testes — see Burn, genital organs, external, male
    third degree T21.30 ☑
    upper back — see Burn, back, upper
    vulva — see Burn, genital organs, external, female
  unspecified site with extent of body surface involved specified
    less than 10 per cent T31.0
    10-19 per cent (0-9 percent third degree) T31.10
      with 10-19 percent third degree T31.11

Burn — continued
    20-29 per cent (0-9 percent third degree) T31.20
      with
        10-19 percent third degree T31.21
        20-29 percent third degree T31.22
    30-39 per cent (0-9 percent third degree) T31.30
      with
        10-19 percent third degree T31.31
        20-29 percent third degree T31.32
        30-39 percent third degree T31.33
    40-49 per cent (0-9 percent third degree) T31.40
      with
        10-19 percent third degree T31.41
        20-29 percent third degree T31.42
        30-39 percent third degree T31.43
        40-49 percent third degree T31.44
    50-59 per cent (0-9 percent third degree) T31.50
      with
        10-19 percent third degree T31.51
        20-29 percent third degree T31.52
        30-39 percent third degree T31.53
        40-49 percent third degree T31.54
        50-59 percent third degree T31.55
    60-69 per cent (0-9 percent third degree) T31.60
      with
        10-19 percent third degree T31.61
        20-29 percent third degree T31.62
        30-39 percent third degree T31.63
        40-49 percent third degree T31.64
        50-59 percent third degree T31.65
        60-69 percent third degree T31.66
    70-79 per cent (0-9 percent third degree) T31.70
      with
        10-19 percent third degree T31.71
        20-29 percent third degree T31.72
        30-39 percent third degree T31.73
        40-49 percent third degree T31.74
        50-59 percent third degree T31.75
        60-69 percent third degree T31.76
        70-79 percent third degree T31.77
    80-89 per cent (0-9 percent third degree) T31.80
      with
        10-19 percent third degree T31.81
        20-29 percent third degree T31.82
        30-39 percent third degree T31.83
        40-49 percent third degree T31.84
        50-59 percent third degree T31.85
        60-69 percent third degree T31.86
        70-79 percent third degree T31.87
        80-89 percent third degree T31.88
    90 per cent or more (0-9 percent third degree) T31.90
      with
        10-19 percent third degree T31.91
        20-29 percent third degree T31.92
        30-39 percent third degree T31.93
        40-49 percent third degree T31.94
        50-59 percent third degree T31.95
        60-69 percent third degree T31.96
        70-79 percent third degree T31.97
        80-89 percent third degree T31.98
        90-99 percent third degree T31.99
  upper limb T22.00 ☑
    above elbow — see Burn, above elbow
    axilla — see Burn, axilla
    elbow — see Burn, elbow
    first degree T22.10 ☑
    forearm — see Burn, forearm
    hand — see Burn, hand
    interscapular region — see Burn, back, upper
    multiple sites T22.099 ☑
      first degree T22.199 ☑
      left T22.092 ☑
        first degree T22.192 ☑
        second degree T22.292 ☑
        third degree T22.392 ☑
      right T22.091 ☑
        first degree T22.191 ☑
        second degree T22.291 ☑
        third degree T22.391 ☑
      second degree T22.299 ☑
      third degree T22.399 ☑
    scapular region — see Burn, scapular region
    second degree T22.20 ☑
    shoulder — see Burn, shoulder

Burn — continued
    third degree T22.30 ☑
    wrist — see Burn, wrist
  uterus T28.3 ☑
  vagina T28.3 ☑
  vulva — see Burn, genital organs, external, female
  wrist T23.079 ☑
    first degree T23.179 ☑
    left T23.072 ☑
      first degree T23.172 ☑
      second degree T23.272 ☑
      third degree T23.372 ☑
    multiple sites with hand T23.099 ☑
      first degree T23.199 ☑
      left T23.092 ☑
        first degree T23.192 ☑
        second degree T23.292 ☑
        third degree T23.392 ☑
      right T23.091 ☑
        first degree T23.191 ☑
        second degree T23.291 ☑
        third degree T23.391 ☑
      second degree T23.299 ☑
      third degree T23.399 ☑
    right T23.071 ☑
      first degree T23.171 ☑
      second degree T23.271 ☑
      third degree T23.371 ☑
    second degree T23.279 ☑
    third degree T23.379 ☑
Burnett's syndrome E83.52
Burning
  feet syndrome E53.9
  sensation R20.8
  tongue K14.6
Burn-out (state) Z73.0
Burns' disease or osteochondrosis — see Osteochondrosis, juvenile, ulna
Bursa — see condition
Bursitis M71.9
  Achilles — see Tendinitis, Achilles
  adhesive — see Bursitis, specified NEC
  ankle — see Enthesopathy, lower limb, ankle, specified type NEC
  calcaneal — see Enthesopathy, foot, specified type NEC
  collateral ligament, tibial — see Bursitis, tibial collateral
  due to use, overuse, pressure (see also Disorder, soft tissue, due to use, specified type NEC)
    specified NEC — see Disorder, soft tissue, due to use, specified NEC
  Duplay's M75.0 ☑
  elbow NEC M70.3- ☑
    olecranon M70.2- ☑
  finger — see Disorder, soft tissue, due to use, specified type NEC, hand
  foot — see Enthesopathy, foot, specified type NEC
  gonococcal A54.49
  gouty — see Gout, idiopathic
  hand M70.1- ☑
  hip NEC M70.7- ☑
    trochanteric M70.6- ☑
  infective NEC M71.10
    abscess — see Abscess, bursa
    ankle M71.17- ☑
    elbow M71.12- ☑
    foot M71.17- ☑
    hand M71.14- ☑
    hip M71.15- ☑
    knee M71.16- ☑
    multiple sites M71.19
    shoulder M71.11- ☑
    specified site NEC M71.18
    wrist M71.13- ☑
  ischial — see Bursitis, hip
  knee NEC M70.5- ☑
    prepatellar M70.4- ☑
  occupational NEC (see also Disorder, soft tissue, due to, use)
  olecranon — see Bursitis, elbow, olecranon
  pharyngeal J39.1
  popliteal — see Bursitis, knee
  prepatellar M70.4- ☑
  radiohumeral M77.8
  rheumatoid M06.20
    ankle M06.27- ☑
    elbow M06.22- ☑
    foot joint M06.27- ☑
    hand joint M06.24- ☑
    hip M06.25- ☑
    knee M06.26- ☑

Bursitis — *continued*
  multiple site M06.29
  shoulder M06.21- ☑
  vertebra M06.28
  wrist M06.23- ☑
 scapulohumeral — *see* Bursitis, shoulder
 semimembranous muscle (knee) — *see* Bursitis, knee
 shoulder M75.5- ☑
  adhesive — *see* Capsulitis, adhesive
 specified NEC M71.50
  ankle M71.57- ☑
  due to use, overuse or pressure — *see* Disorder, soft tissue, due to, use
  elbow M71.52- ☑
  foot M71.57- ☑
  hand M71.54- ☑
  hip M71.55- ☑
  knee M71.56- ☑
  shoulder — *see* Bursitis, shoulder
  specified site NEC M71.58
  tibial collateral M76.4- ☑
  wrist M71.53- ☑
 subacromial — *see* Bursitis, shoulder
 subcoracoid — *see* Bursitis, shoulder
 subdeltoid — *see* Bursitis, shoulder
 syphilitic A52.78
 Thornwaldt, Tornwaldt J39.2
 tibial collateral — *see* Bursitis, tibial collateral
 toe — *see* Enthesopathy, foot, specified type NEC
 trochanteric (area) — *see* Bursitis, hip, trochanteric
 wrist — *see* Bursitis, hand
Bursopathy M71.9
 specified type NEC M71.80
  ankle M71.87- ☑
  elbow M71.82- ☑
  foot M71.87- ☑
  hand M71.84- ☑
  hip M71.85- ☑
  knee M71.86- ☑
  multiple sites M71.89
  shoulder M71.81- ☑
  specified site NEC M71.88
  wrist M71.83- ☑
Burst stitches or sutures (complication of surgery) T81.31 ☑
 external operation wound T81.31 ☑
 internal operation wound T81.32 ☑
Buruli ulcer A31.1
Bury's disease L95.1
Buschke's
 disease B45.3
 scleredema — *see* Sclerosis, systemic
Busse-Buschke disease B45.3
Buttock — *see* condition
Button
 Biskra B55.1
 Delhi B55.1
 oriental B55.1
Buttonhole deformity (finger) — *see* Deformity, finger, boutonniere
Bwamba fever A92.8
Byssinosis J66.0
Bywaters' syndrome T79.5 ☑

C

Cachexia R64
 cancerous R64
 cardiac — *see* Disease, heart
 dehydration E86.0
  with
   hypernatremia E87.0
   hyponatremia E87.1
 due to malnutrition R64
 exophthalmic — *see* Hyperthyroidism
 heart — *see* Disease, heart
 hypophyseal E23.0
 hypopituitary E23.0
 lead — *see* Poisoning, lead
 malignant R64
 marsh — *see* Malaria
 nervous F48.8
 old age R54
 paludal — *see* Malaria
 pituitary E23.0
 renal N28.9
 saturnine — *see* Poisoning, lead

Cachexia — *continued*
 senile R54
 Simmonds' E23.0
 splenica D73.0
 strumipriva E03.4
 tuberculous NEC — *see* Tuberculosis
Café, au lait spots L81.3
Caffey's syndrome Q78.8
Caisson disease T70.3 ☑
Cake kidney Q63.1
Caked breast (puerperal, postpartum) O92.79
Calabar swelling B74.3
Calcaneal spur — *see* Spur, bone, calcaneal
Calcaneo-apophysitis M92.8
Calcareous — *see* condition
Calcicosis J62.8
Calciferol (vitamin D) deficiency E55.9
 with rickets E55.0
Calcification
 adrenal (capsule) (gland) E27.49
  tuberculous E35 [B90.8]
 aorta I70.0
 artery (annular) — *see* Arteriosclerosis
 auricle (ear) — *see* Disorder, pinna, specified type NEC
 basal ganglia G23.8
 bladder N32.89
  due to Schistosoma hematobium B65.0
 brain (cortex) — *see* Calcification, cerebral
 bronchus J98.09
 bursa M71.40
  ankle M71.47- ☑
  elbow M71.42- ☑
  foot M71.47- ☑
  hand M71.44- ☑
  hip M71.45- ☑
  knee M71.46- ☑
  multiple sites M71.49
  shoulder M75.3- ☑
  specified site NEC M71.48
  wrist M71.43- ☑
 cardiac — *see* Degeneration, myocardial
 cerebral (cortex) G93.89
  artery I67.2
 cervix (uteri) N88.8
 choroid plexus G93.89
 conjunctiva — *see* Concretion, conjunctiva
 corpora cavernosa (penis) N48.89
 cortex (brain) — *see* Calcification, cerebral
 dental pulp (nodular) K04.2
 dentinal papilla K00.4
 fallopian tube N83.8
 falx cerebri G96.19
 gallbladder K82.8
 general E83.59
 heart (*see also* Degeneration, myocardial)
  valve — *see* Endocarditis
 idiopathic infantile arterial (IIAC) Q28.8
 intervertebral cartilage or disc (postinfective) — *see* Disorder, disc, specified NEC
 intracranial — *see* Calcification, cerebral
 joint — *see* Disorder, joint, specified type NEC
 kidney N28.89
  tuberculous N29 [B90.1]
 larynx (senile) J38.7
 lens — *see* Cataract, specified NEC
 lung (active) (postinfectional) J98.4
  tuberculous B90.9
 lymph gland or node (postinfectional) I89.8
  tuberculous (*see also* Tuberculosis, lymph gland) B90.8
 mammographic R92.1
 massive (paraplegic) — *see* Myositis, ossificans, in, quadriplegia
 medial — *see* Arteriosclerosis, extremities
 meninges (cerebral) (spinal) G96.19
 metastatic E83.59
 Mönckeberg's — *see* Arteriosclerosis, extremities
 muscle M61.9
  due to burns — *see* Myositis, ossificans, in, burns
  paralytic — *see* Myositis, ossificans, in, quadriplegia
  specified type NEC M61.40
   ankle M61.47- ☑
   foot M61.47- ☑
   forearm M61.43- ☑
   hand M61.44- ☑
   lower leg M61.46- ☑
   multiple sites M61.49
   pelvic region M61.45- ☑
   shoulder region M61.41- ☑

Calcification — *continued*
   specified site NEC M61.48
   thigh M61.45- ☑
   upper arm M61.42- ☑
 myocardium, myocardial — *see* Degeneration, myocardial
 ovary N83.8
 pancreas K86.8
 penis N48.89
 periarticular — *see* Disorder, joint, specified type NEC
 pericardium (*see also* Pericarditis) I31.1
 pineal gland E34.8
 pleura J94.8
  postinfectional J94.8
  tuberculous NEC B90.9
 pulpal (dental) (nodular) K04.2
 sclera H15.89
 spleen D73.89
 subcutaneous L94.2
 suprarenal (capsule) (gland) E27.49
 tendon (sheath) (*see also* Tenosynovitis, specified type NEC)
  with bursitis, synovitis or tenosynovitis — *see* Tendinitis, calcific
 trachea J39.8
 ureter N28.89
 uterus N85.8
 vitreous — *see* Deposit, crystalline
Calcified — *see* Calcification
Calcinosis (interstitial) (tumoral) (universalis) E83.59
 with Raynaud's phenomenon, esophageal dysfunction, sclerodactyly, telangiectasia (CREST syndrome) M34.1
 circumscripta (skin) L94.2
 cutis L94.2
Calciphylaxis (*see also* Calcification, by site) E83.59
Calcium
 deposits — *see* Calcification, by site
 metabolism disorder E83.50
 salts or soaps in vitreous — *see* Deposit, crystalline
Calciuria R82.99
Calculi — *see* Calculus
Calculosis, intrahepatic — *see* Calculus, bile duct
Calculus, calculi, calculous
 ampulla of Vater — *see* Calculus, bile duct
 anuria (impacted) (recurrent) (*see also* Calculus, urinary) N20.9
 appendix K38.1
 bile duct (common) (hepatic) K80.50
  with
   calculus of gallbladder — *see* Calculus, gallbladder and bile duct
   cholangitis K80.30
    with
     cholecystitis — *see* Calculus, bile duct, with cholecystitis
     obstruction K80.31
    acute K80.32
     with
      chronic cholangitis K80.36
       with obstruction K80.37
      obstruction K80.33
    chronic K80.34
     with
      acute cholangitis K80.36
       with obstruction K80.37
      obstruction K80.35
   cholecystitis (with cholangitis) K80.40
    with obstruction K80.41
    acute K80.42
     with
      chronic cholecystitis K80.46
       with obstruction K80.47
      obstruction K80.43
    chronic K80.44
     with
      acute cholecystitis K80.46
       with obstruction K80.47
      obstruction K80.45
   obstruction K80.51
 biliary (*see also* Calculus, gallbladder)
  specified NEC K80.80
   with obstruction K80.81
 bilirubin, multiple — *see* Calculus, gallbladder
 bladder (encysted) (impacted) (urinary) (diverticulum) N21.0
 bronchus J98.09
 calyx (kidney) (renal) — *see* Calculus, kidney
 cholesterol (pure) (solitary) — *see* Calculus, gallbladder

☑ **Additional character required**

Calculus — *continued*
- common duct (bile) — *see* Calculus, bile duct
- conjunctiva — *see* Concretion, conjunctiva
- cystic N21.0
  - duct — *see* Calculus, gallbladder
- dental (subgingival) (supragingival) K03.6
- diverticulum
  - bladder N21.0
  - kidney N20.0
- epididymis N50.8
- gallbladder K80.20
  - with
    - bile duct calculus — *see* Calculus, gallbladder and bile duct
    - cholecystitis K80.10
      - with obstruction K80.11
      - acute K80.00
        - with
          - chronic cholecystitis K80.12
            - with obstruction K80.13
          - obstruction K80.01
      - chronic K80.10
        - with
          - acute cholecystitis K80.12
            - with obstruction K80.13
          - obstruction K80.11
      - specified NEC K80.18
        - with obstruction K80.19
    - obstruction K80.21
- gallbladder and bile duct K80.70
  - with
    - cholecystitis K80.60
      - with obstruction K80.61
      - acute K80.62
        - with
          - chronic cholecystitis K80.66
            - with obstruction K80.67
          - obstruction K80.63
      - chronic K80.64
        - with
          - acute cholecystitis K80.66
            - with obstruction K80.67
          - obstruction K80.65
    - obstruction K80.71
- hepatic (duct) — *see* Calculus, bile duct
- hepatobiliary K80.80
  - with obstruction K80.81
- ileal conduit N21.8
- intestinal (impaction) (obstruction) K56.49
- kidney (impacted) (multiple) (pelvis) (recurrent) (staghorn) N20.0
  - with calculus, ureter N20.2
  - congenital Q63.8
- lacrimal passages — *see* Dacryolith
- liver (impacted) — *see* Calculus, bile duct
- lung J98.4
- mammographic R92.1
- nephritic (impacted) (recurrent) — *see* Calculus, kidney
- nose J34.89
- pancreas (duct) K86.8
- parotid duct or gland K11.5
- pelvis, encysted — *see* Calculus, kidney
- prostate N42.0
- pulmonary J98.4
- pyelitis (impacted) (recurrent) N20.0
  - with hydronephrosis N13.2
- pyelonephritis (impacted) (recurrent)N20
  - with hydronephrosis N13.2
- renal (impacted) (recurrent) — *see* Calculus, kidney
- salivary (duct) (gland) K11.5
- seminal vesicle N50.8
- staghorn — *see* Calculus, kidney
- Stensen's duct K11.5
- stomach K31.89
- sublingual duct or gland K11.5
  - congenital Q38.4
- submandibular duct, gland or region K11.5
- submaxillary duct, gland or region K11.5
- suburethral N21.8
- tonsil J35.8
- tooth, teeth (subgingival) (supragingival) K03.6
- tunica vaginalis N50.8
- ureter (impacted) (recurrent) N20.1
  - with calculus, kidney N20.2
    - with hydronephrosis N13.2
      - with infection N13.6
- urethra (impacted) N21.1
- urinary (duct) (impacted) (passage) (tract) N20.9
  - with hydronephrosis N13.2
    - with infection N13.6

Calculus — *continued*
- in (due to)
  - lower N21.9
    - specified NEC N21.8
  - vagina N89.8
- vesical (impacted) N21.0
- Wharton's duct K11.5
- xanthine E79.8 [N22]

Calicectasis N28.89
Caliectasis N28.89
California
- disease B38.9
- encephalitis A83.5

Caligo cornea — *see* Opacity, cornea, central
Callositas, callosity (infected) L84
Callus (infected) L84
- bone — *see* Osteophyte
  - excessive, following fracture - code as Sequelae of fracture
Calorie deficiency or malnutrition (*see also* Malnutrition) E46
Calvé-Perthes disease — *see* Legg-Calvé-Perthes disease
Calvé's disease — *see* Osteochondrosis, juvenile, spine
Calvities — *see* Alopecia, androgenic
Cameroon fever — *see* Malaria
Camptocormia (hysterical) F44.4
Camurati-Engelmann syndrome Q78.3
Canal (*see also* condition)
- atrioventricular common Q21.2
Canaliculitis (lacrimal) (acute) (subacute) H04.33- ☑
- Actinomyces A42.89
- chronic H04.42- ☑
Canavan's disease E75.29
Canceled procedure (surgical) Z53.9
- because of
  - contraindication Z53.09
    - smoking Z53.01
  - left against medical advice (AMA) Z53.21
  - patient's decision Z53.20
    - for reasons of belief or group pressure Z53.1
    - specified reason NEC Z53.29
  - specified reason NEC Z53.8
Cancer (*see also* Neoplasm, by site, malignant)
- bile duct type liver C22.1
- blood — *see* Leukemia
- breast (*see also* Neoplasm, breast, malignant) C50.91- ☑
- hepatocellular C22.0
- lung (*see also* Neoplasm, lung, malignant) C34.90- ☑
- ovarian (*see also* Neoplasm ovary, malignant) C56.9- ☑
- unspecified site (primary) C80.1
Cancer (o)phobia F45.29
Cancerous — *see* Neoplasm, malignant, by site
Cancrum oris A69.0
Candidiasis, candidal B37.9
- balanitis B37.42
- bronchitis B37.1
- cheilitis B37.83
- congenital P37.5
- cystitis B37.41
- disseminated B37.7
- endocarditis B37.6
- enteritis B37.82
- esophagitis B37.81
- intertrigo B37.2
- lung B37.1
- meningitis B37.5
- mouth B37.0
- nails B37.2
- neonatal P37.5
- onychia B37.2
- oral B37.0
- osteomyelitis B37.89
- otitis externa B37.84
- paronychia B37.2
- perionyxis B37.2
- pneumonia B37.1
- proctitis B37.82
- pulmonary B37.1
- pyelonephritis B37.49
- sepsis B37.7
- skin B37.2
- specified site NEC B37.89
- stomatitis B37.0
- systemic B37.7
- urethritis B37.41
- urogenital site NEC B37.49
- vagina B37.3
- vulva B37.3

Candidiasis — *continued*
- vulvovaginitis B37.3
Candidid L30.2
Candidosis — *see* Candidiasis
Candiru infection or infestation B88.8
Canities (premature) L67.1
- congenital Q84.2
Canker (mouth) (sore) K12.0
- rash A38.9
Cannabinosis J66.2
Canton fever A75.9
Cantrell's syndrome Q87.89
Capillariasis (intestinal) B81.1
- hepatic B83.8
Capillary — *see* condition
Caplan's syndrome — *see* Rheumatoid, lung
Capsule — *see* condition
Capsulitis (joint) (*see also* Enthesopathy)
- adhesive (shoulder) M75.0- ☑
- hepatic K65.8
- labyrinthine — *see* Otosclerosis, specified NEC
- thyroid E06.9
Caput
- crepitus Q75.8
- medusae I86.8
- succedaneum P12.81
Car sickness T75.3 ☑
Carapata (disease) A68.0
Carate — *see* Pinta
Carbon lung J60
Carbuncle L02.93
- abdominal wall L02.231
- anus K61.0
- auditory canal, external — *see* Abscess, ear, external
- auricle ear — *see* Abscess, ear, external
- axilla L02.43- ☑
- back (any part) L02.232
- breast N61
- buttock L02.33
- cheek (external) L02.03
- chest wall L02.233
- chin L02.03
- corpus cavernosum N48.21
- ear (any part) (external) (middle) — *see* Abscess, ear, external
- external auditory canal — *see* Abscess, ear, external
- eyelid — *see* Abscess, eyelid
- face NEC L02.03
- femoral (region) — *see* Carbuncle, lower limb
- finger — *see* Carbuncle, hand
- flank L02.231
- foot L02.63- ☑
- forehead L02.03
- genital — *see* Abscess, genital
- gluteal (region) L02.33
- groin L02.234
- hand L02.53- ☑
- head NEC L02.831
- heel — *see* Carbuncle, foot
- hip — *see* Carbuncle, lower limb
- kidney — *see* Abscess, kidney
- knee — *see* Carbuncle, lower limb
- labium (majus) (minus) N76.4
- lacrimal
  - gland — *see* Dacryoadenitis
  - passages (duct) (sac) — *see* Inflammation, lacrimal, passages, acute
- leg — *see* Carbuncle, lower limb
- lower limb L02.43- ☑
- malignant A22.0
- navel L02.236
- neck L02.13
- nose (external) (septum) J34.0
- orbit, orbital — *see* Abscess, orbit
- palmar (space) — *see* Carbuncle, hand
- partes posteriores L02.33
- pectoral region L02.233
- penis N48.21
- perineum L02.235
- pinna — *see* Abscess, ear, external
- popliteal — *see* Carbuncle, lower limb
- scalp L02.831
- seminal vesicle N49.0
- shoulder — *see* Carbuncle, upper limb
- specified site NEC L02.838
- temple (region) L02.03
- thumb — *see* Carbuncle, hand
- toe — *see* Carbuncle, foot
- trunk L02.239
  - abdominal wall L02.231

☑ **Additional character required**

Carbuncle — *continued*
    back L02.232
    chest wall L02.233
    groin L02.234
    perineum L02.235
    umbilicus L02.236
   umbilicus L02.236
   upper limb L02.43- ☑
   urethra N34.0
   vulva N76.4
Carbunculus — *see* Carbuncle
Carcinoid (tumor) — *see* Tumor, carcinoid
Carcinoidosis E34.0
Carcinoma (malignant) (*see also* Neoplasm, by site, malignant)
   acidophil
    specified site — *see* Neoplasm, malignant, by site
    unspecified site C75.1
   acidophil-basophil, mixed
    specified site — *see* Neoplasm, malignant, by site
    unspecified site C75.1
   adnexal (skin) — *see* Neoplasm, skin, malignant
   adrenal cortical C74.0- ☑
   alveolar — *see* Neoplasm, lung, malignant
    cell — *see* Neoplasm, lung, malignant
   ameloblastic C41.1
    upper jaw (bone) C41.0
   apocrine
    breast — *see* Neoplasm, breast, malignant
    specified site NEC — *see* Neoplasm, skin, malignant
    unspecified site C44.99
   basal cell (pigmented) (*see also* Neoplasm, skin, malignant) C44.91
    fibro-epithelial — *see* Neoplasm, skin, malignant
    morphea — *see* Neoplasm, skin, malignant
    multicentric — *see* Neoplasm, skin, malignant
   basaloid
   basal-squamous cell, mixed — *see* Neoplasm, skin, malignant
   basophil
    specified site — *see* Neoplasm, malignant, by site
    unspecified site C75.1
   basophil-acidophil, mixed
    specified site — *see* Neoplasm, malignant, by site
    unspecified site C75.1
   basosquamous — *see* Neoplasm, skin, malignant
   bile duct
    with hepatocellular, mixed C22.0
    liver C22.1
    specified site NEC — *see* Neoplasm, malignant, by site
    unspecified site C22.1
   branchial or branchiogenic C10.4
   bronchial or bronchogenic — *see* Neoplasm, lung, malignant
   bronchiolar — *see* Neoplasm, lung, malignant
   bronchioloalveolar — *see* Neoplasm, lung, malignant
   C cell
    specified site — *see* Neoplasm, malignant, by site
    unspecified site C73
   ceruminous C44.29- ☑
   cervix uteri
    in situ D06.9
     endocervix D06.0
     exocervix D06.1
     specified site NEC D06.7
   chorionic
    specified site — *see* Neoplasm, malignant, by site
    unspecified site
     female C58
     male C62.90
   chromophobe
    specified site — *see* Neoplasm, malignant, by site
    unspecified site C75.1
   cloacogenic
    specified site — *see* Neoplasm, malignant, by site
    unspecified site C21.2
   diffuse type
    specified site — *see* Neoplasm, malignant, by site
    unspecified site C16.9

Carcinoma — *continued*
   duct (cell)
    with Paget's disease — *see* Neoplasm, breast, malignant
    infiltrating
     with lobular carcinoma (in situ)
      specified site — *see* Neoplasm, malignant, by site
      unspecified site (female) C50.91- ☑
       male C50.92- ☑
     specified site — *see* Neoplasm, malignant, by site
     unspecified site (female) C50.91- ☑
      male C50.92- ☑
   ductal
    with lobular
     specified site — *see* Neoplasm, malignant, by site
     unspecified site (female) C50.91- ☑
      male C50.92- ☑
   ductular, infiltrating
    specified site — *see* Neoplasm, malignant, by site
    unspecified site (female) C50.91- ☑
     male C50.92- ☑
   embryonal
    liver C22.7
   endometrioid
    specified site — *see* Neoplasm, malignant, by site
    unspecified site
     female C56.9
     male C61
   eosinophil
    specified site — *see* Neoplasm, malignant, by site
    unspecified site C75.1
   epidermoid (*see also* Neoplasm, skin malignant)
    in situ, Bowen's type — *see* Neoplasm, skin, in situ
   fibroepithelial, basal cell — *see* Neoplasm, skin, malignant
   follicular
    with papillary (mixed) C73
    moderately differentiated C73
    pure follicle C73
    specified site — *see* Neoplasm, malignant, by site
    trabecular C73
    unspecified site C73
    well differentiated C73
   generalized, with unspecified primary site C80.0
   glycogen-rich — *see* Neoplasm, breast, malignant
   granulosa cell C56- ☑
   hepatic cell C22.0
   hepatocellular C22.0
    with bile duct, mixed C22.0
    fibrolamellar C22.0
   hepatocholangiolitic C22.0
   Hurthle cell C73
   in
    adenomatous
     polyposis coli C18.9
    pleomorphic adenoma — *see* Neoplasm, salivary glands, malignant
    situ — *see* Carcinoma-in-situ
   infiltrating
    duct
     with lobular
      specified site — *see* Neoplasm, malignant, by site
      unspecified site (female) C50.91- ☑
       male C50.92- ☑
     with Paget's disease — *see* Neoplasm, breast, malignant
     specified site — *see* Neoplasm, malignant
     unspecified site (female) C50.91- ☑
      male C50.92- ☑
    ductular
     specified site — *see* Neoplasm, malignant
     unspecified site (female) C50.91- ☑
      male C50.92- ☑
    lobular
     specified site — *see* Neoplasm, malignant
     unspecified site (female) C50.91- ☑
      male C50.92- ☑
   inflammatory
    specified site — *see* Neoplasm, malignant
    unspecified site (female) C50.91- ☑
     male C50.92- ☑
   intestinal type

Carcinoma — *continued*
    specified site — *see* Neoplasm, malignant, by site
    unspecified site C16.9
   intracystic
    noninfiltrating — *see* Neoplasm, in situ, by site
   intraductal (noninfiltrating)
    with Paget's disease — *see* Neoplasm, breast, malignant
    breast D05.1- ☑
    papillary
     with invasion
      specified site — *see* Neoplasm, malignant, by site
      unspecified site (female) C50.91- ☑
       male C50.92- ☑
     breast D05.1- ☑
     specified site NEC — *see* Neoplasm, in situ, by site
     unspecified site (female) D05.1- ☑
    specified site NEC — *see* Neoplasm, in situ, by site
    unspecified site (female) D05.1- ☑
   intraepidermal — *see* Neoplasm, in situ
    squamous cell, Bowen's type — *see* Neoplasm, skin, in situ
   intraepithelial — *see* Neoplasm, in situ, by site
    squamous cell — *see* Neoplasm, in situ, by site
   intraosseous C41.1
    upper jaw (bone) C41.0
   islet cell
    with exocrine, mixed
     specified site — *see* Neoplasm, malignant, by site
     unspecified site C25.9
    pancreas C25.4
    specified site NEC — *see* Neoplasm, malignant, by site
    unspecified site C25.4
   juvenile, breast — *see* Neoplasm, breast, malignant
   large cell
    small cell
     specified site — *see* Neoplasm, malignant, by site
     unspecified site C34.90
   Leydig cell (testis)
    specified site — *see* Neoplasm, malignant, by site
    unspecified site
     female C56.9
     male C62.90
   lipid-rich (female) C50.91- ☑
    male C50.92- ☑
   liver cell C22.0
   liver NEC C22.7
   lobular (infiltrating)
    with intraductal
     specified site — *see* Neoplasm, malignant, by site
     unspecified site (female) C50.91- ☑
      male C50.92- ☑
    noninfiltrating
     breast D05.0- ☑
     specified site NEC — *see* Neoplasm, in situ, by site
     unspecified site D05.0- ☑
    specified site — *see* Neoplasm, malignant, by site
    unspecified site (female) C50.91- ☑
     male C50.92- ☑
   medullary
    with
     amyloid stroma
      specified site — *see* Neoplasm, malignant, by site
      unspecified site C73
     lymphoid stroma
      specified site — *see* Neoplasm, malignant, by site
      unspecified site (female) C50.91- ☑
       male C50.92- ☑
   Merkel cell C4A.9
    anal margin C4A.51
    anal skin C4A.51
    canthus C4A.1- ☑
    ear and external auricular canal C4A.2- ☑
    external auricular canal C4A.2- ☑
    eyelid, including canthus C4A.1- ☑
    face C4A.30
     specified NEC C4A.39
    hip C4A.7- ☑

Carcinoma — *continued*
　lip C4A.0
　lower limb, including hip C4A.7- ☑
　neck C4A.4
　nodal presentation C7B.1
　nose C4A.31
　overlapping sites C4A.8
　perianal skin C4A.51
　scalp C4A.4
　secondary C7B.1
　shoulder C4A.6- ☑
　skin of breast C4A.52
　trunk NEC C4A.59
　upper limb, including shoulder C4A.6- ☑
　visceral metastatic C7B.1
　metastatic — *see* Neoplasm, secondary, by site
　metatypical — *see* Neoplasm, skin, malignant
　morphea, basal cell — *see* Neoplasm, skin,
　　malignant
　mucoid
　　cell
　　　specified site — *see* Neoplasm, malignant,
　　　　by site
　　　unspecified site C75.1
　neuroendocrine (*see also* Tumor, neuroendocrine)
　　high grade, any site C7A.1
　　poorly differentiated, any site C7A.1
　nonencapsulated sclerosing C73
　noninfiltrating
　　intracystic — *see* Neoplasm, in situ, by site
　　intraductal
　　　breast D05.1- ☑
　　　papillary
　　　　breast D05.1- ☑
　　　　specified site NEC — *see* Neoplasm, in situ,
　　　　　by site
　　　　unspecified site D05.1- ☑
　　　specified site — *see* Neoplasm, in situ, by site
　　　unspecified site D05.1- ☑
　　lobular
　　　breast D05.0- ☑
　　　specified site NEC — *see* Neoplasm, in situ,
　　　　by site
　　　unspecified site (female) D05.0- ☑
　oat cell
　　specified site — *see* Neoplasm, malignant, by
　　　site
　　unspecified site C34.90
　odontogenic C41.1
　　upper jaw (bone) C41.0
　papillary
　　with follicular (mixed) C73
　　follicular variant C73
　　intraductal (noninfiltrating)
　　　with invasion
　　　　specified site — *see* Neoplasm, malignant,
　　　　　by site
　　　　unspecified site (female) C50.91- ☑
　　　　　male C50.92- ☑
　　　breast D05.1- ☑
　　　specified site NEC — *see* Neoplasm, in situ,
　　　　by site
　　　unspecified site D05.1- ☑
　　serous
　　　specified site — *see* Neoplasm, malignant,
　　　　by site
　　surface
　　　specified site — *see* Neoplasm, malignant,
　　　　by site
　　　unspecified site C56.9
　　unspecified site C56.9
　papillocystic
　　specified site — *see* Neoplasm, malignant, by
　　　site
　　unspecified site C56.9
　parafollicular cell
　　specified site — *see* Neoplasm, malignant, by
　　　site
　　unspecified site C73
　pilomatrix — *see* Neoplasm, skin, malignant
　pseudomucinous
　　specified site — *see* Neoplasm, malignant, by
　　　site
　　unspecified site C56.9
　renal cell C64- ☑
　Schmincke — *see* Neoplasm, nasopharynx,
　　malignant
　Schneiderian
　　specified site — *see* Neoplasm, malignant, by
　　　site
　　unspecified site C30.0
　sebaceous — *see* Neoplasm, skin, malignant

Carcinoma — *continued*
　secondary (*see also* Neoplasm, secondary, by site)
　　Merkel cell C7B.1
　secretory, breast — *see* Neoplasm, breast,
　　malignant
　serous
　　papillary
　　　specified site — *see* Neoplasm, malignant,
　　　　by site
　　　unspecified site C56.9
　　surface, papillary
　　　specified site — *see* Neoplasm, malignant,
　　　　by site
　　　unspecified site C56.9
　Sertoli cell
　　specified site — *see* Neoplasm, malignant, by
　　　site
　　unspecified site C62.90
　　　female C56.9
　　　male C62.90
　skin appendage — *see* Neoplasm, skin,
　　malignant
　small cell
　　fusiform cell
　　　specified site — *see* Neoplasm, malignant,
　　　　by site
　　　unspecified site C34.90
　　intermediate cell
　　　specified site — *see* Neoplasm, malignant,
　　　　by site
　　　unspecified site C34.90
　　large cell
　　　specified site — *see* Neoplasm, malignant,
　　　　by site
　　　unspecified site C34.90
　solid
　　with amyloid stroma
　　　specified site — *see* Neoplasm, malignant,
　　　　by site
　　　unspecified site C73
　　microinvasive
　　　specified site — *see* Neoplasm, malignant,
　　　　by site
　　　unspecified site C53.9
　sweat gland — *see* Neoplasm, skin, malignant
　theca cell C56.- ☑
　thymic C37
　unspecified site (primary) C80.1
　water-clear cell C75.0
Carcinoma-in-situ (*see also* Neoplasm, in situ, by
　site)
　breast NOS D05.9- ☑
　　specified type NEC D05.8- ☑
　epidermoid (*see also* Neoplasm, in situ, by site)
　　with questionable stromal invasion
　　　cervix D06.9
　　　specified site NEC — *see* Neoplasm, in situ,
　　　　by site
　　　unspecified site D06.9
　　Bowen's type — *see* Neoplasm, skin, in situ
　　intraductal
　　　breast D05.1- ☑
　　　specified site NEC — *see* Neoplasm, in situ,
　　　　by site
　　　unspecified site D05.1- ☑
　lobular
　　with
　　　infiltrating duct
　　　　breast (female) C50.91- ☑
　　　　　male C50.92- ☑
　　　　specified site NEC — *see* Neoplasm,
　　　　　malignant
　　　　unspecified site (female) C50.91- ☑
　　　　　male C50.92- ☑
　　　intraductal
　　　　breast D05.8- ☑
　　　　specified site NEC — *see* Neoplasm, in situ,
　　　　　by site
　　　　unspecified site (female) D05.8- ☑
　　breast D05.0- ☑
　　specified site NEC — *see* Neoplasm, in situ,
　　　by site
　　unspecified site D05.0- ☑
　squamous cell (*see also* Neoplasm, in situ, by site)
　　with questionable stromal invasion
　　　cervix D06.9
　　　specified site NEC — *see* Neoplasm, in situ,
　　　　by site
　　　unspecified site D06.9
Carcinomaphobia F45.29
Carcinomatosis C80.0
　peritonei C78.6

Carcinomatosis — *continued*
　unspecified site (primary) (secondary) C80.0
Carcinosarcoma — *see* Neoplasm, malignant, by
　site
　embryonal — *see* Neoplasm, malignant, by site
Cardia, cardial — *see* condition
Cardiac (*see also* condition)
　death, sudden — *see* Arrest, cardiac
　pacemaker
　　in situ Z95.0
　　management or adjustment Z45.018
　tamponade I31.4
Cardialgia — *see* Pain, precordial
Cardiectasis — *see* Hypertrophy, cardiac
Cardiochalasia K21.9
Cardiomalacia I51.5
Cardiomegalia glycogenica diffusa E74.02 [I43]
Cardiomegaly (*see also* Hypertrophy, cardiac)
　congenital Q24.8
　glycogen E74.02 [I43]
　idiopathic I51.7
Cardiomyoliposis I51.5
Cardiomyopathy (familial) (idiopathic) I42.9
　alcoholic I42.6
　amyloid E85.4 [I43]
　arteriosclerotic — *see* Disease, heart, ischemic,
　　atherosclerotic
　beriberi E51.12
　cobalt-beer I42.6
　congenital I42.4
　congestive I42.0
　constrictive NOS I42.5
　dilated I42.0
　due to
　　alcohol I42.6
　　beriberi E51.12
　　cardiac glycogenosis E74.02 [I43]
　　drugs I42.7
　　external agents NEC I42.7
　　Friedreich's ataxia G11.1
　　myotonia atrophica G71.11 [I43]
　　progressive muscular dystrophy G71.0
　glycogen storage E74.02 [I43]
　hypertensive — *see* Hypertension, heart
　hypertrophic (nonobstructive) I42.2
　　obstructive I42.1
　　　congenital Q24.8
　in
　　Chagas' disease (chronic) B57.2
　　　acute B57.0
　　sarcoidosis D86.85
　ischemic I25.5
　metabolic E88.9 [I43]
　　thyrotoxic E05.90 [I43]
　　　with thyroid storm E05.91 [I43]
　newborn I42.8
　　congenital I42.4
　nutritional E63.9 [I43]
　　beriberi E51.12
　obscure of Africa I42.8
　peripartum O90.3
　postpartum O90.3
　restrictive NEC I42.5
　rheumatic I09.0
　secondary I42.9
　stress induced I51.81
　takotsubo I51.81
　thyrotoxic E05.90 [I43]
　　with thyroid storm E05.91 [I43]
　toxic NEC I42.7
　tuberculous A18.84
　viral B33.24
Cardionephritis — *see* Hypertension, cardiorenal
Cardionephropathy — *see* Hypertension,
　cardiorenal
Cardionephrosis — *see* Hypertension, cardiorenal
Cardiopathia nigra I27.0
Cardiopathy (*see also* Disease, heart) I51.9
　idiopathic I42.9
　mucopolysaccharidosis E76.3 [I52]
Cardiopericarditis — *see* Pericarditis
Cardiophobia F45.29
Cardiorenal — *see* condition
Cardiorrhexis — *see* Infarct, myocardium
Cardiosclerosis — *see* Disease, heart, ischemic,
　atherosclerotic
Cardiosis — *see* Disease, heart
Cardiospasm (esophagus) (reflex) (stomach) K22.0
　congenital Q39.5
　　with megaesophagus Q39.5
Cardiostenosis — *see* Disease, heart
Cardiosymphysis I31.0

☑ **Additional character required**

Cardiovascular — *see* condition
Carditis (acute) (bacterial) (chronic) (subacute)
I51.89
  meningococcal A39.50
  rheumatic — *see* Disease, heart, rheumatic
  rheumatoid — *see* Rheumatoid, carditis
  viral B33.20
Care (of) (for) (following)
  child (routine) Z76.2
  family member (handicapped) (sick)
    creating problem for family Z63.6
    provided away from home for holiday relief
      Z75.5
    unavailable, due to
      absence (person rendering care) (sufferer)
        Z74.2
      inability (any reason) of person rendering
        care Z74.2
  foundling Z76.1
  holiday relief Z75.5
  improper — *see* Maltreatment
  lack of (at or after birth) (infant) — *see*
    Maltreatment, child, neglect
  lactating mother Z39.1
  palliative Z51.5
  postpartum
    immediately after delivery Z39.0
    routine follow-up Z39.2
  respite Z75.5
  unavailable, due to
    absence of person rendering care Z74.2
    inability (any reason) of person rendering care
      Z74.2
  well-baby Z76.2
Caries
  bone NEC A18.03
  dental K02.9
    arrested (coronal) (root) K02.3
    chewing surface
      limited to enamel K02.51
      penetrating into dentin K02.52
      penetrating into pulp K02.53
    coronal surface
      chewing surface
        limited to enamel K02.51
        penetrating into dentin K02.52
        penetrating into pulp K02.53
      pit and fissure surface
        limited to enamel K02.51
        penetrating into dentin K02.52
        penetrating into pulp K02.53
      smooth surface
        limited to enamel K02.61
        penetrating into dentin K02.62
        penetrating into pulp K02.63
    pit and fissure surface
      limited to enamel K02.51
      penetrating into dentin K02.52
      penetrating into pulp K02.53
    root K02.7
    smooth surface
      limited to enamel K02.61
      penetrating into dentin K02.62
      penetrating into pulp K02.63
  external meatus — *see* Disorder, ear, external,
    specified type NEC
  hip (tuberculous) A18.02
  initial (tooth)
    chewing surface K02.51
    pit and fissure surface K02.51
    smooth surface K02.61
  knee (tuberculous) A18.02
  labyrinth H83.8
  limb NEC (tuberculous) A18.03
  mastoid process (chronic) — *see* Mastoiditis,
    chronic
    tuberculous A18.03
  middle ear H74.8
  nose (tuberculous) A18.03
  orbit (tuberculous) A18.03
  ossicles, ear — *see* Abnormal, ear ossicles
  petrous bone — *see* Petrositis
  root (dental) (tooth) K02.7
  sacrum (tuberculous) A18.01
  spine, spinal (column) (tuberculous) A18.01
  syphilitic A52.77
    congenital (early) A50.02 [M90.80]
  tooth, teeth — *see* Caries, dental
  tuberculous A18.03
  vertebra (column) (tuberculous) A18.01
Carious teeth — *see* Caries, dental
Carneous mole O02.0

Carnitine insufficiency E71.40
Carotid body or sinus syndrome G90.01
Carotidynia G90.01
Carotinemia (dietary) E67.1
Carotinosis (cutis) (skin) E67.1
Carpal tunnel syndrome — *see* Syndrome, carpal
  tunnel
Carpenter's syndrome Q87.0
Carpopedal spasm — *see* Tetany
Carr-Barr-Plunkett syndrome Q97.1
Carrier (suspected) of
  amebiasis Z22.1
  bacterial disease NEC Z22.39
    diphtheria Z22.2
    intestinal infectious NEC Z22.1
      typhoid Z22.0
    meningococcal Z22.31
    sexually transmitted Z22.4
    specified NEC Z22.39
    staphylococcal (Methicillin susceptible)
      Z22.321
      Methicillin resistant Z22.322
    streptococcal Z22.338
      group B Z22.330
    typhoid Z22.0
  cholera Z22.1
  diphtheria Z22.2
  gastrointestinal pathogens NEC Z22.1
  genetic Z14.8
    cystic fibrosis Z14.1
    hemophilia A (asymptomatic) Z14.01
      symptomatic Z14.02
  gonorrhea Z22.4
  HAA (hepatitis Australian-antigen) Z22.59
  HB (c)(s)-AG Z22.51
  hepatitis (viral) Z22.50
    Australia-antigen (HAA) Z22.59
    B surface antigen (HBsAg) Z22.51
      with acute delta- (super)infection B17.0
    C Z22.52
    specified NEC Z22.59
  human T-cell lymphotropic virus type-1 (HTLV-1)
    infection Z22.6
  infectious organism Z22.9
    specified NEC Z22.8
  meningococci Z22.31
  Salmonella typhosa Z22.0
  serum hepatitis — *see* Carrier, hepatitis
  staphylococci (Methicillin susceptible) Z22.321
    Methicillin resistant Z22.322
  streptococci Z22.338
    group B Z22.330
  syphilis Z22.4
  typhoid Z22.0
  venereal disease NEC Z22.4
Carrion's disease A44.0
Carter's relapsing fever (Asiatic) A68.1
Cartilage — *see* condition
Caruncle (inflamed)
  conjunctiva (acute) — *see* Conjunctivitis, acute
  labium (majus) (minus) N90.89
  lacrimal — *see* Inflammation, lacrimal, passages
  myrtiform N89.8
  urethral (benign) N36.2
Cascade stomach K31.2
Caseation lymphatic gland (tuberculous) A18.2
Cassidy (-Scholte) syndrome (malignant carcinoid)
  E34.0
Castellani's disease A69.8
Castration, traumatic, male S38.231 ☑
Casts in urine R82.99
Cat
  cry syndrome Q93.4
  ear Q17.3
  eye syndrome Q92.8
Catabolism, senile R54
Catalepsy (hysterical) F44.2
  schizophrenic F20.2
Cataplexy (idiopathic) — *see* - Narcolepsy
Cataract (cortical) (immature) (incipient) H26.9
  with
    neovascularization — *see* Cataract, complicated
  age-related — *see* Cataract, senile
  anterior
    and posterior axial embryonal Q12.0
    pyramidal Q12.0
  associated with
    galactosemia E74.21 [H28]
    myotonic disorders G71.19 [H28]
  blue Q12.0
  central Q12.0
  cerulean Q12.0

Cataract — *continued*
  complicated H26.20
    with
      neovascularization H26.21- ☑
      ocular disorder H26.22- ☑
    glaucomatous flecks H26.23- ☑
  congenital Q12.0
  coraliform Q12.0
  coronary Q12.0
  crystalline Q12.0
  diabetic — *see* Diabetes, cataract
  drug-induced H26.3- ☑
  due to
    ocular disorder — *see* Cataract, complicated
    radiation H26.8
  electric H26.8
  extraction status Z98.4- ☑
  glass-blower's H26.8
  heat ray H26.8
  heterochromic — *see* Cataract, complicated
  hypermature — *see* Cataract, senile, morgagnian
    type
  in (due to)
    chronic iridocyclitis — *see* Cataract,
      complicated
    diabetes — *see* Diabetes, cataract
    endocrine disease E34.9 [H28]
    eye disease — *see* Cataract, complicated
    hypoparathyroidism E20.9 [H28]
    malnutrition-dehydration E46 [H28]
    metabolic disease E88.9 [H28]
    myotonic disorders G71.19 [H28]
    nutritional disease E63.9 [H28]
  infantile — *see* Cataract, presenile
  irradiational — *see* Cataract, specified NEC
  juvenile — *see* Cataract, presenile
  malnutrition-dehydration E46 [H28]
  morgagnian — *see* Cataract, senile, morgagnian
    type
  myotonic G71.19 [H28]
  myxedema E03.9 [H28]
  nuclear
    embryonal Q12.0
    sclerosis — *see* Cataract, senile, nuclear
  presenile H26.00- ☑
    combined forms H26.06- ☑
    cortical H26.01- ☑
    lamellar — *see* Cataract, presenile, cortical
    nuclear H26.03- ☑
    specified NEC H26.09
    subcapsular polar (anterior) H26.04- ☑
      posterior H26.05- ☑
    zonular — *see* Cataract, presenile, cortical
  secondary H26.40
    Soemmering's ring H26.41- ☑
    specified NEC H26.49- ☑
    to eye disease — *see* Cataract, complicated
  senile H25.9
    brunescens — *see* Cataract, senile, nuclear
    combined forms H25.81- ☑
    coronary — *see* Cataract, senile, incipient
    cortical H25.01- ☑
    hypermature — *see* Cataract, senile,
      morgagnian type
    incipient (mature) (total) H25.09- ☑
      cortical — *see* Cataract, senile, cortical
      subcapsular — *see* Cataract, senile,
        subcapsular
    morgagnian type (hypermature) H25.2- ☑
    nuclear (sclerosis) H25.1- ☑
    polar subcapsular (anterior) (posterior) — *see*
      Cataract, senile, incipient
    punctate — *see* Cataract, senile, incipient
    specified NEC H25.89
    subcapsular polar (anterior) H25.03- ☑
      posterior H25.04- ☑
  snowflake — *see* Diabetes, cataract
  specified NEC H26.8
  toxic — *see* Cataract, drug-induced
  traumatic H26.10- ☑
    localized H26.11- ☑
    partially resolved H26.12- ☑
    total H26.13- ☑
  zonular (perinuclear) Q12.0
Cataracta (*see also* Cataract)
  brunescens — *see* Cataract, senile, nuclear
  centralis pulverulenta Q12.0
  cerulea Q12.0
  complicata — *see* Cataract, complicated
  congenita Q12.0
  coralliformis Q12.0
  coronaria Q12.0

☑ **Additional character required**

Cataracta — *continued*
  diabetic — *see* Diabetes, cataract
  membranacea
    accreta — *see* Cataract, secondary
    congenita Q12.0
  nigra — *see* Cataract, senile, nuclear
  sunflower — *see* Cataract, complicated
Catarrh, catarrhal (acute) (febrile) (infectious) (inflammation) (*see also* condition) J00
  bronchial — *see* Bronchitis
  chest — *see* Bronchitis
  chronic J31.0
  due to congenital syphilis A50.03
  enteric — *see* Enteritis
  eustachian H68.009
  fauces — *see* Pharyngitis
  gastrointestinal — *see* Enteritis
  gingivitis K05.00
    nonplaque induced K05.01
    plaque induced K05.00
  hay — *see* Fever, hay
  intestinal — *see* Enteritis
  larynx, chronic J37.0
  liver B15.9
    with hepatic coma B15.0
  lung — *see* Bronchitis
  middle ear, chronic — *see* Otitis, media, nonsuppurative, chronic, serous
  mouth K12.1
  nasal (chronic) — *see* Rhinitis
  nasobronchial J31.1
  nasopharyngeal (chronic) J31.1
    acute J00
  pulmonary — *see* Bronchitis
  spring (eye) (vernal) — *see* Conjunctivitis, acute, atopic
  summer (hay) — *see* Fever, hay
  throat J31.2
  tubotympanal (*see also* Otitis, media, nonsuppurative)
    chronic — *see* Otitis, media, nonsuppurative, chronic, serous
Catatonia (schizophrenic) F20.2
Catatonic
  disorder due to known physiologic condition F06.1
  schizophrenia F20.2
  stupor R40.1
Cat-scratch (*see also* Abrasion)
  disease or fever A28.1
Cauda equina — *see* condition
Cauliflower ear M95.1- ☑
Causalgia (upper limb) G56.4- ☑
  lower limb G57.7- ☑
Cause
  external, general effects T75.89 ☑
Caustic burn — *see* Corrosion, by site
Cavare's disease (familial periodic paralysis) G72.3
Cave-in, injury
  crushing (severe) — *see* Crush
  suffocation — *see* Asphyxia, traumatic, due to low oxygen, due to cave-in
Cavernitis (penis) N48.29
Cavernositis N48.29
Cavernous — *see* condition
Cavitation of lung (*see also* Tuberculosis, pulmonary)
  nontuberculous J98.4
Cavities, dental — *see* Caries, dental
Cavity
  lung — *see* Cavitation of lung
  optic papilla Q14.2
  pulmonary — *see* Cavitation of lung
Cavovarus foot, congenital Q66.1
Cavus foot (congenital) Q66.7
  acquired — *see* Deformity, limb, foot, specified NEC
Cazenave's disease L10.2
Cecitis K52.9
  with perforation, peritonitis, or rupture K65.8
Cecum — *see* condition
Celiac
  artery compression syndrome I77.4
  disease K90.0
  infantilism K90.0
Cell (s), cellular (*see also* condition)
  in urine R82.99
Cellulitis (diffuse) (phlegmonous) (septic) (suppurative) L03.90
  abdominal wall L03.311
  anaerobic A48.0
  ankle — *see* Cellulitis, lower limb
  anus K61.0

Cellulitis — *continued*
  arm — *see* Cellulitis, upper limb
  auricle (ear) — *see* Cellulitis, ear
  axilla L03.11- ☑
  back (any part) L03.312
  broad ligament
    acute N73.0
  buttock L03.317
  cervical (meaning neck) L03.221
  cervix (uteri) — *see* Cervicitis
  cheek (external) L03.211
    internal K12.2
  chest wall L03.313
  chronic L03.90
  clostridial A48.0
  corpus cavernosum N48.22
  digit
    finger — *see* Cellulitis, finger
    toe — *see* Cellulitis, toe
  Douglas' cul-de-sac or pouch
    acute N73.0
  drainage site (following operation) T81.4 ☑
  ear (external) H60.1- ☑
  eosinophilic (granulomatous) L98.3
  erysipelatous — *see* Erysipelas
  external auditory canal — *see* Cellulitis, ear
  eyelid — *see* Abscess, eyelid
  face NEC L03.211
  finger (intrathecal) (periosteal) (subcutaneous) (subcuticular) L03.01- ☑
  foot — *see* Cellulitis, lower limb
  gangrenous — *see* Gangrene
  genital organ NEC
    female (external) N76.4
    male N49.9
      multiple sites N49.8
      specified NEC N49.8
  gluteal (region) L03.317
  gonococcal A54.89
  groin L03.314
  hand — *see* Cellulitis, upper limb
  head NEC L03.811
    face (any part, except ear, eye and nose) L03.211
  heel — *see* Cellulitis, lower limb
  hip — *see* Cellulitis, lower limb
  jaw (region) L03.211
  knee — *see* Cellulitis, lower limb
  labium (majus) (minus) — *see* Vulvitis
  lacrimal passages — *see* Inflammation, lacrimal, passages
  larynx J38.7
  leg — *see* Cellulitis, lower limb
  lip K13.0
  lower limb L03.11- ☑
    toe — *see* Cellulitis, toe
  mouth (floor) K12.2
  multiple sites, so stated L03.90
  nasopharynx J39.1
  navel L03.316
    newborn P38.9
      with mild hemorrhage P38.1
      without hemorrhage P38.9
  neck (region) L03.221
  nose (septum) (external) J34.0
  orbit, orbital H05.01- ☑
  palate (soft) K12.2
  pectoral (region) L03.313
  pelvis, pelvic (chronic)
    female (*see also* Disease, pelvis, inflammatory) N73.2
      acute N73.0
      following ectopic or molar pregnancy O08.0
    male K65.0
  penis N48.22
  perineal, perineum L03.315
  perirectal K61.1
  peritonsillar J36
  periurethral N34.0
  periuterine (*see also* Disease, pelvis, inflammatory) N73.2
    acute N73.0
  pharynx J39.1
  rectum K61.1
  retroperitoneal K68.9
  round ligament
    acute N73.0
  scalp (any part) L03.811
  scrotum N49.2
  seminal vesicle N49.0
  shoulder — *see* Cellulitis, upper limb
  specified site NEC L03.818

Cellulitis — *continued*
  submandibular (region) (space) (triangle) K12.2
    gland K11.3
  submaxillary (region) K12.2
    gland K11.3
  thigh — *see* Cellulitis, lower limb
  thumb (intrathecal) (periosteal) (subcutaneous) (subcuticular) — *see* Cellulitis, finger
  toe (intrathecal) (periosteal) (subcutaneous) (subcuticular) L03.03- ☑
  tonsil J36
  trunk L03.319
    abdominal wall L03.311
    back (any part) L03.312
    buttock L03.317
    chest wall L03.313
    groin L03.314
    perineal, perineum L03.315
    umbilicus L03.316
  tuberculous (primary) A18.4
  umbilicus L03.316
  upper limb L03.11- ☑
    axilla — *see* Cellulitis, axilla
    finger — *see* Cellulitis, finger
    thumb — *see* Cellulitis, finger
  vaccinal T88.0 ☑
  vocal cord J38.3
  vulva — *see* Vulvitis
  wrist — *see* Cellulitis, upper limb
Cementoblastoma, benign — *see* Cyst, calcifying odontogenic
Cementoma — *see* Cyst, calcifying odontogenic
Cementoperiostitis — *see* Periodontitis
Cementosis K03.4
Central auditory processing disorder H93.25
Central pain syndrome G89.0
Cephalematocele, cephal (o)hematocele
  newborn P52.8
    birth injury P10.8
  traumatic — *see* Hematoma, brain
Cephalematoma, cephalhematoma (calcified)
  newborn (birth injury) P12.0
  traumatic — *see* Hematoma, brain
Cephalgia, cephalalgia (*see also* Headache)
  histamine G44.009
    intractable G44.001
    not intractable G44.009
  trigeminal autonomic (TAC) NEC G44.099
    intractable G44.091
    not intractable G44.099
Cephalic — *see* condition
Cephalitis — *see* Encephalitis
Cephalocele — *see* Encephalocele
Cephalomenia N94.89
Cephalopelvic — *see* condition
Cerclage (with cervical incompetence) in pregnancy — *see* Incompetence, cervix, in pregnancy
Cerebellitis — *see* Encephalitis
Cerebellum, cerebellar — *see* condition
Cerebral — *see* condition
Cerebritis — *see* Encephalitis
Cerebro-hepato-renal syndrome Q87.89
Cerebromalacia — *see* Softening, brain
  sequelae of cerebrovascular disease I69.398
Cerebroside lipidosis E75.22
Cerebrospasticity (congenital) G80.1
Cerebrospinal — *see* condition
Cerebrum — *see* condition
Ceroid-lipofuscinosis, neuronal E75.4
Cerumen (accumulation) (impacted) H61.2- ☑
Cervical (*see also* condition)
  auricle Q18.2
  dysplasia in pregnancy — *see* Abnormal, cervix, in pregnancy or childbirth
  erosion in pregnancy — *see* Abnormal, cervix, in pregnancy or childbirth
  fibrosis in pregnancy — *see* Abnormal, cervix, in pregnancy or childbirth
  fusion syndrome Q76.1
  rib Q76.5
  shortening (complicating pregnancy) O26.87- ☑
Cervicalgia M54.2
Cervicitis (acute) (chronic) (nonvenereal) (senile (atrophic)) (subacute) (with ulceration) N72
  with
    abortion — *see* Abortion, by type complicated by genital tract and pelvic infection
    ectopic pregnancy O08.0
    molar pregnancy O08.0
  chlamydial A56.09
  gonococcal A54.03
  herpesviral A60.03

Cervicitis — *continued*
  puerperal (postpartum) O86.11
  syphilitic A52.76
  trichomonal A59.09
  tuberculous A18.16
Cervicocolpitis (emphysematosa) (see also
  Cervicitis) N72
Cervix — *see* condition
Cesarean delivery, previous, affecting management
  of pregnancy O34.21
Céstan (-Chenais) paralysis or syndrome G46.3
Céstan-Raymond syndrome I65.8
Cestode infestation B71.9
  specified type NEC B71.8
Cestodiasis B71.9
Chabert's disease A22.9
Chacaleh E53.8
Chafing L30.4
Chagas' (-Mazza) disease (chronic) B57.2
  with
    cardiovascular involvement NEC B57.2
    digestive system involvement B57.30
      megacolon B57.32
      megaesophagus B57.31
      other specified B57.39
    megacolon B57.32
    megaesophagus B57.31
    myocarditis B57.2
    nervous system involvement B57.40
      meningitis B57.41
      meningoencephalitis B57.42
      other specified B57.49
    specified organ involvement NEC B57.5
  acute (with) B57.1
    cardiovascular NEC B57.0
    myocarditis B57.0
Chagres fever B50.9
Chairridden Z74.09
Chalasia (cardiac sphincter) K21.9
Chalazion H00.19
  left H00.16
    lower H00.15
    upper H00.14
  right H00.13
    lower H00.12
    upper H00.11
Chalcosis (see also Disorder, globe, degenerative,
  chalcosis)
  cornea — see Deposit, cornea
  crystalline lens — see Cataract, complicated
  retina H35.89
Chalicosis (pulmonum) J62.8
Chancre (any genital site) (hard) (hunterian) (mixed)
  (primary) (seronegative) (seropositive) (syphilitic)
  A51.0
  congenital A50.07
  conjunctiva NEC A51.2
  Ducrey's A57
  extragenital A51.2
  eyelid A51.2
  lip A51.2
  nipple A51.2
  Nisbet's A57
  of
    carate A67.0
    pinta A67.0
    yaws A66.0
  palate, soft A51.2
  phagedenic A57
  simple A57
  soft A57
    bubo A57
    palate A51.2
  urethra A51.0
  yaws A66.0
Chancroid (anus) (genital) (penis) (perineum)
  (rectum) (urethra) (vulva) A57
Chandler's disease (osteochondritis dissecans, hip)
  — see Osteochondritis, dissecans, hip
Change (s) (in) (of) (see also Removal)
  arteriosclerotic — see Arteriosclerosis
  bone (see also Disorder, bone)
    diabetic — see Diabetes, bone change
  bowel habit R19.4
  cardiorenal (vascular) — see Hypertension,
    cardiorenal
  cardiovascular — see Disease, cardiovascular
  circulatory I99.9
  cognitive (mild) (organic) R41.89
  color, tooth, teeth
    during formation K00.8
    posteruptive K03.7

Change — *continued*
  contraceptive device Z30.433
  corneal membrane H18.30
    Bowman's membrane fold or rupture H18.31- ☑
    Descemet's membrane
      fold H18.32- ☑
      rupture H18.33- ☑
  coronary — see Disease, heart, ischemic
  degenerative, spine or vertebra — see
    Spondylosis
  dental pulp, regressive K04.2
  dressing (nonsurgical) Z48.00
    surgical Z48.01
  heart — see Disease, heart
  hip joint — see Derangement, joint, hip
  hyperplastic larynx J38.7
  hypertrophic
    nasal sinus J34.89
    turbinate, nasal J34.3
    upper respiratory tract J39.8
  indwelling catheter Z46.6
  inflammatory (see also Inflammation)
    sacroiliac M46.1
  job, anxiety concerning Z56.1
  joint — see Derangement, joint
  life — see Menopause
  mental status R41.82
  minimal (glomerular) (see also N00-N07 with
    fourth character .0) N05.0
  myocardium, myocardial — see Degeneration,
    myocardial
  of life — see Menopause
  pacemaker Z45.018
    pulse generator Z45.010
  personality (enduring) F68.8
    due to (secondary to)
      general medical condition F07.0
    secondary (nonspecific) F60.89
  regressive, dental pulp K04.2
  renal — see Disease, renal
  retina H35.9
    myopic H44.2- ☑
  sacroiliac joint M53.3
  senile (see also condition) R54
  sensory R20.8
  skin R23.9
    acute, due to ultraviolet radiation L56.9
      specified NEC L56.8
    chronic, due to nonionizing radiation L57.9
      specified NEC L57.8
    cyanosis R23.0
    flushing R23.2
    pallor R23.1
    petechiae R23.3
    specified change NEC R23.8
    swelling — see Mass, localized
    texture R23.4
  trophic
    arm — see Mononeuropathy, upper limb
    leg — see Mononeuropathy, lower limb
  vascular I99.9
  vasomotor I73.9
  voice R49.9
    psychogenic F44.4
    specified NEC R49.8
Changing sleep-work schedule, affecting sleep
  G47.26
Changuinola fever A93.1
Chapping skin T69.8 ☑
Charcot-Marie-Tooth disease, paralysis or syndrome
  G60.0
Charcot's
  arthropathy — see Arthropathy, neuropathic
  cirrhosis K74.3
  disease (tabetic arthropathy) A52.16
  joint (disease) (tabetic) A52.16
    diabetic — see Diabetes, with, arthropathy
    syringomyelic G95.0
  syndrome (intermittent claudication) I73.9
CHARGE association Q89.8
Charley-horse (quadriceps) M62.831
  traumatic (quadriceps) S76.11- ☑
Charlouis' disease — see Yaws
Cheadle's disease E54
Checking (of)
  cardiac pacemaker (battery) (electrode(s)) Z45.018
    pulse generator Z45.010
  intrauterine contraceptive device Z30.431
Check-up — see Examination
Chédiak-Higashi (-Steinbrinck) syndrome
  (congenital gigantism of peroxidase granules)
  E70.330

Cheek — *see* condition
Cheese itch B88.0
Cheese-washer's lung J67.8
Cheese-worker's lung J67.8
Cheilitis (acute) (angular) (catarrhal) (chronic)
  (exfoliative) (gangrenous) (glandular) (infectional)
  (suppurative) (ulcerative) (vesicular) K13.0
  actinic (due to sun) L56.8
    other than from sun L59.8
  candidal B37.83
Cheilodynia K13.0
Cheiloschisis — see Cleft, lip
Cheilosis (angular) K13.0
  with pellagra E52
  due to
    vitamin B2 (riboflavin) deficiency E53.0
Cheiromegaly M79.89
Cheiropompholyx L30.1
Cheloid — see Keloid
Chemical burn — see Corrosion, by site
Chemodectoma — see Paraganglioma,
  nonchromaffin
Chemosis, conjunctiva — see Edema, conjunctiva
Chemotherapy (session) (for)
  cancer Z51.11
  neoplasm Z51.11
Cherubism M27.8
Chest — *see* condition
Cheyne-Stokes breathing (respiration) R06.3
Chiari's
  disease or syndrome (hepatic vein thrombosis)
    I82.0
  malformation
    type I G93.5
    type II — see Spina bifida
    net Q24.8
Chicago disease B40.9
Chickenpox — see Varicella
Chiclero ulcer or sore B55.1
Chigger (infestation) B88.0
Chignon (disease) B36.8
  newborn (from vacuum extraction) (birth injury)
    P12.1
Chilaiditi's syndrome (subphrenic displacement,
  colon) Q43.3
Chilblain (s) (lupus) T69.1 ☑
Child
  custody dispute Z65.3
Childbirth — see Delivery
Childhood
  cerebral X-linked adrenoleukodystrophy E71.520
  period of rapid growth Z00.2
Chill (s) R68.83
  with fever R50.9
    congestive in malarial regions B54
  without fever R68.83
Chilomastigiasis A07.8
Chimera 46,XX/46,XY Q99.0
Chin — *see* condition
Chinese dysentery A03.9
Chionophobia F40.228
Chitral fever A93.1
Chlamydia, chlamydial A74.9
  cervicitis A56.09
  conjunctivitis A74.0
  cystitis A56.01
  endometritis A56.11
  epididymitis A56.19
  female
    pelvic inflammatory disease A56.11
    pelviperitonitis A56.11
  orchitis A56.19
  peritonitis A74.81
  pharyngitis A56.4
  proctitis A56.3
  psittaci (infection) A70
  salpingitis A56.11
  sexually-transmitted infection NEC A56.8
  specified NEC A74.89
  urethritis A56.01
  vulvovaginitis A56.02
Chlamydiosis — see Chlamydia
Chloasma (skin) (idiopathic) (symptomatic) L81.1
  eyelid H02.719
    hyperthyroid E05.90 [H02.719]
      with thyroid storm E05.91 [H02.719]
    left H02.716
      lower H02.715
      upper H02.714
    right H02.713
      lower H02.712
      upper H02.711

☑ **Additional character required**

Chloroma C92.3- ☑
Chlorosis D50.9
    Egyptian B76.9 [D63.8]
    miner's B76.9 [D63.8]
Chlorotic anemia D50.8
Chocolate cyst (ovary) N80.1
Choked
    disc or disk — *see* Papilledema
    on food, phlegm, or vomitus NOS — *see* Foreign
        body, by site
    while vomiting NOS — *see* Foreign body, by site
Chokes (resulting from bends) T70.3 ☑
Choking sensation R09.89
Cholangiectasis K83.8
Cholangiocarcinoma
    with hepatocellular carcinoma, combined C22.0
    liver C22.1
    specified site NEC — *see* Neoplasm, malignant,
        by site
    unspecified site C22.1
Cholangiohepatitis K83.8
    due to fluke infestation B66.1
Cholangiohepatoma C22.0
Cholangiolitis (acute) (chronic) (extrahepatic)
    (gangrenous) (intrahepatic) K83.0
    paratyphoidal — *see* Fever, paratyphoid
    typhoidal A01.09
Cholangioma D13.4
    malignant — *see* Cholangiocarcinoma
Cholangitis (ascending) (primary) (recurrent)
    (sclerosing) (secondary) (stenosing) (suppurative)
    K83.0
    with calculus, bile duct — *see* Calculus, bile duct,
        with cholangitis
    chronic nonsuppurative destructive K74.3
Cholecystectasia K82.8
Cholecystitis K81.9
    with
        calculus, stones in
            bile duct (common) (hepatic) — *see* Calculus,
                bile duct, with cholecystitis
            cystic duct — *see* Calculus, gallbladder, with
                cholecystitis
            gallbladder — *see* Calculus, gallbladder, with
                cholecystitis
            choledocholithiasis — *see* Calculus, bile duct,
                with cholecystitis
            cholelithiasis — *see* Calculus, gallbladder, with
                cholecystitis
        acute (emphysematous) (gangrenous)
            (suppurative) K81.0
            with
                calculus, stones in
                    cystic duct — *see* Calculus, gallbladder,
                      with cholecystitis, acute
                  gallbladder — *see* Calculus, gallbladder,
                      with cholecystitis, acute
                  choledocholithiasis — *see* Calculus, bile duct,
                      with cholecystitis, acute
                  cholelithiasis — *see* Calculus, gallbladder,
                      with cholecystitis, acute
        chronic cholecystitis K81.2
            with gallbladder calculus K80.12
                with obstruction K80.13
        chronic K81.1
            with acute cholecystitis K81.2
                with gallbladder calculus K80.12
                  with obstruction K80.13
        emphysematous (acute) — *see* Cholecystitis,
            acute
        gangrenous — *see* Cholecystitis, acute
        paratyphoidal, current A01.4
        suppurative — *see* Cholecystitis, acute
        typhoidal A01.09
Cholecystolithiasis — *see* Calculus, gallbladder
Choledochitis (suppurative) K83.0
Choledocholith — *see* Calculus, bile duct
Choledocholithiasis (common duct) (hepatic duct)
    — *see* Calculus, bile duct
    cystic — *see* Calculus, gallbladder
    typhoidal A01.09
Cholelithiasis (cystic duct) (gallbladder) (impacted)
    (multiple) — *see* Calculus, gallbladder
    bile duct (common) (hepatic) — *see* Calculus,
        bile duct
    hepatic duct — *see* Calculus, bile duct
    specified NEC K80.80
        with obstruction K80.81
Cholemia (*see also* Jaundice)
    familial (simple) (congenital) E80.4
    Gilbert's E80.4
Choleperitoneum, choleperitonitis K65.3

Cholera (Asiatic) (epidemic) (malignant) A00.9
    antimonial — *see* Poisoning, antimony
    classical A00.0
    due to Vibrio cholerae 01 A00.9
        biovar cholerae A00.0
        biovar eltor A00.1
        el tor A00.1
    el tor A00.1
Cholerine — *see* Cholera
Cholestasis NEC K83.1
    with hepatocyte injury K71.0
    due to total parenteral nutrition (TPN) K76.89
    pure K71.0
Cholesteatoma (ear) (middle) (with reaction)
    H71.9- ☑
    attic H71.0- ☑
    external ear (canal) H60.4- ☑
    mastoid H71.2- ☑
    postmastoidectomy cavity (recurrent) — *see*
        Complications, postmastoidectomy,
        recurrent cholesteatoma
    recurrent (postmastoidectomy) — *see*
        Complications, postmastoidectomy,
        recurrent cholesteatoma
    tympanum H71.1- ☑
Cholesteatosis, diffuse H71.3- ☑
Cholesteremia E78.0
Cholesterin in vitreous — *see* Deposit, crystalline
Cholesterol
    deposit
        retina H35.89
        vitreous — *see* Deposit, crystalline
    elevated (high) E78.0
        with elevated (high) triglycerides E78.2
        screening for Z13.220
    imbibition of gallbladder K82.4
Cholesterolemia (essential) (familial) (hereditary)
    (pure) E78.0
Cholesterolosis, cholesterosis (gallbladder) K82.4
    cerebrotendinous E75.5
Cholocolic fistula K82.3
Choluria R82.2
Chondritis M94.8X9
    aurical H61.03- ☑
    costal (Tietze's) M94.0
    external ear H61.03- ☑
    patella, posttraumatic — *see* Chondromalacia,
        patella
    pinna H61.03- ☑
    purulent M94.8X- ☑
    tuberculous NEC A18.02
        intervertebral A18.01
Chondroblastoma (*see also* Neoplasm, bone, benign)
    malignant — *see* Neoplasm, bone, malignant
Chondrocalcinosis M11.20
    ankle M11.27- ☑
    elbow M11.22- ☑
    familial M11.10
        ankle M11.17- ☑
        elbow M11.12- ☑
        foot joint M11.17- ☑
        hand joint M11.14- ☑
        hip M11.15- ☑
        knee M11.16- ☑
        multiple site M11.19
        shoulder M11.11- ☑
        vertebrae M11.18
        wrist M11.13- ☑
    foot joint M11.27- ☑
    hand joint M11.24- ☑
    hip M11.25- ☑
    knee M11.26- ☑
    multiple site M11.29
    shoulder M11.21- ☑
    vertebrae M11.28
    specified type NEC M11.20
        ankle M11.27- ☑
        elbow M11.22- ☑
        foot joint M11.27- ☑
        hand joint M11.24- ☑
        hip M11.25- ☑
        knee M11.26- ☑
        multiple site M11.29
        shoulder M11.21- ☑
        vertebrae M11.28
        wrist M11.23- ☑
    wrist M11.23- ☑
Chondrodermatitis nodularis helicis or anthelicis
    — *see* Perichondritis, ear
Chondrodysplasia Q78.9
    with hemangioma Q78.4
    calcificans congenita Q77.3

Chondrodysplasia — *continued*
    fetalis Q77.4
    metaphyseal (Jansen's) (McKusick's) (Schmid's)
        Q78.5
    punctata Q77.3
Chondrodystrophy, chondrodystrophia (familial)
    (fetalis) (hypoplastic) Q78.9
    calcificans congenita Q77.3
    myotonic (congenital) G71.13
    punctata Q77.3
Chondroectodermal dysplasia Q77.6
Chondrogenesis imperfecta Q77.4
Chondrolysis M94.35- ☑
Chondroma (*see also* Neoplasm, cartilage, benign)
    juxtacortical — *see* Neoplasm, bone, benign
    periosteal — *see* Neoplasm, bone, benign
Chondromalacia (systemic) M94.20
    acromioclavicular joint M94.21- ☑
    ankle M94.27- ☑
    elbow M94.22- ☑
    foot joint M94.27- ☑
    glenohumeral joint M94.21- ☑
    hand joint M94.24- ☑
    hip M94.25- ☑
    knee M94.26- ☑
        patella M22.4- ☑
    multiple sites M94.29
    patella M22.4- ☑
    rib M94.28
    sacroiliac joint M94.259
    shoulder M94.21- ☑
    sternoclavicular joint M94.21- ☑
    vertebral M94.28
    wrist M94.23- ☑
Chondromatosis (*see also* Neoplasm, cartilage,
    uncertain behavior)
    internal Q78.4
Chondromyxosarcoma — *see* Neoplasm, cartilage,
    malignant
Chondro-osteodysplasia (Morquio-Brailsford type)
    E76.219
Chondro-osteodystrophy E76.29
Chondro-osteoma — *see* Neoplasm, bone, benign
Chondropathia tuberosa M94.0
Chondrosarcoma — *see* Neoplasm, cartilage,
    malignant
    juxtacortical — *see* Neoplasm, bone, malignant
    mesenchymal — *see* Neoplasm, connective
        tissue, malignant
    myxoid — *see* Neoplasm, cartilage, malignant
Chordee (nonvenereal) N48.89
    congenital Q54.4
    gonococcal A54.09
Chorditis (fibrinous) (nodosa) (tuberosa) J38.2
Chordoma — *see* Neoplasm, vertebral (column),
    malignant
Chorea (chronic) (gravis) (posthemiplegic) (senile)
    (spasmodic) G25.5
    with
        heart involvement I02.0
            active or acute (conditions in I01-) I02.0
            rheumatic I02.9
                with valvular disorder I02.0
            rheumatic heart disease (chronic) (inactive)
                (quiescent) - code to rheumatic heart
                condition involved
    drug-induced G25.4
    habit F95.8
    hereditary G10
    Huntington's G10
    hysterical F44.4
    minor I02.9
        with heart involvement I02.0
    progressive G25.5
        hereditary G10
    rheumatic (chronic) I02.9
        with heart involvement I02.0
    Sydenham's I02.9
        with heart involvement — *see* Chorea, with
            rheumatic heart disease
        nonrheumatic G25.5
Choreoathetosis (paroxysmal) G25.5
Chorioadenoma (destruens) D39.2
Chorioamnionitis O41.12- ☑
Chorioangioma D26.7
Choriocarcinoma — *see* Neoplasm, malignant, by
    site
    combined with
        embryonal carcinoma — *see* Neoplasm,
            malignant, by site
        other germ cell elements — *see* Neoplasm,
            malignant, by site

Choriocarcinoma — continued
    teratoma — see Neoplasm, malignant, by site
    specified site — see Neoplasm, malignant, by site
    unspecified site
      female C58
      male C62.90
Chorioencephalitis (acute) (lymphocytic) (serous) A87.2
Chorioepithelioma — see Choriocarcinoma
Choriomeningitis (acute) (lymphocytic) (serous) A87.2
Chorionepithelioma — see Choriocarcinoma
Chorioretinitis (see also Inflammation, chorioretinal)
    disseminated (see also Inflammation, chorioretinal, disseminated)
      in neurosyphilis A52.19
    Egyptian B76.9 [D63.8]
    focal (see also Inflammation, chorioretinal, focal)
    histoplasmic B39.9 [H32]
    in (due to)
      histoplasmosis B39.9 [H32]
      syphilis (secondary) A51.43
        late A52.71
      toxoplasmosis (acquired) B58.01
        congenital (active) P37.1 [H32]
      tuberculosis A18.53
    juxtapapillary, juxtapapillaris — see Inflammation, chorioretinal, focal, juxtapapillary
    leprous A30.9 [H32]
    miner's B76.9 [D63.8]
    progressive myopia (degeneration) H44.2- ☑
    syphilitic (secondary) A51.43
      congenital (early) A50.01 [H32]
        late A50.32
      late A52.71
    tuberculous A18.53
Chorioretinopathy, central serous H35.71- ☑
Choroid — see condition
Choroideremia H31.21
Choroiditis — see Chorioretinitis
Choroidopathy — see Disorder, choroid
Choroidoretinitis — see Chorioretinitis
Choroidoretinopathy, central serous — see Chorioretinopathy, central serous
Christian-Weber disease M35.6
Christmas disease D67
Chromaffinoma (see also Neoplasm, benign, by site)
    malignant — see Neoplasm, malignant, by site
Chromatopsia — see Deficiency, color vision
Chromhidrosis, chromidrosis L75.1
Chromoblastomycosis — see Chromomycosis
Chromoconversion R82.91
Chromomycosis B43.9
    brain abscess B43.1
    cerebral B43.1
    cutaneous B43.0
    skin B43.0
    specified NEC B43.8
    subcutaneous abscess or cyst B43.2
Chromophytosis B36.0
Chromosome — see condition by chromosome involved
    D (1) — see condition, chromosome 13
    E (3) — see condition, chromosome 18
    G — see condition, chromosome 21
Chromotrichomycosis B36.8
Chronic — see condition
    fracture — see Fracture, pathological
Churg-Strauss syndrome M30.1
Chyle cyst, mesentery I89.8
Chylocele (nonfilarial) I89.8
    filarial (see also Infestation, filarial) B74.9 [N51]
    tunica vaginalis N50.8
      filarial (see also Infestation, filarial) B74.9 [N51]
Chylomicronemia (fasting) (with hyperprebetalipoproteinemia) E78.3
Chylopericardium I31.3
    acute I30.9
Chylothorax (nonfilarial) I89.8
    filarial (see also Infestation, filarial) B74.9 [J91.8]
Chylous — see condition
Chyluria (nonfilarial) R82.0
    due to
      bilharziasis B65.0
      Brugia (malayi) B74.1
        timori B74.2
      schistosomiasis (bilharziasis) B65.0
      Wuchereria (bancrofti) B74.0
    filarial — see Infestation, filarial
Cicatricial (deformity) — see Cicatrix
Cicatrix (adherent) (contracted) (painful) (vicious) (see also Scar) L90.5

Cicatrix — continued
    adenoid (and tonsil) J35.8
    alveolar process M26.79
    anus K62.89
    auricle — see Disorder, pinna, specified type NEC
    bile duct (common) (hepatic) K83.8
    bladder N32.89
    bone — see Disorder, bone, specified type NEC
    brain G93.89
    cervix (postoperative) (postpartal) N88.1
    common duct K83.8
    cornea H17.9
      tuberculous A18.59
    duodenum (bulb), obstructive K31.5
    esophagus K22.2
    eyelid — see Disorder, eyelid function
    hypopharynx J39.2
    lacrimal passages — see Obstruction, lacrimal
    larynx J38.7
    lung J98.4
    middle ear H74.8
    mouth K13.79
    muscle M62.89
      with contracture — see Contraction, muscle NEC
    nasopharynx J39.2
    palate (soft) K13.79
    penis N48.89
    pharynx J39.2
    prostate N42.89
    rectum K62.89
    retina — see Scar, chorioretinal
    semilunar cartilage — see Derangement, meniscus
    seminal vesicle N50.8
    skin L90.5
      infected L08.89
      postinfective L90.5
      tuberculous B90.8
    specified site NEC L90.5
    throat J39.2
    tongue K14.8
    tonsil (and adenoid) J35.8
    trachea J39.8
    tuberculous NEC B90.9
    urethra N36.8
    uterus N85.8
    vagina N89.8
      postoperative N99.2
    vocal cord J38.3
    wrist, constricting (annular) L90.5
CIDP (chronic inflammatory demyelinating polyneuropathy) G61.81
CIN — see Neoplasia, intraepithelial, cervix
Cinchonism — see Deafness, ototoxic
    correct substance properly administered — see Table of Drugs and Chemicals, by drug, adverse effect
    overdose or wrong substance given or taken — see Table of Drugs and Chemicals, by drug, poisoning
Circle of Willis — see condition
Circular — see condition
Circulating anticoagulants (see also - Disorder, hemorrhagic) D68.318
    due to drugs (see also - Disorder, hemorrhagic) D68.32
    following childbirth O72.3
Circulation
    collateral, any site I99.8
    defective (lower extremity) I99.8
      congenital Q28.9
    embryonic Q28.9
    failure (peripheral) R57.9
      newborn P29.89
    fetal, persistent P29.3
    heart, incomplete Q28.9
Circulatory system — see condition
Circulus senilis (cornea) — see Degeneration, cornea, senile
Circumcision (in absence of medical indication) (ritual) (routine) Z41.2
Circumscribed — see condition
Circumvallate placenta O43.11- ☑
Cirrhosis, cirrhotic (hepatic) (liver) K74.60
    alcoholic K70.30
      with ascites K70.31
    atrophic — see Cirrhosis, liver
    Baumgarten-Cruveilhier K74.69
    biliary (cholangiolitic) (cholangitic) (hypertrophic) (obstructive) (pericholangiolitic) K74.5
      due to

Cirrhosis — continued
    Clonorchiasis B66.1
    flukes B66.3
    primary K74.3
    secondary K74.4
    cardiac (of liver) K76.1
    Charcot's K74.3
    cholangiolitic, cholangitic, cholostatic (primary) K74.3
    congestive K76.1
    Cruveilhier-Baumgarten K74.69
    cryptogenic (liver) K74.69
    due to
      hepatolenticular degeneration E83.01
      Wilson's disease E83.01
      xanthomatosis E78.2
    fatty K76.0
      alcoholic K70.0
    Hanot's (hypertrophic) K74.3
    hepatic — see Cirrhosis, liver
    hypertrophic K74.3
    Indian childhood K74.69
    kidney — see Sclerosis, renal
    Laennec's K70.30
      with ascites K70.31
      alcoholic K70.30
        with ascites K70.31
      nonalcoholic K74.69
    liver K74.60
      alcoholic K70.30
        with ascites K70.31
        fatty K70.0
      congenital P78.81
      syphilitic A52.74
    lung (chronic) J84.10
    macronodular K74.69
      alcoholic K70.30
        with ascites K70.31
    micronodular K74.69
      alcoholic K70.30
        with ascites K70.31
    mixed type K74.69
    monolobular K74.3
    nephritis — see Sclerosis, renal
    nutritional K74.69
      alcoholic K70.30
        with ascites K70.31
    obstructive — see Cirrhosis, biliary
    ovarian N83.8
    pancreas (duct) K86.8
    pigmentary E83.110
    portal K74.69
      alcoholic K70.30
        with ascites K70.31
    postnecrotic K74.69
      alcoholic K70.30
        with ascites K70.31
    pulmonary J84.10
    renal — see Sclerosis, renal
    spleen D73.2
    stasis K76.1
    Todd's K74.3
    unilobar K74.3
    xanthomatous (biliary) K74.5
      due to xanthomatosis (familial) (metabolic) (primary) E78.2
Cistern, subarachnoid R93.0
Citrullinemia E72.23
Citrullinuria E72.23
Civatte's disease or poikiloderma L57.3
Clam digger's itch B65.3
Clammy skin R23.1
Clap — see Gonorrhea
Clarke-Hadfield syndrome (pancreatic infantilism) K86.8
Clark's paralysis G80.9
Clastothrix L67.8
Claude Bernard-Horner syndrome G90.2
    traumatic — see Injury, nerve, cervical sympathetic
Claude's disease or syndrome G46.3
Claudication, intermittent I73.9
    cerebral (artery) G45.9
    spinal cord (arteriosclerotic) G95.19
      syphilitic A52.09
    venous (axillary) I87.8
Claudicatio venosa intermittens I87.8
Claustrophobia F40.240
Clavus (infected) L84
Clawfoot (congenital) Q66.89
    acquired — see Deformity, limb, clawfoot

☑ **Additional character required**

Clawhand (acquired) (see also Deformity, limb, clawhand)
  congenital Q68.1
Clawtoe (congenital) Q66.89
  acquired — see Deformity, toe, specified NEC
Clay eating — see Pica
Cleansing of artificial opening — see Attention to, artificial, opening
Cleft (congenital) (see also Imperfect, closure)
  alveolar process M26.79
  branchial (cyst) (persistent) Q18.2
  cricoid cartilage, posterior Q31.8
  lip (unilateral) Q36.9
    with cleft palate Q37.9
      hard Q37.1
        with soft Q37.5
      soft Q37.3
        with hard Q37.5
    bilateral Q36.0
      with cleft palate Q37.8
        hard Q37.0
          with soft Q37.4
        soft Q37.2
          with hard Q37.4
    median Q36.1
  nose Q30.2
  palate Q35.9
    with cleft lip (unilateral) Q37.9
      bilateral Q37.8
    hard Q35.1
      with
        cleft lip (unilateral) Q37.1
          bilateral Q37.0
        soft Q35.5
          with cleft lip (unilateral) Q37.5
            bilateral Q37.4
    medial Q35.5
    soft Q35.3
      with
        cleft lip (unilateral) Q37.3
          bilateral Q37.2
        hard Q35.5
          with cleft lip (unilateral) Q37.5
            bilateral Q37.4
  penis Q55.69
  scrotum Q55.29
  thyroid cartilage Q31.8
  uvula Q35.7
Cleidocranial dysostosis Q74.0
Cleptomania F63.2
Clicking hip (newborn) R29.4
Climacteric (female) (see also Menopause)
  arthritis (any site) NEC — see Arthritis, specified form NEC
  depression (single episode) F32.8
  male (symptoms) (syndrome) NEC N50.8
  paranoid state F22
  polyarthritis NEC — see Arthritis, specified form NEC
  symptoms (female) N95.1
Clinical research investigation (clinical trial) (control subject) (normal comparison) (participant) Z00.6
Clitoris — see condition
Cloaca (persistent) Q43.7
Clonorchiasis, clonorchis infection (liver) B66.1
Clonus R25.8
Closed bite M26.29
Clostridium (C.) perfringens, as cause of disease classified elsewhere B96.7
Closure
  congenital, nose Q30.0
  cranial sutures, premature Q75.0
  defective or imperfect NEC — see Imperfect, closure
  fistula, delayed — see Fistula
  foramen ovale, imperfect Q21.1
  hymen N89.6
  interauricular septum, defective Q21.1
  interventricular septum, defective Q21.0
  lacrimal duct (see also Stenosis, lacrimal, duct)
    congenital Q10.5
  nose (congenital) Q30.0
    acquired M95.0
  of artificial opening — see Attention to, artificial, opening
  primary angle, without glaucoma damage H40.06- ☑
  vagina N89.5
  valve — see Endocarditis
  vulva N90.5
Clot (blood) (see also Embolism)
  artery (obstruction) (occlusion) — see Embolism

Clot — continued
  bladder N32.89
  brain (intradural or extradural) — see Occlusion, artery, cerebral
  circulation I74.9
  heart (see also Infarct, myocardium)
    not resulting in infarction I24.0
  vein — see Thrombosis
Clouded state R40.1
  epileptic — see Epilepsy, specified NEC
  paroxysmal — see Epilepsy, specified NEC
Cloudy antrum, antra J32.0
Clouston's (hidrotic) ectodermal dysplasia Q82.4
Clubbed nail pachydermoperiostosis M89.40 [L62]
Clubbing of finger (s) (nails) R68.3
Clubfinger R68.3
  congenital Q68.1
Clubfoot (congenital) Q66.89
  acquired — see Deformity, limb, clubfoot
  equinovarus Q66.0
  paralytic — see Deformity, limb, clubfoot
Clubhand (congenital) (radial) Q71.4- ☑
  acquired — see Deformity, limb, clubhand
Clubnail R68.3
  congenital Q84.6
Clump, kidney Q63.1
Clumsiness, clumsy child syndrome F82
Cluttering F80.81
Clutton's joints A50.51 [M12.80]
Coagulation, intravascular (diffuse) (disseminated) (see also Defibrination syndrome)
  complicating abortion — see Abortion, by type, complicated by, intravascular coagulation
  following ectopic or molar pregnancy O08.1
Coagulopathy (see also Defect, coagulation)
  consumption D65
  intravascular D65
    newborn P60
Coalition
  calcaneo-scaphoid Q66.89
  tarsal Q66.89
Coalminer's
  elbow — see Bursitis, elbow, olecranon
  lung or pneumoconiosis J60
Coalworker's lung or pneumoconiosis J60
Coarctation
  aorta (preductal) (postductal) Q25.1
  pulmonary artery Q25.71
Coated tongue K14.3
Coats' disease (exudative retinopathy) — see Retinopathy, exudative
Cocainism — see Dependence, drug, cocaine
Coccidioidomycosis B38.9
  cutaneous B38.3
  disseminated B38.7
  generalized B38.7
  meninges B38.4
  prostate B38.81
  pulmonary B38.2
    acute B38.0
    chronic B38.1
  skin B38.3
  specified NEC B38.89
Coccidioidosis — see Coccidioidomycosis
Coccidiosis (intestinal) A07.3
Coccydynia, coccygodynia M53.3
Coccyx — see condition
Cochin-China diarrhea K90.1
Cockayne's syndrome Q87.1
Cocked up toe — see Deformity, toe, specified NEC
Cock's peculiar tumor L72.3
Codman's tumor — see Neoplasm, bone, benign
Coenurosis B71.8
Coffee-worker's lung J67.8
Cogan's syndrome H16.32- ☑
  oculomotor apraxia H51.8
Coitus, painful (female) N94.1
  male N53.12
  psychogenic F52.6
Cold J00
  with influenza, flu, or grippe — see Influenza, with, respiratory manifestations NEC
  agglutinin disease or hemoglobinuria (chronic) D59.1
  bronchial — see Bronchitis
  chest — see Bronchitis
  common (head) J00
  effects of T69.9 ☑
    specified effect NEC T69.8 ☑
  excessive, effects of T69.9 ☑
    specified effect NEC T69.8 ☑
  exhaustion from T69.8 ☑

Cold — continued
  exposure to T69.9 ☑
    specified effect NEC T69.8 ☑
  head J00
  injury syndrome (newborn) P80.0
  on lung — see Bronchitis
  rose J30.1
  sensitivity, auto-immune D59.1
  virus J00
Coldsore B00.1
Colibacillosis A49.8
  as the cause of other disease (see also Escherichia coli) B96.20
  generalized A41.50
Colic (bilious) (infantile) (intestinal) (recurrent) (spasmodic) R10.83
  abdomen R10.83
    psychogenic F45.8
  appendix, appendicular K38.8
  bile duct — see Calculus, bile duct
  biliary — see Calculus, bile duct
  common duct — see Calculus, bile duct
  cystic duct — see Calculus, gallbladder
  Devonshire NEC — see Poisoning, lead
  gallbladder — see Calculus, gallbladder
  gallstone — see Calculus, gallbladder
    gallbladder or cystic duct — see Calculus, gallbladder
  hepatic (duct) — see Calculus, bile duct
  hysterical F45.8
  kidney N23
  lead NEC — see Poisoning, lead
  mucous K58.9
    with diarrhea K58.0
    psychogenic F54
  nephritic N23
  painter's NEC — see Poisoning, lead
  pancreas K86.8
  psychogenic F45.8
  renal N23
  saturnine NEC — see Poisoning, lead
  ureter N23
  urethral N36.8
    due to calculus N21.1
  uterus NEC N94.89
    menstrual — see Dysmenorrhea
  worm NOS B83.9
Colicystitis — see Cystitis
Colitis (acute) (catarrhal) (chronic) (noninfective) (hemorrhagic) (see also Enteritis) K52.9
  allergic K52.2
  amebic (acute) (see also Amebiasis) A06.0
    nondysenteric A06.2
  anthrax A22.2
  bacillary — see Infection, Shigella
  balantidial A07.0
  Clostridium difficile A04.7
  coccidial A07.3
  collagenous K52.89
  cystica superficialis K52.89
  dietary counseling and surveillance (for) Z71.3
  dietetic K52.2
  drug-induced K52.1
  due to radiation K52.0
  eosinophilic K52.82
  food hypersensitivity K52.2
  giardial A07.1
  granulomatous — see Enteritis, regional, large intestine
  infectious — see Enteritis, infectious
  ischemic K55.9
    acute (fulminant) (subacute) K55.0
    chronic K55.1
    due to mesenteric artery insufficiency K55.1
    fulminant (acute) K55.0
  left sided K51.50
    with
      abscess K51.514
      complication K51.519
        specified NEC K51.518
      fistula K51.513
      obstruction K51.512
      rectal bleeding K51.511
  lymphocytic K52.89
  membranous
    psychogenic F54
  microscopic (collagenous) (lymphocytic) K52.89
  mucous — see Syndrome, irritable, bowel
    psychogenic F54
  noninfective K52.9
    specified NEC K52.89
  polyposa — see Polyp, colon, inflammatory

Colitis — *continued*
  protozoal A07.9
  pseudomembranous A04.7
  pseudomucinous — *see* Syndrome, irritable,
      bowel
  regional — *see* Enteritis, regional, large intestine
  segmental — *see* Enteritis, regional, large
      intestine
  septic — *see* Enteritis, infectious
  spastic K58.9
      with diarrhea K58.0
      psychogenic F54
  staphylococcal A04.8
      foodborne A05.0
  subacute ischemic K55.0
  thromboulcerative K55.0
  toxic NEC K52.1
      due to Clostridium difficile A04.7
  transmural — *see* Enteritis, regional, large
      intestine
  trichomonal A07.8
  tuberculous (ulcerative) A18.32
  ulcerative (chronic) K51.90
      with
          complication K51.919
              abscess K51.914
              fistula K51.913
              obstruction K51.912
              rectal bleeding K51.911
              specified complication NEC K51.918
      enterocolitis — *see* Enterocolitis, ulcerative
      ileocolitis — *see* Ileocolitis, ulcerative
      mucosal proctocolitis — *see* Proctocolitis,
          mucosal
      proctitis — *see* Proctitis, ulcerative
      pseudopolyposis — *see* Polyp, colon,
          inflammatory
      psychogenic F54
      rectosigmoiditis — *see* Rectosigmoiditis,
          ulcerative
      specified type NEC K51.80
          with
              complication K51.819
                  abscess K51.814
                  fistula K51.813
                  obstruction K51.812
                  rectal bleeding K51.811
                  specified complication NEC K51.818
Collagenosis, collagen disease (nonvascular)
    (vascular) M35.9
  cardiovascular I42.8
  reactive perforating L87.1
  specified NEC M35.8
Collapse R55
  adrenal E27.2
  cardiorespiratory R57.0
  cardiovascular R57.0
      newborn P29.89
  circulatory (peripheral) R57.9
      during or after labor and delivery O75.1
      following ectopic or molar pregnancy O08.3
      newborn P29.89
  during or
      after labor and delivery O75.1
      resulting from a procedure, not elsewhere
          classified T81.10 ☑
  external ear canal — *see* Stenosis, external ear
      canal
  general R55
  heart — *see* Disease, heart
  heat T67.1 ☑
  hysterical F44.89
  labyrinth, membranous (congenital) Q16.5
  lung (massive) (*see also* Atelectasis) J98.19
      pressure due to anesthesia (general) (local) or
          other sedation T88.2 ☑
          during labor and delivery O74.1
          in pregnancy O29.02- ☑
          postpartum, puerperal O89.09
  myocardial — *see* Disease, heart
  nervous F48.8
  neurocirculatory F45.8
  nose M95.0
  postoperative T81.10 ☑
  pulmonary (*see also* Atelectasis) J98.19
      newborn — *see* Atelectasis
  trachea J39.8
  tracheobronchial J98.09
  valvular — *see* Endocarditis
  vascular (peripheral) R57.9
      during or after labor and delivery O75.1
      following ectopic or molar pregnancy O08.3

Collapse — *continued*
  newborn P29.89
  vertebra M48.50- ☑
      cervical region M48.52- ☑
      cervicothoracic region M48.53- ☑
      in (due to)
          metastasis — *see* Collapse, vertebra, in,
              specified disease NEC
          osteoporosis (*see also* Osteoporosis) M80.88
              ☑
              cervical region M80.88 ☑
              cervicothoracic region M80.88 ☑
              lumbar region M80.88 ☑
              lumbosacral region M80.88 ☑
              multiple sites M80.88 ☑
              occipito-atlanto-axial region M80.88 ☑
              sacrococcygeal region M80.88 ☑
              thoracic region M80.88 ☑
              thoracolumbar region M80.88 ☑
          specified disease NEC M48.50- ☑
              cervical region M48.52- ☑
              cervicothoracic region M48.53- ☑
              lumbar region M48.56- ☑
              lumbosacral region M48.57- ☑
              occipito-atlanto-axial region M48.51- ☑
              sacrococcygeal region M48.58- ☑
              thoracic region M48.54- ☑
              thoracolumbar region M48.55- ☑
      lumbar region M48.56- ☑
      lumbosacral region M48.57- ☑
      occipito-atlanto-axial region M48.51- ☑
      sacrococcygeal region M48.58- ☑
      thoracic region M48.54- ☑
      thoracolumbar region M48.55- ☑
Collateral (*see also* condition)
  circulation (venous) I87.8
  dilation, veins I87.8
Colles' fracture S52.53- ☑
Collet (-Sicard) syndrome G52.7
Collier's asthma or lung J60
Collodion baby Q80.2
Colloid nodule (of thyroid) (cystic) E04.1
Coloboma (iris) Q13.0
  eyelid Q10.3
  fundus Q14.8
  lens Q12.2
  optic disc (congenital) Q14.2
      acquired H47.31- ☑
Coloenteritis — *see* Enteritis
Colon — *see* condition
Colonization
  MRSA (Methicillin resistant Staphylococcus
      aureus) Z22.322
  MSSA (Methicillin susceptible Staphylococcus
      aureus) Z22.321
  status — *see* Carrier (suspected) of
Coloptosis K63.4
Color blindness — *see* Deficiency, color vision
Colostomy
  attention to Z43.3
  fitting or adjustment Z46.89
  malfunctioning K94.03
  status Z93.3
Colpitis (acute) — *see* Vaginitis
Colpocele N81.5
Colpocystitis — *see* Vaginitis
Colpospasm N94.2
Column, spinal, vertebral — *see* condition
Coma R40.20 ☑
  with
      motor response (none) R40.231 ☑
          abnormal R40.233 ☑
          extension R40.232 ☑
          flexion withdrawal R40.234 ☑
          localizes pain R40.235 ☑
          obeys commands R40.236 ☑
      opening of eyes (never) R40.211 ☑
          in response to
              pain R40.212 ☑
              sound R40.213 ☑
          spontaneous R40.214 ☑
      verbal response (none) R40.221 ☑
          confused conversation R40.224 ☑
          inappropriate words R40.223 ☑
          incomprehensible words R40.222 ☑
          oriented R40.225 ☑
  eclamptic — *see* Eclampsia
  epileptic — *see* Epilepsy
  Glasgow, scale score — *see* Glasgow coma scale
  hepatic — *see* Failure, hepatic, by type, with coma
  hyperglycemic (diabetic) — *see* Diabetes, coma
  hyperosmolar (diabetic) — *see* Diabetes, coma

Coma — *continued*
  hypoglycemic (diabetic) — *see* Diabetes, coma,
      hypoglycemic
      nondiabetic E15
  in diabetes — *see* Diabetes, Coma
  insulin-induced — *see* Coma, hypoglycemic
  myxedematous E03.5
  newborn P91.5
  persistent vegetative state R40.3
  specified NEC, without documented Glasgow
      coma scale score, or with partial Glasgow
      coma scale score reported R40.244 ☑
Comatose — *see* Coma
Combat fatigue F43.0
Combined — *see* condition
Comedo, comedones (giant) L70.0
Comedocarcinoma (*see also* Neoplasm, breast,
    malignant)
  noninfiltrating
      breast D05.8- ☑
      specified site — *see* Neoplasm, in situ, by site
      unspecified site D05.8- ☑
Comedomastitis — *see* Ectasia, mammary duct
Comminuted fracture - code as Fracture, closed
Common
  arterial trunk Q20.0
  atrioventricular canal Q21.2
  atrium Q21.1
  cold (head) J00
  truncus (arteriosus) Q20.0
  variable immunodeficiency — *see*
      Immunodeficiency, common variable
  ventricle Q20.4
Commotio, commotion (current)
  brain — *see* Injury, intracranial, concussion
  cerebri — *see* Injury, intracranial, concussion
  retinae S05.8X- ☑
  spinal cord — *see* Injury, spinal cord, by region
  spinalis — *see* Injury, spinal cord, by region
Communication
  between
      base of aorta and pulmonary artery Q21.4
      left ventricle and right atrium Q20.5
      pericardial sac and pleural sac Q34.8
      pulmonary artery and pulmonary vein,
          congenital Q25.72
  congenital between uterus and digestive or
      urinary tract Q51.7
Compartment syndrome (deep) (posterior)
    (traumatic) T79.A0 ☑
  abdomen T79.A3 ☑
  lower extremity (hip, buttock, thigh, leg, foot,
      toes) T79.A2 ☑
  nontraumatic
      abdomen M79.A3
      lower extremity (hip, buttock, thigh, leg, foot,
          toes) M79.A2- ☑
      specified site NEC M79.A9
      upper extremity (shoulder, arm, forearm, wrist,
          hand, fingers) M79.A1- ☑
  specified site NEC T79.A9 ☑
  upper extremity (shoulder, arm, forearm, wrist,
      hand, fingers) T79.A1 ☑
Compensation
  failure — *see* Disease, heart
  neurosis, psychoneurosis — *see* Disorder,
      factitious
Complaint (*see also* Disease)
  bowel, functional K59.9
      psychogenic F45.8
  intestine, functional K59.9
      psychogenic F45.8
  kidney — *see* Disease, renal
  miners' J60
Complete — *see* condition
Complex
  Addison-Schilder E71.528
  cardiorenal — *see* Hypertension, cardiorenal
  Costen's M26.69
  disseminated mycobacterium avium-
      intracellulare (DMAC) A31.2
  Eisenmenger's (ventricular septal defect) I27.89
  hypersexual F52.8
  jumped process, spine — *see* Dislocation,
      vertebra
  primary, tuberculous A15.7
  Schilder-Addison E71.528
  subluxation (vertebral) M99.19
      abdomen M99.19
      acromioclavicular M99.17
      cervical region M99.11
      cervicothoracic M99.11

☑ **Additional character required**

Complex — *continued*
- costochondral M99.18
- costovertebral M99.18
- head region M99.10
- hip M99.15
- lower extremity M99.16
- lumbar region M99.13
- lumbosacral M99.13
- occipitocervical M99.10
- pelvic region M99.15
- pubic M99.15
- rib cage M99.18
- sacral region M99.14
- sacrococcygeal M99.14
- sacroiliac M99.14
- specified NEC M99.19
- sternochondral M99.18
- sternoclavicular M99.17
- thoracic region M99.12
- thoracolumbar M99.12
- upper extremity M99.17
- Taussig-Bing (transposition, aorta and overriding pulmonary artery) Q20.1

Complication (s) (from) (of)
- accidental puncture or laceration during a procedure (of) — *see* Complications, intraoperative (intraprocedural), puncture or laceration
- amputation stump (surgical) (late) NEC T87.9
  - dehiscence T87.81
  - infection or inflammation T87.40
    - lower limb T87.4- ☑
    - upper limb T87.4- ☑
  - necrosis T87.50
    - lower limb T87.5- ☑
    - upper limb T87.5- ☑
  - neuroma T87.30
    - lower limb T87.3- ☑
    - upper limb T87.3- ☑
  - specified type NEC T87.89
- anastomosis (and bypass) (*see also* Complications, prosthetic device or implant)
  - intestinal (internal) NEC K91.89
    - involving urinary tract N99.89
  - urinary tract (involving intestinal tract) N99.89
  - vascular — *see* Complications, cardiovascular device or implant
- anesthesia, anesthetic (*see also* Anesthesia, complication) T88.59 ☑
  - brain, postpartum, puerperal O89.2
  - cardiac
    - in
      - labor and delivery O74.2
      - pregnancy O29.19- ☑
    - postpartum, puerperal O89.1
  - central nervous system
    - in
      - labor and delivery O74.3
      - pregnancy O29.29- ☑
    - postpartum, puerperal O89.2
  - difficult or failed intubation T88.4 ☑
    - in pregnancy O29.6- ☑
  - failed sedation (conscious) (moderate) during procedure T88.52 ☑
  - hyperthermia, malignant T88.3 ☑
  - hypothermia T88.51 ☑
  - intubation failure T88.4 ☑
  - malignant hyperthermia T88.3 ☑
  - pulmonary
    - in
      - labor and delivery O74.1
      - pregnancy NEC O29.09- ☑
    - postpartum, puerperal O89.09
  - shock T88.2 ☑
  - spinal and epidural
    - in
      - labor and delivery NEC O74.6
        - headache O74.5
      - pregnancy NEC O29.5X- ☑
    - postpartum, puerperal NEC O89.5
      - headache O89.4
- anti-reflux device — *see* Complications, esophageal anti-reflux device
- aortic (bifurcation) graft — *see* Complications, graft, vascular
- aortocoronary (bypass) graft — *see* Complications, coronary artery (bypass) graft
- aortofemoral (bypass) graft — *see* Complications, extremity artery (bypass) graft
- arteriovenous
  - fistula, surgically created T82.9 ☑
    - embolism T82.818 ☑

Complication — *continued*
- fibrosis T82.828 ☑
- hemorrhage T82.838 ☑
- infection or inflammation T82.7 ☑
- mechanical
  - breakdown T82.510 ☑
  - displacement T82.520 ☑
  - leakage T82.530 ☑
  - malposition T82.520 ☑
  - obstruction T82.590 ☑
  - perforation T82.590 ☑
  - protrusion T82.590 ☑
- pain T82.848 ☑
- specified type NEC T82.898 ☑
- stenosis T82.858 ☑
- thrombosis T82.868 ☑
- shunt, surgically created T82.9 ☑
  - embolism T82.818 ☑
  - fibrosis T82.828 ☑
  - hemorrhage T82.838 ☑
  - infection or inflammation T82.7 ☑
  - mechanical
    - breakdown T82.511 ☑
    - displacement T82.521 ☑
    - leakage T82.531 ☑
    - malposition T82.521 ☑
    - obstruction T82.591 ☑
    - perforation T82.591 ☑
    - protrusion T82.591 ☑
  - pain T82.848 ☑
  - specified type NEC T82.898 ☑
  - stenosis T82.858 ☑
  - thrombosis T82.868 ☑
- arthroplasty — *see* Complications, joint prosthesis
- artificial
  - fertilization or insemination N98.9
    - attempted introduction (of)
      - embryo in embryo transfer N98.3
      - ovum following in vitro fertilization N98.2
    - hyperstimulation of ovaries N98.1
    - infection N98.0
    - specified NEC N98.8
  - heart T82.9 ☑
    - embolism T82.817 ☑
    - fibrosis T82.827 ☑
    - hemorrhage T82.837 ☑
    - infection or inflammation T82.7 ☑
    - mechanical
      - breakdown T82.512 ☑
      - displacement T82.522 ☑
      - leakage T82.532 ☑
      - malposition T82.522 ☑
      - obstruction T82.592 ☑
      - perforation T82.592 ☑
      - protrusion T82.592 ☑
    - pain T82.847 ☑
    - specified type NEC T82.897 ☑
    - stenosis T82.857 ☑
    - thrombosis T82.867 ☑
  - opening
    - cecostomy — *see* Complications, colostomy
    - colostomy — *see* Complications, colostomy
    - cystostomy — *see* Complications, cystostomy
    - enterostomy — *see* Complications, enterostomy
    - gastrostomy — *see* Complications, gastrostomy
    - ileostomy — *see* Complications, enterostomy
    - jejunostomy — *see* Complications, enterostomy
    - nephrostomy — *see* Complications, stoma, urinary tract
    - tracheostomy — *see* Complications, tracheostomy
    - ureterostomy — *see* Complications, stoma, urinary tract
    - urethrostomy — *see* Complications, stoma, urinary tract
- balloon implant or device
  - gastrointestinal T85.9 ☑
    - embolism T85.81 ☑
    - fibrosis T85.82 ☑
    - hemorrhage T85.83 ☑
    - infection and inflammation T85.79 ☑
    - pain T85.84 ☑
    - specified type NEC T85.89 ☑
    - stenosis T85.85 ☑
    - thrombosis T85.86 ☑
  - vascular (counterpulsation) T82.9 ☑
    - embolism T82.818 ☑
    - fibrosis T82.828 ☑

Complication — *continued*
- hemorrhage T82.838 ☑
- infection or inflammation T82.7 ☑
- mechanical
  - breakdown T82.513 ☑
  - displacement T82.523 ☑
  - leakage T82.533 ☑
  - malposition T82.523 ☑
  - obstruction T82.593 ☑
  - perforation T82.593 ☑
  - protrusion T82.593 ☑
- pain T82.848 ☑
- specified type NEC T82.898 ☑
- stenosis T82.858 ☑
- thrombosis T82.868 ☑
- bariatric procedure
  - gastric band procedure K95.09
    - infection K95.01
  - specified procedure NEC K95.89
    - infection K95.81
- bile duct implant (prosthetic) T85.9 ☑
  - embolism T85.81 ☑
  - fibrosis T85.82 ☑
  - hemorrhage T85.83 ☑
  - infection and inflammation T85.79 ☑
  - mechanical
    - breakdown T85.510 ☑
    - displacement T85.520 ☑
    - malfunction T85.510 ☑
    - malposition T85.520 ☑
    - obstruction T85.590 ☑
    - perforation T85.590 ☑
    - protrusion T85.590 ☑
    - specified NEC T85.590 ☑
  - pain T85.84 ☑
  - specified type NEC T85.89 ☑
  - stenosis T85.85 ☑
  - thrombosis T85.86 ☑
- bladder device (auxiliary) — *see* Complications, genitourinary, device or implant, urinary system
- bleeding (postoperative) — *see* Complication, postoperative, hemorrhage
  - intraoperative — *see* Complication, intraoperative, hemorrhage
- blood vessel graft — *see* Complications, graft, vascular
- bone
  - device NEC T84.9 ☑
    - embolism T84.81 ☑
    - fibrosis T84.82 ☑
    - hemorrhage T84.83 ☑
    - infection or inflammation T84.7 ☑
    - mechanical
      - breakdown T84.318 ☑
      - displacement T84.328 ☑
      - malposition T84.328 ☑
      - obstruction T84.398 ☑
      - perforation T84.398 ☑
      - protrusion T84.398 ☑
    - pain T84.84 ☑
    - specified type NEC T84.89 ☑
    - stenosis T84.85 ☑
    - thrombosis T84.86 ☑
  - graft — *see* Complications, graft, bone
  - growth stimulator (electrode) — *see* Complications, electronic stimulator device, bone
  - marrow transplant — *see* Complications, transplant, bone, marrow
- brain neurostimulator (electrode) — *see* Complications, electronic stimulator device, brain
- breast implant (prosthetic) T85.9 ☑
  - capsular contracture T85.44 ☑
  - embolism T85.81 ☑
  - fibrosis T85.82 ☑
  - hemorrhage T85.83 ☑
  - infection and inflammation T85.79 ☑
  - mechanical
    - breakdown T85.41 ☑
    - displacement T85.42 ☑
    - leakage T85.43 ☑
    - malposition T85.42 ☑
    - obstruction T85.49 ☑
    - perforation T85.49 ☑
    - protrusion T85.49 ☑
    - specified NEC T85.49 ☑
  - pain T85.84 ☑
  - specified type NEC T85.89 ☑
  - stenosis T85.85 ☑
  - thrombosis T85.86 ☑

Complication

Complication — *continued*
  bypass (*see also* Complications, prosthetic device
    or implant)
    aortocoronary — *see* Complications, coronary
      artery (bypass) graft
    arterial (*see also* Complications, graft, vascular)
      extremity — *see* Complications, extremity
        artery (bypass) graft
  cardiac (*see also* Disease, heart)
    device, implant or graft T82.9 ☑
      embolism T82.817 ☑
      fibrosis T82.827 ☑
      hemorrhage T82.837 ☑
      infection or inflammation T82.7 ☑
        valve prosthesis T82.6 ☑
      mechanical
        breakdown T82.519 ☑
          specified device NEC T82.518 ☑
        displacement T82.529 ☑
          specified device NEC T82.528 ☑
        leakage T82.539 ☑
          specified device NEC T82.538 ☑
        malposition T82.529 ☑
          specified device NEC T82.528 ☑
        obstruction T82.599 ☑
          specified device NEC T82.598 ☑
        perforation T82.599 ☑
          specified device NEC T82.598 ☑
        protrusion T82.599 ☑
          specified device NEC T82.598 ☑
      pain T82.847 ☑
      specified type NEC T82.897 ☑
      stenosis T82.857 ☑
      thrombosis T82.867 ☑
  cardiovascular device, graft or implant T82.9 ☑
    aortic graft — *see* Complications, graft, vascular
    arteriovenous
      fistula, artificial — *see* Complication,
        arteriovenous, fistula, surgically created
      shunt — *see* Complication, arteriovenous,
        shunt, surgically created
    artificial heart — *see* Complication, artificial,
      heart
    balloon (counterpulsation) device — *see*
      Complication, balloon implant, vascular
    carotid artery graft — *see* Complications, graft,
      vascular
    coronary bypass graft — *see* Complication,
      coronary artery (bypass) graft
    dialysis catheter (vascular) — *see* Complication,
      catheter, dialysis
    electronic T82.9 ☑
      electrode T82.9 ☑
        embolism T82.817 ☑
        fibrosis T82.827 ☑
        hemorrhage T82.837 ☑
        infection T82.7 ☑
        mechanical
          breakdown T82.110 ☑
          displacement T82.120 ☑
          leakage T82.190 ☑
          obstruction T82.190 ☑
          perforation T82.190 ☑
          protrusion T82.190 ☑
          specified type NEC T82.190 ☑
        pain T82.847 ☑
        specified NEC T82.897 ☑
        stenosis T82.857 ☑
        thrombosis T82.867 ☑
      embolism T82.817 ☑
      fibrosis T82.827 ☑
      hemorrhage T82.837 ☑
      infection T82.7 ☑
      mechanical
        breakdown T82.119 ☑
        displacement T82.129 ☑
        leakage T82.199 ☑
        obstruction T82.199 ☑
        perforation T82.199 ☑
        protrusion T82.199 ☑
        specified type NEC T82.199 ☑
      pain T82.847 ☑
      pulse generator T82.9 ☑
        embolism T82.817 ☑
        fibrosis T82.827 ☑
        hemorrhage T82.837 ☑
        infection T82.7 ☑
        mechanical
          breakdown T82.111 ☑
          displacement T82.121 ☑
          leakage T82.191 ☑
          obstruction T82.191 ☑

Complication — *continued*
          perforation T82.191 ☑
          protrusion T82.191 ☑
          specified type NEC T82.191 ☑
        pain T82.847 ☑
        specified NEC T82.897 ☑
        stenosis T82.857 ☑
        thrombosis T82.867 ☑
      specified condition NEC T82.897 ☑
      specified device NEC T82.9 ☑
        embolism T82.817 ☑
        fibrosis T82.827 ☑
        hemorrhage T82.837 ☑
        infection T82.7 ☑
        mechanical
          breakdown T82.118 ☑
          displacement T82.128 ☑
          leakage T82.198 ☑
          obstruction T82.198 ☑
          perforation T82.198 ☑
          protrusion T82.198 ☑
          specified type NEC T82.198 ☑
        pain T82.847 ☑
        specified NEC T82.897 ☑
        stenosis T82.857 ☑
        thrombosis T82.867 ☑
      stenosis T82.857 ☑
      thrombosis T82.867 ☑
    extremity artery graft — *see* Complication,
      extremity artery (bypass) graft
    femoral artery graft — *see* Complication,
      extremity artery (bypass) graft
    heart-lung transplant — *see* Complication,
      transplant, heart, with lung
    heart
      transplant — *see* Complication, transplant,
        heart
      valve — *see* Complication, prosthetic device,
        heart valve
        graft — *see* Complication, heart, valve, graft
    infection or inflammation T82.7 ☑
    umbrella device — *see* Complication, umbrella
      device, vascular
    vascular graft (or anastomosis) — *see*
      Complication, graft, vascular
  carotid artery (bypass) graft — *see*
    Complications, graft, vascular
  catheter (device) NEC (*see also* Complications,
    prosthetic device or implant)
    cystostomy T83.9 ☑
      embolism T83.81 ☑
      fibrosis T83.82 ☑
      hemorrhage T83.83 ☑
      infection and inflammation T83.59 ☑
      mechanical
        breakdown T83.010 ☑
        displacement T83.020 ☑
        leakage T83.030 ☑
        malposition T83.020 ☑
        obstruction T83.090 ☑
        perforation T83.090 ☑
        protrusion T83.090 ☑
        specified NEC T83.090 ☑
      pain T83.84 ☑
      specified type NEC T83.89 ☑
      stenosis T83.85 ☑
      thrombosis T83.86 ☑
    dialysis (vascular) T82.9 ☑
      embolism T82.818 ☑
      fibrosis T82.828 ☑
      hemorrhage T82.838 ☑
      infection and inflammation T82.7 ☑
      intraperitoneal — *see* Complications,
        catheter, intraperitoneal
      mechanical
        breakdown T82.41 ☑
        displacement T82.42 ☑
        leakage T82.43 ☑
        malposition T82.42 ☑
        obstruction T82.49 ☑
        perforation T82.49 ☑
        protrusion T82.49 ☑
      pain T82.848 ☑
      specified type NEC T82.898 ☑
      stenosis T82.858 ☑
      thrombosis T82.868 ☑
    epidural infusion T85.9 ☑
      embolism T85.81 ☑
      fibrosis T85.82 ☑
      hemorrhage T85.83 ☑
      infection and inflammation T85.79 ☑
      mechanical

Complication — *continued*
        breakdown T85.610 ☑
        displacement T85.620 ☑
        leakage T85.630 ☑
        malfunction T85.610 ☑
        malposition T85.620 ☑
        obstruction T85.690 ☑
        perforation T85.690 ☑
        protrusion T85.690 ☑
        specified NEC T85.690 ☑
      pain T85.84 ☑
      specified type NEC T85.89 ☑
      stenosis T85.85 ☑
      thrombosis T85.86 ☑
    intraperitoneal dialysis T85.9 ☑
      embolism T85.81 ☑
      fibrosis T85.82 ☑
      hemorrhage T85.83 ☑
      infection and inflammation T85.71 ☑
      mechanical
        breakdown T85.611 ☑
        displacement T85.621 ☑
        leakage T85.631 ☑
        malfunction T85.611 ☑
        malposition T85.621 ☑
        obstruction T85.691 ☑
        perforation T85.691 ☑
        protrusion T85.691 ☑
        specified NEC T85.691 ☑
      pain T85.84 ☑
      specified type NEC T85.89 ☑
      stenosis T85.85 ☑
      thrombosis T85.86 ☑
    intravenous infusion T82.9 ☑
      embolism T82.818 ☑
      fibrosis T82.828 ☑
      hemorrhage T82.838 ☑
      infection or inflammation T82.7 ☑
      mechanical
        breakdown T82.514 ☑
        displacement T82.524 ☑
        leakage T82.534 ☑
        malposition T82.524 ☑
        obstruction T82.594 ☑
        perforation T82.594 ☑
        protrusion T82.594 ☑
      pain T82.848 ☑
      specified type NEC T82.898 ☑
      stenosis T82.858 ☑
      thrombosis T82.868 ☑
    subdural infusion T85.9 ☑
      embolism T85.81 ☑
      fibrosis T85.82 ☑
      hemorrhage T85.83 ☑
      infection and inflammation T85.79 ☑
      mechanical
        breakdown T85.610 ☑
        displacement T85.620 ☑
        leakage T85.630 ☑
        malfunction T85.610 ☑
        malposition T85.620 ☑
        obstruction T85.690 ☑
        perforation T85.690 ☑
        protrusion T85.690 ☑
        specified NEC T85.690 ☑
      pain T85.84 ☑
      specified type NEC T85.89 ☑
      stenosis T85.85 ☑
      thrombosis T85.86 ☑
    urethral, indwelling T83.9 ☑
      displacement T83.028 ☑
      embolism T83.81 ☑
      fibrosis T83.82 ☑
      hemorrhage T83.83 ☑
      infection and inflammation T83.51 ☑
      leakage T83.038 ☑
      malposition T83.028 ☑
      mechanical
        breakdown T83.018 ☑
      obstruction (mechanical) T83.098 ☑
      pain T83.84 ☑
      perforation T83.098 ☑
      protrusion T83.098 ☑
      specified type NEC T83.098 ☑
      stenosis T83.85 ☑
      thrombosis T83.86 ☑
    urinary (indwelling) — *see* Complications,
      catheter, urethral, indwelling
  cecostomy (stoma) — *see* Complications,
    colostomy
  cesarean delivery wound NEC O90.89
    disruption O90.0

☑ **Additional character required**

Complication — *continued*
- hematoma O90.2
  - infection (following delivery) O86.0
- chemotherapy (antineoplastic) NEC T88.7 ☑
- chin implant (prosthetic) — *see* Complication, prosthetic device or implant, specified NEC
- circulatory system I99.8
  - intraoperative I97.88
  - postprocedural I97.89
    - following cardiac surgery I97.19- ☑
      - postcardiotomy syndrome I97.0
    - hypertension I97.3
    - lymphedema after mastectomy I97.2
    - postcardiotomy syndrome I97.0
    - specified NEC I97.89
- colostomy (stoma) K94.00
  - hemorrhage K94.01
  - infection K94.02
  - malfunction K94.03
  - mechanical K94.03
  - specified complication NEC K94.09
- contraceptive device, intrauterine — *see* Complications, intrauterine, contraceptive device
- cord (umbilical) — *see* Complications, umbilical cord
- corneal graft — *see* Complications, graft, cornea
- coronary artery (bypass) graft T82.9 ☑
  - atherosclerosis — *see* Arteriosclerosis, coronary (artery),
  - embolism T82.818 ☑
  - fibrosis T82.828 ☑
  - hemorrhage T82.838 ☑
  - infection and inflammation T82.7 ☑
  - mechanical
    - breakdown T82.211 ☑
    - displacement T82.212 ☑
    - leakage T82.213 ☑
    - malposition T82.212 ☑
    - obstruction T82.218 ☑
    - perforation T82.218 ☑
    - protrusion T82.218 ☑
    - specified NEC T82.218 ☑
  - pain T82.848 ☑
  - specified type NEC T82.897 ☑
  - stenosis T82.858 ☑
  - thrombosis T82.868 ☑
- counterpulsation device (balloon), intra- aortic — *see* Complications, balloon implant, vascular
- cystostomy (stoma) N99.518
  - catheter — *see* Complications, catheter, cystostomy
  - hemorrhage N99.510
  - infection N99.511
  - malfunction N99.512
  - specified type NEC N99.518
- delivery (*see also* Complications, obstetric) O75.9
  - procedure (instrumental) (manual) (surgical) O75.4
  - specified NEC O75.89
- dialysis (peritoneal) (renal) (*see also* Complications, infusion)
  - catheter (vascular) — *see* Complication, catheter, dialysis
  - peritoneal, intraperitoneal — *see* Complications, catheter, intraperitoneal
- dorsal column (spinal) neurostimulator — *see* Complications, electronic stimulator device, spinal cord
- drug NEC T88.7 ☑
- ear procedure (*see also* Disorder, ear)
  - intraoperative H95.88
    - hematoma — *see* Complications, intraoperative, hemorrhage (hematoma) (of), ear
    - hemorrhage — *see* Complications, intraoperative, hemorrhage (hematoma) (of), ear
    - laceration — *see* Complications, intraoperative, puncture or laceration..., ear
    - specified NEC H95.88
  - postoperative H95.89
    - external ear canal stenosis H95.81- ☑
    - hematoma — *see* Complications, postprocedural, hemorrhage (hematoma) (of), ear
    - hemorrhage — *see* Complications, postprocedural, hemorrhage (hematoma) (of), ear
    - postmastoidectomy — *see* Complications, postmastoidectomy

Complication — *continued*
- specified NEC H95.89
- ectopic pregnancy O08.9
  - damage to pelvic organs O08.6
  - embolism O08.2
  - genital infection O08.0
  - hemorrhage (delayed) (excessive) O08.1
  - metabolic disorder O08.5
  - renal failure O08.4
  - shock O08.3
  - specified type NEC O08.0
  - venous complication NEC O08.7
- electronic stimulator device
  - bladder (urinary) — *see* Complications, electronic stimulator device, urinary
  - bone T84.9 ☑
    - breakdown T84.310 ☑
    - displacement T84.320 ☑
    - embolism T84.81 ☑
    - fibrosis T84.82 ☑
    - hemorrhage T84.83 ☑
    - infection or inflammation T84.7 ☑
    - malfunction T84.310 ☑
    - malposition T84.320 ☑
    - mechanical NEC T84.390 ☑
    - obstruction T84.390 ☑
    - pain T84.84 ☑
    - perforation T84.390 ☑
    - protrusion T84.390 ☑
    - specified type NEC T84.89 ☑
    - stenosis T84.85 ☑
    - thrombosis T84.86 ☑
  - brain T85.9 ☑
    - embolism T85.81 ☑
    - fibrosis T85.82 ☑
    - hemorrhage T85.83 ☑
    - infection and inflammation T85.79 ☑
    - mechanical
      - breakdown T85.110 ☑
      - displacement T85.120 ☑
      - leakage T85.190 ☑
      - malposition T85.120 ☑
      - obstruction T85.190 ☑
      - perforation T85.190 ☑
      - protrusion T85.190 ☑
      - specified NEC T85.190 ☑
    - pain T85.84 ☑
    - specified type NEC T85.89 ☑
    - stenosis T85.85 ☑
    - thrombosis T85.86 ☑
  - cardiac (defibrillator) (pacemaker) — *see* Complications, cardiovascular device or implant, electronic
  - muscle T84.9 ☑
    - breakdown T84.418 ☑
    - displacement T84.428 ☑
    - embolism T84.81 ☑
    - fibrosis T84.82 ☑
    - hemorrhage T84.83 ☑
    - infection or inflammation T84.7 ☑
    - mechanical NEC T84.498 ☑
    - pain T84.84 ☑
    - specified type NEC T84.89 ☑
    - stenosis T84.85 ☑
    - thrombosis T84.86 ☑
  - nervous system T85.9 ☑
    - brain — *see* Complications, electronic stimulator device, brain
    - embolism T85.81 ☑
    - fibrosis T85.82 ☑
    - hemorrhage T85.83 ☑
    - infection and inflammation T85.79 ☑
    - mechanical
      - breakdown T85.118 ☑
      - displacement T85.128 ☑
      - leakage T85.199 ☑
      - malposition T85.128 ☑
      - obstruction T85.199 ☑
      - perforation T85.199 ☑
      - protrusion T85.199 ☑
      - specified NEC T85.199 ☑
    - pain T85.84 ☑
    - peripheral nerve — *see* Complications, electronic stimulator device, peripheral nerve
    - specified type NEC T85.89 ☑
    - spinal cord — *see* Complications, electronic stimulator device, spinal cord
    - stenosis T85.85 ☑
    - thrombosis T85.86 ☑
  - peripheral nerve T85.9 ☑
    - embolism T85.81 ☑

Complication — *continued*
- fibrosis T85.82 ☑
- hemorrhage T85.83 ☑
- infection and inflammation T85.79 ☑
- mechanical
  - breakdown T85.111 ☑
  - displacement T85.121 ☑
  - leakage T85.191 ☑
  - malposition T85.121 ☑
  - obstruction T85.191 ☑
  - perforation T85.191 ☑
  - protrusion T85.191 ☑
  - specified NEC T85.191 ☑
- pain T85.84 ☑
- specified type NEC T85.89 ☑
- stenosis T85.85 ☑
- thrombosis T85.86 ☑
  - spinal cord T85.9 ☑
    - embolism T85.81 ☑
    - fibrosis T85.82 ☑
    - hemorrhage T85.83 ☑
    - infection and inflammation T85.79 ☑
    - mechanical
      - breakdown T85.112 ☑
      - displacement T85.122 ☑
      - leakage T85.192 ☑
      - malposition T85.122 ☑
      - obstruction T85.192 ☑
      - perforation T85.192 ☑
      - protrusion T85.192 ☑
      - specified NEC T85.192 ☑
    - pain T85.84 ☑
    - specified type NEC T85.89 ☑
    - stenosis T85.85 ☑
    - thrombosis T85.86 ☑
  - urinary T83.9 ☑
    - embolism T83.81 ☑
    - fibrosis T83.82 ☑
    - hemorrhage T83.83 ☑
    - infection and inflammation T83.59 ☑
    - mechanical
      - breakdown T83.110 ☑
      - displacement T83.120 ☑
      - malposition T83.120 ☑
      - perforation T83.190 ☑
      - protrusion T83.190 ☑
      - specified NEC T83.190 ☑
    - pain T83.84 ☑
    - specified type NEC T83.89 ☑
    - stenosis T83.85 ☑
    - thrombosis T83.86 ☑
- electroshock therapy T88.9 ☑
  - specified NEC T88.8 ☑
- endocrine E34.9
  - postprocedural
    - adrenal hypofunction E89.6
    - hypoinsulinemia E89.1
    - hypoparathyroidism E89.2
    - hypopituitarism E89.3
    - hypothyroidism E89.0
    - ovarian failure E89.40
      - asymptomatic E89.40
      - symptomatic E89.41
    - specified NEC E89.89
    - testicular hypofunction E89.5
- endodontic treatment NEC M27.59
- enterostomy (stoma) K94.10
  - hemorrhage K94.11
  - infection K94.12
  - malfunction K94.13
  - mechanical K94.13
  - specified complication NEC K94.19
- episiotomy, disruption O90.1
- esophageal anti-reflux device T85.9 ☑
  - embolism T85.81 ☑
  - fibrosis T85.82 ☑
  - hemorrhage T85.83 ☑
  - infection and inflammation T85.79 ☑
  - mechanical
    - breakdown T85.511 ☑
    - displacement T85.521 ☑
    - malfunction T85.511 ☑
    - malposition T85.521 ☑
    - obstruction T85.591 ☑
    - perforation T85.591 ☑
    - protrusion T85.591 ☑
    - specified NEC T85.591 ☑
  - pain T85.84 ☑
  - specified type NEC T85.89 ☑
  - stenosis T85.85 ☑
  - thrombosis T85.86 ☑
- esophagostomy K94.30

Complication

Complication — *continued*
- hemorrhage K94.31
- infection K94.32
- malfunction K94.33
- mechanical K94.33
- specified complication NEC K94.39
- extracorporeal circulation T80.90 ☑
- extremity artery (bypass) graft T82.9 ☑
  - arteriosclerosis — *see* Arteriosclerosis, extremities, bypass graft
  - embolism T82.818 ☑
  - fibrosis T82.828 ☑
  - hemorrhage T82.838 ☑
  - infection and inflammation T82.7 ☑
  - mechanical
    - breakdown T82.318 ☑
      - femoral artery T82.312 ☑
    - displacement T82.328 ☑
      - femoral artery T82.322 ☑
    - leakage T82.338 ☑
      - femoral artery T82.332 ☑
    - malposition T82.328 ☑
      - femoral artery T82.322 ☑
    - obstruction T82.398 ☑
      - femoral artery T82.392 ☑
    - perforation T82.398 ☑
      - femoral artery T82.392 ☑
    - protrusion T82.398 ☑
      - femoral artery T82.392 ☑
  - pain T82.848 ☑
  - specified type NEC T82.898 ☑
  - stenosis T82.858 ☑
  - thrombosis T82.868 ☑
- eye H57.9
  - corneal graft — *see* Complications, graft, cornea
  - implant (prosthetic) T85.9 ☑
    - embolism T85.81 ☑
    - fibrosis T85.82 ☑
    - hemorrhage T85.83 ☑
    - infection and inflammation T85.79 ☑
    - mechanical
      - breakdown T85.318 ☑
      - displacement T85.328 ☑
      - leakage T85.398 ☑
      - malposition T85.328 ☑
      - obstruction T85.398 ☑
      - perforation T85.398 ☑
      - protrusion T85.398 ☑
      - specified NEC T85.398 ☑
    - pain T85.84 ☑
    - specified type NEC T85.89 ☑
    - stenosis T85.85 ☑
    - thrombosis T85.86 ☑
  - intraocular lens — *see* Complications, intraocular lens
  - orbital prosthesis — *see* Complications, orbital prosthesis
- female genital N94.9
  - device, implant or graft NEC — *see* Complications, genitourinary, device or implant, genital tract
- femoral artery (bypass) graft — *see* Complication, extremity artery (bypass) graft
- fixation device, internal (orthopedic) T84.9 ☑
  - infection and inflammation T84.60 ☑
    - arm T84.61- ☑
      - humerus T84.61- ☑
      - radius T84.61- ☑
      - ulna T84.61- ☑
    - leg T84.629 ☑
      - femur T84.62- ☑
      - fibula T84.62- ☑
      - tibia T84.62- ☑
    - specified site NEC T84.69 ☑
    - spine T84.63 ☑
  - mechanical
    - breakdown
      - limb T84.119 ☑
        - carpal T84.210 ☑
        - femur T84.11- ☑
        - fibula T84.11- ☑
        - humerus T84.11- ☑
        - metacarpal T84.210 ☑
        - metatarsal T84.213 ☑
        - phalanx
          - foot T84.213 ☑
          - hand T84.210 ☑
        - radius T84.11- ☑
        - tarsal T84.213 ☑
        - tibia T84.11- ☑
        - ulna T84.11- ☑

Complication — *continued*
- specified bone NEC T84.218 ☑
- spine T84.216 ☑
- displacement
  - limb T84.129 ☑
    - carpal T84.220 ☑
    - femur T84.12- ☑
    - fibula T84.12- ☑
    - humerus T84.12- ☑
    - metacarpal T84.220 ☑
    - metatarsal T84.223 ☑
    - phalanx
      - foot T84.223 ☑
      - hand T84.220 ☑
    - radius T84.12- ☑
    - tarsal T84.223 ☑
    - tibia T84.12- ☑
    - ulna T84.12- ☑
  - specified bone NEC T84.228 ☑
  - spine T84.226 ☑
- malposition — *see* Complications, fixation device, internal, mechanical, displacement
- obstruction — *see* Complications, fixation device, internal, mechanical, specified type NEC
- perforation — *see* Complications, fixation device, internal, mechanical, specified type NEC
- protrusion — *see* Complications, fixation device, internal, mechanical, specified type NEC
- specified type NEC
  - limb T84.199 ☑
    - carpal T84.290 ☑
    - femur T84.19- ☑
    - fibula T84.19- ☑
    - humerus T84.19- ☑
    - metacarpal T84.290 ☑
    - metatarsal T84.293 ☑
    - phalanx
      - foot T84.293 ☑
      - hand T84.290 ☑
    - radius T84.19- ☑
    - tarsal T84.293 ☑
    - tibia T84.19- ☑
    - ulna T84.19- ☑
  - specified bone NEC T84.298 ☑
  - vertebra T84.296 ☑
- specified type NEC T84.89 ☑
  - embolism T84.81 ☑
  - fibrosis T84.82 ☑
  - hemorrhage T84.83 ☑
  - pain T84.84 ☑
  - specified complication NEC T84.89 ☑
  - stenosis T84.85 ☑
  - thrombosis T84.86 ☑
- following
  - acute myocardial infarction NEC I23.8
    - aneurysm (false) (of cardiac wall) (of heart wall) (ruptured) I23.3
    - angina I23.7
    - atrial
      - septal defect I23.1
      - thrombosis I23.6
    - cardiac wall rupture I23.3
    - chordae tendinae rupture I23.4
    - defect
      - septal
        - atrial (heart) I23.1
        - ventricular (heart) I23.2
    - hemopericardium I23.0
    - papillary muscle rupture I23.5
    - rupture
      - cardiac wall I23.3
        - with hemopericardium I23.0
      - chordae tendineae I23.4
      - papillary muscle I23.5
    - specified NEC I23.8
    - thrombosis
      - atrium I23.6
      - auricular appendage I23.6
      - ventricle (heart) I23.6
    - ventricular
      - septal defect I23.2
      - thrombosis I23.6
  - ectopic or molar pregnancy O08.9
    - cardiac arrest O08.81
    - sepsis O08.82
    - specified type NEC O08.89
    - urinary tract infection O08.83
  - termination of pregnancy — *see* Abortion

Complication — *continued*
- gastrointestinal K92.9
  - bile duct prosthesis — *see* Complications, bile duct implant
  - esophageal anti-reflux device — *see* Complications, esophageal anti-reflux device
  - postoperative
    - colostomy — *see* Complications, colostomy
    - dumping syndrome K91.1
    - enterostomy — *see* Complications, enterostomy
    - gastrostomy — *see* Complications, gastrostomy
    - malabsorption NEC K91.2
    - obstruction K91.3
    - postcholecystectomy syndrome K91.5
    - specified NEC K91.89
    - vomiting after GI surgery K91.0
  - prosthetic device or implant
    - bile duct prosthesis — *see* Complications, bile duct implant
    - esophageal anti-reflux device — *see* Complications, esophageal anti-reflux device
    - specified type NEC
      - embolism T85.81 ☑
      - fibrosis T85.82 ☑
      - hemorrhage T85.83 ☑
      - mechanical
        - breakdown T85.518 ☑
        - displacement T85.528 ☑
        - malfunction T85.518 ☑
        - malposition T85.528 ☑
        - obstruction T85.598 ☑
        - perforation T85.598 ☑
        - protrusion T85.598 ☑
        - specified NEC T85.598 ☑
      - pain T85.84 ☑
      - specified complication NEC T85.89 ☑
      - stenosis T85.85 ☑
      - thrombosis T85.86 ☑
- gastrostomy (stoma) K94.20
  - hemorrhage K94.21
  - infection K94.22
  - malfunction K94.23
  - mechanical K94.23
  - specified complication NEC K94.29
- genitourinary
  - device or implant T83.9 ☑
    - genital tract T83.9 ☑
      - infection or inflammation T83.6 ☑
      - intrauterine contraceptive device — *see* Complications, intrauterine, contraceptive device
      - mechanical — *see* Complications, by device, mechanical
      - mesh — *see* Complications, mesh
      - penile prosthesis — *see* Complications, prosthetic device, penile
      - specified type NEC T83.89 ☑
        - embolism T83.81 ☑
        - fibrosis T83.82 ☑
        - hemorrhage T83.83 ☑
        - pain T83.84 ☑
        - specified complication NEC T83.89 ☑
        - stenosis T83.85 ☑
        - thrombosis T83.86 ☑
      - vaginal mesh — *see* Complications, mesh
    - urinary system T83.9 ☑
      - cystostomy catheter — *see* Complication, catheter, cystostomy
      - electronic stimulator — *see* Complications, electronic stimulator device, urinary
      - indwelling urethral catheter — *see* Complications, catheter, urethral, indwelling
      - infection or inflammation T83.59 ☑
        - indwelling urinary catheter T83.51 ☑
      - kidney transplant — *see* Complication, transplant, kidney
      - organ graft — *see* Complication, graft, urinary organ
      - specified type NEC T83.89 ☑
        - embolism T83.81 ☑
        - fibrosis T83.82 ☑
        - hemorrhage T83.83 ☑
        - mechanical T83.198 ☑
          - breakdown T83.118 ☑
          - displacement T83.128 ☑
          - malfunction T83.118 ☑
          - malposition T83.128 ☑

☑ **Additional character required**

Complication — *continued*
- obstruction T83.198 ☑
- perforation T83.198 ☑
- protrusion T83.198 ☑
- specified NEC T83.198 ☑
- pain T83.84 ☑
- specified complication NEC T83.89 ☑
- stenosis T83.85 ☑
- thrombosis T83.86 ☑
- sphincter implant — *see* Complications, implant, urinary sphincter
- postprocedural
  - pelvic peritoneal adhesions N99.4
  - renal failure N99.0
  - specified NEC N99.89
  - stoma — *see* Complications, stoma, urinary tract
  - urethral stricture — *see* Stricture, urethra, postprocedural
  - vaginal
    - adhesions N99.2
    - vault prolapse N99.3
- graft (bypass) (patch) (*see also* Complications, prosthetic device or implant)
  - aorta — *see* Complications, graft, vascular
  - arterial — *see* Complication, graft, vascular
  - bone T86.839
    - failure T86.831
    - infection T86.832
    - mechanical T84.318 ☑
      - breakdown T84.318 ☑
      - displacement T84.328 ☑
      - protrusion T84.398 ☑
      - specified type NEC T84.398 ☑
    - rejection T86.830
    - specified type NEC T86.838
  - carotid artery — *see* Complications, graft, vascular
  - cornea T86.849
    - failure T86.841
    - infection T86.842
    - mechanical T85.398 ☑
      - breakdown T85.318 ☑
      - displacement T85.328 ☑
      - protrusion T85.398 ☑
      - specified type NEC T85.398 ☑
    - rejection T86.840
    - retroprosthetic membrane T85.398 ☑
    - specified type NEC T86.848
  - femoral artery (bypass) — *see* Complication, extremity artery (bypass) graft
  - genital organ or tract — *see* Complications, genitourinary, device or implant, genital tract
  - muscle T84.9 ☑
    - breakdown T84.410 ☑
    - displacement T84.420 ☑
    - embolism T84.81 ☑
    - fibrosis T84.82 ☑
    - hemorrhage T84.83 ☑
    - infection and inflammation T84.7 ☑
    - mechanical NEC T84.490 ☑
    - pain T84.84 ☑
    - specified type NEC T84.89 ☑
    - stenosis T84.85 ☑
    - thrombosis T84.86 ☑
  - nerve — *see* Complication, prosthetic device or implant, specified NEC
  - skin — *see* Complications, prosthetic device or implant, skin graft
  - tendon T84.9 ☑
    - breakdown T84.410 ☑
    - displacement T84.420 ☑
    - embolism T84.81 ☑
    - fibrosis T84.82 ☑
    - hemorrhage T84.83 ☑
    - infection and inflammation T84.7 ☑
    - mechanical NEC T84.490 ☑
    - pain T84.84 ☑
    - specified type NEC T84.89 ☑
    - stenosis T84.85 ☑
    - thrombosis T84.86 ☑
  - urinary organ T83.9 ☑
    - embolism T83.81 ☑
    - fibrosis T83.82 ☑
    - hemorrhage T83.83 ☑
    - infection and inflammation T83.59 ☑
      - indwelling urinary catheter T83.51 ☑
    - mechanical
      - breakdown T83.21 ☑
      - displacement T83.22 ☑
      - leakage T83.23 ☑

Complication — *continued*
- malposition T83.22 ☑
- obstruction T83.29 ☑
- perforation T83.29 ☑
- protrusion T83.29 ☑
- specified NEC T83.29 ☑
- pain T83.84 ☑
- specified type NEC T83.89 ☑
- stenosis T83.85 ☑
- thrombosis T83.86 ☑
- vascular T82.9 ☑
  - embolism T82.818 ☑
  - femoral artery — *see* Complication, extremity artery (bypass) graft
  - fibrosis T82.828 ☑
  - hemorrhage T82.838 ☑
  - mechanical
    - breakdown T82.319 ☑
      - aorta (bifurcation) T82.310 ☑
      - carotid artery T82.311 ☑
      - specified vessel NEC T82.318 ☑
    - displacement T82.329 ☑
      - aorta (bifurcation) T82.320 ☑
      - carotid artery T82.321 ☑
      - specified vessel NEC T82.328 ☑
    - leakage T82.339 ☑
      - aorta (bifurcation) T82.330 ☑
      - carotid artery T82.331 ☑
      - specified vessel NEC T82.338 ☑
    - malposition T82.329 ☑
      - aorta (bifurcation) T82.320 ☑
      - carotid artery T82.321 ☑
      - specified vessel NEC T82.328 ☑
    - obstruction T82.399 ☑
      - aorta (bifurcation) T82.390 ☑
      - carotid artery T82.391 ☑
      - specified vessel NEC T82.398 ☑
    - perforation T82.399 ☑
      - aorta (bifurcation) T82.390 ☑
      - carotid artery T82.391 ☑
      - specified vessel NEC T82.398 ☑
    - protrusion T82.399 ☑
      - aorta (bifurcation) T82.390 ☑
      - carotid artery T82.391 ☑
      - specified vessel NEC T82.398 ☑
  - pain T82.848 ☑
  - specified complication NEC T82.898 ☑
  - stenosis T82.858 ☑
  - thrombosis T82.868 ☑
- heart I51.9
  - assist device
    - infection and inflammation T82.7 ☑
  - following acute myocardial infarction — *see* Complications, following, acute myocardial infarction
  - postoperative — *see* Complications, circulatory system
  - transplant — *see* Complication, transplant, heart
  - and lung (s) — *see* Complications, transplant, heart, with lung
  - valve
    - graft (biological) T82.9 ☑
      - embolism T82.817 ☑
      - fibrosis T82.827 ☑
      - hemorrhage T82.837 ☑
      - infection and inflammation T82.7 ☑
      - mechanical T82.228 ☑
        - breakdown T82.221 ☑
        - displacement T82.222 ☑
        - leakage T82.223 ☑
        - malposition T82.222 ☑
        - obstruction T82.228 ☑
        - perforation T82.228 ☑
        - protrusion T82.228 ☑
      - pain T82.847 ☑
      - specified type NEC T82.897 ☑
      - stenosis T82.857 ☑
      - thrombosis T82.867 ☑
    - prosthesis T82.9 ☑
      - embolism T82.817 ☑
      - fibrosis T82.827 ☑
      - hemorrhage T82.837 ☑
      - infection or inflammation T82.6 ☑
      - mechanical T82.09 ☑
        - breakdown T82.01 ☑
        - displacement T82.02 ☑
        - leakage T82.03 ☑
        - malposition T82.02 ☑
        - obstruction T82.09 ☑
        - perforation T82.09 ☑
        - protrusion T82.09 ☑

Complication — *continued*
- pain T82.847 ☑
- specified type NEC T82.897 ☑
  - mechanical T82.09 ☑
- stenosis T82.857 ☑
- thrombosis T82.867 ☑
- hematoma
  - intraoperative — *see* Complication, intraoperative, hemorrhage
  - postprocedural — *see* Complication, postprocedural, hemorrhage
- hemodialysis — *see* Complications, dialysis
- hemorrhage
  - intraoperative — *see* Complication, intraoperative, hemorrhage
  - postprocedural — *see* Complication, postprocedural, hemorrhage
- ileostomy (stoma) — *see* Complications, enterostomy
- immunization (procedure) — *see* Complications, vaccination
- implant (*see also* Complications, by site and type)
  - urinary sphincter T83.9 ☑
    - embolism T83.81 ☑
    - fibrosis T83.82 ☑
    - hemorrhage T83.83 ☑
    - infection and inflammation T83.59 ☑
    - mechanical
      - breakdown T83.111 ☑
      - displacement T83.121 ☑
      - leakage T83.191 ☑
      - malposition T83.121 ☑
      - obstruction T83.191 ☑
      - perforation T83.191 ☑
      - protrusion T83.191 ☑
      - specified NEC T83.191 ☑
    - pain T83.84 ☑
    - specified type NEC T83.89 ☑
    - stenosis T83.85 ☑
    - thrombosis T83.86 ☑
- infusion (procedure) T80.90 ☑
  - air embolism T80.0 ☑
  - blood — *see* Complications, transfusion
  - catheter — *see* Complications, catheter
  - infection T80.29 ☑
  - pump — *see* Complications, cardiovascular, device or implant
  - sepsis T80.29 ☑
  - serum reaction (*see also* Reaction, serum) T80.69 ☑
    - anaphylactic shock (*see also* Shock, anaphylactic) T80.59 ☑
    - specified type NEC T80.89 ☑
- inhalation therapy NEC T81.81 ☑
- injection (procedure) T80.90 ☑
  - drug reaction — *see* Reaction, drug
  - infection T80.29 ☑
  - sepsis T80.29 ☑
  - serum (prophylactic) (therapeutic) — *see* Complications, vaccination
  - specified type NEC T80.89 ☑
  - vaccine (any) — *see* Complications, vaccination
- inoculation (any) — *see* Complications, vaccination
- insulin pump
  - infection and inflammation T85.72 ☑
  - mechanical
    - breakdown T85.614 ☑
    - displacement T85.624 ☑
    - leakage T85.633 ☑
    - malposition T85.624 ☑
    - obstruction T85.694 ☑
    - perforation T85.694 ☑
    - protrusion T85.694 ☑
    - specified NEC T85.694 ☑
- intestinal pouch NEC K91.858
- intraocular lens (prosthetic) T85.9 ☑
  - embolism T85.81 ☑
  - fibrosis T85.82 ☑
  - hemorrhage T85.83 ☑
  - infection and inflammation T85.79 ☑
  - mechanical
    - breakdown T85.21 ☑
    - displacement T85.22 ☑
    - malposition T85.22 ☑
    - obstruction T85.29 ☑
    - perforation T85.29 ☑
    - protrusion T85.29 ☑
    - specified NEC T85.29 ☑
  - pain T85.84 ☑
  - specified type NEC T85.89 ☑
  - stenosis T85.85 ☑

☑ **Additional character required**

Complication

Complication — *continued*
  thrombosis T85.86 ☑
  intraoperative (intraprocedural)
    cardiac arrest
      during cardiac surgery I97.710
      during other surgery I97.711
    cardiac functional disturbance NEC
      during cardiac surgery I97.790
      during other surgery I97.791
    hemorrhage (hematoma) (of)
      circulatory system organ or structure
        during cardiac bypass I97.411
        during cardiac catheterization I97.410
        during other circulatory system procedure I97.418
        during other procedure I97.42
      digestive system organ
        during procedure on digestive system K91.61
        during procedure on other organ K91.62
      ear
        during procedure on ear and mastoid process H95.21
        during procedure on other organ H95.22
      endocrine system organ or structure
        during procedure on endocrine system organ or structure E36.01
        during procedure on other organ E36.02
      eye and adnexa
        during ophthalmic procedure H59.11- ☑
        during other procedure H59.12- ☑
      genitourinary organ or structure
        during procedure on genitourinary organ or structure N99.61
        during procedure on other organ N99.62
      mastoid process
        during procedure on ear and mastoid process H95.21
        during procedure on other organ H95.22
      musculoskeletal structure
        during musculoskeletal surgery M96.810
        during non-orthopedic surgery M96.811
        during orthopedic surgery M96.810
      nervous system
        during a nervous system procedure G97.31
        during other procedure G97.32
      respiratory system
        during other procedure J95.62
        during procedure on respiratory system organ or structure J95.61
      skin and subcutaneous tissue
        during a dermatologic procedure L76.01
        during a procedure on other organ L76.02
      spleen
        during a procedure on other organ D78.02
        during a procedure on the spleen D78.01
    puncture or laceration (accidental) (unintentional) (of)
      brain
        during a nervous system procedure G97.48
        during other procedure G97.49
      circulatory system organ or structure
        during circulatory system procedure I97.51
        during other procedure I97.52
      digestive system
        during procedure on digestive system K91.71
        during procedure on other organ K91.72
      ear
        during procedure on ear and mastoid process H95.31
        during procedure on other organ H95.32
      endocrine system organ or structure
        during procedure on endocrine system organ or structure E36.11
        during procedure on other organ E36.12
      eye and adnexa
        during ophthalmic procedure H59.21- ☑
        during other procedure H59.22- ☑
      genitourinary organ or structure
        during procedure on genitourinary organ or structure N99.71
        during procedure on other organ N99.72
      mastoid process
        during procedure on ear and mastoid process H95.31
        during procedure on other organ H95.32
      musculoskeletal structure
        during musculoskeletal surgery M96.820
        during non-orthopedic surgery M96.821
        during orthopedic surgery M96.820
      nervous system

Complication — *continued*
        during a nervous system procedure G97.48
        during other procedure G97.49
      respiratory system
        during other procedure J95.72
        during procedure on respiratory system organ or structure J95.71
      skin and subcutaneous tissue
        during a dermatologic procedure L76.11
        during a procedure on other organ L76.12
      spleen
        during a procedure on other organ D78.12
        during a procedure on the spleen D78.11
    specified NEC
      circulatory system I97.88
      digestive system K91.81
      ear H95.88
      endocrine system E36.8
      eye and adnexa H59.88
      genitourinary system N99.81
      mastoid process H95.88
      musculoskeletal structure M96.89
      nervous system G97.81
      respiratory system J95.88
      skin and subcutaneous tissue L76.81
      spleen D78.81
  intraperitoneal catheter (dialysis) (infusion) — *see* Complications, catheter, intraperitoneal
  intrauterine
    contraceptive device
      embolism T83.81 ☑
      fibrosis T83.82 ☑
      hemorrhage T83.83 ☑
      infection and inflammation T83.6 ☑
      mechanical
        breakdown T83.31 ☑
        displacement T83.32 ☑
        malposition T83.32 ☑
        obstruction T83.39 ☑
        perforation T83.39 ☑
        protrusion T83.39 ☑
        specified NEC T83.39 ☑
      pain T83.84 ☑
      specified type NEC T83.89 ☑
      stenosis T83.85 ☑
      thrombosis T83.86 ☑
    procedure (fetal), to newborn P96.5
  jejunostomy (stoma) — *see* Complications, enterostomy
  joint prosthesis, internal T84.9 ☑
    breakage (fracture) T84.01- ☑
    dislocation T84.02- ☑
    fracture T84.01- ☑
    infection or inflammation T84.50 ☑
      hip T84.5- ☑
      knee T84.5- ☑
      specified joint NEC T84.59 ☑
    instability T84.02- ☑
    malposition — *see* Complications, joint prosthesis, mechanical, displacement
    mechanical
      breakage, broken T84.01- ☑
      dislocation T84.02- ☑
      fracture T84.01- ☑
      instability T84.02- ☑
      leakage — *see* Complications, joint prosthesis, mechanical, specified NEC
      loosening T84.039 ☑
        hip T84.03- ☑
        knee T84.03- ☑
        specified joint NEC T84.038 ☑
      obstruction — *see* Complications, joint prosthesis, mechanical, specified NEC
      perforation — *see* Complications, joint prosthesis, mechanical, specified NEC
      periprosthetic
        fracture T84.049 ☑
          hip T84.04- ☑
          knee T84.04- ☑
          other specified joint T84.048 ☑
        osteolysis T84.059 ☑
          hip T84.05- ☑
          knee T84.05- ☑
          other specified joint T84.058 ☑
      protrusion — *see* Complications, joint prosthesis, mechanical, specified NEC
      specified complication NEC T84.099 ☑
        hip T84.09- ☑
        knee T84.09- ☑
        other specified joint T84.098 ☑
      subluxation T84.02- ☑
      wear of articular bearing surface T84.069 ☑

Complication — *continued*
      hip T84.06- ☑
      knee T84.06- ☑
      other specified joint T84.068 ☑
    specified joint NEC T84.89 ☑
      embolism T84.81 ☑
      fibrosis T84.82 ☑
      hemorrhage T84.83 ☑
      pain T84.84 ☑
      specified complication NEC T84.89 ☑
      stenosis T84.85 ☑
      thrombosis T84.86 ☑
    subluxation T84.02- ☑
  kidney transplant — *see* Complications, transplant, kidney
  labor O75.9
    specified NEC O75.89
  liver transplant (immune or nonimmune) — *see* Complications, transplant, liver
  lumbar puncture G97.1
    cerebrospinal fluid leak G97.0
    headache or reaction G97.1
  lung transplant — *see* Complications, transplant, lung
    and heart — *see* Complications, transplant, lung, with heart
  male genital N50.9
    device, implant or graft — *see* Complications, genitourinary, device or implant, genital tract
    postprocedural or postoperative — *see* Complications, genitourinary, postprocedural
    specified NEC N99.89
  mastoid (process) procedure
    intraoperative H95.88
      hematoma — *see* Complications, intraoperative, hemorrhage (hematoma) (of), mastoid process
      hemorrhage — *see* Complications, intraoperative, hemorrhage (hematoma) (of), mastoid process
      laceration — *see* Complications, intraoperative, puncture or laceration..., mastoid process
      specified NEC H95.88
    postmastoidectomy — *see* Complications, postmastoidectomy
    postoperative H95.89
      external ear canal stenosis H95.81- ☑
      hematoma — *see* Complications..., postprocedural, hemorrhage (hematoma) (of), mastoid process
      hemorrhage — *see* Complications..., postprocedural, hemorrhage (hematoma) (of), mastoid process
      postmastoidectomy — *see* Complications, postmastoidectomy
      specified NEC H95.89
  mastoidectomy cavity — *see* Complications, postmastoidectomy
  mechanical — *see* Complications, by site and type, mechanical
  medical procedures (*see also* Complication(s), intraoperative) T88.9 ☑
  metabolic E88.9
    postoperative E89.89
    specified NEC E89.89
  molar pregnancy NOS O08.9
    damage to pelvic organs O08.6
    embolism O08.2
    genital infection O08.0
    hemorrhage (delayed) (excessive) O08.1
    metabolic disorder O08.5
    renal failure O08.4
    shock O08.3
    specified type NEC O08.0
    venous complication NEC O08.7
  musculoskeletal system (*see also* Complication, intraoperative (intraprocedural), by site)
    device, implant or graft NEC — *see* Complications, orthopedic, device or implant
    internal fixation (nail) (plate) (rod) — *see* Complications, fixation device, internal
    joint prosthesis — *see* Complications, joint prosthesis
    postoperative (postprocedural) M96.89
      with osteoporosis — *see* Osteoporosis
      fracture following insertion of device — *see* Fracture, following insertion of

Complication — *continued*
    orthopedic implant, joint prosthesis or bone plate
      joint instability after prosthesis removal M96.89
      lordosis M96.4
      postlaminectomy syndrome NEC M96.1
        kyphosis M96.3
      pseudarthrosis M96.0
      specified complication NEC M96.89
      post radiation M96.89
        kyphosis M96.3
        scoliosis M96.5
        specified complication NEC M96.89
  nephrostomy (stoma) — *see* Complications, stoma, urinary tract, external NEC
  nervous system G98.8
    central G96.9
    device, implant or graft (*see also* Complication, prosthetic device or implant, specified NEC)
      electronic stimulator (electrode(s)) — *see* Complications, electronic stimulator device
      ventricular shunt — *see* Complications, ventricular shunt
    electronic stimulator (electrode(s)) — *see* Complications, electronic stimulator device
    postprocedural G97.82
      intracranial hypotension G97.2
      specified NEC G97.82
      spinal fluid leak G97.0
  newborn, due to intrauterine (fetal) procedure P96.5
  nonabsorbable (permanent) sutures — *see* Complication, sutures, permanent
  obstetric O75.9
    procedure (instrumental) (manual) (surgical) specified NEC O75.4
    specified NEC O75.89
    surgical wound NEC O90.89
      hematoma O90.2
      infection O86.0
  ocular lens implant — *see* Complications, intraocular lens
  ophthalmologic
    postprocedural bleb — *see* Blebitis
  orbital prosthesis T85.9 ☑
    embolism T85.81 ☑
    fibrosis T85.82 ☑
    hemorrhage T85.83 ☑
    infection and inflammation T85.79 ☑
    mechanical
      breakdown T85.31- ☑
      displacement T85.32- ☑
      malposition T85.32- ☑
      obstruction T85.39- ☑
      perforation T85.39- ☑
      protrusion T85.39- ☑
      specified NEC T85.39- ☑
    pain T85.84 ☑
    specified type NEC T85.89 ☑
    stenosis T85.85 ☑
    thrombosis T85.86 ☑
  organ or tissue transplant (partial) (total) — *see* Complications, transplant
  orthopedic (*see also* Disorder, soft tissue)
    device or implant T84.9 ☑
      bone
        device or implant — *see* Complication, bone, device NEC
        graft — *see* Complication, graft, bone
      breakdown T84.418 ☑
      displacement T84.428 ☑
      electronic bone stimulator — *see* Complications, electronic stimulator device, bone
      embolism T84.81 ☑
      fibrosis T84.82 ☑
      fixation device — *see* Complication, fixation device, internal
      hemorrhage T84.83 ☑
      infection or inflammation T84.7 ☑
      joint prosthesis — *see* Complication, joint prosthesis, internal
      malfunction T84.418 ☑
      malposition T84.428 ☑
      mechanical NEC T84.498 ☑
      muscle graft — *see* Complications, graft, muscle
      obstruction T84.498 ☑
      pain T84.84 ☑

Complication — *continued*
      perforation T84.498 ☑
      protrusion T84.498 ☑
      specified complication NEC T84.89 ☑
      stenosis T84.85 ☑
      tendon graft — *see* Complications, graft, tendon
      thrombosis T84.86 ☑
    fracture (following insertion of device) — *see* Fracture, following insertion of orthopedic implant, joint prosthesis or bone plate
    postprocedural M96.89
      fracture — *see* Fracture, following insertion of orthopedic implant, joint prosthesis or bone plate
      postlaminectomy syndrome NEC M96.1
        kyphosis M96.3
        lordosis M96.4
      postradiation
        kyphosis M96.2
        scoliosis M96.5
      pseudarthrosis post-fusion M96.0
      specified type NEC M96.89
  pacemaker (cardiac) — *see* Complications, cardiovascular device or implant, electronic
  pancreas transplant — *see* Complications, transplant, pancreas
  penile prosthesis (implant) — *see* Complications, prosthetic device, penile
  perfusion NEC T80.90 ☑
  perineal repair (obstetrical) NEC O90.89
    disruption O90.1
    hematoma O90.2
    infection (following delivery) O86.0
  phototherapy T88.9 ☑
    specified NEC T88.8 ☑
  postmastoidectomy NEC H95.19- ☑
    cyst, mucosal H95.13- ☑
    granulation H95.12- ☑
    inflammation, chronic H95.11- ☑
    recurrent cholesteatoma H95.0- ☑
  postoperative — *see* Complications, postprocedural
    circulatory — *see* Complications, circulatory system
    ear — *see* Complications, ear
    endocrine — *see* Complications, endocrine
    eye — *see* Complications, eye
    lumbar puncture G97.1
      cerebrospinal fluid leak G97.0
    nervous system (central) (peripheral) — *see* Complications, nervous system
    respiratory system — *see* Complications, respiratory system
  postprocedural (*see also* Complications, surgical procedure)
    cardiac arrest
      following cardiac surgery I97.120
      following other surgery I97.121
    cardiac functional disturbance NEC
      following cardiac surgery I97.190
      following other surgery I97.191
    cardiac insufficiency
      following cardiac surgery I97.110
      following other surgery I97.111
    chorioretinal scars following retinal surgery H59.81- ☑
    following cataract surgery
      cataract (lens) fragments H59.02- ☑
      cystoid macular edema H59.03- ☑
      specified NEC H59.09- ☑
      vitreous (touch) syndrome H59.01- ☑
    heart failure
      following cardiac surgery I97.130
      following other surgery I97.131
    hemorrhage (hematoma) (of)
      circulatory system organ or structure
        following a cardiac bypass I97.611
        following a cardiac catheterization I97.610
        following other circulatory system procedure I97.618
        following other procedure I97.62
      digestive system
        following procedure on digestive system K91.840
        following procedure on other organ K91.841
      ear
        following other procedure H95.42
        following procedure on ear and mastoid process H95.41
      endocrine system

Complication — *continued*
        following endocrine system procedure E89.810
        following other procedure E89.811
      eye and adnexa
        following ophthalmic procedure H59.31- ☑
        following other procedure H59.32- ☑
      genitourinary organ or structure
        following procedure on genitourinary organ or structure N99.820
        following procedure on other organ N99.821
      mastoid process
        following other procedure H95.42
        following procedure on ear and mastoid process H95.41
      musculoskeletal structure
        following musculoskeletal surgery M96.830
        following non-orthopedic surgery M96.831
        following orthopedic surgery M96.830
      nervous system
        following a nervous system procedure G97.51
        following other procedure G97.52
      respiratory system
        following other procedure J95.831
        following procedure on respiratory system organ or structure J95.830
      skin and subcutaneous tissue
        following a dermatologic procedure L76.21
        following a procedure on other organ L76.22
      spleen
        following procedure on other organ D78.22
        following procedure on the spleen D78.21
    specified NEC
      circulatory system I97.89
      digestive K91.89
      ear H95.89
      endocrine E89.89
      eye and adnexa H59.89
      genitourinary N99.89
      mastoid process H95.89
      metabolic E89.89
      musculoskeletal structure M96.89
      nervous system G97.82
      respiratory system J95.89
      skin and subcutaneous tissue L76.82
      spleen D78.89
  pregnancy NEC — *see* Pregnancy, complicated by
  prosthetic device or implant T85.9 ☑
    bile duct — *see* Complications, bile duct implant
    breast — *see* Complications, breast implant
    cardiac and vascular NEC — *see* Complications, cardiovascular device or implant
    corneal transplant — *see* Complications, graft, cornea
    electronic nervous system stimulator — *see* Complications, electronic stimulator device
    epidural infusion catheter — *see* Complications, catheter, epidural
    esophageal anti-reflux device — *see* Complications, esophageal anti-reflux device
    genital organ or tract — *see* Complications, genitourinary, device or implant, genital tract
    heart valve — *see* Complications, heart, valve, prosthesis
    infection or inflammation T85.79 ☑
      intestine transplant T86.892
      liver transplant T86.43
      lung transplant T86.812
      pancreas transplant T86.892
      skin graft T86.822
    intraocular lens — *see* Complications, intraocular lens
    intraperitoneal (dialysis) catheter — *see* Complications, catheter, intraperitoneal
    joint — *see* Complications, joint prosthesis, internal
    mechanical NEC T85.698 ☑
      dialysis catheter (vascular) (*see also* Complication, catheter, dialysis, mechanical)
        peritoneal — *see* Complication, catheter, intraperitoneal, mechanical
      gastrointestinal device T85.598 ☑
      ocular device T85.398 ☑
      subdural (infusion) catheter T85.690 ☑

Complication

Complication — *continued*
 suture, permanent T85.692 ☑
  that for bone repair — *see* Complications,
   fixation device, internal (orthopedic),
   mechanical
 ventricular shunt
  breakdown T85.01 ☑
  displacement T85.02 ☑
  leakage T85.03 ☑
  malposition T85.02 ☑
  obstruction T85.09 ☑
  perforation T85.09 ☑
  protrusion T85.09 ☑
  specified NEC T85.09 ☑
 mesh
  erosion (to surrounding organ or tissue)
   T83.718 ☑
   vaginal (into pelvic floor muscles) T83.711
    ☑
  exposure (into surrounding organ or tissue)
   T83.728 ☑
   vaginal (into vagina) (through vaginal wall)
    T83.721 ☑
 orbital — *see* Complications, orbital prosthesis
 penile T83.9 ☑
  embolism T83.81 ☑
  fibrosis T83.82 ☑
  hemorrhage T83.83 ☑
  infection and inflammation T83.6 ☑
  mechanical
   breakdown T83.410 ☑
   displacement T83.420 ☑
   leakage T83.490 ☑
   malposition T83.420 ☑
   obstruction T83.490 ☑
   perforation T83.490 ☑
   protrusion T83.490 ☑
   specified NEC T83.490 ☑
  pain T83.84 ☑
  specified type NEC T83.89 ☑
  stenosis T83.85 ☑
  thrombosis T83.86 ☑
 prosthetic materials NEC
  erosion (to surrounding organ or tissue)
   T83.718 ☑
   vaginal (into pelvic floor muscles) T83.711
    ☑
  exposure (into surrounding organ or tissue)
   T83.728 ☑
   vaginal (into vagina) (through vaginal wall)
    T83.721 ☑
 skin graft T86.829
  artificial skin or decellularized allodermis
   embolism T85.81 ☑
   fibrosis T85.82 ☑
   hemorrhage T85.83 ☑
   infection and inflammation T85.79 ☑
   mechanical
    breakdown T85.613 ☑
    displacement T85.623 ☑
    malfunction T85.613 ☑
    malposition T85.623 ☑
    obstruction T85.693 ☑
    perforation T85.693 ☑
    protrusion T85.693 ☑
    specified NEC T85.693 ☑
   pain T85.84 ☑
   specified type NEC T85.89 ☑
   stenosis T85.85 ☑
   thrombosis T85.86 ☑
  failure T86.821
  infection T86.822
  rejection T86.820
  specified NEC T86.828
 specified NEC T85.9 ☑
  embolism T85.81 ☑
  fibrosis T85.82 ☑
  hemorrhage T85.83 ☑
  infection and inflammation T85.79 ☑
  mechanical
   breakdown T85.618 ☑
   displacement T85.628 ☑
   leakage T85.638 ☑
   malfunction T85.618 ☑
   malposition T85.628 ☑
   obstruction T85.698 ☑
   perforation T85.698 ☑
   protrusion T85.698 ☑
   specified NEC T85.698 ☑
  pain T85.84 ☑
  specified type NEC T85.89 ☑
  stenosis T85.85 ☑

Complication — *continued*
  thrombosis T85.86 ☑
 subdural infusion catheter — *see*
  Complications, catheter, subdural
 sutures — *see* Complications, sutures
 urinary organ or tract NEC — *see*
  Complications, genitourinary, device or
  implant, urinary system
 vascular — *see* Complications, cardiovascular
  device or implant
 ventricular shunt — *see* Complications,
  ventricular shunt (device)
 puerperium — *see* Puerperal
 puncture, spinal G97.1
  cerebrospinal fluid leak G97.0
  headache or reaction G97.1
 pyelogram N99.89
 radiation
  kyphosis M96.2
  scoliosis M96.5
 reattached
  extremity (infection) (rejection)
   lower T87.1X- ☑
   upper T87.0X- ☑
  specified body part NEC T87.2
 reconstructed breast
  asymmetry between native and reconstructed
   breast N65.1
  deformity N65.0
  disproportion between native and
   reconstructed breast N65.1
  excess tissue N65.0
  misshappen N65.0
 reimplant NEC (*see also* Complications, prosthetic
  device or implant)
  limb (infection) (rejection) — *see*
   Complications, reattached, extremity
  organ (partial) (total) — *see* Complications,
   transplant
  prosthetic device NEC — *see* Complications,
   prosthetic device
 renal N28.9
  allograft — *see* Complications, transplant,
   kidney
  dialysis — *see* Complications, dialysis
 respirator
  mechanical J95.850
   specified NEC J95.859
 respiratory system J98.9
  device, implant or graft — *see* Complication,
   prosthetic device or implant, specified NEC
  lung transplant — *see* Complications,
   prosthetic device or implant, lung
   transplant
  postoperative J95.89
   air leak J95.812
   Mendelson's syndrome (chemical
    pneumonitis) J95.4
   pneumothorax J95.811
   pulmonary insufficiency (acute) (after
    nonthoracic surgery) J95.2
    chronic J95.3
    following thoracic surgery J95.1
   respiratory failure (acute) J95.821
    acute and chronic J95.822
   specified NEC J95.89
   subglottic stenosis J95.5
   tracheostomy complication — *see*
    Complications, tracheostomy
  therapy T81.89 ☑
 sedation during labor and delivery O74.9
  cardiac O74.2
  central nervous system O74.3
  pulmonary NEC O74.1
 shunt (*see also* Complications, prosthetic device
  or implant)
  arteriovenous — *see* Complications,
   arteriovenous, shunt
  ventricular (communicating) — *see*
   Complications, ventricular shunt
 skin
  graft T86.829
   failure T86.821
   infection T86.822
   rejection T86.820
   specified type NEC T86.828
 spinal
  anesthesia — *see* Complications, anesthesia,
   spinal
  catheter (epidural) (subdural) — *see*
   Complications, catheter
  puncture or tap G97.1

Complication — *continued*
  cerebrospinal fluid leak G97.0
  headache or reaction G97.1
 stent
  bile duct — *see* Complications, bile duct
   prosthesis
  urinary T83.9 ☑
   embolism T83.81 ☑
   fibrosis T83.82 ☑
   hemorrhage T83.83 ☑
   infection and inflammation T83.59 ☑
   mechanical
    breakdown T83.112 ☑
    displacement T83.122 ☑
    leakage T83.192 ☑
    malposition T83.122 ☑
    obstruction T83.192 ☑
    perforation T83.192 ☑
    protrusion T83.192 ☑
    specified NEC T83.192 ☑
   pain T83.84 ☑
   specified type NEC T83.89 ☑
   stenosis T83.85 ☑
   thrombosis T83.86 ☑
 stoma
  digestive tract
   colostomy — *see* Complications, colostomy
   enterostomy — *see* Complications,
    enterostomy
   esophagostomy — *see* Complications,
    esophagostomy
   gastrostomy — *see* Complications,
    gastrostomy
  urinary tract N99.538
   cystostomy — *see* Complications, cystostomy
   external NOS N99.528
    hemorrhage N99.520
    infection N99.521
    malfunction N99.522
    specified type NEC N99.528
   hemorrhage N99.530
   infection N99.531
   malfunction N99.532
   specified type NEC N99.538
 stomach banding — *see* Complication(s), bariatric
  procedure
 stomach stapling — *see* Complication(s), bariatric
  procedure
 surgical material, nonabsorbable — *see*
  Complication, suture, permanent
 surgical procedure (on) T81.9 ☑
  amputation stump (late) — *see* Complications,
   amputation stump
  cardiac — *see* Complications, circulatory system
  cholesteatoma, recurrent — *see* Complications,
   postmastoidectomy, recurrent
   cholesteatoma
  circulatory (early) — *see* Complications,
   circulatory system
  digestive system — *see* Complications,
   gastrointestinal
  dumping syndrome (postgastrectomy) K91.1
  ear — *see* Complications, ear
  elephantiasis or lymphedema I97.89
   postmastectomy I97.2
  emphysema (surgical) T81.82 ☑
  endocrine — *see* Complications, endocrine
  eye — *see* Complications, eye
  fistula (persistent postoperative) T81.83 ☑
  foreign body inadvertently left in wound
   (sponge) (suture) (swab) — *see* Foreign
   body, accidentally left during a procedure
  gastrointestinal — *see* Complications,
   gastrointestinal
  genitourinary NEC N99.89
  hematoma
   intraoperative — *see* Complication,
    intraoperative, hemorrhage
   postprocedural — *see* Complication,
    postprocedural, hemorrhage
  hemorrhage
   intraoperative — *see* Complication,
    intraoperative, hemorrhage
   postprocedural — *see* Complication,
    postprocedural, hemorrhage
  hepatic failure K91.82
  hyperglycemia (postpancreatectomy) E89.1
  hypoinsulinemia (postpancreatectomy) E89.1
  hypoparathyroidism (postparathyroidectomy)
   E89.2
  hypopituitarism (posthypophysectomy) E89.3
  hypothyroidism (post-thyroidectomy) E89.0

Complication — continued
  intestinal obstruction K91.3
  intracranial hypotension following ventricular
      shunting (ventriculostomy) G97.2
  lymphedema I97.89
      postmastectomy I97.2
  malabsorption (postsurgical) NEC K91.2
      osteoporosis — see Osteoporosis,
          postsurgical malabsorption
  mastoidectomy cavity NEC — see
      Complications, postmastoidectomy
  metabolic E89.89
      specified NEC E89.89
  musculoskeletal — see Complications,
      musculoskeletal system
  nervous system (central) (peripheral) — see
      Complications, nervous system
  ovarian failure E89.40
      asymptomatic E89.40
      symptomatic E89.41
  peripheral vascular — see Complications,
      surgical procedure, vascular
  postcardiotomy syndrome I97.0
  postcholecystectomy syndrome K91.5
  postcommissurotomy syndrome I97.0
  postgastrectomy dumping syndrome K91.1
  postlaminectomy syndrome NEC M96.1
      kyphosis M96.3
  postmastectomy lymphedema syndrome I97.2
  postmastoidectomy cholesteatoma — see
      Complications, postmastoidectomy,
      recurrent cholesteatoma
  postvagotomy syndrome K91.1
  postvalvulotomy syndrome I97.0
  pulmonary insufficiency (acute) J95.2
      chronic J95.3
      following thoracic surgery J95.1
  reattached body part — see Complications,
      reattached
  respiratory — see Complications, respiratory
      system
  shock (hypovolemic) T81.19 ☑
  spleen (postoperative) D78.89
      intraoperative D78.81
  stitch abscess T81.4 ☑
  subglottic stenosis (postsurgical) J95.5
  testicular hypofunction E89.5
  transplant — see Complications, organ or
      tissue transplant
  urinary NEC N99.89
  vaginal vault prolapse (posthysterectomy)
      N99.3
  vascular (peripheral)
      artery T81.719 ☑
          mesenteric T81.710 ☑
          renal T81.711 ☑
          specified NEC T81.718 ☑
      vein T81.72 ☑
  wound infection T81.4 ☑
  suture, permanent (wire) NEC T85.9 ☑
      with repair of bone — see Complications,
          fixation device, internal
      embolism T85.81 ☑
      fibrosis T85.82 ☑
      hemorrhage T85.83 ☑
      infection and inflammation T85.79 ☑
      mechanical
          breakdown T85.612 ☑
          displacement T85.622 ☑
          malfunction T85.612 ☑
          malposition T85.622 ☑
          obstruction T85.692 ☑
          perforation T85.692 ☑
          protrusion T85.692 ☑
          specified NEC T85.692 ☑
      pain T85.84 ☑
      specified type NEC T85.89 ☑
      stenosis T85.85 ☑
      thrombosis T85.86 ☑
  tracheostomy J95.00
      granuloma J95.09
      hemorrhage J95.01
      infection J95.02
      malfunction J95.03
      mechanical J95.03
      obstruction J95.03
      specified type NEC J95.09
      tracheo-esophageal fistula J95.04
  transfusion (blood) (lymphocytes) (plasma)
      T80.92 ☑
      air embolism T80.0 ☑
      circulatory overload E87.71

Complication — continued
  febrile nonhemolytic transfusion reaction
      R50.84
  hemolysis T80.89 ☑
  hemochromatosis E83.111
  hemolytic reaction (antigen unspecified)
      T80.919 ☑
  incompatibility reaction (antigen unspecified)
      T80.919 ☑
      ABO T80.30 ☑
          delayed serologic (DSTR) T80.39 ☑
          hemolytic transfusion reaction (HTR)
              (unspecified time after transfusion)
              T80.319 ☑
          acute (AHTR) (less than 24 hours after
              transfusion) T80.310 ☑
          delayed (DHTR) (24 hours or more after
              transfusion) T80.311 ☑
          specified NEC T80.39 ☑
      acute (antigen unspecified) T80.910 ☑
      delayed (antigen unspecified) T80.911 ☑
      delayed serologic (DSTR) T80.89 ☑
      Non-ABO (minor antigens (Duffy) (Kell) (Kidd)
          (Lewis) (M) (N) (P) (S)) T80.A0 ☑
          delayed serologic (DSTR) T80.A9 ☑
          hemolytic transfusion reaction (HTR)
              (unspecified time after transfusion)
              T80.A19 ☑
          acute (AHTR) (less than 24 hours after
              transfusion) T80.A10 ☑
          delayed (DHTR) (24 hours or more after
              transfusion) T80.A11 ☑
          specified NEC T80.A9 ☑
      Rh (antigens (C) (c) (D) (E) (e)) (factor) T80.40
          ☑
          delayed serologic (DSTR) T80.49 ☑
          hemolytic transfusion reaction (HTR)
              (unspecified time after transfusion)
              T80.419 ☑
          acute (AHTR) (less than 24 hours after
              transfusion) T80.410 ☑
          delayed (DHTR) (24 hours or more after
              transfusion) T80.411 ☑
          specified NEC T80.49 ☑
  infection T80.29 ☑
      acute T80.22 ☑
  reaction NEC T80.89 ☑
  sepsis T80.29 ☑
  shock T80.89 ☑
  transplant T86.90
      bone T86.839
          failure T86.831
          infection T86.832
          rejection T86.830
          specified type NEC T86.838
      bone marrow T86.00
          failure T86.02
          infection T86.03
          rejection T86.01
          specified type NEC T86.09
      cornea T86.849
          failure T86.841
          infection T86.842
          rejection T86.840
          specified type NEC T86.848
      failure T86.92
      heart T86.20
          with lung T86.30
          cardiac allograft vasculopathy T86.290
              failure T86.32
              infection T86.33
              rejection T86.31
              specified type NEC T86.39
          failure T86.22
          infection T86.23
          rejection T86.21
          specified type NEC T86.298
      infection T86.93
      intestine T86.859
          failure T86.851
          infection T86.852
          rejection T86.850
          specified type NEC T86.858
      kidney T86.10
          failure T86.12
          infection T86.13
          rejection T86.11
          specified type NEC T86.19
      liver T86.40
          failure T86.42
          infection T86.43
          rejection T86.41

Complication — continued
      specified type NEC T86.49
      lung T86.819
          with heart T86.30
              failure T86.32
              infection T86.33
              rejection T86.31
              specified type NEC T86.39
          failure T86.811
          infection T86.812
          rejection T86.810
          specified type NEC T86.818
      malignant neoplasm C80.2
      pancreas T86.899
          failure T86.891
          infection T86.892
          rejection T86.890
          specified type NEC T86.898
      peripheral blood stem cells T86.5
      post-transplant lymphoproliferative disorder
          (PTLD) D47.Z1
      rejection T86.91
      skin T86.829
          failure T86.821
          infection T86.822
          rejection T86.820
          specified type NEC T86.828
      specified
          tissue T86.899
              failure T86.891
              infection T86.892
              rejection T86.890
              specified type NEC T86.898
          type NEC T86.99
      stem cell (from peripheral blood) (from
          umbilical cord) T86.5
      umbilical cord stem cells T86.5
  trauma (early) T79.9 ☑
      specified NEC T79.8 ☑
  ultrasound therapy NEC T88.9 ☑
  umbilical cord NEC
      complicating delivery O69.9 ☑
          specified NEC O69.89 ☑
  umbrella device, vascular T82.9 ☑
      embolism T82.818 ☑
      fibrosis T82.828 ☑
      hemorrhage T82.838 ☑
      infection or inflammation T82.7 ☑
      mechanical
          breakdown T82.515 ☑
          displacement T82.525 ☑
          leakage T82.535 ☑
          malposition T82.525 ☑
          obstruction T82.595 ☑
          perforation T82.595 ☑
          protrusion T82.595 ☑
      pain T82.848 ☑
      specified type NEC T82.898 ☑
      stenosis T82.858 ☑
      thrombosis T82.868 ☑
  urethral catheter — see Complications, catheter,
      urethral, indwelling
  vaccination T88.1 ☑
      anaphylaxis NEC T80.52 ☑
      arthropathy — see Arthropathy,
          postimmunization
      cellulitis T88.0 ☑
      encephalitis or encephalomyelitis G04.02
      infection (general) (local) NEC T88.0 ☑
      meningitis G03.8
      myelitis G04.89
      protein sickness T80.62 ☑
      rash T88.1 ☑
      reaction (allergic) T88.1 ☑
          serum T80.62 ☑
      sepsis T88.0 ☑
      serum intoxication, sickness, rash, or other
          serum reaction NEC T80.62 ☑
          anaphylactic shock T80.52 ☑
      shock (allergic) (anaphylactic) T80.52 ☑
      vaccinia (generalized) (localized) T88.1 ☑
  vas deferens device or implant — see
      Complications, genitourinary, device or
      implant, genital tract
  vascular I99.9
      device or implant T82.9 ☑
          embolism T82.818 ☑
          fibrosis T82.828 ☑
          hemorrhage T82.838 ☑
          infection or inflammation T82.7 ☑
          mechanical
              breakdown T82.519 ☑

Complex — *continued*
    specified device NEC T82.518 ☑
    displacement T82.529 ☑
      specified device NEC T82.528 ☑
    leakage T82.539 ☑
      specified device NEC T82.538 ☑
    malposition T82.529 ☑
      specified device NEC T82.528 ☑
    obstruction T82.599 ☑
      specified device NEC T82.598 ☑
    perforation T82.599 ☑
      specified device NEC T82.598 ☑
    protrusion T82.599 ☑
      specified device NEC T82.598 ☑
    pain T82.848 ☑
    specified type NEC T82.898 ☑
    stenosis T82.858 ☑
    thrombosis T82.868 ☑
  dialysis catheter — *see* Complication, catheter, dialysis
  following infusion, therapeutic injection or transfusion T80.1 ☑
  graft T82.9 ☑
    embolism T82.818 ☑
    fibrosis T82.828 ☑
    hemorrhage T82.838 ☑
    mechanical
      breakdown T82.319 ☑
        aorta (bifurcation) T82.310 ☑
        carotid artery T82.311 ☑
        specified vessel NEC T82.318 ☑
      displacement T82.329 ☑
        aorta (bifurcation) T82.320 ☑
        carotid artery T82.321 ☑
        specified vessel NEC T82.328 ☑
      leakage T82.339 ☑
        aorta (bifurcation) T82.330 ☑
        carotid artery T82.331 ☑
        specified vessel NEC T82.338 ☑
      malposition T82.329 ☑
        aorta (bifurcation) T82.320 ☑
        carotid artery T82.321 ☑
        specified vessel NEC T82.328 ☑
      obstruction T82.399 ☑
        aorta (bifurcation) T82.390 ☑
        carotid artery T82.391 ☑
        specified vessel NEC T82.398 ☑
      perforation T82.399 ☑
        aorta (bifurcation) T82.390 ☑
        carotid artery T82.391 ☑
        specified vessel NEC T82.398 ☑
      protrusion T82.399 ☑
        aorta (bifurcation) T82.390 ☑
        carotid artery T82.391 ☑
        specified vessel NEC T82.398 ☑
    pain T82.848 ☑
    specified complication NEC T82.898 ☑
    stenosis T82.858 ☑
    thrombosis T82.868 ☑
  postoperative — *see* Complications, postoperative, circulatory
  vena cava device (filter) (sieve) (umbrella) — *see* Complications, umbrella device, vascular
  ventilation therapy NEC T81.81 ☑
  ventilator
    mechanical J95.850
    specified NEC J95.859
  ventricular (communicating) shunt (device) T85.9 ☑
    embolism T85.81 ☑
    fibrosis T85.82 ☑
    hemorrhage T85.83 ☑
    infection and inflammation T85.79 ☑
    mechanical
      breakdown T85.01 ☑
      displacement T85.02 ☑
      leakage T85.03 ☑
      malposition T85.02 ☑
      obstruction T85.09 ☑
      perforation T85.09 ☑
      protrusion T85.09 ☑
      specified NEC T85.09 ☑
    pain T85.84 ☑
    specified type NEC T85.89 ☑
    stenosis T85.85 ☑
    thrombosis T85.86 ☑
  wire suture, permanent (implanted) — *see* Complications, suture, permanent
Compressed air disease T70.3 ☑
Compression
  with injury - code by Nature of injury
  artery I77.1

Compression — *continued*
  celiac, syndrome I77.4
  brachial plexus G54.0
  brain (stem) G93.5
    due to
      contusion (diffuse) — *see* Injury, intracranial, diffuse
        focal — *see* Injury, intracranial, focal
      injury NEC — *see* Injury, intracranial, diffuse
      traumatic — *see* Injury, intracranial, diffuse
  bronchus J98.09
  cauda equina G83.4
  celiac (artery) (axis) I77.4
  cerebral — *see* Compression, brain
  cervical plexus G54.2
  cord
    spinal — *see* Compression, spinal
    umbilical — *see* Compression, umbilical cord
  cranial nerve G52.9
    eighth H93.3
    eleventh G52.8
    fifth G50.8
    first G52.0
    fourth — *see* Strabismus, paralytic, fourth nerve
    ninth G52.1
    second — *see* Disorder, nerve, optic
    seventh G52.8
    sixth — *see* Strabismus, paralytic, sixth nerve
    tenth G52.2
    third — *see* Strabismus, paralytic, third nerve
    twelfth G52.3
  diver's squeeze T70.3 ☑
  during birth (newborn) P15.9
  esophagus K22.2
  eustachian tube — *see* Obstruction, eustachian tube, cartilaginous
  facies Q67.1
  fracture — *see* Fracture
  heart — *see* Disease, heart
  intestine — *see* Obstruction, intestine
  laryngeal nerve, recurrent G52.2
    with paralysis of vocal cords and larynx J38.00
      bilateral J38.02
      unilateral J38.01
  lumbosacral plexus G54.1
  lung J98.4
  lymphatic vessel I89.0
  medulla — *see* Compression, brain
  nerve (*see also* Disorder, nerve) G58.9
    arm NEC — *see* Mononeuropathy, upper limb
    axillary G54.0
    cranial — *see* Compression, cranial nerve
    leg NEC — *see* Mononeuropathy, lower limb
    median (in carpal tunnel) — *see* Syndrome, carpal tunnel
    optic — *see* Disorder, nerve, optic
    plantar — *see* Lesion, nerve, plantar
    posterior tibial (in tarsal tunnel) — *see* Syndrome, tarsal tunnel
    root or plexus NOS (in) G54.9
      intervertebral disc disorder NEC — *see* Disorder, disc, with, radiculopathy
        with myelopathy — *see* Disorder, disc, with, myelopathy
      neoplastic disease (*see also* Neoplasm) D49.9 [G55]
      spondylosis — *see* Spondylosis, with radiculopathy
    sciatic (acute) — *see* Lesion, nerve, sciatic
    sympathetic G90.8
    traumatic — *see* Injury, nerve
    ulnar — *see* Lesion, nerve, ulnar
    upper extremity NEC — *see* Mononeuropathy, upper limb
  spinal (cord) G95.20
    by displacement of intervertebral disc NEC (*see also* Disorder, disc, with, myelopathy)
    nerve root NOS G54.9
      due to displacement of intervertebral disc NEC — *see* Disorder, disc, with, radiculopathy
        with myelopathy — *see* Disorder, disc, with, myelopathy
    specified NEC G95.29
    spondylogenic (cervical) (lumbar, lumbosacral) (thoracic) — *see* Spondylosis, with myelopathy NEC
    anterior — *see* Syndrome, anterior, spinal artery, compression
    traumatic — *see* Injury, spinal cord, by region
  subcostal nerve (syndrome) — *see* Mononeuropathy, upper limb, specified NEC

Compression — *continued*
  sympathetic nerve NEC G90.8
  syndrome T79.5 ☑
  trachea J39.8
  ulnar nerve (by scar tissue) — *see* Lesion, nerve, ulnar
  umbilical cord
    complicating delivery O69.2 ☑
      cord around neck O69.1 ☑
      prolapse O69.0 ☑
      specified NEC O69.2 ☑
  ureter N13.5
  vein I87.1
  vena cava (inferior) (superior) I87.1
Compulsion, compulsive
  gambling F63.0
  neurosis F42
  personality F60.5
  states F42
  swearing F42
    in Gilles de la Tourette's syndrome F95.2
  tics and spasms F95.9
Concato's disease (pericardial polyserositis) A19.9
  nontubercular I31.1
  pleural — *see* Pleurisy, with effusion
Concavity chest wall M95.4
Concealed penis Q55.69
Concern (normal) about sick person in family Z63.6
Concrescence (teeth) K00.2
Concretio cordis I31.1
  rheumatic I09.2
Concretion (*see also* Calculus)
  appendicular K38.1
  canaliculus — *see* Dacryolith
  clitoris N90.89
  conjunctiva H11.12- ☑
  eyelid — *see* Disorder, eyelid, specified type NEC
  lacrimal passages — *see* Dacryolith
  prepuce (male) N47.8
  salivary gland (any) K11.5
  seminal vesicle N50.8
  tonsil J35.8
Concussion (brain) (cerebral) (current) S06.0X- ☑
  blast (air) (hydraulic) (immersion) (underwater)
    abdomen or thorax — *see* Injury, blast, by site
    ear with acoustic nerve injury — *see* Injury, nerve, acoustic, specified type NEC
  cauda equina S34.3 ☑
  conus medullaris S34.02 ☑
  ocular S05.8X- ☑
  spinal (cord)
    cervical S14.0 ☑
    lumbar S34.01 ☑
    sacral S34.02 ☑
    thoracic S24.0 ☑
  syndrome F07.81
Condition — *see* Disease
Conditions arising in the perinatal period — *see* Newborn, affected by
Conduct disorder — *see* Disorder, conduct
Condyloma A63.0
  acuminatum A63.0
  gonorrheal A54.09
  latum A51.31
  syphilitic A51.31
    congenital A50.07
  venereal, syphilitic A51.31
Conflagration (*see also* Burn)
  asphyxia (by inhalation of gases, fumes or vapors) (*see also* Table of Drugs and Chemicals) T59.9- ☑
Conflict (with) (*see also* Discord)
  family Z73.9
  marital Z63.0
    involving divorce or estrangement Z63.5
  parent-child Z62.820
    parent-adopted child Z62.821
    parent-biological child Z62.820
    parent-foster child Z62.822
  social role NEC Z73.5
Confluent — *see* condition
Confusion, confused R41.0
  epileptic F05
  mental state (psychogenic) F44.89
  psychogenic F44.89
  reactive (from emotional stress, psychological trauma) F44.89
Confusional arousals G47.51
Congelation T69.9 ☑
Congenital (*see also* condition)
  aortic septum Q25.4
  intrinsic factor deficiency D51.0
  malformation — *see* Anomaly

Congestion, congestive
  bladder N32.89
  bowel K63.89
  brain G93.89
  breast N64.59
  bronchial J98.09
  catarrhal J31.0
  chest R09.89
  chill, malarial — *see* Malaria
  circulatory NEC I99.8
  duodenum K31.89
  eye — *see* Hyperemia, conjunctiva
  facial, due to birth injury P15.4
  general R68.89
  glottis J37.0
  heart — *see* Failure, heart, congestive
  hepatic K76.1
  hypostatic (lung) — *see* Edema, lung
  intestine K63.89
  kidney N28.89
  labyrinth H83.8
  larynx J37.0
  liver K76.1
  lung R09.89
    active or acute — *see* Pneumonia
  malaria, malarial — *see* Malaria
  nasal R09.81
  nose R09.81
  orbit, orbital (*see also* Exophthalmos)
    inflammatory (chronic) — *see* Inflammation,
      orbit
  ovary N83.8
  pancreas K86.8
  pelvic, female N94.89
  pleural J94.8
  prostate (active) N42.1
  pulmonary — *see* Congestion, lung
  renal N28.89
  retina H35.81
  seminal vesicle N50.1
  spinal cord G95.19
  spleen (chronic) D73.2
  stomach K31.89
  trachea — *see* Tracheitis
  urethra N36.8
  uterus N85.8
    with subinvolution N85.3
  venous (passive) I87.8
  viscera R68.89
Congestive — *see* Congestion
Conical
  cervix (hypertrophic elongation) N88.4
  cornea — *see* Keratoconus
  teeth K00.2
Conjoined twins Q89.4
Conjugal maladjustment Z63.0
  involving divorce or estrangement Z63.5
Conjunctiva — *see* condition
Conjunctivitis (staphylococcal) (streptococcal) NOS
  H10.9
  Acanthamoeba B60.12
  acute H10.3- ☑
    atopic H10.1- ☑
    mucopurulent H10.02- ☑
      follicular H10.01- ☑
    chemical (*see also* Corrosion, cornea) H10.21- ☑
    pseudomembranous H10.22- ☑
    serous except viral H10.23- ☑
      viral — *see* Conjunctivitis, viral
    toxic H10.21- ☑
  adenoviral (acute) (follicular) B30.1
  allergic (acute) — *see* Conjunctivitis, acute, atopic
    chronic H10.45
      vernal H10.44
  anaphylactic — *see* Conjunctivitis, acute, atopic
  Apollo B30.3
  atopic (acute) — *see* Conjunctivitis, acute, atopic
  Béal's B30.2
  blennorrhagic (gonococcal) (neonatorum) A54.31
  chemical (acute) (*see also* Corrosion, cornea)
    H10.21- ☑
  chlamydial A74.0
    due to trachoma A71.1
    neonatal P39.1
  chronic (nodosa) (petrificans) (phlyctenular)
    H10.40- ☑
    allergic H10.45
      vernal H10.44
    follicular H10.43- ☑
    giant papillary H10.41- ☑
    simple H10.42 ☑
    vernal H10.44

Conjunctivitis — *continued*
  coxsackievirus 24 B30.3
  diphtheritic A36.86
  due to
    dust — *see* Conjunctivitis, acute, atopic
    filariasis B74.9
    mucocutaneous leishmaniasis B55.2
  enterovirus type 70 (hemorrhagic) B30.3
  epidemic (viral) B30.9
    hemorrhagic B30.3
  gonococcal (neonatorum) A54.31
  granular (trachomatous) A71.1
    sequelae (late effect) B94.0
  hemorrhagic (acute) (epidemic) B30.3
  herpes zoster B02.31
  in (due to)
    Acanthamoeba B60.12
    adenovirus (acute) (follicular) B30.1
    Chlamydia A74.0
    coxsackievirus 24 B30.3
    diphtheria A36.86
    enterovirus type 70 (hemorrhagic) B30.3
    filariasis B74.9
    gonococci A54.31
    herpes (simplex) virus B00.53
      zoster B02.31
    infectious disease NEC B99 ☑
    meningococci A39.89
    mucocutaneous leishmaniasis B55.2
    rosacea L71.9
    syphilis (late) A52.71
    zoster B02.31
  inclusion A74.0
  infantile P39.1
    gonococcal A54.31
  Koch-Weeks' — *see* Conjunctivitis, acute,
    mucopurulent
  light — *see* Conjunctivitis, acute, atopic
  ligneous — *see* Blepharoconjunctivitis, ligneous
  meningococcal A39.89
  mucopurulent — *see* Conjunctivitis, acute,
    mucopurulent
  neonatal P39.1
    gonococcal A54.31
  Newcastle B30.8
  of Béal B30.2
  parasitic
    filariasis B74.9
    mucocutaneous leishmaniasis B55.2
  Parinaud's H10.89
  petrificans H10.89
  rosacea L71.9
  specified NEC H10.89
  swimming-pool B30.1
  trachomatous A71.1
    acute A71.0
    sequelae (late effect) B94.0
  traumatic NEC H10.89
  tuberculous A18.59
  tularemic A21.1
  tularensis A21.1
  viral B30.9
    due to
      adenovirus B30.1
      enterovirus B30.3
    specified NEC B30.8
Conjunctivochalasis H11.82- ☑
Connective tissue — *see* condition
Conn's syndrome E26.01
Conradi (-Hunermann) disease Q77.3
Consanguinity Z84.3
  counseling Z71.89
Conscious simulation (of illness) Z76.5
Consecutive — *see* condition
Consolidation lung (base) — *see* Pneumonia, lobar
Constipation (atonic) (neurogenic) (simple) (spastic)
  K59.00
  drug-induced — *see* Table of Drugs and
    Chemicals
  outlet dysfunction K59.02
  psychogenic F45.8
  slow transit K59.01
  specified NEC K59.09
Constitutional (*see also* condition)
  substandard F60.7
Constitutionally substandard F60.7
Constriction (*see also* Stricture)
  auditory canal — *see* Stenosis, external ear canal
  bronchial J98.09
  duodenum K31.5
  esophagus K22.2
  external

Constriction — *continued*
  abdomen, abdominal (wall) S30.841 ☑
  alveolar process S00.542 ☑
  ankle S90.54- ☑
  antecubital space — *see* Constriction, external,
    forearm
  arm (upper) S40.84- ☑
  auricle — *see* Constriction, external, ear
  axilla — *see* Constriction, external, arm
  back, lower S30.840 ☑
  breast S20.14- ☑
  brow S00.84 ☑
  buttock S30.840 ☑
  calf — *see* Constriction, external, leg
  canthus — *see* Constriction, external, eyelid
  cheek S00.84 ☑
    internal S00.542 ☑
  chest wall — *see* Constriction, external, thorax
  chin S00.84 ☑
  clitoris S30.844 ☑
  costal region — *see* Constriction, external,
    thorax
  digit (s)
    foot — *see* Constriction, external, toe
    hand — *see* Constriction, external, finger
  ear S00.44- ☑
  elbow S50.34- ☑
  epididymis S30.843 ☑
  epigastric region S30.841 ☑
  esophagus, cervical S10.14 ☑
  eyebrow — *see* Constriction, external, eyelid
  eyelid S00.24- ☑
  face S00.84 ☑
  finger (s) S60.44- ☑
    index S60.44- ☑
    little S60.44- ☑
    middle S60.44- ☑
    ring S60.44- ☑
  flank S30.841 ☑
  foot (except toe(s) alone) S90.84- ☑
    toe — *see* Constriction, external, toe
  forearm S50.84- ☑
    elbow only — *see* Constriction, external,
      elbow
  forehead S00.84 ☑
  genital organs, external
    female S30.846 ☑
    male S30.845 ☑
  groin S30.841 ☑
  gum S00.542 ☑
  hand S60.54- ☑
  head S00.94 ☑
    ear — *see* Constriction, external, ear
    eyelid — *see* Constriction, external, eyelid
    lip S00.541 ☑
    nose S00.34 ☑
    oral cavity S00.542 ☑
    scalp S00.04 ☑
    specified site NEC S00.84 ☑
  heel — *see* Constriction, external, foot
  hip S70.24- ☑
  inguinal region S30.841 ☑
  interscapular region S20.449 ☑
  jaw S00.84 ☑
  knee S80.24- ☑
  labium (majus) (minus) S30.844 ☑
  larynx S10.14 ☑
  leg (lower) S80.84- ☑
    knee — *see* Constriction, external, knee
    upper — *see* Constriction, external, thigh
  lip S00.541 ☑
  lower back S30.840 ☑
  lumbar region S30.840 ☑
  malar region S00.84 ☑
  mammary — *see* Constriction, external, breast
  mastoid region S00.84 ☑
  mouth S00.542 ☑
  nail
    finger — *see* Constriction, external, finger
    toe — *see* Constriction, external, toe
  nasal S00.34 ☑
  neck S10.94 ☑
    specified site NEC S10.84 ☑
    throat S10.14 ☑
  nose S00.34 ☑
  occipital region S00.04 ☑
  oral cavity S00.542 ☑
  orbital region — *see* Constriction, external,
    eyelid
  palate S00.542 ☑
  palm — *see* Constriction, external, hand
  parietal region S00.04 ☑

☑ **Additional character required**

Constriction — continued
  pelvis S30.840 ☑
  penis S30.842 ☑
  perineum
    female S30.844 ☑
    male S30.840 ☑
  periocular area — see Constriction, external, eyelid
  phalanges
    finger — see Constriction, external, finger
    toe — see Constriction, external, toe
  pharynx S10.14 ☑
  pinna — see Constriction, external, ear
  popliteal space — see Constriction, external, knee
  prepuce S30.842 ☑
  pubic region S30.840 ☑
  pudendum
    female S30.846 ☑
    male S30.845 ☑
  sacral region S30.840 ☑
  scalp S00.04 ☑
  scapular region — see Constriction, external, shoulder
  scrotum S30.843 ☑
  shin — see Constriction, external, leg
  shoulder S40.24- ☑
  sternal region S20.349 ☑
  submaxillary region S00.84 ☑
  submental region S00.84 ☑
  subungual
    finger (s) — see Constriction, external, finger
    toe (s) — see Constriction, external, toe
  supraclavicular fossa S10.84 ☑
  supraorbital S00.84 ☑
  temple S00.84 ☑
  temporal region S00.84 ☑
  testis S30.843 ☑
  thigh S70.34- ☑
  thorax, thoracic (wall) S20.94 ☑
    back S20.44- ☑
    front S20.34- ☑
  throat S10.14 ☑
  thumb S60.34- ☑
  toe (s) (lesser) S90.44- ☑
    great S90.44- ☑
  tongue S00.542 ☑
  trachea S10.14 ☑
  tunica vaginalis S30.843 ☑
  uvula S00.542 ☑
  vagina S30.844 ☑
  vulva S30.844 ☑
  wrist S60.84- ☑
  gallbladder — see Obstruction, gallbladder
  intestine — see Obstruction, intestine
  larynx J38.6
    congenital Q31.8
      specified NEC Q31.8
      subglottic Q31.1
  organ or site, congenital NEC — see Atresia, by site
  prepuce (acquired) (congenital) N47.1
  pylorus (adult hypertrophic) K31.1
    congenital or infantile Q40.0
    newborn Q40.0
  ring dystocia (uterus) O62.4
  spastic (see also Spasm)
    ureter N13.5
  ureter N13.5
    with infection N13.6
  urethra — see Stricture, urethra
  visual field (peripheral) (functional) — see Defect, visual field
Constrictive — see condition
Consultation
  medical — see Counseling, medical
  religious Z71.81
  specified reason NEC Z71.89
  spiritual Z71.81
  without complaint or sickness Z71.9
    feared complaint unfounded Z71.1
    specified reason NEC Z71.89
Consumption — see Tuberculosis
Contact (with) (see also Exposure (to))
  acariasis Z20.7
  AIDS virus Z20.6
  air pollution Z77.110
  algae and algae toxins Z77.121
  algae bloom Z77.121
  anthrax Z20.810
  aromatic amines Z77.020
  aromatic (hazardous) compounds NEC Z77.028

Contact — continued
  aromatic dyes NOS Z77.028
  arsenic Z77.010
  asbestos Z77.090
  bacterial disease NEC Z20.818
  benzene Z77.021
  blue-green algae bloom Z77.121
  body fluids (potentially hazardous) Z77.21
  brown tide Z77.121
  chemicals (chiefly nonmedicinal) (hazardous) NEC Z77.098
  cholera Z20.09
  chromium compounds Z77.018
  communicable disease Z20.9
    bacterial NEC Z20.818
    specified NEC Z20.89
    viral NEC Z20.828
  cyanobacteria bloom Z77.121
  dyes Z77.098
  Escherichia coli (E. coli) Z20.01
  fiberglass — see Table of Drugs and Chemicals, fiberglass
  German measles Z20.4
  gonorrhea Z20.2
  hazardous metals NEC Z77.018
  hazardous substances NEC Z77.29
  hazards in the physical environment NEC Z77.128
  hazards to health NEC Z77.9
  HIV Z20.6
  HTLV-III/LAV Z20.6
  human immunodeficiency virus (HIV) Z20.6
  infection Z20.9
    specified NEC Z20.89
  infestation (parasitic) NEC Z20.7
  intestinal infectious disease NEC Z20.09
    Escherichia coli (E. coli) Z20.01
  lead Z77.011
  meningococcus Z20.811
  mold (toxic) Z77.120
  nickel dust Z77.018
  noise Z77.122
  parasitic disease Z20.7
  pediculosis Z20.7
  pfiesteria piscicida Z77.121
  poliomyelitis Z20.89
  pollution
    air Z77.110
    environmental NEC Z77.118
    soil Z77.112
    water Z77.111
  polycyclic aromatic hydrocarbons Z77.028
  rabies Z20.3
  radiation, naturally occurring NEC Z77.123
  radon Z77.123
  red tide (Florida) Z77.121
  rubella Z20.4
  sexually-transmitted disease Z20.2
  smallpox (laboratory) Z20.89
  syphilis Z20.2
  tuberculosis Z20.1
  uranium Z77.012
  varicella Z20.820
  venereal disease Z20.2
  viral disease NEC Z20.828
  viral hepatitis Z20.5
  water pollution Z77.111
Contamination, food — see Intoxication, foodborne
Contraception, contraceptive
  advice Z30.09
  counseling Z30.09
  device (intrauterine) (in situ) Z97.5
    causing menorrhagia T83.83 ☑
    checking Z30.431
    complications — see Complications, intrauterine, contraceptive device
    in place Z97.5
    initial prescription Z30.014
    reinsertion Z30.433
    removal Z30.432
    replacement Z30.433
  emergency (postcoital) Z30.012
  initial prescription Z30.019
    injectable Z30.013
    intrauterine device Z30.014
    pills Z30.011
    postcoital (emergency) Z30.012
    specified type NEC Z30.018
    subdermal implantable Z30.019
  maintenance Z30.40
    examination Z30.8
    injectable Z30.42
    intrauterine device Z30.431

Contraception — continued
    pills Z30.41
    specified type NEC Z30.49
    subdermal implantable Z30.49
  management Z30.9
    specified NEC Z30.8
  postcoital (emergency) Z30.012
  prescription Z30.019
    repeat Z30.40
  sterilization Z30.2
  surveillance (drug) — see Contraception, maintenance
Contraction (s), contracture, contracted
  Achilles tendon (see also Short, tendon, Achilles)
    congenital Q66.89
  amputation stump (surgical) (flexion) (late) (next proximal joint) T87.89
  anus K59.8
  bile duct (common) (hepatic) K83.8
  bladder N32.89
    neck or sphincter N32.0
  bowel, cecum, colon or intestine, any part — see Obstruction, intestine
  Braxton Hicks — see False, labor
  breast implant, capsular T85.44 ☑
  bronchial J98.09
  burn (old) — see Cicatrix
  cervix — see Stricture, cervix
  cicatricial — see Cicatrix
  conjunctiva, trachomatous, active A71.1
    sequelae (late effect) B94.0
  Dupuytren's M72.0
  eyelid — see Disorder, eyelid function
  fascia (lata) (postural) M72.8
    Dupuytren's M72.0
    palmar M72.0
    plantar M72.2
  finger NEC (see also Deformity, finger)
    congenital Q68.1
    joint — see Contraction, joint, hand
  flaccid — see Contraction, paralytic
  gallbladder K82.0
  heart valve — see Endocarditis
  hip — see Contraction, joint, hip
  hourglass
    bladder N32.89
      congenital Q64.79
    gallbladder K82.0
      congenital Q44.1
    stomach K31.89
      congenital Q40.2
      psychogenic F45.8
    uterus (complicating delivery) O62.4
  hysterical F44.4
  internal os — see Stricture, cervix
  joint (abduction) (acquired) (adduction) (flexion) (rotation) M24.50
    ankle M24.57- ☑
    congenital NEC Q68.8
      hip Q65.89
    elbow M24.52- ☑
    foot joint M24.57- ☑
    hand joint M24.54- ☑
    hip M24.55- ☑
      congenital Q65.89
    hysterical F44.4
    knee M24.56- ☑
    shoulder M24.51- ☑
    wrist M24.53- ☑
  kidney (granular) (secondary) N26.9
    congenital Q63.8
    hydronephritic — see Hydronephrosis Page N26.2
    pyelonephritic — see Pyelitis, chronic
    tuberculous A18.11
  ligament (see also Disorder, ligament)
    congenital Q79.8
  muscle (postinfective) (postural) NEC M62.40
    with contracture of joint — see Contraction, joint
    ankle M62.47- ☑
    congenital Q79.8
      sternocleidomastoid Q68.0
    extraocular — see Strabismus
    eye (extrinsic) — see Strabismus
    foot M62.47- ☑
    forearm M62.43- ☑
    hand M62.44- ☑
    hysterical F44.4
    ischemic (Volkmann's) T79.6 ☑
    lower leg M62.46- ☑
    multiple sites M62.49

☑ Additional character required

Contraction — *continued*
- pelvic region M62.45- ☑
- posttraumatic — *see* Strabismus, paralytic
- psychogenic F45.8
  - conversion reaction F44.4
- shoulder region M62.41- ☑
- specified site NEC M62.48
- thigh M62.45- ☑
- upper arm M62.42- ☑
- neck — *see* Torticollis
- ocular muscle — *see* Strabismus
- organ or site, congenital NEC — *see* Atresia, by site
- outlet (pelvis) — *see* Contraction, pelvis
- palmar fascia M72.0
- paralytic
  - joint — *see* Contraction, joint
  - muscle (*see also* Contraction, muscle NEC)
    - ocular — *see* Strabismus, paralytic
- pelvis (acquired) (general) M95.5
  - with disproportion (fetopelvic) O33.1
    - causing obstructed labor O65.1
    - inlet O33.2
    - mid-cavity O33.3 ☑
    - outlet O33.3 ☑
- plantar fascia M72.2
- premature
  - atrium I49.1
  - auriculoventricular I49.49
  - heart I49.49
  - junctional I49.2
  - supraventricular I49.1
  - ventricular I49.3
- prostate N42.89
- pylorus NEC (*see also* Pylorospasm)
  - psychogenic F45.8
- rectum, rectal (sphincter) K59.8
- ring (Bandl's) (complicating delivery) O62.4
- scar — *see* Cicatrix
- spine — *see* Dorsopathy, deforming
- sternocleidomastoid (muscle), congenital Q68.0
- stomach K31.89
  - hourglass K31.89
    - congenital Q40.2
    - psychogenic F45.8
  - psychogenic F45.8
- tendon (sheath) M62.40
  - with contracture of joint — *see* Contraction, joint
  - Achilles — *see* Short, tendon, Achilles
  - ankle M62.47- ☑
    - Achilles — *see* Short, tendon, Achilles
  - foot M62.47- ☑
  - forearm M62.43- ☑
  - hand M62.44- ☑
  - lower leg M62.46- ☑
  - multiple sites M62.49
  - neck M62.48
  - pelvic region M62.45- ☑
  - shoulder region M62.41- ☑
  - specified site NEC M62.48
  - thigh M62.45- ☑
  - thorax M62.48
  - trunk M62.48
  - upper arm M62.42- ☑
- toe — *see* Deformity, toe, specified NEC
- ureterovesical orifice (postinfectional) N13.5
  - with infection N13.6
- urethra (*see also* Stricture, urethra)
  - orifice N32.0
- uterus N85.8
  - abnormal NEC O62.9
  - clonic (complicating delivery) O62.4
  - dyscoordinate (complicating delivery) O62.4
  - hourglass (complicating delivery) O62.4
  - hypertonic O62.4
  - hypotonic NEC O62.2
  - inadequate
    - primary O62.0
    - secondary O62.1
  - incoordinate (complicating delivery) O62.4
  - poor O62.2
  - tetanic (complicating delivery) O62.4
- vagina (outlet) N89.5
- vesical N32.89
  - neck or urethral orifice N32.0
- visual field — *see* Defect, visual field, generalized
- Volkmann's (ischemic) T79.6 ☑

Contusion (skin surface intact) T14.8
- abdomen, abdominal (muscle) (wall) S30.1 ☑
- adnexa, eye NEC S05.8X- ☑
- adrenal gland S37.812 ☑

Contusion — *continued*
- alveolar process S00.532 ☑
- ankle S90.0- ☑
- antecubital space — *see* Contusion, forearm
- anus S30.3 ☑
- arm (upper) S40.02- ☑
  - lower (with elbow) — *see* Contusion, forearm
- auditory canal — *see* Contusion, ear
- auricle — *see* Contusion, ear
- axilla — *see* Contusion, arm, upper
- back (*see also* Contusion, thorax, back)
  - lower S30.0 ☑
- bile duct S36.13 ☑
- bladder S37.22 ☑
- bone NEC T14.8
- brain (diffuse) — *see* Injury, intracranial, diffuse
  - focal — *see* Injury, intracranial, focal
- brainstem S06.38- ☑
- breast S20.0- ☑
- broad ligament S37.892 ☑
- brow S00.83 ☑
- buttock S30.0 ☑
- canthus, eye S00.1- ☑
- cauda equina S34.3 ☑
- cerebellar, traumatic S06.37- ☑
- cerebral S06.33- ☑
  - left side S06.32- ☑
  - right side S06.31- ☑
- cheek S00.83 ☑
  - internal S00.532 ☑
- chest (wall) — *see* Contusion, thorax
- chin S00.83 ☑
- clitoris S30.23 ☑
- colon — *see* Injury, intestine, large, contusion
- common bile duct S36.13 ☑
- conjunctiva S05.1- ☑
  - with foreign body (in conjunctival sac) — *see* Foreign body, conjunctival sac
- conus medullaris (spine) S34.139 ☑
- cornea — *see* Contusion, eyeball
  - with foreign body — *see* Foreign body, cornea
- corpus cavernosum S30.21 ☑
- cortex (brain) (cerebral) — *see* Injury, intracranial, diffuse
  - focal — *see* Injury, intracranial, focal
- costal region — *see* Contusion, thorax
- cystic duct S36.13 ☑
- diaphragm S27.802 ☑
- duodenum S36.420 ☑
- ear S00.43- ☑
- elbow S50.0- ☑
  - with forearm — *see* Contusion, forearm
- epididymis S30.22 ☑
- epigastric region S30.1 ☑
- epiglottis S10.0 ☑
- esophagus (thoracic) S27.812 ☑
  - cervical S10.0 ☑
- eyeball S05.1- ☑
- eyebrow S00.1- ☑
- eyelid (and periocular area) S00.1- ☑
- face NEC S00.83 ☑
- fallopian tube S37.529 ☑
  - bilateral S37.522 ☑
  - unilateral S37.521 ☑
- femoral triangle S30.1 ☑
- finger (s) S60.00 ☑
  - with damage to nail (matrix) S60.10 ☑
  - index S60.02- ☑
    - with damage to nail S60.12- ☑
  - little S60.05- ☑
    - with damage to nail S60.15- ☑
  - middle S60.03- ☑
    - with damage to nail S60.13- ☑
  - ring S60.04- ☑
    - with damage to nail S60.14- ☑
  - thumb — *see* Contusion, thumb
- flank S30.1 ☑
- foot (except toe(s) alone) S90.3- ☑
  - toe — *see* Contusion, toe
- forearm S50.1- ☑
  - elbow only — *see* Contusion, elbow
- forehead S00.83 ☑
- gallbladder S36.122 ☑
- genital organs, external
  - female S30.202 ☑
  - male S30.201 ☑
- globe (eye) — *see* Contusion, eyeball
- groin S30.1 ☑
- gum S00.532 ☑
- hand S60.22- ☑
  - finger (s) — *see* Contusion, finger
  - wrist — *see* Contusion, wrist

Contusion — *continued*
- head S00.93 ☑
  - ear — *see* Contusion, ear
  - eyelid — *see* Contusion, eyelid
  - lip S00.531 ☑
  - nose S00.33 ☑
  - oral cavity S00.532 ☑
  - scalp S00.03 ☑
  - specified part NEC S00.83 ☑
- heel — *see* Contusion, foot
- hepatic duct S36.13 ☑
- hip S70.0- ☑
- ileum S36.428 ☑
- iliac region S30.1 ☑
- inguinal region S30.1 ☑
- interscapular region S20.229 ☑
- intra-abdominal organ S36.92 ☑
  - colon — *see* Injury, intestine, large, contusion
  - liver S36.112 ☑
  - pancreas — *see* Contusion, pancreas
  - rectum S36.62 ☑
  - small intestine — *see* Injury, intestine, small, contusion
  - specified organ NEC S36.892 ☑
  - spleen — *see* Contusion, spleen
  - stomach S36.32 ☑
- iris (eye) — *see* Contusion, eyeball
- jaw S00.83 ☑
- jejunum S36.428 ☑
- kidney S37.01- ☑
  - major (greater than 2 cm) S37.02- ☑
  - minor (less than 2 cm) S37.01- ☑
- knee S80.0- ☑
- labium (majus) (minus) S30.23 ☑
- lacrimal apparatus, gland or sac S05.8X- ☑
- larynx S10.0 ☑
- leg (lower) S80.1- ☑
  - knee — *see* Contusion, knee
- lens — *see* Contusion, eyeball
- lip S00.531 ☑
- liver S36.112 ☑
- lower back S30.0 ☑
- lumbar region S30.0 ☑
- lung S27.329 ☑
  - bilateral S27.322 ☑
  - unilateral S27.321 ☑
- malar region S00.83 ☑
- mastoid region S00.83 ☑
- membrane, brain — *see* Injury, intracranial, diffuse
  - focal — *see* Injury, intracranial, focal
- mesentery S36.892 ☑
- mesosalpinx S37.892 ☑
- mouth S00.532 ☑
- muscle — *see* Contusion, by site
- nail
  - finger — *see* Contusion, finger, with damage to nail
  - toe — *see* Contusion, toe, with damage to nail
- nasal S00.33 ☑
- neck S10.93 ☑
  - specified site NEC S10.83 ☑
  - throat S10.0 ☑
- nerve — *see* Injury, nerve
- newborn P54.5
- nose S00.33 ☑
- occipital
  - lobe (brain) — *see* Injury, intracranial, diffuse
    - focal — *see* Injury, intracranial, focal
  - region (scalp) S00.03 ☑
- orbit (region) (tissues) S05.1- ☑
- ovary S37.429 ☑
  - bilateral S37.422 ☑
  - unilateral S37.421 ☑
- palate S00.532 ☑
- pancreas S36.229 ☑
  - body S36.221 ☑
  - head S36.220 ☑
  - tail S36.222 ☑
- parietal
  - lobe (brain) — *see* Injury, intracranial, diffuse
    - focal — *see* Injury, intracranial, focal
  - region (scalp) S00.03 ☑
- pelvic organ S37.92 ☑
  - adrenal gland S37.812 ☑
  - bladder S37.22 ☑
  - fallopian tube — *see* Contusion, fallopian tube
  - kidney — *see* Contusion, kidney
  - ovary — *see* Contusion, ovary
  - prostate S37.822 ☑
  - specified organ NEC S37.892 ☑
  - ureter S37.12 ☑

Contusion — *continued*
  urethra S37.32 ☑
  uterus S37.62 ☑
  pelvis S30.0 ☑
  penis S30.21 ☑
  perineum
    female S30.23 ☑
    male S30.0 ☑
  periocular area S00.1- ☑
  peritoneum S36.81 ☑
  periurethral tissue — *see* Contusion, urethra
  pharynx S10.0 ☑
  pinna — *see* Contusion, ear
  popliteal space — *see* Contusion, knee
  prepuce S30.21 ☑
  prostate S37.822 ☑
  pubic region S30.1 ☑
  pudendum
    female S30.202 ☑
    male S30.201 ☑
  quadriceps femoris — *see* Contusion, thigh
  rectum S36.62 ☑
  retroperitoneum S36.892 ☑
  round ligament S37.892 ☑
  sacral region S30.0 ☑
  scalp S00.03 ☑
    due to birth injury P12.3
  scapular region — *see* Contusion, shoulder
  sclera — *see* Contusion, eyeball
  scrotum S30.22 ☑
  seminal vesicle S37.892 ☑
  shoulder S40.01- ☑
  skin NEC T14.8
  small intestine — *see* Injury, intestine, small, contusion
  spermatic cord S30.22 ☑
  spinal cord — *see* Injury, spinal cord, by region
    cauda equina S34.3 ☑
    conus medullaris S34.139 ☑
  spleen S36.029 ☑
    major S36.021 ☑
    minor S36.020 ☑
  sternal region S20.219 ☑
  stomach S36.32 ☑
  subconjunctival S05.1- ☑
  subcutaneous NEC T14.8
  submaxillary region S00.83 ☑
  submental region S00.83 ☑
  subperiosteal NEC T14.8
  subungual
    finger — *see* Contusion, finger, with damage to nail
    toe — *see* Contusion, toe, with damage to nail
  supraclavicular fossa S10.83 ☑
  supraorbital S00.83 ☑
  suprarenal gland S37.812 ☑
  temple (region) S00.83 ☑
  temporal
    lobe (brain) — *see* Injury, intracranial, diffuse
    focal — *see* Injury, intracranial, focal
    region S00.83 ☑
  testis S30.22 ☑
  thigh S70.1- ☑
  thorax (wall) S20.20 ☑
    back S20.22- ☑
    front S20.21- ☑
  throat S10.0 ☑
  thumb S60.01- ☑
    with damage to nail S60.11- ☑
  toe (s) (lesser) S90.12- ☑
    with damage to nail S90.22- ☑
    great S90.11- ☑
      with damage to nail S90.21- ☑
    specified type NEC S90.221 ☑
  tongue S00.532 ☑
  trachea (cervical) S10.0 ☑
    thoracic S27.52 ☑
  tunica vaginalis S30.22 ☑
  tympanum, tympanic membrane — *see* Contusion, ear
  ureter S37.12 ☑
  urethra S37.32 ☑
  urinary organ NEC S37.892 ☑
  uterus S37.62 ☑
  uvula S00.532 ☑
  vagina S30.23 ☑
  vas deferens S37.892 ☑
  vesical S37.22 ☑
  vocal cord (s) S10.0 ☑
  vulva S30.23 ☑
  wrist S60.21- ☑

Conus (congenital) (any type) Q14.8
  cornea — *see* Keratoconus
  medullaris syndrome G95.81
Conversion hysteria, neurosis or reaction F44.9
Converter, tuberculosis (test reaction) R76.11
Conviction (legal), anxiety concerning Z65.0
  with imprisonment Z65.1
Convulsions (idiopathic) (*see also* Seizure(s)) R56.9
  apoplectiform (cerebral ischemia) I67.82
  benign neonatal (familial) — *see* Epilepsy, generalized, idiopathic
  dissociative F44.5
  epileptic — *see* Epilepsy
  epileptiform, epileptoid — *see* Seizure, epileptiform
  ether (anesthetic) — *see* Table of Drugs and Chemicals, by drug
  febrile R56.00
    with status epilepticus G40.901
    complex R56.01
      with status epilepticus G40.901
    simple R56.00
  hysterical F44.5
  infantile P90
    epilepsy — *see* Epilepsy
  jacksonian — *see* Epilepsy, localization-related, symptomatic, with simple partial seizures
  myoclonic G25.3
  neonatal, benign (familial) — *see* Epilepsy, generalized, idiopathic
  newborn P90
  obstetrical (nephritic) (uremic) — *see* Eclampsia
  paretic A52.17
  post traumatic R56.1
  psychomotor — *see* Epilepsy, localization-related, symptomatic, with complex partial seizures
  recurrent R56.9
  reflex R25.8
  scarlatinal A38.8
  tetanus, tetanic — *see* Tetanus
  thymic E32.8
Convulsive (*see also* Convulsions)
Cooley's anemia D56.1
Coolie itch B76.9
Cooper's
  disease — *see* Mastopathy, cystic
  hernia — *see* Hernia, abdomen, specified site NEC
Copra itch B88.0
Coprophagy F50.8
Coprophobia F40.298
Coproporphyria, hereditary E80.29
Cor
  biloculare Q20.8
  bovis, bovinum — *see* Hypertrophy, cardiac
  pulmonale (chronic) I27.81
    acute I26.09
  triatriatum, triatrium Q24.2
  triloculare Q20.8
    biatrium Q20.4
    biventriculare Q21.1
Corbus' disease (gangrenous balanitis) N48.1
Cord (*see also* condition)
  around neck (tightly) (with compression)
    complicating delivery O69.1 ☑
  bladder G95.89
    tabetic A52.19
Cordis ectopia Q24.8
Corditis (spermatic) N49.1
Corectopia Q13.2
Cori's disease (glycogen storage) E74.03
Corkhandler's disease or lung J67.3
Corkscrew esophagus K22.4
Corkworker's disease or lung J67.3
Corn (infected) L84
Cornea (*see also* condition)
  donor Z52.5
  plana Q13.4
Cornelia de Lange syndrome Q87.1
Cornu cutaneum L85.8
Cornual gestation or pregnancy O00.8
Coronary (artery) — *see* condition
Coronavirus, as cause of disease classified elsewhere B97.29
  SARS-associated B97.21
Corpora (*see also* condition)
  amylacea, prostate N42.89
  cavernosa — *see* condition
Corpulence — *see* Obesity
Corpus — *see* condition
Corrected transposition Q20.5
Corrosion (injury) (acid) (caustic) (chemical) (lime) (external) (internal) T30.4

Corrosion — *continued*
  abdomen, abdominal (muscle) (wall) T21.42 ☑
    first degree T21.52 ☑
    second degree T21.62 ☑
    third degree T21.72 ☑
  above elbow T22.439 ☑
    first degree T22.539 ☑
    left T22.432 ☑
      first degree T22.532 ☑
      second degree T22.632 ☑
      third degree T22.732 ☑
    right T22.431 ☑
      first degree T22.531 ☑
      second degree T22.631 ☑
      third degree T22.731 ☑
    second degree T22.639 ☑
    third degree T22.739 ☑
  alimentary tract NEC T28.7 ☑
  ankle T25.419 ☑
    first degree T25.519 ☑
    left T25.412 ☑
      first degree T25.512 ☑
      second degree T25.612 ☑
      third degree T25.712 ☑
    multiple with foot — *see* Corrosion, lower, limb, multiple, ankle and foot
    right T25.411 ☑
      first degree T25.511 ☑
      second degree T25.611 ☑
      third degree T25.711 ☑
    second degree T25.619 ☑
    third degree T25.719 ☑
  anus — *see* Corrosion, buttock
  arm (s) (meaning upper limb(s)) — *see* Corrosion, upper limb
  axilla T22.449 ☑
    first degree T22.549 ☑
    left T22.442 ☑
      first degree T22.542 ☑
      second degree T22.642 ☑
      third degree T22.742 ☑
    right T22.441 ☑
      first degree T22.541 ☑
      second degree T22.641 ☑
      third degree T22.741 ☑
    second degree T22.649 ☑
    third degree T22.749 ☑
  back (lower) T21.44 ☑
    first degree T21.54 ☑
    second degree T21.64 ☑
    third degree T21.74 ☑
    upper T21.43 ☑
      first degree T21.53 ☑
      second degree T21.63 ☑
      third degree T21.73 ☑
  blisters - code as Corrosion, second degree, by site
  breast (s) — *see* Corrosion, chest wall
  buttock (s) T21.45 ☑
    first degree T21.55 ☑
    second degree T21.65 ☑
    third degree T21.75 ☑
  calf T24.439 ☑
    first degree T24.539 ☑
    left T24.432 ☑
      first degree T24.532 ☑
      second degree T24.632 ☑
      third degree T24.732 ☑
    right T24.431 ☑
      first degree T24.531 ☑
      second degree T24.631 ☑
      third degree T24.731 ☑
    second degree T24.639 ☑
    third degree T24.739 ☑
  canthus (eye) — *see* Corrosion, eyelid
  cervix T28.8 ☑
  cheek T20.46 ☑
    first degree T20.56 ☑
    second degree T20.66 ☑
    third degree T20.76 ☑
  chest wall T21.41 ☑
    first degree T21.51 ☑
    second degree T21.61 ☑
    third degree T21.71 ☑
  chin T20.43 ☑
    first degree T20.53 ☑
    second degree T20.63 ☑
    third degree T20.73 ☑
  colon T28.7 ☑
  conjunctiva (and cornea) — *see* Corrosion, cornea
  cornea (and conjunctiva) T26.6- ☑

☑ **Additional character required**

Corrosion — continued
deep necrosis of underlying tissue - code as
  Corrosion, third degree, by site
dorsum of hand T23.469 ☑
  first degree T23.569 ☑
  left T23.462 ☑
    first degree T23.562 ☑
    second degree T23.662 ☑
    third degree T23.762 ☑
  right T23.461 ☑
    first degree T23.561 ☑
    second degree T23.661 ☑
    third degree T23.761 ☑
  second degree T23.669 ☑
  third degree T23.769 ☑
ear (auricle) (external) (canal) T20.41 ☑
  drum T28.91 ☑
  first degree T20.51 ☑
  second degree T20.61 ☑
  third degree T20.71 ☑
elbow T22.429 ☑
  first degree T22.529 ☑
  left T22.422 ☑
    first degree T22.522 ☑
    second degree T22.622 ☑
    third degree T22.722 ☑
  right T22.421 ☑
    first degree T22.521 ☑
    second degree T22.621 ☑
    third degree T22.721 ☑
  second degree T22.629 ☑
  third degree T22.729 ☑
entire body — see Corrosion, multiple body
  regions
epidermal loss - code as Corrosion, second
  degree, by site
epiglottis T27.4 ☑
erythema, erythematous - code as Corrosion,
  first degree, by site
esophagus T28.6 ☑
extent (percentage of body surface)
  less than 10 per cent T32.0
  10-19 per cent (0-9 percent third degree)
    T32.10
    with 10-19 percent third degree T32.11
  20-29 per cent (0-9 percent third degree)
    T32.20
    with
      10-19 percent third degree T32.21
      20-29 percent third degree T32.22
  30-39 per cent (0-9 percent third degree)
    T32.30
    with
      10-19 percent third degree T32.31
      20-29 percent third degree T32.32
      30-39 percent third degree T32.33
  40-49 per cent (0-9 percent third degree)
    T32.40
    with
      10-19 percent third degree T32.41
      20-29 percent third degree T32.42
      30-39 percent third degree T32.43
      40-49 percent third degree T32.44
  50-59 per cent (0-9 percent third degree)
    T32.50
    with
      10-19 percent third degree T32.51
      20-29 percent third degree T32.52
      30-39 percent third degree T32.53
      40-49 percent third degree T32.54
      50-59 percent third degree T32.55
  60-69 per cent (0-9 percent third degree)
    T32.60
    with
      10-19 percent third degree T32.61
      20-29 percent third degree T32.62
      30-39 percent third degree T32.63
      40-49 percent third degree T32.64
      50-59 percent third degree T32.65
      60-69 percent third degree T32.66
  70-79 per cent (0-9 percent third degree)
    T32.70
    with
      10-19 percent third degree T32.71
      20-29 percent third degree T32.72
      30-39 percent third degree T32.73
      40-49 percent third degree T32.74
      50-59 percent third degree T32.75
      60-69 percent third degree T32.76
      70-79 percent third degree T32.77
  80-89 per cent (0-9 percent third degree)
    T32.80

Corrosion — continued
  with
    10-19 percent third degree T32.81
    20-29 percent third degree T32.82
    30-39 percent third degree T32.83
    40-49 percent third degree T32.84
    50-59 percent third degree T32.85
    60-69 percent third degree T32.86
    70-79 percent third degree T32.87
    80-89 percent third degree T32.88
  90 per cent or more (0-9 percent third degree)
    T32.90
    with
      10-19 percent third degree T32.91
      20-29 percent third degree T32.92
      30-39 percent third degree T32.93
      40-49 percent third degree T32.94
      50-59 percent third degree T32.95
      60-69 percent third degree T32.96
      70-79 percent third degree T32.97
      80-89 percent third degree T32.98
      90-99 percent third degree T32.99
extremity — see Corrosion, limb
eye (s) and adnexa T26.9- ☑
  with resulting rupture and destruction of
    eyeball T26.7- ☑
  conjunctival sac — see Corrosion, cornea
  cornea — see Corrosion, cornea
  lid — see Corrosion, eyelid
  periocular area — see Corrosion eyelid
  specified site NEC T26.8- ☑
eyeball — see Corrosion, eye
eyelid (s) T26.5- ☑
face — see Corrosion, head
finger T23.429 ☑
  first degree T23.529 ☑
  left T23.422 ☑
    first degree T23.522 ☑
    second degree T23.622 ☑
    third degree T23.722 ☑
  multiple sites (without thumb) T23.439 ☑
    with thumb T23.449 ☑
      first degree T23.549 ☑
      left T23.442 ☑
        first degree T23.542 ☑
        second degree T23.642 ☑
        third degree T23.742 ☑
      right T23.441 ☑
        first degree T23.541 ☑
        second degree T23.641 ☑
        third degree T23.741 ☑
    second degree T23.649 ☑
    third degree T23.749 ☑
    first degree T23.539 ☑
    left T23.432 ☑
      first degree T23.532 ☑
      second degree T23.632 ☑
      third degree T23.732 ☑
    right T23.431 ☑
      first degree T23.531 ☑
      second degree T23.631 ☑
      third degree T23.731 ☑
    second degree T23.639 ☑
    third degree T23.739 ☑
  right T23.421 ☑
    first degree T23.521 ☑
    second degree T23.621 ☑
    third degree T23.721 ☑
  second degree T23.629 ☑
  third degree T23.729 ☑
flank — see Corrosion, abdomen
foot T25.429 ☑
  first degree T25.529 ☑
  left T25.422 ☑
    first degree T25.522 ☑
    second degree T25.622 ☑
    third degree T25.722 ☑
  multiple with ankle — see Corrosion, lower,
    limb, multiple, ankle and foot
  right T25.421 ☑
    first degree T25.521 ☑
    second degree T25.621 ☑
    third degree T25.721 ☑
  second degree T25.629 ☑
  third degree T25.729 ☑
forearm T22.419 ☑
  first degree T22.519 ☑
  left T22.412 ☑
    first degree T22.512 ☑
    second degree T22.612 ☑
    third degree T22.712 ☑
  right T22.411 ☑

Corrosion — continued
    first degree T22.511 ☑
    second degree T22.611 ☑
    third degree T22.711 ☑
  second degree T22.619 ☑
  third degree T22.719 ☑
forehead T20.46 ☑
  first degree T20.56 ☑
  second degree T20.66 ☑
  third degree T20.76 ☑
fourth degree - code as Corrosion, third degree,
  by site
full thickness skin loss - code as Corrosion, third
  degree, by site
gastrointestinal tract NEC T28.7 ☑
genital organs
  external
    female T21.47 ☑
      first degree T21.57 ☑
      second degree T21.67 ☑
      third degree T21.77 ☑
    male T21.46 ☑
      first degree T21.56 ☑
      second degree T21.66 ☑
      third degree T21.76 ☑
  internal T28.8 ☑
groin — see Corrosion, abdominal wall
hand (s) T23.409 ☑
  back — see Corrosion, dorsum of hand
  finger — see Corrosion, finger
  first degree T23.509 ☑
  left T23.402 ☑
    first degree T23.502 ☑
    second degree T23.602 ☑
    third degree T23.702 ☑
  multiple sites with wrist T23.499 ☑
    first degree T23.599 ☑
    left T23.492 ☑
      first degree T23.592 ☑
      second degree T23.692 ☑
      third degree T23.792 ☑
    right T23.491 ☑
      first degree T23.591 ☑
      second degree T23.691 ☑
      third degree T23.791 ☑
    second degree T23.699 ☑
    third degree T23.799 ☑
  palm — see Corrosion, palm
  right T23.401 ☑
    first degree T23.501 ☑
    second degree T23.601 ☑
    third degree T23.701 ☑
  second degree T23.609 ☑
  third degree T23.709 ☑
  thumb — see Corrosion, thumb
head (and face) (and neck) T20.40 ☑
  cheek — see Corrosion, cheek
  chin — see Corrosion, chin
  ear — see Corrosion, ear
  eye (s) only — see Corrosion, eye
  first degree T20.50 ☑
  forehead — see Corrosion, forehead
  lip — see Corrosion, lip
  multiple sites T20.49 ☑
    first degree T20.59 ☑
    second degree T20.69 ☑
    third degree T20.79 ☑
  neck — see Corrosion, neck
  nose — see Corrosion, nose
  scalp — see Corrosion, scalp
  second degree T20.60 ☑
  third degree T20.70 ☑
hip (s) — see Corrosion, lower, limb
inhalation — see Corrosion, respiratory tract
internal organ (s) (see also Corrosion, by site)
    T28.90 ☑
  alimentary tract T28.7 ☑
    esophagus T28.6 ☑
  esophagus T28.6 ☑
  genitourinary T28.8 ☑
  mouth T28.5 ☑
  pharynx T28.5 ☑
  specified organ NEC T28.99 ☑
interscapular region — see Corrosion, back, upper
intestine (large) (small) T28.7 ☑
knee T24.429 ☑
  first degree T24.529 ☑
  left T24.422 ☑
    first degree T24.522 ☑
    second degree T24.622 ☑
    third degree T24.722 ☑
  right T24.421 ☑

Corrosion

Corrosion — *continued*
    first degree T24.521 ☑
    second degree T24.621 ☑
    third degree T24.721 ☑
  second degree T24.629 ☑
  third degree T24.729 ☑
  labium (majus) (minus) — *see* Corrosion, genital organs, external, female
  lacrimal apparatus, duct, gland or sac — *see* Corrosion, eye, specified site NEC
  larynx T27.4 ☑
    with lung T27.5 ☑
  leg (s) (meaning lower limb(s)) — *see* Corrosion, lower limb
  limb (s)
    lower — *see* Corrosion, lower, limb
    upper — *see* Corrosion, upper limb
  lip (s) T20.42 ☑
    first degree T20.52 ☑
    second degree T20.62 ☑
    third degree T20.72 ☑
  lower
    back — *see* Corrosion, back
    limb T24.409 ☑
      ankle — *see* Corrosion, ankle
      calf — *see* Corrosion, calf
      first degree T24.509 ☑
      foot — *see* Corrosion, foot
      knee — *see* Corrosion, knee
      left T24.402 ☑
        first degree T24.502 ☑
        second degree T24.602 ☑
        third degree T24.702 ☑
      multiple sites, except ankle and foot T24.499 ☑
        ankle and foot T25.499 ☑
          first degree T25.599 ☑
          left T25.492 ☑
            first degree T25.592 ☑
            second degree T25.692 ☑
            third degree T25.792 ☑
          right T25.491 ☑
            first degree T25.591 ☑
            second degree T25.691 ☑
            third degree T25.791 ☑
          second degree T25.699 ☑
          third degree T25.799 ☑
        first degree T24.599 ☑
        left T24.492 ☑
          first degree T24.592 ☑
          second degree T24.692 ☑
          third degree T24.792 ☑
        right T24.491 ☑
          first degree T24.591 ☑
          second degree T24.691 ☑
          third degree T24.791 ☑
        second degree T24.699 ☑
        third degree T24.799 ☑
      right T24.401 ☑
        first degree T24.501 ☑
        second degree T24.601 ☑
        third degree T24.701 ☑
      second degree T24.609 ☑
      hip — *see* Corrosion, thigh
      thigh — *see* Corrosion, thigh
      third degree T24.709 ☑
  lung (with larynx and trachea) T27.5 ☑
  mouth T28.5 ☑
  neck T20.47 ☑
    first degree T20.57 ☑
    second degree T20.67 ☑
    third degree T20.77 ☑
  nose (septum) T20.44 ☑
    first degree T20.54 ☑
    second degree T20.64 ☑
    third degree T20.74 ☑
  ocular adnexa — *see* Corrosion, eye
  orbit region — *see* Corrosion, eyelid
  palm T23.459 ☑
    first degree T23.559 ☑
    left T23.452 ☑
      first degree T23.552 ☑
      second degree T23.652 ☑
      third degree T23.752 ☑
    right T23.451 ☑
      first degree T23.551 ☑
      second degree T23.651 ☑
      third degree T23.751 ☑
    second degree T23.659 ☑
    third degree T23.759 ☑
  partial thickness - code as Corrosion, unspecified degree, by site

Corrosion — *continued*
  pelvis — *see* Corrosion, trunk
  penis — *see* Corrosion, genital organs, external, male
  perineum
    female — *see* Corrosion, genital organs, external, female
    male — *see* Corrosion, genital organs, external, male
  periocular area — *see* Corrosion, eyelid
  pharynx T28.5 ☑
  rectum T28.7 ☑
  respiratory tract T27.7 ☑
    larynx — *see* Corrosion, larynx
    specified part NEC T27.6 ☑
    trachea — *see* Corrosion, larynx
  sac, lacrimal — *see* Corrosion, eye, specified site NEC
  scalp T20.45 ☑
    first degree T20.55 ☑
    second degree T20.65 ☑
    third degree T20.75 ☑
  scapular region T22.469 ☑
    first degree T22.569 ☑
    left T22.462 ☑
      first degree T22.562 ☑
      second degree T22.662 ☑
      third degree T22.762 ☑
    right T22.461 ☑
      first degree T22.561 ☑
      second degree T22.661 ☑
      third degree T22.761 ☑
    second degree T22.669 ☑
    third degree T22.769 ☑
  sclera — *see* Corrosion, eye, specified site NEC
  scrotum — *see* Corrosion, genital organs, external, male
  shoulder T22.459 ☑
    first degree T22.559 ☑
    left T22.452 ☑
      first degree T22.552 ☑
      second degree T22.652 ☑
      third degree T22.752 ☑
    right T22.451 ☑
      first degree T22.551 ☑
      second degree T22.651 ☑
      third degree T22.751 ☑
    second degree T22.659 ☑
    third degree T22.759 ☑
  stomach T28.7 ☑
  temple — *see* Corrosion, head
  testis — *see* Corrosion, genital organs, external, male
  thigh T24.419 ☑
    first degree T24.519 ☑
    left T24.412 ☑
      first degree T24.512 ☑
      second degree T24.612 ☑
      third degree T24.712 ☑
    right T24.411 ☑
      first degree T24.511 ☑
      second degree T24.611 ☑
      third degree T24.711 ☑
    second degree T24.619 ☑
    third degree T24.719 ☑
  thorax (external) — *see* Corrosion, trunk
  throat (meaning pharynx) T28.5 ☑
  thumb (s) T23.419 ☑
    first degree T23.519 ☑
    left T23.412 ☑
      first degree T23.512 ☑
      second degree T23.612 ☑
      third degree T23.712 ☑
    multiple sites with fingers T23.449 ☑
      first degree T23.549 ☑
      left T23.442 ☑
        first degree T23.542 ☑
        second degree T23.642 ☑
        third degree T23.742 ☑
      right T23.441 ☑
        first degree T23.541 ☑
        second degree T23.641 ☑
        third degree T23.741 ☑
      second degree T23.649 ☑
      third degree T23.749 ☑
    right T23.411 ☑
      first degree T23.511 ☑
      second degree T23.611 ☑
      third degree T23.711 ☑
    second degree T23.619 ☑
    third degree T23.719 ☑
  toe T25.439 ☑

Corrosion — *continued*
    first degree T25.539 ☑
    left T25.432 ☑
      first degree T25.532 ☑
      second degree T25.632 ☑
      third degree T25.732 ☑
    right T25.431 ☑
      first degree T25.531 ☑
      second degree T25.631 ☑
      third degree T25.731 ☑
    second degree T25.639 ☑
    third degree T25.739 ☑
  tongue T28.5 ☑
  tonsil (s) T28.5 ☑
  total body — *see* Corrosion, multiple body regions
  trachea T27.4 ☑
    with lung T27.5 ☑
  trunk T21.40 ☑
    abdominal wall — *see* Corrosion, abdominal wall
    anus — *see* Corrosion, buttock
    axilla — *see* Corrosion, upper limb
    back — *see* Corrosion, back
    breast — *see* Corrosion, chest wall
    buttock — *see* Corrosion, buttock
    chest wall — *see* Corrosion, chest wall
    first degree T21.50 ☑
    flank — *see* Corrosion, abdominal wall
    genital
      female — *see* Corrosion, genital organs, external, female
      male — *see* Corrosion, genital organs, external, male
    groin — *see* Corrosion, abdominal wall
    interscapular region — *see* Corrosion, back, upper
    labia — *see* Corrosion, genital organs, external, female
    lower back — *see* Corrosion, back
    penis — *see* Corrosion, genital organs, external, male
    perineum
      female — *see* Corrosion, genital organs, external, female
      male — *see* Corrosion, genital organs, external, male
    scapular region — *see* Corrosion, upper limb
    scrotum — *see* Corrosion, genital organs, external, male
    second degree T21.60 ☑
    shoulder — *see* Corrosion, upper limb
    specified site NEC T21.49 ☑
      first degree T21.59 ☑
      second degree T21.69 ☑
      third degree T21.79 ☑
    testes — *see* Corrosion, genital organs, external, male
    third degree T21.70 ☑
    upper back — *see* Corrosion, back, upper
    vagina T28.8 ☑
    vulva — *see* Corrosion, genital organs, external, female
  unspecified site with extent of body surface involved specified
    less than 10 per cent T32.0
    10-19 per cent (0-9 percent third degree) T32.10
      with 10-19 percent third degree T32.11
    20-29 per cent (0-9 percent third degree) T32.20
      with
        10-19 percent third degree T32.21
        20-29 percent third degree T32.22
    30-39 per cent (0-9 percent third degree) T32.30
      with
        10-19 percent third degree T32.31
        20-29 percent third degree T32.32
        30-39 percent third degree T32.33
    40-49 per cent (0-9 percent third degree) T32.40
      with
        10-19 percent third degree T32.41
        20-29 percent third degree T32.42
        30-39 percent third degree T32.43
        40-49 percent third degree T32.44
    50-59 per cent (0-9 percent third degree) T32.50
      with
        10-19 percent third degree T32.51
        20-29 percent third degree T32.52

☑ **Additional character required**

Corrosion — *continued*
  30-39 percent third degree T32.53
  40-49 percent third degree T32.54
  50-59 percent third degree T32.55
  60-69 per cent (0-9 percent third degree) T32.60
  with
    10-19 percent third degree T32.61
    20-29 percent third degree T32.62
    30-39 percent third degree T32.63
    40-49 percent third degree T32.64
    50-59 percent third degree T32.65
    60-69 percent third degree T32.66
  70-79 per cent (0-9 percent third degree) T32.70
  with
    10-19 percent third degree T32.71
    20-29 percent third degree T32.72
    30-39 percent third degree T32.73
    40-49 percent third degree T32.74
    50-59 percent third degree T32.75
    60-69 percent third degree T32.76
    70-79 percent third degree T32.77
  80-89 per cent (0-9 percent third degree) T32.80
  with
    10-19 percent third degree T32.81
    20-29 percent third degree T32.82
    30-39 percent third degree T32.83
    40-49 percent third degree T32.84
    50-59 percent third degree T32.85
    60-69 percent third degree T32.86
    70-79 percent third degree T32.87
    80-89 percent third degree T32.88
  90 per cent or more (0-9 percent third degree) T32.90
  with
    10-19 percent third degree T32.91
    20-29 percent third degree T32.92
    30-39 percent third degree T32.93
    40-49 percent third degree T32.94
    50-59 percent third degree T32.95
    60-69 percent third degree T32.96
    70-79 percent third degree T32.97
    80-89 percent third degree T32.98
    90-99 percent third degree T32.99
  upper limb (axilla) (scapular region) T22.40 ☑
    above elbow — *see* Corrosion, above elbow
    axilla — *see* Corrosion, axilla
    elbow — *see* Corrosion, elbow
    first degree T22.50 ☑
    forearm — *see* Corrosion, forearm
    hand — *see* Corrosion, hand
    interscapular region — *see* Corrosion, back, upper
    multiple sites T22.499 ☑
      first degree T22.599 ☑
      left T22.492 ☑
        first degree T22.592 ☑
        second degree T22.692 ☑
        third degree T22.792 ☑
      right T22.491 ☑
        first degree T22.591 ☑
        second degree T22.691 ☑
        third degree T22.791 ☑
      second degree T22.699 ☑
      third degree T22.799 ☑
    scapular region — *see* Corrosion, scapular region
    second degree T22.60 ☑
    shoulder — *see* Corrosion, shoulder
    third degree T22.70 ☑
    wrist — *see* Corrosion, hand
  uterus T28.8 ☑
  vagina T28.8 ☑
  vulva — *see* Corrosion, genital organs, external, female
  wrist T23.479 ☑
    first degree T23.579 ☑
    left T23.472 ☑
      first degree T23.572 ☑
      second degree T23.672 ☑
      third degree T23.772 ☑
    multiple sites with hand T23.499 ☑
      first degree T23.599 ☑
      left T23.492 ☑
        first degree T23.592 ☑
        second degree T23.692 ☑
        third degree T23.792 ☑
      right T23.491 ☑
        first degree T23.591 ☑
        second degree T23.691 ☑

Corrosion — *continued*
        third degree T23.791 ☑
      second degree T23.699 ☑
      third degree T23.799 ☑
    right T23.471 ☑
      first degree T23.571 ☑
      second degree T23.671 ☑
      third degree T23.771 ☑
    second degree T23.679 ☑
    third degree T23.779 ☑
Corrosive burn — *see* Corrosion
Corsican fever — *see* Malaria
Cortical — *see* condition
Cortico-adrenal — *see* condition
Coryza (acute) J00
  with grippe or influenza — *see* Influenza, with, respiratory manifestations NEC
  syphilitic
    congenital (chronic) A50.05
Costen's syndrome or complex M26.69
Costiveness — *see* Constipation
Costochondritis M94.0
Cotard's syndrome F22
Cot death R99
Cotia virus B08.8
Cotton wool spots (retinal) H35.81
Cotungo's disease — *see* Sciatica
Cough (affected) (chronic) (epidemic) (nervous) R05
  with hemorrhage — *see* Hemoptysis
  bronchial R05
    with grippe or influenza — *see* Influenza, with, respiratory manifestations NEC
  functional F45.8
  hysterical F45.8
  laryngeal, spasmodic R05
  psychogenic F45.8
  smokers' J41.0
  tea taster's B49
Counseling (for) Z71.9
  abuse NEC
    perpetrator Z69.82
    victim Z69.81
  alcohol abuser Z71.41
    family Z71.42
  child abuse
    nonparental
      perpetrator Z69.021
      victim Z69.020
    parental
      perpetrator Z69.011
      victim Z69.010
  consanguinity Z71.89
  contraceptive Z30.09
  dietary Z71.3
  drug abuser Z71.51
    family member Z71.52
  family Z71.89
  fertility preservation (prior to cancer therapy) (prior to removal of gonads) Z31.62
  for non-attending third party Z71.0
    related to sexual behavior or orientation Z70.2
  genetic NEC Z31.5
  health (advice) (education) (instruction) — *see* Counseling, medical
  human immunodeficiency virus (HIV) Z71.7
  impotence Z70.1
  insulin pump use Z46.81
  medical (for) Z71.9
    boarding school resident Z59.3
    consanguinity Z71.89
    feared complaint and no disease found Z71.1
    human immunodeficiency virus (HIV) Z71.7
    institutional resident Z59.3
    on behalf of another Z71.0
      related to sexual behavior or orientation Z70.2
    person living alone Z60.2
    specified reason NEC Z71.89
  natural family planning
    procreative Z31.61
    to avoid pregnancy Z30.02
  perpetrator (of)
    abuse NEC Z69.82
    child abuse
      non-parental Z69.021
      parental Z69.011
    rape NEC Z69.82
    spousal abuse Z69.12
  procreative NEC Z31.69
    fertility preservation (prior to cancer therapy) (prior to removal of gonads) Z31.62
    using natural family planning Z31.61

Counseling — *continued*
  promiscuity Z70.1
  rape victim Z69.81
  religious Z71.81
  sex, sexual (related to) Z70.9
    attitude (s) Z70.0
    behavior or orientation Z70.1
    combined concerns Z70.3
    non-responsiveness Z70.1
    on behalf of third party Z70.2
    specified reason NEC Z70.8
  specified reason NEC Z71.89
  spiritual Z71.81
  spousal abuse (perpetrator) Z69.12
    victim Z69.11
  substance abuse Z71.89
    alcohol Z71.41
    drug Z71.51
    tobacco Z71.6
  tobacco use Z71.6
  use (of)
    insulin pump Z46.81
  victim (of)
    abuse Z69.81
    child abuse
      by parent Z69.010
      non-parental Z69.020
    rape NEC Z69.81
Coupled rhythm R00.8
Couvelaire syndrome or uterus (complicating delivery) O45.8X- ☑
Cowperitis — *see* Urethritis
Cowper's gland — *see* condition
Cowpox B08.010
  due to vaccination T88.1 ☑
Coxa
  magna M91.4- ☑
  plana M91.2- ☑
  valga (acquired) (*see also* Deformity, limb, specified type NEC, thigh)
    congenital Q65.81
    sequelae (late effect) of rickets E64.3
  vara (acquired) (*see also* Deformity, limb, specified type NEC, thigh)
    congenital Q65.82
    sequelae (late effect) of rickets E64.3
Coxalgia, coxalgic (nontuberculous) (*see also* Pain, joint, hip)
  tuberculous A18.02
Coxitis — *see* Monoarthritis, hip
Coxsackie (virus) (infection) B34.1
  as cause of disease classified elsewhere B97.11
  carditis B33.20
  central nervous system NEC A88.8
  endocarditis B33.21
  enteritis A08.39
  meningitis (aseptic) A87.0
  myocarditis B33.22
  pericarditis B33.23
  pharyngitis B08.5
  pleurodynia B33.0
  specific disease NEC B33.8
Crabs, meaning pubic lice B85.3
Crack baby P04.41
Cracked nipple N64.0
  associated with
    lactation O92.13
    pregnancy O92.11- ☑
    puerperium O92.12
Cracked tooth K03.81
Cradle cap L21.0
Craft neurosis F48.8
Cramp (s) R25.2
  abdominal — *see* Pain, abdominal
  bathing T75.1 ☑
  colic R10.83
    psychogenic F45.8
  due to immersion T75.1 ☑
  fireman T67.2 ☑
  heat T67.2 ☑
  immersion T75.1 ☑
  intestinal — *see* Pain, abdominal
    psychogenic F45.8
  leg, sleep related G47.62
  limb (lower) (upper) NEC R25.2
    sleep related G47.62
  linotypist's F48.8
    organic G25.89
  muscle (limb) (general) R25.2
    due to immersion T75.1 ☑
    psychogenic F45.8
  occupational (hand) F48.8

Cramp — *continued*
  organic G25.89
  salt-depletion E87.1
  sleep related, leg G47.62
  stoker's T67.2 ☑
  swimmer's T75.1 ☑
  telegrapher's F48.8
    organic G25.89
  typist's F48.8
    organic G25.89
  uterus N94.89
    menstrual — *see* Dysmenorrhea
  writer's F48.8
    organic G25.89
Cranial — *see* condition
Craniocleidodysostosis Q74.0
Craniofenestria (skull) Q75.8
Craniolacunia (skull) Q75.8
Craniopagus Q89.4
Craniopathy, metabolic M85.2
Craniopharyngeal — *see* condition
Craniopharyngioma D44.4
Craniorachischisis (totalis) Q00.1
Cranioschisis Q75.8
Craniostenosis Q75.0
Craniosynostosis Q75.0
Craniotabes (cause unknown) M83.8
  neonatal P96.3
  rachitic E64.3
  syphilitic A50.56
Cranium — *see* condition
Craw-craw — *see* Onchocerciasis
Creaking joint — *see* Derangement, joint, specified type NEC
Creeping
  eruption B76.9
  palsy or paralysis G12.22
Crenated tongue K14.8
Creotoxism A05.9
Crepitus
  caput Q75.8
  joint — *see* Derangement, joint, specified type NEC
Crescent or conus choroid, congenital Q14.3
CREST syndrome M34.1
Cretin, cretinism (congenital) (endemic) (nongoitrous) (sporadic) E00.9
  pelvis
    with disproportion (fetopelvic) O33.0
      causing obstructed labor O65.0
  type
    hypothyroid E00.1
    mixed E00.2
    myxedematous E00.1
    neurological E00.0
Creutzfeldt-Jakob disease or syndrome (with dementia) A81.00
  familial A81.09
  iatrogenic A81.09
  specified NEC A81.09
  sporadic A81.09
  variant (vCJD) A81.01
Crib death R99
Cribriform hymen Q52.3
Cri-du-chat syndrome Q93.4
Crigler-Najjar disease or syndrome E80.5
Crime, victim of Z65.4
Crimean hemorrhagic fever A98.0
Criminalism F60.2
Crisis
  abdomen R10.0
  acute reaction F43.0
  addisonian E27.2
  adrenal (cortical) E27.2
  celiac K90.0
  Dietl's N13.8
  emotional (*see also* Disorder, adjustment)
    acute reaction to stress F43.0
    specific to childhood and adolescence F93.8
  glaucomatocyclitic — *see* Glaucoma, secondary, inflammation
  heart — *see* Failure, heart
  nitritoid I95.2
    correct substance properly administered — *see* Table of Drugs and Chemicals, by drug, adverse effect
    overdose or wrong substance given or taken — *see* Table of Drugs and Chemicals, by drug, poisoning
  oculogyric H51.8
    psychogenic F45.8
  Pel's (tabetic) A52.11

Crisis — *continued*
  psychosexual identity F64.2
  renal N28.0
  sickle-cell D57.00
    with
      acute chest syndrome D57.01
      splenic sequestration D57.02
  state (acute reaction) F43.0
  tabetic A52.11
  thyroid — *see* Thyrotoxicosis with thyroid storm
  thyrotoxic — *see* Thyrotoxicosis with thyroid storm
Crocq's disease (acrocyanosis) I73.89
Crohn's disease — *see* Enteritis, regional
Crooked septum, nasal J34.2
Cross syndrome E70.328
Crossbite (anterior) (posterior) M26.24
Cross-eye — *see* Strabismus, convergent concomitant
Croup, croupous (catarrhal) (infectious) (inflammatory) (nondiphtheritic) J05.0
  bronchial J20.9
  diphtheritic A36.2
  false J38.5
  spasmodic J38.5
    diphtheritic A36.2
  stridulous J38.5
    diphtheritic A36.2
Crouzon's disease Q75.1
Crowding, tooth, teeth, fully erupted M26.31
CRST syndrome M34.1
Cruchet's disease A85.8
Cruelty in children (*see also* Disorder, conduct)
Crural ulcer — *see* Ulcer, lower limb
Crush, crushed, crushing T14.8
  abdomen S38.1 ☑
  ankle S97.0- ☑
  arm (upper) (and shoulder) S47.- ☑
  axilla — *see* Crush, arm
  back, lower S38.1 ☑
  buttock S38.I ☑
  cheek S07.0 ☑
  chest S28.0 ☑
  cranium S07.1 ☑
  ear S07.0 ☑
  elbow S57.0- ☑
  extremity
    lower
      ankle — *see* Crush, ankle
      below knee — *see* Crush, leg
      foot — *see* Crush, foot
      hip — *see* Crush, hip
      knee — *see* Crush, knee
      thigh — *see* Crush, thigh
      toe — *see* Crush, toe
    upper
      below elbow S67.9- ☑
      elbow — *see* Crush, elbow
      finger — *see* Crush, finger
      forearm — *see* Crush, forearm
      hand — *see* Crush, hand
      thumb — *see* Crush, thumb
      upper arm — *see* Crush, arm
      wrist — *see* Crush, wrist
  face S07.0 ☑
  finger (s) S67.1- ☑
    with hand (and wrist) — *see* Crush, hand, specified site NEC
    index S67.19- ☑
    little S67.19- ☑
    middle S67.19- ☑
    ring S67.19- ☑
    thumb — *see* Crush, thumb
  foot S97.8- ☑
    toe — *see* Crush, toe
  forearm S57.8- ☑
  genitalia, external
    female S38.002 ☑
      vagina S38.03 ☑
      vulva S38.03 ☑
    male S38.001 ☑
      penis S38.01 ☑
      scrotum S38.02 ☑
      testis S38.02 ☑
  hand (except fingers alone) S67.2- ☑
    with wrist S67.4- ☑
  head S07.9 ☑
    specified NEC S07.8 ☑
  heel — *see* Crush, foot
  hip S77.0- ☑
    with thigh S77.2- ☑

Crush — *continued*
  internal organ (abdomen, chest, or pelvis) NEC T14.8
  knee S87.0- ☑
  labium (majus) (minus) S38.03 ☑
  larynx S17.0 ☑
  leg (lower) S87.8- ☑
    knee — *see* Crush, knee
  lip S07.0 ☑
  lower
    back S38.1 ☑
    leg — *see* Crush, leg
  neck S17.9 ☑
  nerve — *see* Injury, nerve
  nose S07.0 ☑
  pelvis S38.1 ☑
  penis S38.01 ☑
  scalp S07.8 ☑
  scapular region — *see* Crush, arm
  scrotum S38.02 ☑
  severe, unspecified site T14.8
  shoulder (and upper arm) — *see* Crush, arm
  skull S07.1 ☑
  syndrome (complication of trauma) T79.5 ☑
  testis S38.02 ☑
  thigh S77.1- ☑
    with hip S77.2- ☑
  throat S17.8 ☑
  thumb S67.0- ☑
    with hand (and wrist) — *see* Crush, hand, specified site NEC
  toe (s) S97.10- ☑
    great S97.11- ☑
    lesser S97.12- ☑
  trachea S17.0 ☑
  vagina S38.03 ☑
  vulva S38.03 ☑
  wrist S67.3- ☑
    with hand S67.4- ☑
Crusta lactea L21.0
Crusts R23.4
Crutch paralysis — *see* Injury, brachial plexus
Cruveilhier-Baumgarten cirrhosis, disease or syndrome K74.69
Cruveilhier's atrophy or disease G12.8
Crying (constant) (continuous) (excessive)
  child, adolescent, or adult R45.83
  infant (baby) (newborn) R68.11
Cryofibrinogenemia D89.2
Cryoglobulinemia (essential) (idiopathic) (mixed) (primary) (purpura) (secondary) (vasculitis) D89.1
  with lung involvement D89.1 [J99]
Cryptitis (anal) (rectal) K62.89
Cryptococcosis, cryptococcus (infection) (neoformans) B45.9
  bone B45.3
  cerebral B45.1
  cutaneous B45.2
  disseminated B45.7
  generalized B45.7
  meningitis B45.1
  meningocerebralis B45.1
  osseous B45.3
  pulmonary B45.0
  skin B45.2
  specified NEC B45.8
Cryptopapillitis (anus) K62.89
Cryptophthalmos Q11.2
  syndrome Q87.0
Cryptorchid, cryptorchism, cryptorchidism Q53.9
  bilateral Q53.20
    abdominal Q53.21
    perineal Q53.22
  unilateral Q53.10
    abdominal Q53.11
    perineal Q53.12
Cryptosporidiosis A07.2
  hepatobiliary B88.8
  respiratory B88.8
Cryptostromosis J67.6
Crystalluria R82.99
Cubitus
  congenital Q68.8
  valgus (acquired) M21.0- ☑
    congenital Q68.8
    sequelae (late effect) of rickets E64.3
  varus (acquired) M21.1- ☑
    congenital Q68.8
    sequelae (late effect) of rickets E64.3
Cultural deprivation or shock Z60.3
Curling esophagus K22.4
Curling's ulcer — *see* Ulcer, peptic, acute

Curschmann (-Batten) (-Steinert) disease or
   syndrome G71.11
Curse, Ondine's — *see* Apnea, sleep
Curvature
   organ or site, congenital NEC — *see* Distortion
   penis (lateral) Q55.61
   Pott's (spinal) A18.01
   radius, idiopathic, progressive (congenital) Q74.0
   spine (acquired) (angular) (idiopathic) (incorrect)
     (postural) — *see* Dorsopathy, deforming
     congenital Q67.5
     due to or associated with
       Charcot-Marie-Tooth disease (*see also*
         subcategory M49.8) G60.0
       osteitis
         deformans M88.88
         fibrosa cystica (*see also* subcategory M49.8)
           E21.0
       tuberculosis (Pott's curvature) A18.01
     sequelae (late effect) of rickets E64.3
     tuberculous A18.01
Cushingoid due to steroid therapy E24.2
   correct substance properly administered — *see*
     Table of Drugs and Chemicals, by drug,
     adverse effect
   overdose or wrong substance given or taken —
     see Table of Drugs and Chemicals, by drug,
     poisoning
Cushing's
   syndrome or disease E24.9
     drug-induced E24.2
     iatrogenic E24.2
     pituitary-dependent E24.0
     specified NEC E24.8
   ulcer — *see* Ulcer, peptic, acute
Cusp, Carabelli - omit code
Cut (external) (*see also* Laceration)
   muscle — *see* Injury, muscle
Cutaneous (*see also* condition)
   hemorrhage R23.3
   larva migrans B76.9
Cutis (*see also* condition)
   hyperelastica Q82.8
     acquired L57.4
   laxa (hyperelastica) — *see* Dermatolysis
   marmorata R23.8
   osteosis L94.2
   pendula — *see* Dermatolysis
   rhomboidalis nuchae L57.2
   verticis gyrata Q82.8
     acquired L91.8
Cyanosis R23.0
   due to
     patent foramen botalli Q21.1
     persistent foramen ovale Q21.1
   enterogenous D74.8
   paroxysmal digital — *see* Raynaud's disease
     with gangrene I73.01
   retina, retinal H35.89
Cyanotic heart disease I24.9
   congenital Q24.9
Cycle
   anovulatory N97.0
   menstrual, irregular N92.6
Cyclencephaly Q04.9
Cyclical vomiting (*see also* Vomiting, cyclical) G43.A0
   psychogenic F50.8
Cyclitis (*see also* Iridocyclitis) H20.9
   chronic — *see* Iridocyclitis, chronic
   Fuchs' heterochromic H20.81- ☑
   granulomatous — *see* Iridocyclitis, chronic
   lens-induced — *see* Iridocyclitis, lens-induced
   posterior H30.2- ☑
Cycloid personality F34.0
Cyclophoria H50.54
Cyclopia, cyclops Q87.0
Cyclopism Q87.0
Cyclosporiasis A07.4
Cyclothymia F34.0
Cyclothymic personality F34.0
Cyclotropia H50.41- ☑
Cylindroma (*see also* Neoplasm, malignant, by site)
   eccrine dermal — *see* Neoplasm, skin, benign
   skin — *see* Neoplasm, skin, benign
Cylindruria R82.99
Cynanche
   diphtheritic A36.2
   tonsillaris J36
Cynophobia F40.218
Cynorexia R63.2
Cyphosis — *see* Kyphosis
Cyprus fever — *see* Brucellosis

Cyst (colloid) (mucous) (simple) (retention)
   adenoid (infected) J35.8
   adrenal gland E27.8
     congenital Q89.1
   air, lung J98.4
   allantoic Q64.4
   alveolar process (jaw bone) M27.40
   amnion, amniotic O41.8X- ☑
   anterior
     chamber (eye) — *see* Cyst, iris
     nasopalatine K09.1
   antrum J34.1
   anus K62.89
   apical (tooth) (periodontal) K04.8
   appendix K38.8
   arachnoid, brain (acquired) G93.0
     congenital Q04.6
   arytenoid J38.7
   Baker's M71.2- ☑
     ruptured M66.0
     tuberculous A18.02
   Bartholin's gland N75.0
   bile duct (common) (hepatic) K83.5
   bladder (multiple) (trigone) N32.89
   blue dome (breast) — *see* Cyst, breast
   bone (local) NEC M85.60
     aneurysmal M85.50
       ankle M85.57- ☑
       foot M85.57- ☑
       forearm M85.53- ☑
       hand M85.54- ☑
       jaw M27.49
       lower leg M85.56- ☑
       multiple site M85.59
       neck M85.58
       rib M85.58
       shoulder M85.51- ☑
       skull M85.58
       specified site NEC M85.58
       thigh M85.55- ☑
       toe M85.57- ☑
       upper arm M85.52- ☑
       vertebra M85.58
     solitary M85.40
       ankle M85.47- ☑
       fibula M85.46- ☑
       foot M85.47- ☑
       hand M85.44- ☑
       humerus M85.42- ☑
       jaw M27.49
       neck M85.48
       pelvis M85.45- ☑
       radius M85.43- ☑
       rib M85.48
       shoulder M85.41- ☑
       skull M85.48
       specified site NEC M85.48
       tibia M85.46- ☑
       toe M85.47- ☑
       ulna M85.43- ☑
       vertebra M85.48
     specified type NEC M85.60
       ankle M85.67- ☑
       foot M85.67- ☑
       forearm M85.63- ☑
       hand M85.64- ☑
       jaw M27.40
         developmental (nonodontogenic) K09.1
           odontogenic K09.0
         latent M27.0
       lower leg M85.66- ☑
       multiple site M85.69
       neck M85.68
       rib M85.68
       shoulder M85.61- ☑
       skull M85.68
       specified site NEC M85.68
       thigh M85.65- ☑
       toe M85.67- ☑
       upper arm M85.62- ☑
       vertebra M85.68
   brain (acquired) G93.0
     congenital Q04.6
     hydatid B67.99 [G94]
     third ventricle (colloid), congenital Q04.6
   branchial (cleft) Q18.0
   branchiogenic Q18.0
   breast (benign) (blue dome) (pedunculated)
     (solitary) N60.0- ☑
     involution — *see* Dysplasia, mammary,
       specified type NEC

Cyst — *continued*
     sebaceous — *see* Dysplasia, mammary,
       specified type NEC
   broad ligament (benign) N83.8
   bronchogenic (mediastinal) (sequestration) J98.4
     congenital Q33.0
   buccal K09.8
   bulbourethral gland N36.8
   bursa, bursal NEC M71.30
     with rupture — *see* Rupture, synovium
     ankle M71.37- ☑
     elbow M71.32- ☑
     foot M71.37- ☑
     hand M71.34- ☑
     hip M71.35- ☑
     multiple sites M71.39
     pharyngeal J39.2
     popliteal space — *see* Cyst, Baker's
     shoulder M71.31- ☑
     specified site NEC M71.38
     wrist M71.33- ☑
   calcifying odontogenic D16.5
     upper jaw (bone) (maxilla) D16.4
   canal of Nuck (female) N94.89
     congenital Q52.4
   canthus — *see* Cyst, conjunctiva
   carcinomatous — *see* Neoplasm, malignant, by
     site
   cauda equina G95.89
   cavum septi pellucidi — *see* Cyst, brain
   celomic (pericardium) Q24.8
   cerebellopontine (angle) — *see* Cyst, brain
   cerebellum — *see* Cyst, brain
   cerebral — *see* Cyst, brain
   cervical lateral Q18.1
   cervix NEC N88.8
     embryonic Q51.6
     nabothian N88.8
   chiasmal optic NEC — *see* Disorder, optic, chiasm
   chocolate (ovary) N80.1
   choledochus, congenital Q44.4
   chorion O41.8X- ☑
   choroid plexus G93.0
   ciliary body — *see* Cyst, iris
   clitoris N90.7
   colon K63.89
   common (bile) duct K83.5
   congenital NEC Q89.8
     adrenal gland Q89.1
     epiglottis Q31.8
     esophagus Q39.8
     fallopian tube Q50.4
     kidney Q61.00
       more than one (multiple) Q61.02
         specified as polycystic Q61.3
           adult type Q61.2
           infantile type NEC Q61.19
             collecting duct dilation Q61.11
         solitary Q61.01
     larynx Q31.8
     liver Q44.6
     lung Q33.0
     mediastinum Q34.1
     ovary Q50.1
     oviduct Q50.4
     periurethral (tissue) Q64.79
     prepuce Q55.69
     salivary gland (any) Q38.4
     sublingual Q38.6
     submaxillary gland Q38.6
     thymus (gland) Q89.2
     tongue Q38.3
     ureterovesical orifice Q62.8
     vulva Q52.79
   conjunctiva H11.44- ☑
   cornea H18.89- ☑
   corpora quadrigemina G93.0
   corpus
     albicans N83.29
     luteum (hemorrhagic) (ruptured) N83.1
   Cowper's gland (benign) (infected) N36.8
   cranial meninges G93.0
   craniobuccal pouch E23.6
   craniopharyngeal pouch E23.6
   cystic duct K82.8
   Cysticercus — *see* Cysticercosis
   Dandy-Walker Q03.1
     with spina bifida — *see* Spina bifida
   dental (root) K04.8
     developmental K09.0
     eruption K09.0
     primordial K09.0

Cyst — *continued*
dentigerous (mandible) (maxilla) K09.0
dermoid — *see* Neoplasm, benign, by site
  with malignant transformation C56.- ☑
  implantation
    external area or site (skin) NEC L72.0
    iris — *see* Cyst, iris, implantation
    vagina N89.8
    vulva N90.7
  mouth K09.8
  oral soft tissue K09.8
  sacrococcygeal — *see* Cyst, pilonidal
developmental K09.1
  odontogenic K09.0
  oral region (nonodontogenic) K09.1
  ovary, ovarian Q50.1
dura (cerebral) G93.0
  spinal G96.19
ear (external) Q18.1
echinococcal — *see* Echinococcus
embryonic
  cervix uteri Q51.6
  fallopian tube Q50.4
  vagina Q51.6
endometrium, endometrial (uterus) N85.8
  ectopic — *see* Endometriosis
enterogenous Q43.8
epidermal, epidermoid (inclusion) (see also Cyst, skin) L72.0
  mouth K09.8
  oral soft tissue K09.8
epididymis N50.3
epiglottis J38.7
epiphysis cerebri E34.8
epithelial (inclusion) L72.0
epoophoron Q50.5
eruption K09.0
esophagus K22.8
ethmoid sinus J34.1
external female genital organs NEC N90.7
eye NEC H57.8
  congenital Q15.8
eyelid (sebaceous) H02.829
  infected — *see* Hordeolum
  left H02.826
    lower H02.825
    upper H02.824
  right H02.823
    lower H02.822
    upper H02.821
fallopian tube N83.8
  congenital Q50.4
fimbrial (twisted) Q50.4
fissural (oral region) K09.1
follicle (graafian) (hemorrhagic) N83.0
  nabothian N88.8
follicular (atretic) (hemorrhagic) (ovarian) N83.0
  dentigerous K09.0
  odontogenic K09.0
  skin L72.9
    specified NEC L72.8
frontal sinus J34.1
gallbladder K82.8
ganglion — *see* Ganglion
Gartner's duct Q52.4
gingiva K09.0
gland of Moll — *see* Cyst, eyelid
globulomaxillary K09.1
graafian follicle (hemorrhagic) N83.0
granulosal lutein (hemorrhagic) N83.1
hemangiomatous D18.00
  intra-abdominal D18.03
  intracranial D18.02
  skin D18.01
  specified site NEC D18.09
hydatid (see also Echinococcus) B67.90
  brain B67.99 [G94]
  liver (see also Cyst, liver, hydatid) B67.8
  lung NEC B67.99 [J99]
  Morgagni
    female Q50.5
    male (epididymal) Q55.4
      testicular Q55.29
  specified site NEC B67.99
hymen N89.8
  embryonic Q52.4
hypopharynx J39.2
hypophysis, hypophyseal (duct) (recurrent) E23.6
  cerebri E23.6
implantation (dermoid)
  external area or site (skin) NEC L72.0
  iris — *see* Cyst, iris, implantation

Cyst — *continued*
  vagina N89.8
  vulva N90.7
incisive canal K09.1
inclusion (epidermal) (epithelial) (epidermoid) (squamous) L72.0
  not of skin - code under Cyst, by site
intestine (large) (small) K63.89
intracranial — *see* Cyst, brain
intraligamentous (*see also* Disorder, ligament)
  knee — *see* Derangement, knee
intrasellar E23.6
iris H21.309
  exudative H21.31- ☑
  idiopathic H21.30- ☑
  implantation H21.32- ☑
  parasitic H21.33- ☑
  pars plana (primary) H21.34- ☑
    exudative H21.35- ☑
jaw (bone) M27.40
  aneurysmal M27.49
  hemorrhagic M27.49
  traumatic M27.49
  developmental (odontogenic) K09.0
  fissural K09.1
joint NEC — *see* Disorder, joint, specified type NEC
kidney (acquired) N28.1
  calyceal — *see* Hydronephrosis
  congenital Q61.00
  more than one (multiple) Q61.02
    specified as polycystic Q61.3
      adult type (autosomal dominant) Q61.2
      infantile type (autosomal recessive) NEC Q61.19
        collecting duct dilation Q61.11
  pyelogenic — *see* Hydronephrosis
  simple N28.1
  solitary (single) Q61.01
    acquired N28.1
labium (majus) (minus) N90.7
  sebaceous N90.7
lacrimal (*see also* Disorder, lacrimal system, specified NEC)
  gland H04.13- ☑
  passages or sac — *see* Disorder, lacrimal system, specified NEC
larynx J38.7
lateral periodontal K09.0
lens H27.8
  congenital Q12.8
lip (gland) K13.0
liver (idiopathic) (simple) K76.89
  congenital Q44.6
  hydatid B67.8
    granulosus B67.0
    multilocularis B67.5
lung J98.4
  congenital Q33.0
  giant bullous J43.9
lutein N83.1
lymphangiomatous D18.1
lymphoepithelial, oral soft tissue K09.8
macula — *see* Degeneration, macula, hole
malignant — *see* Neoplasm, malignant, by site
mammary gland — *see* Cyst, breast
mandible M27.40
  dentigerous K09.0
  radicular K04.8
maxilla M27.40
  . dentigerous K09.0
  radicular K04.8
medial, face and neck Q18.8
median
  anterior maxillary K09.1
  palatal K09.1
mediastinum, congenital Q34.1
meibomian (gland) — *see* Chalazion
  infected — *see* Hordeolum
membrane, brain G93.0
meninges (cerebral) G93.0
  spinal G96.19
meniscus, knee — *see* Derangement, knee, meniscus, cystic
mesentery, mesenteric K66.8
  chyle I89.8
mesonephric duct
  female Q50.5
  male Q55.4
milk N64.89
Morgagni (hydatid)
  female Q50.5

Cyst — *continued*
  male (epididymal) Q55.4
    testicular Q55.29
mouth K09.8
Müllerian duct Q50.4
  appendix testis Q55.29
  cervix Q51.6
  fallopian tube Q50.4
  female Q50.4
  male Q55.29
  prostatic utricle Q55.4
  vagina (embryonal) Q52.4
multilocular (ovary) D39.10
  benign — *see* Neoplasm, benign, by site
myometrium N85.8
nabothian (follicle) (ruptured) N88.8
nasoalveolar K09.1
nasolabial K09.1
nasopalatine (anterior) (duct) K09.1
nasopharynx J39.2
neoplastic — *see* Neoplasm, uncertain behavior, by site
  benign — *see* Neoplasm, benign, by site
nervous system NEC G96.8
neuroenteric (congenital) Q06.8
nipple — *see* Cyst, breast
nose (turbinates) J34.1
  sinus J34.1
odontogenic, developmental K09.0
omentum (lesser) K66.8
  congenital Q45.8
ora serrata — *see* Cyst, retina, ora serrata
oral
  region K09.9
    developmental (nonodontogenic) K09.1
    specified NEC K09.8
  soft tissue K09.9
    specified NEC K09.8
orbit H05.81- ☑
ovary, ovarian (twisted) N83.20
  adherent N83.20
  chocolate N80.1
  corpus
    albicans N83.29
    luteum (hemorrhagic) N83.1
  dermoid D27.9
  developmental Q50.1
  due to failure of involution NEC N83.20
  endometrial N80.1
  follicular (graafian) (hemorrhagic) N83.0
  hemorrhagic N83.20
  in pregnancy or childbirth O34.8- ☑
    with obstructed labor O65.5
  multilocular D39.10
  pseudomucinous D27.9
  retention N83.29
  serous N83.20
  specified NEC N83.29
  theca lutein (hemorrhagic) N83.1
  tuberculous A18.18
oviduct N83.8
palate (median) (fissural) K09.1
palatine papilla (jaw) K09.1
pancreas, pancreatic (hemorrhagic) (true) K86.2
  congenital Q45.2
  false K86.3
paralabral
  hip M24.85- ☑
  shoulder S43.43- ☑
paramesonephric duct Q50.4
  female Q50.4
  male Q55.29
paranephric N28.1
paraphysis, cerebri, congenital Q04.6
parasitic B89
parathyroid (gland) E21.4
paratubal N83.8
paraurethral duct N36.8
paroophoron Q50.5
parotid gland K11.6
parovarian Q50.5
pelvis, female N94.89
  in pregnancy or childbirth O34.8- ☑
    causing obstructed labor O65.5
penis (sebaceous) N48.89
periapical K04.8
pericardial (congenital) Q24.8
  acquired (secondary) I31.8
pericoronal K09.0
periodontal K04.8
  lateral K09.0
peripelvic (lymphatic) N28.1

☑ **Additional character required**

Cyst — *continued*
  peritoneum K66.8
    chylous I89.8
  periventricular, acquired, newborn P91.1
  pharynx (wall) J39.2
  pilar L72.11
  pilonidal (infected) (rectum) L05.91
    with abscess L05.01
    malignant C44.59- ☑
  pituitary (duct) (gland) E23.6
  placenta O43.19- ☑
  pleura J94.8
  popliteal — *see* Cyst, Baker's
  porencephalic Q04.6
    acquired G93.0
  postanal (infected) — *see* Cyst, pilonidal
  postmastoidectomy cavity (mucosal) — *see*
    Complications, postmastoidectomy, cyst
  preauricular Q18.1
  prepuce N47.4
    congenital Q55.69
  primordial (jaw) K09.0
  prostate N42.83
  pseudomucinous (ovary) D27.9
  pupillary, miotic H21.27- ☑
  radicular (residual) K04.8
  radiculodental K04.8
  ranular K11.8
  Rathke's pouch E23.6
  rectum (epithelium) (mucous) K62.89
  renal — *see* Cyst, kidney
  residual (radicular) K04.8
  retention (ovary) N83.29
    salivary gland K11.6
  retina H33.19- ☑
    ora serrata H33.11- ☑
    parasitic H33.12- ☑
  retroperitoneal K68.9
  sacrococcygeal (dermoid) — *see* Cyst, pilonidal
  salivary gland or duct (mucous extravasation or
    retention) K11.6
  Sampson's N80.1
  sclera H15.89
  scrotum L72.9
    sebaceous L72.3
  sebaceous (duct) (gland) L72.3
    breast — *see* Dysplasia, mammary, specified
      type NEC
    eyelid — *see* Cyst, eyelid
    genital organ NEC
      female N94.89
      male N50.8
    scrotum L72.3
  semilunar cartilage (knee) (multiple) — *see*
    Derangement, knee, meniscus, cystic
  seminal vesicle N50.8
  serous (ovary) N83.20
  sinus (accessory) (nasal) J34.1
  Skene's gland N36.8
  skin L72.9
    breast — *see* Dysplasia, mammary, specified
      type NEC
    epidermal, epidermoid L72.0
    epithelial L72.0
    eyelid — *see* Cyst, eyelid
    genital organ NEC
      female N90.7
      male N50.8
    inclusion L72.0
    scrotum L72.9
    sebaceous L72.3
    sweat gland or duct L74.8
  solitary
    bone — *see* Cyst, bone, solitary
    jaw M27.40
    kidney N28.1
  spermatic cord N50.8
  sphenoid sinus J34.1
  spinal meninges G96.19
  spleen NEC D73.4
    congenital Q89.09
    hydatid (*see also* Echinococcus) B67.99 [D77]
  Stafne's M27.0
  subarachnoid intrasellar R93.0
  subcutaneous, pheomycotic (chromomycotic)
    B43.2
  subdural (cerebral) G93.0
    spinal cord G96.19
  sublingual K11.6
  submandibular gland K11.6
  submaxillary gland K11.6
  suburethral N36.8

Cyst — *continued*
  suprarenal gland E27.8
  suprasellar — *see* Cyst, brain
  sweat gland or duct L74.8
  synovial (*see also* Cyst, bursa)
    ruptured — *see* Rupture, synovium
  tarsal — *see* Chalazion
  tendon (sheath) — *see* Disorder, tendon, specified
    type NEC
  testis N44.2
    tunica albuginea N44.1
  theca lutein (ovary) N83.1
  Thornwaldt's J39.2
  thymus (gland) E32.8
  thyroglossal duct (infected) (persistent) Q89.2
  thyrolingual duct (infected) (persistent) Q89.2
  thyroid (gland) E04.1
  tongue K14.8
  tonsil J35.8
  tooth — *see* Cyst, dental
  Tornwaldt's J39.2
  trichilemmal (proliferating) L72.12
  trichodermal L72.12
  tubal (fallopian) N83.8
    inflammatory — *see* Salpingitis, chronic
  tubo-ovarian N83.8
    inflammatory N70.13
  tunica
    albuginea testis N44.1
    vaginalis N50.8
  turbinate (nose) J34.1
  Tyson's gland N48.89
  urachus, congenital Q64.4
  ureter N28.89
  ureterovesical orifice N28.89
  urethra, urethral (gland) N36.8
  uterine ligament N83.8
  uterus (body) (corpus) (recurrent) N85.8
    embryonic Q51.818
      cervix Q51.6
  vagina, vaginal (implantation) (inclusion)
    (squamous cell) (wall) N89.8
    embryonic Q52.4
  vallecula, vallecular (epiglottis) J38.7
  vesical (orifice) N32.89
  vitreous body H43.89
  vulva (implantation) (inclusion) N90.7
    congenital Q52.79
    sebaceous gland N90.7
  vulvovaginal gland N90.7
  wolffian
    female Q50.5
    male Q55.4
Cystadenocarcinoma — *see* Neoplasm, malignant,
  by site
  bile duct C22.1
  endometrioid — *see* Neoplasm, malignant, by site
    specified site — *see* Neoplasm, malignant, by
      site
    unspecified site
      female C56.9
      male C61
  mucinous
    papillary
      specified site — *see* Neoplasm, malignant,
        by site
      unspecified site C56.9
    specified site — *see* Neoplasm, malignant, by
      site
    unspecified site C56.9
  papillary
    mucinous
      specified site — *see* Neoplasm, malignant,
        by site
      unspecified site C56.9
    pseudomucinous
      specified site — *see* Neoplasm, malignant,
        by site
      unspecified site C56.9
    serous
      specified site — *see* Neoplasm, malignant,
        by site
      unspecified site C56.9
    specified site — *see* Neoplasm, malignant, by
      site
    unspecified site C56.9
  pseudomucinous
    papillary
      specified site — *see* Neoplasm, malignant,
        by site
      unspecified site C56.9

Cystadenocarcinoma — *continued*
    specified site — *see* Neoplasm, malignant, by
      site
    unspecified site C56.9
  serous
    papillary
      specified site — *see* Neoplasm, malignant,
        by site
      unspecified site C56.9
    specified site — *see* Neoplasm, malignant, by
      site
    unspecified site C56.9
Cystadenofibroma
  clear cell — *see* Neoplasm, benign, by site
  endometrioid D27.9
    borderline malignancy D39.1- ☑
    malignant C56.- ☑
  mucinous
    specified site — *see* Neoplasm, benign, by site
    unspecified site D27.9
  serous
    specified site — *see* Neoplasm, benign, by site
    unspecified site D27.9
  specified site — *see* Neoplasm, benign, by site
  unspecified site D27.9
Cystadenoma (*see also* Neoplasm, benign, by site)
  bile duct D13.4
  endometrioid — *see* Neoplasm, benign, by site
    borderline malignancy — *see* Neoplasm,
      uncertain behavior, by site
  malignant — *see* Neoplasm, malignant, by site
  mucinous
    borderline malignancy
      ovary C56.- ☑
      specified site NEC — *see* Neoplasm,
        uncertain behavior, by site
      unspecified site C56.9
    papillary
      borderline malignancy
        ovary C56.- ☑
        specified site NEC — *see* Neoplasm,
          uncertain behavior, by site
        unspecified site C56.9
      specified site — *see* Neoplasm, benign, by
        site
      unspecified site D27.9
    specified site — *see* Neoplasm, benign, by site
    unspecified site D27.9
  papillary
    borderline malignancy
      ovary C56.- ☑
      specified site NEC — *see* Neoplasm,
        uncertain behavior, by site
      unspecified site C56.9
    lymphomatosum
      specified site — *see* Neoplasm, benign, by
        site
      unspecified site D11.9
    mucinous
      borderline malignancy
        ovary C56.- ☑
        specified site NEC — *see* Neoplasm,
          uncertain behavior, by site
        unspecified site C56.9
      specified site — *see* Neoplasm, benign, by
        site
      unspecified site D27.9
    pseudomucinous
      borderline malignancy
        ovary C56.- ☑
        specified site NEC — *see* Neoplasm,
          uncertain behavior, by site
        unspecified site C56.9
      specified site — *see* Neoplasm, benign, by
        site
      unspecified site D27.9
    serous
      borderline malignancy
        ovary C56.- ☑
        specified site NEC — *see* Neoplasm,
          uncertain behavior, by site
        unspecified site C56.9
      specified site — *see* Neoplasm, benign, by
        site
      unspecified site D27.9
    specified site — *see* Neoplasm, benign, by site
    unspecified site D27.9
  pseudomucinous
    borderline malignancy
      ovary C56.- ☑
      specified site NEC — *see* Neoplasm,
        uncertain behavior, by site

Cystadenoma - Czerny's

Cystadenoma — *continued*
    unspecified site C56.9
    papillary
      borderline malignancy
        ovary C56.- ☑
        specified site NEC — *see* Neoplasm,
          uncertain behavior, by site
        unspecified site C56.9
      specified site — *see* Neoplasm, benign, by
        site
      unspecified site D27.9
    specified site — *see* Neoplasm, benign, by site
    unspecified site D27.9
    serous
      borderline malignancy
        ovary C56.- ☑
        specified site NEC — *see* Neoplasm,
          uncertain behavior, by site
        unspecified site C56.9
      papillary
        borderline malignancy
          ovary C56.- ☑
          specified site NEC — *see* Neoplasm,
            uncertain behavior, by site
          unspecified site C56.9
        specified site — *see* Neoplasm, benign, by
          site
        unspecified site D27.9
      specified site — *see* Neoplasm, benign, by site
      unspecified site D27.9
Cystathionine synthase deficiency E72.11
Cystathioninemia E72.19
Cystathioninuria E72.19
Cystic (*see also* condition)
    breast (chronic) — *see* Mastopathy, cystic
    corpora lutea (hemorrhagic) N83.1
    duct — *see* condition
    eyeball (congenital) Q11.0
    fibrosis — *see* Fibrosis, cystic
    kidney (congenital) Q61.9
      adult type Q61.2
      infantile type NEC Q61.19
        collecting duct dilatation Q61.11
      medullary Q61.5
    liver, congenital Q44.6
    lung disease J98.4
      congenital Q33.0
    mastitis, chronic — *see* Mastopathy, cystic
    medullary, kidney Q61.5
    meniscus — *see* Derangement, knee, meniscus,
      cystic
    ovary N83.20
Cysticercosis, cysticerciasis B69.9
    with
      epileptiform fits B69.0
        myositis B69.81
    brain B69.0
    central nervous system B69.0
    cerebral B69.0
    ocular B69.1

Cysticercosis — *continued*
    specified NEC B69.89
Cysticercus cellulose infestation — *see* Cysticercosis
Cystinosis (malignant) E72.04
Cystinuria E72.01
Cystitis (exudative) (hemorrhagic) (septic)
  (suppurative) N30.90
    with
      fibrosis — *see* Cystitis, chronic, interstitial
      hematuria N30.91
      leukoplakia — *see* Cystitis, chronic, interstitial
      malakoplakia — *see* Cystitis, chronic, interstitial
      metaplasia — *see* Cystitis, chronic, interstitial
      prostatitis N41.3
    acute N30.00
      with hematuria N30.01
      of trigone N30.30
        with hematuria N30.31
    allergic — *see* Cystitis, specified type NEC
    amebic A06.81
    bilharzial B65.9 [N33]
    blennorrhagic (gonococcal) A54.01
    bullous — *see* Cystitis, specified type NEC
    calculous N21.0
    chlamydial A56.01
    chronic N30.20
      with hematuria N30.21
      interstitial N30.10
        with hematuria N30.11
      of trigone N30.30
        with hematuria N30.31
      specified NEC N30.20
        with hematuria N30.21
    cystic (a) — *see* Cystitis, specified type NEC
    diphtheritic A36.85
    echinococcal
      granulosus B67.39
      multilocularis B67.69
    emphysematous — *see* Cystitis, specified type
      NEC
    encysted — *see* Cystitis, specified type NEC
    eosinophilic — *see* Cystitis, specified type NEC
    follicular — *see* Cystitis, of trigone
    gangrenous — *see* Cystitis, specified type NEC
    glandularis — *see* Cystitis, specified type NEC
    gonococcal A54.01
    incrusted — *see* Cystitis, specified type NEC
    interstitial (chronic) — *see* Cystitis, chronic,
      interstitial
    irradiation N30.40
      with hematuria N30.41
    irritation — *see* Cystitis, specified type NEC
    malignant — *see* Cystitis, specified type NEC
    of trigone N30.30
      with hematuria N30.31
    panmural — *see* Cystitis, chronic, interstitial
    polyposa — *see* Cystitis, specified type NEC
    prostatic N41.3
    puerperal (postpartum) O86.22
    radiation — *see* Cystitis, irradiation

Cystitis — *continued*
    specified type NEC N30.80
      with hematuria N30.81
    subacute — *see* Cystitis, chronic
    submucous — *see* Cystitis, chronic, interstitial
    syphilitic (late) A52.76
    trichomonal A59.03
    tuberculous A18.12
    ulcerative — *see* Cystitis, chronic, interstitial
Cystocele (-urethrocele)
    female N81.10
      with prolapse of uterus — *see* Prolapse, uterus
      lateral N81.12
      midline N81.11
      paravaginal N81.12
    in pregnancy or childbirth O34.8- ☑
      causing obstructed labor O65.5
    male N32.89
Cystolithiasis N21.0
Cystoma (*see also* Neoplasm, benign, by site)
    endometrial, ovary N80.1
    mucinous
      specified site — *see* Neoplasm, benign, by site
      unspecified site D27.9
    serous
      specified site — *see* Neoplasm, benign, by site
      unspecified site D27.9
    simple (ovary) N83.29
Cystoplegia N31.2
Cystoptosis N32.89
Cystopyelitis — *see* Pyelonephritis
Cystorrhagia N32.89
Cystosarcoma phyllodes D48.6- ☑
    benign D24- ☑
    malignant — *see* Neoplasm, breast, malignant
Cystostomy
    attention to Z43.5
    complication — *see* Complications, cystostomy
    status Z93.50
      appendico-vesicostomy Z93.52
      cutaneous Z93.51
      specified NEC Z93.59
Cystourethritis — *see* Urethritis
Cystourethrocele (*see also* Cystocele)
    female N81.10
      with uterine prolapse — *see* Prolapse, uterus
      lateral N81.12
      midline N81.11
      paravaginal N81.12
    male N32.89
Cytomegalic inclusion disease
    congenital P35.1
Cytomegalovirus infection B25.9
Cytomycosis (reticuloendothelial) B39.4
Cytopenia D75.9
    refractory
      with multilineage dysplasia D46.A
        and ring sideroblasts (RCMD RS) D46.B
Czerny's disease (periodic hydrarthrosis of the knee)
    — *see* Effusion, joint, knee

D

Daae (-Finsen) disease (epidemic pleurodynia) B33.0
Da Costa's syndrome F45.8
Dabney's grip B33.0
Dacryoadenitis, dacryadenitis H04.00- ☑
  acute H04.01- ☑
  chronic H04.02- ☑
Dacryocystitis H04.30- ☑
  acute H04.32- ☑
  chronic H04.41- ☑
  neonatal P39.1
  phlegmonous H04.31- ☑
  syphilitic A52.71
    congenital (early) A50.01
  trachomatous, active A71.1
    sequelae (late effect) B94.0
Dacryocystoblenorrhea — *see* Inflammation, lacrimal, passages, chronic
Dacryocystocele — *see* Disorder, lacrimal system, changes
Dacryolith, dacryolithiasis H04.51- ☑
Dacryoma — *see* Disorder, lacrimal system, changes
Dacryopericystitis — *see* Dacryocystitis
Dacryops H04.11- ☑
Dacryostenosis (*see also* Stenosis, lacrimal)
  congenital Q10.5
Dactylitis
  bone — *see* Osteomyelitis
  sickle-cell D57.00
    Hb C D57.219
    Hb SS D57.00
    specified NEC D57.819
  skin L08.9
  syphilitic A52.77
  tuberculous A18.03
Dactylolysis spontanea (ainhum) L94.6
Dactylosymphysis Q70.9
  fingers — *see* Syndactylism, complex, fingers
  toes — *see* Syndactylism, complex, toes
Damage
  arteriosclerotic — *see* Arteriosclerosis
  brain (nontraumatic) G93.9
    anoxic, hypoxic G93.1
      resulting from a procedure G97.82
    child NEC G80.9
    due to birth injury P11.2
  cardiorenal (vascular) — *see* Hypertension, cardiorenal
  cerebral NEC — *see* Damage, brain
  coccyx, complicating delivery O71.6
  coronary — *see* Disease, heart, ischemic
  eye, birth injury P15.3
  liver (nontraumatic) K76.9
    alcoholic K70.9
    due to drugs — *see* Disease, liver, toxic
    toxic — *see* Disease, liver, toxic
  medication T88.7 ☑
  pelvic
    joint or ligament, during delivery O71.6
    organ NEC
      during delivery O71.5
      following ectopic or molar pregnancy O08.6
  renal — *see* Disease, renal
  subendocardium, subendocardial — *see* Degeneration, myocardial
  vascular I99.9
Dana-Putnam syndrome (subacute combined sclerosis with pernicious anemia) — *see* Degeneration, combined
Danbolt (-Cross) syndrome (acrodermatitis enteropathica) E83.2
Dandruff L21.0
Dandy-Walker syndrome Q03.1
  with spina bifida — *see* Spina bifida
Danlos' syndrome Q79.6
Darier (-White) disease (congenital) Q82.8
  meaning erythema annulare centrifugum L53.1
Darier-Roussy sarcoid D86.3
Darling's disease or histoplasmosis B39.4
Darwin's tubercle Q17.8
Dawson's (inclusion body) encephalitis A81.1
De Beurmann (-Gougerot) disease B42.1
De la Tourette's syndrome F95.2
De Lange's syndrome Q87.1
De Morgan's spots (senile angiomas) I78.1
De Quervain's
  disease (tendon sheath) M65.4
  syndrome E34.51
  thyroiditis (subacute granulomatous thyroiditis) E06.1

De Toni-Fanconi (-Debré) syndrome E72.09
  with cystinosis E72.04
Dead
  fetus, retained (mother) O36.4 ☑
    early pregnancy O02.1
  labyrinth H83.2
  ovum, retained O02.0
Deaf nonspeaking NEC H91.3
Deafmutism (acquired) (congenital) NEC H91.3
  hysterical F44.6
  syphilitic, congenital (*see also* subcategory H94.8) A50.09
Deafness (acquired) (complete) (hereditary) (partial) H91.9- ☑
  with blue sclera and fragility of bone Q78.0
  auditory fatigue — *see* Deafness, specified type NEC
  aviation T70.0 ☑
    nerve injury — *see* Injury, nerve, acoustic, specified type NEC
  boilermaker's H83.3
  central — *see* Deafness, sensorineural
  conductive H90.2
    and sensorineural, mixed H90.8
      bilateral H90.6
    bilateral H90.0
    unilateral H90.1- ☑
  congenital H90.5
    with blue sclera and fragility of bone Q78.0
  due to toxic agents — *see* Deafness, ototoxic
  emotional (hysterical) F44.6
  functional (hysterical) F44.6
  high frequency H91.9- ☑
  hysterical F44.6
  low frequency H91.9- ☑
  mental R48.8
  mixed conductive and sensorineural H90.8
    bilateral H90.6
    unilateral H90.7- ☑
  nerve — *see* Deafness, sensorineural
  neural — *see* Deafness, sensorineural
  noise-induced (*see also* subcategory) H83.3 ☑
    nerve injury — *see* Injury, nerve, acoustic, specified type NEC
  nonspeaking H91.3
  ototoxic H91.0
  perceptive — *see* Deafness, sensorineural
  psychogenic (hysterical) F44.6
  sensorineural H90.5
    and conductive, mixed H90.8
      bilateral H90.6
    bilateral H90.3
    unilateral H90.4- ☑
  sensory — *see* Deafness, sensorineural
  specified type NEC H91.8
  sudden (idiopathic) H91.2- ☑
  syphilitic A52.15
  transient ischemic H93.01- ☑
  traumatic — *see* Injury, nerve, acoustic, specified type NEC
  word (developmental) H93.25
Death (cause unknown) (of) (unexplained) (unspecified cause) R99
  brain G93.82
  cardiac (sudden) (with successful resuscitation) - code to underlying disease
    family history of Z82.41
    personal history of Z86.74
  family member (assumed) Z63.4
Debility (chronic) (general) (nervous) R53.81
  congenital or neonatal NOS P96.9
  nervous R53.81
  old age R54
  senile R54
Débove's disease (splenomegaly) R16.1
Decalcification
  bone — *see* Osteoporosis
  teeth K03.89
Decapsulation, kidney N28.89
Decay
  dental — *see* Caries, dental
  senile R54
  tooth, teeth — *see* Caries, dental
Deciduitis (acute)
  following ectopic or molar pregnancy O08.0
Decline (general) — *see* Debility
  cognitive, age-associated R41.81
Decompensation
  cardiac (acute) (chronic) — *see* Disease, heart
  cardiovascular — *see* Disease, cardiovascular
  heart — *see* Disease, heart
  hepatic — *see* Failure, hepatic

Decompensation — *continued*
  myocardial (acute) (chronic) — *see* Disease, heart
  respiratory J98.8
Decompression sickness T70.3 ☑
Decrease (d)
  absolute neutrophile count — *see* Neutropenia
  blood
    platelets — *see* Thrombocytopenia
    pressure R03.1
      due to shock following
        injury T79.4 ☑
        operation T81.19 ☑
  estrogen E28.39
    postablative E89.40
      asymptomatic E89.40
      symptomatic E89.41
  fragility of erythrocytes D58.8
  function
    lipase (pancreatic) K90.3
    ovary in hypopituitarism E23.0
    parenchyma of pancreas K86.8
    pituitary (gland) (anterior) (lobe) E23.0
    posterior (lobe) E23.0
  functional activity R68.89
  glucose R73.09
  hematocrit R71.0
  hemoglobin R71.0
  leukocytes D72.819
    specified NEC D72.818
  libido R68.82
  lymphocytes D72.810
  platelets D69.6
  respiration, due to shock following injury T79.4 ☑
  sexual desire R68.82
  tear secretion NEC — *see* Syndrome, dry eye
  tolerance
    fat K90.4
    glucose R73.09
    pancreatic K90.3
    salt and water E87.8
  vision NEC H54.7
  white blood cell count D72.819
    specified NEC D72.818
Decubitus (ulcer) — *see* Ulcer, pressure, by site
  cervix N86
Deepening acetabulum — *see* Derangement, joint, specified type NEC, hip
Defect, defective Q89.9
  3-beta-hydroxysteroid dehydrogenase E25.0
  11-hydroxylase E25.0
  21-hydroxylase E25.0
  abdominal wall, congenital Q79.59
  antibody immunodeficiency D80.9
  aorticopulmonary septum Q21.4
  atrial septal (ostium secundum type) Q21.1
    following acute myocardial infarction (current complication) I23.1
    ostium primum type Q21.2
  atrioventricular
    canal Q21.2
    septum Q21.2
  auricular septal Q21.1
  bilirubin excretion NEC E80.6
  biosynthesis, androgen (testicular) E29.1
  bulbar septum Q21.0
  catalase E80.3
  cell membrane receptor complex (CR3) D71
  circulation I99.9
    congenital Q28.9
    newborn Q28.9
  coagulation (factor) (*see also* Deficiency, factor) D68.9
    with
      ectopic pregnancy O08.1
      molar pregnancy O08.1
    acquired D68.4
    antepartum with hemorrhage — *see* Hemorrhage, antepartum, with coagulation defect
    due to
      liver disease D68.4
      vitamin K deficiency D68.4
    hereditary NEC D68.2
    intrapartum O67.0
    newborn, transient P61.6
    postpartum O72.3
    specified type NEC D68.8
  complement system D84.1
  conduction (heart) I45.9
    bone — *see* Deafness, conductive
  congenital, organ or site not listed — *see* Anomaly, by site

Defect - Deficiency

Defect — *continued*
- coronary sinus Q21.1
- cushion, endocardial Q21.2
- degradation, glycoprotein E77.1
- dental bridge, crown, fillings — *see* Defect, dental restoration
- dental restoration K08.50
  - specified NEC K08.59
- dentin (hereditary) K00.5
- Descemet's membrane, congenital Q13.89
- developmental (*see also* Anomaly)
  - cauda equina Q06.3
- diaphragm
  - with elevation, eventration or hernia — *see* Hernia, diaphragm
  - congenital Q79.1
    - with hernia Q79.0
    - gross (with hernia) Q79.0
- ectodermal, congenital Q82.9
- Eisenmenger's Q21.8
- enzyme
  - catalase E80.3
  - peroxidase E80.3
- esophagus, congenital Q39.9
- extensor retinaculum M62.89
- fibrin polymerization D68.2
- filling
  - bladder R93.4
  - kidney R93.4
  - stomach R93.3
  - ureter R93.4
- Gerbode Q21.0
- glycoprotein degradation E77.1
- Hageman (factor) D68.2
- hearing — *see* Deafness
- high grade F70
- interatrial septal Q21.1
- interauricular septal Q21.1
- interventricular septal Q21.0
  - with dextroposition of aorta, pulmonary stenosis and hypertrophy of right ventricle Q21.3
  - in tetralogy of Fallot Q21.3
- learning (specific) — *see* Disorder, learning
- lymphocyte function antigen-1 (LFA-1) D84.0
- lysosomal enzyme, post-translational modification E77.0
- major osseous M89.70
  - ankle M89.77- ☑
  - carpus M89.74- ☑
  - clavicle M89.71- ☑
  - femur M89.75- ☑
  - fibula M89.76- ☑
  - fingers M89.74- ☑
  - foot M89.77- ☑
  - forearm M89.73- ☑
  - hand M89.74- ☑
  - humerus M89.72- ☑
  - lower leg M89.76- ☑
  - metacarpus M89.74- ☑
  - metatarsus M89.77- ☑
  - multiple sites M89.79
  - pelvic region M89.75- ☑
  - pelvis M89.75- ☑
  - radius M89.73- ☑
  - scapula M89.71- ☑
  - shoulder region M89.71- ☑
  - specified NEC M89.78
  - tarsus M89.77- ☑
  - thigh M89.75- ☑
  - tibia M89.76- ☑
  - toes M89.77- ☑
  - ulna M89.73- ☑
- mental — *see* Disability, intellectual
- modification, lysosomal enzymes, post-translational E77.0
- obstructive, congenital
  - renal pelvis Q62.39
  - ureter Q62.39
    - atresia — *see* Atresia, ureter
    - cecoureterocele Q62.32
    - megaureter Q62.2
    - orthotopic ureterocele Q62.31
- osseous, major M89.70
  - ankle M89.77- ☑
  - carpus M89.74- ☑
  - clavicle M89.71- ☑
  - femur M89.75- ☑
  - fibula M89.76- ☑
  - fingers M89.74- ☑
  - foot M89.77- ☑
  - forearm M89.73- ☑

Defect — *continued*
- hand M89.74- ☑
- humerus M89.72- ☑
- lower leg M89.76- ☑
- metacarpus M89.74- ☑
- metatarsus M89.77- ☑
- multiple sites M89.9
- pelvic region M89.75- ☑
- pelvis M89.75- ☑
- radius M89.73- ☑
- scapula M89.71- ☑
- shoulder region M89.71- ☑
- specified NEC M89.78
- tarsus M89.77- ☑
- thigh M89.75- ☑
- tibia M89.76- ☑
- toes M89.77- ☑
- ulna M89.73- ☑
- osteochondral NEC (*see also* Deformity) M95.8
- ostium
  - primum Q21.2
  - secundum Q21.1
- peroxidase E80.3
- placental blood supply — *see* Insufficiency, placental
- platelets, qualitative D69.1
  - constitutional D68.0
- postural NEC, spine — *see* Dorsopathy, deforming
- reduction
  - limb Q73.8
    - lower Q72.9- ☑
      - absence — *see* Agenesis, leg
        - foot — *see* Agenesis, foot
      - longitudinal
        - femur Q72.4- ☑
        - fibula Q72.6- ☑
        - tibia Q72.5- ☑
      - specified type NEC Q72.89- ☑
      - split foot Q72.7- ☑
    - specified type NEC Q73.8
    - upper Q71.9- ☑
      - absence — *see* Agenesis, arm
        - forearm — *see* Agenesis, forearm
        - hand — *see* Agenesis, hand
      - lobster-claw hand Q71.6- ☑
      - longitudinal
        - radius Q71.4- ☑
        - ulna Q71.5- ☑
      - specified type NEC Q71.89- ☑
- renal pelvis Q63.8
  - obstructive Q62.39
- respiratory system, congenital Q34.9
- restoration, dental K08.50
  - specified NEC K08.59
- retinal nerve bundle fibers H35.89
- septal (heart) NOS Q21.9
  - acquired (atrial) (auricular) (ventricular) (old) I51.0
  - atrial Q21.1
    - concurrent with acute myocardial infarction — *see* Infarct, myocardium
    - following acute myocardial infarction (current complication) I23.1
    - ventricular (*see also* Defect, ventricular septal) Q21.0
- sinus venosus Q21.1
- speech R47.9
  - developmental F80.9
  - specified NEC R47.89
- Taussig-Bing (aortic transposition and overriding pulmonary artery) Q20.1
- teeth, wedge K03.1
- vascular (local) I99.9
  - congenital Q27.9
- ventricular septal Q21.0
  - concurrent with acute myocardial infarction — *see* Infarct, myocardium
  - following acute myocardial infarction (current complication) I23.2
  - in tetralogy of Fallot Q21.3
- vision NEC H54.7
- visual field H53.40
  - bilateral
    - heteronymous H53.47
    - homonymous H53.46- ☑
  - generalized contraction H53.48- ☑
  - localized
    - arcuate H53.43- ☑
    - scotoma (central area) H53.41- ☑
      - blind spot area H53.42- ☑
    - sector H53.43- ☑

Defect — *continued*
- specified type NEC H53.45- ☑
- voice R49.9
  - specified NEC R49.8
- wedge, tooth, teeth (abrasion) K03.1

Deferentitis N49.1
- gonorrheal (acute) (chronic) A54.23

Defibrination (syndrome) D65
- antepartum — *see* Hemorrhage, antepartum, with coagulation defect, disseminated intravascular coagulation
- following ectopic or molar pregnancy O08.1
- intrapartum O67.0
- newborn P60
- postpartum O72.3

Deficiency, deficient
- 3-beta hydroxysteroid dehydrogenase E25.0
- 5-alpha reductase (with male pseudohermaphroditism) E29.1
- 11-hydroxylase E25.0
- 21-hydroxylase E25.0
- abdominal muscle syndrome Q79.4
- accelerator globulin (Ac G) (blood) D68.2
- AC globulin (congenital) (hereditary) D68.2
  - acquired D68.4
- acid phosphatase E83.39
- activating factor (blood) D68.2
- adenosine deaminase (ADA) D81.3
- aldolase (hereditary) E74.19
- alpha-1-antitrypsin E88.01
- amino-acids E72.9
- anemia — *see* Anemia
- aneurin E51.9
- antibody with
  - hyperimmunoglobulinemia D80.6
  - near-normal immunoglobins D80.6
- antidiuretic hormone E23.2
- anti-hemophilic
  - factor (A) D66
    - B D67
    - C D68.1
  - globulin (AHG) NEC D66
- antithrombin (antithrombin III) D68.59
- ascorbic acid E54
- attention (disorder) (syndrome) F98.8
  - with hyperactivity — *see* Disorder, attention-deficit hyperactivity
- autoprothrombin
  - I D68.2
  - II D67
  - C D68.2
- beta-glucuronidase E76.29
- biotin E53.8
- biotin-dependent carboxylase D81.819
- biotinidase D81.810
- brancher enzyme (amylopectinosis) E74.03
- calciferol E55.9
  - with
    - adult osteomalacia M83.8
    - rickets — *see* Rickets
- calcium (dietary) E58
- calorie, severe E43
  - with marasmus E41
    - and kwashiorkor E42
- cardiac — *see* Insufficiency, myocardial
- carnitine E71.40
  - due to
    - hemodialysis E71.43
    - inborn errors of metabolism E71.42
    - Valproic acid therapy E71.43
  - iatrogenic E71.43
  - muscle palmityltransferase E71.314
  - primary E71.41
  - secondary E71.448
- carotene E50.9
- central nervous system G96.8
- ceruloplasmin (Wilson) E83.01
- choline E53.8
- Christmas factor D67
- chromium E61.4
- clotting (blood) (*see also* Deficiency, coagulation factor) D68.9
- clotting factor NEC (hereditary) (*see also* Deficiency, factor) D68.2
- coagulation NOS D68.9
  - with
    - ectopic pregnancy O08.1
    - molar pregnancy O08.1
  - acquired (any) D68.4
  - antepartum hemorrhage — *see* Hemorrhage, antepartum, with coagulation defect

☑ **Additional character required**

Deficiency — continued
- clotting factor NEC (see also Deficiency, factor) D68.2
  - due to
    - hyperprothrombinemia D68.4
    - liver disease D68.4
    - vitamin K deficiency D68.4
  - newborn, transient P61.6
  - postpartum O72.3
  - specified NEC D68.8
- cognitive F09
- color vision H53.50
  - achromatopsia H53.51
  - acquired H53.52
  - deuteranomaly H53.53
  - protanomaly H53.54
  - specified type NEC H53.59
  - tritanomaly H53.55
- combined glucocorticoid and mineralocorticoid E27.49
- contact factor D68.2
- copper (nutritional) E61.0
- corticoadrenal E27.40
  - primary E27.1
- craniofacial axis Q75.0
- cyanocobalamin E53.8
- C1 esterase inhibitor (C1-INH) D84.1
- debrancher enzyme (limit dextrinosis) E74.03
- dehydrogenase
  - long chain/very long chain acyl CoA E71.310
  - medium chain acyl CoA E71.311
  - short chain acyl CoA E71.312
- diet E63.9
- dihydropyrimidine dehydrogenase (DPD) E88.89
- disaccharidase E73.9
- edema — see Malnutrition, severe
- endocrine E34.9
- energy-supply — see Malnutrition
- enzymes, circulating NEC E88.09
- ergosterol E55.9
  - with
    - adult osteomalacia M83.8
    - rickets — see Rickets
- essential fatty acid (EFA) E63.0
- factor (see also Deficiency, coagulation)
  - Hageman D68.2
  - I (congenital) (hereditary) D68.2
  - II (congenital) (hereditary) D68.2
  - IX (congenital) (functional) (hereditary) (with functional defect) D67
  - multiple (congenital) D68.8
    - acquired D68.4
  - V (congenital) (hereditary) D68.2
  - VII (congenital) (hereditary) D68.2
  - VIII (congenital) (functional) (hereditary) (with functional defect) D66
    - with vascular defect D68.0
  - X (congenital) (hereditary) D68.2
  - XI (congenital) (hereditary) D68.1
  - XII (congenital) (hereditary) D68.2
  - XIII (congenital) (hereditary) D68.2
- femoral, proximal focal (congenital) — see Defect, reduction, lower limb, longitudinal, femur
- fibrin-stabilizing factor (congenital) (hereditary) D68.2
  - acquired D68.4
- fibrinase D68.2
- fibrinogen (congenital) (hereditary) D68.2
  - acquired D65
- folate E53.8
- folic acid E53.8
- foreskin N47.3
- fructokinase E74.11
- fructose 1,6-diphosphatase E74.19
- fructose-1-phosphate aldolase E74.19
- galactokinase E74.29
- galactose-1-phosphate uridyl transferase E74.29
- gammaglobulin in blood D80.1
  - hereditary D80.0
- glass factor D68.2
- glucocorticoid E27.49
  - mineralocorticoid E27.49
- glucose-6-phosphatase E74.01
- glucose-6-phosphate dehydrogenase anemia D55.0
- glucuronyl transferase E80.5
- glycogen synthetase E74.09
- gonadotropin (isolated) E23.0
- growth hormone (idiopathic) (isolated) E23.0
- Hageman factor D68.2
- hemoglobin D64.9
- hepatophosphorylase E74.09

Deficiency — continued
- homogentisate 1,2-dioxygenase E70.29
- hormone
  - anterior pituitary (partial) NEC E23.0
    - growth E23.0
  - growth (isolated) E23.0
  - pituitary E23.0
  - testicular E29.1
- hypoxanthine- (guanine)-phosphoribosyltransferase (HG- PRT) (total H-PRT) E79.1
- immunity D84.9
  - cell-mediated D84.8
    - with thrombocytopenia and eczema D82.0
  - combined D81.9
  - humoral D80.9
  - IgA (secretory) D80.2
  - IgG D80.3
  - IgM D80.4
- immuno — see Immunodeficiency
- immunoglobulin, selective
  - A (IgA) D80.2
  - G (IgG) (subclasses) D80.3
  - M (IgM) D80.4
- inositol (B complex) E53.8
- intrinsic
  - factor (congenital) D51.0
  - sphincter N36.42
    - with urethral hypermobility N36.43
- iodine E61.8
  - congenital syndrome — see Syndrome, iodine-deficiency, congenital
- iron E61.1
  - anemia D50.9
- kalium E87.6
- kappa-light chain D80.8
- labile factor (congenital) (hereditary) D68.2
  - acquired D68.4
- lacrimal fluid (acquired) (see also Syndrome, dry eye)
  - congenital Q10.6
- lactase
  - congenital E73.0
  - secondary E73.1
- Laki-Lorand factor D68.2
- lecithin cholesterol acyltransferase E78.6
- lipocaic K86.8
- lipoprotein (familial) (high density) E78.6
- liver phosphorylase E74.09
- lysosomal alpha-1, 4 glucosidase E74.02
- magnesium E61.2
- major histocompatibility complex
  - class I D81.6
  - class II D81.7
- manganese E61.3
- menadione (vitamin K) E56.1
  - newborn P53
- mental (familial) (hereditary) — see Disability, intellectual
- methylenetetrahydrofolate reductase (MTHFR) E72.12
- mineral NEC E61.8
- mineralocorticoid E27.49
  - with glucocorticoid E27.49
- molybdenum (nutritional) E61.5
- moral F60.2
- multiple nutrient elements E61.7
- muscle
  - carnitine (palmityltransferase) E71.314
  - phosphofructokinase E74.09
- myoadenylate deaminase E79.2
- myocardial — see Insufficiency, myocardial
- myophosphorylase E74.04
- NADH diaphorase or reductase (congenital) D74.0
- NADH-methemoglobin reductase (congenital) D74.0
- natrium E87.1
- niacin (amide) (-tryptophan) E52
- nicotinamide E52
- nicotinic acid E52
- number of teeth — see Anodontia
- nutrient element E61.9
  - multiple E61.7
  - specified NEC E61.8
- nutrition, nutritional E63.9
  - sequelae — see Sequelae, nutritional deficiency
  - specified NEC E63.8
- ornithine transcarbamylase E72.4
- ovarian E28.39
- oxygen — see Anoxia
- pantothenic acid E53.8

Deficiency — continued
- parathyroid (gland) E20.9
- perineum (female) N81.89
- phenylalanine hydroxylase E70.1
- phosphoenolpyruvate carboxykinase E74.4
- phosphofructokinase E74.19
- phosphomannomutase E74.8
- phosphomannose isomerase E74.8
- phosphomannosyl mutase E74.8
- phosphorylase kinase, liver E74.09
- pituitary hormone (isolated) E23.0
- plasma thromboplastin
  - antecedent (PTA) D68.1
  - component (PTC) D67
- platelet NEC D69.1
  - constitutional D68.0
- polyglandular E31.8
  - autoimmune E31.0
- potassium (K) E87.6
- prepuce N47.3
- proaccelerin (congenital) (hereditary) D68.2
  - acquired D68.4
- proconvertin factor (congenital) (hereditary) D68.2
  - acquired D68.4
- protein (see also Malnutrition) E46
  - anemia D53.0
  - C D68.59
  - S D68.59
- prothrombin (congenital) (hereditary) D68.2
  - acquired D68.4
- Prower factor D68.2
- pseudocholinesterase E88.09
- PTA (plasma thromboplastin antecedent) D68.1
- PTC (plasma thromboplastin component) D67
- purine nucleoside phosphorylase (PNP) D81.5
- pyracin (alpha) (beta) E53.1
- pyridoxal E53.1
- pyridoxamine E53.1
- pyridoxine (derivatives) E53.1
- pyruvate
  - carboxylase E74.4
  - dehydrogenase E74.4
- riboflavin (vitamin B2) E53.0
- salt E87.1
- secretion
  - ovary E28.39
  - salivary gland (any) K11.7
  - urine R34
- selenium (dietary) E59
- serum antitrypsin, familial E88.01
- short stature homeobox gene (SHOX)
  - with
    - dyschondrosteosis Q78.8
    - short stature (idiopathic) E34.3
    - Turner's syndrome Q96.9
- sodium (Na) E87.1
- SPCA (factor VII) D68.2
- sphincter, intrinsic N36.42
  - with urethral hypermobility N36.43
- stable factor (congenital) (hereditary) D68.2
  - acquired D68.4
- Stuart-Prower (factor X) D68.2
- sucrase E74.39
- sulfatase E75.29
- sulfite oxidase E72.19
- thiamin, thiaminic (chloride) E51.9
  - beriberi (dry) E51.11
    - wet E51.12
- thrombokinase D68.2
  - newborn P53
- thyroid (gland) — see Hypothyroidism
- tocopherol E56.0
- tooth bud K00.0
- transcobalamine II (anemia) D51.2
- vanadium E61.6
- vascular I99.9
- vasopressin E23.2
- viosterol — see Deficiency, calciferol
- vitamin (multiple) NOS E56.9
  - A E50.9
    - with
      - Bitot's spot (corneal) E50.1
      - follicular keratosis E50.8
      - keratomalacia E50.4
      - manifestations NEC E50.8
      - night blindness E50.5
      - scar of cornea, xerophthalmic E50.6
      - xeroderma E50.8
      - xerophthalmia E50.7
      - xerosis
        - conjunctival E50.0

Deficiency — *continued*
    and Bitot's spot E50.1
    cornea E50.2
        and ulceration E50.3
    sequelae E64.1
    B (complex) NOS E53.9
        with
            beriberi (dry) E51.11
                wet E51.12
            pellagra E52
    B1 NOS E51.9
        beriberi (dry) E51.11
            with circulatory system manifestations
                E51.11
            wet E51.12
    B12 E53.8
    B2 (riboflavin) E53.0
    B6 E53.1
    C E54
        sequelae E64.2
    D E55.9
        with
            adult osteomalacia M83.8
            rickets — *see* Rickets
        25-hydroxylase E83.32
    E E56.0
    folic acid E53.8
    G E53.0
    group B E53.9
        specified NEC E53.8
    H (biotin) E53.8
    K E56.1
        of newborn P53
    nicotinic E52
    P E56.8
    PP (pellagra-preventing) E52
    specified NEC E56.8
    thiamin E51.9
        beriberi — *see* Beriberi
    zinc, dietary E60
Deficit (*see also* Deficiency)
    attention and concentration R41.840
        disorder — *see* Attention, deficit
    cognitive communication R41.841
    cognitive NEC R41.89
        following
            cerebral infarction I69.31
            cerebrovascular disease I69.91
                specified disease NEC I69.81
            intracerebral hemorrhage I69.11
            nontraumatic intracranial hemorrhage NEC
                I69.21
            subarachnoid hemorrhage I69.01
    concentration R41.840
    executive function R41.844
    frontal lobe R41.844
    neurologic NEC R29.818
        ischemic
            reversible (RIND) I63.9
                prolonged (PRIND) I63.9
    oxygen R09.02
    prolonged reversible ischemic neurologic
        (PRIND) I63.9
    psychomotor R41.843
    visuospatial R41.842
Deflection
    radius — *see* Deformity, limb, specified type NEC,
        forearm
    septum (acquired) (nasal) (nose) J34.2
    spine — *see* Curvature, spine
    turbinate (nose) J34.2
Defluvium
    capillorum — *see* Alopecia
    ciliorum — *see* Madarosis
    unguium L60.8
Deformity Q89.9
    abdomen, congenital Q89.9
    abdominal wall
        acquired M95.8
        congenital Q79.59
    acquired (unspecified site) M95.9
    adrenal gland Q89.1
    alimentary tract, congenital Q45.9
        upper Q40.9
    ankle (joint) (acquired) (*see also* Deformity, limb,
        lower leg)
        abduction — *see* Contraction, joint, ankle
        congenital Q68.8
        contraction — *see* Contraction, joint, ankle
        specified type NEC — *see* Deformity, limb, foot,
            specified NEC
    anus (acquired) K62.89

Deformity — *continued*
    congenital Q43.9
    aorta (arch) (congenital) Q25.4
        acquired I77.89
    aortic
        arch, acquired I77.89
        cusp or valve (congenital) Q23.8
            acquired (*see also* Endocarditis, aortic) I35.8
    arm (acquired) (upper) (*see also* Deformity, limb,
        upper arm)
        congenital Q68.8
        forearm — *see* Deformity, limb, forearm
    artery (congenital) (peripheral) NOS Q27.9
        acquired I77.89
        coronary (acquired) I25.9
            congenital Q24.5
        umbilical Q27.0
    atrial septal Q21.1
    auditory canal (external) (congenital) (*see also*
        Malformation, ear, external)
        acquired — *see* Disorder, ear, external, specified
            type NEC
    auricle
        ear (congenital) (*see also* Malformation, ear,
            external)
            acquired — *see* Disorder, pinna, deformity
    back — *see* Dorsopathy, deforming
    bile duct (common) (congenital) (hepatic) Q44.5
        acquired K83.8
    biliary duct or passage (congenital) Q44.5
        acquired K83.8
    bladder (neck) (trigone) (sphincter) (acquired)
        N32.89
        congenital Q64.79
    bone (acquired) NOS M95.9
        congenital Q79.9
        turbinate M95.0
    brain (congenital) Q04.9
        acquired G93.89
        reduction Q04.3
    breast (acquired) N64.89
        congenital Q83.9
        reconstructed N65.0
    bronchus (congenital) Q32.4
        acquired NEC J98.09
    bursa, congenital Q79.9
    canaliculi (lacrimalis) (acquired) (*see also* Disorder,
        lacrimal system, changes)
        congenital Q10.6
    canthus, acquired — *see* Disorder, eyelid,
        specified type NEC
    capillary (acquired) I78.8
    cardiovascular system, congenital Q28.9
    caruncle, lacrimal (acquired) (*see also* Disorder,
        lacrimal system, changes)
        congenital Q10.6
    cascade, stomach K31.2
    cecum (congenital) Q43.9
        acquired K63.89
    cerebral, acquired G93.89
        congenital Q04.9
    cervix (uterus) (acquired) NEC N88.8
        congenital Q51.9
    cheek (acquired) M95.2
        congenital Q18.9
    chest (acquired) (wall) M95.4
        congenital Q67.8
        sequelae (late effect) of rickets E64.3
    chin (acquired) M95.2
        congenital Q18.9
    choroid (congenital) Q14.3
        acquired H31.8
        plexus Q07.8
            acquired G96.19
    cicatricial — *see* Cicatrix
    cilia, acquired — *see* Disorder, eyelid, specified
        type NEC
    clavicle (acquired) M95.8
        congenital Q68.8
    clitoris (congenital) Q52.6
        acquired N90.89
    clubfoot — *see* Clubfoot
    coccyx (acquired) M43.8
    colon (congenital) Q43.9
        acquired K63.89
    concha (ear), congenital (*see also* Malformation,
        ear, external)
        acquired — *see* Disorder, pinna, deformity
    cornea (acquired) H18.70
        congenital Q13.4
        descemetocele — *see* Descemetocele
        ectasia — *see* Ectasia, cornea

Deformity — *continued*
    specified NEC H18.79- ☑
    staphyloma — *see* Staphyloma, cornea
    coronary artery (acquired) I25.9
        congenital Q24.5
    cranium (acquired) — *see* Deformity, skull
    cricoid cartilage (congenital) Q31.8
        acquired J38.7
    cystic duct (congenital) Q44.5
        acquired K82.8
    Dandy-Walker Q03.1
        with spina bifida — *see* Spina bifida
    diaphragm (congenital) Q79.1
        acquired J98.6
    digestive organ NOS Q45.9
    ductus arteriosus Q25.0
    duodenal bulb K31.89
    duodenum (congenital) Q43.9
        acquired K31.89
    dura — *see* Deformity, meninges
    ear (acquired) (*see also* Disorder, pinna,
        deformity)
        congenital (external) Q17.9
            internal Q16.5
            middle Q16.4
                ossicles Q16.3
            ossicles Q16.3
    ectodermal (congenital) NEC Q84.9
    ejaculatory duct (congenital) Q55.4
        acquired N50.8
    elbow (joint) (acquired) (*see also* Deformity, limb,
        upper arm)
        congenital Q68.8
        contraction — *see* Contraction, joint, elbow
    endocrine gland NEC Q89.2
    epididymis (congenital) Q55.4
        acquired N50.8
    epiglottis (congenital) Q31.8
        acquired J38.7
    esophagus (congenital) Q39.9
        acquired K22.8
    eustachian tube (congenital) NEC Q17.8
    eye, congenital Q15.9
    eyebrow (congenital) Q18.8
    eyelid (acquired) (*see also* Disorder, eyelid,
        specified type NEC)
        congenital Q10.3
    face (acquired) M95.2
        congenital Q18.9
    fallopian tube, acquired N83.8
    femur (acquired) — *see* Deformity, limb, specified
        type NEC, thigh
    fetal
        with fetopelvic disproportion O33.7
        causing obstructed labor O66.3
    finger (acquired) M20.00- ☑
        boutonniere M20.02- ☑
        congenital Q68.1
        flexion contracture — *see* Contraction, joint,
            hand
        mallet finger M20.01- ☑
        specified NEC M20.09- ☑
        swan-neck M20.03- ☑
    flexion (joint) (acquired) (*see also* Deformity, limb,
        flexion) M21.20
        congenital NOS Q74.9
        hip Q65.89
    foot (acquired) (*see also* Deformity, limb, lower
        leg)
        cavovarus (congenital) Q66.1
        congenital NOS Q66.9
            specified type NEC Q66.89
        specified type NEC — *see* Deformity, limb, foot,
            specified NEC
        valgus (congenital) Q66.6
            acquired — *see* Deformity, valgus, ankle
        varus (congenital) NEC Q66.3
            acquired — *see* Deformity, varus, ankle
    forearm (acquired) (*see also* Deformity, limb,
        forearm)
        congenital Q68.8
    forehead (acquired) M95.2
        congenital Q75.8
    frontal bone (acquired) M95.2
        congenital Q75.8
    gallbladder (congenital) Q44.1
        acquired K82.8
    gastrointestinal tract (congenital) NOS Q45.9
        acquired K63.89
    genitalia, genital organ (s) or system NEC
        female (congenital) Q52.9
            acquired N94.89

☑ **Additional character required**

Deformity — *continued*
    external Q52.70
        male (congenital) Q55.9
            acquired N50.8
    globe (eye) (congenital) Q15.8
        acquired H44.89
    gum, acquired NEC K06.8
    hand (acquired) — *see* Deformity, limb, hand
        congenital Q68.1
    head (acquired) M95.2
        congenital Q75.8
    heart (congenital) Q24.9
        septum Q21.9
            auricular Q21.1
            ventricular Q21.0
        valve (congenital) NEC Q24.8
            acquired — *see* Endocarditis
    heel (acquired) — *see* Deformity, foot
    hepatic duct (congenital) Q44.5
        acquired K83.8
    hip (joint) (acquired) (*see also* Deformity, limb, thigh)
        congenital Q65.9
        due to (previous) juvenile osteochondrosis — *see* Coxa, plana
        flexion — *see* Contraction, joint, hip
    hourglass — *see* Contraction, hourglass
    humerus (acquired) M21.82- ☑
        congenital Q74.0
    hypophyseal (congenital) Q89.2
    ileocecal (coil) (valve) (acquired) K63.89
        congenital Q43.9
    ileum (congenital) Q43.9
        acquired K63.89
    ilium (acquired) M95.5
        congenital Q74.2
    integument (congenital) Q84.9
    intervertebral cartilage or disc (acquired) — *see* Disorder, disc, specified NEC
    intestine (large) (small) (congenital) NOS Q43.9
        acquired K63.89
    intrinsic minus or plus (hand) — *see* Deformity, limb, specified type NEC, forearm
    iris (acquired) H21.89
        congenital Q13.2
    ischium (acquired) M95.5
        congenital Q74.2
    jaw (acquired) (congenital) M26.9
    joint (acquired) NEC M21.90
        congenital Q68.8
        elbow M21.92- ☑
        hand M21.94- ☑
        hip M21.95- ☑
        knee M21.96- ☑
        shoulder M21.92- ☑
        wrist M21.93- ☑
    kidney (s) (calyx) (pelvis) (congenital) Q63.9
        acquired N28.89
        artery (congenital) Q27.2
            acquired I77.89
    Klippel-Feil (brevicollis) Q76.1
    knee (acquired) NEC (*see also* Deformity, limb, lower leg)
        congenital Q68.2
    labium (majus) (minus) (congenital) Q52.79
        acquired N90.89
    lacrimal passages or duct (congenital) NEC Q10.6
        acquired — *see* Disorder, lacrimal system, changes
    larynx (muscle) (congenital) Q31.8
        acquired J38.7
        web (glottic) Q31.0
    leg (upper) (acquired) NEC (*see also* Deformity, limb, thigh)
        congenital Q68.8
        lower leg — *see* Deformity, limb, lower leg
    lens (acquired) H27.8
        congenital Q12.9
    lid (fold) (acquired) (*see also* Disorder, eyelid, specified type NEC)
        congenital Q10.3
    ligament (acquired) — *see* Disorder, ligament
        congenital Q79.9
    limb (acquired) M21.90
        clawfoot M21.53- ☑
        clawhand M21.51- ☑
        clubfoot M21.54- ☑
        clubhand M21.52- ☑
        congenital, except reduction deformity Q74.9
        flat foot M21.4- ☑
        flexion M21.20
            ankle M21.27- ☑

Deformity — *continued*
        elbow M21.22- ☑
        finger M21.24- ☑
        hip M21.25- ☑
        knee M21.26- ☑
        shoulder M21.21- ☑
        toe M21.27- ☑
        wrist M21.23- ☑
        foot
            claw — *see* Deformity, limb, clawfoot
            club — *see* Deformity, limb, clubfoot
            drop M21.37- ☑
            flat — *see* Deformity, limb, flat foot
            specified NEC M21.6X- ☑
        forearm M21.93- ☑
        hand M21.94- ☑
        lower leg M21.96- ☑
        specified type NEC M21.80
            forearm M21.83- ☑
            lower leg M21.86- ☑
            thigh M21.85- ☑
            upper arm M21.82- ☑
        thigh M21.95- ☑
        unequal length M21.70
            short site is
                femur M21.75- ☑
                fibula M21.76- ☑
                humerus M21.72- ☑
                radius M21.73- ☑
                tibia M21.76- ☑
                ulna M21.73- ☑
        upper arm M21.92- ☑
        valgus — *see* Deformity, valgus
        varus — *see* Deformity, varus
        wrist drop M21.33- ☑
    lip (acquired) NEC K13.0
        congenital Q38.0
    liver (congenital) Q44.7
        acquired K76.89
    lumbosacral (congenital) (joint) (region) Q76.49
        acquired M43.8
        kyphosis — *see* Kyphosis, congenital
        lordosis — *see* Lordosis, congenital
    lung (congenital) Q33.9
        acquired J98.4
    lymphatic system, congenital Q89.9
    Madelung's (radius) Q74.0
    mandible (acquired) (congenital) M26.9
    maxilla (acquired) (congenital) M26.9
    meninges or membrane (congenital) Q07.9
        cerebral Q04.8
            acquired G96.19
        spinal cord (congenital) G96.19
            acquired G96.19
    metacarpus (acquired) — *see* Deformity, limb, forearm
        congenital Q74.0
    metatarsus (acquired) — *see* Deformity, foot
        congenital Q66.9
    middle ear (congenital) Q16.4
        ossicles Q16.3
    mitral (leaflets) (valve) I05.8
        parachute Q23.2
        stenosis, congenital Q23.2
    mouth (acquired) K13.79
        congenital Q38.6
    multiple, congenital NEC Q89.7
    muscle (acquired) M62.89
        congenital Q79.9
        sternocleidomastoid Q68.0
    musculoskeletal system (acquired) M95.9
        congenital Q79.9
        specified NEC M95.8
    nail (acquired) L60.8
        congenital Q84.6
    nasal — *see* Deformity, nose
    neck (acquired) M95.3
        congenital Q18.9
        sternocleidomastoid Q68.0
    nervous system (congenital) Q07.9
    nipple (congenital) Q83.9
        acquired N64.89
    nose (acquired) (cartilage) M95.0
        bone (turbinate) M95.0
        congenital Q30.9
            bent or squashed Q67.4
        saddle M95.0
            syphilitic A50.57
        septum (acquired) J34.2
            congenital Q30.8
        sinus (wall) (congenital) Q30.8
            acquired M95.0

Deformity — *continued*
    syphilitic (congenital) A50.57
        late A52.73
    ocular muscle (congenital) Q10.3
        acquired — *see* Strabismus, mechanical
    opticociliary vessels (congenital) Q13.2
    orbit (eye) (acquired) H05.30
        atrophy — *see* Atrophy, orbit
        congenital Q10.7
        due to
            bone disease NEC H05.32- ☑
            trauma or surgery H05.33- ☑
        enlargement — *see* Enlargement, orbit
        exostosis — *see* Exostosis, orbit
    organ of Corti (congenital) Q16.5
    ovary (congenital) Q50.39
        acquired N83.8
    oviduct, acquired N83.8
    palate (congenital) Q38.5
        acquired M27.8
        cleft (congenital) — *see* Cleft, palate
    pancreas (congenital) Q45.3
        acquired K86.8
    parathyroid (gland) Q89.2
    parotid (gland) (congenital) Q38.4
        acquired K11.8
    patella (acquired) — *see* Disorder, patella, specified NEC
    pelvis, pelvic (acquired) (bony) M95.5
        with disproportion (fetopelvic) O33.0
            causing obstructed labor O65.0
        congenital Q74.2
        rachitic sequelae (late effect) E64.3
    penis (glans) (congenital) Q55.69
        acquired N48.89
    pericardium (congenital) Q24.8
        acquired — *see* Pericarditis
    pharynx (congenital) Q38.8
        acquired J39.2
    pinna, acquired (*see also* Disorder, pinna, deformity)
        congenital Q17.9
    pituitary (congenital) Q89.2
    posture — *see* Dorsopathy, deforming
    prepuce (congenital) Q55.69
        acquired N47.8
    prostate (congenital) Q55.4
        acquired N42.89
    pupil (congenital) Q13.2
        acquired — *see* Abnormality, pupillary
    pylorus (congenital) Q40.3
        acquired K31.89
    rachitic (acquired), old or healed E64.3
    radius (acquired) (*see also* Deformity, limb, forearm)
        congenital Q68.8
    rectum (congenital) Q43.9
        acquired K62.89
    reduction (extremity) (limb), congenital (*see also* condition and site) Q73.8
        brain Q04.3
        lower — *see* Defect, reduction, lower limb
        upper — *see* Defect, reduction, upper limb
        renal — *see* Deformity, kidney
    respiratory system (congenital) Q34.9
    rib (acquired) M95.4
        congenital Q76.6
        cervical Q76.5
    rotation (joint) (acquired) — *see* Deformity, limb, specified site NEC
        congenital Q74.9
        hip — *see* Deformity, limb, specified type NEC, thigh
            congenital Q65.89
    sacroiliac joint (congenital) Q74.2
        acquired M43.8
    sacrum (acquired) M43.8
    saddle
        back — *see* Lordosis
        nose M95.0
            syphilitic A50.57
    salivary gland or duct (congenital) Q38.4
        acquired K11.8
    scapula (acquired) M95.8
        congenital Q68.8
    scrotum (congenital) (*see also* Malformation, testis and scrotum)
        acquired N50.8
    seminal vesicles (congenital) Q55.4
        acquired N50.8
    septum, nasal (acquired) J34.2

Deformity — *continued*
shoulder (joint) (acquired) — *see* Deformity, limb, upper arm
congenital Q74.0
contraction — *see* Contraction, joint, shoulder
sigmoid (flexure) (congenital) Q43.9
acquired K63.89
skin (congenital) Q82.9
skull (acquired) M95.2
congenital Q75.8
with
anencephaly Q00.0
encephalocele — *see* Encephalocele
hydrocephalus Q03.9
with spina bifida — *see* Spina bifida, by site, with hydrocephalus
microcephaly Q02
soft parts, organs or tissues (of pelvis)
in pregnancy or childbirth NEC O34.8- ☑
causing obstructed labor O65.5
spermatic cord (congenital) Q55.4
acquired N50.8
torsion — *see* Torsion, spermatic cord
spinal — *see* Dorsopathy, deforming
column (acquired) — *see* Dorsopathy, deforming
congenital Q67.5
cord (congenital) Q06.9
acquired G95.89
nerve root (congenital) Q07.9
spine (acquired) (*see also* Dorsopathy, deforming)
congenital Q67.5
rachitic E64.3
specified NEC — *see* Dorsopathy, deforming, specified NEC
spleen
acquired D73.89
congenital Q89.09
Sprengel's (congenital) Q74.0
sternocleidomastoid (muscle), congenital Q68.0
sternum (acquired) M95.4
congenital NEC Q76.7
stomach (congenital) Q40.3
acquired K31.89
submandibular gland (congenital) Q38.4
submaxillary gland (congenital) Q38.4
acquired K11.8
talipes — *see* Talipes
testis (congenital) (*see also* Malformation, testis and scrotum)
acquired N44.8
torsion — *see* Torsion, testis
thigh (acquired) (*see also* Deformity, limb, thigh)
congenital NEC Q68.8
thorax (acquired) (wall) M95.4
congenital Q67.8
sequelae of rickets E64.3
thumb (acquired) (*see also* Deformity, finger)
congenital NEC Q68.1
thymus (tissue) (congenital) Q89.2
thyroid (gland) (congenital) Q89.2
cartilage Q31.8
acquired J38.7
tibia (acquired) (*see also* Deformity, limb, specified type NEC, lower leg)
congenital NEC Q68.8
saber (syphilitic) A50.56
toe (acquired) M20.6- ☑
congenital Q66.9
hallux rigidus M20.2- ☑
hallux valgus M20.1- ☑
hallux varus M20.3- ☑
hammer toe M20.4- ☑
specified NEC M20.5X- ☑
tongue (congenital) Q38.3
acquired K14.8
tooth, teeth K00.2
trachea (rings) (congenital) Q32.1
acquired J39.8
transverse aortic arch (congenital) Q25.4
tricuspid (leaflets) (valve) I07.8
atresia or stenosis Q22.4
Ebstein's Q22.5
trunk (acquired) M95.8
congenital Q89.9
ulna (acquired) (*see also* Deformity, limb, forearm)
congenital NEC Q68.8
urachus, congenital Q64.4
ureter (opening) (congenital) Q62.8
acquired N28.89
urethra (congenital) Q64.79

Deformity — *continued*
acquired N36.8
urinary tract (congenital) Q64.9
urachus Q64.4
uterus (congenital) Q51.9
acquired N85.8
uvula (congenital) Q38.5
vagina (acquired) N89.8
congenital Q52.4
valgus NEC M21.00
ankle M21.07- ☑
elbow M21.02- ☑
hip M21.05- ☑
knee M21.06- ☑
valve, valvular (congenital) (heart) Q24.8
acquired — *see* Endocarditis
varus NEC M21.10
ankle M21.17- ☑
elbow M21.12- ☑
hip M21.15 ☑
knee M21.16- ☑
tibia — *see* Osteochondrosis, juvenile, tibia
vas deferens (congenital) Q55.4
acquired N50.8
vein (congenital) Q27.9
great Q26.9
vertebra — *see* Dorsopathy, deforming
vertical talus (congenital) Q66.80
left foot Q66.82
right foot Q66.81
vesicourethral orifice (acquired) N32.89
congenital NEC Q64.79
vessels of optic papilla (congenital) Q14.2
visual field (contraction) — *see* Defect, visual field
vitreous body, acquired H43.89
vulva (congenital) Q52.79
acquired N90.89
wrist (joint) (acquired) (*see also* Deformity, limb, forearm)
congenital Q68.8
contraction *see* Contraction, joint, wrist
Degeneration, degenerative
adrenal (capsule) (fatty) (gland) (hyaline) (infectional) E27.8
amyloid (*see also* Amyloidosis) E85.9
anterior cornua, spinal cord G12.29
anterior labral S43.49- ☑
aorta, aortic I70.0
fatty I77.89
aortic valve (heart) — *see* Endocarditis, aortic
arteriovascular — *see* Arteriosclerosis
artery, arterial (atheromatous) (calcareous) (*see also* Arteriosclerosis)
cerebral, amyloid E85.4 [I68.0]
medial — *see* Arteriosclerosis, extremities
articular cartilage NEC — *see* Derangement, joint, articular cartilage, by site
atheromatous — *see* Arteriosclerosis
basal nuclei or ganglia G23.9
specified NEC G23.8
bone NEC — *see* Disorder, bone, specified type NEC
brachial plexus G54.0
brain (cortical) (progressive) G31.9
alcoholic G31.2
arteriosclerotic I67.2
childhood G31.9
specified NEC G31.89
cystic G31.89
congenital Q04.6
in
alcoholism G31.2
beriberi E51.2
cerebrovascular disease I67.9
congenital hydrocephalus Q03.9
with spina bifida (*see also* Spina bifida)
Fabry-Anderson disease E75.21
Gaucher's disease E75.22
Hunter's syndrome E76.1
lipidosis
cerebral E75.4
generalized E75.6
mucopolysaccharidosis — *see* Mucopolysaccharidosis
myxedema E03.9 [G32.89]
neoplastic disease (*see also* Neoplasm) D49.6 [G32.89]
Niemann-Pick disease E75.249 [G32.89]
sphingolipidosis E75.3 [G32.89]
vitamin B12 deficiency E53.8 [G32.89]
senile NEC G31.1
breast N64.89

Degeneration — *continued*
Bruch's membrane — *see* Degeneration, choroid
capillaries (fatty) I78.8
amyloid E85.8 [I79.8]
cardiac (*see also* Degeneration, myocardial)
valve, valvular — *see* Endocarditis
cardiorenal — *see* Hypertension, cardiorenal
cardiovascular (*see also* Disease, cardiovascular)
renal — *see* Hypertension, cardiorenal
cerebellar NOS G31.9
alcoholic G31.2
primary (hereditary) (sporadic) G11.9
cerebral — *see* Degeneration, brain
cerebrovascular I67.9
due to hypertension I67.4
cervical plexus G54.2
cervix N88.8
due to radiation (intended effect) N88.8
adverse effect or misadventure N99.89
chamber angle H21.21- ☑
changes, spine or vertebra — *see* Spondylosis
chorioretinal (*see also* Degeneration, choroid)
hereditary H31.20
choroid (colloid) (drusen) H31.10- ☑
atrophy — *see* Atrophy, choroidal
hereditary — *see* Dystrophy, choroidal, hereditary
ciliary body H21.22- ☑
cochlear H83.8
combined (spinal cord) (subacute) E53.8 [G32.0]
with anemia (pernicious) D51.0 [G32.0]
due to dietary vitamin B12 deficiency D51.3 [G32.0]
in (due to)
vitamin B12 deficiency E53.8 [G32.0]
anemia D51.9 [G32.0]
conjunctiva H11.10
concretions — *see* Concretion, conjunctiva
deposits — *see* Deposit, conjunctiva
pigmentations — *see* Pigmentation, conjunctiva
pinguecula — *see* Pinguecula
xerosis — *see* Xerosis, conjunctiva
cornea H18.40
calcerous H18.43
band keratopathy H18.42- ☑
familial, hereditary — *see* Dystrophy, cornea
hyaline (of old scars) H18.49
keratomalacia — *see* Keratomalacia
nodular H18.45- ☑
peripheral H18.46- ☑
senile H18.41- ☑
specified type NEC H18.49
cortical (cerebellar) (parenchymatous) G31.89
alcoholic G31.2
diffuse, due to arteriopathy I67.2
corticobasal G31.85
cutis L98.8
amyloid E85.4 [L99]
dental pulp K04.2
disc disease — *see* Degeneration, intervertebral disc NEC
dorsolateral (spinal cord) — *see* Degeneration, combined
extrapyramidal G25.9
eye, macular (*see also* Degeneration, macula)
congenital or hereditary — *see* Dystrophy, retina
facet joints — *see* Spondylosis
fatty
liver NEC K76.0
alcoholic K70.0
grey matter (brain) (Alpers') G31.81
heart (*see also* Degeneration, myocardial)
amyloid E85.4 [I43]
atheromatous — *see* Disease, heart, ischemic, atherosclerotic
ischemic — *see* Disease, heart, ischemic
hepatolenticular (Wilson's) E83.01
hepatorenal K76.7
hyaline (diffuse) (generalized)
localized — *see* Degeneration, by site
infrapatellar fat pad M79.4
intervertebral disc NOS
with
myelopathy — *see* Disorder, disc, with, myelopathy
radiculitis or radiculopathy — *see* Disorder, disc, with, radiculopathy
cervical, cervicothoracic — *see* Disorder, disc, cervical, degeneration
with

☑ **Additional character required**

Degeneration — *continued*
   myelopathy — *see* Disorder, disc, cervical, with myelopathy
   neuritis, radiculitis or radiculopathy — *see* Disorder, disc, cervical, with neuritis
   lumbar region M51.36
     with
       myelopathy M51.06
       neuritis, radiculitis, radiculopathy or sciatica M51.16
   lumbosacral region M51.37
     with
       neuritis, radiculitis, radiculopathy or sciatica M51.17
   sacrococcygeal region M53.3
   thoracic region M51.34
     with
       myelopathy M51.04
       neuritis, radiculitis, radiculopathy M51.14
   thoracolumbar region M51.35
     with
       myelopathy M51.05
       neuritis, radiculitis, radiculopathy or M51.15
   intestine, amyloid E85.4
   iris (pigmentary) H21.23- ☑
   ischemic — *see* Ischemia
   joint disease — *see* Osteoarthritis
   kidney N28.89
     amyloid E85.4 [N29]
     cystic, congenital Q61.9
     fatty N28.89
     polycystic Q61.3
       adult type (autosomal dominant) Q61.2
       infantile type (autosomal recessive) NEC Q61.19
         collecting duct dilatation Q61.11
   Kuhnt-Junius (*see also* Degeneration, macula) H35.32
   lens — *see* Cataract
   lenticular (familial) (progressive) (Wilson's) (with cirrhosis of liver) E83.01
   liver (diffuse) NEC K76.89
     amyloid E85.4 [K77]
     cystic K76.89
       congenital Q44.6
     fatty NEC K76.0
       alcoholic K70.0
     hypertrophic K76.89
     parenchymatous, acute or subacute K72.00
       with coma K72.01
     pigmentary K76.89
     toxic (acute) K71.9
   lung J98.4
   lymph gland I89.8
     hyaline I89.8
   macula, macular (acquired) (age-related) (senile) H35.30
     angioid streaks H35.33
     atrophic age-related H35.31
     congenital or hereditary — *see* Dystrophy, retina
     cystoid H35.35- ☑
     drusen H35.36- ☑
     exudative H35.32
     hole H35.34- ☑
     nonexudative H35.31
     puckering H35.37- ☑
     toxic H35.38- ☑
   membranous labyrinth, congenital (causing impairment of hearing) Q16.5
   meniscus — *see* Derangement, meniscus
   mitral — *see* Insufficiency, mitral
   Mönckeberg's — *see* Arteriosclerosis, extremities
   motor centers, senile G31.1
   multi-system G90.3
   mural — *see* Degeneration, myocardial
   muscle (fatty) (fibrous) (hyaline) (progressive) M62.89
     heart — *see* Degeneration, myocardial
   myelin, central nervous system G37.9
   myocardial, myocardium (fatty) (hyaline) (senile) I51.5
     with rheumatic fever (conditions in I00) I09.0
       active, acute or subacute I01.2
         with chorea I02.0
       inactive or quiescent (with chorea) I09.0
     hypertensive — *see* Hypertension, heart
     rheumatic — *see* Degeneration, myocardial, with rheumatic fever
     syphilitic A52.06
   nasal sinus (mucosa) J32.9
     frontal J32.1

Degeneration — *continued*
   maxillary J32.0
   nerve — *see* Disorder, nerve
   nervous system G31.9
     alcoholic G31.2
     amyloid E85.4 [G99.8]
     autonomic G90.9
     fatty G31.89
     specified NEC G31.89
   nipple N64.89
   olivopontocerebellar (hereditary) (familial) G23.8
   osseous labyrinth H83.8
   ovary N83.8
     cystic N83.20
     microcystic N83.20
   pallidal pigmentary (progressive) G23.0
   pancreas K86.8
     tuberculous A18.83
   penis N48.89
   pigmentary (diffuse) (general)
     localized — *see* Degeneration, by site
     pallidal (progressive) G23.0
   pineal gland E34.8
   pituitary (gland) E23.6
   popliteal fat pad M79.4
   posterolateral (spinal cord) — *see* Degeneration, combined
   pulmonary valve (heart) I37.8
   pulp (tooth) K04.2
   pupillary margin H21.24- ☑
   renal — *see* Degeneration, kidney
   retina H35.9
     hereditary (cerebroretinal) (congenital) (juvenile) (macula) (peripheral) (pigmentary) — *see* Dystrophy, retina
     Kuhnt-Junius (*see also* Degeneration, macula) H35.32
     macula (cystic) (exudative) (hole) (nonexudative) (pseudohole) (senile) (toxic) — *see* Degeneration, macula
     peripheral H35.40
       lattice H35.41- ☑
       microcystoid H35.42- ☑
       paving stone H35.43- ☑
       secondary
         pigmentary H35.45- ☑
         vitreoretinal H35.46- ☑
       senile reticular H35.44- ☑
     pigmentary (primary) (*see also* Dystrophy, retina)
     secondary — *see* Degeneration, retina, peripheral, secondary
     posterior pole — *see* Degeneration, macula
   saccule, congenital (causing impairment of hearing) Q16.5
   senile R54
     brain G31.1
     cardiac, heart or myocardium — *see* Degeneration, myocardial
     motor centers G31.1
     vascular — *see* Arteriosclerosis
   sinus (cystic) (*see also* Sinusitis)
     polypoid J33.1
   skin L98.8
     amyloid E85.4 [L99]
     colloid L98.8
   spinal (cord) G31.89
     amyloid E85.4 [G32.89]
     combined (subacute) — *see* Degeneration, combined
     dorsolateral — *see* Degeneration, combined
     familial NEC G31.89
     fatty G31.89
     funicular — *see* Degeneration, combined
     posterolateral — *see* Degeneration, combined
     subacute combined — *see* Degeneration, combined
     tuberculous A17.81
   spleen D73.0
     amyloid E85.4 [D77]
   stomach K31.89
   striatonigral G23.2
   suprarenal (capsule) (gland) E27.8
   synovial membrane (pulpy) — *see* Disorder, synovium, specified type NEC
   tapetoretinal — *see* Dystrophy, retina
   thymus (gland) E32.8
     fatty E32.8
   thyroid (gland) E07.89
   tricuspid (heart) (valve) I07.9
   tuberculous NEC — *see* Tuberculosis
   turbinate J34.89

Degeneration — *continued*
   uterus (cystic) N85.8
   vascular (senile) — *see* Arteriosclerosis
     hypertensive — *see* Hypertension
   vitreoretinal, secondary — *see* Degeneration, retina, peripheral, secondary, vitreoretinal
   vitreous (body) H43.81- ☑
   Wallerian — *see* Disorder, nerve
   Wilson's hepatolenticular E83.01
Deglutition
   paralysis R13.0
     hysterical F44.4
   pneumonia J69.0
Degos' disease I77.89
Dehiscence (of)
   amputation stump T87.81
   cesarean wound O90.0
   closure of
     cornea T81.31 ☑
     craniotomy T81.32 ☑
     fascia (muscular) (superficial) T81.32 ☑
     internal organ or tissue T81.32 ☑
     laceration (external) (internal) T81.33 ☑
     ligament T81.32 ☑
     mucosa T81.31 ☑
     muscle or muscle flap T81.32 ☑
     ribs or rib cage T81.32 ☑
     skin and subcutaneous tissue (full-thickness) (superficial) T81.31 ☑
     skull T81.32 ☑
     sternum (sternotomy) T81.32 ☑
     tendon T81.32 ☑
     traumatic laceration (external) (internal) T81.33 ☑
   episiotomy O90.1
   operation wound NEC T81.31 ☑
     external operation wound (superficial) T81.31 ☑
     internal operation wound (deep) T81.32 ☑
   perineal wound (postpartum) O90.1
   traumatic injury wound repair T81.33 ☑
   wound T81.30 ☑
     traumatic repair T81.33 ☑
Dehydration E86.0
   hypertonic E87.0
   hypotonic E87.1
   newborn P74.1
Déjérine-Roussy syndrome G89.0
Déjérine-Sottas disease or neuropathy (hypertrophic) G60.0
Déjérine-Thomas atrophy G23.8
Delay, delayed
   any plane in pelvis
     complicating delivery O66.9
   birth or delivery NOS O63.9
   closure, ductus arteriosus (Botalli) P29.3
   coagulation — *see* Defect, coagulation
   conduction (cardiac) (ventricular) I45.9
   delivery, second twin, triplet, etc O63.2
   development R62.50
     global F88
     intellectual (specific) F81.9
     language F80.9
       due to hearing loss F80.4
     learning F81.9
     pervasive F84.9
     physiological R62.50
       specified stage NEC R62.0
     reading F81.0
     sexual E30.0
     speech F80.9
       due to hearing loss F80.4
     spelling F81.81
   gastric emptying K30
   menarche E30.0
   menstruation (cause unknown) N91.0
   milestone R62.0
   passage of meconium (newborn) P76.0
   primary respiration P28.9
   puberty (constitutional) E30.0
   separation of umbilical cord P96.82
   sexual maturation, female E30.0
   sleep phase syndrome G47.21
   union, fracture — *see* Fracture, by site
   vaccination Z28.9
Deletion (s)
   autosome Q93.9
     identified by fluorescence in situ hybridization (FISH) Q93.89
     identified by in situ hybridization (ISH) Q93.89
   chromosome
     with complex rearrangements NEC Q93.7

Deletion — continued
    part of NEC Q93.5
    seen only at prometaphase Q93.89
    short arm
        4 Q93.3
        5p Q93.4
        22q11.2 Q93.81
    specified NEC Q93.89
    long arm chromosome 18 or 21 Q93.89
        with complex rearrangements NEC Q93.7
    microdeletions NEC Q93.88
Delhi boil or button B55.1
Delinquency (juvenile) (neurotic) F91.8
    group Z72.810
Delinquent immunization status Z28.3
Delirium, delirious (acute or subacute) (not alcohol- or drug-induced) (with dementia) R41.0
    alcoholic (acute) (tremens) (withdrawal) F10.921
        with intoxication F10.921
            in
                abuse F10.121
                dependence F10.221
    due to (secondary to)
        alcohol
            intoxication F10.921
                in
                    abuse F10.121
                    dependence F10.221
            withdrawal F10.231
        amphetamine intoxication F15.921
            in
                abuse F15.121
                dependence F15.221
        anxiolytic
            intoxication F13.921
                in
                    abuse F13.121
                    dependence F13.221
            withdrawal F13.231
        cannabis intoxication (acute) F12.921
            in
                abuse F12.121
                dependence F12.221
        cocaine intoxication (acute) F14.921
            in
                abuse F14.121
                dependence F14.221
        general medical condition F05
        hallucinogen intoxication F16.921
            in
                abuse F16.121
                dependence F16.221
        hypnotic
            intoxication F13.921
                in
                    abuse F13.121
                    dependence F13.221
            withdrawal F13.231
        inhalant intoxication (acute) F18.921
            in
                abuse F18.121
                dependence F18.221
        multiple etiologies F05
        opioid intoxication (acute) F11.921
            in
                abuse F11.121
                dependence F11.221
        phencyclidine intoxication (acute) F16.921
            in
                abuse F16.121
                dependence F16.221
        psychoactive substance NEC intoxication (acute) F19.921
            in
                abuse F19.121
                dependence F19.221
        sedative
            intoxication F13.921
                in
                    abuse F13.121
                    dependence F13.221
            withdrawal F13.231
        unknown etiology F05
    exhaustion F43.0
    hysterical F44.89
    postprocedural (postoperative) F05
    puerperal F05
    thyroid — see Thyrotoxicosis with thyroid storm
    traumatic — see Injury, intracranial
    tremens (alcohol-induced) F10.231
        sedative-induced F13.231
Delivery (childbirth) (labor)

Delivery — continued
    arrested active phase O62.1
    cesarean (for)
        abnormal
            pelvis (bony) (deformity) (major) NEC with disproportion (fetopelvic) O33.0
                with obstructed labor O65.0
            presentation or position O32.9 ☑
        abruptio placentae (see also Abruptio placentae) O45.9- ☑
        acromion presentation O32.2 ☑
        atony, uterus O62.2
        breech presentation O32.1 ☑
            incomplete O32.8 ☑
        brow presentation O32.3 ☑
        cephalopelvic disproportion O33.9
        cerclage O34.3- ☑
        chin presentation O32.3 ☑
        cicatrix of cervix O34.4- ☑
        contracted pelvis (general)
            inlet O33.2
            outlet O33.3 ☑
        cord presentation or prolapse O69.0 ☑
        cystocele O34.8- ☑
        deformity (acquired) (congenital)
            pelvic organs or tissues NEC O34.8- ☑
            pelvis (bony) NEC O33.0
        disproportion NOS O33.9
        eclampsia — see Eclampsia
        face presentation O32.3 ☑
        failed
            forceps O66.5
            induction of labor O61.9
                instrumental O61.1
                mechanical O61.1
                medical O61.0
                specified NEC O61.8
                surgical O61.1
            trial of labor NOS O66.40
                following previous cesarean delivery O66.41
            vacuum extraction O66.5
            ventouse O66.5
        fetal-maternal hemorrhage O43.01- ☑
        hemorrhage (intrapartum) O67.9
            with coagulation defect O67.0
            specified cause NEC O67.8
        high head at term O32.4 ☑
        hydrocephalic fetus O33.6 ☑
        incarceration of uterus O34.51- ☑
        incoordinate uterine action O62.4
        increased size, fetus O33.5 ☑
        inertia, uterus O62.2
            primary O62.0
            secondary O62.1
        lateroversion, uterus O34.59- ☑
        mal lie O32.9 ☑
        malposition
            fetus O32.9 ☑
            pelvic organs or tissues NEC O34.8- ☑
            uterus NEC O34.59- ☑
        malpresentation NOS O32.9 ☑
        oblique presentation O32.2 ☑
        occurring after 37 completed weeks of gestation but before 39 completed weeks gestation due to (spontaneous) onset of labor O75.82
        oversize fetus O33.5 ☑
        pelvic tumor NEC O34.8- ☑
        placenta previa O44.1- ☑
            without hemorrhage O44.0- ☑
        placental insufficiency O36.51- ☑
        planned, occurring after 37 completed weeks of gestation but before 39 completed weeks gestation due to (spontaneous) onset of labor O75.82
        polyp, cervix O34.4- ☑
            causing obstructed labor O65.5
        poor dilatation, cervix O62.0
        pre-eclampsia O14.9- ☑
            mild O14.0- ☑
            moderate O14.0- ☑
            severe
                with hemolysis, elevated liver enzymes and low platelet count (HELLP) O14.2- ☑
        previous
            cesarean delivery O34.21
            surgery (to)
                cervix O34.4- ☑
                gynecological NEC O34.8- ☑
                rectum O34.7- ☑
                uterus O34.29

Delivery — continued
                vagina O34.6- ☑
        prolapse
            arm or hand O32.2 ☑
            uterus O34.52- ☑
        prolonged labor NOS O63.9
        rectocele O34.8- ☑
        retroversion
            uterus O34.53- ☑
        rigid
            cervix O34.4- ☑
            pelvic floor O34.8- ☑
            perineum O34.7- ☑
            vagina O34.6- ☑
            vulva O34.7- ☑
        sacculation, pregnant uterus O34.59- ☑
        scar (s)
            cervix O34.4- ☑
            cesarean delivery O34.21
            uterus O34.29
        Shirodkar suture in situ O34.3- ☑
        shoulder presentation O32.2 ☑
        stenosis or stricture, cervix O34.4- ☑
        streptococcus B carrier state O99.824
        transverse presentation or lie O32.2 ☑
        tumor, pelvic organs or tissues NEC O34.8- ☑
            cervix O34.4- ☑
        umbilical cord presentation or prolapse O69.0 ☑
        without indication O82
    completely normal case O80
    complicated O75.9
        by
            abnormal, abnormality (of)
                forces of labor O62.9
                    specified type NEC O62.8
                glucose O99.814
                uterine contractions NOS O62.9
            abruptio placentae (see also Abruptio placentae) O45.9- ☑
            abuse
                physical O9A.32
                psychological O9A.52
                sexual O9A.42
            adherent placenta O72.0
                without hemorrhage O73.0
            alcohol use O99.314
            anemia (pre-existing) O99.02
            anesthetic death O74.8
            annular detachment of cervix O71.3
            atony, uterus O62.2
            attempted vacuum extraction and forceps O66.5
            Bandl's ring O62.4
            bariatric surgery status O99.844
            biliary tract disorder O26.62
            bleeding — see Delivery, complicated by, hemorrhage
            blood disorder NEC O99.12
            cervical dystocia (hypotonic) O62.2
                primary O62.0
                secondary O62.1
            circulatory system disorder O99.42
            compression of cord (umbilical) NEC O69.2 ☑
            condition NEC O99.89
            contraction, contracted ring O62.4
            cord (umbilical)
                around neck
                    with compression O69.1 ☑
                    without compression O69.81 ☑
                bruising O69.5 ☑
                complication O69.9 ☑
                  specified NEC O69.89 ☑
                compression NEC O69.2 ☑
                entanglement O69.2 ☑
                  without compression O69.82 ☑
                hematoma O69.5 ☑
                presentation O69.0 ☑
                prolapse O69.0 ☑
                short O69.3 ☑
                thrombosis (vessels) O69.5 ☑
                vascular lesion O69.5 ☑
            Couvelaire uterus O45.8X- ☑
            damage to (injury to) NEC
                perineum O71.82
                periurethral tissue O71.82
                vulva O71.82
            delay following rupture of membranes (spontaneous) — see Pregnancy, complicated by, premature rupture of membranes
            depressed fetal heart tones O76

☑ **Additional character required**

Delivery — *continued*

diabetes O24.92
　　gestational O24.429
　　　diet controlled O24.420
　　　insulin controlled O24.424
　　pre-existing O24.32
　　　specified NEC O24.82
　　　type 1 O24.02
　　　type 2 O24.12
diastasis recti (abdominis) O71.89
dilatation
　　bladder O66.8
　　cervix incomplete, poor or slow O62.0
disease NEC O99.89
disruptio uteri — *see* Delivery, complicated
　　by, rupture, uterus
drug use O99.324
dysfunction, uterus NOS O62.9
　　hypertonic O62.4
　　hypotonic O62.2
　　　primary O62.0
　　　secondary O62.1
　　incoordinate O62.4
eclampsia O15.1
embolism (pulmonary) — *see* Embolism,
　　obstetric
endocrine, nutritional or metabolic disease
　　NEC O99.284
failed
　　attempted vaginal birth after previous
　　　cesarean delivery O66.41
　　induction of labor O61.9
　　　instrumental O61.1
　　　mechanical O61.1
　　　medical O61.0
　　　specified NEC O61.8
　　　surgical O61.1
　　trial of labor O66.40
female genital mutilation O65.5
fetal
　　abnormal acid-base balance O68
　　acidemia O68
　　acidosis O68
　　alkalosis O68
　　death, early O02.1
　　deformity O66.3
　　heart rate or rhythm (abnormal) (non-
　　　reassuring) O76
　　hypoxia O77.8
　　stress O77.9
　　　due to drug administration O77.1
　　　electrocardiographic evidence of O77.8
　　　specified NEC O77.8
　　　ultrasound evidence of O77.8
fever during labor O75.2
gastric banding status O99.844
gastric bypass status O99.844
gastrointestinal disease NEC O99.62
gestational diabetes O24.429
　　diet controlled O24.420
　　insulin (and diet) controlled O24.424
gonorrhea O98.22
hematoma O71.7
　　ischial spine O71.7
　　pelvic O71.7
　　vagina O71.7
　　vulva or perineum O71.7
hemorrhage (uterine) O67.9
　　associated with
　　　afibrinogenemia O67.0
　　　coagulation defect O67.0
　　　hyperfibrinolysis O67.0
　　　hypofibrinogenemia O67.0
　　due to
　　　low-lying placenta O44.1- ☑
　　　placenta previa O44.1- ☑
　　　premature separation of placenta
　　　　(normally implanted) (*see also*
　　　　Abruptio placentae) O45.9- ☑
　　　retained placenta O72.0
　　　uterine leiomyoma O67.8
　　placenta NEC O67.8
　　postpartum NEC (atonic) (immediate)
　　　O72.1
　　　with retained or trapped placenta O72.0
　　　delayed O72.2
　　　secondary O72.2
　　　third stage O72.0
hourglass contraction, uterus O62.4
hypertension, hypertensive (pre-existing)
　　— *see* Hypertension, complicated by,
　　childbirth (labor)

Delivery — *continued*

hypotension O26.5- ☑
incomplete dilatation (cervix) O62.0
incoordinate uterus contractions O62.4
inertia, uterus O62.2
　　during latent phase of labor O62.0
　　primary O62.0
　　secondary O62.1
infection (maternal) O98.92
　　carrier state NEC O99.834
　　gonorrhea O98.22
　　human immunodeficiency virus (HIV)
　　　O98.72
　　sexually transmitted NEC O98.32
　　specified NEC O98.82
　　syphilis O98.12
　　tuberculosis O98.02
　　viral hepatitis O98.42
　　viral NEC O98.52
injury (to mother) (*see also* Delivery,
　　complicated, by, damage to) O71.9
　　nonobstetric O9A.22
　　caused by abuse — *see* Delivery,
　　　complicated by, abuse
intrauterine fetal death, early O02.1
inversion, uterus O71.2
laceration (perineal) O70.9
　　anus (sphincter) O70.4
　　　with third degree laceration O70.2
　　　　with mucosa O70.3
　　　without third degree laceration O70.4
　　bladder (urinary) O71.5
　　bowel O71.5
　　cervix (uteri) O71.3
　　fourchette O70.0
　　hymen O70.0
　　labia O70.0
　　pelvic
　　　floor O70.1
　　　organ NEC O71.5
　　perineum, perineal O70.9
　　　first degree O70.0
　　　fourth degree O70.3
　　　muscles O70.1
　　　second degree O70.1
　　　skin O70.0
　　　slight O70.0
　　　third degree O70.2
　　peritoneum (pelvic) O71.5
　　rectovaginal (septum) (without perineal
　　　laceration) O71.4
　　　with perineum O70.2
　　　　with anal or rectal mucosa O70.3
　　specified NEC O71.89
　　sphincter ani — *see* Delivery, complicated,
　　　by, laceration, anus (sphincter)
　　urethra O71.5
　　uterus O71.81
　　　before labor O71.81
　　vagina, vaginal (deep) (high) (without
　　　perineal laceration) O71.4
　　　with perineum O70.0
　　　　muscles, with perineum O70.1
　　vulva O70.0
liver disorder O26.62
malignancy O9A.12
malnutrition O25.2
malposition, malpresentation
　　placenta (with hemorrhage) O44.1- ☑
　　　without hemorrhage O44.0- ☑
　　uterus or cervix O65.5
　　without obstruction (*see also* Delivery,
　　　complicated by, obstruction) O32.9 ☑
　　　breech O32.1 ☑
　　　compound O32.6 ☑
　　　face (brow) (chin) O32.3 ☑
　　　footling O32.8 ☑
　　　high head O32.4 ☑
　　　oblique O32.2 ☑
　　　specified NEC O32.8 ☑
　　　transverse O32.2 ☑
　　　unstable lie O32.0 ☑
meconium in amniotic fluid O77.0
mental disorder NEC O99.344
metrorrhexis — *see* Delivery, complicated by,
　　rupture, uterus
nervous system disorder O99.354
obesity (pre-existing) O99.214
obesity surgery status O99.844
obstetric trauma O71.9
　　specified NEC O71.89
obstructed labor

Delivery — *continued*

due to
　　breech (complete) (frank) presentation
　　　O64.1 ☑
　　　incomplete O64.8 ☑
　　brow presenation O64.3 ☑
　　buttock presentation O64.1 ☑
　　chin presentation O64.2 ☑
　　compound presentation O64.5 ☑
　　contracted pelvis O65.1
　　deep transverse arrest O64.0 ☑
　　deformed pelvis O65.0
　　dystocia (fetal) O66.9
　　　due to
　　　　conjoined twins O66.3
　　　　fetal
　　　　　abnormality NEC O66.3
　　　　　ascites O66.3
　　　　　hydrops O66.3
　　　　　meningomyelocele O66.3
　　　　　sacral teratoma O66.3
　　　　　tumor O66.3
　　　　hydrocephalic fetus O66.3
　　　shoulder O66.0
　　face presentation O64.2 ☑
　　fetopelvic disproportion O65.4
　　footling presentation O64.8 ☑
　　impacted shoulders O66.0
　　incomplete rotation of fetal head O64.0 ☑
　　large fetus O66.2
　　locked twins O66.1
　　malposition O64.9 ☑
　　　specified NEC O64.8 ☑
　　malpresentation O64.9 ☑
　　　specified NEC O64.8 ☑
　　multiple fetuses NEC O66.6
　　pelvic
　　　abnormality (maternal) O65.9
　　　　organ O65.5
　　　　specified NEC O65.8
　　　contraction
　　　　inlet O65.2
　　　　mid-cavity O65.3
　　　　outlet O65.3
　　persistent (position)
　　　occipitoiliac O64.0 ☑
　　　occipitoposterior O64.0 ☑
　　　occipitosacral O64.0 ☑
　　　occipitotransverse O64.0 ☑
　　prolapsed arm O64.4 ☑
　　shoulder presentation O64.4 ☑
　　specified NEC O66.8
pathological retraction ring, uterus O62.4
penetration, pregnant uterus by instrument
　　O71.1
perforation — *see* Delivery, complicated by,
　　laceration
placenta, placental
　　ablatio (*see also* Abruptio placentae)
　　　O45.9- ☑
　　abnormality O43.9- ☑
　　　specified NEC O43.89- ☑
　　abruptio (*see also* Abruptio placentae)
　　　O45.9- ☑
　　accreta O43.21- ☑
　　adherent (with hemorrhage) O72.0
　　　without hemorrhage O73.0
　　detachment (premature) (*see also* Abruptio
　　　placentae) O45.9- ☑
　　disorder O43.9- ☑
　　　specified NEC O43.89- ☑
　　hemorrhage NEC O67.8
　　increta O43.22- ☑
　　low (implantation) O44.1- ☑
　　　without hemorrhage O44.0- ☑
　　malformation O43.10- ☑
　　malposition O44.1- ☑
　　　without hemorrhage O44.0- ☑
　　percreta O43.23- ☑
　　previa (central) (lateral) (low) (marginal)
　　　(partial) (total) O44.1- ☑
　　　without hemorrhage O44.0- ☑
　　retained (with hemorrhage) O72.0
　　　without hemorrhage O73.0
　　separation (premature) O45.9- ☑
　　　specified NEC O45.8X- ☑
　　vicious insertion O44.1- ☑
precipitate labor O62.3
premature rupture, membranes (*see also*
　　Pregnancy, complicated by, premature
　　rupture of membranes) O42.90

Delivery — *continued*
   prolapse
      arm or hand O32.2 ☑
      cord (umbilical) O69.0 ☑
      foot or leg O32.8 ☑
      uterus O34.52- ☑
   prolonged labor O63.9
      first stage O63.0
      second stage O63.1
   protozoal disease (maternal) O98.62
   respiratory disease NEC O99.52
   retained membranes or portions of placenta
      O72.2
      without hemorrhage O73.1
   retarded birth O63.9
   retention of secundines (with hemorrhage)
      O72.0
      without hemorrhage O73.0
      partial O72.2
         without hemorrhage O73.1
   rupture
      bladder (urinary) O71.5
      cervix O71.3
      pelvic organ NEC O71.5
      urethra O71.5
      uterus (during or after labor) O71.1
         before labor O71.0- ☑
   separation, pubic bone (symphysis pubis)
      O71.6
   shock O75.1
   shoulder presentation O64.4 ☑
   skin disorder NEC O99.72
   spasm, cervix O62.4
   stenosis or stricture, cervix O65.5
   streptococcus B carrier state O99.824
   subluxation of symphysis (pubis) O26.72
   syphilis (maternal) O98.12
   tear — *see* Delivery, complicated by,
      laceration
   tetanic uterus O62.4
   trauma (obstetrical) (*see also* Delivery,
      complicated, by, damage to) O71.9
      non-obstetric O9A.22
      periurethral O71.82
      specified NEC O71.89
   tuberculosis (maternal) O98.02
   tumor, pelvic organs or tissues NEC O65.5
   umbilical cord around neck
      with compression O69.1 ☑
      without compression O69.81 ☑
   uterine inertia O62.2
      during latent phase of labor O62.0
      primary O62.0
      secondary O62.1
   vasa previa O69.4 ☑
   velamentous insertion of cord O43.12- ☑
   specified complication NEC O75.89
   delayed NOS O63.9
      following rupture of membranes
         artificial O75.5
      second twin, triplet, etc. O63.2
   forceps, low following failed vacuum extraction
      O66.5
   missed (at or near term) O36.4 ☑
   normal O80
   obstructed — *see* Delivery, complicated by,
      obstruction
   precipitate O62.3
   preterm (*see also* Pregnancy, complicated by,
      preterm labor) O60.10 ☑
   spontaneous O80
   term pregnancy NOS O80
   uncomplicated O80
   vaginal, following previous cesarean delivery
      O34.21
Delusions (paranoid) — *see* Disorder, delusional
Dementia (degenerative (primary)) (old age)
   (persisting) F03.90
   with
      aggressive behavior F03.91
      behavioral disturbance F03.91
      combative behavior F03.91
      Lewy bodies G31.83 [F02.80]
         with behavioral disturbance G31.83 [F02.81]
      Parkinsonism G31.83 [F02.80]
         with behavioral disturbance G31.83 [F02.81]
      Parkinson's disease G20 [F02.80]
         with behavioral disturbance G20 [F02.81]
      violent behavior F03.91
   alcoholic F10.97
      with dependence F10.27
   Alzheimer's type — *see* Disease, Alzheimer's

Dementia — *continued*
   arteriosclerotic — *see* Dementia, vascular
   atypical, Alzheimer's type — *see* Disease,
      Alzheimer's, specified NEC
   congenital — *see* Disability, intellectual
   frontal (lobe) G31.09 [F02.80]
      with behavioral disturbance G31.09 [F02.81]
   frontotemporal G31.09 [F02.80]
      with behavioral disturbance G31.09 [F02.81]
      specified NEC G31.09 [F02.80]
         with behavioral disturbance G31.09 [F02.81]
   in (due to)
      alcohol F10.97
         with dependence F10.27
      Alzheimer's disease — *see* Disease, Alzheimer's
      arteriosclerotic brain disease — *see* Dementia,
         vascular
      cerebral lipidoses E75.- ☑ [F02.80]
         with behavioral disturbance E75.- ☑ [F02.81]
      Creutzfeldt-Jakob disease (*see also* Creutzfeldt-
         Jakob disease or syndrome (with
         dementia)) A81.00
      epilepsy G40.- ☑ [F02.80]
         with behavioral disturbance G40.- ☑ [F02.81]
      hepatolenticular degeneration E83.01 [F02.80]
         with behavioral disturbance E83.01 [F02.81]
      human immunodeficiency virus (HIV) disease
         B20 [F02.80]
         with behavioral disturbance B20 [F02.81]
      Huntington's disease or chorea G10
      hypercalcemia E83.52 [F02.80]
         with behavioral disturbance E83.52 [F02.81]
      hypothyroidism, acquired E03.9 [F02.80]
         with behavioral disturbance E03.9 [F02.81]
         due to iodine deficiency E01.8 [F02.80]
            with behavioral disturbance E01.8 [F02.81]
      inhalants F18.97
         with dependence F18.27
      multiple
         etiologies F03 ☑
         sclerosis G35 [F02.80]
            with behavioral disturbance G35 [F02.81]
      neurosyphilis A52.17 [F02.80]
         with behavioral disturbance A52.17 [F02.81]
         juvenile A50.49 [F02.80]
            with behavioral disturbance A50.49 [F02.81]
      niacin deficiency E52 [F02.80]
         with behavioral disturbance E52 [F02.81]
      paralysis agitans G20 [F02.80]
         with behavioral disturbance G20 [F02.81]
      Parkinson's disease G20 [F02.80]
      pellagra E52 [F02.80]
         with behavioral disturbance E52 [F02.81]
      Pick's G31.01 [F02.80]
         with behavioral disturbance G31.01 [F02.81]
      polyarteritis nodosa M30.0 [F02.80]
         with behavioral disturbance M30.0 [F02.81]
      psychoactive drug F19.97
         with dependence F19.27
         inhalants F18.97
            with dependence F18.27
         sedatives, hypnotics or anxiolytics F13.97
            with dependence F13.27
      sedatives, hypnotics or anxiolytics F13.97
         with dependence F13.27
      systemic lupus erythematosus M32.- ☑ [F02.80]
         with behavioral disturbance M32.- ☑ [F02.81]
      trypanosomiasis
         African B56.9 [F02.80]
            with behavioral disturbance B56.9 [F02.81]
      unknown etiology F03 ☑
      vitamin B12 deficiency E53.8 [F02.80]
         with behavioral disturbance E53.8 [F02.81]
      volatile solvents F18.97
         with dependence F18.27
      with behavioral disturbance G31.83 [F02.81]
   infantile, infantilis F84.3
   Lewy body G31.83 [F02.80]
      with behavioral disturbance G31.83 [F02.81]
   multi-infarct — *see* Dementia, vascular
   paralytica, paralytic (syphilitic) A52.17 [F02.80]
      with behavioral disturbance A52.17 [F02.81]
      juvenilis A50.45
   paretic A52.17
   praecox — *see* Schizophrenia
   presenile F03 ☑
      Alzheimer's type — *see* Disease, Alzheimer's,
         early onset
   primary degenerative F03 ☑
   progressive, syphilitic A52.17
   senile F03 ☑
      with acute confusional state F05

Dementia — *continued*
   Alzheimer's type — *see* Disease, Alzheimer's,
      late onset
   depressed or paranoid type F03 ☑
   vascular (acute onset) (mixed) (multi-infarct)
      (subcortical) F01.50
      with behavioral disturbance F01.51
Demineralization, bone — *see* Osteoporosis
Demodex folliculorum (infestation) B88.0
Demophobia F40.248
Demoralization R45.3
Demyelination, demyelinization
   central nervous system G37.9
      specified NEC G37.8
   corpus callosum (central) G37.1
   disseminated, acute G36.9
      specified NEC G36.8
   global G35
   in optic neuritis G36.0
Dengue (classical) (fever) A90
   hemorrhagic A91
   sandfly A93.1
Dennie-Marfan syphilitic syndrome A50.45
Dens evaginatus, in dente or invaginatus K00.2
Dense breasts R92.2
Density
   increased, bone (disseminated) (generalized)
      (spotted) — *see* Disorder, bone, density and
      structure, specified type NEC
   lung (nodular) J98.4
Dental (*see also* condition)
   examination Z01.20
      with abnormal findings Z01.21
   restoration
      aesthetically inadequate or displeasing K08.56
      defective K08.50
         specified NEC K08.59
      failure of marginal integrity K08.51
      failure of periodontal anatomical integrity
         K08.54
Dentia praecox K00.6
Denticles (pulp) K04.2
Dentigerous cyst K09.0
Dentin
   irregular (in pulp) K04.3
   opalescent K00.5
   secondary (in pulp) K04.3
   sensitive K03.89
Dentinogenesis imperfecta K00.5
Dentinoma — *see* Cyst, calcifying odontogenic
Dentition (syndrome) K00.7
   delayed K00.6
   difficult K00.7
   precocious K00.6
   premature K00.6
   retarded K00.6
Dependence (on) (syndrome) F19.20
   with remission F19.21
   alcohol (ethyl) (methyl) (without remission)
      F10.20
      with
         amnestic disorder, persisting F10.26
         anxiety disorder F10.280
         dementia, persisting F10.27
         intoxication F10.229
            with delirium F10.221
            uncomplicated F10.220
         mood disorder F10.24
         psychotic disorder F10.259
            with
               delusions F10.250
               hallucinations F10.251
         remission F10.21
         sexual dysfunction F10.281
         sleep disorder F10.282
         specified disorder NEC F10.288
         withdrawal F10.239
            with
               delirium F10.231
               perceptual disturbance F10.232
            uncomplicated F10.230
      counseling and surveillance Z71.41
   amobarbital — *see* Dependence, drug, sedative
   amphetamine (s) (type) — *see* Dependence, drug,
      stimulant NEC
   amytal (sodium) — *see* Dependence, drug,
      sedative
   analgesic NEC F55.8
   anesthetic (agent) (gas) (general) (local) NEC —
      see Dependence, drug, psychoactive NEC
   anxiolytic NEC — *see* Dependence, drug, sedative
   barbital (s) — *see* Dependence, drug, sedative

☑ **Additional character required**

Dependence — *continued*
barbiturate (s) (compounds) (drugs classifiable to T42) — *see* Dependence, drug, sedative
benzedrine — *see* Dependence, drug, stimulant NEC
bhang — *see* Dependence, drug, cannabis
bromide (s) NEC — *see* Dependence, drug, sedative
caffeine — *see* Dependence, drug, stimulant NEC
cannabis (sativa) (indica) (resin) (derivatives) (type) — *see* Dependence, drug, cannabis
chloral (betaine) (hydrate) — *see* Dependence, drug, sedative
chlordiazepoxide — *see* Dependence, drug, sedative
coca (leaf) (derivatives) — *see* Dependence, drug, cocaine
cocaine — *see* Dependence, drug, cocaine
codeine — *see* Dependence, drug, opioid
combinations of drugs F19.20
dagga — *see* Dependence, drug, cannabis
demerol — *see* Dependence, drug, opioid
dexamphetamine — *see* Dependence, drug, stimulant NEC
dexedrine — *see* Dependence, drug, stimulant NEC
dextromethorphan — *see* Dependence, drug, opioid
dextromoramide — *see* Dependence, drug, opioid
dextro-nor-pseudo-ephedrine — *see* Dependence, drug, stimulant NEC
dextrorphan — *see* Dependence, drug, opioid
diazepam — *see* Dependence, drug, sedative
dilaudid — *see* Dependence, drug, opioid
D-lysergic acid diethylamide — *see* Dependence, drug, hallucinogen
drug NEC F19.20
   with sleep disorder F19.282
   cannabis F12.20
      with
         anxiety disorder F12.280
         intoxication F12.229
            with
               delirium F12.221
               perceptual disturbance F12.222
            uncomplicated F12.220
         other specified disorder F12.288
         psychosis F12.259
            delusions F12.250
            hallucinations F12.251
         unspecified disorder F12.29
      in remission F12.21
   cocaine F14.20
      with
         anxiety disorder F14.280
         intoxication F14.229
            with
               delirium F14.221
               perceptual disturbance F14.222
            uncomplicated F14.220
         mood disorder F14.24
         other specified disorder F14.288
         psychosis F14.259
            delusions F14.250
            hallucinations F14.251
         sexual dysfunction F14.281
         sleep disorder F14.282
         unspecified disorder F14.29
         withdrawal F14.23
      in remission F14.21
      withdrawal symptoms in newborn P96.1
   counseling and surveillance Z71.51
   hallucinogen F16.20
      with
         anxiety disorder F16.280
         flashbacks F16.283
         intoxication F16.229
            with delirium F16.221
            uncomplicated F16.220
         mood disorder F16.24
         other specified disorder F16.288
         perception disorder, persisting F16.283
         psychosis F16.259
            delusions F16.250
            hallucinations F16.251
         unspecified disorder F16.29
      in remission F16.21
   in remission F19.21
   inhalant F18.20
      with
         anxiety disorder F18.280

Dependence — *continued*
      dementia, persisting F18.27
      intoxication F18.229
         with delirium F18.221
         uncomplicated F18.220
      mood disorder F18.24
      other specified disorder F18.288
      psychosis F18.259
         delusions F18.250
         hallucinations F18.251
      unspecified disorder F18.29
   in remission F18.21
   nicotine F17.200
      with disorder F17.209
      remission F17.201
      specified disorder NEC F17.208
      withdrawal F17.203
      chewing tobacco F17.220
         with disorder F17.229
         remission F17.221
         specified disorder NEC F17.228
         withdrawal F17.223
      cigarettes F17.210
         with disorder F17.219
         remission F17.211
         specified disorder NEC F17.218
         withdrawal F17.213
      specified product NEC F17.290
         with disorder F17.299
         remission F17.291
         specified disorder NEC F17.298
         withdrawal F17.293
   opioid F11.20
      with
         intoxication F11.229
            with
               delirium F11.221
               perceptual disturbance F11.222
            uncomplicated F11.220
         mood disorder F11.24
         other specified disorder F11.288
         psychosis F11.259
            delusions F11.250
            hallucinations F11.251
         sexual dysfunction F11.281
         sleep disorder F11.282
         unspecified disorder F11.29
         withdrawal F11.23
      in remission F11.21
   psychoactive NEC F19.20
      with
         amnestic disorder F19.26
         anxiety disorder F19.280
         dementia F19.27
         intoxication F19.229
            with
               delirium F19.221
               perceptual disturbance F19.222
            uncomplicated F19.220
         mood disorder F19.24
         other specified disorder F19.288
         psychosis F19.259
            delusions F19.250
            hallucinations F19.251
         sexual dysfunction F19.281
         sleep disorder F19.282
         unspecified disorder F19.29
         withdrawal F19.239
            with
               delirium F19.231
               perceptual disturbance F19.232
            uncomplicated F19.230
   sedative, hypnotic or anxiolytic F13.20
      with
         amnestic disorder F13.26
         anxiety disorder F13.280
         dementia, persisting F13.27
         intoxication F13.229
            with delirium F13.221
            uncomplicated F13.220
         mood disorder F13.24
         other specified disorder F13.288
         psychosis F13.259
            delusions F13.250
            hallucinations F13.251
         sexual dysfunction F13.281
         sleep disorder F13.282
         unspecified disorder F13.29
         withdrawal F13.239
            with
               delirium F13.231
               perceptual disturbance F13.232

Dependence — *continued*
         uncomplicated F13.230
      in remission F13.21
   stimulant NEC F15.20
      with
         anxiety disorder F15.280
         intoxication F15.229
            with
               delirium F15.221
               perceptual disturbance F15.222
            uncomplicated F15.220
         mood disorder F15.24
         other specified disorder F15.288
         psychosis F15.259
            delusions F15.250
            hallucinations F15.251
         sexual dysfunction F15.281
         sleep disorder F15.282
         unspecified disorder F15.29
         withdrawal F15.23
      in remission F15.21
   ethyl
      alcohol (without remission) F10.20
         with remission F10.21
      bromide — *see* Dependence, drug, sedative
      carbamate F19.20
      chloride F19.20
      morphine — *see* Dependence, drug, opioid
   ganja — *see* Dependence, drug, cannabis
   glue (airplane) (sniffing) — *see* Dependence, drug, inhalant
   glutethimide — *see* Dependence, drug, sedative
   hallucinogenics — *see* Dependence, drug, hallucinogen
   hashish — *see* Dependence, drug, cannabis
   hemp — *see* Dependence, drug, cannabis
   heroin (salt) (any) — *see* Dependence, drug, opioid
   hypnotic NEC — *see* Dependence, drug, sedative
   Indian hemp — *see* Dependence, drug, cannabis
   inhalants — *see* Dependence, drug, inhalant
   khat — *see* Dependence, drug, stimulant NEC
   laudanum — *see* Dependence, drug, opioid
   LSD (-25) (derivatives) — *see* Dependence, drug, hallucinogen
   luminal — *see* Dependence, drug, sedative
   lysergic acid — *see* Dependence, drug, hallucinogen
   maconha — *see* Dependence, drug, cannabis
   marihuana — *see* Dependence, drug, cannabis
   meprobamate — *see* Dependence, drug, sedative
   mescaline — *see* Dependence, drug, hallucinogen
   methadone — *see* Dependence, drug, opioid
   methamphetamine (s) — *see* Dependence, drug, stimulant NEC
   methaqualone — *see* Dependence, drug, sedative
   methyl
      alcohol (without remission) F10.20
         with remission F10.21
      bromide — *see* Dependence, drug, sedative
      morphine — *see* Dependence, drug, opioid
      phenidate — *see* Dependence, drug, stimulant NEC
      sulfonal — *see* Dependence, drug, sedative
   morphine (sulfate) (sulfite) (type) — *see* Dependence, drug, opioid
   narcotic (drug) NEC — *see* Dependence, drug, opioid
   nembutal — *see* Dependence, drug, sedative
   neraval — *see* Dependence, drug, sedative
   neravan — *see* Dependence, drug, sedative
   neurobarb — *see* Dependence, drug, sedative
   nicotine — *see* Dependence, drug, nicotine
   nitrous oxide F19.20
   nonbarbiturate sedatives and tranquilizers with similar effect — *see* Dependence, drug, sedative
   on
      artificial heart (fully implantable) (mechanical) Z95.812
      aspirator Z99.0
      care provider (because of) Z74.9
         impaired mobility Z74.09
         need for
            assistance with personal care Z74.1
            continuous supervision Z74.3
         no other household member able to render care Z74.2
         specified reason NEC Z74.8
      machine Z99.89
         enabling NEC Z99.89

Dependence — *continued*
    specified type NEC Z99.89
    renal dialysis (hemodialysis) (peritoneal) Z99.2
    respirator Z99.11
    ventilator Z99.11
    wheelchair Z99.3
  opiate — *see* Dependence, drug, opioid
  opioids — *see* Dependence, drug, opioid
  opium (alkaloids) (derivatives) (tincture) — *see* Dependence, drug, opioid
  oxygen (long-term) (supplemental) Z99.81
  paraldehyde — *see* Dependence, drug, sedative
  paregoric — *see* Dependence, drug, opioid
  PCP (phencyclidine) (*see also* Abuse, drug, hallucinogen) F16.20
  pentobarbital — *see* Dependence, drug, sedative
  pentobarbitone (sodium) — *see* Dependence, drug, sedative
  pentothal — *see* Dependence, drug, sedative
  peyote — *see* Dependence, drug, hallucinogen
  phencyclidine (PCP) (and related substances) (*see also* Abuse, drug, hallucinogen) F16.20
  phenmetrazine — *see* Dependence, drug, stimulant NEC
  phenobarbital — *see* Dependence, drug, sedative
  polysubstance F19.20
  psilocibin, psilocin, psilocyn, psilocyline — *see* Dependence, drug, hallucinogen
  psychostimulant NEC — *see* Dependence, drug, stimulant NEC
  secobarbital — *see* Dependence, drug, sedative
  seconal — *see* Dependence, drug, sedative
  sedative NEC — *see* Dependence, drug, sedative
  specified drug NEC — *see* Dependence, drug
  stimulant NEC — *see* Dependence, drug, stimulant NEC
  substance NEC — *see* Dependence, drug
  supplemental oxygen Z99.81
  tobacco — *see* Dependence, drug, nicotine
    counseling and surveillance Z71.6
  tranquilizer NEC — *see* Dependence, drug, sedative
  vitamin B6 E53.1
  volatile solvents — *see* Dependence, drug, inhalant
Dependency
  care-provider Z74.9
  passive F60.7
  reactions (persistent) F60.7
Depersonalization (in neurotic state) (neurotic) (syndrome) F48.1
Depletion
  extracellular fluid E86.9
  plasma E86.1
  potassium E87.6
    nephropathy N25.89
  salt or sodium E87.1
    causing heat exhaustion or prostration T67.4 ☑
    nephropathy N28.9
  volume NOS E86.9
Deployment (current) (military) status Z56.82
  in theater or in support of military war, peacekeeping and humanitarian operations Z56.82
  personal history of Z91.82
    military war, peacekeeping and humanitarian deployment (current or past conflict) Z91.82
  returned from Z91.82
Depolarization, premature I49.40
  atrial I49.1
  junctional I49.2
  specified NEC I49.49
  ventricular I49.3
Deposit
  bone in Boeck's sarcoid D86.89
  calcareous, calcium — *see* Calcification
  cholesterol
    retina H35.89
    vitreous (body) (humor) — *see* Deposit, crystalline
  conjunctiva H11.11- ☑
  cornea H18.00- ☑
    argentous H18.02- ☑
    due to metabolic disorder H18.03- ☑
    Kayser-Fleischer ring H18.04- ☑
    pigmentation — *see* Pigmentation, cornea
  crystalline, vitreous (body) (humor) H43.2- ☑
  hemosiderin in old scars of cornea — *see* Pigmentation, cornea, stromal
  metallic in lens — *see* Cataract, specified NEC
  skin R23.8

Deposit — *continued*
  tooth, teeth (betel) (black) (green) (materia alba) (orange) (tobacco) K03.6
  urate, kidney — *see* Calculus, kidney
Depraved appetite — *see* Pica
Depressed
  HDL cholesterol E78.6
Depression (acute) (mental) F32.9
  agitated (single episode) F32.2
  anaclitic — *see* Disorder, adjustment
  anxiety F41.8
    persistent F34.1
  arches (*see also* Deformity, limb, flat foot)
  atypical (single episode) F32.8
  basal metabolic rate R94.8
  bone marrow D75.89
  central nervous system R09.2
  cerebral R29.818
    newborn P91.4
  cerebrovascular I67.9
  chest wall M95.4
  climacteric (single episode) F32.8
  endogenous (without psychotic symptoms) F33.2
    with psychotic symptoms F33.3
  functional activity R68.89
  hysterical F44.89
  involutional (single episode) F32.8
  major F32.9
    with psychotic symptoms F32.3
    recurrent — *see* Disorder, depressive, recurrent
  manic-depressive — *see* Disorder, depressive, recurrent
  masked (single episode) F32.8
  medullary G93.89
  menopausal (single episode) F32.8
  metatarsus — *see* Depression, arches
  monopolar F33.9
  nervous F34.1
  neurotic F34.1
  nose M95.0
  postnatal F53
  postpartum F53
  post-psychotic of schizophrenia F32.8
  post-schizophrenic F32.8
  psychogenic (reactive) (single episode) F32.9
  psychoneurotic F34.1
  psychotic (single episode) F32.3
    recurrent F33.3
  reactive (psychogenic) (single episode) F32.9
    psychotic (single episode) F32.3
  recurrent — *see* Disorder, depressive, recurrent
  respiratory center G93.89
  seasonal — *see* Disorder, depressive, recurrent
  senile F03 ☑
  severe, single episode F32.2
  situational F43.21
  skull Q67.4
  specified NEC (single episode) F32.8
  sternum M95.4
  visual field — *see* Defect, visual field
  vital (recurrent) (without psychotic symptoms) F33.2
    with psychotic symptoms F33.3
    single episode F32.2
Deprivation
  cultural Z60.3
  effects NOS T73.9 ☑
    specified NEC T73.8 ☑
  emotional NEC Z65.8
    affecting infant or child — *see* Maltreatment, child, psychological
  food T73.0 ☑
  protein — *see* Malnutrition
  sleep Z72.820
  social Z60.4
    affecting infant or child — *see* Maltreatment, child, psychological
  specified NEC T73.8 ☑
  vitamins — *see* Deficiency, vitamin
  water T73.1 ☑
Derangement
  ankle (internal) — *see* Derangement, joint, ankle
  cartilage (articular) NEC — *see* Derangement, joint, articular cartilage, by site
    recurrent — *see* Dislocation, recurrent
  cruciate ligament, anterior, current injury — *see* Sprain, knee, cruciate, anterior
  elbow (internal) — *see* Derangement, joint, elbow
  hip (joint) (internal) (old) — *see* Derangement, joint, hip
  joint (internal) M24.9

Derangement — *continued*
  ankylosis — *see* Ankylosis
  articular cartilage M24.10
    ankle M24.17- ☑
    elbow M24.12- ☑
    foot M24.17- ☑
    hand M24.14- ☑
    hip M24.15- ☑
    knee NEC M23.9- ☑
    loose body — *see* Loose, body
    shoulder M24.11- ☑
    wrist M24.13- ☑
  contracture — *see* Contraction, joint
  current injury (*see also* Dislocation)
    knee, meniscus or cartilage — *see* Tear, meniscus
  dislocation
    pathological — *see* Dislocation, pathological
    recurrent — *see* Dislocation, recurrent
  knee — *see* Derangement, knee
  ligament — *see* Disorder, ligament
  loose body — *see* Loose, body
  recurrent — *see* Dislocation, recurrent
  specified type NEC M24.80
    ankle M24.87- ☑
    elbow M24.82- ☑
    foot joint M24.87- ☑
    hand joint M24.84- ☑
    hip M24.85- ☑
    shoulder M24.81- ☑
    wrist M24.83- ☑
  temporomandibular M26.69
  knee (recurrent) M23.9- ☑
    ligament disruption, spontaneous M23.60- ☑
      anterior cruciate M23.61- ☑
      capsular M23.67- ☑
      instability, chronic M23.5- ☑
      lateral collateral M23.64- ☑
      medial collateral M23.63- ☑
      posterior cruciate M23.62- ☑
    loose body M23.4- ☑
    meniscus M23.30- ☑
      cystic M23.00- ☑
        lateral M23.002
          anterior horn M23.04- ☑
          posterior horn M23.05- ☑
          specified NEC M23.06- ☑
        medial M23.005
          anterior horn M23.01- ☑
          posterior horn M23.02- ☑
          specified NEC M23.03- ☑
      degenerate — *see* Derangement, knee, meniscus, specified NEC
      detached — *see* Derangement, knee, meniscus, specified NEC
      due to old tear or injury M23.20- ☑
        lateral M23.20- ☑
          anterior horn M23.24- ☑
          posterior horn M23.25- ☑
          specified NEC M23.26- ☑
        medial M23.20- ☑
          anterior horn M23.21- ☑
          posterior horn M23.22- ☑
          specified NEC M23.23- ☑
      retained — *see* Derangement, knee, meniscus, specified NEC
      specified NEC M23.30- ☑
        lateral M23.30- ☑
          anterior horn M23.34- ☑
          posterior horn M23.35- ☑
          specified NEC M23.36- ☑
        medial M23.30- ☑
          anterior horn M23.31- ☑
          posterior horn M23.32- ☑
          specified NEC M23.33- ☑
      old M23.8X- ☑
      specified NEC M23.8
  low back NEC — *see* Dorsopathy, specified NEC
  meniscus — *see* Derangement, knee, meniscus
  mental — *see* Psychosis
  patella, specified NEC — *see* Disorder, patella, derangement NEC
  semilunar cartilage (knee) — *see* Derangement, knee, meniscus, specified NEC
  shoulder (internal) — *see* Derangement, joint, shoulder
Dercum's disease E88.2
Derealization (neurotic) F48.1
Dermal — *see* condition
Dermaphytid — *see* Dermatophytosis
Dermatitis (eczematous) L30.9
  ab igne L59.0

☑ **Additional character required**

Dermatitis — *continued*
- acarine B88.0
- actinic (due to sun) L57.8
  - other than from sun L59.8
- allergic — *see* Dermatitis, contact, allergic
- ambustionis, due to burn or scald — *see* Burn
- amebic A06.7
- ammonia L22
- arsenical (ingested) L27.8
- artefacta L98.1
  - psychogenic F54
- atopic L20.9
  - psychogenic F54
  - specified NEC L20.89
- autoimmune progesterone L30.8
- berlock, berloque L56.2
- blastomycotic B40.3
- blister beetle L24.89
- bullous, bullosa L13.9
  - mucosynechial, atrophic L12.1
  - seasonal L30.8
  - specified NEC L13.8
- calorica L59.0
  - due to burn or scald — *see* Burn
- caterpillar L24.89
- cercarial B65.3
- combustionis L59.0
  - due to burn or scald — *see* Burn
- congelationis T69.1 ☑
- contact (occupational) L25.9
  - allergic L23.9
    - due to
      - adhesives L23.1
      - cement L23.5
      - chemical products NEC L23.5
      - chromium L23.0
      - cosmetics L23.2
      - dander (cat) (dog) L23.81
      - drugs in contact with skin L23.3
      - dyes L23.4
      - food in contact with skin L23.6
      - hair (cat) (dog) L23.81
      - insecticide L23.5
      - metals L23.0
      - nickel L23.0
      - plants, non-food L23.7
      - plastic L23.5
      - rubber L23.5
      - specified agent NEC L23.89
    - due to
      - cement L25.3
      - chemical products NEC L25.3
      - cosmetics L25.0
      - dander (cat) (dog) L23.81
      - drugs in contact with skin L25.1
      - dyes L25.2
      - food in contact with skin L25.4
      - hair (cat) (dog) L23.81
      - plants, non-food L25.5
      - specified agent NEC L25.8
  - irritant L24.9
    - due to
      - cement L25.3
      - chemical products NEC L24.5
      - cosmetics L24.3
      - detergents L24.0
      - drugs in contact with skin L24.4
      - food in contact with skin L24.6
      - oils and greases L24.1
      - plants, non-food L24.7
      - solvents L24.2
      - specified agent NEC L24.89
- contusiformis L52
- diabetic — *see* E08-E13 with .620
- diaper L22
- diphtheritica A36.3
- dry skin L85.3
- due to
  - acetone (contact) (irritant) L24.2
  - acids (contact) (irritant) L24.5
  - adhesive (s) (allergic) (contact) (plaster) L23.1
    - irritant L24.5
  - alcohol (irritant) (skin contact) (substances in category T51) L24.2
    - taken internally L27.8
  - alkalis (contact) (irritant) L24.5
  - arsenic (ingested) L27.8
  - carbon disulfide (contact) (irritant) L24.2
  - caustics (contact) (irritant) L24.5
  - cement (contact) L25.3
  - cereal (ingested) L27.2
  - chemical (s) NEC L25.3

Dermatitis — *continued*
- taken internally L27.8
  - chlorocompounds L24.2
  - chromium (contact) (irritant) L24.81
  - coffee (ingested) L27.2
  - cold weather L30.8
  - cosmetics (contact) L25.0
    - allergic L23.2
    - irritant L24.3
  - cyclohexanes L24.2
  - dander (cat) (dog) L23.81
  - Demodex species B88.0
  - Dermanyssus gallinae B88.0
  - detergents (contact) (irritant) L24.0
  - dichromate L24.81
  - drugs and medicaments (generalized) (internal use) L27.0
    - external — *see* Dermatitis, due to, drugs, in contact with skin
    - in contact with skin L25.1
      - allergic L23.3
      - irritant L24.4
    - localized skin eruption L27.1
    - specified substance — *see* Table of Drugs and Chemicals
  - dyes (contact) L25.2
    - allergic L23.4
    - irritant L24.89
  - epidermophytosis — *see* Dermatophytosis
  - esters L24.2
  - external irritant NEC L24.9
  - fish (ingested) L27.2
  - flour (ingested) L27.2
  - food (ingested) L27.2
    - in contact with skin L25.4
  - fruit (ingested) L27.2
  - furs (allergic) (contact) L23.81
  - glues — *see* Dermatitis, due to, adhesives
  - glycols L24.2
  - greases NEC (contact) (irritant) L24.1
  - hair (cat) (dog) L23.81
  - hot
    - objects and materials — *see* Burn
    - weather or places L59.0
  - hydrocarbons L24.2
  - infrared rays L59.8
  - ingestion, ingested substance L27.9
    - chemical NEC L27.8
    - drugs and medicaments — *see* Dermatitis, due to, drugs
    - food L27.2
    - specified NEC L27.8
  - insecticide in contact with skin L24.5
  - internal agent L27.9
    - drugs and medicaments (generalized) — *see* Dermatitis, due to, drugs
    - food L27.2
  - irradiation — *see* Dermatitis, due to, radioactive substance
  - ketones L24.2
  - lacquer tree (allergic) (contact) L23.7
  - light (sun) NEC L57.8
    - acute L56.8
    - other L59.8
  - Liponyssoides sanguineus B88.0
  - low temperature L30.8
  - meat (ingested) L27.2
  - metals, metal salts (contact) (irritant) L24.81
  - milk (ingested) L27.2
  - nickel (contact) (irritant) L24.81
  - nylon (contact) (irritant) L24.5
  - oils NEC (contact) (irritant) L24.1
  - paint solvent (contact) (irritant) L24.2
  - petroleum products (contact) (irritant) (substances in T52.0) L24.2
  - plants NEC (contact) L25.5
    - allergic L23.7
    - irritant L24.7
  - plasters (adhesive) (any) (allergic) (contact) L23.1
    - irritant L24.5
  - plastic L25.3
  - preservatives (contact) — *see* Dermatitis, due to, chemical, in contact with skin
  - primrose (allergic) (contact) L23.7
  - primula (allergic) (contact) L23.7
  - radiation L59.8
    - nonionizing (chronic exposure) L57.8
    - sun NEC L57.8
      - acute L56.8
  - radioactive substance L58.9
    - acute L58.0

Dermatitis — *continued*
- chronic L58.1
  - radium L58.9
    - acute L58.0
    - chronic L58.1
  - ragweed (allergic) (contact) L23.7
  - Rhus (allergic) (contact) (diversiloba) (radicans) (toxicodendron) (venenata) (verniciflua) L23.7
  - rubber (contact) L24.5
  - Senecio jacobaea (allergic) (contact) L23.7
  - solvents (contact) (irritant) (substances in categories T52) L24.2
  - specified agent NEC (contact) L25.8
    - allergic L23.89
    - irritant L24.89
  - sunshine NEC L57.8
    - acute L56.8
  - tetrachlorethylene (contact) (irritant) L24.2
  - toluene (contact) (irritant) L24.2
  - turpentine (contact) L24.2
  - ultraviolet rays (sun NEC) (chronic exposure) L57.8
    - acute L56.8
  - vaccine or vaccination L27.0
    - specified substance — *see* Table of Drugs and Chemicals
  - varicose veins — *see* Varix, leg, with, inflammation
  - X-rays L58.9
    - acute L58.0
    - chronic L58.1
- dyshydrotic L30.1
- dysmenorrheica N94.6
- escharotica — *see* Burn
- exfoliative, exfoliativa (generalized) L26
  - neonatorum L00
- eyelid (*see also* Dermatosis, eyelid)
  - allergic H01.119
    - left H01.116
      - lower H01.115
      - upper H01.114
    - right H01.113
      - lower H01.112
      - upper H01.111
  - contact — *see* Dermatitis, eyelid, allergic
  - due to
    - Demodex species B88.0
    - herpes (zoster) B02.39
      - simplex B00.59
  - eczematous H01.139
    - left H01.136
      - lower H01.135
      - upper H01.134
    - right H01.133
      - lower H01.132
      - upper H01.131
- facta, factitia, factitial L98.1
  - psychogenic F54
- flexural NEC L20.82
- friction L30.4
- fungus B36.9
  - specified type NEC B36.8
- gangrenosa, gangrenous infantum L08.0
- harvest mite B88.0
- heat L59.0
- herpesviral, vesicular (ear) (lip) B00.1
- herpetiformis (bullous) (erythematous) (pustular) (vesicular) L13.0
  - juvenile L12.2
  - senile L12.0
- hiemalis L30.8
- hypostatic, hypostatica — *see* Varix, leg, with, inflammation
- infectious eczematoid L30.3
- infective L30.3
- irritant — *see* Dermatitis, contact, irritant
- Jacquet's (diaper dermatitis) L22
- Leptus B88.0
- lichenified NEC L28.0
- medicamentosa (generalized) (internal use) — *see* Dermatitis, due to drugs
- mite B88.0
- multiformis L13.0
  - juvenile L12.2
- napkin L22
- neurotica L13.0
- nummular L30.0
- papillaris capillitii L73.0
- pellagrous E52
- perioral L71.0
- photocontact L56.2

Dermatitis — *continued*
  polymorpha dolorosa L13.0
  pruriginosa L13.0
  pruritic NEC L30.8
  psychogenic F54
  purulent L08.0
  pustular
    contagious B08.02
    subcorneal L13.1
  pyococcal L08.0
  pyogenica L08.0
  repens L40.2
  Ritter's (exfoliativa) L00
  Schamberg's L81.7
  schistosome B65.3
  seasonal bullous L30.8
  seborrheic L21.9
    infantile L21.1
    specified NEC L21.8
  sensitization NOS L23.9
  septic L08.0
  solare L57.8
  specified NEC L30.8
  stasis I87.2
    with varicose ulcer — *see* Varix, leg, with ulcer,
      with inflammation
    due to postthrombotic syndrome —*see*
      Syndrome, postthrombotic
  suppurative L08.0
  traumatic NEC L30.4
  trophoneurotica L13.0
  ultraviolet (sun) (chronic exposure) L57.8
    acute L56.8
  varicose — *see* Varix, leg, with, inflammation
  vegetans L10.1
  verrucosa B43.0
  vesicular, herpesviral B00.1
Dermatoarthritis, lipoid E78.81
Dermatochalasis, eyelid H02.839
  left H02.836
    lower H02.835
    upper H02.834
  right H02.833
    lower H02.832
    upper H02.831
Dermatofibroma (lenticulare) — *see* Neoplasm, skin,
  benign
  protuberans — *see* Neoplasm, skin, uncertain
    behavior
Dermatofibrosarcoma (pigmented) (protuberans)
  — *see* Neoplasm, skin, malignant
Dermatographia L50.3
Dermatolysis (exfoliativa) (congenital) Q82.8
  acquired L57.4
  eyelids — *see* Blepharochalasis
  palpebrarum — *see* Blepharochalasis
  senile L57.4
Dermatomegaly NEC Q82.8
Dermatomucosomyositis M33.10
  with
    myopathy M33.12
    respiratory involvement M33.11
    specified organ involvement NEC M33.19
Dermatomycosis B36.9
  furfuracea B36.0
  specified type NEC B36.8
Dermatomyositis (acute) (chronic) — *see* also
  Dermatopolymyositis
  in (due to) neoplastic disease (*see also* Neoplasm)
    D49.9 [M36.0]
Dermatoneuritis of children — *see* Poisoning,
  mercury
Dermatophilosis A48.8
Dermatophytid L30.2
Dermatophytide — *see* Dermatophytosis
Dermatophytosis (epidermophyton) (infection)
  (Microsporum) (tinea) (Trichophyton) B35.9
  beard B35.0
  body B35.4
  capitis B35.0
  corporis B35.4
  deep-seated B35.8
  disseminated B35.8
  foot B35.3
  granulomatous B35.8
  groin B35.6
  hand B35.2
  nail B35.1
  perianal (area) B35.6
  scalp B35.0
  specified NEC B35.8
Dermatopolymyositis M33.90

Dermatopolymyositis — *continued*
  with
    myopathy M33.92
    respiratory involvement M33.91
    specified organ involvement NEC M33.99
  in neoplastic disease (*see also* Neoplasm) D49.9
    [M36.0]
  juvenile M33.00
    with
      myopathy M33.02
      respiratory involvement M33.01
      specified organ involvement NEC M33.09
  specified NEC M33.10
    myopathy M33.12
    respiratory involvement M33.11
    specified organ involvement NEC M33.19
Dermatopolyneuritis — *see* Poisoning, mercury
Dermatorrhexis Q79.6
  acquired L57.4
Dermatosclerosis (*see also* Scleroderma)
  localized L94.0
Dermatosis L98.9
  Andrews' L08.89
  Bowen's — *see* Neoplasm, skin, in situ
  bullous L13.9
    specified NEC L13.8
  exfoliativa L26
  eyelid (noninfectious)
    dermatitis — *see* Dermatitis, eyelid
    discoid lupus erythematosus — *see* Lupus,
      erythematosus, eyelid
    xeroderma — *see* Xeroderma, acquired, eyelid
  factitial L98.1
  febrile neutrophilic L98.2
  gonococcal A54.89
  herpetiformis L13.0
    juvenile L12.2
  linear IgA L13.8
  menstrual NEC L98.8
  neutrophilic, febrile L98.2
  occupational — *see* Dermatitis, contact
  papulosa nigra L82.1
  pigmentary L81.9
    progressive L81.7
    Schamberg's L81.7
  psychogenic F54
  purpuric, pigmented L81.7
  pustular, subcorneal L13.1
  transient acantholytic L11.1
Dermographia, dermographism L50.3
Dermographism — *see* Dermographia
Dermoid (cyst) (*see also* Neoplasm, benign, by site)
  with malignant transformation C56- ☑
  due to radiation (nonionizing) L57.8
Dermopathy
  infiltrative with thyrotoxicosis — *see*
    Thyrotoxicosis
  nephrogenic fibrosing L90.8
Dermophytosis — *see* Dermatophytosis
Descemetocele H18.73- ☑
Descemet's membrane — *see* condition
Descending — *see* condition
Descensus uteri — *see* Prolapse, uterus
Desert
  rheumatism B38.0
  sore — *see* Ulcer, skin
Desertion (newborn) — *see* Maltreatment
Desmoid (extra-abdominal) (tumor) — *see*
  Neoplasm, connective tissue, uncertain behavior
  abdominal D48.1
Despondency F32.9
Desquamation, skin R23.4
Destruction, destructive (*see also* Damage)
  articular facet (*see also* Derangement, joint,
    specified type NEC)
    knee M23.8X- ☑
    vertebra — *see* Spondylosis
  bone (*see also* Disorder, bone, specified type
    NEC)
    syphilitic A52.77
  joint (*see also* Derangement, joint, specified type
    NEC)
    sacroiliac M53.3
  rectal sphincter K62.89
  septum (nasal) J34.89
  tuberculous NEC — *see* Tuberculosis
  tympanum, tympanic membrane (nontraumatic)
    — *see* Disorder, tympanic membrane,
    specified NEC
  vertebral disc — *see* Degeneration, intervertebral
    disc
Destructiveness (*see also* Disorder, conduct)
  adjustment reaction — *see* Disorder, adjustment

Desultory labor O62.2
Detachment
  cartilage — *see* Sprain
  cervix, annular N88.8
    complicating delivery O71.3
  choroid (old) (postinfectional) (simple)
    (spontaneous) H31.40- ☑
    hemorrhagic H31.41- ☑
    serous H31.42- ☑
  ligament — *see* Sprain
  meniscus (knee) (*see also* Derangement, knee,
    meniscus, specified NEC)
    current injury — *see* Tear, meniscus
    due to old tear or injury — *see* Derangement,
      knee, meniscus, due to old tear
  retina (without retinal break) (serous) H33.2- ☑
    with retinal:
      break H33.00- ☑
        giant H33.03- ☑
        multiple H33.02- ☑
        single H33.01- ☑
      dialysis H33.04- ☑
    pigment epithelium — *see* Degeneration,
      retina, separation of layers, pigment
      epithelium detachment
    rhegmatogenous — *see* Detachment, retina,
      with retinal, break
    specified NEC H33.8
    total H33.05- ☑
    traction H33.4- ☑
  vitreous (body) H43.81 ☑
Detergent asthma J69.8
Deterioration
  epileptic F06.8
  general physical R53.81
  heart, cardiac — *see* Degeneration, myocardial
  mental — *see* Psychosis
  myocardial, myocardium — *see* Degeneration,
    myocardial
  senile (simple) R54
Deuteranomaly (anomalous trichromat) H53.53
Deuteranopia (complete) (incomplete) H53.53
Development
  abnormal, bone Q79.9
  arrested R62.50
    bone — *see* Arrest, development or growth,
      bone
    child R62.50
    due to malnutrition E45
  defective, congenital (*see also* Anomaly, by site)
    cauda equina Q06.3
    left ventricle Q24.8
      in hypoplastic left heart syndrome Q23.4
    valve Q24.8
      pulmonary Q22.3
  delayed (*see also* Delay, development) R62.50
    arithmetical skills F81.2
    language (skills) (expressive) F80.1
    learning skill F81.9
    mixed skills F88
    motor coordination F82
    reading F81.0
    specified learning skill NEC F81.89
    speech F80.9
    spelling F81.81
    written expression F81.81
  imperfect, congenital (*see also* Anomaly, by site)
    heart Q24.9
    lungs Q33.6
  incomplete
    bronchial tree Q32.4
    organ or site not listed — *see* Hypoplasia, by
      site
    respiratory system Q34.9
  sexual, precocious NEC E30.1
  tardy, mental (*see also* Disability, intellectual) F79
Developmental — *see* condition
  testing, child — *see* Examination, child
Devergie's disease (pityriasis rubra pilaris) L44.0
Deviation (in)
  conjugate palsy (eye) (spastic) H51.0
  esophagus (acquired) K22.8
  eye, skew H51.8
  midline (jaw) (teeth) (dental arch) M26.29
    specified site NEC — *see* Malposition
  nasal septum J34.2
    congenital Q67.4
  opening and closing of the mandible M26.53
  organ or site, congenital NEC — *see* Malposition,
    congenital
  septum (nasal) (acquired) J34.2
    congenital Q67.4

☑ **Additional character required**

Deviation — *continued*
  sexual F65.9
    bestiality F65.89
    erotomania F52.8
    exhibitionism F65.2
    fetishism, fetishistic F65.0
      transvestism F65.1
    frotteurism F65.81
    masochism F65.51
    multiple F65.89
    necrophilia F65.89
    nymphomania F52.8
    pederosis F65.4
    pedophilia F65.4
    sadism, sadomasochism F65.52
    satyriasis F52.8
    specified type NEC F65.89
    transvestism F64.1
    voyeurism F65.3
  teeth, midline M26.29
  trachea J39.8
  ureter, congenital Q62.61
Device
  cerebral ventricle (communicating) in situ Z98.2
  contraceptive — *see* Contraceptive, device
  drainage, cerebrospinal fluid, in situ Z98.2
Devic's disease G36.0
Devil's
  grip B33.0
  pinches (purpura simplex) D69.2
Devitalized tooth K04.99
Devonshire colic — *see* Poisoning, lead
Dextraposition, aorta Q20.3
  in tetralogy of Fallot Q21.3
Dextrinosis, limit (debrancher enzyme deficiency) E74.03
Dextrocardia (true) Q24.0
  with
    complete transposition of viscera Q89.3
    situs inversus Q89.3
Dextrotransposition, aorta Q20.3
d-glycericacidemia E72.59
Dhat syndrome F48.8
Dhobi itch B35.6
Di George's syndrome D82.1
Di Guglielmo's disease C94.0- ☑
Diabetes, diabetic (mellitus) (sugar) E11.9
  with
    amyotrophy E11.44
    arthropathy NEC E11.618
    autonomic (poly)neuropathy E11.43
    cataract E11.36
    Charcot's joints E11.610
    chronic kidney disease E11.22
    circulatory complication NEC E11.59
    complication E11.8
      specified NEC E11.69
    dermatitis E11.620
    foot ulcer E11.621
    gangrene E11.52
    gastroparesis E11.43
    glomerulonephrosis, intracapillary E11.21
    glomerulosclerosis, intercapillary E11.21
    hyperglycemia E11.65
    hyperosmolarity E11.00
      with coma E11.01
    hypoglycemia E11.649
      with coma E11.641
    kidney complications NEC E11.29
    Kimmelstiel-Wilson disease E11.21
    loss of protective sensation (LOPS) — *see* Diabetes, by type, with neuropathy
    mononeuropathy E11.41
    myasthenia E11.44
    necrobiosis lipoidica E11.620
    nephropathy E11.21
    neuralgia E11.42
    neurologic complication NEC E11.49
    neuropathic arthropathy E11.610
    neuropathy E11.40
    ophthalmic complication NEC E11.39
    oral complication NEC E11.638
    periodontal disease E11.630
    peripheral angiopathy E11.51
      with gangrene E11.52
    polyneuropathy E11.42
    renal complication NEC E11.29
    renal tubular degeneration E11.29
    retinopathy E11.319
      with macular edema E11.311
      nonproliferative E11.329
        with macular edema E11.321

Diabetes — *continued*
      mild E11.329
        with macular edema E11.321
      moderate E11.339
        with macular edema E11.331
      severe E11.349
        with macular edema E11.341
      proliferative E11.359
        with macular edema E11.351
    skin complication NEC E11.628
    skin ulcer NEC E11.622
  bronzed E83.110
  complicating pregnancy — *see* Pregnancy, complicated by, diabetes
  dietary counseling and surveillance Z71.3
  due to drug or chemical E09.9
    with
      amyotrophy E09.44
      arthropathy NEC E09.618
      autonomic (poly)neuropathy E09.43
      cataract E09.36
      Charcot's joints E09.610
      chronic kidney disease E09.22
      circulatory complication NEC E09.59
      complication E09.8
        specified NEC E09.69
      dermatitis E09.620
      foot ulcer E09.621
      gangrene E09.52
      gastroparesis E09.43
      glomerulonephrosis, intracapillary E09.21
      glomerulosclerosis, intercapillary E09.21
      hyperglycemia E09.65
      hyperosmolarity E09.00
        with coma E09.01
      hypoglycemia E09.649
        with coma E09.641
      ketoacidosis E09.10
        with coma E09.11
      kidney complications NEC E09.29
      Kimmelstiel-Wilson disease E09.21
      mononeuropathy E09.41
      myasthenia E09.44
      necrobiosis lipoidica E09.620
      nephropathy E09.21
      neuralgia E09.42
      neurologic complication NEC E09.49
      neuropathic arthropathy E09.610
      neuropathy E09.40
      ophthalmic complication NEC E09.39
      oral complication NEC E09.638
      periodontal disease E09.630
      peripheral angiopathy E09.51
        with gangrene E09.52
      polyneuropathy E09.42
      renal complication NEC E09.29
      renal tubular degeneration E09.29
      retinopathy E09.319
        with macular edema E09.311
        nonproliferative E09.329
          with macular edema E09.321
          mild E09.329
            with macular edema E09.321
          moderate E09.339
            with macular edema E09.331
          severe E09.349
            with macular edema E09.341
        proliferative E09.359
          with macular edema E09.351
      skin complication NEC E09.628
      skin ulcer NEC E09.622
  due to underlying condition E08.9
    with
      amyotrophy E08.44
      arthropathy NEC E08.618
      autonomic (poly)neuropathy E08.43
      cataract E08.36
      Charcot's joints E08.610
      chronic kidney disease E08.22
      circulatory complication NEC E08.59
      complication E08.8
        specified NEC E08.69
      dermatitis E08.620
      foot ulcer E08.621
      gangrene E08.52
      gastroparesis E08.43
      glomerulonephrosis, intracapillary E08.21
      glomerulosclerosis, intercapillary E08.21
      hyperglycemia E08.65
      hyperosmolarity E08.00
        with coma E08.01
      hypoglycemia E08.649

Diabetes — *continued*
      with coma E08.641
      ketoacidosis E08.10
        with coma E08.11
      kidney complications NEC E08.29
      Kimmelsteil-WIlson disease E08.21
      mononeuropathy E08.41
      myasthenia E08.44
      necrobiosis lipoidica E08.620
      nephropathy E08.21
      neuralgia E08.42
      neurologic complication NEC E08.49
      neuropathic arthropathy E08.610
      neuropathy E08.40
      ophthalmic complication NEC E08.39
      oral complication NEC E08.638
      periodontal disease E08.630
      peripheral angiopathy E08.51
        with gangrene E08.52
      polyneuropathy E08.42
      renal complication NEC E08.29
      renal tubular degeneration E08.29
      retinopathy E08.319
        with macular edema E08.311
        nonproliferative E08.329
          with macular edema E08.321
          mild E08.329
            with macular edema E08.321
          moderate E08.339
            with macular edema E08.331
          severe E08.349
            with macular edema E08.341
        proliferative E08.359
          with macular edema E08.351
      skin complication NEC E08.628
      skin ulcer NEC E08.622
  gestational (in pregnancy) O24.419
    affecting newborn P70.0
    diet controlled O24.410
    in childbirth O24.429
      diet controlled O24.420
      insulin (and diet) controlled O24.424
    insulin (and diet) controlled O24.414
    puerperal O24.439
      diet controlled O24.430
      insulin (and diet) controlled O24.434
  hepatogenous E13.9
  inadequately controlled - code to Diabetes, by type, with hyperglycemia
  insipidus E23.2
    nephrogenic N25.1
    pituitary E23.2
    vasopressin resistant N25.1
  insulin dependent - code to type of diabetes
  juvenile-onset — *see* Diabetes, type 1
  ketosis-prone — *see* Diabetes, type 1
  latent R73.09
  neonatal (transient) P70.2
  non-insulin dependent - code to type of diabetes
  out of control - code to Diabetes, by type, with hyperglycemia
  phosphate E83.39
  poorly controlled - code to Diabetes, by type, with hyperglycemia
  postpancreatectomy — *see* Diabetes, specified type NEC
  postprocedural — *see* Diabetes, specified type NEC
  secondary diabetes mellitus NEC — *see* Diabetes, specified type NEC
  specified type NEC E13.9
    with
      amyotrophy E13.44
      arthropathy NEC E13.618
      autonomic (poly)neuropathy E13.43
      cataract E13.36
      Charcot's joints E13.610
      chronic kidney disease E13.22
      circulatory complication NEC E13.59
      complication E13.8
        specified NEC E13.69
      dermatitis E13.620
      foot ulcer E13.621
      gangrene E13.52
      gastroparesis E13.43
      glomerulonephrosis, intracapillary E13.21
      glomerulosclerosis, intercapillary E13.21
      hyperglycemia E13.65
      hyperosmolarity E13.00
        with coma E13.01
      hypoglycemia E13.649
        with coma E13.641

Diabetes — *continued*
  ketoacidosis E13.10
    with coma E13.11
  kidney complications NEC E13.29
  Kimmelstiel-Wilson disease E13.21
  mononeuropathy E13.41
  myasthenia E13.44
  necrobiosis lipoidica E13.620
  nephropathy E13.21
  neuralgia E13.42
  neurologic complication NEC E13.49
  neuropathic arthropathy E13.610
  neuropathy E13.40
  ophthalmic complication NEC E13.39
  oral complication NEC E13.638
  periodontal disease E13.630
  peripheral angiopathy E13.51
    with gangrene E13.52
  polyneuropathy E13.42
  renal complication NEC E13.29
  renal tubular degeneration E13.29
  retinopathy E13.319
    with macular edema E13.311
    nonproliferative E13.329
      with macular edema E13.321
      mild E13.329
        with macular edema E13.321
      moderate E13.339
        with macular edema E13.331
      severe E13.349
        with macular edema E13.341
    proliferative E13.359
      with macular edema E13.351
  skin complication NEC E13.628
  skin ulcer NEC E13.622
  steroid-induced — *see* Diabetes, due to, drug or
    chemical
  type 1 E10.9
    with
      amyotrophy E10.44
      arthropathy NEC E10.618
      autonomic (poly)neuropathy E10.43
      cataract E10.36
      Charcot's joints E10.610
      chronic kidney disease E10.22
      circulatory complication NEC E10.59
      complication E10.8
        specified NEC E10.69
      dermatitis E10.620
      foot ulcer E10.621
      gangrene E10.52
      gastroparesis E10.43
      glomerulonephrosis, intracapillary E10.21
      glomerulosclerosis, intercapillary E10.21
      hyperglycemia E10.65
      hypoglycemia E10.649
        with coma E10.641
      ketoacidosis E10.10
        with coma E10.11
      kidney complications NEC E10.29
      Kimmelstiel-Wilson disease E10.21
      mononeuropathy E10.41
      myasthenia E10.44
      necrobiosis lipoidica E10.620
      nephropathy E10.21
      neuralgia E10.42
      neurologic complication NEC E10.49
      neuropathic arthropathy E10.610
      neuropathy E10.40
      ophthalmic complication NEC E10.39
      oral complication NEC E10.638
      periodontal disease E10.630
      peripheral angiopathy E10.51
        with gangrene E10.52
      polyneuropathy E10.42
      renal complication NEC E10.29
      renal tubular degeneration E10.29
      retinopathy E10.319
        with macular edema E10.311
        nonproliferative E10.329
          with macular edema E10.321
          mild E10.329
            with macular edema E10.321
          moderate E10.339
            with macular edema E10.331
          severe E10.349
            with macular edema E10.341
        proliferative E10.359
          with macular edema E10.351
      skin complication NEC E10.628
      skin ulcer NEC E10.622
  type 2 E11.9

Diabetes — *continued*
  with
    amyotrophy E11.44
    arthropathy NEC E11.618
    autonomic (poly)neuropathy E11.43
    cataract E11.36
    Charcot's joints E11.610
    chronic kidney disease E11.22
    circulatory complication NEC E11.59
    complication E11.8
      specified NEC E11.69
    dermatitis E11.620
    foot ulcer E11.621
    gangrene E11.52
    gastroparesis E11.43
    glomerulonephrosis, intracapillary E11.21
    glomerulosclerosis, intercapillary E11.21
    hyperglycemia E11.65
    hyperosmolarity E11.00
      with coma E11.01
    hypoglycemia E11.649
      with coma E11.641
    kidney complications NEC E11.29
    Kimmelstiel-Wilson disease E11.21
    mononeuropathy E11.41
    myasthenia E11.44
    necrobiosis lipoidica E11.620
    nephropathy E11.21
    neuralgia E11.42
    neurologic complication NEC E11.49
    neuropathic arthropathy E11.610
    neuropathy E11.40
    ophthalmic complication NEC E11.39
    oral complication NEC E11.638
    periodontal disease E11.630
    peripheral angiopathy E11.51
      with gangrene E11.52
    polyneuropathy E11.42
    renal complication NEC E11.29
    renal tubular degeneration E11.29
    retinopathy E11.319
      with macular edema E11.311
      nonproliferative E11.329
        with macular edema E11.321
        mild E11.329
          with macular edema E11.321
        moderate E11.339
          with macular edema E11.331
        severe E11.349
          with macular edema E11.341
      proliferative E11.359
        with macular edema E11.351
    skin complication NEC E11.628
    skin ulcer NEC E11.622
Diacyclothrombopathia D69.1
Diagnosis deferred R69
Dialysis (intermittent) (treatment)
  noncompliance (with) Z91.15
  renal (hemodialysis) (peritoneal), status Z99.2
  retina, retinal — *see* Detachment, retina, with
    retinal, dialysis
Diamond-Blackfan anemia (congenital hypoplastic)
  D61.01
Diamond-Gardener syndrome (autoerythrocyte
  sensitization) D69.2
Diaper rash L22
Diaphoresis (excessive) R61
Diaphragm — *see* condition
Diaphragmalgia R07.1
Diaphragmatitis, diaphragmitis J98.6
Diaphysial aclasis Q78.6
Diaphysitis — *see* Osteomyelitis, specified type NEC
Diarrhea, diarrheal (disease) (infantile)
  (inflammatory) R19.7
  achlorhydric K31.83
  allergic K52.2
  amebic (*see also* Amebiasis) A06.0
    with abscess — *see* Abscess, amebic
    acute A06.0
    chronic A06.1
    nondysenteric A06.2
  bacillary — *see* Dysentery, bacillary
  balantidial A07.0
  cachectic NEC K52.89
  Chilomastix A07.8
  choleriformis A00.1
  chronic (noninfectious) K52.9
  coccidial A07.3
  Cochin-China K90.1
    strongyloidiasis B78.0
  Dientamoeba A07.8
  dietetic K52.2

Diarrhea — *continued*
  drug-induced K52.1
  due to
    bacteria A04.9
      specified NEC A04.8
    Campylobacter A04.5
    Capillaria philippinensis B81.1
    Clostridium difficile A04.7
    Clostridium perfringens (C) (F) A04.8
    Cryptosporidium A07.2
    drugs K52.1
    Escherichia coli A04.4
      enteroaggregative A04.4
      enterohemorrhagic A04.3
      enteroinvasive A04.2
      enteropathogenic A04.0
      enterotoxigenic A04.1
      specified NEC A04.4
    food hypersensitivity K52.2
    Necator americanus B76.1
    S. japonicum B65.2
    specified organism NEC A08.8
      bacterial A04.8
      viral A08.39
    Staphylococcus A04.8
    Trichuris trichiuria B79
    virus — *see* Enteritis, viral
    Yersinia enterocolitica A04.6
  dysenteric A09
  endemic A09
  epidemic A09
  flagellate A07.9
  Flexner's (ulcerative) A03.1
  functional K59.1
    following gastrointestinal surgery K91.89
    psychogenic F45.8
  Giardia lamblia A07.1
  giardial A07.1
  hill K90.1
  infectious A09
  malarial — *see* Malaria
  mite B88.0
  mycotic NEC B49
  neonatal (noninfectious) P78.3
  nervous F45.8
  neurogenic K59.1
  noninfectious K52.9
  postgastrectomy K91.1
  postvagotomy K91.1
  protozoal A07.9
    specified NEC A07.8
  psychogenic F45.8
  specified
    bacterium NEC A04.8
    virus NEC A08.39
  strongyloidiasis B78.0
  toxic K52.1
  trichomonal A07.8
  tropical K90.1
  tuberculous A18.32
  viral — *see* Enteritis, viral
Diastasis
  cranial bones M84.88
    congenital NEC Q75.8
  joint (traumatic) — *see* Dislocation
  muscle M62.00
    ankle M62.07- ☑
    congenital Q79.8
    foot M62.07- ☑
    forearm M62.03- ☑
    hand M62.04- ☑
    lower leg M62.06- ☑
    pelvic region M62.05- ☑
    shoulder region M62.01- ☑
    specified site NEC M62.08
    thigh M62.05- ☑
    upper arm M62.02- ☑
  recti (abdomen)
    complicating delivery O71.89
    congenital Q79.59
Diastema, tooth, teeth, fully erupted M26.32
Diastematomyelia Q06.2
Diataxia, cerebral G80.4
Diathesis
  allergic — *see* History, allergy
  bleeding (familial) D69.9
  cystine (familial) E72.00
  gouty — *see* Gout
  hemorrhagic (familial) D69.9
    newborn NEC P53
  spasmophilic R29.0

☑ **Additional character required**

Diaz's disease or osteochondrosis (juvenile) (talus) — *see* Osteochondrosis, juvenile, tarsus
Dibothriocephalus, dibothriocephaliasis (latus) (infection) (infestation) B70.0
  larval B70.1
Dicephalus, dicephaly Q89.4
Dichotomy, teeth K00.2
Dichromat, dichromatopsia (congenital) — *see* Deficiency, color vision
Dichuchwa A65
Dicroceliasis B66.2
Didelphia, didelphys — *see* Double uterus
Didymytis N45.1
  with orchitis N45.3
Dietary
  inadequacy or deficiency E63.9
  surveillance and counseling Z71.3
Dietl's crisis N13.8
Dieulafoy lesion (hemorrhagic)
  duodenum K31.82
  esophagus K22.8
  intestine (colon) K63.81
  stomach K31.82
Difficult, difficulty (in)
  acculturation Z60.3
  feeding R63.3
    newborn P92.9
      breast P92.5
      specified NEC P92.8
    nonorganic (infant or child) F98.29
  intubation, in anesthesia T88.4 ☑
  mechanical, gastroduodenal stoma K91.89
    causing obstruction K91.3
  reading (developmental) F81.0
    secondary to emotional disorders F93.9
  spelling (specific) F81.81
    with reading disorder F81.89
    due to inadequate teaching Z55.8
  swallowing — *see* Dysphagia
  walking R26.2
  work
    conditions NEC Z56.5
    schedule Z56.3
Diffuse — *see* condition
DiGeorge's syndrome (thymic hypoplasia) D82.1
Digestive — *see* condition
Dihydropyrimidine dehydrogenase disease (DPD) E88.89
Diktyoma — *see* Neoplasm, malignant, by site
Dilaceration, tooth K00.4
Dilatation
  anus K59.8
    venule — *see* Hemorrhoids
  aorta (focal) (general) — *see* Ectasia, aorta
    with aneurysm — *see* Aneurysm, aorta
  artery — *see* Aneurysm
  bladder (sphincter) N32.89
    congenital Q64.79
  blood vessel I99.8
  bronchial J47.9
    with
      exacerbation (acute) J47.1
      lower respiratory infection J47.0
  calyx (due to obstruction) — *see* Hydronephrosis
  capillaries I78.8
  cardiac (acute) (chronic) (*see also* Hypertrophy, cardiac)
    congenital Q24.8
      valve NEC Q24.8
        pulmonary Q22.3
      valve — *see* Endocarditis
  cavum septi pellucidi Q06.8
  cervix (uteri) (*see also* Incompetency, cervix)
    incomplete, poor, slow complicating delivery O62.0
  colon K59.3
    congenital Q43.1
    psychogenic F45.8
  common duct (acquired) K83.8
    congenital Q44.5
  cystic duct (acquired) K82.8
    congenital Q44.5
  duct, mammary — *see* Ectasia, mammary duct
  duodenum K59.8
  esophagus K22.8
    congenital Q39.5
    due to achalasia K22.0
  eustachian tube, congenital Q17.8
  gallbladder K82.8
  gastric — *see* Dilatation, stomach
  heart (acute) (chronic) (*see also* Hypertrophy, cardiac)

Dilatation — *continued*
  congenital Q24.8
    valve — *see* Endocarditis
  ileum K59.8
    psychogenic F45.8
  jejunum K59.8
    psychogenic F45.8
  kidney (calyx) (collecting structures) (cystic) (parenchyma) (pelvis) (idiopathic) N28.89
  lacrimal passages or duct — *see* Disorder, lacrimal system, changes
  lymphatic vessel I89.0
  mammary duct — *see* Ectasia, mammary duct
  Meckel's diverticulum (congenital) Q43.0
    malignant — *see* Table of Neoplasms, small intestine, malignant
  myocardium (acute) (chronic) — *see* Hypertrophy, cardiac
  organ or site, congenital NEC — *see* Distortion
  pancreatic duct K86.8
  pericardium — *see* Pericarditis
  pharynx J39.2
  prostate N42.89
  pulmonary
    artery (idiopathic) I28.8
    valve, congenital Q22.3
  pupil H57.04
  rectum K59.3
  saccule, congenital Q16.5
  salivary gland (duct) K11.8
  sphincter ani K62.89
  stomach K31.89
    acute K31.0
    psychogenic F45.8
  submaxillary duct K11.8
  trachea, congenital Q32.1
  ureter (idiopathic) N28.82
    congenital Q62.2
    due to obstruction N13.4
  urethra (acquired) N36.8
  vasomotor I73.9
  vein I86.8
  ventricular, ventricle (acute) (chronic) (*see also* Hypertrophy, cardiac)
    cerebral, congenital Q04.8
  venule NEC I86.8
  vesical orifice N32.89
Dilated, dilation — *see* Dilatation
Diminished, diminution
  hearing (acuity) — *see* Deafness
  sense or sensation (cold) (heat) (tactile) (vibratory) R20.8
  vision NEC H54.7
  vital capacity R94.2
Diminuta taenia B71.0
Dimitri-Sturge-Weber disease Q85.8
Dimple
  parasacral, pilonidal or postanal — *see* Cyst, pilonidal
Dioctophyme renalis (infection) (infestation) B83.8
Dipetalonemiasis B74.4
Diphallus Q55.69
Diphtheria, diphtheritic (gangrenous) (hemorrhagic) A36.9
  carrier (suspected) Z22.2
  cutaneous A36.3
  faucial A36.0
  infection of wound A36.3
  laryngeal A36.2
  myocarditis A36.81
  nasal, anterior A36.89
  nasopharyngeal A36.1
  neurological complication A36.89
  pharyngeal A36.0
  specified site NEC A36.89
  tonsillar A36.0
Diphyllobothriasis (intestine) B70.0
  larval B70.1
Diplacusis H93.22- ☑
Diplegia (upper limbs) G83.0
  congenital (cerebral) G80.8
  facial G51.0
  lower limbs G82.20
  spastic G80.1
Diplococcus, diplococcal — *see* condition
Diplopia H53.2
Dipsomania F10.20
  with
    psychosis — *see* Psychosis, alcoholic
    remission F10.21
Dipylidiasis B71.1
Direction, teeth, abnormal, fully erupted M26.30

Dirofilariasis B74.8
Dirt-eating child F98.3
Disability, disabilities
  heart — *see* Disease, heart
  intellectual F79
    with
      autistic features F84.9
    mild (I.Q.50-69) F70
    moderate (I.Q.35-49) F71
    profound (I.Q. under 20) F73
    severe (I.Q.20-34) F72
    specified level NEC F78
  knowledge acquisition F81.9
  learning F81.9
  limiting activities Z73.6
  spelling, specific F81.81
Disappearance of family member Z63.4
Disarticulation — *see* Amputation
  meaning traumatic amputation — *see* Amputation, traumatic
Discharge (from)
  abnormal finding in — *see* Abnormal, specimen
  breast (female) (male) N64.52
  diencephalic autonomic idiopathic — *see* Epilepsy, specified NEC
  ear (*see also* Otorrhea)
    blood — *see* Otorrhagia
  excessive urine R35.8
  nipple N64.52
  penile R36.9
  postnasal R09.82
  prison, anxiety concerning Z65.2
  urethral R36.9
    without blood R36.0
    hematospermia R36.1
  vaginal N89.8
Discitis, diskitis M46.40
  cervical region M46.42
  cervicothoracic region M46.43
  lumbar region M46.46
  lumbosacral region M46.47
  multiple sites M46.49
  occipito-atlanto-axial region M46.41
  pyogenic — *see* Infection, intervertebral disc, pyogenic
  sacrococcygeal region M46.48
  thoracic region M46.44
  thoracolumbar region M46.45
Discoid
  meniscus (congenital) Q68.6
  semilunar cartilage (congenital) — *see* Derangement, knee, meniscus, specified NEC
Discoloration
  nails L60.8
  teeth (posteruptive) K03.7
    during formation K00.8
Discomfort
  chest R07.89
  visual H53.14- ☑
Discontinuity, ossicles, ear H74.2- ☑
Discord (with)
  boss Z56.4
  classmates Z55.4
  counselor Z64.4
  employer Z56.4
  family Z63.8
  fellow employees Z56.4
  in-laws Z63.1
  landlord Z59.2
  lodgers Z59.2
  neighbors Z59.2
  probation officer Z64.4
  social worker Z64.4
  teachers Z55.4
  workmates Z56.4
Discordant connection
  atrioventricular (congenital) Q20.5
  ventriculoarterial Q20.3
Discrepancy
  centric occlusion maximum intercuspation M26.55
  leg length (acquired) — *see* Deformity, limb, unequal length
    congenital — *see* Defect, reduction, lower limb
  uterine size date O26.84- ☑
Discrimination
  ethnic Z60.5
  political Z60.5
  racial Z60.5
  religious Z60.5
  sex Z60.5

Disease

Disease, diseased (see also Syndrome)
absorbent system I87.8
acid-peptic K30
Acosta's T70.29 ☑
Adams-Stokes (-Morgagni) (syncope with heart block) I45.9
Addison's anemia (pernicious) D51.0
adenoids (and tonsils) J35.9
adrenal (capsule) (cortex) (gland) (medullary) E27.9
  hyperfunction E27.0
  specified NEC E27.8
ainhum L94.6
airway
  obstructive, chronic J44.9
    due to
      cotton dust J66.0
      specific organic dusts NEC J66.8
    reactive — see Asthma
akamushi (scrub typhus) A75.3
Albers-Schönberg (marble bones) Q78.2
Albert's — see Tendinitis, Achilles
alimentary canal K63.9
alligator-skin Q80.9
  acquired L85.0
alpha heavy chain C88.3
alpine T70.29 ☑
altitude T70.20 ☑
alveolar ridge
  edentulous K06.9
    specified NEC K06.8
alveoli, teeth K08.9
Alzheimer's G30.9 [F02.80]
  with behavioral disturbance G30.9 [F02.81]
  early onset G30.0 [F02.80]
    with behavioral disturbance G30.0 [F02.81]
  late onset G30.1 [F02.80]
    with behavioral disturbance G30.1 [F02.81]
  specified NEC G30.8 [F02.80]
    with behavioral disturbance G30.8 [F02.81]
amyloid — see Amyloidosis
Andersen's (glycogenosis IV) E74.09
Andes T70.29 ☑
Andrews' (bacterid) L08.89
angiospastic I73.9
  cerebral G45.9
  vein I87.8
anterior
  chamber H21.9
  horn cell G12.29
antiglomerular basement membrane (anti- GBM) antibody M31.0
  tubulo-interstitial nephritis N12
antral — see Sinusitis, maxillary
anus K62.9
  specified NEC K62.89
aorta (nonsyphilitic) I77.9
  syphilitic NEC A52.02
aortic (heart) (valve) I35.9
  rheumatic I06.9
Apollo B30.3
aponeuroses — see Enthesopathy
appendix K38.9
  specified NEC K38.8
aqueous (chamber) H21.9
Arnold-Chiari — see Arnold-Chiari disease
arterial I77.9
  occlusive — see Occlusion, by site
    due to stricture or stenosis I77.1
arteriocardiorenal — see Hypertension, cardiorenal
arteriolar (generalized) (obliterative) I77.9
arteriorenal — see Hypertension, kidney
arteriosclerotic (see also Arteriosclerosis)
  cardiovascular — see Disease, heart, ischemic, atherosclerotic
  coronary (artery) — see Disease, heart, ischemic, atherosclerotic
  heart — see Disease, heart, ischemic, atherosclerotic
artery I77.9
  cerebral I67.9
  coronary I25.10
    with angina pectoris — see Arteriosclerosis, coronary (artery),
arthropod-borne NOS (viral) A94
  specified type NEC A93.8
atticoantral, chronic H66.20
  left H66.22
    with right H66.23
  right H66.21
    with left H66.23

Disease — continued
auditory canal — see Disorder, ear, external
auricle, ear NEC — see Disorder, pinna
Australian X A83.4
autoimmune (systemic) NOS M35.9
  hemolytic (cold type) (warm type) D59.1
    drug-induced D59.0
  thyroid E06.3
aviator's — see Effect, adverse, high altitude
Ayala's Q78.5
Ayerza's (pulmonary artery sclerosis with pulmonary hypertension) I27.0
Babington's (familial hemorrhagic telangiectasia) I78.0
bacterial A49.9
  specified NEC A48.8
  zoonotic A28.9
    specified type NEC A28.8
Baelz's (cheilitis glandularis apostematosa) K13.0
bagasse J67.1
balloon — see Effect, adverse, high altitude
Bang's (brucella abortus) A23.1
Bannister's T78.3 ☑
barometer makers' — see Poisoning, mercury
Barraquer (-Simons') (progressive lipodystrophy) E88.1
Barrett's — see Barrett's, esophagus
Bartholin's gland N75.9
basal ganglia G25.9
  degenerative G23.9
    specified NEC G23.8
  specified NEC G25.89
Basedow's (exophthalmic goiter) — see Hyperthyroidism, with, goiter (diffuse)
Bateman's B08.1
Batten-Steinert G71.11
Battey A31.0
Beard's (neurasthenia) F48.8
Becker
  idiopathic mural endomyocardial I42.3
  myotonia congenita G71.12
Begbie's (exophthalmic goiter) — see Hyperthyroidism, with, goiter (diffuse)
behavioral, organic F07.9
Beigel's (white piedra) B36.2
Benson's — see Deposit, crystalline
Bernard-Soulier (thrombopathy) D69.1
Bernhardt (-Roth) — see Mononeuropathy, lower limb, meralgia paresthetica
Biermer's (pernicious anemia) D51.0
bile duct (common) (hepatic) K83.9
  with calculus, stones — see Calculus, bile duct
  specified NEC K83.8
biliary (tract) K83.9
  specified NEC K83.8
Billroth's — see Spina bifida
bird fancier's J67.2
black lung J60
bladder N32.9
  in (due to)
    schistosomiasis (bilharziasis) B65.0 [N33]
  specified NEC N32.89
bleeder's D66
blood D75.9
  forming organs D75.9
  vessel I99.9
Bloodgood's — see Mastopathy, cystic
Bodechtel-Guttmann (subacute sclerosing panencephalitis) A81.1
bone (see also Disorder, bone)
  aluminum M83.4
  fibrocystic NEC
    jaw M27.49
bone-marrow D75.9
Borna A83.9
Bornholm (epidemic pleurodynia) B33.0
Bouchard's (myopathic dilatation of the stomach) K31.0
Bouillaud's (rheumatic heart disease) I01.9
Bourneville (-Brissaud) (tuberous sclerosis) Q85.1
Bouveret (-Hoffmann) (paroxysmal tachycardia) I47.9
bowel K63.9
  functional K59.9
    psychogenic F45.8
brain G93.9
  arterial, artery I67.9
  arteriosclerotic I67.2
  congenital Q04.9
  degenerative — see Degeneration, brain
  inflammatory — see Encephalitis
  organic G93.9

Disease — continued
  arteriosclerotic I67.2
  parasitic NEC B71.9 [G94]
  senile NEC G31.1
  specified NEC G93.89
breast (see also Disorder, breast) N64.9
  cystic (chronic) — see Mastopathy, cystic
  fibrocystic — see Mastopathy, cystic
  Paget's
    female, unspecified side C50.91- ☑
    male, unspecified side C50.92- ☑
  specified NEC N64.89
Breda's — see Yaws
Bretonneau's (diphtheritic malignant angina) A36.0
Bright's — see Nephritis
  arteriosclerotic — see Hypertension, kidney
Brill's (recrudescent typhus) A75.1
Brill-Zinsser (recrudescent typhus) A75.1
Brion-Kayser — see Fever, paratyphoid
broad
  beta E78.2
  ligament (noninflammatory) N83.9
    inflammatory — see Disease, pelvis, inflammatory
    specified NEC N83.8
Brocq-Duhring (dermatitis herpetiformis) L13.0
Brocq's
  meaning
    dermatitis herpetiformis L13.0
    prurigo L28.2
bronchopulmonary J98.4
bronchus NEC J98.09
bronze Addison's E27.1
  tuberculous A18.7
budgerigar fancier's J67.2
bullous L13.9
  chronic of childhood L12.2
  specified NEC L13.8
Buerger's (thromboangiitis obliterans) I73.1
Bürger-Grütz (essential familial hyperlipemia) E78.3
bursa — see Bursopathy
caisson T70.3 ☑
California — see Coccidioidomycosis
capillaries I78.9
  specified NEC I78.8
Carapata A68.0
cardiac — see Disease, heart
cardiopulmonary, chronic I27.9
cardiorenal (hepatic) (hypertensive) (vascular) — see Hypertension, cardiorenal
cardiovascular (atherosclerotic) I25.10
  with angina pectoris — see Arteriosclerosis, coronary (artery),
  congenital Q28.9
  newborn P29.9
    specified NEC P29.89
  hypertensive — see Hypertension, heart
  renal (hypertensive) — see Hypertension, cardiorenal
  syphilitic (asymptomatic) A52.00
cartilage — see Disorder, cartilage
Castellani's A69.8
cat-scratch A28.1
Cavare's (familial periodic paralysis) G72.3
cecum K63.9
celiac (adult) (infantile) K90.0
cellular tissue L98.9
central core G71.2
cerebellar, cerebellum — see Disease, brain
cerebral (see also Disease, brain)
  degenerative — see Degeneration, brain
cerebrospinal G96.9
cerebrovascular I67.9
  acute I67.89
    embolic I63.4- ☑
    thrombotic I63.3- ☑
  arteriosclerotic I67.2
  specified NEC I67.89
cervix (uteri) (noninflammatory) N88.9
  inflammatory — see Cervicitis
  specified NEC N88.8
Chabert's A22.9
Chandler's (osteochondritis dissecans, hip) — see Osteochondritis, dissecans, hip
Charlouis — see Yaws
Chédiak-Steinbrinck (-Higashi) (congenital gigantism of peroxidase granules) E70.330
chest J98.9
Chiari's (hepatic vein thrombosis) I82.0
Chicago B40.9

    ☑ **Additional character required**

Disease — *continued*

Chignon B36.8
chigo, chigoe B88.1
childhood granulomatous D71
Chinese liver fluke B66.1
chlamydial A74.9
  specified NEC A74.89
cholecystic K82.9
choroid H31.9
  specified NEC H31.8
Christmas D67
chronic bullous of childhood L12.2
chylomicron retention E78.3
ciliary body H21.9
  specified NEC H21.89
circulatory (system) NEC I99.8
  newborn P29.9
  syphilitic A52.00
    congenital A50.54
coagulation factor deficiency (congenital) — *see*
  Defect, coagulation
coccidioidal — *see* Coccidioidomycosis
cold
  agglutinin or hemoglobinuria D59.1
    paroxysmal D59.6
  hemagglutinin (chronic) D59.1
collagen NOS (nonvascular) (vascular) M35.9
  specified NEC M35.8
colon K63.9
  functional K59.9
    congenital Q43.2
  ischemic K55.0
combined system — *see* Degeneration,
  combined
compressed air T70.3 ☑
Concato's (pericardial polyserositis) A19.9
  nontubercular I31.1
  pleural — *see* Pleurisy, with effusion
conjunctiva H11.9
  chlamydial A74.0
  specified NEC H11.89
  viral B30.9
    specified NEC B30.8
connective tissue, systemic (diffuse) M35.9
  in (due to)
    hypogammaglobulinemia D80.1 [M36.8]
    ochronosis E70.29 [M36.8]
  specified NEC M35.8
Conor and Bruch's (boutonneuse fever) A77.1
Cooper's — *see* Mastopathy, cystic
Cori's (glycogenosis III) E74.03
corkhandler's or corkworker's J67.3
cornea H18.9
  specified NEC H18.89- ☑
coronary (artery) — *see* Disease, heart, ischemic,
  atherosclerotic
  congenital Q24.5
  ostial, syphilitic (aortic) (mitral) (pulmonary)
    A52.03
corpus cavernosum N48.9
  specified NEC N48.89
Cotugno's — *see* Sciatica
coxsackie (virus) NEC B34.1
cranial nerve NOS G52.9
Creutzfeldt-Jakob — *see* Creutzfeldt-Jakob
  disease or syndrome
Crocq's (acrocyanosis) I73.89
Crohn's — *see* Enteritis, regional
Curschmann G71.11
cystic
  breast (chronic) — *see* Mastopathy, cystic
  kidney, congenital Q61.9
  liver, congenital Q44.6
  lung J98.4
    congenital Q33.0
cytomegalic inclusion (generalized) B25.9
  with pneumonia B25.0
  congenital P35.1
cytomegaloviral B25.9
  specified NEC B25.8
Czerny's (periodic hydrarthrosis of the knee) —
  see Effusion, joint, knee
Daae (-Finsen) (epidemic pleurodynia) B33.0
Darling's — *see* Histoplasmosis capsulati
Débove's (splenomegaly) R16.1
deer fly — *see* Tularemia
Degos' I77.89
demyelinating, demyelinizating (nervous system)
  G37.9
  multiple sclerosis G35
  specified NEC G37.8

Disease — *continued*

dense deposit (*see also* N00-N07 with fourth
  character .6) N05.6
deposition, hydroxyapatite — *see* Disease,
  hydroxyapatite deposition
de Quervain's (tendon sheath) M65.4
  thyroid (subacute granulomatous thyroiditis)
    E06.1
Devergie's (pityriasis rubra pilaris) L44.0
Devic's G36.0
diaphorase deficiency D74.0
diaphragm J98.6
diarrheal, infectious NEC A09
digestive system K92.9
  specified NEC K92.89
disc, degenerative — *see* Degeneration,
  intervertebral disc
discogenic (*see also* Displacement, intervertebral
  disc NEC)
  with myelopathy — *see* Disorder, disc, with,
    myelopathy
diverticular — *see* Diverticula
Dubois (thymus) A50.59 [E35]
Duchenne-Griesinger G71.0
Duchenne's
  muscular dystrophy G71.0
  pseudohypertrophy, muscles G71.0
ductless glands E34.9
Duhring's (dermatitis herpetiformis) L13.0
duodenum K31.9
  specified NEC K31.89
Dupré's (meningism) R29.1
Dupuytren's (muscle contracture) M72.0
Durand-Nicholas-Favre (climatic bubo) A55
Duroziez's (congenital mitral stenosis) Q23.2
ear — *see* Disorder, ear
Eberth's — *see* Fever, typhoid
Ebola (virus) A98.4
Ebstein's heart Q22.5
Echinococcus — *see* Echinococcus
echovirus NEC B34.1
Eddowes' (brittle bones and blue sclera) Q78.0
edentulous (alveolar) ridge K06.9
  specified NEC K06.8
Edsall's T67.2 ☑
Eichstedt's (pityriasis versicolor) B36.0
Ellis-van Creveld (chondroectodermal dysplasia)
  Q77.6
end stage renal (ESRD) N18.6
  due to hypertension I12.0
endocrine glands or system NEC E34.9
endomyocardial (eosinophilic) I42.3
English (rickets) E55.0
enteroviral, enterovirus NEC B34.1
  central nervous system NEC A88.8
epidemic B99.9
  specified NEC B99.8
epididymis N50.9
Erb (-Landouzy) G71.0
Erdheim-Chester (ECD) E88.89
esophagus K22.9
  functional K22.4
  psychogenic F45.8
  specified NEC K22.8
Eulenburg's (congenital paramyotonia) G71.19
eustachian tube — *see* Disorder, eustachian tube
external
  auditory canal — *see* Disorder, ear, external
  ear — *see* Disorder, ear, external
extrapyramidal G25.9
  specified NEC G25.89
eye H57.9
  anterior chamber H21.9
  inflammatory NEC H57.8
  muscle (external) — *see* Strabismus
  specified NEC H57.8
  syphilitic — *see* Oculopathy, syphilitic
eyeball H44.9
  specified NEC H44.89
eyelid — *see* Disorder, eyelid
  specified NEC — *see* Disorder, eyelid, specified
    type NEC
eyeworm of Africa B74.3
facial nerve (seventh) G51.9
  newborn (birth injury) P11.3
Fahr (of brain) G23.8
Fahr Volhard (of kidney) I12.- ☑
fallopian tube (noninflammatory) N83.9
  inflammatory — *see* Salpingo-oophoritis
  specified NEC N83.8
familial periodic paralysis G72.3
Fanconi's (congenital pancytopenia) D61.09

Disease — *continued*

fascia NEC (*see also* Disorder, muscle)
  inflammatory — *see* Myositis
  specified NEC M62.89
Fauchard's (periodontitis) — *see* Periodontitis
Favre-Durand-Nicolas (climatic bubo) A55
Fede's K14.0
Feer's — *see* Poisoning, mercury
female pelvic inflammatory (*see also* Disease,
  pelvis, inflammatory) N73.9
  syphilitic (secondary) A51.42
  tuberculous A18.17
Fernels' (aortic aneurysm) I71.9
fibrocaseous of lung — *see* Tuberculosis,
  pulmonary
fibrocystic — *see* Fibrocystic disease
Fiedler's (leptospiral jaundice) A27.0
fifth B08.3
file-cutter's — *see* Poisoning, lead
fish-skin Q80.9
  acquired L85.0
Flajani (-Basedow) (exophthalmic goiter) — *see*
  Hyperthyroidism, with, goiter (diffuse)
flax-dresser's J66.1
fluke — *see* Infestation, fluke
foot and mouth B08.8
foot process N04.9
Forbes' (glycogenosis III) E74.03
Fordyce-Fox (apocrine miliaria) L75.2
Fordyce's (ectopic sebaceous glands) (mouth)
  Q38.6
Forestier's (rhizomelic pseudopolyarthritis) M35.3
  meaning ankylosing hyperostosis — *see*
    Hyperostosis, ankylosing
Fothergill's
  neuralgia — *see* Neuralgia, trigeminal
  scarlatina anginosa A38.9
Fournier (gangrene) N49.3
  female N76.89
fourth B08.8
Fox (-Fordyce) (apocrine miliaria) L75.2
Francis' — *see* Tularemia
Franklin C88.2
Frei's (climatic bubo) A55
Friedreich's
  combined systemic or ataxia G11.1
  myoclonia G25.3
frontal sinus — *see* Sinusitis, frontal
fungus NEC B49
Gaisböck's (polycythemia hypertonica) D75.1
gallbladder K82.9
  calculus — *see* Calculus, gallbladder
  cholecystitis — *see* Cholecystitis
  cholesterolosis K82.4
  fistula — *see* Fistula, gallbladder
  hydrops K82.1
  obstruction — *see* Obstruction, gallbladder
  perforation K82.2
  specified NEC K82.8
gamma heavy chain C88.2
Gamna's (siderotic splenomegaly) D73.2
Gamstorp's (adynamia episodica hereditaria)
  G72.3
Gandy-Nanta (siderotic splenomegaly) D73.2
ganister J62.8
gastric — *see* Disease, stomach
gastroesophageal reflux (GERD) K21.9
  with esophagitis K21.0
gastrointestinal (tract) K92.9
  amyloid E85.4
  functional K59.9
    psychogenic F45.8
  specified NEC K92.89
Gee (-Herter) (-Heubner) (-Thaysen) (nontropical
  sprue) K90.0
genital organs
  female N94.9
  male N50.9
Gerhardt's (erythromelalgia) I73.81
Gibert's (pityriasis rosea) L42
Gierke's (glycogenosis I) E74.01
Gilles de la Tourette's (motor-verbal tic) F95.2
gingiva K06.9
  specified NEC K06.8
gland (lymph) I89.9
Glanzmann's (hereditary hemorrhagic
  thrombasthenia) D69.1
glass-blower's (cataract) — *see* Cataract,
  specified NEC
  salivary gland hypertrophy K11.1
Glisson's — *see* Rickets
globe H44.9

Disease

Disease — *continued*

specified NEC H44.89
glomerular (*see also* Glomerulonephritis)
  with edema — *see* Nephrosis
  acute — *see* Nephritis, acute
  chronic — *see* Nephritis, chronic
  minimal change N05.0
  rapidly progressive N01.9
glycogen storage E74.00
  Andersen's E74.09
  Cori's E74.03
  Forbes' E74.03
  generalized E74.00
  glucose-6-phosphatase deficiency E74.01
  heart E74.02 [I43]
  hepatorenal E74.09
  Hers' E74.09
  liver and kidney E74.09
  McArdle's E74.04
  muscle phosphofructokinase E74.09
  myocardium E74.02 [I43]
  Pompe's E74.02
  Tauri's E74.09
  type 0 E74.09
  type I E74.01
  type II E74.02
  type III E74.03
  type IV E74.09
  type V E74.04
  type VI-XI E74.09
  Von Gierke's E74.01
Goldstein's (familial hemorrhagic telangiectasia) I78.0
gonococcal NOS A54.9
graft-versus-host (GVH) D89.813
  acute D89.810
  acute on chronic D89.812
  chronic D89.811
grainhandler's J67.8
granulomatous (childhood) (chronic) D71
Graves' (exophthalmic goiter) — *see* Hyperthyroidism, with, goiter (diffuse)
Griesinger's — *see* Ancylostomiasis
Grisel's M43.6
Gruby's (tinea tonsurans) B35.0
Guillain-Barré G61.0
Guinon's (motor-verbal tic) F95.2
gum K06.9
gynecological N94.9
H (Hartnup's) E72.02
Haff — *see* Poisoning, mercury
Hageman (congenital factor XII deficiency) D68.2
hair (color) (shaft) L67.9
  follicles L73.9
    specified NEC L73.8
Hamman's (spontaneous mediastinal emphysema) J98.2
hand, foot and mouth B08.4
Hansen's — *see* Leprosy
Hantavirus, with pulmonary manifestations B33.4
  with renal manifestations A98.5
Harada's H30.81- ☑
Hartnup (pellagra-cerebellar ataxia-renal aminoaciduria) E72.02
Hart's (pellagra-cerebellar ataxia-renal aminoaciduria) E72.02
Hashimoto's (struma lymphomatosa) E06.3
Hb — *see* Disease, hemoglobin
heart (organic) I51.9
  with
    pulmonary edema (acute) (*see also* Failure, ventricular, left) I50.1
    rheumatic fever (conditions in I00)
      active I01.9
        with chorea I02.0
        specified NEC I01.8
      inactive or quiescent (with chorea) I09.9
        specified NEC I09.89
  amyloid E85.4 [I43]
  aortic (valve) I35.9
  arteriosclerotic or sclerotic (senile) — *see* Disease, heart, ischemic, atherosclerotic
  artery, arterial — *see* Disease, heart, ischemic, atherosclerotic
  beer drinkers' I42.6
  beriberi (wet) E51.12
  black I27.0
  congenital Q24.9
    cyanotic Q24.9
    specified NEC Q24.8
  coronary — *see* Disease, heart, ischemic
  cryptogenic I51.9

Disease — *continued*

fibroid — *see* Myocarditis
functional I51.89
  psychogenic F45.8
glycogen storage E74.02 [I43]
gonococcal A54.83
hypertensive — *see* Hypertension, heart
hyperthyroid (*see also* Hyperthyroidism) E05.90 [I43]
  with thyroid storm E05.91 [I43]
ischemic (chronic or with a stated duration of over 4 weeks) I25.9
  atherosclerotic (of) I25.10
    with angina pectoris — *see* Arteriosclerosis, coronary (artery)
    coronary artery bypass graft — *see* Arteriosclerosis, coronary (artery), cardiomyopathy I25.5
    diagnosed on ECG or other special investigation, but currently presenting no symptoms I25.6
    silent I25.6
    specified form NEC I25.89
kyphoscoliotic I27.1
meningococcal A39.50
  endocarditis A39.51
  myocarditis A39.52
  pericarditis A39.53
mitral I05.9
  specified NEC I05.8
muscular — *see* Degeneration, myocardial
psychogenic (functional) F45.8
pulmonary (chronic) I27.9
  in schistosomiasis B65.9 [I52]
  specified NEC I27.89
rheumatic (chronic) (inactive) (old) (quiescent) (with chorea) I09.9
  active or acute I01.9
    with chorea (acute) (rheumatic) (Sydenham's) I02.0
  specified NEC I09.89
senile — *see* Myocarditis
syphilitic A52.06
  aortic A52.03
    aneurysm A52.01
  congenital A50.54 [I52]
  thyrotoxic (*see also* Thyrotoxicosis) E05.90 [I43]
    with thyroid storm E05.91 [I43]
  valve, valvular (obstructive) (regurgitant) (*see also* Endocarditis)
    congenital NEC Q24.8
    pulmonary Q22.3
  vascular — *see* Disease, cardiovascular
heavy chain NEC C88.2
  alpha C88.3
  gamma C88.2
  mu C88.2
Hebra's
  pityriasis
    maculata et circinata L42
    rubra pilaris L44.0
  prurigo L28.2
hematopoietic organs D75.9
hemoglobin or Hb
  abnormal (mixed) NEC D58.2
    with thalassemia D56.9
  AS genotype D57.3
  Bart's D56.0
  C (Hb-C) D58.2
    with other abnormal hemoglobin NEC D58.2
    elliptocytosis D58.1
    Hb-S D57.2- ☑
    sickle-cell D57.2- ☑
    thalassemia D56.8
  Constant Spring D58.2
  D (Hb-D) D58.2
  E (Hb-E) D58.2
  E-beta thalassemia D56.5
  elliptocytosis D58.1
  H (Hb-H) (thalassemia) D56.0
    with other abnormal hemoglobin NEC D56.9
    Constant Spring D56.0
  I thalassemia D56.9
  M D74.0
  S or SS D57.1
  SC D57.2- ☑
  SD D57.8- ☑
  SE D57.8- ☑
  spherocytosis D58.0
  unstable, hemolytic D58.2
hemolytic (newborn) P55.9
  autoimmune (cold type) (warm type) D59.1

Disease — *continued*

  drug-induced D59.0
  due to or with
    incompatibility
      ABO (blood group) P55.1
      blood (group) (Duffy) (K(ell)) (Kidd) (Lewis) (M) (S) NEC P55.8
      Rh (blood group) (factor) P55.0
    Rh negative mother P55.0
  specified type NEC P55.8
  unstable hemoglobin D58.2
hemorrhagic D69.9
  newborn P53
Henoch (-Schönlein) (purpura nervosa) D69.0
hepatic — *see* Disease, liver
hepatobiliary K83.9
  toxic K71.9
hepatolenticular E83.01
heredodegenerative NEC
  spinal cord G95.89
herpesviral, disseminated B00.7
Hers' (glycogenosis VI) E74.09
Herter (-Gee) (-Heubner) (nontropical sprue) K90.0
Heubner-Herter (nontropical sprue) K90.0
high fetal gene or hemoglobin thalassemia D56.9
Hildenbrand's — *see* Typhus
hip (joint) M25.9
  congenital Q65.89
  suppurative M00.9
  tuberculous A18.02
His (-Werner) (trench fever) A79.0
Hodgson's I71.2
  ruptured I71.1
Holla — *see* Spherocytosis
hookworm B76.9
  specified NEC B76.8
host-versus-graft D89.813
  acute D89.810
  acute on chronic D89.812
  chronic D89.811
human immunodeficiency virus (HIV) B20
Huntington's G10
Hutchinson's (cheiropompholyx) — *see* Hutchinson's disease
hyaline (diffuse) (generalized)
  membrane (lung) (newborn) P22.0
    adult J80
hydatid — *see* Echinococcus
hydroxyapatite deposition M11.00
  ankle M11.07- ☑
  elbow M11.02- ☑
  foot joint M11.07- ☑
  hand joint M11.04- ☑
  hip M11.05- ☑
  knee M11.06- ☑
  multiple site M11.09
  shoulder M11.01- ☑
  vertebra M11.08
  wrist M11.03- ☑
hyperkinetic — *see* Hyperkinesia
hypertensive — *see* Hypertension
hypophysis E23.7
Iceland G93.3
I-cell E77.0
immune D89.9
immunoproliferative (malignant) C88.9
  small intestinal C88.3
  specified NEC C88.8
inclusion B25.9
  salivary gland B25.9
infectious, infective B99.9
  congenital P37.9
    specified NEC P37.8
    viral P35.9
      specified type NEC P35.8
  specified NEC B99.8
inflammatory
  penis N48.29
    abscess N48.21
    cellulitis N48.22
  prepuce N47.7
    balanoposthitis N47.6
  tubo-ovarian — *see* Salpingo-oophoritis
intervertebral disc (*see also* Disorder, disc)
  with myelopathy — *see* Disorder, disc, with, myelopathy
  cervical, cervicothoracic — *see* Disorder, disc, cervical
    with
      myelopathy — *see* Disorder, disc, cervical, with myelopathy

☑ **Additional character required**

Disease — *continued*

  neuritis, radiculitis or radiculopathy — *see*
    Disorder, disc, cervical, with neuritis
  specified NEC — *see* Disorder, disc, cervical,
    specified type NEC
  lumbar (with)
    myelopathy M51.06
    neuritis, radiculitis, radiculopathy or sciatica
      M51.16
    specified NEC M51.86
  lumbosacral (with)
    neuritis, radiculitis, radiculopathy or sciatica
      M51.17
    specified NEC M51.87
  specified NEC — *see* Disorder, disc, specified
    NEC
  thoracic (with)
    myelopathy M51.04
    neuritis, radiculitis or radiculopathy M51.14
    specified NEC M51.84
  thoracolumbar (with)
    myelopathy M51.05
    neuritis, radiculitis or radiculopathy M51.15
    specified NEC M51.85
intestine K63.9
  functional K59.9
    psychogenic F45.8
    specified NEC K59.8
  organic K63.9
  protozoal A07.9
  specified NEC K63.89
iris H21.9
  specified NEC H21.89
iron metabolism or storage E83.10
island (scrub typhus) A75.3
itai-itai — *see* Poisoning, cadmium
Jakob-Creutzfeldt — *see* Creutzfeldt-Jakob
  disease or syndrome
jaw M27.9
  fibrocystic M27.49
  specified NEC M27.8
jigger B88.1
joint (*see also* Disorder, joint)
  Charcot's — *see* Arthropathy, neuropathic
    (Charcot)
  degenerative — *see* Osteoarthritis
    multiple M15.9
    spine — *see* Spondylosis
  hypertrophic — *see* Osteoarthritis
  sacroiliac M53.3
  specified NEC — *see* Disorder, joint, specified
    type NEC
  spine NEC — *see* Dorsopathy
  suppurative — *see* Arthritis, pyogenic or
    pyemic
Jourdain's (acute gingivitis) K05.00
  nonplaque induced K05.01
  plaque induced K05.00
Kaschin-Beck (endemic polyarthritis) M12.10
  ankle M12.17- ☑
  elbow M12.12- ☑
  foot joint M12.17- ☑
  hand joint M12.14- ☑
  hip M12.15- ☑
  knee M12.16- ☑
  multiple site M12.19
  shoulder M12.11- ☑
  vertebra M12.18
  wrist M12.13- ☑
Katayama B65.2
Kedani (scrub typhus) A75.3
Keshan E59
kidney (functional) (pelvis) N28.9
  chronic N18.9
    hypertensive — *see* Hypertension, kidney
    stage 1 N18.1
    stage 2 (mild) N18.2
    stage 3 (moderate) N18.3
    stage 4 (severe) N18.4
    stage 5 N18.5
  complicating pregnancy — *see* Pregnancy,
    complicated by, renal disease
  cystic (congenital) Q61.9
  diabetic — *see* E08-E13 with .22
  fibrocystic (congenital) Q61.8
  hypertensive — *see* Hypertension, kidney
  in (due to)
    schistosomiasis (bilharziasis) B65.9 [N29]
  multicystic Q61.4
  polycystic Q61.3
    adult type Q61.2
    childhood type NEC Q61.19

Disease — *continued*

  collecting duct dilatation Q61.11
Kimmelstiel (-Wilson) (intercapillary polycystic
  (congenital) glomerulosclerosis) — *see*
  E08-E13 with .21
Kimura D21.9
  specified site (*see* Neoplasm, connective tissue
    benign)
Kinnier Wilson's (hepatolenticular degeneration)
  E83.01
kissing — *see* Mononucleosis, infectious
Klebs' (*see also* Glomerulonephritis) N05.- ☑
Klippel-Feil (brevicollis) Q76.1
Köhler-Pellegrini-Stieda (calcification, knee joint)
  — *see* Bursitis, tibial collateral
Kok Q89.8
König's (osteochondritis dissecans) — *see*
  Osteochondritis, dissecans
Korsakoff's (nonalcoholic) F04
  alcoholic F10.96
    with dependence F10.26
Kostmann's (infantile genetic agranulocytosis)
  D70.0
kuru A81.81
Kyasanur Forest A98.2
labyrinth, ear — *see* Disorder, ear, inner
lacrimal system — *see* Disorder, lacrimal system
Lafora's — *see* Epilepsy, generalized, idiopathic
Lancereaux-Mathieu (leptospiral jaundice) A27.0
Landry's G61.0
Larrey-Weil (leptospiral jaundice) A27.0
larynx J38.7
legionnaires' A48.1
  nonpneumonic A48.2
Lenegre's I44.2
lens H27.9
  specified NEC H27.8
Lev's (acquired complete heart block) I44.2
Lewy body (dementia) G31.83 [F02.80]
  with behavioral disturbance G31.83 [F02.81]
Lichtheim's (subacute combined sclerosis with
  pernicious anemia) D51.0
Lightwood's (renal tubular acidosis) N25.89
Lignac's (cystinosis) E72.04
lip K13.0
lipid-storage E75.6
  specified NEC E75.5
Lipschütz's N76.6
liver (chronic) (organic) K76.9
  alcoholic (chronic) K70.9
    acute — *see* Disease, liver, alcoholic, hepatitis
    cirrhosis K70.30
      with ascites K70.31
    failure K70.40
      with coma K70.41
    fatty liver K70.0
    fibrosis K70.2
    hepatitis K70.10
      with ascites K70.11
    sclerosis K70.2
  cystic, congenital Q44.6
  drug-induced (idiosyncratic) (toxic)
    (predictable) (unpredictable) — *see*
    Disease, liver, toxic
  end stage K72.90
    due to hepatitis — *see* Hepatitis
  fatty, nonalcoholic (NAFLD) K76.0
    alcoholic K70.0
  fibrocystic (congenital) Q44.6
  fluke
    Chinese B66.1
    oriental B66.1
    sheep B66.3
  glycogen storage E74.09 [K77]
  in (due to)
    schistosomiasis (bilharziasis) B65.9 [K77]
  inflammatory K75.9
    alcoholic K70.1 ☑
    specified NEC K75.89
  polycystic (congenital) Q44.6
  toxic K71.9
    with
      cholestasis K71.0
      cirrhosis (liver) K71.7
      fibrosis (liver) K71.7
      focal nodular hyperplasia K71.8
      hepatic granuloma K71.8
      hepatic necrosis K71.10
        with coma K71.11
      hepatitis NEC K71.6
        acute K71.2
        chronic

Disease — *continued*

    active K71.50
      with ascites K71.51
    lobular K71.4
    persistent K71.3
    lupoid K71.50
      with ascites K71.51
    peliosis hepatis K71.8
    veno-occlusive disease (VOD) of liver K71.8
  veno-occlusive K76.5
Lobo's (keloid blastomycosis) B48.0
Lobstein's (brittle bones and blue sclera) Q78.0
Ludwig's (submaxillary cellulitis) K12.2
lumbosacral region M53.87
lung J98.4
  black J60
  congenital Q33.9
  cystic J98.4
    congenital Q33.0
  fibroid (chronic) — *see* Fibrosis, lung
  fluke B66.4
    oriental B66.4
  in
    amyloidosis E85.4 [J99]
    sarcoidosis D86.0
    Sjögren's syndrome M35.02
    systemic
      lupus erythematosus M32.13
      sclerosis M34.81
  interstitial J84.9
    of childhood, specified NEC J84.848
    respiratory bronchiolitis J84.115
    specified NEC J84.89
  obstructive (chronic) J44.9
    with
      acute
        bronchitis J44.0
        exacerbation NEC J44.1
        lower respiratory infection J44.0
      alveolitis, allergic J67.9
      asthma J44.9
      bronchiectasis J47.9
        with
          exacerbation (acute) J47.1
          lower respiratory infection J47.0
      bronchitis J44.9
        with
          exacerbation (acute) J44.1
          lower respiratory infection J44.0
      emphysema J44.9
      hypersensitivity pneumonitis J67.9
    decompensated J44.1
      with
        exacerbation (acute) J44.1
  polycystic J98.4
    congenital Q33.0
  rheumatoid (diffuse) (interstitial) — *see*
    Rheumatoid, lung
Lutembacher's (atrial septal defect with mitral
  stenosis) Q21.1
Lyme A69.20
lymphatic (gland) (system) (channel) (vessel)
  I89.9
lymphoproliferative D47.9
  specified NEC D47.Z9
  T-gamma D47.Z9
  X-linked D82.3
Magitot's M27.2
malarial — *see* Malaria
malignant (*see also* Neoplasm, malignant, by site)
Manson's B65.1
maple bark J67.6
maple-syrup-urine E71.0
Marburg (virus) A98.3
Marion's (bladder neck obstruction) N32.0
Marsh's (exophthalmic goiter) — *see*
  Hyperthyroidism, with, goiter (diffuse)
mastoid (process) — *see* Disorder, ear, middle
Mathieu's (leptospiral jaundice) A27.0
Maxcy's A75.2
McArdle (-Schmid-Pearson) (glycogenosis V)
  E74.04
mediastinum J98.5
medullary center (idiopathic) (respiratory) G93.89
Meige's (chronic hereditary edema) Q82.0
meningococcal — *see* Infection, meningococcal
mental F99
  organic F09
mesenchymal M35.9
mesenteric embolic K55.0
metabolic, metabolism E88.9
  bilirubin E80.7

Disease

Disease — *continued*

metal-polisher's J62.8
metastatic (*see also* Neoplasm, secondary, by site) C79.9
microvascular - code to condition
microvillus
  atrophy Q43.8
  inclusion (MVD) Q43.8
middle ear — *see* Disorder, ear, middle
Mikulicz' (dryness of mouth, absent or decreased lacrimation) K11.8
Milroy's (chronic hereditary edema) Q82.0
Minamata — *see* Poisoning, mercury
minicore G71.2
Minor's G95.19
Minot's (hemorrhagic disease, newborn) P53
Minot-von Willebrand-Jürgens (angiohemophilia) D68.0
Mitchell's (erythromelalgia) I73.81
mitral (valve) I05.9
  nonrheumatic I34.9
mixed connective tissue M35.1
moldy hay J67.0
Monge's T70.29 ☑
Morgagni-Adams-Stokes (syncope with heart block) I45.9
Morgagni's (syndrome) (hyperostosis frontalis interna) M85.2
Morton's (with metatarsalgia) — *see* Lesion, nerve, plantar
Morvan's G60.8
motor neuron (bulbar) (familial) (mixed type) (spinal) G12.20
  amyotrophic lateral sclerosis G12.21
  progressive bulbar palsy G12.22
  specified NEC G12.29
moyamoya I67.5
mu heavy chain disease C88.2
multicore G71.2
muscle (*see also* Disorder, muscle)
  inflammatory — *see* Myositis
  ocular (external) — *see* Strabismus
musculoskeletal system, soft tissue — *see* also Disorder, soft tissue
  specified NEC — *see* Disorder, soft tissue, specified type NEC
mushroom workers' J67.5
mycotic B49
myelodysplastic, not classified C94.6
myeloproliferative, not classified C94.6
  chronic D47.1
myocardium, myocardial (*see also* Degeneration, myocardial) I51.5
  primary (idiopathic) I42.9
myoneural G70.9
Naegeli's D69.1
nails L60.9
  specified NEC L60.8
Nairobi (sheep virus) A93.8
nasal J34.9
nemaline body G71.2
nerve — *see* Disorder, nerve
nervous system G98.8
  autonomic G90.9
  central G96.9
    specified NEC G96.8
  congenital Q07.9
  parasympathetic G90.9
  specified NEC G98.8
  sympathetic G90.9
  vegetative G90.9
neuromuscular system G70.9
Newcastle B30.8
Nicolas (-Durand)-Favre (climatic bubo) A55
nipple N64.9
  Paget's C50.01- ☑
    female C50.01- ☑
    male C50.02- ☑
Nishimoto (-Takeuchi) I67.5
nonarthropod-borne NOS (viral) B34.9
  enterovirus NEC B34.1
nonautoimmune hemolytic D59.4
  drug-induced D59.2
Nonne-Milroy-Meige (chronic hereditary edema) Q82.0
nose J34.9
nucleus pulposus — *see* Disorder, disc
nutritional E63.9
oast-house-urine E72.19
  ocular
    herpesviral B00.50
    zoster B02.30

Disease — *continued*

obliterative vascular I77.1
Ohara's — *see* Tularemia
Opitz's (congestive splenomegaly) D73.2
Oppenheim-Urbach (necrobiosis lipoidica diabeticorum) — *see* E08-E13 with .620
optic nerve NEC — *see* Disorder, nerve, optic
orbit — *see* Disorder, orbit
Oriental liver fluke B66.1
Oriental lung fluke B66.4
Ormond's N13.5
Oropouche virus A93.0
Osler-Rendu (familial hemorrhagic telangiectasia) I78.0
osteofibrocystic E21.0
Otto's M24.7
outer ear — *see* Disorder, ear, external
ovary (noninflammatory) N83.9
  cystic N83.20
  inflammatory — *see* Salpingo-oophoritis
  polycystic E28.2
  specified NEC N83.8
Owren's (congenital) — *see* Defect, coagulation
pancreas K86.9
  cystic K86.2
  fibrocystic E84.9
  specified NEC K86.8
panvalvular I08.9
  specified NEC I08.8
parametrium (noninflammatory) N83.9
parasitic B89
  cerebral NEC B71.9 [G94]
  intestinal NOS B82.9
  mouth B37.0
  skin NOS B88.9
  specified type — *see* Infestation
  tongue B37.0
parathyroid (gland) E21.5
  specified NEC E21.4
Parkinson's G20
parodontal K05.6
Parrot's (syphilitic osteochondritis) A50.02
Parry's (exophthalmic goiter) — *see* Hyperthyroidism, with, goiter (diffuse)
Parson's (exophthalmic goiter) — *see* Hyperthyroidism, with, goiter (diffuse)
Paxton's (white piedra) B36.2
pearl-worker's — *see* Osteomyelitis, specified type NEC
Pellegrini-Stieda (calcification, knee joint) — *see* Bursitis, tibial collateral
pelvis, pelvic
  female NOS N94.9
    specified NEC N94.89
  gonococcal (acute) (chronic) A54.24
  inflammatory (female) N73.9
    acute N73.0
    chronic N73.1
    specified NEC N73.8
    syphilitic (secondary) A51.42
      late A52.76
    tuberculous A18.17
  organ, female N94.9
  peritoneum, female NEC N94.89
penis N48.9
  inflammatory N48.29
    abscess N48.21
    cellulitis N48.22
  specified NEC N48.89
periapical tissues NOS K04.90
periodontal K05.6
  specified NEC K05.5
periosteum — *see* Disorder, bone, specified type NEC
peripheral
  arterial I73.9
  autonomic nervous system G90.9
  nerves — *see* Polyneuropathy
  vascular NOS I73.9
peritoneum K66.9
  pelvic, female NEC N94.89
  specified NEC K66.8
persistent mucosal (middle ear) H66.20
  left H66.22
    with right H66.23
  right H66.21
    with left H66.23
Petit's — *see* Hernia, abdomen, specified site NEC
pharynx J39.2
  specified NEC J39.2
Phocas' — *see* Mastopathy, cystic

Disease — *continued*

photochromogenic (acid-fast bacilli) (pulmonary) A31.0
  nonpulmonary A31.9
Pick's G31.01 [F02.80]
  with behavioral disturbance G31.01 [F02.81]
pigeon fancier's J67.2
pineal gland E34.8
pink — *see* Poisoning, mercury
Pinkus' (lichen nitidus) L44.1
pinworm B80
Piry virus A93.8
pituitary (gland) E23.7
pituitary-snuff-taker's J67.8
pleura (cavity) J94.9
  specified NEC J94.8
pneumatic drill (hammer) T75.21 ☑
Pollitzer's (hidradenitis suppurativa) L73.2
polycystic
  kidney or renal Q61.3
    adult type Q61.2
    childhood type NEC Q61.19
      collecting duct dilatation Q61.11
  liver or hepatic Q44.6
  lung or pulmonary J98.4
    congenital Q33.0
  ovary, ovaries E28.2
  spleen Q89.09
polyethylene T84.05- ☑
Pompe's (glycogenosis II) E74.02
Posadas-Wernicke B38.9
Potain's (pulmonary edema) — *see* Edema, lung
prepuce N47.8
  inflammatory N47.7
    balanoposthitis N47.6
Pringle's (tuberous sclerosis) Q85.1
prion, central nervous system A81.9
  specified NEC A81.89
prostate N42.9
  specified NEC N42.89
protozoal B64
  acanthamebiasis — *see* Acanthamebiasis
  African trypanosomiasis — *see* African trypanosomiasis
  babesiosis B60.0
  Chagas disease — *see* Chagas disease
  intestine, intestinal A07.9
  leishmaniasis — *see* Leishmaniasis
  malaria — *see* Malaria
  naegleriasis B60.2
  pneumocystosis B59
  specified organism NEC B60.8
  toxoplasmosis — *see* Toxoplasmosis
pseudo-Hurler's E77.0
psychiatric F99
psychotic — *see* Psychosis
Puente's (simple glandular cheilitis) K13.0
puerperal (*see also* Puerperal) O90.89
pulmonary (*see also* Disease, lung)
  artery I28.9
  chronic obstructive J44.9
    with
      acute bronchitis J44.0
      exacerbation (acute) J44.1
      lower respiratory infection (acute) J44.0
    decompensated J44.1
      with
        exacerbation (acute) J44.1
  heart I27.9
    specified NEC I27.89
  hypertensive (vascular) I27.0
  valve I37.9
    rheumatic I09.89
pulp (dental) NOS K04.90
pulseless M31.4
Putnam's (subacute combined sclerosis with pernicious anemia) D51.0
Pyle (-Cohn) (craniometaphyseal dysplasia) Q78.5
ragpicker's or ragsorter's A22.1
Raynaud's — *see* Raynaud's disease
reactive airway — *see* Asthma
Reclus' (cystic) — *see* Mastopathy, cystic
rectum K62.9
  specified NEC K62.89
Refsum's (heredopathia atactica polyneuritiformis) G60.1
renal (functional) (pelvis) (*see also* Disease, kidney) N28.9
  with
    edema — *see* Nephrosis
    glomerular lesion — *see* Glomerulonephritis

☑ Additional character required

Disease — continued

with edema — see Nephrosis
interstitial nephritis N12
acute N28.9
chronic (see also Disease, kidney, chronic) N18.9
cystic, congenital Q61.9
diabetic — see E08-E13 with .22
end-stage (failure) N18.6
due to hypertension I12.0
fibrocystic (congenital) Q61.8
hypertensive — see Hypertension, kidney
lupus M32.14
phosphate-losing (tubular) N25.0
polycystic (congenital) Q61.3
adult type Q61.2
childhood type NEC Q61.19
collecting duct dilatation Q61.11
rapidly progressive N01.9
subacute N01.9
Rendu-Osler-Weber (familial hemorrhagic
telangiectasia) I78.0
renovascular (arteriosclerotic) — see
Hypertension, kidney
respiratory (tract) J98.9
acute or subacute NOS J06.9
due to
chemicals, gases, fumes or vapors
(inhalation) J68.3
external agent J70.9
specified NEC J70.8
radiation J70.0
smoke inhalation J70.5
noninfectious J39.8
chronic NOS J98.9
due to
chemicals, gases, fumes or vapors J68.4
external agent J70.9
specified NEC J70.8
radiation J70.1
newborn P27.9
specified NEC P27.8
due to
chemicals, gases, fumes or vapors J68.9
acute or subacute NEC J68.3
chronic J68.4
external agent J70.9
specified NEC J70.8
newborn P28.9
specified type NEC P28.89
upper J39.9
acute or subacute J06.9
noninfectious NEC J39.8
specified NEC J39.8
streptococcal J06.9
retina, retinal H35.9
Batten's or Batten-Mayou E75.4 [H36]
specified NEC H35.89
rheumatoid — see Arthritis, rheumatoid
rickettsial NOS A79.9
specified type NEC A79.89
Riga (-Fede) (cachectic aphthae) K14.0
Riggs' (compound periodontitis) — see
Periodontitis
Ritter's L00
Rivalta's (cervicofacial actinomycosis) A42.2
Robles' (onchocerciasis) B73.01
Roger's (congenital interventricular septal
defect) Q21.0
Rosenthal's (factor XI deficiency) D68.1
Rossbach's (hyperchlorhydria) K30
Ross River B33.1
Rotes Quérol — see Hyperostosis, ankylosing
Roth (-Bernhardt) — see Mononeuropathy, lower
limb, meralgia paresthetica
Runeberg's (progressive pernicious anemia)
D51.0
sacroiliac NEC M53.3
salivary gland or duct K11.9
inclusion B25.9
specified NEC K11.8
virus B25.9
sandworm B76.9
Schimmelbusch's — see Mastopathy, cystic
Schmorl's — see Schmorl's disease or nodes
Schönlein (-Henoch) (purpura rheumatica) D69.0
Schottmüller's — see Fever, paratyphoid
Schultz's (agranulocytosis) — see
Agranulocytosis
Schwalbe-Ziehen-Oppenheim G24.1
Schwartz-Jampel G71.13
sclera H15.9
specified NEC H15.89

Disease — continued

scrofulous (tuberculous) A18.2
scrotum N50.9
sebaceous glands L73.9
semilunar cartilage, cystic (see also Derangement,
knee, meniscus, cystic)
seminal vesicle N50.9
serum NEC (see also Reaction, serum) T80.69 ☑
sexually transmitted A64
anogenital
herpesviral infection — see Herpes,
anogenital
warts A63.0
chancroid A57
chlamydial infection — see Chlamydia
gonorrhea — see Gonorrhea
granuloma inguinale A58
specified organism NEC A63.8
syphilis — see Syphilis
trichomoniasis — see Trichomoniasis
Sézary C84.1- ☑
shimamushi (scrub typhus) A75.3
shipyard B30.0
sickle-cell D57.1
with crisis (vasoocclusive pain) D57.00
with
acute chest syndrome D57.01
splenic sequestration D57.02
elliptocytosis D57.8- ☑
Hb-C D57.20
with crisis (vasoocclusive pain) D57.219
with
acute chest syndrome D57.211
splenic sequestration D57.212
without crisis D57.20
Hb-SD D57.80
with crisis D57.819
with
acute chest syndrome D57.811
splenic sequestration D57.812
Hb-SE D57.80
with crisis D57.819
with
acute chest syndrome D57.811
splenic sequestration D57.812
specified NEC D57.80
with crisis D57.819
with
acute chest syndrome D57.811
splenic sequestration D57.812
spherocytosis D57.80
with crisis D57.819
with
acute chest syndrome D57.811
splenic sequestration D57.812
thalassemia D57.40
with crisis (vasoocclusive pain) D57.419
with
acute chest syndrome D57.411
splenic sequestration D57.412
without crisis D57.40
silo-filler's J68.8
bronchitis J68.0
pneumonitis J68.0
pulmonary edema J68.1
simian B B00.4
Simons' (progressive lipodystrophy) E88.1
sin nombre virus B33.4
sinus — see Sinusitis
Sirkari's B55.0
sixth B08.20
due to human herpesvirus 6 B08.21
due to human herpesvirus 7 B08.22
skin L98.9
due to metabolic disorder NEC E88.9 [L99]
specified NEC L98.8
slim (HIV) B20
small vessel I73.9
Sneddon-Wilkinson (subcorneal pustular
dermatosis) L13.1
South African creeping B88.0
spinal (cord) G95.9
congenital Q06.9
specified NEC G95.89
spine (see also Spondylopathy)
joint — see Dorsopathy
tuberculous A18.01
spinocerebellar (hereditary) G11.9
specified NEC G11.8
spleen D73.9
amyloid E85.4 [D77]
organic D73.9

Disease — continued

polycystic Q89.09
postinfectional D73.89
sponge-diver's — see Toxicity, venom, marine
animal, sea anemone
Startle Q89.8
Steinert's G71.11
Sticker's (erythema infectiosum) B08.3
Stieda's (calcification, knee joint) — see Bursitis,
tibial collateral
Stokes' (exophthalmic goiter) — see
Hyperthyroidism, with, goiter (diffuse)
Stokes-Adams (syncope with heart block) I45.9
stomach K31.9
functional, psychogenic F45.8
specified NEC K31.89
stonemason's J62.8
storage
glycogen — see Disease, glycogen storage
mucopolysaccharide — see
Mucopolysaccharidosis
striatopallidal system NEC G25.89
Stuart-Prower (congenital factor X deficiency)
D68.2
Stuart's (congenital factor X deficiency) D68.2
subcutaneous tissue — see Disease, skin
supporting structures of teeth K08.9
specified NEC K08.8
suprarenal (capsule) (gland) E27.9
hyperfunction E27.0
specified NEC E27.8
sweat glands L74.9
specified NEC L74.8
Sweeley-Klionsky E75.21
Swift (-Feer) — see Poisoning, mercury
swimming-pool granuloma A31.1
Sylvest's (epidemic pleurodynia) B33.0
sympathetic nervous system G90.9
synovium — see Disorder, synovium
syphilitic — see Syphilis
systemic tissue mast cell C96.2
tanapox (virus) B08.71
Tangier E78.6
Tarral-Besnier (pityriasis rubra pilaris) L44.0
Tauri's E74.09
tear duct — see Disorder, lacrimal system
tendon, tendinous (see also Disorder, tendon)
nodular — see Trigger finger
terminal vessel I73.9
testis N50.9
thalassemia Hb-S — see Disease, sickle-cell,
thalassemia
Thaysen-Gee (nontropical sprue) K90.0
Thomsen G71.12
throat J39.2
septic J02.0
thromboembolic — see Embolism
thymus (gland) E32.9
specified NEC E32.8
thyroid (gland) E07.9
heart (see also Hyperthyroidism) E05.90 [I43]
with thyroid storm E05.91 [I43]
specified NEC E07.89
Tietze's M94.0
tongue K14.9
specified NEC K14.8
tonsils, tonsillar (and adenoids) J35.9
tooth, teeth K08.9
hard tissues K03.9
specified NEC K03.89
pulp NEC K04.99
specified NEC K08.8
Tourette's F95.2
trachea NEC J39.8
tricuspid I07.9
nonrheumatic I36.9
triglyceride-storage E75.5
trophoblastic — see Mole, hydatidiform
tsutsugamushi A75.3
tube (fallopian) (noninflammatory) N83.9
inflammatory — see Salpingitis
specified NEC N83.8
tuberculous NEC — see Tuberculosis
tubo-ovarian (noninflammatory) N83.9
inflammatory — see Salpingo-oophoritis
specified NEC N83.8
tubotympanic, chronic — see Otitis, media,
suppurative, chronic, tubotympanic
tubulo-interstitial N15.9
specified NEC N15.8
tympanum — see Disorder, tympanic membrane
Uhl's Q24.8

Disease — continued

Underwood's (sclerema neonatorum) P83.0
Unverricht (-Lundborg) — *see* Epilepsy, generalized, idiopathic
Urbach-Oppenheim (necrobiosis lipoidica diabeticorum) — *see* E08-E13 with .620
ureter N28.9
  in (due to)
    schistosomiasis (bilharziasis) B65.0 [N29]
urethra N36.9
  specified NEC N36.8
urinary (tract) N39.9
  bladder N32.9
    specified NEC N32.89
  specified NEC N39.8
uterus (noninflammatory) N85.9
  infective — *see* Endometritis
  inflammatory — *see* Endometritis
  specified NEC N85.8
uveal tract (anterior) H21.9
  posterior H31.9
vagabond's B85.1
vagina, vaginal (noninflammatory) N89.9
  inflammatory NEC N76.89
  specified NEC N89.8
valve, valvular I38
  multiple I08.9
    specified NEC I08.8
van Creveld-von Gierke (glycogenosis I) E74.01
vas deferens N50.9
vascular I99.9
  arteriosclerotic — *see* Arteriosclerosis
  ciliary body NEC — *see* Disorder, iris, vascular
  hypertensive — *see* Hypertension
  iris NEC — *see* Disorder, iris, vascular
  obliterative I77.1
    peripheral I73.9
  occlusive I99.8
  peripheral (occlusive) I73.9
    in diabetes mellitus — *see* E08-E13 with .51
vasomotor I73.9
vasospastic I73.9
vein I87.9
venereal (*see also* Disease, sexually transmitted) A64
  chlamydial NEC A56.8
    anus A56.3
    genitourinary NOS A56.2
    pharynx A56.4
    rectum A56.3
  fifth A55
  sixth A55
  specified nature or type NEC A63.8
vertebra, vertebral (*see also* Spondylopathy)
  disc — *see* Disorder, disc
vibration — *see* Vibration, adverse effects
viral, virus (*see also* Disease, by type of virus) B34.9
  arbovirus NOS A94
  arthropod-borne NOS A94
  congenital P35.9
    specified NEC P35.8
  Hanta (with renal manifestations) (Dobrava) (Puumala) (Seoul) A98.5
    with pulmonary manifestations (Andes) (Bayou) (Bermejo) (Black Creek Canal) (Choclo) (Juquitiba) (Laguna negra) (Lechiguanas) (New York) (Oran) (Sin nombre) B33.4
  Hantaan (Korean hemorrhagic fever) A98.5
  human immunodeficiency (HIV) B20
  Kunjin A83.4
  nonarthropod-borne NOS B34.9
  Powassan A84.8
  Rocio (encephalitis) A83.6
  Sin nombre (Hantavirus) (cardio)-pulmonary syndrome) B33.4
  Tahyna B33.8
  vesicular stomatitis A93.8
vitreous H43.9
  specified NEC H43.89
vocal cord J38.3
Volkmann's, acquired T79.6 ☑
von Eulenburg's (congenital paramyotonia) G71.19
von Gierke's (glycogenosis I) E74.01
von Graefe's — *see* Strabismus, paralytic, ophthalmoplegia, progressive
von Willebrand (-Jürgens) (angiohemophilia) D68.0
Vrolik's (osteogenesis imperfecta) Q78.0
vulva (noninflammatory) N90.9

Disease — continued

  inflammatory NEC N76.89
  specified NEC N90.89
Wallgren's (obstruction of splenic vein with collateral circulation) I87.8
Wassilieff's (leptospiral jaundice) A27.0
wasting NEC R64
  due to malnutrition E41
Waterhouse-Friderichsen A39.1
Wegner's (syphilitic osteochondritis) A50.02
Weil's (leptospiral jaundice of lung) A27.0
Weir Mitchell's (erythromelalgia) I73.81
Werdnig-Hoffmann G12.0
Wermer's E31.21
Werner-His (trench fever) A79.0
Werner-Schultz (neutropenic splenomegaly) D73.81
Wernicke-Posadas B38.9
whipworm B79
white blood cells D72.9
  specified NEC D72.89
white matter R90.82
white-spot, meaning lichen sclerosus et atrophicus L90.0
  penis N48.0
  vulva N90.4
Wilkie's K55.1
Wilkinson-Sneddon (subcorneal pustular dermatosis) L13.1
Willis' — *see* Diabetes
Wilson's (hepatolenticular degeneration) E83.01
woolsorter's A22.1
yaba monkey tumor B08.72
yaba pox (virus) B08.72
zoonotic, bacterial A28.9
  specified type NEC A28.8
Disfigurement (due to scar) L90.5
Disgerminoma — *see* Dysgerminoma
DISH (diffuse idiopathic skeletal hyperostosis) — *see* Hyperostosis, ankylosing
Disinsertion, retina — *see* Detachment, retina
Dislocatable hip, congenital Q65.6
Dislocation (articular)
  with fracture — *see* Fracture
  acromioclavicular (joint) S43.10- ☑
    with displacement
      100%-200% S43.12- ☑
      more than 200% S43.13- ☑
    inferior S43.14- ☑
    posterior S43.15- ☑
  ankle S93.0- ☑
  astragalus — *see* Dislocation, ankle
  atlantoaxial S13.121 ☑
  atlantooccipital S13.111 ☑
  atloidooccipital S13.111 ☑
  breast bone S23.29 ☑
  capsule, joint - code by site under Dislocation
  carpal (bone) — *see* Dislocation, wrist
  carpometacarpal (joint) NEC S63.05- ☑
    thumb S63.04- ☑
  cartilage (joint) - code by site under Dislocation
  cervical spine (vertebra) — *see* Dislocation, vertebra, cervical
  chronic — *see* Dislocation, recurrent
  clavicle — *see* Dislocation, acromioclavicular joint
  coccyx S33.2 ☑
  congenital NEC Q68.8
  coracoid — *see* Dislocation, shoulder
  costal cartilage S23.29 ☑
  costochondral S23.29 ☑
  cricoarytenoid articulation S13.29 ☑
  cricothyroid articulation S13.29 ☑
  dorsal vertebra — *see* Dislocation, vertebra, thoracic
  ear ossicle — *see* Discontinuity, ossicles, ear
  elbow S53.10- ☑
    congenital Q68.8
    pathological — *see* Dislocation, pathological NEC, elbow
    radial head alone — *see* Dislocation, radial head
    recurrent — *see* Dislocation, recurrent, elbow
    traumatic S53.10- ☑
      anterior S53.11- ☑
      lateral S53.14- ☑
      medial S53.13- ☑
      posterior S53.12- ☑
      specified type NEC S53.19- ☑
  eye, nontraumatic — *see* Luxation, globe
  eyeball, nontraumatic — *see* Luxation, globe
  femur
    distal end — *see* Dislocation, knee
    proximal end — *see* Dislocation, hip

Dislocation — continued

  fibula
    distal end — *see* Dislocation, ankle
    proximal end — *see* Dislocation, knee
  finger S63.25- ☑
    index S63.25- ☑
    interphalangeal S63.27- ☑
      distal S63.29- ☑
        index S63.29- ☑
        little S63.29- ☑
        middle S63.29- ☑
        ring S63.29- ☑
      index S63.27- ☑
      little S63.27- ☑
      middle S63.27- ☑
      proximal S63.28- ☑
        index S63.28- ☑
        little S63.28- ☑
        middle S63.28- ☑
        ring S63.28- ☑
      ring S63.27- ☑
    little S63.25- ☑
    metacarpophalangeal S63.26- ☑
      index S63.26- ☑
      little S63.26- ☑
      middle S63.26- ☑
      ring S63.26- ☑
    middle S63.25- ☑
    recurrent — *see* Dislocation, recurrent, finger
    ring S63.25- ☑
    thumb — *see* Dislocation, thumb
  foot S93.30- ☑
    recurrent — *see* Dislocation, recurrent, foot
    specified site NEC S93.33- ☑
    tarsal joint S93.31- ☑
    tarsometatarsal joint S93.32- ☑
    toe — *see* Dislocation, toe
  fracture — *see* Fracture
  glenohumeral (joint) — *see* Dislocation, shoulder
  glenoid — *see* Dislocation, shoulder
  habitual — *see* Dislocation, recurrent
  hip S73.00- ☑
    anterior S73.03- ☑
      obturator S73.02- ☑
    central S73.04- ☑
    congenital (total) Q65.2
      bilateral Q65.1
      partial Q65.5
        bilateral Q65.4
        unilateral Q65.3- ☑
      unilateral Q65.0- ☑
    developmental M24.85- ☑
    pathological — *see* Dislocation, pathological NEC, hip
    posterior S73.01- ☑
    recurrent — *see* Dislocation, recurrent, hip
  humerus, proximal end — *see* Dislocation, shoulder
  incomplete — *see* Subluxation, by site
  incus — *see* Discontinuity, ossicles, ear
  infracoracoid — *see* Dislocation, shoulder
  innominate (pubic junction) (sacral junction) S33.39 ☑
    acetabulum — *see* Dislocation, hip
  interphalangeal (joint)(s)
    finger S63.279 ☑
      distal S63.29- ☑
        index S63.29- ☑
        little S63.29- ☑
        middle S63.29- ☑
        ring S63.29- ☑
      index S63.27- ☑
      little S63.27- ☑
      middle S63.27- ☑
      proximal S63.28- ☑
        index S63.28- ☑
        little S63.28- ☑
        middle S63.28- ☑
        ring S63.28- ☑
      ring S63.27- ☑
    foot or toe — *see* Dislocation, toe
    thumb S63.12- ☑
      distal joint S63.14- ☑
      proximal joint S63.13- ☑
  jaw (cartilage) (meniscus) S03.0 ☑
  joint prosthesis — *see* Complications, joint prosthesis, mechanical, displacement, by site
  knee S83.106 ☑
    cap — *see* Dislocation, patella
    congenital Q68.2
    old M23.8X- ☑
    patella — *see* Dislocation, patella

☑ **Additional character required**

Dislocation — *continued*
  pathological — *see* Dislocation, pathological
      NEC, knee
    proximal tibia
      anteriorly S83.11- ☑
      laterally S83.14- ☑
      medially S83.13- ☑
      posteriorly S83.12- ☑
    recurrent (*see also* Derangement, knee,
      specified NEC)
    specified type NEC S83.19- ☑
  lacrimal gland H04.16- ☑
  lens (complete) H27.10
    anterior H27.12- ☑
    congenital Q12.1
    ocular implant — *see* Complications,
      intraocular lens
    partial H27.11- ☑
    posterior H27.13- ☑
    traumatic S05.8X- ☑
  ligament - code by site under Dislocation
  lumbar (vertebra) — *see* Dislocation, vertebra,
    lumbar
  lumbosacral (vertebra) (*see also* Dislocation,
    vertebra, lumbar)
    congenital Q76.49
  mandible S03.0 ☑
  meniscus (knee) — *see* Tear, meniscus
    other sites - code by site under Dislocation
  metacarpal (bone)
    distal end — *see* Dislocation, finger
    proximal end S63.06- ☑
  metacarpophalangeal (joint)
    finger S63.26- ☑
      index S63.26- ☑
      little S63.26- ☑
      middle S63.26- ☑
      ring S63.26- ☑
      thumb S63.11- ☑
  metatarsal (bone) — *see* Dislocation, foot
  metatarsophalangeal (joint(s)) — *see* Dislocation,
    toe
  midcarpal (joint) S63.03- ☑
  midtarsal (joint) — *see* Dislocation, foot
  neck S13.20 ☑
    specified site NEC S13.29 ☑
    vertebra — *see* Dislocation, vertebra, cervical
  nose (septal cartilage) S03.1 ☑
  occipitoatloid S13.111 ☑
  old — *see* Derangement, joint, specified type NEC
  ossicles, ear — *see* Discontinuity, ossicles, ear
  partial — *see* Subluxation, by site
  patella S83.006 ☑
    congenital Q74.1
    lateral S83.01- ☑
    recurrent (nontraumatic) M22.0- ☑
      incomplete M22.1- ☑
    specified type NEC S83.09- ☑
  pathological NEC M24.30
    ankle M24.37- ☑
    elbow M24.32- ☑
    foot joint M24.37- ☑
    hand joint M24.34- ☑
    hip M24.35- ☑
    knee M24.36- ☑
    lumbosacral joint M53.2
    pelvic region — *see* Dislocation, pathological,
      hip
    sacroiliac M53.2
    shoulder M24.31- ☑
    wrist M24.33- ☑
  pelvis NEC S33.30 ☑
    specified NEC S33.39 ☑
  phalanx
    finger or hand — *see* Dislocation, finger
    foot or toe — *see* Dislocation, toe
  prosthesis, internal — *see* Complications,
    prosthetic device, by site, mechanical
  radial head S53.006 ☑
    anterior S53.01- ☑
    posterior S53.02- ☑
    specified type NEC S53.09- ☑
  radiocarpal (joint) S63.02- ☑
  radiohumeral (joint) — *see* Dislocation, radial
    head
  radioulnar (joint)
    distal S63.01- ☑
    proximal — *see* Dislocation, elbow
  radius
    distal end — *see* Dislocation, wrist
    proximal end — *see* Dislocation, radial head
  recurrent M24.40

Dislocation — *continued*
    ankle M24.47- ☑
    elbow M24.42- ☑
    finger M24.44- ☑
    foot joint M24.47- ☑
    hand joint M24.44- ☑
    hip M24.45- ☑
    knee M24.46- ☑
      patella — *see* Dislocation, patella, recurrent
    patella — *see* Dislocation, patella, recurrent
    sacroiliac M53.2
    shoulder M24.41- ☑
    toe M24.47- ☑
    vertebra (*see also* subcategory) M43.5 ☑
      atlantoaxial M43.4
        with myelopathy M43.3
    wrist M24.43- ☑
  rib (cartilage) S23.29 ☑
  sacrococcygeal S33.2 ☑
  sacroiliac (joint) (ligament) S33.2 ☑
    congenital Q74.2
    recurrent M53.2
  sacrum S33.2 ☑
  scaphoid (bone) (hand) (wrist) — *see* Dislocation,
    wrist
    foot — *see* Dislocation, foot
  scapula — *see* Dislocation, shoulder, girdle,
    scapula
  semilunar cartilage, knee — *see* Tear, meniscus
  septal cartilage (nose) S03.1 ☑
  septum (nasal) (old) J34.2
  sesamoid bone - code by site under Dislocation
  shoulder (blade) (ligament) (joint) (traumatic)
      S43.006 ☑
    acromioclavicular — *see* Dislocation,
      acromioclavicular
    chronic — *see* Dislocation, recurrent, shoulder
    congenital Q68.8
    girdle S43.30- ☑
      scapula S43.31- ☑
      specified site NEC S43.39- ☑
    humerus S43.00- ☑
      anterior S43.01- ☑
      inferior S43.03- ☑
      posterior S43.02- ☑
    pathological — *see* Dislocation, pathological
      NEC, shoulder
    recurrent — *see* Dislocation, recurrent, shoulder
    specified type NEC S43.08- ☑
  spine
    cervical — *see* Dislocation, vertebra, cervical
    congenital Q76.49
    due to birth trauma P11.5
    lumbar — *see* Dislocation, vertebra, lumbar
    thoracic — *see* Dislocation, vertebra, thoracic
  spontaneous — *see* Dislocation, pathological
  sternoclavicular (joint) S43.206 ☑
    anterior S43.21- ☑
    posterior S43.22- ☑
  sternum S23.29 ☑
  subglenoid — *see* Dislocation, shoulder
  symphysis pubis S33.4 ☑
  talus — *see* Dislocation, ankle
  tarsal (bone(s)) (joint(s)) — *see* Dislocation, foot
  tarsometatarsal (joint(s)) — *see* Dislocation, foot
  temporomandibular (joint) S03.0 ☑
  thigh, proximal end — *see* Dislocation, hip
  thorax S23.20 ☑
    specified site NEC S23.29 ☑
    vertebra — *see* Dislocation, vertebra
  thumb S63.10- ☑
    interphalangeal joint — *see* Dislocation,
      interphalangeal (joint), thumb
    metacarpophalangeal joint — *see* Dislocation,
      metacarpophalangeal (joint), thumb
  thyroid cartilage S13.29 ☑
  tibia
    distal end — *see* Dislocation, ankle
    proximal end — *see* Dislocation, knee
  tibiofibular (joint)
    distal — *see* Dislocation, ankle
    superior — *see* Dislocation, knee
  toe (s) S93.106 ☑
    great S93.10- ☑
      interphalangeal joint S93.11- ☑
      metatarsophalangeal joint S93.12- ☑
    interphalangeal joint S93.119 ☑
    lesser S93.106 ☑
      interphalangeal joint S93.11- ☑
      metatarsophalangeal joint S93.12- ☑
    metatarsophalangeal joint S93.12- ☑
  tooth S03.2 ☑

Dislocation — *continued*
  trachea S23.29 ☑
  ulna
    distal end S63.07- ☑
    proximal end — *see* Dislocation, elbow
  ulnohumeral (joint) — *see* Dislocation, elbow
  vertebra (articular process) (body) (traumatic)
    cervical S13.101 ☑
      atlantoaxial joint S13.121 ☑
      atlantooccipital joint S13.111 ☑
      atloidooccipital joint S13.111 ☑
      joint between
        C0 and C1 S13.111 ☑
        C1 and C2 S13.121 ☑
        C2 and C3 S13.131 ☑
        C3 and C4 S13.141 ☑
        C4 and C5 S13.151 ☑
        C5 and C6 S13.161 ☑
        C6 and C7 S13.171 ☑
        C7 and T1 S13.181 ☑
      occipitoatloid joint S13.111 ☑
    congenital Q76.49
    lumbar S33.101 ☑
      joint between
        L1 and L2 S33.111 ☑
        L2 and L3 S33.121 ☑
        L3 and L4 S33.131 ☑
        L4 and L5 S33.141 ☑
    nontraumatic — *see* Displacement,
      intervertebral disc
    partial — *see* Subluxation, by site
    recurrent NEC M43.5
    thoracic S23.101 ☑
      joint between
        T1 and T2 S23.111 ☑
        T2 and T3 S23.121 ☑
        T3 and T4 S23.123 ☑
        T4 and T5 S23.131 ☑
        T5 and T6 S23.133 ☑
        T6 and T7 S23.141 ☑
        T7 and T8 S23.143 ☑
        T8 and T9 S23.151 ☑
        T9 and T10 S23.153 ☑
        T10 and T11 S23.161 ☑
        T11 and T12 S23.163 ☑
        T12 and L1 S23.171 ☑
  wrist (carpal bone) S63.006 ☑
    carpometacarpal joint — *see* Dislocation,
      carpometacarpal (joint)
    distal radioulnar joint — *see* Dislocation,
      radioulnar (joint), distal
    metacarpal bone, proximal — *see* Dislocation,
      metacarpal (bone), proximal end
    midcarpal — *see* Dislocation, midcarpal (joint)
    radiocarpal joint — *see* Dislocation, radiocarpal
      (joint)
    recurrent — *see* Dislocation, recurrent, wrist
    specified site NEC S63.09- ☑
    ulna — *see* Dislocation, ulna, distal end
  xiphoid cartilage S23.29 ☑
Disorder (of) (*see also* Disease)
  acantholytic L11.9
    specified NEC L11.8
  acute
    psychotic — *see* Psychosis, acute
    stress F43.0
  adjustment (grief) F43.20
    with
      anxiety F43.22
        with depressed mood F43.23
      conduct disturbance F43.24
        with emotional disturbance F43.25
      depressed mood F43.21
        with anxiety F43.23
      other specified symptom F43.29
  adrenal (capsule) (gland) (medullary) E27.9
    specified NEC E27.8
  adrenogenital E25.9
    drug-induced E25.8
    iatrogenic E25.8
    idiopathic E25.8
  adult personality (and behavior) F69
    specified NEC F68.8
  affective (mood) — *see* Disorder, mood
  aggressive, unsocialized F91.1
  alcohol-related F10.99
    with
      amnestic disorder, persisting F10.96
      anxiety disorder F10.980
      dementia, persisting F10.97
      intoxication F10.929
        with delirium F10.921

Disorder

Disorder — *continued*
    uncomplicated F10.920
    mood disorder F10.94
    other specified F10.988
    psychotic disorder F10.959
      with
        delusions F10.950
        hallucinations F10.951
    sexual dysfunction F10.981
    sleep disorder F10.982
  allergic — *see* Allergy
  alveolar NEC J84.09
  amino-acid
    cystathioninuria E72.19
    cystinosis E72.04
    cystinuria E72.01
    glycinuria E72.09
    homocystinuria E72.11
    metabolism — *see* Disturbance, metabolism,
      amino-acid
    specified NEC E72.8
    neonatal, transitory P74.8
    renal transport NEC E72.09
    transport NEC E72.09
  amnesic, amnestic
    alcohol-induced F10.96
      with dependence F10.26
    due to (secondary to) general medical
      condition F04
    psychoactive NEC-induced F19.96
      with
        abuse F19.16
        dependence F19.26
    sedative, hypnotic or anxiolytic-induced F13.96
      with dependence F13.26
  anaerobic glycolysis with anemia D55.2
  anxiety F41.9
    due to (secondary to)
      alcohol F10.980
      amphetamine F15.980
        in
          abuse F15.180
          dependence F15.280
      anxiolytic F13.980
        in
          abuse F13.180
          dependence F13.280
      caffeine F15.980
        in
          abuse F15.180
          dependence F15.280
      cannabis F12.980
        in
          abuse F12.180
          dependence F12.280
      cocaine F14.980
        in
          abuse F14.180
          dependence F14.180
      general medical condition F06.4
      hallucinogen F16.980
        in
          abuse F16.180
          dependence F16.280
      hypnotic F13.980
        in
          abuse F13.180
          dependence F13.280
      inhalant F18.980
        in
          abuse F18.180
          dependence F18.280
      phencyclidine F16.980
        in
          abuse F16.180
          dependence F16.280
      psychoactive substance NEC F19.980
        in
          abuse F19.180
          dependence F19.280
      sedative F13.980
        in
          abuse F13.180
          dependence F13.280
      volatile solvents F18.980
        in
          abuse F18.180
          dependence F18.280
    generalized F41.1
    mixed
      with depression (mild) F41.8
      specified NEC F41.3

Disorder — *continued*
    organic F06.4
    phobic F40.9
      of childhood F40.8
    specified NEC F41.8
  aortic valve — *see* Endocarditis, aortic
  aromatic amino-acid metabolism E70.9
    specified NEC E70.8
  arteriole NEC I77.89
  artery NEC I77.89
  articulation — *see* Disorder, joint
  attachment (childhood)
    disinhibited F94.2
    reactive F94.1
  attention-deficit hyperactivity (adolescent)
    (adult) (child) F90.9
    combined type F90.2
    hyperactive type F90.1
    inattentive type F90.0
    specified type NEC F90.8
  attention-deficit without hyperactivity
    (adolescent) (adult) (child) F90.0
  auditory processing (central) H93.25
  autistic F84.0
  autonomic nervous system G90.9
    specified NEC G90.8
  avoidant, child or adolescent F40.10
  balance
    acid-base E87.8
      mixed E87.4
    electrolyte E87.8
    fluid NEC E87.8
  behavioral (disruptive) — *see* Disorder, conduct
  beta-amino-acid metabolism E72.8
  bile acid and cholesterol metabolism E78.70
    Barth syndrome E78.71
    other specified E78.79
    Smith-Lemli-Opitz syndrome E78.72
  bilirubin excretion E80.6
  binocular
    movement H51.9
      convergence
        excess H51.12
        insufficiency H51.11
      internuclear ophthalmoplegia — *see*
        Ophthalmoplegia, internuclear
      palsy of conjugate gaze H51.0
      specified type NEC H51.8
    vision NEC — *see* Disorder, vision, binocular
  bipolar (I) F31.9
    current episode
      depressed F31.9
        with psychotic features F31.5
        without psychotic features F31.30
          mild F31.31
          moderate F31.32
          severe (without psychotic features) F31.4
            with psychotic features F31.5
      hypomanic F31.0
      manic F31.9
        with psychotic features F31.2
        without psychotic features F31.10
          mild F31.11
          moderate F31.12
          severe (without psychotic features)
            F31.13
            with psychotic features F31.2
      mixed F31.60
        mild F31.61
        moderate F31.62
        severe (without psychotic features) F31.63
          with psychotic features F31.64
      severe depression (without psychotic
        features) F31.4
        with psychotic features F31.5
    in remission (currently) F31.70
      in full remission
        most recent episode
          depressed F31.76
          hypomanic F31.72
          manic F31.74
          mixed F31.78
      in partial remission
        most recent episode
          depressed F31.75
          hypomanic F31.71
          manic F31.73
          mixed F31.77
    specified NEC F31.89
    II F31.81
    organic F06.30
    single manic episode F30.9

Disorder — *continued*
    mild F30.11
    moderate F30.12
    severe (without psychotic symptoms) F30.13
      with psychotic symptoms F30.2
  bladder N32.9
    functional NEC N31.9
    in schistosomiasis B65.0 [N33]
    specified NEC N32.89
  bleeding D68.9
  blood D75.9
    in congenital early syphilis A50.09 [D77]
  body dysmorphic F45.22
  bone M89.9
    continuity M84.9
      specified type NEC M84.80
        ankle M84.87- ☑
        fibula M84.86- ☑
        foot M84.87- ☑
        hand M84.84- ☑
        humerus M84.82- ☑
        neck M84.88
        pelvis M84.859
        radius M84.83- ☑
        rib M84.88
        shoulder M84.81- ☑
        skull M84.88
        thigh M84.85- ☑
        tibia M84.86- ☑
        ulna M84.83- ☑
        vertebra M84.88
    density and structure M85.9
      cyst (*see also* Cyst, bone, specified type NEC)
        aneurysmal — *see* Cyst, bone, aneurysmal
        solitary — *see* Cyst, bone, solitary
      diffuse idiopathic skeletal hyperostosis — *see*
        Hyperostosis, ankylosing
      fibrous dysplasia (monostotic) — *see*
        Dysplasia, fibrous, bone
      fluorosis — *see* Fluorosis, skeletal
      hyperostosis of skull M85.2
      osteitis condensans — *see* Osteitis,
        condensans
      specified type NEC M85.8- ☑
        ankle M85.87- ☑
        foot M85.87- ☑
        forearm M85.83- ☑
        hand M85.84- ☑
        lower leg M85.86- ☑
        multiple sites M85.89
        neck M85.88
        rib M85.88
        shoulder M85.81- ☑
        skull M85.88
        thigh M85.85- ☑
        upper arm M85.82- ☑
        vertebra M85.88
    development and growth NEC M89.20
      carpus M89.24- ☑
      clavicle M89.21- ☑
      femur M89.25- ☑
      fibula M89.26- ☑
      finger M89.24- ☑
      humerus M89.22- ☑
      ilium M89.259
      ischium M89.259
      metacarpus M89.24- ☑
      metatarsus M89.27- ☑
      multiple sites M89.29
      neck M89.28
      radius M89.23- ☑
      rib M89.28
      scapula M89.21- ☑
      skull M89.28
      tarsus M89.27- ☑
      tibia M89.26- ☑
      toe M89.27- ☑
      ulna M89.23- ☑
      vertebra M89.28
    specified type NEC M89.8X- ☑
  brachial plexus G54.0
  branched-chain amino-acid metabolism E71.2
    specified NEC E71.19
  breast N64.9
    agalactia — *see* Agalactia
    associated with
      lactation O92.70
        specified NEC O92.79
      pregnancy O92.20
        specified NEC O92.29
      puerperium O92.20
        specified NEC O92.29

☑ **Additional character required**

Disorder — *continued*
  cracked nipple — *see* Cracked nipple
  galactorrhea — *see* Galactorrhea
  hypogalactia O92.4
  lactation disorder NEC O92.79
  mastitis — *see* Mastitis
  nipple infection — *see* Infection, nipple
  retracted nipple — *see* Retraction, nipple
  specified type NEC N64.89
Briquet's F45.0
bullous, in diseases classified elsewhere L14
cannabis use
  due to drug abuse — *see* Abuse, drug, cannabis
  due to drug dependence — *see* Dependence, drug, cannabis
carbohydrate
  absorption, intestinal NEC E74.39
  metabolism (congenital) E74.9
    specified NEC E74.8
cardiac, functional I51.89
carnitine metabolism E71.40
cartilage M94.9
  articular NEC — *see* Derangement, joint, articular cartilage
    chondrocalcinosis — *see* Chondrocalcinosis
  specified type NEC M94.8X- ☑
    articular — *see* Derangement, joint, articular cartilage
    multiple sites M94.8X0
catatonic
  due to (secondary to) known physiological condition F06.1
  organic F06.1
central auditory processing H93.25
cervical
  region NEC M53.82
  root (nerve) NEC G54.2
character NOS F60.9
childhood disintegrative NEC F84.3
cholesterol and bile acid metabolism E78.70
  Barth syndrome E78.71
  other specified E78.79
  Smith-Lemli-Opitz syndrome E78.72
choroid H31.9
  atrophy — *see* Atrophy, choroid
  degeneration — *see* Degeneration, choroid
  detachment — *see* Detachment, choroid
  dystrophy — *see* Dystrophy, choroid
  hemorrhage — *see* Hemorrhage, choroid
  rupture — *see* Rupture, choroid
  scar — *see* Scar, chorioretinal
  solar retinopathy — *see* Retinopathy, solar
  specified type NEC H31.8
ciliary body — *see* Disorder, iris
  degeneration — *see* Degeneration, ciliary body
coagulation (factor) (*see also* Defect, coagulation) D68.9
  newborn, transient P61.6
coccyx NEC M53.3
cognitive F09
  due to (secondary to) general medical condition F09
  persisting R41.89
    due to
      alcohol F10.97
        with dependence F10.27
      anxiolytics F13.97
        with dependence F13.27
      hypnotics F13.97
        with dependence F13.27
      sedatives F13.97
        with dependence F13.27
      specified substance NEC F19.97
        with
          abuse F19.17
          dependence F19.27
communication F80.9
conduct (childhood) F91.9
  adjustment reaction — *see* Disorder, adjustment
  adolescent onset type F91.2
  childhood onset type F91.1
  compulsive F63.9
  confined to family context F91.0
  depressive F91.8
  group type F91.2
  hyperkinetic — *see* Disorder, attention-deficit hyperactivity
  oppositional defiance F91.3
  socialized F91.2
  solitary aggressive type F91.1
  specified NEC F91.8

Disorder — *continued*
    unsocialized (aggressive) F91.1
conduction, heart I45.9
congenital glycosylation (CDG) E74.8
conjunctiva H11.9
  infection — *see* Conjunctivitis
connective tissue, localized L94.9
  specified NEC L94.8
conversion — *see* Disorder, dissociative
convulsive (secondary) — *see* Convulsions
cornea H18.9
  deformity — *see* Deformity, cornea
  degeneration — *see* Degeneration, cornea
  deposits — *see* Deposit, cornea
  due to contact lens H18.82- ☑
    specified as edema — *see* Edema, cornea
  edema — *see* Edema, cornea
  keratitis — *see* Keratitis
  keratoconjunctivitis — *see* Keratoconjunctivitis
  membrane change — *see* Change, corneal membrane
  neovascularization — *see* Neovascularization, cornea
  scar — *see* Opacity, cornea
  specified type NEC H18.89- ☑
  ulcer — *see* Ulcer, cornea
corpus cavernosum N48.9
cranial nerve — *see* Disorder, nerve, cranial
cyclothymic F34.0
defiant oppositional F91.3
delusional (persistent) (systematized) F22
  induced F24
depersonalization F48.1
depressive F32.9
  major F32.9
    with psychotic symptoms F32.3
    in remission (full) F32.5
      partial F32.4
    recurrent F33.9
    single episode F32.9
      mild F32.0
      moderate F32.1
      severe (without psychotic symptoms) F32.2
        with psychotic symptoms F32.3
  organic F06.31
  recurrent F33.9
    current episode
      mild F33.0
      moderate F33.1
      severe (without psychotic symptoms) F33.2
        with psychotic symptoms F33.3
    in remission F33.40
      full F33.42
      partial F33.41
    specified NEC F33.8
  single episode — *see* Episode, depressive
developmental F89
  arithmetical skills F81.2
  coordination (motor) F82
  expressive writing F81.81
  language F80.9
    expressive F80.1
    mixed receptive and expressive F80.2
    receptive type F80.2
    specified NEC F80.89
  learning F81.9
    arithmetical F81.2
    reading F81.0
  mixed F88
  motor coordination or function F82
  pervasive F84.9
    specified NEC F84.8
  phonological F80.0
  reading F81.0
  scholastic skills (*see also* Disorder, learning)
    mixed F81.89
  specified NEC F88
  speech F80.9
    articulation F80.0
    specified NEC F80.89
  written expression F81.81
diaphragm J98.6
digestive (system) K92.9
  newborn P78.9
    specified NEC P78.89
  postprocedural — *see* Complication, gastrointestinal
  psychogenic F45.8
disc (intervertebral) M51.9
  with
    myelopathy
      cervical region M50.00

Disorder — *continued*
      cervicothoracic region M50.03
      high cervical region M50.01
      lumbar region M51.06
      mid-cervical region M50.02
      sacrococcygeal region M53.3
      thoracic region M51.04
      thoracolumbar region M51.05
    radiculopathy
      cervical region M50.10
      cervicothoracic region M50.13
      high cervical region M50.11
      lumbar region M51.16
      lumbosacral region M51.17
      mid-cervical region M50.12
      sacrococcygeal region M53.3
      thoracic region M51.14
      thoracolumbar region M51.15
  cervical M50.90
    with
      myelopathy M50.00
        C2-C3 M50.01
        C3-C4 M50.01
        C4-C5 M50.02
        C5-C6 M50.02
        C6-C7 M50.02
        C7-T1 M50.03
        cervicothoracic region M50.03
        high cervical region M50.01
        mid-cervical region M50.02
      neuritis, radiculitis or radiculopathy M50.10
        C2-C3 M50.11
        C3-C4 M50.11
        C4-C5 M50.12
        C5-C6 M50.12
        C6-C7 M50.12
        C7-T1 M50.13
        cervicothoracic region M50.13
        high cervical region M50.11
        mid-cervical region M50.12
    C2-C3 M50.91
    C3-C4 M50.91
    C4-C5 M50.92
    C5-C6 M50.92
    C6-C7 M50.92
    C7-T1 M50.93
    cervicothoracic region M50.93
    degeneration M50.30
      C2-C3 M50.31
      C3-C4 M50.31
      C4-C5 M50.32
      C5-C6 M50.32
      C6-C7 M50.32
      C7-T1 M50.33
      cervicothoracic region M50.33
      high cervical region M50.31
      mid-cervical region M50.32
    displacement M50.20
      C2-C3 M50.21
      C3-C4 M50.21
      C4-C5 M50.22
      C5-C6 M50.22
      C6-C7 M50.22
      C7-T1 M50.23
      cervicothoracic region M50.23
      high cervical region M50.21
      mid-cervical region M50.22
    high cervical region M50.91
    mid-cervical region M50.92
    specified type NEC M50.80
      C2-C3 M50.81
      C3-C4 M50.81
      C4-C5 M50.82
      C5-C6 M50.82
      C6-C7 M50.82
      C7-T1 M50.83
      cervicothoracic region M50.83
      high cervical region M50.81
      mid-cervical region M50.82
  specified NEC
    lumbar region M51.86
    lumbosacral region M51.87
    sacrococcygeal region M53.3
    thoracic region M51.84
    thoracolumbar region M51.85
disinhibited attachment (childhood) F94.2
disintegrative, childhood NEC F84.3
disruptive behavior F98.9
dissocial personality F60.2
dissociative F44.9
  affecting
    motor function F44.4

Disorder — continued

and sensation F44.7
sensation F44.6
and motor function F44.7
brief reactive F43.0
due to (secondary to) general medical
condition F06.8
mixed F44.7
organic F06.8
other specified NEC F44.89
double heterozygous sickling — *see* Disease,
sickle-cell
dream anxiety F51.5
drug induced hemorrhagic D68.32
drug related F19.99
abuse — *see* Abuse, drug
dependence — *see* Dependence, drug
dysmorphic body F45.1
dysthymic F34.1
ear H93.9- ☑
bleeding — *see* Otorrhagia
deafness — *see* Deafness
degenerative H93.09- ☑
discharge — *see* Otorrhea
external H61.9- ☑
auditory canal stenosis — *see* Stenosis,
external ear canal
exostosis — *see* Exostosis, external ear canal
impacted cerumen — *see* Impaction,
cerumen
otitis — *see* Otitis, externa
perichondritis — *see* Perichondritis, ear
pinna — *see* Disorder, pinna
specified type NEC H61.89- ☑
in diseases classified elsewhere H62.8X- ☑
inner H83.9- ☑
vestibular dysfunction — *see* Disorder,
vestibular function
middle H74.9- ☑
adhesive H74.1- ☑
ossicle — *see* Abnormal, ear ossicles
polyp — *see* Polyp, ear (middle)
specified NEC, in diseases classified
elsewhere H75.8- ☑
postprocedural — *see* Complications, ear,
procedure
specified NEC, in diseases classified elsewhere
H94.8- ☑
eating (adult) (psychogenic) F50.9
anorexia — *see* Anorexia
bulimia F50.2
child F98.29
pica F98.3
rumination disorder F98.21
pica F50.8
childhood F98.3
electrolyte (balance) NEC E87.8
with
abortion — *see* Abortion by type
complicated by specified condition NEC
ectopic pregnancy O08.5
molar pregnancy O08.5
acidosis (metabolic) (respiratory) E87.2
alkalosis (metabolic) (respiratory) E87.3
elimination, transepidermal L87.9
specified NEC L87.8
emotional (persistent) F34.9
of childhood F93.9
specified NEC F93.8
endocrine E34.9
postprocedural E89.89
specified NEC E89.89
erectile (male) (organic) (*see also* Dysfunction,
sexual, male, erectile) N52.9
nonorganic F52.21
erythematous — *see* Erythema
esophagus K22.9
functional K22.4
psychogenic F45.8
eustachian tube H69.9- ☑
infection — *see* Salpingitis, eustachian
obstruction — *see* Obstruction, eustachian
tube
patulous — *see* Patulous, eustachian tube
specified NEC H69.8- ☑
extrapyramidal G25.9
in diseases classified elsewhereG26
specified type NEC G25.89
eye H57.9
postprocedural — *see* Complication,
postprocedural, eye
eyelid H02.9

Disorder — continued

cyst — *see* Cyst, eyelid
degenerative H02.70
chloasma — *see* Chloasma, eyelid
madarosis — *see* Madarosis
specified type NEC H02.79
vitiligo — *see* Vitiligo, eyelid
xanthelasma — *see* Xanthelasma
dermatochalasis — *see* Dermatochalasis
edema — *see* Edema, eyelid
elephantiasis — *see* Elephantiasis, eyelid
foreign body, retained — *see* Foreign body,
retained, eyelid
function H02.59
abnormal innervation syndrome — *see*
Syndrome, abnormal innervation
blepharochalasis — *see* Blepharochalasis
blepharoclonus — *see* Blepharoclonus
blepharophimosis — *see* Blepharophimosis
blepharoptosis — *see* Blepharoptosis
lagophthalmos — *see* Lagophthalmos
lid retraction — *see* Retraction, lid
hypertrichosis — *see* Hypertrichosis, eyelid
specified type NEC H02.89
vascular H02.879
left H02.876
lower H02.875
upper H02.874
right H02.873
lower H02.872
upper H02.871
factitious F68.10
with predominantly
psychological symptoms F68.11
with physical symptoms F68.13
physical symptoms F68.12
with psychological symptoms F68.13
factor, coagulation — *see* Defect, coagulation
fatty acid
metabolism E71.30
specified NEC E71.39
oxidation
LCAD E71.310
MCAD E71.311
SCAD E71.312
specified deficiency NEC E71.318
feeding (infant or child) (*see also* Disorder, eating)
R63.3
feigned (with obvious motivation) Z76.5
without obvious motivation — *see* Disorder,
factitious
female
hypoactive sexual desire F52.0
orgasmic F52.31
sexual arousal F52.22
fibroblastic M72.9
specified NEC M72.8
fluency
adult onset F98.5
childhood onset F80.81
following
cerebral infarction I69.323
cerebrovascular disease I69.923
specified disease NEC I69.823
intracerebral hemorrhage I69.123
nontraumatic intracranial hemorrhage NEC
I69.223
subarachnoid hemorrhage I69.023
in conditions classified elsewhere R47.82
fluid balance E87.8
follicular (skin) L73.9
specified NEC L73.8
fructose metabolism E74.10
essential fructosuria E74.11
fructokinase deficiency E74.11
fructose-1, 6-diphosphatase deficiency E74.19
hereditary fructose intolerance E74.12
other specified E74.19
functional polymorphonuclear neutrophils D71
gallbladder, biliary tract and pancreas in diseases
classified elsewhere K87
gamma-glutamyl cycle E72.8
gastric (functional) K31.9
motility K30
psychogenic F45.8
secretion K30
gastrointestinal (functional) NOS K92.9
newborn P78.9
psychogenic F45.8
gender-identity or -role F64.9
childhood F64.2
effect on relationship F66

Disorder — continued

of adolescence or adulthood (nontranssexual)
F64.1
specified NEC F64.8
uncertainty F66
genitourinary system
female N94.9
male N50.9
psychogenic F45.8
globe H44.9
degenerated condition H44.50
absolute glaucoma H44.51- ☑
atrophy H44.52- ☑
leucocoria H44.53- ☑
degenerative H44.30
chalcosis H44.31- ☑
myopia H44.2- ☑
siderosis H44.32- ☑
specified type NEC H44.39- ☑
endophthalmitis — *see* Endophthalmitis
foreign body, retained — *see* Foreign body,
intraocular, old, retained
hemophthalmos — *see* Hemophthalmos
hypotony H44.40
due to
ocular fistula H44.42- ☑
specified disorder NEC H44.43- ☑
flat anterior chamber H44.41- ☑
primary H44.44- ☑
luxation — *see* Luxation, globe
specified type NEC H44.89
glomerular (in) N05.9
amyloidosis E85.4 [N08]
cryoglobulinemia D89.1 [N08]
disseminated intravascular coagulation D65
[N08]
Fabry's disease E75.21 [N08]
familial lecithin cholesterol acyltransferase
deficiency E78.6 [N08]
Goodpasture's syndrome M31.0
hemolytic-uremic syndrome D59.3
Henoch (-Schönlein) purpura D69.0 [N08]
malariae malaria B52.0
microscopic polyangiitis M31.7 [N08]
multiple myeloma C90.0- ☑ [N08]
mumps B26.83
schistosomiasis B65.9 [N08]
sepsis NEC A41.- ☑ [N08]
streptococcal A40.- ☑ [N08]
sickle-cell disorders D57.- ☑ [N08]
strongyloidiasis B78.9 [N08]
subacute bacterial endocarditis I33.0 [N08]
syphilis A52.75
systemic lupus erythematosus M32.14
thrombotic thrombocytopenic purpura M31.1
[N08]
Waldenström macroglobulinemia C88.0 [N08]
Wegener's granulomatosis M31.31
gluconeogenesis E74.4
glucosaminoglycan metabolism — *see* Disorder,
metabolism, glucosaminoglycan
glycine metabolism E72.50
d-glycericacidemia E72.59
hyperhydroxyprolinemia E72.59
hyperoxaluria E72.53
hyperprolinemia E72.59
non-ketotic hyperglycinemia E72.51
oxalosis E72.53
oxaluria E72.53
sarcosinemia E72.59
trimethylaminuria E72.52
glycoprotein metabolism E77.9
specified NEC E77.8
habit (and impulse) F63.9
involving sexual behavior NEC F65.9
specified NEC F63.89
heart action I49.9
hematological D75.9
newborn (transient) P61.9
specified NEC P61.8
hematopoietic organs D75.9
hemorrhagic NEC D69.9
drug-induced D68.32
due to
extrinsic circulating anticoagulants D68.32
increase in
anti-IIa D68.32
anti-Xa D68.32
intrinsic
circulating anticoagulants D68.318
increase in
antithrombin D68.318

☑ **Additional character required**

Disorder — continued
                anti-VIIIa D68.318
                anti-IXa D68.318
                anti-XIa D68.318
        following childbirth O72.3
    hemostasis — see Defect, coagulation
    histidine metabolism E70.40
        histidinemia E70.41
        other specified E70.49
    hyperkinetic — see Disorder, attention-deficit
        hyperactivity
    hyperleucine-isoleucinemia E71.19
    hypervalinemia E71.19
    hypoactive sexual desire F52.0
    hypochondriacal F45.22
        body dysmorphic F45.22
        neurosis F45.21
        other specified F45.29
    identity
        dissociative F44.81
        of childhood F93.8
    immune mechanism (immunity) D89.9
        specified type NEC D89.89
    impaired renal tubular function N25.9
        specified NEC N25.89
    impulse (control) F63.9
    inflammatory
        pelvic, in diseases classified elsewhereN74
        penis N48.29
            abscess N48.21
            cellulitis N48.22
    integument, newborn P83.9
        specified NEC P83.8
    intermittent explosive F63.81
    internal secretion pancreas — see Increased,
        secretion, pancreas, endocrine
    intestine, intestinal
        carbohydrate absorption NEC E74.39
            postoperative K91.2
        functional NEC K59.9
            postoperative K91.89
        psychogenic F45.8
        vascular K55.9
            chronic K55.1
            specified NEC K55.8
    intraoperative (intraprocedural) — see
        Complications, intraoperative
    involuntary emotional expression (IEED) F48.2
    iris H21.9
        adhesions — see Adhesions, iris
        atrophy — see Atrophy, iris
        chamber angle recession — see Recession,
            chamber angle
        cyst — see Cyst, iris
        degeneration — see Degeneration, iris
        in diseases classified elsewhere H22
        iridodialysis — see Iridodialysis
        iridoschisis — see Iridoschisis
        miotic pupillary cyst — see Cyst, pupillary
        pupillary
            abnormality — see Abnormality, pupillary
            membrane — see Membrane, pupillary
        specified type NEC H21.89
        vascular NEC H21.1X- ☑
    iron metabolism E83.10
        specified NEC E83.19
    isovaleric acidemia E71.110
    jaw, developmental M27.0
        temporomandibular — see Anomaly,
            dentofacial, temporomandibular joint
    joint M25.9
        derangement — see Derangement, joint
        effusion — see Effusion, joint
        fistula — see Fistula, joint
        hemarthrosis — see Hemarthrosis
        instability — see Instability, joint
        osteophyte — see Osteophyte
        pain — see Pain, joint
        psychogenic F45.8
        specified type NEC M25.80
            ankle M25.87- ☑
            elbow M25.82- ☑
            foot joint M25.87- ☑
            hand joint M25.84- ☑
            hip M25.85- ☑
            knee M25.86- ☑
            shoulder M25.81- ☑
            wrist M25.83- ☑
        stiffness — see Stiffness, joint
    ketone metabolism E71.32
    kidney N28.9
        functional (tubular) N25.9

Disorder — continued
    in
        schistosomiasis B65.9 [N29]
        tubular function N25.9
            specified NEC N25.89
    lacrimal system H04.9
        changes H04.69
            fistula — see Fistula, lacrimal
        gland H04.19
            atrophy — see Atrophy, lacrimal gland
            cyst — see Cyst, lacrimal, gland
            dacryops — see Dacryops
            dislocation — see Dislocation, lacrimal gland
            dry eye syndrome — see Syndrome, dry eye
            infection — see Dacryoadenitis
            granuloma — see Granuloma, lacrimal
            inflammation — see Inflammation, lacrimal
            obstruction — see Obstruction, lacrimal
            specified NEC H04.89
    lactation NEC O92.79
    language (developmental) F80.9
        expressive F80.1
        mixed receptive and expressive F80.2
        receptive F80.2
    late luteal phase dysphoric N94.89
    learning (specific) F81.9
        acalculia R48.8
        alexia R48.0
        mathematics F81.2
        reading F81.0
        specified NEC F81.89
        spelling F81.81
        written expression F81.81
    lens H27.9
        aphakia — see Aphakia
        cataract — see Cataract
        dislocation — see Dislocation, lens
        specified type NEC H27.8
    ligament M24.20
        ankle M24.27- ☑
        attachment, spine — see Enthesopathy, spinal
        elbow M24.22- ☑
        foot joint M24.27- ☑
        hand joint M24.24- ☑
        hip M24.25- ☑
        knee — see Derangement, knee, specified NEC
        shoulder M24.21- ☑
        vertebra M24.28
        wrist M24.23- ☑
    ligamentous attachments (see also
        Enthesopathy)
        spine — see Enthesopathy, spinal
    lipid
        metabolism, congenital E78.9
        storage E75.6
            specified NEC E75.5
    lipoprotein
        deficiency (familial) E78.6
        metabolism E78.9
            specified NEC E78.89
    liver K76.9
        malarial B54 [K77]
    low back (see also Dorsopathy, specified NEC)
    lumbosacral
        plexus G54.1
        root (nerve) NEC G54.4
    lung, interstitial, drug-induced J70.4
        acute J70.2
        chronic J70.3
    lymphoproliferative, post-transplant (PTLD) D47.Z1
    lysine and hydroxylysine metabolism E72.3
    male
        erectile (organic) (see also Dysfunction, sexual,
            male, erectile) N52.9
            nonorganic F52.21
        hypoactive sexual desire F52.0
        orgasmic F52.32
    manic F30.9
        organic F06.33
    mastoid (see also Disorder, ear, middle)
        postprocedural — see Complications, ear,
            procedure
    meniscus — see Derangement, knee, meniscus
    menopausal N95.9
        specified NEC N95.8
    menstrual N92.6
        psychogenic F45.8
        specified NEC N92.5
    mental (or behavioral) (nonpsychotic) F99
        due to (secondary to)
            amphetamine

Disorder — continued
        due to drug abuse — see Abuse, drug,
            stimulant
        due to drug dependence — see
            Dependence, drug, stimulant
        brain disease, damage and dysfunction F09
        caffeine use
            due to drug abuse — see Abuse, drug,
                stimulant
            due to drug dependence — see
                Dependence, drug, stimulant
        cannabis use
            due to drug abuse — see Abuse, drug,
                cannabis
            due to drug dependence — see
                Dependence, drug, cannabis
        general medical condition F09
        sedative or hypnotic use
            due to drug abuse — see Abuse, drug,
                sedative
            due to drug dependence — see
                Dependence, drug, sedative
        tobacco (nicotine) use — see Dependence,
            drug, nicotine
    following organic brain damage F07.9
        frontal lobe syndrome F07.0
        personality change F07.0
        postconcussional syndrome F07.81
        specified NEC F07.89
    infancy, childhood or adolescence F98.9
    neurotic — see Neurosis
    organic or symptomatic F09
    presenile, psychotic F03 ☑
    problem NEC
    psychoneurotic — see Neurosis
    psychotic — see Psychosis
    puerperal F53
    senile, psychotic NEC F03 ☑
    metabolic, amino acid, transitory, newborn P74.8
    metabolism NOS E88.9
        amino-acid E72.9
            aromatic E70.9
                albinism — see Albinism
                histidine E70.40
                    histidinemia E70.41
                    other specified E70.49
                hyperphenylalaninemia E70.1
                    classical phenylketonuria E70.0
                other specified E70.8
                tryptophan E70.5
                tyrosine E70.20
                    hypertyrosinemia E70.21
                    other specified E70.29
            branched chain E71.2
                3-methylglutaconic aciduria E71.111
                hyperleucine-isoleucinemia E71.19
                hypervalinemia E71.19
                isovaleric acidemia E71.110
                maple syrup urine disease E71.0
                methylmalonic acidemia E71.120
                organic aciduria NEC E71.118
                other specified E71.19
                proprionate NEC E71.128
                proprionic acidemia E71.121
            glycine E72.50
                d-glycericacidemia E72.59
                hyperhydroxyprolinemia E72.59
                hyperoxaluria E72.53
                hyperprolinemia E72.59
                non-ketotic hyperglycinemia E72.51
                other specified E72.59
                sarcosinemia E72.59
                trimethylaminuria E72.52
            hydroxylysine E72.3
            lysine E72.3
            ornithine E72.4
            other specified E72.8
                beta-amino acid E72.8
                gamma-glutamyl cycle E72.8
            straight-chain E72.8
            sulfur-bearing E72.10
                homocystinuria E72.11
                methylenetetrahydrofolate reductase
                    deficiency E72.12
                other specified E72.19
        bile acid and cholesterol metabolism E78.70
        bilirubin E80.7
            specified NEC E80.6
        calcium E83.50
            hypercalcemia E83.52
            hypocalcemia E83.51
            other specified E83.59

Disorder

Disorder — *continued*
carbohydrate E74.9
  specified NEC E74.8
cholesterol and bile acid metabolism E78.70
congenital E88.9
copper E83.00
  Wilson's disease E83.01
  specified type NEC E83.09
cystinuria E72.01
fructose E74.10
galactose E74.20
glucosaminoglycan E76.9
  mucopolysaccharidosis — *see*
    Mucopolysaccharidosis
  specified NEC E76.8
glutamine E72.8
glycine E72.50
glycogen storage (hepatorenal) E74.09
glycoprotein E77.9
  specified NEC E77.8
glycosaminoglycan E76.9
  specified NEC E76.8
in labor and delivery O75.89
iron E83.10
isoleucine E71.19
leucine E71.19
lipoid E78.9
lipoprotein E78.9
  specified NEC E78.89
magnesium E83.40
  hypermagnesemia E83.41
  hypomagnesemia E83.42
  other specified E83.49
mineral E83.9
  specified NEC E83.89
mitochondrial E88.40
  MELAS syndrome E88.41
  MERRF syndrome (myoclonic epilepsy
    associated with ragged-red fibers) E88.42
  other specified E88.49
ornithine E72.4
phosphatases E83.30
phosphorus E83.30
  acid phosphatase deficiency E83.39
  hypophosphatasia E83.39
  hypophosphatemia E83.39
    familial E83.31
  other specified E83.39
  pseudovitamin D deficiency E83.32
plasma protein NEC E88.09
porphyrin — *see* Porphyria
postprocedural E89.89
  specified NEC E89.89
purine E79.9
  specified NEC E79.8
pyrimidine E79.9
  specified NEC E79.8
pyruvate E74.4
serine E72.8
sodium E87.8
specified NEC E88.89
threonine E72.8
valine E71.19
zinc E83.2
methylmalonic acidemia E71.120
micturition NEC R39.19
  feeling of incomplete emptying R39.14
  hesitancy R39.11
  poor stream R39.12
  psychogenic F45.8
  split stream R39.13
  straining R39.16
  urgency R39.15
mitochondrial metabolism E88.40
mitral (valve) — *see* Endocarditis, mitral
mixed
  anxiety and depressive F41.8
  of scholastic skills (developmental) F81.89
  receptive expressive language F80.2
mood F39
  bipolar — *see* Disorder, bipolar
  depressive — *see* Disorder, depressive
  due to (secondary to)
    alcohol F10.94
    amphetamine F15.94
      in
        abuse F15.14
        dependence F15.24
    anxiolytic F13.94
      in
        abuse F13.14
        dependence F13.24

Disorder — *continued*
cocaine F14.94
  in
    abuse F14.14
    dependence F14.24
  general medical condition F06.30
  hallucinogen F16.94
    in
      abuse F16.14
      dependence F16.24
  hypnotic F13.94
    in
      abuse F13.14
      dependence F13.24
  inhalant F18.94
    in
      abuse F18.14
      dependence F18.24
  opioid F11.94
    in
      abuse F11.14
      dependence F11.24
  phencyclidine (PCP) F16.94
    in
      abuse F16.14
      dependence F16.24
  physiological condition F06.30
    with
      depressive features F06.31
      major depressive-like episode F06.32
      manic features F06.33
      mixed features F06.34
  psychoactive substance NEC F19.94
    in
      abuse F19.14
      dependence F19.24
  sedative F13.94
    in
      abuse F13.14
      dependence F13.24
  volatile solvents F18.94
    in
      abuse F18.14
      dependence F18.24
manic episode F30.9
  with psychotic symptoms F30.2
  in remission (full) F30.4
    partial F30.3
  specified type NEC F30.8
  without psychotic symptoms F30.10
    mild F30.11
    moderate F30.12
    severe F30.13
organic F06.30
  right hemisphere F07.89
persistent F34.9
  cyclothymia F34.0
  dysthymia F34.1
  specified type NEC F34.8
recurrent F39
right hemisphere organic F07.89
movement G25.9
  drug-induced G25.70
    akathisia G25.71
    specified NEC G25.79
  hysterical F44.4
  in diseases classified elsewhere G26
  periodic limb G47.61
    sleep related G47.61
  specified NEC G25.89
  sleep related NEC G47.69
  stereotyped F98.4
  treatment-induced G25.9
multiple personality F44.81
muscle M62.9
  attachment, spine — *see* Enthesopathy, spinal
  in trichinellosis — *see* Trichinellosis, with
    muscle disorder
  psychogenic F45.8
  specified type NEC M62.89
  tone, newborn P94.9
    specified NEC P94.8
muscular
  attachments (*see also* Enthesopathy)
    spine — *see* Enthesopathy, spinal
  urethra N36.44
musculoskeletal system, soft tissue — *see*
  Disorder, soft tissue
  postprocedural M96.89
  psychogenic F45.8
myoneural G70.9
  due to lead G70.1

Disorder — *continued*
specified NEC G70.89
toxic G70.1
myotonic NEC G71.19
nail, in diseases classified elsewhere L62
neck region NEC — *see* Dorsopathy, specified
  NEC
nerve G58.9
  abducent NEC — *see* Strabismus, paralytic,
    sixth nerve
  accessory G52.8
  acoustic H93.3
  auditory H93.3
  auriculotemporal G50.8
  axillary G54.0
  cerebral — *see* Disorder, nerve, cranial
  cranial G52.9
    eighth H93.3
    eleventh G52.8
    fifth G50.9
    first G52.0
    fourth NEC — *see* Strabismus, paralytic,
      fourth nerve
    multiple G52.7
    ninth G52.1
    second NEC — *see* Disorder, nerve, optic
    seventh NEC G51.8
    sixth NEC — *see* Strabismus, paralytic, sixth
      nerve
    specified NEC G52.8
    tenth G52.2
    third NEC — *see* Strabismus, paralytic, third
      nerve
    twelfth G52.3
  entrapment — *see* Neuropathy, entrapment
  facial G51.9
    specified NEC G51.8
  femoral — *see* Lesion, nerve, femoral
  glossopharyngeal NEC G52.1
  hypoglossal G52.3
  intercostal G58.0
  lateral
    cutaneous of thigh — *see* Mononeuropathy,
      lower limb, meralgia paresthetica
    popliteal — *see* Lesion, nerve, popliteal
  lower limb — *see* Mononeuropathy, lower limb
  medial popliteal — *see* Lesion, nerve, popliteal,
    medial
  median NEC — *see* Lesion, nerve, median
  multiple G58.7
  oculomotor NEC — *see* Strabismus, paralytic,
    third nerve
  olfactory G52.0
  optic NEC H47.09- ☑
    hemorrhage into sheath — *see* Hemorrhage,
      optic nerve
    ischemic H47.01- ☑
  peroneal — *see* Lesion, nerve, popliteal
  phrenic G58.8
  plantar — *see* Lesion, nerve, plantar
  pneumogastric G52.2
  posterior tibial — *see* Syndrome, tarsal tunnel
  radial — *see* Lesion, nerve, radial
  recurrent laryngeal G52.2
  root G54.9
    cervical G54.2
    lumbosacral G54.1
    specified NEC G54.8
    thoracic G54.3
  sciatic NEC — *see* Lesion, nerve, sciatic
  specified NEC G58.8
    lower limb — *see* Mononeuropathy, lower
      limb, specified NEC
    upper limb — *see* Mononeuropathy, upper
      limb, specified NEC
  sympathetic G90.9
  tibial — *see* Lesion, nerve, popliteal, medial
  trigeminal G50.9
    specified NEC G50.8
  trochlear NEC — *see* Strabismus, paralytic,
    fourth nerve
  ulnar — *see* Lesion, nerve, ulnar
  upper limb — *see* Mononeuropathy, upper limb
  vagus G52.2
nervous system G98.8
  autonomic (peripheral) G90.9
    specified NEC G90.8
  central G96.9
    specified NEC G96.8
  parasympathetic G90.9
  specified NEC G98.8
  sympathetic G90.9

☑ **Additional character required**

Disorder — *continued*
vegetative G90.9
neurohypophysis NEC E23.3
neurological NEC R29.818
neuromuscular G70.9
hereditary NEC G71.9
specified NEC G70.89
toxic G70.1
neurotic F48.9
specified NEC F48.8
neutrophil, polymorphonuclear D71
nicotine use — *see* Dependence, drug, nicotine
nightmare F51.5
nose J34.9
specified NEC J34.89
obsessive-compulsive F42
odontogenesis NOS K00.9
opioid use
with
opioid-induced psychotic disorder F11.959
with
delusions F11.950
hallucinations F11.951
due to drug abuse — *see* Abuse, drug, opioid
due to drug dependence — *see* Dependence,
drug, opioid
oppositional defiant F91.3
optic
chiasm H47.49
due to
inflammatory disorder H47.41
neoplasm H47.42
vascular disorder H47.43
disc H47.39- ☑
coloboma — *see* Coloboma, optic disc
drusen — *see* Drusen, optic disc
pseudopapilledema — *see*
Pseudopapilledema
radiations — *see* Disorder, visual, pathway
tracts — *see* Disorder, visual, pathway
orbit H05.9
cyst — *see* Cyst, orbit
deformity — *see* Deformity, orbit
edema — *see* Edema, orbit
enophthalmos — *see* Enophthalmos
exophthalmos — *see* Exophthalmos
hemorrhage — *see* Hemorrhage, orbit
inflammation — *see* Inflammation, orbit
myopathy — *see* Myopathy, extraocular
muscles
retained foreign body — *see* Foreign body,
orbit, old
specified type NEC H05.89
organic
anxiety F06.4
catatonic F06.1
delusional F06.2
dissociative F06.8
emotionally labile (asthenic) F06.8
mood (affective) F06.30
schizophrenia-like F06.2
orgasmic (female) F52.31
male F52.32
ornithine metabolism E72.4
overanxious F41.1
of childhood F93.8
pain
with related psychological factors F45.42
exclusively related to psychological factors
F45.41
pancreatic internal secretion E16.9
specified NEC E16.8
panic F41.0
with agoraphobia F40.01
papulosquamous L44.9
in diseases classified elsewhere L45
specified NEC L44.8
paranoid F22
induced F24
shared F24
parathyroid (gland) E21.5
specified NEC E21.4
parietoalveolar NEC J84.09
paroxysmal, mixed R56.9
patella M22.9- ☑
chondromalacia — *see* Chondromalacia, patella
derangement NEC M22.3X- ☑
recurrent
dislocation — *see* Dislocation, patella,
recurrent
subluxation — *see* Dislocation, patella,
recurrent, incomplete

Disorder — *continued*
specified NEC M22.8X- ☑
patellofemoral M22.2X- ☑
pentose phosphate pathway with anemia D55.1
perception, due to hallucinogens F16.983
in
abuse F16.183
dependence F16.283
peripheral nervous system NEC G64
peroxisomal E71.50
biogenesis
neonatal adrenoleukodystrophy E71.511
specified disorder NEC E71.518
Zellweger syndrome E71.510
rhizomelic chondrodysplasia punctata E71.540
specified form NEC E71.548
group 1 E71.518
group 2 E71.53
group 3 E71.542
X-linked adrenoleukodystrophy E71.529
adolescent E71.521
adrenomyeloneuropathy E71.522
childhood E71.520
specified form NEC E71.528
Zellweger-like syndrome E71.541
persistent
(somatoform) pain F45.41
affective (mood) F34.9
personality (*see also* Personality) F60.9
affective F34.0
aggressive F60.3
amoral F60.2
anankastic F60.5
antisocial F60.2
anxious F60.6
asocial F60.2
asthenic F60.7
avoidant F60.6
borderline F60.3
change (secondary) due to general medical
condition F07.0
compulsive F60.5
cyclothymic F34.0
dependent (passive) F60.7
depressive F34.1
dissocial F60.2
emotional instability F60.3
expansive paranoid F60.0
explosive F60.3
following organic brain damage F07.9
histrionic F60.4
hyperthymic F34.0
hypothymic F34.1
hysterical F60.4
immature F60.89
inadequate F60.7
labile F60.3
mixed (nonspecific) F60.89
moral deficiency F60.2
narcissistic F60.81
negativistic F60.89
obsessional F60.5
obsessive (-compulsive) F60.5
organic F07.9
overconscientious F60.5
paranoid F60.0
passive (-dependent) F60.7
passive-aggressive F60.89
pathological NEC F60.9
pseudosocial F60.2
psychopathic F60.2
schizoid F60.1
schizotypal F21
self-defeating F60.7
specified NEC F60.89
type A F60.5
unstable (emotional) F60.3
pervasive, developmental F84.9
phobic anxiety, childhood F40.8
phosphate-losing tubular N25.0
pigmentation L81.9
choroid, congenital Q14.3
diminished melanin formation L81.6
iron L81.8
specified NEC L81.8
pinna (noninfective) H61.10- ☑
deformity, acquired H61.11- ☑
hematoma H61.12- ☑
perichondritis — *see* Perichondritis, ear
specified type NEC H61.19- ☑
pituitary gland E23.7
iatrogenic (postprocedural) E89.3

Disorder — *continued*
specified NEC E23.6
platelets D69.1
plexus G54.9
specified NEC G54.8
polymorphonuclear neutrophils D71
porphyrin metabolism — *see* Porphyria
postconcussional F07.81
posthallucinogen perception F16.983
in
abuse F16.183
dependence F16.283
postmenopausal N95.9
specified NEC N95.8
postprocedural (postoperative) — *see*
Complications, postprocedural
post-transplant lymphoproliferative D47.Z1
post-traumatic stress (PTSD) F43.10
acute F43.11
chronic F43.12
premenstrual dysphoric (PMDD) N94.3
prepuce N47.8
propionic acidemia E71.121
prostate N42.9
specified NEC N42.89
psychogenic NOS (*see also* condition) F45.9
anxiety F41.8
appetite F50.9
asthenic F48.8
cardiovascular (system) F45.8
compulsive F42
cutaneous F54
depressive F32.9
digestive (system) F45.8
dysmenorrheic F45.8
dyspneic F45.8
endocrine (system) F54
eye NEC F45.8
feeding — *see* Disorder, eating
functional NEC F45.8
gastric F45.8
gastrointestinal (system) F45.8
genitourinary (system) F45.8
heart (function) (rhythm) F45.8
hyperventilatory F45.8
hypochondriacal — *see* Disorder,
hypochondriacal
intestinal F45.8
joint F45.8
learning F81.9
limb F45.8
lymphatic (system) F45.8
menstrual F45.8
micturition F45.8
monoplegic NEC F44.4
motor F44.4
muscle F45.8
musculoskeletal F45.8
neurocirculatory F45.8
obsessive F42
occupational F48.8
organ or part of body NEC F45.8
paralytic NEC F44.4
phobic F40.9
physical NEC F45.8
rectal F45.8
respiratory (system) F45.8
rheumatic F45.8
sexual (function) F52.9
skin (allergic) (eczematous) F54
sleep F51.9
specified part of body NEC F45.8
stomach F45.8
psychological F99
associated with
disease classified elsewhere F54
sexual
development F66
relationship F66
uncertainty about gender identity F66
psychomotor NEC F44.4
hysterical F44.4
psychoneurotic (*see also* Neurosis)
mixed NEC F48.8
psychophysiologic — *see* Disorder, somatoform
psychosexual F65.9
development F66
identity of childhood F64.2
psychosomatic NOS — *see* Disorder, somatoform
multiple F45.0
undifferentiated F45.1
psychotic — *see* Psychosis

Disorder — *continued*
transient (acute) F23
puberty E30.9
specified NEC E30.8
pulmonary (valve) — *see* Endocarditis, pulmonary
purine metabolism E79.9
pyrimidine metabolism E79.9
pyruvate metabolism E74.4
reactive attachment (childhood) F94.1
reading R48.0
developmental (specific) F81.0
receptive language F80.2
receptor, hormonal, peripheral (*see also* Syndrome, androgen insensitivity) E34.50
recurrent brief depressive F33.8
reflex R29.2
refraction H52.7
aniseikonia H52.32
anisometropia H52.31
astigmatism — *see* Astigmatism
hypermetropia — *see* Hypermetropia
myopia — *see* Myopia
presbyopia H52.4
specified NEC H52.6
relationship F68.8
due to sexual orientation F66
REM sleep behavior G47.52
renal function, impaired (tubular) N25.9
resonance R49.9
specified NEC R49.8
respiratory function, impaired (*see also* Failure, respiration)
postprocedural — *see* Complication, postoperative, respiratory system
psychogenic F45.8
retina H35.9
angioid streaks H35.33
changes in vascular appearance H35.01- ☑
degeneration — *see* Degeneration, retina
dystrophy (hereditary) — *see* Dystrophy, retina
edema H35.81
hemorrhage — *see* Hemorrhage, retina
ischemia H35.82
macular degeneration — *see* Degeneration, macula
microaneurysms H35.04- ☑
microvascular abnormality NEC H35.09
neovascularization — *see* Neovascularization, retina
retinopathy — *see* Retinopathy
separation of layers H35.70
central serous chorioretinopathy H35.71- ☑
pigment epithelium detachment (serous) H35.72- ☑
hemorrhagic H35.73- ☑
specified type NEC H35.89
telangiectasis — *see* Telangiectasis, retina
vasculitis — *see* Vasculitis, retina
retroperitoneal K68.9
right hemisphere organic affective F07.89
rumination (infant or child) F98.21
sacrum, sacrococcygeal NEC M53.3
schizoaffective F25.9
bipolar type F25.0
depressive type F25.1
manic type F25.0
mixed type F25.0
specified NEC F25.8
schizoid of childhood F84.5
schizophreniform F20.81
brief F23
schizotypal (personality) F21
secretion, thyrocalcitonin E07.0
seizure (*see also* Epilepsy) G40.909
intractable G40.919
with status epilepticus G40.911
semantic pragmatic F80.89
with autism F84.0
sense of smell R43.1
psychogenic F45.8
separation anxiety, of childhood F93.0
sexual
arousal, female F52.22
aversion F52.1
function, psychogenic F52.9
maturation F66
nonorganic F52.9
preference (*see also* Deviation, sexual) F65.9
fetishistic transvestism F65.1
relationship F66
shyness, of childhood and adolescence F40.10
sibling rivalry F93.8

Disorder — *continued*
sickle-cell (sickling) (homozygous) — *see* Disease, sickle-cell
heterozygous D57.3
specified type NEC D57.8- ☑
trait D57.3
sinus (nasal) J34.9
specified NEC J34.89
skin L98.9
atrophic L90.9
specified NEC L90.8
granulomatous L92.9
specified NEC L92.8
hypertrophic L91.9
specified NEC L91.8
infiltrative NEC L98.6
newborn P83.9
specified NEC P83.8
psychogenic (allergic) (eczematous) F54
sleep G47.9
breathing-related — *see* Apnea, sleep
circadian rhythm G47.20
advance sleep phase type G47.22
delayed sleep phase type G47.21
due to
alcohol
abuse F10.182
dependence F10.282
use F10.982
amphetamines
abuse F15.182
dependence F15.282
use F15.982
caffeine
abuse F15.182
dependence F15.282
use F15.982
cocaine
abuse F14.182
dependence F14.282
use F14.982
drug NEC
abuse F19.182
dependence F19.282
use F19.982
opioid
abuse F11.182
dependence F11.282
use F11.982
psychoactive substance NEC
abuse F19.182
dependence F19.282
use F19.982
sedative, hypnotic, or anxiolytic
abuse F13.182
dependence F13.282
use F13.982
stimulant NEC
abuse F15.182
dependence F15.282
use F15.982
free running type G47.24
in conditions classified elsewhere G47.27
irregular sleep wake type G47.23
jet lag type G47.25
shift work type G47.26
specified NEC G47.29
due to
alcohol
abuse F10.182
dependence F10.282
use F10.982
amphetamine
abuse F15.182
dependence F15.282
use F15.982
anxiolytic
abuse F13.182
dependence F13.282
use F13.982
caffeine
abuse F15.182
dependence F15.282
use F15.982
cocaine
abuse F14.182
dependence F14.282
use F14.982
drug NEC
abuse F19.182
dependence F19.282
use F19.982

Disorder — *continued*
hypnotic
abuse F13.182
dependence F13.282
use F13.982
opioid
abuse F11.182
dependence F11.282
use F11.982
psychoactive substance NEC
abuse F19.182
dependence F19.282
use F19.982
sedative
abuse F13.182
dependence F13.282
use F13.982
stimulant NEC
abuse F15.182
dependence F15.282
use F15.982
emotional F51.9
excessive somnolence — *see* Hypersomnia
hypersomnia type — *see* Hypersomnia
initiating or maintaining — *see* Insomnia
nightmares F51.5
nonorganic F51.9
specified NEC F51.8
parasomnia type G47.50
specified NEC G47.8
terrors F51.4
walking F51.3
sleep-wake pattern or schedule — *see* Disorder, sleep, circadian rhythm
social
anxiety of childhood F40.10
functioning in childhood F94.9
specified NEC F94.8
soft tissue M79.9
ankle M79.9
due to use, overuse and pressure M70.90
ankle M70.97- ☑
bursitis — *see* Bursitis
foot M70.97- ☑
forearm M70.93- ☑
hand M70.94- ☑
lower leg M70.96- ☑
multiple sites M70.99
pelvic region M70.95- ☑
shoulder region M70.91- ☑
specified site NEC M70.98
specified type NEC M70.80
ankle M70.87- ☑
foot M70.87- ☑
forearm M70.83- ☑
hand M70.84- ☑
lower leg M70.86- ☑
multiple sites M70.89
pelvic region M70.85- ☑
shoulder region M70.81- ☑
specified site NEC M70.88
thigh M70.85- ☑
upper arm M70.82- ☑
thigh M70.95- ☑
upper arm M70.92- ☑
foot M79.9
forearm M79.9
hand M79.9
lower leg M79.9
multiple sites M79.9
occupational — *see* Disorder, soft tissue, due to use, overuse and pressure
pelvic region M79.9
shoulder region M79.9
specified type NEC M79.89
thigh M79.9
upper arm M79.9
somatization F45.0
somatoform F45.9
pain (persistent) F45.41
somatization (multiple) (long-lasting) F45.0
specified NEC F45.8
undifferentiated F45.1
somnolence, excessive — *see* Hypersomnia
specific
arithmetical F81.2
developmental, of motor F82
reading F81.0
speech and language F80.9
spelling F81.81
written expression F81.81
speech R47.9

☑ **Additional character required**

Disorder — *continued*

articulation (functional) (specific) F80.0
   developmental F80.9
   specified NEC R47.89
spelling (specific) F81.81
spine (*see also* Dorsopathy)
   ligamentous or muscular attachments,
      peripheral — *see* Enthesopathy, spinal
   specified NEC — *see* Dorsopathy, specified NEC
stereotyped, habit or movement F98.4
stomach (functional) — *see* Disorder, gastric
stress F43.9
   post-traumatic F43.10
      acute F43.11
      chronic F43.12
sulfur-bearing amino-acid metabolism E72.10
sweat gland (eccrine) L74.9
   apocrine L75.9
      specified NEC L75.8
   specified NEC L74.8
synovium M67.90
   acromioclavicular M67.91- ☑
   ankle M67.97- ☑
   elbow M67.92- ☑
   foot M67.97- ☑
   forearm M67.93- ☑
   hand M67.94- ☑
   hip M67.95- ☑
   knee M67.96- ☑
   multiple sites M67.99
   rupture — *see* Rupture, synovium
   shoulder M67.91- ☑
   specified type NEC M67.80
      acromioclavicular M67.81- ☑
      ankle M67.87- ☑
      elbow M67.82- ☑
      foot M67.87- ☑
      hand M67.84- ☑
      hip M67.85- ☑
      knee M67.86- ☑
      multiple sites M67.89
      wrist M67.83- ☑
   synovitis — *see* Synovitis
   upper arm M67.92- ☑
   wrist M67.93- ☑
temperature regulation, newborn P81.9
   specified NEC P81.8
temporomandibular joint — *see* Anomaly,
   dentofacial, temporomandibular joint
tendon M67.90
   acromioclavicular M67.91- ☑
   ankle M67.97- ☑
   contracture — *see* Contracture, tendon
   elbow M67.92- ☑
   foot M67.97- ☑
   forearm M67.93- ☑
   hand M67.94- ☑
   hip M67.95- ☑
   knee M67.96- ☑
   multiple sites M67.99
   rupture — *see* Rupture, tendon
   shoulder M67.91- ☑
   specified type NEC M67.80
      acromioclavicular M67.81- ☑
      ankle M67.87- ☑
      elbow M67.82- ☑
      foot M67.87- ☑
      hand M67.84- ☑
      hip M67.85- ☑
      knee M67.86- ☑
      multiple sites M67.89
      trunk M67.88
      wrist M67.83- ☑
   synovitis — *see* Synovitis
   tendinitis — *see* Tendinitis
   tenosynovitis — *see* Tenosynovitis
   trunk M67.98
   upper arm M67.92- ☑
   wrist M67.93- ☑
thoracic root (nerve) NEC G54.3
thyrocalcitonin hypersecretion E07.0
thyroid (gland) E07.9
   function NEC, neonatal, transitory P72.2
   iodine-deficiency related E01.8
   specified NEC E07.89
tic — *see* Tic
tooth K08.9
   development K00.9
      specified NEC K00.8
   eruption K00.6
Tourette's F95.2
trance and possession F44.89

Disorder — *continued*

tricuspid (valve) — *see* Endocarditis, tricuspid
tryptophan metabolism E70.5
tubular, phosphate-losing N25.0
tubulo-interstitial (in)
   brucellosis A23.9 [N16]
   cystinosis E72.04
   diphtheria A36.84
   glycogen storage disease E74.00 [N16]
   leukemia NEC C95.9- ☑ [N16]
   lymphoma NEC C85.9- ☑ [N16]
   mixed cryoglobulinemia D89.1 [N16]
   multiple myeloma C90.0- ☑ [N16]
   Salmonella infection A02.25
   sarcoidosis D86.84
   sepsis A41.9 [N16]
      streptococcal A40.9 [N16]
   systemic lupus erythematosus M32.15
   toxoplasmosis B58.83
   transplant rejection T86.91 [N16]
   Wilson's disease E83.01 [N16]
tubulo-renal function, impaired N25.9
   specified NEC N25.89
tympanic membrane H73.9- ☑
   atrophy — *see* Atrophy, tympanic membrane
   infection — *see* Myringitis
   perforation — *see* Perforation, tympanum
   specified NEC H73.89- ☑
unsocialized aggressive F91.1
urea cycle metabolism E72.20
   argininemia E72.21
   arginosuccinic aciduria E72.22
   citrullinemia E72.23
   ornithine transcarbamylase deficiency E72.4
   other specified E72.29
ureter (in) N28.9
   schistosomiasis B65.0 [N29]
   tuberculosis A18.11
urethra N36.9
   specified NEC N36.8
urinary system N39.9
   specified NEC N39.8
valve, heart
   aortic — *see* Endocarditis, aortic
   mitral — *see* Endocarditis, mitral
   pulmonary — *see* Endocarditis, pulmonary
   rheumatic
      aortic — *see* Endocarditis, aortic, rheumatic
      mitral — *see* Endocarditis, mitral
      pulmonary — *see* Endocarditis, pulmonary,
         rheumatic
      tricuspid — *see* Endocarditis, tricuspid
   tricuspid — *see* Endocarditis, tricuspid
vestibular function H81.9- ☑
   specified NEC H81.8
      in diseases classified elsewhere H82.- ☑
   vertigo — *see* Vertigo
vision, binocular H53.30
   abnormal retinal correspondence H53.31
   diplopia H53.2
   fusion with defective stereopsis H53.32
   simultaneous perception H53.33
   suppression H53.34
visual
   cortex
      blindness H47.619
         left brain H47.612
         right brain H47.611
      due to
         inflammatory disorder H47.629
            left brain H47.622
            right brain H47.621
         neoplasm H47.639
            left brain H47.632
            right brain H47.631
         vascular disorder H47.649
            left brain H47.642
            right brain H47.641
   pathway H47.9
      due to
         inflammatory disorder H47.51- ☑
         neoplasm H47.52- ☑
         vascular disorder H47.53- ☑
   optic chiasm — *see* Disorder, optic, chiasm
vitreous body H43.9
   crystalline deposits — *see* Deposit, crystalline
   degeneration — *see* Degeneration, vitreous
   hemorrhage — *see* Hemorrhage, vitreous
   opacities — *see* Opacity, vitreous
   prolapse — *see* Prolapse, vitreous
   specified type NEC H43.89
voice R49.9

Disorder — *continued*

specified type NEC R49.8
volatile solvent use
   due to drug abuse — *see* Abuse, drug, inhalant
   due to drug dependence — *see* Dependence,
      drug, inhalant
white blood cells D72.9
   specified NEC D72.89
withdrawing, child or adolescent F40.10
Disorientation R41.0
Displacement, displaced
acquired traumatic of bone, cartilage, joint,
   tendon NEC — *see* Dislocation
adrenal gland (congenital) Q89.1
appendix, retrocecal (congenital) Q43.8
auricle (congenital) Q17.4
bladder (acquired) N32.89
   congenital Q64.19
brachial plexus (congenital) Q07.8
brain stem, caudal (congenital) Q04.8
canaliculus (lacrimalis), congenital Q10.6
cardia through esophageal hiatus (congenital)
   Q40.1
cerebellum, caudal (congenital) Q04.8
cervix — *see* Malposition, uterus
colon (congenital) Q43.3
device, implant or graft (*see also* Complications,
   by site and type, mechanical) T85.628 ☑
   arterial graft NEC — *see* Complication,
      cardiovascular device, mechanical, vascular
   breast (implant) T85.42 ☑
   catheter NEC T85.628 ☑
      dialysis (renal) T82.42 ☑
         intraperitoneal T85.621 ☑
      infusion NEC T82.524 ☑
         spinal (epidural) (subdural) T85.620 ☑
      urinary (indwelling) T83.028 ☑
         cystostomy T83.020 ☑
   electronic (electrode) (pulse generator)
      (stimulator) — *see* Complication, electronic
      stimulator
   fixation, internal (orthopedic) NEC — *see*
      Complication, fixation device, mechanical
   gastrointestinal — *see* Complications,
      prosthetic device, mechanical,
      gastrointestinal device
   genital NEC T83.428 ☑
      intrauterine contraceptive device T83.32 ☑
      penile prosthesis T83.420 ☑
   heart NEC — *see* Complication, cardiovascular
      device, mechanical
   joint prosthesis — *see* Complications, joint
      prosthesis, mechanical
   ocular — *see* Complications, prosthetic device,
      mechanical, ocular device
   orthopedic NEC — *see* Complication,
      orthopedic, device or graft, mechanical
   specified NEC T85.628 ☑
   urinary NEC (*see also* Complication,
      genitourinary, device, urinary, mechanical)
      graft T83.22 ☑
   vascular NEC — *see* Complication,
      cardiovascular device, mechanical
   ventricular intracranial shunt T85.02 ☑
electronic stimulator
   bone T84.320 ☑
   cardiac — *see* Complications, cardiac device,
      electronic
   nervous system — *see* Complication, prosthetic
      device, mechanical, electronic nervous
      system stimulator
   urinary — *see* Complications, electronic
      stimulator, urinary
esophageal mucosa into cardia of stomach,
   congenital Q39.8
esophagus (acquired) K22.8
   congenital Q39.8
eyeball (acquired) (lateral) (old) — *see*
   Displacement, globe
   congenital Q15.8
   current — *see* Avulsion, eye
fallopian tube (acquired) N83.4
   congenital Q50.6
   opening (congenital) Q50.6
gallbladder (congenital) Q44.1
gastric mucosa (congenital) Q40.2
globe (acquired) (old) (lateral) H05.21- ☑
   current — *see* Avulsion, eye
heart (congenital) Q24.8
   acquired I51.89
hymen (upward) (congenital) Q52.4
intervertebral disc NEC

Displacement — *continued*
 with myelopathy — *see* Disorder, disc, with,
 myelopathy
 cervical, cervicothoracic (with) M50.20
 myelopathy — *see* Disorder, disc, cervical,
 with myelopathy
 neuritis, radiculitis or radiculopathy — *see*
 Disorder, disc, cervical, with neuritis
 due to trauma — *see* Dislocation, vertebra
 lumbar region M51.26
 with
 myelopathy M51.06
 neuritis, radiculitis, radiculopathy or
 sciatica M51.16
 lumbosacral region M51.27
 with
 neuritis, radiculitis, radiculopathy or
 sciatica M51.17
 sacrococcygeal region M53.3
 thoracic region M51.24
 with
 myelopathy M51.04
 neuritis, radiculitis, radiculopathy M51.14
 thoracolumbar region M51.25
 with
 myelopathy M51.05
 neuritis, radiculitis, radiculopathy M51.15
 intrauterine device T83.32 ☑
 kidney (acquired) N28.83
 congenital Q63.2
 lachrymal, lacrimal apparatus or duct (congenital)
 Q10.6
 lens, congenital Q12.1
 macula (congenital) Q14.1
 Meckel's diverticulum Q43.0
 malignant — *see* Table of Neoplasms, small
 intestine, malignant
 nail (congenital) Q84.6
 acquired L60.8
 opening of Wharton's duct in mouth Q38.4
 organ or site, congenital NEC — *see* Malposition,
 congenital
 ovary (acquired) N83.4
 congenital Q50.39
 free in peritoneal cavity (congenital) Q50.39
 into hernial sac N83.4
 oviduct (acquired) N83.4
 congenital Q50.6
 parathyroid (gland) E21.4
 parotid gland (congenital) Q38.4
 punctum lacrimale (congenital) Q10.6
 sacro-iliac (joint) (congenital) Q74.2
 current injury S33.2 ☑
 old M53.2
 salivary gland (any) (congenital) Q38.4
 spleen (congenital) Q89.09
 stomach, congenital Q40.2
 sublingual duct Q38.4
 tongue (downward) (congenital) Q38.3
 tooth, teeth, fully erupted M26.30
 horizontal M26.33
 vertical M26.34
 trachea (congenital) Q32.1
 ureter or ureteric opening or orifice (congenital)
 Q62.62
 uterine opening of oviducts or fallopian tubes
 Q50.6
 uterus, uterine — *see* Malposition, uterus
 ventricular septum Q21.0
 with rudimentary ventricle Q20.4
Disproportion
 between native and reconstructed breast N65.1
 fiber-type G71.2
Disruptio uteri — *see* Rupture, uterus
Disruption (of)
 ciliary body NEC H21.89
 closure of
 cornea T81.31 ☑
 craniotomy T81.32 ☑
 fascia (muscular) (superficial) T81.32 ☑
 internal organ or tissue T81.32 ☑
 laceration (external) (internal) T81.33 ☑
 ligament T81.32 ☑
 mucosa T81.31 ☑
 muscle or muscle flap T81.32 ☑
 ribs or rib cage T81.32 ☑
 skin and subcutaneous tissue (full-thickness)
 (superficial) T81.31 ☑
 skull T81.32 ☑
 sternum (sternotomy) T81.32 ☑
 tendon T81.32 ☑

Disruption — *continued*
 traumatic laceration (external) (internal) T81.33
 ☑
 family Z63.8
 due to
 absence of family member due to military
 deployment Z63.31
 absence of family member NEC Z63.32
 alcoholism and drug addiction in family
 Z63.72
 bereavement Z63.4
 death (assumed) or disappearance of family
 member Z63.4
 divorce or separation Z63.5
 drug addiction in family Z63.72
 return of family member from military
 deployment (current or past conflict)
 Z63.71
 stressful life events NEC Z63.79
 iris NEC H21.89
 ligament (s) (*see also* Sprain)
 knee
 current injury — *see* Dislocation, knee
 old (chronic) — *see* Derangement, knee,
 ligament, instability, chronic
 spontaneous NEC — *see* Derangement, knee,
 disruption ligament
 ossicular chain — *see* Discontinuity, ossicles, ear
 pelvic ring (stable) S32.810 ☑
 unstable S32.811 ☑
 wound T81.30 ☑
 episiotomy O90.1
 operation T81.31 ☑
 cesarean O90.0
 external operation wound (superficial)
 T81.31 ☑
 internal operation wound (deep) T81.32 ☑
 perineal (obstetric) O90.1
 traumatic injury repair T81.33 ☑
 traumatic injury wound repair T81.33 ☑
Dissatisfaction with
 employment Z56.9
 school environment Z55.4
Dissecting — *see* condition
Dissection
 aorta I71.00
 abdominal I71.02
 thoracic I71.01
 thoracoabdominal I71.03
 artery
 carotid I77.71
 cerebral (nonruptured) I67.0
 ruptured — *see* Hemorrhage, intracranial,
 subarachnoid
 coronary I25.42
 iliac I77.72
 renal I77.73
 specified NEC I77.79
 vertebral I77.74
 traumatic — *see* Wound, open, by site
 vascular I99.8
 wound — *see* Wound, open
Disseminated — *see* condition
Dissociation
 auriculoventricular or atrioventricular (AV) (any
 degree) (isorhythmic) I45.89
 with heart block I44.2
 interference I45.89
Dissociative reaction, state F44.9
Dissolution, vertebra — *see* Osteoporosis
Distension, distention
 abdomen R14.0
 bladder N32.89
 cecum K63.89
 colon K63.89
 gallbladder K82.8
 intestine K63.89
 kidney N28.89
 liver K76.89
 seminal vesicle N50.8
 stomach K31.89
 acute K31.0
 psychogenic F45.8
 ureter — *see* Dilatation, ureter
 uterus N85.8
Distoma hepaticum infestation B66.3
Distomiasis B66.9
 bile passages B66.3
 hemic B65.9
 hepatic B66.3
 due to Clonorchis sinensis B66.1
 intestinal B66.5

Distomiasis — *continued*
 liver B66.3
 due to Clonorchis sinensis B66.1
 lung B66.4
 pulmonary B66.4
Distomolar (fourth molar) K00.1
Disto-occlusion (Division I) (Division II) M26.212
Distortion (s) (congenital)
 adrenal (gland) Q89.1
 arm NEC Q68.8
 bile duct or passage Q44.5
 bladder Q64.79
 brain Q04.9
 cervix (uteri) Q51.9
 chest (wall) Q67.8
 bones Q76.8
 clavicle Q74.0
 clitoris Q52.6
 coccyx Q76.49
 common duct Q44.5
 coronary Q24.5
 cystic duct Q44.5
 ear (auricle) (external) Q17.3
 inner Q16.5
 middle Q16.4
 ossicles Q16.3
 endocrine NEC Q89.2
 eustachian tube Q17.8
 eye (adnexa) Q15.8
 face bone (s) NEC Q75.8
 fallopian tube Q50.6
 femur NEC Q68.8
 fibula NEC Q68.8
 finger (s) Q68.1
 foot Q66.9
 genitalia, genital organ (s)
 female Q52.8
 external Q52.79
 internal NEC Q52.8
 gyri Q04.8
 hand bone (s) Q68.1
 heart (auricle) (ventricle) Q24.8
 valve (cusp) Q24.8
 hepatic duct Q44.5
 humerus NEC Q68.8
 hymen Q52.4
 intrafamilial communications Z63.8
 jaw NEC M26.89
 labium (majus) (minus) Q52.79
 leg NEC Q68.8
 lens Q12.8
 liver Q44.7
 lumbar spine Q76.49
 with disproportion O33.8
 causing obstructed labor O65.0
 lumbosacral (joint) (region) Q76.49
 kyphosis — *see* Kyphosis, congenital
 lordosis — *see* Lordosis, congenital
 nerve Q07.8
 nose Q30.8
 organ
 of Corti Q16.5
 or site not listed — *see* Anomaly, by site
 ossicles, ear Q16.3
 oviduct Q50.6
 pancreas Q45.3
 parathyroid (gland) Q89.2
 pituitary (gland) Q89.2
 radius NEC Q68.8
 sacroiliac joint Q74.2
 sacrum Q76.49
 scapula Q74.0
 shoulder girdle Q74.0
 skull bone (s) NEC Q75.8
 with
 anencephalus Q00.0
 encephalocele — *see* Encephalocele
 hydrocephalus Q03.9
 with spina bifida — *see* Spina bifida, with
 hydrocephalus
 microcephaly Q02
 spinal cord Q06.8
 spine Q76.49
 kyphosis — *see* Kyphosis, congenital
 lordosis — *see* Lordosis, congenital
 spleen Q89.09
 sternum NEC Q76.7
 thorax (wall) Q67.8
 bony Q76.8
 thymus (gland) Q89.2
 thyroid (gland) Q89.2
 tibia NEC Q68.8

☑ **Additional character required**

Distortion — continued
  toe (s) Q66.9
  tongue Q38.3
  trachea (cartilage) Q32.1
  ulna NEC Q68.8
  ureter Q62.8
  urethra Q64.79
    causing obstruction Q64.39
  uterus Q51.9
  vagina Q52.4
  vertebra Q76.49
    kyphosis — see Kyphosis, congenital
    lordosis — see Lordosis, congenital
  visual (see also Disturbance, vision)
    shape and size H53.15
  vulva Q52.79
  wrist (bones) (joint) Q68.8
Distress
  abdomen — see Pain, abdominal
  acute respiratory (adult) (child) J80
  epigastric R10.13
  fetal P84
    complicating pregnancy — see Stress, fetal
  gastrointestinal (functional) K30
    psychogenic F45.8
  intestinal (functional) NOS K59.9
    psychogenic F45.8
  maternal, during labor and delivery O75.0
  respiratory R06.00
    adult J80
    child J80
    newborn P22.9
      specified NEC P22.8
    orthopnea R06.01
    psychogenic F45.8
    shortness of breath R06.02
    specified type NEC R06.09
Distribution vessel, atypical Q27.9
  coronary artery Q24.5
  precerebral Q28.1
Districhiasis L68.8
Disturbance (s) (see also Disease)
  absorption K90.9
    calcium E58
    carbohydrate K90.4
    fat K90.4
      pancreatic K90.3
    protein K90.4
    starch K90.4
    vitamin — see Deficiency, vitamin
  acid-base equilibrium E87.8
    mixed E87.4
  activity and attention (with hyperkinesis) — see
    Disorder, attention-deficit hyperactivity
  amino acid transport E72.00
  assimilation, food K90.9
  auditory nerve, except deafnessH93.3
  behavior — see Disorder, conduct
  blood clotting (mechanism) (see also Defect,
    coagulation) D68.9
  cerebral
    nerve — see Disorder, nerve, cranial
    status, newborn P91.9
      specified NEC P91.8
  circulatory I99.9
  conduct (see also Disorder, conduct) F91.9
    adjustment reaction — see Disorder,
      adjustment
    compulsive F63.9
    disruptive F91.9
    hyperkinetic — see Disorder, attention-deficit
      hyperactivity
    socialized F91.2
    specified NEC F91.8
    unsocialized F91.1
  coordination R27.8
  cranial nerve — see Disorder, nerve, cranial
  deep sensibility — see Disturbance, sensation
  digestive K30
    psychogenic F45.8
  electrolyte (see also Imbalance, electrolyte)
    newborn, transitory P74.4
      hyperammonemia P74.6
      potassium balance P74.3
      sodium balance P74.2
      specified type NEC P74.4
  emotions specific to childhood and adolescence
    F93.9
    with
      anxiety and fearfulness NEC F93.8
      elective mutism F94.0
      oppositional disorder F91.3

Disturbance — continued
    sensitivity (withdrawal) F40.10
    shyness F40.10
    social withdrawal F40.10
  involving relationship problems F93.8
    mixed F93.8
    specified NEC F93.8
  endocrine (gland) E34.9
    neonatal, transitory P72.9
      specified NEC P72.8
  equilibrium R42
  fructose metabolism E74.10
  gait — see Gait
    hysterical F44.4
    psychogenic F44.4
  gastrointestinal (functional) K30
    psychogenic F45.8
  habit, child F98.9
  hearing, except deafness and tinnitus — see
    Abnormal, auditory perception
  heart, functional (conditions in I44-I50)
    due to presence of (cardiac) prosthesis I97.19-
      ☑
    postoperative I97.89
      cardiac surgery I97.19- ☑
  hormones E34.9
  innervation uterus (parasympathetic)
    (sympathetic) N85.8
  keratinization NEC
    gingiva K05.10
      nonplaque induced K05.11
      plaque induced K05.10
    lip K13.0
    oral (mucosa) (soft tissue) K13.29
    tongue K13.29
  learning (specific) — see Disorder, learning
  memory — see Amnesia
    mild, following organic brain damage F06.8
  mental F99
    associated with diseases classified elsewhere
      F54
  metabolism E88.9
    with
      abortion — see Abortion, by type with other
        specified complication
      ectopic pregnancy O08.5
      molar pregnancy O08.5
    amino-acid E72.9
      aromatic E70.9
      branched-chain E71.2
      straight-chain E72.8
      sulfur-bearing E72.10
    ammonia E72.20
    arginine E72.21
    arginosuccinic acid E72.22
    carbohydrate E74.9
    cholesterol E78.9
    citrulline E72.23
    cystathionine E72.19
    general E88.9
    glutamine E72.8
    histidine E70.40
    homocystine E72.19
    hydroxylysine E72.3
    in labor or delivery O75.89
    iron E83.10
    lipoid E78.9
    lysine E72.3
    methionine E72.19
    neonatal, transitory P74.9
      calcium and magnesium P71.9
        specified type NEC P71.8
      carbohydrate metabolism P70.9
        specified type NEC P70.8
      specified NEC P74.8
    ornithine E72.4
    phosphate E83.39
    sodium NEC E87.8
    threonine E72.8
    tryptophan E70.5
    tyrosine E70.20
    urea cycle E72.20
  motor R29.2
  nervous, functional R45.0
  neuromuscular mechanism (eye), due to syphilis
    A52.15
  nutritional E63.9
    nail L60.3
  ocular motion H51.9
    psychogenic F45.8
  oculogyric H51.8
    psychogenic F45.8

Disturbance — continued
  oculomotor H51.9
    psychogenic F45.8
  olfactory nerve R43.1
  optic nerve NEC — see Disorder, nerve, optic
  oral epithelium, including tongue NEC K13.29
  perceptual due to
    alcohol withdrawal F10.232
    amphetamine intoxication F15.922
      in
        abuse F15.122
        dependence F15.222
    anxiolytic withdrawal F13.232
    cannabis intoxication (acute) F12.922
      in
        abuse F12.122
        dependence F12.222
    cocaine intoxication (acute) F14.922
      in
        abuse F14.122
        dependence F14.222
    hypnotic withdrawal F13.232
    opioid intoxication (acute) F11.922
      in
        abuse F11.122
        dependence F11.222
    phencyclidine intoxication (acute) F19.922
      in
        abuse F19.122
        dependence F19.222
    sedative withdrawal F13.232
  personality (pattern) (trait) (see also Disorder,
    personality) F60.9
    following organic brain damage F07.9
  polyglandular E31.9
    specified NEC E31.8
  potassium balance, newborn P74.3
  psychogenic F45.9
  psychomotor F44.4
  psychophysical visual H53.16
  pupillary — see Anomaly, pupil, function
  reflex R29.2
  rhythm, heart I49.9
  salivary secretion K11.7
  sensation (cold) (heat) (localization) (tactile
    discrimination) (texture) (vibratory) NEC
    R20.9
    hysterical F44.6
    skin R20.9
      anesthesia R20.0
      hyperesthesia R20.3
      hypoesthesia R20.1
      paresthesia R20.2
      specified type NEC R20.8
    smell R43.9
      and taste (mixed) R43.8
      anosmia R43.0
      parosmia R43.1
      specified NEC R43.8
    taste R43.9
      and smell (mixed) R43.8
      parageusia R43.2
      specified NEC R43.8
  sensory — see Disturbance, sensation
  situational (transient) (see also Disorder,
    adjustment)
    acute F43.0
  sleep G47.9
    nonorganic origin F51.9
  smell — see Disturbance, sensation, smell
  sociopathic F60.2
  sodium balance, newborn P74.2
  speech R47.9
    developmental F80.9
    specified NEC R47.89
  stomach (functional) K31.9
  sympathetic (nerve) G90.9
  taste — see Disturbance, sensation, taste
  temperature
    regulation, newborn P81.9
      specified NEC P81.8
    sense R20.8
      hysterical F44.6
  tooth
    eruption K00.6
    formation K00.4
    structure, hereditary NEC K00.5
  touch — see Disturbance, sensation
  vascular I99.9
    arteriosclerotic — see Arteriosclerosis
  vasomotor I73.9
  vasospastic I73.9

Disturbance — *continued*
  vision, visual H53.9
    following
      cerebral infarction I69.398
      cerebrovascular disease I69.998
        specified NEC I69.898
      intracerebral hemorrhage I69.198
      nontraumatic intracranial hemorrhage NEC I69.298
      specified disease NEC I69.898
      subarachnoid hemorrhage I69.098
    psychophysical H53.16
    specified NEC H53.8
    subjective H53.10
      day blindness H53.11
      discomfort H53.14- ☑
      distortions of shape and size H53.15
      loss
        sudden H53.13- ☑
        transient H53.12- ☑
      specified type NEC H53.19
  voice R49.9
    psychogenic F44.4
    specified NEC R49.8
Diuresis R35.8
Diver's palsy, paralysis or squeeze T70.3 ☑
Diverticulitis (acute) K57.92
  bladder — *see* Cystitis
  ileum — *see* Diverticulitis, intestine, small
  intestine K57.92
    with
      abscess, perforation or peritonitis K57.80
        with bleeding K57.81
      bleeding K57.93
    congenital Q43.8
    large K57.32
      with
        abscess, perforation or peritonitis K57.20
          with bleeding K57.21
        bleeding K57.33
        small intestine K57.52
          with
            abscess, perforation or peritonitis K57.40
              with bleeding K57.41
            bleeding K57.53
    small K57.12
      with
        abscess, perforation or peritonitis K57.00
          with bleeding K57.01
        bleeding K57.13
        large intestine K57.52
          with
            abscess, perforation or peritonitis K57.40
              with bleeding K57.41
            bleeding K57.53
Diverticulosis K57.90
  with bleeding K57.91
  large intestine K57.30
    with
      bleeding K57.31
      small intestine K57.50
        with bleeding K57.51
  small intestine K57.10
    with
      bleeding K57.11
      large intestine K57.50
        with bleeding K57.51
Diverticulum, diverticula (multiple) K57.90
  appendix (noninflammatory) K38.2
  bladder (sphincter) N32.3
    congenital Q64.6
  bronchus (congenital) Q32.4
    acquired J98.09
  calyx, calyceal (kidney) N28.89
  cardia (stomach) K31.4
  cecum — *see* Diverticulosis, intestine, large
    congenital Q43.8
  colon — *see* Diverticulosis, intestine, large
    congenital Q43.8
  duodenum — *see* Diverticulosis, intestine, small
    congenital Q43.8
  epiphrenic (esophagus) K22.5
  esophagus (congenital) Q39.6
    acquired (epiphrenic) (pulsion) (traction) K22.5
  eustachian tube — *see* Disorder, eustachian tube, specified NEC
  fallopian tube N83.8
  gastric K31.4
  heart (congenital) Q24.8
  ileum — *see* Diverticulosis, intestine, small

Diverticulum — *continued*
  jejunum — *see* Diverticulosis, intestine, small
  kidney (pelvis) (calyces) N28.89
    with calculus — *see* Calculus, kidney
  Meckel's (displaced) (hypertrophic) Q43.0
    malignant — *see* Table of Neoplasms, small intestine, malignant
  midthoracic K22.5
  organ or site, congenital NEC — *see* Distortion
  pericardium (congenital) (cyst) Q24.8
    acquired I31.8
  pharyngoesophageal (congenital) Q39.6
    acquired K22.5
  pharynx (congenital) Q38.7
  rectosigmoid — *see* Diverticulosis, intestine, large
    congenital Q43.8
  rectum — *see* Diverticulosis, intestine, large
  Rokitansky's K22.5
  seminal vesicle N50.8
  sigmoid — *see* Diverticulosis, intestine, large
    congenital Q43.8
  stomach (acquired) K31.4
    congenital Q40.2
  trachea (acquired) J39.8
  ureter (acquired) N28.89
    congenital Q62.8
  ureterovesical orifice N28.89
  urethra (acquired) N36.1
    congenital Q64.79
  ventricle, left (congenital) Q24.8
  vesical N32.3
    congenital Q64.6
  Zenker's (esophagus) K22.5
Division
  cervix uteri (acquired) N88.8
  glans penis Q55.69
  labia minora (congenital) Q52.79
  ligament (partial or complete) (current) (*see also* Sprain)
    with open wound — *see* Wound, open
  muscle (partial or complete) (current) (*see also* Injury, muscle)
    with open wound — *see* Wound, open
  nerve (traumatic) — *see* Injury, nerve
  spinal cord — *see* Injury, spinal cord, by region
  vein I87.8
Divorce, causing family disruption Z63.5
Dix-Hallpike neurolabyrinthitis — *see* Neuronitis, vestibular
Dizziness R42
  hysterical F44.89
  psychogenic F45.8
DMAC (disseminated mycobacterium avium-intracellulare complex) A31.2
DNR (do not resuscitate) Z66
Doan-Wiseman syndrome (primary splenic neutropenia) — *see* Agranulocytosis
Doehle-Heller aortitis A52.02
Dog bite — *see* Bite
Dohle body panmyelopathic syndrome D72.0
Dolichocephaly Q67.2
Dolichocolon Q43.8
Dolichostenomelia — *see* Syndrome, Marfan's
Donohue's syndrome E34.8
Donor (organ or tissue) Z52.9
  blood (whole) Z52.000
    autologous Z52.010
    specified component (lymphocytes) (platelets) NEC Z52.008
      autologous Z52.018
      specified donor NEC Z52.098
    specified donor NEC Z52.090
  stem cells Z52.001
    autologous Z52.011
    specified donor NEC Z52.091
  bone Z52.20
    autologous Z52.21
    marrow Z52.3
    specified type NEC Z52.29
  cornea Z52.5
  egg (Oocyte) Z52.819
    age 35 and over Z52.812
      anonymous recipient Z52.812
      designated recipient Z52.813
    under age 35 Z52.810
      anonymous recipient Z52.810
      designated recipient Z52.811
  kidney Z52.4
  liver Z52.6
  lung Z52.89
  lymphocyte — *see* Donor, blood, specified components NEC

Donor — *continued*
  Oocyte — *see* Donor, egg
  platelets Z52.008
  potential, examination of Z00.5
  semen Z52.89
  skin Z52.10
    autologous Z52.11
    specified type NEC Z52.19
  specified organ or tissue NEC Z52.89
  sperm Z52.89
Donovanosis A58
Dorsalgia M54.9
  psychogenic F45.41
  specified NEC M54.89
Dorsopathy M53.9
  deforming M43.9
    specified NEC M43.8
  specified NEC M53.80
    cervical region M53.82
    cervicothoracic region M53.83
    lumbar region M53.86
    lumbosacral region M53.87
    occipito-atlanto-axial region M53.81
    sacrococcygeal region M53.88
    thoracic region M53.84
    thoracolumbar region M53.85
Double
  albumin E88.09
  aortic arch Q25.4
  auditory canal Q17.8
  auricle (heart) Q20.8
  bladder Q64.79
  cervix Q51.820
    with doubling of uterus (and vagina) Q51.10
      with obstruction Q51.11
  inlet ventricle Q20.4
  kidney with double pelvis (renal) Q63.0
  meatus urinarius Q64.75
  monster Q89.4
  outlet
    left ventricle Q20.2
    right ventricle Q20.1
  pelvis (renal) with double ureter Q62.5
  tongue Q38.3
  ureter (one or both sides) Q62.5
    with double pelvis (renal) Q62.5
  urethra Q64.74
  urinary meatus Q64.75
  uterus Q51.2
    with
      doubling of cervix (and vagina) Q51.10
        with obstruction Q51.11
    in pregnancy or childbirth O34.59- ☑
      causing obstructed labor O65.5
  vagina Q52.10
    with doubling of uterus (and cervix) Q51.10
      with obstruction Q51.11
  vision H53.2
  vulva Q52.79
Douglas' pouch, cul-de-sac — *see* condition
Down syndrome Q90.9
  meiotic nondisjunction Q90.0
  mitotic nondisjunction Q90.1
  mosaicism Q90.1
  translocation Q90.2
DPD (dihydropyrimidine dehydrogenase deficiency) E88.89
Dracontiasis B72
Dracunculiasis, dracunculosis B72
Dream state, hysterical F44.89
Dreschlera (hawaiiensis) (infection) B43.8
Drepanocytic anemia — *see* Disease, sickle-cell
Dresbach's syndrome (elliptocytosis) D58.1
Dressler's syndrome I24.1
Drift, ulnar — *see* Deformity, limb, specified type NEC, forearm
Drinking (alcohol)
  excessive, to excess NEC (without dependence) F10.10
    habitual (continual) (without remission) F10.20
      with remission F10.21
Drip, postnasal (chronic) R09.82
  due to
    allergic rhinitis — *see* Rhinitis, allergic
    common cold J00
    gastroesophageal reflux — *see* Reflux, gastroesophageal
    nasopharyngitis — *see* Nasopharyngitis
    other know condition - code to condition
    sinusitis — *see* Sinusitis
Droop
  facial R29.810

☑ **Additional character required**

Droop — *continued*
  cerebrovascular disease I69.992
    cerebral infarction I69.392
    intracerebral hemorrhage I69.192
    nontraumatic intracranial hemorrhage NEC I69.292
    specified disease NEC I69.892
    subarachnoid hemorrhage I69.092
Drop (in)
  attack NEC R55
  finger — *see* Deformity, finger
  foot — *see* Deformity, limb, foot, drop
  hematocrit (precipitous) R71.0
  hemoglobin R71.0
  toe — *see* Deformity, toe, specified NEC
  wrist — *see* Deformity, limb, wrist drop
Dropped heart beats I45.9
Dropsy, dropsical (*see also* Hydrops)
  abdomen R18.8
  brain — *see* Hydrocephalus
  cardiac, heart — *see* Failure, heart, congestive
  gangrenous — *see* Gangrene
  heart — *see* Failure, heart, congestive
  kidney — *see* Nephrosis
  lung — *see* Edema, lung
  newborn due to isoimmunization P56.0
  pericardium — *see* Pericarditis
Drowned, drowning (near) T75.1 ☑
Drowsiness R40.0
Drug
  abuse counseling and surveillance Z71.51
  addiction — *see* Dependence
  dependence — *see* Dependence
  habit — *see* Dependence
  harmful use — *see* Abuse, drug
  induced fever R50.2
  overdose — *see* Table of Drugs and Chemicals, by drug, poisoning
  poisoning — *see* Table of Drugs and Chemicals, by drug, poisoning
  resistant organism infection (*see also* Resistant, organism, to, drug) Z16.30
  therapy
    long term (current) (prophylactic) — *see* Therapy, drug long-term (current) (prophylactic)
    short term - omit code
  wrong substance given or taken in error — *see* Table of Drugs and Chemicals, by drug, poisoning
Drunkenness (without dependence) F10.129
  acute in alcoholism F10.229
  chronic (without remission) F10.20
    with remission F10.21
  pathological (without dependence) F10.129
    with dependence F10.229
  sleep F51.9
Drusen
  macula (degenerative) (retina) — *see* Degeneration, macula, drusen
  optic disc H47.32- ☑
Dry, dryness (*see also* condition)
  larynx J38.7
  mouth R68.2
    due to dehydration E86.0
  nose J34.89
  socket (teeth) M27.3
  throat J39.2
DSAP L56.5
Duane's syndrome H50.81- ☑
Dubin-Johnson disease or syndrome E80.6
Dubois' disease (thymus gland) A50.59 [E35]
Dubowitz' syndrome Q87.1
Duchenne-Aran muscular atrophy G12.21
Duchenne-Griesinger disease G71.0
Duchenne's
  disease or syndrome
    motor neuron disease G12.22
    muscular dystrophy G71.0
    locomotor ataxia (syphilitic) A52.11
  paralysis
    birth injury P14.0
    due to or associated with
      motor neuron disease G12.22
      muscular dystrophy G71.0
Ducrey's chancre A57
Duct, ductus — *see* condition
Duhring's disease (dermatitis herpetiformis) L13.0
Dullness, cardiac (decreased) (increased) R01.2
Dumb ague — *see* Malaria
Dumbness — *see* Aphasia
Dumdum fever B55.0

Dumping syndrome (postgastrectomy) K91.1
Duodenitis (nonspecific) (peptic) K29.80
  with bleeding K29.81
Duodenocholangitis — *see* Cholangitis
Duodenum, duodenal — *see* condition
Duplay's bursitis or periarthritis — *see* Tendinitis, calcific, shoulder
Duplication, duplex (*see also* Accessory)
  alimentary tract Q45.8
  anus Q43.4
  appendix (and cecum) Q43.4
  biliary duct (any) Q44.5
  bladder Q64.79
  cecum (and appendix) Q43.4
  cervix Q51.820
  chromosome NEC
    with complex rearrangements NEC Q92.5
    seen only at prometaphase Q92.8
  cystic duct Q44.5
  digestive organs Q45.8
  esophagus Q39.8
  frontonasal process Q75.8
  intestine (large) (small) Q43.4
  kidney Q63.0
  liver Q44.7
  pancreas Q45.3
  penis Q55.69
  respiratory organs NEC Q34.8
  salivary duct Q38.4
  spinal cord (incomplete) Q06.2
  stomach Q40.2
Dupré's disease (meningism) R29.1
Dupuytren's contraction or disease M72.0
Durand-Nicolas-Favre disease A55
Durotomy (inadvertent) (incidental) G97.41
Duroziez's disease (congenital mitral stenosis) Q23.2
Dutton's relapsing fever (West African) A68.1
Dwarfism E34.3
  achondroplastic Q77.4
  congenital E34.3
  constitutional E34.3
  hypochondroplastic Q77.4
  hypophyseal E23.0
  infantile E34.3
  Laron-type E34.3
  Lorain (-Levi) type E23.0
  metatropic Q77.8
  nephrotic-glycosuric (with hypophosphatemic rickets) E72.09
  nutritional E45
  pancreatic K86.8
  pituitary E23.0
  renal N25.0
  thanatophoric Q77.1
Dyke-Young anemia (secondary) (symptomatic) D59.1
Dysacusis — *see* Abnormal, auditory perception
Dysadrenocortism E27.9
  hyperfunction E27.0
Dysarthria R47.1
  following
    cerebral infarction I69.322
    cerebrovascular disease I69.922
      specified disease NEC I69.822
    intracerebral hemorrhage I69.122
    nontraumatic intracranial hemorrhage NEC I69.222
    subarachnoid hemorrhage I69.022
Dysautonomia (familial) G90.1
Dysbarism T70.3 ☑
Dysbasia R26.2
  angiosclerotica intermittens I73.9
  hysterical F44.4
  lordotica (progressiva) G24.1
  nonorganic origin F44.4
  psychogenic F44.4
Dysbetalipoproteinemia (familial) E78.2
Dyscalculia R48.8
  developmental F81.2
Dyschezia K59.00
Dyschondroplasia (with hemangiomata) Q78.4
Dyschromia (skin) L81.9
Dyscollagenosis M35.9
Dyscranio-pygo-phalangy Q87.0
Dyscrasia
  blood (with) D75.9
    antepartum hemorrhage — *see* Hemorrhage, antepartum, with coagulation defect
    newborn P61.9
      specified type NEC P61.8
    intrapartum hemorrhage O67.0

Dyscrasia — *continued*
  puerperal, postpartum O72.3
  polyglandular, pluriglandular E31.9
Dysendocrinism E34.9
Dysentery, dysenteric (catarrhal) (diarrhea) (epidemic) (hemorrhagic) (infectious) (sporadic) (tropical) A09
  abscess, liver A06.4
  amebic (*see also* Amebiasis) A06.0
    with abscess — *see* Abscess, amebic
    acute A06.0
    chronic A06.1
  arthritis (*see also* category M01) A09
    bacillary (*see also* category M01) A03.9
  bacillary A03.9
    arthritis (*see also* category M01) A03.9
    Boyd A03.2
    Flexner A03.1
    Schmitz (-Stutzer) A03.0
    Shiga (-Kruse) A03.0
    Shigella A03.9
      boydii A03.2
      dysenteriae A03.0
      flexneri A03.1
      group A A03.0
      group B A03.1
      group C A03.2
      group D A03.3
      sonnei A03.3
      specified type NEC A03.8
    Sonne A03.3
    specified type NEC A03.8
  balantidial A07.0
  Balantidium coli A07.0
  Boyd's A03.2
  candidal B37.82
  Chilomastix A07.8
  Chinese A03.9
  coccidial A07.3
  Dientamoeba (fragilis) A07.8
  Embadomonas A07.8
  Entamoeba, entamebic — *see* Dysentery, amebic
  Flexner-Boyd A03.2
  Flexner's A03.1
  Giardia lamblia A07.1
  Hiss-Russell A03.1
  Lamblia A07.1
  leishmanial B55.0
  malarial — *see* Malaria
  metazoal B82.0
  monilial B37.82
  protozoal A07.9
  Salmonella A02.0
  schistosomal B65.1
  Schmitz (-Stutzer) A03.0
  Shiga (-Kruse) A03.0
  Shigella NOS — *see* Dysentery, bacillary
  Sonne A03.3
  strongyloidiasis B78.0
  trichomonal A07.8
  viral (*see also* Enteritis, viral) A08.4
Dysequilibrium R42
Dysesthesia R20.8
  hysterical F44.6
Dysfibrinogenemia (congenital) D68.2
Dysfunction
  adrenal E27.9
    hyperfunction E27.0
  autonomic
    due to alcohol G31.2
    somatoform F45.8
  bladder N31.9
    neurogenic NOS — *see* Dysfunction, bladder, neuromuscular
    neuromuscular NOS N31.9
      atonic (motor) (sensory) N31.2
      autonomous N31.2
      flaccid N31.2
      nonreflex N31.2
      reflex N31.1
      specified NEC N31.8
      uninhibited N31.0
  bleeding, uterus N93.8
  cerebral G93.89
  colon K59.9
    psychogenic F45.8
  colostomy K94.03
  cystic duct K82.8
  cystostomy (stoma) — *see* Complications, cystostomy
  ejaculatory N53.19
    anejaculatory orgasm N53.13

Dysfunction — continued
  painful N53.12
  premature F52.4
  retarded N53.11
endocrine NOS E34.9
endometrium N85.8
enterostomy K94.13
gallbladder K82.8
gastrostomy (stoma) K94.23
gland, glandular NOS E34.9
heart I51.89
hemoglobin D75.89
hepatic K76.89
hypophysis E23.7
hypothalamic NEC E23.3
ileostomy (stoma) K94.13
jejunostomy (stoma) K94.13
kidney — see Disease, renal
labyrinthineH83.2
left ventricular, following sudden emotional
    stress I51.81
liver K76.89
male — see Dysfunction, sexual, male
orgasmic (female) F52.31
  male F52.32
ovary E28.9
  specified NEC E28.8
papillary muscle I51.89
parathyroid E21.4
physiological NEC R68.89
  psychogenic F59
pineal gland E34.8
pituitary (gland) E23.3
platelets D69.1
polyglandular E31.9
  specified NEC E31.8
psychophysiologic F59
psychosexual F52.9
  with
    dyspareunia F52.6
    premature ejaculation F52.4
    vaginismus F52.5
pylorus K31.9
rectum K59.9
  psychogenic F45.8
reflex (sympathetic) — see Syndrome, pain,
    complex regional I
segmental — see Dysfunction, somatic
senile R54
sexual (due to) R37
  alcohol F10.981
  amphetamine F15.981
    in
      abuse F15.181
      dependence F15.281
  anxiolytic F13.981
    in
      abuse F13.181
      dependence F13.281
  cocaine F14.981
    in
      abuse F14.181
      dependence F14.281
  excessive sexual drive F52.8
  failure of genital response (male) F52.21
    female F52.22
  female N94.9
    aversion F52.1
    dyspareunia N94.1
      psychogenic F52.6
    frigidity F52.22
    nymphomania F52.8
    orgasmic F52.31
    psychogenic F52.9
      aversion F52.1
      dyspareunia F52.6
      frigidity F52.22
      nymphomania F52.8
      orgasmic F52.31
      vaginismus F52.5
    vaginismus N94.2
      psychogenic F52.5
  hypnotic F13.981
    in
      abuse F13.181
      dependence F13.281
  inhibited orgasm (female) F52.31
    male F52.32
  lack
    of sexual enjoyment F52.1
    or loss of sexual desire F52.0
  male N53.9

Dysfunction — continued
  anejaculatory orgasm N53.13
  ejaculatory N53.19
    painful N53.12
    premature F52.4
    retarded N53.11
  erectile N52.9
    drug induced N52.2
    due to
      disease classified elsewhere N52.1
      drug N52.2
    postoperative (postprocedural) N52.39
      following
        prostatectomy N52.34
          radical N52.31
        radical cystectomy N52.32
        urethral surgery N52.33
    psychogenic F52.21
    specified cause NEC N52.8
    vasculogenic
      arterial insufficiency N52.01
        with corporo-venous occlusive N52.03
      corporo-venous occlusive N52.02
        with arterial insufficiency N52.03
  impotence — see Dysfunction, sexual, male,
    erectile
  psychogenic F52.9
    aversion F52.1
    erectile F52.21
    orgasmic F52.32
    premature ejaculation F52.4
    satyriasis F52.8
    specified type NEC F52.8
    specified type NEC N53.8
  nonorganic F52.9
    specified NEC F52.8
  opioid F11.981
    in
      abuse F11.181
      dependence F11.281
  orgasmic dysfunction (female) F52.31
    male F52.32
  premature ejaculation F52.4
  psychoactive substances NEC F19.981
    in
      abuse F19.181
      dependence F19.281
  psychogenic F52.9
  sedative F13.981
    in
      abuse F13.181
      dependence F13.281
  sexual aversion F52.1
  vaginismus (nonorganic) (psychogenic) F52.5
sinoatrial node I49.5
somatic M99.09
  abdomen M99.09
  acromioclavicular M99.07
  cervical region M99.01
  cervicothoracic M99.01
  costochondral M99.08
  costovertebral M99.08
  head region M99.00
  hip M99.05
  lower extremity M99.06
  lumbar region M99.03
  lumbosacral M99.03
  occipitocervical M99.00
  pelvic region M99.05
  pubic M99.05
  rib cage M99.08
  sacral region M99.04
  sacrococcygeal M99.04
  sacroiliac M99.04
  specified NEC M99.09
  sternochondral M99.08
  sternoclavicular M99.07
  thoracic region M99.02
  thoracolumbar M99.02
  upper extremity M99.07
somatoform autonomic F45.8
stomach K31.89
  psychogenic F45.8
suprarenal E27.9
  hyperfunction E27.0
symbolic R48.9
  specified type NEC R48.8
temporomandibular (joint) M26.69
  joint-pain syndrome M26.62
testicular (endocrine) E29.9
  specified NEC E29.8
thymus E32.9

Dysfunction — continued
  thyroid E07.9
  ureterostomy (stoma) — see Complications,
    stoma, urinary tract
  urethrostomy (stoma) — see Complications,
    stoma, urinary tract
  uterus, complicating delivery O62.9
    hypertonic O62.4
    hypotonic O62.2
      primary O62.0
      secondary O62.1
  ventricular I51.9
    with congestive heart failure I50.9- - left,
      reversible, following sudden emotional
      stress I51.81
Dysgenesis
  gonadal (due to chromosomal anomaly) Q96.9
    pure Q99.1
  renal Q60.5
    bilateral Q60.4
    unilateral Q60.3
  reticular D72.0
  tidal platelet D69.3
Dysgerminoma
  specified site — see Neoplasm, malignant, by site
  unspecified site
    female C56.9
    male C62.90
Dysgeusia R43.2
Dysgraphia R27.8
Dyshidrosis, dysidrosis L30.1
Dyskaryotic cervical smear R87.619
Dyskeratosis L85.8
  cervix — see Dysplasia, cervix
  congenital Q82.8
  uterus NEC N85.8
Dyskinesia G24.9
  biliary (cystic duct or gallbladder) K82.8
  drug induced
    orofacial G24.01
  esophagus K22.4
  hysterical F44.4
  intestinal K59.8
  nonorganic origin F44.4
  orofacial (idiopathic) G24.4
    drug induced G24.01
  psychogenic F44.4
  subacute, drug induced G24.01
  tardive G24.01
    neuroleptic induced G24.01
  trachea J39.8
  tracheobronchial J98.09
Dyslalia (developmental) F80.0
Dyslexia R48.0
  developmental F81.0
Dyslipidemia E78.5
  depressed HDL cholesterol E78.6
  elevated fasting triglycerides E78.1
Dysmaturity (see also Light for dates)
  pulmonary (newborn) (Wilson-Mikity) P27.0
Dysmenorrhea (essential) (exfoliative) N94.6
  congestive (syndrome) N94.6
  primary N94.4
  psychogenic F45.8
  secondary N94.5
Dysmetabolic syndrome X E88.81
Dysmetria R27.8
Dysmorphism (due to)
  alcohol Q86.0
  exogenous cause NEC Q86.8
  hydantoin Q86.1
  warfarin Q86.2
Dysmorphophobia (nondelusional) F45.22
  delusional F22
Dysnomia R47.01
Dysorexia R63.0
  psychogenic F50.8
Dysostosis
  cleidocranial, cleidocranialis Q74.0
  craniofacial Q75.1
  Fairbank's (idiopathic familial generalized
    osteophytosis) Q78.9
  mandibulofacial (incomplete) Q75.4
  multiplex E76.01
  oculomandibular Q75.5
Dyspareunia (female) N94.1
  male N53.12
  nonorganic F52.6
  psychogenic F52.6
  secondary N94.1
Dyspepsia R10.13
  atonic K30

☑ **Additional character required**

Dyspepsia — *continued*
  functional (allergic) (congenital) (gastrointestinal) (occupational) (reflex) K30
  intestinal K59.8
  nervous F45.8
  neurotic F45.8
  psychogenic F45.8
Dysphagia R13.10
  cervical R13.19
  following
    cerebral infarction I69.391
    cerebrovascular disease I69.991
      specified NEC I69.891
    intracerebral hemorrhage I69.191
    nontraumatic intracranial hemorrhage NEC I69.291
    specified disease NEC I69.891
    subarachnoid hemorrhage I69.091
  functional (hysterical) F45.8
  hysterical F45.8
  nervous (hysterical) F45.8
  neurogenic R13.19
  oral phase R13.11
  oropharyngeal phase R13.12
  pharyneal phase R13.13
  pharyngoesophageal phase R13.14
  psychogenic F45.8
  sideropenic D50.1
  spastica K22.4
  specified NEC R13.19
Dysphagocytosis, congenital D71
Dysphasia R47.02
  developmental
    expressive type F80.1
    receptive type F80.2
  following
    cerebrovascular disease I69.921
      cerebral infarction I69.321
      intracerebral hemorrhage I69.121
      nontraumatic intracranial hemorrhage NEC I69.221
      specified disease NEC I69.821
      subarachnoid hemorrhage I69.021
Dysphonia R49.0
  functional F44.4
  hysterical F44.4
  psychogenic F44.4
  spastica J38.3
Dysphoria, postpartal O90.6
Dyspituitarism E23.3
Dysplasia (*see also* Anomaly)
  acetabular, congenital Q65.89
  alveolar capillary, with vein misalignment J84.843
  anus (histologically confirmed) (mild) (moderate) K62.82
    severe D01.3
  arrhythmogenic right ventricular I42.8
  arterial, fibromuscular I77.3
  asphyxiating thoracic (congenital) Q77.2
  brain Q07.9
  bronchopulmonary, perinatal P27.1
  cervix (uteri) N87.9
    mild N87.0
    moderate N87.1
    severe D06.9
  chondroectodermal Q77.6
  colon D12.6
  craniometaphyseal Q78.5
  dentinal K00.5
  diaphyseal, progressive Q78.3
  dystrophic Q77.5
  ectodermal (anhidrotic) (congenital) (hereditary) Q82.4
    hydrotic Q82.8
  epithelial, uterine cervix — *see* Dysplasia, cervix
  eye (congenital) Q11.2
  fibrous
    bone NEC (monostotic) M85.00
      ankle M85.07- ☑
      foot M85.07- ☑
      forearm M85.03- ☑
      hand M85.04- ☑
      lower leg M85.06- ☑
      multiple site M85.09
      neck M85.08
      rib M85.08
      shoulder M85.01- ☑
      skull M85.08
      specified site NEC M85.08
      thigh M85.05- ☑
      toe M85.07- ☑
      upper arm M85.02- ☑

Dysplasia — *continued*
    vertebra M85.08
  diaphyseal, progressive Q78.3
  jaw M27.8
  polyostotic Q78.1
  florid osseous (*see also* Cyst, calcifying odontogenic)
  high grade, focal D12.6
  hip, congenital Q65.89
  joint, congenital Q74.8
  kidney Q61.4
    multicystic Q61.4
  leg Q74.2
  lung, congenital (not associated with short gestation) Q33.6
  mammary (gland) (benign) N60.9- ☑
    cyst (solitary) — *see* Cyst, breast
    cystic — *see* Mastopathy, cystic
    duct ectasia — *see* Ectasia, mammary duct
    fibroadenosis — *see* Fibroadenosis, breast
    fibrosclerosis — *see* Fibrosclerosis, breast
    specified type NEC N60.8- ☑
  metaphyseal (Jansen's) (McKusick's) (Schmid's) Q78.5
  muscle Q79.8
  oculodentodigital Q87.0
  periapical (cemental) (cemento-osseous) — *see* Cyst, calcifying odontogenic
  periosteum — *see* Disorder, bone, specified type NEC
  polyostotic fibrous Q78.1
  prostate (*see also* Neoplasia, intraepithelial, prostate) N42.3
    severe D07.5
  renal Q61.4
    multicystic Q61.4
  retinal, congenital Q14.1
  right ventricular, arrhythmogenic I42.8
  septo-optic Q04.4
  skin L98.8
  spinal cord Q06.1
  spondyloepiphyseal Q77.7
  thymic, with immunodeficiency D82.1
  vagina N89.3
    mild N89.0
    moderate N89.1
    severe NEC D07.2
  vulva N90.3
    mild N90.0
    moderate N90.1
    severe NEC D07.1
Dyspnea (nocturnal) (paroxysmal) R06.00
  asthmatic (bronchial) J45.909
    with
      exacerbation (acute) J45.901
      bronchitis J45.909
        with
          exacerbation (acute) J45.901
          status asthmaticus J45.902
        chronic J44.9
      status asthmaticus J45.902
  cardiac — *see* Failure, ventricular, left
  cardiac — *see* Failure, ventricular, left
  functional F45.8
  hyperventilation R06.4
  hysterical F45.8
  newborn P28.89
  orthopnea R06.01
  psychogenic F45.8
  shortness of breath R06.02
  specified type NEC R06.09
Dyspraxia R27.8
  developmental (syndrome) F82
Dysproteinemia E88.09
Dysreflexia, autonomic G90.4
Dysrhythmia
  cardiac I49.9
    newborn
      bradycardia P29.12
      occurring before birth P03.819
        before onset of labor P03.810
        during labor P03.811
      tachycardia P29.11
    postoperative I97.89
  cerebral or cortical — *see* Epilepsy
Dyssomnia — *see* Disorder, sleep
Dyssynergia
  biliary K83.8
  bladder sphincter N36.44
  cerebellaris myoclonica (Hunt's ataxia) G11.1
Dysthymia F34.1
Dysthyroidism E07.9

Dystocia O66.9
  affecting newborn P03.1
  cervical (hypotonic) O62.2
    affecting newborn P03.6
    primary O62.0
    secondary O62.1
  contraction ring O62.4
  fetal O66.9
    abnormality NEC O66.3
    conjoined twins O66.3
    oversize O66.2
  maternal O66.9
  positional O64.9 ☑
  shoulder (girdle) O66.0
    causing obstructed labor O66.0
  uterine NEC O62.4
Dystonia G24.9
  deformans progressiva G24.1
  drug induced NEC G24.09
    acute G24.02
    specified NEC G24.09
  familial G24.1
  idiopathic G24.1
    familial G24.1
    nonfamilial G24.2
    orofacial G24.4
  lenticularis G24.8
  musculorum deformans G24.1
  neuroleptic induced (acute) G24.02
  orofacial (idiopathic) G24.4
  oromandibular G24.4
    due to drug G24.01
  specified NEC G24.8
  torsion (familial) (idiopathic) G24.1
    acquired G24.8
    genetic G24.1
    symptomatic (nonfamilial) G24.2
Dystonic movements R25.8
Dystrophy, dystrophia
  adiposogenital E23.6
  Becker's type G71.0
  cervical sympathetic G90.2
  choroid (hereditary) H31.20
    central areolar H31.22
    choroideremia H31.21
    gyrate atrophy H31.23
    specified type NEC H31.29
  cornea (hereditary) H18.50
    endothelial H18.51
    epithelial H18.52
    granular H18.53
    lattice H18.54
    macular H18.55
    specified type NEC H18.59
  Duchenne's type G71.0
  due to malnutrition E45
  Erb's G71.0
  Fuchs' H18.51
  Gower's muscular G71.0
  hair L67.8
  infantile neuraxonal G31.89
  Landouzy-Déjérine G71.0
  Leyden-Möbius G71.0
  muscular G71.0
    benign (Becker type) G71.0
    congenital (hereditary) (progressive) (with specific morphological abnormalities of the muscle fiber) G71.0
      myotonic G71.11
    distal G71.0
    Duchenne type G71.0
    Emery-Dreifuss G71.0
    Erb type G71.0
    facioscapulohumeral G71.0
    Gower's G71.0
    hereditary (progressive) G71.0
    Landouzy-Déjérine type G71.0
    limb-girdle G71.0
    myotonic G71.11
    progressive (hereditary) G71.0
      Charcot-Marie (-Tooth) type G60.0
    pseudohypertrophic (infantile) G71.0
    severe (Duchenne type) G71.0
  myocardium, myocardial — *see* Degeneration, myocardial
  myotonic, myotonica G71.11
  nail L60.3
    congenital Q84.6
  nutritional E45
  ocular G71.0
  oculocerebrorenal E72.03
  oculopharyngeal G71.0

Dystrophy — *continued*
  ovarian N83.8
  polyglandular E31.8
  reflex (neuromuscular) (sympathetic) — *see*
    Syndrome, pain, complex regional I
  retinal (hereditary) H35.50
    in
      lipid storage disorders E75.6 [H36]
      systemic lipidoses E75.6 [H36]
    involving
      pigment epithelium H35.54
      sensory area H35.53
    pigmentary H35.52
    vitreoretinal H35.51
  Salzmann's nodular — *see* Degeneration, cornea, nodular
  scapuloperoneal G71.0
  skin NEC L98.8
  sympathetic (reflex) — *see* Syndrome, pain, complex regional I
    cervical G90.2
  tapetoretinal H35.54
  thoracic, asphyxiating Q77.2
  unguium L60.3
    congenital Q84.6
  vitreoretinal H35.51
  vulva N90.4
  yellow (liver) — *see* Failure, hepatic
Dysuria R30.0
  psychogenic F45.8

E

Eales' disease H35.06- ☑
Ear (*see also* condition)
  piercing Z41.3
  tropical B36.8
  wax (impacted) H61.20
    left H61.22
      with right H61.23
    right H61.21
      with left H61.23
Earache H92.0
Early satiety R68.81
Eaton-Lambert syndrome — *see* Syndrome, Lambert-Eaton
Eberth's disease (typhoid fever) A01.00
Ebola virus disease A98.4
Ebstein's anomaly or syndrome (heart) Q22.5
Eccentro-osteochondrodysplasia E76.29
Ecchondroma — *see* Neoplasm, bone, benign
Ecchondrosis D48.0
Ecchymosis R58
  conjunctiva — *see* Hemorrhage, conjunctiva
  eye (traumatic) — *see* Contusion, eyeball
  eyelid (traumatic) — *see* Contusion, eyelid
  newborn P54.5
  spontaneous R23.3
  traumatic — *see* Contusion
Echinococciasis — *see* Echinococcus
Echinococcosis — *see* Echinococcus
Echinococcus (infection) B67.90
  granulosus B67.4
    bone B67.2
    liver B67.0
    lung B67.1
    multiple sites B67.32
    specified site NEC B67.39
    thyroid B67.31 [E35]
  liver NOS B67.8
    granulosus B67.0
    multilocularis B67.5
  lung NEC B67.99
    granulosus B67.1
    multilocularis B67.69
  multilocularis B67.7
    liver B67.5
    multiple sites B67.61
    specified site NEC B67.69
  specified site NEC B67.99
    granulosus B67.39
    multilocularis B67.69
  thyroid NEC B67.99
    granulosus B67.31 [E35]
    multilocularis B67.69 [E35]
Echinorhynchiasis B83.8
Echinostomiasis B66.8
Echolalia R48.8

Echovirus, as cause of disease classified elsewhere B97.12
Eclampsia, eclamptic (coma) (convulsions) (delirium) (with hypertension) NEC O15.9
  during labor and delivery O15.1
  postpartum O15.2
  pregnancy O15.0- ☑
  puerperal O15.2
Economic circumstances affecting care Z59.9
Economo's disease A85.8
Ectasia, ectasis
  annuloaortic I35.8
  aorta I77.819
    with aneurysm — *see* Aneurysm, aorta
      abdominal I77.811
      thoracic I77.810
      thoracoabdominal I77.812
  breast — *see* Ectasia, mammary duct
  capillary I78.8
  cornea H18.71- ☑
  gastric antral vascular (GAVE) K31.819
    with hemorrhage K31.811
    without hemorrhage K31.819
  mammary duct N60.4- ☑
  salivary gland (duct) K11.8
  sclera — *see* Sclerectasia
Ecthyma L08.0
  contagiosum B08.02
  gangrenosum L08.0
  infectiosum B08.02
Ectocardia Q24.8
Ectodermal dysplasia (anhidrotic) Q82.4
Ectodermosis erosiva pluriorificialis L51.1
Ectopic, ectopia (congenital)
  abdominal viscera Q45.8
    due to defect in anterior abdominal wall Q79.59
  ACTH syndrome E24.3
  adrenal gland Q89.1
  anus Q43.5
  atrial beats I49.1
  beats I49.49
    atrial I49.1
    ventricular I49.3
  bladder Q64.10
  bone and cartilage in lung Q33.5
  brain Q04.8
  breast tissue Q83.8
  cardiac Q24.8
  cerebral Q04.8
  cordis Q24.8
  endometrium — *see* Endometriosis
  gastric mucosa Q40.2
  gestation — *see* Pregnancy, by site
  heart Q24.8
  hormone secretion NEC E34.2
  kidney (crossed) (pelvis) Q63.2
  lens, lentis Q12.1
  mole — *see* Pregnancy, by site
  organ or site NEC — *see* Malposition, congenital
  pancreas Q45.3
  pregnancy — *see* Pregnancy, ectopic
  pupil — *see* Abnormality, pupillary
  renal Q63.2
  sebaceous glands of mouth Q38.6
  spleen Q89.09
  testis Q53.00
    bilateral Q53.02
    unilateral Q53.01
  thyroid Q89.2
  tissue in lung Q33.5
  ureter Q62.63
  ventricular beats I49.3
  vesicae Q64.10
Ectromelia Q73.8
  lower limb — *see* Defect, reduction, limb, lower, specified type NEC
  upper limb — *see* Defect, reduction, limb, upper, specified type NEC
Ectropion H02.109
  cervix N86
    with cervicitis N72
  congenital Q10.1
  eyelid (paralytic) H02.109
    cicatricial H02.119
      left H02.116
        lower H02.115
        upper H02.114
      right H02.113
        lower H02.112
        upper H02.111
    congenital Q10.1

Ectropion — *continued*
  left H02.106
    lower H02.105
    upper H02.104
  mechanical H02.129
    left H02.126
      lower H02.125
      upper H02.124
    right H02.123
      lower H02.122
      upper H02.121
  right H02.103
    lower H02.102
    upper H02.101
  senile H02.139
    left H02.136
      lower H02.135
      upper H02.134
    right H02.133
      lower H02.132
      upper H02.131
  spastic H02.149
    left H02.146
      lower H02.145
      upper H02.144
    right H02.143
      lower H02.142
      upper H02.141
  iris H21.89
  lip (acquired) K13.0
    congenital Q38.0
  urethra N36.8
  uvea H21.89
Eczema (acute) (chronic) (erythematous) (fissum) (rubrum) (squamous) (*see also* Dermatitis) L30.9
  contact — *see* Dermatitis, contact
  dyshidrotic L30.1
  external ear — *see* Otitis, externa, acute, eczematoid
  flexural L20.82
  herpeticum B00.0
  hypertrophicum L28.0
  hypostatic — *see* Varix, leg, with, inflammation
  impetiginous L01.1
  infantile (due to any substance) L20.83
    intertriginous L21.1
    seborrheic L21.1
  intertriginous NEC L30.4
    infantile L21.1
  intrinsic (allergic) L20.84
  lichenified NEC L28.0
  marginatum (hebrae) B35.6
  pustular L30.3
  stasis — *see* Varix, leg, with, inflammation
  vaccination, vaccinatum T88.1 ☑
  varicose — *see* Varix, leg, with, inflammation
Eczematid L30.2
Eddowes (-Spurway) syndrome Q78.0
Edema, edematous (infectious) (pitting) (toxic) R60.9
  with nephritis — *see* Nephrosis
  allergic T78.3 ☑
  amputation stump (surgical) (sequelae (late effect)) T87.89
  angioneurotic (allergic) (any site) (with urticaria) T78.3 ☑
    hereditary D84.1
  angiospastic I73.9
  Berlin's (traumatic) S05.8X- ☑
  brain (cytotoxic) (vasogenic) G93.6
    due to birth injury P11.0
    newborn (anoxia or hypoxia) P52.4
      birth injury P11.0
    traumatic — *see* Injury, intracranial, cerebral edema
  cardiac — *see* Failure, heart, congestive
  cardiovascular — *see* Failure, heart, congestive
  cerebral — *see* Edema, brain
  cerebrospinal — *see* Edema, brain
  cervix (uteri) (acute) N88.8
    puerperal, postpartum O90.89
  chronic hereditary Q82.0
  circumscribed, acute T78.3 ☑
    hereditary D84.1
  conjunctiva H11.42- ☑
  cornea H18.2- ☑
    idiopathic H18.22- ☑
    secondary H18.23- ☑
      due to contact lens H18.21- ☑
  due to
    lymphatic obstruction I89.0
    salt retention E87.0
  epiglottis — *see* Edema, glottis

☑ **Additional character required**

Edema — continued
  essential, acute T78.3 ☑
    hereditary D84.1
  extremities, lower — see Edema, legs
  eyelid NEC H02.849
    left H02.846
      lower H02.845
      upper H02.844
    right H02.843
      lower H02.842
      upper H02.841
  familial, hereditary Q82.0
  famine — see Malnutrition, severe
  generalized R60.1
  glottis, glottic, glottidis (obstructive) (passive)
      J38.4
    allergic T78.3 ☑
      hereditary D84.1
  heart — see Failure, heart, congestive
  heat T67.7 ☑
  hereditary Q82.0
  inanition — see Malnutrition, severe
  intracranial G93.6
  iris H21.89
  joint — see Effusion, joint
  larynx — see Edema, glottis
  legs R60.0
    due to venous obstruction I87.1
    hereditary Q82.0
  localized R60.0
    due to venous obstruction I87.1
  lower limbs — see Edema, legs
  lung J81.1
    with heart condition or failure — see Failure,
      ventricular, left
    acute J81.0
    chemical (acute) J68.1
      chronic J68.1
    chronic J81.1
      due to
        chemicals, gases, fumes or vapors
          (inhalation) J68.1
        external agent J70.9
          specified NEC J70.8
        radiation J70.1
      due to
        chemicals, fumes or vapors (inhalation) J68.1
        external agent J70.9
          specified NEC J70.8
        high altitude T70.29 ☑
        near drowning T75.1 ☑
        radiation J70.0
      meaning failure, left ventricle I50.1
  lymphatic I89.0
    due to mastectomy I97.2
  macula H35.81
    cystoid, following cataract surgery — see
      Complications, postprocedural, following
      cataract surgery
    diabetic — see Diabetes, by type, with,
      retinopathy, with macular edema
  malignant — see Gangrene, gas
  Milroy's Q82.0
  nasopharynx J39.2
  newborn P83.30
    hydrops fetalis — see Hydrops, fetalis
    specified NEC P83.39
  nutritional (see also Malnutrition, severe)
    with dyspigmentation, skin and hair E40
  optic disc or nerve — see Papilledema
  orbit H05.22- ☑
  pancreas K86.8
  papilla, optic — see Papilledema
  penis N48.89
  periodic T78.3 ☑
    hereditary D84.1
  pharynx J39.2
  pulmonary — see Edema, lung
  Quincke's T78.3 ☑
    hereditary D84.1
  renal — see Nephrosis
  retina H35.81
    diabetic — see Diabetes, by type, with,
      retinopathy, with macular edema
  salt E87.0
  scrotum N50.8
  seminal vesicle N50.8
  spermatic cord N50.8
  spinal (cord) (vascular) (nontraumatic) G95.19
  starvation — see Malnutrition, severe
  stasis — see Hypertension, venous, (chronic)
  subglottic — see Edema, glottis

Edema — continued
  supraglottic — see Edema, glottis
  testis N44.8
  tunica vaginalis N50.8
  vas deferens N50.8
  vulva (acute) N90.89
Edentulism — see Absence, teeth, acquired
Edsall's disease T67.2 ☑
Educational handicap Z55.9
  specified NEC Z55.8
Edward's syndrome — see Trisomy, 18
Effect, adverse
  abnormal gravitational (G) forces or states T75.81
      ☑
  abuse — see Maltreatment
  air pressure T70.9 ☑
    specified NEC T70.8 ☑
  altitude (high) — see Effect, adverse, high altitude
  anesthesia (see also Anesthesia) T88.59 ☑
    in labor and delivery O74.9
    in pregnancy NEC O29.3- ☑
    local, toxic
      in labor and delivery O74.4
      postpartum, puerperal O89.3
    postpartum, puerperal O89.9
    specified NEC T88.59 ☑
      in labor and delivery O74.8
      postpartum, puerperal O89.8
    spinal and epidural T88.59 ☑
      headache T88.59 ☑
        in labor and delivery O74.5
        postpartum, puerperal O89.4
      specified NEC
        in labor and delivery O74.6
        postpartum, puerperal O89.5
  antitoxin — see Complications, vaccination
  atmospheric pressure T70.9 ☑
    due to explosion T70.8 ☑
    high T70.3 ☑
    low — see Effect, adverse, high altitude
    specified effect NEC T70.8 ☑
  biological, correct substance properly
      administered — see Effect, adverse, drug
  blood (derivatives) (serum) (transfusion) — see
      Complications, transfusion
  chemical substance — see Table of Drugs and
      Chemicals
  cold (temperature) (weather) T69.9 ☑
    chilblains T69.1 ☑
    frostbite — see Frostbite
    specified effect NEC T69.8 ☑
  drugs and medicaments T88.7 ☑
    specified drug — see Table of Drugs and
      Chemicals, by drug, adverse effect
    specified effect - code to condition
  electric current, electricity (shock) T75.4 ☑
    burn — see Burn
  exertion (excessive) T73.3 ☑
  exposure — see Exposure
  external cause NEC T75.89 ☑
  foodstuffs T78.1 ☑
    allergic reaction — see Allergy, food
      causing anaphylaxis — see Shock,
        anaphylactic, due to food
    noxious — see Poisoning, food, noxious
  gases, fumes, or vapors T59.9- ☑
    specified agent — see Table of Drugs and
      Chemicals
  glue (airplane) sniffing
    due to drug abuse — see Abuse, drug, inhalant
    due to drug dependence — see Dependence,
      drug, inhalant
  heat — see Heat
  high altitude NEC T70.29 ☑
    anoxia T70.29 ☑
    on
      ears T70.0 ☑
      sinuses T70.1 ☑
    polycythemia D75.1
  high pressure fluids T70.4 ☑
  hot weather — see Heat
  hunger T73.0 ☑
  immersion, foot — see Immersion
  immunization — see Complications, vaccination
  immunological agents — see Complications,
      vaccination
  infrared (radiation) (rays) NOS T66 ☑
    dermatitis or eczema L59.8
  infusion — see Complications, infusion
  lack of care of infants — see Maltreatment, child
  lightning — see Lightning
  medical care T88.9 ☑

Effect — continued
  specified NEC T88.8 ☑
  medicinal substance, correct, properly
      administered — see Effect, adverse, drug
  motion T75.3 ☑
  noise, on inner ear H83.3
  overheated places — see Heat
  psychosocial, of work environment Z56.5
  radiation (diagnostic) (infrared) (natural source)
      (therapeutic) (ultraviolet) (X-ray) NOS T66 ☑
    dermatitis or eczema — see Dermatitis, due to,
      radiation
    fibrosis of lung J70.1
    pneumonitis J70.0
    pulmonary manifestations
      acute J70.0
      chronic J70.1
    skin L59.9
  radioactive substance NOS
    dermatitis or eczema — see Radiodermatitis
  reduced temperature T69.9 ☑
    immersion foot or hand — see Immersion
    specified effect NEC T69.8 ☑
  serum NEC (see also Reaction, serum) T80.69 ☑
  specified NEC T78.8 ☑
    external cause NEC T75.89 ☑
  strangulation — see Asphyxia, traumatic
  submersion T75.1 ☑
  thirst T73.1 ☑
  toxic — see Toxicity
  transfusion — see Complications, transfusion
  ultraviolet (radiation) (rays) NOS T66 ☑
    burn — see Burn
    dermatitis or eczema — see Dermatitis, due to,
      ultraviolet rays
    acute L56.8
  vaccine (any) — see Complications, vaccination
  vibration — see Vibration, adverse effects
  water pressure NEC T70.9 ☑
    specified NEC T70.8 ☑
  weightlessness T75.82 ☑
  whole blood — see Complications, transfusion
  work environment Z56.5
Effect (s) (of) (from) — see Effect, adverse NEC
Effects, late — see Sequelae
Effluvium
  anagen L65.1
  telogen L65.0
Effort syndrome (psychogenic) F45.8
Effusion
  amniotic fluid — see Pregnancy, complicated by,
      premature rupture of membranes
  brain (serous) G93.6
  bronchial — see Bronchitis
  cerebral G93.6
  cerebrospinal (see also Meningitis)
    vessel G93.6
  chest — see Effusion, pleura
  chylous, chyliform (pleura) J94.0
  intracranial G93.6
  joint M25.40
    ankle M25.47- ☑
    elbow M25.42- ☑
    foot joint M25.47- ☑
    hand joint M25.44- ☑
    hip M25.45- ☑
    knee M25.46- ☑
    shoulder M25.41- ☑
    specified joint NEC M25.48
    wrist M25.43- ☑
  malignant pleural J91.0
  meninges — see Meningitis
  pericardium, pericardial (noninflammatory) I31.3
    acute — see Pericarditis, acute
  peritoneal (chronic) R18.8
  pleura, pleurisy, pleuritic, pleuropericardial J90
    chylous, chyliform J94.0
    due to systemic lupus erythematosis M32.13
    influenzal — see Influenza, with, respiratory
      manifestations NEC
    malignant J91.0
    newborn P28.89
    tuberculous NEC A15.6
      primary (progressive) A15.7
  spinal — see Meningitis
  thorax, thoracic — see Effusion, pleura
Egg shell nails L60.3
  congenital Q84.6
Egyptian splenomegaly B65.1
Ehrlichiosis A77.40
  due to
    E. chafeensis A77.41

Ehrlichiosis — *continued*
 E. sennetsu A79.81
 specified organism NEC A77.49
Ehlers-Danlos syndrome Q79.6
Eichstedt's disease B36.0
Eisenmenger's
 complex or syndrome I27.89
 defect Q21.8
Ejaculation
 painful N53.12
 premature F52.4
 retarded N53.11
 retrograde N53.14
 semen, painful N53.12
 psychogenic F52.6
Ekbom's syndrome (restless legs) G25.81
Ekman's syndrome (brittle bones and blue sclera)
 Q78.0
Elastic skin Q82.8
 acquired L57.4
Elastofibroma — *see* Neoplasm, connective tissue,
 benign
Elastoma (juvenile) Q82.8
 Miescher's L87.2
Elastomyofibrosis I42.4
Elastosis
 actinic, solar L57.8
 atrophicans (senile) L57.4
 perforans serpiginosa L87.2
 senilis L57.4
Elbow — *see* condition
Electric current, electricity, effects (concussion)
 (fatal) (nonfatal) (shock) T75.4 ☑
 burn — *see* Burn
Electric feet syndrome E53.8
Electrocution T75.4 ☑
 from electroshock gun (taser) T75.4 ☑
Electrolyte imbalance E87.8
 with
 abortion — *see* Abortion by type, complicated
 by, electrolyte imbalance
 ectopic pregnancy O08.5
 molar pregnancy O08.5
Elephantiasis (nonfilarial) I89.0
 arabicum — *see* Infestation, filarial
 bancroftian B74.0
 congenital (any site) (hereditary) Q82.0
 due to
 Brugia (malayi) B74.1
 timori B74.2
 mastectomy I97.2
 Wuchereria (bancrofti) B74.0
 eyelid H02.859
 left H02.856
 lower H02.855
 upper H02.854
 right H02.853
 lower H02.852
 upper H02.851
 filarial, filariensis — *see* Infestation, filarial
 glandular I89.0
 graecorum A30.9
 lymphangiectatic I89.0
 lymphatic vessel I89.0
 due to mastectomy I97.2
 scrotum (nonfilarial) I89.0
 streptococcal I89.0
 surgical I97.89
 postmastectomy I97.2
 telangiectodes I89.0
 vulva (nonfilarial) N90.89
Elevated, elevation
 antibody titer R76.0
 basal metabolic rate R94.8
 blood pressure (*see also* Hypertension)
 reading (incidental) (isolated) (nonspecific), no
 diagnosis of hypertension R03.0
 blood sugar R73.9
 body temperature (of unknown origin) R50.9
 C-reactive protein (CRP) R79.82
 cancer antigen 125 [CA 125] R97.1
 carcinoembryonic antigen [CEA] R97.0
 cholesterol E78.0
 with high triglycerides E78.2
 conjugate, eye H51.0
 diaphragm, congenital Q79.1
 erythrocyte sedimentation rate R70.0
 fasting glucose R73.01
 fasting triglycerides E78.1
 finding on laboratory examination — *see*
 Findings, abnormal, inconclusive, without
 diagnosis, by type of exam

Elevated — *continued*
 GFR (glomerular filtration rate) — *see* Findings,
 abnormal, inconclusive, without diagnosis,
 by type of exam
 glucose tolerance (oral) R73.02
 immunoglobulin level R76.8
 indoleacetic acid R82.5
 lactic acid dehydrogenase (LDH) level R74.0
 leukocytes D72.829
 lipoprotein a level E78.8 ☑
 liver function
 study R94.5
 test R79.89
 alkaline phosphatase R74.8
 aminotransferase R74.0
 bilirubin R17
 hepatic enzyme R74.8
 lactate dehydrogenase R74.0
 lymphocytes D72.820
 prostate specific antigen [PSA] R97.2
 Rh titer — *see* Complication(s), transfusion,
 incompatibility reaction, Rh (factor)
 scapula, congenital Q74.0
 sedimentation rate R70.0
 SGOT R74.0
 SGPT R74.0
 transaminase level R74.0
 triglycerides E78.1
 with high cholesterol E78.2
 tumor associated antigens [TAA] NEC R97.8
 tumor specific antigens [TSA] NEC R97.8
 urine level of
 catecholamine R82.5
 indoleacetic acid R82.5
 17-ketosteroids R82.5
 steroids R82.5
 vanillylmandelic acid (VMA) R82.5
 venous pressure I87.8
 white blood cell count D72.829
 specified NEC D72.828
Elliptocytosis (congenital) (hereditary) D58.1
 Hb C (disease) D58.1
 hemoglobin disease D58.1
 sickle-cell (disease) D57.8- ☑
 trait D57.3
Ellison-Zollinger syndrome E16.4
Ellis-van Creveld syndrome (chondroectodermal
 dysplasia) Q77.6
Elongated, elongation (congenital) (*see also*
 Distortion)
 bone Q79.9
 cervix (uteri) Q51.828
 acquired N88.4
 hypertrophic N88.4
 colon Q43.8
 common bile duct Q44.5
 cystic duct Q44.5
 frenulum, penis Q55.69
 labia minora (acquired) N90.6
 ligamentum patellae Q74.1
 petiolus (epiglottidis) Q31.8
 tooth, teeth K00.2
 uvula Q38.6
Eltor cholera A00.1
Emaciation (due to malnutrition) E41
Embadomoniasis A07.8
Embedded tooth, teeth K01.0
 root only K08.3
Embolic — *see* condition
Embolism (multiple) (paradoxical) I74.9
 air (any site) (traumatic) T79.0 ☑
 following
 abortion — *see* Abortion by type
 complicated by embolism
 ectopic pregnancy O08.2
 infusion, therapeutic injection or transfusion
 T80.0 ☑
 molar pregnancy O08.2
 procedure NEC
 artery T81.719 ☑
 mesenteric T81.710 ☑
 renal T81.711 ☑
 specified NEC T81.718 ☑
 vein T81.72 ☑
 in pregnancy, childbirth or puerperium — *see*
 Embolism, obstetric
 amniotic fluid (pulmonary) (*see also* Embolism,
 obstetric)
 following
 abortion — *see* Abortion by type
 complicated by embolism
 ectopic pregnancy O08.2

Embolism — *continued*
 molar pregnancy O08.2
 aorta, aortic I74.10
 abdominal I74.09
 saddle I74.01
 bifurcation I74.09
 saddle I74.01
 thoracic I74.11
 artery I74.9
 auditory, internal I65.8
 basilar — *see* Occlusion, artery, basilar
 carotid (common) (internal) — *see* Occlusion,
 artery, carotid
 cerebellar (anterior inferior) (posterior inferior)
 (superior) I66.3
 cerebral — *see* Occlusion, artery, cerebral
 choroidal (anterior) I66.8
 communicating posterior I66.8
 coronary (*see also* Infarct, myocardium)
 not resulting in infarction I24.0
 extremity I74.4
 lower I74.3
 upper I74.2
 hypophyseal I66.8
 iliac I74.5
 limb I74.4
 lower I74.3
 upper I74.2
 mesenteric (with gangrene) K55.0
 ophthalmic — *see* Occlusion, artery, retina
 peripheral I74.4
 pontine I66.8
 precerebral — *see* Occlusion, artery, precerebral
 pulmonary — *see* Embolism, pulmonary
 renal N28.0
 retinal — *see* Occlusion, artery, retina
 septic I76
 specified NEC I74.8
 vertebral — *see* Occlusion, artery, vertebral
 basilar (artery) I65.1
 blood clot
 following
 abortion — *see* Abortion by type
 complicated by embolism
 ectopic or molar pregnancy O08.2
 in pregnancy, childbirth or puerperium — *see*
 Embolism, obstetric
 brain (*see also* Occlusion, artery, cerebral)
 following
 abortion — *see* Abortion by type
 complicated by embolism
 ectopic or molar pregnancy O08.2
 puerperal, postpartum, childbirth — *see*
 Embolism, obstetric
 capillary I78.8
 cardiac (*see also* Infarct, myocardium)
 not resulting in infarction I24.0
 carotid (artery) (common) (internal) — *see*
 Occlusion, artery, carotid
 cavernous sinus (venous) — *see* Embolism,
 intracranial venous sinus
 cerebral — *see* Occlusion, artery, cerebral
 cholesterol — *see* Atheroembolism
 coronary (artery or vein) (systemic) — *see*
 Occlusion, coronary
 due to device, implant or graft (*see also*
 Complications, by site and type, specified
 NEC)
 arterial graft NEC T82.818 ☑
 breast (implant) T85.81 ☑
 catheter NEC T85.81 ☑
 dialysis (renal) T82.818 ☑
 intraperitoneal T85.81 ☑
 infusion NEC T82.818 ☑
 spinal (epidural) (subdural) T85.81 ☑
 urinary (indwelling) T83.81 ☑
 electronic (electrode) (pulse generator)
 (stimulator)
 bone T84.81 ☑
 cardiac T82.817 ☑
 nervous system (brain) (peripheral nerve)
 (spinal) T85.81 ☑
 urinary T83.81 ☑
 fixation, internal (orthopedic) NEC T84.81 ☑
 gastrointestinal (bile duct) (esophagus) T85.81
 ☑
 genital NEC T83.81 ☑
 heart (graft) (valve) T82.817 ☑
 joint prosthesis T84.81 ☑
 ocular (corneal graft) (orbital implant) T85.81 ☑
 orthopedic (bone graft) NEC T86.838
 specified NEC T85.81 ☑

☑ **Additional character required**

Embolism — *continued*
- urinary (graft) NEC T83.81 ☑
- vascular NEC T82.818 ☑
- ventricular intracranial shunt T85.81 ☑
- extremities
  - lower — *see* Embolism, vein, lower extremity
    - arterial I74.3
  - upper I74.2
- eye H34.9
- fat (cerebral) (pulmonary) (systemic) T79.1 ☑
  - following
    - abortion — *see* Abortion by type complicated by embolism
    - ectopic or molar pregnancy O08.2
  - complicating delivery — *see* Embolism, obstetric
- following
  - abortion — *see* Abortion by type complicated by embolism
  - ectopic or molar pregnancy O08.2
  - infusion, therapeutic injection or transfusion air T80.0 ☑
- heart (fatty) (*see also* Infarct, myocardium)
  - not resulting in infarction I24.0
- hepatic (vein) I82.0
- in pregnancy, childbirth or puerperium — *see* Embolism, obstetric
- intestine (artery) (vein) (with gangrene) K55.0
- intracranial (*see also* Occlusion, artery, cerebral)
  - venous sinus (any) G08
    - nonpyogenic I67.6
- intraspinal venous sinuses or veins G08
  - nonpyogenic G95.19
- kidney (artery) N28.0
- lateral sinus (venous) — *see* Embolism, intracranial, venous sinus
- leg — *see* Embolism, vein, lower extremity
  - arterial I74.3
- longitudinal sinus (venous) — *see* Embolism, intracranial, venous sinus
- lung (massive) — *see* Embolism, pulmonary
- meninges I66.8
- mesenteric (artery) (vein) (with gangrene) K55.0
- obstetric (in) (pulmonary)
  - childbirth O88.82
    - air O88.02
    - amniotic fluid O88.12
    - blood clot O88.22
    - fat O88.82
    - pyemic O88.32
    - septic O88.32
    - specified type NEC O88.82
  - pregnancy O88.81- ☑
    - air O88.01- ☑
    - amniotic fluid O88.11- ☑
    - blood clot O88.21- ☑
    - fat O88.81- ☑
    - pyemic O88.31- ☑
    - septic O88.31- ☑
    - specified type NEC O88.81- ☑
  - puerperal O88.83
    - air O88.03
    - amniotic fluid O88.13
    - blood clot O88.23
    - fat O88.83
    - pyemic O88.33
    - septic O88.33
    - specified type NEC O88.83
- ophthalmic — *see* Occlusion, artery, retina
- penis N48.81
- peripheral artery NOS I74.4
- pituitary E23.6
- popliteal (artery) I74.3
- portal (vein) I81
- postoperative, postprocedural
  - artery T81.719 ☑
    - mesenteric T81.710 ☑
    - renal T81.711 ☑
    - specified NEC T81.718 ☑
  - vein T81.72 ☑
- precerebral artery — *see* Occlusion, artery, precerebral
- puerperal — *see* Embolism, obstetric
- pulmonary (acute) (artery) (vein) I26.99
  - with acute cor pulmonale I26.09
  - chronic I27.82
  - following
    - abortion — *see* Abortion by type complicated by embolism
    - ectopic or molar pregnancy O08.2
  - healed or old Z86.711

Embolism — *continued*
- in pregnancy, childbirth or puerperium — *see* Embolism, obstetric
- personal history of Z86.711
- saddle I26.92
  - with acute cor pulmonale I26.02
- septic I26.90
  - with acute cor pulmonale I26.01
- pyemic (multiple) I76
  - following
    - abortion — *see* Abortion by type complicated by embolism
    - ectopic or molar pregnancy O08.2
  - Hemophilus influenzae A41.3
  - pneumococcal A40.3
    - with pneumonia J13
  - puerperal, postpartum, childbirth (any organism) — *see* Embolism, obstetric
  - specified organism NEC A41.89
  - staphylococcal A41.2
  - streptococcal A40.9
- renal (artery) N28.0
  - vein I82.3
- retina, retinal — *see* Occlusion, artery, retina
- saddle
  - abdominal aorta I74.01
  - pulmonary artery I26.92
    - with acute cor pulmonale I26.02
- septic (arterial) I76
  - complicating abortion — *see* Abortion, by type, complicated by, embolism
- sinus — *see* Embolism, intracranial, venous sinus
- soap complicating abortion — *see* Abortion, by type, complicated by, embolism
- spinal cord G95.19
  - pyogenic origin G06.1
- spleen, splenic (artery) I74.8
- upper extremity I74.2
- vein (acute) I82.90
  - antecubital I82.61- ☑
    - chronic I82.71- ☑
  - axillary I82.A1- ☑
    - chronic I82.A2- ☑
  - basilic I82.61- ☑
    - chronic I82.71- ☑
  - brachial I82.62- ☑
    - chronic I82.72- ☑
  - brachiocephalic (innominate) I82.290
    - chronic I82.291
  - cephalic I82.61- ☑
    - chronic I82.71- ☑
  - chronic I82.91
  - deep (DVT) I82.40- ☑
    - calf I82.4Z- ☑
      - chronic I82.5Z- ☑
    - lower leg I82.4Z- ☑
      - chronic I82.5Z- ☑
    - thigh I82.4Y- ☑
      - chronic I82.5Y- ☑
    - upper leg I82.4Y ☑
      - chronic I82.5y--
  - femoral I82.41- ☑
    - chronic I82.51- ☑
  - iliac (iliofemoral) I82.42- ☑
    - chronic I82.52- ☑
  - innominate I82.290
    - chronic I82.291
  - internal jugular I82.C1- ☑
    - chronic I82.C2- ☑
  - lower extremity
    - deep I82.40- ☑
      - chronic I82.50- ☑
      - specified NEC I82.49- ☑
        - chronic NEC I82.59- ☑
    - distal
      - deep I82.4Z- ☑
    - proximal
      - deep I82.4Y- ☑
        - chronic I82.5Y- ☑
    - superficial I82.81- ☑
  - popliteal I82.43- ☑
    - chronic I82.53- ☑
  - radial I82.62- ☑
    - chronic I82.72- ☑
  - renal I82.3
  - saphenous (greater) (lesser) I82.81- ☑
  - specified NEC I82.890
    - chronic NEC I82.891
  - subclavian I82.B1- ☑
    - chronic I82.B2- ☑
  - thoracic NEC I82.290
    - chronic I82.291

Embolism — *continued*
- tibial I82.44- ☑
  - chronic I82.54- ☑
- ulnar I82.62- ☑
  - chronic I82.72- ☑
- upper extremity I82.60- ☑
  - chronic I82.70- ☑
  - deep I82.62- ☑
    - chronic I82.72- ☑
  - superficial I82.61- ☑
    - chronic I82.71- ☑
- vena cava
  - inferior (acute) I82.220
    - chronic I82.221
  - superior (acute) I82.210
    - chronic I82.211
- venous sinus G08
- vessels of brain — *see* Occlusion, artery, cerebral
Embolus — *see* Embolism
Embryoma (*see also* Neoplasm, uncertain behavior, by site)
- benign — *see* Neoplasm, benign, by site
- kidney C64.- ☑
- liver C22.0
- malignant (*see also* Neoplasm, malignant, by site)
  - kidney C64.- ☑
  - liver C22.0
  - testis C62.9- ☑
    - descended (scrotal) C62.1- ☑
    - undescended C62.0- ☑
- testis C62.9- ☑
  - descended (scrotal) C62.1- ☑
  - undescended C62.0- ☑
Embryonic
- circulation Q28.9
- heart Q28.9
- vas deferens Q55.4
Embryopathia NOS Q89.9
Embryotoxon Q13.4
Emesis — *see* Vomiting
Emotional lability R45.86
Emotionality, pathological F60.3
Emotogenic disease — *see* Disorder, psychogenic
Emphysema (atrophic) (bullous) (chronic) (interlobular) (lung) (obstructive) (pulmonary) (senile) (vesicular) J43.9
- cellular tissue (traumatic) T79.7 ☑
  - surgical T81.82 ☑
- centrilobular J43.2
- compensatory J98.3
- congenital (interstitial) P25.0
- conjunctiva H11.89
- connective tissue (traumatic) T79.7 ☑
  - surgical T81.82 ☑
- due to chemicals, gases, fumes or vapors J68.4
- eyelid (s) — *see* Disorder, eyelid, specified type NEC
  - surgical T81.82 ☑
  - traumatic T79.7 ☑
- interstitial J98.2
  - congenital P25.0
  - perinatal period P25.0
- laminated tissue T79.7 ☑
  - surgical T81.82 ☑
- mediastinal J98.2
  - newborn P25.2
- orbit, orbital — *see* Disorder, orbit, specified type NEC
- panacinar J43.1
- panlobular J43.1
- specified NEC J43.8
- subcutaneous (traumatic) T79.7 ☑
  - nontraumatic J98.2
  - postprocedural T81.82 ☑
    - surgical T81.82 ☑
- surgical T81.82 ☑
- thymus (gland) (congenital) E32.8
- traumatic (subcutaneous) T79.7 ☑
- unilateral J43.0
Empty nest syndrome Z60.0
Empyema (acute) (chest) (double) (pleura) (supradiaphragmatic) (thorax) J86.9
- with fistula J86.0
- accessory sinus (chronic) — *see* Sinusitis
- antrum (chronic) — *see* Sinusitis, maxillary
- brain (any part) — *see* Abscess, brain
- ethmoidal (chronic) (sinus) — *see* Sinusitis, ethmoidal
- extradural — *see* Abscess, extradural
- frontal (chronic) (sinus) — *see* Sinusitis, frontal
- gallbladder K81.0
- mastoid (process) (acute) — *see* Mastoiditis, acute

Empyema - Encephalopathy

Empyema — continued
  maxilla, maxillary M27.2
    sinus (chronic) — see Sinusitis, maxillary
  nasal sinus (chronic) — see Sinusitis
  sinus (accessory) (chronic) (nasal) — see Sinusitis
  sphenoidal (sinus) (chronic) — see Sinusitis,
    sphenoidal
  subarachnoid — see Abscess, extradural
  subdural — see Abscess, subdural
  tuberculous A15.6
  ureter — see Ureteritis
  ventricular — see Abscess, brain
En coup de sabre lesion L94.1
Enamel pearls K00.2
Enameloma K00.2
Enanthema, viral B09
Encephalitis (chronic) (hemorrhagic) (idiopathic)
  (nonepidemic) (spurious) (subacute) G04.90
  acute (see also Encephalitis, viral) A86
    disseminated G04.00
      infectious G04.01
      noninfectious G04.81
      postimmunization (postvaccination) G04.02
      postinfectious G04.01
    inclusion body A85.8
    necrotizing hemorrhagic G04.30
      postimmunization G04.32
      postinfectious G04.31
      specified NEC G04.39
  arboviral, arbovirus NEC A85.2
  arthropod-borne NEC (viral) A85.2
  Australian A83.4
  California (virus) A83.5
  Central European (tick-borne) A84.1
  Czechoslovakian A84.1
  Dawson's (inclusion body) A81.1
  diffuse sclerosing A81.1
  disseminated, acute G04.00
  due to
    cat scratch disease A28.1
    human immunodeficiency virus (HIV) disease
      B20 [G05.3]
    malaria — see Malaria
    rickettsiosis — see Rickettsiosis
    smallpox inoculation G04.02
    typhus — see Typhus
  Eastern equine A83.2
  endemic (viral) A86
  epidemic NEC (viral) A86
  equine (acute) (infectious) (viral) A83.9
    Eastern A83.2
    Venezuelan A92.2
    Western A83.1
  Far Eastern (tick-borne) A84.0
  following vaccination or other immunization
    procedure G04.02
  herpes zoster B02.0
  herpesviral B00.4
    due to herpesvirus 6 B10.01
    due to herpesvirus 7 B10.09
    specified NEC B10.09
  Ilheus (virus) A83.8
  inclusion body A81.1
  in (due to)
    actinomycosis A42.82
    adenovirus A85.1
    African trypanosomiasis B56.9 [G05.3]
    Chagas' disease (chronic) B57.42
    cytomegalovirus B25.8
    enterovirus A85.0
    herpes (simplex) virus B00.4
      due to herpesvirus 6 B10.01
      due to herpesvirus 7 B10.09
      specified NEC B10.09
    infectious disease NEC B99 ☑ [G05.3]
    influenza — see Influenza, with,
      encephalopathy
    listeriosis A32.12
    measles B05.0
    mumps B26.2
    naegleriasis B60.2
    parasitic disease NEC B89 [G05.3]
    poliovirus A80.9 [G05.3]
    rubella B06.01
    syphilis
      congenital A50.42
      late A52.14
    systemic lupus erythematosus M32.19
    toxoplasmosis (acquired) B58.2
      congenital P37.1
    tuberculosis A17.82
    zoster B02.0

Encephalitis — continued
  infectious (acute) (virus) NEC A86
  Japanese (B type) A83.0
  La Crosse A83.5
  lead — see Poisoning, lead
  lethargica (acute) (infectious) A85.8
  louping ill A84.8
  lupus erythematosus, systemic M32.19
  lymphatica A87.2
  Mengo A85.8
  meningococcal A39.81
  Murray Valley A83.4
  otitic NEC H66.40 [G05.3]
  parasitic NOS B71.9
  periaxial G37.0
  periaxialis (concentrica) (diffuse) G37.5
  postchickenpox B01.11
  postexanthematous NEC B09
  postimmunization G04.02
  postinfectious NEC G04.01
  postmeasles B05.0
  postvaccinal G04.02
  postvaricella B01.11
  postviral NEC A86
  Powassan A84.8
  Rasmussen G04.81
  Rio Bravo A85.8
  Russian
    autumnal A83.0
    spring-summer (taiga) A84.0
  saturnine — see Poisoning, lead
  specified NEC G04.81
  St. Louis A83.3
  subacute sclerosing A81.1
  summer A83.0
  suppurative G04.81
  tick-borne A84.9
  Torula, torular (cryptococcal) B45.1
  toxic NEC G92
  trichinosis B75 [G05.3]
  type
    B A83.0
    C A83.3
  van Bogaert's A81.1
  Venezuelan equine A92.2
  Vienna A85.8
  viral, virus A86
    arthropod-borne NEC A85.2
    mosquito-borne A83.9
      Australian X disease A83.4
      California virus A83.5
      Eastern equine A83.2
      Japanese (B type) A83.0
      Murray Valley A83.4
      specified NEC A83.8
      St. Louis A83.3
      type B A83.0
      type C A83.3
      Western equine A83.1
    tick-borne A84.9
      biundulant A84.1
      central European A84.1
      Czechoslovakian A84.1
      diphasic meningoencephalitis A84.1
      Far Eastern A84.0
      Russian spring-summer (taiga) A84.0
      specified NEC A84.8
    specified type NEC A85.8
  Western equine A83.1
Encephalocele Q01.9
  frontal Q01.0
  nasofrontal Q01.1
  occipital Q01.2
  specified NEC Q01.8
Encephalocystocele — see Encephalocele
Encephaloduroarteriomyosynangiosis (EDAMS)
  I67.5
Encephalomalacia (brain) (cerebellar) (cerebral) —
  see Softening, brain
Encephalomeningitis — see Meningoencephalitis
Encephalomeningocele — see Encephalocele
Encephalomeningomyelitis — see
  Meningoencephalitis
Encephalomyelitis (see also Encephalitis) G04.90
  acute disseminated G04.00
    infectious G04.01
    noninfectious G04.81
    postimmunization G04.02
    postinfectious G04.01
  acute necrotizing hemorrhagic G04.30
    postimmunization G04.32
    postinfectious G04.31

Encephalomyelitis — continued
    specified NEC G04.39
  benign myalgic G93.3
  equine A83.9
    Eastern A83.2
    Venezuelan A92.2
    Western A83.1
  in diseases classified elsewhere G05.3
  myalgic, benign G93.3
  postchickenpox B01.11
  postinfectious NEC G04.01
  postmeasles B05.0
  postvaccinal G04.02
  postvaricella B01.11
  rubella B06.01
  specified NEC G04.81
  Venezuelan equine A92.2
Encephalomyelocele — see Encephalocele
Encephalomyelomeningitis — see
  Meningoencephalitis
Encephalomyelopathy G96.9
Encephalomyeloradiculitis (acute) G61.0
Encephalomyeloradiculoneuritis (acute) (Guillain-
  Barré) G61.0
Encephalomyeloradiculopathy G96.9
Encephalopathia hyperbilirubinemica, newborn
  P57.9
  due to isoimmunization (conditions in P55) P57.0
Encephalopathy (acute) G93.40
  acute necrotizing hemorrhagic G04.30
    postimmunization G04.32
    postinfectious G04.31
    specified NEC G04.39
  alcoholic G31.2
  anoxic — see Damage, brain, anoxic
  arteriosclerotic I67.2
  centrolobar progressive (Schilder) G37.0
  congenital Q07.9
  degenerative, in specified disease NEC G32.89
  demyelinating callosal G37.1
  due to
    drugs - (see also Table of Drugs and Chemicals)
      G92
    hepatic — see Failure, hepatic
  hyperbilirubinemic, newborn P57.9
    due to isoimmunization (conditions in P55)
      P57.0
  hypertensive I67.4
  hypoglycemic E16.2
  hypoxic — see Damage, brain, anoxic
  hypoxic ischemic P91.60
    mild P91.61
    moderate P91.62
    severe P91.63
  in (due to) (with)
    birth injury P11.1
    hyperinsulinism E16.1 [G94]
    influenza — see Influenza, with,
      encephalopathy
    lack of vitamin (see also Deficiency, vitamin)
      E56.9 [G32.89]
    neoplastic disease (see also Neoplasm) D49.9
      [G13.1]
    serum (see also Reaction, serum) T80.69 ☑
    syphilis A52.17
    trauma (postconcussional) F07.81
      current injury — see Injury, intracranial
    vaccination G04.02
  lead — see Poisoning, lead
  metabolic G93.41
    drug induced G92
    toxic G92
  myoclonic, early, symptomatic — see Epilepsy,
    generalized, specified NEC
  necrotizing, subacute (Leigh) G31.82
  pellagrous E52 [G32.89]
  portosystemic — see Failure, hepatic
  postcontusional F07.81
    current injury — see Injury, intracranial, diffuse
  posthypoglycemic (coma) E16.1 [G94]
  postradiation G93.89
  saturnine — see Poisoning, lead
  septic G93.41
  specified NEC G93.49
  spongioform, subacute (viral) A81.09
  toxic G92
    metabolic G92
  traumatic (postconcussional) F07.81
    current injury — see Injury, intracranial
  vitamin B deficiency NEC E53.9 [G32.89]
    vitamin B1 E51.2
  Wernicke's E51.2

☑ **Additional character required**

Encephalorrhagia — *see* Hemorrhage, intracranial, intracerebral
Encephalosis, posttraumatic F07.81
Enchondroma (*see also* Neoplasm, bone, benign)
Enchondromatosis (cartilaginous) (multiple) Q78.4
Encopresis R15.9
  functional F98.1
  nonorganic origin F98.1
  psychogenic F98.1
Encounter (with health service) (for) Z76.89
  adjustment and management (of)
    breast implant Z45.81 ☑
    implanted device NEC Z45.89
    myringotomy device (stent) (tube) Z45.82
  administrative purpose only Z02.9
    examination for
      adoption Z02.82
      armed forces Z02.3
      disability determination Z02.71
      driving license Z02.4
      employment Z02.1
      insurance Z02.6
      medical certificate NEC Z02.79
      paternity testing Z02.81
      residential institution admission Z02.2
      school admission Z02.0
      sports Z02.5
      specified reason NEC Z02.89
  aftercare — *see* Aftercare
  antenatal screening Z36
  assisted reproductive fertility procedure cycle Z31.83
  blood typing Z01.83
    Rh typing Z01.83
  breast augmentation or reduction Z41.1
  breast implant exchange (different material) (different size) Z45.81 ☑
  breast reconstruction following mastectomy Z42.1
  check-up — *see* Examination
  chemotherapy for neoplasm Z51.11
  colonoscopy, screening Z12.11
  counseling — *see* Counseling
  delivery, full-term, uncomplicated O80
    cesarean, without indication O82
  ear piercing Z41.3
  examination — *see* Examination
  expectant parent (s) (adoptive) pre-birth pediatrician visit Z76.81
  fertility preservation procedure (prior to cancer therapy) (prior to removal of gonads) Z31.84
  fitting (of) — *see* Fitting (and adjustment) (of)
  genetic
    counseling Z31.5
    testing — *see* Test, genetic
  hearing conservation and treatment Z01.12
  immunotherapy for neoplasm Z51.12
  in vitro fertilization cycle Z31.83
  instruction (in)
    childbirth Z32.2
    child care (postpartal) (prenatal) Z32.3
    natural family planning
      procreative Z31.61
      to avoid pregnancy Z30.02
  insulin pump titration Z46.81
  joint prosthesis insertion following prior explantation of joint prosthesis (staged procedure)
    hip Z47.32
    knee Z47.33
    shoulder Z47.31
  laboratory (as part of a general medical examination) Z00.00
    with abnormal findings Z00.01
  mental health services (for)
    abuse NEC
      perpetrator Z69.82
      victim Z69.81
    child abuse
      nonparental
        perpetrator Z69.021
        victim Z69.020
      parental
        perpetrator Z69.011
        victim Z69.010
    spousal or partner abuse
      perpetrator Z69.12
      victim Z69.11
  observation (for) (ruled out)
    exposure to (suspected)
      anthrax Z03.810
      biological agent NEC Z03.818

Encounter — *continued*
  pediatrician visit, by expectant parent (s) (adoptive) Z76.81
  plastic and reconstructive surgery following medical procedure or healed injury NEC Z42.8
  pregnancy
    supervision of — *see* Pregnancy, supervision of
    test Z32.00
      result negative Z32.02
      result positive Z32.01
  radiation therapy (antineoplastic) Z51.0
  radiological (as part of a general medical examination) Z00.00
    with abnormal findings Z00.01
  reconstructive surgery following medical procedure or healed injury NEC Z42.8
  removal (of) (*see also* Removal)
    artificial
      arm Z44.00- ☑
        complete Z44.01- ☑
        partial Z44.02- ☑
      eye Z44.2- ☑
      leg Z44.10- ☑
        complete Z44.11- ☑
        partial Z44.12- ☑
    breast implant Z45.81 ☑
      tissue expander (without synchronous insertion of permanent implant) Z45.81 ☑
    device Z46.9
      specified NEC Z46.89
    external
      fixation device - code to fracture with seventh character D
      prosthesis, prosthetic device Z44.9
        breast Z44.3- ☑
        specified NEC Z44.8
    implanted device NEC Z45.89
    insulin pump Z46.81
    internal fixation device Z47.2
    myringotomy device (stent) (tube) Z45.82
    nervous system device NEC Z46.2
      brain neuropacemaker Z46.2
      visual substitution device Z46.2
        implanted Z45.31
    non-vascular catheter Z46.82
    orthodontic device Z46.4
    stent
      ureteral Z46.6
    urinary device Z46.6
  repeat cervical smear to confirm findings of recent normal smear following initial abnormal smear Z01.42
  respirator [ventilator] use during power failure Z99.12
  Rh typing Z01.83
  screening — *see* Screening
  specified NEC Z76.89
  sterilization Z30.2
  suspected condition, ruled out
    amniotic cavity and membrane Z03.71
    cervical shortening Z03.75
    fetal anomaly Z03.73
    fetal growth Z03.74
    maternal and fetal conditions NEC Z03.79
    oligohydramnios Z03.71
    placental problem Z03.72
    polyhydramnios Z03.71
  suspected exposure (to), ruled out
    anthrax Z03.810
    biological agents NEC Z03.818
  termination of pregnancy, elective Z33.2
  testing — *see* Test
  therapeutic drug level monitoring Z51.81
  titration, insulin pump Z46.81
  to determine fetal viability of pregnancy O36.80 ☑
  training
    insulin pump Z46.81
  X-ray of chest (as part of a general medical examination) Z00.00
    with abnormal findings Z00.01
Encystment — *see* Cyst
Endarteritis (bacterial, subacute) (infective) I77.6
  brain I67.7
  cerebral or cerebrospinal I67.7
  deformans — *see* Arteriosclerosis
  embolic — *see* Embolism
  obliterans (*see also* Arteriosclerosis)
    pulmonary I28.8
  pulmonary I28.8

Endarteritis — *continued*
  retina — *see* Vasculitis, retina
  senile — *see* Arteriosclerosis
  syphilitic A52.09
    brain or cerebral A52.04
    congenital A50.54 [I79.8]
  tuberculous A18.89
Endemic — *see* condition
Endocarditis (chronic) (marantic) (nonbacterial) (thrombotic) (valvular) I38
  with rheumatic fever (conditions in I00)
    active — *see* Endocarditis, acute, rheumatic
    inactive or quiescent (with chorea) I09.1
  acute or subacute I33.9
    infective I33.0
    rheumatic (aortic) (mitral) (pulmonary) (tricuspid) I01.1
      with chorea (acute) (rheumatic) (Sydenham's) I02.0
  aortic (heart) (nonrheumatic) (valve) I35.8
    with
      mitral disease I08.0
        with tricuspid (valve) disease I08.3
        active or acute I01.1
          with chorea (acute) (rheumatic) (Sydenham's) I02.0
      rheumatic fever (conditions in I00)
        active — *see* Endocarditis, acute, rheumatic
        inactive or quiescent (with chorea) I06.9
      tricuspid (valve) disease I08.2
        with mitral (valve) disease I08.3
    acute or subacute I33.9
    arteriosclerotic I35.8
    rheumatic I06.9
      with mitral disease I08.0
        with tricuspid (valve) disease I08.3
        active or acute I01.1
          with chorea (acute) (rheumatic) (Sydenham's) I02.0
      active or acute I01.1
        with chorea (acute) (rheumatic) (Sydenham's) I02.0
      specified NEC I06.8
    specified cause NEC I35.8
    syphilitic A52.03
  arteriosclerotic I38
  atypical verrucous (Libman-Sacks) M32.11
  bacterial (acute) (any valve) (subacute) I33.0
  candidal B37.6
  congenital Q24.8
  constrictive I33.0
  Coxiella burnetii A78 [I39]
  Coxsackie B33.21
  due to
    prosthetic cardiac valve T82.6 ☑
    Q fever A78 [I39]
    Serratia marcescens I33.0
    typhoid (fever) A01.02
  gonococcal A54.83
  infectious or infective (acute) (any valve) (subacute) I33.0
  lenta (acute) (any valve) (subacute) I33.0
  Libman-Sacks M32.11
  listerial A32.82
  Löffler's I42.3
  malignant (acute) (any valve) (subacute) I33.0
  meningococcal A39.51
  mitral (chronic) (double) (fibroid) (heart) (inactive) (valve) (with chorea) I05.9
    with
      aortic (valve) disease I08.0
        with tricuspid (valve) disease I08.3
        active or acute I01.1
          with chorea (acute) (rheumatic) (Sydenham's) I02.0
      rheumatic fever (conditions in I00)
        active — *see* Endocarditis, acute, rheumatic
        inactive or quiescent (with chorea) I05.9
      tricuspid (valve) disease I08.1
        with aortic (valve) disease I08.3
    active or acute I01.1
      with chorea (acute) (rheumatic) (Sydenham's) I02.0
    bacterial I33.0
    arteriosclerotic I34.8
    nonrheumatic I34.8
      acute or subacute I33.9
    specified NEC I05.8
  monilial B37.6
  multiple valves I08.9

Endocarditis — *continued*
   specified disorders I08.8
   mycotic (acute) (any valve) (subacute) I33.0
   pneumococcal (acute) (any valve) (subacute) I33.0
   pulmonary (chronic) (heart) (valve) I37.8
    with rheumatic fever (conditions in I00)
     active — *see* Endocarditis, acute, rheumatic
     inactive or quiescent (with chorea) I09.89
      with aortic, mitral or tricuspid disease I08.8
   acute or subacute I33.9
    rheumatic I01.1
     with chorea (acute) (rheumatic) (Sydenham's) I02.0
   arteriosclerotic I37.8
   congenital Q22.2
   rheumatic (chronic) (inactive) (with chorea) I09.89
    active or acute I01.1
     with chorea (acute) (rheumatic) (Sydenham's) I02.0
   syphilitic A52.03
   purulent (acute) (any valve) (subacute) I33.0
   Q fever A78 [I39]
   rheumatic (chronic) (inactive) (with chorea) I09.1
    active or acute (aortic) (mitral) (pulmonary) (tricuspid) I01.1
     with chorea (acute) (rheumatic) (Sydenham's) I02.0
   rheumatoid — *see* Rheumatoid, carditis
   septic (acute) (any valve) (subacute) I33.0
   streptococcal (acute) (any valve) (subacute) I33.0
   subacute — *see* Endocarditis, acute
   suppurative (acute) (any valve) (subacute) I33.0
   syphilitic A52.03
   toxic I33.9
   tricuspid (chronic) (heart) (inactive) (rheumatic) (valve) (with chorea) I07.9
    with
     aortic (valve) disease I08.2
      mitral (valve) disease I08.3
     mitral (valve) disease I08.1
      aortic (valve) disease I08.3
     rheumatic fever (conditions in I00)
      active — *see* Endocarditis, acute, rheumatic
      inactive or quiescent (with chorea) I07.8
   active or acute I01.1
    with chorea (acute) (rheumatic) (Sydenham's) I02.0
   arteriosclerotic I36.8
   nonrheumatic I36.8
    acute or subacute I33.9
   specified cause, except rheumatic I36.8
   tuberculous — *see* Tuberculosis, endocarditis
   typhoid A01.02
   ulcerative (acute) (any valve) (subacute) I33.0
   vegetative (acute) (any valve) (subacute) I33.0
   verrucous (atypical) (nonbacterial) (nonrheumatic) M32.11
Endocardium, endocardial (*see also* condition)
   cushion defect Q21.2
Endocervicitis (*see also* Cervicitis)
   due to intrauterine (contraceptive) device T83.6 ☑
   hyperplastic N72
Endocrine — *see* condition
Endocrinopathy, pluriglandular E31.9
Endodontic
   overfill M27.52
   underfill M27.53
Endodontitis K04.0
Endomastoiditis — *see* Mastoiditis
Endometrioma N80.9
Endometriosis N80.9
   appendix N80.5
   bladder N80.8
   bowel N80.5
   broad ligament N80.3
   cervix N80.0
   colon N80.5
   cul-de-sac (Douglas') N80.3
   exocervix N80.0
   fallopian tube N80.2
   female genital organ NEC N80.8
   gallbladder N80.8
   in scar of skin N80.6
   internal N80.0
   intestine N80.5
   lung N80.8
   myometrium N80.0
   ovary N80.1

Endometriosis — *continued*
   parametrium N80.3
   pelvic peritoneum N80.3
   peritoneal (pelvic) N80.3
   rectovaginal septum N80.4
   rectum N80.5
   round ligament N80.3
   skin (scar) N80.6
   specified site NEC N80.8
   stromal D39.0
   umbilicus N80.8
   uterus (internal) N80.0
   vagina N80.4
   vulva N80.8
Endometritis (decidual) (nonspecific) (purulent) (senile) (atrophic) (suppurative) N71.9
   with ectopic pregnancy O08.0
   acute N71.0
   blenorrhagic (gonococcal) (acute) (chronic) A54.24
   cervix, cervical (with erosion or ectropion) (*see also* Cervicitis)
    hyperplastic N72
   chlamydial A56.11
   chronic N71.1
   following
    abortion — *see* Abortion by type complicated by genital infection
    ectopic or molar pregnancy O08.0
   gonococcal, gonorrheal (acute) (chronic) A54.24
   hyperplastic (*see also* Hyperplasia, endometrial) N85.00- ☑
    cervix N72
   puerperal, postpartum, childbirth O86.12
   subacute N71.0
   tuberculous A18.17
Endometrium — *see* condition
Endomyocardiopathy, South African I42.3
Endomyocarditis — *see* Endocarditis
Endomyofibrosis I42.3
Endomyometritis — *see* Endometritis
Endopericarditis — *see* Endocarditis
Endoperineuritis — *see* Disorder, nerve
Endophlebitis — *see* Phlebitis
Endophthalmia — *see* Endophthalmitis, purulent
Endophthalmitis (acute) (infective) (metastatic) (subacute) H44.009
   bleb associated H59.4 — *see also* Bleb, inflamed (infected), postprocedural
   gonorrheal A54.39
   in (due to)
    cysticercosis B69.1
    onchocerciasis B73.01
    toxocariasis B83.0
   panuveitis — *see* Panuveitis
   parasitic H44.12- ☑
   purulent H44.00- ☑
    panophthalmitis — *see* Panophthalmitis
    vitreous abscess H44.02- ☑
   specified NEC H44.19
   sympathetic — *see* Uveitis, sympathetic
Endosalpingioma D28.2
Endosalpingiosis N94.89
Endosteitis — *see* Osteomyelitis
Endothelioma, bone — *see* Neoplasm, bone, malignant
Endotheliosis (hemorrhagic infectional) D69.8
Endotoxemia - code to condition
Endotrachelitis — *see* Cervicitis
Engelmann (-Camurati) syndrome Q78.3
English disease — *see* Rickets
Engman's disease L30.3
Engorgement
   breast N64.59
    newborn P83.4
    puerperal, postpartum O92.79
   lung (passive) — *see* Edema, lung
   pulmonary (passive) — *see* Edema, lung
   stomach K31.89
   venous, retina — *see* Occlusion, retina, vein, engorgement
Enlargement, enlarged (*see also* Hypertrophy)
   adenoids J35.2
    with tonsils J35.3
   alveolar ridge K08.8
    congenital — *see* Anomaly, alveolar
   apertures of diaphragm (congenital) Q79.1
   gingival K06.1
   heart, cardiac — *see* Hypertrophy, cardiac
   lacrimal gland, chronic H04.03- ☑
   liver — *see* Hypertrophy, liver
   lymph gland or node R59.9

Enlargement — *continued*
   generalized R59.1
   localized R59.0
   orbit H05.34- ☑
   organ or site, congenital NEC — *see* Anomaly, by site
   parathyroid (gland) E21.0
   pituitary fossa R93.0
   prostate N40.0
    with lower urinary tract symptoms (LUTS) N40.1
    without lower urinary tract symtpoms (LUTS) N40.0
   sella turcica R93.0
   spleen — *see* Splenomegaly
   thymus (gland) (congenital) E32.0
   thyroid (gland) — *see* Goiter
   tongue K14.8
   tonsils J35.1
    with adenoids J35.3
   uterus N85.2
Enophthalmos H05.40- ☑
   due to
    orbital tissue atrophy H05.41- ☑
    trauma or surgery H05.42- ☑
Enostosis M27.8
Entamebic, entamebiasis — *see* Amebiasis
Entanglement
   umbilical cord (s) O69.2 ☑
    with compression O69.2 ☑
     without compression O69.82 ☑
    around neck (with compression) O69.1 ☑
     without compression O69.81 ☑
    of twins in monoamniotic sac O69.2 ☑
Enteralgia — *see* Pain, abdominal
Enteric — *see* condition
Enteritis (acute) (diarrheal) (hemorrhagic) (noninfective) (septic) K52.9
   adenovirus A08.2
   aertrycke infection A02.0
   allergic K52.2
   amebic (acute) A06.0
    with abscess — *see* Abscess, amebic
    chronic A06.1
     with abscess — *see* Abscess, amebic
     nondysenteric A06.2
    nondysenteric A06.2
   astrovirus A08.32
   bacillary NOS A03.9
   bacterial A04.9
    specified NEC A04.8
   calicivirus A08.31
   candidal B37.82
   Chilomastix A07.8
   choleriformis A00.1
   chronic (noninfectious) K52.9
    ulcerative — *see* Colitis, ulcerative
   cicatrizing (chronic) — *see* Enteritis, regional, small intestine
   Clostridium
    botulinum (food poisoning) A05.1
    difficile A04.7
   coccidial A07.3
   coxsackie virus A08.39
   dietetic K52.2
   drug-induced K52.1
   due to
    astrovirus A08.32
    calicivirus A08.31
    coxsackie virus A08.39
    drugs K52.1
    echovirus A08.39
    enterovirus NEC A08.39
    food hypersensitivity K52.2
    infectious organism (bacterial) (viral) — *see* Enteritis, infectious
    torovirus A08.39
    Yersinia enterocolitica A04.6
   echovirus A08.39
   eltor A00.1
   enterovirus NEC A08.39
   eosinophilic K52.81
   epidemic (infectious) A09
   fulminant K55.0
   gangrenous — *see* Enteritis, infectious
   giardial A07.1
   infectious NOS A09
    due to
     adenovirus A08.2
     Aerobacter aerogenes A04.8
     Arizona (bacillus) A02.0
     bacteria NOS A04.9

☑ **Additional character required**

Enteritis — *continued*
    specified NEC A04.8
    Campylobacter A04.5
    Clostridium difficile A04.7
    Clostridium perfringens A04.8
    Enterobacter aerogenes A04.8
    enterovirus A08.39
    Escherichia coli A04.4
      enteroaggregative A04.4
      enterohemorrhagic A04.3
      enteroinvasive A04.2
      enteropathogenic A04.0
      enterotoxigenic A04.1
      specified NEC A04.4
    specified
      bacteria NEC A04.8
      virus NEC A08.39
    Staphylococcus A04.8
    virus NEC A08.4
      specified type NEC A08.39
    Yersinia enterocolitica A04.6
    specified organism NEC A08.8
  influenzal — *see* Influenza, with, digestive
    manifestations
  ischemic K55.9
    acute K55.0
    chronic K55.1
  microsporidial A07.8
  mucomembranous, myxomembranous — *see*
    Syndrome, irritable bowel
  mucous — *see* Syndrome, irritable bowel
  necroticans A05.2
  necrotizing of newborn — *see* Enterocolitis,
    necrotizing, in newborn
  neurogenic — *see* Syndrome, irritable bowel
  newborn necrotizing — *see* Enterocolitis,
    necrotizing, in newborn
  noninfectious K52.9
  norovirus A08.11
  parasitic NEC B82.9
  paratyphoid (fever) — *see* Fever, paratyphoid
  protozoal A07.9
    specified NEC A07.8
  radiation K52.0
  regional (of) K50.90
    with
      complication K50.919
        abscess K50.914
        fistula K50.913
        intestinal obstruction K50.912
        rectal bleeding K50.911
        specified complication NEC K50.918
    colon — *see* Enteritis, regional, large intestine
    duodenum — *see* Enteritis, regional, small
      intestine
    ileum — *see* Enteritis, regional, small intestine
    jejunum — *see* Enteritis, regional, small
      intestine
    large bowel — *see* Enteritis, regional, large
      intestine
    large intestine (colon) (rectum) K50.10
      with
        complication K50.119
          abscess K50.114
          fistula K50.113
          intestinal obstruction K50.112
          rectal bleeding K50.111
          small intestine (duodenum) (ileum)
            (jejunum) involvement K50.80
            with
              complication K50.819
                abscess K50.814
                fistula K50.813
                intestinal obstruction K50.812
                rectal bleeding K50.811
                specified complication NEC
                  K50.818
          specified complication NEC K50.118
    rectum — *see* Enteritis, regional, large intestine
    small intestine (duodenum) (ileum) (jejunum)
      K50.00
      with
        complication K50.019
          abscess K50.014
          fistula K50.013
          intestinal obstruction K50.012
          large intestine (colon) (rectum)
            involvement K50.80
            with
              complication K50.819
                abscess K50.814
                fistula K50.813

Enteritis — *continued*
                intestinal obstruction K50.812
                rectal bleeding K50.811
                specified complication NEC
                  K50.818
          rectal bleeding K50.011
          specified complication NEC K50.018
  rotaviral A08.0
  Salmonella, salmonellosis (arizonae) (cholerae-
    suis) (enteritidis) (typhimurium) A02.0
  segmental — *see* Enteritis, regional
  septic A09
  Shigella — *see* Infection, Shigella
  small round structured NEC A08.19
  spasmodic, spastic — *see* Syndrome, irritable
    bowel
  staphylococcal A04.8
    due to food A05.0
  torovirus A08.39
  toxic NEC K52.1
    due to Clostridium difficile A04.7
  trichomonal A07.8
  tuberculous A18.32
  typhosa A01.00
  ulcerative (chronic) — *see* Colitis, ulcerative
  viral A08.4
    adenovirus A08.2
    enterovirus A08.39
    Rotavirus A08.0
    small round structured NEC A08.19
    specified NEC A08.39
    virus specified NEC A08.39
Enterobiasis B80
Enterobius vermicularis (infection) (infestation) B80
Enterocele (*see also* Hernia, abdomen)
  pelvic, pelvis (acquired) (congenital) N81.5
  vagina, vaginal (acquired) (congenital) NEC
    N81.5
Enterocolitis (*see also* Enteritis) K52.9
  due to Clostridium difficile A04.7
  fulminant ischemic K55.0
  granulomatous — *see* Enteritis, regional
  hemorrhagic (acute) K55.0
    chronic K55.1
  infectious NEC A09
  ischemic K55.9
  necrotizing
    due to Clostridium difficile A04.7
    in newborn P77.9
      stage 1 (without pneumatosis, without
        perforation) P77.1
      stage 2 (with pneumatosis, without
        perforation) P77.2
      stage 3 (with pneumatosis, with perforation)
        P77.3
  noninfectious K52.9
    newborn — *see* Enterocolitis, necrotizing, in
      newborn
  pseudomembranous (newborn) A04.7
  radiation K52.0
    newborn — *see* Enterocolitis, necrotizing, in
      newborn
  ulcerative (chronic) — *see* Pancolitis, ulcerative
    (chronic)
Enterogastritis — *see* Enteritis
Enteropathy K63.9
  gluten-sensitive K90.0
  hemorrhagic, terminal K55.0
  protein-losing K90.4
Enteroperitonitis — *see* Peritonitis
Enteroptosis K63.4
Enterorrhagia K92.2
Enterospasm (*see also* Syndrome, irritable, bowel)
  psychogenic F45.8
Enterostenosis (*see also* Obstruction, intestine
  K56.69)
Enterostomy
  complication — *see* Complication, enterostomy
  status Z93.4
Enterovirus, as cause of disease classified elsewhere
  B97.10
  coxsackievirus B97.11
  echovirus B97.12
  other specified B97.19
Enthesopathy (peripheral) M77.9
  Achilles tendinitis — *see* Tendinitis, Achilles
  ankle and tarsus M77.9
    specified type NEC — *see* Enthesopathy, foot,
      specified type NEC
  anterior tibial syndrome M76.81- ☑
  calcaneal spur — *see* Spur, bone, calcaneal
  elbow region M77.8

Enthesopathy — *continued*
  lateral epicondylitis — *see* Epicondylitis, lateral
  medial epicondylitis — *see* Epicondylitis,
    medial
  foot NEC M77.9
    metatarsalgia — *see* Metatarsalgia
    specified type NEC M77.5- ☑
  forearm M77.9
  gluteal tendinitis — *see* Tendinitis, gluteal
  hand M77.9
  hip — *see* Enthesopathy, lower limb, specified
    type NEC
  iliac crest spur — *see* Spur, bone, iliac crest
  iliotibial band syndrome — *see* Syndrome,
    iliotibial band
  knee — *see* Enthesopathy, lower limb, lower leg,
    specified type NEC
  lateral epicondylitis — *see* Epicondylitis, lateral
  lower limb (excluding foot) M76.9
    Achilles tendinitis — *see* Tendinitis, Achilles
    anterior tibial syndrome M76.81- ☑
    gluteal tendinitis — *see* Tendinitis, gluteal
    iliac crest spur — *see* Spur, bone, iliac crest
    iliotibial band syndrome — *see* Syndrome,
      iliotibial band
    patellar tendinitis — *see* Tendinitis, patellar
    pelvic region — *see* Enthesopathy, lower limb,
      specified type NEC
    peroneal tendinitis — *see* Tendinitis, peroneal
    posterior tibial syndrome M76.82- ☑
    psoas tendinitis — *see* Tendinitis, psoas
    shoulder M77.9
    specified type NEC M76.89- ☑
    tibial collateral bursitis — *see* Bursitis, tibial
      collateral
  medial epicondylitis — *see* Epicondylitis, medial
  metatarsalgia — *see* Metatarsalgia
  multiple sites M77.9
  patellar tendinitis — *see* Tendinitis, patellar
  pelvis M77.9
  periarthritis of wrist — *see* Periarthritis, wrist
  peroneal tendinitis — *see* Tendinitis, peroneal
  posterior tibial syndrome M76.82- ☑
  psoas tendinitis — *see* Tendinitis, psoas
  shoulder region — *see* Lesion, shoulder
  specified site NEC M77.9
  specified type NEC M77.8
  spinal M46.00
    cervical region M46.02
    cervicothoracic region M46.03
    lumbar region M46.06
    lumbosacral region M46.07
    multiple sites M46.09
    occipito-atlanto-axial region M46.01
    sacrococcygeal region M46.08
    thoracic region M46.04
    thoracolumbar region M46.05
  tibial collateral bursitis — *see* Bursitis, tibial
    collateral
  upper arm M77.9
  wrist and carpus NEC M77.8
    calcaneal spur — *see* Spur, bone, calcaneal
    periarthritis of wrist — *see* Periarthritis, wrist
Entomophobia F40.218
Entomophthoromycosis B46.8
Entrance, air into vein — *see* Embolism, air
Entrapment, nerve — *see* Neuropathy, entrapment
Entropion (eyelid) (paralytic) H02.009
  cicatricial H02.019
    left H02.016
      lower H02.015
      upper H02.014
    right H02.013
      lower H02.012
      upper H02.011
  congenital Q10.2
  left H02.006
    lower H02.005
    upper H02.004
  mechanical H02.029
    left H02.026
      lower H02.025
      upper H02.024
    right H02.023
      lower H02.022
      upper H02.021
  right H02.003
    lower H02.002
    upper H02.001
  senile H02.039
    left H02.036
      lower H02.035

Entropion — continued
    upper H02.034
   right H02.033
    lower H02.032
    upper H02.031
  spastic H02.049
   left H02.046
    lower H02.045
    upper H02.044
   right H02.043
    lower H02.042
    upper H02.041
Enucleated eye (traumatic, current) S05.7- ☑
Enuresis R32
  functional F98.0
  habit disturbance F98.0
  nocturnal N39.44
   psychogenic F98.0
  nonorganic origin F98.0
  psychogenic F98.0
Eosinopenia — see Agranulocytosis
Eosinophilia (allergic) (hereditary) (idiopathic) (secondary) D72.1
  with
   angiolymphoid hyperplasia (ALHE) D18.01
  infiltrative J82
  Löffler's J82
  peritoneal — see Peritonitis, eosinophilic
  pulmonary NEC J82
  tropical (pulmonary) J82
Eosinophilia-myalgia syndrome M35.8
Ependymitis (acute) (cerebral) (chronic) (granular) — see Encephalomyelitis
Ependymoblastoma
  specified site — see Neoplasm, malignant, by site
  unspecified site C71.9
Ependymoma (epithelial) (malignant)
  anaplastic
   specified site — see Neoplasm, malignant, by site
   unspecified site C71.9
  benign
   specified site — see Neoplasm, benign, by site
   unspecified site D33.2
  myxopapillary D43.2
   specified site — see Neoplasm, uncertain behavior, by site
   unspecified site D43.2
  papillary D43.2
   specified site — see Neoplasm, uncertain behavior, by site
   unspecified site D43.2
  specified site — see Neoplasm, malignant, by site
  unspecified site C71.9
Ependymopathy G93.89
Ephelis, ephelides L81.2
Epiblepharon (congenital) Q10.3
Epicanthus, epicanthic fold (eyelid) (congenital) Q10.3
Epicondylitis (elbow)
  lateral M77.1- ☑
  medial M77.0- ☑
Epicystitis — see Cystitis
Epidemic — see condition
Epidermidalization, cervix — see Dysplasia, cervix
Epidermis, epidermal — see condition
Epidermodysplasia verruciformis B07.8
Epidermolysis
  bullosa (congenital) Q81.9
   acquired L12.30
    drug-induced L12.31
    specified cause NEC L12.35
   dystrophica Q81.2
   letalis Q81.1
   simplex Q81.0
   specified NEC Q81.8
  necroticans combustiformis L51.2
   due to drug — see Table of Drugs and Chemicals, by drug
Epidermophytid — see Dermatophytosis
Epidermophytosis (infected) — see Dermatophytosis
Epididymis — see condition
Epididymitis (acute) (nonvenereal) (recurrent) (residual) N45.1
  with orchitis N45.3
  blennorrhagic (gonococcal) A54.23
  caseous (tuberculous) A18.15
  chlamydial A56.19
  filarial (see also Infestation, filarial) B74.9 [N51]
  gonococcal A54.23
  syphilitic A52.76

Epididymitis — continued
  tuberculous A18.15
Epididymo-orchitis (see also Epididymitis) N45.3
Epidural — see condition
Epigastrium, epigastric — see condition
Epigastrocele — see Hernia, ventral
Epiglottis — see condition
Epiglottitis, epiglottiditis (acute) J05.10
  with obstruction J05.11
  chronic J37.0
Epignathus Q89.4
Epilepsia partialis continua (see also Kozhevnikof's epilepsy) G40.1- ☑
Epilepsy, epileptic, epilepsia (attack) (cerebral) (convulsion) (fit) (seizure) G40.909
  Note: the following terms are to be considered equivalent to intractable: pharmacoresistant (pharmacologically resistant), treatment resistant, refractory (medically) and poorly controlled
  with
   complex partial seizures — see Epilepsy, localization-related, symptomatic, with complex partial seizures
   grand mal seizures on awakening — see Epilepsy, generalized, specified NEC
   myoclonic absences — see Epilepsy, generalized, specified NEC
   myoclonic-astatic seizures — see Epilepsy, generalized, specified NEC
   simple partial seizures — see Epilepsy, localization-related, symptomatic, with simple partial seizures
  akinetic — see Epilepsy, generalized, specified NEC
  benign childhood with centrotemporal EEG spikes — see Epilepsy, localization-related, idiopathic
  benign myoclonic in infancy G40.80- ☑
  Bravais-jacksonian — see Epilepsy, localization-related, symptomatic, with simple partial seizures
  childhood
   with occipital EEG paroxysms — see Epilepsy, localization-related, idiopathic
   absence G40.A09
    intractable G40.A19
     with status epilepticus G40.A11
     without status epilepticus G40.A19
    not intractable G40.A09
     with status epilepticus G40.A01
     without status epilepticus G40.A09
  climacteric — see Epilepsy, specified NEC
  cysticercosis B69.0
  deterioration (mental) F06.8
  due to syphilis A52.19
  focal — see Epilepsy, localization-related, symptomatic, with simple partial seizures
  generalized
   idiopathic G40.309
    intractable G40.319
     with status epilepticus G40.311
     without status epilepticus G40.319
    not intractable G40.309
     with status epilepticus G40.301
     without status epilepticus G40.309
   specified NEC G40.409
    intractable G40.419
     with status epilepticus G40.411
     without status epilepticus G40.419
    not intractable G40.409
     with status epilepticus G40.401
     without status epilepticus G40.409
  impulsive petit mal — see Epilepsy, juvenile myoclonic
  intractable G40.919
   with status epilepticus G40.911
   without status epilepticus G40.919
  juvenile absence G40.A09
   intractable G40.A19
    with status epilepticus G40.A11
    without status epilepticus G40.A19
   not intractable G40.A09
    with status epilepticus G40.A01
    without status epilepticus G40.A09
  juvenile myoclonic G40.B09
   intractable G40.B19
    with status epilepticus G40.B11
    without status epilepticus G40.B19
   not intractable G40.B09
    with status epilepticus G40.B01
    without status epilepticus G40.B09

Epilepsy — continued
  localization-related (focal) (partial)
   idiopathic G40.009
    with seizures of localized onset G40.009
     intractable G40.019
      with status epilepticus G40.011
      without status epilepticus G40.019
     not intractable G40.009
      with status epilepticus G40.001
      without status epilepticus G40.009
   symptomatic
    with complex partial seizures G40.209
     intractable G40.219
      with status epilepticus G40.211
      without status epilepticus G40.219
     not intractable G40.209
      with status epilepticus G40.201
      without status epilepticus G40.209
    with simple partial seizures G40.109
     intractable G40.119
      with status epilepticus G40.111
      without status epilepticus G40.119
     not intractable G40.109
      with status epilepticus G40.101
      without status epilepticus G40.109
  myoclonus, myoclonic (progressive) — see Epilepsy, generalized, specified NEC
  not intractable G40.909
   with status epilepticus G40.901
   without status epilepticus G40.909
  on awakening — see Epilepsy, generalized, specified NEC
  parasitic NOS B71.9 [G94]
  partialis continua (see also Kozhevnikof's epilepsy) G40.1- ☑
  peripheral — see Epilepsy, specified NEC
  procursiva — see Epilepsy, localization-related, symptomatic, with simple partial seizures
  progressive (familial) myoclonic — see Epilepsy, generalized, idiopathic
  reflex — see Epilepsy, specified NEC
  related to
   alcohol G40.509
    not intractable G40.509
     with status epilepticus G40.501
     without status epliepticus G40.509
   drugs G40.509
    not intractable G40.509
     with status epilepticus G40.501
     without status epliepticus G40.509
   external causes G40.509
    not intractable G40.509
     with status epilepticus G40.501
     without status epliepticus G40.509
   hormonal changes G40.509
    not intractable G40.509
     with status epilepticus G40.501
     without status epliepticus G40.509
   sleep deprivation G40.509
    not intractable G40.509
     with status epilepticus G40.501
     without status epliepticus G40.509
   stress G40.509
    not intractable G40.509
     with status epilepticus G40.501
     without status epliepticus G40.509
  somatomotor — see Epilepsy, localization-related, symptomatic, with simple partial seizures
  somatosensory — see Epilepsy, localization-related, symptomatic, with simple partial seizures
  spasms G40.822
   intractable G40.824
    with status epilepticus G40.823
    without status epilepticus G40.824
   not intractable G40.822
    with status epilepticus G40.821
    without status epilepticus G40.822
  specified NEC G40.802
   intractable G40.804
    with status epilepticus G40.803
    without status epilepticus G40.804
   not intractable G40.802
    with status epilepticus G40.801
    without status epilepticus G40.802
  syndromes
   generalized
    idiopathic G40.309
     intractable G40.319
      with status epilepticus G40.311
      without status epilepticus G40.319
     not intractable G40.309

☑ **Additional character required**

Epilepsy — *continued*
  with status epilepticus G40.301
  without status epilepticus G40.309
  specified NEC G40.409
    intractable G40.419
      with status epilepticus G40.411
      without status epilepticus G40.419
    not intractable G40.409
      with status epilepticus G40.401
      without status epilepticus G40.409
  localization-related (focal) (partial)
    idiopathic G40.009
      with seizures of localized onset G40.009
        intractable G40.019
          with status epilepticus G40.011
          without status epilepticus G40.019
        not intractable G40.009
          with status epilepticus G40.001
          without status epilepticus G40.009
    symptomatic
      with complex partial seizures G40.209
        intractable G40.219
          with status epilepticus G40.211
          without status epilepticus G40.219
        not intractable G40.209
          with status epilepticus G40.201
          without status epilepticus G40.209
      with simple partial seizures G40.109
        intractable G40.119
          with status epilepticus G40.111
          without status epilepticus G40.119
        not intractable G40.109
          with status epilepticus G40.101
          without status epilepticus G40.109
  specified NEC G40.802
    intractable G40.804
      with status epilepticus G40.803
      without status epilepticus G40.804
    not intractable G40.802
      with status epilepticus G40.801
      without status epilepticus G40.802
  tonic (-clonic) — *see* Epilepsy, generalized, specified NEC
  twilight F05
  uncinate (gyrus) — *see* Epilepsy, localization-related, symptomatic, with complex partial seizures
  Unverricht (-Lundborg) (familial myoclonic) — *see* Epilepsy, generalized, idiopathic
  visceral — *see* Epilepsy, specified NEC
  visual — *see* Epilepsy, specified NEC
Epiloia Q85.1
Epimenorrhea N92.0
Epipharyngitis — *see* Nasopharyngitis
Epiphora H04.20- ☑
  due to
    excess lacrimation H04.21- ☑
    insufficient drainage H04.22- ☑
Epiphyseal arrest — *see* Arrest, epiphyseal
Epiphyseolysis, epiphysiolysis — *see* Osteochondropathy
Epiphysitis (*see also* Osteochondropathy)
  juvenile M92.9
  syphilitic (congenital) A50.02
Epiplocele — *see* Hernia, abdomen
Epiploitis — *see* Peritonitis
Epiplosarcomphalocele — *see* Hernia, umbilicus
Episcleritis (suppurative) H15.10- ☑
  in (due to)
    syphilis A52.71
    tuberculosis A18.51
  nodular H15.12- ☑
  periodica fugax H15.11- ☑
    angioneurotic — *see* Edema, angioneurotic
  syphilitic (late) A52.71
  tuberculous A18.51
Episode
  affective, mixed F39
  depersonalization (in neurotic state) F48.1
  depressive F32.9
    major F32.9
      mild F32.0
      moderate F32.1
      severe (without psychotic symptoms) F32.2
        with psychotic symptoms F32.3
    recurrent F33.9
      brief F33.8
    specified NEC F32.8
  hypomanic F30.8
  manic F30.9
    with
      psychotic symptoms F30.2

Episode — *continued*
  remission (full) F30.4
    partial F30.3
  other specified F30.8
  recurrent F31.89
  without psychotic symptoms F30.10
    mild F30.11
    moderate F30.12
    severe (without psychotic symptoms) F30.13
      with psychotic symptoms F30.2
  psychotic F23
    organic F06.8
  schizophrenic (acute) NEC, brief F23
Epispadias (female) (male) Q64.0
Episplenitis D73.89
Epistaxis (multiple) R04.0
  hereditary I78.0
  vicarious menstruation N94.89
Epithelioma (malignant) — *see also* Neoplasm, malignant, by site
  adenoides cysticum — *see* Neoplasm, skin, benign
  basal cell — *see* Neoplasm, skin, malignant
  benign — *see* Neoplasm, benign, by site
  Bowen's — *see* Neoplasm, skin, in situ
  calcifying, of Malherbe — *see* Neoplasm, skin, benign
  external site — *see* Neoplasm, skin, malignant
  intraepidermal, Jadassohn — *see* Neoplasm, skin, benign
  squamous cell — *see* Neoplasm, malignant, by site
Epitheliomatosis pigmented Q82.1
Epitheliopathy, multifocal placoid pigment H30.14- ☑
Epithelium, epithelial — *see* condition
Epituberculosis (with atelectasis) (allergic) A15.7
Eponychia Q84.6
Epstein's
  nephrosis or syndrome — *see* Nephrosis
  pearl K09.8
Epulis (gingiva) (fibrous) (giant cell) K06.8
Equinia A24.0
Equinovarus (congenital) (talipes) Q66.0
  acquired — *see* Deformity, limb, clubfoot
Equivalent
  convulsive (abdominal) — *see* Epilepsy, specified NEC
  epileptic (psychic) — *see* Epilepsy, localization-related, symptomatic, with complex partial seizures
Erb (-Duchenne) paralysis (birth injury) (newborn) P14.0
Erb-Goldflam disease or syndrome G70.00
  with exacerbation (acute) G70.01
  in crisis G70.01
Erb's
  disease G71.0
  palsy, paralysis (brachial) (birth) (newborn) P14.0
  spinal (spastic) syphilitic A52.17
  pseudohypertrophic muscular dystrophy G71.0
Erdheim's syndrome (acromegalic macrospondylitis) E22.0
Erection, painful (persistent) — *see* Priapism
Ergosterol deficiency (vitamin D) E55.9
  with
    adult osteomalacia M83.8
    rickets — *see* Rickets
Ergotism (*see also* Poisoning, food, noxious, plant)
  from ergot used as drug (migraine therapy) — *see* Table of Drugs and Chemicals
Erosio interdigitalis blastomycetica B37.2
Erosion
  artery I77.2
    without rupture I77.89
  bone — *see* Disorder, bone, density and structure, specified NEC
  bronchus J98.09
  cartilage (joint) — *see* Disorder, cartilage, specified type NEC
  cervix (uteri) (acquired) (chronic) (congenital) N86
    with cervicitis N72
  cornea (nontraumatic) — *see* Ulcer, cornea
    recurrent H18.83- ☑
    traumatic — *see* Abrasion, cornea
  dental (idiopathic) (occupational) (due to diet, drugs or vomiting) K03.2
  duodenum, postpyloric — *see* Ulcer, duodenum
  esophagus K22.10
    with bleeding K22.11
  gastric — *see* Ulcer, stomach

Erosion — *continued*
  gastrojejunal — *see* Ulcer, gastrojejunal
  implanted mesh — *see* Complications, mesh
  intestine K63.3
  lymphatic vessel I89.8
  pylorus, pyloric (ulcer) — *see* Ulcer, stomach
  spine, aneurysmal A52.09
  stomach — *see* Ulcer, stomach
  teeth (idiopathic) (occupational) (due to diet, drugs or vomiting) K03.2
  urethra N36.8
  uterus N85.8
Erotomania F52.8
Error
  metabolism, inborn -- se Disorder, metabolism
  refractive — *see* Disorder, refraction
Eructation R14.2
  nervous or psychogenic F45.8
Eruption
  creeping B76.9
  drug (generalized) (taken internally) L27.0
    fixed L27.1
    in contact with skin — *see* Dermatitis, due to drugs
    localized L27.1
  Hutchinson, summer L56.4
  Kaposi's varicelliform B00.0
  napkin L22
  polymorphous light (sun) L56.4
  recalcitrant pustular L13.8
  ringed R23.8
  skin (nonspecific) R21
    creeping (meaning hookworm) B76.9
    due to inoculation/vaccination (generalized) (*see also* Dermatitis, due to, vaccine) L27.0
      localized L27.1
    erysipeloid A26.0
    feigned L98.1
    Kaposi's varicelliform B00.0
    lichenoid L28.0
    meaning dermatitis — *see* Dermatitis
    toxic NEC L53.0
  tooth, teeth, abnormal (incomplete) (late) (premature) (sequence) K00.6
  vesicular R23.8
Erysipelas (gangrenous) (infantile) (newborn) (phlegmonous) (suppurative) A46
  external ear A46 [H62.40]
  puerperal, postpartum O86.89
Erysipeloid A26.9
  cutaneous (Rosenbach's) A26.0
  disseminated A26.8
  sepsis A26.7
  specified NEC A26.8
Erythema, erythematous (infectional) (inflammation) L53.9
  ab igne L59.0
  annulare (centrifugum) (rheumaticum) L53.1
  arthriticum epidemicum A25.1
  brucellum — *see* Brucellosis
  chronic figurate NEC L53.3
  chronicum migrans (Borrelia burgdorferi) A69.20
  diaper L22
  due to
    chemical NEC L53.0
      in contact with skin L24.5
    drug (internal use) — *see* Dermatitis, due to, drugs
  elevatum diutinum L95.1
  endemic E52
  epidemic, arthritic A25.1
  figuratum perstans L53.3
  gluteal L22
  heat - code by site under Burn, first degree
  ichthyosiforme congenitum bullous Q80.3
  in diseases classified elsewhere L54
  induratum (nontuberculous) L52
    tuberculous A18.4
  infectiosum B08.3
  intertrigo L30.4
  iris L51.9
  marginatum L53.2
    in (due to) acute rheumatic fever I00
  medicamentosum — *see* Dermatitis, due to, drugs
  migrans A26.0
    chronicum A69.20
    tongue K14.1
  multiforme (major) (minor) L51.9
    bullous, bullosum L51.1
    conjunctiva L51.1
    nonbullous L51.0

Erythema — *continued*
  pemphigoides L12.0
    specified NEC L51.8
  napkin L22
  neonatorum P83.8
    toxic P83.1
  nodosum L52
    tuberculous A18.4
  palmar L53.8
  pernio T69.1 ☑
  rash, newborn P83.8
  scarlatiniform (recurrent) (exfoliative) L53.8
  solare L55.0
  specified NEC L53.8
  toxic, toxicum NEC L53.0
    newborn P83.1
  tuberculous (primary) A18.4
Erythematous, erythematosus — *see* condition
Erythermalgia (primary) I73.81
Erythralgia I73.81
Erythrasma L08.1
Erythredema (polyneuropathy) — *see* Poisoning, mercury
Erythremia (acute) C94.0- ☑
  chronic D45
  secondary D75.1
Erythroblastopenia (*see also* Aplasia, red cell) D60.9
  congenital D61.01
Erythroblastophthisis D61.09
Erythroblastosis (fetalis) (newborn) P55.9
  due to
    ABO (antibodies) (incompatibility) (isoimmunization) P55.1
    Rh (antibodies) (incompatibility) (isoimmunization) P55.0
Erythrocyanosis (crurum) I73.89
Erythrocythemia — *see* Erythremia
Erythrocytosis (megalosplenic) (secondary) D75.1
  familial D75.0
  oval, hereditary — *see* Elliptocytosis
  secondary D75.1
  stress D75.1
Erythroderma (secondary) (*see also* Erythema) L53.9
  bullous ichthyosiform, congenital Q80.3
  desquamativum L21.1
  ichthyosiform, congenital (bullous) Q80.3
  neonatorum P83.8
  psoriaticum L40.8
Erythrodysesthesia, palmar plantar (PPE) L27.1
Erythrogenesis imperfecta D61.09
Erythroleukemia C94.0- ☑
Erythromelalgia I73.81
Erythrophagocytosis D75.89
Erythrophobia F40.298
Erythroplakia, oral epithelium, and tongue K13.29
Erythroplasia (Queyrat) D07.4
  specified site — *see* Neoplasm, skin, in situ
  unspecified site D07.4
Escherichia coli (E. coli), as cause of disease classified elsewhere B96.20
  non-O157 Shiga toxin-producing (with known O group) B96.22
  non-Shiga toxin-producing B96.29
  O157 with confirmation of Shiga toxin when H antigen is unknown, or is not H7 B96.21
  O157:H- (nonmotile) with confirmation of Shiga toxin B96.21
  O157:H7 with or without confirmation of Shiga toxin-production B96.21
  Shiga toxin-producing (with unspecified O group) (STEC) B96.23
  O157 B96.21
  O157:H7 with or without confirmation of Shiga toxin-production B96.21
    specified NEC B96.22
  specified NEC B96.29
Esophagismus K22.4
Esophagitis (acute) (alkaline) (chemical) (chronic) (infectional) (necrotic) (peptic) (postoperative) K20.9
  candidal B37.81
  due to gastrointestinal reflux disease K21.0
  eosinophilic K20.0
  reflux K21.0
  specified NEC K20.8
  tuberculous A18.83
  ulcerative K22.10
    with bleeding K22.11
Esophagocele K22.5
Esophagomalacia K22.8
Esophagospasm K22.4
Esophagostenosis K22.2

Esophagostomiasis B81.8
Esophagotracheal — *see* condition
Esophagus — *see* condition
Esophoria H50.51
  convergence, excess H51.12
  divergence, insufficiency H51.8
Esotropia — *see* Strabismus, convergent concomitant
Espundia B55.2
Essential — *see* condition
Esthesioneuroblastoma C30.0
Esthesioneurocytoma C30.0
Esthesioneuroepithelioma C30.0
Esthiomene A55
Estivo-autumnal malaria (fever) B50.9
Estrangement (marital) Z63.5
  parent-child NEC Z62.890
Estriasis — *see* Myiasis
Ethanolism — *see* Alcoholism
Etherism — *see* Dependence, drug, inhalant
Ethmoid, ethmoidal — *see* condition
Ethmoiditis (chronic) (nonpurulent) (purulent) (*see also* Sinusitis, ethmoidal)
  influenzal — *see* Influenza, with, respiratory manifestations NEC
  Woakes' J33.1
Ethylism — *see* Alcoholism
Eulenburg's disease (congenital paramyotonia) G71.19
Eumycetoma B47.0
Eunuchoidism E29.1
  hypogonadotropic E23.0
European blastomycosis — *see* Cryptococcosis
Eustachian — *see* condition
Evaluation (for) (of)
  development state
    adolescent Z00.3
    period of
      delayed growth in childhood Z00.70
        with abnormal findings Z00.71
      rapid growth in childhood Z00.2
    puberty Z00.3
  growth and developmental state (period of rapid growth) Z00.2
    delayed growth Z00.70
      with abnormal findings Z00.71
  mental health (status) Z00.8
    requested by authority Z04.6
  period of
    delayed growth in childhood Z00.70
      with abnormal findings Z00.71
    rapid growth in childhood Z00.2
  suspected condition — *see* Observation
Evans syndrome D69.41
Event, apparent life threatening in newborn and infant (ALTE) R68.13
Eventration (*see also* Hernia, ventral)
  colon into chest — *see* Hernia, diaphragm
  diaphragm (congenital) Q79.1
Eversion
  bladder N32.89
  cervix (uteri) N86
    with cervicitis N72
  foot NEC (*see also* Deformity, valgus, ankle)
    congenital Q66.6
  punctum lacrimale (postinfectional) (senile) H04.52- ☑
  ureter (meatus) N28.89
  urethra (meatus) N36.8
  uterus N81.4
Evidence
  cytologic
    of malignancy on anal smear R85.614
    of malignancy on cervical smear R87.614
    of malignancy on vaginal smear R87.624
Evisceration
  birth injury P15.8
  traumatic NEC
    eye — *see* Enucleated eye
Evulsion — *see* Avulsion
Ewing's sarcoma or tumor - — *see* Neoplasm, bone, malignant
Examination (for) (following) (general) (of) (routine) Z00.00
  with abnormal findings Z00.01
  abuse, physical (alleged), ruled out
    adult Z04.71
    child Z04.72
  adolescent (development state) Z00.3
  alleged rape or sexual assault (victim), ruled out
    adult Z04.41
    child Z04.42

Examination — *continued*
  allergy Z01.82
  annual (adult) (periodic) (physical) Z00.00
    with abnormal findings Z00.01
    gynecological Z01.419
      with abnormal findings Z01.411
  antibody response Z01.84
  blood — *see* Examination, laboratory
  blood pressure Z01.30
    with abnormal findings Z01.31
  cancer staging — *see* Neoplasm, malignant, by site
  cervical Papanicolaou smear Z12.4
    as part of routine gynecological examination Z01.419
    with abnormal findings Z01.411
  child (over 28 days old) Z00.129
    with abnormal findings Z00.121
    under 28 days old — *see* Newborn, examination
  clinical research control or normal comparison (control) (participant) Z00.6
  contraceptive (drug) maintenance (routine) Z30.8
    device (intrauterine) Z30.431
  dental Z01.20
    with abnormal findings Z01.21
  developmental — *see* Examination, child
  donor (potential) Z00.5
  ear Z01.10
    with abnormal findings NEC Z01.118
  eye Z01.00
    with abnormal findings Z01.01
  following
    accident NEC Z04.3
      transport Z04.1
      work Z04.2
    assault, alleged, ruled out
      adult Z04.71
      child Z04.72
    motor vehicle accident Z04.1
    treatment (for) Z09
      combined NEC Z09
        fracture Z09
        malignant neoplasm Z08
      malignant neoplasm Z08
      mental disorder Z09
      specified condition NEC Z09
  follow-up (routine) (following) Z09
    chemotherapy NEC Z09
      malignant neoplasm Z08
    fracture Z09
    malignant neoplasm Z08
    postpartum Z39.2
    psychotherapy Z09
    radiotherapy NEC Z09
      malignant neoplasm Z08
    surgery NEC Z09
      malignant neoplasm Z08
  gynecological Z01.419
    with abnormal findings Z01.411
    for contraceptive maintenance Z30.8
  health — *see* Examination, medical
  hearing Z01.10
    with abnormal findings NEC Z01.118
    following failed hearing screening Z01.110
  immunity status testing Z01.84
  laboratory (as part of a general medical examination) Z00.00
    with abnormal findings Z00.01
    preprocedural Z01.812
  lactating mother Z39.1
  medical (adult) (for) (of) Z00.00
    with abnormal findings Z00.01
    administrative purpose only Z02.9
      specified NEC Z02.89
    admission to
      armed forces Z02.3
      old age home Z02.2
      prison Z02.89
      residential institution Z02.2
      school Z02.0
        following illness or medical treatment Z02.0
      summer camp Z02.89
    adoption Z02.82
    blood alcohol or drug level Z02.83
    camp (summer) Z02.89
    clinical research, normal subject (control) (participant) Z00.6
    control subject in clinical research (normal comparison) (participant) Z00.6
    donor (potential) Z00.5
    driving license Z02.4

☑ **Additional character required**

Examination — *continued*
  general (adult) Z00.00
    with abnormal findings Z00.01
  immigration Z02.89
  insurance purposes Z02.6
  marriage Z02.89
  medicolegal reasons NEC Z04.8
  naturalization Z02.89
  participation in sport Z02.5
  paternity testing Z02.81
  population survey Z00.8
  pre-employment Z02.1
  pre-operative — *see* Examination, pre-
      procedural
  pre-procedural
    cardiovascular Z01.810
    respiratory Z01.811
    specified NEC Z01.818
  preschool children
    for admission to school Z02.0
  prisoners
    for entrance into prison Z02.89
  recruitment for armed forces Z02.3
  specified NEC Z00.8
  sport competition Z02.5
  medicolegal reason NEC Z04.8
  newborn — *see* Newborn, examination
  pelvic (annual) (periodic) Z01.419
    with abnormal findings Z01.411
  period of rapid growth in childhood Z00.2
  periodic (adult) (annual) (routine) Z00.00
    with abnormal findings Z00.01
  physical (adult) (*see also* Examination, medical
      Z00.00)
    sports Z02.5
  postpartum
    immediately after delivery Z39.0
    routine follow-up Z39.2
  prenatal (normal pregnancy) (*see also* Pregnancy,
      normal) Z34.9- ☑
  pre-chemotherapy (antineoplastic) Z01.818
  pre-procedural (pre-operative)
    cardiovascular Z01.810
    laboratory Z01.812
    respiratory Z01.811
    specified NEC Z01.818
  prior to chemotherapy (antineoplastic) Z01.818
  psychiatric NEC Z00.8
    follow-up not needing further care Z09
    requested by authority Z04.6
  radiological (as part of a general medical
      examination) Z00.00
    with abnormal findings Z00.01
  repeat cervical smear to confirm findings
      of recent normal smear following initial
      abnormal smear Z01.42
  skin (hypersensitivity) Z01.82
  special (*see also* Examination, by type) Z01.89
    specified type NEC Z01.89
  specified type or reason NEC Z04.8
  teeth Z01.20
    with abnormal findings Z01.21
  urine — *see* Examination, laboratory
  vision Z01.00
    with abnormal findings Z01.01
Exanthem, exanthema (*see also* Rash)
  with enteroviral vesicular stomatitis B08.4
  Boston A88.0
  epidemic with meningitis A88.0 [G02]
  subitum B08.20
    due to human herpesvirus 6 B08.21
    due to human herpesvirus 7 B08.22
  viral, virus B09
    specified type NEC B08.8
Excess, excessive, excessively
  alcohol level in blood R78.0
  androgen (ovarian) E28.1
  attrition, tooth, teeth K03.0
  carotene, carotin (dietary) E67.1
  cold, effects of T69.9 ☑
    specified effect NEC T69.8 ☑
  convergence H51.12
  crying
    in child, adolescent, or adult R45.83
    in infant R68.11
  development, breast N62
  divergence H51.8
  drinking (alcohol) NEC (without dependence)
      F10.10
    habitual (continual) (without remission) F10.20
  eating R63.2
  estrogen E28.0

Excess — *continued*
  fat (*see also* Obesity)
    in heart — *see* Degeneration, myocardial
    localized E65
  foreskin N47.8
  gas R14.0
  glucagon E16.3
  heat — *see* Heat
  intermaxillary vertical dimension of fully erupted
      teeth M26.37
  interocclusal distance of fully erupted teeth
      M26.37
  kalium E87.5
  large
    colon K59.3
      congenital Q43.8
    infant P08.0
    organ or site, congenital NEC — *see* Anomaly,
        by site
  long
    organ or site, congenital NEC — *see* Anomaly,
        by site
  menstruation (with regular cycle) N92.0
    with irregular cycle N92.1
  napping Z72.821
  natrium E87.0
  number of teeth K00.1
  nutrient (dietary) NEC R63.2
  potassium (K) E87.5
  salivation K11.7
  secretion (*see also* Hypersecretion)
    milk O92.6
    sputum R09.3
    sweat R61
  sexual drive F52.8
  short
    organ or site, congenital NEC — *see* Anomaly,
        by site
    umbilical cord in labor or delivery O69.3 ☑
  skin, eyelid (acquired) — *see* Blepharochalasis
    congenital Q10.3
  sodium (Na) E87.0
  spacing of fully erupted teeth M26.32
  sputum R09.3
  sweating R61
  thirst R63.1
    due to deprivation of water T73.1 ☑
  tuberosity of jaw M26.07
  vitamin
    A (dietary) E67.0
      administered as drug (prolonged intake)
          — *see* Table of Drugs and Chemicals,
          vitamins, adverse effect
      overdose or wrong substance given or taken
          — *see* Table of Drugs and Chemicals,
          vitamins, poisoning
    D (dietary) E67.3
      administered as drug (prolonged intake)
          — *see* Table of Drugs and Chemicals,
          vitamins, adverse effect
      overdose or wrong substance given or taken
          — *see* Table of Drugs and Chemicals,
          vitamins, poisoning
  weight
    gain R63.5
    loss R63.4
Excitability, abnormal, under minor stress
  (personality disorder) F60.3
Excitation
  anomalous atrioventricular I45.6
  psychogenic F30.8
  reactive (from emotional stress, psychological
      trauma) F30.8
Excitement
  hypomanic F30.8
  manic F30.9
  mental, reactive (from emotional stress,
      psychological trauma) F30.8
  state, reactive (from emotional stress,
      psychological trauma) F30.8
Excoriation (traumatic) (*see also* Abrasion)
  neurotic L98.1
Exfoliation
  due to erythematous conditions according to
      extent of body surface involved L49.0
    10-19 percent of body surface L49.1
    20-29 percent of body surface L49.2
    30-39 percent of body surface L49.3
    40-49 percent of body surface L49.4
    50-59 percent of body surface L49.5
    60-69 percent of body surface L49.6
    70-79 percent of body surface L49.7

Exfoliation — *continued*
    80-89 percent of body surface L49.8
    90-99 percent of body surface L49.9
    less than 10 percent of body surface L49.0
  teeth, due to systemic causes K08.0
Exfoliative — *see* condition
Exhaustion, exhaustive (physical NEC) R53.83
  battle F43.0
  cardiac — *see* Failure, heart
  delirium F43.0
  due to
    cold T69.8 ☑
    excessive exertion T73.3 ☑
    exposure T73.2 ☑
    neurasthenia F48.8
  heart — *see* Failure, heart
  heat (*see also* Heat, exhaustion) T67.5 ☑
    due to
      salt depletion T67.4 ☑
      water depletion T67.3 ☑
  maternal, complicating delivery O75.81
  mental F48.8
  myocardium, myocardial — *see* Failure, heart
  nervous F48.8
  old age R54
  psychogenic F48.8
  psychosis F43.0
  senile R54
  vital NEC Z73.0
Exhibitionism F65.2
Exocervicitis — *see* Cervicitis
Exomphalos Q79.2
  meaning hernia — *see* Hernia, umbilicus
Exophoria H50.52
  convergence, insufficiency H51.11
  divergence, excess H51.8
Exophthalmos H05.2- ☑
  congenital Q15.8
  constant NEC H05.24- ☑
  displacement, globe — *see* Displacement, globe
  due to thyrotoxicosis (hyperthyroidism) — *see*
      Hyperthyroidism, with, goiter (diffuse)
  dysthyroid — *see* Hyperthyroidism, with, goiter
      (diffuse)
  goiter — *see* Hyperthyroidism, with, goiter
      (diffuse)
  intermittent NEC H05.25- ☑
  malignant — *see* Hyperthyroidism, with, goiter
      (diffuse)
  orbital
    edema — *see* Edema, orbit
    hemorrhage — *see* Hemorrhage, orbit
  pulsating NEC H05.26- ☑
  thyrotoxic, thyrotropic — *see* Hyperthyroidism,
      with, goiter (diffuse)
Exostosis (*see also* Disorder, bone)
  cartilaginous — *see* Neoplasm, bone, benign
  congenital (multiple) Q78.6
  external ear canal H61.81- ☑
  gonococcal A54.49
  jaw (bone) M27.8
  multiple, congenital Q78.6
  orbit H05.35- ☑
  osteocartilaginous — *see* Neoplasm, bone,
      benign
  syphilitic A52.77
Exotropia — *see* Strabismus, divergent concomitant
Explanation of
  investigation finding Z71.2
  medication Z71.89
Exposure (to) (*see also* Contact, with) T75.89 ☑
  acariasis Z20.7
  AIDS virus Z20.6
  air pollution Z77.110
  algae and algae toxins Z77.121
  algae bloom Z77.121
  anthrax Z20.810
  aromatic amines Z77.020
  aromatic (hazardous) compounds NEC Z77.028
  aromatic dyes NOS Z77.028
  arsenic Z77.010
  asbestos Z77.090
  bacterial disease NEC Z20.818
  benzene Z77.021
  blue-green algae bloom Z77.121
  body fluids (potentially hazardous) Z77.21
  brown tide Z77.121
  chemicals (chiefly nonmedicinal) (hazardous)
      NEC Z77.098
  cholera Z20.09
  chromium compounds Z77.018
  cold, effects of T69.9 ☑

Exposure — *continued*
  specified effect NEC T69.8 ☑
  communicable disease Z20.9
    bacterial NEC Z20.818
    specified NEC Z20.89
    viral NEC Z20.828
  cyanobacteria bloom Z77.121
  disaster Z65.5
  discrimination Z60.5
  dyes Z77.098
  effects of T73.9 ☑
  environmental tobacco smoke (acute) (chronic) Z77.22
  Escherichia coli (E. coli) Z20.01
  exhaustion due to T73.2 ☑
  fiberglass — *see* Table of Drugs and Chemicals, fiberglass
  German measles Z20.4
  gonorrhea Z20.2
  hazardous metals NEC Z77.018
  hazardous substances NEC Z77.29
  hazards in the physical environment NEC Z77.128
  hazards to health NEC Z77.9
  human immunodeficiency virus (HIV) Z20.6
  human T-lymphotropic virus type-1 (HTLV-1) Z20.89
  implanted
    mesh — *see* Complications, mesh
    prosthetic materials NEC — *see* Complications, prosthetic materials NEC
  infestation (parasitic) NEC Z20.7
  intestinal infectious disease NEC Z20.09
    Escherichia coli (E. coli) Z20.01
  lead Z77.011
  meningococcus Z20.811
  mold (toxic) Z77.120
  nickel dust Z77.018
  noise Z77.122
  occupational
    air contaminants NEC Z57.39
    dust Z57.2
    environmental tobacco smoke Z57.31
    extreme temperature Z57.6
    noise Z57.0
    radiation Z57.1
    risk factors Z57.9
      specified NEC Z57.8
    toxic agents (gases) (liquids) (solids) (vapors) in agriculture Z57.4
    toxic agents (gases) (liquids) (solids) (vapors) in industry NEC Z57.5
    vibration Z57.7
  parasitic disease NEC Z20.7
  pediculosis Z20.7
  persecution Z60.5
  pfiesteria piscicida Z77.121
  poliomyelitis Z20.89
  polycyclic aromatic hydrocarbons Z77.028
  pollution
    air Z77.110
    environmental NEC Z77.118
    soil Z77.112
    water Z77.111
  prenatal (drugs) (toxic chemicals) — *see* Newborn, affected by (suspected to be), noxious substances transmitted via placenta or breast milk
  rabies Z20.3
  radiation, naturally occurring NEC Z77.123
  radon Z77.123
  red tide (Florida) Z77.121
  rubella Z20.4
  second hand tobacco smoke (acute) (chronic) Z77.22
    in the perinatal period P96.81
  sexually-transmitted disease Z20.2
  smallpox (laboratory) Z20.89
  syphilis Z20.2
  terrorism Z65.4
  torture Z65.4
  tuberculosis Z20.1
  uranium Z77.012
  varicella Z20.820
  venereal disease Z20.2
  viral disease NEC Z20.828
  war Z65.5
  water pollution Z77.111
Exsanguination — *see* Hemorrhage
Exstrophy
  abdominal contents Q45.8
  bladder Q64.10
    cloacal Q64.12

Exstrophy — *continued*
  specified type NEC Q64.19
  supravesical fissure Q64.11
Extensive — *see* condition
Extra (*see also* Accessory)
  marker chromosomes (normal individual) Q92.61
    in abnormal individual Q92.62
  rib Q76.6
    cervical Q76.5
Extrasystoles (supraventricular) I49.49
  atrial I49.1
  auricular I49.1
  junctional I49.2
  ventricular I49.3
Extrauterine gestation or pregnancy - — *see* Pregnancy, by site
Extravasation
  blood R58
  chyle into mesentery I89.8
  pelvicalyceal N13.8
  pyelosinus N13.8
  urine (from ureter) R39.0
  vesicant agent
    antineoplastic chemotherapy T80.810 ☑
    other agent NEC T80.818 ☑
Extremity — *see* condition, limb
Extrophy — *see* Exstrophy
Extroversion
  bladder Q64.19
  uterus N81.4
    complicating delivery O71.2
    postpartal (old) N81.4
Extruded tooth (teeth) M26.34
Extrusion
  breast implant (prosthetic) T85.42 ☑
  eye implant (globe) (ball) T85.328 ☑
  intervertebral disc — *see* Displacement, intervertebral disc
  ocular lens implant (prosthetic) — *see* Complications, intraocular lens
  vitreous — *see* Prolapse, vitreous
Exudate
  pleural — *see* Effusion, pleura
  retina H35.89
Exudative — *see* condition
Eye, eyeball, eyelid — *see* condition
Eyestrain — *see* Disturbance, vision, subjective
Eyeworm disease of Africa B74.3

F

Faber's syndrome (achlorhydric anemia) D50.9
Fabry (-Anderson) disease E75.21
Faciocephalalgia, autonomic (*see also* Neuropathy, peripheral, autonomic) G90.09
Factor (s)
  psychic, associated with diseases classified elsewhere F54
  psychological
    affecting physical conditions F54
    or behavioral
      affecting general medical condition F54
      associated with disorders or diseases classified elsewhere F54
Fahr disease (of brain) G23.8
Fahr Volhard disease (of kidney) I12.- ☑
Failure, failed
  abortion — *see* Abortion, attempted
  aortic (valve) I35.8
    rheumatic I06.8
  attempted abortion — *see* Abortion, attempted
  biventricular I50.9
  bone marrow — *see* Anemia, aplastic
  cardiac — *see* Failure, heart
  cardiorenal (chronic) I50.9
    hypertensive I13.2
  cardiorespiratory (*see also* Failure, heart) R09.2
  cardiovascular (chronic) — *see* Failure, heart
  cerebrovascular I67.9
  cervical dilatation in labor O62.0
  circulation, circulatory (peripheral) R57.9
    newborn P29.89
  compensation — *see* Disease, heart
  compliance with medical treatment or regimen — *see* Noncompliance
  congestive — *see* Failure, heart, congestive
  dental implant (endosseous) M27.69
    due to
      failure of dental prosthesis M27.63

Failure — *continued*
  lack of attached gingiva M27.62
  occlusal trauma (poor prosthetic design) M27.62
  parafunctional habits M27.62
  periodontal infection (peri-implantitis) M27.62
  poor oral hygiene M27.62
  osseointegration M27.61
    due to
      complications of systemic disease M27.61
      poor bone quality M27.61
    iatrogenic M27.61
    post-osseointegration
      biological M27.62
      due to complications of systemic disease M27.62
      iatrogenic M27.62
      mechanical M27.63
    pre-integration M27.61
    pre-osseointegration M27.61
  specified NEC M27.69
  descent of head (at term) of pregnancy (mother) O32.4 ☑
  endosseous dental implant — *see* Failure, dental implant
  engagement of head (term of pregnancy) (mother) O32.4 ☑
  erection (penile) (*see also* Dysfunction, sexual, male, erectile) N52.9
    nonorgqanic F52.21
  examination (s), anxiety concerning Z55.2
  expansion terminal respiratory units (newborn) (primary) P28.0
  forceps NOS (with subsequent cesarean delivery) O66.5
  gain weight (child over 28 days old) R62.51
    adult R62.7
    newborn P92.6
  genital response (male) F52.21
    female F52.22
  heart (acute) (senile) (sudden) I50.9
    with
      acute pulmonary edema — *see* Failure, ventricular, left
      decompensation — *see* Failure, heart, congestive
      dilatation — *see* Disease, heart
    arteriosclerotic I70.90
    biventricular I50.9
    combined left-right sided I50.9
    compensated I50.9
    complicating
      anesthesia (general) (local) or other sedation in labor and delivery O74.2
        in pregnancy O29.12- ☑
        postpartum, puerperal O89.1
      delivery (cesarean) (instrumental) O75.4
    congestive (compensated) (decompensated) I50.9
      with rheumatic fever (conditions in I00)
        active I01.8
        inactive or quiescent (with chorea) I09.81
      newborn P29.0
      rheumatic (chronic) (inactive) (with chorea) I09.81
        active or acute I01.8
        with chorea I02.0
    decompensated I50.9
    degenerative — *see* Degeneration, myocardial
    diastolic (congestive) I50.30
      acute (congestive) I50.31
        and (on) chronic (congestive) I50.33
      chronic (congestive) I50.32
        and (on) acute (congestive) I50.33
      combined with systolic (congestive) I50.40
        acute (congestive) I50.41
          and (on) chronic (congestive) I50.43
        chronic (congestive) I50.42
          and (on) acute (congestive) I50.43
    due to presence of cardiac prosthesis I97.13- ☑
    following cardiac surgery I97.13- ☑
    high output NOS I50.9
    hypertensive — *see* Hypertension, heart
    left (ventricular) — *see* Failure, ventricular, left
    low output (syndrome) NOS I50.9
    newborn P29.0
    organic — *see* Disease, heart
    peripartum O90.3
    postprocedural I97.13- ☑
    rheumatic (chronic) (inactive) I09.9

☑ **Additional character required**

Failure — *continued*
  right (ventricular) (secondary to left heart
    failure) — *see* Failure, heart, congestive
  systolic (congestive) I50.20
    acute (congestive) I50.21
      and (on) chronic (congestive) I50.23
    chronic (congestive) I50.22
      and (on) acute (congestive) I50.23
    combined with diastolic (congestive) I50.40
      acute (congestive) I50.41
        and (on) chronic (congestive) I50.43
      chronic (congestive) I50.42
        and (on) acute (congestive) I50.43
  thyrotoxic (*see also* Thyrotoxicosis) E05.90 [I43]
    with thyroid storm E05.91 [I43]
  valvular — *see* Endocarditis
  hepatic K72.90
    with coma K72.91
    acute or subacute K72.00
      with coma K72.01
      due to drugs K71.10
        with coma K71.11
    alcoholic (acute) (chronic) (subacute) K70.40
      with coma K70.41
    chronic K72.10
      with coma K72.11
      due to drugs (acute) (subacute) (chronic)
        K71.10
        with coma K71.11
    due to drugs (acute) (subacute) (chronic)
      K71.10
      with coma K71.11
    postprocedural K91.82
  hepatorenal K76.7
  induction (of labor) O61.9
    abortion — *see* Abortion, attempted
    by
      oxytocic drugs O61.0
      prostaglandins O61.0
    instrumental O61.1
    mechanical O61.1
    medical O61.0
    specified NEC O61.8
    surgical O61.1
  intubation during anesthesia T88.4 ☑
    in pregnancy O29.6- ☑
    labor and delivery O74.7
    postpartum, puerperal O89.6
  involution, thymus (gland) E32.0
  kidney (*see also* Disease, kidney, chronic) N19
    acute (*see also* Failure, renal, acute) N17.9- ☑
    diabetic — *see* E08-E13 with .22
  lactation (complete) O92.3
    partial O92.4
  Leydig's cell, adult E29.1
  liver — *see* Failure, hepatic
  menstruation at puberty N91.0
  mitral I05.8
  myocardial, myocardium (*see also* Failure, heart)
    I50.9
    chronic (*see also* Failure, heart, congestive)
      I50.9
    congestive (*see also* Failure, heart, congestive)
      I50.9
  orgasm (female) (psychogenic) F52.31
    male F52.32
  ovarian (primary) E28.39
    iatrogenic E89.40
      asymptomatic E89.40
      symptomatic E89.41
    postprocedural (postablative) (postirradiation)
      (postsurgical) E89.40
      asymptomatic E89.40
      symptomatic E89.41
  ovulation causing infertility N97.0
  polyglandular, autoimmune E31.0
  prosthetic joint implant — *see* Complications,
    joint prosthesis, mechanical, breakdown,
    by site
  renal N19
    with
      tubular necrosis (acute) N17.0
    acute N17.9
      with
        cortical necrosis N17.1
        medullary necrosis N17.2
        tubular necrosis N17.0
      specified NEC N17.8
    chronic N18.9
      hypertensive — *see* Hypertension, kidney
    congenital P96.0
    end stage (chronic) N18.6

Failure — *continued*
  due to hypertension I12.0
  following
    abortion — *see* Abortion by type
      complicated by specified condition NEC
    crushing T79.5 ☑
    ectopic or molar pregnancy O08.4
    labor and delivery (acute) O90.4
  hypertensive — *see* Hypertension, kidney
  postprocedural N99.0
  respiration, respiratory J96.90
    with
      hypercapnia J96.92
      hypoxia J96.91
    acute J96.00
      with
        hypercapnia J96.02
        hypoxia J96.01
    center G93.89
    acute and (on) chronic J96.20
      with
        hypercapnia J96.22
        hypoxia J96.21
    chronic J96.10
      with
        hypercapnia J96.12
        hypoxia J96.11
    newborn P28.5
    postprocedural (acute) J95.821
      acute and chronic J95.822
  rotation
    cecum Q43.3
    colon Q43.3
    intestine Q43.3
    kidney Q63.2
  sedation (conscious) (moderate) during
    procedure T88.52 ☑
    history of Z92.83
  segmentation (*see also* Fusion)
    fingers — *see* Syndactylism, complex, fingers
    vertebra Q76.49
      with scoliosis Q76.3
  seminiferous tubule, adult E29.1
  senile (general) R54
  sexual arousal (male) F52.21
    female F52.22
  testicular endocrine function E29.1
  to thrive (child over 28 days old) R62.51
    adult R62.7
    newborn P92.6
  transplant T86.92
    bone T86.831
      marrow T86.02
    cornea T86.841
    heart T86.22
      with lung (s) T86.32
    intestine T86.851
    kidney T86.12
    liver T86.42
    lung (s) T86.811
      with heart T86.32
    pancreas T86.891
    skin (allograft) (autograft) T86.821
    specified organ or tissue NEC T86.891
    stem cell (peripheral blood) (umbilical cord)
      T86.5
  trial of labor (with subsequent cesarean delivery)
    O66.40
    following previous cesarean delivery O66.41
  tubal ligation N99.89
  urinary — *see* Disease, kidney, chronic
  vacuum extraction NOS (with subsequent
    cesarean delivery) O66.5
  vasectomy N99.89
  ventouse NOS (with subsequent cesarean
    delivery) O66.5
  ventricular (*see also* Failure, heart) I50.9
    left I50.1
      with rheumatic fever (conditions in I00)
        active I01.8
          with chorea I02.0
        inactive or quiescent (with chorea) I09.81
        rheumatic (chronic) (inactive) (with chorea)
          I09.81
        active or acute I01.8
          with chorea I02.0
    right (*see also* Failure, heart, congestive) I50.9
    vital centers, newborn P91.8
Fainting (fit) R55
Fallen arches — *see* Deformity, limb, flat foot
Falling, falls (repeated) R29.6
  any organ or part — *see* Prolapse

Fallopian
  insufflation Z31.41
  tube — *see* condition
Fallot's
  pentalogy Q21.8
  tetrad or tetralogy Q21.3
  triad or trilogy Q22.3
False (*see also* condition)
  croup J38.5
  joint — *see* Nonunion, fracture
  labor (pains) O47.9
    at or after 37 completed weeks of gestation
      O47.1
    before 37 completed weeks of gestation
      O47.0- ☑
  passage, urethra (prostatic) N36.5
  pregnancy F45.8
Family, familial (*see also* condition)
  disruption Z63.8
    involving divorce or separation Z63.5
  Li-Fraumeni (syndrome) Z15.01
  planning advice Z30.09
  problem Z63.9
    specified NEC Z63.8
  retinoblastoma C69.2- ☑
Famine (effects of) T73.0 ☑
  edema — *see* Malnutrition, severe
Fanconi (-de Toni)(-Debré) syndrome E72.09
  with cystinosis E72.04
Fanconi's anemia (congenital pancytopenia) D61.09
Farber's disease or syndrome E75.29
Farcy A24.0
Farmer's
  lung J67.0
  skin L57.8
Farsightedness — *see* Hypermetropia
Fascia — *see* condition
Fasciculation R25.3
Fasciitis M72.9
  diffuse (eosinophilic) M35.4
  infective M72.8
    necrotizing M72.6
  necrotizing M72.6
  nodular M72.4
  perirenal (with ureteral obstruction) N13.5
    with infection N13.6
  plantar M72.2
  specified NEC M72.8
  traumatic (old) M72.8
    current - code by site under Sprain
Fascioliasis B66.3
Fasciolopsis, fasciolopsiasis (intestinal) B66.5
Fascioscapulohumeral myopathy G71.0
Fast pulse R00.0
Fat
  embolism — *see* Embolism, fat
  excessive (*see also* Obesity)
    in heart — *see* Degeneration, myocardial
  in stool R19.5
  localized (pad) E65
    heart — *see* Degeneration, myocardial
    knee M79.4
    retropatellar M79.4
  necrosis
    breast N64.1
    mesentery K65.4
    omentum K65.4
  pad E65
    knee M79.4
Fatigue R53.83
  auditory deafness — *see* Deafness
  chronic R53.82
  combat F43.0
  general R53.83
    psychogenic F48.8
  heat (transient) T67.6 ☑
  muscle M62.89
  myocardium — *see* Failure, heart
  neoplasm-related R53.0
  nervous, neurosis F48.8
  operational F48.8
  psychogenic (general) F48.8
  senile R54
  voice R49.8
Fatness — *see* Obesity
Fatty (*see also* condition)
  apron E65
  degeneration — *see* Degeneration, fatty
  heart (enlarged) — *see* Degeneration, myocardial
  liver NEC K76.0
    alcoholic K70.0
    nonalcoholic K76.0

Fatty — *continued*
necrosis — *see* Degeneration, fatty
Fauces — *see* condition
Fauchard's disease (periodontitis) — *see* Periodontitis
Faucitis J02.9
Favism (anemia) D55.0
Favus — *see* Dermatophytosis
Fazio-Londe disease or syndrome G12.1
Fear complex or reaction F40.9
Fear of — *see* Phobia
Feared complaint unfounded Z71.1
Febris, febrile (*see also* Fever)
flava (*see also* Fever, yellow) A95.9
melitensis A23.0
pestis — *see* Plague
recurrens — *see* Fever, relapsing
rubra A38.9
Fecal
incontinence R15.9
smearing R15.1
soiling R15.1
urgency R15.2
Fecalith (impaction) K56.41
appendix K38.1
congenital P76.8
Fede's disease K14.0
Feeble rapid pulse due to shock following injury T79.4 ☑
Feeble-minded F70
Feeding
difficulties R63.3
problem R63.3
newborn P92.9
specified NEC P92.8
nonorganic (adult) — *see* Disorder, eating
Feeling (of)
foreign body in throat R09.89
Feer's disease — *see* Poisoning, mercury
Feet — *see* condition
Feigned illness Z76.5
Feil-Klippel syndrome (brevicollis) Q76.1
Feinmesser's (hidrotic) ectodermal dysplasia Q82.4
Felon (*see also* Cellulitis, digit)
with lymphangitis — *see* Lymphangitis, acute, digit
Felty's syndrome M05.00
ankle M05.07- ☑
elbow M05.02- ☑
foot joint M05.07- ☑
hand joint M05.04- ☑
hip M05.05- ☑
knee M05.06- ☑
multiple site M05.09
shoulder M05.01- ☑
vertebra — *see* Spondylitis, ankylosing
wrist M05.03- ☑
Female genital cutting status — *see* Female genital mutilation status (FGM)
Female genital mutilation status (FGM) N90.810
specified NEC N90.818
type I (clitorectomy status) N90.811
type II (clitorectomy with excision of labia minora status) N90.812
type III (infibulation status) N90.813
type IV N90.818
Femur, femoral — *see* condition
Fenestration, fenestrated (*see also* Imperfect, closure)
aortico-pulmonary Q21.4
cusps, heart valve NEC Q24.8
pulmonary Q22.3
pulmonic cusps Q22.3
Fernell's disease (aortic aneurysm) I71.9
Fertile eunuch syndrome E23.0
Fetid
breath R19.6
sweat L75.0
Fetishism F65.0
transvestic F65.1
Fetus, fetal (*see also* condition)
alcohol syndrome (dysmorphic) Q86.0
compressus O31.0- ☑
hydantoin syndrome Q86.1
lung tissue P28.0
papyraceous O31.0- ☑
Fever (inanition) (of unknown origin) (persistent) (with chills) (with rigor) R50.9
abortus A23.1
Aden (dengue) A90
African tick-borne A68.1

Fever — *continued*
American
mountain (tick) A93.2
spotted A77.0
aphthous B08.8
arbovirus, arboviral A94
hemorrhagic A94
specified NEC A93.8
Argentinian hemorrhagic A96.0
Assam B55.0
Australian Q A78
Bangkok hemorrhagic A91
Barmah forest A92.8
Bartonella A44.0
bilious, hemoglobinuric B50.8
blackwater B50.8
blister B00.1
Bolivian hemorrhagic A96.1
Bonvale dam T73.3 ☑
boutonneuse A77.1
brain — *see* Encephalitis
Brazilian purpuric A48.4
breakbone A90
Bullis A77.0
Bunyamwera A92.8
Burdwan B55.0
Bwamba A92.8
Cameroon — *see* Malaria
Canton A75.9
catarrhal (acute) J00
chronic J31.0
cat-scratch A28.1
Central Asian hemorrhagic A98.0
cerebral — *see* Encephalitis
cerebrospinal meningococcal A39.0
Chagres B50.9
Chandipura A92.8
Changuinola A93.1
Charcot's (biliary) (hepatic) (intermittent) - — *see* Calculus, bile duct
Chikungunya (viral) (hemorrhagic) A92.0
Chitral A93.1
Colombo — *see* Fever, paratyphoid
Colorado tick (virus) A93.2
congestive (remittent) — *see* Malaria
Congo virus A98.0
continued malarial B50.9
Corsican — *see* Malaria
Crimean-Congo hemorrhagic A98.0
Cyprus — *see* Brucellosis
dandy A90
deer fly — *see* Tularemia
dengue (virus) A90
hemorrhagic A91
sandfly A93.1
desert B38.0
drug induced R50.2
due to
conditions classified elsewhere R50.81
heat T67.0 ☑
enteric A01.00
enteroviral exanthematous (Boston exanthem) A88.0
ephemeral (of unknown origin) R50.9
epidemic hemorrhagic A98.5
erysipelatous — *see* Erysipelas
estivo-autumnal (malarial) B50.9
famine A75.0
five day A79.0
following delivery O86.4
Fort Bragg A27.89
gastroenteric A01.00
gastromalarial — *see* Malaria
Gibraltar — *see* Brucellosis
glandular — *see* Mononucleosis, infectious
Guama (viral) A92.8
Haverhill A25.1
hay (allergic) J30.1
with asthma (bronchial) J45.909
with
exacerbation (acute) J45.901
status asthmaticus J45.902
due to
allergen other than pollen J30.89
pollen, any plant or tree J30.1
heat (effects) T67.0 ☑
hematuric, bilious B50.8
hemoglobinuric (malarial) (bilious) B50.8
hemorrhagic (arthropod-borne) NOS A94
with renal syndrome A98.5
arenaviral A96.9
specified NEC A96.8

Fever — *continued*
Argentinian A96.0
Bangkok A91
Bolivian A96.1
Central Asian A98.0
Chikungunya A92.0
Crimean-Congo A98.0
dengue A91
epidemic A98.5
Junin (virus) A96.0
Korean A98.5
Kyasanur forest A98.2
Machupo (virus) A96.1
mite-borne A93.8
mosquito-borne A92.8
Omsk A98.1
Philippine A91
Russian A98.5
Singapore A91
Southeast Asia A91
Thailand A91
tick-borne NEC A93.8
viral A99
specified NEC A98.8
hepatic — *see* Cholecystitis
herpetic — *see* Herpes
icterohemorrhagic A27.0
Indiana A93.8
infective B99.9
specified NEC B99.8
intermittent (bilious) (*see also* Malaria)
of unknown origin R50.9
pernicious B50.9
iodide R50.2
Japanese river A75.3
jungle (*see also* Malaria)
yellow A95.0
Junin (virus) hemorrhagic A96.0
Katayama B65.2
kedani A75.3
Kenya (tick) A77.1
Kew Garden A79.1
Korean hemorrhagic A98.5
Lassa A96.2
Lone Star A77.0
Machupo (virus) hemorrhagic A96.1
malaria, malarial — *see* Malaria
Malta A23.9
Marseilles A77.1
marsh — *see* Malaria
Mayaro (viral) A92.8
Mediterranean (*see also* Brucellosis) A23.9
familial E85.0
tick A77.1
meningeal — *see* Meningitis
Meuse A79.0
Mexican A75.2
mianeh A68.1
miasmatic — *see* Malaria
mosquito-borne (viral) A92.9
hemorrhagic A92.8
mountain (*see also* Brucellosis)
meaning Rocky Mountain spotted fever A77.0
tick (American) (Colorado) (viral) A93.2
Mucambo (viral) A92.8
mud A27.9
Neapolitan — *see* Brucellosis
neutropenic D70.9
newborn P81.9
environmental P81.0
Nine-Mile A78
non-exanthematous tick A93.2
North Asian tick-borne A77.2
Omsk hemorrhagic A98.1
O'nyong-nyong (viral) A92.1
Oropouche (viral) A93.0
Oroya A44.0
paludal — *see* Malaria
Panama (malarial) B50.9
Pappataci A93.1
paratyphoid A01.4
A A01.1
B A01.2
C A01.3
parrot A70
periodic (Mediterranean) E85.0
persistent (of unknown origin) R50.9
petechial A39.0
pharyngoconjunctival B30.2
Philippine hemorrhagic A91
phlebotomus A93.1
Piry (virus) A93.8

☑ **Additional character required**

Fever — *continued*
Pixuna (viral) A92.8
Plasmodium ovale B53.0
polioviral (nonparalytic) A80.4
Pontiac A48.2
postimmunization R50.83
postoperative R50.82
due to infection T81.4 ☑
posttransfusion R50.84
postvaccination R50.83
presenting with conditions classified elsewhere R50.81
pretibial A27.89
puerperal O86.4
Q A78
quadrilateral A78
quartan (malaria) B52.9
Queensland (coastal) (tick) A77.3
quintan A79.0
rabbit — *see* Tularemia
rat-bite A25.9
due to
Spirillum A25.0
Streptobacillus moniliformis A25.1
recurrent — *see* Fever, relapsing
relapsing (Borrelia) A68.9
Carter's (Asiatic) A68.1
Dutton's (West African) A68.1
Koch's A68.9
louse-borne A68.0
Novy's
louse-borne A68.0
tick-borne A68.1
Obermeyer's (European) A68.0
tick-borne A68.1
remittent (bilious) (congestive) (gastric) — *see* Malaria
rheumatic (active) (acute) (chronic) (subacute) I00
with central nervous system involvement I02.9
active with heart involvement — *see* category I01 ☑
inactive or quiescent with
cardiac hypertrophy I09.89
carditis I09.9
endocarditis I09.1
aortic (valve) I06.9
with mitral (valve) disease I08.0
mitral (valve) I05.9
with aortic (valve) disease I08.0
pulmonary (valve) I09.89
tricuspid (valve) I07.8
heart disease NEC I09.89
heart failure (congestive) (conditions in I50.9) I09.81
left ventricular failure (conditions in I50.1) I09.81
myocarditis, myocardial degeneration (conditions in I51.4) I09.0
pancarditis I09.9
pericarditis I09.2
Rift Valley (viral) A92.4
Rocky Mountain spotted A77.0
rose J30.1
Ross River B33.1
Russian hemorrhagic A98.5
San Joaquin (Valley) B38.0
sandfly A93.1
Sao Paulo A77.0
scarlet A38.9
seven day (leptospirosis) (autumnal) (Japanese) A27.89
dengue A90
shin-bone A79.0
Singapore hemorrhagic A91
solar A90
Songo A98.5
sore B00.1
South African tick-bite A68.1
Southeast Asia hemorrhagic A91
spinal — *see* Meningitis
spirillary A25.0
splenic — *see* Anthrax
spotted A77.9
American A77.0
Brazilian A77.0
cerebrospinal meningitis A39.0
Colombian A77.0
due to Rickettsia
australis A77.3
conorii A77.1
rickettsii A77.0
sibirica A77.2

Fever — *continued*
specified type NEC A77.8
Ehrlichiosis A77.40
due to
E. chafeensis A77.41
specified organism NEC A77.49
Rocky Mountain A77.0
steroid R50.2
streptobacillary A25.1
subtertian B50.9
Sumatran mite A75.3
sun A90
swamp A27.9
swine A02.8
sylvatic, yellow A95.0
Tahyna B33.8
tertian — *see* Malaria, tertian
Thailand hemorrhagic A91
thermic T67.0 ☑
three-day A93.1
tick
American mountain A93.2
Colorado A93.2
Kemerovo A93.8
Mediterranean A77.1
mountain A93.2
nonexanthematous A93.2
Quaranfil A93.8
tick-bite NEC A93.8
tick-borne (hemorrhagic) NEC A93.8
trench A79.0
tsutsugamushi A75.3
typhogastric A01.00
typhoid (abortive) (hemorrhagic) (intermittent) (malignant) A01.00
complicated by
arthritis A01.04
heart involvement A01.02
meningitis A01.01
osteomyelitis A01.05
pneumonia A01.03
specified NEC A01.09
typhomalarial — *see* Malaria
typhus — *see* Typhus (fever)
undulant — *see* Brucellosis
unknown origin R50.9
uveoparotid D86.89
valley B38.0
Venezuelan equine A92.2
vesicular stomatitis A93.8
viral hemorrhagic — *see* Fever, hemorrhagic, by type of virus
Volhynian A79.0
Wesselsbron (viral) A92.8
West
African B50.8
Nile (viral) A92.30
with
complications NEC A92.39
cranial nerve disorders A92.32
encephalitis A92.31
encephalomyelitis A92.31
neurologic manifestation NEC A92.32
optic neuritis A92.32
polyradiculitis A92.32
Whitmore's — *see* Melioidosis
Wolhynian A79.0
worm B83.9
yellow A95.9
jungle A95.0
sylvatic A95.0
urban A95.1
Zika (viral) A92.8
Fibrillation
atrial or auricular (established) I48.91
chronic I48.2
paroxysmal I48.0
permanent I48.2
persistent I48.1
cardiac I49.8
heart I49.8
muscular M62.89
ventricular I49.01
Fibrin
ball or bodies, pleural (sac) J94.1
chamber, anterior (eye) (gelatinous exudate) — *see* Iridocyclitis, acute
Fibrinogenolysis — *see* Fibrinolysis
Fibrinogenopenia D68.8
acquired D65
congenital D68.2
Fibrinolysis (hemorrhagic) (acquired) D65

Fibrinolysis — *continued*
antepartum hemorrhage — *see* Hemorrhage, antepartum, with coagulation defect
following
abortion — *see* Abortion by type complicated by hemorrhage
ectopic or molar pregnancy O08.1
intrapartum O67.0
newborn, transient P60
postpartum O72.3
Fibrinopenia (hereditary) D68.2
acquired D68.4
Fibrinopurulent — *see* condition
Fibrinous — *see* condition
Fibroadenoma
cellular intracanalicular D24- ☑
giant D24- ☑
intracanalicular
cellular D24- ☑
giant D24- ☑
specified site — *see* Neoplasm, benign, by site
unspecified site D24- ☑
juvenile D24- ☑
pericanalicular
specified site — *see* Neoplasm, benign, by site
unspecified site D24- ☑
phyllodes D24- ☑
prostate D29.1
specified site NEC — *see* Neoplasm, benign, by site
unspecified site D24- ☑
Fibroadenosis, breast (chronic) (cystic) (diffuse) (periodic) (segmental) N60.2- ☑
Fibroangioma (*see also* Neoplasm, benign, by site)
juvenile
specified site — *see* Neoplasm, benign, by site
unspecified site D10.6
Fibrochondrosarcoma — *see* Neoplasm, cartilage, malignant
Fibrocystic
disease (*see also* Fibrosis, cystic)
breast — *see* Mastopathy, cystic
jaw M27.49
kidney (congenital) Q61.8
liver Q44.6
pancreas E84.9
kidney (congenital) Q61.8
Fibrodysplasia ossificans progressiva - — *see* Myositis, ossificans, progressiva
Fibroelastosis (cordis) (endocardial) (endomyocardial) I42.4
Fibroid (tumor) (*see also* Neoplasm, connective tissue, benign)
disease, lung (chronic) — *see* Fibrosis, lung
heart (disease) — *see* Myocarditis
in pregnancy or childbirth O34.1- ☑
causing obstructed labor O65.5
induration, lung (chronic) — *see* Fibrosis, lung
lung — *see* Fibrosis, lung
pneumonia (chronic) — *see* Fibrosis, lung
uterus D25.9
Fibrolipoma — *see* Lipoma
Fibroliposarcoma — *see* Neoplasm, connective tissue, malignant
Fibroma (*see also* Neoplasm, connective tissue, benign)
ameloblastic — *see* Cyst, calcifying odontogenic
bone (nonossifying) — *see* Disorder, bone, specified type NEC
ossifying — *see* Neoplasm, bone, benign
cementifying — *see* Neoplasm, bone, benign
chondromyxoid — *see* Neoplasm, bone, benign
desmoplastic — *see* Neoplasm, connective tissue, uncertain behavior
durum — *see* Neoplasm, connective tissue, benign
fascial — *see* Neoplasm, connective tissue, benign
invasive — *see* Neoplasm, connective tissue, uncertain behavior
molle — *see* Lipoma
myxoid — *see* Neoplasm, connective tissue, benign
nasopharynx, nasopharyngeal (juvenile) D10.6
nonosteogenic (nonossifying) — *see* Dysplasia, fibrous
odontogenic (central) — *see* Cyst, calcifying odontogenic
ossifying — *see* Neoplasm, bone, benign
periosteal — *see* Neoplasm, bone, benign
soft — *see* Lipoma

Fibromatosis - Findings

Fibromatosis M72.9
abdominal — see Neoplasm, connective tissue, uncertain behavior
aggressive — see Neoplasm, connective tissue, uncertain behavior
congenital generalized — see Neoplasm, connective tissue, uncertain behavior
Dupuytren's M72.0
gingival K06.1
palmar (fascial) M72.0
plantar (fascial) M72.2
pseudosarcomatous (proliferative) (subcutaneous) M72.4
retroperitoneal D48.3
specified NEC M72.8
Fibromyalgia M79.7
Fibromyoma (see also Neoplasm, connective tissue, benign)
uterus (corpus) (see also Leiomyoma, uterus)
in pregnancy or childbirth — see Fibroid, in pregnancy or childbirth
causing obstructed labor O65.5
Fibromyositis M79.7
Fibromyxolipoma D17.9
Fibromyxoma — see Neoplasm, connective tissue, benign
Fibromyxosarcoma — see Neoplasm, connective tissue, malignant
Fibro-odontoma, ameloblastic — see Cyst, calcifying odontogenic
Fibro-osteoma — see Neoplasm, bone, benign
Fibroplasia, retrolental H35.17- ☑
Fibropurulent — see condition
Fibrosarcoma (see also Neoplasm, connective tissue, malignant)
ameloblastic C41.1
upper jaw (bone) C41.0
congenital — see Neoplasm, connective tissue, malignant
fascial — see Neoplasm, connective tissue, malignant
infantile — see Neoplasm, connective tissue, malignant
odontogenic C41.1
upper jaw (bone) C41.0
periosteal — see Neoplasm, bone, malignant
Fibrosclerosis
breast N60.3- ☑
multifocal M35.5
penis (corpora cavernosa) N48.6
Fibrosis, fibrotic
adrenal (gland) E27.8
amnion O41.8X- ☑
anal papillae K62.89
arteriocapillary — see Arteriosclerosis
bladder N32.89
interstitial — see Cystitis, chronic, interstitial
localized submucosal — see Cystitis, chronic, interstitial
panmural — see Cystitis, chronic, interstitial
breast — see Fibrosclerosis, breast
capillary (see also Arteriosclerosis) I70.90
lung (chronic) — see Fibrosis, lung
cardiac — see Myocarditis
cervix N88.8
chorion O41.8X- ☑
corpus cavernosum (sclerosing) N48.6
cystic (of pancreas) E84.9
with
distal intestinal obstruction syndrome E84.19
fecal impaction E84.19
intestinal manifestations NEC E84.19
pulmonary manifestations E84.0
specified manifestations NEC E84.8
due to device, implant or graft (see also Complications, by site and type, specified NEC) T85.82 ☑
arterial graft NEC T82.828 ☑
breast (implant) T85.82 ☑
catheter NEC T85.82 ☑
dialysis (renal) T82.828 ☑
intraperitoneal T85.82 ☑
infusion NEC T82.828 ☑
spinal (epidural) (subdural) T85.82 ☑
urinary (indwelling) T83.82 ☑
electronic (electrode) (pulse generator) (stimulator)
bone T84.82 ☑
cardiac T82.827 ☑
nervous system (brain) (peripheral nerve) (spinal) T85.82 ☑
urinary T83.82 ☑

Fibrosis — continued
fixation, internal (orthopedic) NEC T84.82 ☑
gastrointestinal (bile duct) (esophagus) T85.82 ☑
genital NEC T83.82 ☑
heart NEC T82.827 ☑
joint prosthesis T84.82 ☑
ocular (corneal graft) (orbital implant) NEC T85.82 ☑
orthopedic NEC T84.82 ☑
specified NEC T85.82 ☑
urinary NEC T83.82 ☑
vascular NEC T82.828 ☑
ventricular intracranial shunt T85.82 ☑
ejaculatory duct N50.8
endocardium — see Endocarditis
endomyocardial (tropical) I42.3
epididymis N50.8
eye muscle — see Strabismus, mechanical
heart — see Myocarditis
hepatic — see Fibrosis, liver
hepatolienal (portal hypertension) K76.6
hepatosplenic (portal hypertension) K76.6
infrapatellar fat pad M79.4
intrascrotal N50.8
kidney N26.9
liver K74.0
with sclerosis K74.2
alcoholic K70.2
lung (atrophic) (chronic) (confluent) (massive) (perialveolar) (peribronchial) J84.10
with
anthracosilicosis J60
anthracosis J60
asbestosis J61
bagassosis J67.1
bauxite J63.1
berylliosis J63.2
byssinosis J66.0
calcicosis J62.8
chalicosis J62.8
dust reticulation J64
farmer's lung J67.0
ganister disease J62.8
graphite J63.3
pneumoconiosis NOS J64
siderosis J63.4
silicosis J62.8
capillary J84.10
congenital P27.8
diffuse (idiopathic) J84.10
chemicals, gases, fumes or vapors (inhalation) J68.4
interstitial J84.10
acute J84.114
talc J62.0
following radiation J70.1
idiopathic J84.112
postinflammatory J84.10
silicotic J62.8
tuberculous — see Tuberculosis, pulmonary
lymphatic gland I89.8
median bar — see Hyperplasia, prostate
mediastinum (idiopathic) J98.5
meninges G96.19
myocardium, myocardial — see Myocarditis
ovary N83.8
oviduct N83.8
pancreas K86.8
penis NEC N48.6
pericardium I31.0
perineum, in pregnancy or childbirth O34.7- ☑
causing obstructed labor O65.5
pleura J94.1
popliteal fat pad M79.4
prostate (chronic) — see Hyperplasia, prostate
pulmonary (see also Fibrosis, lung) J84.10
congenital P27.8
idiopathic J84.112
rectal sphincter K62.89
retroperitoneal, idiopathic (with ureteral obstruction) N13.5
with infection N13.6
sclerosing mesenteric (idiopathic) K65.4
scrotum N50.8
seminal vesicle N50.8
senile R54
skin L90.5
spermatic cord N50.8
spleen D73.89
in schistosomiasis (bilharziasis) B65.9 [D77]

Fibrosis — continued
subepidermal nodular — see Neoplasm, skin, benign
submucous (oral) (tongue) K13.5
testis N44.8
chronic, due to syphilis A52.76
thymus (gland) E32.8
tongue, submucous K13.5
tunica vaginalis N50.8
uterus (non-neoplastic) N85.8
vagina N89.8
valve, heart — see Endocarditis
vas deferens N50.8
vein I87.8
Fibrositis (periarticular) M79.7
nodular, chronic (Jaccoud's) (rheumatoid) — see Arthropathy, postrheumatic, chronic
Fibrothorax J94.1
Fibrotic — see Fibrosis
Fibrous — see condition
Fibroxanthoma (see also Neoplasm, connective tissue, benign)
atypical — see Neoplasm, connective tissue, uncertain behavior
malignant — see Neoplasm, connective tissue, malignant
Fibroxanthosarcoma — see Neoplasm, connective tissue, malignant
Fiedler's
disease (icterohemorrhagic leptospirosis) A27.0
myocarditis (acute) I40.1
Fifth disease B08.3
venereal A55
Filaria, filarial, filariasis — see Infestation, filarial
Filatov's disease — see Mononucleosis, infectious
File-cutter's disease — see Poisoning, lead
Filling defect
biliary tract R93.2
bladder R93.4
duodenum R93.3
gallbladder R93.2
gastrointestinal tract R93.3
intestine R93.3
kidney R93.4
stomach R93.3
ureter R93.4
Fimbrial cyst Q50.4
Financial problem affecting care NOS Z59.9
bankruptcy Z59.8
foreclosure on loan Z59.8
Findings, abnormal, inconclusive, without diagnosis (see also Abnormal)
17-ketosteroids, elevated R82.5
acetonuria R82.4
alcohol in blood R78.0
anisocytosis R71.8
antenatal screening of mother O28.9
biochemical O28.1
chromosomal O28.5
cytological O28.2
genetic O28.5
hematological O28.0
radiological O28.4
specified NEC O28.8
ultrasonic O28.3
antibody titer, elevated R76.0
anticardiolipin antibody R76.0
antiphosphatidylglycerol antibody R76.0
antiphosphatidylinositol antibody R76.0
antiphosphatidylserine antibody R76.0
antiphospholipid antibody R76.0
bacteriuria N39.0
bicarbonate E87.8
bile in urine R82.2
blood sugar R73.09
high R73.9
low (transient) E16.2
body fluid or substance, specified NEC R88.8
casts, urine R82.99
catecholamines R82.5
cells, urine R82.99
chloride E87.8
cholesterol E78.9
high E78.0
with high triglycerides E78.2
chyluria R82.0
cloudy
dialysis effluent R88.0
urine R82.90
creatinine clearance R94.4
crystals, urine R82.99
culture

☑ **Additional character required**

Findings — *continued*

blood R78.81
  positive — *see* Positive, culture
echocardiogram R93.1
electrolyte level, urinary R82.99
function study NEC R94.8
  bladder R94.8
  endocrine NEC R94.7
    thyroid R94.6
  kidney R94.4
  liver R94.5
  pancreas R94.8
  placenta R94.8
  pulmonary R94.2
  spleen R94.8
gallbladder, nonvisualization R93.2
glucose (tolerance test) (non-fasting) R73.09
glycosuria R81
heart
  shadow R93.1
  sounds R01.2
hematinuria R82.3
hematocrit drop (precipitous) R71.0
hemoglobinuria R82.3
human papillomavirus (HPV) DNA test positive
  cervix
    high risk R87.810
    low risk R87.820
  vagina
    high risk R87.811
    low risk R87.821
in blood (of substance not normally found in blood) R78.9
  addictive drug NEC R78.4
  alcohol (excessive level) R78.0
  cocaine R78.2
  hallucinogen R78.3
  heavy metals (abnormal level) R78.79
  lead R78.71
  lithium (abnormal level) R78.89
  opiate drug R78.1
  psychotropic drug R78.5
  specified substance NEC R78.89
  steroid agent R78.6
indoleacetic acid, elevated R82.5
ketonuria R82.4
lactic acid dehydrogenase (LDH) R74.0
liver function test R79.89
mammogram NEC R92.8
  calcification (calculus) R92.1
  inconclusive result (due to dense breasts) R92.2
  microcalcification R92.0
mediastinal shift R93.8
melanin, urine R82.99
myoglobinuria R82.1
neonatal screening P09
nonvisualization of gallbladder R93.2
odor of urine NOS R82.90
Papanicolaou cervix R87.619
  non-atypical endometrial cells R87.618
pneumoencephalogram R93.0
poikilocytosis R71.8
potassium (deficiency) E87.6
  excess E87.5
PPD R76.11
radiologic (X-ray) R93.8
  abdomen R93.5
  biliary tract R93.2
  breast R92.8
  gastrointestinal tract R93.3
  genitourinary organs R93.8
  head R93.0
  inconclusive due to excess body fat of patient R93.9
  intrathoracic organs NEC R93.1
  placenta R93.8
  retroperitoneum R93.5
  skin R93.8
  skull R93.0
  subcutaneous tissue R93.8
red blood cell (count) (morphology) (sickling) (volume) R71.8
scan NEC R94.8
  bladder R94.8
  bone R94.8
  kidney R94.4
  liver R93.2
  lung R94.2
  pancreas R94.8
  placental R94.8
  spleen R94.8
  thyroid R94.6

Findings — *continued*

sedimentation rate, elevated R70.0
SGOT R74.0
SGPT R74.0
sodium (deficiency) E87.1
  excess E87.0
specified body fluid NEC R88.8
stress test R94.39
thyroid (function) (metabolic rate) (scan) (uptake) R94.6
transaminase (level) R74.0
triglycerides E78.9
  high E78.1
    with high cholesterol E78.2
tuberculin skin test (without active tuberculosis) R76.11
urine R82.90
  acetone R82.4
  bacteria N39.0
  bile R82.2
  casts or cells R82.99
  chyle R82.0
  culture positive R82.7
  glucose R81
  hemoglobin R82.3
  ketone R82.4
  sugar R81
vanillylmandelic acid (VMA), elevated R82.5
vectorcardiogram (VCG) R94.39
ventriculogram R93.0
white blood cell (count) (differential) (morphology) D72.9
xerography R92.8

Finger — *see* condition
Fire, Saint Anthony's — *see* Erysipelas
Fire-setting
  pathological (compulsive) F63.1
Fish hook stomach K31.89
Fishmeal-worker's lung J67.8
Fissure, fissured
  anus, anal K60.2
    acute K60.0
    chronic K60.1
    congenital Q43.8
  ear, lobule, congenital Q17.8
  epiglottis (congenital) Q31.8
  larynx J38.7
    congenital Q31.8
  lip K13.0
    congenital — *see* Cleft, lip
  nipple N64.0
    associated with
      lactation O92.13
      pregnancy O92.11- ☑
      puerperium O92.12
  nose Q30.2
  palate (congenital) — *see* Cleft, palate
  skin R23.4
  spine (congenital) (*see also* Spina bifida)
    with hydrocephalus — *see* Spina bifida, by site, with hydrocephalus
  tongue (acquired) K14.5
    congenital Q38.3
Fistula (cutaneous) L98.8
  abdomen (wall) K63.2
    bladder N32.2
    intestine NEC K63.2
    ureter N28.89
    uterus N82.5
  abdominorectal K63.2
  abdominosigmoidal K63.2
  abdominothoracic J86.0
  abdominouterine N82.5
    congenital Q51.7
  abdominovesical N32.2
  accessory sinuses — *see* Sinusitis
  actinomycotic — *see* Actinomycosis
  alveolar antrum — *see* Sinusitis, maxillary
  alveolar process K04.6
  anorectal K60.5
  antrobuccal — *see* Sinusitis, maxillary
  antrum — *see* Sinusitis, maxillary
  anus, anal (recurrent) (infectional) K60.3
    congenital Q43.6
      with absence, atresia and stenosis Q42.2
    tuberculous A18.32
  aorta-duodenal I77.2
  appendix, appendicular K38.3
  arteriovenous (acquired) (nonruptured) I77.0
    brain I67.1
      congenital Q28.2
      ruptured I60.8

Fistula — *continued*

      ruptured I60.8
    cerebral — *see* Fistula, arteriovenous, brain
    congenital (peripheral) (*see also* Malformation, arteriovenous)
      brain Q28.2
        ruptured I60.8
      coronary Q24.5
      pulmonary Q25.72
    coronary I25.41
      congenital Q24.5
    pulmonary I28.0
      congenital Q25.72
    surgically created (for dialysis) Z99.2
      complication — *see* Complication, arteriovenous, fistula, surgically created
    traumatic — *see* Injury, blood vessel
  artery I77.2
  aural (mastoid) — *see* Mastoiditis, chronic
  auricle (*see also* Disorder, pinna, specified type NEC)
    congenital Q18.1
  Bartholin's gland N82.8
  bile duct (common) (hepatic) K83.3
    with calculus, stones — *see* Calculus, bile duct
  biliary (tract) — *see* Fistula, bile duct
  bladder (sphincter) NEC (*see also* Fistula, vesico-) N32.2
    into seminal vesicle N32.2
  bone (*see also* Disorder, bone, specified type NEC)
    with osteomyelitis, chronic — *see* Osteomyelitis, chronic, with draining sinus
  brain G93.89
    arteriovenous (acquired) I67.1
      congenital Q28.2
  branchial (cleft) Q18.0
  branchiogenous Q18.0
  breast N61
    puerperal, postpartum or gestational, due to mastitis (purulent) — *see* Mastitis, obstetric, purulent
  bronchial J86.0
  bronchocutaneous, bronchomediastinal, bronchopleural, bronchopleuromediastinal (infective) J86.0
    tuberculous NEC A15.5
  bronchoesophageal J86.0
    congenital Q39.2
      with atresia of esophagus Q39.1
  bronchovisceral J86.0
  buccal cavity (infective) K12.2
  cecosigmoidal K63.2
  cecum K63.2
  cerebrospinal (fluid) G96.0
  cervical, lateral Q18.1
  cervicoaural Q18.1
  cervicosigmoidal N82.4
  cervicovesical N82.1
  cervix N82.8
  chest (wall) J86.0
  cholecystenteric — *see* Fistula, gallbladder
  cholecystocolic — *see* Fistula, gallbladder
  cholecystocolonic — *see* Fistula, gallbladder
  cholecystoduodenal — *see* Fistula, gallbladder
  cholecystogastric — *see* Fistula, gallbladder
  cholecystointestinal — *see* Fistula, gallbladder
  choledochoduodenal — *see* Fistula, bile duct
  cholocolic K82.3
  coccyx — *see* Sinus, pilonidal
  colon K63.2
  colostomy K94.09
  common duct — *see* Fistula, bile duct
  congenital, site not listed — *see* Anomaly, by site
  coronary, arteriovenous I25.41
    congenital Q24.5
  costal region J86.0
  cul-de-sac, Douglas' N82.8
  cystic duct (*see also* Fistula, gallbladder)
    congenital Q44.5
  dental K04.6
  diaphragm J86.0
  duodenum K31.6
  ear (external) (canal) — *see* Disorder, ear, external, specified type NEC
  enterocolic K63.2
  enterocutaneous K63.2
  enterouterine N82.4
    congenital Q51.7
  enterovaginal N82.4
    congenital Q52.2
    large intestine N82.3

Fistula — *continued*
    small intestine N82.2
  enterovesical N32.1
  epididymis N50.8
    tuberculous A18.15
  esophagobronchial J86.0
    congenital Q39.2
      with atresia of esophagus Q39.1
  esophagocutaneous K22.8
  esophagopleural-cutaneous J86.0
  esophagotracheal J86.0
    congenital Q39.2
      with atresia of esophagus Q39.1
  esophagus K22.8
    congenital Q39.2
      with atresia of esophagus Q39.1
  ethmoid — *see* Sinusitis, ethmoidal
  eyeball (cornea) (sclera) — *see* Disorder, globe, hypotony
  eyelid H01.8
  fallopian tube, external N82.5
  fecal K63.2
    congenital Q43.6
  from periapical abscess K04.6
  frontal sinus — *see* Sinusitis, frontal
  gallbladder K82.3
    with calculus, cholelithiasis, stones — *see* Calculus, gallbladder
  gastric K31.6
  gastrocolic K31.6
    congenital Q40.2
    tuberculous A18.32
  gastroenterocolic K31.6
  gastroesophageal K31.6
  gastrojejunal K31.6
  gastrojejunocolic K31.6
  genital tract (female) N82.9
    specified NEC N82.8
    to intestine NEC N82.4
    to skin N82.5
  hepatic artery-portal vein, congenital Q26.6
  hepatopleural J86.0
  hepatopulmonary J86.0
  ileorectal or ileosigmoidal K63.2
  ileovaginal N82.2
  ileovesical N32.1
  ileum K63.2
  in ano K60.3
    tuberculous A18.32
  inner ear (labyrinth)H83.1
  intestine NEC K63.2
  intestinocolonic (abdominal) K63.2
  intestinoureteral N28.89
  intestinouterine N82.4
  intestinovaginal N82.4
    large intestine N82.3
    small intestine N82.2
  intestinovesical N32.1
  ischiorectal (fossa) K61.3
  jejunum K63.2
  joint M25.10
    ankle M25.17- ☑
    elbow M25.12- ☑
    foot joint M25.17- ☑
    hand joint M25.14- ☑
    hip M25.15- ☑
    knee M25.16- ☑
    shoulder M25.11- ☑
    specified joint NEC M25.18
    tuberculous — *see* Tuberculosis, joint
    vertebrae M25.18
    wrist M25.13- ☑
  kidney N28.89
  labium (majus) (minus) N82.8
  labyrinthH83.1
  lacrimal (gland) (sac) H04.61- ☑
  lacrimonasal duct — *see* Fistula, lacrimal
  laryngotracheal, congenital Q34.8
  larynx J38.7
  lip K13.0
    congenital Q38.0
  lumbar, tuberculous A18.01
  lung J86.0
  lymphatic I89.8
  mammary (gland) N61
  mastoid (process) (region) — *see* Mastoiditis, chronic
  maxillary J32.0
  medial, face and neck Q18.8
  mediastinal J86.0
  mediastinobronchial J86.0
  mediastinocutaneous J86.0

Fistula — *continued*
  middle earH74.8
  mouth K12.2
  nasal J34.89
    sinus — *see* Sinusitis
  nasopharynx J39.2
  nipple N64.0
  nose J34.89
  oral (cutaneous) K12.2
    maxillary J32.0
    nasal (with cleft palate) — *see* Cleft, palate
  orbit, orbital — *see* Disorder, orbit, specified type NEC
  oroantral J32.0
  oviduct, external N82.5
  palate (hard) M27.8
  pancreatic K86.8
  pancreaticoduodenal K86.8
  parotid (gland) K11.4
    region K12.2
  penis N48.89
  perianal K60.3
  pericardium (pleura) (sac) — *see* Pericarditis
  pericecal K63.2
  perineorectal K60.4
  perineosigmoidal K63.2
  perineum, perineal (with urethral involvement) NEC N36.0
    tuberculous A18.13
    ureter N28.89
  perirectal K60.4
    tuberculous A18.32
  peritoneum K65.9
  pharyngoesophageal J39.2
  pharynx J39.2
    branchial cleft (congenital) Q18.0
  pilonidal (infected) (rectum) — *see* Sinus, pilonidal
  pleura, pleural, pleurocutaneous, pleuroperitoneal J86.0
    tuberculous NEC A15.6
  pleuropericardial I31.8
  portal vein-hepatic artery, congenital Q26.6
  postauricular H70.81- ☑
  postoperative, persistent T81.83 ☑
    specified site — *see* Fistula, by site
  preauricular (congenital) Q18.1
  prostate N42.89
  pulmonary J86.0
    arteriovenous I28.0
      congenital Q25.72
    tuberculous — *see* Tuberculosis, pulmonary
  pulmonoperitoneal J86.0
  rectolabial N82.4
  rectosigmoid (intercommunicating) K63.2
  rectoureteral N28.89
  rectourethral N36.0
    congenital Q64.73
  rectouterine N82.4
    congenital Q51.7
  rectovaginal N82.3
    congenital Q52.2
    tuberculous A18.18
  rectovesical N32.1
    congenital Q64.79
  rectovesicovaginal N82.3
  rectovulval N82.4
    congenital Q52.79
  rectum (to skin) K60.4
    congenital Q43.6
      with absence, atresia and stenosis Q42.0
    tuberculous A18.32
  renal N28.89
  retroauricular — *see* Fistula, postauricular
  salivary duct or gland (any) K11.4
    congenital Q38.4
  scrotum (urinary) N50.8
    tuberculous A18.15
  semicircular canalsH83.1
  sigmoid K63.2
    to bladder N32.1
  sinus — *see* Sinusitis
  skin L98.8
    to genital tract (female) N82.5
  splenocolic D73.89
  stercoral K63.2
  stomach K31.6
  sublingual gland K11.4
  submandibular gland K11.4
  submaxillary (gland) K11.4
    region K12.2
  thoracic J86.0

Fistula — *continued*
  duct I89.8
  thoracoabdominal J86.0
  thoracogastric J86.0
  thoracointestinal J86.0
  thorax J86.0
  thyroglossal duct Q89.2
  thyroid E07.89
  trachea, congenital (external) (internal) Q32.1
  tracheoesophageal J86.0
    congenital Q39.2
      with atresia of esophagus Q39.1
    following tracheostomy J95.04
  traumatic arteriovenous — *see* Injury, blood vessel, by site
  tuberculous - code by site under Tuberculosis
  typhoid A01.09
  umbilicourinary Q64.8
  urachus, congenital Q64.4
  ureter (persistent) N28.89
  ureteroabdominal N28.89
  ureterorectal N28.89
  ureterosigmoido-abdominal N28.89
  ureterovaginal N82.1
  ureterovesical N32.2
  urethra N36.0
    congenital Q64.79
    tuberculous A18.13
  urethroperineal N36.0
  urethroperineovesical N32.2
  urethrorectal N36.0
    congenital Q64.73
  urethroscrotal N50.8
  urethrovaginal N82.1
  urethrovesical N32.2
  urinary (tract) (persistent) (recurrent) N36.0
  uteroabdominal N82.5
    congenital Q51.7
  uteroenteric, uterointestinal N82.4
    congenital Q51.7
  uterorectal N82.4
    congenital Q51.7
  uteroureteric N82.1
  uterourethral Q51.7
  uterovaginal N82.8
  uterovesical N82.1
    congenital Q51.7
  uterus N82.8
  vagina (postpartal) (wall) N82.8
  vaginocutaneous (postpartal) N82.5
  vaginointestinal NEC N82.4
    large intestine N82.3
    small intestine N82.2
  vaginoperineal N82.5
  vasocutaneous, congenital Q55.7
  vesical NEC N32.2
  vesicoabdominal N32.2
  vesicocervicovaginal N82.1
  vesicocolic N32.1
  vesicocutaneous N32.2
  vesicoenteric N32.1
  vesicointestinal N32.1
  vesicometrorectal N82.4
  vesicoperineal N32.2
  vesicorectal N32.1
    congenital Q64.79
  vesicosigmoidal N32.1
  vesicosigmoidovaginal N82.3
  vesicoureteral N32.2
  vesicoureterovaginal N82.1
  vesicourethral N32.2
  vesicourethrorectal N32.1
  vesicouterine N82.1
    congenital Q51.7
  vesicovaginal N82.0
  vulvorectal N82.4
    congenital Q52.79
Fit R56.9
  epileptic — *see* Epilepsy
  fainting R55
  hysterical F44.5
  newborn P90
Fitting (and adjustment) (of)
  artificial
    arm — *see* Admission, adjustment, artificial, arm
    breast Z44.3 ☑
    eye Z44.2 ☑
    leg — *see* Admission, adjustment, artificial, leg
  automatic implantable cardiac defibrillator (with synchronous cardiac pacemaker) Z45.02
  brain neuropacemaker Z46.2

☑ **Additional character required**

Fitting — *continued*
  implanted Z45.42
  cardiac defibrillator — *see* Fitting (and adjustment) (of), automatic implantable cardiac defibrillator
  catheter, non-vascular Z46.82
  colostomy belt Z46.89
  contact lenses Z46.0
  cystostomy device Z46.6
  defibrillator, cardiac — *see* Fitting (and adjustment) (of), automatic implantable cardiac defibrillator
  dentures Z46.3
  device NOS Z46.9
    abdominal Z46.89
    gastrointestinal NEC Z46.59
    implanted NEC Z45.89
    nervous system Z46.2
      implanted — *see* Admission, adjustment, device, implanted, nervous system
    orthodontic Z46.4
    orthoptic Z46.0
    orthotic Z46.89
    prosthetic (external) Z44.9
      breast Z44.3 ☑
      dental Z46.3
      eye Z44.2 ☑
      specified NEC Z44.8
    specified NEC Z46.89
    substitution
      auditory Z46.2
        implanted — *see* Admission, adjustment, device, implanted, hearing device
      nervous system Z46.2
        implanted — *see* Admission, adjustment, device, implanted, nervous system
      visual Z46.2
        implanted Z45.31
    urinary Z46.6
  gastric lap band Z46.51
  gastrointestinal appliance NEC Z46.59
  glasses (reading) Z46.0
  hearing aid Z46.1
  ileostomy device Z46.89
  insulin pump Z46.81
  intestinal appliance NEC Z46.89
  myringotomy device (stent) (tube) Z45.82
  neuropacemaker Z46.2
    implanted Z45.42
  non-vascular catheter Z46.82
  orthodontic device Z46.4
  orthopedic device (brace) (cast) (corset) (shoes) Z46.89
  pacemaker (cardiac) Z45.018
    nervous system (brain) (peripheral nerve) (spinal cord) Z46.2
      implanted Z45.42
    pulse generator Z45.010
  portacath (port-a-cath) Z45.2
  prosthesis (external) Z44.9
    arm — *see* Admission, adjustment, artificial, arm
    breast Z44.3 ☑
    dental Z46.3
    eye Z44.2 ☑
    leg — *see* Admission, adjustment, artificial, leg
    specified NEC Z44.8
  spectacles Z46.0
  wheelchair Z46.89
Fitzhugh-Curtis syndrome
  due to
    Chlamydia trachomatis A74.81
    Neisseria gonorrhorea (gonococcal peritonitis) A54.85
Fitz's syndrome (acute hemorrhagic pancreatitis) K85.8
Fixation
  joint — *see* Ankylosis
  larynx J38.7
  stapes — *see* Ankylosis, ear ossicles
    deafness — *see* Deafness, conductive
  uterus (acquired) — *see* Malposition, uterus
  vocal cord J38.3
Flabby ridge K06.8
Flaccid (*see also* condition)
  palate, congenital Q38.5
Flail
  chest S22.5 ☑
    newborn (birth injury) P13.8
  joint (paralytic) M25.20
    ankle M25.27- ☑
    elbow M25.22- ☑

Flail — *continued*
    foot joint M25.27- ☑
    hand joint M25.24- ☑
    hip M25.25- ☑
    knee M25.26- ☑
    shoulder M25.21- ☑
    specified joint NEC M25.28
    wrist M25.23- ☑
Flajani's disease — *see* Hyperthyroidism, with, goiter (diffuse)
Flap, liver K71.3
Flashbacks (residual to hallucinogen use) F16.283
Flat
  chamber (eye) — *see* Disorder, globe, hypotony, flat anterior chamber
  chest, congenital Q67.8
  foot (acquired) (fixed type) (painful) (postural) (*see also* Deformity, limb, flat foot)
    congenital (rigid) (spastic) (everted) Q66.5- ☑
    rachitic sequelae (late effect) E64.3
  organ or site, congenital NEC — *see* Anomaly, by site
  pelvis M95.5
    with disproportion (fetopelvic) O33.0
      causing obstructed labor O65.0
    congenital Q74.2
Flatau-Schilder disease G37.0
Flatback syndrome M40.30
  lumbar region M40.36
  lumbosacral region M40.37
  thoracolumbar region M40.35
Flattening
  head, femur M89.8X5
  hip — *see* Coxa, plana
  lip (congenital) Q18.8
  nose (congenital) Q67.4
    acquired M95.0
Flatulence R14.3
  psychogenic F45.8
Flatus R14.3
  vaginalis N89.8
Flax-dresser's disease J66.1
Flea bite — *see* Injury, bite, by site, superficial, insect
Flecks, glaucomatous (subcapsular) — *see* Cataract, complicated
Fleischer (-Kayser) ring (cornea) H18.04- ☑
Fleshy mole O02.0
Flexibilitas cerea — *see* Catalepsy
Flexion
  amputation stump (surgical) T87.89
  cervix — *see* Malposition, uterus
  contracture, joint — *see* Contraction, joint
  deformity, joint (*see also* Deformity, limb, flexion) M21.20
    hip, congenital Q65.89
  uterus (*see also* Malposition, uterus)
    lateral — *see* Lateroversion, uterus
Flexner-Boyd dysentery A03.2
Flexner's dysentery A03.1
Flexure — *see* Flexion
Flint murmur (aortic insufficiency) I35.1
Floater, vitreous — *see* Opacity, vitreous
Floating
  cartilage (joint) (*see also* Loose, body, joint)
    knee — *see* Derangement, knee, loose body
  gallbladder, congenital Q44.1
  kidney N28.89
    congenital Q63.8
  spleen D73.89
Flooding N92.0
Floor — *see* condition
Floppy
  baby syndrome (nonspecific) P94.2
  iris syndrome (intraoperative) (IFIS) H21.81
  nonrheumatic mitral valve syndrome I34.1
Flu (*see also* Influenza)
  avian (*see also* Influenza, due to, identified novel influenza A virus) J09.X2
  bird (*see also* Influenza, due to, identified novel influenza A virus) J09.X2
  intestinal NEC A08.4
  swine (viruses that normally cause infections in pigs) (*see also* Influenza, due to, identified novel influenza A virus) J09.X2
Fluctuating blood pressure I99.8
Fluid
  abdomen R18.8
  chest J94.8
  heart — *see* Failure, heart, congestive
  joint — *see* Effusion, joint
  loss (acute) E86.9
    with

Fluid — *continued*
    hypernatremia E87.0
    hyponatremia E87.1
  lung — *see* Edema, lung
  overload E87.70
    specified NEC E87.79
  peritoneal cavity R18.8
  pleural cavity J94.8
  retention R60.9
Flukes NEC (*see also* Infestation, fluke)
  blood NEC — *see* Schistosomiasis
  liver B66.3
Fluor (vaginalis) N89.8
  trichomonal or due to Trichomonas (vaginalis) A59.00
Fluorosis
  dental K00.3
  skeletal M85.10
    ankle M85.17- ☑
    foot M85.17- ☑
    forearm M85.13- ☑
    hand M85.14- ☑
    lower leg M85.16- ☑
    multiple site M85.19
    neck M85.18
    rib M85.18
    shoulder M85.11- ☑
    skull M85.18
    specified site NEC M85.18
    thigh M85.15- ☑
    toe M85.17- ☑
    upper arm M85.12- ☑
    vertebra M85.18
Flush syndrome E34.0
Flushing R23.2
  menopausal N95.1
Flutter
  atrial or auricular I48.92
    atypical I48.4
    type I I48.3
    type II I48.4
    typical I48.3
  heart I49.8
    atrial or auricular I48.92
      atypical I48.4
      type I I48.3
      type II I48.4
      typical I48.3
    ventricular I49.02
  ventricular I49.02
FNHTR (febrile nonhemolytic transfusion reaction) R50.84
Fochier's abscess - code by site under Abscess
Focus, Assmann's — *see* Tuberculosis, pulmonary
Fogo selvagem L10.3
Foix-Alajouanine syndrome G95.19
Fold, folds (anomalous) (*see also* Anomaly, by site)
  Descemet's membrane — *see* Change, corneal membrane, Descemet's, fold
  epicanthic Q10.3
  heart Q24.8
Folie deux F24
Follicle
  cervix (nabothian) (ruptured) N88.8
  graafian, ruptured, with hemorrhage N83.0
  nabothian N88.8
Follicular — *see* condition
Folliculitis (superficial) L73.9
  abscedens et suffodiens L66.3
  cyst N83.0
  decalvans L66.2
  deep — *see* Furuncle, by site
  gonococcal (acute) (chronic) A54.01
  keloid, keloidalis L73.0
  pustular L01.02
  ulerythematosa reticulata L66.4
Folliculome lipidique
  specified site — *see* Neoplasm, benign, by site
  unspecified site
    female D27.9
    male D29.20
Følling's disease E70.0
Follow-up — *see* Examination, follow-up
Fong's syndrome (hereditary osteo-onychodysplasia) Q78.5
Food
  allergy L27.2
  asphyxia (from aspiration or inhalation) — *see* Foreign body, by site
  choked on — *see* Foreign body, by site
  deprivation T73.0 ☑
    specified kind of food NEC E63.8

Food — continued
  intoxication — see Poisoning, food
  lack of T73.0 ☑
  poisoning — see Poisoning, food
  rejection NEC — see Disorder, eating
  strangulation or suffocation — see Foreign body, by site
  toxemia — see Poisoning, food
Foot — see condition
Foramen ovale (nonclosure) (patent) (persistent) Q21.1
Forbes' glycogen storage disease E74.03
Fordyce-Fox disease L75.2
Fordyce's disease (mouth) Q38.6
Forearm — see condition
Foreign body
  with
    laceration — see Laceration, by site, with foreign body
    puncture wound — see Puncture, by site, with foreign body
  accidentally left following a procedure T81.509 ☑
  aspiration T81.506 ☑
    resulting in
      adhesions T81.516 ☑
      obstruction T81.526 ☑
      perforation T81.536 ☑
      specified complication NEC T81.596 ☑
  cardiac catheterization T81.505 ☑
    resulting in
      acute reaction T81.60 ☑
        aseptic peritonitis T81.61 ☑
        specified NEC T81.69 ☑
      adhesions T81.515 ☑
      obstruction T81.525 ☑
      perforation T81.535 ☑
      specified complication NEC T81.595 ☑
  causing
    acute reaction T81.60 ☑
      aseptic peritonitis T81.61 ☑
      specified complication NEC T81.69 ☑
    adhesions T81.519 ☑
    aseptic peritonitis T81.61 ☑
    obstruction T81.529 ☑
    perforation T81.539 ☑
    specified complication NEC T81.599 ☑
  endoscopy T81.504 ☑
    resulting in
      adhesions T81.514 ☑
      obstruction T81.524 ☑
      perforation T81.534 ☑
      specified complication NEC T81.594 ☑
  immunization T81.503 ☑
    resulting in
      adhesions T81.513 ☑
      obstruction T81.523 ☑
      perforation T81.533 ☑
      specified complication NEC T81.593 ☑
  infusion T81.501 ☑
    resulting in
      adhesions T81.511 ☑
      obstruction T81.521 ☑
      perforation T81.531 ☑
      specified complication NEC T81.591 ☑
  injection T81.503 ☑
    resulting in
      adhesions T81.513 ☑
      obstruction T81.523 ☑
      perforation T81.533 ☑
      specified complication NEC T81.593 ☑
  kidney dialysis T81.502 ☑
    resulting in
      adhesions T81.512 ☑
      obstruction T81.522 ☑
      perforation T81.532 ☑
      specified complication NEC T81.592 ☑
  packing removal T81.507 ☑
    resulting in
      acute reaction T81.60 ☑
        aseptic peritonitis T81.61 ☑
        specified NEC T81.69 ☑
      adhesions T81.517 ☑
      obstruction T81.527 ☑
      perforation T81.537 ☑
      specified complication NEC T81.597 ☑
  puncture T81.506 ☑
    resulting in
      adhesions T81.516 ☑
      obstruction T81.526 ☑
      perforation T81.536 ☑
      specified complication NEC T81.596 ☑
  specified procedure NEC T81.508 ☑

Foreign — continued
  resulting in
    acute reaction T81.60 ☑
      aseptic peritonitis T81.61 ☑
      specified NEC T81.69 ☑
    adhesions T81.518 ☑
    obstruction T81.528 ☑
    perforation T81.538 ☑
    specified complication NEC T81.598 ☑
  surgical operation T81.500 ☑
    resulting in
      acute reaction T81.60 ☑
        aseptic peritonitis T81.61 ☑
        specified NEC T81.69 ☑
      adhesions T81.510 ☑
      obstruction T81.520 ☑
      perforation T81.530 ☑
      specified complication NEC T81.590 ☑
  transfusion T81.501 ☑
    resulting in
      adhesions T81.511 ☑
      obstruction T81.521 ☑
      perforation T81.531 ☑
      specified complication NEC T81.591 ☑
  alimentary tract T18.9 ☑
    anus T18.5 ☑
    colon T18.4 ☑
    esophagus — see Foreign body, esophagus
    mouth T18.0 ☑
    multiple sites T18.8 ☑
    rectosigmoid (junction) T18.5 ☑
    rectum T18.5 ☑
    small intestine T18.3 ☑
    specified site NEC T18.8 ☑
    stomach T18.2 ☑
  anterior chamber (eye) S05.5- ☑
  auditory canal — see Foreign body, entering through orifice, ear
  bronchus T17.508 ☑
    causing
      asphyxiation T17.500 ☑
        food (bone) (seed) T17.520 ☑
        gastric contents (vomitus) T17.510 ☑
        specified type NEC T17.590 ☑
      injury NEC T17.508 ☑
        food (bone) (seed) T17.528 ☑
        gastric contents (vomitus) T17.518 ☑
        specified type NEC T17.598 ☑
  canthus — see Foreign body, conjunctival sac
  ciliary body (eye) S05.5- ☑
  conjunctival sac T15.1- ☑
  cornea T15.0- ☑
  entering through orifice
    accessory sinus T17.0 ☑
    alimentary canal T18.9 ☑
      multiple parts T18.8 ☑
      specified part NEC T18.8 ☑
    alveolar process T18.0 ☑
    antrum (Highmore's) T17.0 ☑
    anus T18.5 ☑
    appendix T18.4 ☑
    auditory canal — see Foreign body, entering through orifice, ear
    auricle — see Foreign body, entering through orifice, ear
    bladder T19.1 ☑
    bronchioles — see Foreign body, respiratory tract, specified site NEC
    bronchus (main) — see Foreign body, bronchus
    buccal cavity T18.0 ☑
    canthus (inner) — see Foreign body, conjunctival sac
    cecum T18.4 ☑
    cervix (canal) (uteri) T19.3 ☑
    colon T18.4 ☑
    conjunctival sac — see Foreign body, conjunctival sac
    cornea — see Foreign body, cornea
    digestive organ or tract NOS T18.9 ☑
      multiple parts T18.8 ☑
      specified part NEC T18.8 ☑
    duodenum T18.3 ☑
    ear (external) T16.- ☑
    esophagus — see Foreign body, esophagus
    eye (external) NOS T15.9- ☑
      conjunctival sac — see Foreign body, conjunctival sac
      cornea — see Foreign body, cornea
      specified part NEC T15.8- ☑
    eyeball (see also Foreign body, entering through orifice, eye, specified part NEC)

Foreign — continued
  with penetrating wound — see Puncture, eyeball
  eyelid (see also Foreign body, conjunctival sac) with
    laceration — see Laceration, eyelid, with foreign body
    puncture — see Puncture, eyelid, with foreign body
    superficial injury — see Foreign body, superficial, eyelid
  gastrointestinal tract T18.9 ☑
    multiple parts T18.8 ☑
    specified part NEC T18.8 ☑
  genitourinary tract T19.9 ☑
    multiple parts T19.8 ☑
    specified part NEC T19.8 ☑
  globe — see Foreign body, entering through orifice, eyeball
  gum T18.0 ☑
  Highmore's antrum T17.0 ☑
  hypopharynx — see Foreign body, pharynx
  ileum T18.3 ☑
  intestine (small) T18.3 ☑
    large T18.4 ☑
  lacrimal apparatus (punctum) — see Foreign body, entering through orifice, eye, specified part NEC
  large intestine T18.4 ☑
  larynx — see Foreign body, larynx
  lung — see Foreign body, respiratory tract, specified site NEC
  maxillary sinus T17.0 ☑
  mouth T18.0 ☑
  nasal sinus T17.0 ☑
  nasopharynx — see Foreign body, pharynx
  nose (passage) T17.1 ☑
  nostril T17.1 ☑
  oral cavity T18.0 ☑
  palate T18.0 ☑
  penis T19.4 ☑
  pharynx — see Foreign body, pharynx
  piriform sinus — see Foreign body, pharynx
  rectosigmoid (junction) T18.5 ☑
  rectum T18.5 ☑
  respiratory tract — see Foreign body, respiratory tract
  sinus (accessory) (frontal) (maxillary) (nasal) T17.0 ☑
    piriform — see Foreign body, pharynx
  small intestine T18.3 ☑
  stomach T18.2 ☑
  suffocation by — see Foreign body, by site
  tear ducts or glands — see Foreign body, entering through orifice, eye, specified part NEC
  throat — see Foreign body, pharynx
  tongue T18.0 ☑
  tonsil, tonsillar (fossa) — see Foreign body, pharynx
  trachea — see Foreign body, trachea
  ureter T19.8 ☑
  urethra T19.0 ☑
  uterus (any part) T19.3 ☑
  vagina T19.2 ☑
  vulva T19.2 ☑
  esophagus T18.108 ☑
    causing
      injury NEC T18.108 ☑
        food (bone) (seed) T18.128 ☑
        gastric contents (vomitus) T18.118 ☑
        specified type NEC T18.198 ☑
      tracheal compression T18.100 ☑
        food (bone) (seed) T18.120 ☑
        gastric contents (vomitus) T18.110 ☑
        specified type NEC T18.190 ☑
  felling of, in throat R09.89
  fragment — see Retained, foreign body fragments (type of)
  genitourinary tract T19.9 ☑
    bladder T19.1 ☑
    multiple parts T19.8 ☑
    penis T19.4 ☑
    specified site NEC T19.8 ☑
    urethra T19.0 ☑
    uterus T19.3 ☑
      IUD Z97.5
    vagina T19.2 ☑
      contraceptive device Z97.5
    vulva T19.2 ☑
  granuloma (old) (soft tissue) (see also Granuloma, foreign body)

☑ **Additional character required**

Foreign — *continued*
- skin L92.3
- in
  - laceration — *see* Laceration, by site, with foreign body
  - puncture wound — *see* Puncture, by site, with foreign body
  - soft tissue (residual) M79.5
- inadvertently left in operation wound — *see* Foreign body, accidentally left during a procedure
- ingestion, ingested NOS T18.9 ☑
- inhalation or inspiration — *see* Foreign body, by site
- internal organ, not entering through a natural orifice - code as specific injury with foreign body
- intraocular S05.5- ☑
  - old, retained (nonmagnetic) H44.70- ☑
    - anterior chamber H44.71- ☑
    - ciliary body H44.72- ☑
    - iris H44.72- ☑
    - lens H44.73- ☑
    - magnetic H44.60- ☑
      - anterior chamber H44.61- ☑
      - ciliary body H44.62- ☑
      - iris H44.62- ☑
      - lens H44.63- ☑
      - posterior wall H44.64- ☑
      - specified site NEC H44.69- ☑
      - vitreous body H44.65- ☑
    - posterior wall H44.74- ☑
    - specified site NEC H44.79- ☑
    - vitreous body H44.75- ☑
  - iris — *see* Foreign body, intraocular
- lacrimal punctum — *see* Foreign body, entering through orifice, eye, specified part NEC
- larynx T17.308 ☑
  - causing
    - asphyxiation T17.300 ☑
      - food (bone) (seed) T17.320 ☑
      - gastric contents (vomitus) T17.310 ☑
      - specified type NEC T17.390 ☑
    - injury NEC T17.308 ☑
      - food (bone) (seed) T17.328 ☑
      - gastric contents (vomitus) T17.318 ☑
      - specified type NEC T17.398 ☑
- lens — *see* Foreign body, intraocular
- ocular muscle S05.4- ☑
  - old, retained — *see* Foreign body, orbit, old
- old or residual
  - soft tissue (residual) M79.5
- operation wound, left accidentally — *see* Foreign body, accidentally left during a procedure
- orbit S05.4- ☑
  - old, retained H05.5- ☑
- pharynx T17.208 ☑
  - causing
    - asphyxiation T17.200 ☑
      - food (bone) (seed) T17.220 ☑
      - gastric contents (vomitus) T17.210 ☑
      - specified type NEC T17.290 ☑
    - injury NEC T17.208 ☑
      - food (bone) (seed) T17.228 ☑
      - gastric contents (vomitus) T17.218 ☑
      - specified type NEC T17.298 ☑
- respiratory tract T17.908 ☑
  - bronchioles — *see* Foreign body, respiratory tract, specified site NEC
  - bronchus — *see* Foreign body, bronchus
  - causing
    - asphyxiation T17.900 ☑
      - food (bone) (seed) T17.920 ☑
      - gastric contents (vomitus) T17.910 ☑
      - specified type NEC T17.990 ☑
    - injury NEC T17.908 ☑
      - food (bone) (seed) T17.928 ☑
      - gastric contents (vomitus) T17.918 ☑
      - specified type NEC T17.998 ☑
  - larynx — *see* Foreign body, larynx
  - lung — *see* Foreign body, respiratory tract, specified site NEC
  - multiple parts — *see* Foreign body, respiratory tract, specified site NEC
- nasal sinus T17.0
- nasopharynx — *see* Foreign body, pharynx
- nose T17.1 ☑
- nostril T17.1 ☑
- pharynx — *see* Foreign body, pharynx
- specified site NEC T17.808 ☑
  - causing
    - asphyxiation T17.800 ☑

Foreign — *continued*
- food (bone) (seed) T17.820 ☑
- gastric contents (vomitus) T17.810 ☑
- specified type NEC T17.890 ☑
- injury NEC T17.808 ☑
  - food (bone) (seed) T17.828 ☑
  - gastric contents (vomitus) T17.818 ☑
  - specified type NEC T17.898 ☑
- throat — *see* Foreign body, pharynx
- trachea — *see* Foreign body, trachea
- retained (old) (nonmagnetic) (in)
  - anterior chamber (eye) — *see* Foreign body, intraocular, old, retained, anterior chamber
  - magnetic — *see* Foreign body, intraocular, old, retained, magnetic, anterior chamber
  - ciliary body — *see* Foreign body, intraocular, old, retained, ciliary body
  - magnetic — *see* Foreign body, intraocular, old, retained, magnetic, ciliary body
  - eyelid H02.819
    - left H02.816
      - lower H02.815
      - upper H02.814
    - right H02.813
      - lower H02.812
      - upper H02.811
  - fragments — *see* Retained, foreign body fragments (type of)
  - globe — *see* Foreign body, intraocular, old, retained
    - magnetic — *see* Foreign body, intraocular, old, retained, magnetic
  - intraocular — *see* Foreign body, intraocular, old, retained
    - magnetic — *see* Foreign body, intraocular, old, retained, magnetic
  - iris — *see* Foreign body, intraocular, old, retained, iris
    - magnetic — *see* Foreign body, intraocular, old, retained, magnetic, iris
  - lens — *see* Foreign body, intraocular, old, retained, lens
    - magnetic — *see* Foreign body, intraocular, old, retained, magnetic, lens
  - muscle — *see* Foreign body, retained, soft tissue
  - orbit — *see* Foreign body, orbit, old
  - posterior wall of globe — *see* Foreign body, intraocular, old, retained, posterior wall
    - magnetic — *see* Foreign body, intraocular, old, retained, magnetic, posterior wall
  - retrobulbar — *see* Foreign body, orbit, old, retrobulbar
  - soft tissue M79.5
  - vitreous — *see* Foreign body, intraocular, old, retained, vitreous body
    - magnetic — *see* Foreign body, intraocular, old, retained, magnetic, vitreous body
- retina S05.5- ☑
- superficial, without open wound
  - abdomen, abdominal (wall) S30.851 ☑
  - alveolar process S00.552 ☑
  - ankle S90.55- ☑
  - antecubital space — *see* Foreign body, superficial, forearm
  - anus S30.857 ☑
  - arm (upper) S40.85- ☑
  - auditory canal — *see* Foreign body, superficial, ear
  - auricle — *see* Foreign body, superficial, ear
  - axilla — *see* Foreign body, superficial, arm
  - back, lower S30.850 ☑
  - breast S20.15- ☑
  - brow S00.85 ☑
  - buttock S30.850 ☑
  - calf — *see* Foreign body, superficial, leg
  - canthus — *see* Foreign body, superficial, eyelid
  - cheek S00.85 ☑
    - internal S00.552 ☑
  - chest wall — *see* Foreign body, superficial, thorax
  - chin S00.85 ☑
  - clitoris S30.854 ☑
  - costal region — *see* Foreign body, superficial, thorax
  - digit (s)
    - hand — *see* Foreign body, superficial, finger
    - foot — *see* Foreign body, superficial, toe
  - ear S00.45- ☑
  - elbow S50.35- ☑
  - epididymis S30.853 ☑

Foreign — *continued*
- epigastric region S30.851 ☑
- epiglottis S10.15 ☑
- esophagus, cervical S10.15 ☑
- eyebrow — *see* Foreign body, superficial, eyelid
- eyelid S00.25- ☑
- face S00.85 ☑
- finger (s) S60.459 ☑
  - index S60.45- ☑
  - little S60.45- ☑
  - middle S60.45- ☑
  - ring S60.45- ☑
- flank S30.851 ☑
- foot (except toe(s) alone) S90.85- ☑
  - toe — *see* Foreign body, superficial, toe
- forearm S50.85- ☑
  - elbow only — *see* Foreign body, superficial, elbow
- forehead S00.85 ☑
- genital organs, external
  - female S30.856 ☑
  - male S30.855 ☑
- groin S30.851 ☑
- gum S00.552 ☑
- hand S60.55- ☑
- head S00.95 ☑
  - ear — *see* Foreign body, superficial, ear
  - eyelid — *see* Foreign body, superficial, eyelid
  - lip S00.551 ☑
  - nose S00.35 ☑
  - oral cavity S00.552 ☑
  - scalp S00.05 ☑
  - specified site NEC S00.85 ☑
- heel — *see* Foreign body, superficial, foot
- hip S70.25- ☑
- inguinal region S30.851 ☑
- interscapular region S20.459 ☑
- jaw S00.85 ☑
- knee S80.25- ☑
- labium (majus) (minus) S30.854 ☑
- larynx S10.15 ☑
- leg (lower) S80.85- ☑
  - knee — *see* Foreign body, superficial, knee
  - upper — *see* Foreign body, superficial, thigh
- lip S00.551 ☑
- lower back S30.850 ☑
- lumbar region S30.850 ☑
- malar region S00.85 ☑
- mammary — *see* Foreign body, superficial, breast
- mastoid region S00.85 ☑
- mouth S00.552 ☑
- nail
  - finger — *see* Foreign body, superficial, finger
  - toe — *see* Foreign body, superficial, toe
- nape S10.85 ☑
- nasal S00.35 ☑
- neck S10.95 ☑
  - specified site NEC S10.85 ☑
  - throat S10.15 ☑
- nose S00.35 ☑
- occipital region S00.05 ☑
- oral cavity S00.552 ☑
- orbital region — *see* Foreign body, superficial, eyelid
- palate S00.552 ☑
- palm — *see* Foreign body, superficial, hand
- parietal region S00.05 ☑
- pelvis S30.850 ☑
- penis S30.852 ☑
- perineum
  - female S30.854 ☑
  - male S30.850 ☑
- periocular area — *see* Foreign body, superficial, eyelid
- phalanges
  - finger — *see* Foreign body, superficial, finger
  - toe — *see* Foreign body, superficial, toe
- pharynx S10.15 ☑
- pinna — *see* Foreign body, superficial, ear
- popliteal space — *see* Foreign body, superficial, knee
- prepuce S30.852 ☑
- pubic region S30.850 ☑
- pudendum
  - female S30.856 ☑
  - male S30.855 ☑
- sacral region S30.850 ☑
- scalp S00.05 ☑
- scapular region — *see* Foreign body, superficial, shoulder
- scrotum S30.853 ☑

Foreign — *continued*
  shin — *see* Foreign body, superficial, leg
  shoulder S40.25- ☑
  sternal region S20.359 ☑
  submaxillary region S00.85 ☑
  submental region S00.85 ☑
  subungual
    finger (s) — *see* Foreign body, superficial, finger
    toe (s) — *see* Foreign body, superficial, toe
  supraclavicular fossa S10.85 ☑
  supraorbital S00.85 ☑
  temple S00.85 ☑
  temporal region S00.85 ☑
  testis S30.853 ☑
  thigh S70.35- ☑
  thorax, thoracic (wall) S20.95 ☑
    back S20.45- ☑
    front S20.35- ☑
  throat S10.15 ☑
  thumb S60.35- ☑
  toe (s) (lesser) S90.456 ☑
    great S90.45- ☑
  tongue S00.552 ☑
  trachea S10.15 ☑
  tunica vaginalis S30.853 ☑
  tympanum, tympanic membrane — *see* Foreign body, superficial, ear
  uvula S00.552 ☑
  vagina S30.854 ☑
  vocal cords S10.15 ☑
  vulva S30.854 ☑
  wrist S60.85- ☑
  swallowed T18.9 ☑
  trachea T17.408 ☑
    causing
      asphyxiation T17.400 ☑
        food (bone) (seed) T17.420 ☑
        gastric contents (vomitus) T17.410 ☑
        specified type NEC T17.490 ☑
      injury NEC T17.408 ☑
        food (bone) (seed) T17.428 ☑
        gastric contents (vomitus) T17.418 ☑
        specified type NEC T17.498 ☑
  type of fragment — *see* Retained, foreign body fragments (type of)
  vitreous (humor) S05.5- ☑
Forestier's disease (rhizomelic pseudopolyarthritis) M35.3
  meaning ankylosing hyperostosis — *see* Hyperostosis, ankylosing
Formation
  hyalin in cornea — *see* Degeneration, cornea
  sequestrum in bone (due to infection) — *see* Osteomyelitis, chronic
  valve
    colon, congenital Q43.8
    ureter (congenital) Q62.39
Formication R20.2
Fort Bragg fever A27.89
Fossa (*see also* condition)
  pyriform — *see* condition
Foster-Kennedy syndrome H47.14- ☑
Fothergill's
  disease (trigeminal neuralgia) (*see also* Neuralgia, trigeminal)
  scarlatina anginosa A38.9
Foul breath R19.6
Foundling Z76.1
Fournier disease or gangrene N49.3
  female N76.89
Fourth
  cranial nerve — *see* condition
  molar K00.1
Foville's (peduncular) disease or syndrome G46.3
Fox (-Fordyce) disease (apocrine miliaria) L75.2
Fracture, burst — *see* Fracture, traumatic, by site
Fracture, chronic — *see* Fracture, pathological
Fracture, insufficiency — *see* Fracture, pathologic, by site
Fracture, pathological (pathologic) (*see also* Fracture, traumatic M84.40)
  ankle M84.47- ☑
  carpus M84.44- ☑
  clavicle M84.41- ☑
  dental implant M27.63
  dental restorative material K08.539
    with loss of material K08.531
    without loss of material K08.530
  due to
    neoplastic disease NEC (*see also* Neoplasm) M84.50 ☑

Fracture — *continued*
  ankle M84.57- ☑
  carpus M84.54- ☑
  clavicle M84.51- ☑
  femur M84.55- ☑
  fibula M84.56- ☑
  finger M84.54- ☑
  hip M84.559 ☑
  humerus M84.52- ☑
  ilium M84.550 ☑
  ischium M84.550 ☑
  metacarpus M84.54- ☑
  metatarsus M84.57- ☑
  neck M84.58 ☑
  pelvis M84.550 ☑
  radius M84.53- ☑
  rib M84.58 ☑
  scapula M84.51- ☑
  skull M84.58 ☑
  specified site NEC M84.58 ☑
  tarsus M84.57- ☑
  tibia M84.56- ☑
  toe M84.57- ☑
  ulna M84.53- ☑
  vertebra M84.58 ☑
  osteoporosis M80.80 ☑
    disuse — *see* Osteoporosis, specified type NEC, with pathological fracture
    drug-induced — *see* Osteoporosis, drug induced, with pathological fracture
    idiopathic — *see* Osteoporosis, specified type NEC, with pathological fracture
    postmenopausal — *see* Osteoporosis, postmenopausal, with pathological fracture
    postoophorectomy — *see* Osteoporosis, postoophorectomy, with pathological fracture
    postsurgical malabsorption — *see* Osteoporosis, specified type NEC, with pathological fracture
    specified cause NEC — *see* Osteoporosis, specified type NEC, with pathological fracture
  specified disease NEC M84.60 ☑
    ankle M84.67- ☑
    carpus M84.64- ☑
    clavicle M84.61- ☑
    femur M84.65- ☑
    fibula M84.66- ☑
    finger M84.64- ☑
    hip M84.65- ☑
    humerus M84.62- ☑
    ilium M84.650 ☑
    ischium M84.650 ☑
    metacarpus M84.64- ☑
    metatarsus M84.67- ☑
    neck M84.68 ☑
    radius M84.63- ☑
    rib M84.68 ☑
    scapula M84.61- ☑
    skull M84.68 ☑
    tarsus M84.67- ☑
    tibia M84.66- ☑
    toe M84.67- ☑
    ulna M84.63- ☑
    vertebra M84.68 ☑
  femur M84.45- ☑
  fibula M84.46- ☑
  finger M84.44- ☑
  hip M84.459 ☑
  humerus M84.42- ☑
  ilium M84.454 ☑
  ischium M84.454 ☑
  joint prosthesis — *see* Complications, joint prosthesis, mechanical, breakdown, by site
    periprosthetic — *see* Complications, joint prosthesis, mechanical, periprosthesis, fracture, by site
  metacarpus M84.44- ☑
  metatarsus M84.47- ☑
  neck M84.48 ☑
  pelvis M84.454 ☑
  radius M84.43- ☑
  restorative material (dental) K08.539
    with loss of material K08.531
    without loss of material K08.530
  rib M84.48 ☑
  scapula M84.41- ☑
  skull M84.48 ☑
  tarsus M84.47- ☑
  tibia M84.46- ☑

Fracture — *continued*
  toe M84.47- ☑
  ulna M84.43- ☑
  vertebra M84.48 ☑
Fracture, traumatic (abduction) (adduction) (separation) (*see also* Fracture, pathological) T14.8
  acetabulum S32.40- ☑
    column
      anterior (displaced) (iliopubic) S32.43- ☑
        nondisplaced S32.436 ☑
      posterior (displaced) (ilioischial) S32.443 ☑
        nondisplaced S32.44- ☑
    dome (displaced) S32.48- ☑
      nondisplaced S32.48 ☑
    specified NEC S32.49- ☑
    transverse (displaced) S32.45- ☑
      with associated posterior wall fracture (displaced) S32.46- ☑
        nondisplaced S32.46- ☑
      nondisplaced S32.45- ☑
    wall
      anterior (displaced) S32.41- ☑
        nondisplaced S32.41- ☑
      medial (displaced) S32.47- ☑
        nondisplaced S32.47- ☑
      posterior (displaced) S32.42- ☑
        with associated transverse fracture (displaced) S32.46- ☑
          nondisplaced S32.46- ☑
        nondisplaced S32.42- ☑
  acromion — *see* Fracture, scapula, acromial process
  ankle S82.899 ☑
    bimalleolar (displaced) S82.84- ☑
      nondisplaced S82.84- ☑
    lateral malleolus only (displaced) S82.6- ☑
      nondisplaced S82.6- ☑
    medial malleolus (displaced) S82.5- ☑
      associated with Maisonneuve's fracture — *see* Fracture, Maisonneuve's
      nondisplaced S82.5- ☑
    talus — *see* Fracture, tarsal, talus
    trimalleolar (displaced) S82.85- ☑
      nondisplaced S82.85- ☑
  arm (upper) (*see also* Fracture, humerus, shaft)
    humerus — *see* Fracture, humerus
    radius — *see* Fracture, radius
    ulna — *see* Fracture, ulna
  astragalus — *see* Fracture, tarsal, talus
  atlas — *see* Fracture, neck, cervical vertebra, first
  axis — *see* Fracture, neck, cervical vertebra, second
  back — *see* Fracture, vertebra
  Barton's — *see* Barton's fracture
  base of skull — *see* Fracture, skull, base
  basicervical (basal) (femoral) S72.0 ☑
  Bennett's — *see* Bennett's fracture
  bimalleolar — *see* Fracture, ankle, bimalleolar
  blow-out S02.3 ☑
  bone NEC T14.8
    birth injury P13.9
    following insertion of orthopedic implant, joint prosthesis or bone plate — *see* Fracture, following insertion of orthopedic implant, joint prosthesis or bone plate
    in (due to) neoplastic disease NEC — *see* Fracture, pathological, due to, neoplastic disease
    pathological (cause unknown) — *see* Fracture, pathological
  breast bone — *see* Fracture, sternum
  bucket handle (semilunar cartilage) — *see* Tear, meniscus
  burst — *see* Fracture, traumatic, by site
  calcaneus — *see* Fracture, tarsal, calcaneus
  carpal bone (s) S62.10- ☑
    capitate (displaced) S62.13- ☑
      nondisplaced S62.13- ☑
    cuneiform — *see* Fracture, carpal bone, triquetrum
    hamate (body) (displaced) S62.143 ☑
      hook process (displaced) S62.15- ☑
        nondisplaced S62.15- ☑
      nondisplaced S62.14- ☑
    larger multangular — *see* Fracture, carpal bones, trapezium
    lunate (displaced) S62.12- ☑
      nondisplaced S62.12- ☑
    navicular S62.00- ☑
      distal pole (displaced) S62.01- ☑
        nondisplaced S62.01- ☑
      middle third (displaced) S62.02- ☑

☑ **Additional character required**

Fracture — *continued*
- nondisplaced S62.02- ☑
- proximal third (displaced) S62.03- ☑
  - nondisplaced S62.03- ☑
- volar tuberosity — *see* Fracture, carpal bones, navicular, distal pole
- os magnum — *see* Fracture, carpal bones, capitate
- pisiform (displaced) S62.16- ☑
  - nondisplaced S62.16- ☑
- semilunar — *see* Fracture, carpal bones, lunate
- smaller multangular — *see* Fracture, carpal bones, trapezoid
- trapezium (displaced) S62.17- ☑
  - nondisplaced S62.17- ☑
- trapezoid (displaced) S62.18- ☑
  - nondisplaced S62.18- ☑
- triquetrum (displaced) S62.11- ☑
  - nondisplaced S62.11- ☑
- unciform — *see* Fracture, carpal bones, hamate
- cervical — *see* Fracture, vertebra, cervical
- clavicle S42.00- ☑
  - acromial end (displaced) S42.03- ☑
    - nondisplaced S42.03- ☑
  - birth injury P13.4
  - lateral end — *see* Fracture, clavicle, acromial end
  - shaft (displaced) S42.02- ☑
    - nondisplaced S42.02- ☑
  - sternal end (anterior) (displaced) S42.01- ☑
    - nondisplaced S42.01- ☑
    - posterior S42.01- ☑
- coccyx S32.2 ☑
- collapsed — *see* Collapse, vertebra
- collar bone — *see* Fracture, clavicle
- Colles' — *see* Colles' fracture
- compression, not due to trauma — *see* Collapse, vertebra
- coronoid process — *see* Fracture, ulna, upper end, coronoid process
- corpus cavernosum penis S39.840 ☑
- costochondral cartilage S23.41 ☑
- costochondral, costosternal junction — *see* Fracture, rib
- cranium — *see* Fracture, skull
- cricoid cartilage S12.8 ☑
- cuboid (ankle) — *see* Fracture, tarsal, cuboid
- cuneiform
  - foot — *see* Fracture, tarsal, cuneiform
  - wrist — *see* Fracture, carpal, triquetrum
- delayed union — *see* Delay, union, fracture
- dental restorative material K08.539
  - with loss of material K08.531
  - without loss of material K08.530
- due to
  - birth injury — *see* Birth, injury, fracture
  - osteoporosis — *see* Osteoporosis, with fracture
- Dupuytren's — *see* Fracture, ankle, lateral malleolus
- elbow S42.40- ☑
- ethmoid (bone) (sinus) — *see* Fracture, skull, base
- face bone S02.92 ☑
- fatigue (*see also* Fracture, stress)
  - vertebra M48.40 ☑
    - cervical region M48.42 ☑
    - cervicothoracic region M48.43 ☑
    - lumbar region M48.46 ☑
    - lumbosacral region M48.47 ☑
    - occipito-atlanto-axial region M48.41 ☑
    - sacrococcygeal region M48.48 ☑
    - thoracic region M48.44 ☑
    - thoracolumbar region M48.45 ☑
- femur, femoral S72.9- ☑
  - basicervical (basal) S72.0 ☑
  - birth injury P13.2
  - capital epiphyseal S79.01- ☑
  - condyles, epicondyles — *see* Fracture, femur, lower end
  - distal end — *see* Fracture, femur, lower end
  - epiphysis
    - head — *see* Fracture, femur, upper end, epiphysis
    - lower — *see* Fracture, femur, lower end, epiphysis
    - upper — *see* Fracture, femur, upper end, epiphysis
  - following insertion of implant, prosthesis or plate M96.66- ☑
  - head — *see* Fracture, femur, upper end, head
  - intertrochanteric — *see* Fracture, femur, trochanteric

Fracture — *continued*
- intratrochanteric — *see* Fracture, femur, trochanteric
- lower end S72.40- ☑
  - condyle (displaced) S72.41- ☑
    - lateral (displaced) S72.42- ☑
      - nondisplaced S72.42- ☑
    - medial (displaced) S72.43- ☑
      - nondisplaced S72.43- ☑
    - nondisplaced S72.41- ☑
  - epiphysis (displaced) S72.44- ☑
    - nondisplaced S72.44- ☑
  - physeal S79.10- ☑
    - Salter-Harris
      - Type I S79.11- ☑
      - Type II S79.12- ☑
      - Type III S79.13- ☑
      - Type IV S79.14- ☑
    - specified NEC S79.19- ☑
  - specified NEC S72.49- ☑
  - supracondylar (displaced) S72.45- ☑
    - with intracondylar extension (displaced) S72.46- ☑
      - nondisplaced S72.46- ☑
    - nondisplaced S72.45- ☑
  - torus S72.47- ☑
- neck — *see* Fracture, femur, upper end, neck
- pertrochanteric — *see* Fracture, femur, trochanteric
- shaft (lower third) (middle third) (upper third) S72.30- ☑
  - comminuted (displaced) S72.35- ☑
    - nondisplaced S72.35- ☑
  - oblique (displaced) S72.33- ☑
    - nondisplaced S72.33- ☑
  - segmental (displaced) S72.36- ☑
    - nondisplaced S72.36- ☑
  - specified NEC S72.39- ☑
  - spiral (displaced) S72.34- ☑
    - nondisplaced S72.34- ☑
  - transverse (displaced) S72.32- ☑
    - nondisplaced S72.32- ☑
- specified site NEC S72.8
- subcapital (displaced) S72.01- ☑
- subtrochanteric (region) (section) (displaced) S72.2- ☑
  - nondisplaced S72.2- ☑
- transcervical — *see* Fracture, femur, upper end, neck
- transtrochanteric — *see* Fracture, femur, trochanteric
- trochanteric S72.10- ☑
  - apophyseal (displaced) S72.13- ☑
    - nondisplaced S72.13- ☑
  - greater trochanter (displaced) S72.11- ☑
    - nondisplaced S72.11- ☑
  - intertrochanteric (displaced) S72.14- ☑
    - nondisplaced S72.14- ☑
  - lesser trochanter (displaced) S72.12- ☑
    - nondisplaced S72.12- ☑
- upper end S72.00- ☑
  - apophyseal (displaced) S72.13- ☑
    - nondisplaced S72.13- ☑
  - cervicotrochanteric — *see* Fracture, femur, upper end, neck, base
  - epiphysis (displaced) S72.02- ☑
    - nondisplaced S72.02- ☑
  - head S72.05- ☑
    - articular (displaced) S72.06- ☑
      - nondisplaced S72.06- ☑
    - specified NEC S72.09- ☑
  - intertrochanteric (displaced) S72.14- ☑
    - nondisplaced S72.14- ☑
  - intracapsular S72.01- ☑
  - midcervical (displaced) S72.03- ☑
    - nondisplaced S72.03- ☑
  - neck S72.00- ☑
    - base (displaced) S72.04- ☑
      - nondisplaced S72.04- ☑
    - specified NEC S72.09- ☑
  - pertrochanteric — *see* Fracture, femur, upper end, trochanteric
  - physeal S79.00- ☑
    - Salter-Harris type I S79.01- ☑
    - specified NEC S79.09- ☑
  - subcapital (displaced) S72.01- ☑
  - subtrochanteric (displaced) S72.2- ☑
    - nondisplaced S72.2- ☑
  - transcervical — *see* Fracture, femur, upper end, midcervical
  - trochanteric S72.10- ☑
    - greater (displaced) S72.11- ☑

Fracture — *continued*
- nondisplaced S72.11- ☑
  - lesser (displaced) S72.12- ☑
    - nondisplaced S72.12- ☑
- fibula (shaft) (styloid) S82.40- ☑
  - comminuted (displaced) S82.45- ☑
    - nondisplaced S82.45- ☑
  - following insertion of implant, prosthesis or plate M96.67- ☑
  - involving ankle or malleolus — *see* Fracture, fibula, lateral malleolus
  - lateral malleolus (displaced) S82.6- ☑
    - nondisplaced S82.6- ☑
  - lower end
    - physeal S89.30- ☑
      - Salter-Harris
        - Type I S89.31- ☑
        - Type II S89.32- ☑
      - specified NEC S89.39- ☑
    - specified NEC S82.83- ☑
    - torus S82.82- ☑
  - oblique (displaced) S82.43- ☑
    - nondisplaced S82.43- ☑
  - segmental (displaced) S82.46- ☑
    - nondisplaced S82.46- ☑
  - specified NEC S82.49- ☑
  - spiral (displaced) S82.44- ☑
    - nondisplaced S82.44- ☑
  - transverse (displaced) S82.42- ☑
    - nondisplaced S82.42- ☑
  - upper end
    - physeal S89.20- ☑
      - Salter-Harris
        - Type I S89.21- ☑
        - Type II S89.22- ☑
      - specified NEC S89.29- ☑
    - specified NEC S82.83- ☑
    - torus S82.81- ☑
- finger (except thumb) S62.60- ☑
  - distal phalanx (displaced) S62.63- ☑
    - nondisplaced S62.66- ☑
  - index S62.60- ☑
    - distal phalanx (displaced) S62.63- ☑
      - nondisplaced S62.66- ☑
    - medial phalanx (displaced) S62.62- ☑
      - nondisplaced S62.65- ☑
    - proximal phalanx (displaced) S62.61- ☑
      - nondisplaced S62.64- ☑
  - little S62.60- ☑
    - distal phalanx (displaced) S62.63- ☑
      - nondisplaced S62.66- ☑
    - medial phalanx (displaced) S62.62- ☑
      - nondisplaced S62.65- ☑
    - proximal phalanx (displaced) S62.61- ☑
      - nondisplaced S62.64- ☑
  - medial phalanx (displaced) S62.62- ☑
    - nondisplaced S62.65- ☑
  - middle S62.60- ☑
    - distal phalanx (displaced) S62.63- ☑
      - nondisplaced S62.66- ☑
    - medial phalanx (displaced) S62.62- ☑
      - nondisplaced S62.65- ☑
    - proximal phalanx (displaced) S62.61- ☑
      - nondisplaced S62.64- ☑
  - proximal phalanx (displaced) S62.61- ☑
    - nondisplaced S62.64- ☑
  - ring S62.60- ☑
    - distal phalanx (displaced) S62.63- ☑
      - nondisplaced S62.66- ☑
    - medial phalanx (displaced) S62.62- ☑
      - nondisplaced S62.65- ☑
    - proximal phalanx (displaced) S62.61- ☑
      - nondisplaced S62.64- ☑
  - thumb — *see* Fracture, thumb
- following insertion (intraoperative) (postoperative) of orthopedic implant, joint prosthesis or bone plate M96.69
  - femur M96.66- ☑
  - fibula M96.67- ☑
  - humerus M96.62- ☑
  - pelvis M96.65
  - radius M96.63- ☑
  - specified bone NEC M96.69
  - tibia M96.67- ☑
  - ulna M96.63- ☑
- foot S92.90- ☑
  - astragalus — *see* Fracture, tarsal, talus
  - calcaneus — *see* Fracture, tarsal, calcaneus
  - cuboid — *see* Fracture, tarsal, cuboid
  - cuneiform — *see* Fracture, tarsal, cuneiform
  - metatarsal — *see* Fracture, metatarsal
  - navicular — *see* Fracture, tarsal, navicular

Fracture

Fracture — *continued*
 talus — *see* Fracture, tarsal, talus
 tarsal — *see* Fracture, tarsal
 toe — *see* Fracture, toe
 forearm S52.9-
  radius — *see* Fracture, radius
  ulna — *see* Fracture, ulna
 fossa (anterior) (middle) (posterior) S02.19 ☑
 frontal (bone) (skull) S02.0 ☑
  sinus S02.19 ☑
 glenoid (cavity) (scapula) — *see* Fracture, scapula,
   glenoid cavity
 greenstick — *see* Fracture, by site
 hallux — *see* Fracture, toe, great
 hand S62.9-
  carpal — *see* Fracture, carpal bone
  finger (except thumb) — *see* Fracture, finger
  metacarpal — *see* Fracture, metacarpal
  navicular (scaphoid) (hand) — *see* Fracture,
    carpal bone, navicular
  thumb — *see* Fracture, thumb
 healed or old
  with complications - code by Nature of the
    complication
 heel bone — *see* Fracture, tarsal, calcaneus
 Hill-Sachs S42.29- ☑
 hip — *see* Fracture, femur, neck
 humerus S42.30- ☑
  anatomical neck — *see* Fracture, humerus,
    upper end
  articular process — *see* Fracture, humerus,
    lower end
  capitellum — *see* Fracture, humerus, lower end,
    condyle, lateral
  distal end — *see* Fracture, humerus, lower end
  epiphysis
   lower — *see* Fracture, humerus, lower end,
     physeal
   upper — *see* Fracture, humerus, upper end,
     physeal
  external condyle — *see* Fracture, humerus,
    lower end, condyle, lateral
  following insertion of implant, prosthesis or
    plate M96.62- ☑
  great tuberosity — *see* Fracture, humerus,
    upper end, greater tuberosity
  intercondylar — *see* Fracture, humerus, lower
    end
  internal epicondyle — *see* Fracture, humerus,
    lower end, epicondyle, medial
  lesser tuberosity — *see* Fracture, humerus,
    upper end, lesser tuberosity
  lower end S42.40- ☑
   condyle
    lateral (displaced) S42.45- ☑
     nondisplaced S42.45- ☑
    medial (displaced) S42.46- ☑
     nondisplaced S42.46- ☑
   epicondyle
    lateral (displaced) S42.43- ☑
     nondisplaced S42.43- ☑
    medial (displaced) S42.44- ☑
     incarcerated S42.44- ☑
     nondisplaced S42.44- ☑
   physeal S49.10- ☑
    Salter-Harris
     Type I S49.11- ☑
     Type II S49.12- ☑
     Type III S49.13- ☑
     Type IV S49.14- ☑
     specified NEC S49.19- ☑
   specified NEC (displaced) S42.49- ☑
    nondisplaced S42.49- ☑
   supracondylar (simple) (displaced) S42.41- ☑
    comminuted (displaced) S42.42- ☑
     nondisplaced S42.42- ☑
    nondisplaced S42.41- ☑
   torus S42.48- ☑
   transcondylar (displaced) S42.47- ☑
    nondisplaced S42.47- ☑
  proximal end — *see* Fracture, humerus, upper
    end
  shaft S42.30- ☑
   comminuted (displaced) S42.35- ☑
    nondisplaced S42.35- ☑
   greenstick S42.31- ☑
   oblique (displaced) S42.33- ☑
    nondisplaced S42.33- ☑
   segmental (displaced) S42.36- ☑
    nondisplaced S42.36- ☑
   specified NEC S42.39- ☑
   spiral (displaced) S42.34- ☑

Fracture — *continued*
    nondisplaced S42.34- ☑
   transverse (displaced) S42.32- ☑
    nondisplaced S42.32- ☑
  supracondylar — *see* Fracture, humerus, lower
    end
  surgical neck — *see* Fracture, humerus, upper
    end, surgical neck
  trochlea — *see* Fracture, humerus, lower end,
    condyle, medial
  tuberosity — *see* Fracture, humerus, upper end
  upper end S42.20- ☑
   anatomical neck — *see* Fracture, humerus,
     upper end, specified NEC
   articular head — *see* Fracture, humerus,
     upper end, specified NEC
   epiphysis — *see* Fracture, humerus, upper
     end, physeal
   greater tuberosity (displaced) S42.25- ☑
    nondisplaced S42.25- ☑
   lesser tuberosity (displaced) S42.26- ☑
    nondisplaced S42.26- ☑
   physeal S49.00- ☑
    Salter-Harris
     Type I S49.01- ☑
     Type II S49.02- ☑
     Type III S49.03- ☑
     Type IV S49.04- ☑
     specified NEC S49.09- ☑
   specified NEC (displaced) S42.29- ☑
    nondisplaced S42.29- ☑
   surgical neck (displaced) S42.21- ☑
    four-part S42.24- ☑
    nondisplaced S42.21- ☑
    three-part S42.23- ☑
    two-part (displaced) S42.22- ☑
     nondisplaced S42.22- ☑
   torus S42.27- ☑
   transepiphyseal — *see* Fracture, humerus,
     upper end, physeal
 hyoid bone S12.8 ☑
 ilium S32.30- ☑
  with disruption of pelvic ring — *see* Disruption,
    pelvic ring
  avulsion (displaced) S32.31- ☑
   nondisplaced S32.31- ☑
  specified NEC S32.39- ☑
 impaction, impacted - code as Fracture, by site
 innominate bone — *see* Fracture, ilium
 instep — *see* Fracture, foot
 ischium S32.60- ☑
  with disruption of pelvic ring — *see* Disruption,
    pelvic ring
  avulsion (displaced) S32.61- ☑
   nondisplaced S32.61- ☑
  specified NEC S32.69- ☑
 jaw (bone) (lower) — *see* Fracture, mandible
  upper — *see* Fracture, maxilla
 joint prosthesis — *see* Complications, joint
   prosthesis, mechanical, breakdown, by site
  periprosthetic — *see* Complications, joint
    prosthesis, mechanical, periprosthesis,
    fracture, by site
 knee cap — *see* Fracture, patella
 larynx S12.8 ☑
 late effects — *see* Sequelae, fracture
 leg (lower) S82.9- ☑
  ankle — *see* Fracture, ankle
  femur — *see* Fracture, femur
  fibula — *see* Fracture, fibula
  malleolus — *see* Fracture, ankle
  patella — *see* Fracture, patella
  specified site NEC S82.89- ☑
  tibia — *see* Fracture, tibia
 lumbar spine — *see* Fracture, vertebra, lumbar
 lumbosacral spine S32.9 ☑
 Maisonneuve's (displaced) S82.86- ☑
  nondisplaced S82.86- ☑
 malar bone (*see also* Fracture, maxilla) S02.400 ☑
 malleolus — *see* Fracture, ankle
 malunion — *see* Fracture, by site
 mandible (lower jaw) (bone) S02.609 ☑
  alveolus S02.67 ☑
  angle (of jaw) S02.65 ☑
  body, unspecified S02.600 ☑
  condylar process S02.61 ☑
  coronoid process S02.63 ☑
  ramus, unspecified S02.64 ☑
  specified site NEC S02.69 ☑
  subcondylar process S02.62 ☑
  symphysis S02.66 ☑
 manubrium (sterni) S22.21 ☑

Fracture — *continued*
 dissociation from sternum S22.23 ☑
 march — *see* Fracture, traumatic, stress, by site
 maxilla, maxillary (bone) (sinus) (superior) (upper
   jaw) S02.401 ☑
  alveolus S02.42 ☑
  inferior — *see* Fracture, mandible
  LeFort I S02.411 ☑
  LeFort II S02.412 ☑
  LeFort III S02.413 ☑
 metacarpal S62.309 ☑
  base (displaced) S62.319 ☑
   nondisplaced S62.349 ☑
  fifth S62.30- ☑
   base (displaced) S62.31- ☑
    nondisplaced S62.34- ☑
   neck (displaced) S62.33- ☑
    nondisplaced S62.36- ☑
   shaft (displaced) S62.32- ☑
    nondisplaced S62.35- ☑
   specified NEC S62.398 ☑
  first S62.20- ☑
   base NEC (displaced) S62.23- ☑
    nondisplaced S62.23- ☑
   Bennett's — *see* Bennett's fracture
   neck (displaced) S62.25- ☑
    nondisplaced S62.25- ☑
   shaft (displaced) S62.24- ☑
    nondisplaced S62.24- ☑
   specified NEC S62.29- ☑
  fourth S62.30- ☑
   base (displaced) S62.31- ☑
    nondisplaced S62.34- ☑
   neck (displaced) S62.33- ☑
    nondisplaced S62.36- ☑
   shaft (displaced) S62.32- ☑
    nondisplaced S62.35- ☑
   specified NEC S62.39- ☑
  neck (displaced) S62.33- ☑
   nondisplaced S62.36- ☑
  Rolando's — *see* Rolando's fracture
  second S62.30- ☑
   base (displaced) S62.31- ☑
    nondisplaced S62.34- ☑
   neck (displaced) S62.33- ☑
    nondisplaced S62.36- ☑
   shaft (displaced) S62.32- ☑
    nondisplaced S62.35- ☑
   specified NEC S62.39- ☑
  shaft (displaced) S62.32- ☑
   nondisplaced S62.35- ☑
  third S62.30- ☑
   base (displaced) S62.31- ☑
    nondisplaced S62.34- ☑
   neck (displaced) S62.33- ☑
    nondisplaced S62.36- ☑
   shaft (displaced) S62.32- ☑
    nondisplaced S62.35- ☑
   specified NEC S62.39- ☑
  specified NEC S62.399 ☑
 metastatic — *see* Fracture, pathological, due to,
   neoplastic disease (*see also* Neoplasm)
 metatarsal bone S92.30- ☑
  fifth (displaced) S92.35- ☑
   nondisplaced S92.35- ☑
  first (displaced) S92.31- ☑
   nondisplaced S92.31- ☑
  fourth (displaced) S92.34- ☑
   nondisplaced S92.34- ☑
  second (displaced) S92.32- ☑
   nondisplaced S92.32- ☑
  third (displaced) S92.33- ☑
   nondisplaced S92.33- ☑
 Monteggia's — *see* Monteggia's fracture
 multiple
  hand (and wrist) NEC — *see* Fracture, by site
  ribs — *see* Fracture, rib, multiple
 nasal (bone(s)) S02.2 ☑
 navicular (scaphoid) (foot) (*see also* Fracture,
   tarsal, navicular)
  hand — *see* Fracture, carpal, navicular
 neck S12.9 ☑
  cervical vertebra S12.9 ☑
   fifth (displaced) S12.400 ☑
    nondisplaced S12.401 ☑
    specified type NEC (displaced) S12.490 ☑
     nondisplaced S12.491 ☑
   first (displaced) S12.000 ☑
    burst (stable) S12.01 ☑
     unstable S12.02 ☑
    lateral mass (displaced) S12.040 ☑
     nondisplaced S12.041 ☑

☑ **Additional character required**

Fracture — continued
  nondisplaced S12.001 ☑
  posterior arch (displaced) S12.030 ☑
   nondisplaced S12.031 ☑
  specified type NEC (displaced) S12.090 ☑
   nondisplaced S12.091 ☑
  fourth (displaced) S12.300 ☑
   nondisplaced S12.301 ☑
   specified type NEC (displaced) S12.390 ☑
    nondisplaced S12.391 ☑
  second (displaced) S12.100 ☑
   nondisplaced S12.101 ☑
   dens (anterior) (displaced) (type II) S12.110 ☑
    nondisplaced S12.112 ☑
    posterior S12.111 ☑
   specified type NEC (displaced) S12.120 ☑
    nondisplaced S12.121 ☑
  specified type NEC (displaced) S12.190 ☑
   nondisplaced S12.191 ☑
  seventh (displaced) S12.600 ☑
   nondisplaced S12.601 ☑
   specified type NEC (displaced) S12.690 ☑
    displaced S12.691 ☑
  sixth (displaced) S12.500 ☑
   nondisplaced S12.501 ☑
   specified type NEC (displaced) S12.590 ☑
    displaced S12.591 ☑
  third (displaced) S12.200 ☑
   nondisplaced S12.201 ☑
   specified type NEC (displaced) S12.290 ☑
    nondisplaced S12.291 ☑
 hyoid bone S12.8 ☑
 larynx S12.8 ☑
 specified site NEC S12.8 ☑
 thyroid cartilage S12.8 ☑
 trachea S12.8 ☑
neoplastic NEC — see Fracture, pathological, due to, neoplastic disease
neural arch — see Fracture, vertebra
newborn — see Birth, injury, fracture
nontraumatic — see Fracture, pathological
nonunion — see Nonunion, fracture
nose, nasal (bone) (septum) S02.2 ☑
occiput — see Fracture, skull, base, occiput
odontoid process — see Fracture, neck, cervical vertebra, second
olecranon (process) (ulna) — see Fracture, ulna, upper end, olecranon process
orbit, orbital (bone) (region) S02.8 ☑
 floor (blow-out) S02.3 ☑
 roof S02.19 ☑
os
 calcis — see Fracture, tarsal, calcaneus
 magnum — see Fracture, carpal, capitate
 pubis — see Fracture, pubis
palate S02.8 ☑
parietal bone (skull) S02.0 ☑
patella S82.00- ☑
 comminuted (displaced) S82.04- ☑
  nondisplaced S82.04- ☑
 longitudinal (displaced) S82.02- ☑
  nondisplaced S82.02- ☑
 osteochondral (displaced) S82.01- ☑
  nondisplaced S82.01- ☑
 specified NEC S82.09- ☑
 transverse (displaced) S82.03- ☑
  nondisplaced S82.03- ☑
pedicle (of vertebral arch) — see Fracture, vertebra
pelvis, pelvic (bone) S32.9 ☑
 acetabulum — see Fracture, acetabulum
 circle — see Disruption, pelvic ring
 following insertion of implant, prosthesis or plate M96.65
 ilium — see Fracture, ilium
 ischium — see Fracture, ischium
 multiple
  with disruption of pelvic ring (circle) — see Disruption, pelvic ring
  without disruption of pelvic ring (circle) S32.82 ☑
 pubis — see Fracture, pubis
 specified site NEC S32.89 ☑
 sacrum — see Fracture, sacrum
phalanx
 foot — see Fracture, toe
 hand — see Fracture, finger
pisiform — see Fracture, carpal, pisiform
pond — see Fracture, skull
prosthetic device, internal — see Complications, prosthetic device, by site, mechanical

Fracture — continued
 pubis S32.50- ☑
  with disruption of pelvic ring — see Disruption, pelvic ring
  specified site NEC S32.59- ☑
  superior rim S32.51- ☑
 radius S52.9- ☑
  distal end — see Fracture, radius, lower end
  following insertion of implant, prosthesis or plate M96.63- ☑
  head — see Fracture, radius, upper end, head
  lower end S52.50- ☑
   Barton's — see Barton's fracture
   Colles' — see Colles' fracture
   extraarticular NEC S52.55- ☑
   intraarticular NEC S52.57- ☑
   physeal S59.20- ☑
    Salter-Harris
     Type I S59.21- ☑
     Type II S59.22- ☑
     Type III S59.23- ☑
     Type IV S59.24- ☑
    specified NEC S59.29- ☑
   Smith's — see Smith's fracture
   specified NEC S52.59- ☑
   styloid process (displaced) S52.51- ☑
    nondisplaced S52.51- ☑
   torus S52.52- ☑
  neck — see Fracture, radius, upper end
  proximal end — see Fracture, radius, upper end
  shaft S52.30- ☑
   bent bone S52.38- ☑
   comminuted (displaced) S52.35- ☑
    nondisplaced S52.35- ☑
   Galeazzi's — see Galeazzi's fracture
   greenstick S52.31- ☑
   oblique (displaced) S52.33- ☑
    nondisplaced S52.33- ☑
   segmental (displaced) S52.36- ☑
    nondisplaced S52.36- ☑
   specified NEC S52.39- ☑
   spiral (displaced) S52.34- ☑
    nondisplaced S52.34- ☑
   transverse (displaced) S52.32- ☑
    nondisplaced S52.32- ☑
  upper end S52.10- ☑
   head (displaced) S52.12- ☑
    nondisplaced S52.12- ☑
   neck (displaced) S52.13- ☑
    nondisplaced S52.13- ☑
   specified NEC S52.18- ☑
   physeal S59.10- ☑
    Salter-Harris
     Type I S59.11- ☑
     Type II S59.12- ☑
     Type III S59.13- ☑
     Type IV S59.14- ☑
    specified NEC S59.19- ☑
   torus S52.11- ☑
 ramus
  inferior or superior, pubis — see Fracture, pubis
  mandible — see Fracture, mandible
 restorative material (dental) K08.539
  with loss of material K08.531
  without loss of material K08.530
 rib S22.3- ☑
  with flail chest — see Flail, chest
  multiple S22.4- ☑
   with flail chest — see Flail, chest
 root, tooth — see Fracture, tooth
 sacrum S32.10 ☑
  specified NEC S32.19 ☑
  Type
   1 S32.14 ☑
   2 S32.15 ☑
   3 S32.16 ☑
   4 S32.17 ☑
  Zone
   I S32.119 ☑
    displaced (minimally) S32.111 ☑
     severely S32.112 ☑
    nondisplaced S32.110 ☑
   II S32.129 ☑
    displaced (minimally) S32.121 ☑
     severely S32.122 ☑
    nondisplaced S32.120 ☑
   III S32.139 ☑
    displaced (minimally) S32.131 ☑
     severely S32.132 ☑
    nondisplaced S32.130 ☑
 scaphoid (hand) (see also Fracture, carpal, navicular)

Fracture — continued
 foot — see Fracture, tarsal, navicular
 scapula S42.10- ☑
  acromial process (displaced) S42.12- ☑
   nondisplaced S42.12- ☑
  body (displaced) S42.11- ☑
   nondisplaced S42.11- ☑
  coracoid process (displaced) S42.13- ☑
   nondisplaced S42.13- ☑
  glenoid cavity (displaced) S42.14- ☑
   nondisplaced S42.14- ☑
  neck (displaced) S42.15- ☑
   nondisplaced S42.15- ☑
  specified NEC S42.19- ☑
 semilunar bone, wrist — see Fracture, carpal, lunate
 sequelae — see Sequelae, fracture
 sesamoid bone
  hand — see Fracture, carpal
  other - code by site under Fracture
 shepherd's — see Fracture, tarsal, talus
 shoulder (girdle) S42.9- ☑
  blade — see Fracture, scapula
 sinus (ethmoid) (frontal) S02.19 ☑
 skull S02.91 ☑
  base S02.10 ☑
   occiput S02.119 ☑
    condyle S02.113 ☑
    type I S02.110 ☑
    type II S02.111 ☑
    type III S02.112 ☑
   specified NEC S02.118 ☑
   specified NEC S02.19 ☑
  birth injury P13.0
  frontal bone S02.0 ☑
  parietal bone S02.0 ☑
  specified site NEC S02.8 ☑
  temporal bone S02.19 ☑
  vault S02.0 ☑
 Smith's — see Smith's fracture
 sphenoid (bone) (sinus) S02.19 ☑
 spine — see Fracture, vertebra
 spinous process — see Fracture, vertebra
 spontaneous (cause unknown) — see Fracture, pathological
 stave (of thumb) — see Fracture, metacarpal, first
 sternum S22.20 ☑
  with flail chest — see Flail, chest
  body S22.22 ☑
  manubrium S22.21 ☑
  xiphoid (process) S22.24 ☑
 stress M84.30 ☑
  ankle M84.37- ☑
  carpus M84.34- ☑
  clavicle M84.31- ☑
  femoral neck M84.359 ☑
  femur M84.35- ☑
  fibula M84.36- ☑
  finger M84.34- ☑
  hip M84.359 ☑
  humerus M84.32- ☑
  ilium M84.350 ☑
  ischium M84.350 ☑
  metacarpus M84.34- ☑
  metatarsus M84.37- ☑
  neck — see Fracture, fatigue, vertebra
  pelvis M84.350 ☑
  radius M84.33- ☑
  rib M84.38 ☑
  scapula M84.31- ☑
  skull M84.38 ☑
  tarsus M84.37- ☑
  tibia M84.36- ☑
  toe M84.37- ☑
  ulna M84.33- ☑
  vertebra — see Fracture, fatigue, vertebra
 supracondylar, elbow — see Fracture, humerus, lower end, supracondylar
 symphysis pubis — see Fracture, pubis
 talus (ankle bone) — see Fracture, tarsal, talus
 tarsal bone (s) S92.20- ☑
  astragalus — see Fracture, tarsal, talus
  calcaneus S92.00- ☑
   anterior process (displaced) S92.02- ☑
    nondisplaced S92.02- ☑
   body (displaced) S92.01- ☑
    nondisplaced S92.01- ☑
   extraarticular NEC (displaced) S92.05- ☑
    nondisplaced S92.05- ☑
   intraarticular (displaced) S92.06- ☑
    nondisplaced S92.06- ☑
   tuberosity (displaced) S92.04- ☑

Fracture

Fracture — *continued*

avulsion (displaced) S92.03- ☑
  nondisplaced S92.03- ☑
  nondisplaced S92.04- ☑
cuboid (displaced) S92.21- ☑
  nondisplaced S92.21- ☑
cuneiform
  intermediate (displaced) S92.23- ☑
    nondisplaced S92.23- ☑
  lateral (displaced) S92.22- ☑
    nondisplaced S92.22- ☑
  medial (displaced) S92.24- ☑
    nondisplaced S92.24- ☑
navicular (displaced) S92.25- ☑
  nondisplaced S92.25- ☑
scaphoid — *see* Fracture, tarsal, navicular
talus S92.10- ☑
  avulsion (displaced) S92.15- ☑
    nondisplaced S92.15- ☑
  body (displaced) S92.12- ☑
    nondisplaced S92.12- ☑
  dome (displaced) S92.14- ☑
    nondisplaced S92.14- ☑
  head (displaced) S92.12- ☑
    nondisplaced S92.12- ☑
  lateral process (displaced) S92.14- ☑
    nondisplaced S92.14- ☑
  neck (displaced) S92.11- ☑
    nondisplaced S92.11- ☑
  posterior process (displaced) S92.13- ☑
    nondisplaced S92.13- ☑
  specified NEC S92.19- ☑
temporal bone (styloid) S02.19 ☑
thorax (bony) S22.9 ☑
  with flail chest — *see* Flail, chest
  rib S22.3- ☑
    multiple S22.4- ☑
      with flail chest — *see* Flail, chest
  sternum S22.20 ☑
    body S22.22 ☑
    manubrium S22.21 ☑
    xiphoid process S22.24 ☑
  vertebra (displaced) S22.009 ☑
    burst (stable) S22.001 ☑
      unstable S22.002 ☑
    eighth S22.069 ☑
      burst (stable) S22.061 ☑
        unstable S22.062 ☑
      specified type NEC S22.068 ☑
      wedge compression S22.060 ☑
    eleventh S22.089 ☑
      burst (stable) S22.081 ☑
        unstable S22.082 ☑
      specified type NEC S22.088 ☑
      wedge compression S22.080 ☑
    fifth S22.059 ☑
      burst (stable) S22.051 ☑
        unstable S22.052 ☑
      specified type NEC S22.058 ☑
      wedge compression S22.050 ☑
    first S22.019 ☑
      burst (stable) S22.011 ☑
        unstable S22.012 ☑
      specified type NEC S22.018 ☑
      wedge compression S22.010 ☑
    fourth S22.049 ☑
      burst (stable) S22.041 ☑
        unstable S22.042 ☑
      specified type NEC S22.048 ☑
      wedge compression S22.040 ☑
    ninth S22.079 ☑
      burst (stable) S22.071 ☑
        unstable S22.072 ☑
      specified type NEC S22.078 ☑
      wedge compression S22.070 ☑
    nondisplaced S22.001 ☑
    second S22.029 ☑
      burst (stable) S22.021 ☑
        unstable S22.022 ☑
      specified type NEC S22.028 ☑
      wedge compression S22.020 ☑
    seventh S22.069 ☑
      burst (stable) S22.061 ☑
        unstable S22.062 ☑
      specified type NEC S22.068 ☑
      wedge compression S22.060 ☑
    sixth S22.059 ☑
      burst (stable) S22.051 ☑
        unstable S22.052 ☑
      specified type NEC S22.058 ☑
      wedge compression S22.050 ☑
    specified type NEC S22.008 ☑

Fracture — *continued*

tenth S22.079 ☑
  burst (stable) S22.071 ☑
    unstable S22.072 ☑
  specified type NEC S22.078 ☑
  wedge compression S22.070 ☑
third S22.039 ☑
  burst (stable) S22.031 ☑
    unstable S22.032 ☑
  specified type NEC S22.038 ☑
  wedge compression S22.030 ☑
twelfth S22.089 ☑
  burst (stable) S22.081 ☑
    unstable S22.082 ☑
  specified type NEC S22.088 ☑
  wedge compression S22.080 ☑
  wedge compression S22.000 ☑
thumb S62.50- ☑
  distal phalanx (displaced) S62.52- ☑
    nondisplaced S62.52- ☑
  proximal phalanx (displaced) S62.51- ☑
    nondisplaced S62.51- ☑
thyroid cartilage S12.8 ☑
tibia (shaft) S82.20- ☑
  comminuted (displaced) S82.25- ☑
    nondisplaced S82.25- ☑
  condyles — *see* Fracture, tibia, upper end
  distal end — *see* Fracture, tibia, lower end
  epiphysis
    lower — *see* Fracture, tibia, lower end
    upper — *see* Fracture, tibia, upper end
  following insertion of implant, prosthesis or
    plate M96.67- ☑
  head (involving knee joint) — *see* Fracture,
    tibia, upper end
  intercondyloid eminence — *see* Fracture, tibia,
    upper end
  involving ankle or malleolus — *see* Fracture,
    ankle, medial malleolus
  lower end S82.30- ☑
    physeal S89.10- ☑
      Salter-Harris
        Type I S89.11- ☑
        Type II S89.12- ☑
        Type III S89.13- ☑
        Type IV S89.14- ☑
      specified NEC S89.19- ☑
    pilon (displaced) S82.87- ☑
      nondisplaced S82.87- ☑
    specified NEC S82.39- ☑
    torus S82.31- ☑
  malleolus — *see* Fracture, ankle, medial
    malleolus
  oblique (displaced) S82.23- ☑
    nondisplaced S82.23- ☑
  pilon — *see* Fracture, tibia, lower end, pilon
  proximal end — *see* Fracture, tibia, upper end
  segmental (displaced) S82.26- ☑
    nondisplaced S82.26- ☑
  specified NEC S82.29- ☑
  spine — *see* Fracture, upper end, spine
  spiral (displaced) S82.24- ☑
    nondisplaced S82.24- ☑
  transverse (displaced) S82.22- ☑
    nondisplaced S82.22- ☑
  tuberosity — *see* Fracture, tibia, upper end,
    tuberosity
  upper end S82.10- ☑
    bicondylar (displaced) S82.14- ☑
      nondisplaced S82.14- ☑
    lateral condyle (displaced) S82.12- ☑
      nondisplaced S82.12- ☑
    medial condyle (displaced) S82.13- ☑
      nondisplaced S82.13- ☑
    physeal S89.00- ☑
      Salter-Harris
        Type I S89.01- ☑
        Type II S89.02- ☑
        Type III S89.03- ☑
        Type IV S89.04- ☑
      specified NEC S89.09- ☑
    plateau — *see* Fracture, tibia, upper end,
      bicondylar
    spine (displaced) S82.11- ☑
      nondisplaced S82.11- ☑
    torus S82.16- ☑
    specified NEC S82.19- ☑
    tuberosity (displaced) S82.15- ☑
      nondisplaced S82.15- ☑
toe S92.91- ☑
  great (displaced) S92.40- ☑
    distal phalanx (displaced) S92.42- ☑

Fracture — *continued*

    nondisplaced S92.42- ☑
    nondisplaced S92.40- ☑
    proximal phalanx (displaced) S92.41- ☑
      nondisplaced S92.41- ☑
    specified NEC S92.49- ☑
  lesser (displaced) S92.50- ☑
    distal phalanx (displaced) S92.53- ☑
      nondisplaced S92.53- ☑
    medial phalanx (displaced) S92.52- ☑
      nondisplaced S92.52- ☑
    nondisplaced S92.50- ☑
    proximal phalanx (displaced) S92.51- ☑
      nondisplaced S92.51- ☑
    specified NEC S92.59- ☑
tooth (root) S02.5 ☑
trachea (cartilage) S12.8 ☑
transverse process — *see* Fracture, vertebra
trapezium or trapezoid bone — *see* Fracture,
  carpal
trimalleolar — *see* Fracture, ankle, trimalleolar
triquetrum (cuneiform of carpus) — *see* Fracture,
  carpal, triquetrum
trochanter — *see* Fracture, femur, trochanteric
tuberosity (external) - code by site under
  Fracture
ulna (shaft) S52.20- ☑
  bent bone S52.28- ☑
  coronoid process — *see* Fracture, ulna, upper
    end, coronoid process
  distal end — *see* Fracture, ulna, lower end
  following insertion of implant, prosthesis or
    plate M96.63- ☑
  head S52.00- ☑
  lower end S52.60- ☑
    physeal S59.00- ☑
      Salter-Harris
        Type I S59.01- ☑
        Type II S59.02- ☑
        Type III S59.03- ☑
        Type IV S59.04- ☑
      specified NEC S59.09- ☑
    specified NEC S52.69- ☑
    styloid process (displaced) S52.61- ☑
      nondisplaced S52.61- ☑
    torus S52.62- ☑
  proximal end — *see* Fracture, ulna, upper end
  shaft S52.20- ☑
    comminuted (displaced) S52.25- ☑
      nondisplaced S52.25- ☑
    greenstick S52.21- ☑
    Monteggia's — *see* Monteggia's fracture
    oblique (displaced) S52.23- ☑
      nondisplaced S52.23- ☑
    segmental (displaced) S52.26- ☑
      nondisplaced S52.26- ☑
    specified NEC S52.29- ☑
    spiral (displaced) S52.24- ☑
      nondisplaced S52.24- ☑
    transverse (displaced) S52.22- ☑
      nondisplaced S52.22- ☑
  upper end S52.00- ☑
    coronoid process (displaced) S52.04- ☑
      nondisplaced S52.04- ☑
    olecranon process (displaced) S52.02- ☑
      with intraarticular extension S52.03- ☑
      nondisplaced S52.02- ☑
        with intraarticular extension S52.03- ☑
    specified NEC S52.09- ☑
    torus S52.01- ☑
unciform — *see* Fracture, carpal, hamate
vault of skull S02.0 ☑
vertebra, vertebral (arch) (body) (column) (neural
  arch) (pedicle) (spinous process) (transverse
  process)
  atlas — *see* Fracture, neck, cervical vertebra,
    first
  axis — *see* Fracture, neck, cervical vertebra,
    second
  cervical (teardrop) S12.9 ☑
    axis — *see* Fracture, neck, cervical vertebra,
      second
    first (atlas) — *see* Fracture, neck, cervical
      vertebra, first
    second (axis) — *see* Fracture, neck, cervical
      vertebra, second
  chronic M84.48 ☑
  coccyx S32.2 ☑
  dorsal — *see* Fracture, thorax, vertebra
  lumbar S32.009 ☑
    burst (stable) S32.001 ☑
      unstable S32.002 ☑

Fracture — *continued*
fifth S32.059 ☑
burst (stable) S32.051 ☑
unstable S32.052 ☑
specified type NEC S32.058 ☑
wedge compression S32.050 ☑
first S32.019 ☑
burst (stable) S32.011 ☑
unstable S32.012 ☑
specified type NEC S32.018 ☑
wedge compression S32.010 ☑
fourth S32.049 ☑
burst (stable) S32.041 ☑
unstable S32.042 ☑
specified type NEC S32.048 ☑
wedge compression S32.040 ☑
second S32.029 ☑
burst (stable) S32.021 ☑
unstable S32.022 ☑
specified type NEC S32.028 ☑
wedge compression S32.020 ☑
specified type NEC S32.008 ☑
third S32.039 ☑
burst (stable) S32.031 ☑
unstable S32.032 ☑
specified type NEC S32.038 ☑
wedge compression S32.030 ☑
wedge compression S32.000 ☑
metastatic — *see* Collapse, vertebra, in, specified disease NEC (*see also* Neoplasm)
newborn (birth injury) P11.5
sacrum S32.10 ☑
specified NEC S32.19 ☑
Type
1 S32.14 ☑
2 S32.15 ☑
3 S32.16 ☑
4 S32.17 ☑
Zone
I S32.119 ☑
displaced (minimally) S32.111 ☑
severely S32.112 ☑
nondisplaced S32.110 ☑
II S32.129 ☑
displaced (minimally) S32.121 ☑
severely S32.122 ☑
nondisplaced S32.120 ☑
III S32.139 ☑
displaced (minimally) S32.131 ☑
severely S32.132 ☑
nondisplaced S32.130 ☑
thoracic — *see* Fracture, thorax, vertebra
vertex S02.0 ☑
vomer (bone) S02.2 ☑
wrist S62.10- ☑
carpal — *see* Fracture, carpal bone
navicular (scaphoid) (hand) — *see* Fracture, carpal, navicular
xiphisternum, xiphoid (process) S22.24 ☑
zygoma S02.402 ☑
Fragile, fragility
autosomal site Q95.5
bone, congenital (with blue sclera) Q78.0
capillary (hereditary) D69.8
hair L67.8
nails L60.3
non-sex chromosome site Q95.5
X chromosome Q99.2
Fragilitas
crinium L67.8
ossium (with blue sclerae) (hereditary) Q78.0
unguium L60.3
congenital Q84.6
Fragments, cataract (lens), following cataract surgery H59.02- ☑
retained foreign body — *see* Retained, foreign body fragments (type of)
Frailty (frail) R54
mental R41.81
Frambesia, frambesial (tropica) (*see also* Yaws)
initial lesion or ulcer A66.0
primary A66.0
Frambeside
gummatous A66.4
of early yaws A66.2
Frambesioma A66.1
Franceschetti-Klein (-Wildervanck) disease or syndrome Q75.4
Francis' disease — *see* Tularemia
Franklin disease C88.2
Frank's essential thrombocytopenia D69.3
Fraser's syndrome Q87.0

Freckle (s) L81.2
malignant melanoma in — *see* Melanoma
melanotic (Hutchinson's) — *see* Melanoma, in situ
retinal D49.81
Frederickson's hyperlipoproteinemia, type
I and V E78.3
IIA E78.0
IIB and III E78.2
IV E78.1
Freeman Sheldon syndrome Q87.0
Freezing (*see also* Effect, adverse, cold) T69.9 ☑
Freiberg's disease (infraction of metatarsal head or osteochondrosis) — *see* Osteochondrosis, juvenile, metatarsus
Frei's disease A55
Fremitus, friction, cardiac R01.2
Frenum, frenulum
external os Q51.828
tongue (shortening) (congenital) Q38.1
Frequency micturition (nocturnal) R35.0
psychogenic F45.8
Frey's syndrome
auriculotemporal G50.8
hyperhidrosis L74.52
Friction
burn — *see* Burn, by site
fremitus, cardiac R01.2
precordial R01.2
sounds, chest R09.89
Friderichsen-Waterhouse syndrome or disease A39.1
Friedländer's B (bacillus) NEC (*see also* condition) A49.8
Friedreich's
ataxia G11.1
combined systemic disease G11.1
facial hemihypertrophy Q67.4
sclerosis (cerebellum) (spinal cord) G11.1
Frigidity F52.22
Fröhlich's syndrome E23.6
Frontal (*see also* condition)
lobe syndrome F07.0
Frostbite (superficial) T33.90 ☑
with
partial thickness skin loss — *see* Frostbite (superficial), by site
tissue necrosis T34.90 ☑
abdominal wall T33.3 ☑
with tissue necrosis T34.3 ☑
ankle T33.81- ☑
with tissue necrosis T34.81- ☑
arm T33.4- ☑
with tissue necrosis T34.4- ☑
finger (s) — *see* Frostbite, finger
hand — *see* Frostbite, hand
wrist — *see* Frostbite, wrist
ear T33.01- ☑
with tissue necrosis T34.01- ☑
face T33.09 ☑
with tissue necrosis T34.09 ☑
finger T33.53- ☑
with tissue necrosis T34.53- ☑
foot T33.82- ☑
with tissue necrosis T34.82- ☑
hand T33.52- ☑
with tissue necrosis T34.52- ☑
head T33.09 ☑
with tissue necrosis T34.09 ☑
ear — *see* Frostbite, ear
nose — *see* Frostbite, nose
hip (and thigh) T33.6- ☑
with tissue necrosis T34.6- ☑
knee T33.7- ☑
with tissue necrosis T34.7- ☑
leg T33.9- ☑
with tissue necrosis T34.9- ☑
ankle — *see* Frostbite, ankle
foot — *see* Frostbite, foot
knee — *see* Frostbite, knee
lower T33.7- ☑
with tissue necrosis T34.7- ☑
thigh — *see* Frostbite, hip
toe — *see* Frostbite, toe
limb
lower T33.99 ☑
with tissue necrosis T34.99 ☑
upper — *see* Frostbite, arm
neck T33.1 ☑
with tissue necrosis T34.1 ☑
nose T33.02 ☑
with tissue necrosis T34.02 ☑

Frostbite — *continued*
pelvis T33.3 ☑
with tissue necrosis T34.3 ☑
specified site NEC T33.99 ☑
with tissue necrosis T34.99 ☑
thigh — *see* Frostbite, hip
thorax T33.2 ☑
with tissue necrosis T34.2 ☑
toes T33.83- ☑
with tissue necrosis T34.83- ☑
trunk T33.99 ☑
with tissue necrosis T34.99 ☑
wrist T33.51- ☑
with tissue necrosis T34.51- ☑
Frotteurism F65.81
Frozen (*see also* Effect, adverse, cold) T69.9 ☑
pelvis (female) N94.89
male K66.8
shoulder — *see* Capsulitis, adhesive
Fructokinase deficiency E74.11
Fructose 1,6 diphosphatase deficiency E74.19
Fructosemia (benign) (essential) E74.12
Fructosuria (benign) (essential) E74.11
Fuchs'
black spot (myopic) H44.2- ☑
dystrophy (corneal endothelium) H18.51
heterochromic cyclitis — *see* Cyclitis, Fuchs' heterochromic
Fucosidosis E77.1
Fugue R68.89
dissociative F44.1
hysterical (dissociative) F44.1
postictal in epilepsy — *see* Epilepsy
reaction to exceptional stress (transient) F43.0
Fulminant, fulminating — *see* condition
Functional (*see also* condition)
bleeding (uterus) N93.8
Functioning, intellectual, borderline R41.83
Fundus — *see* condition
Fungemia NOS B49
Fungus, fungous
cerebral G93.89
disease NOS B49
infection — *see* Infection, fungus
Funiculitis (acute) (chronic) (endemic) N49.1
gonococcal (acute) (chronic) A54.23
tuberculous A18.15
Funnel
breast (acquired) M95.4
congenital Q67.6
sequelae (late effect) of rickets E64.3
chest (acquired) M95.4
congenital Q67.6
sequelae (late effect) of rickets E64.3
pelvis (acquired) M95.5
with disproportion (fetopelvic) O33.3 ☑
causing obstructed labor O65.3
congenital Q74.2
FUO (fever of unknown origin) R50.9
Furfur L21.0
microsporon B36.0
Furrier's lung J67.8
Furrowed K14.5
nail (s) (transverse) L60.4
congenital Q84.6
tongue K14.5
congenital Q38.3
Furuncle L02.92
abdominal wall L02.221
ankle — *see* Furuncle, lower limb
anus K61.0
antecubital space — *see* Furuncle, upper limb
arm — *see* Furuncle, upper limb
auditory canal, external — *see* Abscess, ear, external
auricle (ear) — *see* Abscess, ear, external
axilla (region) L02.42- ☑
back (any part) L02.222
breast N61
buttock L02.32
cheek (external) L02.02
chest wall L02.223
chin L02.02
corpus cavernosum N48.21
ear, external — *see* Abscess, ear, external
external auditory canal — *see* Abscess, ear, external
eyelid — *see* Abscess, eyelid
face L02.02
femoral (region) — *see* Furuncle, lower limb
finger — *see* Furuncle, hand
flank L02.221

Furuncle — *continued*
  foot L02.62- ☑
  forehead L02.02
  gluteal (region) L02.32
  groin L02.224
  hand L02.52- ☑
  head L02.821
    face L02.02
  hip — *see* Furuncle, lower limb
  kidney — *see* Abscess, kidney
  knee — *see* Furuncle, lower limb
  labium (majus) (minus) N76.4
  lacrimal
    gland — *see* Dacryoadenitis
    passages (duct) (sac) — *see* Inflammation, lacrimal, passages, acute
  leg (any part) — *see* Furuncle, lower limb
  lower limb L02.42- ☑
  malignant A22.0
  mouth K12.2
  navel L02.226
  neck L02.12
  nose J34.0
  orbit, orbital — *see* Abscess, orbit
  palmar (space) — *see* Furuncle, hand
  partes posteriores L02.32
  pectoral region L02.223
  penis N48.21
  perineum L02.225
  pinna — *see* Abscess, ear, external
  popliteal — *see* Furuncle, lower limb
  prepatellar — *see* Furuncle, lower limb
  scalp L02.821
  seminal vesicle N49.0
  shoulder — *see* Furuncle, upper limb
  specified site NEC L02.828
  submandibular K12.2
  temple (region) L02.02
  thumb — *see* Furuncle, hand
  toe — *see* Furuncle, foot
  trunk L02.229
    abdominal wall L02.221
    back L02.222
    chest wall L02.223
    groin L02.224
    perineum L02.225
    umbilicus L02.226
  umbilicus L02.226
  upper limb L02.42- ☑
  vulva N76.4
Furunculosis — *see* Furuncle
Fused — *see* Fusion, fused
Fusion, fused (congenital)
  astragaloscaphoid Q74.2
  atria Q21.1
  auditory canal Q16.1
  auricles, heart Q21.1
  binocular with defective stereopsis H53.32
  bone Q79.8
  cervical spine M43.22
  choanal Q30.0
  commissure, mitral valve Q23.2
  cusps, heart valve NEC Q24.8
    mitral Q23.2
    pulmonary Q22.1
    tricuspid Q22.4
  ear ossicles Q16.3
  fingers Q70.0- ☑
  hymen Q52.3
  joint (acquired) (*see also* Ankylosis)
    congenital Q74.8
  kidneys (incomplete) Q63.1
  labium (majus) (minus) Q52.5
  larynx and trachea Q34.8
  limb, congenital Q74.8
    lower Q74.2
    upper Q74.0
  lobes, lung Q33.8
  lumbosacral (acquired) M43.27
    arthrodesis status Z98.1
    congenital Q76.49
    postprocedural status Z98.1
  nares, nose, nasal, nostril (s) Q30.0
  organ or site not listed — *see* Anomaly, by site
  ossicles Q79.9
    auditory Q16.3
  pulmonic cusps Q22.1
  ribs Q76.6
  sacroiliac (joint) (acquired) M43.28
    arthrodesis status Z98.1
    congenital Q74.2
    postprocedural status Z98.1

Fusion — *continued*
  spine (acquired) NEC M43.20
    arthrodesis status Z98.1
    cervical region M43.22
    cervicothoracic region M43.23
    congenital Q76.49
    lumbar M43.26
    lumbosacral region M43.27
    occipito-atlanto-axial region M43.21
    postoperative status Z98.1
    sacrococcygeal region M43.28
    thoracic region M43.24
    thoracolumbar region M43.25
  sublingual duct with submaxillary duct at opening in mouth Q38.4
  testes Q55.1
  toes Q70.2- ☑
  tooth, teeth K00.2
  trachea and esophagus Q39.8
  twins Q89.4
  vagina Q52.4
  ventricles, heart Q21.0
  vertebra (arch) — *see* Fusion, spine
  vulva Q52.5
Fusospirillosis (mouth) (tongue) (tonsil) A69.1
Fussy baby R68.12

G

Gain in weight (abnormal) (excessive) (*see also* Weight, gain)
Gaisböck's disease (polycythemia hypertonica) D75.1
Gait abnormality R26.9
  ataxic R26.0
  falling R29.6
  hysterical (ataxic) (staggering) F44.4
  paralytic R26.1
  spastic R26.1
  specified type NEC R26.89
  staggering R26.0
  unsteadiness R26.81
  walking difficulty NEC R26.2
Galactocele (breast) N64.89
  puerperal, postpartum O92.79
Galactokinase deficiency E74.29
Galactophoritis N61
  gestational, puerperal, postpartum O91.2- ☑
Galactorrhea O92.6
  not associated with childbirth N64.3
Galactosemia (classic) (congenital) E74.21
Galactosuria E74.29
Galacturia R82.0
  schistosomiasis (bilharziasis) B65.0
Galeazzi's fracture S52.37- ☑
Galen's vein — *see* condition
Galeophobia F40.218
Gall duct — *see* condition
Gallbladder (*see also* condition)
  acute K81.0
Gallop rhythm R00.8
Gallstone (colic) (cystic duct) (gallbladder) (impacted) (multiple) (*see also* Calculus, gallbladder)
  with
    cholecystitis — *see* Calculus, gallbladder, with cholecystitis
    bile duct (common) (hepatic) — *see* Calculus, bile duct
  causing intestinal obstruction K56.3
  specified NEC K80.80
    with obstruction K80.81
Gambling Z72.6
  pathological (compulsive) F63.0
Gammopathy (of undetermined significance [MGUS]) D47.2
  associated with lymphoplasmacytic dyscrasia D47.2
  monoclonal D47.2
  polyclonal D89.0
Gamna's disease (siderotic splenomegaly) D73.1
Gamophobia F40.298
Gampsodactylia (congenital) Q66.7
Gamstorp's disease (adynamia episodica hereditaria) G72.3
Gandy-Nanta disease (siderotic splenomegaly) D73.1
Gang
  membership offenses Z72.810

Gangliocytoma D36.10
Ganglioglioma — *see* Neoplasm, uncertain behavior, by site
Ganglion (compound) (diffuse) (joint) (tendon (sheath)) M67.40
  ankle M67.47- ☑
  foot M67.47- ☑
  forearm M67.43- ☑
  hand M67.44- ☑
  lower leg M67.46- ☑
  multiple sites M67.49
  of yaws (early) (late) A66.6
  pelvic region M67.45- ☑
  periosteal — *see* Periostitis
  shoulder region M67.41- ☑
  specified site NEC M67.48
  thigh region M67.45- ☑
  tuberculous A18.09
  upper arm M67.42- ☑
  wrist M67.43- ☑
Ganglioneuroblastoma — *see* Neoplasm, nerve, malignant
Ganglioneuroma D36.10
  malignant — *see* Neoplasm, nerve, malignant
Ganglioneuromatosis D36.10
Ganglionitis
  fifth nerve — *see* Neuralgia, trigeminal
  gasserian (postherpetic) (postzoster) B02.21
  geniculate G51.1
    newborn (birth injury) P11.3
    postherpetic, postzoster B02.21
  herpes zoster B02.21
  postherpetic geniculate B02.21
Gangliosidosis E75.10
  GM1 E75.19
  GM2 E75.00
    other specified E75.09
    Sandhoff disease E75.01
    Tay-Sachs disease E75.02
  GM3 E75.19
  mucolipidosis IV E75.11
Gangosa A66.5
Gangrene, gangrenous (connective tissue) (dropsical) (dry) (moist) (skin) (ulcer) (*see also* Necrosis) I96
  with diabetes (mellitus) — *see* Diabetes, gangrene
  abdomen (wall) I96
  alveolar M27.3
  appendix K35.80
    with
      perforation or rupture K35.2
      peritoneal abscess K35.3
      peritonitis NEC K35.3
        generalized (with perforation or rupture) K35.2
        localized (with perforation or rupture) K35.3
  arteriosclerotic (general) (senile) — *see* Arteriosclerosis, extremities, with, gangrene
  auricle I96
  Bacillus welchii A48.0
  bladder (infectious) — *see* Cystitis, specified type NEC
  bowel, cecum, or colon — *see* Gangrene, intestine
  Clostridium perfringens or welchii A48.0
  cornea H18.89- ☑
  corpora cavernosa N48.29
    noninfective N48.89
  cutaneous, spreading I96
  decubital — *see* Ulcer, pressure, by site
  diabetic (any site) — *see* Diabetes, gangrene
  epidemic — *see* Poisoning, food, noxious, plant
  epididymis (infectional) N45.1
  erysipelas — *see* Erysipelas
  emphysematous — *see* Gangrene, gas
  extremity (lower) (upper) I96
  Fournier N49.3
    female N76.89
  fusospirochetal A69.0
  gallbladder — *see* Cholecystitis, acute
  gas (bacillus) A48.0
    following
      abortion — *see* Abortion by type complicated by infection
      ectopic or molar pregnancy O08.0
  glossitis K14.0
  hernia — *see* Hernia, by site, with gangrene
  intestine, intestinal (hemorrhagic) (massive) K55.0
    with
      mesenteric embolism K55.0

☑ **Additional character required**

Gangrene — *continued*
　　obstruction — *see* Obstruction, intestine
　laryngitis J04.0
　limb (lower) (upper) I96
　lung J85.0
　　spirochetal A69.8
　lymphangitis I89.1
　Meleney's (synergistic) — *see* Ulcer, skin
　mesentery K55.0
　　with
　　　embolism K55.0
　　　intestinal obstruction — *see* Obstruction,
　　　　intestine
　mouth A69.0
　ovary — *see* Oophoritis
　pancreas K85.9
　penis N48.29
　　noninfective N48.89
　perineum I96
　pharynx (*see also* Pharyngitis)
　　Vincent's A69.1
　presenile I73.1
　progressive synergistic — *see* Ulcer, skin
　pulmonary J85.0
　pulpal (dental) K04.1
　quinsy J36
　Raynaud's (symmetric gangrene) I73.01
　retropharyngeal J39.2
　scrotum N49.3
　　noninfective N50.8
　senile (atherosclerotic) — *see* Arteriosclerosis,
　　extremities, with, gangrene
　spermatic cord N49.1
　　noninfective N50.8
　spine I96
　spirochetal NEC A69.8
　spreading cutaneous I96
　stomatitis A69.0
　symmetrical I73.01
　testis (infectional) N45.2
　　noninfective N44.8
　throat (*see also* Pharyngitis)
　　diphtheritic A36.0
　　Vincent's A69.1
　thyroid (gland) E07.89
　tooth (pulp) K04.1
　tuberculous NEC — *see* Tuberculosis
　tunica vaginalis N49.1
　　noninfective N50.8
　umbilicus I96
　uterus — *see* Endometritis
　uvulitis K12.2
　vas deferens N49.1
　　noninfective N50.8
　vulva N76.89
Ganister disease J62.8
Ganser's syndrome (hysterical) F44.89
Gardner-Diamond syndrome (autoerythrocyte
　sensitization) D69.2
Gargoylism E76.01
Garré's disease, osteitis (sclerosing), osteomyelitis —
　see Osteomyelitis, specified type NEC
Garrod's pad, knuckle M72.1
Gartner's duct
　cyst Q52.4
　persistent Q50.6
Gas R14.3
　asphyxiation, inhalation, poisoning, suffocation
　　NEC — *see* Table of Drugs and Chemicals
　excessive R14.0
　gangrene A48.0
　　following
　　　abortion — *see* Abortion by type
　　　　complicated by infection
　　　ectopic or molar pregnancy O08.0
　on stomach R14.0
　pains R14.1
Gastralgia (*see also* Pain, abdominal)
Gastrectasis K31.0
　psychogenic F45.8
Gastric — *see* condition
Gastrinoma
　malignant
　　pancreas C25.4
　　specified site NEC — *see* Neoplasm, malignant,
　　　by site
　　unspecified site C25.4
　specified site — *see* Neoplasm, uncertain
　　behavior
　unspecified site D37.9
Gastritis (simple) K29.70
　with bleeding K29.71

Gastritis — *continued*
　acute (erosive) K29.00
　　with bleeding K29.01
　alcoholic K29.20
　　with bleeding K29.21
　allergic K29.60
　　with bleeding K29.61
　atrophic (chronic) K29.40
　　with bleeding K29.41
　chronic (antral) (fundal) K29.50
　　with bleeding K29.51
　　atrophic K29.40
　　　with bleeding K29.41
　　superficial K29.30
　　　with bleeding K29.31
　dietary counseling and surveillance Z71.3
　due to diet deficiency E63.9
　eosinophilic K52.81
　giant hypertrophic K29.60
　　with bleeding K29.61
　granulomatous K29.60
　　with bleeding K29.61
　hypertrophic (mucosa) K29.60
　　with bleeding K29.61
　nervous F54
　spastic K29.60
　　with bleeding K29.61
　specified NEC K29.60
　　with bleeding K29.61
　superficial chronic K29.30
　　with bleeding K29.31
　tuberculous A18.83
　viral NEC A08.4
Gastrocarcinoma — *see* Neoplasm, malignant,
　stomach
Gastrocolic — *see* condition
Gastrodisciasis, gastrodiscoidiasis B66.8
Gastroduodenitis K29.90
　with bleeding K29.91
　virus, viral A08.4
　　specified type NEC A08.39
Gastrodynia — *see* Pain, abdominal
Gastroenteritis (acute) (chronic) (noninfectious) (*see
　also* Enteritis) K52.9
　allergic K52.2
　dietetic K52.2
　drug-induced K52.1
　due to
　　Cryptosporidium A07.2
　　drugs K52.1
　　food poisoning — *see* Intoxication, foodborne
　　radiation K52.0
　eosinophilic K52.81
　epidemic (infectious) A09
　food hypersensitivity K52.2
　infectious — *see* Enteritis, infectious
　influenzal — *see* Influenza, with gastroenteritis
　noninfectious K52.9
　　specified NEC K52.89
　rotaviral A08.0
　Salmonella A02.0
　toxic K52.1
　viral NEC A08.4
　　acute infectious A08.39
　　　type Norwalk A08.11
　　infantile (acute) A08.39
　　Norwalk agent A08.11
　　rotaviral A08.0
　　severe of infants A08.39
　　specified type NEC A08.39
Gastroenteropathy (*see also* Gastroenteritis) K52.9
　acute, due to Norwalk agent A08.11
　acute, due to Norovirus A08.11
　infectious A09
Gastroenteroptosis K63.4
Gastroesophageal laceration- hemorrhage
　syndrome K22.6
Gastrointestinal — *see* condition
Gastrojejunal — *see* condition
Gastrojejunitis (*see also* Enteritis) K52.9
Gastrojejunocolic — *see* condition
Gastroliths K31.89
Gastromalacia K31.89
Gastroparalysis K31.84
　diabetic — *see* Diabetes, gastroparalysis
Gastroparesis K31.84
　diabetic — *see* Diabetes, by type, with
　　gastroparesis
Gastropathy K31.9
　congestive portal K31.89
　erythematous K29.70
　exudative K90.89

Gastropathy — *continued*
　portal hypertensive K31.89
Gastroptosis K31.89
Gastrorrhagia K92.2
　psychogenic F45.8
Gastroschisis (congenital) Q79.3
Gastrospasm (neurogenic) (reflex) K31.89
　neurotic F45.8
　psychogenic F45.8
Gastrostaxis — *see* Gastritis, with bleeding
Gastrostenosis K31.89
Gastrostomy
　attention to Z43.1
　status Z93.1
Gastrosuccorrhea (continuous) (intermittent)
　K31.89
　neurotic F45.8
　psychogenic F45.8
Gatophobia F40.218
Gaucher's disease or splenomegaly (adult) (infantile)
　E75.22
Gee (-Herter)(-Thaysen) disease (nontropical sprue)
　K90.0
Gélineau's syndrome G47.419
　with cataplexy G47.411
Gemination, tooth, teeth K00.2
Gemistocytoma
　specified site — *see* Neoplasm, malignant, by site
　unspecified site C71.9
General, generalized — *see* condition
Genetic
　carrier (status)
　　cystic fibrosis Z14.1
　　hemophilia A (asymptomatic) Z14.01
　　　symptomatic Z14.02
　　specified NEC Z14.8
　susceptibility to disease NEC Z15.89
　　malignant neoplasm Z15.09
　　　breast Z15.01
　　　endometrium Z15.04
　　　ovary Z15.02
　　　prostate Z15.03
　　　specified NEC Z15.09
　　multiple endocrine neoplasia Z15.81
Genital — *see* condition
Genito-anorectal syndrome A55
Genitourinary system — *see* condition
Genu
　congenital Q74.1
　extrorsum (acquired) (*see also* Deformity, varus,
　　knee)
　　congenital Q74.1
　　sequelae (late effect) of rickets E64.3
　introrsum (acquired) (*see also* Deformity, valgus,
　　knee)
　　congenital Q74.1
　　sequelae (late effect) of rickets E64.3
　rachitic (old) E64.3
　recurvatum (acquired) (*see also* Deformity, limb,
　　specified type NEC, lower leg)
　　congenital Q68.2
　　sequelae (late effect) of rickets E64.3
　valgum (acquired) (knock-knee) M21.06- ☑
　　congenital Q74.1
　　sequelae (late effect) of rickets E64.3
　varum (acquired) (bowleg) M21.16- ☑
　　congenital Q74.1
　　sequelae (late effect) of rickets E64.3
Geographic tongue K14.1
Geophagia — *see* Pica
Geotrichosis B48.3
　stomatitis B48.3
Gephyrophobia F40.242
Gerbode defect Q21.0
GERD (gastroesophageal reflux disease) K21.9
Gerhardt's
　disease (erythromelalgia) I73.81
　syndrome (vocal cord paralysis) J38.00
　　bilateral J38.02
　　unilateral J38.01
German measles (*see also* Rubella)
　exposure to Z20.4
Germinoblastoma (diffuse) C85.9- ☑
　follicular C82.9- ☑
Germinoma — *see* Neoplasm, malignant, by site
Gerontoxon — *see* Degeneration, cornea, senile
Gerstmann-Sträussler-Scheinker syndrome (GSS)
　A81.82
Gerstmann's syndrome R48.8
　developmental F81.2
Gestation (period) (*see also* Pregnancy)
　ectopic — *see* Pregnancy, by site

Gestation — *continued*
  multiple O30.9- ☑
    greater than quadruplets — *see* Pregnancy, multiple (gestation), specified NEC
    specified NEC — *see* Pregnancy, multiple (gestation), specified NEC
Gestational
  mammary abscess O91.11- ☑
  purulent mastitis O91.11- ☑
  subareolar abscess O91.11- ☑
Ghon tubercle, primary infection A15.7
Ghost
  teeth K00.4
  vessels (cornea) H16.41- ☑
Ghoul hand A66.3
Gianotti-Crosti disease L44.4
Giant
  cell
    epulis K06.8
    peripheral granuloma K06.8
  esophagus, congenital Q39.5
  kidney, congenital Q63.3
  urticaria T78.3 ☑
    hereditary D84.1
Giardiasis A07.1
Gibert's disease or pityriasis L42
Giddiness R42
  hysterical F44.89
  psychogenic F45.8
Gierke's disease (glycogenosis I) E74.01
Gigantism (cerebral) (hypophyseal) (pituitary) E22.0
  constitutional E34.4
Gilbert's disease or syndrome E80.4
Gilchrist's disease B40.9
Gilford-Hutchinson disease E34.8
Gilles de la Tourette's disease or syndrome (motor-verbal tic) F95.2
Gingivitis K05.10
  acute (catarrhal) K05.00
    necrotizing A69.1
    nonplaque induced K05.01
    plaque induced K05.00
  chronic (desquamative) (hyperplastic) (simple marginal) (ulcerative) K05.10
    nonplaque induced K05.11
    plaque induced K05.10
  expulsiva — *see* Periodontitis
  necrotizing ulcerative (acute) A69.1
  pellagrous E52
    acute necrotizing A69.1
  Vincent's A69.1
Gingivoglossitis K14.0
Gingivopericementitis — *see* Periodontitis
Gingivosis — *see* Gingivitis, chronic
Gingivostomatitis K05.10
  herpesviral B00.2
  necrotizing ulcerative (acute) A69.1
Gland, glandular — *see* condition
Glanders A24.0
Glanzmann (-Naegeli) disease or thrombasthenia D69.1
Glasgow coma scale
  total score
    3-8 R40.243 ☑
    9-12 R40.242 ☑
    13-15 R40.241 ☑
Glass-blower's disease (cataract) — *see* Cataract, specified NEC
Glaucoma H40.9
  with
    increased episcleral venous pressure H40.81- ☑
    pseudoexfoliation of lens — *see* Glaucoma, open angle, primary, capsular
  absolute H44.51- ☑
  angle-closure (primary) H40.20- ☑
    acute (attack) (crisis) H40.21- ☑
    chronic H40.22- ☑
    intermittent H40.23- ☑
    residual stage H40.24- ☑
  borderline H40.00- ☑
  capsular (with pseudoexfoliation of lens) — *see* Glaucoma, open angle, primary, capsular
  childhood Q15.0
  closed angle — *see* Glaucoma, angle-closure
  congenital Q15.0
  corticosteroid-induced — *see* Glaucoma, secondary, drugs
  hypersecretion H40.82- ☑
  in (due to)
    amyloidosis E85.4 [H42]
    aniridia Q13.1 [H42]

Glaucoma — *continued*
  concussion of globe — *see* Glaucoma, secondary, trauma
  dislocation of lens — *see* Glaucoma, secondary
  disorder of lens NEC — *see* Glaucoma, secondary
  drugs — *see* Glaucoma, secondary, drugs
  endocrine disease NOS E34.9 [H42]
  eye
    inflammation — *see* Glaucoma, secondary, inflammation
    trauma — *see* Glaucoma, secondary, trauma
  hypermature cataract — *see* Glaucoma, secondary
  iridocyclitis — *see* Glaucoma, secondary, inflammation
  lens disorder — *see* Glaucoma, secondary, Lowe's syndrome E72.03 [H42]
  metabolic disease NOS E88.9 [H42]
  ocular disorders NEC — *see* Glaucoma, secondary
  onchocerciasis B73.02
  pupillary block — *see* Glaucoma, secondary
  retinal vein occlusion — *see* Glaucoma, secondary
  Rieger's anomaly Q13.81 [H42]
  rubeosis of iris — *see* Glaucoma, secondary
  tumor of globe — *see* Glaucoma, secondary
  infantile Q15.0
  low tension — *see* Glaucoma, open angle, primary, low-tension
  malignant H40.83- ☑
  narrow angle — *see* Glaucoma, angle-closure
  newborn Q15.0
  noncongestive (chronic) — *see* Glaucoma, open angle
  nonobstructive — *see* Glaucoma, open angle
  obstructive (*see also* Glaucoma, angle-closure)
    due to lens changes — *see* Glaucoma, secondary
  open angle H40.10- ☑
    primary H40.11- ☑
      capsular (with pseudoexfoliation of lens) H40.14- ☑
      low-tension H40.12- ☑
      pigmentary H40.13- ☑
      residual stage H40.15- ☑
  phacolytic — *see* Glaucoma, secondary
  pigmentary — *see* Glaucoma, open angle, primary, pigmentary
  postinfectious — *see* Glaucoma, secondary, inflammation
  secondary (to) H40.5- ☑
    drugs H40.6- ☑
    inflammation H40.4- ☑
    trauma H40.3- ☑
  simple (chronic) H40.11 ☑
  simplex H40.11 ☑
  specified type NEC H40.89
  suspect H40.00- ☑
  syphilitic A52.71
  traumatic (*see also* Glaucoma, secondary, trauma)
    newborn (birth injury) P15.3
  tuberculous A18.59
Glaucomatous flecks (subcapsular) — *see* Cataract, complicated
Glazed tongue K14.4
Gleet (gonococcal) A54.01
Glénard's disease K63.4
Glioblastoma (multiforme)
  with sarcomatous component
    specified site — *see* Neoplasm, malignant, by site
    unspecified site C71.9
  giant cell
    specified site — *see* Neoplasm, malignant, by site
    unspecified site C71.9
  specified site — *see* Neoplasm, malignant, by site
  unspecified site C71.9
Glioma (malignant)
  astrocytic
    specified site — *see* Neoplasm, malignant, by site
    unspecified site C71.9
  mixed
    specified site — *see* Neoplasm, malignant, by site
    unspecified site C71.9
  nose Q30.8
  specified site NEC — *see* Neoplasm, malignant, by site

Glioma — *continued*
  subependymal D43.2
    specified site — *see* Neoplasm, uncertain behavior, by site
    unspecified site D43.2
  unspecified site C71.9
Gliomatosis cerebri C71.0
Glioneuroma — *see* Neoplasm, uncertain behavior, by site
Gliosarcoma
  specified site — *see* Neoplasm, malignant, by site
  unspecified site C71.9
Gliosis (cerebral) G93.89
  spinal G95.89
Glisson's disease — *see* Rickets
Globinuria R82.3
Globus (hystericus) F45.8
Glomangioma D18.00
  intra-abdominal D18.03
  intracranial D18.02
  skin D18.01
  specified site NEC D18.09
Glomangiomyoma D18.00
  intra-abdominal D18.03
  intracranial D18.02
  skin D18.01
  specified site NEC D18.09
Glomangiosarcoma — *see* Neoplasm, connective tissue, malignant
Glomerular
  disease in syphilis A52.75
  nephritis — *see* Glomerulonephritis
Glomerulitis — *see* Glomerulonephritis
Glomerulonephritis (*see also* Nephritis) N05.9
  with
    edema — *see* Nephrosis
    minimal change N05.0
    minor glomerular abnormality N05.0
  acute N00.9
  chronic N03.9
  crescentic (diffuse) NEC (*see also* N00-N07 with fourth character .7) N05.7
  dense deposit (*see also* N00-N07 with fourth character .6) N05.6
  diffuse
    crescentic (*see also* N00-N07 with fourth character .7) N05.7
    endocapillary proliferative (*see also* N00-N07 with fourth character .4) N05.4
    membranous (*see also* N00-N07 with fourth character .2) N05.2
    mesangial proliferative (*see also* N00-N07 with fourth character .3) N05.3
    mesangiocapillary (*see also* N00-N07 with fourth character .5) N05.5
    sclerosing N05.8
  endocapillary proliferative (diffuse) NEC (*see also* N00-N07 with fourth character .4) N05.4
  extracapillary NEC (*see also* N00-N07 with fourth character .7) N05.7
  focal (and segmental) NEC (*see also* N00-N07 with fourth character .1) N05.1
  hypocomplementemic — *see* Glomerulonephritis, membranoproliferative
  IgA — *see* Nephropathy, IgA
  immune complex (circulating) NEC N05.8
  in (due to)
    amyloidosis E85.4 [N08]
    bilharziasis B65.9 [N08]
    cryoglobulinemia D89.1 [N08]
    defibrination syndrome D65 [N08]
    diabetes mellitus — *see* Diabetes, glomerulosclerosis
    disseminated intravascular coagulation D65 [N08]
    Fabry (-Anderson) disease E75.21 [N08]
    Goodpasture's syndrome M31.0
    hemolytic-uremic syndrome D59.3
    Henoch (-Schönlein) purpura D69.0 [N08]
    lecithin cholesterol acyltransferase deficiency E78.6 [N08]
    microscopic polyangiitis M31.7 [N08]
    multiple myeloma C90.0- ☑ [N08]
    Plasmodium malariae B52.0
    schistosomiasis B65.9 [N08]
    sepsis A41.9 [N08]
      streptococcal A40- ☑ [N08]
    sickle-cell disorders D57.- ☑ [N08]
    strongyloidiasis B78.9 [N08]
    subacute bacterial endocarditis I33.0 [N08]
    syphilis (late) congenital A50.59 [N08]
    systemic lupus erythematosus M32.14

☑ **Additional character required**

Glomerulonephritis - Gougerot-Carteaud

Glomerulonephritis — *continued*
 thrombotic thrombocytopenic purpura M31.1 [N08]
 typhoid fever A01.09
 Waldenström macroglobulinemia C88.0 [N08]
 Wegener's granulomatosis M31.31
 latent or quiescent N03.9
 lobular, lobulonodular — *see* Glomerulonephritis, membranoproliferative
 membranoproliferative (diffuse)(type 1 or 3) (*see also* N00-N07 with fourth character .5) N05.5
  dense deposit (type 2) NEC (*see also* N00-N07 with fourth character .6) N05.6
 membranous (diffuse) NEC (*see also* N00-N07 with fourth character .2) N05.2
 mesangial
  IgA/IgG — *see* Nephropathy, IgA
  proliferative (diffuse) NEC (*see also* N00-N07 with fourth character .3) N05.3
 mesangiocapillary (diffuse) NEC (*see also* N00-N07 with fourth character .5) N05.5
 necrotic, necrotizing NEC (*see also* N00-N07 with fourth character .8) N05.8
 nodular — *see* Glomerulonephritis, membranoproliferative
 poststreptococcal NEC N05.9
  acute N00.9
  chronic N03.9
  rapidly progressive N01.9
 proliferative NEC (*see also* N00-N07 with fourth character .8) N05.8
  diffuse (lupus) M32.14
 rapidly progressive N01.9
 sclerosing, diffuse N05.8
 specified pathology NEC (*see also* N00-N07 with fourth character .8) N05.8
 subacute N01.9
Glomerulopathy — *see* Glomerulonephritis
Glomerulosclerosis (*see also* Sclerosis, renal)
 intercapillary (nodular) (with diabetes) — *see* Diabetes, glomerulosclerosis
 intracapillary — *see* Diabetes, glomerulosclerosis
Glossagra K14.6
Glossalgia K14.6
Glossitis (chronic superficial) (gangrenous) (Moeller's) K14.0
 areata exfoliativa K14.1
 atrophic K14.4
 benign migratory K14.1
 cortical superficial, sclerotic K14.0
 Hunter's D51.0
 interstitial, sclerous K14.0
 median rhomboid K14.2
 pellagrous E52
 superficial, chronic K14.0
Glossocele K14.8
Glossodynia K14.6
 exfoliativa K14.4
Glossoncus K14.8
Glossopathy K14.9
Glossophytia K14.3
Glossoplegia K14.8
Glossoptosis K14.8
Glossopyrosis K14.6
Glossotrichia K14.3
Glossy skin L90.8
Glottis — *see* condition
Glottitis (*see also* Laryngitis) J04.0
Glucagonoma
 pancreas
  benign D13.7
  malignant C25.4
  uncertain behavior D37.8
 specified site NEC
  benign — *see* Neoplasm, benign, by site
  malignant — *see* Neoplasm, malignant, by site
  uncertain behavior — *see* Neoplasm, uncertain behavior, by site
 unspecified site
  benign D13.7
  malignant C25.4
  uncertain behavior D37.8
Glucoglycinuria E72.51
Glucose-galactose malabsorption E74.39
Glue
 ear — *see* Otitis, media, nonsuppurative, chronic, mucoid
 sniffing (airplane) — *see* Abuse, drug, inhalant
 dependence — *see* Dependence, drug, inhalant
Glutaric aciduria E72.3
Glycinemia E72.51
Glycinuria (renal) (with ketosis) E72.09

Glycogen
 infiltration — *see* Disease, glycogen storage
 storage disease — *see* Disease, glycogen storage
Glycogenosis (diffuse) (generalized) (*see also* Disease, glycogen storage)
 cardiac E74.02 [I43]
 diabetic, secondary — *see* Diabetes, glycogenosis, secondary
 pulmonary interstitial J84.842
Glycopenia E16.2
Glycosuria R81
 renal E74.8
Gnathostoma spinigerum (infection) (infestation), gnathostomiasis (wandering swelling) B83.1
Goiter (plunging) (substernal) E04.9
 with
  hyperthyroidism (recurrent) — *see* Hyperthyroidism, with, goiter
  thyrotoxicosis — *see* Hyperthyroidism, with, goiter
 adenomatous — *see* Goiter, nodular
 cancerous C73
 congenital (nontoxic) E03.0
  diffuse E03.0
  parenchymatous E03.0
  transitory, with normal functioning P72.0
 cystic E04.2
  due to iodine-deficiency E01.1
 due to
  enzyme defect in synthesis of thyroid hormone E07.1
  iodine-deficiency (endemic) E01.2
 dyshormonogenetic (familial) E07.1
 endemic (iodine-deficiency) E01.2
  diffuse E01.0
  multinodular E01.1
 exophthalmic — *see* Hyperthyroidism, with, goiter
 iodine-deficiency (endemic) E01.2
  diffuse E01.0
  multinodular E01.1
  nodular E01.1
 lingual Q89.2
 lymphadenoid E06.3
 malignant C73
 multinodular (cystic) (nontoxic) E04.2
  toxic or with hyperthyroidism E05.20
   with thyroid storm E05.21
 neonatal NEC P72.0
 nodular (nontoxic) (due to) E04.9
  with
   hyperthyroidism E05.20
    with thyroid storm E05.21
   thyrotoxicosis E05.20
    with thyroid storm E05.21
  endemic E01.1
  iodine-deficiency E01.1
  sporadic E04.9
  toxic E05.20
   with thyroid storm E05.21
  nontoxic E04.9
   diffuse (colloid) E04.0
   multinodular E04.2
   simple E04.0
   specified NEC E04.8
   uninodular E04.1
 simple E04.0
 toxic — *see* Hyperthyroidism, with, goiter
 uninodular (nontoxic) E04.1
  toxic or with hyperthyroidism E05.10
   with thyroid storm E05.11
Goiter-deafness syndrome E07.1
Goldberg syndrome Q89.8
Goldberg-Maxwell syndrome E34.51
Goldblatt's hypertension or kidney I70.1
Goldenhar (-Gorlin) syndrome Q87.0
Goldflam-Erb disease or syndrome G70.00
 with exacerbation (acute) G70.01
 in crisis G70.01
Goldscheider's disease Q81.8
Goldstein's disease (familial hemorrhagic telangiectasia) I78.0
Golfer's elbow — *see* Epicondylitis, medial
Gonadoblastoma
 specified site — *see* Neoplasm, uncertain behavior, by site
 unspecified site
  female D39.10
  male D40.10
Gonecystitis — *see* Vesiculitis
Gongylonemiasis B83.8

Goniosynechiae — *see* Adhesions, iris, goniosynechiae
Gonococcemia A54.86
Gonococcus, gonococcal (disease) (infection) (*see also* condition) A54.9
 anus A54.6
 bursa, bursitis A54.49
 conjunctiva, conjunctivitis (neonatorum) A54.31
 endocardium A54.83
 eye A54.30
  conjunctivitis A54.31
  iridocyclitis A54.32
  keratitis A54.33
  newborn A54.31
  other specified A54.39
 fallopian tubes (acute) (chronic) A54.24
 genitourinary (organ) (system) (tract) (acute)
  lower A54.00
   with abscess (accessory gland) (periurethral) A54.1
  upper (*see also* condition) A54.29
 heart A54.83
 iridocyclitis A54.32
 joint A54.42
 lymphatic (gland) (node) A54.89
 meninges, meningitis A54.81
 musculoskeletal A54.40
  arthritis A54.42
  osteomyelitis A54.43
  other specified A54.49
  spondylopathy A54.41
 pelviperitonitis A54.24
 pelvis (acute) (chronic) A54.24
 pharynx A54.5
 proctitis A54.6
 pyosalpinx (acute) (chronic) A54.24
 rectum A54.6
 skin A54.89
 specified site NEC A54.89
 tendon sheath A54.49
 throat A54.5
 urethra (acute) (chronic) A54.01
  with abscess (accessory gland) (periurethral) A54.1
 vulva (acute) (chronic) A54.02
Gonocytoma
 specified site — *see* Neoplasm, uncertain behavior, by site
 unspecified site
  female D39.10
  male D40.10
Gonorrhea (acute) (chronic) A54.9
 Bartholin's gland (acute) (chronic) (purulent) A54.02
  with abscess (accessory gland) (periurethral) A54.1
 bladder A54.01
 cervix A54.03
 conjunctiva, conjunctivitis (neonatorum) A54.31
 contact Z20.2
 Cowper's gland (with abscess) A54.1
 exposure to Z20.2
 fallopian tube (acute) (chronic) A54.24
 kidney (acute) (chronic) A54.21
 lower genitourinary tract A54.00
  with abscess (accessory gland) (periurethral) A54.1
 ovary (acute) (chronic) A54.24
 pelvis (acute) (chronic) A54.24
  female pelvic inflammatory disease A54.24
 penis A54.09
 prostate (acute) (chronic) A54.22
 seminal vesicle (acute) (chronic) A54.23
 specified site not listed (*see also* Gonococcus) A54.89
 spermatic cord (acute) (chronic) A54.23
 urethra A54.01
  with abscess (accessory gland) (periurethral) A54.1
 vagina A54.02
 vas deferens (acute) (chronic) A54.23
 vulva A54.02
Goodall's disease A08.19
Goodpasture's syndrome M31.0
Gopalan's syndrome (burning feet) E53.0
Gorlin-Chaudry-Moss syndrome Q87.0
Gottron's papules L94.4
Gougerot's syndrome (trisymptomatic) L81.7
Gougerot-Blum syndrome (pigmented purpuric lichenoid dermatitis) L81.7
Gougerot-Carteaud disease or syndrome (confluent reticulate papillomatosis) L83

Gouley's syndrome (constrictive pericarditis) I31.1
Goundou A66.6
Gout, gouty (acute) (attack) (flare) (see also Gout, chronic) M10.9
  drug-induced M10.20
    ankle M10.27- ☑
    elbow M10.22- ☑
    foot joint M10.27- ☑
    hand joint M10.24- ☑
    hip M10.25- ☑
    knee M10.26- ☑
    multiple site M10.29
    shoulder M10.21- ☑
    vertebrae M10.28
    wrist M10.23- ☑
  idiopathic M10.00
    ankle M10.07- ☑
    elbow M10.02- ☑
    foot joint M10.07- ☑
    hand joint M10.04- ☑
    hip M10.05- ☑
    knee M10.06- ☑
    multiple site M10.09
    shoulder M10.01- ☑
    vertebrae M10.08
    wrist M10.03- ☑
  in (due to) renal impairment M10.30
    ankle M10.37- ☑
    elbow M10.32- ☑
    foot joint M10.37- ☑
    hand joint M10.34- ☑
    hip M10.35- ☑
    knee M10.36- ☑
    multiple site M10.39
    shoulder M10.31- ☑
    vertebrae M10.38
    wrist M10.33- ☑
  lead-induced M10.10
    ankle M10.17- ☑
    elbow M10.12- ☑
    foot joint M10.17- ☑
    hand joint M10.14- ☑
    hip M10.15- ☑
    knee M10.16- ☑
    multiple site M10.19
    shoulder M10.11- ☑
    vertebrae M10.18
    wrist M10.13- ☑
  primary — see Gout, idiopathic
  saturnine — see Gout, lead-induced
  secondary NEC M10.40
    ankle M10.47- ☑
    elbow M10.42- ☑
    foot joint M10.47- ☑
    hand joint M10.44- ☑
    hip M10.45- ☑
    knee M10.46- ☑
    multiple site M10.49
    shoulder M10.41- ☑
    vertebrae M10.48
    wrist M10.43- ☑
  syphilitic (see also subcategory M14.8-) A52.77
  tophi — see Gout, chronic
Gout, chronic (see also Gout, gouty) M1A.9 ☑
  drug-induced M1A.20 ☑
    ankle M1A.27- ☑
    elbow M1A.22- ☑
    foot joint M1A.27- ☑
    hand joint M1A.24- ☑
    hip M1A.25- ☑
    knee M1A.26- ☑
    multiple site M1A.29- ☑
    shoulder M1A.21- ☑
    vertebrae M1A.28 ☑
    wrist M1A.23- ☑
  idiopathic M1A.00 ☑
    ankle M1A.07- ☑
    elbow M1A.02- ☑
    foot joint M1A.07- ☑
    hand joint M1A.04- ☑
    hip M1A.05- ☑
    knee M1A.06- ☑
    multiple site M1A.09 ☑
    shoulder M1A.01- ☑
    vertebrae M1A.08 ☑
    wrist M1A.03- ☑
  in (due to) renal impairment M1A.30 ☑
    ankle M1A.37- ☑
    elbow M1A.32- ☑
    foot joint M1A.37- ☑
    hand joint M1A.34- ☑
    hip M1A.35- ☑

Gout — continued
    knee M1A.36- ☑
    multiple site M1A.39 ☑
    shoulder M1A.31- ☑
    vertebrae M1A.38 ☑
    wrist M1A.33- ☑
  lead-induced M1A.10 ☑
    ankle M1A.17- ☑
    elbow M1A.12- ☑
    foot joint M1A.17- ☑
    hand joint M1A.14- ☑
    hip M1A.15- ☑
    knee M1A.16- ☑
    multiple site M1A.19 ☑
    shoulder M1A.11- ☑
    vertebrae M1A.18 ☑
    wrist M1A.13- ☑
  primary — see Gout, chronic, idiopathic
  saturnine — see Gout, chronic, lead-induced
  secondary NEC M1A.40
    ankle M1A.47- ☑
    elbow M1A.42- ☑
    foot joint M1A.47- ☑
    hand joint M1A.44- ☑
    hip M1A.45- ☑
    knee M1A.46- ☑
    multiple site M1A.49 ☑
    shoulder M1A.41- ☑
    vertebrae M1A.48 ☑
    wrist M1A.43- ☑
  syphilitic (see also subcategory M14.8-) A52.77
  tophi M1A.9 ☑
Gower's
  muscular dystrophy G71.0
  syndrome (vasovagal attack) R55
Gradenigo's syndrome — see Otitis, media, suppurative, acute
Graefe's disease — see Strabismus, paralytic, ophthalmoplegia, progressive
Graft-versus-host disease D89.813
  acute D89.810
  acute on chronic D89.812
  chronic D89.811
Grainhandler's disease or lung J67.8
Grain mite (itch) B88.0
Grand mal — see Epilepsy, generalized, specified NEC
Grand multipara status only (not pregnant) Z64.1
  pregnant — see Pregnancy, complicated by, grand multiparity
Granite worker's lung J62.8
Granular (see also condition)
  inflammation, pharynx J31.2
  kidney (contracting) — see Sclerosis, renal
  liver K74.69
Granulation tissue (abnormal) (excessive) L92.9
  postmastoidectomy cavity — see Complications, postmastoidectomy, granulation
Granulocytopenia (primary) (malignant) — see Agranulocytosis
Granuloma L92.9
  abdomen K66.8
    from residual foreign body L92.3
    pyogenicum L98.0
  actinic L57.5
  annulare (perforating) L92.0
  apical K04.5
  aural — see Otitis, externa, specified NEC
  beryllium (skin) L92.3
  bone
    eosinophilic C96.6
    from residual foreign body — see Osteomyelitis, specified type NEC
    lung C96.6
  brain (any site) G06.0
    schistosomiasis B65.9 [G07]
  canaliculus lacrimalis — see Granuloma, lacrimal
  candidal (cutaneous) B37.2
  cerebral (any site) G06.0
  coccidioidal (primary) (progressive) B38.7
    lung B38.1
    meninges B38.4
  colon K63.89
  conjunctiva H11.22- ☑
  dental K04.5
  ear, middle — see Cholesteatoma
  eosinophilic C96.6
    bone C96.6
    lung C96.6
    oral mucosa K13.4
    skin L92.2
  eyelid H01.8

Granuloma — continued
  facial (e) L92.2
  foreign body (in soft tissue) NEC M60.20
    ankle M60.27- ☑
    foot M60.27- ☑
    forearm M60.23- ☑
    hand M60.24- ☑
    in operation wound — see Foreign body, accidentally left during a procedure
    lower leg M60.26- ☑
    pelvic region M60.25- ☑
    shoulder region M60.21- ☑
    skin L92.3
    specified site NEC M60.28
    subcutaneous tissue L92.3
    thigh M60.25- ☑
    upper arm M60.22- ☑
  gangraenescens M31.2
  genito-inguinale A58
  giant cell (central) (reparative) (jaw) M27.1
    gingiva (peripheral) K06.8
  gland (lymph) I88.8
  hepatic NEC K75.3
    in (due to)
      berylliosis J63.2 [K77]
      sarcoidosis D86.89
  Hodgkin C81.9 ☑
  ileum K63.89
  infectious B99.9
    specified NEC B99.8
  inguinale (Donovan) (venereal) A58
  intestine NEC K63.89
  intracranial (any site) G06.0
  intraspinal (any part) G06.1
  iridocyclitis — see Iridocyclitis, chronic
  jaw (bone) (central) M27.1
    reparative giant cell M27.1
  kidney (see also Infection, kidney) N15.8
  lacrimal H04.81- ☑
  larynx J38.7
  lethal midline (faciale) M31.2
  liver NEC — see Granuloma, hepatic
  lung (infectious) (see also Fibrosis, lung)
    coccidioidal B38.1
    eosinophilic C96.6
  Majocchi's B35.8
  malignant (facial(e)) M31.2
  mandible (central) M27.1
  midline (lethal) M31.2
  monilial (cutaneous) B37.2
  nasal sinus — see Sinusitis
  operation wound T81.89 ☑
    foreign body — see Foreign body, accidentally left during a procedure
    stitch T81.89 ☑
    talc — see Foreign body, accidentally left during a procedure
  oral mucosa K13.4
  orbit, orbital H05.11- ☑
  paracoccidioidal B41.8
  penis, venereal A58
  periapical K04.5
  peritoneum K66.8
    due to ova of helminths NOS (see also Helminthiasis) B83.9 [K67]
  postmastoidectomy cavity — see Complications, postmastoidectomy, recurrent cholesteatoma
  prostate N42.89
  pudendi (ulcerating) A58
  pulp, internal (tooth) K03.3
  pyogenic, pyogenicum (of) (skin) L98.0
    gingiva K06.8
    maxillary alveolar ridge K04.5
    oral mucosa K13.4
  rectum K62.89
  reticulohistiocytic D76.3
  rubrum nasi L74.8
  Schistosoma — see Schistosomiasis
  septic (skin) L98.0
  silica (skin) L92.3
  sinus (accessory) (infective) (nasal) — see Sinusitis
  skin L92.9
    from residual foreign body L92.3
    pyogenicum L98.0
  spine
    syphilitic (epidural) A52.19
    tuberculous A18.01
  stitch (postoperative) T81.89 ☑
  suppurative (skin) L98.0
  swimming pool A31.1
  talc (see also Granuloma, foreign body)

☑ **Additional character required**

Granuloma — *continued*
    in operation wound — *see* Foreign body, accidentally left during a procedure
   telangiectaticum (skin) L98.0
   tracheostomy J95.09
   trichophyticum B35.8
   tropicum A66.4
   umbilicus L92.9
   urethra N36.8
   uveitis — *see* Iridocyclitis, chronic
   vagina A58
   venereum A58
   vocal cord J38.3
Granulomatosis L92.9
   lymphoid C83.8- ☑
   miliary (listerial) A32.89
   necrotizing, respiratory M31.30
   progressive septic D71
   specified NEC L92.8
   Wegener's M31.30
     with renal involvement M31.31
Granulomatous tissue (abnormal) (excessive) L92.9
Granulosis rubra nasi L74.8
Graphite fibrosis (of lung) J63.3
Graphospasm F48.8
   organic G25.89
Grating scapula M89.8X1
Gravel (urinary) — *see* Calculus, urinary
Graves' disease — *see* Hyperthyroidism, with, goiter
Gravis — *see* condition
Grawitz tumor C64.- ☑
Gray syndrome (newborn) P93.0
Grayness, hair (premature) L67.1
   congenital Q84.2
Green sickness D50.8
Greenfield's disease
   meaning
     concentric sclerosis (encephalitis periaxialis concentrica) G37.5
     metachromatic leukodystrophy E75.25
Greenstick fracture - code as Fracture, by site
Grey syndrome (newborn) P93.0
Grief F43.21
   prolonged F43.29
   reaction (*see also* Disorder, adjustment) F43.20
Griesinger's disease B76.9
Grinder's lung or pneumoconiosis J62.8
Grinding, teeth
   psychogenic F45.8
   sleep related G47.63
Grip
   Dabney's B33.0
   devil's B33.0
Grippe, grippal (*see also* Influenza)
   Balkan A78
   summer, of Italy A93.1
Grisel's disease M43.6
Groin — *see* condition
Grooved tongue K14.5
Ground itch B76.9
Grover's disease or syndrome L11.1
Growing pains, children R29.898
Growth (fungoid) (neoplastic) (new) (*see also* Neoplasm)
   adenoid (vegetative) J35.8
   benign — *see* Neoplasm, benign, by site
   malignant — *see* Neoplasm, malignant, by site
   rapid, childhood Z00.2
   secondary — *see* Neoplasm, secondary, by site
Gruby's disease B35.0
Gubler-Millard paralysis or syndrome G46.3
Guerin-Stern syndrome Q74.3
Guidance, insufficient anterior (occlusal) M26.54
Guillain-Barré disease or syndrome G61.0
   sequelae G65.0
Guinea worms (infection) (infestation) B72
Guinon's disease (motor-verbal tic) F95.2
Gull's disease E03.4
Gum — *see* condition
Gumboil K04.7
   with sinus K04.6
Gumma (syphilitic) A52.79
   artery A52.09
     cerebral A52.04
   bone A52.77
     of yaws (late) A66.6
   brain A52.19
   cauda equina A52.19
   central nervous system A52.3
   ciliary body A52.71
   congenital A50.59
   eyelid A52.71

Gumma — *continued*
   heart A52.06
   intracranial A52.19
   iris A52.71
   kidney A52.75
   larynx A52.73
   leptomeninges A52.19
   liver A52.74
   meninges A52.19
   myocardium A52.06
   nasopharynx A52.73
   neurosyphilitic A52.3
   nose A52.73
   orbit A52.71
   palate (soft) A52.79
   penis A52.76
   pericardium A52.06
   pharynx A52.73
   pituitary A52.79
   scrofulous (tuberculous) A18.4
   skin A52.79
   specified site NEC A52.79
   spinal cord A52.19
   tongue A52.79
   tonsil A52.73
   trachea A52.73
   tuberculous A18.4
   ulcerative due to yaws A66.4
   ureter A52.75
   yaws A66.4
     bone A66.6
Gunn's syndrome Q07.8
Gunshot wound (*see also* Wound, open)
   fracture - code as Fracture, by site
   internal organs — *see* Injury, by site
Gynandrism Q56.0
Gynandroblastoma
   specified site — *see* Neoplasm, uncertain behavior, by site
   unspecified site
     female D39.10
     male D40.10
Gynecological examination (periodic) (routine) Z01.419
   with abnormal findings Z01.411
Gynecomastia N62
Gynephobia F40.291
Gyrate scalp Q82.8

H

H (Hartnup's) disease E72.02
Haas' disease or osteochondrosis (juvenile) (head of humerus) — *see* Osteochondrosis, juvenile, humerus
Habit, habituation
   bad sleep Z72.821
   chorea F95.8
   disturbance, child F98.9
   drug — *see* Dependence, drug
   irregular sleep Z72.821
   laxative F55.2
   spasm — *see* Tic
   tic — *see* Tic
Haemophilus (H.) influenzae, as cause of disease classified elsewhere B96.3
Haff disease — *see* Poisoning, mercury
Hageman's factor defect, deficiency or disease D68.2
Haglund's disease or osteochondrosis (juvenile) (os tibiale externum) — *see* Osteochondrosis, juvenile, tarsus
Hailey-Hailey disease Q82.8
Hair (*see also* condition)
   plucking F63.3
     in stereotyped movement disorder F98.4
   tourniquet syndrome (*see also* Constriction, external, by site)
     finger S60.44- ☑
     penis S30.842 ☑
     thumb S60.34- ☑
     toe S90.44- ☑
Hairball in stomach T18.2 ☑
Hair-pulling, pathological (compulsive) F63.3
Hairy black tongue K14.3
Half vertebra Q76.49
Halitosis R19.6
Hallerman-Streiff syndrome Q87.0
Hallervorden-Spatz disease G23.0

Hallopeau's acrodermatitis or disease L40.2
Hallucination R44.3
   auditory R44.0
   gustatory R44.2
   olfactory R44.2
   specified NEC R44.2
   tactile R44.2
   visual R44.1
Hallucinosis (chronic) F28
   alcoholic (acute) F10.951
     in
       abuse F10.151
       dependence F10.251
   drug-induced F19.951
     cannabis F12.951
     cocaine F14.951
     hallucinogen F16.151
     in
       abuse F19.151
         cannabis F12.151
         cocaine F14.151
         hallucinogen F16.151
         inhalant F18.151
         opioid F11.151
         sedative, anxiolytic or hypnotic F13.151
         stimulant NEC F15.151
       dependence F19.251
         cannabis F12.251
         cocaine F14.251
         hallucinogen F16.251
         inhalant F18.251
         opioid F11.251
         sedative, anxiolytic or hypnotic F13.251
         stimulant NEC F15.251
       inhalant F18.951
       opioid F11.951
       sedative, anxiolytic or hypnotic F13.951
       stimulant NEC F15.951
   organic F06.0
Hallux
   deformity (acquired) NEC M20.5X- ☑
   limitus M20.5X- ☑
   malleus (acquired) NEC M20.3- ☑
   rigidus (acquired) M20.2- ☑
     congenital Q74.2
     sequelae (late effect) of rickets E64.3
   valgus (acquired) M20.1- ☑
     congenital Q66.6
   varus (acquired) M20.3- ☑
     congenital Q66.3
Halo, visual H53.19
Hamartoma, hamartoblastoma Q85.9
   epithelial (gingival), odontogenic, central or peripheral — *see* Cyst, calcifying odontogenic
Hamartosis Q85.9
Hamman-Rich syndrome J84.114
Hammer toe (acquired) NEC (*see also* Deformity, toe, hammer toe)
   congenital Q66.89
   sequelae (late effect) of rickets E64.3
Hand — *see* condition
Hand-foot syndrome L27.1
Handicap, handicapped
   educational Z55.9
   specified NEC Z55.8
Hand-Schüller-Christian disease or syndrome C96.5
Hanging (asphyxia) (strangulation) (suffocation) — *see* Asphyxia, traumatic, due to mechanical threat
Hangnail (*see also* Cellulitis, digit)
   with lymphangitis — *see* Lymphangitis, acute, digit
Hangover (alcohol) F10.129
Hanhart's syndrome Q87.0
Hanot-Chauffard (-Troisier) syndrome E83.19
Hanot's cirrhosis or disease K74.3
Hansen's disease — *see* Leprosy
Hantaan virus disease (Korean hemorrhagic fever) A98.5
Hantavirus disease (with renal manifestations) (Dobrava) (Puumala) (Seoul) A98.5
   with pulmonary manifestations (Andes) (Bayou) (Bermejo) (Black Creek Canal) (Choclo) (Juquitiba) (Laguna negra) (Lechiguanas) (New York) (Oran) (Sin nombre) B33.4
Happy puppet syndrome Q93.5
Harada's disease or syndrome H30.81- ☑
Hardening
   artery — *see* Arteriosclerosis
   brain G93.89
Harelip (complete) (incomplete) — *see* Cleft, lip
Harlequin (newborn) Q80.4
Harley's disease D59.6

Harmful use (of)
    alcohol F10.10
    anxiolytics — *see* Abuse, drug, sedative
    cannabinoids — *see* Abuse, drug, cannabis
    cocaine — *see* Abuse, drug, cocaine
    drug — *see* Abuse, drug
    hallucinogens — *see* Abuse, drug, hallucinogen
    hypnotics — *see* Abuse, drug, sedative
    opioids — *see* Abuse, drug, opioid
    PCP (phencyclidine) — *see* Abuse, drug,
        hallucinogen
    sedatives — *see* Abuse, drug, sedative
    stimulants NEC — *see* Abuse, drug, stimulant
Harris' lines — *see* Arrest, epiphyseal
Hartnup's disease E72.02
Harvester's lung J67.0
Harvesting ovum for in vitro fertilization Z31.83
Hashimoto's disease or thyroiditis E06.3
Hashitoxicosis (transient) E06.3
Hassal-Henle bodies or warts (cornea) H18.49
Haut mal — *see* Epilepsy, generalized, specified NEC
Haverhill fever A25.1
Hay fever (*see also* Fever, hay) J30.1
Hayem-Widal syndrome D59.8
Haygarth's nodes M15.8
Haymaker's lung J67.0
Hb (abnormal)
    Bart's disease D56.0
    disease — *see* Disease, hemoglobin
    trait — *see* Trait
Head — *see* condition
Headache R51
    allergic NEC G44.89
    associated with sexual activity G44.82
    chronic daily R51
    cluster G44.009
        chronic G44.029
            intractable G44.021
            not intractable G44.029
        episodic G44.019
            intractable G44.011
            not intractable G44.019
        intractable G44.001
        not intractable G44.009
    cough (primary) G44.83
    daily chronic R51
    drug-induced NEC G44.40
        intractable G44.41
        not intractable G44.40
    exertional (primary) G44.84
    histamine G44.009
        intractable G44.001
        not intractable G44.009
    hypnic G44.81
    lumbar puncture G97.1
    medication overuse G44.40
        intractable G44.41
        not intractable G44.40
    menstrual — *see* Migraine, menstrual
    migraine (type) (*see also* Migraine) G43.909
    nasal septum R51
    neuralgiform, short lasting unilateral, with
        conjunctival injection and tearing (SUNCT)
        G44.059
        intractable G44.051
        not intractable G44.059
    new daily persistent (NDPH) G44.52
    orgasmic G44.82
    periodic syndromes in adults and children G43.
        C0
        with refractory migraine G43.C1
        intractable G43.C1
        not intractable G43.C0
        without refractory migraine G43.C0
    postspinal puncture G97.1
    post-traumatic G44.309
        acute G44.319
            intractable G44.311
            not intractable G44.319
        chronic G44.329
            intractable G44.321
            not intractable G44.329
        intractable G44.301
        not intractable G44.309
    pre-menstrual — *see* Migraine, menstrual
    preorgasmic G44.82
    primary
        cough G44.83
        exertional G44.84
        stabbing G44.85
        thunderclap G44.53
    rebound G44.40

Headache — *continued*
    intractable G44.41
    not intractable G44.40
    short lasting unilateral neuralgiform, with
        conjunctival injection and tearing (SUNCT)
        G44.059
        intractable G44.051
        not intractable G44.059
    specified syndrome NEC G44.89
    spinal and epidural anesthesia - induced
        T88.59 ☑
        in labor and delivery O74.5
        in pregnancy O29.4- ☑
        postpartum, puerperal O89.4
    spinal fluid loss (from puncture) G97.1
    stabbing (primary) G44.85
    tension (-type) G44.209
        chronic G44.229
            intractable G44.221
            not intractable G44.229
        episodic G44.219
            intractable G44.211
            not intractable G44.219
        intractable G44.201
        not intractable G44.209
    thunderclap (primary) G44.53
    vascular NEC G44.1
Healthy
    infant
        accompanying sick mother Z76.3
        receiving care Z76.2
    person accompanying sick person Z76.3
Hearing examination Z01.10
    with abnormal findings NEC Z01.118
    following failed hearing screening Z01.110
    for hearing conservation and treatment Z01.12
Heart — *see* condition
Heart beat
    abnormality R00.9
        specified NEC R00.8
    awareness R00.2
    rapid R00.0
    slow R00.1
Heartburn R12
    psychogenic F45.8
Heat (effects) T67.9 ☑
    apoplexy T67.0 ☑
    burn (*see also* Burn) L55.9
    collapse T67.1 ☑
    cramps T67.2 ☑
    dermatitis or eczema L59.0
    edema T67.7 ☑
    erythema - code by site under Burn, first degree
    excessive T67.9 ☑
        specified effect NEC T67.8 ☑
    exhaustion T67.5 ☑
        anhydrotic T67.3 ☑
        due to
            salt (and water) depletion T67.4 ☑
            water depletion T67.3 ☑
                with salt depletion T67.4 ☑
    fatigue (transient) T67.6 ☑
    fever T67.0 ☑
    hyperpyrexia T67.0 ☑
    prickly L74.0
    prostration — *see* Heat, exhaustion
    pyrexia T67.0 ☑
    rash L74.0
    specified effect NEC T67.8 ☑
    stroke T67.0 ☑
    sunburn — *see* Sunburn
    syncope T67.1 ☑
Heavy-for-dates NEC (infant) (4000g to 4499g)
    P08.1
    exceptionally (4500g or more) P08.0
Hebephrenia, hebephrenic (schizophrenia) F20.1
Heberden's disease or nodes (with arthropathy)
    M15.1
Hebra's
    pityriasis L26
    prurigo L28.2
Heel — *see* condition
Heerfordt's disease D86.89
Hegglin's anomaly or syndrome D72.0
Heilmeyer-Schoner disease D45
Heine-Medin disease A80.9
Heinz body anemia, congenital D58.2
Heliophobia F40.228
Heller's disease or syndrome F84.3
HELLP syndrome (hemolysis, elevated liver enzymes
    and low platelet count) O14.2- ☑

Helminthiasis (*see also* Infestation, helminth)
    Ancylostoma B76.0
    intestinal B82.0
        mixed types (types classifiable to more than
            one of the titles B65.0-B81.3 and B81.8)
            B81.4
        specified type NEC B81.8
    mixed types (intestinal) (types classifiable to
        more than one of the titles B65.0-B81.3 and
        B81.8) B81.4
    Necator (americanus) B76.1
    specified type NEC B83.8
Heloma L84
Hemangioblastoma — *see* Neoplasm, connective
    tissue, uncertain behavior
    malignant — *see* Neoplasm, connective tissue,
        malignant
Hemangioendothelioma (*see also* Neoplasm,
    uncertain behavior, by site)
    benign D18.00
        intra-abdominal D18.03
        intracranial D18.02
        skin D18.01
        specified site NEC D18.09
    bone (diffuse) — *see* Neoplasm, bone, malignant
    epithelioid (*see also* Neoplasm, uncertain
        behavior, by site)
        malignant — *see* Neoplasm, malignant, by site
    malignant — *see* Neoplasm, connective tissue,
        malignant
Hemangiofibroma — *see* Neoplasm, benign, by site
Hemangiolipoma — *see* Lipoma
Hemangioma D18.00
    arteriovenous D18.00
        intra-abdominal D18.03
        intracranial D18.02
        skin D18.01
        specified site NEC D18.09
    capillary D18.00
        intra-abdominal D18.03
        intracranial D18.02
        skin D18.01
        specified site NEC D18.09
    cavernous D18.00
        intra-abdominal D18.03
        intracranial D18.02
        skin D18.01
        specified site NEC D18.09
    epithelioid D18.00
        intra-abdominal D18.03
        intracranial D18.02
        skin D18.01
        specified site NEC D18.09
    histiocytoid D18.00
        intra-abdominal D18.03
        intracranial D18.02
        skin D18.01
        specified site NEC D18.09
    infantile D18.00
        intra-abdominal D18.03
        intracranial D18.02
        skin D18.01
        specified site NEC D18.09
    intra-abdominal D18.03
    intracranial D18.02
    intramuscular D18.00
        intra-abdominal D18.03
        intracranial D18.02
        skin D18.01
        specified site NEC D18.09
    juvenile D18.00
    malignant — *see* Neoplasm,connective tissue,
        malignant
    plexiform D18.00
        intra-abdominal D18.03
        intracranial D18.02
        skin D18.01
        specified site NEC D18.09
    racemose D18.00
        intra-abdominal D18.03
        intracranial D18.02
        skin D18.01
        specified site NEC D18.09
    sclerosing — *see* Neoplasm,skin, benign
    simplex D18.00
        intra-abdominal D18.03
        intracranial D18.02
        skin D18.01
        specified site NEC D18.09
    skin D18.01
    specified site NEC D18.09
    venous D18.00

☑ **Additional character required**

Hemangioma — continued
  intra-abdominal D18.03
  intracranial D18.02
  skin D18.01
  specified site NEC D18.09
  verrucous keratotic D18.00
    intra-abdominal D18.03
    intracranial D18.02
    skin D18.01
    specified site NEC D18.09
Hemangiomatosis (systemic) I78.8
  involving single site — *see* Hemangioma
Hemangiopericytoma (*see also* Neoplasm,
  connective tissue, uncertain behavior)
  benign — *see* Neoplasm, connective tissue,
    benign
  malignant — *see* Neoplasm, connective tissue,
    malignant
Hemangiosarcoma — *see* Neoplasm, connective
  tissue, malignant
Hemarthrosis (nontraumatic) M25.00
  ankle M25.07- ☑
  elbow M25.02- ☑
  foot joint M25.07- ☑
  hand joint M25.04- ☑
  hip M25.05- ☑
  in hemophilic arthropathy — *see* Arthropathy,
    hemophilic
  knee M25.06- ☑
  shoulder M25.01- ☑
  specified joint NEC M25.08
  traumatic — *see* Sprain, by site
  vertebrae M25.08
  wrist M25.03- ☑
Hematemesis K92.0
  with ulcer - code by site under Ulcer, with
    hemorrhage K27.4
  newborn, neonatal P54.0
    due to swallowed maternal blood P78.2
Hematidrosis L74.8
Hematinuria (*see also* Hemoglobinuria)
  malarial B50.8
Hematobilia K83.8
Hematocele
  female NEC N94.89
    with ectopic pregnancy O00.9
    ovary N83.8
  male N50.1
Hematochezia (*see also* Melena) K92.1
Hematochyluria (*see also* Infestation, filarial)
  schistosomiasis (bilharziasis) B65.0
Hematocolpos (with hematometra or
  hematosalpinx) N89.7
Hematocornea — *see* Pigmentation, cornea, stromal
Hematogenous — *see* condition
Hematoma (traumatic) (skin surface intact) (*see also*
  Contusion)
  with
    injury of internal organs — *see* Injury, by site
    open wound — *see* Wound, open
  amputation stump (surgical) (late) T87.89
  aorta, dissecting I71.00
    abdominal I71.02
    thoracic I71.01
    thoracoabdominal I71.03
  aortic intramural — *see* Dissection, aorta
  arterial (complicating trauma) — *see* Injury, blood
    vessel, by site
  auricle — *see* Contusion, ear
    nontraumatic — *see* Disorder, pinna,
      hematoma
  birth injury NEC P15.8
  brain (traumatic)
    with
      cerebral laceration or contusion (diffuse) —
        see Injury, intracranial, diffuse
      focal — *see* Injury, intracranial, focal
    cerebellar, traumatic S06.37- ☑
    newborn NEC P52.4
      birth injury P10.1
    intracerebral, traumatic — *see* Injury,
      intracranial, intracerebral hemorrhage
    nontraumatic — *see* Hemorrhage, intracranial
    subarachnoid, arachnoid, traumatic — *see*
      Injury, intracranial, subarachnoid
      hemorrhage
    subdural, traumatic — *see* Injury, intracranial,
      subdural hemorrhage
  breast (nontraumatic) N64.89
  broad ligament (nontraumatic) N83.7
    traumatic S37.892 ☑
  cerebellar, traumatic S06.37- ☑

Hematoma — continued
  cerebral — *see* Hematoma, brain
  cerebrum S06.36- ☑
    left S06.35- ☑
    right S06.34- ☑
  cesarean delivery wound O90.2
  complicating delivery (perineal) (pelvic) (vagina)
    (vulva) O71.7
  corpus cavernosum (nontraumatic) N48.89
  epididymis (nontraumatic) N50.1
  epidural (traumatic) — *see* Injury, intracranial,
    epidural hemorrhage
    spinal — *see* Injury, spinal cord, by region
  episiotomy O90.2
  face, birth injury P15.4
  genital organ NEC (nontraumatic)
    female (nonobstetric) N94.89
      traumatic S30.202 ☑
    male N50.1
      traumatic S30.201 ☑
  internal organs — *see* Injury, by site
  intracerebral, traumatic — *see* Injury, intracranial,
    intracerebral hemorrhage
  intraoperative — *see* Complications,
    intraoperative, hemorrhage
  labia (nontraumatic) (nonobstetric) N90.89
  liver (subcapsular) (nontraumatic) K76.89
    birth injury P15.0
  mediastinum — *see* Injury, intrathoracic
  mesosalpinx (nontraumatic) N83.7
    traumatic S37.898 ☑
  muscle - code by site under Contusion
  nontraumatic
    muscle M79.81
    soft tissue M79.81
  obstetrical surgical wound O90.2
  orbit, orbital (nontraumatic) (*see also*
    Hemorrhage, orbit)
    traumatic — *see* Contusion, orbit
  pelvis (female) (nontraumatic) (nonobstetric)
    N94.89
    obstetric O71.7
    traumatic — *see* Injury, by site
  penis (nontraumatic) N48.89
    birth injury P15.5
  perianal (nontraumatic) K64.5
  perineal S30.23 ☑
    complicating delivery O71.7
  perirenal — *see* Injury, kidney
  pinna — *see* Contusion, ear
    nontraumatic — *see* Disorder, pinna,
      hematoma
  placenta O43.89- ☑
  postoperative (postprocedural) — *see*
    Complication, postprocedural, hemorrhage
  retroperitoneal (nontraumatic) K66.1
    traumatic S36.892 ☑
  scrotum, superficial S30.22 ☑
    birth injury P15.5
  seminal vesicle (nontraumatic) N50.1
    traumatic S37.892 ☑
  spermatic cord (traumatic) S37.892 ☑
    nontraumatic N50.1
  spinal (cord) (meninges) (*see also* Injury, spinal
    cord, by region)
    newborn (birth injury) P11.5
  spleen D73.5
    intraoperative — *see* Complications,
      intraoperative, hemorrhage, spleen
    postprocedural (postoperative) — *see*
      Complications, postprocedural,
      hemorrhage, spleen
  sternocleidomastoid, birth injury P15.2
  sternomastoid, birth injury P15.2
  subarachnoid (traumatic) — *see* Injury,
    intracranial, subarachnoid hemorrhage
    newborn (nontraumatic) P52.5
      due to birth injury P10.3
    nontraumatic — *see* Hemorrhage, intracranial,
      subarachnoid
  subdural (traumatic) — *see* Injury, intracranial,
    subdural hemorrhage
    newborn (localized) P52.8
      birth injury P10.0
    nontraumatic — *see* Hemorrhage, intracranial,
      subdural
  superficial, newborn P54.5
  testis (nontraumatic) N50.1
    birth injury P15.5
  tunica vaginalis (nontraumatic) N50.1
  umbilical cord, complicating delivery O69.5 ☑
  uterine ligament (broad) (nontraumatic) N83.7

Hematoma — continued
  traumatic S37.892 ☑
  vagina (ruptured) (nontraumatic) N89.8
    complicating delivery O71.7
  vas deferens (nontraumatic) N50.1
    traumatic S37.892 ☑
  vitreous — *see* Hemorrhage, vitreous
  vulva (nontraumatic) (nonobstetric) N90.89
    complicating delivery O71.7
    newborn (birth injury) P15.5
Hematometra N85.7
  with hematocolpos N89.7
Hematomyelia (central) G95.19
  newborn (birth injury) P11.5
  traumatic T14.8
Hematomyelitis G04.90
Hematoperitoneum — *see* Hemoperitoneum
Hematophobia F40.230
Hematopneumothorax (*see* Hemothorax)
Hematopoiesis, cyclic D70.4
Hematoporphyria — *see* Porphyria
Hematorachis, hematorrhachis G95.19
  newborn (birth injury) P11.5
Hematosalpinx N83.6
  with
    hematocolpos N89.7
    hematometra N85.7
      with hematocolpos N89.7
  infectional — *see* Salpingitis
Hematospermia R36.1
Hematothorax (*see* Hemothorax)
Hematuria R31.9
  due to sulphonamide, sulfonamide — *see* Table
    of Drugs and Chemicals, by drug
  benign (familial) (of childhood) (*see also*
    Hematuria, idiopathic)
    essential microscopic R31.1
  endemic (*see also* Schistosomiasis) B65.0
  gross R31.0
  idiopathic N02.9
    with glomerular lesion
      crescentic (diffuse) glomerulonephritis N02.7
      dense deposit disease N02.6
      endocapillary proliferative
        glomerulonephritis N02.4
      focal and segmental hyalinosis or sclerosis
        N02.1
      membranoproliferative (diffuse) N02.5
      membranous (diffuse) N02.2
      mesangial proliferative (diffuse) N02.3
      mesangiocapillary (diffuse) N02.5
      minor abnormality N02.0
      proliferative NEC N02.8
      specified pathology NEC N02.8
  intermittent — *see* Hematuria, idiopathic
  malarial B50.8
  microscopic NEC R31.2
    benign essential R31.1
  paroxysmal (*see also* Hematuria, idiopathic)
    nocturnal D59.5
  persistent — *see* Hematuria, idiopathic
  recurrent — *see* Hematuria, idiopathic
  tropical (*see also* Schistosomiasis) B65.0
  tuberculous A18.13
Hemeralopia (day blindness) H53.11
  vitamin A deficiency E50.5
Hemi-akinesia R41.4
Hemianalgesia R20.0
Hemianencephaly Q00.0
Hemianesthesia R20.0
Hemianopia, hemianopsia (heteronymous) H53.47
  homonymous H53.46- ☑
  syphilitic A52.71
Hemiathetosis R25.8
Hemiatrophy R68.89
  cerebellar G31.9
  face, facial, progressive (Romberg) G51.8
  tongue K14.8
Hemiballism (us) G25.5
Hemicardia Q24.8
Hemicephalus, hemicephaly Q00.0
Hemichorea G25.5
Hemicolitis, left — *see* Colitis, left sided
Hemicrania
  congenital malformation Q00.0
  continua G44.51
  meaning migraine (*see also* Migraine) G43.909
  paroxysmal G44.039
    chronic G44.049
      intractable G44.041
      not intractable G44.049
    episodic G44.039

Hemicrania — *continued*
    intractable G44.031
        not intractable G44.039
    intractable G44.031
    not intractable G44.039
Hemidystrophy — *see* Hemiatrophy
Hemiectromelia Q73.8
Hemihypalgesia R20.8
Hemihypesthesia R20.1
Hemi-inattention R41.4
Hemimelia Q73.8
    lower limb — *see* Defect, reduction, lower limb,
        specified type NEC
    upper limb — *see* Defect, reduction, upper limb,
        specified type NEC
Hemiparalysis — *see* Hemiplegia
Hemiparesis — *see* Hemiplegia
Hemiparesthesia R20.2
Hemiparkinsonism G20
Hemiplegia G81.9- ☑
    alternans facialis G83.89
    ascending NEC G81.90
        spinal G95.89
    congenital (cerebral) G80.8
        spastic G80.2
    embolic (current episode) I63.4- ☑
    flaccid G81.0- ☑
    following
        cerebrovascular disease I69.959
            cerebral infarction I69.35- ☑
            intracerebral hemorrhage I69.15- ☑
            nontraumatic intracranial hemorrhage NEC
                I69.25- ☑
            specified disease NEC I69.85- ☑
            stroke NOS I69.35- ☑
            subarachnoid hemorrhage I69.05- ☑
    hysterical F44.4
    newborn NEC P91.8
        birth injury P11.9
    spastic G81.1- ☑
        congenital G80.2
    thrombotic (current episode) I63.3 ☑
Hemisection, spinal cord — *see* Injury, spinal cord,
    by region
Hemispasm (facial) R25.2
Hemisporosis B48.8
Hemitremor R25.1
Hemivertebra Q76.49
    failure of segmentation with scoliosis Q76.3
    fusion with scoliosis Q76.3
Hemochromatosis E83.119
    with refractory anemia D46.1
    due to repeated red blood cell transfusion
        E83.111
    hereditary (primary) E83.110
    primary E83.110
    specified NEC E83.118
Hemoglobin (*see also* condition)
    abnormal (disease) — *see* Disease, hemoglobin
    AS genotype D57.3
    Constant Spring D58.2
    E-beta thalassemia D56.5
    fetal, hereditary persistence (HPFH) D56.4
    H Constant Spring D56.0
    low NOS D64.9
    S (Hb S), heterozygous D57.3
Hemoglobinemia D59.9
    due to blood transfusion T80.89 ☑
    paroxysmal D59.6
        nocturnal D59.5
Hemoglobinopathy (mixed) D58.2
    with thalassemia D56.8
    sickle-cell D57.1
        with thalassemia D57.40
            with crisis (vasoocclusive pain) D57.419
                with
                    acute chest syndrome D57.411
                    splenic sequestration D57.412
            without crisis D57.40
Hemoglobinuria R82.3
    with anemia, hemolytic, acquired (chronic) NEC
        D59.6
    cold (agglutinin) (paroxysmal) (with Raynaud's
        syndrome) D59.6
    due to exertion or hemolysis NEC D59.6
    intermittent D59.6
    malarial B50.8
    march D59.6
    nocturnal (paroxysmal) D59.5
    paroxysmal (cold) D59.6
        nocturnal D59.5
Hemolymphangioma D18.1

Hemolysis
    intravascular
        with
            abortion — *see* Abortion, by type,
                complicated by, hemorrhage
            ectopic or molar pregnancy O08.1
            hemorrhage
                antepartum — *see* Hemorrhage,
                    antepartum, with coagulation defect
                intrapartum (*see also* Hemorrhage,
                    complicating, delivery) O67.0
        postpartum O72.3
    neonatal (excessive) P58.9
        specified NEC P58.8
Hemolytic — *see* condition
Hemopericardium I31.2
    following acute myocardial infarction (current
        complication) I23.0
    newborn P54.8
    traumatic — *see* Injury, heart, with
        hemopericardium
Hemoperitoneum K66.1
    infectional K65.9
    traumatic S36.899 ☑
        with open wound — *see* Wound, open, with
            penetration into peritoneal cavity
Hemophilia (classical) (familial) (hereditary) D66
    A D66
    B D67
    C D68.1
    acquired D68.311
    autoimmune D68.311
    calcipriva (*see also* Defect, coagulation) D68.4
    nonfamilial (*see also* Defect, coagulation) D68.4
    secondary D68.311
    vascular D68.0
Hemophthalmos H44.81- ☑
Hemopneumothorax (*see also* Hemothorax)
    traumatic S27.2 ☑
Hemoptysis R04.2
    newborn P26.9
    tuberculous — *see* Tuberculosis, pulmonary
Hemorrhage, hemorrhagic (concealed) R58
    abdomen R58
    accidental antepartum — *see* Hemorrhage,
        antepartum
    acute idiopathic pulmonary, in infants R04.81
    adenoid J35.8
    adrenal (capsule) (gland) E27.49
        medulla E27.8
        newborn P54.4
    after delivery — *see* Hemorrhage, postpartum
    alveolar
        lung, newborn P26.8
        process K08.8
    alveolus K08.8
    amputation stump (surgical) T87.89
    anemia (chronic) D50.0
        acute D62
    antepartum (with) O46.90
        with coagulation defect O46.00- ☑
            afibrinogenemia O46.01- ☑
            disseminated intravascular coagulation
                O46.02- ☑
            hypofibrinogenemia O46.01- ☑
            specified defect NEC O46.09- ☑
        before 20 weeks gestation O20.9
            specified type NEC O20.8
            threatened abortion O20.0
        due to
            abruptio placenta (*see also* Abruptio
                placentae) O45.9- ☑
            leiomyoma, uterus — *see* Hemorrhage,
                antepartum, specified cause NEC
            placenta previa O44.1- ☑
        specified cause NECO46.8X-
    anus (sphincter) K62.5
    apoplexy (stroke) — *see* Hemorrhage, intracranial,
        intracerebral
    arachnoid — *see* Hemorrhage, intracranial,
        subarachnoid
    artery R58
        brain — *see* Hemorrhage, intracranial,
            intracerebral
    basilar (ganglion) I61.0
    bladder N32.89
    bowel K92.2
        newborn P54.3
    brain (miliary) (nontraumatic) — *see* Hemorrhage,
        intracranial, intracerebral
        due to
            birth injury P10.1

Hemorrhage — *continued*
    syphilis A52.05
    epidural or extradural (traumatic) — *see* Injury,
        intracranial, epidural hemorrhage
        newborn P52.4
            birth injury P10.1
        subarachnoid — *see* Hemorrhage, intracranial,
            subarachnoid
        subdural — *see* Hemorrhage, intracranial,
            subdural
    brainstem (nontraumatic) I61.3
        traumatic S06.38- ☑
    breast N64.59
    bronchial tube — *see* Hemorrhage, lung
    bronchopulmonary — *see* Hemorrhage, lung
    bronchus — *see* Hemorrhage, lung
    bulbar I61.5
    capillary I78.8
        primary D69.8
    cecum K92.2
    cerebellar, cerebellum (nontraumatic) I61.4
        newborn P52.6
        traumatic S06.37- ☑
    cerebral, cerebrum (*see also* Hemorrhage,
        intracranial, intracerebral)
        newborn (anoxic) P52.4
            birth injury P10.1
        lobe I61.1
    cerebromeningeal I61.8
    cerebrospinal — *see* Hemorrhage, intracranial,
        intracerebral
    cervix (uteri) (stump) NEC N88.8
    chamber, anterior (eye) — *see* Hyphema
    childbirth — *see* Hemorrhage, complicating,
        delivery
    choroid H31.30- ☑
        expulsive H31.31- ☑
    ciliary body — *see* Hyphema
    cochleaH83.8
    colon K92.2
    complicating
        abortion — *see* Abortion, by type, complicated
            by, hemorrhage
        delivery O67.9
            associated with coagulation
                defect (afibrinogenemia) (DIC)
                (hyperfibrinolysis) O67.0
            specified cause NEC O67.8
        surgical procedure — *see* Hemorrhage,
            intraoperative
    conjunctiva H11.3- ☑
        newborn P54.8
    cord, newborn (stump) P51.9
    corpus luteum (ruptured) cyst N83.1
    cortical (brain) I61.1
    cranial — *see* Hemorrhage, intracranial
    cutaneous R23.3
        due to autosensitivity, erythrocyte D69.2
        newborn P54.5
    delayed
        following ectopic or molar pregnancy O08.1
        postpartum O72.2
    diathesis (familial) D69.9
    disease D69.9
        newborn P53
        specified type NEC D69.8
    due to or associated with
        afibrinogenemia or other coagulation defect
            (conditions in categories D65-D69)
            antepartum — *see* Hemorrhage, antepartum,
                with coagulation defect
            intrapartum O67.0
    dental implant M27.61
    device, implant or graft (*see also* Complications,
        by site and type, specified NEC) T85.83 ☑
        arterial graft NEC T82.838 ☑
        breast T85.83 ☑
        catheter NEC T85.83 ☑
            dialysis (renal) T82.838 ☑
                intraperitoneal T85.83 ☑
            infusion NEC T82.838 ☑
                spinal (epidural) (subdural) T85.83 ☑
            urinary (indwelling) T83.83 ☑
        electronic (electrode) (pulse generator)
            (stimulator)
            bone T84.83 ☑
            cardiac T82.837 ☑
            nervous system (brain) (peripheral nerve)
                (spinal) T85.83 ☑
            urinary T83.83 ☑
        fixation, internal (orthopedic) NEC T84.83 ☑

☑ **Additional character required**

Hemorrhage — *continued*

gastrointestinal (bile duct) (esophagus) T85.83 ☑
genital NEC T83.83 ☑
heart NEC T82.837 ☑
joint prosthesis T84.83 ☑
ocular (corneal graft) (orbital implant) NEC T85.83 ☑
orthopedic NEC T84.83 ☑
  bone graft T86.838
specified NEC T85.83 ☑
urinary NEC T83.83 ☑
vascular NEC T82.838 ☑
ventricular intracranial shunt T85.83 ☑
duodenum, duodenal K92.2
ulcer — *see* Ulcer, duodenum, with hemorrhage
dura mater — *see* Hemorrhage, intracranial, subdural
endotracheal — *see* Hemorrhage, lung
epicranial subaponeurotic (massive), birth injury P12.2
epidural (traumatic) (*see also* Injury, intracranial, epidural hemorrhage)
nontraumatic I62.1
esophagus K22.8
varix I85.01
secondary I85.11
excessive, following ectopic gestation (subsequent episode) O08.1
extradural (traumatic) — *see* Injury, intracranial, epidural hemorrhage
birth injury P10.8
newborn (anoxic) (nontraumatic) P52.8
nontraumatic I62.1
eye NEC H57.8
fundus — *see* Hemorrhage, retina
lid — *see* Disorder, eyelid, specified type NEC
fallopian tube N83.6
fibrinogenolysis — *see* Fibrinolysis
fibrinolytic (acquired) — *see* Fibrinolysis
from
  ear (nontraumatic) — *see* Otorrhagia
  tracheostomy stoma J95.01
fundus, eye — *see* Hemorrhage, retina
funis — *see* Hemorrhage, umbilicus, cord
gastric — *see* Hemorrhage, stomach
gastroenteric K92.2
newborn P54.3
gastrointestinal (tract) K92.2
newborn P54.3
genital organ, male N50.1
genitourinary (tract) NOS R31.9
gingiva K06.8
globe (eye) — *see* Hemophthalmos
graafian follicle cyst (ruptured) N83.0
gum K06.8
heart I51.89
hypopharyngeal (throat) R04.1
intermenstrual (regular) N92.3
  irregular N92.1
internal (organs) NEC R58
  capsule I61.0
  ear H83.8
  newborn P54.8
intestine K92.2
  newborn P54.3
intra-abdominal R58
intra-alveolar (lung), newborn P26.8
intracerebral (nontraumatic) — *see* Hemorrhage, intracranial, intracerebral
intracranial (nontraumatic) I62.9
birth injury P10.9
epidural, nontraumatic I62.1
extradural, nontraumatic I62.1
newborn P52.9
  specified NEC P52.8
intracerebral (nontraumatic) (in) I61.9
  brain stem I61.3
  cerebellum I61.4
  newborn P52.4
    birth injury P10.1
  hemisphere I61.2
    cortical (superficial) I61.1
    subcortical (deep) I61.0
  intraoperative
    during a nervous system procedure G97.31
    during other procedure G97.32
  intraventricular I61.5
  multiple localized I61.6
  postprocedural

Hemorrhage — *continued*

following a nervous system procedure G97.51
  following other procedure G97.52
specified NEC I61.8
superficial I61.1
traumatic (diffuse) — *see* Injury, intracranial, diffuse
  focal — *see* Injury, intracranial, focal
subarachnoid (nontraumatic) (from) I60.9
newborn P52.5
  birth injury P10.3
intracranial (cerebral) artery I60.7
  anterior communicating I60.2- ☑
  basilar I60.4
  carotid siphon and bifurcation I60.0- ☑
  communicating I60.7
    anterior I60.2- ☑
    posterior I60.3- ☑
  middle cerebral I60.1- ☑
  posterior communicating I60.3- ☑
  specified artery NEC I60.6
  vertebral I60.5- ☑
specified NEC I60.8
traumatic S06.6X- ☑
subdural (nontraumatic) I62.00
acute I62.01
birth injury P10.0
chronic I62.03
newborn (anoxic) (hypoxic) P52.8
  birth injury P10.0
spinal G95.19
subacute I62.02
traumatic — *see* Injury, intracranial, subdural hemorrhage
traumatic — *see* Injury, intracranial, focal brain injury
intramedullary NEC G95.19
intraocular — *see* Hemophthalmos
intraoperative, intraprocedural — *see* Complication, hemorrhage (hematoma), intraoperative (intraprocedural), by site
intrapartum — *see* Hemorrhage, complicating, delivery
intrapelvic
  female N94.89
  male K66.1
intraperitoneal K66.1
intrapontine I61.3
intraprocedural — *see* Complication, hemorrhage (hematoma), intraoperative (intraprocedural), by site
intrauterine N85.7
complicating delivery (*see also* Hemorrhage, complicating, delivery) O67.9
postpartum — *see* Hemorrhage, postpartum
intraventricular I61.5
newborn (nontraumatic) (*see also* Newborn, affected by, hemorrhage) P52.3
due to birth injury P10.2
grade
  1 P52.0
  2 P52.1
  3 P52.21
  4 P52.22
intravesical N32.89
iris (postinfectional) (postinflammatory) (toxic) — *see* Hyphema
joint (nontraumatic) — *see* Hemarthrosis
kidney N28.89
knee (joint) (nontraumatic) — *see* Hemarthrosis, knee
labyrinth H83.8
lenticular striate artery I61.0
ligature, vessel — *see* Hemorrhage, postoperative
liver K76.89
lung R04.89
newborn P26.9
  massive P26.1
  specified NEC P26.8
tuberculous — *see* Tuberculosis, pulmonary
massive umbilical, newborn P51.0
mediastinum — *see* Hemorrhage, lung
medulla I61.3
membrane (brain) I60.8
  spinal cord — *see* Hemorrhage, spinal cord
meninges, meningeal (brain) (middle) I60.8
  spinal cord — *see* Hemorrhage, spinal cord
mesentery K66.1
metritis — *see* Endometritis
mouth K13.79
mucous membrane NEC R58

Hemorrhage — *continued*

newborn P54.8
muscle M62.89
nail (subungual) L60.8
nasal turbinate R04.0
newborn P54.8
nasal R04.0
newborn P54.9
  specified NEC P54.8
navel, newborn P51.9
newborn P54.9
  specified NEC P54.8
nipple N64.59
nose R04.0
newborn P54.8
omentum K66.1
optic nerve (sheath) H47.02- ☑
orbit, orbital H05.23- ☑
ovary NEC N83.8
oviduct N83.6
pancreas K86.8
parathyroid (gland) (spontaneous) E21.4
parturition — *see* Hemorrhage, complicating, delivery
penis N48.89
pericardium, pericarditis I31.2
peritoneum, peritoneal K66.1
peritonsillar tissue J35.8
  due to infection J36
petechial R23.3
  due to autosensitivity, erythrocyte D69.2
pituitary (gland) E23.6
pleura — *see* Hemorrhage, lung
polioencephalitis, superior E51.2
polymyositis — *see* Polymyositis
pons, pontine I61.3
posterior fossa (nontraumatic) I61.8
newborn P52.6
postmenopausal N95.0
postnasal R04.0
postoperative — *see* Complications, postprocedural, hemorrhage, by site
postpartum NEC (following delivery of placenta) O72.1
delayed or secondary O72.2
retained placenta O72.0
third stage O72.0
pregnancy — *see* Hemorrhage, antepartum
preretinal — *see* Hemorrhage, retina
prostate N42.1
puerperal — *see* Hemorrhage, postpartum
delayed or secondary O72.2
pulmonary R04.89
newborn P26.9
  massive P26.1
  specified NEC P26.8
tuberculous — *see* Tuberculosis, pulmonary
purpura (primary) D69.3
rectum (sphincter) K62.5
newborn P54.2
recurring, following initial hemorrhage at time of injury T79.2 ☑
renal N28.89
respiratory passage or tract R04.9
  specified NEC R04.89
retina, retinal (vessels) H35.6- ☑
diabetic — *see* Diabetes, retinal, hemorrhage
retroperitoneal R58
scalp R58
scrotum N50.1
secondary (nontraumatic) R58
following initial hemorrhage at time of injury T79.2 ☑
seminal vesicle N50.1
skin R23.3
newborn P54.5
slipped umbilical ligature P51.8
spermatic cord N50.1
spinal (cord) G95.19
newborn (birth injury) P11.5
spleen D73.5
intraoperative — *see* Complications, intraoperative, hemorrhage, spleen
postprocedural — *see* Complications, postprocedural, hemorrhage, spleen
stomach K92.2
newborn P54.3
ulcer — *see* Ulcer, stomach, with hemorrhage
subarachnoid (nontraumatic) — *see* Hemorrhage, intracranial, subarachnoid
subconjunctival (*see also* Hemorrhage, conjunctiva)
birth injury P15.3
subcortical (brain) I61.0
subcutaneous R23.3

Hemorrhage — *continued*
  subdiaphragmatic R58
  subdural (acute) (nontraumatic) — *see* Hemorrhage, intracranial, subdural
  subependymal
    newborn P52.0
      with intraventricular extension P52.1
        and intracerebral extension P52.22
  subgaleal P12.1
  subhyaloid — *see* Hemorrhage, retina
  subperiosteal — *see* Disorder, bone, specified type NEC
  subretinal — *see* Hemorrhage, retina
  subtentorial — *see* Hemorrhage, intracranial, subdural
  subungual L60.8
  suprarenal (capsule) (gland) E27.49
    newborn P54.4
  tentorium (traumatic) NEC — *see* Hemorrhage, brain
    newborn (birth injury) P10.4
  testis N50.1
  third stage (postpartum) O72.0
  thorax — *see* Hemorrhage, lung
  throat R04.1
  thymus (gland) E32.8
  thyroid (cyst) (gland) E07.89
  tongue K14.8
  tonsil J35.8
  trachea — *see* Hemorrhage, lung
  tracheobronchial R04.89
    newborn P26.0
  traumatic - code to specific injury
    cerebellar — *see* Hemorrhage, brain
    intracranial — *see* Hemorrhage, brain
    recurring or secondary (following initial hemorrhage at time of injury) T79.2 ☑
  tuberculous NEC (*see also* Tuberculosis, pulmonary) A15.0
  tunica vaginalis N50.1
  ulcer - code by site under Ulcer, with hemorrhage K27.4
  umbilicus, umbilical
    cord
      after birth, newborn P51.9
      complicating delivery O69.5 ☑
    newborn P51.9
      massive P51.0
      slipped ligature P51.8
    stump P51.9
  urethra (idiopathic) N36.8
  uterus, uterine (abnormal) N93.9
    climacteric N92.4
    complicating delivery — *see* Hemorrhage, complicating, delivery
    dysfunctional or functional N93.8
    intermenstrual (regular) N92.3
      irregular N92.1
    postmenopausal N95.0
    postpartum — *see* Hemorrhage, postpartum
    preclimacteric or premenopausal N92.4
    prepubertal N93.8
    pubertal N92.2
  vagina (abnormal) N93.9
    newborn P54.6
  vas deferens N50.1
  vasa previa O69.4 ☑
  ventricular I61.5
  vesical N32.89
  viscera NEC R58
    newborn P54.8
  vitreous (humor) (intraocular) H43.1- ☑
  vulva N90.89
Hemorrhoids (bleeding) (without mention of degree) K64.9
  1st degree (grade/stage I) (without prolapse outside of anal canal) K64.0
  2nd degree (grade/stage II) (that prolapse with straining but retract spontaneously) K64.1
  3rd degree (grade/stage III) (that prolapse with straining and require manual replacement back inside anal canal) K64.2
  4th degree (grade/stage IV) (with prolapsed tissue that cannot be manually replaced) K64.3
  complicating
    pregnancy O22.4 ☑
    puerperium O87.2
  external K64.4
    with
      thrombosis K64.5
  internal (without mention of degree) K64.8

Hemorrhoids — *continued*
  prolapsed K64.8
  skin tags
    anus K64.4
    residual K64.4
  specified NEC K64.8
  strangulated (*see also* Hemorrhoids, by degree) K64.8
  thrombosed (*see also* Hemorrhoids, by degree) K64.5
  ulcerated (*see also* Hemorrhoids, by degree) K64.8
Hemosalpinx N83.6
  with
    hematocolpos N89.7
    hematometra N85.7
      with hematocolpos N89.7
Hemosiderosis (dietary) E83.19
  pulmonary, idiopathic E83.1- ☑ [J84.03]
  transfusion T80.89 ☑
Hemothorax (bacterial) (nontuberculous) J94.2
  newborn P54.8
  traumatic S27.1 ☑
    with pneumothorax S27.2 ☑
  tuberculous NEC A15.6
Henoch (-Schönlein) disease or syndrome (purpura) D69.0
Henpue, henpuye A66.6
Hepar lobatum (syphilitic) A52.74
Hepatalgia K76.89
Hepatitis K75.9
  acute B17.9
    with coma K72.01
    with hepatic failure — *see* Failure, hepatic
    alcoholic — *see* Hepatitis, alcoholic
    infectious B15.9
      with hepatic coma B15.0
    viral B17.9
  alcoholic (acute) (chronic) K70.10
    with ascites K70.11
  amebic — *see* Abscess, liver, amebic
  anicteric, (viral) — *see* Hepatitis, viral
  antigen-associated (HAA) — *see* Hepatitis, B
  Australia-antigen (positive) — *see* Hepatitis, B
  autoimmune K75.4
  B B19.10
    with hepatic coma B19.11
    acute B16.9
      with
        delta-agent (coinfection) (without hepatic coma) B16.1
          with hepatic coma B16.0
        hepatic coma (without delta-agent coinfection) B16.2
    chronic B18.1
      with delta-agent B18.0
  bacterial NEC K75.89
  C (viral) B19.20
    with hepatic coma B19.21
    acute B17.10
      with hepatic coma B17.11
    chronic B18.2
  catarrhal (acute) B15.9
    with hepatic coma B15.0
  cholangiolitic K75.89
  cholestatic K75.89
  chronic K73.9
    active NEC K73.2
    lobular NEC K73.1
    persistent NEC K73.0
    specified NEC K73.8
  cytomegaloviral B25.1
  due to ethanol (acute) (chronic) — *see* Hepatitis, alcoholic
  epidemic B15.9
    with hepatic coma B15.0
  fulminant NEC (viral) — *see* Hepatitis, viral
  neonatal giant cell P59.29
  granulomatous NEC K75.3
  herpesviral B00.81
  history of
    B Z86.19
    C Z86.19
  homologous serum — *see* Hepatitis, viral, type B
  in (due to)
    mumps B26.81
    toxoplasmosis (acquired) B58.1
      congenital (active) P37.1 [K77]
  infectious, infective (acute) (chronic) (subacute) B15.9
    with hepatic coma B15.0
  inoculation — *see* Hepatitis, viral, type B
  interstitial (chronic) K74.69

Hepatitis — *continued*
  lupoid NEC K75.4
  malignant NEC (with hepatic failure) K72.90
    with coma K72.91
  neonatal (idiopathic) (toxic) P59.29
  newborn P59.29
  postimmunization — *see* Hepatitis, viral, type B
  post-transfusion — *see* Hepatitis, viral, type B
  reactive, nonspecific K75.2
  serum — *see* Hepatitis, viral, type B
  specified type NEC
    with hepatic failure — *see* Failure, hepatic
  syphilitic (late) A52.74
    congenital (early) A50.08 [K77]
      late A50.59 [K77]
    secondary A51.45
  toxic (*see also* Disease, liver, toxic) K71.6
  tuberculous A18.83
  viral, virus B19.9
    with hepatic coma B19.0
    acute B17.9
    chronic B18.9
      specified NEC B18.8
    type
      B B18.1
        with delta-agent B18.0
      C B18.2
    congenital P35.3
    coxsackie B33.8 [K77]
    cytomegalic inclusion B25.1
    in remission, any type - code to Hepatitis, chronic, by type
    non-A, non-B B17.8
    specified type NEC (with or without coma) B17.8
    type
      A B15.9
        with hepatic coma B15.0
      B B19.10
        with hepatic coma B19.11
        acute B16.9
          with
            delta-agent (coinfection) (without hepatic coma) B16.1
              with hepatic coma B16.0
            hepatic coma (without delta-agent coinfection) B16.2
        chronic B18.1
          with delta-agent B18.0
      C B19.20
        with hepatic coma B19.21
        acute B17.10
          with hepatic coma B17.11
        chronic B18.2
      E B17.2
    non-A, non-B B17.8
Hepatization lung (acute) — *see* Pneumonia, lobar
Hepatoblastoma C22.2
Hepatocarcinoma C22.0
Hepatocholangiocarcinoma C22.0
Hepatocholangioma, benign D13.4
Hepatocholangitis K75.89
Hepatolenticular degeneration E83.01
Hepatoma (malignant) C22.0
  benign D13.4
  embryonal C22.0
Hepatomegaly (*see also* Hypertrophy, liver)
  with splenomegaly R16.2
  congenital Q44.7
  in mononucleosis
    gammaherpesviral B27.09
    infectious specified NEC B27.89
Hepatoptosis K76.89
Hepatorenal syndrome following labor and delivery O90.4
Hepatosis K76.89
Hepatosplenomegaly R16.2
  hyperlipemic (Bürger-Grütz type) E78.3 [K77]
Hereditary — *see* condition
Heredodegeneration, macular — *see* Dystrophy, retina
Heredopathia atactica polyneuritiformis G60.1
Heredosyphilis — *see* Syphilis, congenital
Herlitz' syndrome Q81.1
Hermansky-Pudlak syndrome E70.331
Hermaphrodite, hermaphroditism (true) Q56.0
  46,XX with streak gonads Q99.1
  46,XX/46,XY Q99.0
  46,XY with streak gonads Q99.1
  chimera 46,XX/46,XY Q99.0
Hernia, hernial (acquired) (recurrent) K46.9
  with

Hernia — *continued*
  gangrene — *see* Hernia, by site, with, gangrene
  incarceration — *see* Hernia, by site, with, obstruction
  irreducible — *see* Hernia, by site, with, obstruction
  obstruction — *see* Hernia, by site, with, obstruction
  strangulation — *see* Hernia, by site, with, obstruction
  abdomen, abdominal K46.9
    with
      gangrene (and obstruction) K46.1
      obstruction K46.0
    femoral — *see* Hernia, femoral
    incisional — *see* Hernia, incisional
    inguinal — *see* Hernia, inguinal
    specified site NEC K45.8
      with
        gangrene (and obstruction) K45.1
        obstruction K45.0
    umbilical — *see* Hernia, umbilical
    wall — *see* Hernia, ventral
  appendix — *see* Hernia, abdomen
  bladder (mucosa) (sphincter)
    congenital (female) (male) Q79.51
    female — *see* Cystocele
    male N32.89
  brain, congenital — *see* Encephalocele
  cartilage, vertebra — *see* Displacement, intervertebral disc
  cerebral, congenital (*see also* Encephalocele)
    endaural Q01.8
  ciliary body (traumatic) S05.2- ☑
  colon — *see* Hernia, abdomen
  Cooper's — *see* Hernia, abdomen, specified site NEC
  crural — *see* Hernia, femoral
  diaphragm, diaphragmatic K44.9
    with
      gangrene (and obstruction) K44.1
      obstruction K44.0
    congenital Q79.0
  direct (inguinal) — *see* Hernia, inguinal
  diverticulum, intestine — *see* Hernia, abdomen
  double (inguinal) — *see* Hernia, inguinal, bilateral
  due to adhesions (with obstruction) K56.5
  epigastric (*see also* Hernia, ventral) K43.9
  esophageal hiatus — *see* Hernia, hiatal
  external (inguinal) — *see* Hernia, inguinal
  fallopian tube N83.4
  fascia M62.89
  femoral K41.90
    with
      gangrene (and obstruction) K41.40
        not specified as recurrent K41.40
        recurrent K41.41
      obstruction K41.30
        not specified as recurrent K41.30
        recurrent K41.31
    bilateral K41.20
      with
        gangrene (and obstruction) K41.10
          not specified as recurrent K41.10
          recurrent K41.11
        obstruction K41.00
          not specified as recurrent K41.00
          recurrent K41.01
      not specified as recurrent K41.20
      recurrent K41.21
    unilateral K41.90
      with
        gangrene (and obstruction) K41.40
          not specified as recurrent K41.40
          recurrent K41.41
        obstruction K41.30
          not specified as recurrent K41.30
          recurrent K41.31
      not specified as recurrent K41.90
      recurrent K41.91
    not specified as recurrent K41.90
    recurrent K41.91
  foramen magnum G93.5
    congenital Q01.8
  funicular (umbilical) (*see also* Hernia, umbilicus)
    spermatic (cord) — *see* Hernia, inguinal
  gastrointestinal tract — *see* Hernia, abdomen
  Hesselbach's — *see* Hernia, femoral, specified site NEC
  hiatal (esophageal) (sliding) K44.9
    with
      gangrene (and obstruction) K44.1

Hernia — *continued*
    obstruction K44.0
    congenital Q40.1
  hypogastric — *see* Hernia, ventral
  incarcerated (*see also* Hernia, by site, with obstruction)
    with gangrene — *see* Hernia, by site, with gangrene
  incisional K43.2
    with
      gangrene (and obstruction) K43.1
      obstruction K43.0
  indirect (inguinal) — *see* Hernia, inguinal
  inguinal (direct) (external) (funicular) (indirect) (internal) (oblique) (scrotal) (sliding) K40.90
    with
      gangrene (and obstruction) K40.40
        not specified as recurrent K40.40
        recurrent K40.41
      obstruction K40.30
        not specified as recurrent K40.30
        recurrent K40.31
    not specified as recurrent K40.90
    recurrent K40.91
    bilateral K40.20
      with
        gangrene (and obstruction) K40.10
          not specified as recurrent K40.10
          recurrent K40.11
        obstruction K40.00
          not specified as recurrent K40.00
          recurrent K40.01
      not specified as recurrent K40.20
      recurrent K40.21
    unilateral K40.90
      with
        gangrene (and obstruction) K40.40
          not specified as recurrent K40.40
          recurrent K40.41
        obstruction K40.30
          not specified as recurrent K40.30
          recurrent K40.31
      not specified as recurrent K40.90
      recurrent K40.91
  internal (*see also* Hernia, abdomen)
    inguinal — *see* Hernia, inguinal
  interstitial — *see* Hernia, abdomen
  intervertebral cartilage or disc — *see* Displacement, intervertebral disc
  intestine, intestinal — *see* Hernia, by site
  intra-abdominal — *see* Hernia, abdomen
  iris (traumatic) S05.2- ☑
  irreducible (*see also* Hernia, by site, with obstruction)
    with gangrene — *see* Hernia, by site, with gangrene
  ischiatic — *see* Hernia, abdomen, specified site NEC
  ischiorectal — *see* Hernia, abdomen, specified site NEC
  lens (traumatic) S05.2- ☑
  linea (alba) (semilunaris) — *see* Hernia, ventral
  Littre's — *see* Hernia, abdomen
  lumbar — *see* Hernia, abdomen, specified site NEC
  lung (subcutaneous) J98.4
  mediastinum J98.5
  mesenteric (internal) — *see* Hernia, abdomen
  midline — *see* Hernia, ventral
  muscle (sheath) M62.89
  nucleus pulposus — *see* Displacement, intervertebral disc
  oblique (inguinal) — *see* Hernia, inguinal
  obstructive (*see also* Hernia, by site, with obstruction)
    with gangrene — *see* Hernia, by site, with gangrene
  obturator — *see* Hernia, abdomen, specified site NEC
  omental — *see* Hernia, abdomen
  ovary N83.4
  oviduct N83.4
  paraesophageal (*see also* Hernia, diaphragm)
    congenital Q40.1
  parastomal K43.5
    with
      gangrene (and obstruction) K43.4
      obstruction K43.3
  paraumbilical — *see* Hernia, umbilicus
  perineal — *see* Hernia, abdomen, specified site NEC
  Petit's — *see* Hernia, abdomen, specified site NEC

Hernia — *continued*
  postoperative — *see* Hernia, incisional
  pregnant uterus — *see* Abnormal, uterus in pregnancy or childbirth
  prevesical N32.89
  properitoneal — *see* Hernia, abdomen, specified site NEC
  pudendal — *see* Hernia, abdomen, specified site NEC
  rectovaginal N81.6
  retroperitoneal — *see* Hernia, abdomen, specified site NEC
  Richter's — *see* Hernia, abdomen, with obstruction
  Rieux's, Riex's — *see* Hernia, abdomen, specified site NEC
  sac condition (adhesion) (dropsy) (inflammation) (laceration) (suppuration) - code by site under Hernia
  sciatic — *see* Hernia, abdomen, specified site NEC
  scrotum, scrotal — *see* Hernia, inguinal
  sliding (inguinal) (*see also* Hernia, inguinal)
    hiatus — *see* Hernia, hiatal
  spigelian — *see* Hernia, ventral
  spinal — *see* Spina bifida
  strangulated (*see also* Hernia, by site, with obstruction)
    with gangrene — *see* Hernia, by site, with gangrene
  subxiphoid — *see* Hernia, ventral
  supra-umbilicus — *see* Hernia, ventral
  tendon — *see* Disorder, tendon, specified type NEC
  Treitz's (fossa) — *see* Hernia, abdomen, specified site NEC
  tunica vaginalis Q55.29
  umbilicus, umbilical K42.9
    with
      gangrene (and obstruction) K42.1
      obstruction K42.0
  ureter N28.89
  urethra, congenital Q64.79
  urinary meatus, congenital Q64.79
  uterus N81.4
    pregnant — *see* Abnormal, uterus in pregnancy or childbirth
  vaginal (anterior) (wall) — *see* Cystocele
  Velpeau's — *see* Hernia, femoral
  ventral K43.9
    with
      gangrene (and obstruction) K43.7
      obstruction K43.6
    recurrent — *see* Hernia, incisional
    incisional K43.2
      with
        gangrene (and obstruction) K43.1
        obstruction K43.0
    specified NEC K43.9
      with
        gangrene (and obstruction) K43.7
        obstruction K43.6
  vesical
    congenital (female) (male) Q79.51
    female — *see* Cystocele
    male N32.89
  vitreous (into wound) S05.2- ☑
    into anterior chamber — *see* Prolapse, vitreous
Herniation (*see also* Hernia)
  brain (stem) G93.5
  cerebral G93.5
  mediastinum J98.5
  nucleus pulposus — *see* Displacement, intervertebral disc
Herpangina B08.5
Herpes, herpesvirus, herpetic B00.9
  anogenital A60.9
    perianal skin A60.1
    rectum A60.1
    urogenital tract A60.00
      cervix A60.03
      male genital organ NEC A60.02
      penis A60.01
      specified site NEC A60.09
      vagina A60.04
      vulva A60.04
  blepharitis (zoster) B02.39
    simplex B00.59
  circinatus B35.4
    bullosus L12.0
  conjunctivitis (simplex) B00.53
    zoster B02.31
  cornea B02.33

Herpes — *continued*
  encephalitis B00.4
    due to herpesvirus 6 B10.01
    due to herpesvirus 7 B10.09
    specified NEC B10.09
  eye (zoster) B02.30
    simplex B00.50
  eyelid (zoster) B02.39
    simplex B00.59
  facialis B00.1
  febrilis B00.1
  geniculate ganglionitis B02.21
  genital, genitalis A60.00
    female A60.09
    male A60.02
  gestational, gestationis O26.4- ☑
  gingivostomatitis B00.2
  human B00.9
    1 — *see* Herpes, simplex
    2 — *see* Herpes, simplex
    3 — *see* Varicella
    4 — *see* Mononucleosis, Epstein-Barr (virus)
    5 — *see* Disease, cytomegalic inclusion (generalized)
    6
      encephalitis B10.01
      specified NEC B10.81
    7
      encephalitis B10.09
      specified NEC B10.82
    8 B10.89
  infection NEC B10.89
    Kaposi's sarcoma associated B10.89
  iridocyclitis (simplex) B00.51
    zoster B02.32
  iris (vesicular erythema multiforme) L51.9
  iritis (simplex) B00.51
  Kaposi's sarcoma associated B10.89
  keratitis (simplex) (dendritic) (disciform) (interstitial) B00.52
    zoster (interstitial) B02.33
  keratoconjunctivitis (simplex) B00.52
    zoster B02.33
  labialis B00.1
  lip B00.1
  meningitis (simplex) B00.3
    zoster B02.1
  ophthalmicus (zoster) NEC B02.30
    simplex B00.50
  penis A60.01
  perianal skin A60.1
  pharyngitis, pharyngotonsillitis B00.2
  rectum A60.1
  scrotum A60.02
  sepsis B00.7
  simplex B00.9
    complicated NEC B00.89
    congenital P35.2
    conjunctivitis B00.53
    external ear B00.1
    eyelid B00.59
    hepatitis B00.81
    keratitis (interstitial) B00.52
    myeliitis B00.82
    specified complication NEC B00.89
    visceral B00.89
  stomatitis B00.2
  tonsurans B35.0
  visceral B00.89
  vulva A60.04
  whitlow B00.89
  zoster (*see also* condition) B02.9
    auricularis B02.21
    complicated NEC B02.8
    conjunctivitis B02.31
    disseminated B02.7
    encephalitis B02.0
    eye (lid) B02.39
    geniculate ganglionitis B02.21
    keratitis (interstitial) B02.33
    meningitis B02.1
    myelitis B02.24
    neuritis, neuralgia B02.29
    ophthalmicus NEC B02.30
    oticus B02.21
    polyneuropathy B02.23
    specified complication NEC B02.8
    trigeminal neuralgia B02.22
Herpesvirus (human) — *see* Herpes
Herpetophobia F40.218
Herrick's anemia — *see* Disease, sickle-cell
Hers' disease E74.09

Herter-Gee syndrome K90.0
Herxheimer's reaction R68.89
Hesitancy
  of micturition R39.11
  urinary R39.11
Hesselbach's hernia — *see* Hernia, femoral, specified site NEC
Heterochromia (congenital) Q13.2
  cataract — *see* Cataract, complicated
  cyclitis (Fuchs) — *see* Cyclitis, Fuchs' heterochromic
  hair L67.1
  iritis — *see* Cyclitis, Fuchs' heterochromic
  retained metallic foreign body (nonmagnetic) — *see* Foreign body, intraocular, old, retained
    magnetic — *see* Foreign body, intraocular, old, retained, magnetic
  uveitis — *see* Cyclitis, Fuchs' heterochromic
Heterophoria — *see* Strabismus, heterophoria
Heterophyes, heterophyiasis (small intestine) B66.8
Heterotopia, heterotopic (*see also* Malposition, congenital)
  cerebralis Q04.8
Heterotropia — *see* Strabismus
Heubner-Herter disease K90.0
Hexadactylism Q69.9
HGSIL (cytology finding) (high grade squamous intraepithelial lesion on cytologic smear) (Pap smear finding)
  anus R85.613
  cervix R87.613
    biopsy (histology) finding - code to CIN II or CIN III
  vagina R87.623
    biopsy (histology) finding - code to VAIN II or VAIN III
Hibernoma — *see* Lipoma
Hiccup, hiccough R06.6
  epidemic B33.0
  psychogenic F45.8
Hidden penis (congenital) Q55.64
  acquired N48.83
Hidradenitis (axillaris) (suppurative) L73.2
Hidradenoma (nodular) (*see also* Neoplasm, skin, benign)
  clear cell — *see* Neoplasm, skin, benign
  papillary — *see* Neoplasm, skin, benign
Hidrocystoma — *see* Neoplasm, skin, benign
High
  altitude effects T70.20 ☑
    anoxia T70.29 ☑
    on
      ears T70.0 ☑
      sinuses T70.1 ☑
    polycythemia D75.1
  arch
    foot Q66.7
    palate, congenital Q38.5
  arterial tension — *see* Hypertension
  basal metabolic rate R94.8
  blood pressure (*see also* Hypertension)
    borderline R03.0
    reading (incidental) (isolated) (nonspecific), without diagnosis of hypertension R03.0
  cholesterol E78.0
    with high triglycerides E78.2
  diaphragm (congenital) Q79.1
  expressed emotional level within family Z63.8
  head at term O32.4 ☑
  palate, congenital Q38.5
  risk
    infant NEC Z76.2
    sexual behavior (heterosexual) Z72.51
      bisexual Z72.53
      homosexual Z72.52
  temperature (of unknown origin) R50.9
  thoracic rib Q76.6
  triglycerides E78.1
    with high cholesterol E78.2
Hildenbrand's disease A75.0
Hilum — *see* condition
Hip — *see* condition
Hippel's disease Q85.8
Hippophobia F40.218
Hippus H57.09
Hirschsprung's disease or megacolon Q43.1
Hirsutism, hirsuties L68.0
Hirudiniasis
  external B88.3
  internal B83.4
Hiss-Russell dysentery A03.1
Histidinemia, histidinuria E70.41

Histiocytoma (*see also* Neoplasm, skin, benign)
  fibrous (*see also* Neoplasm, skin, benign)
    atypical — *see* Neoplasm, connective tissue, uncertain behavior
    malignant — *see* Neoplasm, connective tissue, malignant
Histiocytosis D76.3
  acute differentiated progressive C96.0
  Langerhans' cell NEC C96.6
    multifocal X
      multisystemic (disseminated) C96.0
      unisystemic C96.5
    pulmonary, adult (adult PLCH) J84.82
    unifocal (X) C96.6
  lipid, lipoid D76.3
    essential E75.29
  malignant C96.A
  mononuclear phagocytes NEC D76.1
    Langerhans' cells C96.6
  non-Langerhans cell D76.3
  polyostotic sclerosing D76.3
  sinus, with massive lymphadenopathy D76.3
  syndrome NEC D76.3
  X NEC C96.6
    acute (progressive) C96.0
    chronic C96.6
    multifocal C96.5
    multisystemic C96.0
    unifocal C96.6
Histoplasmosis B39.9
  with pneumonia NEC B39.2
  African B39.5
  American — *see* Histoplasmosis, capsulati
  capsulati B39.4
    disseminated B39.3
    generalized B39.3
    pulmonary B39.2
      acute B39.0
      chronic B39.1
  Darling's B39.4
  duboisii B39.5
  lung NEC B39.2
History
  family (of) (*see also* History, personal (of))
    alcohol abuse Z81.1
    allergy NEC Z84.89
    anemia Z83.2
    arthritis Z82.61
    asthma Z82.5
    blindness Z82.1
    cardiac death (sudden) Z82.41
    carrier of genetic disease Z84.81
    chromosomal anomaly Z82.79
    chronic
      disabling disease NEC Z82.8
      lower respiratory disease Z82.5
    colonic polyps Z83.71
    congenital malformations and deformations Z82.79
      polycystic kidney Z82.71
    consanguinity Z84.3
    deafness Z82.2
    diabetes mellitus Z83.3
    disability NEC Z82.8
    disease or disorder (of)
      allergic NEC Z84.89
      behavioral NEC Z81.8
      blood and blood-forming organs Z83.2
      cardiovascular NEC Z82.49
      chronic disabling NEC Z82.8
      digestive Z83.79
      ear NEC Z83.52
      endocrine NEC Z83.49
      eye NEC Z83.518
        glaucoma Z83.511
      genitourinary NEC Z84.2
      glaucoma Z83.511
      hematological Z83.2
      immune mechanism Z83.2
      infectious NEC Z83.1
      ischemic heart Z82.49
      kidney Z84.1
      mental NEC Z81.8
      metabolic Z83.49
      musculoskeletal NEC Z82.69
      neurological NEC Z82.0
      nutritional Z83.49
      parasitic NEC Z83.1
      psychiatric NEC Z81.8
      respiratory NEC Z83.6
      skin and subcutaneous tissue NEC Z84.0
      specified NEC Z84.89

☑ **Additional character required**

History — *continued*
- drug abuse NEC Z81.3
- epilepsy Z82.0
- genetic disease carrier Z84.81
- glaucoma Z83.511
- hearing loss Z82.2
- human immunodeficiency virus (HIV) infection Z83.0
- Huntington's chorea Z82.0
- intellectual disability Z81.0
- leukemia Z80.6
- malignant neoplasm (of) NOS Z80.9
  - bladder Z80.52
  - breast Z80.3
  - bronchus Z80.1
  - digestive organ Z80.0
  - gastrointestinal tract Z80.0
  - genital organ Z80.49
    - ovary Z80.41
    - prostate Z80.42
    - specified organ NEC Z80.49
    - testis Z80.43
  - hematopoietic NEC Z80.7
  - intrathoracic organ NEC Z80.2
  - kidney Z80.51
  - lung Z80.1
  - lymphatic NEC Z80.7
  - ovary Z80.41
  - prostate Z80.42
  - respiratory organ NEC Z80.2
  - specified site NEC Z80.8
  - testis Z80.43
  - trachea Z80.1
  - urinary organ or tract Z80.59
    - bladder Z80.52
    - kidney Z80.51
- mental
  - disorder NEC Z81.8
- multiple endocrine neoplasia (MEN) syndrome Z83.41
- osteoporosis Z82.62
- polycystic kidney Z82.71
- polyps (colon) Z83.71
- psychiatric disorder Z81.8
- psychoactive substance abuse NEC Z81.3
- respiratory condition Z83.6
  - asthma and other lower respiratory conditions Z82.5
- self-harmful behavior Z81.8
- skin condition Z84.0
- specified condition NEC Z84.89
- stroke (cerebrovascular) Z82.3
- substance abuse NEC Z81.4
  - alcohol Z81.1
  - drug NEC Z81.3
  - psychoactive NEC Z81.3
  - tobacco Z81.2
- sudden cardiac death Z82.41
- tobacco abuse Z81.2
- violence, violent behavior Z81.8
- visual loss Z82.1
- personal (of) (see also History, family (of))
  - abuse
    - childhood Z62.819
      - physical Z62.810
      - psychological Z62.811
      - sexual Z62.810
    - adult Z91.419
      - physical and sexual Z91.410
      - psychological Z91.411
  - alcohol dependence F10.21
  - allergy (to) Z88.9
    - analgesic agent NEC Z88.6
    - anesthetic Z88.4
    - antibiotic agent NEC Z88.1
    - anti-infective agent NEC Z88.3
    - contrast media Z91.041
    - drugs, medicaments and biological substances Z88.9
      - specified NEC Z88.8
    - food Z91.018
      - additives Z91.02
      - eggs Z91.012
      - milk products Z91.011
      - peanuts Z91.010
      - seafood Z91.013
      - specified food NEC Z91.018
    - insect Z91.038
      - bee Z91.030
    - latex Z91.040
    - medicinal agents Z88.9
      - specified NEC Z88.8

- narcotic agent NEC Z88.5
- nonmedicinal agents Z91.048
- penicillin Z88.0
- serum Z88.7
- specified NEC Z91.09
- sulfonamides Z88.2
- vaccine Z88.7
- anaphylactic shock Z87.892
- anaphylaxis Z87.892
- behavioral disorders Z86.59
- benign carcinoid tumor Z86.012
- benign neoplasm Z86.018
  - carcinoid Z86.012
  - brain Z86.011
  - colonic polyps Z86.010
- brain injury (traumatic) Z87.820
- breast implant removal Z98.86
- calculi, renal Z87.442
- cancer — see History, personal (of), malignant neoplasm (of)
- cardiac arrest (death), successfully resuscitated Z86.74
- cerebral infarction without residual deficit Z86.73
- cervical dysplasia Z87.410
- chemotherapy for neoplastic condition Z92.21
- childhood abuse — see History, personal (of), abuse
- cleft lip (corrected) Z87.730
- cleft palate (corrected) Z87.730
- collapsed vertebra (healed) Z87.311
  - due to osteoporosis Z87.310
- combat and operational stress reaction Z86.51
- congenital malformation (corrected) Z87.798
  - circulatory system (corrected) Z87.74
  - digestive system (corrected) NEC Z87.738
  - ear (corrected) Z87.720
  - eye (corrected) Z87.721
  - face and neck (corrected) Z87.790
  - genitourinary system (corrected) NEC Z87.718
  - heart (corrected) Z87.74
  - integument (corrected) Z87.76
  - limb (s) (corrected) Z87.76
  - musculoskeletal system (corrected) Z87.76
  - neck (corrected) Z87.790
  - nervous system (corrected) NEC Z87.728
  - respiratory system (corrected) Z87.75
  - sense organs (corrected) NEC Z87.728
  - specified NEC Z87.798
- contraception Z92.0
- deployment (military) Z91.82
- diabetic foot ulcer Z86.31
- disease or disorder (of) Z87.898
  - blood and blood-forming organs Z86.2
  - circulatory system Z86.79
    - specified condition NEC Z86.79
  - connective tissue NEC Z87.39
  - digestive system Z87.19
    - colonic polyp Z86.010
    - peptic ulcer disease Z87.11
    - specified condition NEC Z87.19
  - ear Z86.69
  - endocrine Z86.39
    - diabetic foot ulcer Z86.31
    - gestational diabetes Z86.32
    - specified type NEC Z86.39
  - eye Z86.69
  - genital (track) system NEC
    - female Z87.42
    - male Z87.438
  - hematological Z86.2
  - Hodgkin Z85.71
  - immune mechanism Z86.2
  - infectious Z86.19
    - malaria Z86.13
    - Methicillin resistant Staphylococcus aureus (MRSA) Z86.14
    - poliomyelitis Z86.12
    - specified NEC Z86.19
    - tuberculosis Z86.11
  - mental NEC Z86.59
  - metabolic Z86.39
    - diabetic foot ulcer Z86.31
    - gestational diabetes Z86.32
    - specified type NEC Z86.39
  - musculoskeletal NEC Z87.39
  - nervous system Z86.69
  - nutritional Z86.39
  - parasitic Z86.19
  - respiratory system NEC Z87.09

- sense organs Z86.69
- skin Z87.2
- specified site or type NEC Z87.898
- subcutaneous tissue Z87.2
- trophoblastic Z87.59
- urinary system NEC Z87.448
- drug dependence — see Dependence, drug, by type, in remission
- drug therapy
  - antineoplastic chemotherapy Z92.21
  - estrogen Z92.23
  - immunosupression Z92.25
  - inhaled steroids Z92.240
  - monoclonal drug Z92.22
  - specified NEC Z92.29
  - steroid Z92.241
  - systemic steroids Z92.241
- dysplasia
  - cervical Z87.410
  - prostatic Z87.430
  - vaginal Z87.411
  - vulvar Z87.412
- embolism (venous) Z86.718
  - pulmonary Z86.711
- encephalitis Z86.61
- estrogen therapy Z92.23
- extracorporeal membrane oxygenation (ECMO) Z92.81
- failed moderate sedation Z92.83
- failed conscious sedation Z92.83
- fall, falling Z91.81
- fracture (healed)
  - fatigue Z87.312
  - fragility Z87.310
  - osteoporosis Z87.310
  - pathological NEC Z87.311
  - stress Z87.312
  - traumatic Z87.81
- gestational diabetes Z86.32
- hepatitis
  - B Z86.19
  - C Z86.19
- Hodgkin disease Z85.71
- hyperthermia, malignant Z88.4
- hypospadias (corrected) Z87.710
- hysterectomy Z90.710
- immunosupression therapy Z92.25
- in situ neoplasm
  - breast Z86.000
  - cervix uteri Z86.001
  - specified NEC Z86.008
- infection NEC Z86.19
  - central nervous system Z86.61
  - Methicillin resistant Staphylococcus aureus (MRSA) Z86.14
  - urinary (recurrent) (tract) Z87.440
- injury NEC Z87.828
- in utero procedure during pregnancy Z98.870
- in utero procedure while a fetus Z98.871
- irradiation Z92.3
- kidney stones Z87.442
- leukemia Z85.6
- lymphoma (non-Hodgkin) Z85.72
- malignant melanoma (skin) Z85.820
- malignant neoplasm (of) Z85.9
  - accessory sinuses Z85.22
  - anus NEC Z85.048
    - carcinoid Z85.040
  - bladder Z85.51
  - bone Z85.830
  - brain Z85.841
  - breast Z85.3
  - bronchus NEC Z85.118
    - carcinoid Z85.110
  - carcinoid — see History, personal (of), malignant neoplasm, by site, carcinoid
  - cervix Z85.41
  - colon NEC Z85.038
    - carcinoid Z85.030
  - digestive organ Z85.00
    - specified NEC Z85.09
  - endocrine gland NEC Z85.858
  - epididymis Z85.48
  - esophagus Z85.01
  - eye Z85.840
  - gastrointestinal tract — see History, malignant neoplasm, digestive organ
  - genital organ
    - female Z85.40
      - specified NEC Z85.44
    - male Z85.45

History — *continued*
    specified NEC Z85.49
  hematopoietic NEC Z85.79
  intrathoracic organ Z85.20
  kidney NEC Z85.528
    carcinoid Z85.520
  large intestine NEC Z85.038
    carcinoid Z85.030
  larynx Z85.21
  liver Z85.05
  lung NEC Z85.118
    carcinoid Z85.110
  mediastinum Z85.29
  Merkel cell Z85.821
  middle ear Z85.22
  nasal cavities Z85.22
  nervous system NEC Z85.848
  oral cavity Z85.819
    specified site NEC Z85.818
  ovary Z85.43
  pancreas Z85.07
  pharynx Z85.819
    specified site NEC Z85.818
  pelvis Z85.53
  pleura Z85.29
  prostate Z85.46
  rectosigmoid junction NEC Z85.048
    carcinoid Z85.040
  rectum NEC Z85.048
    carcinoid Z85.040
  respiratory organ Z85.20
  sinuses, accessory Z85.22
  skin NEC Z85.828
    melanoma Z85.820
    Merkel cell Z85.821
  small intestine NEC Z85.068
    carcinoid Z85.060
  soft tissue Z85.831
  specified site NEC Z85.89
  stomach NEC Z85.028
    carcinoid Z85.020
  testis Z85.47
  thymus NEC Z85.238
    carcinoid Z85.230
  thyroid Z85.850
  tongue Z85.810
  trachea Z85.12
  ureter Z85.54
  urinary organ or tract Z85.50
    specified NEC Z85.59
  uterus Z85.42
 maltreatment Z91.89
 medical treatment NEC Z92.89
 melanoma (malignant) (skin) Z85.820
 meningitis Z86.61
 mental disorder Z86.59
 Merkel cell carcinoma (skin) Z85.821
 Methicillin resistant Staphylococcus aureus (MRSA) Z86.14
 military deployment Z91.82
 military war, peacekeeping and humanitarian deployment (current or past conflict) Z91.82
 myocardial infarction (old) I25.2
 neglect (in)
  adult Z91.412
  childhood Z62.812
 neoplasm
  benign Z86.018
    brain Z86.011
    colon polyp Z86.010
  in situ
    breast Z86.000
    cervix uteri Z86.001
    specified NEC Z86.008
  malignant — *see* History of, malignant neoplasm
  uncertain behavior Z86.03
 nephrotic syndrome Z87.441
 nicotine dependence Z87.891
 noncompliance with medical treatment or regimen — *see* Noncompliance
 nutritional deficiency Z86.39
 obstetric complications Z87.59
  childbirth Z87.59
  pregnancy Z87.59
  pre-term labor Z87.51
  puerperium Z87.59
 osteoporosis fractures Z87.31 ☑
 parasuicide (attempt) Z91.5
 physical trauma NEC Z87.828
  self-harm or suicide attempt Z91.5

History — *continued*
 poisoning NEC Z91.89
  self-harm or suicide attempt Z91.5
 poor personal hygiene Z91.89
 pneumonia (recurrent) Z87.01
 preterm labor Z87.51
 prolonged reversible ischemic neurologic deficit (PRIND) Z86.73
 procedure during pregnancy Z98.870
 procedure while a fetus Z98.871
 prostatic dysplasia Z87.430
 psychological
  abuse
    adult Z91.411
    child Z62.811
  trauma, specified NEC Z91.49
 radiation therapy Z92.3
 removal
  implant
    breast Z98.86
 renal calculi Z87.442
 respiratory condition NEC Z87.09
 retained foreign body fully removed Z87.821
 risk factors NEC Z91.89
 self-harm Z91.5
 self-poisoning attempt Z91.5
 sex reassignment Z87.890
 sleep-wake cycle problem Z72.821
 specified NEC Z87.898
 steroid therapy (systemic) Z92.241
  inhaled Z92.240
 stroke without residual deficits Z86.73
 substance abuse NEC F10-F19 with fifth character 1
 sudden cardiac arrest Z86.74
 sudden cardiac death successfully resuscitated Z86.74
 suicide attempt Z91.5
 surgery NEC Z98.89
  sex reassignment Z87.890
  transplant — *see* Transplant
 thrombophlebitis Z86.72
 thrombosis (venous) Z86.718
  pulmonary Z86.711
 tobacco dependence Z87.891
 transient ischemic attack (TIA) without residual deficits Z86.73
 trauma (physical) NEC Z87.828
  psychological NEC Z91.49
  self-harm Z91.5
 traumatic brain injury Z87.820
 unhealthy sleep-wake cycle Z72.821
 urinary calculi Z87.442
 urinary (recurrent) (tract) infection(s) Z87.440
 vaginal dysplasia Z87.411
 venous thrombosis or embolism Z86.718
  pulmonary Z86.711
 vulvar dysplasia Z87.412
His-Werner disease A79.0
HIV (*see also* Human, immunodeficiency virus) B20
 laboratory evidence (nonconclusive) R75
 positive, seropositive Z21
 nonconclusive test (in infants) R75
Hives (bold) — *see* Urticaria
Hoarseness R49.0
Hobo Z59.0
Hodgkin disease — *see* Lymphoma, Hodgkin
Hodgson's disease I71.2
 ruptured I71.1
Hoffa-Kastert disease E88.89
Hoffa's disease E88.89
Hoffmann-Bouveret syndrome I47.9
Hoffmann's syndrome E03.9 [G73.7]
Hole (round)
 macula H35.34- ☑
 retina (without detachment) — *see* Break, retina, round hole
  with detachment — *see* Detachment, retina, with retinal, break
Holiday relief care Z75.5
Hollenhorst's plaque — *see* Occlusion, artery, retina
Hollow foot (congenital) Q66.7
 acquired — *see* Deformity, limb, foot, specified NEC
Holoprosencephaly Q04.2
Holt-Oram syndrome Q87.2
Homelessness Z59.0
Homesickness — *see* Disorder, adjustment
Homocystinemia, homocystinuria E72.11
Homogentisate 1,2-dioxygenase deficiency E70.29
Homologous serum hepatitis (prophylactic) (therapeutic) — *see* Hepatitis, viral, type B

Honeycomb lung J98.4
 congenital Q33.0
Hooded
 clitoris Q52.6
 penis Q55.69
Hookworm (anemia) (disease) (infection) (infestation) B76.9
 specified NEC B76.8
Hordeolum (eyelid) (externum) (recurrent) H00.019
 internum H00.029
  left H00.026
    lower H00.025
    upper H00.024
  right H00.023
    lower H00.022
    upper H00.021
 left H00.016
  lower H00.015
  upper H00.014
 right H00.013
  lower H00.012
  upper H00.011
Horn
 cutaneous L85.8
 nail L60.2
  congenital Q84.6
Horner (-Claude Bernard) syndrome G90.2
 traumatic — *see* Injury, nerve, cervical sympathetic
Horseshoe kidney (congenital) Q63.1
Horton's headache or neuralgia G44.099
 intractable G44.091
 not intractable G44.099
Hospital hopper syndrome — *see* Disorder, factitious
Hospitalism in children — *see* Disorder, adjustment
Hostility R45.5
 towards child Z62.3
Hot flashes
 menopausal N95.1
Hourglass (contracture) (*see also* Contraction, hourglass)
 stomach K31.89
  congenital Q40.2
  stricture K31.2
Household, housing circumstance affecting care Z59.9
 specified NEC Z59.8
Housemaid's knee — *see* Bursitis, prepatellar
Hudson (-Stähli) line (cornea) — *see* Pigmentation, cornea, anterior
Human
 bite (open wound) (*see also* Bite)
  intact skin surface — *see* Bite, superficial
 herpesvirus — *see* Herpes
 immunodeficiency virus (HIV) disease (infection) B20
  asymptomatic status Z21
  contact Z20.6
  counseling Z71.7
  dementia B20 [F02.80]
    with behavioral disturbance B20 [F02.81]
  exposure to Z20.6
  laboratory evidence R75
  type-2 (HIV 2) as cause of disease classified elsewhere B97.35
 papillomavirus (HPV)
  DNA test positive
    high risk
      cervix R87.810
      vagina R87.811
    low risk
      cervix R87.820
      vagina R87.821
  screening for Z11.51
 T-cell lymphotropic virus
  type-1 (HTLV-I) infection B33.3
    as cause of disease classified elsewhere B97.33
  carrier Z22.6
  type-2 (HTLV-II) as cause of disease classified elsewhere B97.34
Humidifier lung or pneumonitis J67.7
Humiliation (experience) in childhood Z62.898
Humpback (acquired) — *see* Kyphosis
Hunchback (acquired) — *see* Kyphosis
Hunger T73.0 ☑
 air, psychogenic F45.8
Hungry bone syndrome E83.81
Hunner's ulcer — *see* Cystitis, chronic, interstitial
Hunter's
 glossitis D51.0
 syndrome E76.1

☑ **Additional character required**

Huntington's disease or chorea G10
    with dementia G10 [F02.80]
        with behavioral disturbance G10 [F02.81]
Hunt's
    disease or syndrome (herpetic geniculate
        ganglionitis) B02.21
        dyssynergia cerebellaris myoclonica G11.1
        neuralgia B02.21
Hurler (-Scheie) disease or syndrome E76.02
Hurst's disease G36.1
Hurthle cell
    adenocarcinoma C73
    adenoma D34
    carcinoma C73
    tumor D34
Hutchinson-Boeck disease or syndrome — see
    Sarcoidosis
Hutchinson-Gilford disease or syndrome E34.8
Hutchinson's
    disease, meaning
        angioma serpiginosum L81.7
        pompholyx (cheiropompholyx) L30.1
        prurigo estivalis L56.4
        summer eruption or summer prurigo L56.4
    melanotic freckle — see Melanoma, in situ
        malignant melanoma in — see Melanoma
    teeth or incisors (congenital syphilis) A50.52
    triad (congenital syphilis) A50.53
Hyalin plaque, sclera, senile H15.89
Hyaline membrane (disease) (lung) (pulmonary)
    (newborn) P22.0
Hyalinosis
    cutis (et mucosae) E78.89
    focal and segmental (glomerular) (see also
        N00-N07 with fourth character .1) N05.1
Hyalitis, hyalosis, asteroid (see also Deposit,
    crystalline)
    syphilitic (late) A52.71
Hydatid
    cyst or tumor — see Echinococcus
    mole — see Hydatidiform mole
    Morgagni
        female Q50.5
        male (epididymal) Q55.4
        testicular Q55.29
Hydatidiform mole (benign) (complicating
    pregnancy) (delivered) (undelivered) O01.9
    classical O01.0
    complete O01.0
    incomplete O01.1
    invasive D39.2
    malignant D39.2
    partial O01.1
Hydatidosis — see Echinococcus
Hydradenitis (axillaris) (suppurative) L73.2
Hydradenoma — see Hidradenoma
Hydramnios O40.- ☑
Hydrancephaly, hydranencephaly Q04.3
    with spina bifida — see Spina bifida, with
        hydrocephalus
Hydrargyrism NEC — see Poisoning, mercury
Hydrarthrosis (see also Effusion, joint)
    gonococcal A54.42
    intermittent M12.40
        ankle M12.47- ☑
        elbow M12.42- ☑
        foot joint M12.47- ☑
        hand joint M12.44- ☑
        hip M12.45- ☑
        knee M12.46- ☑
        multiple site M12.49
        shoulder M12.41- ☑
        specified joint NEC M12.48
        wrist M12.43- ☑
    of yaws (early) (late) (see also subcategory M14.8-)
        A66.6
    syphilitic (late) A52.77
        congenital A50.55 [M12.80]
Hydremia D64.89
Hydrencephalocele (congenital) — see
    Encephalocele
Hydrencephalomeningocele (congenital) — see
    Encephalocele
Hydroa R23.8
    aestivale L56.4
    vacciniforme L56.4
Hydroadenitis (axillaris) (suppurative) L73.2
Hydrocalycosis — see Hydronephrosis
Hydrocele (spermatic cord) (testis) (tunica vaginalis)
    N43.3
    canal of Nuck N94.89
    communicating N43.2

Hydrocele — continued
    congenital P83.5
    congenital P83.5
    encysted N43.0
    female NEC N94.89
    infected N43.1
    newborn P83.5
    round ligament N94.89
    specified NEC N43.2
    spinalis — see Spina bifida
    vulva N90.89
Hydrocephalus (acquired) (external) (internal)
  (malignant) (recurrent) G91.9
    aqueduct Sylvius stricture Q03.0
    causing disproportion O33.6 ☑
        with obstructed labor O66.3
    communicating G91.0
    congenital (external) (internal) Q03.9
        with spina bifida Q05.4
            cervical Q05.0
            dorsal Q05.1
            lumbar Q05.2
            lumbosacral Q05.2
            sacral Q05.3
            thoracic Q05.1
            thoracolumbar Q05.1
        specified NEC Q03.8
    due to toxoplasmosis (congenital) P37.1
    foramen Magendie block (acquired) G91.1
        congenital (see also Hydrocephalus, congenital)
            Q03.1
    in (due to)
        infectious disease NEC B89 [G91.4]
        neoplastic disease NEC (see also Neoplasm)
            G91.4
        parasitic disease B89 [G91.4]
    newborn Q03.9
        with spina bifida — see Spina bifida, with
            hydrocephalus
    noncommunicating G91.1
    normal pressure G91.2
        secondary G91.0
    obstructive G91.1
    otitic G93.2
    post-traumatic NEC G91.3
    secondary G91.4
        post-traumatic G91.3
    specified NEC G91.8
    syphilitic, congenital A50.49
Hydrocolpos (congenital) N89.8
Hydrocystoma — see Neoplasm, skin, benign
Hydroencephalocele (congenital) — see
    Encephalocele
Hydroencephalomeningocele (congenital) — see
    Encephalocele
Hydrohematopneumothorax — see Hemothorax
Hydromeningitis — see Meningitis
Hydromeningocele (spinal) (see also Spina bifida)
    cranial — see Encephalocele
Hydrometra N85.8
Hydrometrocolpos N89.8
Hydromicrocephaly Q02
Hydromphalos (since birth) Q45.8
Hydromyelia Q06.4
Hydromyelocele — see Spina bifida
Hydronephrosis (atrophic) (early) (functionless)
  (intermittent) (primary) (secondary) NEC N13.30
    with
        infection N13.6
        obstruction (by) (of)
            renal calculus N13.2
                with infection N13.6
            ureteral NEC N13.1
                with infection N13.6
                calculus N13.2
                    with infection N13.6
            ureteropelvic junction (congenital) Q62.0
                with infection N13.6
            ureteral stricture NEC N13.1
                with infection N13.6
    congenital Q62.0
    specified type NEC N13.39
    tuberculous A18.11
Hydropericarditis — see Pericarditis
Hydropericardium — see Pericarditis
Hydroperitoneum R18.8
Hydrophobia — see Rabies
Hydrophthalmos Q15.0
Hydropneumohemothorax — see Hemothorax
Hydropneumopericarditis — see Pericarditis
Hydropneumopericardium — see Pericarditis

Hydropneumothorax J94.8
    traumatic — see Injury, intrathoracic, lung
    tuberculous NEC A15.6
Hydrops R60.9
    abdominis R18.8
    articulorum intermittens — see Hydrarthrosis,
        intermittent
    cardiac — see Failure, heart, congestive
    causing obstructed labor (mother) O66.3
    endolymphatic H81.0- ☑
    fetal — see Pregnancy, complicated by, hydrops,
        fetalis
    fetalis P83.2
        due to
            ABO isoimmunization P56.0
            alpha thalassemia D56.0
            hemolytic disease P56.90
                specified NEC P56.99
            isoimmunization (ABO) (Rh) P56.0
            other specified nonhemolytic disease NEC
                P83.2
            Rh incompatibility P56.0
        during pregnancy — see Pregnancy,
            complicated by, hydrops, fetalis
    gallbladder K82.1
    joint — see Effusion, joint
    labyrinth H81.0- ☑
    newborn (idiopathic) P83.2
        due to
            ABO isoimmunization P56.0
            alpha thalassemia D56.0
            hemolytic disease P56.90
                specified NEC P56.99
            isoimmunization (ABO) (Rh) P56.0
            Rh incompatibility P56.0
    nutritional — see Malnutrition, severe
    pericardium — see Pericarditis
    pleura — see Hydrothorax
    spermatic cord — see Hydrocele
Hydropyonephrosis N13.6
Hydrorachis Q06.4
Hydrorrhea (nasal) J34.89
    pregnancy — see Rupture, membranes,
        premature
Hydrosadenitis (axillaris) (suppurative) L73.2
Hydrosalpinx (fallopian tube) (follicularis) N70.11
Hydrothorax (double) (pleura) J94.8
    chylous (nonfilarial) I89.8
    filarial (see also Infestation, filarial) B74.9 [J91.8]
    traumatic — see Injury, intrathoracic
    tuberculous NEC (non primary) A15.6
Hydroureter (see also Hydronephrosis) N13.4
    with infection N13.6
    congenital Q62.39
Hydroureteronephrosis — see Hydronephrosis
Hydrourethra N36.8
Hydroxykynureninuria E70.8
Hydroxylysinemia E72.3
Hydroxyprolinemia E72.59
Hygiene, sleep
    abuse Z72.821
    inadequate Z72.821
    poor Z72.821
Hygroma (congenital) (cystic) D18.1
    praepatellare, prepatellar — see Bursitis,
        prepatellar
Hymen — see condition
Hymenolepis, hymenolepiasis (diminuta) (infection)
    (infestation) (nana) B71.0
Hypalgesia R20.8
Hyperacidity (gastric) K31.89
    psychogenic F45.8
Hyperactive, hyperactivity F90.9
    basal cell, uterine cervix — see Dysplasia, cervix
    bowel sounds R19.12
    cervix epithelial (basal) — see Dysplasia, cervix
    child F90.9
        attention deficit — see Disorder, attention-
            deficit hyperactivity
    detrusor muscle N32.81
    gastrointestinal K31.89
        psychogenic F45.8
    nasal mucous membrane J34.3
    stomach K31.89
    thyroid (gland) — see Hyperthyroidism
Hyperacusis H93.23- ☑
Hyperadrenalism E27.5
Hyperadrenocorticism E24.9
    congenital E25.0
    iatrogenic E24.2

Hyperadrenocorticism - Hyperostosis

Hyperadrenocorticism — *continued*
    correct substance properly administered — *see* Table of Drugs and Chemicals, by drug, adverse effect
    overdose or wrong substance given or taken — *see* Table of Drugs and Chemicals, by drug, poisoning
    not associated with Cushing's syndrome E27.0
    pituitary-dependent E24.0
Hyperaldosteronism E26.9
    familial (type I) E26.02
    glucocorticoid-remediable E26.02
    primary (due to (bilateral) adrenal hyperplasia) E26.09
    primary NEC E26.09
    secondary E26.1
    specified NEC E26.89
Hyperalgesia R20.8
Hyperalimentation R63.2
    carotene, carotin E67.1
    specified NEC E67.8
    vitamin
      A E67.0
      D E67.3
Hyperaminoaciduria
    arginine E72.21
    cystine E72.01
    lysine E72.3
    ornithine E72.4
Hyperammonemia (congenital) E72.20
Hyperazotemia — *see* Uremia
Hyperbetalipoproteinemia (familial) E78.0
    with prebetalipoproteinemia E78.2
Hyperbilirubinemia
    constitutional E80.6
    familial conjugated E80.6
    neonatal (transient) — *see* Jaundice, newborn
Hypercalcemia, hypocalciuric, familial E83.52
Hypercalciuria, idiopathic E83.52
Hypercapnia R06.89
    newborn P84
Hypercarotenemia, hypercarotinemia (dietary) E67.1
Hypercementosis K03.4
Hyperchloremia E87.8
Hyperchlorhydria K31.89
    neurotic F45.8
    psychogenic F45.8
Hypercholesterinemia — *see* Hypercholesterolemia
Hypercholesterolemia (essential) (familial) (hereditary) (primary) (pure) E78.0
    with hyperglyceridemia, endogenous E78.2
    dietary counseling and surveillance Z71.3
Hyperchylia gastrica, psychogenic F45.8
Hyperchylomicronemia (familial) (primary) E78.3
    with hyperbetalipoproteinemia E78.3
Hypercoagulable (state) D68.59
    activated protein C resistance D68.51
    antithrombin (III) deficiency D68.59
    factor V Leiden mutation D68.51
    primary NEC D68.59
    protein C deficiency D68.59
    protein S deficiency D68.59
    prothrombin gene mutation D68.52
    secondary D68.69
    specified NEC D68.69
Hypercoagulation (state) D68.59
Hypercorticalism, pituitary-dependent E24.0
Hypercorticosolism — *see* Cushing's, syndrome
Hypercorticosteronism E24.2
    correct substance properly administered — *see* Table of Drugs and Chemicals, by drug, adverse effect
    overdose or wrong substance given or taken — *see* Table of Drugs and Chemicals, by drug, poisoning
Hypercortisonism E24.2
    correct substance properly administered — *see* Table of Drugs and Chemicals, by drug, adverse effect
    overdose or wrong substance given or taken — *see* Table of Drugs and Chemicals, by drug, poisoning
Hyperekplexia Q89.8
Hyperelectrolytemia E87.8
Hyperemesis R11.10
    with nausea R11.2
    gravidarum (mild) O21.0
      with
        carbohydrate depletion O21.1
        dehydration O21.1
        electrolyte imbalance O21.1

Hyperemesis — *continued*
      metabolic disturbance O21.1
    severe (with metabolic disturbance) O21.1
    projectile R11.12
    psychogenic F45.8
Hyperemia (acute) (passive) R68.89
    anal mucosa K62.89
    bladder N32.89
    cerebral I67.89
    conjunctiva H11.43- ☑
    ear internal, acute H83.0
    enteric K59.8
    eye — *see* Hyperemia, conjunctiva
    eyelid (active) (passive) — *see* Disorder, eyelid, specified type NEC
    intestine K59.8
    iris — *see* Disorder, iris, vascular
    kidney N28.89
    labyrinth H83.0
    liver (active) K76.89
    lung (passive) — *see* Edema, lung
    pulmonary (passive) — *see* Edema, lung
    renal N28.89
    retina H35.89
    stomach K31.89
Hyperesthesia (body surface) R20.3
    larynx (reflex) J38.7
      hysterical F44.89
    pharynx (reflex) J39.2
      hysterical F44.89
Hyperestrogenism (drug-induced) (iatrogenic) E28.0
Hyperexplexia Q89.8
Hyperfibrinolysis — *see* Fibrinolysis
Hyperfructosemia E74.19
Hyperfunction
    adrenal cortex, not associated with Cushing's syndrome E27.0
      medulla E27.5
        adrenomedullary E27.5
      virilism E25.9
        congenital E25.0
    ovarian E28.8
    pancreas K86.8
    parathyroid (gland) E21.3
    pituitary (gland) (anterior) E22.9
      specified NEC E22.8
    polyglandular E31.1
    testicular E29.0
Hypergammaglobulinemia D89.2
    polyclonal D89.0
    Waldenström D89.0
Hypergastrinemia E16.4
Hyperglobulinemia R77.1
Hyperglycemia, hyperglycemic (transient) R73.9
    coma — *see* Diabetes, by type, with coma
    postpancreatectomy E89.1
Hyperglyceridemia (endogenous) (essential) (familial) (hereditary) (pure) E78.1
    mixed E78.3
Hyperglycinemia (non-ketotic) E72.51
Hypergonadism
    ovarian E28.8
    testicular (primary) (infantile) E29.0
Hyperheparinemia D68.32
Hyperhidrosis, hyperidrosis R61
    focal
      primary L74.519
        axilla L74.510
        face L74.511
        palms L74.512
        soles L74.513
      secondary L74.52
    generalized R61
    localized
      primary L74.519
        axilla L74.510
        face L74.511
        palms L74.512
        soles L74.513
      secondary L74.52
    psychogenic F45.8
    secondary R61
      focal L74.52
Hyperhistidinemia E70.41
Hyperhomocysteinemia E72.11
Hyperhydroxyprolinemia E72.59
Hyperinsulinism (functional) E16.1
    with
      coma (hypoglycemic) E15
      encephalopathy E16.1 [G94]
    ectopic E16.1

Hyperinsulinism — *continued*
    therapeutic misadventure (from administration of insulin) T38.3
Hyperkalemia E87.5
Hyperkeratosis (*see also* Keratosis) L85.9
    cervix N88.0
    due to yaws (early) (late) (palmar or plantar) A66.3
    follicularis Q82.8
      penetrans (in cutem) L87.0
    palmoplantaris climacterica L85.1
    pinta A67.1
    senile (with pruritus) L57.0
    universalis congenita Q80.8
    vocal cord J38.3
    vulva N90.4
Hyperkinesia, hyperkinetic (disease) (reaction) (syndrome) (childhood) (adolescence) (*see also* Disorder, attention-deficit hyperactivity)
    heart I51.89
Hyperleucine-isoleucinemia E71.19
Hyperlipemia, hyperlipidemia E78.5
    combined E78.2
      familial E78.4
    group
      A E78.0
      B E78.1
      C E78.2
      D E78.3
    mixed E78.2
    specified NEC E78.4
Hyperlipidosis E75.6
    hereditary NEC E75.5
Hyperlipoproteinemia E78.5
    Fredrickson's type
      I E78.3
      IIa E78.0
      IIb E78.2
      III E78.2
      IV E78.1
      V E78.3
    low-density-lipoprotein-type (LDL) E78.0
    very-low-density-lipoprotein-type (VLDL) E78.1
Hyperlucent lung, unilateral J43.0
Hyperlysinemia E72.3
Hypermagnesemia E83.41
    neonatal P71.8
Hypermenorrhea N92.0
Hypermethioninemia E72.19
Hypermetropia (congenital) H52.0- ☑
Hypermobility, hypermotility
    cecum — *see* Syndrome, irritable bowel
    coccyx M53.2
    colon — *see* Syndrome, irritable bowel
      psychogenic F45.8
    ileum K58.9
    intestine (*see also* Syndrome, irritable bowel) K58.9
      psychogenic F45.8
    meniscus (knee) — *see* Derangement, knee, meniscus
    scapula — *see* Instability, joint, shoulder
    stomach K31.89
      psychogenic F45.8
    syndrome M35.7
    urethra N36.41
      with intrinsic sphincter deficiency N36.43
Hypernasality R49.21
Hypernatremia E87.0
Hypernephroma C64.- ☑
Hyperopia — *see* Hypermetropia
Hyperorexia nervosa F50.2
Hyperornithinemia E72.4
Hyperosmia R43.1
Hyperosmolality E87.0
Hyperostosis (monomelic) (*see also* Disorder, bone, density and structure, specified NEC)
    ankylosing (spine) M48.10
      cervical region M48.12
      cervicothoracic region M48.13
      lumbar region M48.16
      lumbosacral region M48.17
      multiple sites M48.19
      occipito-atlanto-axial region M48.11
      sacrococcygeal region M48.18
      thoracic region M48.14
      thoracolumbar region M48.15
    cortical (skull) M85.2
      infantile M89.8X- ☑
    frontal, internal of skull M85.2
    interna frontalis M85.2

Hyperostosis — *continued*
  skeletal, diffuse idiopathic — *see* Hyperostosis,
    ankylosing
  skull M85.2
    congenital Q75.8
  vertebral, ankylosing — *see* Hyperostosis,
    ankylosing
Hyperovarism E28.8
Hyperoxaluria (primary) E72.53
Hyperparathyroidism E21.3
  primary E21.0
  secondary (renal) N25.81
    non-renal E21.1
  specified NEC E21.2
  tertiary E21.2
Hyperpathia R20.8
Hyperperistalsis R19.2
  psychogenic F45.8
Hyperpermeability, capillary I78.8
Hyperphagia R63.2
Hyperphenylalaninemia NEC E70.1
Hyperphoria (alternating) H50.53
Hyperphosphatemia E83.39
Hyperpiesis, hyperpiesia — *see* Hypertension
Hyperpigmentation (*see also* Pigmentation)
  melanin NEC L81.4
  postinflammatory L81.0
Hyperpinealism E34.8
Hyperpituitarism E22.9
Hyperplasia, hyperplastic
  adenoids J35.2
  adrenal (capsule) (cortex) (gland) E27.8
    with
      sexual precocity (male) E25.9
        congenital E25.0
      virilism, adrenal E25.9
        congenital E25.0
      virilization (female) E25.9
        congenital E25.0
    congenital E25.0
    salt-losing E25.0
  adrenomedullary E27.5
  angiolymphoid, eosinophilia (ALHE) D18.01
  appendix (lymphoid) K38.0
  artery, fibromuscular I77.3
  bone (*see also* Hypertrophy, bone)
    marrow D75.89
  breast (*see also* Hypertrophy, breast)
    ductal (atypical) N60.9- ☑
  C-cell, thyroid E07.0
  cementation (tooth) (teeth) K03.4
  cervical gland R59.0
  cervix (uteri) (basal cell) (endometrium)
    (polypoid) (*see also* Dysplasia, cervix)
    congenital Q51.828
  clitoris, congenital Q52.6
  denture K06.2
  endocervicitis N72
  endometrium, endometrial (adenomatous)
    (benign) (cystic) (glandular) (glandular-cystic)
    (polypoid) N85.00
    with atypia N85.02
    cervix — *see* Dysplasia, cervix
    complex (without atypia) N85.01
    simple (without atypia) N85.01
  epithelial L85.9
    focal, oral, including tongue K13.29
    nipple N62
    skin L85.9
    tongue K13.29
    vaginal wall N89.3
  erythroid D75.89
  fibromuscular of artery (carotid) (renal) I77.3
  genital
    female NEC N94.89
    male N50.8
  gingiva K06.1
  glandularis cystica uteri (interstitialis) (*see also*
    Hyperplasia, endometrial) N85.00- ☑
  gum K06.1
  hymen, congenital Q52.4
  irritative, edentulous (alveolar) K06.2
  jaw M26.09
    alveolar M26.79
    lower M26.03
      alveolar M26.72
    upper M26.01
      alveolar M26.71
  kidney (congenital) Q63.3
  labia N90.6
    epithelial N90.3
  liver (congenital) Q44.7

Hyperplasia — *continued*
  nodular, focal K76.89
  lymph gland or node R59.9
  mandible, mandibular M26.03
    alveolar M26.72
    unilateral condylar M27.8
  maxilla, maxillary M26.01
    alveolar M26.71
  myometrium, myometrial N85.2
  neuroendocrine cell, of infancy J84.841
  nose
    lymphoid J34.89
    polypoid J33.9
  oral mucosa (irritative) K13.6
  organ or site, congenital NEC — *see* Anomaly,
    by site
  ovary N83.8
  palate, papillary (irritative) K13.6
  pancreatic islet cells E16.9
    alpha E16.8
      with excess
        gastrin E16.4
        glucagon E16.3
    beta E16.1
  parathyroid (gland) E21.0
  pharynx (lymphoid) J39.2
  prostate (adenofibromatous) (nodular) N40.0
    with lower urinary tract symptoms (LUTS)
      N40.1
    without lower urinary tract symtpoms (LUTS)
      N40.0
  renal artery I77.89
  reticulo-endothelial (cell) D75.89
  salivary gland (any) K11.1
  Schimmelbusch's — *see* Mastopathy, cystic
  suprarenal capsule (gland) E27.8
  thymus (gland) (persistent) E32.0
  thyroid (gland) — *see* Goiter
  tonsils (faucial) (infective) (lingual) (lymphoid)
    J35.1
    with adenoids J35.3
  unilateral condylar M27.8
  uterus, uterine N85.2
    endometrium (glandular) (*see also* Hyperplasia,
      endometrial) N85.00- ☑
  vulva N90.6
    epithelial N90.3
Hyperpnea — *see* Hyperventilation
Hyperpotassemia E87.5
Hyperprebetalipoproteinemia (familial) E78.1
Hyperprolactinemia E22.1
Hyperprolinemia (type I) (type II) E72.59
Hyperproteinemia E88.09
Hyperprothrombinemia, causing coagulation
  factor deficiency D68.4
Hyperpyrexia R50.9
  heat (effects) T67.0 ☑
  malignant, due to anesthetic T88.3 ☑
  rheumatic — *see* Fever, rheumatic
  unknown origin R50.9
Hyper-reflexia R29.2
Hypersalivation K11.7
Hypersecretion
  ACTH (not associated with Cushing's syndrome)
    E27.0
    pituitary E24.0
  adrenaline E27.5
  adrenomedullary E27.5
  androgen (testicular) E29.0
    ovarian (drug-induced) (iatrogenic) E28.1
  calcitonin E07.0
  catecholamine E27.5
  corticoadrenal E24.9
  cortisol E24.9
  epinephrine E27.5
  estrogen E28.0
  gastric K31.89
    psychogenic F45.8
  gastrin E16.4
  glucagon E16.3
  hormone (s)
    ACTH (not associated with Cushing's
      syndrome) E27.0
    pituitary E24.0
    antidiuretic E22.2
    growth E22.0
    intestinal NEC E34.1
    ovarian androgen E28.1
    pituitary E22.9
    testicular E29.0
    thyroid stimulating E05.80
      with thyroid storm E05.81

Hypersecretion — *continued*
  insulin — *see* Hyperinsulinism
  lacrimal glands — *see* Epiphora
  medulloadrenal E27.5
  milk O92.6
  ovarian androgens E28.1
  salivary gland (any) K11.7
  thyrocalcitonin E07.0
  upper respiratory J39.8
Hypersegmentation, leukocytic, hereditary D72.0
Hypersensitive, hypersensitiveness, hypersensitivity
  (*see also* Allergy)
  carotid sinus G90.01
  colon — *see* Irritable, colon
  drug T88.7 ☑
  gastrointestinal K52.2
    psychogenic F45.8
  labyrinth H83.2
  pain R20.8
  pneumonitis — *see* Pneumonitis, allergic
  reaction T78.40 ☑
  upper respiratory tract NEC J39.3
Hypersomnia (organic) G47.10
  due to
    alcohol
      abuse F10.182
      dependence F10.282
      use F10.982
    amphetamines
      abuse F15.182
      dependence F15.282
      use F15.982
    caffeine
      abuse F15.182
      dependence F15.282
      use F15.982
    cocaine
      abuse F14.182
      dependence F14.282
      use F14.982
    drug NEC
      abuse F19.182
      dependence F19.282
      use F19.982
    medical condition G47.14
    mental disorder F51.13
    opioid
      abuse F11.182
      dependence F11.282
      use F11.982
    psychoactive substance NEC
      abuse F19.182
      dependence F19.282
      use F19.982
    sedative, hypnotic, or anxiolytic
      abuse F13.182
      dependence F13.282
      use F13.982
    stimulant NEC
      abuse F15.182
      dependence F15.282
      use F15.982
  idiopathic G47.11
    with long sleep time G47.11
    without long sleep time G47.12
  menstrual related G47.13
  nonorganic origin F51.11
    specified NEC F51.19
  not due to a substance or known physiological
    condition F51.11
    specified NEC F51.19
  primary F51.11
  recurrent G47.13
  specified NEC G47.19
Hypersplenia, hypersplenism D73.1
Hyperstimulation, ovaries (associated with induced
  ovulation) N98.1
Hypersusceptibility — *see* Allergy
Hypertelorism (ocular) (orbital) Q75.2
Hypertension, hypertensive (accelerated) (benign)
  (essential) (idiopathic) (malignant) (systemic) I10
  with
    heart involvement (conditions in I51.4- I51.9
      due to hypertension) — *see* Hypertension,
      heart
    kidney involvement — *see* Hypertension,
      kidney
  benign, intracranial G93.2
  borderline R03.0
  cardiorenal (disease) I13.10
    with heart failure I13.0

Hypertension — *continued*

with stage 1 through stage 4 chronic kidney disease I13.0
with stage 5 or end stage renal disease I13.2
without heart failure I13.10
with stage 1 through stage 4 chronic kidney disease I13.10
with stage 5 or end stage renal disease I13.11
cardiovascular
disease (arteriosclerotic) (sclerotic) — *see* Hypertension, heart
renal (disease) — *see* Hypertension, cardiorenal
chronic venous — *see* Hypertension, venous (chronic)
complicating
childbirth (labor) O10.92
with
heart disease O10.12
with renal disease O10.32
renal disease O10.22
with heart disease O10.32
essential O10.02
secondary O10.42
pregnancy O16.- ☑
with edema (*see also* Pre-eclampsia) O14.9- ☑
gestational (pregnancy induced) (transient) (without proteinuria) O13.- ☑
with proteinuria O14.9- ☑
mild pre-eclampsia O14.0- ☑
moderate pre-eclampsia O14.0- ☑
severe pre-eclampsia O14.1- ☑
with hemolysis, elevated liver enzymes and low platelet count (HELLP) O14.2- ☑
pre-existing O10.91- ☑
with
heart disease O10.11- ☑
with renal disease O10.31- ☑
pre-eclampsia O11.- ☑
renal disease O10.21- ☑
with heart disease O10.31- ☑
essential O10.01- ☑
secondary O10.41- ☑
puerperium, pre-existing O10.93
with
heart disease O10.13
with renal disease O10.33
renal disease O10.23
with heart disease O10.33
essential O10.03
pregnancy-induced O13.9
secondary O10.43
due to
endocrine disorders I15.2
pheochromocytoma I15.2
renal disorders NEC I15.1
arterial I15.0
renovascular disorders I15.0
specified disease NEC I15.8
encephalopathy I67.4
gestational (without significant proteinuria) (pregnancy-induced) (transient) O13.- ☑
with significant proteinuria — *see* Pre-eclampsia
Goldblatt's I70.1
heart (disease) (conditions in I51.4-I51.9 due to hypertension) I11.9
with
heart failure (congestive) I11.0
kidney disease (chronic) — *see* Hypertension, cardiorenal
intracranial (benign) G93.2
kidney I12.9
with
heart disease — *see* Hypertension, cardiorenal
stage 5 chronic kidney disease (CKD) or end stage renal disease (ESRD) I12.0
stage 1 through stage 4 chronic kidney disease I12.9
lesser circulation I27.0
newborn P29.2
pulmonary (persistent) P29.3
ocular H40.05- ☑
pancreatic duct - code to underlying condition
with chronic pancreatitis K86.1
portal (due to chronic liver disease) (idiopathic) K76.6
gastropathy K31.89
in (due to) schistosomiasis (bilharziasis) B65.9 [K77]

Hypertension — *continued*

postoperative I97.3
psychogenic F45.8
pulmonary (artery) (secondary) NEC I27.2
with
cor pulmonale (chronic) I27.2
acute I26.09
right heart ventricular strain/failure I27.2
acute I26.09
of newborn (persistent) P29.3
primary (idiopathic) I27.0
renal — *see* Hypertension, kidney
renovascular I15.0
secondary NEC I15.9
due to
endocrine disorders I15.2
pheochromocytoma I15.2
renal disorders NEC I15.1
arterial I15.0
renovascular disorders I15.0
specified NEC I15.8
venous (chronic)
due to
deep vein thrombosis — *see* Syndrome, postthrombotic
idiopathic I87.309
with
inflammation I87.32- ☑
with ulcer I87.33- ☑
specified complication NEC I87.39- ☑
ulcer I87.31- ☑
with inflammation I87.33- ☑
asymptomatic I87.30- ☑
Hypertensive urgency — *see* Hypertension
Hyperthecosis ovary E28.8
Hyperthermia (of unknown origin) (*see also* Hyperpyrexia)
malignant, due to anesthesia T88.3 ☑
newborn P81.9
environmental P81.0
Hyperthyroid (recurrent) — *see* Hyperthyroidism
Hyperthyroidism (latent) (pre-adult) (recurrent) E05.90
with
goiter (diffuse) E05.00
with thyroid storm E05.01
nodular (multinodular) E05.20
with thyroid storm E05.21
uninodular E05.10
with thyroid storm E05.11
storm E05.91
due to ectopic thyroid tissue E05.30
with thyroid storm E05.31
neonatal, transitory P72.1
specified NEC E05.80
with thyroid storm E05.81
Hypertony, hypertonia, hypertonicity
bladder N31.8
congenital P94.1
stomach K31.89
psychogenic F45.8
uterus, uterine (contractions) (complicating delivery) O62.4
Hypertrichosis L68.9
congenital Q84.2
eyelid H02.869
left H02.866
lower H02.865
upper H02.864
right H02.863
lower H02.862
upper H02.861
lanuginosa Q84.2
acquired L68.1
localized L68.2
specified NEC L68.8
Hypertriglyceridemia, essential E78.1
Hypertrophy, hypertrophic
adenofibromatous, prostate — *see* Enlargement, enlarged, prostate
adenoids (infective) J35.2
with tonsils J35.3
adrenal cortex E27.8
alveolar process or ridge — *see* Anomaly, alveolar
anal papillae K62.89
artery I77.89
congenital NEC Q27.8
digestive system Q27.8
lower limb Q27.8
specified site NEC Q27.8
upper limb Q27.8
auricular — *see* Hypertrophy, cardiac

Hypertrophy — *continued*

Bartholin's gland N75.8
bile duct (common) (hepatic) K83.8
bladder (sphincter) (trigone) N32.89
bone M89.30
carpus M89.34- ☑
clavicle M89.31- ☑
femur M89.35- ☑
fibula M89.36- ☑
finger M89.34- ☑
humerus M89.32- ☑
ilium M89.359
ischium M89.359
metacarpus M89.34- ☑
metatarsus M89.37- ☑
multiple sites M89.39
neck M89.38
radius M89.33- ☑
rib M89.38
scapula M89.31- ☑
skull M89.38
tarsus M89.37- ☑
tibia M89.36- ☑
toe M89.37- ☑
ulna M89.33- ☑
vertebra M89.38
brain G93.89
breast N62
cystic — *see* Mastopathy, cystic
newborn P83.4
pubertal, massive N62
puerperal, postpartum — *see* Disorder, breast, specified type NEC
senile (parenchymatous) N62
cardiac (chronic) (idiopathic) I51.7
with rheumatic fever (conditions in I00)
active I01.8
inactive or quiescent (with chorea) I09.89
congenital NEC Q24.8
fatty — *see* Degeneration, myocardial
hypertensive — *see* Hypertension, heart
rheumatic (with chorea) I09.89
active or acute I01.8
with chorea I02.0
valve — *see* Endocarditis
cartilage — *see* Disorder, cartilage, specified type NEC
cecum — *see* Megacolon
cervix (uteri) N88.8
congenital Q51.828
elongation N88.4
clitoris (cirrhotic) N90.89
congenital Q52.6
colon (*see also* Megacolon)
congenital Q43.2
conjunctiva, lymphoid H11.89
corpora cavernosa N48.89
cystic duct K82.8
duodenum K31.89
endometrium (glandular) (*see also* Hyperplasia, endometrial) N85.00- ☑
cervix N88.8
epididymis N50.8
esophageal hiatus (congenital) Q79.1
with hernia — *see* Hernia, hiatal
eyelid — *see* Disorder, eyelid, specified type NEC
fat pad E65
knee (infrapatellar) (popliteal) (prepatellar) (retropatellar) M79.4
foot (congenital) Q74.2
frenulum, frenum (tongue) K14.8
lip K13.0
gallbladder K82.8
gastric mucosa K29.60
with bleeding K29.61
gland, glandular R59.9
generalized R59.1
localized R59.0
gum (mucous membrane) K06.1
heart (idiopathic) (*see also* Hypertrophy, cardiac)
valve (*see also* Endocarditis) I38
hemifacial Q67.4
hepatic — *see* Hypertrophy, liver
hiatus (esophageal) Q79.1
hilus gland R59.0
hymen, congenital Q52.4
ileum K63.89
intestine NEC K63.89
jejunum K63.89
kidney (compensatory) N28.81
congenital Q63.3
labium (majus) (minus) N90.6

☑ **Additional character required**

Hypertrophy — *continued*
- ligament — *see* Disorder, ligament
- lingual tonsil (infective) J35.1
  - with adenoids J35.3
- lip K13.0
  - congenital Q18.6
- liver R16.0
  - acute K76.89
  - congenital Q44.7
  - cirrhotic — *see* Cirrhosis, liver
  - fatty — *see* Fatty, liver
- lymph, lymphatic gland R59.9
  - generalized R59.1
  - localized R59.0
  - tuberculous — *see* Tuberculosis, lymph gland
- mammary gland — *see* Hypertrophy, breast
- Meckel's diverticulum (congenital) Q43.0
  - malignant — *see* Table of Neoplasms, small intestine, malignant
- median bar — *see* Hyperplasia, prostate
- meibomian gland — *see* Chalazion
- meniscus, knee, congenital Q74.1
- metatarsal head — *see* Hypertrophy, bone, metatarsus
- metatarsus — *see* Hypertrophy, bone, metatarsus
- mucous membrane
  - alveolar ridge K06.2
  - gum K06.1
  - nose (turbinate) J34.3
- muscle M62.89
- muscular coat, artery I77.89
- myocardium (*see also* Hypertrophy, cardiac)
  - idiopathic I42.2
- myometrium N85.2
- nail L60.2
  - congenital Q84.5
- nasal J34.89
  - alae J34.89
  - bone J34.89
  - cartilage J34.89
  - mucous membrane (septum) J34.3
  - sinus J34.89
  - turbinate J34.3
- nasopharynx, lymphoid (infectional) (tissue) (wall) J35.2
- nipple N62
- organ or site, congenital NEC — *see* Anomaly, by site
- ovary N83.8
- palate (hard) M27.8
  - soft K13.79
- pancreas, congenital Q45.3
- parathyroid (gland) E21.0
- parotid gland K11.1
- penis N48.89
- pharyngeal tonsil J35.2
- pharynx J39.2
  - lymphoid (infectional) (tissue) (wall) J35.2
- pituitary (anterior) (fossa) (gland) E23.6
- prepuce (congenital) N47.8
  - female N90.89
- prostate — *see* Enlargement, enlarged, prostate
  - congenital Q55.4
- pseudomuscular G71.0
- pylorus (adult) (muscle) (sphincter) K31.1
  - congenital or infantile Q40.0
- rectal, rectum (sphincter) K62.89
- rhinitis (turbinate) J31.0
- salivary gland (any) K11.1
  - congenital Q38.4
- scaphoid (tarsal) — *see* Hypertrophy, bone, tarsus
- scar L91.0
- scrotum N50.8
- seminal vesicle N50.8
- sigmoid — *see* Megacolon
- skin L91.9
  - specified NEC L91.8
- spermatic cord N50.8
- spleen — *see* Splenomegaly
- spondylitis — *see* Spondylosis
- stomach K31.89
- sublingual gland K11.1
- submandibular gland K11.1
- suprarenal cortex (gland) E27.8
- synovial NEC M67.20
  - acromioclavicular M67.21- ☑
  - ankle M67.27- ☑
  - elbow M67.22- ☑
  - foot M67.27- ☑
  - hand M67.24- ☑
  - hip M67.25- ☑
  - knee M67.26- ☑

Hypertrophy — *continued*
- multiple sites M67.29
- specified site NEC M67.28
- wrist M67.23- ☑
- tendon — *see* Disorder, tendon, specified type NEC
- testis N44.8
  - congenital Q55.29
- thymic, thymus (gland) (congenital) E32.0
- thyroid (gland) — *see* Goiter
- toe (congenital) Q74.2
  - acquired (*see also* Deformity, toe, specified NEC)
- tongue K14.8
  - congenital Q38.2
  - papillae (foliate) K14.3
- tonsils (faucial) (infective) (lingual) (lymphoid) J35.1
  - with adenoids J35.3
- tunica vaginalis N50.8
- ureter N28.89
- urethra N36.8
- uterus N85.2
  - neck (with elongation) N88.4
  - puerperal O90.89
- uvula K13.79
- vagina N89.8
- vas deferens N50.8
- vein I87.8
- ventricle, ventricular (heart) (*see also* Hypertrophy, cardiac)
  - congenital Q24.8
  - in tetralogy of Fallot Q21.3
- verumontanum N36.8
- vocal cord J38.3
- vulva N90.6
  - stasis (nonfilarial) N90.6
Hypertropia H50.2- ☑
Hypertyrosinemia E70.21
Hyperuricemia (asymptomatic) E79.0
Hypervalinemia E71.19
Hyperventilation (tetany) R06.4
- hysterical F45.8
- psychogenic F45.8
- syndrome F45.8
Hypervitaminosis (dietary) NEC E67.8
- A E67.0
  - administered as drug (prolonged intake) — *see* Table of Drugs and Chemicals, vitamins, adverse effect
  - overdose or wrong substance given or taken — *see* Table of Drugs and Chemicals, vitamins, poisoning
- B6 E67.2
- D E67.3
  - administered as drug (prolonged intake) — *see* Table of Drugs and Chemicals, vitamins, adverse effect
  - overdose or wrong substance given or taken — *see* Table of Drugs and Chemicals, vitamins, poisoning
- K E67.8
  - administered as drug (prolonged intake) — *see* Table of Drugs and Chemicals, vitamins, adverse effect
  - overdose or wrong substance given or taken — *see* Table of Drugs and Chemicals, vitamins, poisoning
Hypervolemia E87.70
- specified NEC E87.79
Hypesthesia R20.1
- cornea — *see* Anesthesia, cornea
Hyphema H21.0- ☑
- traumatic S05.1- ☑
Hypoacidity, gastric K31.89
- psychogenic F45.8
Hypoadrenalism, hypoadrenia E27.40
- primary E27.1
- tuberculous A18.7
Hypoadrenocorticism E27.40
- pituitary E23.0
- primary E27.1
Hypoalbuminemia E88.09
Hypoaldosteronism E27.40
Hypoalphalipoproteinemia E78.6
Hypobarism T70.29 ☑
Hypobaropathy T70.29 ☑
Hypobetalipoproteinemia (familial) E78.6
Hypocalcemia E83.51
- dietary E58
- neonatal P71.1
  - due to cow's milk P71.0
- phosphate-loading (newborn) P71.1

Hypochloremia E87.8
Hypochlorhydria K31.89
- neurotic F45.8
- psychogenic F45.8
Hypochondria, hypochondriac, hypochondriasis (reaction) F45.21
- sleep F51.03
Hypochondrogenesis Q77.0
Hypochondroplasia Q77.4
Hypochromasia, blood cells D50.8
Hypodontia — *see* Anodontia
Hypoeosinophilia D72.89
Hypoesthesia R20.1
Hypofibrinogenemia D68.8
- acquired D65
- congenital (hereditary) D68.2
Hypofunction
- adrenocortical E27.40
  - drug-induced E27.3
  - postprocedural E89.6
  - primary E27.1
- adrenomedullary, postprocedural E89.6
- cerebral R29.818
- corticoadrenal NEC E27.40
- intestinal K59.8
- labyrinth H83.2
- ovary E28.39
- pituitary (gland) (anterior) E23.0
- testicular E29.1
  - postprocedural (postsurgical) (postirradiation) (iatrogenic) E89.5
Hypogalactia O92.4
Hypogammaglobulinemia (*see also* Agammaglobulinemia) D80.1
- hereditary D80.0
- nonfamilial D80.1
- transient, of infancy D80.7
Hypogenitalism (congenital) — *see* Hypogonadism
Hypoglossia Q38.3
Hypoglycemia (spontaneous) E16.2
- coma E15
  - diabetic — *see* Diabetes, coma
- diabetic — *see* Diabetes, hypoglycemia
- dietary counseling and surveillance Z71.3
- drug-induced E16.0
  - with coma (nondiabetic) E15
- due to insulin E16.0
  - with coma (nondiabetic) E15
  - therapeutic misadventure T38.3
- functional, nonhyperinsulinemic E16.1
- iatrogenic E16.0
  - with coma (nondiabetic) E15
- in infant of diabetic mother P70.1
  - gestational diabetes P70.0
- infantile E16.1
- leucine-induced E71.19
- neonatal (transitory) P70.4
  - iatrogenic P70.3
- reactive (not drug-induced) E16.1
- transitory neonatal P70.4
Hypogonadism
- female E28.39
- hypogonadotropic E23.0
- male E29.1
- ovarian (primary) E28.39
- pituitary E23.0
- testicular (primary) E29.1
Hypohidrosis, hypoidrosis L74.4
Hypoinsulinemia, postprocedural E89.1
Hypokalemia E87.6
Hypoleukocytosis — *see* Agranulocytosis
Hypolipoproteinemia (alpha) (beta) E78.6
Hypomagnesemia E83.42
- neonatal P71.2
Hypomania, hypomanic reaction F30.8
Hypomenorrhea — *see* Oligomenorrhea
Hypometabolism R63.8
Hypomotility
- gastrointestinal (tract) K31.89
  - psychogenic F45.8
- intestine K59.8
  - psychogenic F45.8
- stomach K31.89
  - psychogenic F45.8
Hyponasality R49.22
Hyponatremia E87.1
Hypo-osmolality E87.1
Hypo-ovarianism, hypo-ovarism E28.39
Hypoparathyroidism E20.9
- familial E20.8
- idiopathic E20.0
- neonatal, transitory P71.4

Hypoparathyroidism — *continued*
 postprocedural E89.2
 specified NEC E20.8
Hypoperfusion (in)
 newborn P96.89
Hypopharyngitis — *see* Laryngopharyngitis
Hypophoria H50.53
Hypophosphatemia, hypophosphatasia (acquired) (congenital) (renal) E83.39
 familial E83.31
Hypophyseal, hypophysis (*see also* condition)
 dwarfism E23.0
 gigantism E22.0
Hypopiesis — *see* Hypotension
Hypopinealism E34.8
Hypopituitarism (juvenile) E23.0
 drug-induced E23.1
 due to
  hypophysectomy E89.3
  radiotherapy E89.3
 iatrogenic NEC E23.1
 postirradiation E89.3
 postpartum E23.0
 postprocedural E89.3
Hypoplasia, hypoplastic
 adrenal (gland), congenital Q89.1
 alimentary tract, congenital Q45.8
  upper Q40.8
 anus, anal (canal) Q42.3
  with fistula Q42.2
 aorta, aortic Q25.4
  ascending, in hypoplastic left heart syndrome Q23.4
  valve Q23.1
   in hypoplastic left heart syndrome Q23.4
 areola, congenital Q83.8
 arm (congenital) — *see* Defect, reduction, upper limb
 artery (peripheral) Q27.8
  brain (congenital) Q28.3
  coronary Q24.5
  digestive system Q27.8
  lower limb Q27.8
  pulmonary Q25.79
   functional, unilateral J43.0
  retinal (congenital) Q14.1
  specified site NEC Q27.8
  umbilical Q27.0
  upper limb Q27.8
 auditory canal Q17.8
  causing impairment of hearing Q16.9
 biliary duct or passage Q44.5
 bone NOS Q79.9
  face Q75.8
  marrow D61.9
   megakaryocytic D69.49
  skull — *see* Hypoplasia, skull
 brain Q02
  gyri Q04.3
  part of Q04.3
 breast (areola) N64.82
 bronchus Q32.4
 cardiac Q24.8
 carpus — *see* Defect, reduction, upper limb, specified type NEC
 cartilage hair Q78.5
 cecum Q42.8
 cementum K00.4
 cephalic Q02
 cerebellum Q04.3
 cervix (uteri), congenital Q51.821
 clavicle (congenital) Q74.0
 coccyx Q76.49
 colon Q42.9
  specified NEC Q42.8
 corpus callosum Q04.0
 cricoid cartilage Q31.2
 digestive organ (s) or tract NEC Q45.8
  upper (congenital) Q40.8
 ear (auricle) (lobe) Q17.2
  middle Q16.4
 enamel of teeth (neonatal) (postnatal) (prenatal) K00.4
 endocrine (gland) NEC Q89.2
 endometrium N85.8
 epididymis (congenital) Q55.4
 epiglottis Q31.2
 erythroid, congenital D61.01
 esophagus (congenital) Q39.8
 eustachian tube Q17.8
 eye Q11.2
 eyelid (congenital) Q10.3

Hypoplasia — *continued*
 face Q18.8
  bone (s) Q75.8
 femur (congenital) — *see* Defect, reduction, lower limb, specified type NEC
 fibula (congenital) — *see* Defect, reduction, lower limb, specified type NEC
 finger (congenital) — *see* Defect, reduction, upper limb, specified type NEC
 focal dermal Q82.8
 foot — *see* Defect, reduction, lower limb, specified type NEC
 gallbladder Q44.0
 genitalia, genital organ (s)
  female, congenital Q52.8
   external Q52.79
   internal NEC Q52.8
  in adiposogenital dystrophy E23.6
 glottis Q31.2
 hair Q84.2
 hand (congenital) — *see* Defect, reduction, upper limb, specified type NEC
 heart Q24.8
 humerus (congenital) — *see* Defect, reduction, upper limb, specified type NEC
 intestine (small) Q41.9
  large Q42.9
   specified NEC Q42.8
 jaw M26.09
  alveolar M26.79
  lower M26.04
   alveolar M26.74
  upper M26.02
   alveolar M26.73
 kidney (s) Q60.5
  bilateral Q60.4
  unilateral Q60.3
 labium (majus) (minus), congenital Q52.79
 larynx Q31.2
 left heart syndrome Q23.4
 leg (congenital) — *see* Defect, reduction, lower limb
 limb Q73.8
  lower (congenital) — *see* Defect, reduction, lower limb
  upper (congenital) — *see* Defect, reduction, upper limb
 liver Q44.7
 lung (lobe) (not associated with short gestation) Q33.6
  associated with immaturity, low birth weight, prematurity, or short gestation P28.0
 mammary (areola), congenital Q83.8
 mandible, mandibular M26.04
  alveolar M26.74
  unilateral condylar M27.8
 maxillary M26.02
  alveolar M26.73
 medullary D61.9
 megakaryocytic D69.49
 metacarpus — *see* Defect, reduction, upper limb, specified type NEC
 metatarsus — *see* Defect, reduction, lower limb, specified type NEC
 muscle Q79.8
 nail (s) Q84.6
 nose, nasal Q30.1
 optic nerve H47.03- ☑
 osseous meatus (ear) Q17.8
 ovary, congenital Q50.39
 pancreas Q45.0
 parathyroid (gland) Q89.2
 parotid gland Q38.4
 patella Q74.1
 pelvis, pelvic girdle Q74.2
 penis (congenital) Q55.62
 peripheral vascular system Q27.8
  digestive system Q27.8
  lower limb Q27.8
  specified site NEC Q27.8
  upper limb Q27.8
 pituitary (gland) (congenital) Q89.2
 pulmonary (not associated with short gestation) Q33.6
  artery, functional J43.0
  associated with short gestation P28.0
 radioulnar — *see* Defect, reduction, upper limb, specified type NEC
 radius — *see* Defect, reduction, upper limb
 rectum Q42.1
  with fistula Q42.0
 respiratory system NEC Q34.8

Hypoplasia — *continued*
 rib Q76.6
 right heart syndrome Q22.6
 sacrum Q76.49
 scapula Q74.0
 scrotum Q55.1
 shoulder girdle Q74.0
 skin Q82.8
 skull (bone) Q75.8
  with
   anencephaly Q00.0
   encephalocele — *see* Encephalocele
   hydrocephalus Q03.9
    with spina bifida — *see* Spina bifida, by site, with hydrocephalus
   microcephaly Q02
 spinal (cord) (ventral horn cell) Q06.1
 spine Q76.49
 sternum Q76.7
 tarsus — *see* Defect, reduction, lower limb, specified type NEC
 testis Q55.1
 thymic, with immunodeficiency D82.1
 thymus (gland) Q89.2
  with immunodeficiency D82.1
 thyroid (gland) E03.1
  cartilage Q31.2
 tibiofibular (congenital) — *see* Defect, reduction, lower limb, specified type NEC
 toe — *see* Defect, reduction, lower limb, specified type NEC
 tongue Q38.3
 Turner's K00.4
 ulna (congenital) — *see* Defect, reduction, upper limb
 umbilical artery Q27.0
 unilateral condylar M27.8
 ureter Q62.8
 uterus, congenital Q51.811
 vagina Q52.4
 vascular NEC peripheral Q27.8
  brain Q28.3
  digestive system Q27.8
  lower limb Q27.8
  specified site NEC Q27.8
  upper limb Q27.8
 vein (s) (peripheral) Q27.8
  brain Q28.3
  digestive system Q27.8
  great Q26.8
  lower limb Q27.8
  specified site NEC Q27.8
  upper limb Q27.8
 vena cava (inferior) (superior) Q26.8
 vertebra Q76.49
 vulva, congenital Q52.79
 zonule (ciliary) Q12.8
Hypopotassemia E87.6
Hypoproconvertinemia, congenital (hereditary) D68.2
Hypoproteinemia E77.8
Hypoprothrombinemia (congenital) (hereditary) (idiopathic) D68.2
 acquired D68.4
 newborn, transient P61.6
Hypoptyalism K11.7
Hypopyon (eye) (anterior chamber) — *see* Iridocyclitis, acute, hypopyon
Hypopyrexia R68.0
Hyporeflexia R29.2
Hyposecretion
 ACTH E23.0
 antidiuretic hormone E23.2
 ovary E28.39
 salivary gland (any) K11.7
 vasopressin E23.2
Hyposegmentation, leukocytic, hereditary D72.0
Hyposiderinemia D50.9
Hypospadias Q54.9
 balanic Q54.0
 coronal Q54.0
 glandular Q54.0
 penile Q54.1
 penoscrotal Q54.2
 perineal Q54.3
 specified NEC Q54.8
Hypospermatogenesis — *see* Oligospermia
Hyposplenism D73.0
Hypostasis pulmonary, passive — *see* Edema, lung
Hypostatic — *see* condition
Hyposthenuria N28.89

☑ **Additional character required**

Hypotension (arterial) (constitutional) I95.9
  chronic I95.89
  due to (of) hemodialysis I95.3
  drug-induced I95.2
  iatrogenic I95.89
  idiopathic (permanent) I95.0
  intracranial, following ventricular shunting
    (ventriculostomy) G97.2
  intra-dialytic I95.3
  maternal, syndrome (following labor and
    delivery) O26.5- ☑
  neurogenic, orthostatic G90.3
  orthostatic (chronic) I95.1
    due to drugs I95.2
    neurogenic G90.3
  postoperative I95.81
  postural I95.1
  specified NEC I95.89
Hypothermia (accidental) T68 ☑
  due to anesthesia, anesthetic T88.51 ☑
  low environmental temperature T68 ☑
  neonatal P80.9
    environmental (mild) NEC P80.8
    mild P80.8
    severe (chronic) (cold injury syndrome) P80.0
    specified NEC P80.8
  not associated with low environmental
    temperature R68.0
Hypothyroidism (acquired) E03.9
  congenital (without goiter) E03.1
    with goiter (diffuse) E03.0
  due to
    exogenous substance NEC E03.2
    iodine-deficiency, acquired E01.8
      subclinical E02
    irradiation therapy E89.0
    medicament NEC E03.2
    P-aminosalicylic acid (PAS) E03.2
    phenylbutazone E03.2
    resorcinol E03.2
    sulfonamide E03.2
    surgery E89.0
    thiourea group drugs E03.2
  iatrogenic NEC E03.2
  iodine-deficiency (acquired) E01.8
    congenital — see Syndrome, iodine- deficiency,
      congenital
    subclinical E02
  neonatal, transitory P72.2
  postinfectious E03.3
  postirradiation E89.0
  postprocedural E89.0
  postsurgical E89.0
  specified NEC E03.8
  subclinical, iodine-deficiency related E02
Hypotonia, hypotonicity, hypotony
  bladder N31.2
  congenital (benign) P94.2
  eye — see Disorder, globe, hypotony
Hypotrichosis — see Alopecia
Hypotropia H50.2- ☑
Hypoventilation R06.89
  congenital central alveolar G47.35
  sleep related
    idiopathic nonobstructive alveolar G47.34
    in conditions classified elsewhere G47.36
Hypovitaminosis — see Deficiency, vitamin
Hypovolemia E86.1
  surgical shock T81.19 ☑
  traumatic (shock) T79.4 ☑
Hypoxemia R09.02
  newborn P84
  sleep related, in conditions classified elsewhere
    G47.36
Hypoxia (see also Anoxia) R09.02
  cerebral, during a procedure NEC G97.81
    postprocedural NEC G97.82
  intrauterine P84
  myocardial — see Insufficiency, coronary
  newborn P84
  sleep-related G47.34
Hypsarhythmia — see Epilepsy, generalized,
  specified NEC
Hysteralgia, pregnant uterus O26.89- ☑
Hysteria, hysterical (conversion) (dissociative state)
  F44.9
  anxiety F41.8
  convulsions F44.5
  psychosis, acute F44.9
Hysteroepilepsy F44.5

I

Ichthyoparasitism due to Vandellia cirrhosa B88.8
Ichthyosis (congenital) Q80.9
  acquired L85.0
  fetalis Q80.4
  hystrix Q80.8
  lamellar Q80.2
  lingual K13.29
  palmaris and plantaris Q82.8
  simplex Q80.0
  vera Q80.8
  vulgaris Q80.0
  X-linked Q80.1
Ichthyotoxism — see Poisoning, fish
  bacterial — see Intoxication, foodborne
Icteroanemia, hemolytic (acquired) D59.9
  congenital — see Spherocytosis
Icterus (see also Jaundice)
  conjunctiva R17
  newborn P59.9
  gravis, newborn P55.0
  hematogenous (acquired) D59.9
  hemolytic (acquired) D59.9
    congenital — see Spherocytosis
  hemorrhagic (acute) (leptospiral) (spirochetal)
    A27.0
    newborn P53
  infectious B15.9
    with hepatic coma B15.0
    leptospiral A27.0
    spirochetal A27.0
  neonatorum — see Jaundice, newborn
  spirochetal A27.0
Ictus solaris, solis T67.0 ☑
Ideation
  homicidal R45.850
  suicidal R45.851
Identity disorder (child) F64.9
  gender role F64.2
  psychosexual F64.2
Id reaction (due to bacteria) L30.2
Idioglossia F80.0
Idiopathic — see condition
Idiot, idiocy (congenital) F73
  amaurotic (Bielschowsky(-Jansky)) (family)
    (infantile (late)) (juvenile (late)) (Vogt-
    Spielmeyer) E75.4
  microcephalic Q02
IgE asthma J45.909
IIAC (idiopathic infantile arterial calcification) Q28.8
Ileitis (chronic) (noninfectious) (see also Enteritis)
  K52.9
  backwash — see Pancolitis, ulcerative (chronic)
  infectious A09
  regional (ulcerative) — see Enteritis, regional,
    small intestine
  segmental — see Enteritis, regional
  terminal (ulcerative) — see Enteritis, regional,
    small intestine
Ileocolitis (see also Enteritis) K52.9
  regional — see Enteritis, regional
  infectious A09
Ileostomy
  attention to Z43.2
  malfunctioning K94.13
  status Z93.2
    with complication — see Complications,
      enterostomy
Ileotyphus — see Typhoid
Ileum — see condition
Ileus (bowel) (colon) (inhibitory) (intestine) K56.7
  adynamic K56.0
  due to gallstone (in intestine) K56.3
  duodenal (chronic) K31.5
  gallstone K56.3
  mechanical NEC K56.69
  meconium P76.0
    in cystic fibrosis E84.11
    meaning meconium plug (without cystic
      fibrosis) P76.0
  myxedema K59.8
  neurogenic K56.0
    Hirschsprung's disease or megacolon Q43.1
  newborn
    due to meconium P76.0
      in cystic fibrosis E84.11
      meaning meconium plug (without cystic
        fibrosis) P76.0
    transitory P76.1
  obstructive K56.69

Ileus — continued
  paralytic K56.0
Iliac — see condition
Iliotibial band syndrome M76.3- ☑
Illiteracy Z55.0
Illness (see also Disease) R69
  manic-depressive — see Disorder, bipolar
Imbalance R26.89
  autonomic G90.8
  constituents of food intake E63.1
  electrolyte E87.8
    with
      abortion — see Abortion by type,
        complicated by, electrolyte imbalance
      molar pregnancy O08.5
    due to hyperemesis gravidarum O21.1
    following ectopic or molar pregnancy O08.5
    neonatal, transitory NEC P74.4
      potassium P74.3
      sodium P74.2
  endocrine E34.9
  eye muscle NOS H50.9
  hormone E34.9
  hysterical F44.4
  labyrinth H83.2
  posture R29.3
  protein-energy — see Malnutrition
  sympathetic G90.8
Imbecile, imbecility (I.Q.35-49) F71
Imbedding, intrauterine device T83.39 ☑
Imbibition, cholesterol (gallbladder) K82.4
Imbrication, teeth,, fully erupted M26.30
Imerslund (-Gräsbeck) syndrome D51.1
Immature (see also Immaturity)
  birth (less than 37 completed weeks) — see
    Preterm, newborn
  extremely (less than 28 completed weeks) —
    see Immaturity, extreme
  personality F60.89
Immaturity (less than 37 completed weeks) (see also
  Preterm, newborn)
  extreme of newborn (less than 28 completed
    weeks of gestation) (less than 196 completed
    days of gestation) (unspecified weeks of
    gestation) P07.20
    gestational age
      23 completed weeks (23 weeks, 0 days
        through 23 weeks, 6 days) P07.22
      24 completed weeks (24 weeks, 0 days
        through 24 weeks, 6 days) P07.23
      25 completed weeks (25 weeks, 0 days
        through 25 weeks, 6 days) P07.24
      26 completed weeks (26 weeks, 0 days
        through 26 weeks, 6 days) P07.25
      27 completed weeks (27 weeks, 0 days
        through 27 weeks, 6 days) P07.26
      less than 23 completed weeks P07.21
  fetus or infant light-for-dates — see Light-for-
    dates
  lung, newborn P28.0
  organ or site NEC — see Hypoplasia
  pulmonary, newborn P28.0
  reaction F60.89
  sexual (female) (male), after puberty E30.0
Immersion T75.1 ☑
  hand T69.01- ☑
  foot T69.02- ☑
Immobile, immobility
  complete, due to severe physical disability or
    frailty R53.2
  intestine K59.8
  syndrome (paraplegic) M62.3
Immune reconstitution (inflammatory) syndrome
  [IRIS] D89.3
Immunization (see also Vaccination)
  ABO — see Incompatibility, ABO
    in newborn P55.1
  complication — see Complications, vaccination
  encounter for Z23
  not done (not carried out) Z28.9
    because (of)
      acute illness of patient Z28.01
      allergy to vaccine (or component) Z28.04
      caregiver refusal Z28.82
      chronic illness of patient Z28.02
      contraindication NEC Z28.09
      group pressure Z28.1
      guardian refusal Z28.82
      immune compromised state of patient
        Z28.03
      parent refusal Z28.82
      patient's belief Z28.1

Immunization — *continued*
- patient had disease being vaccinated against Z28.81
- patient refusal Z28.21
- religious beliefs of patient Z28.1
- specified reason NEC Z28.89
  - of patient Z28.29
- unspecified patient reason Z28.20
- Rh factor
  - affecting management of pregnancy NEC O36.09- ☑
    - anti-D antibody O36.01- ☑
  - from transfusion — *see* Complication(s), transfusion, incompatibility reaction, Rh (factor)

Immunocytoma C83.0- ☑

Immunodeficiency D84.9
- with
  - adenosine-deaminase deficiency D81.3
  - antibody defects D80.9
    - specified type NEC D80.8
  - hyperimmunoglobulinemia D80.6
  - increased immunoglobulin M (IgM) D80.5
  - major defect D82.9
    - specified type NEC D82.8
  - partial albinism D82.8
  - short-limbed stature D82.2
  - thrombocytopenia and eczema D82.0
- antibody with
  - hyperimmunoglobulinemia D80.6
  - near-normal immunoglobulins D80.6
- autosomal recessive, Swiss type D80.0
- combined D81.9
  - biotin-dependent carboxylase D81.819
    - biotinidase D81.810
    - holocarboxylase synthetase D81.818
    - specified type NEC D81.818
  - severe (SCID) D81.9
    - with
      - low or normal B-cell numbers D81.2
      - low T- and B-cell numbers D81.1
      - reticular dysgenesis D81.0
    - specified type NEC D81.89
- common variable D83.9
  - with
    - abnormalities of B-cell numbers and function D83.0
    - autoantibodies to B- or T-cells D83.2
    - immunoregulatory T-cell disorders D83.1
  - specified type NEC D83.8
- following hereditary defective response to Epstein-Barr virus (EBV) D82.3
- selective, immunoglobulin
  - A (IgA) D80.2
  - G (IgG) (subclasses) D80.3
  - M (IgM) D80.4
- severe combined (SCID) D81.9
- specified type NEC D84.8
- X-linked, with increased IgM D80.5

Immunotherapy (encounter for)
- antineoplastic Z51.12

Impaction, impacted
- bowel, colon, rectum (*see also* Impaction, fecal) K56.49
  - by gallstone K56.3
- calculus — *see* Calculus
- cerumen (ear) (external) H61.2- ☑
- cuspid — *see* Impaction, tooth
- dental (same or adjacent tooth) K01.1
- fecal, feces K56.41
- fracture — *see* Fracture, by site
- gallbladder — *see* Calculus, gallbladder
- gallstone (s) — *see* Calculus, gallbladder
  - bile duct (common) (hepatic) — *see* Calculus, bile duct
  - cystic duct — *see* Calculus, gallbladder
  - in intestine, with obstruction (any part) K56.3
- intestine (calculous) NEC (*see also* Impaction, fecal) K56.49
  - gallstone, with ileus K56.3
- intrauterine device (IUD) T83.39 ☑
- molar — *see* Impaction, tooth
- shoulder, causing obstructed labor O66.0
- tooth, teeth K01.1
- turbinate J34.89

Impaired, impairment (function)
- auditory discrimination — *see* Abnormal, auditory perception
- cognitive, mild, so stated G31.84
- dual sensory Z73.82
- fasting glucose R73.01
- glucose tolerance (oral) R73.02

Impaired — *continued*
- hearing — *see* Deafness
- heart — *see* Disease, heart
- kidney N28.9
  - disorder resulting from N25.9
    - specified NEC N25.89
- liver K72.90
  - with coma K72.91
- mastication K08.8
- mild cognitive, so stated G31.84
- mobility
  - ear ossicles — *see* Ankylosis, ear ossicles
  - requiring care provider Z74.09
- myocardium, myocardial — *see* Insufficiency, myocardial
- rectal sphincter R19.8
- renal (acute) (chronic) N28.9
  - disorder resulting from N25.9
    - specified NEC N25.89
- vision NEC H54.7
  - both eyes H54.3

Impediment, speech R47.9
- psychogenic (childhood) F98.8
- slurring R47.81
- specified NEC R47.89

Impending
- coronary syndrome I20.0
- delirium tremens F10.239
- myocardial infarction I20.0

Imperception auditory (acquired) (*see also* Deafness)
- congenital H93.25

Imperfect
- aeration, lung (newborn) NEC — *see* Atelectasis
- closure (congenital)
  - alimentary tract NEC Q45.8
    - lower Q43.8
    - upper Q40.8
  - atrioventricular ostium Q21.2
  - atrium (secundum) Q21.1
  - branchial cleft or sinus Q18.0
  - choroid Q14.3
  - cricoid cartilage Q31.8
  - cusps, heart valve NEC Q24.8
    - pulmonary Q22.3
  - ductus
    - arteriosus Q25.0
    - Botalli Q25.0
  - ear drum (causing impairment of hearing) Q16.4
  - esophagus with communication to bronchus or trachea Q39.1
  - eyelid Q10.3
  - foramen
    - botalli Q21.1
    - ovale Q21.1
  - genitalia, genital organ (s) or system
    - female Q52.8
      - external Q52.79
      - internal NEC Q52.8
    - male Q55.8
  - glottis Q31.8
  - interatrial ostium or septum Q21.1
  - interauricular ostium or septum Q21.1
  - interventricular ostium or septum Q21.0
  - larynx Q31.8
  - lip — *see* Cleft, lip
  - nasal septum Q30.3
  - nose Q30.2
  - omphalomesenteric duct Q43.0
  - optic nerve entry Q14.2
  - organ or site not listed — *see* Anomaly, by site
  - ostium
    - interatrial Q21.1
    - interauricular Q21.1
    - interventricular Q21.0
  - palate — *see* Cleft, palate
  - preauricular sinus Q18.1
  - retina Q14.1
  - roof of orbit Q75.8
  - sclera Q13.5
  - septum
    - aorticopulmonary Q21.4
    - atrial (secundum) Q21.1
    - between aorta and pulmonary artery Q21.4
  - heart Q21.9
  - interatrial (secundum) Q21.1
  - interauricular (secundum) Q21.1
  - interventricular Q21.0
    - in tetralogy of Fallot Q21.3
  - nasal Q30.3
  - ventricular Q21.0

Imperfect — *continued*
- with pulmonary stenosis or atresia, dextraposition of aorta, and hypertrophy of right ventricle Q21.3
  - in tetralogy of Fallot Q21.3
- skull Q75.0
  - with
    - anencephaly Q00.0
    - encephalocele — *see* Encephalocele
    - hydrocephalus Q03.9
      - with spina bifida — *see* Spina bifida, by site, with hydrocephalus
    - microcephaly Q02
- spine (with meningocele) — *see* Spina bifida
- trachea Q32.1
- tympanic membrane (causing impairment of hearing) Q16.4
- uterus Q51.818
- vitelline duct Q43.0
- erection — *see* Dysfunction, sexual, male, erectile
- fusion — *see* Imperfect, closure
- inflation, lung (newborn) — *see* Atelectasis
- posture R29.3
- rotation, intestine Q43.3
- septum, ventricular Q21.0

Imperfectly descended testis — *see* Cryptorchid

Imperforate (congenital) (*see also* Atresia)
- anus Q42.3
  - with fistula Q42.2
- cervix (uteri) Q51.828
- esophagus Q39.0
  - with tracheoesophageal fistula Q39.1
- hymen Q52.3
- jejunum Q41.1
- pharynx Q38.8
- rectum Q42.1
  - with fistula Q42.0
- urethra Q64.39
- vagina Q52.4

Impervious (congenital) (*see also* Atresia)
- anus Q42.3
  - with fistula Q42.2
- bile duct Q44.2
- esophagus Q39.0
  - with tracheoesophageal fistula Q39.1
- intestine (small) Q41.9
  - large Q42.9
    - specified NEC Q42.8
- rectum Q42.1
  - with fistula Q42.0
- ureter — *see* Atresia, ureter
- urethra Q64.39

Impetiginization of dermatoses L01.1

Impetigo (any organism) (any site) (circinate) (contagiosa) (simplex) (vulgaris) L01.00
- Bockhart's L01.02
- bullous, bullosa L01.03
- external ear L01.00 [H62.40]
- follicularis L01.02
- furfuracea L30.5
- herpetiformis L40.1
  - nonobstetrical L40.1
- neonatorum L01.03
- nonbullous L01.01
- specified type NEC L01.09
- ulcerative L01.09

Impingement (on teeth)
- soft tissue
  - anterior M26.81
  - posterior M26.82

Implant, endometrial N80.9

Implantation
- anomalous — *see* Anomaly, by site
  - ureter Q62.63
- cyst
  - external area or site (skin) NEC L72.0
  - iris — *see* Cyst, iris, implantation
  - vagina N89.8
  - vulva N90.7
- dermoid (cyst) — *see* Implantation, cyst

Impotence (sexual) N52.9
- counseling Z70.1
- organic origin (*see also* Dysfunction, sexual, male, erectile) N52.9
- psychogenic F52.21

Impression, basilar Q75.8

Imprisonment, anxiety concerning Z65.1

Improper care (child) (newborn) — *see* Maltreatment

Improperly tied umbilical cord (causing hemorrhage) P51.8

Impulsiveness (impulsive) R45.87

Inability to swallow — see Aphagia
Inaccessible, inaccessibility
  health care NEC Z75.3
    due to
      waiting period Z75.2
        for admission to facility elsewhere Z75.1
    other helping agencies Z75.4
Inactive — see condition
Inadequate, inadequacy
  aesthetics of dental restoration K08.56
  biologic, constitutional, functional, or social F60.7
  development
    child R62.50
    genitalia
      after puberty NEC E30.0
      congenital
        female Q52.8
          external Q52.79
          internal Q52.8
        male Q55.8
    lungs Q33.6
      associated with short gestation P28.0
    organ or site not listed — see Anomaly, by site
  diet (causing nutritional deficiency) E63.9
  eating habits Z72.4
  environment, household Z59.1
  family support Z63.8
  food (supply) NEC Z59.4
    hunger effects T73.0 ☑
  functional F60.7
  household care, due to
    family member
      handicapped or ill Z74.2
      on vacation Z75.5
      temporarily away from home Z74.2
    technical defects in home Z59.1
    temporary absence from home of person
      rendering care Z74.2
  housing (heating) (space) Z59.1
  income (financial) Z59.6
  intrafamilial communication Z63.8
  material resources Z59.9
  mental — see Disability, intellectual
  parental supervision or control of child Z62.0
  personality F60.7
  pulmonary
    function R06.89
      newborn P28.5
    ventilation, newborn P28.5
  sample of cytologic smear
    anus R85.615
    cervix R87.615
    vagina R87.625
  social F60.7
    insurance Z59.7
    skills NEC Z73.4
  supervision of child by parent Z62.0
  teaching affecting education Z55.8
  welfare support Z59.7
Inanition R64
  with edema — see Malnutrition, severe
  due to
    deprivation of food T73.0 ☑
    malnutrition — see Malnutrition
  fever R50.9
Inappropriate
  change in quantitative human chorionic
    gonadotropin (hCG) in early pregnancy
    O02.81
  diet or eating habits Z72.4
  level of quantitative human chorionic
    gonadotropin (hCG) for gestational age in
    early pregnancy O02.81
  secretion
    antidiuretic hormone (ADH) (excessive) E22.2
      deficiency E23.2
    pituitary (posterior) E22.2
Inattention at or after birth — see Neglect
Incarceration, incarcerated
  enterocele K46.0
    gangrenous K46.1
  epiplocele K46.0
    gangrenous K46.1
  exophthalmos K42.0
    gangrenous K42.1
  hernia (see also Hernia, by site, with obstruction)
    with gangrene — see Hernia, by site, with
      gangrene
  iris, in wound — see Injury, eye, laceration, with
    prolapse
  lens, in wound — see Injury, eye, laceration, with
    prolapse

Incarceration — continued
  omphalocele K42.0
  prison, anxiety concerning Z65.1
  rupture — see Hernia, by site
  sarcoepiplocele K46.0
    gangrenous K46.1
  sarcoepiplomphalocele K42.0
    with gangrene K42.1
  uterus N85.8
    gravid O34.51- ☑
      causing obstructed labor O65.5
Incised wound
  external — see Laceration
  internal organs — see Injury, by site
Incision, incisional
  hernia K43.2
    with
      gangrene (and obstruction) K43.1
      obstruction K43.0
  surgical, complication — see Complications,
    surgical procedure
  traumatic
    external — see Laceration
    internal organs — see Injury, by site
Inclusion
  azurophilic leukocytic D72.0
  blennorrhea (neonatal) (newborn) P39.1
  gallbladder in liver (congenital) Q44.1
Incompatibility
  ABO
    affecting management of pregnancy
      O36.11- ☑
      anti-A sensitization O36.11- ☑
      anti-B sensitization O36.19- ☑
      specified NEC O36.19- ☑
    infusion or transfusion reaction — see
      Complication(s), transfusion,
      incompatibility reaction, ABO
    newborn P55.1
  blood (group) (Duffy) (K(ell)) (Kidd) (Lewis) (M)
    (S) NEC
    affecting management of pregnancy
      O36.11- ☑
      anti-A sensitization O36.11- ☑
      anti-B sensitization O36.19- ☑
    infusion or transfusion reaction T80.89 ☑
    newborn P55.8
  divorce or estrangement Z63.5
  Rh (blood group) (factor) Z31.82
    affecting management of pregnancy NEC
      O36.09- ☑
      anti-D antibody O36.01- ☑
    infusion or transfusion reaction — see
      Complication(s), transfusion,
      incompatibility reaction, Rh (factor)
    newborn P55.0
  rhesus — see Incompatibility, Rh
Incompetency, incompetent, incompetence
  annular
    aortic (valve) — see Insufficiency, aortic
    mitral (valve) I34.0
    pulmonary valve (heart) I37.1
  aortic (valve) — see Insufficiency, aortic
  cardiac valve — see Endocarditis
  cervix, cervical (os) N88.3
    in pregnancy O34.3- ☑
  chronotropic I45.89
    with
      autonomic dysfunction G90.8
      ischemic heart disease I25.89
      left ventricular dysfunction I51.89
      sinus node dysfunction I49.8
  esophagogastric (junction) (sphincter) K22.0
  mitral (valve) — see Insufficiency, mitral
  pelvic fundus N81.89
  pubocervical tissue N81.82
  pulmonary valve (heart) I37.1
    congenital Q22.3
  rectovaginal tissue N81.83
  tricuspid (annular) (valve) — see Insufficiency,
    tricuspid
  valvular — see Endocarditis
    congenital Q24.8
  vein, venous (saphenous) (varicose) — see Varix,
    leg
Incomplete (see also condition)
  bladder, emptying R33.9
  defecation R15.0
  expansion lungs (newborn) NEC — see
    Atelectasis
  rotation, intestine Q43.3

Inconclusive
  diagnostic imaging due to excess body fat of
    patient R93.9
  findings on diagnostic imaging of breast NEC
    R92.8
  mammogram (due to dense breasts) R92.2
Incontinence R32
  anal sphincter R15.9
  feces R15.9
    nonorganic origin F98.1
  overflow N39.490
  psychogenic F45.8
  rectal R15.9
  reflex N39.498
  stress (female) (male) N39.3
    and urge N39.46
  urethral sphincter R32
  urge N39.41
    and stress (female) (male) N39.46
  urine (urinary) R32
    continuous N39.45
    due to cognitive impairment, or severe physical
      disability or immobility R39.81
    functional R39.81
    mixed (stress and urge) N39.46
    nocturnal N39.44
    nonorganic origin F98.0
    overflow N39.490
    post dribbling N39.43
    reflex N39.498
    specified NEC N39.498
    stress (female) (male) N39.3
      and urge N39.46
    total N39.498
    unaware N39.42
    urge N39.41
      and stress (female) (male) N39.46
Incontinentia pigmenti Q82.3
Incoordinate, incoordination
  esophageal-pharyngeal (newborn) — see
    Dysphagia
  muscular R27.8
  uterus (action) (contractions) (complicating
    delivery) O62.4
Increase, increased
  abnormal, in development R63.8
  androgens (ovarian) E28.1
  anticoagulants (antithrombin) (anti-VIIIa) (anti-
    IXa) (anti-Xa) (anti-XIa) — see Circulating
    anticoagulants
  cold sense R20.8
  estrogen E28.0
  function
    adrenal
      cortex — see Cushing's, syndrome
      medulla E27.5
    pituitary (gland) (anterior) (lobe) E22.9
      posterior E22.2
  heat sense R20.8
  intracranial pressure (benign) G93.2
  permeability, capillaries I78.8
  pressure, intracranial G93.2
  secretion
    gastrin E16.4
    glucagon E16.3
    pancreas, endocrine E16.9
      growth hormone-releasing hormone E16.8
      pancreatic polypeptide E16.8
      somatostatin E16.8
      vasoactive-intestinal polypeptide E16.8
  sphericity, lens Q12.4
  splenic activity D73.1
  venous pressure I87.8
    portal K76.6
Increta placenta O43.22- ☑
Incrustation, cornea, foreign body (lead)(zinc) — see
  Foreign body, cornea
Incyclophoria H50.54
Incyclotropia — see Cyclotropia
Indeterminate sex Q56.4
India rubber skin Q82.8
Indigestion (acid) (bilious) (functional) K30
  catarrhal K31.89
  due to decomposed food NOS A05.9
  nervous F45.8
  psychogenic F45.8
Indirect — see condition
Induratio penis plastica N48.6
Induration, indurated
  brain G93.89
  breast (fibrous) N64.51
    puerperal, postpartum O92.29

Induration — *continued*
  broad ligament N83.8
  chancre
    anus A51.1
    congenital A50.07
    extragenital NEC A51.2
  corpora cavernosa (penis) (plastic) N48.6
  liver (chronic) K76.89
  lung (black) (chronic) (fibroid) (*see also* Fibrosis, lung) J84.10
    essential brown J84.03
  penile (plastic) N48.6
  phlebitic — *see* Phlebitis
  skin R23.4
Inebriety (without dependence) — *see* Alcohol, intoxication
Inefficiency, kidney N28.9
Inelasticity, skin R23.4
Inequality, leg (length) (acquired) (*see also* Deformity, limb, unequal length)
  congenital — *see* Defect, reduction, lower limb
  lower leg — *see* Deformity, limb, unequal length
Inertia
  bladder (neurogenic) N31.2
  stomach K31.89
    psychogenic F45.8
  uterus, uterine during labor O62.2
    during latent phase of labor O62.0
    primary O62.0
    secondary O62.1
  vesical (neurogenic) N31.2
Infancy, infantile, infantilism (*see also* condition)
  celiac K90.0
  genitalia, genitals (after puberty) E30.0
  Herter's (nontropical sprue) K90.0
  intestinal K90.0
  Lorain E23.0
  pancreatic K86.8
  pelvis M95.5
    with disproportion (fetopelvic) O33.1
      causing obstructed labor O65.1
  pituitary E23.0
  renal N25.0
  uterus — *see* Infantile, genitalia
Infant (s) (*see also* Infancy)
  excessive crying R68.11
  irritable child R68.12
  lack of care — *see* Neglect
  liveborn (singleton) Z38.2
    born in hospital Z38.00
      by cesarean Z38.01
    born outside hospital Z38.1
    multiple NEC Z38.8
      born in hospital Z38.68
        by cesarean Z38.69
      born outside hospital Z38.7
    quadruplet Z38.8
      born in hospital Z38.63
        by cesarean Z38.64
      born outside hospital Z38.7
    quintuplet Z38.8
      born in hospital Z38.65
        by cesarean Z38.66
      born outside hospital Z38.7
    triplet Z38.8
      born in hospital Z38.61
        by cesarean Z38.62
      born outside hospital Z38.7
    twin Z38.5
      born in hospital Z38.30
        by cesarean Z38.31
      born outside hospital Z38.4
  of diabetic mother (syndrome of) P70.1
    gestational diabetes P70.0
Infantile (*see also* condition)
  genitalia, genitals E30.0
  os, uterine E30.0
  penis E30.0
  testis E29.1
  uterus E30.0
Infantilism — *see* Infancy
Infarct, infarction
  adrenal (capsule) (gland) E27.49
  appendices epiploicae K55.0
  bowel K55.0
  brain (stem) — *see* Infarct, cerebral
  breast N64.89
  brewer's (kidney) N28.0
  cardiac — *see* Infarct, myocardium
  cerebellar — *see* Infarct, cerebral
  cerebral (*see also* Occlusion, artery cerebral or precerebral, with infarction) I63.9- ☑

Infarct — *continued*
  aborted I63.9
  cortical I63.9
  due to
    cerebral venous thrombosis, nonpyogenic I63.6
    embolism
      cerebral arteries I63.4- ☑
      precerebral arteries I63.1- ☑
    occlusion NEC
      cerebral arteries I63.5- ☑
      precerebral arteries I63.2- ☑
    stenosis NEC
      cerebral arteries I63.5- ☑
      precerebral arteries I63.2- ☑
    thrombosis
      cerebral artery I63.3- ☑
      precerebral artery I63.0- ☑
  intraoperative
    during cardiac surgery I97.810
    during other surgery I97.811
  postprocedural
    following cardiac surgery I97.820
    following other surgery I97.821
  specified NEC I63.8
  colon (acute) (agnogenic) (embolic) (hemorrhagic) (nonocclusive) (nonthrombotic) (occlusive) (segmental) (thrombotic) (with gangrene) K55.0
  coronary artery — *see* Infarct, myocardium
  embolic — *see* Embolism
  fallopian tube N83.8
  gallbladder K82.8
  heart — *see* Infarct, myocardium
  hepatic K76.3
  hypophysis (anterior lobe) E23.6
  impending (myocardium) I20.0
  intestine (acute) (agnogenic) (embolic) (hemorrhagic) (nonocclusive) (nonthrombotic) (occlusive) (thrombotic) (with gangrene) K55.0
  kidney N28.0
  liver K76.3
  lung (embolic) (thrombotic) — *see* Embolism, pulmonary
  lymph node I89.8
  mesentery, mesenteric (embolic) (thrombotic) (with gangrene) K55.0
  muscle (ischemic) M62.20
    ankle M62.27- ☑
    foot M62.27- ☑
    forearm M62.23- ☑
    hand M62.24- ☑
    lower leg M62.26- ☑
    pelvic region M62.25- ☑
    shoulder region M62.21- ☑
    specified site NEC M62.28
    thigh M62.25- ☑
    upper arm M62.22- ☑
  myocardium, myocardial (acute) (with stated duration of 4 weeks or less) I21.3
    diagnosed on ECG, but presenting no symptoms I25.2
    healed or old I25.2
    intraoperative
      during cardiac surgery I97.790
      during other surgery I97.791
    non-Q wave I21.4
    non-ST elevation (NSTEMI) I21.4
      subsequent I22.2
    nontransmural I21.4
    past (diagnosed on ECG or other investigation, but currently presenting no symptoms) I25.2
    postprocedural
      following cardiac surgery I97.190
      following other surgery I97.191
    Q wave (see also, Infarct, myocardium, by site) I21.3
    ST elevation (STEMI) I21.3
      anterior (anteroapical) (anterolateral) (anteroseptal) (Q wave) (wall) I21.09
        subsequent I22.0
      inferior (diaphragmatic) (inferolateral) (inferoposterior) (wall) NEC I21.19
        subsequent I22.1
      inferoposterior transmural (Q wave) I21.11
      involving
        coronary artery of anterior wall NEC I21.09
        coronary artery of inferior wall NEC I21.19
        diagonal coronary artery I21.02

Infarct — *continued*
      left anterior descending coronary artery I21.02
      left circumflex coronary artery I21.21
      left main coronary artery I21.01
      oblique marginal coronary artery I21.21
      right coronary artery I21.11
      lateral (apical-lateral) (basal-lateral) (high) I21.29
        subsequent I22.8
      posterior (posterobasal) (posterolateral) (posteroseptal) (true) I21.29
        subsequent I22.8
      septal I21.29
        subsequent I22.8
      specified NEC I21.29
        subsequent I22.8
      subsequent I22.9
    subsequent (recurrent) (reinfarction) I22.9
      anterior (anteroapical) (anterolateral) (anteroseptal) (wall) I22.0
      diaphragmatic (wall) I22.1
      inferior (diaphragmatic) (inferolateral) (inferoposterior) (wall) I22.1
      lateral (apical-lateral) (basal-lateral) (high) I22.8
      non-ST elevation (NSTEMI) I22.2
      posterior (posterobasal) (posterolateral) (posteroseptal) (true) I22.8
      septal I22.8
      specified NEC I22.8
      ST elevation I22.9
        anterior (anteroapical) (anterolateral) (anteroseptal) (wall) I22.0
        inferior (diaphragmatic) (inferolateral) (inferoposterior) (wall) I22.1
        specified NEC I22.8
      subendocardial I22.2
      transmural I22.9
        anterior (anteroapical) (anterolateral) (anteroseptal) (wall) I22.0
        diaphragmatic (wall) I22.1
        inferior (diaphragmatic) (inferolateral) (inferoposterior) (wall) I22.1
        lateral (apical-lateral) (basal-lateral) (high) I22.8
        posterior (posterobasal) (posterolateral) (posteroseptal) (true) I22.8
        specified NEC I22.8
    syphilitic A52.06
    transmural I21.3
      anterior (anteroapical) (anterolateral) (anteroseptal) (Q wave) (wall) NEC I21.09
      inferior (diaphragmatic) (inferolateral) (inferoposterior) (Q wave) (wall) NEC I21.19
      inferoposterior (Q wave) I21.11
      lateral (apical-lateral) (basal-lateral) (high) NEC I21.29
      posterior (posterobasal) (posterolateral) (posteroseptal) (true) NEC I21.29
      septal NEC I21.29
      specified NEC I21.29
    nontransmural I21.4
  omentum K55.0
  ovary N83.8
  pancreas K86.8
  papillary muscle — *see* Infarct, myocardium
  parathyroid gland E21.4
  pituitary (gland) E23.6
  placenta O43.81- ☑
  prostate N42.89
  pulmonary (artery) (vein) (hemorrhagic) — *see* Embolism, pulmonary
  renal (embolic) (thrombotic) N28.0
  retina, retinal (artery) — *see* Occlusion, artery, retina
  spinal (cord) (acute) (embolic) (nonembolic) G95.11
  spleen D73.5
    embolic or thrombotic I74.8
  subendocardial (acute) (nontransmural) I21.4
  suprarenal (capsule) (gland) E27.49
  testis N50.1
  thrombotic (*see also* Thrombosis)
    artery, arterial — *see* Embolism
  thyroid (gland) E07.89
  ventricle (heart) — *see* Infarct, myocardium
Infecting — *see* condition
Infection, infected, infective (opportunistic) B99.9
  with

Infection — *continued*
  drug resistant organism — *see* Resistance (to),
      drug (*see also* specific organism)
  lymphangitis — *see* Lymphangitis
  organ dysfunction (acute) R65.20
      with septic shock R65.21
  abscess (skin) - code by site under Abscess
  Absidia — *see* Mucormycosis
  Acanthamoeba — *see* Acanthamebiasis
  Acanthocheilonema (perstans) (streptocerca)
      B74.4
  accessory sinus (chronic) — *see* Sinusitis
  achorion — *see* Dermatophytosis
  Acremonium falciforme B47.0
  acromioclavicular M00.9
  Actinobacillus (actinomycetem-comitans) A28.8
      mallei A24.0
      muris A25.1
  Actinomadura B47.1
  Actinomyces (israelii) (*see also* Actinomycosis)
      A42.9
  Actinomycetales — *see* Actinomycosis
  actinomycotic NOS — *see* Actinomycosis
  adenoid (and tonsil) J03.90
      chronic J35.02
  adenovirus NEC
      as cause of disease classified elsewhere B97.0
      unspecified nature or site B34.0
  aerogenes capsulatus A48.0
  aertrycke — *see* Infection, salmonella
  alimentary canal NOS — *see* Enteritis, infectious
  Allescheria boydii B48.2
  Alternaria B48.8
  alveolus, alveolar (process) K04.7
  Ameba, amebic (histolytica) — *see* Amebiasis
  amniotic fluid, sac or cavity O41.10- ☑
      chorioamnionitis O41.12- ☑
      placentitis O41.14- ☑
  amputation stump (surgical) — *see* Complication,
      amputation stump, infection
  Ancylostoma (duodenalis) B76.0
  Anisakiasis, Anisakis larvae B81.0
  anthrax — *see* Anthrax
  antrum (chronic) — *see* Sinusitis, maxillary
  anus, anal (papillae) (sphincter) K62.89
  arbovirus (arbor virus) A94
      specified type NEC A93.8
  artificial insemination N98.0
  Ascaris lumbricoides — *see* Ascariasis
  Ascomycetes B47.0
  Aspergillus (flavus) (fumigatus) (terreus) — *see*
      Aspergillosis
  atypical
      acid-fast (bacilli) — *see* Mycobacterium,
          atypical
      mycobacteria — *see* Mycobacterium, atypical
      virus A81.9
          specified type NEC A81.89
  auditory meatus (external) — *see* Otitis, externa,
      infective
  auricle (ear) — *see* Otitis, externa, infective
  axillary gland (lymph) L04.2
  Bacillus A49.9
      abortus A23.1
      anthracis — *see* Anthrax
      Ducrey's (any location) A57
      Flexner's A03.1
      Friedländer's NEC A49.8
      gas (gangrene) A48.0
      mallei A24.0
      melitensis A23.0
      paratyphoid, paratyphosus A01.4
          A A01.1
          B A01.2
          C A01.3
      Shiga (-Kruse) A03.0
      suipestifer — *see* Infection, salmonella
      swimming pool A31.1
      typhosa A01.00
      welchii — *see* Gangrene, gas
  bacterial NOS A49.9
      as cause of disease classified elsewhere B96.89
          Clostridium perfringens [C. perfringens]
              B96.7
          Bacteroides fragilis [B. fragilis] B96.6
          Enterobacter sakazakii B96.89
          Enterococcus B95.2
          Escherichia coli [E. coli] (*see also* Escherichia
              coli) B96.20
          Helicobacter pylori [H pylori] B96.81
          Hemophilus influenzae [H. influenzae] B96.3

Infection — *continued*
      Klebsiella pneumoniae [K. pneumoniae]
          B96.1
      Mycoplasma pneumoniae [M. pneumoniae]
          B96.0
      Proteus (mirabilis) (morganii) B96.4
      Pseudomonas (aeruginosa) (mallei)
          (pseudomallei) B96.5
      Staphylococcus B95.8
          aureus (methicillin susceptible) (MSSA)
              B95.61
          methicillin resistant (MRSA) B95.62
          specified NEC B95.7
      Streptococcus B95.5
          group A B95.0
          group B B95.1
          pneumoniae B95.3
          specified NEC B95.4
      Vibrio vulnificus B96.82
      specified NEC A48.8
  Bacterium
      paratyphosum A01.4
          A A01.1
          B A01.2
          C A01.3
      typhosum A01.00
  Bacteroides NEC A49.8
      fragilis, as cause of disease classified elsewhere
          B96.6
  Balantidium coli A07.0
  Bartholin's gland N75.8
  Basidiobolus B46.8
  bile duct (common) (hepatic) — *see* Cholangitis
  bladder — *see* Cystitis
  Blastomyces, blastomycotic (*see also*
      Blastomycosis)
      brasiliensis — *see* Paracoccidioidomycosis
      dermatitidis — *see* Blastomycosis
      European — *see* Cryptococcosis
      Loboi B48.0
      North American B40.9
      South American — *see* Paracoccidioidomycosis
  bleb, postprocedure — *see* Blebitis
  bone — *see* Osteomyelitis
  Bordetella — *see* Whooping cough
  Borrelia bergdorfi A69.20
  brain (*see also* Encephalitis) G04.90
      membranes — *see* Meningitis
      septic G06.0
          meninges — *see* Meningitis, bacterial
  branchial cyst Q18.0
  breast — *see* Mastitis
  bronchus — *see* Bronchitis
  Brucella A23.9
      abortus A23.1
      canis A23.3
      melitensis A23.0
      mixed A23.8
      specified NEC A23.8
      suis A23.2
  Brugia (malayi) B74.1
      timori B74.2
  bursa — *see* Bursitis, infective
  buttocks (skin) L08.9
  Campylobacter, intestinal A04.5
      as cause of disease classified elsewhere B96.81
  Candida (albicans) (tropicalis) — *see* Candidiasis
  candiru B88.8
  Capillaria (intestinal) B81.1
      hepatica B83.8
      philippinensis B81.1
  cartilage — *see* Disorder, cartilage, specified type
      NEC
  catheter-related bloodstream (CRBSI) T80.211 ☑
  cat liver fluke B66.0
  cellulitis - code by site under Cellulitis
  central line-associated T80.219 ☑
      bloodstream (CLABSI) T80.211 ☑
      specified NEC T80.218 ☑
  Cephalosporium falciforme B47.0
  cerebrospinal — *see* Meningitis
  cervical gland (lymph) L04.0
  cervix — *see* Cervicitis
  cesarean delivery wound (puerperal) O86.0
  cestodes — *see* Infestation, cestodes
  chest J22
  Chilomastix (intestinal) A07.8
  Chlamydia, chlamydial A74.9
      anus A56.3
      genitourinary tract A56.2
          lower A56.00
          specified NEC A56.19

Infection — *continued*
      lymphogranuloma A55
      pharynx A56.4
      psittaci A70
      rectum A56.3
      sexually transmitted NEC A56.8
  cholera — *see* Cholera
  Cladosporium
      bantianum (brain abscess) B43.1
      carrionii B43.0
      castellanii B36.1
      trichoides (brain abscess) B43.1
      werneckii B36.1
  Clonorchis (sinensis) (liver) B66.1
  Clostridium NEC
      bifermentans A48.0
      botulinum (food poisoning) A05.1
          infant A48.51
          wound A48.52
      difficile
          as cause of disease classified elsewhere
              B96.89
          foodborne (disease) A04.7
          gas gangrene A48.0
          necrotizing enterocolitis A04.7
          sepsis A41.4
      gas-forming NEC A48.0
      histolyticum A48.0
      novyi, causing gas gangrene A48.0
      oedematiens A48.0
      perfringens
          as cause of disease classified elsewhere B96.7
          due to food A05.2
          foodborne (disease) A05.2
          gas gangrene A48.0
          sepsis A41.4
      septicum, causing gas gangrene A48.0
      sordellii, causing gas gangrene A48.0
      welchii
          as cause of disease classified elsewhere B96.7
          foodborne (disease) A05.2
          gas gangrene A48.0
          necrotizing enteritis A05.2
          sepsis A41.4
  Coccidioides (immitis) — *see* Coccidioidomycosis
  colon — *see* Enteritis, infectious
  colostomy K94.02
  common duct — *see* Cholangitis
  congenital P39.9
      Candida (albicans) P37.5
      cytomegalovirus P35.1
      hepatitis, viral P35.3
      herpes simplex P35.2
      infectious or parasitic disease P37.9
          specified NEC P37.8
      listeriosis (disseminated) P37.2
      malaria NEC P37.4
          falciparum P37.3
      Plasmodium falciparum P37.3
      poliomyelitis P35.8
      rubella P35.0
      skin P39.4
      toxoplasmosis (acute) (subacute) (chronic)
          P37.1
      tuberculosis P37.0
      urinary (tract) P39.3
      vaccinia P35.8
      virus P35.9
          specified type NEC P35.8
  Conidiobolus B46.8
  coronavirus NEC B34.2
      as cause of disease classified elsewhere B97.29
      severe acute respiratory syndrome (SARS
          associated) B97.21
  corpus luteum — *see* Salpingo-oophoritis
  Corynebacterium diphtheriae — *see* Diphtheria
  cotia virus B08.8
  Coxiella burnetii A78
  coxsackie — *see* Coxsackie
  Cryptococcus neoformans — *see* Cryptococcosis
  Cryptosporidium A07.2
  Cunninghamella — *see* Mucormycosis
  cyst — *see* Cyst
  cystic duct (*see also* Cholecystitis) K81.9
  Cysticercus cellulosae — *see* Cysticercosis
  cytomegalovirus, cytomegaloviral B25.9
      congenital P35.1
      maternal, maternal care for (suspected)
          damage to fetus O35.3 ☑
      mononucleosis B27.10
          with
              complication NEC B27.19

Infection — continued
    meningitis B27.12
    polyneuropathy B27.11
  delta-agent (acute), in hepatitis B carrier B17.0
  dental (pulpal origin) K04.7
  Deuteromycetes B47.0
  Dicrocoelium dendriticum B66.2
  Dipetalonema (perstans) (streptocerca) B74.4
  diphtherial — see Diphtheria
  Diphyllobothrium (adult) (latum) (pacificum) B70.0
    larval B70.1
  Diplogonoporus (grandis) B71.8
  Dipylidium caninum B67.4
  Dirofilaria B74.8
  Dracunculus medinensis B72
  Drechslera (hawaiiensis) B43.8
  Ducrey Haemophilus (any location) A57
  due to or resulting from
    artificial insemination N98.0
    central venous catheter T80.219 ☑
      bloodstream T80.211 ☑
      exit or insertion site T80.212 ☑
      localized T80.212 ☑
      port or reservoir T80.212 ☑
      specified NEC T80.218 ☑
      tunnel T80.212 ☑
    device, implant or graft (see also Complications, by site and type, infection or inflammation) T85.79 ☑
      arterial graft NEC T82.7 ☑
      breast (implant) T85.79 ☑
      catheter NEC T85.79 ☑
        dialysis (renal) T82.7 ☑
          intraperitoneal T85.71 ☑
        infusion NEC T82.7 ☑
          spinal (epidural) (subdural) T85.79 ☑
        urinary (indwelling) T83.51 ☑
      electronic (electrode) (pulse generator) (stimulator)
        bone T84.7 ☑
        cardiac T82.7 ☑
        nervous system (brain) (peripheral nerve) (spinal) T85.79 ☑
        urinary T83.59 ☑
      fixation, internal (orthopedic) NEC — see Complication, fixation device, infection
      gastrointestinal (bile duct) (esophagus) T85.79 ☑
      genital NEC T83.6 ☑
      heart NEC T82.7 ☑
        valve (prosthesis) T82.6 ☑
          graft T82.7 ☑
      joint prosthesis — see Complication, joint prosthesis, infection
      ocular (corneal graft) (orbital implant) NEC T85.79 ☑
      orthopedic NEC T84.7 ☑
      specified NEC T85.79 ☑
      urinary NEC T83.59 ☑
      vascular NEC T82.7 ☑
      ventricular intracranial shunt T85.79 ☑
    Hickman catheter T80.219 ☑
      bloodstream T80.211 ☑
      localized T80.212 ☑
      specified NEC T80.218 ☑
    immunization or vaccination T88.0 ☑
    infusion, injection or transfusion NEC T80.29 ☑
      acute T80.22 ☑
    injury NEC - code by site under Wound, open
    peripherally inserted central catheter (PICC) T80.219 ☑
      bloodstream T80.211 ☑
      localized T80.212 ☑
      specified NEC T80.218 ☑
    portacath (port-a-cath) T80.219 ☑
      bloodstream T80.211 ☑
      localized T80.212 ☑
      specified NEC T80.218 ☑
    surgery T81.4 ☑
    triple lumen catheter T80.219 ☑
      bloodstream T80.211 ☑
      localized T80.212 ☑
      specified NEC T80.218 ☑
    umbilical venous catheter T80.219 ☑
      bloodstream T80.211 ☑
      localized T80.212 ☑
      specified NEC T80.218 ☑
  during labor NEC O75.3
  ear (middle) (see also Otitis media)
    external — see Otitis, externa, infective
    inner H83.0

Infection — continued
  Eberthella typhosa A01.00
  Echinococcus — see Echinococcus
  echovirus
    as cause of disease classified elsewhere B97.12
    unspecified nature or site B34.1
  endocardium I33.0
  endocervix — see Cervicitis
  Entamoeba — see Amebiasis
  enteric — see Enteritis, infectious
  Enterobacter sakazakii B96.89
  Enterobius vermicularis B80
  enterostomy K94.12
  enterovirus B34.1
    as cause of disease classified elsewhere B97.10
      coxsackievirus B97.11
      echovirus B97.12
      specified NEC B97.19
  Entomophthora B46.8
  Epidermophyton — see Dermatophytosis
  epididymis — see Epididymitis
  episiotomy (puerperal) O86.0
  Erysipelothrix (insidiosa) (rhusiopathiae) — see Erysipeloid
  erythema infectiosum B08.3
  Escherichia (E.) coli NEC A49.8
    as cause of disease classified elsewhere (see also Escherichia coli) B96.20
    congenital P39.8
      sepsis P36.4
    generalized A41.51
    intestinal — see Enteritis, infectious, due to, Escherichia coli
  ethmoidal (chronic) (sinus) — see Sinusitis, ethmoidal
  eustachian tube (ear) — see Salpingitis, eustachian
  external auditory canal (meatus) NEC — see Otitis, externa, infective
  eye (purulent) — see Endophthalmitis, purulent
  eyelid — see Inflammation, eyelid
  fallopian tube — see Salpingo-oophoritis
  Fasciola (gigantica) (hepatica) (indica) B66.3
  Fasciolopsis (buski) B66.5
  filarial — see Infestation, filarial
  finger (skin) L08.9
    nail L03.01- ☑
      fungus B35.1
  fish tapeworm B70.0
    larval B70.1
  flagellate, intestinal A07.9
  fluke — see Infestation, fluke
  focal
    teeth (pulpal origin) K04.7
    tonsils J35.01
  Fonsecaea (compactum) (pedrosoi) B43.0
  food — see Intoxication, foodborne
  foot (skin) L08.9
    dermatophytic fungus B35.3
  Francisella tularensis — see Tularemia
  frontal (sinus) (chronic) — see Sinusitis, frontal
  fungus NOS B49
    beard B35.0
    dermatophytic — see Dermatophytosis
    foot B35.3
    groin B35.6
    hand B35.2
    nail B35.1
    pathogenic to compromised host only B48.8
    perianal (area) B35.6
    scalp B35.0
    skin B36.9
      foot B35.3
      hand B35.2
      toenails B35.1
  Fusarium B48.8
  gallbladder — see Cholecystitis
  gas bacillus — see Gangrene, gas
  gastrointestinal — see Enteritis, infectious
  generalized NEC — see Sepsis
  genital organ or tract
    female — see Disease, pelvis, inflammatory
    male N49.9
      multiple sites N49.8
      specified NEC N49.8
  Ghon tubercle, primary A15.7
  Giardia lamblia A07.1
  gingiva (chronic) K05.10
    acute K05.00
      nonplaque induced K05.01
      plaque induced K05.00
    nonplaque induced K05.11

Infection — continued
    plaque induced K05.10
  glanders A24.0
  glenosporopsis B48.0
  Gnathostoma (spinigerum) B83.1
  Gongylonema B83.8
  gonococcal — see Gonococcus
  gram-negative bacilli NOS A49.9
  guinea worm B72
  gum (chronic) K05.10
    acute K05.00
      nonplaque induced K05.01
      plaque induced K05.00
    nonplaque induced K05.11
    plaque induced K05.10
  Haemophilus — see Infection, Hemophilus
  heart — see Carditis
  Helicobacter pylori A04.8
    as cause of disease classified elsewhere B96.81
  helminths B83.9
    intestinal B82.0
      mixed (types classifiable to more than one of the titles B65.0-B81.3 and B81.8) B81.4
      specified type NEC B81.8
    specified type NEC B83.8
  Hemophilus
    aegyptius, systemic A48.4
    ducrey (any location) A57
    influenzae NEC A49.2
      as cause of disease classified elsewhere B96.3
    generalized A41.3
  herpes (simplex) (see also Herpes)
    congenital P35.2
    disseminated B00.7
    zoster B02.9
  herpesvirus, herpesviral — see Herpes
  hip (joint) NEC M00.9
    due to internal joint prosthesis
      left T84.52 ☑
      right T84.51 ☑
    skin NEC L08.9
  Heterophyes (heterophyes) B66.8
  Histoplasma — see Histoplasmosis
    American B39.4
    capsulatum B39.4
  hookworm B76.9
  human
    papilloma virus A63.0
    T-cell lymphotropic virus type-1 (HTLV-1) B33.3
  hydrocele N43.0
  Hymenolepis B71.0
  hypopharynx — see Pharyngitis
  inguinal (lymph) glands L04.1
    due to soft chancre A57
  intervertebral disc, pyogenic M46.30
    cervical region M46.32
    cervicothoracic region M46.33
    lumbar region M46.36
    lumbosacral region M46.37
    multiple sites M46.39
    occipito-atlanto-axial region M46.31
    sacrococcygeal region M46.38
    thoracic region M46.34
    thoracolumbar region M46.35
  intestine, intestinal — see Enteritis, infectious
    specified NEC A08.8
  intra-amniotic affecting newborn NEC P39.2
  Isospora belli or hominis A07.3
  Japanese B encephalitis A83.0
  jaw (bone) (lower) (upper) M27.2
  joint NEC M00.9
    due to internal joint prosthesis T84.50 ☑
  kidney (cortex) (hematogenous) N15.9
    with calculus N20.0
      with hydronephrosis N13.6
    following ectopic gestation O08.83
    pelvis and ureter (cystic) N28.85
    puerperal (postpartum) O86.21
    specified NEC N15.8
  Klebsiella (K.) pneumoniae NEC A49.8
    as cause of disease classified elsewhere B96.1
  knee (joint) NEC M00.9
    joint M00.9
    due to internal joint prosthesis
      left T84.54 ☑
      right T84.53 ☑
    skin L08.9
  Koch's — see Tuberculosis
  labia (majora) (minora) (acute) — see Vulvitis
  lacrimal
    gland — see Dacryoadenitis

☑ **Additional character required**

Infection — *continued*

passages (duct) (sac) — *see* Inflammation, lacrimal, passages
lancet fluke B66.2
larynx NEC J38.7
leg (skin) NOS L08.9
Legionella pneumophila A48.1
    nonpneumonic A48.2
Leishmania (*see also* Leishmaniasis)
    aethiopica B55.1
    braziliensis B55.2
    chagasi B55.0
    donovani B55.0
    infantum B55.0
    major B55.1
    mexicana B55.1
    tropica B55.1
lentivirus, as cause of disease classified elsewhere B97.31
Leptosphaeria senegalensis B47.0
Leptospira interrogans A27.9
    autumnalis A27.89
    canicola A27.89
    hebdomadis A27.89
    icterohaemorrhagiae A27.0
    pomona A27.89
    specified type NEC A27.89
leptospirochetal NEC — *see* Leptospirosis
Listeria monocytogenes (*see also* Listeriosis)
    congenital P37.2
Loa loa B74.3
    with conjunctival infestation B74.3
    eyelid B74.3
Loboa loboi B48.0
local, skin (staphylococcal) (streptococcal) L08.9
    abscess - code by site under Abscess
    cellulitis - code by site under Cellulitis
    specified NEC L08.89
    ulcer — *see* Ulcer, skin
Loefflerella mallei A24.0
lung (*see also* Pneumonia) J18.9
    atypical Mycobacterium A31.0
    spirochetal A69.8
    tuberculous — *see* Tuberculosis, pulmonary
    virus — *see* Pneumonia, viral
lymph gland (*see also* Lymphadenitis, acute)
    mesenteric I88.0
lymphoid tissue, base of tongue or posterior pharynx, NEC (chronic) J35.03
Madurella (grisea) (mycetomii) B47.0
major
    following ectopic or molar pregnancy O08.0
    puerperal, postpartum, childbirth O85
Malassezia furfur B36.0
Malleomyces
    mallei A24.0
    pseudomallei (whitmori) — *see* Melioidosis
mammary gland N61
Mansonella (ozzardi) (perstans) (streptocerca) B74.4
mastoid — *see* Mastoiditis
maxilla, maxillary M27.2
    sinus (chronic) — *see* Sinusitis, maxillary
mediastinum J98.5
Medina (worm) B72
meibomian cyst or gland — *see* Hordeolum
meninges — *see* Meningitis, bacterial
meningococcal (*see also* condition) A39.9
    adrenals A39.1
    brain A39.81
    cerebrospinal A39.0
    conjunctiva A39.89
    endocardium A39.51
    heart A39.50
        endocardium A39.51
        myocardium A39.52
        pericardium A39.53
    joint A39.83
    meninges A39.0
    meningococcemia A39.4
        acute A39.2
        chronic A39.3
    myocardium A39.52
    pericardium A39.53
    retrobulbar neuritis A39.82
    specified site NEC A39.89
mesenteric lymph nodes or glands NEC I88.0
Metagonimus B66.8
metatarsophalangeal M00.9
methicillin
    resistant Staphylococcus aureus (MRSA) A49.02

Infection — *continued*

susceptible Staphylococcus aureus (MSSA) A49.01
Microsporum, microsporic — *see* Dermatophytosis
mixed flora (bacterial) NEC A49.8
Monilia — *see* Candidiasis
Monosporium apiospermum B48.2
mouth, parasitic B37.0
Mucor — *see* Mucormycosis
muscle NEC — *see* Myositis, infective
mycelium NOS B49
mycetoma B47.9
    actinomycotic NEC B47.1
    mycotic NEC B47.0
Mycobacterium, mycobacterial — *see* Mycobacterium
Mycoplasma NEC A49.3
    pneumoniae, as cause of disease classified elsewhere B96.0
mycotic NOS B49
    pathogenic to compromised host only B48.8
    skin NOS B36.9
myocardium NEC I40.0
nail (chronic)
    with lymphangitis — *see* Lymphangitis, acute, digit
    finger L03.01- ☑
        fungus B35.1
    ingrowing L60.0
    toe L03.03- ☑
        fungus B35.1
nasal sinus (chronic) — *see* Sinusitis
nasopharynx — *see* Nasopharyngitis
navel L08.82
Necator americanus B76.1
Neisseria — *see* Gonococcus
Neotestudina rosatii B47.0
newborn P39.9
    intra-amniotic NEC P39.2
    skin P39.4
    specified type NEC P39.8
nipple N61
    associated with
        lactation O91.03
        pregnancy O91.01- ☑
        puerperium O91.02
Nocardia — *see* Nocardiosis
obstetrical surgical wound (puerperal) O86.0
Oesophagostomum (apiostomum) B81.8
Oestrus ovis — *see* Myiasis
Oidium albicans B37.9
Onchocerca (volvulus) — *see* Onchocerciasis
oncovirus, as cause of disease classified elsewhere B97.32
operation wound T81.4 ☑
Opisthorchis (felineus) (viverrini) B66.0
orbit, orbital — *see* Inflammation, orbit
orthopoxvirus NEC B08.09
ovary — *see* Salpingo-oophoritis
Oxyuris vermicularis B80
pancreas (acute) K85.9
    abscess — *see* Pancreatitis, acute
    specified NEC K85.8
papillomavirus, as cause of disease classified elsewhere B97.7
papovavirus NEC B34.4
Paracoccidioides brasiliensis — *see* Paracoccidioidomycosis
Paragonimus (westermani) B66.4
parainfluenza virus B34.8
parameningococcus NOS A39.9
parapoxvirus B08.60
    specified NEC B08.69
parasitic B89
Parastrongylus
    cantonensis B83.2
    costaricensis B81.3
    paratyphoid A01.4
        Type A A01.1
        Type B A01.2
        Type C A01.3
paraurethral ducts N34.2
parotid gland — *see* Sialoadenitis
parvovirus NEC B34.3
    as cause of disease classified elsewhere B97.6
Pasteurella NEC A28.0
    multocida A28.0
    pestis — *see* Plague
    pseudotuberculosis A28.0
    septica (cat bite) (dog bite) A28.0
    tularensis — *see* Tularemia

Infection — *continued*

pelvic, female — *see* Disease, pelvis, inflammatory
Penicillium (marneffei) B48.4
penis (glans) (retention) NEC N48.29
periapical K04.5
peridental, periodontal K05.20
    generalized K05.22
    localized K05.21
perinatal period P39.9
    specified type NEC P39.8
perineal repair (puerperal) O86.0
periorbital — *see* Inflammation, orbit
perirectal K62.89
perirenal — *see* Infection, kidney
peritoneal — *see* Peritonitis
periureteral N28.89
Petriellidium boydii B48.2
pharynx (*see also* Pharyngitis)
    coxsackievirus B08.5
    posterior, lymphoid (chronic) J35.03
Phialophora
    gougerotii (subcutaneous abscess or cyst) B43.2
    jeanselmei (subcutaneous abscess or cyst) B43.2
    verrucosa (skin) B43.0
Piedraia hortae B36.3
pinta A67.9
    intermediate A67.1
    late A67.2
    mixed A67.3
    primary A67.0
pinworm B80
pityrosporum furfur B36.0
pleuro-pneumonia-like organism (PPLO) NEC A49.3
    as cause of disease classified elsewhere B96.0
pneumococcus, pneumococcal NEC A49.1
    as cause of disease classified elsewhere B95.3
    generalized (purulent) A40.3
        with pneumonia J13
Pneumocystis carinii (pneumonia) B59
Pneumocystis jiroveci (pneumonia) B59
port or reservoir T80.212 ☑
postoperative T81.4 ☑
postoperative wound T81.4 ☑
postprocedural T81.4 ☑
postvaccinal T88.0 ☑
prepuce NEC N47.7
    with penile inflammation N47.6
prion — *see* Disease, prion, central nervous system
prostate (capsule) — *see* Prostatitis
Proteus (mirabilis) (morganii) (vulgaris) NEC A49.8
    as cause of disease classified elsewhere B96.4
protozoal NEC B64
    intestinal A07.9
        specified NEC A07.8
    specified NEC B60.8
Pseudoallescheria boydii B48.2
Pseudomonas NEC A49.8
    as cause of disease classified elsewhere B96.5
    mallei A24.0
    pneumonia J15.1
    pseudomallei — *see* Melioidosis
puerperal O86.4
    genitourinary tract NEC O86.89
    major or generalized O85
    minor O86.4
    specified NEC O86.89
pulmonary — *see* Infection, lung
purulent — *see* Abscess
Pyrenochaeta romeroi B47.0
Q fever A78
rectum (sphincter) K62.89
renal (*see also* Infection, kidney)
    pelvis and ureter (cystic) N28.85
reovirus, as cause of disease classified elsewhere B97.5
respiratory (tract) NEC J98.8
    acute J22
    chronic J98.8
    influenzal (upper) (acute) — *see* Influenza, with, respiratory manifestations NEC
    lower (acute) J22
        chronic — *see* Bronchitis, chronic
    rhinovirus J00
    syncytial virus, as cause of disease classified elsewhere B97.4
    upper (acute) NOS J06.9
        chronic J39.8
        streptococcal J06.9

Infection

Infection — *continued*
 viral NOS J06.9
 resulting from
  presence of internal prosthesis, implant, graft
   — *see* Complications, by site and type,
   infection
 retortamoniasis A07.8
 retroperitoneal NEC K68.9
 retrovirus B33.3
  as cause of disease classified elsewhere B97.30
   human
    immunodeficiency, type 2 (HIV 2) B97.35
    T-cell lymphotropic
     type I (HTLV-I) B97.33
     type II (HTLV-II) B97.34
   lentivirus B97.31
   oncovirus B97.32
   specified NEC B97.39
 Rhinosporidium (seeberi) B48.1
 rhinovirus
  as cause of disease classified elsewhere B97.89
  unspecified nature or site B34.8
 Rhizopus — *see* Mucormycosis
 rickettsial NOS A79.9
 roundworm (large) NEC B82.0
  Ascariasis (*see also* Ascariasis) B77.9
 rubella — *see* Rubella
 Saccharomyces — *see* Candidiasis
 salivary duct or gland (any) — *see* Sialoadenitis
 Salmonella (aertrycke) (arizonae) (callinarum)
   (cholerae-suis) (enteritidis) (suipestifer)
   (typhimurium) A02.9
  with
   (gastro)enteritis A02.0
   sepsis A02.1
   specified manifestation NEC A02.8
  due to food (poisoning) A02.9
  hirschfeldii A01.3
  localized A02.20
   arthritis A02.23
   meningitis A02.21
   osteomyelitis A02.24
   pneumonia A02.22
   pyelonephritis A02.25
   specified NEC A02.29
  paratyphi A01.4
   A A01.1
   B A01.2
   C A01.3
  schottmuelleri A01.2
  typhi, typhosa — *see* Typhoid
 Sarcocystis A07.8
 scabies B86
 Schistosoma — *see* Infestation, Schistosoma
 scrotum (acute) NEC N49.2
 seminal vesicle — *see* Vesiculitis
 septic
  localized, skin — *see* Abscess
 sheep liver fluke B66.3
 Shigella A03.9
  boydii A03.2
  dysenteriae A03.0
  flexneri A03.1
  group
   A A03.0
   B A03.1
   C A03.2
   D A03.3
  Schmitz (-Stutzer) A03.0
  schmitzii A03.0
  shigae A03.0
  sonnei A03.3
  specified NEC A03.8
 shoulder (joint) NEC M00.9
  due to internal joint prosthesis T84.59 ☑
  skin NEC L08.9
 sinus (accessory) (chronic) (nasal) (*see also*
   Sinusitis)
  pilonidal — *see* Sinus, pilonidal
  skin NEC L08.89
 Skene's duct or gland — *see* Urethritis
 skin (local) (staphylococcal) (streptococcal) L08.9
  abscess - code by site under Abscess
  cellulitis - code by site under Cellulitis
  due to fungus B36.9
   specified type NEC B36.8
  mycotic B36.9
   specified type NEC B36.8
  newborn P39.4
  ulcer — *see* Ulcer, skin
 slow virus A81.9
  specified NEC A81.89

Infection — *continued*
 Sparganum (mansoni) (proliferum) (baxteri) B70.1
 specific (*see also* Syphilis)
  to perinatal period — *see* Infection, congenital
 specified NEC B99.8
 spermatic cord NEC N49.1
 sphenoidal (sinus) — *see* Sinusitis, sphenoidal
 spinal cord NOS (*see also* Myelitis) G04.91
  abscess G06.1
  meninges — *see* Meningitis
  streptococcal G04.89
 Spirillum A25.0
 spirochetal NOS A69.9
  lung A69.8
  specified NEC A69.8
 Spirometra larvae B70.1
 spleen D73.89
 Sporotrichum, Sporothrix (schenckii) — *see*
   Sporotrichosis
 staphylococcal, unspecified site
  aureus (methicillin susceptible) (MSSA) A49.01
   methicillin resistant (MRSA) A49.02
  as cause of disease classified elsewhere B95.8
   aureus (methicillin susceptible) (MSSA)
    B95.61
    methicillin resistant (MRSA) B95.62
   specified NEC B95.7
  food poisoning A05.0
  generalized (purulent) A41.2
  pneumonia — *see* Pneumonia, staphylococcal
 Stellantchasmus falcatus B66.8
 streptobacillus moniliformis A25.1
 streptococcal NEC A49.1
  as cause of disease classified elsewhere B95.5
   B genitourinary complicating
    childbirth O98.82
    pregnancy O98.81- ☑
    puerperium O98.83
  congenital
   sepsis P36.10
    group B P36.0
    specified NEC P36.19
  generalized (purulent) A40.9
 Streptomyces B47.1
 Strongyloides (stercoralis) — *see* Strongyloidiasis
 stump (amputation) (surgical) — *see*
   Complication, amputation stump, infection
 subcutaneous tissue, local L08.9
 suipestifer — *see* Infection, salmonella
 swimming pool bacillus A31.1
 Taenia — *see* Infestation, Taenia
 Taeniarhynchus saginatus B68.1
 tapeworm — *see* Infestation, tapeworm
 tendon (sheath) — *see* Tenosynovitis, infective
   NEC
 Ternidens diminutus B81.8
 testis — *see* Orchitis
 threadworm B80
 throat — *see* Pharyngitis
 thyroglossal duct K14.8
 toe (skin) L08.9
  cellulitis L03.03- ☑
   fungus B35.1
  nail L03.03- ☑
   fungus B35.1
 tongue NEC K14.0
  parasitic B37.0
 tonsil (and adenoid) (faucial) (lingual)
   (pharyngeal) — *see* Tonsillitis
 tooth, teeth K04.7
  periapical K04.7
  peridental, periodontal K05.20
   generalized K05.22
   localized K05.21
  pulp K04.0
  socket M27.3
 TORCH — *see* Infection, congenital
  without active infection P00.2
 Torula histolytica — *see* Cryptococcosis
 Toxocara (canis) (cati) (felis) B83.0
 Toxoplasma gondii — *see* Toxoplasma
 trachea, chronic J42
 trematode NEC — *see* Infestation, fluke
 trench fever A79.0
 Treponema pallidum — *see* Syphilis
 Trichinella (spiralis) B75
 Trichomonas A59.9
  cervix A59.09
  intestine A07.8
  prostate A59.02
  specified site NEC A59.8
  urethra A59.03

Infection — *continued*
 urogenitalis A59.00
  vagina A59.01
  vulva A59.01
 Trichophyton, trichophytic — *see*
   Dermatophytosis
 Trichosporon (beigelii) cutaneum B36.2
 Trichostrongylus B81.2
 Trichuris (trichiura) B79
 Trombicula (irritans) B88.0
 Trypanosoma
  brucei
   gambiense B56.0
   rhodesiense B56.1
  cruzi — *see* Chagas' disease
 tubal — *see* Salpingo-oophoritis
 tuberculous NEC — *see* Tuberculosis
 tubo-ovarian — *see* Salpingo-oophoritis
 tunnel T80.212 ☑
 tunica vaginalis N49.1
 tympanic membrane NEC — *see* Myringitis
 typhoid (abortive) (ambulant) (bacillus) — *see*
   Typhoid
 typhus A75.9
  flea-borne A75.2
  mite-borne A75.3
  recrudescent A75.1
  tick-borne A77.9
   African A77.1
   North Asian A77.2
 umbilicus L08.82
 ureter N28.86
 urethra — *see* Urethritis
 urinary (tract) N39.0
  bladder — *see* Cystitis
  complicating
   pregnancy O23.4- ☑
    specified type NEC O23.3- ☑
  kidney — *see* Infection, kidney
  newborn P39.3
  puerperal (postpartum) O86.20
  tuberculous A18.13
  urethra — *see* Urethritis
 uterus, uterine — *see* Endometritis
 vaccination T88.0 ☑
 vaccinia not from vaccination B08.011
 vagina (acute) — *see* Vaginitis
 varicella B01.9
 varicose veins — *see* Varix
 vas deferens NEC N49.1
 vesical — *see* Cystitis
 Vibrio
  cholerae A00.0
   El Tor A00.1
  parahaemolyticus (food poisoning) A05.3
  vulnificus
   as cause of disease classified elsewhere
    B96.82
   foodborne intoxication A05.5
 Vincent's (gum) (mouth) (tonsil) A69.1
 virus, viral NOS B34.9
  adenovirus
   as cause of disease classified elsewhere B97.0
   unspecified nature or site B34.0
  arbovirus, arbovirus arthropod-borne A94
  as cause of disease classified elsewhere B97.89
   adenovirus B97.0
   coronavirus B97.29
    SARS-associated B97.21
   coxsackievirus B97.11
   echovirus B97.12
   enterovirus B97.10
    coxsackievirus B97.11
    echovirus B97.12
    specified NEC B97.19
   human
    immunodeficiency, type 2 (HIV 2) B97.35
    T-cell lymphotropic,
     type I (HTLV-I) B97.33
     type II (HTLV-II) B97.34
    metapneumovirus B97.81
   papillomavirus B97.7
   parvovirus B97.6
   reovirus B97.5
   respiratory syncytial B97.4
   retrovirus B97.30
    human
     immunodeficiency, type 2 (HIV 2) B97.35
     T-cell lymphotropic,
      type I (HTLV-I) B97.33
      type II (HTLV-II) B97.34
    lentivirus B97.31

☑ **Additional character required**

Infection — *continued*
oncovirus B97.32
specified NEC B97.39
specified NEC B97.89
central nervous system A89
atypical A81.9
specified NEC A81.89
enterovirus NEC A88.8
meningitis A87.0
slow virus A81.9
specified NEC A81.89
specified NEC A88.8
chest J98.8
cotia B08.8
coxsackie (*see also* Infection, coxsackie) B34.1
as cause of disease classified elsewhere
B97.11
ECHO
as cause of disease classified elsewhere
B97.12
unspecified nature or site B34.1
encephalitis, tick-borne A84.9
enterovirus, as cause of disease classified
elsewhere B97.10
coxsackievirus B97.11
echovirus B97.12
specified NEC B97.19
exanthem NOS B09
human papilloma as cause of disease classified
elsewhere B97.7
human metapneumovirus as cause of disease
classified elsewhere B97.81
intestine — *see* Enteritis, viral
respiratory syncytial
as cause of disease classified elsewhere B97.4
bronchopneumonia J12.1
common cold syndrome J00
nasopharyngitis (acute) J00
rhinovirus
as cause of disease classified elsewhere
B97.89
unspecified nature or site B34.8
slow A81.9
specified NEC A81.89
specified type NEC B33.8
as cause of disease classified elsewhere
B97.89
unspecified nature or site B34.8
unspecified nature or site B34.9
West Nile — *see* Virus, West Nile
vulva (acute) — *see* Vulvitis
West Nile — *see* Virus, West Nile
whipworm B79
worms B83.9
specified type NEC B83.8
Wuchereria (bancrofti) B74.0
malayi B74.1
yatapoxvirus B08.70
specified NEC B08.79
yeast (*see also* Candidiasis) B37.9
yellow fever — *see* Fever, yellow
Yersinia
enterocolitica (intestinal) A04.6
pestis — *see* Plague
pseudotuberculosis A28.2
Zeis' gland — *see* Hordeolum
zoonotic bacterial NOS A28.9
Zopfia senegalensis B47.0
Infective, infectious — *see* condition
Infertility
female N97.9
age-related N97.8
associated with
anovulation N97.0
cervical (mucus) disease or anomaly N88.3
congenital anomaly
cervix N88.3
fallopian tube N97.1
uterus N97.2
vagina N97.8
dysmucorrhea N88.3
fallopian tube disease or anomaly N97.1
pituitary-hypothalamic origin E23.0
specified origin NEC N97.8
Stein-Leventhal disease E28.2
uterine disease or anomaly N97.2
vaginal disease or anomaly N97.8
due to
cervical anomaly N88.3
fallopian tube anomaly N97.1
ovarian failure E28.39
Stein-Leventhal syndrome E28.2

Infertility — *continued*
uterine anomaly N97.2
vaginal anomaly N97.8
nonimplantation N97.2
origin
cervical N88.3
tubal (block) (occlusion) (stenosis) N97.1
uterine N97.2
vaginal N97.8
male N46.9
azoospermia N46.01
extratesticular cause N46.029
drug therapy N46.021
efferent duct obstruction N46.023
infection N46.022
radiation N46.024
specified cause NEC N46.029
systemic disease N46.025
oligospermia N46.11
extratesticular cause N46.129
drug therapy N46.121
efferent duct obstruction N46.123
infection N46.122
radiation N46.124
specified cause NEC N46.129
systemic disease N46.125
specified type NEC N46.8
Infestation B88.9
Acanthocheilonema (perstans) (streptocerca)
B74.4
Acariasis B88.0
demodex folliculorum B88.0
sarcoptes scabiei B86
trombiculae B88.0
Agamofilaria streptocerca B74.4
Ancylostoma, ankylostoma (braziliense)
(caninum) (ceylanicum) (duodenale) B76.0
americanum B76.1
new world B76.1
Anisakis larvae, anisakiasis B81.0
arthropod NEC B88.2
Ascaris lumbricoides — *see* Ascariasis
Balantidium coli A07.0
beef tapeworm B68.1
Bothriocephalus (latus) B70.0
larval B70.1
broad tapeworm B70.0
larval B70.1
Brugia (malayi) B74.1
timori B74.2
candiru B88.8
Capillaria
hepatica B83.8
philippinensis B81.1
cat liver fluke B66.0
cestodes B71.9
diphyllobothrium — *see* Infestation,
diphyllobothrium
dipylidiasis B71.1
hymenolepiasis B71.0
specified type NEC B71.8
chigger B88.0
chigo, chigoe B88.1
Clonorchis (sinensis) (liver) B66.1
coccidial A07.3
crab-lice B85.3
Cysticercus cellulosae — *see* Cysticercosis
Demodex (folliculorum) B88.0
Dermanyssus gallinae B88.0
Dermatobia (hominis) — *see* Myiasis
Dibothriocephalus (latus) B70.0
larval B70.1
Dicrocoelium dendriticum B66.2
Diphyllobothrium (adult) (latum) (intestinal)
(pacificum) B70.0
larval B70.1
Diplogonoporus (grandis) B71.8
Dipylidium caninum B67.4
Distoma hepaticum B66.3
dog tapeworm B67.4
Dracunculus medinensis B72
dragon worm B72
dwarf tapeworm B71.0
Echinococcus — *see* Echinococcus
Echinostomum ilocanum B66.8
Entamoeba (histolytica) — *see* Infection, Ameba
Enterobius vermicularis B80
eyelid
in (due to)
leishmaniasis B55.1
loiasis B74.3
onchocerciasis B73.09

Infestation — *continued*
phthiriasis B85.3
parasitic NOS B89
eyeworm B74.3
Fasciola (gigantica) (hepatica) (indica) B66.3
Fasciolopsis (buski) (intestine) B66.5
filarial B74.9
bancroftian B74.0
conjunctiva B74.9
due to
Acanthocheilonema (perstans) (streptocerca)
B74.4
Brugia (malayi) B74.1
timori B74.2
Dracunculus medinensis B72
guinea worm B72
loa loa B74.3
Mansonella (ozzardi) (perstans) (streptocerca)
B74.4
Onchocerca volvulus B73.00
eye B73.00
eyelid B73.09
Wuchereria (bancrofti) B74.0
Malayan B74.1
ozzardi B74.4
specified type NEC B74.8
fish tapeworm B70.0
larval B70.1
fluke B66.9
blood NOS — *see* Schistosomiasis
cat liver B66.0
intestinal B66.5
liver (sheep) B66.3
cat B66.0
Chinese B66.1
due to clonorchiasis B66.1
oriental B66.1
lancet B66.2
lung (oriental) B66.4
sheep liver B66.3
specified type NEC B66.8
fly larvae — *see* Myiasis
Gasterophilus (intestinalis) — *see* Myiasis
Gastrodiscoides hominis B66.8
Giardia lamblia A07.1
Gnathostoma (spinigerum) B83.1
Gongylonema B83.8
guinea worm B72
helminth B83.9
angiostrongyliasis B83.2
intestinal B81.3
gnathostomiasis B83.1
hirudiniasis, internal B83.4
intestinal B82.0
angiostrongyliasis B81.3
anisakiasis B81.0
ascariasis — *see* Ascariasis
capillariasis B81.1
cysticercosis — *see* Cysticercosis
diphyllobothriasis — *see* Infestation,
diphyllobothriasis
dracunculiasis B72
echinococcus — *see* Echinococcosis
enterobiasis B80
filariasis - — *see* Infestation, filarial
fluke — *see* Infestation, fluke
hookworm — *see* Infestation, hookworm
mixed (types classifiable to more than one of
the titles B65.0-B81.3 and B81.8) B81.4
onchocerciasis — *see* Onchocerciasis
schistosomiasis — *see* Infestation,
schistosoma
specified
cestode NEC — *see* Infestation, cestode
type NEC B81.8
strongyloidiasis — *see* Strongyloidiasis
taenia — *see* Infestation, taenia
trichinellosis B75
trichostrongyliasis B81.2
trichuriasis B79
specified type NEC B83.8
syngamiasis B83.3
visceral larva migrans B83.0
Heterophyes (heterophyes) B66.8
hookworm B76.9
ancylostomiasis B76.0
necatoriasis B76.1
specified type NEC B76.8
Hymenolepis (diminuta) (nana) B71.0
intestinal NEC B82.9
leeches (aquatic) (land) — *see* Hirudiniasis
Leishmania — *see* Leishmaniasis

Infestation — continued
lice, louse — see Infestation, Pediculus
Linguatula B88.8
Liponyssoides sanguineus B88.0
Loa loa B74.3
  conjunctival B74.3
  eyelid B74.3
louse — see Infestation, Pediculus
maggots — see Myiasis
Mansonella (ozzardi) (perstans) (streptocerca) B74.4
Medina (worm) B72
Metagonimus (yokogawai) B66.8
microfilaria streptocerca — see Onchocerciasis
  eye B73.00
  eyelid B73.09
mites B88.9
  scabic B86
Monilia (albicans) — see Candidiasis
mouth B37.0
Necator americanus B76.1
nematode NEC (intestinal) B82.0
  Ancylostoma B76.0
  conjunctiva NEC B83.9
  Enterobius vermicularis B80
  Gnathostoma spinigerum B83.1
  physaloptera B80
  specified NEC B81.8
  trichostrongylus B81.2
  trichuris (trichuria) B79
Oesophagostomum (apiostomum) B81.8
Oestrus ovis (see also Myiasis) B87.9
Onchocerca (volvulus) — see Onchocerciasis
Opisthorchis (felineus) (viverrini) B66.0
orbit, parasitic NOS B89
Oxyuris vermicularis B80
Paragonimus (westermani) B66.4
parasite, parasitic B89
  eyelid B89
  intestinal NOS B82.9
  mouth B37.0
  skin B88.9
  tongue B37.0
Parastrongylus
  cantonensis B83.2
  costaricensis B81.3
Pediculus B85.2
  body B85.1
  capitis (humanus) (any site) B85.0
  corporis (humanus) (any site) B85.1
  head B85.0
  mixed (classifiable to more than one of the titles B85.0-B85.3) B85.4
  pubis (any site) B85.3
Pentastoma B88.8
Phthirus (pubis) (any site) B85.3
  with any infestation classifiable to B85.0-B85.2 B85.4
pinworm B80
pork tapeworm (adult) B68.0
protozoal NEC B64
  intestinal A07.9
    specified NEC A07.8
  specified NEC B60.8
pubic, louse B85.3
rat tapeworm B71.0
red bug B88.0
roundworm (large) NEC B82.0
  Ascariasis (see also Ascariasis) B77.9
sandflea B88.1
Sarcoptes scabiei B86
scabies B86
Schistosoma B65.9
  bovis B65.8
  cercariae B65.3
  haematobium B65.0
  intercalatum B65.8
  japonicum B65.2
  mansoni B65.1
  mattheei B65.8
  mekongi B65.8
  specified type NEC B65.8
  spindale B65.8
screw worms — see Myiasis
skin NOS B88.9
Sparganum (mansoni) (proliferum) (baxteri) B70.1
  larval B70.1
specified type NEC B88.8
Spirometra larvae B70.1
Stellantchasmus falcatus B66.8
Strongyloides stercoralis — see Strongyloidiasis
Taenia B68.9

Infestation — continued
diminuta B71.0
echinococcus — see Echinococcus
mediocanellata B68.1
nana B71.0
saginata B68.1
solium (intestinal form) B68.0
  larval form — see Cysticercosis
Taeniarhynchus saginatus B68.1
tapeworm B71.9
  beef B68.1
  broad B70.0
    larval B70.1
  dog B67.4
  dwarf B71.0
  fish B70.0
    larval B70.1
  pork B68.0
  rat B71.0
Ternidens diminutus B81.8
Tetranychus molestissimus B88.0
threadworm B80
tongue B37.0
Toxocara (canis) (cati) (felis) B83.0
trematode (s) NEC — see Infestation, fluke
Trichinella (spiralis) B75
Trichocephalus B79
Trichomonas — see Trichomoniasis
Trichostrongylus B81.2
Trichuris (trichiura) B79
Trombicula (irritans) B88.0
Tunga penetrans B88.1
Uncinaria americana B76.1
Vandellia cirrhosa B88.8
whipworm B79
worms B83.9
  intestinal B82.0
Wuchereria (bancrofti) B74.0
Infiltrate, infiltration
amyloid (generalized) (localized) — see Amyloidosis
calcareous NEC R89.7
  localized — see Degeneration, by site
calcium salt R89.7
cardiac
  fatty — see Degeneration, myocardial
  glycogenic E74.02 [I43]
corneal — see Edema, cornea
eyelid — see Inflammation, eyelid
glycogen, glycogenic — see Disease, glycogen storage
heart, cardiac
  fatty — see Degeneration, myocardial
  glycogenic E74.02 [I43]
inflammatory in vitreous H43.89
kidney N28.89
leukemic — see Leukemia
liver K76.89
  fatty — see Fatty, liver NEC
  glycogen (see also Disease, glycogen storage) E74.03 [K77]
lung R91.8
  eosinophilic J82
lymphatic (see also Leukemia, lymphatic) C91.9- ☑
  gland I88.9
muscle, fatty M62.89
myocardium, myocardial
  fatty — see Degeneration, myocardial
  glycogenic E74.02 [I43]
on chest x-ray R91.8
pulmonary R91.8
  with eosinophilia J82
skin (lymphocytic) L98.6
thymus (gland) (fatty) E32.8
urine R39.0
vesicant agent
  antineoplastic chemotherapy T80.810 ☑
  other agent NEC T80.818 ☑
vitreous body H43.89
Infirmity R68.89
senile R54
Inflammation, inflamed, inflammatory (with exudation)
abducent (nerve) — see Strabismus, paralytic, sixth nerve
accessory sinus (chronic) — see Sinusitis
adrenal (gland) E27.8
alveoli, teeth M27.3
  scorbutic E54
anal canal, anus K62.89
antrum (chronic) — see Sinusitis, maxillary

Inflammation — continued
appendix — see Appendicitis
arachnoid — see Meningitis
areola
  puerperal, postpartum or gestational — see Infection, nipple
areolar tissue NOS L08.9
artery — see Arteritis
auditory meatus (external) — see Otitis, externa
Bartholin's gland N75.8
bile duct (common) (hepatic) or passage — see Cholangitis
bladder — see Cystitis
bone — see Osteomyelitis
brain (see also Encephalitis)
  membrane — see Meningitis
breast N61
  puerperal, postpartum, gestational — see Mastitis, obstetric
broad ligament — see Disease, pelvis, inflammatory
bronchi — see Bronchitis
catarrhal J00
cecum — see Appendicitis
cerebral (see also Encephalitis)
  membrane — see Meningitis
cerebrospinal
  meningococcal A39.0
cervix (uteri) — see Cervicitis
chest J98.8
chorioretinal H30.9- ☑
  cyclitis — see Cyclitis
  disseminated H30.10- ☑
    generalized H30.13- ☑
    peripheral H30.12- ☑
    posterior pole H30.11- ☑
  epitheliopathy — see Epitheliopathy
  focal H30.00- ☑
    juxtapapillary H30.01- ☑
    macular H30.04- ☑
    paramacular — see Inflammation, chorioretinal, focal, macular
    peripheral H30.03- ☑
    posterior pole H30.02- ☑
  specified type NEC H30.89- ☑
choroid — see Inflammation, chorioretinal
chronic, postmastoidectomy cavity — see Complications, postmastoidectomy, inflammation
colon — see Enteritis
connective tissue (diffuse) NEC — see Disorder, soft tissue, specified type NEC
cornea — see Keratitis
corpora cavernosa N48.29
cranial nerve — see Disorder, nerve, cranial
Douglas' cul-de-sac or pouch (chronic) N73.0
due to device, implant or graft (see also Complications, by site and type, infection or inflammation)
  arterial graft T82.7 ☑
  breast (implant) T85.79 ☑
  catheter T85.79 ☑
    dialysis (renal) T82.7 ☑
      intraperitoneal T85.71 ☑
    infusion T82.7 ☑
      spinal (epidural) (subdural) T85.79 ☑
    urinary (indwelling) T83.51 ☑
  electronic (electrode) (pulse generator) (stimulator)
    bone T84.7 ☑
    cardiac T82.7 ☑
    nervous system (brain) (peripheral nerve) (spinal) T85.79 ☑
    urinary T83.59 ☑
  fixation, internal (orthopedic) NEC — see Complication, fixation device, infection
  gastrointestinal (bile duct) (esophagus) T85.79 ☑
  genital NEC T83.6 ☑
  heart NEC T82.7 ☑
    valve (prosthesis) T82.6 ☑
      graft T82.7 ☑
  joint prosthesis — see Complication, joint prosthesis, infection
  ocular (corneal graft) (orbital implant) NEC T85.79 ☑
  orthopedic NEC T84.7 ☑
  specified NEC T85.79 ☑
  urinary NEC T83.59 ☑
  vascular NEC T82.7 ☑
  ventricular intracranial shunt T85.79 ☑
duodenum K29.80

☑ **Additional character required**

Inflammation — *continued*
- with bleeding K29.81
- dura mater — *see* Meningitis
- ear (middle) (*see also* Otitis, media)
  - external — *see* Otitis, externa
  - innerH83.0
- epididymis — *see* Epididymitis
- esophagus K20.9
- ethmoidal (sinus) (chronic) — *see* Sinusitis, ethmoidal
- eustachian tube (catarrhal) — *see* Salpingitis, eustachian
- eyelid H01.9
  - abscess — *see* Abscess, eyelid
  - blepharitis — *see* Blepharitis
  - chalazion — *see* Chalazion
  - dermatosis (noninfectious) — *see* Dermatosis, eyelid
  - hordeolum — *see* Hordeolum
  - specified NEC H01.8
- fallopian tube — *see* Salpingo-oophoritis
- fascia — *see* Myositis
- follicular, pharynx J31.2
- frontal (sinus) (chronic) — *see* Sinusitis, frontal
- gallbladder — *see* Cholecystitis
- gastric — *see* Gastritis
- gastrointestinal — *see* Enteritis
- genital organ (internal) (diffuse)
  - female — *see* Disease, pelvis, inflammatory
  - male N49.9
    - multiple sites N49.8
    - specified NEC N49.8
- gland (lymph) — *see* Lymphadenitis
- glottis — *see* Laryngitis
- granular, pharynx J31.2
- gum K05.10
  - nonplaque induced K05.11
  - plaque induced K05.10
- heart — *see* Carditis
- hepatic duct — *see* Cholangitis
- ileoanal (internal) pouch K91.850
- ileum (*see also* Enteritis)
  - regional or terminal — *see* Enteritis, regional
- intestine (any part) — *see* Enteritis
- intestinal pouch K91.850
- jaw (acute) (bone) (chronic) (lower) (suppurative) (upper) M27.2
- joint NEC — *see* Arthritis
  - sacroiliac M46.1
- kidney — *see* Nephritis
- knee (joint) M13.169
  - tuberculous A18.02
- labium (majus) (minus) — *see* Vulvitis
- lacrimal
  - gland — *see* Dacryoadenitis
  - passages (duct) (sac) (*see also* Dacryocystitis)
    - canaliculitis — *see* Canaliculitis, lacrimal
- larynx — *see* Laryngitis
- leg NOS L08.9
- lip K13.0
- liver (capsule) (*see also* Hepatitis)
  - chronic K73.9
  - suppurative K75.0
- lung (acute) (*see also* Pneumonia)
  - chronic J98.4
- lymph gland or node — *see* Lymphadenitis
- lymphatic vessel — *see* Lymphangitis
- maxilla, maxillary M27.2
  - sinus (chronic) — *see* Sinusitis, maxillary
- membranes of brain or spinal cord — *see* Meningitis
- meninges — *see* Meningitis
- mouth K12.1
- muscle — *see* Myositis
- myocardium — *see* Myocarditis
- nasal sinus (chronic) — *see* Sinusitis
- nasopharynx — *see* Nasopharyngitis
- navel L08.82
- nerve NEC — *see* Neuralgia
- nipple N61
  - puerperal, postpartum or gestational — *see* Infection, nipple
- nose — *see* Rhinitis
- oculomotor (nerve) — *see* Strabismus, paralytic, third nerve
- optic nerve — *see* Neuritis, optic
- orbit (chronic) H05.10
  - acute H05.00
    - abscess — *see* Abscess, orbit
    - cellulitis — *see* Cellulitis, orbit
    - osteomyelitis — *see* Osteomyelitis, orbit
    - periostitis — *see* Periostitis, orbital

Inflammation — *continued*
- tenonitis — *see* Tenonitis, eye
- granuloma — *see* Granuloma, orbit
- myositis — *see* Myositis, orbital
- ovary — *see* Salpingo-oophoritis
- oviduct — *see* Salpingo-oophoritis
- pancreas (acute) — *see* Pancreatitis
- parametrium N73.0
- parotid region L08.9
- pelvis, female — *see* Disease, pelvis, inflammatory
- penis (corpora cavernosa) N48.29
- perianal K62.89
- pericardium — *see* Pericarditis
- perineum (female) (male) L08.9
- perirectal K62.89
- peritoneum — *see* Peritonitis
- periuterine — *see* Disease, pelvis, inflammatory
- perivesical — *see* Cystitis
- petrous bone (acute) (chronic) — *see* Petrositis
- pharynx (acute) — *see* Pharyngitis
- pia mater — *see* Meningitis
- pleura — *see* Pleurisy
- polyp, colon (*see also* Polyp, colon, inflammatory) K51.40
- prostate (*see also* Prostatitis)
  - specified type NEC N41.8
- rectosigmoid — *see* Rectosigmoiditis
- rectum (*see also* Proctitis) K62.89
- respiratory, upper (*see also* Infection, respiratory, upper) J06.9
  - acute, due to radiation J70.0
  - chronic, due to external agent — *see* condition, respiratory, chronic, due to
  - due to
    - chemicals, gases, fumes or vapors (inhalation) J68.2
    - radiation J70.1
- retina — *see* Chorioretinitis
- retrocecal — *see* Appendicitis
- retroperitoneal — *see* Peritonitis
- salivary duct or gland (any) (suppurative) — *see* Sialoadenitis
- scorbutic, alveoli, teeth E54
- scrotum N49.2
- seminal vesicle — *see* Vesiculitis
- sigmoid — *see* Enteritis
- sinus — *see* Sinusitis
- Skene's duct or gland — *see* Urethritis
- skin L08.9
- spermatic cord N49.1
- sphenoidal (sinus) — *see* Sinusitis, sphenoidal
- spinal
  - cord — *see* Encephalitis
  - membrane — *see* Meningitis
  - nerve — *see* Disorder, nerve
- spine — *see* Spondylopathy, inflammatory
- spleen (capsule) D73.89
- stomach — *see* Gastritis
- subcutaneous tissue L08.9
- suprarenal (gland) E27.8
- synovial — *see* Tenosynovitis
- tendon (sheath) NEC — *see* Tenosynovitis
- testis — *see* Orchitis
- throat (acute) — *see* Pharyngitis
- thymus (gland) E32.8
- thyroid (gland) — *see* Thyroiditis
- tongue K14.0
- tonsil — *see* Tonsillitis
- trachea — *see* Tracheitis
- trochlear (nerve) — *see* Strabismus, paralytic, fourth nerve
- tubal — *see* Salpingo-oophoritis
- tuberculous NEC — *see* Tuberculosis
- tubo-ovarian — *see* Salpingo-oophoritis
- tunica vaginalis N49.1
- tympanic membrane — *see* Tympanitis
- umbilicus, umbilical L08.82
- uterine ligament — *see* Disease, pelvis, inflammatory
- uterus (catarrhal) — *see* Endometritis
- uveal tract (anterior) NOS (*see also* Iridocyclitis)
  - posterior — *see* Chorioretinitis
- vagina — *see* Vaginitis
- vas deferens N49.1
- vein (*see also* Phlebitis)
  - intracranial or intraspinal (septic) G08
  - thrombotic I80.9
    - leg — *see* Phlebitis, leg
    - lower extremity — *see* Phlebitis, leg
- vocal cord J38.3
- vulva — *see* Vulvitis
- Wharton's duct (suppurative) — *see* Sialoadenitis

Inflation, lung, imperfect (newborn) — *see* Atelectasis

Influenza (bronchial) (epidemic) (respiratory (upper)) (unidentified influenza virus) J11.1
- with
  - digestive manifestations J11.2
  - encephalopathy J11.81
  - enteritis J11.2
  - gastroenteritis J11.2
  - gastrointestinal manifestations J11.2
  - laryngitis J11.1
  - myocarditis J11.82
  - otitis media J11.83
  - pharyngitis J11.1
  - pneumonia J11.00
    - specified type J11.08
  - respiratory manifestations NEC J11.1
  - specified manifestation NEC J11.89
- A/H5N1 (*see also* Influenza, due to, identified novel influenza A virus) J09.X2
- avian (*see also* Influenza, due to, identified novel influenza A virus) J09.X2
- bird (*see also* Influenza, due to, identified novel influenza A virus) J09.X2
- novel (2009) H1N1 influenza (*see also* Influenza, due to, identified influenza virus NEC) J10.1
- novel influenza A/H1N1 (*see also* Influenza, due to, identified influenza virus NEC) J10.1
- due to
  - avian (*see also* Influenza, due to, identified novel influenza A virus) J09.X2
  - identified influenza virus NEC J10.1
    - with
      - digestive manifestations J10.2
      - encephalopathy J10.81
      - enteritis J10.2
      - gastroenteritis J10.2
      - gastrointestinal manifestations J10.2
      - laryngitis J10.1
      - myocarditis J10.82
      - otitis media J10.83
      - pharyngitis J10.1
      - pneumonia (unspecified type) J10.00
        - with same identified influenza virus J10.01
        - specified type NEC J10.08
      - respiratory manifestations NEC J10.1
      - specified manifestation NEC J10.89
  - identified novel influenza A virus J09.X2
    - with
      - digestive manifestations J09.X3
      - encephalopathy J09.X9
      - enteritis J09.X3
      - gastroenteritis J09.X3
      - gastrointestinal manifestations J09.X3
      - laryngitis J09.X2
      - myocarditis J09.X9
      - otitis media J09.X9
      - pharyngitis J09.X2
      - pneumonia J09.X1
      - respiratory manifestations NEC J09.X2
      - specified manifestation NEC J09.X9
      - upper respiratory symptoms J09.X2
  - of other animal origin, not bird or swine (*see also* Influenza, due to, identified novel influenza A virus) J09.X2
  - swine (viruses that normally cause infections in pigs) (*see also* Influenza, due to, identified novel influenza A virus) J09.X2

Influenza-like disease — *see* Influenza

Influenzal — *see* Influenza

Infraction, Freiberg's (metatarsal head) — *see* Osteochondrosis, juvenile, metatarsus

Infraeruption of tooth (teeth) M26.34

Infusion complication, misadventure, or reaction — *see* Complications, infusion

Ingestion
- chemical — *see* Table of Drugs and Chemicals, by substance, poisoning
- drug or medicament
  - correct substance properly administered — *see* Table of Drugs and Chemicals, by drug, adverse effect
  - overdose or wrong substance given or taken — *see* Table of Drugs and Chemicals, by drug, poisoning
- foreign body — *see* Foreign body, alimentary tract
- tularemia A21.3

Ingrowing
- hair (beard) L73.1
- nail (finger) (toe) L60.0

Inguinal (see also condition)
  testicle Q53.9
    bilateral Q53.21
    unilateral Q53.11
Inhalation
  anthrax A22.1
  flame T27.3 ☑
  food or foreign body — see Foreign body, by site
  gases, fumes, or vapors NEC T59.9- ☑
    specified agent — see Table of Drugs and
      Chemicals, by substance
  liquid or vomitus — see Asphyxia
  meconium (newborn) P24.00
    with
      pneumonia (pneumonitis) P24.01
      with respiratory symptoms P24.01
  mucus — see Asphyxia, mucus
  oil or gasoline (causing suffocation) — see
    Foreign body, by site
  smoke J70.5
    due to chemicals, gases, fumes and vapors
      J68.9
  steam — see Toxicity, vapors
  stomach contents or secretions — see Foreign
    body, by site
    due to anesthesia (general) (local) or other
      sedation T88.59 ☑
      in labor and delivery O74.0
      in pregnancy O29.01- ☑
      postpartum, puerperal O89.01
Inhibition, orgasm
  female F52.31
  male F52.32
Inhibitor, systemic lupus erythematosus (presence
  of) D68.62
Iniencephalus, iniencephaly Q00.2
Injection, traumatic jet (air) (industrial) (water)
  (paint or dye) T70.4 ☑
Injury (see also specified injury type) T14.90
  abdomen, abdominal S39.91 ☑
    blood vessel — see Injury, blood vessel,
      abdomen
    cavity — see Injury, intra-abdominal
    contusion S30.1 ☑
    internal — see Injury, intra-abdominal
    intra-abdominal organ — see Injury, intra-
      abdominal
    nerve — see Injury, nerve, abdomen
    open — see Wound, open, abdomen
    specified NEC S39.81 ☑
    superficial — see Injury, superficial, abdomen
  Achilles tendon S86.00- ☑
    laceration S86.02- ☑
    specified type NEC S86.09- ☑
    strain S86.01- ☑
  acoustic, resulting in deafness — see Injury,
    nerve, acoustic
  adrenal (gland) S37.819 ☑
    contusion S37.812 ☑
    laceration S37.813 ☑
    specified type NEC S37.818 ☑
  alveolar (process) S09.93 ☑
  ankle S99.91- ☑
    contusion — see Contusion, ankle
    dislocation — see Dislocation, ankle
    fracture — see Fracture, ankle
    nerve — see Injury, nerve, ankle
    open — see Wound, open, ankle
    specified type NEC S99.81- ☑
    sprain — see Sprain, ankle
    superficial — see Injury, superficial, ankle
  anterior chamber, eye — see Injury, eye, specified
    site NEC
  anus — see Injury, abdomen
  aorta (thoracic) S25.00 ☑
    abdominal S35.00 ☑
      laceration (minor) (superficial) S35.01 ☑
        major S35.02 ☑
      specified type NEC S35.09 ☑
    laceration (minor) (superficial) S25.01 ☑
      major S25.02 ☑
    specified type NEC S25.09 ☑
  arm (upper) S49.9- ☑
    blood vessel — see Injury, blood vessel, arm
    contusion — see Contusion, arm, upper
    fracture — see Fracture, humerus
    lower — see Injury, forearm
    muscle — see Injury, muscle, shoulder
    nerve — see Injury, nerve, arm
    open — see Wound, open, arm
    specified type NEC S49.8- ☑
    superficial — see Injury, superficial, arm

Injury — continued
  artery (complicating trauma) (see also Injury,
    blood vessel, by site)
    cerebral or meningeal — see Injury, intracranial
  auditory canal (external) (meatus) S09.91 ☑
  auricle, auris, ear S09.91
  axilla — see Injury, shoulder
  back — see Injury, back, lower
  bile duct S36.13 ☑
  birth (see also Birth, injury) P15.9
  bladder (sphincter) S37.20 ☑
    at delivery O71.5
    contusion S37.22 ☑
    laceration S37.23 ☑
    obstetrical trauma O71.5
    specified type NEC S37.29 ☑
  blast (air) (hydraulic) (immersion) (underwater)
    NEC T14.8
    acoustic nerve trauma — see Injury, nerve,
      acoustic
    bladder — see Injury, bladder
    brain — see Concussion
    colon — see Injury, intestine, large, blast injury
    ear (primary) S09.31- ☑
      secondary S09.39- ☑
    generalized T70.8 ☑
    lung — see Injury, intrathoracic, lung, blast
      injury
    multiple body organs T70.8 ☑
    peritoneum S36.81 ☑
    rectum S36.61 ☑
    retroperitoneum S36.898 ☑
    small intestine S36.419 ☑
      duodenum S36.410 ☑
      specified site NEC S36.418 ☑
    specified
      intra-abdominal organ NEC S36.898 ☑
      pelvic organ NEC S37.899 ☑
  blood vessel NEC T14.8
    abdomen S35.9- ☑
      aorta — see Injury, aorta, abdominal
      celiac artery — see Injury, blood vessel, celiac
        artery
      iliac vessel — see Injury, blood vessel, iliac
      laceration S35.91 ☑
      mesenteric vessel — see Injury, mesenteric
      portal vein — see Injury, blood vessel, portal
        vein
      renal vessel — see Injury, blood vessel, renal
      specified vessel NEC S35.8X- ☑
      splenic vessel — see Injury, blood vessel,
        splenic
      vena cava — see Injury, vena cava, inferior
    ankle — see Injury, blood vessel, foot
    aorta (abdominal) (thoracic) — see Injury, aorta
    arm (upper) NEC S45.90- ☑
      forearm — see Injury, blood vessel, forearm
      laceration S45.91- ☑
      specified
        site NEC S45.80- ☑
          laceration S45.81- ☑
          specified type NEC S45.89- ☑
        type NEC S45.99- ☑
      superficial vein S45.30- ☑
        laceration S45.31- ☑
        specified type NEC S45.39- ☑
    axillary
      artery S45.00- ☑
        laceration S45.01- ☑
        specified type NEC S45.09- ☑
      vein S45.20- ☑
        laceration S45.21- ☑
        specified type NEC S45.29- ☑
    azygos vein — see Injury, blood vessel, thoracic,
      specified site NEC
    brachial
      artery S45.10- ☑
        laceration S45.11- ☑
        specified type NEC S45.19- ☑
      vein S45.20- ☑
        laceration S45.219 ☑
        specified type NEC S45.29- ☑
    carotid artery (common) (external) (internal,
      extracranial) S15.00- ☑
      internal, intracranial S06.8- ☑
      laceration (minor) (superficial) S15.01- ☑
        major S15.02- ☑
      specified type NEC S15.09- ☑
    celiac artery S35.219 ☑
      branch S35.299 ☑
        laceration (minor) (superficial) S35.291 ☑
        major S35.292 ☑

Injury — continued
    specified NEC S35.298 ☑
    laceration (minor) (superficial) S35.211 ☑
      major S35.212 ☑
    specified type NEC S35.218 ☑
  cerebral — see Injury, intracranial
  deep plantar — see Injury, blood vessel, plantar
    artery
  digital (hand) — see Injury, blood vessel, finger
  dorsal
    artery (foot) S95.00- ☑
      laceration S95.01- ☑
      specified type NEC S95.09- ☑
    vein (foot) S95.20- ☑
      laceration S95.21- ☑
      specified type NEC S95.29- ☑
  due to accidental laceration during procedure
    — see Laceration, accidental complicating
    surgery
  extremity — see Injury, blood vessel, limb
  femoral
    artery (common) (superficial) S75.00- ☑
      laceration (minor) (superficial) S75.01- ☑
        major S75.02- ☑
      specified type NEC S75.09- ☑
    vein (hip level) (thigh level) S75.10- ☑
      laceration (minor) (superficial) S75.11- ☑
        major S75.12- ☑
      specified type NEC S75.19- ☑
  finger S65.50- ☑
    index S65.50- ☑
      laceration S65.51- ☑
      specified type NEC S65.59- ☑
    laceration S65.51- ☑
    little S65.50- ☑
      laceration S65.51- ☑
      specified type NEC S65.59- ☑
    middle S65.50- ☑
      laceration S65.51- ☑
      specified type NEC S65.59- ☑
    specified type NEC S65.59- ☑
    thumb — see Injury, blood vessel, thumb
  foot S95.90- ☑
    dorsal
      artery — see Injury, blood vessel, dorsal,
        artery
      vein — see Injury, blood vessel, dorsal, vein
    laceration S95.91- ☑
    plantar artery — see Injury, blood vessel,
      plantar artery
    specified
      site NEC S95.80- ☑
        laceration S95.81- ☑
        specified type NEC S95.89- ☑
      specified type NEC S95.99- ☑
  forearm S55.90- ☑
    laceration S55.91- ☑
    radial artery — see Injury, blood vessel, radial
      artery
    specified
      site NEC S55.80- ☑
        laceration S55.81- ☑
        specified type NEC S55.89- ☑
      type NEC S55.99- ☑
    ulnar artery — see Injury, blood vessel, ulnar
      artery
    vein S55.20- ☑
      laceration S55.21- ☑
      specified type NEC S55.29- ☑
  gastric
    artery — see Injury, mesenteric, artery,
      branch
    vein — see Injury, blood vessel, abdomen
  gastroduodenal artery — see Injury,
    mesenteric, artery, branch
  greater saphenous vein (lower leg level)
    S85.30- ☑
    hip (and thigh) level S75.20- ☑
      laceration (minor) (superficial) S75.21- ☑
        major S75.22- ☑
      specified type NEC S75.29- ☑
    laceration S85.31- ☑
    specified type NEC S85.39- ☑
  hand (level) S65.90- ☑
    finger — see Injury, blood vessel, finger
    laceration S65.91- ☑
    palmar arch — see Injury, blood vessel,
      palmar arch
    radial artery — see Injury, blood vessel, radial
      artery, hand
    specified
      site NEC S65.80- ☑

Injury — *continued*
  laceration S65.81- ☑
  specified type NEC S65.89- ☑
  type NEC S65.99- ☑
 thumb — *see* Injury, blood vessel, thumb
 ulnar artery — *see* Injury, blood vessel, ulnar artery, hand
head S09.0 ☑
 intracranial — *see* Injury, intracranial
 multiple S09.0 ☑
hepatic
 artery — *see* Injury, mesenteric, artery
 vein — *see* Injury, vena cava, inferior
hip S75.90- ☑
 femoral artery — *see* Injury, blood vessel, femoral, artery
 femoral vein — *see* Injury, blood vessel, femoral, vein
 greater saphenous vein — *see* Injury, blood vessel, greater saphenous, hip level
 laceration S75.91- ☑
 specified
  site NEC S75.80- ☑
   laceration S75.81- ☑
   specified type NEC S75.89- ☑
  type NEC S75.99- ☑
hypogastric (artery) (vein) — *see* Injury, blood vessel, iliac
iliac S35.5- ☑
 artery S35.51- ☑
 specified vessel NEC S35.5- ☑
 uterine vessel — *see* Injury, blood vessel, uterine
 vein S35.51- ☑
innominate — *see* Injury, blood vessel, thoracic, innominate
intercostal (artery) (vein) — *see* Injury, blood vessel, thoracic, intercostal
jugular vein (external) S15.20- ☑
 internal S15.30- ☑
  laceration (minor) (superficial) S15.31- ☑
  major S15.32- ☑
  specified type NEC S15.39- ☑
 laceration (minor) (superficial) S15.21- ☑
 major S15.22- ☑
 specified type NEC S15.29- ☑
leg (level) (lower) S85.90- ☑
 greater saphenous — *see* Injury, blood vessel, greater saphenous
 laceration S85.91- ☑
 lesser saphenous — *see* Injury, blood vessel, lesser saphenous
 peroneal artery — *see* Injury, blood vessel, peroneal artery
 popliteal
  artery — *see* Injury, blood vessel, popliteal, artery
  vein — *see* Injury, blood vessel, popliteal, vein
 specified
  site NEC S85.80- ☑
   laceration S85.81- ☑
   specified type NEC S85.89- ☑
  type NEC S85.99- ☑
 thigh — *see* Injury, blood vessel, hip
 tibial artery — *see* Injury, blood vessel, tibial artery
lesser saphenous vein (lower leg level) S85.40- ☑
 laceration S85.41- ☑
 specified type NEC S85.49- ☑
limb
 lower — *see* Injury, blood vessel, leg
 upper — *see* Injury, blood vessel, arm
lower back — *see* Injury, blood vessel, abdomen
 specified NEC — *see* Injury, blood vessel, abdomen, specified, site NEC
mammary (artery) (vein) — *see* Injury, blood vessel, thoracic, specified site NEC
mesenteric (inferior) (superior)
 artery — *see* Injury, mesenteric, artery
 vein — *see* Injury, mesenteric, vein
neck S15.9 ☑
 specified site NEC S15.8 ☑
ovarian (artery) (vein)S35.8

pelvis — *see* Injury, blood vessel, abdomen
 specified NEC — *see* Injury, blood vessel, abdomen, specified, site NEC
peroneal artery S85.20- ☑
 laceration S85.21- ☑
 specified type NEC S85.29- ☑
plantar artery (deep) (foot) S95.10- ☑
 laceration S95.11- ☑
 specified type NEC S95.19- ☑
popliteal
 artery S85.00- ☑
  laceration S85.01- ☑
  specified type NEC S85.09- ☑
 vein S85.50- ☑
  laceration S85.51- ☑
  specified type NEC S85.59- ☑
portal vein S35.319 ☑
 laceration S35.311 ☑
 specified type NEC S35.318 ☑
precerebral — *see* Injury, blood vessel, neck
pulmonary (artery) (vein) — *see* Injury, blood vessel, thoracic, pulmonary
radial artery (forearm level) S55.10- ☑
 hand and wrist (level) S65.10- ☑
  laceration S65.11- ☑
  specified type NEC S65.19- ☑
 laceration S55.11- ☑
 specified type NEC S55.19- ☑
renal
 artery S35.40- ☑
  laceration S35.41- ☑
  specified NEC S35.49- ☑
 vein S35.40- ☑
  laceration S35.41- ☑
  specified NEC S35.49- ☑
saphenous vein (greater) (lower leg level) — *see* Injury, blood vessel, greater saphenous
 hip and thigh level — *see* Injury, blood vessel, greater saphenous, hip level
 lesser — *see* Injury, blood vessel, lesser saphenous
shoulder
 specified NEC — *see* Injury, blood vessel, arm, specified site NEC
 superficial vein — *see* Injury, blood vessel, arm, superficial vein
specified NEC T14.8
splenic
 artery — *see* Injury, blood vessel, celiac artery, branch
 vein S35.329 ☑
  laceration S35.321 ☑
  specified NEC S35.328 ☑
subclavian — *see* Injury, blood vessel, thoracic, innominate
thigh — *see* Injury, blood vessel, hip
thoracic S25.90 ☑
 aorta S25.00 ☑
  laceration (minor) (superficial) S25.01 ☑
  major S25.02 ☑
  specified type NEC S25.09 ☑
 azygos vein — *see* Injury, blood vessel, thoracic, specified, site NEC
 innominate
  artery S25.10- ☑
   laceration (minor) (superficial) S25.11- ☑
   major S25.12- ☑
   specified type NEC S25.19- ☑
  vein S25.30- ☑
   laceration (minor) (superficial) S25.31- ☑
   major S25.32- ☑
   specified type NEC S25.39- ☑
 intercostal S25.50- ☑
  laceration S25.51- ☑
  specified type NEC S25.59- ☑
 laceration S25.91 ☑
 mammary vessel — *see* Injury, blood vessel, thoracic, specified, site NEC
 pulmonary S25.40- ☑
  laceration (minor) (superficial) S25.41- ☑
  major S25.42- ☑
  specified type NEC S25.49- ☑
 specified
  site NEC S25.80- ☑
   laceration S25.81- ☑
   specified type NEC S25.89- ☑
  type NEC S25.99 ☑
 subclavian — *see* Injury, blood vessel, thoracic, innominate
 vena cava (superior) S25.20 ☑
  laceration (minor) (superficial) S25.21 ☑

major S25.22 ☑
 specified type NEC S25.29 ☑
thumb S65.40- ☑
 laceration S65.41- ☑
 specified type NEC S65.49- ☑
tibial artery S85.10- ☑
 anterior S85.13- ☑
  laceration S85.14- ☑
  specified injury NEC S85.15- ☑
 laceration S85.11- ☑
 posterior S85.16- ☑
  laceration S85.17- ☑
  specified injury NEC S85.18- ☑
 specified injury NEC S85.12- ☑
ulnar artery (forearm level) S55.00- ☑
 hand and wrist (level) S65.00- ☑
  laceration S65.01- ☑
  specified type NEC S65.09- ☑
 laceration S55.01- ☑
 specified type NEC S55.09- ☑
upper arm (level) — *see* Injury, blood vessel, arm
 superficial vein — *see* Injury, blood vessel, arm, superficial vein
uterine S35.5- ☑
 artery S35.53- ☑
 vein S35.53- ☑
vena cava — *see* Injury, vena cava
vertebral artery S15.10- ☑
 laceration (minor) (superficial) S15.11- ☑
 major S15.12- ☑
 specified type NEC S15.19- ☑
wrist (level) — *see* Injury, blood vessel, hand
brachial plexus S14.3 ☑
 newborn P14.3
brain (traumatic) S06.9- ☑
 diffuse (axonal) S06.2X- ☑
 focal S06.30- ☑
 traumaticS06
brainstem S06.38- ☑
breast NOS S29.9 ☑
broad ligament — *see* Injury, pelvic organ, specified site NEC
bronchus, bronchi — *see* Injury, intrathoracic, bronchus
brow S09.90 ☑
buttock S39.92 ☑
canthus, eye S05.90 ☑
cardiac plexus — *see* Injury, nerve, thorax, sympathetic
cauda equina S34.3 ☑
cavernous sinus — *see* Injury, intracranial
cecum — *see* Injury, colon
celiac ganglion or plexus — *see* Injury, nerve, lumbosacral, sympathetic
cerebellum — *see* Injury, intracranial
cerebral — *see* Injury, intracranial
cervix (uteri) — *see* Injury, uterus
cheek (wall) S09.93 ☑
chest — *see* Injury, thorax
childbirth (newborn) (*see also* Birth, injury)
 maternal NEC O71.9
chin S09.93 ☑
choroid (eye) — *see* Injury, eye, specified site NEC
clitoris S39.94 ☑
coccyx (*see also* Injury, back, lower)
 complicating delivery O71.6
colon — *see* Injury, intestine, large
common bile duct — *see* Injury, liver
conjunctiva (superficial) — *see* Injury, eye, conjunctiva
conus medullaris — *see* Injury, spinal, sacral
cord
 spermatic (pelvic region) S37.898 ☑
  scrotal region S39.848 ☑
 spinal — *see* Injury, spinal cord, by region
cornea — *see* Injury, eye, specified site NEC
 abrasion — *see* Injury, eye, cornea, abrasion
cortex (cerebral) (*see also* Injury, intracranial)
 visual — *see* Injury, nerve, optic
costal region NEC S29.9 ☑
costochondral NEC S29.9 ☑
cranial
 cavity — *see* Injury, intracranial
 nerve — *see* Injury, nerve, cranial
crushing — *see* Crush
cutaneous sensory nerve
cystic duct — *see* Injury, liver
deep tissue — *see* Contusion, by site
 meaning pressure ulcer — *see* Ulcer, pressure, unstageable, by site

Injury

Injury — continued
  delivery (newborn) P15.9
    maternal NEC O71.9
  Descemet's membrane — see Injury, eyeball,
    penetrating
  diaphragm — see Injury, intrathoracic, diaphragm
  duodenum — see Injury, intestine, small,
    duodenum
  ear (auricle) (external) (canal) S09.91 ☑
    abrasion — see Abrasion, ear
    bite — see Bite, ear
    blister — see Blister, ear
    bruise — see Contusion, ear
    contusion — see Contusion, ear
    external constriction — see Constriction,
      external, ear
    hematoma — see Hematoma, ear
    inner — see Injury, ear, middle
    laceration — see Laceration, ear
    middle S09.30- ☑
      blast — see Injury, blast, ear
      specified NEC S09.39- ☑
    puncture — see Puncture, ear
    superficial — see Injury, superficial, ear
  eighth cranial nerve (acoustic or auditory) — see
    Injury, nerve, acoustic
  elbow S59.90- ☑
    contusion — see Contusion, elbow
    dislocation — see Dislocation, elbow
    fracture — see Fracture, ulna, upper end
    open — see Wound, open, elbow
    specified NEC S59.80- ☑
    sprain — see Sprain, elbow
    superficial — see Injury, superficial, elbow
  eleventh cranial nerve (accessory) — see Injury,
    nerve, accessory
  epididymis S39.94 ☑
  epigastric region S39.91 ☑
  epiglottis NEC S19.89 ☑
  esophageal plexus — see Injury, nerve, thorax,
    sympathetic
  esophagus (thoracic part) (see also Injury,
    intrathoracic, esophagus)
    cervical NEC S19.85 ☑
  eustachian tube S09.30- ☑
  eye S05.9- ☑
    avulsion S05.7- ☑
    ball — see Injury, eyeball
    conjunctiva S05.0- ☑
    cornea
      abrasion S05.0- ☑
      laceration S05.3- ☑
        with prolapse S05.2- ☑
    lacrimal apparatus S05.8X- ☑
    orbit penetration S05.4- ☑
    specified site NEC S05.8X- ☑
  eyeball S05.8X- ☑
    contusion S05.1- ☑
    penetrating S05.6- ☑
      with
        foreign body S05.5- ☑
        prolapse or loss of intraocular tissue
          S05.2- ☑
        without prolapse or loss of intraocular tissue
          S05.3- ☑
    specified type NEC S05.8- ☑
  eyebrow S09.93 ☑
  eyelid S09.93 ☑
    abrasion — see Abrasion, eyelid
    contusion — see Contusion, eyelid
    open — see Wound, open, eyelid
  face S09.93 ☑
  fallopian tube S37.509 ☑
    bilateral S37.502 ☑
      blast injury S37.512 ☑
      contusion S37.522 ☑
      laceration S37.532 ☑
      specified type NEC S37.592 ☑
    blast injury (primary) S37.519 ☑
      bilateral S37.512 ☑
      secondary — see Injury, fallopian tube,
        specified type NEC
      unilateral S37.511 ☑
    contusion S37.529 ☑
      bilateral S37.522 ☑
      unilateral S37.521 ☑
    laceration S37.539 ☑
      bilateral S37.532 ☑
      unilateral S37.531 ☑
    specified type NEC S37.599 ☑
      bilateral S37.592 ☑
      unilateral S37.591 ☑

Injury — continued
    unilateral S37.501 ☑
      blast injury S37.511 ☑
      contusion S37.521 ☑
      laceration S37.531 ☑
      specified type NEC S37.591 ☑
  fascia — see Injury, muscle
  fifth cranial nerve (trigeminal) — see Injury, nerve,
    trigeminal
  finger (nail) S69.9- ☑
    blood vessel — see Injury, blood vessel, finger
    contusion — see Contusion, finger
    dislocation — see Dislocation, finger
    fracture — see Fracture, finger
    muscle — see Injury, muscle, finger
    nerve — see Injury, nerve, digital, finger
    open — see Wound, open, finger
    specified NEC S69.8- ☑
    sprain — see Sprain, finger
    superficial — see Injury, superficial, finger
  first cranial nerve (olfactory) — see Injury, nerve,
    olfactory
  flank — see Injury, abdomen
  foot S99.92- ☑
    blood vessel — see Injury, blood vessel, foot
    contusion — see Contusion, foot
    dislocation — see Dislocation, foot
    fracture — see Fracture, foot
    muscle — see Injury, muscle, foot
    open — see Wound, open, foot
    specified type NEC S99.82- ☑
    sprain — see Sprain, foot
    superficial — see Injury, superficial, foot
  forceps NOS P15.9
  forearm S59.91- ☑
    blood vessel — see Injury, blood vessel, forearm
    contusion — see Contusion, forearm
    fracture — see Fracture, forearm
    muscle — see Injury, muscle, forearm
    nerve — see Injury, nerve, forearm
    open — see Wound, open, forearm
    specified NEC S59.81- ☑
    superficial — see Injury, superficial, forearm
  forehead S09.90 ☑
  fourth cranial nerve (trochlear) — see Injury,
    nerve, trochlear
  gallbladder S36.129 ☑
    contusion S36.122 ☑
    laceration S36.123 ☑
    specified NEC S36.128 ☑
  ganglion
    celiac, coeliac — see Injury, nerve, lumbosacral,
      sympathetic
    gasserian — see Injury, nerve, trigeminal
    stellate — see Injury, nerve, thorax, sympathetic
    thoracic sympathetic — see Injury, nerve,
      thorax, sympathetic
  gasserian ganglion — see Injury, nerve, trigeminal
  gastric artery — see Injury, blood vessel, celiac
    artery, branch
  gastroduodenal artery — see Injury, blood vessel,
    celiac artery, branch
  gastrointestinal tract — see Injury, intra-
    abdominal
    with open wound into abdominal cavity —
      see Wound, open, with penetration into
      peritoneal cavity
    colon — see Injury, intestine, large
    rectum — see Injury, intestine, large, rectum
      with open wound into abdominal cavity
        S36.61 ☑
    specified site NEC — see Injury, intra-
      abdominal, specified, site NEC
    stomach — see Injury, stomach
    small intestine — see Injury, intestine, small
  genital organ (s)
    external S39.94 ☑
      specified NEC S39.848 ☑
    internal S37.90 ☑
      fallopian tube — see Injury, fallopian tube
      ovary — see Injury, ovary
      prostate — see Injury, prostate
      seminal vesicle — see Injury, pelvis, organ,
        specified site NEC
      uterus — see Injury, uterus
      vas deferens — see Injury, pelvis, organ,
        specified site NEC
    obstetrical trauma O71.9
  gland
    lacrimal laceration — see Injury, eye, specified
      site NEC
    salivary S09.90 ☑

Injury — continued
  thyroid NEC S19.84 ☑
  globe (eye) S05.90 ☑
    specified NEC S05.8X- ☑
  groin — see Injury, abdomen
  gum S09.90 ☑
  hand S69.9- ☑
    blood vessel — see Injury, blood vessel, hand
    contusion — see Contusion, hand
    fracture — see Fracture, hand
    muscle — see Injury, muscle, hand
    nerve — see Injury, nerve, hand
    open — see Wound, open, hand
    specified NEC S69.8- ☑
    sprain — see Sprain, hand
    superficial — see Injury, superficial, hand
  head S09.90 ☑
    with loss of consciousness S06.9- ☑
    specified NEC S09.8 ☑
  heart S26.90 ☑
    with hemopericardium S26.00 ☑
      contusion S26.01 ☑
      laceration (mild) S26.020 ☑
        moderate S26.021 ☑
        major S26.022 ☑
      specified type NEC S26.09 ☑
    contusion S26.91 ☑
    laceration S26.92 ☑
    specified type NEC S26.99 ☑
    without hemopericardium S26.10 ☑
      contusion S26.11 ☑
      laceration S26.12 ☑
      specified type NEC S26.19 ☑
  heel — see Injury, foot
  hepatic
    artery — see Injury, blood vessel, celiac artery,
      branch
    duct — see Injury, liver
    vein — see Injury, vena cava, inferior
  hip S79.91- ☑
    blood vessel — see Injury, blood vessel, hip
    contusion — see Contusion, hip
    dislocation — see Dislocation, hip
    fracture — see Fracture, femur, neck
    muscle — see Injury, muscle, hip
    nerve — see Injury, nerve, hip
    open — see Wound, open, hip
    sprain — see Sprain, hip
    superficial — see Injury, superficial, hip
    specified NEC S79.81- ☑
  hymen S39.94 ☑
  hypogastric
    blood vessel — see Injury, blood vessel, iliac
    plexus — see Injury, nerve, lumbosacral,
      sympathetic
  ileum — see Injury, intestine, small
  iliac region S39.91 ☑
  instrumental (during surgery) — see Laceration,
    accidental complicating surgery
    birth injury — see Birth, injury
    nonsurgical — see Injury, by site
    obstetrical O71.9
      bladder O71.5
      cervix O71.3
      high vaginal O71.4
      perineal NOS O70.9
      urethra O71.5
      uterus O71.5
        with rupture or perforation O71.1
  internal T14.8
    aorta — see Injury, aorta
    bladder (sphincter) — see Injury, bladder
      with
        ectopic or molar pregnancy O08.6
        following ectopic or molar pregnancy O08.6
        obstetrical trauma O71.5
    bronchus, bronchi — see Injury, intrathoracic,
      bronchus
    cecum — see Injury, intestine, large
    cervix (uteri) (see also Injury, uterus)
      with ectopic or molar pregnancy O08.6
      following ectopic or molar pregnancy O08.6
      obstetrical trauma O71.3
    chest — see Injury, intrathoracic
    gastrointestinal tract — see Injury, intra-
      abdominal
    heart — see Injury, heart
    intestine NEC — see Injury, intestine
    intrauterine — see Injury, uterus
    mesentery — see Injury, intra-abdominal,
      specified, site NEC
    pelvis, pelvic (organ) S37.90 ☑

Injury — *continued*
- following ectopic or molar pregnancy (subsequent episode) O08.6
- obstetrical trauma NEC O71.5
- rupture or perforation O71.1
- specified NEC S39.83 ☑
- rectum — *see* Injury, intestine, large, rectum
- stomach — *see* Injury, stomach
- ureter — *see* Injury, ureter
- urethra (sphincter) following ectopic or molar pregnancy O08.6
- uterus — *see* Injury, uterus
- interscapular area — *see* Injury, thorax
- intestine
  - large S36.509 ☑
    - ascending (right) S36.500 ☑
      - blast injury (primary) S36.510 ☑
        - secondary S36.590 ☑
      - contusion S36.520 ☑
      - laceration S36.530 ☑
      - specified type NEC S36.590 ☑
    - blast injury (primary) S36.519 ☑
      - ascending (right) S36.510 ☑
      - descending (left) S36.512 ☑
      - rectum S36.61 ☑
      - sigmoid S36.513 ☑
      - specified site NEC S36.518 ☑
      - transverse S36.511 ☑
    - contusion S36.529 ☑
      - ascending (right) S36.520 ☑
      - descending (left) S36.522 ☑
      - rectum S36.62 ☑
      - sigmoid S36.523 ☑
      - specified site NEC S36.528 ☑
      - transverse S36.521 ☑
    - descending (left) S36.502 ☑
      - blast injury (primary) S36.512 ☑
        - secondary S36.592 ☑
      - contusion S36.522 ☑
      - laceration S36.532 ☑
      - specified type NEC S36.592 ☑
    - laceration S36.539 ☑
      - ascending (right) S36.530 ☑
      - descending (left) S36.532 ☑
      - rectum S36.63 ☑
      - sigmoid S36.533 ☑
      - specified site NEC S36.538 ☑
      - transverse S36.531 ☑
    - rectum S36.60 ☑
      - blast injury (primary) S36.61 ☑
        - secondary S36.69 ☑
      - contusion S36.62 ☑
      - laceration S36.63 ☑
      - specified type NEC S36.69 ☑
    - sigmoid S36.503 ☑
      - blast injury (primary) S36.513 ☑
        - secondary S36.593 ☑
      - contusion S36.523 ☑
      - laceration S36.533 ☑
      - specified type NEC S36.593 ☑
    - specified
      - site NEC S36.508 ☑
        - blast injury (primary) S36.518 ☑
          - secondary S36.598 ☑
        - contusion S36.528 ☑
        - laceration S36.538 ☑
        - specified type NEC S36.598 ☑
      - type NEC S36.509 ☑
        - ascending (right) S36.590 ☑
        - descending (left) S36.592 ☑
        - rectum S36.69 ☑
        - sigmoid S36.593 ☑
        - specified site NEC S36.598 ☑
        - transverse S36.591 ☑
    - transverse S36.501 ☑
      - blast injury (primary) S36.511 ☑
        - secondary S36.591 ☑
      - contusion S36.521 ☑
      - laceration S36.531 ☑
      - specified type NEC S36.591 ☑
  - small S36.409 ☑
    - blast injury (primary) S36.419 ☑
      - duodenum S36.410 ☑
      - secondary S36.499 ☑
        - duodenum S36.490 ☑
        - specified site NEC S36.498 ☑
      - specified site NEC S36.418 ☑
    - contusion S36.429 ☑
      - duodenum S36.420 ☑
      - specified site NEC S36.428 ☑
    - duodenum S36.400 ☑
      - blast injury (primary) S36.410 ☑

- secondary S36.490 ☑
- contusion S36.420 ☑
- laceration S36.430 ☑
  - specified NEC S36.490 ☑
- laceration S36.439 ☑
  - duodenum S36.430 ☑
  - specified site NEC S36.438 ☑
- specified
  - type NEC S36.499 ☑
    - duodenum S36.490 ☑
    - specified site NEC S36.498 ☑
  - site NEC S36.408 ☑
- intra-abdominal S36.90 ☑
  - adrenal gland — *see* Injury, adrenal gland
  - bladder — *see* Injury, bladder
  - colon — *see* Injury, intestine, large
  - contusion S36.92 ☑
  - fallopian tube — *see* Injury, fallopian tube
  - gallbladder — *see* Injury, gallbladder
  - intestine — *see* Injury, intestine
  - laceration S36.93 ☑
  - liver — *see* Injury, liver
  - kidney — *see* Injury, kidney
  - ovary — *see* Injury, ovary
  - pancreas — *see* Injury, pancreas
  - pelvic NOS S37.90 ☑
  - peritoneum — *see* Injury, intra-abdominal, specified, site NEC
  - prostate — *see* Injury, prostate
  - rectum — *see* Injury, intestine, large, rectum
  - retroperitoneum — *see* Injury, intra-abdominal, specified, site NEC
  - seminal vesicle — *see* Injury, pelvis, organ, specified site NEC
  - small intestine — *see* Injury, intestine, small
  - specified
    - site NEC S36.899 ☑
      - contusion S36.892 ☑
      - laceration S36.893 ☑
      - specified type NEC S36.898 ☑
    - type NEC S36.99 ☑
  - pelvic S37.90 ☑
    - specified
      - site NEC S37.899 ☑
        - specified type NEC S37.898 ☑
      - type NEC S37.99 ☑
  - spleen — *see* Injury, spleen
  - stomach — *see* Injury, stomach
  - ureter — *see* Injury, ureter
  - urethra — *see* Injury, urethra
  - uterus — *see* Injury, uterus
  - vas deferens — *see* Injury, pelvis, organ, specified site NEC
- intracranial (traumatic) S06.9- ☑
  - cerebellar hemorrhage, traumatic — *see* Injury, intracranial, focal
  - cerebral edema, traumatic S06.1X- ☑
    - diffuse S06.1X- ☑
    - focal S06.1X- ☑
  - diffuse (axonal) S06.2X- ☑
  - epidural hemorrhage (traumatic) S06.4X- ☑
  - focal brain injury S06.30- ☑
    - contusion — *see* Contusion, cerebral
    - laceration — *see* Laceration, cerebral
    - intracerebral hemorrhage, traumatic S06.36- ☑
      - left side S06.35- ☑
      - right side S06.34- ☑
    - subarachnoid hemorrhage, traumatic S06.6X- ☑
    - subdural hemorrhage, traumatic S06.5X- ☑
  - intraocular — *see* Injury, eyeball, penetrating
- intrathoracic S27.9 ☑
  - bronchus S27.409 ☑
    - bilateral S27.402 ☑
    - blast injury (primary) S27.419 ☑
      - bilateral S27.412 ☑
      - secondary — *see* Injury, intrathoracic, bronchus, specified type NEC
      - unilateral S27.411 ☑
    - contusion S27.429 ☑
      - bilateral S27.422 ☑
      - unilateral S27.421 ☑
    - laceration S27.439 ☑
      - bilateral S27.432 ☑
      - unilateral S27.431 ☑
    - specified type NEC S27.499 ☑
      - bilateral S27.492 ☑
      - unilateral S27.491 ☑
      - unilateral S27.401 ☑
  - diaphragm S27.809 ☑
    - contusion S27.802 ☑

- laceration S27.803 ☑
- specified type NEC S27.808 ☑
- esophagus (thoracic) S27.819 ☑
  - contusion S27.812 ☑
  - laceration S27.813 ☑
  - specified type NEC S27.818 ☑
- heart — *see* Injury, heart
- hemopneumothorax S27.2 ☑
- hemothorax S27.1 ☑
- lung S27.309 ☑
  - aspiration J69.0
  - bilateral S27.302 ☑
  - blast injury (primary) S27.319 ☑
    - bilateral S27.312 ☑
    - secondary — *see* Injury, intrathoracic, lung, specified type NEC
    - unilateral S27.311 ☑
  - contusion S27.329 ☑
    - bilateral S27.322 ☑
    - unilateral S27.321 ☑
  - laceration S27.339 ☑
    - bilateral S27.332 ☑
    - unilateral S27.331 ☑
  - specified type NEC S27.399 ☑
    - bilateral S27.392 ☑
    - unilateral S27.391 ☑
  - unilateral S27.301 ☑
- pleura S27.60 ☑
  - laceration S27.63 ☑
  - specified type NEC S27.69 ☑
- pneumothorax S27.0 ☑
- specified organ NEC S27.899 ☑
  - contusion S27.892 ☑
  - laceration S27.893 ☑
  - specified type NEC S27.898 ☑
- thoracic duct — *see* Injury, intrathoracic, specified organ NEC
- thymus gland — *see* Injury, intrathoracic, specified organ NEC
- trachea, thoracic S27.50 ☑
  - blast (primary) S27.51 ☑
  - contusion S27.52 ☑
  - laceration S27.53 ☑
  - specified type NEC S27.59 ☑
- iris — *see* Injury, eye, specified site NEC
  - penetrating — *see* Injury, eyeball, penetrating
- jaw S09.93 ☑
- jejunum — *see* Injury, intestine, small
- joint NOS T14.8
  - old or residual — *see* Disorder, joint, specified type NEC
- kidney S37.00- ☑
  - acute (nontraumatic) N17.9
  - contusion — *see* Contusion, kidney
  - laceration — *see* Laceration, kidney
  - specified NEC S37.09- ☑
- knee S89.9- ☑
  - contusion — *see* Contusion, knee
  - dislocation — *see* Dislocation, knee
  - meniscus (lateral) (medial) — *see* Sprain, knee, specified site NEC
    - old injury or tear — *see* Derangement, knee, meniscus, due to old injury
  - open — *see* Wound, open, knee
  - specified NEC S89.8- ☑
  - sprain — *see* Sprain, knee
  - superficial — *see* Injury, superficial, knee
- labium (majus) (minus) S39.94 ☑
- labyrinth, ear S09.30- ☑
- lacrimal apparatus, duct, gland, or sac — *see* Injury, eye, specified site NEC
- larynx NEC S19.81 ☑
- leg (lower) S89.9- ☑
  - blood vessel — *see* Injury, blood vessel, leg
  - contusion — *see* Contusion, leg
  - fracture — *see* Fracture, leg
  - muscle — *see* Injury, muscle, leg
  - nerve — *see* Injury, nerve, leg
  - open — *see* Wound, open, leg
  - specified NEC S89.8- ☑
  - superficial — *see* Injury, superficial, leg
- lens, eye — *see* Injury, eye, specified site NEC
  - penetrating — *see* Injury, eyeball, penetrating
- limb NEC T14.8
- lip S09.93 ☑
- liver S36.119 ☑
  - contusion S36.112 ☑
  - laceration S36.113 ☑
    - major (stellate) S36.116 ☑
    - minor S36.114 ☑
    - moderate S36.115 ☑

Injury — *continued*
    specified NEC S36.118 ☑
  lower back S39.92 ☑
    specified NEC S39.82 ☑
  lumbar, lumbosacral (region) S39.92 ☑
    plexus — *see* Injury, lumbosacral plexus
  lumbosacral plexus S34.4 ☑
  lung (*see also* Injury, intrathoracic, lung)
    aspiration J69.0
    transfusion-related (TRALI) J95.84
  lymphatic thoracic duct — *see* Injury,
    intrathoracic, specified organ NEC
  malar region S09.93 ☑
  mastoid region S09.90 ☑
  maxilla S09.93 ☑
  mediastinum — *see* Injury, intrathoracic, specified
    organ NEC
  membrane, brain — *see* Injury, intracranial
  meningeal artery — *see* Injury, intracranial,
    subdural hemorrhage
  meninges (cerebral) — *see* Injury, intracranial
  mesenteric
    artery
      branch S35.299 ☑
        laceration (minor) (superficial) S35.291 ☑
          major S35.292 ☑
        specified NEC S35.298 ☑
      inferior S35.239 ☑
        laceration (minor) (superficial) S35.231 ☑
          major S35.232 ☑
        specified NEC S35.238 ☑
      superior S35.229 ☑
        laceration (minor) (superficial) S35.221 ☑
          major S35.222 ☑
        specified NEC S35.228 ☑
      plexus (inferior) (superior) — *see* Injury, nerve,
        lumbosacral, sympathetic
    vein
      inferior S35.349 ☑
        laceration S35.341 ☑
        specified NEC S35.348 ☑
      superior S35.339 ☑
        laceration S35.331 ☑
        specified NEC S35.338 ☑
  mesentery — *see* Injury, intra-abdominal,
    specified site NEC
  mesosalpinx — *see* Injury, pelvic organ, specified
    site NEC
  middle ear S09.30- ☑
  midthoracic region NOS S29.9 ☑
  mouth S09.93 ☑
  multiple NOS T07
  muscle (and fascia) (and tendon)
    abdomen S39.001 ☑
      laceration S39.021 ☑
      specified type NEC S39.091 ☑
      strain S39.011 ☑
    abductor
      thumb, forearm level — *see* Injury, muscle,
        thumb, abductor
    adductor
      thigh S76.20- ☑
        laceration S76.22- ☑
        specified type NEC S76.29- ☑
        strain S76.21- ☑
    ankle — *see* Injury, muscle, foot
    anterior muscle group, at leg level (lower)
      S86.20- ☑
      laceration S86.22- ☑
      specified type NEC S86.29- ☑
      strain S86.21- ☑
    arm (upper) — *see* Injury, muscle, shoulder
    biceps (parts NEC) S46.20- ☑
      laceration S46.22- ☑
      long head S46.10- ☑
        laceration S46.12- ☑
        strain S46.11- ☑
        specified type NEC S46.19- ☑
      specified type NEC S46.29- ☑
      strain S46.21- ☑
    extensor
      finger (s) (other than thumb) — *see* Injury,
        muscle, finger by site, extensor
      forearm level, specified NEC — *see* Injury,
        muscle, forearm, extensor
      thumb — *see* Injury, muscle, thumb, extensor
      toe (large) (ankle level) (foot level) — *see*
        Injury, muscle, toe, extensor
    finger
      extensor (forearm level) S56.40- ☑
        hand level S66.309 ☑
          laceration S66.329 ☑

Injury — *continued*
          specified type NEC S66.399 ☑
          strain S66.319 ☑
        laceration S56.429 ☑
        specified type NEC S56.499 ☑
        strain S56.419 ☑
      flexor (forearm level) S56.10- ☑
        hand level S66.109 ☑
          laceration S66.129 ☑
          specified type NEC S66.199 ☑
          strain S66.119 ☑
        laceration S56.129 ☑
        specified type NEC S56.199 ☑
        strain S56.119 ☑
      intrinsic S66.509 ☑
        laceration S66.529 ☑
        specified type NEC S66.599 ☑
        strain S66.519 ☑
      index
        extensor (forearm level)
          hand level S66.308 ☑
            laceration S66.32- ☑
            specified type NEC S66.39- ☑
            strain S66.31- ☑
          specified type NEC S56.492- ☑
        flexor (forearm level)
          hand level S66.108 ☑
            laceration S66.12- ☑
            specified type NEC S66.19- ☑
            strain S66.11- ☑
          specified type NEC S56.19- ☑
          strain S56.11- ☑
        intrinsic S66.50- ☑
          laceration S66.52- ☑
          specified type NEC S66.59- ☑
          strain S66.51- ☑
      little
        extensor (forearm level)
          hand level S66.30- ☑
            laceration S66.32- ☑
            specified type NEC S66.39- ☑
            strain S66.31- ☑
          laceration S56.42- ☑
          specified type NEC S56.49- ☑
          strain S56.41- ☑
        flexor (forearm level)
          hand level S66.10- ☑
            laceration S66.12- ☑
            specified type NEC S66.19- ☑
            strain S66.11- ☑
          laceration S56.12- ☑
          specified type NEC S56.19- ☑
          strain S56.11- ☑
        intrinsic S66.50- ☑
          laceration S66.52- ☑
          specified type NEC S66.59- ☑
          strain S66.51- ☑
      middle
        extensor (forearm level)
          hand level S66.30- ☑
            laceration S66.32- ☑
            specified type NEC S66.39- ☑
            strain S66.31- ☑
          laceration S56.42- ☑
          specified type NEC S56.49- ☑
          strain S56.41- ☑
        flexor (forearm level)
          hand level S66.10- ☑
            laceration S66.12- ☑
            specified type NEC S66.19- ☑
            strain S66.11- ☑
          laceration S56.12- ☑
          specified type NEC S56.19- ☑
          strain S56.11- ☑
        intrinsic S66.50- ☑
          laceration S66.52- ☑
          specified type NEC S66.59- ☑
          strain S66.51- ☑
      ring
        extensor (forearm level)
          hand level S66.30- ☑
            laceration S66.32- ☑
            specified type NEC S66.39- ☑
            strain S66.31- ☑
          laceration S56.42- ☑
          specified type NEC S56.49- ☑
          strain S56.41- ☑
        flexor (forearm level)
          hand level S66.10- ☑
            laceration S66.12- ☑
            specified type NEC S66.19- ☑
            strain S66.11- ☑

Injury — *continued*
        laceration S56.12- ☑
        specified type NEC S56.19- ☑
        strain S56.11- ☑
      intrinsic S66.50- ☑
        laceration S66.52- ☑
        specified type NEC S66.59- ☑
        strain S66.51- ☑
    flexor
      finger (s) (other than thumb) — *see* Injury,
        muscle, finger
      forearm level, specified NEC — *see* Injury,
        muscle, forearm, flexor
      thumb — *see* Injury, muscle, thumb, flexor
      toe (long) (ankle level) (foot level) — *see*
        Injury, muscle, toe, flexor
    foot S96.90- ☑
      intrinsic S96.20- ☑
        laceration S96.22- ☑
        specified type NEC S96.29- ☑
        strain S96.21- ☑
      laceration S96.92- ☑
      long extensor, toe — *see* Injury, muscle, toe,
        extensor
      long flexor, toe — *see* Injury, muscle, toe,
        flexor
      specified
        site NEC S96.80- ☑
          laceration S96.82- ☑
          specified type NEC S96.89- ☑
          strain S96.81- ☑
        type NEC S96.99- ☑
      strain S96.91- ☑
    forearm (level) S56.90- ☑
      extensor S56.50- ☑
        laceration S56.52- ☑
        specified type NEC S56.59- ☑
        strain S56.51- ☑
      flexor S56.20- ☑
        laceration S56.22- ☑
        specified type NEC S56.29- ☑
        strain S56.21- ☑
      laceration S56.92- ☑
      specified S56.99- ☑
        site NEC S56.80- ☑
          laceration S56.82- ☑
          strain S56.81- ☑
          type NEC S56.89- ☑
        strain S56.91- ☑
    hand (level) S66.90- ☑
      laceration S66.92- ☑
      specified
        site NEC S66.80- ☑
          laceration S66.82- ☑
          specified type NEC S66.89- ☑
          strain S66.81- ☑
        type NEC S66.99- ☑
      strain S66.91- ☑
    head S09.10 ☑
      laceration S09.12 ☑
      specified type NEC S09.19 ☑
      strain S09.11 ☑
    hip NEC S76.00- ☑
      laceration S76.02- ☑
      specified type NEC S76.09- ☑
      strain S76.01- ☑
    intrinsic
      ankle and foot level — *see* Injury, muscle,
        foot, intrinsic
      finger (other than thumb) — *see* Injury,
        muscle, finger by site, intrinsic
      foot (level) — *see* Injury, muscle, foot, intrinsic
      thumb — *see* Injury, muscle, thumb, intrinsic
    leg (level) (lower) S86.90- ☑
      Achilles tendon — *see* Injury, Achilles tendon
      anterior muscle group — *see* Injury, muscle,
        anterior muscle group
      laceration S86.92- ☑
      peroneal muscle group — *see* Injury, muscle,
        peroneal muscle group
      posterior muscle group — *see* Injury, muscle,
        posterior muscle group, leg level
      specified
        site NEC S86.80- ☑
          laceration S86.82- ☑
          specified type NEC S86.89- ☑
          strain S86.81- ☑
        type NEC S86.99- ☑
      strain S86.91- ☑
    long
      extensor toe, at ankle and foot level — *see*
        Injury, muscle, toe, extensor

☑ **Additional character required**

Injury — continued

flexor, toe, at ankle and foot level — see Injury, muscle, toe, flexor
head, biceps — see Injury, muscle, biceps, long head
lower back S39.002 ☑
  laceration S39.022 ☑
  specified type NEC S39.092 ☑
  strain S39.012 ☑
neck (level) S16.9 ☑
  laceration S16.2 ☑
  specified type NEC S16.8 ☑
  strain S16.1 ☑
pelvis S39.003 ☑
  laceration S39.023 ☑
  specified type NEC S39.093 ☑
  strain S39.013 ☑
peroneal muscle group, at leg level (lower) S86.30- ☑
  laceration S86.32- ☑
  specified type NEC S86.39- ☑
  strain S86.31- ☑
posterior muscle (group)
  leg level (lower) S86.10- ☑
   laceration S86.12- ☑
   specified type NEC S86.19- ☑
   strain S86.11- ☑
  thigh level S76.30- ☑
   laceration S76.32- ☑
   specified type NEC S76.39- ☑
   strain S76.31- ☑
quadriceps (thigh) S76.10- ☑
  laceration S76.12- ☑
  specified type NEC S76.19- ☑
  strain S76.11- ☑
shoulder S46.90- ☑
  laceration S46.92- ☑
  rotator cuff — see Injury, rotator cuff
  specified site NEC S46.80- ☑
   laceration S46.82- ☑
   strain S46.81- ☑
   specified type NEC S46.89- ☑
  strain S46.91- ☑
  specified type NEC S46.99- ☑
thigh NEC (level) S76.90- ☑
  adductor — see Injury, muscle, adductor, thigh
  laceration S76.92- ☑
  posterior muscle (group) — see Injury, muscle, posterior muscle, thigh level
  quadriceps — see Injury, muscle, quadriceps
  specified
   site NEC S76.80- ☑
    laceration S76.82- ☑
    specified type NEC S76.89- ☑
    strain S76.81- ☑
   type NEC S76.99- ☑
  strain S76.91- ☑
thorax (level) S29.009 ☑
  back wall S29.002 ☑
  front wall S29.001 ☑
  laceration S29.029 ☑
   back wall S29.022 ☑
   front wall S29.021 ☑
  specified type NEC S29.099 ☑
   back wall S29.092 ☑
   front wall S29.091 ☑
  strain S29.019 ☑
   back wall S29.012 ☑
   front wall S29.011 ☑
thumb
  abductor (forearm level) S56.30- ☑
   laceration S56.32- ☑
   specified type NEC S56.39- ☑
   strain S56.31- ☑
  extensor (forearm level) S56.30- ☑
   hand level S66.20- ☑
    laceration S66.22- ☑
    specified type NEC S66.29- ☑
    strain S66.21- ☑
   laceration S56.32- ☑
   specified type NEC S56.39- ☑
   strain S56.31- ☑
  flexor (forearm level) S56.00- ☑
   hand level S66.00- ☑
    laceration S66.02- ☑
    specified type NEC S66.09- ☑
    strain S66.01- ☑
   laceration S56.02- ☑
   specified type NEC S56.09- ☑
   strain S56.01- ☑

Injury — continued

wrist level — see Injury, muscle, thumb, flexor, hand level
intrinsic S66.40- ☑
  laceration S66.42- ☑
  specified type NEC S66.49- ☑
  strain S66.41- ☑
toe (see also Injury, muscle, foot)
  extensor, long S96.10- ☑
   laceration S96.12- ☑
   specified type NEC S96.19- ☑
   strain S96.11- ☑
  flexor, long S96.00- ☑
   laceration S96.02- ☑
   specified type NEC S96.09- ☑
   strain S96.01- ☑
  triceps S46.30- ☑
   laceration S46.32- ☑
   specified type NEC S46.39- ☑
   strain S46.31- ☑
wrist (and hand) level — see Injury, muscle, hand
musculocutaneous nerve — see Injury, nerve, musculocutaneous
myocardium — see Injury, heart
nape — see Injury, neck
nasal (septum) (sinus) S09.92 ☑
nasopharynx S09.92 ☑
neck S19.9 ☑
  specified NEC S19.80 ☑
  specified site NEC S19.89 ☑
nerve NEC T14.8
  abdomen S34.9 ☑
   peripheral S34.6 ☑
   specified site NEC S34.8 ☑
  abducens S04.4- ☑
   contusion S04.4- ☑
   laceration S04.4- ☑
   specified type NEC S04.4- ☑
  abducent — see Injury, nerve, abducens
  accessory S04.7- ☑
   contusion S04.7- ☑
   laceration S04.7- ☑
   specified type NEC S04.7- ☑
  acoustic S04.6- ☑
   contusion S04.6- ☑
   laceration S04.6- ☑
   specified type NEC S04.6- ☑
  ankle S94.9- ☑
   cutaneous sensory S94.3- ☑
   specified site NEC S94.8
  anterior crural, femoral — see Injury, nerve, femoral
  arm (upper) S44.9- ☑
   axillary — see Injury, nerve, axillary
   cutaneous — see Injury, nerve, cutaneous, arm
   median — see Injury, nerve, median, upper arm
   musculocutaneous — see Injury, nerve, musculocutaneous
   radial — see Injury, nerve, radial, upper arm
   specified site NEC S44.8
   ulnar — see Injury, nerve, ulnar, arm
  auditory — see Injury, nerve, acoustic
  axillary S44.3- ☑
  brachial plexus — see Injury, brachial plexus
  cervical sympathetic S14.5 ☑
  cranial S04.9 ☑
   contusion S04.9 ☑
   eighth (acoustic or auditory) — see Injury, nerve, acoustic
   eleventh (accessory) — see Injury, nerve, accessory
   fifth (trigeminal) — see Injury, nerve, trigeminal
   first (olfactory) — see Injury, nerve, olfactory
   fourth (trochlear) — see Injury, nerve, trochlear
   laceration S04.9 ☑
   ninth (glossopharyngeal) — see Injury, nerve, glossopharyngeal
   second (optic) — see Injury, nerve, optic
   seventh (facial) — see Injury, nerve, facial
   sixth (abducent) — see Injury, nerve, abducens
   specified
    nerve NEC S04.89- ☑
     contusion S04.89- ☑
     laceration S04.89- ☑
     specified type NEC S04.89- ☑
    type NEC S04.9 ☑

Injury — continued

tenth (pneumogastric or vagus) — see Injury, nerve, vagus
third (oculomotor) — see Injury, nerve, oculomotor
twelfth (hypoglossal) — see Injury, nerve, hypoglossal
cutaneous sensory
  ankle (level) S94.3- ☑
  arm (upper) (level) S44.5- ☑
  foot (level) — see Injury, nerve, cutaneous sensory, ankle
  forearm (level) S54.3- ☑
  hip (level) S74.2- ☑
  leg (lower level) S84.2- ☑
  shoulder (level) — see Injury, nerve, cutaneous sensory, arm
  thigh (level) — see Injury, nerve, cutaneous sensory, hip
deep peroneal — see Injury, nerve, peroneal, foot
digital
  finger S64.4- ☑
   index S64.49- ☑
   little S64.49- ☑
   middle S64.49- ☑
   ring S64.49- ☑
  thumb S64.3- ☑
  toe — see Injury, nerve, ankle, specified site NEC
eighth cranial (acoustic or auditory) — see Injury, nerve, acoustic
eleventh cranial (accessory) — see Injury, nerve, accessory
facial S04.5- ☑
  contusion S04.5- ☑
  laceration S04.5- ☑
  newborn P11.3
  specified type NEC S04.5- ☑
femoral (hip level) (thigh level) S74.1- ☑
fifth cranial (trigeminal) — see Injury, nerve, trigeminal
finger (digital) — see Injury, nerve, digital, finger
first cranial (olfactory) — see Injury, nerve, olfactory
foot S94.9- ☑
  cutaneous sensory S94.3- ☑
  deep peroneal S94.2- ☑
  lateral plantar S94.0- ☑
  medial plantar S94.1- ☑
  specified site NEC S94.8
forearm (level) S54.9- ☑
  cutaneous sensory — see Injury, nerve, cutaneous sensory, forearm
  median — see Injury, nerve, median
  radial — see Injury, nerve, radial
  specified site NEC S54.8
  ulnar — see Injury, nerve, ulnar
fourth cranial (trochlear) — see Injury, nerve, trochlear
glossopharyngeal S04.89- ☑
  specified type NEC S04.89- ☑
hand S64.9- ☑
  median — see Injury, nerve, median, hand
  radial — see Injury, nerve, radial, hand
  specified NEC S64.8
  ulnar — see Injury, nerve, ulnar, hand
hip (level) S74.9- ☑
  cutaneous sensory — see Injury, nerve, cutaneous sensory, hip
  femoral — see Injury, nerve, femoral
  sciatic — see Injury, nerve, sciatic
  specified site NEC S74.8
hypoglossal S04.89- ☑
  specified type NEC S04.89- ☑
lateral plantar S94.0- ☑
leg (lower) S84.9- ☑
  cutaneous sensory — see Injury, nerve, cutaneous sensory, leg
  peroneal — see Injury, nerve, peroneal
  specified site NEC S84.8
  tibial — see Injury, nerve, tibial
  upper — see Injury, nerve, thigh
lower
  back — see Injury, nerve, abdomen, specified site NEC
  peripheral — see Injury, nerve, abdomen, peripheral
  limb — see Injury, nerve, leg
lumbar spinal — see Injury, nerve, spinal, lumbar

Injury

Injury — *continued*

lumbar plexus — *see* Injury, nerve, lumbosacral, sympathetic
lumbosacral
  plexus — *see* Injury, nerve, lumbosacral, sympathetic
  sympathetic S34.5 ☑
medial plantar S94.1- ☑
median (forearm level) S54.1- ☑
  hand (level) S64.1- ☑
  upper arm (level) S44.1- ☑
  wrist (level) — *see* Injury, nerve, median, hand
musculocutaneous S44.4- ☑
musculospiral (upper arm level) — *see* Injury, nerve, radial, upper arm
neck S14.9 ☑
  peripheral S14.4 ☑
  specified site NEC S14.8 ☑
  sympathetic S14.5 ☑
ninth cranial (glossopharyngeal) — *see* Injury, nerve, glossopharyngeal
oculomotor S04.1- ☑
  contusion S04.1- ☑
  laceration S04.1- ☑
  specified type NEC S04.1- ☑
olfactory S04.81- ☑
  specified type NEC S04.81- ☑
optic S04.01- ☑
  contusion S04.01- ☑
  laceration S04.01- ☑
  specified type NEC S04.01- ☑
pelvic girdle — *see* Injury, nerve, hip
pelvis — *see* Injury, nerve, abdomen, specified site NEC
  peripheral — *see* Injury, nerve, abdomen, peripheral
peripheral NEC T14.8
  abdomen — *see* Injury, nerve, abdomen, peripheral
  lower back — *see* Injury, nerve, abdomen, peripheral
  neck — *see* Injury, nerve, neck, peripheral
  pelvis — *see* Injury, nerve, abdomen, peripheral
  specified NEC T14.8
peroneal (lower leg level) S84.1- ☑
  foot S94.2- ☑
plexus
  brachial — *see* Injury, brachial plexus
  celiac, coeliac — *see* Injury, nerve, lumbosacral, sympathetic
  mesenteric, inferior — *see* Injury, nerve, lumbosacral, sympathetic
  sacral — *see* Injury, lumbosacral plexus
  spinal
    brachial — *see* Injury, brachial plexus
    lumbosacral — *see* Injury, lumbosacral plexus
  pneumogastric — *see* Injury, nerve, vagus
radial (forearm level) S54.2- ☑
  hand (level) S64.2- ☑
  upper arm (level) S44.2- ☑
  wrist (level) — *see* Injury, nerve, radial, hand
root — *see* Injury, nerve, spinal, root
sacral plexus — *see* Injury, lumbosacral plexus
sacral spinal — *see* Injury, nerve, spinal, sacral
sciatic (hip level) (thigh level) S74.0- ☑
second cranial (optic) — *see* Injury, nerve, optic
seventh cranial (facial) — *see* Injury, nerve, facial
shoulder — *see* Injury, nerve, arm
sixth cranial (abducent) — *see* Injury, nerve, abducens
spinal
  plexus — *see* Injury, nerve, plexus, spinal
  root
    cervical S14.2 ☑
    dorsal S24.2 ☑
    lumbar S34.21 ☑
    sacral S34.22 ☑
    thoracic — *see* Injury, nerve, spinal, root, dorsal
splanchnic — *see* Injury, nerve, lumbosacral, sympathetic
sympathetic NEC — *see* Injury, nerve, lumbosacral, sympathetic
  cervical — *see* Injury, nerve, cervical, sympathetic
tenth cranial (pneumogastric or vagus) — *see* Injury, nerve, vagus
thigh (level) — *see* Injury, nerve, hip

Injury — *continued*

cutaneous sensory — *see* Injury, nerve, cutaneous sensory, hip
  femoral — *see* Injury, nerve, femoral
  sciatic — *see* Injury, nerve, sciatic
  specified NEC — *see* Injury, nerve, hip
third cranial (oculomotor) — *see* Injury, nerve, oculomotor
thorax S24.9 ☑
  peripheral S24.3 ☑
  specified site NEC S24.8 ☑
  sympathetic S24.4 ☑
thumb, digital — *see* Injury, nerve, digital, thumb
tibial (lower leg level) (posterior) S84.0- ☑
toe — *see* Injury, nerve, ankle
trigeminal S04.3- ☑
  contusion S04.3- ☑
  laceration S04.3- ☑
  specified type NEC S04.3- ☑
trochlear S04.2- ☑
  contusion S04.2- ☑
  laceration S04.2- ☑
  specified type NEC S04.2- ☑
twelfth cranial (hypoglossal) — *see* Injury, nerve, hypoglossal
ulnar (forearm level) S54.0- ☑
  arm (upper) (level) S44.0- ☑
  hand (level) S64.0- ☑
  wrist (level) — *see* Injury, nerve, ulnar, hand
vagus S04.89- ☑
  specified type NEC S04.89- ☑
wrist (level) — *see* Injury, nerve, hand
ninth cranial nerve (glossopharyngeal) — *see* Injury, nerve, glossopharyngeal
nose (septum) S09.92 ☑
obstetrical O71.9
  specified NEC O71.89
occipital (region) (scalp) S09.90 ☑
  lobe — *see* Injury, intracranial
optic chiasm S04.02 ☑
optic radiation S04.03- ☑
optic tract and pathways S04.03- ☑
orbit, orbital (region) — *see* Injury, eye
  penetrating (with foreign body) — *see* Injury, eye, orbit, penetrating
  specified NEC — *see* Injury, eye, specified site NEC
ovary, ovarian S37.409 ☑
  bilateral S37.402 ☑
    contusion S37.422 ☑
    laceration S37.432 ☑
    specified type NEC S37.492 ☑
  blood vessel — *see* Injury, blood vessel, ovarian
  contusion S37.429 ☑
    bilateral S37.422 ☑
    unilateral S37.421 ☑
  laceration S37.439 ☑
    bilateral S37.432 ☑
    unilateral S37.431 ☑
  specified type NEC S37.499 ☑
    bilateral S37.492 ☑
    unilateral S37.491 ☑
  unilateral S37.401 ☑
    contusion S37.421 ☑
    laceration S37.431 ☑
    specified type NEC S37.491 ☑
palate (hard) (soft) S09.93 ☑
pancreas S36.209 ☑
  body S36.201 ☑
    contusion S36.221 ☑
    laceration S36.231 ☑
      major S36.261 ☑
      minor S36.241 ☑
      moderate S36.251 ☑
    specified type NEC S36.291 ☑
  contusion S36.229 ☑
  head S36.200 ☑
    contusion S36.220 ☑
    laceration S36.230 ☑
      major S36.260 ☑
      minor S36.240 ☑
      moderate S36.250 ☑
    specified type NEC S36.290 ☑
  laceration S36.239 ☑
    major S36.269 ☑
    minor S36.249 ☑
    moderate S36.259 ☑
  specified type NEC S36.299 ☑
  tail S36.202 ☑
    contusion S36.222 ☑
    laceration S36.232 ☑

Injury — *continued*

      major S36.262 ☑
      minor S36.242 ☑
      moderate S36.252 ☑
    specified type NEC S36.292 ☑
parietal (region) (scalp) S09.90 ☑
  lobe — *see* Injury, intracranial
patellar ligament (tendon) S76.10- ☑
  laceration S76.12- ☑
  specified NEC S76.19- ☑
  strain S76.11- ☑
pelvis, pelvic (floor) S39.93 ☑
  complicating delivery O70.1
  joint or ligament, complicating delivery O71.6
  organ S37.90 ☑
    with ectopic or molar pregnancy O08.6
    complication of abortion — *see* Abortion
    contusion S37.92 ☑
    following ectopic or molar pregnancy O08.6
    laceration S37.93 ☑
    obstetrical trauma NEC O71.5
    specified
      site NEC S37.899 ☑
        contusion S37.892 ☑
        laceration S37.893 ☑
        specified type NEC S37.898 ☑
      type NEC S37.99 ☑
  specified NEC S39.83 ☑
penis S39.94 ☑
perineum S39.94 ☑
peritoneum S36.81 ☑
  laceration S36.893 ☑
periurethral tissue — *see* Injury, urethra
  complicating delivery O71.82
phalanges
  foot — *see* Injury, foot
  hand — *see* Injury, hand
pharynx NEC S19.85 ☑
pleura — *see* Injury, intrathoracic, pleura
plexus
  brachial — *see* Injury, brachial plexus
  cardiac — *see* Injury, nerve, thorax, sympathetic
  celiac, coeliac — *see* Injury, nerve, lumbosacral, sympathetic
  esophageal — *see* Injury, nerve, thorax, sympathetic
  hypogastric — *see* Injury, nerve, lumbosacral, sympathetic
  lumbar, lumbosacral — *see* Injury, lumbosacral plexus
  mesenteric — *see* Injury, nerve, lumbosacral, sympathetic
  pulmonary — *see* Injury, nerve, thorax, sympathetic
postcardiac surgery (syndrome) I97.0
prepuce S39.94 ☑
prostate S37.829 ☑
  contusion S37.822 ☑
  laceration S37.823 ☑
  specified type NEC S37.828 ☑
pubic region S39.94 ☑
pudendum S39.94 ☑
pulmonary plexus — *see* Injury, nerve, thorax, sympathetic
rectovaginal septum NEC S39.83 ☑
rectum — *see* Injury, intestine, large, rectum
retina — *see* Injury, eye, specified site NEC
  penetrating — *see* Injury, eyeball, penetrating
retroperitoneal — *see* Injury, intra-abdominal, specified site NEC
rotator cuff (muscle(s)) (tendon(s)) S46.00- ☑
  laceration S46.02- ☑
  specified type NEC S46.09- ☑
  strain S46.01- ☑
round ligament — *see* Injury, pelvic organ, specified site NEC
sacral plexus — *see* Injury, lumbosacral plexus
salivary duct or gland S09.93 ☑
scalp S09.90 ☑
  newborn (birth injury) P12.9
    due to monitoring (electrode) (sampling incision) P12.4
    specified NEC P12.89
      caput succedaneum P12.81
scapular region — *see* Injury, shoulder
sclera — *see* Injury, eye, specified site NEC
  penetrating — *see* Injury, eyeball, penetrating
scrotum S39.94 ☑
second cranial nerve (optic) — *see* Injury, nerve, optic
seminal vesicle — *see* Injury, pelvic organ, specified site NEC

Injury — *continued*
- seventh cranial nerve (facial) — *see* Injury, nerve, facial
- shoulder S49.9- ☑
  - blood vessel — *see* Injury, blood vessel, arm
  - contusion — *see* Contusion, shoulder
  - dislocation — *see* Dislocation, shoulder
  - fracture — *see* Fracture, shoulder
  - muscle — *see* Injury, muscle, shoulder
  - nerve — *see* Injury, nerve, shoulder
  - open — *see* Wound, open, shoulder
  - specified type NEC S49.8- ☑
  - sprain — *see* Sprain, shoulder girdle
  - superficial — *see* Injury, superficial, shoulder
- sinus
  - cavernous — *see* Injury, intracranial
  - nasal S09.92 ☑
- sixth cranial nerve (abducent) — *see* Injury, nerve, abducens
- skeleton, birth injury P13.9
  - specified part NEC P13.8
- skin NEC T14.8
  - surface intact — *see* Injury, superficial
- skull NEC S09.90 ☑
- specified NEC T14.8
- spermatic cord (pelvic region) S37.898 ☑
  - scrotal region S39.848 ☑
- spinal (cord)
  - cervical (neck) S14.109 ☑
    - anterior cord syndrome S14.139 ☑
      - C1 level S14.131 ☑
      - C2 level S14.132 ☑
      - C3 level S14.133 ☑
      - C4 level S14.134 ☑
      - C5 level S14.135 ☑
      - C6 level S14.136 ☑
      - C7 level S14.137 ☑
      - C8 level S14.138 ☑
    - Brown-Séquard syndrome S14.149 ☑
      - C1 level S14.141 ☑
      - C2 level S14.142 ☑
      - C3 level S14.143 ☑
      - C4 level S14.144 ☑
      - C5 level S14.145 ☑
      - C6 level S14.146 ☑
      - C7 level S14.147 ☑
      - C8 level S14.148 ☑
    - C1 level S14.101 ☑
    - C2 level S14.102 ☑
    - C3 level S14.103 ☑
    - C4 level S14.104 ☑
    - C5 level S14.105 ☑
    - C6 level S14.106 ☑
    - C7 level S14.107 ☑
    - C8 level S14.108 ☑
    - central cord syndrome S14.129 ☑
      - C1 level S14.121 ☑
      - C2 level S14.122 ☑
      - C3 level S14.123 ☑
      - C4 level S14.124 ☑
      - C5 level S14.125 ☑
      - C6 level S14.126 ☑
      - C7 level S14.127 ☑
      - C8 level S14.128 ☑
    - complete lesion S14.119 ☑
      - C1 level S14.111 ☑
      - C2 level S14.112 ☑
      - C3 level S14.113 ☑
      - C4 level S14.114 ☑
      - C5 level S14.115 ☑
      - C6 level S14.116 ☑
      - C7 level S14.117 ☑
      - C8 level S14.118 ☑
    - concussion S14.0 ☑
    - edema S14.0 ☑
    - incomplete lesion specified NEC S14.159 ☑
      - C1 level S14.151 ☑
      - C2 level S14.152 ☑
      - C3 level S14.153 ☑
      - C4 level S14.154 ☑
      - C5 level S14.155 ☑
      - C6 level S14.156 ☑
      - C7 level S14.157 ☑
      - C8 level S14.158 ☑
    - posterior cord syndrome S14.159 ☑
      - C1 level S14.151 ☑
      - C2 level S14.152 ☑
      - C3 level S14.153 ☑
      - C4 level S14.154 ☑
      - C5 level S14.155 ☑
      - C6 level S14.156 ☑
      - C7 level S14.157 ☑

Injury — *continued*
- C8 level S14.158 ☑
- dorsal — *see* Injury, spinal, thoracic
- lumbar S34.109 ☑
  - complete lesion S34.119 ☑
    - L1 level S34.111 ☑
    - L2 level S34.112 ☑
    - L3 level S34.113 ☑
    - L4 level S34.114 ☑
    - L5 level S34.115 ☑
  - concussion S34.01 ☑
  - edema S34.01 ☑
  - incomplete lesion S34.129 ☑
    - L1 level S34.121 ☑
    - L2 level S34.122 ☑
    - L3 level S34.123 ☑
    - L4 level S34.124 ☑
    - L5 level S34.125 ☑
  - L1 level S34.101 ☑
  - L2 level S34.102 ☑
  - L3 level S34.103 ☑
  - L4 level S34.104 ☑
  - L5 level S34.105 ☑
- nerve root NEC
  - cervical — *see* Injury, nerve, spinal, root, cervical
  - dorsal — *see* Injury, nerve, spinal, root, dorsal
  - lumbar S34.21 ☑
  - sacral S34.22 ☑
  - thoracic — *see* Injury, nerve, spinal, root, dorsal
- plexus
  - brachial — *see* Injury, brachial plexus
  - lumbosacral — *see* Injury, lumbosacral plexus
- sacral S34.139 ☑
  - complete lesion S34.131 ☑
  - incomplete lesion S34.132 ☑
- thoracic S24.109 ☑
  - anterior cord syndrome S24.139 ☑
    - T1 level S24.131 ☑
    - T2-T6 level S24.132 ☑
    - T7-T10 level S24.133 ☑
    - T11-T12 level S24.134 ☑
  - Brown-Séquard syndrome S24.149 ☑
    - T1 level S24.141 ☑
    - T2-T6 level S24.142 ☑
    - T7-T10 level S24.143 ☑
    - T11-T12 level S24.144 ☑
  - complete lesion S24.119 ☑
    - T1 level S24.111 ☑
    - T2-T6 level S24.112 ☑
    - T7-T10 level S24.113 ☑
    - T11-T12 level S24.114 ☑
  - concussion S24.0 ☑
  - edema S24.0 ☑
  - incomplete lesion specified NEC S24.159 ☑
    - T1 level S24.151 ☑
    - T2-T6 level S24.152 ☑
    - T7-T10 level S24.153 ☑
    - T11-T12 level S24.154 ☑
  - posterior cord syndrome S24.159 ☑
    - T1 level S24.151 ☑
    - T2-T6 level S24.152 ☑
    - T7-T10 level S24.153 ☑
    - T11-T12 level S24.154 ☑
  - T1 level S24.101 ☑
  - T2-T6 level S24.102 ☑
  - T7-T10 level S24.103 ☑
  - T11-T12 level S24.104 ☑
- splanchnic nerve — *see* Injury, nerve, lumbosacral, sympathetic
- spleen S36.00 ☑
  - contusion S36.029 ☑
    - major S36.021 ☑
    - minor S36.020 ☑
  - laceration S36.039 ☑
    - major (massive) (stellate) S36.032 ☑
    - moderate S36.031 ☑
    - superficial (capsular) (minor) S36.030 ☑
  - specified type NEC S36.09 ☑
- splenic artery — *see* Injury, blood vessel, celiac artery, branch
- stellate ganglion — *see* Injury, nerve, thorax, sympathetic
- sternal region S29.9 ☑
- stomach S36.30 ☑
  - contusion S36.32 ☑
  - laceration S36.33 ☑
  - specified type NEC S36.39 ☑
- subconjunctival — *see* Injury, eye, conjunctiva
- subcutaneous NEC T14.8
- submaxillary region S09.93 ☑

Injury — *continued*
- submental region S09.93 ☑
- subungual
  - fingers — *see* Injury, hand
  - toes — *see* Injury, foot
- superficial NEC T14.8
  - abdomen, abdominal (wall) S30.92 ☑
    - abrasion S30.811 ☑
    - bite S30.871 ☑
      - insect S30.861 ☑
    - contusion S30.1 ☑
    - external constriction S30.841 ☑
    - foreign body S30.851 ☑
  - abrasion — *see* Abrasion, by site
  - adnexa, eye NEC — *see* Injury, eye, specified site NEC
  - alveolar process — *see* Injury, superficial, oral cavity
  - ankle S90.91- ☑
    - abrasion — *see* Abrasion, ankle
    - blister — *see* Blister, ankle
    - bite — *see* Bite, ankle
    - contusion — *see* Contusion, ankle
    - external constriction — *see* Constriction, external, ankle
    - foreign body — *see* Foreign body, superficial, ankle
  - anus S30.98 ☑
  - arm (upper) S40.92- ☑
    - abrasion — *see* Abrasion, arm
    - bite — *see* Bite, superficial, arm
    - blister — *see* Blister, arm (upper)
    - contusion — *see* Contusion, arm
    - external constriction — *see* Constriction, external, arm
    - foreign body — *see* Foreign body, superficial, arm
  - auditory canal (external) (meatus) — *see* Injury, superficial, ear
  - auricle — *see* Injury, superficial, ear
  - axilla — *see* Injury, superficial, arm
  - back (*see also* Injury, superficial, thorax, back)
    - lower S30.91 ☑
      - abrasion S30.810 ☑
      - contusion S30.0 ☑
      - external constriction S30.840 ☑
      - superficial
        - bite NEC S30.870 ☑
          - insect S30.860 ☑
        - foreign body S30.850 ☑
  - bite NEC — *see* Bite, superficial NEC, by site
  - blister — *see* Blister, by site
  - breast S20.10- ☑
    - abrasion — *see* Abrasion, breast
    - bite — *see* Bite, superficial, breast
    - contusion — *see* Contusion, breast
    - external constriction — *see* Constriction, external, breast
    - foreign body — *see* Foreign body, superficial, breast
  - brow — *see* Injury, superficial, head, specified NEC
  - buttock S30.91 ☑
  - calf — *see* Injury, superficial, leg
  - canthus, eye — *see* Injury, superficial, periocular area
  - cheek (external) — *see* Injury, superficial, head, specified NEC
    - internal — *see* Injury, superficial, oral cavity
  - chest wall — *see* Injury, superficial, thorax
  - chin — *see* Injury, superficial, head NEC
  - clitoris S30.95 ☑
  - conjunctiva — *see* Injury, eye, conjunctiva
    - with foreign body (in conjunctival sac) — *see* Foreign body, conjunctival sac
  - contusion — *see* Contusion, by site
  - costal region — *see* Injury, superficial, thorax
  - digit (s)
    - hand — *see* Injury, superficial, finger
  - ear (auricle) (canal) (external) S00.40- ☑
    - abrasion — *see* Abrasion, ear
    - bite — *see* Bite, superficial, ear
    - contusion — *see* Contusion, ear
    - external constriction — *see* Constriction, external, ear
    - foreign body — *see* Foreign body, superficial, ear
  - elbow S50.90- ☑
    - abrasion — *see* Abrasion, elbow
    - bite — *see* Bite, superficial, elbow
    - blister — *see* Blister, elbow
    - contusion — *see* Contusion, elbow

Injury

Injury — *continued*

external constriction — *see* Constriction, external, elbow
foreign body — *see* Foreign body, superficial, elbow
epididymis S30.94 ☑
epigastric region S30.92 ☑
epiglottis — *see* Injury, superficial, throat
esophagus
  cervical — *see* Injury, superficial, throat
external constriction — *see* Constriction, external, by site
extremity NEC T14.8
eyeball NEC — *see* Injury, eye, specified site NEC
eyebrow — *see* Injury, superficial, periocular area
eyelid S00.20- ☑
  abrasion — *see* Abrasion, eyelid
  bite — *see* Bite, superficial, eyelid
  contusion — *see* Contusion, eyelid
  external constriction — *see* Constriction, external, eyelid
  foreign body — *see* Foreign body, superficial, eyelid
face NEC — *see* Injury, superficial, head, specified NEC
finger (s) S60.949 ☑
  abrasion — *see* Abrasion, finger
  bite — *see* Bite, superficial, finger
  blister — *see* Blister, finger
  contusion — *see* Contusion, finger
  external constriction — *see* Constriction, external, finger
  foreign body — *see* Foreign body, superficial, finger
  insect bite — *see* Bite, by site, superficial, insect
  index S60.94- ☑
  little S60.94- ☑
  middle S60.94- ☑
  ring S60.94- ☑
flank S30.92 ☑
foot S90.92- ☑
  abrasion — *see* Abrasion, foot
  bite — *see* Bite, foot
  blister — *see* Blister, foot
  contusion — *see* Contusion, foot
  external constriction — *see* Constriction, external, foot
  foreign body — *see* Foreign body, superficial, foot
forearm S50.91- ☑
  abrasion — *see* Abrasion, forearm
  bite — *see* Bite, forearm, superficial
  blister — *see* Blister, forearm
  contusion — *see* Contusion, forearm
  elbow only — *see* Injury, superficial, elbow
  external constriction — *see* Constriction, external, forearm
  foreign body — *see* Foreign body, superficial, forearm
forehead — *see* Injury, superficial, head NEC
foreign body — *see* Foreign body, superficial
genital organs, external
  female S30.97 ☑
  male S30.96 ☑
globe (eye) — *see* Injury, eye, specified site NEC
groin S30.92 ☑
gum — *see* Injury, superficial, oral cavity
hand S60.92- ☑
  abrasion — *see* Abrasion, hand
  bite — *see* Bite, superficial, hand
  contusion — *see* Contusion, hand
  external constriction — *see* Constriction, external, hand
  foreign body — *see* Foreign body, superficial, hand
head S00.90 ☑
  ear — *see* Injury, superficial, ear
  eyelid — *see* Injury, superficial, eyelid
  nose S00.30 ☑
  oral cavity S00.502 ☑
  scalp S00.00 ☑
  specified site NEC S00.80 ☑
heel — *see* Injury, superficial, foot
hip S70.91- ☑
  abrasion — *see* Abrasion, hip
  bite — *see* Bite, superficial, hip
  blister — *see* Blister, hip
  contusion — *see* Contusion, hip

Injury — *continued*

external constriction — *see* Constriction, external, hip
foreign body — *see* Foreign body, superficial, hip
iliac region — *see* Injury, superficial, abdomen
inguinal region — *see* Injury, superficial, abdomen
insect bite — *see* Bite, by site, superficial, insect
interscapular region — *see* Injury, superficial, thorax, back
jaw — *see* Injury, superficial, head, specified NEC
knee S80.91- ☑
  abrasion — *see* Abrasion, knee
  bite — *see* Bite, superficial, knee
  blister — *see* Blister, knee
  contusion — *see* Contusion, knee
  external constriction — *see* Constriction, external, knee
  foreign body — *see* Foreign body, superficial, knee
labium (majus) (minus) S30.95 ☑
lacrimal (apparatus) (gland) (sac) — *see* Injury, eye, specified site NEC
larynx — *see* Injury, superficial, throat
leg (lower) S80.92- ☑
  abrasion — *see* Abrasion, leg
  bite — *see* Bite, superficial, leg
  contusion — *see* Contusion, leg
  external constriction — *see* Constriction, external, leg
  foreign body — *see* Foreign body, superficial, leg
  knee — *see* Injury, superficial, knee
limb NEC T14.8
lip S00.501 ☑
lower back S30.91 ☑
lumbar region S30.91 ☑
malar region — *see* Injury, superficial, head, specified NEC
mammary — *see* Injury, superficial, breast
mastoid region — *see* Injury, superficial, head, specified NEC
mouth — *see* Injury, superficial, oral cavity
muscle NEC T14.8
nail NEC T14.8
  finger — *see* Injury, superficial, finger
  toe — *see* Injury, superficial, toe
nasal (septum) — *see* Injury, superficial, nose
neck S10.90 ☑
  specified site NEC S10.80 ☑
nose (septum) S00.30 ☑
occipital region — *see* Injury, superficial, scalp
oral cavity S00.502 ☑
orbital region — *see* Injury, superficial, periocular area
palate — *see* Injury, superficial, oral cavity
palm — *see* Injury, superficial, hand
parietal region — *see* Injury, superficial, scalp
pelvis S30.91 ☑
  girdle — *see* Injury, superficial, hip
penis S30.93 ☑
perineum
  female S30.95 ☑
  male S30.91 ☑
periocular area S00.20- ☑
  abrasion — *see* Abrasion, eyelid
  bite — *see* Bite, superficial, eyelid
  contusion — *see* Contusion, eyelid
  external constriction — *see* Constriction, external, eyelid
  foreign body — *see* Foreign body, superficial, eyelid
phalanges
  finger — *see* Injury, superficial, finger
  toe — *see* Injury, superficial, toe
pharynx — *see* Injury, superficial, throat
pinna — *see* Injury, superficial, ear
popliteal space — *see* Injury, superficial, knee
prepuce S30.93 ☑
pubic region S30.91 ☑
pudendum
  female S30.97 ☑
  male S30.96 ☑
sacral region S30.91 ☑
scalp S00.00 ☑
scapular region — *see* Injury, superficial, shoulder
sclera — *see* Injury, eye, specified site NEC
scrotum S30.94 ☑
shin — *see* Injury, superficial, leg

Injury — *continued*

shoulder S40.91- ☑
  abrasion — *see* Abrasion, shoulder
  bite — *see* Bite, superficial, shoulder
  blister — *see* Blister, shoulder
  contusion — *see* Contusion, shoulder
  external constriction — *see* Constriction, external, shoulder
  foreign body — *see* Foreign body, superficial, shoulder
skin NEC T14.8
sternal region — *see* Injury, superficial, thorax, front
subconjunctival — *see* Injury, eye, specified site NEC
subcutaneous NEC T14.8
submaxillary region — *see* Injury, superficial, head, specified NEC
submental region — *see* Injury, superficial, head, specified NEC
subungual
  finger (s) — *see* Injury, superficial, finger
  toe (s) — *see* Injury, superficial, toe
supraclavicular fossa — *see* Injury, superficial, neck
supraorbital — *see* Injury, superficial, head, specified NEC
temple — *see* Injury, superficial, head, specified NEC
temporal region — *see* Injury, superficial, head, specified NEC
testis S30.94 ☑
thigh S70.92- ☑
  abrasion — *see* Abrasion, thigh
  bite — *see* Bite, superficial, thigh
  blister — *see* Blister, thigh
  contusion — *see* Contusion, thigh
  external constriction — *see* Constriction, external, thigh
  foreign body — *see* Foreign body, superficial, thigh
thorax, thoracic (wall) S20.90 ☑
  abrasion — *see* Abrasion, thorax
  back S20.40- ☑
  bite — *see* Bite, thorax, superficial
  blister — *see* Blister, thorax
  contusion — *see* Contusion, thorax
  external constriction — *see* Constriction, external, thorax
  foreign body — *see* Foreign body, superficial, thorax
  front S20.30- ☑
throat S10.10 ☑
  abrasion S10.11 ☑
  bite S10.17 ☑
    insect S10.16 ☑
  blister S10.12 ☑
  contusion S10.0 ☑
  external constriction S10.14 ☑
  foreign body S10.15 ☑
thumb S60.93- ☑
  abrasion — *see* Abrasion, thumb
  bite — *see* Bite, superficial, thumb
  blister — *see* Blister, thumb
  contusion — *see* Contusion, thumb
  external constriction — *see* Constriction, external, thumb
  foreign body — *see* Foreign body, superficial, thumb
  insect bite — *see* Bite, by site, superficial, insect
  specified type NEC S60.39- ☑
toe (s) S90.93- ☑
  abrasion — *see* Abrasion, toe
  bite — *see* Bite, toe
  blister — *see* Blister, toe
  contusion — *see* Contusion, toe
  external constriction — *see* Constriction, external, toe
  foreign body — *see* Foreign body, superficial, toe
  great S90.93- ☑
tongue — *see* Injury, superficial, oral cavity
tooth, teeth — *see* Injury, superficial, oral cavity
trachea S10.10 ☑
tunica vaginalis S30.94 ☑
tympanum, tympanic membrane — *see* Injury, superficial, ear
uvula — *see* Injury, superficial, oral cavity
vagina S30.95 ☑
vocal cords — *see* Injury, superficial, throat
vulva S30.95 ☑

☑ **Additional character required**

Injury — continued

wrist S60.91- ☑
supraclavicular region — see Injury, neck
supraorbital S09.93 ☑
suprarenal gland (multiple) — see Injury, adrenal
surgical complication (external or internal site)
— see Laceration, accidental complicating
surgery
temple S09.90 ☑
temporal region S09.90 ☑
tendon (see also Injury, muscle, by site)
abdomen — see Injury, muscle, abdomen
Achilles — see Injury, Achilles tendon
lower back — see Injury, muscle, lower back
pelvic organs — see Injury, muscle, pelvis
tenth cranial nerve (pneumogastric or vagus) —
see Injury, nerve, vagus
testis S39.94 ☑
thigh S79.92- ☑
blood vessel — see Injury, blood vessel, hip
contusion — see Contusion, thigh
fracture — see Fracture, femur
muscle — see Injury, muscle, thigh
nerve — see Injury, nerve, thigh
open — see Wound, open, thigh
specified NEC S79.82- ☑
superficial — see Injury, superficial, thigh
third cranial nerve (oculomotor) — see Injury,
nerve, oculomotor
thorax, thoracic S29.9 ☑
blood vessel — see Injury, blood vessel, thorax
cavity — see Injury, intrathoracic
dislocation — see Dislocation, thorax
external (wall) S29.9 ☑
contusion — see Contusion, thorax
nerve — see Injury, nerve, thorax
open — see Wound, open, thorax
specified NEC S29.8 ☑
sprain — see Sprain, thorax
superficial — see Injury, superficial, thorax
fracture — see Fracture, thorax
internal — see Injury, intrathoracic
intrathoracic organ — see Injury, intrathoracic
sympathetic ganglion — see Injury, nerve,
thorax, sympathetic
throat (see also Injury, neck) S19.9 ☑
thumb S69.9- ☑
blood vessel — see Injury, blood vessel, thumb
contusion — see Contusion, thumb
dislocation — see Dislocation, thumb
fracture — see Fracture, thumb
muscle — see Injury, muscle, thumb
nerve — see Injury, nerve, digital, thumb
open — see Wound, open, thumb
specified NEC S69.8- ☑
sprain — see Sprain, thumb
superficial — see Injury, superficial, thumb
thymus (gland) — see Injury, intrathoracic,
specified organ NEC
thyroid (gland) NEC S19.84 ☑
toe S99.92- ☑
contusion — see Contusion, toe
dislocation — see Dislocation, toe
fracture — see Fracture, toe
muscle — see Injury, muscle, toe
open — see Wound, open, toe
specified type NEC S99.82- ☑
sprain — see Sprain, toe
superficial — see Injury, superficial, toe
tongue S09.93 ☑
tonsil S09.93 ☑
tooth S09.93 ☑
trachea (cervical) NEC S19.82 ☑
thoracic — see Injury, intrathoracic, trachea,
thoracic
transfusion-related acute lung (TRALI) J95.84
tunica vaginalis S39.94 ☑
twelfth cranial nerve (hypoglossal) — see Injury,
nerve, hypoglossal
ureter S37.10 ☑
contusion S37.12 ☑
laceration S37.13 ☑
specified type NEC S37.19 ☑
urethra (sphincter) S37.30 ☑
at delivery O71.5
contusion S37.32 ☑
laceration S37.33 ☑
specified type NEC S37.39 ☑
urinary organ S37.90 ☑
contusion S37.92 ☑
laceration S37.93 ☑
specified

Injury — continued

site NEC S37.899 ☑
contusion S37.892 ☑
laceration S37.893 ☑
specified type NEC S37.898 ☑
type NEC S37.99 ☑
uterus, uterine S37.60 ☑
with ectopic or molar pregnancy O08.6
blood vessel — see Injury, blood vessel, iliac
contusion S37.62 ☑
laceration S37.63 ☑
cervix at delivery O71.3
rupture associated with obstetrics — see
Rupture, uterus
specified type NEC S37.69 ☑
uvula S09.93 ☑
vagina S39.93 ☑
abrasion S30.814 ☑
bite S31.45 ☑
insect S30.864 ☑
superficial NEC S30.874 ☑
contusion S30.23 ☑
crush S38.03 ☑
during delivery — see Laceration, vagina,
during delivery
external constriction S30.844 ☑
insect bite S30.864 ☑
laceration S31.41 ☑
with foreign body S31.42 ☑
open wound S31.40 ☑
puncture S31.43 ☑
with foreign body S31.44 ☑
superficial S30.95 ☑
foreign body S30.854 ☑
vas deferens — see Injury, pelvic organ, specified
site NEC
vascular NEC T14.8
vein — see Injury, blood vessel
vena cava (superior) S25.20 ☑
inferior S35.10 ☑
laceration (minor) (superficial) S35.11 ☑
major S35.12 ☑
specified type NEC S35.19 ☑
laceration (minor) (superficial) S25.21 ☑
major S25.22 ☑
specified type NEC S25.29 ☑
vesical (sphincter) — see Injury, bladder
visual cortex S04.04- ☑
vitreous (humor) S05.90 ☑
specified NEC S05.8X- ☑
vocal cord NEC S19.83 ☑
vulva S39.94 ☑
abrasion S30.814 ☑
bite S31.45 ☑
insect S30.864 ☑
superficial NEC S30.874 ☑
contusion S30.23 ☑
crush S38.03 ☑
during delivery — see Laceration, perineum,
female, during delivery
external constriction S30.844 ☑
insect bite S30.864 ☑
laceration S31.41 ☑
with foreign body S31.42 ☑
open wound S31.40 ☑
puncture S31.43 ☑
with foreign body S31.44 ☑
superficial S30.95 ☑
foreign body S30.854 ☑
whiplash (cervical spine) S13.4 ☑
wrist S69.9- ☑
blood vessel — see Injury, blood vessel, hand
contusion — see Contusion, wrist
dislocation — see Dislocation, wrist
fracture — see Fracture, wrist
muscle — see Injury, muscle, hand
nerve — see Injury, nerve, hand
open — see Wound, open, wrist
specified NEC S69.8- ☑
sprain — see Sprain, wrist
superficial — see Injury, superficial, wrist
Inoculation (see also Vaccination)
complication or reaction — see Complications,
vaccination
Insanity, insane (see also Psychosis)
adolescent — see Schizophrenia
confusional F28
acute or subacute F05
delusional F22
senile F03 ☑
Insect
bite — see Bite, by site, superficial, insect

Insect — continued
venomous, poisoning NEC (by) — see Venom,
arthropod
Insensitivity
adrenocorticotropin hormone (ACTH) E27.49
androgen E34.50
complete E34.51
partial E34.52
Insertion
cord (umbilical) lateral or velamentous O43.12- ☑
intrauterine contraceptive device (encounter for)
— see Intrauterine contraceptive device
Insolation (sunstroke) T67.0 ☑
Insomnia (organic) G47.00
adjustment F51.02
adjustment disorder F51.02
behavioral, of childhood Z73.819
combined type Z73.812
limit setting type Z73.811
sleep-onset association type Z73.810
childhood Z73.819
chronic F51.04
somatized tension F51.04
conditioned F51.04
due to
alcohol
abuse F10.182
dependence F10.282
use F10.982
amphetamines
abuse F15.182
dependence F15.282
use F15.982
anxiety disorder F51.05
caffeine
abuse F15.182
dependence F15.282
use F15.982
cocaine
abuse F14.182
dependence F14.282
use F14.982
depression F51.05
drug NEC
abuse F19.182
dependence F19.282
use F19.982
medical condition G47.01
mental disorder NEC F51.05
opioid
abuse F11.182
dependence F11.282
use F11.982
psychoactive substance NEC
abuse F19.182
dependence F19.282
use F19.982
sedative, hypnotic, or anxiolytic
abuse F13.182
dependence F13.282
use F13.982
stimulant NEC
abuse F15.182
dependence F15.282
use F15.982
fatal familial (FFI) A81.83
idiopathic F51.01
learned F51.3
nonorganic origin F51.01
not due to a substance or known physiological
condition F51.01
specified NEC F51.09
paradoxical F51.03
primary F51.01
psychiatric F51.05
psychophysiologic F51.04
related to psychopathology F51.05
short-term F51.02
specified NEC G47.09
stress-related F51.02
transient F51.02
without objective findings F51.02
Inspiration
food or foreign body — see Foreign body, by site
mucus — see Asphyxia, mucus
Inspissated bile syndrome (newborn) P59.1
Instability
emotional (excessive) F60.3
joint (post-traumatic) M25.30
ankle M25.37- ☑
due to old ligament Injury — see Disorder,
ligament

Instability — *continued*
elbow M25.32- ☑
flail — *see* Flail, joint
foot M25.37- ☑
hand M25.34- ☑
hip M25.35- ☑
knee M25.36- ☑
lumbosacralM53.2
prosthesis — *see* Complications, joint
  prosthesis, mechanical, displacement, by
  site
sacroiliacM53.2
secondary to
  old ligament injury — *see* Disorder, ligament
  removal of joint prosthesis M96.89
shoulder (region) M25.31- ☑
spineM53.2
wrist M25.33- ☑
knee (chronic) M23.5- ☑
lumbosacralM53.2
nervous F48.8
personality (emotional) F60.3
spine — *see* Instability, joint, spine
vasomotor R55
Institutional syndrome (childhood) F94.2
Institutionalization, affecting child Z62.22
disinhibited attachment F94.2
Insufficiency, insufficient
accommodation, old age H52.4
adrenal (gland) E27.40
  primary E27.1
adrenocortical E27.40
  drug-induced E27.3
  iatrogenic E27.3
  primary E27.1
anterior (occlusal) guidance M26.54
anus K62.89
aortic (valve) I35.1
  with
    mitral (valve) disease I08.0
      with tricuspid (valve) disease I08.3
    stenosis I35.2
    tricuspid (valve) disease I08.2
      with mitral (valve) disease I08.3
  congenital Q23.1
  rheumatic I06.1
    with
      mitral (valve) disease I08.0
        with tricuspid (valve) disease I08.3
      stenosis I06.2
        with mitral (valve) disease I08.0
          with tricuspid (valve) disease I08.3
      tricuspid (valve) disease I08.2
        with mitral (valve) disease I08.3
  specified cause NEC I35.1
  syphilitic A52.03
arterial I77.1
  basilar G45.0
  carotid (hemispheric) G45.1
  cerebral I67.81
  coronary (acute or subacute) I24.8
  mesenteric K55.1
  peripheral I73.9
  precerebral (multiple) (bilateral) G45.2
  vertebral G45.0
arteriovenous I99.8
biliary K83.8
cardiac (*see also* Insufficiency, myocardial)
  due to presence of (cardiac) prosthesis I97.11-
    ☑
  postprocedural I97.11- ☑
cardiorenal, hypertensive I13.2
cardiovascular — *see* Disease, cardiovascular
cerebrovascular (acute) I67.81
  with transient focal neurological signs and
    symptoms G45.8
circulatory NEC I99.8
  newborn P29.89
convergence H51.11
coronary (acute or subacute) I24.8
  chronic or with a stated duration of over 4
    weeks I25.89
corticoadrenal E27.40
  primary E27.1
dietary E63.9
divergence H51.8
food T73.0 ☑
gastroesophageal K22.8
gonadal
  ovary E28.39
  testis E29.1
heart (*see also* Insufficiency, myocardial)

Insufficiency — *continued*
newborn P29.0
valve — *see* Endocarditis
hepatic — *see* Failure, hepatic
idiopathic autonomic G90.09
interocclusal distance of fully erupted teeth
  (ridge) M26.36
kidney N28.9
  acute N28.9
  chronic N18.9
lacrimal (secretion) H04.12- ☑
  passages — *see* Stenosis, lacrimal
liver — *see* Failure, hepatic
lung — *see* Insufficiency, pulmonary
mental (congenital) — *see* Disability, intellectual
mesenteric K55.1
mitral (valve) I34.0
  with
    aortic valve disease I08.0
      with tricuspid (valve) disease I08.3
    obstruction or stenosis I05.2
      with aortic valve disease I08.0
    tricuspid (valve) disease I08.1
      with aortic (valve) disease I08.3
  congenital Q23.3
  rheumatic I05.1
    with
      aortic valve disease I08.0
        with tricuspid (valve) disease I08.3
      obstruction or stenosis I05.2
        with aortic valve disease I08.0
          with tricuspid (valve) disease I08.3
      tricuspid (valve) disease I08.1
        with aortic (valve) disease I08.3
    active or acute I01.1
      with chorea, rheumatic (Sydenham's) I02.0
  specified cause, except rheumatic I34.0
muscle (*see also* Disease, muscle)
  heart — *see* Insufficiency, myocardial
  ocular NEC H50.9
myocardial, myocardium (with arteriosclerosis)
  I50.9
  with
    rheumatic fever (conditions in I00) I09.0
      active, acute or subacute I01.2
        with chorea I02.0
      inactive or quiescent (with chorea) I09.0
  congenital Q24.8
  hypertensive — *see* Hypertension, heart
  newborn P29.0
  rheumatic I09.0
    active, acute, or subacute I01.2
  syphilitic A52.06
nourishment T73.0 ☑
pancreatic K86.8
parathyroid (gland) E20.9
peripheral vascular (arterial) I73.9
pituitary E23.0
placental (mother) O36.51- ☑
platelets D69.6
prenatal care affecting management of
  pregnancy O09.3- ☑
progressive pluriglandular E31.0
pulmonary J98.4
  acute, following surgery (nonthoracic) J95.2
    thoracic J95.1
  chronic, following surgery J95.3
  following
    shock J98.4
    trauma J98.4
  newborn P28.5
  valve I37.1
    with stenosis I37.2
    congenital Q22.2
    rheumatic I09.89
      with aortic, mitral or tricuspid (valve)
        disease I08.8
pyloric K31.89
renal (acute) N28.9
  chronic N18.9
respiratory R06.89
  newborn P28.5
rotation — *see* Malrotation
sleep syndrome F51.12
social insurance Z59.7
suprarenal E27.40
  primary E27.1
tarso-orbital fascia, congenital Q10.3
testis E29.1
thyroid (gland) (acquired) E03.9
  congenital E03.1
tricuspid (valve) (rheumatic) I07.1

Insufficiency — *continued*
  with
    aortic (valve) disease I08.2
      with mitral (valve) disease I08.3
    mitral (valve) disease I08.1
      with aortic (valve) disease I08.3
    obstruction or stenosis I07.2
      with aortic (valve) disease I08.2
      with mitral (valve) disease I08.3
  congenital Q22.8
  nonrheumatic I36.1
    with stenosis I36.2
urethral sphincter R32
valve, valvular (heart) — *see* Endocarditis
  congenital Q24.8
vascular I99.8
  intestine K55.9
    acute K55.0
  mesenteric K55.1
  peripheral I73.9
  renal — *see* Hypertension, kidney
velopharyngeal
  acquired K13.79
  congenital Q38.8
venous (chronic) (peripheral) I87.2
ventricular — *see* Insufficiency, myocardial
welfare support Z59.7
Insufflation, fallopian Z31.41
Insular — *see* condition
Insulinoma
pancreas
  benign D13.7
  malignant C25.4
  uncertain behavior D37.8
specified site
  benign — *see* Neoplasm, by site, benign
  malignant — *see* Neoplasm, by site, malignant
  uncertain behavior — *see* Neoplasm, by site,
    uncertain behavior
unspecified site
  benign D13.7
  malignant C25.4
  uncertain behavior D37.8
Insuloma — *see* Insulinoma
Interference
balancing side M26.56
non-working side M26.56
Intermenstrual — *see* condition
Intermittent — *see* condition
Internal — *see* condition
Interrogation
cardiac defibrillator (automatic) (implantable)
  Z45.02
cardiac pacemaker Z45.018
cardiac (event) (loop) recorder Z45.09
infusion pump (implanted) (intrathecal) Z45.1
neurostimulator Z46.2
Interruption
bundle of His I44.30
phase-shift, sleep cycle — *see* Disorder, sleep,
  circadian rhythm
sleep phase-shift, or 24 hour sleep-wake cycle —
  see Disorder, sleep, circadian rhythm
Interstitial — *see* condition
Intertrigo L30.4
labialis K13.0
Intervertebral disc — *see* condition
Intestine, intestinal — *see* condition
Intolerance
carbohydrate K90.4
disaccharide, hereditary E73.0
fat NEC K90.4
  pancreatic K90.3
food K90.4
  dietary counseling and surveillance Z71.3
fructose E74.10
  hereditary E74.12
glucose (-galactose) E74.39
gluten K90.0
lactose E73.9
  specified NEC E73.8
lysine E72.3
milk NEC K90.4
  lactose E73.9
protein K90.4
starch NEC K90.4
sucrose (-isomaltose) E74.31
Intoxicated NEC (without dependence) — *see*
  Alcohol, intoxication
Intoxication
acid E87.2

☑ **Additional character required**

Intoxication — *continued*
  alcoholic (acute) (without dependence) — *see*
    Alcohol, intoxication
  alimentary canal K52.1
  amphetamine (without dependence) — *see*
    Abuse, drug, stimulant, with intoxication
    with dependence — *see* Dependence, drug,
      stimulant, with intoxication
  anxiolytic (acute) (without dependence) — *see*
    Abuse, drug, sedative, with intoxication
    with dependence — *see* Dependence, drug,
      sedative, with intoxication
  caffeine (acute) (without dependence) — *see*
    Abuse, drug, stimulant, with intoxication
    with dependence — *see* Dependence, drug,
      stimulant, with intoxication
  cannabinoids (acute) (without dependence) —
    see Abuse, drug, cannabis, with intoxication
    with dependence — *see* Dependence, drug,
      cannabis, with intoxication
  chemical — *see* Table of Drugs and Chemicals
    via placenta or breast milk — *see* - Absorption,
      chemical, through placenta
  cocaine (acute) (without dependence) — *see*
    Abuse, drug, cocaine, with intoxication
    with dependence — *see* Dependence, drug,
      cocaine, with intoxication
  drug
    acute (without dependence) — *see* Abuse,
      drug, by type with intoxication
      with dependence — *see* Dependence, drug,
        by type with intoxication
    addictive
      via placenta or breast milk — *see* Absorption,
        drug, addictive, through placenta
    newborn P93.8
      gray baby syndrome P93.0
    overdose or wrong substance given or taken —
      see Table of Drugs and Chemicals, by drug,
      poisoning
  enteric K52.1
  foodborne A05.9
    bacterial A05.9
    classical (Clostridium botulinum) A05.1
    due to
      Bacillus cereus A05.4
      bacterium A05.9
        specified NEC A05.8
      Clostridium
        botulinum A05.1
        perfringens A05.2
        welchii A05.2
      Salmonella A02.9
        with
          (gastro)enteritis A02.0
          localized infection (s) A02.20
            arthritis A02.23
            meningitis A02.21
            osteomyelitis A02.24
            pneumonia A02.22
            pyelonephritis A02.25
            specified NEC A02.29
          sepsis A02.1
          specified manifestation NEC A02.8
      Staphylococcus A05.0
      Vibrio
        parahaemolyticus A05.3
        vulnificus A05.5
    enterotoxin, staphylococcal A05.0
    noxious — *see* Poisoning, food, noxious
  gastrointestinal K52.1
  hallucinogenic (without dependence) — *see*
    Abuse, drug, hallucinogen, with intoxication
    with dependence — *see* Dependence, drug,
      hallucinogen, with intoxication
  hypnotic (acute) (without dependence) — *see*
    Abuse, drug, sedative, with intoxication
    with dependence — *see* Dependence, drug,
      sedative, with intoxication
  inhalant (acute) (without dependence) — *see*
    Abuse, drug, inhalant, with intoxication
    with dependence — *see* Dependence, drug,
      inhalant, with intoxication
  meaning
    inebriationF10
    poisoning — *see* Table of Drugs and Chemicals
  methyl alcohol (acute) (without dependence) —
    see Alcohol, intoxication
  opioid (acute) (without dependence) — *see*
    Abuse, drug, opioid, with intoxication
    with dependence — *see* Dependence, drug,
      opioid, with intoxication

Intoxication — *continued*
  pathologic NEC (without dependence) — *see*
    Alcohol, intoxication
  phencyclidine (without dependence) — *see*
    Abuse, drug, psychoactive NEC, with
    intoxication
    with dependence — *see* Dependence, drug,
      psychoactive NEC, with intoxication
  potassium (K) E87.5
  psychoactive substance NEC (without
    dependence) — *see* Abuse, drug,
    psychoactive NEC, with intoxication
    with dependence — *see* Dependence, drug,
      psychoactive NEC, with intoxication
  sedative (acute) (without dependence) — *see*
    Abuse, drug, sedative, with intoxication
    with dependence — *see* Dependence, drug,
      sedative, with intoxication
  serum (*see also* Reaction, serum) T80.69 ☑
  uremic — *see* Uremia
  volatile solvents (acute) (without dependence) —
    see Abuse, drug, inhalant, with intoxication
    with dependence — *see* Dependence, drug,
      inhalant, with intoxication
  water E87.79
Intracranial — *see* condition
Intrahepatic gallbladder Q44.1
Intraligamentous — *see* condition
Intrathoracic (*see also* condition)
  kidney Q63.2
Intrauterine contraceptive device
  checking Z30.431
  insertion Z30.430
    immediately following removal Z30.433
  in situ Z97.5
  management Z30.431
  reinsertion Z30.433
  removal Z30.432
  replacement Z30.433
  retention in pregnancy O26.3- ☑
Intraventricular — *see* condition
Intrinsic deformity — *see* Deformity
Intubation, difficult or failed T88.4 ☑
Intumescence, lens (eye) (cataract) — *see* Cataract
Intussusception (bowel) (colon) (enteric) (ileocecal)
  (ileocolic) (intestine) (rectum) K56.1
  appendix K38.8
  congenital Q43.8
  ureter (with obstruction) N13.5
Invagination (bowel, colon, intestine or rectum)
  K56.1
Inversion
  albumin-globulin (A-G) ratio E88.09
  bladder N32.89
  cecum — *see* Intussusception
  cervix N88.8
  chromosome in normal individual Q95.1
  circadian rhythm — *see* Disorder, sleep, circadian
    rhythm
  nipple N64.59
    congenital Q83.8
    gestational — *see* Retraction, nipple
    puerperal, postpartum — *see* Retraction, nipple
  nyctohemeral rhythm — *see* Disorder, sleep,
    circadian rhythm
  optic papilla Q14.2
  organ or site, congenital NEC — *see* Anomaly,
    by site
  sleep rhythm — *see* Disorder, sleep, circadian
    rhythm
  testis (congenital) Q55.29
  uterus (chronic) (postinfectional) (postpartal,
    old) N85.5
    postpartum O71.2
  vagina (posthysterectomy) N99.3
  ventricular Q20.5
Investigation (*see also* Examination) Z04.9
  clinical research subject (control) (normal
    comparison) (participant) Z00.6
Involuntary movement, abnormal R25.9
Involution, involutional (*see also* condition)
  breast, cystic — *see* Dysplasia, mammary,
    specified type NEC
  depression (single episode) F32.8
    recurrent episode F33.9
  melancholia (recurrent episode) (single episode)
    F32.8
  ovary, senile — *see* Atrophy, ovary
  thymus failure E32.8
I.Q.
  under 20 F73
  20-34 F72

I.Q. — *continued*
  35-49 F71
  50-69 F70
IRDS (type I) P22.0
  type II P22.1
Irideremia Q13.1
Iridis rubeosis — *see* Disorder, iris, vascular
Iridochoroiditis (panuveitis) — *see* Panuveitis
Iridocyclitis H20.9
  acute H20.0- ☑
    hypopyon H20.05- ☑
    primary H20.01- ☑
    recurrent H20.02- ☑
    secondary (noninfectious) H20.04- ☑
      infectious H20.03- ☑
  chronic H20.1- ☑
  due to allergy — *see* Iridocyclitis, acute,
    secondary
  endogenous — *see* Iridocyclitis, acute, primary
  Fuchs' — *see* Cyclitis, Fuchs' heterochromic
  gonococcal A54.32
  granulomatous — *see* Iridocyclitis, chronic
  herpes, herpetic (simplex) B00.51
    zoster B02.32
  hypopyon — *see* Iridocyclitis, acute, hypopyon
  in (due to)
    ankylosing spondylitis M45.9
    gonococcal infection A54.32
    herpes (simplex) virus B00.51
      zoster B02.32
    infectious disease NOS B99 ☑
    parasitic disease NOS B89 [H22]
    sarcoidosis D86.83
    syphilis A51.43
    tuberculosis A18.54
    zoster B02.32
  lens-induced H20.2- ☑
  nongranulomatous — *see* Iridocyclitis, acute
  recurrent — *see* Iridocyclitis, acute, recurrent
  rheumatic — *see* Iridocyclitis, chronic
  subacute — *see* Iridocyclitis, acute
  sympathetic — *see* Uveitis, sympathetic
  syphilitic (secondary) A51.43
  tuberculous (chronic) A18.54
  Vogt-Koyanagi H20.82- ☑
Iridocyclochoroiditis (panuveitis) — *see* Panuveitis
Iridodialysis H21.53- ☑
Iridodonesis H21.89
Iridoplegia (complete) (partial) (reflex) H57.09
Iridoschisis H21.25- ☑
Iris (*see also* condition)
  bombé — *see* Membrane, pupillary
Iritis (*see also* Iridocyclitis)
  chronic — *see* Iridocyclitis, chronic
  diabetic — *see* E08-E13 with .39
  due to
    herpes simplex B00.51
    leprosy A30.9 [H22]
  gonococcal A54.32
  gouty M10.9
  granulomatous — *see* Iridocyclitis, chronic
  lens induced — *see* Iridocyclitis, lens-induced
  papulosa (syphilitic) A52.71
  rheumatic — *see* Iridocyclitis, chronic
  syphilitic (secondary) A51.43
    congenital (early) A50.01
    late A52.71
  tuberculous A18.54
Iron — *see* condition
Iron-miner's lung J63.4
Irradiated enamel (tooth, teeth) K03.89
Irradiation effects, adverse T66 ☑
Irreducible, irreducibility — *see* condition
Irregular, irregularity
  action, heart I49.9
  alveolar process K08.8
  bleeding N92.6
  breathing R06.89
  contour of cornea (acquired) — *see* Deformity,
    cornea
    congenital Q13.4
  contour, reconstructed breast N65.0
  dentin (in pulp) K04.3
  eye movements H55.89
    nystagmus — *see* Nystagmus
    saccadic H55.81
  labor O62.2
  menstruation (cause unknown) N92.6
  periods N92.6
  prostate N42.9
  pupil — *see* Abnormality, pupillary
  reconstructed breast N65.0

Irregular — *continued*
  respiratory R06.89
  septum (nasal) J34.2
  shape, organ or site, congenital NEC — *see*
    Distortion
  sleep-wake pattern (rhythm) G47.23
Irritable, irritability R45.4
  bladder N32.89
  bowel (syndrome) K58.9
    with diarrhea K58.0
    psychogenic F45.8
  bronchial — *see* Bronchitis
  cerebral, in newborn P91.3
  colon K58.9
    with diarrhea K58.0
    psychogenic F45.8
  duodenum K59.8
  heart (psychogenic) F45.8
  hip — *see* Derangement, joint, specified type
    NEC, hip
  ileum K59.8
  infant R68.12
  jejunum K59.8
  rectum K59.8
  stomach K31.89
    psychogenic F45.8
  sympathetic G90.8
  urethra N36.8
Irritation
  anus K62.89
  axillary nerve G54.0
  bladder N32.89
  brachial plexus G54.0
  bronchial — *see* Bronchitis
  cervical plexus G54.2
  cervix — *see* Cervicitis
  choroid, sympathetic — *see* Endophthalmitis
  cranial nerve — *see* Disorder, nerve, cranial
  gastric K31.89
    psychogenic F45.8
  globe, sympathetic — *see* Uveitis, sympathetic
  labyrinth H83.2
  lumbosacral plexus G54.1
  meninges (traumatic) — *see* Injury, intracranial
    nontraumatic — *see* Meningismus
  nerve — *see* Disorder, nerve
  nervous R45.0
  penis N48.89
  perineum NEC L29.3
  peripheral autonomic nervous system G90.8
  peritoneum — *see* Peritonitis
  pharynx J39.2
  plantar nerve — *see* Lesion, nerve, plantar
  spinal (cord) (traumatic) (*see also* Injury, spinal
    cord, by region)
    nerve G58.9
      root NEC — *see* Radiculopathy
    nontraumatic — *see* Myelopathy
  stomach K31.89
    psychogenic F45.8
  sympathetic nerve NEC G90.8
  ulnar nerve — *see* Lesion, nerve, ulnar
  vagina N89.8
Ischemia, ischemic I99.8
  brain — *see* Ischemia, cerebral
  bowel (transient)
    acute K55.0
    chronic K55.1
    due to mesenteric artery insufficiency K55.1
  cardiac (see Disease, heart, ischemic)
  cardiomyopathy I25.5
  cerebral (chronic) (generalized) I67.82
    arteriosclerotic I67.2
    intermittent G45.9
    newborn P91.0
    recurrent focal G45.8
    transient G45.9
  colon chronic (due to mesenteric artery
    insufficiency) K55.1
  coronary — *see* Disease, heart, ischemic
  demand (coronary) (*see also* Angina) I24.8
  heart (chronic or with a stated duration of over 4
    weeks) I25.9
    acute or with a stated duration of 4 weeks or
      less I24.9
    subacute I24.9
  infarction, muscle — *see* Infarct, muscle
  intestine (large) (small) (transient) K55.9
    acute K55.0
    chronic K55.1
    due to mesenteric artery insufficiency K55.1
  kidney N28.0

Ischemia — *continued*
  mesenteric, acute K55.0
  muscle, traumatic T79.6 ☑
  myocardium, myocardial (chronic or with a stated
    duration of over 4 weeks) I25.9
    acute, without myocardial infarction I24.0
    silent (asymptomatic) I25.6
    transient of newborn P29.4
  renal N28.0
  retina, retinal — *see* Occlusion, artery, retina
  small bowel
    acute K55.0
    chronic K55.1
    due to mesenteric artery insufficiency K55.1
  spinal cord G95.11
  subendocardial — *see* Insufficiency, coronary
  supply (coronary) (*see also* Angina) I25.9
    due to vasospasm I20.1
Ischial spine — *see* condition
Ischialgia — *see* Sciatica
Ischiopagus Q89.4
Ischium, ischial — *see* condition
Ischuria R34
Iselin's disease or osteochondrosis — *see*
  Osteochondrosis, juvenile, metatarsus
Islands of
  parotid tissue in
    lymph nodes Q38.6
    neck structures Q38.6
  submaxillary glands in
    fascia Q38.6
    lymph nodes Q38.6
    neck muscles Q38.6
Islet cell tumor, pancreas D13.7
Isoimmunization NEC (*see also* Incompatibility)
  affecting management of pregnancy (ABO) (with
    hydrops fetalis) O36.11- ☑
    anti-A sensitization O36.11- ☑
    anti-B sensitization O36.19- ☑
    anti-c sensitization O36.09- ☑
    anti-C sensitization O36.09- ☑
    anti-e sensitization O36.09- ☑
    anti-E sensitization O36.09- ☑
    Rh NEC O36.09- ☑
      anti-D antibody O36.01- ☑
    specified NEC O36.19- ☑
  newborn P55.9
    with
      hydrops fetalis P56.0
      kernicterus P57.0
    ABO (blood groups) P55.1
    Rhesus (Rh) factor P55.0
    specified type NEC P55.8
Isolation, isolated
  dwelling Z59.8
  family Z63.79
  social Z60.4
Isoleucinosis E71.19
Isomerism atrial appendages (with asplenia or
  polysplenia) Q20.6
Isosporiasis, isosporosis A07.3
Isovaleric acidemia E71.110
Issue of
  medical certificate Z02.79
    for disability determination Z02.71
  repeat prescription (appliance) (glasses)
    (medicinal substance, medicament,
    medicine) Z76.0
    contraception — *see* Contraception
Itch, itching (*see also* Pruritus)
  baker's L23.6
  barber's B35.0
  bricklayer's L24.5
  cheese B88.0
  clam digger's B65.3
  coolie B76.9
  copra B88.0
  dew B76.9
  dhobi B35.6
  filarial — *see* Infestation, filarial
  grain B88.0
  grocer's B88.0
  ground B76.9
  harvest B88.0
  jock B35.6
  Malabar B35.5
    beard B35.0
    foot B35.3
    scalp B35.0
  meaning scabies B86
  Norwegian B86
  perianal L29.0

Itch — *continued*
  poultrymen's B88.0
  sarcoptic B86
  scabies B86
  scrub B88.0
  straw B88.0
  swimmer's B65.3
  water B76.9
  winter L29.8
Ivemark's syndrome (asplenia with congenital heart
  disease) Q89.01
Ivory bones Q78.2
Ixodiasis NEC B88.8

J

Jaccoud's syndrome — *see* Arthropathy,
  postrheumatic, chronic
Jackson's
  membrane Q43.3
  paralysis or syndrome G83.89
  veil Q43.3
Jacquet's dermatitis (diaper dermatitis) L22
Jadassohn-Pellizari's disease or anetoderma L90.2
Jadassohn's
  blue nevus — *see* Nevus
  intraepidermal epithelioma — *see* Neoplasm,
    skin, benign
Jaffe-Lichtenstein (-Uehlinger) syndrome — *see*
  Dysplasia, fibrous, bone NEC
Jakob-Creutzfeldt disease or syndrome — *see*
  Creutzfeldt-Jakob disease or syndrome
Jaksch-Luzet disease D64.89
Jamaican
  neuropathy G92
  paraplegic tropical ataxic-spastic syndrome G92
Janet's disease F48.8
Janiceps Q89.4
Jansky-Bielschowsky amaurotic idiocy E75.4
Japanese
  B-type encephalitis A83.0
  river fever A75.3
Jaundice (yellow) R17
  acholuric (familial) (splenomegalic) (*see also*
    Spherocytosis)
    acquired D59.8
  breast-milk (inhibitor) P59.3
  catarrhal (acute) B15.9
    with hepatic coma B15.0
  cholestatic (benign) R17
  due to or associated with
    delayed conjugation P59.8
      associated with (due to) preterm delivery
        P59.0
    preterm delivery P59.0
  epidemic (catarrhal) B15.9
    with hepatic coma B15.0
    leptospiral A27.0
    spirochetal A27.0
  familial nonhemolytic (congenital) (Gilbert) E80.4
    Crigler-Najjar E80.5
  febrile (acute) B15.9
    with hepatic coma B15.0
    leptospiral A27.0
    spirochetal A27.0
  hematogenous D59.9
  hemolytic (acquired) D59.9
    congenital — *see* Spherocytosis
  hemorrhagic (acute) (leptospiral) (spirochetal)
    A27.0
  infectious (acute) (subacute) B15.9
    with hepatic coma B15.0
    leptospiral A27.0
    spirochetal A27.0
  leptospiral (hemorrhagic) A27.0
  malignant (without coma) K72.90
    with coma K72.91
  newborn P59.9
    due to or associated with
      ABO
        antibodies P55.1
        incompatibility, maternal/fetal P55.1
        isoimmunization P55.1
      absence or deficiency of enzyme system for
        bilirubin conjugation (congenital) P59.8
      bleeding P58.1
      breast milk inhibitors to conjugation P59.3
        associated with preterm delivery P59.0
      bruising P58.0

☑ **Additional character required**

Jaundice — continued
- Crigler-Najjar syndrome E80.5
- delayed conjugation P59.8
  - associated with preterm delivery P59.0
- drugs or toxins
  - given to newborn P58.42
  - transmitted from mother P58.41
- excessive hemolysis P58.9
  - due to
    - bleeding P58.1
    - bruising P58.0
    - drugs or toxins
      - given to newborn P58.42
      - transmitted from mother P58.41
    - infection P58.2
    - polycythemia P58.3
    - swallowed maternal blood P58.5
  - specified type NEC P58.8
- galactosemia E74.21
- Gilbert syndrome E80.4
- hemolytic disease P55.9
  - ABO isoimmunization P55.1
  - Rh isoimmunization P55.0
  - specified NEC P55.8
- hepatocellular damage P59.20
  - specified NEC P59.29
- hereditary hemolytic anemia P58.8
- hypothyroidism, congenital E03.1
- incompatibility, maternal/fetal NOS P55.9
- infection P58.2
- inspissated bile syndrome P59.1
- isoimmunization NOS P55.9
- mucoviscidosis E84.9
- polycythemia P58.3
- preterm delivery P59.0
- Rh
  - antibodies P55.0
  - incompatibility, maternal/fetal P55.0
  - isoimmunization P55.0
- specified cause NEC P59.8
- swallowed maternal blood P58.5
- spherocytosis (congenital) D58.0
- neonatal — see Jaundice, newborn
- nonhemolytic congenital familial (Gilbert) E80.4
- nuclear, newborn (see also Kernicterus of newborn) P57.9
- obstructive (see also Obstruction, bile duct) K83.1
- post-immunization — see Hepatitis, viral, type, B
- post-transfusion — see Hepatitis, viral, type, B
- regurgitation (see also Obstruction, bile duct) K83.1
- serum (homologous) (prophylactic) (therapeutic) — see Hepatitis, viral, type, B
- spirochetal (hemorrhagic) A27.0
- symptomatic R17
  - newborn P59.9
Jaw — see condition
Jaw-winking phenomenon or syndrome Q07.8
Jealousy
- alcoholic F10.988
- childhood F93.8
- sibling F93.8
Jejunitis — see Enteritis
Jejunostomy status Z93.4
Jejunum, jejunal — see condition
Jensen's disease — see Inflammation, chorioretinal, focal, juxtapapillary
Jerks, myoclonic G25.3
Jervell-Lange-Nielsen syndrome I45.81
Jeune's disease Q77.2
Jigger disease B88.1
Job's syndrome (chronic granulomatous disease) D71
Joint (see also condition)
- mice — see Loose, body, joint
  - knee M23.4- ☑
Jordan's anomaly or syndrome D72.0
Joseph-Diamond-Blackfan anemia (congenital hypoplastic) D61.01
Jungle yellow fever A95.0
Jüngling's disease — see Sarcoidosis
Juvenile — see condition

K

Kahler's disease C90.0- ☑
Kakke E51.11
Kala-azar B55.0
Kallmann's syndrome E23.0

Kanner's syndrome (autism) — see Psychosis, childhood
Kaposi's
- dermatosis (xeroderma pigmentosum) Q82.1
- lichen ruber L44.0
  - acuminatus L44.0
- sarcoma
  - colon C46.4
  - connective tissue C46.1
  - gastrointestinal organ C46.4
  - lung C46.5- ☑
  - lymph node (multiple) C46.3
  - palate (hard) (soft) C46.2
  - rectum C46.4
  - skin (multiple sites) C46.0
  - specified site NEC C46.7
  - stomach C46.4
  - unspecified site C46.9
- varicelliform eruption B00.0
  - vaccinia T88.1 ☑
Kartagener's syndrome or triad (sinusitis, bronchiectasis, situs inversus) Q89.3
Karyotype
- with abnormality except Iso (Xq) Q96.2
- 45,X Q96.0
- 46,X
  - iso (Xq) Q96.1
- 46,XX Q98.3
  - with streak gonads Q50.32
  - hermaphrodite (true) Q99.1
  - male Q98.3
- 46,XY
  - with streak gonads Q56.1
  - female Q97.3
  - hermaphrodite (true) Q99.1
- 47,XXX Q97.0
- 47,XXY Q98.0
- 47,XYY Q98.5
Kaschin-Beck disease — see Disease, Kaschin-Beck
Katayama's disease or fever B65.2
Kawasaki's syndrome M30.3
Kayser-Fleischer ring (cornea) (pseudosclerosis) H18.04- ☑
Kaznelson's syndrome (congenital hypoplastic anemia) D61.01
Kearns-Sayre syndrome H49.81- ☑
Kedani fever A75.3
Kelis L91.0
Kelly (-Patterson) syndrome (sideropenic dysphagia) D50.1
Keloid, cheloid L91.0
- acne L73.0
- Addison's L94.0
- cornea — see Opacity, cornea
- Hawkin's L91.0
- scar L91.0
Keloma L91.0
Kenya fever A77.1
Keratectasia (see also Ectasia, cornea)
- congenital Q13.4
Keratinization of alveolar ridge mucosa
- excessive K13.23
- minimal K13.22
Keratinized residual ridge mucosa
- excessive K13.23
- minimal K13.22
Keratitis (nodular) (nonulcerative) (simple) (zonular) H16.9
- with ulceration (central) (marginal) (perforated) (ring) — see Ulcer, cornea
- actinic — see Photokeratitis
- arborescens (herpes simplex) B00.52
- areolar H16.11- ☑
- bullosa H16.8
- deep H16.309
  - specified type NEC H16.399
- dendritic (a) (herpes simplex) B00.52
- disciform (is) (herpes simplex) B00.52
  - varicella B01.81
- filamentary H16.12- ☑
- gonococcal (congenital or prenatal) A54.33
- herpes, herpetic (simplex) B00.52
  - zoster B02.33
- in (due to)
  - acanthamebiasis B60.13
  - adenovirus B30.0
  - exanthema (see also Exanthem) B09
  - herpes (simplex) virus B00.52
  - measles B05.81
  - syphilis A50.31
  - tuberculosis A18.52
  - zoster B02.33

Keratitis — continued
- interstitial (nonsyphilitic) H16.30- ☑
  - diffuse H16.32- ☑
  - herpes, herpetic (simplex) B00.52
    - zoster B02.33
  - sclerosing H16.33- ☑
  - specified type NEC H16.39- ☑
  - syphilitic (congenital) (late) A50.31
  - tuberculous A18.52
- macular H16.11- ☑
- nummular H16.11- ☑
- oyster shuckers' H16.8
- parenchymatous — see Keratitis, interstitial
- petrifaciens H16.8
- postmeasles B05.81
- punctata
  - leprosa A30.9 [H16.14-]
  - syphilitic (profunda) A50.31
- punctate H16.14- ☑
- purulent H16.8
- rosacea L71.8
- sclerosing H16.33- ☑
- specified type NEC H16.8
- stellate H16.11- ☑
- striate H16.11- ☑
- superficial H16.10- ☑
  - with conjunctivitis — see Keratoconjunctivitis
  - due to light — see Photokeratitis
- suppurative H16.8
- syphilitic (congenital) (prenatal) A50.31
- trachomatous A71.1
  - sequelae B94.0
- tuberculous A18.52
- vesicular H16.8
- xerotic (see also Keratomalacia) H16.8
  - vitamin A deficiency E50.4
Keratoacanthoma L85.8
Keratocele — see Descemetocele
Keratoconjunctivitis H16.20- ☑
- Acanthamoeba B60.13
- adenoviral B30.0
- epidemic B30.0
- exposure H16.21- ☑
- herpes, herpetic (simplex) B00.52
  - zoster B02.33
- in exanthema (see also Exanthem) B09
- infectious B30.0
- lagophthalmic — see Keratoconjunctivitis, specified type NEC
- neurotrophic H16.23- ☑
- phlyctenular H16.25- ☑
- postmeasles B05.81
- shipyard B30.0
- sicca (Sjogren's) M35.0- ☑
  - not Sjogren's H16.22- ☑
- specified type NEC H16.29- ☑
- tuberculous (phlyctenular) A18.52
- vernal H16.26- ☑
Keratoconus H18.60- ☑
- congenital Q13.4
- stable H18.61- ☑
- unstable H18.62- ☑
Keratocyst (dental) (odontogenic) — see Cyst, calcifying odontogenic
Keratoderma, keratodermia (congenital) (palmaris et plantaris) (symmetrical) Q82.8
- acquired L85.1
  - in diseases classified elsewhere L86
- climactericum L85.1
- gonococcal A54.89
- gonorrheal A54.89
- punctata L85.2
- Reiter's — see Reiter's disease
Keratodermatocele — see Descemetocele
Keratoglobus H18.79 ☑
- congenital Q15.8
  - with glaucoma Q15.0
Keratohemia — see Pigmentation, cornea, stromal
Keratoiritis (see also Iridocyclitis)
- syphilitic A50.39
- tuberculous A18.54
Keratoma L57.0
- palmaris and plantaris hereditarium Q82.8
- senile L57.0
Keratomalacia H18.44- ☑
- vitamin A deficiency E50.4
Keratomegaly Q13.4
Keratomycosis B49
- nigrans, nigricans (palmaris) B36.1
Keratopathy H18.9
- band H18.42- ☑
- bullous H18.1- ☑

Keratopathy - Laceration

Keratopathy — *continued*
  bullous (aphakic), following cataract surgery H59.01- ☑
Keratoscleritis, tuberculous A18.52
Keratosis L57.0
  actinic L57.0
  arsenical L85.8
  congenital, specified NEC Q80.8
  female genital NEC N94.89
  follicularis Q82.8
    acquired L11.0
    congenita Q82.8
    et parafollicularis in cutem penetrans L87.0
    spinulosa (decalvans) Q82.8
    vitamin A deficiency E50.8
  gonococcal A54.89
  male genital (external) N50.8
  nigricans L83
  obturans, external ear (canal) — *see* Cholesteatoma, external ear
  palmaris et plantaris (inherited) (symmetrical) Q82.8
    acquired L85.1
  penile N48.89
  pharynx J39.2
  pilaris, acquired L85.8
  punctata (palmaris et plantaris) L85.2
  scrotal N50.8
  seborrheic L82.1
    inflamed L82.0
  senile L57.0
  solar L57.0
  tonsillaris J35.8
  vagina N89.4
  vegetans Q82.8
  vitamin A deficiency E50.8
  vocal cord J38.3
Kerato-uveitis — *see* Iridocyclitis
Kerunoparalysis T75.09 ☑
Kerion (celsi) B35.0
Kernicterus of newborn (not due to isoimmunization) P57.9
  due to isoimmunization (conditions in P55.0-P55.9) P57.0
  specified type NEC P57.8
Keshan disease E59
Ketoacidosis E87.2
  diabetic — *see* Diabetes, by type, with ketoacidosis
Ketonuria R82.4
Ketosis NEC E88.89
  diabetic — *see* Diabetes, by type, with with ketoacidosis
Kew Garden fever A79.1
Kidney — *see* condition
Kienböck's disease (*see also* Osteochondrosis, juvenile, hand, carpal lunate)
  adult M93.1
Kimmelstiel (-Wilson) disease — *see* Diabetes, Kimmelstiel (-Wilson) disease
Kimura disease D21.9
  specified site (*see* Neoplasm, connective tissue benign)
Kink, kinking
  artery I77.1
  hair (acquired) L67.8
  ileum or intestine — *see* Obstruction, intestine
  Lane's — *see* Obstruction, intestine
  organ or site, congenital NEC — *see* Anomaly, by site
  ureter (pelvic junction) N13.5
    with
      hydronephrosis N13.1
        with infection N13.6
      pyelonephritis (chronic) N11.1
    congenital Q62.39
  vein (s) I87.8
    caval I87.1
    peripheral I87.1
Kinnier Wilson's disease (hepatolenticular degeneration) E83.01
Kissing spine M48.20
  cervical region M48.22
  cervicothoracic region M48.23
  lumbar region M48.26
  lumbosacral region M48.27
  occipito-atlanto-axial region M48.21
  thoracic region M48.24
  thoracolumbar region M48.25
Klatskin's tumor C24.0
Klauder's disease A26.8
Klebs' disease (*see also* Glomerulonephritis) N05.- ☑

Klebsiella (K.) pneumoniae, as cause of disease classified elsewhere B96.1
Klein (e)-Levin syndrome G47.13
Kleptomania F63.2
Klinefelter's syndrome Q98.4
  karyotype 47,XXY Q98.0
  male with more than two X chromosomes Q98.1
Klippel-Feil deficiency, disease, or syndrome (brevicollis) Q76.1
Klippel's disease I67.2
Klippel-Trenaunay (-Weber) syndrome Q87.2
Klumpke (-Déjerine) palsy, paralysis (birth) (newborn) P14.1
Knee — *see* condition
Knock knee (acquired) M21.06- ☑
  congenital Q74.1
Knot (s)
  intestinal, syndrome (volvulus) K56.2
  surfer S89.8- ☑
  umbilical cord (true) O69.2 ☑
Knotting (of)
  hair L67.8
  intestine K56.2
Knuckle pad (Garrod's) M72.1
Koch's
  infection — *see* Tuberculosis
  relapsing fever A68.9
Koch-Weeks' conjunctivitis — *see* Conjunctivitis, acute, mucopurulent
Köebner's syndrome Q81.8
Köenig's disease (osteochondritis dissecans) — *see* Osteochondritis, dissecans
Köhler-Pellegrini-Steida disease or syndrome (calcification, knee joint) — *see* Bursitis, tibial collateral
Köhler's disease
  patellar — *see* Osteochondrosis, juvenile, patella
  tarsal navicular — *see* Osteochondrosis, juvenile, tarsus
Koilonychia L60.3
  congenital Q84.6
Kojevnikov's, epilepsy — *see* Kozhevnikof's epilepsy
Koplik's spots B05.9
Kopp's asthma E32.8
Korsakoff's (Wernicke) disease, psychosis or syndrome (alcoholic) F10.96
  with dependence F10.26
  drug-induced
    due to drug abuse — *see* Abuse, drug, by type, with amnestic disorder
    due to drug dependence — *see* Dependence, drug, by type, with amnestic disorder
  nonalcoholic F04
Korsakov's disease, psychosis or syndrome — *see* Korsakoff's disease
Korsakow's disease, psychosis or syndrome — *see* Korsakoff's disease
Kostmann's disease or syndrome (infantile genetic agranulocytosis) — *see* Agranulocytosis
Kozhevnikof's epilepsy G40.109
  intractable G40.119
    with status epilepticus G40.111
    without status epilepticus G40.119
  not intractable G40.109
    with status epilepticus G40.101
    without status epilepticus G40.109
Krabbe's
  disease E75.23
  syndrome, congenital muscle hypoplasia Q79.8
Kraepelin-Morel disease — *see* Schizophrenia
Kraft-Weber-Dimitri disease Q85.8
Kraurosis
  ani K62.89
  penis N48.0
  vagina N89.8
  vulva N90.4
Kreotoxism A05.9
Krukenberg's
  spindle — *see* Pigmentation, cornea, posterior
  tumor C79.6- ☑
Kufs' disease E75.4
Kugelberg-Welander disease G12.1
Kuhnt-Junius degeneration (*see also* Degeneration, macula) H35.32
Kümmell's disease or spondylitis — *see* Spondylopathy, traumatic
Kupffer cell sarcoma C22.3
Kuru A81.81
Kussmaul's
  disease M30.0
  respiration E87.2

Kussmaul's — *continued*
  in diabetic acidosis — *see* Diabetes, by type, with ketoacidosis
Kwashiorkor E40
  marasmic, marasmus type E42
Kyasanur Forest disease A98.2
Kyphoscoliosis, kyphoscoliotic (acquired) (*see also* Scoliosis) M41.9
  congenital Q67.5
  heart (disease) I27.1
  sequelae of rickets E64.3
  tuberculous A18.01
Kyphosis, kyphotic (acquired) M40.209
  cervical region M40.202
  cervicothoracic region M40.203
  congenital Q76.419
    cervical region Q76.412
    cervicothoracic region Q76.413
    occipito-atlanto-axial region Q76.411
    thoracic region Q76.414
    thoracolumbar region Q76.415
  Morquio-Brailsford type (spinal) (*see also* subcategory M49.8) E76.219
  postlaminectomy M96.3
  postradiation therapy M96.2
  postural (adolescent) M40.00
    cervicothoracic region M40.03
    thoracic region M40.04
    thoracolumbar region M40.05
  secondary NEC M40.10
    cervical region M40.12
    cervicothoracic region M40.13
    thoracic region M40.14
    thoracolumbar region M40.15
  sequelae of rickets E64.3
  specified type NEC M40.299
    cervical region M40.292
    cervicothoracic region M40.293
    thoracic region M40.294
    thoracolumbar region M40.295
  syphilitic, congenital A50.56
  thoracic region M40.204
  thoracolumbar region M40.205
  tuberculous A18.01
Kyrle disease L87.0

L

Labia, labium — *see* condition
Labile
  blood pressure R09.89
  vasomotor system I73.9
Labioglossal paralysis G12.29
Labium leporinum — *see* Cleft, lip
Labor — *see* Delivery
Labored breathing — *see* Hyperventilation
Labyrinthitis (circumscribed) (destructive) (diffuse) (inner ear) (latent) (purulent) (suppurative) (*see also* subcategory) H83.0 ☑
  syphilitic A52.79
Laceration
  with abortion — *see* Abortion, by type, complicated by laceration of pelvic organs
  abdomen, abdominal
    wall S31.119 ☑
      with
        foreign body S31.129 ☑
        penetration into peritoneal cavity S31.619 ☑
          with foreign body S31.629 ☑
      epigastric region S31.112 ☑
        with
          foreign body S31.122 ☑
          penetration into peritoneal cavity S31.612 ☑
            with foreign body S31.622 ☑
      left
        lower quadrant S31.114 ☑
          with
            foreign body S31.124 ☑
            penetration into peritoneal cavity S31.614 ☑
              with foreign body S31.624 ☑
        upper quadrant S31.111 ☑
          with
            foreign body S31.121 ☑
            penetration into peritoneal cavity S31.611 ☑
              with foreign body S31.621 ☑

☑ **Additional character required**

Laceration — *continued*

periumbilic region S31.115 ☑
  with
    foreign body S31.125 ☑
    penetration into peritoneal cavity
      S31.615 ☑
      with foreign body S31.625 ☑
  right
    lower quadrant S31.113 ☑
      with
        foreign body S31.123 ☑
        penetration into peritoneal cavity
          S31.613 ☑
          with foreign body S31.623 ☑
    upper quadrant S31.110 ☑
      with
        foreign body S31.120 ☑
        penetration into peritoneal cavity
          S31.610 ☑
          with foreign body S31.620 ☑
accidental, complicating surgery — *see*
  Complications, surgical, accidental puncture
  or laceration
Achilles tendon S86.02- ☑
adrenal gland S37.813 ☑
alveolar (process) — *see* Laceration, oral cavity
ankle S91.01- ☑
  with
    foreign body S91.02- ☑
antecubital space — *see* Laceration, elbow
anus (sphincter) S31.831 ☑
  with
    ectopic or molar pregnancy O08.6
    foreign body S31.832 ☑
  complicating delivery — *see* Delivery,
    complicated, by, laceration, anus
    (sphincter)
  following ectopic or molar pregnancy O08.6
  nontraumatic, nonpuerperal — *see* Fissure,
    anus
arm (upper) S41.11- ☑
  with foreign body S41.12- ☑
  lower — *see* Laceration, forearm
auditory canal (external) (meatus) — *see*
  Laceration, ear
auricle, ear — *see* Laceration, ear
axilla — *see* Laceration, arm
back (*see also* Laceration, thorax, back)
  lower S31.010 ☑
    with
      foreign body S31.020 ☑
        with penetration into retroperitoneal
          space S31.021 ☑
      penetration into retroperitoneal space
        S31.011 ☑
bile duct S36.13 ☑
bladder S37.23 ☑
  with ectopic or molar pregnancy O08.6
  following ectopic or molar pregnancy O08.6
  obstetrical trauma O71.5
blood vessel — *see* Injury, blood vessel
bowel (*see also* Laceration, intestine)
  with ectopic or molar pregnancy O08.6
  complicating abortion — *see* Abortion, by type,
    complicated by, specified condition NEC
  following ectopic or molar pregnancy O08.6
  obstetrical trauma O71.5
brain (any part) (cortex) (diffuse) (membrane) (*see*
  also Injury, intracranial, diffuse)
  during birth P10.8
    with hemorrhage P10.1
  focal — *see* Injury, intracranial, focal brain injury
brainstem S06.38- ☑
breast S21.01- ☑
  with foreign body S21.02- ☑
broad ligament S37.893 ☑
  with ectopic or molar pregnancy O08.6
  following ectopic or molar pregnancy O08.6
  laceration syndrome N83.8
  obstetrical trauma O71.6
  syndrome (laceration) N83.8
buttock S31.801 ☑
  with foreign body S31.802 ☑
  left S31.821 ☑
    with foreign body S31.822 ☑
  right S31.811 ☑
    with foreign body S31.812 ☑
calf — *see* Laceration, leg
canaliculus lacrimalis — *see* Laceration, eyelid
canthus, eye — *see* Laceration, eyelid
capsule, joint — *see* Sprain
causing eversion of cervix uteri (old) N86

Laceration — *continued*

central (perineal), complicating delivery O70.9
cerebellum, traumatic S06.37- ☑
cerebral S06.33- ☑
  left side S06.32- ☑
  during birth P10.8
    with hemorrhage P10.1
  right side S06.31- ☑
cervix (uteri)
  with ectopic or molar pregnancy O08.6
  following ectopic or molar pregnancy O08.6
  nonpuerperal, nontraumatic N88.1
  obstetrical trauma (current) O71.3
  old (postpartal) N88.1
  traumatic S37.63 ☑
cheek (external) S01.41- ☑
  with foreign body S01.42- ☑
  internal — *see* Laceration, oral cavity
chest wall — *see* Laceration, thorax
chin — *see* Laceration, head, specified site NEC
chordae tendinae NEC I51.1
  concurrent with acute myocardial infarction —
    see Infarct, myocardium
  following acute myocardial infarction (current
    complication) I23.4
clitoris — *see* Laceration, vulva
colon — *see* Laceration, intestine, large, colon
common bile duct S36.13 ☑
cortex (cerebral) — *see* Injury, intracranial, diffuse
costal region — *see* Laceration, thorax
cystic duct S36.13 ☑
diaphragm S27.803 ☑
digit (s)
  hand — *see* Laceration, finger
  foot — *see* Laceration, toe
duodenum S36.430 ☑
ear (canal) (external) S01.31- ☑
  with foreign body S01.32- ☑
  drum S09.2- ☑
elbow S51.01- ☑
  with
    foreign body S51.02- ☑
epididymis — *see* Laceration, testis
epigastric region — *see* Laceration, abdomen,
  wall, epigastric region
esophagus K22.8
  traumatic
    cervical S11.21 ☑
      with foreign body S11.22 ☑
    thoracic S27.813 ☑
eye (ball) S05.3- ☑
  with prolapse or loss of intraocular tissue
    S05.2- ☑
  penetrating S05.6- ☑
eyebrow — *see* Laceration, eyelid
eyelid S01.11- ☑
  with foreign body S01.12- ☑
face NEC — *see* Laceration, head, specified site
  NEC
fallopian tube S37.539 ☑
  bilateral S37.532 ☑
  unilateral S37.531 ☑
finger (s) S61.219 ☑
  with
    damage to nail S61.319 ☑
      with
        foreign body S61.329 ☑
    foreign body S61.229 ☑
  index S61.218 ☑
    with
      damage to nail S61.318 ☑
        with
          foreign body S61.328 ☑
      foreign body S61.228 ☑
    left S61.211 ☑
      with
        damage to nail S61.311 ☑
          with
            foreign body S61.321 ☑
        foreign body S61.221 ☑
    right S61.210 ☑
      with
        damage to nail S61.310 ☑
          with
            foreign body S61.320 ☑
        foreign body S61.220 ☑
  little S61.218 ☑
    with
      damage to nail S61.318 ☑
        with
          foreign body S61.328 ☑
      foreign body S61.228 ☑

Laceration — *continued*

    left S61.217 ☑
      with
        damage to nail S61.317 ☑
          with
            foreign body S61.327 ☑
        foreign body S61.227 ☑
    right S61.216 ☑
      with
        damage to nail S61.316 ☑
          with
            foreign body S61.326 ☑
        foreign body S61.226 ☑
  middle S61.218 ☑
    with
      damage to nail S61.318 ☑
        with
          foreign body S61.328 ☑
      foreign body S61.228 ☑
    left S61.213 ☑
      with
        damage to nail S61.313 ☑
          with
            foreign body S61.323 ☑
        foreign body S61.223 ☑
    right S61.212 ☑
      with
        damage to nail S61.312 ☑
          with
            foreign body S61.322 ☑
        foreign body S61.222 ☑
  ring S61.218 ☑
    with
      damage to nail S61.318 ☑
        with
          foreign body S61.328 ☑
      foreign body S61.228 ☑
    left S61.215 ☑
      with
        damage to nail S61.315 ☑
          with
            foreign body S61.325 ☑
        foreign body S61.225 ☑
    right S61.214 ☑
      with
        damage to nail S61.314 ☑
          with
            foreign body S61.324 ☑
        foreign body S61.224 ☑
flank S31.119 ☑
  with foreign body S31.129 ☑
foot (except toe(s) alone) S91.319 ☑
  with foreign body S91.329 ☑
  left S91.312 ☑
    with foreign body S91.322 ☑
  right S91.311 ☑
    with foreign body S91.321 ☑
  toe — *see* Laceration, toe
forearm S51.819 ☑
  with
    foreign body S51.829 ☑
  elbow only — *see* Laceration, elbow
  left S51.812 ☑
    with
      foreign body S51.822 ☑
  right S51.811 ☑
    with
      foreign body S51.821 ☑
forehead S01.81 ☑
  with foreign body S01.82 ☑
fourchette O70.0
  with ectopic or molar pregnancy O08.6
  complicating delivery O70.0
  following ectopic or molar pregnancy O08.6
gallbladder S36.123 ☑
genital organs, external
  female S31.512 ☑
    with foreign body S31.522 ☑
    vagina — *see* Laceration, vagina
    vulva — *see* Laceration, vulva
  male S31.511 ☑
    with foreign body S31.521 ☑
    penis — *see* Laceration, penis
    scrotum — *see* Laceration, scrotum
    testis — *see* Laceration, testis
groin — *see* Laceration, abdomen, wall
gum — *see* Laceration, oral cavity
hand S61.419 ☑
  with
    foreign body S61.429 ☑
  finger — *see* Laceration, finger
  left S61.412 ☑

Laceration — *continued*
  with
    foreign body S61.422 ☑
  right S61.411 ☑
    with
      foreign body S61.421 ☑
  thumb — *see* Laceration, thumb
  head S01.91 ☑
    with foreign body S01.92 ☑
    cheek — *see* Laceration, cheek
    ear — *see* Laceration, ear
    eyelid — *see* Laceration, eyelid
    lip — *see* Laceration, lip
    nose — *see* Laceration, nose
    oral cavity — *see* Laceration, oral cavity
    scalp S01.01 ☑
      with foreign body S01.02 ☑
    specified site NEC S01.81 ☑
      with foreign body S01.82 ☑
    temporomandibular area — *see* Laceration, cheek
  heart — *see* Injury, heart, laceration
  heel — *see* Laceration, foot
  hepatic duct S36.13 ☑
  hip S71.019 ☑
    with foreign body S71.029 ☑
    left S71.012 ☑
      with foreign body S71.022 ☑
    right S71.011 ☑
      with foreign body S71.021 ☑
  hymen — *see* Laceration, vagina
  hypochondrium — *see* Laceration, abdomen, wall
  hypogastric region — *see* Laceration, abdomen, wall
  ileum S36.438 ☑
  inguinal region — *see* Laceration, abdomen, wall
  instep — *see* Laceration, foot
  internal organ — *see* Injury, by site
  interscapular region — *see* Laceration, thorax, back
  intestine
    large
      colon S36.539 ☑
        ascending S36.530 ☑
        descending S36.532 ☑
        sigmoid S36.533 ☑
        specified site NEC S36.538 ☑
      rectum S36.63 ☑
      transverse S36.531 ☑
    small S36.439 ☑
      duodenum S36.430 ☑
      specified site NEC S36.438 ☑
  intra-abdominal organ S36.93 ☑
    intestine — *see* Laceration, intestine
    liver — *see* Laceration, liver
    pancreas — *see* Laceration, pancreas
    peritoneum S36.81 ☑
    specified site NEC S36.893 ☑
    spleen — *see* Laceration, spleen
    stomach — *see* Laceration, stomach
  intracranial NEC (*see also* Injury, intracranial, diffuse)
    birth injury P10.9
  jaw — *see* Laceration, head, specified site NEC
  jejunum S36.438 ☑
  joint capsule — *see* Sprain, by site
  kidney S37.03- ☑
    major (greater than 3 cm) (massive) (stellate) S37.06- ☑
    minor (less than 1 cm) S37.04- ☑
    moderate (1 to 3 cm) S37.05- ☑
    multiple S37.06- ☑
  knee S81.01- ☑
    with foreign body S81.02- ☑
  labium (majus) (minus) — *see* Laceration, vulva
  lacrimal duct — *see* Laceration, eyelid
  large intestine — *see* Laceration, intestine, large
  larynx S11.011 ☑
    with foreign body S11.012 ☑
  leg (lower) S81.819 ☑
    with foreign body S81.829 ☑
    foot — *see* Laceration, foot
    knee — *see* Laceration, knee
    left S81.812 ☑
      with foreign body S81.822 ☑
    right S81.811 ☑
      with foreign body S81.821 ☑
    upper — *see* Laceration, thigh
  ligament — *see* Sprain
  lip S01.511 ☑
    with foreign body S01.521 ☑
  liver S36.113 ☑

Laceration — *continued*
    major (stellate) S36.116 ☑
    minor S36.114 ☑
    moderate S36.115 ☑
  loin — *see* Laceration, abdomen, wall
  lower back — *see* Laceration, back, lower
  lumbar region — *see* Laceration, back, lower
  lung S27.339 ☑
    bilateral S27.332 ☑
    unilateral S27.331 ☑
  malar region — *see* Laceration, head, specified site NEC
  mammary — *see* Laceration, breast
  mastoid region — *see* Laceration, head, specified site NEC
  meninges — *see* Injury, intracranial, diffuse
  meniscus — *see* Tear, meniscus
  mesentery S36.893 ☑
  mesosalpinx S37.893 ☑
  mouth — *see* Laceration, oral cavity
  muscle — *see* Injury, muscle, by site, laceration
  nail
    finger — *see* Laceration, finger, with damage to nail
    toe — *see* Laceration, toe, with damage to nail
  nasal (septum) (sinus) — *see* Laceration, nose
  nasopharynx — *see* Laceration, head, specified site NEC
  neck S11.91 ☑
    with foreign body S11.92 ☑
    involving
      cervical esophagus S11.21 ☑
        with foreign body S11.22 ☑
      larynx — *see* Laceration, larynx
      pharynx — *see* Laceration, pharynx
      thyroid gland — *see* Laceration, thyroid gland
      trachea — *see* Laceration, trachea
    specified site NEC S11.81 ☑
      with foreign body S11.82 ☑
  nerve — *see* Injury, nerve
  nose (septum) (sinus) S01.21 ☑
    with foreign body S01.22 ☑
  ocular NOS S05.3- ☑
    adnexa NOS S01.11- ☑
  oral cavity S01.512 ☑
    with foreign body S01.522 ☑
  orbit (eye) — *see* Wound, open, ocular, orbit
  ovary S37.439 ☑
    bilateral S37.432 ☑
    unilateral S37.431 ☑
  palate — *see* Laceration, oral cavity
  palm — *see* Laceration, hand
  pancreas S36.239 ☑
    body S36.231 ☑
      major S36.261 ☑
      minor S36.241 ☑
      moderate S36.251 ☑
    head S36.230 ☑
      major S36.260 ☑
      minor S36.240 ☑
      moderate S36.250 ☑
    major S36.269 ☑
    minor S36.249 ☑
    moderate S36.259 ☑
    tail S36.232 ☑
      major S36.262 ☑
      minor S36.242 ☑
      moderate S36.252 ☑
  pelvic S31.010 ☑
    with
      foreign body S31.020 ☑
        penetration into retroperitoneal cavity S31.021 ☑
      penetration into retroperitoneal cavity S31.011 ☑
    floor (*see also* Laceration, back, lower)
      with ectopic or molar pregnancy O08.6
      complicating delivery O70.1
      following ectopic or molar pregnancy O08.6
      old (postpartal) N81.89
    organ S37.93 ☑
      with ectopic or molar pregnancy O08.6
      adrenal gland S37.813 ☑
      bladder S37.23 ☑
      fallopian tube — *see* Laceration, fallopian tube
      following ectopic or molar pregnancy O08.6
      kidney — *see* Laceration, kidney
      obstetrical trauma O71.5
      ovary — *see* Laceration, ovary
      prostate S37.823 ☑
      specified site NEC S37.893 ☑

Laceration — *continued*
    ureter S37.13 ☑
    urethra S37.33 ☑
    uterus S37.63 ☑
  penis S31.21 ☑
    with foreign body S31.22 ☑
  perineum
    female S31.41 ☑
      with
        ectopic or molar pregnancy O08.6
        foreign body S31.42 ☑
      during delivery O70.9
        first degree O70.0
        fourth degree O70.3
        second degree O70.1
        third degree O70.2
      old (postpartal) N81.89
      postpartal N81.89
      secondary (postpartal) O90.1
    male S31.119 ☑
      with foreign body S31.129 ☑
  periocular area (with or without lacrimal passages) — *see* Laceration, eyelid
  peritoneum S36.893 ☑
  periumbilic region — *see* Laceration, abdomen, wall, periumbilic
  periurethral tissue — *see* Laceration, urethra
  phalanges
    finger — *see* Laceration, finger
    toe — *see* Laceration, toe
  pharynx S11.21 ☑
    with foreign body S11.22 ☑
  pinna — *see* Laceration, ear
  popliteal space — *see* Laceration, knee
  prepuce — *see* Laceration, penis
  prostate S37.823 ☑
  pubic region S31.119 ☑
    with foreign body S31.129 ☑
  pudendum — *see* Laceration, genital organs, external
  rectovaginal septum — *see* Laceration, vagina
  rectum S36.63 ☑
  retroperitoneum S36.893 ☑
  round ligament S37.893 ☑
  sacral region — *see* Laceration, back, lower
  sacroiliac region — *see* Laceration, back, lower
  salivary gland — *see* Laceration, oral cavity
  scalp S01.01 ☑
    with foreign body S01.02 ☑
  scapular region — *see* Laceration, shoulder
  scrotum S31.31 ☑
    with foreign body S31.32 ☑
  seminal vesicle S37.893 ☑
  shin — *see* Laceration, leg
  shoulder S41.019 ☑
    with foreign body S41.029 ☑
    left S41.012 ☑
      with foreign body S41.022 ☑
    right S41.011 ☑
      with foreign body S41.021 ☑
  small intestine — *see* Laceration, intestine, small
  spermatic cord — *see* Laceration, testis
  spinal cord (meninges) (*see also* Injury, spinal cord, by region)
    due to injury at birth P11.5
    newborn (birth injury) P11.5
  spleen S36.039 ☑
    major (massive) (stellate) S36.032 ☑
    moderate S36.031 ☑
    superficial (minor) S36.030 ☑
  sternal region — *see* Laceration, thorax, front
  stomach S36.33 ☑
  submaxillary region — *see* Laceration, head, specified site NEC
  submental region — *see* Laceration, head, specified site NEC
  subungual
    finger (s) — *see* Laceration, finger, with damage to nail
    toe (s) — *see* Laceration, toe, with damage to nail
  suprarenal gland — *see* Laceration, adrenal gland
  temple, temporal region — *see* Laceration, head, specified site NEC
  temporomandibular area — *see* Laceration, cheek
  tendon — *see* Injury, muscle, by site, laceration
    Achilles S86.02- ☑
  tentorium cerebelli — *see* Injury, intracranial, diffuse
  testis S31.31 ☑
    with foreign body S31.32 ☑
  thigh S71.11- ☑

☑ **Additional character required**

Laceration — *continued*
  with foreign body S71.12- ☑
  thorax, thoracic (wall) S21.91 ☑
   with foreign body S21.92 ☑
    back S21.22- ☑
     with penetration into thoracic cavity
       S21.42- ☑
    front S21.12- ☑
     with penetration into thoracic cavity
       S21.32- ☑
    back S21.21- ☑
     with
       foreign body S21.22- ☑
        with penetration into thoracic cavity
          S21.42- ☑
       penetration into thoracic cavity S21.41- ☑
    breast — *see* Laceration, breast
    front S21.11- ☑
     with
       foreign body S21.12- ☑
        with penetration into thoracic cavity
          S21.32- ☑
       penetration into thoracic cavity S21.31- ☑
  thumb S61.019 ☑
   with
    damage to nail S61.119 ☑
     with
       foreign body S61.129 ☑
    foreign body S61.029 ☑
    left S61.012 ☑
     with
       damage to nail S61.112 ☑
        with
          foreign body S61.122 ☑
       foreign body S61.022 ☑
    right S61.011 ☑
     with
       damage to nail S61.111 ☑
        with
          foreign body S61.121 ☑
       foreign body S61.021 ☑
  thyroid gland S11.11 ☑
   with foreign body S11.12 ☑
  toe (s) S91.119 ☑
   with
    damage to nail S91.219 ☑
     with
       foreign body S91.229 ☑
    foreign body S91.129 ☑
    great S91.113 ☑
     with
       damage to nail S91.213 ☑
        with
          foreign body S91.223 ☑
       foreign body S91.123 ☑
    left S91.112 ☑
     with
       damage to nail S91.212 ☑
        with
          foreign body S91.222 ☑
       foreign body S91.122 ☑
    right S91.111 ☑
     with
       damage to nail S91.211 ☑
        with
          foreign body S91.221 ☑
       foreign body S91.121 ☑
    lesser S91.116 ☑
     with
       damage to nail S91.216 ☑
        with
          foreign body S91.226 ☑
       foreign body S91.126 ☑
    left S91.115 ☑
     with
       damage to nail S91.215 ☑
        with
          foreign body S91.225 ☑
       foreign body S91.125 ☑
    right S91.114 ☑
     with
       damage to nail S91.214 ☑
        with
          foreign body S91.224 ☑
       foreign body S91.124 ☑
  tongue — *see* Laceration, oral cavity
  trachea S11.021 ☑
   with foreign body S11.022 ☑
  tunica vaginalis — *see* Laceration, testis
  tympanum, tympanic membrane — *see*
    Laceration, ear, drum
  umbilical region S31.115 ☑

Laceration — *continued*
  with foreign body S31.125 ☑
  ureter S37.13 ☑
  urethra S37.33 ☑
   with or following ectopic or molar pregnancy
     O08.6
   obstetrical trauma O71.5
  urinary organ NEC S37.893 ☑
  uterus S37.63 ☑
   with ectopic or molar pregnancy O08.6
   following ectopic or molar pregnancy O08.6
   nonpuerperal, nontraumatic N85.8
   obstetrical trauma NEC O71.81
   old (postpartal) N85.8
  uvula — *see* Laceration, oral cavity
  vagina S31.41 ☑
   with
     ectopic or molar pregnancy O08.6
     foreign body S31.42 ☑
   during delivery O71.4
     with perineal laceration — *see* Laceration,
       perineum, female, during delivery
   following ectopic or molar pregnancy O08.6
   nonpuerperal, nontraumatic N89.8
   old (postpartal) N89.8
  vas deferens S37.893 ☑
  vesical — *see* Laceration, bladder
  vocal cords S11.031 ☑
   with foreign body S11.032 ☑
  vulva S31.41 ☑
   with
     ectopic or molar pregnancy O08.6
     foreign body S31.42 ☑
   complicating delivery O70.0
   following ectopic or molar pregnancy O08.6
   nonpuerperal, nontraumatic N90.89
   old (postpartal) N90.89
  wrist S61.519 ☑
   with
     foreign body S61.529 ☑
   left S61.512 ☑
     with
       foreign body S61.522 ☑
   right S61.511 ☑
     with
       foreign body S61.521 ☑
Lack of
  achievement in school Z55.3
  adequate
   food Z59.4
   intermaxillary vertical dimension of fully
     erupted teeth M26.36
   sleep Z72.820
  appetite (see Anorexia) R63.0
  awareness R41.9
  care
   in home Z74.2
   of infant (at or after birth) T76.02 ☑
     confirmed T74.02 ☑
  cognitive functions R41.9
  coordination R27.9
   ataxia R27.0
   specified type NEC R27.8
  development (physiological) R62.50
   failure to thrive (child over 28 days old) R62.51
     adult R62.7
     newborn P92.6
   short stature R62.52
   specified type NEC R62.59
  energy R53.83
  financial resources Z59.6
  food T73.0 ☑
  growth R62.52
  heating Z59.1
  housing (permanent) (temporary) Z59.0
   adequate Z59.1
  learning experiences in childhood Z62.898
  leisure time (affecting life-style) Z73.2
  material resources Z59.9
  memory (see also Amnesia)
   mild, following organic brain damage F06.8
  ovulation N97.0
  parental supervision or control of child Z62.0
  person able to render necessary care Z74.2
  physical exercise Z72.3
  play experience in childhood Z62.898
  posterior occlusal support M26.57
  relaxation (affecting life-style) Z73.2
  sexual
   desire F52.0
   enjoyment F52.1
  shelter Z59.0

Lack of — *continued*
  sleep (adequate) Z72.820
  supervision of child by parent Z62.0
  support, posterior occlusal M26.57
  water T73.1 ☑
Lacrimal — *see* condition
Lacrimation, abnormal — *see* Epiphora
Lacrimonasal duct — *see* condition
Lactation, lactating (breast) (puerperal, postpartum)
  associated
   cracked nipple O92.13
   retracted nipple O92.03
  defective O92.4
  disorder NEC O92.79
  excessive O92.6
  failed (complete) O92.3
   partial O92.4
  mastitis NEC — *see* Mastitis, obstetric
  mother (care and/or examination) Z39.1
  nonpuerperal N64.3
Lacticemia, excessive E87.2
Lacunar skull Q75.8
Laennec's cirrhosis K74.69
  alcoholic K70.30
   with ascites K70.31
Lafora's disease — *see* Epilepsy, generalized,
   idiopathic
Lag, lid (nervous) — *see* Retraction, lid
Lagophthalmos (eyelid) (nervous) H02.209
  cicatricial H02.219
   left H02.216
     lower H02.215
     upper H02.214
   right H02.213
     lower H02.212
     upper H02.211
  keratoconjunctivitis — *see* Keratoconjunctivitis
  left H02.206
   lower H02.205
   upper H02.204
  mechanical H02.229
   left H02.226
     lower H02.225
     upper H02.224
   right H02.223
     lower H02.222
     upper H02.221
  paralytic H02.239
   left H02.236
     lower H02.235
     upper H02.234
   right H02.233
     lower H02.232
     upper H02.231
  right H02.203
   lower H02.202
   upper H02.201
Laki-Lorand factor deficiency — *see* Defect,
   coagulation, specified type NEC
Lalling F80.0
Lambert-Eaton syndrome — *see* Syndrome,
   Lambert-Eaton
Lambliasis, lambliosis A07.1
Landau-Kleffner syndrome — *see* Epilepsy,
   specified NEC
Landouzy-Déjérine dystrophy or
   facioscapulohumeral atrophy G71.0
Landouzy's disease (icterohemorrhagic
   leptospirosis) A27.0
Landry-Guillain-Barré, syndrome or paralysis G61.0
Landry's disease or paralysis G61.0
Lane's
  band Q43.3
  kink — *see* Obstruction, intestine
  syndrome K90.2
Langdon Down syndrome — *see* Trisomy, 21
Lapsed immunization schedule status Z28.3
Large
  baby (regardless of gestational age) (4000g to
   4499g) P08.1
  ear, congenital Q17.1
  physiological cup Q14.2
  stature R68.89
Large-for-dates NEC (infant) (4000g to 4499g) P08.1
  affecting management of pregnancy O36.6- ☑
  exceptionally (4500g or more) P08.0
Larsen-Johansson disease orosteochondrosis — *see*
   Osteochondrosis, juvenile, patella
Larsen's syndrome (flattened facies and multiple
   congenital dislocations) Q74.8
Larva migrans
  cutaneous B76.9

Larva — *continued*
    Ancylostoma B76.0
    visceral B83.0
Laryngeal — *see* condition
Laryngismus (stridulus) J38.5
    congenital P28.89
    diphtheritic A36.2
Laryngitis (acute) (edematous) (fibrinous)
    (infective) (infiltrative) (malignant)
    (membranous) (phlegmonous) (pneumococcal)
    (pseudomembranous) (septic) (subglottic)
    (suppurative) (ulcerative) J04.0
    with
        influenza, flu, or grippe — *see* Influenza, with,
            laryngitis
        tracheitis (acute) — *see* Laryngotracheitis
    atrophic J37.0
    catarrhal J37.0
    chronic J37.0
        with tracheitis (chronic) J37.1
    diphtheritic A36.2
    due to external agent — *see* Inflammation,
        respiratory, upper, due to
    Hemophilus influenzae J04.0
    H. influenzae J04.0
    hypertrophic J37.0
    influenzal — *see* Influenza, with, respiratory
        manifestations NEC
    obstructive J05.0
    sicca J37.0
    spasmodic J05.0
        acute J04.0
    streptococcal J04.0
    stridulous J05.0
    syphilitic (late) A52.73
        congenital A50.59 [J99]
            early A50.03 [J99]
    tuberculous A15.5
    Vincent's A69.1
Laryngocele (congenital) (ventricular) Q31.3
Laryngofissure J38.7
    congenital Q31.8
Laryngomalacia (congenital) Q31.5
Laryngopharyngitis (acute) J06.0
    chronic J37.0
    due to external agent — *see* Inflammation,
        respiratory, upper, due to
Laryngoplegia J38.00
    bilateral J38.02
    unilateral J38.01
Laryngoptosis J38.7
Laryngospasm J38.5
Laryngostenosis J38.6
Laryngotracheitis (acute) (Infectional) (infective)
    (viral) J04.2
    atrophic J37.1
    catarrhal J37.1
    chronic J37.1
    diphtheritic A36.2
    due to external agent — *see* Inflammation,
        respiratory, upper, due to
    Hemophilus influenzae J04.2
    hypertrophic J37.1
    influenzal — *see* Influenza, with, respiratory
        manifestations NEC
    pachydermic J38.7
    sicca J37.1
    spasmodic J38.5
        acute J05.0
    streptococcal J04.2
    stridulous J38.5
    syphilitic (late) A52.73
        congenital A50.59 [J99]
            early A50.03 [J99]
    tuberculous A15.5
    Vincent's A69.1
Laryngotracheobronchitis — *see* Bronchitis
Larynx, laryngeal — *see* condition
Lassa fever A96.2
Lassitude — *see* Weakness
Late
    talker R62.0
    walker R62.0
Late effect (s) — *see* Sequelae
Latent — *see* condition
Laterocession — *see* Lateroversion
Lateroflexion — *see* Lateroversion
Lateroversion
    cervix — *see* Lateroversion, uterus
    uterus, uterine (cervix) (postinfectional)
        (postpartal, old) N85.4
        congenital Q51.818

Lateroversion — *continued*
    in pregnancy or childbirth O34.59- ☑
Lathyrism — *see* Poisoning, food, noxious, plant
Launois' syndrome (pituitary gigantism) E22.0
Launois-Bensaude adenolipomatosis E88.89
Laurence-Moon (-Bardet)-Biedl syndrome Q87.89
Lax, laxity (*see also* Relaxation)
    ligament (ous) (*see also* Disorder, ligament)
        familial M35.7
        knee — *see* Derangement, knee
    skin (acquired) L57.4
        congenital Q82.8
Laxative habit F55.2
Lazy leukocyte syndrome D70.8
Lead miner's lung J63.6
Leak, leakage
    air NEC J93.82
        postprocedural J95.812
    amniotic fluid — *see* Rupture, membranes,
        premature
    blood (microscopic), fetal, into maternal
        circulation affecting management of
        pregnancy — *see* Pregnancy, complicated by
    cerebrospinal fluid G96.0
        from spinal (lumbar) puncture G97.0
    device, implant or graft (*see also* Complications,
        by site and type, mechanical)
        arterial graft NEC — *see* Complication,
            cardiovascular device, mechanical, vascular
        breast (implant) T85.43 ☑
        catheter NEC T85.638 ☑
            urinary, indwelling T83.038 ☑
                cystostomy T83.030 ☑
            dialysis (renal) T82.43 ☑
                intraperitoneal T85.631 ☑
            infusion NEC T82.534 ☑
                spinal (epidural) (subdural) T85.630 ☑
        gastrointestinal — *see* Complications,
            prosthetic device, mechanical,
            gastrointestinal device
        genital NEC T83.498 ☑
            penile prosthesis T83.490 ☑
        heart NEC — *see* Complication, cardiovascular
            device, mechanical
        joint prosthesis — *see* Complications, joint
            prosthesis, mechanical, specified NEC, by
            site
        ocular NEC — *see* Complications, prosthetic
            device, mechanical, ocular device
        orthopedic NEC — *see* Complication,
            orthopedic, device, mechanical
        persistent air J93.82
        specified NEC T85.638 ☑
        urinary NEC (*see also* Complication,
            genitourinary, device, urinary, mechanical)
            graft T83.23 ☑
        vascular NEC — *see* Complication,
            cardiovascular device, mechanical
        ventricular intracranial shunt T85.03 ☑
    urine — *see* Incontinence
Leaky heart — *see* Endocarditis
Learning defect (specific) F81.9
Leather bottle stomach C16.9
Leber's
    congenital amaurosis H35.50
    optic atrophy (hereditary) H47.22
Lederer's anemia D59.1
Leeches (external) — *see* Hirudiniasis
Leg — *see* condition
Legg (-Calvé)-Perthes disease, syndrome or
    osteochondrosis M91.1- ☑
Legionellosis A48.1
    nonpneumonic A48.2
Legionnaires'
    disease A48.1
        nonpneumonic A48.2
    pneumonia A48.1
Leigh's disease G31.82
Leiner's disease L21.1
Leiofibromyoma — *see* Leiomyoma
Leiomyoblastoma — *see* Neoplasm, connective
    tissue, benign
Leiomyofibroma (*see also* Neoplasm, connective
    tissue, benign)
    uterus (cervix) (corpus) D25.9
Leiomyoma (*see also* Neoplasm, connective tissue,
    benign)
    bizarre — *see* Neoplasm, connective tissue,
        benign
    cellular — *see* Neoplasm, connective tissue,
        benign

Leiomyoma — *continued*
    epithelioid — *see* Neoplasm, connective tissue,
        benign
    uterus (cervix) (corpus) D25.9
        intramural D25.1
        submucous D25.0
        subserosal D25.2
    vascular — *see* Neoplasm, connective tissue,
        benign
Leiomyoma, leiomyomatosis (intravascular) — *see*
    Neoplasm, connective tissue, uncertain behavior
Leiomyosarcoma (*see also* Neoplasm, connective
    tissue, malignant)
    epithelioid — *see* Neoplasm, connective tissue,
        malignant
    myxoid — *see* Neoplasm, connective tissue,
        malignant
Leishmaniasis B55.9
    American (mucocutaneous) B55.2
        cutaneous B55.1
    Asian Desert B55.1
    Brazilian B55.2
    cutaneous (any type) B55.1
    dermal (*see also* Leishmaniasis, cutaneous)
        post-kala-azar B55.0
    eyelid B55.1
    infantile B55.0
    Mediterranean B55.0
    mucocutaneous (American) (New World) B55.2
    naso-oral B55.2
    nasopharyngeal B55.2
    old world B55.1
    tegumentaria diffusa B55.1
    visceral B55.0
Leishmanoid, dermal (*see also* Leishmaniasis,
    cutaneous)
    post-kala-azar B55.0
Lenegre's disease I44.2
Lengthening, leg — *see* Deformity, limb, unequal
    length
Lennert's lymphoma — *see* Lymphoma, Lennert's
Lennox-Gastaut syndrome G40.812
    intractable G40.814
        with status epilepticus G40.813
        without status epilepticus G40.814
    not intractable G40.812
        with status epilepticus G40.811
        without status epilepticus G40.812
Lens — *see* condition
Lenticonus (anterior) (posterior) (congenital) Q12.8
Lenticular degeneration, progressive E83.01
Lentiglobus (posterior) (congenital) Q12.8
Lentigo (congenital) L81.4
    maligna (*see also* Melanoma, in situ)
        melanoma — *see* Melanoma
Lentivirus, as cause of disease classified elsewhere
    B97.31
Leontiasis
    ossium M85.2
    syphilitic (late) A52.78
        congenital A50.59
Lepothrix A48.8
Lepra — *see* Leprosy
Leprechaunism E34.8
Leprosy A30.- ☑
    with muscle disorder A30.9 [M63.80]
        ankle A30.9 [M63.87-]
        foot A30.9 [M63.87-]
        forearm A30.9 [M63.83-]
        hand A30.9 [M63.84-]
        lower leg A30.9 [M63.86-]
        multiple sites A30.9 [M63.89]
        pelvic region A30.9 [M63.85-]
        shoulder region A30.9 [M63.81-]
        specified site NEC A30.9 [M63.88]
        thigh A30.9 [M63.85-]
        upper arm A30.9 [M63.82-]
    anesthetic A30.9
    BB A30.3
    BL A30.4
    borderline (infiltrated) (neuritic) A30.3
        lepromatous A30.4
        tuberculoid A30.2
    BT A30.2
    dimorphous (infiltrated) (neuritic) A30.3
    I A30.0
    indeterminate (macular) (neuritic) A30.0
    lepromatous (diffuse) (infiltrated) (macular)
        (neuritic) (nodular) A30.5
    LL A30.5
    macular (early) (neuritic) (simple) A30.9
    maculoanesthetic A30.9

☑ **Additional character required**

Leprosy — *continued*
  mixed A30.3
  neural A30.9
  nodular A30.5
  primary neuritic A30.3
  specified type NEC A30.8
  TT A30.1
  tuberculoid (major) (minor) A30.1
Leptocytosis, hereditary D56.9
Leptomeningitis (chronic) (circumscribed) (hemorrhagic) (nonsuppurative) — *see* Meningitis
Leptomeningopathy G96.19
Leptospiral — *see* condition
Leptospirochetal — *see* condition
Leptospirosis A27.9
  canicola A27.89
  due to Leptospira interrogans serovar
    icterohaemorrhagiae A27.0
  icterohemorrhagica A27.0
  pomona A27.89
  Weil's disease A27.0
Leptus dermatitis B88.0
Leriche's syndrome (aortic bifurcation occlusion) I74.09
Leri's pleonosteosis Q78.8
Leri-Weill syndrome Q77.8
Lermoyez' syndrome — *see* Vertigo, peripheral NEC
Lesch-Nyhan syndrome E79.1
Leser-Trélat disease L82.1
  inflamed L82.0
Lesion (s) (nontraumatic)
  abducens nerve — *see* Strabismus, paralytic, sixth nerve
  alveolar process K08.9
  angiocentric immunoproliferative D47.Z9
  anorectal K62.9
  aortic (valve) I35.9
  auditory nerve H93.3
  basal ganglion G25.9
  bile duct — *see* Disease, bile duct
  biomechanical M99.9
    specified type NEC M99.89
      abdomen M99.89
      acromioclavicular M99.87
      cervical region M99.81
      cervicothoracic M99.81
      costochondral M99.88
      costovertebral M99.88
      head region M99.80
      hip M99.85
      lower extremity M99.86
      lumbar region M99.83
      lumbosacral M99.83
      occipitocervical M99.80
      pelvic region M99.85
      pubic M99.85
      rib cage M99.88
      sacral region M99.84
      sacrococcygeal M99.84
      sacroiliac M99.84
      specified NEC M99.89
      sternochondral M99.88
      sternoclavicular M99.87
      thoracic region M99.82
      thoracolumbar M99.82
      upper extremity M99.87
  bladder N32.9
  bone — *see* Disorder, bone
  brachial plexus G54.0
  brain G93.9
    congenital Q04.9
    vascular I67.9
      degenerative I67.9
      hypertensive I67.4
  buccal cavity K13.79
  calcified — *see* Calcification
  canthus — *see* Disorder, eyelid
  carate — *see* Pinta, lesions
  cardia K22.9
  cardiac (*see also* Disease, heart) I51.9
    congenital Q24.9
    valvular — *see* Endocarditis
  cauda equina G83.4
  cecum K63.9
  cerebral — *see* Lesion, brain
  cerebrovascular I67.9
    degenerative I67.9
    hypertensive I67.4
  cervical (nerve) root NEC G54.2
  chiasmal — *see* Disorder, optic, chiasm
  chorda tympani G51.8
  coin, lung R91.1

Lesion — *continued*
  colon K63.9
  congenital — *see* Anomaly, by site
  conjunctiva H11.9
  conus medullaris — *see* Injury, conus medullaris
  coronary artery — *see* Ischemia, heart
  cranial nerve G52.9
    eighth — *see* Disorder, ear
    eleventh G52.9
    fifth G50.9
    first G52.0
    fourth — *see* Strabismus, paralytic, fourth nerve
    seventh G51.9
    sixth — *see* Strabismus, paralytic, sixth nerve
    tenth G52.2
    twelfth G52.3
  cystic — *see* Cyst
  degenerative — *see* Degeneration
  duodenum K31.9
  edentulous (alveolar) ridge, associated with trauma, due to traumatic occlusion K06.2
  en coup de sabre L94.1
  eyelid — *see* Disorder, eyelid
  gasserian ganglion G50.8
  gastric K31.9
  gastroduodenal K31.9
  gastrointestinal K63.9
  gingiva, associated with trauma K06.2
  glomerular
    focal and segmental (*see also* N00-N07 with fourth character .1) N05.1
    minimal change (*see also* N00-N07 with fourth character .0) N05.0
  heart (organic) — *see* Disease, heart
  hyperchromic, due to pinta (carate) A67.1
  hyperkeratotic — *see* Hyperkeratosis
  hypothalamic E23.7
  ileocecal K63.9
  ileum K63.9
  iliohypogastric nerve G57.8- ☑
  inflammatory — *see* Inflammation
  intestine K63.9
  intracerebral — *see* Lesion, brain
  intrachiasmal (optic) — *see* Disorder, optic, chiasm
  intracranial, space-occupying R90.0
  joint — *see* Disorder, joint
    sacroiliac (old) M53.3
  keratotic — *see* Keratosis
  kidney — *see* Disease, renal
  laryngeal nerve (recurrent) G52.2
  lip K13.0
  liver K76.9
  lumbosacral
    plexus G54.1
    root (nerve) NEC G54.4
  lung (coin) R91.1
  maxillary sinus J32.0
  mitral I05.9
  Morel-Lavallée — *see* Hematoma, by site
  motor cortex NEC G93.89
  mouth K13.79
  nerve G58.9
    femoral G57.2- ☑
    median G56.1- ☑
      carpal tunnel syndrome — *see* Syndrome, carpal tunnel
    plantar G57.6- ☑
    popliteal (lateral) G57.3- ☑
      medial G57.4- ☑
    radial G56.3- ☑
    sciatic G57.0- ☑
    spinal — *see* Injury, nerve, spinal
    ulnar G56.2- ☑
  nervous system, congenital Q07.9
  nonallopathic — *see* Lesion, biomechanical
  nose (internal) J34.89
  obstructive — *see* Obstruction
  obturator nerve G57.8- ☑
  oral mucosa K13.70
  organ or site NEC — *see* Disease, by site
  osteolytic — *see* Osteolysis
  peptic K27.9
  periodontal, due to traumatic occlusion K05.5
  pharynx J39.2
  pigment, pigmented (skin) L81.9
  pinta — *see* Pinta, lesions
  polypoid — *see* Polyp
  prechiasmal (optic) — *see* Disorder, optic, chiasm
  primary (*see also* Syphilis, primary) A51.0
    carate A67.0
    pinta A67.0

Lesion — *continued*
  yaws A66.0
  pulmonary J98.4
    valve I37.9
  pylorus K31.9
  rectosigmoid K63.9
  retina, retinal H35.9
  sacroiliac (joint) (old) M53.3
  salivary gland K11.9
    benign lymphoepithelial K11.8
  saphenous nerve G57.8- ☑
  sciatic nerve G57.0- ☑
  secondary — *see* Syphilis, secondary
  shoulder (region) M75.9- ☑
    specified NEC M75.8- ☑
  sigmoid K63.9
  sinus (accessory) (nasal) J34.89
  skin L98.9
    suppurative L08.0
  SLAP S43.43- ☑
  spinal cord G95.9
    congenital Q06.9
  spleen D73.89
  stomach K31.9
  superior glenoid labrum S43.43- ☑
  syphilitic — *see* Syphilis
  tertiary — *see* Syphilis, tertiary
  thoracic root (nerve) NEC G54.3
  tonsillar fossa J35.9
  tooth, teeth K08.9
    white spot
      chewing surface K02.51
      pit and fissure surface K02.51
      smooth surface K02.61
  traumatic — *see* specific type of injury by site
  tricuspid (valve) I07.9
    nonrheumatic I36.9
  trigeminal nerve G50.9
  ulcerated or ulcerative — *see* Ulcer, skin
  uterus N85.9
  vagus nerve G52.2
  valvular — *see* Endocarditis
  vascular I99.9
    affecting central nervous system I67.9
    following trauma NEC T14.8
    umbilical cord, complicating delivery O69.5 ☑
  warty — *see* Verruca
  white spot (tooth)
    chewing surface K02.51
    pit and fissure surface K02.51
    smooth surface K02.61
Lethargic — *see* condition
Lethargy R53.83
Letterer-Siwe's disease C96.0
Leukemia, leukemic C95.9- ☑
  acute basophilic C94.8- ☑
  acute bilineal C95.0- ☑
  acute erythroid C94.0- ☑
  acute lymphoblastic C91.0- ☑
  acute megakaryoblastic C94.2- ☑
  acute megakaryocytic C94.2- ☑
  acute mixed lineage C95.0- ☑
  acute monoblastic (monoblastic/monocytic) C93.0- ☑
  acute monocytic (monoblastic/monocytic) C93.0- ☑
  acute myeloblastic (minimal differentiation) (with maturation) C92.0- ☑
  acute myeloid
    with
      11q23-abnormality C92.6- ☑
      dysplasia of remaining hematopoesis and/or myelodysplastic disease in its history C92.A- ☑
      multilineage dysplasia C92.A- ☑
      variation of MLL-gene C92.6- ☑
    M6 (a)(b) C94.0- ☑
    M7 C94.2- ☑
  acute myelomonocytic C92.5- ☑
  acute promyelocytic C92.4- ☑
  adult T-cell (HTLV-1-associated) (acute variant) (chronic variant) (lymphomatoid variant) (smouldering variant) C91.5- ☑
  aggressive NK-cell C94.8- ☑
  AML (1/ETO) (M0) (M1) (M2) (without a FAB classification) C92.0- ☑
  AML M3 C92.4- ☑
  AML M4 (Eo with inv(16) or t(16;16)) C92.5- ☑
  AML M5 C93.0- ☑
  AML M5a C93.0- ☑
  AML M5b C93.0- ☑
  AML Me with t (15;17) and variants C92.4- ☑

☑ **Additional character required**

Leukemia — *continued*
  atypical chronic myeloid, BCR/ABL-negative
    C92.2- ☑
  biphenotypic acute C95.0- ☑
  blast cell C95.0- ☑
  Burkitt-type, mature B-cell C91.A- ☑
  chronic lymphocytic, of B-cell type C91.1- ☑
  chronic monocytic C93.1- ☑
  chronic myelogenous (Philadelphia chromosome
    (Ph1) positive) (t(9;22)) (q34;q11) (with crisis
    of blast cells) C92.1- ☑
  chronic myeloid, BCR/ABL-positive C92.1- ☑
    atypical, BCR/ABL-negative C92.2- ☑
  chronic myelomonocytic C93.1- ☑
  chronic neutrophilic D47.1
  CMML (-1) (-2) (with eosinophilia) C93.1- ☑
  granulocytic (*see also* Category C92) C92.9- ☑
  hairy cell C91.4- ☑
  juvenile myelomonocytic C93.3- ☑
  lymphoid C91.9- ☑
    specified NEC C91.Z- ☑
  mast cell C94.3- ☑
  mature B-cell, Burkitt-type C91.A- ☑
  monocytic (subacute) C93.9- ☑
    specified NEC C93.Z- ☑
  myelogenous (*see also* Category C92) C92.9- ☑
  myeloid C92.9- ☑
    specified NEC C92.Z- ☑
  plasma cell C90.1- ☑
  plasmacytic C90.1- ☑
  prolymphocytic
    of B-cell type C91.3- ☑
    of T-cell type C91.6- ☑
  specified NEC C94.8- ☑
  stem cell, of unclear lineage C95.0- ☑
  subacute lymphocytic C91.9- ☑
  T-cell large granular lymphocytic C91.Z- ☑
  unspecified cell type C95.9- ☑
    acute C95.0- ☑
    chronic C95.1- ☑
Leukemoid reaction (*see also* Reaction, leukemoid)
  D72.823- ☑
Leukoaraiosis (hypertensive) I67.81
Leukoariosis — *see* Leukoaraiosis
Leukocoria — *see* Disorder, globe, degenerated
  condition, leucocoria
Leukocytopenia D72.819
Leukocytosis D72.829
  eosinophilic D72.1
Leukoderma, leukodermia NEC L81.5
  syphilitic A51.39
    late A52.79
Leukodystrophy E75.29
Leukoedema, oral epithelium K13.29
Leukoencephalitis G04.81
  acute (subacute) hemorrhagic G36.1
    postimmunization or postvaccinal G04.02
  postinfectious G04.01
  subacute sclerosing A81.1
  van Bogaert's (sclerosing) A81.1
Leukoencephalopathy (*see also* Encephalopathy)
  G93.49
  Binswanger's I67.3
  heroin vapor G92
  metachromatic E75.25
  multifocal (progressive) A81.2
  postimmunization and postvaccinal G04.02
  progressive multifocal A81.2
  reversible, posterior G93.6
  van Bogaert's (sclerosing) A81.1
  vascular, progressive I67.3
Leukoerythroblastosis D75.9
Leukokeratosis (*see also* Leukoplakia)
  mouth K13.21
  nicotina palati K13.24
  oral mucosa K13.21
  tongue K13.21
  vocal cord J38.3
Leukokraurosis vulva (e) N90.4
Leukoma (cornea) (*see also* Opacity, cornea)
  adherent H17.0- ☑
  interfering with central vision — *see* Opacity,
    cornea, central
Leukomalacia, cerebral, newborn P91.2
  periventricular P91.2
Leukomelanopathy, hereditary D72.0
Leukonychia (punctata) (striata) L60.8
  congenital Q84.4
Leukopathia unguium L60.8
  congenital Q84.4
Leukopenia D72.819
  basophilic D72.818

Leukopenia — *continued*
  chemotherapy (cancer) induced D70.1
  congenital D70.0
  cyclic D70.0
  drug induced NEC D70.2
    due to cytoreductive cancer chemotherapy
    D70.1
  eosinophilic D72.818
  familial D70.0
  infantile genetic D70.0
  malignant D70.9
  periodic D70.0
  transitory neonatal P61.5
Leukopenic — *see* condition
Leukoplakia
  anus K62.89
  bladder (postinfectional) N32.89
  buccal K13.21
  cervix (uteri) N88.0
  esophagus K22.8
  gingiva K13.21
  hairy (oral mucosa) (tongue) K13.3
  kidney (pelvis) N28.89
  larynx J38.7
  lip K13.21
  mouth K13.21
  oral epithelium, including tongue (mucosa)
    K13.21
  palate K13.21
  pelvis (kidney) N28.89
  penis (infectional) N48.0
  rectum K62.89
  syphilitic (late) A52.79
  tongue K13.21
  ureter (postinfectional) N28.89
  urethra (postinfectional) N36.8
  uterus N85.8
  vagina N89.4
  vocal cord J38.3
  vulva N90.4
Leukorrhea N89.8
  due to Trichomonas (vaginalis) A59.00
  trichomonal A59.00
Leukosarcoma C85.9- ☑
Levocardia (isolated) Q24.1
  with situs inversus Q89.3
Levotransposition Q20.5
Lev's disease or syndrome (acquired complete heart
  block) I44.2
Levulosuria — *see* Fructosuria
Levurid L30.2
Lewy body (ies) (dementia) (disease) G31.83
Leyden-Moebius dystrophy G71.0
Leydig cell
  carcinoma
    specified site — *see* Neoplasm, malignant, by
      site
    unspecified site
      female C56.9
      male C62.9- ☑
  tumor
    benign
      specified site — *see* Neoplasm, benign, by
        site
      unspecified site
        female C27.- ☑
        male D29.2- ☑
    malignant
      specified site — *see* Neoplasm, malignant,
        by site
      unspecified site
        female C56.- ☑
        male C62.9- ☑
    specified site — *see* Neoplasm, uncertain
      behavior, by site
    unspecified site
      female D39.1- ☑
      male D40.1- ☑
Leydig-Sertoli cell tumor
  specified site — *see* Neoplasm, benign, by site
  unspecified site
    female D27.- ☑
    male D29.2- ☑
LGSIL (Low grade squamous intraepithelial lesion on
  cytologic smear of)
  anus R85.612
  cervix R87.612
  vagina R87.622
Liar, pathologic F60.2
Libido
  decreased R68.82
Libman-Sacks disease M32.11

Lice (infestation) B85.2
  body (Pediculus corporis) B85.1
  crab B85.3
  head (Pediculus capitis) B85.0
  mixed (classifiable to more than one of the titles
    B85.0-B85.3) B85.4
  pubic (Phthirus pubis) B85.3
Lichen L28.0
  albus L90.0
    penis N48.0
    vulva N90.4
  amyloidosis E85.4 [L99]
  atrophicus L90.0
    penis N48.0
    vulva N90.4
  congenital Q82.8
  myxedematosus L98.5
  nitidus L44.1
  pilaris Q82.8
    acquired L85.8
  planopilaris L66.1
  planus (chronicus) L43.9
    annularis L43.8
    bullous L43.1
    follicular L66.1
    hypertrophic L43.0
    moniliformis L44.3
    of Wilson L43.9
    specified NEC L43.8
    subacute (active) L43.3
    tropicus L43.3
  ruber
    acuminatus L44.0
    moniliformis L44.3
    planus L43.9
  sclerosus (et atrophicus) L90.0
    penis N48.0
    vulva N90.4
  scrofulosus (primary) (tuberculous) A18.4
  simplex (chronicus) (circumscriptus) L28.0
  striatus L44.2
  urticatus L28.2
Lichenification L28.0
Lichenoides tuberculosis (primary) A18.4
Lichtheim's disease or syndrome — *see*
  Degeneration, combined
Lien migrans D73.89
Ligament — *see* condition
Light
  for gestational age — *see* Light for dates
  headedness R42
Light-for-dates (infant) P05.00
  with weight of
    499 grams or less P05.01
    500-749 grams P05.02
    750-999 grams P05.03
    1000-1249 grams P05.04
    1250-1499 grams P05.05
    1500-1749 grams P05.06
    1750-1999 grams P05.07
    2000-2499 grams P05.08
  and small-for-dates — *see* Small for dates
  affecting management of pregnancy O36.59- ☑
Lightning (effects) (stroke) (struck by) T75.00 ☑
  burn — *see* Burn
  foot E53.8
  shock T75.01 ☑
  specified effect NEC T75.09 ☑
Lightwood-Albright syndrome N25.89
Lightwood's disease or syndrome (renal tubular
  acidosis) N25.89
Lignac (-de Toni) (-Fanconi) (-Debré) disease or
  syndrome E72.09
  with cystinosis E72.04
Ligneous thyroiditis E06.5
Likoff's syndrome I20.8
Limb — *see* condition
Limbic epilepsy personality syndrome F07.0
Limitation, limited
  activities due to disability Z73.6
  cardiac reserve — *see* Disease, heart
  eye muscle duction, traumatic — *see* Strabismus,
    mechanical
  mandibular range of motion M26.52
Lindau (-von Hippel) disease Q85.8
Line (s)
  Beau's L60.4
  Harris' — *see* Arrest, epiphyseal
  Hudson's (cornea) — *see* Pigmentation, cornea,
    anterior
  Stähli's (cornea) — *see* Pigmentation, cornea,
    anterior

Linea corneae senilis — *see* Change, cornea, senile
Lingua
  geographica K14.1
  nigra (villosa) K14.3
  plicata K14.5
  tylosis K13.29
Lingual — *see* condition
Linguatulosis B88.8
Linitis (gastric) plasticaC16.9
Lip — *see* condition
Lipedema — *see* Edema
Lipemia (*see also* Hyperlipidemia)
  retina, retinalis E78.3
Lipidosis E75.6
  cerebral (infantile) (juvenile) (late) E75.4
  cerebroretinal E75.4
  cerebroside E75.22
  cholesterol (cerebral) E75.5
  glycolipid E75.21
  hepatosplenomegalic E78.3
  sphingomyelin — *see* Niemann-Pick disease or
    syndrome
  sulfatide E75.29
Lipoadenoma — *see* Neoplasm, benign, by site
Lipoblastoma — *see* Lipoma
Lipoblastomatosis — *see* Lipoma
Lipochondrodystrophy E76.01
Lipodermatosclerosis — *see* Varix, leg, with,
  inflammation
  ulcerated — *see* Varix, leg, with, ulcer, with
    inflammation by site
Lipochrome histiocytosis (familial) D71
Lipodystrophia progressiva E88.1
Lipodystrophy (progressive) E88.1
  insulin E88.1
  intestinal K90.81
  mesenteric K65.4
Lipofibroma — *see* Lipoma
Lipofuscinosis, neuronal (with ceroidosis) E75.4
Lipogranuloma, sclerosing L92.8
Lipogranulomatosis E78.89
Lipoid (*see also* condition)
  histiocytosis D76.3
    essential E75.29
  nephrosis N04.9
  proteinosis of Urbach E78.89
Lipoidemia — *see* Hyperlipidemia
Lipoidosis — *see* Lipidosis
Lipoma D17.9
  fetal D17.9
    fat cell D17.9
  infiltrating D17.9
  intramuscular D17.9
  pleomorphic D17.9
  site classification
    arms (skin) (subcutaneous) D17.2- ☑
    connective tissue D17.30
      intra-abdominal D17.5
      intrathoracic D17.4
      peritoneum D17.79
      retroperitoneum D17.79
      specified site NEC D17.39
      spermatic cord D17.6
    face (skin) (subcutaneous) D17.0
    genitourinary organ NEC D17.72
    head (skin) (subcutaneous) D17.0
    intra-abdominal D17.5
    intrathoracic D17.4
    kidney D17.71
    legs (skin) (subcutaneous) D17.2- ☑
    neck (skin) (subcutaneous) D17.0
    peritoneum D17.79
    retroperitoneum D17.79
    skin D17.30
      specified site NEC D17.39
    specified site NEC D17.79
    spermatic cord D17.6
    subcutaneous D17.30
      specified site NEC D17.39
    trunk (skin) (subcutaneous) D17.1
    unspecified D17.9
  spindle cell D17.9
Lipomatosis E88.2
  dolorosa (Dercum) E88.2
  fetal — *see* Lipoma
  Launois-Bensaude E88.89
Lipomyoma — *see* Lipoma
Lipomyxoma — *see* Lipoma
Lipomyxosarcoma — *see* Neoplasm, connective
  tissue, malignant
Lipoprotein metabolism disorder E78.9
Lipoproteinemia E78.5

  broad-beta E78.2
  floating-beta E78.2
  hyper-pre-beta E78.1
Liposarcoma (*see also* Neoplasm, connective tissue,
  malignant)
  dedifferentiated — *see* Neoplasm, connective
    tissue, malignant
  differentiated type — *see* Neoplasm, connective
    tissue, malignant
  embryonal — *see* Neoplasm, connective tissue,
    malignant
  mixed type — *see* Neoplasm, connective tissue,
    malignant
  myxoid — *see* Neoplasm, connective tissue,
    malignant
  pleomorphic — *see* Neoplasm, connective tissue,
    malignant
  round cell — *see* Neoplasm, connective tissue,
    malignant
  well differentiated type — *see* Neoplasm,
    connective tissue, malignant
Liposynovitis prepatellaris E88.89
Lipping, cervix N86
Lipschütz disease or ulcer N76.6
Lipuria R82.0
  schistosomiasis (bilharziasis) B65.0
Lisping F80.0
Lissauer's paralysis A52.17
Lissencephalia, lissencephaly Q04.3
Listeriosis, listerellosis A32.9
  congenital (disseminated) P37.2
  cutaneous A32.0
  neonatal, newborn (disseminated) P37.2
  oculoglandular A32.81
  specified NEC A32.89
Lithemia E79.0
Lithiasis — *see* Calculus
Lithosis J62.8
Lithuria R82.99
Litigation, anxiety concerning Z65.3
Little leaguer's elbow — *see* Epicondylitis, medial
Little's disease G80.9
Littre's
  gland — *see* condition
  hernia — *see* Hernia, abdomen
Littritis — *see* Urethritis
Livedo (annularis) (racemosa) (reticularis) R23.1
Liver — *see* condition
Living alone (problems with) Z60.2
  with handicapped person Z74.2
Lloyd's syndrome — *see* Adenomatosis, endocrine
Loa loa, loaiasis, loasis B74.3
Lobar — *see* condition
Lobomycosis B48.0
Lobo's disease B48.0
Lobotomy syndrome F07.0
Lobstein (-Ekman) disease or syndrome Q78.0
Lobster-claw hand Q71.6- ☑
Lobulation (congenital) (*see also* Anomaly, by site)
  kidney, Q63.1
  liver, abnormal Q44.7
  spleen Q89.09
Lobule, lobular — *see* condition
Local, localized — *see* condition
Locked-in state G83.5
Locked twins causing obstructed labor O66.1
Locking
  joint — *see* Derangement, joint, specified type
    NEC
  knee — *see* Derangement, knee
Lockjaw — *see* Tetanus
Löffler's
  endocarditis I42.3
  eosinophilia J82
  pneumonia J82
  syndrome (eosinophilic pneumonitis) J82
Loiasis (with conjunctival infestation) (eyelid) B74.3
Lone Star fever A77.0
Long
  labor O63.9
    first stage O63.0
    second stage O63.1
  QT syndrome I45.81
Long-term (current) (prophylactic) drug therapy
  (use of)
  agents affecting estrogen receptors and estrogen
    levels NEC Z79.818
  anastrozole (Arimidex) Z79.811
  antibiotics Z79.2
    short-term use - omit code
  anticoagulants Z79.01
  anti-inflammatory, non-steroidal (NSAID) Z79.1

Long-term — *continued*
  antiplatelet Z79.02
  antithrombotics Z79.02
  aromatase inhibitors Z79.811
  aspirin Z79.82
  birth control pill or patch Z79.3
  bisphosphonates Z79.83
  contraceptive, oral Z79.3
  drug, specified NEC Z79.899
  estrogen receptor downregulators Z79.818
  Evista Z79.810
  exemestane (Aromasin) Z79.811
  Fareston Z79.810
  fulvestrant (Faslodex) Z79.818
  gonadotropin-releasing hormone (GnRH) agonist
    Z79.818
  goserelin acetate (Zoladex) Z79.818
  hormone replacement (postmenopausal)
    Z79.890
  insulin Z79.4
  letrozole (Femara) Z79.811
  leuprolide acetate (leuprorelin) (Lupron) Z79.818
  megestrol acetate (Megace) Z79.818
  methadone for pain management Z79.891
  Nolvadex Z79.810
  non-steroidal anti-inflammatories (NSAID) Z79.1
  opiate analgesic Z79.891
  oral contraceptive Z79.3
  raloxifene (Evista) Z79.810
  selective estrogen receptor modulators (SERMs)
    Z79.810
  steroids
    inhaled Z79.51
    systemic Z79.52
  tamoxifen (Nolvadex) Z79.810
  toremifene (Fareston) Z79.810
Longitudinal stripes or grooves, nails L60.8
  congenital Q84.6
Loop
  intestine — *see* Volvulus
  vascular on papilla (optic) Q14.2
Loose (*see also* condition)
  body
    joint M24.00
      ankle M24.07- ☑
      elbow M24.02- ☑
      hand M24.04- ☑
      hip M24.05- ☑
      knee M23.4- ☑
      shoulder (region) M24.01- ☑
      specified site NEC M24.08
      vertebra M24.08
      toe M24.07- ☑
      wrist M24.03- ☑
    knee M23.4- ☑
    sheath, tendon — *see* Disorder, tendon,
      specified type NEC
  cartilage — *see* Loose, body, joint
  tooth, teeth K08.8
Loosening
  aseptic
    joint prosthesis — *see* Complications, joint
      prosthesis, mechanical, loosening, by site
    epiphysis — *see* Osteochondropathy
  mechanical
    joint prosthesis — *see* Complications, joint
      prosthesis, mechanical, loosening, by site
Looser-Milkman (-Debray) syndrome M83.8
Lop ear (deformity) Q17.3
Lorain (-Levi) short stature syndrome E23.0
Lordosis M40.50
  acquired — *see* Lordosis, specified type NEC
  congenital Q76.429
    lumbar region Q76.426
    lumbosacral region Q76.427
    sacral region Q76.428
    sacrococcygeal region Q76.428
    thoracolumbar region Q76.425
  lumbar region M40.56
  lumbosacral region M40.57
  postsurgical M96.4
  postural — *see* Lordosis, specified type NEC
  rachitic (late effect) (sequelae) E64.3
  sequelae of rickets E64.3
  specified type NEC M40.40
    lumbar region M40.46
    lumbosacral region M40.47
    thoracolumbar region M40.45
  thoracolumbar region M40.55
  tuberculous A18.01
Loss (of)
  appetite (see Anorexia) R63.0

Loss - Lymphadenopathy

Loss — *continued*
hysterical F50.8
nonorganic origin F50.8
psychogenic F50.8
blood — *see* Hemorrhage
control, sphincter, rectum R15.9
nonorganic origin F98.1
consciousness, transient R55
traumatic — *see* Injury, intracranial
elasticity, skin R23.4
family (member) in childhood Z62.898
fluid (acute) E86.9
with
hypernatremia E87.0
hyponatremia E87.1
function of labyrinth H83.2
hair, nonscarring — *see* Alopecia
hearing (*see also* Deafness)
central NOS H90.5
neural NOS H90.5
perceptive NOS H90.5
sensorineural NOS H90.5
sensory NOS H90.5
height R29.890
limb or member, traumatic, current — *see*
Amputation, traumatic
love relationship in childhood Z62.898
memory (*see also* Amnesia)
mild, following organic brain damage F06.8
mind — *see* Psychosis
occlusal vertical dimension of fully erupted teeth
M26.37
organ or part — *see* Absence, by site, acquired
ossicles, ear (partial) H74.32- ☑
parent in childhood Z63.4
pregnancy, recurrent N96
care in current pregnancy O26.2- ☑
without current pregnancy N96
recurrent pregnancy — *see* Loss, pregnancy,
recurrent
self-esteem, in childhood Z62.898
sense of
smell — *see* Disturbance, sensation, smell
taste — *see* Disturbance, sensation, taste
touch R20.8
sensory R44.9
dissociative F44.6
sexual desire F52.0
sight (acquired) (complete) (congenital) — *see*
Blindness
substance of
bone — *see* Disorder, bone, density and
structure, specified NEC
cartilage — *see* Disorder, cartilage, specified
type NEC
auricle (ear) — *see* Disorder, pinna, specified
type NEC
vitreous (humor) H15.89
tooth, teeth — *see* Absence, teeth, acquired
vision, visual H54.7
both eyes H54.3
one eye H54.60
left (normal vision on right) H54.62
right (normal vision on left) H54.61
specified as blindness — *see* Blindness
subjective
sudden H53.13- ☑
transient H53.12- ☑
vitreous — *see* Prolapse, vitreous
voice — *see* Aphonia
weight (abnormal) (cause unknown) R63.4
Louis-Bar syndrome (ataxia-telangiectasia) G11.3
Louping ill (encephalitis) A84.8
Louse, lousiness — *see* Lice
Low
achiever, school Z55.3
back syndrome M54.5
basal metabolic rate R94.8
birthweight (2499 grams or less) P07.10
with weight of
1000-1249 grams P07.14
1250-1499 grams P07.15
1500-1749 grams P07.16
1750-1999 grams P07.17
2000-2499 grams P07.18
extreme (999 grams or less) P07.00
with weight of
499 grams or less P07.01
500-749 grams P07.02
750-999 grams P07.03
for gestational age — *see* Light for dates
blood pressure (*see also* Hypotension)

Low — *continued*
reading (incidental) (isolated) (nonspecific)
R03.1
cardiac reserve — *see* Disease, heart
function (*see also* Hypofunction)
kidney N28.9
hematocrit D64.9
hemoglobin D64.9
income Z59.6
level of literacy Z55.0
lying
kidney N28.89
organ or site, congenital — *see* Malposition,
congenital
output volume (cardiac) — *see* Failure, heart
platelets (blood) — *see* Thrombocytopenia
reserve, kidney N28.89
salt syndrome E87.1
self esteem R45.81
set ears Q17.4
vision H54.2
one eye (other eye normal) H54.50
left (normal vision on right) H54.52
other eye blind — *see* Blindness
right (normal vision on left) H54.51
Low-density-lipoprotein-type (LDL)
hyperlipoproteinemia E78.0
Lowe's syndrome E72.03
Lown-Ganong-Levine syndrome I45.6
LSD reaction (acute) (without dependence) F16.90
with dependence F16.20
L-shaped kidney Q63.8
Ludwig's angina or disease K12.2
Lues (venerea), luetic — *see* Syphilis
Luetscher's syndrome (dehydration) E86.0
Lumbago, lumbalgia M54.5
with sciatica M54.4- ☑
due to intervertebral disc disorder M51.17
due to displacement, intervertebral disc M51.27
with sciatica M51.17
Lumbar — *see* condition
Lumbarization, vertebra, congenital Q76.49
Lumbermen's itch B88.0
Lump — *see* Mass
Lunacy — *see* Psychosis
Lung — *see* condition
Lupoid (miliary) of Boeck D86.3
Lupus
anticoagulant D68.62
with
hemorrhagic disorder D68.312
hypercoagulable state D68.62
finding without diagnosis R76.0
discoid (local) L93.0
erythematosus (discoid) (local) L93.0
disseminated — *see* Lupus, erythematosus,
systemic
eyelid H01.129
left H01.126
lower H01.125
upper H01.124
right H01.123
lower H01.122
upper H01.121
profundus L93.2
specified NEC L93.2
subacute cutaneous L93.1
systemic M32.9
with organ or system involvement M32.10
endocarditis M32.11
lung M32.13
pericarditis M32.12
renal (glomerular) M32.14
tubulo-interstitial M32.15
specified organ or system NEC M32.19
drug-induced M32.0
inhibitor (presence of) D68.62
with
hemorrhagic disorder D68.312
hypercoagulable state D68.62
finding without diagnosis R76.0
specified NEC M32.8
exedens A18.4
hydralazine M32.0
correct substance properly administered — *see*
Table of Drugs and Chemicals, by drug,
adverse effect
overdose or wrong substance given or taken —
see Table of Drugs and Chemicals, by drug,
poisoning
nephritis (chronic) M32.14
nontuberculous, not disseminated L93.0

Lupus — *continued*
panniculitis L93.2
pernio (Besnier) D86.3
systemic — *see* Lupus, erythematosus, systemic
tuberculous A18.4
eyelid A18.4
vulgaris A18.4
eyelid A18.4
Luteinoma D27.- ☑
Lutembacher's disease or syndrome (atrial septal
defect with mitral stenosis) Q21.1
Luteoma D27.- ☑
Lutz (-Splendore-de Almeida) disease — *see*
Paracoccidioidomycosis
Luxation (*see also* Dislocation)
eyeball (nontraumatic) — *see* Luxation, globe
birth injury P15.3
globe, nontraumatic H44.82- ☑
lacrimal gland — *see* Dislocation, lacrimal gland
lens (old) (partial) (spontaneous)
congenital Q12.1
syphilitic A50.39
Lycanthropy F22
Lyell's syndrome L51.2
due to drug L51.2
correct substance properly administered — *see*
Table of Drugs and Chemicals, by drug,
adverse effect
overdose or wrong substance given or taken —
see Table of Drugs and Chemicals, by drug,
poisoning
Lyme disease A69.20
Lymph
gland or node — *see* condition
scrotum — *see* Infestation, filarial
Lymphadenitis I88.9
with ectopic or molar pregnancy O08.0
acute L04.9
axilla L04.2
face L04.0
head L04.0
hip L04.3
limb
lower L04.3
upper L04.2
neck L04.0
shoulder L04.2
specified site NEC L04.8
trunk L04.1
anthracosis (occupational) J60
any site, except mesenteric I88.9
chronic I88.1
subacute I88.1
breast
gestational — *see* Mastitis, obstetric
puerperal, postpartum (nonpurulent) O91.22
chancroidal (congenital) A57
chronic I88.1
mesenteric I88.0
due to
Brugia (malayi) B74.1
timori B74.2
chlamydial lymphogranuloma A55
diphtheria (toxin) A36.89
lymphogranuloma venereum A55
Wuchereria bancrofti B74.0
following ectopic or molar pregnancy O08.0
gonorrheal A54.89
infective — *see* Lymphadenitis, acute
mesenteric (acute) (chronic) (nonspecific)
(subacute) I88.0
due to Salmonella typhi A01.09
tuberculous A18.39
mycobacterial A31.8
purulent — *see* Lymphadenitis, acute
pyogenic — *see* Lymphadenitis, acute
regional, nonbacterial I88.8
septic — *see* Lymphadenitis, acute
subacute, unspecified site I88.1
suppurative — *see* Lymphadenitis, acute
syphilitic (early) (secondary) A51.49
late A52.79
tuberculous — *see* Tuberculosis, lymph gland
venereal (chlamydial) A55
Lymphadenoid goiter E06.3
Lymphadenopathy (generalized) R59.1
angioimmunoblastic, with dysproteinemia (AILD)
C86.5
due to toxoplasmosis (acquired) B58.89
congenital (acute) (subacute) (chronic) P37.1
localized R59.0
syphilitic (early) (secondary) A51.49

☑ **Additional character required**

Lymphadenosis R59.1
Lymphangiectasis I89.0
  conjunctiva H11.89
  postinfectional I89.0
  scrotum I89.0
Lymphangiectatic elephantiasis, nonfilarial I89.0
Lymphangioendothelioma D18.1
  malignant — *see* Neoplasm, connective tissue, malignant
Lymphangioleiomyomatosis J84.81
Lymphangioma D18.1
  capillary D18.1
  cavernous D18.1
  cystic D18.1
  malignant — *see* Neoplasm, connective tissue, malignant
Lymphangiomyoma D18.1
Lymphangiomyomatosis J84.81
Lymphangiosarcoma — *see* Neoplasm, connective tissue, malignant
Lymphangitis I89.1
  with
    abscess - code by site under Abscess
    cellulitis - code by site under Cellulitis
    ectopic or molar pregnancy O08.0
  acute L03.91
    abdominal wall L03.321
    ankle — *see* Lymphangitis, acute, lower limb
    arm — *see* Lymphangitis, acute, upper limb
    auricle (ear) — *see* Lymphangitis, acute, ear
    axilla L03.12- ☑
    back (any part) L03.322
    buttock L03.327
    cervical (meaning neck) L03.222
    cheek (external) L03.212
    chest wall L03.323
    digit
      finger — *see* Lymphangitis, acute, finger
      toe — *see* Lymphangitis, acute, toe
    ear (external) H60.1- ☑
    external auditory canal — *see* Lymphangitis, acute, ear
    eyelid — *see* Abscess, eyelid
    face NEC L03.212
    finger (intrathecal) (periosteal) (subcutaneous) (subcuticular) L03.02- ☑
    foot — *see* Lymphangitis, acute, lower limb
    gluteal (region) L03.327
    groin L03.324
    hand — *see* Lymphangitis, acute, upper limb
    head NEC L03.891
      face (any part, except ear, eye and nose) L03.212
    heel — *see* Lymphangitis, acute, lower limb
    hip — *see* Lymphangitis, acute, lower limb
    jaw (region) L03.212
    knee — *see* Lymphangitis, acute, lower limb
    leg — *see* Lymphangitis, acute, lower limb
    lower limb L03.12- ☑
      toe — *see* Lymphangitis, acute, toe
    navel L03.326
    neck (region) L03.222
    orbit, orbital — *see* Cellulitis, orbit
    pectoral (region) L03.323
    perineal, perineum L03.325
    scalp (any part) L03.891
    shoulder — *see* Lymphangitis, acute, upper limb
    specified site NEC L03.898
    thigh — *see* Lymphangitis, acute, lower limb
    thumb (intrathecal) (periosteal) (subcutaneous) (subcuticular) — *see* Lymphangitis, acute, finger
    toe (intrathecal) (periosteal) (subcutaneous) (subcuticular) L03.04- ☑
    trunk L03.329
      abdominal wall L03.321
      back (any part) L03.322
      buttock L03.327
      chest wall L03.323
      groin L03.324
      perineal, perineum L03.325
      umbilicus L03.326
    umbilicus L03.326
    upper limb L03.12- ☑
      axilla — *see* Lymphangitis, acute, axilla
      finger — *see* Lymphangitis, acute, finger
      thumb — *see* Lymphangitis, acute, finger
    wrist — *see* Lymphangitis, acute, upper limb
  breast
    gestational — *see* Mastitis, obstetric
  chancroidal A57

Lymphangitis — *continued*
  chronic (any site) I89.1
  due to
    Brugia (malayi) B74.1
      timori B74.2
    Wuchereria bancrofti B74.0
  following ectopic or molar pregnancy O08.89
  penis
    acute N48.29
    gonococcal (acute) (chronic) A54.09
  puerperal, postpartum, childbirth O86.89
  strumous, tuberculous A18.2
  subacute (any site) I89.1
  tuberculous — *see* Tuberculosis, lymph gland
Lymphatic (vessel) — *see* condition
Lymphatism E32.8
Lymphectasia I89.0
Lymphedema (acquired) (*see also* Elephantiasis)
  congenital Q82.0
  hereditary (chronic) (idiopathic) Q82.0
  postmastectomy I97.2
  praecox I89.0
  secondary I89.0
  surgical NEC I97.89
    postmastectomy (syndrome) I97.2
Lymphoblastic — *see* condition
Lymphoblastoma (diffuse) — *see* Lymphoma, lymphoblastic (diffuse)
  giant follicular — *see* Lymphoma, lymphoblastic (diffuse)
  macrofollicular — *see* Lymphoma, lymphoblastic (diffuse)
Lymphocele I89.8
Lymphocytic
  chorioencephalitis (acute) (serous) A87.2
  choriomeningitis (acute) (serous) A87.2
  meningoencephalitis A87.2
Lymphocytoma, benign cutis L98.8
Lymphocytopenia D72.810
Lymphocytosis (symptomatic) D72.820
  infectious (acute) B33.8
Lymphoepithelioma — *see* Neoplasm, malignant, by site
Lymphogranuloma (malignant) (*see also* Lymphoma, Hodgkin)
  chlamydial A55
  inguinale A55
  venereum (any site) (chlamydial) (with stricture of rectum) A55
Lymphogranulomatosis (malignant) (*see also* Lymphoma, Hodgkin)
  benign (Boeck's sarcoid) (Schaumann's) D86.1
Lymphohistiocytosis, hemophagocytic (familial) D76.1
Lymphoid — *see* condition
Lymphoma (of) (malignant) C85.90
  adult T-cell (HTLV-1-associated) (acute variant) (chronic variant) (lymphomatoid variant) (smouldering variant) C91.5- ☑
  anaplastic large cell
    ALK-negative C84.7- ☑
    ALK-positive C84.6- ☑
    CD30-positive C84.6- ☑
    primary cutaneous C86.6
  angioimmunoblastic T-cell C86.5
  BALT C88.4
  B-cell C85.1- ☑
  B-precursor C83.5- ☑
  blastic NK-cell C86.4
  bronchial-associated lymphoid tissue [BALT-lymphoma] C88.4
  Burkitt (atypical) C83.7- ☑
  Burkitt-like C83.7- ☑
  centrocytic C83.1- ☑
  cutaneous follicle center C82.6- ☑
  cutaneous T-cell C84.A- ☑
  diffuse follicle center C82.5- ☑
  diffuse large cell C83.3- ☑
    anaplastic C83.3- ☑
    B-cell C83.3- ☑
    CD30-positive C83.3- ☑
    centroblastic C83.3- ☑
    immunoblastic C83.3- ☑
    plasmablastic C83.3- ☑
    subtype not specified C83.3- ☑
    T-cell rich C83.3- ☑
  enteropathy-type (associated) (intestinal) T-cell C86.2
  extranodal NK/T-cell, nasal type C86.0
  extranodal marginal zone B-cell lymphoma of mucosa-associated lymphoid tissue [MALT-lymphoma] C88.4

Lymphoma — *continued*
  follicular C82.9- ☑
    grade
      I C82.0- ☑
      II C82.1- ☑
      III C82.2- ☑
      IIIa C82.3- ☑
      IIIb C82.4- ☑
    specified NEC C82.8- ☑
  hepatosplenic T-cell (alpha-beta) (gamma-delta) C86.1
  histiocytic C85.9- ☑
    true C96.A
  Hodgkin C81.9- ☑
    classical C81.7- ☑
      lymphocyte-rich C81.4- ☑
      lymphocyte depleted C81.3- ☑
      mixed cellularity C81.2- ☑
      nodular sclerosis C81.1- ☑
      specified NEC C81.7- ☑
    lymphocyte-rich classical C81.4- ☑
    lymphocyte depleted classical C81.3- ☑
    mixed cellularity classical C81.2- ☑
    nodular
      lymphocyte predominant C81.0- ☑
      sclerosis classical C81.1- ☑
  intravascular large B-cell C83.8- ☑
  Lennert's C84.4- ☑
  lymphoblastic B-cell C83.5- ☑
  lymphoblastic (diffuse) C83.5- ☑
  lymphoblastic T-cell C83.5- ☑
  lymphoepithelioid C84.4- ☑
  lymphoplasmacytic C83.0- ☑
    with IgM-production C88.0
  MALT C88.4
  mantle cell C83.1- ☑
  mature T-cell NEC C84.4- ☑
  mature T/NK-cell C84.9- ☑
    specified NEC C84.Z- ☑
  mediastinal (thymic) large B-cell C85.2- ☑
  Mediterranean C88.3
  mucosa-associated lymphoid tissue [MALT-lymphoma] C88.4
  NK/T cell C84.9- ☑
  nodal marginal zone C83.0- ☑
  non-follicular (diffuse) C83.9- ☑
    specified NEC C83.8- ☑
  non-Hodgkin (*see also* Lymphoma, by type) C85.9- ☑
    specified NEC C85.8- ☑
  non-leukemic variant of B-CLL C83.0- ☑
  peripheral T-cell, not classified C84.4- ☑
  primary cutaneous
    anaplastic large cell C86.6
    CD30-positive large T-cell C86.6
  primary effusion B-cell C83.8- ☑
  SALT C88.4
  skin-associated lymphoid tissue [SALT-lymphoma] C88.4
  small cell B-cell C83.0- ☑
  splenic marginal zone C83.0- ☑
  subcutaneous panniculitis-like T-cell C86.3
  T-precursor C83.5- ☑
  true histiocytic C96.A
Lymphomatosis — *see* Lymphoma
Lymphopathia venereum, veneris A55
Lymphopenia D72.810
Lymphoplasmacytic leukemia — *see* Leukemia, chronic lymphocytic, B-cell type
Lymphoproliferation, X-linked disease D82.3
Lymphoreticulosis, benign (of inoculation) A28.1
Lymphorrhea I89.8
Lymphosarcoma (diffuse) (*see also* Lymphoma) C85.9- ☑
Lymphostasis I89.8
Lypemania — *see* Melancholia
Lysine and hydroxylysine metabolism disorder E72.3
Lyssa — *see* Rabies

M

Macacus ear Q17.3
Maceration, wet feet, tropical (syndrome) T69.02- ☑
MacLeod's syndrome J43.0
Macrocephalia, macrocephaly Q75.3
Macrocheilia, macrochilia (congenital) Q18.6
Macrocolon (see also Megacolon) Q43.1
Macrocornea Q15.8
　　with glaucoma Q15.0
Macrocytic — see condition
Macrocytosis D75.89
Macrodactylia, macrodactylism (fingers) (thumbs) Q74.0
　　toes Q74.2
Macrodontia K00.2
Macrogenia M26.05
Macrogenitosomia (adrenal) (male) (praecox) E25.9
　　congenital E25.0
Macroglobulinemia (idiopathic) (primary) C88.0
　　monoclonal (essential) D47.2
　　Waldenström C88.0
Macroglossia (congenital) Q38.2
　　acquired K14.8
Macrognathia, macrognathism (congenital) (mandibular) (maxillary) M26.09
Macrogyria (congenital) Q04.8
Macrohydrocephalus — see Hydrocephalus
Macromastia — see Hypertrophy, breast
Macrophthalmos Q11.3
　　in congenital glaucoma Q15.0
Macropsia H53.15
Macrosigmoid K59.3
　　congenital Q43.2
Macrospondylitis, acromegalic E22.0
Macrostomia (congenital) Q18.4
Macrotia (external ear) (congenital) Q17.1
Macula
　　cornea, corneal — see Opacity, cornea
　　degeneration (atrophic) (exudative) (senile) (see also Degeneration, macula)
　　　　hereditary — see Dystrophy, retina
Maculae ceruleae -- B85.1
Maculopathy, toxic — see Degeneration, macula, toxic
Madarosis (eyelid) H02.729
　　left H02.726
　　　　lower H02.725
　　　　upper H02.724
　　right H02.723
　　　　lower H02.722
　　　　upper H02.721
Madelung's
　　deformity (radius) Q74.0
　　disease
　　　　radial deformity Q74.0
　　　　symmetrical lipomas, neck E88.89
Madness — see Psychosis
Madura
　　foot B47.9
　　　　actinomycotic B47.1
　　　　mycotic B47.0
Maduromycosis B47.0
Maffucci's syndrome Q78.4
Magnesium metabolism disorder — see Disorder, metabolism, magnesium
Main en griffe (acquired) (see also Deformity, limb, clawhand)
　　congenital Q74.0
Maintenance (encounter for)
　　antineoplastic chemotherapy Z51.11
　　antineoplastic radiation therapy Z51.0
　　methadone F11.20
Majocchi's
　　disease L81.7
　　granuloma B35.8
Major — see condition
Malabar itch (any site) B35.5
Malabsorption K90.9
　　calcium K90.89
　　carbohydrate K90.4
　　disaccharide E73.9
　　fat K90.4
　　galactose E74.20
　　glucose (-galactose) E74.39
　　intestinal K90.9
　　　　specified NEC K90.89
　　isomaltose E74.31
　　lactose E73.9
　　methionine E72.19
　　monosaccharide E74.39

Malabsorption — continued
　　postgastrectomy K91.2
　　postsurgical K91.2
　　protein K90.4
　　starch K90.4
　　sucrose E74.39
　　syndrome K90.9
　　　　postsurgical K91.2
Malacia, bone (adult) M83.9
　　juvenile — see Rickets
Malacoplakia
　　bladder N32.89
　　pelvis (kidney) N28.89
　　ureter N28.89
　　urethra N36.8
Malacosteon, juvenile — see Rickets
Maladaptation — see Maladjustment
Maladie de Roger Q21.0
Maladjustment
　　conjugal Z63.0
　　　　involving divorce or estrangement Z63.5
　　educational Z55.4
　　family Z63.9
　　marital Z63.0
　　　　involving divorce or estrangement Z63.5
　　occupational NEC Z56.89
　　simple, adult — see Disorder, adjustment
　　situational — see Disorder, adjustment
　　social Z60.9
　　　　due to
　　　　　　acculturation difficulty Z60.3
　　　　　　discrimination and persecution (perceived) Z60.5
　　　　　　exclusion and isolation Z60.4
　　　　　　life-cycle (phase of life) transition Z60.0
　　　　　　rejection Z60.4
　　　　　　specified reason NEC Z60.8
Malaise R53.81
Malakoplakia — see Malacoplakia
Malaria, malarial (fever) B54
　　with
　　　　blackwater fever B50.8
　　　　　　hemoglobinuric (bilious) B50.8
　　　　　　hemoglobinuria B50.8
　　accidentally induced (therapeutically) - code by type under Malaria
　　algid B50.9
　　cerebral B50.0 [G94]
　　clinically diagnosed (without parasitological confirmation) B54
　　congenital NEC P37.4
　　　　falciparum P37.3
　　congestion, congestive B54
　　continued (fever) B50.9
　　estivo-autumnal B50.9
　　falciparum B50.9
　　　　with complications NEC B50.8
　　　　　　cerebral B50.0 [G94]
　　　　severe B50.8
　　hemorrhagic B54
　　malariae B52.9
　　　　with
　　　　　　complications NEC B52.8
　　　　　　glomerular disorder B52.0
　　malignant (tertian) — see Malaria, falciparum
　　mixed infections - code to first listed type in B50-B53
　　ovale B53.0
　　parasitologically confirmed NEC B53.8
　　pernicious, acute — see Malaria, falciparum
　　Plasmodium (P.)
　　　　falciparum NEC — see Malaria, falciparum
　　　　malariae NEC B52.9
　　　　　　with Plasmodium
　　　　　　　　falciparum (and or vivax) — see Malaria, falciparum
　　　　　　　　vivax (see also Malaria, vivax)
　　　　　　　　　　and falciparum — see Malaria, falciparum
　　　　ovale B53.0
　　　　　　with Plasmodium malariae (see also Malaria, malariae)
　　　　　　and vivax (see also Malaria, vivax)
　　　　　　　　and falciparum — see Malaria, falciparum
　　　　simian B53.1
　　　　　　with Plasmodium malariae (see also Malaria, malariae)
　　　　　　and vivax (see also Malaria, vivax)
　　　　　　　　and falciparum — see Malaria, falciparum
　　　　vivax NEC B51.9
　　　　　　with Plasmodium falciparum — see Malaria, falciparum
　　quartan — see Malaria, malariae

Malaria — continued
　　quotidian — see Malaria, falciparum
　　recurrent B54
　　remittent B54
　　specified type NEC (parasitologically confirmed) B53.8
　　spleen B54
　　subtertian (fever) — see Malaria, falciparum
　　tertian (benign) (see also Malaria, vivax)
　　　　malignant B50.9
　　tropical B50.9
　　typhoid B54
　　vivax B51.9
　　　　with
　　　　　　complications NEC B51.8
　　　　　　ruptured spleen B51.0
Malassimilation K90.9
Malassez's disease (cystic) N50.8
Mal de los pintos — see Pinta
Mal de mer T75.3 ☑
Maldescent, testis Q53.9
　　bilateral Q53.20
　　　　abdominal Q53.21
　　　　perineal Q53.22
　　unilateral Q53.10
　　　　abdominal Q53.11
　　　　perineal Q53.12
Maldevelopment (see also Anomaly)
　　brain Q07.9
　　colon Q43.9
　　hip Q74.2
　　　　congenital dislocation Q65.2
　　　　　　bilateral Q65.1
　　　　　　unilateral Q65.0- ☑
　　mastoid process Q75.8
　　middle ear Q16.4
　　　　except ossicles Q16.4
　　　　ossicles Q16.3
　　ossicles Q16.3
　　spine Q76.49
　　toe Q74.2
Male type pelvis Q74.2
　　with disproportion (fetopelvic) O33.3 ☑
　　　　causing obstructed labor O65.3
Malformation (congenital) (see also Anomaly)
　　adrenal gland Q89.1
　　affecting multiple systems with skeletal changes NEC Q87.5
　　alimentary tract Q45.9
　　　　specified type NEC Q45.8
　　　　upper Q40.9
　　　　　　specified type NEC Q40.8
　　aorta Q25.9
　　　　atresia Q25.2
　　　　coarctation (preductal) (postductal) Q25.1
　　　　patent ductus arteriosus Q25.0
　　　　specified type NEC Q25.4
　　　　stenosis (supravalvular) Q25.3
　　aortic valve Q23.9
　　　　specified NEC Q23.8
　　arteriovenous, aneurysmatic (congenital) Q27.30
　　　　brain Q28.2
　　　　cerebral Q28.2
　　　　peripheral Q27.30
　　　　　　digestive system Q27.33
　　　　　　lower limb Q27.32
　　　　　　other specified site Q27.39
　　　　　　renal vessel Q27.34
　　　　　　upper limb Q27.31
　　　　precerebral vessels (nonruptured) Q28.0
　　auricle
　　　　ear (congenital) Q17.3
　　　　　　acquired H61.119
　　　　　　　　left H61.112
　　　　　　　　　　with right H61.113
　　　　　　　　right H61.111
　　　　　　　　　　with left H61.113
　　bile duct Q44.5
　　bladder Q64.79
　　　　aplasia Q64.5
　　　　diverticulum Q64.6
　　　　exstrophy — see Exstrophy, bladder
　　　　neck obstruction Q64.31
　　bone Q79.9
　　　　face Q75.9
　　　　　　specified type NEC Q75.8
　　　　skull Q75.9
　　　　　　specified type NEC Q75.8
　　brain (multiple) Q04.9
　　　　arteriovenous Q28.2
　　　　specified type NEC Q04.8
　　branchial cleft Q18.2

☑ **Additional character required**

Malformation — *continued*
breast Q83.9
  specified type NEC Q83.8
broad ligament Q50.6
bronchus Q32.4
bursa Q79.9
cardiac
  chambers Q20.9
    specified type NEC Q20.8
  septum Q21.9
    specified type NEC Q21.8
cerebral Q04.9
  vessels Q28.3
cervix uteri Q51.9
  specified type NEC Q51.828
Chiari
  Type I G93.5
  Type II Q07.01
choroid (congenital) Q14.3
  plexus Q07.8
circulatory system Q28.9
cochlea Q16.5
cornea Q13.4
coronary vessels Q24.5
corpus callosum (congenital) Q04.0
diaphragm Q79.1
digestive system NEC, specified type NEC Q45.8
dura Q07.9
  brain Q04.9
  spinal Q06.9
ear Q17.9
  causing impairment of hearing Q16.9
  external Q17.9
    accessory auricle Q17.0
    causing impairment of hearing Q16.9
      absence of
        auditory canal Q16.1
        auricle Q16.0
    macrotia Q17.1
    microtia Q17.2
    misplacement Q17.4
    misshapen NEC Q17.3
    prominence Q17.5
    specified type NEC Q17.8
  inner Q16.5
  middle Q16.4
    absence of eustachian tube Q16.2
    ossicles (fusion) Q16.3
  ossicles Q16.3
  specified type NEC Q17.8
epididymis Q55.4
esophagus Q39.9
  specified type NEC Q39.8
eye Q15.9
  lid Q10.3
  specified NEC Q15.8
fallopian tube Q50.6
genital organ — *see* Anomaly, genitalia
great
  artery Q25.9
    aorta — *see* Malformation, aorta
    pulmonary artery — *see* Malformation,
      pulmonary, artery
    specified type NEC Q25.8
  vein Q26.9
    anomalous
      portal venous connection Q26.5
      pulmonary venous connection Q26.4
        partial Q26.3
        total Q26.2
    persistent left superior vena cava Q26.1
    portal vein-hepatic artery fistula Q26.6
    specified type NEC Q26.8
    vena cava stenosis, congenital Q26.0
gum Q38.6
hair Q84.2
heart Q24.9
  specified type NEC Q24.8
integument Q84.9
  specified type NEC Q84.8
internal ear Q16.5
intestine Q43.9
  specified type NEC Q43.8
iris Q13.2
joint Q74.9
  ankle Q74.2
  lumbosacral Q76.49
  sacroiliac Q74.2
  specified type NEC Q74.8
kidney Q63.9
  accessory Q63.0
  giant Q63.3

Malformation — *continued*
  horseshoe Q63.1
  hydronephrosis Q62.0
  malposition Q63.2
  specified type NEC Q63.8
lacrimal apparatus Q10.6
lip Q38.0
lingual Q38.3
liver Q44.7
lung Q33.9
meninges or membrane (congenital) Q07.9
  cerebral Q04.8
  spinal (cord) Q06.9
middle ear Q16.4
  ossicles Q16.3
mitral valve Q23.9
  specified NEC Q23.8
Mondini's (congenital) (malformation, cochlea)
  Q16.5
mouth (congenital) Q38.6
multiple types NEC Q89.7
musculoskeletal system Q79.9
myocardium Q24.8
nail Q84.6
nervous system (central) Q07.9
nose Q30.9
  specified type NEC Q30.8
optic disc Q14.2
orbit Q10.7
ovary Q50.39
palate Q38.5
parathyroid gland Q89.2
pelvic organs or tissues NEC
  in pregnancy or childbirth O34.8- ☑
    causing obstructed labor O65.5
penis Q55.69
  aplasia Q55.5
  curvature (lateral) Q55.61
  hypoplasia Q55.62
pericardium Q24.8
peripheral vascular system Q27.9
  specified type NEC Q27.8
pharynx Q38.8
precerebral vessels Q28.1
prostate Q55.4
pulmonary
  arteriovenous Q25.72
  artery Q25.9
    atresia Q25.5
    specified type NEC Q25.79
    stenosis Q25.6
  valve Q22.3
renal artery Q27.2
respiratory system Q34.9
retina Q14.1
scrotum — *see* Malformation, testis and scrotum
seminal vesicles Q55.4
sense organs NEC Q07.9
skin Q82.9
specified NEC Q89.8
spinal
  cord Q06.9
  nerve root Q07.8
spine Q76.49
  kyphosis — *see* Kyphosis, congenital
  lordosis — *see* Lordosis, congenital
spleen Q89.09
stomach Q40.3
  specified type NEC Q40.2
teeth, tooth K00.9
tendon Q79.9
testis and scrotum Q55.20
  aplasia Q55.0
  hypoplasia Q55.1
  polyorchism Q55.21
  retractile testis Q55.22
  scrotal transposition Q55.23
  specified NEC Q55.29
throat Q38.8
thorax, bony Q76.9
thyroid gland Q89.2
tongue (congenital) Q38.3
  hypertrophy Q38.2
  tie Q38.1
trachea Q32.1
tricuspid valve Q22.9
  specified type NEC Q22.8
umbilical cord NEC (complicating delivery)
  O69.89 ☑
umbilicus O89.9
ureter Q62.8
  agenesis Q62.4

Malformation — *continued*
  duplication Q62.5
  malposition — *see* Malposition, congenital,
    ureter
  obstructive defect — *see* Defect, obstructive,
    ureter
  vesico-uretero-renal reflux Q62.7
urethra Q64.79
  aplasia Q64.5
  duplication Q64.74
  posterior valves Q64.2
  prolapse Q64.71
  stricture Q64.32
urinary system Q64.9
uterus Q51.9
  specified type NEC Q51.818
vagina Q52.4
vascular system, peripheral Q27.9
vas deferens Q55.4
  atresia Q55.3
venous — *see* Anomaly, vein(s)
vulva Q52.70
Malfunction (*see also* Dysfunction)
cardiac electronic device T82.119 ☑
  electrode T82.110 ☑
  pulse generator T82.111 ☑
  specified type NEC T82.118 ☑
catheter device NEC T85.618 ☑
  cystostomy T83.010 ☑
  dialysis (renal) (vascular) T82.41 ☑
    intraperitoneal T85.611 ☑
  infusion NEC T82.514 ☑
    spinal (epidural) (subdural) T85.610 ☑
  urinary, indwelling T83.018 ☑
colostomy K94.03
  valve K94.03
cystostomy (stoma) N99.512
  catheter T83.010 ☑
enteric stoma K94.13
enterostomy K94.13
esophagostomy K94.33
gastroenteric K31.89
gastrostomy K94.23
ileostomy K94.13
  valve K94.13
jejunostomy K94.13
pacemaker — *see* Malfunction, cardiac electronic
  device
prosthetic device, internal — *see* Complications,
  prosthetic device, by site, mechanical
tracheostomy J95.03
urinary device NEC — *see* Complication,
  genitourinary, device, urinary, mechanical
valve
  colostomy K94.03
  heart T82.09 ☑
  ileostomy K94.13
vascular graft or shunt NEC — *see* Complication,
  cardiovascular device, mechanical, vascular
ventricular (communicating shunt) T85.01 ☑
Malherbe's tumor — *see* Neoplasm, skin, benign
Malibu disease L98.8
Malignancy (*see also* Neoplasm, malignant, by site)
  unspecified site (primary) C80.1
Malignant — *see* condition
Malingerer, malingering Z76.5
Mallet finger (acquired) — *see* Deformity, finger,
  mallet finger
  congenital Q74.0
  sequelae of rickets E64.3
Malleus A24.0
Mallory's bodies R89.7
Mallory-Weiss syndrome K22.6
Malnutrition E46
degree
  first E44.1
    mild (protein) E44.1
    moderate (protein) E44.0
  second E44.0
    severe (protein-energy) E43
      intermediate form E42
        with
          kwashiorkor (and marasmus) E42
          marasmus E41
  third E43
following gastrointestinal surgery K91.2
intrauterine
  light-for-dates — *see* Light for dates
  small-for-dates — *see* Small for dates
lack of care, or neglect (child) (infant) T76.02 ☑
  confirmed T74.02 ☑
malignant E40

Malnutrition — *continued*
   protein E46
      calorie E46
         mild E44.1
         moderate E44.0
         severe E43
            intermediate form E42
               with
                  kwashiorkor (and marasmus) E42
                  marasmus E41
      energy E46
         mild E44.1
         moderate E44.0
         severe E43
            intermediate form E42
               with
                  kwashiorkor (and marasmus) E42
                  marasmus E41
      severe (protein-energy) E43
         with
            kwashiorkor (and marasmus) E42
            marasmus E41
Malocclusion (teeth) M26.4
   Angle's M26.219
      class I M26.211
      class II M26.212
      class III M26.213
   due to
      abnormal swallowing M26.59
      mouth breathing M26.59
      tongue, lip or finger habits M26.59
   temporomandibular (joint) M26.69
Malposition
   cervix — *see* Malposition, uterus
   congenital
      adrenal (gland) Q89.1
      alimentary tract Q45.8
         lower Q43.8
         upper Q40.8
      aorta Q25.4
      appendix Q43.8
      arterial trunk Q20.0
      artery (peripheral) Q27.8
         coronary Q24.5
         digestive system Q27.8
         lower limb Q27.8
         pulmonary Q25.79
         specified site NEC Q27.8
         upper limb Q27.8
      auditory canal Q17.8
         causing impairment of hearing Q16.9
      auricle (ear) Q17.4
         causing impairment of hearing Q16.9
         cervical Q18.2
      biliary duct or passage Q44.5
      bladder (mucosa) — *see* Exstrophy, bladder
      brachial plexus Q07.8
      brain tissue Q04.8
      breast Q83.8
      bronchus Q32.4
      cecum Q43.8
      clavicle Q74.0
      colon Q43.8
      digestive organ or tract NEC Q45.8
         lower Q43.8
         upper Q40.8
      ear (auricle) (external) Q17.4
         ossicles Q16.3
      endocrine (gland) NEC Q89.2
      epiglottis Q31.8
      eustachian tube Q17.8
      eye Q15.8
      facial features Q18.8
      fallopian tube Q50.6
      finger (s) Q68.1
         supernumerary Q69.0
      foot Q66.9
      gallbladder Q44.1
      gastrointestinal tract Q45.8
      genitalia, genital organ (s) or tract
         female Q52.8
            external Q52.79
            internal NEC Q52.8
         male Q55.8
      glottis Q31.8
      hand Q68.1
      heart Q24.8
         dextrocardia Q24.0
            with complete transposition of viscera
               Q89.3
      hepatic duct Q44.5
      hip (joint) Q65.89

Malposition — *continued*
   intestine (large) (small) Q43.8
      with anomalous adhesions, fixation or
         malrotation Q43.3
   joint NEC Q68.8
   kidney Q63.2
   larynx Q31.8
   limb Q68.8
      lower Q68.8
      upper Q68.8
   liver Q44.7
   lung (lobe) Q33.8
   nail (s) Q84.6
   nerve Q07.8
   nervous system NEC Q07.8
   nose, nasal (septum) Q30.8
   organ or site not listed — *see* Anomaly, by site
   ovary Q50.39
   pancreas Q45.3
   parathyroid (gland) Q89.2
   patella Q74.1
   peripheral vascular system Q27.8
   pituitary (gland) Q89.2
   respiratory organ or system NEC Q34.8
   rib (cage) Q76.6
      supernumerary in cervical region Q76.5
   scapula Q74.0
   shoulder Q74.0
   spinal cord Q06.8
   spleen Q89.09
   sternum NEC Q76.7
   stomach Q40.2
   symphysis pubis Q74.2
   thymus (gland) Q89.2
   thyroid (gland) (tissue) Q89.2
      cartilage Q31.8
   toe (s) Q66.9
      supernumerary Q69.2
   tongue Q38.3
   trachea Q32.1
   ureter Q62.60
      deviation Q62.61
      displacement Q62.62
      ectopia Q62.63
      specified type NEC Q62.69
   uterus Q51.818
   vein (s) (peripheral) Q27.8
      great Q26.8
   vena cava (inferior) (superior) Q26.8
   device, implant or graft (*see also* Complications,
      by site and type, mechanical) T85.628 ☑
      arterial graft NEC — *see* Complication,
         cardiovascular device, mechanical, vascular
      breast (implant) T85.42 ☑
      catheter NEC T85.628 ☑
         cystostomy T83.020 ☑
         dialysis (renal) T82.42 ☑
            intraperitoneal T85.621 ☑
         infusion NEC T82.524 ☑
            spinal (epidural) (subdural) T85.620 ☑
         urinary, indwelling T83.028 ☑
      electronic (electrode) (pulse generator)
         (stimulator)
         bone T84.320 ☑
         cardiac T82.129 ☑
            electrode T82.120 ☑
            pulse generator T82.121 ☑
            specified type NEC T82.128 ☑
         nervous system — *see* Complication,
            prosthetic device, mechanical, electronic
            nervous system stimulator
         urinary — *see* Complication, genitourinary,
            device, urinary, mechanical
      fixation, internal (orthopedic) NEC — *see*
         Complication, fixation device, mechanical
      gastrointestinal — *see* Complications,
         prosthetic device, mechanical,
         gastrointestinal device
      genital NEC T83.428 ☑
         intrauterine contraceptive device T83.32 ☑
         penile prosthesis T83.420 ☑
      heart NEC — *see* Complication, cardiovascular
         device, mechanical
      joint prosthesis — *see* Complication, joint
         prosthesis, mechanical
      ocular NEC — *see* Complications, prosthetic
         device, mechanical, ocular device
      orthopedic NEC — *see* Complication,
         orthopedic, device, mechanical
      specified NEC T85.628 ☑
      urinary NEC (*see also* Complication,
         genitourinary, device, urinary, mechanical)

Malposition — *continued*
   graft T83.22 ☑
   vascular NEC — *see* Complication,
      cardiovascular device, mechanical
   ventricular intracranial shunt T85.02 ☑
   fetus — *see* Pregnancy, complicated by
      (management affected by), presentation,
      fetal
   gallbladder K82.8
   gastrointestinal tract, congenital Q45.8
   heart, congenital NEC Q24.8
   joint prosthesis — *see* Complications, joint
      prosthesis, mechanical, displacement, by site
   stomach K31.89
      congenital Q40.2
   tooth, teeth, fully erupted M26.30
   uterus (acute) (acquired) (adherent)
      (asymptomatic) (postinfectional) (postpartal,
      old) N85.4
      anteflexion or anteversion N85.4
         congenital Q51.818
      flexion N85.4
         lateral — *see* Lateroversion, uterus
      inversion N85.5
      lateral (flexion) (version) — *see* Lateroversion,
         uterus
         in pregnancy or childbirth O34.5
      retroflexion or retroversion — *see* Retroversion,
         uterus
Malposture R29.3
Malrotation
   cecum Q43.3
   colon Q43.3
   intestine Q43.3
   kidney Q63.2
Maltreatment
   adult
      abandonment
         confirmed T74.01 ☑
         suspected T76.01 ☑
      confirmed T74.91 ☑
      history of Z91.419
      neglect
         confirmed T74.01 ☑
         suspected T76.01 ☑
      physical abuse
         confirmed T74.11 ☑
         suspected T76.11 ☑
      psychological abuse
         confirmed T74.31 ☑
         suspected T76.31 ☑
         history of Z91.411
      sexual abuse
         confirmed T74.21 ☑
         suspected T76.21 ☑
      suspected T76.91 ☑
   child
      abandonment
         confirmed T74.02 ☑
         suspected T76.02 ☑
      confirmed T74.92 ☑
      history of — *see* History, personal (of), abuse
      neglect
         confirmed T74.02 ☑
         history of — *see* History, personal (of), abuse
         suspected T76.02 ☑
      physical abuse
         confirmed T74.12 ☑
         history of — *see* History, personal (of), abuse
         suspected T76.12 ☑
      psychological abuse
         confirmed T74.32 ☑
         history of — *see* History, personal (of), abuse
         suspected T76.32 ☑
      sexual abuse
         confirmed T74.22 ☑
         history of — *see* History, personal (of), abuse
         suspected T76.22 ☑
      suspected T76.92 ☑
   personal history of Z91.89
Malta fever — *see* Brucellosis
Maltworker's lung J67.4
Malunion, fracture — *see* Fracture, by site
Mammillitis N61
   puerperal, postpartum O91.02
Mammitis — *see* Mastitis
Mammogram (examination) Z12.39
   routine Z12.31
Mammoplasia N62
Management (of)
   bone conduction hearing device (implanted)
      Z45.320

Management — *continued*
cardiac pacemaker NEC Z45.018
cerebrospinal fluid drainage device Z45.41
cochlear device (implanted) Z45.321
contraceptive Z30.9
specified NEC Z30.8
implanted device Z45.9
specified NEC Z45.89
infusion pump Z45.1
procreative Z31.9
male factor infertility in female Z31.81
specified NEC Z31.89
prosthesis (external) (*see also* Fitting) Z44.9
implanted Z45.9
specified NEC Z45.89
renal dialysis catheter Z49.01
vascular access device Z45.2
Mangled — *see* specified injury by site
Mania (monopolar) (*see also* Disorder, mood, manic episode)
with psychotic symptoms F30.2
without psychotic symptoms F30.10
mild F30.11
moderate F30.12
severe F30.13
Bell's F30.8
chronic (recurrent) F31.89
hysterical F44.89
puerperal F30.8
recurrent F31.89
Manic-depressive insanity, psychosis, or syndrome — *see* Disorder, bipolar
Mannosidosis E77.1
Mansonelliasis, mansonellosis B74.4
Manson's
disease B65.1
schistosomiasis B65.1
Manual — *see* condition
Maple-bark-stripper's lung (disease) J67.6
Maple-syrup-urine disease E71.0
Marable's syndrome (celiac artery compression) I77.4
Marasmus E41
due to malnutrition E41
intestinal E41
nutritional E41
senile R54
tuberculous NEC — *see* Tuberculosis
Marble
bones Q78.2
skin R23.8
Marburg virus disease A98.3
March
fracture — *see* Fracture, traumatic, stress, by site
hemoglobinuria D59.6
Marchesani (-Weill) syndrome Q87.0
Marchiafava (-Bignami) syndrome or disease G37.1
Marchiafava-Micheli syndrome D59.5
Marcus Gunn's syndrome Q07.8
Marfan's syndrome — *see* Syndrome, Marfan's
Marie-Bamberger disease — *see* Osteoarthropathy, hypertrophic, specified NEC
Marie-Charcot-Tooth neuropathic muscular atrophy G60.0
Marie's
cerebellar ataxia (late-onset) G11.2
disease or syndrome (acromegaly) E22.0
Marie-Strümpell arthritis, disease or spondylitis — *see* Spondylitis, ankylosing
Marion's disease (bladder neck obstruction) N32.0
Marital conflict Z63.0
Mark
port wine Q82.5
raspberry Q82.5
strawberry Q82.5
stretch L90.6
tattoo L81.8
Marker heterochromatin — *see* Extra, marker chromosomes
Maroteaux-Lamy syndrome (mild) (severe) E76.29
Marrow (bone)
arrest D61.9
poor function D75.89
Marseilles fever A77.1
Marsh fever — *see* Malaria
Marshall's (hidrotic) ectodermal dysplasia Q82.4
Marsh's disease (exophthalmic goiter) E05.00
with storm E05.01
Masculinization (female) with adrenal hyperplasia E25.9
congenital E25.0
Masculinovoblastoma D27.- ☑

Masochism (sexual) F65.51
Mason's lung J62.8
Mass
abdominal R19.00
epigastric R19.06
generalized R19.07
left lower quadrant R19.04
left upper quadrant R19.02
periumbilic R19.05
right lower quadrant R19.03
right upper quadrant R19.01
specified site NEC R19.09
breast N63
chest R22.2
cystic — *see* Cyst
ear H93.8- ☑
head R22.0
intra-abdominal (diffuse) (generalized) — *see* Mass, abdominal
kidney N28.89
liver R16.0
localized (skin) R22.9
chest R22.2
head R22.0
limb
lower R22.4- ☑
upper R22.3- ☑
neck R22.1
trunk R22.2
lung R91.8
malignant — *see* Neoplasm, malignant, by site
neck R22.1
pelvic (diffuse) (generalized) — *see* Mass, abdominal
specified organ NEC — *see* Disease, by site
splenic R16.1
substernal thyroid — *see* Goiter
superficial (localized) R22.9
umbilical (diffuse) (generalized) R19.09
Massive — *see* condition
Mast cell
disease, systemic tissue D47.0
leukemia C94.3- ☑
sarcoma C96.2
tumor D47.0
malignant C96.2
Mastalgia N64.4
Masters-Allen syndrome N83.8
Mastitis (acute) (diffuse) (nonpuerperal) (subacute) N61
chronic (cystic) — *see* Mastopathy, cystic
cystic (Schimmelbusch's type) — *see* Mastopathy, cystic
fibrocystic — *see* Mastopathy, cystic
infective N61
newborn P39.0
interstitial, gestational or puerperal — *see* Mastitis, obstetric
neonatal (noninfective) P83.4
infective P39.0
obstetric (interstitial) (nonpurulent)
associated with
lactation O91.23
pregnancy O91.21- ☑
puerperium O91.22
purulent
associated with
lactation O91.13
pregnancy O91.11- ☑
puerperium O91.12
periductal — *see* Ectasia, mammary duct
phlegmonous — *see* Mastopathy, cystic
plasma cell — *see* Ectasia, mammary duct
Mastocytoma D47.0
malignant C96.2
Mastocytosis Q82.2
aggressive systemic C96.2
indolent systemic D47.0
malignant C96.2
systemic, associated with clonal hematopoetic non-mast-cell disease (SM-AHNMD) D47.0
Mastodynia N64.4
Mastoid — *see* condition
Mastoidalgia H92.0
Mastoiditis (coalescent) (hemorrhagic) (suppurative) H70.9- ☑
acute, subacute H70.00- ☑
complicated NEC H70.09- ☑
subperiosteal H70.01- ☑
chronic (necrotic) (recurrent) H70.1- ☑
in (due to)
infectious disease NEC B99 ☑ [H75.0- ☑]

Mastoiditis — *continued*
parasitic disease NEC B89 [H75.0- ☑]
tuberculosis A18.03
petrositis — *see* Petrositis
postauricular fistula — *see* Fistula, postauricular
specified NEC H70.89- ☑
tuberculous A18.03
Mastopathy, mastopathia N64.9
chronica cystica — *see* Mastopathy, cystic
cystic (chronic) (diffuse) N60.1- ☑
with epithelial proliferation N60.3- ☑
diffuse cystic — *see* Mastopathy, cystic
estrogenic, oestrogenica N64.89
ovarian origin N64.89
Mastoplasia, mastoplastia N62
Masturbation (excessive) F98.8
Maternal care (for) — *see* Pregnancy (complicated by) (management affected by)
Matheiu's disease (leptospiral jaundice) A27.0
Mauclaire's disease or osteochondrosis — *see* Osteochondrosis, juvenile, hand, metacarpal
Maxcy's disease A75.2
Maxilla, maxillary — *see* condition
May (-Hegglin) anomaly or syndrome D72.0
McArdle (-Schmid)(-Pearson) disease (glycogen storage) E74.04
McCune-Albright syndrome Q78.1
McQuarrie's syndrome (idiopathic familial hypoglycemia) E16.2
Meadow's syndrome Q86.1
Measles (black) (hemorrhagic) (suppressed) B05.9
with
complications NEC B05.89
encephalitis B05.0
intestinal complications B05.4
keratitis (keratoconjunctivitis) B05.81
meningitis B05.1
otitis media B05.3
pneumonia B05.2
French — *see* Rubella
German — *see* Rubella
Liberty — *see* Rubella
Meatitis, urethral — *see* Urethritis
Meatus, meatal — *see* condition
Meat-wrappers' asthma J68.9
Meckel-Gruber syndrome Q61.9
Meckel's diverticulitis, diverticulum (displaced) (hypertrophic) Q43.0
malignant — *see* Table of Neoplasms, small intestine, malignant
Meconium
ileus, newborn P76.0
in cystic fibrosis E84.11
meaning meconium plug (without cystic fibrosis) P76.0
obstruction, newborn P76.0
due to fecaliths P76.0
in mucoviscidosis E84.11
peritonitis P78.0
plug syndrome (newborn) NEC P76.0
Median (*see also* condition)
arcuate ligament syndrome I77.4
bar (prostate) (vesical orifice) — *see* Hyperplasia, prostate
rhomboid glossitis K14.2
Mediastinal shift R93.8
Mediastinitis (acute) (chronic) J98.5
syphilitic A52.73
tuberculous A15.8
Mediastinopericarditis (*see also* Pericarditis)
acute I30.9
adhesive I31.0
chronic I31.8
rheumatic I09.2
Mediastinum, mediastinal — *see* condition
Medicine poisoning — *see* Table of Drugs and Chemicals, by drug, poisoning
Mediterranean
fever — *see* Brucellosis
familial E85.0
tick A77.1
kala-azar B55.0
leishmaniasis B55.0
tick fever A77.1
Medulla — *see* condition
Medullary cystic kidney Q61.5
Medullated fibers
optic (nerve) Q14.8
retina Q14.1
Medulloblastoma
desmoplastic C71.6
specified site — *see* Neoplasm, malignant, by site

Medulloblastoma — *continued*
  unspecified site C71.6
Medulloepithelioma (*see also* Neoplasm, malignant, by site)
  teratoid — *see* Neoplasm, malignant, by site
Medullomyoblastoma
  specified site — *see* Neoplasm, malignant, by site
  unspecified site C71.6
Meekeren-Ehlers-Danlos syndrome Q79.6
Megacolon (acquired) (functional) (not Hirschsprung's disease) (in) K59.3
  Chagas' disease B57.32
  congenital, congenitum (aganglionic) Q43.1
  Hirschsprung's (disease) Q43.1
  toxic NEC K59.3
    due to Clostridium difficile A04.7
Megaesophagus (functional) K22.0
  congenital Q39.5
  in (due to) Chagas' disease B57.31
Megalencephaly Q04.5
Megalerythema (epidemic) B08.3
Megaloappendix Q43.8
Megalocephalus, megalocephaly NEC Q75.3
Megalocornea Q15.8
  with glaucoma Q15.0
Megalocytic anemia D53.1
Megalodactylia (fingers) (thumbs) (congenital) Q74.0
  toes Q74.2
Megaloduodenum Q43.8
Megaloesophagus (functional) K22.0
  congenital Q39.5
Megalogastria (acquired) K31.89
  congenital Q40.2
Megalophthalmos Q11.3
Megalopsia H53.15
Megalosplenia — *see* Splenomegaly
Megaloureter N28.82
  congenital Q62.2
Megarectum K62.89
Megasigmoid K59.3
  congenital Q43.2
Megaureter N28.82
  congenital Q62.2
Megavitamin-B6 syndrome E67.2
Megrim — *see* Migraine
Meibomian
  cyst, infected — *see* Hordeolum
  gland — *see* condition
  sty, stye — *see* Hordeolum
Meibomitis — *see* Hordeolum
Meige-Milroy disease (chronic hereditary edema) Q82.0
Meige's syndrome Q82.0
Melalgia, nutritional E53.8
Melancholia F32.9
  climacteric (single episode) F32.8
    recurrent episode F33.9
  hypochondriac F45.29
  intermittent (single episode) F32.8
    recurrent episode F33.9
  involutional (single episode) F32.8
    recurrent episode F33.9
  menopausal (single episode) F32.8
    recurrent episode F33.9
  puerperal F32.8
  reactive (emotional stress or trauma) F32.3
  recurrent F33.9
  senile F03 ☑
  stuporous (single episode) F32.8
    recurrent episode F33.9
Melanemia R79.89
Melanoameloblastoma — *see* Neoplasm, bone, benign
Melanoblastoma — *see* Melanoma
Melanocarcinoma — *see* Melanoma
Melanocytoma, eyeball D31.4- ☑
Melanocytosis, neurocutaneous Q82.8
Melanoderma, melanodermia L81.4
Melanodontia, infantile K03.89
Melanodontoclasia K03.89
Melanoepithelioma — *see* Melanoma
Melanoma (malignant) C43.9
  acral lentiginous, malignant — *see* Melanoma, skin, by site
  amelanotic — *see* Melanoma, skin, by site
  balloon cell — *see* Melanoma, skin, by site
  benign — *see* Nevus
  desmoplastic, malignant — *see* Melanoma, skin, by site
  epithelioid cell — *see* Melanoma, skin, by site

Melanoma — *continued*
  with spindle cell, mixed — *see* Melanoma, skin, by site
  in
    giant pigmented nevus — *see* Melanoma, skin, by site
    Hutchinson's melanotic freckle — *see* Melanoma, skin, by site
    junctional nevus — *see* Melanoma, skin, by site
    precancerous melanosis — *see* Melanoma, skin, by site
  in situ D03.9
    abdominal wall D03.59
    ala nasi D03.39
    ankle D03.7- ☑
    anus, anal (margin) (skin) D03.51
    arm D03.6- ☑
    auditory canal D03.2- ☑
    auricle (ear) D03.2- ☑
    auricular canal (external) D03.2- ☑
    axilla, axillary fold D03.59
    back D03.59
    breast D03.52
    brow D03.39
    buttock D03.59
    canthus (eye) D03.1- ☑
    cheek (external) D03.39
    chest wall D03.59
    chin D03.39
    choroid D03.8
    conjunctiva D03.8
    ear (external) D03.2- ☑
    external meatus (ear) D03.2- ☑
    eye D03.8
    eyebrow D03.39
    eyelid (lower) (upper) D03.1- ☑
    face D03.30
      specified NEC D03.39
    female genital organ (external) NEC D03.8
    finger D03.6- ☑
    flank D03.59
    foot D03.7- ☑
    forearm D03.6- ☑
    forehead D03.39
    foreskin D03.8
    gluteal region D03.59
    groin D03.59
    hand D03.6- ☑
    heel D03.7- ☑
    helix D03.2- ☑
    hip D03.7- ☑
    interscapular region D03.59
    iris D03.8
    jaw D03.39
    knee D03.7- ☑
    labium (majus) (minus) D03.8
    lacrimal gland D03.8
    leg D03.7- ☑
    lip (lower) (upper) D03.0
    lower limb NEC D03.7- ☑
    male genital organ (external) NEC D03.8
    nail D03.9
      finger D03.6- ☑
      toe D03.7- ☑
    neck D03.4
    nose (external) D03.39
    orbit D03.8
    penis D03.8
    perianal skin D03.51
    perineum D03.51
    pinna D03.2- ☑
    popliteal fossa or space D03.7- ☑
    prepuce D03.8
    pudendum D03.8
    retina D03.8
    retrobulbar D03.8
    scalp D03.4
    scrotum D03.8
    shoulder D03.6- ☑
    specified site NEC D03.8
    submammary fold D03.52
    temple D03.39
    thigh D03.7- ☑
    toe D03.7- ☑
    trunk NEC D03.59
    umbilicus D03.59
    upper limb NEC D03.6- ☑
    vulva D03.8
  juvenile — *see* Nevus
  malignant, of soft parts except skin — *see* Neoplasm, connective tissue, malignant
  metastatic

Melanoma — *continued*
  breast C79.81
  genital organ C79.82
  specified site NEC C79.89
  neurotropic, malignant — *see* Melanoma, skin, by site
  nodular — *see* Melanoma, skin, by site
  regressing, malignant — *see* Melanoma, skin, by site
  skin C43.9
    abdominal wall C43.59
    ala nasi C43.31
    ankle C43.7- ☑
    anus, anal (skin) C43.51
    arm C43.6- ☑
    auditory canal (external) C43.2- ☑
    auricle (ear) C43.2- ☑
    auricular canal (external) C43.2- ☑
    axilla, axillary fold C43.59
    back C43.59
    breast (female) (male) C43.52
    brow C43.39
    buttock C43.59
    canthus (eye) C43.1- ☑
    cheek (external) C43.39
    chest wall C43.59
    chin C43.39
    ear (external) C43.2- ☑
    elbow C43.6- ☑
    external meatus (ear) C43.2- ☑
    eyebrow C43.39
    eyelid (lower) (upper) C43.1- ☑
    face C43.39
      specified NEC C43.39
    female genital organ (external) NEC C51.9
    finger C43.6- ☑
    flank C43.59
    foot C43.7- ☑
    forearm C43.6- ☑
    forehead C43.39
    foreskin C60.0
    glabella C43.39
    gluteal region C43.59
    groin C43.59
    hand C43.6- ☑
    heel C43.7- ☑
    helix C43.2- ☑
    hip C43.7- ☑
    interscapular region C43.59
    jaw (external) C43.39
    knee C43.7- ☑
    labium C51.9
      majus C51.0
      minus C51.1
    leg C43.7- ☑
    lip (lower) (upper) C43.0
    lower limb NEC C43.7- ☑
    male genital organ (external) NEC C63.9
    nail
      finger C43.6- ☑
      toe C43.7- ☑
    nasolabial groove C43.39
    nates C43.59
    neck C43.4
    nose (external) C43.31
    overlapping site C43.8
    palpebra C43.1- ☑
    penis C60.9
    perianal skin C43.51
    perineum C43.51
    pinna C43.2- ☑
    popliteal fossa or space C43.7- ☑
    prepuce C60.0
    pudendum C51.9
    scalp C43.4
    scrotum C63.2
    shoulder C43.6- ☑
    skin NEC C43.9
    submammary fold C43.52
    temple C43.39
    thigh C43.7- ☑
    toe C43.7- ☑
    trunk NEC C43.59
    umbilicus C43.59
    upper limb NEC C43.6- ☑
    vulva C51.9
      overlapping sites C51.8
  spindle cell
    with epithelioid, mixed — *see* Melanoma, skin, by site
    type A C69.4- ☑
    type B C69.4- ☑

☑ **Additional character required**

Melanoma — *continued*
  superficial spreading — *see* Melanoma, skin, by
    site
Melanosarcoma (*see also* Melanoma)
  epithelioid cell — *see* Melanoma
Melanosis L81.4
  addisonian E27.1
    tuberculous A18.7
  adrenal E27.1
  colon K63.89
  conjunctiva — *see* Pigmentation, conjunctiva
    congenital Q13.89
  cornea (presenile) (senile) (*see also* Pigmentation,
    cornea)
    congenital Q13.4
  eye NEC H57.8
    congenital Q15.8
  lenticularis progressiva Q82.1
  liver K76.89
  precancerous (*see also* Melanoma, in situ)
    malignant melanoma in — *see* Melanoma
  Riehl's L81.4
  sclera H15.89
    congenital Q13.89
  suprarenal E27.1
  tar L81.4
  toxic L81.4
Melanuria R82.99
MELAS syndrome E88.41
Melasma L81.1
  adrenal (gland) E27.1
  suprarenal (gland) E27.1
Melena K92.1
  with ulcer - code by site under Ulcer, with
    hemorrhage K27.4
  due to swallowed maternal blood P78.2
  newborn, neonatal P54.1
    due to swallowed maternal blood P78.2
Meleney's
  gangrene (cutaneous) — *see* Ulcer, skin
  ulcer (chronic undermining) — *see* Ulcer, skin
Melioidosis A24.9
  acute A24.1
  chronic A24.2
  fulminating A24.1
  pneumonia A24.1
  pulmonary (chronic) A24.2
    acute A24.1
    subacute A24.2
  sepsis A24.1
  specified NEC A24.3
  subacute A24.2
Melitensis, febris A23.0
Melkersson (-Rosenthal) syndrome G51.2
Mellitus, diabetes — *see* Diabetes
Melorheostosis (bone) — *see* Disorder, bone,
  density and structure, specified NEC
Meloschisis Q18.4
Melotia Q17.4
Membrana
  capsularis lentis posterior Q13.89
  epipapillaris Q14.2
Membranacea placenta O43.19- ☑
Membranaceous uterus N85.8
Membrane (s), membranous (*see also* condition)
  cyclitic — *see* Membrane, pupillary
  folds, congenital — *see* Web
  Jackson's Q43.3
  over face of newborn P28.9
  premature rupture — *see* Rupture, membranes,
    premature
  pupillary H21.4- ☑
    persistent Q13.89
  retained (with hemorrhage) (complicating
    delivery) O72.2
    without hemorrhage O73.1
  secondary cataract — *see* Cataract, secondary
  unruptured (causing asphyxia) — *see* Asphyxia,
    newborn
  vitreous — *see* Opacity, vitreous, membranes and
    strands
Membranitis — *see* Chorioamnionitis
Memory disturbance, lack or loss (*see also* Amnesia)
  mild, following organic brain damage F06.8
Menadione deficiency E56.1
Menarche
  delayed E30.0
  precocious E30.1
Mendacity, pathologic F60.2
Mendelson's syndrome (due to anesthesia) J95.4
  in labor and delivery O74.0
  in pregnancy O29.01- ☑

Mendelson's — *continued*
  obstetric O74.0
  postpartum, puerperal O89.01
Ménétrier's disease or syndrome K29.60
  with bleeding K29.61
Ménière's disease, syndrome or vertigo H81.0- ☑
Meninges, meningeal — *see* condition
Meningioma (*see also* Neoplasm, meninges, benign)
  angioblastic — *see* Neoplasm, meninges, benign
  angiomatous — *see* Neoplasm, meninges, benign
  endotheliomatous — *see* Neoplasm, meninges,
    benign
  fibroblastic — *see* Neoplasm, meninges, benign
  fibrous — *see* Neoplasm, meninges, benign
  hemangioblastic — *see* Neoplasm, meninges,
    benign
  hemangiopericytic — *see* Neoplasm, meninges,
    benign
  malignant — *see* Neoplasm, meninges, malignant
  meningiothelial — *see* Neoplasm, meninges,
    benign
  meningotheliomatous — *see* Neoplasm,
    meninges, benign
  mixed — *see* Neoplasm, meninges, benign
  multiple — *see* Neoplasm, meninges, uncertain
    behavior
  papillary — *see* Neoplasm, meninges, uncertain
    behavior
  psammomatous — *see* Neoplasm, meninges,
    benign
  syncytial — *see* Neoplasm, meninges, benign
  transitional — *see* Neoplasm, meninges, benign
Meningiomatosis (diffuse) — *see* Neoplasm,
  meninges, uncertain behavior
Meningism — *see* Meningismus
Meningismus (infectional) (pneumococcal) R29.1
  due to serum or vaccine R29.1
  influenzal — *see* Influenza, with, manifestations
    NEC
Meningitis (basal) (basic) (brain) (cerebral) (cervical)
  (congestive) (diffuse) (hemorrhagic) (infantile)
  (membranous) (metastatic) (nonspecific)
  (pontine) (progressive) (simple) (spinal) (subacute)
  (sympathetic) (toxic) G03.9
  abacterial G03.0
  actinomycotic A42.81
  adenoviral A87.1
  arbovirus A87.8
  aseptic (acute) G03.0
  bacterial G00.9
    Escherichia coli (E. coli) G00.8
    Friedländer (bacillus) G00.8
    gram-negative A39.9
    H. influenzae G00.0
    Klebsiella G00.8
    pneumococcal G00.1
    specified organism NEC G00.8
    staphylococcal G00.3
    streptococcal (acute) G00.2
  benign recurrent (Mollaret) G03.2
  candidal B37.5
  caseous (tuberculous) A17.0
  cerebrospinal A39.0
  chronic NEC G03.1
  clear cerebrospinal fluid NEC G03.0
  coxsackievirus A87.0
  cryptococcal B45.1
  diplococcal (gram positive) A39.0
  echovirus A87.0
  enteroviral A87.0
  eosinophilic B83.2
  epidemic NEC A39.0
  Escherichia coli (E. coli) G00.8
  fibrinopurulent G00.9
    specified organism NEC G00.8
  Friedländer (bacillus) G00.8
  gonococcal A54.81
  gram-negative cocci G00.9
  gram-positive cocci G00.9
  Haemophilus (influenzae) G00.0
  H. influenzae G00.0
  in (due to)
    adenovirus A87.1
    African trypanosomiasis B56.9 [G02]
    anthrax A22.8
    bacterial disease NEC A48.8 [G01]
    Chagas' disease (chronic) B57.41
    chickenpox B01.0
    coccidioidomycosis B38.4
    Diplococcus pneumoniae G00.1
    enterovirus A87.0
    herpes (simplex) virus B00.3

Meningitis — *continued*
    zoster B02.1
  infectious mononucleosis B27.92
  leptospirosis A27.81
  Listeria monocytogenes A32.11
  Lyme disease A69.21
  measles B05.1
  mumps (virus) B26.1
  neurosyphilis (late) A52.13
  parasitic disease NEC B89 [G02]
  poliovirus A80.9 [G02]
  preventive immunization, inoculation or
    vaccination G03.8
  rubella B06.02
  Salmonella infection A02.21
  specified cause NEC G03.8
  typhoid fever A01.01
  varicella B01.0
  viral disease NEC A87.8
  whooping cough A37.90
  zoster B02.1
  infectious G00.9
  influenzal (H. influenzae) G00.0
  Klebsiella G00.8
  leptospiral (aseptic) A27.81
  lymphocytic (acute) (benign) (serous) A87.2
  meningococcal A39.0
  Mima polymorpha G00.8
  Mollaret (benign recurrent) G03.2
  monilial B37.5
  mycotic NEC B49 [G02]
  Neisseria A39.0
  nonbacterial G03.0
  nonpyogenic NEC G03.0
  ossificans G96.19
  pneumococcal G00.1
  poliovirus A80.9 [G02]
  postmeasles B05.1
  purulent G00.9
    specified organism NEC G00.8
  pyogenic G00.9
    specified organism NEC G00.8
  Salmonella (arizonae) (Cholerae-Suis) (enteritidis)
    (typhimurium) A02.21
  septic G00.9
    specified organism NEC G00.8
  serosa circumscripta NEC G03.0
  serous NEC G93.2
  specified organism NEC G00.8
  sporotrichosis B42.81
  staphylococcal G00.3
  sterile G03.0
  streptococcal (acute) G00.2
  suppurative G00.9
    specified organism NEC G00.8
  syphilitic (late) (tertiary) A52.13
    acute A51.41
    congenital A50.41
    secondary A51.41
  Torula histolytica (cryptococcal) B45.1
  traumatic (complication of injury) T79.8 ☑
  tuberculous A17.0
  typhoid A01.01
  viral NEC A87.9
  Yersinia pestis A20.3
Meningocele (spinal) (*see also* Spina bifida)
  with hydrocephalus — *see* Spina bifida, by site,
    with hydrocephalus
  acquired (traumatic) G96.19
  cerebral — *see* Encephalocele
Meningocerebritis — *see* Meningoencephalitis
Meningococcemia A39.4
  acute A39.2
  chronic A39.3
Meningococcus, meningococcal (*see also* condition)
  A39.9
  adrenalitis, hemorrhagic A39.1
  carrier (suspected) of Z22.31
  meningitis (cerebrospinal) A39.0
Meningoencephalitis (*see also* Encephalitis) G04.90
  acute NEC (*see also* Encephalitis, viral) A86
  bacterial NEC G04.2
  California A83.5
  diphasic A84.1
  eosinophilic B83.2
  epidemic A39.81
  herpesviral, herpetic B00.4
    due to herpesvirus 6 B10.01
    due to herpesvirus 7 B10.09
    specified NEC B10.09
  in (due to)
    blastomycosis NEC B40.81

Meningoencephalitis — continued
  diseases classified elsewhere G05.3
  free-living amebae B60.2
  Hemophilus influenzae (H .influenzae) G04.2
  herpes B00.4
    due to herpesvirus 6 B10.01
    due to herpesvirus 7 B10.09
    specified NEC B10.09
  H. influenzae G00.0
  Lyme disease A69.22
  mercuryT56.1
  mumps B26.2
  Naegleria (amebae) (organisms) (fowleri) B60.2
  Parastrongylus cantonensis B83.2
  toxoplasmosis (acquired) B58.2
    congenital P37.1
  infectious (acute) (viral) A86
  influenzal (H. influenzae) G04.2
  Listeria monocytogenes A32.12
  lymphocytic (serous) A87.2
  mumps B26.2
  parasitic NEC B89 [G05.3]
  pneumococcal G00.1
  primary ambic B60.2
  specific (syphilitic) A52.14
  specified organism NEC G04.81
  staphylococcal G04.2
  streptococcal G04.2
  syphilitic A52.14
  toxic NEC G92
    due to mercuryT56.1
  tuberculous A17.82
  virus NEC A86
Meningoencephalocele (see also Encephalocele)
  syphilitic A52.19
    congenital A50.49
Meningoencephalomyelitis (see also
  Meningoencephalitis)
  acute NEC (viral) A86
    disseminated G04.00
      postimmunization or postvaccination G04.02
      postinfectious G04.01
    due to
      actinomycosis A42.82
      Torula B45.1
      Toxoplasma or toxoplasmosis (acquired) B58.2
        congenital P37.1
    postimmunization or postvaccination G04.02
Meningoencephalomyelopathy G96.9
Meningoencephalopathy G96.9
Meningomyelitis (see also Meningoencephalitis)
  bacterial NEC G04.2
  blastomycotic NEC B40.81
  cryptococcal B45.1
  in diseases classified elsewhere G05.4
  meningococcal A39.81
  syphilitic A52.14
  tuberculous A17.82
Meningomyelocele (see also Spina bifida)
  syphilitic A52.19
Meningomyeloneuritis — see Meningoencephalitis
Meningoradiculitis — see Meningitis
Meningovascular — see condition
Menkes' disease or syndrome E83.09
  meaning maple-syrup-urine disease E71.0
Menometrorrhagia N92.1
Menopause, menopausal (asymptomatic) (state)
  Z78.0
  arthritis (any site) NEC — see Arthritis, specified
    form NEC
  bleeding N92.4
  depression (single episode) F32.8
    agitated (single episode) F32.2
      recurrent episode F33.9
    psychotic (single episode) F32.8
      recurrent episode F33.9
    recurrent episode F33.9
  melancholia (single episode) F32.8
    recurrent episode F33.9
  paranoid state F22
  premature E28.319
    asymptomatic E28.319
      postirradiation E89.40
      postsurgical E89.40
    symptomatic E28.310
      postirradiation E89.41
      postsurgical E89.41
  psychosis NEC F28
  symptomatic N95.1
  toxic polyarthritis NEC — see Arthritis, specified
    form NEC

Menorrhagia (primary) N92.0
  climacteric N92.4
    menopausal N92.4
  menopausal N92.4
  postclimacteric N95.0
  postmenopausal N95.0
  preclimacteric or premenopausal N92.4
  pubertal (menses retained) N92.2
Menostaxis N92.0
Menses, retention N94.89
Menstrual — see Menstruation
Menstruation
  absent — see Amenorrhea
  anovulatory N97.0
  cycle, irregular N92.6
  delayed N91.0
  disorder N93.9
    psychogenic F45.8
  during pregnancy O20.8
  excessive (with regular cycle) N92.0
    with irregular cycle N92.1
    at puberty N92.2
  frequent N92.0
  infrequent — see Oligomenorrhea
  irregular N92.6
    specified NEC N92.5
  latent N92.5
  membranous N92.5
  painful (see also Dysmenorrhea) N94.6
    primary N94.4
    psychogenic F45.8
    secondary N94.5
  passage of clots N92.0
  precocious E30.1
  protracted N92.5
  rare — see Oligomenorrhea
  retained N94.89
  retrograde N92.5
  scanty — see Oligomenorrhea
  suppression N94.89
  vicarious (nasal) N94.89
Mental (see also condition)
  deficiency — see Disability, intellectual
  deterioration — see Psychosis
  disorder — see Disorder, mental
  exhaustion F48.8
  insufficiency (congenital) — see Disability,
    intellectual
  observation without need for further medical
    care Z03.89
  retardation — see Disability, intellectual
  subnormality — see Disability, intellectuall
  upset — see Disorder, mental
Meralgia paresthetica G57.1- ☑
Mercurial — see condition
MercurialismT56.1
MERRF syndrome (myoclonic epilepsy associated
  with ragged-red fiber) E88.42
Merkel cell tumor — see Carcinoma, Merkel cell
Merocele — see Hernia, femoral
Meromelia
  lower limb — see Defect, reduction, lower limb
    intercalary
      femur — see Defect, reduction, lower limb,
        specified type NEC
        tibiofibular (complete) (incomplete) — see
          Defect, reduction, lower limb
  upper limb — see Defect, reduction, upper limb
    intercalary, humeral, radioulnar — see Agenesis,
      arm, with hand present
Merzbacher-Pelizaeus disease E75.29
Mesaortitis — see Aortitis
Mesarteritis — see Arteritis
Mesencephalitis — see Encephalitis
Mesenchymoma (see also Neoplasm, connective
  tissue, uncertain behavior)
  benign — see Neoplasm, connective tissue,
    benign
  malignant — see Neoplasm, connective tissue,
    malignant
Mesenteritis
  retractile K65.4
  sclerosing K65.4
Mesentery, mesenteric — see condition
Mesiodens, mesiodentes K00.1
Mesio-occlusion M26.213
Mesocolon — see condition
Mesonephroma (malignant) — see Neoplasm,
  malignant, by site
  benign — see Neoplasm, benign, by site
Mesophlebitis — see Phlebitis
Mesostromal dysgenesis Q13.89

Mesothelioma (malignant) C45.9
  benign
    mesentery D19.1
    mesocolon D19.1
    omentum D19.1
    peritoneum D19.1
    pleura D19.0
    specified site NEC D19.7
    unspecified site D19.9
  biphasic C45.9
    benign
      mesentery D19.1
      mesocolon D19.1
      omentum D19.1
      peritoneum D19.1
      pleura D19.0
      specified site NEC D19.7
      unspecified site D19.9
  cystic D48.4
  epithelioid C45.9
    benign
      mesentery D19.1
      mesocolon D19.1
      omentum D19.1
      peritoneum D19.1
      pleura D19.0
      specified site NEC D19.7
      unspecified site D19.9
  fibrous C45.9
    benign
      mesentery D19.1
      mesocolon D19.1
      omentum D19.1
      peritoneum D19.1
      pleura D19.0
      specified site NEC D19.7
      unspecified site D19.9
  site classification
    liver C45.7
    lung C45.7
    mediastinum C45.7
    mesentery C45.1
    mesocolon C45.1
    omentum C45.1
    pericardium C45.2
    peritoneum C45.1
    pleura C45.0
      parietal C45.0
    retroperitoneum C45.7
    specified site NEC C45.7
    unspecified C45.9
Metabolic syndrome E88.81
Metagonimiasis B66.8
Metagonimus infestation (intestine) B66.8
Metal
  pigmentation L81.8
  polisher's disease J62.8
Metamorphopsia H53.15
Metaplasia
  apocrine (breast) — see Dysplasia, mammary,
    specified type NEC
  cervix (squamous) — see Dysplasia, cervix
  endometrium (squamous) (uterus) N85.8
  esophagus
  kidney (pelvis) (squamous) N28.89
  myelogenous D73.1
  myeloid (agnogenic) (megakaryocytic) D73.1
  spleen D73.1
  squamous cell, bladder N32.89
Metastasis, metastatic
  abscess — see Abscess
  calcification E83.59
  cancer
    from specified site — see Neoplasm, malignant,
      by site
    to specified site — see Neoplasm, secondary,
      by site
  deposits (in) — see Neoplasm, secondary, by site
  disease (see also Neoplasm, secondary, by site)
    C79.9
  spread (to) — see Neoplasm, secondary, by site
Metastrongyliasis B83.8
Metatarsalgia M77.4- ☑
  anterior G57.6- ☑
  Morton's G57.6- ☑
Metatarsus, metatarsal (see also condition)
  valgus (abductus), congenital Q66.6
  varus (adductus) (congenital) Q66.2
Methadone use F11.20
Methemoglobinemia D74.9
  acquired (with sulfhemoglobinemia) D74.8
  congenital D74.0

☑ **Additional character required**

Methemoglobinemia — *continued*
- enzymatic (congenital) D74.0
- Hb M disease D74.0
- hereditary D74.0
- toxic D74.8

Methemoglobinuria — *see* Hemoglobinuria
Methioninemia E72.19
Methylmalonic acidemia E71.120
Metritis (catarrhal) (hemorrhagic) (septic) (suppurative) (*see also* Endometritis)
- cervical — *see* Cervicitis

Metropathia hemorrhagica N93.8
Metroperitonitis — *see* Peritonitis, pelvic, female
Metrorrhagia N92.1
- climacteric N92.4
- menopausal N92.4
- postpartum NEC (atonic) (following delivery of placenta) O72.1
  - delayed or secondary O72.2
- preclimacteric or premenopausal N92.4
- psychogenic F45.8

Metrorrhexis — *see* Rupture, uterus
Metrosalpingitis N70.91
Metrostaxis N93.8
Metrovaginitis — *see* Endometritis
Meyer-Schwickerath and Weyers syndrome Q87.0
Meynert's amentia (nonalcoholic) F04
- alcoholic F10.96
- with dependence F10.26

Mibelli's disease (porokeratosis) Q82.8
Mice, joint — *see* Loose, body, joint
- knee M23.4- ☑

Micrencephalon, micrencephaly Q02
Microalbuminuria R80.9
Microaneurysm, retinal (*see also* Disorder, retina, microaneurysms)
- diabetic — *see* E08-E13 with .31

Microangiopathy (peripheral) I73.9
- thrombotic M31.1

Microcalcifications, breast R92.0
Microcephalus, microcephalic, microcephaly Q02
- due to toxoplasmosis (congenital) P37.1

Microcheilia Q18.7
Microcolon (congenital) Q43.8
Microcornea (congenital) Q13.4
Microcytic — *see* condition
Microdeletions NEC Q93.88
Microdontia K00.2
Microdrepanocytosis D57.40
- with crisis (vasoocclusive pain) D57.419
  - with
    - acute chest syndrome D57.411
    - splenic sequestration D57.412

Microembolism
- atherothrombotic — *see* Atheroembolism
- retinal — *see* Occlusion, artery, retina

Microencephalon Q02
Microfilaria streptocerca infestation — *see* Onchocerciasis
Microgastria (congenital) Q40.2
Microgenia M26.06
Microgenitalia, congenital
- female Q52.8
- male Q55.8

Microglioma — *see* Lymphoma, non-Hodgkin, specified NEC
Microglossia (congenital) Q38.3
Micrognathia, micrognathism (congenital) (mandibular) (maxillary) M26.09
Microgyria (congenital) Q04.3
Microinfarct of heart — *see* Insufficiency, coronary
Microlentia (congenital) Q12.8
Microlithiasis, alveolar, pulmonary J84.02
Micromastia N64.82
Micromyelia (congenital) Q06.8
Micropenis Q55.62
Microphakia (congenital) Q12.8
Microphthalmos, microphthalmia (congenital) Q11.2
- due to toxoplasmosis P37.1

Micropsia H53.15
Microscopic polyangiitis (polyarteritis) M31.7
Microsporidiosis B60.8
- intestinal A07.8

Microsporon furfur infestation B36.0
Microsporosis (*see also* Dermatophytosis)
- nigra B36.1

Microstomia (congenital) Q18.5
Microtia (congenital) (external ear) Q17.2
Microtropia H50.40
Microvillus inclusion disease (MVD) (MVID) Q43.8

Micturition
- disorder NEC R39.19
  - psychogenic F45.8
- frequency R35.0
  - psychogenic F45.8
- hesitancy R39.11
- incomplete emptying R39.14
- nocturnal R35.1
- painful R30.9
  - dysuria R30.0
  - psychogenic F45.8
  - tenesmus R30.1
- poor stream R39.12
- split stream R39.13
- straining R39.16
- urgency R39.15

Mid plane — *see* condition
Middle
- ear — *see* condition
- lobe (right) syndrome J98.19

Miescher's elastoma L87.2
Mietens' syndrome Q87.2
Migraine (idiopathic) G43.909
- with refractory migraine G43.919
  - with status migrainosus G43.911
  - without status migrainosus G43.919
- with aura (acute-onset) (prolonged) (typical) (without headache) G43.109
  - with refractory migraine G43.119
    - with status migrainosus G43.111
    - without status migrainosus G43.119
  - intractable G43.119
    - with status migrainosus G43.111
    - without status migrainosus G43.119
  - not intractable G43.109
    - with status migrainosus G43.101
    - without status migrainosus G43.109
  - persistent G43.509
    - with cerebral infarction G43.609
      - with refractory migraine G43.619
        - with status migrainosus G43.611
        - without status migrainosus G43.619
      - intractable G43.619
        - with status migrainosus G43.611
        - without status migrainosus G43.619
      - not intractable G43.609
        - with status migrainosus G43.601
        - without status migrainosus G43.609
      - without refractory migraine G43.609
        - with status migrainosus G43.601
        - without status migrainosus G43.609
    - without cerebral infarction G43.509
      - with refractory migraine G43.519
        - with status migrainosus G43.511
        - without status migrainosus G43.519
      - intractable G43.519
        - with status migrainosus G43.511
        - without status migrainosus G43.519
      - not intractable G43.509
        - with status migrainosus G43.501
        - without status migrainosus G43.509
      - without refractory migraine G43.509
        - with status migrainosus G43.501
        - without status migrainosus G43.509
  - without mention of refractory migraine G43.109
    - with status migrainosus G43.101
    - without status migrainosus G43.109
- abdominal G43.D0
  - with refractory migraine G43.D1
  - intractable G43.D1
  - not intractable G43.D0
  - without refractory migraine G43.D0
- basilar — *see* Migraine, with aura
- classical — *see* Migraine, with aura
- common — *see* Migraine, without aura
- complicated G43.109
- equivalents — *see* Migraine, with aura
- familiar — *see* Migraine, hemiplegic
- hemiplegic G43.409
  - with refractory migraine G43.419
    - with status migrainosus G43.411
    - without status migrainosus G43.419
  - intractable G43.419
    - with status migrainosus G43.411
    - without status migrainosus G43.419
  - not intractable G43.409
    - with status migrainosus G43.401
    - without status migrainosus G43.409
  - without refractory migraine G43.409
    - with status migrainosus G43.401
    - without status migrainosus G43.409

Migraine — *continued*
- intractable G43.919
  - with status migrainosus G43.911
  - without status migrainosus G43.919
- menstrual G43.829
  - with refractory migraine G43.839
    - with status migrainosus G43.831
    - without status migrainosus G43.839
  - intractable G43.839
    - with status migrainosus G43.831
    - without status migrainosus G43.839
  - not intractable 4G43.829
    - with status migrainosus G43.821
    - without status migrainosus G43.829
  - without refractory migraine G43.829
    - with status migrainosus G43.821
    - without status migrainosus G43.829
- menstrually related — *see* Migraine, menstrual
- not intractable G43.909
  - with status migrainosus G43.901
  - without status migrainosus G43.919
- ophthalmoplegic G43.B0
  - with refractory migraine G43.B1
  - intractable G43.B1
  - not intractable G43.B0
  - without refractory migraine G43.B0
- persistent aura (with, without) cerebral infarction — *see* Migraine, with aura, persistent
- preceded or accompanied by transient focal neurological phenomena — *see* Migraine, with aura
- pre-menstrual — *see* Migraine, menstrual
- pure menstrual — *see* Migraine, menstrual
- retinal — *see* Migraine, with aura
- specified NEC G43.809
  - intractable G43.819
    - with status migrainosus G43.811
    - without status migrainosus G43.819
  - not intractable G43.809
    - with status migrainosus G43.801
    - without status migrainosus G43.809
- sporadic — *see* Migraine, hemiplegic
- transformed — *see* Migraine, without aura, chronic
- triggered seizures — *see* Migraine, with aura
- without aura G43.009
  - with refractory migraine G43.019
    - with status migrainosus G43.011
    - without status migrainosus G43.019
  - chronic G43.709
    - with refractory migraine G43.719
      - with status migrainosus G43.711
      - without status migrainosus G43.719
    - intractable
      - with status migrainosus G43.711
      - without status migrainosus G43.719
    - not intractable
      - with status migrainosus G43.701
      - without status migrainosus G43.709
    - without refractory migraine G43.709
      - with status migrainosus G43.701
      - without status migrainosus G43.709
  - intractable
    - with status migrainosus G43.011
    - without status migrainosus G43.019
  - not intractable
    - with status migrainosus G43.001
    - without status migrainosus G43.009
  - without mention of refractory migraine G43.009
    - with status migrainosus G43.001
    - without status migrainosus G43.009
- without refractory migraineG43.909
  - with status migrainosus G43.901
  - without status migrainosus G43.919

Migrant, social Z59.0
Migration, anxiety concerning Z60.3
Migratory, migrating (*see also* condition)
- person Z59.0
- testis Q55.29

Mikity-Wilson disease or syndrome P27.0
Mikulicz' disease or syndrome K11.8
Miliaria L74.3
- alba L74.1
- apocrine L75.2
- crystallina L74.1
- profunda L74.2
- rubra L74.0
- tropicalis L74.2

Miliary — *see* condition
Milium L72.0
- colloid L57.8

Milk
- crust L21.0
- excessive secretion O92.6
- poisoning — *see* Poisoning, food, noxious
- retention O92.79
- sickness — *see* Poisoning, food, noxious
- spots I31.0

Milk-alkali disease or syndrome E83.52

Milk-leg (deep vessels) (nonpuerperal) — *see* Embolism, vein, lower extremity
- complicating pregnancy O22.3-
- puerperal, postpartum, childbirth O87.1

Milkman's disease or syndrome M83.8

Milky urine — *see* Chyluria

Millard-Gubler (-Foville) paralysis or syndrome G46.3

Millar's asthma J38.5

Miller Fisher syndrome G61.0

Mills' disease — *see* Hemiplegia

Millstone maker's pneumoconiosis J62.8

Milroy's disease (chronic hereditary edema) Q82.0

Minamata disease T26.1- ☑

Miners' asthma or lung J60

Minkowski-Chauffard syndrome — *see* Spherocytosis

Minor — *see* condition

Minor's disease (hematomyelia) G95.19

Minot's disease (hemorrhagic disease), newborn P53

Minot-von Willebrand-Jurgens disease or syndrome (angiohemophilia) D68.0

Minus (and plus) hand (intrinsic) — *see* Deformity, limb, specified type NEC, forearm

Miosis (pupil) H57.03

Mirizzi's syndrome (hepatic duct stenosis) K83.1

Mirror writing F81.0

Misadventure (of) (prophylactic) (therapeutic) (*see also* Complications) T88.9 ☑
- administration of insulin (by accident)T38.3
- infusion — *see* Complications, infusion
- local applications (of fomentations, plasters, etc.) T88.9 ☑
  - burn or scald — *see* Burn
  - specified NEC T88.8 ☑
- medical care (early) (late) T88.9 ☑
  - adverse effect of drugs or chemicals — *see* Table of Drugs and Chemicals
- medical care (early) (late)
  - burn or scald — *see* Burn
  - specified NEC T88.8 ☑
- specified NEC T88.8 ☑
- surgical procedure (early) (late) — *see* Complications, surgical procedure
- transfusion — *see* Complications, transfusion
- vaccination or other immunological procedure — *see* Complications, vaccination

Miscarriage O03.9

Misdirection, aqueous H40.83- ☑

Misperception, sleep state F51.02

Misplaced, misplacement
- ear Q17.4
- kidney (acquired) N28.89
  - congenital Q63.2
- organ or site, congenital NEC — *see* Malposition, congenital

Missed
- abortion O02.1
- delivery O36.4 ☑

Missing — *see* Absence

Misuse of drugs F19.99

Mitchell's disease (erythromelalgia) I73.81

Mite (s) (infestation) B88.9
- diarrhea B88.0
- grain (itch) B88.0
- hair follicle (itch) B88.0
- in sputum B88.0

Mitral — *see* condition

Mittelschmerz N94.0

Mixed — *see* condition

MNGIE (Mitochondrial Neurogastrointestinal Encephalopathy) syndrome E88.49

Mobile, mobility
- cecum Q43.3
- excessive — *see* Hypermobility
- gallbladder, congenital Q44.1
- kidney N28.89
- organ or site, congenital NEC — *see* Malposition, congenital

Mobitz heart block (atrioventricular) I44.1

Moebius, Möbius
- disease (ophthalmoplegic migraine) — *see* Migraine, ophthalmoplegic
- syndrome Q87.0

Moebius — *continued*
- congenital oculofacial paralysis (with other anomalies) Q87.0
- ophthalmoplegic migraine — *see* Migraine, ophthalmoplegic

Moeller's glossitis K14.0

Mohr's syndrome (Types I and II) Q87.0

Mola destruens D39.2

Molar pregnancy O02.0

Molarization of premolars K00.2

Molding, head (during birth) - omit code

Mole (pigmented) (*see also* Nevus)
- blood O02.0
- Breus' O02.0
- cancerous — *see* Melanoma
- carneous O02.0
- destructive D39.2
- fleshy O02.0
- hydatid, hydatidiform (benign) (complicating pregnancy) (delivered) (undelivered) O01.9
  - classical O01.0
  - complete O01.0
  - incomplete O01.1
  - invasive D39.2
  - malignant D39.2
  - partial O01.1
- intrauterine O02.0
- invasive (hydatidiform) D39.2
- malignant
  - meaning
    - malignant hydatidiform mole D39.2
    - melanoma — *see* Melanoma
- nonhydatidiform — *see* Nevus
- nonpigmented — *see* Nevus
- pregnancy NEC O02.0
- skin — *see* Nevus
- tubal O00.1
- vesicular — *see* Mole, hydatidiform

Molimen, molimina (menstrual) N94.3

Molluscum contagiosum (epitheliale) B08.1

Mönckeberg's arteriosclerosis, disease, or sclerosis — *see* Arteriosclerosis, extremities

Mondini's malformation (cochlea) Q16.5

Mondor's disease I80.8

Monge's disease T70.29 ☑

Monilethrix (congenital) Q84.1

Moniliasis (*see also* Candidiasis) B37.9
- neonatal P37.5

Monitoring (encounter for)
- therapeutic drug level Z51.81

Monkey malaria B53.1

Monkeypox B04

Monoarthritis M13.10
- ankle M13.17- ☑
- elbow M13.12- ☑
- foot joint M13.17- ☑
- hand joint M13.14- ☑
- hip M13.15- ☑
- knee M13.16- ☑
- shoulder M13.11- ☑
- wrist M13.13- ☑

Monoblastic — *see* condition

Monochromat (ism), monochromatopsia (acquired) (congenital) H53.51

Monocytic — *see* condition

Monocytopenia D72.818

Monocytosis (symptomatic) D72.821

Monomania — *see* Psychosis

Mononeuritis G58.9
- cranial nerve — *see* Disorder, nerve, cranial
- femoral nerve G57.2- ☑
- lateral
  - cutaneous nerve of thigh G57.1- ☑
  - popliteal nerve G57.3- ☑
- lower limb G57.9- ☑
  - specified nerve NEC G57.8- ☑
- medial popliteal nerve G57.4- ☑
- median nerve G56.1- ☑
- multiplex G58.7
- plantar nerve G57.6- ☑
- posterior tibial nerve G57.5- ☑
- radial nerve G56.3- ☑
- sciatic nerve G57.0- ☑
- specified NEC G58.8
- tibial nerve G57.4- ☑
- ulnar nerve G56.2- ☑
- upper limb G56.9- ☑
  - specified nerve NEC G56.8- ☑
- vestibularH93.3

Mononeuropathy G58.9
- carpal tunnel syndrome — *see* Syndrome, carpal tunnel

Mononeuropathy — *continued*
- diabetic NEC — *see* E08-E13 with .41
- femoral nerve — *see* Lesion, nerve, femoral
- ilioinguinal nerve G57.8- ☑
- in diseases classified elsewhereG59
- intercostal G58.0
- lower limb G57.9- ☑
  - causalgia — *see* Causalgia, lower limb
  - femoral nerve — *see* Lesion, nerve, femoral
  - meralgia paresthetica G57.1- ☑
  - plantar nerve — *see* Lesion, nerve, plantar
  - popliteal nerve — *see* Lesion, nerve, popliteal
  - sciatic nerve — *see* Lesion, nerve, sciatic
  - specified NEC G57.8- ☑
  - tarsal tunnel syndrome — *see* Syndrome, tarsal tunnel
- median nerve — *see* Lesion, nerve, median
- multiplex G58.7
- obturator nerve G57.8- ☑
- popliteal nerve — *see* Lesion, nerve, popliteal
- radial nerve — *see* Lesion, nerve, radial
- saphenous nerve G57.8- ☑
- specified NEC G58.8
- tarsal tunnel syndrome — *see* Syndrome, tarsal tunnel
- tuberculous A17.83
- ulnar nerve — *see* Lesion, nerve, ulnar
- upper limb G56.9- ☑
  - carpal tunnel syndrome — *see* Syndrome, carpal tunnel
  - causalgia — *see* Causalgia
  - median nerve — *see* Lesion, nerve, median
  - radial nerve — *see* Lesion, nerve, radial
  - specified site NEC G56.8- ☑
  - ulnar nerve — *see* Lesion, nerve, ulnar

Mononucleosis, infectious B27.90
- with
  - complication NEC B27.99
  - meningitis B27.92
  - polyneuropathy B27.91
- cytomegaloviral B27.10
  - with
    - complication NEC B27.19
    - meningitis B27.12
    - polyneuropathy B27.11
- Epstein-Barr (virus) B27.00
  - with
    - complication NEC B27.09
    - meningitis B27.02
    - polyneuropathy B27.01
- gammaherpesviral B27.00
  - with
    - complication NEC B27.09
    - meningitis B27.02
    - polyneuropathy B27.01
- specified NEC B27.80
  - with
    - complication NEC B27.89
    - meningitis B27.82
    - polyneuropathy B27.81

Monoplegia G83.3- ☑
- congenital (cerebral) G80.8
  - spastic G80.1
- embolic (current episode) I63.4 ☑
- following
  - cerebrovascular disease
    - cerebral infarction
      - lower limb I69.34- ☑
      - upper limb I69.33- ☑
    - intracerebral hemorrhage
      - lower limb I69.14- ☑
      - upper limb I69.13- ☑
    - lower limb I69.94- ☑
    - nontraumatic intracranial hemorrhage NEC
      - lower limb I69.24- ☑
      - upper limb I69.23- ☑
    - specified disease NEC
      - lower limb I69.84- ☑
      - upper limb I69.83- ☑
    - stroke NOS
      - lower limb I69.34- ☑
      - upper limb I69.33- ☑
    - subarachnoid hemorrhage
      - lower limb I69.04- ☑
      - upper limb I69.03- ☑
    - upper limb I69.93- ☑
- hysterical (transient) F44.4
- lower limb G83.1- ☑
- psychogenic (conversion reaction) F44.4
- thrombotic (current episode) I63.3 ☑
- transient R29.818
- upper limb G83.2- ☑

☑ **Additional character required**

Monorchism, monorchidism Q55.0
Monosomy (see also Deletion, chromosome) Q93.9
  specified NEC Q93.89
  whole chromosome
    meiotic nondisjunction Q93.0
    mitotic nondisjunction Q93.1
    mosaicism Q93.1
    X Q96.9
Monster, monstrosity (single) Q89.7
  acephalic Q00.0
  twin Q89.4
Monteggia's fracture (-dislocation) S52.27- ☑
Mooren's ulcer (cornea) — see Ulcer, cornea, Mooren's
Moore's syndrome — see Epilepsy, specified NEC
Mooser-Neill reaction A75.2
Mooser's bodies A75.2
Morbidity not stated or unknown R69
Morbilli — see Measles
Morbus (see also Disease)
  angelicus, anglorum E55.0
  Beigel B36.2
  caducus — see Epilepsy
  celiacus K90.0
  comitialis — see Epilepsy
  cordis (see also Disease, heart) I51.9
    valvulorum — see Endocarditis
  coxae senilis M16.9
    tuberculous A18.02
  hemorrhagicus neonatorum P53
  maculosus neonatorum P54.5
Morel (-Stewart)(-Morgagni) syndrome M85.2
Morel-Kraepelin disease — see Schizophrenia
Morel-Moore syndrome M85.2
Morgagni's
  cyst, organ, hydatid, or appendage
    female Q50.5
    male (epididymal) Q55.4
      testicular Q55.29
  syndrome M85.2
Morgagni-Stokes-Adams syndrome I45.9
Morgagni-Stewart-Morel syndrome M85.2
Morgagni-Turner (-Albright) syndrome Q96.9
Moria F07.0
Moron (I.Q.50-69) F70
Morphea L94.0
Morphinism (without remission) F11.20
  with remission F11.21
Morphinomania (without remission) F11.20
  with remission F11.21
Morquio (-Ullrich)(-Brailsford) disease or syndrome — see Mucopolysaccharidosis
Mortification (dry) (moist) — see Gangrene
Morton's metatarsalgia (neuralgia)(neuroma) (syndrome) G57.6- ☑
Morvan's disease or syndrome G60.8
Mosaicism, mosaic (autosomal) (chromosomal)
  45,X/other cell lines NEC with abnormal sex chromosome Q96.4
  45,X/46,XX Q96.3
  sex chromosome
    female Q97.8
    lines with various numbers of X chromosomes Q97.2
    male Q98.7
    XY Q96.3
Moschowitz' disease M31.1
Mother yaw A66.0
Motion sickness (from travel, any vehicle) (from roundabouts or swings) T75.3 ☑
Mottled, mottling, teeth (enamel) (endemic) (nonendemic) K00.3
Mounier-Kuhn syndrome Q32.4
  with bronchiectasis J47.9
    exacerbation (acute) J47.1
    lower respiratory infection J47.0
  acquired J98.09
    with bronchiectasis J47.9
      with
        exacerbation (acute) J47.1
        lower respiratory infection J47.0
Mountain
  sickness T70.29 ☑
    with polycythemia , acquired (acute) D75.1
  tick fever A93.2
Mouse, joint — see Loose, body, joint
  knee M23.4- ☑
Mouth — see condition
Movable
  coccyx M53.2
  kidney N28.89
    congenital Q63.8

Movable — continued
  spleen D73.89
Movements, dystonic R25.8
Moyamoya disease I67.5
MRSA (Methicillin resistant Staphylococcus aureus)
  infection A49.02
    as the cause of diseases classified elsewhere B95.62
  sepsis A41.02
MSSA (Methicillin susceptible Staphylococcus aureus)
  infection A49.01
    as the cause of diseases classified elsewhere B95.61
  sepsis A41.01
Mucha-Habermann disease L41.0
Mucinosis (cutaneous) (focal) (papular) (reticular erythematous) (skin) L98.5
  oral K13.79
Mucocele
  appendix K38.8
  buccal cavity K13.79
  gallbladder K82.1
  lacrimal sac, chronic H04.43- ☑
  nasal sinus J34.1
  nose J34.1
  salivary gland (any) K11.6
  sinus (accessory) (nasal) J34.1
  turbinate (bone) (middle) (nasal) J34.1
  uterus N85.8
Mucolipidosis
  I E77.1
  II, III E77.0
  IV E75.11
Mucopolysaccharidosis E76.3
  beta-gluduronidase deficiency E76.29
  cardiopathy E76.3 [I52]
  Hunter's syndrome E76.1
  Hurler's syndrome E76.01
  Hurler-Scheie syndrome E76.02
  Maroteaux-Lamy syndrome E76.29
  Morquio syndrome E76.219
    A E76.210
    B E76.211
    classic E76.210
  Sanfilippo syndrome E76.22
  Scheie's syndrome E76.03
  specified NEC E76.29
  type
    I
      Hurler's syndrome E76.01
      Hurler-Scheie syndrome E76.02
      Scheie's syndrome E76.03
    II E76.1
    III E76.22
    IV E76.219
    IVA E76.210
    IVB E76.211
    VI E76.29
    VII E76.29
Mucormycosis B46.5
  cutaneous B46.3
  disseminated B46.4
  gastrointestinal B46.2
  generalized B46.4
  pulmonary B46.0
  rhinocerebral B46.1
  skin B46.3
  subcutaneous B46.3
Mucositis (ulcerative) K12.30
  due to drugs NEC K12.32
  gastrointestinal K92.81
  mouth (oral) (oropharyngeal) K12.30
    due to antineoplastic therapy K12.31
    due to drugs NEC K12.32
    due to radiation K12.33
    specified NEC K12.39
    viral K12.39
  nasal J34.81
  oral cavity — see Mucositis, mouth
  oral soft tissues — see Mucositis, mouth
  vagina and vulva N76.81
Mucositis necroticans agranulocytica — see Agranulocytosis
Mucous (see also condition)
  patches (syphilitic) A51.39
    congenital A50.07
Mucoviscidosis E84.9
  with meconium obstruction E84.11
Mucus
  asphyxia or suffocation — see Asphyxia, mucus
  in stool R19.5

Mucus — continued
  plug — see Asphyxia, mucus
Muguet B37.0
Mulberry molars (congenital syphilis) A50.52
Müllerian mixed tumor
  specified site — see Neoplasm, malignant, by site
  unspecified site C54.9
Multicystic kidney (development) Q61.4
Multiparity (grand) Z64.1
  affecting management of pregnancy, labor and delivery (supervision only) O09.4- ☑
  requiring contraceptive management — see Contraception
Multipartita placenta O43.19- ☑
Multiple, multiplex (see also condition)
  digits (congenital) Q69.9
  endocrine neoplasia — see Neoplasia, endocrine, multiple (MEN)
  personality F44.81
Mumps B26.9
  arthritis B26.85
  complication NEC B26.89
  encephalitis B26.2
  hepatitis B26.81
  meningitis (aseptic) B26.1
  meningoencephalitis B26.2
  myocarditis B26.82
  oophoritis B26.89
  orchitis B26.0
  pancreatitis B26.3
  polyneuropathy B26.84
Mumu (see also Infestation, filarial) B74.9 [N51]
Münchhausen's syndrome — see Disorder, factitious
Münchmeyer's syndrome — see Myositis, ossificans, progressiva
Mural — see condition
Murmur (cardiac) (heart) (organic) R01.1
  abdominal R19.15
  aortic (valve) — see Endocarditis, aortic
  benign R01.0
  diastolic — see Endocarditis
  Flint I35.1
  functional R01.0
  Graham Steell I37.1
  innocent R01.0
  mitral (valve) — see Insufficiency, mitral
  nonorganic R01.0
  presystolic, mitral — see Insufficiency, mitral
  pulmonic (valve) I37.8
  systolic (valvular) — see Endocarditis
  tricuspid (valve) I07.9
  valvular — see Endocarditis
Murri's disease (intermittent hemoglobinuria) D59.6
Muscle, muscular (see also condition)
  carnitine (palmityltransferase) deficiency E71.314
Musculoneuralgia — see Neuralgia
Mushroom-workers' (pickers') disease or lung J67.5
Mushrooming hip — see Derangement, joint, specified NEC, hip
Mutation (s)
  factor V Leiden D68.51
  surfactant, of lung J84.83
  prothrombin gene D68.52
Mutism (see also Aphasia)
  deaf (acquired) (congenital) NEC H91.3
  elective (adjustment reaction) (childhood) F94.0
  hysterical F44.4
  selective (childhood) F94.0
MVD (microvillus inclusion disease) Q43.8
MVID (microvillus inclusion disease) Q43.8
Myalgia M79.1
  epidemic (cervical) B33.0
  traumatic NEC T14.8
Myasthenia G70.9
  congenital G70.2
  cordis — see Failure, heart
  developmental G70.2
  gravis G70.00
    with exacerbation (acute) G70.01
    in crisis G70.01
    neonatal, transient P94.0
    pseudoparalytica G70.00
      with exacerbation (acute) G70.01
      in crisis G70.01
  stomach, psychogenic F45.8
  syndrome
    in
      diabetes mellitus — see E08-E13 with .44
      neoplastic disease (see also Neoplasm) D49.9 [G73.3]
      pernicious anemia D51.0 [G73.3]
      thyrotoxicosis E05.90 [G73.3]

Myasthenia - Myocarditis

Myasthenia — *continued*
  with thyroid storm E05.91 [G73.3]
Myasthenic M62.81
Mycelium infection B49
Mycetismus — *see* Poisoning, food, noxious, mushroom
Mycetoma B47.9
  actinomycotic B47.1
  bone (mycotic) B47.9 [M90.80]
  eumycotic B47.0
  foot B47.9
    actinomycotic B47.1
    mycotic B47.0
  madurae NEC B47.9
    mycotic B47.0
  maduromycotic B47.0
  mycotic B47.0
  nocardial B47.1
Mycobacteriosis — *see* Mycobacterium
Mycobacterium, mycobacterial (infection) A31.9
  anonymous A31.9
  atypical A31.9
    cutaneous A31.1
    pulmonary A31.0
      tuberculous — *see* Tuberculosis, pulmonary
    specified site NEC A31.8
  avium (intracellulare complex) A31.0
  balnei A31.1
  Battey A31.0
  chelonei A31.8
  cutaneous A31.1
  extrapulmonary systemic A31.8
  fortuitum A31.8
  intracellulare (Battey bacillus) A31.0
  kansasii (yellow bacillus) A31.0
  kakaferifu A31.8
  kasongo A31.8
  leprae (*see also* Leprosy) A30.9
  luciflavum A31.1
  marinum (M. balnei) A31.1
  nonspecific — *see* Mycobacterium, atypical
  pulmonary (atypical) A31.0
    tuberculous — *see* Tuberculosis, pulmonary
  scrofulaceum A31.8
  simiae A31.8
  systemic, extrapulmonary A31.8
  szulgai A31.8
  terrae A31.8
  triviale A31.8
  tuberculosis (human, bovine) - see Tuberculosis
  ulcerans A31.1
  xenopi A31.8
Mycoplasma (M.) pneumoniae, as cause of disease classified elsewhere B96.0
Mycosis, mycotic B49
  cutaneous NEC B36.9
  ear B36.8
  fungoides (extranodal) (solid organ) C84.0- ☑
  mouth B37.0
  nails B35.1
  opportunistic B48.8
  skin NEC B36.9
  specified NEC B48.8
  stomatitis B37.0
  vagina, vaginitis (candidal) B37.3
Mydriasis (pupil) H57.04
Myelatelia Q06.1
Myelinolysis, pontine, central G37.2
Myelitis (acute) (ascending) (childhood) (chronic) (descending) (diffuse) (disseminated) (idiopathic) (pressure) (progressive) (spinal cord) (subacute) (*see also* Encephalitis) G04.91
  herpes simplex B00.82
  herpes zoster B02.24
  in diseases classified elsewhere G05.4
  necrotizing, subacute G37.4
  optic neuritis in G36.0
  postchickenpox B01.12
  postherpetic B02.24
  postimmunization G04.02
  postinfectious NEC G04.89
  postvaccinal G04.02
  specified NEC G04.89
  syphilitic (transverse) A52.14
  toxic G92
  transverse (in demyelinating diseases of central nervous system) G37.3
  tuberculous A17.82
  varicella B01.12
Myeloblastic — *see* condition
Myeloblastoma
  granular cell (*see also* Neoplasm, connective tissue)

Myeloblastoma — *continued*
  malignant — *see* Neoplasm, connective tissue, malignant
  tongue D10.1
Myelocele — *see* Spina bifida
Myelocystocele — *see* Spina bifida
Myelocytic — *see* condition
Myelodysplasia D46.9
  specified NEC D46.Z
  spinal cord (congenital) Q06.1
Myelodysplastic syndrome D46.9
  with
    5q deletion D46.C
    isolated del (5q) chromosomal abnormality D46.C
  specified NEC D46.Z
Myeloencephalitis — *see* Encephalitis
Myelofibrosis D75.81
  with myeloid metaplasia D47.4
  acute C94.4- ☑
  idiopathic (chronic) D47.4
  primary D47.1
  secondary D75.81
    in myeloproliferative disease D47.4
Myelogenous — *see* condition
Myeloid — *see* condition
Myelokathexis D70.9
Myeloleukodystrophy E75.29
Myelolipoma — *see* Lipoma
Myeloma (multiple) C90.0- ☑
  monostotic C90.3 ☑
    plasma cell C90.0- ☑
  plasma cell C90.0- ☑
  solitary (*see also* Plasmacytoma, solitary) C90.3- ☑
Myelomalacia G95.89
Myelomatosis C90.0- ☑
Myelomeningitis — *see* Meningoencephalitis
Myelomeningocele (spinal cord) — *see* Spina bifida
Myelo-osteo-musculodysplasia hereditaria Q79.8
Myelopathic
  anemia D64.89
  muscle atrophy — *see* Atrophy, muscle, spinal
  pain syndrome G89.0
Myelopathy (spinal cord) G95.9
  drug-induced G95.89
  in (due to)
    degeneration or displacement, intervertebral disc NEC — *see* Disorder, disc, with, myelopathy
    infection — *see* Encephalitis
    intervertebral disc disorder (*see also* Disorder, disc, with, myelopathy)
    mercury T56.1
    neoplastic disease (*see also* Neoplasm) D49.9 [G99.2]
    pernicious anemia D51.0 [G99.2]
    spondylosis — *see* Spondylosis, with myelopathy NEC
  necrotic (subacute) (vascular) G95.19
  radiation-induced G95.89
  spondylogenic NEC — *see* Spondylosis, with myelopathy NEC
  toxic G95.89
  transverse, acute G37.3
  vascular G95.19
  vitamin B12 E53.8 [G32.0]
Myelophthisis D61.82
Myeloradiculitis G04.91
Myeloradiculodysplasia (spinal) Q06.1
Myelosarcoma C92.3- ☑
Myelosclerosis D75.89
  with myeloid metaplasia D47.4
  disseminated, of nervous system G35
  megakaryocytic D47.4
    with myeloid metaplasia D47.4
Myelosis
  acute C92.0- ☑
  aleukemic C92.9- ☑
  chronic D47.1
  erythremic (acute) C94.0- ☑
  megakaryocytic C94.2- ☑
  nonleukemic D72.828
  subacute C92.9- ☑
Myiasis (cavernous) B87.9
  aural B87.4
  creeping B87.0
  cutaneous B87.0
  dermal B87.0
  ear (external) (middle) B87.4
  eye B87.2
  genitourinary B87.81

Myiasis — *continued*
  intestinal B87.82
  laryngeal B87.3
  nasopharyngeal B87.3
  ocular B87.2
  orbit B87.2
  skin B87.0
  specified site NEC B87.89
  traumatic B87.1
  wound B87.1
Myoadenoma, prostate — *see* Hyperplasia, prostate
Myoblastoma
  granular cell (*see also* Neoplasm, connective tissue, benign)
    malignant — *see* Neoplasm, connective tissue, malignant
  tongue D10.1
Myocardial — *see* condition
Myocardiopathy (congestive) (constrictive) (familial) (hypertrophic nonobstructive) (idiopathic) (infiltrative) (obstructive) (primary) (restrictive) (sporadic) (*see also* Cardiomyopathy) I42.9
  alcoholic I42.6
  cobalt-beer I42.6
  glycogen storage E74.02 [I43]
  hypertrophic obstructive I42.1
  in (due to)
    beriberi E51.12
    cardiac glycogenosis E74.02 [I43]
    Friedreich's ataxia G11.1 [I43]
    myotonia atrophica G71.11 [I43]
    progressive muscular dystrophy G71.0 [I43]
  obscure (African) I42.8
  secondary I42.9
  thyrotoxic E05.90 [I43]
    with storm E05.91 [I43]
  toxic NEC I42.7
Myocarditis (with arteriosclerosis)(chronic)(fibroid) (interstitial) (old) (progressive) (senile) I51.4
  with
    rheumatic fever (conditions in I00) I09.0
      active — *see* Myocarditis, acute, rheumatic
      inactive or quiescent (with chorea) I09.0
  active I40.9
    rheumatic I01.2
      with chorea (acute) (rheumatic) (Sydenham's) I02.0
  acute or subacute (interstitial) I40.9
    due to
      streptococcus (beta-hemolytic) I01.2
    idiopathic I40.1
    rheumatic I01.2
      with chorea (acute) (rheumatic) (Sydenham's) I02.0
    specified NEC I40.8
  aseptic of newborn B33.22
  bacterial (acute) I40.0
  Coxsackie (virus) B33.22
  diphtheritic A36.81
  eosinophilic I40.1
  epidemic of newborn (Coxsackie) B33.22
  Fiedler's (acute) (isolated) I40.1
  giant cell (acute) (subacute) I40.1
  gonococcal A54.83
  granulomatous (idiopathic) (isolated) (nonspecific) I40.1
  hypertensive — *see* Hypertension, heart
  idiopathic (granulomatous) I40.1
  in (due to)
    diphtheria A36.81
    epidemic louse-borne typhus A75.0 [I41]
    Lyme disease A69.29
    sarcoidosis D86.85
    scarlet fever A38.1
    toxoplasmosis (acquired) B58.81
    typhoid A01.02
    typhus NEC A75.9 [I41]
  infective I40.0
  influenzal — *see* Influenza, with, myocarditis
  isolated (acute) I40.1
  meningococcal A39.52
  mumps B26.82
  nonrheumatic, active I40.9
  parenchymatous I40.9
  pneumococcal I40.0
  rheumatic (chronic) (inactive) (with chorea) I09.0
    active or acute I01.2
      with chorea (acute) (rheumatic) (Sydenham's) I02.0
  rheumatoid — *see* Rheumatoid, carditis
  septic I40.0
  staphylococcal I40.0

☑ **Additional character required**

Myocarditis — *continued*
  suppurative I40.0
  syphilitic (chronic) A52.06
  toxic I40.8
    rheumatic — *see* Myocarditis, acute, rheumatic
  tuberculous A18.84
  typhoid A01.02
  valvular — *see* Endocarditis
  virus, viral I40.0
    of newborn (Coxsackie) B33.22
Myocardium, myocardial — *see* condition
Myocardosis — *see* Cardiomyopathy
Myoclonus, myoclonic, myoclonia (familial)
  (essential) (multifocal) (simplex) G25.3
    drug-induced G25.3
    epilepsy (*see also* Epilepsy, generalized, specified
      NEC) G40.4- ☑
      familial (progressive) G25.3
    epileptica G40.409
      with status epilepticus G40.401
    facial G51.3
    familial progressive G25.3
    Friedreich's G25.3
    jerks G25.3
    massive G25.3
    palatal G25.3
    pharyngeal G25.3
Myocytolysis I51.5
Myodiastasis — *see* Diastasis, muscle
Myoendocarditis — *see* Endocarditis
Myoepithelioma — *see* Neoplasm, benign, by site
Myofasciitis (acute) — *see* Myositis
Myofibroma (*see also* Neoplasm, connective tissue,
  benign)
    uterus (cervix) (corpus) — *see* Leiomyoma
Myofibromatosis D48.1
  infantile Q89.8
Myofibrosis M62.89
  heart — *see* Myocarditis
  scapulohumeral — *see* Lesion, shoulder, specified
    NEC
Myofibrositis M79.7
  scapulohumeral — *see* Lesion, shoulder, specified
    NEC
Myoglobulinuria, myoglobinuria (primary) R82.1
Myokymia, facial G51.4
Myolipoma — *see* Lipoma
Myoma (*see also* Neoplasm, connective tissue,
  benign)
    malignant — *see* Neoplasm, connective tissue,
      malignant
    prostate D29.1
    uterus (cervix) (corpus) — *see* Leiomyoma
Myomalacia M62.89
Myometritis — *see* Endometritis
Myometrium — *see* condition
Myonecrosis, clostridial A48.0
Myopathy G72.9
  acute
    necrotizing G72.81
    quadriplegic G72.81
  alcoholic G72.1
  benign congenital G71.2
  central core G71.2
  centronuclear G71.2
  congenital (benign) G71.2
  critical illness G72.81
  distal G71.0
  drug-induced G72.0
  endocrine NEC E34.9 [G73.7]
  extraocular muscles H05.82- ☑
  facioscapulohumeral G71.0
  hereditary G71.9
    specified NEC G71.8
  immune NEC G72.49
  in (due to)
    Addison's disease E27.1 [G73.7]
    alcohol G72.1
    amyloidosis E85.0 [G73.7]
    cretinism E00.9 [G73.7]
    Cushing's syndrome E24.9 [G73.7]
    drugs G72.0
    endocrine disease NEC E34.9 [G73.7]
    giant cell arteritis M31.6 [G73.7]
    glycogen storage disease E74.00 [G73.7]
    hyperadrenocorticism E24.9 [G73.7]
    hyperparathyroidism NEC E21.3 [G73.7]
    hypoparathyroidism E20.9 [G73.7]
    hypopituitarism E23.0 [G73.7]
    hypothyroidism E03.9 [G73.7]
    infectious disease NEC B99 ☑ [G73.7]
    lipid storage disease E75.6 [G73.7]

Myopathy — *continued*
  metabolic disease NEC E88.9 [G73.7]
  myxedema E03.9 [G73.7]
  parasitic disease NEC B89 [G73.7]
  polyarteritis nodosa M30.0 [G73.7]
  rheumatoid arthritis — *see* Rheumatoid,
    myopathy
  sarcoidosis D86.87
  scleroderma M34.82
  sicca syndrome M35.03
  Sjögren's syndrome M35.03
  systemic lupus erythematosus M32.19
  thyrotoxicosis (hyperthyroidism) E05.90 [G73.7]
    with thyroid storm E05.91 [G73.7]
  toxic agent NEC G72.2
inflammatory NEC G72.49
intensive care (ICU) G72.81
limb-girdle G71.0
mitochondrial NEC G71.3
myotonic, proximal (PROMM) G71.11
myotubular G71.2
nemaline G71.2
ocular G71.0
oculopharyngeal G71.0
of critical illness G72.81
primary G71.9
  specified NEC G71.8
progressive NEC G72.89
proximal myotonic (PROMM) G71.11
rod G71.2
scapulohumeral G71.0
specified NEC G72.89
toxic G72.2
Myopericarditis (*see also* Pericarditis)
  chronic rheumatic I09.2
Myopia (axial) (congenital) H52.1- ☑
  degenerative (malignant) H44.2- ☑
  malignant H44.2- ☑
  pernicious H44.2- ☑
  progressive high (degenerative) H44.2- ☑
Myosarcoma — *see* Neoplasm, connective tissue,
  malignant
Myosis (pupil) H57.03
  stromal (endolymphatic) D39.0
Myositis M60.9
  clostridial A48.0
  due to posture — *see* Myositis, specified type NEC
  epidemic B33.0
  fibrosa or fibrous (chronic), Volkmann's T79.6 ☑
  foreign body granuloma — *see* Granuloma,
    foreign body
  in (due to)
    bilharziasis B65.9 [M63.8- ☑]
    cysticercosis B69.81
    leprosy A30.9 [M63.8- ☑]
    mycosis B49 [M63.8- ☑]
    sarcoidosis D86.87
    schistosomiasis B65.9 [M63.8- ☑]
    syphilis
      late A52.78
      secondary A51.49
    toxoplasmosis (acquired) B58.82
    trichinellosis B75 [M63.8- ☑]
    tuberculosis A18.09
  inclusion body [IBM] G72.41
  infective M60.009
    arm M60.002
      left M60.001
      right M60.000
    leg M60.005
      left M60.004
      right M60.003
    lower limb M60.005
      ankle M60.07- ☑
      foot M60.07- ☑
      lower leg M60.06- ☑
      thigh M60.05- ☑
      toe M60.07- ☑
    multiple sites M60.09
    specified site NEC M60.08
    upper limb M60.002
      finger M60.04- ☑
      forearm M60.03- ☑
      hand M60.04- ☑
      shoulder region M60.01- ☑
      upper arm M60.02- ☑
  interstitial M60.10
    ankle M60.17- ☑
    foot M60.17- ☑
    forearm M60.13- ☑
    hand M60.14- ☑
    lower leg M60.16- ☑

Myositis — *continued*
    multiple sites M60.19
    shoulder region M60.11- ☑
    specified site NEC M60.18
    thigh M60.15- ☑
    upper arm M60.12- ☑
  mycotic B49 [M63.8- ☑]
  orbital, chronic H05.12- ☑
  ossificans or ossifying (circumscripta) (*see also*
    Ossification, muscle, specified NEC)
    in (due to)
      burns M61.30
        ankle M61.37- ☑
        foot M61.37- ☑
        forearm M61.33- ☑
        hand M61.34- ☑
        lower leg M61.36- ☑
        multiple sites M61.39
        pelvic region M61.35- ☑
        shoulder region M61.31- ☑
        specified site NEC M61.38
        thigh M61.35- ☑
        upper arm M61.32- ☑
      quadriplegia or paraplegia M61.20
        ankle M61.27- ☑
        foot M61.27- ☑
        forearm M61.23- ☑
        hand M61.24- ☑
        lower leg M61.26- ☑
        multiple sites M61.29
        pelvic region M61.25- ☑
        shoulder region M61.21- ☑
        specified site NEC M61.28
        thigh M61.25- ☑
        upper arm M61.22- ☑
    progressiva M61.10
      ankle M61.17- ☑
      finger M61.14- ☑
      foot M61.17- ☑
      forearm M61.13- ☑
      hand M61.14- ☑
      lower leg M61.16- ☑
      multiple sites M61.19
      pelvic region M61.15- ☑
      shoulder region M61.11- ☑
      specified site NEC M61.18
      thigh M61.15- ☑
      toe M61.17- ☑
      upper arm M61.12- ☑
    traumatica M61.00
      ankle M61.07- ☑
      foot M61.07- ☑
      forearm M61.03- ☑
      hand M61.04- ☑
      lower leg M61.06- ☑
      multiple sites M61.09
      pelvic region M61.05- ☑
      shoulder region M61.01- ☑
      specified site NEC M61.08
      thigh M61.05- ☑
      upper arm M61.02- ☑
  purulent — *see* Myositis, infective
  specified type NEC M60.80
    ankle M60.87- ☑
    foot M60.87- ☑
    forearm M60.83- ☑
    hand M60.84- ☑
    lower leg M60.86- ☑
    multiple sites M60.89
    pelvic region M60.85- ☑
    shoulder region M60.81- ☑
    specified site NEC M60.88
    thigh M60.85- ☑
    upper arm M60.82- ☑
  suppurative — *see* Myositis, infective
  traumatic (old) — *see* Myositis, specified type NEC
Myospasia impulsiva F95.2
Myotonia (acquisita) (intermittens) M62.89
  atrophica G71.11
  chondrodystrophic G71.13
  congenita (acetazolamide responsive)
    (dominant) (recessive) G71.12
  drug-induced G71.14
  dystrophica G71.11
  fluctuans G71.19
  levior G71.12
  permanens G71.19
  symptomatic G71.19
Myotonic pupil — *see* Anomaly, pupil, function,
  tonic pupil
Myriapodiasis B88.2

Myringitis H73.2- ☑
  with otitis media — *see* Otitis, media
  acute H73.00- ☑
    bullous H73.01- ☑
    specified NEC H73.09- ☑
  bullous — *see* Myringitis, acute, bullous
  chronic H73.1- ☑
Mysophobia F40.228
Mytilotoxism — *see* Poisoning, fish
Myxadenitis labialis K13.0
Myxedema (adult) (idiocy) (infantile) (*see also* Hypothyroidism) E03.9
  circumscribed E05.90
    with storm E05.91
  coma E03.5
  congenital E00.1
  cutis L98.5
  localized (pretibial) E05.90
    with storm E05.91
  papular L98.5
Myxochondrosarcoma — *see* Neoplasm, cartilage, malignant
Myxofibroma — *see* Neoplasm, connective tissue, benign
  odontogenic — *see* Cyst, calcifying odontogenic
Myxofibrosarcoma — *see* Neoplasm, connective tissue, malignant
Myxolipoma D17.9
Myxoliposarcoma — *see* Neoplasm, connective tissue, malignant
Myxoma (*see also* Neoplasm, connective tissue, benign)
  nerve sheath — *see* Neoplasm, nerve, benign
  odontogenic — *see* Cyst, calcifying odontogenic
Myxosarcoma — *see* Neoplasm, connective tissue, malignant

N

Naegeli's
  disease Q82.8
  leukemia, monocytic C93.1- ☑
Naegleriasis (with meningoencephalitis) B60.2
Naffziger's syndrome G54.0
Naga sore — *see* Ulcer, skin
Nägele's pelvis M95.5
  with disproportion (fetopelvic) O33.0
    causing obstructed labor O65.0
Nail (*see also* condition)
  biting F98.8
  patella syndrome Q87.2
Nanism, nanosomia — *see* Dwarfism
Nanophyetiasis B66.8
Nanukayami A27.89
Napkin rash L22
Narcolepsy G47.419
  with cataplexy G47.411
  in conditions classified elsewhere G47.429
    with cataplexy G47.421
Narcosis R06.89
Narcotism — *see* Dependence
NARP (Neuropathy, Ataxia and Retinitis pigmentosa) syndrome E88.49
Narrow
  anterior chamber angle H40.03- ☑
  pelvis — *see* Contraction, pelvis
Narrowing (*see also* Stenosis)
  artery I77.1
    auditory, internal I65.8
    basilar — *see* Occlusion, artery, basilar
    carotid — *see* Occlusion, artery, carotid
    cerebellar — *see* Occlusion, artery, cerebellar
    cerebral — *see* Occlusion artery, cerebral
    choroidal — *see* Occlusion, artery, cerebral, specified NEC
    communicating posterior — *see* Occlusion, artery, cerebral, specified NEC
    coronary (*see also* Disease, heart, ischemic, atherosclerotic)
      congenital Q24.5
        syphilitic A50.54 [I52]
      due to syphilis NEC A52.06
    hypophyseal — *see* Occlusion, artery, cerebral, specified NEC
    pontine — *see* Occlusion, artery, cerebral, specified NEC
    precerebral — *see* Occlusion, artery, precerebral
    vertebral — *see* Occlusion, artery, vertebral

Narrowing — *continued*
  auditory canal (external) — *see* Stenosis, external ear canal
  eustachian tube — *see* Obstruction, eustachian tube
  eyelid — *see* Disorder, eyelid function
  larynx J38.6
  mesenteric artery K55.0
  palate M26.89
  palpebral fissure — *see* Disorder, eyelid function
  ureter N13.5
    with infection N13.6
  urethra — *see* Stricture, urethra
Narrowness, abnormal, eyelid Q10.3
Nasal — *see* condition
Nasolachrymal, nasolacrimal — *see* condition
Nasopharyngeal (*see also* condition)
  pituitary gland Q89.2
  torticollis M43.6
Nasopharyngitis (acute) (infective) (streptococcal) (subacute) J00
  chronic (suppurative) (ulcerative) J31.1
Nasopharynx, nasopharyngeal — *see* condition
Natal tooth, teeth K00.6
Nausea (without vomiting) R11.0
  with vomiting R11.2
  gravidarum — *see* Hyperemesis, gravidarum
  marina T75.3 ☑
  navalis T75.3 ☑
Navel — *see* condition
Neapolitan fever — *see* Brucellosis
Near drowning T75.1 ☑
Nearsightedness — *see* Myopia
Near-syncope R55
Nebula, cornea — *see* Opacity, cornea
Necator americanus infestation B76.1
Necatoriasis B76.1
Neck — *see* condition
Necrobiosis R68.89
  lipoidica NEC L92.1
    with diabetes — *see* E08-E13 with .620
Necrolysis, toxic epidermal L51.2
  due to drug
    correct substance properly administered — *see* Table of Drugs and Chemicals, by drug, adverse effect
    overdose or wrong substance given or taken — *see* Table of Drugs and Chemicals, by drug, poisoning
Necrophilia F65.89
Necrosis, necrotic (ischemic) (*see also* Gangrene)
  adrenal (capsule) (gland) E27.49
  amputation stump (surgical) (late) T87.50
    arm T87.5- ☑
    leg T87.5- ☑
  antrum J32.0
  aorta (hyaline) (*see also* Aneurysm, aorta)
    cystic medial — *see* Dissection, aorta
  artery I77.5
  bladder (aseptic) (sphincter) N32.89
  bone (*see also* Osteonecrosis) M87.9
    aseptic or avascular — *see* Osteonecrosis
      idiopathic M87.00
    ethmoid J32.2
    jaw M27.2
    tuberculous — *see* Tuberculosis, bone
  brain I67.89
  breast (aseptic) (fat) (segmental) N64.1
  bronchus J98.09
  central nervous system NEC I67.89
  cerebellar I67.89
  cerebral I67.89
  colon K55.0
  cornea H18.40
  cortical (acute) (renal) N17.1
  cystic medial (aorta) — *see* Dissection, aorta
  dental pulp K04.1
  esophagus K22.8
  ethmoid (bone) J32.2
  eyelid — *see* Disorder, eyelid, degenerative
  fat, fatty (generalized) (*see also* Disorder, soft tissue, specified type NEC)
    abdominal wall K65.4
    breast (aseptic) (segmental) N64.1
    localized — *see* Degeneration, by site, fatty
    mesentery K65.4
    omentum K65.4
    pancreas K86.8
    peritoneum K65.4
  skin (subcutaneous), newborn P83.0
  subcutaneous, due to birth injury P15.6
  gallbladder — *see* Cholecystitis, acute

Necrosis — *continued*
  heart — *see* Infarct, myocardium
  hip, aseptic or avascular — *see* Osteonecrosis, by type, femur
  intestine (acute) (hemorrhagic) (massive) K55.0
  jaw M27.2
  kidney (bilateral) N28.0
    acute N17.9
    cortical (acute) (bilateral) N17.1
      with ectopic or molar pregnancy O08.4
    medullary (bilateral) (in acute renal failure) (papillary) N17.2
    papillary (bilateral) (in acute renal failure) N17.2
    tubular N17.0
      with ectopic or molar pregnancy O08.4
      complicating
        abortion — *see* Abortion, by type, complicated by, tubular necrosis
        ectopic or molar pregnancy O08.4
        pregnancy — *see* Pregnancy, complicated by, diseases of, specified type or system NEC
      following ectopic or molar pregnancy O08.4
      traumatic T79.5 ☑
  larynx J38.7
  liver (with hepatic failure) (cell) — *see* Failure, hepatic
    hemorrhagic, central K76.2
  lung J85.0
  lymphatic gland — *see* Lymphadenitis, acute
  mammary gland (fat) (segmental) N64.1
  mastoid (chronic) — *see* Mastoiditis, chronic
  medullary (acute) (renal) N17.2
  mesentery K55.0
    fat K65.4
  mitral valve — *see* Insufficiency, mitral
  myocardium, myocardial — *see* Infarct, myocardium
  nose J34.0
  omentum (with mesenteric infarction) K55.0
    fat K65.4
  orbit, orbital — *see* Osteomyelitis, orbit
  ossicles, ear — *see* Abnormal, ear ossicles
  ovary N70.92
  pancreas (aseptic) (duct) (fat) K86.8
    acute (infective) — *see* Pancreatitis, acute
    infective — *see* Pancreatitis, acute
  papillary (acute) (renal) N17.2
  perineum N90.89
  peritoneum (with mesenteric infarction) K55.0
    fat K65.4
  pharynx J02.9
    in granulocytopenia — *see* Neutropenia
    Vincent's A69.1
  phosphorus T54.2
  pituitary (gland) (postpartum) (Sheehan) E23.0
  pressure — *see* Ulcer, pressure, by site
  pulmonary J85.0
  pulp (dental) K04.1
  radiation — *see* Necrosis, by site
  radium — *see* Necrosis, by site
  renal — *see* Necrosis, kidney
  sclera H15.89
  scrotum N50.8
  skin or subcutaneous tissue NEC I96
  spine, spinal (column) (*see also* Osteonecrosis, by type, vertebra)
    cord G95.19
  spleen D73.5
  stomach K31.89
  stomatitis (ulcerative) A69.0
  subcutaneous fat, newborn P83.8
  subendocardial (acute) I21.4
    chronic I25.89
  suprarenal (capsule) (gland) E27.49
  testis N50.8
  thymus (gland) E32.8
  tonsil J35.8
  trachea J39.8
  tuberculous NEC — *see* Tuberculosis
  tubular (acute) (anoxic) (renal) (toxic) N17.0
    postprocedural N99.0
  vagina N89.8
  vertebra (*see also* Osteonecrosis, by type, vertebra)
    tuberculous A18.01
  vulva N90.89
  X-ray — *see* Necrosis, by site
Necrospermia — *see* Infertility, male
Need (for)
  care provider because (of)
    assistance with personal care Z74.1

☑ **Additional character required**

Need — *continued*
- continuous supervision required Z74.3
- impaired mobility Z74.09
- no other household member able to render care Z74.2
- specified reason NEC Z74.8
- immunization — *see* Vaccination
- vaccination — *see* Vaccination

Neglect
- adult
  - confirmed T74.01 ☑
  - history of Z91.412
  - suspected T76.01 ☑
- child (childhood)
  - confirmed T74.02 ☑
  - history of Z62.812
  - suspected T76.02 ☑
- emotional, in childhood Z62.898
- hemispatial R41.4
- left-sided R41.4
- sensory R41.4
- visuospatial R41.4

Neisserian infection NEC — *see* Gonococcus
Nelaton's syndrome G60.8
Nelson's syndrome E24.1
Nematodiasis (intestinal) B82.0
- Ancylostoma B76.0

Neonatal (*see also* Newborn)
- acne L70.4
- bradycardia P29.12
- tachycardia P29.11
- screening, abnormal findings on P09
- tooth, teeth K00.6

Neonatorum — *see* condition
Neoplasia
- endocrine, multiple (MEN) E31.20
  - type I E31.21
  - type IIA E31.22
  - type IIB E31.23
- intraepithelial (histologically confirmed)
  - anal (AIN) (histologically confirmed) K62.82
    - grade I K62.82
    - grade II K62.82
    - severe D01.3
  - cervical glandular (histologically confirmed) D06.9
  - cervix (uteri) (CIN) (histologically confirmed) N87.9
    - glandular D06.9
    - grade I N87.0
    - grade II N87.1
    - grade III (severe dysplasia) (*see also* Carcinoma, cervix uteri, in situ) D06.9
  - prostate (histologically confirmed) (PIN I) (PIN II) N42.3
    - grade I N42.3
    - grade II N42.3
    - severe D07.5
  - vagina (histologically confirmed) (VAIN) N89.3
    - grade I N89.0
    - grade II N89.1
    - grade III (severe dysplasia) D07.2
  - vulva (histologically confirmed) (VIN) N90.3
    - grade I N90.0
    - grade II N90.1
    - grade III (severe dysplasia) D07.1

Neoplasm, neoplastic (*see also* Table of Neoplasms)
- lipomatous, benign — *see* Lipoma

Neovascularization
- ciliary body — *see* Disorder, iris, vascular
- cornea H16.40- ☑
  - deep H16.44- ☑
  - ghost vessels — *see* Ghost, vessels
  - localized H16.43- ☑
  - pannus — *see* Pannus
- iris — *see* Disorder, iris, vascular
- retina H35.05- ☑

Nephralgia N23
Nephritis, nephritic (albuminuric) (azotemic) (congenital) (disseminated) (epithelial) (familial) (focal) (granulomatous) (hemorrhagic) (infantile) (nonsuppurative, excretory) (uremic) N05.9
- with
  - dense deposit disease N05.6
  - diffuse
    - crescentic glomerulonephritis N05.7
    - endocapillary proliferative glomerulonephritis N05.4
    - membranous glomerulonephritis N05.2
    - mesangial proliferative glomerulonephritis N05.3
    - mesangiocapillary glomerulonephritis N05.5

Nephritis — *continued*
- edema — *see* Nephrosis
- focal and segmental glomerular lesions N05.1
- foot process disease N04.9
- glomerular lesion
  - diffuse sclerosing N05.8
  - hypocomplementemic — *see* Nephritis, membranoproliferative
  - IgA — *see* Nephropathy, IgA
  - lobular, lobulonodular — *see* Nephritis, membranoproliferative
  - nodular — *see* Nephritis, membranoproliferative
- lesion of
  - glomerulonephritis, proliferative N05.8
  - renal necrosis N05.9
- minor glomerular abnormality N05.0
- specified morphological changes NEC N05.8
- acute N00.9
  - with
    - dense deposit disease N00.6
    - diffuse
      - crescentic glomerulonephritis N00.7
      - endocapillary proliferative glomerulonephritis N00.4
      - membranous glomerulonephritis N00.2
      - mesangial proliferative glomerulonephritis N00.3
      - mesangiocapillary glomerulonephritis N00.5
    - focal and segmental glomerular lesions N00.1
    - minor glomerular abnormality N00.0
    - specified morphological changes NEC N00.8
- amyloid E85.4 [N08]
- antiglomerular basement membrane (anti-GBM) antibody NEC
  - in Goodpasture's syndrome M31.0
- antitubular basement membrane (tubulo-interstitial) NEC N12
  - toxic — *see* Nephropathy, toxic
- arteriolar — *see* Hypertension, kidney
- arteriosclerotic — *see* Hypertension, kidney
- ascending — *see* Nephritis, tubulo-interstitial
- atrophic N03.9
- Balkan (endemic) N15.0
- calculous, calculus — *see* Calculus, kidney
- cardiac — *see* Hypertension, kidney
- cardiovascular — *see* Hypertension, kidney
- chronic N03.9
  - with
    - dense deposit disease N03.6
    - diffuse
      - crescentic glomerulonephritis N03.7
      - endocapillary proliferative glomerulonephritis N03.4
      - membranous glomerulonephritis N03.2
      - mesangial proliferative glomerulonephritis N03.3
      - mesangiocapillary glomerulonephritis N03.5
    - focal and segmental glomerular lesions N03.1
    - minor glomerular abnormality N03.0
    - specified morphological changes NEC N03.8
  - arteriosclerotic — *see* Hypertension, kidney
- cirrhotic N26.9
- complicating pregnancy O26.83- ☑
- croupous N00.9
- degenerative — *see* Nephrosis
- diffuse sclerosing N05.8
- due to
  - diabetes mellitus — *see* E08-E13 with .21
  - subacute bacterial endocarditis I33.0
  - systemic lupus erythematosus (chronic) M32.14
  - typhoid fever A01.09
- gonococcal (acute) (chronic) A54.21
- hypocomplementemic — *see* Nephritis, membranoproliferative
- IgA — *see* Nephropathy, IgA
- immune complex (circulating) NEC N05.8
- infective — *see* Nephritis, tubulo-interstitial
- interstitial — *see* Nephritis, tubulo-interstitial
- lead N14.3
- membranoproliferative (diffuse) (type 1 or 3) (*see also* N00-N07 with fourth character .5) N05.5
  - type 2 (*see also* N00-N07 with fourth character .6) N05.6
- minimal change N05.0
- necrotic, necrotizing NEC (*see also* N00-N07 with fourth character .8) N05.8
- nephrotic — *see* Nephrosis

Nephritis — *continued*
- nodular — *see* Nephritis, membranoproliferative
- polycystic Q61.3
  - adult type Q61.2
  - autosomal
    - dominant Q61.2
    - recessive NEC Q61.19
  - childhood type NEC Q61.19
  - infantile type NEC Q61.19
- poststreptococcal N05.9
  - acute N00.9
  - chronic N03.9
  - rapidly progressive N01.9
- proliferative NEC (*see also* N00-N07 with fourth character .8) N05.8
- purulent — *see* Nephritis, tubulo-interstitial
- rapidly progressive N01.9
  - with
    - dense deposit disease N01.6
    - diffuse
      - crescentic glomerulonephritis N01.7
      - endocapillary proliferative glomerulonephritis N01.4
      - membranous glomerulonephritis N01.2
      - mesangial proliferative glomerulonephritis N01.3
      - mesangiocapillary glomerulonephritis N01.5
    - focal and segmental glomerular lesions N01.1
    - minor glomerular abnormality N01.0
    - specified morphological changes NEC N01.8
- salt losing or wasting NEC N28.89
- saturnine N14.3
- sclerosing, diffuse N05.8
- septic — *see* Nephritis, tubulo-interstitial
- specified pathology NEC (*see also* N00-N07 with fourth character .8) N05.8
- subacute N01.9
- suppurative — *see* Nephritis, tubulo-interstitial
- syphilitic (late) A52.75
  - congenital A50.59 [N08]
  - early (secondary) A51.44
- toxic — *see* Nephropathy, toxic
- tubal, tubular — *see* Nephritis, tubulo-interstitial
- tuberculous A18.11
- tubulo-interstitial (in) N12
  - acute (infectious) N10
  - chronic (infectious) N11.9
    - nonobstructive N11.8
      - reflux-associated N11.0
    - obstructive N11.1
    - specified NEC N11.8
  - due to
    - brucellosis A23.9 [N16]
    - cryoglobulinemia D89.1 [N16]
    - glycogen storage disease E74.00 [N16]
    - Sjögren's syndrome M35.04
- vascular — *see* Hypertension, kidney
- war N00.9

Nephroblastoma (epithelial) (mesenchymal) C64- ☑
Nephrocalcinosis E83.59 [N29]
Nephrocystitis, pustular — *see* Nephritis, tubulo-interstitial
Nephrolithiasis (congenital) (pelvis) (recurrent) (*see also* Calculus, kidney)
Nephroma C64- ☑
- mesoblastic D41.0- ☑
Nephronephritis — *see* Nephrosis
Nephronophthisis Q61.5
Nephropathia epidemica A98.5
Nephropathy (*see also* Nephritis) N28.9
- with
  - edema — *see* Nephrosis
  - glomerular lesion — *see* Glomerulonephritis
- amyloid, hereditary E85.0
- analgesic N14.0
  - with medullary necrosis, acute N17.2
- Balkan (endemic) N15.0
- chemical — *see* Nephropathy, toxic
- diabetic — *see* E08-E13 with .21
- drug-induced N14.2
  - specified NEC N14.1
- focal and segmental hyalinosis or sclerosis N02.1
- heavy metal-induced N14.3
- hereditary NEC N07.9
  - with
    - dense deposit disease N07.6
    - diffuse
      - crescentic glomerulonephritis N07.7
      - endocapillary proliferative glomerulonephritis N07.4

Nephropathy — *continued*
    membranous glomerulonephritis N07.2
    mesangial proliferative glomerulonephritis N07.3
    mesangiocapillary glomerulonephritis N07.5
    focal and segmental glomerular lesions N07.1
    minor glomerular abnormality N07.0
    specified morphological changes NEC N07.8
  hypercalcemic N25.89
  hypertensive — *see* Hypertension, kidney
  hypokalemic (vacuolar) N25.89
  IgA N02.8
    with glomerular lesion N02.9
      focal and segmental hyalinosis or sclerosis N02.1
      membranoproliferative (diffuse) N02.5
      membranous (diffuse) N02.2
      mesangial proliferative (diffuse) N02.3
      mesangiocapillary (diffuse) N02.5
      proliferative NEC N02.8
      specified pathology NEC N02.8
  lead N14.3
  membranoproliferative (diffuse) N02.5
  membranous (diffuse) N02.2
  mesangial (IgA/IgG) — *see* Nephropathy, IgA
    proliferative (diffuse) N02.3
  mesangiocapillary (diffuse) N02.5
  obstructive N13.8
  phenacetin N17.2
  phosphate-losing N25.0
  potassium depletion N25.89
  pregnancy-related O26.83- ☑
  proliferative NEC (*see also* N00-N07 with fourth character .8) N05.8
  protein-losing N25.89
  saturnine N14.3
  sickle-cell D57.- ☑ [N08]
  toxic NEC N14.4
    due to
      drugs N14.2
        analgesic N14.0
        specified NEC N14.1
      heavy metals N14.3
  vasomotor N17.0
  water-losing N25.89
Nephroptosis N28.83
Nephropyosis — *see* Abscess, kidney
Nephrorrhagia N28.89
Nephrosclerosis (arteriolar)(arteriosclerotic) (chronic) (hyaline) (*see also* Hypertension, kidney)
  hyperplastic — *see* Hypertension, kidney
  senile N26.9
Nephrosis, nephrotic (Epstein's) (syndrome) (congenital) N04.9
  with
    foot process disease N04.9
    glomerular lesion N04.1
    hypocomplementemic N04.5
  acute N04.9
  anoxic — *see* Nephrosis, tubular
  chemical — *see* Nephrosis, tubular
  cholemic K76.7
  diabetic — *see* E08-E13 with .21
  Finnish type (congenital) Q89.8
  hemoglobin N10
  hemoglobinuric — *see* Nephrosis, tubular
  in
    amyloidosis E85.4 [N08]
    diabetes mellitus — *see* E08-E13 with .21
    epidemic hemorrhagic fever A98.5
    malaria (malariae) B52.0
  ischemic — *see* Nephrosis, tubular
  lipoid N04.9
  lower nephron — *see* Nephrosis, tubular
  malarial (malariae) B52.0
  minimal change N04.0
  myoglobin N10
  necrotizing — *see* Nephrosis, tubular
  osmotic (sucrose) N25.89
  radiation N04.9
  syphilitic (late) A52.75
  toxic — *see* Nephrosis, tubular
  tubular (acute) N17.0
    postprocedural N99.0
    radiation N04.9
Nephrosonephritis, hemorrhagic (endemic) A98.5
Nephrostomy
  attention to Z43.6
  status Z93.6

Nerve (*see also* condition)
  injury — *see* Injury, nerve, by body site
Nerves R45.0
Nervous (*see also* condition) R45.0
  heart F45.8
  stomach F45.8
  tension R45.0
Nervousness R45.0
Nesidioblastoma
  pancreas D13.7
  specified site NEC — *see* Neoplasm, benign, by site
  unspecified site D13.7
Nettleship's syndrome Q82.2
Neumann's disease or syndrome L10.1
Neuralgia, neuralgic (acute) M79.2
  accessory (nerve) G52.8
  acoustic (nerve) H93.3
  auditory (nerve) H93.3
  ciliary G44.009
    intractable G44.001
    not intractable G44.009
  cranial
    nerve (*see also* Disorder, nerve, cranial)
      fifth or trigeminal — *see* Neuralgia, trigeminal
      postherpetic, postzoster B02.29
  ear H92.0
  facialis vera G51.1
  Fothergill's — *see* Neuralgia, trigeminal
  glossopharyngeal (nerve) G52.1
  Horton's G44.099
    intractable G44.091
    not intractable G44.099
  Hunt's B02.21
  hypoglossal (nerve) G52.3
  infraorbital — *see* Neuralgia, trigeminal
  malarial — *see* Malaria
  migrainous G44.009
    intractable G44.001
    not intractable G44.009
  Morton's G57.6- ☑
  nerve, cranial — *see* Disorder, nerve, cranial
  nose G52.0
  occipital M54.81
  olfactory G52.0
  penis N48.9
  perineum R10.2
  postherpetic NEC B02.29
    trigeminal B02.22
  pubic region R10.2
  scrotum R10.2
  Sluder's G44.89
  specified nerve NEC G58.8
  spermatic cord R10.2
  sphenopalatine (ganglion) G90.09
  trifacial — *see* Neuralgia, trigeminal
  trigeminal G50.0
    postherpetic, postzoster B02.22
  vagus (nerve) G52.2
  writer's F48.8
    organic G25.89
Neurapraxia — *see* Injury, nerve
Neurasthenia F48.8
  cardiac F45.8
  gastric F45.8
  heart F45.8
Neurilemmoma (*see also* Neoplasm, nerve, benign)
  acoustic (nerve) D33.3
  malignant (*see also* Neoplasm, nerve, malignant)
    acoustic (nerve) C72.4- ☑
Neurilemmosarcoma — *see* Neoplasm, nerve, malignant
Neurinoma — *see* Neoplasm, nerve, benign
Neurinomatosis — *see* Neoplasm, nerve, uncertain behavior
Neuritis (rheumatoid) M79.2
  abducens (nerve) — *see* Strabismus, paralytic, sixth nerve
  accessory (nerve) G52.8
  acoustic (nerve) (*see also* subcategory) H93.3 ☑
    in (due to)
      infectious disease NEC B99 ☑ [H94.0- ☑]
      parasitic disease NEC B89 [H94.0- ☑]
      syphilitic A52.15
  alcoholic G62.1
    with psychosis — *see* Psychosis, alcoholic
  amyloid, any site E85.4 [G63]
  auditory (nerve) H93.3
  brachial — *see* Radiculopathy
    due to displacement, intervertebral disc — *see* Disorder, disc, cervical, with neuritis
  cranial nerve

Neuritis — *continued*
  due to Lyme disease A69.22
  eighth or acoustic or auditory H93.3
  eleventh or accessory G52.8
  fifth or trigeminal G51.0
  first or olfactory G52.0
  fourth or trochlear — *see* Strabismus, paralytic, fourth nerve
  second or optic — *see* Neuritis, optic
  seventh or facial G51.8
    newborn (birth injury) P11.3
  sixth or abducent — *see* Strabismus, paralytic, sixth nerve
  tenth or vagus G52.2
  third or oculomotor — *see* Strabismus, paralytic, third nerve
  twelfth or hypoglossal G52.3
  Déjérine-Sottas G60.0
  diabetic (mononeuropathy) — *see* E08-E13 with .41
    polyneuropathy — *see* E08-E13 with .42
  due to
    beriberi E51.11
    displacement, prolapse or rupture, intervertebral disc — *see* Disorder, disc, with, radiculopathy
    herniation, nucleus pulposus M51.9 [G55]
  endemic E51.11
  facial G51.8
    newborn (birth injury) P11.3
  general — *see* Polyneuropathy
  geniculate ganglion G51.1
    due to herpes (zoster) B02.21
  gouty M10.00 [G63]
  hypoglossal (nerve) G52.3
  ilioinguinal (nerve) G57.9- ☑
  infectious (multiple) NEC G61.0
  interstitial hypertrophic progressive G60.0
  lumbar M54.16
  lumbosacral M54.17
  multiple (*see also* Polyneuropathy)
    endemic E51.11
    infective, acute G61.0
  multiplex endemica E51.11
  nerve root — *see* Radiculopathy
  oculomotor (nerve) — *see* Strabismus, paralytic, third nerve
  olfactory nerve G52.0
  optic (nerve) (hereditary) (sympathetic) H46.9
    with demyelination G36.0
      in myelitis G36.0
    nutritional H46.2
    papillitis — *see* Papillitis, optic
    retrobulbar H46.1- ☑
    specified type NEC H46.8
    toxic H46.3
  peripheral (nerve) G62.9
    multiple — *see* Polyneuropathy
    single — *see* Mononeuritis
  pneumogastric (nerve) G52.2
  postherpetic, postzoster B02.29
  progressive hypertrophic interstitial G60.0
  retrobulbar (*see also* Neuritis, optic, retrobulbar)
    in (due to)
      late syphilis A52.15
      meningococcal infection A39.82
    meningococcal A39.82
    syphilitic A52.15
  sciatic (nerve) (*see also* Sciatica)
    due to displacement of intervertebral disc — *see* Disorder, disc, with, radiculopathy
  serum (*see also* Reaction, serum) T80.69 ☑
  shoulder-girdle G54.5
  specified nerve NEC G58.8
  spinal (nerve) root — *see* Radiculopathy
  syphilitic A52.15
  thenar (median) G56.1- ☑
  thoracic M54.14
  toxic NEC G62.2
  trochlear (nerve) — *see* Strabismus, paralytic, fourth nerve
  vagus (nerve) G52.2
Neuroastrocytoma — *see* Neoplasm, uncertain behavior, by site
Neuroavitaminosis E56.9 [G99.8]
Neuroblastoma
  olfactory C30.0
  specified site — *see* Neoplasm, malignant, by site
  unspecified site C74.90
Neurochorioretinitis — *see* Chorioretinitis
Neurocirculatory asthenia F45.8
Neurocysticercosis B69.0

Neurocytoma — *see* Neoplasm, benign, by site
Neurodermatitis (circumscribed) (circumscripta) (local) L28.0
  atopic L20.81
  diffuse (Brocq) L20.81
  disseminated L20.81
Neuroencephalomyelopathy, optic G36.0
Neuroepithelioma (*see also* Neoplasm, malignant, by site)
  olfactory C30.0
Neurofibroma (*see also* Neoplasm, nerve, benign)
  melanotic — *see* Neoplasm, nerve, benign
  multiple — *see* Neurofibromatosis
  plexiform — *see* Neoplasm, nerve, benign
Neurofibromatosis (multiple) (nonmalignant) Q85.00
  acoustic Q85.02
  malignant — *see* Neoplasm, nerve, malignant
  specified NEC Q85.09
  type 1 (von Recklinghausen) Q85.01
  type 2 Q85.02
Neurofibrosarcoma — *see* Neoplasm, nerve, malignant
Neurogenic (*see also* condition)
  bladder (*see also* Dysfunction, bladder, neuromuscular) N31.9
    cauda equina syndrome G83.4
  bowel NEC K59.2
  heart F45.8
Neuroglioma — *see* Neoplasm, uncertain behavior, by site
Neurolabyrinthitis (of Dix and Hallpike) — *see* Neuronitis, vestibular
Neurolathyrism — *see* Poisoning, food, noxious, plant
Neuroleprosy A30.9
Neuroma (*see also* Neoplasm, nerve, benign)
  acoustic (nerve) D33.3
  amputation (stump) (traumatic) (surgical complication) (late) T87.3- ☑
    arm T87.3- ☑
    leg T87.3- ☑
  digital (toe) G57.6- ☑
  interdigital (toe) G58.8
    lower limb G57.8- ☑
    upper limb G56.8- ☑
  intermetatarsal G57.8- ☑
  Morton's G57.6- ☑
  nonneoplastic
    arm G56.9- ☑
    leg G57.9- ☑
    lower extremity G57.9- ☑
    upper extremity G56.9- ☑
  optic (nerve) D33.3
  plantar G57.6- ☑
  plexiform — *see* Neoplasm, nerve, benign
  surgical (nonneoplastic)
    arm G56.9- ☑
    leg G57.9- ☑
    lower extremity G57.9- ☑
    upper extremity G56.9- ☑
Neuromyalgia — *see* Neuralgia
Neuromyasthenia (epidemic) (postinfectious) G93.3
Neuromyelitis G36.9
  ascending G61.0
  optica G36.0
Neuromyopathy G70.9
  paraneoplastic D49.9 [G13.0]
Neuromyotonia (Isaacs) G71.19
Neuronevus — *see* Nevus
Neuronitis G58.9
  ascending (acute) G57.2- ☑
  vestibular H81.2- ☑
Neuroparalytic — *see* condition
Neuropathy, neuropathic G62.9
  acute motor G62.81
  alcoholic G62.1
    with psychosis — *see* Psychosis, alcoholic
  arm G56.9- ☑
  autonomic, peripheral — *see* Neuropathy, peripheral, autonomic
  axillary G56.9- ☑
  bladder N31.9
    atonic (motor) (sensory) N31.2
    autonomous N31.2
    flaccid N31.2
    nonreflex N31.2
    reflex N31.1
    uninhibited N31.0
  brachial plexus G54.0
  cervical plexus G54.2
  chronic

Neuropathy — *continued*
  progressive segmentally demyelinating G62.89
  relapsing demyelinating G62.89
  Déjérine-Sottas G60.0
  diabetic — *see* E08-E13 with .40
    mononeuropathy — *see* E08-E13 with .41
    polyneuropathy — *see* E08-E13 with .42
  entrapment G58.9
    iliohypogastric nerve G57.8- ☑
    ilioinguinal nerve G57.8- ☑
    lateral cutaneous nerve of thigh G57.1- ☑
    median nerve G56.0- ☑
    obturator nerve G57.8- ☑
    peroneal nerve G57.3- ☑
    posterior tibial nerve G57.5- ☑
    saphenous nerve G57.8- ☑
    ulnar nerve G56.2- ☑
  facial nerve G51.9
  hereditary G60.9
    motor and sensory (types I-IV) G60.0
    sensory G60.8
    specified NEC G60.8
  hypertrophic G60.0
    Charcot-Marie-Tooth G60.0
    Déjérine-Sottas G60.0
    interstitial progressive G60.0
    of infancy G60.0
    Refsum G60.1
  idiopathic G60.9
    progressive G60.3
    specified NEC G60.8
  in association with hereditary ataxia G60.2
  intercostal G58.0
  ischemic — *see* Disorder, nerve
  Jamaica (ginger) G62.2
  leg NEC G57.9- ☑
  lower extremity G57.9- ☑
  lumbar plexus G54.1
  median nerve G56.1- ☑
  motor and sensory (*see also* Polyneuropathy)
    hereditary (types I-IV) G60.0
  multiple (acute) (chronic) — *see* Polyneuropathy
  optic (nerve) (*see also* Neuritis, optic)
    ischemic H47.01- ☑
  paraneoplastic (sensorial) (Denny Brown) D49.9 [G13.0]
  peripheral (nerve) (*see also* Polyneuropathy) G62.9
    autonomic G90.9
      idiopathic G90.09
      in (due to)
        amyloidosis E85.4 [G99.0]
        diabetes mellitus — *see* E08-E13 with .43
        endocrine disease NEC E34.9 [G99.0]
        gout M10.00 [G99.0]
        hyperthyroidism E05.90 [G99.0]
          with thyroid storm E05.91 [G99.0]
        metabolic disease NEC E88.9 [G99.0]
    idiopathic G60.9
      progressive G60.3
    in (due to)
      antitetanus serum G62.0
      arsenic G62.2
      drugs NEC G62.0
      lead G62.2
      organophosphate compounds G62.2
      toxic agent NEC G62.2
  plantar nerves G57.6- ☑
  progressive
    hypertrophic interstitial G60.0
    inflammatory G62.81
  radicular NEC — *see* Radiculopathy
  sacral plexus G54.1
  sciatic G57.0- ☑
  serum G61.1
  toxic NEC G62.2
  trigeminal sensory G50.8
  ulnar nerve G56.2- ☑
  uremic N18.9 [G63]
  vitamin B12 E53.8 [G63]
    with anemia (pernicious) D51.0 [G63]
    due to dietary deficiency D51.3 [G63]
Neurophthisis (*see also* Disorder, nerve)
  peripheral, diabetic — *see* E08-E13 with .42
Neuroretinitis — *see* Chorioretinitis
Neuroretinopathy, hereditary optic H47.22
Neurosarcoma — *see* Neoplasm, nerve, malignant
Neurosclerosis — *see* Disorder, nerve
Neurosis, neurotic F48.9
  anankastic F42
  anxiety (state) F41.1
    panic type F41.0

Neurosis — *continued*
  asthenic F48.8
  bladder F45.8
  cardiac (reflex) F45.8
  cardiovascular F45.8
  character F60.9
  colon F45.8
  compensation F68.1 ☑
  compulsive, compulsion F42
  conversion F44.9
  craft F48.8
  cutaneous F45.8
  depersonalization F48.1
  depressive (reaction) (type) F34.1
  environmental F48.8
  excoriation L98.1
  fatigue F48.8
  functional — *see* Disorder, somatoform
  gastric F45.8
  gastrointestinal F45.8
  heart F45.8
  hypochondriacal F45.21
  hysterical F44.9
  incoordination F45.8
    larynx F45.8
    vocal cord F45.8
  intestine F45.8
  larynx (sensory) F45.8
    hysterical F44.4
  mixed NEC F48.8
  musculoskeletal F45.8
  obsessional F42
  obsessive-compulsive F42
  occupational F48.8
  ocular NEC F45.8
  organ — *see* Disorder, somatoform
  pharynx F45.8
  phobic F40.9
  posttraumatic (situational) F43.10
    acute F43.11
    chronic F43.12
  psychasthenic (type) F48.8
  railroad F48.8
  rectum F45.8
  respiratory F45.8
  rumination F45.8
  sexual F65.9
  situational F48.8
  social F40.10
    generalized F40.11
  specified type NEC F48.8
  state F48.9
    with depersonalization episode F48.1
  stomach F45.8
  traumatic F43.10
    acute F43.11
    chronic F43.12
  vasomotor F45.8
  visceral F45.8
  war F48.8
Neurospongioblastosis diffusa Q85.1
Neurosyphilis (arrested) (early) (gumma) (late) (latent) (recurrent) (relapse) A52.3
  with ataxia (cerebellar) (locomotor) (spastic) (spinal) A52.19
  aneurysm (cerebral) A52.05
  arachnoid (adhesive) A52.13
  arteritis (any artery) (cerebral) A52.04
  asymptomatic A52.2
  congenital A50.40
  dura (mater) A52.13
  general paresis A52.17
  hemorrhagic A52.05
  juvenile (asymptomatic) (meningeal) A50.40
  leptomeninges (aseptic) A52.13
  meningeal, meninges (adhesive) A52.13
  meningitis A52.13
  meningovascular (diffuse) A52.13
  optic atrophy A52.15
  parenchymatous (degenerative) A52.19
  paresis, paretic A52.17
    juvenile A50.45
  remission in (sustained) A52.3
  serological (without symptoms) A52.2
  specified nature or site NEC A52.19
  tabes, tabetic (dorsalis) A52.11
    juvenile A50.45
  taboparesis A52.17
    juvenile A50.45
  thrombosis (cerebral) A52.05
  vascular (cerebral) NEC A52.05
Neurothekeoma — *see* Neoplasm, nerve, benign

Neurotic — *see* Neurosis
Neurotoxemia — *see* Toxemia
Neuroclusion M26.211
Neutropenia, neutropenic (chronic) (genetic) (idiopathic) (immune) (infantile) (malignant) (pernicious) (splenic) D70.9
　congenital (primary) D70.0
　cyclic D70.4
　cytoreductive cancer chemotherapy sequela D70.1
　drug-induced D70.2
　　due to cytoreductive cancer chemotherapy D70.1
　due to infection D70.3
　fever D70.9
　neonatal, transitory (isoimmune) (maternal transfer) P61.5
　periodic D70.4
　secondary (cyclic) (periodic) (splenic) D70.4
　　drug-induced D70.2
　　　due to cytoreductive cancer chemotherapy D70.1
　toxic D70.8
Neutrophilia, hereditary giant D72.0
Nevocarcinoma — *see* Melanoma
Nevus D22.9
　achromic — *see* Neoplasm, skin, benign
　amelanotic — *see* Neoplasm, skin, benign
　angiomatousD18.00
　　intra-abdominal D18.03
　　intracranial D18.02
　　skin D18.01
　　specified site NEC D18.09
　araneus I78.1
　balloon cell — *see* Neoplasm, skin, benign
　bathing trunk D48.5
　blue — *see* Neoplasm, skin, benign
　　cellular — *see* Neoplasm, skin, benign
　　giant — *see* Neoplasm, skin, benign
　　Jadassohn's — *see* Neoplasm, skin, benign
　　malignant — *see* Melanoma
　capillary D18.00
　　intra-abdominal D18.03
　　intracranial D18.02
　　skin D18.01
　　specified site NEC D18.09
　cavernous D18.00
　　intra-abdominal D18.03
　　intracranial D18.02
　　skin D18.01
　　specified site NEC D18.09
　cellular — *see* Neoplasm, skin, benign
　　blue — *see* Neoplasm, skin, benign
　choroid D31.3- ☑
　comedonicus Q82.5
　conjunctiva D31.0- ☑
　dermal — *see* Neoplasm, skin, benign
　　with epidermal nevus — *see* Neoplasm, skin, benign
　dysplastic — *see* Neoplasm, skin, benign
　eye D31.9- ☑
　flammeus Q82.5
　hemangiomatous D18.00
　　intra-abdominal D18.03
　　intracranial D18.02
　　skin D18.01
　　specified site NEC D18.09
　iris D31.4- ☑
　lacrimal gland D31.5- ☑
　lymphatic D18.1
　magnocellular
　　specified site — *see* Neoplasm, benign, by site
　　unspecified site D31.40
　malignant — *see* Melanoma
　meaning hemangioma D18.00
　　intra-abdominal D18.03
　　intracranial D18.02
　　skin D18.01
　　specified site NEC D18.09
　mouth (mucosa) D10.30
　　specified site NEC D10.39
　　white sponge Q38.6
　multiplex Q85.1
　non-neoplastic I78.1
　oral mucosa D10.30
　　specified site NEC D10.39
　　white sponge Q38.6
　orbit D31.6- ☑
　pigmented
　　giant (*see also* Neoplasm, skin, uncertain behavior) D48.5
　　　malignant melanoma in — *see* Melanoma

Nevus — *continued*
　portwine Q82.5
　retina D31.2- ☑
　retrobulbar D31.6- ☑
　sanguineous Q82.5
　senile I78.1
　skin D22.9
　　abdominal wall D22.5
　　ala nasi D22.39
　　ankle D22.7- ☑
　　anus, anal D22.5
　　arm D22.6- ☑
　　auditory canal (external) D22.2- ☑
　　auricle (ear) D22.2- ☑
　　auricular canal (external) D22.2- ☑
　　axilla, axillary fold D22.5
　　back D22.5
　　breast D22.5
　　brow D22.39
　　buttock D22.5
　　canthus (eye) D22.1- ☑
　　cheek (external) D22.39
　　chest wall D22.5
　　chin D22.39
　　ear (external) D22.2- ☑
　　external meatus (ear) D22.2- ☑
　　eyebrow D22.39
　　eyelid (lower) (upper) D22.1- ☑
　　face D22.30
　　　specified NEC D22.39
　　female genital organ (external) NEC D28.0
　　finger D22.6- ☑
　　flank D22.5
　　foot D22.7- ☑
　　forearm D22.6- ☑
　　forehead D22.39
　　foreskin D29.0
　　genital organ (external) NEC
　　　female D28.0
　　　male D29.9
　　gluteal region D22.5
　　groin D22.5
　　hand D22.6- ☑
　　heel D22.7- ☑
　　helix D22.2- ☑
　　hip D22.7- ☑
　　interscapular region D22.5
　　jaw D22.39
　　knee D22.7- ☑
　　labium (majus) (minus) D28.0
　　leg D22.7- ☑
　　lip (lower) (upper) D22.0
　　lower limb D22.7- ☑
　　male genital organ (external) D29.9
　　nail D22.9
　　　finger D22.6- ☑
　　　toe D22.7- ☑
　　nasolabial groove D22.39
　　nates D22.5
　　neck D22.4
　　nose (external) D22.39
　　palpebra D22.1- ☑
　　penis D29.0
　　perianal skin D22.5
　　perineum D22.5
　　pinna D22.2- ☑
　　popliteal fossa or space D22.7- ☑
　　prepuce D29.0
　　pudendum D28.0
　　scalp D22.4
　　scrotum D29.4
　　shoulder D22.6- ☑
　　submammary fold D22.5
　　temple D22.39
　　thigh D22.7- ☑
　　toe D22.7- ☑
　　trunk NEC D22.5
　　umbilicus D22.5
　　upper limb D22.6- ☑
　　vulva D28.0
　specified site NEC — *see* Neoplasm, by site, benign
　spider I78.1
　stellar I78.1
　strawberry Q82.5
　Sutton's — *see* Neoplasm, skin, benign
　unius lateris Q82.5
　Unna's Q82.5
　vascular Q82.5
　verrucous Q82.5
Newborn (infant) (liveborn) (singleton) Z38.2
　acne L70.4

Newborn — *continued*
　abstinence syndrome P96.1
　affected by (suspected to be)
　　abnormalities of membranes P02.9
　　　specified NEC P02.8
　　abruptio placenta P02.1
　　amino-acid metabolic disorder, transitory P74.8
　　amniocentesis (while in utero) P00.6
　　amnionitis P02.7
　　apparent life threatening event (ALTE) R68.13
　　bleeding (into)
　　　cerebral cortex P52.22
　　　germinal matrix P52.0
　　　ventricles P52.1
　　breech delivery P03.0
　　cardiac arrest P29.81
　　cardiomyopathy I42.8
　　　congenital I42.4
　　cerebral ischemia P91.0
　　Cesarean delivery P03.4
　　chemotherapy agents P04.1
　　chorioamnionitis P02.7
　　cocaine (crack) P04.41
　　complications of labor and delivery P03.9
　　　specified NEC P03.89
　　compression of umbilical cord NEC P02.5
　　contracted pelvis P03.1
　　delivery P03.9
　　　Cesarean P03.4
　　　forceps P03.2
　　　vacuum extractor P03.3
　　environmental chemicals P04.6
　　entanglement (knot) in umbilical cord P02.5
　　fetal (intrauterine)
　　　growth retardation P05.9
　　　malnutrition not light or small for gestational age P05.2
　　forceps delivery P03.2
　　heart rate abnormalities
　　　bradycardia P29.12
　　　intrauterine P03.819
　　　　before onset of labor P03.810
　　　　during labor P03.811
　　　tachycardia P29.11
　　hemorrhage (antepartum) P02.1
　　　cerebellar (nontraumatic) P52.6
　　　intracerebral (nontraumatic) P52.4
　　　intracranial (nontraumatic) P52.9
　　　　specified NEC P52.8
　　　intraventricular (nontraumatic) P52.3
　　　　grade 1 P52.0
　　　　grade 2 P52.1
　　　　grade 3 P52.21
　　　　grade 4 P52.22
　　　posterior fossa (nontraumatic) P52.6
　　　subarachnoid (nontraumatic) P52.5
　　　subependymal P52.0
　　　　with intracerebral extension P52.22
　　　　with intraventricular extension P52.1
　　　　　with enlargment of ventricles P52.21
　　　　without intraventricular extension P52.0
　　hypoxic ischemic encephalopathy [HIE] P91.60
　　　mild P91.61
　　　moderate P91.62
　　　severe P91.63
　　induction of labor P03.89
　　intestinal perforation P78.0
　　intrauterine (fetal) blood loss P50.9
　　　due to (from)
　　　　cut end of co-twin cord P50.5
　　　　hemorrhage into
　　　　　co-twin P50.3
　　　　　maternal circulation P50.4
　　　　placenta P50.2
　　　　ruptured cord blood P50.1
　　　　vasa previa P50.0
　　　specified NEC P50.8
　　intrauterine (fetal) hemorrhage P50.9
　　intrauterine (in utero) procedure P96.5
　　malpresentation (malposition) NEC P03.1
　　maternal (complication of) (use of)
　　　alcohol P04.3
　　　analgesia (maternal) P04.0
　　　anesthesia (maternal) P04.0
　　　blood loss P02.1
　　　circulatory disease P00.3
　　　condition P00.9
　　　　specified NEC P00.89
　　　delivery P03.9
　　　　Cesarean P03.4
　　　　forceps P03.2
　　　　vacuum extractor P03.3

☑ **Additional character required**

Newborn — *continued*
- diabetes mellitus (pre-existing) P70.1
- disorder P00.9
  - specified NEC P00.89
- drugs (addictive) (illegal) NEC P04.49
- ectopic pregnancy P01.4
- gestational diabetes P70.0
- hemorrhage P02.1
- hypertensive disorder P00.0
- incompetent cervix P01.0
- infectious disease P00.2
- injury P00.5
- labor and delivery P03.9
- malpresentation before labor P01.7
- maternal death P01.6
- medical procedure P00.7
- medication P04.1
- multiple pregnancy P01.5
- nutritional disorder P00.4
- oligohydramnios P01.2
- parasitic disease P00.2
- periodontal disease P00.81
- placenta previa P02.0
- polyhydramnios P01.3
- precipitate delivery P03.5
- pregnancy P01.9
  - specified P01.8
- premature rupture of membranes P01.1
- renal disease P00.1
- respiratory disease P00.3
- surgical procedure P00.6
- urinary tract disease P00.1
- uterine contraction (abnormal) P03.6
- meconium peritonitis P78.0
- medication (legal) (maternal use) (prescribed) P04.1
- membrane abnormalities P02.9
  - specified NEC P02.8
- membranitis P02.7
- methamphetamine (s) P04.49
- mixed metabolic and respiratory acidosis P84
- neonatal abstinence syndrome P96.1
- noxious substances transmitted via placenta or breast milk P04.9
  - specified NEC P04.8
- nutritional supplements P04.5
- placenta previa P02.0
- placental
  - abnormality (functional) (morphological) P02.20
    - specified NEC P02.29
  - dysfunction P02.29
  - infarction P02.29
  - insufficiency P02.29
  - separation NEC P02.1
  - transfusion syndromes P02.3
- placentitis P02.7
- precipitate delivery P03.5
- prolapsed cord P02.4
- respiratory arrest P28.81
- slow intrauterine growth P05.9
- tobacco P04.2
- twin to twin transplacental transfusion P02.3
- umbilical cord (tightly) around neck P02.5
- umbilical cord condition P02.60
  - short cord P02.69
  - specified NEC P02.69
- uterine contractions (abnormal) P03.6
- vasa previa P02.69
  - from intrauterine blood loss P50.0
- apnea P28.3
  - primary P28.3
  - obstructive P28.4
  - specified P28.4
- born in hospital Z38.00
  - by cesarean Z38.01
- born outside hospital Z38.1
- breast buds P96.89
- breast engorgement P83.4
- check-up — *see* Newborn, examination
- convulsion P90
- dehydration P74.1
- examination
  - 8 to 28 days old Z00.111
  - under 8 days old Z00.110
- fever P81.9
  - environmentally-induced P81.0
- hyperbilirubinemia P59.9
  - of prematurity P59.0
- hypernatremia P74.2
- hyponatremia P74.2
- infection P39.9

Newborn — *continued*
- candidal P37.5
  - specified NEC P39.8
  - urinary tract P39.3
- jaundice P59.8
  - due to
    - breast milk inhibitor P59.3
    - hepatocellular damage P59.20
      - specified NEC P59.29
    - preterm delivery P59.0
  - of prematurity P59.0
  - specified NEC P59.8
- late metabolic acidosis P74.0
- mastitis P39.0
  - infective P39.0
  - noninfective P83.4
- multiple born NEC Z38.8
  - born in hospital Z38.68
    - by cesarean Z38.69
  - born outside hospital Z38.7
- omphalitis P38.9
  - with mild hemorrhage P38.1
  - without hemorrhage P38.9
- post-term P08.21
- prolonged gestation (over 42 completed weeks) P08.22
- quadruplet Z38.8
  - born in hospital Z38.63
    - by cesarean Z38.64
  - born outside hospital Z38.7
- quintuplet Z38.8
  - born in hospital Z38.65
    - by cesarean Z38.66
  - born outside hospital Z38.7
- seizure P90
- sepsis (congenital) P36.9
  - due to
    - anaerobes NEC P36.5
    - Escherichia coli P36.4
    - Staphylococcus P36.30
      - aureus P36.2
      - specified NEC P36.39
    - Streptococcus P36.10
      - group B P36.0
      - specified NEC P36.19
  - specified NEC P36.8
- triplet Z38.8
  - born in hospital Z38.61
    - by cesarean Z38.62
  - born outside hospital Z38.7
- twin Z38.5
  - born in hospital Z38.30
    - by cesarean Z38.31
  - born outside hospital Z38.4
- vomiting P92.09
  - bilious P92.01
- weight check Z00.111

Newcastle conjunctivitis or disease B30.8
Nezelof's syndrome (pure alymphocytosis) D81.4
Niacin (amide) deficiency E52
Nicolas (-Durand)-Favre disease A55
Nicotine — *see* Tobacco
Nicotinic acid deficiency E52
Niemann-Pick disease or syndrome E75.249
- specified NEC E75.248
- type
  - A E75.240
  - B E75.241
  - C E75.242
  - D E75.243

Night
- blindness — *see* Blindness, night
- sweats R61
- terrors (child) F51.4
Nightmares (REM sleep type) F51.5
Nipple — *see* condition
Nisbet's chancre A57
Nishimoto (-Takeuchi) disease I67.5
Nitritoid crisis or reaction — *see* Crisis, nitritoid
Nitrosohemoglobinemia D74.8
Njovera A65
Nocardiosis, nocardiasis A43.9
- cutaneous A43.1
- lung A43.0
- pneumonia A43.0
- pulmonary A43.0
- specified site NEC A43.8
Nocturia R35.1
- psychogenic F45.8
Nocturnal — *see* condition
Nodal rhythm I49.8
Node (s) (*see also* Nodule)

Node — *continued*
- Bouchard's (with arthropathy) M15.2
- Haygarth's M15.8
- Heberden's (with arthropathy) M15.1
- larynx J38.7
- lymph — *see* condition
- milker's B08.03
- Osler's I33.0
- Schmorl's — *see* Schmorl's disease
- singer's J38.2
- teacher's J38.2
- tuberculous — *see* Tuberculosis, lymph gland
- vocal cord J38.2
Nodule (s), nodular
- actinomycotic — *see* Actinomycosis
- breast NEC N63
- colloid (cystic), thyroid E04.1
- cutaneous — *see* Swelling, localized
- endometrial (stromal) D26.1
- Haygarth's M15.8
- inflammatory — *see* Inflammation
- juxta-articular
  - syphilitic A52.77
  - yaws A66.7
- larynx J38.2
- lung, solitary (subsegmental branch of the bronchial tree) R91.1
  - multiple R91.8
- milker's B08.03
- prostate N40.2
  - with lower urinary tract symptoms (LUTS) N40.3
  - without lower urinary tract symtpoms (LUTS) N40.2
- pulmonary, solitary (subsegmental branch of the bronchial tree) R91.1
- retrocardiac R09.89
- rheumatoid M06.30
  - ankle M06.37- ☑
  - elbow M06.32- ☑
  - foot joint M06.37- ☑
  - hand joint M06.34- ☑
  - hip M06.35- ☑
  - knee M06.36- ☑
  - multiple site M06.39
  - shoulder M06.31- ☑
  - vertebra M06.38
  - wrist M06.33- ☑
- scrotum (inflammatory) N49.2
- singer's J38.2
- solitary, lung (subsegmental branch of the bronchial tree) R91.1
  - multiple R91.8
- subcutaneous — *see* Swelling, localized
- teacher's J38.2
- thyroid (cold) (gland) (nontoxic) E04.1
  - with thyrotoxicosis E05.20
    - with thyroid storm E05.21
  - toxic or with hyperthyroidism E05.20
    - with thyroid storm E05.21
- vocal cord J38.2
Noma (gangrenous) (hospital) (infective) A69.0
- auricle I96
- mouth A69.0
- pudendi N76.89
- vulvae N76.89
Nomad, nomadism Z59.0
Nonautoimmune hemolytic anemia D59.4
- drug-induced D59.2
Nonclosure (*see also* Imperfect, closure)
- ductus arteriosus (Botallo's) Q25.0
- foramen
  - botalli Q21.1
  - ovale Q21.1
Noncompliance Z91.19
- with
  - dietary regimen Z91.11
  - dialysis Z91.15
  - medical treatment Z91.19
  - medication regimen NEC Z91.14
    - underdosing (*see also* Table of Drugs and Chemicals, categories T36-T50, with final character 6) Z91.14
    - intentional NEC Z91.128
      - due to financial hardship of patient Z91.120
    - unintentional NEC Z91.138
      - due to patient's age related debility Z91.130
  - renal dialysis Z91.15
Nondescent (congenital) (*see also* Malposition, congenital)

Nondescent — *continued*
  cecum Q43.3
  colon Q43.3
  testicle Q53.9
    bilateral Q53.20
      abdominal Q53.21
      perineal Q53.22
    unilateral Q53.10
      abdominal Q53.11
      perineal Q53.12
Nondevelopment
  brain Q02
    part of Q04.3
  heart Q24.8
  organ or site, congenital NEC — *see* Hypoplasia
Nonengagement
  head NEC O32.4 ☑
    in labor, causing obstructed labor O64.8 ☑
Nonexanthematous tick fever A93.2
Nonexpansion, lung (newborn) P28.0
Nonfunctioning
  cystic duct (*see also* Disease, gallbladder) K82.8
  gallbladder (*see also* Disease, gallbladder) K82.8
  kidney N28.9
  labyrinth H83.2
Non-Hodgkin lymphoma NEC — *see* Lymphoma, non-Hodgkin
Non-working side interference M26.56
Nonimplantation, ovum N97.2
Noninsufflation, fallopian tube N97.1
Non-ketotic hyperglycinemia E72.51
Nonne-Milroy syndrome Q82.0
Nonovulation N97.0
Nonpatent fallopian tube N97.1
Nonpneumatization, lung NEC P28.0
Nonrotation — *see* Malrotation
Nonsecretion, urine — *see* Anuria
Nonunion
  fracture — *see* Fracture, by site
  organ or site, congenital NEC — *see* Imperfect, closure
  symphysis pubis, congenital Q74.2
Nonvisualization, gallbladder R93.2
Nonvital, nonvitalized tooth K04.99
Noonan's syndrome Q87.1
Normocytic anemia (infectional) due to blood loss (chronic) D50.0
  acute D62
Norrie's disease (congenital) Q15.8
North American blastomycosis B40.9
Norwegian itch B86
Nose, nasal — *see* condition
Nosebleed R04.0
Nose-picking F98.8
Nosomania F45.21
Nosophobia F45.22
Nostalgia F43.20
Notch of iris Q13.2
Notching nose, congenital (tip) Q30.2
Nothnagel's
  syndrome — *see* Strabismus, paralytic, third nerve
  vasomotor acroparesthesia I73.89
Novy's relapsing fever A68.9
  louse-borne A68.0
  tick-borne A68.1
Noxious
  foodstuffs, poisoning by — *see* Poisoning, food, noxious, plant
  substances transmitted through placenta or breast milk P04.9
Nucleus pulposus — *see* condition
Numbness R20.0
Nuns' knee — *see* Bursitis, prepatellar
Nursemaid's elbow S53.03- ☑
Nutcracker esophagus K22.4
Nutmeg liver K76.1
Nutrient element deficiency E61.9
  specified NEC E61.8
Nutrition deficient or insufficient (*see also* Malnutrition) E46
  due to
    insufficient food T73.0 ☑
    lack of
      care (child) T76.02 ☑
        adult T76.01 ☑
      food T73.0 ☑
Nutritional stunting E45
Nyctalopia (night blindness) — *see* Blindness, night
Nycturia R35.1
  psychogenic F45.8
Nymphomania F52.8

Nystagmus H55.00
  benign paroxysmal — *see* Vertigo, benign paroxysmal
  central positional H81.4- ☑
  congenital H55.01
  dissociated H55.04
  latent H55.02
  miners' H55.09
  positional
    benign paroxysmal H81.4- ☑
    central H81.4- ☑
  specified form NEC H55.09
  visual deprivation H55.03

O

Obermeyer's relapsing fever (European) A68.0
Obesity E66.9
  with alveolar hyperventilation E66.2
  adrenal E27.8
  complicating
    childbirth O99.214
    pregnancy O99.21- ☑
    puerperium O99.215
  constitutional E66.8
  dietary counseling and surveillance Z71.3
  drug-induced E66.1
  due to
    drug E66.1
    excess calories E66.09
      morbid E66.01
      severe E66.01
  endocrine E66.8
  endogenous E66.8
  familial E66.8
  glandular E66.8
  hypothyroid — *see* Hypothyroidism
  morbid E66.01
    with alveolar hypoventilation E66.2
    due to excess calories E66.01
  nutritional E66.09
  pituitary E23.6
  severe E66.01
  specified type NEC E66.8
Oblique — *see* condition
Obliteration
  appendix (lumen) K38.8
  artery I77.1
  bile duct (noncalculous) K83.1
  common duct (noncalculous) K83.1
  cystic duct — *see* Obstruction, gallbladder
  disease, arteriolar I77.1
  endometrium N85.8
  eye, anterior chamber — *see* Disorder, globe, hypotony
  fallopian tube N97.1
  lymphatic vessel I89.0
    due to mastectomy I97.2
  organ or site, congenital NEC — *see* Atresia, by site
  ureter N13.5
    with infection N13.6
  urethra — *see* Stricture, urethra
  vein I87.8
  vestibule (oral) K08.8
Observation (following) (for) (without need for further medical care) Z04.9
  accident NEC Z04.3
    at work Z04.2
    transport Z04.1
  adverse effect of drug Z03.6
  alleged rape or sexual assault (victim), ruled out
    adult Z04.41
    child Z04.42
  criminal assault Z04.8
  development state
    adolescent Z00.3
    period of rapid growth in childhood Z00.2
    puberty Z00.3
  disease, specified NEC Z03.89
  following work accident Z04.2
  growth and development state — *see* Observation, development state
  injuries (accidental) NEC (*see also* Observation, accident)
  newborn (for suspected condition, ruled out) — *see* - Newborn, affected by (suspected to be), maternal (complication of) (use of)
  postpartum

Observation — *continued*
  immediately after delivery Z39.0
  routine follow-up Z39.2
  pregnancy (normal) (without complication) Z34.9- ☑
    high risk O09.9- ☑
  suicide attempt, alleged NEC Z03.89
    self-poisoning Z03.6
  suspected, ruled out (*see also* Suspected condition, ruled out)
    abuse, physical
      adult Z04.71
      child Z04.72
    accident at work Z04.2
    adult battering victim Z04.71
    child battering victim Z04.72
    condition NEC Z03.89
      newborn — *see* - Newborn, affected by (suspected to be), maternal (complication of) (use of)
    drug poisoning or adverse effect Z03.6
    exposure (to)
      anthrax Z03.810
      biological agent NEC Z03.818
    inflicted injury NEC Z04.8
    suicide attempt, alleged Z03.89
      self-poisoning Z03.6
    toxic effects from ingested substance (drug) (poison) Z03.6
  toxic effects from ingested substance (drug) (poison) Z03.6
Obsession, obsessional state F42
Obsessive-compulsive neurosis or reaction F42
Obstetric embolism, septic — *see* Embolism, obstetric, septic
Obstetrical trauma (complicating delivery) O71.9
  with or following ectopic or molar pregnancy O08.6
  specified type NEC O71.89
Obstipation — *see* Constipation
Obstruction, obstructed, obstructive
  airway J98.8
    with
      allergic alveolitis J67.9
      asthma J45.909
        with
          exacerbation (acute) J45.901
          status asthmaticus J45.902
      bronchiectasis J47.9
        with
          exacerbation (acute) J47.1
          lower respiratory infection J47.0
      bronchitis (chronic) J44.9
      emphysema J43.9
    chronic J44.9
      with
        allergic alveolitis — *see* Pneumonitis, hypersensitivity
        bronchiectasis J47.9
          with
            exacerbation (acute) J47.1
            lower respiratory infection J47.0
    due to
      foreign body — *see* Foreign body, by site, causing asphyxia
      inhalation of fumes or vapors J68.9
      laryngospasm J38.5
  ampulla of Vater K83.1
  aortic (heart) (valve) — *see* Stenosis, aortic
  aortoiliac I74.09
  aqueduct of Sylvius G91.1
    congenital Q03.0
      with spina bifida — *see* Spina bifida, by site, with hydrocephalus
  Arnold-Chiari — *see* Arnold-Chiari disease
  artery (*see also* Embolism, artery) I74.9
    basilar (complete) (partial) — *see* Occlusion, artery, basilar
    carotid (complete) (partial) — *see* Occlusion, artery, carotid
    cerebellar (complete) (partial) — *see* Occlusion, artery, cerebellar
    cerebral (anterior) (middle) (posterior) — *see* Occlusion, artery, cerebral
    precerebral — *see* Occlusion, artery, precerebral
    renal N28.0
    retinal NEC — *see* Occlusion, artery, retina
    vertebral (complete) (partial) — *see* Occlusion, artery, vertebral
  band (intestinal) K56.69
  bile duct or passage (common) (hepatic) (noncalculous) K83.1
    with calculus K80.51

☑ **Additional character required**

Obstruction — *continued*
    congenital (causing jaundice) Q44.3
  biliary (duct) (tract) K83.1
    gallbladder K82.0
  bladder-neck (acquired) N32.0
    congenital Q64.31
    due to hyperplasia (hypertrophy) of prostate — *see* Hyperplasia, prostate
  bowel — *see* Obstruction, intestine
  bronchus J98.09
  canal, ear — *see* Stenosis, external ear canal
  cardia K22.2
  caval veins (inferior) (superior) I87.1
  cecum — *see* Obstruction, intestine
  circulatory I99.8
  colon — *see* Obstruction, intestine
  common duct (noncalculous) K83.1
  coronary (artery) — *see* Occlusion, coronary
  cystic duct (*see also* Obstruction, gallbladder)
    with calculus K80.21
  device, implant or graft (*see also* Complications, by site and type, mechanical) T85.698 ☑
    arterial graft NEC — *see* Complication, cardiovascular device, mechanical, vascular
    catheter NEC T85.628 ☑
      cystostomy T83.090 ☑
      dialysis (renal) T82.49 ☑
        intraperitoneal T85.691 ☑
      infusion NEC T82.594 ☑
        spinal (epidural) (subdural) T85.690 ☑
      urinary, indwelling T83.098 ☑
      due to infection T85.79 ☑
    gastrointestinal — *see* Complications, prosthetic device, mechanical, gastrointestinal device
    genital NEC T83.498 ☑
      intrauterine contraceptive device T83.39 ☑
      penile prosthesis T83.490 ☑
    heart NEC — *see* Complication, cardiovascular device, mechanical
    joint prosthesis — *see* Complications, joint prosthesis, mechanical, specified NEC, by site
    orthopedic NEC — *see* Complication, orthopedic, device, mechanical
    specified NEC T85.628 ☑
    urinary NEC (*see also* Complication, genitourinary, device, urinary, mechanical)
      graft T83.29 ☑
    vascular NEC — *see* Complication, cardiovascular device, mechanical
    ventricular intracranial shunt T85.09 ☑
  due to foreign body accidentally left in operative wound T81.529 ☑
  duodenum K31.5
  ejaculatory duct N50.8
  esophagus K22.2
  eustachian tube (complete) (partial) H68.10- ☑
    cartilagenous (extrinsic) H68.13- ☑
      intrinsic H68.12- ☑
    osseous H68.11- ☑
  fallopian tube (bilateral) N97.1
  fecal K56.41
    with hernia — *see* Hernia, by site, with obstruction
  foramen of Monro (congenital) Q03.8
    with spina bifida — *see* Spina bifida, by site, with hydrocephalus
  foreign body — *see* Foreign body
  gallbladder K82.0
    with calculus, stones K80.21
    congenital Q44.1
  gastric outlet K31.1
  gastrointestinal — *see* Obstruction, intestine
  hepatic K76.89
    duct (noncalculous) K83.1
  hepatobiliary K83.1
  ileum — *see* Obstruction, intestine
  iliofemoral (artery) I74.5
  intestine K56.60
    with
      adhesions (intestinal) (peritoneal) K56.5
    adynamic K56.0
    by gallstone K56.3
    congenital (small) Q41.9
      large Q42.9
        specified part NEC Q42.8
    neurogenic K56.0
      Hirschsprung's disease or megacolon Q43.1
    newborn P76.9
      due to
        fecaliths P76.8

Obstruction — *continued*
    inspissated milk P76.2
    meconium (plug) P76.0
      in mucoviscidosis E84.11
    specified NEC P76.8
    postoperative K91.3
    reflex K56.0
    specified NEC K56.69
    volvulus K56.2
  intracardiac ball valve prosthesis T82.09 ☑
  jejunum — *see* Obstruction, intestine
  joint prosthesis — *see* Complications, joint prosthesis, mechanical, specified NEC, by site
  kidney (calices) N28.89
  labor — *see* Delivery
  lacrimal (passages) (duct)
    by
      dacryolith — *see* Dacryolith
      stenosis — *see* Stenosis, lacrimal
    congenital Q10.5
    neonatal H04.53- ☑
  lacrimonasal duct — *see* Obstruction, lacrimal
  lacteal, with steatorrhea K90.2
  laryngitis — *see* Laryngitis
  larynx NEC J38.6
    congenital Q31.8
  lung J98.4
    disease, chronic J44.9
  lymphatic I89.0
  meconium (plug)
    newborn P76.0
      due to fecaliths P76.0
      in mucoviscidosis E84.11
  mitral — *see* Stenosis, mitral
  nasal J34.89
  nasolacrimal duct (*see also* Obstruction, lacrimal)
    congenital Q10.5
  nasopharynx J39.2
  nose J34.89
  organ or site, congenital NEC — *see* Atresia, by site
  pancreatic duct K86.8
  parotid duct or gland K11.8
  pelviureteral junction N13.5
    congenital Q62.39
  pharynx J39.2
  portal (circulation) (vein) I81
  prostate (*see also* Hyperplasia, prostate)
    valve (urinary) N32.0
  pulmonary valve (heart) I37.0
  pyelonephritis (chronic) N11.1
  pylorus
    adult K31.1
    congenital or infantile Q40.0
  rectosigmoid — *see* Obstruction, intestine
  rectum K62.4
  renal N28.89
    outflow N13.8
    pelvis, congenital Q62.39
  respiratory J98.8
    chronic J44.9
  retinal (vessels) H34.9
  salivary duct (any) K11.8
    with calculus K11.5
  sigmoid — *see* Obstruction, intestine
  sinus (accessory) (nasal) J34.89
  Stensen's duct K11.8
  stomach NEC K31.89
    acute K31.0
    congenital Q40.2
    due to pylorospasm K31.3
  submandibular duct K11.8
  submaxillary gland K11.8
    with calculus K11.5
  thoracic duct I89.0
  thrombotic — *see* Thrombosis
  trachea J39.8
  tracheostomy airway J95.03
  tricuspid (valve) — *see* Stenosis, tricuspid
  upper respiratory, congenital Q34.8
  ureter (functional) (pelvic junction) NEC N13.5
    with
      hydronephrosis N13.1
        with infection N13.6
      pyelonephritis (chronic) N11.1
    congenital Q62.39
    due to calculus — *see* Calculus, ureter
  urethra NEC N36.8
    congenital Q64.39
  urinary (moderate) N13.9
    due to hyperplasia (hypertrophy) of prostate — *see* Hyperplasia, prostate

Obstruction — *continued*
    organ or tract (lower) N13.9
    prostatic valve N32.0
    specified NEC N13.8
  uropathy N13.9
  uterus N85.8
  vagina N89.5
  valvular — *see* Endocarditis
  vein, venous I87.1
    caval (inferior) (superior) I87.1
    thrombotic — *see* Thrombosis
  vena cava (inferior) (superior) I87.1
  vesical NEC N32.0
  vesicourethral orifice N32.0
    congenital Q64.31
  vessel NEC I99.8
Obturator — *see* condition
Occlusal wear, teeth K03.0
Occlusio pupillae — *see* Membrane, pupillary
Occlusion, occluded
  anus K62.4
    congenital Q42.3
      with fistula Q42.2
  aortoiliac (chronic) I74.09
  aqueduct of Sylvius G91.1
    congenital Q03.0
      with spina bifida — *see* Spina bifida, by site, with hydrocephalus
  artery (*see also* Embolism, artery) I74.9
    auditory, internal I65.8
    basilar I65.1
      with
        infarction I63.22
        due to
          embolism I63.12
          thrombosis I63.02
    brain or cerebral I66.9
      with infarction (due to) I63.5 ☑
        embolism I63.4 ☑
        thrombosis I63.3 ☑
    carotid I65.2- ☑
      with
        infarction I63.23- ☑
        due to
          embolism I63.13- ☑
          thrombosis I63.03- ☑
    cerebellar (anterior inferior) (posterior inferior) (superior) I66.3
      with infarction I63.54- ☑
        due to
          embolism I63.44- ☑
          thrombosis I63.34- ☑
    cerebral I66.9
      with infarction I63.50
        due to
          embolism I63.40
            specified NEC I63.49
          thrombosis I63.30
            specified NEC I63.39
      anterior I66.1- ☑
        with infarction I63.52- ☑
          due to
            embolism I63.42- ☑
            thrombosis I63.32- ☑
      middle I66.0- ☑
        with infarction I63.51- ☑
          due to
            embolism I63.41- ☑
            thrombosis I63.31- ☑
      posterior I66.2- ☑
        with infarction I63.53- ☑
          due to
            embolism I63.43- ☑
            thrombosis I63.33- ☑
      specified NEC I66.8
        with infarction I63.59
          due to
            embolism I63.4 ☑
            thrombosis I63.3 ☑
    choroidal (anterior) — *see* Occlusion, artery, precerebral, specified NEC
    communicating posterior — *see* Occlusion, artery, cerebral, specified NEC
  complete
    coronary I25.82
    extremities I70.92
  coronary (acute) (thrombotic) (without myocardial infarction) I24.0
    with myocardial infarction — *see* Infarction, myocardium
    chronic total I25.82
    complete I25.82

Occlusion — *continued*
  healed or old I25.2
    total (chronic) I25.82
  hypophyseal — *see* Occlusion, artery, precerebral, specified NEC
  iliac I74.5
  lower extremities due to stenosis or stricture I77.1
  mesenteric (embolic) (thrombotic) K55.0
  perforating — *see* Occlusion, artery, cerebral, specified NEC
  peripheral I77.9
    thrombotic or embolic I74.4
  pontine — *see* Occlusion, artery, cerebral, specified NEC
  precerebral I65.9
    with infarction I63.20
      specified NEC I63.29
      due to
        embolism I63.10
          specified NEC I63.19
        thrombosis I63.00
          specified NEC I63.09
    basilar — *see* Occlusion, artery, basilar
    carotid — *see* Occlusion, artery, carotid
    puerperal O88.23
    specified NEC I65.8
      with infarction I63.29
      due to
        embolism I63.19
        thrombosis I63.00
    vertebral — *see* Occlusion, artery, vertebral
  renal N28.0
  retinal
    central H34.1- ☑
    partial H34.21- ☑
    branch H34.23- ☑
    transient H34.0- ☑
  spinal — *see* Occlusion, artery, precerebral, vertebral
  total (chronic)
    coronary I25.82
    extremities I70.92
  vertebral I65.0- ☑
    with
      infarction I63.21- ☑
      due to
        embolism I63.11- ☑
        thrombosis I63.01- ☑
  basilar artery — *see* Occlusion, artery, basilar
  bile duct (common) (hepatic) (noncalculous) K83.1
  bowel — *see* Obstruction, intestine
  carotid (artery) (common) (internal) — *see* Occlusion, artery, carotid
  centric (of teeth) M26.59
    maximum intercuspation discrepancy M26.55
  cerebellar (artery) — *see* Occlusion, artery, cerebellar
  cerebral (artery) — *see* Occlusion, artery, cerebral
  cerebrovascular (*see also* Occlusion, artery, cerebral)
    with infarction I63.5 ☑
  cervical canal — *see* Stricture, cervix
  cervix (uteri) — *see* Stricture, cervix
  choanal Q30.0
  choroidal (artery) — *see* Occlusion, artery, precerebral, specified NEC
  colon — *see* Obstruction, intestine
  communicating posterior artery — *see* Occlusion, artery, precerebral, specified NEC
  coronary (artery) (vein) (thrombotic) (*see also* Infarct, myocardium)
    chronic total I25.82
    healed or old I25.2
    not resulting in infarction I24.0
    total (chronic) I25.82
  cystic duct — *see* Obstruction, gallbladder
  embolic — *see* Embolism
  fallopian tube N97.1
    congenital Q50.6
  gallbladder (*see also* Obstruction, gallbladder)
    congenital (causing jaundice) Q44.1
  gingiva, traumatic K06.2
  hymen N89.6
    congenital Q52.3
  hypophyseal (artery) — *see* Occlusion, artery, precerebral, specified NEC
  iliac artery I74.5
  intestine — *see* Obstruction, intestine
  lacrimal passages — *see* Obstruction, lacrimal
  lung J98.4

Occlusion — *continued*
  lymph or lymphatic channel I89.0
  mammary duct N64.89
  mesenteric artery (embolic) (thrombotic) K55.0
  nose J34.89
    congenital Q30.0
  organ or site, congenital NEC — *see* Atresia, by site
  oviduct N97.1
    congenital Q50.6
  peripheral arteries
    due to stricture or stenosis I77.1
    upper extremity I74.2
  pontine (artery) — *see* Occlusion, artery, precerebral, specified NEC
  posterior lingual, of mandibular teeth M26.29
  precerebral artery — *see* Occlusion, artery, precerebral
  punctum lacrimale — *see* Obstruction, lacrimal
  pupil — *see* Membrane, pupillary
  pylorus, adult (*see also* Stricture, pylorus) K31.1
  renal artery N28.0
  retina, retinal
    artery — *see* Occlusion, artery, retinal
    vein (central) H34.81- ☑
      engorgement H34.82- ☑
      tributary H34.83- ☑
    vessels H34.9
  spinal artery — *see* Occlusion, artery, precerebral, vertebral
  teeth (mandibular) (posterior lingual) M26.29
  thoracic duct I89.0
  thrombotic — *see* Thrombosis, artery
  traumatic
    edentulous (alveolar) ridge K06.2
    gingiva K06.2
    periodontal K05.5
  tubal N97.1
  ureter (complete) (partial) N13.5
    congenital Q62.10
  ureteropelvic junction N13.5
    congenital Q62.10
  ureterovesical orifice N13.5
    congenital Q62.12
  urethra — *see* Stricture, urethra
  uterus N85.8
  vagina N89.5
  vascular NEC I99.8
  vein — *see* Thrombosis
    retinal — *see* Occlusion, retinal, vein
  vena cava (inferior) (superior) — *see* Embolism, vena cava
  ventricle (brain) NEC G91.1
  vertebral (artery) — *see* Occlusion, artery, vertebral
  vessel (blood) I99.8
  vulva N90.5
Occult
  blood in feces (stools) R19.5
Occupational
  problems NEC Z56.89
Ochlophobia — *see* Agoraphobia
Ochronosis (endogenous) E70.29
Ocular muscle — *see* condition
Oculogyric crisis or disturbance H51.8
  psychogenic F45.8
Oculomotor syndrome H51.9
Oculopathy
  syphilitic NEC A52.71
    congenital
      early A50.01
      late A50.30
    early (secondary) A51.43
    late A52.71
Oddi's sphincter spasm K83.4
Odontalgia K08.8
Odontoameloblastoma — *see* Cyst, calcifying odontogenic
Odontoclasia K03.89
Odontodysplasia, regional K00.4
Odontogenesis imperfecta K00.5
Odontoma (ameloblastic) (complex) (compound) (fibroameloblastic) — *see* Cyst, calcifying odontogenic
Odontomyelitis (closed) (open) K04.0
Odontorrhagia K08.8
Odontosarcoma, ameloblastic C41.1
  upper jaw (bone) C41.0
Oestriasis — *see* Myiasis
Oguchi's disease H53.63
Ohara's disease — *see* Tularemia
Oidiomycosis — *see* Candidiasis

Oidium albicans infection — *see* Candidiasis
Old age (without mention of debility) R54
  dementia F03 ☑
Old (previous) myocardial infarction I25.2
Olfactory — *see* condition
Oligemia — *see* Anemia
Oligoastrocytoma
  specified site — *see* Neoplasm, malignant, by site
  unspecified site C71.9
Oligocythemia D64.9
Oligodendroblastoma
  specified site — *see* Neoplasm, malignant
  unspecified site C71.9
Oligodendroglioma
  anaplastic type
    specified site — *see* Neoplasm, malignant, by site
    unspecified site C71.9
  specified site — *see* Neoplasm, malignant, by site
  unspecified site C71.9
Oligodontia — *see* Anodontia
Oligoencephalon Q02
Oligohidrosis L74.4
Oligohydramnios O41.0- ☑
Oligohydrosis L74.4
Oligomenorrhea N91.5
  primary N91.3
  secondary N91.4
Oligophrenia (*see also* Disability, intellectual)
  phenylpyruvic E70.0
Oligospermia N46.11
  due to
    drug therapy N46.121
    efferent duct obstruction N46.123
    infection N46.122
    radiation N46.124
    specified cause NEC N46.129
    systemic disease N46.125
Oligotrichia — *see* Alopecia
Oliguria R34
  with, complicating or following ectopic or molar pregnancy O08.4
  postprocedural N99.0
Ollier's disease Q78.4
Omentitis — *see* Peritonitis
Omenotocele — *see* Hernia, abdomen, specified site NEC
Omentum, omental — *see* condition
Omphalitis (congenital) (newborn) P38.9
  with mild hemorrhage P38.1
  without hemorrhage P38.9
  not of newborn L08.82
  tetanus A33
Omphalocele Q79.2
Omphalomesenteric duct, persistent Q43.0
Omphalorrhagia, newborn P51.9
Omsk hemorrhagic fever A98.1
Onanism (excessive) F98.8
Onchocerciasis, onchocercosis B73.1
  with
    eye disease B73.00
      endophthalmitis B73.01
      eyelid B73.09
      glaucoma B73.02
      specified NEC B73.09
    eye NEC B73.00
    eyelid B73.09
Oncocytoma — *see* Neoplasm, benign, by site
Oncovirus, as cause of disease classified elsewhere B97.32
Ondine's curse — *see* Apnea, sleep
Oneirophrenia F23
Onychauxis L60.2
  congenital Q84.5
Onychia (*see also* Cellulitis, digit)
  with lymphangitis — *see* Lymphangitis, acute, digit
  candidal B37.2
  dermatophytic B35.1
Onychitis (*see also* Cellulitis, digit)
  with lymphangitis — *see* Lymphangitis, acute, digit
Onychocryptosis L60.0
Onychodystrophy L60.3
  congenital Q84.6
Onychogryphosis, onychogryposis L60.2
Onycholysis L60.1
Onychomadesis L60.8
Onychomalacia L60.3
Onychomycosis (finger) (toe) B35.1
Onycho-osteodysplasia Q79.8
Onychophagia F98.8

☑ **Additional character required**

ICD-10-CM 2015   ICD-10-CM INDEX TO DISEASES AND INJURIES

Onychophosis - Osteitis

Onychophosis L60.8
Onychoptosis L60.8
Onychorrhexis L60.3
  congenital Q84.6
Onychoschizia L60.3
Onyxis (finger) (toe) L60.0
Onyxitis (see also Cellulitis, digit)
  with lymphangitis — see Lymphangitis, acute, digit
Oophoritis (cystic) (infectional) (interstitial) N70.92
  with salpingitis N70.93
  acute N70.02
    with salpingitis N70.03
  chronic N70.12
    with salpingitis N70.13
  complicating abortion — see Abortion, by type, complicated by, oophoritis
Oophorocele N83.4
Opacity, opacities
  cornea H17.- ☑
    central H17.1- ☑
    congenital Q13.3
    degenerative — see Degeneration, cornea
    hereditary — see Dystrophy, cornea
    inflammatory — see Keratitis
    minor H17.81- ☑
    peripheral H17.82- ☑
    sequelae of trachoma (healed) B94.0
    specified NEC H17.89
  enamel (teeth) (fluoride) (nonfluoride) K00.3
  lens — see Cataract
  snowball — see Deposit, crystalline
  vitreous (humor) NEC H43.39- ☑
    congenital Q14.0
    membranes and strands H43.31- ☑
Opalescent dentin (hereditary) K00.5
Open, opening
  abnormal, organ or site, congenital — see Imperfect, closure
  angle with
    borderline
      findings
        high risk H40.02- ☑
        low risk H40.01- ☑
      intraocular pressure H40.00- ☑
    cupping of discs H40.01- ☑
    glaucoma (primary) — see Glaucoma, open angle
  bite
    anterior M26.220
    posterior M26.221
  false — see Imperfect, closure
  margin on tooth restoration K08.51
  restoration margins of tooth K08.51
  wound — see Wound, open
Operational fatigue F48.8
Operative — see condition
Operculitis — see Periodontitis
Operculum — see Break, retina
Ophiasis L63.2
Ophthalmia (see also Conjunctivitis) H10.9
  actinic rays — see Photokeratitis
  allergic (acute) — see Conjunctivitis, acute, atopic
  blennorrhagic (gonococcal) (neonatorum) A54.31
  diphtheritic A36.86
  Egyptian A71.1
  electrica — see Photokeratitis
  gonococcal (neonatorum) A54.31
  metastatic — see Endophthalmitis, purulent
  migraine — see Migraine, ophthalmoplegic
  neonatorum, newborn P39.1
    gonococcal A54.31
  nodosa H16.24- ☑
  purulent — see Conjunctivitis, acute, mucopurulent
  spring — see Conjunctivitis, acute, atopic
  sympathetic — see Uveitis, sympathetic
Ophthalmitis — see Ophthalmia
Ophthalmocele (congenital) Q15.8
Ophthalmoneuromyelitis G36.0
Ophthalmoplegia (see also Strabismus, paralytic)
  anterior internuclear — see Ophthalmoplegia, internuclear
  ataxia-areflexia G61.0
  diabetic — see E08-E13 with .39
  exophthalmic E05.00
    with thyroid storm E05.01
  external H49.88- ☑
    progressive H49.4- ☑
      with pigmentary retinopathy — see Kearns-Sayre syndrome
    total H49.3- ☑

Ophthalmoplegia — continued
  internal (complete) (total) H52.51- ☑
  internuclear H51.2- ☑
  migraine — see Migraine, ophthalmoplegic
  Parinaud's H49.88- ☑
  progressive external — see Ophthalmoplegia, external, progressive
  supranuclear, progressive G23.1
  total (external) — see Ophthalmoplegia, external, total
Opioid(s)
  abuse — see Abuse, drug, opioids
  dependence — see Dependence, drug, opioids
Opisthognathism M26.09
Opisthorchiasis (felineus) (viverrini) B66.0
Opitz' disease D73.2
Opiumism — see Dependence, drug, opioid
Oppenheim's disease G70.2
Oppenheim-Urbach disease (necrobiosis lipoidica diabeticorum) — see E08-E13 with .620
Optic nerve — see condition
Orbit — see condition
Orchioblastoma C62.9- ☑
Orchitis (gangrenous) (nonspecific) (septic) (suppurative) N45.2
  blennorrhagic (gonococcal) (acute) (chronic) A54.23
  chlamydial A56.19
  filarial (see also Infestation, filarial) B74.9 [N51]
  gonococcal (acute) (chronic) A54.23
  mumps B26.0
  syphilitic A52.76
  tuberculous A18.15
Orf (virus disease) B08.02
Organic (see also condition)
  brain syndrome F09
  heart — see Disease, heart
  mental disorder F09
  psychosis F09
Orgasm
  anejaculatory N53.13
Oriental
  bilharziasis B65.2
  schistosomiasis B65.2
Orifice — see condition
Origin of both great vessels from right ventricle Q20.1
Ormond's disease (with ureteral obstruction) N13.5
  with infection N13.6
Ornithine metabolism disorder E72.4
Ornithinemia (Type I) (Type II) E72.4
Ornithosis A70
Orotaciduria, oroticaciduria (congenital) (hereditary) (pyrimidine deficiency) E79.8
  anemia D53.0
Orthodontics
  adjustment Z46.4
  fitting Z46.4
Orthopnea R06.01
Orthopoxvirus B08.09
  specified NEC B08.09
Os, uterus — see condition
Osgood-Schlatter disease or osteochondrosis — see Osteochondrosis, juvenile, tibia
Osler (-Weber)-Rendu disease I78.0
Osler's nodes I33.0
Osmidrosis L75.0
Osseous — see condition
Ossification
  artery — see Arteriosclerosis
  auricle (ear) — see Disorder, pinna, specified type NEC
  bronchial J98.09
  cardiac — see Degeneration, myocardial
  cartilage (senile) — see Disorder, cartilage, specified type NEC
  coronary (artery) — see Disease, heart, ischemic, atherosclerotic
  diaphragm J98.6
  ear, middle — see Otosclerosis
  falx cerebri G96.19
  fontanel, premature Q75.0
  heart (see also Degeneration, myocardial)
    valve — see Endocarditis
  larynx J38.7
  ligament — see Disorder, tendon, specified type NEC
    posterior longitudinal — see Spondylopathy, specified NEC
  meninges (cerebral) (spinal) G96.19
  multiple, eccentric centers — see Disorder, bone, development or growth

Ossification — continued
  muscle (see also Calcification, muscle)
    due to burns — see Myositis, ossificans, in, burns
    paralytic — see Myositis, ossificans, in, quadriplegia
    progressive — see Myositis, ossificans, progressiva
    specified NEC M61.50
      ankle M61.57- ☑
      foot M61.57- ☑
      forearm M61.53- ☑
      hand M61.54- ☑
      lower leg M61.56- ☑
      multiple sites M61.59
      pelvic region M61.55- ☑
      shoulder region M61.51- ☑
      specified site NEC M61.58
      thigh M61.55- ☑
      upper arm M61.52- ☑
    traumatic — see Myositis, ossificans, traumatica
  myocardium, myocardial — see Degeneration, myocardial
  penis N48.89
  periarticular — see Disorder, joint, specified type NEC
  pinna — see Disorder, pinna, specified type NEC
  rider's bone — see Ossification, muscle, specified NEC
  sclera H15.89
  subperiosteal, post-traumatic M89.8X- ☑
  tendon — see Disorder, tendon, specified type NEC
  trachea J39.8
  tympanic membrane — see Disorder, tympanic membrane, specified NEC
  vitreous (humor) — see Deposit, crystalline
Osteitis (see also Osteomyelitis)
  alveolar M27.3
  condensans M85.30
    ankle M85.37- ☑
    foot M85.37- ☑
    forearm M85.33- ☑
    hand M85.34- ☑
    lower leg M85.36- ☑
    multiple site M85.39
    neck M85.38
    rib M85.38
    shoulder M85.31- ☑
    skull M85.38
    specified site NEC M85.38
    thigh M85.35- ☑
    toe M85.37- ☑
    upper arm M85.32- ☑
    vertebra M85.38
  deformans M88.9
    in (due to)
      malignant neoplasm of bone C41.9 [M90.60]
      neoplastic disease (see also Neoplasm) D49.9 [M90.60]
        carpus D49.9 [M90.64- ☑]
        clavicle D49.9 [M90.61- ☑]
        femur D49.9 [M90.65- ☑]
        fibula D49.9 [M90.66- ☑]
        finger D49.9 [M90.64- ☑]
        humerus D49.9 [M90.62- ☑]
        ilium D49.9 [M90.65- ☑]
        ischium D49.9 [M90.65- ☑]
        metacarpus D49.9 [M90.64- ☑]
        metatarsus D49.9 [M90.67- ☑]
        multiple sites D49.9 [M90.69]
        neck D49.9 [M90.68]
        radius D49.9 [M90.63- ☑]
        rib D49.9 [M90.68]
        scapula D49.9 [M90.61- ☑]
        skull D49.9 [M90.68]
        tarsus D49.9 [M90.67- ☑]
        tibia D49.9 [M90.66- ☑]
        toe D49.9 [M90.67- ☑]
        ulna D49.9 [M90.63- ☑]
        vertebra D49.9 [M90.68]
    skull M88.0
    specified NEC — see Paget's disease, bone, by site
    vertebra M88.1
  due to yaws A66.6
  fibrosa NEC — see Cyst, bone, by site
    circumscripta — see Dysplasia, fibrous, bone NEC
    cystica (generalisata) E21.0
    disseminata Q78.1
    osteoplastica E21.0

ICD-10-CM 2015   ICD-10-CM INDEX TO DISEASES AND INJURIES

Osteitis - Osteochondrosis

Osteitis — *continued*
 fragilitans Q78.0
 Garr's (sclerosing) — *see* Osteomyelitis, specified type NEC
 jaw (acute) (chronic) (lower) (suppurative) (upper) M27.2
 parathyroid E21.0
 petrous bone (acute) (chronic) — *see* Petrositis
 sclerotic, nonsuppurative — *see* Osteomyelitis, specified type NEC
 tuberculosa A18.09
  cystica D86.89
  multiplex cystoides D86.89
Osteoarthritis M19.90
 ankle M19.07- ☑
 elbow M19.02- ☑
 foot joint M19.07- ☑
 generalized M15.9
  erosive M15.4
  primary M15.0
  specified NEC M15.8
 hand joint M19.04- ☑
  first carpometacarpal joint M18.9
 hip M16.1- ☑
  bilateral M16.0
  due to hip dysplasia (unilateral) M16.3- ☑
   bilateral M16.2
 interphalangeal
  distal (Heberden) M15.1
  proximal (Bouchard) M15.2
 knee M17.9
  bilateral M17.0
 shoulder M19.01- ☑
 spine — *see* Spondylosis
 wrist M19.03- ☑
 post-traumatic NEC M19.92
  ankle M19.17- ☑
  elbow M19.12- ☑
  foot joint M19.17- ☑
  hand joint M19.14- ☑
   first carpometacarpal joint M18.3- ☑
    bilateral M18.2
  hip M16.5- ☑
   bilateral M16.4
  knee M17.3- ☑
   bilateral M17.2
  shoulder M19.11- ☑
  wrist M19.13- ☑
 primary M19.91
  ankle M19.07- ☑
  elbow M19.02- ☑
  foot joint M19.07- ☑
  hand joint M19.04- ☑
   first carpometacarpal joint M18.1- ☑
    bilateral M18.0
  hip M16.1- ☑
   bilateral M16.0
  knee M17.1- ☑
   bilateral M17.0
  shoulder M19.01- ☑
  spine — *see* Spondylosis
  wrist M19.03- ☑
 secondary M19.93
  ankle M19.27- ☑
  elbow M19.22- ☑
  foot joint M19.27- ☑
  hand joint M19.24- ☑
   first carpometacarpal joint M18.5- ☑
    bilateral M18.4
  hip M16.7
   bilateral M16.6
  knee M17.5
   bilateral M17.4
  multiple M15.3
  shoulder M19.21- ☑
  spine — *see* Spondylosis
  wrist M19.23- ☑
Osteoarthropathy (hypertrophic) M19.90
 ankle — *see* Osteoarthritis, primary, ankle
 elbow — *see* Osteoarthritis, primary, elbow
 foot joint — *see* Osteoarthritis, primary, foot
 hand joint — *see* Osteoarthritis, primary, hand joint
 knee joint — *see* Osteoarthritis, primary, knee
 multiple site — *see* Osteoarthritis, primary, multiple joint
 pulmonary (*see also* Osteoarthropathy, specified type NEC)
  hypertrophic — *see* Osteoarthropathy, hypertrophic, specified type NEC
  secondary hypertrophic — *see* Osteoarthropathy, specified type NEC

Osteoarthropathy — *continued*
 shoulder — *see* Osteoarthritis, primary, shoulder
 specified joint NEC — *see* Osteoarthritis, primary, specified joint NEC
 specified type NEC M89.40
  carpus M89.44- ☑
  clavicle M89.41- ☑
  femur M89.45- ☑
  fibula M89.46- ☑
  finger M89.44- ☑
  humerus M89.42- ☑
  ilium M89.459
  ischium M89.459
  metacarpus M89.44- ☑
  metatarsus M89.47- ☑
  multiple sites M89.49
  neck M89.48
  radius M89.43- ☑
  rib M89.48
  scapula M89.41- ☑
  skull M89.48
  tarsus M89.47- ☑
  tibia M89.46- ☑
  toe M89.47- ☑
  ulna M89.43- ☑
  vertebra M89.48
 secondary — *see* Osteoarthropathy, specified type NEC
 spine — *see* Spondylosis
 wrist — *see* Osteoarthritis, primary, wrist
Osteoarthrosis (degenerative) (hypertrophic) (joint) (*see also* Osteoarthritis)
 deformans alkaptonurica E70.29 [M36.8]
 erosive M15.4
 generalized M15.9
  primary M15.0
 polyarticular M15.9
 spine — *see* Spondylosis
Osteoblastoma — *see* Neoplasm, bone, benign
 aggressive — *see* Neoplasm, bone, uncertain behavior
Osteochondroarthrosis deformans endemica — *see* Disease, Kaschin-Beck
Osteochondritis (*see also* Osteochondropathy, by site)
 Brailsford's — *see* Osteochondrosis, juvenile, radius
 dissecans M93.20
  ankle M93.27- ☑
  elbow M93.22- ☑
  foot M93.27- ☑
  hand M93.24- ☑
  hip M93.25- ☑
  knee M93.26- ☑
  multiple sites M93.29
  shoulder joint M93.21- ☑
  specified site NEC M93.28
  wrist M93.23- ☑
 juvenile M92.9
  patellar — *see* Osteochondrosis, juvenile, patella
 syphilitic (congenital) (early) A50.02 [M90.80]
  ankle A50.02 [M90.87- ☑]
  elbow A50.02 [M90.82- ☑]
  foot A50.02 [M90.87- ☑]
  forearm A50.02 [M90.83- ☑]
  hand A50.02 [M90.84- ☑]
  hip A50.02 [M90.85- ☑]
  knee A50.02 [M90.86- ☑]
  multiple sites A50.02 [M90.89]
  shoulder joint A50.02 [M90.81- ☑]
  specified site NEC A50.02 [M90.88]
Osteochondrodysplasia Q78.9
 with defects of growth of tubular bones and spine Q77.9
 specified NEC Q77.8
 specified NEC Q78.8
Osteochondrodystrophy E78.9
Osteochondrolysis — *see* Osteochondritis, dissecans
Osteochondroma — *see* Neoplasm, bone, benign
Osteochondromatosis D48.0
 syndrome Q78.4
Osteochondromyxosarcoma — *see* Neoplasm, bone, malignant
Osteochondropathy M93.90
 ankle M93.97- ☑
 elbow M93.92- ☑
 foot M93.97- ☑
 hand M93.94- ☑
 hip M93.95- ☑
 Kienböck's disease of adults M93.1

Osteochondropathy — *continued*
 knee M93.96- ☑
 multiple joints M93.99
 osteochondritis dissecans — *see* Osteochondritis, dissecans
 osteochondrosis — *see* Osteochondrosis
 shoulder region M93.91- ☑
 slipped upper femoral epiphysis — *see* Slipped, epiphysis, upper femoral
 specified joint NEC M93.98
 specified type NEC M93.80
  ankle M93.87- ☑
  elbow M93.82- ☑
  foot M93.87- ☑
  hand M93.84- ☑
  hip M93.85- ☑
  knee M93.86- ☑
  multiple joints M93.89
  shoulder region M93.81- ☑
  specified joint NEC M93.88
  wrist M93.83- ☑
 syphilitic, congenital
  early A50.02 [M90.80]
  late A50.56 [M90.80]
 wrist M93.93- ☑
Osteochondrosarcoma — *see* Neoplasm, bone, malignant
Osteochondrosis (*see also* Osteochondropathy, by site)
 acetabulum (juvenile) M91.0
 adult — *see* Osteochondropathy, specified type NEC, by site
 astragalus (juvenile) — *see* Osteochondrosis, juvenile, tarsus
 Blount's — *see* Osteochondrosis, juvenile, tibia
 Buchanan's M91.0
 Burns' — *see* Osteochondrosis, juvenile, ulna
 calcaneus (juvenile) — *see* Osteochondrosis, juvenile, tarsus
 capitular epiphysis (femur) (juvenile) — *see* Legg-Calvé-Perthes disease
 carpal (juvenile) (lunate) (scaphoid) — *see* Osteochondrosis, juvenile, hand, carpal lunate
 adult M93.1
 coxae juvenilis — *see* Legg-Calvé-Perthes disease
 deformans juvenilis, coxae — *see* Legg-Calvé-Perthes disease
 Diaz's — *see* Osteochondrosis, juvenile, tarsus
 dissecans (knee) (shoulder) — *see* Osteochondritis, dissecans
 femoral capital epiphysis (juvenile) — *see* Legg-Calvé-Perthes disease
 femur (head), juvenile — *see* Legg-Calvé-Perthes disease
 fibula (juvenile) — *see* Osteochondrosis, juvenile, fibula
 foot NEC (juvenile) M92.8
 Freiberg's — *see* Osteochondrosis, juvenile, metatarsus
 Haas' (juvenile) — *see* Osteochondrosis, juvenile, humerus
 Haglund's — *see* Osteochondrosis, juvenile, tarsus
 hip (juvenile) — *see* Legg-Calvé-Perthes disease
 humerus (capitulum) (head) (juvenile) — *see* Osteochondrosis, juvenile, humerus
 ilium, iliac crest (juvenile) M91.0
 ischiopubic synchondrosis M91.0
 Iselin's — *see* Osteochondrosis, juvenile, metatarsus
 juvenile, juvenilis M92.9
  after congenital dislocation of hip reduction — *see* Osteochondrosis, juvenile, hip, specified NEC
  arm — *see* Osteochondrosis, juvenile, upper limb NEC
  capitular epiphysis (femur) — *see* Legg-Calvé-Perthes disease
  clavicle, sternal epiphysis — *see* Osteochondrosis, juvenile, upper limb NEC
  coxae — *see* Legg-Calvé-Perthes disease
  deformans M92.9
  fibula M92.5- ☑
  foot NEC M92.8
  hand M92.20- ☑
   carpal lunate M92.21- ☑
   metacarpal head M92.22- ☑
   specified site NEC M92.29- ☑
  head of femur — *see* Legg-Calvé-Perthes disease
  hip and pelvis M91.9- ☑

Osteochondrosis — *continued*
    coxa plana — *see* Coxa, plana
    femoral head — *see* Legg-Calvé-Perthes
      disease
    pelvis M91.0
    pseudocoxalgia — *see* Pseudocoxalgia
    specified NEC M91.8- ☑
    humerus M92.0- ☑
    limb
      lower NEC M92.8
      upper NEC — *see* Osteochondrosis, juvenile,
        upper limb NEC
    medial cuneiform bone — *see* Osteochondrosis,
      juvenile, tarsus
    metatarsus M92.7- ☑
    patella M92.4- ☑
    radius M92.1- ☑
    specified site NEC M92.8
    spine M42.00
      cervical region M42.02
      cervicothoracic region M42.03
      lumbar region M42.06
      lumbosacral region M42.07
      multiple sites M42.09
      occipito-atlanto-axial region M42.01
      sacrococcygeal region M42.08
      thoracic region M42.04
      thoracolumbar region M42.05
    tarsus M92.6- ☑
    tibia M92.5- ☑
    ulna M92.1- ☑
    upper limb NEC M92.3- ☑
    vertebra (body) (epiphyseal plates) (Calvé's)
      (Scheuermann's) — *see* Osteochondrosis,
      juvenile, spine
  Kienböck's — *see* Osteochondrosis, juvenile,
    hand, carpal lunate
    adult M93.1
  Köhler's
    patellar — *see* Osteochondrosis, juvenile,
      patella
    tarsal navicular — *see* Osteochondrosis,
      juvenile, tarsus
  Legg-Perthes (-Calvé)(-Waldenström) — *see* Legg-
    Calvé-Perthes disease
  limb
    lower NEC (juvenile) M92.8
    upper NEC (juvenile) — *see* Osteochondrosis,
      juvenile, upper limb NEC
  lunate bone (carpal) (juvenile) (*see also*
    Osteochondrosis, juvenile, hand, carpal
    lunate)
    adult M93.1
  Mauclaire's — *see* Osteochondrosis, juvenile,
    hand, metacarpal
  metacarpal (head) (juvenile) — *see*
    Osteochondrosis, juvenile, hand, metacarpal
  metatarsus (fifth) (head) (juvenile) (second) — *see*
    Osteochondrosis, juvenile, metatarsus
  navicular (juvenile) — *see* Osteochondrosis,
    juvenile, tarsus
  os
    calcis (juvenile) — *see* Osteochondrosis,
      juvenile, tarsus
    tibiale externum (juvenile) — *see*
      Osteochondrosis, juvenile, tarsus
  Osgood-Schlatter — *see* Osteochondrosis,
    juvenile, tibia
  Panner's — *see* Osteochondrosis, juvenile,
    humerus
  patellar center (juvenile) (primary) (secondary) —
    see Osteochondrosis, juvenile, patella
  pelvis (juvenile) M91.0
  Pierson's M91.0
  radius (head) (juvenile) — *see* Osteochondrosis,
    juvenile, radius
  Scheuermann's — *see* Osteochondrosis, juvenile,
    spine
  Sever's — *see* Osteochondrosis, juvenile, tarsus
  Sinding-Larsen — *see* Osteochondrosis, juvenile,
    patella
  spine M42.9
    adult M42.10
      cervical region M42.12
      cervicothoracic region M42.13
      lumbar region M42.16
      lumbosacral region M42.17
      multiple sites M42.19
      occipito-atlanto-axial region M42.11
      sacrococcygeal region M42.18
      thoracic region M42.14
      thoracolumbar region M42.15

Osteochondrosis — *continued*
  juvenile — *see* Osteochondrosis, juvenile, spine
  symphysis pubis (juvenile) M91.0
  syphilitic (congenital) A50.02
  talus (juvenile) — *see* Osteochondrosis, juvenile,
    tarsus
  tarsus (navicular) (juvenile) — *see*
    Osteochondrosis, juvenile, tarsus
  tibia (proximal) (tubercle) (juvenile) — *see*
    Osteochondrosis, juvenile, tibia
  tuberculous — *see* Tuberculosis, bone
  ulna (lower) (juvenile) — *see* Osteochondrosis,
    juvenile, ulna
  van Neck's M91.0
  vertebral — *see* Osteochondrosis, spine
Osteoclastoma D48.0
  malignant — *see* Neoplasm, bone, malignant
Osteodynia — *see* Disorder, bone, specified type
  NEC
Osteodystrophy Q78.9
  azotemic N25.0
  congenital Q78.9
  parathyroid, secondary E21.1
  renal N25.0
Osteofibroma — *see* Neoplasm, bone, benign
Osteofibrosarcoma — *see* Neoplasm, bone,
  malignant
Osteogenesis imperfecta Q78.0
Osteogenic — *see* condition
Osteolysis M89.50
  carpus M89.54- ☑
  clavicle M89.51- ☑
  femur M89.55- ☑
  fibula M89.56- ☑
  finger M89.54- ☑
  humerus M89.52- ☑
  ilium M89.559
  ischium M89.559
  joint prosthesis (periprosthetic) — *see*
    Complications, joint prosthesis, mechanical,
    periprosthetic, osteolysis, by site
  metacarpus M89.54- ☑
  metatarsus M89.57- ☑
  multiple sites M89.59
  neck M89.58
  periprosthetic — *see* Complications, joint
    prosthesis, mechanical, periprosthetic,
    osteolysis, by site
  radius M89.53- ☑
  rib M89.58
  scapula M89.51- ☑
  skull M89.58
  tarsus M89.57- ☑
  tibia M89.56- ☑
  toe M89.57- ☑
  ulna M89.53- ☑
  vertebra M89.58
Osteoma (*see also* Neoplasm, bone, benign)
  osteoid (*see also* Neoplasm, bone, benign)
  giant — *see* Neoplasm, bone, benign
Osteomalacia M83.9
  adult M83.9
    drug-induced NEC M83.5
    due to
      malabsorption (postsurgical) M83.2
      malnutrition M83.3
    specified NEC M83.8
  aluminium-induced M83.4
  infantile — *see* Rickets
  juvenile — *see* Rickets
  oncogenic E83.89
  pelvis M83.8
  puerperal M83.0
  senile M83.1
  vitamin-D-resistant in adults E83.31 [M90.8- ☑]
    carpus E83.31 [M90.84- ☑]
    clavicle E83.31 [M90.81- ☑]
    femur E83.31 [M90.85- ☑]
    fibula E83.31 [M90.86- ☑]
    finger E83.31 [M90.84- ☑]
    humerus E83.31 [M90.82- ☑]
    ilium E83.31 [M90.859]
    ischium E83.31 [M90.859]
    metacarpus E83.31 [M90.84- ☑]
    metatarsus E83.31 [M90.87- ☑]
    multiple sites E83.31 [M90.89]
    neck E83.31 [M90.88]
    radius E83.31 [M90.83- ☑]
    rib E83.31 [M90.88]
    scapula E83.31 [M90.819]
    skull E83.31 [M90.88]
    tarsus E83.31 [M90.879]

Osteomalacia — *continued*
  tibia E83.31 [M90.869]
  toe E83.31 [M90.879]
  ulna E83.31 [M90.839]
  vertebra E83.31 [M90.88]
Osteomyelitis (general) (infective) (localized)
  (neonatal) (purulent) (septic) (staphylococcal)
  (streptococcal) (suppurative) (with periostitis)
  M86.9
  acute M86.10
    carpus M86.14- ☑
    clavicle M86.11- ☑
    femur M86.15- ☑
    fibula M86.16- ☑
    finger M86.14- ☑
    hematogenous M86.00
      carpus M86.04- ☑
      clavicle M86.01- ☑
      femur M86.05- ☑
      fibula M86.06- ☑
      finger M86.04- ☑
      humerus M86.02- ☑
      ilium M86.059
      ischium M86.059
      mandible M27.2
      metacarpus M86.04- ☑
      metatarsus M86.07- ☑
      multiple sites M86.09
      neck M86.08
      orbit H05.02- ☑
      petrous bone — *see* Petrositis
      radius M86.03- ☑
      rib M86.08
      scapula M86.01- ☑
      skull M86.08
      tarsus M86.07- ☑
      tibia M86.06- ☑
      toe M86.07- ☑
      ulna M86.03- ☑
      vertebra — *see* Osteomyelitis, vertebra
    humerus M86.12- ☑
    ilium M86.159
    ischium M86.159
    mandible M27.2
    metacarpus M86.14- ☑
    metatarsus M86.17- ☑
    multiple sites M86.19
    neck M86.18
    orbit H05.02- ☑
    petrous bone — *see* Petrositis
    radius M86.13- ☑
    rib M86.18
    scapula M86.11- ☑
    skull M86.18
    tarsus M86.17- ☑
    tibia M86.16- ☑
    toe M86.17- ☑
    ulna M86.13- ☑
    vertebra — *see* Osteomyelitis, vertebra
  chronic (or old) M86.60
    with draining sinus M86.40
      carpus M86.44- ☑
      clavicle M86.41- ☑
      femur M86.45- ☑
      fibula M86.46- ☑
      finger M86.44- ☑
      humerus M86.42- ☑
      ilium M86.459
      ischium M86.459
      mandible M27.2
      metacarpus M86.44- ☑
      metatarsus M86.47- ☑
      multiple sites M86.49
      neck M86.48
      orbit H05.02- ☑
      petrous bone — *see* Petrositis
      radius M86.43- ☑
      rib M86.48
      scapula M86.41- ☑
      skull M86.48
      tarsus M86.47- ☑
      tibia M86.46- ☑
      toe M86.47- ☑
      ulna M86.43- ☑
      vertebra — *see* Osteomyelitis, vertebra
    carpus M86.64- ☑
    clavicle M86.61- ☑
    femur M86.65- ☑
    fibula M86.66- ☑
    finger M86.64- ☑
    hematogenous NEC M86.50
      carpus M86.54- ☑

Osteomyelitis — *continued*
  clavicle M86.51- ☑
  femur M86.55- ☑
  fibula M86.56- ☑
  finger M86.54- ☑
  humerus M86.52- ☑
  ilium M86.559
  ischium M86.559
  mandible M27.2
  metacarpus M86.54- ☑
  metatarsus M86.57- ☑
  multifocal M86.30
    carpus M86.34- ☑
    clavicle M86.31- ☑
    femur M86.35- ☑
    fibula M86.36- ☑
    finger M86.34- ☑
    humerus M86.32- ☑
    ilium M86.359
    ischium M86.359
    metacarpus M86.34- ☑
    metatarsus M86.37- ☑
    multiple sites M86.39
    neck M86.38
    radius M86.33- ☑
    rib M86.38
    scapula M86.31- ☑
    skull M86.38
    tarsus M86.37- ☑
    tibia M86.36- ☑
    toe M86.37- ☑
    ulna M86.33- ☑
    vertebra — *see* Osteomyelitis, vertebra
  multiple sites M86.59
  neck M86.58
  orbit H05.02- ☑
  petrous bone — *see* Petrositis
  radius M86.53- ☑
  rib M86.58
  scapula M86.51- ☑
  skull M86.58
  tarsus M86.57- ☑
  tibia M86.56- ☑
  toe M86.57- ☑
  ulna M86.53- ☑
  vertebra — *see* Osteomyelitis, vertebra
  humerus M86.62- ☑
  ilium M86.659
  ischium M86.659
  mandible M27.2
  metacarpus M86.64- ☑
  metatarsus M86.67- ☑
  multifocal — *see* Osteomyelitis, chronic,
      hematogenous, multifocal
  multiple sites M86.69
  neck M86.68
  orbit H05.02- ☑
  petrous bone — *see* Petrositis
  radius M86.63- ☑
  rib M86.68
  scapula M86.61- ☑
  skull M86.68
  tarsus M86.67- ☑
  tibia M86.66- ☑
  toe M86.67- ☑
  ulna M86.63- ☑
  vertebra — *see* Osteomyelitis, vertebra
echinococcal B67.2
Garr's — *see* Osteomyelitis, specified type NEC
jaw (acute) (chronic) (lower) (neonatal)
    (suppurative) (upper) M27.2
nonsuppurating — *see* Osteomyelitis, specified
    type NEC
orbit H05.02- ☑
petrous bone — *see* Petrositis
Salmonella (arizonae) (cholerae-suis) (enteritidis)
    (typhimurium) A02.24
sclerosing, nonsuppurative — *see* Osteomyelitis,
    specified type NEC
specified type NEC (*see also* subcategory)
    M86.8X- ☑
  mandible M27.2
  orbit H05.02- ☑
  petrous bone — *see* Petrositis
  vertebra — *see* Osteomyelitis, vertebra
subacute M86.20
  carpus M86.24- ☑
  clavicle M86.21- ☑
  femur M86.25- ☑
  fibula M86.26- ☑
  finger M86.24- ☑
  humerus M86.22- ☑

Osteomyelitis — *continued*
  mandible M27.2
  metacarpus M86.24- ☑
  metatarsus M86.27- ☑
  multiple sites M86.29
  neck M86.28
  orbit H05.02- ☑
  petrous bone — *see* Petrositis
  radius M86.23- ☑
  rib M86.28
  scapula M86.21- ☑
  skull M86.28
  tarsus M86.27- ☑
  tibia M86.26- ☑
  toe M86.27- ☑
  ulna M86.23- ☑
  vertebra — *see* Osteomyelitis, vertebra
syphilitic A52.77
  congenital (early) A50.02 [M90.80]
tuberculous — *see* Tuberculosis, bone
typhoid A01.05
vertebra M46.20
  cervical region M46.22
  cervicothoracic region M46.23
  lumbar region M46.26
  lumbosacral region M46.27
  occipito-atlanto-axial region M46.21
  sacrococcygeal region M46.28
  thoracic region M46.24
  thoracolumbar region M46.25
Osteomyelofibrosis D75.89
Osteomyelosclerosis D75.89
Osteonecrosis M87.9
  due to
    drugs — *see* Osteonecrosis, secondary, due
        to, drugs
    trauma — *see* Osteonecrosis, secondary, due
        to, trauma
  idiopathic aseptic M87.00
    ankle M87.07- ☑
    carpus M87.03- ☑
    clavicle M87.01- ☑
    femur M87.05- ☑
    fibula M87.06- ☑
    finger M87.04- ☑
    humerus M87.02- ☑
    ilium M87.050
    ischium M87.050
    metacarpus M87.04- ☑
    metatarsus M87.07- ☑
    multiple sites M87.09
    neck M87.08
    pelvis M87.050
    radius M87.03- ☑
    rib M87.08
    scapula M87.01- ☑
    skull M87.08
    tarsus M87.07- ☑
    tibia M87.06- ☑
    toe M87.07- ☑
    ulna M87.03- ☑
    vertebra M87.08
  secondary NEC M87.30
    carpus M87.33- ☑
    clavicle M87.31- ☑
    due to
      drugs M87.10
        carpus M87.13- ☑
        clavicle M87.11- ☑
        femur M87.15- ☑
        fibula M87.16- ☑
        finger M87.14- ☑
        humerus M87.12- ☑
        ilium M87.159
        ischium M87.159
        jaw M87.180
        metacarpus M87.14- ☑
        metatarsus M87.17- ☑
        multiple sites M87.19
        neck M87.18
        radius M87.13- ☑
        rib M87.18
        scapula M87.11- ☑
        skull M87.18
        tarsus M87.17- ☑
        tibia M87.16- ☑
        toe M87.17- ☑
        ulna M87.13- ☑
        vertebra M87.18
      hemoglobinopathy NEC D58.2 [M90.50]
        carpus D58.2 [M90.54- ☑]
        clavicle D58.2 [M90.51- ☑]

Osteonecrosis — *continued*
    femur D58.2 [M90.55- ☑]
    fibula D58.2 [M90.56- ☑]
    finger D58.2 [M90.54- ☑]
    humerus D58.2 [M90.52- ☑]
    ilium D58.2 [M90.55- ☑]
    ischium D58.2 [M90.55- ☑]
    metacarpus D58.2 [M90.54- ☑]
    metatarsus D58.2 [M90.57- ☑]
    multiple sites D58.2 [M90.58]
    neck D58.2 [M90.58]
    radius D58.2 [M90.53- ☑]
    rib D58.2 [M90.58]
    scapula D58.2 [M90.51- ☑]
    skull D58.2 [M90.58]
    tarsus D58.2 [M90.57- ☑]
    tibia D58.2 [M90.56- ☑]
    toe D58.2 [M90.57- ☑]
    ulna D58.2 [M90.53- ☑]
    vertebra D58.2 [M90.58]
  trauma (previous) M87.20
    carpus M87.23- ☑
    clavicle M87.21- ☑
    femur M87.25- ☑
    fibula M87.26- ☑
    finger M87.24- ☑
    humerus M87.22- ☑
    ilium M87.25- ☑
    ischium M87.25- ☑
    metacarpus M87.24- ☑
    metatarsus M87.27- ☑
    multiple sites M87.29
    neck M87.28
    radius M87.23- ☑
    rib M87.28
    scapula M87.21- ☑
    skull M87.28
    tarsus M87.27- ☑
    tibia M87.26- ☑
    toe M87.27- ☑
    ulna M87.23- ☑
    vertebra M87.28
  femur M87.35- ☑
  fibula M87.36- ☑
  finger M87.34- ☑
  humerus M87.32- ☑
  ilium M87.350
  in
    caisson disease T70.3 ☑ [M90.50]
      carpus T70.3 ☑ [M90.54- ☑]
      clavicle T70.3 ☑ [M90.51- ☑]
      femur T70.3 ☑ [M90.55- ☑]
      fibula T70.3 ☑ [M90.56- ☑]
      finger T70.3 ☑ [M90.54- ☑]
      humerus T70.3 ☑ [M90.52- ☑]
      ilium T70.3 ☑ [M90.55- ☑]
      ischium T70.3 ☑ [M90.55- ☑]
      metacarpus T70.3 ☑ [M90.54- ☑]
      metatarsus T70.3 ☑ [M90.57- ☑]
      multiple sites T70.3 ☑ [M90.59]
      neck T70.3 ☑ [M90.58]
      radius T70.3 ☑ [M90.53- ☑]
      rib T70.3 ☑ [M90.58]
      scapula T70.3 ☑ [M90.51- ☑]
      skull T70.3 ☑ [M90.58]
      tarsus T70.3 ☑ [M90.57- ☑]
      tibia T70.3 ☑ [M90.56- ☑]
      toe T70.3 ☑ [M90.57- ☑]
      ulna T70.3 ☑ [M90.53- ☑]
      vertebra T70.3 ☑ [M90.58]
  ischium M87.350
  metacarpus M87.34- ☑
  metatarsus M87.37- ☑
  multiple site M87.39
  neck M87.38
  radius M87.33- ☑
  rib M87.38
  scapula M87.319
  skull M87.38
  tarsus M87.379
  tibia M87.366
  toe M87.379
  ulna M87.33- ☑
  vertebra M87.38
  specified type NEC M87.80
    carpus M87.83- ☑
    clavicle M87.81- ☑
    femur M87.85- ☑
    fibula M87.86- ☑
    finger M87.84- ☑
    humerus M87.82- ☑
    ilium M87.85- ☑

Osteonecrosis — *continued*
- ischium M87.85- ☑
- metacarpus M87.84- ☑
- metatarsus M87.87- ☑
- multiple sites M87.89
- neck M87.88
- radius M87.83- ☑
- rib M87.88
- scapula M87.81- ☑
- skull M87.88
- tarsus M87.87- ☑
- tibia M87.86- ☑
- toe M87.87- ☑
- ulna M87.83- ☑
- vertebra M87.88

Osteo-onycho-arthro-dysplasia Q79.8
Osteo-onychodysplasia, hereditary Q79.8
Osteopathia condensans disseminata Q78.8
Osteopathy (*see also* Osteomyelitis, Osteonecrosis, Osteoporosis)
- after poliomyelitis M89.60
  - carpus M89.64- ☑
  - clavicle M89.61- ☑
  - femur M89.65- ☑
  - fibula M89.66- ☑
  - finger M89.64- ☑
  - humerus M89.62- ☑
  - ilium M89.659
  - ischium M89.659
  - metacarpus M89.64- ☑
  - metatarsus M89.67- ☑
  - multiple sites M89.69
  - neck M89.68
  - radius M89.63- ☑
  - rib M89.68
  - scapula M89.61- ☑
  - skull M89.68
  - tarsus M89.67- ☑
  - tibia M89.66- ☑
  - toe M89.67- ☑
  - ulna M89.63- ☑
  - vertebra M89.68
- in (due to)
  - renal osteodystrophy N25.0
  - specified diseases classified elsewhere M90.8

Osteopenia M85.8- ☑
- borderline M85.8- ☑
Osteoperiostitis — *see* Osteomyelitis, specified type NEC
Osteopetrosis (familial) Q78.2
Osteophyte M25.70
- ankle M25.77- ☑
- elbow M25.72- ☑
- foot joint M25.77- ☑
- hand joint M25.74- ☑
- hip M25.75- ☑
- knee M25.76- ☑
- shoulder M25.71- ☑
- spine M25.78
- vertebrae M25.78
- wrist M25.73- ☑
Osteopoikilosis Q78.8
Osteoporosis (female) (male) M81.0
- with current pathological fracture M80.00 ☑
- age-related M81.0
  - with current pathologic fracture M80.00 ☑
    - carpus M80.04- ☑
    - clavicle M80.01- ☑
    - fibula M80.06- ☑
    - finger M80.04- ☑
    - humerus M80.02- ☑
    - ilium M80.05- ☑
    - ischium M80.05- ☑
    - metacarpus M80.04- ☑
    - metatarsus M80.07- ☑
    - pelvis M80.05- ☑
    - radius M80.03- ☑
    - scapula M80.01- ☑
    - tarsus M80.07- ☑
    - tibia M80.06- ☑
    - toe M80.07- ☑
    - ulna M80.03- ☑
    - vertebra M80.08 ☑
- disuse M81.8
  - with current pathological fracture M80.80 ☑
    - carpus M80.84- ☑
    - clavicle M80.81- ☑
    - fibula M80.86- ☑
    - finger M80.84- ☑
    - humerus M80.82- ☑
    - ilium M80.85- ☑
    - ischium M80.85- ☑

Osteoporosis — *continued*
- metacarpus M80.84- ☑
- metatarsus M80.87- ☑
- pelvis M80.85- ☑
- radius M80.83- ☑
- scapula M80.81- ☑
- tarsus M80.87- ☑
- tibia M80.86- ☑
- toe M80.87- ☑
- ulna M80.83- ☑
- vertebra M80.88 ☑
- drug-induced — *see* Osteoporosis, specified type NEC
- idiopathic — *see* Osteoporosis, specified type NEC
- involutional — *see* Osteoporosis, age-related
- Lequesne M81.6
- localized M81.6
- postmenopausal M81.0
  - with pathological fracture M80.00 ☑
    - carpus M80.04- ☑
    - clavicle M80.01- ☑
    - fibula M80.06- ☑
    - finger M80.04- ☑
    - humerus M80.02- ☑
    - ilium M80.05- ☑
    - ischium M80.05- ☑
    - metacarpus M80.04- ☑
    - metatarsus M80.07- ☑
    - pelvis M80.05- ☑
    - radius M80.03- ☑
    - scapula M80.01- ☑
    - tarsus M80.07- ☑
    - tibia M80.06- ☑
    - toe M80.07- ☑
    - ulna M80.03- ☑
    - vertebra M80.08 ☑
- postoophorectomy — *see* Osteoporosis, specified type NEC
- postsurgical malabsorption — *see* Osteoporosis, specified type NEC
- post-traumatic — *see* Osteoporosis, specified type NEC
- senile — *see* Osteoporosis, age-related
- specified type NEC M81.8
  - with pathological fracture M80.80 ☑
    - carpus M80.84- ☑
    - clavicle M80.81- ☑
    - fibula M80.86- ☑
    - finger M80.84- ☑
    - humerus M80.82- ☑
    - ilium M80.85- ☑
    - ischium M80.85- ☑
    - metacarpus M80.84- ☑
    - metatarsus M80.87- ☑
    - pelvis M80.85- ☑
    - radius M80.83- ☑
    - scapula M80.81- ☑
    - tarsus M80.87- ☑
    - tibia M80.86- ☑
    - toe M80.87- ☑
    - ulna M80.83- ☑
    - vertebra M80.88 ☑
Osteopsathyrosis (idiopathica) Q78.0
Osteoradionecrosis, jaw (acute) (chronic) (lower) (suppurative) (upper) M27.2
Osteosarcoma (any form) — *see* Neoplasm, bone, malignant
Osteosclerosis Q78.2
- acquired M85.8- ☑
- congenita Q77.4
- fragilitas (generalisata) Q78.2
- myelofibrosis D75.81
Osteosclerotic anemia D64.89
Osteosis
- cutis L94.2
- renal fibrocystic N25.0
Österreicher-Turner syndrome Q87.2
Ostium
- atrioventriculare commune Q21.2
- primum (arteriosum) (defect) (persistent) Q21.2
- secundum (arteriosum) (defect) (patent) (persistent) Q21.1
Ostrum-Furst syndrome Q75.8
Otalgia H92.0
Otitis (acute) H66.90
- with effusion (*see also* Otitis, media, nonsuppurative)
  - purulent — *see* Otitis, media, suppurative
- adhesive H74.1
- chronic (*see also* Otitis, media, chronic)

Otitis — *continued*
- with effusion (*see also* Otitis, media, nonsuppurative, chronic)
- externa H60.9- ☑
  - abscess — *see* Abscess, ear, external
  - acute (noninfective) H60.50- ☑
    - actinic H60.51- ☑
    - chemical H60.52- ☑
    - contact H60.53- ☑
    - eczematoid H60.54- ☑
    - infective — *see* Otitis, externa, infective
    - reactive H60.55- ☑
    - specified NEC H60.59- ☑
  - cellulitis — *see* Cellulitis, ear
  - chronic H60.6- ☑
  - diffuse — *see* Otitis, externa, infective, diffuse
  - hemorrhagic — *see* Otitis, externa, infective, hemorrhagic
  - in (due to)
    - aspergillosis B44.89
    - candidiasis B37.84
    - erysipelas A46 [H62.40]
    - herpes (simplex) virus infection B00.1
      - zoster B02.8
    - impetigo L01.00 [H62.40]
    - infectious disease NEC B99 ☑ [H62.4- ☑]
    - mycosis NEC B36.9 [H62.40]
    - parasitic disease NEC B89 [H62.40]
    - viral disease NEC B34.9 [H62.40]
    - zoster B02.8
  - infective NEC H60.39- ☑
    - abscess — *see* Abscess, ear, external
    - cellulitis — *see* Cellulitis, ear
    - diffuse H60.31- ☑
    - hemorrhagic H60.32- ☑
    - swimmer's ear — *see* Swimmer's, ear
  - malignant H60.2- ☑
  - mycotic B36.9 [H62.40]
  - necrotizing — *see* Otitis, externa, malignant
  - Pseudomonas aeruginosa — *see* Otitis, externa, malignant
  - reactive — *see* Otitis, externa, acute, reactive
  - specified NEC H60.8
  - tropical B36.8
- insidiosa — *see* Otosclerosis
- interna H83.0
- media (hemorrhagic) (staphylococcal) (streptococcal) H66.9- ☑
  - with effusion (nonpurulent) — *see* Otitis, media, nonsuppurative
  - acute, subacute H66.90
    - allergic — *see* Otitis, media, nonsuppurative, acute, allergic
    - exudative — *see* Otitis, media, nonsuppurative, acute
    - mucoid — *see* Otitis, media, nonsuppurative, acute
    - necrotizing (*see also* Otitis, media, suppurative, acute)
      - in
        - measles B05.3
        - scarlet fever A38.0
    - nonsuppurative NEC — *see* Otitis, media, nonsuppurative, acute
    - purulent — *see* Otitis, media, suppurative, acute
    - sanguinous — *see* Otitis, media, nonsuppurative, acute
    - secretory — *see* Otitis, media, nonsuppurative, acute, serous
    - seromucinous — *see* Otitis, media, nonsuppurative, acute
    - serous — *see* Otitis, media, nonsuppurative, acute, serous
    - suppurative — *see* Otitis, media, suppurative, acute
  - allergic — *see* Otitis, media, nonsuppurative
  - catarrhal — *see* Otitis, media, nonsuppurative
  - chronic H66.90
    - with effusion (nonpurulent) — *see* Otitis, media, nonsuppurative, chronic
    - allergic — *see* Otitis, media, nonsuppurative, chronic, allergic
    - benign suppurative — *see* Otitis, media, suppurative, chronic, tubotympanic
    - catarrhal — *see* Otitis, media, nonsuppurative, chronic, serous
    - exudative — *see* Otitis, media, nonsuppurative, chronic
    - mucinous — *see* Otitis, media, nonsuppurative, chronic, mucoid

Otitis — *continued*
    mucoid — *see* Otitis, media, nonsuppurative, chronic, mucoid
    nonsuppurative NEC — *see* Otitis, media, nonsuppurative, chronic
    purulent — *see* Otitis, media, suppurative, chronic
    secretory — *see* Otitis, media, nonsuppurative, chronic, mucoid
    seromucinous — *see* Otitis, media, nonsuppurative, chronic
    serous — *see* Otitis, media, nonsuppurative, chronic, serous
    suppurative — *see* Otitis, media, suppurative, chronic
    transudative — *see* Otitis, media, nonsuppurative, chronic, mucoid
  exudative — *see* Otitis, media, nonsuppurative
  in (due to) (with)
    influenza — *see* Influenza, with, otitis media
    measles B05.3
    scarlet fever A38.0
    tuberculosis A18.6
    viral disease NEC B34.- ☑ [H67.- ☑]
  mucoid — *see* Otitis, media, nonsuppurative
  nonsuppurative H65.9- ☑
    acute or subacute NEC H65.19- ☑
      allergic H65.11- ☑
        recurrent H65.11- ☑
      recurrent H65.19- ☑
      secretory — *see* Otitis, media, nonsuppurative, serous
      serous H65.0- ☑
        recurrent H65.0- ☑
    chronic H65.49- ☑
      allergic H65.41- ☑
      mucoid H65.3- ☑
      serous H65.2- ☑
    postmeasles B05.3
  purulent — *see* Otitis, media, suppurative
  secretory — *see* Otitis, media, nonsuppurative
  seromucinous — *see* Otitis, media, nonsuppurative
  serous — *see* Otitis, media, nonsuppurative
  suppurative H66.4- ☑
    acute H66.00- ☑
      with rupture of ear drum H66.01- ☑
      recurrent H66.00- ☑
        with rupture of ear drum H66.01- ☑
    chronic (*see also* subcategory) H66.3 ☑
      atticoantral H66.2- ☑
      benign — *see* Otitis, media, suppurative, chronic, tubotympanic
      tubotympanic H66.1- ☑
    transudative — *see* Otitis, media, nonsuppurative
    tuberculous A18.6
Otocephaly Q18.2
Otolith syndrome H81.8
Otomycosis (diffuse) NEC B36.9 [H62.40]
  in
    aspergillosis B44.89
    candidiasis B37.84
    moniliasis B37.84
Otoporosis — *see* Otosclerosis
Otorrhagia (nontraumatic) H92.2- ☑
  traumatic - code by Type of injury
Otorrhea H92.1- ☑ ✓
  cerebrospinal G96.0
Otosclerosis (general) H80.9- ☑
  cochlear (endosteal) H80.2- ☑
  involving
    otic capsule — *see* Otosclerosis, cochlear
    oval window
      nonobliterative H80.0- ☑
      obliterative H80.1- ☑
    round window — *see* Otosclerosis, cochlear
  nonobliterative — *see* Otosclerosis, involving, oval window, nonobliterative
  obliterative — *see* Otosclerosis, involving, oval window, obliterative
  specified NEC H80.8- ☑
Otospongiosis — *see* Otosclerosis
Otto's disease or pelvis M24.7
Outcome of delivery Z37.9
  multiple births Z37.9
    all liveborn Z37.50
      quadruplets Z37.52
      quintuplets Z37.53
      sextuplets Z37.54
      specified number NEC Z37.59
      triplets Z37.51

Outcome — *continued*
    all stillborn Z37.7
    some liveborn Z37.60
      quadruplets Z37.62
      quintuplets Z37.63
      sextuplets Z37.64
      specified number NEC Z37.69
      triplets Z37.61
  single NEC Z37.9
    liveborn Z37.0
    stillborn Z37.1
  twins NEC Z37.9
    both liveborn Z37.2
    both stillborn Z37.4
    one liveborn, one stillborn Z37.3
Outlet — *see* condition
Ovalocytosis (congenital) (hereditary) — *see* Elliptocytosis
Ovarian — *see* Condition
Ovariocele N83.4
Ovaritis (cystic) — *see* Oophoritis
Ovary, ovarian (*see also* condition)
  resistant syndrome E28.39
  vein syndrome N13.8
Overactive (*see also* Hyperfunction)
  adrenal cortex NEC E27.0
  bladder N32.81
  hypothalamus E23.3
  thyroid — *see* Hyperthyroidism
Overactivity R46.3
  child — *see* Disorder, attention-deficit hyperactivity
Overbite (deep) (excessive) (horizontal) (vertical) M26.29
Overbreathing — *see* Hyperventilation
Overconscientious personality F60.5
Overdevelopment — *see* Hypertrophy
Overdistension — *see* Distension
Overdose, overdosage (drug) — *see* Table of Drugs and Chemicals, by drug, poisoning
Overeating R63.2
  nonorganic origin F50.8
  psychogenic F50.8
Overexertion (effects) (exhaustion) T73.3 ☑
Overexposure (effects) T73.9 ☑
  exhaustion T73.2 ☑
Overfeeding — *see* Overeating
  newborn P92.4
Overfill, endodontic M27.52
Overgrowth, bone — *see* Hypertrophy, bone
Overhanging of dental restorative material (unrepairable) K08.52
Overheated (places) (effects) — *see* Heat
Overjet (excessive horizontal) M26.23
Overlaid, overlying (suffocation) — *see* Asphyxia, traumatic, due to mechanical threat
Overlap, excessive horizontal (teeth) M26.23
Overlapping toe (acquired) (*see also* Deformity, toe, specified NEC)
  congenital (fifth toe) Q66.89
Overload
  circulatory, due to transfusion (blood) (blood components) (TACO) E87.71
  fluid E87.70
    due to transfusion (blood) (blood components) E87.71
    specified NEC E87.79
  iron, due to repeated red blood cell transfusions E83.111
  potassium (K) E87.5
  sodium (Na) E87.0
Overnutrition — *see* Hyperalimentation
Overproduction (*see also* Hypersecretion)
  ACTH E27.0
  catecholamine E27.5
  growth hormone E22.0
Overprotection, child by parent Z62.1
Overriding
  aorta Q25.4
  finger (acquired) — *see* Deformity, finger
    congenital Q68.1
  toe (acquired) (*see also* Deformity, toe, specified NEC)
    congenital Q66.89
Overstrained R53.83
  heart — *see* Hypertrophy, cardiac
Overuse, muscle NEC M70.8- ☑
Overweight E66.3
Overworked R53.83
Oviduct — *see* condition
Ovotestis Q56.0

Ovulation (cycle)
  failure or lack of N97.0
  pain N94.0
Ovum — *see* condition
Owren's disease or syndrome (parahemophilia) D68.2
Ox heart — *see* Hypertrophy, cardiac
Oxalosis E72.53
Oxaluria E72.53
Oxycephaly, oxycephalic Q75.0
  syphilitic, congenital A50.02
Oxyuriasis B80
Oxyuris vermicularis (infestation) B80
Ozena J31.0

P

Pachyderma, pachydermia L85.9
  larynx (verrucosa) J38.7
Pachydermatocele (congenital) Q82.8
Pachydermoperiostosis (*see also* Osteoarthropathy, hypertrophic, specified type NEC)
  clubbed nail M89.40 [L62]
Pachygyria Q04.3
Pachymeningitis (adhesive) (basal) (brain) (cervical) (chronic)(circumscribed) (external) (fibrous) (hemorrhagic) (hypertrophic) (internal) (purulent) (spinal) (suppurative) — *see* Meningitis
Pachyonychia (congenital) Q84.5
Pacinian tumor — *see* Neoplasm, skin, benign
Pad, knuckle or Garrod's M72.1
Paget-Schroetter syndrome I82.890
Paget's disease
  with infiltrating duct carcinoma — *see* Neoplasm, breast, malignant
  bone M88.9
    carpus M88.84- ☑
    clavicle M88.81- ☑
    femur M88.85- ☑
    fibula M88.86- ☑
    finger M88.84- ☑
    humerus M88.82- ☑
    ilium M88.85- ☑
    in neoplastic disease — *see* Osteitis, deformans, in neoplastic disease
    ischium M88.85- ☑
    metacarpus M88.84- ☑
    metatarsus M88.87- ☑
    multiple sites M88.89
    neck M88.88
    radius M88.83- ☑
    rib M88.88
    scapula M88.81- ☑
    skull M88.0
    tarsus M88.87- ☑
    tibia M88.86- ☑
    toe M88.87- ☑
    ulna M88.83- ☑
    vertebra M88.88
  breast (female) C50.01- ☑
    male C50.02- ☑
  extramammary (*see also* Neoplasm, skin, malignant)
    anus C21.0
      margin C44.590
      skin C44.590
  intraductal carcinoma — *see* Neoplasm, breast, malignant
  malignant — *see* Neoplasm, skin, malignant
    breast (female) C50.01- ☑
      male C50.02- ☑
    unspecified site (female) C50.01- ☑
      male C50.02- ☑
  mammary — *see* Paget's disease, breast
  nipple — *see* Paget's disease, breast
  osteitis deformans — *see* Paget's disease, bone
Pain (s) (*see also* Painful) R52
  abdominal R10.9
    colic R10.83
    generalized R10.84
      with acute abdomen R10.0
    lower R10.30
      left quadrant R10.32
      pelvic or perineal R10.2
      periumbilical R10.33
      right quadrant R10.31
    rebound — *see* Tenderness, abdominal, rebound
    severe with abdominal rigidity R10.0

☑ **Additional character required**

Pain — *continued*
 tenderness — *see* Tenderness, abdominal
 upper R10.10
  epigastric R10.13
  left quadrant R10.12
  right quadrant R10.11
 acute R52
  due to trauma G89.11
  neoplasm related G89.3
  postprocedural NEC G89.18
  post-thoracotomy G89.12
  specified by site - code to Pain, by site
 adnexa (uteri) R10.2
 anginoid — *see* Pain, precordial
 anus K62.89
 arm — *see* Pain, limb, upper
 axillary (axilla) M79.62- ☑
 back (postural) M54.9
 bladder R39.89
  associated with micturition — *see* Micturition, painful
 bone — *see* Disorder, bone, specified type NEC
 breast N64.4
 broad ligament R10.2
 cancer associated (acute) (chronic) G89.3
 cecum — *see* Pain, abdominal
 cervicobrachial M53.1
 chest (central) R07.9
  anterior wall R07.89
  atypical R07.89
  ischemic I20.9
  musculoskeletal R07.89
  non-cardiac R07.89
  on breathing R07.1
  pleurodynia R07.81
  precordial R07.2
  wall (anterior) R07.89
 chronic G89.29
  associated with significant psychosocial dysfunction G89.4
  due to trauma G89.21
  neoplasm related G89.3
  postoperative NEC G89.28
  postprocedural NEC G89.28
  post-thoracotomy G89.22
  specified NEC G89.29
 coccyx M53.3
 colon — *see* Pain, abdominal
 coronary — *see* Angina
 costochondral R07.1
 diaphragm R07.1
 due to cancer G89.3
 due to device, implant or graft (*see also* Complications, by site and type, specified NEC) T85.84 ☑
  arterial graft NEC T82.848 ☑
  breast (implant) T85.84 ☑
  catheter NEC T85.84 ☑
   dialysis (renal) T82.848 ☑
    intraperitoneal T85.84 ☑
   infusion NEC T82.848 ☑
    spinal (epidural) (subdural) T85.84 ☑
   urinary (indwelling) T83.84 ☑
  electronic (electrode) (pulse generator) (stimulator)
   bone T84.84 ☑
   cardiac T82.847 ☑
   nervous system (brain) (peripheral nerve) (spinal) T85.84 ☑
   urinary T83.84 ☑
  fixation, internal (orthopedic) NEC T84.84 ☑
  gastrointestinal (bile duct) (esophagus) T85.84 ☑
  genital NEC T83.84 ☑
  heart NEC T82.847 ☑
  infusion NEC T85.84 ☑
  joint prosthesis T84.84 ☑
  ocular (corneal graft) (orbital implant) NEC T85.84 ☑
  orthopedic NEC T84.84 ☑
  specified NEC T85.84 ☑
  urinary NEC T83.84 ☑
  vascular NEC T82.848 ☑
  ventricular intracranial shunt T85.84 ☑
 due to malignancy (primary) (secondary) G89.3
 ear H92.0
 epigastric, epigastrium R10.13
 eye — *see* Pain, ocular
 face, facial R51
  atypical G50.1
 female genital organs NEC N94.89
 finger — *see* Pain, limb, upper

Pain — *continued*
 flank — *see* Pain, abdominal
 foot — *see* Pain, limb, lower
 gallbladder K82.9
 gas (intestinal) R14.1
 gastric — *see* Pain, abdominal
 generalized NOS R52
 genital organ
  female N94.89
  male N50.8
 groin — *see* Pain, abdominal, lower
 hand — *see* Pain, limb, upper
 head — *see* Headache
 heart — *see* Pain, precordial
 infra-orbital — *see* Neuralgia, trigeminal
 intercostal R07.82
 intermenstrual N94.0
 jaw R68.84
 joint M25.50
  ankle M25.57- ☑
  elbow M25.52- ☑
  finger M79.64- ☑
  foot M25.57- ☑
  hand M79.64- ☑
  hip M25.55- ☑
  knee M25.56- ☑
  shoulder M25.51- ☑
  toe M25.57- ☑
  wrist M25.53- ☑
 kidney N23
 laryngeal R07.0
 leg — *see* Pain, limb, lower
 limb M79.609
  lower M79.60- ☑
   foot M79.67- ☑
   lower leg M79.66- ☑
   thigh M79.65- ☑
   toe M79.67- ☑
  upper M79.60- ☑
   axilla M79.62- ☑
   finger M79.64- ☑
   forearm M79.63- ☑
   hand M79.64- ☑
   upper arm M79.62- ☑
 loin M54.5
 low back M54.5
 lumbar region M54.5
 mandibular R68.84
 mastoid H92.0
 maxilla R68.84
 menstrual (*see also* Dysmenorrhea) N94.6
 metacarpophalangeal (joint) — *see* Pain, joint, hand
 metatarsophalangeal (joint) — *see* Pain, joint, foot
 mouth K13.79
 muscle — *see* Myalgia
 musculoskeletal (*see also* Pain, by site) M79.1
 myofascial M79.1
 nasal J34.89
 nasopharynx J39.2
 neck NEC M54.2
 nerve NEC — *see* Neuralgia
 neuromuscular — *see* Neuralgia
 nose J34.89
 ocular H57.1- ☑
 ophthalmic — *see* Pain, ocular
 orbital region — *see* Pain, ocular
 ovary N94.89
 over heart — *see* Pain, precordial
 ovulation N94.0
 pelvic (female) R10.2
 penis N48.89
 pericardial — *see* Pain, precordial
 perineal, perineum R10.2
 pharynx J39.2
 pleura, pleural, pleuritic R07.81
 postoperative NOS G89.18
 postprocedural NOS G89.18
 post-thoracotomy G89.12
 precordial (region) R07.2
 premenstrual N94.3
 psychogenic (persistent) (any site) F45.41
 radicular (spinal) — *see* Radiculopathy
 rectum K62.89
 respiration R07.1
 retrosternal R07.2
 rheumatoid, muscular — *see* Myalgia
 rib R07.81
 root (spinal) — *see* Radiculopathy
 round ligament (stretch) R10.2
 sacroiliac M53.3

Pain — *continued*
 sciatic — *see* Sciatica
 scrotum N50.8
 seminal vesicle N50.8
 shoulder M25.51- ☑
 spermatic cord N50.8
 spinal root — *see* Radiculopathy
 spine M54.9
  cervical M54.2
  low back M54.5
   with sciatica M54.4- ☑
  thoracic M54.6
 stomach — *see* Pain, abdominal
 substernal R07.2
 temporomandibular (joint) M26.62
 testis N50.8
 thoracic spine M54.6
  with radicular and visceral pain M54.14
 throat R07.0
 tibia — *see* Pain, limb, lower
 toe — *see* Pain, limb, lower
 tongue K14.6
 tooth K08.8
 trigeminal — *see* Neuralgia, trigeminal
 tumor associated G89.3
 ureter N23
 urinary (organ) (system) N23
 uterus NEC N94.89
 vagina R10.2
 vertebrogenic (syndrome) M54.89
 vesical R39.89
  associated with micturition — *see* Micturition, painful
 vulva R10.2
Painful (*see also* Pain)
 coitus
  female N94.1
  male N53.12
  psychogenic F52.6
 ejaculation (semen) N53.12
  psychogenic F52.6
 erection — *see* Priapism
 feet syndrome E53.8
 joint replacement (hip) (knee) T84.84 ☑
 menstruation — *see* Dysmenorrhea
  psychogenic F45.8
 micturition — *see* Micturition, painful
 respiration R07.1
 scar NEC L90.5
 wire sutures T81.89 ☑
Painter's colic T56.0
Palate — *see* condition
Palatoplegia K13.79
Palatoschisis — *see* Cleft, palate
Palilalia R48.8
Palliative care Z51.5
Pallor R23.1
 optic disc, temporal — *see* Atrophy, optic
Palmar (*see also* condition)
 fascia — *see* condition
Palpable
 cecum K63.89
 kidney N28.89
 ovary N83.8
 prostate N42.9
 spleen — *see* Splenomegaly
Palpitations (heart) R00.2
 psychogenic F45.8
Palsy (*see also* Paralysis) G83.9
 atrophic diffuse (progressive) G12.22
 Bell's (*see also* Palsy, facial)
  newborn P11.3
 brachial plexus NEC G54.0
  newborn (birth injury) P14.3
 brain — *see* Palsy, cerebral
 bulbar (progressive) (chronic) G12.22
  of childhood (Fazio-Londe) G12.1
  pseudo NEC G12.29
  supranuclear (progressive) G23.1
 cerebral (congenital) G80.9
  ataxic G80.4
  athetoid G80.3
  choreathetoid G80.3
  diplegic G80.8
   spastic G80.1
  dyskinetic G80.3
   athetoid G80.3
   choreathetoid G80.3
   distonic G80.3
  dystonic G80.3
  hemiplegic G80.8
   spastic G80.2

Palsy — continued
  mixed G80.8
  monoplegic G80.8
    spastic G80.1
  paraplegic G80.8
    spastic G80.1
  quadriplegic G80.8
    spastic G80.0
  spastic G80.1
    diplegic G80.1
    hemiplegic G80.2
    monoplegic G80.1
    quadriplegic G80.0
    specified NEC G80.1
    tetrapelgic G80.0
  specified NEC G80.8
  syphilitic A52.12
    congenital A50.49
  tetraplegic G80.8
    spastic G80.0
  cranial nerve (see also Disorder, nerve, cranial)
    multiple G52.7
      in
        infectious disease B99 ☑ [G53]
        neoplastic disease (see also Neoplasm)
          D49.9 [G53]
        parasitic disease B89 [G53]
        sarcoidosis D86.82
  creeping G12.22
  diver's T70.3 ☑
  Erb's P14.0
  facial G51.0
    newborn (birth injury) P11.3
  glossopharyngeal G52.1
  Klumpke (-Déjérine) P14.1
  lead T56.0
  median nerve (tardy) G56.1- ☑
  nerve G58.9
    specified NEC G58.8
  peroneal nerve (acute) (tardy) G57.3- ☑
  progressive supranuclear G23.1
  pseudobulbar NEC G12.29
  radial nerve (acute) G56.3- ☑
  seventh nerve (see also Palsy, facial)
    newborn P11.3
  shaking — see Parkinsonism
  spastic (cerebral) (spinal) G80.1
  ulnar nerve (tardy) G56.2- ☑
  wasting G12.29
Paludism — see Malaria
Panangiitis M30.0
Panaris, panaritium (see also Cellulitis, digit)
  with lymphangitis — see Lymphangitis, acute,
    digit
Panarteritis nodosa M30.0
  brain or cerebral I67.7
Pancake heart R93.1
  with cor pulmonale (chronic) I27.81
Pancarditis (acute) (chronic) I51.89
  rheumatic I09.89
    active or acute I01.8
Pancoast's syndrome or tumor C34.1- ☑
Pancolitis, ulcerative (chronic) K51.00
  with
    complication K51.019
    abscess K51.014
    fistula K51.013
    obstruction K51.012
    rectal bleeding K51.011
    specified complication NEC K51.018
Pancreas, pancreatic — see condition
Pancreatitis (annular) (apoplectic) (calcareous)
  (edematous) (hemorrhagic) (malignant) (recurrent)
  (subacute) (suppurative) K85.9
  acute K85.9
    alcohol induced K85.2
    biliary K85.1
    drug induced K85.3
    gallstone K85.1
    idiopathic K85.0
    specified NEC K85.8
  chronic (infectious) K86.1
    alcohol-induced K86.0
    recurrent K86.1
    relapsing K86.1
  cystic (chronic) K86.1
  cytomegaloviral B25.2
  fibrous (chronic) K86.1
  gangrenous K85.8
  gallstone K85.1
  interstitial (chronic) K86.1
    acute K85.8

Pancreatitis — continued
  mumps B26.3
  recurrent (chronic) K86.1
  relapsing, chronic K86.1
  syphilitic A52.74
Pancreatoblastoma — see Neoplasm, pancreas,
  malignant
Pancreolithiasis K86.8
Pancytolysis D75.89
Pancytopenia (acquired) D61.818
  with
    malformations D61.09
    myelodysplastic syndrome — see Syndrome,
      myelodysplastic
  antineoplastic chemotherapy induced D61.810
  congenital D61.09
  drug-induced NEC D61.811
Panencephalitis, subacute, sclerosing A81.1
Panhematopenia D61.9
  congenital D61.09
  constitutional D61.09
  splenic, primary D73.1
Panhemocytopenia D61.9
  congenital D61.09
  constitutional D61.09
Panhypogonadism E29.1
Panhypopituitarism E23.0
  prepubertal E23.0
Panic (attack) (state) F41.0
  reaction to exceptional stress (transient) F43.0
Panmyelopathy, familial, constitutional D61.09
Panmyelophthisis D61.82
  congenital D61.09
Panmyelosis (acute) (with myelofibrosis) C94.4- ☑
Panner's disease — see Osteochondrosis, juvenile,
  humerus
Panneuritis endemica E51.11
Panniculitis (nodular) (nonsuppurative) M79.3
  back M54.00
    cervical region M54.02
    cervicothoracic region M54.03
    lumbar region M54.06
    lumbosacral region M54.07
    multiple sites M54.09
    occipito-atlanto-axial region M54.01
    sacrococcygeal region M54.08
    thoracic region M54.04
    thoracolumbar region M54.05
  lupus L93.2
  mesenteric K65.4
  neck M54.02
    cervicothoracic region M54.03
    occipito-atlanto-axial region M54.01
  relapsing M35.6
Panniculus adiposus (abdominal) E65
Pannus (allergic) (cornea) (degenerativus) (keratic)
  H16.42- ☑
  abdominal (symptomatic) E65
  trachomatosus, trachomatous (active) A71.1
Panophthalmitis H44.01- ☑
Pansinusitis (chronic) (hyperplastic) (nonpurulent)
  (purulent) J32.4
  acute J01.40
    recurrent J01.41
  tuberculous A15.8
Panuveitis (sympathetic) H44.11- ☑
Panvalvular disease I08.9
  specified NEC I08.8
Papanicolaou smear, cervix Z12.4
  as part of routine gynecological examination
    Z01.419
    with abnormal findings Z01.411
  for suspected neoplasm Z12.4
  nonspecific abnormal finding R87.619
  routine Z01.419
    with abnormal findings Z01.411
Papilledema (choked disc) H47.10
  associated with
    decreased ocular pressure H47.12
    increased intracranial pressure H47.11
    retinal disorder H47.13
  Foster-Kennedy syndrome H47.14- ☑
Papillitis H46.00
  anus K62.89
  chronic lingual K14.4
  necrotizing, kidney N17.2
  optic H46.0- ☑
  rectum K62.89
  renal, necrotizing N17.2
  tongue K14.0
Papilloma (see also Neoplasm, benign, by site)
  acuminatum (female) (male) (anogenital) A63.0

Papilloma — continued
  benign pinta (primary) A67.0
  bladder (urinary) (transitional cell) D41.4
  choroid plexus (lateral ventricle) (third ventricle)
    D33.0
    anaplastic C71.5
    fourth ventricle D33.1
    malignant C71.5
  renal pelvis (transitional cell) D41.1- ☑
    benign D30.1- ☑
  Schneiderian
    specified site — see Neoplasm, benign, by site
    unspecified site D14.0
  serous surface
    borderline malignancy
      specified site — see Neoplasm, uncertain
        behavior, by site
      unspecified site D39.10
    specified site — see Neoplasm, benign, by site
    unspecified site D27.9
  transitional (cell)
    bladder (urinary) D41.4
    inverted type — see Neoplasm, uncertain
      behavior, by site
    renal pelvis D41.1- ☑
    ureter D41.2- ☑
  ureter (transitional cell) D41.2- ☑
    benign D30.2- ☑
  urothelial — see Neoplasm, uncertain behavior,
    by site
  villous — see Neoplasm, uncertain behavior, by
    site
    adenocarcinoma in — see Neoplasm,
      malignant, by site
    in situ — see Neoplasm, in situ
  yaws, plantar or palmar A66.1
Papillomata, multiple, of yaws A66.1
Papillomatosis (see also Neoplasm, benign, by site)
  confluent and reticulated L83
  cystic, breast — see Mastopathy, cystic
  ductal, breast — see Mastopathy, cystic
  intraductal (diffuse) — see Neoplasm, benign,
    by site
  subareolar duct D24- ☑
Papillomavirus, as cause of disease classified
  elsewhere B97.7
Papillon-Léage and Psaume syndrome Q87.0
Papule (s) R23.8
  carate (primary) A67.0
  fibrous, of nose D22.39
  Gottron's L94.4
  pinta (primary) A67.0
Papulosis
  lymphomatoid C86.6
  malignant I77.89
Papyraceous fetus O31.0- ☑
Para-albuminemia E88.09
Paracephalus Q89.7
Parachute mitral valve Q23.2
Paracoccidioidomycosis B41.9
  disseminated B41.7
  generalized B41.7
  mucocutaneous-lymphangitic B41.8
  pulmonary B41.0
  specified NEC B41.8
  visceral B41.8
Paradentosis K05.4
Paraffinoma T88.8 ☑
Paraganglioma D44.7
  adrenal D35.0- ☑
    malignant C74.1- ☑
  aortic body D44.7
    malignant C75.5
  carotid body D44.6
    malignant C75.4
  chromaffin (see also Neoplasm, benign, by site)
    malignant — see Neoplasm, malignant, by site
  extra-adrenal D44.7
    malignant C75.5
      specified site — see Neoplasm, malignant,
        by site
      unspecified site C75.5
    specified site — see Neoplasm, uncertain
      behavior, by site
    unspecified site D44.7
  gangliocytic D13.2
    specified site — see Neoplasm, benign, by site
    unspecified site D13.2
  glomus jugulare D44.7
    malignant C75.5
  jugular D44.7
  malignant C75.5

☑ **Additional character required**

Paraganglioma — continued
　specified site — *see* Neoplasm, malignant, by site
　unspecified site C75.5
　nonchromaffin D44.7
　　malignant C75.5
　　　specified site — *see* Neoplasm, malignant, by site
　　　unspecified site C75.5
　　specified site — *see* Neoplasm, uncertain behavior, by site
　　unspecified site D44.7
　parasympathetic D44.7
　　specified site — *see* Neoplasm, uncertain behavior, by site
　　unspecified site D44.7
　specified site — *see* Neoplasm, uncertain behavior, by site
　sympathetic D44.7
　　specified site — *see* Neoplasm, uncertain behavior, by site
　　unspecified site D44.7
　unspecified site D44.7
Parageusia R43.2
　psychogenic F45.8
Paragonimiasis B66.4
Paragranuloma, Hodgkin — *see* Lymphoma, Hodgkin, classical, specified NEC
Parahemophilia (*see also* Defect, coagulation) D68.2
Parakeratosis R23.4
　variegata L41.0
Paralysis, paralytic (complete) (incomplete) G83.9
　with
　　syphilis A52.17
　abducens, abducent (nerve) — *see* Strabismus, paralytic, sixth nerve
　abductor, lower extremity G57.9- ☑
　accessory nerve G52.8
　accommodation (*see also* Paresis, of accommodation)
　　hysterical F44.89
　acoustic nerve (except Deafness)H93.3
　agitans (*see also* Parkinsonism) G20
　　arteriosclerotic G21.4
　alternating (oculomotor) G83.89
　amyotrophic G12.21
　ankle G57.9- ☑
　anus (sphincter) K62.89
　arm — *see* Monoplegia, upper limb
　ascending (spinal), acute G61.0
　association G12.29
　asthenic bulbar G70.00
　　with exacerbation (acute) G70.01
　　in crisis G70.01
　ataxic (hereditary) G11.9
　　general (syphilitic) A52.17
　atrophic G58.9
　　infantile, acute — *see* Poliomyelitis, paralytic
　　progressive G12.22
　　spinal (acute) — *see* Poliomyelitis, paralytic
　axillary G54.0
　Babinski-Nageotte's G83.89
　Bell's G51.0
　　newborn P11.3
　Benedikt's G46.3
　birth injury P14.9
　　spinal cord P11.5
　bladder (neurogenic) (sphincter) N31.2
　bowel, colon or intestine K56.0
　brachial plexus G54.0
　　birth injury P14.3
　　newborn (birth injury) P14.3
　brain G83.9
　　diplegia G83.0
　　triplegia G83.89
　bronchial J98.09
　Brown-Séquard G83.81
　bulbar (chronic) (progressive) G12.22
　　infantile — *see* Poliomyelitis, paralytic
　　poliomyelitic — *see* Poliomyelitis, paralytic
　　pseudo G12.29
　bulbospinal G70.00
　　with exacerbation (acute) G70.01
　　in crisis G70.01
　cardiac (*see also* Failure, heart) I50.9
　cerebrocerebellar, diplegic G80.1
　cervical
　　plexus G54.2
　　sympathetic G90.09
　Céstan-Chenais G46.3
　Charcot-Marie-Tooth type G60.0
　Clark's G80.9

Paralysis — continued
　colon K56.0
　compressed air T70.3 ☑
　compression
　　arm G56.9- ☑
　　leg G57.9- ☑
　　lower extremity G57.9- ☑
　　upper extremity G56.9- ☑
　congenital (cerebral) — *see* Palsy, cerebral
　conjugate movement (gaze) (of eye) H51.0
　　cortical (nuclear) (supranuclear) H51.0
　cordis — *see* Failure, heart
　cranial or cerebral nerve G52.9
　creeping G12.22
　crossed leg G83.89
　crutch — *see* Injury, brachial plexus
　deglutition R13.0
　　hysterical F44.4
　dementia A52.17
　descending (spinal) NEC G12.29
　diaphragm (flaccid) J98.6
　　due to accidental dissection of phrenic nerve during procedure — *see* Puncture, accidental complicating surgery
　digestive organs NEC K59.8
　diplegic — *see* Diplegia
　divergence (nuclear) H51.8
　diver's T70.3 ☑
　Duchenne's
　　birth injury P14.0
　　due to or associated with
　　　motor neuron disease G12.22
　　　muscular dystrophy G71.0
　　due to intracranial or spinal birth injury — *see* Palsy, cerebral
　embolic (current episode) I63.4 ☑
　Erb (-Duchenne) (birth) (newborn) P14.0
　Erb's syphilitic spastic spinal A52.17
　esophagus K22.8
　eye muscle (extrinsic) H49.9
　　intrinsic (*see also* Paresis, of accommodation)
　facial (nerve) G51.0
　　birth injury P11.3
　　congenital P11.3
　　following operation NEC — *see* Puncture, accidental complicating surgery
　　newborn (birth injury) P11.3
　familial (recurrent) (periodic) G72.3
　　spastic G11.4
　fauces J39.2
　finger G56.9- ☑
　gait R26.1
　gastric nerve (nondiabetic) G52.2
　gaze, conjugate H51.0
　general (progressive) (syphilitic) A52.17
　　juvenile A50.45
　glottis J38.00
　　bilateral J38.02
　　unilateral J38.01
　gluteal G54.1
　Gubler (-Millard) G46.3
　hand — *see* Monoplegia, upper limb
　heart — *see* Arrest, cardiac
　hemiplegic — *see* Hemiplegia
　hyperkalemic periodic (familial) G72.3
　hypoglossal (nerve) G52.3
　hypokalemic periodic G72.3
　hysterical F44.4
　ileus K56.0
　infantile (*see also* Poliomyelitis, paralytic) A80.30
　　bulbar — *see* Poliomyelitis, paralytic
　　cerebral — *see* Palsy, cerebral
　　spastic — *see* Palsy, cerebral, spastic
　infective — *see* Poliomyelitis, paralytic
　inferior nuclear G83.9
　internuclear — *see* Ophthalmoplegia, internuclear
　intestine K56.0
　iris H57.09
　　due to diphtheria (toxin) A36.89
　ischemic, Volkmann's (complicating trauma) T79.6 ☑
　Jackson's G83.89
　jake — *see* Poisoning, food, noxious, plant
　Jamaica ginger (jake) G62.2
　juvenile general A50.45
　Klumpke (-Déjérine) (birth) (newborn) P14.1
　labioglossal (laryngeal) (pharyngeal) G12.29
　Landry's G61.0
　laryngeal nerve (recurrent) (superior) (unilateral) J38.00
　　bilateral J38.02

Paralysis — continued
　　unilateral J38.01
　larynx J38.00
　　bilateral J38.02
　　due to diphtheria (toxin) A36.2
　　unilateral J38.01
　lateral G12.21
　leadT56.0
　left side — *see* Hemiplegia
　leg G83.1- ☑
　　both — *see* Paraplegia
　　crossed G83.89
　　hysterical F44.4
　　psychogenic F44.4
　　transient or transitory R29.818
　　　traumatic NEC — *see* Injury, nerve, leg
　levator palpebrae superioris — *see* Blepharoptosis, paralytic
　limb — *see* Monoplegia
　lip K13.0
　Lissauer's A52.17
　lower limb — *see* Monoplegia, lower limb
　　both — *see* Paraplegia
　lung J98.4
　median nerve G56.1- ☑
　medullary (tegmental) G83.89
　mesencephalic NEC G83.89
　　tegmental G83.89
　middle alternating G83.89
　Millard-Gubler-Foville G46.3
　monoplegic — *see* Monoplegia
　motor G83.9
　muscle, muscular NEC G72.89
　　due to nerve lesion G58.9
　　eye (extrinsic) H49.9
　　　intrinsic — *see* Paresis, of accommodation
　　oblique — *see* Strabismus, paralytic, fourth nerve
　　iris sphincter H21.9
　　ischemic (Volkmann's) (complicating trauma) T79.6 ☑
　　progressive G12.21
　　pseudohypertrophic G71.0
　musculocutaneous nerve G56.9- ☑
　musculospiral G56.9- ☑
　nerve (*see also* Disorder, nerve)
　　abducent — *see* Strabismus, paralytic, sixth nerve
　　accessory G52.8
　　auditory (except Deafness)H93.3
　　birth injury P14.9
　　cranial or cerebral G52.9
　　facial G51.0
　　　birth injury P11.3
　　　congenital P11.3
　　　newborn (birth injury) P11.3
　　fourth or trochlear — *see* Strabismus, paralytic, fourth nerve
　　newborn (birth injury) P14.9
　　oculomotor — *see* Strabismus, paralytic, third nerve
　　phrenic (birth injury) P14.2
　　radial G56.3- ☑
　　seventh or facial G51.0
　　　newborn (birth injury) P11.3
　　sixth or abducent — *see* Strabismus, paralytic, sixth nerve
　　syphilitic A52.15
　　third or oculomotor — *see* Strabismus, paralytic, third nerve
　　trigeminal G50.9
　　trochlear — *see* Strabismus, paralytic, fourth nerve
　　ulnar G56.2- ☑
　normokalemic periodic G72.3
　ocular H49.9
　　alternating G83.89
　oculofacial, congenital (Moebius) Q87.0
　oculomotor (external bilateral) (nerve) — *see* Strabismus, paralytic, third nerve
　palate (soft) K13.79
　paratrigeminal G50.9
　periodic (familial) (hyperkalemic) (hypokalemic) (myotonic) (normokalemic) (potassium sensitive) (secondary) G72.3
　peripheral autonomic nervous system — *see* Neuropathy, peripheral, autonomic
　peroneal (nerve) G57.3- ☑
　pharynx J39.2
　phrenic nerve G56.8- ☑
　plantar nerve (s) G57.6- ☑
　pneumogastric nerve G52.2

Paralysis — continued
  poliomyelitis (current) — see Poliomyelitis,
    paralytic
  popliteal nerve G57.3- ☑
  postepileptic transitory G83.84
  progressive (atrophic) (bulbar) (spinal) G12.22
    general A52.17
    infantile acute — see Poliomyelitis, paralytic
    supranuclear G23.1
  pseudobulbar G12.29
  pseudohypertrophic (muscle) G71.0
  psychogenic F44.4
  quadriceps G57.9- ☑
  quadriplegic — see Tetraplegia
  radial nerve G56.3- ☑
  rectus muscle (eye) H49.9
  recurrent isolated sleep G47.53
  respiratory (muscle) (system) (tract) R06.81
    center NEC G93.89
    congenital P28.89
    newborn P28.89
  right side — see Hemiplegia
  saturnine T56.0
  sciatic nerve G57.0- ☑
  senile G83.9
  shaking — see Parkinsonism
  shoulder G56.9- ☑
  sleep, recurrent isolated G47.53
  spastic G83.9
    cerebral — see Palsy, cerebral, spastic
    congenital (cerebral) — see Palsy, cerebral,
      spastic
    familial G11.4
    hereditary G11.4
    quadriplegic G80.0
    syphilitic (spinal) A52.17
  sphincter, bladder — see Paralysis, bladder
  spinal (cord) G83.9
    accessory nerve G52.8
    acute — see Poliomyelitis, paralytic
    ascending acute G61.0
    atrophic (acute) (see also Poliomyelitis,
      paralytic)
      spastic, syphilitic A52.17
    congenital NEC — see Palsy, cerebral
    infantile — see Poliomyelitis, paralytic
    hereditary G95.89
    progressive G12.21
    sequelae NEC G83.89
  sternomastoid G52.8
  stomach K31.84
    diabetic — see Diabetes, by type, with
      gastroparesis
    nerve G52.2
      diabetic — see Diabetes, by type, with
        gastroparesis
  stroke — see Infarct, brain
  subcapsularis G56.8- ☑
  supranuclear (progressive) G23.1
  sympathetic G90.8
    cervical G90.09
    nervous system — see Neuropathy, peripheral,
      autonomic
  syndrome G83.9
    specified NEC G83.89
  syphilitic spastic spinal (Erb's) A52.17
  thigh G57.9- ☑
  throat J39.2
    diphtheritic A36.0
    muscle J39.2
  thrombotic (current episode) I63.3 ☑
  thumb G56.9- ☑
  tick — see Toxicity, venom, arthropod, specified
    NEC
  Todd's (postepileptic transitory paralysis) G83.84
  toe G57.6- ☑
  tongue K14.8
  transient R29.5
    arm or leg NEC R29.818
    traumatic NEC — see Injury, nerve
  trapezius G52.8
  traumatic, transient NEC — see Injury, nerve
  trembling — see Parkinsonism
  triceps brachii G56.9- ☑
  trigeminal nerve G50.9
  trochlear (nerve) — see Strabismus, paralytic,
    fourth nerve
  ulnar nerve G56.2- ☑
  upper limb — see Monoplegia, upper limb
  uremic N18.9 [G99.8]
  uveoparotitic D86.89
  uvula K13.79

Paralysis — continued
    postdiphtheritic A36.0
  vagus nerve G52.2
  vasomotor NEC G90.8
  velum palati K13.79
  vesical — see Paralysis, bladder
  vestibular nerve (except Vertigo) H93.3
  vocal cords J38.00
    bilateral J38.02
    unilateral J38.01
  Volkmann's (complicating trauma) T79.6 ☑
  wasting G12.29
  Weber's G46.3
  wrist G56.9- ☑
Paramedial urethrovesical orifice Q64.79
Paramenia N92.6
Parametritis (see also Disease, pelvis, inflammatory)
  N73.2
  acute N73.0
  complicating abortion — see Abortion, by type,
    complicated by, parametritis
Parametrium, parametric — see condition
Paramnesia — see Amnesia
Paramolar K00.1
Paramyloidosis E85.8
Paramyoclonus multiplex G25.3
Paramyotonia (congenita) G71.19
Parangi — see Yaws
Paranoia (querulans) F22
  senile F03 ☑
Paranoid
  dementia (senile) F03 ☑
    praecox — see Schizophrenia
  personality F60.0
  psychosis (climacteric) (involutional)
    (menopausal) F22
    psychogenic (acute) F23
    senile F03 ☑
  reaction (acute) F23
    chronic F22
  schizophrenia F20.0
  state (climacteric) (involutional) (menopausal)
    (simple) F22
    senile F03 ☑
  tendencies F60.0
  traits F60.0
  trends F60.0
  type, psychopathic personality F60.0
Paraparesis — see Paraplegia
Paraphasia R47.02
Paraphilia F65.9
Paraphimosis (congenital) N47.2
  chancroidal A57
Paraphrenia, paraphrenic (late) F22
  schizophrenia F20.0
Paraplegia (lower) G82.20
  ataxic — see Degeneration, combined, spinal
    cord
  complete G82.21
  congenital (cerebral) G80.8
    spastic G80.1
  familial spastic G11.4
  functional (hysterical) F44.4
  hereditary, spastic G11.4
  hysterical F44.4
  incomplete G82.22
  Pott's A18.01
  psychogenic F44.4
  spastic
    Erb's spinal, syphilitic A52.17
    hereditary G11.4
    tropical G04.1
  syphilitic (spastic) A52.17
  tropical spastic G04.1
Parapoxvirus B08.60
  specified NEC B08.69
Paraproteinemia D89.2
  benign (familial) D89.2
  monoclonal D47.2
  secondary to malignant disease D47.2
Parapsoriasis L41.9
  en plaques L41.4
  guttata L41.1
  large plaque L41.4
  retiform, retiformis L41.5
  small plaque L41.3
  specified NEC L41.8
  varioliformis (acuta) L41.0
Parasitic (see also condition)
  disease NEC B89
  stomatitis B37.0
  sycosis (beard) (scalp) B35.0

Parasitic — continued
  twin Q89.4
Parasitism B89
  intestinal B82.9
  skin B88.9
  specified — see Infestation
Parasitophobia F40.218
Parasomnia G47.50
  due to
    alcohol
      abuse F10.182
      dependence F10.282
      use F10.982
    amphetamines
      abuse F15.182
      dependence F15.282
      use F15.982
    caffeine
      abuse F15.182
      dependence F15.282
      use F15.982
    cocaine
      abuse F14.182
      dependence F14.282
      use F14.982
    drug NEC
      abuse F19.182
      dependence F19.282
      use F19.982
    opioid
      abuse F11.182
      dependence F11.282
      use F11.982
    psychoactive substance NEC
      abuse F19.182
      dependence F19.282
      use F19.982
    sedative, hypnotic, or anxiolytic
      abuse F13.182
      dependence F13.282
      use F13.982
    stimulant NEC
      abuse F15.182
      dependence F15.282
      use F15.982
  in conditions classified elsewhere G47.54
  nonorganic origin F51.8
  organic G47.50
  specified NEC G47.59
Paraspadias Q54.9
Paraspasmus facialis G51.8
Parasuicide (attempt)
  history of (personal) Z91.5
    in family Z81.8
Parathyroid gland — see condition
Parathyroid tetany E20.9
Paratrachoma A74.0
Paratyphilitis — see Appendicitis
Paratyphoid (fever) — see Fever, paratyphoid
Paratyphus — see Fever, paratyphoid
Paraurethral duct Q64.79
  nonorganic origin F51.5
Paraurethritis (see also Urethritis)
  gonococcal (acute) (chronic) (with abscess) A54.1
Paravaccinia NEC B08.04
Paravaginitis — see Vaginitis
Parencephalitis (see also Encephalitis)
  sequelae G09
Parent-child conflict — see Conflict, parent-child
  estrangement NEC Z62.890
Paresis (see also Paralysis)
  accommodation — see Paresis, of
    accommodation
  Bernhardt's G57.1- ☑
  bladder (sphincter) (see also Paralysis, bladder)
    tabetic A52.17
  bowel, colon or intestine K56.0
  extrinsic muscle, eye H49.9
  general (progressive) (syphilitic) A52.17
    juvenile A50.45
  heart — see Failure, heart
  insane (syphilitic) A52.17
  juvenile (general) A50.45
  of accommodation H52.52- ☑
  peripheral progressive (idiopathic) G60.3
  pseudohypertrophic G71.0
  senile G83.9
  syphilitic (general) A52.17
    congenital A50.45
  vesical NEC N31.2
Paresthesia (see also Disturbance, sensation)
  Bernhardt G57.1- ☑

Paretic — *see* condition
Parinaud's
  conjunctivitis H10.89
  oculoglandular syndrome H10.89
  ophthalmoplegia H49.88- ☑
Parkinsonism (idiopathic) (primary) G20
  with neurogenic orthostatic hypotension
    (symptomatic) G90.3
  arteriosclerotic G21.4
  dementia G31.83 [F02.80]
    with behavioral disturbance G31.83 [F02.81]
  due to
    drugs NEC G21.19
      neuroleptic G21.11
  neuroleptic induced G21.11
  postencephalitic G21.3
  secondary G21.9
    due to
      arteriosclerosis G21.4
      drugs NEC G21.19
        neuroleptic G21.11
      encephalitis G21.3
      external agents NEC G21.2
      syphilis A52.19
    specified NEC G21.8
    syphilitic A52.19
    treatment-induced NEC G21.19
    vascular G21.4
Parkinson's disease, syndrome or tremor — *see*
  Parkinsonism
Parodontitis — *see* Periodontitis
Parodontosis K05.4
Paronychia (*see also* Cellulitis, digit)
  with lymphangitis — *see* Lymphangitis, acute,
    digit
  candidal (chronic) B37.2
  tuberculous (primary) A18.4
Parorexia (psychogenic) F50.8
Parosmia R43.1
  psychogenic F45.8
Parotid gland — *see* condition
Parotitis, parotiditis (allergic)(nonspecific toxic)
  (purulent) (septic) (suppurative) (*see also*
  Sialoadenitis)
  epidemic — *see* Mumps
  infectious — *see* Mumps
  postoperative K91.89
  surgical K91.89
Parrot fever A70
Parrot's disease (early congenital syphilitic
  pseudoparalysis) A50.02
Parry-Romberg syndrome G51.8
Parry's disease or syndrome E05.00
  with thyroid storm E05.01
Pars planitis — *see* Cyclitis
Parsonage (-Aldren)-Turner syndrome G54.5
Parson's disease (exophthalmic goiter) E05.00
  with thyroid storm E05.01
Particolored infant Q82.8
Parturition — *see* Delivery
Parulis K04.7
  with sinus K04.6
Parvovirus, as cause of disease classified elsewhere
  B97.6
Pasini and Pierini's atrophoderma L90.3
Passage
  false, urethra N36.5
  meconium (newborn) during delivery P03.82
  of sounds or bougies — *see* Attention to, artificial,
    opening
Passive — *see* condition
  smoking Z77.22
Pasteurella septica A28.0
Pasteurellosis — *see* Infection, Pasteurella
PAT (paroxysmal atrial tachycardia) I47.1
Patau's syndrome — *see* Trisomy, 13
Patches
  mucous (syphilitic) A51.39
    congenital A50.07
  smokers' (mouth) K13.24
Patellar — *see* condition
Patent (*see also* Imperfect, closure)
  canal of Nuck Q52.4
  cervix N88.3
  ductus arteriosus or Botallo's Q25.0
  foramen
    botalli Q21.1
    ovale Q21.1
  interauricular septum Q21.1
  interventricular septum Q21.0
  omphalomesenteric duct Q43.0
  os (uteri) — *see* Patent, cervix

Patent — *continued*
  ostium secundum Q21.1
  urachus Q64.4
  vitelline duct Q43.0
Paterson (-Brown)(-Kelly) syndrome or web D50.1
Pathologic, pathological (*see also* condition)
  asphyxia R09.01
  fire-setting F63.1
  gambling F63.0
  ovum O02.0
  resorption, tooth K03.3
  stealing F63.2
Pathology (of) — *see* Disease
  periradicular, associated with previous
    endodontic treatment NEC M27.59
Pattern, sleep-wake, irregular G47.23
Patulous, (*see also* Imperfect, closure (congenital))
  alimentary tract Q45.8
    lower Q43.8
    upper Q40.8
  eustachian tube H69.0- ☑
Pause, sinoatrial I49.5
Paxton's disease B36.2
Pearl (s)
  enamel K00.2
  Epstein's K09.8
Pearl-worker's disease — *see* Osteomyelitis,
  specified type NEC
Pectenosis K62.4
Pectoral — *see* condition
Pectus
  carinatum (congenital) Q67.7
    acquired M95.4
    rachitic sequelae (late effect) E64.3
  excavatum (congenital) Q67.6
    acquired M95.4
    rachitic sequelae (late effect) E64.3
  recurvatum (congenital) Q67.6
Pedatrophia E41
Pederosis F65.4
Pediculosis (infestation) B85.2
  capitis (head-louse) (any site) B85.0
  corporis (body-louse) (any site) B85.1
  eyelid B85.0
  mixed (classifiable to more than one of the titles
    B85.0-B85.3) B85.4
  pubis (pubic louse) (any site) B85.3
  vestimenti B85.1
  vulvae B85.3
Pediculus (infestation) — *see* Pediculosis
Pedophilia F65.4
Peg-shaped teeth K00.2
Pelade — *see* Alopecia, areata
Pelger-Huët anomaly or syndrome D72.0
Peliosis (rheumatica) D69.0
  hepatis K76.4
    with toxic liver disease K71.8
Pelizaeus-Merzbacher disease E75.29
Pellagra (alcoholic) (with polyneuropathy) E52
Pellagra-cerebellar-ataxia-renal aminoaciduria
  syndrome E72.02
Pellegrini (-Stieda) disease or syndrome — *see*
  Bursitis, tibial collateral
Pellizzi's syndrome E34.8
Pel's crisis A52.11
Pelvic (*see also* condition)
  examination (periodic) (routine) Z01.419
    with abnormal findings Z01.411
  kidney, congenital Q63.2
Pelviolithiasis — *see* Calculus, kidney
Pelviperitonitis (*see also* Peritonitis, pelvic)
  gonococcal A54.24
  puerperal O85
Pelvis — *see* condition or type
Pemphigoid L12.9
  benign, mucous membrane L12.1
  bullous L12.0
  cicatricial L12.1
  juvenile L12.2
  ocular L12.1
  specified NEC L12.8
Pemphigus L10.9
  benign familial (chronic) Q82.8
  Brazilian L10.3
  circinatus L13.0
  conjunctiva L12.1
  drug-induced L10.5
  erythematosus L10.4
  foliaceous L10.2
  gangrenous — *see* Gangrene
  neonatorum L01.03
  ocular L12.1

Pemphigus — *continued*
  paraneoplastic L10.81
  specified NEC L10.89
  syphilitic (congenital) A50.06
  vegetans L10.1
  vulgaris L10.0
  wildfire L10.3
Pendred's syndrome E07.1
Pendulous
  abdomen, in pregnancy — *see* Pregnancy,
    complicated by, abnormal, pelvic organs or
    tissues NEC
  breast N64.89
Penetrating wound (*see also* Puncture)
  with internal injury — *see* Injury, by site
  eyeball — *see* Puncture, eyeball
  orbit (with or without foreign body) — *see*
    Puncture, orbit
  uterus by instrument with or following ectopic or
    molar pregnancy O08.6
Penicillosis B48.4
Penis — *see* condition
Penitis N48.29
Pentalogy of Fallot Q21.8
Pentasomy X syndrome Q97.1
Pentosuria (essential) E74.8
Percreta placenta O43.23- ☑
Peregrinating patient — *see* Disorder, factitious
Perforation, perforated (nontraumatic) (of)
  accidental during procedure (blood vessel)
    (nerve) (organ) — *see* Complication,
    accidental puncture or laceration
  antrum — *see* Sinusitis, maxillary
  appendix K35.2
  atrial septum, multiple Q21.1
  attic, ear — *see* Perforation, tympanum, attic
  bile duct (common) (hepatic) K83.2
    cystic K82.2
  bladder (urinary)
    with or following ectopic or molar pregnancy
      O08.6
    obstetrical trauma O71.5
    traumatic S37.29 ☑
      at delivery O71.5
  bowel K63.1
    with or following ectopic or molar pregnancy
      O08.6
    newborn P78.0
    obstetrical trauma O71.5
    traumatic — *see* Laceration, intestine
  broad ligament N83.8
    with or following ectopic or molar pregnancy
      O08.6
    obstetrical trauma O71.6
  by
    device, implant or graft (*see also* Complications,
      by site and type, mechanical) T85.628 ☑
      arterial graft NEC — *see* Complication,
        cardiovascular device, mechanical,
        vascular
      breast (implant) T85.49 ☑
      catheter NEC T85.698 ☑
        cystostomy T83.090 ☑
        dialysis (renal) T82.49 ☑
          intraperitoneal T85.691 ☑
        infusion NEC T82.594 ☑
          spinal (epidural) (subdural) T85.690 ☑
        urinary, indwelling T83.098 ☑
      electronic (electrode) (pulse generator)
        (stimulator)
        bone T84.390 ☑
        cardiac T82.199 ☑
          electrode T82.190 ☑
          pulse generator T82.191 ☑
          specified type NEC T82.198 ☑
        nervous system — *see* Complication,
          prosthetic device, mechanical,
          electronic nervous system stimulator
        urinary — *see* Complication, genitourinary,
          device, urinary, mechanical
      fixation, internal (orthopedic) NEC —
        see Complication, fixation device,
        mechanical
      gastrointestinal — *see* Complications,
        prosthetic device, mechanical,
        gastrointestinal device
      genital NEC T83.498 ☑
        intrauterine contraceptive device T83.39 ☑
        penile prosthesis T83.490 ☑
      heart NEC — *see* Complication,
        cardiovascular device, mechanical

Perforation - Peridiverticulitis

Perforation — *continued*
- joint prosthesis — *see* Complications, joint prosthesis, mechanical, specified NEC, by site
- ocular NEC — *see* Complications, prosthetic device, mechanical, ocular device
- orthopedic NEC — *see* Complication, orthopedic, device, mechanical
  - specified NEC T85.628 ☑
- urinary NEC (*see also* Complication, genitourinary, device, urinary, mechanical)
  - graft T83.29 ☑
- vascular NEC — *see* Complication, cardiovascular device, mechanical
- ventricular intracranial shunt T85.09 ☑
- foreign body left accidentally in operative wound T81.539 ☑
- instrument (any) during a procedure, accidental — *see* Puncture, accidental complicating surgery
- cecum K35.2
- cervix (uteri) N88.8
  - with or following ectopic or molar pregnancy O08.6
  - obstetrical trauma O71.3
- colon K63.1
  - newborn P78.0
  - obstetrical trauma O71.5
  - traumatic — *see* Laceration, intestine, large
- common duct (bile) K83.2
- cornea (due to ulceration) — *see* Ulcer, cornea, perforated
- cystic duct K82.2
- diverticulum (intestine) K57.80
  - with bleeding K57.81
  - large intestine K57.20
    - with
      - bleeding K57.21
      - small intestine K57.40
        - with bleeding K57.41
  - small intestine K57.00
    - with
      - bleeding K57.01
      - large intestine K57.40
        - with bleeding K57.41
- ear drum — *see* Perforation, tympanum
- esophagus K22.3
- ethmoidal sinus — *see* Sinusitis, ethmoidal
- frontal sinus — *see* Sinusitis, frontal
- gallbladder K82.2
- heart valve — *see* Endocarditis
- ileum K63.1
  - newborn P78.0
  - obstetrical trauma O71.5
  - traumatic — *see* Laceration, intestine, small
- instrumental, surgical (accidental) (blood vessel) (nerve) (organ) — *see* Puncture, accidental complicating surgery
- intestine NEC K63.1
  - with ectopic or molar pregnancy O08.6
  - newborn P78.0
  - obstetrical trauma O71.5
  - traumatic — *see* Laceration, intestine
  - ulcerative NEC K63.1
    - newborn P78.0
- jejunum, jejunal K63.1
  - obstetrical trauma O71.5
  - traumatic — *see* Laceration, intestine, small
  - ulcer — *see* Ulcer, gastrojejunal, with perforation
- joint prosthesis — *see* Complications, joint prosthesis, mechanical, specified NEC, by site
- mastoid (antrum) (cell) — *see* Disorder, mastoid, specified NEC
- maxillary sinus — *see* Sinusitis, maxillary
- membrana tympani — *see* Perforation, tympanum
- nasal
  - septum J34.89
    - congenital Q30.3
    - syphilitic A52.73
  - sinus J34.89
    - congenital Q30.8
    - due to sinusitis — *see* Sinusitis
- palate (*see also* Cleft, palate) Q35.9
  - syphilitic A52.79
- palatine vault (*see also* Cleft, palate, hard) Q35.1
  - syphilitic A52.79
  - congenital A50.59
- pars flaccida (ear drum) — *see* Perforation, tympanum, attic

Perforation — *continued*
- pelvic
  - floor S31.030 ☑
    - with
      - ectopic or molar pregnancy O08.6
      - penetration into retroperitoneal space S31.031 ☑
      - retained foreign body S31.040 ☑
        - with penetration into retroperitoneal space S31.041 ☑
    - following ectopic or molar pregnancy O08.6
    - obstetrical trauma O70.1
  - organ S37.99 ☑
    - adrenal gland S37.818 ☑
    - bladder — *see* Perforation, bladder
    - fallopian tube S37.599 ☑
      - bilateral S37.592 ☑
      - unilateral S37.591 ☑
    - kidney S37.09- ☑
      - obstetrical trauma O71.5
    - ovary S37.499 ☑
      - bilateral S37.492 ☑
      - unilateral S37.491 ☑
    - prostate S37.828 ☑
    - specified organ NEC S37.898 ☑
    - ureter — *see* Perforation, ureter
    - urethra — *see* Perforation, urethra
    - uterus — *see* Perforation, uterus
- perineum — *see* Laceration, perineum
- pharynx J39.2
- rectum K63.1
  - newborn P78.0
  - obstetrical trauma O71.5
  - traumatic S36.63 ☑
- root canal space due to endodontic treatment M27.51
- sigmoid K63.1
  - newborn P78.0
  - obstetrical trauma O71.5
  - traumatic S36.533 ☑
- sinus (accessory) (chronic) (nasal) J34.89
- sphenoidal sinus — *see* Sinusitis, sphenoidal
- surgical (accidental) (by instrument) (blood vessel) (nerve) (organ) — *see* Puncture, accidental complicating surgery
- traumatic
  - external — *see* Puncture
  - eye — *see* Puncture, eyeball
  - internal organ — *see* Injury, by site
- tympanum, tympanic (membrane) (persistent post-traumatic) (postinflammatory) H72.9- ☑
  - attic H72.1- ☑
    - multiple — *see* Perforation, tympanum, multiple
    - total — *see* Perforation, tympanum, total
  - central H72.0- ☑
    - multiple — *see* Perforation, tympanum, multiple
    - total — *see* Perforation, tympanum, total
  - marginal NEC H72.2
  - multiple H72.81- ☑
  - pars flaccida — *see* Perforation, tympanum, attic
  - total H72.82- ☑
  - traumatic, current episode S09.2- ☑
- typhoid, gastrointestinal — *see* Typhoid
- ulcer — *see* Ulcer, by site, with perforation
- ureter N28.89
  - traumatic S37.19 ☑
- urethra N36.8
  - with ectopic or molar pregnancy O08.6
  - following ectopic or molar pregnancy O08.6
  - obstetrical trauma O71.5
  - traumatic S37.39 ☑
    - at delivery O71.5
- uterus
  - with ectopic or molar pregnancy O08.6
  - by intrauterine contraceptive device T83.39 ☑
  - following ectopic or molar pregnancy O08.6
  - obstetrical trauma O71.1
  - traumatic S37.69 ☑
    - obstetric O71.1
- uvula K13.79
  - syphilitic A52.79
- vagina
  - obstetrical trauma O71.4
  - other trauma — *see* Puncture, vagina
- **Periadenitis** mucosa necrotica recurrens K12.0
- **Periappendicitis** (acute) — *see* Appendicitis
- **Periarteritis** nodosa (disseminated) (infectious) (necrotizing) M30.0
- **Periarthritis** (joint) (*see also* Enthesopathy)

Periarthritis — *continued*
- Duplay's M75.0- ☑
- gonococcal A54.42
- humeroscapularis — *see* Capsulitis, adhesive
- scapulohumeral — *see* Capsulitis, adhesive
- shoulder — *see* Capsulitis, adhesive
- wrist M77.2- ☑
- **Periarthrosis** (angioneural) — *see* Enthesopathy
- **Pericapsulitis**, adhesive (shoulder) — *see* Capsulitis, adhesive
- **Pericarditis** (with decompensation) (with effusion) I31.9
  - with rheumatic fever (conditions in I00)
    - active — *see* Pericarditis, rheumatic
    - inactive or quiescent I09.2
  - acute (hemorrhagic) (nonrheumatic) (Sicca) I30.9
    - with chorea (acute) (rheumatic) (Sydenham's) I02.0
  - benign I30.8
  - nonspecific I30.0
  - rheumatic I01.0
    - with chorea (acute) (Sydenham's) I02.0
  - adhesive or adherent (chronic) (external) (internal) I31.0
    - acute — *see* Pericarditis, acute
    - rheumatic I09.2
  - bacterial (acute) (subacute) (with serous or seropurulent effusion) I30.1
  - calcareous I31.1
  - cholesterol (chronic) I31.8
    - acute I30.9
  - chronic (nonrheumatic) I31.9
    - rheumatic I09.2
  - constrictive (chronic) I31.1
  - coxsackie B33.23
  - fibrinocaseous (tuberculous) A18.84
  - fibrinopurulent I30.1
  - fibrinous I30.8
  - fibrous I31.0
  - gonococcal A54.83
  - idiopathic I30.0
  - in systemic lupus erythematosus M32.12
  - infective I30.1
  - meningococcal A39.53
  - neoplastic (chronic) I31.8
    - acute I30.9
  - obliterans, obliterating I31.0
  - plastic I31.0
  - pneumococcal I30.1
  - postinfarction I24.1
  - purulent I30.1
  - rheumatic (active) (acute) (with effusion) (with pneumonia) I01.0
    - with chorea (acute) (rheumatic) (Sydenham's) I02.0
    - chronic or inactive (with chorea) I09.2
  - rheumatoid — *see* Rheumatoid, carditis
  - septic I30.1
  - serofibrinous I30.8
  - staphylococcal I30.1
  - streptococcal I30.1
  - suppurative I30.1
  - syphilitic A52.06
  - tuberculous A18.84
  - uremic N18.9 [I32]
  - viral I30.1
- **Pericardium, pericardial** — *see* condition
- **Pericellulitis** — *see* Cellulitis
- **Pericementitis** (chronic) (suppurative) (*see also* Periodontitis)
  - acute K05.20
    - generalized K05.22
    - localized K05.21
- **Perichondritis**
  - auricle — *see* Perichondritis, ear
  - bronchus J98.09
  - ear (external) H61.00- ☑
    - acute H61.01- ☑
    - chronic H61.02- ☑
  - external auditory canal — *see* Perichondritis, ear
  - larynx J38.7
    - syphilitic A52.73
    - typhoid A01.09
  - nose J34.89
  - pinna — *see* Perichondritis, ear
  - trachea J39.8
- **Periclasia** K05.4
- **Pericoronitis** — *see* Periodontitis
- **Pericystitis** N30.90
  - with hematuria N30.91
- **Peridiverticulitis** (intestine) K57.92
  - cecum — *see* Diverticulitis, intestine, large

☑ **Additional character required**

Peridiverticulitis — *continued*
  colon — *see* Diverticulitis, intestine, large
  duodenum — *see* Diverticulitis, intestine, small
  intestine — *see* Diverticulitis, intestine
  jejunum — *see* Diverticulitis, intestine, small
  rectosigmoid — *see* Diverticulitis, intestine, large
  rectum — *see* Diverticulitis, intestine, large
  sigmoid — *see* Diverticulitis, intestine, large
Periendocarditis — *see* Endocarditis
Periepididymitis N45.1
Perifolliculitis L01.02
  abscedens, caput, scalp L66.3
  capitis, abscedens (et suffodiens) L66.3
  superficial pustular L01.02
Perihepatitis K65.8
Perilabyrinthitis (acute)H83.0
Perimeningitis — *see* Meningitis
Perimetritis — *see* Endometritis
Perimetrosalpingitis — *see* Salpingo-oophoritis
Perineocele N81.81
Perinephric, perinephritic — *see* condition
Perinephritis (*see also* Infection, kidney)
  purulent — *see* Abscess, kidney
Perineum, perineal — *see* condition
Perineuritis NEC — *see* Neuralgia
Periodic — *see* condition
Periodontitis (chronic) (complex) (compound)
  (local) (simplex) K05.30
  acute K05.20
    generalized K05.22
    localized K05.21
  apical K04.5
    acute (pulpal origin) K04.4
  generalized K05.32
  localized K05.31
Periodontoclasia K05.4
Periodontosis (juvenile) K05.4
Periods (*see also* Menstruation)
  heavy N92.0
  irregular N92.6
  shortened intervals (irregular) N92.1
Perionychia (*see also* Cellulitis, digit)
  with lymphangitis — *see* Lymphangitis, acute,
    digit
Perioophoritis — *see* Salpingo-oophoritis
Periorchitis N45.2
Periosteum, periosteal — *see* condition
Periostitis (albuminosa) (circumscribed) (diffuse)
  (infective) (monomelic) (*see also* Osteomyelitis)
  alveolar M27.3
  alveolodental M27.3
  dental M27.3
  gonorrheal A54.43
  jaw (lower) (upper) M27.2
  orbit H05.03- ☑
  syphilitic A52.77
    congenital (early) A50.02 [M90.80]
    secondary A51.46
  tuberculous — *see* Tuberculosis, bone
  yaws (hypertrophic) (early) (late) A66.6 [M90.80]
Periostosis (hyperplastic) (*see also* Disorder, bone,
  specified type NEC)
  with osteomyelitis — *see* Osteomyelitis, specified
    type NEC
Peripartum
  cardiomyopathy O90.3
Periphlebitis — *see* Phlebitis
Periproctitis K62.89
Periprostatitis — *see* Prostatitis
Perirectal — *see* condition
Perirenal — *see* condition
Perisalpingitis — *see* Salpingo-oophoritis
Perisplenitis (infectional) D73.89
Peristalsis, visible or reversed R19.2
Peritendinitis — *see* Enthesopathy
Peritoneum, peritoneal — *see* condition
Peritonitis (adhesive) (bacterial) (fibrinous)
  (hemorrhagic) (idiopathic) (localized) (perforative)
  (primary) (with adhesions) (with effusion) K65.9
  with or following
    abscess K65.1
    appendicitis K35.2
      with perforation or rupture K35.2
      generalized K35.2
      localized K35.3
    diverticular disease (intestine) K57.80
      with bleeding K57.81
      large intestine K57.20
        with
          bleeding K57.21
          small intestine K57.40
            with bleeding K57.41

Peritonitis — *continued*
  small intestine K57.00
    with
      bleeding K57.01
      large intestine K57.40
        with bleeding K57.41
    ectopic or molar pregnancy O08.0
  acute (generalized) K65.0
  aseptic T81.61 ☑
  bile, biliary K65.3
  chemical T81.61 ☑
  chlamydial A74.81
  complicating abortion — *see* Abortion, by type,
    complicated by, pelvic peritonitis
  congenital P78.1
  chronic proliferative K65.8
  diaphragmatic K65.0
  diffuse K65.0
  diphtheritic A36.89
  disseminated K65.0
  due to
    bile K65.3
    foreign
      body or object accidentally left during a
        procedure (instrument) (sponge) (swab)
        T81.599 ☑
      substance accidentally left during a
        procedure (chemical) (powder) (talc)
        T81.61 ☑
    talc T81.61 ☑
    urine K65.8
  eosinophilic K65.8
    acute K65.0
  fibrocaseous (tuberculous) A18.31
  fibropurulent K65.0
  following ectopic or molar pregnancy O08.0
  general (ized) K65.0
  gonococcal A54.85
  meconium (newborn) P78.0
  neonatal P78.1
    meconium P78.0
  pancreatic K65.0
  paroxysmal, familial E85.0
    benign E85.0
  pelvic
    female N73.5
      acute N73.3
      chronic N73.4
        with adhesions N73.6
    male K65.0
  periodic, familial E85.0
  proliferative, chronic K65.8
  puerperal, postpartum, childbirth O85
  purulent K65.0
  septic K65.0
  specified NEC K65.8
  spontaneous bacterial K65.2
  subdiaphragmatic K65.0
  subphrenic K65.0
  suppurative K65.0
  syphilitic A52.74
    congenital (early) A50.08 [K67]
  talc T81.61 ☑
  tuberculous A18.31
  urine K65.8
Peritonsillar — *see* condition
Peritonsillitis J36
Perityphlitis K37
Periureteritis N28.89
Periurethral — *see* condition
Periurethritis (gangrenous) — *see* Urethritis
Periuterine — *see* condition
Perivaginitis — *see* Vaginitis
Perivasculitis, retinal H35.06- ☑
Perivasitis (chronic) N49.1
Perivesiculitis (seminal) — *see* Vesiculitis
Perlèche NEC K13.0
  due to
    candidiasis B37.83
    moniliasis B37.83
    riboflavin deficiency E53.0
    vitamin B2 (riboflavin) deficiency E53.0
Pernicious — *see* condition
Pernio, perniosis T69.1 ☑
Perpetrator (of abuse) — *see* Index to External
  Causes of Injury, Perpetrator
Persecution
  delusion F22
  social Z60.5
Perseveration (tonic) R48.8
Persistence, persistent (congenital)
  anal membrane Q42.3

Persistence — *continued*
  with fistula Q42.2
  arteria stapedia Q16.3
  atrioventricular canal Q21.2
  branchial cleft Q18.0
  bulbus cordis in left ventricle Q21.8
  canal of Cloquet Q14.0
  capsule (opaque) Q12.8
  cilioretinal artery or vein Q14.8
  cloaca Q43.7
  communication — *see* Fistula, congenital
  convolutions
    aortic arch Q25.4
    fallopian tube Q50.6
    oviduct Q50.6
    uterine tube Q50.6
  double aortic arch Q25.4
  ductus arteriosus (Botalli) Q25.0
  fetal
    circulation P29.3
    form of cervix (uteri) Q51.828
    hemoglobin, hereditary (HPFH) D56.4
  foramen
    Botalli Q21.1
    ovale Q21.1
  Gartner's duct Q52.4
  hemoglobin, fetal (hereditary) (HPFH) D56.4
  hyaloid
    artery (generally incomplete) Q14.0
    system Q14.8
  hymen, in pregnancy or childbirth — *see*
    Pregnancy, complicated by, abnormal, vulva
  lanugo Q84.2
  left
    posterior cardinal vein Q26.8
    root with right arch of aorta Q25.4
    superior vena cava Q26.1
  Meckel's diverticulum Q43.0
    malignant — *see* Table of Neoplasms, small
      intestine, malignant
  mucosal disease (middle ear) — *see* Otitis, media,
    suppurative, chronic, tubotympanic
  nail (s), anomalous Q84.6
  omphalomesenteric duct Q43.0
  organ or site not listed — *see* Anomaly, by site
  ostium
    atrioventriculare commune Q21.2
    primum Q21.2
    secundum Q21.1
  ovarian rests in fallopian tube Q50.6
  pancreatic tissue in intestinal tract Q43.8
  primary (deciduous)
    teeth K00.6
    vitreous hyperplasia Q14.0
  pupillary membrane Q13.89
  right aortic arch Q25.4
  rhesus (Rh) titer — *see* Complication(s),
    transfusion, incompatibility reaction, Rh
    (factor)
  sinus
    urogenitalis
      female Q52.8
      male Q55.8
    venosus with imperfect incorporation in right
      auricle Q26.8
  thymus (gland) (hyperplasia) E32.0
  thyroglossal duct Q89.2
  thyrolingual duct Q89.2
  truncus arteriosus or communis Q20.0
  tunica vasculosa lentis Q12.2
  umbilical sinus Q64.4
  urachus Q64.4
  vitelline duct Q43.0
Person (with)
  admitted for clinical research, as a control subject
    (normal comparison) (participant) Z00.6
  awaiting admission to adequate facility
    elsewhere Z75.1
  concern (normal) about sick person in family
    Z63.6
  consulting on behalf of another Z71.0
  feigning illness Z76.5
  living (in)
    alone Z60.2
    boarding school Z59.3
    residential institution Z59.3
    without
      adequate housing (heating) (space) Z59.1
      housing (permanent) (temporary) Z59.0
      person able to render necessary care Z74.2
      shelter Z59.0
  on waiting list Z75.1

Person — *continued*
  sick or handicapped in family Z63.6
Personality (disorder) F60.9
  accentuation of traits (type A pattern) Z73.1
  affective F34.0
  aggressive F60.3
  amoral F60.2
  anacastic, anankastic F60.5
  antisocial F60.2
  anxious F60.6
  asocial F60.2
  asthenic F60.7
  avoidant F60.6
  borderline F60.3
  change due to organic condition (enduring) F07.0
  compulsive F60.5
  cycloid F34.0
  cyclothymic F34.0
  dependent F60.7
  depressive F34.1
  dissocial F60.2
  dual F44.81
  eccentric F60.89
  emotionally unstable F60.3
  expansive paranoid F60.0
  explosive F60.3
  fanatic F60.0
  haltose type F60.89
  histrionic F60.4
  hyperthymic F34.0
  hypothymic F34.1
  hysterical F60.4
  immature F60.89
  inadequate F60.7
  labile (emotional) F60.3
  mixed (nonspecific) F60.81
  morally defective F60.2
  multiple F44.81
  narcissistic F60.81
  obsessional F60.5
  obsessive (-compulsive) F60.5
  organic F07.0
  overconscientious F60.5
  paranoid F60.0
  passive (-dependent) F60.7
  passive-aggressive F60.89
  pathologic F60.9
  pattern defect or disturbance F60.9
  pseudopsychopathic (organic) F07.0
  pseudoretarded (organic) F07.0
  psychoinfantile F60.4
  psychoneurotic NEC F60.89
  psychopathic F60.2
  querulant F60.0
  sadistic F60.89
  schizoid F60.1
  self-defeating F60.7
  sensitive paranoid F60.0
  sociopathic (amoral) (antisocial) (asocial) (dissocial) F60.2
  specified NEC F60.89
  type A Z73.1
  unstable (emotional) F60.3
Perthes' disease — *see* Legg-Calvé-Perthes disease
Pertussis (*see also* Whooping cough) A37.90
Perversion, perverted
  appetite F50.8
    psychogenic F50.8
  function
    pituitary gland E23.2
      posterior lobe E22.2
  sense of smell and taste R43.8
    psychogenic F45.8
  sexual — *see* Deviation, sexual
Pervious, congenital (*see also* Imperfect, closure)
  ductus arteriosus Q25.0
Pes (congenital) (*see also* Talipes)
  acquired (*see also* Deformity, limb, foot, specified NEC)
    planus — *see* Deformity, limb, flat foot
  adductus Q66.89
  cavus Q66.7
  deformity NEC, acquired — *see* Deformity, limb, foot, specified NEC
  planus (acquired) (any degree) (*see also* Deformity, limb, flat foot)
    rachitic sequelae (late effect) E64.3
  valgus Q66.6
Pest, pestis — *see* Plague
Petechia, petechiae R23.3
  newborn P54.5

Petechial typhus A75.9
Peter's anomaly Q13.4
Petit mal seizure — *see* Epilepsy, generalized, specified NEC
Petit's hernia — *see* Hernia, abdomen, specified site NEC
Petrellidosis B48.2
Petrositis H70.20- ☑
  acute H70.21- ☑
  chronic H70.22- ☑
Peutz-Jeghers disease or syndrome Q85.8
Peyronie's disease N48.6
Pfeiffer's disease — *see* Mononucleosis, infectious
Phagedena (dry) (moist) (sloughing) (*see also* Gangrene)
  geometric L88
  penis N48.29
  tropical — *see* Ulcer, skin
  vulva N76.6
Phagedenic — *see* condition
Phakoma H35.89
Phakomatosis (*see also* specific eponymous syndromes) Q85.9
  Bourneville's Q85.1
  specified NEC Q85.8
Phantom limb syndrome (without pain) G54.7
  with pain G54.6
Pharyngeal pouch syndrome D82.1
Pharyngitis (acute) (catarrhal)(gangrenous) (infective) (malignant) (membranous) (phlegmonous) (pseudomembranous) (simple) (subacute) (suppurative) (ulcerative) (viral) J02.9
  with influenza, flu, or grippe — *see* Influenza, with, pharyngitis
  aphthous B08.5
  atrophic J31.2
  chlamydial A56.4
  chronic (atrophic) (granular) (hypertrophic) J31.2
  coxsackievirus B08.5
  diphtheritic A36.0
  enteroviral vesicular B08.5
  follicular (chronic) J31.2
  fusospirochetal A69.1
  gonococcal A54.5
  granular (chronic) J31.2
  herpesviral B00.2
  hypertrophic J31.2
  infectional, chronic J31.2
  influenzal — *see* Influenza, with, respiratory manifestations NEC
  lymphonodular, acute (enteroviral) B08.8
  pneumococcal J02.8
  purulent J02.9
  putrid J02.9
  septic J02.0
  sicca J31.2
  specified organism NEC J02.8
  staphylococcal J02.8
  streptococcal J02.0
  syphilitic, congenital (early) A50.03
  tuberculous A15.8
  vesicular, enteroviral B08.5
  viral NEC J02.8
Pharyngoconjunctivitis, viral B30.2
Pharyngolaryngitis (acute) J06.0
  chronic J37.0
Pharyngoplegia J39.2
Pharyngotonsillitis, herpesviral B00.2
Pharyngotracheitis, chronic J42
Pharynx, pharyngeal — *see* condition
Phenomenon
  Arthus' — *see* Arthus' phenomenon
  jaw-winking Q07.8
  lupus erythematosus (LE) cell M32.9
  Raynaud's (secondary) I73.00
    with gangrene I73.01
  vasomotor R55
  vasospastic I73.9
  vasovagal R55
  Wenckebach's I44.1
Phenylketonuria E70.1
  classical E70.0
  maternal E70.1
Pheochromoblastoma
  specified site — *see* Neoplasm, malignant, by site
  unspecified site C74.10
Pheochromocytoma
  malignant
    specified site — *see* Neoplasm, malignant, by site
    unspecified site C74.10
  specified site — *see* Neoplasm, benign, by site

Pheochromocytoma — *continued*
  unspecified site D35.00
Pheohyphomycosis — *see* Chromomycosis
Pheomycosis — *see* Chromomycosis
Phimosis (congenital) (due to infection) N47.1
  chancroidal A57
Phlebectasia (*see also* Varix)
  congenital Q27.4
Phlebitis (infective) (pyemic) (septic) (suppurative) I80.9
  antepartum — *see* Thrombophlebitis, antepartum
  blue — *see* Phlebitis, leg, deep
  breast, superficial I80.8
  cavernous (venous) sinus — *see* Phlebitis, intracranial (venous) sinus
  cerebral (venous) sinus — *see* Phlebitis, intracranial (venous) sinus
  chest wall, superficial I80.8
  cranial (venous) sinus — *see* Phlebitis, intracranial (venous) sinus
  deep (vessels) — *see* Phlebitis, leg, deep
  due to implanted device — *see* Complications, by site and type, specified NEC
  during or resulting from a procedure T81.72 ☑
  femoral vein (superficial) I80.1- ☑
  femoropopliteal vein I80.0- ☑
  gestational — *see* Phlebopathy, gestational
  hepatic veins I80.8
  iliofemoral — *see* Phlebitis, femoral vein
  intracranial (venous) sinus (any) G08
    nonpyogenic I67.6
  intraspinal venous sinuses and veins G08
    nonpyogenic G95.19
  lateral (venous) sinus — *see* Phlebitis, intracranial (venous) sinus
  leg I80.3
    antepartum — *see* Thrombophlebitis, antepartum
    deep (vessels) NEC I80.20- ☑
      iliac I80.21- ☑
      popliteal vein I80.22- ☑
      specified vessel NEC I80.29- ☑
      tibial vein I80.23- ☑
    femoral vein (superficial) I80.1- ☑
    superficial (vessels) I80.0- ☑
  longitudinal sinus — *see* Phlebitis, intracranial (venous) sinus
  lower limb — *see* Phlebitis, leg
  migrans, migrating (superficial) I82.1
  pelvic
    with ectopic or molar pregnancy O08.0
    following ectopic or molar pregnancy O08.0
    puerperal, postpartum O87.1
  popliteal vein — *see* Phlebitis, leg, deep, popliteal
  portal (vein) K75.1
  postoperative T81.72 ☑
  pregnancy — *see* Thrombophlebitis, antepartum
  puerperal, postpartum, childbirth O87.0
    deep O87.1
    pelvic O87.1
    superficial O87.0
  retina — *see* Vasculitis, retina
  saphenous (accessory) (great) (long) (small) — *see* Phlebitis, leg, superficial
  sinus (meninges) — *see* Phlebitis, intracranial (venous) sinus
  specified site NEC I80.8
  syphilitic A52.09
  tibial vein — *see* Phlebitis, leg, deep, tibial
  ulcerative I80.9
    leg — *see* Phlebitis, leg
  umbilicus I80.8
  uterus (septic) — *see* Endometritis
  varicose (leg) (lower limb) — *see* Varix, leg, with, inflammation
Phlebofibrosis I87.8
Pheboliths I87.8
Phlebopathy,
  gestational O22.9- ☑
  puerperal O87.9
Phlebosclerosis I87.8
Phlebothrombosis (*see also* Thrombosis)
  antepartum — *see* Thrombophlebitis, antepartum
  pregnancy — *see* Thrombophlebitis, antepartum
  puerperal — *see* Thrombophlebitis, puerperal
Phlebotomus fever A93.1
Phlegmasia
  alba dolens O87.1
    nonpuerperal — *see* Phlebitis, femoral vein
  cerulea dolens — *see* Phlebitis, leg, deep

☑ **Additional character required**

Phlegmon — *see* Abscess
Phlegmonous — *see* condition
Phlyctenulosis (allergic) (keratoconjunctivitis) (nontuberculous) (*see also* Keratoconjunctivitis)
  cornea — *see* Keratoconjunctivitis
  tuberculous A18.52
Phobia, phobic F40.9
  animal F40.218
    spiders F40.210
  examination F40.298
  reaction F40.9
  simple F40.298
  social F40.10
    generalized F40.11
  specific (isolated) F40.298
    animal F40.218
      spiders F40.210
    blood F40.230
    injection F40.231
    injury F40.233
    men F40.290
    natural environment F40.228
      thunderstorms F40.220
    situational F40.248
      bridges F40.242
      closed in spaces F40.240
      flying F40.243
      heights F40.241
    specified focus NEC F40.298
    transfusion F40.231
    women F40.291
  specified NEC F40.8
    medical care NEC F40.232
  state F40.9
Phocas' disease — *see* Mastopathy, cystic
Phocomelia Q73.1
  lower limb — *see* Agenesis, leg, with foot present
  upper limb — *see* Agenesis, arm, with hand present
Phoria H50.50
Phosphate-losing tubular disorder N25.0
Phosphatemia E83.39
Phosphaturia E83.39
Photodermatitis (sun) L56.8
  chronic L57.8
  due to drug L56.8
  light other than sun L59.8
Photokeratitis H16.13- ☑
Photophobia H53.14- ☑
Photophthalmia — *see* Photokeratitis
Photopsia H53.19
Photoretinitis — *see* Retinopathy, solar
Photosensitivity, photosensitization (sun) skin L56.8
  light other than sun L59.8
Phrenitis — *see* Encephalitis
Phrynoderma (vitamin A deficiency) E50.8
Phthiriasis (pubis) B85.3
  with any infestation classifiable to B85.0-B85.2 B85.4
Phthirus infestation — *see* Phthiriasis
Phthisis (*see also* Tuberculosis)
  bulbi (infectional) — *see* Disorder, globe, degenerated condition, atrophy
  eyeball (due to infection) — *see* Disorder, globe, degenerated condition, atrophy
Phycomycosis — *see* Zygomycosis
Physalopteriasis B81.8
Physical restraint status Z78.1
Phytobezoar T18.9 ☑
  intestine T18.3 ☑
  stomach T18.2 ☑
Pian — *see* Yaws
Pianoma A66.1
Pica F50.8
  in adults F50.8
  infant or child F98.3
Picking, nose F98.8
Pick-Niemann disease — *see* Niemann-Pick disease or syndrome
Pick's
  cerebral atrophy G31.01 [F02.80]
    with behavioral disturbance G31.01 [F02.81]
  disease or syndrome (brain) G31.01 [F02.80]
    with behavioral disturbance G31.01 [F02.81]
Pickwickian syndrome E66.2
Piebaldism E70.39
Piedra (beard) (scalp) B36.8
  black B36.3
  white B36.2
Pierre Robin deformity or syndrome Q87.0
Pierson's disease or osteochondrosis M91.0

Pig-bel A05.2
Pigeon
  breast or chest (acquired) M95.4
    congenital Q67.7
    rachitic sequelae (late effect) E64.3
  breeder's disease or lung J67.2
  fancier's disease or lung J67.2
  toe — *see* Deformity, toe, specified NEC
Pigmentation (abnormal) (anomaly) L81.9
  conjunctiva H11.13- ☑
  cornea (anterior) H18.01- ☑
    posterior H18.05- ☑
    stromal H18.06- ☑
  diminished melanin formation NEC L81.6
  iron L81.8
  lids, congenital Q82.8
  limbus corneae — *see* Pigmentation, cornea
  metals L81.8
  optic papilla, congenital Q14.2
  retina, congenital (grouped) (nevoid) Q14.1
  scrotum, congenital Q82.8
  tattoo L81.8
Piles (*see also* Hemorrhoids) K64.9
Pili
  annulati or torti (congenital) Q84.1
  incarnati L73.1
Pill roller hand (intrinsic) — *see* Parkinsonism
Pilomatrixoma — *see* Neoplasm, skin, benign
  malignant — *see* Neoplasm, skin, malignant
Pilonidal — *see* condition
Pimple R23.8
Pinched nerve — *see* Neuropathy, entrapment
Pindborg tumor — *see* Cyst, calcifying odontogenic
Pineal body or gland — *see* condition
Pinealoblastoma C75.3
Pinealoma D44.5
  malignant C75.3
Pineoblastoma C75.3
Pineocytoma D44.5
Pinguecula H11.15- ☑
Pingueculitis H10.81- ☑
Pinhole meatus (*see also* Stricture, urethra) N35.9
Pink
  disease T56.1
  eye — *see* Conjunctivitis, acute, mucopurulent
Pinkus' disease (lichen nitidus) L44.1
Pinpoint
  meatus — *see* Stricture, urethra
  os (uteri) — *see* Stricture, cervix
Pins and needles R20.2
Pinta A67.9
  cardiovascular lesions A67.2
  chancre (primary) A67.0
  erythematous plaques A67.1
  hyperchromic lesions A67.1
  hyperkeratosis A67.1
  lesions A67.9
    cardiovascular A67.2
    hyperchromic A67.1
    intermediate A67.1
    late A67.2
    mixed A67.3
    primary A67.0
    skin (achromic) (cicatricial) (dyschromic) A67.2
      hyperchromic A67.1
      mixed (achromic and hyperchromic) A67.3
  papule (primary) A67.0
  skin lesions (achromic) (cicatricial) (dyschromic) A67.2
    hyperchromic A67.1
    mixed (achromic and hyperchromic) A67.3
  vitiligo A67.2
Pintids A67.1
Pinworm (disease) (infection) (infestation) B80
Piroplasmosis B60.0
Pistol wound — *see* Gunshot wound
Pitchers' elbow — *see* Derangement, joint, specified type NEC, elbow
Pithecoid pelvis Q74.2
  with disproportion (fetopelvic) O33.0
    causing obstructed labor O65.0
Pithiatism F48.8
Pitted — *see* Pitting
Pitting (*see also* Edema) R60.9
  lip R60.0
  nail L60.8
  teeth K00.4
Pituitary gland — *see* condition
Pituitary-snuff-taker's disease J67.8
Pityriasis (capitis) L21.0
  alba L30.5
  circinata (et maculata) L42

Pityriasis — *continued*
  furfuracea L21.0
  Hebra's L26
  lichenoides L41.0
    chronica L41.1
    et varioliformis (acuta) L41.0
  maculata (et circinata) L30.5
  nigra B36.1
  pilaris, Hebra's L44.0
  rosea L42
  rotunda L44.8
  rubra (Hebra) pilaris L44.0
  simplex L30.5
  specified type NEC L30.5
  streptogenes L30.5
  versicolor (scrotal) B36.0
Placenta, placental — *see* Pregnancy, complicated by (care of) (management affected by), specified condition
Placentitis O41.14- ☑
Plagiocephaly Q67.3
Plague A20.9
  abortive A20.8
  ambulatory A20.8
  asymptomatic A20.8
  bubonic A20.0
  cellulocutaneous A20.1
  cutaneobubonic A20.1
  lymphatic gland A20.0
  meningitis A20.3
  pharyngeal A20.8
  pneumonic (primary) (secondary) A20.2
  pulmonary, pulmonic A20.2
  septicemic A20.7
  tonsillar A20.8
    septicemic A20.7
Planning, family
  contraception Z30.9
  procreation Z31.69
Plaque (s)
  artery, arterial — *see* Arteriosclerosis
  calcareous — *see* Calcification
  coronary, lipid rich I25.83
  epicardial I31.8
  erythematous, of pinta A67.1
  Hollenhorst's — *see* Occlusion, artery, retina
  lipid rich, coronary I25.83
  pleural (without asbestos) J92.9
    with asbestos J92.0
  tongue K13.29
Plasmacytoma C90.3- ☑
  extramedullary C90.2- ☑
  medullary C90.0- ☑
  solitary C90.3- ☑
Plasmacytopenia D72.818
Plasmacytosis D72.822
Plaster ulcer — *see* Ulcer, pressure, by site
Plateau iris syndrome (post-iridectomy) (postprocedural) (without glaucoma) H21.82
  with glaucoma H40.22- ☑
Platybasia Q75.8
Platyonychia (congenital) Q84.6
  acquired L60.8
Platypelloid pelvis M95.5
  with disproportion (fetopelvic) O33.0
    causing obstructed labor O65.0
  congenital Q74.2
Platyspondylisis Q76.49
Plaut (-Vincent) disease (*see also* Vincent's) A69.1
Plethora R23.2
  newborn P61.1
Pleura, pleural — *see* condition
Pleuralgia R07.81
Pleurisy (acute) (adhesive) (chronic) (costal) (diaphragmatic) (double) (dry) (fibrinous) (fibrous) (interlobar) (latent) (plastic) (primary) (residual) (sicca) (sterile) (subacute) (unresolved) R09.1
  with
    adherent pleura J86.0
    effusion J90
      chylous, chyliform J94.0
      tuberculous (non primary) A15.6
        primary (progressive) A15.7
      tuberculosis — *see* Pleurisy, tuberculous (non primary)
  encysted — *see* Pleurisy, with effusion
  exudative — *see* Pleurisy, with effusion
  fibrinopurulent, fibropurulent — *see* Pyothorax
  hemorrhagic — *see* Hemothorax
  pneumococcal J90
  purulent — *see* Pyothorax
  septic — *see* Pyothorax

Pleurisy - Pneumonia

Pleurisy — *continued*
  serofibrinous — *see* Pleurisy, with effusion
  seropurulent — *see* Pyothorax
  serous — *see* Pleurisy, with effusion
  staphylococcal J86.9
  streptococcal J90
  suppurative — *see* Pyothorax
  traumatic (post) (current) — *see* Injury,
    intrathoracic, pleura
  tuberculous (with effusion) (non primary) A15.6
    primary (progressive) A15.7
Pleuritis sicca — *see* Pleurisy
Pleurobronchopneumonia — *see* Pneumonia,
  broncho-
Pleurodynia R07.81
  epidemic B33.0
  viral B33.0
Pleuropericarditis (*see also* Pericarditis)
  acute I30.9
Pleuropneumonia (acute) (bilateral) (double)
  (septic) (*see also* Pneumonia) J18.8
  chronic — *see* Fibrosis, lung
Pleuro-pneumonia-like-organism (PPLO), as cause
  of disease classified elsewhere B96.0
Pleurorrhea — *see* Pleurisy, with effusion
Plexitis, brachial G54.0
Plica
  polonica B85.0
  syndrome, knee M67.5- ☑
  tonsil J35.8
Plicated tongue K14.5
Plug
  bronchus NEC J98.09
  meconium (newborn) NEC syndrome P76.0
  mucus — *see* Asphyxia, mucus
Plumbism T56.0
Plummer's disease E05.20
  with thyroid storm E05.21
Plummer-Vinson syndrome D50.1
Pluricarential syndrome of infancy E40
Plus (and minus) hand (intrinsic) — *see* Deformity,
  limb, specified type NEC, forearm
Pneumathemia — *see* Air, embolism
Pneumatic hammer (drill) syndrome T75.21 ☑
Pneumatocele (lung) J98.4
  intracranial G93.89
  tension J44.9
Pneumatosis
  cystoides intestinalis K63.89
  intestinalis K63.89
  peritonei K66.8
Pneumaturia R39.89
Pneumoblastoma — *see* Neoplasm, lung, malignant
Pneumocephalus G93.89
Pneumococcemia A40.3
Pneumococcus, pneumococcal — *see* condition
Pneumoconiosis (due to) (inhalation of) J64
  with tuberculosis (any type in A15) J65
  aluminum J63.0
  asbestos J61
  bagasse, bagassosis J67.1
  bauxite J63.1
  beryllium J63.2
  coal miners' (simple) J60
  coalworkers' (simple) J60
  collier's J60
  cotton dust J66.0
  diatomite (diatomaceous earth) J62.8
  dust
    inorganic NEC J63.6
    lime J62.8
    marble J62.8
    organic NEC J66.8
  fumes or vapors (from silo) J68.9
  graphite J63.3
  grinder's J62.8
  kaolin J62.8
  mica J62.8
  millstone maker's J62.8
  mineral fibers NEC J61
  miner's J60
  moldy hay J67.0
  potter's J62.8
  rheumatoid — *see* Rheumatoid, lung
  sandblaster's J62.8
  silica, silicate NEC J62.8
    with carbon J60
  stonemason's J62.8
  talc (dust) J62.0
Pneumocystis carinii pneumonia B59
Pneumocystis jiroveci (pneumonia) B59
Pneumocystosis (with pneumonia) B59

Pneumohemopericardium I31.2
Pneumohemothorax J94.2
  traumatic S27.2 ☑
Pneumohydropericardium — *see* Pericarditis
Pneumohydrothorax — *see* Hydrothorax
Pneumomediastinum J98.2
  congenital or perinatal P25.2
Pneumomycosis B49 [J99]
Pneumonia (acute) (double) (migratory) (purulent)
  (septic) (unresolved) J18.9
  with
    lung abscess J85.1
      due to specified organism — *see* Pneumonia,
        in (due to)
    influenza — *see* Influenza, with, pneumonia
  adenoviral J12.0
  adynamic J18.2
  alba A50.04
  allergic (eosinophilic) J82
  alveolar — *see* Pneumonia, lobar
  anaerobes J15.8
  anthrax A22.1
  apex, apical — *see* Pneumonia, lobar
  Ascaris B77.81
  aspiration J69.0
    due to
      aspiration of microorganisms
        bacterial J15.9
        viral J12.9
      food (regurgitated) J69.0
      gastric secretions J69.0
      milk (regurgitated) J69.0
      oils, essences J69.1
      solids, liquids NEC J69.8
      vomitus J69.0
    newborn P24.81
      amniotic fluid (clear) P24.11
      blood P24.21
      liquor (amnii) P24.11
      meconium P24.01
      milk P24.31
      mucus P24.11
      food (regurgitated) P24.31
      specified NEC P24.81
      stomach contents P24.31
    postprocedural J95.4
  atypical NEC J18.9
  bacillus J15.9
    specified NEC J15.8
  bacterial J15.9
    specified NEC J15.8
  Bacteroides (fragilis) (oralis) (melaninogenicus)
    J15.8
  basal, basic, basilar — *see* Pneumonia, by type
  bronchiolitis obliterans organized (BOOP) J84.89
  broncho-, bronchial (confluent) (croupous)
    (diffuse) (disseminated) (hemorrhagic)
    (involving lobes) (lobar) (terminal) J18.0
    allergic (eosinophilic) J82
    aspiration — *see* Pneumonia, aspiration
    bacterial J15.9
      specified NEC J15.8
    chronic — *see* Fibrosis, lung
    diplococcal J13
    Eaton's agent J15.7
    Escherichia coli (E. coli) J15.5
    Friedländer's bacillus J15.0
    Hemophilus influenzae J14
    hypostatic J18.2
    inhalation (*see also* Pneumonia, aspiration)
      due to fumes or vapors (chemical) J68.0
      of oils or essences J69.1
    Klebsiella (pneumoniae) J15.0
    lipid, lipoid J69.1
      endogenous J84.89
    Mycoplasma (pneumoniae) J15.7
    pleuro-pneumonia-like-organisms (PPLO) J15.7
    pneumococcal J13
    Proteus J15.6
    Pseudomonas J15.1
    Serratia marcescens J15.6
    specified organism NEC J16.8
    staphylococcal — *see* Pneumonia,
      staphylococcal
    streptococcal NEC J15.4
      group B J15.3
      pneumoniae J13
    viral, virus — *see* Pneumonia, viral
  Butyrivibrio (fibriosolvens) J15.8
  Candida B37.1
  caseous — *see* Tuberculosis, pulmonary
  catarrhal — *see* Pneumonia, broncho

Pneumonia — *continued*
  chlamydial J16.0
    congenital P23.1
  cholesterol J84.89
  cirrhotic (chronic) — *see* Fibrosis, lung
  Clostridium (haemolyticum) (novyi) J15.8
  confluent — *see* Pneumonia, broncho
  congenital (infective) P23.9
    due to
      bacterium NEC P23.6
      Chlamydia P23.1
      Escherichia coli P23.4
      Haemophilus influenzae P23.6
      infective organism NEC P23.8
      Klebsiella pneumoniae P23.6
      Mycoplasma P23.6
      Pseudomonas P23.5
      Staphylococcus P23.2
      Streptococcus (except group B) P23.6
        group B P23.3
      viral agent P23.0
    specified NEC P23.8
  croupous — *see* Pneumonia, lobar
  cryptogenic organizing J84.116
  cytomegalic inclusion B25.0
  cytomegaloviral B25.0
  deglutition — *see* Pneumonia, aspiration
  desquamative interstitial J84.117
  diffuse — *see* Pneumonia, broncho
  diplococcal, diplococcus (broncho-) (lobar) J13
  disseminated (focal) — *see* Pneumonia, broncho
  Eaton's agent J15.7
  embolic, embolism — *see* Embolism, pulmonary
  Enterobacter J15.6
  eosinophilic J82
  Escherichia coli (E. coli) J15.5
  Eubacterium J15.8
  fibrinous — *see* Pneumonia, lobar
  fibroid, fibrous (chronic) — *see* Fibrosis, lung
  Friedländer's bacillus J15.0
  Fusobacterium (nucleatum) J15.8
  gangrenous J85.0
  giant cell (measles) B05.2
  gonococcal A54.84
  gram-negative bacteria NEC J15.6
    anaerobic J15.8
  Hemophilus influenzae (broncho) (lobar) J14
  human metapneumovirus J12.3
  hypostatic (broncho) (lobar) J18.2
  in (due to)
    actinomycosis A42.0
    adenovirus J12.0
    anthrax A22.1
    ascariasis B77.81
    aspergillosis B44.9
    Bacillus anthracis A22.1
    Bacterium anitratum J15.6
    candidiasis B37.1
    chickenpox B01.2
    Chlamydia J16.0
      neonatal P23.1
    coccidioidomycosis B38.2
      acute B38.0
      chronic B38.1
    cytomegalovirus disease B25.0
    Diplococcus (pneumoniae) J13
    Eaton's agent J15.7
    Enterobacter J15.6
    Escherichia coli (E. coli) J15.5
    Friedländer's bacillus J15.0
    fumes and vapors (chemical) (inhalation) J68.0
    gonorrhea A54.84
    Hemophilus influenzae (H. influenzae) J14
    Herellea J15.6
    histoplasmosis B39.2
      acute B39.0
      chronic B39.1
    human metapneumovirus J12.3
    Klebsiella (pneumoniae) J15.0
    measles B05.2
    Mycoplasma (pneumoniae) J15.7
    nocardiosis, nocardiasis A43.0
    ornithosis A70
    parainfluenza virus J12.2
    pleuro-pneumonia-like-organism (PPLO) J15.7
    pneumococcus J13
    pneumocystosis (Pneumocystis carinii)
      (Pneumocystis jiroveci) B59
    Proteus J15.6
    Pseudomonas NEC J15.1
      pseudomallei A24.1
    psittacosis A70

☑ **Additional character required**

Pneumonia — continued
　　Q fever A78
　　respiratory syncytial virus J12.1
　　rheumatic fever I00 [J17]
　　rubella B06.81
　　Salmonella (infection) A02.22
　　　　typhi A01.03
　　schistosomiasis B65.9 [J17]
　　Serratia marcescens J15.6
　　specified
　　　　bacterium NEC J15.8
　　　　organism NEC J16.8
　　spirochetal NEC A69.8
　　Staphylococcus J15.20
　　　　aureus (methicillin susceptible) (MSSA)
　　　　　　J15.211
　　　　　　methicillin resistant (MRSA) J15.212
　　　　specified NEC J15.29
　　Streptococcus J15.4
　　　　group B J15.3
　　　　pneumoniae J13
　　　　specified NEC J15.4
　　toxoplasmosis B58.3
　　tularemia A21.2
　　typhoid (fever) A01.03
　　varicella B01.2
　　virus — see Pneumonia, viral
　　whooping cough A37.91
　　　　due to
　　　　　　Bordetella parapertussis A37.11
　　　　　　Bordetella pertussis A37.01
　　　　　　specified NEC A37.81
　　Yersinia pestis A20.2
　　inhalation of food or vomit — see Pneumonia,
　　　　aspiration
　　interstitial J84.9
　　　　chronic J84.111
　　　　desquamative J84.117
　　　　due to
　　　　　　collagen vascular disease J84.17
　　　　　　known underlying cause J84.17
　　　　idiopathic NOS J84.111
　　　　in disease classified elsewhere J84.17
　　　　lymphocytic (due to collagen vascular disease)
　　　　　　(in diseases classified elsewhere) J84.17
　　　　lymphoid J84.2
　　　　non-specific J84.89
　　　　　　due to
　　　　　　　　collagen vascular disease J84.17
　　　　　　　　known underlying cause J84.17
　　　　　　idiopathic J84.113
　　　　　　in diseases classified elsewhere J84.17
　　　　plasma cell B59
　　　　pseudomonas J15.1
　　　　usual J84.112
　　　　　　due to collagen vascular disease J84.17
　　　　　　idiopathic J84.112
　　　　　　in diseases classified elsewhere J84.17
　　Klebsiella (pneumoniae) J15.0
　　lipid, lipoid (exogenous) J69.1
　　　　endogenous J84.89
　　lobar (disseminated) (double) (interstitial) J18.1
　　　　bacterial J15.9
　　　　　　specified NEC J15.8
　　　　chronic — see Fibrosis, lung
　　　　Escherichia coli (E. coli) J15.5
　　　　Friedländer's bacillus J15.0
　　　　Hemophilus influenzae J14
　　　　hypostatic J18.2
　　　　Klebsiella (pneumoniae) J15.0
　　　　pneumococcal J13
　　　　Proteus J15.6
　　　　Pseudomonas J15.1
　　　　specified organism NEC J16.8
　　　　staphylococcal — see Pneumonia,
　　　　　　staphylococcal
　　　　streptococcal NEC J15.4
　　　　Streptococcus pneumoniae J13
　　　　viral, virus — see Pneumonia, viral
　　lobular — see Pneumonia, broncho
　　Löffler's J82
　　lymphoid interstitial J84.2
　　massive — see Pneumonia, lobar
　　meconium P24.01
　　MSSA (methicillin susceptible Staphylococcus
　　　　aureus) J15.211
　　multilobar — see Pneumonia, by type
　　Mycoplasma (pneumoniae) J15.7
　　necrotic J85.0
　　neonatal P23.9
　　　　aspiration — see Aspiration, by substance, with
　　　　　　pneumonia

Pneumonia — continued
　　nitrogen dioxide J68.9
　　organizing J84.89
　　　　due to
　　　　　　collagen vascular disease J84.17
　　　　　　known underlying cause J84.17
　　　　in diseases classified elsewhere J84.17
　　orthostatic J18.2
　　parainfluenza virus J12.2
　　parenchymatous — see Fibrosis, lung
　　passive J18.2
　　patchy — see Pneumonia, broncho
　　Peptococcus J15.8
　　Peptostreptococcus J15.8
　　plasma cell (of infants) B59
　　pleurolobar — see Pneumonia, lobar
　　pleuro-pneumonia-like organism (PPLO) J15.7
　　pneumococcal (broncho) (lobar) J13
　　Pneumocystis (carinii) (jiroveci) B59
　　postinfectional NEC B99 ☑ [J17]
　　postmeasles B05.2
　　Proteus J15.6
　　Pseudomonas J15.1
　　psittacosis A70
　　radiation J70.0
　　respiratory syncytial virus J12.1
　　resulting from a procedure J95.89
　　rheumatic I00 [J17]
　　Salmonella (arizonae) (cholerae-suis) (enteritidis)
　　　　(typhimurium) A02.22
　　　　typhi A01.03
　　　　typhoid fever A01.03
　　SARS-associated coronavirus J12.81
　　segmented, segmental — see Pneumonia,
　　　　broncho-
　　Serratia marcescens J15.6
　　specified NEC J18.8
　　　　bacterium NEC J15.8
　　　　organism NEC J16.8
　　　　virus NEC J12.89
　　spirochetal NEC A69.8
　　staphylococcal (broncho) (lobar) J15.20
　　　　aureus (methicillin susceptible) (MSSA) J15.211
　　　　　　methicillin resistant (MRSA) J15.212
　　　　specified NEC J15.29
　　static, stasis J18.2
　　streptococcal NEC (broncho) (lobar) J15.4
　　　　group
　　　　　　A J15.4
　　　　　　B J15.3
　　　　　　specified NEC J15.4
　　Streptococcus pneumoniae J13
　　syphilitic, congenital (early) A50.04
　　traumatic (complication) (early) (secondary)
　　　　T79.8 ☑
　　tuberculous (any) — see Tuberculosis, pulmonary
　　tularemic A21.2
　　varicella B01.2
　　Veillonella J15.8
　　ventilator associated J95.851
　　viral, virus (broncho) (interstitial) (lobar) J12.9
　　　　adenoviral J12.0
　　　　congenital P23.0
　　　　human metapneumovirus J12.3
　　　　parainfluenza J12.2
　　　　respiratory syncytial J12.1
　　　　SARS-associated coronavirus J12.81
　　　　specified NEC J12.89
　　white (congenital) A50.04
Pneumonic — see condition
Pneumonitis (acute) (primary) (see also Pneumonia)
　　air-conditioner J67.7
　　allergic (due to) J67.9
　　　　organic dust NEC J67.8
　　　　red cedar dust J67.8
　　　　sequoiosis J67.8
　　　　wood dust J67.8
　　aspiration J69.0
　　　　due to
　　　　　　anesthesia J95.4
　　　　　　　　during
　　　　　　　　　　labor and delivery O74.0
　　　　　　　　　　pregnancy O29.01- ☑
　　　　　　　　　　puerperium O89.01
　　　　　　fumes or gases J68.0
　　　　obstetric O74.0
　　chemical (due to gases, fumes or vapors)
　　　　(inhalation) J68.0
　　　　due to anesthesia J95.4
　　cholesterol J84.89
　　crack (cocaine) J68.0
　　chronic — see Fibrosis, lung

Pneumonitis — continued
　　congenital rubella P35.0
　　due to
　　　　beryllium J68.0
　　　　cadmium J68.0
　　　　crack (cocaine) J68.0
　　　　detergent J69.8
　　　　fluorocarbon-polymer J68.0
　　　　food, vomit (aspiration) J69.0
　　　　fumes or vapors J68.0
　　　　gases, fumes or vapors (inhalation) J68.0
　　　　inhalation
　　　　　　blood J69.8
　　　　　　essences J69.1
　　　　　　food (regurgitated), milk, vomit J69.0
　　　　　　oils, essences J69.1
　　　　　　saliva J69.0
　　　　　　solids, liquids NEC J69.8
　　　　manganese J68.0
　　　　nitrogen dioxide J68.0
　　　　oils, essences J69.1
　　　　solids, liquids NEC J69.8
　　　　toxoplasmosis (acquired) B58.3
　　　　　　congenital P37.1
　　　　vanadium J68.0
　　　　ventilator J95.851
　　eosinophilic J82
　　hypersensitivity J67.9
　　　　air conditioner lung J67.7
　　　　bagassosis J67.1
　　　　bird fancier's lung J67.2
　　　　farmer's lung J67.0
　　　　maltworker's lung J67.4
　　　　maple bark-stripper's lung J67.6
　　　　mushroom worker's lung J67.5
　　　　specified organic dust NEC J67.8
　　　　suberosis J67.3
　　interstitial (chronic) J84.89
　　　　acute J84.114
　　　　lymphoid J84.2
　　　　non-specific J84.89
　　　　　　idiopathic J84.113
　　lymphoid, interstitial J84.2
　　meconium P24.01
　　postanesthetic J95.4
　　　　correct substance properly administered — see
　　　　　　Table of Drugs and Chemicals, by drug,
　　　　　　adverse effect
　　　　in labor and delivery O74.0
　　　　in pregnancy O29.01- ☑
　　　　obstetric O74.0
　　　　overdose or wrong substance given or taken
　　　　　　(by accident) — see Table of Drugs and
　　　　　　Chemicals, by drug, poisoning
　　　　postpartum, puerperal O89.01
　　postoperative J95.4
　　　　obstetric O74.0
　　radiation J70.0
　　rubella, congenital P35.0
　　ventilation (air-conditioning) J67.7
　　ventilator associated J95.851
　　wood-dust J67.8
Pneumonoconiosis — see Pneumoconiosis
Pneumoparotid K11.8
Pneumopathy NEC J98.4
　　alveolar J84.09
　　due to organic dust NEC J66.8
　　parietoalveolar J84.09
Pneumopericarditis (see also Pericarditis)
　　acute I30.9
Pneumopericardium (see also Pericarditis)
　　congenital P25.3
　　newborn P25.3
　　traumatic (post) — see Injury, heart
Pneumophagia (psychogenic) F45.8
Pneumopleurisy, pneumopleuritis (see also
　　Pneumonia) J18.8
Pneumopyopericardium I30.1
Pneumopyothorax — see Pyopneumothorax
　　with fistula J86.0
Pneumorrhagia (see also Hemorrhage, lung)
　　tuberculous — see Tuberculosis, pulmonary
Pneumothorax NOS J93.9
　　acute J93.83
　　chronic J93.81
　　congenital P25.1
　　perinatal period P25.1
　　postprocedural J95.811
　　specified NEC J93.83
　　spontaneous NOS J93.83
　　　　newborn P25.1
　　　　primary J93.11

Pneumothorax — *continued*
secondary J93.12
tension J93.0
tense valvular, infectional J93.0
tension (spontaneous) J93.0
traumatic S27.0 ☑
with hemothorax S27.2 ☑
tuberculous — *see* Tuberculosis, pulmonary
Podagra (*see also* Gout) M10.9
Podencephalus Q01.9
Poikilocytosis R71.8
Poikiloderma L81.6
Civatte's L57.3
congenital Q82.8
vasculare atrophicans L94.5
Poikilodermatomyositis M33.10
with
myopathy M33.12
respiratory involvement M33.11
specified organ involvement NEC M33.19
Pointed ear (congenital) Q17.3
Poison ivy, oak, sumac or other plant dermatitis (allergic) (contact) L23.7
Poisoning (acute) (*see also* Table of Drugs and Chemicals)
algae and toxins T65.82- ☑
Bacillus B (aertrycke) (cholerae (suis)) (paratyphosus) (suipestifer) A02.9
botulinus A05.1
bacterial toxins A05.9
berries, noxious — *see* Poisoning, food, noxious, berries
botulism A05.1
ciguatera fish T61.0- ☑
Clostridium botulinum A05.1
death-cap (Amanita phalloides) (Amanita verna) — *see* Poisoning, food, noxious, mushrooms
drug — *see* Table of Drugs and Chemicals, by drug, poisoning
epidemic, fish (noxious) — *see* Poisoning, seafood
bacterial A05.9
fava bean D55.0
fish (noxious) T61.9- ☑
bacterial — *see* Intoxication, foodborne, by agent
ciguatera fish — *see* Poisoning, ciguatera fish
scombroid fish — *see* Poisoning, scombroid fish
specified type NEC T61.77- ☑
food (acute) (diseased) (infected) (noxious) NEC T62.9- ☑
bacterial — *see* Intoxication, foodborne, by agent
due to
Bacillus (aertrycke) (choleraesuis) (paratyphosus) (suipestifer) A02.9
botulinus A05.1
Clostridium (perfringens) (Welchii) A05.2
salmonella (aertrycke) (callinarum) (choleraesuis) (enteritidis) (paratyphi) (suipestifer) A02.9
with
gastroenteritis A02.0
sepsis A02.1
staphylococcus A05.0
Vibrio
parahaemolyticus A05.3
vulnificus A05.5
noxious or naturally toxic T62.9- ☑
berriesT62.1-
fish — *see* Poisoning, seafood
mushroomsT62.0X-
plants NECT62.2X-
seafood — *see* Poisoning, seafood
specified NECT62.8X-
ichthyotoxism — *see* Poisoning, seafood
kreotoxism, food A05.9
latex T65.81- ☑
lead T56.0- ☑
mushroom — *see* Poisoning, food, noxious, mushroom
mussels (*see also* Poisoning, shellfish)
bacterial — *see* Intoxication, foodborne, by agent
nicotine (tobacco) T65.2- ☑
noxious foodstuffs — *see* Poisoning, food, noxious
plants, noxious — *see* Poisoning, food, noxious, plants NEC
ptomaine — *see* Poisoning, food
radiation J70.0
Salmonella (arizonae) (cholerae-suis) (enteritidis) (typhimurium) A02.9

Poisoning — *continued*
scombroid fish T61.1- ☑
seafood (noxious) T61.9- ☑
bacterial — *see* Intoxication, foodborne, by agent
fish — *see* Poisoning, fish
shellfish — *see* Poisoning, shellfish
specified NECT61.8X-
shellfish (amnesic) (azaspiracid) (diarrheic) (neurotoxic) (noxious) (paralytic) T61.78- ☑
bacterial — *see* Intoxication, foodborne, by agent
ciguatera mollusk — *see* Poisoning, ciguatera fish
specified substance NEC T65.891 ☑
Staphylococcus, food A05.0
tobacco (nicotine) T65.2- ☑
water E87.79
Poker spine — *see* Spondylitis, ankylosing
Poland syndrome Q79.8
Polioencephalitis (acute) (bulbar) A80.9
inferior G12.22
influenzal — *see* Influenza, with, encephalopathy
superior hemorrhagic (acute) (Wernicke's) E51.2
Wernicke's E51.2
Polioencephalomyelitis (acute) (anterior) A80.9
with beriberi E51.2
Polioencephalopathy, superior hemorrhagic E51.2
with
beriberi E51.11
pellagra E52
Poliomeningoencephalitis — *see* Meningoencephalitis
Poliomyelitis (acute) (anterior) (epidemic) A80.9
with paralysis (bulbar) — *see* Poliomyelitis, paralytic
abortive A80.4
ascending (progressive) — *see* Poliomyelitis, paralytic
bulbar (paralytic) — *see* Poliomyelitis, paralytic
congenital P35.8
nonepidemic A80.9
nonparalytic A80.4
paralytic A80.30
specified NEC A80.39
vaccine-associated A80.0
wild virus
imported A80.1
indigenous A80.2
spinal, acute A80.9
Poliosis (eyebrow) (eyelashes) L67.1
circumscripta, acquired L67.1
Pollakiuria R35.0
psychogenic F45.8
Pollinosis J30.1
Pollitzer's disease L73.2
Polyadenitis (*see also* Lymphadenitis)
malignant A20.0
Polyalgia M79.89
Polyangiitis M30.0
microscopic M31.7
overlap syndrome M30.8
Polyarteritis
microscopic M31.7
nodosa M30.0
with lung involvement M30.1
juvenile M30.2
related condition NEC M30.8
Polyarthralgia — *see* Pain, joint
Polyarthritis, polyarthropathy (*see also* Arthritis) M13.0
due to or associated with other specified conditions — *see* Arthritis
epidemic (Australian) (with exanthema) B33.1
infective — *see* Arthritis, pyogenic or pyemic
inflammatory M06.4
juvenile (chronic) (seronegative) M08.3
migratory — *see* Fever, rheumatic
rheumatic, acute — *see* Fever, rheumatic
Polyarthrosis M15.9
post-traumatic M15.3
primary M15.0
specified NEC M15.8
Polycarential syndrome of infancy E40
Polychondritis (atrophic) (chronic) (*see also* Disorder, cartilage, specified type NEC)
relapsing M94.1
Polycoria Q13.2
Polycystic (disease)
degeneration, kidney Q61.3
autosomal dominant (adult type) Q61.2

Polycystic — *continued*
autosomal recessive (infantile type) NEC Q61.19
kidney Q61.3
autosomal
dominant Q61.2
recessive NEC Q61.19
autosomal dominant (adult type) Q61.2
autosomal recessive (childhood type) NEC Q61.19
infantile type NEC Q61.19
liver Q44.6
lung J98.4
congenital Q33.0
ovary, ovaries E28.2
spleen Q89.09
Polycythemia (secondary) D75.1
acquired D75.1
benign (familial) D75.0
due to
donor twin P61.1
erythropoietin D75.1
fall in plasma volume D75.1
high altitude D75.1
maternal-fetal transfusion P61.1
stress D75.1
emotional D75.1
erythropoietin D75.1
familial (benign) D75.0
Gaisböck's (hypertonica) D75.1
high altitude D75.1
hypertonica D75.1
hypoxemic D75.1
neonatorum P61.1
nephrogenous D75.1
relative D75.1
secondary D75.1
spurious D75.1
stress D75.1
vera D45
Polycytosis cryptogenica D75.1
Polydactylism, polydactyly Q69.9
toes Q69.2
Polydipsia R63.1
Polydystrophy, pseudo-Hurler E77.0
Polyembryoma — *see* Neoplasm, malignant, by site
Polyglandular
deficiency E31.0
dyscrasia E31.9
dysfunction E31.9
syndrome E31.8
Polyhydramnios O40.- ☑
Polymastia Q83.1
Polymenorrhea N92.0
Polymyalgia M35.3
arteritica, giant cell M31.5
rheumatica M35.3
with giant cell arteritis M31.5
Polymyositis (acute) (chronic) (hemorrhagic) M33.20
with
myopathy M33.22
respiratory involvement M33.21
skin involvement — *see* Dermatopolymyositis
specified organ involvement NEC M33.29
ossificans (generalisata) (progressiva) — *see* Myositis, ossificans, progressiva
Polyneuritis, polyneuritic (*see also* Polyneuropathy)
acute (post-)infective G61.0
alcoholic G62.1
cranialis G52.7
demyelinating, chronic inflammatory (CIDP) G61.81
diabetic — *see* Diabetes, polyneuropathy
diphtheritic A36.83
due to lack of vitamin NEC E56.9 [G63]
endemic E51.11
erythredemaT56.1
febrile, acute G61.0
hereditary ataxic G60.1
idiopathic, acute G61.0
infective (acute) G61.0
inflammatory, chronic demyelinating (CIDP) G61.81
nutritional E63.9 [G63]
postinfective (acute) G61.0
specified NEC G62.89
Polyneuropathy (peripheral) G62.9
alcoholic G62.1
amyloid (Portuguese) E85.1 [G63]
arsenical G62.2
critical illness G62.81

Polyneuropathy — *continued*
demyelinating, chronic inflammatory (CIDP) G61.81
diabetic — *see* Diabetes, polyneuropathy
drug-induced G62.0
hereditary G60.9
specified NEC G60.8
idiopathic G60.9
progressive G60.3
in (due to)
alcohol G62.1
sequelae G65.2
amyloidosis, familial (Portuguese) E85.1 [G63]
antitetanus serum G61.1
arsenic G62.2
sequelae G65.2
avitaminosis NEC E56.9 [G63]
beriberi E51.11
collagen vascular disease NEC M35.9 [G63]
deficiency (of)
B (-complex) vitamins E53.9 [G63]
vitamin B6 E53.1 [G63]
diabetes — *see* Diabetes, polyneuropathy
diphtheria A36.83
drug or medicament G62.0
correct substance properly administered — *see* Table of Drugs and Chemicals, by drug, adverse effect
overdose or wrong substance given or taken — *see* Table of Drugs and Chemicals, by drug, poisoning
endocrine disease NEC E34.9 [G63]
herpes zoster B02.23
hypoglycemia E16.2 [G63]
infectious
disease NEC B99 ☑ [G63]
mononucleosis B27.91
lack of vitamin NEC E56.9 [G63]
lead G62.2
sequelae G65.2
leprosy A30.9 [G63]
Lyme disease A69.22
metabolic disease NEC E88.9 [G63]
microscopic polyangiitis M31.7 [G63]
mumps B26.84
neoplastic disease (*see also* Neoplasm) D49.9 [G63]
nutritional deficiency NEC E63.9 [G63]
organophosphate compounds G62.2
sequelae G65.2
parasitic disease NEC B89 [G63]
pellagra E52 [G63]
polyarteritis nodosa M30.0
porphyria E80.20 [G63]
radiation G62.82
rheumatoid arthritis — *see* Rheumatoid, polyneuropathy
sarcoidosis D86.89
serum G61.1
syphilis (late) A52.15
congenital A50.43
systemic
connective tissue disorder M35.9 [G63]
lupus erythematosus M32.19
toxic agent NEC G62.2
sequelae G65.2
triorthocresyl phosphate G62.2
sequelae G65.2
tuberculosis A17.89
uremia N18.9 [G63]
vitamin B12 deficiency E53.8 [G63]
with anemia (pernicious) D51.0 [G63]
due to dietary deficiency D51.3 [G63]
zoster B02.23
inflammatory G61.9
chronic demyelinating (CIDP) G61.81
sequelae G65.1
specified NEC G61.89
lead G62.2
sequelae G65.2
nutritional NEC E63.9 [G63]
postherpetic (zoster) B02.23
progressive G60.3
radiation-induced G62.82
sensory (hereditary) (idiopathic) G60.8
specified NEC G62.89
syphilitic (late) A52.15
congenital A50.43
Polyopia H53.8
Polyorchism, polyorchidism Q55.21
Polyosteoarthritis (*see also* Osteoarthritis, generalized) M15.9- ☑
Polyosteoarthritis — *continued*
post-traumatic M15.3
specified NEC M15.8
Polyostotic fibrous dysplasia Q78.1
Polyotia Q17.0
Polyp, polypus
accessory sinus J33.8
adenocarcinoma in — *see* Neoplasm, malignant, by site
adenocarcinoma in situ in — *see* Neoplasm, in situ, by site
adenoid tissue J33.0
adenomatous (*see also* Neoplasm, benign, by site)
adenocarcinoma in — *see* Neoplasm, malignant, by site
adenocarcinoma in situ in — *see* Neoplasm, in situ, by site
carcinoma in — *see* Neoplasm, malignant, by site
carcinoma in situ in — *see* Neoplasm, in situ, by site
multiple — *see* Neoplasm, benign
adenocarcinoma in — *see* Neoplasm, malignant, by site
adenocarcinoma in situ in — *see* Neoplasm, in situ, by site
antrum J33.8
anus, anal (canal) K62.0
Bartholin's gland N84.3
bladder D41.4
carcinoma in — *see* Neoplasm, malignant, by site
carcinoma in situ in — *see* Neoplasm, in situ, by site
cecum D12.0
cervix (uteri) N84.1
in pregnancy or childbirth — *see* Pregnancy, complicated by, abnormal, cervix
mucous N84.1
nonneoplastic N84.1
choanal J33.0
cholesterol K82.4
clitoris N84.3
colon K63.5
adenomatous D12.6
ascending D12.2
cecum D12.0
descending D12.4
inflammatory K51.40
with
abscess K51.414
complication K51.419
specified NEC K51.418
fistula K51.413
intestinal obstruction K51.412
rectal bleeding K51.411
sigmoid D12.5
transverse D12.3
corpus uteri N84.0
dental K04.0
duodenum K31.7
ear (middle) H74.4- ☑
endometrium N84.0
ethmoidal (sinus) J33.8
fallopian tube N84.8
female genital tract N84.9
specified NEC N84.8
frontal (sinus) J33.8
gallbladder K82.4
gingiva, gum K06.8
labia, labium (majus) (minus) N84.3
larynx (mucous) J38.1
adenomatous D14.1
malignant — *see* Neoplasm, malignant, by site
maxillary (sinus) J33.8
middle ear — *see* Polyp, ear (middle)
myometrium N84.0
nares
anterior J33.9
posterior J33.0
nasal (mucous) J33.9
cavity J33.0
septum J33.0
nasopharyngeal J33.0
nose (mucous) J33.9
oviduct N84.8
pharynx J39.2
placenta O90.89
prostate — *see* Enlargement, enlarged, prostate
pudenda, pudendum N84.3
pulpal (dental) K04.0
rectum (nonadenomatous) K62.1
adenomatous — *see* Polyp, adenomatous
Polyp — *continued*
septum (nasal) J33.0
sinus (accessory) (ethmoidal) (frontal) (maxillary) (sphenoidal) J33.8
sphenoidal (sinus) J33.8
stomach K31.7
adenomatous D13.1
tube, fallopian N84.8
turbinate, mucous membrane J33.8
umbilical, newborn P83.6
ureter N28.89
urethra N36.2
uterus (body) (corpus) (mucous) N84.0
cervix N84.1
in pregnancy or childbirth — *see* Pregnancy, complicated by, tumor, uterus
vagina N84.2
vocal cord (mucous) J38.1
vulva N84.3
Polyphagia R63.2
Polyploidy Q92.7
Polypoid — *see* condition
Polyposis (*see also* Polyp)
coli (adenomatous) D12.6
adenocarcinoma in C18.9
adenocarcinoma in situ in — *see* Neoplasm, in situ, by site
carcinoma in C18.9
colon (adenomatous) D12.6
familial D12.6
adenocarcinoma in situ in — *see* Neoplasm, in situ, by site
intestinal (adenomatous) D12.6
malignant lymphomatous C83.1- ☑
multiple, adenomatous (*see also* Neoplasm, benign) D36.9
Polyradiculitis — *see* Polyneuropathy
Polyradiculoneuropathy (acute) (postinfective) (segmentally demyelinating) G61.0
Polyserositis
due to pericarditis I31.1
pericardial I31.1
periodic, familial E85.0
tuberculous A19.9
acute A19.1
chronic A19.8
Polysplenia syndrome Q89.09
Polysyndactyly (*see also* Syndactylism, syndactyly) Q70.4
Polytrichia L68.3
Polyunguia Q84.6
Polyuria R35.8
nocturnal R35.1
psychogenic F45.8
Pompe's disease (glycogen storage) E74.02
Pompholyx L30.1
Poncet's disease (tuberculous rheumatism) A18.09
Pond fracture — *see* Fracture, skull
Ponos B55.0
Pons, pontine — *see* condition
Poor
aesthetic of existing restoration of tooth K08.56
contractions, labor O62.2
gingival margin to tooth restoration K08.51
personal hygiene R46.0
prenatal care, affecting management of pregnancy — *see* Pregnancy, complicated by, insufficient, prenatal care
sucking reflex (newborn) R29.2
urinary stream R39.12
vision NEC H54.7
Poradenitis, nostras inguinalis or venerea A55
Porencephaly (congenital) (developmental) (true) Q04.6
acquired G93.0
nondevelopmental G93.0
traumatic (post) F07.89
Porocephaliasis B88.8
Porokeratosis Q82.8
Poroma, eccrine — *see* Neoplasm, skin, benign
Porphyria (South African) E80.20
acquired E80.20
acute intermittent (hepatic) (Swedish) E80.21
cutanea tarda (hereditary) (symptomatic) E80.1
due to drugs E80.20
correct substance properly administered — *see* Table of Drugs and Chemicals, by drug, adverse effect
overdose or wrong substance given or taken — *see* Table of Drugs and Chemicals, by drug, poisoning
erythropoietic (congenital) (hereditary) E80.0

Porphyria — *continued*
  hepatocutaneous type E80.1
  secondary E80.20
  toxic NEC E80.20
  variegata E80.20
Porphyrinuria — *see* Porphyria
Porphyruria — *see* Porphyria
Portal — *see* condition
Port wine nevus, mark, or stain Q82.5
Posadas-Wernicke disease B38.9
Positive
  culture (nonspecific)
    blood R78.81
    bronchial washings R84.5
    cerebrospinal fluid R83.5
    cervix uteri R87.5
    nasal secretions R84.5
    nipple discharge R89.5
    nose R84.5
      staphylococcus (Methicillin susceptible) Z22.321
        Methicillin resistant Z22.322
    peritoneal fluid R85.5
    pleural fluid R84.5
    prostatic secretions R86.5
    saliva R85.5
    seminal fluid R86.5
    sputum R84.5
    synovial fluid R89.5
    throat scrapings R84.5
    urine R82.7
    vagina R87.5
    vulva R87.5
    wound secretions R89.5
  PPD (skin test) R76.11
  serology for syphilis A53.0
    false R76.8
    with signs or symptoms - code as Syphilis, by site and stage
  skin test, tuberculin (without active tuberculosis) R76.11
  test, human immunodeficiency virus (HIV) R75
  VDRL A53.0
    with signs or symptoms - code by site and stage under Syphilis A53.9
  Wassermann reaction A53.0
Postcardiotomy syndrome I97.0
Postcaval ureter Q62.62
Postcholecystectomy syndrome K91.5
Postclimacteric bleeding N95.0
Postcommissurotomy syndrome I97.0
Postconcussional syndrome F07.81
Postcontusional syndrome F07.81
Postcricoid region — *see* condition
Post-dates (40-42 weeks) (pregnancy) (mother) O48.0
  more than 42 weeks gestation O48.1
Postencephalitic syndrome F07.89
Posterior — *see* condition
Posterolateral sclerosis (spinal cord) — *see* Degeneration, combined
Postexanthematous — *see* condition
Postfebrile — *see* condition
Postgastrectomy dumping syndrome K91.1
Posthemiplegic chorea — *see* Monoplegia
Posthemorrhagic anemia (chronic) D50.0
  acute D62
  newborn P61.3
Postherpetic neuralgia (zoster) B02.29
  trigeminal B02.22
Posthitis N47.7
Postimmunization complication or reaction — *see* Complications, vaccination
Postinfectious — *see* condition
Postlaminectomy syndrome NEC M96.1
Postleukotomy syndrome F07.0
Postmastectomy lymphedema (syndrome) I97.2
Postmaturity, postmature (over 42 weeks)
  maternal (over 42 weeks gestation) O48.1
  newborn P08.22
Postmeasles complication NEC (*see also* condition) B05.89
Postmenopausal
  endometrium (atrophic) N95.8
    suppurative (*see also* Endometritis) N71.9
  osteoporosis — *see* Osteoporosis, postmenopausal
Postnasal drip R09.82
  due to
    allergic rhinitis — *see* Rhinitis, allergic
    common cold J00

Postnasal — *continued*
    gastroesophageal reflux — *see* Reflux, gastroesophageal
    nasopharyngitis — *see* Nasopharyngitis
    other know condition - code to condition
    sinusitis — *see* Sinusitis
Postnatal — *see* condition
Postoperative (postprocedural) — *see* Complication, postoperative
  pneumothorax, therapeutic Z98.3
  state NEC Z98.89
Postpancreatectomy hyperglycemia E89.1
Postpartum — *see* Puerperal
Postphlebitic syndrome — *see* Syndrome, postthrombotic
Postpoliomyelitic (*see also* condition)
  osteopathy — *see* Osteopathy, after poliomyelitis
Postpolio (myelitic) syndrome G14
Postprocedural (*see also* Postoperative)
  hypoinsulinemia E89.1
Postschizophrenic depression F32.8
Postsurgery status (*see also* Status (post))
  pneumothorax, therapeutic Z98.3
Post-term (40-42 weeks) (pregnancy) (mother) O48.0
  infant P08.21
  more than 42 weeks gestation (mother) O48.1
Post-traumatic brain syndrome, nonpsychotic F07.81
Post-typhoid abscess A01.09
Postures, hysterical F44.2
Postvaccinal reaction or complication — *see* Complications, vaccination
Postvalvulotomy syndrome I97.0
Potain's
  disease (pulmonary edema) — *see* Edema, lung
  syndrome (gastrectasis with dyspepsia) K31.0
Potter's
  asthma J62.8
  facies Q60.6
  lung J62.8
  syndrome (with renal agenesis) Q60.6
Pott's
  curvature (spinal) A18.01
  disease or paraplegia A18.01
  spinal curvature A18.01
  tumor, puffy — *see* Osteomyelitis, specified type NEC
Pouch
  bronchus Q32.4
  Douglas' — *see* condition
  esophagus, esophageal, congenital Q39.6
    acquired K22.5
  gastric K31.4
  Hartmann's K82.8
  pharynx, pharyngeal (congenital) Q38.7
Pouchitis K91.850
Poultrymen's itch B88.0
Poverty NEC Z59.6
  extreme Z59.5
Poxvirus NEC B08.8
Prader-Willi syndrome Q87.1
Preauricular appendage or tag Q17.0
Prebetalipoproteinemia (acquired) (essential) (familial) (hereditary) (primary) (secondary) E78.1
  with chylomicronemia E78.3
Precipitate labor or delivery O62.3
Preclimacteric bleeding (menorrhagia) N92.4
Precocious
  adrenarche E30.1
  menarche E30.1
  menstruation E30.1
  pubarche E30.1
  puberty E30.1
    central E22.8
  sexual development NEC E30.1
  thelarche E30.8
Precocity, sexual (constitutional) (cryptogenic) (female) (idiopathic) (male) E30.1
  with adrenal hyperplasia E25.9
    congenital E25.0
Precordial pain R07.2
Predeciduous teeth K00.2
Prediabetes, prediabetic R73.09
  complicating
    pregnancy — *see* Pregnancy, complicated by, diseases of, specified type or system NEC
    puerperium O99.89
Predislocation status of hip at birth Q65.6
Pre-eclampsia O14.9- ☑

Pre-eclampsia — *continued*
  with pre-existing hypertension — *see* Hypertension, complicating pregnancy, pre-existing, with, pre-eclampsia
  mild O14.0- ☑
  moderate O14.0- ☑
  severe O14.1- ☑
    with hemolysis, elevated liver enzymes and low platelet count (HELLP) O14.2- ☑
Pre-eruptive color change, teeth, tooth K00.8
Pre-excitation atrioventricular conduction I45.6
Preglaucoma H40.00- ☑
Pregnancy (single) (uterine) (*see also* Delivery and Puerperal)
  Note: The Tabular must be reviewed for assignment of the appropriate character indicating the trimester of the pregnancy
  Note: The Tabular must be reviewed for assignment of appropriate seventh character for multiple gestation codes in Chapter 15
  abdominal (ectopic) O00.0
    with viable fetus O36.7- ☑
  ampullar O00.1
  biochemical O02.81
  broad ligament O00.8
  cervical O00.8
  chemical O02.81
  complicated NOS O26.9- ☑
  complicated by (care of) (management affected by)
    abnormal, abnormality
      cervix O34.4- ☑
        causing obstructed labor O65.5
      cord (umbilical) O69.9 ☑
      findings on antenatal screening of mother O28.9
        biochemical O28.1
        cytological O28.2
        chromosomal O28.5
        genetic O28.5
        hematological O28.0
        radiological O28.4
        specified NEC O28.8
        ultrasonic O28.3
      glucose (tolerance) NEC O99.810
      pelvic organs O34.9- ☑
        specified NEC O34.8- ☑
          causing obstructed labor O65.5
      pelvis (bony) (major) NEC O33.0
      perineum O34.7- ☑
      position
        placenta O44.1- ☑
          without hemorrhage O44.0- ☑
        uterus O34.59- ☑
      uterus O34.59- ☑
        causing obstructed labor O65.5
        congenital O34.0- ☑
      vagina O34.6- ☑
        causing obstructed labor O65.5
      vulva O34.7- ☑
        causing obstructed labor O65.5
    abruptio placentae — *see* Abruptio placentae
    abscess or cellulitis
      bladder O23.1- ☑
      breast O91.11- ☑
      genital organ or tract O23.9- ☑
    abuse
      physical O9A.31- ☑
      psychological O9A.51- ☑
      sexual O9A.41- ☑
    adverse effect anesthesia O29.9- ☑
      aspiration pneumonitis O29.01- ☑
      cardiac arrest O29.11- ☑
      cardiac complication NEC O29.19- ☑
      cardiac failure O29.12- ☑
      central nervous system complication NEC O29.29- ☑
      cerebral anoxia O29.21- ☑
      failed or difficult intubation O29.6- ☑
      inhalation of stomach contents or secretions NOS O29.01- ☑
      local, toxic reaction O29.3X ☑
      Mendelson's syndrome O29.01- ☑
      pressure collapse of lung O29.02- ☑
      pulmonary complications NEC O29.09- ☑
      specified NEC O29.8X- ☑
      spinal and epidural type NEC O29.5X ☑
        induced headache O29.4- ☑
    albuminuria O12.1- ☑
    alcohol use O99.31- ☑
    amnionitis O41.12- ☑

☑ **Additional character required**

Pregnancy — *continued*

anaphylactoid syndrome of pregnancy O88.01- ☑
anemia (conditions in D50-D64) (pre-existing) O99.01- ☑
　complicating the puerperium O99.03
antepartum hemorrhage O46.9- ☑
　with coagulation defect — *see* Hemorrhage, antepartum, with coagulation defect
　specified NEC O46.8X- ☑
appendicitis O99.61- ☑
atrophy (yellow) (acute) liver (subacute) O26.61- ☑
bariatric surgery status O99.84- ☑
bicornis or bicornuate uterus O34.59- ☑
biliary tract problems O26.61- ☑
breech presentation O32.1 ☑
cardiovascular diseases (conditions in I00-I09, I20-I52, I70-I99) O99.41- ☑
cerebrovascular disorders (conditions in I60-I69) O99.41- ☑
cervical shortening O26.87- ☑
cervicitis O23.51- ☑
chloasma (gravidarum) O26.89- ☑
cholestasis (intrahepatic) O26.61- ☑
cholecystitis O99.61- ☑
chorioamnionitis O41.12- ☑
circulatory system disorder (conditions in I00-I09, I20-I99, O99.41-)
compound presentation O32.6 ☑
conjoined twins O30.02- ☑
connective system disorders (conditions in M00-M99) O99.89
contracted pelvis (general) O33.1
　inlet O33.2
　outlet O33.3
convulsions (eclamptic) (uremic) (*see also* Eclampsia) O15.9- ☑
cracked nipple O92.11- ☑
cystitis O23.1- ☑
cystocele O34.8- ☑
death of fetus (near term) O36.4 ☑
　early pregnancy O02.1
　of one fetus or more in multiple gestation O31.2- ☑
deciduitis O41.14- ☑
decreased fetal movement O36.81- ☑
dental problems O99.61- ☑
diabetes (mellitus) O24.91- ☑
　gestational (pregnancy induced) — *see* - Diabetes, gestational
　pre-existing O24.31- ☑
　　specified NEC O24.81- ☑
　　type 1 O24.01- ☑
　　type 2 O24.11- ☑
digestive system disorders (conditions in K00-K93) O99.61- ☑
diseases of — *see* Pregnancy, complicated by, specified body system disease
　biliary tract O26.61- ☑
　blood NEC (conditions in D65-D77) O99.11- ☑
　liver O26.61- ☑
　specified NEC O99.89
disorders of — *see* Pregnancy, complicated by, specified body system disorder
　amniotic fluid and membranes O41.9- ☑
　　specified NEC O41.8X- ☑
　biliary tract O26.61- ☑
　ear and mastoid process (conditions in H60-H95) O99.89
　eye and adnexa (conditions in H00-H59) O99.89
　liver O26.61- ☑
　skin (conditions in L00-L99) O99.71- ☑
　specified NEC O99.89
displacement, uterus NEC O34.59- ☑
　causing obstructed labor O65.5
disproportion (due to) O33.9
　fetal deformities NEC O33.7
　generally contracted pelvis O33.1
　hydrocephalic fetus O33.6
　inlet contraction of pelvis O33.2
　mixed maternal and fetal origin O33.4 ☑
　specified NEC O33.8
double uterus O34.59- ☑
　causing obstructed labor O65.5
drug use (conditions in F11-F19) O99.32- ☑
eclampsia, eclamptic (coma) (convulsions) (delirium) (nephritis) (uremia) (*see also* Eclampsia) O15.- ☑
ectopic pregnancy — *see* Pregnancy, ectopic

Pregnancy — *continued*

edema O12.0- ☑
　with
　　gestational hypertension, mild (*see also* Pre-eclampsia) O14.0- ☑
　　proteinuria O12.2- ☑
effusion, amniotic fluid — *see* Pregnancy, complicated by, premature rupture of membranes
elderly
　multigravida O09.52- ☑
　primigravida O09.51- ☑
embolism (*see also* Embolism, obstetric, pregnancy) O88.- ☑
endocrine diseases NEC O99.28- ☑
endometritis O86.12
excessive weight gain O26.0- ☑
exhaustion O26.81- ☑
　during labor and delivery O75.81
face presentation O32.3 ☑
failed induction of labor O61.9
　instrumental O61.1
　mechanical O61.1
　medical O61.0
　specified NEC O61.8
　surgical O61.1
failed or difficult intubation for anesthesia O29.6- ☑
false labor (pains) O47.9
　at or after 37 completed weeks of pregnancy O47.1
　before 37 completed weeks of pregnancy O47.0- ☑
fatigue O26.81- ☑
　during labor and delivery O75.81
fatty metamorphosis of liver O26.61- ☑
female genital mutilation O34.8- [N90.81- ☑]
fetal (maternal care for)
　abnormality or damage O35.9 ☑
　　acid-base balance O68
　　specified type NEC O35.8 ☑
　acidemia O68
　acidosis O68
　alkalosis O68
　anemia and thrombocytopenia O36.82- ☑
　anencephaly O35.0 ☑
　chromosomal abnormality (conditions in Q90-Q99) O35.1 ☑
　conjoined twins O30.02- ☑
　damage from
　　amniocentesis O35.7 ☑
　　biopsy procedures O35.7 ☑
　　drug addiction O35.5 ☑
　　hematological investigation O35.7 ☑
　　intrauterine contraceptive device O35.7 ☑
　　maternal
　　　alcohol addiction O35.4 ☑
　　　cytomegalovirus infection O35.3 ☑
　　　disease NEC O35.8 ☑
　　　drug addiction O35.5 ☑
　　　listeriosis O35.8 ☑
　　　rubella O35.3 ☑
　　　toxoplasmosis O35.8 ☑
　　　viral infection O35.3 ☑
　　medical procedure NEC O35.7 ☑
　　radiation O35.6 ☑
　death (near term) O36.4 ☑
　　early pregnancy O02.1
　decreased movement O36.81- ☑
　disproportion due to deformity (fetal) O33.7
　excessive growth (large for dates) O36.6- ☑
　growth retardation O36.59- ☑
　　light for dates O36.59- ☑
　　small for dates O36.59- ☑
　heart rate irregularity (bradycardia) (decelerations) (tachycardia) O76
　hereditary disease O35.2 ☑
　hydrocephalus O35.0 ☑
　intrauterine death O36.4 ☑
　poor growth O36.59- ☑
　　light for dates O36.59- ☑
　　small for dates O36.59- ☑
　problem O36.9- ☑
　　specified NEC O36.89- ☑
　reduction (elective) O31.3- ☑
　selective termination O31.3- ☑
　spina bifida O35.0 ☑
　thrombocytopenia O36.82- ☑
fibroid (tumor) (uterus) O34.1- ☑
fissure of nipple O92.11- ☑
gallstones O99.61- ☑
gastric banding status O99.84- ☑

Pregnancy — *continued*

gastric bypass status O99.84- ☑
genital herpes (asymptomatic) (history of) (inactive) O98.51- ☑
genital tract infection O23.9- ☑
glomerular diseases (conditions in N00-N07) O26.83- ☑
　with hypertension, pre-existing — *see* Hypertension, complicating, pregnancy, pre-existing, with, renal disease
gonorrhea O98.21- ☑
grand multiparity O09.4 ☑
habitual aborter — *see* Pregnancy, complicated by, recurrent pregnancy loss
HELLP syndrome (hemolysis, elevated liver enzymes and low platelet count) O14.2- ☑
hemorrhage
　antepartum — *see* Hemorrhage, antepartum
　before 20 completed weeks gestation O20.9
　　specified NEC O20.8
　due to premature separation, placenta (*see also* Abruptio placentae) O45.9- ☑
　early O20.9
　　specified NEC O20.8
　threatened abortion O20.0
hemorrhoids O22.4- ☑
hepatitis (viral) O98.41- ☑
herniation of uterus O34.59- ☑
high
　head at term O32.4 ☑
　risk — *see* Supervision (of) (for), high-risk
history of in utero procedure during previous pregnancy O09.82- ☑
HIV O98.71- ☑
human immunodeficiency virus (HIV) disease O98.71- ☑
hydatidiform mole (*see also* Mole, hydatidiform) O01.9- ☑
hydramnios O40.- ☑
hydrocephalic fetus (disproportion) O33.6
hydrops
　amnii O40.- ☑
　fetalis O36.2- ☑
　　associated with isoimmunization (*see also* Pregnancy, complicated by, isoimmunization) O36.11- ☑
hydrorrhea O42.90
hyperemesis (gravidarum) (mild) (*see also* Hyperemesis, gravidarum) O21.0- ☑
hypertension — *see* Hypertension, complicating pregnancy
hypertensive
　heart and renal disease, pre-existing — *see* Hypertension, complicating, pregnancy, pre-existing, with, heart disease, with renal disease
　heart disease, pre-existing — *see* Hypertension, complicating, pregnancy, pre-existing, with, heart disease
　renal disease, pre-existing — *see* Hypertension, complicating, pregnancy, pre-existing, with, renal disease
hypotension O26.5- ☑
immune disorders NEC (conditions in D80-D89) O99.11- ☑
incarceration, uterus O34.51- ☑
incompetent cervix O34.3- ☑
inconclusive fetal viability O36.80 ☑
infection (s) O98.91- ☑
　amniotic fluid or sac O41.10- ☑
　bladder O23.1- ☑
　carrier state NEC O99.830
　　streptococcus B O99.820
　genital organ or tract O23.9- ☑
　　specified NEC O23.59- ☑
　genitourinary tract O23.9- ☑
　gonorrhea O98.21- ☑
　hepatitis (viral) O98.41- ☑
　HIV O98.71- ☑
　human immunodeficiency virus (HIV) O98.71- ☑
　kidney O23.0- ☑
　nipple O91.01- ☑
　parasitic disease O98.91- ☑
　　specified NEC O98.81- ☑
　protozoal disease O98.61- ☑
　sexually transmitted NEC O98.31- ☑
　specified type NEC O98.81- ☑
　syphilis O98.11- ☑
　tuberculosis O98.01- ☑
　urethra O23.2- ☑
　urinary (tract) O23.4- ☑

Pregnancy

Pregnancy — *continued*
  specified NEC O23.3- ☑
  viral disease O98.51- ☑
  injury or poisoning (conditions in S00-T88)
      O9A.21- ☑
      due to abuse
          physical O9A.31- ☑
          psychological O9A.51- ☑
          sexual O9A.41- ☑
  insufficient
      prenatal care O09.3- ☑
      weight gain O26.1- ☑
  insulin resistance O26.89 ☑
  intrauterine fetal death (near term) O36.4 ☑
      early pregnancy O02.1
      multiple gestation (one fetus or more)
          O31.2- ☑
  isoimmunization O36.11- ☑
      anti-A sensitization O36.11- ☑
      anti-B sensitization O36.19- ☑
      Rh O36.09- ☑
          anti-D antibody O36.01- ☑
      specified NEC O36.19- ☑
  laceration of uterus NEC O71.81
  malformation
      placenta, placental (vessel) O43.10- ☑
          specified NEC O43.19- ☑
      uterus (congenital) O34.0- ☑
  malnutrition (conditions in E40-E46) O25.1- ☑
  maternal hypotension syndrome O26.5- ☑
  mental disorders (conditions in F01-F09,
      F20-F99) O99.34- ☑
      alcohol use O99.31- ☑
      drug use O99.32- ☑
      smoking O99.33- ☑
  mentum presentation O32.3 ☑
  metabolic disorders O99.28- ☑
  missed
      abortion O02.1
      delivery O36.4 ☑
  multiple gestations O30.9- ☑
      conjoined twins O30.02- ☑
      specified number of multiples NEC — *see*
          Pregnancy, multiple (gestation), specified
          NEC
      quadruplet — *see* Pregnancy, quadruplet
      specified complication NEC O31.8X- ☑
      triplet — *see* Pregnancy, triplet
      twin — *see* Pregnancy, twin
  musculoskeletal condition (conditions is
      M00-M99) O99.89
  necrosis, liver (conditions in K72) O26.61- ☑
  neoplasm
      benign
          cervix O34.4- ☑
          corpus uteri O34.1- ☑
          uterus O34.1- ☑
      malignant O9A.11- ☑
  nephropathy NEC O26.83- ☑
  nervous system condition (conditions in
      G00-G99) O99.35- ☑
  nutritional diseases NEC O99.28- ☑
  obesity (pre-existing) O99.21- ☑
  obesity surgery status O99.84- ☑
  oblique lie or presentation O32.2 ☑
  older mother — *see* Pregnancy, complicated
      by, elderly
  oligohydramnios O41.0- ☑
      with premature rupture of membranes
          (*see also* Pregnancy, complicated by,
          premature rupture of membranes)
          O42.- ☑
  onset (spontaneous) of labor after 37
      completed weeks of gestation but before
      39 completed weeks gestation, with
      delivery by (planned) cesarean section
      O75.82
  oophoritis O23.52- ☑
  overdose, drug (*see also* Table of Drugs and
      Chemicals, by drug, poisoning) O9A.21- ☑
  oversize fetus O33.5 ☑
  papyraceous fetus O31.0- ☑
  pelvic inflammatory disease O99.89
  periodontal disease O99.61- ☑
  peripheral neuritis O26.82- ☑
  peritoneal (pelvic) adhesions O99.89
  phlebitis O22.9- ☑
  phlebopathy O22.9- ☑
  phlebothrombosis (superficial) O22.2- ☑
      deep O22.3- ☑
  placenta accreta O43.21- ☑
  placenta increta O43.22- ☑

Pregnancy — *continued*
  placenta percreta O43.23- ☑
  placenta previa O44.1- ☑
      without hemorrhage O44.0- ☑
  placental disorder O43.9- ☑
      specified NEC O43.89- ☑
  placental dysfunction O43.89- ☑
  placental infarction O43.81- ☑
  placental insufficiency O36.51- ☑
  placental transfusion syndromes
      fetomaternal O43.01- ☑
      fetus to fetus O43.02- ☑
      maternofetal O43.01- ☑
  placentitis O41.14- ☑
  pneumonia O99.51- ☑
  poisoning (*see also* Table of Drugs and
      Chemicals) O9A.21- ☑
  polyhydramnios O40- ☑
  polymorphic eruption of pregnancy O26.86
  poor obstetric history NEC O09.29- ☑
  postmaturity (post-term) (40 to 42 weeks)
      O48.0
      more than 42 completed weeks gestation
          (prolonged) O48.1
  pre-eclampsia O14.9- ☑
      mild O14.0- ☑
      moderate O14.0- ☑
      severe O14.1- ☑
          with hemolysis, elevated liver enzymes and
              low platelet count (HELLP) O14.2- ☑
  premature labor — *see* Pregnancy, complicated
      by, preterm labor
  premature rupture of membranes O42.90
      full-term O42.92
      with onset of labor
          within 24 hours O42.00
              after 37 weeks gestation O42.02
              pre-term (before 37 completed weeks of
                  gestation) O42.01- ☑
          after 24 hours O42.10
              after 37 weeks gestation O42.12
              pre-term (before 37 completed weeks of
                  gestation) O42.11- ☑
          after 37 weeks gestation O42.92
          pre-term (before 37 completed weeks of
              gestation) O42.91- ☑
  premature separation of placenta (*see also*
      Abruptio placentae) O45.9- ☑
  presentation, fetal - — *see* Delivery,
      complicated by, malposition
  preterm delivery O60.10 ☑
  preterm labor
      with delivery O60.10 ☑
          preterm O60.10 ☑
          term O60.20 ☑
      second trimester
          with term delivery O60.22 ☑
          without delivery O60.02
          with preterm delivery
              second trimester O60.12 ☑
              third trimester O60.13 ☑
      third trimester
          with term delivery O60.23 ☑
          without delivery O60.03
          with third trimester preterm delivery
              O60.14 ☑
      without delivery O60.00
          second trimester O60.02
          third trimester O60.03
  previous history of — *see* Pregnancy,
      supervision of, high-risk
  prolapse, uterus O34.52- ☑
  proteinuria (gestational) O12.1- ☑
      with edema O12.2- ☑
  pruritic urticarial papules and plaques of
      pregnancy (PUPPP) O26.86
  pruritus (neurogenic) O26.89- ☑
  psychosis or psychoneurosis (puerperal) F53
  ptyalism O26.89- ☑
  PUPPP (pruritic urticarial papules and plaques
      of pregnancy) O26.86
  pyelitis O23.0- ☑
  recurrent pregnancy loss O26.2- ☑
  renal disease or failure NEC O26.83- ☑
      with secondary hypertension, pre-existing
          — *see* Hypertension, complicating,
          pregnancy, pre-existing, secondary
      hypertensive, pre-existing — *see*
          Hypertension, complicating, pregnancy,
          pre-existing, with, renal disease
  respiratory condition (conditions in J00-J99)
      O99.51- ☑

Pregnancy — *continued*
  retained, retention
      dead ovum O02.0
      intrauterine contraceptive device O26.3- ☑
  retroversion, uterus O34.53- ☑
  Rh immunization, incompatibility or
      sensitization NEC O36.09- ☑
      anti-D antibody O36.01- ☑
  rupture
      amnion (premature) (*see also* Pregnancy,
          complicated by, premature rupture of
          membranes) O42- ☑
      membranes (premature) (*see also* Pregnancy,
          complicated by, premature rupture of
          membranes) O42- ☑
      uterus (during labor) O71.1
          before onset of labor O71.0- ☑
  salivation (excessive) O26.89- ☑
  salpingitis O23.52- ☑
  salpingo-oophoritis O23.52- ☑
  sepsis (conditions in A40, A41) O98.81- ☑
  size date discrepancy (uterine) O26.84- ☑
  skin condition (conditions in L00-L99) O99.71-
      ☑
  smoking (tobacco) O99.33- ☑
  social problem O09.7- ☑
  specified condition NEC O26.89- ☑
  spotting O26.85- ☑
  streptococcus B carrier state O99.820
  subluxation of symphysis (pubis) O26.71- ☑
  syphilis (conditions in A50-A53) O98.11- ☑
  threatened
      abortion O20.0
      labor O47.9
          at or after 37 completed weeks of gestation
              O47.1
          before 37 completed weeks of gestation
              O47.0- ☑
  thrombophlebitis (superficial) O22.2- ☑
  thrombosis O22.9- ☑
      cerebral venous O22.5- ☑
      cerebrovascular sinus O22.5- ☑
      deep O22.3- ☑
  torsion of uterus O34.59- ☑
  toxemia O14.9- ☑
  transverse lie or presentation O32.2 ☑
  tuberculosis (conditions in A15-A19) O98.01- ☑
  tumor (benign)
      cervix O34.4- ☑
      malignant O9A.11- ☑
      uterus O34.1- ☑
  unstable lie O32.0 ☑
  upper respiratory infection O99.51- ☑
  urethritis O23.2- ☑
  uterine size date discrepancy O26.84- ☑
  vaginitis or vulvitis O23.59- ☑
  varicose veins (lower extremities) O22.0- ☑
      genitals O22.1- ☑
      legs O22.0- ☑
      perineal O22.1- ☑
      vaginal or vulval O22.1- ☑
  venereal disease NEC (conditions in A63.8)
      O98.31- ☑
  venous disorders O22.9- ☑
      specified NEC O22.8X- ☑
  viral diseases (conditions in A80-B09, B25-B34)
      O98.51- ☑
  very young mother — *see* Pregnancy,
      complicated by, young mother
  vomiting O21.9
      due to diseases classified elsewhere O21.8
      hyperemesis gravidarum (mild) (*see also*
          Hyperemesis, gravidarum) O21.0- ☑
      late (occurring after 20 weeks of gestation)
          O21.2
  young mother
      multigravida O09.62- ☑
      primigravida O09.61- ☑
  concealed O09.3- ☑
  continuing following
      elective fetal reduction of one or more fetus
          O31.3- ☑
      intrauterine death of one or more fetus O31.2-
          ☑
      spontaneous abortion of one or more fetus
          O31.1- ☑
  cornual O00.8
  ectopic (ruptured) O00.9
      abdominal O00.0
          with viable fetus O36.7- ☑
      cervical O00.8
      complicated (by) O08.9

☑ **Additional character required**

Pregnancy — *continued*
  afibrinogenemia O08.1
  cardiac arrest O08.81
  chemical damage of pelvic organ (s) O08.6
  circulatory collapse O08.3
  defibrination syndrome O08.1
  electrolyte imbalance O08.5
  embolism (amniotic fluid) (blood clot)
      (pulmonary) (septic) O08.2
  endometritis O08.0
  genital tract and pelvic infection O08.0
  hemorrhage (delayed) (excessive) O08.1
  infection
      genital tract or pelvic O08.0
      kidney O08.83
      urinary tract O08.83
  intravascular coagulation O08.1
  laceration of pelvic organ (s) O08.6
  metabolic disorder O08.5
  oliguria O08.4
  oophoritis O08.0
  parametritis O08.0
  pelvic peritonitis O08.0
  perforation of pelvic organ (s) O08.6
  renal failure or shutdown O08.4
  salpingitis or salpingo-oophoritis O08.0
  sepsis O08.82
  shock O08.83
      septic O08.82
  specified condition NEC O08.89
  tubular necrosis (renal) O08.4
  uremia O08.4
  urinary infection O08.83
  venous complication NEC O08.7
      embolism O08.2
  cornual O00.8
  intraligamentous O00.8
  mural O00.8
  ovarian O00.2
  specified site NEC O00.8
  tubal (ruptured) O00.1
  examination (normal) Z34.9- ☑
  high-risk — *see* Pregnancy, supervision of,
      high-risk
  first Z34.0- ☑
  specified Z34.8- ☑
  extrauterine — *see* Pregnancy, ectopic
  fallopian O00.1
  false F45.8
  hidden O09.3- ☑
  high-risk — *see* Pregnancy, supervision of,
      high-risk
  incidental finding Z33.1
  interstitial O00.8
  intraligamentous O00.8
  intramural O00.8
  intraperitoneal O00.0
  isthmian O00.1
  mesometric (mural) O00.8
  molar NEC O02.0
      complicated (by) O08.9
          afibrinogenemia O08.1
          cardiac arrest O08.81
          chemical damage of pelvic organ (s) O08.6
          circulatory collapse O08.3
          defibrination syndrome O08.1
          electrolyte imbalance O08.5
          embolism (amniotic fluid) (blood clot)
              (pulmonary) (septic) O08.2
          endometritis O08.0
          genital tract and pelvic infection O08.0
          hemorrhage (delayed) (excessive) O08.1
          infection
              genital tract or pelvic O08.0
              kidney O08.83
              urinary tract O08.83
          intravascular coagulation O08.1
          laceration of pelvic organ (s) O08.6
          metabolic disorder O08.5
          oliguria O08.4
          oophoritis O08.0
          parametritis O08.0
          pelvic peritonitis O08.0
          perforation of pelvic organ (s) O08.6
          renal failure or shutdown O08.4
          salpingitis or salpingo-oophoritis O08.0
          sepsis O08.82
          shock O08.3
              septic O08.82
          specified condition NEC O08.89
          tubular necrosis (renal) O08.4
          uremia O08.4

Pregnancy — *continued*
  urinary infection O08.83
  venous complication NEC O08.7
      embolism O08.2
  hydatidiform (*see also* Mole, hydatidiform)
      O01.9- ☑
  multiple (gestation) O30.9- ☑
      greater than quadruplets — *see* Pregnancy,
          multiple (gestation), specified NEC
      specified NEC O30.80- ☑
          with
              two or more monoamniotic fetuses
                  O30.82- ☑
              two or more monochorionic fetuses
                  O30.81- ☑
          two or more monoamniotic fetuses O30.82-
              ☑
          two or more monochorionic fetuses O30.81-
              ☑
          unable to determine number of placenta and
              number of amniotic sacs O30.89- ☑
          unspecified number of placenta and
              unspecified number of amniotic sacs
              O30.80- ☑
  mural O00.8
  normal (supervision of) Z34.9- ☑
      high-risk — *see* Pregnancy, supervision of,
          high-risk
      first Z34.0- ☑
      specified Z34.8- ☑
  ovarian O00.2
  postmature (40 to 42 weeks) O48.0
      more than 42 weeks gestation O48.1
  post-term (40 to 42 weeks) O48.0
  prenatal care only Z34.9- ☑
      high-risk — *see* Pregnancy, supervision of,
          high-risk
      first Z34.0- ☑
      specified Z34.8- ☑
  prolonged (more than 42 weeks gestation) O48.1
  quadruplet O30.20- ☑
      with
          two or more monoamniotic fetuses O30.22-
              ☑
          two or more monochorionic fetuses O30.21-
              ☑
      two or more monoamniotic fetuses O30.22- ☑
      two or more monochorionic fetuses O30.21- ☑
      unable to determine number of placenta and
          number of amniotic sacs O30.29- ☑
      unspecified number of placenta and
          unspecified number of amniotic sacs
          O30.20- ☑
  quintuplet — *see* Pregnancy, multiple (gestation),
      specified NEC
  sextuplet — *see* Pregnancy, multiple (gestation),
      specified NEC
  supervision of
      concealed pregnancy O09.3- ☑
      elderly mother
          multigravida O09.52- ☑
          primigravida O09.51- ☑
      hidden pregnancy O09.3- ☑
      high-risk O09.9- ☑
          due to (history of)
              ectopic pregnancy O09.1- ☑
              elderly — *see* Pregnancy, supervision,
                  elderly mother
              grand multiparity O09.4 ☑
              infertility O09.0- ☑
              insufficient prenatal care O09.3- ☑
              in utero procedure during previous
                  pregnancy O09.82- ☑
              in vitro fertilization O09.81- ☑
              molar pregnancy O09.1- ☑
              multiple previous pregnancies O09.4- ☑
              older mother — *see* Pregnancy, supervision
                  of, elderly mother
              poor reproductive or obstetric history NEC
                  O09.29- ☑
              pre-term labor O09.21- ☑
              previous
                  neonatal death O09.29- ☑
              social problems O09.7- ☑
              specified NEC O09.89- ☑
              very young mother — *see* Pregnancy,
                  supervision, young mother
          resulting from in vitro fertilization O09.81- ☑
      normal Z34.9- ☑
          first Z34.0- ☑
          specified NEC Z34.8- ☑
      young mother

Pregnancy — *continued*
  multigravida O09.62- ☑
  primigravida O09.61- ☑
  triplet O30.10- ☑
      with
          two or more monoamniotic fetuses O30.12-
              ☑
          two or more monochrorionic fetuses O30.11-
              ☑
      two or more monoamniotic fetuses O30.12- ☑
      two or more monochrorionic fetuses O30.11-
          ☑
      unable to determine number of placenta and
          number of amniotic sacs O30.19- ☑
      unspecified number of placenta and
          unspecified number of amniotic sacs
          O30.10- ☑
  tubal (with abortion) (with rupture) O00.1
  twin O30.00- ☑
      conjoined O30.02- ☑
      dichorionic/diamniotic (two placenta, two
          amniotic sacs) O30.04- ☑
      monochorionic/diamniotic (one placenta, two
          amniotic sacs) O30.03- ☑
      monochorionic/monoamniotic (one placenta,
          one amniotic sac) O30.01- ☑
      unable to determine number of placenta and
          number of amniotic sacs O30.09- ☑
      unspecified number of placenta and
          unspecified number of amniotic sacs
          O30.00- ☑
  unwanted Z64.0
  weeks of gestation
      8 weeks Z3A.08
      9 weeks Z3A.09
      10 weeks Z3A.10
      11 weeks Z3A.11
      12 weeks Z3A.12
      13 weeks Z3A.13
      14 weeks Z3A.14
      15 weeks Z3A.15
      16 weeks Z3A.16
      17 weeks Z3A.17
      18 weeks Z3A.18
      19 weeks Z3A.19
      20 weeks Z3A.20
      21 weeks Z3A.21
      22 weeks Z3A.22
      23 weeks Z3A.23
      24 weeks Z3A.24
      25 weeks Z3A.25
      26 weeks Z3A.26
      27 weeks Z3A.27
      28 weeks Z3A.28
      29 weeks Z3A.29
      30 weeks Z3A.30
      31 weeks Z3A.31
      32 weeks Z3A.32
      33 weeks Z3A.33
      34 weeks Z3A.34
      35 weeks Z3A.35
      36 weeks Z3A.36
      37 weeks Z3A.37
      38 weeks Z3A.38
      39 weeks Z3A.39
      40 weeks Z3A.40
      41 weeks Z3A.41
      42 weeks Z3A.42
      greater than 42 weeks Z3A.49
      less than 8 weeks Z3A.01
      not specified Z3A.00
Preiser's disease — *see* Osteonecrosis, secondary,
  due to, trauma, metacarpus
Pre-kwashiorkor — *see* Malnutrition, severe
Preleukemia (syndrome) D46.9
Preluxation, hip, congenital Q65.6
Premature (*see also* condition)
  adrenarche E27.0
  aging E34.8
  beats I49.40
      atrial I49.1
      auricular I49.1
      supraventricular I49.1
  birth NEC — *see* Preterm, newborn
  closure, foramen ovale Q21.8
  contraction
      atrial I49.1
      atrioventricular I49.2
      auricular I49.1
      auriculoventricular I49.49
      heart (extrasystole) I49.49
      junctional I49.2

Premature — continued
  ventricular I49.3
  delivery (see also Pregnancy, complicated by, preterm labor) O60.10 ☑
  ejaculation F52.4
  infant NEC — see Preterm, newborn
    light-for-dates — see Light for dates
  labor — see Pregnancy, complicated by, preterm labor
  lungs P28.0
  menopause E28.319
    asymptomatic E28.319
    symptomatic E28.310
  newborn
    extreme (less than 28 completed weeks) — see Immaturity, extreme
    less than 37 completed weeks — see Preterm, newborn
  puberty E30.1
  rupture membranes or amnion — see Pregnancy, complicated by, premature rupture of membranes
  senility E34.8
  thelarche E30.8
  ventricular systole I49.3
Prematurity NEC (less than 37 completed weeks) — see Preterm, newborn
  extreme (less than 28 completed weeks) — see Immaturity, extreme
Premenstrual
  dysphoric disorder (PMDD) N94.3
  tension (syndrome) N94.3
Premolarization, cuspids K00.2
Prenatal
  care, normal pregnancy — see Pregnancy, normal
  screening of mother Z36
  teeth K00.6
Preparatory care for subsequent treatment NEC for dialysis Z49.01
  peritoneal Z49.02
Prepartum — see condition
Preponderance, left or right ventricular I51.7
Prepuce — see condition
PRES (posterior reversible encephalopathy syndrome) I67.83
Presbycardia R54
Presbycusis, presbyacusia H91.1- ☑
Presbyesophagus K22.8
Presbyophrenia F03 ☑
Presbyopia H52.4
Prescription of contraceptives (initial) Z30.019
  emergency (postcoital) Z30.012
  implantable subdermal Z30.019
  injectable Z30.013
  intrauterine contraceptive device Z30.014
  pills Z30.011
  postcoital (emergency) Z30.012
  repeat Z30.40
    implantable subdermal Z30.49
    injectable Z30.42
    pills Z30.41
    specified type NEC Z30.49
  specified type NEC Z30.018
Presence (of)
  ankle-joint implant (functional) (prosthesis) Z96.66- ☑
  aortocoronary (bypass) graft Z95.1
  arterial-venous shunt (dialysis) Z99.2
  artificial
    eye (globe) Z97.0
    heart (fully implantable) (mechanical) Z95.812
      valve Z95.2
    larynx Z96.3
    lens (intraocular) Z96.1
    limb (complete) (partial) Z97.1- ☑
      arm Z97.1- ☑
        bilateral Z97.15
      leg Z97.1- ☑
        bilateral Z97.16
  audiological implant (functional) Z96.29
  bladder implant (functional) Z96.0
  bone
    conduction hearing device Z96.29
    implant (functional) NEC Z96.7
    joint (prosthesis) — see Presence, joint implant
  cardiac
    defibrillator (functional) (with synchronous cardiac pacemaker) Z95.810
    implant or graft Z95.9
      specified type NEC Z95.818
    pacemaker Z95.0
  cerebrospinal fluid drainage device Z98.2

Presence — continued
  cochlear implant (functional) Z96.21
  contact lens (es) Z97.3
  coronary artery graft or prosthesis Z95.5
  CSF shunt Z98.2
  dental prosthesis device Z97.2
  dentures Z97.2
  device (external) NEC Z97.8
    cardiac NEC Z95.818
    heart assist Z95.811
    implanted (functional) Z96.9
      specified NEC Z96.89
    prosthetic Z97.8
  ear implant Z96.20
    cochlear implant Z96.21
    myringotomy tube Z96.22
    specified type NEC Z96.29
  elbow-joint implant (functional) (prosthesis) Z96.62- ☑
  endocrine implant (functional) NEC Z96.49
  eustachian tube stent or device (functional) Z96.29
  external hearing-aid or device Z97.4
  finger-joint implant (functional) (prosthetic) Z96.69- ☑
  functional implant Z96.9
    specified NEC Z96.89
  graft
    cardiac NEC Z95.818
    vascular NEC Z95.828
  hearing-aid or device (external) Z97.4
    implant (bone) (cochlear) (functional) Z96.21
  heart assist device Z95.811
  heart valve implant (functional) Z95.2
    prosthetic Z95.2
    specified type NEC Z95.4
    xenogenic Z95.3
  hip-joint implant (functional) (prosthesis) Z96.64- ☑
  implanted device (artificial) (functional) (prosthetic) Z96.9
    automatic cardiac defibrillator (with synchronous cardiac pacemaker) Z95.810
    cardiac pacemaker Z95.0
    cochlear Z96.21
    dental Z96.5
    heart Z95.812
    heart valve Z95.2
      prosthetic Z95.2
      specified NEC Z95.4
      xenogenic Z95.3
    insulin pump Z96.41
    intraocular lens Z96.1
    joint Z96.60
      ankle Z96.66- ☑
      elbow Z96.62- ☑
      finger Z96.69- ☑
      hip Z96.64- ☑
      knee Z96.65- ☑
      shoulder Z96.61- ☑
      specified NEC Z96.698
      wrist Z96.63- ☑
    larynx Z96.3
    myringotomy tube Z96.22
    otological Z96.20
      cochlear Z96.21
      eustachian stent Z96.29
      myringotomy Z96.22
      specified NEC Z96.29
      stapes Z96.29
    skin Z96.81
    skull plate Z96.7
    specified NEC Z96.89
    urogenital Z96.0
  insulin pump (functional) Z96.41
  intestinal bypass or anastomosis Z98.0
  intraocular lens (functional) Z96.1
  intrauterine contraceptive device (IUD) Z97.5
  intravascular implant (functional) (prosthetic) NEC Z95.9
    coronary artery Z95.5
    defibrillator (with synchronous cardiac pacemaker) Z95.810
    peripheral vessel (with angioplasty) Z95.820
  joint implant (prosthetic) (any) Z96.60
    ankle — see Presence, ankle joint implant
    elbow — see Presence, elbow joint implant
    finger — see Presence, finger joint implant
    hip — see Presence, hip joint implant
    knee — see Presence, knee joint implant
    shoulder — see Presence, shoulder joint implant

Presence — continued
    specified joint NEC Z96.698
    wrist — see Presence, wrist joint implant
  knee-joint implant (functional) (prosthesis) Z96.65- ☑
  laryngeal implant (functional) Z96.3
  mandibular implant (dental) Z96.5
  myringotomy tube (s) Z96.22
  orthopedic-joint implant (prosthetic) (any) — see Presence, joint implant
  otological implant (functional) Z96.29
  shoulder-joint implant (functional) (prosthesis) Z96.61- ☑
  skull-plate implant Z96.7
  spectacles Z97.3
  stapes implant (functional) Z96.29
  systemic lupus erythematosus [SLE] inhibitor D68.62
  tendon implant (functional) (graft) Z96.7
  tooth root (s) implant Z96.5
  ureteral stent Z96.0
  urethral stent Z96.0
  urogenital implant (functional) Z96.0
  vascular implant or device Z95.9
    access port device Z95.828
    specified type NEC Z95.828
  wrist-joint implant (functional) (prosthesis) Z96.63- ☑
Presenile (see also condition)
  dementia F03 ☑
  premature aging E34.8
Presentation, fetal — see Delivery , complicated by, malposition
Prespondylolisthesis (congenital) Q76.2
Pressure
  area, skin — see Ulcer, pressure, by site
  brachial plexus G54.0
  brain G93.5
    injury at birth NEC P11.1
  cerebral — see Pressure, brain
  chest R07.89
  cone, tentorial G93.5
  hyposystolic (see also Hypotension)
    incidental reading, without diagnosis of hypotension R03.1
  increased
    intracranial (benign) G93.2
      injury at birth P11.0
    intraocular H40.05- ☑
  lumbosacral plexus G54.1
  mediastinum J98.5
  necrosis (chronic) — see Ulcer, pressure, by site
  parental, inappropriate (excessive) Z62.6
  sore (chronic) — see Ulcer, pressure, by site
  spinal cord G95.20
  ulcer (chronic) — see Ulcer, pressure, by site
  venous, increased I87.8
Pre-syncope R55
Preterm
  delivery (see also Pregnancy, complicated by, preterm labor) O60.10 ☑
  labor — see Pregnancy, complicated by, preterm labor
  newborn (infant) P07.30
    gestational age
      28 completed weeks (28 weeks, 0 days through 28 weeks, 6 days) P07.31
      29 completed weeks (29 weeks, 0 days through 29 weeks, 6 days) P07.32
      30 completed weeks (30 weeks, 0 days through 30 weeks, 6 days) P07.33
      31 completed weeks (31 weeks, 0 days through 31 weeks, 6 days) P07.34
      32 completed weeks (32 weeks, 0 days through 32 weeks, 6 days) P07.35
      33 completed weeks (33 weeks, 0 days through 33 weeks, 6 days) P07.36
      34 completed weeks (34 weeks, 0 days through 34 weeks, 6 days) P07.37
      35 completed weeks (35 weeks, 0 days through 35 weeks, 6 days) P07.38
      36 completed weeks (36 weeks, 0 days through 36 weeks, 6 days) P07.39
Previa
  placenta (low) (marginal) (partial) (total) (with hemorrhage) O44.1- ☑
    without hemorrhage O44.0- ☑
  vasa O69.4 ☑
Priapism N48.30
  due to
    disease classified elsewhere N48.32
    drug N48.33

Priapism — *continued*
  specified cause NEC N48.39
  trauma N48.31
Prickling sensation (skin) R20.2
Prickly heat L74.0
Primary — *see* condition
Primigravida
  elderly, affecting management of pregnancy, labor and delivery (supervision only) — *see* Pregnancy, complicated by, elderly, primigravida
  older, affecting management of pregnancy, labor and delivery (supervision only) — *see* Pregnancy, complicated by, elderly, primigravida
  very young, affecting management of pregnancy, labor and delivery (supervision only) — *see* Pregnancy, complicated by, young mother, primigravida
Primipara
  elderly, affecting management of pregnancy, labor and delivery (supervision only) — *see* Pregnancy, complicated by, elderly, primigravida
  older, affecting management of pregnancy, labor and delivery (supervision only) — *see* Pregnancy, complicated by, elderly, primigravida
  very young, affecting management of pregnancy, labor and delivery (supervision only) — *see* Pregnancy, complicated by, young mother, primigravida
Primus varus (bilateral) Q66.2
PRIND (Prolonged reversible ischemic neurologic deficit) I63.9
Pringle's disease (tuberous sclerosis) Q85.1
Prinzmetal angina I20.1
Prizefighter ear — *see* Cauliflower ear
Problem (with) (related to)
  academic Z55.8
  acculturation Z60.3
  adjustment (to)
   change of job Z56.1
   life-cycle transition Z60.0
   pension Z60.0
   retirement Z60.0
  adopted child Z62.821
  alcoholism in family Z63.72
  atypical parenting situation Z62.9
  bankruptcy Z59.8
  behavioral (adult) F69
   drug seeking Z72.89
  birth of sibling affecting child Z62.898
  care (of)
   provider dependency Z74.9
    specified NEC Z74.8
   sick or handicapped person in family or household Z63.6
  child
   abuse (affecting the child) — *see* Maltreatment, child
   custody or support proceedings Z65.3
   in welfare custody Z62.21
   in care of non-parental family member Z62.21
   in foster care Z62.21
   living in orphanage or group home Z62.22
  child-rearing Z62.9
   specified NEC Z62.898
  communication (developmental) F80.9
  conflict or discord (with)
   boss Z56.4
   classmates Z55.4
   counselor Z64.4
   employer Z56.4
   family Z63.9
    specified NEC Z63.8
   probation officer Z64.4
   social worker Z64.4
   teachers Z55.4
   workmates Z56.4
  conviction in legal proceedings Z65.0
   with imprisonment Z65.1
  counselor Z64.4
  creditors Z59.8
  digestive K92.9
  drug addict in family Z63.72
  ear — *see* Disorder, ear
  economic Z59.9
   affecting care Z59.9
   specified NEC Z59.8
  education Z55.9
   specified NEC Z55.8

Problem — *continued*
  employment Z56.9
   change of job Z56.1
   discord Z56.4
   environment Z56.5
   sexual harassment Z56.81
   specified NEC Z56.89
   stress NEC Z56.6
   stressful schedule Z56.3
   threat of job loss Z56.2
   unemployment Z56.0
  enuresis, child F98.0
  eye H57.9
  failed examinations (school) Z55.2
  falling Z91.81
  family (*see also* Disruption, family) Z63.9- ☑
   specified NEC Z63.8
  feeding (elderly) (infant) R63.3
   newborn P92.9
    breast P92.5
    overfeeding P92.4
    slow P92.2
    specified NEC P92.8
    underfeeding P92.3
   nonorganic F50.8
  finance Z59.9
   specified NEC Z59.8
  foreclosure on loan Z59.8
  foster child Z62.822
  frightening experience (s) in childhood Z62.898
  genital NEC
   female N94.9
   male N50.9
  health care Z75.9
   specified NEC Z75.8
  hearing — *see* Deafness
  homelessness Z59.0
  housing Z59.9
   inadequate Z59.1
   isolated Z59.8
   specified NEC Z59.8
  identity (of childhood) F93.8
  illegitimate pregnancy (unwanted) Z64.0
  illiteracy Z55.0
  impaired mobility Z74.09
  imprisonment or incarceration Z65.1
  inadequate teaching affecting education Z55.8
  inappropriate (excessive) parental pressure Z62.6
  influencing health status NEC Z78.9
  in-law Z63.1
  institutionalization, affecting child Z62.22
  intrafamilial communication Z63.8
  jealousy, child F93.8
  landlord Z59.2
  language (developmental) F80.9
  learning (developmental) F81.9
  legal Z65.3
   conviction without imprisonment Z65.0
   imprisonment Z65.1
   release from prison Z65.2
  life-management Z73.9
   specified NEC Z73.89
  life-style Z72.9
   gambling Z72.6
   high-risk sexual behavior (heterosexual) Z72.51
    bisexual Z72.53
    homosexual Z72.52
   inappropriate eating habits Z72.4
   self-damaging behavior NEC Z72.89
   specified NEC Z72.89
   tobacco use Z72.0
  literacy Z55.9
   low level Z55.0
   specified NEC Z55.8
  living alone Z60.2
  lodgers Z59.2
  loss of love relationship in childhood Z62.898
  marital Z63.0
   involving
    divorce Z63.5
    estrangement Z63.5
    gender identity F66
  mastication K08.8
  medical
   care, within family Z63.6
   facilities Z75.9
    specified NEC Z75.8
  mental F48.9
  multiparity Z64.1
  negative life events in childhood Z62.9
   altered pattern of family relationships Z62.898
   frightening experience Z62.898

Problem — *continued*
  loss of
   love relationship Z62.898
   self-esteem Z62.898
   physical abuse (alleged) — *see* Maltreatment, child
   removal from home Z62.29
   specified event NEC Z62.898
  neighbor Z59.2
  neurological NEC R29.818
  new step-parent affecting child Z62.898
  none (feared complaint unfounded) Z71.1
  occupational NEC Z56.89
  parent-child — *see* Conflict, parent-child
  personal hygiene Z91.89
  personality F69
  phase-of-life transition, adjustment Z60.0
  presence of sick or disabled person in family or household Z63.79
   needing care Z63.6
  primary support group (family) Z63.9
   specified NEC Z63.8
  probation officer Z64.4
  psychiatric F99
  psychosexual (development) F66
  psychosocial Z65.9
   specified NEC Z65.8
  relationship Z63.9
   childhood F93.8
  release from prison Z65.2
  removal from home affecting child Z62.29
  seeking and accepting known hazardous and harmful
   behavioral or psychological interventions Z65.8
   chemical, nutritional or physical interventions Z65.8
  sexual function (nonorganic) F52.9
  sight H54.7
  sleep disorder, child F51.9
  smell — *see* Disturbance, sensation, smell
  social
   environment Z60.9
    specified NEC Z60.8
   exclusion and rejection Z60.4
   worker Z64.4
  speech R47.9
   developmental F80.9
   specified NEC R47.89
  swallowing — *see* Dysphagia
  taste — *see* Disturbance, sensation, taste
  tic, child F95.0
  underachievement in school Z55.3
  unemployment Z56.0
   threatened Z56.2
  unwanted pregnancy Z64.0
  upbringing Z62.9
   specified NEC Z62.898
  urinary N39.9
  voice production R47.89
  work schedule (stressful) Z56.3
Procedure (surgical)
  for purpose other than remedying health state Z41.9
   specified NEC Z41.8
  not done Z53.9
   because of
    administrative reasons Z53.8
    contraindication Z53.09
     smoking Z53.01
    patient's decision Z53.20
     for reasons of belief or group pressure Z53.1
     left against medical advice (AMA) Z53.21
     specified reason NEC Z53.29
    specified reason NEC Z53.8
Procidentia (uteri) N81.3
Proctalgia K62.89
  fugax K59.4
  spasmodic K59.4
Proctitis K62.89
  amebic (acute) A06.0
  chlamydial A56.3
  gonococcal A54.6
  granulomatous — *see* Enteritis, regional, large intestine
  herpetic A60.1
  radiation K62.7
  tuberculous A18.32
  ulcerative (chronic) K51.20
   with
    complication K51.219
     abscess K51.214

Proctitis — continued
    fistula K51.213
    obstruction K51.212
    rectal bleeding K51.211
    specified NEC K51.218
Proctocele
  female (without uterine prolapse) N81.6
    with uterine prolapse N81.2
      complete N81.3
  male K62.3
Proctocolitis, mucosal — *see* Rectosigmoiditis, ulcerative
Proctoptosis K62.3
Proctorrhagia K62.5
Proctosigmoiditis K63.89
  ulcerative (chronic) — *see* Rectosigmoiditis, ulcerative
Proctospasm K59.4
  psychogenic F45.8
Profichet's disease — *see* Disorder, soft tissue, specified type NEC
Progeria E34.8
Prognathism (mandibular) (maxillary) M26.19
Progonoma (melanotic) — *see* Neoplasm, benign, by site
Progressive — *see* condition
Prolactinoma
  specified site — *see* Neoplasm, benign, by site
  unspecified site D35.2
Prolapse, prolapsed
  anus, anal (canal) (sphincter) K62.2
  arm or hand O32.2 ☑
    causing obstructed labor O64.4 ☑
  bladder (mucosa) (sphincter) (acquired)
    congenital Q79.4
    female — *see* Cystocele
    male N32.89
  breast implant (prosthetic) T85.49 ☑
  cecostomy K94.09
  cecum K63.4
  cervix, cervical (hypertrophied) N81.2
    anterior lip, obstructing labor O65.5
    congenital Q51.828
    postpartal, old N81.2
    stump N81.85
  ciliary body (traumatic) — *see* Laceration, eye(ball), with prolapse or loss of interocular tissue
  colon (pedunculated) K63.4
  colostomy K94.09
  disc (intervertebral) — *see* Displacement, intervertebral disc
  eye implant (orbital) T85.398 ☑
    lens (ocular) — *see* Complications, intraocular lens
  fallopian tube N83.4
  gastric (mucosa) K31.89
  genital, female N81.9
    specified NEC N81.89
  globe, nontraumatic — *see* Luxation, globe
  ileostomy bud K94.19
  intervertebral disc — *see* Displacement, intervertebral disc
  intestine (small) K63.4
  iris (traumatic) — *see* Laceration, eye(ball), with prolapse or loss of interocular tissue
    nontraumatic H21.89
  kidney N28.83
    congenital Q63.2
  laryngeal muscles or ventricle J38.7
  liver K76.89
  meatus urinarius N36.8
  mitral (valve) I34.1
  ocular lens implant — *see* Complications, intraocular lens
  organ or site, congenital NEC — *see* Malposition, congenital
  ovary N83.4
  pelvic floor, female N81.89
  perineum, female N81.89
  rectum (mucosa) (sphincter) K62.3
    due to trichuris trichuria B79
  spleen D73.89
  stomach K31.89
  umbilical cord
    complicating delivery O69.0 ☑
  urachus, congenital Q64.4
  ureter N28.89
    with obstruction N13.5
      with infection N13.6
  ureterovesical orifice N28.89
  urethra (acquired) (infected) (mucosa) N36.8

Prolapse — continued
  congenital Q64.71
  urinary meatus N36.8
    congenital Q64.72
  uterovaginal N81.4
    complete N81.3
    incomplete N81.2
  uterus (with prolapse of vagina) N81.4
    complete N81.3
    congenital Q51.818
    first degree N81.2
    in pregnancy or childbirth — *see* Pregnancy, complicated by, abnormal, uterus
    incomplete N81.2
    postpartal (old) N81.4
    second degree N81.2
    third degree N81.3
  uveal (traumatic) — *see* Laceration, eye(ball), with prolapse or loss of interocular tissue
  vagina (anterior) (wall) — *see* Cystocele
    with prolapse of uterus N81.4
      complete N81.3
      incomplete N81.2
    posterior wall N81.6
    posthysterectomy N99.3
  vitreous (humor) H43.0-
    in wound — *see* Laceration, eye(ball), with prolapse or loss of interocular tissue
  womb — *see* Prolapse, uterus
Prolapsus, female N81.9
  specified NEC N81.89
Proliferation (s)
  primary cutaneous CD30-positive large T-cell C86.6
Proliferative — *see* condition
Prolonged, prolongation (of)
  bleeding (time) (idiopathic) R79.1
  coagulation (time) R79.1
  gestation (over 42 completed weeks)
    mother O48.1
    newborn P08.22
  interval I44.0
  labor O63.9
    first stage O63.0
    second stage O63.1
  partial thromboplastin time (PTT) R79.1
  pregnancy (more than 42 weeks gestation) O48.1
  prothrombin time R79.1
  QT interval I45.81
  uterine contractions in labor O62.4
Prominence, prominent
  auricle (congenital) (ear) Q17.5
  ischial spine or sacral promontory
    with disproportion (fetopelvic) O33.0
      causing obstructed labor O65.0
  nose (congenital) acquired M95.0
Promiscuity — *see* High, risk, sexual behavior
Pronation
  ankle — *see* Deformity, limb, foot, specified NEC
  foot (*see also* Deformity, limb, foot, specified NEC)
    congenital Q74.2
Prophylactic
  administration of
    antibiotics, long-term Z79.2
      short-term use - omit code
    drug (*see also* Long-term (current) drug therapy (use of)) Z79.899- ☑
    medication Z79.899
    organ removal (for neoplasia management) Z40.00
      breast Z40.01
      ovary Z40.02
      specified site NEC Z40.09
    surgery Z40.9
      for risk factors related to malignant neoplasm — *see* Prophylactic, organ removal
      specified NEC Z40.8
    vaccination Z23
Propionic acidemia E71.121
Proptosis (ocular) (*see also* Exophthalmos)
  thyroid — *see* Hyperthyroidism, with goiter
Prosecution, anxiety concerning Z65.3
Prosopagnosia R48.3
Prostadynia N42.81
Prostate, prostatic — *see* condition
Prostatism — *see* Hyperplasia, prostate
Prostatitis (congestive) (suppurative) (with cystitis) N41.9
  acute N41.0
  cavitary N41.8
  chronic N41.1
  diverticular N41.8

Prostatitis — continued
  due to Trichomonas (vaginalis) A59.02
  fibrous N41.1
  gonococcal (acute) (chronic) A54.22
  granulomatous N41.4
  hypertrophic N41.1
  subacute N41.1
  trichomonal A59.02
  tuberculous A18.14
Prostatocystitis N41.3
Prostatorrhea N42.89
Prostatosis N42.82
Prostration R53.83
  heat (*see also* Heat, exhaustion)
    anhydrotic T67.3 ☑
    due to
      salt (and water) depletion T67.4 ☑
      water depletion T67.3 ☑
  nervous F48.8
  senile R54
Protanomaly (anomalous trichromat) H53.54
Protanopia (complete) (incomplete) H53.54
Protection (against) (from) — *see* Prophylactic
Protein
  deficiency NEC — *see* Malnutrition
  malnutrition — *see* Malnutrition
  sickness (*see also* Reaction, serum) T80.69 ☑
Proteinemia R77.9
Proteinosis
  alveolar (pulmonary) J84.01
  lipid or lipoid (of Urbach) E78.89
Proteinuria R80.9
  Bence Jones R80.3
  complicating pregnancy — *see* Proteinuria, gestational
  gestational O12.1- ☑
    with edema O12.2- ☑
  idiopathic R80.0
  isolated R80.0
    with glomerular lesion N06.9
      dense deposit disease N06.6
      diffuse
        crescentic glomerulonephritis N06.7
        endocapillary proliferative glomerulonephritis N06.4
        mesangiocapillary glomerulonephritis N06.5
      focal and segmental hyalinosis or sclerosis N06.1
      membranous (diffuse) N06.2
      mesangial proliferative (diffuse) N06.3
      minimal change N06.0
      specified pathology NEC N06.8
  orthostatic R80.2
    with glomerular lesion — *see* Proteinuria, isolated, with glomerular lesion
  persistent R80.1
    with glomerular lesion — *see* Proteinuria, isolated, with glomerular lesion
  postural R80.2
    with glomerular lesion — *see* Proteinuria, isolated, with glomerular lesion
  pre-eclamptic — *see* Pre-eclampsia
  specified type NEC R80.8
Proteolysis, pathologic D65
Proteus (mirabilis) (morganii), as cause of disease classified elsewhere B96.4
Prothrombin gene mutation D68.52
Protoporphyria, erythropoietic E80.0
Protozoal (*see also* condition)
  disease B64
  specified NEC B60.8
Protrusion, protrusio
  acetabuli M24.7
  acetabulum (into pelvis) M24.7
  device, implant or graft (*see also* Complications, by site and type, mechanical) T85.698 ☑
    arterial graft NEC — *see* Complication, cardiovascular device, mechanical, vascular
    breast (implant) T85.49 ☑
    catheter NEC T85.698 ☑
      cystostomy T83.090 ☑
      dialysis (renal) T82.49 ☑
        intraperitoneal T85.691 ☑
      infusion NEC T82.594 ☑
        spinal (epidural) (subdural) T85.690 ☑
      urinary, indwelling T83.098 ☑
    electronic (electrode) (pulse generator) (stimulator)
      bone T84.390 ☑

☑ **Additional character required**

Protrusion — *continued*
　　nervous system — *see* Complication, prosthetic device, mechanical, electronic nervous system stimulator
　　fixation, internal (orthopedic) NEC — *see* Complication, fixation device, mechanical
　　gastrointestinal — *see* Complications, prosthetic device, mechanical, gastrointestinal device
　　genital NEC T83.498 ☑
　　　　intrauterine contraceptive device T83.39 ☑
　　　　penile prosthesis T83.490 ☑
　　heart NEC — *see* Complication, cardiovascular device, mechanical
　　joint prosthesis — *see* Complications, joint prosthesis, mechanical, specified NEC, by site
　　ocular NEC — *see* Complications, prosthetic device, mechanical, ocular device
　　orthopedic NEC — *see* Complication, orthopedic, device, mechanical
　　specified NEC T85.628 ☑
　　urinary NEC (*see also* Complication, genitourinary, device, urinary, mechanical) graft T83.29 ☑
　　vascular NEC — *see* Complication, cardiovascular device, mechanical
　　ventricular intracranial shunt T85.09 ☑
　　intervertebral disc — *see* Displacement, intervertebral disc
　　joint prosthesis — *see* Complications, joint prosthesis, mechanical, specified NEC, by site
　　nucleus pulposus — *see* Displacement, intervertebral disc
Prune belly (syndrome) Q79.4
Prurigo (ferox) (gravis) (Hebrae) (Hebra's) (mitis) (simplex) L28.2
　　Besnier's L20.0
　　estivalis L56.4
　　nodularis L28.1
　　psychogenic F45.8
Pruritus, pruritic (essential) L29.9
　　ani, anus L29.0
　　　　psychogenic F45.8
　　anogenital L29.3
　　　　psychogenic F45.8
　　due to onchocerca volvulus B73.1
　　gravidarum — *see* Pregnancy, complicated by, specified pregnancy-related condition NEC
　　hiemalis L29.8
　　neurogenic (any site) F45.8
　　perianal L29.0
　　psychogenic (any site) F45.8
　　scroti, scrotum L29.1
　　　　psychogenic F45.8
　　senile, senilis L29.8
　　specified NEC L29.8
　　　　psychogenic F45.8
　　Trichomonas A59.9
　　vulva, vulvae L29.2
　　　　psychogenic F45.8
Pseudarthrosis, pseudoarthrosis (bone) — *see* Nonunion, fracture
　　clavicle, congenital Q74.0
　　joint, following fusion or arthrodesis M96.0
Pseudoaneurysm — *see* Aneurysm
Pseudoangioma I81
Pseudoangina (pectoris) — *see* Angina
Pseudoarteriosus Q28.8
Pseudoarthrosis — *see* Pseudarthrosis
Pseudobulbar affect (PBA) F48.2
Pseudochromhidrosis L67.8
Pseudocirrhosis, liver, pericardial I31.1
Pseudocowpox B08.03
Pseudocoxalgia M91.3- ☑
Pseudocroup J38.5
Pseudo-Cushing's syndrome, alcohol-induced E24.4
Pseudocyesis F45.8
Pseudocyst
　　lung J98.4
　　pancreas K86.3
　　retina — *see* Cyst, retina
Pseudoelephantiasis neuroarthritica Q82.0
Pseudoexfoliation, capsule (lens) — *see* Cataract, specified NEC
Pseudofolliculitis barbae L73.1
Pseudoglioma H44.89
Pseudohemophilia (Bernuth's) (hereditary) (type B) D68.0
　　Type A D69.8
　　vascular D69.8

Pseudohermaphroditism Q56.3
　　adrenal E25.8
　　female Q56.2
　　　　with adrenocortical disorder E25.8
　　　　without adrenocortical disorder Q56.2
　　　　adrenal, congenital E25.0
　　male Q56.1
　　　　with
　　　　　　adrenocortical disorder E25.8
　　　　　　androgen resistance E34.51
　　　　　　cleft scrotum Q56.1
　　　　　　feminizing testis E34.51
　　　　　　5-alpha-reductase deficiency E29.1
　　　　without gonadal disorder Q56.1
　　　　adrenal E25.8
Pseudo-Hurler's polydystrophy E77.0
Pseudohydrocephalus G93.2
Pseudohypertrophic muscular dystrophy (Erb's) G71.0
Pseudohypertrophy, muscle G71.0
Pseudohypoparathyroidism E20.1
Pseudoinsomnia F51.03
Pseudoleukemia, infantile D64.89
Pseudomembranous — *see* condition
Pseudomenses (newborn) P54.6
Pseudomenstruation (newborn) P54.6
Pseudomeningocele (cerebral) (infective) (post-traumatic) G96.19
　　postprocedural (spinal) G97.82
Pseudomonas
　　aeruginosa, as cause of disease classified elsewhere B96.5
　　mallei infection A24.0
　　　　as cause of disease classified elsewhere B96.5
　　pseudomallei, as cause of disease classified elsewhere B96.5
Pseudomyotonia G71.19
Pseudomyxoma peritonei C78.6
Pseudoneuritis, optic (nerve) (disc) (papilla), congenital Q14.2
Pseudo-obstruction intestine (acute) (chronic) (idiopathic) (intermittent secondary) (primary) K59.8
Pseudopapilledema H47.33- ☑
　　congenital Q14.2
Pseudoparalysis
　　arm or leg R29.818
　　atonic, congenital P94.2
Pseudopelade L66.0
Pseudophakia Z96.1
Pseudopolyarthritis, rhizomelic M35.3
Pseudopolycythemia D75.1
Pseudopseudohypoparathyroidism E20.1
Pseudopterygium H11.81- ☑
Pseudoptosis (eyelid) — *see* Blepharochalasis
Pseudopuberty, precocious
　　female heterosexual E25.8
　　male isosexual E25.8
Pseudorickets (renal) N25.0
Pseudorubella B08.20
Pseudosclerema, newborn P83.8
Pseudosclerosis (brain)
　　of Westphal (Strümpell) E83.01
　　Jakob's — *see* Creutzfeldt-Jakob disease or syndrome
　　spastic — *see* Creutzfeldt-Jakob disease or syndrome
Pseudotetanus — *see* Convulsions
Pseudotetany R29.0
　　hysterical F44.5
Pseudotruncus arteriosus Q25.4
Pseudotuberculosis A28.2
　　enterocolitis A04.8
　　pasteurella (infection) A28.0
Pseudotumor
　　cerebri G93.2
　　orbital H05.11- ☑
Pseudoxanthoma elasticum Q82.8
Psilosis (sprue) (tropical) K90.1
　　nontropical K90.0
Psittacosis A70
Psoitis M60.88
Psoriasis L40.9
　　arthropathic L40.50
　　　　arthritis mutilans L40.52
　　　　distal interphalangeal L40.51
　　　　juvenile L40.54
　　　　other specified L40.59
　　　　spondylitis L40.53
　　buccal K13.29
　　flexural L40.8
　　guttate L40.4

Psoriasis — *continued*
　　mouth K13.29
　　nummular L40.0
　　plaque L40.0
　　psychogenic F54
　　pustular (generalized) L40.1
　　　　palmaris et plantaris L40.3
　　specified NEC L40.8
　　vulgaris L40.0
Psychasthenia F48.8
Psychiatric disorder or problem F99
Psychogenic (*see also* condition)
　　factors associated with physical conditions F54
Psychological and behavioral factors affecting medical condition F59
Psychoneurosis, psychoneurotic (*see also* Neurosis)
　　anxiety (state) F41.1
　　depersonalization F48.1
　　hypochondriacal F45.21
　　hysteria F44.9
　　neurasthenic F48.8
　　personality NEC F60.89
Psychopathy, psychopathic
　　affectionless F94.2
　　autistic F84.5
　　constitution, post-traumatic F07.81
　　personality — *see* Disorder, personality
　　sexual — *see* Deviation, sexual
　　state F60.2
Psychosexual identity disorder of childhood F64.2
Psychosis, psychotic F29
　　acute (transient) F23
　　　　hysterical F44.9
　　affective — *see* Disorder, mood
　　alcoholic F10.959
　　　　with
　　　　　　abuse F10.159
　　　　　　anxiety disorder F10.980
　　　　　　　　with
　　　　　　　　　　abuse F10.180
　　　　　　　　　　dependence F10.280
　　　　　　delirium tremens F10.231
　　　　　　delusions F10.950
　　　　　　　　with
　　　　　　　　　　abuse F10.150
　　　　　　　　　　dependence F10.250
　　　　　　dementia F10.97
　　　　　　　　with dependence F10.27
　　　　　　dependence F10.259
　　　　　　hallucinosis F10.951
　　　　　　　　with
　　　　　　　　　　abuse F10.151
　　　　　　　　　　dependence F10.251
　　　　　　mood disorder F10.94
　　　　　　　　with
　　　　　　　　　　abuse F10.14
　　　　　　　　　　dependence F10.24
　　　　　　paranoia F10.950
　　　　　　　　with
　　　　　　　　　　abuse F10.150
　　　　　　　　　　dependence F10.250
　　　　　　persisting amnesia F10.96
　　　　　　　　with dependence F10.26
　　　　　　amnestic confabulatory F10.96
　　　　　　　　with dependence F10.26
　　　　　　delirium tremens F10.231
　　　　　　Korsakoff's, Korsakov's, Korsakow's F10.26
　　　　　　paranoid type F10.950
　　　　　　　　with
　　　　　　　　　　abuse F10.150
　　　　　　　　　　dependence F10.250
　　anergastic — *see* Psychosis, organic
　　arteriosclerotic (simple type) (uncomplicated) F01.50
　　　　with behavioral disturbance F01.51
　　childhood F84.0
　　　　atypical F84.8
　　climacteric — *see* Psychosis, involutional
　　confusional F29
　　　　acute or subacute F05
　　　　reactive F23
　　cycloid F23
　　depressive — *see* Disorder, depressive
　　disintegrative (childhood) F84.3
　　drug-induced — *see* F11-F19 with .x59
　　　　paranoid and hallucinatory states — *see* F11-F19 with .x50 or .x51
　　due to or associated with
　　　　addiction, drug — *see* F11-F19 with .x59
　　　　dependence
　　　　　　alcohol F10.259
　　　　　　drug — *see* F11-F19 with .x59

Psychosis — *continued*
- epilepsy F06.8
- Huntington's chorea F06.8
- ischemia, cerebrovascular (generalized) F06.8
- multiple sclerosis F06.8
- physical disease F06.8
- presenile dementia F03 ☑
- senile dementia F03 ☑
- vascular disease (arteriosclerotic) (cerebral) F01.50
  - with behavioral disturbance F01.51
- epileptic F06.8
- episode F23
  - due to or associated with physical condition F06.8
- exhaustive F43.0
- hallucinatory, chronic F28
- hypomanic F30.8
- hysterical (acute) F44.9
- induced F24
- infantile F84.0
  - atypical F84.8
- infective (acute) (subacute) F05
- involutional F28
  - depressive — *see* Disorder, depressive
  - melancholic — *see* Disorder, depressive
  - paranoid (state) F22
- Korsakoff's, Korsakov's, Korsakow's (nonalcoholic) F04
  - alcoholic F10.96
    - in dependence F10.26
  - induced by other psychoactive substance — *see* categories F11-F19 with .x5x
- mania, manic (single episode) F30.2
  - recurrent type F31.89
- manic-depressive — *see* Disorder, mood
- menopausal — *see* Psychosis, involutional
- mixed schizophrenic and affective F25.8
- multi-infarct (cerebrovascular) F01.50
  - with behavioral disturbance F01.51
- nonorganic F29
  - specified NEC F28
- organic F09
  - due to or associated with
    - arteriosclerosis (cerebral) — *see* Psychosis, arteriosclerotic
    - cerebrovascular disease, arteriosclerotic — *see* Psychosis, arteriosclerotic
    - childbirth — *see* Psychosis, puerperal
    - Creutzfeldt-Jakob disease or syndrome — *see* Creutzfeldt-Jakob disease or syndrome
    - dependence, alcohol F10.259
    - disease
      - alcoholic liver F10.259
      - brain, arteriosclerotic — *see* Psychosis, arteriosclerotic
      - cerebrovascular F01.50
        - with behavioral disturbance F01.51
      - Creutzfeldt-Jakob — *see* Creutzfeldt-Jakob disease or syndrome
      - endocrine or metabolic F06.8
        - acute or subacute F05
      - liver, alcoholic F10.259
    - epilepsy transient (acute) F05
    - infection
      - brain (intracranial) F06.8
        - acute or subacute F05
    - intoxication
      - alcoholic (acute) F10.259
      - drug F19 with .x59 F11- ☑
    - ischemia, cerebrovascular (generalized) — *see* Psychosis, arteriosclerotic
    - puerperium — *see* Psychosis, puerperal
    - trauma, brain (birth) (from electric current) (surgical) F06.8
      - acute or subacute F05
  - infective F06.8
    - acute or subacute F05
  - post-traumatic F06.8
    - acute or subacute F05
- paranoiac F22
- paranoid (climacteric) (involutional) (menopausal) F22
  - psychogenic (acute) F23
  - schizophrenic F20.0
  - senile F03 ☑
- postpartum F53
- presbyophrenic (type) F03 ☑
- presenile F03 ☑
- psychogenic (paranoid) F23
  - depressive F32.3
- puerperal F53

Psychosis — *continued*
- specified type — *see* Psychosis, by type
- reactive (brief) (transient) (emotional stress) (psychological trauma) F23
  - depressive F32.3
    - recurrent F33.3
  - excitative type F30.8
- schizoaffective F25.9
  - depressive type F25.1
  - manic type F25.0
- schizophrenia, schizophrenic — *see* Schizophrenia
- schizophrenia-like, in epilepsy F06.2
- schizophreniform F20.81
  - affective type F25.9
  - brief F23
  - confusional type F23
  - depressive type F25.1
  - manic type F25.0
  - mixed type F25.0
- senile NEC F03 ☑
  - depressed or paranoid type F03 ☑
  - simple deterioration F03 ☑
  - specified type - code to condition
- shared F24
- situational (reactive) F23
- symbiotic (childhood) F84.3
- symptomatic F09
Psychosomatic — *see* Disorder, psychosomatic
Psychosyndrome, organic F07.9
Psychotic episode due to or associated with physical condition F06.8
Pterygium (eye) H11.00- ☑
- amyloid H11.01- ☑
- central H11.02- ☑
- colli Q18.3
- double H11.03- ☑
- peripheral
  - progressive H11.05- ☑
  - stationary H11.04- ☑
- recurrent H11.06- ☑
Ptilosis (eyelid) — *see* Madarosis
Ptomaine (poisoning) — *see* Poisoning, food
Ptosis (*see also* Blepharoptosis)
- adiposa (false) — *see* Blepharoptosis
- breast N64.81
- cecum K63.4
- colon K63.4
- congenital (eyelid) Q10.0
  - specified site NEC — *see* Anomaly, by site
- eyelid — *see* Blepharoptosis
  - congenital Q10.0
- gastric K31.89
- intestine K63.4
- kidney N28.83
- liver K76.89
- renal N28.83
- splanchnic K63.4
- spleen D73.89
- stomach K31.89
- viscera K63.4
PTP D69.51
Ptyalism (periodic) K11.7
- hysterical F45.8
- pregnancy — *see* Pregnancy, complicated by, specified pregnancy-related condition NEC
- psychogenic F45.8
Ptyalolithiasis K11.5
Pubarche, precocious E30.1
Pubertas praecox E30.1
Puberty (development state) Z00.3
- bleeding (excessive) N92.2
- delayed E30.0
- precocious (constitutional) (cryptogenic) (idiopathic) E30.1
  - central E22.8
  - due to
    - ovarian hyperfunction E28.1
      - estrogen E28.0
    - testicular hyperfunction E29.0
- premature E30.1
  - due to
    - adrenal cortical hyperfunction E25.8
    - pineal tumor E34.8
    - pituitary (anterior) hyperfunction E22.8
Puckering, macula — *see* Degeneration, macula, puckering
Pudenda, pudendum — *see* condition
Puerperal, puerperium (complicated by, complications)
- abnormal glucose (tolerance test) O99.815

Puerperal — *continued*
- abscess
  - areola O91.02
    - associated with lactation O91.03
  - Bartholin's gland O86.19
  - breast O91.12
    - associated with lactation O91.13
  - cervix (uteri) O86.11
  - genital organ NEC O86.19
  - kidney O86.21
  - mammary O91.12
    - associated with lactation O91.13
  - nipple O91.02
    - associated with lactation O91.03
  - peritoneum O85
  - subareolar O91.12
    - associated with lactation O91.13
  - urinary tract — *see* Puerperal, infection, urinary
  - uterus O86.12
  - vagina (wall) O86.13
  - vaginorectal O86.13
  - vulvovaginal gland O86.13
- adnexitis O86.19
- afibrinogenemia, or other coagulation defect O72.3
- albuminuria (acute) (subacute) — *see* Proteinuria, gestational
- alcohol use O99.315
- anemia O90.81
  - pre-existing (pre-pregnancy) O99.03
- anesthetic death O89.8
- apoplexy O99.43
- bariatric surgery status O99.845
- blood disorder NEC O99.13
- blood dyscrasia O72.3
- cardiomyopathy O90.3
- cerebrovascular disorder (conditions in I60-I69) O99.43
- cervicitis O86.11
- circulatory system disorder O99.43
- coagulopathy (any) O72.3
- complications O90.9
  - specified NEC O90.89
- convulsions — *see* Eclampsia
- cystitis O86.22
- cystopyelitis O86.29
- delirium NEC F05
- diabetes O24.93
  - gestational — *see* Puerperal, gestational diabetes
  - pre-existing O24.33
    - specified NEC O24.83
    - type 1 O24.03
    - type 2 O24.13
- digestive system disorder O99.63
- disease O90.9
  - breast NEC O92.29
  - cerebrovascular (acute) O99.43
  - nonobstetric NEC O99.89
  - tubo-ovarian O86.19
  - Valsuani's O99.03
- disorder O90.9
  - biliary tract O26.63
  - lactation O92.70
  - liver O26.63
  - nonobstetric NEC O99.89
- disruption
  - cesarean wound O90.0
  - episiotomy wound O90.1
  - perineal laceration wound O90.1
- drug use O99.325
- eclampsia (with pre-existing hypertension) O15.2
- embolism (pulmonary) (blood clot) — *see* Embolism, obstetric, puerperal
- endocrine, nutritional or metabolic disease NEC O99.285
- endophlebitis — *see* Puerperal, phlebitis
- endotrachelitis O86.11
- failure
  - lactation (complete) O92.3
    - partial O92.4
  - renal, acute O90.4
- fever (of unknown origin) O86.4
  - septic O85
- fissure, nipple O92.12
  - associated with lactation O92.13
- fistula
  - breast (due to mastitis) O91.12
    - associated with lactation O91.13
  - nipple O91.02
    - associated with lactation O91.03
- galactophoritis O91.22

☑ **Additional character required**

Puerperal — *continued*
  associated with lactation O91.23
galactorrhea O92.6
gastric banding status O99.845
gastric bypass status O99.845
gastrointestinal disease NEC O99.63
gestational diabetes O24.439
  diet controlled O24.430
  insulin (and diet) controlled O24.434
gonorrhea O98.23
hematoma, subdural O99.43
hemiplegia, cerebral O99.355
  due to cerbrovascular disorder O99.43
hemorrhage O72.1
  brain O99.43
  bulbar O99.43
  cerebellar O99.43
  cerebral O99.43
  cortical O99.43
  delayed or secondary O72.2
  extradural O99.43
  internal capsule O99.43
  intracranial O99.43
  intrapontine O99.43
  meningeal O99.43
  pontine O99.43
  retained placenta O72.0
  subarachnoid O99.43
  subcortical O99.43
  subdural O99.43
  third stage O72.0
  uterine, delayed O72.2
  ventricular O99.43
hemorrhoids O87.2
hepatorenal syndrome O90.4
hypertension — *see* Hypertension, complicating, puerperium
hypertrophy, breast O92.29
induration breast (fibrous) O92.29
infection O86.4
  cervix O86.11
  generalized O85
  genital tract NEC O86.19
    obstetric surgical wound O86.0
  kidney (bacillus coli) O86.21
  maternal O98.93
    carrier state NEC O99.835
    gonorrhea O98.23
    human immunodeficiency virus (HIV) O98.73
    protozoal O98.63
    sexually transmitted NEC O98.33
    specified NEC O98.83
    streptococcus B carrier state O99.825
    syphilis O98.13
    tuberculosis O98.03
    viral hepatitis O98.43
    viral NEC O98.53
  nipple O91.02
    associated with lactation O91.03
  peritoneum O85
  renal O86.21
  specified NEC O86.89
  urinary (asymptomatic) (tract) NEC O86.20
    bladder O86.22
    kidney O86.21
    specified site NEC O86.29
    urethra O86.22
  vagina O86.13
  vein — *see* Puerperal, phlebitis
ischemia, cerebral O99.43
lymphangitis O86.89
  breast O91.22
    associated with lactation O91.23
malignancy O9A.13
malnutrition O25.3
mammillitis O91.02
  associated with lactation O91.03
mammitis O91.22
  associated with lactation O91.23
mania F30.8
mastitis O91.22
  associated with lactation O91.23
  purulent O91.12
    associated with lactation O91.13
melancholia — *see* Disorder, depressive
mental disorder NEC O99.345
metroperitonitis O85
metrorrhagia — *see* Hemorrhage, postpartum
metrosalpingitis O86.19
metrovaginitis O86.13
milk leg O87.1
monoplegia, cerebral O99.43

Puerperal — *continued*
mood disturbance O90.6
necrosis, liver (acute) (subacute) (conditions in subcategory K72.0) O26.63
  with renal failure O90.4
nervous system disorder O99.355
neuritis O90.89
obesity (pre-existing prior to pregnancy) O99.215
obesity surgery status O99.845
occlusion, precerebral artery O99.43
paralysis
  bladder (sphincter) O90.89
  cerebral O99.43
paralytic stroke O99.43
parametritis O85
paravaginitis O86.13
pelviperitonitis O85
perimetritis O86.12
perimetrosalpingitis O86.19
perinephritis O86.21
periphlebitis — *see* Puerperal phlebitis
peritoneal infection O85
peritonitis (pelvic) O85
perivaginitis O86.13
phlebitis O87.0
  deep O87.1
  pelvic O87.1
  superficial O87.0
phlebothrombosis, deep O87.1
phlegmasia alba dolens O87.1
placental polyp O90.89
pneumonia, embolic — *see* Embolism, obstetric, puerperal
pre-eclampsia — *see* Pre-eclampsia
psychosis F53
pyelitis O86.21
pyelocystitis O86.29
pyelonephritis O86.21
pyelonephrosis O86.21
pyemia O85
pyocystitis O86.29
pyohemia O85
pyometra O86.12
pyonephritis O86.21
pyosalpingitis O86.19
pyrexia (of unknown origin) O86.4
renal
  disease NEC O90.89
  failure O90.4
respiratory disease NEC O99.53
retention
  decidua — *see* Retention, decidua
  placenta O72.0
  secundines — *see* Retention, secundines
retrated nipple O92.02
salpingo-ovaritis O86.19
salpingoperitonitis O85
secondary perineal tear O90.1
sepsis (pelvic) O85
sepsis O85
septic thrombophlebitis O86.81
skin disorder NEC O99.73
specified condition NEC O99.89
stroke O99.43
subinvolution (uterus) O90.89
subluxation of symphysis (pubis) O26.73
suppuration — *see* Puerperal, abscess
tetanus A34
thelitis O91.02
  associated with lactation O91.03
thrombocytopenia O90.89
thrombophlebitis (superficial) O87.0
  deep O87.1
  pelvic O87.1
  septic O86.81
thrombosis (venous) — *see* Thrombosis, puerperal
thyroiditis O90.5
toxemia (eclamptic) (pre-eclamptic) (with convulsions) O15.2
trauma, non-obstetric O9A.23
  caused by abuse (physical) (suspected) O9A.33
    confirmed O9A.33
    psychological (suspected) O9A.53
      confirmed O9A.53
    sexual (suspected) O9A.43
      confirmed O9A.43
uremia (due to renal failure) O90.4
urethritis O86.22
vaginitis O86.13
varicose veins (legs) O87.4
  vulva or perineum O87.8

Puerperal — *continued*
venous O87.9
vulvitis O86.19
vulvovaginitis O86.13
white leg O87.1
Puerperium — *see* Puerperal
Pulmolithiasis J98.4
Pulmonary — *see* condition
Pulpitis (acute) (anachoretic) (chronic) (hyperplastic) (irreversible) (putrescent) (reversible) (suppurative) (ulcerative) K04.0
Pulpless tooth K04.99
Pulse
  alternating R00.8
  bigeminal R00.8
  fast R00.0
  feeble, rapid due to shock following injury T79.4 ☑
  rapid R00.0
  weak R09.89
Pulsus alternans or trigeminus R00.8
Punch drunk F07.81
Punctum lacrimale occlusion — *see* Obstruction, lacrimal
Puncture
  abdomen, abdominal
    wall S31.139 ☑
      with
        foreign body S31.149 ☑
        penetration into peritoneal cavity S31.639 ☑
          with foreign body S31.649 ☑
    epigastric region S31.132 ☑
      with
        foreign body S31.142 ☑
        penetration into peritoneal cavity S31.632 ☑
          with foreign body S31.642 ☑
    left
      lower quadrant S31.134 ☑
        with
          foreign body S31.144 ☑
          penetration into peritoneal cavity S31.634 ☑
            with foreign body S31.644 ☑
      upper quadrant S31.131 ☑
        with
          foreign body S31.141 ☑
          penetration into peritoneal cavity S31.631 ☑
            with foreign body S31.641 ☑
    periumbilic region S31.135 ☑
      with
        foreign body S31.145 ☑
        penetration into peritoneal cavity S31.635 ☑
          with foreign body S31.645 ☑
    right
      lower quadrant S31.133 ☑
        with
          foreign body S31.143 ☑
          penetration into peritoneal cavity S31.633 ☑
            with foreign body S31.643 ☑
      upper quadrant S31.130 ☑
        with
          foreign body S31.140 ☑
          penetration into peritoneal cavity S31.630 ☑
            with foreign body S31.640 ☑
  accidental, complicating surgery — *see* Complication, accidental puncture or laceration
  alveolar (process) — *see* Puncture, oral cavity
  ankle S91.039 ☑
    with
      foreign body S91.049 ☑
    left S91.032 ☑
      with
        foreign body S91.042 ☑
    right S91.031 ☑
      with
        foreign body S91.041 ☑
  anus S31.833 ☑
    with foreign body S31.834 ☑
  arm (upper) S41.139 ☑
    with foreign body S41.149 ☑
    left S41.132 ☑
      with foreign body S41.142 ☑
    lower — *see* Puncture, forearm
    right S41.131 ☑
      with foreign body S41.141 ☑

Puncture

Puncture — continued

auditory canal (external) (meatus) — see Puncture, ear
auricle, ear — see Puncture, ear
axilla — see Puncture, arm
back (see also Puncture, thorax, back)
    lower S31.030 ☑
      with
        foreign body S31.040 ☑
          with penetration into retroperitoneal
            space S31.041 ☑
          penetration into retroperitoneal space
            S31.031 ☑
bladder (traumatic) S37.29 ☑
    nontraumatic N32.89
breast S21.039 ☑
    with foreign body S21.049 ☑
    left S21.032 ☑
      with foreign body S21.042 ☑
    right S21.031 ☑
      with foreign body S21.041 ☑
buttock S31.803 ☑
    with foreign body S31.804 ☑
    left S31.823 ☑
      with foreign body S31.824 ☑
    right S31.813 ☑
      with foreign body S31.814 ☑
by
    device, implant or graft — see Complications,
      by site and type, mechanical
    foreign body left accidentally in operative
      wound T81.539 ☑
    instrument (any) during a procedure,
      accidental — see Puncture, accidental
      complicating surgery
calf — see Puncture, leg
canaliculus lacrimalis — see Puncture, eyelid
canthus, eye — see Puncture, eyelid
cervical esophagus S11.23 ☑
    with foreign body S11.24 ☑
cheek (external) S01.439 ☑
    with foreign body S01.449 ☑
    left S01.432 ☑
      with foreign body S01.442 ☑
    right S01.431 ☑
      with foreign body S01.441 ☑
    internal — see Puncture, oral cavity
chest wall — see Puncture, thorax
chin — see Puncture, head, specified site NEC
clitoris — see Puncture, vulva
costal region — see Puncture, thorax
digit (s)
    hand — see Puncture, finger
    foot — see Puncture, toe
ear (canal) (external) S01.339 ☑
    with foreign body S01.349 ☑
    left S01.332 ☑
      with foreign body S01.342 ☑
    right S01.331 ☑
      with foreign body S01.341 ☑
    drum S09.2- ☑
elbow S51.039 ☑
    with
      foreign body S51.049 ☑
    left S51.032 ☑
      with
        foreign body S51.042 ☑
    right S51.031 ☑
      with
        foreign body S51.041 ☑
epididymis — see Puncture, testis
epigastric region — see Puncture, abdomen, wall,
    epigastric
epiglottis S11.83 ☑
    with foreign body S11.84 ☑
esophagus
    cervical S11.23 ☑
      with foreign body S11.24 ☑
    thoracic S27.818 ☑
eyeball S05.6- ☑
    with foreign body S05.5- ☑
eyebrow — see Puncture, eyelid
eyelid S01.13- ☑
    with foreign body S01.14- ☑
    left S01.132 ☑
      with foreign body S01.142 ☑
    right S01.131 ☑
      with foreign body S01.141 ☑
face NEC — see Puncture, head, specified site NEC
finger (s) S61.239 ☑
    with
      damage to nail S61.339 ☑

Puncture — continued

    with
      foreign body S61.349 ☑
    foreign body S61.249 ☑
    index S61.238 ☑
      with
        damage to nail S61.338 ☑
          with
            foreign body S61.348 ☑
        foreign body S61.248 ☑
      left S61.231 ☑
        with
          damage to nail S61.331 ☑
            with
              foreign body S61.341 ☑
          foreign body S61.241 ☑
      right S61.230 ☑
        with
          damage to nail S61.330 ☑
            with
              foreign body S61.340 ☑
          foreign body S61.240 ☑
    little S61.238 ☑
      with
        damage to nail S61.338 ☑
          with
            foreign body S61.348 ☑
        foreign body S61.248 ☑
      left S61.237 ☑
        with
          damage to nail S61.337 ☑
            with
              foreign body S61.347 ☑
          foreign body S61.247 ☑
      right S61.236 ☑
        with
          damage to nail S61.336 ☑
            with
              foreign body S61.346 ☑
          foreign body S61.246 ☑
    middle S61.238 ☑
      with
        damage to nail S61.338 ☑
          with
            foreign body S61.348 ☑
        foreign body S61.248 ☑
      left S61.233 ☑
        with
          damage to nail S61.333 ☑
            with
              foreign body S61.343 ☑
          foreign body S61.243 ☑
      right S61.232 ☑
        with
          damage to nail S61.332 ☑
            with
              foreign body S61.342 ☑
          foreign body S61.242 ☑
    ring S61.238 ☑
      with
        damage to nail S61.338 ☑
          with
            foreign body S61.348 ☑
        foreign body S61.248 ☑
      left S61.235 ☑
        with
          damage to nail S61.335 ☑
            with
              foreign body S61.345 ☑
          foreign body S61.245 ☑
      right S61.234 ☑
        with
          damage to nail S61.334 ☑
            with
              foreign body S61.344 ☑
          foreign body S61.244 ☑
flank S31.139 ☑
    with foreign body S31.149 ☑
foot (except toe(s) alone) S91.339 ☑
    with foreign body S91.349 ☑
    left S91.332 ☑
      with foreign body S91.342 ☑
    right S91.331 ☑
      with foreign body S91.341 ☑
    toe — see Puncture, toe
forearm S51.839 ☑
    with
      foreign body S51.849 ☑
    elbow only — see Puncture, elbow
    left S51.832 ☑
      with
        foreign body S51.842 ☑

Puncture — continued

    right S51.831 ☑
      with
        foreign body S51.841 ☑
forehead — see Puncture, head, specified site
    NEC
genital organs, external
    female S31.532 ☑
      with foreign body S31.542 ☑
      vagina — see Puncture, vagina
      vulva — see Puncture, vulva
    male S31.531 ☑
      with foreign body S31.541 ☑
      penis — see Puncture, penis
      scrotum — see Puncture, scrotum
      testis — see Puncture, testis
groin — see Puncture, abdomen, wall
gum — see Puncture, oral cavity
hand S61.439 ☑
    with
      foreign body S61.449 ☑
    finger — see Puncture, finger
    left S61.432 ☑
      with
        foreign body S61.442 ☑
    right S61.431 ☑
      with
        foreign body S61.441 ☑
    thumb — see Puncture, thumb
head S01.93 ☑
    with foreign body S01.94 ☑
    cheek — see Puncture, cheek
    ear — see Puncture, ear
    eyelid — see Puncture, eyelid
    lip — see Puncture, oral cavity
    nose — see Puncture, nose
    oral cavity — see Puncture, oral cavity
    scalp S01.03 ☑
      with foreign body S01.04 ☑
    specified site NEC S01.83 ☑
      with foreign body S01.84 ☑
    temporomandibular area — see Puncture,
      cheek
heart S26.99 ☑
    with hemopericardium S26.09 ☑
    without hemopericardium S26.19 ☑
heel — see Puncture, foot
hip S71.039 ☑
    with foreign body S71.049 ☑
    left S71.032 ☑
      with foreign body S71.042 ☑
    right S71.031 ☑
      with foreign body S71.041 ☑
hymen — see Puncture, vagina
hypochondrium — see Puncture, abdomen, wall
hypogastric region — see Puncture, abdomen,
    wall
inguinal region — see Puncture, abdomen, wall
instep — see Puncture, foot
internal organs — see Injury, by site
interscapular region — see Puncture, thorax, back
intestine
    large
      colon S36.599 ☑
        ascending S36.590 ☑
        descending S36.592 ☑
        sigmoid S36.593 ☑
        specified site NEC S36.598 ☑
        transverse S36.591 ☑
      rectum S36.69 ☑
    small S36.499 ☑
      duodenum S36.490 ☑
      specified site NEC S36.498 ☑
intra-abdominal organ S36.99 ☑
    gallbladder S36.128 ☑
    intestine — see Puncture, intestine
    liver S36.118 ☑
    pancreas — see Puncture, pancreas
    peritoneum S36.81 ☑
    specified site NEC S36.898 ☑
    spleen S36.09 ☑
    stomach S36.39 ☑
jaw — see Puncture, head, specified site NEC
knee S81.039 ☑
    with foreign body S81.049 ☑
    left S81.032 ☑
      with foreign body S81.042 ☑
    right S81.031 ☑
      with foreign body S81.041 ☑
labium (majus) (minus) — see Puncture, vulva
lacrimal duct — see Puncture, eyelid
larynx S11.013 ☑

☑ **Additional character required**

Puncture — *continued*

with foreign body S11.014 ☑
leg (lower) S81.839 ☑
  with foreign body S81.849 ☑
  foot — *see* Puncture, foot
  knee — *see* Puncture, knee
  left S81.832 ☑
    with foreign body S81.842 ☑
  right S81.831 ☑
    with foreign body S81.841 ☑
  upper — *see* Puncture, thigh
lip S01.531 ☑
  with foreign body S01.541 ☑
loin — *see* Puncture, abdomen, wall
lower back — *see* Puncture, back, lower
lumbar region — *see* Puncture, back, lower
malar region — *see* Puncture, head, specified site NEC
mammary — *see* Puncture, breast
mastoid region — *see* Puncture, head, specified site NEC
mouth — *see* Puncture, oral cavity
nail
  finger — *see* Puncture, finger, with damage to nail
  toe — *see* Puncture, toe, with damage to nail
nasal (septum) (sinus) — *see* Puncture, nose
nasopharynx — *see* Puncture, head, specified site NEC
neck S11.93 ☑
  with foreign body S11.94 ☑
  involving
    cervical esophagus — *see* Puncture, cervical esophagus
    larynx — *see* Puncture, larynx
    pharynx — *see* Puncture, pharynx
    thyroid gland — *see* Puncture, thyroid gland
    trachea — *see* Puncture, trachea
  specified site NEC S11.83 ☑
    with foreign body S11.84 ☑
nose (septum) (sinus) S01.23 ☑
  with foreign body S01.24 ☑
ocular — *see* Puncture, eyeball
oral cavity S01.532 ☑
  with foreign body S01.542 ☑
orbit S05.4- ☑
palate — *see* Puncture, oral cavity
palm — *see* Puncture, hand
pancreas S36.299 ☑
  body S36.291 ☑
  head S36.290 ☑
  tail S36.292 ☑
pelvis — *see* Puncture, back, lower
penis S31.23 ☑
  with foreign body S31.24 ☑
perineum
  female S31.43 ☑
    with foreign body S31.44 ☑
  male S31.139 ☑
    with foreign body S31.149 ☑
periocular area (with or without lacrimal passages) — *see* Puncture, eyelid
phalanges
  finger — *see* Puncture, finger
  toe — *see* Puncture, toe
pharynx S11.23 ☑
  with foreign body S11.24 ☑
pinna — *see* Puncture, ear
popliteal space — *see* Puncture, knee
prepuce — *see* Puncture, penis
pubic region S31.139 ☑
  with foreign body S31.149 ☑
pudendum — *see* Puncture, genital organs, external
rectovaginal septum — *see* Puncture, vagina
sacral region — *see* Puncture, back, lower
sacroiliac region — *see* Puncture, back, lower
salivary gland — *see* Puncture, oral cavity
scalp S01.03 ☑
  with foreign body S01.04 ☑
scapular region — *see* Puncture, shoulder
scrotum S31.33 ☑
  with foreign body S31.34 ☑
shin — *see* Puncture, leg
shoulder S41.039 ☑
  with foreign body S41.049 ☑
  left S41.032 ☑
    with foreign body S41.042 ☑
  right S41.031 ☑
    with foreign body S41.041 ☑
spermatic cord — *see* Puncture, testis
sternal region — *see* Puncture, thorax, front

Puncture — *continued*

submaxillary region — *see* Puncture, head, specified site NEC
submental region — *see* Puncture, head, specified site NEC
subungual
  finger (s) — *see* Puncture, finger, with damage to nail
  toe — *see* Puncture, toe, with damage to nail
supraclavicular fossa — *see* Puncture, neck, specified site NEC
temple, temporal region — *see* Puncture, head, specified site NEC
temporomandibular area — *see* Puncture, cheek
testis S31.33 ☑
  with foreign body S31.34 ☑
thigh S71.139 ☑
  with foreign body S71.149 ☑
  left S71.132 ☑
    with foreign body S71.142 ☑
  right S71.131 ☑
    with foreign body S71.141 ☑
thorax, thoracic (wall) S21.93 ☑
  with foreign body S21.94 ☑
  back S21.23- ☑
    with
      foreign body S21.24- ☑
        with penetration S21.44 ☑
      penetration S21.43 ☑
  breast — *see* Puncture, breast
  front S21.13- ☑
    with
      foreign body S21.14- ☑
        with penetration S21.34 ☑
      penetration S21.33 ☑
throat — *see* Puncture, neck
thumb S61.039 ☑
  with
    damage to nail S61.139 ☑
      with
        foreign body S61.149 ☑
    foreign body S61.049 ☑
  left S61.032 ☑
    with
      damage to nail S61.132 ☑
        with
          foreign body S61.142 ☑
      foreign body S61.042 ☑
  right S61.031 ☑
    with
      damage to nail S61.131 ☑
        with
          foreign body S61.141 ☑
      foreign body S61.041 ☑
thyroid gland S11.13 ☑
  with foreign body S11.14 ☑
toe (s) S91.139 ☑
  with
    damage to nail S91.239 ☑
      with
        foreign body S91.249 ☑
    foreign body S91.149 ☑
  great S91.133 ☑
    with
      damage to nail S91.233 ☑
        with
          foreign body S91.243 ☑
      foreign body S91.143 ☑
    left S91.132 ☑
      with
        damage to nail S91.232 ☑
          with
            foreign body S91.242 ☑
        foreign body S91.142 ☑
    right S91.131 ☑
      with
        damage to nail S91.231 ☑
          with
            foreign body S91.241 ☑
        foreign body S91.141 ☑
  lesser S91.136 ☑
    with
      damage to nail S91.236 ☑
        with
          foreign body S91.246 ☑
      foreign body S91.146 ☑
    left S91.135 ☑
      with
        damage to nail S91.235 ☑
          with
            foreign body S91.245 ☑
        foreign body S91.145 ☑

Puncture — *continued*

right S91.134 ☑
  with
    damage to nail S91.234 ☑
      with
        foreign body S91.244 ☑
    foreign body S91.144 ☑
tongue — *see* Puncture, oral cavity
trachea S11.023 ☑
  with foreign body S11.024 ☑
tunica vaginalis — *see* Puncture, testis
tympanum, tympanic membrane S09.2- ☑
umbilical region S31.135 ☑
  with foreign body S31.145 ☑
uvula — *see* Puncture, oral cavity
vagina S31.43 ☑
  with foreign body S31.44 ☑
vocal cords S11.033 ☑
  with foreign body S11.034 ☑
vulva S31.43 ☑
  with foreign body S31.44 ☑
wrist S61.539 ☑
  with
    foreign body S61.549 ☑
  left S61.532 ☑
    with
      foreign body S61.542 ☑
  right S61.531 ☑
    with
      foreign body S61.541 ☑
PUO (pyrexia of unknown origin) R50.9
Pupillary membrane (persistent) Q13.89
Pupillotonia — *see* Anomaly, pupil, function, tonic pupil
Purpura D69.2
abdominal D69.0
allergic D69.0
anaphylactoid D69.0
annularis telangiectodes L81.7
arthritic D69.0
autoerythrocyte sensitization D69.2
autoimmune D69.0
bacterial D69.0
Bateman's (senile) D69.2
capillary fragility (hereditary) (idiopathic) D69.8
cryoglobulinemic D89.1
Devil's pinches D69.2
fibrinolytic — *see* Fibrinolysis
fulminans, fulminous D65
gangrenous D65
hemorrhagic, hemorrhagica D69.3
  not due to thrombocytopenia D69.0
Henoch (-Schönlein) (allergic) D69.0
hypergammaglobulinemic (benign) (Waldenström) D89.0
idiopathic (thrombocytopenic) D69.3
  nonthrombocytopenic D69.0
immune thrombocytopenic D69.3
infectious D69.0
malignant D69.0
neonatorum P54.5
nervosa D69.0
newborn P54.5
nonthrombocytopenic D69.2
  hemorrhagic D69.0
  idiopathic D69.0
nonthrombopenic D69.2
peliosis rheumatica D69.0
posttransfusion (post-transfusion) (from (fresh) whole blood or blood products) D69.51
primary D69.49
red cell membrane sensitivity D69.2
rheumatica D69.0
Schönlein (-Henoch) (allergic) D69.0
scorbutic E54 [D77]
senile D69.2
simplex D69.2
symptomatica D69.0
telangiectasia annularis L81.7
thrombocytopenic D69.49
  congenital D69.42
  hemorrhagic D69.3
  hereditary D69.42
  idiopathic D69.3
  immune D69.3
  neonatal, transitory P61.0
  thrombotic M31.1
thrombohemolytic — *see* Fibrinolysis
thrombolytic — *see* Fibrinolysis
thrombopenic D69.49
thrombotic, thrombocytopenic M31.1
toxic D69.0

Purpura — *continued*
  vascular D69.0
  visceral symptoms D69.0
Purpuric spots R23.3
Purulent — *see* condition
Pus
  in
    stool R19.5
    urine N39.0
  tube (rupture) — *see* Salpingo-oophoritis
Pustular rash L08.0
Pustule (nonmalignant) L08.9
  malignant A22.0
Pustulosis palmaris et plantaris L40.3
Putnam (-Dana) disease or syndrome — *see* Degeneration, combined
Putrescent pulp (dental) K04.1
Pyarthritis, pyarthrosis — *see* Arthritis, pyogenic or pyemic
  tuberculous — *see* Tuberculosis, joint
Pyelectasis — *see* Hydronephrosis
Pyelitis (congenital) (uremic) (*see also* Pyelonephritis)
  with
    calculusN20
      with hydronephrosis N13.2
    contracted kidney N11.9
  acute N10
  chronic N11.9
    with calculusN20
      with hydronephrosis N13.2
  cystica N28.84
  puerperal (postpartum) O86.21
  tuberculous A18.11
Pyelocystitis — *see* Pyelonephritis
Pyelonephritis (*see also* Nephritis, tubulo-interstitial)
  with
    calculusN20
      with hydronephrosis N13.2
    contracted kidney N11.9
  acute N10
  calculousN20
    with hydronephrosis N13.2
  chronic N11.9
    with calculusN20
      with hydronephrosis N13.2
    associated with ureteral obstruction or stricture N11.1
    nonobstructive N11.8
      with reflux (vesicoureteral) N11.0
    obstructive N11.1
    specified NEC N11.8
  in (due to)
    brucellosis A23.9 [N16]
    cryoglobulinemia (mixed) D89.1 [N16]
    cystinosis E72.04
    diphtheria A36.84
    glycogen storage disease E74.09 [N16]
    leukemia NEC C95.9- ☑ [N16]
    lymphoma NEC C85.90 [N16]
    multiple myeloma C90.0- ☑ [N16]
    obstruction N11.1
    Salmonella infection A02.25
    sarcoidosis D86.84
    sepsis A41.9 [N16]
    Sjögren's disease M35.04
    toxoplasmosis B58.83
    transplant rejection T86.91 [N16]
    Wilson's disease E83.01 [N16]
  nonobstructive N12
    with reflux (vesicoureteral) N11.0
    chronic N11.8
  syphilitic A52.75
Pyelonephrosis (obstructive) N11.1
  chronic N11.9
Pyelophlebitis I80.8
Pyeloureteritis cystica N28.85
Pyemia, pyemic (fever) (infection) (purulent) (*see also* Sepsis)
  joint — *see* Arthritis, pyogenic or pyemic
  liver K75.1
  pneumococcal A40.3
  portal K75.1
  postvaccinal T88.0 ☑
  puerperal, postpartum, childbirth O85
  specified organism NEC A41.89
  tuberculous — *see* Tuberculosis, miliary
Pygopagus Q89.4
Pyknoepilepsy (idiopathic) — *see* Pyknolepsy
Pyknolepsy G40.A09
  intractable G40.A19

Pyknolepsy — *continued*
  with status epilepticus G40.A11
  without status epilepticus G40.A19
  not intractable G40.A09
    with status epilepticus G40.A01
    without status epilepticus G40.A09
Pylephlebitis K75.1
Pyle's syndrome Q78.5
Pylethrombophlebitis K75.1
Pylethrombosis K75.1
Pyloritis K29.90
  with bleeding K29.91
Pylorospasm (reflex) NEC K31.3
  congenital or infantile Q40.0
  newborn Q40.0
  neurotic F45.8
  psychogenic F45.8
Pylorus, pyloric — *see* condition
Pyoarthrosis — *see* Arthritis, pyogenic or pyemic
Pyocele
  mastoid — *see* Mastoiditis, acute
  sinus (accessory) — *see* Sinusitis
  turbinate (bone) J32.9
  urethra (*see also* Urethritis) N34.0
Pyocolpos — *see* Vaginitis
Pyocystitis N30.80
  with hematuria N30.81
Pyoderma, pyodermia L08.0
  gangrenosum L88
  newborn P39.4
  phagedenic L88
  vegetans L08.81
Pyodermatitis L08.0
  vegetans L08.81
Pyogenic — *see* condition
Pyohydronephrosis N13.6
Pyometra, pyometrium, pyometritis — *see* Endometritis
Pyomyositis (tropical) — *see* Myositis, infective
Pyonephritis N12
Pyonephrosis N13.6
  tuberculous A18.11
Pyo-oophoritis — *see* Salpingo-oophoritis
Pyo-ovarium — *see* Salpingo-oophoritis
Pyopericarditis, pyopericardium I30.1
Pyophlebitis — *see* Phlebitis
Pyopneumopericardium I30.1
Pyopneumothorax (infective) J86.9
  with fistula J86.0
  tuberculous NEC A15.6
Pyosalpinx, pyosalpingitis (*see also* Salpingo-oophoritis)
Pyothorax J86.9
  with fistula J86.0
  tuberculous NEC A15.6
Pyoureter N28.89
  tuberculous A18.11
Pyramidopallidonigral syndrome G20
Pyrexia (of unknown origin) R50.9
  atmospheric T67.0 ☑
  during labor NEC O75.2
  heat T67.0 ☑
  newborn P81.9
    environmentally-induced P81.0
  persistent R50.9
  puerperal O86.4
Pyroglobulinemia NEC E88.09
Pyromania F63.1
Pyrosis R12
Pyuria (bacterial) N39.0

Q

Q fever A78
  with pneumonia A78
Quadricuspid aortic valve Q23.8
Quadrilateral fever A78
Quadriparesis — *see* Quadriplegia
  meaning muscle weakness M62.81
Quadriplegia G82.50
  complete
    C1-C4 level G82.51
    C5-C7 level G82.53
  congenital (cerebral) (spinal) G80.8
    spastic G80.0
  embolic (current episode) I63.4 ☑
  functional R53.2
  incomplete
    C1-C4 level G82.52

Quadriplegia — *continued*
    C5-C7 level G82.54
  thrombotic (current episode) I63.3 ☑
  traumatic -- code to injury with seventh character S
    current episode — *see* Injury, spinal (cord), cervical
Quadruplet, pregnancy — *see* Pregnancy, quadruplet
Quarrelsomeness F60.3
Queensland fever A77.3
Quervain's disease M65.4
  thyroid E06.1
Queyrat's erythroplasia D07.4
  penis D07.4
  specified site — *see* Neoplasm, skin, in situ
  unspecified site D07.4
Quincke's disease or edema T78.3 ☑
  hereditary D84.1
Quinsy (gangrenous) J36
Quintan fever A79.0
Quintuplet, pregnancy — *see* Pregnancy, quintuplet

R

Rabbit fever — *see* Tularemia
Rabies A82.9
  contact Z20.3
  exposure to Z20.3
  inoculation reaction — *see* Complications, vaccination
  sylvatic A82.0
  urban A82.1
Rachischisis — *see* Spina bifida
Rachitic (*see also* condition)
  deformities of spine (late effect) (sequelae) E64.3
  pelvis (late effect) (sequelae) E64.3
    with disproportion (fetopelvic) O33.0
      causing obstructed labor O65.0
Rachitis, rachitism (acute) (tarda) (*see also* Rickets)
  renalis N25.0
  sequelae E64.3
Radial nerve — *see* condition
Radiation
  burn — *see* Burn
  effects NOS T66 ☑
  sickness NOS T66 ☑
  therapy, encounter for Z51.0
Radiculitis (pressure) (vertebrogenic) — *see* Radiculopathy
Radiculomyelitis (*see also* Encephalitis)
  toxic, due to
    Clostridium tetani A35
    Corynebacterium diphtheriae A36.82
Radiculopathy M54.10
  cervical region M54.12
  cervicothoracic region M54.13
  due to
    disc disorder
      C3 M50.11
      C4 M50.11
      C5 M50.12
      C6 M50.12
      C7 M50.12
      C8 M50.13
    displacement of intervertebral disc — *see* Disorder, disc, with, radiculopathy
  leg M54.1- ☑
  lumbar region M54.16
  lumbosacral region M54.17
  occipito-atlanto-axial region M54.11
  postherpetic B02.29
  sacrococcygeal region M54.18
  syphilitic A52.11
  thoracic region (with visceral pain) M54.14
  thoracolumbar region M54.15
Radiodermal burns (acute, chronic, or occupational) — *see* Burn
Radiodermatitis L58.9
  acute L58.0
  chronic L58.1
Radiotherapy session Z51.0
Rage, meaning rabies — *see* Rabies
Ragpicker's disease A22.1
Ragsorter's disease A22.1
Raillietiniasis B71.8
Railroad neurosis F48.8
Railway spine F48.8
Raised (*see also* Elevated)
  antibody titer R76.0

☑ **Additional character required**

Rake teeth, tooth M26.39
Rales R09.89
Ramifying renal pelvis Q63.8
Ramsay-Hunt disease or syndrome (*see also* Hunt's disease) B02.21
   meaning dyssynergia cerebellaris myoclonica G11.1
Ranula K11.6
   congenital Q38.4
Rape
   adult
      confirmed T74.21 ☑
      suspected T76.21 ☑
   alleged, observation or examination, ruled out
      adult Z04.41
      child Z04.42
   child
      confirmed T74.22 ☑
      suspected T76.22 ☑
Rapid
   feeble pulse, due to shock, following injury T79.4 ☑
   heart (beat) R00.0
      psychogenic F45.8
   second stage (delivery) O62.3
   time-zone change syndrome — *see* Disorder, sleep, circadian rhythm, psychogenic
Rarefaction, bone — *see* Disorder, bone, density and structure, specified NEC
Rash (toxic) R21
   canker A38.9
   diaper L22
   drug (internal use) L27.0
      contact (*see also* Dermatitis, due to, drugs, external) L25.1
   following immunization T88.1 ☑
   food — *see* Dermatitis, due to, food
   heat L74.0
   napkin (psoriasiform) L22
   nettle — *see* Urticaria
   pustular L08.0
   rose R21
      epidemic B06.9
   scarlet A38.9
   serum (*see also* Reaction, serum) T80.69 ☑
   wandering tongue K14.1
Rasmussen aneurysm — *see* Tuberculosis, pulmonary
Rasmussen encephalitis G04.81
Rat-bite fever A25.9
   due to Streptobacillus moniliformis A25.1
   spirochetal (morsus muris) A25.0
Rathke's pouch tumor D44.3
Raymond (-Céstan) syndrome I65.8
Raynaud's disease, phenomenon or syndrome (secondary) I73.00
   with gangrene (symmetric) I73.01
RDS (newborn) (type I) P22.0
   type II P22.1
Reaction (*see also* Disorder)
   adaptation — *see* Disorder, adjustment
   adjustment (anxiety) (conduct disorder) (depressiveness) (distress) — *see* Disorder, adjustment
      with
         mutism, elective (child) (adolescent) F94.0
   adverse
      food (any) (ingested) NEC T78.1 ☑
         anaphylactic — *see* Shock, anaphylactic, due to food
   affective — *see* Disorder, mood
   allergic — *see* Allergy
   anaphylactic — *see* Shock, anaphylactic
   anaphylactoid — *see* Shock, anaphylactic
   anesthesia — *see* Anesthesia, complication
   antitoxin (prophylactic) (therapeutic) — *see* Complications, vaccination
   anxiety F41.1
   Arthus — *see* Arthus' phenomenon
   asthenic F48.8
   combat and operational stress F43.0
   compulsive F42
   conversion F44.9
   crisis, acute F43.0
   deoxyribonuclease (DNA) (DNase) hypersensitivity D69.2
   depressive (single episode) F32.9
      affective (single episode) F31.4
         recurrent episode F33.9
      neurotic F34.1
      psychoneurotic F34.1
      psychotic F32.3

Reaction — *continued*
      recurrent — *see* Disorder, depressive, recurrent
   dissociative F44.9
   drug NEC T88.7 ☑
      addictive — *see* Dependence, drug
         transmitted via placenta or breast milk — *see* Absorption, drug, addictive, through placenta
      allergic — *see* Allergy, drug
      lichenoid L43.2
      newborn P93.8
         gray baby syndrome P93.0
      overdose or poisoning (by accident) — *see* Table of Drugs and Chemicals, by drug, poisoning
      photoallergic L56.1
      phototoxic L56.0
      withdrawal — *see* Dependence, by drug, with, withdrawal
         infant of dependent mother P96.1
         newborn P96.1
      wrong substance given or taken (by accident) — *see* Table of Drugs and Chemicals, by drug, poisoning
   fear F40.9
      child (abnormal) F93.8
   febrile nonhemolytic transfusion (FNHTR) R50.84
   fluid loss, cerebrospinal G97.1
   foreign
      body NEC — *see* Granuloma, foreign body
         in operative wound (inadvertently left) — *see* Foreign body, accidentally left during a procedure
      substance accidentally left during a procedure (chemical) (powder) (talc) T81.60 ☑
         aseptic peritonitis T81.61 ☑
         body or object (instrument) (sponge) (swab) — *see* Foreign body, accidentally left during a procedure
         specified reaction NEC T81.69 ☑
   grief — *see* Disorder, adjustment
   Herxheimer's R68.89
   hyperkinetic — *see* Hyperkinesia
   hypochondriacal F45.20
   hypoglycemic, due to insulin E16.0
      with coma (diabetic) — *see* Diabetes, coma
         nondiabetic E15
      therapeutic misadventure T38.3
   hypomanic F30.8
   hysterical F44.9
   immunization — *see* Complications, vaccination
   incompatibility
      ABO blood group (infusion) (transfusion) — *see* Complication(s), transfusion, incompatibility reaction, ABO
      delayed serologic T80.39 ☑
      minor blood group (Duffy) (E) (K(ell)) (Kidd) (Lewis) (M) (N) (P) (S) T80.89 ☑
      Rh (factor) (infusion) (transfusion) — *see* Complication(s), transfusion, incompatibility reaction, Rh (factor)
   inflammatory — *see* Infection
   infusion — *see* Complications, infusion
   inoculation (immune serum) — *see* Complications, vaccination
   insulin T38.3- ☑
   involutional psychotic — *see* Disorder, depressive
   leukemoid D72.823
      basophilic D72.823
      lymphocytic D72.823
      monocytic D72.823
      myelocytic D72.823
      neutrophilic D72.823
   LSD (acute)
      due to drug abuse — *see* Abuse, drug, hallucinogen
      due to drug dependence — *see* Dependence, drug, hallucinogen
   lumbar puncture G97.1
   manic-depressive — *see* Disorder, bipolar
   neurasthenic F48.8
   neurogenic — *see* Neurosis
   neurotic F48.9
   neurotic-depressive F34.1
   nitritoid — *see* Crisis, nitritoid
   nonspecific
      to
         cell mediated immunity measurement of gamma interferon antigen response without active tuberculosis R76.12
         QuantiFERON-TB test (QFT) without active tuberculosis R76.12

Reaction — *continued*
      tuberculin test (*see also* Reaction, tuberculin skin test) R76.11
   obsessive-compulsive F42
   organic, acute or subacute — *see* Delirium
   paranoid (acute) F23
      chronic F22
      senile F03 ☑
   passive dependency F60.7
   phobic F40.9
   post-traumatic stress, uncomplicated Z73.3
   psychogenic F99
   psychoneurotic (*see also* Neurosis)
      compulsive F42
      depersonalization F48.1
      depressive F34.1
      hypochondriacal F45.20
      neurasthenic F48.8
      obsessive F42
   psychophysiologic — *see* Disorder, somatoform
   psychosomatic — *see* Disorder, somatoform
   psychotic — *see* Psychosis
   scarlet fever toxin — *see* Complications, vaccination
   schizophrenic F23
      acute (brief) (undifferentiated) F23
      latent F21
      undifferentiated (acute) (brief) F23
   serological for syphilis — *see* Serology for syphilis
   serum T80.69 ☑
      anaphylactic (immediate) (*see also* Shock, anaphylactic) T80.59 ☑
      specified reaction NEC
         due to
            administration of blood and blood products T80.61 ☑
            immunization T80.62 ☑
            serum specified NEC T80.69 ☑
            vaccination T80.62 ☑
   situational — *see* Disorder, adjustment
   somatization — *see* Disorder, somatoform
   spinal puncture G97.1
   stress (severe) F43.9
      acute (agitation) ("daze") (disorientation) (disturbance of consciousness) (flight reaction) (fugue) F43.0
      specified NEC F43.8
   surgical procedure — *see* Complications, surgical procedure
   tetanus antitoxin — *see* Complications, vaccination
   toxic, to local anesthesia T81.89 ☑
      in labor and delivery O74.4
      in pregnancy O29.3X- ☑
      postpartum, puerperal O89.3
   toxin-antitoxin — *see* Complications, vaccination
   transfusion (blood) (bone marrow) (lymphocytes) (allergic) — *see* Complications, transfusion
   tuberculin skin test, abnormal R76.11
   vaccination (any) — *see* Complications, vaccination
   withdrawing, child or adolescent F93.8
Reactive airway disease — *see* Asthma
Reactive depression — *see* Reaction, depressive
Rearrangement
   chromosomal
      balanced (in) Q95.9
         abnormal individual (autosomal) Q95.2
         non-sex (autosomal) chromosomes Q95.2
         sex/non-sex chromosomes Q95.3
         specified NEC Q95.8
Recalcitrant patient — *see* Noncompliance
Recanalization, thrombus — *see* Thrombosis
Recession, receding
   chamber angle (eye) H21.55- ☑
   chin M26.09
   gingival (generalized) (localized) (postinfective) (postoperative) K06.0
Recklinghausen disease Q85.01
   bones E21.0
Reclus' disease (cystic) — *see* Mastopathy, cystic
Recrudescent typhus (fever) A75.1
Recruitment, auditory H93.21- ☑
Rectalgia K62.89
Rectitis K62.89
Rectocele
   female (without uterine prolapse) N81.6
      with uterine prolapse N81.4
         incomplete N81.2
   in pregnancy — *see* Pregnancy, complicated by, abnormal, pelvic organs or tissues NEC
   male K62.3

Rectosigmoid junction — *see* condition
Rectosigmoiditis K63.89
  ulcerative (chronic) K51.30
    with
      complication K51.319
        abscess K51.314
        fistula K51.313
        obstruction K51.312
        rectal bleeding K51.311
        specified NEC K51.318
Rectourethral — *see* condition
Rectovaginal — *see* condition
Rectovesical — *see* condition
Rectum, rectal — *see* condition
Recurrent — *see* condition
  pregnancy loss — *see* Loss (of), pregnancy, recurrent
Red bugs B88.0
Red-cedar lung or pneumonitis J67.8
Red tide (*see also* Table of Drugs and Chemicals) T65.82- ☑
Reduced
  mobility Z74.09
  ventilatory or vital capacity R94.2
Redundant, redundancy
  anus (congenital) Q43.8
  clitoris N90.89
  colon (congenital) Q43.8
  foreskin (congenital) N47.8
  intestine (congenital) Q43.8
  labia N90.6
  organ or site, congenital NEC — *see* Accessory
  panniculus (abdominal) E65
  prepuce (congenital) N47.8
  pylorus K31.89
  rectum (congenital) Q43.8
  scrotum N50.8
  sigmoid (congenital) Q43.8
  skin (of face) L57.4
    eyelids — *see* Blepharochalasis
  stomach K31.89
Reduplication — *see* Duplication
Reflex R29.2
  hyperactive gag J39.2
  pupillary, abnormal — *see* Anomaly, pupil, function
  vasoconstriction I73.9
  vasovagal R55
Reflux K21.9
  acid K21.9
  esophageal K21.9
    with esophagitis K21.0
      newborn P78.83
  gastroesophageal K21.9
    with esophagitis K21.0
  mitral — *see* Insufficiency, mitral
  ureteral — *see* Reflux, vesicoureteral
  vesicoureteral (with scarring) N13.70
    with
      nephropathy N13.729
        with hydroureter N13.739
          bilateral N13.732
          unilateral N13.731
        bilateral N13.722
        unilateral N13.721
        without hydroureter N13.729
          bilateral N13.722
          unilateral N13.721
      pyelonephritis (chronic) N11.0
    congenital Q62.7
    without nephropathy N13.71
Reforming, artificial openings — *see* Attention to, artificial, opening
Refractive error — *see* Disorder, refraction
Refsum's disease or syndrome G60.1
Refusal of
  food, psychogenic F50.8
  treatment (because of) Z53.20
    left against medical advice (AMA) Z53.21
    patient's decision NEC Z53.29
    reasons of belief or group pressure Z53.1
Regional — *see* condition
Regurgitation R11.10
  aortic (valve) — *see* Insufficiency, aortic
  food (*see also* Vomiting)
    with reswallowing — *see* Rumination
    newborn P92.1
  gastric contents — *see* Vomiting
  heart — *see* Endocarditis
  mitral (valve) — *see* Insufficiency, mitral
    congenital Q23.3
  myocardial — *see* Endocarditis

Regurgitation — *continued*
  pulmonary (valve) (heart) I37.1
    congenital Q22.2
    syphilitic A52.03
  tricuspid — *see* Insufficiency, tricuspid
  valve, valvular — *see* Endocarditis
    congenital Q24.8
  vesicoureteral — *see* Reflux, vesicoureteral
Reifenstein syndrome E34.52
Reinsertion, contraceptive device Z30.433
Reiter's disease, syndrome, or urethritis M02.30
  ankle M02.37- ☑
  elbow M02.32- ☑
  foot joint M02.37- ☑
  hand joint M02.34- ☑
  hip M02.35- ☑
  knee M02.36- ☑
  multiple site M02.39
  shoulder M02.31- ☑
  vertebra M02.38
  wrist M02.33- ☑
Reichmann's disease or syndrome K31.89
Rejection
  food, psychogenic F50.8
  transplant T86.91
    bone T86.830
      marrow T86.01
    cornea T86.840
    heart T86.21
      with lung (s) T86.31
    intestine T86.850
    kidney T86.11
    liver T86.41
    lung (s) T86.810
      with heart T86.31
    organ (immune or nonimmune cause) T86.91
    pancreas T86.890
    skin (allograft) (autograft) T86.820
    specified NEC T86.890
    stem cell (peripheral blood) (umbilical cord) T86.5
Relapsing fever A68.9
  Carter's (Asiatic) A68.1
  Dutton's (West African) A68.1
  Koch's A68.9
  louse-borne (epidemic) A68.0
  Novy's (American) A68.1
  Obermeyers's (European) A68.0
  Spirillum A68.9
  tick-borne (endemic) A68.1
Relationship
  occlusal
    open anterior M26.220
    open posterior M26.221
Relaxation
  anus (sphincter) K62.89
    psychogenic F45.8
  arch (foot) (*see also* Deformity, limb, flat foot)
  back ligaments — *see* Instability, joint, spine
  bladder (sphincter) N31.2
  cardioesophageal K21.9
  cervix — *see* Incompetency, cervix
  diaphragm J98.6
  joint (capsule) (ligament) (paralytic) — *see* Flail, joint
    congenital NEC Q74.8
  lumbosacral (joint) M53.2
  pelvic floor N81.89
  perineum N81.89
  posture R29.3
  rectum (sphincter) K62.89
  sacroiliac (joint) M53.2
  scrotum N50.8
  urethra (sphincter) N36.44
  vesical N31.2
Release from prison, anxiety concerning Z65.2
Remains
  canal of Cloquet Q14.0
  capsule (opaque) Q14.8
Remittent fever (malarial) B54
Remnant
  canal of Cloquet Q14.0
  capsule (opaque) Q14.8
  cervix, cervical stump (acquired) (postoperative) N88.8
  cystic duct, postcholecystectomy K91.5
  fingernail L60.8
    congenital Q84.6
  meniscus, knee — *see* Derangement, knee, meniscus, specified NEC
  thyroglossal duct Q89.2
  tonsil J35.8

Remnant — *continued*
  infected (chronic) J35.01
  urachus Q64.4
Removal (from) (of)
  artificial
    arm Z44.00- ☑
      complete Z44.01- ☑
      partial Z44.02- ☑
    eye Z44.2- ☑
    leg Z44.10- ☑
      complete Z44.11- ☑
      partial Z44.12- ☑
  breast implant Z45.81 ☑
  cardiac pulse generator (battery) (end-of-life) Z45.010
  catheter (urinary) (indwelling) Z46.6
    from artificial opening — *see* Attention to, artificial, opening
    non-vascular Z46.82
    vascular NEC Z45.2
  drains Z48.03
  device Z46.9
    contraceptive Z30.432
    implanted NEC Z45.89
    specified NEC Z46.89
  dressing (nonsurgical) Z48.00
    surgical Z48.01
  external
    fixation device - code to fracture with seventh character D
    prosthesis, prosthetic device Z44.9
      breast Z44.3- ☑
      specified NEC Z44.8
  home in childhood (to foster home or institution) Z62.29
  ileostomy Z43.2
  insulin pump Z46.81
  myringotomy device (stent) (tube) Z45.82
  nervous system device NEC Z46.2
    brain neuropacemaker Z46.2
    visual substitution device Z46.2
      implanted Z45.31
  non-vascular catheter Z46.82
  orthodontic device Z46.4
  organ, prophylactic (for neoplasia management) — *see* Prophylactic, organ removal
  staples Z48.02
  stent
    ureteral Z46.6
  suture Z48.02
  urinary device Z46.6
  vascular access device or catheter Z45.2
Ren
  arcuatus Q63.1
  mobile, mobilis N28.89
    congenital Q63.8
  unguliformis Q63.1
Renal — *see* condition
Rendu-Osler-Weber disease or syndrome I78.0
Reninoma D41.0- ☑
Renon-Delille syndrome E23.3
Reovirus, as cause of disease classified elsewhere B97.5
Repeated falls NEC R29.6
Replaced chromosome by dicentric ring Q93.2
Replacement by artificial or mechanical device or prosthesis of
  bladder Z96.0
  blood vessel NEC Z95.828
  bone NEC Z96.7
  cochlea Z96.21
  coronary artery Z95.5
  eustachian tube Z96.29
  eye globe Z97.0
  heart Z95.812
    valve Z95.2
      prosthetic Z95.2
      specified NEC Z95.4
      xenogenic Z95.3
  intestine Z96.89
  joint Z96.60
    hip — *see* Presence, hip joint implant
    knee — *see* Presence, knee joint implant
    specified site NEC Z96.698
  larynx Z96.3
  lens Z96.1
  limb (s) — *see* Presence, artificial, limb
  mandible NEC (for tooth root implant(s)) Z96.5
  organ NEC Z96.89
  peripheral vessel NEC Z95.828
  stapes Z96.29
  teeth Z97.2

Replacement — continued
tendon Z96.7
tissue NEC Z96.89
tooth root (s) Z96.5
vessel NEC Z95.828
coronary (artery) Z95.5
Request for expert evidence Z04.8
Reserve, decreased or low
cardiac — see Disease, heart
kidney N28.89
Residual (see also condition)
ovary syndrome N99.83
state, schizophrenic F20.5
urine R39.19
Resistance, resistant (to)
activated protein C D68.51
complicating pregnancy O26.89 ☑
insulin E88.81
organism (s)
to
drug
aminoglycosides Z16.29
amoxicillin Z16.11
ampicillin Z16.11
antibiotic (s) Z16.20
multiple Z16.24
specified NEC Z16.29
antifungal Z16.32
antimicrobial (single) Z16.30
multiple Z16.35
specified NEC Z16.39
antimycbacterial (single) Z16.341
multiple Z16.342
antiparasitic Z16.31
antiviral Z16.33
beta lactam antibiotics Z16.10
specified NEC Z16.19
cephalosporins Z16.19
extended beta lactamase (ESBL) Z16.12
fluoroquinolones Z16.23
macrolides Z16.29
methicillin — see MRSA
multiple drugs (MDRO)
antibiotics Z16.24
penicillins Z16.11
quinine (and related compounds) Z16.31
quinolones Z16.23
sulfonamides Z16.29
tetracyclines Z16.29
tuberculostatics (single) Z16.341
multiple Z16.342
vancomycin Z16.21
related antibiotics Z16.22
thyroid hormone E07.89
Resorption
dental (roots) K03.3
alveoli M26.79
teeth (external) (internal) (pathological) (roots)
K03.3
Respiration
Cheyne-Stokes R06.3
decreased due to shock, following injury T79.4 ☑
disorder of, psychogenic F45.8
insufficient, or poor R06.89
newborn P28.5
painful R07.1
sighing, psychogenic F45.8
Respiratory (see also condition)
distress syndrome (newborn) (type I) P22.0
type II P22.1
syncytial virus, as cause of disease classified
elsewhere B97.4
Respite care Z75.5
Response (drug)
photoallergic L56.1
phototoxic L56.0
Restless legs (syndrome) G25.81
Restlessness R45.1
Restriction of housing space Z59.1
Restoration (of)
dental
aesthetically inadequate or displeasing K08.56
defective K08.50
specified NEC K08.59
failure of marginal integrity K08.51
failure of periodontal anatomical intergrity
K08.54
organ continuity from previous sterilization
(tuboplasty) (vasoplasty) Z31.0
aftercare Z31.42
tooth (existing)

Restoration — continued
contours biologically incompatible with oral
health K08.54
open margins K08.51
overhanging K08.52
poor aesthetic K08.56
poor gingival margins K08.51
unsatisfactory, of tooth K08.50
specified NEC K08.59
Restorative material (dental)
allergy to K08.55
fractured K08.539
with loss of material K08.531
without loss of material K08.530
unrepairable overhanging of K08.52
Rests, ovarian, in fallopian tube Q50.6
Restzustand (schizophrenic) F20.5
Retained (see also Retention)
cholelithiasis following cholecystectomy K91.86
foreign body fragments (type of) Z18.9
acrylics Z18.2
animal quill (s) or spines Z18.31
cement Z18.83
concrete Z18.83
crystalline Z18.83
depleted isotope Z18.09
depleted uranium Z18.01
diethylhexylphthalates Z18.2
glass Z18.81
isocyanate Z18.2
magnetic metal Z18.11
metal Z18.10
nonmagnectic metal Z18.12
nontherapeutic radioactive Z18.09
organic NEC Z18.39
plastic Z18.2
quill (s) (animal) Z18.31
radioactive (nontherapeutic) NEC Z18.09
specified NEC Z18.89
spine (s) (animal) Z18.31
stone Z18.83
tooth (teeth) Z18.32
wood Z18.33
fragments (type of) Z18.9
acrylics Z18.2
animal quill (s) or spines Z18.31
cement Z18.83
concrete Z18.83
crystalline Z18.83
depleted isotope Z18.09
depleted uranium Z18.01
diethylhexylphthalates Z18.2
glass Z18.81
isocyanate Z18.2
magnetic metal Z18.11
metal Z18.10
nonmagnectic metal Z18.12
nontherapeutic radioactive Z18.09
organic NEC Z18.39
plastic Z18.2
quill (s) (animal) Z18.31
radioactive (nontherapeutic) NEC Z18.09
specified NEC Z18.89
spine (s) (animal) Z18.31
stone Z18.83
tooth (teeth) Z18.32
wood Z18.33
gallstones, following cholecystectomy K91.86
Retardation
development, developmental, specific — see
Disorder, developmental
endochondral bone growth — see Disorder,
bone, development or growth
growth R62.50
due to malnutrition E45
mental — see Disability, intellectual
motor function, specific F82
physical (child) R62.52
due to malnutrition E45
reading (specific) F81.0
spelling (specific) (without reading disorder)
F81.81
Retching — see Vomiting
Retention (see also Retained)
bladder — see Retention, urine
carbon dioxide E87.2
cholelithiasis following cholecystectomy K91.86
cyst — see Cyst
dead
fetus (at or near term) (mother) O36.4 ☑
early fetal death O02.1
ovum O02.0

Retention — continued
decidua (fragments) (following delivery) (with
hemorrhage) O72.2
without hemorrhage O73.1
deciduous tooth K00.6
dental root K08.3
fecal — see Constipation
fetus
dead O36.4 ☑
early O02.1
fluid R60.9
foreign body (see also Foreign body, retained)
current trauma - code as Foreign body, by site
or type
gallstones, following cholecystectomy K91.86
gastric K31.89
intrauterine contraceptive device, in pregnancy
— see Pregnancy, complicated by, retention,
intrauterine device
membranes (complicating delivery) (with
hemorrhage) O72.2
with abortion — see Abortion, by type
without hemorrhage O73.1
meniscus — see Derangement, meniscus
menses N94.89
milk (puerperal, postpartum) O92.79
nitrogen, extrarenal R39.2
ovary syndrome N99.83
placenta (total) (with hemorrhage) O72.0
without hemorrhage O73.0
portions or fragments (with hemorrhage)
O72.2
without hemorrhage O73.1
products of conception
early pregnancy (dead fetus) O02.1
following
delivery (with hemorrhage) O72.2
without hemorrhage O73.1
secundines (following delivery) (with
hemorrhage) O72.2
without hemorrhage O73.0
complicating puerperium (delayed
hemorrhage) O72.2
partial O72.2
without hemorrhage O73.1
smegma, clitoris N90.89
urine R33.9
due to hyperplasia (hypertrophy) of prostate —
see Hyperplasia, prostate
drug-induced R33.0
organic R33.8
drug-induced R33.0
psychogenic F45.8
specified NEC R33.8
water (in tissues) — see Edema
Reticular erythematous mucinosis L98.5
Reticulation, dust — see Pneumoconiosis
Reticulocytosis R70.1
Reticuloendotheliosis
acute infantile C96.0
leukemic C91.4- ☑
malignant C96.9
nonlipid C96.0
Reticulohistiocytoma (giant-cell) D76.3
Reticuloid, actinic L57.1
Reticulosis (skin)
acute of infancy C96.0
hemophagocytic, familial D76.1
histiocytic medullary C96.9
lipomelanotic I89.8
malignant (midline) C86.0
nonlipid C96.0
polymorphic C86.0
Sézary — see Sézary disease
Retina, retinal (see also condition)
dark area D49.81
Retinitis (see also Inflammation, chorioretinal)
albuminurica N18.9 [H32]
diabetic — see Diabetes, retinitis
disciformis — see Degeneration, macula
focal — see Inflammation, chorioretinal, focal
gravidarum — see Pregnancy, complicated by,
specified pregnancy-related condition NEC
juxtapapillaris — see Inflammation, chorioretinal,
focal, juxtapapillary
luetic — see Retinitis, syphilitic
pigmentosa H35.52
proliferans — see Disorder, globe, degenerative,
specified type NEC
proliferating — see Disorder, globe, degenerative,
specified type NEC
renal N18.9 [H32]

Retinitis — *continued*
- syphilitic (early) (secondary) A51.43
  - central, recurrent A52.71
  - congenital (early) A50.01 [H32]
  - late A52.71
- tuberculous A18.53

Retinoblastoma C69.2- ☑
- differentiated C69.2- ☑
- undifferentiated C69.2- ☑

Retinochoroiditis (*see also* Inflammation, chorioretinal)
- disseminated — *see* Inflammation, chorioretinal, disseminated
  - syphilitic A52.71
- focal — *see* Inflammation, chorioretinal
- juxtapapillaris — *see* Inflammation, chorioretinal, focal, juxtapapillary

Retinopathy (background) H35.00
- arteriosclerotic I70.8 [H35.0- ☑]
- atherosclerotic I70.8 [H35.0- ☑]
- central serous — *see* Chorioretinopathy, central serous
- Coats H35.02- ☑
- diabetic — *see* Diabetes, retinopathy
- exudative H35.02- ☑
- hypertensive H35.03- ☑
- in (due to)
  - diabetes — *see* Diabetes, retinopathy
  - sickle-cell disorders D57.- ☑ [H36]
- of prematurity H35.10- ☑
  - stage 0 H35.11- ☑
  - stage 1 H35.12- ☑
  - stage 2 H35.13- ☑
  - stage 3 H35.14- ☑
  - stage 4 H35.15- ☑
  - stage 5 H35.16- ☑
- pigmentary, congenital — *see* Dystrophy, retina
- proliferative NEC H35.2- ☑
  - diabetic — *see* Diabetes, retinopathy, proliferative
  - sickle-cell D57.- ☑ [H36]
- solar H31.02- ☑

Retinoschisis H33.10- ☑
- congenital Q14.1
- specified type NEC H33.19- ☑

Retortamoniasis A07.8

Retractile testis Q55.22

Retraction
- cervix — *see* Retroversion, uterus
- drum (membrane) — *see* Disorder, tympanic membrane, specified NEC
- finger — *see* Deformity, finger
- lid H02.539
  - left H02.536
    - lower H02.535
    - upper H02.534
  - right H02.533
    - lower H02.532
    - upper H02.531
- lung J98.4
- mediastinum J98.5
- nipple N64.53
  - associated with
    - lactation O92.03
    - pregnancy O92.01- ☑
    - puerperium O92.02
  - congenital Q83.8
- palmar fascia M72.0
- pleura — *see* Pleurisy
- ring, uterus (Bandl's) (pathological) O62.4
- sternum (congenital) Q76.7
  - acquired M95.4
- uterus — *see* Retroversion, uterus
- valve (heart) — *see* Endocarditis

Retrobulbar — *see* condition

Retrocecal — *see* condition

Retrocession — *see* Retroversion

Retrodisplacement — *see* Retroversion

Retroflection, retroflexion — *see* Retroversion

Retrognathia, retrognathism (mandibular) (maxillary) M26.19

Retrograde menstruation N92.5

Retroperineal — *see* condition

Retroperitoneal — *see* condition

Retroperitonitis K68.9

Retropharyngeal — *see* condition

Retroplacental — *see* condition

Retroposition — *see* Retroversion

Retroprosthetic membrane T85.398 ☑

Retrosternal thyroid (congenital) Q89.2

Retroversion, retroverted
- cervix — *see* Retroversion, uterus

Retroversion — *continued*
- female NEC — *see* Retroversion, uterus
- iris H21.89
- testis (congenital) Q55.29
- uterus (acquired) (acute) (any degree) (asymptomatic) (cervix) (postinfectional) (postpartal, old) N85.4
  - congenital Q51.818
  - in pregnancy O34.53- ☑

Retrovirus, as cause of disease classified elsewhere B97.30
- human
  - immunodeficiency, type 2 (HIV 2) B97.35
  - T-cell lymphotropic
    - type I (HTLV-I) B97.33
    - type II (HTLV-II) B97.34
  - lentivirus B97.31
  - oncovirus B97.32
  - specified NEC B97.39

Retrusion, premaxilla (developmental) M26.09

Rett's disease or syndrome F84.2

Reverse peristalsis R19.2

Reye's syndrome G93.7

Rh (factor)
- hemolytic disease (newborn) P55.0
- incompatibility, immunization or sensitization
  - affecting management of pregnancy NEC O36.09- ☑
    - anti-D antibody O36.01- ☑
  - newborn P55.0
  - transfusion reaction — *see* Complication(s), transfusion, incompatibility reaction, Rh (factor)
- negative mother affecting newborn P55.0
- titer elevated — *see* Complication(s), transfusion, incompatibility reaction, Rh (factor)
- transfusion reaction — *see* Complication(s), transfusion, incompatibility reaction, Rh (factor)

Rhabdomyolysis (idiopathic) NEC M62.82
- traumatic T79.6 ☑

Rhabdomyoma (*see also* Neoplasm, connective tissue, benign)
- adult — *see* Neoplasm, connective tissue, benign
- fetal — *see* Neoplasm, connective tissue, benign
- glycogenic — *see* Neoplasm, connective tissue, benign

Rhabdomyosarcoma (any type) — *see* Neoplasm, connective tissue, malignant

Rhabdosarcoma — *see* Rhabdomyosarcoma

Rhesus (factor) incompatibility — *see* Rh, incompatibility

Rheumatic (acute) (subacute) (chronic)
- adherent pericardium I09.2
- coronary arteritis I01.9
- degeneration, myocardium I09.0
- fever (acute) — *see* Fever, rheumatic
- heart — *see* Disease, heart, rheumatic
- myocardial degeneration — *see* Degeneration, myocardium
- myocarditis (chronic) (inactive) (with chorea) I09.0
  - active or acute I01.2
    - with chorea (acute) (rheumatic) (Sydenham's) I02.0
- pancarditis, acute I01.8
  - with chorea (acute) (rheumatic) Sydenham's) I02.0
- pericarditis (active) (acute) (with effusion) (with pneumonia) I01.0
  - with chorea (acute) (rheumatic) (Sydenham's) I02.0
- chronic or inactive I09.2
- pneumonia I00 [J17]
- torticollis M43.6
- typhoid fever A01.09

Rheumatism (articular) (neuralgic) (nonarticular) M79.0
- gout — *see* Arthritis, rheumatoid
- intercostal, meaning Tietze's disease M94.0
- palindromic (any site) M12.30
  - ankle M12.37- ☑
  - elbow M12.32- ☑
  - foot joint M12.37- ☑
  - hand joint M12.34- ☑
  - hip M12.35- ☑
  - knee M12.36- ☑
  - multiple site M12.39
  - shoulder M12.31- ☑
  - specified joint NEC M12.38
  - vertebrae M12.38
  - wrist M12.33- ☑

Rheumatism — *continued*
- sciatic M54.4- ☑

Rheumatoid (*see also* condition)
- arthritis (*see also* Arthritis, rheumatoid)
  - with involvement of organs NEC M05.60
    - ankle M05.67- ☑
    - elbow M05.62- ☑
    - foot joint M05.618
    - hand joint M05.64- ☑
    - hip M05.65- ☑
    - knee M05.66- ☑
    - multiple site M05.69
    - shoulder M05.61- ☑
    - vertebra — *see* Spondylitis, ankylosing
    - wrist M05.63- ☑
  - seronegative — *see* Arthritis, rheumatoid, seronegative
  - seropositive — *see* Arthritis, rheumatoid, seropositive
- carditis M05.30
  - ankle M05.37- ☑
  - elbow M05.32- ☑
  - foot joint M05.37- ☑
  - hand joint M05.34- ☑
  - hip M05.35- ☑
  - knee M05.36- ☑
  - multiple site M05.39
  - shoulder M05.31- ☑
  - vertebra — *see* Spondylitis, ankylosing
  - wrist M05.33- ☑
- endocarditis — *see* Rheumatoid, carditis
- lung (disease) M05.10
  - ankle M05.17- ☑
  - elbow M05.12- ☑
  - foot joint M05.17- ☑
  - hand joint M05.14- ☑
  - hip M05.15- ☑
  - knee M05.16- ☑
  - multiple site M05.19
  - shoulder M05.11- ☑
  - vertebra — *see* Spondylitis, ankylosing
  - wrist M05.13- ☑
- myocarditis — *see* Rheumatoid, carditis
- myopathy M05.40
  - ankle M05.47- ☑
  - elbow M05.42- ☑
  - foot joint M05.47- ☑
  - hand joint M05.44- ☑
  - hip M05.45- ☑
  - knee M05.46- ☑
  - multiple site M05.49
  - shoulder M05.41- ☑
  - vertebra — *see* Spondylitis, ankylosing
  - wrist M05.43- ☑
- pericarditis — *see* Rheumatoid, carditis
- polyarthritis — *see* Arthritis, rheumatoid
- polyneuropathy M05.50
  - ankle M05.57- ☑
  - elbow M05.52- ☑
  - foot joint M05.57- ☑
  - hand joint M05.54- ☑
  - hip M05.55- ☑
  - knee M05.56- ☑
  - multiple site M05.59
  - shoulder M05.51- ☑
  - vertebra — *see* Spondylitis, ankylosing
  - wrist M05.53- ☑
- vasculitis M05.20
  - ankle M05.27- ☑
  - elbow M05.22- ☑
  - foot joint M05.27- ☑
  - hand joint M05.24- ☑
  - hip M05.25- ☑
  - knee M05.26- ☑
  - multiple site M05.29
  - shoulder M05.21- ☑
  - vertebra — *see* Spondylitis, ankylosing
  - wrist M05.23- ☑

Rhinitis (atrophic) (catarrhal) (chronic) (croupous) (fibrinous) (granulomatous) (hyperplastic) (hypertrophic) (membranous) (obstructive) (purulent) (suppurative) (ulcerative) J31.0
- with
  - sore throat — *see* Nasopharyngitis
- acute J00
- allergic J30.9
  - with asthma J45.909
    - with
      - exacerbation (acute) J45.901
      - status asthmaticus J45.902
  - due to
    - food J30.5

☑ **Additional character required**

Rhinitis — *continued*
pollen J30.1
nonseasonal J30.89
perennial J30.89
seasonal NEC J30.2
specified NEC J30.89
infective J00
pneumococcal J00
syphilitic A52.73
congenital A50.05 [J99]
tuberculous A15.8
vasomotor J30.0
Rhinoantritis (chronic) — *see* Sinusitis, maxillary
Rhinodacryolith — *see* Dacryolith
Rhinolith (nasal sinus) J34.89
Rhinomegaly J34.89
Rhinopharyngitis (acute) (subacute) (*see also* Nasopharyngitis)
chronic J31.1
destructive ulcerating A66.5
mutilans A66.5
Rhinophyma L71.1
Rhinorrhea J34.89
cerebrospinal (fluid) G96.0
paroxysmal — *see* Rhinitis, allergic
spasmodic — *see* Rhinitis, allergic
Rhinosalpingitis — *see* Salpingitis, eustachian
Rhinoscleroma A48.8
Rhinosporidiosis B48.1
Rhinovirus infection NEC B34.8
Rhizomelic chondrodysplasia punctata E71.540
Rhythm
atrioventricular nodal I49.8
disorder I49.9
coronary sinus I49.8
ectopic I49.8
nodal I49.8
escape I49.9
heart, abnormal I49.9
idioventricular I44.2
nodal I49.8
sleep, inversion G47.2- ☑
nonorganic origin — *see* Disorder, sleep, circadian rhythm, psychogenic
Rhytidosis facialis L98.8
Rib (*see also* condition)
cervical Q76.5
Riboflavin deficiency E53.0
Rice bodies (*see also* Loose, body, joint)
knee M23.4- ☑
Richter syndrome — *see* Leukemia, chronic lymphocytic, B-cell type
Richter's hernia — *see* Hernia, abdomen, with obstruction
Ricinism — *see* Poisoning, food, noxious, plant
Rickets (active) (acute) (adolescent) (chest wall) (congenital) (current) (infantile) (intestinal) E55.0
adult — *see* Osteomalacia
celiac K90.0
hypophosphatemic with nephrotic-glycosuric dwarfism E72.09
inactive E64.3
kidney N25.0
renal N25.0
sequelae, any E64.3
vitamin-D-resistant E83.31 [M90.80]
Rickettsial disease A79.9
specified type NEC A79.89
Rickettsialpox (Rickettsia akari) A79.1
Rickettsiosis A79.9
due to
Ehrlichia sennetsu A79.81
Rickettsia akari (rickettsialpox) A79.1
specified type NEC A79.89
tick-borne A77.9
vesicular A79.1
Rider's bone — *see* Ossification, muscle, specified NEC
Ridge, alveolus (*see also* condition)
flabby K06.8
Ridged ear, congenital Q17.3
Riedel's
lobe, liver Q44.7
struma, thyroiditis or disease E06.5
Rieger's anomaly or syndrome Q13.81
Riehl's melanosis L81.4
Rietti-Greppi-Micheli anemia D56.9
Rieux's hernia — *see* Hernia, abdomen, specified site NEC
Riga (-Fede) disease K14.0
Riggs' disease — *see* Periodontitis
Right middle lobe syndrome J98.11

Rigid, rigidity (*see also* condition)
abdominal R19.30
with severe abdominal pain R10.0
epigastric R19.36
generalized R19.37
left lower quadrant R19.34
left upper quadrant R19.32
periumbilic R19.35
right lower quadrant R19.33
right upper quadrant R19.31
articular, multiple, congenital Q68.8
cervix (uteri) in pregnancy — *see* Pregnancy, complicated by, abnormal, cervix
hymen (acquired) (congenital) N89.6
nuchal R29.1
pelvic floor in pregnancy — *see* Pregnancy, complicated by, abnormal, pelvic organs or tissues NEC
perineum or vulva in pregnancy — *see* Pregnancy, complicated by, abnormal, vulva
spine — *see* Dorsopathy, specified NEC
vagina in pregnancy — *see* Pregnancy, complicated by, abnormal, vagina
Rigors R68.89
with fever R50.9
Riley-Day syndrome G90.1
RIND (reversible ischemic neurologic deficit) I63.9
Ring (s)
aorta (vascular) Q25.4
Bandl's O62.4
contraction, complicating delivery O62.4
esophageal, lower (muscular) K22.2
Fleischer's (cornea) H18.04- ☑
hymenal, tight (acquired) (congenital) N89.6
Kayser-Fleischer (cornea) H18.04- ☑
retraction, uterus, pathological O62.4
Schatzki's (esophagus) (lower) K22.2
congenital Q39.3
Soemmerring's — *see* Cataract, secondary
vascular (congenital) Q25.8
aorta Q25.4
Ringed hair (congenital) Q84.1
Ringworm B35.9
beard B35.0
black dot B35.0
body B35.4
Burmese B35.5
corporeal B35.4
foot B35.3
groin B35.6
hand B35.2
honeycomb B35.0
nails B35.1
perianal (area) B35.6
scalp B35.0
specified NEC B35.8
Tokelau B35.5
Rise, venous pressure I87.8
Risk, suicidal
meaning personal history of attempted suicide Z91.5
meaning suicidal ideation — *see* Ideation, suicidal
Ritter's disease L00
Rivalry, sibling Z62.891
Rivalta's disease A42.2
River blindness B73.01
Robert's pelvis Q74.2
with disproportion (fetopelvic) O33.0
causing obstructed labor O65.0
Robin (-Pierre) syndrome Q87.0
Robinow-Silvermann-Smith syndrome Q87.1
Robinson's (hidrotic) ectodermal dysplasia or syndrome Q82.4
Robles' disease B73.01
Rocky Mountain (spotted) fever A77.0
Roetheln — *see* Rubella
Roger's disease Q21.0
Rokitansky-Aschoff sinuses (gallbladder) K82.8
Rolando's fracture (displaced) S62.22- ☑
nondisplaced S62.22- ☑
Romano-Ward (prolonged QT interval) syndrome I45.81
Romberg's disease or syndrome G51.8
Roof, mouth — *see* condition
Rosacea L71.9
acne L71.9
keratitis L71.8
specified NEC L71.8
Rosary, rachitic E55.0
Rose
cold J30.1
fever J30.1

Rose — *continued*
rash R21
epidemic B06.9
Rosenbach's erysipeloid A26.0
Rosenthal's disease or syndrome D68.1
Roseola B09
infantum B08.20
due to human herpesvirus 6 B08.21
due to human herpesvirus 7 B08.22
Rossbach's disease K31.89
psychogenic F45.8
Ross River disease or fever B33.1
Rostan's asthma (cardiac) — *see* Failure, ventricular, left
Rotation
anomalous, incomplete or insufficient, intestine Q43.3
cecum (congenital) Q43.3
colon (congenital) Q43.3
spine, incomplete or insufficient — *see* Dorsopathy, deforming, specified NEC
tooth, teeth, fully erupted M26.35
vertebra, incomplete or insufficient — *see* Dorsopathy, deforming, specified NEC
Rotes Quérol disease or syndrome — *see* Hyperostosis, ankylosing
Roth (-Bernhardt) disease or syndrome — *see* Meralgia paraesthetica
Rothmund (-Thomson) syndrome Q82.8
Rotor's disease or syndrome E80.6
Round
back (with wedging of vertebrae) — *see* Kyphosis
sequelae (late effect) of rickets E64.3
worms (large) (infestation) NEC B82.0
Ascariasis (*see also* Ascariasis) B77.9
Roussy-Lévy syndrome G60.0
Rubella (German measles) B06.9
complication NEC B06.09
neurological B06.00
congenital P35.0
contact Z20.4
exposure to Z20.4
maternal
manifest rubella in infant P35.0
care for (suspected) damage to fetus O35.3 ☑
suspected damage to fetus affecting management of pregnancy O35.3 ☑
specified complications NEC B06.89
Rubeola (meaning measles) — *see* Measles
meaning rubella — *see* Rubella
Rubeosis, iris — *see* Disorder, iris, vascular
Rubinstein-Taybi syndrome Q87.2
Rudimentary (congenital) (*see also* Agenesis)
arm — *see* Defect, reduction, upper limb
bone Q79.9
cervix uteri Q51.828
eye Q11.2
lobule of ear Q17.3
patella Q74.1
respiratory organs in thoracopagus Q89.4
tracheal bronchus Q32.4
uterus Q51.818
in male Q56.1
vagina Q52.0
Ruled out condition — *see* Observation, suspected
Rumination R11.10
with nausea R11.2
disorder of infancy F98.21
neurotic F42
newborn P92.1
obsessional F42
psychogenic F42
Runeberg's disease D51.0
Runny nose R09.89
Rupia (syphilitic) A51.39
congenital A50.06
tertiary A52.79
Rupture, ruptured
abscess (spontaneous) - code by site under Abscess
aneurysm — *see* Aneurysm
anus (sphincter) — *see* Laceration, anus
aorta, aortic I71.8
abdominal I71.3
arch I71.1
ascending I71.1
descending I71.8
abdominal I71.3
thoracic I71.1
syphilitic A52.01
thoracoabdominal I71.5
thorax, thoracic I71.1

Rupture — continued
- transverse I71.1
  - traumatic — *see* Injury, aorta, laceration, major
  - valve or cusp (*see also* Endocarditis, aortic) I35.8
- appendix (with peritonitis) K35.2
- arteriovenous fistula, brain I60.8
- artery I77.2
  - brain — *see* Hemorrhage, intracranial, intracerebral
  - coronary — *see* Infarct, myocardium
  - heart — *see* Infarct, myocardium
  - pulmonary I28.8
  - traumatic (complication) — *see* Injury, blood vessel
- bile duct (common) (hepatic) K83.2
  - cystic K82.2
- bladder (sphincter) (nontraumatic) (spontaneous) N32.89
  - following ectopic or molar pregnancy O08.6
  - obstetrical trauma O71.5
  - traumatic S37.29 ☑
- blood vessel (*see also* Hemorrhage)
  - brain — *see* Hemorrhage, intracranial, intracerebral
  - heart — *see* Infarct, myocardium
  - traumatic (complication) — *see* Injury, blood vessel, laceration, major, by site
- bone — *see* Fracture
- bowel (nontraumatic) K63.1
- brain
  - aneurysm (congenital) (*see also* Hemorrhage, intracranial, subarachnoid)
    - syphilitic A52.05
  - hemorrhagic — *see* Hemorrhage, intracranial, intracerebral
- capillaries I78.8
- cardiac (auricle) (ventricle) (wall) I23.3
  - with hemopericardium I23.0
  - infectional I40.9
  - traumatic — *see* Injury, heart
- cartilage (articular) (current) (*see also* Sprain)
  - knee S83.3- ☑
  - semilunar — *see* Tear, meniscus
- cecum (with peritonitis) K65.0
  - with peritoneal abscess K35.3
  - traumatic S36.598 ☑
- celiac artery, traumatic — *see* Injury, blood vessel, celiac artery, laceration, major
- cerebral aneurysm (congenital) (see Hemorrhage, intracranial, subarachnoid)
- cervix (uteri)
  - with ectopic or molar pregnancy O08.6
  - following ectopic or molar pregnancy O08.6
  - obstetrical trauma O71.3
  - traumatic S37.69 ☑
- chordae tendineae NEC I51.1
  - concurrent with acute myocardial infarction — *see* Infarct, myocardium
  - following acute myocardial infarction (current complication) I23.4
- choroid (direct) (indirect) (traumatic) H31.32- ☑
- circle of Willis I60.6
- colon (nontraumatic) K63.1
  - traumatic — *see* Injury, intestine, large
- cornea (traumatic) — *see* Injury, eye, laceration
- coronary (artery) (thrombotic) — *see* Infarct, myocardium
- corpus luteum (infected) (ovary) N83.1
- cyst — *see* Cyst
- cystic duct K82.2
- Descemet's membrane — *see* Change, corneal membrane, Descemet's, rupture
  - traumatic — *see* Injury, eye, laceration
- diaphragm, traumatic — *see* Injury, intrathoracic, diaphragm
- disc — *see* Rupture, intervertebral disc
- diverticulum (intestine) K57.80
  - with bleeding K57.81
  - bladder N32.3
  - large intestine K57.20
    - with
      - bleeding K57.21
      - small intestine K57.40
        - with bleeding K57.41
  - small intestine K57.00
    - with
      - bleeding K57.01
      - large intestine K57.40
        - with bleeding K57.41
- duodenal stump K31.89
- ear drum (nontraumatic) (*see also* Perforation, tympanum)

Rupture — continued
- traumatic S09.2- ☑
  - due to blast injury — *see* Injury, blast, ear
- esophagus K22.3
- eye (without prolapse or loss of intraocular tissue) — *see* Injury, eye, laceration
- fallopian tube NEC (nonobstetric) (nontraumatic) N83.8
  - due to pregnancy O00.1
- fontanel P13.1
- gallbladder K82.2
  - traumatic S36.128 ☑
- gastric (*see also* Rupture, stomach)
  - vessel K92.2
- globe (eye) (traumatic) — *see* Injury, eye, laceration
- graafian follicle (hematoma) N83.0
- heart — *see* Rupture, cardiac
- hymen (nontraumatic) (nonintentional) N89.8
- internal organ, traumatic — *see* Injury, by site
- intervertebral disc — *see* Displacement, intervertebral disc
  - traumatic — *see* Rupture, traumatic, intervertebral disc
- intestine NEC (nontraumatic) K63.1
  - traumatic — *see* Injury, intestine
- iris (*see also* Abnormality, pupillary)
  - traumatic — *see* Injury, eye, laceration
- joint capsule, traumatic — *see* Sprain
- kidney (traumatic) S37.06- ☑
  - birth injury P15.8
  - nontraumatic N28.89
- lacrimal duct (traumatic) — *see* Injury, eye, specified site NEC
- lens (cataract) (traumatic) — *see* Cataract, traumatic
- ligament, traumatic — *see* Rupture, traumatic, ligament, by site
- liver S36.116 ☑
  - birth injury P15.0
- lymphatic vessel I89.8
- marginal sinus (placental) (with hemorrhage) — *see* Hemorrhage, antepartum, specified cause NEC
- membrana tympani (nontraumatic) — *see* Perforation, tympanum
- membranes (spontaneous)
  - artificial
    - delayed delivery following O75.5
    - delayed delivery following — *see* Pregnancy, complicated by, premature rupture of membranes
- meningeal artery I60.8
- meniscus (knee) (*see also* Tear, meniscus)
  - old — *see* Derangement, meniscus
  - site other than knee - code as Sprain
- mesenteric artery, traumatic — *see* Injury, mesenteric, artery, laceration, major
- mesentery (nontraumatic) K66.8
  - traumatic — *see* Injury, intra-abdominal, specified, site NEC
- mitral (valve) I34.8
- muscle (traumatic) (*see also* Strain)
  - diastasis — *see* Diastasis, muscle
  - nontraumatic M62.10
    - ankle M62.17- ☑
    - foot M62.17- ☑
    - forearm M62.13- ☑
    - hand M62.14- ☑
    - lower leg M62.16- ☑
    - pelvic region M62.15- ☑
    - shoulder region M62.11- ☑
    - specified site NEC M62.18
    - thigh M62.15- ☑
    - upper arm M62.12- ☑
  - traumatic — *see* Strain, by site
- musculotendinous junction NEC, nontraumatic — *see* Rupture, tendon, spontaneous
- mycotic aneurysm causing cerebral hemorrhage — *see* Hemorrhage, intracranial, subarachnoid
- myocardium, myocardial — *see* Rupture, cardiac
  - traumatic — *see* Injury, heart
- nontraumatic, meaning hernia — *see* Hernia
  - obstructed — *see* Hernia, by site, obstructed
- operation wound — *see* Disruption, wound, operation
- ovary, ovarian N83.8
  - corpus luteum cyst N83.1
  - follicle (graafian) N83.0
- oviduct (nonobstetric) (nontraumatic) N83.8
  - due to pregnancy O00.1

Rupture — continued
- pancreas (nontraumatic) K86.8
  - traumatic S36.299 ☑
- papillary muscle NEC I51.2
  - following acute myocardial infarction (current complication) I23.5
- pelvic
  - floor, complicating delivery O70.1
  - organ NEC, obstetrical trauma O71.5
- perineum (nonobstetric) (nontraumatic) N90.89
  - complicating delivery — *see* Delivery, complicated, by, laceration, anus (sphincter)
- postoperative wound — *see* Disruption, wound, operation
- prostate (traumatic) S37.828 ☑
- pulmonary
  - artery I28.8
  - valve (heart) I37.8
  - vein I28.8
  - vessel I28.8
- pus tube — *see* Salpingitis
- pyosalpinx — *see* Salpingitis
- rectum (nontraumatic) K63.1
  - traumatic S36.69 ☑
- retina, retinal (traumatic) (without detachment) (*see also* Break, retina)
  - with detachment — *see* Detachment, retina, with retinal, break
- rotator cuff (nontraumatic) M75.10- ☑
  - complete M75.12- ☑
  - incomplete M75.11- ☑
- sclera — *see* Injury, eye, laceration
- sigmoid (nontraumatic) K63.1
  - traumatic S36.593 ☑
- spinal cord (*see also* Injury, spinal cord, by region)
  - due to injury at birth P11.5
  - newborn (birth injury) P11.5
- spleen (traumatic) S36.09 ☑
  - birth injury P15.1
  - congenital (birth injury) P15.1
  - due to P. vivax malaria B51.0
  - nontraumatic D73.5
  - spontaneous D73.5
- splenic vein R58
  - traumatic — *see* Injury, blood vessel, splenic vein
- stomach (nontraumatic) (spontaneous) K31.89
  - traumatic S36.39 ☑
- supraspinatus (complete) (incomplete) (nontraumatic) — *see* Tear, rotator cuff
- symphysis pubis
  - obstetric O71.6
  - traumatic S33.4 ☑
- synovium (cyst) M66.10
  - ankle M66.17- ☑
  - elbow M66.12- ☑
  - finger M66.14- ☑
  - foot M66.17- ☑
  - forearm M66.13- ☑
  - hand M66.14- ☑
  - pelvic region M66.15- ☑
  - shoulder region M66.11- ☑
  - specified site NEC M66.18
  - thigh M66.15- ☑
  - toe M66.17- ☑
  - upper arm M66.12- ☑
  - wrist M66.13- ☑
- tendon (traumatic) — *see* Strain
  - nontraumatic (spontaneous) M66.9
    - ankle M66.87- ☑
    - extensor M66.20
      - ankle M66.27- ☑
      - foot M66.27- ☑
      - forearm M66.23- ☑
      - hand M66.24- ☑
      - lower leg M66.26- ☑
      - multiple sites M66.29
      - pelvic region M66.25- ☑
      - shoulder region M66.21- ☑
      - specified site NEC M66.28
      - thigh M66.25- ☑
      - upper arm M66.22- ☑
    - flexor M66.30
      - ankle M66.37- ☑
      - foot M66.37- ☑
      - forearm M66.33- ☑
      - hand M66.34- ☑
      - lower leg M66.36- ☑
      - multiple sites M66.39
      - pelvic region M66.35- ☑
      - shoulder region M66.31- ☑

☑ **Additional character required**

Rupture — *continued*
  specified site NEC M66.38
    thigh M66.35- ☑
    upper arm M66.32- ☑
  foot M66.87- ☑
  forearm M66.83- ☑
  hand M66.84- ☑
  lower leg M66.86- ☑
  multiple sites M66.89
  pelvic region M66.85- ☑
  shoulder region M66.81- ☑
  specified
    site NEC M66.88
    tendon M66.80
  thigh M66.85- ☑
  upper arm M66.82- ☑
thoracic duct I89.8
tonsil J35.8
traumatic
  aorta — *see* Injury, aorta, laceration, major
  diaphragm — *see* Injury, intrathoracic, diaphragm
  external site — *see* Wound, open, by site
  eye — *see* Injury, eye, laceration
  internal organ — *see* Injury, by site
  intervertebral disc
    cervical S13.0 ☑
    lumbar S33.0 ☑
    thoracic S23.0 ☑
  kidney S37.06- ☑
  ligament (*see also* Sprain)
    ankle — *see* Sprain, ankle
    carpus — *see* Rupture, traumatic, ligament, wrist
    collateral (hand) — *see* Rupture, traumatic, ligament, finger, collateral
    finger (metacarpophalangeal) (interphalangeal) S63.40- ☑
      collateral S63.41- ☑
        index S63.41- ☑
        little S63.41- ☑
        middle S63.41- ☑
        ring S63.41- ☑
      index S63.40- ☑
      little S63.40- ☑
      middle S63.40- ☑
      palmar S63.42- ☑
        index S63.42- ☑
        little S63.42- ☑
        middle S63.42- ☑
        ring S63.42- ☑
      ring S63.40- ☑
      specified site NEC S63.499 ☑
        index S63.49- ☑
        little S63.49- ☑
        middle S63.49- ☑
        ring S63.49- ☑
      volar plate S63.43- ☑
        index S63.43- ☑
        little S63.43- ☑
        middle S63.43- ☑
        ring S63.43- ☑
    foot — *see* Sprain, foot
    radial collateral S53.2- ☑
    radiocarpal — *see* Rupture, traumatic, ligament, wrist, radiocarpal
    ulnar collateral S53.3- ☑
    ulnocarpal — *see* Rupture, traumatic, ligament, wrist, ulnocarpal
    wrist S63.30- ☑
      collateral S63.31- ☑
      radiocarpal S63.32- ☑
      specified site NEC S63.39- ☑
      ulnocarpal (palmar) S63.33- ☑
  liver S36.116 ☑
  membrana tympani — *see* Rupture, ear drum, traumatic
  muscle or tendon — *see* Strain
  myocardium — *see* Injury, heart
  pancreas S36.299 ☑
  rectum S36.69 ☑
  sigmoid S36.593 ☑
  spleen S36.09 ☑
  stomach S36.39 ☑
  symphysis pubis S33.4 ☑
  tympanum, tympanic (membrane) — *see* Rupture, ear drum, traumatic
  ureter S37.19 ☑
  uterus S37.69 ☑
  vagina — *see* Injury, vagina
  vena cava — *see* Injury, vena cava, laceration, major

Rupture — *continued*
  tricuspid (heart) (valve) I07.8
  tube, tubal (nonobstetric) (nontraumatic) N83.8
    abscess — *see* Salpingitis
    due to pregnancy O00.1
  tympanum, tympanic (membrane) (nontraumatic) (*see also* Perforation, tympanic membrane) H72.9- ☑
    traumatic — *see* Rupture, ear drum, traumatic
  umbilical cord, complicating delivery O69.89 ☑
  ureter (traumatic) S37.19 ☑
    nontraumatic N28.89
  urethra (nontraumatic) N36.8
    with ectopic or molar pregnancy O08.6
    following ectopic or molar pregnancy O08.6
    obstetrical trauma O71.5
    traumatic S37.39 ☑
  uterosacral ligament (nonobstetric) (nontraumatic) N83.8
  uterus (traumatic) S37.69 ☑
    before labor O71.0- ☑
    during or after labor O71.1
    nonpuerperal, nontraumatic N85.8
    pregnant (during labor) O71.1
      before labor O71.0- ☑
  vagina — *see* Injury, vagina
  valve, valvular (heart) — *see* Endocarditis
  varicose vein — *see* Varix
  varix — *see* Varix
  vena cava R58
    traumatic — *see* Injury, vena cava, laceration, major
  vesical (urinary) N32.89
  vessel (blood) R58
    pulmonary I28.8
    traumatic — *see* Injury, blood vessel
  viscus R19.8
  vulva complicating delivery O70.0
Russell-Silver syndrome Q87.1
Russian spring-summer type encephalitis A84.0
Rust's disease (tuberculous cervical spondylitis) A18.01
Ruvalcaba-Myhre-Smith syndrome E71.440
Rytand-Lipsitch syndrome I44.2

S

Saber, sabre shin or tibia (syphilitic) A50.56 [M90.8- ☑]
Sac lacrimal — *see* condition
Saccharomyces infection B37.9
Saccharopinuria E72.3
Saccular — *see* condition
Sacculation
  aorta (nonsyphilitic) — *see* Aneurysm, aorta
  bladder N32.3
  intralaryngeal (congenital) (ventricular) Q31.3
  larynx (congenital) (ventricular) Q31.3
  organ or site, congenital — *see* Distortion
  pregnant uterus — *see* Pregnancy, complicated by, abnormal, uterus
  ureter N28.89
  urethra N36.1
  vesical N32.3
Sachs' amaurotic familial idiocy or disease E75.02
Sachs-Tay disease E75.02
Sacks-Libman disease M32.11
Sacralgia M53.3
Sacralization Q76.49
Sacrodynia M53.3
Sacroiliac joint — *see* condition
Sacroiliitis NEC M46.1
Sacrum — *see* condition
Saddle
  back — *see* Lordosis
  embolus
    abdominal aorta I74.01
    pulmonary artery I26.92
      with acute cor pulmonale I26.02
  injury - code to condition
  nose M95.0
    due to syphilis A50.57
Sadism (sexual) F65.52
Sadness, postpartal O90.6
Sadomasochism F65.50
Saemisch's ulcer (cornea) — *see* Ulcer, cornea, central
Sahib disease B55.0
Sailors' skin L57.8

Saint
  Anthony's fire — *see* Erysipelas
  triad — *see* Hernia, diaphragm
  Vitus' dance — *see* Chorea, Sydenham's
Salaam
  attack (s) — *see* Epilepsy, spasms
  tic R25.8
Salicylism
  abuse F55.8
  overdose or wrong substance given — *see* Table of Drugs and Chemicals, by drug, poisoning
Salivary duct or gland — *see* condition
Salivation, excessive K11.7
Salmonella — *see* Infection, Salmonella
Salmonellosis A02.0
Salpingitis (catarrhal) (fallopian tube) (nodular) (pseudofollicular) (purulent) (septic) N70.91
  with oophoritis N70.93
  acute N70.01
    with oophoritis N70.03
  chlamydial A56.11
  chronic N70.11
    with oophoritis N70.13
  complicating abortion — *see* Abortion, by type, complicated by, salpingitis
  ear — *see* Salpingitis, eustachian
  eustachian (tube) H68.00- ☑
    acute H68.01- ☑
    chronic H68.02- ☑
  follicularis N70.11
    with oophoritis N70.13
  gonococcal (acute) (chronic) A54.24
  interstitial, chronic N70.11
    with oophoritis N70.13
  isthmica nodosa N70.11
    with oophoritis N70.13
  specific (gonococcal) (acute) (chronic) A54.24
  tuberculous (acute) (chronic) A18.17
  venereal (gonococcal) (acute) (chronic) A54.24
Salpingocele N83.4
Salpingo-oophoritis (catarrhal) (purulent) (ruptured) (septic) (suppurative) N70.93
  acute N70.03
    with ectopic or molar pregnancy O08.0
    following ectopic or molar pregnancy O08.0
    gonococcal A54.24
  chronic N70.13
  following ectopic or molar pregnancy O08.0
  gonococcal (acute) (chronic) A54.24
  puerperal O86.19
  specific (gonococcal) (acute) (chronic) A54.24
  subacute N70.03
  tuberculous (acute) (chronic) A18.17
  venereal (gonococcal) (acute) (chronic) A54.24
Salpingo-ovaritis — *see* Salpingo-oophoritis
Salpingoperitonitis — *see* Salpingo-oophoritis
Salzmann's nodular dystrophy — *see* Degeneration, cornea, nodular
Sampson's cyst or tumor N80.1
San Joaquin (Valley) fever B38.0
Sandblaster's asthma, lung or pneumoconiosis J62.8
Sander's disease (paranoia) F22
Sandfly fever A93.1
Sandhoff's disease E75.01
Sanfilippo (Type B) (Type C) (Type D) syndrome E76.22
Sanger-Brown ataxia G11.2
Sao Paulo fever or typhus A77.0
Saponification, mesenteric K65.8
Sarcocele (benign)
  syphilitic A52.76
    congenital A50.59
Sarcocystosis A07.8
Sarcoepiplocele — *see* Hernia
Sarcoepiplomphalocele Q79.2
Sarcoid (*see also* Sarcoidosis)
  arthropathy D86.86
  Boeck's D86.9
  Darier-Roussy D86.3
  iridocyclitis D86.83
  meningitis D86.81
  myocarditis D86.85
  myositis D86.87
  pyelonephritis D86.84
  Spiegler-Fendt L08.89
Sarcoidosis D86.9
  with
    cranial nerve palsies D86.82
    hepatic granuloma D86.89
    polyarthritis D86.86
    tubulo-interstitial nephropathy D86.84

Sarcoidosis — *continued*
  combined sites NEC D86.89
  lung D86.0
    and lymph nodes D86.2
  lymph nodes D86.1
    and lung D86.2
  meninges D86.81
  skin D86.3
  specified type NEC D86.89
Sarcoma (of) (*see also* Neoplasm, connective tissue, malignant)
  alveolar soft part — *see* Neoplasm, connective tissue, malignant
  ameloblastic C41.1
    upper jaw (bone) C41.0
  botryoid — *see* Neoplasm, connective tissue, malignant
  botryoides — *see* Neoplasm, connective tissue, malignant
  cerebellar C71.6
    circumscribed (arachnoidal) C71.6
  circumscribed (arachnoidal) cerebellar C71.6
  clear cell (*see also* Neoplasm, connective tissue, malignant)
    kidney C64.- ☑
  dendritic cells (accessory cells) C96.4
  embryonal — *see* Neoplasm, connective tissue, malignant
  endometrial (stromal) C54.1
    isthmus C54.0
  epithelioid (cell) — *see* Neoplasm, connective tissue, malignant
  Ewing's — *see* Neoplasm, bone, malignant
  follicular dendritic cell C96.4
  germinoblastic (diffuse) — *see* Lymphoma, diffuse large cell
    follicular — *see* Lymphoma, follicular, specified NEC
  giant cell (except of bone) (*see also* Neoplasm, connective tissue, malignant)
    bone — *see* Neoplasm, bone, malignant
  glomoid — *see* Neoplasm, connective tissue, malignant
  granulocytic C92.3- ☑
  hemangioendothelial — *see* Neoplasm, connective tissue, malignant
  hemorrhagic, multiple — *see* Sarcoma, Kaposi's
  histiocytic C96.A
  Hodgkin — *see* Lymphoma, Hodgkin
  immunoblastic (diffuse) — *see* Lymphoma, diffuse large cell
  interdigitating dendritic cell C96.4
  Kaposi's
    colon C46.4
    connective tissue C46.1
    gastrointestinal organ C46.4
    lung C46.5- ☑
    lymph node (s) C46.3
    palate (hard) (soft) C46.2
    rectum C46.4
    skin C46.0
    specified site NEC C46.7
    stomach C46.4
    unspecified site C46.9
  Kupffer cell C22.3
  Langerhans cell C96.4
  leptomeningeal — *see* Neoplasm, meninges, malignant
  liver NEC C22.4
  lymphangioendothelial — *see* Neoplasm, connective tissue, malignant
  lymphoblastic — *see* Lymphoma, lymphoblastic (diffuse)
  lymphocytic — *see* Lymphoma, small cell B-cell
  mast cell C96.2
  melanotic — *see* Melanoma
  meningeal — *see* Neoplasm, meninges, malignant
  meningothelial — *see* Neoplasm, meninges, malignant
  mesenchymal (*see also* Neoplasm, connective tissue, malignant)
    mixed — *see* Neoplasm, connective tissue, malignant
  mesothelial — *see* Mesothelioma
  monstrocellular
    specified site — *see* Neoplasm, malignant, by site
    unspecified site C71.9
  myeloid C92.3- ☑
  neurogenic — *see* Neoplasm, nerve, malignant
  odontogenic C41.1

Sarcoma — *continued*
  upper jaw (bone) C41.0
  osteoblastic — *see* Neoplasm, bone, malignant
  osteogenic (*see also* Neoplasm, bone, malignant)
    juxtacortical — *see* Neoplasm, bone, malignant
    periosteal — *see* Neoplasm, bone, malignant
  periosteal (*see also* Neoplasm, bone, malignant)
    osteogenic — *see* Neoplasm, bone, malignant
  pleomorphic cell — *see* Neoplasm, connective tissue, malignant
  reticulum cell (diffuse) — *see* Lymphoma, diffuse large cell
    nodular — *see* Lymphoma, follicular
    pleomorphic cell type — *see* Lymphoma, diffuse large cell
  rhabdoid — *see* Neoplasm, malignant, by site
  round cell — *see* Neoplasm, connective tissue, malignant
  small cell — *see* Neoplasm, connective tissue, malignant
  soft tissue — *see* Neoplasm, connective tissue, malignant
  spindle cell — *see* Neoplasm, connective tissue, malignant
  stromal (endometrial) C54.1
    isthmus C54.0
  synovial (*see also* Neoplasm, connective tissue, malignant)
    biphasic — *see* Neoplasm, connective tissue, malignant
    epithelioid cell — *see* Neoplasm, connective tissue, malignant
    spindle cell — *see* Neoplasm, connective tissue, malignant
Sarcomatosis
  meningeal — *see* Neoplasm, meninges, malignant
  specified site NEC — *see* Neoplasm, connective tissue, malignant
  unspecified site C80.1
Sarcosinemia E72.59
Sarcosporidiosis (intestinal) A07.8
Satiety, early R68.81
Saturnine — *see* condition
Saturnism
  overdose or wrong substance given or taken — *see* Table of Drugs and Chemicals, by drug, poisoning
Satyriasis F52.8
Sauriasis — *see* Ichthyosis
SBE (subacute bacterial endocarditis) I33.0
Scabs R23.4
Scabies (any site) B86
Scaglietti-Dagnini syndrome E22.0
Scald — *see* Burn
Scalenus anticus (anterior) syndrome G54.0
Scales R23.4
Scaling, skin R23.4
Scalp — *see* condition
Scapegoating affecting child Z62.3
Scaphocephaly Q75.0
Scapulalgia M89.8X1
Scapulohumeral myopathy G71.0
Scar, scarring (*see also* Cicatrix) L90.5
  adherent L90.5
  atrophic L90.5
  cervix
    in pregnancy or childbirth — *see* Pregnancy, complicated by, abnormal cervix
  cheloid L91.0
  chorioretinal H31.00- ☑
    posterior pole macula H31.01- ☑
    postsurgical H59.81- ☑
    solar retinopathy H31.02- ☑
    specified type NEC H31.09- ☑
  choroid — *see* Scar, chorioretinal
  conjunctiva H11.24- ☑
  cornea H17.9
    xerophthalmic (*see also* Opacity, cornea)
      vitamin A deficiency E50.6
  duodenum, obstructive K31.5
  hypertrophic L91.0
  keloid L91.0
  labia N90.89
  lung (base) J98.4
  macula — *see* Scar, chorioretinal, posterior pole
  muscle M62.89
  myocardium, myocardial I25.2
  painful L90.5
  posterior pole (eye) — *see* Scar, chorioretinal, posterior pole
  retina — *see* Scar, chorioretinal

Scar — *continued*
  trachea J39.8
  uterus N85.8
    in pregnancy O34.29
  vagina N89.8
    postoperative N99.2
  vulva N90.89
Scarabiasis B88.2
Scarlatina (anginosa) (maligna) (ulcerosa) A38.9
  myocarditis (acute) A38.1
    old — *see* Myocarditis
  otitis media A38.0
Scarlet fever (albuminuria) (angina) A38.9
Schamberg's disease (progressive pigmentary dermatosis) L81.7
Schatzki's ring (acquired) (esophagus) (lower) K22.2
  congenital Q39.3
Schaufenster krankheit I20.8
Schaumann's
  benign lymphogranulomatosis D86.1
  disease or syndrome — *see* Sarcoidosis
Scheie's syndrome E76.03
Schenck's disease B42.1
Scheuermann's disease or osteochondrosis — *see* Osteochondrosis, juvenile, spine
Schilder (-Flatau) disease G37.0
Schilling-type monocytic leukemia C93.0- ☑
Schimmelbusch's disease, cystic mastitis, or hyperplasia — *see* Mastopathy, cystic
Schistosoma infestation — *see* Infestation, Schistosoma
Schistosomiasis B65.9
  with muscle disorder B65.9 [M63.80]
    ankle B65.9 [M63.87- ☑]
    foot B65.9 [M63.87- ☑]
    forearm B65.9 [M63.83- ☑]
    hand B65.9 [M63.84- ☑]
    lower leg B65.9 [M63.86- ☑]
    multiple sites B65.9 [M63.89]
    pelvic region B65.9 [M63.85- ☑]
    shoulder region B65.9 [M63.81- ☑]
    specified site NEC B65.9 [M63.88]
    thigh B65.9 [M63.85- ☑]
    upper arm B65.9 [M63.82- ☑]
  Asiatic B65.2
  bladder B65.0
  chestermani B65.8
  colon B65.1
  cutaneous B65.3
  due to
    S. haematobium B65.0
    S. japonicum B65.2
    S. mansoni B65.1
    S. mattheii B65.8
  Eastern B65.2
  genitourinary tract B65.0
  intestinal B65.1
  lung NEC B65.9 [J99]
    pneumonia B65.9 [J17]
  Manson's (intestinal) B65.1
  oriental B65.2
  pulmonary NEC B65.9 [J99]
    pneumonia B65.9
  Schistosoma
    haematobium B65.0
    japonicum B65.2
    mansoni B65.1
  specified type NEC B65.8
  urinary B65.0
  vesical B65.0
Schizencephaly Q04.6
Schizoaffective psychosis F25.9
Schizodontia K00.2
Schizoid personality F60.1
Schizophrenia, schizophrenic F20.9
  acute (brief) (undifferentiated) F23
  atypical (form) F20.3
  borderline F21
  catalepsy F20.2
  catatonic (type) (excited) (withdrawn) F20.2
  cenesthopathic, cenesthesiopathic F20.89
  childhood type F84.5
  chronic undifferentiated F20.5
  cyclic F25.0
  disorganized (type) F20.1
  flexibilitas cerea F20.2
  hebephrenic (type) F20.1
  incipient F21
  latent F21
  negative type F20.5
  paranoid (type) F20.0
  paraphrenic F20.0

☑ **Additional character required**

Schizophrenia — continued
  post-psychotic depression F32.8
  prepsychotic F21
  prodromal F21
  pseudoneurotic F21
  pseudopsychopathic F21
  reaction F23
  residual (state) (type) F20.5
  restzustand F20.5
  schizoaffective (type) — see Psychosis,
    schizoaffective
  simple (type) F20.89
  simplex F20.89
  specified type NEC F20.89
  stupor F20.2
  syndrome of childhood F84.5
  undifferentiated (type) F20.3
    chronic F20.5
Schizothymia (persistent) F60.1
Schlatter-Osgood disease or osteochondrosis — see
  Osteochondrosis, juvenile, tibia
Schlatter's tibia — see Osteochondrosis, juvenile,
  tibia
Schmidt's syndrome (polyglandular, autoimmune)
  E31.0
Schmincke's carcinoma or tumor — see Neoplasm,
  nasopharynx, malignant
Schmitz (-Stutzer) dysentery A03.0
Schmorl's disease or nodes
  lumbar region M51.46
  lumbosacral region M51.47
  sacrococcygeal region M53.3
  thoracic region M51.44
  thoracolumbar region M51.45
Schneiderian
  papilloma — see Neoplasm, nasopharynx, benign
    specified site — see Neoplasm, benign, by site
    unspecified site D14.0
  specified site — see Neoplasm, malignant, by site
    unspecified site C30.0
Scholte's syndrome (malignant carcinoid) E34.0
Scholz (-Bielchowsky-Henneberg) disease or
  syndrome E75.25
Schönlein (-Henoch) disease or purpura (primary)
  (rheumatic) D69.0
Schottmuller's disease A01.4
Schroeder's syndrome (endocrine hypertensive)
  E27.0
Schüller-Christian disease or syndrome C96.5
Schultze's type acroparesthesia, simple I73.89
Schultz's disease or syndrome — see
  Agranulocytosis
Schwalbe-Ziehen-Oppenheim disease G24.1
Schwannoma (see also Neoplasm, nerve, benign)
  malignant (see also Neoplasm, nerve, malignant)
    with rhabdomyoblastic differentiation — see
      Neoplasm, nerve, malignant
  melanocytic — see Neoplasm, nerve, benign
  pigmented — see Neoplasm, nerve, benign
Schwannomatosis Q85.03
Schwartz (-Jampel) syndrome G71.13
Schwartz-Bartter syndrome E22.2
Schweniger-Buzzi anetoderma L90.1
Sciatic — see condition
Sciatica (infective)
  with lumbago M54.4- ☑
    due to intervertebral disc disorder — see
      Disorder, disc, with, radiculopathy
  due to displacement of intervertebral disc
    (with lumbago) — see Disorder, disc, with,
    radiculopathy
  wallet M54.3- ☑
Scimitar syndrome Q26.8
Sclera — see condition
Sclerectasia H15.84- ☑
Scleredema
  adultorum — see Sclerosis, systemic
  Buschke's — see Sclerosis, systemic
  newborn P83.0
Sclerema (adiposum) (edematosum) (neonatorum)
  (newborn) P83.0
  adultorum — see Sclerosis, systemic
Scleriasis — see Scleroderma
Scleritis H15.00- ☑
  with corneal involvement H15.04- ☑
  anterior H15.01- ☑
  brawny H15.02- ☑
  in (due to) zoster B02.34
  posterior H15.03- ☑
  specified type NEC H15.09- ☑
  syphilitic A52.71
  tuberculous (nodular) A18.51

Sclerochoroiditis H31.8
Scleroconjunctivitis — see Scleritis
Sclerocystic ovary syndrome E28.2
Sclerodactyly, sclerodactylia L94.3
Scleroderma, sclerodermia (acrosclerotic) (diffuse)
  (generalized) (progressive) (pulmonary) (see also
  Sclerosis, systemic) M34.9- ☑
  circumscribed L94.0
  linear L94.1
  localized L94.0
  newborn P83.8
  systemic M34.9
Sclerokeratitis H16.8
  tuberculous A18.52
Scleroma nasi A48.8
Scleromalacia (perforans) H15.05- ☑
Scleromyxedema L98.5
Sclérose en plaques G35
Sclerosis, sclerotic
  adrenal (gland) E27.8
  Alzheimer's — see Disease, Alzheimer's
  amyotrophic (lateral) G12.21
  aorta, aortic I70.0
    valve — see Endocarditis, aortic
  artery, arterial, arteriolar, arteriovascular — see
    Arteriosclerosis
  ascending multiple G35
  brain (generalized) (lobular) G37.9
    artery, arterial I67.2
    diffuse G37.0
    disseminated G35
    insular G35
    Krabbe's E75.23
    miliary G35
    multiple G35
    presenile (Alzheimer's) — see Disease,
      Alzheimer's, early onset
    senile (arteriosclerotic) I67.2
    stem, multiple G35
    tuberous Q85.1
  bulbar, multiple G35
  bundle of His I44.39
  cardiac — see Disease, heart, ischemic,
    atherosclerotic
  cardiorenal — see Hypertension, cardiorenal
  cardiovascular (see also Disease, cardiovascular)
    renal — see Hypertension, cardiorenal
  cerebellar — see Sclerosis, brain
  cerebral — see Sclerosis, brain
  cerebrospinal (disseminated) (multiple) G35
  cerebrovascular I67.2
  choroid — see Degeneration, choroid
  combined (spinal cord) (see also Degeneration,
    combined)
    multiple G35
  concentric (Balo) G37.5
  cornea — see Opacity, cornea
  coronary (artery) I25.10
    with angina pectoris — see Arteriosclerosis,
      coronary (artery),
  corpus cavernosum
    female N90.89
    male N48.6
  diffuse (brain) (spinal cord) G37.0
  disseminated G35
  dorsal G35
  dorsolateral (spinal cord) — see Degeneration,
    combined
  endometrium N85.5
  extrapyramidal G25.9
  eye, nuclear (senile) — see Cataract, senile,
    nuclear
  focal and segmental (glomerular) (see also
    N00-N07 with fourth character .1) N05.1
  Friedreich's (spinal cord) G11.1
  funicular (spermatic cord) N50.8
  general (vascular) — see Arteriosclerosis
  gland (lymphatic) I89.8
  hepatic K74.1
    alcoholic K70.2
  hereditary
    cerebellar G11.9
    spinal (Friedreich's ataxia) G11.1
  hippocampal G93.81
  insular G35
  kidney — see Sclerosis, renal
  larynx J38.7
  lateral (amyotrophic) (descending) (primary)
    (spinal) G12.21
  lens, senile nuclear — see Cataract, senile, nuclear
  liver K74.1
    with fibrosis K74.2

Sclerosis — continued
  alcoholic K70.2
  alcoholic K70.2
  cardiac K76.1
  lung — see Fibrosis, lung
  mastoid — see Mastoiditis, chronic
  mesial temporal G93.81
  mitral I05.8
  Mönckeberg's (medial) — see Arteriosclerosis,
    extremities
  multiple (brain stem) (cerebral) (generalized)
    (spinal cord) G35
  myocardium, myocardial — see Disease, heart,
    ischemic, atherosclerotic
  nuclear (senile), eye — see Cataract, senile,
    nuclear
  ovary N83.8
  pancreas K86.8
  penis N48.6
  peripheral arteries — see Arteriosclerosis,
    extremities
  plaques G35
  pluriglandular E31.8
  polyglandular E31.8
  posterolateral (spinal cord) — see Degeneration,
    combined
  presenile (Alzheimer's) — see Disease,
    Alzheimer's, early onset
  primary, lateral G12.29
  progressive, systemic M34.0
  pulmonary — see Fibrosis, lung
    artery I27.0
    valve (heart) — see Endocarditis, pulmonary
  renal N26.9
    with
      cystine storage disease E72.09
      hypertensive heart disease (conditions in I11)
        — see Hypertension, cardiorenal
      arteriolar (hyaline) (hyperplastic) — see
        Hypertension, kidney
  retina (senile) (vascular) H35.00
  senile (vascular) — see Arteriosclerosis
  spinal (cord) (progressive) G95.89
    ascending G61.0
    combined (see also Degeneration, combined)
      multiple G35
      syphilitic A52.11
    disseminated G35
    dorsolateral — see Degeneration, combined
    hereditary (Friedreich's) (mixed form) G11.1
    lateral (amyotrophic) G12.21
    multiple G35
    posterior (syphilitic) A52.11
  stomach K31.89
  subendocardial, congenital I42.4
  systemic M34.9
    with
      lung involvement M34.81
      myopathy M34.82
      polyneuropathy M34.83
    drug-induced M34.2
    due to chemicals NEC M34.2
    progressive M34.0
    specified NEC M34.89
  temporal (mesial) G93.81
  tricuspid (heart) (valve) I07.8
  tuberous (brain) Q85.1
  tympanic membrane — see Disorder, tympanic
    membrane, specified NEC
  valve, valvular (heart) — see Endocarditis
  vascular — see Arteriosclerosis
  vein I87.8
Scoliosis (acquired) (postural) M41.9
  adolescent (idiopathic) — see Scoliosis,
    idiopathic, juvenile
  congenital Q67.5
    due to bony malformation Q76.3
    failure of segmentation (hemivertebra) Q76.3
    hemivertebra fusion Q76.3
    postural Q67.5
  idiopathic M41.20
    adolescent M41.129
      cervical region M41.122
      cervicothoracic region M41.123
      lumbar region M41.126
      lumbosacral region M41.127
      thoracic region M41.124
      thoracolumbar region M41.125
    cervical region M41.22
    cervicothoracic region M41.23
    infantile M41.00
      cervical region M41.02

Scoliosis — *continued*
    cervicothoracic region M41.03
    lumbar region M41.06
    lumbosacral region M41.07
    sacrococcygeal region M41.08
    thoracic region M41.04
    thoracolumbar region M41.05
  juvenile M41.119
    cervical region M41.112
    cervicothoracic region M41.113
    lumbar region M41.116
    lumbosacral region M41.117
    thoracic region M41.114
    thoracolumbar region M41.115
  lumbar region M41.26
  lumbosacral region M41.27
  thoracic region M41.24
  thoracolumbar region M41.25
  neuromuscular M41.40
    cervical region M41.42
    cervicothoracic region M41.43
    lumbar region M41.46
    lumbosacral region M41.47
    occipito-atlanto-axial region M41.41
    thoracic region M41.44
    thoracolumbar region M41.45
  paralytic — *see* Scoliosis, neuromuscular
  postradiation therapy M96.5
  rachitic (late effect or sequelae) E64.3 [M49.80]
    cervical region E64.3 [M49.82]
    cervicothoracic region E64.3 [M49.83]
    lumbar region E64.3 [M49.86]
    lumbosacral region E64.3 [M49.87]
    multiple sites E64.3 [M49.89]
    occipito-atlanto-axial region E64.3 [M49.81]
    sacrococcygeal region E64.3 [M49.88]
    thoracic region E64.3 [M49.84]
    thoracolumbar region E64.3 [M49.85]
  sciatic M54.4- ☑
  secondary (to) NEC M41.50
    cerebral palsy, Friedreich's ataxia, poliomyelitis,
      neuromuscular disorders — *see* Scoliosis,
      neuromuscular
    cervical region M41.52
    cervicothoracic region M41.53
    lumbar region M41.56
    lumbosacral region M41.57
    thoracic region M41.54
    thoracolumbar region M41.55
  specified form NEC M41.80
    cervical region M41.82
    cervicothoracic region M41.83
    lumbar region M41.86
    lumbosacral region M41.87
    thoracic region M41.84
    thoracolumbar region M41.85
  thoracogenic M41.30
    thoracic region M41.34
    thoracolumbar region M41.35
  tuberculous A18.01
Scoliotic pelvis
  with disproportion (fetopelvic) O33.0
    causing obstructed labor O65.0
Scorbutus, scorbutic (*see also* Scurvy)
  anemia D53.2
Scotoma (arcuate) (Bjerrum) (central) (ring) (*see also*
  Defect, visual field, localized, scotoma)
  scintillating H53.19
Scratch — *see* Abrasion
Scratchy throat R09.89
Screening (for) Z13.9
  alcoholism Z13.89
  anemia Z13.0
  anomaly, congenital Z13.89
  antenatal, of mother Z36
  arterial hypertension Z13.6
  arthropod-borne viral disease NEC Z11.59
  bacteriuria, asymptomatic Z13.89
  behavioral disorder Z13.89
  brain injury, traumatic Z13.850
  bronchitis, chronic Z13.83
  brucellosis Z11.2
  cardiovascular disorder Z13.6
  cataract Z13.5
  chlamydial diseases Z11.8
  cholera Z11.0
  chromosomal abnormalities (nonprocreative)
    NEC Z13.79
  colonoscopy Z12.11
  congenital
    dislocation of hip Z13.89
    eye disorder Z13.5

Screening — *continued*
  malformation or deformation Z13.89
  contamination NEC Z13.88
  cystic fibrosis Z13.228
  dengue fever Z11.59
  dental disorder Z13.84
  depression Z13.89
  developmental handicap Z13.4
    in early childhood Z13.4
  diabetes mellitus Z13.1
  diphtheria Z11.2
  disability, intellectual Z13.4
  disease or disorder Z13.9
    bacterial NEC Z11.2
      intestinal infectious Z11.0
      respiratory tuberculosis Z11.1
    blood or blood-forming organ Z13.0
    cardiovascular Z13.6
    Chagas' Z11.6
    chlamydial Z11.8
    dental Z13.89
    developmental Z13.4
    digestive tract NEC Z13.818
      lower GI Z13.811
      upper GI Z13.810
    ear Z13.5
    endocrine Z13.29
    eye Z13.5
    genitourinary Z13.89
    heart Z13.6
    human immunodeficiency virus (HIV) infection
      Z11.4
    immunity Z13.0
    infection
      intestinal Z11.0
      specified NEC Z11.6
    infectious Z11.9
    mental Z13.89
    metabolic Z13.228
    neurological Z13.89
    nutritional Z13.21
      metabolic Z13.228
      lipoid disorders Z13.220
    protozoal Z11.6
      intestinal Z11.0
    respiratory Z13.83
    rheumatic Z13.828
    rickettsial Z11.8
    sexually-transmitted NEC Z11.3
      human immunodeficiency virus (HIV) Z11.4
    sickle-cell (trait) Z13.0
    skin Z13.89
    specified NEC Z13.89
    spirochetal Z11.8
    thyroid Z13.29
    vascular Z13.6
    venereal Z11.3
    viral NEC Z11.59
      human immunodeficiency virus (HIV) Z11.4
      intestinal Z11.0
  elevated titer Z13.89
  emphysema Z13.83
  encephalitis, viral (mosquito- or tick-borne)
    Z11.59
  exposure to contaminants (toxic) Z13.88
  fever
    dengue Z11.59
    hemorrhagic Z11.59
    yellow Z11.59
  filariasis Z11.6
  galactosemia Z13.228
  gastrointestinal condition Z13.818
  genetic (nonprocreative) - for procreative
    management — *see* Testing, genetic, for
    procreative management
    disease carrier status (nonprocreative) Z13.71
    specified NEC (nonprocreative) Z13.79
  genitourinary condition Z13.89
  glaucoma Z13.5
  gonorrhea Z11.3
  gout Z13.89
  helminthiasis (intestinal) Z11.6
  hematopoietic malignancy Z12.89
  hemoglobinopathies NEC Z13.0
  hemorrhagic fever Z11.59
  Hodgkin disease Z12.89
  human immunodeficiency virus (HIV) Z11.4
  human papillomavirus Z11.51
  hypertension Z13.6
  immunity disorders Z13.0
  infection
    mycotic Z11.8

Screening — *continued*
  parasitic Z11.8
  ingestion of radioactive substance Z13.88
  intellectual disability Z13.4
  intestinal
    helminthiasis Z11.6
    infectious disease Z11.0
  leishmaniasis Z11.6
  leprosy Z11.2
  leptospirosis Z11.8
  leukemia Z12.89
  lymphoma Z12.89
  malaria Z11.6
  malnutrition Z13.29
    metabolic Z13.228
    nutritional Z13.21
  measles Z11.59
  mental disorder Z13.89
  metabolic errors, inborn Z13.228
  multiphasic Z13.89
  musculoskeletal disorder Z13.828
    osteoporosis Z13.820
  mycoses Z11.8
  myocardial infarction (acute) Z13.6
  neoplasm (malignant) (of) Z12.9
    bladder Z12.6
    blood Z12.89
    breast Z12.39
      routine mammogram Z12.31
    cervix Z12.4
    colon Z12.11
    genitourinary organs NEC Z12.79
      bladder Z12.6
      cervix Z12.4
      ovary Z12.73
      prostate Z12.5
      testis Z12.71
      vagina Z12.72
    hematopoietic system Z12.89
    intestinal tract Z12.10
      colon Z12.11
      rectum Z12.12
      small intestine Z12.13
    lung Z12.2
    lymph (glands) Z12.89
    nervous system Z12.82
    oral cavity Z12.81
    prostate Z12.5
    rectum Z12.12
    respiratory organs Z12.2
    skin Z12.83
    small intestine Z12.13
    specified site NEC Z12.89
    stomach Z12.0
  nephropathy Z13.89
  nervous system disorders NEC Z13.858
  neurological condition Z13.89
  osteoporosis Z13.820
  parasitic infestation Z11.9
    specified NEC Z11.8
  phenylketonuria Z13.228
  plague Z11.2
  poisoning (chemical) (heavy metal) Z13.88
  poliomyelitis Z11.59
  postnatal, chromosomal abnormalities Z13.89
  prenatal, of mother Z36
  protozoal disease Z11.6
    intestinal Z11.0
  pulmonary tuberculosis Z11.1
  radiation exposure Z13.88
  respiratory condition Z13.83
  respiratory tuberculosis Z11.1
  rheumatoid arthritis Z13.828
  rubella Z11.59
  schistosomiasis Z11.6
  sexually-transmitted disease NEC Z11.3
    human immunodeficiency virus (HIV) Z11.4
  sickle-cell disease or trait Z13.0
  skin condition Z13.89
  sleeping sickness Z11.6
  special Z13.9
    specified NEC Z13.89
  syphilis Z11.3
  tetanus Z11.2
  trachoma Z11.8
  traumatic brain injury Z13.850
  trypanosomiasis Z11.6
  tuberculosis, respiratory Z11.1
  venereal disease Z11.3
  viral encephalitis (mosquito- or tick-borne)
    Z11.59
  whooping cough Z11.2

☑ **Additional character required**

Screening — *continued*
- worms, intestinal Z11.6
- yaws Z11.8
- yellow fever Z11.59

Scrofula, scrofulosis (tuberculosis of cervical lymph glands) A18.2

Scrofulide (primary) (tuberculous) A18.4

Scrofuloderma, scrofulodermia (any site) (primary) A18.4

Scrofulosus lichen (primary) (tuberculous) A18.4

Scrofulous — *see* condition

Scrotal tongue K14.5

Scrotum — *see* condition

Scurvy, scorbutic E54
- anemia D53.2
- gum E54
- infantile E54
- rickets E55.0 [M90.80]

Sealpox B08.62

Seasickness T75.3 ☑

Seatworm (infection) (infestation) B80

Sebaceous (*see also* condition)
- cyst — *see* Cyst, sebaceous

Seborrhea, seborrheic L21.9
- capillitii R23.8
- capitis L21.0
- dermatitis L21.9
  - infantile L21.1
- eczema L21.9
  - infantile L21.1
- sicca L21.0

Seckel's syndrome Q87.1

Seclusion, pupil — *see* Membrane, pupillary

Second hand tobacco smoke exposure (acute) (chronic) Z77.22
- in the perinatal period P96.81

Secondary
- dentin (in pulp) K04.3
- neoplasm, secondaries — *see* Table of Neoplasms, secondary

Secretion
- antidiuretic hormone, inappropriate E22.2
- catecholamine, by pheochromocytoma E27.5
- hormone
  - antidiuretic, inappropriate (syndrome) E22.2
  - by
    - carcinoid tumor E34.0
    - pheochromocytoma E27.5
  - ectopic NEC E34.2
- urinary
  - excessive R35.8
  - suppression R34

Section
- nerve, traumatic — *see* Injury, nerve

Segmentation, incomplete (congenital) (*see also* Fusion)
- bone NEC Q78.8
- lumbosacral (joint) (vertebra) Q76.49

Seitelberger's syndrome (infantile neuraxonal dystrophy) G31.89

Seizure (s) (*see also* Convulsions) R56.9
- akinetic — *see* Epilepsy, generalized, specified NEC
- atonic — *see* Epilepsy, generalized, specified NEC
- autonomic (hysterical) F44.5
- convulsive — *see* Convulsions
- cortical (focal) (motor) — *see* Epilepsy, localization-related, symptomatic, with simple partial seizures
- disorder (*see also* Epilepsy) G40.909
- due to stroke — *see* Sequelae (of), disease, cerebrovascular, by type, specified NEC
- epileptic — *see* Epilepsy
- febrile (simple) R56.00
  - with status epilepticus G40.901
  - complex (atypical) (complicated) R56.01
    - with status epilepticus G40.901
- grand mal G40.409
  - intractable G40.419
    - with status epilepticus G40.411
    - without status epilepticus G40.419
  - not intractable G40.409
    - with status epilepticus G40.401
    - without status epilepticus G40.409
- heart — *see* Disease, heart
- hysterical F44.5
- intractable G40.919
  - with status epilepticus G40.911
- Jacksonian (focal) (motor type) (sensory type) — *see* Epilepsy, localization-related, symptomatic, with simple partial seizures
- newborn P90

Seizure — *continued*
- nonspecific epileptic
  - atonic — *see* Epilepsy, generalized, specified NEC
  - clonic — *see* Epilepsy, generalized, specified NEC
  - myoclonic — *see* Epilepsy, generalized, specified NEC
  - tonic — *see* Epilepsy, generalized, specified NEC
  - tonic-clonic — *see* Epilepsy, generalized, specified NEC
- partial, developing into secondarily generalized seizures
  - complex — *see* Epilepsy, localization-related, symptomatic, with complex partial seizures
  - simple — *see* Epilepsy, localization-related, symptomatic, with simple partial seizures
- petit mal G40.409
  - intractable G40.419
    - with status epilepticus G40.411
    - without status epilepticus G40.419
  - not intractable G40.409
    - with status epilepticus G40.401
    - without status epilepticus G40.409
- post traumatic R56.1
- recurrent G40.909
- specified NEC G40.89
- uncinate — *see* Epilepsy, localization-related, symptomatic, with complex partial seizures

Selenium deficiency, dietary E59

Self-damaging behavior (life-style) Z72.89

Self-harm (attempted)
- history (personal) Z91.5
  - in family Z81.8

Self-mutilation (attempted)
- history (personal) Z91.5
  - in family Z81.8

Self-poisoning
- history (personal) Z91.5
  - in family Z81.8
- observation following (alleged) attempt Z03.6

Semicoma R40.1

Seminal vesiculitis N49.0

Seminoma C62.9- ☑
- specified site — *see* Neoplasm, malignant, by site

Senear-Usher disease or syndrome L10.4

Senectus R54

Senescence (without mention of psychosis) R54

Senile, senility (*see also* condition) R41.81
- with
  - acute confusional state F05
  - mental changes NOS F03 ☑
  - psychosis NEC — *see* Psychosis, senile
- asthenia R54
- cervix (atrophic) N88.8
- debility R54
- endometrium (atrophic) N85.8
- fallopian tube (atrophic) — *see* Atrophy, fallopian tube
- heart (failure) R54
- ovary (atrophic) — *see* Atrophy, ovary
- premature E34.8
- vagina, vaginitis (atrophic) N95.2
- wart L82.1

Sensation
- burning (skin) R20.8
  - tongue K14.6
- loss of R20.8
- prickling (skin) R20.2
- tingling (skin) R20.2

Sense loss
- smell — *see* Disturbance, sensation, smell
- taste — *see* Disturbance, sensation, taste
- touch R20.8

Sensibility disturbance (cortical) (deep) (vibratory) R20.9

Sensitive, sensitivity (*see also* Allergy)
- carotid sinus G90.01
- child (excessive) F93.8
- cold, autoimmune D59.1
- dentin K03.89
- latex Z91.040
- methemoglobin D74.8
- tuberculin, without clinical or radiological symptoms R76.11
- visual
  - glare H53.71
  - impaired contrast H53.72

Sensitiver Beziehungswahn F22

Sensitization, auto-erythrocytic D69.2

Separation
- anxiety, abnormal (of childhood) F93.0

Separation — *continued*
- apophysis, traumatic - code as Fracture, by site
- choroid — *see* Detachment, choroid
- epiphysis, epiphyseal
  - nontraumatic (*see also* Osteochondropathy, specified type NEC)
    - upper femoral — *see* Slipped, epiphysis, upper femoral
  - traumatic - code as Fracture, by site
- fracture — *see* Fracture
- infundibulum cardiac from right ventricle by a partition Q24.3
- joint (traumatic) (current) - code by site under Dislocation
- pubic bone, obstetrical trauma O71.6
- retina, retinal — *see* Detachment, retina
- symphysis pubis, obstetrical trauma O71.6
- tracheal ring, incomplete, congenital Q32.1

Sepsis (generalized) (unspecified organism) A41.9
- with
  - organ dysfunction (acute) (multiple) R65.20
    - with septic shock R65.21
- actinomycotic A42.7
- adrenal hemorrhage syndrome (meningococcal) A39.1
- anaerobic A41.4
- Bacillus anthracis A22.7
- Brucella (*see also* Brucellosis) A23.9
- candidal B37.7
- cryptogenic A41.9
- due to device, implant or graft T85.79 ☑
  - arterial graft NEC T82.7 ☑
  - breast (implant) T85.79 ☑
  - catheter NEC T85.79 ☑
    - dialysis (renal) T82.7 ☑
      - intraperitoneal T85.71 ☑
    - infusion NEC T82.7 ☑
      - spinal (epidural) (subdural) T85.79 ☑
    - urinary (indwelling) T83.51 ☑
- ectopic or molar pregnancy O08.82
- electronic (electrode) (pulse generator) (stimulator)
  - bone T84.7 ☑
  - cardiac T82.7 ☑
  - nervous system (brain) (peripheral nerve) (spinal) T85.79 ☑
  - urinary T83.59 ☑
- fixation, internal (orthopedic) — *see* Complication, fixation device, infection
- gastrointestinal (bile duct) (esophagus) T85.79 ☑
- genital T83.6 ☑
- heart NEC T82.7 ☑
  - valve (prosthesis) T82.6 ☑
    - graft T82.7 ☑
- joint prosthesis — *see* Complication, joint prosthesis, infection
- ocular (corneal graft) (orbital implant) T85.79 ☑
- orthopedic NEC T84.7 ☑
  - fixation device, internal — *see* Complication, fixation device, infection
- specified NEC T85.79 ☑
- vascular T82.7 ☑
- ventricular intracranial shunt T85.79 ☑
- during labor O75.3
- Enterococcus A41.81
- Erysipelothrix (rhusiopathiae) (erysipeloid) A26.7
- Escherichia coli (E. coli) A41.5 ☑
- extraintestinal yersiniosis A28.2
- following
  - abortion (subsequent episode) O08.0
    - current episode — *see* Abortion
  - ectopic or molar pregnancy O08.82
  - immunization T88.0 ☑
  - infusion, therapeutic injection or transfusion NEC T80.29 ☑
- gangrenous A41.9
- gonococcal A54.86
- Gram-negative (organism) A41.5 ☑
  - anaerobic A41.4
- Haemophilus influenzae A41.3
- herpesviral B00.7
- intra-abdominal K65.1
- intraocular — *see* Endophthalmitis, purulent
- Listeria monocytogenes A32.7
- localized - code to specific localized infection
  - in operation wound T81.4 ☑
  - skin — *see* Abscess
- malleus A24.0
- melioidosis A24.1
- meningeal — *see* Meningitis
- meningococcal A39.4

Sepsis - Sequelae

ICD-10-CM INDEX TO DISEASES AND INJURIES

Sepsis — *continued*
  acute A39.2
  chronic A39.3
  MSSA (Methicillin susceptible Staphylococcus aureus) A41.01
  newborn P36.9
    due to
      anaerobes NEC P36.5
      Escherichia coli P36.4
      Staphylococcus P36.30
        aureus P36.2
        specified NEC P36.39
      Streptococcus P36.10
        group B P36.0
        specified NEC P36.19
    specified NEC P36.8
  Pasteurella multocida A28.0
  pelvic, puerperal, postpartum, childbirth O85
  postprocedural T81.4 ☑
  pneumococcal A40.3
  puerperal, postpartum, childbirth (pelvic) O85
  Salmonella (arizonae) (cholerae-suis) (enteritidis) (typhimurium) A02.1
  severe R65.20
    with septic shock R65.21
  skin, localized — *see* Abscess
  Shigella (*see also* Dysentery, bacillary) A03.9
  specified organism NEC A41.89
  Staphylococcus, staphylococcal A41.2
    aureus (methicillin susceptible) (MSSA) A41.01
      methicillin resistant (MRSA) A41.02
    coagulase-negative A41.1
    specified NEC A41.1
  Streptococcus, streptococcal A40.9
    agalactiae A40.1
    group
      A A40.0
      B A40.1
      D A41.81
    neonatal P36.10
      group B P36.0
      specified NEC P36.19
    pneumoniae A40.3
    pyogenes A40.0
    specified NEC A40.8
  tracheostomy stoma J95.02
  tularemic A21.7
  umbilical, umbilical cord (newborn) — *see* Sepsis, newborn
  Yersinia pestis A20.7
Septate — *see* Septum
Septic — *see* condition
  arm — *see* Cellulitis, upper limb
    with lymphangitis — *see* Lymphangitis, acute, upper limb
  embolus — *see* Embolism
  finger — *see* Cellulitis, digit
    with lymphangitis — *see* Lymphangitis, acute, digit
  foot — *see* Cellulitis, lower limb
    with lymphangitis — *see* Lymphangitis, acute, lower limb
  gallbladder (acute) K81.0
  hand — *see* Cellulitis, upper limb
    with lymphangitis — *see* Lymphangitis, acute, upper limb
  joint — *see* Arthritis, pyogenic or pyemic
  leg — *see* Cellulitis, lower limb
    with lymphangitis — *see* Lymphangitis, acute, lower limb
  nail (*see also* Cellulitis, digit)
    with lymphangitis — *see* Lymphangitis, acute, digit
  sore (*see also* Abscess)
    throat J02.0
      streptococcal J02.0
  spleen (acute) D73.89
  teeth, tooth (pulpal origin) K04.4
  throat — *see* Pharyngitis
  thrombus — *see* Thrombosis
  toe — *see* Cellulitis, digit
    with lymphangitis — *see* Lymphangitis, acute, digit
  tonsils, chronic J35.01
    with adenoiditis J35.03
  uterus — *see* Endometritis
Septicemia A41.9
  meaning sepsis — *see* Sepsis
Septum, septate (congenital) (*see also* Anomaly, by site)
  anal Q42.3
    with fistula Q42.2

Septum — *continued*
  aqueduct of Sylvius Q03.0
    with spina bifida — *see* Spina bifida, by site, with hydrocephalus
  uterus (complete) (partial) Q51.2
  vagina Q52.10
    in pregnancy — *see* Pregnancy, complicated by, abnormal vagina
    causing obstructed labor O65.5
    longitudinal (with or without obstruction) Q52.12
    transverse Q52.11
Sequelae (of) (*see also* condition)
  abscess, intracranial or intraspinal (conditions in G06) G09
  amputation -- code to injury with seventh character S
  burn and corrosion -- code to injury with seventh character S
  calcium deficiency E64.8
  cerebrovascular disease — *see* Sequelae, disease, cerebrovascular
  childbirth O94
  contusion -- code to injury with seventh character S
  corrosion — *see* Sequelae, burn and corrosion
  crushing injury -- code to injury with seventh character S
  disease
    cerebrovascular I69.90
      alteration of sensation I69.998
      aphasia I69.920
      apraxia I69.990
      ataxia I69.993
      cognitive deficits I69.91
      disturbance of vision I69.998
      dysarthria I69.922
      dysphagia I69.991
      dysphasia I69.921
      facial droop I69.992
      facial weakness I69.992
      fluency disorder I69.923
      hemiplegia I69.95- ☑
      hemorrhage
        intracerebral — *see* Sequelae, hemorrhage, intracerebral
        intracranial, nontraumatic NEC — *see* Sequelae, hemorrhage, intracranial, nontraumatic
        subarachnoid — *see* Sequelae, hemorrhage, subarachnoid
      language deficit I69.928
      monoplegia
        lower limb I69.84- ☑
        upper limb I69.93- ☑
      paralytic syndrome I69.96- ☑
      specified effect NEC I69.998
    specified type NEC I69.80
      alteration of sensation I69.898
      aphasia I69.820
      apraxia I69.890
      ataxia I69.893
      cognitive deficits I69.81
      disturbance of vision I69.898
      dysarthria I69.822
      dysphagia I69.891
      dysphasia I69.821
      facial droop I69.892
      facial weakness I69.892
      fluency disorder I69.823
      hemiplegia I69.85- ☑
      language deficit I69.828
      monoplegia
        lower limb I69.84- ☑
        upper limb I69.83- ☑
      paralytic syndrome I69.86- ☑
      specified effect NEC I69.898
    speech deficit I69.928
    speech deficit I69.828
    stroke NOS — *see* Sequelae, stroke NOS
  dislocation -- code to injury with seventh character S
  encephalitis or encephalomyelitis (conditions in G04) G09
    in infectious disease NEC B94.8
    viral B94.1
  external cause -- code to injury with seventh character S
  foreign body entering natural orifice -- code to injury with seventh character S
  fracture -- code to injury with seventh character S

Sequelae — *continued*
  frostbite -- code to injury with seventh character S
  Hansen's disease B92
  hemorrhage
    intracerebral I69.10
      alteration of sensation I69.198
      aphasia I69.120
      apraxia I69.190
      ataxia I69.193
      cognitive deficits I69.11
      disturbance of vision I69.198
      dysarthria I69.122
      dysphagia I69.191
      dysphasia I69.121
      facial droop I69.192
      facial weakness I69.192
      fluency disorder I69.123
      hemiplegia I69.15- ☑
      language deficit NEC I69.128
      monoplegia
        lower limb I69.14- ☑
        upper limb I69.13- ☑
      paralytic syndrome I69.16- ☑
      specified effect NEC I69.198
      speech deficit NEC I69.128
    intracranial, nontraumatic NEC I69.20
      alteration of sensation I69.298
      aphasia I69.220
      apraxia I69.290
      ataxia I69.293
      cognitive deficits I69.21
      disturbance of vision I69.298
      dysarthria I69.222
      dysphagia I69.291
      dysphasia I69.221
      facial droop I69.292
      facial weakness I69.292
      fluency disorder I69.223
      hemiplegia I69.25- ☑
      language deficit NEC I69.228
      monoplegia
        lower limb I69.24- ☑
        upper limb I69.23- ☑
      paralytic syndrome I69.26- ☑
      specified effect NEC I69.298
      speech deficit NEC I69.228
    subarachnoid I69.00
      alteration of sensation I69.098
      aphasia I69.020
      apraxia I69.090
      ataxia I69.093
      cognitive deficits I69.01
      disturbance of vision I69.098
      dysarthria I69.022
      dysphagia I69.091
      dysphasia I69.021
      facial droop I69.092
      facial weakness I69.092
      fluency disorder I69.023
      hemiplegia I69.05- ☑
      language deficit NEC I69.028
      monoplegia
        lower limb I69.04- ☑
        upper limb I69.03- ☑
      paralytic syndrome I69.06- ☑
      specified effect NEC I69.098
      speech deficit NEC I69.028
  hepatitis, viral B94.2
  hyperalimentation E68
  infarction
    cerebral I69.30
      alteration of sensation I69.398
      aphasia I69.320
      apraxia I69.390
      ataxia I69.393
      cognitive deficits I69.31
      disturbance of vision I69.398
      dysarthria I69.322
      dysphagia I69.391
      dysphasia I69.321
      facial droop I69.392
      facial weakness I69.392
      fluency disorder I69.323
      hemiplegia I69.35- ☑
      language deficit NEC I69.328
      monoplegia
        lower limb I69.34- ☑
        upper limb I69.33- ☑
      paralytic syndrome I69.36- ☑
      specified effect NEC I69.398
      speech deficit NEC I69.328

☑ **Additional character required**

Sequelae — *continued*
  infection, pyogenic, intracranial or intraspinal
    G09
  infectious disease B94.9
    specified NEC B94.8
  injury -- code to injury with seventh character S
  leprosy B92
  meningitis
    bacterial (conditions in G00) G09
    other or unspecified cause (conditions in G03)
      G09
  muscle (and tendon) injury -- code to injury with
    seventh character S
  myelitis — *see* Sequelae, encephalitis
  niacin deficiency E64.8
  nutritional deficiency E64.9
    specified NEC E64.8
  obstetrical condition O94
  parasitic disease B94.9
  phlebitis or thrombophlebitis of intracranial
    or intraspinal venous sinuses and veins
    (conditions in G08) G09
  poisoning -- code to poisoning with seventh
    character S
    nonmedicinal substance — *see* Sequelae, toxic-
      effect, nonmedicinal substance
  poliomyelitis (acute) B91
  pregnancy O94
  protein-energy malnutrition E64.0
  puerperium O94
  rickets E64.3
  selenium deficiency E64.8
  sprain and strain -- code to injury with seventh
    character S
  stroke NOS I69.30
    alteration in sensation I69.398
    aphasia I69.320
    apraxia I69.390
    ataxia I69.393
    cognitive deficits I69.31
    disturbance of vision I69.398
    dysarthria I69.322
    dysphagia I69.391
    dysphasia I69.321
    facial droop I69.392
    facial weakness I69.392
    hemiplegia I69.35-☑
    language deficit NEC I69.328
    monoplegia
      lower limb I69.34-☑
      upper limb I69.33-☑
    paralytic syndrome I69.36-☑
    specified effect NEC I69.398
    speech deficit NEC I69.328
  tendon and muscle injury -- code to injury with
    seventh character S
  thiamine deficiency E64.8
  trachoma B94.0
  tuberculosis B90.9
    bones and joints B90.2
    central nervous system B90.0
    genitourinary B90.1
    pulmonary (respiratory) B90.9
    specified organs NEC B90.8
  viral
    encephalitis B94.1
    hepatitis B94.2
  vitamin deficiency NEC E64.8
    A E64.1
    B E64.8
    C E64.2
  wound, open -- code to injury with seventh
    character S
Sequestration (*see also* Sequestrum)
  lung, congenital Q33.2
Sequestrum
  bone — *see* Osteomyelitis, chronic
  dental M27.2
  jaw bone M27.2
  orbit — *see* Osteomyelitis, orbit
  sinus (accessory) (nasal) — *see* Sinusitis
Sequoiosis lung or pneumonitis J67.8
Serology for syphilis
  doubtful
    with signs or symptoms - code by site and
      stage under Syphilis
    follow-up of latent syphilis — *see* Syphilis,
      latent
  negative, with signs or symptoms - code by site
    and stage under Syphilis
  positive A53.0

Serology — *continued*
  with signs or symptoms - code by site and
    stage under Syphilis
  reactivated A53.0
Seroma (*see also* Hematoma)
  traumatic, secondary and recurrent T79.2☑
Seropurulent — *see* condition
Serositis, multiple K65.8
  pericardial I31.1
  peritoneal K65.8
Serous — *see* condition
Sertoli cell
  adenoma
    specified site — *see* Neoplasm, benign, by site
    unspecified site
      female D27.9
      male D29.20
  carcinoma
    specified site — *see* Neoplasm, malignant, by
      site
    unspecified site (male) C62.9-☑
      female C56.9
  tumor
    with lipid storage
      specified site — *see* Neoplasm, benign, by
        site
      unspecified site
        female D27.9
        male D29.20
    specified site — *see* Neoplasm, benign, by site
    unspecified site
      female D27.9
      male D29.20
Sertoli-Leydig cell tumor — *see* Neoplasm, benign,
  by site
  specified site — *see* Neoplasm, benign, by site
  unspecified site
    female D27.9
    male D29.20
Serum
  allergy, allergic reaction (*see also* Reaction, serum)
    T80.69☑
    shock (*see also* Shock, anaphylactic) T80.59☑
  arthritis (*see also* Reaction, serum) T80.69☑
  complication or reaction NEC (*see also* Reaction,
    serum) T80.69☑
  disease NEC (*see also* Reaction, serum) T80.69☑
  hepatitis (*see also* Hepatitis, viral, type B)
    carrier (suspected) of Z22.51
  intoxication (*see also* Reaction, serum) T80.69☑
  neuritis (*see also* Reaction, serum) T80.69☑
  neuropathy G61.1
  poisoning NEC (*see also* Reaction, serum) T80.69
    ☑
  rash NEC (*see also* Reaction, serum) T80.69☑
  reaction NEC (*see also* Reaction, serum) T80.69☑
  sickness NEC (*see also* Reaction, serum) T80.69☑
  urticaria (*see also* Reaction, serum) T80.69☑
Sesamoiditis M25.8-☑
Sever's disease or osteochondrosis — *see*
  Osteochondrosis, juvenile, tarsus
Severe sepsis R65.20
  with septic shock R65.21
Sex
  chromosome mosaics Q97.8
    lines with various numbers of X chromosomes
      Q97.2
  education Z70.8
  reassignment surgery status Z87.890
Sextuplet pregnancy — *see* Pregnancy, sextuplet
Sexual
  function, disorder of (psychogenic) F52.9
  immaturity (female) (male) E30.0
  impotence (psychogenic) organic origin NEC —
    see Dysfunction, sexual, male
  precocity (constitutional) (cryptogenic)(female)
    (idiopathic) (male) E30.1
Sexuality, pathologic — *see* Deviation, sexual
Sézary disease C84.1-☑
Shadow, lung R91.8
Shaking palsy or paralysis — *see* Parkinsonism
Shallowness, acetabulum — *see* Derangement,
  joint, specified type NEC, hip
Shaver's disease J63.1
Sheath (tendon) — *see* condition
Sheathing, retinal vessels H35.01-☑
Shedding
  nail L60.8
  premature, primary (deciduous) teeth K00.6
Sheehan's disease or syndrome E23.0
Shelf, rectal K62.89
Shell teeth K00.5

Shellshock (current) F43.0
  lasting state — *see* Disorder, post-traumatic stress
Shield kidney Q63.1
Shift
  auditory threshold (temporary) H93.24-☑
  mediastinal R93.8
Shifting sleep-work schedule (affecting sleep)
  G47.26
Shiga (-Kruse) dysentery A03.0
Shiga's bacillus A03.0
Shigella (dysentery) — *see* Dysentery, bacillary
Shigellosis A03.9
  Group A A03.0
  Group B A03.1
  Group C A03.2
  Group D A03.3
Shin splints S86.89☑
Shingles — *see* Herpes, zoster
Shipyard disease or eye B30.0
Shirodkar suture, in pregnancy — *see* Pregnancy,
  complicated by, incompetent cervix
Shock R57.9
  with ectopic or molar pregnancy O08.3
  adrenal (cortical) (Addisonian) E27.2
  adverse food reaction (anaphylactic) — *see*
    Shock, anaphylactic, due to food
  allergic — *see* Shock, anaphylactic
  anaphylactic T78.2☑
    chemical — *see* Table of Drugs and Chemicals
    due to drug or medicinal substance
      correct substance properly administered
        T88.6☑
      overdose or wrong substance given or taken
        (by accident) — *see* Table of Drugs and
        Chemicals, by drug, poisoning
    due to food (nonpoisonous) T78.00☑
      additives T78.06☑
      dairy products T78.07☑
      eggs T78.08☑
      fish T78.03☑
        shellfish T78.02☑
      fruit T78.04☑
      milk T78.07☑
      nuts T78.05☑
        peanuts T78.01☑
      peanuts T78.01☑
      seeds T78.05☑
      specified type NEC T78.09☑
      vegetable T78.04☑
    following sting (s) — *see* Venom
    immunization T80.52☑
    serum T80.59☑
      blood and blood products T80.51☑
      immunization T80.52☑
      specified NEC T80.59☑
      vaccination T80.52☑
  anaphylactoid — *see* Shock, anaphylactic
  anesthetic
    correct substance properly administered T88.2
      ☑
    overdose or wrong substance given or taken —
      see Table of Drugs and Chemicals, by drug,
      poisoning
      specified anesthetic — *see* Table of Drugs
        and Chemicals, by drug, poisoning
  cardiogenic R57.0
  chemical substance — *see* Table of Drugs and
    Chemicals
  complicating ectopic or molar pregnancy O08.3
  culture — *see* Disorder, adjustment
  drug
    due to correct substance properly administered
      T88.6☑
    overdose or wrong substance given or taken
      (by accident) — *see* Table of Drugs and
      Chemicals, by drug, poisoning
  during or after labor and delivery O75.1
  electric T75.4☑
    (taser) T75.4☑
  endotoxic R65.21
    postprocedural (during or resulting from a
      procedure, not elsewhere classified) T81.12
      ☑
  following
    ectopic or molar pregnancy O08.3
    injury (immediate) (delayed) T79.4☑
    labor and delivery O75.1
  food (anaphylactic) — *see* Shock, anaphylactic,
    due to food
  from electroshock gun (taser) T75.4☑
  gram-negative R65.21

Shock — *continued*
  postprocedural (during or resulting from a procedure, not elsewhere classified) T81.12 ☑
  hematologic R57.8
  hemorrhagic
    surgery (intraoperative) (postoperative) T81.19 ☑
    trauma T79.4 ☑
  hypovolemic R57.1
    surgical T81.19 ☑
    traumatic T79.4 ☑
  insulin E15
    therapeutic misadventureT38.3
  kidney N17.0
    traumatic (following crushing) T79.5 ☑
  lightning T75.01 ☑
  lung J80
  obstetric O75.1
    with ectopic or molar pregnancy O08.3
    following ectopic or molar pregnancy O08.3
  pleural (surgical) T81.19 ☑
    due to trauma T79.4 ☑
  postprocedural (postoperative) T81.10 ☑
    with ectopic or molar pregnancy O08.3
    cardiogenic T81.11 ☑
    endotoxic T81.12 ☑
    following ectopic or molar pregnancy O08.3
    gram-negative T81.12 ☑
    hypovolemic T81.19 ☑
    septic T81.12 ☑
    specified type NEC T81.19 ☑
  psychic F43.0
  septic (due to severe sepsis) R65.21
  specified NEC R57.8
  surgical T81.10 ☑
  taser gun (taser) T75.4 ☑
  therapeutic misadventure NEC T81.10 ☑
  thyroxin
    overdose or wrong substance given or taken — *see* Table of Drugs and Chemicals, by drug, poisoning
  toxic, syndrome A48.3
  transfusion — *see* Complications, transfusion
  traumatic (immediate) (delayed) T79.4 ☑
Shoemaker's chest M95.4
Short, shortening, shortness
  arm (acquired) (*see also* Deformity, limb, unequal length)
    congenital Q71.81- ☑
    forearm — *see* Deformity, limb, unequal length
  bowel syndrome K91.2
  breath R06.02
  cervical (complicating pregnancy) O26.87- ☑
    non-gravid uterus N88.3
  common bile duct, congenital Q44.5
  cord (umbilical), complicating delivery O69.3 ☑
  cystic duct, congenital Q44.5
  esophagus (congenital) Q39.8
  femur (acquired) — *see* Deformity, limb, unequal length, femur
    congenital — *see* Defect, reduction, lower limb, longitudinal, femur
  frenum, frenulum, linguae (congenital) Q38.1
  hip (acquired) (*see also* Deformity, limb, unequal length)
    congenital Q65.89
  leg (acquired) (*see also* Deformity, limb, unequal length)
    congenital Q72.81- ☑
    lower leg (*see also* Deformity, limb, unequal length)
  limbed stature, with immunodeficiency D82.2
  lower limb (acquired) (*see also* Deformity, limb, unequal length)
    congenital Q72.81- ☑
  organ or site, congenital NEC — *see* Distortion
  palate, congenital Q38.5
  radius (acquired) (*see also* Deformity, limb, unequal length)
    congenital — *see* Defect, reduction, upper limb, longitudinal, radius
  rib syndrome Q77.2
  stature (child) (hereditary) (idiopathic) NEC R62.52
    constitutional E34.3
    due to endocrine disorder E34.3
    Laron-type E34.3
  tendon (*see also* Contraction, tendon)
    with contracture of joint — *see* Contraction, joint
    Achilles (acquired) M67.0- ☑

Short — *continued*
  congenital Q66.89
  congenital Q79.8
  thigh (acquired) (*see also* Deformity, limb, unequal length, femur)
    congenital — *see* Defect, reduction, lower limb, longitudinal, femur
  tibialis anterior (tendon) — *see* Contraction, tendon
  umbilical cord
    complicating delivery O69.3 ☑
  upper limb, congenital — *see* Defect, reduction, upper limb, specified type NEC
  urethra N36.8
  uvula, congenital Q38.5
  vagina (congenital) Q52.4
Shortsightedness — *see* Myopia
Shoshin (acute fulminating beriberi) E51.11
Shoulder — *see* condition
Shovel-shaped incisors K00.2
Shower, thromboembolic — *see* Embolism
Shunt
  arterial-venous (dialysis) Z99.2
  arteriovenous, pulmonary (acquired) I28.0
    congenital Q25.72
  cerebral ventricle (communicating) in situ Z98.2
  surgical, prosthetic, with complications — *see* Complications, cardiovascular, device or implant
Shutdown, renal N28.9
Shy-Drager syndrome G90.3
Sialadenitis, sialadenosis (any gland) (chronic) (periodic) (suppurative) — *see* Sialoadenitis
Sialectasia K11.8
Sialidosis E77.1
Sialitis, silitis (any gland) (chronic) (suppurative) — *see* Sialoadenitis
Sialoadenitis (any gland) (periodic) (suppurative) K11.20
  acute K11.21
    recurrent K11.22
  chronic K11.23
Sialoadenopathy K11.9
Sialoangitis — *see* Sialoadenitis
Sialodochitis (fibrinosa) — *see* Sialoadenitis
Sialodocholithiasis K11.5
Sialolithiasis K11.5
Sialometaplasia, necrotizing K11.8
Sialorrhea (*see also* Ptyalism)
  periodic — *see* Sialoadenitis
Sialosis K11.7
Siamese twin Q89.4
Sibling rivalry Z62.891
Sicard's syndrome G52.7
Sicca syndrome M35.00
  with
    keratoconjunctivitis M35.01
    lung involvement M35.02
    myopathy M35.03
    renal tubulo-interstitial disorders M35.04
    specified organ involvement NEC M35.09
Sick R69
  or handicapped person in family Z63.79
    needing care at home Z63.6
  sinus (syndrome) I49.5
Sick-euthyroid syndrome E07.81
Sickle-cell
  anemia — *see* Disease, sickle-cell
  trait D57.3
Sicklemia (*see also* Disease, sickle-cell)
  trait D57.3
Sickness
  air (travel) T75.3 ☑
  airplane T75.3 ☑
  alpine T70.29 ☑
  altitude T70.20 ☑
  Andes T70.29 ☑
  aviator's T70.29 ☑
  balloon T70.29 ☑
  car T75.3 ☑
  compressed air T70.3 ☑
  decompression T70.3 ☑
  green D50.8
  milk — *see* Poisoning, food, noxious
  motion T75.3 ☑
  mountain T70.29 ☑
    acute D75.1
  protein (*see also* Reaction, serum) T80.69 ☑
  radiation T66 ☑
  roundabout (motion) T75.3 ☑
  sea T75.3 ☑
  serum NEC (*see also* Reaction, serum) T80.69 ☑

Sickness — *continued*
  sleeping (African) B56.9
    by Trypanosoma B56.9
    brucei
      gambiense B56.0
      rhodesiense B56.1
    East African B56.1
    Gambian B56.0
    Rhodesian B56.1
    West African B56.0
  swing (motion) T75.3 ☑
  train (railway) (travel) T75.3 ☑
  travel (any vehicle) T75.3 ☑
Sideropenia — *see* Anemia, iron deficiency
Siderosilicosis J62.8
Siderosis (lung) J63.4
  eye (globe) — *see* Disorder, globe, degenerative, siderosis
Siemens' syndrome (ectodermal dysplasia) Q82.8
Sighing R06.89
  psychogenic F45.8
Sigmoid (*see also* condition)
  flexure — *see* condition
  kidney Q63.1
Sigmoiditis (*see also* Enteritis) K52.9
  infectious A09
  noninfectious K52.9
Silfversköld's syndrome Q78.9
Silicosiderosis J62.8
Silicosis, silicotic (simple) (complicated) J62.8
  with tuberculosis J65
Silicotuberculosis J65
Silo-fillers' disease J68.8
  bronchitis J68.0
  pneumonitis J68.0
  pulmonary edema J68.1
Silver's syndrome Q87.1
Simian malaria B53.1
Simmonds' cachexia or disease E23.0
Simons' disease or syndrome (progressive lipodystrophy) E88.1
Simple, simplex — *see* condition
Simulation, conscious (of illness) Z76.5
Simultanagnosia (asimultagnosia) R48.3
Sin Nombre virus disease (Hantavirus) (cardio)-pulmonary syndrome) B33.4
Sinding-Larsen disease or osteochondrosis — *see* Osteochondrosis, juvenile, patella
Singapore hemorrhagic fever A91
Singer's node or nodule J38.2
Single
  atrium Q21.2
  coronary artery Q24.5
  umbilical artery Q27.0
  ventricle Q20.4
Singultus R06.6
  epidemicus B33.0
Sinus (*see also* Fistula)
  abdominal K63.89
  arrest I45.5
  arrhythmia I49.8
  bradycardia R00.1
  branchial cleft (internal) (external) Q18.0
  coccygeal — *see* Sinus, pilonidal
  dental K04.6
  dermal (congenital) Q06.8
    with abscess Q06.8
    coccygeal, pilonidal — *see* Sinus, coccygeal
  infected, skin NEC L08.89
  marginal, ruptured or bleeding — *see* Hemorrhage, antepartum, specified cause NEC
  medial, face and neck Q18.8
  pause I45.5
  pericranii Q01.9
  pilonidal (infected) (rectum) L05.92
    with abscess L05.02
  preauricular Q18.1
  rectovaginal N82.3
  Rokitansky-Aschoff (gallbladder) K82.8
  sacrococcygeal (dermoid) (infected) — *see* Sinus, pilonidal
  tachycardia R00.0
    paroxysmal I47.1
  tarsi syndrome - M25.57- ☑
  testis N50.8
  tract (postinfective) — *see* Fistula
  urachus Q64.4
Sinusitis (accessory) (chronic) (hyperplastic) (nasal) (nonpurulent) (purulent) J32.9
  acute J01.90
    ethmoidal J01.20

Sinusitis — *continued*
  recurrent J01.21
    frontal J01.10
      recurrent J01.11
    involving more than one sinus, other than
      pansinusitis J01.80
        recurrent J01.81
    maxillary J01.00
      recurrent J01.01
    pansinusitis J01.40
      recurrent J01.41
    recurrent J01.91
    specified NEC J01.80
      recurrent J01.81
    sphenoidal J01.30
      recurrent J01.31
  allergic — *see* Rhinitis, allergic
  due to high altitude T70.1 ☑
  ethmoidal J32.2
    acute J01.20
      recurrent J01.21
  frontal J32.1
    acute J01.10
      recurrent J01.11
  influenzal — *see* Influenza, with, respiratory
    manifestations NEC
  involving more than one sinus but not
    pansinusitis J32.8
      acute J01.80
        recurrent J01.81
  maxillary J32.0
    acute J01.00
      recurrent J01.01
  sphenoidal J32.3
    acute J01.30
      recurrent J01.31
  tuberculous, any sinus A15.8
Sinusitis-bronchiectasis-situs inversus (syndrome)
  (triad) Q89.3
Sipple's syndrome E31.22
Sirenomelia (syndrome) Q87.2
Siriasis T67.0 ☑
Sirkari's disease B55.0
Siti A65
Situation, psychiatric F99
Situational
  disturbance (transient) — *see* Disorder,
    adjustment
    acute F43.0
  maladjustment — *see* Disorder, adjustment
  reaction — *see* Disorder, adjustment
    acute F43.0
Situs inversus or transversus (abdominalis) (thoracis)
  Q89.3
Sixth disease B08.20
  due to human herpesvirus 6 B08.21
  due to human herpesvirus 7 B08.22
Sjögren-Larsson syndrome Q87.1
Sjögren's syndrome or disease — *see* Sicca
  syndrome
Skeletal — *see* condition
Skene's gland — *see* condition
Skenitis — *see* Urethritis
Skerljevo A65
Skevas-Zerfus disease — *see* Toxicity, venom,
  marine animal, sea anemone
Skin (*see also* condition)
  clammy R23.1
  donor — *see* Donor, skin
  hidebound M35.9
Slate-dressers' or slate-miners' lung J62.8
Sleep
  apnea — *see* Apnea, sleep
  deprivation Z72.820
  disorder or disturbance G47.9
    child F51.9
    nonorganic origin F51.9
    specified NEC G47.8
  disturbance G47.9
    nonorganic origin F51.9
  drunkenness F51.9
  rhythm inversion G47.2- ☑
  terrors F51.4
  walking F51.3
    hysterical F44.89
Sleep hygiene
  abuse Z72.821
  inadequate Z72.821
  poor Z72.821
Sleeping sickness — *see* Sickness, sleeping
Sleeplessness — *see* Insomnia
  menopausal N95.1

Sleep-wake schedule disorder G47.20
Slim disease (in HIV infection) B20
Slipped, slipping
  epiphysis (traumatic) (*see also*
    Osteochondropathy, specified type NEC)
    capital femoral (traumatic)
      acute (on chronic) S79.01- ☑
      current traumatic - code as Fracture, by site
    upper femoral (nontraumatic) M93.00- ☑
      acute M93.01- ☑
        on chronic M93.03- ☑
      chronic M93.02- ☑
  intervertebral disc — *see* Displacement,
    intervertebral disc
  ligature, umbilical P51.8
  patella — *see* Disorder, patella, derangement NEC
  rib M89.8X8
  sacroiliac joint M53.2
  tendon — *see* Disorder, tendon
  ulnar nerve, nontraumatic — *see* Lesion, nerve,
    ulnar
  vertebra NEC — *see* Spondylolisthesis
Slocumb's syndrome E27.0
Sloughing (multiple) (phagedena) (skin) (*see also*
  Gangrene)
  abscess — *see* Abscess
  appendix K38.8
  fascia — *see* Disorder, soft tissue, specified type
    NEC
  scrotum N50.8
  tendon — *see* Disorder, tendon
  transplanted organ — *see* Rejection, transplant
  ulcer — *see* Ulcer, skin
Slow
  feeding, newborn P92.2
  flow syndrome, coronary I20.8
  heart (beat) R00.1
Slowing, urinary stream R39.19
Sluder's neuralgia (syndrome) G44.89
Slurred, slurring speech R47.81
Small (ness)
  for gestational age — *see* Small for dates
  introitus, vagina N89.6
  kidney (unknown cause) N27.9
    bilateral N27.1
    unilateral N27.0
  ovary (congenital) Q50.39
  pelvis
    with disproportion (fetopelvic) O33.1
      causing obstructed labor O65.1
  uterus N85.8
  white kidney N03.9
Small-and-light-for-dates — *see* Small for dates
Small-for-dates (infant) P05.10
  with weight of
    499 grams or less P05.11
    500-749 grams P05.12
    750-999 grams P05.13
    1000-1249 grams P05.14
    1250-1499 grams P05.15
    1500-1749 grams P05.16
    1750-1999 grams P05.17
    2000-2499 grams P05.18
Smallpox B03
Smearing, fecal R15.1
Smith-Lemli-Opitz syndrome E78.72
Smith's fracture S52.54- ☑
Smoker — *see* Dependence, drug, nicotine
Smoker's
  bronchitis J41.0
  cough J41.0
  palate K13.24
  throat J31.2
  tongue K13.24
Smoking
  passive Z77.22
Smothering spells R06.81
Snaggle teeth, tooth M26.39
Snapping
  finger — *see* Trigger finger
  hip — *see* Derangement, joint, specified type
    NEC, hip
    involving the iliotiblial band M76.3- ☑
  knee — *see* Derangement, knee
    involving the iliotiblial band M76.3- ☑
Sneddon-Wilkinson disease or syndrome (subcorneal pustular dermatosis) L13.1
Sneezing (intractable) R06.7
Sniffing
  cocaine
    abuse — *see* Abuse, drug, cocaine
    dependence — *see* Dependence, drug, cocaine

Sniffing — *continued*
  gasoline
    abuse — *see* Abuse, drug, inhalant
    dependence — *see* Dependence, drug, inhalant
  glue (airplane)
    abuse — *see* Abuse, drug, inhalant
    drug dependence — *see* Dependence, drug,
      inhalant
Sniffles
  newborn P28.89
Snoring R06.83
Snow blindness — *see* Photokeratitis
Snuffles (non-syphilitic) R06.5
  newborn P28.89
  syphilitic (infant) A50.05 [J99]
Social
  exclusion Z60.4
    due to discrimination or persecution
      (perceived) Z60.5
  migrant Z59.0
    acculturation difficulty Z60.3
  rejection Z60.4
    due to discrimination or persecution Z60.5
  role conflict NEC Z73.5
  skills inadequacy NEC Z73.4
  transplantation Z60.3
Sodoku A25.0
Soemmerring's ring — *see* Cataract, secondary
Soft (*see also* condition)
  nails L60.3
Softening
  bone — *see* Osteomalacia
  brain (necrotic) (progressive) G93.89
    congenital Q04.8
    embolic I63.4 ☑
    hemorrhage — *see* Hemorrhage, intracranial,
      intracerebral
    occlusive I63.5 ☑
    thrombotic I63.3 ☑
  cartilage M94.2- ☑
    patella M22.4- ☑
  cerebellar — *see* Softening, brain
  cerebral — *see* Softening, brain
  cerebrospinal — *see* Softening, brain
  myocardial, heart — *see* Degeneration,
    myocardial
  spinal cord G95.89
  stomach K31.89
Soldier's
  heart F45.8
  patches I31.0
Solitary
  cyst, kidney N28.1
  kidney, congenital Q60.0
Solvent abuse — *see* Abuse, drug, inhalant
  dependence — *see* Dependence, drug, inhalant
Somatization reaction, somatic reaction — *see*
  Disorder, somatoform
Somnambulism F51.3
  hysterical F44.89
Somnolence R40.0
  nonorganic origin F51.11
Sonne dysentery A03.3
Soor B37.0
Sore
  bed — *see* Ulcer, pressure, by site
  chiclero B55.1
  Delhi B55.1
  desert — *see* Ulcer, skin
  eye H57.1- ☑
  Lahore B55.1
  mouth K13.79
    canker K12.0
  muscle M79.1
  Naga — *see* Ulcer, skin
  of skin — *see* Ulcer, skin
  oriental B55.1
  pressure — *see* Ulcer, pressure, by site
  skin L98.9
  soft A57
  throat (acute) (*see also* Pharyngitis)
    with influenza, flu, or grippe — *see* Influenza,
      with, respiratory manifestations NEC
    chronic J31.2
    coxsackie (virus) B08.5
    diphtheritic A36.0
    herpesviral B00.2
    influenzal — *see* Influenza, with, respiratory
      manifestations NEC
    septic J02.0
    streptococcal (ulcerative) J02.0
    viral NEC J02.8

Sore — *continued*
- coxsackie B08.5
- tropical — *see* Ulcer, skin
- veldt — *see* Ulcer, skin

Soto's syndrome (cerebral gigantism) Q87.3

South African cardiomyopathy syndrome I42.8

Southeast Asian hemorrhagic fever A91

Spacing
- abnormal, tooth, teeth, fully erupted M26.30
- excessive, tooth, fully erupted M26.32

Spade-like hand (congenital) Q68.1

Spading nail L60.8
- congenital Q84.6

Spanish collar N47.1

Sparganosis B70.1

Spasm (s), spastic, spasticity (*see also* condition) R25.2
- accommodation — *see* Spasm, of accommodation
- ampulla of Vater K83.4
- anus, ani (sphincter) (reflex) K59.4
  - psychogenic F45.8
- artery I73.9
  - cerebral G45.9
- Bell's G51.3
- bladder (sphincter, external or internal) N32.89
  - psychogenic F45.8
- bronchus, bronchiole J98.01
- cardia K22.0
- cardiac I20.1
- carpopedal — *see* Tetany
- cerebral (arteries) (vascular) G45.9
- cervix, complicating delivery O62.4
- ciliary body (of accommodation) — *see* Spasm, of accommodation
- colon K58.9
  - with diarrhea K58.0
  - psychogenic F45.8
- common duct K83.8
- compulsive — *see* Tic
- conjugate H51.8
- coronary (artery) I20.1
- diaphragm (reflex) R06.6
  - epidemic B33.0
  - psychogenic F45.8
- duodenum K59.8
- epidemic diaphragmatic (transient) B33.0
- esophagus (diffuse) K22.4
  - psychogenic F45.8
- facial G51.3
- fallopian tube N83.8
- gastrointestinal (tract) K31.89
  - psychogenic F45.8
- glottis J38.5
  - hysterical F44.4
  - psychogenic F45.8
    - conversion reaction F44.4
  - reflex through recurrent laryngeal nerve J38.5
- habit — *see* Tic
- heart I20.1
- hemifacial (clonic) G51.3
- hourglass — *see* Contraction, hourglass
- hysterical F44.4
- infantile — *see* Epilepsy, spasms
- inferior oblique, eye H51.8
- intestinal (*see also* Syndrome, irritable bowel) K58.9
  - psychogenic F45.8
- larynx, laryngeal J38.5
  - hysterical F44.4
  - psychogenic F45.8
    - conversion reaction F44.4
- levator palpebrae superioris — *see* Disorder, eyelid function
- muscle NEC M62.838
  - back M62.830
- nerve, trigeminal G51.0
- nervous F45.8
- nodding F98.4
- occupational F48.8
- oculogyric H51.8
  - psychogenic F45.8
- of accommodation H52.53- ☑
- ophthalmic artery — *see* Occlusion, artery, retina
- perineal, female N94.89
- peroneo-extensor (*see also* Deformity, limb, flat foot)
- pharynx (reflex) J39.2
  - hysterical F45.8
  - psychogenic F45.8
- psychogenic F45.8
- pylorus NEC K31.3

Spasm — *continued*
- adult hypertrophic K31.89
- congenital or infantile Q40.0
- psychogenic F45.8
- rectum (sphincter) K59.4
  - psychogenic F45.8
- retinal (artery) — *see* Occlusion, artery, retina
- sigmoid (*see also* Syndrome, irritable bowel) K58.9
  - psychogenic F45.8
- sphincter of Oddi K83.4
- stomach K31.89
  - neurotic F45.8
- throat J39.2
  - hysterical F45.8
  - psychogenic F45.8
- tic F95.9
  - chronic F95.1
  - transient of childhood F95.0
- tongue K14.8
- torsion (progressive) G24.1
- trigeminal nerve — *see* Neuralgia, trigeminal
- ureter N13.5
- urethra (sphincter) N35.9
- uterus N85.8
  - complicating labor O62.4
- vagina N94.2
  - psychogenic F52.5
- vascular I73.9
- vasomotor I73.9
- vein NEC I87.8
- viscera — *see* Pain, abdominal

Spasmodic — *see* condition

Spasmophilia — *see* Tetany

Spasmus nutans F98.4

Spastic, spasticity (*see also* Spasm)
- child (cerebral) (congenital) (paralysis) G80.1

Speaker's throat R49.8

Specific, specified — *see* condition

Speech
- defect, disorder, disturbance, impediment R47.9
  - psychogenic, in childhood and adolescence F98.8
  - slurring R47.81
  - specified NEC R47.89

Spencer's disease A08.19

Spens' syndrome (syncope with heart block) I45.9

Sperm counts (fertility testing) Z31.41
- postvasectomy Z30.8
- reversal Z31.42

Spermatic cord — *see* condition

Spermatocele N43.40
- congenital Q55.4
- multiple N43.42
- single N43.41

Spermatocystitis N49.0

Spermatocytoma C62.9- ☑
- specified site — *see* Neoplasm, malignant, by site

Spermatorrhea N50.8

Sphacelus — *see* Gangrene

Sphenoidal — *see* condition

Sphenoiditis (chronic) — *see* Sinusitis, sphenoidal

Sphenopalatine ganglion neuralgia G90.09

Sphericity, increased, lens (congenital) Q12.4

Spherocytosis (congenital) (familial) (hereditary) D58.0
- hemoglobin disease D58.0
- sickle-cell (disease) D57.8- ☑

Spherophakia Q12.4

Sphincter — *see* condition

Sphincteritis, sphincter of Oddi — *see* Cholangitis

Sphingolipidosis E75.3
- specified NEC E75.29

Sphingomyelinosis E75.3

Spicule tooth K00.2

Spider
- bite — *see* Toxicity, venom, spider
- fingers — *see* Syndrome, Marfan's
- nevus I78.1
- toes — *see* Syndrome, Marfan's
- vascular I78.1

Spiegler-Fendt
- benign lymphocytoma L98.8
- sarcoid L08.89

Spielmeyer-Vogt disease E75.4

Spina bifida (aperta) Q05.9
- with hydrocephalus NEC Q05.4
- cervical Q05.5
  - with hydrocephalus Q05.0
- dorsal Q05.6
  - with hydrocephalus Q05.1
- lumbar Q05.7

Spina — *continued*
- with hydrocephalus Q05.2
- lumbosacral Q05.7
  - with hydrocephalus Q05.2
- occulta Q76.0
- sacral Q05.8
  - with hydrocephalus Q05.3
- thoracic Q05.6
  - with hydrocephalus Q05.1
- thoracolumbar Q05.6
  - with hydrocephalus Q05.1

Spindle, Krukenberg's — *see* Pigmentation, cornea, posterior

Spine, spinal — *see* condition

Spiradenoma (eccrine) — *see* Neoplasm, skin, benign

Spirillosis A25.0

Spirillum
- minus A25.0
- obermeieri infection A68.0

Spirochetal — *see* condition

Spirochetosis A69.9
- arthritic, arthritica A69.9
- bronchopulmonary A69.8
- icterohemorrhagic A27.0
- lung A69.8

Spirometrosis B70.1

Spitting blood — *see* Hemoptysis

Splanchnoptosis K63.4

Spleen, splenic — *see* condition

Splenectasis — *see* Splenomegaly

Splenitis (interstitial) (malignant) (nonspecific) D73.89
- malarial (*see also* Malaria) B54 [D77]
- tuberculous A18.85

Splenocele D73.89

Splenomegaly, splenomegalia (Bengal) (cryptogenic) (idiopathic) (tropical) R16.1
- with hepatomegaly R16.2
- cirrhotic D73.2
- congenital Q89.09
- congestive, chronic D73.2
- Egyptian B65.1
- Gaucher's E75.22
- malarial (*see also* Malaria) B54 [D77]
- neutropenic D73.81
- Niemann-Pick — *see* Niemann-Pick disease or syndrome
- siderotic D73.2
- syphilitic A52.79
  - congenital (early) A50.08 [D77]

Splenopathy D73.9

Splenoptosis D73.89

Splenosis D73.89

Splinter — *see* Foreign body, superficial, by site

Split, splitting
- foot Q72.7- ☑
- heart sounds R01.2
- lip, congenital — *see* Cleft, lip
- nails L60.3
- urinary stream R39.13

Spondylarthrosis — *see* Spondylosis

Spondylitis (chronic) (*see also* Spondylopathy, inflammatory)
- ankylopoietica — *see* Spondylitis, ankylosing
- ankylosing (chronic) M45.9
  - with lung involvement M45.9 [J99]
  - cervical region M45.2
  - cervicothoracic region M45.3
  - juvenile M08.1
  - lumbar region M45.6
  - lumbosacral region M45.7
  - multiple sites M45.0
  - occipito-atlanto-axial region M45.1
  - sacrococcygeal region M45.8
  - thoracic region M45.4
  - thoracolumbar region M45.5
- atrophic (ligamentous) — *see* Spondylitis, ankylosing
- deformans (chronic) — *see* Spondylosis
- gonococcal A54.41
- gouty M10.08
- in (due to)
  - brucellosis A23.9 [M49.80]
    - cervical region A23.9 [M49.82]
    - cervicothoracic region A23.9 [M49.83]
    - lumbar region A23.9 [M49.86]
    - lumbosacral region A23.9 [M49.87]
    - multiple sites A23.9 [M49.89]
    - occipito-atlanto-axial region A23.9 [M49.81]
    - sacrococcygeal region A23.9 [M49.88]
    - thoracic region A23.9 [M49.84]

☑ **Additional character required**

Spondylitis — *continued*
  thoracolumbar region A23.9 [M49.85]
  enterobacteria (*see also* subcategory M49.8) A04.9
  tuberculosis A18.01
  infectious NEC — *see* Spondylopathy, infective
  juvenile ankylosing (chronic) M08.1
  Kümmell's — *see* Spondylopathy, traumatic
  Marie-Strümpell — *see* Spondylitis, ankylosing
  muscularis — *see* Spondylopathy, specified NEC
  psoriatic L40.53
  rheumatoid — *see* Spondylitis, ankylosing
  rhizomelica — *see* Spondylitis, ankylosing
  sacroiliac NEC M46.1
  senescent, senile — *see* Spondylosis
  traumatic (chronic) or post-traumatic — *see* Spondylopathy, traumatic
  tuberculous A18.01
  typhosa A01.05
Spondylolisthesis (acquired) (degenerative) M43.10
  with disproportion (fetopelvic) O33.0
    causing obstructed labor O65.0
  cervical region M43.12
  cervicothoracic region M43.13
  congenital Q76.2
  lumbar region M43.16
  lumbosacral region M43.17
  multiple sites M43.19
  occipito-atlanto-axial region M43.11
  sacrococcygeal region M43.18
  thoracic region M43.14
  thoracolumbar region M43.15
  traumatic (old) M43.10
    acute
      fifth cervical (displaced) S12.430 ☑
        nondisplaced S12.431 ☑
        specified type NEC (displaced) S12.450 ☑
          nondisplaced S12.451 ☑
        type III S12.44 ☑
      fourth cervical (displaced) S12.330 ☑
        nondisplaced S12.331 ☑
        specified type NEC (displaced) S12.350 ☑
          nondisplaced S12.351 ☑
        type III S12.34 ☑
      second cervical (displaced) S12.130 ☑
        nondisplaced S12.131 ☑
        specified type NEC (displaced) S12.150 ☑
          nondisplaced S12.151 ☑
        type III S12.14 ☑
      seventh cervical (displaced) S12.630 ☑
        nondisplaced S12.631 ☑
        specified type NEC (displaced) S12.650 ☑
          nondisplaced S12.651 ☑
        type III S12.64 ☑
      sixth cervical (displaced) S12.530 ☑
        nondisplaced S12.531 ☑
        specified type NEC (displaced) S12.550 ☑
          nondisplaced S12.551 ☑
        type III S12.54 ☑
      third cervical (displaced) S12.230 ☑
        nondisplaced S12.231 ☑
        specified type NEC (displaced) S12.250 ☑
          nondisplaced S12.251 ☑
        type III S12.24 ☑
Spondylolysis (acquired) M43.00
  cervical region M43.02
  cervicothoracic region M43.03
  congenital Q76.2
  lumbar region M43.06
  lumbosacral region M43.07
    with disproportion (fetopelvic) O33.0
      causing obstructed labor O65.8
  multiple sites M43.09
  occipito-atlanto-axial region M43.01
  sacrococcygeal region M43.08
  thoracic region M43.04
  thoracolumbar region M43.05
Spondylopathy M48.9
  infective NEC M46.50
    cervical region M46.52
    cervicothoracic region M46.53
    lumbar region M46.56
    lumbosacral region M46.57
    multiple sites M46.59
    occipito-atlanto-axial region M46.51
    sacrococcygeal region M46.58
    thoracic region M46.54
    thoracolumbar region M46.55
  inflammatory M46.90
    cervical region M46.92
    cervicothoracic region M46.93
    lumbar region M46.96

Spondylopathy — *continued*
    lumbosacral region M46.97
    multiple sites M46.99
    occipito-atlanto-axial region M46.91
    sacrococcygeal region M46.98
    specified type NEC M46.80
      cervical region M46.82
      cervicothoracic region M46.83
      lumbar region M46.86
      lumbosacral region M46.87
      multiple sites M46.89
      occipito-atlanto-axial region M46.81
      sacrococcygeal region M46.88
      thoracic region M46.84
      thoracolumbar region M46.85
    thoracic region M46.94
    thoracolumbar region M46.95
  neuropathic, in
    syringomyelia and syringobulbia G95.0
    tabes dorsalis A52.11
  specified NEC M48.8
  traumatic M48.30
    cervical region M48.32
    cervicothoracic region M48.33
    lumbar region M48.36
    lumbosacral region M48.37
    occipito-atlanto-axial region M48.31
    sacrococcygeal region M48.38
    thoracic region M48.34
    thoracolumbar region M48.35
Spondylosis M47.9
  with
    disproportion (fetopelvic) O33.0
      causing obstructed labor O65.0
    myelopathy NEC M47.10
      cervical region M47.12
      cervicothoracic region M47.13
      lumbar region M47.16
      occipito-atlanto-axial region M47.11
      thoracic region M47.14
      thoracolumbar region M47.15
    radiculopathy M47.20
      cervical region M47.22
      cervicothoracic region M47.23
      lumbar region M47.26
      lumbosacral region M47.27
      occipito-atlanto-axial region M47.21
      sacrococcygeal region M47.28
      thoracic region M47.24
      thoracolumbar region M47.25
  specified NEC M47.899
    cervical region M47.892
    cervicothoracic region M47.893
    lumbar region M47.896
    lumbosacral region M47.897
    occipito-atlanto-axial region M47.891
    sacrococcygeal region M47.898
    thoracic region M47.894
    thoracolumbar region M47.895
  traumatic — *see* Spondylopathy, traumatic
  without myelopathy or radiculopathy M47.819
    cervical region M47.812
    cervicothoracic region M47.813
    lumbar region M47.816
    lumbosacral region M47.817
    occipito-atlanto-axial region M47.811
    sacrococcygeal region M47.818
    thoracic region M47.814
    thoracolumbar region M47.815
Sponge
  inadvertently left in operation wound — *see* Foreign body, accidentally left during a procedure
  kidney (medullary) Q61.5
Sponge-diver's disease — *see* Toxicity, venom, marine animal, sea anemone
Spongioblastoma (any type) — *see* Neoplasm, malignant, by site
  specified site — *see* Neoplasm, malignant, by site
  unspecified site C71.9
Spongioneuroblastoma — *see* Neoplasm, malignant, by site
Spontaneous (*see also* condition)
  fracture (cause unknown) — *see* Fracture, pathological
Spoon nail L60.3
  congenital Q84.6
Sporadic — *see* condition
Sporothrix schenckii infection — *see* Sporotrichosis
Sporotrichosis B42.9
  arthritis B42.82
  disseminated B42.7

Sporotrichosis — *continued*
  generalized B42.7
  lymphocutaneous (fixed) (progressive) B42.1
  pulmonary B42.0
  specified NEC B42.89
Spots, spotting (in) (of)
  Bitot's (*see also* Pigmentation, conjunctiva)
    in the young child E50.1
    vitamin A deficiency E50.1
  café, au lait L81.3
  Cayenne pepper I78.1
  cotton wool, retina — *see* Occlusion, artery, retina
  de Morgan's (senile angiomas) I78.1
  Fuchs' black (myopic) H44.2- ☑
  intermenstrual (regular) N92.0
    irregular N92.1
  Koplik's B05.9
  liver L81.4
  pregnancy O26.85- ☑
  purpuric R23.3
  ruby I78.1
Spotted fever — *see* Fever, spotted N92.3
Sprain (joint) (ligament)
  acromioclavicular joint or ligament S43.5- ☑
  ankle S93.40- ☑
    calcaneofibular ligament S93.41- ☑
    deltoid ligament S93.42- ☑
    internal collateral ligament — *see* Sprain, ankle, specified ligament NEC
    specified ligament NEC S93.49- ☑
    talofibular ligament — *see* Sprain, ankle, specified ligament NEC
    tibiofibular ligament S93.43- ☑
  anterior longitudinal, cervical S13.4 ☑
  atlas, atlanto-axial, atlanto-occipital S13.4 ☑
  breast bone — *see* Sprain, sternum
  calcaneofibular — *see* Sprain, ankle
  carpal — *see* Sprain, wrist
  carpometacarpal — *see* Sprain, hand, specified site NEC
  cartilage
    costal S23.41 ☑
    semilunar (knee) — *see* Sprain, knee, specified site NEC
      with current tear — *see* Tear, meniscus
    thyroid region S13.5 ☑
    xiphoid — *see* Sprain, sternum
  cervical, cervicodorsal, cervicothoracic S13.4 ☑
  chondrosternal S23.421 ☑
  coracoclavicular S43.8- ☑
  coracohumeral S43.41- ☑
  coronary, knee — *see* Sprain, knee, specified site NEC
  costal cartilage S23.41 ☑
  cricoarytenoid articulation or ligament S13.5 ☑
  cricothyroid articulation S13.5 ☑
  cruciate, knee — *see* Sprain, knee, cruciate
  deltoid, ankle — *see* Sprain, ankle
  dorsal (spine) S23.3 ☑
  elbow S53.40- ☑
    radial collateral ligament S53.43- ☑
    radiohumeral S53.41- ☑
    rupture
      radial collateral ligament — *see* Rupture, traumatic, ligament, radial collateral
      ulnar collateral ligament — *see* Rupture, traumatic, ligament, ulnar collateral
    specified type NEC S53.49- ☑
    ulnar collateral ligament S53.44- ☑
    ulnohumeral S53.42- ☑
  femur, head — *see* Sprain, hip
  fibular collateral, knee — *see* Sprain, knee, collateral
  fibulocalcaneal — *see* Sprain, ankle
  finger (s) S63.61- ☑
    index S63.61- ☑
    interphalangeal (joint) S63.63- ☑
      index S63.63- ☑
      little S63.63- ☑
      middle S63.63- ☑
      ring S63.63- ☑
    little S63.61- ☑
    middle S63.61- ☑
    ring S63.61- ☑
    metacarpophalangeal (joint) S63.65- ☑
    specified site NEC S63.69- ☑
      index S63.69- ☑
      little S63.69- ☑
      middle S63.69- ☑
      ring S63.69- ☑
  foot S93.60- ☑
    specified ligament NEC S93.69- ☑

Sprain — *continued*
  tarsal ligament S93.61- ☑
  tarsometatarsal ligament S93.62- ☑
  toe — *see* Sprain, toe
  hand S63.9- ☑
    finger — *see* Sprain, finger
    specified site NECS63.8
    thumb — *see* Sprain, thumb
  head S03.9 ☑
  hip S73.10- ☑
    iliofemoral ligament S73.11- ☑
    ischiocapsular (ligament) S73.12- ☑
    specified NEC S73.19- ☑
  iliofemoral — *see* Sprain, hip
  innominate
    acetabulum — *see* Sprain, hip
    sacral junction S33.6 ☑
  internal
    collateral, ankle — *see* Sprain, ankle
    semilunar cartilage — *see* Sprain, knee,
      specified site NEC
  interphalangeal
    finger — *see* Sprain, finger, interphalangeal
      (joint)
    toe — *see* Sprain, toe, interphalangeal joint
  ischiocapsular — *see* Sprain, hip
  ischiofemoral — *see* Sprain, hip
  jaw (articular disc) (cartilage) (meniscus) S03.4 ☑
    old M26.69
  knee S83.9- ☑
    collateral ligament S83.40- ☑
      lateral (fibular) S83.42- ☑
      medial (tibial) S83.41- ☑
    cruciate ligament S83.50- ☑
      anterior S83.51- ☑
      posterior S83.52- ☑
    lateral (fibular) collateral ligament S83.42- ☑
    medial (tibial) collateral ligament S83.41- ☑
    patellar ligament S76.11- ☑
    specified site NEC S83.8X- ☑
    superior tibiofibular joint (ligament) S83.6- ☑
  lateral collateral, knee — *see* Sprain, knee,
    collateral
  lumbar (spine) S33.5 ☑
  lumbosacral S33.9 ☑
  mandible (articular disc) S03.4 ☑
    old M26.69
  medial collateral, knee — *see* Sprain, knee,
    collateral
  meniscus
    jaw S03.4 ☑
      old M26.69
    knee — *see* Sprain, knee, specified site NEC
      with current tear — *see* Tear, meniscus
        old — *see* Derangement, knee, meniscus,
          due to old tear
    mandible S03.4 ☑
      old M26.69
  metacarpal (distal) (proximal) — *see* Sprain, hand,
    specified site NEC
  metacarpophalangeal — *see* Sprain, finger,
    metacarpophalangeal (joint)
  metatarsophalangeal — *see* Sprain, toe,
    metatarsophalangeal joint
  midcarpal — *see* Sprain, hand, specified site NEC
  midtarsal — *see* Sprain, foot, specified site NEC
  neck S13.9 ☑
    anterior longitudinal cervical ligament S13.4 ☑
    atlanto-axial joint S13.4 ☑
    atlanto-occipital joint S13.4 ☑
    cervical spine S13.4 ☑
    cricoarytenoid ligament S13.5 ☑
    cricothyroid ligament S13.5 ☑
    specified site NEC S13.8 ☑
    thyroid region (cartilage) S13.5 ☑
  nose S03.8 ☑
  orbicular, hip — *see* Sprain, hip
  patella — *see* Sprain, knee, specified site NEC
  patellar ligament S76.11- ☑
  pelvis NEC S33.8 ☑
  phalanx
    finger — *see* Sprain, finger
    toe — *see* Sprain, toe
  pubofemoral — *see* Sprain, hip
  radiocarpal — *see* Sprain, wrist
  radiohumeral — *see* Sprain, elbow
  radius, collateral — *see* Rupture, traumatic,
    ligament, radial collateral
  rib (cage) S23.41 ☑
  rotator cuff (capsule) S43.42- ☑
  sacroiliac (region)
    chronic or oldM53.2

Sprain — *continued*
  joint S33.6 ☑
  scaphoid (hand) — *see* Sprain, hand, specified
    site NEC
  scapula (r) — *see* Sprain, shoulder girdle,
    specified site NEC
  semilunar cartilage (knee) — *see* Sprain, knee,
    specified site NEC
    with current tear — *see* Tear, meniscus
      old — *see* Derangement, knee, meniscus, due
        to old tear
  shoulder joint S43.40- ☑
    acromioclavicular joint (ligament) — *see* Sprain,
      acromioclavicular joint
    blade — *see* Sprain, shoulder, girdle, specified
      site NEC
    coracoclavicular joint (ligament) — *see* Sprain,
      coracoclavicular joint
    coracohumeral ligament — *see* Sprain,
      coracohumeral joint
    girdle S43.9- ☑
      specified site NEC S43.8- ☑
    rotator cuff — *see* Sprain, rotator cuff
    specified site NEC S43.49- ☑
    sternoclavicular joint (ligament) — *see* Sprain,
      sternoclavicular joint
  spine
    cervical S13.4 ☑
    lumbar S33.5 ☑
    thoracic S23.3 ☑
  sternoclavicular joint S43.6- ☑
  sternum S23.429 ☑
    chondrosternal joint S23.421 ☑
    specified site NEC S23.428 ☑
    sternoclavicular (joint) (ligament) S23.420 ☑
  symphysis
    jaw S03.4 ☑
      old M26.69
    mandibular S03.4 ☑
      old M26.69
  talofibular — *see* Sprain, ankle
  tarsal — *see* Sprain, foot, specified site NEC
  tarsometatarsal — *see* Sprain, foot, specified site
    NEC
  temporomandibular S03.4 ☑
    old M26.69
  thorax S23.9 ☑
    ribs S23.41 ☑
    specified site NEC S23.8 ☑
    spine S23.3 ☑
    sternum — *see* Sprain, sternum
  thumb S63.60- ☑
    interphalangeal (joint) S63.62- ☑
    metacarpophalangeal (joint) S63.64- ☑
    specified site NEC S63.68- ☑
  thyroid cartilage or region S13.5 ☑
  tibia (proximal end) — *see* Sprain, knee, specified
    site NEC
  tibial collateral, knee — *see* Sprain, knee,
    collateral
  tibiofibular
    distal — *see* Sprain, ankle
    superior — *see* Sprain, knee, specified site NEC
  toe (s) S93.50- ☑
    great S93.50- ☑
    interphalangeal joint S93.51- ☑
      great S93.51- ☑
      lesser S93.51- ☑
    lesser S93.50- ☑
    metatarsophalangeal joint S93.52- ☑
      great S93.52- ☑
      lesser S93.52- ☑
  ulna, collateral — *see* Rupture, traumatic,
    ligament, ulnar collateral
  ulnohumeral — *see* Sprain, elbow
  wrist S63.50- ☑
    carpal S63.51- ☑
    radiocarpal S63.52- ☑
    specified site NEC S63.59- ☑
  xiphoid cartilage — *see* Sprain, sternum
Sprengel's deformity (congenital) Q74.0
Sprue (tropical) K90.1
  celiac K90.0
  idiopathic K90.0
  meaning thrush B37.0
  nontropical K90.0
Spur, bone (*see also* Enthesopathy)
  calcaneal M77.3-
  iliac crest M76.2- ☑
  nose (septum) J34.89
Spurway's syndrome Q78.0

Sputum
  abnormal (amount) (color) (odor) (purulent) R09.3
  blood-stained R04.2
  excessive (cause unknown) R09.3
Squamous (*see also* condition)
  epithelium in
    cervical canal (congenital) Q51.828
    uterine mucosa (congenital) Q51.818
Squashed nose M95.0
  congenital Q67.4
Squeeze, diver's T70.3 ☑
Squint (*see also* Strabismus)
  accommodative — *see* Strabismus, convergent
    concomitant
St. Hubert's disease A82.9
Stab (*see also* Laceration)
  internal organs — *see* Injury, by site
Stafne's cyst or cavity M27.0
Staggering gait R26.0
  hysterical F44.4
Staghorn calculus — *see* Calculus, kidney
Stähli's line (cornea) (pigment) — *see* Pigmentation,
  cornea, anterior
Stain, staining
  meconium (newborn) P96.83
  port wine Q82.5
  tooth, teeth (hard tissues) (extrinsic) K03.6
    due to
      accretions K03.6
      deposits (betel) (black) (green) (materia alba)
        (orange) (soft) (tobacco) K03.6
      metals (copper) (silver) K03.7
      nicotine K03.6
      pulpal bleeding K03.7
      tobacco K00.8
    intrinsic K00.0
Stammering (*see also* Disorder, fluency) F80.81
Standstill
  auricular I45.5
  cardiac — *see* Arrest, cardiac
  sinoatrial I45.5
  ventricular — *see* Arrest, cardiac
Stannosis J63.5
Stanton's disease — *see* Melioidosis
Staphylitis (acute) (catarrhal) (chronic) (gangrenous)
  (membranous) (suppurative) (ulcerative) K12.2
Staphylococcal scalded skin syndrome L00
Staphylococcemia A41.2
Staphylococcus, staphylococcal (*see also* condition)
  as cause of disease classified elsewhere B95.8
    aureus (methicillin susceptible) (MSSA) B95.61
      methicillin resistant (MRSA) B95.62
    specified NEC, as cause of disease classified
      elsewhere B95.7
Staphyloma (sclera)
  cornea H18.72- ☑
  equatorial H15.81- ☑
  localized (anterior) H15.82- ☑
  posticum H15.83- ☑
  ring H15.85- ☑
Stargardt's disease — *see* Dystrophy, retina
Starvation (inanition) (due to lack of food) T73.0 ☑
  edema — *see* Malnutrition, severe
Stasis
  bile (noncalculous) K83.1
  bronchus J98.09
    with infection — *see* Bronchitis
  cardiac — *see* Failure, heart, congestive
  cecum K59.8
  colon K59.8
  dermatitis — *see* Varix, leg, with, inflammation
  duodenal K31.5
  eczema — *see* Varix, leg, with, inflammation
  edema — *see* Hypertension, venous (chronic),
    idiopathic
  foot T69.0- ☑
  ileocecal coil K59.8
  ileum K59.8
  intestinal K59.8
  jejunum K59.8
  kidney N19
  liver (cirrhotic) K76.1
  lymphatic I89.8
  pneumonia J18.2
  pulmonary — *see* Edema, lung
  rectal K59.8
  renal N19
    tubular N17.0
  ulcer — *see* Varix, leg, with, ulcer
    without varicose veins I87.2
  urine — *see* Retention, urine
  venous I87.8

☑ **Additional character required**

State (of)
  affective and paranoid, mixed, organic psychotic
    F06.8
  agitated R45.1
    acute reaction to stress F43.0
  anxiety (neurotic) F41.1
  apprehension F41.1
  burn-out Z73.0
  climacteric, female Z78.0
    symptomatic N95.1
  compulsive F42
    mixed with obsessional thoughts F42
  confusional (psychogenic) F44.89
    acute (*see also* Delirium)
      with
        arteriosclerotic dementia F01.50
          with behavioral disturbance F01.51
        senility or dementia F05
      alcoholic F10.231
    epileptic F05
    reactive (from emotional stress, psychological
      trauma) F44.89
    subacute — *see* Delirium
  convulsive — *see* Convulsions
  crisis F43.0
  depressive F32.9
    neurotic F34.1
  dissociative F44.9
  emotional shock (stress) R45.7
  hypercoagulation — *see* Hypercoagulable
  locked-in G83.5
  menopausal Z78.0
    symptomatic N95.1
  neurotic F48.9
    with depersonalization F48.1
  obsessional F42
  oneiroid (schizophrenia-like) F23
  organic
    hallucinatory (nonalcoholic) F06.0
    paranoid (-hallucinatory) F06.2
  panic F41.0
  paranoid F22
    climacteric F22
    involutional F22
    menopausal F22
    organic F06.2
    senile F03 ☑
    simple F22
  persistent vegetative R40.3
  phobic F40.9
  postleukotomy F07.0
  pregnant, incidental Z33.1
  psychogenic, twilight F44.89
  psychopathic (constitutional) F60.2
  psychotic, organic (*see also* Psychosis, organic)
    mixed paranoid and affective F06.8
    senile or presenile F03 ☑
    transient NEC F06.8
      with
        hallucinations F06.0
        depression F06.31
  residual schizophrenic F20.5
  restlessness R45.1
  stress (emotional) R45.7
  tension (mental) F48.9
    specified NEC F48.8
  transient organic psychotic NEC F06.8
    depressive type F06.31
    hallucinatory type F06.30
  twilight
    epileptic F05
    psychogenic F44.89
  vegetative, persistent R40.3
  vital exhaustion Z73.0
  withdrawal, — *see* Withdrawal, state
Status (post) (*see also* Presence (of))
  absence, epileptic — *see* Epilepsy, by type, with
    status epilepticus
  administration of tPA (rtPA) in a different facility
    within the last 24 hours prior to admission to
    current facility Z92.82
  adrenalectomy (unilateral) (bilateral) E89.6
  anastomosis Z98.0
  angioplasty (peripheral) Z98.62
    with implant Z95.820
    coronary artery Z98.61
      with implant Z95.5
  anginosus I20.9
  aortocoronary bypass Z95.1
  arthrodesis Z98.1
  artificial opening (of) Z93.9
    gastrointestinal tract Z93.4

Status — *continued*
    specified NEC Z93.8
    urinary tract Z93.6
    vagina Z93.8
  asthmaticus — *see* Asthma, by type, with status
    asthmaticus
  awaiting organ transplant Z76.82
  bariatric surgery Z98.84
  bed confinement Z74.01
  bleb, filtering (vitreous), after glaucoma surgery
    Z98.83
  breast implant Z98.82
    removal Z98.86
  cataract extraction Z98.4- ☑
  cholecystectomy Z90.49
  clitorectomy N90.811
    with excision of labia minora N90.812
  colectomy (complete) (partial) Z90.49
  colonization — *see* Carrier (suspected) of
  colostomy Z93.3
  convulsivus idiopathicus — *see* Epilepsy, by type,
    with status epilepticus
  coronary artery angioplasty — *see* Status,
    angioplasty, coronary artery
  cystectomy (urinary bladder) Z90.6
  cystostomy Z93.50
    appendico-vesicostomy Z93.52
    cutaneous Z93.51
    specified NEC Z93.59
  delinquent immunization Z28.3
  dental Z98.818
    crown Z98.811
    fillings Z98.811
    restoration Z98.811
    sealant Z98.810
    specified NEC Z98.818
  deployment (current) (military) Z56.82
  dialysis (hemodialysis) (peritoneal) Z99.2
  do not resuscitate (DNR) Z66
  donor — *see* Donor
  embedded fragments — *see* Retained, foreign
    body fragments (type of)
  embedded splinter — *see* Retained, foreign body
    fragments (type of)
  enterostomy Z93.4
  epileptic, epilepticus (*see also* Epilepsy, by type,
    with status epilepticus) G40.901
  estrogen receptor
    negative Z17.1
    positive Z17.0
  female genital cutting — *see* Female genital
    mutilation status
  female genital mutilation — *see* Female genital
    mutilation status
  filtering (vitreous) bleb after glaucoma surgery
    Z98.83
  gastrectomy (complete) (partial) Z90.3
  gastric banding Z98.84
  gastric bypass for obesity Z98.84
  gastrostomy Z93.1
  human immunodeficiency virus (HIV) infection,
    asymptomatic Z21
  hysterectomy (complete) (total) Z90.710
    partial (with remaining cervial stump) Z90.711
  ileostomy Z93.2
  implant
    breast Z98.82
  infibulation N90.813
  intestinal bypass Z98.0
  jejunostomy Z93.4
  laryngectomy Z90.02
  lapsed immunization schedule Z28.3
  lymphaticus E32.8
  marmoratus G80.3
  mastectomy (unilateral) (bilateral) Z90.1- ☑
  military deployment status (current) Z56.82
    in theater or in support of military war,
      peacekeeping and humanitarian
      operations Z56.82
  nephrectomy (unilateral) (bilateral) Z90.5
  nephrostomy Z93.6
  obesity surgery Z98.84
  oophorectomy
    bilateral Z90.722
    unilateral Z90.721
  organ replacement
    by artificial or mechanical device or prosthesis
      of
      artery Z95.828
      bladder Z96.0
      blood vessel Z95.828
      breast Z97.8

Status — *continued*
    eye globe Z97.0
    heart Z95.812
      valve Z95.2
    intestine Z97.8
    joint Z96.60
      hip — *see* Presence, hip joint implant
      knee — *see* Presence, knee joint implant
      specified site NEC Z96.698
    kidney Z97.8
    larynx Z96.3
    lens Z96.1
    limbs — *see* Presence, artificial, limb
    liver Z97.8
    lung Z97.8
    pancreas Z97.8
    by organ transplant (heterologous)
      (homologous) — *see* Transplant
  pacemaker
    brain Z96.89
    cardiac Z95.0
    specified NEC Z96.89
  pancreatectomy Z90.410
    complete Z90.410
    partial Z90.411
    total Z90.410
  physical restraint Z78.1
  pneumonectomy (complete) (partial) Z90.2
  pneumothorax, therapeutic Z98.3
  postcommotio cerebri F07.81
  postoperative (postprocedural) NEC Z98.89
    breast implant Z98.82
    dental Z98.818
      crown Z98.811
      fillings Z98.811
      restoration Z98.811
      sealant Z98.810
      specified NEC Z98.818
    pneumothorax, therapeutic Z98.3
  postpartum (routine follow-up) Z39.2
    care immediately after delivery Z39.0
  postsurgical (postprocedural) NEC Z98.89
    pneumothorax, therapeutic Z98.3
  pregnancy, incidental Z33.1
  prosthesis coronary angioplasty Z95.5
  pseudophakia Z96.1
  renal dialysis (hemodialysis) (peritoneal) Z99.2
  retained foreign body — *see* Retained, foreign
    body fragments (type of)
  reversed jejunal transposition (for bypass) Z98.0
  salpingo-oophorectomy
    bilateral Z90.722
    unilateral Z90.721
  sex reassignment surgery status Z87.890
  shunt
    arteriovenous (for dialysis) Z99.2
    cerebrospinal fluid Z98.2
    ventricular (communicating) (for drainage)
      Z98.2
  splenectomy Z90.81
  thymicolymphaticus E32.8
  thymicus E32.8
  thymolymphaticus E32.8
  thyroidectomy (hypothyroidism) E89.0
  tooth (teeth) extraction (*see also* Absence, teeth,
    acquired) K08.409
  tPA (rtPA) administration in a different facility
    within the last 24 hours prior to admission to
    current facility Z92.82
  tracheostomy Z93.0
  transplant — *see* Transplant
    organ removed Z98.85
  tubal ligation Z98.51
  underimmunization Z28.3
  ureterostomy Z93.6
  urethrostomy Z93.6
  vagina, artificial Z93.8
  vasectomy Z98.52
  wheelchair confinement Z99.3
Stealing
  child problem F91.8
    in company with others Z72.810
  pathological (compulsive) F63.2
Steam burn — *see* Burn
Steatocystoma multiplex L72.2
Steatohepatitis (nonalcoholic) (NASH) K75.81
Steatoma L72.3
  eyelid (cystic) — *see* Dermatosis, eyelid
    infected — *see* Hordeolum
Steatorrhea (chronic) K90.4
  with lacteal obstruction K90.2
  idiopathic (adult) (infantile) K90.0

Steatorrhea — *continued*
  pancreatic K90.3
  primary K90.0
  tropical K90.1
Steatosis E88.89
  heart — *see* Degeneration, myocardial
  kidney N28.89
  liver NEC K76.0
Steele-Richardson-Olszewski disease or syndrome
    G23.1
Steinbrocker's syndrome G90.8
Steinert's disease G71.11
Stein-Leventhal syndrome E28.2
Stein's syndrome E28.2
STEMI (*see also* - Infarct, myocardium, ST elevation)
    I21.3
Stenocardia I20.8
Stenocephaly Q75.8
Stenosis, stenotic (cicatricial) (*see also* Stricture)
  ampulla of Vater K83.1
  anus, anal (canal) (sphincter) K62.4
    and rectum K62.4
    congenital Q42.3
      with fistula Q42.2
  aorta (ascending) (supraventricular) (congenital)
      Q25.3
  arteriosclerotic I70.0
  calcified I70.0
  aortic (valve) I35.0
    with insufficiency I35.2
    congenital Q23.0
    rheumatic I06.0
      with
        incompetency, insufficiency or
          regurgitation I06.2
          with mitral (valve) disease I08.0
            with tricuspid (valve) disease I08.3
          mitral (valve) disease I08.0
            with tricuspid (valve) disease I08.3
          tricuspid (valve) disease I08.2
            with mitral (valve) disease I08.3
    specified cause NEC I35.0
    syphilitic A52.03
  aqueduct of Sylvius (congenital) Q03.0
    with spina bifida — *see* Spina bifida, by site,
      with hydrocephalus
    acquired G91.1
  artery NEC (*see also* Arteriosclerosis) I77.1
    celiac I77.4
    cerebral — *see* Occlusion, artery, cerebral
    extremities — *see* Arteriosclerosis, extremities
    precerebral — *see* Occlusion, artery, precerebral
    pulmonary (congenital) Q25.6
      acquired I28.8
    renal I70.1
  bile duct (common) (hepatic) K83.1
    congenital Q44.3
  bladder-neck (acquired) N32.0
    congenital Q64.31
  brain G93.89
  bronchus J98.09
    congenital Q32.3
    syphilitic A52.72
  cardia (stomach) K22.2
    congenital Q39.3
  cardiovascular — *see* Disease, cardiovascular
  caudal M48.08
  cervix, cervical (canal) N88.2
    congenital Q51.828
    in pregnancy or childbirth — *see* Pregnancy,
      complicated by, abnormal cervix
  colon (*see also* Obstruction, intestine)
    congenital Q42.9
      specified NEC Q42.8
  colostomy K94.03
  common (bile) duct K83.1
    congenital Q44.3
  coronary (artery) — *see* Disease, heart, ischemic,
    atherosclerotic
  cystic duct — *see* Obstruction, gallbladder
  due to presence of device, implant or graft
      (*see also* Complications, by site and type,
      specified NEC) T85.85 ☑
    arterial graft NEC T82.858 ☑
    breast (implant) T85.85 ☑
    catheter T85.85 ☑
      dialysis (renal) T82.858 ☑
        intraperitoneal T85.85 ☑
      infusion NEC T82.858 ☑
        spinal (epidural) (subdural) T85.85 ☑
      urinary (indwelling) T83.85 ☑
    fixation, internal (orthopedic) NEC T84.85 ☑

Stenosis — *continued*
  gastrointestinal (bile duct) (esophagus)
      T85.85 ☑
    genital NEC T83.85 ☑
    heart NEC T82.857 ☑
    joint prosthesis T84.85 ☑
    ocular (corneal graft) (orbital implant) NEC
      T85.85 ☑
    orthopedic NEC T84.85 ☑
    specified NEC T85.85 ☑
    urinary NEC T83.85 ☑
    vascular NEC T82.858 ☑
    ventricular intracranial shunt T85.85 ☑
  duodenum K31.5
    congenital Q41.0
  ejaculatory duct NEC N50.8
  endocervical os — *see* Stenosis, cervix
  enterostomy K94.13
  esophagus K22.2
    congenital Q39.3
    syphilitic A52.79
      congenital A50.59 [K23]
  eustachian tube — *see* Obstruction, eustachian
    tube
  external ear canal (acquired) H61.30- ☑
    congenital Q16.1
    due to
      inflammation H61.32- ☑
      trauma H61.31- ☑
    postprocedural H95.81- ☑
    specified cause NEC H61.39- ☑
  gallbladder — *see* Obstruction, gallbladder
  glottis J38.6
  heart valve (congenital) Q24.8
    aortic Q23.0
    mitral Q23.2
    pulmonary Q22.1
    tricuspid Q22.4
  hepatic duct K83.1
  hymen N89.6
  hypertrophic subaortic (idiopathic) I42.1
  ileum K56.69
    congenital Q41.2
  infundibulum cardia Q24.3
  intervertebral foramina (*see also* Lesion,
      biomechanical, specified NEC)
    connective tissue M99.79
      abdomen M99.79
      cervical region M99.71
      cervicothoracic M99.71
      head region M99.70
      lumbar region M99.73
      lumbosacral M99.73
      occipitocervical M99.70
      sacral region M99.74
      sacrococcygeal M99.74
      sacroiliac M99.74
      specified NEC M99.79
      thoracic region M99.72
      thoracolumbar M99.72
    disc M99.79
      abdomen M99.79
      cervical region M99.71
      cervicothoracic M99.71
      head region M99.70
      lower extremity M99.76
      lumbar region M99.73
      lumbosacral M99.73
      occipitocervical M99.70
      pelvic M99.75
      rib cage M99.78
      sacral region M99.74
      sacrococcygeal M99.74
      sacroiliac M99.74
      specified NEC M99.79
      thoracic region M99.72
      thoracolumbar M99.72
      upper extremity M99.77
    osseous M99.69
      abdomen M99.69
      cervical region M99.61
      cervicothoracic M99.61
      head region M99.60
      lower extremity M99.66
      lumbar region M99.63
      lumbosacral M99.63
      occipitocervical M99.60
      pelvic M99.65
      rib cage M99.68
      sacral region M99.64
      sacrococcygeal M99.64
      sacroiliac M99.64

Stenosis — *continued*
    specified NEC M99.69
    thoracic region M99.62
    thoracolumbar M99.62
    upper extremity M99.67
  subluxation — *see* Stenosis, intervertebral
    foramina, osseous
  intestine (*see also* Obstruction, intestine)
    congenital (small) Q41.9
      large Q42.9
        specified NEC Q42.8
      specified NEC Q41.8
    jejunum K56.69
      congenital Q41.1
  lacrimal (passage)
    canaliculi H04.54- ☑
    congenital Q10.5
    duct H04.55- ☑
    punctum H04.56- ☑
    sac H04.57- ☑
  lacrimonasal duct — *see* Stenosis, lacrimal, duct
    congenital Q10.5
  larynx J38.6
    congenital NEC Q31.8
    subglottic Q31.1
    syphilitic A52.73
      congenital A50.59 [J99]
  mitral (chronic) (inactive) (valve) I05.0
    with
      aortic valve disease I08.0
      incompetency, insufficiency or regurgitation
        I05.2
    active or acute I01.1
      with rheumatic or Sydenham's chorea I02.0
    congenital Q23.2
    specified cause, except rheumatic I34.2
    syphilitic A52.03
  myocardium, myocardial (*see also* Degeneration,
    myocardial)
    hypertrophic subaortic (idiopathic) I42.1
  nares (anterior) (posterior) J34.89
    congenital Q30.0
  nasal duct (*see also* Stenosis, lacrimal, duct)
    congenital Q10.5
  nasolacrimal duct (*see also* Stenosis, lacrimal,
    duct)
    congenital Q10.5
  neural canal (*see also* Lesion, biomechanical,
    specified NEC)
    connective tissue M99.49
      abdomen M99.49
      cervical region M99.41
      cervicothoracic M99.41
      head region M99.40
      lower extremity M99.46
      lumbar region M99.43
      lumbosacral M99.43
      occipitocervical M99.40
      pelvic M99.45
      rib cage M99.48
      sacral region M99.44
      sacrococcygeal M99.44
      sacroiliac M99.44
      specified NEC M99.49
      thoracic region M99.42
      thoracolumbar M99.42
      upper extremity M99.47
    intervertebral disc M99.59
      abdomen M99.59
      cervical region M99.51
      cervicothoracic M99.51
      head region M99.50
      lower extremity M99.56
      lumbar region M99.53
      lumbosacral M99.53
      occipitocervical M99.50
      pelvic M99.55
      rib cage M99.58
      sacral region M99.54
      sacrococcygeal M99.54
      sacroiliac M99.54
      specified NEC M99.59
      thoracic region M99.52
      thoracolumbar M99.52
      upper extremity M99.57
    osseous M99.39
      abdomen M99.39
      cervical region M99.31
      cervicothoracic M99.31
      head region M99.30
      lower extremity M99.36
      lumbar region M99.33

☑ **Additional character required**

Stenosis — continued
- lumbosacral M99.33
- pelvic M99.35
- rib cage M99.38
- occipitocervical M99.30
- sacral region M99.34
- sacrococcygeal M99.34
- sacroiliac M99.34
- specified NEC M99.39
- thoracic region M99.32
- thoracolumbar M99.32
- upper extremity M99.37
- subluxation M99.29
  - cervical region M99.21
  - cervicothoracic M99.21
  - head region M99.20
  - lower extremity M99.26
  - lumbar region M99.23
  - lumbosacral M99.23
  - occipitocervical M99.20
  - pelvic M99.25
  - rib cage M99.28
  - sacral region M99.24
  - sacrococcygeal M99.24
  - sacroiliac M99.24
  - specified NEC M99.29
  - thoracic region M99.22
  - thoracolumbar M99.22
  - upper extremity M99.27
- organ or site, congenital NEC — see Atresia, by site
- papilla of Vater K83.1
- pulmonary (artery) (congenital) Q25.6
  - with ventricular septal defect, transposition of aorta, and hypertrophy of right ventricle Q21.3
  - acquired I28.8
  - in tetralogy of Fallot Q21.3
  - infundibular Q24.3
  - subvalvular Q24.3
  - supravalvular Q25.6
  - valve I37.0
    - with insufficiency I37.2
    - congenital Q22.1
    - rheumatic I09.89
      - with aortic, mitral or tricuspid (valve) disease I08.8
  - vein, acquired I28.8
  - vessel NEC I28.8
- pulmonic (congenital) Q22.1
  - infundibular Q24.3
  - subvalvular Q24.3
- pylorus (hypertrophic) (acquired) K31.1
  - adult K31.1
  - congenital Q40.0
  - infantile Q40.0
- rectum (sphincter) — see Stricture, rectum
- renal artery I70.1
  - congenital Q27.1
- salivary duct (any) K11.8
- sphincter of Oddi K83.1
- spinal M48.00
  - cervical region M48.02
  - cervicothoracic region M48.03
  - lumbar region M48.06
  - lumbosacral region M48.07
  - occipito-atlanto-axial region M48.01
  - sacrococcygeal region M48.08
  - thoracic region M48.04
  - thoracolumbar region M48.05
- stomach, hourglass K31.2
- subaortic (congenital) Q24.4
  - hypertrophic (idiopathic) I42.1
- subglottic J38.6
  - congenital Q31.1
  - postprocedural J95.5
- trachea J39.8
  - congenital Q32.1
  - syphilitic A52.73
  - tuberculous NEC A15.5
- tracheostomy J95.03
- tricuspid (valve) I07.0
  - with
    - aortic (valve) disease I08.2
    - incompetency, insufficiency or regurgitation I07.2
      - with aortic (valve) disease I08.2
        - with mitral (valve) disease I08.3
      - mitral (valve) disease I08.1
        - with aortic (valve) disease I08.3
  - congenital Q22.4
  - nonrheumatic I36.0

Stenosis — continued
- with insufficiency I36.2
- tubal N97.1
- ureter — see Atresia, ureter
- ureteropelvic junction, congenital Q62.11
- ureterovesical orifice, congenital Q62.12
- urethra (valve) (see also Stricture, urethra)
  - congenital Q64.32
- urinary meatus, congenital Q64.33
- vagina N89.5
  - congenital Q52.4
  - in pregnancy — see Pregnancy, complicated by, abnormal vagina
    - causing obstructed labor O65.5
- valve (cardiac) (heart) (see also Endocarditis) I38
  - congenital Q24.8
    - aortic Q23.0
    - mitral Q23.2
    - pulmonary Q22.1
    - tricuspid Q22.4
- vena cava (inferior) (superior) I87.1
  - congenital Q26.0
- vesicourethral orifice Q64.31
- vulva N90.5

Stent jail T82.897 ☑
Stercolith (impaction) K56.41
- appendix K38.1
Stercoraceous, stercoral ulcer K63.3
- anus or rectum K62.6
Stereotypies NEC F98.4
Sterility — see Infertility
Sterilization — see Encounter (for), sterilization
Sternalgia — see Angina
Sternopagus Q89.4
Sternum bifidum Q76.7
Steroid
- effects (adverse) (adrenocortical) (iatrogenic)
  - cushingoid E24.2
    - correct substance properly administered — see Table of Drugs and Chemicals, by drug, adverse effect
    - overdose or wrong substance given or taken — see Table of Drugs and Chemicals, by drug, poisoning
  - diabetes E09
    - correct substance properly administered — see Table of Drugs and Chemicals, by drug, adverse effect
    - overdose or wrong substance given or taken — see Table of Drugs and Chemicals, by drug, poisoning
  - fever R50.2
  - insufficiency E27.3
    - correct substance properly administered — see Table of Drugs and Chemicals, by drug, adverse effect
    - overdose or wrong substance given or taken — see Table of Drugs and Chemicals, by drug, poisoning
  - responder H40.04- ☑
Stevens-Johnson disease or syndrome L51.1
- toxic epidermal necrolysis overlap L51.3
Stewart-Morel syndrome M85.2
Sticker's disease B08.3
Sticky eye — see Conjunctivitis, acute, mucopurulent
Stieda's disease — see Bursitis, tibial collateral
Stiff neck — see Torticollis
Stiff-man syndrome G25.82
Stiffness, joint NEC M25.60- ☑
- ankle M25.67- ☑
- ankylosis — see Ankylosis, joint
- contracture — see Contraction, joint
- elbow M25.62- ☑
- foot M25.67- ☑
- hand M25.64- ☑
- hip M25.65- ☑
- knee M25.66- ☑
- shoulder M25.61- ☑
- wrist M25.63- ☑
Stigmata congenital syphilis A50.59
Stillbirth P95
Still-Felty syndrome — see Felty's syndrome
Still's disease or syndrome (juvenile) M08.20
- adult-onset M06.1
- ankle M08.27- ☑
- elbow M08.22- ☑
- foot joint M08.27- ☑
- hand joint M08.24- ☑
- hip M08.25- ☑
- knee M00.26 ☑
- multiple site M08.29
- shoulder M08.21- ☑

Still's — continued
- vertebra M08.28
- wrist M08.23- ☑
Stimulation, ovary E28.1
Sting (venomous) (with allergic or anaphylactic shock) — see Table of Drugs and Chemicals, by animal or substance, poisoning
Stippled epiphyses Q78.8
Stitch
- abscess T81.4 ☑
- burst (in operation wound) — see Disruption, wound, operation
Stokes-Adams disease or syndrome I45.9
Stokes' disease E05.00
- with thyroid storm E05.01
Stokvis (-Talma) disease D74.8
Stoma malfunction
- colostomy K94.03
- enterostomy K94.13
- gastrostomy K94.23
- ileostomy K94.13
- tracheostomy J95.03
Stomach — see condition
Stomatitis (denture) (ulcerative) K12.1
- angular K13.0
  - due to dietary or vitamin deficiency E53.0
- aphthous K12.0
- bovine B08.61
- candidal B37.0
- catarrhal K12.1
- diphtheritic A36.89
- due to
  - dietary deficiency E53.0
  - thrush B37.0
  - vitamin deficiency
    - B group NEC E53.9
    - B2 (riboflavin) E53.0
- epidemic B08.8
- epizootic B08.8
- follicular K12.1
- gangrenous A69.0
- Geotrichum B48.3
- herpesviral, herpetic B00.2
- herpetiformis K12.0
- malignant K12.1
- membranous acute K12.1
- monilial B37.0
- mycotic B37.0
- necrotizing ulcerative A69.0
- parasitic B37.0
- septic K12.1
- spirochetal A69.1
- suppurative (acute) K12.2
- ulceromembranous A69.1
- vesicular K12.1
  - with exanthem (enteroviral) B08.4
  - virus disease A93.8
- Vincent's A69.1
Stomatocytosis D58.8
Stomatomycosis B37.0
Stomatorrhagia K13.79
Stone (s) (see also Calculus)
- bladder (diverticulum) N21.0
- cystine E72.09
- heart syndrome I50.1
- kidney N20.0
- prostate N42.0
- pulpal (dental) K04.2
- renal N20.0
- salivary gland or duct (any) K11.5
- urethra (impacted) N21.1
- urinary (duct) (impacted) (passage) N20.9
  - bladder (diverticulum) N21.0
  - lower tract N21.9
  - specified NEC N21.8
- xanthine E79.8 [N22]
Stonecutter's lung J62.8
Stonemason's asthma, disease, lung or pneumoconiosis J62.8
Stoppage
- heart — see Arrest, cardiac
- urine — see Retention, urine
Storm, thyroid — see Thyrotoxicosis
Strabismus (congenital) (nonparalytic) H50.9
- concomitant H50.40
  - convergent — see Strabismus, convergent concomitant
  - divergent — see Strabismus, divergent concomitant
- convergent concomitant H50.00
  - accommodative component H50.43
  - alternating H50.05

Strabismus — *continued*
  with
    A pattern H50.06
    specified nonconcomitances NEC H50.08
    V pattern H50.07
  monocular H50.01- ☑
    with
      A pattern H50.02- ☑
      specified nonconcomitances NEC
        H50.04- ☑
      V pattern H50.03- ☑
    intermittent H50.31- ☑
      alternating H50.32
  cyclotropia H50.1- ☑
  divergent concomitant H50.10
    alternating H50.15
    with
      A pattern H50.16
      specified noncomitances NEC H50.18
      V pattern H50.17
  monocular H50.11- ☑
    with
      A pattern H50.12- ☑
      specified noncomitances NEC H50.14- ☑
      V pattern H50.13- ☑
    intermittent H50.33 ☑
      alternating H50.34
  Duane's syndrome H50.81- ☑
  due to adhesions, scars H50.69
  heterophoria H50.50
    alternating H50.55
    cyclophoria H50.54
    esophoria H50.51
    exophoria H50.52
    vertical H50.53
  heterotropia H50.40
    intermittent H50.30
  hypertropia H50.2- ☑
  hypotropia — *see* Hypertropia
  latent H50.50
  mechanical H50.60
    Brown's sheath syndrome H50.61- ☑
    specified type NEC H50.69
  monofixation syndrome H50.42
  paralytic H49.9
    abducens nerve H49.2- ☑
    fourth nerve H49.1- ☑
    Kearns-Sayre syndrome H49.81- ☑
    ophthalmoplegia (external)
      progressive H49.4- ☑
        with pigmentary retinopathy H49.81- ☑
      total H49.3- ☑
    sixth nerve H49.2- ☑
    specified type NEC H49.88- ☑
    third nerve H49.0- ☑
    trochlear nerve H49.1- ☑
  specified type NEC H50.89
  vertical H50.2- ☑
Strain
  back S39.012 ☑
  cervical S16.1 ☑
  eye NEC — *see* Disturbance, vision, subjective
  heart — *see* Disease, heart
  low back S39.012 ☑
  mental NOS Z73.3
    work-related Z56.6
  muscle (tendon) — *see* Injury, muscle, by site,
    strain
  neck S16.1 ☑
  postural (*see also* Disorder, soft tissue, due to use)
  physical NOS Z73.3
    work-related Z56.6
  psychological NEC Z73.3
  tendon — *see* Injury, muscle, by site, strain
Straining, on urination R39.16
Strand, vitreous — *see* Opacity, vitreous, membranes
  and strands
Strangulation, strangulated (*see also* Asphyxia,
  traumatic)
  appendix K38.8
  bladder-neck N32.0
  bowel or colon K56.2
  food or foreign body — *see* Foreign body, by site
  hemorrhoids — *see* Hemorrhoids, with
    complication
  hernia (*see also* Hernia, by site, with obstruction)
    with gangrene — *see* Hernia, by site, with
      gangrene
  intestine (large) (small) K56.2
    with hernia (*see also* Hernia, by site, with
      obstruction)

Strangulation — *continued*
    with gangrene — *see* Hernia, by site, with
      gangrene
  mesentery K56.2
  mucus — *see* Asphyxia, mucus
  omentum K56.2
  organ or site, congenital NEC — *see* Atresia, by
    site
  ovary — *see* Torsion, ovary
  penis N48.89
    foreign body T19.4 ☑
  rupture — *see* Hernia, by site, with obstruction
  stomach due to hernia (*see also* Hernia, by site,
    with obstruction)
    with gangrene — *see* Hernia, by site, with
      gangrene
  vesicourethral orifice N32.0
Strangury R30.0
Straw itch B88.0
Strawberry
  gallbladder K82.4
  mark Q82.5
  tongue (red) (white) K14.3
Streak (s)
  macula, angioid H35.33
  ovarian Q50.32
Strephosymbolia F81.0
  secondary to organic lesion R48.8
Streptobacillary fever A25.1
Streptobacillosis A25.1
Streptobacillus moniliformis A25.1
Streptococcus, streptococcal (*see also* condition)
  as cause of disease classified elsewhere B95.5
  group
    A, as cause of disease classified elsewhere
      B95.0
    B, as cause of disease classified elsewhere B95.1
    D, as cause of disease classified elsewhere
      B95.2
    pneumoniae, as cause of disease classified
      elsewhere B95.3
    specified NEC, as cause of disease classified
      elsewhere B95.4
Streptomycosis B47.1
Streptotrichosis A48.8
Stress F43.9
  family — *see* Disruption, family
  fetal P84
    complicating pregnancy O77.9
      due to drug administration O77.1
  mental NEC Z73.3
    work-related Z56.6
  physical NEC Z73.3
    work-related Z56.6
  polycythemia D75.1
  reaction (*see also* Reaction, stress) F43.9
  work schedule Z56.3
Stretching, nerve — *see* Injury, nerve
Striae albicantes, atrophicae or distensae (cutis)
  L90.6
Stricture (*see also* Stenosis)
  ampulla of Vater K83.1
  anus (sphincter) K62.4
    congenital Q42.3
      with fistula Q42.2
    infantile Q42.3
      with fistula Q42.2
  aorta (ascending) (congenital) Q25.3
    arteriosclerotic I70.0
    calcified I70.0
    supravalvular, congenital Q25.3
  aortic (valve) — *see* Stenosis, aortic
  aqueduct of Sylvius (congenital) Q03.0
    with spina bifida — *see* Spina bifida, by site,
      with hydrocephalus
    acquired G91.1
  artery I77.1
    basilar — *see* Occlusion, artery, basilar
    carotid — *see* Occlusion, artery, carotid
    celiac I77.4
    congenital (peripheral) Q27.8
      cerebral Q28.3
      coronary Q24.5
      digestive system Q27.8
      lower limb Q27.8
      retinal Q14.1
      specified site NEC Q27.8
      umbilical Q27.0
      upper limb Q27.8
    coronary — *see* Disease, heart, ischemic,
      atherosclerotic
      congenital Q24.5

Stricture — *continued*
  precerebral — *see* Occlusion, artery, precerebral
  pulmonary (congenital) Q25.6
    acquired I28.8
  renal I70.1
  vertebral — *see* Occlusion, artery, vertebral
  auditory canal (external) (congenital)
    acquired — *see* Stenosis, external ear canal
  bile duct (common) (hepatic) K83.1
    congenital Q44.3
    postoperative K91.89
  bladder N32.89
    neck N32.0
  bowel — *see* Obstruction, intestine
  brain G93.89
  bronchus J98.09
    congenital Q32.3
    syphilitic A52.72
  cardia (stomach) K22.2
    congenital Q39.3
  cardiac (*see also* Disease, heart)
    orifice (stomach) K22.2
  cecum — *see* Obstruction, intestine
  cervix, cervical (canal) N88.2
    congenital Q51.828
    in pregnancy — *see* Pregnancy, complicated by,
      abnormal cervix
        causing obstructed labor O65.5
  colon (*see also* Obstruction, intestine)
    congenital Q42.9
    specified NEC Q42.8
  colostomy K94.03
  common (bile) duct K83.1
  coronary (artery) — *see* Disease, heart, ischemic,
    atherosclerotic
  cystic duct — *see* Obstruction, gallbladder
  digestive organs NEC, congenital Q45.8
  duodenum K31.5
    congenital Q41.0
  ear canal (external) (congenital) Q16.1
    acquired — *see* Stricture, auditory canal,
      acquired
  ejaculatory duct N50.8
  enterostomy K94.13
  esophagus K22.2
    congenital Q39.3
    syphilitic A52.79
      congenital A50.59 [K23]
  eustachian tube (*see also* Obstruction, eustachian
    tube)
    congenital Q17.8
  fallopian tube N97.1
    gonococcal A54.24
    tuberculous A18.17
  gallbladder — *see* Obstruction, gallbladder
  glottis J38.6
  heart (*see also* Disease, heart)
    valve (*see also* Endocarditis) I38
      aortic Q23.0
      mitral Q23.4
      pulmonary Q22.1
      tricuspid Q22.4
  hepatic duct K83.1
  hourglass, of stomach K31.2
  hymen N89.6
  hypopharynx J39.2
  ileum K56.69
    congenital Q41.2
  intestine (*see also* Obstruction, intestine)
    congenital (small) Q41.9
      large Q42.9
        specified NEC Q42.8
      specified NEC Q41.8
    ischemic K55.1
  jejunum K56.69
    congenital Q41.1
  lacrimal passages (*see also* Stenosis, lacrimal)
    congenital Q10.5
  larynx J38.6
    congenital NEC Q31.8
      subglottic Q31.1
    syphilitic A52.73
      congenital A50.59 [J99]
  meatus
    ear (congenital) Q16.1
      acquired — *see* Stricture, auditory canal,
        acquired
    osseous (ear) (congenital) Q16.1
      acquired — *see* Stricture, auditory canal,
        acquired
  urinarius (*see also* Stricture, urethra)
    congenital Q64.33

Stricture — continued
mitral (valve) — see Stenosis, mitral
myocardium, myocardial I51.5
hypertrophic subaortic (idiopathic) I42.1
nares (anterior) (posterior) J34.89
congenital Q30.0
nasal duct (see also Stenosis, lacrimal, duct)
congenital Q10.5
nasolacrimal duct (see also Stenosis, lacrimal, duct)
congenital Q10.5
nasopharynx J39.2
syphilitic A52.73
nose J34.89
congenital Q30.0
nostril (anterior) (posterior) J34.89
congenital Q30.0
syphilitic A52.73
congenital A50.59 [J99]
organ or site, congenital NEC — see Atresia, by site
os uteri — see Stricture, cervix
osseous meatus (ear) (congenital) Q16.1
acquired — see Stricture, auditory canal, acquired
oviduct — see Stricture, fallopian tube
pelviureteric junction (congenital) Q62.11
penis, by foreign body T19.4 ☑
pharynx J39.2
prostate N42.89
pulmonary, pulmonic
artery (congenital) Q25.6
acquired I28.8
noncongenital I28.8
infundibulum (congenital) Q24.3
valve I37.0
congenital Q22.1
vein, acquired I28.8
vessel NEC I28.8
punctum lacrimale (see also Stenosis, lacrimal, punctum)
congenital Q10.5
pylorus (hypertrophic) K31.1
adult K31.1
congenital Q40.0
infantile Q40.0
rectosigmoid K56.69
rectum (sphincter) K62.4
congenital Q42.1
with fistula Q42.0
due to
chlamydial lymphogranuloma A55
irradiation K91.89
lymphogranuloma venereum A55
gonococcal A54.6
inflammatory (chlamydial) A55
syphilitic A52.74
tuberculous A18.32
renal artery I70.1
congenital Q27.1
salivary duct or gland (any) K11.8
sigmoid (flexure) — see Obstruction, intestine
spermatic cord N50.8
stoma (following) (of)
colostomy K94.03
enterostomy K94.13
gastrostomy K94.23
ileostomy K94.13
tracheostomy J95.03
stomach K31.89
congenital Q40.2
hourglass K31.2
subaortic Q24.4
hypertrophic (acquired) (idiopathic) I42.1
subglottic J38.6
syphilitic NEC A52.79
trachea J39.8
congenital Q32.1
syphilitic A52.73
tuberculous NEC A15.5
tracheostomy J95.03
tricuspid (valve) — see Stenosis, tricuspid
tunica vaginalis N50.8
ureter (postoperative) N13.5
with
hydronephrosis N13.1
with infection N13.6
pyelonephritis (chronic) N11.1
congenital — see Atresia, ureter
tuberculous A18.11
ureteropelvic junction (congenital) Q62.11
ureterovesical orifice N13.5

Stricture — continued
with infection N13.6
urethra (organic) (spasmodic) N35.9
associated with schistosomiasis B65.0 [N37]
congenital Q64.39
valvular (posterior) Q64.2
due to
infection — see Stricture, urethra, postinfective
trauma — see Stricture, urethra, post-traumatic
gonococcal, gonorrheal A54.01
infective NEC — see Stricture, urethra, postinfective
late effect (sequelae) of injury — see Stricture, urethra, post-traumatic
postcatheterization — see Stricture, urethra, postprocedural
postinfective NEC
female N35.12
male N35.119
anterior urethra N35.114
bulbous urethra N35.112
meatal N35.111
membranous urethra N35.113
postobstetric N35.021
postoperative — see Stricture, urethra, postprocedural
postprocedural
female N99.12
male N99.114
anterior urethra N99.113
bulbous urethra N99.111
meatal N99.110
membranous urethra N99.112
post-traumatic
female N35.028
due to childbirth N35.021
male N35.014
anterior urethra N35.013
bulbous urethra N35.011
meatal N35.010
membranous urethra N35.012
sequela (late effect) of
childbirth N35.021
injury — see Stricture, urethra, post-traumatic
specified cause NEC N35.8
syphilitic A52.76
traumatic — see Stricture, urethra, post-traumatic
valvular (posterior), congenital Q64.2
urinary meatus — see Stricture, urethra
uterus, uterine (synechiae) N85.6
os (external) (internal) — see Stricture, cervix
vagina (outlet) — see Stenosis, vagina
valve (cardiac) (heart) (see also Endocarditis)
congenital
aortic Q23.0
mitral Q23.2
pulmonary Q22.1
tricuspid Q22.4
vas deferens N50.8
congenital Q55.4
vein I87.1
vena cava (inferior) (superior) NEC I87.1
congenital Q26.0
vesicourethral orifice N32.0
congenital Q64.31
vulva (acquired) N90.5
Stridor R06.1
congenital (larynx) P28.89
Stridulous — see condition
Stroke (apoplectic) (brain) (embolic) (ischemic) (paralytic) (thrombotic) I63.9
epileptic — see Epilepsy
heat T67.0 ☑
in evolution I63.9
intraoperative
during cardiac surgery I97.810
during other surgery I97.811
lightning — see Lightning
meaning
cerebral hemorrhage - code to Hemorrhage, intracranial
cerebral infarction - code to Infarction, cerebral
postprocedural
following cardiac surgery I97.820
following other surgery I97.821
unspecified (NOS) I63.9
Stromatosis, endometrial D39.0
Strongyloidiasis, strongyloidosis B78.9
cutaneous B78.1

Strongyloidiasis — continued
disseminated B78.7
intestinal B78.0
Strophulus pruriginosus L28.2
Struck by lightning — see Lightning
Struma (see also Goiter)
Hashimoto E06.3
lymphomatosa E06.3
nodosa (simplex) E04.9
endemic E01.2
multinodular E01.1
multinodular E01.1
iodine-deficiency related E01.1
toxic or with hyperthyroidism E05.20
with thyroid storm E05.21
multinodular E05.20
with thyroid storm E05.21
uninodular E05.10
with thyroid storm E05.11
toxicosa E05.20
with thyroid storm E05.21
multinodular E05.20
with thyroid storm E05.21
uninodular E05.10
with thyroid storm E05.11
uninodular E04.1
ovarii D27.- ☑
Riedel's E06.5
Strumipriva cachexia E03.4
Strümpell-Marie spine — see Spondylitis, ankylosing
Strümpell-Westphal pseudosclerosis E83.01
Stuart deficiency disease (factor X) D68.2
Stuart-Prower factor deficiency (factor X) D68.2
Student's elbow — see Bursitis, elbow, olecranon
Stump — see Amputation
Stunting, nutritional E45
Stupor (catatonic) R40.1
depressive F32.8
dissociative F44.2
manic F30.2
manic-depressive F31.89
psychogenic (anergic) F44.2
reaction to exceptional stress (transient) F43.0
Sturge (-Weber) (-Dimitri) (-Kalischer) disease or syndrome Q85.8
Stuttering F80.81
adult onset F98.5
childhood onset F80.81
following cerebrovascular disease — see Disorder, fluency. following cerebrovascular disease
in conditions classified elsewhere R47.82
Sty, stye (external) (internal) (meibomian) (zeisian) — see Hordeolum
Subacidity, gastric K31.89
psychogenic F45.8
Subacute — see condition
Subarachnoid — see condition
Subcortical — see condition
Subcostal syndrome, nerve compression — see Mononeuropathy, upper limb, specified site NEC
Subcutaneous, subcuticular — see condition
Subdural — see condition
Subendocardium — see condition
Subependymoma
specified site — see Neoplasm, uncertain behavior, by site
unspecified site D43.2
Suberosis J67.3
Subglossitis — see Glossitis
Subhemophilia D66
Subinvolution
breast (postlactational) (postpuerperal) N64.89
puerperal O90.89
uterus (chronic) (nonpuerperal) N85.3
puerperal O90.89
Sublingual — see condition
Sublinguitis — see Sialoadenitis
Subluxatable hip Q65.6
Subluxation (see also Dislocation)
acromioclavicular S43.11- ☑
ankle S93.0- ☑
atlantoaxial, recurrent M43.4
with myelopathy M43.3
carpometacarpal (joint) NEC S63.05- ☑
thumb S63.04- ☑
complex, vertebral — see Complex, subluxation
congenital (see also Malposition, congenital)
hip — see Dislocation, hip, congenital, partial
joint (excluding hip)
lower limb Q68.8
shoulder Q68.8

Subluxation — *continued*
    upper limb Q68.8
    elbow (traumatic) S53.10- ☑
      anterior S53.11- ☑
      lateral S53.14- ☑
      medial S53.13- ☑
      posterior S53.12- ☑
      specified type NEC S53.19- ☑
    finger S63.20- ☑
      index S63.20- ☑
      interphalangeal S63.22- ☑
        distal S63.24- ☑
          index S63.24- ☑
          little S63.24- ☑
          middle S63.24- ☑
          ring S63.24- ☑
        index S63.22- ☑
        little S63.22- ☑
        middle S63.22- ☑
        proximal S63.23- ☑
          index S63.23- ☑
          little S63.23- ☑
          middle S63.23- ☑
          ring S63.23- ☑
        ring S63.22- ☑
      little S63.20- ☑
      metacarpophalangeal S63.21- ☑
        index S63.21- ☑
        little S63.21- ☑
        middle S63.21- ☑
        ring S63.21- ☑
      middle S63.20- ☑
      ring S63.20- ☑
    foot S93.30- ☑
      specified site NEC S93.33- ☑
      tarsal joint S93.31- ☑
      tarsometatarsal joint S93.32- ☑
      toe — *see* Subluxation, toe
    hip S73.00- ☑
      anterior S73.03- ☑
      obturator S73.02- ☑
      central S73.04- ☑
      posterior S73.01- ☑
    interphalangeal (joint)
      finger S63.22- ☑
        distal joint S63.24- ☑
          index S63.24- ☑
          little S63.24- ☑
          middle S63.24- ☑
          ring S63.24- ☑
        index S63.22- ☑
        little S63.22- ☑
        middle S63.22- ☑
        proximal joint S63.23- ☑
          index S63.23- ☑
          little S63.23- ☑
          middle S63.23- ☑
          ring S63.23- ☑
        ring S63.22- ☑
      thumb S63.12- ☑
        distal joint S63.14- ☑
        proximal joint S63.13- ☑
      toe S93.13- ☑
        great S93.13- ☑
        lesser S93.13- ☑
    joint prosthesis — *see* Complications, joint
      prosthesis, mechanical, displacement, by site
    knee S83.10- ☑
      cap — *see* Subluxation, patella
      patella — *see* Subluxation, patella
      proximal tibia
        anteriorly S83.11- ☑
        laterally S83.14- ☑
        medially S83.13- ☑
        posteriorly S83.12- ☑
      specified type NEC S83.19- ☑
    lens — *see* Dislocation, lens, partial
    ligament, traumatic — *see* Sprain, by site
    metacarpal (bone)
      proximal end S63.06- ☑
    metacarpophalangeal (joint)
      finger S63.21- ☑
        index S63.21- ☑
        little S63.21- ☑
        middle S63.21- ☑
        ring S63.21- ☑
        thumb S63.11- ☑
    metatarsophalangeal joint S93.14- ☑
      great toe S93.14- ☑
      lesser toe S93.14- ☑
    midcarpal (joint) S63.03- ☑
    patella S83.00- ☑

Subluxation — *continued*
    lateral S83.01- ☑
    recurrent (nontraumatic) — *see* Dislocation,
      patella, recurrent, incomplete
    specified type NEC S83.09- ☑
    pathological — *see* Dislocation, pathological
    radial head S53.00- ☑
      anterior S53.01- ☑
      nursemaid's elbow S53.03- ☑
      posterior S53.02- ☑
      specified type NEC S53.09- ☑
    radiocarpal (joint) S63.02- ☑
    radioulnar (joint)
      distal S63.01- ☑
      proximal — *see* Subluxation, elbow
    shoulder
      congenital Q68.8
      girdle S43.30- ☑
        scapula S43.31- ☑
        specified site NEC S43.39- ☑
      traumatic S43.00- ☑
        anterior S43.01- ☑
        inferior S43.03- ☑
        posterior S43.02- ☑
        specified type NEC S43.08- ☑
    sternoclavicular (joint) S43.20- ☑
      anterior S43.21- ☑
      posterior S43.22- ☑
    symphysis (pubis)
    thumb S63.103
      interphalangeal joint — *see* Subluxation,
        interphalangeal (joint), thumb
      metacarpophalangeal joint — *see* Subluxation,
        metacarpophalangeal (joint), thumb
    toe (s) S93.10- ☑
      great S93.10- ☑
        interphalangeal joint S93.13- ☑
        metatarsophalangeal joint S93.14- ☑
      interphalangeal joint S93.13- ☑
      lesser S93.10- ☑
        interphalangeal joint S93.13- ☑
        metatarsophalangeal joint S93.14- ☑
      metatarsophalangeal joint S93.149
    ulnohumeral joint — *see* Subluxation, elbow
    vertebral
      recurrent NEC M43.5
      traumatic
        cervical S13.100 ☑
          atlantoaxial joint S13.120 ☑
          atlantooccipital joint S13.110 ☑
          atloidooccipital joint S13.110 ☑
          joint between
            C0 and C1 S13.110 ☑
            C1 and C2 S13.120 ☑
            C2 and C3 S13.130 ☑
            C3 and C4 S13.140 ☑
            C4 and C5 S13.150 ☑
            C5 and C6 S13.160 ☑
            C6 and C7 S13.170 ☑
            C7 and T1 S13.180 ☑
          occipitoatloid joint S13.110 ☑
        lumbar S33.100 ☑
          joint between
            L1 and L2 S33.110 ☑
            L2 and L3 S33.120 ☑
            L3 and L4 S33.130 ☑
            L4 and L5 S33.140 ☑
        thoracic S23.100 ☑
          joint between
            T1 and T2 S23.110 ☑
            T2 and T3 S23.120 ☑
            T3 and T4 S23.122 ☑
            T4 and T5 S23.130 ☑
            T5 and T6 S23.132 ☑
            T6 and T7 S23.140 ☑
            T7 and T8 S23.142 ☑
            T8 and T9 S23.150 ☑
            T9 and T10 S23.152 ☑
            T10 and T11 S23.160 ☑
            T11 and T12 S23.162 ☑
            T12 and L1 S23.170 ☑
    ulna
      distal end S63.07- ☑
      proximal end — *see* Subluxation, elbow
    wrist (carpal bone) S63.00- ☑
      carpometacarpal joint — *see* Subluxation,
        carpometacarpal (joint)
      distal radioulnar joint — *see* Subluxation,
        radioulnar (joint), distal
      metacarpal bone, proximal   *see* Subluxation,
        metacarpal (bone), proximal end
      midcarpal — *see* Subluxation, midcarpal (joint)

Subluxation — *continued*
    radiocarpal joint — *see* Subluxation,
      radiocarpal (joint)
    recurrent — *see* Dislocation, recurrent, wrist
    specified site NEC S63.09- ☑
    ulna — *see* Subluxation, ulna, distal end
Submaxillary — *see* condition
Submersion (fatal) (nonfatal) T75.1 ☑
Submucous — *see* condition
Subnormal, subnormality
    accommodation (old age) H52.4
    mental — *see* Disability, intellectual
    temperature (accidental) T68
Subphrenic — *see* condition
Subscapular nerve — *see* condition
Subseptus uterus Q51.2
Subsiding appendicitis K36
Substernal thyroid E04.9
    congenital Q89.2
Substitution disorder F44.9
Subtentorial — *see* condition
Subthyroidism (acquired) (*see also* Hypothyroidism)
    congenital E03.1
Succenturiate placenta O43.19- ☑
Sucking thumb, child (excessive) F98.8
Sudamen, sudamina L74.1
Sudanese kala-azar B55.0
Sudden
    heart failure — *see* Failure, heart
    hearing loss — *see* Deafness, sudden
Sudeck's atrophy, disease, or syndrome — *see*
    Algoneurodystrophy
Suffocation — *see* Asphyxia, traumatic
Sugar
    blood
      high (transient) R73.9
      low (transient) E16.2
    in urine R81
Suicide, suicidal (attempted) T14.91
    by poisoning — *see* Table of Drugs and Chemicals
    history of (personal) Z91.5
      in family Z81.8
    ideation — *see* Ideation, suicidal
    risk
      meaning personal history of attempted suicide
        Z91.5
      meaning suicidal ideation — *see* Ideation,
        suicidal
    tendencies
      meaning personal history of attempted suicide
        Z91.5
      meaning suicidal ideation — *see* Ideation,
        suicidal
    trauma — *see* nature of injury by site
Suipestifer infection — *see* Infection, salmonella
Sulfhemoglobinemia, sulphemoglobinemia
    (acquired) (with methemoglobinemia) D74.8
Sumatran mite fever A75.3
Summer — *see* condition
Sunburn L55.9
    first degree L55.0
    second degree L55.1
    third degree L55.2
SUNCT (short lasting unilateral neuralgiform
    headache with conjunctival injection and tearing)
    G44.059
    intractable G44.051
    not intractable G44.059
Sunken acetabulum — *see* Derangement, joint,
    specified type NEC, hip
Sunstroke T67.0 ☑
Superfecundation — *see* Pregnancy, multiple
Superfetation — *see* Pregnancy, multiple
Superinvolution (uterus) N85.8
Supernumerary (congenital)
    aortic cusps Q23.8
    auditory ossicles Q16.3
    bone Q79.8
    breast Q83.1
    carpal bones Q74.0
    cusps, heart valve NEC Q24.8
      aortic Q23.8
      mitral Q23.2
      pulmonary Q22.3
    digit (s) Q69.9
    ear (lobule) Q17.0
    fallopian tube Q50.6
    finger Q69.0
    hymen Q52.4
    kidney Q63.0
    lacrimonasal duct Q10.6
    lobule (ear) Q17.0

☑ **Additional character required**

Supernumerary — *continued*
- mitral cusps Q23.2
- muscle Q79.8
- nipple (s) Q83.3
- organ or site not listed — *see* Accessory
- ossicles, auditory Q16.3
- ovary Q50.31
- oviduct Q50.6
- pulmonary, pulmonic cusps Q22.3
- rib Q76.6
  - cervical or first (syndrome) Q76.5
- roots (of teeth) K00.2
- spleen Q89.09
- tarsal bones Q74.2
- teeth K00.1
- testis Q55.29
- thumb Q69.1
- toe Q69.2
- uterus Q51.2
- vagina Q52.1 ☑
- vertebra Q76.49

Supervision (of)
- contraceptive — *see* Prescription, contraceptives
- dietary (for) Z71.3
  - allergy (food) Z71.3
  - colitis Z71.3
  - diabetes mellitus Z71.3
  - food allergy or intolerance Z71.3
  - gastritis Z71.3
  - hypercholesterolemia Z71.3
  - hypoglycemia Z71.3
  - intolerance (food) Z71.3
  - obesity Z71.3
  - specified NEC Z71.3
- healthy infant or child Z76.2
  - foundling Z76.1
- high-risk pregnancy — *see* Pregnancy, complicated by, high, risk
- lactation Z39.1
- pregnancy — *see* Pregnancy, supervision of

Supplemental teeth K00.1

Suppression
- binocular vision H53.34
- lactation O92.5
- menstruation N94.89
- ovarian secretion E28.39
- renal N28.9
- urine, urinary secretion R34

Suppuration, suppurative (*see also* condition)
- accessory sinus (chronic) — *see* Sinusitis
- adrenal gland
- antrum (chronic) — *see* Sinusitis, maxillary
- bladder — *see* Cystitis
- brain G06.0
  - sequelae G09
- breast N61
  - puerperal, postpartum or gestational — *see* Mastitis, obstetric, purulent
- dental periosteum M27.3
- ear (middle) (*see also* Otitis, media)
  - external NEC — *see* Otitis, externa, infective
  - internalH83.0
- ethmoidal (chronic) (sinus) — *see* Sinusitis, ethmoidal
- fallopian tube — *see* Salpingo-oophoritis
- frontal (chronic) (sinus) — *see* Sinusitis, frontal
- gallbladder (acute) K81.0
- gum K05.20
  - generalized K05.22
  - localized K05.21
- intracranial G06.0
- joint — *see* Arthritis, pyogenic or pyemic
- labyrinthineH83.0
- lung — *see* Abscess, lung
- mammary gland N61
  - puerperal, postpartum O91.12
    - associated with lactation O91.13
- maxilla, maxillary M27.2
  - sinus (chronic) — *see* Sinusitis, maxillary
- muscle — *see* Myositis, infective
- nasal sinus (chronic) — *see* Sinusitis
- pancreas, acute K85.8
- parotid gland — *see* Sialoadenitis
- pelvis, pelvic
  - female — *see* Disease, pelvis, inflammatory
  - male K65.0
- pericranial — *see* Osteomyelitis
- salivary duct or gland (any) — *see* Sialoadenitis
- sinus (accessory) (chronic) (nasal) — *see* Sinusitis
- sphenoidal sinus (chronic) — *see* Sinusitis, sphenoidal
- thymus (gland) E32.1

Suppuration — *continued*
- thyroid (gland) E06.0
- tonsil — *see* Tonsillitis
- uterus — *see* Endometritis

Supraeruption of tooth (teeth) M26.34

Supraglottitis J04.30
- with obstruction J04.31

Suprarenal (gland) — *see* condition

Suprascapular nerve — *see* condition

Suprasellar — *see* condition

Surfer's knots or nodules S89.8- ☑

Surgical
- emphysema T81.82 ☑
- procedures, complication or misadventure — *see* Complications, surgical procedures
- shock T81.10 ☑

Surveillance (of) (for) (*see also* Observation)
- alcohol abuse Z71.41
- contraceptive — *see* Prescription, contraceptives
- dietary Z71.3
- drug abuse Z71.51

Susceptibility to disease, genetic Z15.89
- malignant neoplasm Z15.09
  - breast Z15.01
  - endometrium Z15.04
  - ovary Z15.02
  - prostate Z15.03
  - specified NEC Z15.09
- multiple endocrine neoplasia Z15.81

Suspected condition, ruled out (*see also* Observation, suspected)
- amniotic cavity and membrane Z03.71
- cervical shortening Z03.75
- fetal anomaly Z03.73
- fetal growth Z03.74
- maternal and fetal conditions NEC Z03.79
- oligohydramnios Z03.71
- placental problem Z03.72
- polyhydramnios Z03.71

Suspended uterus
- in pregnancy or childbirth — *see* Pregnancy, complicated by, abnormal uterus

Sutton's nevus D22.9

Suture
- burst (in operation wound) T81.31 ☑
  - external operation wound T81.31 ☑
  - internal operation wound T81.32 ☑
- inadvertently left in operation wound — *see* Foreign body, accidentally left during a procedure
- removal Z48.02

Swab inadvertently left in operation wound — *see* Foreign body, accidentally left during a procedure

Swallowed, swallowing
- difficulty — *see* Dysphagia
- foreign body — *see* Foreign body, alimentary tract

Swan-neck deformity (finger) — *see* Deformity, finger, swan-neck

Swearing, compulsive F42
- in Gilles de la Tourette's syndrome F95.2

Sweat, sweats
- fetid L75.0
- night R61

Sweating, excessive R61

Sweeley-Klionsky disease E75.21

Sweet's disease or dermatosis L98.2

Swelling (of) R60.9
- abdomen, abdominal (not referable to any particular organ) — *see* Mass, abdominal
- ankle — *see* Effusion, joint, ankle
- arm M79.89
  - forearm M79.89
- breast N63
- Calabar B74.3
- cervical gland R59.0
- chest, localized R22.2
- ear H93.8- ☑
- extremity (lower) (upper) — *see* Disorder, soft tissue, specified type NEC
- finger M79.89
- foot M79.89
- glands R59.9
  - generalized R59.1
  - localized R59.0
- hand M79.89
- head (localized) R22.0
- inflammatory — *see* Inflammation
- intra-abdominal — *see* Mass, abdominal
- joint — *see* Effusion, joint
- leg M79.89
  - lower M79.89

Swelling — *continued*
- limb — *see* Disorder, soft tissue, specified type NEC
- localized (skin) R22.9
  - chest R22.2
  - head R22.0
  - limb
    - lower — *see* Mass, localized, limb, lower
    - upper — *see* Mass, localized, limb, upper
  - neck R22.1
  - trunk R22.2
- neck (localized) R22.1
- pelvic — *see* Mass, abdominal
- scrotum N50.8
- splenic — *see* Splenomegaly
- testis N50.8
- toe M79.89
- umbilical R19.09
- wandering, due to Gnathostoma (spinigerum) B83.1
- white — *see* Tuberculosis, arthritis

Swift (-Feer) disease
- overdose or wrong substance given or taken — *see* Table of Drugs and Chemicals, by drug, poisoning

Swimmer's
- cramp T75.1 ☑
- ear H60.33- ☑
- itch B65.3

Swimming in the head R42

Swollen — *see* Swelling

Swyer syndrome Q99.1

Sycosis L73.8
- barbae (not parasitic) L73.8
- contagiosa (mycotic) B35.0
- lupoides L73.8
- mycotic B35.0
- parasitic B35.0
- vulgaris L73.8

Sydenham's chorea — *see* Chorea, Sydenham's

Sylvatic yellow fever A95.0

Sylvest's disease B33.0

Symblepharon H11.23- ☑
- congenital Q10.3

Symond's syndrome G93.2

Sympathetic — *see* condition

Sympatheticotonia G90.8

Sympathicoblastoma
- specified site — *see* Neoplasm, malignant, by site
- unspecified site C74.90

Sympathogonioma — *see* Sympathicoblastoma

Symphalangy (fingers) (toes) Q70.9

Symptoms NEC R68.89
- breast NEC N64.59
- development NEC R63.8
- factitious, self-induced — *see* Disorder, factitious
- genital organs, female R10.2
- involving
  - abdomen NEC R19.8
  - appearance NEC R46.89
  - awareness R41.9
    - altered mental status R41.82
    - amnesia — *see* Amnesia
    - borderline intellectual functioning R41.83
    - coma — *see* Coma
    - disorientation R41.0
    - neurologic neglect syndrome R41.4
    - senile cognitive decline R41.81
    - specified symptom NEC R41.89
  - behavior NEC R46.89
  - cardiovascular system NEC R09.89
  - chest NEC R09.89
  - circulatory system NEC R09.89
  - cognitive functions R41.9
    - altered mental status R41.82
    - amnesia — *see* Amnesia
    - borderline intellectual functioning R41.83
    - coma — *see* Coma
    - disorientation R41.0
    - neurologic neglect syndrome R41.4
    - senile cognitive decline R41.81
    - specified symptom NEC R41.89
  - development NEC R62.50
  - digestive system NEC R19.8
  - emotional state NEC R45.89
    - emotional lability R45.86
  - food and fluid intake R63.8
  - general perceptions and sensations R44.9
    - specified NEC R44.8
  - musculoskeletal system R29.91
    - specified NEC R29.898
  - nervous system R29.90

Symptoms — *continued*
    specified NEC R29.818
    pelvis NEC R19.8
    respiratory system NEC R09.89
    skin and integument R23.9
    urinary system R39.9
  menopausal N95.1
  metabolism NEC R63.8
  neurotic F48.8
  of infancy R68.19
  pelvis NEC, female R10.2
  skin and integument NEC R23.9
  subcutaneous tissue NEC R23.9
Sympus Q74.2
Syncephalus Q89.4
Synchondrosis
  abnormal (congenital) Q78.8
  ischiopubic M91.0
Synchysis (scintillans) (senile) (vitreous body) H43.89
Syncope (near) (pre-) R55
  anginosa I20.8
  bradycardia R00.1
  cardiac R55
  carotid sinus G90.01
  due to spinal (lumbar) puncture G97.1
  heart R55
  heat T67.1 ☑
  laryngeal R05
  psychogenic F48.8
  tussive R05
  vasoconstriction R55
  vasodepressor R55
  vasomotor R55
  vasovagal R55
Syndactylism, syndactyly Q70.9
  complex (with synostosis)
    fingers Q70.0- ☑
    toes Q70.2- ☑
  simple (without synostosis)
    fingers Q70.1- ☑
    toes Q70.3- ☑
Syndrome (*see also* Disease)
  5q minus NOS D46.C
  48,XXXX Q97.1
  49,XXXXX Q97.1
  abdominal
    acute R10.0
    muscle deficiency Q79.4
  abnormal innervation H02.519
    left H02.516
      lower H02.515
      upper H02.514
    right H02.513
      lower H02.512
      upper H02.511
  abstinence, neonatal P96.1
  acid pulmonary aspiration, obstetric O74.0
  acquired immunodeficiency — *see* Human, immunodeficiency virus (HIV) disease
  acute abdominal R10.0
  acute respiratory distress (adult) (child) J80
  Adair-Dighton Q78.0
  Adams-Stokes (-Morgagni) I45.9
  adiposogenital E23.6
  adrenal
    hemorrhage (meningococcal) A39.1
    meningococcic A39.1
  adrenocortical — *see* Cushing's, syndrome
  adrenogenital E25.9
    congenital, associated with enzyme deficiency E25.0
  afferent loop NEC K91.89
  Alagille's Q44.7
  alcohol withdrawal (without convulsions) — *see* Dependence, alcohol, with, withdrawal
  Alder's D72.0
  Aldrich (-Wiskott) D82.0
  alien hand R41.4
  Alport Q87.81
  alveolar hypoventilation E66.2
  alveolocapillary block J84.10
  amnesic, amnestic (confabulatory) (due to) — *see* Disorder, amnesic
  amyostatic (Wilson's disease) E83.01
  androgen insensitivity E34.50
    complete E34.51
    partial E34.52
  androgen resistance (*see also* Syndrome, androgen insensitivity) E34.50
  Angelman Q93.5
  anginal — *see* Angina
  ankyloglossia superior Q38.1

Syndrome — *continued*
  anterior
    chest wall R07.89
    cord G83.82
    spinal artery G95.19
      compression M47.019
        cervical region M47.012
        cervicothoracic region M47.013
        lumbar region M47.016
        occipito-atlanto-axial region M47.011
        thoracic region M47.014
        thoracolumbar region M47.015
    tibial M76.81- ☑
  antibody deficiency D80.9
    agammaglobulinemic D80.1
      hereditary D80.0
    congenital D80.0
    hypogammaglobulinemic D80.1
      hereditary D80.0
  anticardiolipin (-antibody) D68.61
  antiphospholipid (-antibody) D68.61
  aortic
    arch M31.4
    bifurcation I74.09
  aortomesenteric duodenum occlusion K31.5
  apical ballooning (transient left ventricular) I51.81
  arcuate ligament I77.4
  argentaffin, argintaffinoma E34.0
  Arnold-Chiari — *see* Arnold-Chiari disease
  Arrillaga-Ayerza I27.0
  Asherman's N85.6
  aspiration, of newborn — *see* Aspiration, by substance, with pneumonia
    meconium P24.01
  ataxia-telangiectasia G11.3
  auriculotemporal G50.8
  autoerythrocyte sensitization (Gardner-Diamond) D69.2
  autoimmune polyglandular E31.0
  autoimmune lymphoproliferative [ALPS] D89.82
  autosomal — *see* Abnormal, autosomes
  Avellis' G46.8
  Ayerza (-Arrillaga) I27.0
  Babinski-Nageotte G83.89
  Bakwin-Krida Q79.8
  bare lymphocyte D81.6
  Barré-Guillain G61.0
  Barré-Liéou M53.0
  Barrett's — *see* Barrett's, esophagus
  Barsony-Polgar K22.4
  Barsony-Teschendorf K22.4
  Barth E78.71
  Bartter's E26.81
  basal cell nevus Q87.89
  Basedow's E05.00
    with thyroid storm E05.01
  basilar artery G45.0
  Batten-Steinert G71.11
  battered
    baby or child — *see* Maltreatment, child, physical abuse
    spouse — *see* Maltreatment, adult, physical abuse
  Beals Q87.40
  Beau's I51.5
  Beck's I65.8
  Benedikt's G46.3
  Bernhardt-Roth — *see* Meralgia paresthetica
  Bernheim's I50.9
  Béquez César (-Steinbrinck-Chédiak-Higashi) E70.330
  big spleen D73.1
  bilateral polycystic ovarian E28.2
  Bing-Horton's — *see* Horton's headache
  Birt-Hogg-Dube syndrome Q87.89
  Björck (-Thorsen) E34.0
  black
    lung J60
    widow spider bite — *see* Toxicity, venom, spider, black widow
  Blackfan-Diamond D61.01
  blind loop K90.2
    congenital Q43.8
    postsurgical K91.2
  blue sclera E78.0
  blue toe I75.02- ☑
  Boder-Sedgewick G11.3
  Boerhaave's K22.3
  Borjeson Forssman Lehmann Q89.8
  Bouillaud's I01.9
  Bourneville (-Pringle) Q85.1

Syndrome — *continued*
  Bouveret (-Hoffman) I47.9
  brachial plexus G54.0
  bradycardia-tachycardia I49.5
  brain (nonpsychotic) F09
    with psychosis, psychotic reaction F09
    acute or subacute — *see* Delirium
    congenital — *see* Disability, intellectual
    organic F09
      post-traumatic (nonpsychotic) F07.81
        psychotic F09
    personality change F07.0
    postcontusional F07.81
    post-traumatic, nonpsychotic F07.81
    psycho-organic F09
    psychotic F06.8
  brain stem stroke G46.3
  Brandt's (acrodermatitis enteropathica) E83.2
  broad ligament laceration N83.8
  Brock's J98.11
  bronze baby P83.8
  Brown-Sequard G83.81
  bubbly lung P27.0
  Buchem's M85.2
  Budd-Chiari I82.0
  bulbar (progressive) G12.22
  Bürger-Grütz E78.3
  Burke's K86.8
  Burnett's (milk-alkali) E83.52
  burning feet E53.9
  Bywaters' T79.5 ☑
  Call-Fleming I67.841
  carbohydrate-deficient glycoprotein (CDGS) E77.8
  carcinogenic thrombophlebitis I82.1
  carcinoid E34.0
  cardiac asthma I50.1
  cardiacos negros I27.0
  cardiofaciocutaneous Q87.89
  cardiopulmonary-obesity E66.2
  cardiorenal — *see* Hypertension, cardiorenal
  cardiorespiratory distress (idiopathic), newborn P22.0
  cardiovascular renal — *see* Hypertension, cardiorenal
  carotid
    artery (hemispheric) (internal) G45.1
    body G90.01
    sinus G90.01
  carpal tunnel G56.0- ☑
  Cassidy (-Scholte) E34.0
  cat cry Q93.4
  cat eye Q92.8
  cauda equina G83.4
  causalgia — *see* Causalgia
  celiac K90.0
    artery compression I77.4
    axis I77.4
  central pain G89.0
  cerebellar
    hereditary G11.9
    stroke G46.4
  cerebellomedullary malformation — *see* Spina bifida
  cerebral
    artery
      anterior G46.1
      middle G46.0
      posterior G46.2
    gigantism E22.0
  cervical (root) M53.1
    disc — *see* Disorder, disc, cervical, with neuritis
    fusion Q76.1
    posterior, sympathicus M53.0
    rib Q76.5
    sympathetic paralysis G90.2
  cervicobrachial (diffuse) M53.1
  cervicocranial M53.0
  cervicodorsal outlet G54.2
  cervicothoracic outlet G54.0
  Céstan (-Raymond) I65.8
  Charcot's (angina cruris) (intermittent claudication) I73.9
  Charcot-Weiss-Baker G90.09
  CHARGE Q89.8
  Chédiak-Higashi (-Steinbrinck) E70.330
  chest wall R07.1
  Chiari's (hepatic vein thrombosis) I82.0
  Chilaiditi's Q43.3
  child maltreatment — *see* Maltreatment, child
  chondrocostal junction M94.0
  chondroectodermal dysplasia Q77.6

☑ **Additional character required**

Syndrome — *continued*
chromosome 4 short arm deletion Q93.3
chromosome 5 short arm deletion Q93.4
chronic
  pain G89.4
    personality F68.8
Clarke-Hadfield K86.8
Clerambault's automatism G93.89
Clouston's (hidrotic ectodermal dysplasia) Q82.4
clumsiness, clumsy child F82
cluster headache G44.009
  intractable G44.001
  not intractable G44.009
Coffin-Lowry Q89.8
cold injury (newborn) P80.0
combined immunity deficiency D81.9
compartment (deep) (posterior) (traumatic) T79.
    A0 ☑
  abdomen T79.A3 ☑
  lower extremity (hip, buttock, thigh, leg, foot,
      toes) T79.A2 ☑
  nontraumatic
    abdomen M79.A3
    lower extremity (hip, buttock, thigh, leg, foot,
        toes) M79.A2- ☑
    specified site NEC M79.A9
    upper extremity (shoulder, arm, forearm,
        wrist, hand, fingers) M79.A1- ☑
  postprocedural — *see* Syndrome,
      compartment, nontraumatic
  specified site NEC T79.A9 ☑
  upper extremity (shoulder, arm, forearm, wrist,
      hand, fingers) T79.A1 ☑
complex regional pain — *see* Syndrome, pain,
    complex regional
compression T79.5 ☑
  anterior spinal — *see* Syndrome, anterior, spinal
      artery, compression
  cauda equina G83.4
  celiac artery I77.4
  vertebral artery M47.029
    occipito-atlanto-axial region M47.021
    cervical region M47.022
concussion F07.81
congenital
  affecting multiple systems NEC Q87.89
  central alveolar hypoventilation G47.35
  facial diplegia Q87.0
  muscular hypertrophy-cerebral Q87.89
  oculo-auriculovertebral Q87.0
  oculofacial diplegia (Moebius) Q87.0
  rubella (manifest) P35.0
congestion-fibrosis (pelvic), female N94.89
congestive dysmenorrhea N94.6
Conn's E26.01
connective tissue M35.9
  overlap NEC M35.1
conus medullaris G95.81
cord
  anterior G83.82
  posterior G83.83
coronary
  acute NEC I24.9
  insufficiency or intermediate I20.0
  slow flow I20.8
Costen's (complex) M26.69
costochondral junction M94.0
costoclavicular G54.0
costovertebral E22.0
Cowden Q85.8
craniovertebral M53.0
Creutzfeldt-Jakob — *see* Creutzfeldt-Jakob
    disease or syndrome
cri-du-chat Q93.4
crib death R99
cricopharyngeal — *see* Dysphagia
croup J05.0
CRPS I — *see* Syndrome, pain, complex regional I
crush T79.5 ☑
cubital tunnel — *see* Lesion, nerve, ulnar
Curschmann (-Batten) (-Steinert) G71.11
Cushing's E24.9
  alcohol-induced E24.4
  due to
    alcohol
    drugs E24.2
    ectopic ACTH E24.3
    overproduction of pituitary ACTH E24.0
  drug-induced E24.2
  overdose or wrong substance given or taken —
      see Table of Drugs and Chemicals, by drug,
      poisoning

Syndrome — *continued*
  pituitary-dependent E24.0
    specified type NEC E24.8
cryptophthalmos Q87.0
cystic duct stump K91.5
Dana-Putnam D51.0
Danbolt (-Cross) (acrodermatitis enteropathica)
    E83.2
Dandy-Walker Q03.1
  with spina bifida Q07.01
Danlos' Q79.8
defibrination (*see also* Fibrinolysis)
  with
    antepartum hemorrhage — *see* Hemorrhage,
      antepartum, with coagulation defect
    intrapartum hemorrhage — *see* Hemorrhage,
      complicating, delivery
  newborn P60
  postpartum O72.3
Degos' I77.89
Déjérine-Roussy G89.0
delayed sleep phase G47.21
demyelinating G37.9
dependence — *see* F10-F19 with fourth character
    .2
depersonalization (-derealization) F48.1
De Quervain E34.51
de Toni-Fanconi (-Debré) E72.09
  with cystinosis E72.04
diabetes mellitus-hypertension-nephrosis — *see*
    Diabetes, nephrosis
diabetes mellitus in newborn infant P70.2
diabetes-nephrosis — *see* Diabetes, nephrosis
diabetic amyotrophy — *see* Diabetes,
    amyotrophy
Diamond-Blackfan D61.01
Diamond-Gardener D69.2
DIC (diffuse or disseminated intravascular
    coagulopathy) D65
di George's D82.1
Dighton's Q78.0
disequilibrium E87.8
Döhle body-panmyelopathic D72.0
dorsolateral medullary G46.4
double athetosis G80.3
Down (*see also* Down syndrome) Q90.9
Dresbach's (elliptocytosis) D58.1
Dressler's (postmyocardial infarction) I24.1
  postcardiotomy I97.0
drug withdrawal, infant of dependent mother
    P96.1
dry eye H04.12- ☑
due to abnormality
  chromosomal Q99.9
    sex
      female phenotype Q97.9
      male phenotype Q98.9
    specified NEC Q99.8
dumping (postgastrectomy) K91.1
  nonsurgical K31.89
Dupré's (meningism) R29.1
dysmetabolic X E88.81
dyspraxia, developmental F82
Eagle-Barrett Q79.4
Eaton-Lambert — *see* Syndrome, Lambert-Eaton
Ebstein's Q22.5
ectopic ACTH E24.3
eczema-thrombocytopenia D82.0
Eddowes' Q78.0
effort (psychogenic) F45.8
Eisenmenger's I27.89
Ehlers-Danlos Q79.6
Ekman's Q78.0
electric feet E53.8
Ellis-van Creveld Q77.6
empty nest Z60.0
endocrine-hypertensive E27.0
entrapment — *see* Neuropathy, entrapment
eosinophilia-myalgia M35.8
epileptic (*see also* Epilepsy, by type)
  absence G40.A09
    intractable G40.A19
      with status epilepticus G40.A11
      without status epilepticus G40.A19
    not intractable G40.A09
      with status epilepticus G40.A01
      without status epilepticus G40.A09
Erdheim-Chester (ECD) E88.89
Erdheim's E22.0
erythrocyte fragmentation D59.4
Evans D69.41
exhaustion F48.8

Syndrome — *continued*
extrapyramidal G25.9
  specified NEC G25.89
eye retraction — *see* Strabismus
eyelid-malar-mandible Q87.0
Faber's D50.9
facial pain, paroxysmal G50.0
Fallot's Q21.3
familial eczema-thrombocytopenia (Wiskott-
    Aldrich) D82.0
Fanconi (-de Toni) (-Debré) E72.09
  with cystinosis E72.04
Fanconi's (anemia) (congenital pancytopenia)
    D61.09
fatigue
  chronic R53.82
  psychogenic F48.8
faulty bowel habit K59.3
Feil-Klippel (brevicollis) Q76.1
Felty's — *see* Felty's syndrome
fertile eunuch E23.0
fetal
  alcohol (dysmorphic) Q86.0
  hydantoin Q86.1
Fiedler's I40.1
first arch Q87.0
fish odor E72.8
Fisher's G61.0
Fitzhugh-Curtis
  due to
    Chlamydia trachomatis A74.81
    Neisseria gonorrhorea (gonococcal
        peritonitis) A54.85
Fitz's K85.8
Flajani (-Basedow) E05.00
  with thyroid storm E05.01
flatback — *see* Flatback syndrome
floppy
  baby P94.2
  iris (intraoperative) (IFIS) H21.81
  mitral valve I34.1
flush E34.0
Foix-Alajouanine G95.19
Fong's Q79.8
foramen magnum G93.5
Foster-Kennedy H47.14- ☑
Foville's (peduncular) G46.3
fragile X Q99.2
Franceschetti Q75.4
Frey's
  auriculotemporal G50.8
  hyperhidrosis L74.52
Friderichsen-Waterhouse A39.1
Froin's G95.89
frontal lobe F07.0
Fukuhara E88.49
functional
  bowel K59.9
  prepubertal castrate E29.1
Gaisböck's D75.1
ganglion (basal ganglia brain) G25.9
  geniculi G51.1
Gardner-Diamond D69.2
gastroesophageal
  junction K22.0
  laceration-hemorrhage K22.6
gastrojejunal loop obstruction K91.89
Gee-Herter-Heubner K90.0
Gelineau's G47.419
  with cataplexy G47.411
genito-anorectal A55
Gerstmann-Sträussler-Scheinker (GSS) A81.82
Gianotti-Crosti L44.4
giant platelet (Bernard-Soulier) D69.1
Gilles de la Tourette's F95.2
goiter-deafness E07.1
Goldberg Q89.8
Goldberg-Maxwell E34.51
Good's D83.8
Gopalan' (burning feet) E53.8
Gorlin's Q87.89
Gougerot-Blum L81.7
Gouley's I31.1
Gower's R55
gray or grey (newborn) P93.0
  platelet D69.1
Gubler-Millard G46.3
Guillain-Barré (-Strohl) G61.0
gustatory sweating G50.8
Hadfield-Clarke K86.8
hair tourniquet — *see* Constriction, external, by
    site

Syndrome

Syndrome — *continued*
- Hamman's J98.19
- hand-foot L27.1
- hand-shoulder G90.8
- hantavirus (cardio)-pulmonary (HPS) (HCPS) B33.4
- happy puppet Q93.5
- Harada's H30.81- ☑
- Hayem-Faber D50.9
- headache NEC G44.89
  - complicated NEC G44.59
- Heberden's I20.8
- Hedinger's E34.0
- Hegglin's D72.0
- HELLP (hemolysis, elevated liver enzymes and low platelet count) O14.2- ☑
- hemolytic-uremic D59.3
- hemophagocytic, infection-associated D76.2
- Henoch-Schönlein D69.0
- hepatic flexure K59.8
- hepatopulmonary K76.81
- hepatorenal K76.7
  - following delivery O90.4
  - postoperative or postprocedural K91.83
  - postpartum, puerperal O90.4
- hepatourologic K76.7
- Herter (-Gee) (nontropical sprue) K90.0
- Heubner-Herter K90.0
- Heyd's K76.7
- Hilger's G90.09
- histamine-like (fish poisoning) — *see* Poisoning, fish
- histiocytic D76.3
- histiocytosis NEC D76.3
- HIV infection, acute B20
- Hoffmann-Werdnig G12.0
- Hollander-Simons E88.1
- Hoppe-Goldflam G70.00
  - with exacerbation (acute) G70.01
  - in crisis G70.01
- Horner's G90.2
- hungry bone E83.81
- hunterian glossitis D51.0
- Hutchinson's triad A50.53
- hyperabduction G54.0
- hyperammonemia-hyperornithinemia-homocitrullinemia E72.4
- hypereosinophilic (idiopathic) D72.1
- hyperimmunoglobulin E (IgE) D82.4
- hyperkalemic E87.5
- hyperkinetic — *see* Hyperkinesia
- hypermobility M35.7
- hypernatremia E87.0
- hyperosmolarity E87.0
- hyperperfusion G97.82
- hypersplenic D73.1
- hypertransfusion, newborn P61.1
- hyperventilation F45.8
- hyperviscosity (of serum)
  - polycythemic D75.1
  - sclerothymic D58.8
- hypoglycemic (familial) (neonatal) E16.2
- hypokalemic E87.6
- hyponatremic E87.1
- hypopituitarism E23.0
- hypoplastic left-heart Q23.4
- hypopotassemia E87.6
- hyposmolality E87.1
- hypotension, maternal O26.5- ☑
- hypothenar hammer I73.89
- ICF (intravascular coagulation-fibrinolysis) D65
- idiopathic
  - cardiorespiratory distress, newborn P22.0
  - nephrotic (infantile) N04.9
- iliotibial band M76.3- ☑
- immobility, immobilization (paraplegic) M62.3
- immune reconstitution D89.3
- immune reconstitution inflammatory [IRIS] D89.3
- immunity deficiency, combined D81.9
- immunodeficiency
  - acquired — *see* Human, immunodeficiency virus (HIV) disease
  - combined D81.9
- impending coronary I20.0
- impingement, shoulder M75.4- ☑
- inappropriate secretion of antidiuretic hormone E22.2
- infant
  - of diabetic mother P70.1
  - gestational diabetes P70.0
- infantilism (pituitary) E23.0
- inferior vena cava I87.1

Syndrome — *continued*
- inspissated bile (newborn) P59.1
- institutional (childhood) F94.2
- insufficient sleep F51.12
- intermediate coronary (artery) I20.0
- interspinous ligament — *see* Spondylopathy, specified NEC
- intestinal
  - carcinoid E34.0
  - knot K56.2
- intravascular coagulation-fibrinolysis (ICF) D65
- iodine-deficiency, congenital E00.9
  - type
    - mixed E00.2
    - myxedematous E00.1
    - neurological E00.0
- IRDS (idiopathic respiratory distress, newborn) P22.0
- irritable
  - bowel K58.9
    - with diarrhea K58.0
    - psychogenic F45.8
  - heart (psychogenic) F45.8
  - weakness F48.8
- ischemic bowel (transient) K55.9
  - chronic K55.1
  - due to mesenteric artery insufficiency K55.1
- IVC (intravascular coagulopathy) D65
- Ivemark's Q89.01
- Jaccoud's — *see* Arthropathy, postrheumatic, chronic
- Jackson's G83.89
- Jakob-Creutzfeldt — *see* Creutzfeldt-Jakob disease or syndrome
- jaw-winking Q07.8
- Jervell-Lange-Nielsen I45.81
- jet lag G47.25
- Job's D71
- Joseph-Diamond-Blackfan D61.01
- jugular foramen G52.7
- Kabuki Q89.8
- Kanner's (autism) F84.0
- Kartagener's Q89.3
- Kelly's D50.1
- Kimmelstiel-Wilson — *see* Diabetes, specified type, with Kimmelstiel-Wilson disease
- Klein (e)-Levine G47.13
- Klippel-Feil (brevicollis) Q76.1
- Köhler-Pellegrini-Steida — *see* Bursitis, tibial collateral
- König's K59.8
- Korsakoff (-Wernicke) (nonalcoholic) F04
  - alcoholic F10.26
- Kostmann's D70.0
- Krabbe's congenital muscle hypoplasia Q79.8
- labyrinthineH83.2
- lacunar NEC G46.7
- Lambert-Eaton G70.80
  - in
    - neoplastic disease G73.1
    - specified disease NEC G70.81
- Landau-Kleffner — *see* Epilepsy, specified NEC
- Larsen's Q74.8
- lateral
  - cutaneous nerve of thigh G57.1- ☑
  - medullary G46.4
- Launois' E22.0
- lazy
  - leukocyte D70.8
  - posture M62.3
- Lemiere I80.8
- Lennox-Gastaut G40.812
  - intractable G40.814
    - with status epilepticus G40.813
    - without status epilepticus G40.814
  - not intractable G40.812
    - with status epilepticus G40.811
    - without status epilepticus G40.812
- lenticular, progressive E83.01
- Leopold-Levi's E05.90
- Lev's I44.2
- Li-Fraumeni Z15.01
- Lichtheim's D51.0
- Lightwood's N25.89
- Lignac (de Toni) (-Fanconi) (-Debré) E72.09
  - with cystinosis E72.04
- Likoff's I20.8
- limbic epilepsy personality F07.0
- liver-kidney K76.7
- lobotomy F07.0
- Loffler's J82
- long arm 18 or 21 deletion Q93.89

Syndrome — *continued*
- long QT I45.81
- Louis-Barré G11.3
- low
  - atmospheric pressure T70.29 ☑
  - back M54.5
  - output (cardiac) I50.9
- lower radicular, newborn (birth injury) P14.8
- Luetscher's (dehydration) E86.0
- Lupus anticoagulant D68.62
- Lutembacher's Q21.1
- macrophage activation D76.1
  - due to infection D76.2
- magnesium-deficiency R29.0
- Mal de Debarquement R42
- malabsorption K90.9
  - postsurgical K91.2
- malformation, congenital, due to
  - alcohol Q86.0
  - exogenous cause NEC Q86.8
  - hydantoin Q86.1
  - warfarin Q86.2
- malignant
  - carcinoid E34.0
  - neuroleptic G21.0
- Mallory-Weiss K22.6
- mandibulofacial dysostosis Q75.4
- manic-depressive — *see* Disorder, bipolar, affective
- maple-syrup-urine E71.0
- Marable's I77.4
- Marfan's Q87.40
  - with
    - cardiovascular manifestations Q87.418
      - aortic dilation Q87.410
    - ocular manifestations Q87.42
    - skeletal manifestations Q87.43
- Marie's (acromegaly) E22.0
- maternal hypotension — *see* Syndrome, hypotension, maternal
- May (-Hegglin) D72.0
- McArdle (-Schmidt) (-Pearson) E74.04
- McQuarrie's E16.2
- meconium plug (newborn) P76.0
- median arcuate ligament I77.4
- Meekeren-Ehlers-Danlos Q79.6
- megavitamin-B6 E67.2
- Meige G24.4
- MELAS E88.41
- Mendelson O74.0
- MERRF (myoclonic epilepsy associated with ragged-red fibers) E88.42
- mesenteric
  - artery (superior) K55.1
  - vascular insufficiency K55.1
- metabolic E88.81
- metastatic carcinoid E34.0
- micrognathia-glossoptosis Q87.0
- midbrain NEC G93.89
- middle lobe (lung) J98.19
- middle radicular G54.0
- migraine (*see also* Migraine) G43.909- ☑
- Mikulicz' K11.8
- milk-alkali E83.52
- Millard-Gubler G46.3
- Miller-Dieker Q93.88
- Miller-Fisher G61.0
- Minkowski-Chauffard D58.0
- Mirizzi's K83.1
- MNGIE (Mitochondrial Neurogastrointestinal Encephalopathy) E88.49
- Möbius, ophthalmoplegic migraine — *see* Migraine, ophthalmoplegic
- monofixation H50.42
- Morel-Moore M85.2
- Morel-Morgagni M85.2
- Morgagni (-Morel) (-Stewart) M85.2
- Morgagni-Adams-Stokes I45.9
- mucocutaneous lymph node (acute febrile) (MCLS) M30.3
- multiple endocrine neoplasia (MEN) — *see* Neoplasia, endocrine, multiple (MEN)
- multiple operations — *see* Disorder, factitious
- Mounier-Kuhn Q32.4
  - with bronchiectasis J47.9
    - with
      - exacerbation (acute) J47.1
      - lower respiratory infection J47.0
  - acquired J98.09
    - with bronchiectasis J47.9
      - with
        - exacerbation (acute) J47.1

☑ **Additional character required**

Syndrome — *continued*
        lower respiratory infection J47.0
  myasthenic G70.9
    in
      diabetes mellitus — *see* Diabetes,
        amyotrophy
      endocrine disease NEC E34.9 [G73.3]
      neoplastic disease (*see also* Neoplasm) D49.9
        [G73.3]
      thyrotoxicosis (hyperthyroidism) E05.90
        [G73.3]
        with thyroid storm E05.91 [G73.3]
  myelodysplastic D46.9
    with
      5q deletion D46.C
      isolated del (5q) chromosomal abnormality
        D46.C
    lesions, low grade D46.20
    specified NEC D46.Z
  myelopathic pain G89.0
  myeloproliferative (chronic) D47.1
  myofascial pain M79.1
  Naffziger's G54.0
  nail patella Q87.2
  NARP (Neuropathy, Ataxia and Retinitis
    pigmentosa) E88.49
  neonatal abstinence P96.1
  nephritic (*see also* Nephritis)
    with edema — *see* Nephrosis
    acute N00.9
    chronic N03.9
    rapidly progressive N01.9
  nephrotic (congenital) (*see also* Nephrosis) N04.9
    with
      dense deposit disease N04.6
      diffuse
        crescentic glomerulonephritis N04.7
        endocapillary proliferative
          glomerulonephritis N04.4
        membranous glomerulonephritis N04.2
        mesangial proliferative glomerulonephritis
          N04.3
        mesangiocapillary glomerulonephritis
          N04.5
      focal and segmental glomerular lesions
        N04.1
      minor glomerular abnormality N04.0
      specified morphological changes NEC N04.8
    diabetic — *see* Diabetes, nephrosis
  neurologic neglect R41.4
  Nezelof's D81.4
  Nonne-Milroy-Meige Q82.0
  Nothnagel's vasomotor acroparesthesia I73.89
  oculomotor H51.9
  ophthalmoplegia-cerebellar ataxia — *see*
    Strabismus, paralytic, third nerve
  oral-facial-digital Q87.0
  organic
    affective F06.30
    amnesic (not alcohol- or drug-induced) F04
    brain F09
    depressive F06.31
    hallucinosis F06.0
    personality F07.0
  Ormond's N13.5
  oro-facial-digital Q87.0
  os trigonum Q68.8
  Osler-Weber-Rendu I78.0
  osteoporosis-osteomalacia M83.8
  Osterreicher-Turner Q79.8
  otolith H81.8
  oto-palatal-digital Q87.0
  outlet (thoracic) G54.0
  ovary
    polycystic E28.2
    resistant E28.39
    sclerocystic E28.2
  Owren's D68.2
  Paget-Schroetter I82.890
  pain (*see also* Pain)
    complex regional I G90.50
      lower limb G90.52- ☑
      specified site NEC G90.59
      upper limb G90.51- ☑
    complex regional II — *see* Causalgia
  painful
    bruising D69.2
    feet E53.8
    prostate N42.81
  paralysis agitans — *see* Parkinsonism
  paralytic G83.9
    specified NEC G83.89

Syndrome — *continued*
  Parinaud's H51.0
  parkinsonian — *see* Parkinsonism
  Parkinson's — *see* Parkinsonism
  paroxysmal facial pain G50.0
  Parry's E05.00
    with thyroid storm E05.01
  Parsonage (-Aldren)-Turner G54.5
  patella clunk M25.86- ☑
  Paterson (-Brown) (-Kelly) D50.1
  pectoral girdle I77.89
  pectoralis minor I77.89
  Pelger-Huet D72.0
  pellagra-cerebellar ataxia-renal aminoaciduria
    E72.02
  pellagroid E52
  Pellegrini-Stieda — *see* Bursitis, tibial collateral
  pelvic congestion-fibrosis, female N94.89
  penta X Q97.1
  peptic ulcer — *see* Ulcer, peptic
  perabduction I77.89
  periodic headache, in adults and children — *see*
    Headache, periodic syndromes in adults and
    children
  periurethral fibrosis N13.5
  phantom limb (without pain) G54.7
    with pain G54.6
  pharyngeal pouch D82.1
  Pick's (heart) (liver) I31.1
  Pickwickian E66.2
  PIE (pulmonary infiltration with eosinophilia) J82
  pigmentary pallidal degeneration (progressive)
    G23.0
  pineal E34.8
  pituitary E22.0
  plantar fascia M72.2
  placental transfusion — *see* Pregnancy,
    complicated by, placental transfusion
    syndromes
  plateau iris (post-iridectomy) (postprocedural)
    H21.82
  Plummer-Vinson D50.1
  pluricarential of infancy E40
  plurideficiency E40
  pluriglandular (compensatory) E31.8
    autoimmune E31.0
  pneumatic hammer T75.21 ☑
  polyangiitis overlap M30.8
  polycarential of infancy E40
  polyglandular E31.8
    autoimmune E31.0
  polysplenia Q89.09
  pontine NEC G93.89
  popliteal
    artery entrapment I77.89
    web Q87.89
  postcardiac injury
    postcardiotomy I97.0
    postmyocardial infarction I24.1
  postcardiotomy I97.0
  post chemoembolization - code to associated
    conditions
  postcholecystectomy K91.5
  postcommissurotomy I97.0
  postconcussional F07.81
  postcontusional F07.81
  postencephalitic F07.89
  posterior
    cervical sympathetic M53.0
    cord G83.83
    fossa compression G93.5
    reversible encephalopathy (PRES) I67.83
  postgastrectomy (dumping) K91.1
  postgastric surgery K91.1
  postinfarction I24.1
  postlaminectomy NEC M96.1
  postleukotomy F07.0
  postmastectomy lymphedema I97.2
  postmyocardial infarction I24.1
  postoperative NEC T81.9 ☑
    blind loop K90.2
  postpartum panhypopituitary (Sheehan) E23.0
  postpolio (myelitic) G14
  postthrombotic I87.009
    with
      inflammation I87.02- ☑
        with ulcer I87.03- ☑
      specified complication NEC I87.09- ☑
      ulcer I87.01- ☑
        with inflammation I87.03- ☑
    asymptomatic I87.00- ☑
  postvagotomy K91.1

Syndrome — *continued*
  postvalvulotomy I97.0
  postviral NEC G93.3
    fatigue G93.3
  Potain's K31.0
  potassium intoxication E87.5
  precerebral artery (multiple) (bilateral) G45.2
  preinfarction I20.0
  preleukemic D46.9
  premature senility E34.8
  premenstrual dysphoric N94.3
  premenstrual tension N94.3
  Prinzmetal-Massumi R07.1
  prune belly Q79.4
  pseudocarpal tunnel (sublimis) — *see* Syndrome,
    carpal tunnel
  pseudoparalytica G70.00
    with exacerbation (acute) G70.01
    in crisis G70.01
  pseudo -Turner's Q87.1
  psycho-organic (nonpsychotic severity) F07.9
    acute or subacute F05
    depressive type F06.31
    hallucinatory type F06.0
    nonpsychotic severity F07.0
    specified NEC F07.89
  pulmonary
    arteriosclerosis I27.0
    dysmaturity (Wilson-Mikity) P27.0
    hypoperfusion (idiopathic) P22.0
    renal (hemorrhagic) (Goodpasture's) M31.0
  pure
    motor lacunar G46.5
    sensory lacunar G46.6
  Putnam-Dana D51.0
  pyramidopallidonigral G20
  pyriformis — *see* Lesion, nerve, sciatic
  QT interval prolongation I45.81
  radicular NEC — *see* Radiculopathy
    upper limbs, newborn (birth injury) P14.3
  rapid time-zone change G47.25
  Rasmussen G04.81
  Raymond (-Céstan) I65.8
  Raynaud's I73.00
    with gangrene I73.01
  RDS (respiratory distress syndrome, newborn)
    P22.0
  reactive airways dysfunction J68.3
  Refsum's G60.1
  Reifenstein E34.52
  renal glomerulohyalinosis-diabetic — *see*
    Diabetes, nephrosis
  Rendu-Osler-Weber I78.0
  residual ovary N99.83
  resistant ovary E28.39
  respiratory
    distress
      acute J80
      adult J80
      child J80
      newborn (idiopathic) (type I) P22.0
      type II P22.1
  restless legs G25.81
  retinoblastoma (familial) C69.2 ☑
  retroperitoneal fibrosis N13.5
  retroviral seroconversion (acute) Z21
  Reye's G93.7
  Richter — *see* Leukemia, chronic lymphocytic,
    B-cell type
  Ridley's I50.1
  right
    heart, hypoplastic Q22.6
    ventricular obstruction — *see* Failure, heart,
      congestive
  Romano-Ward (prolonged QT interval) I45.81
  rotator cuff, shoulder (*see also* Tear, rotator cuff)
    M75.10- ☑
  Rotes Quérol — *see* Hyperostosis, ankylosing
  Roth — *see* Meralgia paresthetica
  rubella (congenital) P35.0
  Ruvalcaba-Myhre-Smith E71.440
  Rytand-Lipsitch I44.2
  salt
    depletion E87.1
      due to heat NEC T67.8 ☑
        causing heat exhaustion or prostration
          T67.4 ☑
    low E87.1
  salt-losing N28.89
  Scaglietti-Dagnini E22.0
  scalenus anticus (anterior) G54.0

Syndrome — *continued*
scapulocostal — *see* Mononeuropathy, upper limb, specified site NEC
scapuloperoneal G71.0
schizophrenic, of childhood NEC F84.5
Schnitzler D47.2
Scholte's E34.0
Schroeder's E27.0
Schüller-Christian C96.5
Schwachman's — *see* Syndrome, Shwachman's
Schwartz (-Jampel) G71.13
Schwartz-Bartter E22.2
scimitar Q26.8
sclerocystic ovary E28.2
Seitelberger's G31.89
septicemic adrenal hemorrhage A39.1
seroconversion, retroviral (acute) Z21
serous meningitis G93.2
severe acute respiratory (SARS) J12.81
shaken infant T74.4 ☑
shock (traumatic) T79.4 ☑
  kidney N17.0
    following crush injury T79.5 ☑
  toxic A48.3
shock-lung J80
Shone's - code to specific anomalies
short
  bowel K91.2
  rib Q77.2
shoulder-hand — *see* Algoneurodystrophy
Shwachman's D70.4
sicca — *see* Sicca syndrome
sick
  cell E87.1
  sinus I49.5
sick-euthyroid E07.81
sideropenic D50.1
Siemens' ectodermal dysplasia Q82.4
Silfversköld's Q78.9
Simons' E88.1
sinus tarsi - M25.57- ☑
sinusitis-bronchiectasis-situs inversus Q89.3
Sipple's E31.22
sirenomelia Q87.2
Slocumb's E27.0
slow flow, coronary I20.8
Sluder's G44.89
Smith-Magenis Q93.88
Sneddon-Wilkinson L13.1
Sotos' E22.0
South African cardiomyopathy I42.8
spasmodic
  upward movement, eyes H51.8
  winking F95.8
Spen's I45.9
splenic
  agenesis Q89.01
  flexure K59.8
  neutropenia D73.81
Spurway's Q78.0
staphylococcal scalded skin L00
Stein-Leventhal E28.2
Stein's E28.2
Stevens-Johnson syndrome L51.1
  toxic epidermal necrolysis overlap L51.3
Stewart-Morel M85.2
Stickler Q89.8
stiff baby Q89.8
stiff man G25.82
Still-Felty — *see* Felty's syndrome
Stokes (-Adams) I45.9
stone heart I50.1
straight back, congenital Q76.49
subclavian steal G45.8
subcoracoid-pectoralis minor G54.0
subcostal nerve compression I77.89
subphrenic interposition Q43.3
superior
  cerebellar artery I63.8
  mesenteric artery K55.1
  semi-circular canal dehiscence H83.8X- ☑
  vena cava I87.1
supine hypotensive (maternal) — *see* Syndrome, hypotension, maternal
suprarenal cortical E27.0
supraspinatus (*see also* Tear, rotator cuff) M75.10- ☑
Susac G93.49
swallowed blood P78.2
sweat retention L74.0
Swyer Q99.1
Symond's G93.2

Syndrome — *continued*
sympathetic
  cervical paralysis G90.2
  pelvic, female N94.89
systemic inflammatory response (SIRS), of non-infectious origin (without organ dysfunction) R65.10
  with acute organ dysfunction R65.11
tachycardia-bradycardia I49.5
takotsubo I51.81
TAR (thrombocytopenia with absent radius) Q87.2
tarsal tunnel G57.5- ☑
teething K00.7
tegmental G93.89
telangiectasic-pigmentation-cataract Q82.8
temporal pyramidal apex — *see* Otitis, media, suppurative, acute
temporomandibular joint-pain-dysfunction M26.62
Terry's H44.2- ☑
testicular feminization (*see also* Syndrome, androgen insensitivity) E34.51
thalamic pain (hyperesthetic) G89.0
thoracic outlet (compression) G54.0
Thorson-Björck E34.0
thrombocytopenia with absent radius (TAR) Q87.2
thyroid-adrenocortical insufficiency E31.0
tibial
  anterior M76.81- ☑
  posterior M76.82- ☑
Tietze's M94.0
time-zone (rapid) G47.25
Toni-Fanconi E72.09
  with cystinosis E72.04
Touraine's Q79.8
tourniquet — *see* Constriction, external, by site
toxic shock A48.3
transient left ventricular apical ballooning I51.81
traumatic vasospastic T75.22 ☑
Treacher Collins Q75.4
triple X, female Q97.0
trisomy Q92.9
  13 Q91.7
    meiotic nondisjunction Q91.4
    mitotic nondisjunction Q91.5
    mosaicism Q91.5
    translocation Q91.6
  18 Q91.3
    meiotic nondisjunction Q91.0
    mitotic nondisjunction Q91.1
    mosaicism Q91.1
    translocation Q91.2
  20 (q)(p) Q92.8
  21 Q90.9
    meiotic nondisjunction Q90.0
    mitotic nondisjunction Q90.1
    mosaicism Q90.1
    translocation Q90.2
  22 Q92.8
tropical wet feet T69.0- ☑
Trousseau's I82.1
tumor lysis (following antineoplastic chemotherapy) (spontaneous) NEC E88.3
Twiddler's (due to)
  automatic implantable defibrillator T82.198 ☑
  cardiac pacemaker T82.198 ☑
Unverricht (-Lundborg) — *see* Epilepsy, generalized, idiopathic
upward gaze H51.8
uremia, chronic (*see also* Disease, kidney, chronic) N18.9
urethral N34.3
urethro-oculo-articular — *see* Reiter's disease
urohepatic K76.7
vago-hypoglossal G52.7
vascular NEC in cerebrovascular disease G46.8
vasoconstriction, reversible cerebrovascular I67.841
vasomotor I73.9
vasospastic (traumatic) T75.22 ☑
vasovagal R55
van Buchem's M85.2
van der Hoeve's Q78.0
VATER Q87.2
velo-cardio-facial Q93.81
vena cava (inferior) (superior) (obstruction) I87.1
vertebral
  artery G45.0
    compression — *see* Syndrome, anterior, spinal artery, compression

Syndrome — *continued*
steal G45.0
vertebro-basilar artery G45.0
vertebrogenic (pain) M54.89
vertiginous — *see* Disorder, vestibular function
Vinson-Plummer D50.1
virus B34.9
visceral larva migrans B83.0
visual disorientation H53.8
vitamin B6 deficiency E53.1
vitreal corneal H59.01- ☑
vitreous (touch) H59.01- ☑
Vogt-Koyanagi H20.82- ☑
Volkmann's T79.6 ☑
von Schroetter's I82.890
von Willebrand (-Jürgen) D68.0
Waldenström-Kjellberg D50.1
Wallenberg's G46.3
water retention E87.79
Waterhouse (-Friderichsen) A39.1
Weber-Gubler G46.3
Weber-Leyden G46.3
Weber's G46.3
Wegener's M31.30
  with
    kidney involvement M31.31
    lung involvement M31.30
      with kidney involvement M31.31
Weingarten's (tropical eosinophilia) J82
Weiss-Baker G90.09
Werdnig-Hoffman G12.0
Wermer's E31.21
Werner's E34.8
Wernicke-Korsakoff (nonalcoholic) F04
  alcoholic F10.26
West's — *see* Epilepsy, spasms
Westphal-Strümpell E83.01
wet
  feet (maceration) (tropical) T69.0- ☑
  lung, newborn P22.1
whiplash S13.4 ☑
whistling face Q87.0
Wilkie's K55.1
Wilkinson-Sneddon L13.1
Willebrand (-Jürgens) D68.0
Wilson's (hepatolenticular degeneration) E83.01
Wiskott-Aldrich D82.0
withdrawal — *see* Withdrawal, state
  drug
    infant of dependent mother P96.1
    therapeutic use, newborn P96.2
Woakes' (ethmoiditis) J33.1
Wright's (hyperabduction) I77.89
X I20.9
XXXX Q97.1
XXXXX Q97.1
XXXXY Q98.1
XXY Q98.0
yellow nail L60.5
Zahorsky's B08.5
Zellweger syndrome E71.510
Zellweger-like syndrome E71.541
Synechia (anterior) (iris) (posterior) (pupil) (*see also* Adhesions, iris)
  intra-uterine (traumatic) N85.6
Synesthesia R20.8
Syngamiasis, syngamosis B83.3
Synodontia K00.2
Synorchidism, synorchism Q55.1
Synostosis (congenital) Q78.8
  astragalo-scaphoid Q74.2
  radioulnar Q74.0
Synovial sarcoma — *see* Neoplasm, connective tissue, malignant
Synovioma (malignant) (*see also* Neoplasm, connective tissue, malignant)
  benign — *see* Neoplasm, connective tissue, benign
Synoviosarcoma — *see* Neoplasm, connective tissue, malignant
Synovitis (*see also* Tenosynovitis)
  crepitant
    hand M70.0- ☑
    wrist M70.03- ☑
  gonococcal A54.49
  gouty — *see* Gout, idiopathic
  in (due to)
    crystals M65.8- ☑
    gonorrhea A54.49
    syphilis (late) A52.78
    use, overuse, pressure — *see* Disorder, soft tissue, due to use

☑ **Additional character required**

Synovitis — *continued*
 infective NEC — *see* Tenosynovitis, infective NEC
 specified NEC — *see* Tenosynovitis, specified
  type NEC
 syphilitic A52.78
  congenital (early) A50.02
 toxic — *see* Synovitis, transient
 transient M67.3- ☑
  ankle M67.37- ☑
  elbow M67.32- ☑
  foot joint M67.37- ☑
  hand joint M67.34- ☑
  hip M67.35- ☑
  knee M67.36- ☑
  multiple site M67.39
  pelvic region M67.35- ☑
  shoulder M67.31- ☑
  specified joint NEC M67.38
  wrist M67.33- ☑
 traumatic, current — *see* Sprain
 tuberculous — *see* Tuberculosis, synovitis
 villonodular (pigmented) M12.2- ☑
  ankle M12.27- ☑
  elbow M12.22- ☑
  foot joint M12.27- ☑
  hand joint M12.24- ☑
  hip M12.25- ☑
  knee M12.26- ☑
  multiple site M12.29
  pelvic region M12.25- ☑
  shoulder M12.21- ☑
  specified joint NEC M12.28
  vertebrae M12.28
  wrist M12.23- ☑
Syphilid A51.39
 congenital A50.06
 newborn A50.06
 tubercular (late) A52.79
Syphilis, syphilitic (acquired) A53.9
 abdomen (late) A52.79
 acoustic nerve A52.15
 adenopathy (secondary) A51.49
 adrenal (gland) (with cortical hypofunction)
  A52.79
 age under 2 years NOS (*see also* Syphilis,
  congenital, early)
  acquired A51.9
 alopecia (secondary) A51.32
 anemia (late) A52.79 [D63.8]
 aneurysm (aorta) (ruptured) A52.01
  central nervous system A52.05
  congenital A50.54 [I79.0]
 anus (late) A52.74
  primary A51.1
  secondary A51.39
 aorta (arch) (abdominal) (thoracic) A52.02
  aneurysm A52.01
 aortic (insufficiency) (regurgitation) (stenosis)
  A52.03
  aneurysm A52.01
 arachnoid (adhesive) (cerebral) (spinal) A52.13
 asymptomatic — *see* Syphilis, latent
 ataxia (locomotor) A52.11
 atrophoderma maculatum A51.39
 auricular fibrillation A52.06
 bladder (late) A52.76
 bone A52.77
  secondary A51.46
 brain A52.17
 breast (late) A52.79
 bronchus (late) A52.72
 bubo (primary) A51.0
 bulbar palsy A52.19
 bursa (late) A52.78
 cardiac decompensation A52.06
 cardiovascular A52.00
 central nervous system (late) (recurrent) (relapse)
  (tertiary) A52.3
  with
   ataxia A52.11
   general paralysis A52.17
    juvenile A50.45
   paresis (general) A52.17
    juvenile A50.45
   tabes (dorsalis) A52.11
    juvenile A50.45
   taboparesis A52.17
    juvenile A50.45
  aneurysm A52.05
  congenital A50.40
  juvenile A50.40
  remission in (sustained) A52.3

Syphilis — *continued*
 serology doubtful, negative, or positive A52.3
 specified nature or site NEC A52.19
 vascular A52.05
 cerebral A52.17
  meningovascular A52.13
  nerves (multiple palsies) A52.15
  sclerosis A52.17
  thrombosis A52.05
 cerebrospinal (tabetic type) A52.12
 cerebrovascular A52.05
 cervix (late) A52.76
 chancre (multiple) A51.0
  extragenital A51.2
  Rollet's A51.0
 Charcot's joint A52.16
 chorioretinitis A51.43
  congenital A50.01
  late A52.71
  prenatal A50.01
 choroiditis — *see* Syphilitic chorioretinitis
 choroidoretinitis — *see* Syphilitic chorioretinitis
 ciliary body (secondary) A51.43
  late A52.71
 colon (late) A52.74
 combined spinal sclerosis A52.11
 condyloma (latum) A51.31
 congenital A50.9
  with
   paresis (general) A50.45
   tabes (dorsalis) A50.45
   taboparesis A50.45
  chorioretinitis, choroiditis A50.01 [H32]
  early, or less than 2 years after birth NEC A50.2
   with manifestations — *see* Syphilis,
    congenital, early, symptomatic
   latent (without manifestations) A50.1
    negative spinal fluid test A50.1
    serology positive A50.1
   symptomatic A50.09
    cutaneous A50.06
    mucocutaneous A50.07
    oculopathy A50.01
    osteochondropathy A50.02
    pharyngitis A50.03
    pneumonia A50.04
    rhinitis A50.05
    visceral A50.08
  interstitial keratitis A50.31
  juvenile neurosyphilis A50.45
  late, or 2 years or more after birth NEC A50.7
   chorioretinitis, choroiditis A50.32
   interstitial keratitis A50.31
   juvenile neurosyphilis A50.45
   latent (without manifestations) A50.6
    negative spinal fluid test A50.6
    serology positive A50.6
   symptomatic or with manifestations NEC
    A50.59
    arthropathy A50.55
    cardiovascular A50.54
    Clutton's joints A50.51
    Hutchinson's teeth A50.52
    Hutchinson's triad A50.53
    osteochondropathy A50.56
    saddle nose A50.57
 conjugal A53.9
  tabes A52.11
 conjunctiva (late) A52.71
 contact Z20.2
 cord bladder A52.19
 cornea, late A52.71
 coronary (artery) (sclerosis) A52.06
 coryza, congenital A50.05
 cranial nerve A52.15
  multiple palsies A52.15
 cutaneous — *see* Syphilis, skin
 dacryocystitis (late) A52.71
 degeneration, spinal cord A52.12
 dementia paralytica A52.17
  juvenilis A50.45
 destruction of bone A52.77
 dilatation, aorta A52.01
 due to blood transfusion A53.9
 dura mater A52.13
 ear A52.79
  inner A52.79
   nerve (eighth) A52.15
   neurorecurrence A52.15
 early A51.9
  cardiovascular A52.00
  central nervous system A52.3

Syphilis — *continued*
 latent (without manifestations) (less than 2
   years after infection) A51.5
  negative spinal fluid test A51.5
  serological relapse after treatment A51.5
  serology positive A51.5
 relapse (treated, untreated) A51.9
 skin A51.39
 symptomatic A51.9
  extragenital chancre A51.2
  primary, except extragenital chancre A51.0
  secondary (*see also* Syphilis, secondary)
   A51.39
   relapse (treated, untreated) A51.49
 ulcer A51.39
 eighth nerve (neuritis) A52.15
 endemic A65
 endocarditis A52.03
  aortic A52.03
  pulmonary A52.03
 epididymis (late) A52.76
 epiglottis (late) A52.73
 epiphysitis (congenital) (early) A50.02
 episcleritis (late) A52.71
 esophagus A52.79
 eustachian tube A52.73
 exposure to Z20.2
 eye A52.71
 eyelid (late) (with gumma) A52.71
 fallopian tube (late) A52.76
 fracture A52.77
 gallbladder (late) A52.74
 gastric (polyposis) (late) A52.74
 general A53.9
  paralysis A52.17
   juvenile A50.45
 genital (primary) A51.0
 glaucoma A52.71
 gumma NEC A52.79
  cardiovascular system A52.00
  central nervous system A52.3
  congenital A50.59
 heart (block) (decompensation) (disease) (failure)
  A52.06 [I52]
  valve NEC A52.03
 hemianesthesia A52.19
 hemianopsia A52.71
 hemiparesis A52.17
 hemiplegia A52.17
 hepatic artery A52.09
 hepatis A52.74
 hepatomegaly, congenital A50.08
 hereditaria tarda — *see* Syphilis, congenital, late
 hereditary — *see* Syphilis, congenital
 Hutchinson's teeth A50.52
 hyalitis A52.71
 inactive — *see* Syphilis, latent
 infantum — *see* Syphilis, congenital
 inherited — *see* Syphilis, congenital
 internal ear A52.79
 intestine (late) A52.74
 iris, iritis (secondary) A51.43
  late A52.71
 joint (late) A52.77
 keratitis (congenital) (interstitial) (late) A50.31
 kidney (late) A52.75
 lacrimal passages (late) A52.71
 larynx (late) A52.73
 late A52.9
  cardiovascular A52.00
  central nervous system A52.3
  kidney A52.75
  latent or 2 years or more after infection
   (without manifestations) A52.8
   negative spinal fluid test A52.8
   serology positive A52.8
  paresis A52.17
  specified site NEC A52.79
  symptomatic or with manifestations A52.79
  tabes A52.11
 latent A53.0
  with signs or symptoms - code by site and
   stage under Syphilis
  central nervous system A52.2
  date of infection unspecified A53.0
  early, or less than 2 years after infection A51.5
  follow-up of latent syphilis A53.0
   date of infection unspecified A53.0
   late, or 2 years or more after infection A52.8
  late, or 2 years or more after infection A52.8
  positive serology (only finding) A53.0
   date of infection unspecified A53.0

Syphilis — *continued*

      early, or less than 2 years after infection A51.5
      late, or 2 years or more after infection A52.8
  lens (late) A52.71
  leukoderma A51.39
    late A52.79
  lienitis A52.79
  lip A51.39
    chancre (primary) A51.2
    late A52.79
  Lissauer's paralysis A52.17
  liver A52.74
  locomotor ataxia A52.11
  lung A52.72
  lymph gland (early) (secondary) A51.49
    late A52.79
  lymphadenitis (secondary) A51.49
  macular atrophy of skin A51.39
    striated A52.79
  mediastinum (late) A52.73
  meninges (adhesive) (brain) (spinal cord) A52.13
  meningitis A52.13
    acute (secondary) A51.41
    congenital A50.41
  meningoencephalitis A52.14
  meningovascular A52.13
    congenital A50.41
  mesarteritis A52.09
    brain A52.04
  middle ear A52.77
  mitral stenosis A52.03
  monoplegia A52.17
  mouth (secondary) A51.39
    late A52.79
  mucocutaneous (secondary) A51.39
    late A52.79
  mucous
    membrane (secondary) A51.39
      late A52.79
    patches A51.39
      congenital A50.07
  mulberry molars A50.52
  muscle A52.78
  myocardium A52.06
  nasal sinus (late) A52.73
  neonatorum — *see* Syphilis, congenital
  nephrotic syndrome (secondary) A51.44
  nerve palsy (any cranial nerve) A52.15
    multiple A52.15
  nervous system, central A52.3
  neuritis A52.15
    acoustic A52.15
  neurorecidive of retina A52.19
  neuroretinitis A52.19
  newborn — *see* Syphilis, congenital
  nodular superficial (late) A52.79
  nonvenereal A65
  nose (late) A52.73
    saddle back deformity A50.57
  occlusive arterial disease A52.09
  oculopathy A52.71
  ophthalmic (late) A52.71
  optic nerve (atrophy) (neuritis) (papilla) A52.15
  orbit (late) A52.71
  organic A53.9
  osseous (late) A52.77
  osteochondritis (congenital) (early) A50.02
    [M90.80]
  osteoporosis A52.77
  ovary (late) A52.76
  oviduct (late) A52.76
  palate (late) A52.79
  pancreas (late) A52.74
  paralysis A52.17
    general A52.17
      juvenile A50.45
  paresis (general) A52.17
    juvenile A50.45
  paresthesia A52.19
  Parkinson's disease or syndrome A52.19
  paroxysmal tachycardia A52.06
  pemphigus (congenital) A50.06
  penis (chancre) A51.0
    late A52.76
  pericardium A52.06
  perichondritis, larynx (late) A52.73
  periosteum (late) A52.77
    congenital (early) A50.02 [M90.80]
    early (secondary) A51.46
  peripheral nerve A52.79
  petrous bone (late) A52.77
  pharynx (late) A52.73
    secondary A51.39

Syphilis — *continued*

  pituitary (gland) A52.79
  pleura (late) A52.73
  pneumonia, white A50.04
  pontine lesion A52.17
  portal vein A52.09
  primary A51.0
    anal A51.1
    and secondary — *see* Syphilis, secondary
    central nervous system A52.3
    extragenital chancre NEC A51.2
    fingers A51.2
    genital A51.0
    lip A51.2
    specified site NEC A51.2
    tonsils A51.2
  prostate (late) A52.76
  ptosis (eyelid) A52.71
  pulmonary (late) A52.72
    artery A52.09
  pyelonephritis (late) A52.75
  recently acquired, symptomatic A51.9
  rectum (late) A52.74
  respiratory tract (late) A52.73
  retina, late A52.71
  retrobulbar neuritis A52.15
  salpingitis A52.76
  sclera (late) A52.71
  sclerosis
    cerebral A52.17
    coronary A52.06
    multiple A52.11
  scotoma (central) A52.71
  scrotum (late) A52.76
  secondary (and primary) A51.49
    adenopathy A51.49
    anus A51.39
    bone A51.46
    chorioretinitis, choroiditis A51.43
    hepatitis A51.45
    liver A51.45
    lymphadenitis A51.49
    meningitis (acute) A51.41
    mouth A51.39
    mucous membranes A51.39
    periosteum, periostitis A51.46
    pharynx A51.39
    relapse (treated, untreated) A51.49
    skin A51.39
    specified form NEC A51.49
    tonsil A51.39
    ulcer A51.39
    viscera NEC A51.49
    vulva A51.39
  seminal vesicle (late) A52.76
  seronegative with signs or symptoms - code by
    site and stage under Syphilis
  seropositive
    with signs or symptoms - code by site and
      stage under Syphilis
    follow-up of latent syphilis — *see* Syphilis,
      latent
    only finding — *see* Syphilis, latent
  seventh nerve (paralysis) A52.15
  sinus, sinusitis (late) A52.73
  skeletal system A52.77
  skin (with ulceration) (early) (secondary) A51.39
    late or tertiary A52.79
  small intestine A52.74
  spastic spinal paralysis A52.17
  spermatic cord (late) A52.76
  spinal (cord) A52.12
  spleen A52.79
  splenomegaly A52.79
  spondylitis A52.77
  staphyloma A52.71
  stigmata (congenital) A50.59
  stomach A52.74
  synovium A52.78
  tabes dorsalis (late) A52.11
    juvenile A50.45
  tabetic type A52.11
    juvenile A50.45
  taboparesis A52.17
    juvenile A50.45
  tachycardia A52.06
  tendon (late) A52.78
  tertiary A52.9
    with symptoms NEC A52.79
    cardiovascular A52.00
    central nervous system A52.3
    multiple NEC A52.79
    specified site NEC A52.79

Syphilis — *continued*

  testis A52.76
  thorax A52.73
  throat A52.73
  thymus (gland) (late) A52.79
  thyroid (late) A52.79
  tongue (late) A52.79
  tonsil (lingual) (late) A52.73
    primary A51.2
    secondary A51.39
  trachea (late) A52.73
  tunica vaginalis (late) A52.76
  ulcer (any site) (early) (secondary) A51.39
    late A52.79
    perforating A52.79
      foot A52.11
  urethra (late) A52.76
  urogenital (late) A52.76
  uterus (late) A52.76
  uveal tract (secondary) A51.43
    late A52.71
  uveitis (secondary) A51.43
    late A52.71
  uvula (late) (perforated) A52.79
  vagina A51.0
    late A52.76
  valvulitis NEC A52.03
  vascular A52.00
    brain (cerebral) A52.05
  ventriculi A52.74
  vesicae urinariae (late) A52.76
  viscera (abdominal) (late) A52.74
    secondary A51.49
  vitreous (opacities) (late) A52.71
    hemorrhage A52.71
  vulva A51.0
    late A52.76
    secondary A51.39
Syphiloma A52.79
  cardiovascular system A52.00
  central nervous system A52.3
  circulatory system A52.00
  congenital A50.59
Syphilophobia F45.29
Syringadenoma (*see also* Neoplasm, skin, benign)
  papillary — *see* Neoplasm, skin, benign
Syringobulbia G95.0
Syringocystadenoma — *see* Neoplasm, skin, benign
  papillary — *see* Neoplasm, skin, benign
Syringoma (*see also* Neoplasm, skin, benign)
  chondroid — *see* Neoplasm, skin, benign
Syringomyelia G95.0
Syringomyelitis — *see* Encephalitis
Syringomyelocele — *see* Spina bifida
Syringopontia G95.0
System, systemic (*see also* condition)
  disease, combined — *see* Degeneration,
    combined
  inflammatory response syndrome (SIRS) of non-
    infectious origin (without organ dysfunction)
    R65.10
    with acute organ dysfunction R65.11
  lupus erythematosus M32.9
    inhibitor present D68.62

T

Tabacism, tabacosis, tabagism (*see also* Poisoning, tobacco)
  meaning dependence (without remission) F17.200
    with
      disorder F17.299
        remission F17.211
        specified disorder NEC F17.298
        withdrawal F17.203
Tabardillo A75.9
  flea-borne A75.2
  louse-borne A75.0
Tabes, tabetic A52.10
  with
    central nervous system syphilis A52.10
    Charcot's joint A52.16
    cord bladder A52.19
    crisis, viscera (any) A52.19
    paralysis, general A52.17
    paresis (general) A52.17
    perforating ulcer (foot) A52.19
  arthropathy (Charcot) A52.16
  bladder A52.19
  bone A52.11
  cerebrospinal A52.12
  congenital A50.45
  conjugal A52.10
  dorsalis A52.11
    juvenile A50.49
  juvenile A50.49
  latent A52.19
  mesenterica A18.39
  paralysis, insane, general A52.17
  spasmodic A52.17
  syphilis (cerebrospinal) A52.12
Taboparalysis A52.17
Taboparesis (remission) A52.17
  juvenile A50.45
TAC (trigeminal autonomic cephalgia) NEC G44.099
  intractable G44.091
  not intractable G44.099
Tache noir S60.22- ☑
Tachyalimentation K91.2
Tachyarrhythmia, tachyrhythmia — *see* Tachycardia
Tachycardia R00.0
  atrial (paroxysmal) I47.1
  auricular I47.1
  AV nodal re-entry (re-entrant) I47.1
  junctional (paroxysmal) I47.1
  newborn P29.11
  nodal (paroxysmal) I47.1
  non-paroxysmal AV nodal I45.89
  paroxysmal (sustained) (nonsustained) I47.9
    with sinus bradycardia I49.5
    atrial (PAT) I47.1
    atrioventricular (AV) (re-entrant) I47.1
      psychogenic F54
    junctional I47.1
      ectopic I47.1
    nodal I47.1
    psychogenic (atrial) (supraventricular) (ventricular) F54
    supraventricular (sustained) I47.1
      psychogenic F54
    ventricular I47.2
      psychogenic F54
  psychogenic F45.8
  sick sinus I49.5
  sinoauricular NOS R00.0
    paroxysmal I47.1
  sinus [sinusal] NOS R00.0
    paroxysmal I47.1
  supraventricular I47.1
  ventricular (paroxysmal) (sustained) I47.2
    psychogenic F54
Tachygastria K31.89
Tachypnea R06.82
  hysterical F45.8
  newborn (idiopathic) (transitory) P22.1
  psychogenic F45.8
  transitory, of newborn P22.1
Taenia (infection) (infestation) B68.9
  diminuta B71.0
  echinococcal infestation B67.90
  mediocanellata B68.1
  nana B71.0
  saginata B68.1
  solium (intestinal form) B68.0
    larval form — *see* Cysticercosis

Taeniasis (intestine) — *see* Taenia
TACO (transfusion associated circulatory overload) E87.71
Tag (hypertrophied skin) (infected) L91.8
  adenoid J35.8
  anus K64.4
  hemorrhoidal K64.4
  hymen N89.8
  perineal N90.89
  preauricular Q17.0
  sentinel K64.4
  skin L91.8
    accessory (congenital) Q82.8
    anus K64.4
    congenital Q82.8
    preauricular Q17.0
  tonsil J35.8
  urethra, urethral N36.8
  vulva N90.89
Tahyna fever B33.8
Takahara's disease E80.3
Takayasu's disease or syndrome M31.4
Talcosis (pulmonary) J62.0
Talipes (congenital) Q66.89
  acquired, planus — *see* Deformity, limb, flat foot
  asymmetric Q66.89
  calcaneovalgus Q66.4
  calcaneovarus Q66.1
  calcaneus Q66.89
  cavus Q66.7
  equinovalgus Q66.6
  equinovarus Q66.0
  equinus Q66.89
  percavus Q66.7
  planovalgus Q66.6
  planus (acquired) (any degree) (*see also* Deformity, limb, flat foot)
    congenital Q66.5- ☑
    due to rickets (sequelae) E64.3
  valgus Q66.6
  varus Q66.3
Tall stature, constitutional E34.4
Talma's disease M62.89
Talon noir S90.3- ☑
  hand S60.22- ☑
  heel S90.3- ☑
  toe S90.1- ☑
Tamponade, heart I31.4
Tanapox (virus disease) B08.71
Tangier disease E78.6
Tantrum, child problem F91.8
Tapeworm (infection) (infestation) — *see* Infestation, tapeworm
Tapia's syndrome G52.7
TAR (thrombocytopenia with absent radius) syndrome Q87.2
Tarral-Besnier disease L44.0
Tarsal tunnel syndrome — *see* Syndrome, tarsal tunnel
Tarsalgia — *see* Pain, limb, lower
Tarsitis (eyelid) H01.8
  syphilitic A52.71
  tuberculous A18.4
Tartar (teeth) (dental calculus) K03.6
Tattoo (mark) L81.8
Tauri's disease E74.09
Taurodontism K00.2
Taussig-Bing syndrome Q20.1
Taybi's syndrome Q87.2
Tay-Sachs amaurotic familial idiocy or disease E75.02
TBI (traumatic brain injury) S06
Teacher's node or nodule J38.2
Tear, torn (traumatic) (*see also* Laceration)
  with abortion — *see* Abortion
  annular fibrosis M51.35
  anus, anal (sphincter) S31.831 ☑
    complicating delivery
      with third degree perineal laceration O70.2
        with mucosa O70.3
      without third degree perineal laceration O70.4
    nontraumatic (healed) (old) K62.81
  articular cartilage, old — *see* Derangement, joint, articular cartilage, by site
  bladder
    with ectopic or molar pregnancy O08.6
    following ectopic or molar pregnancy O08.6
    obstetrical O71.5
    traumatic — *see* Injury, bladder
  bowel
    with ectopic or molar pregnancy O08.6

Tear — *continued*
    following ectopic or molar pregnancy O08.6
    obstetrical trauma O71.5
  broad ligament
    with ectopic or molar pregnancy O08.6
    following ectopic or molar pregnancy O08.6
    obstetrical trauma O71.6
  bucket handle (knee) (meniscus) — *see* Tear, meniscus
  capsule, joint — *see* Sprain
  cartilage (*see also* Sprain)
    articular, old — *see* Derangement, joint, articular cartilage, by site
  cervix
    with ectopic or molar pregnancy O08.6
    following ectopic or molar pregnancy O08.6
    obstetrical trauma (current) O71.3
    old N88.1
    traumatic — *see* Injury, uterus
  dural G97.41
    nontraumatic G96.11
  internal organ — *see* Injury, by site
  knee cartilage
    articular (current) S83.3- ☑
    old — *see* Derangement, knee, meniscus, due to old tear
  ligament — *see* Sprain
  meniscus (knee) (current injury) S83.209 ☑
    bucket-handle S83.20- ☑
    lateral
      bucket-handle S83.25- ☑
      complex S83.27- ☑
      peripheral S83.26- ☑
      specified type NEC S83.28- ☑
    medial
      bucket-handle S83.21- ☑
      complex S83.23- ☑
      peripheral S83.22- ☑
      specified type NEC S83.24- ☑
    old — *see* Derangement, knee, meniscus, due to old tear
    site other than knee - code as Sprain
    specified type NEC S83.20- ☑
  muscle — *see* Strain
  pelvic
    floor, complicating delivery O70.1
    organ NEC, obstetrical trauma O71.5
      with ectopic or molar pregnancy O08.6
      following ectopic or molar pregnancy O08.6
  perineal, secondary O90.1
  periurethral tissue, obstetrical trauma O71.82
    with ectopic or molar pregnancy O08.6
    following ectopic or molar pregnancy O08.6
  rectovaginal septum — *see* Laceration, vagina
  retina, retinal (without detachment) (horseshoe) (*see also* Break, retina, horseshoe)
    with detachment — *see* Detachment, retina, with retinal, break
  rotator cuff (nontraumatic) M75.10- ☑
    complete M75.12- ☑
    incomplete M75.11- ☑
    traumatic S46.01- ☑
    capsule S43.42- ☑
  semilunar cartilage, knee — *see* Tear, meniscus
  supraspinatus (complete) (incomplete) (nontraumatic) (*see also* Tear, rotator cuff) M75.10- ☑
  tendon — *see* Strain
  tentorial, at birth P10.4
  umbilical cord
    complicating delivery O69.89 ☑
  urethra
    with ectopic or molar pregnancy O08.6
    following ectopic or molar pregnancy O08.6
    obstetrical trauma O71.5
  uterus — *see* Injury, uterus
  vagina — *see* Laceration, vagina
  vessel, from catheter — *see* Puncture, accidental complicating surgery
  vulva, complicating delivery O70.0
Tear-stone — *see* Dacryolith
Teeth (*see also* condition)
  grinding
    psychogenic F45.8
    sleep related G47.63
Teething (syndrome) K00.7
Telangiectasia, telangiectasis (verrucous) I78.1
  ataxic (cerebellar) (Louis-Bar) G11.3
  familial I78.0
  hemorrhagic, hereditary (congenital) (senile) I78.0

Telangiectasia — *continued*
  hereditary, hemorrhagic (congenital) (senile) I78.0
  juxtafoveal H35.07- ☑
  macular H35.07- ☑
  parafoveal H35.07- ☑
  retinal (idiopathic) (juxtafoveal) (macular) (parafoveal) H35.07- ☑
  spider I78.1
Telephone scatologia F65.89
Telescoped bowel or intestine K56.1
  congenital Q43.8
Temperature
  body, high (of unknown origin) R50.9
  cold, trauma from T69.9 ☑
    newborn P80.0
    specified effect NEC T69.8 ☑
Temple — *see* condition
Temporal — *see* condition
Temporomandibular joint pain-dysfunction syndrome M26.62
Temporosphenoidal — *see* condition
Tendency
  bleeding — *see* Defect, coagulation
  suicide
    meaning personal history of attempted suicide Z91.5
    meaning suicidal ideation — *see* Ideation, suicidal
  to fall R29.6
Tenderness, abdominal R10.819
  epigastric R10.816
  generalized R10.817
  left lower quadrant R10.814
  left upper quadrant R10.812
  periumbilic R10.815
  right lower quadrant R10.813
  right upper quadrant R10.811
  rebound R10.829
    epigastric R10.826
    generalized R10.827
    left lower quadrant R10.824
    left upper quadrant R10.822
    periumbilic R10.825
    right lower quadrant R10.823
    right upper quadrant R10.821
Tendinitis, tendonitis (*see also* Enthesopathy)
  Achilles M76.6- ☑
  adhesive — *see* Tenosynovitis, specified type NEC
    shoulder — *see* Capsulitis, adhesive
  bicipital M75.2- ☑
  calcific M65.2- ☑
    ankle M65.27- ☑
    foot M65.27- ☑
    forearm M65.23- ☑
    hand M65.24- ☑
    lower leg M65.26- ☑
    multiple sites M65.29
    pelvic region M65.25- ☑
    shoulder M75.3- ☑
    specified site NEC M65.28
    thigh M65.25- ☑
    upper arm M65.22- ☑
  due to use, overuse, pressure (*see also* Disorder, soft tissue, due to use)
    specified NEC — *see* Disorder, soft tissue, due to use, specified NEC
  gluteal M76.0- ☑
  patellar M76.5- ☑
  peroneal M76.7- ☑
  psoas M76.1- ☑
  tibial (posterior) M76.82- ☑
    anterior M76.81- ☑
  trochanteric — *see* Bursitis, hip, trochanteric
Tendon — *see* condition
Tendosynovitis — *see* Tenosynovitis
Tenesmus (rectal) R19.8
  vesical R30.1
Tennis elbow — *see* Epicondylitis, lateral
Tenonitis (*see also* Tenosynovitis)
  eye (capsule) H05.04- ☑
Tenontosynovitis — *see* Tenosynovitis
Tenontothecitis — *see* Tenosynovitis
Tenophyte — *see* Disorder, synovium, specified type NEC
Tenosynovitis (*see also* Synovitis) M65.9
  adhesive — *see* Tenosynovitis, specified type NEC
    shoulder — *see* Capsulitis, adhesive
  bicipital (calcifying) — *see* Tendinitis, bicipital
  gonococcal A54.49
  in (due to)
    crystals M65.8- ☑

Tenosynovitis — *continued*
  gonorrhea A54.49
  syphilis (late) A52.78
  use, overuse, pressure (*see also* Disorder, soft tissue, due to use)
    specified NEC — *see* Disorder, soft tissue, due to use, specified NEC
  infective NEC M65.1- ☑
    ankle M65.17- ☑
    foot M65.17- ☑
    forearm M65.13- ☑
    hand M65.14- ☑
    lower leg M65.16- ☑
    multiple sites M65.19
    pelvic region M65.15- ☑
    shoulder region M65.11- ☑
    specified site NEC M65.18
    thigh M65.15- ☑
    upper arm M65.12- ☑
  radial styloid M65.4
  shoulder region M65.81- ☑
    adhesive — *see* Capsulitis, adhesive
  specified type NEC M65.88
    ankle M65.87- ☑
    foot M65.87- ☑
    forearm M65.83- ☑
    hand M65.84- ☑
    lower leg M65.86- ☑
    multiple sites M65.89
    pelvic region M65.85- ☑
    shoulder region M65.81- ☑
    specified site NEC M65.88
    thigh M65.85- ☑
    upper arm M65.82- ☑
  tuberculous — *see* Tuberculosis, tenosynovitis
Tenovaginitis — *see* Tenosynovitis
Tension
  arterial, high (*see also* Hypertension)
    without diagnosis of hypertension R03.0
  headache G44.209
    intractable G44.201
    not intractable G44.209
  nervous R45.0
  pneumothorax J93.0
  premenstrual N94.3
  state (mental) F48.9
Tentorium — *see* condition
Teratencephalus Q89.8
Teratism Q89.7
Teratoblastoma (malignant) — *see* Neoplasm, malignant, by site
Teratocarcinoma (*see also* Neoplasm, malignant, by site)
  liver C22.7
Teratoma (solid) (*see also* Neoplasm, uncertain behavior, by site)
  with embryonal carcinoma, mixed — *see* Neoplasm, malignant, by site
  with malignant transformation — *see* Neoplasm, malignant, by site
  adult (cystic) — *see* Neoplasm, benign, by site
  benign — *see* Neoplasm, benign, by site
  combined with choriocarcinoma — *see* Neoplasm, malignant, by site
  cystic (adult) — *see* Neoplasm, benign, by site
  differentiated — *see* Neoplasm, benign, by site
  embryonal (*see also* Neoplasm, malignant, by site)
    liver C22.7
  immature — *see* Neoplasm, malignant, by site
  liver C22.7
    adult, benign, cystic, differentiated type or mature D13.4
  malignant (*see also* Neoplasm, malignant, by site)
    anaplastic — *see* Neoplasm, malignant, by site
    intermediate — *see* Neoplasm, malignant, by site
    specified site — *see* Neoplasm, malignant, by site
    unspecified site C62.90
    undifferentiated — *see* Neoplasm, malignant, by site
  mature — *see* Neoplasm, uncertain behavior, by site
    malignant — *see* Neoplasm, by site, malignant, by site
  ovary D27.- ☑
    embryonal, immature or malignant C56- ☑
  solid — *see* Neoplasm, uncertain behavior, by site
  testis C62.9- ☑
    adult, benign, cystic, differentiated type or mature D29.2- ☑

Teratoma — *continued*
    scrotal C62.1- ☑
    undescended C62.0- ☑
Termination
  anomalous (*see also* Malposition, congenital)
    right pulmonary vein Q26.3
  pregnancy, elective Z33.2
Ternidens diminutus infestation B81.8
Ternidensiasis B81.8
Terror (s) night (child) F51.4
Terrorism, victim of Z65.4
Terry's syndrome H44.2- ☑
Tertiary — *see* condition
Test, tests, testing (for)
  adequacy (for dialysis)
    hemodialysis Z49.31
    peritoneal Z49.32
  blood pressure Z01.30
    abnormal reading — *see* Blood, pressure
  blood-alcohol Z04.8
    positive — *see* Findings, abnormal, in blood
  blood-drug Z04.8
    positive — *see* Findings, abnormal, in blood
  blood typing Z01.83
    Rh typing Z01.83
  cardiac pulse generator (battery) Z45.010
  fertility Z31.41
  genetic
    disease carrier status for procreative management
      female Z31.430
      male Z31.440
    male partner of patient with recurrent pregnancy loss Z31.441
    procreative management NEC
      female Z31.438
      male Z31.448
  hearing Z01.10
    with abnormal findings NEC Z01.118
  HIV (human immunodeficiency virus)
    nonconclusive (in infants) R75
    positive Z21
    seropositive Z21
  immunity status Z01.84
  intelligence NEC Z01.89
  laboratory (as part of a general medical examination) Z00.00
    with abnormal finding Z00.01
    for medicolegal reason NEC Z04.8
  male partner of patient with recurrent pregnancy loss Z31.441
  Mantoux (for tuberculosis) Z11.1
    abnormal result R76.11
  pregnancy, positive first pregnancy — *see* Pregnancy, normal, first
  procreative Z31.49
    fertility Z31.41
  skin, diagnostic
    allergy Z01.82
    special screening examination — *see* Screening, by name of disease
    Mantoux Z11.1
    tuberculin Z11.1
  specified NEC Z01.89
  tuberculin Z11.1
    abnormal result R76.11
  vision Z01.00
    with abnormal findings Z01.01
  Wassermann Z11.3
    positive — *see* Serology for syphilis, positive
Testicle, testicular, testis (*see also* condition)
  feminization syndrome (*see also* Syndrome, androgen insensitivity) E34.51
  migrans Q55.29
Tetanus, tetanic (cephalic) (convulsions) A35
  with
    abortion A34
    ectopic or molar pregnancy O08.0
  following ectopic or molar pregnancy O08.0
  inoculation reaction (due to serum) — *see* Complications, vaccination
  neonatorum A33
  obstetrical A34
  puerperal, postpartum, childbirth A34
Tetany (due to) R29.0
  alkalosis E87.3
  associated with rickets E55.0
  convulsions R29.0
    hysterical F44.5
  functional (hysterical) F44.5
  hyperkinetic R29.0
    hysterical F44.5

☑ **Additional character required**

Tetany — continued
  hyperpnea R06.4
    hysterical F44.5
    psychogenic F45.8
  hyperventilation (see also Hyperventilation) R06.4
    hysterical F44.5
  neonatal (without calcium or magnesium
      deficiency) P71.3
  parathyroid (gland) E20.9
  parathyroprival E89.2
  post- (para)thyroidectomy E89.2
  postoperative E89.2
  pseudotetany R29.0
  psychogenic (conversion reaction) F44.5
Tetralogy of Fallot Q21.3
Tetraplegia (chronic) (see also Quadriplegia) G82.50
Thailand hemorrhagic fever A91
Thalassanemia — see Thalassemia
Thalassemia (anemia) (disease) D56.9
  with other hemoglobinopathy D56.8
  alpha (major) (severe) (triple gene defect) D56.0
    minor D56.3
    silent carrier D56.3
    trait D56.3
  beta (severe) D56.1
    homozygous D56.1
    major D56.1
    minor D56.3
    trait D56.3
  delta-beta (homozygous) D56.2
    minor D56.3
    trait D56.3
  dominant D56.8
  hemoglobin
    C D56.8
    E-beta D56.5
  intermedia D56.1
  major D56.1
  minor D56.3
  mixed D56.8
  sickle-cell — see Disease, sickle-cell, thalassemia
  specified type NEC D56.8
  trait D56.3
  variants D56.8
Thanatophoric dwarfism or short stature Q77.1
Thaysen-Gee disease (nontropical sprue) K90.0
Thaysen's disease K90.0
Thecoma D27- ☑
  luteinized D27- ☑
  malignant C56- ☑
Thelarche, premature E30.8
Thelaziasis B83.8
Thelitis N61
  puerperal, postpartum or gestational — see
      Infection, nipple
Therapeutic — see condition
Therapy
  drug, long-term (current) (prophylactic)
    agents affecting estrogen receptors and
        estrogen levels NEC Z79.818
    anastrozole (Arimidex) Z79.811
    antibiotics Z79.2
      short-term use - omit code
    anticoagulants Z79.01
    anti-inflammatory Z79.1
    antiplatelet Z79.02
    antithrombotics Z79.02
    aromatase inhibitors Z79.811
    aspirin Z79.82
    birth control pill or patch Z79.3
    bisphosphonates Z79.83
    contraceptive, oral Z79.3
    drug, specified NEC Z79.899
    estrogen receptor downregulators Z79.818
    Evista Z79.810
    exemestane (Aromasin) Z79.811
    Fareston Z79.810
    fulvestrant (Faslodex) Z79.818
    gonadotropin-releasing hormone (GnRH)
        agonist Z79.818
    goserelin acetate (Zoladex) Z79.818
    hormone replacement (postmenopausal)
        Z79.890
    insulin Z79.4
    letrozole (Femara) Z79.811
    leuprolide acetate (leuprorelin) (Lupron)
        Z79.818
    megestrol acetate (Megace) Z79.818
    methadone
      for pain management Z79.891
      maintenance therapy F11.20
    Nolvadex Z79.810

Therapy — continued
    opiate analgesic Z79.891
    oral contraceptive Z79.3
    raloxifene (Evista) Z79.810
    selective estrogen receptor modulators
        (SERMs) Z79.810
    short term - omit code
    steroids
      inhaled Z79.51
      systemic Z79.52
    tamoxifen (Nolvadex) Z79.810
    toremifene (Fareston) Z79.810
Thermic — see condition
Thermography (abnormal) (see also Abnormal,
    diagnostic imaging) R93.8
  breast R92.8
Thermoplegia T67.0 ☑
Thesaurismosis, glycogen — see Disease, glycogen
    storage
Thiamin deficiency E51.9
  specified NEC E51.8
Thiaminic deficiency with beriberi E51.11
Thibierge-Weissenbach syndrome — see Sclerosis,
    systemic
Thickening
  bone — see Hypertrophy, bone
  breast N64.59
  endometrium R93.8
  epidermal L85.9
    specified NEC L85.8
  hymen N89.6
  larynx J38.7
  nail L60.2
    congenital Q84.5
  periosteal — see Hypertrophy, bone
  pleura J92.9
    with asbestos J92.0
  skin R23.4
  subepiglottic J38.7
  tongue K14.8
  valve, heart — see Endocarditis
Thigh — see condition
Thinning vertebra — see Spondylopathy, specified
    NEC
Thirst, excessive R63.1
  due to deprivation of water T73.1 ☑
Thomsen disease G71.12
Thoracic (see also condition)
  kidney Q63.2
  outlet syndrome G54.0
Thoracogastroschisis (congenital) Q79.8
Thoracopagus Q89.4
Thorax — see condition
Thorn's syndrome N28.89
Thorson-Björck syndrome E34.0
Threadworm (infection) (infestation) B80
Threatened
  abortion O20.0
    with subsequent abortion O03.9
  job loss, anxiety concerning Z56.2
  labor (without delivery) O47.9
    after 37 completed weeks of gestation O47.1
    before 37 completed weeks of gestation
        O47.0- ☑
  loss of job, anxiety concerning Z56.2
  miscarriage O20.0
  unemployment, anxiety concerning Z56.2
Three-day fever A93.1
Threshers' lung J67.0
Thrix annulata (congenital) Q84.1
Throat — see condition
Thrombasthenia (Glanzmann) (hemorrhagic)
    (hereditary) D69.1
Thromboangiitis I73.1
  obliterans (general) I73.1
    cerebral I67.89
    vessels
      brain I67.89
      spinal cord I67.89
Thromboarteritis — see Arteritis
Thromboasthenia (Glanzmann) (hemorrhagic)
    (hereditary) D69.1
Thrombocytasthenia (Glanzmann) D69.1
Thrombocythemia (essential) (hemorrhagic)
    (idiopathic) (primary) D47.3
Thrombocytopathy (dystrophic) (granulopenic)
    D69.1
Thrombocytopenia, thrombocytopenic D69.6
  with absent radius (TAR) Q87.2
  congenital D69.42
  dilutional D69.59
  due to

Thrombocytopenia — continued
    drugs D69.59
    extracorporeal circulation of blood D69.59
    (massive) blood transfusion D69.59
    platelet alloimmunization D69.59
  essential D69.3
  heparin induced (HIT) D75.82
  hereditary D69.42
  idiopathic D69.3
  neonatal, transitory P61.0
    due to
      exchange transfusion P61.0
      idiopathic maternal thrombocytopenia P61.0
      isoimmunization P61.0
  primary NEC D69.49
    idiopathic D69.3
  puerperal, postpartum O72.3
  secondary D69.59
  transient neonatal P61.0
Thrombocytosis, essential D47.3
  primary D47.3
Thromboembolism — see Embolism
Thrombopathy (Bernard-Soulier) D69.1
  constitutional D68.0
  Willebrand-Jurgens D68.0
Thrombopenia — see Thrombocytopenia
Thrombophilia D68.59
  primary NEC D68.59
  secondary NEC D68.69
  specified NEC D68.69
Thrombophlebitis I80.9
  antepartum O22.2- ☑
    deep O22.3- ☑
    superficial O22.2- ☑
  cavernous (venous) sinus G08
    complicating pregnancy O22.5- ☑
    nonpyogenic I67.6
  cerebral (sinus) (vein) G08
    nonpyogenic I67.6
    sequelae G09
  due to implanted device — see Complications, by
      site and type, specified NEC
  during or resulting from a procedure NEC T81.72
      ☑
  femoral vein (superficial) I80.1- ☑
  femoropopliteal vein I80.0- ☑
  hepatic (vein) I80.8
  idiopathic, recurrent I82.1
  iliofemoral I80.1- ☑
  intracranial venous sinus (any) G08
    nonpyogenic I67.6
    sequelae G09
  intraspinal venous sinuses and veins G08
    nonpyogenic G95.19
  lateral (venous) sinus G08
    nonpyogenic I67.6
  leg I80.299
    superficial I80.0- ☑
  longitudinal (venous) sinus G08
    nonpyogenic I67.6
  lower extremity I80.299
  migrans, migrating I82.1
  pelvic
    with ectopic or molar pregnancy O08.0
    following ectopic or molar pregnancy O08.0
    puerperal O87.1
  popliteal vein — see Phlebitis, leg, deep, popliteal
  portal (vein) K75.1
  postoperative T81.72 ☑
  pregnancy — see Thrombophlebitis, antepartum
  puerperal, postpartum, childbirth O87.0
    deep O87.1
    pelvic O87.1
    septic O86.81
    superficial O87.0
  saphenous (greater) (lesser) I80.0- ☑
  sinus (intracranial) G08
    nonpyogenic I67.6
  specified site NEC I80.8
  tibial vein I80.23- ☑
Thrombosis, thrombotic (bland) (multiple)
    (progressive) (silent) (vessel) I82.90
  anal K64.5
  antepartum — see Thrombophlebitis,
      antepartum
  aorta, aortic I74.10
    abdominal I74.09
      saddle I74.01
    bifurcation I74.09
      saddle I74.01
    specified site NEC I74.19
    terminal I74.09

Thrombosis — *continued*
 thoracic I74.11
 valve — *see* Endocarditis, aortic
apoplexy I63.3 ☑
artery, arteries (postinfectional) I74.9
 auditory, internal — *see* Occlusion, artery, precerebral, specified NEC
 basilar — *see* Occlusion, artery, basilar
 carotid (common) (internal) — *see* Occlusion, artery, carotid
 cerebellar (anterior inferior) (posterior inferior) (superior) — *see* Occlusion, artery, cerebellar
 cerebral — *see* Occlusion, artery, cerebral
 choroidal (anterior) — *see* Occlusion, artery, cerebral, specified NEC
 communicating, posterior — *see* Occlusion, artery, cerebral, specified NEC
 coronary (*see also* Infarct, myocardium)
  not resulting in infarction I24.0
 hepatic I74.8
 hypophyseal — *see* Occlusion, artery, cerebral, specified NEC
 iliac I74.5
 limb I74.4
  lower I74.3
  upper I74.2
 meningeal, anterior or posterior — *see* Occlusion, artery, cerebral, specified NEC
 mesenteric (with gangrene) K55.0
 ophthalmic — *see* Occlusion, artery, retina
 pontine — *see* Occlusion, artery, cerebral, specified NEC
 precerebral — *see* Occlusion, artery, precerebral
 pulmonary (iatrogenic) — *see* Embolism, pulmonary
 renal N28.0
 retinal — *see* Occlusion, artery, retina
 spinal, anterior or posterior G95.11
 traumatic NEC T14.8
 vertebral — *see* Occlusion, artery, vertebral
atrium, auricular (*see also* Infarct, myocardium)
 following acute myocardial infarction (current complication) I23.6
 not resulting in infarction I24.0
basilar (artery) — *see* Occlusion, artery, basilar
brain (artery) (stem) (*see also* Occlusion, artery, cerebral)
 due to syphilis A52.05
 puerperal O99.43
 sinus — *see* Thrombosis, intracranial venous sinus
capillary I78.8
cardiac (*see also* Infarct, myocardium)
 not resulting in infarction I24.0
 valve — *see* Endocarditis
carotid (artery) (common) (internal) — *see* Occlusion, artery, carotid
cavernous (venous) sinus — *see* Thrombosis, intracranial venous sinus
cerebellar artery (anterior inferior) (posterior inferior) (superior) I66.3
cerebral (artery) — *see* Occlusion, artery, cerebral
cerebrovenous sinus (*see also* Thrombosis, intracranial venous sinus)
 puerperium O87.3
chronic I82.91
coronary (artery) (vein) (*see also* Infarct, myocardium)
 not resulting in infarction I24.0
corpus cavernosum N48.89
cortical I66.9
deep — *see* Embolism, vein, lower extremity
due to device, implant or graft (*see also* Complications, by site and type, specified NEC) T85.86 ☑
 arterial graft NEC T82.868 ☑
 breast (implant) T85.86 ☑
 catheter NEC T85.86 ☑
  dialysis (renal) T82.868 ☑
   intraperitoneal T85.86 ☑
  infusion NEC T82.868 ☑
   spinal (epidural) (subdural) T85.86 ☑
  urinary (indwelling) T83.86 ☑
 electronic (electrode) (pulse generator) (stimulator)
  bone T84.86 ☑
  cardiac T82.867 ☑
  nervous system (brain) (peripheral nerve) (spinal) T85.86 ☑
  urinary T83.86 ☑
 fixation, internal (orthopedic) NEC T84.86 ☑

Thrombosis — *continued*
 gastrointestinal (bile duct) (esophagus) T85.86 ☑
 genital NEC T83.86 ☑
 heart T82.867 ☑
 joint prosthesis T84.86 ☑
 ocular (corneal graft) (orbital implant) NEC T85.86 ☑
 orthopedic NEC T84.86 ☑
 specified NEC T85.86 ☑
 urinary NEC T83.86 ☑
 vascular NEC T82.868 ☑
 ventricular intracranial shunt T85.86 ☑
during the puerperium — *see* Thrombosis, puerperal
endocardial (*see also* Infarct, myocardium)
 not resulting in infarction I24.0
eye — *see* Occlusion, retina
genital organ
 female NEC N94.89
  pregnancy — *see* Thrombophlebitis, antepartum
 male N50.1
gestational — *see* Phlebopathy, gestational
heart (chamber) (*see also* Infarct, myocardium)
 not resulting in infarction I24.0
hepatic (vein) I82.0
 artery I74.8
history (of) Z86.718
intestine (with gangrene) K55.0
intracardiac NEC (apical) (atrial) (auricular) (ventricular) (old) I51.3
intracranial (arterial) I66.9
 venous sinus (any) G08
  nonpyogenic origin I67.6
  puerperium O87.3
intramural (*see also* Infarct, myocardium)
 not resulting in infarction I24.0
intraspinal venous sinuses and veins G08
 nonpyogenic G95.19
kidney (artery) N28.0
lateral (venous) sinus — *see* Thrombosis, intracranial venous sinus
leg — *see* Thrombosis, vein, lower extremity
 arterial I74.3
liver (venous) I82.0
 artery I74.8
 portal vein I81
longitudinal (venous) sinus — *see* Thrombosis, intracranial venous sinus
lower limb — *see* Thrombosis, vein, lower extremity
lung (iatrogenic) (postoperative) — *see* Embolism, pulmonary
meninges (brain) (arterial) I66.8
mesenteric (artery) (with gangrene) K55.0
 vein (inferior) (superior) I81
mitral I34.8
mural (*see also* Infarct, myocardium)
 due to syphilis A52.06
 not resulting in infarction I24.0
omentum (with gangrene) K55.0
ophthalmic — *see* Occlusion, retina
pampiniform plexus (male) N50.1
parietal (*see also* Infarct, myocardium)
 not resulting in infarction I24.0
penis, superficial vein N48.81
perianal venous K64.5
peripheral arteries I74.4
 upper I74.2
personal history (of) Z86.718
portal I81
 due to syphilis A52.09
precerebral artery — *see* Occlusion, artery, precerebral
puerperal, postpartum O87.0
 brain (artery) O99.43
  venous (sinus) O87.3
 cardiac O99.43
 cerebral (artery) O99.43
  venous (sinus) O87.3
 superficial O87.0
pulmonary (artery) (iatrogenic) (postoperative) (vein) — *see* Embolism, pulmonary
renal (artery) N28.0
 vein I82.3
resulting from presence of device, implant or graft — *see* Complications, by site and type, specified NEC
retina, retinal — *see* Occlusion, retina
scrotum N50.1
seminal vesicle N50.1

Thrombosis — *continued*
 sigmoid (venous) sinus — *see* Thrombosis, intracranial venous sinus
 sinus, intracranial (any) — *see* Thrombosis, intracranial venous sinus
 specified site NEC I82.890
  chronic I82.891
 spermatic cord N50.1
 spinal cord (arterial) G95.11
  due to syphilis A52.09
  pyogenic origin G06.1
 spleen, splenic D73.5
  artery I74.8
 testis N50.1
 tumor — *see* Neoplasm, unspecified behavior, by site
 traumatic NEC T14.8
 tricuspid I07.8
 tunica vaginalis N50.1
 umbilical cord (vessels), complicating delivery O69.5 ☑
 vas deferens N50.1
 vein (acute) I82.90
  antecubital I82.61- ☑
   chronic I82.71- ☑
  axillary I82.A1- ☑
   chronic I82.A2- ☑
  basilic I82.61- ☑
   chronic I82.71- ☑
  brachial I82.62- ☑
   chronic I82.72- ☑
  brachiocephalic (innominate) I82.290
   chronic I82.291
  cerebral, nonpyogenic I67.6
  cephalic I82.61- ☑
   chronic I82.71- ☑
  chronic I82.91
  deep (DVT) I82.40- ☑
   calf I82.4Z- ☑
    chronic I82.5Z- ☑
   lower leg I82.4Z- ☑
    chronic I82.5Z- ☑
   thigh I82.4Y- ☑
    chronic I82.5Y- ☑
   upper leg I82.4Y ☑
    chronic I82.5y--
  femoral I82.41- ☑
   chronic I82.51- ☑
  iliac (iliofemoral) I82.42- ☑
   chronic I82.52- ☑
  innominate I82.290
   chronic I82.291
  internal jugular I82.C1- ☑
   chronic I82.C2- ☑
  lower extremity
   deep I82.40- ☑
    chronic I82.50- ☑
    specified NEC I82.49- ☑
     chronic NEC I82.59- ☑
   distal
    deep I82.4Z- ☑
   proximal
    deep I82.4Y- ☑
     chronic I82.5Y- ☑
   superficial I82.81- ☑
  perianal K64.5
  popliteal I82.43- ☑
   chronic I82.53- ☑
  radial I82.62- ☑
   chronic I82.72- ☑
  renal I82.3
  saphenous (greater) (lesser) I82.81- ☑
  specified NEC I82.890
   chronic NEC I82.891
  subclavian I82.B1- ☑
   chronic I82.B2- ☑
  thoracic NEC I82.290
   chronic I82.291
  tibial I82.44- ☑
   chronic I82.54- ☑
  ulnar I82.62- ☑
   chronic I82.72- ☑
  upper extremity I82.60- ☑
   chronic I82.70- ☑
   deep I82.62- ☑
    chronic I82.72- ☑
   superficial I82.61- ☑
    chronic I82.71- ☑
 vena cava
  inferior I82.220
   chronic I82.221
  superior I82.210

☑ **Additional character required**

Thrombosis — *continued*
    chronic I82.211
    venous, perianal K64.5
    ventricle (*see also* Infarct, myocardium)
      following acute myocardial infarction (current complication) I23.6
      not resulting in infarction I24.0
Thrombus — *see* Thrombosis
Thrush (*see also* Candidiasis)
    oral B37.0
    newborn P37.5
    vaginal B37.3
Thumb (*see also* condition)
    sucking (child problem) F98.8
Thymitis E32.8
Thymoma (benign) D15.0
    malignant C37
Thymus, thymic (gland) — *see* condition
Thyrocele — *see* Goiter
Thyroglossal (*see also* condition)
    cyst Q89.2
    duct, persistent Q89.2
Thyroid (gland) (body) (*see also* condition)
    hormone resistance E07.89
    lingual Q89.2
    nodule (cystic) (nontoxic) (single) E04.1
Thyroiditis E06.9
    acute (nonsuppurative) (pyogenic) (suppurative) E06.0
    autoimmune E06.3
    chronic (nonspecific) (sclerosing) E06.5
      with thyrotoxicosis, transient E06.2
      fibrous E06.5
      lymphadenoid E06.3
      lymphocytic E06.3
      lymphoid E06.3
    de Quervain's E06.1
    drug-induced E06.4
    fibrous (chronic) E06.5
    giant-cell (follicular) E06.1
    granulomatous (de Quervain) (subacute) E06.1
    Hashimoto's (struma lymphomatosa) E06.3
    iatrogenic E06.4
    ligneous E06.5
    lymphocytic (chronic) E06.3
    lymphoid E06.3
    lymphomatous E06.3
    nonsuppurative E06.1
    postpartum, puerperal O90.5
    pseudotuberculous E06.1
    pyogenic E06.0
    radiation E06.4
    Riedel's E06.5
    subacute (granulomatous) E06.1
    suppurative E06.0
    tuberculous A18.81
    viral E06.1
    woody E06.5
Thyrolingual duct, persistent Q89.2
Thyromegaly E01.0
Thyrotoxic
    crisis — *see* Thyrotoxicosis
    heart disease or failure (*see also* Thyrotoxicosis) E05.90 [I43]
      with thyroid storm E05.91 [I43]
    storm — *see* Thyrotoxicosis
Thyrotoxicosis (recurrent) E05.90
    with
      goiter (diffuse) E05.00
        with thyroid storm E05.01
        adenomatous uninodular E05.10
          with thyroid storm E05.11
        multinodular E05.20
          with thyroid storm E05.21
        nodular E05.20
          with thyroid storm E05.21
        uninodular E05.10
          with thyroid storm E05.11
      infiltrative
        dermopathy E05.00
          with thyroid storm E05.01
        ophthalmopathy E05.00
          with thyroid storm E05.01
      single thyroid nodule E05.10
        with thyroid storm E05.11
      thyroid storm E05.91
    due to
      ectopic thyroid nodule or tissue E05.30
        with thyroid storm E05.31
      ingestion of (excessive) thyroid material E05.40
        with thyroid storm E05.41

Thyrotoxicosis — *continued*
      overproduction of thyroid-stimulating hormone E05.80
        with thyroid storm E05.81
      specified cause NEC E05.80
        with thyroid storm E05.81
    factitia E05.40
      with thyroid storm E05.41
    heart E05.90 [I43]
      with thyroid storm E05.91 [I43]
      failure E05.90 [I43]
    neonatal (transient) P72.1
    transient with chronic thyroiditis E06.2
Tibia vara — *see* Osteochondrosis, juvenile, tibia
Tic (disorder) F95.9
    breathing F95.8
    child problem F95.0
    compulsive F95.1
    de la Tourette F95.2
    degenerative (generalized) (localized) G25.69
      facial G25.69
    disorder
      chronic
        motor F95.1
        vocal F95.1
      combined vocal and multiple motor F95.2
      transient F95.0
    douloureux G50.0
      atypical G50.1
      postherpetic, postzoster B02.22
    drug-induced G25.61
    eyelid F95.8
    habit F95.9
      chronic F95.1
      transient of childhood F95.0
    lid, transient of childhood F95.0
    motor-verbal F95.2
    occupational F48.8
    orbicularis F95.8
      transient of childhood F95.0
    organic origin G25.69
    postchoreic G25.69
    psychogenic, compulsive F95.1
    salaam R25.8
    spasm (motor or vocal) F95.9
      chronic F95.1
      transient of childhood F95.0
    specified NEC F95.8
Tick-borne — *see* condition
Tietze's disease or syndrome M94.0
Tight, tightness
    anus K62.89
    chest R07.89
    fascia (lata) M62.89
    foreskin (congenital) N47.1
    hymen, hymenal ring N89.6
    introitus (acquired) (congenital) N89.6
    rectal sphincter K62.89
    tendon — *see* Short, tendon
    urethral sphincter N35.9
Tilting vertebra — *see* Dorsopathy, deforming, specified NEC
Timidity, child F93.8
Tin-miner's lung J63.5
Tinea (intersecta) (tarsi) B35.9
    amiantacea L44.8
    asbestina B35.0
    barbae B35.0
    beard B35.0
    black dot B35.0
    blanca B36.2
    capitis B35.0
    corporis B35.4
    cruris B35.6
    flava B36.0
    foot B35.3
    furfuracea B36.0
    imbricata (Tokelau) B35.5
    kerion B35.0
    manuum B35.2
    microsporic — *see* Dermatophytosis
    nigra B36.1
    nodosa — *see* Piedra
    pedis B35.3
    scalp B35.0
    specified site NEC B35.8
    sycosis B35.0
    tonsurans B35.0
    trichophytic — *see* Dermatophytosis
    unguium B35.1
    versicolor B36.0
Tingling sensation (skin) R20.2

Tinnitus (audible) (aurium) (subjective) H93.1
Tipped tooth (teeth) M26.33
Tipping
    pelvis M95.5
      with disproportion (fetopelvic) O33.0
        causing obstructed labor O65.0
    tooth (teeth), fully erupted M26.33
Tiredness R53.83
Tissue — *see* condition
Tobacco (nicotine)
    dependence — *see* Dependence, drug, nicotine
    harmful use Z72.0
    heart — *see* Tobacco, toxic effect
    maternal use, affecting newborn P04.2
    toxic effect — *see* Table of Drugs and Chemicals, by substance, poisoning
      chewing tobacco — *see* Table of Drugs and Chemicals, by substance, poisoning
      cigarettes — *see* Table of Drugs and Chemicals, by substance, poisoning
    use Z72.0
      complicating
        childbirth O99.334
        pregnancy O99.33- ☑
        puerperium O99.335
      counseling and surveillance Z71.6
    withdrawal state — *see* Dependence, drug, nicotine
Tocopherol deficiency E56.0
Todd's
    cirrhosis K74.3
    paralysis (postepileptic) (transitory) G83.84
Toe — *see* condition
Toilet, artificial opening — *see* Attention to, artificial, opening
Tokelau (ringworm) B35.5
Tollwut — *see* Rabies
Tommaselli's disease R31.9
    correct substance properly administered — *see* Table of Drugs and Chemicals, by drug, adverse effect
    overdose or wrong substance given or taken — *see* Table of Drugs and Chemicals, by drug, poisoning
Tongue (*see also* condition)
    tie Q38.1
Tonic pupil — *see* Anomaly, pupil, function, tonic pupil
Toni-Fanconi syndrome (cystinosis) E72.09
    with cystinosis E72.04
Tonsil — *see* condition
Tonsillitis (acute) (catarrhal) (croupous) (follicular) (gangrenous) (infective) (lacunar) (lingual) (malignant) (membranous) (parenchymatous) (phlegmonous) (pseudomembranous) (purulent) (septic) (subacute) (suppurative) (toxic) (ulcerative) (vesicular) (viral) J03.90
    chronic J35.01
      with adenoiditis J35.03
    diphtheritic A36.0
    hypertrophic J35.01
      with adenoiditis J35.03
    recurrent J03.91
    specified organism NEC J03.80
      recurrent J03.81
    staphylococcal J03.80
      recurrent J03.81
    streptococcal J03.00
      recurrent J03.01
    tuberculous A15.8
    Vincent's A69.1
Tooth, teeth — *see* condition
Toothache K08.8
Topagnosis R20.8
Tophi — *see* Gout, chronic
TORCH infection — *see* Infection, congenital without active infection P00.2
Torn — *see* Tear
Tornwaldt's cyst or disease J39.2
Torsion
    accessory tube — *see* Torsion, fallopian tube
    adnexa (female) — *see* Torsion, fallopian tube
    aorta, acquired I77.1
    appendix epididymis N44.04
    appendix testis N44.03
    bile duct (common) (hepatic) K83.8
      congenital Q44.5
    bowel, colon or intestine K56.2
    cervix — *see* Malposition, uterus
    cystic duct K82.8
    dystonia — *see* Dystonia, torsion
    epididymis (appendix) N44.04

Torsion — *continued*
　fallopian tube N83.52
　　with ovary N83.53
　gallbladder K82.8
　　congenital Q44.1
　hydatid of Morgagni
　　female N83.52
　　male N44.03
　kidney (pedicle) (leading to infarction) N28.0
　Meckel's diverticulum (congenital) Q43.0
　　malignant — *see* Table of Neoplasms, small
　　　intestine, malignant
　mesentery K56.2
　omentum K56.2
　organ or site, congenital NEC — *see* Anomaly,
　　by site
　ovary (pedicle) N83.51
　　with fallopian tube N83.53
　　congenital Q50.2
　oviduct — *see* Torsion, fallopian tube
　penis (acquired) N48.82
　　congenital Q55.63
　spasm — *see* Dystonia, torsion
　spermatic cord N44.02
　　extravaginal N44.01
　　intravaginal N44.02
　spleen D73.5
　testis, testicle N44.00
　　appendix N44.03
　tibia — *see* Deformity, limb, specified type NEC,
　　lower leg
　uterus — *see* Malposition, uterus
Torticollis (intermittent) (spastic) M43.6
　congenital (sternomastoid) Q68.0
　due to birth injury P15.8
　hysterical F44.4
　ocular R29.891
　psychogenic F45.8
　　conversion reaction F44.4
　rheumatic M43.6
　rheumatoid M06.88
　spasmodic G24.3
　traumatic, current S13.4 ☑
Tortipelvis G24.1
Tortuous
　artery I77.1
　organ or site, congenital NEC — *see* Distortion
　retinal vessel, congenital Q14.1
　ureter N13.8
　urethra N36.8
　vein — *see* Varix
Torture, victim of Z65.4
Torula, torular (histolytica) (infection) — *see*
　Cryptococcosis
Torulosis — *see* Cryptococcosis
Torus (mandibularis) (palatinus) M27.0
　fracture — *see* Fracture, by site, torus
Touraine's syndrome Q79.8
Tourette's syndrome F95.2
Tourniquet syndrome — *see* Constriction, external,
　by site
Tower skull Q75.0
　with exophthalmos Q87.0
Toxemia R68.89
　bacterial — *see* Sepsis
　burn — *see* Burn
　eclamptic (with pre-existing hypertension) — *see*
　　Eclampsia
　erysipelatous — *see* Erysipelas
　fatigue R68.89
　food — *see* Poisoning, food
　gastrointestinal K52.1
　intestinal K52.1
　kidney — *see* Uremia
　malarial — *see* Malaria
　myocardial — *see* Myocarditis, toxic
　of pregnancy — *see* Pre-eclampsia
　pre-eclamptic — *see* Pre-eclampsia
　small intestine K52.1
　staphylococcal, due to food A05.0
　stasis R68.89
　uremic — *see* Uremia
　urinary — *see* Uremia
Toxemica cerebropathia psychica (nonalcoholic) F04
　alcoholic — *see* Alcohol, amnestic disorder
Toxic (poisoning) (*see also* condition) T65.91 ☑
　effect — *see* Table of Drugs and Chemicals, by
　　substance, poisoning
　shock syndrome A48.3
　thyroid (gland) — *see* Thyrotoxicosis
Toxicemia — *see* Toxemia

Toxicity — *see* Table of Drugs and Chemicals, by
　substance, poisoning
　fava bean D55.0
　food, noxious — *see* Poisoning, food
　from drug or nonmedicinal substance — *see*
　　Table of Drugs and Chemicals, by drug
Toxicosis (*see also* Toxemia)
　capillary, hemorrhagic D69.0
Toxinfection, gastrointestinal K52.1
Toxocariasis B83.0
Toxoplasma, toxoplasmosis (acquired) B58.9
　with
　　hepatitis B58.1
　　meningoencephalitis B58.2
　　ocular involvement B58.00
　　other organ involvement B58.89
　　pneumonia, pneumonitis B58.3
　congenital (acute) (subacute) (chronic) P37.1
　maternal, manifest toxoplasmosis in infant
　　(acute) (subacute) (chronic) P37.1
tPA (rtPA) administration in a different facility within
　the last 24 hours prior to admission to current
　facility Z92.82
Trabeculation, bladder N32.89
Trachea — *see* condition
Tracheitis (catarrhal) (infantile) (membranous)
　(plastic) (septal) (suppurative) (viral) J04.10
　with
　　bronchitis (15 years of age and above) J40
　　　acute or subacute — *see* Bronchitis, acute
　　　chronic J42
　　　tuberculous NEC A15.5
　　　under 15 years of age J20.9
　　laryngitis (acute) J04.2
　　　chronic J37.1
　　　tuberculous NEC A15.5
　acute J04.10
　　with obstruction J04.11
　chronic J42
　　with
　　　bronchitis (chronic) J42
　　　laryngitis (chronic) J37.1
　diphtheritic (membranous) A36.89
　due to external agent — *see* Inflammation,
　　respiratory, upper, due to
　syphilitic A52.73
　tuberculous A15.5
Trachelitis (nonvenereal) — *see* Cervicitis
Tracheobronchial — *see* condition
Tracheobronchitis (15 years of age and above) (*see
　also* Bronchitis)
　due to
　　Bordetella bronchiseptica A37.80
　　　with pneumonia A37.81
　　Francisella tularensis A21.8
Tracheobronchomegaly Q32.4
　with bronchiectasis J47.9
　　with
　　　exacerbation (acute) J47.1
　　　lower respiratory infection J47.0
　acquired J98.09
　　with bronchiectasis J47.9
　　　with
　　　　exacerbation (acute) J47.1
　　　　lower respiratory infection J47.0
Tracheobronchopneumonitis — *see* Pneumonia,
　broncho-
Tracheocele (external) (internal) J39.8
　congenital Q32.1
Tracheomalacia J39.8
　congenital Q32.0
Tracheopharyngitis (acute) J06.9
　chronic J42
　due to external agent — *see* Inflammation,
　　respiratory, upper, due to
Tracheostenosis J39.8
Tracheostomy
　complication — *see* Complication, tracheostomy
　status Z93.0
　　attention to Z43.0
　　malfunctioning J95.03
Trachoma, trachomatous A71.9
　active (stage) A71.1
　contraction of conjunctiva A71.1
　dubium A71.0
　initial (stage) A71.0
　healed or sequelae B94.0
　pannus A71.1
　Türck's J37.0
Traction, vitreomacular H43.82- ☑
Train sickness T75.3 ☑

Trait (s)
　Hb-S D57.3
　hemoglobin
　　abnormal NEC D58.2
　　　with thalassemia D56.3
　　C — *see* Disease, hemoglobin C
　　S (Hb-S) D57.3
　Lepore D56.3
　personality, accentuated Z73.1
　sickle-cell D57.3
　　with elliptocytosis or spherocytosis D57.3
　type A personality Z73.1
Tramp Z59.0
Trance R41.89
　hysterical F44.89
Transection
　abdomen (partial) S38.3 ☑
　aorta (incomplete) (*see also* Injury, aorta)
　　complete — *see* Injury, aorta, laceration, major
　carotid artery (incomplete) (*see also* Injury, blood
　　vessel, carotid, laceration)
　　complete — *see* Injury, blood vessel, carotid,
　　　laceration, major
　celiac artery (incomplete) S35.211 ☑
　　branch (incomplete) S35.291 ☑
　　　complete S35.292 ☑
　　complete S35.212 ☑
　innominate
　　artery (incomplete) (*see also* Injury, blood
　　　vessel, thoracic, innominate, artery,
　　　laceration)
　　complete — *see* Injury, blood vessel, thoracic,
　　　innominate, artery, laceration, major
　　vein (incomplete) (*see also* Injury, blood vessel,
　　　thoracic, innominate, vein, laceration)
　　complete — *see* Injury, blood vessel, thoracic,
　　　innominate, vein, laceration, major
　jugular vein (external) (incomplete) (*see also*
　　Injury, blood vessel, jugular vein, laceration)
　　complete — *see* Injury, blood vessel, jugular
　　　vein, laceration, major
　　internal (incomplete) (*see also* Injury, blood
　　　vessel, jugular vein, internal, laceration)
　　complete — *see* Injury, blood vessel, jugular
　　　vein, internal, laceration, major
　mesenteric artery (incomplete) (*see also* Injury,
　　mesenteric, artery, laceration)
　　complete — *see* Injury, mesenteric artery,
　　　laceration, major
　pulmonary vessel (incomplete) (*see also* Injury,
　　blood vessel, thoracic, pulmonary, laceration)
　　complete — *see* Injury, blood vessel, thoracic,
　　　pulmonary, laceration, major
　subclavian — *see* Transection, innominate
　vena cava (incomplete) (*see also* Injury, vena cava)
　　complete — *see* Injury, vena cava, laceration,
　　　major
　vertebral artery (incomplete) (*see also* Injury,
　　blood vessel, vertebral, laceration)
　　complete — *see* Injury, blood vessel, vertebral,
　　　laceration, major
Transaminasemia R74.0
Transfusion
　associated (red blood cell) hemochromatosis
　　E83.111
　blood
　　ABO incompatible — *see* Complication(s),
　　　transfusion, incompatibility reaction, ABO
　　minor blood group (Duffy) (E) (K(ell)) (Kidd)
　　　(Lewis) (M) (N) (P) (S) T80.89 ☑
　　reaction or complication — *see* Complications,
　　　transfusion
　　fetomaternal (mother) — *see* Pregnancy,
　　　complicated by, placenta, transfusion
　　　syndrome
　　maternofetal (mother) — *see* Pregnancy,
　　　complicated by, placenta, transfusion
　　　syndrome
　　placental (syndrome) (mother) — *see* Pregnancy,
　　　complicated by, placenta, transfusion
　　　syndrome
　　reaction (adverse) — *see* Complications,
　　　transfusion
　　related acute lung injury (TRALI) J95.84
　　twin-to-twin — *see* Pregnancy, complicated by,
　　　placenta, transfusion syndrome, fetus to
　　　fetus
Transient (meaning homeless) (*see also* condition)
　Z59.0
Translocation
　balanced autosomal Q95.9
　　in normal individual Q95.0

☑ **Additional character required**

Translocation — *continued*
  chromosomes NEC Q99.8
    balanced and insertion in normal individual
      Q95.0
    Down syndrome Q90.2
    trisomy
      13 Q91.6
      18 Q91.2
      21 Q90.2
Translucency, iris — *see* Degeneration, iris
Transmission of chemical substances through the
  placenta — *see* Absorption, chemical, through
  placenta
Transparency, lung, unilateral J43.0
Transplant (ed) (status) Z94.9
  awaiting organ Z76.82
  bone Z94.6
    marrow Z94.81
  candidate Z76.82
  complication — *see* Complication, transplant
  cornea Z94.7
  heart Z94.1
    and lung (s) Z94.3
    valve Z95.2
      prosthetic Z95.2
      specified NEC Z95.4
      xenogenic Z95.3
  intestine Z94.82
  kidney Z94.0
  liver Z94.4
  lung (s) Z94.2
    and heart Z94.3
  organ (failure) (infection) (rejection) Z94.9
    removal status Z98.85
  pancreas Z94.83
  skin Z94.5
  social Z60.3
  specified organ or tissue NEC Z94.89
  stem cells Z94.84
  tissue Z94.9
Transplants, ovarian, endometrial N80.1
Transposed — *see* Transposition
Transposition (congenital) (*see also* Malposition,
  congenital)
  abdominal viscera Q89.3
  aorta (dextra) Q20.3
  appendix Q43.8
  colon Q43.8
  corrected Q20.5
  great vessels (complete) (partial) Q20.3
  heart Q24.0
    with complete transposition of viscera Q89.3
  intestine (large) (small) Q43.8
  reversed jejunal (for bypass) (status) Z98.0
  scrotum Q55.23
  stomach Q40.2
    with general transposition of viscera Q89.3
  tooth, teeth, fully erupted M26.30
  vessels, great (complete) (partial) Q20.3
  viscera (abdominal) (thoracic) Q89.3
Transsexualism F64.1
Transverse (*see also* condition)
  arrest (deep), in labor O64.0 ☑
  lie (mother) O32.2 ☑
    causing obstructed labor O64.8 ☑
Transvestism, transvestitism (dual-role) F64.1
  fetishistic F65.1
Trapped placenta (with hemorrhage) O72.0
  without hemorrhage O73.0
Trauma, traumatism (*see also* Injury)
  acoustic H83.3
  birth — *see* Birth, injury
  complicating ectopic or molar pregnancy O08.6
  during delivery O71.9
  following ectopic or molar pregnancy O08.6
  obstetric O71.9
    specified NEC O71.89
Traumatic (*see also* condition)
  brain injury S06
Treacher Collins syndrome Q75.4
Treitz's hernia — *see* Hernia, abdomen, specified
  site NEC
Trematode infestation — *see* Infestation, fluke
Trematodiasis — *see* Infestation, fluke
Trembling paralysis — *see* Parkinsonism
Tremor (s) R25.1
  drug induced G25.1
  essential (benign) G25.0
  familial G25.0
  hereditary G25.0
  hysterical F44.4
  intention G25.2

Tremor — *continued*
  medication induced postural G25.1
  mercurial T56.1
  Parkinson's — *see* Parkinsonism
  psychogenic (conversion reaction) F44.4
  senilis R54
  specified type NEC G25.2
Trench
  fever A79.0
  foot — *see* Immersion, foot
  mouth A69.1
Treponema pallidum infection — *see* Syphilis
Treponematosis
  due to
    T. pallidum — *see* Syphilis
    T. pertenue — *see* Yaws
Triad
  Hutchinson's (congenital syphilis) A50.53
  Kartagener's Q89.3
  Saint's — *see* Hernia, diaphragm
Trichiasis (eyelid) H02.059
  with entropion — *see* Entropion
  left H02.056
    lower H02.055
    upper H02.054
  right H02.053
    lower H02.052
    upper H02.051
Trichinella spiralis (infection) (infestation) B75
Trichinellosis, trichiniasis, trichinelliasis, trichinosis
  B75
  with muscle disorder B75 [M63.80]
    ankle B75 [M63.87- ☑]
    foot B75 [M63.87- ☑]
    forearm B75 [M63.83- ☑]
    hand B75 [M63.84- ☑]
    lower leg B75 [M63.86- ☑]
    multiple sites B75 [M63.89]
    pelvic region B75 [M63.85- ☑]
    shoulder region B75 [M63.81- ☑]
    specified site NEC B75 [M63.88]
    thigh B75 [M63.85- ☑]
    upper arm B75 [M63.82- ☑]
Trichobezoar T18.9 ☑
  intestine T18.3 ☑
  stomach T18.2 ☑
Trichocephaliasis, trichocephalosis B79
Trichocephalus infestation B79
Trichoclasis L67.8
Trichoepithelioma (*see also* Neoplasm, skin, benign)
  malignant — *see* Neoplasm, skin, malignant
Trichofolliculoma — *see* Neoplasm, skin, benign
Tricholemmoma — *see* Neoplasm, skin, benign
Trichomoniasis A59.9
  bladder A59.03
  cervix A59.09
  intestinal A07.8
  prostate A59.02
  seminal vesicles A59.09
  specified site NEC A59.8
  urethra A59.03
  urogenitalis A59.00
  vagina A59.01
  vulva A59.01
Trichomycosis
  axillaris A48.8
  nodosa, nodularis B36.8
Trichonodosis L67.8
Trichophytid, trichophyton infection — *see*
  Dermatophytosis
Trichophytobezoar T18.9 ☑
  intestine T18.3 ☑
  stomach T18.2 ☑
Trichophytosis — *see* Dermatophytosis
Trichoptilosis L67.8
Trichorrhexis (nodosa) (invaginata) L67.0
Trichosis axillaris A48.8
Trichosporosis nodosa B36.2
Trichostasis spinulosa (congenital) Q84.1
Trichostrongyliasis, trichostrongylosis (small
  intestine) B81.2
Trichostrongylus infection B81.2
Trichotillomania F63.3
Trichromat, trichromatopsia, anomalous
  (congenital) H53.55
Trichuriasis B79
Trichuris trichiura (infection) (infestation) (any site)
  B79
Tricuspid (valve) — *see* condition
Trifid (*see also* Accessory)
  kidney (pelvis) Q63.8
  tongue Q38.3

Trigeminal neuralgia — *see* Neuralgia, trigeminal
Trigeminy R00.8
Trigger finger (acquired) M65.30
  congenital Q74.0
  index finger M65.32- ☑
  little finger M65.35- ☑
  middle finger M65.33- ☑
  ring finger M65.34- ☑
  thumb M65.31- ☑
Trigonitis (bladder) (chronic) (pseudomembranous)
  N30.30
  with hematuria N30.31
Trigonocephaly Q75.0
Trilocular heart — *see* Cor triloculare
Trimethylaminuria E72.52
Tripartite placenta O43.19- ☑
Triphalangeal thumb Q74.0
Triple (*see also* Accessory)
  kidneys Q63.0
  uteri Q51.818
  X, female Q97.0
Triplegia G83.89
  congenital G80.8
Triplet (newborn) (*see also* Newborn, triplet)
  complicating pregnancy — *see* Pregnancy, triplet
Triplication — *see* Accessory
Triploidy Q92.7
Trismus R25.2
  neonatorum A33
  newborn A33
Trisomy (syndrome) Q92.9
  autosomes Q92.9
  chromosome specified NEC Q92.8
    partial Q92.2
      due to unbalanced translocation Q92.5
    whole (nonsex chromosome)
      meiotic nondisjunction Q92.0
      mitotic nondisjunction Q92.1
      mosaicism Q92.1
    specified NEC Q92.8
  due to
    dicentrics — *see* Extra, marker chromosomes
    extra rings — *see* Extra, marker chromosomes
    isochromosomes — *see* Extra, marker
      chromosomes
  specified NEC Q92.8
  whole chromosome Q92.9
    meiotic nondisjunction Q92.0
    mitotic nondisjunction Q92.1
    mosaicism Q92.1
    partial Q92.9
    specified NEC Q92.8
  13 (partial) Q91.7
    meiotic nondisjunction Q91.4
    mitotic nondisjunction Q91.5
    mosaicism Q91.5
    translocation Q91.6
  18 (partial) Q91.3
    meiotic nondisjunction Q91.0
    mitotic nondisjunction Q91.1
    mosaicism Q91.1
    translocation Q91.2
  20 Q92.8
  21 (partial) Q90.9
    meiotic nondisjunction Q90.0
    mitotic nondisjunction Q90.1
    mosaicism Q90.1
    translocation Q90.2
  22 Q92.8
Tritanomaly, tritanopia H53.55
Trombiculosis, trombiculiasis, trombidiosis B88.0
Trophedema (congenital) (hereditary) Q82.0
Trophoblastic disease (*see also* Mole, hydatidiform)
  O01.9
Tropholymphedema Q82.0
Trophoneurosis NEC G96.8
  disseminated M34.9
Tropical — *see* condition
Trouble (*see also* Disease)
  heart — *see* Disease, heart
  kidney — *see* Disease, renal
  nervous R45.0
  sinus — *see* Sinusitis
Trousseau's syndrome (thrombophlebitis migrans)
  I82.1
Truancy, childhood
  from school Z72.810
Truncus
  arteriosus (persistent) Q20.0
  communis Q20.0
Trunk — *see* condition

Trypanosomiasis - Tuberculosis

Trypanosomiasis
  African B56.9
    by Trypanosoma brucei
      gambiense B56.0
      rhodesiense B56.1
  American — see Chagas' disease
  Brazilian — see Chagas' disease
  by Trypanosoma
    brucei gambiense B56.0
    brucei rhodesiense B56.1
    cruzi — see Chagas' disease
  gambiensis, Gambian B56.0
  rhodesiensis, Rhodesian B56.1
  South American — see Chagas' disease
  where
    African trypanosomiasis is prevalent B56.9
    Chagas' disease is prevalent B57.2
T-shaped incisors K00.2
Tsutsugamushi (disease) (fever) A75.3
Tube, tubal, tubular — see condition
Tubercle (see also Tuberculosis)
  brain, solitary A17.81
  Darwin's Q17.8
  Ghon, primary infection A15.7
Tuberculid, tuberculide (indurating, subcutaneous) (lichenoid) (miliary) (papulonecrotic) (primary) (skin) A18.4
Tuberculoma (see also Tuberculosis)
  brain A17.81
  meninges (cerebral) (spinal) A17.1
  spinal cord A17.81
Tuberculosis, tubercular, tuberculous (calcification) (calcified) (caseous) (chromogenic acid-fast bacilli) (degeneration) (fibrocaseous) (fistula) (interstitial) (isolated circumscribed lesions) (necrosis) (parenchymatous) (ulcerative) A15.9
  with pneumoconiosis (any condition in J60-J64) J65
  abdomen (lymph gland) A18.39
  abscess (respiratory) A15.9
    bone A18.03
      hip A18.02
      knee A18.02
      sacrum A18.01
      specified site NEC A18.03
      spinal A18.01
      vertebra A18.01
    brain A17.81
    breast A18.89
    Cowper's gland A18.15
    dura (mater) (cerebral) (spinal) A17.81
    epidural (cerebral) (spinal) A17.81
    female pelvis A18.17
    frontal sinus A15.8
    genital organs NEC A18.10
    genitourinary A18.10
    gland (lymphatic) — see Tuberculosis, lymph gland
    hip A18.02
    intestine A18.32
    ischiorectal A18.32
    joint NEC A18.02
      hip A18.02
      knee A18.02
      specified NEC A18.02
      vertebral A18.01
    kidney A18.11
    knee A18.02
    latent R76.11
    lumbar (spine) A18.01
    lung — see Tuberculosis, pulmonary
    meninges (cerebral) (spinal) A17.0
    muscle A18.09
    perianal (fistula) A18.32
    perinephritic A18.11
    perirectal A18.32
    rectum A18.32
    retropharyngeal A15.8
    sacrum A18.01
    scrofulous A18.2
    scrotum A18.15
    skin (primary) A18.4
    spinal cord A17.81
    spine or vertebra (column) A18.01
    subdiaphragmatic A18.31
    testis A18.15
    urinary A18.13
    uterus A18.17
  accessory sinus — see Tuberculosis, sinus
  Addison's disease A18.7
  adenitis — see Tuberculosis, lymph gland
  adenoids A15.8

Tuberculosis — continued
  adenopathy — see Tuberculosis, lymph gland
  adherent pericardium A18.84
  adnexa (uteri) A18.17
  adrenal (capsule) (gland) A18.7
  alimentary canal A18.32
  anemia A18.89
  ankle (joint) (bone) A18.02
  anus A18.32
  apex, apical — see Tuberculosis, pulmonary
  appendicitis, appendix A18.32
  arachnoid A17.0
  artery, arteritis A18.89
    cerebral A18.89
  arthritis (chronic) (synovial) A18.02
    spine or vertebra (column) A18.01
  articular — see Tuberculosis, joint
  ascites A18.31
  asthma — see Tuberculosis, pulmonary
  axilla, axillary (gland) A18.2
  bladder A18.12
  bone A18.03
    hip A18.02
    knee A18.02
    limb NEC A18.03
    sacrum A18.01
    spine or vertebral column A18.01
  bowel (miliary) A18.32
  brain A17.81
  breast A18.89
  broad ligament A18.17
  bronchi, bronchial, bronchus A15.5
    ectasia, ectasis (bronchiectasis) — see Tuberculosis, pulmonary
    fistula A15.5
      primary (progressive) A15.7
    gland or node A15.4
      primary (progressive) A15.7
    lymph gland or node A15.4
      primary (progressive) A15.7
  bronchiectasis — see Tuberculosis, pulmonary
  bronchitis A15.5
  bronchopleural A15.6
  bronchopneumonia, bronchopneumonic — see Tuberculosis, pulmonary
  bronchorrhagia A15.5
  bronchotracheal A15.5
  bronze disease A18.7
  buccal cavity A18.83
  bulbourethral gland A18.15
  bursa A18.09
  cachexia A15.9
  cardiomyopathy A18.84
  caries — see Tuberculosis, bone
  cartilage A18.02
    intervertebral A18.01
  catarrhal — see Tuberculosis, respiratory
  cecum A18.32
  cellulitis (primary) A18.4
  cerebellum A17.81
  cerebral, cerebrum A17.81
  cerebrospinal A17.81
    meninges A17.0
  cervical (lymph gland or node) A18.2
  cervicitis, cervix (uteri) A18.16
  chest — see Tuberculosis, respiratory
  chorioretinitis A18.53
  choroid, choroiditis A18.53
  ciliary body A18.54
  colitis A18.32
  collier's J65
  colliquativa (primary) A18.4
  colon A18.32
  complex, primary A15.7
  congenital P37.0
  conjunctiva A18.59
  connective tissue (systemic) A18.89
  contact Z20.1
  cornea (ulcer) A18.52
  Cowper's gland A18.15
  coxae A18.02
  coxalgia A18.02
  cul-de-sac of Douglas A18.17
  curvature, spine A18.01
  cutis (colliquativa) (primary) A18.4
  cyst, ovary A18.18
  cystitis A18.12
  dactylitis A18.03
  diarrhea A18.32
  diffuse — see Tuberculosis, miliary
  digestive tract A18.32
  disseminated — see Tuberculosis, miliary

Tuberculosis — continued
  duodenum A18.32
  dura (mater) (cerebral) (spinal) A17.0
    abscess (cerebral) (spinal) A17.81
  dysentery A18.32
  ear (inner) (middle) A18.6
    bone A18.03
    external (primary) A18.4
    skin (primary) A18.4
  elbow A18.02
  emphysema — see Tuberculosis, pulmonary
  empyema A15.6
  encephalitis A17.82
  endarteritis A18.89
  endocarditis A18.84
    aortic A18.84
    mitral A18.84
    pulmonary A18.84
    tricuspid A18.84
  endocrine glands NEC A18.82
  endometrium A18.17
  enteric, enterica, enteritis A18.32
  enterocolitis A18.32
  epididymis, epididymitis A18.15
  epidural abscess (cerebral) (spinal) A17.81
  epiglottis A15.5
  episcleritis A18.51
  erythema (induratum) (nodosum) (primary) A18.4
  esophagus A18.83
  eustachian tube A18.6
  exposure (to) Z20.1
  exudative — see Tuberculosis, pulmonary
  eye A18.50
  eyelid (primary) (lupus) A18.4
  fallopian tube (acute) (chronic) A18.17
  fascia A18.09
  fauces A15.8
  female pelvic inflammatory disease A18.17
  finger A18.03
  first infection A15.7
  gallbladder A18.83
  ganglion A18.09
  gastritis A18.83
  gastrocolic fistula A18.32
  gastroenteritis A18.32
  gastrointestinal tract A18.32
  general, generalized — see Tuberculosis, miliary
  genital organs A18.10
  genitourinary A18.10
  genu A18.02
  glandula suprarenalis A18.7
  glandular, general A18.2
  glottis A15.5
  grinder's J65
  gum A18.83
  hand A18.03
  heart A18.84
  hematogenous — see Tuberculosis, miliary
  hemoptysis — see Tuberculosis, pulmonary
  hemorrhage NEC — see Tuberculosis, pulmonary
  hemothorax A15.6
  hepatitis A18.83
  hilar lymph nodes A15.4
    primary (progressive) A15.7
  hip (joint) (disease) (bone) A18.02
  hydropneumothorax A15.6
  hydrothorax A15.6
  hypoadrenalism A18.7
  hypopharynx A15.8
  ileocecal (hyperplastic) A18.32
  ileocolitis A18.32
  ileum A18.32
  iliac spine (superior) A18.03
  immunological findings only A15.7
  indurativa (primary) A18.4
  infantile A15.7
  infection A15.9
    without clinical manifestations A15.7
  infraclavicular gland A18.2
  inguinal gland A18.2
  inguinalis A18.2
  intestine (any part) A18.32
  iridocyclitis A18.54
  iris, iritis A18.54
  ischiorectal A18.32
  jaw A18.03
  jejunum A18.32
  joint A18.02
    vertebral A18.01
  keratitis (interstitial) A18.52
  keratoconjunctivitis A18.52

☑ **Additional character required**

Tuberculosis — *continued*
kidney A18.11
knee (joint) A18.02
kyphosis, kyphoscoliosis A18.01
laryngitis A15.5
larynx A15.5
latent R76.11
leptomeninges, leptomeningitis (cerebral) (spinal) A17.0
lichenoides (primary) A18.4
linguae A18.83
lip A18.83
liver A18.83
lordosis A18.01
lung — *see* Tuberculosis, pulmonary
lupus vulgaris A18.4
lymph gland or node (peripheral) A18.2
abdomen A18.39
bronchial A15.4
primary (progressive) A15.7
cervical A18.2
hilar A15.4
primary (progressive) A15.7
intrathoracic A15.4
primary (progressive) A15.7
mediastinal A15.4
primary (progressive) A15.7
mesenteric A18.39
retroperitoneal A18.39
tracheobronchial A15.4
primary (progressive) A15.7
lymphadenitis — *see* Tuberculosis, lymph gland
lymphangitis — *see* Tuberculosis, lymph gland
lymphatic (gland) (vessel) — *see* Tuberculosis, lymph gland
mammary gland A18.89
marasmus A15.9
mastoiditis A18.03
mediastinal lymph gland or node A15.4
primary (progressive) A15.7
mediastinitis A15.8
primary (progressive) A15.7
mediastinum A15.8
primary (progressive) A15.7
medulla A17.81
melanosis, Addisonian A18.7
meninges, meningitis (basilar) (cerebral) (cerebrospinal) (spinal) A17.0
meningoencephalitis A17.82
mesentery, mesenteric (gland or node) A18.39
miliary A19.9
acute A19.2
multiple sites A19.1
single specified site A19.0
chronic A19.8
specified NEC A19.8
millstone makers' J65
miner's J65
molder's J65
mouth A18.83
multiple A19.9
acute A19.1
chronic A19.8
muscle A18.09
myelitis A17.82
myocardium, myocarditis A18.84
nasal (passage) (sinus) A15.8
nasopharynx A15.5
neck gland A18.2
nephritis A18.11
nerve (mononeuropathy) A17.83
nervous system A17.9
nose (septum) A15.8
ocular A18.50
omentum A18.31
oophoritis (acute) (chronic) A18.17
optic (nerve trunk) (papilla) A18.59
orbit A18.59
orchitis A18.15
organ, specified NEC A18.89
osseous — *see* Tuberculosis, bone
osteitis — *see* Tuberculosis, bone
osteomyelitis — *see* Tuberculosis, bone
otitis media A18.6
ovary, ovaritis (acute) (chronic) A18.17
oviduct (acute) (chronic) A18.17
pachymeningitis A17.0
palate (soft) A18.83
pancreas A18.83
papulonecrotic (a) (primary) A18.4
parathyroid glands A18.82
paronychia (primary) A18.4

Tuberculosis — *continued*
parotid gland or region A18.83
pelvis (bony) A18.03
penis A18.15
peribronchitis A15.5
pericardium, pericarditis A18.84
perichondritis, larynx A15.5
periostitis — *see* Tuberculosis, bone
perirectal fistula A18.32
peritoneum NEC A18.31
peritonitis A18.31
pharynx, pharyngitis A15.8
phlyctenulosis (keratoconjunctivitis) A18.52
phthisis NEC — *see* Tuberculosis, pulmonary
pituitary gland A18.82
pleura, pleural, pleurisy, pleuritis (fibrinous) (obliterative) (purulent) (simple plastic) (with effusion) A15.6
primary (progressive) A15.7
pneumonia, pneumonic — *see* Tuberculosis, pulmonary
pneumothorax (spontaneous) (tense valvular) — *see* Tuberculosis, pulmonary
polyneuropathy A17.89
polyserositis A19.9
acute A19.1
chronic A19.8
potter's J65
prepuce A18.15
primary (complex) A15.7
proctitis A18.32
prostate, prostatitis A18.14
pulmonalis — *see* Tuberculosis, pulmonary
pulmonary (cavitated) (fibrotic) (infiltrative) (nodular) A15.0
childhood type or first infection A15.7
primary (complex) A15.7
pyelitis A18.11
pyelonephritis A18.11
pyemia — *see* Tuberculosis, miliary
pyonephrosis A18.11
pyopneumothorax A15.6
pyothorax A15.6
rectum (fistula) (with abscess) A18.32
reinfection stage — *see* Tuberculosis, pulmonary
renal A18.11
renis A18.11
respiratory A15.9
primary A15.7
specified site NEC A15.8
retina, retinitis A18.53
retroperitoneal (lymph gland or node) A18.39
rheumatism NEC A18.09
rhinitis A15.8
sacroiliac (joint) A18.01
sacrum A18.01
salivary gland A18.83
salpingitis (acute) (chronic) A18.17
sandblaster's J65
sclera A18.51
scoliosis A18.01
scrofulous A18.2
scrotum A18.15
seminal tract or vesicle A18.15
senile A15.9
septic — *see* Tuberculosis, miliary
shoulder (joint) A18.02
blade A18.03
sigmoid A18.32
sinus (any nasal) A15.8
bone A18.03
epididymis A18.15
skeletal NEC A18.03
skin (any site) (primary) A18.4
small intestine A18.32
soft palate A18.83
spermatic cord A18.15
spine, spinal (column) A18.01
cord A17.81
medulla A17.81
membrane A17.0
meninges A17.0
spleen, splenitis A18.85
spondylitis A18.01
sternoclavicular joint A18.02
stomach A18.83
stonemason's J65
subcutaneous tissue (cellular) (primary) A18.4
subcutis (primary) A18.4
subdeltoid bursa A18.83
submaxillary (region) A18.83
supraclavicular gland A18.2

Tuberculosis — *continued*
suprarenal (capsule) (gland) A18.7
swelling, joint (see also category M01) (see also Tuberculosis, joint) A18.02
symphysis pubis A18.02
synovitis A18.09
articular A18.02
spine or vertebra A18.01
systemic — *see* Tuberculosis, miliary
tarsitis A18.4
tendon (sheath) — *see* Tuberculosis, tenosynovitis
tenosynovitis A18.09
spine or vertebra A18.01
testis A18.15
throat A15.8
thymus gland A18.82
thyroid gland A18.81
tongue A18.83
tonsil, tonsillitis A15.8
trachea, tracheal A15.5
lymph gland or node A15.4
primary (progressive) A15.7
tracheobronchial A15.5
lymph gland or node A15.4
primary (progressive) A15.7
tubal (acute) (chronic) A18.17
tunica vaginalis A18.15
ulcer (skin) (primary) A18.4
bowel or intestine A18.32
specified NEC - code under Tuberculosis, by site
unspecified site A15.9
ureter A18.11
urethra, urethral (gland) A18.13
urinary organ or tract A18.13
uterus A18.17
uveal tract A18.54
uvula A18.83
vagina A18.18
vas deferens A18.15
verruca, verrucosa (cutis) (primary) A18.4
vertebra (column) A18.01
vesiculitis A18.15
vulva A18.18
wrist (joint) A18.02
Tuberculum
Carabelli — *see* Note at K00.2
occlusal — *see* Note at K00.2
paramolare K00.2
Tuberosity, enitre maxillary M26.07
Tuberous sclerosis (brain) Q85.1
Tubo-ovarian — *see* condition
Tuboplasty, after previous sterilization Z31.0
aftercare Z31.42
Tubotympanitis, catarrhal (chronic) — *see* Otitis, media, nonsuppurative, chronic, serous
Tularemia A21.9
with
conjunctivitis A21.1
pneumonia A21.2
abdominal A21.3
bronchopneumonic A21.2
conjunctivitis A21.1
cryptogenic A21.3
enteric A21.3
gastrointestinal A21.3
generalized A21.7
ingestion A21.3
intestinal A21.3
oculoglandular A21.1
ophthalmic A21.1
pneumonia (any), pneumonic A21.2
pulmonary A21.2
sepsis A21.7
specified NEC A21.8
typhoidal A21.7
ulceroglandular A21.0
Tularensis conjunctivitis A21.1
Tumefaction (see also Swelling)
liver — *see* Hypertrophy, liver
Tumor (see also Neoplasm, unspecified behavior, by site)
acinar cell — *see* Neoplasm, uncertain behavior, by site
acinic cell — *see* Neoplasm, uncertain behavior, by site
adenocarcinoid — *see* Neoplasm, malignant, by site
adenomatoid (see also Neoplasm, benign, by site)
odontogenic — *see* Cyst, calcifying odontogenic

Tumor

Tumor — *continued*
adnexal (skin) — *see* Neoplasm, skin, benign,
   by site
adrenal
   cortical (benign) D35.0- ☑
      malignant C74.0- ☑
   rest — *see* Neoplasm, benign, by site
alpha-cell
   malignant
      pancreas C25.4
      specified site NEC — *see* Neoplasm,
        malignant, by site
      unspecified site C25.4
   pancreas D13.7
   specified site NEC — *see* Neoplasm, benign,
      by site
   unspecified site D13.7
aneurysmal — *see* Aneurysm
aortic body D44.7
   malignant C75.5
Askin's — *see* Neoplasm, connective tissue,
   malignant
basal cell (*see also* Neoplasm, skin, uncertain
   behavior) D48.5
Bednar — *see* Neoplasm, skin, malignant
benign (unclassified) — *see* Neoplasm, benign,
   by site
beta-cell
   malignant
      pancreas C25.4
      specified site NEC — *see* Neoplasm,
        malignant, by site
      unspecified site C25.4
   pancreas D13.7
   specified site NEC — *see* Neoplasm, benign,
      by site
   unspecified site D13.7
Brenner D27.9
   borderline malignancy D39.1- ☑
   malignant C56- ☑
   proliferating D39.1- ☑
bronchial alveolar, intravascular D38.1
Brooke's — *see* Neoplasm, skin, benign
brown fat — *see* Lipoma
Burkitt — *see* Lymphoma, Burkitt
calcifying epithelial odontogenic — *see* Cyst,
   calcifying odontogenic
carcinoid
   benign D3A.00
      appendix D3A.020
      ascending colon D3A.022
      bronchus (lung) D3A.090
      cecum D3A.021
      colon D3A.029
      descending colon D3A.024
      duodenum D3A.010
      foregut NOS D3A.094
      hindgut NOS D3A.096
      ileum D3A.012
      jejunum D3A.011
      kidney D3A.093
      large intestine D3A.029
      lung (bronchus) D3A.090
      midgut NOS D3A.095
      rectum D3A.026
      sigmoid colon D3A.025
      small intestine D3A.019
      specified NEC D3A.098
      stomach D3A.092
      thymus D3A.091
      transverse colon D3A.023
   malignant C7A.00
      appendix C7A.020
      ascending colon C7A.022
      bronchus (lung) C7A.090
      cecum C7A.021
      colon C7A.029
      descending colon C7A.024
      duodenum C7A.010
      foregut NOS C7A.094
      hindgut NOS C7A.096
      ileum C7A.012
      jejunum C7A.011
      kidney C7A.093
      large intestine C7A.029
      lung (bronchus) C7A.090
      midgut NOS C7A.095
      rectum C7A.026
      sigmoid colon C7A.025
      small intestine C7A.019
      specified NEC C7A.098
      stomach C7A.092

Tumor — *continued*
      thymus C7A.091
      transverse colon C7A.023
   mesentary metastasis C7B.04
   secondary C7B.00
      bone C7B.03
      distant lymph nodes C7B.01
      liver C7B.02
      peritoneum C7B.04
      specified NEC C7B.09
carotid body D44.6
   malignant C75.4
cells (*see also* Neoplasm, unspecified behavior,
   by site)
   benign — *see* Neoplasm, benign, by site
   malignant — *see* Neoplasm, malignant, by site
   uncertain whether benign or malignant — *see*
      Neoplasm, uncertain behavior, by site
cervix, in pregnancy or childbirth — *see*
   Pregnancy, complicated by, tumor, cervix
chondromatous giant cell — *see* Neoplasm, bone,
   benign
chromaffin (*see also* Neoplasm, benign, by site)
   malignant — *see* Neoplasm, malignant, by site
Cock's peculiar L72.3
Codman's — *see* Neoplasm, bone, benign
dentigerous, mixed — *see* Cyst, calcifying
   odontogenic
dermoid — *see* Neoplasm, benign, by site
   with malignant transformation C56- ☑
desmoid (extra-abdominal) (*see also* Neoplasm,
   connective tissue, uncertain behavior)
   abdominal — *see* Neoplasm, connective tissue,
      uncertain behavior
embolus — *see* Neoplasm, secondary, by site
embryonal (mixed) (*see also* Neoplasm, uncertain
   behavior, by site)
   liver C22.7
endodermal sinus
   specified site — *see* Neoplasm, malignant, by
      site
   unspecified site
      female C56.- ☑
      male C62.90
epithelial
   benign — *see* Neoplasm, benign, by site
   malignant — *see* Neoplasm, malignant, by site
Ewing's — *see* Neoplasm, bone, malignant, by site
fatty — *see* Lipoma
fibroid — *see* Leiomyoma
G cell
   malignant
      pancreas C25.4
      specified site NEC — *see* Neoplasm,
        malignant, by site
      unspecified site C25.4
   specified site — *see* Neoplasm, uncertain
      behavior, by site
   unspecified site D37.8
germ cell (*see also* Neoplasm, malignant, by site)
   mixed — *see* Neoplasm, malignant, by site
ghost cell, odontogenic — *see* Cyst, calcifying
   odontogenic
giant cell (*see also* Neoplasm, uncertain behavior,
   by site)
   bone D48.0
      malignant — *see* Neoplasm, bone, malignant
   chondromatous — *see* Neoplasm, bone, benign
   malignant — *see* Neoplasm, malignant, by site
   soft parts — *see* Neoplasm, connective tissue,
      uncertain behavior
      malignant — *see* Neoplasm, connective
        tissue, malignant
glomus D18.00
   intra-abdominal D18.03
   intracranial D18.02
   jugulare D44.7
      malignant C75.5
   skin D18.01
   specified site NEC D18.09
gonadal stromal — *see* Neoplasm, uncertain
   behavior, by site
granular cell (*see also* Neoplasm, connective
   tissue, benign)
   malignant — *see* Neoplasm, connective tissue,
      malignant
granulosa cell D39.1- ☑
   juvenile D39.1- ☑
   malignant C56- ☑
granulosa cell-theca cell D39.1- ☑
   malignant C56- ☑
Grawitz's C64- ☑

Tumor — *continued*
hemorrhoidal — *see* Hemorrhoids
hilar cell D27- ☑
hilus cell D27- ☑
Hurthle cell (benign) D34
   malignant C73
hydatid — *see* Echinococcus
hypernephroid (*see also* Neoplasm, uncertain
   behavior, by site)
interstitial cell (*see also* Neoplasm, uncertain
   behavior, by site)
   benign — *see* Neoplasm, benign, by site
   malignant — *see* Neoplasm, malignant, by site
intravascular bronchial alveolar D38.1
islet cell — *see* Neoplasm, benign, by site
   malignant — *see* Neoplasm, malignant, by site
      pancreas C25.4
      specified site NEC — *see* Neoplasm,
        malignant, by site
      unspecified site C25.4
   pancreas D13.7
   specified site NEC — *see* Neoplasm, benign,
      by site
   unspecified site D13.7
juxtaglomerular D41.0- ☑
Klatskin's C24.0
Krukenberg's C79.6- ☑
Leydig cell — *see* Neoplasm, uncertain behavior,
   by site
   benign — *see* Neoplasm, benign, by site
      specified site — *see* Neoplasm, benign, by
        site
      unspecified site
        female D27.9
        male D29.20
   malignant — *see* Neoplasm, malignant, by site
      specified site — *see* Neoplasm, malignant,
        by site
      unspecified site
        female C56.9
        male C62.90
   specified site — *see* Neoplasm, uncertain
      behavior, by site
   unspecified site
      female D39.10
      male D40.10
lipid cell, ovary D27- ☑
lipoid cell, ovary D27- ☑
malignant (*see also* Neoplasm, malignant, by
   site) C80.1
   fusiform cell (type) C80.1
   giant cell (type) C80.1
   localized, plasma cell — *see* Plasmacytoma,
      solitary
   mixed NEC C80.1
   small cell (type) C80.1
   spindle cell (type) C80.1
   unclassified C80.1
mast cell D47.0
   malignant C96.2
melanotic, neuroectodermal — *see* Neoplasm,
   benign, by site
Merkel cell — *see* Carcinoma, Merkel cell
mesenchymal
   malignant — *see* Neoplasm, connective tissue,
      malignant
   mixed — *see* Neoplasm, connective tissue,
      uncertain behavior
mesodermal, mixed (*see also* Neoplasm,
   malignant, by site)
   liver C22.4
mesonephric (*see also* Neoplasm, uncertain
   behavior, by site)
   malignant — *see* Neoplasm, malignant, by site
metastatic
   from specified site — *see* Neoplasm, malignant,
      by site
   of specified site — *see* Neoplasm, malignant,
      by site
   to specified site — *see* Neoplasm, secondary,
      by site
mixed NEC (*see also* Neoplasm, benign, by site)
   malignant — *see* Neoplasm, malignant, by site
mucinous of low malignant potential
   specified site — *see* Neoplasm, malignant, by
      site
   unspecified site C56.9
mucocarcinoid
   specified site — *see* Neoplasm, malignant, by
      site
   unspecified site C18.1

☑ **Additional character required**

Tumor — *continued*
  mucoepidermoid — *see* Neoplasm, uncertain behavior, by site
  Müllerian, mixed
    specified site — *see* Neoplasm, malignant, by site
    unspecified site C54.9
  myoepithelial — *see* Neoplasm, benign, by site
  neuroectodermal (peripheral) — *see* Neoplasm, malignant, by site
    primitive
      specified site — *see* Neoplasm, malignant, by site
      unspecified site C71.9
  neuroendocrine D3A.8
    malignant poorly differentiated C7A.1
    secondary NEC C7B.8
    specified NEC C7A.8
  neurogenic olfactory C30.0
  nonencapsulated sclerosing C73
  odontogenic (adenomatoid) (benign) (calcifying epithelial) (keratocystic) (squamous) — *see* Cyst, calcifying odontogenic
    malignant C41.1
      upper jaw (bone) C41.0
  ovarian stromal D39.1- ☑
  ovary, in pregnancy — *see* Pregnancy, complicated by
  pacinian — *see* Neoplasm, skin, benign
  Pancoast's — *see* Pancoast's syndrome
  papillary (*see also* Papilloma)
    cystic D37.9
      mucinous of low malignant potential C56- ☑
        specified site — *see* Neoplasm, malignant, by site
        unspecified site C56.9
      serous of low malignant potential
        specified site — *see* Neoplasm, malignant, by site
        unspecified site C56.9
  pelvic, in pregnancy or childbirth — *see* Pregnancy, complicated by
  phantom F45.8
  phyllodes D48.6- ☑
    benign D24- ☑
    malignant — *see* Neoplasm, breast, malignant
  Pindborg — *see* Cyst, calcifying odontogenic
  placental site trophoblastic D39.2
  plasma cell (malignant) (localized) — *see* Plasmacytoma, solitary
  polyvesicular vitelline
    specified site — *see* Neoplasm, malignant, by site
    unspecified site
      female C56.9
      male C62.90
  Pott's puffy — *see* Osteomyelitis, specified NEC
  Rathke's pouch D44.3
  retinal anlage — *see* Neoplasm, benign, by site
  salivary gland type, mixed — *see* Neoplasm, salivary gland, benign
    malignant — *see* Neoplasm, salivary gland, malignant
  Sampson's N80.1
  Schmincke's — *see* Neoplasm, nasopharynx, malignant
  sclerosing stromal D27- ☑
  sebaceous — *see* Cyst, sebaceous
  secondary — *see* Neoplasm, secondary, by site
    carcinoid C7B.00
      bone C7B.03
      distant lymph nodes C7B.01
      liver C7B.02
      peritoneum C7B.04
      specified NEC C7B.09
    neuroendocrine NEC C7B.8
  serous of low malignant potential
    specified site — *see* Neoplasm, malignant, by site
    unspecified site C56.9
  Sertoli cell — *see* Neoplasm, benign, by site
    with lipid storage
      specified site — *see* Neoplasm, benign, by site
      unspecified site
        female D27.9
        male D29.20
    specified site — *see* Neoplasm, benign, by site
    unspecified site
      female D27.9
      male D29.20

Tumor — *continued*
  Sertoli-Leydig cell — *see* Neoplasm, benign, by site
    specified site — *see* Neoplasm, benign, by site
    unspecified site
      female D27.9
      male D29.20
  sex cord (-stromal) — *see* Neoplasm, uncertain behavior, by site
    with annular tubules D39.1- ☑
  skin appendage — *see* Neoplasm, skin, benign
  smooth muscle — *see* Neoplasm, connective tissue, uncertain behavior
  soft tissue
    benign — *see* Neoplasm, connective tissue, benign
    malignant — *see* Neoplasm, connective tissue, malignant
  sternomastoid (congenital) Q68.0
  stromal
    endometrial D39.0
    gastric D48.1
      benign D21.4
      malignant C16.9
      uncertain behavior D48.1
    gastrointestinal
      benign D21.4
      malignant C49.4
      uncertain behavior D48.1
    intestine
      benign D21.4
      malignant C49.4
      uncertain behavior D48.1
    ovarian D39.1- ☑
    stomach
      benign D21.4
      malignant C16.9
      uncertain behavior D48.1
  testicular D40.10
  sweat gland (*see also* Neoplasm, skin, uncertain behavior)
    benign — *see* Neoplasm, skin, benign
    malignant — *see* Neoplasm, skin, malignant
  syphilitic, brain A52.17
  testicular stromal D40.1- ☑
  theca cell D27.- ☑
  theca cell-granulosa cell D39.1- ☑
  Triton, malignant — *see* Neoplasm, nerve, malignant
  trophoblastic, placental site D39.2
  turban D23.4
  uterus (body), in pregnancy or childbirth — *see* Pregnancy, complicated by, tumor, uterus
  vagina, in pregnancy or childbirth — *see* Pregnancy, complicated by
  varicose — *see* Varix
  von Recklinghausen's — *see* Neurofibromatosis
  vulva or perineum, in pregnancy or childbirth — *see* Pregnancy, complicated by
    causing obstructed labor O65.5
  Warthin's — *see* Neoplasm, salivary gland, benign
  Wilms' C64- ☑
  yolk sac — *see* Neoplasm, malignant, by site
    specified site — *see* Neoplasm, malignant, by site
    unspecified site
      female C56.9
      male C62.90
Tumor lysis syndrome (following antineoplastic chemotherapy) (spontaneous) NEC E88.3
Tumorlet — *see* Neoplasm, uncertain behavior, by site
Tungiasis B88.1
Tunica vasculosa lentis Q12.2
Turban tumor D23.4
Türck's trachoma J37.0
Turner-Kieser syndrome Q79.8
Turner-like syndrome Q87.1
Turner's
  hypoplasia (tooth) K00.4
  syndrome Q96.9
    specified NEC Q96.8
  tooth K00.4
Turner-Ullrich syndrome Q96.9
Tussis convulsiva — *see* Whooping cough
Twiddler's syndrome (due to)
  automatic implantable defibrillator T82.198 ☑
  cardiac pacemaker T82.198 ☑
Twilight state
  epileptic F05
  psychogenic F44.89

Twin (newborn) (*see also* Newborn, twin)
  conjoined Q89.4
  pregnancy — *see* Pregnancy, twin, conjoined
Twinning, teeth K00.2
Twist, twisted
  bowel, colon or intestine K56.2
  hair (congenital) Q84.1
  mesentery K56.2
  omentum K56.2
  organ or site, congenital NEC — *see* Anomaly, by site
  ovarian pedicle — *see* Torsion, ovary
Twitching R25.3
Tylosis (acquired) L84
  buccalis K13.29
  linguae K13.29
  palmaris et plantaris (congenital) (inherited) Q82.8
    acquired L85.1
Tympanism R14.0
Tympanites (abdominal) (intestinal) R14.0
Tympanitis — *see* Myringitis
Tympanosclerosis H74.0
Tympanum — *see* condition
Tympany
  abdomen R14.0
  chest R09.89
Type A behavior pattern Z73.1
Typhlitis — *see* Appendicitis
Typhoenteritis — *see* Typhoid
Typhoid (abortive) (ambulant) (any site) (clinical) (fever) (hemorrhagic) (infection) (intermittent) (malignant) (rheumatic) (Widal negative) A01.00
  with pneumonia A01.03
  abdominal A01.09
  arthritis A01.04
  carrier (suspected) of Z22.0
  cholecystitis (current) A01.09
  endocarditis A01.02
  heart involvement A01.02
  inoculation reaction — *see* Complications, vaccination
  meningitis A01.01
  mesenteric lymph nodes A01.09
  myocarditis A01.02
  osteomyelitis A01.05
  perichondritis, larynx A01.09
  pneumonia A01.03
  spine A01.05
  specified NEC A01.09
  ulcer (perforating) A01.09
Typhomalaria (fever) — *see* Malaria
Typhomania A01.00
Typhoperitonitis A01.09
Typhus (fever) A75.9
  abdominal, abdominalis — *see* Typhoid
  African tick A77.1
  amarillic A95.9
  brain A75.9 [G94]
  cerebral A75.9 [G94]
  classical A75.0
  due to Rickettsia
    prowazekii A75.0
      recrudescent A75.1
    tsutsugamushi A75.3
    typhi A75.2
  endemic (flea-borne) A75.2
  epidemic (louse-borne) A75.0
  exanthematic NEC A75.0
  exanthematicus SAI A75.0
    brillii SAI A75.1
    mexicanus SAI A75.2
    typhus murinus A75.2
  flea-borne A75.2
  India tick A77.1
  Kenya (tick) A77.1
  louse-borne A75.0
  Mexican A75.2
  mite-borne A75.3
  murine A75.2
  North Asian tick-borne A77.2
  petechial A75.9
  Queensland tick A77.3
  rat A75.2
  recrudescent A75.1
  recurrens — *see* Fever, relapsing
  Sao Paulo A77.0
  scrub (China) (India) (Malaysia) (New Guinea) A75.3
  shop (of Malaysia) A75.2
  Siberian tick A77.2
  tick-borne A77.9

Typhus — *continued*
tropical (mite-borne) A75.3
Tyrosinemia E70.21
newborn, transitory P74.5
Tyrosinosis E70.21
Tyrosinuria E70.29

U

Uhl's anomaly or disease Q24.8
Ulcer, ulcerated, ulcerating, ulceration, ulcerative
alveolar process M27.3
amebic (intestine) A06.1
skin A06.7
anastomotic — *see* Ulcer, gastrojejunal
anorectal K62.6
antral — *see* Ulcer, stomach
anus (sphincter) (solitary) K62.6
aorta — *see* Aneurysm
aphthous (oral) (recurrent) K12.0
genital organ (s)
female N76.6
male N50.8
artery I77.2
atrophic — *see* Ulcer, skin
decubitus — *see* Ulcer, pressure, by site
back L98.429
with
bone necrosis L98.424
exposed fat layer L98.422
muscle necrosis L98.423
skin breakdown only L98.421
Barrett's (esophagus) K22.10
with bleeding K22.11
bile duct (common) (hepatic) K83.8
bladder (solitary) (sphincter) NEC N32.89
bilharzial B65.9 [N33]
in schistosomiasis (bilharzial) B65.9 [N33]
submucosal — *see* Cystitis, interstitial
tuberculous A18.12
bleeding K27.4
bone — *see* Osteomyelitis, specified type NEC
bowel — *see* Ulcer, intestine
breast N61
bronchus J98.09
buccal (cavity) (traumatic) K12.1
Buruli A31.1
buttock L98.419
with
bone necrosis L98.414
exposed fat layer L98.412
muscle necrosis L98.413
skin breakdown only L98.411
cancerous — *see* Neoplasm, malignant, by site
cardia K22.10
with bleeding K22.11
cardioesophageal (peptic) K22.10
with bleeding K22.11
cecum — *see* Ulcer, intestine
cervix (uteri) (decubitus) (trophic) N86
with cervicitis N72
chancroidal A57
chiclero B55.1
chronic (cause unknown) — *see* Ulcer, skin
Cochin-China B55.1
colon — *see* Ulcer, intestine
conjunctiva H10.89
cornea H16.00- ☑
with hypopyon H16.03- ☑
central H16.01- ☑
dendritic (herpes simplex) B00.52
marginal H16.04- ☑
Mooren's H16.05- ☑
mycotic H16.06- ☑
perforated H16.07- ☑
ring H16.02- ☑
tuberculous (phlyctenular) A18.52
corpus cavernosum (chronic) N48.5
crural — *see* Ulcer, lower limb
Curling's — *see* Ulcer, peptic, acute
Cushing's — *see* Ulcer, peptic, acute
cystic duct K82.8
cystitis (interstitial) — *see* Cystitis, interstitial
decubitus — *see* Ulcer, pressure, by site
dendritic, cornea (herpes simplex) B00.52
diabetes, diabetic — *see* Diabetes, ulcer
Dieulafoy's K25.0
due to
infection NEC — *see* Ulcer, skin

Ulcer — *continued*
radiation NEC L59.8
trophic disturbance (any region) — *see* Ulcer, skin
X-ray L58.1
duodenum, duodenal (eroded) (peptic) K26.9
with
hemorrhage K26.4
and perforation K26.6
perforation K26.5
acute K26.3
with
hemorrhage K26.0
and perforation K26.2
perforation K26.1
chronic K26.7
with
hemorrhage K26.4
and perforation K26.6
perforation K26.5
dysenteric A09
elusive — *see* Cystitis, interstitial
endocarditis (acute) (chronic) (subacute) I28.8
epiglottis J38.7
esophagus (peptic) K22.10
with bleeding K22.11
due to
aspirin K22.10
with bleeding K22.11
gastrointestinal reflux disease K21.0
ingestion of chemical or medicament K22.10
with bleeding K22.11
fungal K22.10
with bleeding K22.11
infective K22.10
with bleeding K22.11
varicose — *see* Varix, esophagus
eyelid (region) H01.8
fauces J39.2
Fenwick (-Hunner) (solitary) — *see* Cystitis, interstitial
fistulous — *see* Ulcer, skin
foot (indolent) (trophic) — *see* Ulcer, lower limb
frambesial, initial A66.0
frenum (tongue) K14.0
gallbladder or duct K82.8
gangrenous — *see* Gangrene
gastric — *see* Ulcer, stomach
gastrocolic — *see* Ulcer, gastrojejunal
gastroduodenal — *see* Ulcer, peptic
gastroesophageal — *see* Ulcer, stomach
gastrointestinal — *see* Ulcer, gastrojejunal
gastrojejunal (peptic) K28.9
with
hemorrhage K28.4
and perforation K28.6
perforation K28.5
acute K28.3
with
hemorrhage K28.0
and perforation K28.2
perforation K28.1
chronic K28.7
with
hemorrhage K28.4
and perforation K28.6
perforation K28.5
gastrojejunocolic — *see* Ulcer, gastrojejunal
gingiva K06.8
gingivitis K05.10
nonplaque induced K05.11
plaque induced K05.10
glottis J38.7
granuloma of pudenda A58
gum K06.8
gumma, due to yaws A66.4
heel — *see* Ulcer, lower limb
hemorrhoid (*see also* Hemorrhoids, by degree) K64.8
Hunner's — *see* Cystitis, interstitial
hypopharynx J39.2
hypopyon (chronic) (subacute) — *see* Ulcer, cornea, with hypopyon
hypostaticum — *see* Ulcer, varicose
ileum — *see* Ulcer, intestine
intestine, intestinal K63.3
with perforation K63.1
amebic A06.1
duodenal — *see* Ulcer, duodenum
granulocytopenic (with hemorrhage) — *see* Neutropenia
marginal — *see* Ulcer, gastrojejunal

Ulcer — *continued*
perforating K63.1
newborn P78.0
primary, small intestine K63.3
rectum K62.6
stercoraceous, stercoral K63.3
tuberculous A18.32
typhoid (fever) — *see* Typhoid
varicose I86.8
jejunum, jejunal — *see* Ulcer, gastrojejunal
keratitis — *see* Ulcer, cornea
knee — *see* Ulcer, lower limb
labium (majus) (minus) N76.6
laryngitis — *see* Laryngitis
larynx (aphthous) (contact) J38.7
diphtheritic A36.2
leg — *see* Ulcer, lower limb
lip K13.0
Lipschütz's N76.6
lower limb (atrophic) (chronic) (neurogenic) (perforating) (pyogenic) (trophic) (tropical) L97.909
with
bone necrosis L97.904
exposed fat layer L97.902
muscle necrosis L97.903
skin breakdown only L97.901
ankle L97.309
with
bone necrosis L97.304
exposed fat layer L97.302
muscle necrosis L97.303
skin breakdown only L97.301
left L97.329
with
bone necrosis L97.324
exposed fat layer L97.322
muscle necrosis L97.323
skin breakdown only L97.321
right L97.319
with
bone necrosis L97.314
exposed fat layer L97.312
muscle necrosis L97.313
skin breakdown only L97.311
calf L97.209
with
bone necrosis L97.204
exposed fat layer L97.202
muscle necrosis L97.203
skin breakdown only L97.201
left L97.229
with
bone necrosis L97.224
exposed fat layer L97.222
muscle necrosis L97.223
skin breakdown only L97.221
right L97.219
with
bone necrosis L97.214
exposed fat layer L97.212
muscle necrosis L97.213
skin breakdown only L97.211
decubitus — *see* Ulcer, pressure, by site
foot specified NEC L97.509
with
bone necrosis L97.504
exposed fat layer L97.502
muscle necrosis L97.503
skin breakdown only L97.501
left L97.529
with
bone necrosis L97.524
exposed fat layer L97.522
muscle necrosis L97.523
skin breakdown only L97.521
right L97.519
with
bone necrosis L97.514
exposed fat layer L97.512
muscle necrosis L97.513
skin breakdown only L97.511
heel L97.409
with
bone necrosis L97.404
exposed fat layer L97.402
muscle necrosis L97.403
skin breakdown only L97.401
left L97.429
with
bone necrosis L97.424
exposed fat layer L97.422

☑ **Additional character required**

Ulcer — *continued*
    muscle necrosis L97.423
    skin breakdown only L97.421
  right L97.419
    with
      bone necrosis L97.414
      exposed fat layer L97.412
      muscle necrosis L97.413
      skin breakdown only L97.411
  left L97.929
    with
      bone necrosis L97.924
      exposed fat layer L97.922
      muscle necrosis L97.923
      skin breakdown only L97.921
  lower leg NOS L97.909
    with
      bone necrosis L97.904
      exposed fat layer L97.902
      muscle necrosis L97.903
      skin breakdown only L97.901
    left L97.929
      with
        bone necrosis L97.924
        exposed fat layer L97.922
        muscle necrosis L97.923
        skin breakdown only L97.921
    right L97.919
      with
        bone necrosis L97.914
        exposed fat layer L97.912
        muscle necrosis L97.913
        skin breakdown only L97.911
  specified site NEC L97.809
    with
      bone necrosis L97.804
      exposed fat layer L97.802
      muscle necrosis L97.803
      skin breakdown only L97.801
    left L97.829
      with
        bone necrosis L97.824
        exposed fat layer L97.822
        muscle necrosis L97.823
        skin breakdown only L97.821
    right L97.819
      with
        bone necrosis L97.814
        exposed fat layer L97.812
        muscle necrosis L97.813
        skin breakdown only L97.811
  midfoot L97.409
    with
      bone necrosis L97.404
      exposed fat layer L97.402
      muscle necrosis L97.403
      skin breakdown only L97.401
    left L97.429
      with
        bone necrosis L97.424
        exposed fat layer L97.422
        muscle necrosis L97.423
        skin breakdown only L97.421
    right L97.419
      with
        bone necrosis L97.414
        exposed fat layer L97.412
        muscle necrosis L97.413
        skin breakdown only L97.411
  right L97.919
    with
      bone necrosis L97.914
      exposed fat layer L97.912
      muscle necrosis L97.913
      skin breakdown only L97.911
  thigh L97.109
    with
      bone necrosis L97.104
      exposed fat layer L97.102
      muscle necrosis L97.103
      skin breakdown only L97.101
    left L97.129
      with
        bone necrosis L97.124
        exposed fat layer L97.122
        muscle necrosis L97.123
        skin breakdown only L97.121
    right L97.119
      with
        bone necrosis L97.114
        exposed fat layer L97.112
        muscle necrosis L97.113

Ulcer — *continued*
      skin breakdown only L97.111
  toe L97.509
    with
      bone necrosis L97.504
      exposed fat layer L97.502
      muscle necrosis L97.503
      skin breakdown only L97.501
    left L97.529
      with
        bone necrosis L97.524
        exposed fat layer L97.522
        muscle necrosis L97.523
        skin breakdown only L97.521
    right L97.519
      with
        bone necrosis L97.514
        exposed fat layer L97.512
        muscle necrosis L97.513
        skin breakdown only L97.511
  leprous A30.1
  syphilitic A52.19
  varicose — *see* Varix, leg, with, ulcer
  luetic — *see* Ulcer, syphilitic
  lung J98.4
    tuberculous — *see* Tuberculosis, pulmonary
  malignant — *see* Neoplasm, malignant, by site
  marginal NEC — *see* Ulcer, gastrojejunal
  meatus (urinarius) N34.2
  Meckel's diverticulum Q43.0
    malignant — *see* Table of Neoplasms, small
      intestine, malignant
  Meleney's (chronic undermining) — *see* Ulcer,
    skin
  Mooren's (cornea) — *see* Ulcer, cornea, Mooren's
  mycobacterial (skin) A31.1
  nasopharynx J39.2
  neck, uterus N86
  neurogenic NEC — *see* Ulcer, skin
  nose, nasal (passage) (infective) (septum) J34.0
    skin — *see* Ulcer, skin
    spirochetal A69.8
    varicose (bleeding) I86.8
  oral mucosa (traumatic) K12.1
  palate (soft) K12.1
  penis (chronic) N48.5
  peptic (site unspecified) K27.9
    with
      hemorrhage K27.4
        and perforation K27.6
      perforation K27.5
    acute K27.3
      with
        hemorrhage K27.0
          and perforation K27.2
        perforation K27.1
    chronic K27.7
      with
        hemorrhage K27.4
          and perforation K27.6
        perforation K27.5
    esophagus K22.10
      with bleeding K22.11
    newborn P78.82
    perforating K27.5
  skin — *see* Ulcer, skin
  peritonsillar J35.8
  phagedenic (tropical) — *see* Ulcer, skin
  pharynx J39.2
  phlebitis — *see* Phlebitis
  plaster — *see* Ulcer, pressure, by site
  popliteal space — *see* Ulcer, lower limb
  postpyloric — *see* Ulcer, duodenum
  prepuce N47.7
  prepyloric — *see* Ulcer, stomach
  pressure (pressure area) L89.9- ☑
    ankle L89.5- ☑
    back L89.1- ☑
    buttock L89.3- ☑
    coccyx L89.15- ☑
    contiguous site of back, buttock, hip L89.4- ☑
    elbow L89.0- ☑
    face L89.81- ☑
    head L89.81- ☑
    heel L89.6- ☑
    hip L89.2- ☑
    sacral region (tailbone) L89.15- ☑
    specified site NEC L89.89- ☑
    stage 1 (healing) (pre-ulcer skin changes
      limited to persistent focal edema)
      ankle L89.5- ☑
      back L89.1- ☑

Ulcer — *continued*
    buttock L89.3- ☑
    coccyx L89.15- ☑
    contiguous site of back, buttock, hip
      L89.4- ☑
    elbow L89.0- ☑
    face L89.81- ☑
    head L89.81- ☑
    heel L89.6- ☑
    hip L89.2- ☑
    sacral region (tailbone) L89.15- ☑
    specified site NEC L89.89- ☑
    stage 2 (healing) (abrasion, blister, partial
      thickness skin loss involving epidermis
      and/or dermis)
      ankle L89.5- ☑
      back L89.1- ☑
      buttock L89.3- ☑
      coccyx L89.15- ☑
      contiguous site of back, buttock, hip
        L89.4- ☑
      elbow L89.0- ☑
      face L89.81- ☑
      head L89.81- ☑
      heel L89.6- ☑
      hip L89.2- ☑
      sacral region (tailbone) L89.15- ☑
      specified site NEC L89.89- ☑
    stage 3 (healing) (full thickness skin loss
      involving damage or necrosis of
      subcutaneous tissue)
      ankle L89.5- ☑
      back L89.1- ☑
      buttock L89.3- ☑
      coccyx L89.15- ☑
      contiguous site of back, buttock, hip
        L89.4- ☑
      elbow L89.0- ☑
      face L89.81- ☑
      head L89.81- ☑
      heel L89.6- ☑
      hip L89.2- ☑
      sacral region (tailbone) L89.15- ☑
      specified site NEC L89.89- ☑
    stage 4 (healing) (necrosis of soft tissues
      through to underlying muscle, tendon, or
      bone)
      ankle L89.5- ☑
      back L89.1- ☑
      buttock L89.3- ☑
      coccyx L89.15- ☑
      contiguous site of back, buttock, hip
        L89.4- ☑
      elbow L89.0- ☑
      face L89.81- ☑
      head L89.81- ☑
      heel L89.6- ☑
      hip L89.2- ☑
      sacral region (tailbone) L89.15- ☑
      specified site NEC L89.89- ☑
    unspecified stage
      ankle L89.5- ☑
      back L89.1- ☑
      buttock L89.3- ☑
      coccyx L89.15- ☑
      contiguous site of back, buttock, hip
        L89.4- ☑
      elbow L89.0- ☑
      face L89.81- ☑
      head L89.81- ☑
      heel L89.6- ☑
      hip L89.2- ☑
      sacral region (tailbone) L89.15- ☑
      specified site NEC L89.89- ☑
    unstageable
      ankle L89.5- ☑
      back L89.1- ☑
      buttock L89.3- ☑
      coccyx L89.15- ☑
      contiguous site of back, buttock, hip
        L89.4- ☑
      elbow L89.0- ☑
      face L89.81- ☑
      head L89.81- ☑
      heel L89.6- ☑
      hip L89.2- ☑
      sacral region (tailbone) L89.15- ☑
      specified site NEC L89.89- ☑
  primary of intestine K63.3
    with perforation K63.1
  prostate N41.9
  pyloric — *see* Ulcer, stomach

Ulcer — *continued*
  rectosigmoid K63.3
    with perforation K63.1
  rectum (sphincter) (solitary) K62.6
    stercoraceous, stercoral K62.6
  retina — *see* Inflammation, chorioretinal
  rodent (*see also* Neoplasm, skin, malignant)
  sclera — *see* Scleritis
  scrofulous (tuberculous) A18.2
  scrotum N50.8
    tuberculous A18.15
    varicose I86.1
  seminal vesicle N50.8
  sigmoid — *see* Ulcer, intestine
  skin (atrophic) (chronic) (neurogenic) (non-
    healing) (perforating) (pyogenic) (trophic)
    (tropical) L98.499
    with gangrene — *see* Gangrene
    amebic A06.7
    back — *see* Ulcer, back
    buttock — *see* Ulcer, buttock
    decubitus — *see* Ulcer, pressure
    lower limb — *see* Ulcer, lower limb
    mycobacterial A31.1
    specified site NEC L98.499
      with
        bone necrosis L98.494
        exposed fat layer L98.492
        muscle necrosis L98.493
        skin breakdown only L98.491
    tuberculous (primary) A18.4
    varicose — *see* Ulcer, varicose
  sloughing — *see* Ulcer, skin
  solitary, anus or rectum (sphincter) K62.6
  sore throat J02.9
    streptococcal J02.0
  spermatic cord N50.8
  spine (tuberculous) A18.01
  stasis (venous) — *see* Varix, leg, with, ulcer
    without varicose veins I87.2
  stercoraceous, stercoral K63.3
    with perforation K63.1
    anus or rectum K62.6
  stoma, stomal — *see* Ulcer, gastrojejunal
  stomach (eroded) (peptic) (round) K25.9
    with
      hemorrhage K25.4
        and perforation K25.6
      perforation K25.5
    acute K25.3
      with
        hemorrhage K25.0
          and perforation K25.2
        perforation K25.1
    chronic K25.7
      with
        hemorrhage K25.4
          and perforation K25.6
        perforation K25.5
  stomal — *see* Ulcer, gastrojejunal
  stomatitis K12.1
  stress — *see* Ulcer, peptic
  strumous (tuberculous) A18.2
  submucosal, bladder — *see* Cystitis, interstitial
  syphilitic (any site) (early) (secondary) A51.39
    late A52.79
    perforating A52.79
      foot A52.11
  testis N50.8
  thigh — *see* Ulcer, lower limb
  throat J39.2
    diphtheritic A36.0
  toe — *see* Ulcer, lower limb
  tongue (traumatic) K14.0
  tonsil J35.8
    diphtheritic A36.0
  trachea J39.8
  trophic — *see* Ulcer, skin
  tropical — *see* Ulcer, skin
  tuberculous — *see* Tuberculosis, ulcer
  tunica vaginalis N50.8
  turbinate J34.89
  typhoid (perforating) — *see* Typhoid
  unspecified site — *see* Ulcer, skin
  urethra (meatus) — *see* Urethritis
  uterus N85.8
    cervix N86
      with cervicitis N72
    neck N86
      with cervicitis N72
  vagina N76.5
    in Behçet's disease M35.2 [N77.0]

Ulcer — *continued*
  pessary N89.8
  valve, heart I33.0
  varicose (lower limb, any part) (*see also* Varix, leg,
    with, ulcer)
    broad ligament I86.2
    esophagus — *see* Varix, esophagus
    inflamed or infected — *see* Varix, leg, with ulcer,
      with inflammation
    nasal septum I86.8
    perineum I86.3
    scrotum I86.1
    specified site NEC I86.8
    sublingual I86.0
    vulva I86.3
  vas deferens N50.8
  vulva (acute) (infectional) N76.6
    in (due to)
      Behçet's disease M35.2 [N77.0]
      herpesviral (herpes simplex) infection A60.04
      tuberculosis A18.18
  vulvobuccal, recurring N76.6
  X-ray L58.1
  yaws A66.4
Ulcerosa scarlatina A38.8
Ulcus (*see also* Ulcer)
  cutis tuberculosum A18.4
  duodeni — *see* Ulcer, duodenum
  durum (syphilitic) A51.0
    extragenital A51.2
  gastrojejunale — *see* Ulcer, gastrojejunal
  hypostaticum — *see* Ulcer, varicose
  molle (cutis) (skin) A57
  serpens corneae — *see* Ulcer, cornea, central
  ventriculi — *see* Ulcer, stomach
Ulegyria Q04.8
Ulerythema
  ophryogenes, congenital Q84.2
  sycosiforme L73.8
Ullrich (-Bonnevie)(-Turner) syndrome Q87.1
Ullrich-Feichtiger syndrome Q87.0
Ulnar — *see* condition
Ulorrhagia, ulorrhea K06.8
Umbilicus, umbilical — *see* condition
Unacceptable
  contours of tooth K08.54
  morphology of tooth K08.54
Unavailability (of)
  bed at medical facility Z75.1
  health service-related agencies Z75.4
  medical facilities (at) Z75.3
    due to
      investigation by social service agency Z75.2
      lack of services at home Z75.0
      remoteness from facility Z75.3
      waiting list Z75.1
    home Z75.0
    outpatient clinic Z75.3
  schooling Z55.1
  social service agencies Z75.4
Uncinaria americana infestation B76.1
Uncinariasis B76.9
Uncongenial work Z56.5
Unconscious (ness) — *see* Coma
Under observation — *see* Observation
Underachievement in school Z55.3
Underdevelopment (*see also* Undeveloped)
  nose Q30.1
  sexual E30.0
Underdosing (*see also* Table of Drugs and
  Chemicals, categories T36-T50, with final character
  6) Z91.14
  intentional NEC Z91.128
    due to financial hardship of patient Z91.120
  unintentional NEC Z91.138
    due to patient's age related debility Z91.130
Underfeeding, newborn P92.3
Underfill, endodontic M27.53
Underimmunization status Z28.3
Undernourishment — *see* Malnutrition
Undernutrition — *see* Malnutrition
Underweight R63.6
  for gestational age — *see* Light for dates
Underwood's disease P83.0
Undescended (*see also* Malposition, congenital)
  cecum Q43.3
  colon Q43.3
  testicle — *see* Cryptorchid
Undeveloped, undevelopment (*see also* Hypoplasia)
  brain (congenital) Q02
  cerebral (congenital) Q02
  heart Q24.8

Undeveloped — *continued*
  lung Q33.6
  testis E29.1
  uterus E30.0
Undiagnosed (disease) R69
Undulant fever — *see* Brucellosis
Undulant fever — *see* Brucellosis
Unemployment, anxiety concerning Z56.0
  threatened Z56.2
Unequal length (acquired) (limb) (*see also* Deformity,
  limb, unequal length)
  leg (*see also* Deformity, limb, unequal length)
    congenital Q72.9- ☑
Unextracted dental root K08.3
Unguis incarnatus L60.0
Unhappiness R45.2
Unicornate uterus Q51.4
Unilateral (*see also* condition)
  development, breast N64.89
  organ or site, congenital NEC — *see* Agenesis,
    by site
Unilocular heart Q20.8
Union, abnormal (*see also* Fusion)
  larynx and trachea Q34.8
Universal mesentery Q43.3
Unrepairable overhanging of dental restorative
  materials K08.52
Unsatisfactory
  restoration of tooth K08.50
    specified NEC K08.59
  sample of cytologic smear
    anus R85.615
    cervix R87.615
    vagina R87.625
    surroundings Z59.1
    work Z56.5
Unsoundness of mind — *see* Psychosis
Unstable
  back NEC — *see* Instability, joint, spine
  hip (congenital) Q65.6
    acquired — *see* Derangement, joint, specified
      type NEC, hip
  joint — *see* Instability, joint
    secondary to removal of joint prosthesis
      M96.89
  lie (mother) O32.0 ☑
  lumbosacral joint (congenital)
    acquiredM53.2
  sacroiliacM53.2
  spine NEC — *see* Instability, joint, spine
Unsteadiness on feet R26.81
Untruthfulness, child problem F91.8
Unverricht (-Lundborg) disease or epilepsy — *see*
  Epilepsy, generalized, idiopathic
Unwanted pregnancy Z64.0
Upbringing, institutional Z62.22
  away from parents NEC Z62.29
  in care of non-parental family member Z62.21
  in foster care Z62.21
  in orphanage or group home Z62.22
  in welfare custody Z62.21
Upper respiratory — *see* condition
Upset
  gastric K30
  gastrointestinal K30
    psychogenic F45.8
  intestinal (large) (small) K59.9
    psychogenic F45.8
  menstruation N93.9
  mental F48.9
  stomach K30
    psychogenic F45.8
Urachus (*see also* condition)
  patent or persistent Q64.4
Urbach-Oppenheim disease (necrobiosis lipoidica
  diabeticorum) — *see* E08-E13 with .620
Urbach's lipoid proteinosis E78.89
Urbach-Wiethe disease E78.89
Urban yellow fever A95.1
Urea
  blood, high — *see* Uremia
  cycle metabolism disorder — *see* Disorder, urea
    cycle metabolism
Uremia, uremic N19
  with
    ectopic or molar pregnancy O08.4
    polyneuropathy N18.9 [G63]
  chronic (*see also* Disease, kidney, chronic) N18.9
    due to hypertension — *see* Hypertensive,
      kidney
  complicating
    ectopic or molar pregnancy O08.4
  congenital P96.0

☑ **Additional character required**

Uremia — continued
  extrarenal R39.2
  following ectopic or molar pregnancy O08.4
  newborn P96.0
  prerenal R39.2
Ureter, ureteral — see condition
Ureteralgia N23
Ureterectasis — see Hydroureter
Ureteritis N28.89
  cystica N28.86
  due to calculus N20.1
    with calculus, kidney N20.2
      with hydronephrosis N13.2
  gonococcal (acute) (chronic) A54.21
  nonspecific N28.89
Ureterocele N28.89
  congenital (orthotopic) Q62.31
    ectopic Q62.32
Ureterolith, ureterolithiasis — see Calculus, ureter
Ureterostomy
  attention to Z43.6
  status Z93.6
Urethra, urethral — see condition
Urethralgia R39.89
Urethritis (anterior) (posterior) N34.2
  calculous N21.1
  candidal B37.41
  chlamydial A56.01
  diplococcal (gonococcal) A54.01
    with abscess (accessory gland) (periurethral) A54.1
  gonococcal A54.01
    with abscess (accessory gland) (periurethral) A54.1
  nongonococcal N34.1
    Reiter's — see Reiter's disease
  nonspecific N34.1
  nonvenereal N34.1
  postmenopausal N34.2
  puerperal O86.22
  Reiter's — see Reiter's disease
  specified NEC N34.2
  trichomonal or due to Trichomonas (vaginalis) A59.03
Urethrocele N81.0
  with
    cystocele — see Cystocele
    prolapse of uterus — see Prolapse, uterus
Urethrolithiasis (with colic or infection) N21.1
Urethrorectal — see condition
Urethrorrhagia N36.8
Urethrorrhea R36.9
Urethrostomy
  attention to Z43.6
  status Z93.6
Urethrotrigonitis — see Trigonitis
Urethrovaginal — see condition
Urgency
  fecal R15.2
  hypertensive — see Hypertension
  urinary N39.41
Urhidrosis, uridrosis L74.8
Uric acid in blood (increased) E79.0
Uricacidemia (asymptomatic) E79.0
Uricemia (asymptomatic) E79.0
Uricosuria R82.99
Urinary — see condition
Urination
  frequent R35.0
  painful R30.9
Urine
  blood in — see Hematuria
  discharge, excessive R35.8
  enuresis, nonorganic origin F98.0
  extravasation R39.0
  frequency R35.0
  incontinence R32
    nonorganic origin F98.0
  intermittent stream R39.19
  pus in N39.0
  retention or stasis R33.9
    organic R33.8
      drug-induced R33.0
    psychogenic F45.8
  secretion
    deficient R34
    excessive R35.8
    frequency R35.0
  stream
    intermittent R39.19
    slowing R39.19
    splitting R39.13

Urine — continued
  weak R39.12
Urinemia — see Uremia
Urinoma, urethra N36.8
Uroarthritis, infectious (Reiter's) — see Reiter's disease
Urodialysis R34
Urolithiasis — see Calculus, urinary
Uronephrosis — see Hydronephrosis
Uropathy N39.9
  obstructive N13.9
    specified NEC N13.8
  reflux N13.9
    specified NEC N13.8
  vesicoureteral reflux-associated — see Reflux, vesicoureteral
Urosepsis - code to condition
Urticaria L50.9
  with angioneurotic edema T78.3 ☑
    hereditary D84.1
  allergic L50.0
  cholinergic L50.5
  chronic L50.8
  cold, familial L50.2
  contact L50.6
  dermatographic L50.3
  due to
    cold or heat L50.2
    drugs L50.0
    food L50.0
    inhalants L50.0
    plants L50.6
    serum (see also Reaction, serum) T80.69 ☑
  factitial L50.3
  giant T78.3 ☑
    hereditary D84.1
  gigantea T78.3 ☑
  idiopathic L50.1
  larynx T78.3 ☑
    hereditary D84.1
  neonatorum P83.8
  nonallergic L50.1
  papulosa (Hebra) L28.2
  pigmentosa Q82.2
  recurrent periodic L50.8
  serum (see also Reaction, serum) T80.69 ☑
  solar L56.3
  specified type NEC L50.8
  thermal (cold) (heat) L50.2
  vibratory L50.4
  xanthelasmoidea Q82.2
Use (of)
  alcohol F10.99
    with sleep disorder F10.982
    harmful — see Abuse, alcohol
  amphetamines — see Use, stimulant NEC
  caffeine — see Use, stimulant NEC
  cannabis F12.90
    with
      anxiety disorder F12.980
      intoxication F12.929
        with
          delirium F12.921
          perceptual disturbance F12.922
        uncomplicated F12.920
      other specified disorder F12.988
      psychosis F12.959
        delusions F12.950
        hallucinations F12.951
      unspecified disorder F12.99
  cocaine F14.90
    with
      anxiety disorder F14.980
      intoxication F14.929
        with
          delirium F14.921
          perceptual disturbance F14.922
        uncomplicated F14.920
      other specified disorder F14.988
      psychosis F14.959
        delusions F14.950
        hallucinations F14.951
      sexual dysfunction F14.981
      sleep disorder F14.982
      unspecified disorder F14.99
    harmful — see Abuse, drug, cocaine
  drug (s) NEC F19.90
    with sleep disorder F19.982
    harmful — see Abuse, drug, by type
  hallucinogen NEC F16.90
    with
      anxiety disorder F16.980

Use — continued
      intoxication F16.929
        with
          delirium F16.921
        uncomplicated F16.920
      mood disorder F16.94
      other specified disorder F16.988
      perception disorder (flashbacks) F16.983
      psychosis F16.959
        delusions F16.950
        hallucinations F16.951
      unspecified disorder F16.99
    harmful — see Abuse, drug, hallucinogen NEC
  inhalants F18.90
    with
      anxiety disorder F18.980
      intoxication F18.929
        with delirium F18.921
        uncomplicated F18.920
      mood disorder F18.94
      other specified disorder F18.988
      persisting dementia F18.97
      psychosis F18.959
        delusions F18.950
        hallucinations F18.951
      unspecified disorder F18.99
    harmful — see Abuse, drug, inhalant
  methadone F11.20
  nonprescribed drugs F19.90
    harmful — see Abuse, non-psychoactive substance
  opioid F11.90
    with
      disorder F11.99
        mood F11.94
        sleep F11.982
        specified type NEC F11.988
      intoxication F11.929
        with
          delirium F11.921
          perceptual disturbance F11.922
        uncomplicated F11.920
      withdrawal F11.93
    harmful — see Abuse, drug, opioid
  patent medicines F19.90
    harmful — see Abuse, non-psychoactive substance
  psychoactive drug NEC F19.90
    with
      anxiety disorder F19.980
      intoxication F19.929
        with
          delirium F19.921
          perceptual disturbance F19.922
        uncomplicated F19.920
      mood disorder F19.94
      other specified disorder F19.988
      persisting
        amnestic disorder F19.96
        dementia F19.97
      psychosis F19.959
        delusions F19.950
        hallucinations F19.951
      sexual dysfunction F19.981
      sleep disorder F19.982
      unspecified disorder F19.99
      withdrawal F19.939
        with
          delirium F19.931
          perceptual disturbance F19.932
        uncomplicated F19.930
    harmful — see Abuse, drug NEC, psychoactive NEC
  sedative, hypnotic, or anxiolytic F13.90
    with
      anxiety disorder F13.980
      intoxication F13.929
        with
          delirium F13.921
        uncomplicated F13.920
      other specified disorder F13.988
      persisting
        amnestic disorder F13.96
        dementia F13.97
      psychosis F13.959
        delusions F13.950
        hallucinations F13.951
      sexual dysfunction F13.981
      sleep disorder F13.982
      unspecified disorder F13.99
    harmful — see Abuse, drug, sedative, hypnotic, or anxiolytic

Use — *continued*
  stimulant NEC F15.90
    with
      anxiety disorder F15.980
      intoxication F15.929
        with
          delirium F15.921
          perceptual disturbance F15.922
        uncomplicated F15.920
      mood disorder F15.94
      other specified disorder F15.988
      psychosis F15.959
        delusions F15.950
        hallucinations F15.951
      sexual dysfunction F15.981
      sleep disorder F15.982
      unspecified disorder F15.99
      withdrawal F15.93
    harmful — *see* Abuse, drug, stimulant NEC
  volatile solvents (*see also* Use, inhalant) F18.90
    harmful — *see* Abuse, drug, inhalant
  tobacco Z72.0
    with dependence — *see* Dependence, drug,
      nicotine
Usher-Senear disease or syndrome L10.4
Uta B55.1
Uteromegaly N85.2
Uterovaginal — *see* condition
Uterovesical — *see* condition
Uveal — *see* condition
Uveitis (anterior) (*see also* Iridocyclitis)
  acute — *see* Iridocyclitis, acute
  chronic — *see* Iridocyclitis, chronic
  due to toxoplasmosis (acquired) B58.09
    congenital P37.1
  granulomatous — *see* Iridocyclitis, chronic
  heterochromic — *see* Cyclitis, Fuchs'
    heterochromic
  lens-induced — *see* Iridocyclitis, lens-induced
  posterior — *see* Chorioretinitis
  sympathetic H44.13- ☑
  syphilitic (secondary) A51.43
    congenital (early) A50.01
    late A52.71
  tuberculous A18.54
Uveoencephalitis — *see* Inflammation, chorioretinal
Uveokeratitis — *see* Iridocyclitis
Uveoparotitis D86.89
Uvula — *see* condition
Uvulitis (acute) (catarrhal) (chronic) (membranous)
  (suppurative) (ulcerative) K12.2

V

Vaccination (prophylactic)
  complication or reaction — *see* Complications,
    vaccination
  delayed Z28.9
  encounter for Z23
  not done — *see* Immunization, not done, because
    (of)
Vaccinia (generalized) (localized) T88.1 ☑
  congenital P35.8
  without vaccination B08.011
Vacuum, in sinus (accessory) (nasal) J34.89
Vagabond, vagabondage Z59.0
Vagabond's disease B85.1
Vagina, vaginal — *see* condition
Vaginalitis (tunica) (testis) N49.1
Vaginismus (reflex) N94.2
  functional F52.5
  nonorganic F52.5
  psychogenic F52.5
  secondary N94.2
Vaginitis (acute) (circumscribed) (diffuse)
  (emphysematous) (nonvenereal) (ulcerative) N76.0
  with ectopic or molar pregnancy O08.0
  amebic A06.82
  atrophic, postmenopausal N95.2
  bacterial N76.0
  blennorrhagic (gonococcal) A54.02
  candidal B37.3
  chlamydial A56.02
  chronic N76.1
  due to Trichomonas (vaginalis) A59.01
  following ectopic or molar pregnancy O08.0
  gonococcal A54.02
    with abscess (accessory gland) (periurethral)
      A54.1

Vaginitis — *continued*
  granuloma A58
  in (due to)
    candidiasis B37.3
    herpesviral (herpes simplex) infection A60.04
    pinworm infection B80 [N77.1]
  monilial B37.3
  mycotic (candidal) B37.3
  postmenopausal atrophic N95.2
  puerperal (postpartum) O86.13
  senile (atrophic) N95.2
  subacute or chronic N76.1
  syphilitic (early) A51.0
    late A52.76
  trichomonal A59.01
  tuberculous A18.18
Vaginosis — *see* Vaginitis
Vagotonia G52.2
Vagrancy Z59.0
VAIN — *see* Neoplasia, intraepithelial, vagina
Vallecula — *see* condition
Valley fever B38.0
Valsuani's disease — *see* Anemia, obstetric
Valve, valvular (formation) (*see also* condition)
  cerebral ventricle (communicating) in situ Z98.2
  cervix, internal os Q51.828
  congenital NEC — *see* Atresia, by site
  ureter (pelvic junction) (vesical orifice) Q62.39
  urethra (congenital) (posterior) Q64.2
Valvulitis (chronic) — *see* Endocarditis
Valvulopathy — *see* Endocarditis
Van Bogaert's leukoencephalopathy (sclerosing)
  (subacute) A81.1
Van Bogaert-Scherer-Epstein disease or syndrome
  E75.5
Van Buchem's syndrome M85.2
Van Creveld-von Gierke disease E74.01
Van der Hoeve (-de Kleyn) syndrome Q78.0
Van der Woude's syndrome Q38.0
Van Neck's disease or osteochondrosis M91.0
Vanishing lung J44.9
Vapor asphyxia or suffocation T59.9 ☑
  specified agent — *see* Table of Drugs and
    Chemicals
Variance, lethal ball, prosthetic heart valve T82.09 ☑
Variants, thalassemic D56.8
Variations in hair color L67.1
Varicella B01.9
  with
    complications NEC B01.89
    encephalitis B01.11
    encephalomyelitis B01.11
    meningitis B01.0
    myelitis B01.12
    pneumonia B01.2
  congenital P35.8
Varices — *see* Varix
Varicocele (scrotum) (thrombosed) I86.1
  ovary I86.2
  perineum I86.3
  spermatic cord (ulcerated) I86.1
Varicose
  aneurysm (ruptured) I77.0
  dermatitis — *see* Varix, leg, with, inflammation
  eczema — *see* Varix, leg, with, inflammation
  phlebitis — *see* Varix, with, inflammation
  tumor — *see* Varix
  ulcer (lower limb, any part) (*see also* Varix, leg,
    with, ulcer)
    anus (*see also* Hemorrhoids) K64.8
    esophagus — *see* Varix, esophagus
    inflamed or infected — *see* Varix, leg, with ulcer,
      with inflammation
    nasal septum I86.8
    perineum I86.3
    scrotum I86.1
    specified site NEC I86.8
  vein — *see* Varix
  vessel — *see* Varix, leg
Varicosis, varicosities, varicosity — *see* Varix
Variola (major) (minor) B03
Varioloid B03
Varix (lower limb) (ruptured) I83.90
  with
    edema I83.899
    inflammation I83.10
      with ulcer (venous) I83.209
    pain I83.819
    specified complication NEC I83.899
    stasis dermatitis I83.10
      with ulcer (venous) I83.209
    swelling I83.899

Varix — *continued*
  ulcer I83.009
    with inflammation I83.209
  aneurysmal I77.0
  asymptomatic I83.9- ☑
  bladder I86.2
  broad ligament I86.2
  complicating
    childbirth (lower extremity) O87.4
      anus or rectum O87.2
      genital (vagina, vulva or perineum) O87.8
    pregnancy (lower extremity) O22.0- ☑
      anus or rectum O22.4- ☑
      genital (vagina, vulva or perineum) O22.1- ☑
    puerperium (lower extremity) O87.4
      anus or rectum O87.2
      genital (vagina, vulva, perineum) O87.8
  congenital (any site) Q27.8
  esophagus (idiopathic) (primary) (ulcerated)
    I85.00
    bleeding I85.01
    congenital Q27.8
    in (due to)
      alcoholic liver disease I85.10
        bleeding I85.11
      cirrhosis of liver I85.10
        bleeding I85.11
      portal hypertension I85.10
        bleeding I85.11
      schistosomiasis I85.10
        bleeding I85.11
      toxic liver disease I85.10
        bleeding I85.11
    secondary I85.10
      bleeding I85.11
  gastric I86.4
  inflamed or infected I83.10
    ulcerated I83.209
  labia (majora) I86.3
  leg (asymptomatic) I83.90
    with
      edema I83.899
      inflammation I83.10
        with ulcer — *see* Varix, leg, with, ulcer, with
          inflammation by site
      pain I83.819
      specified complication NEC I83.899
      swelling I83.899
      ulcer I83.009
        with inflammation I83.209
        ankle I83.003
          with inflammation I83.203
        calf I83.002
          with inflammation I83.202
        foot NEC I83.005
          with inflammation I83.205
        heel I83.004
          with inflammation I83.204
        lower leg NEC I83.008
          with inflammation I83.208
        midfoot I83.004
          with inflammation I83.204
        thigh I83.001
          with inflammation I83.201
    bilateral (asymptomatic) I83.93
      with
        edema I83.893
        pain I83.813
        specified complication NEC I83.893
        swelling I83.893
        ulcer I83.009
          with inflammation I83.209
    left (asymptomatic) I83.92
      with
        edema I83.892
        pain I83.812
        specified complication NEC I83.892
        swelling I83.892
        inflammation I83.12
          with ulcer — *see* Varix, leg, with, ulcer,
            with inflammation by site
        ulcer I83.029
          with inflammation I83.229
          ankle I83.023
            with inflammation I83.223
          calf I83.022
            with inflammation I83.222
          foot NEC I83.025
            with inflammation I83.225
          heel I83.024
            with inflammation I83.224
          lower leg NEC I83.028

Varix — *continued*
  with inflammation I83.228
    midfoot I83.024
      with inflammation I83.224
    thigh I83.021
      with inflammation I83.221
  right (asymptomatic) I83.91
    with
      edema I83.891
      pain I83.811
      specified complication NEC I83.891
      swelling I83.891
      inflammation I83.11
        with ulcer — *see* Varix, leg, with, ulcer, with inflammation by site
      ulcer I83.019
        with inflammation I83.219
        ankle I83.013
          with inflammation I83.213
        calf I83.012
          with inflammation I83.212
        foot NEC I83.015
          with inflammation I83.215
        heel I83.014
          with inflammation I83.214
        lower leg NEC I83.018
          with inflammation I83.218
        midfoot I83.014
          with inflammation I83.214
        thigh I83.011
          with inflammation I83.211
  nasal septum I86.8
  orbit I86.8
    congenital Q27.8
  ovary I86.2
  papillary I78.1
  pelvis I86.2
  perineum I86.3
  pharynx I86.8
  placenta O43.89- ☑
  renal papilla I86.8
  retina H35.09
  scrotum (ulcerated) I86.1
  sigmoid colon I86.8
  specified site NEC I86.8
  spinal (cord) (vessels) I86.8
  spleen, splenic (vein) (with phlebolith) I86.8
  stomach I86.4
  sublingual I86.0
  ulcerated I83.009
    inflamed or infected I83.209
  uterine ligament I86.2
  vagina I86.8
  vocal cord I86.8
  vulva I86.3
Vas deferens — *see* condition
Vas deferentitis N49.1
Vasa previa O69.4 ☑
  hemorrhage from, affecting newborn P50.0
Vascular (*see also* condition)
  loop on optic papilla Q14.2
  spasm I73.9
  spider I78.1
Vascularization, cornea — *see* Neovascularization, cornea
Vasculitis I77.6
  allergic D69.0
  cryoglobulinemic D89.1
  disseminated I77.6
  hypocomplementemic M31.8
  kidney I77.89
  livedoid L95.0
  nodular L95.8
  retina H35.06- ☑
  rheumatic — *see* Fever, rheumatic
  rheumatoid — *see* Rheumatoid, vasculitis
  skin (limited to) L95.9
    specified NEC L95.8
Vasculopathy, necrotizing M31.9
  cardiac allograft T86.290
  specified NEC M31.8
Vasitis (nodosa) N49.1
  tuberculous A18.15
Vasodilation I73.9
Vasomotor — *see* condition
Vasoplasty, after previous sterilization Z31.0
  aftercare Z31.42
Vasospasm (vasoconstriction) I73.9
  cerebral (cerebrovascular) (artery) I67.848
    reversible I67.841
  coronary I20.1
  nerve

Vasospasm — *continued*
  arm — *see* Mononeuropathy, upper limb
  brachial plexus G54.0
  cervical plexus G54.2
  leg — *see* Mononeuropathy, lower limb
  peripheral NOS I73.9
  retina (artery) — *see* Occlusion, artery, retina
Vasospastic — *see* condition
Vasovagal attack (paroxysmal) R55
  psychogenic F45.8
VATER syndrome Q87.2
Vater's ampulla — *see* condition
Vegetation, vegetative
  adenoid (nasal fossa) J35.8
  endocarditis (acute) (any valve) (subacute) I33.0
  heart (mycotic) (valve) I33.0
Veil
  Jackson's Q43.3
Vein, venous — *see* condition
Veldt sore — *see* Ulcer, skin
Velpeau's hernia — *see* Hernia, femoral
Venereal
  bubo A55
  disease A64
  granuloma inguinale A58
  lymphogranuloma (Durand-Nicolas-Favre) A55
Venofibrosis I87.8
Venom, venomous — *see* Table of Drugs and Chemicals, by animal or substance, poisoning
Venous — *see* condition
Ventilator lung, newborn P27.8
Ventral — *see* condition
Ventricle, ventricular (*see also* condition)
  escape I49.3
  inversion Q20.5
Ventriculitis (cerebral) (*see also* Encephalitis) G04.90
Ventriculostomy status Z98.2
Vernet's syndrome G52.7
Verneuil's disease (syphilitic bursitis) A52.78
Verruca (due to HPV) (filiformis) (simplex) (viral) (vulgaris) B07.9
  acuminata A63.0
  necrogenica (primary) (tuberculosa) A18.4
  plana B07.8
  plantaris B07.0
  seborrheica L82.1
    inflamed L82.0
  senile (seborrheic) L82.1
    inflamed L82.0
  tuberculosa (primary) A18.4
  venereal A63.0
Verrucosities — *see* Verruca
Verruga peruana, peruviana A44.1
Version
  with extraction
  cervix — *see* Malposition, uterus
  uterus (postinfectional) (postpartal, old) — *see* Malposition, uterus
Vertebra, vertebral — *see* condition
Vertical talus (congenital) Q66.80
  left foot Q66.82
  right foot Q66.81
Vertigo R42
  auditory — *see* Vertigo, aural
  aural H81.31- ☑
  benign paroxysmal (positional) H81.1- ☑
  central (origin) H81.4- ☑
  cerebral H81.4- ☑
  Dix and Hallpike (epidemic) — *see* Neuronitis, vestibular
  due to infrasound T75.23 ☑
  epidemic A88.1
    Dix and Hallpike — *see* Neuronitis, vestibular
    Pedersen's — *see* Neuronitis, vestibular
    vestibular neuronitis — *see* Neuronitis, vestibular
  hysterical F44.89
  infrasound T75.23 ☑
  labyrinthine H81.0
  laryngeal R05
  malignant positional H81.4- ☑
  Ménière's H81.0
  menopausal N95.1
  otogenic — *see* Vertigo, aural
  paroxysmal positional, benign — *see* Vertigo, benign paroxysmal
  Pedersen's (epidemic) — *see* Neuronitis, vestibular
  peripheral NEC H81.39- ☑
  positional
    benign paroxysmal — *see* Vertigo, benign paroxysmal

Vertigo — *continued*
  malignant H81.4- ☑
Very-low-density-lipoprotein-type (VLDL) hyperlipoproteinemia E78.1
Vesania — *see* Psychosis
Vesical — *see* condition
Vesicle
  cutaneous R23.8
  seminal — *see* condition
  skin R23.8
Vesicocolic — *see* condition
Vesicoperineal — *see* condition
Vesicorectal — *see* condition
Vesicourethrorectal — *see* condition
Vesicovaginal — *see* condition
Vesicular — *see* condition
Vesiculitis (seminal) N49.0
  amebic A06.82
  gonorrheal (acute) (chronic) A54.23
  trichomonal A59.09
  tuberculous A18.15
Vestibulitis (ear) (*see also* subcategory) H83.0 ☑
  nose (external) J34.89
  vulvar N94.810
Vestibulopathy, acute peripheral (recurrent) — *see* Neuronitis, vestibular
Vestige, vestigial (*see also* Persistence)
  branchial Q18.0
  structures in vitreous Q14.0
Vibration
  adverse effects T75.20 ☑
    pneumatic hammer syndrome T75.21 ☑
    specified effect NEC T75.29 ☑
    vasospastic syndrome T75.22 ☑
    vertigo from infrasound T75.23 ☑
  exposure (occupational) Z57.7
  vertigo T75.23 ☑
Vibriosis A28.9
Victim (of)
  crime Z65.4
  disaster Z65.5
  terrorism Z65.4
  torture Z65.4
  war Z65.5
Vidal's disease L28.0
Villaret's syndrome G52.7
Villous — *see* condition
VIN — *see* Neoplasia, intraepithelial, vulva
Vincent's infection (angina) (gingivitis) A69.1
  stomatitis NEC A69.1
Vinson-Plummer syndrome D50.1
Violence, physical R45.6
Viosterol deficiency — *see* Deficiency, calciferol
Vipoma — *see* Neoplasm, malignant, by site
Viremia B34.9
Virilism (adrenal) E25.9
  congenital E25.0
Virilization (female) (suprarenal) E25.9
  congenital E25.0
  isosexual E28.2
Virulent bubo A57
Virus, viral (*see also* condition)
  as cause of disease classified elsewhere B97.89
  cytomegalovirus B25.9
  human immunodeficiency (HIV) — *see* Human, immunodeficiency virus (HIV) disease
  infection — *see* Infection, virus
  specified NEC B34.8
  swine influenza (viruses that normally cause infections in pigs) (*see also* Influenza, due to, identified novel influenza A virus) J09.X2
  West Nile (fever) A92.30
    with
      complications NEC A92.39
      cranial nerve disorders A92.32
      encephalitis A92.31
      encephalomyelitis A92.31
      neurologic manifestation NEC A92.32
      optic neuritis A92.32
      polyradiculitis A92.32
Viscera, visceral — *see* condition
Visceroptosis K63.4
Visible peristalsis R19.2
Vision, visual
  binocular, suppression H53.34
  blurred, blurring H53.8
    hysterical F44.6
  defect, defective NEC H54.7
  disorientation (syndrome) H53.8
  disturbance H53.9
    hysterical F44.6
  double H53.2

Vision — *continued*
  examination Z01.00
    with abnormal findings Z01.01
  field, limitation (defect) — *see* Defect, visual field
  hallucinations R44.1
  halos H53.19
  loss — *see* Loss, vision
    sudden — *see* Disturbance, vision, subjective,
      loss, sudden
  low (both eyes) — *see* Low, vision
  perception, simultaneous without fusion H53.33
Vitality, lack or want of R53.83
  newborn P96.89
Vitamin deficiency — *see* Deficiency, vitamin
Vitelline duct, persistent Q43.0
Vitiligo L80
  eyelid H02.739
    left H02.736
      lower H02.735
      upper H02.734
    right H02.733
      lower H02.732
      upper H02.731
  pinta A67.2
  vulva N90.89
Vitreal corneal syndrome H59.01- ☑
Vitreoretinopathy, proliferative (*see also*
  Retinopathy, proliferative)
  with retinal detachment — *see* Detachment,
    retina, traction
Vitreous (*see also* condition)
  touch syndrome — *see* Complication,
    postprocedural, following cataract surgery
Vocal cord — *see* condition
Vogt-Koyanagi syndrome H20.82- ☑
Vogt's disease or syndrome G80.3
Vogt-Spielmeyer amaurotic idiocy or disease E75.4
Voice
  change R49.9
    specified NEC R49.8
  loss — *see* Aphonia
Volhynian fever A79.0
Volkmann's ischemic contracture or paralysis
  (complicating trauma) T79.6 ☑
Volvulus (bowel) (colon) (duodenum) (intestine)
  K56.2
  with perforation K56.2
  congenital Q43.8
  fallopian tube — *see* Torsion, fallopian tube
  oviduct — *see* Torsion, fallopian tube
  stomach (due to absence of gastrocolic ligament)
    K31.89
Vomiting R11.10
  with nausea R11.2
  asphyxia — *see* Foreign body, by site, causing
    asphyxia, gastric contents
  bilious (cause unknown) R11.14
    in newborn P92.01
    following gastro-intestinal surgery K91.0
  blood — *see* Hematemesis
  causing asphyxia, choking, or suffocation — *see*
    Foreign body, by site
  cyclical G43.A0
    with refractory migraine G43.A1
    intractable G43.A1
    not intractable G43.A0
    psychogenic F50.8
    without refractory migraine G43.A0
  fecal mater R11.13
  following gastrointestinal surgery K91.0
    psychogenic F50.8
  functional K31.89
  hysterical F50.8
  nervous F50.8
  neurotic F50.8
  newborn NEC P92.09
    bilious P92.01
  periodic R11.10
    psychogenic F50.8
  projectile R11.12
  psychogenic F50.8
  uremic — *see* Uremia
  without nausea R11.11
Vomito negro — *see* Fever, yellow
Von Bezold's abscess — *see* Mastoiditis, acute
Von Economo-Cruchet disease A85.8
Von Eulenburg's disease G71.19
Von Gierke's disease E74.01
Von Hippel (-Lindau) disease or syndrome Q85.8
Von Jaksch's anemia or disease D64.89
Von Recklinghausen
  disease (neurofibromatosis) Q85.01

Von — *continued*
  bones E21.0
Von Schroetter's syndrome I82.890
Von Willebrand (-Jurgens)(-Minot) disease or
  syndrome D68.0
Von Zumbusch's disease L40.1
Voyeurism F65.3
Vrolik's disease Q78.0
Vulva — *see* condition
Vulvismus N94.2
Vulvitis (acute) (allergic) (atrophic) (hypertrophic)
  (intertriginous) (senile) N76.2
  with ectopic or molar pregnancy O08.0
  adhesive, congenital Q52.79
  blennorrhagic (gonococcal) A54.02
  candidal B37.3
  chlamydial A56.02
  due to Haemophilus ducreyi A57
  following ectopic or molar pregnancy O08.0
  gonococcal A54.02
    with abscess (accessory gland) (periurethral)
      A54.1
  herpesviral A60.04
  leukoplakic N90.4
  monilial B37.3
  puerperal (postpartum) O86.19
  subacute or chronic N76.3
  syphilitic (early) A51.0
    late A52.76
  trichomonal A59.01
  tuberculous A18.18
Vulvodynia N94.819
  specified NEC N94.818
Vulvorectal — *see* condition
Vulvovaginitis (acute) — *see* Vaginitis

W

Waiting list, person on Z75.1
  for organ transplant Z76.82
  undergoing social agency investigation Z75.2
Waldenström-Kjellberg syndrome D50.1
Waldenström
  hypergammaglobulinemia D89.0
  syndrome or macroglobulinemia C88.0
Walking
  difficulty R26.2
    psychogenic F44.4
  sleep F51.3
    hysterical F44.89
Wall, abdominal — *see* condition
Wallenberg's disease or syndrome G46.3
Wallgren's disease I87.8
Wandering
  gallbladder, congenital Q44.1
  in diseases classified elsewhere Z91.83
  kidney, congenital Q63.8
  organ or site, congenital NEC — *see* Malposition,
    congenital, by site
  pacemaker (heart) I49.8
  spleen D73.89
War neurosis F48.8
Wart (due to HPV) (filiform) (infectious) (viral) B07.9
  anogenital region (venereal) A63.0
  common B07.8
  external genital organs (venereal) A63.0
  flat B07.8
  Hassal-Henle's (of cornea) H18.49
  Peruvian A44.1
  plantar B07.0
  prosector (tuberculous) A18.4
  seborrheic L82.1
    inflamed L82.0
  senile (seborrheic) L82.1
    inflamed L82.0
  tuberculous A18.4
  venereal A63.0
Warthin's tumor — *see* Neoplasm, salivary gland,
  benign
Wassilieff's disease A27.0
Wasting
  disease R64
    due to malnutrition E41
    extreme (due to malnutrition) E41
  muscle NEC — *see* Atrophy, muscle
Water
  clefts (senile cataract) — *see* Cataract, senile,
    incipient
  deprivation of T73.1 ☑

Water — *continued*
  intoxication E87.79
  itch B76.9
  lack of T73.1 ☑
  loading E87.70
  on
    brain — *see* Hydrocephalus
    chest J94.8
  poisoning E87.79
Waterbrash R12
Waterhouse (-Friderichsen) syndrome or disease
  (meningococcal) A39.1
Water-losing nephritis N25.89
Watermelon stomach K31.819
  with hemorrhage K31.811
  without hemorrhage K31.819
Watsoniasis B66.8
Wax in ear — *see* Impaction, cerumen
Weak, weakening, weakness (generalized) R53.1
  arches (acquired) (*see also* Deformity, limb, flat
    foot)
  bladder (sphincter) R32
  facial R29.810
    following
      cerebrovascular disease I69.992
        cerebral infarction I69.392
        intracerebral hemorrhage I69.192
        nontraumatic intracranial hemorrhage NEC
          I69.292
        specified disease NEC I69.892
        stroke I69.392
        subarachnoid hemorrhage I69.092
  foot (double) — *see* Weak, arches
  heart, cardiac — *see* Failure, heart
  mind F70
  muscle M62.81
  myocardium — *see* Failure, heart
  newborn P96.89
  pelvic fundus N81.89
  pubocervical tissue N81.82
  senile R54
  rectovaginal tissue N81.83
  urinary stream R39.12
  valvular — *see* Endocarditis
Wear, worn (with normal or routine use)
  articular bearing surface of internal joint
    prosthesis — *see* Complications, joint
    prosthesis, mechanical, wear of articular
    bearing surfaces, by site
  device, implant or graft — *see* Complications, by
    site, mechanical complication
  tooth, teeth (approximal) (hard tissues)
    (interproximal) (occlusal) K03.0
Weather, weathered
  effects of
    cold T69.9 ☑
      specified effect NEC T69.8 ☑
    hot — *see* Heat
  skin L57.8
Weaver's syndrome Q87.3
Web, webbed (congenital)
  duodenal Q43.8
  esophagus Q39.4
  fingers Q70.1- ☑
  larynx (glottic) (subglottic) Q31.0
  neck (pterygium colli) Q18.3
  Paterson-Kelly D50.1
  popliteal syndrome Q87.89
  toes Q70.3- ☑
Weber-Christian disease M35.6
Weber-Cockayne syndrome (epidermolysis bullosa)
  Q81.8
Weber-Gubler syndrome G46.3
Weber-Leyden syndrome G46.3
Weber-Osler syndrome I78.0
Weber's paralysis or syndrome G46.3
Wedge-shaped or wedging vertebra — *see* Collapse,
  vertebra NEC
Wegener's granulomatosis or syndrome M31.30
  with
    kidney involvement M31.31
    lung involvement M31.30
      with kidney involvement M31.31
Wegner's disease A50.02
Weight
  1000-2499 grams at birth (low) — *see* Low,
    birthweight
  999 grams or less at birth (extremely low) — *see*
    Low, birthweight, extreme
  gain (abnormal) (excessive) R63.5
    in pregnancy — *see* Pregnancy, complicated by,
      excessive weight gain

☑ **Additional character required**

Weight — continued
  low — see Pregnancy, complicated by, insufficient, weight gain
  loss (abnormal) (cause unknown) R63.4
Weightlessness (effect of) T75.82 ☑
Weil (I)-Marchesani syndrome Q87.1
Weil's disease A27.0
Weingarten's syndrome J82
Weir Mitchell's disease I73.81
Weiss-Baker syndrome G90.09
Wells' disease L98.3
Wen — see Cyst, sebaceous
Wenckebach's block or phenomenon I44.1
Werdnig-Hoffmann syndrome (muscular atrophy) G12.0
Werlhof's disease D69.3
Wermer's disease or syndrome E31.21
Werner-His disease A79.0
Werner's disease or syndrome E34.8
Wernicke-Korsakoff's syndrome or psychosis (alcoholic) F10.96
  with dependence F10.26
  drug-induced
    due to drug abuse — see Abuse, drug, by type, with amnestic disorder
    due to drug dependence — see Dependence, drug, by type, with amnestic disorder
  nonalcoholic F04
Wernicke-Posadas disease B38.9
Wernicke's
  developmental aphasia F80.2
  disease or syndrome E51.2
  encephalopathy E51.2
  polioencephalitis, superior E51.2
West African fever B50.8
Westphal-Strümpell syndrome E83.01
West's syndrome — see Epilepsy, spasms
Wet
  feet, tropical (maceration) (syndrome) — see Immersion, foot
  lung (syndrome), newborn P22.1
Wharton's duct — see condition
Wheal — see Urticaria
Wheezing R06.2
Whiplash injury S13.4 ☑
Whipple's disease (see also subcategory M14.8-) K90.81
Whipworm (disease) (infection) (infestation) B79
Whistling face Q87.0
White (see also condition)
  kidney, small N03.9
  leg, puerperal, postpartum, childbirth O87.1
  mouth B37.0
  patches of mouth K13.29
  spot lesions, teeth
    chewing surface K02.51
    pit and fissure surface K02.51
    smooth surface K02.61
Whitehead L70.0
Whitlow (see also Cellulitis, digit)
  with lymphangitis — see Lymphangitis, acute, digit
  herpesviral B00.89
Whitmore's disease or fever — see Melioidosis
Whooping cough A37.90
  with pneumonia A37.91
    due to Bordetella
      bronchiseptica A37.81
      parapertussis A37.11
      pertussis A37.01
      specified organism NEC A37.81
  due to
    Bordetella
      bronchiseptica A37.80
        with pneumonia A37.81
      parapertussis A37.10
        with pneumonia A37.11
      pertussis A37.00
        with pneumonia A37.01
      specified NEC A37.80
        with pneumonia A37.81
Wichman's asthma J38.5
Wide cranial sutures, newborn P96.3
Widening aorta — see Ectasia, aorta
  with aneurysm — see Aneurysm, aorta
Wilkie's disease or syndrome K55.1
Wilkinson-Sneddon disease or syndrome L13.1
Willebrand (-Jürgens) thrombopathy D68.0
Willige-Hunt disease or syndrome G23.1
Wilms' tumor C64- ☑
Wilson-Mikity syndrome P27.0

Wilson's
  disease or syndrome E83.01
  hepatolenticular degeneration E83.01
  lichen ruber L43.9
Window (see also Imperfect, closure)
  aorticopulmonary Q21.4
Winter — see condition
Wiskott-Aldrich syndrome D82.0
Withdrawal state (see also Dependence, drug by type, with withdrawal)
  newborn
    correct therapeutic substance properly administered P96.2
    infant of dependent mother P96.1
    therapeutic substance, neonatal P96.2
Witts' anemia D50.8
Witzelsucht F07.0
Woakes' ethmoiditis or syndrome J33.1
Wolff-Hirschorn syndrome Q93.3
Wolff-Parkinson-White syndrome I45.6
Wolhynian fever A79.0
Wolman's disease E75.5
Wood lung or pneumonitis J67.8
Woolly, wooly hair (congenital) (nevus) Q84.1
Woolsorter's disease A22.1
Word
  blindness (congenital) (developmental) F81.0
  deafness (congenital) (developmental) H93.25
Worm (s) (infection) (infestation) (see also Infestation, helminth)
  guinea B72
  in intestine NEC B82.0
Worm-eaten soles A66.3
Worn out — see Exhaustion
  cardiac
    defibrillator (with synchronous cardiac pacemaker) Z45.02
    pacemaker
      battery Z45.010
      lead Z45.018
  device, implant or graft — see Complications, by site, mechanical
Worried well Z71.1
Worries R45.82
Wound, open
  abdomen, abdominal
    wall S31.109 ☑
      with penetration into peritoneal cavity S31.609 ☑
      bite — see Bite, abdomen, wall
      epigastric region S31.102 ☑
        with penetration into peritoneal cavity S31.602 ☑
        bite — see Bite, abdomen, wall, epigastric region
        laceration — see Laceration, abdomen, wall, epigastric region
        puncture — see Puncture, abdomen, wall, epigastric region
      laceration — see Laceration, abdomen, wall
      left
        lower quadrant S31.104 ☑
          with penetration into peritoneal cavity S31.604 ☑
          bite — see Bite, abdomen, wall, left, lower quadrant
          laceration — see Laceration, abdomen, wall, left, lower quadrant
          puncture — see Puncture, abdomen, wall, left, lower quadrant
        upper quadrant S31.101 ☑
          with penetration into peritoneal cavity S31.601 ☑
          bite — see Bite, abdomen, wall, left, upper quadrant
          laceration — see Laceration, abdomen, wall, left, upper quadrant
          puncture — see Puncture, abdomen, wall, left, upper quadrant
      periumbilic region S31.105 ☑
        with penetration into peritoneal cavity S31.605 ☑
        bite — see Bite, abdomen, wall, periumbilic region
        laceration — see Laceration, abdomen, wall, periumbilic region
        puncture — see Puncture, abdomen, wall, periumbilic region
      puncture — see Puncture, abdomen, wall
      right
        lower quadrant S31.103 ☑

Wound — continued
        with penetration into peritoneal cavity S31.603 ☑
        bite — see Bite, abdomen, wall, right, lower quadrant
        laceration — see Laceration, abdomen, wall, right, lower quadrant
        puncture — see Puncture, abdomen, wall, right, lower quadrant
      upper quadrant S31.100 ☑
        with penetration into peritoneal cavity S31.600 ☑
        bite — see Bite, abdomen, wall, right, upper quadrant
        laceration — see Laceration, abdomen, wall, right, upper quadrant
        puncture — see Puncture, abdomen, wall, right, upper quadrant
  alveolar (process) — see Wound, open, oral cavity
  ankle S91.00- ☑
    bite — see Bite, ankle
    laceration — see Laceration, ankle
    puncture — see Puncture, ankle
  antecubital space — see Wound, open, elbow
  anterior chamber, eye — see Wound, open, ocular
  anus S31.839 ☑
    bite S31.835 ☑
    laceration — see Laceration, anus
    puncture — see Puncture, anus
  arm (upper) S41.10- ☑
    with amputation — see Amputation, traumatic, arm
    bite — see Bite, arm
    forearm — see Wound, open, forearm
    laceration — see Laceration, arm
    puncture — see Puncture, arm
  auditory canal (external) (meatus) — see Wound, open, ear
  auricle, ear — see Wound, open, ear
  axilla — see Wound, open, arm
  back (see also Wound, open, thorax, back)
    lower S31.000 ☑
      with penetration into retroperitoneal space S31.001 ☑
      bite — see Bite, back, lower
      laceration — see Laceration, back, lower
      puncture — see Puncture, back, lower
  bite — see Bite
  blood vessel — see Injury, blood vessel
  breast S21.00- ☑
    with amputation — see Amputation, traumatic, breast
    bite — see Bite, breast
    laceration — see Laceration, breast
    puncture — see Puncture, breast
  buttock S31.809 ☑
    bite — see Bite, buttock
    laceration — see Laceration, buttock
    left S31.829 ☑
    puncture — see Puncture, buttock
    right S31.819 ☑
  calf — see Wound, open, leg
  canaliculus lacrimalis — see Wound, open, eyelid
  canthus, eye — see Wound, open, eyelid
  cervical esophagus S11.20 ☑
    bite S11.25 ☑
    laceration — see Laceration, esophagus, traumatic, cervical
    puncture — see Puncture, cervical esophagus
  cheek (external) S01.40- ☑
    bite — see Bite, cheek
    laceration — see Laceration, cheek
    puncture — see Puncture, cheek
    internal — see Wound, open, oral cavity
  chest wall — see Wound, open, thorax
  chin — see Wound, open, head, specified site NEC
  choroid — see Wound, open, ocular
  ciliary body (eye) — see Wound, open, ocular
  clitoris S31.40 ☑
    with amputation — see Amputation, traumatic, clitoris
    bite S31.45 ☑
    laceration — see Laceration, vulva
    puncture — see Puncture, vulva
  conjunctiva — see Wound, open, ocular
  cornea — see Wound, open, ocular
  costal region — see Wound, open, thorax
  Descemet's membrane — see Wound, open, ocular
  digit (s)
    foot — see Wound, open, toe
    hand — see Wound, open, finger

Wound — *continued*

ear (canal) (external) S01.30- ☑
  with amputation — *see* Amputation, traumatic, ear
  bite — *see* Bite, ear
  laceration — *see* Laceration, ear
  puncture — *see* Puncture, ear
  drum S09.2- ☑
elbow S51.00- ☑
  bite — *see* Bite, elbow
  laceration — *see* Laceration, elbow
  puncture — *see* Puncture, elbow
epididymis — *see* Wound, open, testis
epigastric region S31.102 ☑
  with penetration into peritoneal cavity S31.602 ☑
  bite — *see* Bite, abdomen, wall, epigastric region
  laceration — *see* Laceration, abdomen, wall, epigastric region
  puncture — *see* Puncture, abdomen, wall, epigastric region
epiglottis — *see* Wound, open, neck, specified site NEC
esophagus (thoracic) S27.819 ☑
  cervical — *see* Wound, open, cervical esophagus
  laceration S27.813 ☑
  specified type NEC S27.818 ☑
eye — *see* Wound, open, ocular
eyeball — *see* Wound, open, ocular
eyebrow — *see* Wound, open, eyelid
eyelid S01.10- ☑
  bite — *see* Bite, eyelid
  laceration — *see* Laceration, eyelid
  puncture — *see* Puncture, eyelid
face NEC — *see* Wound, open, head, specified site NEC
finger (s) S61.209 ☑
  with
    amputation — *see* Amputation, traumatic, finger
    damage to nail S61.309 ☑
  bite — *see* Bite, finger
  index S61.208 ☑
    with
      damage to nail S61.308 ☑
    left S61.201 ☑
      with
        damage to nail S61.301 ☑
    right S61.200 ☑
      with
        damage to nail S61.300 ☑
  laceration — *see* Laceration, finger
  little S61.208 ☑
    with
      damage to nail S61.308 ☑
    left S61.207 ☑
      with damage to nail S61.307 ☑
    right S61.206 ☑
      with damage to nail S61.306 ☑
  middle S61.208 ☑
    with
      damage to nail S61.308 ☑
    left S61.203 ☑
      with damage to nail S61.303 ☑
    right S61.202 ☑
      with damage to nail S61.302 ☑
  puncture — *see* Puncture, finger
  ring S61.208 ☑
    with
      damage to nail S61.308 ☑
    left S61.205 ☑
      with damage to nail S61.305 ☑
    right S61.204 ☑
      with damage to nail S61.304 ☑
flank — *see* Wound, open, abdomen, wall
foot (except toe(s) alone) S91.30- ☑
  with amputation — *see* Amputation, traumatic, foot
  bite — *see* Bite, foot
  laceration — *see* Laceration, foot
  puncture — *see* Puncture, foot
  toe — *see* Wound, open, toe
forearm S51.80- ☑
  with
    amputation — *see* Amputation, traumatic, forearm
  bite — *see* Bite, forearm
  elbow only — *see* Wound, open, elbow
  laceration — *see* Laceration, forearm
  puncture — *see* Puncture, forearm

Wound — *continued*

forehead — *see* Wound, open, head, specified site NEC
genital organs, external
  with amputation — *see* Amputation, traumatic, genital organs
  bite — *see* Bite, genital organ
  female S31.502 ☑
    vagina S31.40 ☑
    vulva S31.40 ☑
  laceration — *see* Laceration, genital organ
  male S31.501 ☑
    penis S31.20 ☑
    scrotum S31.30 ☑
    testes S31.30 ☑
  puncture — *see* Puncture, genital organ
globe (eye) — *see* Wound, open, ocular
groin — *see* Wound, open, abdomen, wall
gum — *see* Wound, open, oral cavity
hand S61.40- ☑
  with
    amputation — *see* Amputation, traumatic, hand
  bite — *see* Bite, hand
  finger (s) — *see* Wound, open, finger
  laceration — *see* Laceration, hand
  puncture — *see* Puncture, hand
  thumb — *see* Wound, open, thumb
head S01.90 ☑
  bite — *see* Bite, head
  cheek — *see* Wound, open, cheek
  ear — *see* Wound, open, ear
  eyelid — *see* Wound, open, eyelid
  laceration — *see* Laceration, head
  lip — *see* Wound, open, lip
  nose S01.20 ☑
  oral cavity — *see* Wound, open, oral cavity
  puncture — *see* Puncture, head
  scalp — *see* Wound, open, scalp
  specified site NEC S01.80 ☑
  temporomandibular area — *see* Wound, open, cheek
heel — *see* Wound, open, foot
hip S71.00- ☑
  with amputation — *see* Amputation, traumatic, hip
  bite — *see* Bite, hip
  laceration — *see* Laceration, hip
  puncture — *see* Puncture, hip
hymen S31.40 ☑
  bite — *see* Bite, vulva
  laceration — *see* Laceration, vagina
  puncture — *see* Puncture, vagina
hypochondrium S31.109 ☑
  bite — *see* Bite, hypochondrium
  laceration — *see* Laceration, hypochondrium
  puncture — *see* Puncture, hypochondrium
hypogastric region S31.109 ☑
  bite — *see* Bite, hypogastric region
  laceration — *see* Laceration, hypogastric region
  puncture — *see* Puncture, hypogastric region
iliac (region) — *see* Wound, open, inguinal region
inguinal region S31.109 ☑
  bite — *see* Bite, abdomen, wall, lower quadrant
  laceration — *see* Laceration, inguinal region
  puncture — *see* Puncture, inguinal region
instep — *see* Wound, open, foot
interscapular region — *see* Wound, open, thorax, back
intraocular — *see* Wound, open, ocular
iris — *see* Wound, open, ocular
jaw — *see* Wound, open, head, specified site NEC
knee S81.00- ☑
  bite — *see* Bite, knee
  laceration — *see* Laceration, knee
  puncture — *see* Puncture, knee
labium (majus) (minus) — *see* Wound, open, vulva
laceration — *see* Laceration, by site
lacrimal duct — *see* Wound, open, eyelid
larynx S11.019 ☑
  bite — *see* Bite, larynx
  laceration — *see* Laceration, larynx
  puncture — *see* Puncture, larynx
left
  lower quadrant S31.104 ☑
    with penetration into peritoneal cavity S31.604 ☑
    bite — *see* Bite, abdomen, wall, left, lower quadrant
    laceration — *see* Laceration, abdomen, wall, left, lower quadrant

Wound — *continued*

    puncture — *see* Puncture, abdomen, wall, left, lower quadrant
  upper quadrant S31.101 ☑
    with penetration into peritoneal cavity S31.601 ☑
    bite — *see* Bite, abdomen, wall, left, upper quadrant
    laceration — *see* Laceration, abdomen, wall, left, upper quadrant
    puncture — *see* Puncture, abdomen, wall, left, upper quadrant
leg (lower) S81.80- ☑
  with amputation — *see* Amputation, traumatic, leg
  ankle — *see* Wound, open, ankle
  bite — *see* Bite, leg
  foot — *see* Wound, open, foot
  knee — *see* Wound, open, knee
  laceration — *see* Laceration, leg
  puncture — *see* Puncture, leg
  toe — *see* Wound, open, toe
  upper — *see* Wound, open, thigh
lip S01.501 ☑
  bite — *see* Bite, lip
  laceration — *see* Laceration, lip
  puncture — *see* Puncture, lip
loin S31.109 ☑
  bite — *see* Bite, abdomen, wall
  laceration — *see* Laceration, loin
  puncture — *see* Puncture, loin
lower back — *see* Wound, open, back, lower
lumbar region — *see* Wound, open, back, lower
malar region — *see* Wound, open, head, specified site NEC
mammary — *see* Wound, open, breast
mastoid region — *see* Wound, open, head, specified site NEC
mouth — *see* Wound, open, oral cavity
nail
  finger — *see* Wound, open, finger, with damage to nail
  toe — *see* Wound, open, toe, with damage to nail
nape (neck) — *see* Wound, open, neck
nasal (septum) (sinus) — *see* Wound, open, nose
nasopharynx — *see* Wound, open, head, specified site NEC
neck S11.90 ☑
  bite — *see* Bite, neck
  involving
    cervical esophagus S11.20 ☑
    larynx — *see* Wound, open, larynx
    pharynx S11.20 ☑
    thyroid S11.10 ☑
    trachea (cervical) S11.029 ☑
      bite — *see* Bite, trachea
      laceration S11.021 ☑
        with foreign body S11.022 ☑
      puncture S11.023 ☑
        with foreign body S11.024 ☑
  laceration — *see* Laceration, neck
  puncture — *see* Puncture, neck
  specified site NEC S11.80 ☑
  specified type NEC S11.89 ☑
nose (septum) (sinus) S01.20 ☑
  with amputation — *see* Amputation, traumatic, nose
  bite — *see* Bite, nose
  laceration — *see* Laceration, nose
  puncture — *see* Puncture, nose
ocular S05.90 ☑
  avulsion (traumatic enucleation) S05.7- ☑
  eyeball S05.6- ☑
    with foreign body S05.5- ☑
  eyelid — *see* Wound, open, eyelid
  laceration and rupture S05.3- ☑
    with prolapse or loss of intraocular tissue S05.2- ☑
  orbit (penetrating) (with or without foreign body) S05.4- ☑
  periocular area — *see* Wound, open, eyelid
  specified NEC S05.8X- ☑
oral cavity S01.502 ☑
  bite S01.552 ☑
  laceration — *see* Laceration, oral cavity
  puncture — *see* Puncture, oral cavity
orbit — *see* Wound, open, ocular, orbit
palate — *see* Wound, open, oral cavity
palm — *see* Wound, open, hand
pelvis, pelvic (*see also* Wound, open, back, lower)
  girdle — *see* Wound, open, hip

☑ **Additional character required**

Wound — continued
  penetrating — see Puncture, by site
  penis S31.20 ☑
    with amputation — see Amputation, traumatic, penis
    bite S31.25 ☑
    laceration — see Laceration, penis
    puncture — see Puncture, penis
  perineum
    bite — see Bite, perineum
    female S31.502 ☑
    laceration — see Laceration, perineum
    male S31.501 ☑
    puncture — see Puncture, perineum
  periocular area (with or without lacrimal passages) — see Wound, open, eyelid
  periumbilic region S31.105 ☑
    with penetration into peritoneal cavity S31.605 ☑
    bite — see Bite, abdomen, wall, periumbilic region
    laceration — see Laceration, abdomen, wall, periumbilic region
    puncture — see Puncture, abdomen, wall, periumbilic region
  phalanges
    finger — see Wound, open, finger
    toe — see Wound, open, toe
  pharynx S11.20 ☑
  pinna — see Wound, open, ear
  popliteal space — see Wound, open, knee
  prepuce — see Wound, open, penis
  pubic region — see Wound, open, back, lower
  pudendum — see Wound, open, genital organs, external
  puncture wound — see Puncture
  rectovaginal septum — see Wound, open, vagina
  right
    lower quadrant S31.103 ☑
      with penetration into peritoneal cavity S31.603 ☑
      bite — see Bite, abdomen, wall, right, lower quadrant
      laceration — see Laceration, abdomen, wall, right, lower quadrant
      puncture — see Puncture, abdomen, wall, right, lower quadrant
    upper quadrant S31.100 ☑
      with penetration into peritoneal cavity S31.600 ☑
      bite — see Bite, abdomen, wall, right, upper quadrant
      laceration — see Laceration, abdomen, wall, right, upper quadrant
      puncture — see Puncture, abdomen, wall, right, upper quadrant
  sacral region — see Wound, open, back, lower
  sacroiliac region — see Wound, open, back, lower
  salivary gland — see Wound, open, oral cavity
  scalp S01.00 ☑
    bite S01.05 ☑
    laceration — see Laceration, scalp
    puncture — see Puncture, scalp
  scalpel, newborn (birth injury) P15.8
  scapular region — see Wound, open, shoulder
  sclera — see Wound, open, ocular
  scrotum S31.30 ☑
    with amputation — see Amputation, traumatic, scrotum
    bite S31.35 ☑
    laceration — see Laceration, scrotum
    puncture — see Puncture, scrotum
  shin — see Wound, open, leg
  shoulder S41.00- ☑
    with amputation — see Amputation, traumatic, arm
    bite — see Bite, shoulder
    laceration — see Laceration, shoulder
    puncture — see Puncture, shoulder
  skin NOS T14.8
  spermatic cord — see Wound, open, testis
  sternal region — see Wound, open, thorax, front wall
  submaxillary region — see Wound, open, head, specified site NEC
  submental region — see Wound, open, head, specified site NEC
  subungual
    finger (s) — see Wound, open, finger
    toe (s) — see Wound, open, toe
  supraclavicular region — see Wound, open, neck, specified site NEC

Wound — continued
  temple, temporal region — see Wound, open, head, specified site NEC
  temporomandibular area — see Wound, open, cheek
  testis S31.30 ☑
    with amputation — see Amputation, traumatic, testes
    bite S31.35 ☑
    laceration — see Laceration, testis
    puncture — see Puncture, testis
  thigh S71.10- ☑
    with amputation — see Amputation, traumatic, hip
    bite — see Bite, thigh
    laceration — see Laceration, thigh
    puncture — see Puncture, thigh
  thorax, thoracic (wall) S21.90 ☑
    back S21.20- ☑
      with penetration S21.40 ☑
    bite — see Bite, thorax
    breast — see Wound, open, breast
    front S21.10- ☑
      with penetration S21.30 ☑
    laceration — see Laceration, thorax
    puncture — see Puncture, thorax
  throat — see Wound, open, neck
  thumb S61.009 ☑
    with
      amputation — see Amputation, traumatic, thumb
      damage to nail S61.109 ☑
    bite — see Bite, thumb
    laceration — see Laceration, thumb
    left S61.002 ☑
      with
        damage to nail S61.102 ☑
    puncture — see Puncture, thumb
    right S61.001 ☑
      with
        damage to nail S61.101 ☑
  thyroid (gland) — see Wound, open, neck, thyroid
  toe (s) S91.109 ☑
    with
      amputation — see Amputation, traumatic, toe
      damage to nail S91.209 ☑
    bite — see Bite, toe
    great S91.103 ☑
      with
        damage to nail S91.203 ☑
      left S91.102 ☑
        with
          damage to nail S91.202 ☑
      right S91.101 ☑
        with
          damage to nail S91.201 ☑
    laceration — see Laceration, toe
    lesser S91.106 ☑
      with
        damage to nail S91.206 ☑
      left S91.105 ☑
        with
          damage to nail S91.205 ☑
      right S91.104 ☑
        with
          damage to nail S91.204 ☑
    puncture — see Puncture, toe
  tongue — see Wound, open, oral cavity
  trachea (cervical region) — see Wound, open, neck, trachea
  tunica vaginalis — see Wound, open, testis
  tympanum, tympanic membrane S09.2- ☑
    laceration — see Laceration, ear, drum
    puncture — see Puncture, tympanum
  umbilical region — see Wound, open, abdomen, wall, periumbilic region
  uvula — see Wound, open, oral cavity
  vagina S31.40 ☑
    bite S31.45 ☑
    laceration — see Laceration, vagina
    puncture — see Puncture, vagina
  vocal cord S11.039 ☑
    bite — see Bite, vocal cord
    laceration S11.031 ☑
      with foreign body S11.032 ☑
    puncture S11.033 ☑
      with foreign body S11.034 ☑
  vitreous (humor) — see Wound, open, ocular
  vulva S31.40 ☑
    with amputation — see Amputation, traumatic, vulva

Wound — continued
  bite S31.45 ☑
  laceration — see Laceration, vulva
  puncture — see Puncture, vulva
  wrist S61.50- ☑
    bite — see Bite, wrist
    laceration — see Laceration, wrist
    puncture — see Puncture, wrist
Wound, superficial — see Injury (see also specified injury type)
Wright's syndrome G54.0
Wrist — see condition
Wrong drug (by accident) (given in error) — see Table of Drugs and Chemicals, by drug, poisoning
Wry neck — see Torticollis
Wuchereria (bancrofti) infestation B74.0
Wuchereriasis B74.0
Wuchernde Struma Langhans C73

X

Xanthelasma (eyelid) (palpebrarum) H02.60
  left H02.66
    lower H02.65
    upper H02.64
  right H02.63
    lower H02.62
    upper H02.61
Xanthelasmatosis (essential) E78.2
Xanthinuria, hereditary E79.8
Xanthoastrocytoma
  specified site — see Neoplasm, malignant, by site
  unspecified site C71.9
Xanthofibroma — see Neoplasm, connective tissue, benign
Xanthogranuloma D76.3
Xanthoma (s), xanthomatosis (primary) (familial) (hereditary) E75.5
  with
    hyperlipoproteinemia
      Type I E78.3
      Type III E78.2
      Type IV E78.1
      Type V E78.3
  bone (generalisata) C96.5
  cerebrotendinous E75.5
  cutaneotendinous E75.5
  disseminatum (skin) E78.2
  eruptive E78.2
  hypercholesterinemic E78.0
  hypercholesterolemic E78.0
  hyperlipidemic E78.5
  joint E75.5
  multiple (skin) E78.2
  tendon (sheath) E75.5
  tubo-eruptive E78.2
  tuberosum E78.2
  tuberous E78.2
  verrucous, oral mucosa K13.4
Xanthosis R23.8
Xenophobia F40.10
Xeroderma (see also Ichthyosis)
  acquired L85.0
  eyelid H01.149
    left H01.146
      lower H01.145
      upper H01.144
    right H01.143
      lower H01.142
      upper H01.141
  pigmentosum Q82.1
  vitamin A deficiency E50.8
Xerophthalmia (vitamin A deficiency) E50.7
  unrelated to vitamin A deficiency — see Keratoconjunctivitis
Xerosis
  conjunctiva H11.14- ☑
    with Bitot's spots (see also Pigmentation, conjunctiva)
      vitamin A deficiency E50.1
    vitamin A deficiency E50.0
  cornea H18.89- ☑
    with ulceration — see Ulcer, cornea
      vitamin A deficiency E50.3
    vitamin A deficiency E50.2
  cutis L85.3
  skin L85.3
Xerostomia K11.7
Xiphopagus Q89.4

XO syndrome Q96.9
X-ray (of)
  abnormal findings — *see* Abnormal, diagnostic
    imaging
  breast (mammogram) (routine) Z12.31
  chest
    routine (as part of a general medical
      examination) Z00.00
      with abnormal findings Z00.01
    routine (as part of a general medical
      examination) Z00.00
      with abnormal findings Z00.01
XXXXY syndrome Q98.1
XXY syndrome Q98.0

Y

Yaba pox (virus disease) B08.72
Yatapoxvirus B08.70
  specified NEC B08.79
Yawning R06.89
  psychogenic F45.8
Yaws A66.9
  bone lesions A66.6
  butter A66.1
  chancre A66.0
  cutaneous, less than five years after infection A66.2
  early (cutaneous) (macular) (maculopapular)
    (micropapular) (papular) A66.2

Yaws — *continued*
  frambeside A66.2
  skin lesions NEC A66.2
  eyelid A66.2
  ganglion A66.6
  gangosis, gangosa A66.5
  gumma, gummata A66.4
    bone A66.6
  gummatous
    frambeside A66.4
    osteitis A66.6
    periostitis A66.6
  hydrarthrosis (*see also* subcategory M14.8-) A66.6
  hyperkeratosis (early) (late) A66.3
  initial lesions A66.0
  joint lesions (*see also* subcategory M14.8-) A66.6
  juxta-articular nodules A66.7
  late nodular (ulcerated) A66.4
  latent (without clinical manifestations) (with
    positive serology) A66.8
  mother A66.0
  mucosal A66.7
  multiple papillomata A66.1
  nodular, late (ulcerated) A66.4
  osteitis A66.6
  papilloma, plantar or palmar A66.1
  periostitis (hypertrophic) A66.6
  specified NEC A66.7
  ulcers A66.4
  wet crab A66.1
Yeast infection (*see also* Candidiasis) B37.9

Yellow
  atrophy (liver) — *see* Failure, hepatic
  fever — *see* Fever, yellow
  jack — *see* Fever, yellow
  jaundice — *see* Jaundice
  nail syndrome L60.5
Yersiniosis (*see also* Infection, Yersinia)
  extraintestinal A28.2
  intestinal A04.6

Z

Zahorsky's syndrome (herpangina) B08.5
Zellweger's syndrome Q87.89
Zenker's diverticulum (esophagus) K22.5
Ziehen-Oppenheim disease G24.1
Zieve's syndrome K70.0
Zinc
  deficiency, dietary E60
  metabolism disorder E83.2
Zollinger-Ellison syndrome E16.4
Zona — *see* Herpes, zoster
Zoophobia F40.218
Zoster (herpes) — *see* Herpes, zoster
Zygomycosis B46.9
  specified NEC B46.8
Zymotic — *see* condition

☑ **Additional character required**

ICD-10-CM Table of Neoplasms

The list below gives the code numbers for neoplasms by anatomical site. For each site, there are six possible code numbers according to whether the neoplasm in question is malignant, benign, in situ, of uncertain behavior, or of unspecified nature. The description of the neoplasm will often indicate which of the six columns is appropriate; e.g., malignant melanoma of skin, benign fibroadenoma of breast, carcinoma in situ of cervix uteri.

Where such descriptors are not present, the remainder of the Index to Diseases and Injuries should be consulted where guidance is given to the appropriate column for each morphological (histological) variety listed; e.g., Mesonephroma—*see* Neoplasm, malignant; Embryoma—*see also* Neoplasm, uncertain behavior; Disease, Bowen's—*see* Neoplasm, skin, in situ. However, the guidance in the Index to Diseases and Injuries can be overridden if one of the descriptors mentioned above are present; e.g., malignant adenoma of colon is coded to C18.9 and not to D12.6 as the adjective "malignant" overrides the Index entry "Adenoma—*see also* Neoplasm, benign."

Codes listed with a dash -, following the code have a required additional character for laterality. The tabular must be reviewed for the complete code.

Neoplasm Index	Malignant Primary	Malignant Secondary	Ca in situ	Benign	Uncertain Behavior	Unspecified Behavior
Neoplasm, neoplastic	**C80.1**	**C79.9**	**D09.9**	**D36.9**	**D48.9**	**D49.9**
abdomen, abdominal	C76.2	C79.8-	D09.8	D36.7	D48.7	D49.89
cavity	C76.2	C79.8-	D09.8	D36.7	D48.7	D49.89
organ	C76.2	C79.8-	D09.8	D36.7	D48.7	D49.89
viscera	C76.2	C79.8-	D09.8	D36.7	D48.7	D49.89
wall (*see also* Neoplasm, abdomen, wall, skin)	C44.509	C79.2-	D04.5	D23.5	D48.5	D49.2
connective tissue	C49.4	C79.8-	-	D21.4	D48.1	D49.2
skin	C44.509					
basal cell carcinoma	C44.519	-	-	-	-	-
specified type NEC	C44.599	-	-	-	-	-
squamous cell carcinoma	C44.529	-	-	-	-	-
abdominopelvic	C76.8	C79.8-		D36.7	D48.7	D49.89
accessory sinus—*see* Neoplasm, sinus						
acoustic nerve	C72.4-	C79.49	-	D33.3	D43.3	D49.7
adenoid(pharynx) (tissue)	C11.1	C79.89	D00.08	D10.6	D37.05	D49.0
adipose tissue (*see also* Neoplasm, connective tissue)	C49.4	C79.89	-	D21.9	D48.1	D49.2
adnexa(uterine)	C57.4	C79.89	D07.39	D28.7	D39.8	D49.5
adrenal	C74.9-	C79.7-	D09.3	D35.0-	D44.1-	D49.7
capsule	C74.9-	C79.7-	D09.3	D35.0-	D44.1-	D49.7
cortex	C74.0-	C79.7-	D09.3	D35.0-	D44.1-	D49.7
gland	C74.9-	C79.7-	D09.3	D35.0-	D44.1-	D49.7
medulla	C74.1-	C79.7-	D09.3	D35.0-	D44.1-	D49.7
ala nasi(external) (*see also* Neoplasm, skin, nose)	C44.301	C79.2	D04.39	D23.39	D48.5	D49.2
alimentary canal or tract NEC	C26.9	C78.80	D01.9	D13.9	D37.9	D49.0
alveolar	C03.9	C79.89	D00.03	D10.39	D37.09	D49.0
mucosa	C03.9	C79.89	D00.03	D10.39	D37.09	D49.0
lower	C03.1	C79.89	D00.03	D10.39	D37.09	D49.0
upper	C03.0	C79.89	D00.03	D10.39	D37.09	D49.0
ridge or process	C41.1	C79.51	-	D16.5-	D48.0	D49.2
carcinoma	C03.9	C79.8-	-	-	-	-
lower	C03.1	C79.8-	-	-	-	-
upper	C03.0	C79.8-	-	-	-	-
lower	C41.1	C79.51	-	D16.5-	D48.0	D49.2
mucosa	C03.9	C79.89	D00.03	D10.39	D37.09	D49.0
lower	C03.1	C79.89	D00.03	D10.39	D37.09	D49.0
upper	C03.0	C79.89	D00.03	D10.39	D37.09	D49.0
upper	C41.0	C79.51	-	D16.4-	D48.0	D49.2

Neoplasm Index	Malignant Primary	Malignant Secondary	Ca in situ	Benign	Uncertain Behavior	Unspecified Behavior
ridge or process — *continued*						
sulcus	C06.1	C79.89	D00.02	D10.39	D37.09	D49.0
alveolus	C03.9	C79.89	D00.03	D10.39	D37.09	D49.0
lower	C03.1	C79.89	D00.03	D10.39	D37.09	D49.0
upper	C03.0	C79.89	D00.03	D10.39	D37.09	D49.0
ampulla of Vater	C24.1	C78.89	D01.5	D13.5	D37.6	D49.0
ankle NEC	C76.5-	C79.89	D04.7-	D36.7	D48.7	D49.89
anorectum, anorectal(junction)	C21.8	C78.5	D01.3	D12.9	D37.8	D49.0
antecubital fossa or space	C76.4-	C79.89	D04.6-	D36.7	D48.7	D49.89
antrum(Highmore) (maxillary)	C31.0	C78.39	D02.3	D14.0	D38.5	D49.1
pyloric	C16.3	C78.89	D00.2	D13.1	D37.1	D49.0
tympanicum	C30.1	C78.39	D02.3	D14.0	D38.5	D49.1
anus, anal	C21.0	C78.5	D01.3	D12.9	D37.8	D49.0
canal	C21.1	C78.5	D01.3	D12.9	D37.8	D49.0
cloacogenic zone	C21.2	C78.5	D01.3	D12.9	D37.8	D49.0
margin (*see also* Neoplasm, anus, skin)	C44.500	C79.2	D04.5	D23.5	D48.5	D49.2
overlapping lesion with rectosigmoid junction or rectum	C21.8	-	-	-	-	-
skin	C44.500	C79.2	D04.5	D23.5	D48.5	D49.2
basal cell carcinoma	C44.510	-	-	-	-	-
specified type NEC	C44.590	-	-	-	-	-
squamous cell carcinoma	C44.520	-	-	-	-	-
sphincter	C21.1	C78.5	D01.3	D12.9	D37.8	D49.0
aorta(thoracic)	C49.3	C79.89	-	D21.3	D48.1	D49.2
abdominal	C49.4	C79.89	-	D21.4	D48.1	D49.2
aortic body	C75.5	C79.89	-	D35.6	D44.7	D49.7
aponeurosis	C49.9	C79.89	-	D21.9	D48.1	D49.2
palmar	C49.1-	C79.89	-	D21.1-	D48.1	D49.2
plantar	C49.2-	C79.89	-	D21.2-	D48.1	D49.2
appendix	C18.1	C78.5	D01.0	D12.1	D37.3	D49.0
arachnoid	C70.9	C79.49	-	D32.9	D42.9	D49.7
cerebral	C70.0	C79.32	-	D32.0	D42.0	D49.7
spinal	C70.1	C79.49	-	D32.1	D42.1	D49.7
areola	C50.0-	C79.81	D05.-	D24.-	D48.6-	D49.3
arm NEC	C76.4-	C79.89	D04.6-	D36.7	D48.7	D49.89
artery—*see* Neoplasm, connective tissue						
aryepiglottic fold	C13.1	C79.89	D00.08	D10.7	D37.05	D49.0
hypopharyngeal aspect	C13.1	C79.89	D00.08	D10.7	D37.05	D49.0
laryngeal aspect	C32.1	C78.39	D02.0	D14.1	D38.0	D49.1
marginal zone	C13.1	C79.89	D00.08	D10.7	D37.05	D49.0
arytenoid(cartilage)	C32.3	C78.39	D02.0	D14.1	D38.0	D49.1
fold—*see* Neoplasm, aryepiglottic						
associated with transplanted organ	C80.2	-	-	-	-	-
atlas	C41.2	C79.51	-	D16.6	D48.0	D49.2
atrium, cardiac	C38.0	C79.89	-	D15.1	D48.7	D49.89
auditory						
canal(external) (skin) A81	C44.20-	C79.2	D04.2-	D23.2-	D48.5	D49.2
internal	C30.1	C78.39	D02.3	D14.0	D38.5	D49.1
nerve	C72.4-	C79.49	-	D33.3	D43.3	D49.7
tube	C30.1	C78.39	D02.3	D14.0	D38.5	D49.1
opening	C11.2	C79.89	D00.08	D10.6	D37.05	D49.0
auricle, ear (*see also* Neoplasm, skin, ear)	C44.20-	C79.2	D04.2-	D23.2-	D48.5	D49.2

auricular - bone(periosteum)

Neoplasm Index	Malignant Primary	Malignant Secondary	Ca in situ	Benign	Uncertain Behavior	Unspecified Behavior
auricular canal(external) (see also Neoplasm, skin, ear)	C44.20-	C79.2	D04.2-	D23.2-	D48.5	D49.2
internal	C30.1	C78.39	D02.3	D14.0	D38.5	D49.2
autonomic nerve or nervous system NEC (see also Neoplasm, nerve, peripheral)						
axilla, axillary	C76.1	C79.89	D09.8	D36.7	D48.7	D49.89
fold (see also Neoplasm, skin, trunk)	C44.509	C79.2	D04.5	D23.5	D48.5	D49.2
back NEC	C76.8	C79.89	D04.5	D36.7	D48.7	D49.89
Bartholin's gland	C51.0	C79.82	D07.1	D28.0	D39.8	D49.5
basal ganglia	C71.0	C79.31	-	D33.0	D43.0	D49.6
basis pedunculi	C71.7	C79.31	-	D33.1	D43.1	D49.6
bile or biliary(tract)	C24.9	C78.89	D01.5	D13.5	D37.6	D49.0
canaliculi(biliferi) (intrahepatic)	C22.1	C78.7	D01.5	D13.4	D37.6	D49.0
canals, interlobular	C22.1	C78.89	D01.5	D13.4	D37.6	D49.0
duct or passage(common) (cystic) (extrahepatic)	C24.0	C78.89	D01.5	D13.5	D37.6	D49.0
interlobular	C22.1	C78.89	D01.5	D13.4	D37.6	D49.0
intrahepatic	C22.1	C78.7	D01.5	D13.4	D37.6	D49.0
and extrahepatic	C24.8	C78.89	D01.5	D13.5	D37.6	D49.0
bladder(urinary)	C67.9	C79.11	D09.0	D30.3	D41.4	D49.4
dome	C67.1	C79.11	D09.0	D30.3	D41.4	D49.4
neck	C67.5	C79.11	D09.0	D30.3	D41.4	D49.4
orifice	C67.9	C79.11	D09.0	D30.3	D41.4	D49.4
ureteric	C67.6	C79.11	D09.0	D30.3	D41.4	D49.4
urethral	C67.5	C79.11	D09.0	D30.3	D41.4	D49.4
overlapping lesion	C67.8	-	-	-	-	-
sphincter	C67.8	C79.11	D09.0	D30.3	D41.4	D49.4
trigone	C67.0	C79.11	D09.0	D30.3	D41.4	D49.4
urachus	C67.7	C79.11	D09.0	D30.3	D41.4	D49.4
wall	C67.9	C79.11	D09.0	D30.3	D41.4	D49.4
anterior	C67.3	C79.11	D09.0	D30.3	D41.4	D49.4
lateral	C67.2	C79.11	D09.0	D30.3	D41.4	D49.4
posterior	C67.4	C79.11	D09.0	D30.3	D41.4	D49.4
blood vessel—see Neoplasm, connective tissue						
bone(periosteum)	C41.9	C79.51	-	D16.9-	D48.0	D49.2
acetabulum	C41.4	C79.51	-	D16.8-	D48.0	D49.2
ankle	C40.3-	C79.51	-	D16.3-	-	-
arm NEC	C40.0-	C79.51	-	D16.0-	-	-
astragalus	C40.3-	C79.51	-	D16.3-	-	-
atlas	C41.2	C79.51	-	D16.6-	D48.0	D49.2
axis	C41.2	C79.51	-	D16.6-	D48.0	D49.2
back NEC	C41.2	C79.51	-	D16.6-	D48.0	D49.2
calcaneus	C40.3-	C79.51	-	D16.3-	-	-
calvarium	C41.0	C79.51	-	D16.4-	D48.0	D49.2
carpus(any)	C40.1-	C79.51	-	D16.1-	-	-
cartilage NEC	C41.9	C79.51	-	D16.9-	D48.0	D49.2
clavicle	C41.3	C79.51	-	D16.7-	D48.0	D49.2
clivus	C41.0	C79.51	-	D16.4-	D48.0	D49.2
coccygeal vertebra	C41.4	C79.51	-	D16.8-	D48.0	D49.2
coccyx	C41.4	C79.51	-	D16.8-	D48.0	D49.2
costal cartilage	C41.3	C79.51	-	D16.7-	D48.0	D49.2
costovertebral joint	C41.3	C79.51	-	D16.7-	D48.0	D49.2
cranial	C41.0	C79.51	-	D16.4-	D48.0	D49.2
cuboid	C40.3-	C79.51	-	D16.3-	-	-
cuneiform	C41.9	C79.51	-	D16.9-	D48.0	D49.2
elbow	C40.0-	C79.51	-	D16.0-	-	-

Neoplasm Index	Malignant Primary	Malignant Secondary	Ca in situ	Benign	Uncertain Behavior	Unspecified Behavior
bone(periosteum) — continued						
ethmoid(labyrinth)	C41.0	C79.51	-	D16.4-	D48.0	D49.2
face	C41.0	C79.51	-	D16.4-	D48.0	D49.2
femur(any part)	C40.2-	C79.51	-	D16.2-	-	-
fibula(any part)	C40.2-	C79.51	-	D16.2-	-	-
finger(any)	C40.1-	C79.51	-	D16.1-	-	-
foot	C40.3-	C79.51	-	D16.3-	-	-
forearm	C40.0-	C79.51	-	D16.0-	-	-
frontal	C41.0	C79.51	-	D16.4-	D48.0	D49.2
hand	C40.1-	C79.51	-	D16.1-	-	-
heel	C40.3-	C79.51	-	D16.3-	-	-
hip	C41.4	C79.51	-	D16.8-	D48.0	D49.2
humerus(any part)	C40.0-	C79.51	-	D16.0-	-	-
hyoid	C41.0	C79.51	-	D16.4-	D48.0	D49.2
ilium	C41.4	C79.51	-	D16.8-	D48.0	D49.2
innominate	C41.4	C79.51	-	D16.8-	D48.0	D49.2
intervertebral cartilage or disc	C41.2	C79.51	-	D16.6-	D48.0	D49.2
ischium	C41.4	C79.51	-	D16.8-	D48.0	D49.2
jaw(lower)	C41.1	C79.51	-	D16.5-	D48.0	D49.2
knee	C40.2-	C79.51	-	D16.2-	-	-
leg NEC	C40.2-	C79.51	-	D16.2-	-	-
limb NEC	C40.9-	C79.51	-	D16.9-	-	-
lower(long bones)	C40.2-	C79.51	-	D16.2-	-	-
short bones	C40.3-	C79.51	-	D16.3-	-	-
upper(long bones)	C40.0-	C79.51	-	D16.0-	-	-
short bones	C40.1-	C79.51	-	D16.1-	-	-
malar	C41.0	C79.51	-	D16.4-	D48.0	D49.2
mandible	C41.1	C79.51	-	D16.5-	D48.0	D49.2
marrow NEC(any bone)	C96.9	C79.52	-	-	D47.9	D49.89
mastoid	C41.0	C79.51	-	D16.4-	D48.0	D49.2
maxilla, maxillary(superior)	C41.0	C79.51	-	D16.4-	D48.0	D49.2
inferior	C41.1	C79.51	-	D16.5-	D48.0	D49.2
metacarpus(any)	C40.1-	C79.51	-	D16.1-	-	-
metatarsus(any)	C40.3-	C79.51	-	D16.3-	-	-
overlapping sites	C40.8-	-	-	-	-	-
navicular						
ankle	C40.3-	C79.51	-	-	-	-
hand	C40.1-	C79.51	-	-	-	-
nose, nasal	C41.0	C79.51	-	D16.4-	D48.0	D49.2
occipital	C41.0	C79.51	-	D16.4-	D48.0	D49.2
orbit	C41.0	C79.51	-	D16.4-	D48.0	D49.2
parietal	C41.0	C79.51	-	D16.4-	D48.0	D49.2
patella	C40.2-	C79.51	-	-	-	-
pelvic	C41.4	C79.51	-	D16.8	D48.0	D49.2
phalanges						
foot	C40.3-	C79.51	-	-	-	-
hand	C40.1-	C79.51	-	-	-	-
pubic	C41.4	C79.51	-	D16.8	D48.0	D49.2
radius(any part)	C40.0-	C79.51	-	D16.0-	-	-
rib	C41.3	C79.51	-	D16.7	D48.0	D49.2
sacral vertebra	C41.4	C79.51	-	D16.8	D48.0	D49.2
sacrum	C41.4	C79.51	-	D16.8	D48.0	D49.2
scaphoid	-	-				
of ankle	C40.3-	C79.51	-	-	-	-
of hand	C40.1-	C79.51	-	-	-	-
scapula(any part)	C40.0-	C79.51	-	D16.0-	-	-
sella turcica	C41.0	C79.51	-	D16.4-	D48.0	D49.2
shoulder	C40.0-	C79.51	-	D16.0-	-	-
skull	C41.0	C79.51	-	D16.4-	D48.0	D49.2
sphenoid	C41.0	C79.51	-	D16.4-	D48.0	D49.2
spine, spinal(column)	C41.2	C79.51	-	D16.6	D48.0	D49.2

Neoplasm Index	Malignant Primary	Malignant Secondary	Ca in situ	Benign	Uncertain Behavior	Unspecified Behavior
bone(periosteum) — *continued*						
spine, spinal(column) — *continued*						
coccyx	C41.4	C79.51	-	D16.8	D48.0	D49.2
sacrum	C41.4	C79.51	-	D16.8	D48.0	D49.2
sternum	C41.3	C79.51	-	D16.7	D48.0	D49.2
tarsus(any)	C40.3-	C79.51	-	-	-	-
temporal	C41.0	C79.51	-	D16.4-	D48.0	D49.2
thumb	C40.1-	C79.51	-	-	-	-
tibia(any part)	C40.2-	C79.51	-	-	-	-
toe(any)	C40.3-	C79.51	-	-	-	-
trapezium	C40.1-	C79.51	-	-	-	-
trapezoid	C40.1-	C79.51	-	-	-	-
turbinate	C41.0	C79.51	-	D16.4-	D48.0	D49.2
ulna(any part)	C40.0-	C79.51	-	D16.0-	-	-
unciform	C40.1-	C79.51	-	-	-	-
vertebra(column)	C41.2	C79.51	-	D16.6	D48.0	D49.2
coccyx	C41.4	C79.51	-	D16.8	D48.0	D49.2
sacrum	C41.4	C79.51	-	D16.8	D48.0	D49.2
vomer	C41.0	C79.51	-	D16.4-	D48.0	D49.2
wrist	C40.1-	C79.51	-	-	-	-
xiphoid process	C41.3	C79.51	-	D16.7	D48.0	D49.2
zygomatic	C41.0	C79.51	-	D16.4-	D48.0	D49.2
book-leaf(mouth)	C06.89	C79.89	D00.00	D10.39	D37.09	D49.0
bowel—*see* Neoplasm, intestine						
brachial plexus	C47.1-	C79.89	-	D36.12	D48.2	D49.2
brain NEC	C71.9	C79.31	-	D33.2	D43.2	D49.6
basal ganglia	C71.0	C79.31	-	D33.0	D43.0	D49.6
cerebellopontine angle	C71.6	C79.31	-	D33.1	D43.1	D49.6
cerebellum NOS	C71.6	C79.31	-	D33.1	D43.1	D49.6
cerebrum	C71.0	C79.31	-	D33.0	D43.0	D49.6
choroid plexus	C71.7	C79.31	-	D33.1	D43.1	D49.6
corpus callosum	C71.8	C79.31	-	D33.2	D43.2	D49.6
corpus striatum	C71.0	C79.31	-	D33.0	D43.0	D49.6
cortex(cerebral)	C71.0	C79.31	-	D33.0	D43.0	D49.6
frontal lobe	C71.1	C79.31	-	D33.0	D43.0	D49.6
globus pallidus	C71.0	C79.31	-	D33.0	D43.0	D49.6
hippocampus	C71.2	C79.31	-	D33.0	D43.0	D49.6
hypothalamus	C71.0	C79.31	-	D33.0	D43.0	D49.6
internal capsule	C71.0	C79.31	-	D33.0	D43.0	D49.6
medulla oblongata	C71.7	C79.31	-	D33.1	D43.1	D49.6
meninges	C70.0	C79.32	-	D32.0	D42.0	D49.7
midbrain	C71.7	C79.31	-	D33.1	D43.1	D49.6
occipital lobe	C71.4	C79.31	-	D33.0	D43.0	D49.6
overlapping lesion	C71.8	C79.31	-	-	-	-
parietal lobe	C71.3	C79.31	-	D33.0	D43.0	D49.6
peduncle	C71.7	C79.31	-	D33.1	D43.1	D49.6
pons	C71.7	C79.31	-	D33.1	D43.1	D49.6
stem	C71.7	C79.31	-	D33.1	D43.1	D49.6
tapetum	C71.8	C79.31	-	D33.2	D43.2	D49.6
temporal lobe	C71.2	C79.31	-	D33.0	D43.0	D49.6
thalamus	C71.0	C79.31	-	D33.0	D43.0	D49.6
uncus	C71.2	C79.31	-	D33.0	D43.0	D49.6
ventricle(floor)	C71.5	C79.31	-	D33.0	D43.0	D49.6
fourth	C71.7	C79.31	-	D33.1	D43.1	D49.6
branchial(cleft) (cyst) (vestiges)	C10.4	C79.89	D00.08	D10.5	D37.05	D49.0
breast(connective tissue) (glandular tissue) (soft parts)	C50.9-	C79.81	D05.-	D24.-	D48.6-	D49.3
areola	C50.0-	C79.81	D05.-	D24.-	D48.6-	D49.3
axillary tail	C50.6-	C79.81	D05.-	D24.-	D48.6-	D49.3

Neoplasm Index	Malignant Primary	Malignant Secondary	Ca in situ	Benign	Uncertain Behavior	Unspecified Behavior
breast(connective tissue) (glandular tissue) (soft parts) — *continued*						
central portion	C50.1-	C79.81	D05.-	D24.-	D48.6-	D49.3
inner	C50.8-	C79.81	D05.-	D24.-	D48.6-	D49.3
lower	C50.8-	C79.81	D05.-	D24.-	D48.6-	D49.3
lower-inner quadrant	C50.3-	C79.81	D05.-	D24.-	D48.6-	D49.3
lower-outer quadrant	C50.5-	C79.81	D05.-	D24.-	D48.6-	D49.3
mastectomy site(skin) (*see also* Neoplasm, breast, skin)	C44.501	C79.2	-	-	-	-
specified as breast tissue	C50.8-	C79.81	-	-	-	-
midline	C50.8-	C79.81	D05.-	D24.-	D48.6-	D49.3
nipple	C50.0-	C79.81	D05.-	D24.-	D48.6-	D49.3
outer	C50.8-	C79.81	D05.-	D24.-	D48.6-	D49.3
overlapping lesion	C50.8-	-	-	-	-	-
skin	C44.501	C79.2	D04.5	D23.5	D48.5	D49.2
basal cell carcinoma	C44.511	-	-	-	-	-
specified type NEC	C44.591	-	-	-	-	-
squamous cell carcinoma	C44.521	-	-	-	-	-
tail(axillary)	C50.6-	C79.81	D05.-	D24.-	D48.6-	D49.3
upper	C50.8-	C79.81	D05.-	D24.-	D48.6-	D49.3
upper-inner quadrant	C50.2-	C79.81	D05.-	D24.-	D48.6-	D49.3
upper-outer quadrant	C50.4-	C79.81	D05.-	D24.-	D48.6-	D49.3
broad ligament	C57.1	C79.82	D07.39	D28.2	D39.8	D49.5
bronchiogenic, bronchogenic(lung)	C34.9-	C78.0-	D02.2-	D14.3-	D38.1	D49.1
bronchiole	C34.9-	C78.0-	D02.2-	D14.3-	D38.1	D49.1
bronchus	C34.9-	C78.0-	D02.2-	D14.3-	D38.1	D49.1
carina	C34.0-	C78.0-	D02.2-	D14.3-	D38.1	D49.1
lower lobe of lung	C34.3-	C78.0-	D02.2-	D14.3-	D38.1	D49.1
main	C34.0-	C78.0-	D02.2-	D14.3-	D38.1	D49.1
middle lobe of lung	C34.2	C78.0-	D02.21	D14.31	D38.1	D49.1
overlapping lesion	C34.8-	-	-	-	-	-
upper lobe of lung	C34.1-	C78.0-	D02.2-	D14.3-	D38.1	D49.1
brow	C44.309	C79.2	D04.39	D23.39	D48.5	D49.2
basal cell carcinoma	C44.319	-	-	-	-	-
specified type NEC	C44.399	-	-	-	-	-
squamous cell carcinoma	C44.329	-	-	-	-	-
buccal(cavity)	C06.9	C79.89	D00.00	D10.39	D37.09	D49.0
commissure	C06.0	C79.89	D00.02	D10.39	D37.09	D49.0
groove(lower) (upper)	C06.1	C79.89	D00.02	D10.39	D37.09	D49.0
mucosa	C06.0	C79.89	D00.02	D10.39	D37.09	D49.0
sulcus(lower) (upper)	C06.1	C79.89	D00.02	D10.39	D37.09	D49.0
bulbourethral gland	C68.0	C79.19	D09.19	D30.4	D41.3	D49.5
bursa—*see* Neoplasm, connective tissue						
buttock NEC	C76.3	C79.89	D04.5	D36.7	D48.7	D49.89
calf	C76.5-	C79.89	D04.7-	D36.7	D48.7	D49.89
calvarium	C41.0	C79.51	-	D16.4-	D48.0	D49.2
calyx, renal	C65.-	C79.0-	D09.19	D30.1-	D41.1-	D49.5
canal						
anal	C21.1	C78.5	D01.3	D12.9	D37.8	D49.0
auditory(external) (*see also* Neoplasm, skin, ear)	C44.20-	C79.2	D04.2-	D23.2-	D48.5	D49.2
auricular(external) (*see also* Neoplasm, skin, ear)	C44.20-	C79.2	D04.2-	D23.2-	D48.5	D49.2
canaliculi, biliary(biliferi) (intrahepatic)	C22.1	C78.7	D01.5	D13.4	D37.6	D49.0

Neoplasm Index	Malignant Primary	Malignant Secondary	Ca in situ	Benign	Uncertain Behavior	Unspecified Behavior
canthus(eye) (inner) (outer)	C44.10-	C79.2	D04.1-	D23.1-	D48.5	D49.2
basal cell carcinoma	C44.11-	-	-	-	-	-
specified type NEC	C44.19-	-	-	-	-	-
squamous cell carcinoma	C44.12-	-	-	-	-	-
capillary—see Neoplasm, connective tissue						
caput coli	C18.0	C78.5	D01.0	D12.0	D37.4	D49.0
carcinoid—see Tumor, carcinoid						
cardia(gastric)	C16.0	C78.89	D00.2	D13.1	D37.1	D49.0
cardiac orifice(stomach)	C16.0	C78.89	D00.2	D13.1	D37.1	D49.0
cardio-esophageal junction	C16.0	C78.89	D00.2	D13.1	D37.1	D49.0
cardio-esophagus	C16.0	C78.89	D00.2	D13.1	D37.1	D49.0
carina(bronchus)	C34.0-	C78.0-	D02.2-	D14.3-	D38.1	D49.1
carotid(artery)	C49.0	C79.89	-	D21.0	D48.1	D49.2
body	C75.4	C79.89	-	D35.5	D44.6	D49.7
carpus(any bone)	C40.1-	C79.51	-	D16.1-	-	-
cartilage(articular) (joint) NEC (see also Neoplasm, bone)	C41.9	C79.51	-	D16.9-	D48.0	D49.2
arytenoid	C32.3	C78.39	D02.0	D14.1	D38.0	D49.1
auricular	C49.0	C79.89	-	D21.0	D48.1	D49.2
bronchi	C34.0-	C78.39	-	D14.3-	D38.1	D49.1
costal	C41.3	C79.51	-	D16.7	D48.0	D49.2
cricoid	C32.3	C78.39	D02.0	D14.1	D38.0	D49.1
cuneiform	C32.3	C78.39	D02.0	D14.1	D38.0	D49.1
ear(external)	C49.0	C79.89	-	D21.0	D48.1	D49.2
ensiform	C41.3	C79.51	-	D16.7	D48.0	D49.2
epiglottis	C32.1	C78.39	D02.0	D14.1	D38.0	D49.1
anterior surface	C10.1	C79.89	D00.08	D10.5	D37.05	D49.0
eyelid	C49.0	C79.89	-	D21.0	D48.1	D49.2
intervertebral	C41.2	C79.51	-	D16.6	D48.0	D49.2
larynx, laryngeal	C32.3	C78.39	D02.0	D14.1	D38.0	D49.1
nose, nasal	C30.0	C78.39	D02.3	D14.0	D38.5	D49.1
pinna	C49.0	C79.89	-	D21.0	D48.1	D49.2
rib	C41.3	C79.51	-	D16.7	D48.0	D49.2
semilunar(knee)	C40.2-	C79.51	-	D16.2-	D48.0	D49.2
thyroid	C32.3	C78.39	D02.0	D14.1	D38.0	D49.1
trachea	C33	C78.39	D02.1	D14.2	D38.1	D49.1
cauda equina	C72.1	C79.49	-	D33.4	D43.4	D49.7
cavity						
buccal	C06.9	C79.89	D00.00	D10.30	D37.09	D49.0
nasal	C30.0	C78.39	D02.3	D14.0	D38.5	D49.1
oral	C06.9	C79.89	D00.00	D10.30	D37.09	D49.0
peritoneal	C48.2	C78.6	-	D20.1	D48.4	D49.0
tympanic	C30.1	C78.39	D02.3	D14.0	D38.5	D49.1
cecum	C18.0	C78.5	D01.0	D12.0	D37.4	D49.0
central nervous system	C72.9	C79.40	-	-	-	-
cerebellopontine(angle)	C71.6	C79.31	-	D33.1	D43.1	D49.6
cerebellum, cerebellar	C71.6	C79.31	-	D33.1	D43.1	D49.6
cerebrum, cerebral(cortex) (hemisphere) (white matter)	C71.0	C79.31	-	D33.0	D43.0	D49.6
meninges	C70.0	C79.32	-	D32.0	D42.0	D49.7
peduncle	C71.7	C79.31	-	D33.1	D43.1	D49.6
ventricle	C71.5	C79.31	-	D33.0	D43.0	D49.6
fourth	C71.7	C79.31	-	D33.1	D43.1	D49.6
cervical region	C76.0	C79.89	D09.8	D36.7	D48.7	D49.89
cervix(cervical) (uteri) (uterus)	C53.9	C79.82	D06.9	D26.0	D39.0	D49.5
canal	C53.0	C79.82	D06.0	D26.0	D39.0	D49.5

Neoplasm Index	Malignant Primary	Malignant Secondary	Ca in situ	Benign	Uncertain Behavior	Unspecified Behavior
cervix(cervical) (uteri) (uterus) — continued						
endocervix(canal) (gland)	C53.0	C79.82	D06.0	D26.0	D39.0	D49.5
exocervix	C53.1	C79.82	D06.1	D26.0	D39.0	D49.5
external os	C53.1	C79.82	D06.1	D26.0	D39.0	D49.5
internal os	C53.0	C79.82	D06.0	D26.0	D39.0	D49.5
nabothian gland	C53.0	C79.82	D06.0	D26.0	D39.0	D49.5
overlapping lesion	C53.8	-	-	-	-	-
squamocolumnar junction	C53.8	C79.82	D06.7	D26.0	D39.0	D49.5
stump	C53.8	C79.82	D06.7	D26.0	D39.0	D49.5
cheek	C76.0	C79.89	D09.8	D36.7	D48.7	D49.89
external	C44.309	C79.2	D04.39	D23.39	D48.5	D49.2
basal cell carcinoma	C44.319	-	-	-	-	-
specified type NEC	C44.399	-	-	-	-	-
squamous cell carcinoma	C44.329	-	-	-	-	-
inner aspect	C06.0	C79.89	D00.02	D10.39	D37.09	D49.0
internal	C06.0	C79.89	D00.02	D10.39	D37.09	D49.0
mucosa	C06.0	C79.89	D00.02	D10.39	D37.09	D49.0
chest(wall) NEC	C76.1	C79.89	D09.8	D36.7	D48.7	D49.89
chiasma opticum	C72.3-	C79.49	-	D33.3	D43.3	D49.7
chin	C44.309	C79.2	D04.39	D23.39	D48.5	D49.2
basal cell carcinoma	C44.319	-	-	-	-	-
specified type NEC	C44.399	-	-	-	-	-
squamous cell carcinoma	C44.329	-	-	-	-	-
choana	C11.3	C79.89	D00.08	D10.6	D37.05	D49.0
cholangiole	C22.1	C78.89	D01.5	D13.4	D37.6	D49.0
choledochal duct	C24.0	C78.89	D01.5	D13.5	D37.6	D49.0
choroid	C69.3-	C79.49	D09.2-	D31.3-	D48.7	D49.81
plexus	C71.5	C79.31	-	D33.0	D43.0	D49.6
ciliary body	C69.4-	C79.49	D09.2-	D31.4-	D48.7	D49.89
clavicle	C41.3	C79.51	-	D16.7	D48.0	D49.2
clitoris	C51.2	C79.82	D07.1	D28.0	D39.8	D49.5
clivus	C41.0	C79.51	-	D16.4-	D48.0	D49.2
cloacogenic zone	C21.2	C78.5	D01.3	D12.9	D37.8	D49.0
coccygeal						
body or glomus	C49.5	C79.89	-	D21.5	D48.1	D49.2
vertebra	C41.4	C79.51	-	D16.8	D48.0	D49.2
coccyx	C41.4	C79.51	-	D16.8	D48.0	D49.2
colon (see also Neoplasm, intestine, large)	C18.9	C78.5	-	-	-	-
with rectum	C19	C78.5	D01.1	D12.7	D37.5	D49.0
column, spinal—see Neoplasm, spine						
columnella (see also Neoplasm, skin, face)	C44.390	C79.2	D04.39	D23.39	D48.5	D49.2
commissure						
labial, lip	C00.6	C79.89	D00.01	D10.39	D37.01	D49.0
laryngeal	C32.0	C78.39	D02.0	D14.1	D38.0	D49.1
common(bile) duct	C24.0	C78.89	D01.5	D13.5	D37.6	D49.0
concha (see also Neoplasm, skin, ear)	C44.20-	C79.2	D04.2-	D23.2-	D48.5	D49.2
nose	C30.0	C78.39	D02.3	D14.0	D38.5	D49.1
conjunctiva	C69.0-	C79.49	D09.2-	D31.0-	D48.7	D49.89

Neoplasm Index	Malignant Primary	Malignant Secondary	Ca in situ	Benign	Uncertain Behavior	Unspecified Behavior
connective tissue NEC	C49.9	C79.89	-	D21.9	D48.1	D49.2

Note: For neoplasms of connective tissue(blood vessel, bursa, fascia, ligament, muscle, peripheral nerves, sympathetic and parasympathetic nerves and ganglia, synovia, tendon, etc.) or of morphological types that indicate connective tissue, code according to the list under "Neoplasm, connective tissue". For sites that do not appear in this list, code to neoplasm of that site; e.g., fibrosarcoma, pancreas (C25.9)

Note: Morphological types that indicate connective tissue appear in their proper place in the alphabetic index with the instruction "see Neoplasm, connective tissue ...."

Neoplasm Index	Malignant Primary	Malignant Secondary	Ca in situ	Benign	Uncertain Behavior	Unspecified Behavior
abdomen	C49.4	C79.89	-	D21.4	D48.1	D49.2
abdominal wall	C49.4	C79.89	-	D21.4	D48.1	D49.2
ankle	C49.2-	C79.89	-	D21.2-	D48.1	D49.2
antecubital fossa or space	C49.1-	C79.89	-	D21.1-	D48.1	D49.2
arm	C49.1-	C79.89	-	D21.1-	D48.1	D49.2
auricle(ear)	C49.0	C79.89	-	D21.0	D48.1	D49.2
axilla	C49.3	C79.89	-	D21.3	D48.1	D49.2
back	C49.6	C79.89	-	D21.6	D48.1	D49.2
breast—see Neoplasm, breast						
buttock	C49.5	C79.89	-	D21.5	D48.1	D49.2
calf	C49.2-	C79.89	-	D21.2-	D48.1	D49.2
cervical region	C49.0	C79.89	-	D21.0	D48.1	D49.2
cheek	C49.0	C79.89	-	D21.0	D48.1	D49.2
chest(wall)	C49.3	C79.89	-	D21.3	D48.1	D49.2
chin	C49.0	C79.89	-	D21.0	D48.1	D49.2
diaphragm	C49.3	C79.89	-	D21.3	D48.1	D49.2
ear(external)	C49.0	C79.89	-	D21.0	D48.1	D49.2
elbow	C49.1-	C79.89	-	D21.1-	D48.1	D49.2
extrarectal	C49.5	C79.89	-	D21.5	D48.1	D49.2
extremity	C49.9	C79.89	-	D21.9	D48.1	D49.2
lower	C49.2-	C79.89	-	D21.2-	D48.1	D49.2
upper	C49.1-	C79.89	-	D21.1-	D48.1	D49.2
eyelid	C49.0	C79.89	-	D21.0	D48.1	D49.2
face	C49.0	C79.89	-	D21.0	D48.1	D49.2
finger	C49.1-	C79.89	-	D21.1-	D48.1	D49.2
flank	C49.6	C79.89	-	D21.6	D48.1	D49.2
foot	C49.2-	C79.89	-	D21.2-	D48.1	D49.2
forearm	C49.1-	C79.89	-	D21.1-	D48.1	D49.2
forehead	C49.0	C79.89	-	D21.0	D48.1	D49.2
gastric	C49.4	C79.89	-	D21.4	D48.1	D49.2
gastrointestinal	C49.4	C79.89	-	D21.4	D48.1	D49.2
gluteal region	C49.5	C79.89	-	D21.5	D48.1	D49.2
great vessels NEC	C49.3	C79.89	-	D21.3	D48.1	D49.2
groin	C49.5	C79.89	-	D21.5	D48.1	D49.2
hand	C49.1-	C79.89	-	D21.1-	D48.1	D49.2
head	C49.0	C79.89	-	D21.0	D48.1	D49.2
heel	C49.2-	C79.89	-	D21.2-	D48.1	D49.2
hip	C49.2-	C79.89	-	D21.2-	D48.1	D49.2
hypochondrium	C49.4	C79.89	-	D21.4	D48.1	D49.2
iliopsoas muscle	C49.5	C79.89	-	D21.5	D48.1	D49.2
infraclavicular region	C49.3	C79.89	-	D21.3	D48.1	D49.2
inguinal(canal) (region)	C49.5	C79.89	-	D21.5	D48.1	D49.2
intestinal	C49.4	C79.89	-	D21.4	D48.1	D49.2
intrathoracic	C49.3	C79.89	-	D21.3	D48.1	D49.2
ischiorectal fossa	C49.5	C79.89	-	D21.5	D48.1	D49.2
jaw	C03.9	C79.89	D00.03	D10.39	D48.1	D49.0
knee	C49.2-	C79.89	-	D21.2-	D48.1	D49.2
leg	C49.2-	C79.89	-	D21.2-	D48.1	D49.2
limb NEC	C49.9	C79.89	-	D21.9	D48.1	D49.2
lower	C49.2-	C79.89	-	D21.2-		

Neoplasm Index	Malignant Primary	Malignant Secondary	Ca in situ	Benign	Uncertain Behavior	Unspecified Behavior
connective tissue NEC — continued						
limb NEC — continued						
upper	C49.1-	C79.89	-	D21.1-	D48.1	D49.2
nates	C49.5	C79.89	-	D21.5	D48.1	D49.2
neck	C49.0	C79.89	-	D21.0	D48.1	D49.2
orbit	C69.6-	C79.49	D09.2-	D31.6-	D48.1	D49.89
overlapping lesion	C49.8	-	-	-	-	-
pararectal	C49.5	C79.89	-	D21.5	D48.1	D49.2
para-urethral	C49.5	C79.89	-	D21.5	D48.1	D49.2
paravaginal	C49.5	C79.89	-	D21.5	D48.1	D49.2
pelvis(floor)	C49.5	C79.89	-	D21.5	D48.1	D49.2
pelvo-abdominal	C49.8	C79.89	-	D21.6	D48.1	D49.2
perineum	C49.5	C79.89	-	D21.5	D48.1	D49.2
perirectal(tissue)	C49.5	C79.89	-	D21.5	D48.1	D49.2
periurethral(tissue)	C49.5	C79.89	-	D21.5	D48.1	D49.2
popliteal fossa or space	C49.2-	C79.89	-	D21.2-	D48.1	D49.2
presacral	C49.5	C79.89	-	D21.5	D48.1	D49.2
psoas muscle	C49.4	C79.89	-	D21.4	D48.1	D49.2
pterygoid fossa	C49.0	C79.89	-	D21.0	D48.1	D49.2
rectovaginal septum or wall	C49.5	C79.89	-	D21.5	D48.1	D49.2
rectovesical	C49.5	C79.89	-	D21.5	D48.1	D49.2
retroperitoneum	C48.0	C78.6	-	D20.0	D48.3	D49.0
sacrococcygeal region	C49.5	C79.89	-	D21.5	D48.1	D49.2
scalp	C49.0	C79.89	-	D21.0	D48.1	D49.2
scapular region	C49.3	C79.89	-	D21.3	D48.1	D49.2
shoulder	C49.1-	C79.89	-	D21.1-	D48.1	D49.2
skin(dermis) NEC (see also Neoplasm, skin, by site)	C44.90	C79.2	D04.9	D23.9	D48.5	D49.2
stomach	C49.4	C79.89	-	D21.4	D48.1	D49.2
submental	C49.0	C79.89	-	D21.0	D48.1	D49.2
supraclavicular region	C49.0	C79.89	-	D21.0	D48.1	D49.2
temple	C49.0	C79.89	-	D21.0	D48.1	D49.2
temporal region	C49.0	C79.89	-	D21.0	D48.1	D49.2
thigh	C49.2-	C79.89	-	D21.2-	D48.1	D49.2
thoracic(duct) (wall)	C49.3	C79.89	-	D21.3	D48.1	D49.2
thorax	C49.3	C79.89	-	D21.3	D48.1	D49.2
thumb	C49.1-	C79.89	-	D21.1-	D48.1	D49.2
toe	C49.2-	C79.89	-	D21.2-	D48.1	D49.2
trunk	C49.6	C79.89	-	D21.6	D48.1	D49.2
umbilicus	C49.4	C79.89	-	D21.4	D48.1	D49.2
vesicorectal	C49.5	C79.89	-	D21.5	D48.1	D49.2
wrist	C49.1-	C79.89	-	D21.1-	D48.1	D49.2
conus medullaris	C72.0	C79.49	-	D33.4	D43.4	D49.7
cord(true) (vocal)	C32.0	C78.39	D02.0	D14.1	D38.0	D49.1
false	C32.1	C78.39	D02.0	D14.1	D38.0	D49.1
spermatic	C63.1-	C79.82	D07.69	D29.8	D40.8	D49.5
spinal(cervical) (lumbar) (thoracic)	C72.0	C79.49	-	D33.4	D43.4	D49.7
cornea(limbus)	C69.1-	C79.49	D09.2-	D31.1-	D48.7	D49.89
corpus						
albicans	C56.-	C79.6-	D07.39	D27.-	D39.1-	D49.5
callosum, brain	C71.0	C79.31	-	D33.2	D43.2	D49.6
cavernosum	C60.2	C79.82	D07.4	D29.0	D40.8	D49.5
gastric	C16.2	C78.89	D00.2	D13.1	D37.1	D49.0
overlapping sites	C54.8	-	-	-	-	-
penis	C60.2	C79.82	D07.4	D29.0	D40.8	D49.5
striatum, cerebrum	C71.0	C79.31	-	D33.0	D43.0	D49.6
uteri	C54.9	C79.82	D07.0	D26.1	D39.0	D49.5
isthmus	C54.0	C79.82	D07.0	D26.1	D39.0	D49.5
cortex						
adrenal	C74.0	C79.7	D09.3	D35.0	D44.1	D49.7

Neoplasm Index	Malignant Primary	Malignant Secondary	Ca in situ	Benign	Uncertain Behavior	Unspecified Behavior
cortex — *continued*						
cerebral	C71.0	C79.31	-	D33.0	D43.0	D49.6
costal cartilage	C41.3	C79.51	-	D16.7	D48.0	D49.2
costovertebral joint	C41.3	C79.51	-	D16.7	D48.0	D49.2
Cowper's gland	C68.0	C79.19	D09.19	D30.4	D41.3	D49.5
cranial(fossa, any)	C71.9	C79.31	-	D33.2	D43.2	D49.6
meninges	C70.0	C79.32	-	D32.0	D42.0	D49.7
nerve	C72.50	C79.49	-	D33.3	D43.3	D49.7
specified NEC	C72.59	C79.49	-	D33.3	D43.3	D49.7
craniobuccal pouch	C75.2	C79.89	D09.3	D35.2	D44.3	D49.7
craniopharyngeal(duct) (pouch)	C75.2	C79.89	D09.3	D35.3	D44.4	D49.7
cricoid	C13.0	C79.89	D00.08	D10.7	D37.05	D49.0
cartilage	C32.3	C78.39	D02.0	D14.1	D38.0	D49.1
cricopharynx	C13.0	C79.89	D00.08	D10.7	D37.05	D49.0
crypt of Morgagni	C21.8	C78.5	D01.3	D12.9	D37.8	D49.0
crystalline lens	C69.4-	C79.49	D09.2-	D31.4-	D48.7	D49.89
cul-de-sac(Douglas')	C48.1	C78.6	-	D20.1	D48.4	D49.0
cuneiform cartilage	C32.3	C78.39	D02.0	D14.1	D38.0	D49.1
cutaneous—*see* Neoplasm, skin						
cutis—*see* Neoplasm, skin						
cystic(bile) duct (common)	C24.0	C78.89	D01.5	D13.5	D37.6	D49.0
dermis—*see* Neoplasm, skin						
diaphragm	C49.3	C79.89	-	D21.3	D48.1	D49.2
digestive organs, system, tube, or tract NEC	C26.9	C78.89	D01.9	D13.9	D37.9	D49.0
disc, intervertebral	C41.2	C79.51	-	D16.6	D48.0	D49.2
disease, generalized	C80.0	-	-	-	-	-
disseminated	C80.0	-	-	-	-	-
Douglas' cul-de-sac or pouch	C48.1	C78.6	-	D20.1	D48.4	D49.0
duodenojejunal junction	C17.8	C78.4	D01.49	D13.39	D37.2	D49.0
duodenum	C17.0	C78.4	D01.49	D13.2	D37.2	D49.0
dura(cranial) (mater)	C70.9	C79.49	-	D32.9	D42.9	D49.7
cerebral	C70.0	C79.32	-	D32.0	D42.0	D49.7
spinal	C70.1	C79.49	-	D32.1	D42.1	D49.7
ear(external) *(see also* Neoplasm, skin, ear)	C44.20-	C79.2	D04.2-	D23.2-	D48.5	D49.2
auricle or auris *(see also* Neoplasm, skin, ear)	C44.20-	C79.2	D04.2-	D23.2-	D48.5	D49.2
canal, external *(see also* Neoplasm, skin, ear)	C44.20-	C79.2	D04.2-	D23.2-	D48.5	D49.2
cartilage	C49.0	C79.89	-	D21.0	D48.1	D49.2
external meatus *(see also* Neoplasm, skin, ear)	C44.20-	C79.2	D04.2-	D23.2-	D48.5	D49.2
inner	C30.1	C78.39	D02.3	D14.0	D38.5	D49.1
lobule *(see also* Neoplasm, skin, ear)	C44.20-	C79.2	D04.2-	D23.2-	D48.5	D49.2
middle	C30.1	C78.39	D02.3	D14.0	D38.5	D49.1
overlapping lesion with accessory sinuses	C31.8	-	-	-	-	-
skin	C44.20-	C79.2	D04.2-	D23.2-	D48.5	D49.2
basal cell carcinoma	C44.21-	-	-	-	-	-
specified type NEC	C44.29-	-	-	-	-	-
squamous cell carcinoma	C44.22-	-	-	-	-	-
earlobe	C44.20-	C79.2	D04.2-	D23.2-	D48.5	D49.2
basal cell carcinoma	C44.21-	-	-	-	-	-
specified type NEC	C44.29-	-	-	-	-	-
squamous cell carcinoma	C44.22-	-	-	-	-	-

Neoplasm Index	Malignant Primary	Malignant Secondary	Ca in situ	Benign	Uncertain Behavior	Unspecified Behavior
earlobe — *continued*						
ejaculatory duct	C63.7	C79.82	D07.69	D29.8	D40.8	D49.5
elbow NEC	C76.4-	C79.89	D04.6-	D36.7	D48.7	D49.89
endocardium	C38.0	C79.89	-	D15.1	D48.7	D49.89
endocervix(canal) (gland)	C53.0	C79.82	D06.0	D26.0	D39.0	D49.5
endocrine gland NEC	C75.9	C79.89	D09.3	D35.9	D44.9	D49.7
pluriglandular	C75.8	C79.89	D09.3	D35.7	D44.9	D49.7
endometrium(gland) (stroma)	C54.1	C79.82	D07.0	D26.1	D39.0	D49.5
ensiform cartilage	C41.3	C79.51	-	D16.7	D48.0	D49.2
enteric—*see* Neoplasm, intestine						
ependyma(brain)	C71.5	C79.31	-	D33.0	D43.0	D49.6
fourth ventricle	C71.7	C79.31	-	D33.1	D43.1	D49.6
epicardium	C38.0	C79.89	-	D15.1	D48.7	D49.89
epididymis	C63.0-	C79.82	D07.69	D29.3-	D40.8	D49.5
epidural	C72.9	C79.49	-	D33.9	D43.9	D49.7
epiglottis	C32.1	C78.39	D02.0	D14.1	D38.0	D49.1
anterior aspect or surface	C10.1	C79.89	D00.08	D10.5	D37.05	D49.0
cartilage	C32.3	C78.39	D02.0	D14.1	D38.0	D49.1
free border(margin)	C10.1	C79.89	D00.08	D10.5	D37.05	D49.0
junctional region	C10.8	C79.89	D00.08	D10.5	D37.05	D49.0
posterior(laryngeal) surface	C32.1	C78.39	D02.0	D14.1	D38.0	D49.1
suprahyoid portion	C32.1	C78.39	D02.0	D14.1	D38.0	D49.1
esophagogastric junction	C16.0	C78.89	D00.2	D13.1	D37.1	D49.0
esophagus	C15.9	C78.89	D00.1	D13.0	D37.8	D49.0
abdominal	C15.5	C78.89	D00.1	D13.0	D37.8	D49.0
cervical	C15.3	C78.89	D00.1	D13.0	D37.8	D49.0
distal(third)	C15.5	C78.89	D00.1	D13.0	D37.8	D49.0
lower(third)	C15.5	C78.89	D00.1	D13.0	D37.8	D49.0
middle(third)	C15.4	C78.89	D00.1	D13.0	D37.8	D49.0
overlapping lesion	C15.8	-	-	-	-	-
proximal(third)	C15.3	C78.89	D00.1	D13.0	D37.8	D49.0
thoracic	C15.4	C78.89	D00.1	D13.0	D37.8	D49.0
upper(third)	C15.3	C78.89	D00.1	D13.0	D37.8	D49.0
ethmoid(sinus)	C31.1	C78.39	D02.3	D14.0	D38.5	D49.1
bone or labyrinth	C41.0	C79.51	-	D16.4-	D48.0	D49.2
eustachian tube	C30.1	C78.39	D02.3	D14.0	D38.5	D49.1
exocervix	C53.1	C79.82	D06.1	D26.0	D39.0	D49.5
external						
meatus(ear) *(see also* Neoplasm, skin, ear)	C44.20-	C79.2	D04.2-	D23.2-	D48.5	D49.2
os, cervix uteri	C53.1	C79.82	D06.1	D26.0	D39.0	D49.5
extradural	C72.9	C79.49	-	D33.9	D43.9	D49.7
extrahepatic(bile) duct	C24.0	C78.89	D01.5	D13.5	D37.6	D49.0
overlapping lesion with gallbladder	C24.8	-	-	-	-	-
extraocular muscle	C69.6-	C79.49	D09.2-	D31.6-	D48.7	D49.89
extrarectal	C76.3	C79.89	D09.8	D36.7	D48.7	D49.89
extremity	C76.8	C79.89	D04.8	D36.7	D48.7	D49.89
lower	C76.5-	C79.89	D04.7-	D36.7	D48.7	D49.89
upper	C76.4-	C79.89	D04.6-	D36.7	D48.7	D49.89
eye NEC	C69.9-	C79.49	D09.2	D31.9	D48.7	D49.89
overlapping sites	C69.8	-	-	-	-	-
eyeball	C69.9-	C79.49	D09.2-	D31.9-	D48.7	D49.89
eyebrow	C44.309	C79.2	D04.39	D23.39	D48.5	D49.2
basal cell carcinoma	C44.319	-	-	-	-	-
specified type NEC	C44.399	-	-	-	-	-
squamous cell carcinoma	C44.329	-	-	-	-	-
eyelid(lower) (skin) (upper)	C44.10-					

Neoplasm Index	Malignant Primary	Malignant Secondary	Ca in situ	Benign	Uncertain Behavior	Unspecified Behavior
eyelid(lower) (skin) (upper) — *continued*						
basal cell carcinoma	C44.11-	-	-	-	-	-
specified type NEC	C44.19-	-	-	-	-	-
squamous cell carcinoma	C44.12-	-	-	-	-	-
cartilage	C49.0	C79.89	-	D21.0	D48.1	D49.2
face NEC	C76.0	C79.89	D04.39	D36.7	D48.7	D49.89
fallopian tube(accessory)	C57.0-	C79.82	D07.39	D28.2	D39.8	D49.5
falx(cerebella) (cerebri)	C70.0	C79.32	-	D32.0	D42.0	D49.7
fascia (*see also* Neoplasm, connective tissue)						
palmar	C49.1-	C79.89	-	D21.1-	D48.1	D49.2
plantar	C49.2-	C79.89	-	D21.2-	D48.1	D49.2
fatty tissue—*see* Neoplasm, connective tissue						
fauces, faucial NEC	C10.9	C79.89	D00.08	D10.5	D37.05	D49.0
pillars	C09.1	C79.89	D00.08	D10.5	D37.05	D49.0
tonsil	C09.9	C79.89	D00.08	D10.4	D37.05	D49.0
femur(any part)	C40.2-	-	-	D16.2-	-	-
fetal membrane	C58	C79.82	D07.0	D26.7	D39.2	D49.5
fibrous tissue—*see* Neoplasm, connective tissue						
fibula(any part)	C40.2-	C79.51	-	D16.2-	-	-
filum terminale	C72.0	C79.49	-	D33.4	D43.4	D49.7
finger NEC	C76.4-	C79.89	D04.6-	D36.7	D48.7	D49.89
flank NEC	C76.8	C79.89	D04.5	D36.7	D48.7	D49.89
follicle, nabothian	C53.0	C79.82	D06.0	D26.0	D39.0	D49.5
foot NEC	C76.5-	C79.89	D04.7-	D36.7	D48.7	D49.89
forearm NEC	C76.4-	C79.89	D04.6-	D36.7	D48.7	D49.89
forehead(skin)	C44.309	C79.2	D04.39	D23.39	D48.5	D49.2
basal cell carcinoma	C44.319	-	-	-	-	-
specified type NEC	C44.399	-	-	-	-	-
squamous cell carcinoma	C44.329	-	-	-	-	-
foreskin	C60.0	C79.82	D07.4	D29.0	D40.8	D49.5
fornix						
pharyngeal	C11.3	C79.89	D00.08	D10.6	D37.05	D49.0
vagina	C52	C79.82	D07.2	D28.1	D39.8	D49.5
fossa(of)						
anterior(cranial)	C71.9	C79.31	-	D33.2	D43.2	D49.6
cranial	C71.9	C79.31	-	D33.2	D43.2	D49.6
ischiorectal	C76.3	C79.89	D09.8	D36.7	D48.7	D49.89
middle(cranial)	C71.9	C79.31	-	D33.2	D43.2	D49.6
piriform	C12	C79.89	D00.08	D10.7	D37.05	D49.0
pituitary	C75.1	C79.89	D09.3	D35.2	D44.3	D49.7
posterior(cranial)	C71.9	C79.31	-	D33.2	D43.2	D49.6
pterygoid	C49.0	C79.89	-	D21.0	D48.1	D49.2
pyriform	C12	C79.89	D00.08	D10.7	D37.05	D49.0
Rosenmuller	C11.2	C79.89	D00.08	D10.6	D37.05	D49.0
tonsillar	C09.0	C79.89	D00.08	D10.5	D37.05	D49.0
fourchette	C51.9	C79.82	D07.1	D28.0	D39.8	D49.5
frenulum						
labii—*see* Neoplasm, lip, internal						
linguae	C02.2	C79.89	D00.07	D10.1	D37.02	D49.0
frontal						
bone	C41.0	C79.51	-	D16.4-	D48.0	D49.2
lobe, brain	C71.1	C79.31	-	D33.0	D43.0	D49.6
pole	C71.1	C79.31	-	D33.0	D43.0	D49.6
sinus	C31.2	C78.39	D02.3	D14.0	D38.5	D49.1
fundus						

Neoplasm Index	Malignant Primary	Malignant Secondary	Ca in situ	Benign	Uncertain Behavior	Unspecified Behavior
fundus — *continued*						
stomach	C16.1	C78.89	D00.2	D13.1	D37.1	D49.0
uterus	C54.3	C79.82	D07.0	D26.1	D39.0	D49.5
gall duct(extrahepatic)	C24.0	C78.89	D01.5	D13.5	D37.6	D49.0
intrahepatic	C22.1	C78.7	D01.5	D13.4	D37.6	D49.0
gallbladder	C23	C78.89	D01.5	D13.5	D37.6	D49.0
overlapping lesion with extrahepatic bile ducts	C24.8	-	-	-	-	-
ganglia (*see also* Neoplasm, nerve, peripheral)	C47.9	C79.89	-	D36.10	D48.2	D49.2
basal	C71.0	C79.31	-	D33.0	D43.0	D49.6
cranial nerve	C72.50	C79.49	-	D33.3	D43.3	D49.7
Gartner's duct	C52	C79.82	D07.2	D28.1	D39.8	D49.5
gastric—*see* Neoplasm, stomach						
gastrocolic	C26.9	C78.89	D01.9	D13.9	D37.9	D49.0
gastroesophageal junction	C16.0	C78.89	D00.2	D13.1	D37.1	D49.0
gastrointestinal(tract) NEC	C26.9	C78.89	D01.9	D13.9	D37.9	D49.0
generalized	C80.0	-	-	-	-	-
genital organ or tract						
female NEC	C57.9	C79.82	D07.30	D28.9	D39.9	D49.5
overlapping lesion	C57.8	-	-	-	-	-
specified site NEC	C57.7	C79.82	D07.39	D28.7	D39.8	D49.5
male NEC	C63.9	C79.82	D07.60	D29.9	D40.9	D49.5
overlapping lesion	C63.8	-	-	-	-	-
specified site NEC	C63.7	C79.82	D07.69	D29.8	D40.8	D49.5
genitourinary tract						
female	C57.9	C79.82	D07.30	D28.9	D39.9	D49.5
male	C63.9	C79.82	D07.60	D29.9	D40.9	D49.5
gingiva(alveolar) (marginal)	C03.9	C79.89	D00.03	D10.39	D37.09	D49.0
lower	C03.1	C79.89	D00.03	D10.39	D37.09	D49.0
mandibular	C03.1	C79.89	D00.03	D10.39	D37.09	D49.0
maxillary	C03.0	C79.89	D00.03	D10.39	D37.09	D49.0
upper	C03.0	C79.89	D00.03	D10.39	D37.09	D49.0
gland, glandular(lymphatic) (system) (*see also* Neoplasm, lymph gland)						
endocrine NEC	C75.9	C79.89	D09.3	D35.9	D44.9	D49.7
salivary—*see* Neoplasm, salivary gland						
glans penis	C60.1	C79.82	D07.4	D29.0	D40.8	D49.5
globus pallidus	C71.0	C79.31	-	D33.0	D43.0	D49.6
glomus						
coccygeal	C49.5	C79.89	-	D21.5	D48.1	D49.2
jugularis	C75.5	C79.89	-	D35.6	D44.7	D49.7
glosso-epiglottic fold(s)	C10.1	C79.89	D00.08	D10.5	D37.05	D49.0
glossopalatine fold	C09.1	C79.89	D00.08	D10.5	D37.05	D49.0
glossopharyngeal sulcus	C09.0	C79.89	D00.08	D10.5	D37.05	D49.0
glottis	C32.0	C78.39	D02.0	D14.1	D38.0	D49.1
gluteal region	C76.3	C79.89	D04.5	D36.7	D48.7	D49.89
great vessels NEC	C49.3	C79.89	-	D21.3	D48.1	D49.2
groin NEC	C76.3	C79.89	D04.5	D36.7	D48.7	D49.89
gum	C03.9	C79.89	D00.03	D10.39	D37.09	D49.0
lower	C03.1	C79.89	D00.03	D10.39	D37.09	D49.0
upper	C03.0	C79.89	D00.03	D10.39	D37.09	D49.0
hand NEC	C76.4-	C79.89	D04.6-	D36.7	D48.7	D49.89
head NEC	C76.0	C79.89	D04.4	D36.7	D48.7	D49.89
heart	C38.0	C79.89	-	D15.1	D48.7	D49.89

Neoplasm Index	Malignant Primary	Malignant Secondary	Ca in situ	Benign	Uncertain Behavior	Unspecified Behavior
heel NEC	C76.5-	C79.89	D04.7-	D36.7	D48.7	D49.89
helix (see also Neoplasm, skin, ear)	C44.20-	C79.2	D04.2-	D23.2-	D48.5	D49.2
hematopoietic, hemopoietic tissue NEC	C96.9	-	-	-	-	-
specified NEC	C96.Z	-	-	-	-	-
hemisphere, cerebral	C71.0	C79.31	-	D33.0	D43.0	D49.6
hemorrhoidal zone	C21.1	C78.5	D01.3	D12.9	D37.8	D49.0
hepatic (see also Index to disease, by histology)	C22.9	C78.7	D01.5	D13.4	D37.6	D49.0
duct(bile)	C24.0	C78.89	D01.5	D13.5	D37.6	D49.0
flexure(colon)	C18.3	C78.5	D01.0	D12.3	D37.4	D49.0
primary	C22.8	C78.7	D01.5	D13.4	D37.6	D49.0
hepatobiliary	C24.9	C78.89	D01.5	D13.5	D37.6	D49.0
hepatoblastoma	C22.2	C78.7	D01.5	D13.4	D37.6	D49.0
hepatoma	C22.0	C78.7	D01.5	D13.4	D37.6	D49.0
hilus of lung	C34.0-	C78.0-	D02.2-	D14.3-	D38.1	D49.1
hip NEC	C76.5-	C79.89	D04.7-	D36.7	D48.7	D49.89
hippocampus, brain	C71.2	C79.31	-	D33.0	D43.0	D49.6
humerus(any part)	C40.0-	C79.51	-	D16.0-	-	-
hymen	C52	C79.82	D07.2	D28.1	D39.8	D49.5
hypopharynx, hypopharyngeal NEC	C13.9	C79.89	D00.08	D10.7	D37.05	D49.0
overlapping lesion	C13.8	-	-	-	-	-
postcricoid region	C13.0	C79.89	D00.08	D10.7	D37.05	D49.0
posterior wall	C13.2	C79.89	D00.08	D10.7	D37.05	D49.0
pyriform fossa(sinus)	C12	C79.89	D00.08	D10.7	D37.05	D49.0
hypophysis	C75.1	C79.89	D09.3	D35.2	D44.3	D49.7
hypothalamus	C71.0	C79.31	-	D33.0	D43.0	D49.6
ileocecum, ileocecal(coil) (junction) (valve)	C18.0	C78.5	D01.0	D12.0	D37.4	D49.0
ileum	C17.2	C78.4	D01.49	D13.39	D37.2	D49.0
ilium	C41.4	C79.51	-	D16.8	D48.0	D49.2
immunoproliferative NEC	C88.9	-	-	-	-	-
infraclavicular(region)	C76.1	C79.89	D04.5	D36.7	D48.7	D49.89
inguinal(region)	C76.3	C79.89	D04.5	D36.7	D48.7	D49.89
insula	C71.0	C79.31	-	D33.0	D43.0	D49.6
insular tissue(pancreas)	C25.4	C78.89	D01.7	D13.7	D37.8	D49.0
brain	C71.0	C79.31	-	D33.0	D43.0	D49.6
interarytenoid fold	C13.1	C79.89	D00.08	D10.7	D37.05	D49.0
hypopharyngeal aspect	C13.1	C79.89	D00.08	D10.7	D37.05	D49.0
laryngeal aspect	C32.1	C78.39	D02.0	D14.1	D38.0	D49.1
marginal zone	C13.1	C79.89	D00.08	D10.7	D37.05	D49.0
interdental papillae	C03.9	C79.89	D00.03	D10.39	D37.09	D49.0
lower	C03.1	C79.89	D00.03	D10.39	D37.09	D49.0
upper	C03.0	C79.89	D00.03	D10.39	D37.09	D49.0
internal						
capsule	C71.0	C79.31	-	D33.0	D43.0	D49.6
os(cervix)	C53.0	C79.82	D06.0	D26.0	D39.0	D49.5
intervertebral cartilage or disc	C41.2	C79.51	-	D16.6	D48.0	D49.2
intestine, intestinal	C26.0	C78.80	D01.40	D13.9	D37.8	D49.0
large	C18.9	C78.5	D01.0	D12.6	D37.4	D49.0
appendix	C18.1	C78.5	D01.0	D12.1	D37.3	D49.0
caput coli	C18.0	C78.5	D01.0	D12.0	D37.4	D49.0
cecum	C18.0	C78.5	D01.0	D12.0	D37.4	D49.0
colon	C18.9	C78.5	D01.0	D12.6	D37.4	D49.0
and rectum	C19	C78.5	D01.1	D12.7	D37.5	D49.0
ascending	C18.2	C78.5	D01.0	D12.2	D37.4	D49.0
caput	C18.0	C78.5	D01.0	D12.0	D37.4	D49.0
descending	C18.6	C78.5	D01.0	D12.4	D37.4	D49.0
distal	C18.6	C78.5	D01.0	D12.4	D37.4	D49.0
left	C18.6	C78.5	D01.0	D12.4	D37.4	D49.0

Neoplasm Index	Malignant Primary	Malignant Secondary	Ca in situ	Benign	Uncertain Behavior	Unspecified Behavior
intestine, intestinal — continued						
large — continued						
colon — continued						
overlapping lesion	C18.8	-	-	-	-	-
pelvic	C18.7	C78.5	D01.0	D12.5	D37.4	D49.0
right	C18.2	C78.5	D01.0	D12.2	D37.4	D49.0
sigmoid(flexure)	C18.7	C78.5	D01.0	D12.5	D37.4	D49.0
transverse	C18.4	C78.5	D01.0	D12.3	D37.4	D49.0
hepatic flexure	C18.3	C78.5	D01.0	D12.3	D37.4	D49.0
ileocecum, ileocecal(coil) (valve)	C18.0	C78.5	D01.0	D12.0	D37.4	D49.0
overlapping lesion	C18.8	-	-	-	-	-
sigmoid flexure(lower) (upper)	C18.7	C78.5	D01.0	D12.5	D37.4	D49.0
splenic flexure	C18.5	C78.5	D01.0	D12.3	D37.4	D49.0
small	C17.9	C78.4	D01.40	D13.30	D37.2	D49.0
duodenum	C17.0	C78.4	D01.49	D13.2	D37.2	D49.0
ileum	C17.2	C78.4	D01.49	D13.39	D37.2	D49.0
jejunum	C17.1	C78.4	D01.49	D13.39	D37.2	D49.0
overlapping lesion	C17.8	-	-	-	-	-
tract NEC	C26.0	C78.89	D01.40	D13.9	D37.8	D49.0
intra-abdominal	C76.2	C79.89	D09.8	D36.7	D48.7	D49.89
intracranial NEC	C71.9	C79.31	-	D33.2	D43.2	D49.6
intrahepatic(bile) duct	C22.1	C78.7	D01.5	D13.4	D37.6	D49.0
intraocular	C69.9-	C79.49	D09.2-	D31.9-	D48.7	D49.89
intraorbital	C69.6-	C79.49	D09.2-	D31.6-	D48.7	D49.89
intrasellar	C75.1	C79.89	D09.3	D35.2	D44.3	D49.7
intrathoracic(cavity) (organs)	C76.1	C79.89	D09.8	D15.9	D48.7	D49.89
specified NEC	C76.1	C79.89	D09.8	D15.7	-	-
iris	C69.4-	C79.49	D09.2-	D31.4-	D48.7	D49.89
ischiorectal(fossa)	C76.3	C79.89	D09.8	D36.7	D48.7	D49.89
ischium	C41.4	C79.51	-	D16.8	D48.0	D49.2
island of Reil	C71.0	C79.31	-	D33.0	D43.0	D49.6
islands or islets of Langerhans	C25.4	C78.89	D01.7	D13.7	D37.8	D49.0
isthmus uteri	C54.0	C79.82	D07.0	D26.1	D39.0	D49.5
jaw	C76.0	C79.89	D09.8	D36.7	D48.7	D49.89
bone	C41.1	C79.51	-	D16.5-	D48.0	D49.2
lower	C41.1	C79.51	-	D16.5-	-	-
upper	C41.0	C79.51	-	D16.4-	-	-
carcinoma(any type) (lower) (upper)	C76.0	C79.89				
skin (see also Neoplasm, skin, face)	C44.309	C79.2	D04.39	D23.39	D48.5	D49.2
soft tissues	C03.9	C79.89	D00.03	D10.39	D37.09	D49.0
lower	C03.1	C79.89	D00.03	D10.39	D37.09	D49.0
upper	C03.0	C79.89	D00.03	D10.39	D37.09	D49.0
jejunum	C17.1	C78.4	D01.49	D13.39	D37.2	D49.0
joint NEC (see also Neoplasm, bone)	C41.9	C79.51	-	D16.9-	D48.0	D49.2
acromioclavicular	C40.0-	C79.51	-	D16.0-	-	-
bursa or synovial membrane— see Neoplasm, connective tissue						
costovertebral	C41.3	C79.51	-	D16.7	D48.0	D49.2
sternocostal	C41.3	C79.51	-	D16.7	D48.0	D49.2
temporomandibular	C41.1	C79.51	-	D16.5-	D48.0	D49.2
junction						
anorectal	C21.8	C78.5	D01.3	D12.9	D37.8	D49.0
cardioesophageal	C16.0	C78.89	D00.2	D13.1	D37.1	D49.0
esophagogastric	C16.0	C78.89	D00.2	D13.1	D37.1	D49.0

Neoplasm Index	Malignant Primary	Malignant Secondary	Ca in situ	Benign	Uncertain Behavior	Unspecified Behavior
intestine, intestinal — *continued*						
gastroesophageal	C16.0	C78.89	D00.2	D13.1	D37.1	D49.0
hard and soft palate	C05.9	C79.89	D00.00	D10.39	D37.09	D49.0
ileocecal	C18.0	C78.5	D01.0	D12.0	D37.4	D49.0
pelvirectal	C19	C78.5	D01.1	D12.7	D37.5	D49.0
pelviureteric	C65.-	C79.0-	D09.19	D30.1-	D41.1-	D49.5
rectosigmoid	C19	C78.5	D01.1	D12.7	D37.5	D49.0
squamocolumnar, of cervix	C53.8	C79.82	D06.7	D26.0	D39.0	D49.5
Kaposi's sarcoma—*see* Kaposi's, sarcoma						
kidney(parenchymal)	C64.-	C79.0-	D09.19	D30.0-	D41.0-	D49.5
calyx	C65.-	C79.0-	D09.19	D30.1-	D41.1-	D49.5
hilus	C65.-	C79.0-	D09.19	D30.1-	D41.1-	D49.5
pelvis	C65.-	C79.0-	D09.19	D30.1-	D41.1-	D49.5
knee NEC	C76.5-	C79.89	D04.7-	D36.7	D48.7	D49.89
labia(skin)	C51.9	C79.82	D07.1	D28.0	D39.8	D49.5
majora	C51.0	C79.82	D07.1	D28.0	D39.8	D49.5
minora	C51.1	C79.82	D07.1	D28.0	D39.8	D49.5
labial (*see also* Neoplasm, lip)	C00.9	C79.89	D00.01	D10.0	D37.01	D49.0
sulcus(lower) (upper)	C06.1	C79.89	D00.02	D10.39	D37.09	D49.0
labium(skin)	C51.9	C79.82	D07.1	D28.0	D39.8	D49.5
majus	C51.0	C79.82	D07.1	D28.0	D39.8	D49.5
minus	C51.1	C79.82	D07.1	D28.0	D39.8	D49.5
lacrimal						
canaliculi	C69.5-	C79.49	D09.2-	D31.5-	D48.7	D49.89
duct(nasal)	C69.5-	C79.49	D09.2-	D31.5-	D48.7	D49.89
gland	C69.5-	C79.49	D09.2-	D31.5-	D48.7	D49.89
punctum	C69.5-	C79.49	D09.2-	D31.5-	D48.7	D49.89
sac	C69.5-	C79.49	D09.2-	D31.5-	D48.7	D49.89
Langerhans, islands or islets	C25.4	C78.89	D01.7	D13.7	D37.8	D49.0
laryngopharynx	C13.9	C79.89	D00.08	D10.7	D37.05	D49.0
larynx, laryngeal NEC	C32.9	C78.39	D02.0	D14.1	D38.0	D49.1
aryepiglottic fold	C32.1	C78.39	D02.0	D14.1	D38.0	D49.1
cartilage(arytenoid) (cricoid) (cuneiform) (thyroid)	C32.3	C78.39	D02.0	D14.1	D38.0	D49.1
commissure(anterior) (posterior)	C32.0	C78.39	D02.0	D14.1	D38.0	D49.1
extrinsic NEC	C32.1	C78.39	D02.0	D14.1	D38.0	D49.1
meaning hypopharynx	C13.9	C79.89	D00.08	D10.7	D37.05	D49.0
interarytenoid fold	C32.1	C78.39	D02.0	D14.1	D38.0	D49.1
intrinsic	C32.0	C78.39	D02.0	D14.1	D38.0	D49.1
overlapping lesion	C32.8	-	-	-	-	-
ventricular band	C32.1	C78.39	D02.0	D14.1	D38.0	D49.1
leg NEC	C76.5-	C79.89	D04.7-	D36.7	D48.7	D49.89
lens, crystalline	C69.4-	C79.49	D09.2-	D31.4-	D48.7	D49.89
lid(lower) (upper)	C44.10-	C79.2	D04.1-	D23.1-	D48.5	D49.2
basal cell carcinoma	C44.11-	-	-	-	-	-
specified type NEC	C44.19-	-	-	-	-	-
squamous cell carcinoma	C44.12-	-	-	-	-	-
ligament (*see also* Neoplasm, connective tissue)						
broad	C57.1	C79.82	D07.39	D28.2	D39.8	D49.5
Mackenrodt's	C57.7	C79.82	D07.39	D28.7	D39.8	D49.5
non-uterine—*see* Neoplasm, connective tissue						
round	C57.2	C79.82	-	D28.2	D39.8	D49.5

Neoplasm Index	Malignant Primary	Malignant Secondary	Ca in situ	Benign	Uncertain Behavior	Unspecified Behavior
ligament (*see also* Neoplasm, connective tissue) — *continued*						
sacro-uterine	C57.3	C79.82	-	D28.2	D39.8	D49.5
uterine	C57.3	C79.82	-	D28.2	D39.8	D49.5
utero-ovarian	C57.7	C79.82	D07.39	D28.2	D39.8	D49.5
uterosacral	C57.3	C79.82	-	D28.2	D39.8	D49.5
limb	C76.8	C79.89	D04.8	D36.7	D48.7	D49.89
lower	C76.5-	C79.89	D04.7-	D36.7	D48.7	D49.89
upper	C76.4-	C79.89	D04.6-	D36.7	D48.7	D49.89
limbus of cornea	C69.1-	C79.49	D09.2-	D31.1-	D48.7	D49.89
lingual NEC (*see also* Neoplasm, tongue)	C02.9	C79.89	D00.07	D10.1	D37.02	D49.0
lingula, lung	C34.1-	C78.0-	D02.2-	D14.3-	D38.1	D49.1
lip	C00.9	C79.89	D00.01	D10.0	D37.01	D49.0
buccal aspect—*see* Neoplasm, lip, internal						
commissure	C00.6	C79.89	D00.01	D10.0	D37.01	D49.0
external	C00.2	C79.89	D00.01	D10.0	D37.01	D49.0
lower	C00.1	C79.89	D00.01	D10.0	D37.01	D49.0
upper	C00.0	C79.89	D00.01	D10.0	D37.01	D49.0
frenulum—*see* Neoplasm, lip, internal						
inner aspect—*see* Neoplasm, lip, internal						
internal	C00.5	C79.89	D00.01	D10.0	D37.01	D49.0
lower	C00.4	C79.89	D00.01	D10.0	D37.01	D49.0
upper	C00.3	C79.89	D00.01	D10.0	D37.01	D49.0
lipstick area	C00.2	C79.89	D00.01	D10.0	D37.01	D49.0
lower	C00.1	C79.89	D00.01	D10.0	D37.01	D49.0
upper	C00.0	C79.89	D00.01	D10.0	D37.01	D49.0
lower	C00.1	C79.89	D00.01	D10.0	D37.01	D49.0
internal	C00.4	C79.89	D00.01	D10.0	D37.01	D49.0
mucosa—*see* Neoplasm, lip, internal						
oral aspect—*see* Neoplasm, lip, internal						
overlapping lesion	C00.8	-	-	-	-	-
with oral cavity or pharynx	C14.8	-	-	-	-	-
skin(commissure) (lower) (upper)	C44.00	C79.2	D04.0	D23.0	D48.5	D49.2
basal cell carcinoma	C44.01	-	-	-	-	-
specified type NEC	C44.09	-	-	-	-	-
squamous cell carcinoma	C44.02	-	-	-	-	-
upper	C00.0	C79.89	D00.01	D10.0	D37.01	D49.0
internal	C00.3	C79.89	D00.01	D10.0	D37.01	D49.0
vermilion border	C00.2	C79.89	D00.01	D10.0	D37.01	D49.0
lower	C00.1	C79.89	D00.01	D10.0	D37.01	D49.0
upper	C00.0	C79.89	D00.01	D10.0	D37.01	D49.0
lipomatous—*see* Lipoma, by site						
liver (*see also* Index to disease, by histology)	C22.9	C78.7	D01.5	D13.4	D37.6	D49.0
primary	C22.8	C78.7	D01.5	D13.4	D37.6	D49.0
lumbosacral plexus	C47.5	C79.89	-	D36.16	D48.2	D49.2
lung	C34.9-	C78.0-	D02.2-	D14.3-	D38.1	D49.1
azygos lobe	C34.1-	C78.0-	D02.2-	D14.3-	D38.1	D49.1
carina	C34.0-	C78.0-	D02.2-	D14.3-	D38.1	D49.1

Neoplasm Index	Malignant Primary	Malignant Secondary	Ca in situ	Benign	Uncertain Behavior	Unspecified Behavior
lung — *continued*						
hilus	C34.0-	C78.0-	D02.2-	D14.3-	D38.1	D49.1
lingula	C34.1-	C78.0-	D02.2-	D14.3-	D38.1	D49.1
lobe NEC	C34.9-	C78.0-	D02.2-	D14.3-	D38.1	D49.1
lower lobe	C34.3-	C78.0-	D02.2-	D14.3-	D38.1	D49.1
main bronchus	C34.0-	C78.0-	D02.2-	D14.3-	D38.1	D49.1
mesothelioma—*see* Mesothelioma						
middle lobe	C34.2	C78.0-	D02.21	D14.31	D38.1	D49.1
overlapping lesion	C34.8-	-	-	-	-	-
upper lobe	C34.1-	C78.0-	D02.2-	D14.3-	D38.1	D49.1
lymph, lymphatic channel NEC	C49.9	C79.89	-	D21.9	D48.1	D49.2
gland(secondary)	-	C77.9	-	D36.0	D48.7	D49.89
abdominal	-	C77.2	-	D36.0	D48.7	D49.89
aortic	-	C77.2	-	D36.0	D48.7	D49.89
arm	-	C77.3	-	D36.0	D48.7	D49.89
auricular(anterior) (posterior)	-	C77.0	-	D36.0	D48.7	D49.89
axilla, axillary	-	C77.3	-	D36.0	D48.7	D49.89
brachial	-	C77.3	-	D36.0	D48.7	D49.89
bronchial	-	C77.1	-	D36.0	D48.7	D49.89
bronchopulmonary	-	C77.1	-	D36.0	D48.7	D49.89
celiac	-	C77.2	-	D36.0	D48.7	D49.89
cervical	-	C77.0	-	D36.0	D48.7	D49.89
cervicofacial	-	C77.0	-	D36.0	D48.7	D49.89
Cloquet	-	C77.4	-	D36.0	D48.7	D49.89
colic	-	C77.2	-	D36.0	D48.7	D49.89
common duct	-	C77.2	-	D36.0	D48.7	D49.89
cubital	-	C77.3	-	D36.0	D48.7	D49.89
diaphragmatic	-	C77.1	-	D36.0	D48.7	D49.89
epigastric, inferior	-	C77.1	-	D36.0	D48.7	D49.89
epitrochlear	-	C77.3	-	D36.0	D48.7	D49.89
esophageal	-	C77.1	-	D36.0	D48.7	D49.89
face	-	C77.0	-	D36.0	D48.7	D49.89
femoral	-	C77.4	-	D36.0	D48.7	D49.89
gastric	-	C77.2	-	D36.0	D48.7	D49.89
groin	-	C77.4	-	D36.0	D48.7	D49.89
head	-	C77.0	-	D36.0	D48.7	D49.89
hepatic	-	C77.2	-	D36.0	D48.7	D49.89
hilar(pulmonary)	-	C77.1	-	D36.0	D48.7	D49.89
splenic	-	C77.2	-	D36.0	D48.7	D49.89
hypogastric	-	C77.5	-	D36.0	D48.7	D49.89
ileocolic	-	C77.2	-	D36.0	D48.7	D49.89
iliac	-	C77.5	-	D36.0	D48.7	D49.89
infraclavicular	-	C77.3	-	D36.0	D48.7	D49.89
inguina, inguinal	-	C77.4	-	D36.0	D48.7	D49.89
innominate	-	C77.1	-	D36.0	D48.7	D49.89
intercostal	-	C77.1	-	D36.0	D48.7	D49.89
intestinal	-	C77.2	-	D36.0	D48.7	D49.89
intrabdominal	-	C77.2	-	D36.0	D48.7	D49.89
intrapelvic	-	C77.5	-	D36.0	D48.7	D49.89
intrathoracic	-	C77.1	-	D36.0	D48.7	D49.89
jugular	-	C77.0	-	D36.0	D48.7	D49.89
leg	-	C77.4	-	D36.0	D48.7	D49.89
limb						
lower	-	C77.4	-	D36.0	D48.7	D49.89
upper	-	C77.3	-	D36.0	D48.7	D49.89
lower limb	-	C77.4	-	D36.0	D48.7	D49.89
lumbar	-	C77.2	-	D36.0	D48.7	D49.89
mandibular	-	C77.0	-	D36.0	D48.7	D49.89
mediastinal	-	C77.1	-	D36.0	D48.7	D49.89
mesenteric(inferior) (superior)	-	C77.2	-	D36.0	D48.7	D49.89
Neoplasm Index	Malignant Primary	Malignant Secondary	Ca in situ	Benign	Uncertain Behavior	Unspecified Behavior
lymph, lymphatic channel NEC — *continued*						
gland(secondary) — *continued*						
midcolic	-	C77.2	-	D36.0	D48.7	D49.89
multiple sites in categories C77.0 - C77.5	-	C77.8	-	D36.0	D48.7	D49.89
neck	-	C77.0	-	D36.0	D48.7	D49.89
obturator	-	C77.5	-	D36.0	D48.7	D49.89
occipital	-	C77.0	-	D36.0	D48.7	D49.89
pancreatic	-	C77.2	-	D36.0	D48.7	D49.89
para-aortic	-	C77.2	-	D36.0	D48.7	D49.89
paracervical	-	C77.5	-	D36.0	D48.7	D49.89
parametrial	-	C77.5	-	D36.0	D48.7	D49.89
parasternal	-	C77.1	-	D36.0	D48.7	D49.89
parotid	-	C77.0	-	D36.0	D48.7	D49.89
pectoral	-	C77.3	-	D36.0	D48.7	D49.89
pelvic	-	C77.5	-	D36.0	D48.7	D49.89
peri-aortic	-	C77.2	-	D36.0	D48.7	D49.89
peripancreatic	-	C77.2	-	D36.0	D48.7	D49.89
popliteal	-	C77.4	-	D36.0	D48.7	D49.89
porta hepatis	-	C77.2	-	D36.0	D48.7	D49.89
portal	-	C77.2	-	D36.0	D48.7	D49.89
preauricular	-	C77.0	-	D36.0	D48.7	D49.89
prelaryngeal	-	C77.0	-	D36.0	D48.7	D49.89
presymphysial	-	C77.5	-	D36.0	D48.7	D49.89
pretracheal	-	C77.0	-	D36.0	D48.7	D49.89
primary(any site) NEC	C96.9	-	-	-	-	-
pulmonary(hiler)	-	C77.1	-	D36.0	D48.7	D49.89
pyloric	-	C77.2	-	D36.0	D48.7	D49.89
retroperitoneal	-	C77.2	-	D36.0	D48.7	D49.89
retropharyngeal	-	C77.0	-	D36.0	D48.7	D49.89
Rosenmuller's	-	C77.4	-	D36.0	D48.7	D49.89
sacral	-	C77.5	-	D36.0	D48.7	D49.89
scalene	-	C77.0	-	D36.0	D48.7	D49.89
site NEC	-	C77.9	-	D36.0	D48.7	D49.89
splenic(hilar)	-	C77.2	-	D36.0	D48.7	D49.89
subclavicular	-	C77.3	-	D36.0	D48.7	D49.89
subinguinal	-	C77.4	-	D36.0	D48.7	D49.89
sublingual	-	C77.0	-	D36.0	D48.7	D49.89
submandibular	-	C77.0	-	D36.0	D48.7	D49.89
submaxillary	-	C77.0	-	D36.0	D48.7	D49.89
submental	-	C77.0	-	D36.0	D48.7	D49.89
subscapular	-	C77.3	-	D36.0	D48.7	D49.89
supraclavicular	-	C77.0	-	D36.0	D48.7	D49.89
thoracic	-	C77.1	-	D36.0	D48.7	D49.89
tibial	-	C77.4	-	D36.0	D48.7	D49.89
tracheal	-	C77.1	-	D36.0	D48.7	D49.89
tracheobronchial	-	C77.1	-	D36.0	D48.7	D49.89
upper limb	-	C77.3	-	D36.0	D48.7	D49.89
Virchow's	-	C77.0	-	D36.0	D48.7	D49.89
node (*see also* Neoplasm, lymph gland)						
primary NEC	C96.9	-	-	-	-	-
vessel (*see also* Neoplasm, connective tissue)	C49.9	C79.89	-	D21.9	D48.1	D49.2
Mackenrodt's ligament	C57.7	C79.82	D07.39	D28.7	D39.8	D49.5
malar	C41.0	C79.51	-	D16.4-	D48.0	D49.2
region—*see* Neoplasm, cheek						

Neoplasm Index	Malignant Primary	Malignant Secondary	Ca in situ	Benign	Uncertain Behavior	Unspecified Behavior
mammary gland—see Neoplasm, breast						
mandible	C41.1	C79.51	-	D16.5-	D48.0	D49.2
alveolar						
mucosa(carcinoma)	C03.1	C79.89	D00.03	D10.39	D37.09	D49.0
ridge or process	C41.1	C79.51	-	D16.5-	D48.0	D49.2
marrow(bone) NEC	C96.9	C79.52	-		D47.9	D49.89
mastectomy site(skin)	C44.501	C79.2	-	-	-	-
(see also Neoplasm, breast, skin)						
specified as breast tissue	C50.8-	C79.81	-	-	-	-
mastoid(air cells) (antrum) (cavity)	C30.1	C78.39	D02.3	D14.0	D38.5	D49.1
bone or process	C41.0	C79.51	-	D16.4-	D48.0	D49.2
maxilla, maxillary(superior)	C41.0	C79.51	-	D16.4-	D48.0	D49.2
alveolar						
mucosa	C03.0	C79.89	D00.03	D10.39	D37.09	D49.0
ridge or process(carcinoma)	C41.0	C79.51	-	D16.4-	D48.0	D49.2
antrum	C31.0	C78.39	D02.3	D14.0	D38.5	D49.1
carcinoma	C03.0	C79.51	-	-	-	-
inferior—see Neoplasm, mandible						
sinus	C31.0	C78.39	D02.3	D14.0	D38.5	D49.1
meatus external(ear) (see also Neoplasm, skin, ear)	C44.20-	C79.2	D04.2-	D23.2-	D48.5	D49.2
Meckel diverticulum, malignant	C17.3	C78.4	D01.49	D13.39	D37.2	D49.0
mediastinum, mediastinal	C38.3	C78.1	-	D15.2	D38.3	D49.89
anterior	C38.1	C78.1	-	D15.2	D38.3	D49.89
posterior	C38.2	C78.1	-	D15.2	D38.3	D49.89
medulla						
adrenal	C74.1-	C79.7-	D09.3	D35.0-	D44.1-	D49.7
oblongata	C71.7	C79.31	-	D33.1	D43.1	D49.6
meibomian gland	C44.10-	C79.2	D04.1-	D23.1-	D48.5	D49.2
basal cell carcinoma	C44.11-	-	-	-	-	-
specified type NEC	C44.19-	-	-	-	-	-
squamous cell carcinoma	C44.12-	-	-	-	-	-
melanoma—see Melanoma						
meninges	C70.9	C79.49	-	D32.9	D42.9	D49.7
brain	C70.0	C79.32	-	D32.0	D42.0	D49.7
cerebral	C70.0	C79.32	-	D32.0	D42.0	D49.7
crainial	C70.0	C79.32	-	D32.0	D42.0	D49.7
intracranial	C70.0	C79.32	-	D32.0	D42.0	D49.7
spinal(cord)	C70.1	C79.49	-	D32.1	D42.1	D49.7
meniscus, knee joint(lateral) (medial)	C40.2-	C79.51	-	D16.2-	D48.0	D49.2
Merkel cell—see Carcinoma, Merkel cell						
mesentery, mesenteric	C48.1	C78.6	-	D20.1	D48.4	D49.0
mesoappendix	C48.1	C78.6	-	D20.1	D48.4	D49.0
mesocolon	C48.1	C78.6	-	D20.1	D48.4	D49.0
mesopharynx— see Neoplasm, oropharynx						
mesosalpinx	C57.1	C79.82	D07.39	D28.2	D39.8	D49.5
mesothelial tissue—see Mesothelioma						

Neoplasm Index	Malignant Primary	Malignant Secondary	Ca in situ	Benign	Uncertain Behavior	Unspecified Behavior
mesothelioma—see Mesothelioma						
mesovarium	C57.1	C79.82	D07.39	D28.2	D39.8	D49.5
metacarpus(any bone)	C40.1-	C79.51	-	D16.1-	-	-
metastatic NEC (see also Neoplasm, by site, secondary)	-	C79.9				
metatarsus(any bone)	C40.3-	C79.51	-	D16.3-	-	-
midbrain	C71.7	C79.31	-	D33.1	D43.1	D49.6
milk duct—see Neoplasm, breast						
mons						
pubis	C51.9	C79.82	D07.1	D28.0	D39.8	D49.5
veneris	C51.9	C79.82	D07.1	D28.0	D39.8	D49.5
motor tract	C72.9	C79.49	-	D33.9	D43.9	D49.7
brain	C71.9	C79.31	-	D33.2	D43.2	D49.6
cauda equina	C72.1	C79.49	-	D33.4	D43.4	D49.7
spinal	C72.0	C79.49	-	D33.4	D43.4	D49.7
mouth	C06.9	C79.89	D00.00	D10.30	D37.09	D49.0
book-leaf	C06.89	C79.89				
floor	C04.9	C79.89	D00.06	D10.2	D37.09	D49.0
anterior portion	C04.0	C79.89	D00.06	D10.2	D37.09	D49.0
lateral portion	C04.1	C79.89	D00.06	D10.2	D37.09	D49.0
overlapping lesion	C04.8	-	-	-	-	-
overlapping NEC	C06.80	-		-	-	-
roof	C05.9	C79.89	D00.00	D10.39	D37.09	D49.0
specified part NEC	C06.89	C79.89	D00.00	D10.39	D37.09	D49.0
vestibule	C06.1	C79.89	D00.00	D10.39	D37.09	D49.0
mucosa						
alveolar(ridge or process)	C03.9	C79.89	D00.03	D10.39	D37.09	D49.0
lower	C03.1	C79.89	D00.03	D10.39	D37.09	D49.0
upper	C03.0	C79.89	D00.03	D10.39	D37.09	D49.0
buccal	C06.0	C79.89	D00.02	D10.39	D37.09	D49.0
cheek	C06.0	C79.89	D00.02	D10.39	D37.09	D49.0
lip—see Neoplasm, lip, internal						
nasal	C30.0	C78.39	D02.3	D14.0	D38.5	D49.1
oral	C06.0	C79.89	D00.02	D10.39	D37.09	D49.0
Mullerian duct						
female	C57.7	C79.82	D07.39	D28.7	D39.8	D49.5
male	C63.7	C79.82	D07.69	D29.8	D40.8	D49.5
muscle (see also Neoplasm, connective tissue)						
extraocular	C69.6-	C79.49	D09.2-	D31.6-	D48.7	D49.89
myocardium	C38.0	C79.89	-	D15.1	D48.7	D49.89
myometrium	C54.2	C79.82	D07.0	D26.1	D39.0	D49.5
myopericardium	C38.0	C79.89	-	D15.1	D48.7	D49.89
nabothian gland(follicle)	C53.0	C79.82	D06.0	D26.0	D39.0	D49.5
nail (see also Neoplasm, skin, limb)	C44.90	C79.2	D04.9	D23.9	D48.5	D49.2
finger (see also Neoplasm, skin, limb, upper)	C44.60-	C79.2	D04.6-	D23.6-	D48.5	D49.2
toe (see also Neoplasm, skin, limb, lower)	C44.70-	C79.2	D04.7-	D23.7-	D48.5	D49.2
nares, naris(anterior) (posterior)	C30.0	C78.39	D02.3	D14.0	D38.5	D49.1
nasal—see Neoplasm, nose						
nasolabial groove (see also Neoplasm, skin, face)	C44.309	C79.2	D04.39	D23.39	D48.5	D49.2
nasolacrimal duct	C69.5-	C79.49	D09.2-	D31.5-	D48.7	D49.89

Neoplasm Index	Malignant Primary	Malignant Secondary	Ca in situ	Benign	Uncertain Behavior	Unspecified Behavior
nasopharynx, nasopharyngeal	C11.9	C79.89	D00.08	D10.6	D37.05	D49.0
floor	C11.3	C79.89	D00.08	D10.6	D37.05	D49.0
overlapping lesion	C11.8	-	-	-	-	-
roof	C11.0	C79.89	D00.08	D10.6	D37.05	D49.0
wall	C11.9	C79.89	D00.08	D10.6	D37.05	D49.0
anterior	C11.3	C79.89	D00.08	D10.6	D37.05	D49.0
lateral	C11.2	C79.89	D00.08	D10.6	D37.05	D49.0
posterior	C11.1	C79.89	D00.08	D10.6	D37.05	D49.0
superior	C11.0	C79.89	D00.08	D10.6	D37.05	D49.0
nates (see also Neoplasm, skin, trunk)	C44.509	C79.2	D04.5	D23.5	D48.5	D49.2
neck NEC	C76.0	C79.89	D09.8	D36.7	D48.7	D49.89
skin	C44.40	-	-	-	-	-
basal cell carcinoma	C44.41	-	-	-	-	-
specified type NEC	C44.49	-	-	-	-	-
squamous cell carcinoma	C44.42	-	-	-	-	-
nerve(ganglion)	C47.9	C79.89	-	D36.10	D48.2	D49.2
abducens	C72.59	C79.49	-	D33.3	D43.3	D49.7
accessory(spinal)	C72.59	C79.49	-	D33.3	D43.3	D49.7
acoustic	C72.4-	C79.49	-	D33.3	D43.3	D49.7
auditory	C72.4-	C79.49	-	D33.3	D43.3	D49.7
autonomic NEC (see also Neoplasm, nerve, peripheral)	C47.9	C79.89	-	D36.10	D48.2	D49.2
brachial	C47.1-	C79.89	-	D36.12	D48.2	D49.2
cranial	C72.50	C79.49	-	D33.3	D43.3	D49.7
specified NEC	C72.59	C79.49	-	D33.3	D43.3	D49.7
facial	C72.59	C79.49	-	D33.3	D43.3	D49.7
femoral	C47.2-	C79.89	-	D36.13	D48.2	D49.2
ganglion NEC (see also Neoplasm, nerve, peripheral)	C47.9	C79.89	-	D36.10	D48.2	D49.2
glossopharyngeal	C72.59	C79.49	-	D33.3	D43.3	D49.7
hypoglossal	C72.59	C79.49	-	D33.3	D43.3	D49.7
intercostal	C47.3	C79.89	-	D36.14	D48.2	D49.2
lumbar	C47.6	C79.89	-	D36.17	D48.2	D49.2
median	C47.1-	C79.89	-	D36.12	D48.2	D49.2
obturator	C47.2-	C79.89	-	D36.13	D48.2	D49.2
oculomotor	C72.59	C79.49	-	D33.3	D43.3	D49.7
olfactory	C47.2-	C79.49	-	D33.3	D43.3	D49.7
optic	C72.3-	C79.49	-	D33.3	D43.3	D49.7
parasympathetic NEC	C47.9	C79.89	-	D36.10	D48.2	D49.2
peripheral NEC	C47.9	C79.89	-	D36.10	D48.2	D49.2
abdomen	C47.4	C79.89	-	D36.15	D48.2	D49.2
abdominal wall	C47.4	C79.89	-	D36.15	D48.2	D49.2
ankle	C47.2-	C79.89	-	D36.13	D48.2	D49.2
antecubital fossa or space	C47.1-	C79.89	-	D36.12	D48.2	D49.2
arm	C47.1-	C79.89	-	D36.12	D48.2	D49.2
auricle(ear)	C47.0	C79.89	-	D36.11	D48.2	D49.2
axilla	C47.3	C79.89	-	D36.12	D48.2	D49.2
back	C47.6	C79.89	-	D36.17	D48.2	D49.2
buttock	C47.5	C79.89	-	D36.16	D48.2	D49.2
calf	C47.2-	C79.89	-	D36.13	D48.2	D49.2
cervical region	C47.0	C79.89	-	D36.11	D48.2	D49.2
cheek	C47.0	C79.89	-	D36.11	D48.2	D49.2
chest(wall)	C47.3	C79.89	-	D36.14	D48.2	D49.2
chin	C47.0	C79.89	-	D36.11	D48.2	D49.2
ear(external)	C47.0	C79.89	-	D36.11	D48.2	D49.2
elbow	C47.1-	C79.89	-	D36.12	D48.2	D49.2
extrarectal	C47.5	C79.89	-	D36.16	D48.2	D49.2
extremity	C47.9	C79.89	-	D36.10	D48.2	D49.2

Neoplasm Index	Malignant Primary	Malignant Secondary	Ca in situ	Benign	Uncertain Behavior	Unspecified Behavior
nerve(ganglion) — continued						
peripheral NEC — continued						
extremity — continued						
lower	C47.2-	C79.89	-	D36.13	D48.2	D49.2
upper	C47.1-	C79.89	-	D36.12	D48.2	D49.2
eyelid	C47.0	C79.89	-	D36.11	D48.2	D49.2
face	C47.0	C79.89	-	D36.11	D48.2	D49.2
finger	C47.1-	C79.89	-	D36.12	D48.2	D49.2
flank	C47.6	C79.89	-	D36.17	D48.2	D49.2
foot	C47.2-	C79.89	-	D36.13	D48.2	D49.2
forearm	C47.1-	C79.89	-	D36.12	D48.2	D49.2
forehead	C47.0	C79.89	-	D36.11	D48.2	D49.2
gluteal region	C47.5	C79.89	-	D36.16	D48.2	D49.2
groin	C47.5	C79.89	-	D36.16	D48.2	D49.2
hand	C47.1-	C79.89	-	D36.12	D48.2	D49.2
head	C47.0	C79.89	-	D36.11	D48.2	D49.2
heel	C47.2-	C79.89	-	D36.13	D48.2	D49.2
hip	C47.2-	C79.89	-	D36.13	D48.2	D49.2
infraclavicular region	C47.3	C79.89	-	D36.14	D48.2	D49.2
inguinal(canal) (region)	C47.5	C79.89	-	D36.16	D48.2	D49.2
intrathoracic	C47.3	C79.89	-	D36.14	D48.2	D49.2
ischiorectal fossa	C47.5	C79.89	-	D36.16	D48.2	D49.2
knee	C47.2-	C79.89	-	D36.13	D48.2	D49.2
leg	C47.2-	C79.89	-	D36.13	D48.2	D49.2
limb NEC	C47.9	C79.89	-	D36.10	D48.2	D49.2
lower	C47.2-	C79.89	-	D36.13	D48.2	D49.2
upper	C47.1-	C79.89	-	D36.12	D48.2	D49.2
nates	C47.5	C79.89	-	D36.16	D48.2	D49.2
neck	C47.0	C79.89	-	D36.11	D48.2	D49.2
orbit	C69.6-	C79.49	-	D31.6-	D48.7	D49.2
pararectal	C47.5	C79.89	-	D36.16	D48.2	D49.2
paraurethral	C47.5	C79.89	-	D36.16	D48.2	D49.2
paravaginal	C47.5	C79.89	-	D36.16	D48.2	D49.2
pelvis(floor)	C47.5	C79.89	-	D36.16	D48.2	D49.2
pelvoabdominal	C47.8	C79.89	-	D36.17	D48.2	D49.2
perineum	C47.5	C79.89	-	D36.16	D48.2	D49.2
perirectal(tissue)	C47.5	C79.89	-	D36.16	D48.2	D49.2
periurethral(tissue)	C47.5	C79.89	-	D36.16	D48.2	D49.2
popliteal fossa or space	C47.2-	C79.89	-	D36.13	D48.2	D49.2
presacral	C47.5	C79.89	-	D36.16	D48.2	D49.2
pterygoid fossa	C47.0	C79.89	-	D36.11	D48.2	D49.2
rectovaginal septum or wall	C47.5	C79.89	-	D36.16	D48.2	D49.2
rectovesical	C47.5	C79.89	-	D36.16	D48.2	D49.2
sacrococcygeal region	C47.5	C79.89	-	D36.16	D48.2	D49.2
scalp	C47.0	C79.89	-	D36.11	D48.2	D49.2
scapular region	C47.3	C79.89	-	D36.14	D48.2	D49.2
shoulder	C47.1-	C79.89	-	D36.12	D48.2	D49.2
submental	C47.0	C79.89	-	D36.11	D48.2	D49.2
supraclavicular region	C47.0	C79.89	-	D36.11	D48.2	D49.2
temple	C47.0	C79.89	-	D36.11	D48.2	D49.2
temporal region	C47.0	C79.89	-	D36.11	D48.2	D49.2
thigh	C47.2-	C79.89	-	D36.13	D48.2	D49.2
thoracic(duct) (wall)	C47.3	C79.89	-	D36.14	D48.2	D49.2
thorax	C47.3	C79.89	-	D36.14	D48.2	D49.2
thumb	C47.1-	C79.89	-	D36.12	D48.2	D49.2
toe	C47.2-	C79.89	-	D36.13	D48.2	D49.2
trunk	C47.6	C79.89	-	D36.17	D48.2	D49.2
umbilicus	C47.4	C79.89	-	D36.15	D48.2	D49.2
vesicorectal	C47.5	C79.89	-	D36.16	D48.2	D49.2

Neoplasm Index	Malignant Primary	Malignant Secondary	Ca in situ	Benign	Uncertain Behavior	Unspecified Behavior
nerve(ganglion) — *continued*						
peripheral NEC — *continued*						
wrist	C47.1-	C79.89	-	D36.12	D48.2	D49.2
radial	C47.1-	C79.89	-	D36.12	D48.2	D49.2
sacral	C47.5	C79.89	-	D36.16	D48.2	D49.2
sciatic	C47.2-	C79.89	-	D36.13	D48.2	D49.2
spinal NEC	C47.9	C79.89	-	D36.10	D48.2	D49.2
accessory	C72.59	C79.49	-	D33.3	D43.3	D49.7
sympathetic NEC (*see also* Neoplasm, nerve, peripheral)	C47.9	C79.89	-	D36.10	D48.2	D49.2
trigeminal	C72.59	C79.49	-	D33.3	D43.3	D49.7
trochlear	C72.59	C79.49	-	D33.3	D43.3	D49.7
ulnar	C47.1-	C79.89	-	D36.12	D48.2	D49.2
vagus	C72.59	C79.49	-	D33.3	D43.3	D49.7
nervous system(central)	C72.9	C79.40	-	D33.9	D43.9	D49.7
autonomic—*see* Neoplasm, nerve, peripheral						
parasympathetic—*see* Neoplasm, nerve, peripheral						
specified site NEC	-	C79.49	-	D33.7	D43.8	-
sympathetic—*see* Neoplasm, nerve, peripheral						
nevus—*see* Nevus						
nipple	C50.0-	C79.81	D05.-	D24.-	-	-
nose, nasal	C76.0	C79.89	D09.8	D36.7	D48.7	D49.89
ala(external) (nasi) (*see also* Neoplasm, nose, skin)	C44.301	C79.2	D04.39	D23.39	D48.5	D49.2
bone	C41.0	C79.51	-	D16.4-	D48.0	D49.2
cartilage	C30.0	C78.39	D02.3	D14.0	D38.5	D49.1
cavity	C30.0	C78.39	D02.3	D14.0	D38.5	D49.1
choana	C11.3	C79.89	D00.08	D10.6	D37.05	D49.0
external(skin) (*see also* Neoplasm, nose, skin)	C44.301	C79.2	D04.39	D23.39	D48.5	D49.2
fossa	C30.0	C78.39	D02.3	D14.0	D38.5	D49.1
internal	C30.0	C78.39	D02.3	D14.0	D38.5	D49.1
mucosa	C30.0	C78.39	D02.3	D14.0	D38.5	D49.1
septum	C30.0	C78.39	D02.3	D14.0	D38.5	D49.1
posterior margin	C11.3	C79.89	D00.08	D10.6	D37.05	D49.0
sinus—*see* Neoplasm, sinus						
skin	C44.301	C79.2	D04.39	D23.39	D48.5	D49.2
basal cell carcinoma	C44.311	-	-	-	-	-
specified type NEC	C44.391	-	-	-	-	-
squamous cell carcinoma	C44.321	-	-	-	-	-
turbinate(mucosa)	C30.0	C78.39	D02.3	D14.0	D38.5	D49.1
bone	C41.0	C79.51	-	D16.4-	D48.0	D49.2
vestibule	C30.0	C78.39	D02.3	D14.0	D38.5	D49.1
nostril	C30.0	C78.39	D02.3	D14.0	D38.5	D49.1
nucleus pulposus	C41.2	C79.51	-	D16.6	D48.0	D49.2
occipital						
bone	C41.0	C79.51	-	D16.4-	D48.0	D49.2
lobe or pole, brain	C71.4	C79.31	-	D33.0	D43.0	D49.6
odontogenic—*see* Neoplasm, jaw bone						
olfactory nerve or bulb	C72.2-	C79.49	-	D33.3	D43.3	D49.7
olive(brain)	C71.7	C79.31	-	D33.1	D43.1	D49.6
omentum	C48.1	C78.6	-	D20.1	D48.4	D49.0
operculum(brain)	C71.0	C79.31	-	D33.0	D43.0	D49.6
optic nerve, chiasm, or tract	C72.3-	C79.49	-	D33.3	D43.3	D49.7
oral(cavity)	C06.9	C79.89	D00.00	D10.30	D37.09	D49.0
ill-defined	C14.8	C79.89	D00.00	D10.30	D37.09	D49.0
mucosa	C06.0	C79.89	D00.02	D10.39	D37.09	D49.0
orbit	C69.6-	C79.49	D09.2-	D31.6-	D48.7	D49.89
autonomic nerve	C69.6-	C79.49	-	D31.6-	D48.7	D49.2
bone	C41.0	C79.51	-	D16.4-	D48.0	D49.2
eye	C69.6-	C79.49	D09.2-	D31.6-	D48.7	D49.89
peripheral nerves	C69.6-	C79.49	-	D31.6-	D48.7	D49.2
soft parts	C69.6-	C79.49	D09.2-	D31.6-	D48.7	D49.89
organ of Zuckerkandl	C75.5	C79.89	-	D35.6	D44.7	D49.7
oropharynx	C10.9	C79.89	D00.08	D10.5	D37.05	D49.0
branchial cleft(vestige)	C10.4	C79.89	D00.08	D10.5	D37.05	D49.0
junctional region	C10.8	C79.89	D00.08	D10.5	D37.05	D49.0
lateral wall	C10.2	C79.89	D00.08	D10.5	D37.05	D49.0
overlapping lesion	C10.8	-	-	-	-	-
pillars or fauces	C09.1	C79.89	D00.08	D10.5	D37.05	D49.0
posterior wall	C10.3	C79.89	D00.08	D10.5	D37.05	D49.0
vallecula	C10.0	C79.89	D00.08	D10.5	D37.05	D49.0
os						
external	C53.1	C79.82	D06.1	D26.0	D39.0	D49.5
internal	C53.0	C79.82	D06.0	D26.0	D39.0	D49.5
ovary	C56.-	C79.6-	D07.39	D27.-	D39.1-	D49.5
oviduct	C57.0-	C79.82	D07.39	D28.2	D39.8	D49.5
palate	C05.9	C79.89	D00.00	D10.39	D37.09	D49.0
hard	C05.0	C79.89	D00.05	D10.39	D37.09	D49.0
junction of hard and soft palate	C05.9	C79.89	D00.00	D10.39	D37.09	D49.0
overlapping lesions	C05.8	-	-	-	-	-
soft	C05.1	C79.89	D00.04	D10.39	D37.09	D49.0
nasopharyngeal surface	C11.3	C79.89	D00.08	D10.6	D37.05	D49.0
posterior surface	C11.3	C79.89	D00.08	D10.6	D37.05	D49.0
superior surface	C11.3	C79.89	D00.08	D10.6	D37.05	D49.0
palatoglossal arch	C09.1	C79.89	D00.00	D10.5	D37.09	D49.0
palatopharyngeal arch	C09.1	C79.89	D00.00	D10.5	D37.09	D49.0
pallium	C71.0	C79.31	-	D33.0	D43.0	D49.6
palpebra	C44.10-	C79.2	D04.1-	D23.1-	D48.5	D49.2
basal cell carcinoma	C44.11-	-	-	-	-	-
specified type NEC	C44.19-	-	-	-	-	-
squamous cell carcinoma	C44.12-	-	-	-	-	-
pancreas	C25.9	C78.89	D01.7	D13.6	D37.8	D49.0
body	C25.1	C78.89	D01.7	D13.6	D37.8	D49.0
duct(of Santorini) (of Wirsung)	C25.3	C78.89	D01.7	D13.6	D37.8	D49.0
ectopic tissue	C25.7	C78.89	-	D13.6	D37.8	D49.0
head	C25.0	C78.89	D01.7	D13.6	D37.8	D49.0
islet cells	C25.4	C78.89	D01.7	D13.7	D37.8	D49.0
neck	C25.7	C78.89	D01.7	D13.6	D37.8	D49.0
overlapping lesion	C25.8	-	-	-	-	-
tail	C25.2	C78.89	D01.7	D13.6	D37.8	D49.0
para-aortic body	C75.5	C79.89	-	D35.6	D44.7	D49.7
paraganglion NEC	C75.5	C79.89	-	D35.6	D44.7	D49.7
parametrium	C57.3	C79.82	-	D28.2	D39.8	D49.5
paranephric	C48.0	C78.6	-	D20.0	D48.3	D49.0
pararectal	C76.3	C79.89	-	D36.7	D48.7	D49.89
parasagittal(region)	C76.0	C79.89	D09.8	D36.7	D48.7	D49.89
parasellar	C72.9	C79.49	-	D33.9	D43.8	D49.7
parathyroid(gland)	C75.0	C79.89	D09.3	D35.1	D44.2	D49.7
paraurethral	C76.3	C79.89	-	D36.7	D48.7	D49.89
gland	C68.1	C79.19	D09.19	D30.8	D41.8	D49.5

Neoplasm Index	Malignant Primary	Malignant Secondary	Ca in situ	Benign	Uncertain Behavior	Unspecified Behavior
paravaginal	C76.3	C79.89	-	D36.7	D48.7	D49.89
parenchyma, kidney	C64.-	C79.0-	D09.19	D30.0-	D41.0-	D49.5
parietal						
bone	C41.0	C79.51	-	D16.4-	D48.0	D49.2
lobe, brain	C71.3	C79.31	-	D33.0	D43.0	D49.6
paroophoron	C57.1	C79.82	D07.39	D28.2	D39.8	D49.5
parotid(duct) (gland)	C07	C79.89	D00.00	D11.0	D37.030	D49.0
parovarium	C57.1	C79.82	D07.39	D28.2	D39.8	D49.5
patella	C40.20	C79.51	-	-	-	-
peduncle, cerebral	C71.7	C79.31	-	D33.1	D43.1	D49.6
pelvirectal junction	C19	C78.5	D01.1	D12.7	D37.5	D49.0
pelvis, pelvic	C76.3	C79.89	D09.8	D36.7	D48.7	D49.89
bone	C41.4	C79.51	-	D16.8	D48.0	D49.2
floor	C76.3	C79.89	D09.8	D36.7	D48.7	D49.89
renal	C65.-	C79.0-	D09.19	D30.1-	D41.1-	D49.5
viscera	C76.3	C79.89	D09.8	D36.7	D48.7	D49.89
wall	C76.3	C79.89	D09.8	D36.7	D48.7	D49.89
pelvo-abdominal	C76.8	C79.89	D09.8	D36.7	D48.7	D49.89
penis	C60.9	C79.82	D07.4	D29.0	D40.8	D49.5
body	C60.2	C79.82	D07.4	D29.0	D40.8	D49.5
corpus(cavernosum)	C60.2	C79.82	D07.4	D29.0	D40.8	D49.5
glans	C60.1	C79.82	D07.4	D29.0	D40.8	D49.5
overlapping sites	C60.8	-	-	-	-	-
skin NEC	C60.9	C79.82	D07.4	D29.0	D40.8	D49.5
periadrenal(tissue)	C48.0	C78.6	-	D20.0	D48.3	D49.0
perianal(skin) (*see also* Neoplasm, anus, skin)	C44.500	C79.2	D04.5	D23.5	D48.5	D49.2
pericardium	C38.0	C79.89	-	D15.1	D48.7	D49.89
perinephric	C48.0	C78.6	-	D20.0	D48.3	D49.0
perineum	C76.3	C79.89	D09.8	D36.7	D48.7	D49.89
periodontal tissue NEC	C03.9	C79.89	D00.03	D10.39	D37.09	D49.0
periosteum—*see* Neoplasm, bone						
peripancreatic	C48.0	C78.6	-	D20.0	D48.3	D49.0
peripheral nerve NEC	C47.9	C79.89	-	D36.10	D48.2	D49.2
perirectal(tissue)	C76.3	C79.89	-	D36.7	D48.7	D49.89
perirenal(tissue)	C48.0	C78.6	-	D20.0	D48.3	D49.0
peritoneum, peritoneal(cavity)	C48.2	C78.6	-	D20.1	D48.4	D49.0
benign mesothelial tissue—*see* Mesothelioma, benign						
overlapping lesion	C48.8	-	-	-	-	-
with digestive organs	C26.9	-	-	-	-	-
parietal	C48.1	C78.6	-	D20.1	D48.4	D49.0
pelvic	C48.1	C78.6	-	D20.1	D48.4	D49.0
specified part NEC	C48.1	C78.6	-	D20.1	D48.4	D49.0
peritonsillar(tissue)	C76.0	C79.89	D09.8	D36.7	D48.7	D49.89
periurethral tissue	C76.3	C79.89	-	D36.7	D48.7	D49.89
phalanges						
foot	C40.3-	C79.51	-	D16.3-	-	-
hand	C40.1-	C79.51	-	D16.1-	-	-
pharynx, pharyngeal	C14.0	C79.89	D00.08	D10.9	D37.05	D49.0
bursa	C11.1	C79.89	D00.08	D10.6	D37.05	D49.0
fornix	C11.3	C79.89	D00.08	D10.6	D37.05	D49.0
recess	C11.2	C79.89	D00.08	D10.6	D37.05	D49.0
region	C14.0	C79.89	D00.08	D10.9	D37.05	D49.0
tonsil	C11.1	C79.89	D00.08	D10.6	D37.05	D49.0
wall(lateral) (posterior)	C14.0	C79.89	D00.08	D10.9	D37.05	D49.0
pia mater	C70.9	C79.40	-	D32.9	D42.9	D49.7
cerebral	C70.0	C79.32	-	D32.0	D42.0	D49.7
cranial	C70.0	C79.32	-	D32.0	D42.0	D49.7
spinal	C70.1	C79.49	-	D32.1	D42.1	D49.7

Neoplasm Index	Malignant Primary	Malignant Secondary	Ca in situ	Benign	Uncertain Behavior	Unspecified Behavior
pillars of fauces	C09.1	C79.89	D00.08	D10.5	D37.05	D49.0
pineal(body) (gland)	C75.3	C79.89	D09.3	D35.4	D44.5	D49.7
pinna(ear) NEC (*see also* Neoplasm, skin, ear)	C44.20-	C79.2	D04.2-	D23.2-	D48.5	D49.2
piriform fossa or sinus	C12	C79.89	D00.08	D10.7	D37.05	D49.0
pituitary(body) (fossa) (gland) (lobe)	C75.1	C79.89	D09.3	D35.2	D44.3	D49.7
placenta	C58	C79.82	D07.0	D26.7	D39.2	D49.5
pleura, pleural(cavity)	C38.4	C78.2	-	D19.0	D38.2	D49.1
overlapping lesion with heart or mediastinum	C38.8	-	-	-	-	-
parietal	C38.4	C78.2	-	D19.0	D38.2	D49.1
visceral	C38.4	C78.2	-	D19.0	D38.2	D49.1
plexus						
brachial	C47.1-	C79.89	-	D36.12	D48.2	D49.2
cervical	C47.0	C79.89	-	D36.11	D48.2	D49.2
choroid	C71.5	C79.31	-	D33.0	D43.0	D49.6
lumbosacral	C47.5	C79.89	-	D36.16	D48.2	D49.2
sacral	C47.5	C79.89	-	D36.16	D48.2	D49.2
pluriendocrine	C75.8	C79.89	D09.3	D35.7	D44.9	D49.7
pole						
frontal	C71.1	C79.31	-	D33.0	D43.0	D49.6
occipital	C71.4	C79.31	-	D33.0	D43.0	D49.6
pons(varolii)	C71.7	C79.31	-	D33.1	D43.1	D49.6
popliteal fossa or space	C76.5-	C79.89	D04.7-	D36.7	D48.7	D49.89
postcricoid(region)	C13.0	C79.89	D00.08	D10.7	D37.05	D49.0
posterior fossa(cranial)	C71.9	C79.31	-	D33.2	D43.2	D49.6
postnasal space	C11.9	C79.89	D00.08	D10.6	D37.05	D49.0
prepuce	C60.0	C79.82	D07.4	D29.0	D40.8	D49.5
prepylorus	C16.4	C78.89	D00.2	D13.1	D37.1	D49.0
presacral(region)	C76.3	C79.89	-	D36.7	D48.7	D49.89
prostate(gland)	C61	C79.82	D07.5	D29.1	D40.0	D49.5
utricle	C68.0	C79.19	D09.19	D30.4	D41.3	D49.5
pterygoid fossa	C49.0	C79.89	-	D21.0	D48.1	D49.2
pubic bone	C41.4	C79.51	-	D16.8	D48.0	D49.2
pudenda, pudendum(femaie)	C51.9	C79.82	D07.1	D28.0	D39.8	D49.5
pulmonary (*see also* Neoplasm, lung)	C34.9-	C78.0-	D02.2-	D14.3-	D38.1	D49.1
putamen	C71.0	C79.31	-	D33.0	D43.0	D49.6
pyloric						
antrum	C16.3	C78.89	D00.2	D13.1	D37.1	D49.0
canal	C16.4	C78.89	D00.2	D13.1	D37.1	D49.0
pylorus	C16.4	C78.89	D00.2	D13.1	D37.1	D49.0
pyramid(brain)	C71.7	C79.31	-	D33.1	D43.1	D49.6
pyriform fossa or sinus	C12	C79.89	D00.08	D10.7	D37.05	D49.0
radius(any part)	C40.0-	C79.51	-	D16.0-	-	-
Rathke's pouch	C75.1	C79.89	D09.3	D35.2	D44.3	D49.7
rectosigmoid(junction)	C19	C78.5	D01.1	D12.7	D37.5	D49.0
overlapping lesion with anus or rectum	C21.8	-	-	-	-	-
rectouterine pouch	C48.1	C78.6	-	D20.1	D48.4	D49.0
rectovaginal septum or wall	C76.3	C79.89	D09.8	D36.7	D48.7	D49.89
rectovesical septum	C76.3	C79.89	D09.8	D36.7	D48.7	D49.89
rectum(ampulla)	C20	C78.5	D01.2	D12.8	D37.5	D49.0
and colon	C19	C78.5	D01.1	D12.7	D37.5	D49.0
overlapping lesion with anus or rectosigmoid junction	C21.8	-	-	-	-	-
renal	C64.-	C79.0-	D09.19	D30.0-	D41.0-	D49.5
calyx	C65.	C79.0	D09.19	D30.1-	D41.1-	D49.5
hilus	C65.-	C79.0-	D09.19	D30.1-	D41.1-	D49.5

Neoplasm Index	Malignant Primary	Malignant Secondary	Ca in situ	Benign	Uncertain Behavior	Unspecified Behavior
renal — *continued*						
parenchyma	C64.-	C79.0-	D09.19	D30.0-	D41.0-	D49.5
pelvis	C65.-	C79.0-	D09.19	D30.1-	D41.1-	D49.5
respiratory						
organs or system NEC	C39.9	C78.30	D02.4	D14.4	D38.6	D49.1
tract NEC	C39.9	C78.30	D02.4	D14.4	D38.5	D49.1
upper	C39.0	C78.30	D02.4	D14.4	D38.5	D49.1
retina	C69.2-	C79.49	D09.2-	D31.2-	D48.7	D49.81
retrobulbar	C69.6-	C79.49	-	D31.6-	D48.7	D49.89
retrocecal	C48.0	C78.6	-	D20.0	D48.3	D49.0
retromolar(area) (triangle) (trigone)	C06.2	C79.89	D00.00	D10.39	D37.09	D49.0
retro-orbital	C76.0	C79.89	D09.8	D36.7	D48.7	D49.89
retroperitoneal(space) (tissue)	C48.0	C78.6	-	D20.0	D48.3	D49.0
retroperitoneum	C48.0	C78.6	-	D20.0	D48.3	D49.0
retropharyngeal	C14.0	C79.89	D00.08	D10.9	D37.05	D49.0
retrovesical(septum)	C76.3	C79.89	D09.8	D36.7	D48.7	D49.89
rhinencephalon	C71.0	C79.31	-	D33.0	D43.0	D49.6
rib	C41.3	C79.51	-	D16.7	D48.0	D49.2
Rosenmuller's fossa	C11.2	C79.89	D00.08	D10.6	D37.05	D49.0
round ligament	C57.2	C79.82	-	D28.2	D39.8	D49.5
sacrococcyx, sacrococcygeal	C41.4	C79.51	D16.8	D48.0	D49.2	
region	C76.3	C79.89	D09.8	D36.7	D48.7	D49.89
sacrouterine ligament	C57.3	C79.82	-	D28.2	D39.8	D49.5
sacrum, sacral(vertebra)	C41.4	C79.51	-	D16.8	D48.0	D49.2
salivary gland or duct(major)	C08.9	C79.89	D00.00	D11.9	D37.039	D49.0
minor NEC	C06.9	C79.89	D00.00	D10.39	D37.04	D49.0
overlapping lesion	C08.9	-	-	-	-	-
parotid	C07	C79.89	D00.00	D11.0	D37.030	D49.0
pluriglandular	C08.9	C79.89	D00.00	D11.9	D37.039	D49.0
sublingual	C08.1	C79.89	D00.00	D11.7	D37.031	D49.0
submandibular	C08.0	C79.89	D00.00	D11.7	D37.032	D49.0
submaxillary	C08.0	C79.89	D00.00	D11.7	D37.032	D49.0
salpinx(uterine)	C57.0-	C79.82	D07.39	D28.2	D39.8	D49.5
Santorini's duct	C25.3	C78.89	D01.7	D13.6	D37.8	D49.0
scalp	C44.40	C79.2	D04.4	D23.4	D48.5	D49.2
basal cell carcinoma	C44.41	-	-	-	-	-
specified type NEC	C44.49	-	-	-	-	-
squamous cell carcinoma	C44.42	-	-	-	-	-
scapula(any part)	C40.0-	C79.51	-	D16.0-	-	-
scapular region	C76.1	C79.89	D09.8	D36.7	D48.7	D49.89
scar NEC (*see also* Neoplasm, skin, by site)	C44.90	C79.2	D04.9	D23.9	D48.5	D49.2
sciatic nerve	C47.2-	C79.89	-	D36.13	D48.2	D49.2
sclera	C69.4-	C79.49	D09.2-	D31.4-	D48.7	D49.89
scrotum(skin)	C63.2	C79.82	D07.61	D29.4	D40.8	D49.5
sebaceous gland—*see* Neoplasm, skin						
sella turcica	C75.1	C79.89	D09.3	D35.2	D44.3	D49.7
bone	C41.0	C79.51	-	D16.4-	D48.0	D49.2
semilunar cartilage(knee)	C40.2-	C79.51	-	D16.2-	D48.0	D49.2
seminal vesicle	C63.7	C79.82	D07.69	D29.8	D40.8	D49.5
septum						
nasal	C30.0	C78.39	D02.3	D14.0	D38.5	D49.1
posterior margin	C11.3	C79.89	D00.08	D10.6	D37.05	D49.0
rectovaginal	C76.3	C79.89	D09.8	D36.7	D48.7	D49.89
rectovesical	C76.3	C79.89	D09.8	D36.7	D48.7	D49.89
urethrovaginal	C57.9	C79.82	D07.30	D28.9	D39.9	D49.5
vesicovaginal	C57.9	C79.82	D07.30	D28.9	D39.9	D49.5

Neoplasm Index	Malignant Primary	Malignant Secondary	Ca in situ	Benign	Uncertain Behavior	Unspecified Behavior
shoulder NEC	C76.4-	C79.89	D04.6-	D36.7	D48.7	D49.89
sigmoid flexure(lower) (upper)	C18.7	C78.5	D01.0	D12.5	D37.4	D49.0
sinus(accessory)	C31.9	C78.39	D02.3	D14.0	D38.5	D49.1
bone(any)	C41.0	C79.51	-	D16.4-	D48.0	D49.2
ethmoidal	C31.1	C78.39	D02.3	D14.0	D38.5	D49.1
frontal	C31.2	C78.39	D02.3	D14.0	D38.5	D49.1
maxillary	C31.0	C78.39	D02.3	D14.0	D38.5	D49.1
nasal, paranasal NEC	C31.9	C78.39	D02.3	D14.0	D38.5	D49.1
overlapping lesion	C31.8	-	-	-	-	-
sinus(accessory) — *continued*						
pyriform	C12	C79.89	D00.08	D10.7	D37.05	D49.0
sphenoid	C31.3	C78.39	D02.3	D14.0	D38.5	D49.1
skeleton, skeletal NEC	C41.9	C79.51	-	D16.9-	D48.0	D49.2
Skene's gland	C68.1	C79.19	D09.19	D30.8	D41.8	D49.5
skin NOS	C44.90	C79.2	D04.9	D23.9	D48.5	D49.2
abdominal wall	C44.509	C79.2	D04.5	D23.5	D48.5	D49.2
basal cell carcinoma	C44.519	-	-	-	-	-
specified type NEC	C44.599	-	-	-	-	-
squamous cell carcinoma	C44.529	-	-	-	-	-
ala nasi (*see also* Neoplasm, nose, skin)	C44.301	C79.2	D04.39	D23.39	D48.5	D49.2
ankle (*see also* Neoplasm, skin, limb, lower)	C44.70-	C79.2	D04.7-	D23.7-	D48.5	D49.2
antecubital space (*see also* Neoplasm, skin, limb, upper)	C44.60-	C79.2	D04.6-	D23.6-	D48.5	D49.2
anus	C44.500	C79.2	D04.5	D23.5	D48.5	D49.2
basal cell carcinoma	C44.510	-	-	-	-	-
specified type NEC	C44.590	-	-	-	-	-
squamous cell carcinoma	C44.520	-	-	-	-	-
arm (*see also* Neoplasm, skin, limb, upper)	C44.60-	C79.2	D04.6-	D23.6-	D48.5	D49.2
auditory canal(external) (*see also* Neoplasm, skin, ear)	C44.20-	C79.2	D04.2-	D23.2-	D48.5	D49.2
auricle(ear) (*see also* Neoplasm, skin, ear)	C44.20-	C79.2	D04.2-	D23.2-	D48.5	D49.2
auricular canal(external) (*see also* Neoplasm, skin, ear)	C44.20-	C79.2	D04.2-	D23.2-	D48.5	D49.2
axilla, axillary fold (*see also* Neoplasm, skin, trunk)	C44.509	C79.2	D04.5	D23.5	D48.5	D49.2
back (*see also* Neoplasm, skin, trunk)	C44.509	C79.2	D04.5	D23.5	D48.5	D49.2
basal cell carcinoma	C44.91					
breast	C44.501	C79.2	D04.5	D23.5	D48.5	D49.2
basal cell carcinoma	C44.511	-	-	-	-	-
specified type NEC	C44.591	-	-	-	-	-
squamous cell carcinoma	C44.521	-	-	-	-	-
brow (*see also* Neoplasm, skin, face)	C44.309	C79.2	D04.39	D23.39	D48.5	D49.2
buttock (*see also* Neoplasm, skin, trunk)	C44.509	C79.2	D04.5	D23.5	D48.5	D49.2
calf (*see also* Neoplasm, skin, limb, lower)	C44.70-	C79.2	D04.7-	D23.7-	D48.5	D49.2

Neoplasm Index	Malignant Primary	Malignant Secondary	Ca in situ	Benign	Uncertain Behavior	Unspecified Behavior
skin NOS — *continued*						
canthus(eye) (inner) (outer)	C44.10-	C79.2	D04.1-	D23.1-	D48.5	D49.2
basal cell carcinoma	C44.11-	-	-	-	-	-
specified type NEC	C44.19-	-	-	-	-	-
squamous cell carcinoma	C44.12-	-	-	-	-	-
cervical region (*see also* Neoplasm, skin, neck)	C44.40	C79.2	D04.4	D23.4	D48.5	D49.2
cheek(external) (*see also* Neoplasm, skin, face)	C44.309	C79.2	D04.39	D23.39	D48.5	D49.2
chest(wall) (*see also* Neoplasm, skin, trunk)	C44.509	C79.2	D04.5	D23.5	D48.5	D49.2
chin (*see also* Neoplasm, skin, face)	C44.309	C79.2	D04.39	D23.39	D48.5	D49.2
clavicular area (*see also* Neoplasm, skin, trunk)	C44.509	C79.2	D04.5	D23.5	D48.5	D49.2
clitoris	C51.2	C79.82	D07.1	D28.0	D39.8	D49.5
columnella (*see also* Neoplasm, skin, face)	C44.309	C79.2	D04.39	D23.39	D48.5	D49.2
concha (*see also* Neoplasm, skin, ear)	C44.20-	C79.2	D04.2-	D23.2-	D48.5	D49.2
ear(external)	C44.20-	C79.2	D04.2-	D23.2-	D48.5	D49.2
basal cell carcinoma	C44.21-	-	-	-	-	-
specified type NEC	C44.29-	-	-	-	-	-
squamous cell carcinoma	C44.22-	-	-	-	-	-
elbow (*see also* Neoplasm, skin, limb, upper)	C44.60-	C79.2	D04.6-	D23.6-	D48.5	D49.2
eyebrow (*see also* Neoplasm, skin, face)	C44.309	C79.2	D04.39	D23.39	D48.5	D49.2
eyelid	C44.10-	C79.2	D04.1-	D23.1-	D48.5	D49.2
basal cell carcinoma	C44.11-	-	-	-	-	-
specified type NEC	C44.19-	-	-	-	-	-
squamous cell carcinoma	C44.12-	-	-	-	-	-
face NOS	C44.300	C79.2	D04.30	D23.30	D48.5	D49.2
basal cell carcinoma	C44.310	-	-	-	-	-
specified type NEC	C44.390	-	-	-	-	-
squamous cell carcinoma	C44.320	-	-	-	-	-
female genital organs(external)	C51.9	C79.82	D07.1	D28.0	D39.8	D49.5
clitoris	C51.2	C79.82	D07.1	D28.0	D39.8	D49.5
labium NEC	C51.9	C79.82	D07.1	D28.0	D39.8	D49.5
majus	C51.0	C79.82	D07.1	D28.0	D39.8	D49.5
minus	C51.1	C79.82	D07.1	D28.0	D39.8	D49.5
pudendum	C51.9	C79.82	D07.1	D28.0	D39.8	D49.5
vulva	C51.9	C79.82	D07.1	D28.0	D39.8	D49.5
finger (*see also* Neoplasm, skin, limb, upper)	C44.60-	C79.2	D04.6-	D23.6-	D48.5	D49.2
flank (*see also* Neoplasm, skin, trunk)	C44.509	C79.2	D04.5	D23.5	D48.5	D49.2
foot (*see also* Neoplasm, skin, limb, lower)	C44.70-	C79.2	D04.7-	D23.7-	D48.5	D49.2
skin NOS — *continued*						
forearm (*see also* Neoplasm, skin, limb, upper)	C44.60-	C79.2	D04.6-	D23.6-	D48.5	D49.2
forehead (*see also* Neoplasm, skin, face)	C44.309	C79.2	D04.39	D23.39	D48.5	D49.2
glabella (*see also* Neoplasm, skin, face)	C44.309	C79.2	D04.39	D23.39	D48.5	D49.2
gluteal region (*see also* Neoplasm, skin, trunk)	C44.509	C79.2	D04.5	D23.5	D48.5	D49.2
groin (*see also* Neoplasm, skin, trunk)	C44.509	C79.2	D04.5	D23.5	D48.5	D49.2
hand (*see also* Neoplasm, skin, limb, upper)	C44.60-	C79.2	D04.6-	D23.6-	D48.5	D49.2
head NEC (*see also* Neoplasm, skin, scalp)	C44.40	C79.2	D04.4	D23.4	D48.5	D49.2
heel (*see also* Neoplasm, skin, limb, lower)	C44.70-	C79.2	D04.7-	D23.7-	D48.5	D49.2
helix (*see also* Neoplasm, skin, ear)	C44.20-	C79.2	D04.2-	D23.2-	D48.5	D49.2
hip (*see also* Neoplasm, skin, limb, lower)	C44.70-	C79.2	D04.7-	D23.7-	D48.5	D49.2
infraclavicular region (*see also* Neoplasm, skin, trunk)	C44.509	C79.2	D04.5	D23.5	D48.5	D49.2
inguinal region (*see also* Neoplasm, skin, trunk)	C44.509	C79.2	D04.5	D23.5	D48.5	D49.2
jaw (*see also* Neoplasm, skin, face)	C44.309	C79.2	D04.39	D23.39	D48.5	D49.2
Kaposi's sarcoma—*see* Kaposi's, sarcoma, skin						
knee (*see also* Neoplasm, skin, limb, lower)	C44.70-	C79.2	D04.7-	D23.7-	D48.5	D49.2
labia						
majora	C51.0	C79.82	D07.1	D28.0	D39.8	D49.5
minora	C51.1	C79.82	D07.1	D28.0	D39.8	D49.5
leg (*see also* Neoplasm, skin, limb, lower)	C44.70-	C79.2	D04.7-	D23.7-	D48.5	D49.2
lid(lower) (upper)	C44.10-	C79.2	D04.1-	D23.1-	D48.5	D49.2
basal cell carcinoma	C44.11-	-	-	-	-	-
specified type NEC	C44.19-	-	-	-	-	-
squamous cell carcinoma	C44.12-	-	-	-	-	-
limb NEC	C44.90	C79.2	D04.9	D23.9	D48.5	D49.2
basal cell carcinoma	C44.91					
lower	C44.70-	C79.2	D04.7-	D23.7-	D48.5	D49.2
basal cell carcinoma	C44.71-	-	-	-	-	-
specified type NEC	C44.79-	-	-	-	-	-
squamous cell carcinoma	C44.72-	-	-	-	-	-
upper	C44.60-	C79.2	D04.6-	D23.6-	D48.5	D49.2
basal cell carcinoma	C44.61-	-	-	-	-	-
specified type NEC	C44.69-	-	-	-	-	-
squamous cell carcinoma	C44.62-	-	-	-	-	-
lip(lower) (upper)	C44.00	C79.2	D04.0	D23.0	D48.5	D49.2
basal cell carcinoma	C44.01	-	-	-	-	-

Neoplasm Index	Malignant Primary	Malignant Secondary	Ca in situ	Benign	Uncertain Behavior	Unspecified Behavior
skin NOS — *continued*						
lip(lower) (upper) — *continued*						
specified type NEC	C44.09	-	-	-	-	-
squamous cell carcinoma	C44.02	-	-	-	-	-
male genital organs	C63.9	C79.82	D07.60	D29.9	D40.8	D49.5
penis	C60.9	C79.82	D07.4	D29.0	D40.8	D49.5
prepuce	C60.0	C79.82	D07.4	D29.0	D40.8	D49.5
scrotum	C63.2	C79.82	D07.61	D29.4	D40.8	D49.5
mastectomy site(skin) (*see also* Neoplasm, skin, breast)	C44.501	C79.2	-	-	-	-
specified as breast tissue	C50.8-	C79.81	-	-	-	-
meatus, acoustic(external) (*see also* Neoplasm, skin, ear)	C44.20-	C79.2	D04.2-	D23.2-	D48.5	D49.2
melanotic—*see* Melanoma						
Merkel cell—*see* Carcinoma, Merkel cell						
nates (*see also* Neoplasm, skin, trunk)	C44.509	C79.2	D04.5	D23.5	D48.5	D49.2
neck	C44.40	C79.2	D04.4	D23.4	D48.5	D49.2
basal cell carcinoma	C44.41	-	-	-	-	-
specified type NEC	C44.49	-	-	-	-	-
squamous cell carcinoma	C44.42	-	-	-	-	-
nevus—*see* Nevus, skin						
nose(external) (*see also* Neoplasm, nose, skin)	C44.301	C79.2	D04.39	D23.39	D48.5	D49.2
overlapping lesion	C44.80	-	-	-	-	-
basal cell carcinoma	C44.81	-	-	-	-	-
specified type NEC	C44.89	-	-	-	-	-
squamous cell carcinoma	C44.82	-	-	-	-	-
palm (*see also* Neoplasm, skin, limb, upper)	C44.60-	C79.2	D04.6-	D23.6-	D48.5	D49.2
palpebra	C44.10-	C79.2	D04.1-	D23.1-	D48.5	D49.2
basal cell carcinoma	C44.11-	-	-	-	-	-
specified type NEC	C44.19-	-	-	-	-	-
squamous cell carcinoma	C44.12-	-	-	-	-	-
penis NEC	C60.9	C79.82	D07.4	D29.0	D40.8	D49.5
perianal (*see also* Neoplasm, skin, anus)	C44.500	C79.2	D04.5	D23.5	D48.5	D49.2
perineum (*see also* Neoplasm, skin, anus)	C44.500	C79.2	D04.5	D23.5	D48.5	D49.2
pinna (*see also* Neoplasm, skin, ear)	C44.20-	C79.2	D04.2-	D23.2-	D48.5	D49.2
plantar (*see also* Neoplasm, skin, limb, lower)	C44.70-	C79.2	D04.7-	D23.7-	D48.5	D49.2
popliteal fossa or space (*see also* Neoplasm, skin, limb, lower)	C44.70-	C79.2	D04.7-	D23.7-	D48.5	D49.2
prepuce	C60.0	C79.82	D07.4	D29.0	D40.8	D49.5

Neoplasm Index	Malignant Primary	Malignant Secondary	Ca in situ	Benign	Uncertain Behavior	Unspecified Behavior
skin NOS — *continued*						
pubes (*see also* Neoplasm, skin, trunk)	C44.509	C79.2	D04.5	D23.5	D48.5	D49.2
sacrococcygeal region (*see also* Neoplasm, skin, trunk)	C44.509	C79.2	D04.5	D23.5	D48.5	D49.2
scalp	C44.40	C79.2	D04.4	D23.4	D48.5	D49.2
basal cell carcinoma	C44.41	-	-	-	-	-
specified type NEC	C44.49	-	-	-	-	-
squamous cell carcinoma	C44.42	-	-	-	-	-
scapular region (*see also* Neoplasm, skin, trunk)	C44.509	C79.2	D04.5	D23.5	D48.5	D49.2
scrotum	C63.2	C79.82	D07.61	D29.4	D40.8	D49.5
shoulder (*see also* Neoplasm, skin, limb, upper)	C44.60-	C79.2	D04.6-	D23.6-	D48.5	D49.2
sole(foot) (*see also* Neoplasm, skin, limb, lower)	C44.70-	C79.2	D04.7-	D23.7-	D48.5	D49.2
specified sites NEC	C44.80	C79.2	D04.8	D23.9	D48.5	D49.2
basal cell carcinoma	C44.81	-	-	-	-	-
specified type NEC	C44.89	-	-	-	-	-
squamous cell carcinoma	C44.82	-	-	-	-	-
specified type NEC	C44.99	-	-	-	-	-
squamous cell carcinoma	C44.92	-	-	-	-	-
submammary fold (*see also* Neoplasm, skin, trunk)	C44.509	C79.2	D04.5	D23.5	D48.5	D49.2
supraclavicular region (*see also* Neoplasm, skin, neck)	C44.40	C79.2	D04.4	D23.4	D48.5	D49.2
temple (*see also* Neoplasm, skin, face)	C44.309	C79.2	D04.39	D23.39	D48.5	D49.2
thigh (*see also* Neoplasm, skin, limb, lower)	C44.70-	C79.2	D04.7-	D23.7-	D48.5	D49.2
thoracic wall (*see also* Neoplasm, skin, trunk)	C44.509	C79.2	D04.5	D23.5	D48.5	D49.2
thumb (*see also* Neoplasm, skin, limb, upper)	C44.60-	C79.2	D04.6-	D23.6-	D48.5	D49.2
toe (*see also* Neoplasm, skin, limb, lower)	C44.70-	C79.2	D04.7-	D23.7-	D48.5	D49.2
tragus (*see also* Neoplasm, skin, ear)	C44.20-	C79.2	D04.2-	D23.2-	D48.5	D49.2
trunk	C44.509	C79.2	D04.5	D23.5	D48.5	D49.2
basal cell carcinoma	C44.519	-	-	-	-	-
specified type NEC	C44.599	-	-	-	-	-
squamous cell carcinoma	C44.529	-	-	-	-	-
umbilicus (*see also* Neoplasm, skin, trunk)	C44.509	C79.2	D04.5	D23.5	D48.5	D49.2
vulva	C51.9	C79.82	D07.1	D28.0	D39.8	D49.5
overlapping lesion	C51.8	-	-	-	-	-
wrist (*see also* Neoplasm, skin, limb, upper)	C44.60-	C79.2	D04.6-	D23.6-	D48.5	D49.2

Neoplasm Index	Malignant Primary	Malignant Secondary	Ca in situ	Benign	Uncertain Behavior	Unspecified Behavior
skull	C41.0	C79.51	-	D16.4-	D48.0	D49.2
soft parts or tissues—see Neoplasm, connective tissue						
specified site NEC	C76.8	C79.89	D09.8	D36.7	D48.7	D49.89
spermatic cord	C63.1-	C79.82	D07.69	D29.8	D40.8	D49.5
sphenoid	C31.3	C78.39	D02.3	D14.0	D38.5	D49.1
bone	C41.0	C79.51	-	D16.4-	D48.0	D49.2
sinus	C31.3	C78.39	D02.3	D14.0	D38.5	D49.1
sphincter						
anal	C21.1	C78.5	D01.3	D12.9	D37.8	D49.0
of Oddi	C24.0	C78.89	D01.5	D13.5	D37.6	D49.0
spine, spinal(column)	C41.2	C79.51	-	D16.6	D48.0	D49.2
bulb	C71.7	C79.31	-	D33.1	D43.1	D49.6
coccyx	C41.4	C79.51	-	D16.8	D48.0	D49.2
cord(cervical) (lumbar) (sacral) (thoracic)	C72.0	C79.49	-	D33.4	D43.4	D49.7
dura mater	C70.1	C79.49	-	D32.1	D42.1	D49.7
lumbosacral	C41.2	C79.51	-	D16.6	D48.0	D49.2
marrow NEC	C96.9	C79.52	-	-	D47.9	D49.89
membrane	C70.1	C79.49	-	D32.1	D42.1	D49.7
meninges	C70.1	C79.49	-	D32.1	D42.1	D49.7
nerve(root)	C47.9	C79.89	-	D36.10	D48.2	D49.2
pia mater	C70.1	C79.49	-	D32.1	D42.1	D49.7
root	C47.9	C79.89	-	D36.10	D48.2	D49.2
sacrum	C41.4	C79.51	-	D16.8	D48.0	D49.2
spleen, splenic NEC	C26.1	C78.89	D01.7	D13.9	D37.8	D49.0
flexure(colon)	C18.5	C78.5	D01.0	D12.3	D37.4	D49.0
stem, brain	C71.7	C79.31	-	D33.1	D43.1	D49.6
Stensen's duct	C07	C79.89	D00.00	D11.0	D37.030	D49.0
sternum	C41.3	C79.51	-	D16.7	D48.0	D49.2
stomach	C16.9	C78.89	D00.2	D13.1	D37.1	D49.0
antrum(pyloric)	C16.3	C78.89	D00.2	D13.1	D37.1	D49.0
body	C16.2	C78.89	D00.2	D13.1	D37.1	D49.0
cardia	C16.0	C78.89	D00.2	D13.1	D37.1	D49.0
cardiac orifice	C16.0	C78.89	D00.2	D13.1	D37.1	D49.0
corpus	C16.2	C78.89	D00.2	D13.1	D37.1	D49.0
fundus	C16.1	C78.89	D00.2	D13.1	D37.1	D49.0
greater curvature NEC	C16.6	C78.89	D00.2	D13.1	D37.1	D49.0
lesser curvature NEC	C16.5	C78.89	D00.2	D13.1	D37.1	D49.0
overlapping lesion	C16.8	-	-	-	-	-
prepylorus	C16.4	C78.89	D00.2	D13.1	D37.1	D49.0
pylorus	C16.4	C78.89	D00.2	D13.1	D37.1	D49.0
wall NEC	C16.9	C78.89	D00.2	D13.1	D37.1	D49.0
anterior NEC	C16.8	C78.89	D00.2	D13.1	D37.1	D49.0
posterior NEC	C16.8	C78.89	D00.2	D13.1	D37.1	D49.0
stroma, endometrial	C54.1	C79.82	D07.0	D26.1	D39.0	D49.5
stump, cervical	C53.8	C79.82	D06.7	D26.0	D39.0	D49.5
subcutaneous(nodule) (tissue) NEC—see Neoplasm, connective tissue						
subdural	C70.9	C79.32	-	D32.9	D42.9	D49.7
subglottis, subglottic	C32.2	C78.39	D02.0	D14.1	D38.0	D49.1
sublingual	C04.9	C79.89	D00.06	D10.2	D37.09	D49.0
gland or duct	C08.1	C79.89	D00.00	D11.7	D37.031	D49.0
submandibular gland	C08.0	C79.89	D00.00	D11.7	D37.032	D49.0
submaxillary gland or duct	C08.0	C79.89	D00.00	D11.7	D37.032	D49.0
submental	C76.0	C79.89	D09.8	D36.7	D48.7	D49.89
subpleural	C34.9-	C78.0-	D02.2-	D14.3-	D38.1	D49.1
substernal	C38.1	C78.1	-	D15.2	D38.3	D49.89
sudoriferous, sudoriparous gland, site unspecified	C44.90	C79.2	D04.9	D23.9	D48.5	D49.2

Neoplasm Index	Malignant Primary	Malignant Secondary	Ca in situ	Benign	Uncertain Behavior	Unspecified Behavior
sudoriferous, sudoriparous gland, site unspecified — continued						
specified site—see Neoplasm, skin						
supraclavicular region	C76.0	C79.89	D09.8	D36.7	D48.7	D49.89
supraglottis	C32.1	C78.39	D02.0	D14.1	D38.0	D49.1
suprarenal	C74.9-	C79.7-	D09.3	D35.0-	D44.1-	D49.7
capsule	C74.9-	C79.7-	D09.3	D35.0-	D44.1-	D49.7
cortex	C74.0-	C79.7-	D09.3	D35.0-	D44.1-	D49.7
gland	C74.9-	C79.7-	D09.3	D35.0-	D44.1-	D49.7
medulla	C74.1-	C79.7-	D09.3	D35.0-	D44.1-	D49.7
suprasellar(region)	C71.9	C79.31	-	D33.2	D43.2	D49.6
supratentorial(brain) NEC	C71.0	C79.31	-	D33.0	D43.0	D49.6
sweat gland(apocrine) (eccrine), site unspecified	C44.90	C79.2	D04.9	D23.9	D48.5	D49.2
specified site—see Neoplasm, skin						
sympathetic nerve or nervous system NEC	C47.9	C79.89	-	D36.10	D48.2	D49.2
symphysis pubis	C41.4	C79.51	-	D16.8	D48.0	D49.2
synovial membrane—see Neoplasm, connective tissue						
tapetum, brain	C71.8	C79.31	-	D33.2	D43.2	D49.6
tarsus(any bone)	C40.3-	C79.51	-	D16.3-	-	-
temple(skin) (see also Neoplasm, skin, face)	C44.309	C79.2	D04.39	D23.39	D48.5	D49.2
temporal						
bone	C41.0	C79.51	-	D16.4-	D48.0	D49.2
lobe or pole	C71.2	C79.31	-	D33.0	D43.0	D49.6
region	C76.0	C79.89	D09.8	D36.7	D48.7	D49.89
skin (see also Neoplasm, skin, face)	C44.309	C79.2	D04.39	D23.39	D48.5	D49.2
tendon(sheath)—see Neoplasm, connective tissue						
tentorium(cerebelli)	C70.0	C79.32	-	D32.0	D42.0	D49.7
testis, testes	C62.9-	C79.82	D07.69	D29.2-	D40.1-	D49.5
descended	C62.1-	C79.82	D07.69	D29.2-	D40.1-	D49.5
ectopic	C62.0-	C79.82	D07.69	D29.2-	D40.1-	D49.5
retained	C62.0-	C79.82	D07.69	D29.2-	D40.1-	D49.5
scrotal	C62.1-	C79.82	D07.69	D29.2-	D40.1-	D49.5
undescended	C62.0-	C79.82	D07.69	D29.2-	D40.1-	D49.5
unspecified whether descended or undescended	C62.9-	C79.82	D07.69	D29.2-	D40.1-	D49.5
thalamus	C71.0	C79.31	-	D33.0	D43.0	D49.6
thigh NEC	C76.5-	C79.89	D04.7-	D36.7	D48.7	D49.89
thorax, thoracic(cavity) (organs NEC)	C76.1	C79.89	D09.8	D36.7	D48.7	D49.89
duct	C49.3	C79.89	-	D21.3	D48.1	D49.2
wall NEC	C76.1	C79.89	D09.8	D36.7	D48.7	D49.89
throat	C14.0	C79.89	D00.08	D10.9	D37.05	D49.0
thumb NEC	C76.4-	C79.89	D04.6-	D36.7	D48.7	D49.89
thymus(gland)	C37	C79.89	D09.3	D15.0	D38.4	D49.89
thyroglossal duct	C73	C79.89	D09.3	D34	D44.0	D49.7
thyroid(gland)	C73	C79.89	D09.3	D34	D44.0	D49.7
cartilage	C32.3	C78.39	D02.0	D14.1	D38.0	D49.1
tibia(any part)	C40.2-	C79.51	-	D16.2-	-	-
toe NEC	C76.5-	C79.89	D04.7	D36.7	D48.7	D49.89
tongue	C02.9	C79.89	D00.07	D10.1	D37.02	D49.0

Neoplasm Index	Malignant Primary	Malignant Secondary	Ca in situ	Benign	Uncertain Behavior	Unspecified Behavior
tongue — continued						
anterior(two-thirds) NEC	C02.3	C79.89	D00.07	D10.1	D37.02	D49.0
dorsal surface	C02.0	C79.89	D00.07	D10.1	D37.02	D49.0
ventral surface	C02.2	C79.89	D00.07	D10.1	D37.02	D49.0
base(dorsal surface)	C01	C79.89	D00.07	D10.1	D37.02	D49.0
border(lateral)	C02.1	C79.89	D00.07	D10.1	D37.02	D49.0
dorsal surface NEC	C02.0	C79.89	D00.07	D10.1	D37.02	D49.0
fixed part NEC	C01	C79.89	D00.07	D10.1	D37.02	D49.0
foreamen cecum	C02.0	C79.89	D00.07	D10.1	D37.02	D49.0
frenulum linguae	C02.2	C79.89	D00.07	D10.1	D37.02	D49.0
junctional zone	C02.8	C79.89	D00.07	D10.1	D37.02	D49.0
margin(lateral)	C02.1	C79.89	D00.07	D10.1	D37.02	D49.0
midline NEC	C02.0	C79.89	D00.07	D10.1	D37.02	D49.0
mobile part NEC	C02.3	C79.89	D00.07	D10.1	D37.02	D49.0
overlapping lesion	C02.8	-	-	-	-	-
posterior(third)	C01	C79.89	D00.07	D10.1	D37.02	D49.0
root	C01	C79.89	D00.07	D10.1	D37.02	D49.0
surface(dorsal)	C02.0	C79.89	D00.07	D10.1	D37.02	D49.0
base	C01	C79.89	D00.07	D10.1	D37.02	D49.0
ventral	C02.2	C79.89	D00.07	D10.1	D37.02	D49.0
tip	C02.1	C79.89	D00.07	D10.1	D37.02	D49.0
tonsil	C02.4	C79.89	D00.07	D10.1	D37.02	D49.0
tonsil	C09.9	C79.89	D00.08	D10.4	D37.05	D49.0
fauces, faucial	C09.9	C79.89	D00.08	D10.4	D37.05	D49.0
lingual	C02.4	C79.89	D00.07	D10.1	D37.02	D49.0
overlapping sites	C09.8	-	-	-	-	-
palatine	C09.9	C79.89	D00.08	D10.4	D37.05	D49.0
pharyngeal	C11.1	C79.89	D00.08	D10.6	D37.05	D49.0
pillar(anterior) (posterior)	C09.1	C79.89	D00.08	D10.5	D37.05	D49.0
tonsillar fossa	C09.0	C79.89	D00.08	D10.5	D37.05	D49.0
tooth socket NEC	C03.9	C79.89	D00.03	D10.39	D37.09	D49.0
trachea(cartilage) (mucosa)	C33	C78.39	D02.1	D14.2	D38.1	D49.1
overlapping lesion with bronchus or lung	C34.8-	-	-	-	-	-
tracheobronchial	C34.8-	C78.39	D02.1	D14.2	D38.1	D49.1
overlapping lesion with lung	C34.8-	-	-	-	-	-
tragus (see also Neoplasm, skin, ear)	C44.20-	C79.2	D04.2-	D23.2-	D48.5	D49.2
trunk NEC	C76.8	C79.89	D04.5	D36.7	D48.7	D49.89
tubo-ovarian	C57.8	C79.82	D07.39	D28.7	D39.8	D49.5
tunica vaginalis	C63.7	C79.82	D07.69	D29.8	D40.8	D49.5
turbinate(bone)	C41.0	C79.51	-	D16.4-	D48.0	D49.2
nasal	C30.0	C78.39	D02.3	D14.0	D38.5	D49.1
tympanic cavity	C30.1	C78.39	D02.3	D14.0	D38.5	D49.1
ulna(any part)	C40.0-	C79.51	-	D16.0-	-	-
umbilicus, umbilical (see also Neoplasm, skin, trunk)	C44.509	C79.2	D04.5	D23.5	D48.5	D49.2
uncus, brain	C71.2	C79.31	-	D33.0	D43.0	D49.6
unknown site or unspecified	C80.1	C79.9	D09.9	D36.9	D48.9	D49.9
urachus	C67.7	C79.11	D09.0	D30.3	D41.4	D49.4
ureter, ureteral	C66.-	C79.19	D09.19	D30.2-	D41.2-	D49.5
orifice(bladder)	C67.6	C79.11	D09.0	D30.3	D41.4	D49.4
ureter-bladder(junction)	C67.6	C79.11	D09.0	D30.3	D41.4	D49.4
urethra, urethral(gland)	C68.0	C79.19	D09.19	D30.4	D41.3	D49.5
orifice, internal	C67.5	C79.11	D09.0	D30.3	D41.4	D49.4
urethrovaginal(septum)	C57.9	C79.82	D07.30	D28.9	D39.8	D49.5
urinary organ or system	C68.9	C79.10	D09.10	D30.9	D41.9	D49.5
bladder—see Neoplasm, bladder						

Neoplasm Index	Malignant Primary	Malignant Secondary	Ca in situ	Benign	Uncertain Behavior	Unspecified Behavior
urinary organ or system — continued						
bladder—see Neoplasm, bladder — continued						
overlapping lesion	C68.8	-	-	-	-	-
specified sites NEC	C68.8	C79.19	D09.19	D30.8	D41.8	D49.5
utero-ovarian	C57.8	C79.82	D07.39	D28.7	D39.8	D49.5
ligament	C57.1	C79.82	D07.39	D28.2	D39.8	D49.5
uterosacral ligament	C57.3	C79.82	-	D28.2	D39.8	D49.5
uterus, uteri, uterine	C55	C79.82	D07.0	D26.9	D39.0	D49.5
adnexa NEC	C57.4	C79.82	D07.39	D28.7	D39.8	D49.5
body	C54.9	C79.82	D07.0	D26.1	D39.0	D49.5
cervix	C53.9	C79.82	D06.9	D26.0	D39.0	D49.5
cornu	C54.9	C79.82	D07.0	D26.1	D39.0	D49.5
corpus	C54.9	C79.82	D07.0	D26.1	D39.0	D49.5
endocervix(canal) (gland)	C53.0	C79.82	D06.0	D26.0	D39.0	D49.5
endometrium	C54.1	C79.82	D07.0	D26.1	D39.0	D49.5
exocervix	C53.1	C79.82	D06.1	D26.0	D39.0	D49.5
external os	C53.1	C79.82	D06.1	D26.0	D39.0	D49.5
fundus	C54.3	C79.82	D07.0	D26.1	D39.0	D49.5
internal os	C53.0	C79.82	D06.0	D26.0	D39.0	D49.5
isthmus	C54.0	C79.82	D07.0	D26.1	D39.0	D49.5
ligament	C57.3	C79.82	-	D28.2	D39.8	D49.5
broad	C57.1	C79.82	D07.39	D28.2	D39.8	D49.5
round	C57.2	C79.82	-	D28.2	D39.8	D49.5
lower segment	C54.0	C79.82	D07.0	D26.1	D39.0	D49.5
myometrium	C54.2	C79.82	D07.0	D26.1	D39.0	D49.5
overlapping sites	C54.8	-	-	-	-	-
squamocolumnar junction	C53.8	C79.82	D06.7	D26.0	D39.0	D49.5
tube	C57.0-	C79.82	D07.39	D28.2	D39.8	D49.5
utricle, prostatic	C68.0	C79.19	D09.19	D30.4	D41.3	D49.5
uveal tract	C69.4-	C79.49	D09.2-	D31.4-	D48.7	D49.89
uvula	C05.2	C79.89	D00.04	D10.39	D37.09	D49.0
vagina, vaginal(fornix) (vault) (wall)	C52	C79.82	D07.2	D28.1	D39.8	D49.5
vaginovesical	C57.9	C79.82	D07.30	D28.9	D39.9	D49.5
septum	C57.9	C79.82	D07.30	D28.9	D39.9	D49.5
vallecula(epigiottis)	C10.0	C79.89	D00.08	D10.5	D37.05	D49.0
vas deferens	C63.1-	C79.82	D07.69	D29.8	D40.8	D49.5
vascular—see Neoplasm, connective tissue						
Vater's ampulla	C24.1	C78.89	D01.5	D13.5	D37.6	D49.0
vein, venous—see Neoplasm, connective tissue						
vena cava(abdominal) (inferior)	C49.4	C79.89	-	D21.4	D48.1	D49.2
superior	C49.3	C79.89	-	D21.3	D48.1	D49.2
ventricle(cerebral) (floor) (lateral) (third)	C71.5	C79.31	-	D33.0	D43.0	D49.6
cardiac(left) (right)	C38.0	C79.89	-	D15.1	D48.7	D49.89
fourth	C71.7	C79.31	-	D33.1	D43.1	D49.6
ventricular band of larynx	C32.1	C78.39	D02.0	D14.1	D38.0	D49.1
ventriculus—see Neoplasm, stomach						
vermillion border—see Neoplasm, lip						
vermis, cerebellum	C71.6	C79.31	-	D33.1	D43.1	D49.6
vertebra(column)	C41.2	C79.51	-	D16.6	D48.0	D49.2
coccyx	C41.4	C79.51	-	D16.8-	D48.0	D49.2
marrow NEC	C96.9	C79.52	-	-	D47.9	D49.89
sacrum	C41.4	C79.51	-	D16.8-	D48.0	D49.2

Neoplasm Index	Malignant Primary	Malignant Secondary	Ca in situ	Benign	Uncertain Behavior	Unspecified Behavior
vesical—*see* Neoplasm, bladder						
vesicle, seminal	C63.7	C79.82	D07.69	D29.8	D40.8	D49.5
vesicocervical tissue	C57.9	C79.82	D07.30	D28.9	D39.9	D49.5
vesicorectal	C76.3	C79.82	D09.8	D36.7	D48.7	D49.89
vesicovaginal	C57.9	C79.82	D07.30	D28.9	D39.9	D49.5
septum	C57.9	C79.82	D07.30	D28.9	D39.8	D49.5
vessel(blood)—*see* Neoplasm, connective tissue						
vestibular gland, greater	C51.0	C79.82	D07.1	D28.0	D39.8	D49.5
vestibule						
mouth	C06.1	C79.89	D00.00	D10.39	D37.09	D49.0
nose	C30.0	C78.39	D02.3	D14.0	D38.5	D49.1
Virchow's gland	C77.0	C77.0	-	D36.0	D48.7	D49.89
viscera NEC	C76.8	C79.89	D09.8	D36.7	D48.7	D49.89
vocal cords(true)	C32.0	C78.39	D02.0	D14.1	D38.0	D49.1
false	C32.1	C78.39	D02.0	D14.1	D38.0	D49.1
vomer	C41.0	C79.51	-	D16.4-	D48.0	D49.2
vulva	C51.9	C79.82	D07.1	D28.0	D39.8	D49.5
vulvovaginal gland	C51.0	C79.82	D07.1	D28.0	D39.8	D49.5
Waldeyer's ring	C14.2	C79.89	D00.08	D10.9	D37.05	D49.0
Wharton's duct	C08.0	C79.89	D00.00	D11.7	D37.032	D49.0
white matter(central) (cerebral)	C71.0	C79.31	-	D33.0	D43.0	D49.6
windpipe	C33	C78.39	D02.1	D14.2	D38.1	D49.1
Wirsung's duct	C25.3	C78.89	D01.7	D13.6	D37.8	D49.0
wolffian(body) (duct)						
female	C57.7	C79.82	D07.39	D28.7	D39.8	D49.5
male	C63.7	C79.82	D07.69	D29.8	D40.8	D49.5
womb—*see* Neoplasm, uterus						
wrist NEC	C76.4-	C79.89	D04.6-	D36.7	D48.7	D49.89
xiphoid process	C41.3	C79.51	-	D16.7	D48.0	D49.2
Zuckerkandl organ	C75.5	C79.89	-	D35.6	D44.7	D49.7

ICD-10-CM Table of Drugs and Chemicals

Substance	Poisoning, Accidental (unintentional)	Poisoning, Intentional self-harm	Poisoning, Assault	Poisoning, Undetermined	Adverse effect	Underdosing
1-propanol	T51.3X1	T51.3X2	T51.3X3	T51.3X4	—	—
2-propanol	T51.2X1	T51.2X2	T51.2X3	T51.2X4	—	—
2,4-D (dichlorophen-oxyacetic acid)	T60.3X1	T60.3X2	T60.3X3	T60.3X4	—	—
2,4-toluene diisocyanate	T65.0X1	T65.0X2	T65.0X3	T65.0X4	—	—
2,4,5-T (trichloro-phenoxyacetic acid)	T60.1X1	T60.1X2	T60.1X3	T60.1X4	—	—
14-hydroxydihydro-morphinone	T40.2X1	T40.2X2	T40.2X3	T40.2X4	T40.2X5	T40.2X6
A						
ABOB	T37.5X1	T37.5X2	T37.5X3	T37.5X4	T37.5X5	T37.5X6
Abrine	T62.2X1	T62.2X2	T62.2X3	T62.2X4	—	—
Abrus (seed)	T62.2X1	T62.2X2	T62.2X3	T62.2X4	—	—
Absinthe	T51.0X1	T51.0X2	T51.0X3	T51.0X4	—	—
beverage	T51.0X1	T51.0X2	T51.0X3	T51.0X4	—	—
Acaricide	T60.8X1	T60.8X2	T60.8X3	T60.8X4	—	—
Acebutolol	T44.7X1	T44.7X2	T44.7X3	T44.7X4	T44.7X5	T44.7X6
Acecarbromal	T42.6X1	T42.6X2	T42.6X3	T42.6X4	T42.6X5	T42.6X6
Aceclidine	T44.1X1	T44.1X2	T44.1X3	T44.1X4	T44.1X5	T44.1X6
Acedapsone	T37.0X1	T37.0X2	T37.0X3	T37.0X4	T37.0X5	T37.0X6
Acefylline piperazine	T48.6X1	T48.6X2	T48.6X3	T48.6X4	T48.6X5	T48.6X6
Acemorphan	T40.2X1	T40.2X2	T40.2X3	T40.2X4	T40.2X5	T40.2X6
Acenocoumarin	T45.511	T45.512	T45.513	T45.514	T45.515	T45.516
Acenocoumarol	T45.511	T45.512	T45.513	T45.514	T45.515	T45.516
Acepifylline	T48.6X1	T48.6X2	T48.6X3	T48.6X4	T48.6X5	T48.6X6
Acepromazine	T43.3X1	T43.3X2	T43.3X3	T43.3X4	T43.3X5	T43.3X6
Acesulfamethoxypyridazine	T37.0X1	T37.0X2	T37.0X3	T37.0X4	T37.0X5	T37.0X6
Acetal	T52.8X1	T52.8X2	T52.8X3	T52.8X4	—	—
Acetaldehyde (vapor)	T52.8X1	T52.8X2	T52.8X3	T52.8X4	—	—
liquid	T65.891	T65.892	T65.893	T65.894	—	—
P-Acetamidophenol	T39.1X1	T39.1X2	T39.1X3	T39.1X4	T39.1X5	T39.1X6
Acetaminophen	T39.1X1	T39.1X2	T39.1X3	T39.1X4	T39.1X5	T39.1X6
Acetaminosalol	T39.1X1	T39.1X2	T39.1X3	T39.1X4	T39.1X5	T39.1X6
Acetanilide	T39.1X1	T39.1X2	T39.1X3	T39.1X4	T39.1X5	T39.1X6
Acetarsol	T37.3X1	T37.3X2	T37.3X3	T37.3X4	T37.3X5	T37.3X6
Acetazolamide	T50.2X1	T50.2X2	T50.2X3	T50.2X4	T50.2X5	T50.2X6
Acetiamine	T45.2X1	T45.2X2	T45.2X3	T45.2X4	T45.2X5	T45.2X6
Acetic						
acid	T54.2X1	T54.2X2	T54.2X3	T54.2X4	—	—
with sodium acetate (ointment)	T49.3X1	T49.3X2	T49.3X3	T49.3X4	T49.3X5	T49.3X6
ester (solvent) (vapor)	T52.8X1	T52.8X2	T52.8X3	T52.8X4	—	—
irrigating solution	T50.3X1	T50.3X2	T50.3X3	T50.3X4	T50.3X5	T50.3X6
medicinal (lotion)	T49.2X1	T49.2X2	T49.2X3	T49.2X4	T49.2X5	T49.2X6
anhydride	T65.891	T65.892	T65.893	T65.894	—	—
ether (vapor)	T52.8X1	T52.8X2	T52.8X3	T52.8X4	—	—
Acetohexamide	T38.3X1	T38.3X2	T38.3X3	T38.3X4	T38.3X5	T38.3X6
Acetohydroxamic acid	T50.991	T50.992	T50.993	T50.994	T50.995	T50.996
Acetomenaphthone	T45.7X1	T45.7X2	T45.7X3	T45.7X4	T45.7X5	T45.7X6
Acetomorphine	T40.1X1	T40.1X2	T40.1X3	T40.1X4	—	—
Acetone (oils)	T52.4X1	T52.4X2	T52.4X3	T52.4X4	—	—
chlorinated	T52.4X1	T52.4X2	T52.4X3	T52.4X4	—	—
vapor	T52.4X1	T52.4X2	T52.4X3	T52.4X4	—	—
Acetonitrile	T52.8X1	T52.8X2	T52.8X3	T52.8X4	—	—
Acetophenazine	T43.3X1	T43.3X2	T43.3X3	T43.3X4	T43.3X5	T43.3X6
Acetophenetedin	T39.1X1	T39.1X2	T39.1X3	T39.1X4	T39.1X5	T39.1X6
Acetophenone	T52.4X1	T52.4X2	T52.4X3	T52.4X4	—	—
Acetorphine	T40.2X1	T40.2X2	T40.2X3	T40.2X4	—	—

Substance	Poisoning, Accidental (unintentional)	Poisoning, Intentional self-harm	Poisoning, Assault	Poisoning, Undetermined	Adverse effect	Underdosing
Acetosulfone (sodium)	T37.1X1	T37.1X2	T37.1X3	T37.1X4	T37.1X5	T37.1X6
Acetrizoate (sodium)	T50.8X1	T50.8X2	T50.8X3	T50.8X4	T50.8X5	T50.8X6
Acetrizoic acid	T50.8X1	T50.8X2	T50.8X3	T50.8X4	T50.8X5	T50.8X6
Acetyl						
bromide	T53.6X1	T53.6X2	T53.6X3	T53.6X4	—	—
chloride	T53.6X1	T53.6X2	T53.6X3	T53.6X4	—	—
Acetylcarbromal	T42.6X1	T42.6X2	T42.6X3	T42.6X4	T42.6X5	T42.6X6
Acetylcholine						
chloride	T44.1X1	T44.1X2	T44.1X3	T44.1X4	T44.1X5	T44.1X6
derivative	T44.1X1	T44.1X2	T44.1X3	T44.1X4	T44.1X5	T44.1X6
Acetylcysteine	T48.4X1	T48.4X2	T48.4X3	T48.4X4	T48.4X5	T48.4X6
Acetyldigitoxin	T46.0X1	T46.0X2	T46.0X3	T46.0X4	T46.0X5	T46.0X6
Acetyldigoxin	T46.0X1	T46.0X2	T46.0X3	T46.0X4	T46.0X5	T46.0X6
Acetyldihydrocodeine	T40.2X1	T40.2X2	T40.2X3	T40.2X4	—	—
Acetyldihydrocodeinone	T40.2X1	T40.2X2	T40.2X3	T40.2X4	—	—
Acetylene (gas)	T59.891	T59.892	T59.893	T59.894	—	—
dichloride	T53.6X1	T53.6X2	T53.6X3	T53.6X4	—	—
incomplete combustion of	T58.11	T58.12	T58.13	T58.14	—	—
industrial	T59.891	T59.892	T59.893	T59.894	—	—
tetrachloride	T53.6X1	T53.6X2	T53.6X3	T53.6X4	—	—
vapor	T53.6X1	T53.6X2	T53.6X3	T53.6X4	—	—
Acetylpheneturide	T42.6X1	T42.6X2	T42.6X3	T42.6X4	T42.6X5	T42.6X6
Acetylphenylhydrazine	T39.8X1	T39.8X2	T39.8X3	T39.8X4	T39.8X5	T39.8X6
Acetylsalicylic acid (salts)	T39.011	T39.012	T39.013	T39.014	T39.015	T39.016
enteric coated	T39.011	T39.012	T39.013	T39.014	T39.015	T39.016
Acetylsulfamethoxypyridazine	T37.0X1	T37.0X2	T37.0X3	T37.0X4	T37.0X5	T37.0X6
Achromycin	T36.4X1	T36.4X2	T36.4X3	T36.4X4	T36.4X5	T36.4X6
ophthalmic preparation	T49.5X1	T49.5X2	T49.5X3	T49.5X4	T49.5X5	T49.5X6
topical NEC	T49.0X1	T49.0X2	T49.0X3	T49.0X4	T49.0X5	T49.0X6
Aciclovir	T37.5X1	T37.5X2	T37.5X3	T37.5X4	T37.5X5	T37.5X6
Acid (corrosive) NEC	T54.2X1	T54.2X2	T54.2X3	T54.2X4	—	—
Acidifying agent NEC	T50.901	T50.902	T50.903	T50.904	T50.905	T50.906
Acipimox	T46.6X1	T46.6X2	T46.6X3	T46.6X4	T46.6X5	T46.6X6
Acitretin	T50.991	T50.992	T50.993	T50.994	T50.995	T50.996
Aclarubicin	T45.1X1	T45.1X2	T45.1X3	T45.1X4	T45.1X5	T45.1X6
Aclatonium napadisilate	T48.1X1	T48.1X2	T48.1X3	T48.1X4	T48.1X5	T48.1X6
Aconite (wild)	T46.991	T46.992	T46.993	T46.994	T46.995	T46.996
Aconitine	T46.991	T46.992	T46.993	T46.994	T46.995	T46.996
Aconitum ferox	T46.991	T46.992	T46.993	T46.994	T46.995	T46.996
Acridine	T65.6X1	T65.6X2	T65.6X3	T65.6X4	—	—
vapor	T59.891	T59.892	T59.893	T59.894	—	—
Acriflavine	T37.91	T37.92	T37.93	T37.94	T37.95	T37.96
Acriflavinium chloride	T49.0X1	T49.0X2	T49.0X3	T49.0X4	T49.0X5	T49.0X6
Acrinol	T49.0X1	T49.0X2	T49.0X3	T49.0X4	T49.0X5	T49.0X6
Acrisorcin	T49.0X1	T49.0X2	T49.0X3	T49.0X4	T49.0X5	T49.0X6
Acrivastine	T45.0X1	T45.0X2	T45.0X3	T45.0X4	T45.0X5	T45.0X6
Acrolein (gas)	T59.891	T59.892	T59.893	T59.894	—	—
liquid	T54.1X1	T54.1X2	T54.1X3	T54.1X4	—	—
Acrylamide	T65.891	T65.892	T65.893	T65.894	—	—
Acrylic resin	T49.3X1	T49.3X2	T49.3X3	T49.3X4	T49.3X5	T49.3X6
Acrylonitrile	T65.891	T65.892	T65.893	T65.894	—	—
Actaea spicata	T62.2X1	T62.2X2	T62.2X3	T62.2X4	—	—
berry	T62.1X1	T62.1X2	T62.1X3	T62.1X4	—	—
Acterol	T37.3X1	T37.3X2	T37.3X3	T37.3X4	T37.3X5	T37.3X6
ACTH	T38.811	T38.812	T38.813	T38.814	T38.815	T38.816
Actinomycin C	T45.1X1	T45.1X2	T45.1X3	T45.1X4	T45.1X5	T45.1X6
Actinomycin D	T45.1X1	T45.1X2	T45.1X3	T45.1X4	T45.1X5	T45.1X6

Activated charcoal - Alglucerase

Substance	Poisoning, Accidental (unintentional)	Poisoning, Intentional self-harm	Poisoning, Assault	Poisoning, Undetermined	Adverse effect	Underdosing
Activated charcoal— *see also Charcoal, medicinal*	T47.6X1	T47.6X2	T47.6X3	T47.6X4	T47.6X5	T47.6X6
Acyclovir	T37.5X1	T37.5X2	T37.5X3	T37.5X4	T37.5X5	T37.5X6
Adenine	T45.2X1	T45.2X2	T45.2X3	T45.2X4	T45.2X5	T45.2X6
arabinoside	T37.5X1	T37.5X2	T37.5X3	T37.5X4	T37.5X5	T37.5X6
Adenosine (phosphate)	T46.2X1	T46.2X2	T46.2X3	T46.2X4	T46.2X5	T46.2X6
ADH	T38.891	T38.892	T38.893	T38.894	T38.895	T38.896
Adhesive NEC	T65.891	T65.892	T65.893	T65.894		
Adicillin	T36.0X1	T36.0X2	T36.0X3	T36.0X4	T36.0X5	T36.0X6
Adiphenine	T44.3X1	T44.3X2	T44.3X3	T44.3X4	T44.3X5	T44.3X6
Adipiodone	T50.8X1	T50.8X2	T50.8X3	T50.8X4	T50.8X5	T50.8X6
Adjunct, pharmaceutical	T50.901	T50.902	T50.903	T50.904	T50.905	T50.906
Adrenal (extract, cortex or medulla) (glucocorticoids) (hormones) (mineralocorticoids)	T38.0X1	T38.0X2	T38.0X3	T38.0X4	T38.0X5	T38.0X6
ENT agent	T49.6X1	T49.6X2	T49.6X3	T49.6X4	T49.6X5	T49.6X6
ophthalmic preparation	T49.5X1	T49.5X2	T49.5X3	T49.5X4	T49.5X5	T49.5X6
topical NEC	T49.0X1	T49.0X2	T49.0X3	T49.0X4	T49.0X5	T49.0X6
Adrenaline	T44.5X1	T44.5X2	T44.5X3	T44.5X4	T44.5X5	T44.5X6
Adrenalin—*see Adrenaline*						
Adrenergic NEC	T44.901	T44.902	T44.903	T44.904	T44.905	T44.906
blocking agent NEC	T44.8X1	T44.8X2	T44.8X3	T44.8X4	T44.8X5	T44.8X6
beta, heart	T44.7X1	T44.7X2	T44.7X3	T44.7X4	T44.7X5	T44.7X6
specified NEC	T44.991	T44.992	T44.993	T44.994	T44.995	T44.996
Adrenochrome						
(mono) semicarbazone	T46.991	T46.992	T46.993	T46.994	T46.995	T46.996
derivative	T46.991	T46.992	T46.993	T46.994	T46.995	T46.996
Adrenocorticotrophic hormone	T38.811	T38.812	T38.813	T38.814	T38.815	T38.816
Adrenocorticotrophin	T38.811	T38.812	T38.813	T38.814	T38.815	T38.816
Adriamycin	T45.1X1	T45.1X2	T45.1X3	T45.1X4	T45.1X5	T45.1X6
Aerosol spray NEC	T65.91	T65.92	T65.93	T65.94	—	—
Aerosporin	T36.8X1	T36.8X2	T36.8X3	T36.8X4	T36.8X5	T36.8X6
ENT agent	T49.6X1	T49.6X2	T49.6X3	T49.6X4	T49.6X5	T49.6X6
ophthalmic preparation	T49.5X1	T49.5X2	T49.5X3	T49.5X4	T49.5X5	T49.5X6
topical NEC	T49.0X1	T49.0X2	T49.0X3	T49.0X4	T49.0X5	T49.0X6
Aethusa cynapium	T62.2X1	T62.2X2	T62.2X3	T62.2X4	—	—
Afghanistan black	T40.7X1	T40.7X2	T40.7X3	T40.7X4	T40.7X5	T40.7X6
Aflatoxin	T64.01	T64.02	T64.03	T64.04		
Afloqualone	T42.8X1	T42.8X2	T42.8X3	T42.8X4	T42.8X5	T42.8X6
African boxwood	T62.2X1	T62.2X2	T62.2X3	T62.2X4	—	—
Agar	T47.4X1	T47.4X2	T47.4X3	T47.4X4	T47.4X5	T47.4X6
Agonist						
predominantly						
alpha-adrenoreceptor	T44.4X1	T44.4X2	T44.4X3	T44.4X4	T44.4X5	T44.4X6
beta-adrenoreceptor	T44.5X1	T44.5X2	T44.5X3	T44.5X4	T44.5X5	T44.5X6
Agricultural agent NEC	T65.91	T65.92	T65.93	T65.94	—	—
Agrypnal	T42.3X1	T42.3X2	T42.3X3	T42.3X4	T42.3X5	T42.3X6
AHLG	T50.Z11	T50.Z12	T50.Z13	T50.Z14	T50.Z15	T50.Z16
Air contaminant (s), source/type NOS	T65.91	T65.92	T65.93	T65.94	—	—
Ajmaline	T46.2X1	T46.2X2	T46.2X3	T46.2X4	T46.2X5	T46.2X6
Akee	T62.1X1	T62.1X2	T62.1X3	T62.1X4	—	—
Akrinol	T49.0X1	T49.0X2	T49.0X3	T49.0X4	T49.0X5	T49.0X6
Akritoin	T37.8X1	T37.8X2	T37.8X3	T37.8X4	T37.8X5	T37.8X6
Alacepril	T46.4X1	T46.4X2	T46.4X3	T46.4X4	T46.4X5	T46.4X6
Alantolactone	T37.4X1	T37.4X2	T37.4X3	T37.4X4	T37.4X5	T37.4X6

Substance	Poisoning, Accidental (unintentional)	Poisoning, Intentional self-harm	Poisoning, Assault	Poisoning, Undetermined	Adverse effect	Underdosing
Albamycin	T36.8X1	T36.8X2	T36.8X3	T36.8X4	T36.8X5	T36.8X6
Albendazole	T37.4X1	T37.4X2	T37.4X3	T37.4X4	T37.4X5	T37.4X6
Albumin						
bovine	T45.8X1	T45.8X2	T45.8X3	T45.8X4	T45.8X5	T45.8X6
human serum	T45.8X1	T45.8X2	T45.8X3	T45.8X4	T45.8X5	T45.8X6
salt-poor	T45.8X1	T45.8X2	T45.8X3	T45.8X4	T45.8X5	T45.8X6
normal human serum	T45.8X1	T45.8X2	T45.8X3	T45.8X4	T45.8X5	T45.8X6
Albuterol	T48.6X1	T48.6X2	T48.6X3	T48.6X4	T48.6X5	T48.6X6
Albutoin	T42.0X1	T42.0X2	T42.0X3	T42.0X4	T42.0X5	T42.0X6
Alclometasone	T49.0X1	T49.0X2	T49.0X3	T49.0X4	T49.0X5	T49.0X6
Alcohol	T51.91	T51.92	T51.93	T51.94	—	—
absolute	T51.0X1	T51.0X2	T51.0X3	T51.0X4	—	—
beverage	T51.0X1	T51.0X2	T51.0X3	T51.0X4		
allyl	T51.8X1	T51.8X2	T51.8X3	T51.8X4	—	—
amyl	T51.3X1	T51.3X2	T51.3X3	T51.3X4	—	—
antifreeze	T51.1X1	T51.1X2	T51.1X3	T51.1X4	—	—
beverage	T51.0X1	T51.0X2	T51.0X3	T51.0X4		
butyl	T51.3X1	T51.3X2	T51.3X3	T51.3X4	—	—
dehydrated	T51.0X1	T51.0X2	T51.0X3	T51.0X4	—	—
beverage	T51.0X1	T51.0X2	T51.0X3	T51.0X4		
denatured	T51.0X1	T51.0X2	T51.0X3	T51.0X4	—	—
deterrent NEC	T50.6X1	T50.6X2	T50.6X3	T50.6X4	T50.6X5	T50.6X6
diagnostic (gastric function)	T50.8X1	T50.8X2	T50.8X3	T50.8X4	T50.8X5	T50.8X6
ethyl	T51.0X1	T51.0X2	T51.0X3	T51.0X4	—	—
beverage	T51.0X1	T51.0X2	T51.0X3	T51.0X4		
grain	T51.0X1	T51.0X2	T51.0X3	T51.0X4	—	—
beverage	T51.0X1	T51.0X2	T51.0X3	T51.0X4		
industrial	T51.0X1	T51.0X2	T51.0X3	T51.0X4	—	—
isopropyl	T51.2X1	T51.2X2	T51.2X3	T51.2X4	—	—
methyl	T51.1X1	T51.1X2	T51.1X3	T51.1X4	—	—
preparation for consumption	T51.0X1	T51.0X2	T51.0X3	T51.0X4		
propyl	T51.3X1	T51.3X2	T51.3X3	T51.3X4	—	—
secondary	T51.2X1	T51.2X2	T51.2X3	T51.2X4	—	—
radiator	T51.1X1	T51.1X2	T51.1X3	T51.1X4	—	—
rubbing	T51.2X1	T51.2X2	T51.2X3	T51.2X4	—	—
specified type NEC	T51.8X1	T51.8X2	T51.8X3	T51.8X4	—	—
surgical	T51.0X1	T51.0X2	T51.0X3	T51.0X4	—	—
vapor (from any type of Alcohol)	T59.891	T59.892	T59.893	T59.894		
wood	T51.1X1	T51.1X2	T51.1X3	T51.1X4	—	—
Alcuronium (chloride)	T48.1X1	T48.1X2	T48.1X3	T48.1X4	T48.1X5	T48.1X6
Aldactone	T50.0X1	T50.0X2	T50.0X3	T50.0X4	T50.0X5	T50.0X6
Aldesulfone sodium	T37.1X1	T37.1X2	T37.1X3	T37.1X4	T37.1X5	T37.1X6
Aldicarb	T60.0X1	T60.0X2	T60.0X3	T60.0X4	—	—
Aldomet	T46.5X1	T46.5X2	T46.5X3	T46.5X4	T46.5X5	T46.5X6
Aldosterone	T50.0X1	T50.0X2	T50.0X3	T50.0X4	T50.0X5	T50.0X6
Aldrin (dust)	T60.1X1	T60.1X2	T60.1X3	T60.1X4	—	—
Aleve—*see Naproxen*						
Alexitol sodium	T47.1X1	T47.1X2	T47.1X3	T47.1X4	T47.1X5	T47.1X6
Alfacalcidol	T45.2X1	T45.2X2	T45.2X3	T45.2X4	T45.2X5	T45.2X6
Alfadolone	T41.1X1	T41.1X2	T41.1X3	T41.1X4	T41.1X5	T41.1X6
Alfaxalone	T41.1X1	T41.1X2	T41.1X3	T41.1X4	T41.1X5	T41.1X6
Alfentanil	T40.4X1	T40.4X2	T40.4X3	T40.4X4	T40.4X5	T40.4X6
Alfuzosin (hydrochloride)	T44.8X1	T44.8X2	T44.8X3	T44.8X4	T44.8X5	T44.8X6
Algae (harmful) (toxin)	T65.821	T65.822	T65.823	T65.824	—	—
Algeldrate	T47.1X1	T47.1X2	T47.1X3	T47.1X4	T47.1X5	T47.1X6
Algin	T47.8X1	T47.8X2	T47.8X3	T47.8X4	T47.8X5	T47.8X6
Alglucerase	T45.3X1	T45.3X2	T45.3X3	T45.3X4	T45.3X5	T45.3X6

Substance	Poisoning, Accidental (unintentional)	Poisoning, Intentional self-harm	Poisoning, Assault	Poisoning, Undetermined	Adverse effect	Underdosing
Alidase	T45.3X1	T45.3X2	T45.3X3	T45.3X4	T45.3X5	T45.3X6
Alimemazine	T43.3X1	T43.3X2	T43.3X3	T43.3X4	T43.3X5	T43.3X6
Aliphatic thiocyanates	T65.0X1	T65.0X2	T65.0X3	T65.0X4	—	—
Alizapride	T45.0X1	T45.0X2	T45.0X3	T45.0X4	T45.0X5	T45.0X6
Alkali (caustic)	T54.3X1	T54.3X2	T54.3X3	T54.3X4	—	—
Alkaline antiseptic solution (aromatic)	T49.6X1	T49.6X2	T49.6X3	T49.6X4	T49.6X5	T49.6X6
Alkalinizing agents (medicinal)	T50.901	T50.902	T50.903	T50.904	T50.905	T50.906
Alkalizing agent NEC	T50.901	T50.902	T50.903	T50.904	T50.905	T50.906
Alka-seltzer	T39.011	T39.012	T39.013	T39.014	T39.015	T39.016
Alkavervir	T46.5X1	T46.5X2	T46.5X3	T46.5X4	T46.5X5	T46.5X6
Alkonium (bromide)	T49.0X1	T49.0X2	T49.0X3	T49.0X4	T49.0X5	T49.0X6
Alkylating drug NEC	T45.1X1	T45.1X2	T45.1X3	T45.1X4	T45.1X5	T45.1X6
antimyeloproliferative	T45.1X1	T45.1X2	T45.1X3	T45.1X4	T45.1X5	T45.1X6
lymphatic	T45.1X1	T45.1X2	T45.1X3	T45.1X4	T45.1X5	T45.1X6
Alkylisocyanate	T65.0X1	T65.0X2	T65.0X3	T65.0X4	—	—
Allantoin	T49.4X1	T49.4X2	T49.4X3	T49.4X4	T49.4X5	T49.4X6
Allegron	T43.011	T43.012	T43.013	T43.014	T43.015	T43.016
Allethrin	T49.0X1	T49.0X2	T49.0X3	T49.0X4	T49.0X5	T49.0X6
Allobarbital	T42.3X1	T42.3X2	T42.3X3	T42.3X4	T42.3X5	T42.3X6
Allopurinol	T50.4X1	T50.4X2	T50.4X3	T50.4X4	T50.4X5	T50.4X6
Allyl						
Alcohol	T51.8X1	T51.8X2	T51.8X3	T51.8X4	—	—
disulfide	T46.6X1	T46.6X2	T46.6X3	T46.6X4	T46.6X5	T46.6X6
Allylestrenol	T38.5X1	T38.5X2	T38.5X3	T38.5X4	T38.5X5	T38.5X6
Allylisopropylacetylurea	T42.6X1	T42.6X2	T42.6X3	T42.6X4	T42.6X5	T42.6X6
Allylisopropylmalonylurea	T42.3X1	T42.3X2	T42.3X3	T42.3X4	T42.3X5	T42.3X6
Allylthiourea	T49.3X1	T49.3X2	T49.3X3	T49.3X4	T49.3X5	T49.3X6
Allyltribromide	T42.6X1	T42.6X2	T42.6X3	T42.6X4	T42.6X5	T42.6X6
Allypropymal	T42.3X1	T42.3X2	T42.3X3	T42.3X4	T42.3X5	T42.3X6
Almagate	T47.1X1	T47.1X2	T47.1X3	T47.1X4	T47.1X5	T47.1X6
Almasilate	T47.1X1	T47.1X2	T47.1X3	T47.1X4	T47.1X5	T47.1X6
Almitrine	T50.7X1	T50.7X2	T50.7X3	T50.7X4	T50.7X5	T50.7X6
Aloes	T47.2X1	T47.2X2	T47.2X3	T47.2X4	T47.2X5	T47.2X6
Aloglutamol	T47.1X1	T47.1X2	T47.1X3	T47.1X4	T47.1X5	T47.1X6
Aloin	T47.2X1	T47.2X2	T47.2X3	T47.2X4	T47.2X5	T47.2X6
Aloxidone	T42.2X1	T42.2X2	T42.2X3	T42.2X4	T42.2X5	T42.2X6
Alpha						
acetyldigoxin	T46.0X1	T46.0X2	T46.0X3	T46.0X4	T46.0X5	T46.0X6
adrenergic blocking drug	T44.6X1	T44.6X2	T44.6X3	T44.6X4	T44.6X5	T44.6X6
amylase	T45.3X1	T45.3X2	T45.3X3	T45.3X4	T45.3X5	T45.3X6
tocoferol (acetate)	T45.2X1	T45.2X2	T45.2X3	T45.2X4	T45.2X5	T45.2X6
tocopherol	T45.2X1	T45.2X2	T45.2X3	T45.2X4	T45.2X5	T45.2X6
Alphadolone	T41.1X1	T41.1X2	T41.1X3	T41.1X4	T41.1X5	T41.1X6
Alphaprodine	T40.4X1	T40.4X2	T40.4X3	T40.4X4	T40.4X5	T40.4X6
Alphaxalone	T41.1X1	T41.1X2	T41.1X3	T41.1X4	T41.1X5	T41.1X6
Alprazolam	T42.4X1	T42.4X2	T42.4X3	T42.4X4	T42.4X5	T42.4X6
Alprenolol	T44.7X1	T44.7X2	T44.7X3	T44.7X4	T44.7X5	T44.7X6
Alprostadil	T46.7X1	T46.7X2	T46.7X3	T46.7X4	T46.7X5	T46.7X6
Alsactide	T38.811	T38.812	T38.813	T38.814	T38.815	T38.816
Alseroxylon	T46.5X1	T46.5X2	T46.5X3	T46.5X4	T46.5X5	T46.5X6
Alteplase	T45.611	T45.612	T45.613	T45.614	T45.615	T45.616
Altizide	T50.2X1	T50.2X2	T50.2X3	T50.2X4	T50.2X5	T50.2X6
Altretamine	T45.1X1	T45.1X2	T45.1X3	T45.1X4	T45.1X5	T45.1X6
Alum (medicinal)	T49.4X1	T49.4X2	T49.4X3	T49.4X4	T49.4X5	T49.4X6
nonmedicinal (ammonium) (potassium)	T56.891	T56.892	T56.893	T56.894	—	—

Substance	Poisoning, Accidental (unintentional)	Poisoning, Intentional self-harm	Poisoning, Assault	Poisoning, Undetermined	Adverse effect	Underdosing
Aluminium, aluminum						
acetate	T49.2X1	T49.2X2	T49.2X3	T49.2X4	T49.2X5	T49.2X6
solution	T49.0X1	T49.0X2	T49.0X3	T49.0X4	T49.0X5	T49.0X6
aspirin	T39.011	T39.012	T39.013	T39.014	T39.015	T39.016
bis (acetylsalicylate)	T39.011	T39.012	T39.013	T39.014	T39.015	T39.016
carbonate (gel, basic)	T47.1X1	T47.1X2	T47.1X3	T47.1X4	T47.1X5	T47.1X6
chlorhydroxide-complex	T47.1X1	T47.1X2	T47.1X3	T47.1X4	T47.1X5	T47.1X6
chloride	T49.2X1	T49.2X2	T49.2X3	T49.2X4	T49.2X5	T49.2X6
clofibrate	T46.6X1	T46.6X2	T46.6X3	T46.6X4	T46.6X5	T46.6X6
diacetate	T49.2X1	T49.2X2	T49.2X3	T49.2X4	T49.2X5	T49.2X6
glycinate	T47.1X1	T47.1X2	T47.1X3	T47.1X4	T47.1X5	T47.1X6
hydroxide (gel)	T47.1X1	T47.1X2	T47.1X3	T47.1X4	T47.1X5	T47.1X6
hydroxide-magnesium carb. gel	T47.1X1	T47.1X2	T47.1X3	T47.1X4	T47.1X5	T47.1X6
magnesium silicate	T47.1X1	T47.1X2	T47.1X3	T47.1X4	T47.1X5	T47.1X6
nicotinate	T46.7X1	T46.7X2	T46.7X3	T46.7X4	T46.7X5	T46.7X6
ointment (surgical) (topical)	T49.3X1	T49.3X2	T49.3X3	T49.3X4	T49.3X5	T49.3X6
phosphate	T47.1X1	T47.1X2	T47.1X3	T47.1X4	T47.1X5	T47.1X6
salicylate	T39.091	T39.092	T39.093	T39.094	T39.095	T39.096
silicate	T47.1X1	T47.1X2	T47.1X3	T47.1X4	T47.1X5	T47.1X6
sodium silicate	T47.1X1	T47.1X2	T47.1X3	T47.1X4	T47.1X5	T47.1X6
subacetate	T49.2X1	T49.2X2	T49.2X3	T49.2X4	T49.2X5	T49.2X6
sulfate	T49.0X1	T49.0X2	T49.0X3	T49.0X4	T49.0X5	T49.0X6
tannate	T47.6X1	T47.6X2	T47.6X3	T47.6X4	T47.6X5	T47.6X6
topical NEC	T49.3X1	T49.3X2	T49.3X3	T49.3X4	T49.3X5	T49.3X6
Alurate	T42.3X1	T42.3X2	T42.3X3	T42.3X4	T42.3X5	T42.3X6
Alverine	T44.3X1	T44.3X2	T44.3X3	T44.3X4	T44.3X5	T44.3X6
Alvodine	T40.2X1	T40.2X2	T40.2X3	T40.2X4	T40.2X5	T40.2X6
Amanita phalloides	T62.0X1	T62.0X2	T62.0X3	T62.0X4	—	—
Amanitine	T62.0X1	T62.0X2	T62.0X3	T62.0X4	—	—
Amantadine	T42.8X1	T42.8X2	T42.8X3	T42.8X4	T42.8X5	T42.8X6
Ambazone	T49.6X1	T49.6X2	T49.6X3	T49.6X4	T49.6X5	T49.6X6
Ambenonium (chloride)	T44.0X1	T44.0X2	T44.0X3	T44.0X4	T44.0X5	T44.0X6
Ambroxol	T48.4X1	T48.4X2	T48.4X3	T48.4X4	T48.4X5	T48.4X6
Ambuphylline	T48.6X1	T48.6X2	T48.6X3	T48.6X4	T48.6X5	T48.6X6
Ambutonium bromide	T44.3X1	T44.3X2	T44.3X3	T44.3X4	T44.3X5	T44.3X6
Amcinonide	T49.0X1	T49.0X2	T49.0X3	T49.0X4	T49.0X5	T49.0X6
Amdinocilline	T36.0X1	T36.0X2	T36.0X3	T36.0X4	T36.0X5	T36.0X6
Ametazole	T50.8X1	T50.8X2	T50.8X3	T50.8X4	T50.8X5	T50.8X6
Amethocaine	T41.3X1	T41.3X2	T41.3X3	T41.3X4	T41.3X5	T41.3X6
regional	T41.3X1	T41.3X2	T41.3X3	T41.3X4	T41.3X5	T41.3X6
spinal	T41.3X1	T41.3X2	T41.3X3	T41.3X4	T41.3X5	T41.3X6
Amethopterin	T45.1X1	T45.1X2	T45.1X3	T45.1X4	T45.1X5	T45.1X6
Amezinium metilsulfate	T44.991	T44.992	T44.993	T44.994	T44.995	T44.996
Amfebutamone	T43.291	T43.292	T43.293	T43.294	T43.295	T43.296
Amfepramone	T50.5X1	T50.5X2	T50.5X3	T50.5X4	T50.5X5	T50.5X6
Amfetamine	T43.621	T43.622	T43.623	T43.624	T43.625	T43.626
Amfetaminil	T43.621	T43.622	T43.623	T43.624	T43.625	T43.626
Amfomycin	T36.8X1	T36.8X2	T36.8X3	T36.8X4	T36.8X5	T36.8X6
Amidefrine mesilate	T48.5X1	T48.5X2	T48.5X3	T48.5X4	T48.5X5	T48.5X6
Amidone	T40.3X1	T40.3X2	T40.3X3	T40.3X4	T40.3X5	T40.3X6
Amidopyrine	T39.2X1	T39.2X2	T39.2X3	T39.2X4	T39.2X5	T39.2X6
Amidotrizoate	T50.8X1	T50.8X2	T50.8X3	T50.8X4	T50.8X5	T50.8X6
Amiflamine	T43.1X1	T43.1X2	T43.1X3	T43.1X4	T43.1X5	T43.1X6
Amikacin	T36.5X1	T36.5X2	T36.5X3	T36.5X4	T36.5X5	T36.5X6
Amikhelline	T46.3X1	T46.3X2	T46.3X3	T46.3X4	T46.3X5	T46.3X6
Amiloride	T50.2X1	T50.2X2	T50.2X3	T50.2X4	T50.2X5	T50.2X6
Aminacrine	T49.0X1	T49.0X2	T49.0X3	T49.0X4	T49.0X5	T49.0X6

Amineptine - Anemone pulsatilla

Substance	Poisoning, Accidental (unintentional)	Poisoning, Intentional self-harm	Poisoning, Assault	Poisoning, Undetermined	Adverse effect	Underdosing
Amineptine	T43.011	T43.012	T43.013	T43.014	T43.015	T43.016
Aminitrozole	T37.3X1	T37.3X2	T37.3X3	T37.3X4	T37.3X5	T37.3X6
Amino acids	T50.3X1	T50.3X2	T50.3X3	T50.3X4	T50.3X5	T50.3X6
Aminoacetic acid (derivatives)	T50.3X1	T50.3X2	T50.3X3	T50.3X4	T50.3X5	T50.3X6
Aminoacridine	T49.0X1	T49.0X2	T49.0X3	T49.0X4	T49.0X5	T49.0X6
Aminobenzoic acid (-p)	T49.3X1	T49.3X2	T49.3X3	T49.3X4	T49.3X5	T49.3X6
4-Aminobutyric acid	T43.8X1	T43.8X2	T43.8X3	T43.8X4	T43.8X5	T43.8X6
Aminocaproic acid	T45.621	T45.622	T45.623	T45.624	T45.625	T45.626
Aminoethylisothiourium	T45.8X1	T45.8X2	T45.8X3	T45.8X4	T45.8X5	T45.8X6
Aminofenazone	T39.2X1	T39.2X2	T39.2X3	T39.2X4	T39.2X5	T39.2X6
Aminoglutethimide	T45.1X1	T45.1X2	T45.1X3	T45.1X4	T45.1X5	T45.1X6
Aminohippuric acid	T50.8X1	T50.8X2	T50.8X3	T50.8X4	T50.8X5	T50.8X6
Aminomethylbenzoic acid	T45.691	T45.692	T45.693	T45.694	T45.695	T45.696
Aminometradine	T50.2X1	T50.2X2	T50.2X3	T50.2X4	T50.2X5	T50.2X6
Aminopentamide	T44.3X1	T44.3X2	T44.3X3	T44.3X4	T44.3X5	T44.3X6
Aminophenazone	T39.2X1	T39.2X2	T39.2X3	T39.2X4	T39.2X5	T39.2X6
Aminophenol	T54.0X1	T54.0X2	T54.0X3	T54.0X4	—	—
4-Aminophenol derivatives	T39.1X1	T39.1X2	T39.1X3	T39.1X4	T39.1X5	T39.1X6
Aminophenylpyridone	T43.591	T43.592	T43.593	T43.594	T43.595	T43.596
Aminophylline	T48.6X1	T48.6X2	T48.6X3	T48.6X4	T48.6X5	T48.6X6
Aminopterin sodium	T45.1X1	T45.1X2	T45.1X3	T45.1X4	T45.1X5	T45.1X6
Aminopyrine	T39.2X1	T39.2X2	T39.2X3	T39.2X4	T39.2X5	T39.2X6
8-Aminoquinoline drugs	T37.2X1	T37.2X2	T37.2X3	T37.2X4	T37.2X5	T37.2X6
Aminorex	T50.5X1	T50.5X2	T50.5X3	T50.5X4	T50.5X5	T50.5X6
Aminosalicylic acid	T37.1X1	T37.1X2	T37.1X3	T37.1X4	T37.1X5	T37.1X6
Aminosalylum	T37.1X1	T37.1X2	T37.1X3	T37.1X4	T37.1X5	T37.1X6
Amiodarone	T46.2X1	T46.2X2	T46.2X3	T46.2X4	T46.2X5	T46.2X6
Amiphenazole	T50.7X1	T50.7X2	T50.7X3	T50.7X4	T50.7X5	T50.7X6
Amiquinsin	T46.5X1	T46.5X2	T46.5X3	T46.5X4	T46.5X5	T46.5X6
Amisometradine	T50.2X1	T50.2X2	T50.2X3	T50.2X4	T50.2X5	T50.2X6
Amisulpride	T43.591	T43.592	T43.593	T43.594	T43.595	T43.596
Amitriptyline	T43.011	T43.012	T43.013	T43.014	T43.015	T43.016
Amitriptylinoxide	T43.011	T43.012	T43.013	T43.014	T43.015	T43.016
Amlexanox	T48.6X1	T48.6X2	T48.6X3	T48.6X4	T48.6X5	T48.6X6
Ammonia (fumes) (gas) (vapor)	T59.891	T59.892	T59.893	T59.894	—	—
aromatic spirit	T48.991	T48.992	T48.993	T48.994	T48.995	T48.996
liquid (household)	T54.3X1	T54.3X2	T54.3X3	T54.3X4	—	—
Ammoniated mercury	T49.0X1	T49.0X2	T49.0X3	T49.0X4	T49.0X5	T49.0X6
Ammonium						
acid tartrate	T49.5X1	T49.5X2	T49.5X3	T49.5X4	T49.5X5	T49.5X6
bromide	T42.6X1	T42.6X2	T42.6X3	T42.6X4	T42.6X5	T42.6X6
carbonate	T54.3X1	T54.3X2	T54.3X3	T54.3X4	—	—
chloride	T50.991	T50.992	T50.993	T50.994	T50.995	T50.996
expectorant	T48.4X1	T48.4X2	T48.4X3	T48.4X4	T48.4X5	T48.4X6
compounds (household) NEC	T54.3X1	T54.3X2	T54.3X3	T54.3X4	—	—
fumes (any usage)	T59.891	T59.892	T59.893	T59.894	—	—
industrial	T54.3X1	T54.3X2	T54.3X3	T54.3X4	—	—
ichthyosulronate	T49.4X1	T49.4X2	T49.4X3	T49.4X4	T49.4X5	T49.4X6
mandelate	T37.91	T37.92	T37.93	T37.94	T37.95	T37.96
sulfamate	T60.3X1	T60.3X2	T60.3X3	T60.3X4	—	—
sulfonate resin	T47.8X1	T47.8X2	T47.8X3	T47.8X4	T47.8X5	T47.8X6
Amobarbital (sodium)	T42.3X1	T42.3X2	T42.3X3	T42.3X4	T42.3X5	T42.3X6
Amodiaquine	T37.2X1	T37.2X2	T37.2X3	T37.2X4	T37.2X5	T37.2X6
Amopyroquin (e)	T37.2X1	T37.2X2	T37.2X3	T37.2X4	T37.2X5	T37.2X6
Amoxapine	T43.011	T43.012	T43.013	T43.014	T43.015	T43.016
Amoxicillin	T36.0X1	T36.0X2	T36.0X3	T36.0X4	T36.0X5	T36.0X6

Substance	Poisoning, Accidental (unintentional)	Poisoning, Intentional self-harm	Poisoning, Assault	Poisoning, Undetermined	Adverse effect	Underdosing
Amperozide	T43.591	T43.592	T43.593	T43.594	T43.595	T43.596
Amphenidone	T43.591	T43.592	T43.593	T43.594	T43.595	T43.596
Amphetamine NEC	T43.621	T43.622	T43.623	T43.624	T43.625	T43.626
Amphomycin	T36.8X1	T36.8X2	T36.8X3	T36.8X4	T36.8X5	T36.8X6
Amphotalide	T37.4X1	T37.4X2	T37.4X3	T37.4X4	T37.4X5	T37.4X6
Amphotericin B	T36.7X1	T36.7X2	T36.7X3	T36.7X4	T36.7X5	T36.7X6
topical	T49.0X1	T49.0X2	T49.0X3	T49.0X4	T49.0X5	T49.0X6
Ampicillin	T36.0X1	T36.0X2	T36.0X3	T36.0X4	T36.0X5	T36.0X6
Amprotropine	T44.3X1	T44.3X2	T44.3X3	T44.3X4	T44.3X5	T44.3X6
Amsacrine	T45.1X1	T45.1X2	T45.1X3	T45.1X4	T45.1X5	T45.1X6
Amygdaline	T62.2X1	T62.2X2	T62.2X3	T62.2X4	—	—
Amyl						
acetate	T52.8X1	T52.8X2	T52.8X3	T52.8X4	—	—
vapor	T59.891	T59.892	T59.893	T59.894	—	—
alcohol	T51.3X1	T51.3X2	T51.3X3	T51.3X4	—	—
chloride	T53.6X1	T53.6X2	T53.6X3	T53.6X4	—	—
formate	T52.8X1	T52.8X2	T52.8X3	T52.8X4	—	—
nitrite	T46.3X1	T46.3X2	T46.3X3	T46.3X4	T46.3X5	T46.3X6
propionate	T65.891	T65.892	T65.893	T65.894	—	—
Amylase	T47.5X1	T47.5X2	T47.5X3	T47.5X4	T47.5X5	T47.5X6
Amyleine, regional	T41.3X1	T41.3X2	T41.3X3	T41.3X4	T41.3X5	T41.3X6
Amylene						
dichloride	T53.6X1	T53.6X2	T53.6X3	T53.6X4	—	—
hydrate	T51.3X1	T51.3X2	T51.3X3	T51.3X4	—	—
Amylmetacresol	T49.6X1	T49.6X2	T49.6X3	T49.6X4	T49.6X5	T49.6X6
Amylobarbitone	T42.3X1	T42.3X2	T42.3X3	T42.3X4	T42.3X5	T42.3X6
Amylocaine, regional	T41.3X1	T41.3X2	T41.3X3	T41.3X4	T41.3X5	T41.3X6
infiltration (subcutaneous)	T41.3X1	T41.3X2	T41.3X3	T41.3X4	T41.3X5	T41.3X6
nerve block (peripheral) (plexus)	T41.3X1	T41.3X2	T41.3X3	T41.3X4	T41.3X5	T41.3X6
spinal	T41.3X1	T41.3X2	T41.3X3	T41.3X4	T41.3X5	T41.3X6
topical (surface)	T41.3X1	T41.3X2	T41.3X3	T41.3X4	T41.3X5	T41.3X6
Amylopectin	T47.6X1	T47.6X2	T47.6X3	T47.6X4	T47.6X5	T47.6X6
Amytal (sodium)	T42.3X1	T42.3X2	T42.3X3	T42.3X4	T42.3X5	T42.3X6
Anabolic steroid	T38.7X1	T38.7X2	T38.7X3	T38.7X4	T38.7X5	T38.7X6
Analeptic NEC	T50.7X1	T50.7X2	T50.7X3	T50.7X4	T50.7X5	T50.7X6
Analgesic	T39.91	T39.92	T39.93	T39.94	T39.95	T39.96
anti-inflammatory NEC	T39.91	T39.92	T39.93	T39.94	T39.95	T39.96
propionic acid derivative	T39.311	T39.312	T39.313	T39.314	T39.315	T39.316
antirheumatic NEC	T39.4X1	T39.4X2	T39.4X3	T39.4X4	T39.4X5	T39.4X6
aromatic NEC	T39.1X1	T39.1X2	T39.1X3	T39.1X4	T39.1X5	T39.1X6
narcotic NEC	T40.601	T40.602	T40.603	T40.604	T40.605	T40.606
combination	T40.601	T40.602	T40.603	T40.604	T40.605	T40.606
obstetric	T40.601	T40.602	T40.603	T40.604	T40.605	T40.606
non-narcotic NEC	T39.91	T39.92	T39.93	T39.94	T39.95	T39.96
combination	T39.91	T39.92	T39.93	T39.94	T39.95	T39.96
pyrazole	T39.2X1	T39.2X2	T39.2X3	T39.2X4	T39.2X5	T39.2X6
specified NEC	T39.8X1	T39.8X2	T39.8X3	T39.8X4	T39.8X5	T39.8X6
Analgin	T39.2X1	T39.2X2	T39.2X3	T39.2X4	T39.2X5	T39.2X6
Anamirta cocculus	T62.1X1	T62.1X2	T62.1X3	T62.1X4	—	—
Ancillin	T36.0X1	T36.0X2	T36.0X3	T36.0X4	T36.0X5	T36.0X6
Ancrod	T45.691	T45.692	T45.693	T45.694	T45.695	T45.696
Androgen	T38.7X1	T38.7X2	T38.7X3	T38.7X4	T38.7X5	T38.7X6
Androgen-estrogen mixture	T38.7X1	T38.7X2	T38.7X3	T38.7X4	T38.7X5	T38.7X6
Androstalone	T38.7X1	T38.7X2	T38.7X3	T38.7X4	T38.7X5	T38.7X6
Androstanolone	T38.7X1	T38.7X2	T38.7X3	T38.7X4	T38.7X5	T38.7X6
Androsterone	T38.7X1	T38.7X2	T38.7X3	T38.7X4	T38.7X5	T38.7X6
Anemone pulsatilla	T62.2X1	T62.2X2	T62.2X3	T62.2X4	—	—

Substance	Poisoning, Accidental (unintentional)	Poisoning, Intentional self-harm	Poisoning, Assault	Poisoning, Undetermined	Adverse effect	Underdosing
Anesthesia						
caudal	T41.3X1	T41.3X2	T41.3X3	T41.3X4	T41.3X5	T41.3X6
endotracheal	T41.0X1	T41.0X2	T41.0X3	T41.0X4	T41.0X5	T41.0X6
epidural	T41.3X1	T41.3X2	T41.3X3	T41.3X4	T41.3X5	T41.3X6
inhalation	T41.0X1	T41.0X2	T41.0X3	T41.0X4	T41.0X5	T41.0X6
local	T41.3X1	T41.3X2	T41.3X3	T41.3X4	T41.3X5	T41.3X6
mucosal	T41.3X1	T41.3X2	T41.3X3	T41.3X4	T41.3X5	T41.3X6
muscle relaxation	T48.1X1	T48.1X2	T48.1X3	T48.1X4	T48.1X5	T48.1X6
nerve blocking	T41.3X1	T41.3X2	T41.3X3	T41.3X4	T41.3X5	T41.3X6
plexus blocking	T41.3X1	T41.3X2	T41.3X3	T41.3X4	T41.3X5	T41.3X6
potentiated	T41.201	T41.202	T41.203	T41.204	T41.205	T41.206
rectal	T41.201	T41.202	T41.203	T41.204	T41.205	T41.206
general	T41.201	T41.202	T41.203	T41.204	T41.205	T41.206
local	T41.3X1	T41.3X2	T41.3X3	T41.3X4	T41.3X5	T41.3X6
regional	T41.3X1	T41.3X2	T41.3X3	T41.3X4	T41.3X5	T41.3X6
surface	T41.3X1	T41.3X2	T41.3X3	T41.3X4	T41.3X5	T41.3X6
Anesthetic NEC—*see also* Anesthesia	T41.41	T41.42	T41.43	T41.44	T41.45	T41.46
with muscle relaxant	T41.201	T41.202	T41.203	T41.204	T41.205	T41.206
general	T41.201	T41.202	T41.203	T41.204	T41.205	T41.206
local	T41.3X1	T41.3X2	T41.3X3	T41.3X4	T41.3X5	T41.3X6
gaseous NEC	T41.0X1	T41.0X2	T41.0X3	T41.0X4	T41.0X5	T41.0X6
general NEC	T41.201	T41.202	T41.203	T41.204	T41.205	T41.206
halogenated hydrocarbon derivatives NEC	T41.0X1	T41.0X2	T41.0X3	T41.0X4	T41.0X5	T41.0X6
infiltration NEC	T41.3X1	T41.3X2	T41.3X3	T41.3X4	T41.3X5	T41.3X6
intravenous NEC	T41.1X1	T41.1X2	T41.1X3	T41.1X4	T41.1X5	T41.1X6
local NEC	T41.3X1	T41.3X2	T41.3X3	T41.3X4	T41.3X5	T41.3X6
rectal	T41.201	T41.202	T41.203	T41.204	T41.205	T41.206
general	T41.201	T41.202	T41.203	T41.204	T41.205	T41.206
local	T41.3X1	T41.3X2	T41.3X3	T41.3X4	T41.3X5	T41.3X6
regional NEC	T41.3X1	T41.3X2	T41.3X3	T41.3X4	T41.3X5	T41.3X6
spinal NEC	T41.3X1	T41.3X2	T41.3X3	T41.3X4	T41.3X5	T41.3X6
thiobarbiturate	T41.1X1	T41.1X2	T41.1X3	T41.1X4	T41.1X5	T41.1X6
topical	T41.3X1	T41.3X2	T41.3X3	T41.3X4	T41.3X5	T41.3X6
Aneurine	T45.2X1	T45.2X2	T45.2X3	T45.2X4	T45.2X5	T45.2X6
Angio-Conray	T50.8X1	T50.8X2	T50.8X3	T50.8X4	T50.8X5	T50.8X6
Angiotensin	T44.5X1	T44.5X2	T44.5X3	T44.5X4	T44.5X5	T44.5X6
Angiotensinamide	T44.991	T44.992	T44.993	T44.994	T44.995	T44.996
Anhydrohydroxy-progesterone	T38.5X1	T38.5X2	T38.5X3	T38.5X4	T38.5X5	T38.5X6
Anhydron	T50.2X1	T50.2X2	T50.2X3	T50.2X4	T50.2X5	T50.2X6
Anileridine	T40.4X1	T40.4X2	T40.4X3	T40.4X4	T40.4X5	T40.4X6
Aniline (dye) (liquid)	T65.3X1	T65.3X2	T65.3X3	T65.3X4	—	—
analgesic	T39.1X1	T39.1X2	T39.1X3	T39.1X4	T39.1X5	T39.1X6
derivatives, therapeutic NEC	T39.1X1	T39.1X2	T39.1X3	T39.1X4	T39.1X5	T39.1X6
vapor	T65.3X1	T65.3X2	T65.3X3	T65.3X4	—	—
Aniscoropine	T44.3X1	T44.3X2	T44.3X3	T44.3X4	T44.3X5	T44.3X6
Anise oil	T47.5X1	T47.5X2	T47.5X3	T47.5X4	T47.5X5	T47.5X6
Anisidine	T65.3X1	T65.3X2	T65.3X3	T65.3X4	—	—
Anisindione	T45.511	T45.512	T45.513	T45.514	T45.515	T45.516
Anisotropine methyl-bromide	T44.3X1	T44.3X2	T44.3X3	T44.3X4	T44.3X5	T44.3X6
Anistreplase	T45.611	T45.612	T45.613	T45.614	T45.615	T45.616
Anorexiant (central)	T50.5X1	T50.5X2	T50.5X3	T50.5X4	T50.5X5	T50.5X6
Anorexic agents	T50.5X1	T50.5X2	T50.5X3	T50.5X4	T50.5X5	T50.5X6
Ansamycin	T36.6X1	T36.6X2	T36.6X3	T36.6X4	T36.6X5	T36.6X6
Ant (bite) (sting)	T63.421	T63.422	T63.423	T63.424	—	—

Substance	Poisoning, Accidental (unintentional)	Poisoning, Intentional self-harm	Poisoning, Assault	Poisoning, Undetermined	Adverse effect	Underdosing
Ant poison—*see* Insecticide						
Antabuse	T50.6X1	T50.6X2	T50.6X3	T50.6X4	T50.6X5	T50.6X6
Antacid NEC	T47.1X1	T47.1X2	T47.1X3	T47.1X4	T47.1X5	T47.1X6
Antagonist						
Aldosterone	T50.0X1	T50.0X2	T50.0X3	T50.0X4	T50.0X5	T50.0X6
alpha-adrenoreceptor	T44.6X1	T44.6X2	T44.6X3	T44.6X4	T44.6X5	T44.6X6
anticoagulant	T45.7X1	T45.7X2	T45.7X3	T45.7X4	T45.7X5	T45.7X6
beta-adrenoreceptor	T44.7X1	T44.7X2	T44.7X3	T44.7X4	T44.7X5	T44.7X6
extrapyramidal NEC	T44.3X1	T44.3X2	T44.3X3	T44.3X4	T44.3X5	T44.3X6
folic acid	T45.1X1	T45.1X2	T45.1X3	T45.1X4	T45.1X5	T45.1X6
H2 receptor	T47.0X1	T47.0X2	T47.0X3	T47.0X4	T47.0X5	T47.0X6
heavy metal	T45.8X1	T45.8X2	T45.8X3	T45.8X4	T45.8X5	T45.8X6
narcotic analgesic	T50.7X1	T50.7X2	T50.7X3	T50.7X4	T50.7X5	T50.7X6
opiate	T50.7X1	T50.7X2	T50.7X3	T50.7X4	T50.7X5	T50.7X6
pyrimidine	T45.1X1	T45.1X2	T45.1X3	T45.1X4	T45.1X5	T45.1X6
serotonin	T46.5X1	T46.5X2	T46.5X3	T46.5X4	T46.5X5	T46.5X6
Antazolin (e)	T45.0X1	T45.0X2	T45.0X3	T45.0X4	T45.0X5	T45.0X6
Anterior pituitary hormone NEC	T38.811	T38.812	T38.813	T38.814	T38.815	T38.816
Anthelmintic NEC	T37.4X1	T37.4X2	T37.4X3	T37.4X4	T37.4X5	T37.4X6
Anthiolimine	T37.4X1	T37.4X2	T37.4X3	T37.4X4	T37.4X5	T37.4X6
Anthralin	T49.4X1	T49.4X2	T49.4X3	T49.4X4	T49.4X5	T49.4X6
Anthramycin	T45.1X1	T45.1X2	T45.1X3	T45.1X4	T45.1X5	T45.1X6
Antiadrenergic NEC	T44.8X1	T44.8X2	T44.8X3	T44.8X4	T44.8X5	T44.8X6
Antiallergic NEC	T45.0X1	T45.0X2	T45.0X3	T45.0X4	T45.0X5	T45.0X6
Anti-anemic (drug) (preparation)	T45.8X1	T45.8X2	T45.8X3	T45.8X4	T45.8X5	T45.8X6
Antiandrogen NEC	T38.6X1	T38.6X2	T38.6X3	T38.6X4	T38.6X5	T38.6X6
Antianxiety drug NEC	T43.501	T43.502	T43.503	T43.504	T43.505	T43.506
Antiaris toxicaria	T65.891	T65.892	T65.893	T65.894	—	—
Antiarteriosclerotic drug	T46.6X1	T46.6X2	T46.6X3	T46.6X4	T46.6X5	T46.6X6
Antiasthmatic drug NEC	T48.6X1	T48.6X2	T48.6X3	T48.6X4	T48.6X5	T48.6X6
Antibiotic NEC	T36.91	T36.92	T36.93	T36.94	T36.95	T36.96
aminoglycoside	T36.5X1	T36.5X2	T36.5X3	T36.5X4	T36.5X5	T36.5X6
anticancer	T45.1X1	T45.1X2	T45.1X3	T45.1X4	T45.1X5	T45.1X6
antifungal	T36.7X1	T36.7X2	T36.7X3	T36.7X4	T36.7X5	T36.7X6
antimycobacterial	T36.5X1	T36.5X2	T36.5X3	T36.5X4	T36.5X5	T36.5X6
antineoplastic	T45.1X1	T45.1X2	T45.1X3	T45.1X4	T45.1X5	T45.1X6
cephalosporin (group)	T36.1X1	T36.1X2	T36.1X3	T36.1X4	T36.1X5	T36.1X6
chloramphenicol (group)	T36.2X1	T36.2X2	T36.2X3	T36.2X4	T36.2X5	T36.2X6
ENT	T49.6X1	T49.6X2	T49.6X3	T49.6X4	T49.6X5	T49.6X6
eye	T49.5X1	T49.5X2	T49.5X3	T49.5X4	T49.5X5	T49.5X6
fungicidal (local)	T49.0X1	T49.0X2	T49.0X3	T49.0X4	T49.0X5	T49.0X6
intestinal	T36.8X1	T36.8X2	T36.8X3	T36.8X4	T36.8X5	T36.8X6
b-lactam NEC	T36.1X1	T36.1X2	T36.1X3	T36.1X4	T36.1X5	T36.1X6
local	T49.0X1	T49.0X2	T49.0X3	T49.0X4	T49.0X5	T49.0X6
macrolides	T36.3X1	T36.3X2	T36.3X3	T36.3X4	T36.3X5	T36.3X6
polypeptide	T36.8X1	T36.8X2	T36.8X3	T36.8X4	T36.8X5	T36.8X6
specified NEC	T36.8X1	T36.8X2	T36.8X3	T36.8X4	T36.8X5	T36.8X6
tetracycline (group)	T36.4X1	T36.4X2	T36.4X3	T36.4X4	T36.4X5	T36.4X6
throat	T49.6X1	T49.6X2	T49.6X3	T49.6X4	T49.6X5	T49.6X6
Anticancer agents NEC	T45.1X1	T45.1X2	T45.1X3	T45.1X4	T45.1X5	T45.1X6
Anticholesterolemic drug NEC	T46.6X1	T46.6X2	T46.6X3	T46.6X4	T46.6X5	T46.6X6
Anticholinergic NEC	T44.3X1	T44.3X2	T44.3X3	T44.3X4	T44.3X5	T44.3X6
Anticholinesterase	T44.0X1	T44.0X2	T44.0X3	T44.0X4	T44.0X5	T44.0X6
organophosphorus	T44.0X1	T44.0X2	T44.0X3	T44.0X4	T44.0X5	T44.0X6
insecticide	T60.0X1	T60.0X2	T60.0X3	T60.0X4	—	—
nerve gas	T59.891	T59.892	T59.893	T59.894	—	—

Anticholinesterase - Antimitotic agent

Substance	Poisoning, Accidental (unintentional)	Poisoning, Intentional self-harm	Poisoning, Assault	Poisoning, Undetermined	Adverse effect	Underdosing
Anticholinesterase — *continued*						
reversible	T44.0X1	T44.0X2	T44.0X3	T44.0X4	T44.0X5	T44.0X6
ophthalmological	T49.5X1	T49.5X2	T49.5X3	T49.5X4	T49.5X5	T49.5X6
Anticoagulant NEC	T45.511	T45.512	T45.513	T45.514	T45.515	T45.516
Antagonist	T45.7X1	T45.7X2	T45.7X3	T45.7X4	T45.7X5	T45.7X6
Anti-common-cold drug NEC	T48.5X1	T48.5X2	T48.5X3	T48.5X4	T48.5X5	T48.5X6
Anticonvulsant	T42.71	T42.72	T42.73	T42.74	T42.75	T42.76
barbiturate	T42.3X1	T42.3X2	T42.3X3	T42.3X4	T42.3X5	T42.3X6
combination (with barbiturate)	T42.3X1	T42.3X2	T42.3X3	T42.3X4	T42.3X5	T42.3X6
hydantoin	T42.0X1	T42.0X2	T42.0X3	T42.0X4	T42.0X5	T42.0X6
hypnotic NEC	T42.6X1	T42.6X2	T42.6X3	T42.6X4	T42.6X5	T42.6X6
oxazolidinedione	T42.2X1	T42.2X2	T42.2X3	T42.2X4	T42.2X5	T42.2X6
pyrimidinedione	T42.6X1	T42.6X2	T42.6X3	T42.6X4	T42.6X5	T42.6X6
specified NEC	T42.6X1	T42.6X2	T42.6X3	T42.6X4	T42.6X5	T42.6X6
succinimide	T42.2X1	T42.2X2	T42.2X3	T42.2X4	T42.2X5	T42.2X6
Anti-D immunoglobulin (human)	T50.Z11	T50.Z12	T50.Z13	T50.Z14	T50.Z15	T50.Z16
Antidepressant	T43.201	T43.202	T43.203	T43.204	T43.205	T43.206
monoamine oxidase inhibitor	T43.1X1	T43.1X2	T43.1X3	T43.1X4	T43.1X5	T43.1X6
selective serotonin norepinephrine reuptake inhibitor	T43.211	T43.212	T43.213	T43.214	T43.215	T43.216
selective serotonin reuptake inhibitor	T43.221	T43.222	T43.223	T43.224	T43.225	T43.226
specified NEC	T43.291	T43.292	T43.293	T43.294	T43.295	T43.296
tetracyclic	T43.021	T43.022	T43.023	T43.024	T43.025	T43.026
triazolopyridine	T43.211	T43.212	T43.213	T43.214	T43.215	T43.216
tricyclic	T43.011	T43.012	T43.013	T43.014	T43.015	T43.016
Antidiabetic NEC	T38.3X1	T38.3X2	T38.3X3	T38.3X4	T38.3X5	T38.3X6
biguanide	T38.3X1	T38.3X2	T38.3X3	T38.3X4	T38.3X5	T38.3X6
and sulfonyl combined	T38.3X1	T38.3X2	T38.3X3	T38.3X4	T38.3X5	T38.3X6
combined	T38.3X1	T38.3X2	T38.3X3	T38.3X4	T38.3X5	T38.3X6
sulfonylurea	T38.3X1	T38.3X2	T38.3X3	T38.3X4	T38.3X5	T38.3X6
Antidiarrheal drug NEC	T47.6X1	T47.6X2	T47.6X3	T47.6X4	T47.6X5	T47.6X6
absorbent	T47.6X1	T47.6X2	T47.6X3	T47.6X4	T47.6X5	T47.6X6
Antidiphtheria serum	T50.Z11	T50.Z12	T50.Z13	T50.Z14	T50.Z15	T50.Z16
Antidiuretic hormone	T38.891	T38.892	T38.893	T38.894	T38.895	T38.896
Antidote NEC	T50.6X1	T50.6X2	T50.6X3	T50.6X4	T50.6X5	T50.6X6
heavy metal	T45.8X1	T45.8X2	T45.8X3	T45.8X4	T45.8X5	T45.8X6
Antidysrhythmic NEC	T46.2X1	T46.2X2	T46.2X3	T46.2X4	T46.2X5	T46.2X6
Antiemetic drug	T45.0X1	T45.0X2	T45.0X3	T45.0X4	T45.0X5	T45.0X6
Antiepilepsy agent	T42.71	T42.72	T42.73	T42.74	T42.75	T42.76
combination	T42.5X1	T42.5X2	T42.5X3	T42.5X4	T42.5X5	T42.5X6
mixed	T42.5X1	T42.5X2	T42.5X3	T42.5X4	T42.5X5	T42.5X6
specified, NEC	T42.6X1	T42.6X2	T42.6X3	T42.6X4	T42.6X5	T42.6X6
Antiestrogen NEC	T38.6X1	T38.6X2	T38.6X3	T38.6X4	T38.6X5	T38.6X6
Antifertility pill	T38.4X1	T38.4X2	T38.4X3	T38.4X4	T38.4X5	T38.4X6
Antifibrinolytic drug	T45.621	T45.622	T45.623	T45.624	T45.625	T45.626
Antifilarial drug	T37.4X1	T37.4X2	T37.4X3	T37.4X4	T37.4X5	T37.4X6
Antiflatulent	T47.5X1	T47.5X2	T47.5X3	T47.5X4	T47.5X5	T47.5X6
Antifreeze	T65.91	T65.92	T65.93	T65.94	—	—
alcohol	T51.1X1	T51.1X2	T51.1X3	T51.1X4	—	—
ethylene glycol	T51.8X1	T51.8X2	T51.8X3	T51.8X4	—	—
Antifungal						
antibiotic (systemic)	T36.7X1	T36.7X2	T36.7X3	T36.7X4	T36.7X5	T36.7X6
anti-infective NEC	T37.91	T37.92	T37.93	T37.94	T37.95	T37.96

Substance	Poisoning, Accidental (unintentional)	Poisoning, Intentional self-harm	Poisoning, Assault	Poisoning, Undetermined	Adverse effect	Underdosing
Antifungal — *continued*						
disinfectant, local	T49.0X1	T49.0X2	T49.0X3	T49.0X4	T49.0X5	T49.0X6
nonmedicinal (spray)	T60.3X1	T60.3X2	T60.3X3	T60.3X4	—	—
topical	T49.0X1	T49.0X2	T49.0X3	T49.0X4	T49.0X5	T49.0X6
Anti-gastric-secretion drug NEC	T47.1X1	T47.1X2	T47.1X3	T47.1X4	T47.1X5	T47.1X6
Antigonadotrophin NEC	T38.6X1	T38.6X2	T38.6X3	T38.6X4	T38.6X5	T38.6X6
Antihallucinogen	T43.501	T43.502	T43.503	T43.504	T43.505	T43.506
Antihelmintics	T37.4X1	T37.4X2	T37.4X3	T37.4X4	T37.4X5	T37.4X6
Antihemophilic						
factor	T45.8X1	T45.8X2	T45.8X3	T45.8X4	T45.8X5	T45.8X6
fraction	T45.8X1	T45.8X2	T45.8X3	T45.8X4	T45.8X5	T45.8X6
globulin concentrate	T45.7X1	T45.7X2	T45.7X3	T45.7X4	T45.7X5	T45.7X6
human plasma	T45.8X1	T45.8X2	T45.8X3	T45.8X4	T45.8X5	T45.8X6
plasma, dried	T45.7X1	T45.7X2	T45.7X3	T45.7X4	T45.7X5	T45.7X6
Antihemorrhoidal preparation	T49.2X1	T49.2X2	T49.2X3	T49.2X4	T49.2X5	T49.2X6
Antiheparin drug	T45.7X1	T45.7X2	T45.7X3	T45.7X4	T45.7X5	T45.7X6
Antihistamine	T45.0X1	T45.0X2	T45.0X3	T45.0X4	T45.0X5	T45.0X6
Antihookworm drug	T37.4X1	T37.4X2	T37.4X3	T37.4X4	T37.4X5	T37.4X6
Anti-human lymphocytic globulin	T50.Z11	T50.Z12	T50.Z13	T50.Z14	T50.Z15	T50.Z16
Antihyperlipidemic drug	T46.6X1	T46.6X2	T46.6X3	T46.6X4	T46.6X5	T46.6X6
Antihypertensive drug NEC	T46.5X1	T46.5X2	T46.5X3	T46.5X4	T46.5X5	T46.5X6
Anti-infective NEC	T37.91	T37.92	T37.93	T37.94	T37.95	T37.96
anthelmintic	T37.4X1	T37.4X2	T37.4X3	T37.4X4	T37.4X5	T37.4X6
antibiotics	T36.91	T36.92	T36.93	T36.94	T36.95	T36.96
specified NEC	T36.8X1	T36.8X2	T36.8X3	T36.8X4	T36.8X5	T36.8X6
antimalarial	T37.2X1	T37.2X2	T37.2X3	T37.2X4	T37.2X5	T37.2X6
antimycobacterial NEC	T37.1X1	T37.1X2	T37.1X3	T37.1X4	T37.1X5	T37.1X6
antibiotics	T36.5X1	T36.5X2	T36.5X3	T36.5X4	T36.5X5	T36.5X6
antiprotozoal NEC	T37.3X1	T37.3X2	T37.3X3	T37.3X4	T37.3X5	T37.3X6
blood	T37.2X1	T37.2X2	T37.2X3	T37.2X4	T37.2X5	T37.2X6
antiviral	T37.5X1	T37.5X2	T37.5X3	T37.5X4	T37.5X5	T37.5X6
arsenical	T37.8X1	T37.8X2	T37.8X3	T37.8X4	T37.8X5	T37.8X6
bismuth, local	T49.0X1	T49.0X2	T49.0X3	T49.0X4	T49.0X5	T49.0X6
ENT	T49.6X1	T49.6X2	T49.6X3	T49.6X4	T49.6X5	T49.6X6
eye NEC	T49.5X1	T49.5X2	T49.5X3	T49.5X4	T49.5X5	T49.5X6
heavy metals NEC	T37.8X1	T37.8X2	T37.8X3	T37.8X4	T37.8X5	T37.8X6
local NEC	T49.0X1	T49.0X2	T49.0X3	T49.0X4	T49.0X5	T49.0X6
specified NEC	T49.0X1	T49.0X2	T49.0X3	T49.0X4	T49.0X5	T49.0X6
mixed	T37.91	T37.92	T37.93	T37.94	T37.95	T37.96
ophthalmic preparation	T49.5X1	T49.5X2	T49.5X3	T49.5X4	T49.5X5	T49.5X6
topical NEC	T49.0X1	T49.0X2	T49.0X3	T49.0X4	T49.0X5	T49.0X6
Anti-inflammatory drug NEC	T39.391	T39.392	T39.393	T39.394	T39.395	T39.396
local	T49.0X1	T49.0X2	T49.0X3	T49.0X4	T49.0X5	T49.0X6
nonsteroidal NEC	T39.391	T39.392	T39.393	T39.394	T39.395	T39.396
propionic acid derivative	T39.311	T39.312	T39.313	T39.314	T39.315	T39.316
specified NEC	T39.391	T39.392	T39.393	T39.394	T39.395	T39.396
Antikaluretic	T50.3X1	T50.3X2	T50.3X3	T50.3X4	T50.3X5	T50.3X6
Antiknock (tetraethyl lead)	T56.0X1	T56.0X2	T56.0X3	T56.0X4	—	—
Antilipemic drug NEC	T46.6X1	T46.6X2	T46.6X3	T46.6X4	T46.6X5	T46.6X6
Antimalarial	T37.2X1	T37.2X2	T37.2X3	T37.2X4	T37.2X5	T37.2X6
prophylactic NEC	T37.2X1	T37.2X2	T37.2X3	T37.2X4	T37.2X5	T37.2X6
pyrimidine derivative	T37.2X1	T37.2X2	T37.2X3	T37.2X4	T37.2X5	T37.2X6
Antimetabolite	T45.1X1	T45.1X2	T45.1X3	T45.1X4	T45.1X5	T45.1X6
Antimitotic agent	T45.1X1	T45.1X2	T45.1X3	T45.1X4	T45.1X5	T45.1X6

Substance	Poisoning, Accidental (unintentional)	Poisoning, Intentional self-harm	Poisoning, Assault	Poisoning, Undetermined	Adverse effect	Underdosing
Antimony (compounds) (vapor) NEC	T56.891	T56.892	T56.893	T56.894	—	—
anti-infectives	T37.8X1	T37.8X2	T37.8X3	T37.8X4	T37.8X5	T37.8X6
dimercaptosuccinate	T37.3X1	T37.3X2	T37.3X3	T37.3X4	T37.3X5	T37.3X6
hydride	T56.891	T56.892	T56.893	T56.894	—	—
pesticide (vapor)	T60.8X1	T60.8X2	T60.8X3	T60.8X4	—	—
potassium (sodium) tartrate	T37.8X1	T37.8X2	T37.8X3	T37.8X4	T37.8X5	T37.8X6
sodium dimercaptosuccinate	T37.3X1	T37.3X2	T37.3X3	T37.3X4	T37.3X5	T37.3X6
tartrated	T37.8X1	T37.8X2	T37.8X3	T37.8X4	T37.8X5	T37.8X6
Antimuscarinic NEC	T44.3X1	T44.3X2	T44.3X3	T44.3X4	T44.3X5	T44.3X6
Antimycobacterial drug NEC	T37.1X1	T37.1X2	T37.1X3	T37.1X4	T37.1X5	T37.1X6
antibiotics	T36.5X1	T36.5X2	T36.5X3	T36.5X4	T36.5X5	T36.5X6
combination	T37.1X1	T37.1X2	T37.1X3	T37.1X4	T37.1X5	T37.1X6
Antinausea drug	T45.0X1	T45.0X2	T45.0X3	T45.0X4	T45.0X5	T45.0X6
Antinematode drug	T37.4X1	T37.4X2	T37.4X3	T37.4X4	T37.4X5	T37.4X6
Antineoplastic NEC	T45.1X1	T45.1X2	T45.1X3	T45.1X4	T45.1X5	T45.1X6
alkaloidal	T45.1X1	T45.1X2	T45.1X3	T45.1X4	T45.1X5	T45.1X6
antibiotics	T45.1X1	T45.1X2	T45.1X3	T45.1X4	T45.1X5	T45.1X6
combination	T45.1X1	T45.1X2	T45.1X3	T45.1X4	T45.1X5	T45.1X6
estrogen	T38.5X1	T38.5X2	T38.5X3	T38.5X4	T38.5X5	T38.5X6
steroid	T38.7X1	T38.7X2	T38.7X3	T38.7X4	T38.7X5	T38.7X6
Antiparasitic drug (systemic)	T37.91	T37.92	T37.93	T37.94	T37.95	T37.96
local	T49.0X1	T49.0X2	T49.0X3	T49.0X4	T49.0X5	T49.0X6
specified NEC	T37.8X1	T37.8X2	T37.8X3	T37.8X4	T37.8X5	T37.8X6
Antiparkinsonism drug NEC	T42.8X1	T42.8X2	T42.8X3	T42.8X4	T42.8X5	T42.8X6
Antiperspirant NEC	T49.2X1	T49.2X2	T49.2X3	T49.2X4	T49.2X5	T49.2X6
Antiphlogistic NEC	T39.4X1	T39.4X2	T39.4X3	T39.4X4	T39.4X5	T39.4X6
Antiplatyhelmintic drug	T37.4X1	T37.4X2	T37.4X3	T37.4X4	T37.4X5	T37.4X6
Antiprotozoal drug NEC	T37.3X1	T37.3X2	T37.3X3	T37.3X4	T37.3X5	T37.3X6
blood	T37.2X1	T37.2X2	T37.2X3	T37.2X4	T37.2X5	T37.2X6
local	T49.0X1	T49.0X2	T49.0X3	T49.0X4	T49.0X5	T49.0X6
Antipruritic drug NEC	T49.1X1	T49.1X2	T49.1X3	T49.1X4	T49.1X5	T49.1X6
Antipsychotic drug	T43.501	T43.502	T43.503	T43.504	T43.505	T43.506
specified NEC	T43.591	T43.592	T43.593	T43.594	T43.595	T43.596
Antipyretic	T39.91	T39.92	T39.93	T39.94	T39.95	T39.96
specified NEC	T39.8X1	T39.8X2	T39.8X3	T39.8X4	T39.8X5	T39.8X6
Antipyrine	T39.2X1	T39.2X2	T39.2X3	T39.2X4	T39.2X5	T39.2X6
Antirabies hyperimmune serum	T50.Z11	T50.Z12	T50.Z13	T50.Z14	T50.Z15	T50.Z16
Antirheumatic NEC	T39.4X1	T39.4X2	T39.4X3	T39.4X4	T39.4X5	T39.4X6
Antirigidity drug NEC	T42.8X1	T42.8X2	T42.8X3	T42.8X4	T42.8X5	T42.8X6
Antischistosomal drug	T37.4X1	T37.4X2	T37.4X3	T37.4X4	T37.4X5	T37.4X6
Antiscorpion sera	T50.Z11	T50.Z12	T50.Z13	T50.Z14	T50.Z15	T50.Z16
Antiseborrheics	T49.4X1	T49.4X2	T49.4X3	T49.4X4	T49.4X5	T49.4X6
Antiseptics (external) (medicinal)	T49.0X1	T49.0X2	T49.0X3	T49.0X4	T49.0X5	T49.0X6
Antistine	T45.0X1	T45.0X2	T45.0X3	T45.0X4	T45.0X5	T45.0X6
Antitapeworm drug	T37.4X1	T37.4X2	T37.4X3	T37.4X4	T37.4X5	T37.4X6
Antitetanus immunoglobulin	T50.Z11	T50.Z12	T50.Z13	T50.Z14	T50.Z15	T50.Z16
Antithyroid drug NEC	T38.2X1	T38.2X2	T38.2X3	T38.2X4	T38.2X5	T38.2X6
Antitoxin	T50.Z11	T50.Z12	T50.Z13	T50.Z14	T50.Z15	T50.Z16
diphtheria	T50.Z11	T50.Z12	T50.Z13	T50.Z14	T50.Z15	T50.Z16
gas gangrene	T50.Z11	T50.Z12	T50.Z13	T50.Z14	T50.Z15	T50.Z16
tetanus	T50.Z11	T50.Z12	T50.Z13	T50.Z14	T50.Z15	T50.Z16
Antitrichomonal drug	T37.3X1	T37.3X2	T37.3X3	T37.3X4	T37.3X5	T37.3X6
Antituberculars	T37.1X1	T37.1X2	T37.1X3	T37.1X4	T37.1X5	T37.1X6
antibiotics	T36.5X1	T36.5X2	T36.5X3	T36.5X4	T36.5X5	T36.5X6
Antitussive NEC	T48.3X1	T48.3X2	T48.3X3	T48.3X4	T48.3X5	T48.3X6
codeine mixture	T40.2X1	T40.2X2	T40.2X3	T40.2X4	T40.2X5	T40.2X6
opiate	T40.2X1	T40.2X2	T40.2X3	T40.2X4	T40.2X5	T40.2X6
Antivaricose drug	T46.8X1	T46.8X2	T46.8X3	T46.8X4	T46.8X5	T46.8X6
Antivenin, antivenom (sera)	T50.Z11	T50.Z12	T50.Z13	T50.Z14	T50.Z15	T50.Z16
crotaline	T50.Z11	T50.Z12	T50.Z13	T50.Z14	T50.Z15	T50.Z16
spider bite	T50.Z11	T50.Z12	T50.Z13	T50.Z14	T50.Z15	T50.Z16
Antivertigo drug	T45.0X1	T45.0X2	T45.0X3	T45.0X4	T45.0X5	T45.0X6
Antiviral drug NEC	T37.5X1	T37.5X2	T37.5X3	T37.5X4	T37.5X5	T37.5X6
eye	T49.5X1	T49.5X2	T49.5X3	T49.5X4	T49.5X5	T49.5X6
Antiwhipworm drug	T37.4X1	T37.4X2	T37.4X3	T37.4X4	T37.4X5	T37.4X6
Antrol—*see also by specific chemical substance*	T60.91	T60.92	T60.93	T60.94	—	—
fungicide	T60.91	T60.92	T60.93	T60.94	—	—
ANTU (alpha naphthylthiourea)	T60.4X1	T60.4X2	T60.4X3	T60.4X4	—	—
Apalcillin	T36.0X1	T36.0X2	T36.0X3	T36.0X4	T36.0X5	T36.0X6
APC	T48.5X1	T48.5X2	T48.5X3	T48.5X4	T48.5X5	T48.5X6
Aplonidine	T44.4X1	T44.4X2	T44.4X3	T44.4X4	T44.4X5	T44.4X6
Apomorphine	T47.7X1	T47.7X2	T47.7X3	T47.7X4	T47.7X5	T47.7X6
Appetite depressants, central	T50.5X1	T50.5X2	T50.5X3	T50.5X4	T50.5X5	T50.5X6
Apraclonidine (hydrochloride)	T44.4X1	T44.4X2	T44.4X3	T44.4X4	T44.4X5	T44.4X6
Apresoline	T46.5X1	T46.5X2	T46.5X3	T46.5X4	T46.5X5	T46.5X6
Aprindine	T46.2X1	T46.2X2	T46.2X3	T46.2X4	T46.2X5	T46.2X6
Aprobarbital	T42.3X1	T42.3X2	T42.3X3	T42.3X4	T42.3X5	T42.3X6
Apronalide	T42.6X1	T42.6X2	T42.6X3	T42.6X4	T42.6X5	T42.6X6
Aprotinin	T45.621	T45.622	T45.623	T45.624	T45.625	T45.626
Aptocaine	T41.3X1	T41.3X2	T41.3X3	T41.3X4	T41.3X5	T41.3X6
Aqua fortis	T54.2X1	T54.2X2	T54.2X3	T54.2X4	—	—
Ara-A	T37.5X1	T37.5X2	T37.5X3	T37.5X4	T37.5X5	T37.5X6
Ara-C	T45.1X1	T45.1X2	T45.1X3	T45.1X4	T45.1X5	T45.1X6
Arachis oil	T49.3X1	T49.3X2	T49.3X3	T49.3X4	T49.3X5	T49.3X6
cathartic	T47.4X1	T47.4X2	T47.4X3	T47.4X4	T47.4X5	T47.4X6
Aralen	T37.2X1	T37.2X2	T37.2X3	T37.2X4	T37.2X5	T37.2X6
Arecoline	T44.1X1	T44.1X2	T44.1X3	T44.1X4	T44.1X5	T44.1X6
Arginine	T50.991	T50.992	T50.993	T50.994	T50.995	T50.996
glutamate	T50.991	T50.992	T50.993	T50.994	T50.995	T50.996
Argyrol	T49.0X1	T49.0X2	T49.0X3	T49.0X4	T49.0X5	T49.0X6
ENT agent	T49.6X1	T49.6X2	T49.6X3	T49.6X4	T49.6X5	T49.6X6
ophthalmic preparation	T49.5X1	T49.5X2	T49.5X3	T49.5X4	T49.5X5	T49.5X6
Aristocort	T38.0X1	T38.0X2	T38.0X3	T38.0X4	T38.0X5	T38.0X6
ENT agent	T49.6X1	T49.6X2	T49.6X3	T49.6X4	T49.6X5	T49.6X6
ophthalmic preparation	T49.5X1	T49.5X2	T49.5X3	T49.5X4	T49.5X5	T49.5X6
topical NEC	T49.0X1	T49.0X2	T49.0X3	T49.0X4	T49.0X5	T49.0X6
Aromatics, corrosive	T54.1X1	T54.1X2	T54.1X3	T54.1X4	—	—
disinfectants	T54.1X1	T54.1X2	T54.1X3	T54.1X4	—	—
Arsenate of lead	T57.0X1	T57.0X2	T57.0X3	T57.0X4	—	—
herbicide	T57.0X1	T57.0X2	T57.0X3	T57.0X4	—	—
Arsenic, arsenicals (compounds) (dust) (vapor) NEC	T57.0X1	T57.0X2	T57.0X3	T57.0X4	—	—
anti-infectives	T37.8X1	T37.8X2	T37.8X3	T37.8X4	T37.8X5	T37.8X6
pesticide (dust) (fumes)	T57.0X1	T57.0X2	T57.0X3	T57.0X4	—	—
Arsine (gas)	T57.0X1	T57.0X2	T57.0X3	T57.0X4	—	—
Arsphenamine (silver)	T37.8X1	T37.8X2	T37.8X3	T37.8X4	T37.8X5	T37.8X6

Substance	Poisoning, Accidental (unintentional)	Poisoning, Intentional self-harm	Poisoning, Assault	Poisoning, Undetermined	Adverse effect	Underdosing
Arsthinol	T37.3X1	T37.3X2	T37.3X3	T37.3X4	T37.3X5	T37.3X6
Artane	T44.3X1	T44.3X2	T44.3X3	T44.3X4	T44.3X5	T44.3X6
Arthropod (venomous) NEC	T63.481	T63.482	T63.483	T63.484	—	—
Articaine	T41.3X1	T41.3X2	T41.3X3	T41.3X4	T41.3X5	T41.3X6
Asbestos	T57.8X1	T57.8X2	T57.8X3	T57.8X4	—	—
Ascaridole	T37.4X1	T37.4X2	T37.4X3	T37.4X4	T37.4X5	T37.4X6
Ascorbic acid	T45.2X1	T45.2X2	T45.2X3	T45.2X4	T45.2X5	T45.2X6
Asiaticoside	T49.0X1	T49.0X2	T49.0X3	T49.0X4	T49.0X5	T49.0X6
Asparaginase	T45.1X1	T45.1X2	T45.1X3	T45.1X4	T45.1X5	T45.1X6
Aspidium (oleoresin)	T37.4X1	T37.4X2	T37.4X3	T37.4X4	T37.4X5	T37.4X6
Aspirin (aluminum) (soluble)	T39.011	T39.012	T39.013	T39.014	T39.015	T39.016
Aspoxicillin	T36.0X1	T36.0X2	T36.0X3	T36.0X4	T36.0X5	T36.0X6
Astemizole	T45.0X1	T45.0X2	T45.0X3	T45.0X4	T45.0X5	T45.0X6
Astringent (local)	T49.2X1	T49.2X2	T49.2X3	T49.2X4	T49.2X5	T49.2X6
specified NEC	T49.2X1	T49.2X2	T49.2X3	T49.2X4	T49.2X5	T49.2X6
Astromicin	T36.5X1	T36.5X2	T36.5X3	T36.5X4	T36.5X5	T36.5X6
Ataractic drug NEC	T43.501	T43.502	T43.503	T43.504	T43.505	T43.506
Atenolol	T44.7X1	T44.7X2	T44.7X3	T44.7X4	T44.7X5	T44.7X6
Atonia drug, intestinal	T47.4X1	T47.4X2	T47.4X3	T47.4X4	T47.4X5	T47.4X6
Atophan	T50.4X1	T50.4X2	T50.4X3	T50.4X4	T50.4X5	T50.4X6
Atracurium besilate	T48.1X1	T48.1X2	T48.1X3	T48.1X4	T48.1X5	T48.1X6
Atropine	T44.3X1	T44.3X2	T44.3X3	T44.3X4	T44.3X5	T44.3X6
derivative	T44.3X1	T44.3X2	T44.3X3	T44.3X4	T44.3X5	T44.3X6
methonitrate	T44.3X1	T44.3X2	T44.3X3	T44.3X4	T44.3X5	T44.3X6
Attapulgite	T47.6X1	T47.6X2	T47.6X3	T47.6X4	T47.6X5	T47.6X6
Auramine	T65.891	T65.892	T65.893	T65.894	—	—
dye	T65.6X1	T65.6X2	T65.6X3	T65.6X4	—	—
fungicide	T60.3X1	T60.3X2	T60.3X3	T60.3X4	—	—
Auranofin	T39.4X1	T39.4X2	T39.4X3	T39.4X4	T39.4X5	T39.4X6
Aurantiin	T46.991	T46.992	T46.993	T46.994	T46.995	T46.996
Aureomycin	T36.4X1	T36.4X2	T36.4X3	T36.4X4	T36.4X5	T36.4X6
ophthalmic preparation	T49.5X1	T49.5X2	T49.5X3	T49.5X4	T49.5X5	T49.5X6
topical NEC	T49.0X1	T49.0X2	T49.0X3	T49.0X4	T49.0X5	T49.0X6
Aurothioglucose	T39.4X1	T39.4X2	T39.4X3	T39.4X4	T39.4X5	T39.4X6
Aurothioglycanide	T39.4X1	T39.4X2	T39.4X3	T39.4X4	T39.4X5	T39.4X6
Aurothiomalate sodium	T39.4X1	T39.4X2	T39.4X3	T39.4X4	T39.4X5	T39.4X6
Aurotioprol	T39.4X1	T39.4X2	T39.4X3	T39.4X4	T39.4X5	T39.4X6
Automobile fuel	T52.0X1	T52.0X2	T52.0X3	T52.0X4	—	—
Autonomic nervous system agent NEC	T44.901	T44.902	T44.903	T44.904	T44.905	T44.906
Avlosulfon	T37.1X1	T37.1X2	T37.1X3	T37.1X4	T37.1X5	T37.1X6
Avomine	T42.6X1	T42.6X2	T42.6X3	T42.6X4	T42.6X5	T42.6X6
Axerophthol	T45.2X1	T45.2X2	T45.2X3	T45.2X4	T45.2X5	T45.2X6
Azacitidine	T45.1X1	T45.1X2	T45.1X3	T45.1X4	T45.1X5	T45.1X6
Azacyclonol	T43.591	T43.592	T43.593	T43.594	T43.595	T43.596
Azadirachta	T60.2X1	T60.2X2	T60.2X3	T60.2X4	—	—
Azanidazole	T37.3X1	T37.3X2	T37.3X3	T37.3X4	T37.3X5	T37.3X6
Azapetine	T46.7X1	T46.7X2	T46.7X3	T46.7X4	T46.7X5	T46.7X6
Azapropazone	T39.2X1	T39.2X2	T39.2X3	T39.2X4	T39.2X5	T39.2X6
Azaribine	T45.1X1	T45.1X2	T45.1X3	T45.1X4	T45.1X5	T45.1X6
Azaserine	T45.1X1	T45.1X2	T45.1X3	T45.1X4	T45.1X5	T45.1X6
Azatadine	T45.0X1	T45.0X2	T45.0X3	T45.0X4	T45.0X5	T45.0X6
Azatepa	T45.1X1	T45.1X2	T45.1X3	T45.1X4	T45.1X5	T45.1X6
Azathioprine	T45.1X1	T45.1X2	T45.1X3	T45.1X4	T45.1X5	T45.1X6
Azelaic acid	T49.0X1	T49.0X2	T49.0X3	T49.0X4	T49.0X5	T49.0X6
Azelastine	T45.0X1	T45.0X2	T45.0X3	T45.0X4	T45.0X5	T45.0X6
Azidocillin	T36.0X1	T36.0X2	T36.0X3	T36.0X4	T36.0X5	T36.0X6
Azidothymidine	T37.5X1	T37.5X2	T37.5X3	T37.5X4	T37.5X5	T37.5X6
Azinphos (ethyl) (methyl)	T60.0X1	T60.0X2	T60.0X3	T60.0X4	—	—

Substance	Poisoning, Accidental (unintentional)	Poisoning, Intentional self-harm	Poisoning, Assault	Poisoning, Undetermined	Adverse effect	Underdosing
Aziridine (chelating)	T54.1X1	T54.1X2	T54.1X3	T54.1X4	—	—
Azithromycin	T36.3X1	T36.3X2	T36.3X3	T36.3X4	T36.3X5	T36.3X6
Azlocillin	T36.0X1	T36.0X2	T36.0X3	T36.0X4	T36.0X5	T36.0X6
Azobenzene smoke	T65.3X1	T65.3X2	T65.3X3	T65.3X4	—	—
acaricide	T60.8X1	T60.8X2	T60.8X3	T60.8X4	—	—
Azosulfamide	T37.0X1	T37.0X2	T37.0X3	T37.0X4	T37.0X5	T37.0X6
AZT	T37.5X1	T37.5X2	T37.5X3	T37.5X4	T37.5X5	T37.5X6
Aztreonam	T36.1X1	T36.1X2	T36.1X3	T36.1X4	T36.1X5	T36.1X6
Azulfidine	T37.0X1	T37.0X2	T37.0X3	T37.0X4	T37.0X5	T37.0X6
Azuresin	T50.8X1	T50.8X2	T50.8X3	T50.8X4	T50.8X5	T50.8X6
B						
Bacampicillin	T36.0X1	T36.0X2	T36.0X3	T36.0X4	T36.0X5	T36.0X6
Bacillus						
lactobacillus	T47.8X1	T47.8X2	T47.8X3	T47.8X4	T47.8X5	T47.8X6
subtilis	T47.6X1	T47.6X2	T47.6X3	T47.6X4	T47.6X5	T47.6X6
Bacimycin	T49.0X1	T49.0X2	T49.0X3	T49.0X4	T49.0X5	T49.0X6
ophthalmic preparation	T49.5X1	T49.5X2	T49.5X3	T49.5X4	T49.5X5	T49.5X6
Bacitracin zinc	T49.0X1	T49.0X2	T49.0X3	T49.0X4	T49.0X5	T49.0X6
with neomycin	T49.0X1	T49.0X2	T49.0X3	T49.0X4	T49.0X5	T49.0X6
ENT agent	T49.6X1	T49.6X2	T49.6X3	T49.6X4	T49.6X5	T49.6X6
ophthalmic preparation	T49.5X1	T49.5X2	T49.5X3	T49.5X4	T49.5X5	T49.5X6
topical NEC	T49.0X1	T49.0X2	T49.0X3	T49.0X4	T49.0X5	T49.0X6
Baclofen	T42.8X1	T42.8X2	T42.8X3	T42.8X4	T42.8X5	T42.8X6
Baking soda	T50.991	T50.992	T50.993	T50.994	T50.995	T50.996
BAL	T45.8X1	T45.8X2	T45.8X3	T45.8X4	T45.8X5	T45.8X6
Bambuterol	T48.6X1	T48.6X2	T48.6X3	T48.6X4	T48.6X5	T48.6X6
Bamethan (sulfate)	T46.7X1	T46.7X2	T46.7X3	T46.7X4	T46.7X5	T46.7X6
Bamifylline	T48.6X1	T48.6X2	T48.6X3	T48.6X4	T48.6X5	T48.6X6
Bamipine	T45.0X1	T45.0X2	T45.0X3	T45.0X4	T45.0X5	T45.0X6
Baneberry—see Actaea spicata						
Banewort—see Belladonna						
Barbenyl	T42.3X1	T42.3X2	T42.3X3	T42.3X4	T42.3X5	T42.3X6
Barbexaclone	T42.6X1	T42.6X2	T42.6X3	T42.6X4	T42.6X5	T42.6X6
Barbital	T42.3X1	T42.3X2	T42.3X3	T42.3X4	T42.3X5	T42.3X6
sodium	T42.3X1	T42.3X2	T42.3X3	T42.3X4	T42.3X5	T42.3X6
Barbitone	T42.3X1	T42.3X2	T42.3X3	T42.3X4	T42.3X5	T42.3X6
Barbiturate NEC	T42.3X1	T42.3X2	T42.3X3	T42.3X4	T42.3X5	T42.3X6
with tranquilizer	T42.3X1	T42.3X2	T42.3X3	T42.3X4	T42.3X5	T42.3X6
anesthetic (intravenous)	T41.1X1	T41.1X2	T41.1X3	T41.1X4	T41.1X5	T41.1X6
Barium (carbonate) (chloride) (sulfite)	T57.8X1	T57.8X2	T57.8X3	T57.8X4	—	—
diagnostic agent	T50.8X1	T50.8X2	T50.8X3	T50.8X4	T50.8X5	T50.8X6
pesticide	T60.4X1	T60.4X2	T60.4X3	T60.4X4	—	—
rodenticide	T60.4X1	T60.4X2	T60.4X3	T60.4X4	—	—
sulfate (medicinal)	T50.8X1	T50.8X2	T50.8X3	T50.8X4	T50.8X5	T50.8X6
Barrier cream	T49.3X1	T49.3X2	T49.3X3	T49.3X4	T49.3X5	T49.3X6
Basic fuchsin	T49.0X1	T49.0X2	T49.0X3	T49.0X4	T49.0X5	T49.0X6
Battery acid or fluid	T54.2X1	T54.2X2	T54.2X3	T54.2X4	—	—
Bay rum	T51.8X1	T51.8X2	T51.8X3	T51.8X4	—	—
BCG (vaccine)	T50.A91	T50.A92	T50.A93	T50.A94	T50.A95	T50.A96
BCNU	T45.1X1	T45.1X2	T45.1X3	T45.1X4	T45.1X5	T45.1X6
Bearsfoot	T62.2X1	T62.2X2	T62.2X3	T62.2X4	—	—
Beclamide	T42.6X1	T42.6X2	T42.6X3	T42.6X4	T42.6X5	T42.6X6
Beclomethasone	T44.5X1	T44.5X2	T44.5X3	T44.5X4	T44.5X5	T44.5X6
Bee (sting) (venom)	T63.441	T63.442	T63.443	T63.444	—	—
Befunolol	T49.5X1	T49.5X2	T49.5X3	T49.5X4	T49.5X5	T49.5X6
Bekanamycin	T36.5X1	T36.5X2	T36.5X3	T36.5X4	T36.5X5	T36.5X6

Substance	Poisoning, Accidental (unintentional)	Poisoning, Intentional self-harm	Poisoning, Assault	Poisoning, Undetermined	Adverse effect	Underdosing
Belladonna—see also Nightshade						
alkaloids	T44.3X1	T44.3X2	T44.3X3	T44.3X4	T44.3X5	T44.3X6
extract	T44.3X1	T44.3X2	T44.3X3	T44.3X4	T44.3X5	T44.3X6
herb	T44.3X1	T44.3X2	T44.3X3	T44.3X4	T44.3X5	T44.3X6
Bemegride	T50.7X1	T50.7X2	T50.7X3	T50.7X4	T50.7X5	T50.7X6
Benactyzine	T44.3X1	T44.3X2	T44.3X3	T44.3X4	T44.3X5	T44.3X6
Benadryl	T45.0X1	T45.0X2	T45.0X3	T45.0X4	T45.0X5	T45.0X6
Benaprizine	T44.3X1	T44.3X2	T44.3X3	T44.3X4	T44.3X5	T44.3X6
Benazepril	T46.4X1	T46.4X2	T46.4X3	T46.4X4	T46.4X5	T46.4X6
Bencyclane	T46.7X1	T46.7X2	T46.7X3	T46.7X4	T46.7X5	T46.7X6
Bendazol	T46.3X1	T46.3X2	T46.3X3	T46.3X4	T46.3X5	T46.3X6
Bendrofluazide	T50.2X1	T50.2X2	T50.2X3	T50.2X4	T50.2X5	T50.2X6
Bendroflumethiazide	T50.2X1	T50.2X2	T50.2X3	T50.2X4	T50.2X5	T50.2X6
Benemid	T50.4X1	T50.4X2	T50.4X3	T50.4X4	T50.4X5	T50.4X6
Benethamine penicillin	T36.0X1	T36.0X2	T36.0X3	T36.0X4	T36.0X5	T36.0X6
Benexate	T47.1X1	T47.1X2	T47.1X3	T47.1X4	T47.1X5	T47.1X6
Benfluorex	T46.6X1	T46.6X2	T46.6X3	T46.6X4	T46.6X5	T46.6X6
Benfotiamine	T45.2X1	T45.2X2	T45.2X3	T45.2X4	T45.2X5	T45.2X6
Benisone	T49.0X1	T49.0X2	T49.0X3	T49.0X4	T49.0X5	T49.0X6
Benomyl	T60.0X1	T60.0X2	T60.0X3	T60.0X4	—	—
Benoquin	T49.8X1	T49.8X2	T49.8X3	T49.8X4	T49.8X5	T49.8X6
Benoxinate	T41.3X1	T41.3X2	T41.3X3	T41.3X4	T41.3X5	T41.3X6
Benperidol	T43.4X1	T43.4X2	T43.4X3	T43.4X4	T43.4X5	T43.4X6
Benproperine	T48.3X1	T48.3X2	T48.3X3	T48.3X4	T48.3X5	T48.3X6
Benserazide	T42.8X1	T42.8X2	T42.8X3	T42.8X4	T42.8X5	T42.8X6
Bentazepam	T42.4X1	T42.4X2	T42.4X3	T42.4X4	T42.4X5	T42.4X6
Bentiromide	T50.8X1	T50.8X2	T50.8X3	T50.8X4	T50.8X5	T50.8X6
Bentonite	T49.3X1	T49.3X2	T49.3X3	T49.3X4	T49.3X5	T49.3X6
Benzalbutyramide	T46.6X1	T46.6X2	T46.6X3	T46.6X4	T46.6X5	T46.6X6
Benzalkonium (chloride)	T49.0X1	T49.0X2	T49.0X3	T49.0X4	T49.0X5	T49.0X6
ophthalmic preparation	T49.5X1	T49.5X2	T49.5X3	T49.5X4	T49.5X5	T49.5X6
Benzamidosalicylate (calcium)	T37.1X1	T37.1X2	T37.1X3	T37.1X4	T37.1X5	T37.1X6
Benzamine	T41.3X1	T41.3X2	T41.3X3	T41.3X4	T41.3X5	T41.3X6
lactate	T49.1X1	T49.1X2	T49.1X3	T49.1X4	T49.1X5	T49.1X6
Benzamphetamine	T50.5X1	T50.5X2	T50.5X3	T50.5X4	T50.5X5	T50.5X6
Benzapril hydrochloride	T46.5X1	T46.5X2	T46.5X3	T46.5X4	T46.5X5	T46.5X6
Benzathine benzylpenicillin	T36.0X1	T36.0X2	T36.0X3	T36.0X4	T36.0X5	T36.0X6
Benzathine penicillin	T36.0X1	T36.0X2	T36.0X3	T36.0X4	T36.0X5	T36.0X6
Benzatropine	T42.8X1	T42.8X2	T42.8X3	T42.8X4	T42.8X5	T42.8X6
Benzbromarone	T50.4X1	T50.4X2	T50.4X3	T50.4X4	T50.4X5	T50.4X6
Benzcarbimine	T45.1X1	T45.1X2	T45.1X3	T45.1X4	T45.1X5	T45.1X6
Benzedrex	T44.991	T44.992	T44.993	T44.994	T44.995	T44.996
Benzedrine (amphetamine)	T43.621	T43.622	T43.623	T43.624	T43.625	T43.626
Benzenamine	T65.3X1	T65.3X2	T65.3X3	T65.3X4	—	—
Benzene	T52.1X1	T52.1X2	T52.1X3	T52.1X4	—	—
homologues (acetyl) (dimethyl) (methyl) (solvent)	T52.2X1	T52.2X2	T52.2X3	T52.2X4	—	—
Benzethonium (chloride)	T49.0X1	T49.0X2	T49.0X3	T49.0X4	T49.0X5	T49.0X6
Benzfetamine	T50.5X1	T50.5X2	T50.5X3	T50.5X4	T50.5X5	T50.5X6
Benzhexol	T44.3X1	T44.3X2	T44.3X3	T44.3X4	T44.3X5	T44.3X6
Benzhydramine (chloride)	T45.0X1	T45.0X2	T45.0X3	T45.0X4	T45.0X5	T45.0X6
Benzidine	T65.891	T65.892	T65.893	T65.894	—	—
Benzilonium bromide	T44.3X1	T44.3X2	T44.3X3	T44.3X4	T44.3X5	T44.3X6
Benzimidazole	T60.3X1	T60.3X2	T60.3X3	T60.3X4	—	—
Benzin (e)—see Ligroin						
Benziodarone	T46.3X1	T46.3X2	T46.3X3	T46.3X4	T46.3X5	T46.3X6
Benznidazole	T37.3X1	T37.3X2	T37.3X3	T37.3X4	T37.3X5	T37.3X6
Benzocaine	T41.3X1	T41.3X2	T41.3X3	T41.3X4	T41.3X5	T41.3X6
Benzodiapin	T42.4X1	T42.4X2	T42.4X3	T42.4X4	T42.4X5	T42.4X6
Benzodiazepine NEC	T42.4X1	T42.4X2	T42.4X3	T42.4X4	T42.4X5	T42.4X6
Benzoic acid	T49.0X1	T49.0X2	T49.0X3	T49.0X4	T49.0X5	T49.0X6
with salicylic acid	T49.0X1	T49.0X2	T49.0X3	T49.0X4	T49.0X5	T49.0X6
Benzoin (tincture)	T48.5X1	T48.5X2	T48.5X3	T48.5X4	T48.5X5	T48.5X6
Benzol (benzene)	T52.1X1	T52.1X2	T52.1X3	T52.1X4	—	—
vapor	T52.0X1	T52.0X2	T52.0X3	T52.0X4	—	—
Benzomorphan	T40.2X1	T40.2X2	T40.2X3	T40.2X4	T40.2X5	T40.2X6
Benzonatate	T48.3X1	T48.3X2	T48.3X3	T48.3X4	T48.3X5	T48.3X6
Benzophenones	T49.3X1	T49.3X2	T49.3X3	T49.3X4	T49.3X5	T49.3X6
Benzopyrone	T46.991	T46.992	T46.993	T46.994	T46.995	T46.996
Benzothiadiazides	T50.2X1	T50.2X2	T50.2X3	T50.2X4	T50.2X5	T50.2X6
Benzoxonium chloride	T49.0X1	T49.0X2	T49.0X3	T49.0X4	T49.0X5	T49.0X6
Benzoyl peroxide	T49.0X1	T49.0X2	T49.0X3	T49.0X4	T49.0X5	T49.0X6
Benzoylpas calcium	T37.1X1	T37.1X2	T37.1X3	T37.1X4	T37.1X5	T37.1X6
Benzperidin	T43.591	T43.592	T43.593	T43.594	T43.595	T43.596
Benzperidol	T43.591	T43.592	T43.593	T43.594	T43.595	T43.596
Benzphetamine	T50.5X1	T50.5X2	T50.5X3	T50.5X4	T50.5X5	T50.5X6
Benzpyrinium bromide	T44.1X1	T44.1X2	T44.1X3	T44.1X4	T44.1X5	T44.1X6
Benzquinamide	T45.0X1	T45.0X2	T45.0X3	T45.0X4	T45.0X5	T45.0X6
Benzthiazide	T50.2X1	T50.2X2	T50.2X3	T50.2X4	T50.2X5	T50.2X6
Benztropine						
anticholinergic	T44.3X1	T44.3X2	T44.3X3	T44.3X4	T44.3X5	T44.3X6
antiparkinson	T42.8X1	T42.8X2	T42.8X3	T42.8X4	T42.8X5	T42.8X6
Benzydamine	T49.0X1	T49.0X2	T49.0X3	T49.0X4	T49.0X5	T49.0X6
Benzyl						
acetate	T52.8X1	T52.8X2	T52.8X3	T52.8X4	—	—
alcohol	T49.0X1	T49.0X2	T49.0X3	T49.0X4	T49.0X5	T49.0X6
benzoate	T49.0X1	T49.0X2	T49.0X3	T49.0X4	T49.0X5	T49.0X6
Benzoic acid	T49.0X1	T49.0X2	T49.0X3	T49.0X4	T49.0X5	T49.0X6
morphine	T40.2X1	T40.2X2	T40.2X3	T40.2X4	—	—
nicotinate	T46.6X1	T46.6X2	T46.6X3	T46.6X4	T46.6X5	T46.6X6
penicillin	T36.0X1	T36.0X2	T36.0X3	T36.0X4	T36.0X5	T36.0X6
Benzylhydrochlorthiazide	T50.2X1	T50.2X2	T50.2X3	T50.2X4	T50.2X5	T50.2X6
Benzylpenicillin	T36.0X1	T36.0X2	T36.0X3	T36.0X4	T36.0X5	T36.0X6
Benzylthiouracil	T38.2X1	T38.2X2	T38.2X3	T38.2X4	T38.2X5	T38.2X6
Bephenium hydroxynaphthoate	T37.4X1	T37.4X2	T37.4X3	T37.4X4	T37.4X5	T37.4X6
Bepridil	T46.1X1	T46.1X2	T46.1X3	T46.1X4	T46.1X5	T46.1X6
Bergamot oil	T65.891	T65.892	T65.893	T65.894	—	—
Bergapten	T50.991	T50.992	T50.993	T50.994	T50.995	T50.996
Berries, poisonous	T62.1X1	T62.1X2	T62.1X3	T62.1X4	—	—
Beryllium (compounds)	T56.7X1	T56.7X2	T56.7X3	T56.7X4	—	—
b-acetyldigoxin	T46.0X1	T46.0X2	T46.0X3	T46.0X4	T46.0X5	T46.0X6
beta adrenergic blocking agent, heart	T44.7X1	T44.7X2	T44.7X3	T44.7X4	T44.7X5	T44.7X6
b-benzalbutyramide	T46.6X1	T46.6X2	T46.6X3	T46.6X4	T46.6X5	T46.6X6
Betacarotene	T45.2X1	T45.2X2	T45.2X3	T45.2X4	T45.2X5	T45.2X6
b-eucaine	T49.1X1	T49.1X2	T49.1X3	T49.1X4	T49.1X5	T49.1X6
Beta-Chlor	T42.6X1	T42.6X2	T42.6X3	T42.6X4	T42.6X5	T42.6X6
b-galactosidase	T47.5X1	T47.5X2	T47.5X3	T47.5X4	T47.5X5	T47.5X6
Betahistine	T46.7X1	T46.7X2	T46.7X3	T46.7X4	T46.7X5	T46.7X6
Betaine	T47.5X1	T47.5X2	T47.5X3	T47.5X4	T47.5X5	T47.5X6
Betamethasone	T49.0X1	T49.0X2	T49.0X3	T49.0X4	T49.0X5	T49.0X6
topical	T49.0X1	T49.0X2	T49.0X3	T49.0X4	T49.0X5	T49.0X6
Betamicin	T36.8X1	T36.8X2	T36.8X3	T36.8X4	T36.8X5	T36.8X6
Betanidine	T46.5X1	T46.5X2	T46.5X3	T46.5X4	T46.5X5	T46.5X6

Substance	Poisoning, Accidental (unintentional)	Poisoning, Intentional self-harm	Poisoning, Assault	Poisoning, Undetermined	Adverse effect	Underdosing
b-sitosterol (s)	T46.6X1	T46.6X2	T46.6X3	T46.6X4	T46.6X5	T46.6X6
Betaxolol	T44.7X1	T44.7X2	T44.7X3	T44.7X4	T44.7X5	T44.7X6
Betazole	T50.8X1	T50.8X2	T50.8X3	T50.8X4	T50.8X5	T50.8X6
Bethanechol	T44.1X1	T44.1X2	T44.1X3	T44.1X4	T44.1X5	T44.1X6
chloride	T44.1X1	T44.1X2	T44.1X3	T44.1X4	T44.1X5	T44.1X6
Bethanidine	T46.5X1	T46.5X2	T46.5X3	T46.5X4	T46.5X5	T46.5X6
Betoxycaine	T41.3X1	T41.3X2	T41.3X3	T41.3X4	T41.3X5	T41.3X6
Betula oil	T49.3X1	T49.3X2	T49.3X3	T49.3X4	T49.3X5	T49.3X6
Bevantolol	T44.7X1	T44.7X2	T44.7X3	T44.7X4	T44.7X5	T44.7X6
Bevonium metilsulfate	T44.3X1	T44.3X2	T44.3X3	T44.3X4	T44.3X5	T44.3X6
Bezafibrate	T46.6X1	T46.6X2	T46.6X3	T46.6X4	T46.6X5	T46.6X6
Bezitramide	T40.4X1	T40.4X2	T40.4X3	T40.4X4	T40.4X5	T40.4X6
BHA	T50.991	T50.992	T50.993	T50.994	T50.995	T50.996
Bhang	T40.7X1	T40.7X2	T40.7X3	T40.7X4	T40.7X5	T40.7X6
BHC (medicinal)	T49.0X1	T49.0X2	T49.0X3	T49.0X4	T49.0X5	T49.0X6
nonmedicinal (vapor)	T53.6X1	T53.6X2	T53.6X3	T53.6X4	—	—
Bialamicol	T37.3X1	T37.3X2	T37.3X3	T37.3X4	T37.3X5	T37.3X6
Bibenzonium bromide	T48.3X1	T48.3X2	T48.3X3	T48.3X4	T48.3X5	T48.3X6
Bibrocathol	T49.5X1	T49.5X2	T49.5X3	T49.5X4	T49.5X5	T49.5X6
Bichloride of mercury— *see* Mercury, chloride						
Bichromates (calcium) (potassium) (sodium) (crystals)	T57.8X1	T57.8X2	T57.8X3	T57.8X4	—	—
fumes	T56.2X1	T56.2X2	T56.2X3	T56.2X4	—	—
Biclotymol	T49.6X1	T49.6X2	T49.6X3	T49.6X4	T49.6X5	T49.6X6
Bicucculine	T50.7X1	T50.7X2	T50.7X3	T50.7X4	T50.7X5	T50.7X6
Bifemelane	T43.291	T43.292	T43.293	T43.294	T43.295	T43.296
Biguanide derivatives, oral	T38.3X1	T38.3X2	T38.3X3	T38.3X4	T38.3X5	T38.3X6
Bile salts	T47.5X1	T47.5X2	T47.5X3	T47.5X4	T47.5X5	T47.5X6
Biligrafin	T50.8X1	T50.8X2	T50.8X3	T50.8X4	T50.8X5	T50.8X6
Bilopaque	T50.8X1	T50.8X2	T50.8X3	T50.8X4	T50.8X5	T50.8X6
Binifibrate	T46.6X1	T46.6X2	T46.6X3	T46.6X4	T46.6X5	T46.6X6
Binitrobenzol	T65.3X1	T65.3X2	T65.3X3	T65.3X4	—	—
Bioflavonoid (s)	T46.991	T46.992	T46.993	T46.994	T46.995	T46.996
Biological substance NEC	T50.901	T50.902	T50.903	T50.904	T50.905	T50.906
Biotin	T45.2X1	T45.2X2	T45.2X3	T45.2X4	T45.2X5	T45.2X6
Biperiden	T44.3X1	T44.3X2	T44.3X3	T44.3X4	T44.3X5	T44.3X6
Bisacodyl	T47.2X1	T47.2X2	T47.2X3	T47.2X4	T47.2X5	T47.2X6
Bisbentiamine	T45.2X1	T45.2X2	T45.2X3	T45.2X4	T45.2X5	T45.2X6
Bisbutiamine	T45.2X1	T45.2X2	T45.2X3	T45.2X4	T45.2X5	T45.2X6
Bisdequalinium (salts) (diacetate)	T49.6X1	T49.6X2	T49.6X3	T49.6X4	T49.6X5	T49.6X6
Bishydroxycoumarin	T45.511	T45.512	T45.513	T45.514	T45.515	T45.516
Bismarsen	T37.8X1	T37.8X2	T37.8X3	T37.8X4	T37.8X5	T37.8X6
Bismuth salts	T47.6X1	T47.6X2	T47.6X3	T47.6X4	T47.6X5	T47.6X6
aluminate	T47.1X1	T47.1X2	T47.1X3	T47.1X4	T47.1X5	T47.1X6
anti-infectives	T37.8X1	T37.8X2	T37.8X3	T37.8X4	T37.8X5	T37.8X6
formic iodide	T49.0X1	T49.0X2	T49.0X3	T49.0X4	T49.0X5	T49.0X6
glycolylarsenate	T49.0X1	T49.0X2	T49.0X3	T49.0X4	T49.0X5	T49.0X6
nonmedicinal (compounds) NEC	T65.91	T65.92	T65.93	T65.94	—	—
subcarbonate	T47.6X1	T47.6X2	T47.6X3	T47.6X4	T47.6X5	T47.6X6
subsalicylate	T37.8X1	T37.8X2	T37.8X3	T37.8X4	T37.8X5	T37.8X6
sulfarsphenamine	T37.8X1	T37.8X2	T37.8X3	T37.8X4	T37.8X5	T37.8X6
Bisoprolol	T44.7X1	T44.7X2	T44.7X3	T44.7X4	T44.7X5	T44.7X6
Bisoxatin	T47.2X1	T47.2X2	T47.2X3	T47.2X4	T47.2X5	T47.2X6
Bisulepin (hydrochloride)	T45.0X1	T45.0X2	T45.0X3	T45.0X4	T45.0X5	T45.0X6
Bithionol	T37.8X1	T37.8X2	T37.8X3	T37.8X4	T37.8X5	T37.8X6
anthelminthic	T37.4X1	T37.4X2	T37.4X3	T37.4X4	T37.4X5	T37.4X6
Bitolterol	T48.6X1	T48.6X2	T48.6X3	T48.6X4	T48.6X5	T48.6X6

Substance	Poisoning, Accidental (unintentional)	Poisoning, Intentional self-harm	Poisoning, Assault	Poisoning, Undetermined	Adverse effect	Underdosing
Bitoscanate	T37.4X1	T37.4X2	T37.4X3	T37.4X4	T37.4X5	T37.4X6
Bitter almond oil	T62.8X1	T62.8X2	T62.8X3	T62.8X4	—	—
Bittersweet	T62.2X1	T62.2X2	T62.2X3	T62.2X4	—	—
Black						
flag	T60.91	T60.92	T60.93	T60.94		
henbane	T62.2X1	T62.2X2	T62.2X3	T62.2X4		
leaf (40)	T60.91	T60.92	T60.93	T60.94		
widow spider (bite)	T63.311	T63.312	T63.313	T63.314		
antivenin	T50.Z11	T50.Z12	T50.Z13	T50.Z14	T50.Z15	T50.Z16
Blast furnace gas (carbon monoxide from)	T58.8X1	T58.8X2	T58.8X3	T58.8X4		
Bleach	T54.91	T54.92	T54.93	T54.94	—	—
Bleaching agent (medicinal)	T49.4X1	T49.4X2	T49.4X3	T49.4X4	T49.4X5	T49.4X6
Bleomycin	T45.1X1	T45.1X2	T45.1X3	T45.1X4	T45.1X5	T45.1X6
Blockain	T41.3X1	T41.3X2	T41.3X3	T41.3X4	T41.3X5	T41.3X6
infiltration (subcutaneous)	T41.3X1	T41.3X2	T41.3X3	T41.3X4	T41.3X5	T41.3X6
nerve block (peripheral) (plexus)	T41.3X1	T41.3X2	T41.3X3	T41.3X4	T41.3X5	T41.3X6
topical (surface)	T41.3X1	T41.3X2	T41.3X3	T41.3X4	T41.3X5	T41.3X6
Blockers, calcium channel	T46.1X1	T46.1X2	T46.1X3	T46.1X4	T46.1X5	T46.1X6
Blood (derivatives) (natural) (plasma) (whole)	T45.8X1	T45.8X2	T45.8X3	T45.8X4	T45.8X5	T45.8X6
dried	T45.8X1	T45.8X2	T45.8X3	T45.8X4	T45.8X5	T45.8X6
drug affecting NEC	T45.91	T45.92	T45.93	T45.94	T45.95	T45.96
expander NEC	T45.8X1	T45.8X2	T45.8X3	T45.8X4	T45.8X5	T45.8X6
fraction NEC	T45.8X1	T45.8X2	T45.8X3	T45.8X4	T45.8X5	T45.8X6
substitute (macromolecular)	T45.8X1	T45.8X2	T45.8X3	T45.8X4	T45.8X5	T45.8X6
Blue velvet	T40.2X1	T40.2X2	T40.2X3	T40.2X4	—	—
Bone meal	T62.8X1	T62.8X2	T62.8X3	T62.8X4	—	—
Bonine	T45.0X1	T45.0X2	T45.0X3	T45.0X4	T45.0X5	T45.0X6
Bopindolol	T44.7X1	T44.7X2	T44.7X3	T44.7X4	T44.7X5	T44.7X6
Boracic acid	T49.0X1	T49.0X2	T49.0X3	T49.0X4	T49.0X5	T49.0X6
ENT agent	T49.6X1	T49.6X2	T49.6X3	T49.6X4	T49.6X5	T49.6X6
ophthalmic preparation	T49.5X1	T49.5X2	T49.5X3	T49.5X4	T49.5X5	T49.5X6
Borane complex	T57.8X1	T57.8X2	T57.8X3	T57.8X4	—	—
Borate (s)	T57.8X1	T57.8X2	T57.8X3	T57.8X4	—	—
buffer	T50.991	T50.992	T50.993	T50.994	T50.995	T50.996
cleanser	T54.91	T54.92	T54.93	T54.94	—	—
sodium	T57.8X1	T57.8X2	T57.8X3	T57.8X4	—	—
Borax (cleanser)	T54.91	T54.92	T54.93	T54.94	—	—
Bordeaux mixture	T60.3X1	T60.3X2	T60.3X3	T60.3X4	—	—
Boric acid	T49.0X1	T49.0X2	T49.0X3	T49.0X4	T49.0X5	T49.0X6
ENT agent	T49.6X1	T49.6X2	T49.6X3	T49.6X4	T49.6X5	T49.6X6
ophthalmic preparation	T49.5X1	T49.5X2	T49.5X3	T49.5X4	T49.5X5	T49.5X6
Bornaprine	T44.3X1	T44.3X2	T44.3X3	T44.3X4	T44.3X5	T44.3X6
Boron	T57.8X1	T57.8X2	T57.8X3	T57.8X4	—	—
hydride NEC	T57.8X1	T57.8X2	T57.8X3	T57.8X4	—	—
fumes or gas	T57.8X1	T57.8X2	T57.8X3	T57.8X4	—	—
trifluoride	T59.891	T59.892	T59.893	T59.894	—	—
Botox	T48.291	T48.292	T48.293	T48.294	T48.295	T48.296
Botulinus anti-toxin (type A, B)	T50.Z11	T50.Z12	T50.Z13	T50.Z14	T50.Z15	T50.Z16
Brake fluid vapor	T59.891	T59.892	T59.893	T59.894		
Brallobarbital	T42.3X1	T42.3X2	T42.3X3	T42.3X4	T42.3X5	T42.3X6
Bran (wheat)	T47.4X1	T47.4X2	T47.4X3	T47.4X4	T47.4X5	T47.4X6

Substance	Poisoning, Accidental (unintentional)	Poisoning, Intentional self-harm	Poisoning, Assault	Poisoning, Undetermined	Adverse effect	Underdosing
Brass (fumes)	T56.891	T56.892	T56.893	T56.894	—	—
Brasso	T52.0X1	T52.0X2	T52.0X3	T52.0X4	—	—
Bretylium tosilate	T46.2X1	T46.2X2	T46.2X3	T46.2X4	T46.2X5	T46.2X6
Brevital (sodium)	T41.1X1	T41.1X2	T41.1X3	T41.1X4	T41.1X5	T41.1X6
Brinase	T45.3X1	T45.3X2	T45.3X3	T45.3X4	T45.3X5	T45.3X6
British antilewisite	T45.8X1	T45.8X2	T45.8X3	T45.8X4	T45.8X5	T45.8X6
Brodifacoum	T60.4X1	T60.4X2	T60.4X3	T60.4X4		
Bromal (hydrate)	T42.6X1	T42.6X2	T42.6X3	T42.6X4	T42.6X5	T42.6X6
Bromazepam	T42.4X1	T42.4X2	T42.4X3	T42.4X4	T42.4X5	T42.4X6
Bromazine	T45.0X1	T45.0X2	T45.0X3	T45.0X4	T45.0X5	T45.0X6
Brombenzylcyanide	T59.3X1	T59.3X2	T59.3X3	T59.3X4	—	—
Bromelains	T45.3X1	T45.3X2	T45.3X3	T45.3X4	T45.3X5	T45.3X6
Bromethalin	T60.4X1	T60.4X2	T60.4X3	T60.4X4		
Bromhexine	T48.4X1	T48.4X2	T48.4X3	T48.4X4	T48.4X5	T48.4X6
Bromide salts	T42.6X1	T42.6X2	T42.6X3	T42.6X4	T42.6X5	T42.6X6
Bromindione	T45.511	T45.512	T45.513	T45.514	T45.515	T45.516
Bromine						
compounds (medicinal)	T42.6X1	T42.6X2	T42.6X3	T42.6X4	T42.6X5	T42.6X6
sedative	T42.6X1	T42.6X2	T42.6X3	T42.6X4	T42.6X5	T42.6X6
vapor	T59.891	T59.892	T59.893	T59.894	—	—
Bromisoval	T42.6X1	T42.6X2	T42.6X3	T42.6X4	T42.6X5	T42.6X6
Bromisovalum	T42.6X1	T42.6X2	T42.6X3	T42.6X4	T42.6X5	T42.6X6
Bromobenzylcyanide	T59.3X1	T59.3X2	T59.3X3	T59.3X4	—	—
Bromochlorosalicylani-lide	T49.0X1	T49.0X2	T49.0X3	T49.0X4	T49.0X5	T49.0X6
Bromocriptine	T42.8X1	T42.8X2	T42.8X3	T42.8X4	T42.8X5	T42.8X6
Bromodiphenhydramine	T45.0X1	T45.0X2	T45.0X3	T45.0X4	T45.0X5	T45.0X6
Bromoform	T42.6X1	T42.6X2	T42.6X3	T42.6X4	T42.6X5	T42.6X6
Bromophenol blue reagent	T50.991	T50.992	T50.993	T50.994	T50.995	T50.996
Bromopride	T47.8X1	T47.8X2	T47.8X3	T47.8X4	T47.8X5	T47.8X6
Bromosalicylchloranitide	T49.0X1	T49.0X2	T49.0X3	T49.0X4	T49.0X5	T49.0X6
Bromosalicylhydroxamic acid	T37.1X1	T37.1X2	T37.1X3	T37.1X4	T37.1X5	T37.1X6
Bromo-seltzer	T39.1X1	T39.1X2	T39.1X3	T39.1X4	T39.1X5	T39.1X6
Bromoxynil	T60.3X1	T60.3X2	T60.3X3	T60.3X4	—	—
Bromperidol	T43.4X1	T43.4X2	T43.4X3	T43.4X4	T43.4X5	T43.4X6
Brompheniramine	T45.0X1	T45.0X2	T45.0X3	T45.0X4	T45.0X5	T45.0X6
Bromsulfophthalein	T50.8X1	T50.8X2	T50.8X3	T50.8X4	T50.8X5	T50.8X6
Bromural	T42.6X1	T42.6X2	T42.6X3	T42.6X4	T42.6X5	T42.6X6
Bromvaletone	T42.6X1	T42.6X2	T42.6X3	T42.6X4	T42.6X5	T42.6X6
Bronchodilator NEC	T48.6X1	T48.6X2	T48.6X3	T48.6X4	T48.6X5	T48.6X6
Brotizolam	T42.4X1	T42.4X2	T42.4X3	T42.4X4	T42.4X5	T42.4X6
Brovincamine	T46.7X1	T46.7X2	T46.7X3	T46.7X4	T46.7X5	T46.7X6
Brown recluse spider (bite) (venom)	T63.331	T63.332	T63.333	T63.334	—	—
Brown spider (bite) (venom)	T63.391	T63.392	T63.393	T63.394	—	—
Broxaterol	T48.6X1	T48.6X2	T48.6X3	T48.6X4	T48.6X5	T48.6X6
Broxuridine	T45.1X1	T45.1X2	T45.1X3	T45.1X4	T45.1X5	T45.1X6
Broxyquinoline	T37.8X1	T37.8X2	T37.8X3	T37.8X4	T37.8X5	T37.8X6
Bruceine	T48.291	T48.292	T48.293	T48.294	T48.295	T48.296
Brucia	T62.2X1	T62.2X2	T62.2X3	T62.2X4	—	—
Brucine	T65.1X1	T65.1X2	T65.1X3	T65.1X4	—	—
Brunswick green—see Copper						
Bruten—see Ibuprofen						
Bryonia	T47.2X1	T47.2X2	T47.2X3	T47.2X4	T47.2X5	T47.2X6
Buclizine	T45.0X1	T45.0X2	T45.0X3	T45.0X4	T45.0X5	T45.0X6
Buclosamide	T49.0X1	T49.0X2	T49.0X3	T49.0X4	T49.0X5	T49.0X6

Substance	Poisoning, Accidental (unintentional)	Poisoning, Intentional self-harm	Poisoning, Assault	Poisoning, Undetermined	Adverse effect	Underdosing
Budesonide	T44.5X1	T44.5X2	T44.5X3	T44.5X4	T44.5X5	T44.5X6
Budralazine	T46.5X1	T46.5X2	T46.5X3	T46.5X4	T46.5X5	T46.5X6
Bufferin	T39.011	T39.012	T39.013	T39.014	T39.015	T39.016
Buflomedil	T46.7X1	T46.7X2	T46.7X3	T46.7X4	T46.7X5	T46.7X6
Buformin	T38.3X1	T38.3X2	T38.3X3	T38.3X4	T38.3X5	T38.3X6
Bufotenine	T40.991	T40.992	T40.993	T40.994	—	—
Bufrolin	T48.6X1	T48.6X2	T48.6X3	T48.6X4	T48.6X5	T48.6X6
Bufylline	T48.6X1	T48.6X2	T48.6X3	T48.6X4	T48.6X5	T48.6X6
Bulk filler	T50.5X1	T50.5X2	T50.5X3	T50.5X4	T50.5X5	T50.5X6
cathartic	T47.4X1	T47.4X2	T47.4X3	T47.4X4	T47.4X5	T47.4X6
Bumetanide	T50.1X1	T50.1X2	T50.1X3	T50.1X4	T50.1X5	T50.1X6
Bunaftine	T46.2X1	T46.2X2	T46.2X3	T46.2X4	T46.2X5	T46.2X6
Bunamiodyl	T50.8X1	T50.8X2	T50.8X3	T50.8X4	T50.8X5	T50.8X6
Bunazosin	T44.6X1	T44.6X2	T44.6X3	T44.6X4	T44.6X5	T44.6X6
Bunitrolol	T44.7X1	T44.7X2	T44.7X3	T44.7X4	T44.7X5	T44.7X6
Buphenine	T46.7X1	T46.7X2	T46.7X3	T46.7X4	T46.7X5	T46.7X6
Bupivacaine	T41.3X1	T41.3X2	T41.3X3	T41.3X4	T41.3X5	T41.3X6
infiltration (subcutaneous)	T41.3X1	T41.3X2	T41.3X3	T41.3X4	T41.3X5	T41.3X6
nerve block (peripheral) (plexus)	T41.3X1	T41.3X2	T41.3X3	T41.3X4	T41.3X5	T41.3X6
spinal	T41.3X1	T41.3X2	T41.3X3	T41.3X4	T41.3X5	T41.3X6
Bupranolol	T44.7X1	T44.7X2	T44.7X3	T44.7X4	T44.7X5	T44.7X6
Buprenorphine	T40.4X1	T40.4X2	T40.4X3	T40.4X4	T40.4X5	T40.4X6
Bupropion	T43.291	T43.292	T43.293	T43.294	T43.295	T43.296
Burimamide	T47.1X1	T47.1X2	T47.1X3	T47.1X4	T47.1X5	T47.1X6
Buserelin	T38.891	T38.892	T38.893	T38.894	T38.895	T38.896
Buspirone	T43.591	T43.592	T43.593	T43.594	T43.595	T43.596
Busulfan, busulphan	T45.1X1	T45.1X2	T45.1X3	T45.1X4	T45.1X5	T45.1X6
Butabarbital (sodium)	T42.3X1	T42.3X2	T42.3X3	T42.3X4	T42.3X5	T42.3X6
Butabarbitone	T42.3X1	T42.3X2	T42.3X3	T42.3X4	T42.3X5	T42.3X6
Butabarpal	T42.3X1	T42.3X2	T42.3X3	T42.3X4	T42.3X5	T42.3X6
Butacaine	T41.3X1	T41.3X2	T41.3X3	T41.3X4	T41.3X5	T41.3X6
Butalamine	T46.7X1	T46.7X2	T46.7X3	T46.7X4	T46.7X5	T46.7X6
Butalbital	T42.3X1	T42.3X2	T42.3X3	T42.3X4	T42.3X5	T42.3X6
Butallylonal	T42.3X1	T42.3X2	T42.3X3	T42.3X4	T42.3X5	T42.3X6
Butamben	T41.3X1	T41.3X2	T41.3X3	T41.3X4	T41.3X5	T41.3X6
Butamirate	T48.3X1	T48.3X2	T48.3X3	T48.3X4	T48.3X5	T48.3X6
Butane (distributed in mobile container)	T59.891	T59.892	T59.893	T59.894	—	—
distributed through pipes	T59.891	T59.892	T59.893	T59.894	—	—
incomplete combustion	T58.11	T58.12	T58.13	T58.14		
Butanilicaine	T41.3X1	T41.3X2	T41.3X3	T41.3X4	T41.3X5	T41.3X6
Butanol	T51.3X1	T51.3X2	T51.3X3	T51.3X4		
Butanone, 2-butanone	T52.4X1	T52.4X2	T52.4X3	T52.4X4	—	—
Butantrone	T49.4X1	T49.4X2	T49.4X3	T49.4X4	T49.4X5	T49.4X6
Butaperazine	T43.3X1	T43.3X2	T43.3X3	T43.3X4	T43.3X5	T43.3X6
Butazolidin	T39.2X1	T39.2X2	T39.2X3	T39.2X4	T39.2X5	T39.2X6
Butetamate	T48.6X1	T48.6X2	T48.6X3	T48.6X4	T48.6X5	T48.6X6
Butethal	T42.3X1	T42.3X2	T42.3X3	T42.3X4	T42.3X5	T42.3X6
Butethamate	T44.3X1	T44.3X2	T44.3X3	T44.3X4	T44.3X5	T44.3X6
Buthalitone (sodium)	T41.1X1	T41.1X2	T41.1X3	T41.1X4	T41.1X5	T41.1X6
Butisol (sodium)	T42.3X1	T42.3X2	T42.3X3	T42.3X4	T42.3X5	T42.3X6
Butizide	T50.2X1	T50.2X2	T50.2X3	T50.2X4	T50.2X5	T50.2X6
Butobarbital	T42.3X1	T42.3X2	T42.3X3	T42.3X4	T42.3X5	T42.3X6
sodium	T42.3X1	T42.3X2	T42.3X3	T42.3X4	T42.3X5	T42.3X6
Butobarbitone	T42.3X1	T42.3X2	T42.3X3	T42.3X4	T42.3X5	T42.3X6

Butoconazole - Carbamate

Substance	Poisoning, Accidental (unintentional)	Poisoning, Intentional self-harm	Poisoning, Assault	Poisoning, Undetermined	Adverse effect	Underdosing
Butoconazole (nitrate)	T49.0X1	T49.0X2	T49.0X3	T49.0X4	T49.0X5	T49.0X6
Butorphanol	T40.4X1	T40.4X2	T40.4X3	T40.4X4	T40.4X5	T40.4X6
Butriptyline	T43.011	T43.012	T43.013	T43.014	T43.015	T43.016
Butropium bromide	T44.3X1	T44.3X2	T44.3X3	T44.3X4	T44.3X5	T44.3X6
Butter of antimony—*see Antimony*						
Buttercups	T62.2X1	T62.2X2	T62.2X3	T62.2X4	—	—
Butyl						
acetate (secondary)	T52.8X1	T52.8X2	T52.8X3	T52.8X4	—	—
alcohol	T51.3X1	T51.3X2	T51.3X3	T51.3X4	—	—
aminobenzoate	T41.3X1	T41.3X2	T41.3X3	T41.3X4	T41.3X5	T41.3X6
butyrate	T52.8X1	T52.8X2	T52.8X3	T52.8X4	—	—
carbinol	T51.3X1	T51.3X2	T51.3X3	T51.3X4	—	—
carbitol	T52.3X1	T52.3X2	T52.3X3	T52.3X4	—	—
cellosolve	T52.3X1	T52.3X2	T52.3X3	T52.3X4	—	—
chloral (hydrate)	T42.6X1	T42.6X2	T42.6X3	T42.6X4	T42.6X5	T42.6X6
formate	T52.8X1	T52.8X2	T52.8X3	T52.8X4	—	—
lactate	T52.8X1	T52.8X2	T52.8X3	T52.8X4	—	—
propionate	T52.8X1	T52.8X2	T52.8X3	T52.8X4	—	—
scopolamine bromide	T44.3X1	T44.3X2	T44.3X3	T44.3X4	T44.3X5	T44.3X6
thiobarbital sodium	T41.1X1	T41.1X2	T41.1X3	T41.1X4	T41.1X5	T41.1X6
Butylated hydroxy-anisole	T50.991	T50.992	T50.993	T50.994	T50.995	T50.996
Butylchloral hydrate	T42.6X1	T42.6X2	T42.6X3	T42.6X4	T42.6X5	T42.6X6
Butyltoluene	T52.2X1	T52.2X2	T52.2X3	T52.2X4	—	—
Butyn	T41.3X1	T41.3X2	T41.3X3	T41.3X4	T41.3X5	T41.3X6
Butyrophenone (based tranquilizers)	T43.4X1	T43.4X2	T43.4X3	T43.4X4	T43.4X5	T43.4X6
C						
Cabergoline	T42.8X1	T42.8X2	T42.8X3	T42.8X4	T42.8X5	T42.8X6
Cacodyl, cacodylic acid	T57.0X1	T57.0X2	T57.0X3	T57.0X4	—	—
Cactinomycin	T45.1X1	T45.1X2	T45.1X3	T45.1X4	T45.1X5	T45.1X6
Cade oil	T49.4X1	T49.4X2	T49.4X3	T49.4X4	T49.4X5	T49.4X6
Cadexomer iodine	T49.0X1	T49.0X2	T49.0X3	T49.0X4	T49.0X5	T49.0X6
Cadmium (chloride) (fumes) (oxide)	T56.3X1	T56.3X2	T56.3X3	T56.3X4		
sulfide (medicinal) NEC	T49.4X1	T49.4X2	T49.4X3	T49.4X4	T49.4X5	T49.4X6
Cadralazine	T46.5X1	T46.5X2	T46.5X3	T46.5X4	T46.5X5	T46.5X6
Caffeine	T43.611	T43.612	T43.613	T43.614	T43.615	T43.616
Calabar bean	T62.2X1	T62.2X2	T62.2X3	T62.2X4	—	—
Caladium seguinum	T62.2X1	T62.2X2	T62.2X3	T62.2X4	—	—
Calamine (lotion)	T49.3X1	T49.3X2	T49.3X3	T49.3X4	T49.3X5	T49.3X6
Calcifediol	T45.2X1	T45.2X2	T45.2X3	T45.2X4	T45.2X5	T45.2X6
Calciferol	T45.2X1	T45.2X2	T45.2X3	T45.2X4	T45.2X5	T45.2X6
Calcitonin	T50.991	T50.992	T50.993	T50.994	T50.995	T50.996
Calcitriol	T45.2X1	T45.2X2	T45.2X3	T45.2X4	T45.2X5	T45.2X6
Calcium	T50.3X1	T50.3X2	T50.3X3	T50.3X4	T50.3X5	T50.3X6
actylsalicylate	T39.011	T39.012	T39.013	T39.014	T39.015	T39.016
benzamidosalicylate	T37.1X1	T37.1X2	T37.1X3	T37.1X4	T37.1X5	T37.1X6
bromide	T42.6X1	T42.6X2	T42.6X3	T42.6X4	T42.6X5	T42.6X6
bromolactobionate	T42.6X1	T42.6X2	T42.6X3	T42.6X4	T42.6X5	T42.6X6
carbaspirin	T39.011	T39.012	T39.013	T39.014	T39.015	T39.016
carbimide	T50.6X1	T50.6X2	T50.6X3	T50.6X4	T50.6X5	T50.6X6
carbonate	T47.1X1	T47.1X2	T47.1X3	T47.1X4	T47.1X5	T47.1X6
chloride	T50.991	T50.992	T50.993	T50.994	T50.995	T50.996
anhydrous	T50.991	T50.992	T50.993	T50.994	T50.995	T50.996
cyanide	T57.8X1	T57.8X2	T57.8X3	T57.8X4	—	—
dioctyl sulfosuccinate	T47.4X1	T47.4X2	T47.4X3	T47.4X4	T47.4X5	T47.4X6
disodium cdathamil	T45.8X1	T45.8X2	T45.8X3	T45.8X4	T45.8X5	T45.8X6
disodium edetate	T45.8X1	T45.8X2	T45.8X3	T45.8X4	T45.8X5	T45.8X6
dobesilate	T46.991	T46.992	T46.993	T46.994	T46.995	T46.996

Substance	Poisoning, Accidental (unintentional)	Poisoning, Intentional self-harm	Poisoning, Assault	Poisoning, Undetermined	Adverse effect	Underdosing
Calcium — *continued*						
EDTA	T45.8X1	T45.8X2	T45.8X3	T45.8X4	T45.8X5	T45.8X6
ferrous citrate	T45.4X1	T45.4X2	T45.4X3	T45.4X4	T45.4X5	T45.4X6
folinate	T45.8X1	T45.8X2	T45.8X3	T45.8X4	T45.8X5	T45.8X6
glubionate	T50.3X1	T50.3X2	T50.3X3	T50.3X4	T50.3X5	T50.3X6
gluconate	T50.3X1	T50.3X2	T50.3X3	T50.3X4	T50.3X5	T50.3X6
gluconogalactogluc-onate	T50.3X1	T50.3X2	T50.3X3	T50.3X4	T50.3X5	T50.3X6
hydrate, hydroxide	T54.3X1	T54.3X2	T54.3X3	T54.3X4	—	—
hypochlorite	T54.3X1	T54.3X2	T54.3X3	T54.3X4	—	—
iodide	T48.4X1	T48.4X2	T48.4X3	T48.4X4	T48.4X5	T48.4X6
ipodate	T50.8X1	T50.8X2	T50.8X3	T50.8X4	T50.8X5	T50.8X6
lactate	T50.3X1	T50.3X2	T50.3X3	T50.3X4	T50.3X5	T50.3X6
leucovorin	T45.8X1	T45.8X2	T45.8X3	T45.8X4	T45.8X5	T45.8X6
mandelate	T37.91	T37.92	T37.93	T37.94	T37.95	T37.96
oxide	T54.3X1	T54.3X2	T54.3X3	T54.3X4	—	—
pantothenate	T45.2X1	T45.2X2	T45.2X3	T45.2X4	T45.2X5	T45.2X6
phosphate	T50.3X1	T50.3X2	T50.3X3	T50.3X4	T50.3X5	T50.3X6
salicylate	T39.091	T39.092	T39.093	T39.094	T39.095	T39.096
salts	T50.3X1	T50.3X2	T50.3X3	T50.3X4	T50.3X5	T50.3X6
Calculus-dissolving drug	T50.991	T50.992	T50.993	T50.994	T50.995	T50.996
Calomel	T49.0X1	T49.0X2	T49.0X3	T49.0X4	T49.0X5	T49.0X6
Caloric agent	T50.3X1	T50.3X2	T50.3X3	T50.3X4	T50.3X5	T50.3X6
Calusterone	T38.7X1	T38.7X2	T38.7X3	T38.7X4	T38.7X5	T38.7X6
Camazepam	T42.4X1	T42.4X2	T42.4X3	T42.4X4	T42.4X5	T42.4X6
Camomile	T49.0X1	T49.0X2	T49.0X3	T49.0X4	T49.0X5	T49.0X6
Camoquin	T37.2X1	T37.2X2	T37.2X3	T37.2X4	T37.2X5	T37.2X6
Camphor						
insecticide	T60.2X1	T60.2X2	T60.2X3	T60.2X4	—	—
medicinal	T49.8X1	T49.8X2	T49.8X3	T49.8X4	T49.8X5	T49.8X6
Camylofin	T44.3X1	T44.3X2	T44.3X3	T44.3X4	T44.3X5	T44.3X6
Cancer chemotherapy drug regimen	T45.1X1	T45.1X2	T45.1X3	T45.1X4	T45.1X5	T45.1X6
Candeptin	T49.0X1	T49.0X2	T49.0X3	T49.0X4	T49.0X5	T49.0X6
Candicidin	T49.0X1	T49.0X2	T49.0X3	T49.0X4	T49.0X5	T49.0X6
Cannabinol	T40.7X1	T40.7X2	T40.7X3	T40.7X4	T40.7X5	T40.7X6
Cannabis (derivatives)	T40.7X1	T40.7X2	T40.7X3	T40.7X4	T40.7X5	T40.7X6
Canned heat	T51.1X1	T51.1X2	T51.1X3	T51.1X4	—	—
Canrenoic acid	T50.0X1	T50.0X2	T50.0X3	T50.0X4	T50.0X5	T50.0X6
Canrenone	T50.0X1	T50.0X2	T50.0X3	T50.0X4	T50.0X5	T50.0X6
Cantharides, cantharidin, cantharis	T49.8X1	T49.8X2	T49.8X3	T49.8X4	T49.8X5	T49.8X6
Canthaxanthin	T50.991	T50.992	T50.993	T50.994	T50.995	T50.996
Capillary-active drug NEC	T46.901	T46.902	T46.903	T46.904	T46.905	T46.906
Capreomycin	T36.8X1	T36.8X2	T36.8X3	T36.8X4	T36.8X5	T36.8X6
Capsicum	T49.4X1	T49.4X2	T49.4X3	T49.4X4	T49.4X5	T49.4X6
Captafol	T60.3X1	T60.3X2	T60.3X3	T60.3X4	—	—
Captan	T60.3X1	T60.3X2	T60.3X3	T60.3X4	—	—
Captodiame, captodiamine	T43.591	T43.592	T43.593	T43.594	T43.595	T43.596
Captopril	T46.4X1	T46.4X2	T46.4X3	T46.4X4	T46.4X5	T46.4X6
Caramiphen	T44.3X1	T44.3X2	T44.3X3	T44.3X4	T44.3X5	T44.3X6
Carazolol	T44.7X1	T44.7X2	T44.7X3	T44.7X4	T44.7X5	T44.7X6
Carbachol	T44.1X1	T44.1X2	T44.1X3	T44.1X4	T44.1X5	T44.1X6
Carbacrylamine (resin)	T50.3X1	T50.3X2	T50.3X3	T50.3X4	T50.3X5	T50.3X6
Carbamate (insecticide)	T60.0X1	T60.0X2	T60.0X3	T60.0X4	—	—
Carbamate (sedative)	T42.6X1	T42.6X2	T42.6X3	T42.6X4	T42.6X5	T42.6X6
herbicide	T60.0X1	T60.0X2	T60.0X3	T60.0X4	—	—
insecticide	T60.0X1	T60.0X2	T60.0X3	T60.0X4	—	—

Substance	Poisoning, Accidental (unintentional)	Poisoning, Intentional self-harm	Poisoning, Assault	Poisoning, Undetermined	Adverse effect	Underdosing
Carbamazepine	T42.1X1	T42.1X2	T42.1X3	T42.1X4	T42.1X5	T42.1X6
Carbamide	T47.3X1	T47.3X2	T47.3X3	T47.3X4	T47.3X5	T47.3X6
peroxide	T49.0X1	T49.0X2	T49.0X3	T49.0X4	T49.0X5	T49.0X6
topical	T49.8X1	T49.8X2	T49.8X3	T49.8X4	T49.8X5	T49.8X6
Carbamylcholine chloride	T44.1X1	T44.1X2	T44.1X3	T44.1X4	T44.1X5	T44.1X6
Carbaril	T60.0X1	T60.0X2	T60.0X3	T60.0X4	—	—
Carbarsone	T37.3X1	T37.3X2	T37.3X3	T37.3X4	T37.3X5	T37.3X6
Carbaryl	T60.0X1	T60.0X2	T60.0X3	T60.0X4	—	—
Carbaspirin	T39.011	T39.012	T39.013	T39.014	T39.015	T39.016
Carbazochrome (salicylate) (sodium sulfonate)	T49.4X1	T49.4X2	T49.4X3	T49.4X4	T49.4X5	T49.4X6
Carbenicillin	T36.0X1	T36.0X2	T36.0X3	T36.0X4	T36.0X5	T36.0X6
Carbenoxolone	T47.1X1	T47.1X2	T47.1X3	T47.1X4	T47.1X5	T47.1X6
Carbetapentane	T48.3X1	T48.3X2	T48.3X3	T48.3X4	T48.3X5	T48.3X6
Carbethyl salicylate	T39.091	T39.092	T39.093	T39.094	T39.095	T39.096
Carbidopa (with levodopa)	T42.8X1	T42.8X2	T42.8X3	T42.8X4	T42.8X5	T42.8X6
Carbimazole	T38.2X1	T38.2X2	T38.2X3	T38.2X4	T38.2X5	T38.2X6
Carbinol	T51.1X1	T51.1X2	T51.1X3	T51.1X4	—	—
Carbinoxamine	T45.0X1	T45.0X2	T45.0X3	T45.0X4	T45.0X5	T45.0X6
Carbiphene	T39.8X1	T39.8X2	T39.8X3	T39.8X4	T39.8X5	T39.8X6
Carbitol	T52.3X1	T52.3X2	T52.3X3	T52.3X4	—	—
Carbo medicinalis	T47.6X1	T47.6X2	T47.6X3	T47.6X4	T47.6X5	T47.6X6
Carbocaine	T41.3X1	T41.3X2	T41.3X3	T41.3X4	T41.3X5	T41.3X6
infiltration (subcutaneous)	T41.3X1	T41.3X2	T41.3X3	T41.3X4	T41.3X5	T41.3X6
nerve block (peripheral) (plexus)	T41.3X1	T41.3X2	T41.3X3	T41.3X4	T41.3X5	T41.3X6
topical (surface)	T41.3X1	T41.3X2	T41.3X3	T41.3X4	T41.3X5	T41.3X6
Carbocisteine	T48.4X1	T48.4X2	T48.4X3	T48.4X4	T48.4X5	T48.4X6
Carbocromen	T46.3X1	T46.3X2	T46.3X3	T46.3X4	T46.3X5	T46.3X6
Carbol fuchsin	T49.0X1	T49.0X2	T49.0X3	T49.0X4	T49.0X5	T49.0X6
Carbolic acid—see also Phenol	T54.0X1	T54.0X2	T54.0X3	T54.0X4	—	—
Carbolonium (bromide)	T48.1X1	T48.1X2	T48.1X3	T48.1X4	T48.1X5	T48.1X6
Carbomycin	T36.8X1	T36.8X2	T36.8X3	T36.8X4	T36.8X5	T36.8X6
Carbon						
bisulfide (liquid)	T65.4X1	T65.4X2	T65.4X3	T65.4X4	—	—
vapor	T65.4X1	T65.4X2	T65.4X3	T65.4X4	—	—
dioxide (gas)	T59.7X1	T59.7X2	T59.7X3	T59.7X4	—	—
medicinal	T41.5X1	T41.5X2	T41.5X3	T41.5X4	T41.5X5	T41.5X6
nonmedicinal	T59.7X1	T59.7X2	T59.7X3	T59.7X4	—	—
snow	T49.4X1	T49.4X2	T49.4X3	T49.4X4	T49.4X5	T49.4X6
disulfide (liquid)	T65.4X1	T65.4X2	T65.4X3	T65.4X4	—	—
vapor	T65.4X1	T65.4X2	T65.4X3	T65.4X4	—	—
monoxide (from incomplete combustion)	T58.91	T58.92	T58.93	T58.94	—	—
blast furnace gas	T58.8X1	T58.8X2	T58.8X3	T58.8X4	—	—
butane (distributed in mobile container)	T58.11	T58.12	T58.13	T58.14	—	—
distributed through pipes	T58.11	T58.12	T58.13	T58.14	—	—
charcoal fumes	T58.2X1	T58.2X2	T58.2X3	T58.2X4	—	—
coal	T58.2X1	T58.2X2	T58.2X3	T58.2X4	—	—
coke (in domestic stoves, fireplaces)	T58.2X1	T58.2X2	T58.2X3	T58.2X4	—	—
gas (piped)	T58.11	T58.12	T58.13	T58.14	—	—

Substance	Poisoning, Accidental (unintentional)	Poisoning, Intentional self-harm	Poisoning, Assault	Poisoning, Undetermined	Adverse effect	Underdosing
Carbon — *continued*						
monoxide (from incomplete combustion) — *continued*						
solid (in domestic stoves, fireplaces)	T58.2X1	T58.2X2	T58.2X3	T58.2X4	—	—
exhaust gas (motor) not in transit	T58.01	T58.02	T58.03	T58.04	—	—
combustion engine, any not in watercraft	T58.01	T58.02	T58.03	T58.04	—	—
farm tractor, not in transit	T58.01	T58.02	T58.03	T58.04	—	—
gas engine	T58.01	T58.02	T58.03	T58.04	—	—
motor pump	T58.01	T58.02	T58.03	T58.04	—	—
motor vehicle, not in transit	T58.01	T58.02	T58.03	T58.04	—	—
fuel (in domestic use)	T58.2X1	T58.2X2	T58.2X3	T58.2X4	—	—
gas (piped)	T58.11	T58.12	T58.13	T58.14	—	—
in mobile container	T58.11	T58.12	T58.13	T58.14	—	—
piped (natural)	T58.11	T58.12	T58.13	T58.14	—	—
utility	T58.11	T58.12	T58.13	T58.14	—	—
in mobile container	T58.11	T58.12	T58.13	T58.14	—	—
illuminating gas	T58.11	T58.12	T58.13	T58.14	—	—
industrial fuels or gases, any	T58.8X1	T58.8X2	T58.8X3	T58.8X4	—	—
kerosene (in domestic stoves, fireplaces)	T58.2X1	T58.2X2	T58.2X3	T58.2X4	—	—
kiln gas or vapor	T58.8X1	T58.8X2	T58.8X3	T58.8X4	—	—
motor exhaust gas, not in transit	T58.01	T58.02	T58.03	T58.04	—	—
piped gas (manufactured) (natural)	T58.11	T58.12	T58.13	T58.14	—	—
producer gas	T58.8X1	T58.8X2	T58.8X3	T58.8X4	—	—
propane (distributed in mobile container)	T58.11	T58.12	T58.13	T58.14	—	—
distributed through pipes	T58.11	T58.12	T58.13	T58.14	—	—
specified source NEC	T58.8X1	T58.8X2	T58.8X3	T58.8X4	—	—
stove gas	T58.11	T58.12	T58.13	T58.14	—	—
piped	T58.11	T58.12	T58.13	T58.14	—	—
utility gas	T58.11	T58.12	T58.13	T58.14	—	—
piped	T58.11	T58.12	T58.13	T58.14	—	—
water gas	T58.11	T58.12	T58.13	T58.14	—	—
wood (in domestic stoves, fireplaces)	T58.2X1	T58.2X2	T58.2X3	T58.2X4	—	—
tetrachloride (vapor) NEC	T53.0X1	T53.0X2	T53.0X3	T53.0X4	—	—
liquid (cleansing agent) NEC	T53.0X1	T53.0X2	T53.0X3	T53.0X4	—	—
solvent	T53.0X1	T53.0X2	T53.0X3	T53.0X4	—	—
Carbonic acid gas	T59.7X1	T59.7X2	T59.7X3	T59.7X4	—	—
anhydrase inhibitor NEC	T50.2X1	T50.2X2	T50.2X3	T50.2X4	T50.2X5	T50.2X6
Carbophenothion	T60.0X1	T60.0X2	T60.0X3	T60.0X4	—	—
Carboplatin	T45.1X1	T45.1X2	T45.1X3	T45.1X4	T45.1X5	T45.1X6
Carboprost	T48.0X1	T48.0X2	T48.0X3	T48.0X4	T48.0X5	T48.0X6
Carboquone	T45.1X1	T45.1X2	T45.1X3	T45.1X4	T45.1X5	T45.1X6
Carbowax	T49.3X1	T49.3X2	T49.3X3	T49.3X4	T49.3X5	T49.3X6

Carboxymethyl-cellulose - Central nervous system

Substance	Poisoning, Accidental (unintentional)	Poisoning, Intentional self-harm	Poisoning, Assault	Poisoning, Undetermined	Adverse effect	Underdosing
Carboxymethyl-cellulose	T47.4X1	T47.4X2	T47.4X3	T47.4X4	T47.4X5	T47.4X6
S-Carboxymethyl-cysteine	T48.4X1	T48.4X2	T48.4X3	T48.4X4	T48.4X5	T48.4X6
Carbrital	T42.3X1	T42.3X2	T42.3X3	T42.3X4	T42.3X5	T42.3X6
Carbromal	T42.6X1	T42.6X2	T42.6X3	T42.6X4	T42.6X5	T42.6X6
Carbutamide	T38.3X1	T38.3X2	T38.3X3	T38.3X4	T38.3X5	T38.3X6
Carbuterol	T48.6X1	T48.6X2	T48.6X3	T48.6X4	T48.6X5	T48.6X6
Cardiac						
depressants	T46.2X1	T46.2X2	T46.2X3	T46.2X4	T46.2X5	T46.2X6
rhythm regulator	T46.2X1	T46.2X2	T46.2X3	T46.2X4	T46.2X5	T46.2X6
specified NEC	T46.2X1	T46.2X2	T46.2X3	T46.2X4	T46.2X5	T46.2X6
Cardiografin	T50.8X1	T50.8X2	T50.8X3	T50.8X4	T50.8X5	T50.8X6
Cardio-green	T50.8X1	T50.8X2	T50.8X3	T50.8X4	T50.8X5	T50.8X6
Cardiotonic (glycoside) NEC	T46.0X1	T46.0X2	T46.0X3	T46.0X4	T46.0X5	T46.0X6
Cardiovascular drug NEC	T46.901	T46.902	T46.903	T46.904	T46.905	T46.906
Cardrase	T50.2X1	T50.2X2	T50.2X3	T50.2X4	T50.2X5	T50.2X6
Carfecillin	T36.0X1	T36.0X2	T36.0X3	T36.0X4	T36.0X5	T36.0X6
Carfenazine	T43.3X1	T43.3X2	T43.3X3	T43.3X4	T43.3X5	T43.3X6
Carfusin	T49.0X1	T49.0X2	T49.0X3	T49.0X4	T49.0X5	T49.0X6
Carindacillin	T36.0X1	T36.0X2	T36.0X3	T36.0X4	T36.0X5	T36.0X6
Carisoprodol	T42.8X1	T42.8X2	T42.8X3	T42.8X4	T42.8X5	T42.8X6
Carmellose	T47.4X1	T47.4X2	T47.4X3	T47.4X4	T47.4X5	T47.4X6
Carminative	T47.5X1	T47.5X2	T47.5X3	T47.5X4	T47.5X5	T47.5X6
Carmofur	T45.1X1	T45.1X2	T45.1X3	T45.1X4	T45.1X5	T45.1X6
Carmustine	T45.1X1	T45.1X2	T45.1X3	T45.1X4	T45.1X5	T45.1X6
Carotene	T45.2X1	T45.2X2	T45.2X3	T45.2X4	T45.2X5	T45.2X6
Carphenazine	T43.3X1	T43.3X2	T43.3X3	T43.3X4	T43.3X5	T43.3X6
Carpipramine	T42.4X1	T42.4X2	T42.4X3	T42.4X4	T42.4X5	T42.4X6
Carprofen	T39.311	T39.312	T39.313	T39.314	T39.315	T39.316
Carpronium chloride	T44.3X1	T44.3X2	T44.3X3	T44.3X4	T44.3X5	T44.3X6
Carrageenan	T47.8X1	T47.8X2	T47.8X3	T47.8X4	T47.8X5	T47.8X6
Carteolol	T44.7X1	T44.7X2	T44.7X3	T44.7X4	T44.7X5	T44.7X6
Carter's Little Pills	T47.2X1	T47.2X2	T47.2X3	T47.2X4	T47.2X5	T47.2X6
Cascara (sagrada)	T47.2X1	T47.2X2	T47.2X3	T47.2X4	T47.2X5	T47.2X6
Cassava	T62.2X1	T62.2X2	T62.2X3	T62.2X4	—	—
Castellani's paint	T49.0X1	T49.0X2	T49.0X3	T49.0X4	T49.0X5	T49.0X6
Castor						
bean	T62.2X1	T62.2X2	T62.2X3	T62.2X4	—	—
oil	T47.2X1	T47.2X2	T47.2X3	T47.2X4	T47.2X5	T47.2X6
Catalase	T45.3X1	T45.3X2	T45.3X3	T45.3X4	T45.3X5	T45.3X6
Caterpillar (sting)	T63.431	T63.432	T63.433	T63.434	—	—
Catha (edulis) (tea)	T43.691	T43.692	T43.693	T43.694	—	—
Cathartic NEC	T47.4X1	T47.4X2	T47.4X3	T47.4X4	T47.4X5	T47.4X6
anthacene derivative	T47.2X1	T47.2X2	T47.2X3	T47.2X4	T47.2X5	T47.2X6
bulk	T47.4X1	T47.4X2	T47.4X3	T47.4X4	T47.4X5	T47.4X6
contact	T47.2X1	T47.2X2	T47.2X3	T47.2X4	T47.2X5	T47.2X6
emollient NEC	T47.4X1	T47.4X2	T47.4X3	T47.4X4	T47.4X5	T47.4X6
irritant NEC	T47.2X1	T47.2X2	T47.2X3	T47.2X4	T47.2X5	T47.2X6
mucilage	T47.4X1	T47.4X2	T47.4X3	T47.4X4	T47.4X5	T47.4X6
saline	T47.3X1	T47.3X2	T47.3X3	T47.3X4	T47.3X5	T47.3X6
vegetable	T47.2X1	T47.2X2	T47.2X3	T47.2X4	T47.2X5	T47.2X6
Cathine	T50.5X1	T50.5X2	T50.5X3	T50.5X4	T50.5X5	T50.5X6
Cathomycin	T36.8X1	T36.8X2	T36.8X3	T36.8X4	T36.8X5	T36.8X6
Cation exchange resin	T50.3X1	T50.3X2	T50.3X3	T50.3X4	T50.3X5	T50.3X6
Caustic (s) NEC	T54.91	T54.92	T54.93	T54.94	—	—
alkali	T54.3X1	T54.3X2	T54.3X3	T54.3X4	—	—
hydroxide	T54.3X1	T54.3X2	T54.3X3	T54.3X4	—	—
potash	T54.3X1	T54.3X2	T54.3X3	T54.3X4		
soda	T54.3X1	T54.3X2	T54.3X3	T54.3X4	—	—
specified NEC	T54.91	T54.92	T54.93	T54.94	—	—

Substance	Poisoning, Accidental (unintentional)	Poisoning, Intentional self-harm	Poisoning, Assault	Poisoning, Undetermined	Adverse effect	Underdosing
Ceepryn	T49.0X1	T49.0X2	T49.0X3	T49.0X4	T49.0X5	T49.0X6
ENT agent	T49.6X1	T49.6X2	T49.6X3	T49.6X4	T49.6X5	T49.6X6
lozenges	T49.6X1	T49.6X2	T49.6X3	T49.6X4	T49.6X5	T49.6X6
Cefacetrile	T36.1X1	T36.1X2	T36.1X3	T36.1X4	T36.1X5	T36.1X6
Cefaclor	T36.1X1	T36.1X2	T36.1X3	T36.1X4	T36.1X5	T36.1X6
Cefadroxil	T36.1X1	T36.1X2	T36.1X3	T36.1X4	T36.1X5	T36.1X6
Cefalexin	T36.1X1	T36.1X2	T36.1X3	T36.1X4	T36.1X5	T36.1X6
Cefaloglycin	T36.1X1	T36.1X2	T36.1X3	T36.1X4	T36.1X5	T36.1X6
Cefaloridine	T36.1X1	T36.1X2	T36.1X3	T36.1X4	T36.1X5	T36.1X6
Cefalosporins	T36.1X1	T36.1X2	T36.1X3	T36.1X4	T36.1X5	T36.1X6
Cefalotin	T36.1X1	T36.1X2	T36.1X3	T36.1X4	T36.1X5	T36.1X6
Cefamandole	T36.1X1	T36.1X2	T36.1X3	T36.1X4	T36.1X5	T36.1X6
Cefamycin antibiotic	T36.1X1	T36.1X2	T36.1X3	T36.1X4	T36.1X5	T36.1X6
Cefapirin	T36.1X1	T36.1X2	T36.1X3	T36.1X4	T36.1X5	T36.1X6
Cefatrizine	T36.1X1	T36.1X2	T36.1X3	T36.1X4	T36.1X5	T36.1X6
Cefazedone	T36.1X1	T36.1X2	T36.1X3	T36.1X4	T36.1X5	T36.1X6
Cefazolin	T36.1X1	T36.1X2	T36.1X3	T36.1X4	T36.1X5	T36.1X6
Cefbuperazone	T36.1X1	T36.1X2	T36.1X3	T36.1X4	T36.1X5	T36.1X6
Cefetamet	T36.1X1	T36.1X2	T36.1X3	T36.1X4	T36.1X5	T36.1X6
Cefixime	T36.1X1	T36.1X2	T36.1X3	T36.1X4	T36.1X5	T36.1X6
Cefmenoxime	T36.1X1	T36.1X2	T36.1X3	T36.1X4	T36.1X5	T36.1X6
Cefmetazole	T36.1X1	T36.1X2	T36.1X3	T36.1X4	T36.1X5	T36.1X6
Cefminox	T36.1X1	T36.1X2	T36.1X3	T36.1X4	T36.1X5	T36.1X6
Cefonicid	T36.1X1	T36.1X2	T36.1X3	T36.1X4	T36.1X5	T36.1X6
Cefoperazone	T36.1X1	T36.1X2	T36.1X3	T36.1X4	T36.1X5	T36.1X6
Ceforanide	T36.1X1	T36.1X2	T36.1X3	T36.1X4	T36.1X5	T36.1X6
Cefotaxime	T36.1X1	T36.1X2	T36.1X3	T36.1X4	T36.1X5	T36.1X6
Cefotetan	T36.1X1	T36.1X2	T36.1X3	T36.1X4	T36.1X5	T36.1X6
Cefotiam	T36.1X1	T36.1X2	T36.1X3	T36.1X4	T36.1X5	T36.1X6
Cefoxitin	T36.1X1	T36.1X2	T36.1X3	T36.1X4	T36.1X5	T36.1X6
Cefpimizole	T36.1X1	T36.1X2	T36.1X3	T36.1X4	T36.1X5	T36.1X6
Cefpiramide	T36.1X1	T36.1X2	T36.1X3	T36.1X4	T36.1X5	T36.1X6
Cefradine	T36.1X1	T36.1X2	T36.1X3	T36.1X4	T36.1X5	T36.1X6
Cefroxadine	T36.1X1	T36.1X2	T36.1X3	T36.1X4	T36.1X5	T36.1X6
Cefsulodin	T36.1X1	T36.1X2	T36.1X3	T36.1X4	T36.1X5	T36.1X6
Ceftazidime	T36.1X1	T36.1X2	T36.1X3	T36.1X4	T36.1X5	T36.1X6
Cefteram	T36.1X1	T36.1X2	T36.1X3	T36.1X4	T36.1X5	T36.1X6
Ceftezole	T36.1X1	T36.1X2	T36.1X3	T36.1X4	T36.1X5	T36.1X6
Ceftizoxime	T36.1X1	T36.1X2	T36.1X3	T36.1X4	T36.1X5	T36.1X6
Ceftriaxone	T36.1X1	T36.1X2	T36.1X3	T36.1X4	T36.1X5	T36.1X6
Cefuroxime	T36.1X1	T36.1X2	T36.1X3	T36.1X4	T36.1X5	T36.1X6
Cefuzonam	T36.1X1	T36.1X2	T36.1X3	T36.1X4	T36.1X5	T36.1X6
Celestone	T38.0X1	T38.0X2	T38.0X3	T38.0X4	T38.0X5	T38.0X6
topical	T49.0X1	T49.0X2	T49.0X3	T49.0X4	T49.0X5	T49.0X6
Celiprolol	T44.7X1	T44.7X2	T44.7X3	T44.7X4	T44.7X5	T44.7X6
Cell stimulants and proliferants	T49.8X1	T49.8X2	T49.8X3	T49.8X4	T49.8X5	T49.8X6
Cellosolve	T52.91	T52.92	T52.93	T52.94	—	—
Cellulose						
cathartic	T47.4X1	T47.4X2	T47.4X3	T47.4X4	T47.4X5	T47.4X6
hydroxyethyl	T47.4X1	T47.4X2	T47.4X3	T47.4X4	T47.4X5	T47.4X6
nitrates (topical)	T49.3X1	T49.3X2	T49.3X3	T49.3X4	T49.3X5	T49.3X6
oxidized	T49.4X1	T49.4X2	T49.4X3	T49.4X4	T49.4X5	T49.4X6
Centipede (bite)	T63.411	T63.412	T63.413	T63.414	—	—
Central nervous system						
depressants	T42.71	T42.72	T42.73	T42.74	T42.75	T42.76
anesthetic (general) NEC	T41.201	T41.202	T41.203	T41.204	T41.205	T41.206
gases NEC	T41.0X1	T41.0X2	T41.0X3	T41.0X4	T41.0X5	T41.0X6
intravenous	T41.1X1	T41.1X2	T41.1X3	T41.1X4	T41.1X5	T41.1X6
barbiturates	T42.3X1	T42.3X2	T42.3X3	T42.3X4	T42.3X5	T42.3X6

Substance	Poisoning, Accidental (unintentional)	Poisoning, Intentional self-harm	Poisoning, Assault	Poisoning, Undetermined	Adverse effect	Underdosing
Central nervous system — *continued*						
depressants — *continued*						
benzodiazepines	T42.4X1	T42.4X2	T42.4X3	T42.4X4	T42.4X5	T42.4X6
bromides	T42.6X1	T42.6X2	T42.6X3	T42.6X4	T42.6X5	T42.6X6
cannabis sativa	T40.7X1	T40.7X2	T40.7X3	T40.7X4	T40.7X5	T40.7X6
chloral hydrate	T42.6X1	T42.6X2	T42.6X3	T42.6X4	T42.6X5	T42.6X6
ethanol	T51.0X1	T51.0X2	T51.0X3	T51.0X4	T51.0X4	
hallucinogenics	T40.901	T40.902	T40.903	T40.904	T40.905	T40.906
hypnotics	T42.71	T42.72	T42.73	T42.74	T42.75	T42.76
specified NEC	T42.6X1	T42.6X2	T42.6X3	T42.6X4	T42.6X5	T42.6X6
muscle relaxants	T42.8X1	T42.8X2	T42.8X3	T42.8X4	T42.8X5	T42.8X6
paraldehyde	T42.6X1	T42.6X2	T42.6X3	T42.6X4	T42.6X5	T42.6X6
sedatives; sedative-hypnotics	T42.71	T42.72	T42.73	T42.74	T42.75	T42.76
mixed NEC	T42.6X1	T42.6X2	T42.6X3	T42.6X4	T42.6X5	T42.6X6
specified NEC	T42.6X1	T42.6X2	T42.6X3	T42.6X4	T42.6X5	T42.6X6
muscle-tone depressants	T42.8X1	T42.8X2	T42.8X3	T42.8X4	T42.8X5	T42.8X6
stimulants	T43.601	T43.602	T43.603	T43.604	T43.605	T43.606
amphetamines	T43.621	T43.622	T43.623	T43.624	T43.625	T43.626
analeptics	T50.7X1	T50.7X2	T50.7X3	T50.7X4	T50.7X5	T50.7X6
antidepressants	T43.201	T43.202	T43.203	T43.204	T43.205	T43.206
opiate antagonists	T50.7X1	T50.7X2	T50.7X3	T50.7X4	T50.7X5	T50.7X6
specified NEC	T43.691	T43.692	T43.693	T43.694	T43.695	T43.696
Cephalexin	T36.1X1	T36.1X2	T36.1X3	T36.1X4	T36.1X5	T36.1X6
Cephaloglycin	T36.1X1	T36.1X2	T36.1X3	T36.1X4	T36.1X5	T36.1X6
Cephaloridine	T36.1X1	T36.1X2	T36.1X3	T36.1X4	T36.1X5	T36.1X6
Cephalosporins	T36.1X1	T36.1X2	T36.1X3	T36.1X4	T36.1X5	T36.1X6
N (adicillin)	T36.0X1	T36.0X2	T36.0X3	T36.0X4	T36.0X5	T36.0X6
Cephalothin	T36.1X1	T36.1X2	T36.1X3	T36.1X4	T36.1X5	T36.1X6
Cephalotin	T36.1X1	T36.1X2	T36.1X3	T36.1X4	T36.1X5	T36.1X6
Cephradine	T36.1X1	T36.1X2	T36.1X3	T36.1X4	T36.1X5	T36.1X6
Cerbera (odallam)	T62.2X1	T62.2X2	T62.2X3	T62.2X4	—	—
Cerberin	T46.0X1	T46.0X2	T46.0X3	T46.0X4	T46.0X5	T46.0X6
Cerebral stimulants	T43.601	T43.602	T43.603	T43.604	T43.605	T43.606
psychotherapeutic	T43.601	T43.602	T43.603	T43.604	T43.605	T43.606
specified NEC	T43.691	T43.692	T43.693	T43.694	T43.695	T43.696
Cerium oxalate	T45.0X1	T45.0X2	T45.0X3	T45.0X4	T45.0X5	T45.0X6
Cerous oxalate	T45.0X1	T45.0X2	T45.0X3	T45.0X4	T45.0X5	T45.0X6
Ceruletide	T50.8X1	T50.8X2	T50.8X3	T50.8X4	T50.8X5	T50.8X6
Cetalkonium (chloride)	T49.0X1	T49.0X2	T49.0X3	T49.0X4	T49.0X5	T49.0X6
Cethexonium chloride	T49.0X1	T49.0X2	T49.0X3	T49.0X4	T49.0X5	T49.0X6
Cetiedil	T46.7X1	T46.7X2	T46.7X3	T46.7X4	T46.7X5	T46.7X6
Cetirizine	T45.0X1	T45.0X2	T45.0X3	T45.0X4	T45.0X5	T45.0X6
Cetomacrogol	T50.991	T50.992	T50.993	T50.994	T50.995	T50.996
Cetotiamine	T45.2X1	T45.2X2	T45.2X3	T45.2X4	T45.2X5	T45.2X6
Cetoxime	T45.0X1	T45.0X2	T45.0X3	T45.0X4	T45.0X5	T45.0X6
Cetraxate	T47.1X1	T47.1X2	T47.1X3	T47.1X4	T47.1X5	T47.1X6
Cetrimide	T49.0X1	T49.0X2	T49.0X3	T49.0X4	T49.0X5	T49.0X6
Cetrimonium (bromide)	T49.0X1	T49.0X2	T49.0X3	T49.0X4	T49.0X5	T49.0X6
Cetylpyridinium chloride	T49.0X1	T49.0X2	T49.0X3	T49.0X4	T49.0X5	T49.0X6
ENT agent	T49.6X1	T49.6X2	T49.6X3	T49.6X4	T49.6X5	T49.6X6
lozenges	T49.6X1	T49.6X2	T49.6X3	T49.6X4	T49.6X5	T49.6X6
Cevadilla—*see Sabadilla*						
Cevitamic acid	T45.2X1	T45.2X2	T45.2X3	T45.2X4	T45.2X5	T45.2X6
Chalk, precipitated	T47.1X1	T47.1X2	T47.1X3	T47.1X4	T47.1X5	T47.1X6
Chamomile	T49.0X1	T49.0X2	T49.0X3	T49.0X4	T49.0X5	T49.0X6
Ch'an su	T46.0X1	T46.0X2	T46.0X3	T46.0X4	T46.0X5	T46.0X6

Substance	Poisoning, Accidental (unintentional)	Poisoning, Intentional self-harm	Poisoning, Assault	Poisoning, Undetermined	Adverse effect	Underdosing
Charcoal	T47.6X1	T47.6X2	T47.6X3	T47.6X4	T47.6X5	T47.6X6
activated—*see also Charcoal, medicinal*	T47.6X1	T47.6X2	T47.6X3	T47.6X4	T47.6X5	T47.6X6
fumes (Carbon monoxide)	T58.2X1	T58.2X2	T58.2X3	T58.2X4	—	—
industrial	T58.8X1	T58.8X2	T58.8X3	T58.8X4	—	—
medicinal (activated)	T47.6X1	T47.6X2	T47.6X3	T47.6X4	T47.6X5	T47.6X6
antidiarrheal	T47.6X1	T47.6X2	T47.6X3	T47.6X4	T47.6X5	T47.6X6
poison control	T47.8X1	T47.8X2	T47.8X3	T47.8X4	T47.8X5	T47.8X6
specified use other than for diarrhea	T47.8X1	T47.8X2	T47.8X3	T47.8X4	T47.8X5	T47.8X6
topical	T49.8X1	T49.8X2	T49.8X3	T49.8X4	T49.8X5	T49.8X6
Chaulmosulfone	T37.1X1	T37.1X2	T37.1X3	T37.1X4	T37.1X5	T37.1X6
Chelating agent NEC	T50.6X1	T50.6X2	T50.6X3	T50.6X4	T50.6X5	T50.6X6
Chelidonium majus	T62.2X1	T62.2X2	T62.2X3	T62.2X4	—	—
Chemical substance NEC	T65.91	T65.92	T65.93	T65.94	—	—
Chenodeoxycholic acid	T47.5X1	T47.5X2	T47.5X3	T47.5X4	T47.5X5	T47.5X6
Chenodiol	T47.5X1	T47.5X2	T47.5X3	T47.5X4	T47.5X5	T47.5X6
Chenopodium	T37.4X1	T37.4X2	T37.4X3	T37.4X4	T37.4X5	T37.4X6
Cherry laurel	T62.2X1	T62.2X2	T62.2X3	T62.2X4	—	—
Chinidin (e)	T46.2X1	T46.2X2	T46.2X3	T46.2X4	T46.2X5	T46.2X6
Chiniofon	T37.8X1	T37.8X2	T37.8X3	T37.8X4	T37.8X5	T37.8X6
Chlophedianol	T48.3X1	T48.3X2	T48.3X3	T48.3X4	T48.3X5	T48.3X6
Chloral	T42.6X1	T42.6X2	T42.6X3	T42.6X4	T42.6X5	T42.6X6
derivative	T42.6X1	T42.6X2	T42.6X3	T42.6X4	T42.6X5	T42.6X6
hydrate	T42.6X1	T42.6X2	T42.6X3	T42.6X4	T42.6X5	T42.6X6
Chloralamide	T42.6X1	T42.6X2	T42.6X3	T42.6X4	T42.6X5	T42.6X6
Chloralodol	T42.6X1	T42.6X2	T42.6X3	T42.6X4	T42.6X5	T42.6X6
Chloralose	T60.4X1	T60.4X2	T60.4X3	T60.4X4	—	—
Chlorambucil	T45.1X1	T45.1X2	T45.1X3	T45.1X4	T45.1X5	T45.1X6
Chloramine	T57.8X1	T57.8X2	T57.8X3	T57.8X4	—	—
T	T49.0X1	T49.0X2	T49.0X3	T49.0X4	T49.0X5	T49.0X6
topical	T49.0X1	T49.0X2	T49.0X3	T49.0X4	T49.0X5	T49.0X6
Chloramphenicol	T36.2X1	T36.2X2	T36.2X3	T36.2X4	T36.2X5	T36.2X6
ENT agent	T49.6X1	T49.6X2	T49.6X3	T49.6X4	T49.6X5	T49.6X6
ophthalmic preparation	T49.5X1	T49.5X2	T49.5X3	T49.5X4	T49.5X5	T49.5X6
topical NEC	T49.0X1	T49.0X2	T49.0X3	T49.0X4	T49.0X5	T49.0X6
Chlorate (potassium) (sodium) NEC	T60.3X1	T60.3X2	T60.3X3	T60.3X4	—	—
herbicide	T60.3X1	T60.3X2	T60.3X3	T60.3X4	—	—
Chlorazanil	T50.2X1	T50.2X2	T50.2X3	T50.2X4	T50.2X5	T50.2X6
Chlorbenzene, chlorbenzol	T53.7X1	T53.7X2	T53.7X3	T53.7X4	—	—
Chlorbenzoxamine	T44.3X1	T44.3X2	T44.3X3	T44.3X4	T44.3X5	T44.3X6
Chlorbutol	T42.6X1	T42.6X2	T42.6X3	T42.6X4	T42.6X5	T42.6X6
Chlorcyclizine	T45.0X1	T45.0X2	T45.0X3	T45.0X4	T45.0X5	T45.0X6
Chlordan (e) (dust)	T60.1X1	T60.1X2	T60.1X3	T60.1X4	—	—
Chlordantoin	T49.0X1	T49.0X2	T49.0X3	T49.0X4	T49.0X5	T49.0X6
Chlordiazepoxide	T42.4X1	T42.4X2	T42.4X3	T42.4X4	T42.4X5	T42.4X6
Chlordiethyl benzamide	T49.3X1	T49.3X2	T49.3X3	T49.3X4	T49.3X5	T49.3X6
Chloresium	T49.8X1	T49.8X2	T49.8X3	T49.8X4	T49.8X5	T49.8X6
Chlorethiazol	T42.6X1	T42.6X2	T42.6X3	T42.6X4	T42.6X5	T42.6X6
Chlorethyl—*see Ethyl chloride*						
Chloretone	T42.6X1	T42.6X2	T42.6X3	T42.6X4	T42.6X5	T42.6X6
Chlorex	T53.6X1	T53.6X2	T53.6X3	T53.6X4	—	—
insecticide	T60.1X1	T60.1X2	T60.1X3	T60.1X4	—	—
Chlorfenvinphos	T60.0X1	T60.0X2	T60.0X3	T60.0X4	—	—
Chlorhexadol	T42.6X1	T42.6X2	T42.6X3	T42.6X4	T42.6X5	T42.6X6
Chlorhexamide	T45.1X1	T45.1X2	T45.1X3	T45.1X4	T45.1X5	T45.1X6
Chlorhexidine	T49.0X1	T49.0X2	T49.0X3	T49.0X4	T49.0X5	T49.0X6

Chlorhydroxyquinolin - Cholebrine

Substance	Poisoning, Accidental (unintentional)	Poisoning, Intentional self-harm	Poisoning, Assault	Poisoning, Undetermined	Adverse effect	Underdosing
Chlorhydroxyquinolin	T49.0X1	T49.0X2	T49.0X3	T49.0X4	T49.0X5	T49.0X6
Chloride of lime (bleach)	T54.3X1	T54.3X2	T54.3X3	T54.3X4	—	—
Chlorimipramine	T43.011	T43.012	T43.013	T43.014	T43.015	T43.016
Chlorinated						
camphene	T53.6X1	T53.6X2	T53.6X3	T53.6X4	—	—
diphenyl	T53.7X1	T53.7X2	T53.7X3	T53.7X4	—	—
hydrocarbons NEC	T53.91	T53.92	T53.93	T53.94	—	—
solvents	T53.91	T53.92	T53.93	T53.94	—	—
lime (bleach)	T54.3X1	T54.3X2	T54.3X3	T54.3X4	—	—
and boric acid solution	T49.0X1	T49.0X2	T49.0X3	T49.0X4	T49.0X5	T49.0X6
naphthalene (insecticide)	T60.1X1	T60.1X2	T60.1X3	T60.1X4	—	—
industrial (non-pesticide)	T53.7X1	T53.7X2	T53.7X3	T53.7X4	—	—
pesticide NEC	T60.8X1	T60.8X2	T60.8X3	T60.8X4	—	—
soda—see also sodium hypochlorite						
solution	T49.0X1	T49.0X2	T49.0X3	T49.0X4	T49.0X5	T49.0X6
Chlorine (fumes) (gas)	T59.4X1	T59.4X2	T59.4X3	T59.4X4	—	—
bleach	T54.3X1	T54.3X2	T54.3X3	T54.3X4	—	—
compound gas NEC	T59.4X1	T59.4X2	T59.4X3	T59.4X4	—	—
disinfectant	T59.4X1	T59.4X2	T59.4X3	T59.4X4	—	—
releasing agents NEC	T59.4X1	T59.4X2	T59.4X3	T59.4X4	—	—
Chlorisondamine chloride	T46.991	T46.992	T46.993	T46.994	T46.995	T46.996
Chlormadinone	T38.5X1	T38.5X2	T38.5X3	T38.5X4	T38.5X5	T38.5X6
Chlormephos	T60.0X1	T60.0X2	T60.0X3	T60.0X4	—	—
Chlormerodrin	T50.2X1	T50.2X2	T50.2X3	T50.2X4	T50.2X5	T50.2X6
Chlormethiazole	T42.6X1	T42.6X2	T42.6X3	T42.6X4	T42.6X5	T42.6X6
Chlormethine	T45.1X1	T45.1X2	T45.1X3	T45.1X4	T45.1X5	T45.1X6
Chlormethylenecycline	T36.4X1	T36.4X2	T36.4X3	T36.4X4	T36.4X5	T36.4X6
Chlormezanone	T42.6X1	T42.6X2	T42.6X3	T42.6X4	T42.6X5	T42.6X6
Chloroacetic acid	T60.3X1	T60.3X2	T60.3X3	T60.3X4	—	—
Chloroacetone	T59.3X1	T59.3X2	T59.3X3	T59.3X4	—	—
Chloroacetophenone	T59.3X1	T59.3X2	T59.3X3	T59.3X4	—	—
Chloroaniline	T53.7X1	T53.7X2	T53.7X3	T53.7X4	—	—
Chlorobenzene, chlorobenzol	T53.7X1	T53.7X2	T53.7X3	T53.7X4	—	—
Chlorobromomethane (fire extinguisher)	T53.6X1	T53.6X2	T53.6X3	T53.6X4	—	—
Chlorobutanol	T49.0X1	T49.0X2	T49.0X3	T49.0X4	T49.0X5	T49.0X6
Chlorocresol	T49.0X1	T49.0X2	T49.0X3	T49.0X4	T49.0X5	T49.0X6
Chlorodehydro-methyltestosterone	T38.7X1	T38.7X2	T38.7X3	T38.7X4	T38.7X5	T38.7X6
Chlorodinitrobenzene	T53.7X1	T53.7X2	T53.7X3	T53.7X4	—	—
dust or vapor	T53.7X1	T53.7X2	T53.7X3	T53.7X4	—	—
Chlorodiphenyl	T53.7X1	T53.7X2	T53.7X3	T53.7X4	—	—
Chloroethane—see Ethyl chloride						
Chloroethylene	T53.6X1	T53.6X2	T53.6X3	T53.6X4	—	—
Chlorofluorocarbons	T53.5X1	T53.5X2	T53.5X3	T53.5X4	—	—
Chloroform (fumes) (vapor)	T53.1X1	T53.1X2	T53.1X3	T53.1X4	—	—
anesthetic	T41.0X1	T41.0X2	T41.0X3	T41.0X4	T41.0X5	T41.0X6
solvent	T53.1X1	T53.1X2	T53.1X3	T53.1X4	—	—
water, concentrated	T41.0X1	T41.0X2	T41.0X3	T41.0X4	T41.0X5	T41.0X6
Chloroguanide	T37.2X1	T37.2X2	T37.2X3	T37.2X4	T37.2X5	T37.2X6
Chloromycetin	T36.2X1	T36.2X2	T36.2X3	T36.2X4	T36.2X5	T36.2X6
ENT agent	T49.6X1	T49.6X2	T49.6X3	T49.6X4	T49.6X5	T49.6X6
ophthalmic preparation	T49.5X1	T49.5X2	T49.5X3	T49.5X4	T49.5X5	T49.5X6
Chloromycetin — continued						
otic solution	T49.6X1	T49.6X2	T49.6X3	T49.6X4	T49.6X5	T49.6X6
topical NEC	T49.0X1	T49.0X2	T49.0X3	T49.0X4	T49.0X5	T49.0X6
Chloronitrobenzene	T53.7X1	T53.7X2	T53.7X3	T53.7X4	—	—
dust or vapor	T53.7X1	T53.7X2	T53.7X3	T53.7X4	—	—
Chlorophacinone	T60.4X1	T60.4X2	T60.4X3	T60.4X4	—	—
Chlorophenol	T53.7X1	T53.7X2	T53.7X3	T53.7X4	—	—
Chlorophenothane	T60.1X1	T60.1X2	T60.1X3	T60.1X4	—	—
Chlorophyll	T50.991	T50.992	T50.993	T50.994	T50.995	T50.996
Chloropicrin (fumes)	T53.6X1	T53.6X2	T53.6X3	T53.6X4	—	—
fumigant	T60.8X1	T60.8X2	T60.8X3	T60.8X4	—	—
fungicide	T60.3X1	T60.3X2	T60.3X3	T60.3X4	—	—
pesticide	T60.8X1	T60.8X2	T60.8X3	T60.8X4	—	—
Chloroprocaine	T41.3X1	T41.3X2	T41.3X3	T41.3X4	T41.3X5	T41.3X6
infiltration (subcutaneous)	T41.3X1	T41.3X2	T41.3X3	T41.3X4	T41.3X5	T41.3X6
nerve block (peripheral) (plexus)	T41.3X1	T41.3X2	T41.3X3	T41.3X4	T41.3X5	T41.3X6
spinal	T41.3X1	T41.3X2	T41.3X3	T41.3X4	T41.3X5	T41.3X6
Chloroptic	T49.5X1	T49.5X2	T49.5X3	T49.5X4	T49.5X5	T49.5X6
Chloropurine	T45.1X1	T45.1X2	T45.1X3	T45.1X4	T45.1X5	T45.1X6
Chloropyramine	T45.0X1	T45.0X2	T45.0X3	T45.0X4	T45.0X5	T45.0X6
Chloropyrifos	T60.0X1	T60.0X2	T60.0X3	T60.0X4	—	—
Chloropyrilene	T45.0X1	T45.0X2	T45.0X3	T45.0X4	T45.0X5	T45.0X6
Chloroquine	T37.2X1	T37.2X2	T37.2X3	T37.2X4	T37.2X5	T37.2X6
Chlorothalonil	T60.3X1	T60.3X2	T60.3X3	T60.3X4	—	—
Chlorothen	T45.0X1	T45.0X2	T45.0X3	T45.0X4	T45.0X5	T45.0X6
Chlorothiazide	T50.2X1	T50.2X2	T50.2X3	T50.2X4	T50.2X5	T50.2X6
Chlorothymol	T49.4X1	T49.4X2	T49.4X3	T49.4X4	T49.4X5	T49.4X6
Chlorotrianisene	T38.5X1	T38.5X2	T38.5X3	T38.5X4	T38.5X5	T38.5X6
Chlorovinyldichloro-arsine, not in war	T57.0X1	T57.0X2	T57.0X3	T57.0X4		
Chloroxine	T49.4X1	T49.4X2	T49.4X3	T49.4X4	T49.4X5	T49.4X6
Chloroxylenol	T49.0X1	T49.0X2	T49.0X3	T49.0X4	T49.0X5	T49.0X6
Chlorphenamine	T45.0X1	T45.0X2	T45.0X3	T45.0X4	T45.0X5	T45.0X6
Chlorphenesin	T42.8X1	T42.8X2	T42.8X3	T42.8X4	T42.8X5	T42.8X6
topical (antifungal)	T49.0X1	T49.0X2	T49.0X3	T49.0X4	T49.0X5	T49.0X6
Chlorpheniramine	T45.0X1	T45.0X2	T45.0X3	T45.0X4	T45.0X5	T45.0X6
Chlorphenoxamine	T45.0X1	T45.0X2	T45.0X3	T45.0X4	T45.0X5	T45.0X6
Chlorphentermine	T50.5X1	T50.5X2	T50.5X3	T50.5X4	T50.5X5	T50.5X6
Chlorprocaine—see Chloroprocaine						
Chlorproguanil	T37.2X1	T37.2X2	T37.2X3	T37.2X4	T37.2X5	T37.2X6
Chlorpromazine	T43.3X1	T43.3X2	T43.3X3	T43.3X4	T43.3X5	T43.3X6
Chlorpropamide	T38.3X1	T38.3X2	T38.3X3	T38.3X4	T38.3X5	T38.3X6
Chlorprothixene	T43.4X1	T43.4X2	T43.4X3	T43.4X4	T43.4X5	T43.4X6
Chlorquinaldol	T49.0X1	T49.0X2	T49.0X3	T49.0X4	T49.0X5	T49.0X6
Chlorquinol	T49.0X1	T49.0X2	T49.0X3	T49.0X4	T49.0X5	T49.0X6
Chlortalidone	T50.2X1	T50.2X2	T50.2X3	T50.2X4	T50.2X5	T50.2X6
Chlortetracycline	T36.4X1	T36.4X2	T36.4X3	T36.4X4	T36.4X5	T36.4X6
Chlorthalidone	T50.2X1	T50.2X2	T50.2X3	T50.2X4	T50.2X5	T50.2X6
Chlorthiophos	T60.0X1	T60.0X2	T60.0X3	T60.0X4	—	—
Chlortrianisene	T38.5X1	T38.5X2	T38.5X3	T38.5X4	T38.5X5	T38.5X6
Chlor-Trimeton	T45.0X1	T45.0X2	T45.0X3	T45.0X4	T45.0X5	T45.0X6
Chlorthion	T60.0X1	T60.0X2	T60.0X3	T60.0X4	—	—
Chlorzoxazone	T42.8X1	T42.8X2	T42.8X3	T42.8X4	T42.8X5	T42.8X6
Choke damp	T59.7X1	T59.7X2	T59.7X3	T59.7X4	—	—
Cholagogues	T47.5X1	T47.5X2	T47.5X3	T47.5X4	T47.5X5	T47.5X6
Cholebrine	T50.8X1	T50.8X2	T50.8X3	T50.8X4	T50.8X5	T50.8X6

Substance	Poisoning, Accidental (unintentional)	Poisoning, Intentional self-harm	Poisoning, Assault	Poisoning, Undetermined	Adverse effect	Underdosing
Cholecalciferol	T45.2X1	T45.2X2	T45.2X3	T45.2X4	T45.2X5	T45.2X6
Cholecystokinin	T50.8X1	T50.8X2	T50.8X3	T50.8X4	T50.8X5	T50.8X6
Cholera vaccine	T50.A91	T50.A92	T50.A93	T50.A94	T50.A95	T50.A96
Choleretic	T47.5X1	T47.5X2	T47.5X3	T47.5X4	T47.5X5	T47.5X6
Cholesterol-lowering agents	T46.6X1	T46.6X2	T46.6X3	T46.6X4	T46.6X5	T46.6X6
Cholestyramine (resin)	T46.6X1	T46.6X2	T46.6X3	T46.6X4	T46.6X5	T46.6X6
Cholic acid	T47.5X1	T47.5X2	T47.5X3	T47.5X4	T47.5X5	T47.5X6
Choline	T48.6X1	T48.6X2	T48.6X3	T48.6X4	T48.6X5	T48.6X6
chloride	T50.991	T50.992	T50.993	T50.994	T50.995	T50.996
dihydrogen citrate	T50.991	T50.992	T50.993	T50.994	T50.995	T50.996
salicylate	T39.091	T39.092	T39.093	T39.094	T39.095	T39.096
theophyllinate	T48.6X1	T48.6X2	T48.6X3	T48.6X4	T48.6X5	T48.6X6
Cholinergic (drug) NEC	T44.1X1	T44.1X2	T44.1X3	T44.1X4	T44.1X5	T44.1X6
muscle tone enhancer	T44.1X1	T44.1X2	T44.1X3	T44.1X4	T44.1X5	T44.1X6
organophosphorus	T44.0X1	T44.0X2	T44.0X3	T44.0X4	T44.0X5	T44.0X6
insecticide	T60.0X1	T60.0X2	T60.0X3	T60.0X4	—	—
nerve gas	T59.891	T59.892	T59.893	T59.894	—	—
trimethyl ammonium propanediol	T44.1X1	T44.1X2	T44.1X3	T44.1X4	T44.1X5	T44.1X6
Cholinesterase reactivator	T50.6X1	T50.6X2	T50.6X3	T50.6X4	T50.6X5	T50.6X6
Cholografin	T50.8X1	T50.8X2	T50.8X3	T50.8X4	T50.8X5	T50.8X6
Chorionic gonadotropin	T38.891	T38.892	T38.893	T38.894	T38.895	T38.896
Chromate	T56.2X1	T56.2X2	T56.2X3	T56.2X4	—	—
dust or mist	T56.2X1	T56.2X2	T56.2X3	T56.2X4	—	—
lead—see also lead	T56.0X1	T56.0X2	T56.0X3	T56.0X4	—	—
paint	T56.0X1	T56.0X2	T56.0X3	T56.0X4	—	—
Chromic						
acid	T56.2X1	T56.2X2	T56.2X3	T56.2X4	—	—
dust or mist	T56.2X1	T56.2X2	T56.2X3	T56.2X4	—	—
phosphate 32P	T45.1X1	T45.1X2	T45.1X3	T45.1X4	T45.1X5	T45.1X6
Chromium	T56.2X1	T56.2X2	T56.2X3	T56.2X4	—	—
compounds—see Chromate						
sesquioxide	T50.8X1	T50.8X2	T50.8X3	T50.8X4	T50.8X5	T50.8X6
Chromomycin A3	T45.1X1	T45.1X2	T45.1X3	T45.1X4	T45.1X5	T45.1X6
Chromonar	T46.3X1	T46.3X2	T46.3X3	T46.3X4	T46.3X5	T46.3X6
Chromyl chloride	T56.2X1	T56.2X2	T56.2X3	T56.2X4	—	—
Chrysarobin	T49.4X1	T49.4X2	T49.4X3	T49.4X4	T49.4X5	T49.4X6
Chrysazin	T47.2X1	T47.2X2	T47.2X3	T47.2X4	T47.2X5	T47.2X6
Chymar	T45.3X1	T45.3X2	T45.3X3	T45.3X4	T45.3X5	T45.3X6
ophthalmic preparation	T49.5X1	T49.5X2	T49.5X3	T49.5X4	T49.5X5	T49.5X6
Chymopapain	T45.3X1	T45.3X2	T45.3X3	T45.3X4	T45.3X5	T45.3X6
Chymotrypsin	T45.3X1	T45.3X2	T45.3X3	T45.3X4	T45.3X5	T45.3X6
ophthalmic preparation	T49.5X1	T49.5X2	T49.5X3	T49.5X4	T49.5X5	T49.5X6
Cianidanol	T50.991	T50.992	T50.993	T50.994	T50.995	T50.996
Cianopramine	T43.011	T43.012	T43.013	T43.014	T43.015	T43.016
Cibenzoline	T46.2X1	T46.2X2	T46.2X3	T46.2X4	T46.2X5	T46.2X6
Ciclacillin	T36.0X1	T36.0X2	T36.0X3	T36.0X4	T36.0X5	T36.0X6
Ciclobarbital—see Hexobarbital						
Ciclonicate	T46.7X1	T46.7X2	T46.7X3	T46.7X4	T46.7X5	T46.7X6
Ciclopirox (olamine)	T49.0X1	T49.0X2	T49.0X3	T49.0X4	T49.0X5	T49.0X6
Ciclosporin	T45.1X1	T45.1X2	T45.1X3	T45.1X4	T45.1X5	T45.1X6
Cicuta maculata or virosa	T62.2X1	T62.2X2	T62.2X3	T62.2X4	—	—
Cicutoxin	T62.2X1	T62.2X2	T62.2X3	T62.2X4	—	—
Cigarette lighter fluid	T52.0X1	T52.0X2	T52.0X3	T52.0X4	—	—
Cigarettes (tobacco)	T65.221	T65.222	T65.223	T65.224		

Substance	Poisoning, Accidental (unintentional)	Poisoning, Intentional self-harm	Poisoning, Assault	Poisoning, Undetermined	Adverse effect	Underdosing
Ciguatoxin	T61.01	T61.02	T61.03	T61.04	—	—
Cilazapril	T46.4X1	T46.4X2	T46.4X3	T46.4X4	T46.4X5	T46.4X6
Cimetidine	T47.0X1	T47.0X2	T47.0X3	T47.0X4	T47.0X5	T47.0X6
Cimetropium bromide	T44.3X1	T44.3X2	T44.3X3	T44.3X4	T44.3X5	T44.3X6
Cinchocaine	T41.3X1	T41.3X2	T41.3X3	T41.3X4	T41.3X5	T41.3X6
topical (surface)	T41.3X1	T41.3X2	T41.3X3	T41.3X4	T41.3X5	T41.3X6
Cinchona	T37.2X1	T37.2X2	T37.2X3	T37.2X4	T37.2X5	T37.2X6
Cinchonine alkaloids	T37.2X1	T37.2X2	T37.2X3	T37.2X4	T37.2X5	T37.2X6
Cinchophen	T50.4X1	T50.4X2	T50.4X3	T50.4X4	T50.4X5	T50.4X6
Cinepazide	T46.7X1	T46.7X2	T46.7X3	T46.7X4	T46.7X5	T46.7X6
Cinnamedrine	T48.5X1	T48.5X2	T48.5X3	T48.5X4	T48.5X5	T48.5X6
Cinnarizine	T45.0X1	T45.0X2	T45.0X3	T45.0X4	T45.0X5	T45.0X6
Cinoxacin	T37.8X1	T37.8X2	T37.8X3	T37.8X4	T37.8X5	T37.8X6
Ciprofibrate	T46.6X1	T46.6X2	T46.6X3	T46.6X4	T46.6X5	T46.6X6
Ciprofloxacin	T36.8X1	T36.8X2	T36.8X3	T36.8X4	T36.8X5	T36.8X6
Cisapride	T47.8X1	T47.8X2	T47.8X3	T47.8X4	T47.8X5	T47.8X6
Cisplatin	T45.1X1	T45.1X2	T45.1X3	T45.1X4	T45.1X5	T45.1X6
Citalopram	T43.221	T43.222	T43.223	T43.224	T43.225	T43.226
Citanest	T41.3X1	T41.3X2	T41.3X3	T41.3X4	T41.3X5	T41.3X6
infiltration (subcutaneous)	T41.3X1	T41.3X2	T41.3X3	T41.3X4	T41.3X5	T41.3X6
nerve block (peripheral) (plexus)	T41.3X1	T41.3X2	T41.3X3	T41.3X4	T41.3X5	T41.3X6
Citric acid	T47.5X1	T47.5X2	T47.5X3	T47.5X4	T47.5X5	T47.5X6
Citrovorum (factor)	T45.8X1	T45.8X2	T45.8X3	T45.8X4	T45.8X5	T45.8X6
Claviceps purpurea	T62.2X1	T62.2X2	T62.2X3	T62.2X4	—	—
Clavulanic acid	T36.1X1	T36.1X2	T36.1X3	T36.1X4	T36.1X5	T36.1X6
Cleaner, cleansing agent, type not specified	T65.891	T65.892	T65.893	T65.894	—	—
of paint or varnish	T52.91	T52.92	T52.93	T52.94	—	—
specified type NEC	T65.891	T65.892	T65.893	T65.894	—	—
Clebopride	T47.8X1	T47.8X2	T47.8X3	T47.8X4	T47.8X5	T47.8X6
Clefamide	T37.3X1	T37.3X2	T37.3X3	T37.3X4	T37.3X5	T37.3X6
Clemastine	T45.0X1	T45.0X2	T45.0X3	T45.0X4	T45.0X5	T45.0X6
Clematis vitalba	T62.2X1	T62.2X2	T62.2X3	T62.2X4	—	—
Clemizole	T45.0X1	T45.0X2	T45.0X3	T45.0X4	T45.0X5	T45.0X6
penicillin	T36.0X1	T36.0X2	T36.0X3	T36.0X4	T36.0X5	T36.0X6
Clenbuterol	T48.6X1	T48.6X2	T48.6X3	T48.6X4	T48.6X5	T48.6X6
Clidinium bromide	T44.3X1	T44.3X2	T44.3X3	T44.3X4	T44.3X5	T44.3X6
Clindamycin	T36.8X1	T36.8X2	T36.8X3	T36.8X4	T36.8X5	T36.8X6
Clinofibrate	T46.6X1	T46.6X2	T46.6X3	T46.6X4	T46.6X5	T46.6X6
Clioquinol	T37.8X1	T37.8X2	T37.8X3	T37.8X4	T37.8X5	T37.8X6
Cliradon	T40.2X1	T40.2X2	T40.2X3	T40.2X4	—	—
Clobazam	T42.4X1	T42.4X2	T42.4X3	T42.4X4	T42.4X5	T42.4X6
Clobenzorex	T50.5X1	T50.5X2	T50.5X3	T50.5X4	T50.5X5	T50.5X6
Clobetasol	T49.0X1	T49.0X2	T49.0X3	T49.0X4	T49.0X5	T49.0X6
Clobetasone	T49.0X1	T49.0X2	T49.0X3	T49.0X4	T49.0X5	T49.0X6
Clobutinol	T48.3X1	T48.3X2	T48.3X3	T48.3X4	T48.3X5	T48.3X6
Clocortolone	T38.0X1	T38.0X2	T38.0X3	T38.0X4	T38.0X5	T38.0X6
Clodantoin	T49.0X1	T49.0X2	T49.0X3	T49.0X4	T49.0X5	T49.0X6
Clodronic acid	T50.991	T50.992	T50.993	T50.994	T50.995	T50.996
Clofazimine	T37.1X1	T37.1X2	T37.1X3	T37.1X4	T37.1X5	T37.1X6
Clofedanol	T48.3X1	T48.3X2	T48.3X3	T48.3X4	T48.3X5	T48.3X6
Clofenamide	T50.2X1	T50.2X2	T50.2X3	T50.2X4	T50.2X5	T50.2X6
Clofenotane	T49.0X1	T49.0X2	T49.0X3	T49.0X4	T49.0X5	T49.0X6
Clofezone	T39.2X1	T39.2X2	T39.2X3	T39.2X4	T39.2X5	T39.2X6
Clofibrate	T46.6X1	T46.6X2	T46.6X3	T46.6X4	T46.6X5	T46.6X6
Clofibride	T46.6X1	T46.6X2	T46.6X3	T46.6X4	T46.6X5	T46.6X6
Cloforex	T50.5X1	T50.5X2	T50.5X3	T50.5X4	T50.5X5	T50.5X6
Clomethiazole	T42.6X1	T42.6X2	T42.6X3	T42.6X4	T42.6X5	T42.6X6

Clometocillin - Convallaria majalis

Substance	Poisoning, Accidental (unintentional)	Poisoning, Intentional self-harm	Poisoning, Assault	Poisoning, Undetermined	Adverse effect	Underdosing
Clometocillin	T36.0X1	T36.0X2	T36.0X3	T36.0X4	T36.0X5	T36.0X6
Clomifene	T38.5X1	T38.5X2	T38.5X3	T38.5X4	T38.5X5	T38.5X6
Clomiphene	T38.5X1	T38.5X2	T38.5X3	T38.5X4	T38.5X5	T38.5X6
Clomipramine	T43.011	T43.012	T43.013	T43.014	T43.015	T43.016
Clomocycline	T36.4X1	T36.4X2	T36.4X3	T36.4X4	T36.4X5	T36.4X6
Clonazepam	T42.4X1	T42.4X2	T42.4X3	T42.4X4	T42.4X5	T42.4X6
Clonidine	T46.5X1	T46.5X2	T46.5X3	T46.5X4	T46.5X5	T46.5X6
Clonixin	T39.8X1	T39.8X2	T39.8X3	T39.8X4	T39.8X5	T39.8X6
Clopamide	T50.2X1	T50.2X2	T50.2X3	T50.2X4	T50.2X5	T50.2X6
Clopenthixol	T43.4X1	T43.4X2	T43.4X3	T43.4X4	T43.4X5	T43.4X6
Cloperastine	T48.3X1	T48.3X2	T48.3X3	T48.3X4	T48.3X5	T48.3X6
Clophedianol	T48.3X1	T48.3X2	T48.3X3	T48.3X4	T48.3X5	T48.3X6
Cloponone	T36.2X1	T36.2X2	T36.2X3	T36.2X4	T36.2X5	T36.2X6
Cloprednol	T38.0X1	T38.0X2	T38.0X3	T38.0X4	T38.0X5	T38.0X6
Cloral betaine	T42.6X1	T42.6X2	T42.6X3	T42.6X4	T42.6X5	T42.6X6
Cloramfenicol	T36.2X1	T36.2X2	T36.2X3	T36.2X4	T36.2X5	T36.2X6
Clorazepate (dipotassium)	T42.4X1	T42.4X2	T42.4X3	T42.4X4	T42.4X5	T42.4X6
Clorexolone	T50.2X1	T50.2X2	T50.2X3	T50.2X4	T50.2X5	T50.2X6
Clorfenamine	T45.0X1	T45.0X2	T45.0X3	T45.0X4	T45.0X5	T45.0X6
Clorgiline	T43.1X1	T43.1X2	T43.1X3	T43.1X4	T43.1X5	T43.1X6
Clorotepine	T44.3X1	T44.3X2	T44.3X3	T44.3X4	T44.3X5	T44.3X6
Clorox (bleach)	T54.91	T54.92	T54.93	T54.94	—	—
Clorprenaline	T48.6X1	T48.6X2	T48.6X3	T48.6X4	T48.6X5	T48.6X6
Clortermine	T50.5X1	T50.5X2	T50.5X3	T50.5X4	T50.5X5	T50.5X6
Clotiapine	T43.591	T43.592	T43.593	T43.594	T43.595	T43.596
Clotiazepam	T42.4X1	T42.4X2	T42.4X3	T42.4X4	T42.4X5	T42.4X6
Clotibric acid	T46.6X1	T46.6X2	T46.6X3	T46.6X4	T46.6X5	T46.6X6
Clotrimazole	T49.0X1	T49.0X2	T49.0X3	T49.0X4	T49.0X5	T49.0X6
Cloxacillin	T36.0X1	T36.0X2	T36.0X3	T36.0X4	T36.0X5	T36.0X6
Cloxazolam	T42.4X1	T42.4X2	T42.4X3	T42.4X4	T42.4X5	T42.4X6
Cloxiquine	T49.0X1	T49.0X2	T49.0X3	T49.0X4	T49.0X5	T49.0X6
Clozapine	T42.4X1	T42.4X2	T42.4X3	T42.4X4	T42.4X5	T42.4X6
Coagulant NEC	T45.7X1	T45.7X2	T45.7X3	T45.7X4	T45.7X5	T45.7X6
Coal (carbon monoxide from)—see also Carbon, monoxide, coal oil—see Kerosene	T58.2X1	T58.2X2	T58.2X3	T58.2X4	—	—
tar	T49.1X1	T49.1X2	T49.1X3	T49.1X4	T49.1X5	T49.1X6
fumes	T59.891	T59.892	T59.893	T59.894		
medicinal (ointment)	T49.4X1	T49.4X2	T49.4X3	T49.4X4	T49.4X5	T49.4X6
analgesics NEC	T39.2X1	T39.2X2	T39.2X3	T39.2X4	T39.2X5	T39.2X6
naphtha (solvent)	T52.0X1	T52.0X2	T52.0X3	T52.0X4		
Cobalamine	T45.2X1	T45.2X2	T45.2X3	T45.2X4	T45.2X5	T45.2X6
Cobalt (nonmedicinal) (fumes) (industrial)	T56.891	T56.892	T56.893	T56.894	—	—
medicinal (trace) (chloride)	T45.8X1	T45.8X2	T45.8X3	T45.8X4	T45.8X5	T45.8X6
Cobra (venom)	T63.041	T63.042	T63.043	T63.044	—	—
Coca (leaf)	T40.5X1	T40.5X2	T40.5X3	T40.5X4	T40.5X5	T40.5X6
Cocaine	T40.5X1	T40.5X2	T40.5X3	T40.5X4	T40.5X5	T40.5X6
topical anesthetic	T41.3X1	T41.3X2	T41.3X3	T41.3X4	T41.3X5	T41.3X6
Cocarboxylase	T45.3X1	T45.3X2	T45.3X3	T45.3X4	T45.3X5	T45.3X6
Coccidioidin	T50.8X1	T50.8X2	T50.8X3	T50.8X4	T50.8X5	T50.8X6
Cocculus indicus	T62.1X1	T62.1X2	T62.1X3	T62.1X4	—	—
Cochineal	T65.6X1	T65.6X2	T65.6X3	T65.6X4	—	—
medicinal products	T50.991	T50.992	T50.993	T50.994	T50.995	T50.996
Codeine	T40.2X1	T40.2X2	T40.2X3	T40.2X4	T40.2X5	T40.2X6
Cod-liver oil	T45.2X1	T45.2X2	T45.2X3	T45.2X4	T45.2X5	T45.2X6
Coenzyme A	T50.991	T50.992	T50.993	T50.994	T50.995	T50.996
Coffee	T62.8X1	T62.8X2	T62.8X3	T62.8X4	—	—

Substance	Poisoning, Accidental (unintentional)	Poisoning, Intentional self-harm	Poisoning, Assault	Poisoning, Undetermined	Adverse effect	Underdosing
Cogalactoiso-merase	T50.991	T50.992	T50.993	T50.994	T50.995	T50.996
Cogentin	T44.3X1	T44.3X2	T44.3X3	T44.3X4	T44.3X5	T44.3X6
Coke fumes or gas (carbon monoxide)	T58.2X1	T58.2X2	T58.2X3	T58.2X4	—	—
industrial use	T58.8X1	T58.8X2	T58.8X3	T58.8X4	—	—
Colace	T47.4X1	T47.4X2	T47.4X3	T47.4X4	T47.4X5	T47.4X6
Colaspase	T45.1X1	T45.1X2	T45.1X3	T45.1X4	T45.1X5	T45.1X6
Colchicine	T50.4X1	T50.4X2	T50.4X3	T50.4X4	T50.4X5	T50.4X6
Colchicum	T62.2X1	T62.2X2	T62.2X3	T62.2X4	—	—
Cold cream	T49.3X1	T49.3X2	T49.3X3	T49.3X4	T49.3X5	T49.3X6
Colecalciferol	T45.2X1	T45.2X2	T45.2X3	T45.2X4	T45.2X5	T45.2X6
Colestipol	T46.6X1	T46.6X2	T46.6X3	T46.6X4	T46.6X5	T46.6X6
Colestyramine	T46.6X1	T46.6X2	T46.6X3	T46.6X4	T46.6X5	T46.6X6
Colimycin	T36.8X1	T36.8X2	T36.8X3	T36.8X4	T36.8X5	T36.8X6
Colistimethate	T36.8X1	T36.8X2	T36.8X3	T36.8X4	T36.8X5	T36.8X6
Colistin	T36.8X1	T36.8X2	T36.8X3	T36.8X4	T36.8X5	T36.8X6
sulfate (eye preparation)	T49.5X1	T49.5X2	T49.5X3	T49.5X4	T49.5X5	T49.5X6
Collagen	T50.991	T50.992	T50.993	T50.994	T50.995	T50.996
Collagenase	T49.4X1	T49.4X2	T49.4X3	T49.4X4	T49.4X5	T49.4X6
Collodion	T49.3X1	T49.3X2	T49.3X3	T49.3X4	T49.3X5	T49.3X6
Colocynth	T47.2X1	T47.2X2	T47.2X3	T47.2X4	T47.2X5	T47.2X6
Colophony adhesive	T49.3X1	T49.3X2	T49.3X3	T49.3X4	T49.3X5	T49.3X6
Colorant—see also Dye	T50.991	T50.992	T50.993	T50.994	T50.995	T50.996
Coloring matter—see Dye(s)						
Combustion gas (after combustion)—see Carbon, monoxide						
prior to combustion	T59.891	T59.892	T59.893	T59.894	—	—
Compazine	T43.3X1	T43.3X2	T43.3X3	T43.3X4	T43.3X5	T43.3X6
Compound						
42 (warfarin)	T60.4X1	T60.4X2	T60.4X3	T60.4X4		
269 (endrin)	T60.1X1	T60.1X2	T60.1X3	T60.1X4		
497 (dieldrin)	T60.1X1	T60.1X2	T60.1X3	T60.1X4		
1080 (sodium fluoroacetate)	T60.4X1	T60.4X2	T60.4X3	T60.4X4		
3422 (parathion)	T60.0X1	T60.0X2	T60.0X3	T60.0X4		
3911 (phorate)	T60.0X1	T60.0X2	T60.0X3	T60.0X4		
3956 (toxaphene)	T60.1X1	T60.1X2	T60.1X3	T60.1X4		
4049 (malathion)	T60.0X1	T60.0X2	T60.0X3	T60.0X4		
4069 (malathion)	T60.0X1	T60.0X2	T60.0X3	T60.0X4		
4124 (dicapthon)	T60.0X1	T60.0X2	T60.0X3	T60.0X4		
E (cortisone)	T38.0X1	T38.0X2	T38.0X3	T38.0X4	T38.0X5	T38.0X6
F (hydrocortisone)	T38.0X1	T38.0X2	T38.0X3	T38.0X4	T38.0X5	T38.0X6
Congener, anabolic	T38.7X1	T38.7X2	T38.7X3	T38.7X4	T38.7X5	T38.7X6
Congo red	T50.8X1	T50.8X2	T50.8X3	T50.8X4	T50.8X5	T50.8X6
Coniine, conine	T62.2X1	T62.2X2	T62.2X3	T62.2X4	—	—
Conium (maculatum)	T62.2X1	T62.2X2	T62.2X3	T62.2X4	—	—
Conjugated estrogenic substances	T38.5X1	T38.5X2	T38.5X3	T38.5X4	T38.5X5	T38.5X6
Contac	T48.5X1	T48.5X2	T48.5X3	T48.5X4	T48.5X5	T48.5X6
Contact lens solution	T49.5X1	T49.5X2	T49.5X3	T49.5X4	T49.5X5	T49.5X6
Contraceptive (oral)	T38.4X1	T38.4X2	T38.4X3	T38.4X4	T38.4X5	T38.4X6
vaginal	T49.8X1	T49.8X2	T49.8X3	T49.8X4	T49.8X5	T49.8X6
Contrast medium, radiography	T50.8X1	T50.8X2	T50.8X3	T50.8X4	T50.8X5	T50.8X6
Convallaria glycosides	T46.0X1	T46.0X2	T46.0X3	T46.0X4	T46.0X5	T46.0X6
Convallaria majalis	T62.2X1	T62.2X2	T62.2X3	T62.2X4	—	—
berry	T62.1X1	T62.1X2	T62.1X3	T62.1X4	—	—

Substance	Poisoning, Accidental (unintentional)	Poisoning, Intentional self-harm	Poisoning, Assault	Poisoning, Undetermined	Adverse effect	Underdosing
Copper (dust) (fumes) (nonmedicinal) NEC	T56.4X1	T56.4X2	T56.4X3	T56.4X4	—	—
arsenate, arsenite	T57.0X1	T57.0X2	T57.0X3	T57.0X4	—	—
insecticide	T60.2X1	T60.2X2	T60.2X3	T60.2X4	—	—
emetic	T47.7X1	T47.7X2	T47.7X3	T47.7X4	T47.7X5	T47.7X6
fungicide	T60.3X1	T60.3X2	T60.3X3	T60.3X4	—	—
gluconate	T49.0X1	T49.0X2	T49.0X3	T49.0X4	T49.0X5	T49.0X6
insecticide	T60.2X1	T60.2X2	T60.2X3	T60.2X4	—	—
medicinal (trace)	T45.8X1	T45.8X2	T45.8X3	T45.8X4	T45.8X5	T45.8X6
oleate	T49.0X1	T49.0X2	T49.0X3	T49.0X4	T49.0X5	T49.0X6
sulfate	T56.4X1	T56.4X2	T56.4X3	T56.4X4	—	—
cupric	T56.4X1	T56.4X2	T56.4X3	T56.4X4	—	—
fungicide	T60.3X1	T60.3X2	T60.3X3	T60.3X4	—	—
medicinal						
ear	T49.6X1	T49.6X2	T49.6X3	T49.6X4	T49.6X5	T49.6X6
emetic	T47.7X1	T47.7X2	T47.7X3	T47.7X4	T47.7X5	T47.7X6
eye	T49.5X1	T49.5X2	T49.5X3	T49.5X4	T49.5X5	T49.5X6
cuprous	T56.4X1	T56.4X2	T56.4X3	T56.4X4	—	—
fungicide	T60.3X1	T60.3X2	T60.3X3	T60.3X4	—	—
medicinal						
ear	T49.6X1	T49.6X2	T49.6X3	T49.6X4	T49.6X5	T49.6X6
emetic	T47.7X1	T47.7X2	T47.7X3	T47.7X4	T47.7X5	T47.7X6
eye	T49.5X1	T49.5X2	T49.5X3	T49.5X4	T49.5X5	T49.5X6
Copperhead snake (bite) (venom)	T63.061	T63.062	T63.063	T63.064	—	—
Coral (sting)	T63.691	T63.692	T63.693	T63.694	—	—
snake (bite) (venom)	T63.021	T63.022	T63.023	T63.024	—	—
Corbadrine	T49.6X1	T49.6X2	T49.6X3	T49.6X4	T49.6X5	T49.6X6
Cordite	T65.891	T65.892	T65.893	T65.894	—	—
vapor	T59.891	T59.892	T59.893	T59.894	—	—
Cordran	T49.0X1	T49.0X2	T49.0X3	T49.0X4	T49.0X5	T49.0X6
Corn cures	T49.4X1	T49.4X2	T49.4X3	T49.4X4	T49.4X5	T49.4X6
Corn starch	T49.3X1	T49.3X2	T49.3X3	T49.3X4	T49.3X5	T49.3X6
Cornhusker's lotion	T49.3X1	T49.3X2	T49.3X3	T49.3X4	T49.3X5	T49.3X6
Coronary vasodilator NEC	T46.3X1	T46.3X2	T46.3X3	T46.3X4	T46.3X5	T46.3X6
Corrosive NEC	T54.91	T54.92	T54.93	T54.94	—	—
acid NEC	T54.2X1	T54.2X2	T54.2X3	T54.2X4	—	—
aromatics	T54.1X1	T54.1X2	T54.1X3	T54.1X4	—	—
disinfectant	T54.1X1	T54.1X2	T54.1X3	T54.1X4	—	—
fumes NEC	T54.91	T54.92	T54.93	T54.94	—	—
specified NEC	T54.91	T54.92	T54.93	T54.94	—	—
sublimate	T56.1X1	T56.1X2	T56.1X3	T56.1X4	—	—
Cortate	T38.0X1	T38.0X2	T38.0X3	T38.0X4	T38.0X5	T38.0X6
Cort-Dome	T38.0X1	T38.0X2	T38.0X3	T38.0X4	T38.0X5	T38.0X6
ENT agent	T49.6X1	T49.6X2	T49.6X3	T49.6X4	T49.6X5	T49.6X6
ophthalmic preparation	T49.5X1	T49.5X2	T49.5X3	T49.5X4	T49.5X5	T49.5X6
topical NEC	T49.0X1	T49.0X2	T49.0X3	T49.0X4	T49.0X5	T49.0X6
Cortef	T38.0X1	T38.0X2	T38.0X3	T38.0X4	T38.0X5	T38.0X6
ENT agent	T49.6X1	T49.6X2	T49.6X3	T49.6X4	T49.6X5	T49.6X6
ophthalmic preparation	T49.5X1	T49.5X2	T49.5X3	T49.5X4	T49.5X5	T49.5X6
topical NEC	T49.0X1	T49.0X2	T49.0X3	T49.0X4	T49.0X5	T49.0X6
Corticosteroid	T38.0X1	T38.0X2	T38.0X3	T38.0X4	T38.0X5	T38.0X6
ENT agent	T49.6X1	T49.6X2	T49.6X3	T49.6X4	T49.6X5	T49.6X6
mineral	T50.0X1	T50.0X2	T50.0X3	T50.0X4	T50.0X5	T50.0X6
ophthalmic	T49.5X1	T49.5X2	T49.5X3	T49.5X4	T49.5X5	T49.5X6
topical NEC	T49.0X1	T49.0X2	T49.0X3	T49.0X4	T49.0X5	T49.0X6
Corticotropin	T38.811	T38.812	T38.813	T38.814	T38.815	T38.816
Cortisol	T49.0X1	T49.0X2	T49.0X3	T49.0X4	T49.0X5	T49.0X6
ENT agent	T49.6X1	T49.6X2	T49.6X3	T49.6X4	T49.6X5	T49.6X6

Substance	Poisoning, Accidental (unintentional)	Poisoning, Intentional self-harm	Poisoning, Assault	Poisoning, Undetermined	Adverse effect	Underdosing
Cortisol — *continued*						
ophthalmic preparation	T49.5X1	T49.5X2	T49.5X3	T49.5X4	T49.5X5	T49.5X6
topical NEC	T49.0X1	T49.0X2	T49.0X3	T49.0X4	T49.0X5	T49.0X6
Cortisone (acetate)	T38.0X1	T38.0X2	T38.0X3	T38.0X4	T38.0X5	T38.0X6
ENT agent	T49.6X1	T49.6X2	T49.6X3	T49.6X4	T49.6X5	T49.6X6
ophthalmic preparation	T49.5X1	T49.5X2	T49.5X3	T49.5X4	T49.5X5	T49.5X6
topical NEC	T49.0X1	T49.0X2	T49.0X3	T49.0X4	T49.0X5	T49.0X6
Cortivazol	T38.0X1	T38.0X2	T38.0X3	T38.0X4	T38.0X5	T38.0X6
Cortogen	T38.0X1	T38.0X2	T38.0X3	T38.0X4	T38.0X5	T38.0X6
ENT agent	T49.6X1	T49.6X2	T49.6X3	T49.6X4	T49.6X5	T49.6X6
ophthalmic preparation	T49.5X1	T49.5X2	T49.5X3	T49.5X4	T49.5X5	T49.5X6
Cortone	T38.0X1	T38.0X2	T38.0X3	T38.0X4	T38.0X5	T38.0X6
ENT agent	T49.6X1	T49.6X2	T49.6X3	T49.6X4	T49.6X5	T49.6X6
ophthalmic preparation	T49.5X1	T49.5X2	T49.5X3	T49.5X4	T49.5X5	T49.5X6
Cortril	T38.0X1	T38.0X2	T38.0X3	T38.0X4	T38.0X5	T38.0X6
ENT agent	T49.6X1	T49.6X2	T49.6X3	T49.6X4	T49.6X5	T49.6X6
ophthalmic preparation	T49.5X1	T49.5X2	T49.5X3	T49.5X4	T49.5X5	T49.5X6
topical NEC	T49.0X1	T49.0X2	T49.0X3	T49.0X4	T49.0X5	T49.0X6
Corynebacterium parvum	T45.1X1	T45.1X2	T45.1X3	T45.1X4	T45.1X5	T45.1X6
Cosmetic preparation	T49.8X1	T49.8X2	T49.8X3	T49.8X4	T49.8X5	T49.8X6
Cosmetics	T49.8X1	T49.8X2	T49.8X3	T49.8X4	T49.8X5	T49.8X6
Cosyntropin	T38.811	T38.812	T38.813	T38.814	T38.815	T38.816
Cotarnine	T45.7X1	T45.7X2	T45.7X3	T45.7X4	T45.7X5	T45.7X6
Co-trimoxazole	T36.8X1	T36.8X2	T36.8X3	T36.8X4	T36.8X5	T36.8X6
Cottonseed oil	T49.3X1	T49.3X2	T49.3X3	T49.3X4	T49.3X5	T49.3X6
Cough mixture (syrup)	T48.4X1	T48.4X2	T48.4X3	T48.4X4	T48.4X5	T48.4X6
containing opiates	T40.2X1	T40.2X2	T40.2X3	T40.2X4	T40.2X5	T40.2X6
expectorants	T48.4X1	T48.4X2	T48.4X3	T48.4X4	T48.4X5	T48.4X6
Coumadin	T45.511	T45.512	T45.513	T45.514	T45.515	T45.516
rodenticide	T60.4X1	T60.4X2	T60.4X3	T60.4X4	—	—
Coumaphos	T60.0X1	T60.0X2	T60.0X3	T60.0X4	—	—
Coumarin	T45.511	T45.512	T45.513	T45.514	T45.515	T45.516
Coumetarol	T45.511	T45.512	T45.513	T45.514	T45.515	T45.516
Cowbane	T62.2X1	T62.2X2	T62.2X3	T62.2X4	—	—
Cozyme	T45.2X1	T45.2X2	T45.2X3	T45.2X4	T45.2X5	T45.2X6
Crack	T40.5X1	T40.5X2	T40.5X3	T40.5X4	—	—
Crataegus extract	T46.0X1	T46.0X2	T46.0X3	T46.0X4	T46.0X5	T46.0X6
Creolin	T54.1X1	T54.1X2	T54.1X3	T54.1X4	—	—
disinfectant	T54.1X1	T54.1X2	T54.1X3	T54.1X4	—	—
Creosol (compound)	T49.0X1	T49.0X2	T49.0X3	T49.0X4	T49.0X5	T49.0X6
Creosote (coal tar) (beechwood)	T49.0X1	T49.0X2	T49.0X3	T49.0X4	T49.0X5	T49.0X6
medicinal (expectorant)	T48.4X1	T48.4X2	T48.4X3	T48.4X4	T48.4X5	T48.4X6
syrup	T48.4X1	T48.4X2	T48.4X3	T48.4X4	T48.4X5	T48.4X6
Cresol (s)	T49.0X1	T49.0X2	T49.0X3	T49.0X4	T49.0X5	T49.0X6
and soap solution	T49.0X1	T49.0X2	T49.0X3	T49.0X4	T49.0X5	T49.0X6
Cresyl acetate	T49.0X1	T49.0X2	T49.0X3	T49.0X4	T49.0X5	T49.0X6
Cresylic acid	T49.0X1	T49.0X2	T49.0X3	T49.0X4	T49.0X5	T49.0X6
Crimidine	T60.4X1	T60.4X2	T60.4X3	T60.4X4	—	—
Croconazole	T37.8X1	T37.8X2	T37.8X3	T37.8X4	T37.8X5	T37.8X6
Cromoglicic acid	T48.6X1	T48.6X2	T48.6X3	T48.6X4	T48.6X5	T48.6X6
Cromolyn	T48.6X1	T48.6X2	T48.6X3	T48.6X4	T48.6X5	T48.6X6
Cromonar	T46.3X1	T46.3X2	T46.3X3	T46.3X4	T46.3X5	T46.3X6
Cropropamide	T39.8X1	T39.8X2	T39.8X3	T39.8X4	T39.8X5	T39.8X6
with crotethamide	T50.7X1	T50.7X2	T50.7X3	T50.7X4	T50.7X5	T50.7X6
Crotamiton	T49.0X1	T49.0X2	T49.0X3	T49.0X4	T49.0X5	T49.0X6
Crotethamide	T39.8X1	T39.8X2	T39.8X3	T39.8X4	T39.8X5	T39.8X6
with cropropamide	T50.7X1	T50.7X2	T50.7X3	T50.7X4	T50.7X5	T50.7X6
Croton (oil)	T47.2X1	T47.2X2	T47.2X3	T47.2X4	T47.2X5	T47.2X6
chloral	T42.6X1	T42.6X2	T42.6X3	T42.6X4	T42.6X5	T42.6X6

Substance	Poisoning, Accidental (unintentional)	Poisoning, Intentional self-harm	Poisoning, Assault	Poisoning, Undetermined	Adverse effect	Underdosing
Crude oil	T52.0X1	T52.0X2	T52.0X3	T52.0X4	—	—
Cryogenine	T39.8X1	T39.8X2	T39.8X3	T39.8X4	T39.8X5	T39.8X6
Cryolite (vapor)	T60.1X1	T60.1X2	T60.1X3	T60.1X4	—	—
insecticide	T60.1X1	T60.1X2	T60.1X3	T60.1X4	—	—
Cryptenamine (tannates)	T46.5X1	T46.5X2	T46.5X3	T46.5X4	T46.5X5	T46.5X6
Crystal violet	T49.0X1	T49.0X2	T49.0X3	T49.0X4	T49.0X5	T49.0X6
Cuckoopint	T62.2X1	T62.2X2	T62.2X3	T62.2X4	—	—
Cumetharol	T45.511	T45.512	T45.513	T45.514	T45.515	T45.516
Cupric						
acetate	T60.3X1	T60.3X2	T60.3X3	T60.3X4	—	—
acetoarsenite	T57.0X1	T57.0X2	T57.0X3	T57.0X4	—	—
arsenate	T57.0X1	T57.0X2	T57.0X3	T57.0X4	—	—
gluconate	T49.0X1	T49.0X2	T49.0X3	T49.0X4	T49.0X5	T49.0X6
oleate	T49.0X1	T49.0X2	T49.0X3	T49.0X4	T49.0X5	T49.0X6
sulfate	T56.4X1	T56.4X2	T56.4X3	T56.4X4	—	—
Cuprous sulfate—see also Copper sulfate	T56.4X1	T56.4X2	T56.4X3	T56.4X4	—	—
Curare, curarine	T48.1X1	T48.1X2	T48.1X3	T48.1X4	T48.1X5	T48.1X6
Cyamemazine	T43.3X1	T43.3X2	T43.3X3	T43.3X4	T43.3X5	T43.3X6
Cyamopsis tetragono-loba	T46.6X1	T46.6X2	T46.6X3	T46.6X4	T46.6X5	T46.6X6
Cyanacetyl hydrazide	T37.1X1	T37.1X2	T37.1X3	T37.1X4	T37.1X5	T37.1X6
Cyanic acid (gas)	T59.891	T59.892	T59.893	T59.894	—	—
Cyanide (s) (compounds) (potassium) (sodium) NEC	T65.0X1	T65.0X2	T65.0X3	T65.0X4		
dust or gas (inhalation) NEC	T57.3X1	T57.3X2	T57.3X3	T57.3X4	—	—
fumigant	T65.0X1	T65.0X2	T65.0X3	T65.0X4	—	—
hydrogen	T57.3X1	T57.3X2	T57.3X3	T57.3X4	—	—
mercuric—see Mercury						
pesticide (dust) (fumes)	T65.0X1	T65.0X2	T65.0X3	T65.0X4	—	—
Cyanoacrylate adhesive	T49.3X1	T49.3X2	T49.3X3	T49.3X4	T49.3X5	T49.3X6
Cyanocobalamin	T45.8X1	T45.8X2	T45.8X3	T45.8X4	T45.8X5	T45.8X6
Cyanogen (chloride) (gas) NEC	T59.891	T59.892	T59.893	T59.894		—
Cyclacillin	T36.0X1	T36.0X2	T36.0X3	T36.0X4	T36.0X5	T36.0X6
Cyclaine	T41.3X1	T41.3X2	T41.3X3	T41.3X4	T41.3X5	T41.3X6
Cyclamate	T50.991	T50.992	T50.993	T50.994	T50.995	T50.996
Cyclamen europaeum	T62.2X1	T62.2X2	T62.2X3	T62.2X4	—	—
Cyclandelate	T46.7X1	T46.7X2	T46.7X3	T46.7X4	T46.7X5	T46.7X6
Cyclazocine	T50.7X1	T50.7X2	T50.7X3	T50.7X4	T50.7X5	T50.7X6
Cyclizine	T45.0X1	T45.0X2	T45.0X3	T45.0X4	T45.0X5	T45.0X6
Cyclobarbital	T42.3X1	T42.3X2	T42.3X3	T42.3X4	T42.3X5	T42.3X6
Cyclobarbitone	T42.3X1	T42.3X2	T42.3X3	T42.3X4	T42.3X5	T42.3X6
Cyclobenzaprine	T48.1X1	T48.1X2	T48.1X3	T48.1X4	T48.1X5	T48.1X6
Cyclodrine	T44.3X1	T44.3X2	T44.3X3	T44.3X4	T44.3X5	T44.3X6
Cycloguanil embonate	T37.2X1	T37.2X2	T37.2X3	T37.2X4	T37.2X5	T37.2X6
Cyclohexane	T52.8X1	T52.8X2	T52.8X3	T52.8X4	—	—
Cyclohexanol	T51.8X1	T51.8X2	T51.8X3	T51.8X4	—	—
Cyclohexanone	T52.4X1	T52.4X2	T52.4X3	T52.4X4	—	—
Cycloheximide	T60.3X1	T60.3X2	T60.3X3	T60.3X4	—	—
Cyclohexyl acetate	T52.8X1	T52.8X2	T52.8X3	T52.8X4	—	—
Cycloleucin	T45.1X1	T45.1X2	T45.1X3	T45.1X4	T45.1X5	T45.1X6
Cyclomethycaine	T41.3X1	T41.3X2	T41.3X3	T41.3X4	T41.3X5	T41.3X6
Cyclopentamine	T44.4X1	T44.4X2	T44.4X3	T44.4X4	T44.4X5	T44.4X6
Cyclopenthiazide	T50.2X1	T50.2X2	T50.2X3	T50.2X4	T50.2X5	T50.2X6
Cyclopentolate	T44.3X1	T44.3X2	T44.3X3	T44.3X4	T44.3X5	T44.3X6
Cyclophosphamide	T45.1X1	T45.1X2	T45.1X3	T45.1X4	T45.1X5	T45.1X6
Cycloplegic drug	T49.5X1	T49.5X2	T49.5X3	T49.5X4	T49.5X5	T49.5X6
Cyclopropane	T41.291	T41.292	T41.293	T41.294	T41.295	T41.296
Cyclopyrabital	T39.8X1	T39.8X2	T39.8X3	T39.8X4	T39.8X5	T39.8X6
Cycloserine	T37.1X1	T37.1X2	T37.1X3	T37.1X4	T37.1X5	T37.1X6
Cyclosporin	T45.1X1	T45.1X2	T45.1X3	T45.1X4	T45.1X5	T45.1X6
Cyclothiazide	T50.2X1	T50.2X2	T50.2X3	T50.2X4	T50.2X5	T50.2X6
Cycrimine	T44.3X1	T44.3X2	T44.3X3	T44.3X4	T44.3X5	T44.3X6
Cyhalothrin	T60.1X1	T60.1X2	T60.1X3	T60.1X4	—	—
Cymarin	T46.0X1	T46.0X2	T46.0X3	T46.0X4	T46.0X5	T46.0X6
Cypermethrin	T60.1X1	T60.1X2	T60.1X3	T60.1X4	—	—
Cyphenothrin	T60.2X1	T60.2X2	T60.2X3	T60.2X4	—	—
Cyproheptadine	T45.0X1	T45.0X2	T45.0X3	T45.0X4	T45.0X5	T45.0X6
Cyproterone	T38.6X1	T38.6X2	T38.6X3	T38.6X4	T38.6X5	T38.6X6
Cysteamine	T50.6X1	T50.6X2	T50.6X3	T50.6X4	T50.6X5	T50.6X6
Cytarabine	T45.1X1	T45.1X2	T45.1X3	T45.1X4	T45.1X5	T45.1X6
Cytisus						
laburnum	T62.2X1	T62.2X2	T62.2X3	T62.2X4	—	—
scoparius	T62.2X1	T62.2X2	T62.2X3	T62.2X4	—	—
Cytochrome C	T47.5X1	T47.5X2	T47.5X3	T47.5X4	T47.5X5	T47.5X6
Cytomel	T38.1X1	T38.1X2	T38.1X3	T38.1X4	T38.1X5	T38.1X6
Cytosine arabinoside	T45.1X1	T45.1X2	T45.1X3	T45.1X4	T45.1X5	T45.1X6
Cytoxan	T45.1X1	T45.1X2	T45.1X3	T45.1X4	T45.1X5	T45.1X6
Cytozyme	T45.7X1	T45.7X2	T45.7X3	T45.7X4	T45.7X5	T45.7X6
2,4-D	T60.3X1	T60.3X2	T60.3X3	T60.3X4	—	—
D						
Dacarbazine	T45.1X1	T45.1X2	T45.1X3	T45.1X4	T45.1X5	T45.1X6
Dactinomycin	T45.1X1	T45.1X2	T45.1X3	T45.1X4	T45.1X5	T45.1X6
DADPS	T37.1X1	T37.1X2	T37.1X3	T37.1X4	T37.1X5	T37.1X6
Dakin's solution	T49.0X1	T49.0X2	T49.0X3	T49.0X4	T49.0X5	T49.0X6
Dalapon (sodium)	T60.3X1	T60.3X2	T60.3X3	T60.3X4		
Dalmane	T42.4X1	T42.4X2	T42.4X3	T42.4X4	T42.4X5	T42.4X6
Danazol	T38.6X1	T38.6X2	T38.6X3	T38.6X4	T38.6X5	T38.6X6
Danilone	T45.511	T45.512	T45.513	T45.514	T45.515	T45.516
Danthron	T47.2X1	T47.2X2	T47.2X3	T47.2X4	T47.2X5	T47.2X6
Dantrolene	T42.8X1	T42.8X2	T42.8X3	T42.8X4	T42.8X5	T42.8X6
Dantron	T47.2X1	T47.2X2	T47.2X3	T47.2X4	T47.2X5	T47.2X6
Daphne (gnidium) (mezereum)	T62.2X1	T62.2X2	T62.2X3	T62.2X4	—	—
berry	T62.1X1	T62.1X2	T62.1X3	T62.1X4	—	—
Dapsone	T37.1X1	T37.1X2	T37.1X3	T37.1X4	T37.1X5	T37.1X6
Daraprim	T37.2X1	T37.2X2	T37.2X3	T37.2X4	T37.2X5	T37.2X6
Darnel	T62.2X1	T62.2X2	T62.2X3	T62.2X4	—	—
Darvon	T39.8X1	T39.8X2	T39.8X3	T39.8X4	T39.8X5	T39.8X6
Daunomycin	T45.1X1	T45.1X2	T45.1X3	T45.1X4	T45.1X5	T45.1X6
Daunorubicin	T45.1X1	T45.1X2	T45.1X3	T45.1X4	T45.1X5	T45.1X6
DBI	T38.3X1	T38.3X2	T38.3X3	T38.3X4	T38.3X5	T38.3X6
D-Con	T60.91	T60.92	T60.93	T60.94	—	—
insecticide	T60.2X1	T60.2X2	T60.2X3	T60.2X4	—	—
rodenticide	T60.4X1	T60.4X2	T60.4X3	T60.4X4	—	—
DDAVP	T38.891	T38.892	T38.893	T38.894	T38.895	T38.896
DDE (bis(chlorophenyl) dichloroethylene)	T60.2X1	T60.2X2	T60.2X3	T60.2X4	—	—
DDS	T37.1X1	T37.1X2	T37.1X3	T37.1X4	T37.1X5	T37.1X6
DDT (dust)	T60.1X1	T60.1X2	T60.1X3	T60.1X4	—	—
Deadly nightshade—see also Belladonna	T62.2X1	T62.2X2	T62.2X3	T62.2X4	—	—
berry	T62.1X1	T62.1X2	T62.1X3	T62.1X4	—	—
Deamino-D-arginine vasopressin	T38.891	T38.892	T38.893	T38.894	T38.895	T38.896
Deanol (aceglumate)	T50.991	T50.992	T50.993	T50.994	T50.995	T50.996
Debrisoquine	T46.5X1	T46.5X2	T46.5X3	T46.5X4	T46.5X5	T46.5X6
Decaborane	T57.8X1	T57.8X2	T57.8X3	T57.8X4	—	—
fumes	T59.891	T59.892	T59.893	T59.894	—	—

Decadron - Dextromoramide

Substance	Poisoning, Accidental (unintentional)	Poisoning, Intentional self-harm	Poisoning, Assault	Poisoning, Undetermined	Adverse effect	Underdosing
Decadron	T38.0X1	T38.0X2	T38.0X3	T38.0X4	T38.0X5	T38.0X6
ENT agent	T49.6X1	T49.6X2	T49.6X3	T49.6X4	T49.6X5	T49.6X6
ophthalmic preparation	T49.5X1	T49.5X2	T49.5X3	T49.5X4	T49.5X5	T49.5X6
topical NEC	T49.0X1	T49.0X2	T49.0X3	T49.0X4	T49.0X5	T49.0X6
Decahydronaphthalene	T52.8X1	T52.8X2	T52.8X3	T52.8X4	—	—
Decalin	T52.8X1	T52.8X2	T52.8X3	T52.8X4	—	—
Decamethonium (bromide)	T48.1X1	T48.1X2	T48.1X3	T48.1X4	T48.1X5	T48.1X6
Decholin	T47.5X1	T47.5X2	T47.5X3	T47.5X4	T47.5X5	T47.5X6
Declomycin	T36.4X1	T36.4X2	T36.4X3	T36.4X4	T36.4X5	T36.4X6
Decongestant, nasal (mucosa)	T48.5X1	T48.5X2	T48.5X3	T48.5X4	T48.5X5	T48.5X6
combination	T48.5X1	T48.5X2	T48.5X3	T48.5X4	T48.5X5	T48.5X6
Deet	T60.8X1	T60.8X2	T60.8X3	T60.8X4	—	—
Deferoxamine	T45.8X1	T45.8X2	T45.8X3	T45.8X4	T45.8X5	T45.8X6
Deflazacort	T38.0X1	T38.0X2	T38.0X3	T38.0X4	T38.0X5	T38.0X6
Deglycyrrhizinized extract of licorice	T48.4X1	T48.4X2	T48.4X3	T48.4X4	T48.4X5	T48.4X6
Dehydrocholic acid	T47.5X1	T47.5X2	T47.5X3	T47.5X4	T47.5X5	T47.5X6
Dehydroemetine	T37.3X1	T37.3X2	T37.3X3	T37.3X4	T37.3X5	T37.3X6
Dekalin	T52.8X1	T52.8X2	T52.8X3	T52.8X4	—	—
Delalutin	T38.5X1	T38.5X2	T38.5X3	T38.5X4	T38.5X5	T38.5X6
Delorazepam	T42.4X1	T42.4X2	T42.4X3	T42.4X4	T42.4X5	T42.4X6
Delphinium	T62.2X1	T62.2X2	T62.2X3	T62.2X4	—	—
Deltamethrin	T60.1X1	T60.1X2	T60.1X3	T60.1X4	—	—
Deltasone	T38.0X1	T38.0X2	T38.0X3	T38.0X4	T38.0X5	T38.0X6
Deltra	T38.0X1	T38.0X2	T38.0X3	T38.0X4	T38.0X5	T38.0X6
Delvinal	T42.3X1	T42.3X2	T42.3X3	T42.3X4	T42.3X5	T42.3X6
Demecarium (bromide)	T49.5X1	T49.5X2	T49.5X3	T49.5X4	T49.5X5	T49.5X6
Demeclocycline	T36.4X1	T36.4X2	T36.4X3	T36.4X4	T36.4X5	T36.4X6
Demecolcine	T45.1X1	T45.1X2	T45.1X3	T45.1X4	T45.1X5	T45.1X6
Demegestone	T38.5X1	T38.5X2	T38.5X3	T38.5X4	T38.5X5	T38.5X6
Demelanizing agents	T49.8X1	T49.8X2	T49.8X3	T49.8X4	T49.8X5	T49.8X6
Demephion O and S	T60.0X1	T60.0X2	T60.0X3	T60.0X4		
Demerol	T40.2X1	T40.2X2	T40.2X3	T40.2X4	T40.2X5	T40.2X6
Demethylchlortetracycline	T36.4X1	T36.4X2	T36.4X3	T36.4X4	T36.4X5	T36.4X6
Demethyltetracycline	T36.4X1	T36.4X2	T36.4X3	T36.4X4	T36.4X5	T36.4X6
Demeton O and S	T60.0X1	T60.0X2	T60.0X3	T60.0X4		
Demulcent (external)	T49.3X1	T49.3X2	T49.3X3	T49.3X4	T49.3X5	T49.3X6
specified NEC	T49.3X1	T49.3X2	T49.3X3	T49.3X4	T49.3X5	T49.3X6
Demulen	T38.4X1	T38.4X2	T38.4X3	T38.4X4	T38.4X5	T38.4X6
Denatured alcohol	T51.0X1	T51.0X2	T51.0X3	T51.0X4		
Dendrid	T49.5X1	T49.5X2	T49.5X3	T49.5X4	T49.5X5	T49.5X6
Dental drug, topical application NEC	T49.7X1	T49.7X2	T49.7X3	T49.7X4	T49.7X5	T49.7X6
Dentifrice	T49.7X1	T49.7X2	T49.7X3	T49.7X4	T49.7X5	T49.7X6
Deodorant spray (feminine hygiene)	T49.8X1	T49.8X2	T49.8X3	T49.8X4	T49.8X5	T49.8X6
Deoxycortone	T50.0X1	T50.0X2	T50.0X3	T50.0X4	T50.0X5	T50.0X6
2-Deoxy-5-fluorouridine	T45.1X1	T45.1X2	T45.1X3	T45.1X4	T45.1X5	T45.1X6
5-Deoxy-5-fluorouridine	T45.1X1	T45.1X2	T45.1X3	T45.1X4	T45.1X5	T45.1X6
Deoxyribonuclease (pancreatic)	T45.3X1	T45.3X2	T45.3X3	T45.3X4	T45.3X5	T45.3X6
Depilatory	T49.4X1	T49.4X2	T49.4X3	T49.4X4	T49.4X5	T49.4X6
Deprenalin	T42.8X1	T42.8X2	T42.8X3	T42.8X4	T42.8X5	T42.8X6
Deprenyl	T42.8X1	T42.8X2	T42.8X3	T42.8X4	T42.8X5	T42.8X6
Depressant, appetite	T50.5X1	T50.5X2	T50.5X3	T50.5X4	T50.5X5	T50.5X6
Depressant						
appetite (central)	T50.5X1	T50.5X2	T50.5X3	T50.5X4	T50.5X5	T50.5X6
cardiac	T46.2X1	T46.2X2	T46.2X3	T46.2X4	T46.2X5	T46.2X6

Substance	Poisoning, Accidental (unintentional)	Poisoning, Intentional self-harm	Poisoning, Assault	Poisoning, Undetermined	Adverse effect	Underdosing
Depressant — *continued*						
central nervous system (anesthetic)—*see also Central nervous system, depressants*	T42.71	T42.72	T42.73	T42.74	T42.75	T42.76
general anesthetic	T41.201	T41.202	T41.203	T41.204	T41.205	T41.206
muscle tone	T42.8X1	T42.8X2	T42.8X3	T42.8X4	T42.8X5	T42.8X6
muscle tone, central	T42.8X1	T42.8X2	T42.8X3	T42.8X4	T42.8X5	T42.8X6
psychotherapeutic	T43.501	T43.502	T43.503	T43.504	T43.505	T43.506
Deptropine	T45.0X1	T45.0X2	T45.0X3	T45.0X4	T45.0X5	T45.0X6
Dequalinium (chloride)	T49.0X1	T49.0X2	T49.0X3	T49.0X4	T49.0X5	T49.0X6
Derris root	T60.2X1	T60.2X2	T60.2X3	T60.2X4	—	—
Deserpidine	T46.5X1	T46.5X2	T46.5X3	T46.5X4	T46.5X5	T46.5X6
Desferrioxamine	T45.8X1	T45.8X2	T45.8X3	T45.8X4	T45.8X5	T45.8X6
Desipramine	T43.011	T43.012	T43.013	T43.014	T43.015	T43.016
Deslanoside	T46.0X1	T46.0X2	T46.0X3	T46.0X4	T46.0X5	T46.0X6
Desloughing agent	T49.4X1	T49.4X2	T49.4X3	T49.4X4	T49.4X5	T49.4X6
Desmethylimipramine	T43.011	T43.012	T43.013	T43.014	T43.015	T43.016
Desmopressin	T38.891	T38.892	T38.893	T38.894	T38.895	T38.896
Desocodeine	T40.2X1	T40.2X2	T40.2X3	T40.2X4	T40.2X5	T40.2X6
Desogestrel	T38.5X1	T38.5X2	T38.5X3	T38.5X4	T38.5X5	T38.5X6
Desomorphine	T40.2X1	T40.2X2	T40.2X3	T40.2X4	—	—
Desonide	T49.0X1	T49.0X2	T49.0X3	T49.0X4	T49.0X5	T49.0X6
Desoximetasone	T49.0X1	T49.0X2	T49.0X3	T49.0X4	T49.0X5	T49.0X6
Desoxycorticosteroid	T50.0X1	T50.0X2	T50.0X3	T50.0X4	T50.0X5	T50.0X6
Desoxycortone	T50.0X1	T50.0X2	T50.0X3	T50.0X4	T50.0X5	T50.0X6
Desoxyephedrine	T43.621	T43.622	T43.623	T43.624	T43.625	T43.626
Detaxtran	T46.6X1	T46.6X2	T46.6X3	T46.6X4	T46.6X5	T46.6X6
Detergent	T49.2X1	T49.2X2	T49.2X3	T49.2X4	T49.2X5	T49.2X6
external medication	T49.2X1	T49.2X2	T49.2X3	T49.2X4	T49.2X5	T49.2X6
local	T49.2X1	T49.2X2	T49.2X3	T49.2X4	T49.2X5	T49.2X6
medicinal	T49.2X1	T49.2X2	T49.2X3	T49.2X4	T49.2X5	T49.2X6
nonmedicinal	T55.1X1	T55.1X2	T55.1X3	T55.1X4	—	—
specified NEC	T55.1X1	T55.1X2	T55.1X3	T55.1X4	—	—
Deterrent, alcohol	T50.6X1	T50.6X2	T50.6X3	T50.6X4	T50.6X5	T50.6X6
Detoxifying agent	T50.6X1	T50.6X2	T50.6X3	T50.6X4	T50.6X5	T50.6X6
Detrothyronine	T38.1X1	T38.1X2	T38.1X3	T38.1X4	T38.1X5	T38.1X6
Dettol (external medication)	T49.0X1	T49.0X2	T49.0X3	T49.0X4	T49.0X5	T49.0X6
Dexamethasone	T38.0X1	T38.0X2	T38.0X3	T38.0X4	T38.0X5	T38.0X6
ENT agent	T49.6X1	T49.6X2	T49.6X3	T49.6X4	T49.6X5	T49.6X6
ophthalmic preparation	T49.5X1	T49.5X2	T49.5X3	T49.5X4	T49.5X5	T49.5X6
topical NEC	T49.0X1	T49.0X2	T49.0X3	T49.0X4	T49.0X5	T49.0X6
Dexamfetamine	T43.621	T43.622	T43.623	T43.624	T43.625	T43.626
Dexamphetamine	T43.621	T43.622	T43.623	T43.624	T43.625	T43.626
Dexbrompheniramine	T45.0X1	T45.0X2	T45.0X3	T45.0X4	T45.0X5	T45.0X6
Dexchlorpheniramine	T45.0X1	T45.0X2	T45.0X3	T45.0X4	T45.0X5	T45.0X6
Dexedrine	T43.621	T43.622	T43.623	T43.624	T43.625	T43.626
Dexetimide	T44.3X1	T44.3X2	T44.3X3	T44.3X4	T44.3X5	T44.3X6
Dexfenfluramine	T50.5X1	T50.5X2	T50.5X3	T50.5X4	T50.5X5	T50.5X6
Dexpanthenol	T45.2X1	T45.2X2	T45.2X3	T45.2X4	T45.2X5	T45.2X6
Dextran (40) (70) (150)	T45.8X1	T45.8X2	T45.8X3	T45.8X4	T45.8X5	T45.8X6
Dextriferron	T45.4X1	T45.4X2	T45.4X3	T45.4X4	T45.4X5	T45.4X6
Dextro calcium pantothenate	T45.2X1	T45.2X2	T45.2X3	T45.2X4	T45.2X5	T45.2X6
Dextro pantothenyl alcohol	T45.2X1	T45.2X2	T45.2X3	T45.2X4	T45.2X5	T45.2X6
Dextroamphetamine	T43.621	T43.622	T43.623	T43.624	T43.625	T43.626
Dextromethorphan	T48.3X1	T48.3X2	T48.3X3	T48.3X4	T48.3X5	T48.3X6
Dextromoramide	T40.4X1	T40.4X2	T40.4X3	T40.4X4	—	—
topical	T49.8X1	T49.8X2	T49.8X3	T49.8X4	T49.8X5	T49.8X6

Dextropropoxyphene - Diethylene

Substance	Poisoning, Accidental (unintentional)	Poisoning, Intentional self-harm	Poisoning, Assault	Poisoning, Undetermined	Adverse effect	Underdosing
Dextropropoxyphene	T40.4X1	T40.4X2	T40.4X3	T40.4X4	T40.4X5	T40.4X6
Dextrorphan	T40.2X1	T40.2X2	T40.2X3	T40.2X4	T40.2X5	T40.2X6
Dextrose	T50.3X1	T50.3X2	T50.3X3	T50.3X4	T50.3X5	T50.3X6
concentrated solution, intravenous	T46.8X1	T46.8X2	T46.8X3	T46.8X4	T46.8X5	T46.8X6
Dextrothyroxin	T38.1X1	T38.1X2	T38.1X3	T38.1X4	T38.1X5	T38.1X6
Dextrothyroxine sodium	T38.1X1	T38.1X2	T38.1X3	T38.1X4	T38.1X5	T38.1X6
DFP	T44.0X1	T44.0X2	T44.0X3	T44.0X4	T44.0X5	T44.0X6
DHE	T37.3X1	T37.3X2	T37.3X3	T37.3X4	T37.3X5	T37.3X6
45	T46.5X1	T46.5X2	T46.5X3	T46.5X4	T46.5X5	T46.5X6
Diabinese	T38.3X1	T38.3X2	T38.3X3	T38.3X4	T38.3X5	T38.3X6
Diacetone alcohol	T52.4X1	T52.4X2	T52.4X3	T52.4X4	—	—
Diacetyl monoxime	T50.991	T50.992	T50.993	T50.994	—	—
Diacetylmorphine	T40.1X1	T40.1X2	T40.1X3	T40.1X4	—	—
Diachylon plaster	T49.4X1	T49.4X2	T49.4X3	T49.4X4	T49.4X5	T49.4X6
Diaethylstilboestrolum	T38.5X1	T38.5X2	T38.5X3	T38.5X4	T38.5X5	T38.5X6
Diagnostic agent NEC	T50.8X1	T50.8X2	T50.8X3	T50.8X4	T50.8X5	T50.8X6
Dial (soap)	T49.2X1	T49.2X2	T49.2X3	T49.2X4	T49.2X5	T49.2X6
sedative	T42.3X1	T42.3X2	T42.3X3	T42.3X4	T42.3X5	T42.3X6
Dialkyl carbonate	T52.91	T52.92	T52.93	T52.94	—	—
Diallylbarbituric acid	T42.3X1	T42.3X2	T42.3X3	T42.3X4	T42.3X5	T42.3X6
Diallymal	T42.3X1	T42.3X2	T42.3X3	T42.3X4	T42.3X5	T42.3X6
Dialysis solution (intraperitoneal)	T50.3X1	T50.3X2	T50.3X3	T50.3X4	T50.3X5	T50.3X6
Diaminodiphenylsulfone	T37.1X1	T37.1X2	T37.1X3	T37.1X4	T37.1X5	T37.1X6
Diamorphine	T40.1X1	T40.1X2	T40.1X3	T40.1X4	—	—
Diamox	T50.2X1	T50.2X2	T50.2X3	T50.2X4	T50.2X5	T50.2X6
Diamthazole	T49.0X1	T49.0X2	T49.0X3	T49.0X4	T49.0X5	T49.0X6
Dianthone	T47.2X1	T47.2X2	T47.2X3	T47.2X4	T47.2X5	T47.2X6
Diaphenylsulfone	T37.0X1	T37.0X2	T37.0X3	T37.0X4	T37.0X5	T37.0X6
Diasone (sodium)	T37.1X1	T37.1X2	T37.1X3	T37.1X4	T37.1X5	T37.1X6
Diastase	T47.5X1	T47.5X2	T47.5X3	T47.5X4	T47.5X5	T47.5X6
Diatrizoate	T50.8X1	T50.8X2	T50.8X3	T50.8X4	T50.8X5	T50.8X6
Diazepam	T42.4X1	T42.4X2	T42.4X3	T42.4X4	T42.4X5	T42.4X6
Diazinon	T60.0X1	T60.0X2	T60.0X3	T60.0X4	—	—
Diazomethane (gas)	T59.891	T59.892	T59.893	T59.894	—	—
Diazoxide	T46.5X1	T46.5X2	T46.5X3	T46.5X4	T46.5X5	T46.5X6
Dibekacin	T36.5X1	T36.5X2	T36.5X3	T36.5X4	T36.5X5	T36.5X6
Dibenamine	T44.6X1	T44.6X2	T44.6X3	T44.6X4	T44.6X5	T44.6X6
Dibenzepin	T43.011	T43.012	T43.013	T43.014	T43.015	T43.016
Dibenzheptropine	T45.0X1	T45.0X2	T45.0X3	T45.0X4	T45.0X5	T45.0X6
Dibenzyline	T44.6X1	T44.6X2	T44.6X3	T44.6X4	T44.6X5	T44.6X6
Diborane (gas)	T59.891	T59.892	T59.893	T59.894	—	—
Dibromochloropropane	T60.8X1	T60.8X2	T60.8X3	T60.8X4	—	—
Dibromodulcitol	T45.1X1	T45.1X2	T45.1X3	T45.1X4	T45.1X5	T45.1X6
Dibromoethane	T53.6X1	T53.6X2	T53.6X3	T53.6X4	—	—
Dibromomannitol	T45.1X1	T45.1X2	T45.1X3	T45.1X4	T45.1X5	T45.1X6
Dibromopropamidine isethionate	T49.0X1	T49.0X2	T49.0X3	T49.0X4	T49.0X5	T49.0X6
Dibrompropamidine	T49.0X1	T49.0X2	T49.0X3	T49.0X4	T49.0X5	T49.0X6
Dibucaine	T41.3X1	T41.3X2	T41.3X3	T41.3X4	T41.3X5	T41.3X6
topical (surface)	T41.3X1	T41.3X2	T41.3X3	T41.3X4	T41.3X5	T41.3X6
Dibunate sodium	T48.3X1	T48.3X2	T48.3X3	T48.3X4	T48.3X5	T48.3X6
Dibutoline sulfate	T44.3X1	T44.3X2	T44.3X3	T44.3X4	T44.3X5	T44.3X6
Dicamba	T60.3X1	T60.3X2	T60.3X3	T60.3X4	—	—
Dicapthon	T60.0X1	T60.0X2	T60.0X3	T60.0X4	—	—
Dichlobenil	T60.3X1	T60.3X2	T60.3X3	T60.3X4	—	—
Dichlone	T60.3X1	T60.3X2	T60.3X3	T60.3X4	—	—
Dichloralphenozone	T42.6X1	T42.6X2	T42.6X3	T42.6X4	T42.6X5	T42.6X6
Dichlorbenzidine	T65.3X1	T65.3X2	I65.3X3	T65.3X4	—	—

Substance	Poisoning, Accidental (unintentional)	Poisoning, Intentional self-harm	Poisoning, Assault	Poisoning, Undetermined	Adverse effect	Underdosing
Dichlorhydrin	T52.8X1	T52.8X2	T52.8X3	T52.8X4	—	—
Dichlorhydroxyquinoline	T37.8X1	T37.8X2	T37.8X3	T37.8X4	T37.8X5	T37.8X6
Dichlorobenzene	T53.7X1	T53.7X2	T53.7X3	T53.7X4	—	—
Dichlorobenzyl alcohol	T49.6X1	T49.6X2	T49.6X3	T49.6X4	T49.6X5	T49.6X6
Dichlorodifluoromethane	T53.5X1	T53.5X2	T53.5X3	T53.5X4	—	—
Dichloroethane	T52.8X1	T52.8X2	T52.8X3	T52.8X4	—	—
Sym-Dichloroethyl ether	T53.6X1	T53.6X2	T53.6X3	T53.6X4	—	—
Dichloroethyl sulfide, not in war	T59.891	T59.892	T59.893	T59.894	—	—
Dichloroethylene	T53.6X1	T53.6X2	T53.6X3	T53.6X4	—	—
Dichloroformoxine, not in war	T59.891	T59.892	T59.893	T59.894	—	—
Dichlorohydrin, alpha-dichlorohydrin	T52.8X1	T52.8X2	T52.8X3	T52.8X4	—	—
Dichloromethane (solvent)	T53.4X1	T53.4X2	T53.4X3	T53.4X4	—	—
vapor	T53.4X1	T53.4X2	T53.4X3	T53.4X4	—	—
Dichloronaphthoquinone	T60.3X1	T60.3X2	T60.3X3	T60.3X4	—	—
Dichlorophen	T37.4X1	T37.4X2	T37.4X3	T37.4X4	T37.4X5	T37.4X6
2,4-Dichlorophenoxyacetic acid	T60.3X1	T60.3X2	T60.3X3	T60.3X4	—	—
Dichloropropene	T60.3X1	T60.3X2	T60.3X3	T60.3X4	—	—
Dichloropropionic acid	T60.3X1	T60.3X2	T60.3X3	T60.3X4	—	—
Dichlorphenamide	T50.2X1	T50.2X2	T50.2X3	T50.2X4	T50.2X5	T50.2X6
Dichlorvos	T60.0X1	T60.0X2	T60.0X3	T60.0X4	—	—
Diclofenac	T39.391	T39.392	T39.393	T39.394	T39.395	T39.396
Diclofenamide	T50.2X1	T50.2X2	T50.2X3	T50.2X4	T50.2X5	T50.2X6
Diclofensine	T43.291	T43.292	T43.293	T43.294	T43.295	T43.296
Diclonixine	I39.8X1	T39.8X2	T39.8X3	T39.8X4	T39.8X5	T39.8X6
Dicloxacillin	T36.0X1	T36.0X2	T36.0X3	T36.0X4	T36.0X5	T36.0X6
Dicophane	T49.0X1	T49.0X2	T49.0X3	T49.0X4	T49.0X5	T49.0X6
Dicoumarol, dicoumarin, dicumarol	T45.511	T45.512	T45.513	T45.514	T45.515	T45.516
Dicrotophos	T60.0X1	T60.0X2	T60.0X3	T60.0X4	—	—
Dicyanogen (gas)	T65.0X1	T65.0X2	T65.0X3	T65.0X4	—	—
Dicyclomine	T44.3X1	T44.3X2	T44.3X3	T44.3X4	T44.3X5	T44.3X6
Dicycloverine	T44.3X1	T44.3X2	T44.3X3	T44.3X4	T44.3X5	T44.3X6
Dideoxycytidine	T37.5X1	T37.5X2	T37.5X3	T37.5X4	T37.5X5	T37.5X6
Dideoxyinosine	T37.5X1	T37.5X2	T37.5X3	T37.5X4	T37.5X5	T37.5X6
Dieldrin (vapor)	T60.1X1	T60.1X2	T60.1X3	T60.1X4	—	—
Diemal	T42.3X1	T42.3X2	T42.3X3	T42.3X4	T42.3X5	T42.3X6
Dienestrol	T38.5X1	T38.5X2	T38.5X3	T38.5X4	T38.5X5	T38.5X6
Dienoestrol	T38.5X1	T38.5X2	T38.5X3	T38.5X4	T38.5X5	T38.5X6
Dietetic drug NEC	T50.901	T50.902	T50.903	T50.904	T50.905	T50.906
Diethazine	T42.8X1	T42.8X2	T42.8X3	T42.8X4	T42.8X5	T42.8X6
Diethyl						
barbituric acid	T42.3X1	T42.3X2	T42.3X3	T42.3X4	T42.3X5	T42.3X6
carbamazine	T37.4X1	T37.4X2	T37.4X3	T37.4X4	T37.4X5	T37.4X6
carbinol	T51.3X1	T51.3X2	T51.3X3	T51.3X4	—	—
carbonate	T52.8X1	T52.8X2	T52.8X3	T52.8X4	—	—
ether (vapor)—see also ether	T41.0X1	T41.0X2	T41.0X3	T41.0X4	T41.0X5	T41.0X6
oxide	T52.8X1	T52.8X2	T52.8X3	T52.8X4	—	—
propion	T50.5X1	T50.5X2	T50.5X3	T50.5X4	T50.5X5	T50.5X6
stilbestrol	T38.5X1	T38.5X2	T38.5X3	T38.5X4	T38.5X5	T38.5X6
toluamide (nonmedicinal)	T60.8X1	T60.8X2	T60.8X3	T60.8X4	—	—
medicinal	T49.3X1	T49.3X2	T49.3X3	T49.3X4	T49.3X5	T49.3X6
Diethylcarbamazine	T37.4X1	T37.4X2	T37.4X3	T37.4X4	T37.4X5	T37.4X6
Diethylene						

Substance	Poisoning, Accidental (unintentional)	Poisoning, Intentional self-harm	Poisoning, Assault	Poisoning, Undetermined	Adverse effect	Underdosing
Diethylene — *continued*						
dioxide	T52.8X1	T52.8X2	T52.8X3	T52.8X4	—	—
glycol (monoacetate) (monobutyl ether) (monoethyl ether)	T52.3X1	T52.3X2	T52.3X3	T52.3X4	—	—
Diethylhexylphthalate	T65.891	T65.892	T65.893	T65.894	—	—
Diethylpropion	T50.5X1	T50.5X2	T50.5X3	T50.5X4	T50.5X5	T50.5X6
Diethylstilbestrol	T38.5X1	T38.5X2	T38.5X3	T38.5X4	T38.5X5	T38.5X6
Diethylstilboestrol	T38.5X1	T38.5X2	T38.5X3	T38.5X4	T38.5X5	T38.5X6
Diethylsulfone-diethylmethane	T42.6X1	T42.6X2	T42.6X3	T42.6X4	T42.6X5	T42.6X6
Diethyltoluamide	T49.0X1	T49.0X2	T49.0X3	T49.0X4	T49.0X5	T49.0X6
Diethyltryptamine (DET)	T40.991	T40.992	T40.993	T40.994	—	—
Difebarbamate	T42.3X1	T42.3X2	T42.3X3	T42.3X4	T42.3X5	T42.3X6
Difencloxazine	T40.2X1	T40.2X2	T40.2X3	T40.2X4	T40.2X5	T40.2X6
Difenidol	T45.0X1	T45.0X2	T45.0X3	T45.0X4	T45.0X5	T45.0X6
Difenoxin	T47.6X1	T47.6X2	T47.6X3	T47.6X4	T47.6X5	T47.6X6
Difetarsone	T37.3X1	T37.3X2	T37.3X3	T37.3X4	T37.3X5	T37.3X6
Diffusin	T45.3X1	T45.3X2	T45.3X3	T45.3X4	T45.3X5	T45.3X6
Diflorasone	T49.0X1	T49.0X2	T49.0X3	T49.0X4	T49.0X5	T49.0X6
Diflos	T44.0X1	T44.0X2	T44.0X3	T44.0X4	T44.0X5	T44.0X6
Diflubenzuron	T60.1X1	T60.1X2	T60.1X3	T60.1X4	—	—
Diflucortolone	T49.0X1	T49.0X2	T49.0X3	T49.0X4	T49.0X5	T49.0X6
Diflunisal	T39.091	T39.092	T39.093	T39.094	T39.095	T39.096
Difluoromethyldopa	T42.8X1	T42.8X2	T42.8X3	T42.8X4	T42.8X5	T42.8X6
Difluorophate	T44.0X1	T44.0X2	T44.0X3	T44.0X4	T44.0X5	T44.0X6
Digestant NEC	T47.5X1	T47.5X2	T47.5X3	T47.5X4	T47.5X5	T47.5X6
Digitalin (e)	T46.0X1	T46.0X2	T46.0X3	T46.0X4	T46.0X5	T46.0X6
Digitalis (leaf) (glycoside)	T46.0X1	T46.0X2	T46.0X3	T46.0X4	T46.0X5	T46.0X6
lanata	T46.0X1	T46.0X2	T46.0X3	T46.0X4	T46.0X5	T46.0X6
purpurea	T46.0X1	T46.0X2	T46.0X3	T46.0X4	T46.0X5	T46.0X6
Digitoxin	T46.0X1	T46.0X2	T46.0X3	T46.0X4	T46.0X5	T46.0X6
Digitoxose	T46.0X1	T46.0X2	T46.0X3	T46.0X4	T46.0X5	T46.0X6
Digoxin	T46.0X1	T46.0X2	T46.0X3	T46.0X4	T46.0X5	T46.0X6
Digoxine	T46.0X1	T46.0X2	T46.0X3	T46.0X4	T46.0X5	T46.0X6
Dihydralazine	T46.5X1	T46.5X2	T46.5X3	T46.5X4	T46.5X5	T46.5X6
Dihydrazine	T46.5X1	T46.5X2	T46.5X3	T46.5X4	T46.5X5	T46.5X6
Dihydrocodeine	T40.2X1	T40.2X2	T40.2X3	T40.2X4	T40.2X5	T40.2X6
Dihydrocodeinone	T40.2X1	T40.2X2	T40.2X3	T40.2X4	T40.2X5	T40.2X6
Dihydroergocornine	T46.7X1	T46.7X2	T46.7X3	T46.7X4	T46.7X5	T46.7X6
Dihydroergocristine (mesilate)	T46.7X1	T46.7X2	T46.7X3	T46.7X4	T46.7X5	T46.7X6
Dihydroergokryptine	T46.7X1	T46.7X2	T46.7X3	T46.7X4	T46.7X5	T46.7X6
Dihydroergotamine	T46.5X1	T46.5X2	T46.5X3	T46.5X4	T46.5X5	T46.5X6
Dihydroergotoxine	T46.7X1	T46.7X2	T46.7X3	T46.7X4	T46.7X5	T46.7X6
mesilate	T46.7X1	T46.7X2	T46.7X3	T46.7X4	T46.7X5	T46.7X6
Dihydrohydroxycodeinone	T40.2X1	T40.2X2	T40.2X3	T40.2X4	T40.2X5	T40.2X6
Dihydrohydroxymorphinone	T40.2X1	T40.2X2	T40.2X3	T40.2X4	T40.2X5	T40.2X6
Dihydroisocodeine	T40.2X1	T40.2X2	T40.2X3	T40.2X4	T40.2X5	T40.2X6
Dihydromorphine	T40.2X1	T40.2X2	T40.2X3	T40.2X4	—	—
Dihydromorphinone	T40.2X1	T40.2X2	T40.2X3	T40.2X4	T40.2X5	T40.2X6
Dihydrostreptomycin	T36.5X1	T36.5X2	T36.5X3	T36.5X4	T36.5X5	T36.5X6
Dihydrotachysterol	T45.2X1	T45.2X2	T45.2X3	T45.2X4	T45.2X5	T45.2X6
Dihydroxyaluminum aminoacetate	T47.1X1	T47.1X2	T47.1X3	T47.1X4	T47.1X5	T47.1X6
Dihydroxyaluminum sodium carbonate	T47.1X1	T47.1X2	T47.1X3	T47.1X4	T47.1X5	T47.1X6
Dihydroxyanthraquinone	T47.2X1	T47.2X2	T47.2X3	T47.2X4	T47.2X5	T47.2X6
Dihydroxycodeinone	T40.2X1	T40.2X2	T40.2X3	T40.2X4	T40.2X5	T40.2X6
Dihydroxypropyl theophylline	T50.2X1	T50.2X2	T50.2X3	T50.2X4	T50.2X5	T50.2X6
Diiodohydroxyquin	T37.8X1	T37.8X2	T37.8X3	T37.8X4	T37.8X5	T37.8X6
topical	T49.0X1	T49.0X2	T49.0X3	T49.0X4	T49.0X5	T49.0X6
Diiodohydroxyquinoline	T37.8X1	T37.8X2	T37.8X3	T37.8X4	T37.8X5	T37.8X6
Diiodotyrosine	T38.2X1	T38.2X2	T38.2X3	T38.2X4	T38.2X5	T38.2X6
Diisopromine	T44.3X1	T44.3X2	T44.3X3	T44.3X4	T44.3X5	T44.3X6
Diisopropylamine	T46.3X1	T46.3X2	T46.3X3	T46.3X4	T46.3X5	T46.3X6
Diisopropylfluorophos-phonate	T44.0X1	T44.0X2	T44.0X3	T44.0X4	T44.0X5	T44.0X6
Dilantin	T42.0X1	T42.0X2	T42.0X3	T42.0X4	T42.0X5	T42.0X6
Dilaudid	T40.2X1	T40.2X2	T40.2X3	T40.2X4	T40.2X5	T40.2X6
Dilazep	T46.3X1	T46.3X2	T46.3X3	T46.3X4	T46.3X5	T46.3X6
Dill	T47.5X1	T47.5X2	T47.5X3	T47.5X4	T47.5X5	T47.5X6
Diloxanide	T37.3X1	T37.3X2	T37.3X3	T37.3X4	T37.3X5	T37.3X6
Diltiazem	T46.1X1	T46.1X2	T46.1X3	T46.1X4	T46.1X5	T46.1X6
Dimazole	T49.0X1	T49.0X2	T49.0X3	T49.0X4	T49.0X5	T49.0X6
Dimefline	T50.7X1	T50.7X2	T50.7X3	T50.7X4	T50.7X5	T50.7X6
Dimefox	T60.0X1	T60.0X2	T60.0X3	T60.0X4	—	—
Dimemorfan	T48.3X1	T48.3X2	T48.3X3	T48.3X4	T48.3X5	T48.3X6
Dimenhydrinate	T45.0X1	T45.0X2	T45.0X3	T45.0X4	T45.0X5	T45.0X6
Dimercaprol (British anti-lewisite)	T45.8X1	T45.8X2	T45.8X3	T45.8X4	T45.8X5	T45.8X6
Dimercaptopropanol	T45.8X1	T45.8X2	T45.8X3	T45.8X4	T45.8X5	T45.8X6
Dimestrol	T38.5X1	T38.5X2	T38.5X3	T38.5X4	T38.5X5	T38.5X6
Dimetane	T45.0X1	T45.0X2	T45.0X3	T45.0X4	T45.0X5	T45.0X6
Dimethicone	T47.1X1	T47.1X2	T47.1X3	T47.1X4	T47.1X5	T47.1X6
Dimethindene	T45.0X1	T45.0X2	T45.0X3	T45.0X4	T45.0X5	T45.0X6
Dimethisoquin	T49.1X1	T49.1X2	T49.1X3	T49.1X4	T49.1X5	T49.1X6
Dimethisterone	T38.5X1	T38.5X2	T38.5X3	T38.5X4	T38.5X5	T38.5X6
Dimethoate	T60.0X1	T60.0X2	T60.0X3	T60.0X4	—	—
Dimethocaine	T41.3X1	T41.3X2	T41.3X3	T41.3X4	T41.3X5	T41.3X6
Dimethoxanate	T48.3X1	T48.3X2	T48.3X3	T48.3X4	T48.3X5	T48.3X6
Dimethyl						
arsine, arsinic acid	T57.0X1	T57.0X2	T57.0X3	T57.0X4		
carbinol	T51.2X1	T51.2X2	T51.2X3	T51.2X4		
carbonate	T52.8X1	T52.8X2	T52.8X3	T52.8X4	—	—
diguanide	T38.3X1	T38.3X2	T38.3X3	T38.3X4	T38.3X5	T38.3X6
ketone	T52.4X1	T52.4X2	T52.4X3	T52.4X4		
vapor	T52.4X1	T52.4X2	T52.4X3	T52.4X4		
meperidine	T40.2X1	T40.2X2	T40.2X3	T40.2X4	T40.2X5	T40.2X6
parathion	T60.0X1	T60.0X2	T60.0X3	T60.0X4		
phthlate	T49.3X1	T49.3X2	T49.3X3	T49.3X4	T49.3X5	T49.3X6
polysiloxane	T47.8X1	T47.8X2	T47.8X3	T47.8X4	T47.8X5	T47.8X6
sulfate (fumes)	T59.891	T59.892	T59.893	T59.894		
liquid	T65.891	T65.892	T65.893	T65.894		
sulfoxide (nonmedicinal)	T52.8X1	T52.8X2	T52.8X3	T52.8X4		
medicinal	T49.4X1	T49.4X2	T49.4X3	T49.4X4	T49.4X5	T49.4X6
tryptamine	T40.991	T40.992	T40.993	T40.994	—	—
tubocurarine	T48.1X1	T48.1X2	T48.1X3	T48.1X4	T48.1X5	T48.1X6
Dimethylamine sulfate	T49.4X1	T49.4X2	T49.4X3	T49.4X4	T49.4X5	T49.4X6
Dimethylformamide	T52.8X1	T52.8X2	T52.8X3	T52.8X4		
Dimethyltubocurarinium chloride	T48.1X1	T48.1X2	T48.1X3	T48.1X4	T48.1X5	T48.1X6
Dimeticone	T47.1X1	T47.1X2	T47.1X3	T47.1X4	T47.1X5	T47.1X6
Dimetilan	T60.0X1	T60.0X2	T60.0X3	T60.0X4	—	—
Dimetindene	T45.0X1	T45.0X2	T45.0X3	T45.0X4	T45.0X5	T45.0X6
Dimetotiazine	T43.3X1	T43.3X2	T43.3X3	T43.3X4	T43.3X5	T43.3X6
Dimorpholamine	T50.7X1	T50.7X2	T50.7X3	T50.7X4	T50.7X5	T50.7X6
Dimoxyline	T46.3X1	T46.3X2	T46.3X3	T46.3X4	T46.3X5	T46.3X6
Dinitrobenzene	T65.3X1	T65.3X2	T65.3X3	T65.3X4	—	—
vapor	T59.891	T59.892	T59.893	T59.894	—	—

Substance	Poisoning, Accidental (unintentional)	Poisoning, Intentional self-harm	Poisoning, Assault	Poisoning, Undetermined	Adverse effect	Underdosing
Dinitrobenzol	T65.3X1	T65.3X2	T65.3X3	T65.3X4	—	—
vapor	T59.891	T59.892	T59.893	T59.894	—	—
Dinitrobutylphenol	T65.3X1	T65.3X2	T65.3X3	T65.3X4	—	—
Dinitro (-ortho-)cresol (pesticide) (spray)	T65.3X1	T65.3X2	T65.3X3	T65.3X4	—	—
Dinitrocyclohexylphenol	T65.3X1	T65.3X2	T65.3X3	T65.3X4	—	—
Dinitrophenol	T65.3X1	T65.3X2	T65.3X3	T65.3X4	—	—
Dinoprost	T48.0X1	T48.0X2	T48.0X3	T48.0X4	T48.0X5	T48.0X6
Dinoprostone	T48.0X1	T48.0X2	T48.0X3	T48.0X4	T48.0X5	T48.0X6
Dinoseb	T60.3X1	T60.3X2	T60.3X3	T60.3X4	—	—
Dioctyl sulfosuccinate (calcium) (sodium)	T47.4X1	T47.4X2	T47.4X3	T47.4X4	T47.4X5	T47.4X6
Diodone	T50.8X1	T50.8X2	T50.8X3	T50.8X4	T50.8X5	T50.8X6
Diodoquin	T37.8X1	T37.8X2	T37.8X3	T37.8X4	T37.8X5	T37.8X6
Dionin	T40.2X1	T40.2X2	T40.2X3	T40.2X4	T40.2X5	T40.2X6
Diosmin	T46.991	T46.992	T46.993	T46.994	T46.995	T46.996
Dioxane	T52.8X1	T52.8X2	T52.8X3	T52.8X4	—	—
Dioxathion	T60.0X1	T60.0X2	T60.0X3	T60.0X4	—	—
Dioxin	T53.7X1	T53.7X2	T53.7X3	T53.7X4	—	—
Dioxopromethazine	T43.3X1	T43.3X2	T43.3X3	T43.3X4	T43.3X5	T43.3X6
Dioxyline	T46.3X1	T46.3X2	T46.3X3	T46.3X4	T46.3X5	T46.3X6
Dipentene	T52.8X1	T52.8X2	T52.8X3	T52.8X4	—	—
Diperodon	T41.3X1	T41.3X2	T41.3X3	T41.3X4	T41.3X5	T41.3X6
Diphacinone	T60.4X1	T60.4X2	T60.4X3	T60.4X4	—	—
Diphemanil	T44.3X1	T44.3X2	T44.3X3	T44.3X4	T44.3X5	T44.3X6
metilsulfate	T44.3X1	T44.3X2	T44.3X3	T44.3X4	T44.3X5	T44.3X6
Diphenadione	T45.511	T45.512	T45.513	T45.514	T45.515	T45.516
rodenticide	T60.4X1	T60.4X2	T60.4X3	T60.4X4		
Diphenhydramine	T45.0X1	T45.0X2	T45.0X3	T45.0X4	T45.0X5	T45.0X6
Diphenidol	T45.0X1	T45.0X2	T45.0X3	T45.0X4	T45.0X5	T45.0X6
Diphenoxylate	T47.6X1	T47.6X2	T47.6X3	T47.6X4	T47.6X5	T47.6X6
Diphenylamine	T65.3X1	T65.3X2	T65.3X3	T65.3X4	—	—
Diphenylbutazone	T39.2X1	T39.2X2	T39.2X3	T39.2X4	T39.2X5	T39.2X6
Diphenylchloroarsine, not in war	T57.0X1	T57.0X2	T57.0X3	T57.0X4	—	—
Diphenylhydantoin	T42.0X1	T42.0X2	T42.0X3	T42.0X4	T42.0X5	T42.0X6
Diphenylmethane dye	T52.1X1	T52.1X2	T52.1X3	T52.1X4	—	—
Diphenylpyraline	T45.0X1	T45.0X2	T45.0X3	T45.0X4	T45.0X5	T45.0X6
Diphtheria						
antitoxin	T50.Z11	T50.Z12	T50.Z13	T50.Z14	T50.Z15	T50.Z16
toxoid	T50.A91	T50.A92	T50.A93	T50.A94	T50.A95	T50.A96
with tetanus toxoid	T50.A21	T50.A22	T50.A23	T50.A24	T50.A25	T50.A26
with pertussis component	T50.A11	T50.A12	T50.A13	T50.A14	T50.A15	T50.A16
vaccine	T50.A91	T50.A92	T50.A93	T50.A94	T50.A95	T50.A96
combination						
including pertussis	T50.A11	T50.A12	T50.A13	T50.A14	T50.A15	T50.A16
without pertussis	T50.A21	T50.A22	T50.A23	T50.A24	T50.A25	T50.A26
Diphylline	T50.2X1	T50.2X2	T50.2X3	T50.2X4	T50.2X5	T50.2X6
Dipipanone	T40.4X1	T40.4X2	T40.4X3	T40.4X4	—	—
Dipivefrine	T49.5X1	T49.5X2	T49.5X3	T49.5X4	T49.5X5	T49.5X6
Diplovax	T50.B91	T50.B92	T50.B93	T50.B94	T50.B95	T50.B96
Diprophylline	T50.2X1	T50.2X2	T50.2X3	T50.2X4	T50.2X5	T50.2X6
Dipropyline	T48.291	T48.292	T48.293	T48.294	T48.295	T48.296
Dipyridamole	T46.3X1	T46.3X2	T46.3X3	T46.3X4	T46.3X5	T46.3X6
Dipyrone	T39.2X1	T39.2X2	T39.2X3	T39.2X4	T39.2X5	T39.2X6

Substance	Poisoning, Accidental (unintentional)	Poisoning, Intentional self-harm	Poisoning, Assault	Poisoning, Undetermined	Adverse effect	Underdosing
Diquat (dibromide)	T60.3X1	T60.3X2	T60.3X3	T60.3X4	—	—
Disinfectant	T65.891	T65.892	T65.893	T65.894	—	—
alkaline	T54.3X1	T54.3X2	T54.3X3	T54.3X4	—	—
aromatic	T54.1X1	T54.1X2	T54.1X3	T54.1X4	—	—
intestinal	T37.8X1	T37.8X2	T37.8X3	T37.8X4	T37.8X5	T37.8X6
Disipal	T42.8X1	T42.8X2	T42.8X3	T42.8X4	T42.8X5	T42.8X6
Disodium edetate	T50.6X1	T50.6X2	T50.6X3	T50.6X4	T50.6X5	T50.6X6
Disoprofol	T41.291	T41.292	T41.293	T41.294	T41.295	T41.296
Disopyramide	T46.2X1	T46.2X2	T46.2X3	T46.2X4	T46.2X5	T46.2X6
Distigmine (bromide)	T44.0X1	T44.0X2	T44.0X3	T44.0X4	T44.0X5	T44.0X6
Disulfamide	T50.2X1	T50.2X2	T50.2X3	T50.2X4	T50.2X5	T50.2X6
Disulfanilamide	T37.0X1	T37.0X2	T37.0X3	T37.0X4	T37.0X5	T37.0X6
Disulfiram	T50.6X1	T50.6X2	T50.6X3	T50.6X4	T50.6X5	T50.6X6
Disulfoton	T60.0X1	T60.0X2	T60.0X3	T60.0X4	—	—
Dithiazanine iodide	T37.4X1	T37.4X2	T37.4X3	T37.4X4	T37.4X5	T37.4X6
Dithiocarbamate	T60.0X1	T60.0X2	T60.0X3	T60.0X4	—	—
Dithranol	T49.4X1	T49.4X2	T49.4X3	T49.4X4	T49.4X5	T49.4X6
Diucardin	T50.2X1	T50.2X2	T50.2X3	T50.2X4	T50.2X5	T50.2X6
Diupres	T50.2X1	T50.2X2	T50.2X3	T50.2X4	T50.2X5	T50.2X6
Diuretic NEC	T50.2X1	T50.2X2	T50.2X3	T50.2X4	T50.2X5	T50.2X6
benzothiadiazine	T50.2X1	T50.2X2	T50.2X3	T50.2X4	T50.2X5	T50.2X6
carbonic acid anhydrase inhibitors	T50.2X1	T50.2X2	T50.2X3	T50.2X4	T50.2X5	T50.2X6
furfuryl NEC	T50.2X1	T50.2X2	T50.2X3	T50.2X4	T50.2X5	T50.2X6
loop (high-ceiling)	T50.1X1	T50.1X2	T50.1X3	T50.1X4	T50.1X5	T50.1X6
mercurial NEC	T50.2X1	T50.2X2	T50.2X3	T50.2X4	T50.2X5	T50.2X6
osmotic	T50.2X1	T50.2X2	T50.2X3	T50.2X4	T50.2X5	T50.2X6
purine NEC	T50.2X1	T50.2X2	T50.2X3	T50.2X4	T50.2X5	T50.2X6
saluretic NEC	T50.2X1	T50.2X2	T50.2X3	T50.2X4	T50.2X5	T50.2X6
sulfonamide	T50.2X1	T50.2X2	T50.2X3	T50.2X4	T50.2X5	T50.2X6
thiazide NEC	T50.2X1	T50.2X2	T50.2X3	T50.2X4	T50.2X5	T50.2X6
xanthine	T50.2X1	T50.2X2	T50.2X3	T50.2X4	T50.2X5	T50.2X6
Diurgin	T50.2X1	T50.2X2	T50.2X3	T50.2X4	T50.2X5	T50.2X6
Diuril	T50.2X1	T50.2X2	T50.2X3	T50.2X4	T50.2X5	T50.2X6
Diuron	T60.3X1	T60.3X2	T60.3X3	T60.3X4	—	—
Divalproex	T42.6X1	T42.6X2	T42.6X3	T42.6X4	T42.6X5	T42.6X6
Divinyl ether	T41.0X1	T41.0X2	T41.0X3	T41.0X4	T41.0X5	T41.0X6
Dixanthogen	T49.0X1	T49.0X2	T49.0X3	T49.0X4	T49.0X5	T49.0X6
Dixyrazine	T43.3X1	T43.3X2	T43.3X3	T43.3X4	T43.3X5	T43.3X6
D-lysergic acid diethylamide	T40.8X1	T40.8X2	T40.8X3	T40.8X4	—	—
DMCT	T36.4X1	T36.4X2	T36.4X3	T36.4X4	T36.4X5	T36.4X6
DMSO—see Dimethyl sulfoxide						
DNBP	T60.3X1	T60.3X2	T60.3X3	T60.3X4	—	—
DNOC	T65.3X1	T65.3X2	T65.3X3	T65.3X4	—	—
Dobutamine	T44.5X1	T44.5X2	T44.5X3	T44.5X4	T44.5X5	T44.5X6
DOCA	T38.0X1	T38.0X2	T38.0X3	T38.0X4	T38.0X5	T38.0X6
Docusate sodium	T47.4X1	T47.4X2	T47.4X3	T47.4X4	T47.4X5	T47.4X6
Dodicin	T49.0X1	T49.0X2	T49.0X3	T49.0X4	T49.0X5	T49.0X6
Dofamium chloride	T49.0X1	T49.0X2	T49.0X3	T49.0X4	T49.0X5	T49.0X6
Dolophine	T40.3X1	T40.3X2	T40.3X3	T40.3X4	T40.3X5	T40.3X6
Doloxene	T39.8X1	T39.8X2	T39.8X3	T39.8X4	T39.8X5	T39.8X6
Domestic gas (after combustion)—see Gas, utility						
prior to combustion	T59.891	T59.892	T59.893	T59.894	—	—
Domiodol	T48.4X1	T48.4X2	T48.4X3	T48.4X4	T48.4X5	T48.4X6
Domiphen (bromide)	T49.0X1	T49.0X2	T49.0X3	T49.0X4	T49.0X5	T49.0X6
Domperidone	T45.0X1	T45.0X2	T45.0X3	T45.0X4	T45.0X5	T45.0X6

Substance	Poisoning, Accidental (unintentional)	Poisoning, Intentional self-harm	Poisoning, Assault	Poisoning, Undetermined	Adverse effect	Underdosing
Dopa	T42.8X1	T42.8X2	T42.8X3	T42.8X4	T42.8X5	T42.8X6
Dopamine	T44.991	T44.992	T44.993	T44.994	T44.995	T44.996
Doriden	T42.6X1	T42.6X2	T42.6X3	T42.6X4	T42.6X5	T42.6X6
Dormiral	T42.3X1	T42.3X2	T42.3X3	T42.3X4	T42.3X5	T42.3X6
Dormison	T42.6X1	T42.6X2	T42.6X3	T42.6X4	T42.6X5	T42.6X6
Dornase	T48.4X1	T48.4X2	T48.4X3	T48.4X4	T48.4X5	T48.4X6
Dorsacaine	T41.3X1	T41.3X2	T41.3X3	T41.3X4	T41.3X5	T41.3X6
Dosulepin	T43.011	T43.012	T43.013	T43.014	T43.015	T43.016
Dothiepin	T43.011	T43.012	T43.013	T43.014	T43.015	T43.016
Doxantrazole	T48.6X1	T48.6X2	T48.6X3	T48.6X4	T48.6X5	T48.6X6
Doxapram	T50.7X1	T50.7X2	T50.7X3	T50.7X4	T50.7X5	T50.7X6
Doxazosin	T44.6X1	T44.6X2	T44.6X3	T44.6X4	T44.6X5	T44.6X6
Doxepin	T43.011	T43.012	T43.013	T43.014	T43.015	T43.016
Doxifluridine	T45.1X1	T45.1X2	T45.1X3	T45.1X4	T45.1X5	T45.1X6
Doxorubicin	T45.1X1	T45.1X2	T45.1X3	T45.1X4	T45.1X5	T45.1X6
Doxycycline	T36.4X1	T36.4X2	T36.4X3	T36.4X4	T36.4X5	T36.4X6
Doxylamine	T45.0X1	T45.0X2	T45.0X3	T45.0X4	T45.0X5	T45.0X6
Dramamine	T45.0X1	T45.0X2	T45.0X3	T45.0X4	T45.0X5	T45.0X6
Drano (drain cleaner)	T54.3X1	T54.3X2	T54.3X3	T54.3X4	—	—
Dressing, live pulp	T49.7X1	T49.7X2	T49.7X3	T49.7X4	T49.7X5	T49.7X6
Drocode	T40.2X1	T40.2X2	T40.2X3	T40.2X4	T40.2X5	T40.2X6
Dromoran	T40.2X1	T40.2X2	T40.2X3	T40.2X4	T40.2X5	T40.2X6
Dromostanolone	T38.7X1	T38.7X2	T38.7X3	T38.7X4	T38.7X5	T38.7X6
Dronabinol	T40.7X1	T40.7X2	T40.7X3	T40.7X4	T40.7X5	T40.7X6
Droperidol	T43.591	T43.592	T43.593	T43.594	T43.595	T43.596
Dropropizine	T48.3X1	T48.3X2	T48.3X3	T48.3X4	T48.3X5	T48.3X6
Drostanolone	T38.7X1	T38.7X2	T38.7X3	T38.7X4	T38.7X5	T38.7X6
Drotaverine	T44.3X1	T44.3X2	T44.3X3	T44.3X4	T44.3X5	T44.3X6
Drotrecogin alfa	T45.511	T45.512	T45.513	T45.514	T45.515	T45.516
Drug NEC	T50.901	T50.902	T50.903	T50.904	T50.905	T50.906
specified NEC	T50.991	T50.992	T50.993	T50.994	T50.995	T50.996
DTIC	T45.1X1	T45.1X2	T45.1X3	T45.1X4	T45.1X5	T45.1X6
Duboisine	T44.3X1	T44.3X2	T44.3X3	T44.3X4	T44.3X5	T44.3X6
Dulcolax	T47.2X1	T47.2X2	T47.2X3	T47.2X4	T47.2X5	T47.2X6
Duponol (C) (EP)	T49.2X1	T49.2X2	T49.2X3	T49.2X4	T49.2X5	T49.2X6
Durabolin	T38.7X1	T38.7X2	T38.7X3	T38.7X4	T38.7X5	T38.7X6
Dyclone	T41.3X1	T41.3X2	T41.3X3	T41.3X4	T41.3X5	T41.3X6
Dyclonine	T41.3X1	T41.3X2	T41.3X3	T41.3X4	T41.3X5	T41.3X6
Dydrogesterone	T38.5X1	T38.5X2	T38.5X3	T38.5X4	T38.5X5	T38.5X6
Dye NEC	T65.6X1	T65.6X2	T65.6X3	T65.6X4	—	—
antiseptic	T49.0X1	T49.0X2	T49.0X3	T49.0X4	T49.0X5	T49.0X6
diagnostic agents	T50.8X1	T50.8X2	T50.8X3	T50.8X4	T50.8X5	T50.8X6
pharmaceutical NEC	T50.901	T50.902	T50.903	T50.904	T50.905	T50.906
Dyflos	T44.0X1	T44.0X2	T44.0X3	T44.0X4	T44.0X5	T44.0X6
Dymelor	T38.3X1	T38.3X2	T38.3X3	T38.3X4	T38.3X5	T38.3X6
Dynamite	T65.3X1	T65.3X2	T65.3X3	T65.3X4	—	—
fumes	T59.891	T59.892	T59.893	T59.894	—	—
Dyphylline	T44.3X1	T44.3X2	T44.3X3	T44.3X4	T44.3X5	T44.3X6
E						
Ear drug NEC	T49.6X1	T49.6X2	T49.6X3	T49.6X4	T49.6X5	T49.6X6
Ear preparations	T49.6X1	T49.6X2	T49.6X3	T49.6X4	T49.6X5	T49.6X6
Echothiophate, echothiopate, ecothiopate	T49.5X1	T49.5X2	T49.5X3	T49.5X4	T49.5X5	T49.5X6
Econazole	T49.0X1	T49.0X2	T49.0X3	T49.0X4	T49.0X5	T49.0X6
Ecothiopate iodide	T49.5X1	T49.5X2	T49.5X3	T49.5X4	T49.5X5	T49.5X6
Ecstasy	T43.621	T43.622	T43.623	T43.624	T43.625	T43.626
Ectylurea	T42.6X1	T42.6X2	T42.6X3	T42.6X4	T42.6X5	T42.6X6
Edathamil disodium	T45.8X1	T45.8X2	T45.8X3	T45.8X4	T45.8X5	T45.8X6
Edecrin	T50.1X1	T50.1X2	T50.1X3	T50.1X4	T50.1X5	T50.1X6

Substance	Poisoning, Accidental (unintentional)	Poisoning, Intentional self-harm	Poisoning, Assault	Poisoning, Undetermined	Adverse effect	Underdosing
Edetate, disodium (calcium)	T45.8X1	T45.8X2	T45.8X3	T45.8X4	T45.8X5	T45.8X6
Edoxudine	T49.5X1	T49.5X2	T49.5X3	T49.5X4	T49.5X5	T49.5X6
Edrophonium	T44.0X1	T44.0X2	T44.0X3	T44.0X4	T44.0X5	T44.0X6
chloride	T44.0X1	T44.0X2	T44.0X3	T44.0X4	T44.0X5	T44.0X6
EDTA	T50.6X1	T50.6X2	T50.6X3	T50.6X4	T50.6X5	T50.6X6
Eflornithine	T37.2X1	T37.2X2	T37.2X3	T37.2X4	T37.2X5	T37.2X6
Efloxate	T46.3X1	T46.3X2	T46.3X3	T46.3X4	T46.3X5	T46.3X6
Elase	T49.8X1	T49.8X2	T49.8X3	T49.8X4	T49.8X5	T49.8X6
Elastase	T47.5X1	T47.5X2	T47.5X3	T47.5X4	T47.5X5	T47.5X6
Elaterium	T47.2X1	T47.2X2	T47.2X3	T47.2X4	T47.2X5	T47.2X6
Elcatonin	T50.991	T50.992	T50.993	T50.994	T50.995	T50.996
Elder	T62.2X1	T62.2X2	T62.2X3	T62.2X4	—	—
berry, (unripe)	T62.1X1	T62.1X2	T62.1X3	T62.1X4	—	—
Electrolyte balance drug	T50.3X1	T50.3X2	T50.3X3	T50.3X4	T50.3X5	T50.3X6
Electrolytes NEC	T50.3X1	T50.3X2	T50.3X3	T50.3X4	T50.3X5	T50.3X6
Electrolytic agent NEC	T50.3X1	T50.3X2	T50.3X3	T50.3X4	T50.3X5	T50.3X6
Elemental diet	T50.901	T50.902	T50.903	T50.904	T50.905	T50.906
Elliptinium acetate	T45.1X1	T45.1X2	T45.1X3	T45.1X4	T45.1X5	T45.1X6
Embramine	T45.0X1	T45.0X2	T45.0X3	T45.0X4	T45.0X5	T45.0X6
Emepronium (salts)	T44.3X1	T44.3X2	T44.3X3	T44.3X4	T44.3X5	T44.3X6
bromide	T44.3X1	T44.3X2	T44.3X3	T44.3X4	T44.3X5	T44.3X6
Emetic NEC	T47.7X1	T47.7X2	T47.7X3	T47.7X4	T47.7X5	T47.7X6
Emetine	T37.3X1	T37.3X2	T37.3X3	T37.3X4	T37.3X5	T37.3X6
Emollient NEC	T49.3X1	T49.3X2	T49.3X3	T49.3X4	T49.3X5	T49.3X6
Emorfazone	T39.8X1	T39.8X2	T39.8X3	T39.8X4	T39.8X5	T39.8X6
Emylcamate	T43.591	T43.592	T43.593	T43.594	T43.595	T43.596
Enalapril	T46.4X1	T46.4X2	T46.4X3	T46.4X4	T46.4X5	T46.4X6
Enalaprilat	T46.4X1	T46.4X2	T46.4X3	T46.4X4	T46.4X5	T46.4X6
Encainide	T46.2X1	T46.2X2	T46.2X3	T46.2X4	T46.2X5	T46.2X6
Endocaine	T41.3X1	T41.3X2	T41.3X3	T41.3X4	T41.3X5	T41.3X6
Endosulfan	T60.2X1	T60.2X2	T60.2X3	T60.2X4	—	—
Endothall	T60.3X1	T60.3X2	T60.3X3	T60.3X4	—	—
Endralazine	T46.5X1	T46.5X2	T46.5X3	T46.5X4	T46.5X5	T46.5X6
Endrin	T60.1X1	T60.1X2	T60.1X3	T60.1X4	—	—
Enflurane	T41.0X1	T41.0X2	T41.0X3	T41.0X4	T41.0X5	T41.0X6
Enhexymal	T42.3X1	T42.3X2	T42.3X3	T42.3X4	T42.3X5	T42.3X6
Enocitabine	T45.1X1	T45.1X2	T45.1X3	T45.1X4	T45.1X5	T45.1X6
Enovid	T38.4X1	T38.4X2	T38.4X3	T38.4X4	T38.4X5	T38.4X6
Enoxacin	T36.8X1	T36.8X2	T36.8X3	T36.8X4	T36.8X5	T36.8X6
Enoxaparin (sodium)	T45.511	T45.512	T45.513	T45.514	T45.515	T45.516
Enpiprazole	T43.591	T43.592	T43.593	T43.594	T43.595	T43.596
Enprofylline	T48.6X1	T48.6X2	T48.6X3	T48.6X4	T48.6X5	T48.6X6
Enprostil	T47.1X1	T47.1X2	T47.1X3	T47.1X4	T47.1X5	T47.1X6
ENT preparations (anti-infectives)	T49.6X1	T49.6X2	T49.6X3	T49.6X4	T49.6X5	T49.6X6
Enterogastrone	T38.891	T38.892	T38.893	T38.894	T38.895	T38.896
Enviomycin	T36.8X1	T36.8X2	T36.8X3	T36.8X4	T36.8X5	T36.8X6
Enzodase	T45.3X1	T45.3X2	T45.3X3	T45.3X4	T45.3X5	T45.3X6
Enzyme NEC	T45.3X1	T45.3X2	T45.3X3	T45.3X4	T45.3X5	T45.3X6
depolymerizing	T49.8X1	T49.8X2	T49.8X3	T49.8X4	T49.8X5	T49.8X6
fibrolytic	T45.3X1	T45.3X2	T45.3X3	T45.3X4	T45.3X5	T45.3X6
gastric	T47.5X1	T47.5X2	T47.5X3	T47.5X4	T47.5X5	T47.5X6
intestinal	T47.5X1	T47.5X2	T47.5X3	T47.5X4	T47.5X5	T47.5X6
local action	T49.4X1	T49.4X2	T49.4X3	T49.4X4	T49.4X5	T49.4X6
proteolytic	T49.4X1	T49.4X2	T49.4X3	T49.4X4	T49.4X5	T49.4X6
thrombolytic	T45.3X1	T45.3X2	T45.3X3	T45.3X4	T45.3X5	T45.3X6
EPAB	T41.3X1	T41.3X2	T41.3X3	T41.3X4	T41.3X5	T41.3X6
Epanutin	T42.0X1	T42.0X2	T42.0X3	T42.0X4	T42.0X5	T42.0X6
Ephedra	T44.991	T44.992	T44.993	T44.994	T44.995	T44.996

Substance	Poisoning, Accidental (unintentional)	Poisoning, Intentional self-harm	Poisoning, Assault	Poisoning, Undetermined	Adverse effect	Underdosing
Ephedrine	T44.991	T44.992	T44.993	T44.994	T44.995	T44.996
Epichlorhydrin, epichlorohydrin	T52.8X1	T52.8X2	T52.8X3	T52.8X4	—	—
Epicillin	T36.0X1	T36.0X2	T36.0X3	T36.0X4	T36.0X5	T36.0X6
Epiestriol	T38.5X1	T38.5X2	T38.5X3	T38.5X4	T38.5X5	T38.5X6
Epilim—see Sodium valproate						
Epimestrol	T38.5X1	T38.5X2	T38.5X3	T38.5X4	T38.5X5	T38.5X6
Epinephrine	T44.5X1	T44.5X2	T44.5X3	T44.5X4	T44.5X5	T44.5X6
Epirubicin	T45.1X1	T45.1X2	T45.1X3	T45.1X4	T45.1X5	T45.1X6
Epitiostanol	T38.7X1	T38.7X2	T38.7X3	T38.7X4	T38.7X5	T38.7X6
Epitizide	T50.2X1	T50.2X2	T50.2X3	T50.2X4	T50.2X5	T50.2X6
EPN	T60.0X1	T60.0X2	T60.0X3	T60.0X4	—	—
EPO	T45.8X1	T45.8X2	T45.8X3	T45.8X4	T45.8X5	T45.8X6
Epoetin alpha	T45.8X1	T45.8X2	T45.8X3	T45.8X4	T45.8X5	T45.8X6
Epomediol	T50.991	T50.992	T50.993	T50.994	T50.995	T50.996
Epoprostenol	T45.521	T45.522	T45.523	T45.524	T45.525	T45.526
Epoxy resin	T65.891	T65.892	T65.893	T65.894	—	—
Eprazinone	T48.4X1	T48.4X2	T48.4X3	T48.4X4	T48.4X5	T48.4X6
Epsilon amino-caproic acid	T45.621	T45.622	T45.623	T45.624	T45.625	T45.626
Epsom salt	T47.3X1	T47.3X2	T47.3X3	T47.3X4	T47.3X5	T47.3X6
Eptazocine	T40.4X1	T40.4X2	T40.4X3	T40.4X4	T40.4X5	T40.4X6
Equanil	T43.591	T43.592	T43.593	T43.594	T43.595	T43.596
Equisetum	T62.2X1	T62.2X2	T62.2X3	T62.2X4	—	—
diuretic	T50.2X1	T50.2X2	T50.2X3	T50.2X4	T50.2X5	T50.2X6
Ergobasine	T48.0X1	T48.0X2	T48.0X3	T48.0X4	T48.0X5	T48.0X6
Ergocalciferol	T45.2X1	T45.2X2	T45.2X3	T45.2X4	T45.2X5	T45.2X6
Ergoloid mesylates	T46.7X1	T46.7X2	T46.7X3	T46.7X4	T46.7X5	T46.7X6
Ergometrine	T48.0X1	T48.0X2	T48.0X3	T48.0X4	T48.0X5	T48.0X6
Ergonovine	T48.0X1	T48.0X2	T48.0X3	T48.0X4	T48.0X5	T48.0X6
Ergot NEC	T64.81	T64.82	T64.83	T64.84	—	—
derivative	T48.0X1	T48.0X2	T48.0X3	T48.0X4	T48.0X5	T48.0X6
medicinal (alkaloids)	T48.0X1	T48.0X2	T48.0X3	T48.0X4	T48.0X5	T48.0X6
prepared	T48.0X1	T48.0X2	T48.0X3	T48.0X4	T48.0X5	T48.0X6
Ergotamine	T46.5X1	T46.5X2	T46.5X3	T46.5X4	T46.5X5	T46.5X6
Ergotocine	T48.0X1	T48.0X2	T48.0X3	T48.0X4	T48.0X5	T48.0X6
Ergotrate	T48.0X1	T48.0X2	T48.0X3	T48.0X4	T48.0X5	T48.0X6
Eritrityl tetranitrate	T46.3X1	T46.3X2	T46.3X3	T46.3X4	T46.3X5	T46.3X6
Erythrityl tetranitrate	T46.3X1	T46.3X2	T46.3X3	T46.3X4	T46.3X5	T46.3X6
Erythrol tetranitrate	T46.3X1	T46.3X2	T46.3X3	T46.3X4	T46.3X5	T46.3X6
Erythromycin (salts)	T36.3X1	T36.3X2	T36.3X3	T36.3X4	T36.3X5	T36.3X6
ophthalmic preparation	T49.5X1	T49.5X2	T49.5X3	T49.5X4	T49.5X5	T49.5X6
topical NEC	T49.0X1	T49.0X2	T49.0X3	T49.0X4	T49.0X5	T49.0X6
Erythropoietin	T45.8X1	T45.8X2	T45.8X3	T45.8X4	T45.8X5	T45.8X6
human	T45.8X1	T45.8X2	T45.8X3	T45.8X4	T45.8X5	T45.8X6
Escin	T46.991	T46.992	T46.993	T46.994	T46.995	T46.996
Esculin	T45.2X1	T45.2X2	T45.2X3	T45.2X4	T45.2X5	T45.2X6
Esculoside	T45.2X1	T45.2X2	T45.2X3	T45.2X4	T45.2X5	T45.2X6
ESDT (ether-soluble tar distillate)	T49.1X1	T49.1X2	T49.1X3	T49.1X4	T49.1X5	T49.1X6
Eserine	T49.5X1	T49.5X2	T49.5X3	T49.5X4	T49.5X5	T49.5X6
Esflurbiprofen	T39.311	T39.312	T39.313	T39.314	T39.315	T39.316
Eskabarb	T42.3X1	T42.3X2	T42.3X3	T42.3X4	T42.3X5	T42.3X6
Eskalith	T43.8X1	T43.8X2	T43.8X3	T43.8X4	T43.8X5	T43.8X6
Esmolol	T44.7X1	T44.7X2	T44.7X3	T44.7X4	T44.7X5	T44.7X6
Estanozolol	T38.7X1	T38.7X2	T38.7X3	T38.7X4	T38.7X5	T38.7X6
Estazolam	T42.4X1	T42.4X2	T42.4X3	T42.4X4	T42.4X5	T42.4X6
Estradiol	T38.5X1	T38.5X2	T38.5X3	T38.5X4	T38.5X5	T38.5X6
with testosterone	T38.7X1	T38.7X2	T38.7X3	T38.7X4	T38.7X5	T38.7X6
benzoate	T38.5X1	T38.5X2	T38.5X3	T38.5X4	T38.5X5	T38.5X6

Substance	Poisoning, Accidental (unintentional)	Poisoning, Intentional self-harm	Poisoning, Assault	Poisoning, Undetermined	Adverse effect	Underdosing
Estramustine	T45.1X1	T45.1X2	T45.1X3	T45.1X4	T45.1X5	T45.1X6
Estriol	T38.5X1	T38.5X2	T38.5X3	T38.5X4	T38.5X5	T38.5X6
Estrogen	T38.5X1	T38.5X2	T38.5X3	T38.5X4	T38.5X5	T38.5X6
with progesterone	T38.5X1	T38.5X2	T38.5X3	T38.5X4	T38.5X5	T38.5X6
conjugated	T38.5X1	T38.5X2	T38.5X3	T38.5X4	T38.5X5	T38.5X6
Estrone	T38.5X1	T38.5X2	T38.5X3	T38.5X4	T38.5X5	T38.5X6
Estropipate	T38.5X1	T38.5X2	T38.5X3	T38.5X4	T38.5X5	T38.5X6
Etacrynate sodium	T50.1X1	T50.1X2	T50.1X3	T50.1X4	T50.1X5	T50.1X6
Etacrynic acid	T50.1X1	T50.1X2	T50.1X3	T50.1X4	T50.1X5	T50.1X6
Etafedrine	T48.6X1	T48.6X2	T48.6X3	T48.6X4	T48.6X5	T48.6X6
Etafenone	T46.3X1	T46.3X2	T46.3X3	T46.3X4	T46.3X5	T46.3X6
Etambutol	T37.1X1	T37.1X2	T37.1X3	T37.1X4	T37.1X5	T37.1X6
Etamiphyllin	T48.6X1	T48.6X2	T48.6X3	T48.6X4	T48.6X5	T48.6X6
Etamivan	T50.7X1	T50.7X2	T50.7X3	T50.7X4	T50.7X5	T50.7X6
Etamsylate	T45.7X1	T45.7X2	T45.7X3	T45.7X4	T45.7X5	T45.7X6
Etebenecid	T50.4X1	T50.4X2	T50.4X3	T50.4X4	T50.4X5	T50.4X6
Ethacridine	T49.0X1	T49.0X2	T49.0X3	T49.0X4	T49.0X5	T49.0X6
Ethacrynic acid	T50.1X1	T50.1X2	T50.1X3	T50.1X4	T50.1X5	T50.1X6
Ethadione	T42.2X1	T42.2X2	T42.2X3	T42.2X4	T42.2X5	T42.2X6
Ethambutol	T37.1X1	T37.1X2	T37.1X3	T37.1X4	T37.1X5	T37.1X6
Ethamide	T50.2X1	T50.2X2	T50.2X3	T50.2X4	T50.2X5	T50.2X6
Ethamivan	T50.7X1	T50.7X2	T50.7X3	T50.7X4	T50.7X5	T50.7X6
Ethamsylate	T45.7X1	T45.7X2	T45.7X3	T45.7X4	T45.7X5	T45.7X6
Ethanol	T51.0X1	T51.0X2	T51.0X3	T51.0X4	—	—
beverage	T51.0X1	T51.0X2	T51.0X3	T51.0X4	—	—
Ethanolamine oleate	T46.8X1	T46.8X2	T46.8X3	T46.8X4	T46.8X5	T46.8X6
Ethaverine	T44.3X1	T44.3X2	T44.3X3	T44.3X4	T44.3X5	T44.3X6
Ethchlorvynol	T42.6X1	T42.6X2	T42.6X3	T42.6X4	T42.6X5	T42.6X6
Ethebenecid	T50.4X1	T50.4X2	T50.4X3	T50.4X4	T50.4X5	T50.4X6
Ether (vapor)	T41.0X1	T41.0X2	T41.0X3	T41.0X4	T41.0X5	T41.0X6
anesthetic	T41.0X1	T41.0X2	T41.0X3	T41.0X4	T41.0X5	T41.0X6
divinyl	T41.0X1	T41.0X2	T41.0X3	T41.0X4	T41.0X5	T41.0X6
ethyl (medicinal)	T41.0X1	T41.0X2	T41.0X3	T41.0X4	T41.0X5	T41.0X6
nonmedicinal	T52.8X1	T52.8X2	T52.8X3	T52.8X4	—	—
petroleum—see Ligroin						
solvent	T52.8X1	T52.8X2	T52.8X3	T52.8X4	—	—
Ethiazide	T50.2X1	T50.2X2	T50.2X3	T50.2X4	T50.2X5	T50.2X6
Ethidium chloride (vapor)	T59.891	T59.892	T59.893	T59.894	—	—
Ethinamate	T42.6X1	T42.6X2	T42.6X3	T42.6X4	T42.6X5	T42.6X6
Ethinylestradiol, ethinyloestradiol	T38.5X1	T38.5X2	T38.5X3	T38.5X4	T38.5X5	T38.5X6
with						
levonorgestrel	T38.4X1	T38.4X2	T38.4X3	T38.4X4	T38.4X5	T38.4X6
norethisterone	T38.4X1	T38.4X2	T38.4X3	T38.4X4	T38.4X5	T38.4X6
Ethiodized oil (131 I)	T50.8X1	T50.8X2	T50.8X3	T50.8X4	T50.8X5	T50.8X6
Ethion	T60.0X1	T60.0X2	T60.0X3	T60.0X4	—	—
Ethionamide	T37.1X1	T37.1X2	T37.1X3	T37.1X4	T37.1X5	T37.1X6
Ethioniamide	T37.1X1	T37.1X2	T37.1X3	T37.1X4	T37.1X5	T37.1X6
Ethisterone	T38.5X1	T38.5X2	T38.5X3	T38.5X4	T38.5X5	T38.5X6
Ethobral	T42.3X1	T42.3X2	T42.3X3	T42.3X4	T42.3X5	T42.3X6
Ethocaine (infiltration) (topical)	T41.3X1	T41.3X2	T41.3X3	T41.3X4	T41.3X5	T41.3X6
nerve block (peripheral) (plexus)	T41.3X1	T41.3X2	T41.3X3	T41.3X4	T41.3X5	T41.3X6
spinal	T41.3X1	T41.3X2	T41.3X3	T41.3X4	T41.3X5	T41.3X6
Ethoheptazine	T40.4X1	T40.4X2	T40.4X3	T40.4X4	T40.4X5	T40.4X6
Ethopropazine	T44.3X1	T44.3X2	T44.3X3	T44.3X4	T44.3X5	T44.3X6
Ethosuximide	T42.2X1	T42.2X2	T42.2X3	T42.2X4	T42.2X5	T42.2X6
Ethotoin	T42.0X1	T42.0X2	T42.0X3	T42.0X4	T42.0X5	T42.0X6
Ethoxazene	T37.91	T37.92	T37.93	T37.94	T37.95	T37.96

Substance	Poisoning, Accidental (unintentional)	Poisoning, Intentional self-harm	Poisoning, Assault	Poisoning, Undetermined	Adverse effect	Underdosing
Ethoxazorutoside	T46.991	T46.992	T46.993	T46.994	T46.995	T46.996
2-Ethoxyethanol	T52.3X1	T52.3X2	T52.3X3	T52.3X4	—	—
Ethoxzolamide	T50.2X1	T50.2X2	T50.2X3	T50.2X4	T50.2X5	T50.2X6
Ethyl						
acetate	T52.8X1	T52.8X2	T52.8X3	T52.8X4	—	—
alcohol	T51.0X1	T51.0X2	T51.0X3	T51.0X4	—	—
beverage	T51.0X1	T51.0X2	T51.0X3	T51.0X4	—	—
aldehyde (vapor)	T59.891	T59.892	T59.893	T59.894	—	—
liquid	T52.8X1	T52.8X2	T52.8X3	T52.8X4	—	—
aminobenzoate	T41.3X1	T41.3X2	T41.3X3	T41.3X4	T41.3X5	T41.3X6
aminophenothiazine	T43.3X1	T43.3X2	T43.3X3	T43.3X4	T43.3X5	T43.3X6
benzoate	T52.8X1	T52.8X2	T52.8X3	T52.8X4	—	—
biscoumacetate	T45.511	T45.512	T45.513	T45.514	T45.515	T45.516
bromide (anesthetic)	T41.0X1	T41.0X2	T41.0X3	T41.0X4	T41.0X5	T41.0X6
carbamate	T45.1X1	T45.1X2	T45.1X3	T45.1X4	T45.1X5	T45.1X6
carbinol	T51.3X1	T51.3X2	T51.3X3	T51.3X4	—	—
carbonate	T52.8X1	T52.8X2	T52.8X3	T52.8X4	—	—
chaulmoograte	T37.1X1	T37.1X2	T37.1X3	T37.1X4	T37.1X5	T37.1X6
chloride (anesthetic)	T41.0X1	T41.0X2	T41.0X3	T41.0X4	T41.0X5	T41.0X6
anesthetic (local)	T41.3X1	T41.3X2	T41.3X3	T41.3X4	T41.3X5	T41.3X6
inhaled	T41.0X1	T41.0X2	T41.0X3	T41.0X4	T41.0X5	T41.0X6
local	T49.4X1	T49.4X2	T49.4X3	T49.4X4	T49.4X5	T49.4X6
solvent	T53.6X1	T53.6X2	T53.6X3	T53.6X4	—	—
dibunate	T48.3X1	T48.3X2	T48.3X3	T48.3X4	T48.3X5	T48.3X6
dichloroarsine (vapor)	T57.0X1	T57.0X2	T57.0X3	T57.0X4	—	—
estranol	T38.7X1	T38.7X2	T38.7X3	T38.7X4	T38.7X5	T38.7X6
ether—see also ether	T52.8X1	T52.8X2	T52.8X3	T52.8X4	—	—
formate NEC (solvent)	T52.0X1	T52.0X2	T52.0X3	T52.0X4	—	—
fumarate	T49.4X1	T49.4X2	T49.4X3	T49.4X4	T49.4X5	T49.4X6
hydroxyisobutyrate NEC (solvent)	T52.8X1	T52.8X2	T52.8X3	T52.8X4	—	—
iodoacetate	T59.3X1	T59.3X2	T59.3X3	T59.3X4	—	—
lactate NEC (solvent)	T52.8X1	T52.8X2	T52.8X3	T52.8X4	—	—
loflazepate	T42.4X1	T42.4X2	T42.4X3	T42.4X4	T42.4X5	T42.4X6
mercuric chloride	T56.1X1	T56.1X2	T56.1X3	T56.1X4	—	—
methylcarbinol	T51.8X1	T51.8X2	T51.8X3	T51.8X4	—	—
morphine	T40.2X1	T40.2X2	T40.2X3	T40.2X4	T40.2X5	T40.2X6
noradrenaline	T48.6X1	T48.6X2	T48.6X3	T48.6X4	T48.6X5	T48.6X6
oxybutyrate NEC (solvent)	T52.8X1	T52.8X2	T52.8X3	T52.8X4	—	—
Ethylene (gas)	T59.891	T59.892	T59.893	T59.894	—	—
anesthetic (general)	T41.0X1	T41.0X2	T41.0X3	T41.0X4	T41.0X5	T41.0X6
chlorohydrin	T52.8X1	T52.8X2	T52.8X3	T52.8X4	—	—
vapor	T53.6X1	T53.6X2	T53.6X3	T53.6X4	—	—
dichloride	T52.8X1	T52.8X2	T52.8X3	T52.8X4	—	—
vapor	T53.6X1	T53.6X2	T53.6X3	T53.6X4	—	—
dinitrate	T52.3X1	T52.3X2	T52.3X3	T52.3X4	—	—
glycol (s)	T52.8X1	T52.8X2	T52.8X3	T52.8X4	—	—
dinitrate	T52.3X1	T52.3X2	T52.3X3	T52.3X4	—	—
monobutyl ether	T52.3X1	T52.3X2	T52.3X3	T52.3X4	—	—
imine	T54.1X1	T54.1X2	T54.1X3	T54.1X4	—	—
oxide (fumigant) (nonmedicinal)	T59.891	T59.892	T59.893	T59.894	—	—
medicinal	T49.0X1	T49.0X2	T49.0X3	T49.0X4	T49.0X5	T49.0X6
Ethylenediamine theophylline	T48.6X1	T48.6X2	T48.6X3	T48.6X4	T48.6X5	T48.6X6
Ethylenediaminetetra-acetic acid	T50.6X1	T50.6X2	T50.6X3	T50.6X4	T50.6X5	T50.6X6
Ethylenedinitrilotetra-acetate	T50.6X1	T50.6X2	T50.6X3	T50.6X4	T50.6X5	T50.6X6
Ethylestrenol	T38.7X1	T38.7X2	T38.7X3	T38.7X4	T38.7X5	T38.7X6

Substance	Poisoning, Accidental (unintentional)	Poisoning, Intentional self-harm	Poisoning, Assault	Poisoning, Undetermined	Adverse effect	Underdosing
Ethylhydroxycellulose	T47.4X1	T47.4X2	T47.4X3	T47.4X4	T47.4X5	T47.4X6
Ethylidene						
chloride NEC	T53.6X1	T53.6X2	T53.6X3	T53.6X4	—	—
diacetate	T60.3X1	T60.3X2	T60.3X3	T60.3X4	—	—
dicoumarin	T45.511	T45.512	T45.513	T45.514	T45.515	T45.516
dicoumarol	T45.511	T45.512	T45.513	T45.514	T45.515	T45.516
diethyl ether	T52.0X1	T52.0X2	T52.0X3	T52.0X4	—	—
Ethylmorphine	T40.2X1	T40.2X2	T40.2X3	T40.2X4	T40.2X5	T40.2X6
Ethylnorepinephrine	T48.6X1	T48.6X2	T48.6X3	T48.6X4	T48.6X5	T48.6X6
Ethylparachlorophen-oxyisobutyrate	T46.6X1	T46.6X2	T46.6X3	T46.6X4	T46.6X5	T46.6X6
Ethynodiol	T38.4X1	T38.4X2	T38.4X3	T38.4X4	T38.4X5	T38.4X6
with mestranol diacetate	T38.4X1	T38.4X2	T38.4X3	T38.4X4	T38.4X5	T38.4X6
Etidocaine	T41.3X1	T41.3X2	T41.3X3	T41.3X4	T41.3X5	T41.3X6
infiltration (subcutaneous)	T41.3X1	T41.3X2	T41.3X3	T41.3X4	T41.3X5	T41.3X6
nerve (peripheral) (plexus)	T41.3X1	T41.3X2	T41.3X3	T41.3X4	T41.3X5	T41.3X6
Etidronate	T50.991	T50.992	T50.993	T50.994	T50.995	T50.996
Etidronic acid (disodium salt)	T50.991	T50.992	T50.993	T50.994	T50.995	T50.996
Etifoxine	T42.6X1	T42.6X2	T42.6X3	T42.6X4	T42.6X5	T42.6X6
Etilefrine	T44.4X1	T44.4X2	T44.4X3	T44.4X4	T44.4X5	T44.4X6
Etilfen	T42.3X1	T42.3X2	T42.3X3	T42.3X4	T42.3X5	T42.3X6
Etinodiol	T38.4X1	T38.4X2	T38.4X3	T38.4X4	T38.4X5	T38.4X6
Etiroxate	T46.6X1	T46.6X2	T46.6X3	T46.6X4	T46.6X5	T46.6X6
Etizolam	T42.4X1	T42.4X2	T42.4X3	T42.4X4	T42.4X5	T42.4X6
Etodolac	T39.391	T39.392	T39.393	T39.394	T39.395	T39.396
Etofamide	T37.3X1	T37.3X2	T37.3X3	T37.3X4	T37.3X5	T37.3X6
Etofibrate	T46.6X1	T46.6X2	T46.6X3	T46.6X4	T46.6X5	T46.6X6
Etofylline	T46.7X1	T46.7X2	T46.7X3	T46.7X4	T46.7X5	T46.7X6
clofibrate	T46.6X1	T46.6X2	T46.6X3	T46.6X4	T46.6X5	T46.6X6
Etoglucid	T45.1X1	T45.1X2	T45.1X3	T45.1X4	T45.1X5	T45.1X6
Etomidate	T41.1X1	T41.1X2	T41.1X3	T41.1X4	T41.1X5	T41.1X6
Etomide	T39.8X1	T39.8X2	T39.8X3	T39.8X4	T39.8X5	T39.8X6
Etomidoline	T44.3X1	T44.3X2	T44.3X3	T44.3X4	T44.3X5	T44.3X6
Etoposide	T45.1X1	T45.1X2	T45.1X3	T45.1X4	T45.1X5	T45.1X6
Etorphine	T40.2X1	T40.2X2	T40.2X3	T40.2X4	T40.2X5	T40.2X6
Etoval	T42.3X1	T42.3X2	T42.3X3	T42.3X4	T42.3X5	T42.3X6
Etozolin	T50.1X1	T50.1X2	T50.1X3	T50.1X4	T50.1X5	T50.1X6
Etretinate	T50.991	T50.992	T50.993	T50.994	T50.995	T50.996
Etryptamine	T43.691	T43.692	T43.693	T43.694	T43.695	T43.696
Etybenzatropine	T44.3X1	T44.3X2	T44.3X3	T44.3X4	T44.3X5	T44.3X6
Etynodiol	T38.4X1	T38.4X2	T38.4X3	T38.4X4	T38.4X5	T38.4X6
Eucaine	T41.3X1	T41.3X2	T41.3X3	T41.3X4	T41.3X5	T41.3X6
Eucalyptus oil	T49.7X1	T49.7X2	T49.7X3	T49.7X4	T49.7X5	T49.7X6
Eucatropine	T49.5X1	T49.5X2	T49.5X3	T49.5X4	T49.5X5	T49.5X6
Eucodal	T40.2X1	T40.2X2	T40.2X3	T40.2X4	T40.2X5	T40.2X6
Euneryl	T42.3X1	T42.3X2	T42.3X3	T42.3X4	T42.3X5	T42.3X6
Euphthalmine	T44.3X1	T44.3X2	T44.3X3	T44.3X4	T44.3X5	T44.3X6
Eurax	T49.0X1	T49.0X2	T49.0X3	T49.0X4	T49.0X5	T49.0X6
Euresol	T49.4X1	T49.4X2	T49.4X3	T49.4X4	T49.4X5	T49.4X6
Euthroid	T38.1X1	T38.1X2	T38.1X3	T38.1X4	T38.1X5	T38.1X6
Evans blue	T50.8X1	T50.8X2	T50.8X3	T50.8X4	T50.8X5	T50.8X6
Evipal	T42.3X1	T42.3X2	T42.3X3	T42.3X4	T42.3X5	T42.3X6
sodium	T41.1X1	T41.1X2	T41.1X3	T41.1X4	T41.1X5	T41.1X6
Evipan	T42.3X1	T42.3X2	T42.3X3	T42.3X4	T42.3X5	T42.3X6
sodium	T41.1X1	T41.1X2	T41.1X3	T41.1X4	T41.1X5	T41.1X6
Exalamide	T49.0X1	T49.0X2	T49.0X3	T49.0X4	T49.0X5	T49.0X6
Exalgin	T39.1X1	T39.1X2	T39.1X3	T39.1X4	T39.1X5	T39.1X6

Excipients, pharmaceutical - Flomoxef

Substance	Poisoning, Accidental (unintentional)	Poisoning, Intentional self-harm	Poisoning, Assault	Poisoning, Undetermined	Adverse effect	Underdosing
Excipients, pharmaceutical	T50.901	T50.902	T50.903	T50.904	T50.905	T50.906
Exhaust gas (engine) (motor vehicle)	T58.01	T58.02	T58.03	T58.04	—	—
Ex-Lax (phenolphthalein)	T47.2X1	T47.2X2	T47.2X3	T47.2X4	T47.2X5	T47.2X6
Expectorant NEC	T48.4X1	T48.4X2	T48.4X3	T48.4X4	T48.4X5	T48.4X6
Extended insulin zinc suspension	T38.3X1	T38.3X2	T38.3X3	T38.3X4	T38.3X5	T38.3X6
External medications (skin) (mucous membrane)	T49.91	T49.92	T49.93	T49.94	T49.95	T49.96
dental agent	T49.7X1	T49.7X2	T49.7X3	T49.7X4	T49.7X5	T49.7X6
ENT agent	T49.6X1	T49.6X2	T49.6X3	T49.6X4	T49.6X5	T49.6X6
ophthalmic preparation	T49.5X1	T49.5X2	T49.5X3	T49.5X4	T49.5X5	T49.5X6
specified NEC	T49.8X1	T49.8X2	T49.8X3	T49.8X4	T49.8X5	T49.8X6
Extrapyramidal antagonist NEC	T44.3X1	T44.3X2	T44.3X3	T44.3X4	T44.3X5	T44.3X6
Eye agents (anti-infective)	T49.5X1	T49.5X2	T49.5X3	T49.5X4	T49.5X5	T49.5X6
Eye drug NEC	T49.5X1	T49.5X2	T49.5X3	T49.5X4	T49.5X5	T49.5X6
F						
FAC (fluorouracil + doxorubicin + cyclophosphamide)	T45.1X1	T45.1X2	T45.1X3	T45.1X4	T45.1X5	T45.1X6
Factor						
I (fibrinogen)	T45.8X1	T45.8X2	T45.8X3	T45.8X4	T45.8X5	T45.8X6
III (thromboplastin)	T45.8X1	T45.8X2	T45.8X3	T45.8X4	T45.8X5	T45.8X6
VIII (antihemophilic Factor) (concentrate)	T45.8X1	T45.8X2	T45.8X3	T45.8X4	T45.8X5	T45.8X6
IX complex	T45.7X1	T45.7X2	T45.7X3	T45.7X4	T45.7X5	T45.7X6
human	T45.8X1	T45.8X2	T45.8X3	T45.8X4	T45.8X5	T45.8X6
Famotidine	T47.0X1	T47.0X2	T47.0X3	T47.0X4	T47.0X5	T47.0X6
Fat suspension, intravenous	T50.991	T50.992	T50.993	T50.994	T50.995	T50.996
Fazadinium bromide	T48.1X1	T48.1X2	T48.1X3	T48.1X4	T48.1X5	T48.1X6
Febarbamate	T42.3X1	T42.3X2	T42.3X3	T42.3X4	T42.3X5	T42.3X6
Fecal softener	T47.4X1	T47.4X2	T47.4X3	T47.4X4	T47.4X5	T47.4X6
Fedrilate	T48.3X1	T48.3X2	T48.3X3	T48.3X4	T48.3X5	T48.3X6
Felodipine	T46.1X1	T46.1X2	T46.1X3	T46.1X4	T46.1X5	T46.1X6
Felypressin	T38.891	T38.892	T38.893	T38.894	T38.895	T38.896
Femoxetine	T43.221	T43.222	T43.223	T43.224	T43.225	T43.226
Fenalcomine	T46.3X1	T46.3X2	T46.3X3	T46.3X4	T46.3X5	T46.3X6
Fenamisal	T37.1X1	T37.1X2	T37.1X3	T37.1X4	T37.1X5	T37.1X6
Fenazone	T39.2X1	T39.2X2	T39.2X3	T39.2X4	T39.2X5	T39.2X6
Fenbendazole	T37.4X1	T37.4X2	T37.4X3	T37.4X4	T37.4X5	T37.4X6
Fenbutrazate	T50.5X1	T50.5X2	T50.5X3	T50.5X4	T50.5X5	T50.5X6
Fencamfamine	T43.691	T43.692	T43.693	T43.694	T43.695	T43.696
Fendiline	T46.1X1	T46.1X2	T46.1X3	T46.1X4	T46.1X5	T46.1X6
Fenetylline	T43.691	T43.692	T43.693	T43.694	T43.695	T43.696
Fenflumizole	T39.391	T39.392	T39.393	T39.394	T39.395	T39.396
Fenfluramine	T50.5X1	T50.5X2	T50.5X3	T50.5X4	T50.5X5	T50.5X6
Fenobarbital	T42.3X1	T42.3X2	T42.3X3	T42.3X4	T42.3X5	T42.3X6
Fenofibrate	T46.6X1	T46.6X2	T46.6X3	T46.6X4	T46.6X5	T46.6X6
Fenoprofen	T39.311	T39.312	T39.313	T39.314	T39.315	T39.316
Fenoterol	T48.6X1	T48.6X2	T48.6X3	T48.6X4	T48.6X5	T48.6X6
Fenoverine	T44.3X1	T44.3X2	T44.3X3	T44.3X4	T44.3X5	T44.3X6
Fenoxazoline	T48.5X1	T48.5X2	T48.5X3	T48.5X4	T48.5X5	T48.5X6
Fenproporex	T50.5X1	T50.5X2	T50.5X3	T50.5X4	T50.5X5	T50.5X6
Fenquizone	T50.2X1	T50.2X2	T50.2X3	T50.2X4	T50.2X5	T50.2X6
Fentanyl	T40.4X1	T40.4X2	T40.4X3	T40.4X4	T40.4X5	T40.4X6
Fentazin	T43.3X1	T43.3X2	T43.3X3	T43.3X4	T43.3X5	T43.3X6

Substance	Poisoning, Accidental (unintentional)	Poisoning, Intentional self-harm	Poisoning, Assault	Poisoning, Undetermined	Adverse effect	Underdosing
Fenthion	T60.0X1	T60.0X2	T60.0X3	T60.0X4	—	—
Fenticlor	T49.0X1	T49.0X2	T49.0X3	T49.0X4	T49.0X5	T49.0X6
Fenylbutazone	T39.2X1	T39.2X2	T39.2X3	T39.2X4	T39.2X5	T39.2X6
Feprazone	T39.2X1	T39.2X2	T39.2X3	T39.2X4	T39.2X5	T39.2X6
Fer de lance (bite) (venom)	T63.061	T63.062	T63.063	T63.064		
Ferric—see also Iron						
chloride	T45.4X1	T45.4X2	T45.4X3	T45.4X4	T45.4X5	T45.4X6
citrate	T45.4X1	T45.4X2	T45.4X3	T45.4X4	T45.4X5	T45.4X6
hydroxide						
colloidal	T45.4X1	T45.4X2	T45.4X3	T45.4X4	T45.4X5	T45.4X6
polymaltose	T45.4X1	T45.4X2	T45.4X3	T45.4X4	T45.4X5	T45.4X6
pyrophosphate	T45.4X1	T45.4X2	T45.4X3	T45.4X4	T45.4X5	T45.4X6
Ferritin	T45.4X1	T45.4X2	T45.4X3	T45.4X4	T45.4X5	T45.4X6
Ferrocholinate	T45.4X1	T45.4X2	T45.4X3	T45.4X4	T45.4X5	T45.4X6
Ferrodextrane	T45.4X1	T45.4X2	T45.4X3	T45.4X4	T45.4X5	T45.4X6
Ferropolimaler	T45.4X1	T45.4X2	T45.4X3	T45.4X4	T45.4X5	T45.4X6
Ferrous—see also Iron						
phosphate	T45.4X1	T45.4X2	T45.4X3	T45.4X4	T45.4X5	T45.4X6
salt	T45.4X1	T45.4X2	T45.4X3	T45.4X4	T45.4X5	T45.4X6
with folic acid	T45.4X1	T45.4X2	T45.4X3	T45.4X4	T45.4X5	T45.4X6
Ferrous fumerate, gluconate, lactate, salt NEC, sulfate (medicinal)	T45.4X1	T45.4X2	T45.4X3	T45.4X4	T45.4X5	T45.4X6
Ferrovanadium (fumes)	T59.891	T59.892	T59.893	T59.894	—	—
Ferrum—see Iron						
Fertilizers NEC	T65.891	T65.892	T65.893	T65.894	—	—
with herbicide mixture	T60.3X1	T60.3X2	T60.3X3	T60.3X4	—	—
Fetoxilate	T47.6X1	T47.6X2	T47.6X3	T47.6X4	T47.6X5	T47.6X6
Fiber, dietary	T47.4X1	T47.4X2	T47.4X3	T47.4X4	T47.4X5	T47.4X6
Fiberglass	T65.831	T65.832	T65.833	T65.834	—	—
Fibrinogen (human)	T45.8X1	T45.8X2	T45.8X3	T45.8X4	T45.8X5	T45.8X6
Fibrinolysin (human)	T45.691	T45.692	T45.693	T45.694	T45.695	T45.696
Fibrinolysis						
affecting drug	T45.601	T45.602	T45.603	T45.604	T45.605	T45.606
inhibitor NEC	T45.621	T45.622	T45.623	T45.624	T45.625	T45.626
Fibrinolytic drug	T45.611	T45.612	T45.613	T45.614	T45.615	T45.616
Filix mas	T37.4X1	T37.4X2	T37.4X3	T37.4X4	T37.4X5	T37.4X6
Filtering cream	T49.3X1	T49.3X2	T49.3X3	T49.3X4	T49.3X5	T49.3X6
Fiorinal	T39.011	T39.012	T39.013	T39.014	T39.015	T39.016
Firedamp	T59.891	T59.892	T59.893	T59.894	—	—
Fish, noxious, nonbacterial	T61.91	T61.92	T61.93	T61.94	—	—
ciguatera	T61.01	T61.02	T61.03	T61.04	—	—
scombroid	T61.11	T61.12	T61.13	T61.14	—	—
shell	T61.781	T61.782	T61.783	T61.784	—	—
specified NEC	T61.771	T61.772	T61.773	T61.774	—	—
Flagyl	T37.3X1	T37.3X2	T37.3X3	T37.3X4	T37.3X5	T37.3X6
Flavine adenine dinucleotide	T45.2X1	T45.2X2	T45.2X3	T45.2X4	T45.2X5	T45.2X6
Flavodic acid	T46.991	T46.992	T46.993	T46.994	T46.995	T46.996
Flavoxate	T44.3X1	T44.3X2	T44.3X3	T44.3X4	T44.3X5	T44.3X6
Flaxedil	T48.1X1	T48.1X2	T48.1X3	T48.1X4	T48.1X5	T48.1X6
Flaxseed (medicinal)	T49.3X1	T49.3X2	T49.3X3	T49.3X4	T49.3X5	T49.3X6
Flecainide	T46.2X1	T46.2X2	T46.2X3	T46.2X4	T46.2X5	T46.2X6
Fleroxacin	T36.8X1	T36.8X2	T36.8X3	T36.8X4	T36.8X5	T36.8X6
Floctafenine	T39.8X1	T39.8X2	T39.8X3	T39.8X4	T39.8X5	T39.8X6
Flomax	T44.6X1	T44.6X2	T44.6X3	T44.6X4	T44.6X5	T44.6X6
Flomoxef	T36.1X1	T36.1X2	T36.1X3	T36.1X4	T36.1X5	T36.1X6

Substance	Poisoning, Accidental (unintentional)	Poisoning, Intentional self-harm	Poisoning, Assault	Poisoning, Undetermined	Adverse effect	Underdosing
Flopropione	T44.3X1	T44.3X2	T44.3X3	T44.3X4	T44.3X5	T44.3X6
Florantyrone	T47.5X1	T47.5X2	T47.5X3	T47.5X4	T47.5X5	T47.5X6
Floraquin	T37.8X1	T37.8X2	T37.8X3	T37.8X4	T37.8X5	T37.8X6
Florinef	T38.0X1	T38.0X2	T38.0X3	T38.0X4	T38.0X5	T38.0X6
ENT agent	T49.6X1	T49.6X2	T49.6X3	T49.6X4	T49.6X5	T49.6X6
ophthalmic preparation	T49.5X1	T49.5X2	T49.5X3	T49.5X4	T49.5X5	T49.5X6
topical NEC	T49.0X1	T49.0X2	T49.0X3	T49.0X4	T49.0X5	T49.0X6
Flowers of sulfur	T49.4X1	T49.4X2	T49.4X3	T49.4X4	T49.4X5	T49.4X6
Floxuridine	T45.1X1	T45.1X2	T45.1X3	T45.1X4	T45.1X5	T45.1X6
Fluanisone	T43.4X1	T43.4X2	T43.4X3	T43.4X4	T43.4X5	T43.4X6
Flubendazole	T37.4X1	T37.4X2	T37.4X3	T37.4X4	T37.4X5	T37.4X6
Fluclorolone acetonide	T49.0X1	T49.0X2	T49.0X3	T49.0X4	T49.0X5	T49.0X6
Flucloxacillin	T36.0X1	T36.0X2	T36.0X3	T36.0X4	T36.0X5	T36.0X6
Fluconazole	T37.8X1	T37.8X2	T37.8X3	T37.8X4	T37.8X5	T37.8X6
Flucytosine	T37.8X1	T37.8X2	T37.8X3	T37.8X4	T37.8X5	T37.8X6
Fludeoxyglucose (18F)	T50.8X1	T50.8X2	T50.8X3	T50.8X4	T50.8X5	T50.8X6
Fludiazepam	T42.4X1	T42.4X2	T42.4X3	T42.4X4	T42.4X5	T42.4X6
Fludrocortisone	T50.0X1	T50.0X2	T50.0X3	T50.0X4	T50.0X5	T50.0X6
ENT agent	T49.6X1	T49.6X2	T49.6X3	T49.6X4	T49.6X5	T49.6X6
ophthalmic preparation	T49.5X1	T49.5X2	T49.5X3	T49.5X4	T49.5X5	T49.5X6
topical NEC	T49.0X1	T49.0X2	T49.0X3	T49.0X4	T49.0X5	T49.0X6
Fludroxycortide	T49.0X1	T49.0X2	T49.0X3	T49.0X4	T49.0X5	T49.0X6
Flufenamic acid	T39.391	T39.392	T39.393	T39.394	T39.395	T39.396
Fluindione	T45.511	T45.512	T45.513	T45.514	T45.515	T45.516
Flumequine	T37.8X1	T37.8X2	T37.8X3	T37.8X4	T37.8X5	T37.8X6
Flumethasone	T49.0X1	T49.0X2	T49.0X3	T49.0X4	T49.0X5	T49.0X6
Flumethiazide	T50.2X1	T50.2X2	T50.2X3	T50.2X4	T50.2X5	T50.2X6
Flumidin	T37.5X1	T37.5X2	T37.5X3	T37.5X4	T37.5X5	T37.5X6
Flunarizine	T46.7X1	T46.7X2	T46.7X3	T46.7X4	T46.7X5	T46.7X6
Flunidazole	T37.8X1	T37.8X2	T37.8X3	T37.8X4	T37.8X5	T37.8X6
Flunisolide	T48.6X1	T48.6X2	T48.6X3	T48.6X4	T48.6X5	T48.6X6
Flunitrazepam	T42.4X1	T42.4X2	T42.4X3	T42.4X4	T42.4X5	T42.4X6
Fluocinolone (acetonide)	T49.0X1	T49.0X2	T49.0X3	T49.0X4	T49.0X5	T49.0X6
Fluocinonide	T49.0X1	T49.0X2	T49.0X3	T49.0X4	T49.0X5	T49.0X6
Fluocortin (butyl)	T49.0X1	T49.0X2	T49.0X3	T49.0X4	T49.0X5	T49.0X6
Fluocortolone	T49.0X1	T49.0X2	T49.0X3	T49.0X4	T49.0X5	T49.0X6
Fluohydrocortisone	T38.0X1	T38.0X2	T38.0X3	T38.0X4	T38.0X5	T38.0X6
ENT agent	T49.6X1	T49.6X2	T49.6X3	T49.6X4	T49.6X5	T49.6X6
ophthalmic preparation	T49.5X1	T49.5X2	T49.5X3	T49.5X4	T49.5X5	T49.5X6
topical NEC	T49.0X1	T49.0X2	T49.0X3	T49.0X4	T49.0X5	T49.0X6
Fluonid	T49.0X1	T49.0X2	T49.0X3	T49.0X4	T49.0X5	T49.0X6
Fluopromazine	T43.3X1	T43.3X2	T43.3X3	T43.3X4	T43.3X5	T43.3X6
Fluoracetate	T60.8X1	T60.8X2	T60.8X3	T60.8X4	—	—
Fluorescein	T50.8X1	T50.8X2	T50.8X3	T50.8X4	T50.8X5	T50.8X6
Fluorhydrocortisone	T50.0X1	T50.0X2	T50.0X3	T50.0X4	T50.0X5	T50.0X6
Fluoride (nonmedicinal) (pesticide) (sodium) NEC	T60.8X1	T60.8X2	T60.8X3	T60.8X4	—	—
hydrogen—see Hydrofluoric acid						
medicinal NEC	T50.991	T50.992	T50.993	T50.994	T50.995	T50.996
dental use	T49.7X1	T49.7X2	T49.7X3	T49.7X4	T49.7X5	T49.7X6
not pesticide NEC	T54.91	T54.92	T54.93	T54.94	—	—
stannous	T49.7X1	T49.7X2	T49.7X3	T49.7X4	T49.7X5	T49.7X6
Fluorinated corticosteroids	T38.0X1	T38.0X2	T38.0X3	T38.0X4	T38.0X5	T38.0X6
Fluorine (gas)	T59.5X1	T59.5X2	T59.5X3	T59.5X4	—	—
salt—see Fluoride(s)						
Fluoristan	T49.7X1	T49.7X2	T49.7X3	T49.7X4	T49.7X5	T49.7X6
Fluormetholone	T49.0X1	T49.0X2	T49.0X3	T49.0X4	T49.0X5	T49.0X6
Fluoroacetate	T60.8X1	T60.8X2	T60.8X3	T60.8X4	—	—

Substance	Poisoning, Accidental (unintentional)	Poisoning, Intentional self-harm	Poisoning, Assault	Poisoning, Undetermined	Adverse effect	Underdosing
Fluorocarbon monomer	T53.6X1	T53.6X2	T53.6X3	T53.6X4	—	—
Fluorocytosine	T37.8X1	T37.8X2	T37.8X3	T37.8X4	T37.8X5	T37.8X6
Fluorodeoxyuridine	T45.1X1	T45.1X2	T45.1X3	T45.1X4	T45.1X5	T45.1X6
Fluorometholone	T49.0X1	T49.0X2	T49.0X3	T49.0X4	T49.0X5	T49.0X6
ophthalmic preparation	T49.5X1	T49.5X2	T49.5X3	T49.5X4	T49.5X5	T49.5X6
Fluorophosphate insecticide	T60.0X1	T60.0X2	T60.0X3	T60.0X4	—	—
Fluorosol	T46.3X1	T46.3X2	T46.3X3	T46.3X4	T46.3X5	T46.3X6
Fluorouracil	T45.1X1	T45.1X2	T45.1X3	T45.1X4	T45.1X5	T45.1X6
Fluorphenylalanine	T49.5X1	T49.5X2	T49.5X3	T49.5X4	T49.5X5	T49.5X6
Fluothane	T41.0X1	T41.0X2	T41.0X3	T41.0X4	T41.0X5	T41.0X6
Fluoxetine	T43.221	T43.222	T43.223	T43.224	T43.225	T43.226
Fluoxymesterone	T38.7X1	T38.7X2	T38.7X3	T38.7X4	T38.7X5	T38.7X6
Flupenthixol	T43.4X1	T43.4X2	T43.4X3	T43.4X4	T43.4X5	T43.4X6
Flupentixol	T43.4X1	T43.4X2	T43.4X3	T43.4X4	T43.4X5	T43.4X6
Fluphenazine	T43.3X1	T43.3X2	T43.3X3	T43.3X4	T43.3X5	T43.3X6
Fluprednidene	T49.0X1	T49.0X2	T49.0X3	T49.0X4	T49.0X5	T49.0X6
Fluprednisolone	T38.0X1	T38.0X2	T38.0X3	T38.0X4	T38.0X5	T38.0X6
Fluradoline	T39.8X1	T39.8X2	T39.8X3	T39.8X4	T39.8X5	T39.8X6
Flurandrenolide	T49.0X1	T49.0X2	T49.0X3	T49.0X4	T49.0X5	T49.0X6
Flurandrenolone	T49.0X1	T49.0X2	T49.0X3	T49.0X4	T49.0X5	T49.0X6
Flurazepam	T42.4X1	T42.4X2	T42.4X3	T42.4X4	T42.4X5	T42.4X6
Flurbiprofen	T39.311	T39.312	T39.313	T39.314	T39.315	T39.316
Flurobate	T49.0X1	T49.0X2	T49.0X3	T49.0X4	T49.0X5	T49.0X6
Fluroxene	T41.0X1	T41.0X2	T41.0X3	T41.0X4	T41.0X5	T41.0X6
Fluspirilene	T43.591	T43.592	T43.593	T43.594	T43.595	T43.596
Flutamide	T38.6X1	T38.6X2	T38.6X3	T38.6X4	T38.6X5	T38.6X6
Flutazolam	T42.4X1	T42.4X2	T42.4X3	T42.4X4	T42.4X5	T42.4X6
Fluticasone propionate	T49.1X1	T49.1X2	T49.1X3	T49.1X4	T49.1X5	T49.1X6
Flutoprazepam	T42.4X1	T42.4X2	T42.4X3	T42.4X4	T42.4X5	T42.4X6
Flutropium bromide	T48.6X1	T48.6X2	T48.6X3	T48.6X4	T48.6X5	T48.6X6
Fluvoxamine	T43.221	T43.222	T43.223	T43.224	T43.225	T43.226
Folacin	T45.8X1	T45.8X2	T45.8X3	T45.8X4	T45.8X5	T45.8X6
Folic acid	T45.8X1	T45.8X2	T45.8X3	T45.8X4	T45.8X5	T45.8X6
with ferrous salt	T45.2X1	T45.2X2	T45.2X3	T45.2X4	T45.2X5	T45.2X6
antagonist	T45.1X1	T45.1X2	T45.1X3	T45.1X4	T45.1X5	T45.1X6
Folinic acid	T45.8X1	T45.8X2	T45.8X3	T45.8X4	T45.8X5	T45.8X6
Folium stramoniae	T48.6X1	T48.6X2	T48.6X3	T48.6X4	T48.6X5	T48.6X6
Follicle-stimulating hormone, human	T38.811	T38.812	T38.813	T38.814	T38.815	T38.816
Folpet	T60.3X1	T60.3X2	T60.3X3	T60.3X4	—	—
Fominoben	T48.3X1	T48.3X2	T48.3X3	T48.3X4	T48.3X5	T48.3X6
Food, foodstuffs, noxious, nonbacterial, NEC	T62.91	T62.92	T62.93	T62.94	—	—
berries	T62.1X1	T62.1X2	T62.1X3	T62.1X4	—	—
fish—see also Fish	T61.91	T61.92	T61.93	T61.94	—	—
mushrooms	T62.0X1	T62.0X2	T62.0X3	T62.0X4	—	—
plants	T62.2X1	T62.2X2	T62.2X3	T62.2X4	—	—
seafood	T61.91	T61.92	T61.93	T61.94	—	—
specified NEC	T61.8X1	T61.8X2	T61.8X3	T61.8X4	—	—
seeds	T62.2X1	T62.2X2	T62.2X3	T62.2X4	—	—
shellfish	T61.781	T61.782	T61.783	T61.784	—	—
specified NEC	T62.8X1	T62.8X2	T62.8X3	T62.8X4	—	—
Fool's parsley	T62.2X1	T62.2X2	T62.2X3	T62.2X4	—	—
Formaldehyde (solution), gas or vapor	T59.2X1	T59.2X2	T59.2X3	T59.2X4	—	—
fungicide	T60.3X1	T60.3X2	T60.3X3	T60.3X4	—	—
Formalin	T59.2X1	T59.2X2	T59.2X3	T59.2X4	—	—
fungicide	T60.3X1	T60.3X2	T60.3X3	T60.3X4	—	—
vapor	T59.2X1	T59.2X2	T59.2X3	T59.2X4	—	—

Formic acid - Gamimune

Substance	Poisoning, Accidental (unintentional)	Poisoning, Intentional self-harm	Poisoning, Assault	Poisoning, Undetermined	Adverse effect	Underdosing
Formic acid	T54.2X1	T54.2X2	T54.2X3	T54.2X4	—	—
vapor	T59.891	T59.892	T59.893	T59.894	—	—
Foscarnet sodium	T37.5X1	T37.5X2	T37.5X3	T37.5X4	T37.5X5	T37.5X6
Fosfestrol	T38.5X1	T38.5X2	T38.5X3	T38.5X4	T38.5X5	T38.5X6
Fosfomycin	T36.8X1	T36.8X2	T36.8X3	T36.8X4	T36.8X5	T36.8X6
Fosfonet sodium	T37.5X1	T37.5X2	T37.5X3	T37.5X4	T37.5X5	T37.5X6
Fosinopril	T46.4X1	T46.4X2	T46.4X3	T46.4X4	T46.4X5	T46.4X6
sodium	T46.4X1	T46.4X2	T46.4X3	T46.4X4	T46.4X5	T46.4X6
Fowler's solution	T57.0X1	T57.0X2	T57.0X3	T57.0X4	—	—
Foxglove	T62.2X1	T62.2X2	T62.2X3	T62.2X4	—	—
Framycetin	T36.5X1	T36.5X2	T36.5X3	T36.5X4	T36.5X5	T36.5X6
Frangula	T47.2X1	T47.2X2	T47.2X3	T47.2X4	T47.2X5	T47.2X6
extract	T47.2X1	T47.2X2	T47.2X3	T47.2X4	T47.2X5	T47.2X6
Frei antigen	T50.8X1	T50.8X2	T50.8X3	T50.8X4	T50.8X5	T50.8X6
Freon	T53.5X1	T53.5X2	T53.5X3	T53.5X4	—	—
Fructose	T50.3X1	T50.3X2	T50.3X3	T50.3X4	T50.3X5	T50.3X6
Frusemide	T50.1X1	T50.1X2	T50.1X3	T50.1X4	T50.1X5	T50.1X6
FSH	T38.811	T38.812	T38.813	T38.814	T38.815	T38.816
Ftorafur	T45.1X1	T45.1X2	T45.1X3	T45.1X4	T45.1X5	T45.1X6
Fuel						
automobile	T52.0X1	T52.0X2	T52.0X3	T52.0X4	—	—
exhaust gas, not in transit	T58.01	T58.02	T58.03	T58.04	—	—
vapor NEC	T52.0X1	T52.0X2	T52.0X3	T52.0X4	—	—
gas (domestic use)— see also Carbon, monoxide, fuel, utility	T59.891	T59.892	T59.893	T59.894	—	—
utility	T59.891	T59.892	T59.893	T59.894	—	—
in mobile container	T59.891	T59.892	T59.893	T59.894	—	—
incomplete combustion of—see Carbon, monoxide, fuel, utility						
piped (natural)	T59.891	T59.892	T59.893	T59.894	—	—
industrial, incomplete combustion	T58.8X1	T58.8X2	T58.8X3	T58.8X4	—	—
Fugillin	T36.8X1	T36.8X2	T36.8X3	T36.8X4	T36.8X5	T36.8X6
Fulminate of mercury	T56.1X1	T56.1X2	T56.1X3	T56.1X4	—	—
Fulvicin	T36.7X1	T36.7X2	T36.7X3	T36.7X4	T36.7X5	T36.7X6
Fumadil	T36.8X1	T36.8X2	T36.8X3	T36.8X4	T36.8X5	T36.8X6
Fumagillin	T36.8X1	T36.8X2	T36.8X3	T36.8X4	T36.8X5	T36.8X6
Fumaric acid	T49.4X1	T49.4X2	T49.4X3	T49.4X4	T49.4X5	T49.4X6
Fumes (from)	T59.91	T59.92	T59.93	T59.94	—	—
carbon monoxide—see Carbon, monoxide						
charcoal (domestic use)—see Charcoal, fumes						
chloroform—see Chloroform						
coke (in domestic stoves, fireplaces)— see Coke fumes						
corrosive NEC	T54.91	T54.92	T54.93	T54.94	—	—
ether—see ether						
freons	T53.5X1	T53.5X2	T53.5X3	T53.5X4	—	—
hydrocarbons	T59.891	T59.892	T59.893	T59.894	—	—
petroleum (liquefied)	T59.891	T59.892	T59.893	T59.894	—	—

Substance	Poisoning, Accidental (unintentional)	Poisoning, Intentional self-harm	Poisoning, Assault	Poisoning, Undetermined	Adverse effect	Underdosing
Fumes (from) — *continued*						
hydrocarbons — *continued*						
petroleum (liquefied) — *continued*						
distributed through pipes (pure or mixed with air)	T59.891	T59.892	T59.893	T59.894	—	—
lead—*see lead*						
metal—*see Metals, or the specified metal*						
nitrogen dioxide	T59.0X1	T59.0X2	T59.0X3	T59.0X4	—	—
pesticides—*see Pesticides*						
petroleum (liquefied)	T59.891	T59.892	T59.893	T59.894	—	—
distributed through pipes (pure or mixed with air)	T59.891	T59.892	T59.893	T59.894	—	—
polyester	T59.891	T59.892	T59.893	T59.894	—	—
specified source NEC— *see also substance specified*	T59.891	T59.892	T59.893	T59.894	—	—
sulfur dioxide	T59.1X1	T59.1X2	T59.1X3	T59.1X4	—	—
Fumigant NEC	T60.91	T60.92	T60.93	T60.94	—	—
Fungi, noxious, used as food	T62.0X1	T62.0X2	T62.0X3	T62.0X4	—	—
Fungicide NEC (nonmedicinal)	T60.3X1	T60.3X2	T60.3X3	T60.3X4	—	—
Fungizone	T36.7X1	T36.7X2	T36.7X3	T36.7X4	T36.7X5	T36.7X6
topical	T49.0X1	T49.0X2	T49.0X3	T49.0X4	T49.0X5	T49.0X6
Furacin	T49.0X1	T49.0X2	T49.0X3	T49.0X4	T49.0X5	T49.0X6
Furadantin	T37.91	T37.92	T37.93	T37.94	T37.95	T37.96
Furazolidone	T37.8X1	T37.8X2	T37.8X3	T37.8X4	T37.8X5	T37.8X6
Furazolium chloride	T49.0X1	T49.0X2	T49.0X3	T49.0X4	T49.0X5	T49.0X6
Furfural	T52.8X1	T52.8X2	T52.8X3	T52.8X4	—	—
Furnace (coal burning) (domestic), gas from	T58.2X1	T58.2X2	T58.2X3	T58.2X4	—	—
industrial	T58.8X1	T58.8X2	T58.8X3	T58.8X4	—	—
Furniture polish	T65.891	T65.892	T65.893	T65.894	—	—
Furosemide	T50.1X1	T50.1X2	T50.1X3	T50.1X4	T50.1X5	T50.1X6
Furoxone	T37.91	T37.92	T37.93	T37.94	T37.95	T37.96
Fursultiamine	T45.2X1	T45.2X2	T45.2X3	T45.2X4	T45.2X5	T45.2X6
Fusafungine	T36.8X1	T36.8X2	T36.8X3	T36.8X4	T36.8X5	T36.8X6
Fusel oil (any) (amyl) (butyl) (propyl), vapor	T51.3X1	T51.3X2	T51.3X3	T51.3X4	—	—
Fusidate (ethanolamine) (sodium)	T36.8X1	T36.8X2	T36.8X3	T36.8X4	T36.8X5	T36.8X6
Fusidic acid	T36.8X1	T36.8X2	T36.8X3	T36.8X4	T36.8X5	T36.8X6
Fytic acid, nonasodium	T50.6X1	T50.6X2	T50.6X3	T50.6X4	T50.6X5	T50.6X6
G						
GABA	T43.8X1	T43.8X2	T43.8X3	T43.8X4	T43.8X5	T43.8X6
Gadopentetic acid	T50.8X1	T50.8X2	T50.8X3	T50.8X4	T50.8X5	T50.8X6
Galactose	T50.3X1	T50.3X2	T50.3X3	T50.3X4	T50.3X5	T50.3X6
b-Galactosidase	T47.5X1	T47.5X2	T47.5X3	T47.5X4	T47.5X5	T47.5X6
Galantamine	T44.0X1	T44.0X2	T44.0X3	T44.0X4	T44.0X5	T44.0X6
Gallamine (triethiodide)	T48.1X1	T48.1X2	T48.1X3	T48.1X4	T48.1X5	T48.1X6
Gallium citrate	T50.991	T50.992	T50.993	T50.994	T50.995	T50.996
Gallopamil	T46.1X1	T46.1X2	T46.1X3	T46.1X4	T46.1X5	T46.1X6
Gamboge	T47.2X1	T47.2X2	T47.2X3	T47.2X4	T47.2X5	T47.2X6
Gamimune	T50.Z11	T50.Z12	T50.Z13	T50.Z14	T50.Z15	T50.Z16

Substance	Poisoning, Accidental (unintentional)	Poisoning, Intentional self-harm	Poisoning, Assault	Poisoning, Undetermined	Adverse effect	Underdosing
Gamma globulin	T50.Z11	T50.Z12	T50.Z13	T50.Z14	T50.Z15	T50.Z16
Gamma-aminobutyric acid	T43.8X1	T43.8X2	T43.8X3	T43.8X4	T43.8X5	T43.8X6
Gamma-benzene hexachloride (medicinal)	T49.0X1	T49.0X2	T49.0X3	T49.0X4	T49.0X5	T49.0X6
nonmedicinal, vapor	T53.6X1	T53.6X2	T53.6X3	T53.6X4	—	—
Gamma-BHC (medicinal)—*see also Gamma-benzene hexachloride*	T49.0X1	T49.0X2	T49.0X3	T49.0X4	T49.0X5	T49.0X6
Gamulin	T50.Z11	T50.Z12	T50.Z13	T50.Z14	T50.Z15	T50.Z16
Ganciclovir (sodium)	T37.5X1	T37.5X2	T37.5X3	T37.5X4	T37.5X5	T37.5X6
Ganglionic blocking drug NEC	T44.2X1	T44.2X2	T44.2X3	T44.2X4	T44.2X5	T44.2X6
specified NEC	T44.2X1	T44.2X2	T44.2X3	T44.2X4	T44.2X5	T44.2X6
Ganja	T40.7X1	T40.7X2	T40.7X3	T40.7X4	T40.7X5	T40.7X6
Garamycin	T36.5X1	T36.5X2	T36.5X3	T36.5X4	T36.5X5	T36.5X6
ophthalmic preparation	T49.5X1	T49.5X2	T49.5X3	T49.5X4	T49.5X5	T49.5X6
topical NEC	T49.0X1	T49.0X2	T49.0X3	T49.0X4	T49.0X5	T49.0X6
Gardenal	T42.3X1	T42.3X2	T42.3X3	T42.3X4	T42.3X5	T42.3X6
Gardepanyl	T42.3X1	T42.3X2	T42.3X3	T42.3X4	T42.3X5	T42.3X6
Gas	T59.91	T59.92	T59.93	T59.94	—	—
acetylene	T59.891	T59.892	T59.893	T59.894	—	—
incomplete combustion of	T58.11	T58.12	T58.13	T58.14	—	—
air contaminants, source or type not specified	T59.91	T59.92	T59.93	T59.94	—	—
anesthetic	T41.0X1	T41.0X2	T41.0X3	T41.0X4	T41.0X5	T41.0X6
blast furnace	T58.8X1	T58.8X2	T58.8X3	T58.8X4	—	—
butane—*see butane*						
carbon monoxide—*see Carbon, monoxide*						
chlorine	T59.4X1	T59.4X2	T59.4X3	T59.4X4	—	—
coal	T58.2X1	T58.2X2	T58.2X3	T58.2X4	—	—
cyanide	T57.3X1	T57.3X2	T57.3X3	T57.3X4	—	—
dicyanogen	T65.0X1	T65.0X2	T65.0X3	T65.0X4	—	—
domestic—*see Domestic gas*						
exhaust	T58.01	T58.02	T58.03	T58.04	—	—
from utility (for cooking, heating, or lighting) (after combustion)—*see Carbon, monoxide, fuel, utility*						
prior to combustion	T59.891	T59.892	T59.893	T59.894	—	—
from wood- or coal-burning stove or fireplace	T58.2X1	T58.2X2	T58.2X3	T58.2X4	—	—
fuel (domestic use) (after combustion)—*see also Carbon, monoxide, fuel*						
industrial use	T58.8X1	T58.8X2	T58.8X3	T58.8X4	—	—
prior to combustion	T59.891	T59.892	T59.893	T59.894	—	—
utility	T59.891	T59.892	T59.893	T59.894	—	—
in mobile container	T59.891	T59.892	T59.893	T59.894	—	—

Substance	Poisoning, Accidental (unintentional)	Poisoning, Intentional self-harm	Poisoning, Assault	Poisoning, Undetermined	Adverse effect	Underdosing
Gas — *continued*						
fuel (domestic use) (after combustion)— *see also Carbon, monoxide, fuel* — *continued*						
utility — *continued*						
incomplete combustion of—*see Carbon, monoxide, fuel, utility*						
piped (natural)	T59.891	T59.892	T59.893	T59.894	—	—
garage	T58.01	T58.02	T58.03	T58.04	—	—
hydrocarbon NEC	T59.891	T59.892	T59.893	T59.894	—	—
incomplete combustion of—*see Carbon, monoxide, fuel, utility*						
liquefied—*see butane*						
piped	T59.891	T59.892	T59.893	T59.894	—	—
hydrocyanic acid	T65.0X1	T65.0X2	T65.0X3	T65.0X4	—	—
illuminating (after combustion)	T58.11	T58.12	T58.13	T58.14	—	—
prior to combustion	T59.891	T59.892	T59.893	T59.894	—	—
incomplete combustion, any—*see Carbon, monoxide*						
kiln	T58.8X1	T58.8X2	T58.8X3	T58.8X4	—	—
lacrimogenic	T59.3X1	T59.3X2	T59.3X3	T59.3X4	—	—
liquefied petroleum— *see butane*						
marsh	T59.891	T59.892	T59.893	T59.894	—	—
motor exhaust, not in transit	T58.01	T58.02	T58.03	T58.04	—	—
mustard, not in war	T59.891	T59.892	T59.893	T59.894	—	—
natural	T59.891	T59.892	T59.893	T59.894	—	—
nerve, not in war	T59.91	T59.92	T59.93	T59.94	—	—
oil	T52.0X1	T52.0X2	T52.0X3	T52.0X4	—	—
petroleum (liquefied) (distributed in mobile containers)	T59.891	T59.892	T59.893	T59.894	—	—
piped (pure or mixed with air)	T59.891	T59.892	T59.893	T59.894	—	—
piped (manufactured) (natural) NEC	T59.891	T59.892	T59.893	T59.894	—	—
producer	T58.8X1	T58.8X2	T58.8X3	T58.8X4	—	—
propane—*see propane*						
refrigerant (chlorofluoro-carbon)	T53.5X1	T53.5X2	T53.5X3	T53.5X4	—	—
not chlorofluoro-carbon	T59.891	T59.892	T59.893	T59.894	—	—
sewer	T59.91	T59.92	T59.93	T59.94	—	—
specified source NEC	T59.91	T59.92	T59.93	T59.94	—	—
stove (after combustion)	T58.11	T58.12	T58.13	T58.14	—	—
prior to combustion	T59.891	T59.892	T59.893	T59.894	—	—

Substance	Poisoning, Accidental (unintentional)	Poisoning, Intentional self-harm	Poisoning, Assault	Poisoning, Undetermined	Adverse effect	Underdosing
Gas — *continued*						
tear	T59.3X1	T59.3X2	T59.3X3	T59.3X4	—	—
therapeutic	T41.5X1	T41.5X2	T41.5X3	T41.5X4	T41.5X5	T41.5X6
utility (for cooking, heating, or lighting) (piped) NEC	T59.891	T59.892	T59.893	T59.894	—	—
in mobile container	T59.891	T59.892	T59.893	T59.894	—	—
incomplete combustion of—*see Carbon, monoxide, fuel, utilty*						
piped (natural)	T59.891	T59.892	T59.893	T59.894	—	—
water	T58.11	T58.12	T58.13	T58.14	—	—
incomplete combustion of—*see Carbon, monoxide, fuel, utility*						
Gaseous substance—*see Gas*						
Gasoline	T52.0X1	T52.0X2	T52.0X3	T52.0X4	—	—
vapor	T52.0X1	T52.0X2	T52.0X3	T52.0X4	—	—
Gastric enzymes	T47.5X1	T47.5X2	T47.5X3	T47.5X4	T47.5X5	T47.5X6
Gastrografin	T50.8X1	T50.8X2	T50.8X3	T50.8X4	T50.8X5	T50.8X6
Gastrointestinal drug	T47.91	T47.92	T47.93	T47.94	T47.95	T47.96
biological	T47.8X1	T47.8X2	T47.8X3	T47.8X4	T47.8X5	T47.8X6
specified NEC	T47.8X1	T47.8X2	T47.8X3	T47.8X4	T47.8X5	T47.8X6
Gaultheria procumbens	T62.2X1	T62.2X2	T62.2X3	T62.2X4	—	—
Gefarnate	T44.3X1	T44.3X2	T44.3X3	T44.3X4	T44.3X5	T44.3X6
Gelatin (intravenous)	T45.8X1	T45.8X2	T45.8X3	T45.8X4	T45.8X5	T45.8X6
absorbable (sponge)	T45.7X1	T45.7X2	T45.7X3	T45.7X4	T45.7X5	T45.7X6
Gelfilm	T49.8X1	T49.8X2	T49.8X3	T49.8X4	T49.8X5	T49.8X6
Gelfoam	T45.7X1	T45.7X2	T45.7X3	T45.7X4	T45.7X5	T45.7X6
Gelsemine	T50.991	T50.992	T50.993	T50.994	T50.995	T50.996
Gelsemium (sempervirens)	T62.2X1	T62.2X2	T62.2X3	T62.2X4	—	—
Gemeprost	T48.0X1	T48.0X2	T48.0X3	T48.0X4	T48.0X5	T48.0X6
Gemfibrozil	T46.6X1	T46.6X2	T46.6X3	T46.6X4	T46.6X5	T46.6X6
Gemonil	T42.3X1	T42.3X2	T42.3X3	T42.3X4	T42.3X5	T42.3X6
Gentamicin	T36.5X1	T36.5X2	T36.5X3	T36.5X4	T36.5X5	T36.5X6
ophthalmic preparation	T49.5X1	T49.5X2	T49.5X3	T49.5X4	T49.5X5	T49.5X6
topical NEC	T49.0X1	T49.0X2	T49.0X3	T49.0X4	T49.0X5	T49.0X6
Gentian	T47.5X1	T47.5X2	T47.5X3	T47.5X4	T47.5X5	T47.5X6
violet	T49.0X1	T49.0X2	T49.0X3	T49.0X4	T49.0X5	T49.0X6
Gepefrine	T44.4X1	T44.4X2	T44.4X3	T44.4X4	T44.4X5	T44.4X6
Gestonorone caproate	T38.5X1	T38.5X2	T38.5X3	T38.5X4	T38.5X5	T38.5X6
Gexane	T49.0X1	T49.0X2	T49.0X3	T49.0X4	T49.0X5	T49.0X6
Gila monster (venom)	T63.111	T63.112	T63.113	T63.114	—	—
Ginger	T47.5X1	T47.5X2	T47.5X3	T47.5X4	T47.5X5	T47.5X6
Jamaica—*see Jamaica, ginger*						
Gitalin	T46.0X1	T46.0X2	T46.0X3	T46.0X4	T46.0X5	T46.0X6
amorphous	T46.0X1	T46.0X2	T46.0X3	T46.0X4	T46.0X5	T46.0X6
Gitaloxin	T46.0X1	T46.0X2	T46.0X3	T46.0X4	T46.0X5	T46.0X6
Gitoxin	T46.0X1	T46.0X2	T46.0X3	T46.0X4	T46.0X5	T46.0X6
Glafenine	T39.8X1	T39.8X2	T39.8X3	T39.8X4	T39.8X5	T39.8X6
Glandular extract (medicinal) NEC	T50.Z91	T50.Z92	T50.Z93	T50.Z94	T50.Z95	T50.Z96
Glaucarubin	T37.3X1	T37.3X2	T37.3X3	T37.3X4	T37.3X5	T37.3X6
Glibenclamide	T38.3X1	T38.3X2	T38.3X3	T38.3X4	T38.3X5	T38.3X6

Substance	Poisoning, Accidental (unintentional)	Poisoning, Intentional self-harm	Poisoning, Assault	Poisoning, Undetermined	Adverse effect	Underdosing
Glibornuride	T38.3X1	T38.3X2	T38.3X3	T38.3X4	T38.3X5	T38.3X6
Gliclazide	T38.3X1	T38.3X2	T38.3X3	T38.3X4	T38.3X5	T38.3X6
Glimidine	T38.3X1	T38.3X2	T38.3X3	T38.3X4	T38.3X5	T38.3X6
Glipizide	T38.3X1	T38.3X2	T38.3X3	T38.3X4	T38.3X5	T38.3X6
Gliquidone	T38.3X1	T38.3X2	T38.3X3	T38.3X4	T38.3X5	T38.3X6
Glisolamide	T38.3X1	T38.3X2	T38.3X3	T38.3X4	T38.3X5	T38.3X6
Glisoxepide	T38.3X1	T38.3X2	T38.3X3	T38.3X4	T38.3X5	T38.3X6
Globin zinc insulin	T38.3X1	T38.3X2	T38.3X3	T38.3X4	T38.3X5	T38.3X6
Globulin						
antilymphocytic	T50.Z11	T50.Z12	T50.Z13	T50.Z14	T50.Z15	T50.Z16
antirhesus	T50.Z11	T50.Z12	T50.Z13	T50.Z14	T50.Z15	T50.Z16
antivenin	T50.Z11	T50.Z12	T50.Z13	T50.Z14	T50.Z15	T50.Z16
antiviral	T50.Z11	T50.Z12	T50.Z13	T50.Z14	T50.Z15	T50.Z16
Glucagon	T38.3X1	T38.3X2	T38.3X3	T38.3X4	T38.3X5	T38.3X6
Glucocorticoids	T38.0X1	T38.0X2	T38.0X3	T38.0X4	T38.0X5	T38.0X6
Glucocorticosteroid	T38.0X1	T38.0X2	T38.0X3	T38.0X4	T38.0X5	T38.0X6
Gluconic acid	T50.991	T50.992	T50.993	T50.994	T50.995	T50.996
Glucosamine sulfate	T39.4X1	T39.4X2	T39.4X3	T39.4X4	T39.4X5	T39.4X6
Glucose	T50.3X1	T50.3X2	T50.3X3	T50.3X4	T50.3X5	T50.3X6
with sodium chloride	T50.3X1	T50.3X2	T50.3X3	T50.3X4	T50.3X5	T50.3X6
Glucosulfone sodium	T37.1X1	T37.1X2	T37.1X3	T37.1X4	T37.1X5	T37.1X6
Glucurolactone	T47.8X1	T47.8X2	T47.8X3	T47.8X4	T47.8X5	T47.8X6
Glue NEC	T52.8X1	T52.8X2	T52.8X3	T52.8X4	—	—
Glutamic acid	T47.5X1	T47.5X2	T47.5X3	T47.5X4	T47.5X5	T47.5X6
Glutaral (medicinal)	T49.0X1	T49.0X2	T49.0X3	T49.0X4	T49.0X5	T49.0X6
nonmedicinal	T65.891	T65.892	T65.893	T65.894	—	—
Glutaraldehyde (nonmedicinal)	T65.891	T65.892	T65.893	T65.894	—	—
medicinal	T49.0X1	T49.0X2	T49.0X3	T49.0X4	T49.0X5	T49.0X6
Glutathione	T50.6X1	T50.6X2	T50.6X3	T50.6X4	T50.6X5	T50.6X6
Glutethimide	T42.6X1	T42.6X2	T42.6X3	T42.6X4	T42.6X5	T42.6X6
Glyburide	T38.3X1	T38.3X2	T38.3X3	T38.3X4	T38.3X5	T38.3X6
Glycerin	T47.4X1	T47.4X2	T47.4X3	T47.4X4	T47.4X5	T47.4X6
Glycerol	T47.4X1	T47.4X2	T47.4X3	T47.4X4	T47.4X5	T47.4X6
borax	T49.6X1	T49.6X2	T49.6X3	T49.6X4	T49.6X5	T49.6X6
intravenous	T50.3X1	T50.3X2	T50.3X3	T50.3X4	T50.3X5	T50.3X6
iodinated	T48.4X1	T48.4X2	T48.4X3	T48.4X4	T48.4X5	T48.4X6
Glycerophosphate	T50.991	T50.992	T50.993	T50.994	T50.995	T50.996
Glyceryl						
gualacolate	T48.4X1	T48.4X2	T48.4X3	T48.4X4	T48.4X5	T48.4X6
nitrate	T46.3X1	T46.3X2	T46.3X3	T46.3X4	T46.3X5	T46.3X6
triacetate (topical)	T49.0X1	T49.0X2	T49.0X3	T49.0X4	T49.0X5	T49.0X6
trinitrate	T46.3X1	T46.3X2	T46.3X3	T46.3X4	T46.3X5	T46.3X6
Glycine	T50.3X1	T50.3X2	T50.3X3	T50.3X4	T50.3X5	T50.3X6
Glyclopyramide	T38.3X1	T38.3X2	T38.3X3	T38.3X4	T38.3X5	T38.3X6
Glycobiarsol	T37.3X1	T37.3X2	T37.3X3	T37.3X4	T37.3X5	T37.3X6
Glycols (ether)	T52.3X1	T52.3X2	T52.3X3	T52.3X4	—	—
Glyconiazide	T37.1X1	T37.1X2	T37.1X3	T37.1X4	T37.1X5	T37.1X6
Glycopyrrolate	T44.3X1	T44.3X2	T44.3X3	T44.3X4	T44.3X5	T44.3X6
Glycopyrronium	T44.3X1	T44.3X2	T44.3X3	T44.3X4	T44.3X5	T44.3X6
bromide	T44.3X1	T44.3X2	T44.3X3	T44.3X4	T44.3X5	T44.3X6
Glycoside, cardiac (stimulant)	T46.0X1	T46.0X2	T46.0X3	T46.0X4	T46.0X5	T46.0X6
Glycyclamide	T38.3X1	T38.3X2	T38.3X3	T38.3X4	T38.3X5	T38.3X6
Glycyrrhiza extract	T48.4X1	T48.4X2	T48.4X3	T48.4X4	T48.4X5	T48.4X6
Glycyrrhizic acid	T48.4X1	T48.4X2	T48.4X3	T48.4X4	T48.4X5	T48.4X6
Glycyrrhizinate potassium	T48.4X1	T48.4X2	T48.4X3	T48.4X4	T48.4X5	T48.4X6
Glymidine sodium	T38.3X1	T38.3X2	T38.3X3	T38.3X4	T38.3X5	T38.3X6
Glyphosate	T60.3X1	T60.3X2	T60.3X3	T60.3X4	—	—
Glyphylline	T48.6X1	T48.6X2	T48.6X3	T48.6X4	T48.6X5	T48.6X6

Substance	Poisoning, Accidental (unintentional)	Poisoning, Intentional self-harm	Poisoning, Assault	Poisoning, Undetermined	Adverse effect	Underdosing
Gold						
colloidal (l98Au)	T45.1X1	T45.1X2	T45.1X3	T45.1X4	T45.1X5	T45.1X6
salts	T39.4X1	T39.4X2	T39.4X3	T39.4X4	T39.4X5	T39.4X6
Golden sulfide of antimony	T56.891	T56.892	T56.893	T56.894	—	—
Goldylocks	T62.2X1	T62.2X2	T62.2X3	T62.2X4	—	—
Gonadal tissue extract	T38.901	T38.902	T38.903	T38.904	T38.905	T38.906
female	T38.5X1	T38.5X2	T38.5X3	T38.5X4	T38.5X5	T38.5X6
male	T38.7X1	T38.7X2	T38.7X3	T38.7X4	T38.7X5	T38.7X6
Gonadorelin	T38.891	T38.892	T38.893	T38.894	T38.895	T38.896
Gonadotropin	T38.891	T38.892	T38.893	T38.894	T38.895	T38.896
chorionic	T38.891	T38.892	T38.893	T38.894	T38.895	T38.896
pituitary	T38.811	T38.812	T38.813	T38.814	T38.815	T38.816
Goserelin	T45.1X1	T45.1X2	T45.1X3	T45.1X4	T45.1X5	T45.1X6
Grain alcohol	T51.0X1	T51.0X2	T51.0X3	T51.0X4	—	—
Gramicidin	T49.0X1	T49.0X2	T49.0X3	T49.0X4	T49.0X5	T49.0X6
Granisetron	T45.0X1	T45.0X2	T45.0X3	T45.0X4	T45.0X5	T45.0X6
Gratiola officinalis	T62.2X1	T62.2X2	T62.2X3	T62.2X4	—	—
Grease	T65.891	T65.892	T65.893	T65.894	—	—
Green hellebore	T62.2X1	T62.2X2	T62.2X3	T62.2X4	—	—
Green soap	T49.2X1	T49.2X2	T49.2X3	T49.2X4	T49.2X5	T49.2X6
Grifulvin	T36.7X1	T36.7X2	T36.7X3	T36.7X4	T36.7X5	T36.7X6
Griseofulvin	T36.7X1	T36.7X2	T36.7X3	T36.7X4	T36.7X5	T36.7X6
Growth hormone	T38.811	T38.812	T38.813	T38.814	T38.815	T38.816
Guaiac reagent	T50.991	T50.992	T50.993	T50.994	T50.995	T50.996
Guaiacol derivatives	T48.4X1	T48.4X2	T48.4X3	T48.4X4	T48.4X5	T48.4X6
Guaifenesin	T48.4X1	T48.4X2	T48.4X3	T48.4X4	T48.4X5	T48.4X6
Guaimesal	T48.4X1	T48.4X2	T48.4X3	T48.4X4	T48.4X5	T48.4X6
Guaiphenesin	T48.4X1	T48.4X2	T48.4X3	T48.4X4	T48.4X5	T48.4X6
Guamecycline	T36.4X1	T36.4X2	T36.4X3	T36.4X4	T36.4X5	T36.4X6
Guanabenz	T46.5X1	T46.5X2	T46.5X3	T46.5X4	T46.5X5	T46.5X6
Guanacline	T46.5X1	T46.5X2	T46.5X3	T46.5X4	T46.5X5	T46.5X6
Guanadrel	T46.5X1	T46.5X2	T46.5X3	T46.5X4	T46.5X5	T46.5X6
Guanatol	T37.2X1	T37.2X2	T37.2X3	T37.2X4	T37.2X5	T37.2X6
Guanethidine	T46.5X1	T46.5X2	T46.5X3	T46.5X4	T46.5X5	T46.5X6
Guanfacine	T46.5X1	T46.5X2	T46.5X3	T46.5X4	T46.5X5	T46.5X6
Guano	T65.891	T65.892	T65.893	T65.894	—	—
Guanochlor	T46.5X1	T46.5X2	T46.5X3	T46.5X4	T46.5X5	T46.5X6
Guanoclor	T46.5X1	T46.5X2	T46.5X3	T46.5X4	T46.5X5	T46.5X6
Guanoctine	T46.5X1	T46.5X2	T46.5X3	T46.5X4	T46.5X5	T46.5X6
Guanoxabenz	T46.5X1	T46.5X2	T46.5X3	T46.5X4	T46.5X5	T46.5X6
Guanoxan	T46.5X1	T46.5X2	T46.5X3	T46.5X4	T46.5X5	T46.5X6
Guar gum (medicinal)	T46.6X1	T46.6X2	T46.6X3	T46.6X4	T46.6X5	T46.6X6
H						
Hachimycin	T36.7X1	T36.7X2	T36.7X3	T36.7X4	T36.7X5	T36.7X6
Hair						
dye	T49.4X1	T49.4X2	T49.4X3	T49.4X4	T49.4X5	T49.4X6
preparation NEC	T49.4X1	T49.4X2	T49.4X3	T49.4X4	T49.4X5	T49.4X6
Halazepam	T42.4X1	T42.4X2	T42.4X3	T42.4X4	T42.4X5	T42.4X6
Halcinolone	T49.0X1	T49.0X2	T49.0X3	T49.0X4	T49.0X5	T49.0X6
Halcinonide	T49.0X1	T49.0X2	T49.0X3	T49.0X4	T49.0X5	T49.0X6
Halethazole	T49.0X1	T49.0X2	T49.0X3	T49.0X4	T49.0X5	T49.0X6
Hallucinogen NEC	T40.901	T40.902	T40.903	T40.904	T40.905	T40.906
Halofantrine	T37.2X1	T37.2X2	T37.2X3	T37.2X4	T37.2X5	T37.2X6
Halofenate	T46.6X1	T46.6X2	T46.6X3	T46.6X4	T46.6X5	T46.6X6
Halometasone	T49.0X1	T49.0X2	T49.0X3	T49.0X4	T49.0X5	T49.0X6
Haloperidol	T43.4X1	T43.4X2	T43.4X3	T43.4X4	T43.4X5	T43.4X6
Haloprogin	T49.0X1	T49.0X2	T49.0X3	T49.0X4	T49.0X5	T49.0X6
Halotex	T49.0X1	T49.0X2	T49.0X3	T49.0X4	T49.0X5	T49.0X6
Halothane	T41.0X1	T41.0X2	T41.0X3	T41.0X4	T41.0X5	T41.0X6

Substance	Poisoning, Accidental (unintentional)	Poisoning, Intentional self-harm	Poisoning, Assault	Poisoning, Undetermined	Adverse effect	Underdosing
Haloxazolam	T42.4X1	T42.4X2	T42.4X3	T42.4X4	T42.4X5	T42.4X6
Halquinols	T49.0X1	T49.0X2	T49.0X3	T49.0X4	T49.0X5	T49.0X6
Hamamelis	T49.2X1	T49.2X2	T49.2X3	T49.2X4	T49.2X5	T49.2X6
Haptendextran	T45.8X1	T45.8X2	T45.8X3	T45.8X4	T45.8X5	T45.8X6
Harmonyl	T46.5X1	T46.5X2	T46.5X3	T46.5X4	T46.5X5	T46.5X6
Hartmann's solution	T50.3X1	T50.3X2	T50.3X3	T50.3X4	T50.3X5	T50.3X6
Hashish	T40.7X1	T40.7X2	T40.7X3	T40.7X4	T40.7X5	T40.7X6
Hawaiian Woodrose seeds	T40.991	T40.992	T40.993	T40.994	—	—
HCB	T60.3X1	T60.3X2	T60.3X3	T60.3X4		
HCH	T53.6X1	T53.6X2	T53.6X3	T53.6X4		
medicinal	T49.0X1	T49.0X2	T49.0X3	T49.0X4	T49.0X5	T49.0X6
HCN	T57.3X1	T57.3X2	T57.3X3	T57.3X4		
Headache cures, drugs, powders NEC	T50.901	T50.902	T50.903	T50.904	T50.905	T50.906
Heavenly Blue (morning glory)	T40.991	T40.992	T40.993	T40.994	—	—
Heavy metal antidote	T45.8X1	T45.8X2	T45.8X3	T45.8X4	T45.8X5	T45.8X6
Hedaquinium	T49.0X1	T49.0X2	T49.0X3	T49.0X4	T49.0X5	T49.0X6
Hedge hyssop	T62.2X1	T62.2X2	T62.2X3	T62.2X4	—	—
Heet	T49.8X1	T49.8X2	T49.8X3	T49.8X4	T49.8X5	T49.8X6
Helenin	T37.4X1	T37.4X2	T37.4X3	T37.4X4	T37.4X5	T37.4X6
Helium (nonmedicinal) NEC	T59.891	T59.892	T59.893	T59.894	—	—
medicinal	T48.991	T48.992	T48.993	T48.994	T48.995	T48.996
Hellebore (black) (green) (white)	T62.2X1	T62.2X2	T62.2X3	T62.2X4	—	—
Hematin	T45.8X1	T45.8X2	T45.8X3	T45.8X4	T45.8X5	T45.8X6
Hematinic preparation	T45.8X1	T45.8X2	T45.8X3	T45.8X4	T45.8X5	T45.8X6
Hematological agent	T45.91	T45.92	T45.93	T45.94	T45.95	T45.96
specified NEC	T45.8X1	T45.8X2	T45.8X3	T45.8X4	T45.8X5	T45.8X6
Hemlock	T62.2X1	T62.2X2	T62.2X3	T62.2X4	—	—
Hemostatic	T45.621	T45.622	T45.623	T45.624	T45.625	T45.626
drug, systemic	T45.621	T45.622	T45.623	T45.624	T45.625	T45.626
Hemostyptic	T49.4X1	T49.4X2	T49.4X3	T49.4X4	T49.4X5	T49.4X6
Henbane	T62.2X1	T62.2X2	T62.2X3	T62.2X4	—	—
Heparin (sodium)	T45.511	T45.512	T45.513	T45.514	T45.515	T45.516
action reverser	T45.7X1	T45.7X2	T45.7X3	T45.7X4	T45.7X5	T45.7X6
Heparin-fraction	T45.511	T45.512	T45.513	T45.514	T45.515	T45.516
Heparinoid (systemic)	T45.511	T45.512	T45.513	T45.514	T45.515	T45.516
Hepatic secretion stimulant	T47.8X1	T47.8X2	T47.8X3	T47.8X4	T47.8X5	T47.8X6
Hepatitis B						
immune globulin	T50.Z11	T50.Z12	T50.Z13	T50.Z14	T50.Z15	T50.Z16
vaccine	T50.B91	T50.B92	T50.B93	T50.B94	T50.B95	T50.B96
Hepronicate	T46.7X1	T46.7X2	T46.7X3	T46.7X4	T46.7X5	T46.7X6
Heptabarb	T42.3X1	T42.3X2	T42.3X3	T42.3X4	T42.3X5	T42.3X6
Heptabarbital	T42.3X1	T42.3X2	T42.3X3	T42.3X4	T42.3X5	T42.3X6
Heptabarbitone	T42.3X1	T42.3X2	T42.3X3	T42.3X4	T42.3X5	T42.3X6
Heptachlor	T60.1X1	T60.1X2	T60.1X3	T60.1X4	—	—
Heptalgin	T40.2X1	T40.2X2	T40.2X3	T40.2X4	T40.2X5	T40.2X6
Heptaminol	T46.3X1	T46.3X2	T46.3X3	T46.3X4	T46.3X5	T46.3X6
Herbicide NEC	T60.3X1	T60.3X2	T60.3X3	T60.3X4	—	—
Heroin	T40.1X1	T40.1X2	T40.1X3	T40.1X4	—	—
Herplex	T49.5X1	T49.5X2	T49.5X3	T49.5X4	T49.5X5	T49.5X6
HES	T45.8X1	T45.8X2	T45.8X3	T45.8X4	T45.8X5	T45.8X6
Hesperidin	T46.991	T46.992	T46.993	T46.994	T46.995	T46.996
Hetacillin	T36.0X1	T36.0X2	T36.0X3	T36.0X4	T36.0X5	T36.0X6
Hetastarch	T45.8X1	T45.8X2	T45.8X3	T45.8X4	T45.8X5	T45.8X6
HETP	T60.0X1	T60.0X2	T60.0X3	T60.0X4	—	—

Hexachlorobenzene - Hydrocarbon gas

Substance	Poisoning, Accidental (unintentional)	Poisoning, Intentional self-harm	Poisoning, Assault	Poisoning, Undetermined	Adverse effect	Underdosing
Hexachlorobenzene (vapor)	T60.3X1	T60.3X2	T60.3X3	T60.3X4	—	—
Hexachlorocyclohexane	T53.6X1	T53.6X2	T53.6X3	T53.6X4	—	—
Hexachlorophene	T49.0X1	T49.0X2	T49.0X3	T49.0X4	T49.0X5	T49.0X6
Hexadiline	T46.3X1	T46.3X2	T46.3X3	T46.3X4	T46.3X5	T46.3X6
Hexadimethrine (bromide)	T45.7X1	T45.7X2	T45.7X3	T45.7X4	T45.7X5	T45.7X6
Hexadylamine	T46.3X1	T46.3X2	T46.3X3	T46.3X4	T46.3X5	T46.3X6
Hexaethyl tetraphosphate	T60.0X1	T60.0X2	T60.0X3	T60.0X4	—	—
Hexafluorenium bromide	T48.1X1	T48.1X2	T48.1X3	T48.1X4	T48.1X5	T48.1X6
Hexafluronium (bromide)	T48.1X1	T48.1X2	T48.1X3	T48.1X4	T48.1X5	T48.1X6
Hexa-germ	T49.2X1	T49.2X2	T49.2X3	T49.2X4	T49.2X5	T49.2X6
Hexahydrobenzol	T52.8X1	T52.8X2	T52.8X3	T52.8X4	—	—
Hexahydrocresol (s)	T51.8X1	T51.8X2	T51.8X3	T51.8X4	—	—
arsenide	T57.0X1	T57.0X2	T57.0X3	T57.0X4	—	—
arseniurated	T57.0X1	T57.0X2	T57.0X3	T57.0X4	—	—
cyanide	T57.3X1	T57.3X2	T57.3X3	T57.3X4	—	—
gas	T59.891	T59.892	T59.893	T59.894	—	—
Fluoride (liquid)	T57.8X1	T57.8X2	T57.8X3	T57.8X4	—	—
vapor	T59.891	T59.892	T59.893	T59.894	—	—
phophorated	T60.0X1	T60.0X2	T60.0X3	T60.0X4	—	—
sulfate	T57.8X1	T57.8X2	T57.8X3	T57.8X4	—	—
sulfide (gas)	T59.6X1	T59.6X2	T59.6X3	T59.6X4	—	—
arseniurated	T57.0X1	T57.0X2	T57.0X3	T57.0X4	—	—
sulfurated	T57.8X1	T57.8X2	T57.8X3	T57.8X4	—	—
Hexahydrophenol	T51.8X1	T51.8X2	T51.8X3	T51.8X4	—	—
Hexalen	T51.8X1	T51.8X2	T51.8X3	T51.8X4	—	—
Hexamethonium bromide	T44.2X1	T44.2X2	T44.2X3	T44.2X4	T44.2X5	I44.2X6
Hexamethylene	T52.8X1	T52.8X2	T52.8X3	T52.8X4	—	—
Hexamethylmelamine	T45.1X1	T45.1X2	T45.1X3	T45.1X4	T45.1X5	T45.1X6
Hexamidine	T49.0X1	T49.0X2	T49.0X3	T49.0X4	T49.0X5	T49.0X6
Hexamine (mandelate)	T37.8X1	T37.8X2	T37.8X3	T37.8X4	T37.8X5	T37.8X6
Hexanone, 2-hexanone	T52.4X1	T52.4X2	T52.4X3	T52.4X4	—	—
Hexanuorenium	T48.1X1	T48.1X2	T48.1X3	T48.1X4	T48.1X5	T48.1X6
Hexapropymate	T42.6X1	T42.6X2	T42.6X3	T42.6X4	T42.6X5	T42.6X6
Hexasonium iodide	T44.3X1	T44.3X2	T44.3X3	T44.3X4	T44.3X5	T44.3X6
Hexcarbacholine bromide	T48.1X1	T48.1X2	T48.1X3	T48.1X4	T48.1X5	T48.1X6
Hexemal	T42.3X1	T42.3X2	T42.3X3	T42.3X4	T42.3X5	T42.3X6
Hexestrol	T38.5X1	T38.5X2	T38.5X3	T38.5X4	T38.5X5	T38.5X6
Hexethal (sodium)	T42.3X1	T42.3X2	T42.3X3	T42.3X4	T42.3X5	T42.3X6
Hexetidine	T37.8X1	T37.8X2	T37.8X3	T37.8X4	T37.8X5	T37.8X6
Hexobarbital	T42.3X1	T42.3X2	T42.3X3	T42.3X4	T42.3X5	T42.3X6
rectal	T41.291	T41.292	T41.293	T41.294	T41.295	T41.296
sodium	T41.1X1	T41.1X2	T41.1X3	T41.1X4	T41.1X5	T41.1X6
Hexobendine	T46.3X1	T46.3X2	T46.3X3	T46.3X4	T46.3X5	T46.3X6
Hexocyclium	T44.3X1	T44.3X2	T44.3X3	T44.3X4	T44.3X5	T44.3X6
metilsulfate	T44.3X1	T44.3X2	T44.3X3	T44.3X4	T44.3X5	T44.3X6
Hexoestrol	T38.5X1	T38.5X2	T38.5X3	T38.5X4	T38.5X5	T38.5X6
Hexone	T52.4X1	T52.4X2	T52.4X3	T52.4X4	—	—
Hexoprenaline	T48.6X1	T48.6X2	T48.6X3	T48.6X4	T48.6X5	T48.6X6
Hexylcaine	T41.3X1	T41.3X2	T41.3X3	T41.3X4	T41.3X5	T41.3X6
Hexylresorcinol	T52.2X1	T52.2X2	T52.2X3	T52.2X4	—	—
HGH (human growth hormone)	T38.811	T38.812	T38.813	T38.814	T38.815	T38.816
Hinkle's pills	T47.2X1	T47.2X2	T47.2X3	T47.2X4	T47.2X5	T47.2X6
Histalog	T50.8X1	T50.8X2	T50.8X3	T50.8X4	T50.8X5	T50.8X6
Histamine (phosphate)	T50.8X1	T50.8X2	T50.8X3	T50.8X4	T50.8X5	T50.8X6

Substance	Poisoning, Accidental (unintentional)	Poisoning, Intentional self-harm	Poisoning, Assault	Poisoning, Undetermined	Adverse effect	Underdosing
Histoplasmin	T50.8X1	T50.8X2	T50.8X3	T50.8X4	T50.8X5	T50.8X6
Holly berries	T62.2X1	T62.2X2	T62.2X3	T62.2X4	—	—
Homatropine	T44.3X1	T44.3X2	T44.3X3	T44.3X4	T44.3X5	T44.3X6
methylbromide	T44.3X1	T44.3X2	T44.3X3	T44.3X4	T44.3X5	T44.3X6
Homochlorcyclizine	T45.0X1	T45.0X2	T45.0X3	T45.0X4	T45.0X5	T45.0X6
Homosalate	T49.3X1	T49.3X2	T49.3X3	T49.3X4	T49.3X5	T49.3X6
Homo-tet	T50.Z11	T50.Z12	T50.Z13	T50.Z14	T50.Z15	T50.Z16
Hormone	T38.801	T38.802	T38.803	T38.804	T38.805	T38.806
adrenal cortical steroids	T38.0X1	T38.0X2	T38.0X3	T38.0X4	T38.0X5	T38.0X6
androgenic	T38.7X1	T38.7X2	T38.7X3	T38.7X4	T38.7X5	T38.7X6
anterior pituitary NEC	T38.811	T38.812	T38.813	T38.814	T38.815	T38.816
antidiabetic agents	T38.3X1	T38.3X2	T38.3X3	T38.3X4	T38.3X5	T38.3X6
antidiuretic	T38.891	T38.892	T38.893	T38.894	T38.895	T38.896
cancer therapy	T45.1X1	T45.1X2	T45.1X3	T45.1X4	T45.1X5	T45.1X6
follicle stimulating	T38.811	T38.812	T38.813	T38.814	T38.815	T38.816
gonadotropic	T38.891	T38.892	T38.893	T38.894	T38.895	T38.896
pituitary	T38.811	T38.812	T38.813	T38.814	T38.815	T38.816
growth	T38.811	T38.812	T38.813	T38.814	T38.815	T38.816
luteinizing	T38.811	T38.812	T38.813	T38.814	T38.815	T38.816
ovarian	T38.5X1	T38.5X2	T38.5X3	T38.5X4	T38.5X5	T38.5X6
oxytocic	T48.0X1	T48.0X2	T48.0X3	T48.0X4	T48.0X5	T48.0X6
parathyroid (derivatives)	T50.991	T50.992	T50.993	T50.994	T50.995	T50.996
pituitary (posterior) NEC	T38.891	T38.892	T38.893	T38.894	T38.895	T38.896
anterior	T38.811	T38.812	T38.813	T38.814	T38.815	T38.816
specified, NEC	T38.891	T38.892	T38.893	T38.894	T38.895	T38.896
thyroid	T38.1X1	T38.1X2	T38.1X3	T38.1X4	T38.1X5	T38.1X6
Hornet (sting)	T63.451	T63.452	T63.453	T63.454	—	—
Horse anti-human lymphocytic serum	T50.Z11	T50.Z12	T50.Z13	T50.Z14	T50.Z15	T50.Z16
Horticulture agent NEC	T65.91	T65.92	T65.93	T65.94	—	—
with pesticide	T60.91	T60.92	T60.93	T60.94	—	—
Human						
albumin	T45.8X1	T45.8X2	T45.8X3	T45.8X4	T45.8X5	T45.8X6
growth hormone (HGH)	T38.811	T38.812	T38.813	T38.814	T38.815	T38.816
immune serum	T50.Z11	T50.Z12	T50.Z13	T50.Z14	T50.Z15	T50.Z16
Hyaluronidase	T45.3X1	T45.3X2	T45.3X3	T45.3X4	T45.3X5	T45.3X6
Hyazyme	T45.3X1	T45.3X2	T45.3X3	T45.3X4	T45.3X5	T45.3X6
Hycodan	T40.2X1	T40.2X2	T40.2X3	T40.2X4	T40.2X5	T40.2X6
Hydantoin derivative NEC	T42.0X1	T42.0X2	T42.0X3	T42.0X4	T42.0X5	T42.0X6
Hydeltra	T38.0X1	T38.0X2	T38.0X3	T38.0X4	T38.0X5	T38.0X6
Hydergine	T44.6X1	T44.6X2	T44.6X3	T44.6X4	T44.6X5	T44.6X6
Hydrabamine penicillin	T36.0X1	T36.0X2	T36.0X3	T36.0X4	T36.0X5	T36.0X6
Hydralazine	T46.5X1	T46.5X2	T46.5X3	T46.5X4	T46.5X5	T46.5X6
Hydrargaphen	T49.0X1	T49.0X2	T49.0X3	T49.0X4	T49.0X5	T49.0X6
Hydrargyri amino-chloridum	T49.0X1	T49.0X2	T49.0X3	T49.0X4	T49.0X5	T49.0X6
Hydrastine	T48.291	T48.292	T48.293	T48.294	T48.295	T48.296
Hydrazine	T54.1X1	T54.1X2	T54.1X3	T54.1X4	—	—
monoamine oxidase inhibitors	T43.1X1	T43.1X2	T43.1X3	T43.1X4	T43.1X5	T43.1X6
Hydrazoic acid, azides	T54.2X1	T54.2X2	T54.2X3	T54.2X4	—	—
Hydriodic acid	T48.4X1	T48.4X2	T48.4X3	T48.4X4	T48.4X5	T48.4X6
Hydrocarbon gas	T59.891	T59.892	T59.893	T59.894	—	—
incomplete combustion of—see Carbon, monoxide, fuel, utility						

Substance	Poisoning, Accidental (unintentional)	Poisoning, Intentional self-harm	Poisoning, Assault	Poisoning, Undetermined	Adverse effect	Underdosing
Hydrocarbon gas — *continued*						
liquefied (mobile container)	T59.891	T59.892	T59.893	T59.894	—	—
piped (natural)	T59.891	T59.892	T59.893	T59.894	—	—
Hydrochloric acid (liquid)	T54.2X1	T54.2X2	T54.2X3	T54.2X4	—	—
medicinal (digestant)	T47.5X1	T47.5X2	T47.5X3	T47.5X4	T47.5X5	T47.5X6
vapor	T59.891	T59.892	T59.893	T59.894	—	—
Hydrochlorothiazide	T50.2X1	T50.2X2	T50.2X3	T50.2X4	T50.2X5	T50.2X6
Hydrocodone	T40.2X1	T40.2X2	T40.2X3	T40.2X4	T40.2X5	T40.2X6
Hydrocortisone (derivatives)	T49.0X1	T49.0X2	T49.0X3	T49.0X4	T49.0X5	T49.0X6
aceponate	T49.0X1	T49.0X2	T49.0X3	T49.0X4	T49.0X5	T49.0X6
ENT agent	T49.6X1	T49.6X2	T49.6X3	T49.6X4	T49.6X5	T49.6X6
ophthalmic preparation	T49.5X1	T49.5X2	T49.5X3	T49.5X4	T49.5X5	T49.5X6
topical NEC	T49.0X1	T49.0X2	T49.0X3	T49.0X4	T49.0X5	T49.0X6
Hydrocortone	T38.0X1	T38.0X2	T38.0X3	T38.0X4	T38.0X5	T38.0X6
ENT agent	T49.6X1	T49.6X2	T49.6X3	T49.6X4	T49.6X5	T49.6X6
ophthalmic preparation	T49.5X1	T49.5X2	T49.5X3	T49.5X4	T49.5X5	T49.5X6
topical NEC	T49.0X1	T49.0X2	T49.0X3	T49.0X4	T49.0X5	T49.0X6
Hydrocyanic acid (liquid)	T57.3X1	T57.3X2	T57.3X3	T57.3X4	—	—
gas	T65.0X1	T65.0X2	T65.0X3	T65.0X4	—	—
Hydroflumethiazide	T50.2X1	T50.2X2	T50.2X3	T50.2X4	T50.2X5	T50.2X6
Hydrofluoric acid (liquid)	T54.2X1	T54.2X2	T54.2X3	T54.2X4	—	—
vapor	T59.891	T59.892	T59.893	T59.894	—	—
Hydrogen	T59.891	T59.892	T59.893	T59.894	—	—
arsenide	T57.0X1	T57.0X2	T57.0X3	T57.0X4	—	—
arseniureted	T57.0X1	T57.0X2	T57.0X3	T57.0X4	—	—
chloride	T57.8X1	T57.8X2	T57.8X3	T57.8X4	—	—
cyanide (salts)	T57.3X1	T57.3X2	T57.3X3	T57.3X4	—	—
gas	T57.3X1	T57.3X2	T57.3X3	T57.3X4	—	—
Fluoride	T59.5X1	T59.5X2	T59.5X3	T59.5X4	—	—
vapor	T59.5X1	T59.5X2	T59.5X3	T59.5X4	—	—
peroxide	T49.0X1	T49.0X2	T49.0X3	T49.0X4	T49.0X5	T49.0X6
phosphureted	T57.1X1	T57.1X2	T57.1X3	T57.1X4	—	—
sulfide	T59.6X1	T59.6X2	T59.6X3	T59.6X4	—	—
arseniureted	T57.0X1	T57.0X2	T57.0X3	T57.0X4	—	—
sulfureted	T59.6X1	T59.6X2	T59.6X3	T59.6X4	—	—
Hydromethylpyridine	T46.7X1	T46.7X2	T46.7X3	T46.7X4	T46.7X5	T46.7X6
Hydromorphinol	T40.2X1	T40.2X2	T40.2X3	T40.2X4	—	—
Hydromorphinone	T40.2X1	T40.2X2	T40.2X3	T40.2X4	T40.2X5	T40.2X6
Hydromorphone	T40.2X1	T40.2X2	T40.2X3	T40.2X4	T40.2X5	T40.2X6
Hydromox	T50.2X1	T50.2X2	T50.2X3	T50.2X4	T50.2X5	T50.2X6
Hydrophilic lotion	T49.3X1	T49.3X2	T49.3X3	T49.3X4	T49.3X5	T49.3X6
Hydroquinidine	T46.2X1	T46.2X2	T46.2X3	T46.2X4	T46.2X5	T46.2X6
Hydroquinone	T52.2X1	T52.2X2	T52.2X3	T52.2X4	—	—
vapor	T59.891	T59.892	T59.893	T59.894	—	—
Hydrosulfuric acid (gas)	T59.6X1	T59.6X2	T59.6X3	T59.6X4	—	—
Hydrotalcite	T47.1X1	T47.1X2	T47.1X3	T47.1X4	T47.1X5	T47.1X6
Hydrous wool fat	T49.3X1	T49.3X2	T49.3X3	T49.3X4	T49.3X5	T49.3X6
Hydroxide, caustic	T54.3X1	T54.3X2	T54.3X3	T54.3X4	—	—
Hydroxocobalamin	T45.8X1	T45.8X2	T45.8X3	T45.8X4	T45.8X5	T45.8X6
Hydroxyamphetamine	T49.5X1	T49.5X2	T49.5X3	T49.5X4	T49.5X5	T49.5X6
Hydroxycarbamide	T45.1X1	T45.1X2	T45.1X3	T45.1X4	T45.1X5	T45.1X6
Hydroxychloroquine	T37.8X1	T37.8X2	T37.8X3	T37.8X4	T37.8X5	T37.8X6
Hydroxydihydrocodeinone	T40.2X1	T40.2X2	T40.2X3	T40.2X4	T40.2X5	T40.2X6
Hydroxyestrone	T38.5X1	T38.5X2	T38.5X3	T38.5X4	T38.5X5	T38.5X6
Hydroxyethyl starch	T45.8X1	T45.8X2	T45.8X3	T45.8X4	T45.8X5	T45.8X6
Hydroxymethylpenta-none	T52.4X1	T52.4X2	T52.4X3	T52.4X4	—	—
Hydroxyphenamate	T43.591	T43.592	T43.593	T43.594	T43.595	T43.596

Substance	Poisoning, Accidental (unintentional)	Poisoning, Intentional self-harm	Poisoning, Assault	Poisoning, Undetermined	Adverse effect	Underdosing
Hydroxyphenylbutazone	T39.2X1	T39.2X2	T39.2X3	T39.2X4	T39.2X5	T39.2X6
Hydroxyprogesterone	T38.5X1	T38.5X2	T38.5X3	T38.5X4	T38.5X5	T38.5X6
caproate	T38.5X1	T38.5X2	T38.5X3	T38.5X4	T38.5X5	T38.5X6
Hydroxyquinoline (derivatives) NEC	T37.8X1	T37.8X2	T37.8X3	T37.8X4	T37.8X5	T37.8X6
Hydroxystilbamidine	T37.3X1	T37.3X2	T37.3X3	T37.3X4	T37.3X5	T37.3X6
Hydroxytoluene (nonmedicinal)	T54.0X1	T54.0X2	T54.0X3	T54.0X4	—	—
medicinal	T49.0X1	T49.0X2	T49.0X3	T49.0X4	T49.0X5	T49.0X6
Hydroxyurea	T45.1X1	T45.1X2	T45.1X3	T45.1X4	T45.1X5	T45.1X6
Hydroxyzine	T43.591	T43.592	T43.593	T43.594	T43.595	T43.596
Hyoscine	T44.3X1	T44.3X2	T44.3X3	T44.3X4	T44.3X5	T44.3X6
Hyoscyamine	T44.3X1	T44.3X2	T44.3X3	T44.3X4	T44.3X5	T44.3X6
Hyoscyamus	T44.3X1	T44.3X2	T44.3X3	T44.3X4	T44.3X5	T44.3X6
dry extract	T44.3X1	T44.3X2	T44.3X3	T44.3X4	T44.3X5	T44.3X6
Hypaque	T50.8X1	T50.8X2	T50.8X3	T50.8X4	T50.8X5	T50.8X6
Hypertussis	T50.Z11	T50.Z12	T50.Z13	T50.Z14	T50.Z15	T50.Z16
Hypnotic	T42.71	T42.72	T42.73	T42.74	T42.75	T42.76
anticonvulsant	T42.71	T42.72	T42.73	T42.74	T42.75	T42.76
specified NEC	T42.6X1	T42.6X2	T42.6X3	T42.6X4	T42.6X5	T42.6X6
Hypochlorite	T49.0X1	T49.0X2	T49.0X3	T49.0X4	T49.0X5	T49.0X6
Hypophysis, posterior	T38.891	T38.892	T38.893	T38.894	T38.895	T38.896
Hypotensive NEC	T46.5X1	T46.5X2	T46.5X3	T46.5X4	T46.5X5	T46.5X6
Hypromellose	T49.5X1	T49.5X2	T49.5X3	T49.5X4	T49.5X5	T49.5X6
Ibacitabine	T37.5X1	T37.5X2	T37.5X3	T37.5X4	T37.5X5	T37.5X6
Ibopamine	T44.991	T44.992	T44.993	T44.994	T44.995	T44.996
Ibufenac	T39.311	T39.312	T39.313	T39.314	T39.315	T39.316
Ibuprofen	T39.311	T39.312	T39.313	T39.314	T39.315	T39.316
Ibuproxam	T39.311	T39.312	T39.313	T39.314	T39.315	T39.316
Ibuterol	T48.6X1	T48.6X2	T48.6X3	T48.6X4	T48.6X5	T48.6X6
Ichthammol	T49.0X1	T49.0X2	T49.0X3	T49.0X4	T49.0X5	T49.0X6
Ichthyol	T49.4X1	T49.4X2	T49.4X3	T49.4X4	T49.4X5	T49.4X6
Idarubicin	T45.1X1	T45.1X2	T45.1X3	T45.1X4	T45.1X5	T45.1X6
Idrocilamide	T42.8X1	T42.8X2	T42.8X3	T42.8X4	T42.8X5	T42.8X6
Ifenprodil	T46.7X1	T46.7X2	T46.7X3	T46.7X4	T46.7X5	T46.7X6
Ifosfamide	T45.1X1	T45.1X2	T45.1X3	T45.1X4	T45.1X5	T45.1X6
Iletin	T38.3X1	T38.3X2	T38.3X3	T38.3X4	T38.3X5	T38.3X6
Ilex	T62.2X1	T62.2X2	T62.2X3	T62.2X4	—	—
Illuminating gas (after combustion)	T58.11	T58.12	T58.13	T58.14	—	—
prior to combustion	T59.891	T59.892	T59.893	T59.894	—	—
Ilopan	T45.2X1	T45.2X2	T45.2X3	T45.2X4	T45.2X5	T45.2X6
Iloprost	T46.7X1	T46.7X2	T46.7X3	T46.7X4	T46.7X5	T46.7X6
Ilotycin	T36.3X1	T36.3X2	T36.3X3	T36.3X4	T36.3X5	T36.3X6
ophthalmic preparation	T49.5X1	T49.5X2	T49.5X3	T49.5X4	T49.5X5	T49.5X6
topical NEC	T49.0X1	T49.0X2	T49.0X3	T49.0X4	T49.0X5	T49.0X6
Imidazole-4-carboxamide	T45.1X1	T45.1X2	T45.1X3	T45.1X4	T45.1X5	T45.1X6
Imipenem	T36.0X1	T36.0X2	T36.0X3	T36.0X4	T36.0X5	T36.0X6
Imipramine	T43.011	T43.012	T43.013	T43.014	T43.015	T43.016
Iminostilbene	T42.1X1	T42.1X2	T42.1X3	T42.1X4	T42.1X5	T42.1X6
Immu-G	T50.Z11	T50.Z12	T50.Z13	T50.Z14	T50.Z15	T50.Z16
Immuglobin	T50.Z11	T50.Z12	T50.Z13	T50.Z14	T50.Z15	T50.Z16
Immune						
globulin	T50.Z11	T50.Z12	T50.Z13	T50.Z14	T50.Z15	T50.Z16
serum globulin	T50.Z11	T50.Z12	T50.Z13	T50.Z14	T50.Z15	T50.Z16
Immunoglobin human (intravenous) (normal)	T50.Z11	T50.Z12	T50.Z13	T50.Z14	T50.Z15	T50.Z16
unmodified	T50.Z11	T50.Z12	T50.Z13	T50.Z14	T50.Z15	T50.Z16

Immunosuppressive drug - Iodipamide

Substance	Poisoning, Accidental (unintentional)	Poisoning, Intentional self-harm	Poisoning, Assault	Poisoning, Undetermined	Adverse effect	Underdosing
Immunosuppressive drug	T45.1X1	T45.1X2	T45.1X3	T45.1X4	T45.1X5	T45.1X6
Immu-tetanus	T50.Z11	T50.Z12	T50.Z13	T50.Z14	T50.Z15	T50.Z16
Indalpine	T43.221	T43.222	T43.223	T43.224	T43.225	T43.226
Indanazoline	T48.5X1	T48.5X2	T48.5X3	T48.5X4	T48.5X5	T48.5X6
Indandione (derivatives)	T45.511	T45.512	T45.513	T45.514	T45.515	T45.516
Indapamide	T46.5X1	T46.5X2	T46.5X3	T46.5X4	T46.5X5	T46.5X6
Indendione (derivatives)	T45.511	T45.512	T45.513	T45.514	T45.515	T45.516
Indenolol	T44.7X1	T44.7X2	T44.7X3	T44.7X4	T44.7X5	T44.7X6
Inderal	T44.7X1	T44.7X2	T44.7X3	T44.7X4	T44.7X5	T44.7X6
Indian						
hemp	T40.7X1	T40.7X2	T40.7X3	T40.7X4	T40.7X5	T40.7X6
tobacco	T62.2X1	T62.2X2	T62.2X3	T62.2X4	—	—
Indigo carmine	T50.8X1	T50.8X2	T50.8X3	T50.8X4	T50.8X5	T50.8X6
Indobufen	T45.521	T45.522	T45.523	T45.524	T45.525	T45.526
Indocin	T39.2X1	T39.2X2	T39.2X3	T39.2X4	T39.2X5	T39.2X6
Indocyanine green	T50.8X1	T50.8X2	T50.8X3	T50.8X4	T50.8X5	T50.8X6
Indometacin	T39.391	T39.392	T39.393	T39.394	T39.395	T39.396
Indomethacin	T39.391	T39.392	T39.393	T39.394	T39.395	T39.396
farnesil	T39.4X1	T39.4X2	T39.4X3	T39.4X4	T39.4X5	T39.4X6
Indoramin	T44.6X1	T44.6X2	T44.6X3	T44.6X4	T44.6X5	T44.6X6
Industrial						
alcohol	T51.0X1	T51.0X2	T51.0X3	T51.0X4	—	—
fumes	T59.891	T59.892	T59.893	T59.894	—	—
solvents (fumes) (vapors)	T52.91	T52.92	T52.93	T52.94	—	—
Influenza vaccine	T50.B91	T50.B92	T50.B93	T50.B94	T50.B95	T50.B96
Ingested substance NEC	T65.91	T65.92	T65.93	T65.94		
INH	T37.1X1	T37.1X2	T37.1X3	T37.1X4	T37.1X5	T37.1X6
Inhalation, gas (noxious)—see Gas						
Inhibitor						
angiotensin-converting enzyme	T46.4X1	T46.4X2	T46.4X3	T46.4X4	T46.4X5	T46.4X6
carbonic anhydrase	T50.2X1	T50.2X2	T50.2X3	T50.2X4	T50.2X5	T50.2X6
fibrinolysis	T45.621	T45.622	T45.623	T45.624	T45.625	T45.626
monoamine oxidase NEC	T43.1X1	T43.1X2	T43.1X3	T43.1X4	T43.1X5	T43.1X6
hydrazine	T43.1X1	T43.1X2	T43.1X3	T43.1X4	T43.1X5	T43.1X6
postsynaptic	T43.8X1	T43.8X2	T43.8X3	T43.8X4	T43.8X5	T43.8X6
prothrombin synthesis	T45.511	T45.512	T45.513	T45.514	T45.515	T45.516
Ink	T65.891	T65.892	T65.893	T65.894	—	—
Inorganic substance NEC	T57.91	T57.92	T57.93	T57.94	—	—
Inosine pranobex	T37.5X1	T37.5X2	T37.5X3	T37.5X4	T37.5X5	T37.5X6
Inositol	T50.991	T50.992	T50.993	T50.994	T50.995	T50.996
nicotinate	T46.7X1	T46.7X2	T46.7X3	T46.7X4	T46.7X5	T46.7X6
Inproquone	T45.1X1	T45.1X2	T45.1X3	T45.1X4	T45.1X5	T45.1X6
Insect (sting), venomous	T63.481	T63.482	T63.483	T63.484	—	—
ant	T63.421	T63.422	T63.423	T63.424	—	—
bee	T63.441	T63.442	T63.443	T63.444	—	—
caterpillar	T63.431	T63.432	T63.433	T63.434	—	—
hornet	T63.451	T63.452	T63.453	T63.454	—	—
wasp	T63.461	T63.462	T63.463	T63.464	—	—
Insecticide NEC	T60.91	T60.92	T60.93	T60.94	—	—
carbamate	T60.0X1	T60.0X2	T60.0X3	T60.0X4	—	—
chlorinated	T60.1X1	T60.1X2	T60.1X3	T60.1X4	—	—
mixed	T60.91	T60.92	T60.93	T60.94	—	—
organochlorine	T60.1X1	T60.1X2	T60.1X3	T60.1X4	—	—
organophosphorus	T60.0X1	T60.0X2	T60.0X3	T60.0X4	—	—
Insular tissue extract	T38.3X1	T38.3X2	T38.3X3	T38.3X4	T38.3X5	T38.3X6

Substance	Poisoning, Accidental (unintentional)	Poisoning, Intentional self-harm	Poisoning, Assault	Poisoning, Undetermined	Adverse effect	Underdosing
Insulin (amorphous) (globin) (isophane) (Lente) (NPH) (Semilente) (Ultralente)	T38.3X1	T38.3X2	T38.3X3	T38.3X4	T38.3X5	T38.3X6
defalan	T38.3X1	T38.3X2	T38.3X3	T38.3X4	T38.3X5	T38.3X6
human	T38.3X1	T38.3X2	T38.3X3	T38.3X4	T38.3X5	T38.3X6
injection, soluble	T38.3X1	T38.3X2	T38.3X3	T38.3X4	T38.3X5	T38.3X6
biphasic	T38.3X1	T38.3X2	T38.3X3	T38.3X4	T38.3X5	T38.3X6
intermediate acting	T38.3X1	T38.3X2	T38.3X3	T38.3X4	T38.3X5	T38.3X6
protamine zinc	T38.3X1	T38.3X2	T38.3X3	T38.3X4	T38.3X5	T38.3X6
slow acting	T38.3X1	T38.3X2	T38.3X3	T38.3X4	T38.3X5	T38.3X6
zinc						
protamine injection	T38.3X1	T38.3X2	T38.3X3	T38.3X4	T38.3X5	T38.3X6
suspension (amorphous) (crystalline)	T38.3X1	T38.3X2	T38.3X3	T38.3X4	T38.3X5	T38.3X6
Interferon (alpha) (beta) (gamma)	T37.5X1	T37.5X2	T37.5X3	T37.5X4	T37.5X5	T37.5X6
Intestinal motility control drug	T47.6X1	T47.6X2	T47.6X3	T47.6X4	T47.6X5	T47.6X6
biological	T47.8X1	T47.8X2	T47.8X3	T47.8X4	T47.8X5	T47.8X6
Intranarcon	T41.1X1	T41.1X2	T41.1X3	T41.1X4	T41.1X5	T41.1X6
Intravenous						
amino acids	T50.991	T50.992	T50.993	T50.994	T50.995	T50.996
fat suspension	T50.991	T50.992	T50.993	T50.994	T50.995	T50.996
Inulin	T50.8X1	T50.8X2	T50.8X3	T50.8X4	T50.8X5	T50.8X6
Invert sugar	T50.3X1	T50.3X2	T50.3X3	T50.3X4	T50.3X5	T50.3X6
Inza—see Naproxen						
Iobenzamic acid	T50.8X1	T50.8X2	T50.8X3	T50.8X4	T50.8X5	T50.8X6
Iocarmic acid	T50.8X1	T50.8X2	T50.8X3	T50.8X4	T50.8X5	T50.8X6
Iocetamic acid	T50.8X1	T50.8X2	T50.8X3	T50.8X4	T50.8X5	T50.8X6
Iodamide	T50.8X1	T50.8X2	T50.8X3	T50.8X4	T50.8X5	T50.8X6
Iodide NEC—see also Iodine	T49.0X1	T49.0X2	T49.0X3	T49.0X4	T49.0X5	T49.0X6
mercury (ointment)	T49.0X1	T49.0X2	T49.0X3	T49.0X4	T49.0X5	T49.0X6
methylate	T49.0X1	T49.0X2	T49.0X3	T49.0X4	T49.0X5	T49.0X6
potassium (expectorant) NEC	T48.4X1	T48.4X2	T48.4X3	T48.4X4	T48.4X5	T48.4X6
Iodinated						
contrast medium	T50.8X1	T50.8X2	T50.8X3	T50.8X4	T50.8X5	T50.8X6
glycerol	T48.4X1	T48.4X2	T48.4X3	T48.4X4	T48.4X5	T48.4X6
human serum albumin (131I)	T50.8X1	T50.8X2	T50.8X3	T50.8X4	T50.8X5	T50.8X6
Iodine (antiseptic, external) (tincture) NEC	T49.0X1	T49.0X2	T49.0X3	T49.0X4	T49.0X5	T49.0X6
125—see also Radiation sickness, and Exposure to radioactivce isotopes	T50.8X1	T50.8X2	T50.8X3	T50.8X4	T50.8X5	T50.8X6
therapeutic	T50.991	T50.992	T50.993	T50.994	T50.995	T50.996
131—see also Radiation sickness, and Exposure to radioactivce isotopes	T50.8X1	T50.8X2	T50.8X3	T50.8X4	T50.8X5	T50.8X6
therapeutic	T38.2X1	T38.2X2	T38.2X3	T38.2X4	T38.2X5	T38.2X6
diagnostic	T50.8X1	T50.8X2	T50.8X3	T50.8X4	T50.8X5	T50.8X6
for thyroid conditions (antithyroid)	T38.2X1	T38.2X2	T38.2X3	T38.2X4	T38.2X5	T38.2X6
solution	T49.0X1	T49.0X2	T49.0X3	T49.0X4	T49.0X5	T49.0X6
vapor	T59.891	T59.892	T59.893	T59.894	—	—
Iodipamide	T50.8X1	T50.8X2	T50.8X3	T50.8X4	T50.8X5	T50.8X6

Substance	Poisoning, Accidental (unintentional)	Poisoning, Intentional self-harm	Poisoning, Assault	Poisoning, Undetermined	Adverse effect	Underdosing
Iodized (poppy seed) oil	T50.8X1	T50.8X2	T50.8X3	T50.8X4	T50.8X5	T50.8X6
Iodobismitol	T37.8X1	T37.8X2	T37.8X3	T37.8X4	T37.8X5	T37.8X6
Iodochlorhydroxyquin	T37.8X1	T37.8X2	T37.8X3	T37.8X4	T37.8X5	T37.8X6
topical	T49.0X1	T49.0X2	T49.0X3	T49.0X4	T49.0X5	T49.0X6
Iodochlorhydroxyquinoline	T37.8X1	T37.8X2	T37.8X3	T37.8X4	T37.8X5	T37.8X6
Iodocholesterol (131I)	T50.8X1	T50.8X2	T50.8X3	T50.8X4	T50.8X5	T50.8X6
Iodoform	T49.0X1	T49.0X2	T49.0X3	T49.0X4	T49.0X5	T49.0X6
Iodohippuric acid	T50.8X1	T50.8X2	T50.8X3	T50.8X4	T50.8X5	T50.8X6
Iodopanoic acid	T50.8X1	T50.8X2	T50.8X3	T50.8X4	T50.8X5	T50.8X6
Iodophthalein (sodium)	T50.8X1	T50.8X2	T50.8X3	T50.8X4	T50.8X5	T50.8X6
Iodopyracet	T50.8X1	T50.8X2	T50.8X3	T50.8X4	T50.8X5	T50.8X6
Iodoquinol	T37.8X1	T37.8X2	T37.8X3	T37.8X4	T37.8X5	T37.8X6
Iodoxamic acid	T50.8X1	T50.8X2	T50.8X3	T50.8X4	T50.8X5	T50.8X6
Iofendylate	T50.8X1	T50.8X2	T50.8X3	T50.8X4	T50.8X5	T50.8X6
Ioglycamic acid	T50.8X1	T50.8X2	T50.8X3	T50.8X4	T50.8X5	T50.8X6
Iohexol	T50.8X1	T50.8X2	T50.8X3	T50.8X4	T50.8X5	T50.8X6
Ion exchange resin						
anion	T47.8X1	T47.8X2	T47.8X3	T47.8X4	T47.8X5	T47.8X6
cation	T50.3X1	T50.3X2	T50.3X3	T50.3X4	T50.3X5	T50.3X6
cholestyramine	T46.6X1	T46.6X2	T46.6X3	T46.6X4	T46.6X5	T46.6X6
intestinal	T47.8X1	T47.8X2	T47.8X3	T47.8X4	T47.8X5	T47.8X6
Iopamidol	T50.8X1	T50.8X2	T50.8X3	T50.8X4	T50.8X5	T50.8X6
Iopanoic acid	T50.8X1	T50.8X2	T50.8X3	T50.8X4	T50.8X5	T50.8X6
Iophenoic acid	T50.8X1	T50.8X2	T50.8X3	T50.8X4	T50.8X5	T50.8X6
Iopodate, sodium	T50.8X1	T50.8X2	T50.8X3	T50.8X4	T50.8X5	T50.8X6
Iopodic acid	T50.8X1	T50.8X2	T50.8X3	T50.8X4	T50.8X5	T50.8X6
Iopromide	T50.8X1	T50.8X2	T50.8X3	T50.8X4	T50.8X5	T50.8X6
Iopydol	T50.8X1	T50.8X2	T50.8X3	T50.8X4	T50.8X5	T50.8X6
Iotalamic acid	T50.8X1	T50.8X2	T50.8X3	T50.8X4	T50.8X5	T50.8X6
Iothalamate	T50.8X1	T50.8X2	T50.8X3	T50.8X4	T50.8X5	T50.8X6
Iothiouracil	T38.2X1	T38.2X2	T38.2X3	T38.2X4	T38.2X5	T38.2X6
Iotrol	T50.8X1	T50.8X2	T50.8X3	T50.8X4	T50.8X5	T50.8X6
Iotrolan	T50.8X1	T50.8X2	T50.8X3	T50.8X4	T50.8X5	T50.8X6
Iotroxate	T50.8X1	T50.8X2	T50.8X3	T50.8X4	T50.8X5	T50.8X6
Iotroxic acid	T50.8X1	T50.8X2	T50.8X3	T50.8X4	T50.8X5	T50.8X6
Ioversol	T50.8X1	T50.8X2	T50.8X3	T50.8X4	T50.8X5	T50.8X6
Ioxaglate	T50.8X1	T50.8X2	T50.8X3	T50.8X4	T50.8X5	T50.8X6
Ioxaglic acid	T50.8X1	T50.8X2	T50.8X3	T50.8X4	T50.8X5	T50.8X6
Ioxitalamic acid	T50.8X1	T50.8X2	T50.8X3	T50.8X4	T50.8X5	T50.8X6
Ipecac	T47.7X1	T47.7X2	T47.7X3	T47.7X4	T47.7X5	T47.7X6
Ipecacuanha	T48.4X1	T48.4X2	T48.4X3	T48.4X4	T48.4X5	T48.4X6
Ipodate, calcium	T50.8X1	T50.8X2	T50.8X3	T50.8X4	T50.8X5	T50.8X6
Ipral	T42.3X1	T42.3X2	T42.3X3	T42.3X4	T42.3X5	T42.3X6
Ipratropium (bromide)	T48.6X1	T48.6X2	T48.6X3	T48.6X4	T48.6X5	T48.6X6
Ipriflavone	T46.3X1	T46.3X2	T46.3X3	T46.3X4	T46.3X5	T46.3X6
Iprindole	T43.011	T43.012	T43.013	T43.014	T43.015	T43.016
Iproclozide	T43.1X1	T43.1X2	T43.1X3	T43.1X4	T43.1X5	T43.1X6
Iprofenin	T50.8X1	T50.8X2	T50.8X3	T50.8X4	T50.8X5	T50.8X6
Iproheptine	T49.2X1	T49.2X2	T49.2X3	T49.2X4	T49.2X5	T49.2X6
Iproniazid	T43.1X1	T43.1X2	T43.1X3	T43.1X4	T43.1X5	T43.1X6
Iproplatin	T45.1X1	T45.1X2	T45.1X3	T45.1X4	T45.1X5	T45.1X6
Iproveratril	T46.1X1	T46.1X2	T46.1X3	T46.1X4	T46.1X5	T46.1X6
Iron (compounds) (medicinal) NEC	T45.4X1	T45.4X2	T45.4X3	T45.4X4	T45.4X5	T45.4X6
ammonium	T45.4X1	T45.4X2	T45.4X3	T45.4X4	T45.4X5	T45.4X6
dextran injection	T45.4X1	T45.4X2	T45.4X3	T45.4X4	T45.4X5	T45.4X6
nonmedicinal	T56.891	T56.892	T56.893	T56.894	—	—
salts	T45.4X1	T45.4X2	T45.4X3	T45.4X4	T45.4X5	T45.4X6
sorbitex	T45.4X1	T45.4X2	T45.4X3	T45.4X4	T45.4X5	T45.4X6
sorbitol citric acid complex	T45.4X1	T45.4X2	T45.4X3	T45.4X4	T45.4X5	T45.4X6
Irrigating fluid (vaginal)	T49.8X1	T49.8X2	T49.8X3	T49.8X4	T49.8X5	T49.8X6
eye	T49.5X1	T49.5X2	T49.5X3	T49.5X4	T49.5X5	T49.5X6
Isepamicin	T36.5X1	T36.5X2	T36.5X3	T36.5X4	T36.5X5	T36.5X6
Isoaminile (citrate)	T48.3X1	T48.3X2	T48.3X3	T48.3X4	T48.3X5	T48.3X6
Isoamyl nitrite	T46.3X1	T46.3X2	T46.3X3	T46.3X4	T46.3X5	T46.3X6
Isobenzan	T60.1X1	T60.1X2	T60.1X3	T60.1X4	—	—
Isobutyl acetate	T52.8X1	T52.8X2	T52.8X3	T52.8X4	—	—
Isocarboxazid	T43.1X1	T43.1X2	T43.1X3	T43.1X4	T43.1X5	T43.1X6
Isoconazole	T49.0X1	T49.0X2	T49.0X3	T49.0X4	T49.0X5	T49.0X6
Isocyanate	T65.0X1	T65.0X2	T65.0X3	T65.0X4	—	—
Isoephedrine	T44.991	T44.992	T44.993	T44.994	T44.995	T44.996
Isoetarine	T48.6X1	T48.6X2	T48.6X3	T48.6X4	T48.6X5	T48.6X6
Isoethadione	T42.2X1	T42.2X2	T42.2X3	T42.2X4	T42.2X5	T42.2X6
Isoetharine	T44.5X1	T44.5X2	T44.5X3	T44.5X4	T44.5X5	T44.5X6
Isoflurane	T41.0X1	T41.0X2	T41.0X3	T41.0X4	T41.0X5	T41.0X6
Isoflurophate	T44.0X1	T44.0X2	T44.0X3	T44.0X4	T44.0X5	T44.0X6
Isomaltose, ferric complex	T45.4X1	T45.4X2	T45.4X3	T45.4X4	T45.4X5	T45.4X6
Isometheptene	T44.3X1	T44.3X2	T44.3X3	T44.3X4	T44.3X5	T44.3X6
Isoniazid	T37.1X1	T37.1X2	T37.1X3	T37.1X4	T37.1X5	T37.1X6
with						
rifampicin	T36.6X1	T36.6X2	T36.6X3	T36.6X4	T36.6X5	T36.6X6
thioacetazone	T37.1X1	T37.1X2	T37.1X3	T37.1X4	T37.1X5	T37.1X6
Isonicotinic acid hydrazide	T37.1X1	T37.1X2	T37.1X3	T37.1X4	T37.1X5	T37.1X6
Isonipecaine	T40.4X1	T40.4X2	T40.4X3	T40.4X4	T40.4X5	T40.4X6
Isopentaquine	T37.2X1	T37.2X2	T37.2X3	T37.2X4	T37.2X5	T37.2X6
Isophane insulin	T38.3X1	T38.3X2	T38.3X3	T38.3X4	T38.3X5	T38.3X6
Isophorone	T65.891	T65.892	T65.893	T65.894	—	—
Isophosphamide	T45.1X1	T45.1X2	T45.1X3	T45.1X4	T45.1X5	T45.1X6
Isopregnenone	T38.5X1	T38.5X2	T38.5X3	T38.5X4	T38.5X5	T38.5X6
Isoprenaline	T48.6X1	T48.6X2	T48.6X3	T48.6X4	T48.6X5	T48.6X6
Isopromethazine	T43.3X1	T43.3X2	T43.3X3	T43.3X4	T43.3X5	T43.3X6
Isopropamide	T44.3X1	T44.3X2	T44.3X3	T44.3X4	T44.3X5	T44.3X6
iodide	T44.3X1	T44.3X2	T44.3X3	T44.3X4	T44.3X5	T44.3X6
Isopropanol	T51.2X1	T51.2X2	T51.2X3	T51.2X4	—	—
Isopropyl						
acetate	T52.8X1	T52.8X2	T52.8X3	T52.8X4	—	—
alcohol	T51.2X1	T51.2X2	T51.2X3	T51.2X4	—	—
medicinal	T49.4X1	T49.4X2	T49.4X3	T49.4X4	T49.4X5	T49.4X6
ether	T52.8X1	T52.8X2	T52.8X3	T52.8X4	—	—
Isopropylaminophenazone	T39.2X1	T39.2X2	T39.2X3	T39.2X4	T39.2X5	T39.2X6
Isoproterenol	T48.6X1	T48.6X2	T48.6X3	T48.6X4	T48.6X5	T48.6X6
Isosorbide dinitrate	T46.3X1	T46.3X2	T46.3X3	T46.3X4	T46.3X5	T46.3X6
Isothipendyl	T45.0X1	T45.0X2	T45.0X3	T45.0X4	T45.0X5	T45.0X6
Isotretinoin	T50.991	T50.992	T50.993	T50.994	T50.995	T50.996
Isoxazolyl penicillin	T36.0X1	T36.0X2	T36.0X3	T36.0X4	T36.0X5	T36.0X6
Isoxicam	T39.391	T39.392	T39.393	T39.394	T39.395	T39.396
Isoxsuprine	T46.7X1	T46.7X2	T46.7X3	T46.7X4	T46.7X5	T46.7X6
Ispagula	T47.4X1	T47.4X2	T47.4X3	T47.4X4	T47.4X5	T47.4X6
husk	T47.4X1	T47.4X2	T47.4X3	T47.4X4	T47.4X5	T47.4X6
Isradipine	T46.1X1	T46.1X2	T46.1X3	T46.1X4	T46.1X5	T46.1X6
I-thyroxine sodium	T38.1X1	T38.1X2	T38.1X3	T38.1X4	T38.1X5	T38.1X6
Itraconazole	T37.8X1	T37.8X2	T37.8X3	T37.8X4	T37.8X5	T37.8X6
Itramin tosilate	T46.3X1	T46.3X2	T46.3X3	T46.3X4	T46.3X5	T46.3X6
Ivermectin	T37.4X1	T37.4X2	T37.4X3	T37.4X4	T37.4X5	T37.4X6
Izoniazid	T37.1X1	T37.1X2	T37.1X3	T37.1X4	T37.1X5	T37.1X6
with thioacetazone	T37.1X1	T37.1X2	T37.1X3	T37.1X4	T37.1X5	T37.1X6

Substance	Poisoning, Accidental (unintentional)	Poisoning, Intentional self-harm	Poisoning, Assault	Poisoning, Undetermined	Adverse effect	Underdosing
J						
Jalap	T47.2X1	T47.2X2	T47.2X3	T47.2X4	T47.2X5	T47.2X6
Jamaica						
dogwood (bark)	T39.8X1	T39.8X2	T39.8X3	T39.8X4	T39.8X5	T39.8X6
ginger	T65.891	T65.892	T65.893	T65.894	—	—
root	T62.2X1	T62.2X2	T62.2X3	T62.2X4	—	—
Jatropha	T62.2X1	T62.2X2	T62.2X3	T62.2X4	—	—
curcas	T62.2X1	T62.2X2	T62.2X3	T62.2X4	—	—
Jectofer	T45.4X1	T45.4X2	T45.4X3	T45.4X4	T45.4X5	T45.4X6
Jellyfish (sting)	T63.621	T63.622	T63.623	T63.624	—	—
Jequirity (bean)	T62.2X1	T62.2X2	T62.2X3	T62.2X4	—	—
Jimson weed (stramonium)	T62.2X1	T62.2X2	T62.2X3	T62.2X4	—	—
seeds	T62.2X1	T62.2X2	T62.2X3	T62.2X4	—	—
Josamycin	T36.3X1	T36.3X2	T36.3X3	T36.3X4	T36.3X5	T36.3X6
Juniper tar	T49.1X1	T49.1X2	T49.1X3	T49.1X4	T49.1X5	T49.1X6
K						
Kallidinogenase	T46.7X1	T46.7X2	T46.7X3	T46.7X4	T46.7X5	T46.7X6
Kallikrein	T46.7X1	T46.7X2	T46.7X3	T46.7X4	T46.7X5	T46.7X6
Kanamycin	T36.5X1	T36.5X2	T36.5X3	T36.5X4	T36.5X5	T36.5X6
Kantrex	T36.5X1	T36.5X2	T36.5X3	T36.5X4	T36.5X5	T36.5X6
Kaolin	T47.6X1	T47.6X2	T47.6X3	T47.6X4	T47.6X5	T47.6X6
light	T47.6X1	T47.6X2	T47.6X3	T47.6X4	T47.6X5	T47.6X6
Karaya (gum)	T47.4X1	T47.4X2	T47.4X3	T47.4X4	T47.4X5	T47.4X6
Kebuzone	T39.2X1	T39.2X2	T39.2X3	T39.2X4	T39.2X5	T39.2X6
Kelevan	T60.1X1	T60.1X2	T60.1X3	T60.1X4	—	—
Kemithal	T41.1X1	T41.1X2	T41.1X3	T41.1X4	T41.1X5	T41.1X6
Kenacort	T38.0X1	T38.0X2	T38.0X3	T38.0X4	T38.0X5	T38.0X6
Keratolytic drug NEC	T49.4X1	T49.4X2	T49.4X3	T49.4X4	T49.4X5	T49.4X6
anthracene	T49.4X1	T49.4X2	T49.4X3	T49.4X4	T49.4X5	T49.4X6
Keratoplastic NEC	T49.4X1	T49.4X2	T49.4X3	T49.4X4	T49.4X5	T49.4X6
Kerosene, kerosine (fuel) (solvent) NEC	T52.0X1	T52.0X2	T52.0X3	T52.0X4	—	—
insecticide	T52.0X1	T52.0X2	T52.0X3	T52.0X4	—	—
vapor	T52.0X1	T52.0X2	T52.0X3	T52.0X4	—	—
Ketamine	T41.291	T41.292	T41.293	T41.294	T41.295	T41.296
Ketazolam	T42.4X1	T42.4X2	T42.4X3	T42.4X4	T42.4X5	T42.4X6
Ketazon	T39.2X1	T39.2X2	T39.2X3	T39.2X4	T39.2X5	T39.2X6
Ketobemidone	T40.4X1	T40.4X2	T40.4X3	T40.4X4	—	—
Ketoconazole	T49.0X1	T49.0X2	T49.0X3	T49.0X4	T49.0X5	T49.0X6
Ketols	T52.4X1	T52.4X2	T52.4X3	T52.4X4	—	—
Ketone oils	T52.4X1	T52.4X2	T52.4X3	T52.4X4	—	—
Ketoprofen	T39.311	T39.312	T39.313	T39.314	T39.315	T39.316
Ketorolac	T39.8X1	T39.8X2	T39.8X3	T39.8X4	T39.8X5	T39.8X6
Ketotifen	T45.0X1	T45.0X2	T45.0X3	T45.0X4	T45.0X5	T45.0X6
Khat	T43.691	T43.692	T43.693	T43.694	—	—
Khellin	T46.3X1	T46.3X2	T46.3X3	T46.3X4	T46.3X5	T46.3X6
Khelloside	T46.3X1	T46.3X2	T46.3X3	T46.3X4	T46.3X5	T46.3X6
Kiln gas or vapor (carbon monoxide)	T58.8X1	T58.8X2	T58.8X3	T58.8X4	—	—
Kitasamycin	T36.3X1	T36.3X2	T36.3X3	T36.3X4	T36.3X5	T36.3X6
Konsyl	T47.4X1	T47.4X2	T47.4X3	T47.4X4	T47.4X5	T47.4X6
Kosam seed	T62.2X1	T62.2X2	T62.2X3	T62.2X4	—	—
Krait (venom)	T63.091	T63.092	T63.093	T63.094	—	—
Kwell (insecticide)	T60.1X1	T60.1X2	T60.1X3	T60.1X4	—	—
anti-infective (topical)	T49.0X1	T49.0X2	T49.0X3	T49.0X4	T49.0X5	T49.0X6
L						
Labetalol	T44.8X1	T44.8X2	T44.8X3	T44.8X4	T44.8X5	T44.8X6
Laburnum (seeds)	T62.2X1	T62.2X2	T62.2X3	T62.2X4	—	—
leaves	T62.2X1	T62.2X2	T62.2X3	T62.2X4	—	—
Lachesine	T49.5X1	T49.5X2	T49.5X3	T49.5X4	T49.5X5	T49.5X6
Lacidipine	T46.5X1	T46.5X2	T46.5X3	T46.5X4	T46.5X5	T46.5X6
Lacquer	T65.6X1	T65.6X2	T65.6X3	T65.6X4	—	—
Lacrimogenic gas	T59.3X1	T59.3X2	T59.3X3	T59.3X4	—	—
Lactated potassic saline	T50.3X1	T50.3X2	T50.3X3	T50.3X4	T50.3X5	T50.3X6
Lactic acid	T49.8X1	T49.8X2	T49.8X3	T49.8X4	T49.8X5	T49.8X6
Lactobacillus						
acidophilus	T47.6X1	T47.6X2	T47.6X3	T47.6X4	T47.6X5	T47.6X6
compound	T47.6X1	T47.6X2	T47.6X3	T47.6X4	T47.6X5	T47.6X6
bifidus, lyophilized	T47.6X1	T47.6X2	T47.6X3	T47.6X4	T47.6X5	T47.6X6
bulgaricus	T47.6X1	T47.6X2	T47.6X3	T47.6X4	T47.6X5	T47.6X6
sporogenes	T47.6X1	T47.6X2	T47.6X3	T47.6X4	T47.6X5	T47.6X6
Lactoflavin	T45.2X1	T45.2X2	T45.2X3	T45.2X4	T45.2X5	T45.2X6
Lactose (as excipient)	T50.901	T50.902	T50.903	T50.904	T50.905	T50.906
Lactuca (virosa) (extract)	T42.6X1	T42.6X2	T42.6X3	T42.6X4	T42.6X5	T42.6X6
Lactucarium	T42.6X1	T42.6X2	T42.6X3	T42.6X4	T42.6X5	T42.6X6
Lactulose	T47.3X1	T47.3X2	T47.3X3	T47.3X4	T47.3X5	T47.3X6
Laevo—*see* Levo						
Lanatosides	T46.0X1	T46.0X2	T46.0X3	T46.0X4	T46.0X5	T46.0X6
Lanolin	T49.3X1	T49.3X2	T49.3X3	T49.3X4	T49.3X5	T49.3X6
Largactil	T43.3X1	T43.3X2	T43.3X3	T43.3X4	T43.3X5	T43.3X6
Larkspur	T62.2X1	T62.2X2	T62.2X3	T62.2X4	—	—
Laroxyl	T43.011	T43.012	T43.013	T43.014	T43.015	T43.016
Lasix	T50.1X1	T50.1X2	T50.1X3	T50.1X4	T50.1X5	T50.1X6
Lassar's paste	T49.4X1	T49.4X2	T49.4X3	T49.4X4	T49.4X5	T49.4X6
Latamoxef	T36.1X1	T36.1X2	T36.1X3	T36.1X4	T36.1X5	T36.1X6
Latex	T65.811	T65.812	T65.813	T65.814	—	—
Lathyrus (seed)	T62.2X1	T62.2X2	T62.2X3	T62.2X4	—	—
Laudanum	T40.0X1	T40.0X2	T40.0X3	T40.0X4	T40.0X5	T40.0X6
Laudexium	T48.1X1	T48.1X2	T48.1X3	T48.1X4	T48.1X5	T48.1X6
Laughing gas	T41.0X1	T41.0X2	T41.0X3	T41.0X4	T41.0X5	T41.0X6
Laurel, black or cherry	T62.2X1	T62.2X2	T62.2X3	T62.2X4	—	—
Laurolinium	T49.0X1	T49.0X2	T49.0X3	T49.0X4	T49.0X5	T49.0X6
Lauryl sulfoacetate	T49.2X1	T49.2X2	T49.2X3	T49.2X4	T49.2X5	T49.2X6
Laxative NEC	T47.4X1	T47.4X2	T47.4X3	T47.4X4	T47.4X5	T47.4X6
osmotic	T47.3X1	T47.3X2	T47.3X3	T47.3X4	T47.3X5	T47.3X6
saline	T47.3X1	T47.3X2	T47.3X3	T47.3X4	T47.3X5	T47.3X6
stimulant	T47.2X1	T47.2X2	T47.2X3	T47.2X4	T47.2X5	T47.2X6
L-dopa	T42.8X1	T42.8X2	T42.8X3	T42.8X4	T42.8X5	T42.8X6
Lead (dust) (fumes) (vapor) NEC	T56.0X1	T56.0X2	T56.0X3	T56.0X4	—	—
acetate	T49.2X1	T49.2X2	T49.2X3	T49.2X4	T49.2X5	T49.2X6
alkyl (fuel additive)	T56.0X1	T56.0X2	T56.0X3	T56.0X4	—	—
anti-infectives	T37.8X1	T37.8X2	T37.8X3	T37.8X4	T37.8X5	T37.8X6
antiknock compound (tetraethyl)	T56.0X1	T56.0X2	T56.0X3	T56.0X4	—	—
arsenate, arsenite (dust) (herbicide) (insecticide) (vapor)	T57.0X1	T57.0X2	T57.0X3	T57.0X4	—	—
carbonate	T56.0X1	T56.0X2	T56.0X3	T56.0X4	—	—
paint	T56.0X1	T56.0X2	T56.0X3	T56.0X4	—	—
chromate	T56.0X1	T56.0X2	T56.0X3	T56.0X4	—	—
paint	T56.0X1	T56.0X2	T56.0X3	T56.0X4	—	—
dioxide	T56.0X1	T56.0X2	T56.0X3	T56.0X4	—	—
inorganic	T56.0X1	T56.0X2	T56.0X3	T56.0X4	—	—
iodide	T56.0X1	T56.0X2	T56.0X3	T56.0X4	—	—
pigment (paint)	T56.0X1	T56.0X2	T56.0X3	T56.0X4	—	—
monoxide (dust)	T56.0X1	T56.0X2	T56.0X3	T56.0X4	—	—
paint	T56.0X1	T56.0X2	T56.0X3	T56.0X4	—	—
organic	T56.0X1	T56.0X2	T56.0X3	T56.0X4	—	—

Substance	Poisoning, Accidental (unintentional)	Poisoning, Intentional self-harm	Poisoning, Assault	Poisoning, Undetermined	Adverse effect	Underdosing
Lead (dust) (fumes) (vapor) NEC — *continued*						
oxide	T56.0X1	T56.0X2	T56.0X3	T56.0X4	—	—
paint	T56.0X1	T56.0X2	T56.0X3	T56.0X4	—	—
paint	T56.0X1	T56.0X2	T56.0X3	T56.0X4	—	—
salts	T56.0X1	T56.0X2	T56.0X3	T56.0X4	—	—
specified compound NEC	T56.0X1	T56.0X2	T56.0X3	T56.0X4	—	—
tetra-ethyl	T56.0X1	T56.0X2	T56.0X3	T56.0X4	—	—
Lebanese red	T40.7X1	T40.7X2	T40.7X3	T40.7X4	T40.7X5	T40.7X6
Lefetamine	T39.8X1	T39.8X2	T39.8X3	T39.8X4	T39.8X5	T39.8X6
Lenperone	T43.4X1	T43.4X2	T43.4X3	T43.4X4	T43.4X5	T43.4X6
Lente lietin (insulin)	T38.3X1	T38.3X2	T38.3X3	T38.3X4	T38.3X5	T38.3X6
Leptazol	T50.7X1	T50.7X2	T50.7X3	T50.7X4	T50.7X5	T50.7X6
Leptophos	T60.0X1	T60.0X2	T60.0X3	T60.0X4	—	—
Leritine	T40.2X1	T40.2X2	T40.2X3	T40.2X4	T40.2X5	T40.2X6
Letosteine	T48.4X1	T48.4X2	T48.4X3	T48.4X4	T48.4X5	T48.4X6
Letter	T38.1X1	T38.1X2	T38.1X3	T38.1X4	T38.1X5	T38.1X6
Lettuce opium	T42.6X1	T42.6X2	T42.6X3	T42.6X4	T42.6X5	T42.6X6
Leucinocaine	T41.3X1	T41.3X2	T41.3X3	T41.3X4	T41.3X5	T41.3X6
Leucocianidol	T46.991	T46.992	T46.993	T46.994	T46.995	T46.996
Leucovorin (factor)	T45.8X1	T45.8X2	T45.8X3	T45.8X4	T45.8X5	T45.8X6
Leukeran	T45.1X1	T45.1X2	T45.1X3	T45.1X4	T45.1X5	T45.1X6
Leuprolide	T38.891	T38.892	T38.893	T38.894	T38.895	T38.896
Levalbuterol	T48.6X1	T48.6X2	T48.6X3	T48.6X4	T48.6X5	T48.6X6
Levallorphan	T50.7X1	T50.7X2	T50.7X3	T50.7X4	T50.7X5	T50.7X6
Levamisole	T37.4X1	T37.4X2	T37.4X3	T37.4X4	T37.4X5	T37.4X6
Levanil	T42.6X1	T42.6X2	T42.6X3	T42.6X4	T42.6X5	T42.6X6
Levarterenol	T44.4X1	T44.4X2	T44.4X3	T44.4X4	T44.4X5	T44.4X6
Levdropropizine	T48.3X1	T48.3X2	T48.3X3	T48.3X4	T48.3X5	T48.3X6
Levobunolol	T49.5X1	T49.5X2	T49.5X3	T49.5X4	T49.5X5	T49.5X6
Levocabastine (hydrochloride)	T45.0X1	T45.0X2	T45.0X3	T45.0X4	T45.0X5	T45.0X6
Levocarnitine	T50.991	T50.992	T50.993	T50.994	T50.995	T50.996
Levodopa	T42.8X1	T42.8X2	T42.8X3	T42.8X4	T42.8X5	T42.8X6
with carbidopa	T42.8X1	T42.8X2	T42.8X3	T42.8X4	T42.8X5	T42.8X6
Levo-dromoran	T40.2X1	T40.2X2	T40.2X3	T40.2X4	T40.2X5	T40.2X6
Levoglutamide	T50.991	T50.992	T50.993	T50.994	T50.995	T50.996
Levoid	T38.1X1	T38.1X2	T38.1X3	T38.1X4	T38.1X5	T38.1X6
Levo-iso-methadone	T40.3X1	T40.3X2	T40.3X3	T40.3X4	T40.3X5	T40.3X6
Levomepromazine	T43.3X1	T43.3X2	T43.3X3	T43.3X4	T43.3X5	T43.3X6
Levonordefrin	T49.6X1	T49.6X2	T49.6X3	T49.6X4	T49.6X5	T49.6X6
Levonorgestrel	T38.4X1	T38.4X2	T38.4X3	T38.4X4	T38.4X5	T38.4X6
with ethinylestradiol	T38.5X1	T38.5X2	T38.5X3	T38.5X4	T38.5X5	T38.5X6
Levopromazine	T43.3X1	T43.3X2	T43.3X3	T43.3X4	T43.3X5	T43.3X6
Levoprome	T42.6X1	T42.6X2	T42.6X3	T42.6X4	T42.6X5	T42.6X6
Levopropoxyphene	T40.4X1	T40.4X2	T40.4X3	T40.4X4	T40.4X5	T40.4X6
Levopropylhexedrine	T50.5X1	T50.5X2	T50.5X3	T50.5X4	T50.5X5	T50.5X6
Levoproxyphylline	T48.6X1	T48.6X2	T48.6X3	T48.6X4	T48.6X5	T48.6X6
Levorphanol	T40.4X1	T40.4X2	T40.4X3	T40.4X4	T40.4X5	T40.4X6
Levothyroxine	T38.1X1	T38.1X2	T38.1X3	T38.1X4	T38.1X5	T38.1X6
sodium	T38.1X1	T38.1X2	T38.1X3	T38.1X4	T38.1X5	T38.1X6
Levsin	T44.3X1	T44.3X2	T44.3X3	T44.3X4	T44.3X5	T44.3X6
Levulose	T50.3X1	T50.3X2	T50.3X3	T50.3X4	T50.3X5	T50.3X6
Lewisite (gas), not in war	T57.0X1	T57.0X2	T57.0X3	T57.0X4	—	—
Librium	T42.4X1	T42.4X2	T42.4X3	T42.4X4	T42.4X5	T42.4X6
Lidex	T49.0X1	T49.0X2	T49.0X3	T49.0X4	T49.0X5	T49.0X6
Lidocaine	T41.3X1	T41.3X2	T41.3X3	T41.3X4	T41.3X5	T41.3X6
regional	T41.3X1	T41.3X2	T41.3X3	T41.3X4	T41.3X5	T41.3X6
spinal	T41.3X1	T41.3X2	T41.3X3	T41.3X4	T41.3X5	T41.3X6

Substance	Poisoning, Accidental (unintentional)	Poisoning, Intentional self-harm	Poisoning, Assault	Poisoning, Undetermined	Adverse effect	Underdosing
Lidofenin	T50.8X1	T50.8X2	T50.8X3	T50.8X4	T50.8X5	T50.8X6
Lidoflazine	T46.1X1	T46.1X2	T46.1X3	T46.1X4	T46.1X5	T46.1X6
Lighter fluid	T52.0X1	T52.0X2	T52.0X3	T52.0X4	—	—
Lignin hemicellulose	T47.6X1	T47.6X2	T47.6X3	T47.6X4	T47.6X5	T47.6X6
Lignocaine	T41.3X1	T41.3X2	T41.3X3	T41.3X4	T41.3X5	T41.3X6
regional	T41.3X1	T41.3X2	T41.3X3	T41.3X4	T41.3X5	T41.3X6
spinal	T41.3X1	T41.3X2	T41.3X3	T41.3X4	T41.3X5	T41.3X6
Ligroin (e) (solvent)	T52.0X1	T52.0X2	T52.0X3	T52.0X4	—	—
vapor	T59.891	T59.892	T59.893	T59.894	—	—
Ligustrum vulgare	T62.2X1	T62.2X2	T62.2X3	T62.2X4	—	—
Lily of the valley	T62.2X1	T62.2X2	T62.2X3	T62.2X4	—	—
Lime (chloride)	T54.3X1	T54.3X2	T54.3X3	T54.3X4	—	—
Limonene	T52.8X1	T52.8X2	T52.8X3	T52.8X4	—	—
Lincomycin	T36.8X1	T36.8X2	T36.8X3	T36.8X4	T36.8X5	T36.8X6
Lindane (insecticide) (nonmedicinal) (vapor)	T53.6X1	T53.6X2	T53.6X3	T53.6X4	—	—
medicinal	T49.0X1	T49.0X2	T49.0X3	T49.0X4	T49.0X5	T49.0X6
Liniments NEC	T49.91	T49.92	T49.93	T49.94	T49.95	T49.96
Linoleic acid	T46.6X1	T46.6X2	T46.6X3	T46.6X4	T46.6X5	T46.6X6
Linolenic acid	T46.6X1	T46.6X2	T46.6X3	T46.6X4	T46.6X5	T46.6X6
Linseed	T47.4X1	T47.4X2	T47.4X3	T47.4X4	T47.4X5	T47.4X6
Liothyronine	T38.1X1	T38.1X2	T38.1X3	T38.1X4	T38.1X5	T38.1X6
Liotrix	T38.1X1	T38.1X2	T38.1X3	T38.1X4	T38.1X5	T38.1X6
Lipancreatin	T47.5X1	T47.5X2	T47.5X3	T47.5X4	T47.5X5	T47.5X6
Lipo-alprostadil	T46.7X1	T46.7X2	T46.7X3	T46.7X4	T46.7X5	T46.7X6
Lipo-Lutin	T38.5X1	T38.5X2	T38.5X3	T38.5X4	T38.5X5	T38.5X6
Lipotropic drug NEC	T50.901	T50.902	T50.903	T50.904	T50.905	T50.906
Liquefied petroleum gases	T59.891	T59.892	T59.893	T59.894	—	—
piped (pure or mixed with air)	T59.891	T59.892	T59.893	T59.894	—	—
Liquid						
paraffin	T47.4X1	T47.4X2	T47.4X3	T47.4X4	T47.4X5	T47.4X6
petrolatum	T47.4X1	T47.4X2	T47.4X3	T47.4X4	T47.4X5	T47.4X6
topical	T49.3X1	T49.3X2	T49.3X3	T49.3X4	T49.3X5	T49.3X6
specified NEC	T65.891	T65.892	T65.893	T65.894	—	—
substance	T65.91	T65.92	T65.93	T65.94	—	—
Liquor creosolis compositus	T65.891	T65.892	T65.893	T65.894	—	—
Liquorice	T48.4X1	T48.4X2	T48.4X3	T48.4X4	T48.4X5	T48.4X6
extract	T47.8X1	T47.8X2	T47.8X3	T47.8X4	T47.8X5	T47.8X6
Lisinopril	T46.4X1	T46.4X2	T46.4X3	T46.4X4	T46.4X5	T46.4X6
Lisuride	T42.8X1	T42.8X2	T42.8X3	T42.8X4	T42.8X5	T42.8X6
Lithane	T43.8X1	T43.8X2	T43.8X3	T43.8X4	T43.8X5	T43.8X6
Lithium	T56.891	T56.892	T56.893	T56.894	—	—
gluconate	T43.591	T43.592	T43.593	T43.594	T43.595	T43.596
salts (carbonate)	T43.591	T43.592	T43.593	T43.594	T43.595	T43.596
Lithonate	T43.8X1	T43.8X2	T43.8X3	T43.8X4	T43.8X5	T43.8X6
Liver						
extract	T45.8X1	T45.8X2	T45.8X3	T45.8X4	T45.8X5	T45.8X6
for parenteral use	T45.8X1	T45.8X2	T45.8X3	T45.8X4	T45.8X5	T45.8X6
fraction 1	T45.8X1	T45.8X2	T45.8X3	T45.8X4	T45.8X5	T45.8X6
hydrolysate	T45.8X1	T45.8X2	T45.8X3	T45.8X4	T45.8X5	T45.8X6
Lizard (bite) (venom)	T63.121	T63.122	T63.123	T63.124	—	—
LMD	T45.8X1	T45.8X2	T45.8X3	T45.8X4	T45.8X5	T45.8X6
Lobelia	T62.2X1	T62.2X2	T62.2X3	T62.2X4	—	—
Lobeline	T50.7X1	T50.7X2	T50.7X3	T50.7X4	T50.7X5	T50.7X6
Local action drug NEC	T49.8X1	T49.8X2	T49.8X3	T49.8X4	T49.8X5	T49.8X6
Locorten	T49.0X1	T49.0X2	T49.0X3	T49.0X4	T49.0X5	T49.0X6
Lofepramine	T43.011	T43.012	T43.013	T43.014	T43.015	T43.016
Lollum temulentum	T62.2X1	T62.2X2	T62.2X3	T62.2X4	—	—
Lomotil	T47.6X1	T47.6X2	T47.6X3	T47.6X4	T47.6X5	T47.6X6

Substance	Poisoning, Accidental (unintentional)	Poisoning, Intentional self-harm	Poisoning, Assault	Poisoning, Undetermined	Adverse effect	Underdosing
Lomustine	T45.1X1	T45.1X2	T45.1X3	T45.1X4	T45.1X5	T45.1X6
Lonidamine	T45.1X1	T45.1X2	T45.1X3	T45.1X4	T45.1X5	T45.1X6
Loperamide	T47.6X1	T47.6X2	T47.6X3	T47.6X4	T47.6X5	T47.6X6
Loprazolam	T42.4X1	T42.4X2	T42.4X3	T42.4X4	T42.4X5	T42.4X6
Lorajmine	T46.2X1	T46.2X2	T46.2X3	T46.2X4	T46.2X5	T46.2X6
Loratidine	T45.0X1	T45.0X2	T45.0X3	T45.0X4	T45.0X5	T45.0X6
Lorazepam	T42.4X1	T42.4X2	T42.4X3	T42.4X4	T42.4X5	T42.4X6
Lorcainide	T46.2X1	T46.2X2	T46.2X3	T46.2X4	T46.2X5	T46.2X6
Lormetazepam	T42.4X1	T42.4X2	T42.4X3	T42.4X4	T42.4X5	T42.4X6
Lotions NEC	T49.91	T49.92	T49.93	T49.94	T49.95	T49.96
Lotusate	T42.3X1	T42.3X2	T42.3X3	T42.3X4	T42.3X5	T42.3X6
Lovastatin	T46.6X1	T46.6X2	T46.6X3	T46.6X4	T46.6X5	T46.6X6
Lowila	T49.2X1	T49.2X2	T49.2X3	T49.2X4	T49.2X5	T49.2X6
Loxapine	T43.591	T43.592	T43.593	T43.594	T43.595	T43.596
Lozenges (throat)	T49.6X1	T49.6X2	T49.6X3	T49.6X4	T49.6X5	T49.6X6
LSD	T40.8X1	T40.8X2	T40.8X3	T40.8X4	—	—
L-Tryptophan—see amino acid						
Lubricant, eye	T49.5X1	T49.5X2	T49.5X3	T49.5X4	T49.5X5	T49.5X6
Lubricating oil NEC	T52.0X1	T52.0X2	T52.0X3	T52.0X4	—	—
Lucanthone	T37.4X1	T37.4X2	T37.4X3	T37.4X4	T37.4X5	T37.4X6
Luminal	T42.3X1	T42.3X2	T42.3X3	T42.3X4	T42.3X5	T42.3X6
Lung irritant (gas) NEC	T59.91	T59.92	T59.93	T59.94		
Luteinizing hormone	T38.811	T38.812	T38.813	T38.814	T38.815	T38.816
Lutocylol	T38.5X1	T38.5X2	T38.5X3	T38.5X4	T38.5X5	T38.5X6
Lutromone	T38.5X1	T38.5X2	T38.5X3	T38.5X4	T38.5X5	T38.5X6
Lututrin	T48.291	T48.292	T48.293	T48.294	T48.295	T48.296
Lye (concentrated)	T54.3X1	T54.3X2	T54.3X3	T54.3X4	—	—
Lygranum (skin test)	T50.8X1	T50.8X2	T50.8X3	T50.8X4	T50.8X5	T50.8X6
Lymecycline	T36.4X1	T36.4X2	T36.4X3	I36.4X4	T36.4X5	T36.4X6
Lymphogranuloma venereum antigen	T50.8X1	T50.8X2	T50.8X3	T50.8X4	T50.8X5	T50.8X6
Lynestrenol	T38.4X1	T38.4X2	T38.4X3	T38.4X4	T38.4X5	T38.4X6
Lyovac Sodium Edecrin	T50.1X1	T50.1X2	T50.1X3	T50.1X4	T50.1X5	T50.1X6
Lypressin	T38.891	T38.892	T38.893	T38.894	T38.895	T38.896
Lysergic acid diethylamide	T40.8X1	T40.8X2	T40.8X3	T40.8X4	—	—
Lysergide	T40.8X1	T40.8X2	T40.8X3	T40.8X4	—	—
Lysine vasopressin	T38.891	T38.892	T38.893	T38.894	T38.895	T38.896
Lysol	T54.1X1	T54.1X2	T54.1X3	T54.1X4	—	—
Lysozyme	T49.0X1	T49.0X2	T49.0X3	T49.0X4	T49.0X5	T49.0X6
Lytta (vitatta)	T49.8X1	T49.8X2	T49.8X3	T49.8X4	T49.8X5	T49.8X6
M						
Mace	T59.3X1	T59.3X2	T59.3X3	T59.3X4	—	—
Macrogol	T50.991	T50.992	T50.993	T50.994	T50.995	T50.996
Macrolide						
anabolic drug	T38.7X1	T38.7X2	T38.7X3	T38.7X4	T38.7X5	T38.7X6
antibiotic	T36.3X1	T36.3X2	T36.3X3	T36.3X4	T36.3X5	T36.3X6
Mafenide	T49.0X1	T49.0X2	T49.0X3	T49.0X4	T49.0X5	T49.0X6
Magaldrate	T47.1X1	T47.1X2	T47.1X3	T47.1X4	T47.1X5	T47.1X6
Magic mushroom	T40.991	T40.992	T40.993	T40.994	—	—
Magnamycin	T36.8X1	T36.8X2	T36.8X3	T36.8X4	T36.8X5	T36.8X6
Magnesia magma	T47.1X1	T47.1X2	T47.1X3	T47.1X4	T47.1X5	T47.1X6
Magnesium NEC	T56.891	T56.892	T56.893	T56.894	—	—
carbonate	T47.1X1	T47.1X2	T47.1X3	T47.1X4	T47.1X5	T47.1X6
citrate	T47.4X1	T47.4X2	T47.4X3	T47.4X4	T47.4X5	T47.4X6
hydroxide	T47.1X1	T47.1X2	T47.1X3	T47.1X4	T47.1X5	T47.1X6
oxide	T47.1X1	T47.1X2	T47.1X3	T47.1X4	T47.1X5	T47.1X6
peroxide	T49.0X1	T49.0X2	T49.0X3	T49.0X4	T49.0X5	T49.0X6
salicylate	T39.091	T39.092	T39.093	T39.094	T39.095	T39.096

Substance	Poisoning, Accidental (unintentional)	Poisoning, Intentional self-harm	Poisoning, Assault	Poisoning, Undetermined	Adverse effect	Underdosing
Magnesium NEC — continued						
silicofluoride	T50.3X1	T50.3X2	T50.3X3	T50.3X4	T50.3X5	T50.3X6
sulfate	T47.4X1	T47.4X2	T47.4X3	T47.4X4	T47.4X5	T47.4X6
thiosulfate	T45.0X1	T45.0X2	T45.0X3	T45.0X4	T45.0X5	T45.0X6
trisilicate	T47.1X1	T47.1X2	T47.1X3	T47.1X4	T47.1X5	T47.1X6
Malathion (medicinal)	T49.0X1	T49.0X2	T49.0X3	T49.0X4	T49.0X5	T49.0X6
insecticide	T60.0X1	T60.0X2	T60.0X3	T60.0X4	—	—
Male fern extract	T37.4X1	T37.4X2	T37.4X3	T37.4X4	T37.4X5	T37.4X6
M-AMSA	T45.1X1	T45.1X2	T45.1X3	T45.1X4	T45.1X5	T45.1X6
Mandelic acid	T37.8X1	T37.8X2	T37.8X3	T37.8X4	T37.8X5	T37.8X6
Manganese (dioxide) (salts)	T57.2X1	T57.2X2	T57.2X3	T57.2X4	—	—
medicinal	T50.991	T50.992	T50.993	T50.994	T50.995	T50.996
Mannitol	T47.3X1	T47.3X2	T47.3X3	T47.3X4	T47.3X5	T47.3X6
hexanitrate	T46.3X1	T46.3X2	T46.3X3	T46.3X4	T46.3X5	T46.3X6
Mannomustine	T45.1X1	T45.1X2	T45.1X3	T45.1X4	T45.1X5	T45.1X6
MAO inhibitors	T43.1X1	T43.1X2	T43.1X3	T43.1X4	T43.1X5	T43.1X6
Mapharsen	T37.8X1	T37.8X2	T37.8X3	T37.8X4	T37.8X5	T37.8X6
Maphenide	T49.0X1	T49.0X2	T49.0X3	T49.0X4	T49.0X5	T49.0X6
Maprotiline	T43.021	T43.022	T43.023	T43.024	T43.025	T43.026
Marcaine	T41.3X1	T41.3X2	T41.3X3	T41.3X4	T41.3X5	T41.3X6
infiltration (subcutaneous)	T41.3X1	T41.3X2	T41.3X3	T41.3X4	T41.3X5	T41.3X6
nerve block (peripheral) (plexus)	T41.3X1	T41.3X2	T41.3X3	T41.3X4	T41.3X5	T41.3X6
Marezine	T45.0X1	T45.0X2	T45.0X3	T45.0X4	T45.0X5	T45.0X6
Marihuana	T40.7X1	T40.7X2	T40.7X3	T40.7X4	T40.7X5	T40.7X6
Marijuana	T40.7X1	T40.7X2	T40.7X3	T40.7X4	I40./X5	T40.7X6
Marine (sting)	T63.691	T63.692	T63.693	T63.694	—	—
animals (sting)	T63.691	T63.692	T63.693	T63.694	—	—
plants (sting)	T63.711	T63.712	T63.713	T63.714	—	—
Marplan	T43.1X1	T43.1X2	T43.1X3	T43.1X4	T43.1X5	T43.1X6
Marsh gas	T59.891	T59.892	T59.893	T59.894	—	—
Marsilid	T43.1X1	T43.1X2	T43.1X3	T43.1X4	T43.1X5	T43.1X6
Matulane	T45.1X1	T45.1X2	T45.1X3	T45.1X4	T45.1X5	T45.1X6
Mazindol	T50.5X1	T50.5X2	T50.5X3	T50.5X4	T50.5X5	T50.5X6
MCPA	T60.3X1	T60.3X2	T60.3X3	T60.3X4	—	—
MDMA	T43.621	T43.622	T43.623	T43.624	T43.625	T43.626
Meadow saffron	T62.2X1	T62.2X2	T62.2X3	T62.2X4	—	—
Measles virus vaccine (attenuated)	T50.B91	T50.B92	T50.B93	T50.B94	T50.B95	T50.B96
Meat, noxious	T62.8X1	T62.8X2	T62.8X3	T62.8X4	—	—
Meballymal	T42.3X1	T42.3X2	T42.3X3	T42.3X4	T42.3X5	T42.3X6
Mebanazine	T43.1X1	T43.1X2	T43.1X3	T43.1X4	T43.1X5	T43.1X6
Mebaral	T42.3X1	T42.3X2	T42.3X3	T42.3X4	T42.3X5	T42.3X6
Mebendazole	T37.4X1	T37.4X2	T37.4X3	T37.4X4	T37.4X5	T37.4X6
Mebeverine	T44.3X1	T44.3X2	T44.3X3	T44.3X4	T44.3X5	T44.3X6
Mebhydrolin	T45.0X1	T45.0X2	T45.0X3	T45.0X4	T45.0X5	T45.0X6
Mebumal	T42.3X1	T42.3X2	T42.3X3	T42.3X4	T42.3X5	T42.3X6
Mebutamate	T43.591	T43.592	T43.593	T43.594	T43.595	T43.596
Mecamylamine	T44.2X1	T44.2X2	T44.2X3	T44.2X4	T44.2X5	T44.2X6
Mechlorethamine	T45.1X1	T45.1X2	T45.1X3	T45.1X4	T45.1X5	T45.1X6
Mecillinam	T36.0X1	T36.0X2	T36.0X3	T36.0X4	T36.0X5	T36.0X6
Meclizine (hydrochloride)	T45.0X1	T45.0X2	T45.0X3	T45.0X4	T45.0X5	T45.0X6
Meclocycline	T36.4X1	T36.4X2	T36.4X3	T36.4X4	T36.4X5	T36.4X6
Meclofenamate	T39.391	T39.392	T39.393	T39.394	T39.395	T39.396
Meclofenamic acid	T39.391	T39.392	T39.393	T39.394	T39.395	T39.396
Meclofenoxate	T43.691	T43.692	T43.693	T43.694	T43.695	T43.696
Meclozine	T45.0X1	T45.0X2	T45.0X3	T45.0X4	T45.0X5	T45.0X6

Mecobalamin - Mesterolone

Substance	Poisoning, Accidental (unintentional)	Poisoning, Intentional self-harm	Poisoning, Assault	Poisoning, Undetermined	Adverse effect	Underdosing
Mecobalamin	T45.8X1	T45.8X2	T45.8X3	T45.8X4	T45.8X5	T45.8X6
Mecoprop	T60.3X1	T60.3X2	T60.3X3	T60.3X4	—	—
Mecrilate	T49.3X1	T49.3X2	T49.3X3	T49.3X4	T49.3X5	T49.3X6
Mecysteine	T48.4X1	T48.4X2	T48.4X3	T48.4X4	T48.4X5	T48.4X6
Medazepam	T42.4X1	T42.4X2	T42.4X3	T42.4X4	T42.4X5	T42.4X6
Medicament NEC	T50.901	T50.902	T50.903	T50.904	T50.905	T50.906
Medinal	T42.3X1	T42.3X2	T42.3X3	T42.3X4	T42.3X5	T42.3X6
Medomin	T42.3X1	T42.3X2	T42.3X3	T42.3X4	T42.3X5	T42.3X6
Medrogestone	T38.5X1	T38.5X2	T38.5X3	T38.5X4	T38.5X5	T38.5X6
Medroxalol	T44.8X1	T44.8X2	T44.8X3	T44.8X4	T44.8X5	T44.8X6
Medroxyprogesterone acetate (depot)	T38.5X1	T38.5X2	T38.5X3	T38.5X4	T38.5X5	T38.5X6
Medrysone	T49.0X1	T49.0X2	T49.0X3	T49.0X4	T49.0X5	T49.0X6
Mefenamic acid	T39.391	T39.392	T39.393	T39.394	T39.395	T39.396
Mefenorex	T50.5X1	T50.5X2	T50.5X3	T50.5X4	T50.5X5	T50.5X6
Mefloquine	T37.2X1	T37.2X2	T37.2X3	T37.2X4	T37.2X5	T37.2X6
Mefruside	T50.2X1	T50.2X2	T50.2X3	T50.2X4	T50.2X5	T50.2X6
Megahallucinogen	T40.901	T40.902	T40.903	T40.904	T40.905	T40.906
Megestrol	T38.5X1	T38.5X2	T38.5X3	T38.5X4	T38.5X5	T38.5X6
Meglumine						
antimoniate	T37.8X1	T37.8X2	T37.8X3	T37.8X4	T37.8X5	T37.8X6
diatrizoate	T50.8X1	T50.8X2	T50.8X3	T50.8X4	T50.8X5	T50.8X6
iodipamide	T50.8X1	T50.8X2	T50.8X3	T50.8X4	T50.8X5	T50.8X6
iotroxate	T50.8X1	T50.8X2	T50.8X3	T50.8X4	T50.8X5	T50.8X6
MEK (methyl ethyl ketone)	T52.4X1	T52.4X2	T52.4X3	T52.4X4	—	—
Meladinin	T49.3X1	T49.3X2	T49.3X3	T49.3X4	T49.3X5	T49.3X6
Meladrazine	T44.3X1	T44.3X2	T44.3X3	T44.3X4	T44.3X5	T44.3X6
Melaleuca alternifolia oil	T49.0X1	T49.0X2	T49.0X3	T49.0X4	T49.0X5	T49.0X6
Melanizing agents	T49.3X1	T49.3X2	T49.3X3	T49.3X4	T49.3X5	T49.3X6
Melanocyte-stimulating hormone	T38.891	T38.892	T38.893	T38.894	T38.895	T38.896
Melarsonyl potassium	T37.3X1	T37.3X2	T37.3X3	T37.3X4	T37.3X5	T37.3X6
Melarsoprol	T37.3X1	T37.3X2	T37.3X3	T37.3X4	T37.3X5	T37.3X6
Melia azedarach	T62.2X1	T62.2X2	T62.2X3	T62.2X4	—	—
Melitracen	T43.011	T43.012	T43.013	T43.014	T43.015	T43.016
Mellaril	T43.3X1	T43.3X2	T43.3X3	T43.3X4	T43.3X5	T43.3X6
Meloxine	T49.3X1	T49.3X2	T49.3X3	T49.3X4	T49.3X5	T49.3X6
Melperone	T43.4X1	T43.4X2	T43.4X3	T43.4X4	T43.4X5	T43.4X6
Melphalan	T45.1X1	T45.1X2	T45.1X3	T45.1X4	T45.1X5	T45.1X6
Memantine	T43.8X1	T43.8X2	T43.8X3	T43.8X4	T43.8X5	T43.8X6
Menadiol	T45.7X1	T45.7X2	T45.7X3	T45.7X4	T45.7X5	T45.7X6
sodium sulfate	T45.7X1	T45.7X2	T45.7X3	T45.7X4	T45.7X5	T45.7X6
Menadione	T45.7X1	T45.7X2	T45.7X3	T45.7X4	T45.7X5	T45.7X6
sodium bisulfite	T45.7X1	T45.7X2	T45.7X3	T45.7X4	T45.7X5	T45.7X6
Menaphthone	T45.7X1	T45.7X2	T45.7X3	T45.7X4	T45.7X5	T45.7X6
Menaquinone	T45.7X1	T45.7X2	T45.7X3	T45.7X4	T45.7X5	T45.7X6
Menatetrenone	T45.7X1	T45.7X2	T45.7X3	T45.7X4	T45.7X5	T45.7X6
Meningococcal vaccine	T50.A91	T50.A92	T50.A93	T50.A94	T50.A95	T50.A96
Menningovax (AC) (C)	T50.A91	T50.A92	T50.A93	T50.A94	T50.A95	T50.A96
Menotropins	T38.811	T38.812	T38.813	T38.814	T38.815	T38.816
Menthol	T48.5X1	T48.5X2	T48.5X3	T48.5X4	T48.5X5	T48.5X6
Mepacrine	T37.2X1	T37.2X2	T37.2X3	T37.2X4	T37.2X5	T37.2X6
Meparfynol	T42.6X1	T42.6X2	T42.6X3	T42.6X4	T42.6X5	T42.6X6
Mepartricin	T36.7X1	T36.7X2	T36.7X3	T36.7X4	T36.7X5	T36.7X6
Mepazine	T43.3X1	T43.3X2	T43.3X3	T43.3X4	T43.3X5	T43.3X6
Mepenzolate	T44.3X1	T44.3X2	T44.3X3	T44.3X4	T44.3X5	T44.3X6
bromide	T44.3X1	T44.3X2	T44.3X3	T44.3X4	T44.3X5	T44.3X6
Meperidine	T40.4X1	T40.4X2	T40.4X3	T40.4X4	T40.4X5	T40.4X6
Mephebarbital	T42.3X1	T42.3X2	T42.3X3	T42.3X4	T42.3X5	T42.3X6

Substance	Poisoning, Accidental (unintentional)	Poisoning, Intentional self-harm	Poisoning, Assault	Poisoning, Undetermined	Adverse effect	Underdosing
Mephenamin (e)	T42.8X1	T42.8X2	T42.8X3	T42.8X4	T42.8X5	T42.8X6
Mephenesin	T42.8X1	T42.8X2	T42.8X3	T42.8X4	T42.8X5	T42.8X6
Mephenhydramine	T45.0X1	T45.0X2	T45.0X3	T45.0X4	T45.0X5	T45.0X6
Mephenoxalone	T42.8X1	T42.8X2	T42.8X3	T42.8X4	T42.8X5	T42.8X6
Mephentermine	T44.991	T44.992	T44.993	T44.994	T44.995	T44.996
Mephenytoin	T42.0X1	T42.0X2	T42.0X3	T42.0X4	T42.0X5	T42.0X6
with phenobarbital	T42.3X1	T42.3X2	T42.3X3	T42.3X4	T42.3X5	T42.3X6
Mephobarbital	T42.3X1	T42.3X2	T42.3X3	T42.3X4	T42.3X5	T42.3X6
Mephosfolan	T60.0X1	T60.0X2	T60.0X3	T60.0X4	—	—
Mepindolol	T44.7X1	T44.7X2	T44.7X3	T44.7X4	T44.7X5	T44.7X6
Mepiperphenidol	T44.3X1	T44.3X2	T44.3X3	T44.3X4	T44.3X5	T44.3X6
Mepitiostane	T38.7X1	T38.7X2	T38.7X3	T38.7X4	T38.7X5	T38.7X6
Mepivacaine	T41.3X1	T41.3X2	T41.3X3	T41.3X4	T41.3X5	T41.3X6
epidural	T41.3X1	T41.3X2	T41.3X3	T41.3X4	T41.3X5	T41.3X6
Meprednisone	T38.0X1	T38.0X2	T38.0X3	T38.0X4	T38.0X5	T38.0X6
Meprobam	T43.591	T43.592	T43.593	T43.594	T43.595	T43.596
Meprobamate	T43.591	T43.592	T43.593	T43.594	T43.595	T43.596
Meproscillarin	T46.0X1	T46.0X2	T46.0X3	T46.0X4	T46.0X5	T46.0X6
Meprylcaine	T41.3X1	T41.3X2	T41.3X3	T41.3X4	T41.3X5	T41.3X6
Meptazinol	T39.8X1	T39.8X2	T39.8X3	T39.8X4	T39.8X5	T39.8X6
Mepyramine	T45.0X1	T45.0X2	T45.0X3	T45.0X4	T45.0X5	T45.0X6
Mequitazine	T43.3X1	T43.3X2	T43.3X3	T43.3X4	T43.3X5	T43.3X6
Meralluride	T50.2X1	T50.2X2	T50.2X3	T50.2X4	T50.2X5	T50.2X6
Merbaphen	T50.2X1	T50.2X2	T50.2X3	T50.2X4	T50.2X5	T50.2X6
Merbromin	T49.0X1	T49.0X2	T49.0X3	T49.0X4	T49.0X5	T49.0X6
Mercaptobenzothiazole salts	T49.0X1	T49.0X2	T49.0X3	T49.0X4	T49.0X5	T49.0X6
Mercaptomerin	T50.2X1	T50.2X2	T50.2X3	T50.2X4	T50.2X5	T50.2X6
Mercaptopurine	T45.1X1	T45.1X2	T45.1X3	T45.1X4	T45.1X5	T45.1X6
Mercumatilin	T50.2X1	T50.2X2	T50.2X3	T50.2X4	T50.2X5	T50.2X6
Mercuramide	T50.2X1	T50.2X2	T50.2X3	T50.2X4	T50.2X5	T50.2X6
Mercurochrome	T49.0X1	T49.0X2	T49.0X3	T49.0X4	T49.0X5	T49.0X6
Mercurophylline	T50.2X1	T50.2X2	T50.2X3	T50.2X4	T50.2X5	T50.2X6
Mercury, mercurial, mercuric, mercurous (compounds) (cyanide) (fumes) (nonmedicinal) (vapor) NEC	T56.1X1	T56.1X2	T56.1X3	T56.1X4	—	—
ammoniated	T49.0X1	T49.0X2	T49.0X3	T49.0X4	T49.0X5	T49.0X6
anti-infective						
local	T49.0X1	T49.0X2	T49.0X3	T49.0X4	T49.0X5	T49.0X6
systemic	T37.8X1	T37.8X2	T37.8X3	T37.8X4	T37.8X5	T37.8X6
topical	T49.0X1	T49.0X2	T49.0X3	T49.0X4	T49.0X5	T49.0X6
chloride (ammoniated)	T49.0X1	T49.0X2	T49.0X3	T49.0X4	T49.0X5	T49.0X6
fungicide	T56.1X1	T56.1X2	T56.1X3	T56.1X4	—	—
diuretic NEC	T50.2X1	T50.2X2	T50.2X3	T50.2X4	T50.2X5	T50.2X6
fungicide	T56.1X1	T56.1X2	T56.1X3	T56.1X4	—	—
organic (fungicide)	T56.1X1	T56.1X2	T56.1X3	T56.1X4	—	—
oxide, yellow	T49.0X1	T49.0X2	T49.0X3	T49.0X4	T49.0X5	T49.0X6
Mersalyl	T50.2X1	T50.2X2	T50.2X3	T50.2X4	T50.2X5	T50.2X6
Merthiolate	T49.0X1	T49.0X2	T49.0X3	T49.0X4	T49.0X5	T49.0X6
ophthalmic preparation	T49.5X1	T49.5X2	T49.5X3	T49.5X4	T49.5X5	T49.5X6
Meruvax	T50.B91	T50.B92	T50.B93	T50.B94	T50.B95	T50.B96
Mesalazine	T47.8X1	T47.8X2	T47.8X3	T47.8X4	T47.8X5	T47.8X6
Mescal buttons	T40.991	T40.992	T40.993	T40.994	—	—
Mescaline	T40.991	T40.992	T40.993	T40.994	—	—
Mesna	T48.4X1	T48.4X2	T48.4X3	T48.4X4	T48.4X5	T48.4X6
Mesoglycan	T46.6X1	T46.6X2	T46.6X3	T46.6X4	T46.6X5	T46.6X6
Mesoridazine	T43.3X1	T43.3X2	T43.3X3	T43.3X4	T43.3X5	T43.3X6
Mestanolone	T38.7X1	T38.7X2	T38.7X3	T38.7X4	T38.7X5	T38.7X6
Mesterolone	T38.7X1	T38.7X2	T38.7X3	T38.7X4	T38.7X5	T38.7X6

Substance	Poisoning, Accidental (unintentional)	Poisoning, Intentional self-harm	Poisoning, Assault	Poisoning, Undetermined	Adverse effect	Underdosing
Mestranol	T38.5X1	T38.5X2	T38.5X3	T38.5X4	T38.5X5	T38.5X6
Mesulergine	T42.8X1	T42.8X2	T42.8X3	T42.8X4	T42.8X5	T42.8X6
Mesulfen	T49.0X1	T49.0X2	T49.0X3	T49.0X4	T49.0X5	T49.0X6
Mesuximide	T42.2X1	T42.2X2	T42.2X3	T42.2X4	T42.2X5	T42.2X6
Metabutethamine	T41.3X1	T41.3X2	T41.3X3	T41.3X4	T41.3X5	T41.3X6
Metactesylacetate	T49.0X1	T49.0X2	T49.0X3	T49.0X4	T49.0X5	T49.0X6
Metacycline	T36.4X1	T36.4X2	T36.4X3	T36.4X4	T36.4X5	T36.4X6
Metaldehyde (snail killer) NEC	T60.8X1	T60.8X2	T60.8X3	T60.8X4	—	—
Metals (heavy) (nonmedicinal)	T56.91	T56.92	T56.93	T56.94	—	—
dust, fumes, or vapor NEC	T56.91	T56.92	T56.93	T56.94	—	—
light NEC	T56.91	T56.92	T56.93	T56.94	—	—
dust, fumes, or vapor NEC	T56.91	T56.92	T56.93	T56.94	—	—
specified NEC	T56.891	T56.892	T56.893	T56.894	—	—
thallium	T56.811	T56.812	T56.813	T56.814	—	—
Metamfetamine	T43.621	T43.622	T43.623	T43.624	T43.625	T43.626
Metamizole sodium	T39.2X1	T39.2X2	T39.2X3	T39.2X4	T39.2X5	T39.2X6
Metampicillin	T36.0X1	T36.0X2	T36.0X3	T36.0X4	T36.0X5	T36.0X6
Metamucil	T47.4X1	T47.4X2	T47.4X3	T47.4X4	T47.4X5	T47.4X6
Metandienone	T38.7X1	T38.7X2	T38.7X3	T38.7X4	T38.7X5	T38.7X6
Metandrostenolone	T38.7X1	T38.7X2	T38.7X3	T38.7X4	T38.7X5	T38.7X6
Metaphen	T49.0X1	T49.0X2	T49.0X3	T49.0X4	T49.0X5	T49.0X6
Metaphos	T60.0X1	T60.0X2	T60.0X3	T60.0X4		
Metapramine	T43.011	T43.012	T43.013	T43.014	T43.015	T43.016
Metaproterenol	T48.291	T48.292	T48.293	T48.294	T48.295	T48.296
Metaraminol	T44.4X1	T44.4X2	T44.4X3	T44.4X4	T44.4X5	T44.4X6
Metaxalone	T42.8X1	T42.8X2	T42.8X3	T42.8X4	T42.8X5	T42.8X6
Metenolone	T38.7X1	T38.7X2	T38.7X3	T38.7X4	T38.7X5	T38.7X6
Metergoline	T42.8X1	T42.8X2	T42.8X3	T42.8X4	T42.8X5	T42.8X6
Metescufylline	T46.991	T46.992	T46.993	T46.994	T46.995	T46.996
Meteteoin	T42.0X1	T42.0X2	T42.0X3	T42.0X4	T42.0X5	T42.0X6
Metformin	T38.3X1	T38.3X2	T38.3X3	T38.3X4	T38.3X5	T38.3X6
Methacholine	T44.1X1	T44.1X2	T44.1X3	T44.1X4	T44.1X5	T44.1X6
Methacycline	T36.4X1	T36.4X2	T36.4X3	T36.4X4	T36.4X5	T36.4X6
Methadone	T40.3X1	T40.3X2	T40.3X3	T40.3X4	T40.3X5	T40.3X6
Methallenestril	T38.5X1	T38.5X2	T38.5X3	T38.5X4	T38.5X5	T38.5X6
Methallenoestril	T38.5X1	T38.5X2	T38.5X3	T38.5X4	T38.5X5	T38.5X6
Methamphetamine	T43.621	T43.622	T43.623	T43.624	T43.625	T43.626
Methampyrone	T39.2X1	T39.2X2	T39.2X3	T39.2X4	T39.2X5	T39.2X6
Methandienone	T38.7X1	T38.7X2	T38.7X3	T38.7X4	T38.7X5	T38.7X6
Methandriol	T38.7X1	T38.7X2	T38.7X3	T38.7X4	T38.7X5	T38.7X6
Methandrostenolone	T38.7X1	T38.7X2	T38.7X3	T38.7X4	T38.7X5	T38.7X6
Methane	T59.891	T59.892	T59.893	T59.894	—	—
Methanethiol	T59.891	T59.892	T59.893	T59.894	—	—
Methaniazide	T37.1X1	T37.1X2	T37.1X3	T37.1X4	T37.1X5	T37.1X6
Methanol (vapor)	T51.1X1	T51.1X2	T51.1X3	T51.1X4	—	—
Methantheline	T44.3X1	T44.3X2	T44.3X3	T44.3X4	T44.3X5	T44.3X6
Methanthelinium bromide	T44.3X1	T44.3X2	T44.3X3	T44.3X4	T44.3X5	T44.3X6
Methaphenilene	T45.0X1	T45.0X2	T45.0X3	T45.0X4	T45.0X5	T45.0X6
Methapyrilene	T45.0X1	T45.0X2	T45.0X3	T45.0X4	T45.0X5	T45.0X6
Methaqualone (compound)	T42.6X1	T42.6X2	T42.6X3	T42.6X4	T42.6X5	T42.6X6
Metharbital	T42.3X1	T42.3X2	T42.3X3	T42.3X4	T42.3X5	T42.3X6
Methazolamide	T50.2X1	T50.2X2	T50.2X3	T50.2X4	T50.2X5	T50.2X6
Methdilazine	T43.3X1	T43.3X2	T43.3X3	T43.3X4	T43.3X5	T43.3X6
Methedrine	T43.621	T43.622	T43.623	T43.624	T43.625	T43.626

Substance	Poisoning, Accidental (unintentional)	Poisoning, Intentional self-harm	Poisoning, Assault	Poisoning, Undetermined	Adverse effect	Underdosing
Methenamine (mandelate)	T37.8X1	T37.8X2	T37.8X3	T37.8X4	T37.8X5	T37.8X6
Methenolone	T38.7X1	T38.7X2	T38.7X3	T38.7X4	T38.7X5	T38.7X6
Methergine	T48.0X1	T48.0X2	T48.0X3	T48.0X4	T48.0X5	T48.0X6
Methetoin	T42.0X1	T42.0X2	T42.0X3	T42.0X4	T42.0X5	T42.0X6
Methiacil	T38.2X1	T38.2X2	T38.2X3	T38.2X4	T38.2X5	T38.2X6
Methicillin	T36.0X1	T36.0X2	T36.0X3	T36.0X4	T36.0X5	T36.0X6
Methimazole	T38.2X1	T38.2X2	T38.2X3	T38.2X4	T38.2X5	T38.2X6
Methiodal sodium	T50.8X1	T50.8X2	T50.8X3	T50.8X4	T50.8X5	T50.8X6
Methionine	T50.991	T50.992	T50.993	T50.994	T50.995	T50.996
Methisazone	T37.5X1	T37.5X2	T37.5X3	T37.5X4	T37.5X5	T37.5X6
Methisoprinol	T37.5X1	T37.5X2	T37.5X3	T37.5X4	T37.5X5	T37.5X6
Methitural	T42.3X1	T42.3X2	T42.3X3	T42.3X4	T42.3X5	T42.3X6
Methixene	T44.3X1	T44.3X2	T44.3X3	T44.3X4	T44.3X5	T44.3X6
Methobarbital, methobarbitone	T42.3X1	T42.3X2	T42.3X3	T42.3X4	T42.3X5	T42.3X6
Methocarbamol	T42.8X1	T42.8X2	T42.8X3	T42.8X4	T42.8X5	T42.8X6
skeletal muscle relaxant	T48.1X1	T48.1X2	T48.1X3	T48.1X4	T48.1X5	T48.1X6
Methohexital	T41.1X1	T41.1X2	T41.1X3	T41.1X4	T41.1X5	T41.1X6
Methohexitone	T41.1X1	T41.1X2	T41.1X3	T41.1X4	T41.1X5	T41.1X6
Methoin	T42.0X1	T42.0X2	T42.0X3	T42.0X4	T42.0X5	T42.0X6
Methopholine	T39.8X1	T39.8X2	T39.8X3	T39.8X4	T39.8X5	T39.8X6
Methopromazine	T43.3X1	T43.3X2	T43.3X3	T43.3X4	T43.3X5	T43.3X6
Methorate	T48.3X1	T48.3X2	T48.3X3	T48.3X4	T48.3X5	T48.3X6
Methoserpidine	T46.5X1	T46.5X2	T46.5X3	T46.5X4	T46.5X5	T46.5X6
Methotrexate	T45.1X1	T45.1X2	T45.1X3	T45.1X4	T45.1X5	T45.1X6
Methotrimeprazine	T43.3X1	T43.3X2	T43.3X3	T43.3X4	T43.3X5	T43.3X6
Methoxa-Dome	T49.3X1	T49.3X2	T49.3X3	T49.3X4	T49.3X5	T49.3X6
Methoxamine	T44.4X1	T44.4X2	144.4X3	T44.4X4	T44.4X5	T44.4X6
Methoxsalen	T50.991	T50.992	T50.993	T50.994	T50.995	T50.996
Methoxyaniline	T65.3X1	T65.3X2	T65.3X3	T65.3X4	—	—
Methoxybenzyl penicillin	T36.0X1	T36.0X2	T36.0X3	T36.0X4	T36.0X5	T36.0X6
Methoxychlor	T53.7X1	T53.7X2	T53.7X3	T53.7X4	—	—
Methoxy-DDT	T53.7X1	T53.7X2	T53.7X3	T53.7X4	—	—
2-Methoxyethanol	T52.3X1	T52.3X2	T52.3X3	T52.3X4	—	—
Methoxyflurane	T41.0X1	T41.0X2	T41.0X3	T41.0X4	T41.0X5	T41.0X6
Methoxyphenamine	T48.6X1	T48.6X2	T48.6X3	T48.6X4	T48.6X5	T48.6X6
Methoxypromazine	T43.3X1	T43.3X2	T43.3X3	T43.3X4	T43.3X5	T43.3X6
5-Methoxypsoralen (5-MOP)	T50.991	T50.992	T50.993	T50.994	T50.995	T50.996
8-Methoxypsoralen (8-MOP)	T50.991	T50.992	T50.993	T50.994	T50.995	T50.996
Methscopolamine bromide	T44.3X1	T44.3X2	T44.3X3	T44.3X4	T44.3X5	T44.3X6
Methsuximide	T42.2X1	T42.2X2	T42.2X3	T42.2X4	T42.2X5	T42.2X6
Methyclothiazide	T50.2X1	T50.2X2	T50.2X3	T50.2X4	T50.2X5	T50.2X6
Methyl						
acetate	T52.4X1	T52.4X2	T52.4X3	T52.4X4	—	—
acetone	T52.4X1	T52.4X2	T52.4X3	T52.4X4	—	—
acrylate	T65.891	T65.892	T65.893	T65.894	—	—
alcohol	T51.1X1	T51.1X2	T51.1X3	T51.1X4	—	—
aminophenol	T65.3X1	T65.3X2	T65.3X3	T65.3X4	—	—
amphetamine	T43.621	T43.622	T43.623	T43.624	T43.625	T43.626
androstanolone	T38.7X1	T38.7X2	T38.7X3	T38.7X4	T38.7X5	T38.7X6
atropine	T44.3X1	T44.3X2	T44.3X3	T44.3X4	T44.3X5	T44.3X6
benzene	T52.2X1	T52.2X2	T52.2X3	T52.2X4	—	—
benzoate	T52.8X1	T52.8X2	T52.8X3	T52.8X4	—	—
benzol	T52.2X1	T52.2X2	T52.2X3	T52.2X4	—	—
bromide (gas)	T59.891	T59.892	T59.893	T59.894	—	—
fumigant	T60.8X1	T60.8X2	T60.8X3	T60.8X4	—	—

Methyl - Mevinphos

Substance	Poisoning, Accidental (unintentional)	Poisoning, Intentional self-harm	Poisoning, Assault	Poisoning, Undetermined	Adverse effect	Underdosing
Methyl — *continued*						
butanol	T51.3X1	T51.3X2	T51.3X3	T51.3X4	—	—
carbinol	T51.1X1	T51.1X2	T51.1X3	T51.1X4	—	—
carbonate	T52.8X1	T52.8X2	T52.8X3	T52.8X4	—	—
CCNU	T45.1X1	T45.1X2	T45.1X3	T45.1X4	T45.1X5	T45.1X6
cellosolve	T52.91	T52.92	T52.93	T52.94		
cellulose	T47.4X1	T47.4X2	T47.4X3	T47.4X4	T47.4X5	T47.4X6
chloride (gas)	T59.891	T59.892	T59.893	T59.894	—	—
chloroformate	T59.3X1	T59.3X2	T59.3X3	T59.3X4	—	—
cyclohexane	T52.8X1	T52.8X2	T52.8X3	T52.8X4	—	—
cyclohexanol	T51.8X1	T51.8X2	T51.8X3	T51.8X4	—	—
cyclohexanone	T52.8X1	T52.8X2	T52.8X3	T52.8X4	—	—
cyclohexyl acetate	T52.8X1	T52.8X2	T52.8X3	T52.8X4	—	—
demeton	T60.0X1	T60.0X2	T60.0X3	T60.0X4	—	—
dihydromorphinone	T40.2X1	T40.2X2	T40.2X3	T40.2X4	T40.2X5	T40.2X6
ergometrine	T48.0X1	T48.0X2	T48.0X3	T48.0X4	T48.0X5	T48.0X6
ergonovine	T48.0X1	T48.0X2	T48.0X3	T48.0X4	T48.0X5	T48.0X6
ethyl ketone	T52.4X1	T52.4X2	T52.4X3	T52.4X4	—	—
glucamine antimonate	T37.8X1	T37.8X2	T37.8X3	T37.8X4	T37.8X5	T37.8X6
hydrazine	T65.891	T65.892	T65.893	T65.894	—	—
iodide	T65.891	T65.892	T65.893	T65.894	—	—
isobutyl ketone	T52.4X1	T52.4X2	T52.4X3	T52.4X4	—	—
isothiocyanate	T60.3X1	T60.3X2	T60.3X3	T60.3X4	—	—
mercaptan	T59.891	T59.892	T59.893	T59.894	—	—
morphine NEC	T40.2X1	T40.2X2	T40.2X3	T40.2X4	T40.2X5	T40.2X6
nicotinate	T49.4X1	T49.4X2	T49.4X3	T49.4X4	T49.4X5	T49.4X6
paraben	T49.0X1	T49.0X2	T49.0X3	T49.0X4	T49.0X5	T49.0X6
parafynol	T42.6X1	T42.6X2	T42.6X3	T42.6X4	T42.6X5	T42.6X6
parathion	T60.0X1	T60.0X2	T60.0X3	T60.0X4	—	—
peridol	T43.4X1	T43.4X2	T43.4X3	T43.4X4	T43.4X5	T43.4X6
phenidate	T43.631	T43.632	T43.633	T43.634	T43.635	T43.636
prednisolone	T38.0X1	T38.0X2	T38.0X3	T38.0X4	T38.0X5	T38.0X6
ENT agent	T49.6X1	T49.6X2	T49.6X3	T49.6X4	T49.6X5	T49.6X6
ophthalmic preparation	T49.5X1	T49.5X2	T49.5X3	T49.5X4	T49.5X5	T49.5X6
topical NEC	T49.0X1	T49.0X2	T49.0X3	T49.0X4	T49.0X5	T49.0X6
propylcarbinol	T51.3X1	T51.3X2	T51.3X3	T51.3X4	—	—
rosaniline NEC	T49.0X1	T49.0X2	T49.0X3	T49.0X4	T49.0X5	T49.0X6
salicylate	T49.2X1	T49.2X2	T49.2X3	T49.2X4	T49.2X5	T49.2X6
sulfate (fumes)	T59.891	T59.892	T59.893	T59.894	—	—
liquid	T52.8X1	T52.8X2	T52.8X3	T52.8X4	—	—
sulfonal	T42.6X1	T42.6X2	T42.6X3	T42.6X4	T42.6X5	T42.6X6
testosterone	T38.7X1	T38.7X2	T38.7X3	T38.7X4	T38.7X5	T38.7X6
thiouracil	T38.2X1	T38.2X2	T38.2X3	T38.2X4	T38.2X5	T38.2X6
Methylamphetamine	T43.621	T43.622	T43.623	T43.624	T43.625	T43.626
Methylated spirit	T51.1X1	T51.1X2	T51.1X3	T51.1X4		
Methylatropine nitrate	T44.3X1	T44.3X2	T44.3X3	T44.3X4	T44.3X5	T44.3X6
Methylbenactyzium bromide	T44.3X1	T44.3X2	T44.3X3	T44.3X4	T44.3X5	T44.3X6
Methylbenzethonium chloride	T49.0X1	T49.0X2	T49.0X3	T49.0X4	T49.0X5	T49.0X6
Methylcellulose	T47.4X1	T47.4X2	T47.4X3	T47.4X4	T47.4X5	T47.4X6
laxative	T47.4X1	T47.4X2	T47.4X3	T47.4X4	T47.4X5	T47.4X6
Methylchlorophenoxy-acetic acid	T60.3X1	T60.3X2	T60.3X3	T60.3X4	—	—
Methyldopa	T46.5X1	T46.5X2	T46.5X3	T46.5X4	T46.5X5	T46.5X6
Methyldopate	T46.5X1	T46.5X2	T46.5X3	T46.5X4	T46.5X5	T46.5X6
Methylene						
blue	T50.6X1	T50.6X2	T50.6X3	T50.6X4	T50.6X5	T50.6X6

Substance	Poisoning, Accidental (unintentional)	Poisoning, Intentional self-harm	Poisoning, Assault	Poisoning, Undetermined	Adverse effect	Underdosing
chloride or dichloride (solvent) NEC	T53.4X1	T53.4X2	T53.4X3	T53.4X4	—	—
Methylenedioxyamphet-amine	T43.621	T43.622	T43.623	T43.624	T43.625	T43.626
Methylenedioxy methamphetamine	T43.621	T43.622	T43.623	T43.624	T43.625	T43.626
Methylergometrine	T48.0X1	T48.0X2	T48.0X3	T48.0X4	T48.0X5	T48.0X6
Methylergonovine	T48.0X1	T48.0X2	T48.0X3	T48.0X4	T48.0X5	T48.0X6
Methylestrenolone	T38.5X1	T38.5X2	T38.5X3	T38.5X4	T38.5X5	T38.5X6
Methylethyl cellulose	T50.991	T50.992	T50.993	T50.994	T50.995	T50.996
Methylhexabital	T42.3X1	T42.3X2	T42.3X3	T42.3X4	T42.3X5	T42.3X6
Methylmorphine	T40.2X1	T40.2X2	T40.2X3	T40.2X4	T40.2X5	T40.2X6
Methylparaben (ophthalmic)	T49.5X1	T49.5X2	T49.5X3	T49.5X4	T49.5X5	T49.5X6
Methylparafynol	T42.6X1	T42.6X2	T42.6X3	T42.6X4	T42.6X5	T42.6X6
Methylpentynol, methylpenthynol	T42.6X1	T42.6X2	T42.6X3	T42.6X4	T42.6X5	T42.6X6
Methylphenidate	T43.631	T43.632	T43.633	T43.634	T43.635	T43.636
Methylphenobarbital	T42.3X1	T42.3X2	T42.3X3	T42.3X4	T42.3X5	T42.3X6
Methylpolysiloxane	T47.1X1	T47.1X2	T47.1X3	T47.1X4	T47.1X5	T47.1X6
Methylprednisolone— *see Methyl, prednisolone*						
Methylrosaniline	T49.0X1	T49.0X2	T49.0X3	T49.0X4	T49.0X5	T49.0X6
Methylrosanilinium chloride	T49.0X1	T49.0X2	T49.0X3	T49.0X4	T49.0X5	T49.0X6
Methyltestosterone	T38.7X1	T38.7X2	T38.7X3	T38.7X4	T38.7X5	T38.7X6
Methylthionine chloride	T50.6X1	T50.6X2	T50.6X3	T50.6X4	T50.6X5	T50.6X6
Methylthioninium chloride	T50.6X1	T50.6X2	T50.6X3	T50.6X4	T50.6X5	T50.6X6
Methylthiouracil	T38.2X1	T38.2X2	T38.2X3	T38.2X4	T38.2X5	T38.2X6
Methyprylon	T42.6X1	T42.6X2	T42.6X3	T42.6X4	T42.6X5	T42.6X6
Methysergide	T46.5X1	T46.5X2	T46.5X3	T46.5X4	T46.5X5	T46.5X6
Metiamide	T47.1X1	T47.1X2	T47.1X3	T47.1X4	T47.1X5	T47.1X6
Meticillin	T36.0X1	T36.0X2	T36.0X3	T36.0X4	T36.0X5	T36.0X6
Meticrane	T50.2X1	T50.2X2	T50.2X3	T50.2X4	T50.2X5	T50.2X6
Metildigoxin	T46.0X1	T46.0X2	T46.0X3	T46.0X4	T46.0X5	T46.0X6
Metipranolol	T49.5X1	T49.5X2	T49.5X3	T49.5X4	T49.5X5	T49.5X6
Metirosine	T46.5X1	T46.5X2	T46.5X3	T46.5X4	T46.5X5	T46.5X6
Metisazone	T37.5X1	T37.5X2	T37.5X3	T37.5X4	T37.5X5	T37.5X6
Metixene	T44.3X1	T44.3X2	T44.3X3	T44.3X4	T44.3X5	T44.3X6
Metizoline	T48.5X1	T48.5X2	T48.5X3	T48.5X4	T48.5X5	T48.5X6
Metoclopramide	T45.0X1	T45.0X2	T45.0X3	T45.0X4	T45.0X5	T45.0X6
Metofenazate	T43.3X1	T43.3X2	T43.3X3	T43.3X4	T43.3X5	T43.3X6
Metofoline	T39.8X1	T39.8X2	T39.8X3	T39.8X4	T39.8X5	T39.8X6
Metolazone	T50.2X1	T50.2X2	T50.2X3	T50.2X4	T50.2X5	T50.2X6
Metopon	T40.2X1	T40.2X2	T40.2X3	T40.2X4	T40.2X5	T40.2X6
Metoprine	T45.1X1	T45.1X2	T45.1X3	T45.1X4	T45.1X5	T45.1X6
Metoprolol	T44.7X1	T44.7X2	T44.7X3	T44.7X4	T44.7X5	T44.7X6
Metrifonate	T60.0X1	T60.0X2	T60.0X3	T60.0X4	—	—
Metrizamide	T50.8X1	T50.8X2	T50.8X3	T50.8X4	T50.8X5	T50.8X6
Metrizoic acid	T50.8X1	T50.8X2	T50.8X3	T50.8X4	T50.8X5	T50.8X6
Metronidazole	T37.8X1	T37.8X2	T37.8X3	T37.8X4	T37.8X5	T37.8X6
Metycaine	T41.3X1	T41.3X2	T41.3X3	T41.3X4	T41.3X5	T41.3X6
infiltration (subcutaneous)	T41.3X1	T41.3X2	T41.3X3	T41.3X4	T41.3X5	T41.3X6
nerve block (peripheral) (plexus)	T41.3X1	T41.3X2	T41.3X3	T41.3X4	T41.3X5	T41.3X6
topical (surface)	T41.3X1	T41.3X2	T41.3X3	T41.3X4	T41.3X5	T41.3X6
Metyrapone	T50.8X1	T50.8X2	T50.8X3	T50.8X4	T50.8X5	T50.8X6
Mevinphos	T60.0X1	T60.0X2	T60.0X3	T60.0X4		

Substance	Poisoning, Accidental (unintentional)	Poisoning, Intentional self-harm	Poisoning, Assault	Poisoning, Undetermined	Adverse effect	Underdosing
Mexazolam	T42.4X1	T42.4X2	T42.4X3	T42.4X4	T42.4X5	T42.4X6
Mexenone	T49.3X1	T49.3X2	T49.3X3	T49.3X4	T49.3X5	T49.3X6
Mexiletine	T46.2X1	T46.2X2	T46.2X3	T46.2X4	T46.2X5	T46.2X6
Mezereon	T62.2X1	T62.2X2	T62.2X3	T62.2X4	—	—
berries	T62.1X1	T62.1X2	T62.1X3	T62.1X4	—	—
Mezlocillin	T36.0X1	T36.0X2	T36.0X3	T36.0X4	T36.0X5	T36.0X6
Mianserin	T43.021	T43.022	T43.023	T43.024	T43.025	T43.026
Micatin	T49.0X1	T49.0X2	T49.0X3	T49.0X4	T49.0X5	T49.0X6
Miconazole	T49.0X1	T49.0X2	T49.0X3	T49.0X4	T49.0X5	T49.0X6
Micronomicin	T36.5X1	T36.5X2	T36.5X3	T36.5X4	T36.5X5	T36.5X6
Midazolam	T42.4X1	T42.4X2	T42.4X3	T42.4X4	T42.4X5	T42.4X6
Midecamycin	T36.3X1	T36.3X2	T36.3X3	T36.3X4	T36.3X5	T36.3X6
Mifepristone	T38.6X1	T38.6X2	T38.6X3	T38.6X4	T38.6X5	T38.6X6
Milk of magnesia	T47.1X1	T47.1X2	T47.1X3	T47.1X4	T47.1X5	T47.1X6
Millipede (tropical) (venomous)	T63.411	T63.412	T63.413	T63.414	—	—
Miltown	T43.591	T43.592	T43.593	T43.594	T43.595	T43.596
Milverine	T44.3X1	T44.3X2	T44.3X3	T44.3X4	T44.3X5	T44.3X6
Minaprine	T43.291	T43.292	T43.293	T43.294	T43.295	T43.296
Minaxolone	T41.291	T41.292	T41.293	T41.294	T41.295	T41.296
Mineral						
acids	T54.2X1	T54.2X2	T54.2X3	T54.2X4	—	—
oil (laxative) (medicinal)	T47.4X1	T47.4X2	T47.4X3	T47.4X4	T47.4X5	T47.4X6
emulsion	T47.2X1	T47.2X2	T47.2X3	T47.2X4	T47.2X5	T47.2X6
nonmedicinal	T52.0X1	T52.0X2	T52.0X3	T52.0X4	—	—
topical	T49.3X1	T49.3X2	T49.3X3	T49.3X4	T49.3X5	T49.3X6
salt NEC	T50.3X1	T50.3X2	T50.3X3	T50.3X4	T50.3X5	T50.3X6
spirits	T52.0X1	T52.0X2	T52.0X3	T52.0X4	—	—
Mineralocorticosteroid	T50.0X1	T50.0X2	T50.0X3	T50.0X4	T50.0X5	T50.0X6
Minocycline	T36.4X1	T36.4X2	T36.4X3	T36.4X4	T36.4X5	T36.4X6
Minoxidil	T46.7X1	T46.7X2	T46.7X3	T46.7X4	T46.7X5	T46.7X6
Miokamycin	T36.3X1	T36.3X2	T36.3X3	T36.3X4	T36.3X5	T36.3X6
Miotic drug	T49.5X1	T49.5X2	T49.5X3	T49.5X4	T49.5X5	T49.5X6
Mipafox	T60.0X1	T60.0X2	T60.0X3	T60.0X4	—	—
Mirex	T60.1X1	T60.1X2	T60.1X3	T60.1X4	—	—
Mirtazapine	T43.021	T43.022	T43.023	T43.024	T43.025	T43.026
Misonidazole	T37.3X1	T37.3X2	T37.3X3	T37.3X4	T37.3X5	T37.3X6
Misoprostol	T47.1X1	T47.1X2	T47.1X3	T47.1X4	T47.1X5	T47.1X6
Mithramycin	T45.1X1	T45.1X2	T45.1X3	T45.1X4	T45.1X5	T45.1X6
Mitobronitol	T45.1X1	T45.1X2	T45.1X3	T45.1X4	T45.1X5	T45.1X6
Mitoguazone	T45.1X1	T45.1X2	T45.1X3	T45.1X4	T45.1X5	T45.1X6
Mitolactol	T45.1X1	T45.1X2	T45.1X3	T45.1X4	T45.1X5	T45.1X6
Mitomycin	T45.1X1	T45.1X2	T45.1X3	T45.1X4	T45.1X5	T45.1X6
Mitopodozide	T45.1X1	T45.1X2	T45.1X3	T45.1X4	T45.1X5	T45.1X6
Mitotane	T45.1X1	T45.1X2	T45.1X3	T45.1X4	T45.1X5	T45.1X6
Mitoxantrone	T45.1X1	T45.1X2	T45.1X3	T45.1X4	T45.1X5	T45.1X6
Mivacurium chloride	T48.1X1	T48.1X2	T48.1X3	T48.1X4	T48.1X5	T48.1X6
Miyari bacteria	T47.6X1	T47.6X2	T47.6X3	T47.6X4	T47.6X5	T47.6X6
Moclobemide	T43.1X1	T43.1X2	T43.1X3	T43.1X4	T43.1X5	T43.1X6
Moderil	T46.5X1	T46.5X2	T46.5X3	T46.5X4	T46.5X5	T46.5X6
Mofebutazone	T39.2X1	T39.2X2	T39.2X3	T39.2X4	T39.2X5	T39.2X6
Mogadon—see Nitrazepam						
Molindone	T43.591	T43.592	T43.593	T43.594	T43.595	T43.596
Molsidomine	T46.3X1	T46.3X2	T46.3X3	T46.3X4	T46.3X5	T46.3X6
Mometasone	T49.0X1	T49.0X2	T49.0X3	T49.0X4	T49.0X5	T49.0X6
Monistat	T49.0X1	T49.0X2	T49.0X3	T49.0X4	T49.0X5	T49.0X6
Monkshood	T62.2X1	T62.2X2	T62.2X3	T62.2X4	—	—
Monoamine oxidase inhibitor NEC	T43.1X1	T43.1X2	T43.1X3	T43.1X4	T43.1X5	T43.1X6
hydrazine	T43.1X1	T43.1X2	T43.1X3	T43.1X4	T43.1X5	T43.1X6

Substance	Poisoning, Accidental (unintentional)	Poisoning, Intentional self-harm	Poisoning, Assault	Poisoning, Undetermined	Adverse effect	Underdosing
Monobenzone	T49.4X1	T49.4X2	T49.4X3	T49.4X4	T49.4X5	T49.4X6
Monochloroacetic acid	T60.3X1	T60.3X2	T60.3X3	T60.3X4	—	—
Monochlorobenzene	T53.7X1	T53.7X2	T53.7X3	T53.7X4	—	—
Monoethanolamine	T46.8X1	T46.8X2	T46.8X3	T46.8X4	T46.8X5	T46.8X6
oleate	T46.8X1	T46.8X2	T46.8X3	T46.8X4	T46.8X5	T46.8X6
Monooctanoin	T50.991	T50.992	T50.993	T50.994	T50.995	T50.996
Monophenylbutazone	T39.2X1	T39.2X2	T39.2X3	T39.2X4	T39.2X5	T39.2X6
Monosodium glutamate	T65.891	T65.892	T65.893	T65.894	—	—
Monosulfiram	T49.0X1	T49.0X2	T49.0X3	T49.0X4	T49.0X5	T49.0X6
Monoxide, carbon—see Carbon, monoxide						
Monoxidine hydrochloride	T46.1X1	T46.1X2	T46.1X3	T46.1X4	T46.1X5	T46.1X6
Monuron	T60.3X1	T60.3X2	T60.3X3	T60.3X4	—	—
Moperone	T43.4X1	T43.4X2	T43.4X3	T43.4X4	T43.4X5	T43.4X6
Mopidamol	T45.1X1	T45.1X2	T45.1X3	T45.1X4	T45.1X5	T45.1X6
MOPP (mechloreth-amine + vincristine + prednisone + procarba-zine)	T45.1X1	T45.1X2	T45.1X3	T45.1X4	T45.1X5	T45.1X6
Morfin	T40.2X1	T40.2X2	T40.2X3	T40.2X4	T40.2X5	T40.2X6
Morinamide	T37.1X1	T37.1X2	T37.1X3	T37.1X4	T37.1X5	T37.1X6
Morning glory seeds	T40.991	T40.992	T40.993	T40.994	—	—
Moroxydine	T37.5X1	T37.5X2	T37.5X3	T37.5X4	T37.5X5	T37.5X6
Morphazinamide	T37.1X1	T37.1X2	T37.1X3	T37.1X4	T37.1X5	T37.1X6
Morphine	T40.2X1	T40.2X2	T40.2X3	T40.2X4	T40.2X5	T40.2X6
antagonist	T50.7X1	T50.7X2	T50.7X3	T50.7X4	T50.7X5	T50.7X6
Morpholinylethylmorphine	T40.2X1	T40.2X2	T40.2X3	T40.2X4	—	—
Morsuximide	T42.2X1	T42.2X2	T42.2X3	T42.2X4	T42.2X5	T42.2X6
Mosapramine	T43.591	T43.592	T43.593	T43.594	T43.595	T43.596
Moth balls—see also Pesticides	T60.2X1	T60.2X2	T60.2X3	T60.2X4	—	—
naphthalene	T60.2X1	T60.2X2	T60.2X3	T60.2X4	—	—
paradichlorobenzene	T60.1X1	T60.1X2	T60.1X3	T60.1X4	—	—
Motor exhaust gas	T58.01	T58.02	T58.03	T58.04	—	—
Mouthwash (antiseptic) (zinc chloride)	T49.6X1	T49.6X2	T49.6X3	T49.6X4	T49.6X5	T49.6X6
Moxastine	T45.0X1	T45.0X2	T45.0X3	T45.0X4	T45.0X5	T45.0X6
Moxaverine	T44.3X1	T44.3X2	T44.3X3	T44.3X4	T44.3X5	T44.3X6
Moxisylyte	T46.7X1	T46.7X2	T46.7X3	T46.7X4	T46.7X5	T46.7X6
Mucilage, plant	T47.4X1	T47.4X2	T47.4X3	T47.4X4	T47.4X5	T47.4X6
Mucolytic drug	T48.4X1	T48.4X2	T48.4X3	T48.4X4	T48.4X5	T48.4X6
Mucomyst	T48.4X1	T48.4X2	T48.4X3	T48.4X4	T48.4X5	T48.4X6
Mucous membrane agents (external)	T49.91	T49.92	T49.93	T49.94	T49.95	T49.96
specified NEC	T49.8X1	T49.8X2	T49.8X3	T49.8X4	T49.8X5	T49.8X6
Mumps						
immune globulin (human)	T50.Z11	T50.Z12	T50.Z13	T50.Z14	T50.Z15	T50.Z16
skin test antigen	T50.8X1	T50.8X2	T50.8X3	T50.8X4	T50.8X5	T50.8X6
vaccine	T50.B91	T50.B92	T50.B93	T50.B94	T50.B95	T50.B96
Mumpsvax	T50.B91	T50.B92	T50.B93	T50.B94	T50.B95	T50.B96
Mupirocin	T49.0X1	T49.0X2	T49.0X3	T49.0X4	T49.0X5	T49.0X6
Muriatic acid—see Hydrochloric acid						
Muromonab-CD3	T45.1X1	T45.1X2	T45.1X3	T45.1X4	T45.1X5	T45.1X6
Muscle-action drug NEC	T48.201	T48.202	T48.203	T48.204	T48.205	T48.206
Muscle affecting agents NEC	T48.201	T48.202	T48.203	T48.204	T48.205	T48.206
oxytocic	T48.0X1	T48.0X2	T48.0X3	T48.0X4	T48.0X5	T48.0X6
relaxants	T48.201	T48.202	T48.203	T48.204	T48.205	T48.206

Muscle affecting agents NEC - Neostigmine bromide

Substance	Poisoning, Accidental (unintentional)	Poisoning, Intentional self-harm	Poisoning, Assault	Poisoning, Undetermined	Adverse effect	Underdosing
Muscle affecting agents NEC — *continued*						
relaxants — *continued*						
central nervous system	T42.8X1	T42.8X2	T42.8X3	T42.8X4	T42.8X5	T42.8X6
skeletal	T48.1X1	T48.1X2	T48.1X3	T48.1X4	T48.1X5	T48.1X6
smooth	T44.3X1	T44.3X2	T44.3X3	T44.3X4	T44.3X5	T44.3X6
Muscle relaxant—*see Relaxant, muscle*						
Muscle-tone depressant, central NEC	T42.8X1	T42.8X2	T42.8X3	T42.8X4	T42.8X5	T42.8X6
specified NEC	T42.8X1	T42.8X2	T42.8X3	T42.8X4	T42.8X5	T42.8X6
Mushroom, noxious	T62.0X1	T62.0X2	T62.0X3	T62.0X4	—	—
Mussel, noxious	T61.781	T61.782	T61.783	T61.784	—	—
Mustard (emetic)	T47.7X1	T47.7X2	T47.7X3	T47.7X4	T47.7X5	T47.7X6
black	T47.7X1	T47.7X2	T47.7X3	T47.7X4	T47.7X5	T47.7X6
gas, not in war	T59.91	T59.92	T59.93	T59.94	—	—
nitrogen	T45.1X1	T45.1X2	T45.1X3	T45.1X4	T45.1X5	T45.1X6
Mustine	T45.1X1	T45.1X2	T45.1X3	T45.1X4	T45.1X5	T45.1X6
M-vac	T45.1X1	T45.1X2	T45.1X3	T45.1X4	T45.1X5	T45.1X6
Mycifradin	T36.5X1	T36.5X2	T36.5X3	T36.5X4	T36.5X5	T36.5X6
topical	T49.0X1	T49.0X2	T49.0X3	T49.0X4	T49.0X5	T49.0X6
Mycitracin	T36.8X1	T36.8X2	T36.8X3	T36.8X4	T36.8X5	T36.8X6
ophthalmic preparation	T49.5X1	T49.5X2	T49.5X3	T49.5X4	T49.5X5	T49.5X6
Mycostatin	T36.7X1	T36.7X2	T36.7X3	T36.7X4	T36.7X5	T36.7X6
topical	T49.0X1	T49.0X2	T49.0X3	T49.0X4	T49.0X5	T49.0X6
Mycotoxins	T64.81	T64.82	T64.83	T64.84	—	—
aflatoxin	T64.01	T64.02	T64.03	T64.04	—	—
specified NEC	T64.81	T64.82	T64.83	T64.84	—	—
Mydriacyl	T44.3X1	T44.3X2	T44.3X3	T44.3X4	T44.3X5	T44.3X6
Mydriatic drug	T49.5X1	T49.5X2	T49.5X3	T49.5X4	T49.5X5	T49.5X6
Myelobromal	T45.1X1	T45.1X2	T45.1X3	T45.1X4	T45.1X5	T45.1X6
Myleran	T45.1X1	T45.1X2	T45.1X3	T45.1X4	T45.1X5	T45.1X6
Myochrysin (e)	T39.2X1	T39.2X2	T39.2X3	T39.2X4	T39.2X5	T39.2X6
Myoneural blocking agents	T48.1X1	T48.1X2	T48.1X3	T48.1X4	T48.1X5	T48.1X6
Myralact	T49.0X1	T49.0X2	T49.0X3	T49.0X4	T49.0X5	T49.0X6
Myristica fragrans	T62.2X1	T62.2X2	T62.2X3	T62.2X4	—	—
Myristicin	T65.891	T65.892	T65.893	T65.894	—	—
Mysoline	T42.3X1	T42.3X2	T42.3X3	T42.3X4	T42.3X5	T42.3X6
N						
Nabilone	T40.7X1	T40.7X2	T40.7X3	T40.7X4	T40.7X5	T40.7X6
Nabumetone	T39.391	T39.392	T39.393	T39.394	T39.395	T39.396
Nadolol	T44.7X1	T44.7X2	T44.7X3	T44.7X4	T44.7X5	T44.7X6
Nafcillin	T36.0X1	T36.0X2	T36.0X3	T36.0X4	T36.0X5	T36.0X6
Nafoxidine	T38.6X1	T38.6X2	T38.6X3	T38.6X4	T38.6X5	T38.6X6
Naftazone	T46.991	T46.992	T46.993	T46.994	T46.995	T46.996
Naftidrofuryl (oxalate)	T46.7X1	T46.7X2	T46.7X3	T46.7X4	T46.7X5	T46.7X6
Naftifine	T49.0X1	T49.0X2	T49.0X3	T49.0X4	T49.0X5	T49.0X6
Nail polish remover	T52.91	T52.92	T52.93	T52.94	—	—
Nalbuphine	T40.4X1	T40.4X2	T40.4X3	T40.4X4	T40.4X5	T40.4X6
Naled	T60.0X1	T60.0X2	T60.0X3	T60.0X4	—	—
Nalidixic acid	T37.8X1	T37.8X2	T37.8X3	T37.8X4	T37.8X5	T37.8X6
Nalorphine	T50.7X1	T50.7X2	T50.7X3	T50.7X4	T50.7X5	T50.7X6
Naloxone	T50.7X1	T50.7X2	T50.7X3	T50.7X4	T50.7X5	T50.7X6
Naltrexone	T50.7X1	T50.7X2	T50.7X3	T50.7X4	T50.7X5	T50.7X6
Namenda	T43.8X1	T43.8X2	T43.8X3	T43.8X4	T43.8X5	T43.8X6
Nandrolone	T38.7X1	T38.7X2	T38.7X3	T38.7X4	T38.7X5	T38.7X6
Naphazoline	T48.5X1	T48.5X2	T48.5X3	T48.5X4	T48.5X5	T48.5X6
Naphtha (painters') (petroleum)	T52.0X1	T52.0X2	T52.0X3	T52.0X4	—	—

Substance	Poisoning, Accidental (unintentional)	Poisoning, Intentional self-harm	Poisoning, Assault	Poisoning, Undetermined	Adverse effect	Underdosing
Naphtha (painters') (petroleum) — *continued*						
solvent	T52.0X1	T52.0X2	T52.0X3	T52.0X4	—	—
vapor	T52.0X1	T52.0X2	T52.0X3	T52.0X4	—	—
Naphthalene (non-chlorinated)	T60.2X1	T60.2X2	T60.2X3	T60.2X4	—	—
chlorinated	T60.1X1	T60.1X2	T60.1X3	T60.1X4	—	—
vapor	T60.1X1	T60.1X2	T60.1X3	T60.1X4	—	—
insecticide or moth repellent	T60.2X1	T60.2X2	T60.2X3	T60.2X4	—	—
chlorinated	T60.1X1	T60.1X2	T60.1X3	T60.1X4	—	—
vapor	T60.2X1	T60.2X2	T60.2X3	T60.2X4	—	—
chlorinated	T60.1X1	T60.1X2	T60.1X3	T60.1X4	—	—
Naphthol	T65.891	T65.892	T65.893	T65.894	—	—
Naphthylamine	T65.891	T65.892	T65.893	T65.894	—	—
Naphthylthiourea (ANTU)	T60.4X1	T60.4X2	T60.4X3	T60.4X4	—	—
Naprosyn—*see Naproxen*						
Naproxen	T39.311	T39.312	T39.313	T39.314	T39.315	T39.316
Narcotic (drug)	T40.601	T40.602	T40.603	T40.604	T40.605	T40.606
analgesic NEC	T40.601	T40.602	T40.603	T40.604	T40.605	T40.606
antagonist	T50.7X1	T50.7X2	T50.7X3	T50.7X4	T50.7X5	T50.7X6
specified NEC	T40.691	T40.692	T40.693	T40.694	T40.695	T40.696
synthetic	T40.4X1	T40.4X2	T40.4X3	T40.4X4	T40.4X5	T40.4X6
Narcotine	T48.3X1	T48.3X2	T48.3X3	T48.3X4	T48.3X5	T48.3X6
Nardil	T43.1X1	T43.1X2	T43.1X3	T43.1X4	T43.1X5	T43.1X6
Nasal drug NEC	T49.6X1	T49.6X2	T49.6X3	T49.6X4	T49.6X5	T49.6X6
Natamycin	T49.0X1	T49.0X2	T49.0X3	T49.0X4	T49.0X5	T49.0X6
Natrium cyanide—*see Cyanide(s)*						
Natural						
blood (product)	T45.8X1	T45.8X2	T45.8X3	T45.8X4	T45.8X5	T45.8X6
gas (piped)	T59.891	T59.892	T59.893	T59.894	—	—
incomplete combustion	T58.11	T58.12	T58.13	T58.14	—	—
Nealbarbital	T42.3X1	T42.3X2	T42.3X3	T42.3X4	T42.3X5	T42.3X6
Nectadon	T48.3X1	T48.3X2	T48.3X3	T48.3X4	T48.3X5	T48.3X6
Nedocromil	T48.6X1	T48.6X2	T48.6X3	T48.6X4	T48.6X5	T48.6X6
Nefopam	T39.8X1	T39.8X2	T39.8X3	T39.8X4	T39.8X5	T39.8X6
Nematocyst (sting)	T63.691	T63.692	T63.693	T63.694	—	—
Nembutal	T42.3X1	T42.3X2	T42.3X3	T42.3X4	T42.3X5	T42.3X6
Nemonapride	T43.591	T43.592	T43.593	T43.594	T43.595	T43.596
Neoarsphenamine	T37.8X1	T37.8X2	T37.8X3	T37.8X4	T37.8X5	T37.8X6
Neocinchophen	T50.4X1	T50.4X2	T50.4X3	T50.4X4	T50.4X5	T50.4X6
Neomycin (derivatives)	T36.5X1	T36.5X2	T36.5X3	T36.5X4	T36.5X5	T36.5X6
with						
bacitracin	T49.0X1	T49.0X2	T49.0X3	T49.0X4	T49.0X5	T49.0X6
neostigmine	T44.0X1	T44.0X2	T44.0X3	T44.0X4	T44.0X5	T44.0X6
ENT agent	T49.6X1	T49.6X2	T49.6X3	T49.6X4	T49.6X5	T49.6X6
ophthalmic preparation	T49.5X1	T49.5X2	T49.5X3	T49.5X4	T49.5X5	T49.5X6
topical NEC	T49.0X1	T49.0X2	T49.0X3	T49.0X4	T49.0X5	T49.0X6
Neonal	T42.3X1	T42.3X2	T42.3X3	T42.3X4	T42.3X5	T42.3X6
Neoprontosil	T37.0X1	T37.0X2	T37.0X3	T37.0X4	T37.0X5	T37.0X6
Neosalvarsan	T37.8X1	T37.8X2	T37.8X3	T37.8X4	T37.8X5	T37.8X6
Neosilversalvarsan	T37.8X1	T37.8X2	T37.8X3	T37.8X4	T37.8X5	T37.8X6
Neosporin	T36.8X1	T36.8X2	T36.8X3	T36.8X4	T36.8X5	T36.8X6
ENT agent	T49.6X1	T49.6X2	T49.6X3	T49.6X4	T49.6X5	T49.6X6
opthalmic preparation	T49.5X1	T49.5X2	T49.5X3	T49.5X4	T49.5X5	T49.5X6
topical NEC	T49.0X1	T49.0X2	T49.0X3	T49.0X4	T49.0X5	T49.0X6
Neostigmine bromide	T44.0X1	T44.0X2	T44.0X3	T44.0X4	T44.0X5	T44.0X6

Substance	Poisoning, Accidental (unintentional)	Poisoning, Intentional self-harm	Poisoning, Assault	Poisoning, Undetermined	Adverse effect	Underdosing
Neraval	T42.3X1	T42.3X2	T42.3X3	T42.3X4	T42.3X5	T42.3X6
Neravan	T42.3X1	T42.3X2	T42.3X3	T42.3X4	T42.3X5	T42.3X6
Nerium oleander	T62.2X1	T62.2X2	T62.2X3	T62.2X4	—	—
Nerve gas, not in war	T59.91	T59.92	T59.93	T59.94	—	—
Nesacaine	T41.3X1	T41.3X2	T41.3X3	T41.3X4	T41.3X5	T41.3X6
infiltration (subcutaneous)	T41.3X1	T41.3X2	T41.3X3	T41.3X4	T41.3X5	T41.3X6
nerve block (peripheral) (plexus)	T41.3X1	T41.3X2	T41.3X3	T41.3X4	T41.3X5	T41.3X6
Netilmicin	T36.5X1	T36.5X2	T36.5X3	T36.5X4	T36.5X5	T36.5X6
Neurobarb	T42.3X1	T42.3X2	T42.3X3	T42.3X4	T42.3X5	T42.3X6
Neuroleptic drug NEC	T43.501	T43.502	T43.503	T43.504	T43.505	T43.506
Neuromuscular blocking drug	T48.1X1	T48.1X2	T48.1X3	T48.1X4	T48.1X5	T48.1X6
Neutral insulin injection	T38.3X1	T38.3X2	T38.3X3	T38.3X4	T38.3X5	T38.3X6
Neutral spirits	T51.0X1	T51.0X2	T51.0X3	T51.0X4	—	—
beverage	T51.0X1	T51.0X2	T51.0X3	T51.0X4	—	—
Niacin	T46.7X1	T46.7X2	T46.7X3	T46.7X4	T46.7X5	T46.7X6
Niacinamide	T45.2X1	T45.2X2	T45.2X3	T45.2X4	T45.2X5	T45.2X6
Nialamide	T43.1X1	T43.1X2	T43.1X3	T43.1X4	T43.1X5	T43.1X6
Niaprazine	T42.6X1	T42.6X2	T42.6X3	T42.6X4	T42.6X5	T42.6X6
Nicametate	T46.7X1	T46.7X2	T46.7X3	T46.7X4	T46.7X5	T46.7X6
Nicardipine	T46.1X1	T46.1X2	T46.1X3	T46.1X4	T46.1X5	T46.1X6
Nicergoline	T46.7X1	T46.7X2	T46.7X3	T46.7X4	T46.7X5	T46.7X6
Nickel (carbonyl) (tetra-carbonyl) (fumes) (vapor)	T56.891	T56.892	T56.893	T56.894	—	—
Nickelocene	T56.891	T56.892	T56.893	T56.894	—	—
Niclosamide	T37.4X1	T37.4X2	T37.4X3	T37.4X4	T37.4X5	T37.4X6
Nicofuranose	T46.7X1	T46.7X2	T46.7X3	T46.7X4	T46.7X5	T46.7X6
Nicomorphine	T40.2X1	T40.2X2	T40.2X3	T40.2X4	—	—
Nicorandil	T46.3X1	T46.3X2	T46.3X3	T46.3X4	T46.3X5	T46.3X6
Nicotiana (plant)	T62.2X1	T62.2X2	T62.2X3	T62.2X4	—	—
Nicotinamide	T45.2X1	T45.2X2	T45.2X3	T45.2X4	T45.2X5	T45.2X6
Nicotine (insecticide) (spray) (sulfate) NEC	T60.2X1	T60.2X2	T60.2X3	T60.2X4	—	—
from tobacco	T65.291	T65.292	T65.293	T65.294	—	—
cigarettes	T65.221	T65.222	T65.223	T65.224	—	—
not insecticide	T65.291	T65.292	T65.293	T65.294	—	—
Nicotinic acid	T46.7X1	T46.7X2	T46.7X3	T46.7X4	T46.7X5	T46.7X6
Nicotinyl alcohol	T46.7X1	T46.7X2	T46.7X3	T46.7X4	T46.7X5	T46.7X6
Nicoumalone	T45.511	T45.512	T45.513	T45.514	T45.515	T45.516
Nifedipine	T46.1X1	T46.1X2	T46.1X3	T46.1X4	T46.1X5	T46.1X6
Nifenazone	T39.2X1	T39.2X2	T39.2X3	T39.2X4	T39.2X5	T39.2X6
Nifuraldezone	T37.91	T37.92	T37.93	T37.94	T37.95	T37.96
Nifuratel	T37.8X1	T37.8X2	T37.8X3	T37.8X4	T37.8X5	T37.8X6
Nifurtimox	T37.3X1	T37.3X2	T37.3X3	T37.3X4	T37.3X5	T37.3X6
Nifurtoinol	T37.8X1	T37.8X2	T37.8X3	T37.8X4	T37.8X5	T37.8X6
Nightshade, deadly (solanum)—*see also* *Belladonna*	T62.2X1	T62.2X2	T62.2X3	T62.2X4	—	—
berry	T62.1X1	T62.1X2	T62.1X3	T62.1X4	—	—
Nikethamide	T50.7X1	T50.7X2	T50.7X3	T50.7X4	T50.7X5	T50.7X6
Nilstat	T36.7X1	T36.7X2	T36.7X3	T36.7X4	T36.7X5	T36.7X6
topical	T49.0X1	T49.0X2	T49.0X3	T49.0X4	T49.0X5	T49.0X6
Nilutamide	T38.6X1	T38.6X2	T38.6X3	T38.6X4	T38.6X5	T38.6X6
Nimesulide	T39.391	T39.392	T39.393	T39.394	T39.395	T39.396
Nimetazepam	T42.4X1	T42.4X2	T42.4X3	T42.4X4	T42.4X5	T42.4X6
Nimodipine	T46.1X1	T46.1X2	T46.1X3	T46.1X4	T46.1X5	T46.1X6
Nimorazole	T37.3X1	T37.3X2	T37.3X3	T37.3X4	T37.3X5	T37.3X6
Nimustine	T45.1X1	T45.1X2	T45.1X3	T45.1X4	T45.1X5	T45.1X6

Substance	Poisoning, Accidental (unintentional)	Poisoning, Intentional self-harm	Poisoning, Assault	Poisoning, Undetermined	Adverse effect	Underdosing
Niridazole	T37.4X1	T37.4X2	T37.4X3	T37.4X4	T37.4X5	T37.4X6
Nisentil	T40.2X1	T40.2X2	T40.2X3	T40.2X4	T40.2X5	T40.2X6
Nisoldipine	T46.1X1	T46.1X2	T46.1X3	T46.1X4	T46.1X5	T46.1X6
Nitramine	T65.3X1	T65.3X2	T65.3X3	T65.3X4	—	—
Nitrate, organic	T46.3X1	T46.3X2	T46.3X3	T46.3X4	T46.3X5	T46.3X6
Nitrazepam	T42.4X1	T42.4X2	T42.4X3	T42.4X4	T42.4X5	T42.4X6
Nitrefazole	T50.6X1	T50.6X2	T50.6X3	T50.6X4	T50.6X5	T50.6X6
Nitrendipine	T46.1X1	T46.1X2	T46.1X3	T46.1X4	T46.1X5	T46.1X6
Nitric						
acid (liquid)	T54.2X1	T54.2X2	T54.2X3	T54.2X4	—	—
vapor	T59.891	T59.892	T59.893	T59.894	—	—
oxide (gas)	T59.0X1	T59.0X2	T59.0X3	T59.0X4	—	—
Nitrimidazine	T37.3X1	T37.3X2	T37.3X3	T37.3X4	T37.3X5	T37.3X6
Nitrite, amyl (medicinal) (vapor)	T46.3X1	T46.3X2	T46.3X3	T46.3X4	T46.3X5	T46.3X6
Nitroaniline	T65.3X1	T65.3X2	T65.3X3	T65.3X4	—	—
vapor	T59.891	T59.892	T59.893	T59.894	—	—
Nitrobenzene, nitrobenzol	T65.3X1	T65.3X2	T65.3X3	T65.3X4	—	—
vapor	T65.3X1	T65.3X2	T65.3X3	T65.3X4	—	—
Nitrocellulose	T65.891	T65.892	T65.893	T65.894	—	—
lacquer	T65.891	T65.892	T65.893	T65.894	—	—
Nitrodiphenyl	T65.3X1	T65.3X2	T65.3X3	T65.3X4	—	—
Nitrofural	T49.0X1	T49.0X2	T49.0X3	T49.0X4	T49.0X5	T49.0X6
Nitrofurantoin	T37.8X1	T37.8X2	T37.8X3	T37.8X4	T37.8X5	T37.8X6
Nitrofurazone	T49.0X1	T49.0X2	T49.0X3	T49.0X4	T49.0X5	T49.0X6
Nitrogen	T59.0X1	T59.0X2	T59.0X3	T59.0X4	—	—
mustard	T45.1X1	T45.1X2	T45.1X3	T45.1X4	T45.1X5	T45.1X6
Nitroglycerin, nitro-glycerol (medicinal)	T46.3X1	T46.3X2	T46.3X3	T46.3X4	T46.3X5	T46.3X6
nonmedicinal	T65.5X1	T65.5X2	T65.5X3	T65.5X4	—	—
fumes	T65.5X1	T65.5X2	T65.5X3	T65.5X4	—	—
Nitroglycol	T52.3X1	T52.3X2	T52.3X3	T52.3X4	—	—
Nitrohydrochloric acid	T54.2X1	T54.2X2	T54.2X3	T54.2X4	—	—
Nitromersol	T49.0X1	T49.0X2	T49.0X3	T49.0X4	T49.0X5	T49.0X6
Nitronaphthalene	T65.891	T65.892	T65.893	T65.894	—	—
Nitrophenol	T54.0X1	T54.0X2	T54.0X3	T54.0X4	—	—
Nitropropane	T52.8X1	T52.8X2	T52.8X3	T52.8X4	—	—
Nitroprusside	T46.5X1	T46.5X2	T46.5X3	T46.5X4	T46.5X5	T46.5X6
Nitrosodimethylamine	T65.3X1	T65.3X2	T65.3X3	T65.3X4	—	—
Nitrothiazol	T37.4X1	T37.4X2	T37.4X3	T37.4X4	T37.4X5	T37.4X6
Nitrotoluene, nitrotoluol	T65.3X1	T65.3X2	T65.3X3	T65.3X4	—	—
vapor	T65.3X1	T65.3X2	T65.3X3	T65.3X4	—	—
Nitrous						
acid (liquid)	T54.2X1	T54.2X2	T54.2X3	T54.2X4	—	—
fumes	T59.891	T59.892	T59.893	T59.894	—	—
ether spirit	T46.3X1	T46.3X2	T46.3X3	T46.3X4	T46.3X5	T46.3X6
oxide	T41.0X1	T41.0X2	T41.0X3	T41.0X4	T41.0X5	T41.0X6
Nitroxoline	T37.8X1	T37.8X2	T37.8X3	T37.8X4	T37.8X5	T37.8X6
Nitrozone	T49.0X1	T49.0X2	T49.0X3	T49.0X4	T49.0X5	T49.0X6
Nizatidine	T47.0X1	T47.0X2	T47.0X3	T47.0X4	T47.0X5	T47.0X6
Nizofenone	T43.8X1	T43.8X2	T43.8X3	T43.8X4	T43.8X5	T43.8X6
Noctec	T42.6X1	T42.6X2	T42.6X3	T42.6X4	T42.6X5	T42.6X6
Noludar	T42.6X1	T42.6X2	T42.6X3	T42.6X4	T42.6X5	T42.6X6
Nomegestrol	T38.5X1	T38.5X2	T38.5X3	T38.5X4	T38.5X5	T38.5X6
Nomifensine	T43.291	T43.292	T43.293	T43.294	T43.295	T43.296
Nonoxinol	T49.8X1	T49.8X2	T49.8X3	T49.8X4	T49.8X5	T49.8X6
Nonylphenoxy (polyethoxy-ethanol)	T49.8X1	T49.8X2	T49.8X3	T49.8X4	T49.8X5	T49.8X6
Noptil	T42.3X1	T42.3X2	T42.3X3	T42.3X4	T42.3X5	T42.3X6
Noradrenaline	T44.4X1	T44.4X2	T44.4X3	T44.4X4	T44.4X5	T44.4X6

Substance	Poisoning, Accidental (unintentional)	Poisoning, Intentional self-harm	Poisoning, Assault	Poisoning, Undetermined	Adverse effect	Underdosing
Noramidopyrine	T39.2X1	T39.2X2	T39.2X3	T39.2X4	T39.2X5	T39.2X6
methanesulfonate sodium	T39.2X1	T39.2X2	T39.2X3	T39.2X4	T39.2X5	T39.2X6
Norbormide	T60.4X1	T60.4X2	T60.4X3	T60.4X4	—	—
Nordazepam	T42.4X1	T42.4X2	T42.4X3	T42.4X4	T42.4X5	T42.4X6
Norepinephrine	T44.4X1	T44.4X2	T44.4X3	T44.4X4	T44.4X5	T44.4X6
Norethandrolone	T38.7X1	T38.7X2	T38.7X3	T38.7X4	T38.7X5	T38.7X6
Norethindrone	T38.4X1	T38.4X2	T38.4X3	T38.4X4	T38.4X5	T38.4X6
Norethisterone (acetate) (enantate)	T38.4X1	T38.4X2	T38.4X3	T38.4X4	T38.4X5	T38.4X6
with ethinylestradiol	T38.5X1	T38.5X2	T38.5X3	T38.5X4	T38.5X5	T38.5X6
Noretynodrel	T38.5X1	T38.5X2	T38.5X3	T38.5X4	T38.5X5	T38.5X6
Norfenefrine	T44.4X1	T44.4X2	T44.4X3	T44.4X4	T44.4X5	T44.4X6
Norfloxacin	T36.8X1	T36.8X2	T36.8X3	T36.8X4	T36.8X5	T36.8X6
Norgestrel	T38.4X1	T38.4X2	T38.4X3	T38.4X4	T38.4X5	T38.4X6
Norgestrienone	T38.4X1	T38.4X2	T38.4X3	T38.4X4	T38.4X5	T38.4X6
Norlestrin	T38.4X1	T38.4X2	T38.4X3	T38.4X4	T38.4X5	T38.4X6
Norlutin	T38.4X1	T38.4X2	T38.4X3	T38.4X4	T38.4X5	T38.4X6
Normal serum albumin (human), salt-poor	T45.8X1	T45.8X2	T45.8X3	T45.8X4	T45.8X5	T45.8X6
Normethandrone	T38.5X1	T38.5X2	T38.5X3	T38.5X4	T38.5X5	T38.5X6
Normison—see Benzodiazepines						
Normorphine	T40.2X1	T40.2X2	T40.2X3	T40.2X4	—	—
Norpseudoephedrine	T50.5X1	T50.5X2	T50.5X3	T50.5X4	T50.5X5	T50.5X6
Nortestosterone (furanpropionate)	T38.7X1	T38.7X2	T38.7X3	T38.7X4	T38.7X5	T38.7X6
Nortriptyline	T43.011	T43.012	T43.013	T43.014	T43.015	T43.016
Noscapine	T48.3X1	T48.3X2	T48.3X3	T48.3X4	T48.3X5	T48.3X6
Nose preparations	T49.6X1	T49.6X2	T49.6X3	T49.6X4	T49.6X5	T49.6X6
Novobiocin	T36.5X1	T36.5X2	T36.5X3	T36.5X4	T36.5X5	T36.5X6
Novocain (infiltration) (topical)	T41.3X1	T41.3X2	T41.3X3	T41.3X4	T41.3X5	T41.3X6
nerve block (peripheral) (plexus)	T41.3X1	T41.3X2	T41.3X3	T41.3X4	T41.3X5	T41.3X6
spinal	T41.3X1	T41.3X2	T41.3X3	T41.3X4	T41.3X5	T41.3X6
Noxious foodstuff	T62.91	T62.92	T62.93	T62.94	—	—
specified NEC	T62.8X1	T62.8X2	T62.8X3	T62.8X4	—	—
Noxiptiline	T43.011	T43.012	T43.013	T43.014	T43.015	T43.016
Noxytiolin	T49.0X1	T49.0X2	T49.0X3	T49.0X4	T49.0X5	T49.0X6
NPH Iletin (insulin)	T38.3X1	T38.3X2	T38.3X3	T38.3X4	T38.3X5	T38.3X6
Numorphan	T40.2X1	T40.2X2	T40.2X3	T40.2X4	T40.2X5	T40.2X6
Nunol	T42.3X1	T42.3X2	T42.3X3	T42.3X4	T42.3X5	T42.3X6
Nupercaine (spinal anesthetic)	T41.3X1	T41.3X2	T41.3X3	T41.3X4	T41.3X5	T41.3X6
topical (surface)	T41.3X1	T41.3X2	T41.3X3	T41.3X4	T41.3X5	T41.3X6
Nutmeg oil (liniment)	T49.3X1	T49.3X2	T49.3X3	T49.3X4	T49.3X5	T49.3X6
Nutritional supplement	T50.901	T50.902	T50.903	T50.904	T50.905	T50.906
Nux vomica	T65.1X1	T65.1X2	T65.1X3	T65.1X4	—	—
Nydrazid	T37.1X1	T37.1X2	T37.1X3	T37.1X4	T37.1X5	T37.1X6
Nylidrin	T46.7X1	T46.7X2	T46.7X3	T46.7X4	T46.7X5	T46.7X6
Nystatin	T36.7X1	T36.7X2	T36.7X3	T36.7X4	T36.7X5	T36.7X6
topical	T49.0X1	T49.0X2	T49.0X3	T49.0X4	T49.0X5	T49.0X6
Nytol	T45.0X1	T45.0X2	T45.0X3	T45.0X4	T45.0X5	T45.0X6
O						
Obidoxime chloride	T50.6X1	T50.6X2	T50.6X3	T50.6X4	T50.6X5	T50.6X6
Octafonium (chloride)	T49.3X1	T49.3X2	T49.3X3	T49.3X4	T49.3X5	T49.3X6
Octamethyl pyrophosphoramide	T60.0X1	T60.0X2	T60.0X3	T60.0X4	—	—
Octanoin	T50.991	T50.992	T50.993	T50.994	T50.995	T50.996

Substance	Poisoning, Accidental (unintentional)	Poisoning, Intentional self-harm	Poisoning, Assault	Poisoning, Undetermined	Adverse effect	Underdosing
Octatropine methyl-bromide	T44.3X1	T44.3X2	T44.3X3	T44.3X4	T44.3X5	T44.3X6
Octotiamine	T45.2X1	T45.2X2	T45.2X3	T45.2X4	T45.2X5	T45.2X6
Octoxinol (9)	T49.8X1	T49.8X2	T49.8X3	T49.8X4	T49.8X5	T49.8X6
Octreotide	T38.991	T38.992	T38.993	T38.994	T38.995	T38.996
Octyl nitrite	T46.3X1	T46.3X2	T46.3X3	T46.3X4	T46.3X5	T46.3X6
Oestradiol	T38.5X1	T38.5X2	T38.5X3	T38.5X4	T38.5X5	T38.5X6
Oestriol	T38.5X1	T38.5X2	T38.5X3	T38.5X4	T38.5X5	T38.5X6
Oestrogen	T38.5X1	T38.5X2	T38.5X3	T38.5X4	T38.5X5	T38.5X6
Oestrone	T38.5X1	T38.5X2	T38.5X3	T38.5X4	T38.5X5	T38.5X6
Ofloxacin	T36.8X1	T36.8X2	T36.8X3	T36.8X4	T36.8X5	T36.8X6
Oil (of)	T65.891	T65.892	T65.893	T65.894	—	—
bitter almond	T62.8X1	T62.8X2	T62.8X3	T62.8X4	—	—
cloves	T49.7X1	T49.7X2	T49.7X3	T49.7X4	T49.7X5	T49.7X6
colors	T65.6X1	T65.6X2	T65.6X3	T65.6X4	—	—
fumes	T59.891	T59.892	T59.893	T59.894	—	—
lubricating	T52.0X1	T52.0X2	T52.0X3	T52.0X4	—	—
Niobe	T52.8X1	T52.8X2	T52.8X3	T52.8X4	—	—
vitriol (liquid)	T54.2X1	T54.2X2	T54.2X3	T54.2X4	—	—
fumes	T54.2X1	T54.2X2	T54.2X3	T54.2X4	—	—
wintergreen (bitter) NEC	T49.3X1	T49.3X2	T49.3X3	T49.3X4	T49.3X5	T49.3X6
Oily preparation (for skin)	T49.3X1	T49.3X2	T49.3X3	T49.3X4	T49.3X5	T49.3X6
Ointment NEC	T49.3X1	T49.3X2	T49.3X3	T49.3X4	T49.3X5	T49.3X6
Olanzapine	T43.591	T43.592	T43.593	T43.594	T43.595	T43.596
Oleander	T62.2X1	T62.2X2	T62.2X3	T62.2X4	—	—
Oleandomycin	T36.3X1	T36.3X2	T36.3X3	T36.3X4	T36.3X5	T36.3X6
Oleandrin	T46.0X1	T46.0X2	T46.0X3	T46.0X4	T46.0X5	T46.0X6
Oleic acid	T46.6X1	T46.6X2	T46.6X3	T46.6X4	T46.6X5	T46.6X6
Oleovitamin A	T45.2X1	T45.2X2	T45.2X3	T45.2X4	T45.2X5	T45.2X6
Oleum ricini	T47.2X1	T47.2X2	T47.2X3	T47.2X4	T47.2X5	T47.2X6
Olive oil (medicinal) NEC	T47.4X1	T47.4X2	T47.4X3	T47.4X4	T47.4X5	T47.4X6
Olivomycin	T45.1X1	T45.1X2	T45.1X3	T45.1X4	T45.1X5	T45.1X6
Olsalazine	T47.8X1	T47.8X2	T47.8X3	T47.8X4	T47.8X5	T47.8X6
Omeprazole	T47.1X1	T47.1X2	T47.1X3	T47.1X4	T47.1X5	T47.1X6
OMPA	T60.0X1	T60.0X2	T60.0X3	T60.0X4	—	—
Oncovin	T45.1X1	T45.1X2	T45.1X3	T45.1X4	T45.1X5	T45.1X6
Ondansetron	T45.0X1	T45.0X2	T45.0X3	T45.0X4	T45.0X5	T45.0X6
Ophthaine	T41.3X1	T41.3X2	T41.3X3	T41.3X4	T41.3X5	T41.3X6
Ophthetic	T41.3X1	T41.3X2	T41.3X3	T41.3X4	T41.3X5	T41.3X6
Opiate NEC	T40.601	T40.602	T40.603	T40.604	T40.605	T40.606
antagonists	T50.7X1	T50.7X2	T50.7X3	T50.7X4	T50.7X5	T50.7X6
Opioid NEC	T40.2X1	T40.2X2	T40.2X3	T40.2X4	T40.2X5	T40.2X6
Opipramol	T43.011	T43.012	T43.013	T43.014	T43.015	T43.016
Opium alkaloids (total)	T40.0X1	T40.0X2	T40.0X3	T40.0X4	T40.0X5	T40.0X6
standardized powdered	T40.0X1	T40.0X2	T40.0X3	T40.0X4	T40.0X5	T40.0X6
tincture (camphorated)	T40.0X1	T40.0X2	T40.0X3	T40.0X4	T40.0X5	T40.0X6
Oracon	T38.4X1	T38.4X2	T38.4X3	T38.4X4	T38.4X5	T38.4X6
Oragrafin	T50.8X1	T50.8X2	T50.8X3	T50.8X4	T50.8X5	T50.8X6
Oral contraceptives	T38.4X1	T38.4X2	T38.4X3	T38.4X4	T38.4X5	T38.4X6
Oral rehydration salts	T50.3X1	T50.3X2	T50.3X3	T50.3X4	T50.3X5	T50.3X6
Orazamide	T50.991	T50.992	T50.993	T50.994	T50.995	T50.996
Orciprenaline	T48.291	T48.292	T48.293	T48.294	T48.295	T48.296
Organidin	T48.4X1	T48.4X2	T48.4X3	T48.4X4	T48.4X5	T48.4X6
Organonitrate NEC	T46.3X1	T46.3X2	T46.3X3	T46.3X4	T46.3X5	T46.3X6
Organophosphates	T60.0X1	T60.0X2	T60.0X3	T60.0X4	—	—
Orimune	T50.B91	T50.B92	T50.B93	T50.B94	T50.B95	T50.B96
Orinase	T38.3X1	T38.3X2	T38.3X3	T38.3X4	T38.3X5	T38.3X6
Ormeloxifene	T38.6X1	T38.6X2	T38.6X3	T38.6X4	T38.6X5	T38.6X6
Ornidazole	T37.3X1	T37.3X2	T37.3X3	T37.3X4	T37.3X5	T37.3X6
Ornithine aspartate	T50.991	T50.992	T50.993	T50.994	T50.995	T50.996

Substance	Poisoning, Accidental (unintentional)	Poisoning, Intentional self-harm	Poisoning, Assault	Poisoning, Undetermined	Adverse effect	Underdosing
Ornoprostil	T47.1X1	T47.1X2	T47.1X3	T47.1X4	T47.1X5	T47.1X6
Orphenadrine (hydrochloride)	T42.8X1	T42.8X2	T42.8X3	T42.8X4	T42.8X5	T42.8X6
Ortal (sodium)	T42.3X1	T42.3X2	T42.3X3	T42.3X4	T42.3X5	T42.3X6
Orthoboric acid	T49.0X1	T49.0X2	T49.0X3	T49.0X4	T49.0X5	T49.0X6
ENT agent	T49.6X1	T49.6X2	T49.6X3	T49.6X4	T49.6X5	T49.6X6
ophthalmic preparation	T49.5X1	T49.5X2	T49.5X3	T49.5X4	T49.5X5	T49.5X6
Orthocaine	T41.3X1	T41.3X2	T41.3X3	T41.3X4	T41.3X5	T41.3X6
Orthodichlorobenzene	T53.7X1	T53.7X2	T53.7X3	T53.7X4	—	—
Ortho-Novum	T38.4X1	T38.4X2	T38.4X3	T38.4X4	T38.4X5	T38.4X6
Orthotolidine (reagent)	T54.2X1	T54.2X2	T54.2X3	T54.2X4	—	—
Osmic acid (liquid)	T54.2X1	T54.2X2	T54.2X3	T54.2X4	—	—
fumes	T54.2X1	T54.2X2	T54.2X3	T54.2X4	—	—
Osmotic diuretics	T50.2X1	T50.2X2	T50.2X3	T50.2X4	T50.2X5	T50.2X6
Otilonium bromide	T44.3X1	T44.3X2	T44.3X3	T44.3X4	T44.3X5	T44.3X6
Otorhinolaryngological drug NEC	T49.6X1	T49.6X2	T49.6X3	T49.6X4	T49.6X5	T49.6X6
Ouabain (e)	T46.0X1	T46.0X2	T46.0X3	T46.0X4	T46.0X5	T46.0X6
Ovarian						
hormone	T38.5X1	T38.5X2	T38.5X3	T38.5X4	T38.5X5	T38.5X6
stimulant	T38.5X1	T38.5X2	T38.5X3	T38.5X4	T38.5X5	T38.5X6
Ovral	T38.4X1	T38.4X2	T38.4X3	T38.4X4	T38.4X5	T38.4X6
Ovulen	T38.4X1	T38.4X2	T38.4X3	T38.4X4	T38.4X5	T38.4X6
Oxacillin	T36.0X1	T36.0X2	T36.0X3	T36.0X4	T36.0X5	T36.0X6
Oxalic acid	T54.2X1	T54.2X2	T54.2X3	T54.2X4	—	—
ammonium salt	T50.991	T50.992	T50.993	T50.994	T50.995	T50.996
Oxamniquine	T37.4X1	T37.4X2	T37.4X3	T37.4X4	T37.4X5	T37.4X6
Oxanamide	T43.591	T43.592	T43.593	T43.594	T43.595	T43.596
Oxandrolone	T38.7X1	T38.7X2	T38.7X3	T38.7X4	T38.7X5	T38.7X6
Oxantel	T37.4X1	T37.4X2	T37.4X3	T37.4X4	T37.4X5	T37.4X6
Oxapium iodide	T44.3X1	T44.3X2	T44.3X3	T44.3X4	T44.3X5	T44.3X6
Oxaprotiline	T43.021	T43.022	T43.023	T43.024	T43.025	T43.026
Oxaprozin	T39.311	T39.312	T39.313	T39.314	T39.315	T39.316
Oxatomide	T45.0X1	T45.0X2	T45.0X3	T45.0X4	T45.0X5	T45.0X6
Oxazepam	T42.4X1	T42.4X2	T42.4X3	T42.4X4	T42.4X5	T42.4X6
Oxazimedrine	T50.5X1	T50.5X2	T50.5X3	T50.5X4	T50.5X5	T50.5X6
Oxazolam	T42.4X1	T42.4X2	T42.4X3	T42.4X4	T42.4X5	T42.4X6
Oxazolidine derivatives	T42.2X1	T42.2X2	T42.2X3	T42.2X4	T42.2X5	T42.2X6
Oxazolidinedione (derivative)	T42.2X1	T42.2X2	T42.2X3	T42.2X4	T42.2X5	T42.2X6
Ox bile extract	T47.5X1	T47.5X2	T47.5X3	T47.5X4	T47.5X5	T47.5X6
Oxcarbazepine	T42.1X1	T42.1X2	T42.1X3	T42.1X4	T42.1X5	T42.1X6
Oxedrine	T44.4X1	T44.4X2	T44.4X3	T44.4X4	T44.4X5	T44.4X6
Oxeladin (citrate)	T48.3X1	T48.3X2	T48.3X3	T48.3X4	T48.3X5	T48.3X6
Oxendolone	T38.5X1	T38.5X2	T38.5X3	T38.5X4	T38.5X5	T38.5X6
Oxetacaine	T41.3X1	T41.3X2	T41.3X3	T41.3X4	T41.3X5	T41.3X6
Oxethazine	T41.3X1	T41.3X2	T41.3X3	T41.3X4	T41.3X5	T41.3X6
Oxetorone	T39.8X1	T39.8X2	T39.8X3	T39.8X4	T39.8X5	T39.8X6
Oxiconazole	T49.0X1	T49.0X2	T49.0X3	T49.0X4	T49.0X5	T49.0X6
Oxidizing agent NEC	T54.91	T54.92	T54.93	T54.94	—	—
Oxipurinol	T50.4X1	T50.4X2	T50.4X3	T50.4X4	T50.4X5	T50.4X6
Oxitriptan	T43.291	T43.292	T43.293	T43.294	T43.295	T43.296
Oxitropium bromide	T48.6X1	T48.6X2	T48.6X3	T48.6X4	T48.6X5	T48.6X6
Oxodipine	T46.1X1	T46.1X2	T46.1X3	T46.1X4	T46.1X5	T46.1X6
Oxolamine	T48.3X1	T48.3X2	T48.3X3	T48.3X4	T48.3X5	T48.3X6
Oxolinic acid	T37.8X1	T37.8X2	T37.8X3	T37.8X4	T37.8X5	T37.8X6
Oxomemazine	T43.3X1	T43.3X2	T43.3X3	T43.3X4	T43.3X5	T43.3X6
Oxophenarsine	T37.3X1	T37.3X2	T37.3X3	T37.3X4	T37.3X5	T37.3X6
Oxprenolol	T44.7X1	T44.7X2	T44.7X3	T44.7X4	T44.7X5	T44.7X6
Oxsoralen	T49.3X1	T49.3X2	T49.3X3	T49.3X4	T49.3X5	T49.3X6

Substance	Poisoning, Accidental (unintentional)	Poisoning, Intentional self-harm	Poisoning, Assault	Poisoning, Undetermined	Adverse effect	Underdosing
Oxtriphylline	T48.6X1	T48.6X2	T48.6X3	T48.6X4	T48.6X5	T48.6X6
Oxybate sodium	T41.291	T41.292	T41.293	T41.294	T41.295	T41.296
Oxybuprocaine	T41.3X1	T41.3X2	T41.3X3	T41.3X4	T41.3X5	T41.3X6
Oxybutynin	T44.3X1	T44.3X2	T44.3X3	T44.3X4	T44.3X5	T44.3X6
Oxychlorosene	T49.0X1	T49.0X2	T49.0X3	T49.0X4	T49.0X5	T49.0X6
Oxycodone	T40.2X1	T40.2X2	T40.2X3	T40.2X4	T40.2X5	T40.2X6
Oxyfedrine	T46.3X1	T46.3X2	T46.3X3	T46.3X4	T46.3X5	T46.3X6
Oxygen	T41.5X1	T41.5X2	T41.5X3	T41.5X4	T41.5X5	T41.5X6
Oxylone	T49.0X1	T49.0X2	T49.0X3	T49.0X4	T49.0X5	T49.0X6
ophthalmic preparation	T49.5X1	T49.5X2	T49.5X3	T49.5X4	T49.5X5	T49.5X6
Oxymesterone	T38.7X1	T38.7X2	T38.7X3	T38.7X4	T38.7X5	T38.7X6
Oxymetazoline	T48.5X1	T48.5X2	T48.5X3	T48.5X4	T48.5X5	T48.5X6
Oxymetholone	T38.7X1	T38.7X2	T38.7X3	T38.7X4	T38.7X5	T38.7X6
Oxymorphone	T40.2X1	T40.2X2	T40.2X3	T40.2X4	T40.2X5	T40.2X6
Oxypertine	T43.591	T43.592	T43.593	T43.594	T43.595	T43.596
Oxyphenbutazone	T39.2X1	T39.2X2	T39.2X3	T39.2X4	T39.2X5	T39.2X6
Oxyphencyclimine	T44.3X1	T44.3X2	T44.3X3	T44.3X4	T44.3X5	T44.3X6
Oxyphenisatine	T47.2X1	T47.2X2	T47.2X3	T47.2X4	T47.2X5	T47.2X6
Oxyphenonium bromide	T44.3X1	T44.3X2	T44.3X3	T44.3X4	T44.3X5	T44.3X6
Oxypolygelatin	T45.8X1	T45.8X2	T45.8X3	T45.8X4	T45.8X5	T45.8X6
Oxyquinoline (derivatives)	T37.8X1	T37.8X2	T37.8X3	T37.8X4	T37.8X5	T37.8X6
Oxytetracycline	T36.4X1	T36.4X2	T36.4X3	T36.4X4	T36.4X5	T36.4X6
Oxytocic drug NEC	T48.0X1	T48.0X2	T48.0X3	T48.0X4	T48.0X5	T48.0X6
Oxytocin (synthetic)	T48.0X1	T48.0X2	T48.0X3	T48.0X4	T48.0X5	T48.0X6
Ozone	T59.891	T59.892	T59.893	T59.894	—	—
P						
PABA	T49.3X1	T49.3X2	T49.3X3	T49.3X4	T49.3X5	T49.3X6
Packed red cells	T45.8X1	T45.8X2	T45.8X3	T45.8X4	T45.8X5	T45.8X6
Padimate	T49.3X1	T49.3X2	T49.3X3	T49.3X4	T49.3X5	T49.3X6
Paint NEC	T65.6X1	T65.6X2	T65.6X3	T65.6X4	—	—
cleaner	T52.91	T52.92	T52.93	T52.94	—	—
fumes NEC	T59.891	T59.892	T59.893	T59.894	—	—
lead (fumes)	T56.0X1	T56.0X2	T56.0X3	T56.0X4	—	—
solvent NEC	T52.8X1	T52.8X2	T52.8X3	T52.8X4	—	—
stripper	T52.8X1	T52.8X2	T52.8X3	T52.8X4	—	—
Palfium	T40.2X1	T40.2X2	T40.2X3	T40.2X4	—	—
Palm kernel oil	T50.991	T50.992	T50.993	T50.994	T50.995	T50.996
Paludrine	T37.2X1	T37.2X2	T37.2X3	T37.2X4	T37.2X5	T37.2X6
PAM (pralidoxime)	T50.6X1	T50.6X2	T50.6X3	T50.6X4	T50.6X5	T50.6X6
Pamaquine (naphthoute)	T37.2X1	T37.2X2	T37.2X3	T37.2X4	T37.2X5	T37.2X6
Panadol	T39.1X1	T39.1X2	T39.1X3	T39.1X4	T39.1X5	T39.1X6
Pancreatic						
digestive secretion stimulant	T47.8X1	T47.8X2	T47.8X3	T47.8X4	T47.8X5	T47.8X6
dornase	T45.3X1	T45.3X2	T45.3X3	T45.3X4	T45.3X5	T45.3X6
Pancreatin	T47.5X1	T47.5X2	T47.5X3	T47.5X4	T47.5X5	T47.5X6
Pancrelipase	T47.5X1	T47.5X2	T47.5X3	T47.5X4	T47.5X5	T47.5X6
Pancuronium (bromide)	T48.1X1	T48.1X2	T48.1X3	T48.1X4	T48.1X5	T48.1X6
Pangamic acid	T45.2X1	T45.2X2	T45.2X3	T45.2X4	T45.2X5	T45.2X6
Panthenol	T45.2X1	T45.2X2	T45.2X3	T45.2X4	T45.2X5	T45.2X6
topical	T49.8X1	T49.8X2	T49.8X3	T49.8X4	T49.8X5	T49.8X6
Pantopon	T40.0X1	T40.0X2	T40.0X3	T40.0X4	T40.0X5	T40.0X6
Pantothenic acid	T45.2X1	T45.2X2	T45.2X3	T45.2X4	T45.2X5	T45.2X6
Panwarfin	T45.511	T45.512	T45.513	T45.514	T45.515	T45.516
Papain	T47.5X1	T47.5X2	T47.5X3	T47.5X4	T47.5X5	T47.5X6
digestant	T47.5X1	T47.5X2	T47.5X3	T47.5X4	T47.5X5	T47.5X6
Papaveretum	T40.0X1	T40.0X2	T40.0X3	T40.0X4	T40.0X5	T40.0X6
Papaverine	T44.3X1	T44.3X2	T44.3X3	T44.3X4	T44.3X5	T44.3X6
Para-acetamidophenol	T39.1X1	T39.1X2	T39.1X3	T39.1X4	T39.1X5	T39.1X6

Substance	Poisoning, Accidental (unintentional)	Poisoning, Intentional self-harm	Poisoning, Assault	Poisoning, Undetermined	Adverse effect	Underdosing
Para-aminobenzoic acid	T49.3X1	T49.3X2	T49.3X3	T49.3X4	T49.3X5	T49.3X6
Para-aminophenol derivatives	T39.1X1	T39.1X2	T39.1X3	T39.1X4	T39.1X5	T39.1X6
Para-aminosalicylic acid	T37.1X1	T37.1X2	T37.1X3	T37.1X4	T37.1X5	T37.1X6
Paracetaldehyde	T42.6X1	T42.6X2	T42.6X3	T42.6X4	T42.6X5	T42.6X6
Paracetamol	T39.1X1	T39.1X2	T39.1X3	T39.1X4	T39.1X5	T39.1X6
Parachlorophenol (camphorated)	T49.0X1	T49.0X2	T49.0X3	T49.0X4	T49.0X5	T49.0X6
Paracodin	T40.2X1	T40.2X2	T40.2X3	T40.2X4	T40.2X5	T40.2X6
Paradione	T42.2X1	T42.2X2	T42.2X3	T42.2X4	T42.2X5	T42.2X6
Paraffin (s) (wax)	T52.0X1	T52.0X2	T52.0X3	T52.0X4	—	—
liquid (medicinal)	T47.4X1	T47.4X2	T47.4X3	T47.4X4	T47.4X5	T47.4X6
nonmedicinal	T52.0X1	T52.0X2	T52.0X3	T52.0X4	—	—
Paraformaldehyde	T60.3X1	T60.3X2	T60.3X3	T60.3X4	—	—
Paraldehyde	T42.6X1	T42.6X2	T42.6X3	T42.6X4	T42.6X5	T42.6X6
Paramethadione	T42.2X1	T42.2X2	T42.2X3	T42.2X4	T42.2X5	T42.2X6
Paramethasone	T38.0X1	T38.0X2	T38.0X3	T38.0X4	T38.0X5	T38.0X6
acetate	T49.0X1	T49.0X2	T49.0X3	T49.0X4	T49.0X5	T49.0X6
Paraoxon	T60.0X1	T60.0X2	T60.0X3	T60.0X4	—	—
Paraquat	T60.3X1	T60.3X2	T60.3X3	T60.3X4	—	—
Parasympatholytic NEC	T44.3X1	T44.3X2	T44.3X3	T44.3X4	T44.3X5	T44.3X6
Parasympathomimetic drug NEC	T44.1X1	T44.1X2	T44.1X3	T44.1X4	T44.1X5	T44.1X6
Parathion	T60.0X1	T60.0X2	T60.0X3	T60.0X4	—	—
Parathormone	T50.991	T50.992	T50.993	T50.994	T50.995	T50.996
Parathyroid extract	T50.991	T50.992	T50.993	T50.994	T50.995	T50.996
Paratyphoid vaccine	T50.A91	T50.A92	T50.A93	T50.A94	T50.A95	T50.A96
Paredrine	T44.4X1	T44.4X2	T44.4X3	T44.4X4	T44.4X5	T44.4X6
Paregoric	T40.0X1	T40.0X2	T40.0X3	T40.0X4	T40.0X5	T40.0X6
Pargyline	T46.5X1	T46.5X2	T46.5X3	T46.5X4	T46.5X5	T46.5X6
Paris green	T57.0X1	T57.0X2	T57.0X3	T57.0X4	—	—
insecticide	T57.0X1	T57.0X2	T57.0X3	T57.0X4	—	—
Parnate	T43.1X1	T43.1X2	T43.1X3	T43.1X4	T43.1X5	T43.1X6
Paromomycin	T36.5X1	T36.5X2	T36.5X3	T36.5X4	T36.5X5	T36.5X6
Paroxypropione	T45.1X1	T45.1X2	T45.1X3	T45.1X4	T45.1X5	T45.1X6
Parzone	T40.2X1	T40.2X2	T40.2X3	T40.2X4	T40.2X5	T40.2X6
PAS	T37.1X1	T37.1X2	T37.1X3	T37.1X4	T37.1X5	T37.1X6
Pasiniazid	T37.1X1	T37.1X2	T37.1X3	T37.1X4	T37.1X5	T37.1X6
PBB (polybrominated biphenyls)	T65.891	T65.892	T65.893	T65.894	—	—
PCB	T65.891	T65.892	T65.893	T65.894	—	—
PCP						
meaning pentachlorophenol	T60.1X1	T60.1X2	T60.1X3	T60.1X4	—	—
fungicide	T60.3X1	T60.3X2	T60.3X3	T60.3X4	—	—
herbicide	T60.3X1	T60.3X2	T60.3X3	T60.3X4	—	—
insecticide	T60.1X1	T60.1X2	T60.1X3	T60.1X4	—	—
meaning phencyclidine	T40.991	T40.992	T40.993	T40.994	—	—
Peach kernel oil (emulsion)	T47.4X1	T47.4X2	T47.4X3	T47.4X4	T47.4X5	T47.4X6
Peanut oil (emulsion) NEC	T47.4X1	T47.4X2	T47.4X3	T47.4X4	T47.4X5	T47.4X6
topical	T49.3X1	T49.3X2	T49.3X3	T49.3X4	T49.3X5	T49.3X6
Pearly Gates (morning glory seeds)	T40.991	T40.992	T40.993	T40.994	—	—
Pecazine	T43.3X1	T43.3X2	T43.3X3	T43.3X4	T43.3X5	T43.3X6
Pectin	T47.6X1	T47.6X2	T47.6X3	T47.6X4	T47.6X5	T47.6X6
Pefloxacin	T37.8X1	T37.8X2	T37.8X3	T37.8X4	T37.8X5	T37.8X6
Pegademase, bovine	T50.Z91	T50.Z92	T50.Z93	T50.Z94	T50.Z95	T50.Z96
Pelletierine tannate	T37.4X1	T37.4X2	T37.4X3	T37.4X4	T37.4X5	T37.4X6
Pemirolast (potassium)	T48.6X1	T48.6X2	T48.6X3	T48.6X4	T48.6X5	T48.6X6

Substance	Poisoning, Accidental (unintentional)	Poisoning, Intentional self-harm	Poisoning, Assault	Poisoning, Undetermined	Adverse effect	Underdosing
Pemoline	T50.7X1	T50.7X2	T50.7X3	T50.7X4	T50.7X5	T50.7X6
Pempidine	T44.2X1	T44.2X2	T44.2X3	T44.2X4	T44.2X5	T44.2X6
Penamecillin	T36.0X1	T36.0X2	T36.0X3	T36.0X4	T36.0X5	T36.0X6
Penbutolol	T44.7X1	T44.7X2	T44.7X3	T44.7X4	T44.7X5	T44.7X6
Penethamate	T36.0X1	T36.0X2	T36.0X3	T36.0X4	T36.0X5	T36.0X6
Penfluridol	T43.591	T43.592	T43.593	T43.594	T43.595	T43.596
Penflutizide	T50.2X1	T50.2X2	T50.2X3	T50.2X4	T50.2X5	T50.2X6
Pengitoxin	T46.0X1	T46.0X2	T46.0X3	T46.0X4	T46.0X5	T46.0X6
Penicillamine	T50.6X1	T50.6X2	T50.6X3	T50.6X4	T50.6X5	T50.6X6
Penicillin (any)	T36.0X1	T36.0X2	T36.0X3	T36.0X4	T36.0X5	T36.0X6
Penicillinase	T45.3X1	T45.3X2	T45.3X3	T45.3X4	T45.3X5	T45.3X6
Penicilloyl polylysine	T50.8X1	T50.8X2	T50.8X3	T50.8X4	T50.8X5	T50.8X6
Penimepicycline	T36.4X1	T36.4X2	T36.4X3	T36.4X4	T36.4X5	T36.4X6
Pentachloroethane	T53.6X1	T53.6X2	T53.6X3	T53.6X4	—	—
Pentachloronaphthalene	T53.7X1	T53.7X2	T53.7X3	T53.7X4	—	—
Pentachlorophenol (pesticide)	T60.1X1	T60.1X2	T60.1X3	T60.1X4	—	—
fungicide	T60.3X1	T60.3X2	T60.3X3	T60.3X4	—	—
herbicide	T60.3X1	T60.3X2	T60.3X3	T60.3X4	—	—
insecticide	T60.1X1	T60.1X2	T60.1X3	T60.1X4	—	—
Pentaerythritol	T46.3X1	T46.3X2	T46.3X3	T46.3X4	T46.3X5	T46.3X6
chloral	T42.6X1	T42.6X2	T42.6X3	T42.6X4	T42.6X5	T42.6X6
tetranitrate NEC	T46.3X1	T46.3X2	T46.3X3	T46.3X4	T46.3X5	T46.3X6
Pentaerythrityl tetranitrate	T46.3X1	T46.3X2	T46.3X3	T46.3X4	T46.3X5	T46.3X6
Pentagastrin	T50.8X1	T50.8X2	T50.8X3	T50.8X4	T50.8X5	T50.8X6
Pentalin	T53.6X1	T53.6X2	T53.6X3	T53.6X4	—	—
Pentamethonium bromide	T44.2X1	T44.2X2	T44.2X3	T44.2X4	T44.2X5	T44.2X6
Pentamidine	T37.3X1	T37.3X2	T37.3X3	T37.3X4	T37.3X5	T37.3X6
Pentanol	T51.3X1	T51.3X2	T51.3X3	T51.3X4	—	—
Pentapyrrolinium (bitartrate)	T44.2X1	T44.2X2	T44.2X3	T44.2X4	T44.2X5	T44.2X6
Pentaquine	T37.2X1	T37.2X2	T37.2X3	T37.2X4	T37.2X5	T37.2X6
Pentazocine	T40.4X1	T40.4X2	T40.4X3	T40.4X4	T40.4X5	T40.4X6
Pentetrazole	T50.7X1	T50.7X2	T50.7X3	T50.7X4	T50.7X5	T50.7X6
Penthienate bromide	T44.3X1	T44.3X2	T44.3X3	T44.3X4	T44.3X5	T44.3X6
Pentifylline	T46.7X1	T46.7X2	T46.7X3	T46.7X4	T46.7X5	T46.7X6
Pentobarbital	T42.3X1	T42.3X2	T42.3X3	T42.3X4	T42.3X5	T42.3X6
sodium	T42.3X1	T42.3X2	T42.3X3	T42.3X4	T42.3X5	T42.3X6
Pentobarbitone	T42.3X1	T42.3X2	T42.3X3	T42.3X4	T42.3X5	T42.3X6
Pentolonium tartrate	T44.2X1	T44.2X2	T44.2X3	T44.2X4	T44.2X5	T44.2X6
Pentosan polysulfate (sodium)	T39.8X1	T39.8X2	T39.8X3	T39.8X4	T39.8X5	T39.8X6
Pentostatin	T45.1X1	T45.1X2	T45.1X3	T45.1X4	T45.1X5	T45.1X6
Pentothal	T41.1X1	T41.1X2	T41.1X3	T41.1X4	T41.1X5	T41.1X6
Pentoxifylline	T46.7X1	T46.7X2	T46.7X3	T46.7X4	T46.7X5	T46.7X6
Pentoxyverine	T48.3X1	T48.3X2	T48.3X3	T48.3X4	T48.3X5	T48.3X6
Pentrinat	T46.3X1	T46.3X2	T46.3X3	T46.3X4	T46.3X5	T46.3X6
Pentylenetetrazole	T50.7X1	T50.7X2	T50.7X3	T50.7X4	T50.7X5	T50.7X6
Pentylsalicylamide	T37.1X1	T37.1X2	T37.1X3	T37.1X4	T37.1X5	T37.1X6
Pentymal	T42.3X1	T42.3X2	T42.3X3	T42.3X4	T42.3X5	T42.3X6
Peplomycin	T45.1X1	T45.1X2	T45.1X3	T45.1X4	T45.1X5	T45.1X6
Peppermint (oil)	T47.5X1	T47.5X2	T47.5X3	T47.5X4	T47.5X5	T47.5X6
Pepsin	T47.5X1	T47.5X2	T47.5X3	T47.5X4	T47.5X5	T47.5X6
digestant	T47.5X1	T47.5X2	T47.5X3	T47.5X4	T47.5X5	T47.5X6
Pepstatin	T47.1X1	T47.1X2	T47.1X3	T47.1X4	T47.1X5	T47.1X6
Peptavlon	T50.8X1	T50.8X2	T50.8X3	T50.8X4	T50.8X5	T50.8X6
Perazine	T43.3X1	T43.3X2	T43.3X3	T43.3X4	T43.3X5	T43.3X6
Percaine (spinal)	T41.3X1	T41.3X2	T41.3X3	T41.3X4	T41.3X5	T41.3X6
topical (surface)	T41.3X1	T41.3X2	T41.3X3	T41.3X4	T41.3X5	T41.3X6

Perchloroethylene - Phenoctide

Substance	Poisoning, Accidental (unintentional)	Poisoning, Intentional self-harm	Poisoning, Assault	Poisoning, Undetermined	Adverse effect	Underdosing
Perchloroethylene	T53.3X1	T53.3X2	T53.3X3	T53.3X4	—	—
medicinal	T37.4X1	T37.4X2	T37.4X3	T37.4X4	T37.4X5	T37.4X6
vapor	T53.3X1	T53.3X2	T53.3X3	T53.3X4	—	—
Percodan	T40.2X1	T40.2X2	T40.2X3	T40.2X4	T40.2X5	T40.2X6
Percogesic—*see also acetaminophen*	T45.0X1	T45.0X2	T45.0X3	T45.0X4	T45.0X5	T45.0X6
Percorten	T38.0X1	T38.0X2	T38.0X3	T38.0X4	T38.0X5	T38.0X6
Pergolide	T42.8X1	T42.8X2	T42.8X3	T42.8X4	T42.8X5	T42.8X6
Pergonal	T38.811	T38.812	T38.813	T38.814	T38.815	T38.816
Perhexilene	T46.3X1	T46.3X2	T46.3X3	T46.3X4	T46.3X5	T46.3X6
Perhexiline (maleate)	T46.3X1	T46.3X2	T46.3X3	T46.3X4	T46.3X5	T46.3X6
Periactin	T45.0X1	T45.0X2	T45.0X3	T45.0X4	T45.0X5	T45.0X6
Periciazine	T43.3X1	T43.3X2	T43.3X3	T43.3X4	T43.3X5	T43.3X6
Periclor	T42.6X1	T42.6X2	T42.6X3	T42.6X4	T42.6X5	T42.6X6
Perindopril	T46.4X1	T46.4X2	T46.4X3	T46.4X4	T46.4X5	T46.4X6
Perisoxal	T39.8X1	T39.8X2	T39.8X3	T39.8X4	T39.8X5	T39.8X6
Peritoneal dialysis solution	T50.3X1	T50.3X2	T50.3X3	T50.3X4	T50.3X5	T50.3X6
Peritrate	T46.3X1	T46.3X2	T46.3X3	T46.3X4	T46.3X5	T46.3X6
Perlapine	T42.4X1	T42.4X2	T42.4X3	T42.4X4	T42.4X5	T42.4X6
Permanganate	T65.891	T65.892	T65.893	T65.894	—	—
Permethrin	T60.1X1	T60.1X2	T60.1X3	T60.1X4	—	—
Pernocton	T42.3X1	T42.3X2	T42.3X3	T42.3X4	T42.3X5	T42.3X6
Pernoston	T42.3X1	T42.3X2	T42.3X3	T42.3X4	T42.3X5	T42.3X6
Peronine	T40.2X1	T40.2X2	T40.2X3	T40.2X4	—	—
Perphenazine	T43.3X1	T43.3X2	T43.3X3	T43.3X4	T43.3X5	T43.3X6
Pertofrane	T43.011	T43.012	T43.013	T43.014	T43.015	T43.016
Pertussis						
immune serum (human)	T50.Z11	T50.Z12	T50.Z13	T50.Z14	T50.Z15	T50.Z16
vaccine (with diphtheria toxoid) (with tetanus toxoid)	T50.A11	T50.A12	T50.A13	T50.A14	T50.A15	T50.A16
Peruvian balsam	T49.0X1	T49.0X2	T49.0X3	T49.0X4	T49.0X5	T49.0X6
Peruvoside	T46.0X1	T46.0X2	T46.0X3	T46.0X4	T46.0X5	T46.0X6
Pesticide (dust) (fumes) (vapor) NEC	T60.91	T60.92	T60.93	T60.94	—	—
arsenic	T57.0X1	T57.0X2	T57.0X3	T57.0X4	—	—
chlorinated	T60.1X1	T60.1X2	T60.1X3	T60.1X4	—	—
cyanide	T65.0X1	T65.0X2	T65.0X3	T65.0X4	—	—
kerosene	T52.0X1	T52.0X2	T52.0X3	T52.0X4	—	—
mixture (of compounds)	T60.91	T60.92	T60.93	T60.94	—	—
naphthalene	T60.2X1	T60.2X2	T60.2X3	T60.2X4	—	—
organochlorine (compounds)	T60.1X1	T60.1X2	T60.1X3	T60.1X4	—	—
petroleum (distillate) (products) NEC	T60.8X1	T60.8X2	T60.8X3	T60.8X4	—	—
specified ingredient NEC	T60.8X1	T60.8X2	T60.8X3	T60.8X4	—	—
strychnine	T65.1X1	T65.1X2	T65.1X3	T65.1X4	—	—
thallium	T60.4X1	T60.4X2	T60.4X3	T60.4X4	—	—
Pethidine	T40.4X1	T40.4X2	T40.4X3	T40.4X4	T40.4X5	T40.4X6
Petrichloral	T42.6X1	T42.6X2	T42.6X3	T42.6X4	T42.6X5	T42.6X6
Petrol	T52.0X1	T52.0X2	T52.0X3	T52.0X4	—	—
vapor	T52.0X1	T52.0X2	T52.0X3	T52.0X4	—	—
Petrolatum	T49.3X1	T49.3X2	T49.3X3	T49.3X4	T49.3X5	T49.3X6
hydrophilic	T49.3X1	T49.3X2	T49.3X3	T49.3X4	T49.3X5	T49.3X6
liquid	T47.4X1	T47.4X2	T47.4X3	T47.4X4	T47.4X5	T47.4X6
topical	T49.3X1	T49.3X2	T49.3X3	T49.3X4	T49.3X5	T49.3X6

Substance	Poisoning, Accidental (unintentional)	Poisoning, Intentional self-harm	Poisoning, Assault	Poisoning, Undetermined	Adverse effect	Underdosing
Petrolatum — *continued*						
nonmedicinal	T52.0X1	T52.0X2	T52.0X3	T52.0X4	—	—
red veterinary	T49.3X1	T49.3X2	T49.3X3	T49.3X4	T49.3X5	T49.3X6
white	T49.3X1	T49.3X2	T49.3X3	T49.3X4	T49.3X5	T49.3X6
Petroleum (products) NEC	T52.0X1	T52.0X2	T52.0X3	T52.0X4	—	—
benzine (s)—*see Ligroin*						
ether—*see Ligroin*						
jelly—*see Petrolatum*						
naphtha—*see Ligroin*						
pesticide	T60.8X1	T60.8X2	T60.8X3	T60.8X4	—	—
solids	T52.0X1	T52.0X2	T52.0X3	T52.0X4	—	—
solvents	T52.0X1	T52.0X2	T52.0X3	T52.0X4	—	—
vapor	T52.0X1	T52.0X2	T52.0X3	T52.0X4	—	—
Peyote	T40.991	T40.992	T40.993	T40.994	—	—
Phanodorm, phanodorn	T42.3X1	T42.3X2	T42.3X3	T42.3X4	T42.3X5	T42.3X6
Phanquinone	T37.3X1	T37.3X2	T37.3X3	T37.3X4	T37.3X5	T37.3X6
Phanquone	T37.3X1	T37.3X2	T37.3X3	T37.3X4	T37.3X5	T37.3X6
Pharmaceutical						
adjunct NEC	T50.901	T50.902	T50.903	T50.904	T50.905	T50.906
excipient NEC	T50.901	T50.902	T50.903	T50.904	T50.905	T50.906
sweetener	T50.901	T50.902	T50.903	T50.904	T50.905	T50.906
viscous agent	T50.901	T50.902	T50.903	T50.904	T50.905	T50.906
Phemitone	T42.3X1	T42.3X2	T42.3X3	T42.3X4	T42.3X5	T42.3X6
Phenacaine	T41.3X1	T41.3X2	T41.3X3	T41.3X4	T41.3X5	T41.3X6
Phenacemide	T42.6X1	T42.6X2	T42.6X3	T42.6X4	T42.6X5	T42.6X6
Phenacetin	T39.1X1	T39.1X2	T39.1X3	T39.1X4	T39.1X5	T39.1X6
Phenadoxone	T40.2X1	T40.2X2	T40.2X3	T40.2X4	—	—
Phenaglycodol	T43.591	T43.592	T43.593	T43.594	T43.595	T43.596
Phenantoin	T42.0X1	T42.0X2	T42.0X3	T42.0X4	T42.0X5	T42.0X6
Phenaphthazine reagent	T50.991	T50.992	T50.993	T50.994	T50.995	T50.996
Phenazocine	T40.4X1	T40.4X2	T40.4X3	T40.4X4	T40.4X5	T40.4X6
Phenazone	T39.2X1	T39.2X2	T39.2X3	T39.2X4	T39.2X5	T39.2X6
Phenazopyridine	T39.8X1	T39.8X2	T39.8X3	T39.8X4	T39.8X5	T39.8X6
Phenbenicillin	T36.0X1	T36.0X2	T36.0X3	T36.0X4	T36.0X5	T36.0X6
Phenbutrazate	T50.5X1	T50.5X2	T50.5X3	T50.5X4	T50.5X5	T50.5X6
Phencyclidine	T40.991	T40.992	T40.993	T40.994	T40.995	T40.996
Phendimetrazine	T50.5X1	T50.5X2	T50.5X3	T50.5X4	T50.5X5	T50.5X6
Phenelzine	T43.1X1	T43.1X2	T43.1X3	T43.1X4	T43.1X5	T43.1X6
Phenemal	T42.3X1	T42.3X2	T42.3X3	T42.3X4	T42.3X5	T42.3X6
Phenergan	T42.6X1	T42.6X2	T42.6X3	T42.6X4	T42.6X5	T42.6X6
Pheneticillin	T36.0X1	T36.0X2	T36.0X3	T36.0X4	T36.0X5	T36.0X6
Pheneturide	T42.6X1	T42.6X2	T42.6X3	T42.6X4	T42.6X5	T42.6X6
Phenformin	T38.3X1	T38.3X2	T38.3X3	T38.3X4	T38.3X5	T38.3X6
Phenglutarimide	T44.3X1	T44.3X2	T44.3X3	T44.3X4	T44.3X5	T44.3X6
Phenicarbazide	T39.8X1	T39.8X2	T39.8X3	T39.8X4	T39.8X5	T39.8X6
Phenindamine	T45.0X1	T45.0X2	T45.0X3	T45.0X4	T45.0X5	T45.0X6
Phenindione	T45.511	T45.512	T45.513	T45.514	T45.515	T45.516
Pheniprazine	T43.1X1	T43.1X2	T43.1X3	T43.1X4	T43.1X5	T43.1X6
Pheniramine	T45.0X1	T45.0X2	T45.0X3	T45.0X4	T45.0X5	T45.0X6
Phenisatin	T47.2X1	T47.2X2	T47.2X3	T47.2X4	T47.2X5	T47.2X6
Phenmetrazine	T50.5X1	T50.5X2	T50.5X3	T50.5X4	T50.5X5	T50.5X6
Phenobal	T42.3X1	T42.3X2	T42.3X3	T42.3X4	T42.3X5	T42.3X6
Phenobarbital	T42.3X1	T42.3X2	T42.3X3	T42.3X4	T42.3X5	T42.3X6
with						
mephenytoin	T42.3X1	T42.3X2	T42.3X3	T42.3X4	T42.3X5	T42.3X6
phenytoin	T42.3X1	T42.3X2	T42.3X3	T42.3X4	T42.3X5	T42.3X6
sodium	T42.3X1	T42.3X2	T42.3X3	T42.3X4	T42.3X5	T42.3X6
Phenobarbitone	T42.3X1	T42.3X2	T42.3X3	T42.3X4	T42.3X5	T42.3X6
Phenobutiodil	T50.8X1	T50.8X2	T50.8X3	T50.8X4	T50.8X5	T50.8X6
Phenoctide	T49.0X1	T49.0X2	T49.0X3	T49.0X4	T49.0X5	T49.0X6

Substance	Poisoning, Accidental (unintentional)	Poisoning, Intentional self-harm	Poisoning, Assault	Poisoning, Undetermined	Adverse effect	Underdosing
Phenol	T49.0X1	T49.0X2	T49.0X3	T49.0X4	T49.0X5	T49.0X6
disinfectant	T54.0X1	T54.0X2	T54.0X3	T54.0X4	—	—
in oil injection	T46.8X1	T46.8X2	T46.8X3	T46.8X4	T46.8X5	T46.8X6
medicinal	T49.1X1	T49.1X2	T49.1X3	T49.1X4	T49.1X5	T49.1X6
nonmedicinal NEC	T54.0X1	T54.0X2	T54.0X3	T54.0X4	—	—
pesticide	T60.8X1	T60.8X2	T60.8X3	T60.8X4	—	—
red	T50.8X1	T50.8X2	T50.8X3	T50.8X4	T50.8X5	T50.8X6
Phenolic preparation	T49.1X1	T49.1X2	T49.1X3	T49.1X4	T49.1X5	T49.1X6
Phenolphthalein	T47.2X1	T47.2X2	T47.2X3	T47.2X4	T47.2X5	T47.2X6
Phenolsulfonphthalein	T50.8X1	T50.8X2	T50.8X3	T50.8X4	T50.8X5	T50.8X6
Phenomorphan	T40.2X1	T40.2X2	T40.2X3	T40.2X4	—	—
Phenonyl	T42.3X1	T42.3X2	T42.3X3	T42.3X4	T42.3X5	T42.3X6
Phenoperidine	T40.4X1	T40.4X2	T40.4X3	T40.4X4	—	—
Phenopyrazone	T46.991	T46.992	T46.993	T46.994	T46.995	T46.996
Phenoquin	T50.4X1	T50.4X2	T50.4X3	T50.4X4	T50.4X5	T50.4X6
Phenothiazine (psychotropic) NEC	T43.3X1	T43.3X2	T43.3X3	T43.3X4	T43.3X5	T43.3X6
insecticide	T60.2X1	T60.2X2	T60.2X3	T60.2X4	—	—
Phenothrin	T49.0X1	T49.0X2	T49.0X3	T49.0X4	T49.0X5	T49.0X6
Phenoxybenzamine	T46.7X1	T46.7X2	T46.7X3	T46.7X4	T46.7X5	T46.7X6
Phenoxyethanol	T49.0X1	T49.0X2	T49.0X3	T49.0X4	T49.0X5	T49.0X6
Phenoxymethyl penicillin	T36.0X1	T36.0X2	T36.0X3	T36.0X4	T36.0X5	T36.0X6
Phenprobamate	T42.8X1	T42.8X2	T42.8X3	T42.8X4	T42.8X5	T42.8X6
Phenprocoumon	T45.511	T45.512	T45.513	T45.514	T45.515	T45.516
Phensuximide	T42.2X1	T42.2X2	T42.2X3	T42.2X4	T42.2X5	T42.2X6
Phentermine	T50.5X1	T50.5X2	T50.5X3	T50.5X4	T50.5X5	T50.5X6
Phenthicillin	T36.0X1	T36.0X2	T36.0X3	T36.0X4	T36.0X5	T36.0X6
Phentolamine	T46.7X1	T46.7X2	T46.7X3	T46.7X4	T46.7X5	T46.7X6
Phenyl						
butazone	T39.2X1	T39.2X2	T39.2X3	T39.2X4	T39.2X5	T39.2X6
enediamine	T65.3X1	T65.3X2	T65.3X3	T65.3X4	—	—
hydrazine	T65.3X1	T65.3X2	T65.3X3	T65.3X4	—	—
antineoplastic	T45.1X1	T45.1X2	T45.1X3	T45.1X4	T45.1X5	T45.1X6
mercuric compounds— *see Mercury*						
salicylate	T49.3X1	T49.3X2	T49.3X3	T49.3X4	T49.3X5	T49.3X6
Phenylalanine mustard	T45.1X1	T45.1X2	T45.1X3	T45.1X4	T45.1X5	T45.1X6
Phenylbutazone	T39.2X1	T39.2X2	T39.2X3	T39.2X4	T39.2X5	T39.2X6
Phenylenediamine	T65.3X1	T65.3X2	T65.3X3	T65.3X4	—	—
Phenylephrine	T44.4X1	T44.4X2	T44.4X3	T44.4X4	T44.4X5	T44.4X6
Phenylethylbiguanide	T38.3X1	T38.3X2	T38.3X3	T38.3X4	T38.3X5	T38.3X6
Phenylmercuric						
acetate	T49.0X1	T49.0X2	T49.0X3	T49.0X4	T49.0X5	T49.0X6
borate	T49.0X1	T49.0X2	T49.0X3	T49.0X4	T49.0X5	T49.0X6
nitrate	T49.0X1	T49.0X2	T49.0X3	T49.0X4	T49.0X5	T49.0X6
Phenylmethylbarbitone	T42.3X1	T42.3X2	T42.3X3	T42.3X4	T42.3X5	T42.3X6
Phenylpropanol	T47.5X1	T47.5X2	T47.5X3	T47.5X4	T47.5X5	T47.5X6
Phenylpropanolamine	T44.991	T44.992	T44.993	T44.994	T44.995	T44.996
Phenylsulfthion	T60.0X1	T60.0X2	T60.0X3	T60.0X4	—	—
Phenyltoloxamine	T45.0X1	T45.0X2	T45.0X3	T45.0X4	T45.0X5	T45.0X6
Phenyramidol, phenyramidon	T39.8X1	T39.8X2	T39.8X3	T39.8X4	T39.8X5	T39.8X6
Phenytoin	T42.0X1	T42.0X2	T42.0X3	T42.0X4	T42.0X5	T42.0X6
with Phenobarbital	T42.3X1	T42.3X2	T42.3X3	T42.3X4	T42.3X5	T42.3X6
pHisoHex	T49.2X1	T49.2X2	T49.2X3	T49.2X4	T49.2X5	T49.2X6
Pholcodine	T48.3X1	T48.3X2	T48.3X3	T48.3X4	T48.3X5	T48.3X6
Pholedrine	T46.991	T46.992	T46.993	T46.994	T46.995	T46.996
Phorate	T60.0X1	T60.0X2	T60.0X3	T60.0X4	—	—
Phosdrin	T60.0X1	T60.0X2	T60.0X3	T60.0X4	—	—
Phosfolan	T60.0X1	T60.0X2	T60.0X3	T60.0X4	—	—

Substance	Poisoning, Accidental (unintentional)	Poisoning, Intentional self-harm	Poisoning, Assault	Poisoning, Undetermined	Adverse effect	Underdosing
Phosgene (gas)	T59.891	T59.892	T59.893	T59.894	—	—
Phosphamidon	T60.0X1	T60.0X2	T60.0X3	T60.0X4	—	—
Phosphate	T65.891	T65.892	T65.893	T65.894	—	—
laxative	T47.4X1	T47.4X2	T47.4X3	T47.4X4	T47.4X5	T47.4X6
organic	T60.0X1	T60.0X2	T60.0X3	T60.0X4	—	—
solvent	T52.91	T52.92	T52.93	T52.94	—	—
tricresyl	T65.891	T65.892	T65.893	T65.894	—	—
Phosphine	T57.1X1	T57.1X2	T57.1X3	T57.1X4	—	—
fumigant	T57.1X1	T57.1X2	T57.1X3	T57.1X4	—	—
Phospholine	T49.5X1	T49.5X2	T49.5X3	T49.5X4	T49.5X5	T49.5X6
Phosphoric acid	T54.2X1	T54.2X2	T54.2X3	T54.2X4	—	—
Phosphorus (compound) NEC	T57.1X1	T57.1X2	T57.1X3	T57.1X4	—	—
pesticide	T60.0X1	T60.0X2	T60.0X3	T60.0X4	—	—
Phthalates	T65.891	T65.892	T65.893	T65.894	—	—
Phthalic anhydride	T65.891	T65.892	T65.893	T65.894	—	—
Phthalimidoglutarimide	T42.6X1	T42.6X2	T42.6X3	T42.6X4	T42.6X5	T42.6X6
Phthalylsulfathiazole	T37.0X1	T37.0X2	T37.0X3	T37.0X4	T37.0X5	T37.0X6
Phylloquinone	T45.7X1	T45.7X2	T45.7X3	T45.7X4	T45.7X5	T45.7X6
Physeptone	T40.3X1	T40.3X2	T40.3X3	T40.3X4	T40.3X5	T40.3X6
Physostigma venenosum	T62.2X1	T62.2X2	T62.2X3	T62.2X4	—	—
Physostigmine	T49.5X1	T49.5X2	T49.5X3	T49.5X4	T49.5X5	T49.5X6
Phytolacca decandra	T62.2X1	T62.2X2	T62.2X3	T62.2X4	—	—
berries	T62.1X1	T62.1X2	T62.1X3	T62.1X4	—	—
Phytomenadione	T45.7X1	T45.7X2	T45.7X3	T45.7X4	T45.7X5	T45.7X6
Phytonadione	T45.7X1	T45.7X2	T45.7X3	T45.7X4	T45.7X5	T45.7X6
Picoperine	T48.3X1	T48.3X2	T48.3X3	T48.3X4	T48.3X5	T48.3X6
Picosulfate (sodium)	T47.2X1	T47.2X2	T47.2X3	T47.2X4	T47.2X5	T47.2X6
Picric (acid)	T54.2X1	T54.2X2	T54.2X3	T54.2X4	—	—
Picrotoxin	T50.7X1	T50.7X2	T50.7X3	T50.7X4	T50.7X5	T50.7X6
Piketoprofen	T49.0X1	T49.0X2	T49.0X3	T49.0X4	T49.0X5	T49.0X6
Pilocarpine	T44.1X1	T44.1X2	T44.1X3	T44.1X4	T44.1X5	T44.1X6
Pilocarpus (jaborandi) extract	T44.1X1	T44.1X2	T44.1X3	T44.1X4	T44.1X5	T44.1X6
Pilsicainide (hydrochloride)	T46.2X1	T46.2X2	T46.2X3	T46.2X4	T46.2X5	T46.2X6
Pimaricin	T36.7X1	T36.7X2	T36.7X3	T36.7X4	T36.7X5	T36.7X6
Pimeclone	T50.7X1	T50.7X2	T50.7X3	T50.7X4	T50.7X5	T50.7X6
Pimelic ketone	T52.8X1	T52.8X2	T52.8X3	T52.8X4	—	—
Pimethixene	T45.0X1	T45.0X2	T45.0X3	T45.0X4	T45.0X5	T45.0X6
Piminodine	T40.2X1	T40.2X2	T40.2X3	T40.2X4	T40.2X5	T40.2X6
Pimozide	T43.591	T43.592	T43.593	T43.594	T43.595	T43.596
Pinacidil	T46.5X1	T46.5X2	T46.5X3	T46.5X4	T46.5X5	T46.5X6
Pinaverium bromide	T44.3X1	T44.3X2	T44.3X3	T44.3X4	T44.3X5	T44.3X6
Pinazepam	T42.4X1	T42.4X2	T42.4X3	T42.4X4	T42.4X5	T42.4X6
Pindolol	T44.7X1	T44.7X2	T44.7X3	T44.7X4	T44.7X5	T44.7X6
Pindone	T60.4X1	T60.4X2	T60.4X3	T60.4X4	—	—
Pine oil (disinfectant)	T65.891	T65.892	T65.893	T65.894	—	—
Pinkroot	T37.4X1	T37.4X2	T37.4X3	T37.4X4	T37.4X5	T37.4X6
Pipadone	T40.2X1	T40.2X2	T40.2X3	T40.2X4	—	—
Pipamazine	T45.0X1	T45.0X2	T45.0X3	T45.0X4	T45.0X5	T45.0X6
Pipamperone	T43.4X1	T43.4X2	T43.4X3	T43.4X4	T43.4X5	T43.4X6
Pipazetate	T48.3X1	T48.3X2	T48.3X3	T48.3X4	T48.3X5	T48.3X6
Pipemidic acid	T37.8X1	T37.8X2	T37.8X3	T37.8X4	T37.8X5	T37.8X6
Pipenzolate bromide	T44.3X1	T44.3X2	T44.3X3	T44.3X4	T44.3X5	T44.3X6
Piperacetazine	T43.3X1	T43.3X2	T43.3X3	T43.3X4	T43.3X5	T43.3X6
Piperacillin	T36.0X1	T36.0X2	T36.0X3	T36.0X4	T36.0X5	T36.0X6
Piperazine	T37.4X1	T37.4X2	T37.4X3	T37.4X4	T37.4X5	T37.4X6
estrone sulfate	T38.5X1	T38.5X2	T38.5X3	T38.5X4	T38.5X5	T38.5X6
Piper cubeba	T62.2X1	T62.2X2	T62.2X3	T62.2X4	—	—
Piperidione	T48.3X1	T48.3X2	T48.3X3	T48.3X4	T48.3X5	T48.3X6

Piperidolate - Potassic saline injection

Substance	Poisoning, Accidental (unintentional)	Poisoning, Intentional self-harm	Poisoning, Assault	Poisoning, Undetermined	Adverse effect	Underdosing
Piperidolate	T44.3X1	T44.3X2	T44.3X3	T44.3X4	T44.3X5	T44.3X6
Piperocaine	T41.3X1	T41.3X2	T41.3X3	T41.3X4	T41.3X5	T41.3X6
infiltration (subcutaneous)	T41.3X1	T41.3X2	T41.3X3	T41.3X4	T41.3X5	T41.3X6
nerve block (peripheral) (plexus)	T41.3X1	T41.3X2	T41.3X3	T41.3X4	T41.3X5	T41.3X6
topical (surface)	T41.3X1	T41.3X2	T41.3X3	T41.3X4	T41.3X5	T41.3X6
Piperonyl butoxide	T60.8X1	T60.8X2	T60.8X3	T60.8X4	—	—
Pipethanate	T44.3X1	T44.3X2	T44.3X3	T44.3X4	T44.3X5	T44.3X6
Pipobroman	T45.1X1	T45.1X2	T45.1X3	T45.1X4	T45.1X5	T45.1X6
Pipotiazine	T43.3X1	T43.3X2	T43.3X3	T43.3X4	T43.3X5	T43.3X6
Pipoxizine	T45.0X1	T45.0X2	T45.0X3	T45.0X4	T45.0X5	T45.0X6
Pipradrol	T43.691	T43.692	T43.693	T43.694	T43.695	T43.696
Piprinhydrinate	T45.0X1	T45.0X2	T45.0X3	T45.0X4	T45.0X5	T45.0X6
Pirarubicin	T45.1X1	T45.1X2	T45.1X3	T45.1X4	T45.1X5	T45.1X6
Pirazinamide	T37.1X1	T37.1X2	T37.1X3	T37.1X4	T37.1X5	T37.1X6
Pirbuterol	T48.6X1	T48.6X2	T48.6X3	T48.6X4	T48.6X5	T48.6X6
Pirenzepine	T47.1X1	T47.1X2	T47.1X3	T47.1X4	T47.1X5	T47.1X6
Piretanide	T50.1X1	T50.1X2	T50.1X3	T50.1X4	T50.1X5	T50.1X6
Piribedil	T42.8X1	T42.8X2	T42.8X3	T42.8X4	T42.8X5	T42.8X6
Piridoxilate	T46.3X1	T46.3X2	T46.3X3	T46.3X4	T46.3X5	T46.3X6
Piritramide	T40.4X1	T40.4X2	T40.4X3	T40.4X4		
Piromidic acid	T37.8X1	T37.8X2	T37.8X3	T37.8X4	T37.8X5	T37.8X6
Piroxicam	T39.391	T39.392	T39.393	T39.394	T39.395	T39.396
beta-cyclodextrin complex	T39.8X1	T39.8X2	T39.8X3	T39.8X4	T39.8X5	T39.8X6
Pirozadil	T46.6X1	T46.6X2	T46.6X3	T46.6X4	T46.6X5	T46.6X6
Piscidia (bark) (erythrina)	T39.8X1	T39.8X2	T39.8X3	T39.8X4	T39.8X5	T39.8X6
Pitch	T65.891	T65.892	T65.893	T65.894	—	—
Pitkin's solution	T41.3X1	T41.3X2	T41.3X3	T41.3X4	T41.3X5	T41.3X6
Pitocin	T48.0X1	T48.0X2	T48.0X3	T48.0X4	T48.0X5	T48.0X6
Pitressin (tannate)	T38.891	T38.892	T38.893	T38.894	T38.895	T38.896
Pituitary extracts (posterior)	T38.891	T38.892	T38.893	T38.894	T38.895	T38.896
anterior	T38.811	T38.812	T38.813	T38.814	T38.815	T38.816
Pituitrin	T38.891	T38.892	T38.893	T38.894	T38.895	T38.896
Pivampicillin	T36.0X1	T36.0X2	T36.0X3	T36.0X4	T36.0X5	T36.0X6
Pivmecillinam	T36.0X1	T36.0X2	T36.0X3	T36.0X4	T36.0X5	T36.0X6
Placental hormone	T38.891	T38.892	T38.893	T38.894	T38.895	T38.896
Placidyl	T42.6X1	T42.6X2	T42.6X3	T42.6X4	T42.6X5	T42.6X6
Plague vaccine	T50.A91	T50.A92	T50.A93	T50.A94	T50.A95	T50.A96
Plant						
food or fertilizer NEC	T65.891	T65.892	T65.893	T65.894	—	—
containing herbicide	T60.3X1	T60.3X2	T60.3X3	T60.3X4	—	—
noxious, used as food	T62.2X1	T62.2X2	T62.2X3	T62.2X4	—	—
berries	T62.1X1	T62.1X2	T62.1X3	T62.1X4	—	—
seeds	T62.2X1	T62.2X2	T62.2X3	T62.2X4	—	—
specified type NEC	T62.2X1	T62.2X2	T62.2X3	T62.2X4	—	—
Plasma	T45.8X1	T45.8X2	T45.8X3	T45.8X4	T45.8X5	T45.8X6
expander NEC	T45.8X1	T45.8X2	T45.8X3	T45.8X4	T45.8X5	T45.8X6
protein fraction (human)	T45.8X1	T45.8X2	T45.8X3	T45.8X4	T45.8X5	T45.8X6
Plasmanate	T45.8X1	T45.8X2	T45.8X3	T45.8X4	T45.8X5	T45.8X6
Plasminogen (tissue) activator	T45.611	T45.612	T45.613	T45.614	T45.615	T45.616
Plaster dressing	T49.3X1	T49.3X2	T49.3X3	T49.3X4	T49.3X5	T49.3X6
Plastic dressing	T49.3X1	T49.3X2	T49.3X3	T49.3X4	T49.3X5	T49.3X6
Plegicil	T43.3X1	T43.3X2	T43.3X3	T43.3X4	T43.3X5	T43.3X6
Plicamycin	T45.1X1	T45.1X2	T45.1X3	T45.1X4	T45.1X5	T45.1X6
Podophyllotoxin	T49.8X1	T49.8X2	T49.8X3	T49.8X4	T49.8X5	T49.8X6

Substance	Poisoning, Accidental (unintentional)	Poisoning, Intentional self-harm	Poisoning, Assault	Poisoning, Undetermined	Adverse effect	Underdosing
Podophyllum (resin)	T49.4X1	T49.4X2	T49.4X3	T49.4X4	T49.4X5	T49.4X6
Poison NEC	T65.91	T65.92	T65.93	T65.94	—	—
Poisonous berries	T62.1X1	T62.1X2	T62.1X3	T62.1X4	—	—
Pokeweed (any part)	T62.2X1	T62.2X2	T62.2X3	T62.2X4	—	—
Poldine metilsulfate	T44.3X1	T44.3X2	T44.3X3	T44.3X4	T44.3X5	T44.3X6
Polidexide (sulfate)	T46.6X1	T46.6X2	T46.6X3	T46.6X4	T46.6X5	T46.6X6
Polidocanol	T46.8X1	T46.8X2	T46.8X3	T46.8X4	T46.8X5	T46.8X6
Poliomyelitis vaccine	T50.B91	T50.B92	T50.B93	T50.B94	T50.B95	T50.B96
Polish (car) (floor) (furni-ture) (metal) (porcelain) (silver)	T65.891	T65.892	T65.893	T65.894	—	—
abrasive	T65.891	T65.892	T65.893	T65.894	—	—
porcelain	T65.891	T65.892	T65.893	T65.894	—	—
Poloxalkol	T47.4X1	T47.4X2	T47.4X3	T47.4X4	T47.4X5	T47.4X6
Poloxamer	T47.4X1	T47.4X2	T47.4X3	T47.4X4	T47.4X5	T47.4X6
Polyaminostyrene resins	T50.3X1	T50.3X2	T50.3X3	T50.3X4	T50.3X5	T50.3X6
Polycarbophil	T47.4X1	T47.4X2	T47.4X3	T47.4X4	T47.4X5	T47.4X6
Polychlorinated biphenyl	T65.891	T65.892	T65.893	T65.894	—	—
Polycycline	T36.4X1	T36.4X2	T36.4X3	T36.4X4	T36.4X5	T36.4X6
Polyester fumes	T59.891	T59.892	T59.893	T59.894	—	—
Polyester resin hardener	T52.91	T52.92	T52.93	T52.94	—	—
fumes	T59.891	T59.892	T59.893	T59.894	—	—
Polyestradiol phosphate	T38.5X1	T38.5X2	T38.5X3	T38.5X4	T38.5X5	T38.5X6
Polyethanolamine alkyl sulfate	T49.2X1	T49.2X2	T49.2X3	T49.2X4	T49.2X5	T49.2X6
Polyethylene adhesive	T49.3X1	T49.3X2	T49.3X3	T49.3X4	T49.3X5	T49.3X6
Polyferose	T45.4X1	T45.4X2	T45.4X3	T45.4X4	I45.4X5	I45.4X6
Polygeline	T45.8X1	T45.8X2	T45.8X3	T45.8X4	T45.8X5	T45.8X6
Polymyxin	T36.8X1	T36.8X2	T36.8X3	T36.8X4	T36.8X5	T36.8X6
B	T36.8X1	T36.8X2	T36.8X3	T36.8X4	T36.8X5	T36.8X6
ENT agent	T49.6X1	T49.6X2	T49.6X3	T49.6X4	T49.6X5	T49.6X6
ophthalmic preparation	T49.5X1	T49.5X2	T49.5X3	T49.5X4	T49.5X5	T49.5X6
topical NEC	T49.0X1	T49.0X2	T49.0X3	T49.0X4	T49.0X5	T49.0X6
E sulfate (eye preparation)	T49.5X1	T49.5X2	T49.5X3	T49.5X4	T49.5X5	T49.5X6
Polynoxylin	T49.0X1	T49.0X2	T49.0X3	T49.0X4	T49.0X5	T49.0X6
Polyoestradiol phosphate	T38.5X1	T38.5X2	T38.5X3	T38.5X4	T38.5X5	T38.5X6
Polyoxymethyleneurea	T49.0X1	T49.0X2	T49.0X3	T49.0X4	T49.0X5	T49.0X6
Polysilane	T47.8X1	T47.8X2	T47.8X3	T47.8X4	T47.8X5	T47.8X6
Polytetrafluoroethylene (inhaled)	T59.891	T59.892	T59.893	T59.894	—	—
Polythiazide	T50.2X1	T50.2X2	T50.2X3	T50.2X4	T50.2X5	T50.2X6
Polyvidone	T45.8X1	T45.8X2	T45.8X3	T45.8X4	T45.8X5	T45.8X6
Polyvinylpyrrolidone	T45.8X1	T45.8X2	T45.8X3	T45.8X4	T45.8X5	T45.8X6
Pontocaine (hydrochloride) (infiltration) (topical)	T41.3X1	T41.3X2	T41.3X3	T41.3X4	T41.3X5	T41.3X6
nerve block (peripheral) (plexus)	T41.3X1	T41.3X2	T41.3X3	T41.3X4	T41.3X5	T41.3X6
spinal	T41.3X1	T41.3X2	T41.3X3	T41.3X4	T41.3X5	T41.3X6
Porfiromycin	T45.1X1	T45.1X2	T45.1X3	T45.1X4	T45.1X5	T45.1X6
Posterior pituitary hormone NEC	T38.891	T38.892	T38.893	T38.894	T38.895	T38.896
Pot	T40.7X1	T40.7X2	T40.7X3	T40.7X4	T40.7X5	T40.7X6
Potash (caustic)	T54.3X1	T54.3X2	T54.3X3	T54.3X4	—	—
Potassic saline injection (lactated)	T50.3X1	T50.3X2	T50.3X3	T50.3X4	T50.3X5	T50.3X6

Substance	Poisoning, Accidental (unintentional)	Poisoning, Intentional self-harm	Poisoning, Assault	Poisoning, Undetermined	Adverse effect	Underdosing
Potassium (salts) NEC	T50.3X1	T50.3X2	T50.3X3	T50.3X4	T50.3X5	T50.3X6
aminobenzoate	T45.8X1	T45.8X2	T45.8X3	T45.8X4	T45.8X5	T45.8X6
aminosalicylate	T37.1X1	T37.1X2	T37.1X3	T37.1X4	T37.1X5	T37.1X6
antimony ' tartrate'	T37.8X1	T37.8X2	T37.8X3	T37.8X4	T37.8X5	T37.8X6
arsenite (solution)	T57.0X1	T57.0X2	T57.0X3	T57.0X4	—	—
bichromate	T56.2X1	T56.2X2	T56.2X3	T56.2X4	—	—
bisulfate	T47.3X1	T47.3X2	T47.3X3	T47.3X4	T47.3X5	T47.3X6
bromide	T42.6X1	T42.6X2	T42.6X3	T42.6X4	T42.6X5	T42.6X6
canrenoate	T50.0X1	T50.0X2	T50.0X3	T50.0X4	T50.0X5	T50.0X6
carbonate	T54.3X1	T54.3X2	T54.3X3	T54.3X4	—	—
chlorate NEC	T65.891	T65.892	T65.893	T65.894	—	—
chloride	T50.3X1	T50.3X2	T50.3X3	T50.3X4	T50.3X5	T50.3X6
citrate	T50.991	T50.992	T50.993	T50.994	T50.995	T50.996
cyanide	T65.0X1	T65.0X2	T65.0X3	T65.0X4	—	—
ferric hexacyanoferrate (medicinal)	T50.6X1	T50.6X2	T50.6X3	T50.6X4	T50.6X5	T50.6X6
nonmedicinal	T65.891	T65.892	T65.893	T65.894	—	—
Fluoride	T57.8X1	T57.8X2	T57.8X3	T57.8X4	—	—
glucaldrate	T47.1X1	T47.1X2	T47.1X3	T47.1X4	T47.1X5	T47.1X6
hydroxide	T54.3X1	T54.3X2	T54.3X3	T54.3X4	—	—
iodate	T49.0X1	T49.0X2	T49.0X3	T49.0X4	T49.0X5	T49.0X6
iodide	T48.4X1	T48.4X2	T48.4X3	T48.4X4	T48.4X5	T48.4X6
nitrate	T57.8X1	T57.8X2	T57.8X3	T57.8X4	—	—
oxalate	T65.891	T65.892	T65.893	T65.894	—	—
perchlorate (nonmedicinal) NEC	T65.891	T65.892	T65.893	T65.894	—	—
antithyroid	T38.2X1	T38.2X2	T38.2X3	T38.2X4	T38.2X5	T38.2X6
medicinal	T38.2X1	T38.2X2	T38.2X3	T38.2X4	T38.2X5	T38.2X6
Permanganate (nonmedicinal)	T65.891	T65.892	T65.893	T65.894	—	—
medicinal	T49.0X1	T49.0X2	T49.0X3	T49.0X4	T49.0X5	T49.0X6
sulfate	T47.2X1	T47.2X2	T47.2X3	T47.2X4	T47.2X5	T47.2X6
Potassium-removing resin	T50.3X1	T50.3X2	T50.3X3	T50.3X4	T50.3X5	T50.3X6
Potassium-retaining drug	T50.3X1	T50.3X2	T50.3X3	T50.3X4	T50.3X5	T50.3X6
Povidone	T45.8X1	T45.8X2	T45.8X3	T45.8X4	T45.8X5	T45.8X6
iodine	T49.0X1	T49.0X2	T49.0X3	T49.0X4	T49.0X5	T49.0X6
Practolol	T44.7X1	T44.7X2	T44.7X3	T44.7X4	T44.7X5	T44.7X6
Prajmalium bitartrate	T46.2X1	T46.2X2	T46.2X3	T46.2X4	T46.2X5	T46.2X6
Pralidoxime (iodide)	T50.6X1	T50.6X2	T50.6X3	T50.6X4	T50.6X5	T50.6X6
chloride	T50.6X1	T50.6X2	T50.6X3	T50.6X4	T50.6X5	T50.6X6
Pramiverine	T44.3X1	T44.3X2	T44.3X3	T44.3X4	T44.3X5	T44.3X6
Pramocaine	T49.1X1	T49.1X2	T49.1X3	T49.1X4	T49.1X5	T49.1X6
Pramoxine	T49.1X1	T49.1X2	T49.1X3	T49.1X4	T49.1X5	T49.1X6
Prasterone	T38.7X1	T38.7X2	T38.7X3	T38.7X4	T38.7X5	T38.7X6
Pravastatin	T46.6X1	T46.6X2	T46.6X3	T46.6X4	T46.6X5	T46.6X6
Prazepam	T42.4X1	T42.4X2	T42.4X3	T42.4X4	T42.4X5	T42.4X6
Praziquantel	T37.4X1	T37.4X2	T37.4X3	T37.4X4	T37.4X5	T37.4X6
Prazitone	T43.291	T43.292	T43.293	T43.294	T43.295	T43.296
Prazosin	T44.6X1	T44.6X2	T44.6X3	T44.6X4	T44.6X5	T44.6X6
Prednicarbate	T49.0X1	T49.0X2	T49.0X3	T49.0X4	T49.0X5	T49.0X6
Prednimustine	T45.1X1	T45.1X2	T45.1X3	T45.1X4	T45.1X5	T45.1X6
Prednisolone	T38.0X1	T38.0X2	T38.0X3	T38.0X4	T38.0X5	T38.0X6
ENT agent	T49.6X1	T49.6X2	T49.6X3	T49.6X4	T49.6X5	T49.6X6
ophthalmic preparation	T49.5X1	T49.5X2	T49.5X3	T49.5X4	T49.5X5	T49.5X6
steaglate	T49.0X1	T49.0X2	T49.0X3	T49.0X4	T49.0X5	T49.0X6
topical NEC	T49.0X1	T49.0X2	T49.0X3	T49.0X4	T49.0X5	T49.0X6
Prednisone	T38.0X1	T38.0X2	T38.0X3	T38.0X4	T38.0X5	T38.0X6
Prednylidene	T38.0X1	T38.0X2	T38.0X3	T38.0X4	T38.0X5	T38.0X6
Pregnandiol	T38.5X1	T38.5X2	T38.5X3	T38.5X4	T38.5X5	T38.5X6
Pregneninolone	T38.5X1	T38.5X2	T38.5X3	T38.5X4	T38.5X5	T38.5X6
Preludin	T43.691	T43.692	T43.693	T43.694	T43.695	T43.696
Premarin	T38.5X1	T38.5X2	T38.5X3	T38.5X4	T38.5X5	T38.5X6
Premedication anesthetic	T41.201	T41.202	T41.203	T41.204	T41.205	T41.206
Prenalterol	T44.5X1	T44.5X2	T44.5X3	T44.5X4	T44.5X5	T44.5X6
Prenoxdiazine	T48.3X1	T48.3X2	T48.3X3	T48.3X4	T48.3X5	T48.3X6
Prenylamine	T46.3X1	T46.3X2	T46.3X3	T46.3X4	T46.3X5	T46.3X6
Preparation H	T49.8X1	T49.8X2	T49.8X3	T49.8X4	T49.8X5	T49.8X6
Preparation, local	T49.4X1	T49.4X2	T49.4X3	T49.4X4	T49.4X5	T49.4X6
Preservative (nonmedicinal)	T65.891	T65.892	T65.893	T65.894	—	—
medicinal	T50.901	T50.902	T50.903	T50.904	T50.905	T50.906
wood	T60.91	T60.92	T60.93	T60.94	—	—
Prethcamide	T50.7X1	T50.7X2	T50.7X3	T50.7X4	T50.7X5	T50.7X6
Pride of China	T62.2X1	T62.2X2	T62.2X3	T62.2X4	—	—
Pridinol	T44.3X1	T44.3X2	T44.3X3	T44.3X4	T44.3X5	T44.3X6
Prifinium bromide	T44.3X1	T44.3X2	T44.3X3	T44.3X4	T44.3X5	T44.3X6
Prilocaine	T41.3X1	T41.3X2	T41.3X3	T41.3X4	T41.3X5	T41.3X6
infiltration (subcutaneous)	T41.3X1	T41.3X2	T41.3X3	T41.3X4	T41.3X5	T41.3X6
nerve block (peripheral) (plexus)	T41.3X1	T41.3X2	T41.3X3	T41.3X4	T41.3X5	T41.3X6
regional	T41.3X1	T41.3X2	T41.3X3	T41.3X4	T41.3X5	T41.3X6
Primaquine	T37.2X1	T37.2X2	T37.2X3	T37.2X4	T37.2X5	T37.2X6
Primidone	T42.6X1	T42.6X2	T42.6X3	T42.6X4	T42.6X5	T42.6X6
Primula (veris)	T62.2X1	T62.2X2	T62.2X3	T62.2X4	—	—
Prinadol	T40.2X1	T40.2X2	T40.2X3	T40.2X4	T40.2X5	T40.2X6
Priscol, Priscoline	T44.6X1	T44.6X2	T44.6X3	T44.6X4	T44.6X5	T44.6X6
Pristinamycin	T36.3X1	T36.3X2	T36.3X3	T36.3X4	T36.3X5	T36.3X6
Privet	T62.2X1	T62.2X2	T62.2X3	T62.2X4	—	—
berries	T62.1X1	T62.1X2	T62.1X3	T62.1X4	—	—
Privine	T44.4X1	T44.4X2	T44.4X3	T44.4X4	T44.4X5	T44.4X6
Pro-Banthine	T44.3X1	T44.3X2	T44.3X3	T44.3X4	T44.3X5	T44.3X6
Probarbital	T42.3X1	T42.3X2	T42.3X3	T42.3X4	T42.3X5	T42.3X6
Probenecid	T50.4X1	T50.4X2	T50.4X3	T50.4X4	T50.4X5	T50.4X6
Probucol	T46.6X1	T46.6X2	T46.6X3	T46.6X4	T46.6X5	T46.6X6
Procainamide	T46.2X1	T46.2X2	T46.2X3	T46.2X4	T46.2X5	T46.2X6
Procaine	T41.3X1	T41.3X2	T41.3X3	T41.3X4	T41.3X5	T41.3X6
benzylpenicillin	T36.0X1	T36.0X2	T36.0X3	T36.0X4	T36.0X5	T36.0X6
nerve block (periphreal) (plexus)	T41.3X1	T41.3X2	T41.3X3	T41.3X4	T41.3X5	T41.3X6
penicillin G	T36.0X1	T36.0X2	T36.0X3	T36.0X4	T36.0X5	T36.0X6
regional	T41.3X1	T41.3X2	T41.3X3	T41.3X4	T41.3X5	T41.3X6
spinal	T41.3X1	T41.3X2	T41.3X3	T41.3X4	T41.3X5	T41.3X6
Procalmidol	T43.591	T43.592	T43.593	T43.594	T43.595	T43.596
Procarbazine	T45.1X1	T45.1X2	T45.1X3	T45.1X4	T45.1X5	T45.1X6
Procaterol	T44.5X1	T44.5X2	T44.5X3	T44.5X4	T44.5X5	T44.5X6
Prochlorperazine	T43.3X1	T43.3X2	T43.3X3	T43.3X4	T43.3X5	T43.3X6
Procyclidine	T44.3X1	T44.3X2	T44.3X3	T44.3X4	T44.3X5	T44.3X6
Producer gas	T58.8X1	T58.8X2	T58.8X3	T58.8X4	—	—
Profadol	T40.4X1	T40.4X2	T40.4X3	T40.4X4	T40.4X5	T40.4X6
Profenamine	T44.3X1	T44.3X2	T44.3X3	T44.3X4	T44.3X5	T44.3X6
Profenil	T44.3X1	T44.3X2	T44.3X3	T44.3X4	T44.3X5	T44.3X6
Proflavine	T49.0X1	T49.0X2	T49.0X3	T49.0X4	T49.0X5	T49.0X6
Progabide	T42.6X1	T42.6X2	T42.6X3	T42.6X4	T42.6X5	T42.6X6
Progesterone	T38.5X1	T38.5X2	T38.5X3	T38.5X4	T38.5X5	T38.5X6
Progestin	T38.5X1	T38.5X2	T38.5X3	T38.5X4	T38.5X5	T38.5X6
oral contraceptive	T38.4X1	T38.4X2	T38.4X3	T38.4X4	T38.4X5	T38.4X6
Progestogen NEC	T38.5X1	T38.5X2	T38.5X3	T38.5X4	T38.5X5	T38.5X6
Progestone	T38.5X1	T38.5X2	T38.5X3	T38.5X4	T38.5X5	T38.5X6

Substance	Poisoning, Accidental (unintentional)	Poisoning, Intentional self-harm	Poisoning, Assault	Poisoning, Undetermined	Adverse effect	Underdosing
Proglumide	T47.1X1	T47.1X2	T47.1X3	T47.1X4	T47.1X5	T47.1X6
Proguanil	T37.2X1	T37.2X2	T37.2X3	T37.2X4	T37.2X5	T37.2X6
Prolactin	T38.811	T38.812	T38.813	T38.814	T38.815	T38.816
Prolintane	T43.691	T43.692	T43.693	T43.694	T43.695	T43.696
Proloid	T38.1X1	T38.1X2	T38.1X3	T38.1X4	T38.1X5	T38.1X6
Proluton	T38.5X1	T38.5X2	T38.5X3	T38.5X4	T38.5X5	T38.5X6
Promacetin	T37.1X1	T37.1X2	T37.1X3	T37.1X4	T37.1X5	T37.1X6
Promazine	T43.3X1	T43.3X2	T43.3X3	T43.3X4	T43.3X5	T43.3X6
Promedol	T40.2X1	T40.2X2	T40.2X3	T40.2X4	—	—
Promegestone	T38.5X1	T38.5X2	T38.5X3	T38.5X4	T38.5X5	T38.5X6
Promethazine (teoclate)	T43.3X1	T43.3X2	T43.3X3	T43.3X4	T43.3X5	T43.3X6
Promin	T37.1X1	T37.1X2	T37.1X3	T37.1X4	T37.1X5	T37.1X6
Pronase	T45.3X1	T45.3X2	T45.3X3	T45.3X4	T45.3X5	T45.3X6
Pronestyl (hydrochloride)	T46.2X1	T46.2X2	T46.2X3	T46.2X4	T46.2X5	T46.2X6
Pronetalol	T44.7X1	T44.7X2	T44.7X3	T44.7X4	T44.7X5	T44.7X6
Prontosil	T37.0X1	T37.0X2	T37.0X3	T37.0X4	T37.0X5	T37.0X6
Propachlor	T60.3X1	T60.3X2	T60.3X3	T60.3X4	—	—
Propafenone	T46.2X1	T46.2X2	T46.2X3	T46.2X4	T46.2X5	T46.2X6
Propallylonal	T42.3X1	T42.3X2	T42.3X3	T42.3X4	T42.3X5	T42.3X6
Propamidine	T49.0X1	T49.0X2	T49.0X3	T49.0X4	T49.0X5	T49.0X6
Propane (distributed in mobile container)	T59.891	T59.892	T59.893	T59.894	—	—
distributed through pipes	T59.891	T59.892	T59.893	T59.894	—	—
incomplete combustion	T58.11	T58.12	T58.13	T58.14	—	—
Propanidid	T41.291	T41.292	T41.293	T41.294	T41.295	T41.296
Propanil	T60.3X1	T60.3X2	T60.3X3	T60.3X4	—	—
1-Propanol	T51.3X1	T51.3X2	T51.3X3	T51.3X4	—	—
2-Propanol	T51.2X1	T51.2X2	T51.2X3	T51.2X4	—	—
Propantheline	T44.3X1	T44.3X2	T44.3X3	T44.3X4	T44.3X5	T44.3X6
bromide	I44.3X1	I44.3X2	I44.3X3	I44.3X4	I44.3X5	I44.3X6
Proparacaine	T41.3X1	T41.3X2	T41.3X3	T41.3X4	T41.3X5	T41.3X6
Propatylnitrate	T46.3X1	T46.3X2	T46.3X3	T46.3X4	T46.3X5	T46.3X6
Propicillin	T36.0X1	T36.0X2	T36.0X3	T36.0X4	T36.0X5	T36.0X6
Propiolactone	T49.0X1	T49.0X2	T49.0X3	T49.0X4	T49.0X5	T49.0X6
Propiomazine	T45.0X1	T45.0X2	T45.0X3	T45.0X4	T45.0X5	T45.0X6
Propionaldehyde (medicinal)	T42.6X1	T42.6X2	T42.6X3	T42.6X4	T42.6X5	T42.6X6
Propionate (calcium) (sodium)	T49.0X1	T49.0X2	T49.0X3	T49.0X4	T49.0X5	T49.0X6
Propion gel	T49.0X1	T49.0X2	T49.0X3	T49.0X4	T49.0X5	T49.0X6
Propitocaine	T41.3X1	T41.3X2	T41.3X3	T41.3X4	T41.3X5	T41.3X6
infiltration (subcutaneous)	T41.3X1	T41.3X2	T41.3X3	T41.3X4	T41.3X5	T41.3X6
nerve block (peripheral) (plexus)	T41.3X1	T41.3X2	T41.3X3	T41.3X4	T41.3X5	T41.3X6
Propofol	T41.291	T41.292	T41.293	T41.294	T41.295	T41.296
Propoxur	T60.0X1	T60.0X2	T60.0X3	T60.0X4	—	—
Propoxycaine	T41.3X1	T41.3X2	T41.3X3	T41.3X4	T41.3X5	T41.3X6
infiltration (subcutaneous)	T41.3X1	T41.3X2	T41.3X3	T41.3X4	T41.3X5	T41.3X6
nerve block (peripheral) (plexus)	T41.3X1	T41.3X2	T41.3X3	T41.3X4	T41.3X5	T41.3X6
topical (surface)	T41.3X1	T41.3X2	T41.3X3	T41.3X4	T41.3X5	T41.3X6
Propoxyphene	T40.4X1	T40.4X2	T40.4X3	T40.4X4	T40.4X5	T40.4X6
Propranolol	T44.7X1	T44.7X2	T44.7X3	T44.7X4	T44.7X5	T44.7X6
Propyl						
alcohol	T51.3X1	T51.3X2	T51.3X3	T51.3X4	—	—
carbinol	T51.3X1	T51.3X2	T51.3X3	T51.3X4	—	—
hexadrine	T44.4X1	T44.4X2	T44.4X3	T44.4X4	T44.4X5	T44.4X6
iodone	T50.8X1	T50.8X2	T50.8X3	T50.8X4	T50.8X5	T50.8X6
thiouracil	T38.2X1	T38.2X2	T38.2X3	T38.2X4	T38.2X5	T38.2X6

Substance	Poisoning, Accidental (unintentional)	Poisoning, Intentional self-harm	Poisoning, Assault	Poisoning, Undetermined	Adverse effect	Underdosing
Propylaminopheno-thiazine	T43.3X1	T43.3X2	T43.3X3	T43.3X4	T43.3X5	T43.3X6
Propylene	T59.891	T59.892	T59.893	T59.894	—	—
Propylhexedrine	T48.5X1	T48.5X2	T48.5X3	T48.5X4	T48.5X5	T48.5X6
Propyliodone	T50.8X1	T50.8X2	T50.8X3	T50.8X4	T50.8X5	T50.8X6
Propylparaben (ophthalmic)	T49.5X1	T49.5X2	T49.5X3	T49.5X4	T49.5X5	T49.5X6
Propylthiouracil	T38.2X1	T38.2X2	T38.2X3	T38.2X4	T38.2X5	T38.2X6
Propyphenazone	T39.2X1	T39.2X2	T39.2X3	T39.2X4	T39.2X5	T39.2X6
Proquazone	T39.391	T39.392	T39.393	T39.394	T39.395	T39.396
Proscillaridin	T46.0X1	T46.0X2	T46.0X3	T46.0X4	T46.0X5	T46.0X6
Prostacyclin	T45.521	T45.522	T45.523	T45.524	T45.525	T45.526
Prostaglandin (I2)	T45.521	T45.522	T45.523	T45.524	T45.525	T45.526
E1	T46.7X1	T46.7X2	T46.7X3	T46.7X4	T46.7X5	T46.7X6
E2	T48.0X1	T48.0X2	T48.0X3	T48.0X4	T48.0X5	T48.0X6
F2 alpha	T48.0X1	T48.0X2	T48.0X3	T48.0X4	T48.0X5	T48.0X6
Prostigmin	T44.0X1	T44.0X2	T44.0X3	T44.0X4	T44.0X5	T44.0X6
Prosultiamine	T45.2X1	T45.2X2	T45.2X3	T45.2X4	T45.2X5	T45.2X6
Protamine sulfate	T45.7X1	T45.7X2	T45.7X3	T45.7X4	T45.7X5	T45.7X6
zinc insulin	T38.3X1	T38.3X2	T38.3X3	T38.3X4	T38.3X5	T38.3X6
Protease	T47.5X1	T47.5X2	T47.5X3	T47.5X4	T47.5X5	T47.5X6
Protectant, skin NEC	T49.3X1	T49.3X2	T49.3X3	T49.3X4	T49.3X5	T49.3X6
Protein hydrolysate	T50.991	T50.992	T50.993	T50.994	T50.995	T50.996
Prothiaden—see Dothiepin hydrochloride						
Prothionamide	T37.1X1	T37.1X2	T37.1X3	T37.1X4	T37.1X5	T37.1X6
Prothipendyl	T43.591	T43.592	T43.593	T43.594	T43.595	T43.596
Prothoate	T60.0X1	T60.0X2	T60.0X3	T60.0X4	—	—
Prothrombin						
activator	T45.7X1	T45.7X2	T45.7X3	T45.7X4	T45.7X5	T45.7X6
synthesis inhibitor	T45.511	T45.512	T45.513	T45.514	T45.515	T45.516
Protionamide	T37.1X1	T37.1X2	T37.1X3	T37.1X4	T37.1X5	T37.1X6
Protirelin	T38.891	T38.892	T38.893	T38.894	T38.895	T38.896
Protokylol	T48.6X1	T48.6X2	T48.6X3	T48.6X4	T48.6X5	T48.6X6
Protopam	T50.6X1	T50.6X2	T50.6X3	T50.6X4	T50.6X5	T50.6X6
Protoveratrine (s) (A) (B)	T46.5X1	T46.5X2	T46.5X3	T46.5X4	T46.5X5	T46.5X6
Protriptyline	T43.011	T43.012	T43.013	T43.014	T43.015	T43.016
Provera	T38.5X1	T38.5X2	T38.5X3	T38.5X4	T38.5X5	T38.5X6
Provitamin A	T45.2X1	T45.2X2	T45.2X3	T45.2X4	T45.2X5	T45.2X6
Proxibarbal	T42.3X1	T42.3X2	T42.3X3	T42.3X4	T42.3X5	T42.3X6
Proxymetacaine	T41.3X1	T41.3X2	T41.3X3	T41.3X4	T41.3X5	T41.3X6
Proxyphylline	T48.6X1	T48.6X2	T48.6X3	T48.6X4	T48.6X5	T48.6X6
Prozac—see Fluoxetine hydrochloride						
Prunus						
laurocerasus	T62.2X1	T62.2X2	T62.2X3	T62.2X4	—	—
virginiana	T62.2X1	T62.2X2	T62.2X3	T62.2X4	—	—
Prussian blue						
commercial	T65.891	T65.892	T65.893	T65.894	—	—
therapeutic	T50.6X1	T50.6X2	T50.6X3	T50.6X4	T50.6X5	T50.6X6
Prussic acid	T65.0X1	T65.0X2	T65.0X3	T65.0X4	—	—
vapor	T57.3X1	T57.3X2	T57.3X3	T57.3X4	—	—
Pseudoephedrine	T44.991	T44.992	T44.993	T44.994	T44.995	T44.996
Psilocin	T40.991	T40.992	T40.993	T40.994	—	—
Psilocybin	T40.991	T40.992	T40.993	T40.994	—	—
Psilocybine	T40.991	T40.992	T40.993	T40.994	—	—
Psoralene (nonmedicinal)	T65.891	T65.892	T65.893	T65.894	—	—
Psoralens (medicinal)	T50.991	T50.992	T50.993	T50.994	T50.995	T50.996
PSP (phenolsulfonphthalein)	T50.8X1	T50.8X2	T50.8X3	T50.8X4	T50.8X5	T50.8X6
Psychodysleptic drug NEC	T40.901	T40.902	T40.903	T40.904	T40.905	T40.906

Substance	Poisoning, Accidental (unintentional)	Poisoning, Intentional self-harm	Poisoning, Assault	Poisoning, Undetermined	Adverse effect	Underdosing
Psychostimulant	T43.601	T43.602	T43.603	T43.604	T43.605	T43.606
amphetamine	T43.621	T43.622	T43.623	T43.624	T43.625	T43.626
caffeine	T43.611	T43.612	T43.613	T43.614	T43.615	T43.616
methylphenidate	T43.631	T43.632	T43.633	T43.634	T43.635	T43.636
specified NEC	T43.691	T43.692	T43.693	T43.694	T43.695	T43.696
Psychotherapeutic drug NEC	T43.91	T43.92	T43.93	T43.94	T43.95	T43.96
antidepressants—see also Antidepressant	T43.201	T43.202	T43.203	T43.204	T43.205	T43.206
specified NEC	T43.8X1	T43.8X2	T43.8X3	T43.8X4	T43.8X5	T43.8X6
tranquilizers NEC	T43.501	T43.502	T43.503	T43.504	T43.505	T43.506
Psychotomimetic agents	T40.901	T40.902	T40.903	T40.904	T40.905	T40.906
Psychotropic drug NEC	T43.91	T43.92	T43.93	T43.94	T43.95	T43.96
specified NEC	T43.8X1	T43.8X2	T43.8X3	T43.8X4	T43.8X5	T43.8X6
Psyllium hydrophilic mucilloid	T47.4X1	T47.4X2	T47.4X3	T47.4X4	T47.4X5	T47.4X6
Pteroylglutamic acid	T45.8X1	T45.8X2	T45.8X3	T45.8X4	T45.8X5	T45.8X6
Pteroyltriglutamate	T45.1X1	T45.1X2	T45.1X3	T45.1X4	T45.1X5	T45.1X6
PTFE—see Polytetrafluoroethylene						
Pulp						
devitalizing paste	T49.7X1	T49.7X2	T49.7X3	T49.7X4	T49.7X5	T49.7X6
dressing	T49.7X1	T49.7X2	T49.7X3	T49.7X4	T49.7X5	T49.7X6
Pulsatilla	T62.2X1	T62.2X2	T62.2X3	T62.2X4	—	—
Pumpkin seed extract	T37.4X1	T37.4X2	T37.4X3	T37.4X4	T37.4X5	T37.4X6
Purex (bleach)	T54.91	T54.92	T54.93	T54.94		
Purgative NEC—see also Cathartic	T47.4X1	T47.4X2	T47.4X3	T47.4X4	T47.4X5	T47.4X6
Purine analogue (antineoplastic)	T45.1X1	T45.1X2	T45.1X3	T45.1X4	T45.1X5	T45.1X6
Purine diuretics	T50.2X1	T50.2X2	T50.2X3	T50.2X4	T50.2X5	T50.2X6
Purinethol	T45.1X1	T45.1X2	T45.1X3	T45.1X4	T45.1X5	T45.1X6
PVP	T45.8X1	T45.8X2	T45.8X3	T45.8X4	T45.8X5	T45.8X6
Pyrabital	T39.8X1	T39.8X2	T39.8X3	T39.8X4	T39.8X5	T39.8X6
Pyramidon	T39.2X1	T39.2X2	T39.2X3	T39.2X4	T39.2X5	T39.2X6
Pyrantel	T37.4X1	T37.4X2	T37.4X3	T37.4X4	T37.4X5	T37.4X6
Pyrathiazine	T45.0X1	T45.0X2	T45.0X3	T45.0X4	T45.0X5	T45.0X6
Pyrazinamide	T37.1X1	T37.1X2	T37.1X3	T37.1X4	T37.1X5	T37.1X6
Pyrazinoic acid (amide)	T37.1X1	T37.1X2	T37.1X3	T37.1X4	T37.1X5	T37.1X6
Pyrazole (derivatives)	T39.2X1	T39.2X2	T39.2X3	T39.2X4	T39.2X5	T39.2X6
Pyrazolone analgesic NEC	T39.2X1	T39.2X2	T39.2X3	T39.2X4	T39.2X5	T39.2X6
Pyrethrin, pyrethrum (nonmedicinal)	T60.2X1	T60.2X2	T60.2X3	T60.2X4	—	—
Pyrethrum extract	T49.0X1	T49.0X2	T49.0X3	T49.0X4	T49.0X5	T49.0X6
Pyribenzamine	T45.0X1	T45.0X2	T45.0X3	T45.0X4	T45.0X5	T45.0X6
Pyridine	T52.8X1	T52.8X2	T52.8X3	T52.8X4		
aldoxime methiodide	T50.6X1	T50.6X2	T50.6X3	T50.6X4	T50.6X5	T50.6X6
aldoxime methyl chloride	T50.6X1	T50.6X2	T50.6X3	T50.6X4	T50.6X5	T50.6X6
vapor	T59.891	T59.892	T59.893	T59.894	—	—
Pyridium	T39.8X1	T39.8X2	T39.8X3	T39.8X4	T39.8X5	T39.8X6
Pyridostigmine bromide	T44.0X1	T44.0X2	T44.0X3	T44.0X4	T44.0X5	T44.0X6
Pyridoxal phosphate	T45.2X1	T45.2X2	T45.2X3	T45.2X4	T45.2X5	T45.2X6
Pyridoxine	T45.2X1	T45.2X2	T45.2X3	T45.2X4	T45.2X5	T45.2X6
Pyrilamine	T45.0X1	T45.0X2	T45.0X3	T45.0X4	T45.0X5	T45.0X6
Pyrimethamine	T37.2X1	T37.2X2	T37.2X3	T37.2X4	T37.2X5	T37.2X6
with sulfadoxine	T37.2X1	T37.2X2	T37.2X3	T37.2X4	T37.2X5	T37.2X6
Pyrimidine antagonist	T45.1X1	T45.1X2	T45.1X3	T45.1X4	T45.1X5	T45.1X6
Pyriminil	T60.4X1	T60.4X2	T60.4X3	T60.4X4	—	—
Pyrithione zinc	T49.4X1	T49.4X2	T49.4X3	T49.4X4	I49.4X5	I49.4X6
Pyrithyldione	T42.6X1	T42.6X2	T42.6X3	T42.6X4	T42.6X5	T42.6X6

Substance	Poisoning, Accidental (unintentional)	Poisoning, Intentional self-harm	Poisoning, Assault	Poisoning, Undetermined	Adverse effect	Underdosing
Pyrogallic acid	T49.0X1	T49.0X2	T49.0X3	T49.0X4	T49.0X5	T49.0X6
Pyrogallol	T49.0X1	T49.0X2	T49.0X3	T49.0X4	T49.0X5	T49.0X6
Pyroxylin	T49.3X1	T49.3X2	T49.3X3	T49.3X4	T49.3X5	T49.3X6
Pyrrobutamine	T45.0X1	T45.0X2	T45.0X3	T45.0X4	T45.0X5	T45.0X6
Pyrrolizidine alkaloids	T62.8X1	T62.8X2	T62.8X3	T62.8X4	—	—
Pyrvinium chloride	T37.4X1	T37.4X2	T37.4X3	T37.4X4	T37.4X5	T37.4X6
PZI	T38.3X1	T38.3X2	T38.3X3	T38.3X4	T38.3X5	T38.3X6
Q						
Quaalude	T42.6X1	T42.6X2	T42.6X3	T42.6X4	T42.6X5	T42.6X6
Quarternary ammonium						
anti-infective	T49.0X1	T49.0X2	T49.0X3	T49.0X4	T49.0X5	T49.0X6
ganglion blocking	T44.2X1	T44.2X2	T44.2X3	T44.2X4	T44.2X5	T44.2X6
parasympatholytic	T44.3X1	T44.3X2	T44.3X3	T44.3X4	T44.3X5	T44.3X6
Quazepam	T42.4X1	T42.4X2	T42.4X3	T42.4X4	T42.4X5	T42.4X6
Quicklime	T54.3X1	T54.3X2	T54.3X3	T54.3X4	—	—
Quillaja extract	T48.4X1	T48.4X2	T48.4X3	T48.4X4	T48.4X5	T48.4X6
Quinacrine	T37.2X1	T37.2X2	T37.2X3	T37.2X4	T37.2X5	T37.2X6
Quinaglute	T46.2X1	T46.2X2	T46.2X3	T46.2X4	T46.2X5	T46.2X6
Quinalbarbital	T42.3X1	T42.3X2	T42.3X3	T42.3X4	T42.3X5	T42.3X6
Quinalbarbitone sodium	T42.3X1	T42.3X2	T42.3X3	T42.3X4	T42.3X5	T42.3X6
Quinalphos	T60.0X1	T60.0X2	T60.0X3	T60.0X4		
Quinapril	T46.4X1	T46.4X2	T46.4X3	T46.4X4	T46.4X5	T46.4X6
Quinestradiol	T38.5X1	T38.5X2	T38.5X3	T38.5X4	T38.5X5	T38.5X6
Quinestradol	T38.5X1	T38.5X2	T38.5X3	T38.5X4	T38.5X5	T38.5X6
Quinestrol	T38.5X1	T38.5X2	T38.5X3	T38.5X4	T38.5X5	T38.5X6
Quinethazone	T50.2X1	T50.2X2	T50.2X3	T50.2X4	T50.2X5	T50.2X6
Quingestanol	T38.4X1	T38.4X2	T38.4X3	T38.4X4	T38.4X5	T38.4X6
Quinidine	T46.2X1	T46.2X2	T46.2X3	T46.2X4	T46.2X5	T46.2X6
Quinine	T37.2X1	T37.2X2	T37.2X3	T37.2X4	T37.2X5	T37.2X6
Quiniobine	T37.8X1	T37.8X2	T37.8X3	T37.8X4	T37.8X5	T37.8X6
Quinisocaine	T49.1X1	T49.1X2	T49.1X3	T49.1X4	T49.1X5	T49.1X6
Quinocide	T37.2X1	T37.2X2	T37.2X3	T37.2X4	T37.2X5	T37.2X6
Quinoline (derivatives) NEC	T37.8X1	T37.8X2	T37.8X3	T37.8X4	T37.8X5	T37.8X6
Quinupramine	T43.011	T43.012	T43.013	T43.014	T43.015	T43.016
Quotane	T41.3X1	T41.3X2	T41.3X3	T41.3X4	T41.3X5	T41.3X6
R						
Rabies						
immune globulin (human)	T50.Z11	T50.Z12	T50.Z13	T50.Z14	T50.Z15	T50.Z16
vaccine	T50.B91	T50.B92	T50.B93	T50.B94	T50.B95	T50.B96
Racemoramide	T40.2X1	T40.2X2	T40.2X3	T40.2X4		
Racemorphan	T40.2X1	T40.2X2	T40.2X3	T40.2X4	T40.2X5	T40.2X6
Racepinefrin	T44.5X1	T44.5X2	T44.5X3	T44.5X4	T44.5X5	T44.5X6
Raclopride	T43.591	T43.592	T43.593	T43.594	T43.595	T43.596
Radiator alcohol	T51.1X1	T51.1X2	T51.1X3	T51.1X4		
Radioactive drug NEC	T50.8X1	T50.8X2	T50.8X3	T50.8X4	T50.8X5	T50.8X6
Radio-opaque (drugs) (materials)	T50.8X1	T50.8X2	T50.8X3	T50.8X4	T50.8X5	T50.8X6
Ramifenazone	T39.2X1	T39.2X2	T39.2X3	T39.2X4	T39.2X5	T39.2X6
Ramipril	T46.4X1	T46.4X2	T46.4X3	T46.4X4	T46.4X5	T46.4X6
Ranitidine	T47.0X1	T47.0X2	T47.0X3	T47.0X4	T47.0X5	T47.0X6
Ranunculus	T62.2X1	T62.2X2	T62.2X3	T62.2X4	—	—
Rat poison NEC	T60.4X1	T60.4X2	T60.4X3	T60.4X4	—	—
Rattlesnake (venom)	T63.011	T63.012	T63.013	T63.014	—	—
Raubasine	T46.7X1	T46.7X2	T46.7X3	T46.7X4	T46.7X5	T46.7X6
Raudixin	T46.5X1	T46.5X2	T46.5X3	T46.5X4	T46.5X5	T46.5X6
Rautensin	T46.5X1	T46.5X2	T46.5X3	T46.5X4	T46.5X5	T46.5X6
Rautina	T46.5X1	T46.5X2	T46.5X3	T46.5X4	T46.5X5	T46.5X6
Rautotal	T46.5X1	T46.5X2	T46.5X3	T46.5X4	T46.5X5	T46.5X6
Rauwiloid	T46.5X1	T46.5X2	T46.5X3	T46.5X4	T46.5X5	T46.5X6

Substance	Poisoning, Accidental (unintentional)	Poisoning, Intentional self-harm	Poisoning, Assault	Poisoning, Undetermined	Adverse effect	Underdosing
Rauwoldin	T46.5X1	T46.5X2	T46.5X3	T46.5X4	T46.5X5	T46.5X6
Rauwolfia (alkaloids)	T46.5X1	T46.5X2	T46.5X3	T46.5X4	T46.5X5	T46.5X6
Razoxane	T45.1X1	T45.1X2	T45.1X3	T45.1X4	T45.1X5	T45.1X6
Realgar	T57.0X1	T57.0X2	T57.0X3	T57.0X4	—	—
Recombinant (R)—*see specific protein*						
Red blood cells, packed	T45.8X1	T45.8X2	T45.8X3	T45.8X4	T45.8X5	T45.8X6
Red squill (scilliroside)	T60.4X1	T60.4X2	T60.4X3	T60.4X4	—	—
Reducing agent, industrial NEC	T65.891	T65.892	T65.893	T65.894	—	—
Refrigerant gas (chlorofluoro-carbon)	T53.5X1	T53.5X2	T53.5X3	T53.5X4	—	—
not chlorofluoro-carbon	T59.891	T59.892	T59.893	T59.894	—	—
Regroton	T50.2X1	T50.2X2	T50.2X3	T50.2X4	T50.2X5	T50.2X6
Rehydration salts (oral)	T50.3X1	T50.3X2	T50.3X3	T50.3X4	T50.3X5	T50.3X6
Rela	T42.8X1	T42.8X2	T42.8X3	T42.8X4	T42.8X5	T42.8X6
Relaxant, muscle						
anesthetic	T48.1X1	T48.1X2	T48.1X3	T48.1X4	T48.1X5	T48.1X6
central nervous system	T42.8X1	T42.8X2	T42.8X3	T42.8X4	T42.8X5	T42.8X6
skeletal NEC	T48.1X1	T48.1X2	T48.1X3	T48.1X4	T48.1X5	T48.1X6
smooth NEC	T44.3X1	T44.3X2	T44.3X3	T44.3X4	T44.3X5	T44.3X6
Remoxipride	T43.591	T43.592	T43.593	T43.594	T43.595	T43.596
Renese	T50.2X1	T50.2X2	T50.2X3	T50.2X4	T50.2X5	T50.2X6
Renografin	T50.8X1	T50.8X2	T50.8X3	T50.8X4	T50.8X5	T50.8X6
Replacement solution	T50.3X1	T50.3X2	T50.3X3	T50.3X4	T50.3X5	T50.3X6
Reproterol	T48.6X1	T48.6X2	T48.6X3	T48.6X4	T48.6X5	T48.6X6
Rescinnamine	T46.5X1	T46.5X2	T46.5X3	T46.5X4	T46.5X5	T46.5X6
Reserpin (e)	T46.5X1	T46.5X2	T46.5X3	T46.5X4	T46.5X5	T46.5X6
Resorcin, resorcinol (nonmedicinal)	T65.891	T65.892	T65.893	T65.894	—	—
medicinal	T49.4X1	T49.4X2	T49.4X3	T49.4X4	T49.4X5	T49.4X6
Respaire	T48.4X1	T48.4X2	T48.4X3	T48.4X4	T48.4X5	T48.4X6
Respiratory drug NEC	T48.901	T48.902	T48.903	T48.904	T48.905	T48.906
antiasthmatic NEC	T48.6X1	T48.6X2	T48.6X3	T48.6X4	T48.6X5	T48.6X6
anti-common-cold NEC	T48.5X1	T48.5X2	T48.5X3	T48.5X4	T48.5X5	T48.5X6
expectorant NEC	T48.4X1	T48.4X2	T48.4X3	T48.4X4	T48.4X5	T48.4X6
stimulant	T48.901	T48.902	T48.903	T48.904	T48.905	T48.906
Retinoic acid	T49.0X1	T49.0X2	T49.0X3	T49.0X4	T49.0X5	T49.0X6
Retinol	T45.2X1	T45.2X2	T45.2X3	T45.2X4	T45.2X5	T45.2X6
Rh (D) immune globulin (human)	T50.Z11	T50.Z12	T50.Z13	T50.Z14	T50.Z15	T50.Z16
Rhodine	T39.011	T39.012	T39.013	T39.014	T39.015	T39.016
RhoGAM	T50.Z11	T50.Z12	T50.Z13	T50.Z14	T50.Z15	T50.Z16
Rhubarb						
dry extract	T47.2X1	T47.2X2	T47.2X3	T47.2X4	T47.2X5	T47.2X6
tincture, compound	T47.2X1	T47.2X2	T47.2X3	T47.2X4	T47.2X5	T47.2X6
Ribavirin	T37.5X1	T37.5X2	T37.5X3	T37.5X4	T37.5X5	T37.5X6
Riboflavin	T45.2X1	T45.2X2	T45.2X3	T45.2X4	T45.2X5	T45.2X6
Ribostamycin	T36.5X1	T36.5X2	T36.5X3	T36.5X4	T36.5X5	T36.5X6
Ricin	T62.2X1	T62.2X2	T62.2X3	T62.2X4	—	—
Ricinus communis	T62.2X1	T62.2X2	T62.2X3	T62.2X4	—	—
Rickettsial vaccine NEC	T50.A91	T50.A92	T50.A93	T50.A94	T50.A95	T50.A96
Rifabutin	T36.6X1	T36.6X2	T36.6X3	T36.6X4	T36.6X5	T36.6X6
Rifamide	T36.6X1	T36.6X2	T36.6X3	T36.6X4	T36.6X5	T36.6X6
Rifampicin	T36.6X1	T36.6X2	T36.6X3	T36.6X4	T36.6X5	T36.6X6
with isoniazid	T37.1X1	T37.1X2	T37.1X3	T37.1X4	T37.1X5	T37.1X6
Rifampin	T36.6X1	T36.6X2	T36.6X3	T36.6X4	T36.6X5	T36.6X6
Rifamycin	T36.6X1	T36.6X2	T36.6X3	T36.6X4	T36.6X5	T36.6X6
Rifaximin	T36.6X1	T36.6X2	T36.6X3	T36.6X4	T36.6X5	T36.6X6
Rimantadine	T37.5X1	T37.5X2	T37.5X3	T37.5X4	T37.5X5	T37.5X6
Rimazolium metilsulfate	T39.8X1	T39.8X2	T39.8X3	T39.8X4	T39.8X5	T39.8X6

Substance	Poisoning, Accidental (unintentional)	Poisoning, Intentional self-harm	Poisoning, Assault	Poisoning, Undetermined	Adverse effect	Underdosing
Rimifon	T37.1X1	T37.1X2	T37.1X3	T37.1X4	T37.1X5	T37.1X6
Rimiterol	T48.6X1	T48.6X2	T48.6X3	T48.6X4	T48.6X5	T48.6X6
Ringer (lactate) solution	T50.3X1	T50.3X2	T50.3X3	T50.3X4	T50.3X5	T50.3X6
Ristocetin	T36.8X1	T36.8X2	T36.8X3	T36.8X4	T36.8X5	T36.8X6
Ritalin	T43.631	T43.632	T43.633	T43.634	T43.635	T43.636
Ritodrine	T44.5X1	T44.5X2	T44.5X3	T44.5X4	T44.5X5	T44.5X6
Roach killer—*see Insecticide*						
Rociverine	T44.3X1	T44.3X2	T44.3X3	T44.3X4	T44.3X5	T44.3X6
Rocky Mountain spotted fever vaccine	T50.A91	T50.A92	T50.A93	T50.A94	T50.A95	T50.A96
Rodenticide NEC	T60.4X1	T60.4X2	T60.4X3	T60.4X4	—	—
Rohypnol	T42.4X1	T42.4X2	T42.4X3	T42.4X4	T42.4X5	T42.4X6
Rokitamycin	T36.3X1	T36.3X2	T36.3X3	T36.3X4	T36.3X5	T36.3X6
Rolaids	T47.1X1	T47.1X2	T47.1X3	T47.1X4	T47.1X5	T47.1X6
Rolitetracycline	T36.4X1	T36.4X2	T36.4X3	T36.4X4	T36.4X5	T36.4X6
Romilar	T48.3X1	T48.3X2	T48.3X3	T48.3X4	T48.3X5	T48.3X6
Ronifibrate	T46.6X1	T46.6X2	T46.6X3	T46.6X4	T46.6X5	T46.6X6
Rosaprostol	T47.1X1	T47.1X2	T47.1X3	T47.1X4	T47.1X5	T47.1X6
Rose bengal sodium (131I)	T50.8X1	T50.8X2	T50.8X3	T50.8X4	T50.8X5	T50.8X6
Rose water ointment	T49.3X1	T49.3X2	T49.3X3	T49.3X4	T49.3X5	T49.3X6
Rosoxacin	T37.8X1	T37.8X2	T37.8X3	T37.8X4	T37.8X5	T37.8X6
Rotenone	T60.2X1	T60.2X2	T60.2X3	T60.2X4	—	—
Rotoxamine	T45.0X1	T45.0X2	T45.0X3	T45.0X4	T45.0X5	T45.0X6
Rough-on-rats	T60.4X1	T60.4X2	T60.4X3	T60.4X4	—	—
Roxatidine	T47.0X1	T47.0X2	T47.0X3	T47.0X4	T47.0X5	T47.0X6
Roxithromycin	T36.3X1	T36.3X2	T36.3X3	T36.3X4	T36.3X5	T36.3X6
Rt-PA	T45.611	T45.612	T45.613	T45.614	T45.615	T45.616
Rubbing alcohol	T51.2X1	T51.2X2	T51.2X3	T51.2X4	—	—
Rubefacient	T49.4X1	T49.4X2	T49.4X3	T49.4X4	T49.4X5	T49.4X6
Rubella vaccine	T50.B91	T50.B92	T50.B93	T50.B94	T50.B95	T50.B96
Rubeola vaccine	T50.B91	T50.B92	T50.B93	T50.B94	T50.B95	T50.B96
Rubidium chloride Rb82	T50.8X1	T50.8X2	T50.8X3	T50.8X4	T50.8X5	T50.8X6
Rubidomycin	T45.1X1	T45.1X2	T45.1X3	T45.1X4	T45.1X5	T45.1X6
Rue	T62.2X1	T62.2X2	T62.2X3	T62.2X4	—	—
Rufocromomycin	T45.1X1	T45.1X2	T45.1X3	T45.1X4	T45.1X5	T45.1X6
Russel's viper venin	T45.7X1	T45.7X2	T45.7X3	T45.7X4	T45.7X5	T45.7X6
Ruta (graveolens)	T62.2X1	T62.2X2	T62.2X3	T62.2X4	—	—
Rutinum	T46.991	T46.992	T46.993	T46.994	T46.995	T46.996
Rutoside	T46.991	T46.992	T46.993	T46.994	T46.995	T46.996
S						
Sabadilla (plant)	T62.2X1	T62.2X2	T62.2X3	T62.2X4	—	—
pesticide	T60.2X1	T60.2X2	T60.2X3	T60.2X4	—	—
Saccharated iron oxide	T45.8X1	T45.8X2	T45.8X3	T45.8X4	T45.8X5	T45.8X6
Saccharin	T50.901	T50.902	T50.903	T50.904	T50.905	T50.906
Saccharomyces boulardii	T47.6X1	T47.6X2	T47.6X3	T47.6X4	T47.6X5	T47.6X6
Safflower oil	T46.6X1	T46.6X2	T46.6X3	T46.6X4	T46.6X5	T46.6X6
Safrazine	T43.1X1	T43.1X2	T43.1X3	T43.1X4	T43.1X5	T43.1X6
Salazosulfapyridine	T37.0X1	T37.0X2	T37.0X3	T37.0X4	T37.0X5	T37.0X6
Salbutamol	T48.6X1	T48.6X2	T48.6X3	T48.6X4	T48.6X5	T48.6X6
Salicylamide	T39.091	T39.092	T39.093	T39.094	T39.095	T39.096
Salicylate NEC	T39.091	T39.092	T39.093	T39.094	T39.095	T39.096
methyl	T49.3X1	T49.3X2	T49.3X3	T49.3X4	T49.3X5	T49.3X6
theobromine calcium	T50.2X1	T50.2X2	T50.2X3	T50.2X4	T50.2X5	T50.2X6
Salicylazosulfapyridine	T37.0X1	T37.0X2	T37.0X3	T37.0X4	T37.0X5	T37.0X6
Salicylhydroxamic acid	T49.0X1	T49.0X2	T49.0X3	T49.0X4	T49.0X5	T49.0X6
Salicylic acid	T49.4X1	T49.4X2	T49.4X3	T49.4X4	T49.4X5	T49.4X6
with benzoic acid	T49.4X1	T49.4X2	T49.4X3	T49.4X4	T49.4X5	T49.4X6
congeners	T39.091	T39.092	T39.093	T39.094	T39.095	T39.096
derivative	T39.091	T39.092	T39.093	T39.094	T39.095	T39.096
salts	T39.091	T39.092	T39.093	T39.094	T39.095	T39.096

Substance	Poisoning, Accidental (unintentional)	Poisoning, Intentional self-harm	Poisoning, Assault	Poisoning, Undetermined	Adverse effect	Underdosing
Salinazid	T37.1X1	T37.1X2	T37.1X3	T37.1X4	T37.1X5	T37.1X6
Salmeterol	T48.6X1	T48.6X2	T48.6X3	T48.6X4	T48.6X5	T48.6X6
Salol	T49.3X1	T49.3X2	T49.3X3	T49.3X4	T49.3X5	T49.3X6
Salsalate	T39.091	T39.092	T39.093	T39.094	T39.095	T39.096
Salt substitute	T50.901	T50.902	T50.903	T50.904	T50.905	T50.906
Salt-replacing drug	T50.901	T50.902	T50.903	T50.904	T50.905	T50.906
Salt-retaining mineralocorticoid	T50.0X1	T50.0X2	T50.0X3	T50.0X4	T50.0X5	T50.0X6
Saluretic NEC	T50.2X1	T50.2X2	T50.2X3	T50.2X4	T50.2X5	T50.2X6
Saluron	T50.2X1	T50.2X2	T50.2X3	T50.2X4	T50.2X5	T50.2X6
Salvarsan 606 (neosilver) (silver)	T37.8X1	T37.8X2	T37.8X3	T37.8X4	T37.8X5	T37.8X6
Sambucus canadensis	T62.2X1	T62.2X2	T62.2X3	T62.2X4	—	—
berry	T62.1X1	T62.1X2	T62.1X3	T62.1X4	—	—
Sandril	T46.5X1	T46.5X2	T46.5X3	T46.5X4	T46.5X5	T46.5X6
Sanguinaria canadensis	T62.2X1	T62.2X2	T62.2X3	T62.2X4	—	—
Saniflush (cleaner)	T54.2X1	T54.2X2	T54.2X3	T54.2X4	—	—
Santonin	T37.4X1	T37.4X2	T37.4X3	T37.4X4	T37.4X5	T37.4X6
Santyl	T49.8X1	T49.8X2	T49.8X3	T49.8X4	T49.8X5	T49.8X6
Saralasin	T46.5X1	T46.5X2	T46.5X3	T46.5X4	T46.5X5	T46.5X6
Sarcolysin	T45.1X1	T45.1X2	T45.1X3	T45.1X4	T45.1X5	T45.1X6
Sarkomycin	T45.1X1	T45.1X2	T45.1X3	T45.1X4	T45.1X5	T45.1X6
Saroten	T43.011	T43.012	T43.013	T43.014	T43.015	T43.016
Saturnine—see Lead						
Savin (oil)	T49.4X1	T49.4X2	T49.4X3	T49.4X4	T49.4X5	T49.4X6
Scammony	T47.2X1	T47.2X2	T47.2X3	T47.2X4	T47.2X5	T47.2X6
Scarlet red	T49.8X1	T49.8X2	T49.8X3	T49.8X4	T49.8X5	T49.8X6
Scheele's green	T57.0X1	T57.0X2	T57.0X3	T57.0X4	—	—
insecticide	T57.0X1	T57.0X2	T57.0X3	T57.0X4	—	—
Schizontozide (blood) (tissue)	T37.2X1	T37.2X2	T37.2X3	T37.2X4	T37.2X5	T37.2X6
Schradan	T60.0X1	T60.0X2	T60.0X3	T60.0X4	—	—
Schweinfurth green	T57.0X1	T57.0X2	T57.0X3	T57.0X4	—	—
insecticide	T57.0X1	T57.0X2	T57.0X3	T57.0X4	—	—
Scilla, rat poison	T60.4X1	T60.4X2	T60.4X3	T60.4X4	—	—
Scillaren	T60.4X1	T60.4X2	T60.4X3	T60.4X4	—	—
Sclerosing agent	T46.8X1	T46.8X2	T46.8X3	T46.8X4	T46.8X5	T46.8X6
Scombrotoxin	T61.11	T61.12	T61.13	T61.14	—	—
Scopolamine	T44.3X1	T44.3X2	T44.3X3	T44.3X4	T44.3X5	T44.3X6
Scopolia extract	T44.3X1	T44.3X2	T44.3X3	T44.3X4	T44.3X5	T44.3X6
Scouring powder	T65.891	T65.892	T65.893	T65.894	—	—
Sea						
anemone (sting)	T63.631	T63.632	T63.633	T63.634	—	—
cucumber (sting)	T63.691	T63.692	T63.693	T63.694	—	—
snake (bite) (venom)	T63.091	T63.092	T63.093	T63.094	—	—
urchin spine (puncture)	T63.691	T63.692	T63.693	T63.694	—	—
Seafood	T61.91	T61.92	T61.93	T61.94	—	—
specified NEC	T61.8X1	T61.8X2	T61.8X3	T61.8X4	—	—
Secbutabarbital	T42.3X1	T42.3X2	T42.3X3	T42.3X4	T42.3X5	T42.3X6
Secbutabarbitone	T42.3X1	T42.3X2	T42.3X3	T42.3X4	T42.3X5	T42.3X6
Secnidazole	T37.3X1	T37.3X2	T37.3X3	T37.3X4	T37.3X5	T37.3X6
Secobarbital	T42.3X1	T42.3X2	T42.3X3	T42.3X4	T42.3X5	T42.3X6
Seconal	T42.3X1	T42.3X2	T42.3X3	T42.3X4	T42.3X5	T42.3X6
Secretin	T50.8X1	T50.8X2	T50.8X3	T50.8X4	T50.8X5	T50.8X6
Sedative NEC	T42.71	T42.72	T42.73	T42.74	T42.75	T42.76
mixed NEC	T42.6X1	T42.6X2	T42.6X3	T42.6X4	T42.6X5	T42.6X6
Sedormid	T42.6X1	T42.6X2	T42.6X3	T42.6X4	T42.6X5	T42.6X6
Seed disinfectant or dressing	T60.8X1	T60.8X2	T60.8X3	T60.8X4	—	—
Seeds (poisonous)	T62.2X1	T62.2X2	T62.2X3	T62.2X4	—	—
Selegiline	T42.8X1	T42.8X2	T42.8X3	T42.8X4	T42.8X5	T42.8X6
Selenium NEC	T56.891	T56.892	T56.893	T56.894	—	—
disulfide or sulfide	T49.4X1	T49.4X2	T49.4X3	T49.4X4	T49.4X5	T49.4X6
fumes	T59.891	T59.892	T59.893	T59.894	—	—
sulfide	T49.4X1	T49.4X2	T49.4X3	T49.4X4	T49.4X5	T49.4X6
Selenomethionine (75Se)	T50.8X1	T50.8X2	T50.8X3	T50.8X4	T50.8X5	T50.8X6
Selsun	T49.4X1	T49.4X2	T49.4X3	T49.4X4	T49.4X5	T49.4X6
Semustine	T45.1X1	T45.1X2	T45.1X3	T45.1X4	T45.1X5	T45.1X6
Senega syrup	T48.4X1	T48.4X2	T48.4X3	T48.4X4	T48.4X5	T48.4X6
Senna	T47.2X1	T47.2X2	T47.2X3	T47.2X4	T47.2X5	T47.2X6
Sennoside A+B	T47.2X1	T47.2X2	T47.2X3	T47.2X4	T47.2X5	T47.2X6
Septisol	T49.2X1	T49.2X2	T49.2X3	T49.2X4	T49.2X5	T49.2X6
Seractide	T38.811	T38.812	T38.813	T38.814	T38.815	T38.816
Serax	T42.4X1	T42.4X2	T42.4X3	T42.4X4	T42.4X5	T42.4X6
Serenesil	T42.6X1	T42.6X2	T42.6X3	T42.6X4	T42.6X5	T42.6X6
Serenium (hydrochloride)	T37.91	T37.92	T37.93	T37.94	T37.95	T37.96
Serepax—see Oxazepam						
Sermorelin	T38.891	T38.892	T38.893	T38.894	T38.895	T38.896
Sernyl	T41.1X1	T41.1X2	T41.1X3	T41.1X4	T41.1X5	T41.1X6
Serotonin	T50.991	T50.992	T50.993	T50.994	T50.995	T50.996
Serpasil	T46.5X1	T46.5X2	T46.5X3	T46.5X4	T46.5X5	T46.5X6
Serrapeptase	T45.3X1	T45.3X2	T45.3X3	T45.3X4	T45.3X5	T45.3X6
Serum						
antibotulinus	T50.Z11	T50.Z12	T50.Z13	T50.Z14	T50.Z15	T50.Z16
anticytotoxic	T50.Z11	T50.Z12	T50.Z13	T50.Z14	T50.Z15	T50.Z16
antidiphtheria	T50.Z11	T50.Z12	T50.Z13	T50.Z14	T50.Z15	T50.Z16
antimeningococcus	T50.Z11	T50.Z12	T50.Z13	T50.Z14	T50.Z15	T50.Z16
anti-Rh	T50.Z11	T50.Z12	T50.Z13	T50.Z14	T50.Z15	T50.Z16
anti-snake-bite	T50.Z11	T50.Z12	T50.Z13	T50.Z14	T50.Z15	T50.Z16
antitetanic	T50.Z11	T50.Z12	T50.Z13	T50.Z14	T50.Z15	T50.Z16
antitoxic	T50.Z11	T50.Z12	T50.Z13	T50.Z14	T50.Z15	T50.Z16
complement (inhibitor)	T45.8X1	T45.8X2	T45.8X3	T45.8X4	T45.8X5	T45.8X6
convalescent	T50.Z11	T50.Z12	T50.Z13	T50.Z14	T50.Z15	T50.Z16
hemolytic complement	T45.8X1	T45.8X2	T45.8X3	T45.8X4	T45.8X5	T45.8X6
immune (human)	T50.Z11	T50.Z12	T50.Z13	T50.Z14	T50.Z15	T50.Z16
protective NEC	T50.Z11	T50.Z12	T50.Z13	T50.Z14	T50.Z15	T50.Z16
Setastine	T45.0X1	T45.0X2	T45.0X3	T45.0X4	T45.0X5	T45.0X6
Setoperone	T43.591	T43.592	T43.593	T43.594	T43.595	T43.596
Sewer gas	T59.91	T59.92	T59.93	T59.94	—	—
Shampoo	T55.0X1	T55.0X2	T55.0X3	T55.0X4	—	—
Shellfish, noxious, nonbacterial	T61.781	T61.782	T61.783	T61.784	—	—
Sildenafil	T46.7X1	T46.7X2	T46.7X3	T46.7X4	T46.7X5	T46.7X6
Silibinin	T50.991	T50.992	T50.993	T50.994	T50.995	T50.996
Silicone NEC	T65.891	T65.892	T65.893	T65.894	—	—
medicinal	T49.3X1	T49.3X2	T49.3X3	T49.3X4	T49.3X5	T49.3X6
Silvadene	T49.0X1	T49.0X2	T49.0X3	T49.0X4	T49.0X5	T49.0X6
Silver	T49.0X1	T49.0X2	T49.0X3	T49.0X4	T49.0X5	T49.0X6
anti-infectives	T49.0X1	T49.0X2	T49.0X3	T49.0X4	T49.0X5	T49.0X6
arsphenamine	T37.8X1	T37.8X2	T37.8X3	T37.8X4	T37.8X5	T37.8X6
colloidal	T49.0X1	T49.0X2	T49.0X3	T49.0X4	T49.0X5	T49.0X6
nitrate	T49.0X1	T49.0X2	T49.0X3	T49.0X4	T49.0X5	T49.0X6
ophthalmic preparation	T49.5X1	T49.5X2	T49.5X3	T49.5X4	T49.5X5	T49.5X6
toughened (keratolytic)	T49.4X1	T49.4X2	T49.4X3	T49.4X4	T49.4X5	T49.4X6
nonmedicinal (dust)	T56.891	T56.892	T56.893	T56.894	—	—
protein	T49.5X1	T49.5X2	T49.5X3	T49.5X4	T49.5X5	T49.5X6
salvarsan	T37.8X1	T37.8X2	T37.8X3	T37.8X4	T37.8X5	T37.8X6
sulfadiazine	T49.4X1	T49.4X2	T49.4X3	T49.4X4	T49.4X5	T49.4X6

Substance	Poisoning, Accidental (unintentional)	Poisoning, Intentional self-harm	Poisoning, Assault	Poisoning, Undetermined	Adverse effect	Underdosing
Silymarin	T50.991	T50.992	T50.993	T50.994	T50.995	T50.996
Simaldrate	T47.1X1	T47.1X2	T47.1X3	T47.1X4	T47.1X5	T47.1X6
Simazine	T60.3X1	T60.3X2	T60.3X3	T60.3X4	—	—
Simethicone	T47.1X1	T47.1X2	T47.1X3	T47.1X4	T47.1X5	T47.1X6
Simfibrate	T46.6X1	T46.6X2	T46.6X3	T46.6X4	T46.6X5	T46.6X6
Simvastatin	T46.6X1	T46.6X2	T46.6X3	T46.6X4	T46.6X5	T46.6X6
Sincalide	T50.8X1	T50.8X2	T50.8X3	T50.8X4	T50.8X5	T50.8X6
Sinequan	T43.011	T43.012	T43.013	T43.014	T43.015	T43.016
Singoserp	T46.5X1	T46.5X2	T46.5X3	T46.5X4	T46.5X5	T46.5X6
Sintrom	T45.511	T45.512	T45.513	T45.514	T45.515	T45.516
Sisomicin	T36.5X1	T36.5X2	T36.5X3	T36.5X4	T36.5X5	T36.5X6
Sitosterols	T46.6X1	T46.6X2	T46.6X3	T46.6X4	T46.6X5	T46.6X6
Skeletal muscle relaxants	T48.1X1	T48.1X2	T48.1X3	T48.1X4	T48.1X5	T48.1X6
Skin						
agents (external)	T49.91	T49.92	T49.93	T49.94	T49.95	T49.96
specified NEC	T49.8X1	T49.8X2	T49.8X3	T49.8X4	T49.8X5	T49.8X6
test antigen	T50.8X1	T50.8X2	T50.8X3	T50.8X4	T50.8X5	T50.8X6
Sleep-eze	T45.0X1	T45.0X2	T45.0X3	T45.0X4	T45.0X5	T45.0X6
Sleeping draught, pill	T42.71	T42.72	T42.73	T42.74	T42.75	T42.76
Smallpox vaccine	T50.B11	T50.B12	T50.B13	T50.B14	T50.B15	T50.B16
Smelter fumes NEC	T56.91	T56.92	T56.93	T56.94	—	—
Smog	T59.1X1	T59.1X2	T59.1X3	T59.1X4	—	—
Smoke NEC	T59.811	T59.812	T59.813	T59.814	—	—
Smooth muscle relaxant	T44.3X1	T44.3X2	T44.3X3	T44.3X4	T44.3X5	T44.3X6
Snail killer NEC	T60.8X1	T60.8X2	T60.8X3	T60.8X4	—	—
Snake venom or bite	T63.001	T63.002	T63.003	T63.004	—	—
hemocoagulase	T45.7X1	T45.7X2	T45.7X3	T45.7X4	T45.7X5	T45.7X6
Snuff	T65.211	T65.212	T65.213	T65.214	—	—
Soap (powder) (product)	T55.0X1	T55.0X2	T55.0X3	T55.0X4	—	—
enema	T47.4X1	T47.4X2	T47.4X3	T47.4X4	T47.4X5	T47.4X6
medicinal, soft	T49.2X1	T49.2X2	T49.2X3	T49.2X4	T49.2X5	T49.2X6
superfatted	T49.2X1	T49.2X2	T49.2X3	T49.2X4	T49.2X5	T49.2X6
Sobrerol	T48.4X1	T48.4X2	T48.4X3	T48.4X4	T48.4X5	T48.4X6
Soda (caustic)	T54.3X1	T54.3X2	T54.3X3	T54.3X4	—	—
bicarb	T47.1X1	T47.1X2	T47.1X3	T47.1X4	T47.1X5	T47.1X6
chlorinated—*see Sodium, hypochlorite*						
Sodium						
acetosulfone	T37.1X1	T37.1X2	T37.1X3	T37.1X4	T37.1X5	T37.1X6
acetrizoate	T50.8X1	T50.8X2	T50.8X3	T50.8X4	T50.8X5	T50.8X6
acid phosphate	T50.3X1	T50.3X2	T50.3X3	T50.3X4	T50.3X5	T50.3X6
alginate	T47.8X1	T47.8X2	T47.8X3	T47.8X4	T47.8X5	T47.8X6
amidotrizoate	T50.8X1	T50.8X2	T50.8X3	T50.8X4	T50.8X5	T50.8X6
aminopterin	T45.1X1	T45.1X2	T45.1X3	T45.1X4	T45.1X5	T45.1X6
amylosulfate	T47.8X1	T47.8X2	T47.8X3	T47.8X4	T47.8X5	T47.8X6
amytal	T42.3X1	T42.3X2	T42.3X3	T42.3X4	T42.3X5	T42.3X6
antimony gluconate	T37.3X1	T37.3X2	T37.3X3	T37.3X4	T37.3X5	T37.3X6
arsenate	T57.0X1	T57.0X2	T57.0X3	T57.0X4	—	—
aurothiomalate	T39.4X1	T39.4X2	T39.4X3	T39.4X4	T39.4X5	T39.4X6
aurothiosulfate	T39.4X1	T39.4X2	T39.4X3	T39.4X4	T39.4X5	T39.4X6
barbiturate	T42.3X1	T42.3X2	T42.3X3	T42.3X4	T42.3X5	T42.3X6
basic phosphate	T47.4X1	T47.4X2	T47.4X3	T47.4X4	T47.4X5	T47.4X6
bicarbonate	T47.1X1	T47.1X2	T47.1X3	T47.1X4	T47.1X5	T47.1X6
bichromate	T57.8X1	T57.8X2	T57.8X3	T57.8X4	—	—
biphosphate	T50.3X1	T50.3X2	T50.3X3	T50.3X4	T50.3X5	T50.3X6
bisulfate	T65.891	T65.892	T65.893	T65.894	—	—
borate						
cleanser	T57.8X1	T57.8X2	T57.8X3	T57.8X4	—	—
eye	T49.5X1	T49.5X2	T49.5X3	T49.5X4	T49.5X5	T49.5X6
therapeutic	T49.8X1	T49.8X2	T49.8X3	T49.8X4	T49.8X5	T49.8X6

Substance	Poisoning, Accidental (unintentional)	Poisoning, Intentional self-harm	Poisoning, Assault	Poisoning, Undetermined	Adverse effect	Underdosing
Sodium — *continued*						
bromide	T42.6X1	T42.6X2	T42.6X3	T42.6X4	T42.6X5	T42.6X6
cacodylate (nonmedicinal) NEC	T50.8X1	T50.8X2	T50.8X3	T50.8X4	T50.8X5	T50.8X6
anti-infective	T37.8X1	T37.8X2	T37.8X3	T37.8X4	T37.8X5	T37.8X6
herbicide	T60.3X1	T60.3X2	T60.3X3	T60.3X4	—	—
calcium edetate	T45.8X1	T45.8X2	T45.8X3	T45.8X4	T45.8X5	T45.8X6
carbonate NEC	T54.3X1	T54.3X2	T54.3X3	T54.3X4	—	—
chlorate NEC	T65.891	T65.892	T65.893	T65.894	—	—
herbicide	T54.91	T54.92	T54.93	T54.94	—	—
chloride	T50.3X1	T50.3X2	T50.3X3	T50.3X4	T50.3X5	T50.3X6
with glucose	T50.3X1	T50.3X2	T50.3X3	T50.3X4	T50.3X5	T50.3X6
chromate	T65.891	T65.892	T65.893	T65.894	—	—
citrate	T50.991	T50.992	T50.993	T50.994	T50.995	T50.996
cromoglicate	T48.6X1	T48.6X2	T48.6X3	T48.6X4	T48.6X5	T48.6X6
cyanide	T65.0X1	T65.0X2	T65.0X3	T65.0X4	—	—
cyclamate	T50.3X1	T50.3X2	T50.3X3	T50.3X4	T50.3X5	T50.3X6
dehydrocholate	T45.8X1	T45.8X2	T45.8X3	T45.8X4	T45.8X5	T45.8X6
diatrizoate	T50.8X1	T50.8X2	T50.8X3	T50.8X4	T50.8X5	T50.8X6
dibunate	T48.4X1	T48.4X2	T48.4X3	T48.4X4	T48.4X5	T48.4X6
dioctyl sulfosuccinate	T47.4X1	T47.4X2	T47.4X3	T47.4X4	T47.4X5	T47.4X6
dipantoyl ferrate	T45.8X1	T45.8X2	T45.8X3	T45.8X4	T45.8X5	T45.8X6
edetate	T45.8X1	T45.8X2	T45.8X3	T45.8X4	T45.8X5	T45.8X6
ethacrynate	T50.1X1	T50.1X2	T50.1X3	T50.1X4	T50.1X5	T50.1X6
feredetate	T45.8X1	T45.8X2	T45.8X3	T45.8X4	T45.8X5	T45.8X6
Fluoride—*see Fluoride*						
fluoroacetate (dust) (pesticide)	T60.4X1	T60.4X2	T60.4X3	T60.4X4		
free salt	T50.3X1	T50.3X2	T50.3X3	T50.3X4	T50.3X5	T50.3X6
fusidate	T36.8X1	T36.8X2	T36.8X3	T36.8X4	T36.8X5	T36.8X6
glucaldrate	T47.1X1	T47.1X2	T47.1X3	T47.1X4	T47.1X5	T47.1X6
glucosulfone	T37.1X1	T37.1X2	T37.1X3	T37.1X4	T37.1X5	T37.1X6
glutamate	T45.8X1	T45.8X2	T45.8X3	T45.8X4	T45.8X5	T45.8X6
hydrogen carbonate	T50.3X1	T50.3X2	T50.3X3	T50.3X4	T50.3X5	T50.3X6
hydroxide	T54.3X1	T54.3X2	T54.3X3	T54.3X4	—	—
hypochlorite (bleach) NEC	T54.3X1	T54.3X2	T54.3X3	T54.3X4	—	—
disinfectant	T54.3X1	T54.3X2	T54.3X3	T54.3X4	—	—
medicinal (anti-infective) (external)	T49.0X1	T49.0X2	T49.0X3	T49.0X4	T49.0X5	T49.0X6
vapor	T54.3X1	T54.3X2	T54.3X3	T54.3X4	—	—
hyposulfite	T49.0X1	T49.0X2	T49.0X3	T49.0X4	T49.0X5	T49.0X6
indigotin disulfonate	T50.8X1	T50.8X2	T50.8X3	T50.8X4	T50.8X5	T50.8X6
iodide	T50.991	T50.992	T50.993	T50.994	T50.995	T50.996
I-131	T50.8X1	T50.8X2	T50.8X3	T50.8X4	T50.8X5	T50.8X6
therapeutic	T38.2X1	T38.2X2	T38.2X3	T38.2X4	T38.2X5	T38.2X6
iodohippurate (131I)	T50.8X1	T50.8X2	T50.8X3	T50.8X4	T50.8X5	T50.8X6
iopodate	T50.8X1	T50.8X2	T50.8X3	T50.8X4	T50.8X5	T50.8X6
iothalamate	T50.8X1	T50.8X2	T50.8X3	T50.8X4	T50.8X5	T50.8X6
iron edetate	T45.4X1	T45.4X2	T45.4X3	T45.4X4	T45.4X5	T45.4X6
lactate (compound solution)	T45.8X1	T45.8X2	T45.8X3	T45.8X4	T45.8X5	T45.8X6
lauryl (sulfate)	T49.2X1	T49.2X2	T49.2X3	T49.2X4	T49.2X5	T49.2X6
L-triiodothyronine	T38.1X1	T38.1X2	T38.1X3	T38.1X4	T38.1X5	T38.1X6
magnesium citrate	T50.991	T50.992	T50.993	T50.994	T50.995	T50.996
mersalate	T50.2X1	T50.2X2	T50.2X3	T50.2X4	T50.2X5	T50.2X6
metasilicate	T65.891	T65.892	T65.893	T65.894	—	—
metrizoate	T50.8X1	T50.8X2	T50.8X3	T50.8X4	T50.8X5	T50.8X6
monofluoroacetate (pesticide)	T60.1X1	T60.1X2	T60.1X3	T60.1X4		

Substance	Poisoning, Accidental (unintentional)	Poisoning, Intentional self-harm	Poisoning, Assault	Poisoning, Undetermined	Adverse effect	Underdosing
Sodium — *continued*						
morrhuate	T46.8X1	T46.8X2	T46.8X3	T46.8X4	T46.8X5	T46.8X6
nafcillin	T36.0X1	T36.0X2	T36.0X3	T36.0X4	T36.0X5	T36.0X6
nitrate (oxidizing agent)	T65.891	T65.892	T65.893	T65.894	—	—
nitrite	T50.6X1	T50.6X2	T50.6X3	T50.6X4	T50.6X5	T50.6X6
nitroferricyanide	T46.5X1	T46.5X2	T46.5X3	T46.5X4	T46.5X5	T46.5X6
nitroprusside	T46.5X1	T46.5X2	T46.5X3	T46.5X4	T46.5X5	T46.5X6
oxalate	T65.891	T65.892	T65.893	T65.894	—	—
oxide/peroxide	T65.891	T65.892	T65.893	T65.894	—	—
oxybate	T41.291	T41.292	T41.293	T41.294	T41.295	T41.296
para-aminohippurate	T50.8X1	T50.8X2	T50.8X3	T50.8X4	T50.8X5	T50.8X6
perborate (nonmedicinal) NEC	T65.891	T65.892	T65.893	T65.894	—	—
medicinal	T49.0X1	T49.0X2	T49.0X3	T49.0X4	T49.0X5	T49.0X6
soap	T55.0X1	T55.0X2	T55.0X3	T55.0X4	—	—
percarbonate—*see Sodium, perborate*						
pertechnetate Tc99m	T50.8X1	T50.8X2	T50.8X3	T50.8X4	T50.8X5	T50.8X6
phosphate						
cellulose	T45.8X1	T45.8X2	T45.8X3	T45.8X4	T45.8X5	T45.8X6
dibasic	T47.2X1	T47.2X2	T47.2X3	T47.2X4	T47.2X5	T47.2X6
monobasic	T47.2X1	T47.2X2	T47.2X3	T47.2X4	T47.2X5	T47.2X6
phytate	T50.6X1	T50.6X2	T50.6X3	T50.6X4	T50.6X5	T50.6X6
picosulfate	T47.2X1	T47.2X2	T47.2X3	T47.2X4	T47.2X5	T47.2X6
polyhydroxyaluminium monocarbonate	T47.1X1	T47.1X2	T47.1X3	T47.1X4	T47.1X5	T47.1X6
polystyrene sulfonate	T50.3X1	T50.3X2	T50.3X3	T50.3X4	T50.3X5	T50.3X6
propionate	T49.0X1	T49.0X2	T49.0X3	T49.0X4	T49.0X5	T49.0X6
propyl hydroxybenzoate	T50.991	T50.992	T50.993	T50.994	T50.995	T50.996
psylliate	T46.8X1	T46.8X2	T46.8X3	T46.8X4	T46.8X5	T46.8X6
removing resins	T50.3X1	T50.3X2	T50.3X3	T50.3X4	T50.3X5	T50.3X6
salicylate	T39.091	T39.092	T39.093	T39.094	T39.095	T39.096
salt NEC	T50.3X1	T50.3X2	T50.3X3	T50.3X4	T50.3X5	T50.3X6
selenate	T60.2X1	T60.2X2	T60.2X3	T60.2X4	—	—
stibogluconate	T37.3X1	T37.3X2	T37.3X3	T37.3X4	T37.3X5	T37.3X6
sulfate	T47.4X1	T47.4X2	T47.4X3	T47.4X4	T47.4X5	T47.4X6
sulfoxone	T37.1X1	T37.1X2	T37.1X3	T37.1X4	T37.1X5	T37.1X6
tetradecyl sulfate	T46.8X1	T46.8X2	T46.8X3	T46.8X4	T46.8X5	T46.8X6
thiopental	T41.1X1	T41.1X2	T41.1X3	T41.1X4	T41.1X5	T41.1X6
thiosalicylate	T39.091	T39.092	T39.093	T39.094	T39.095	T39.096
thiosulfate	T50.6X1	T50.6X2	T50.6X3	T50.6X4	T50.6X5	T50.6X6
tolbutamide	T38.3X1	T38.3X2	T38.3X3	T38.3X4	T38.3X5	T38.3X6
(L)triiodothyronine	T38.1X1	T38.1X2	T38.1X3	T38.1X4	T38.1X5	T38.1X6
tyropanoate	T50.8X1	T50.8X2	T50.8X3	T50.8X4	T50.8X5	T50.8X6
valproate	T42.6X1	T42.6X2	T42.6X3	T42.6X4	T42.6X5	T42.6X6
versenate	T50.6X1	T50.6X2	T50.6X3	T50.6X4	T50.6X5	T50.6X6
Sodium-free salt	T50.901	T50.902	T50.903	T50.904	T50.905	T50.906
Sodium-removing resin	T50.3X1	T50.3X2	T50.3X3	T50.3X4	T50.3X5	T50.3X6
Soft soap	T55.0X1	T55.0X2	T55.0X3	T55.0X4	—	—
Solanine	T62.2X1	T62.2X2	T62.2X3	T62.2X4	—	—
berries	T62.1X1	T62.1X2	T62.1X3	T62.1X4	—	—
Solanum dulcamara	T62.2X1	T62.2X2	T62.2X3	T62.2X4	—	—
berries	T62.1X1	T62.1X2	T62.1X3	T62.1X4	—	—
Solapsone	T37.1X1	T37.1X2	T37.1X3	T37.1X4	T37.1X5	T37.1X6
Solar lotion	T49.3X1	T49.3X2	T49.3X3	T49.3X4	T49.3X5	T49.3X6
Solasulfone	T37.1X1	T37.1X2	T37.1X3	T37.1X4	T37.1X5	T37.1X6
Soldering fluid	T65.891	T65.892	T65.893	T65.894	—	—
Solid substance	T65.91	T65.92	T65.93	T65.94	—	—
specified NEC	T65.891	T65.892	T65.893	T65.894	—	—

Substance	Poisoning, Accidental (unintentional)	Poisoning, Intentional self-harm	Poisoning, Assault	Poisoning, Undetermined	Adverse effect	Underdosing
Solvent, industrial NEC	T52.91	T52.92	T52.93	T52.94	—	—
naphtha	T52.0X1	T52.0X2	T52.0X3	T52.0X4	—	—
petroleum	T52.0X1	T52.0X2	T52.0X3	T52.0X4	—	—
specified NEC	T52.8X1	T52.8X2	T52.8X3	T52.8X4	—	—
Soma	T42.8X1	T42.8X2	T42.8X3	T42.8X4	T42.8X5	T42.8X6
Somatorelin	T38.891	T38.892	T38.893	T38.894	T38.895	T38.896
Somatostatin	T38.991	T38.992	T38.993	T38.994	T38.995	T38.996
Somatotropin	T38.811	T38.812	T38.813	T38.814	T38.815	T38.816
Somatrem	T38.811	T38.812	T38.813	T38.814	T38.815	T38.816
Somatropin	T38.811	T38.812	T38.813	T38.814	T38.815	T38.816
Sominex	T45.0X1	T45.0X2	T45.0X3	T45.0X4	T45.0X5	T45.0X6
Somnos	T42.6X1	T42.6X2	T42.6X3	T42.6X4	T42.6X5	T42.6X6
Somonal	T42.3X1	T42.3X2	T42.3X3	T42.3X4	T42.3X5	T42.3X6
Soneryl	T42.3X1	T42.3X2	T42.3X3	T42.3X4	T42.3X5	T42.3X6
Soothing syrup	T50.901	T50.902	T50.903	T50.904	T50.905	T50.906
Sopor	T42.6X1	T42.6X2	T42.6X3	T42.6X4	T42.6X5	T42.6X6
Soporific	T42.71	T42.72	T42.73	T42.74	T42.75	T42.76
Soporific drug	T42.71	T42.72	T42.73	T42.74	T42.75	T42.76
specified type NEC	T42.6X1	T42.6X2	T42.6X3	T42.6X4	T42.6X5	T42.6X6
Sorbide nitrate	T46.3X1	T46.3X2	T46.3X3	T46.3X4	T46.3X5	T46.3X6
Sorbitol	T47.4X1	T47.4X2	T47.4X3	T47.4X4	T47.4X5	T47.4X6
Sotalol	T44.7X1	T44.7X2	T44.7X3	T44.7X4	T44.7X5	T44.7X6
Sotradecol	T46.8X1	T46.8X2	T46.8X3	T46.8X4	T46.8X5	T46.8X6
Soysterol	T46.6X1	T46.6X2	T46.6X3	T46.6X4	T46.6X5	T46.6X6
Spacoline	T44.3X1	T44.3X2	T44.3X3	T44.3X4	T44.3X5	T44.3X6
Spanish fly	T49.8X1	T49.8X2	T49.8X3	T49.8X4	T49.8X5	T49.8X6
Sparine	T43.3X1	T43.3X2	T43.3X3	T43.3X4	T43.3X5	T43.3X6
Sparteine	T48.0X1	T48.0X2	T48.0X3	T48.0X4	T48.0X5	T48.0X6
Spasmolytic						
anticholinergics	T44.3X1	T44.3X2	T44.3X3	T44.3X4	T44.3X5	T44.3X6
autonomic	T44.3X1	T44.3X2	T44.3X3	T44.3X4	T44.3X5	T44.3X6
bronchial NEC	T48.6X1	T48.6X2	T48.6X3	T48.6X4	T48.6X5	T48.6X6
quaternary ammonium	T44.3X1	T44.3X2	T44.3X3	T44.3X4	T44.3X5	T44.3X6
skeletal muscle NEC	T48.1X1	T48.1X2	T48.1X3	T48.1X4	T48.1X5	T48.1X6
Spectinomycin	T36.5X1	T36.5X2	T36.5X3	T36.5X4	T36.5X5	T36.5X6
Speed	T43.621	T43.622	T43.623	T43.624	T43.625	T43.626
Spermicide	T49.8X1	T49.8X2	T49.8X3	T49.8X4	T49.8X5	T49.8X6
Spider (bite) (venom)	T63.391	T63.392	T63.393	T63.394	—	—
antivenin	T50.Z11	T50.Z12	T50.Z13	T50.Z14	T50.Z15	T50.Z16
Spigelia (root)	T37.4X1	T37.4X2	T37.4X3	T37.4X4	T37.4X5	T37.4X6
Spindle inactivator	T50.4X1	T50.4X2	T50.4X3	T50.4X4	T50.4X5	T50.4X6
Spiperone	T43.4X1	T43.4X2	T43.4X3	T43.4X4	T43.4X5	T43.4X6
Spiramycin	T36.3X1	T36.3X2	T36.3X3	T36.3X4	T36.3X5	T36.3X6
Spirapril	T46.4X1	T46.4X2	T46.4X3	T46.4X4	T46.4X5	T46.4X6
Spirilene	T43.591	T43.592	T43.593	T43.594	T43.595	T43.596
Spirit (s) (neutral) NEC	T51.0X1	T51.0X2	T51.0X3	T51.0X4	—	—
beverage	T51.0X1	T51.0X2	T51.0X3	T51.0X4	—	—
industrial	T51.0X1	T51.0X2	T51.0X3	T51.0X4	—	—
mineral	T52.0X1	T52.0X2	T52.0X3	T52.0X4	—	—
of salt—*see Hydrochloric acid*						
surgical	T51.0X1	T51.0X2	T51.0X3	T51.0X4	—	—
Spironolactone	T50.0X1	T50.0X2	T50.0X3	T50.0X4	T50.0X5	T50.0X6
Spiroperidol	T43.4X1	T43.4X2	T43.4X3	T43.4X4	T43.4X5	T43.4X6
Sponge, absorbable (gelatin)	T45.7X1	T45.7X2	T45.7X3	T45.7X4	T45.7X5	T45.7X6
Sporostacin	T49.0X1	T49.0X2	T49.0X3	T49.0X4	T49.0X5	T49.0X6
Spray (aerosol)	T65.91	T65.92	T65.93	T65.94	—	—
cosmetic	T65.891	T65.892	T65.893	T65.894	—	—
medicinal NEC	T50.901	T50.902	T50.903	T50.904	T50.905	T50.906

Substance	Poisoning, Accidental (unintentional)	Poisoning, Intentional self-harm	Poisoning, Assault	Poisoning, Undetermined	Adverse effect	Underdosing
Spray (aerosol) — *continued*						
pesticides—*see Pesticides*						
specified content—*see specific substance*						
Spurge flax	T62.2X1	T62.2X2	T62.2X3	T62.2X4	—	—
Spurges	T62.2X1	T62.2X2	T62.2X3	T62.2X4	—	—
Sputum viscosity-lowering drug	T48.4X1	T48.4X2	T48.4X3	T48.4X4	T48.4X5	T48.4X6
Squill	T46.0X1	T46.0X2	T46.0X3	T46.0X4	T46.0X5	T46.0X6
rat poison	T60.4X1	T60.4X2	T60.4X3	T60.4X4	—	—
Squirting cucumber (cathartic)	T47.2X1	T47.2X2	T47.2X3	T47.2X4	T47.2X5	T47.2X6
Stains	T65.6X1	T65.6X2	T65.6X3	T65.6X4	—	—
Stannous fluoride	T49.7X1	T49.7X2	T49.7X3	T49.7X4	T49.7X5	T49.7X6
Stanolone	T38.7X1	T38.7X2	T38.7X3	T38.7X4	T38.7X5	T38.7X6
Stanozolol	T38.7X1	T38.7X2	T38.7X3	T38.7X4	T38.7X5	T38.7X6
Staphisagria or stavesacre (pediculicide)	T49.0X1	T49.0X2	T49.0X3	T49.0X4	T49.0X5	T49.0X6
Starch	T50.901	T50.902	T50.903	T50.904	T50.905	T50.906
Stelazine	T43.3X1	T43.3X2	T43.3X3	T43.3X4	T43.3X5	T43.3X6
Stemetil	T43.3X1	T43.3X2	T43.3X3	T43.3X4	T43.3X5	T43.3X6
Stepronin	T48.4X1	T48.4X2	T48.4X3	T48.4X4	T48.4X5	T48.4X6
Sterculia	T47.4X1	T47.4X2	T47.4X3	T47.4X4	T47.4X5	T47.4X6
Sternutator gas	T59.891	T59.892	T59.893	T59.894	—	—
Steroid	T38.0X1	T38.0X2	T38.0X3	T38.0X4	T38.0X5	T38.0X6
anabolic	T38.7X1	T38.7X2	T38.7X3	T38.7X4	T38.7X5	T38.7X6
androgenic	T38.7X1	T38.7X2	T38.7X3	T38.7X4	T38.7X5	T38.7X6
antineoplastic, hormone	T38.7X1	T38.7X2	T38.7X3	T38.7X4	T38.7X5	T38.7X6
estrogen	T38.5X1	T38.5X2	T38.5X3	T38.5X4	T38.5X5	T38.5X6
ENT agent	T49.6X1	T49.6X2	T49.6X3	T49.6X4	T49.6X5	T49.6X6
ophthalmic preparation	T49.5X1	T49.5X2	T49.5X3	T49.5X4	T49.5X5	T49.5X6
topical NEC	T49.0X1	T49.0X2	T49.0X3	T49.0X4	T49.0X5	T49.0X6
Stibine	T56.891	T56.892	T56.893	T56.894		
Stibogluconate	T37.3X1	T37.3X2	T37.3X3	T37.3X4	T37.3X5	T37.3X6
Stibophen	T37.4X1	T37.4X2	T37.4X3	T37.4X4	T37.4X5	T37.4X6
Stilbamidine (isetionate)	T37.3X1	T37.3X2	T37.3X3	T37.3X4	T37.3X5	T37.3X6
Stilbestrol	T38.5X1	T38.5X2	T38.5X3	T38.5X4	T38.5X5	T38.5X6
Stilboestrol	T38.5X1	T38.5X2	T38.5X3	T38.5X4	T38.5X5	T38.5X6
Stimulant						
central nervous system—*see also Psychostimulant*	T43.601	T43.602	T43.603	T43.604	T43.605	T43.606
analeptics	T50.7X1	T50.7X2	T50.7X3	T50.7X4	T50.7X5	T50.7X6
opiate antagonist	T50.7X1	T50.7X2	T50.7X3	T50.7X4	T50.7X5	T50.7X6
psychotherapeutic NEC—*see also Psychotherapeutic drug*	T43.601	T43.602	T43.603	T43.604	T43.605	T43.606
specified NEC	T43.691	T43.692	T43.693	T43.694	T43.695	T43.696
respiratory	T48.901	T48.902	T48.903	T48.904	T48.905	T48.906
Stone-dissolving drug	T50.901	T50.902	T50.903	T50.904	T50.905	T50.906
Storage battery (cells) (acid)	T54.2X1	T54.2X2	T54.2X3	T54.2X4	—	—
Stovaine	T41.3X1	T41.3X2	T41.3X3	T41.3X4	T41.3X5	T41.3X6
infiltration (subcutaneous)	T41.3X1	T41.3X2	T41.3X3	T41.3X4	T41.3X5	T41.3X6

Substance	Poisoning, Accidental (unintentional)	Poisoning, Intentional self-harm	Poisoning, Assault	Poisoning, Undetermined	Adverse effect	Underdosing
Stovaine — *continued*						
nerve block (peripheral) (plexus)	T41.3X1	T41.3X2	T41.3X3	T41.3X4	T41.3X5	T41.3X6
spinal	T41.3X1	T41.3X2	T41.3X3	T41.3X4	T41.3X5	T41.3X6
topical (surface)	T41.3X1	T41.3X2	T41.3X3	T41.3X4	T41.3X5	T41.3X6
Stovarsal	T37.8X1	T37.8X2	T37.8X3	T37.8X4	T37.8X5	T37.8X6
Stove gas—*see Gas, stove*						
Stoxil	T49.5X1	T49.5X2	T49.5X3	T49.5X4	T49.5X5	T49.5X6
Stramonium	T48.6X1	T48.6X2	T48.6X3	T48.6X4	T48.6X5	T48.6X6
natural state	T62.2X1	T62.2X2	T62.2X3	T62.2X4	—	—
Streptodornase	T45.3X1	T45.3X2	T45.3X3	T45.3X4	T45.3X5	T45.3X6
Streptoduocin	T36.5X1	T36.5X2	T36.5X3	T36.5X4	T36.5X5	T36.5X6
Streptokinase	T45.611	T45.612	T45.613	T45.614	T45.615	T45.616
Streptomycin (derivative)	T36.5X1	T36.5X2	T36.5X3	T36.5X4	T36.5X5	T36.5X6
Streptonivicin	T36.5X1	T36.5X2	T36.5X3	T36.5X4	T36.5X5	T36.5X6
Streptovarycin	T36.5X1	T36.5X2	T36.5X3	T36.5X4	T36.5X5	T36.5X6
Streptozocin	T45.1X1	T45.1X2	T45.1X3	T45.1X4	T45.1X5	T45.1X6
Streptozotocin	T45.1X1	T45.1X2	T45.1X3	T45.1X4	T45.1X5	T45.1X6
Stripper (paint) (solvent)	T52.8X1	T52.8X2	T52.8X3	T52.8X4	—	—
Strobane	T60.1X1	T60.1X2	T60.1X3	T60.1X4	—	—
Strofantina	T46.0X1	T46.0X2	T46.0X3	T46.0X4	T46.0X5	T46.0X6
Strophanthin (g) (k)	T46.0X1	T46.0X2	T46.0X3	T46.0X4	T46.0X5	T46.0X6
Strophanthus	T46.0X1	T46.0X2	T46.0X3	T46.0X4	T46.0X5	T46.0X6
Strophantin	T46.0X1	T46.0X2	T46.0X3	T46.0X4	T46.0X5	T46.0X6
Strophantin-g	T46.0X1	T46.0X2	T46.0X3	T46.0X4	T46.0X5	T46.0X6
Strychnine (nonmedicinal) (pesticide) (salts)	T65.1X1	T65.1X2	T65.1X3	T65.1X4		
medicinal	T48.291	T48.292	T48.293	T48.294	T48.295	T48.296
Strychnos (ignatii)—*see Strychnine*						
Styramate	T42.8X1	T42.8X2	T42.8X3	T42.8X4	T42.8X5	T42.8X6
Styrene	T65.891	T65.892	T65.893	T65.894	—	—
Succinimide, antiepileptic or anticonvulsant	T42.2X1	T42.2X2	T42.2X3	T42.2X4	T42.2X5	T42.2X6
mercuric—*see Mercury*						
Succinylcholine	T48.1X1	T48.1X2	T48.1X3	T48.1X4	T48.1X5	T48.1X6
Succinylsulfathiazole	T37.0X1	T37.0X2	T37.0X3	T37.0X4	T37.0X5	T37.0X6
Sucralfate	T47.1X1	T47.1X2	T47.1X3	T47.1X4	T47.1X5	T47.1X6
Sucrose	T50.3X1	T50.3X2	T50.3X3	T50.3X4	T50.3X5	T50.3X6
Sufentanil	T40.4X1	T40.4X2	T40.4X3	T40.4X4	T40.4X5	T40.4X6
Sulbactam	T36.0X1	T36.0X2	T36.0X3	T36.0X4	T36.0X5	T36.0X6
Sulbenicillin	T36.0X1	T36.0X2	T36.0X3	T36.0X4	T36.0X5	T36.0X6
Sulbentine	T49.0X1	T49.0X2	T49.0X3	T49.0X4	T49.0X5	T49.0X6
Sulfacetamide	T49.0X1	T49.0X2	T49.0X3	T49.0X4	T49.0X5	T49.0X6
ophthalmic preparation	T49.5X1	T49.5X2	T49.5X3	T49.5X4	T49.5X5	T49.5X6
Sulfachlorpyridazine	T37.0X1	T37.0X2	T37.0X3	T37.0X4	T37.0X5	T37.0X6
Sulfacitine	T37.0X1	T37.0X2	T37.0X3	T37.0X4	T37.0X5	T37.0X6
Sulfadiasulfone sodium	T37.0X1	T37.0X2	T37.0X3	T37.0X4	T37.0X5	T37.0X6
Sulfadiazine	T37.0X1	T37.0X2	T37.0X3	T37.0X4	T37.0X5	T37.0X6
silver (topical)	T49.0X1	T49.0X2	T49.0X3	T49.0X4	T49.0X5	T49.0X6
Sulfadimethoxine	T37.0X1	T37.0X2	T37.0X3	T37.0X4	T37.0X5	T37.0X6
Sulfadimidine	T37.0X1	T37.0X2	T37.0X3	T37.0X4	T37.0X5	T37.0X6
Sulfadoxine	T37.0X1	T37.0X2	T37.0X3	T37.0X4	T37.0X5	T37.0X6
with pyrimethamine	T37.2X1	T37.2X2	T37.2X3	T37.2X4	T37.2X5	T37.2X6
Sulfaethidole	T37.0X1	T37.0X2	T37.0X3	T37.0X4	T37.0X5	T37.0X6
Sulfafurazole	T37.0X1	T37.0X2	T37.0X3	T37.0X4	T37.0X5	T37.0X6
Sulfaguanidine	T37.0X1	T37.0X2	T37.0X3	T37.0X4	T37.0X5	T37.0X6
Sulfalene	T37.0X1	T37.0X2	T37.0X3	T37.0X4	T37.0X5	T37.0X6

Substance	Poisoning, Accidental (unintentional)	Poisoning, Intentional self-harm	Poisoning, Assault	Poisoning, Undetermined	Adverse effect	Underdosing
Sulfaloxate	T37.0X1	T37.0X2	T37.0X3	T37.0X4	T37.0X5	T37.0X6
Sulfaloxic acid	T37.0X1	T37.0X2	T37.0X3	T37.0X4	T37.0X5	T37.0X6
Sulfamazone	T39.2X1	T39.2X2	T39.2X3	T39.2X4	T39.2X5	T39.2X6
Sulfamerazine	T37.0X1	T37.0X2	T37.0X3	T37.0X4	T37.0X5	T37.0X6
Sulfameter	T37.0X1	T37.0X2	T37.0X3	T37.0X4	T37.0X5	T37.0X6
Sulfamethazine	T37.0X1	T37.0X2	T37.0X3	T37.0X4	T37.0X5	T37.0X6
Sulfamethizole	T37.0X1	T37.0X2	T37.0X3	T37.0X4	T37.0X5	T37.0X6
Sulfamethoxazole	T37.0X1	T37.0X2	T37.0X3	T37.0X4	T37.0X5	T37.0X6
with trimethoprim	T36.8X1	T36.8X2	T36.8X3	T36.8X4	T36.8X5	T36.8X6
Sulfamethoxydiazine	T37.0X1	T37.0X2	T37.0X3	T37.0X4	T37.0X5	T37.0X6
Sulfamethoxypyridazine	T37.0X1	T37.0X2	T37.0X3	T37.0X4	T37.0X5	T37.0X6
Sulfamethylthiazole	T37.0X1	T37.0X2	T37.0X3	T37.0X4	T37.0X5	T37.0X6
Sulfametoxydiazine	T37.0X1	T37.0X2	T37.0X3	T37.0X4	T37.0X5	T37.0X6
Sulfamidopyrine	T39.2X1	T39.2X2	T39.2X3	T39.2X4	T39.2X5	T39.2X6
Sulfamonomethoxine	T37.0X1	T37.0X2	T37.0X3	T37.0X4	T37.0X5	T37.0X6
Sulfamoxole	T37.0X1	T37.0X2	T37.0X3	T37.0X4	T37.0X5	T37.0X6
Sulfamylon	T49.0X1	T49.0X2	T49.0X3	T49.0X4	T49.0X5	T49.0X6
Sulfan blue (diagnostic dye)	T50.8X1	T50.8X2	T50.8X3	T50.8X4	T50.8X5	T50.8X6
Sulfanilamide	T37.0X1	T37.0X2	T37.0X3	T37.0X4	T37.0X5	T37.0X6
Sulfanilylguanidine	T37.0X1	T37.0X2	T37.0X3	T37.0X4	T37.0X5	T37.0X6
Sulfaperin	T37.0X1	T37.0X2	T37.0X3	T37.0X4	T37.0X5	T37.0X6
Sulfaphenazole	T37.0X1	T37.0X2	T37.0X3	T37.0X4	T37.0X5	T37.0X6
Sulfaphenylthiazole	T37.0X1	T37.0X2	T37.0X3	T37.0X4	T37.0X5	T37.0X6
Sulfaproxyline	T37.0X1	T37.0X2	T37.0X3	T37.0X4	T37.0X5	T37.0X6
Sulfapyridine	T37.0X1	T37.0X2	T37.0X3	T37.0X4	T37.0X5	T37.0X6
Sulfapyrimidine	T37.0X1	T37.0X2	T37.0X3	T37.0X4	T37.0X5	T37.0X6
Sulfarsphenamine	T37.8X1	T37.8X2	T37.8X3	T37.8X4	T37.8X5	T37.8X6
Sulfasalazine	T37.0X1	T37.0X2	T37.0X3	T37.0X4	T37.0X5	T37.0X6
Sulfasuxidine	T37.0X1	T37.0X2	T37.0X3	T37.0X4	T37.0X5	T37.0X6
Sulfasymazine	T37.0X1	T37.0X2	T37.0X3	T37.0X4	T37.0X5	T37.0X6
Sulfated amylopectin	T47.8X1	T47.8X2	T47.8X3	T47.8X4	T47.8X5	T47.8X6
Sulfathiazole	T37.0X1	T37.0X2	T37.0X3	T37.0X4	T37.0X5	T37.0X6
Sulfatostearate	T49.2X1	T49.2X2	T49.2X3	T49.2X4	T49.2X5	T49.2X6
Sulfinpyrazone	T50.4X1	T50.4X2	T50.4X3	T50.4X4	T50.4X5	T50.4X6
Sulfiram	T49.0X1	T49.0X2	T49.0X3	T49.0X4	T49.0X5	T49.0X6
Sulfisomidine	T37.0X1	T37.0X2	T37.0X3	T37.0X4	T37.0X5	T37.0X6
Sulfisoxazole	T37.0X1	T37.0X2	T37.0X3	T37.0X4	T37.0X5	T37.0X6
ophthalmic preparation	T49.5X1	T49.5X2	T49.5X3	T49.5X4	T49.5X5	T49.5X6
Sulfobromophthalein (sodium)	T50.8X1	T50.8X2	T50.8X3	T50.8X4	T50.8X5	T50.8X6
Sulfobromphthalein	T50.8X1	T50.8X2	T50.8X3	T50.8X4	T50.8X5	T50.8X6
Sulfogaiacol	T48.4X1	T48.4X2	T48.4X3	T48.4X4	T48.4X5	T48.4X6
Sulfomyxin	T36.8X1	T36.8X2	T36.8X3	T36.8X4	T36.8X5	T36.8X6
Sulfonal	T42.6X1	T42.6X2	T42.6X3	T42.6X4	T42.6X5	T42.6X6
Sulfonamide NEC	T37.0X1	T37.0X2	T37.0X3	T37.0X4	T37.0X5	T37.0X6
eye	T49.5X1	T49.5X2	T49.5X3	T49.5X4	T49.5X5	T49.5X6
Sulfonazide	T37.1X1	T37.1X2	T37.1X3	T37.1X4	T37.1X5	T37.1X6
Sulfones	T37.1X1	T37.1X2	T37.1X3	T37.1X4	T37.1X5	T37.1X6
Sulfonethylmethane	T42.6X1	T42.6X2	T42.6X3	T42.6X4	T42.6X5	T42.6X6
Sulfonmethane	T42.6X1	T42.6X2	T42.6X3	T42.6X4	T42.6X5	T42.6X6
Sulfonphthal, sulfonphthol	T50.8X1	T50.8X2	T50.8X3	T50.8X4	T50.8X5	T50.8X6
Sulfonylurea derivatives, oral	T38.3X1	T38.3X2	T38.3X3	T38.3X4	T38.3X5	T38.3X6
Sulforidazine	T43.3X1	T43.3X2	T43.3X3	T43.3X4	T43.3X5	T43.3X6
Sulfoxone	T37.1X1	T37.1X2	T37.1X3	T37.1X4	T37.1X5	T37.1X6
Sulfur, sulfurated, sulfuric, sulfurous, sulfuryl (compounds NEC) (medicinal)	T49.4X1	T49.4X2	T49.4X3	T49.4X4	T49.4X5	T49.4X6

Substance	Poisoning, Accidental (unintentional)	Poisoning, Intentional self-harm	Poisoning, Assault	Poisoning, Undetermined	Adverse effect	Underdosing
Sulfur, sulfurated, sulfuric, sulfurous, sulfuryl (compounds NEC) (medicinal) — *continued*						
acid	T54.2X1	T54.2X2	T54.2X3	T54.2X4	—	—
dioxide (gas)	T59.1X1	T59.1X2	T59.1X3	T59.1X4	—	—
ether—*see Ether(s)*						
hydrogen	T59.6X1	T59.6X2	T59.6X3	T59.6X4	—	—
medicinal (keratolytic) (ointment) NEC	T49.4X1	T49.4X2	T49.4X3	T49.4X4	T49.4X5	T49.4X6
ointment	T49.0X1	T49.0X2	T49.0X3	T49.0X4	T49.0X5	T49.0X6
pesticide (vapor)	T60.91	T60.92	T60.93	T60.94	—	—
vapor NEC	T59.891	T59.892	T59.893	T59.894	—	—
Sulfuric acid	T54.2X1	T54.2X2	T54.2X3	T54.2X4	—	—
Sulglicotide	T47.1X1	T47.1X2	T47.1X3	T47.1X4	T47.1X5	T47.1X6
Sulindac	T39.391	T39.392	T39.393	T39.394	T39.395	T39.396
Sulisatin	T47.2X1	T47.2X2	T47.2X3	T47.2X4	T47.2X5	T47.2X6
Sulisobenzone	T49.3X1	T49.3X2	T49.3X3	T49.3X4	T49.3X5	T49.3X6
Sulkowitch's reagent	T50.8X1	T50.8X2	T50.8X3	T50.8X4	T50.8X5	T50.8X6
Sulmetozine	T44.3X1	T44.3X2	T44.3X3	T44.3X4	T44.3X5	T44.3X6
Suloctidil	T46.7X1	T46.7X2	T46.7X3	T46.7X4	T46.7X5	T46.7X6
Sulph—*see also Sulf*						
Sulphadiazine	T37.0X1	T37.0X2	T37.0X3	T37.0X4	T37.0X5	T37.0X6
Sulphadimethoxine	T37.0X1	T37.0X2	T37.0X3	T37.0X4	T37.0X5	T37.0X6
Sulphadimidine	T37.0X1	T37.0X2	T37.0X3	T37.0X4	T37.0X5	T37.0X6
Sulphadione	T37.1X1	T37.1X2	T37.1X3	T37.1X4	T37.1X5	T37.1X6
Sulphafurazole	T37.0X1	T37.0X2	T37.0X3	T37.0X4	T37.0X5	T37.0X6
Sulphamethizole	T37.0X1	T37.0X2	T37.0X3	T37.0X4	T37.0X5	T37.0X6
Sulphamethoxazole	T37.0X1	T37.0X2	T37.0X3	T37.0X4	T37.0X5	T37.0X6
Sulphan blue	T50.8X1	T50.8X2	T50.8X3	T50.8X4	T50.8X5	T50.8X6
Sulphaphenazole	T37.0X1	T37.0X2	T37.0X3	T37.0X4	T37.0X5	T37.0X6
Sulphapyridine	T37.0X1	T37.0X2	T37.0X3	T37.0X4	T37.0X5	T37.0X6
Sulphasalazine	T37.0X1	T37.0X2	T37.0X3	T37.0X4	T37.0X5	T37.0X6
Sulphinpyrazone	T50.4X1	T50.4X2	T50.4X3	T50.4X4	T50.4X5	T50.4X6
Sulpiride	T43.591	T43.592	T43.593	T43.594	T43.595	T43.596
Sulprostone	T48.0X1	T48.0X2	T48.0X3	T48.0X4	T48.0X5	T48.0X6
Sulpyrine	T39.2X1	T39.2X2	T39.2X3	T39.2X4	T39.2X5	T39.2X6
Sultamicillin	T36.0X1	T36.0X2	T36.0X3	T36.0X4	T36.0X5	T36.0X6
Sulthiame	T42.6X1	T42.6X2	T42.6X3	T42.6X4	T42.6X5	T42.6X6
Sultiame	T42.6X1	T42.6X2	T42.6X3	T42.6X4	T42.6X5	T42.6X6
Sultopride	T43.591	T43.592	T43.593	T43.594	T43.595	T43.596
Sumatriptan	T39.8X1	T39.8X2	T39.8X3	T39.8X4	T39.8X5	T39.8X6
Sunflower seed oil	T46.6X1	T46.6X2	T46.6X3	T46.6X4	T46.6X5	T46.6X6
Superinone	T48.4X1	T48.4X2	T48.4X3	T48.4X4	T48.4X5	T48.4X6
Suprofen	T39.311	T39.312	T39.313	T39.314	T39.315	T39.316
Suramin (sodium)	T37.4X1	T37.4X2	T37.4X3	T37.4X4	T37.4X5	T37.4X6
Surfacaine	T41.3X1	T41.3X2	T41.3X3	T41.3X4	T41.3X5	T41.3X6
Surital	T41.1X1	T41.1X2	T41.1X3	T41.1X4	T41.1X5	T41.1X6
Sutilains	T45.3X1	T45.3X2	T45.3X3	T45.3X4	T45.3X5	T45.3X6
Suxamethonium (chloride)	T48.1X1	T48.1X2	T48.1X3	T48.1X4	T48.1X5	T48.1X6
Suxethonium (chloride)	T48.1X1	T48.1X2	T48.1X3	T48.1X4	T48.1X5	T48.1X6
Suxibuzone	T39.2X1	T39.2X2	T39.2X3	T39.2X4	T39.2X5	T39.2X6
Sweet niter spirit	T46.3X1	T46.3X2	T46.3X3	T46.3X4	T46.3X5	T46.3X6
Sweet oil (birch)	T49.3X1	T49.3X2	T49.3X3	T49.3X4	T49.3X5	T49.3X6
Sweetener	T50.901	T50.902	T50.903	T50.904	T50.905	T50.906
Sym-dichloroethyl ether	T53.6X1	T53.6X2	T53.6X3	T53.6X4	—	—
Sympatholytic NEC	T44.8X1	T44.8X2	T44.8X3	T44.8X4	T44.8X5	T44.8X6
haloalkylamine	T44.8X1	T44.8X2	T44.8X3	T44.8X4	T44.8X5	T44.8X6

Sympathomimetic NEC - Tetracosactide

Substance	Poisoning, Accidental (unintentional)	Poisoning, Intentional self-harm	Poisoning, Assault	Poisoning, Undetermined	Adverse effect	Underdosing
Sympathomimetic NEC	T44.901	T44.902	T44.903	T44.904	T44.905	T44.906
anti-common-cold	T48.5X1	T48.5X2	T48.5X3	T48.5X4	T48.5X5	T48.5X6
bronchodilator	T48.6X1	T48.6X2	T48.6X3	T48.6X4	T48.6X5	T48.6X6
specified NEC	T44.991	T44.992	T44.993	T44.994	T44.995	T44.996
Synagis	T50.B91	T50.B92	T50.B93	T50.B94	T50.B95	T50.B96
Synalar	T49.0X1	T49.0X2	T49.0X3	T49.0X4	T49.0X5	T49.0X6
Synthroid	T38.1X1	T38.1X2	T38.1X3	T38.1X4	T38.1X5	T38.1X6
Syntocinon	T48.0X1	T48.0X2	T48.0X3	T48.0X4	T48.0X5	T48.0X6
Syrosingopine	T46.5X1	T46.5X2	T46.5X3	T46.5X4	T46.5X5	T46.5X6
Systemic drug	T45.91	T45.92	T45.93	T45.94	T45.95	T45.96
specified NEC	T45.8X1	T45.8X2	T45.8X3	T45.8X4	T45.8X5	T45.8X6
2,4,5-T	T60.3X1	T60.3X2	T60.3X3	T60.3X4	—	—
T						
Tablets—*see also specified substance*	T50.901	T50.902	T50.903	T50.904	T50.905	T50.906
Tace	T38.5X1	T38.5X2	T38.5X3	T38.5X4	T38.5X5	T38.5X6
Tacrine	T44.0X1	T44.0X2	T44.0X3	T44.0X4	T44.0X5	T44.0X6
Tadalafil	T46.7X1	T46.7X2	T46.7X3	T46.7X4	T46.7X5	T46.7X6
Talampicillin	T36.0X1	T36.0X2	T36.0X3	T36.0X4	T36.0X5	T36.0X6
Talbutal	T42.3X1	T42.3X2	T42.3X3	T42.3X4	T42.3X5	T42.3X6
Talc powder	T49.3X1	T49.3X2	T49.3X3	T49.3X4	T49.3X5	T49.3X6
Talcum	T49.3X1	T49.3X2	T49.3X3	T49.3X4	T49.3X5	T49.3X6
Taleranol	T38.6X1	T38.6X2	T38.6X3	T38.6X4	T38.6X5	T38.6X6
Tamoxifen	T38.6X1	T38.6X2	T38.6X3	T38.6X4	T38.6X5	T38.6X6
Tamsulosin	T44.6X1	T44.6X2	T44.6X3	T44.6X4	T44.6X5	T44.6X6
Tandearil, tanderil	T39.2X1	T39.2X2	T39.2X3	T39.2X4	T39.2X5	T39.2X6
Tannic acid	T49.2X1	T49.2X2	T49.2X3	T49.2X4	T49.2X5	T49.2X6
medicinal (astringent)	T49.2X1	T49.2X2	T49.2X3	T49.2X4	T49.2X5	T49.2X6
Tannin—*see Tannic acid*						
Tansy	T62.2X1	T62.2X2	T62.2X3	T62.2X4	—	—
TAO	T36.3X1	T36.3X2	T36.3X3	T36.3X4	T36.3X5	T36.3X6
Tapazole	T38.2X1	T38.2X2	T38.2X3	T38.2X4	T38.2X5	T38.2X6
Tar NEC	T52.0X1	T52.0X2	T52.0X3	T52.0X4	—	—
camphor	T60.1X1	T60.1X2	T60.1X3	T60.1X4	—	—
distillate	T49.1X1	T49.1X2	T49.1X3	T49.1X4	T49.1X5	T49.1X6
fumes	T59.891	T59.892	T59.893	T59.894	—	—
medicinal	T49.1X1	T49.1X2	T49.1X3	T49.1X4	T49.1X5	T49.1X6
ointment	T49.1X1	T49.1X2	T49.1X3	T49.1X4	T49.1X5	T49.1X6
Taractan	T43.591	T43.592	T43.593	T43.594	T43.595	T43.596
Tarantula (venomous)	T63.321	T63.322	T63.323	T63.324	—	—
Tartar emetic	T37.8X1	T37.8X2	T37.8X3	T37.8X4	T37.8X5	T37.8X6
Tartaric acid	T65.891	T65.892	T65.893	T65.894	—	—
Tartrate, laxative	T47.4X1	T47.4X2	T47.4X3	T47.4X4	T47.4X5	T47.4X6
Tartrated antimony (anti-infective)	T37.8X1	T37.8X2	T37.8X3	T37.8X4	T37.8X5	T37.8X6
Tauromustine	T45.1X1	T45.1X2	T45.1X3	T45.1X4	T45.1X5	T45.1X6
TCA—*see Trichloroacetic acid*						
TCDD	T53.7X1	T53.7X2	T53.7X3	T53.7X4	—	—
TDI (vapor)	T65.0X1	T65.0X2	T65.0X3	T65.0X4	—	—
Tear						
gas	T59.3X1	T59.3X2	T59.3X3	T59.3X4	—	—
solution	T49.5X1	T49.5X2	T49.5X3	T49.5X4	T49.5X5	T49.5X6
Teclothiazide	T50.2X1	T50.2X2	T50.2X3	T50.2X4	T50.2X5	T50.2X6
Teclozan	T37.3X1	T37.3X2	T37.3X3	T37.3X4	T37.3X5	T37.3X6
Tegafur	T45.1X1	T45.1X2	T45.1X3	T45.1X4	T45.1X5	T45.1X6
Tegretol	T42.1X1	T42.1X2	T42.1X3	T42.1X4	T42.1X5	T42.1X6
Teicoplanin	T36.8X1	T36.8X2	T36.8X3	T36.8X4	T36.8X5	T36.8X6
Telepaque	T50.8X1	T50.8X2	T50.8X3	T50.8X4	T50.8X5	T50.8X6

Substance	Poisoning, Accidental (unintentional)	Poisoning, Intentional self-harm	Poisoning, Assault	Poisoning, Undetermined	Adverse effect	Underdosing
Tellurium	T56.891	T56.892	T56.893	T56.894	—	—
fumes	T56.891	T56.892	T56.893	T56.894	—	—
TEM	T45.1X1	T45.1X2	T45.1X3	T45.1X4	T45.1X5	T45.1X6
Temazepam	T42.4X1	T42.4X2	T42.4X3	T42.4X4	T42.4X5	T42.4X6
Temocillin	T36.0X1	T36.0X2	T36.0X3	T36.0X4	T36.0X5	T36.0X6
Tenamfetamine	T43.621	T43.622	T43.623	T43.624	T43.625	T43.626
Teniposide	T45.1X1	T45.1X2	T45.1X3	T45.1X4	T45.1X5	T45.1X6
Tenitramine	T46.3X1	T46.3X2	T46.3X3	T46.3X4	T46.3X5	T46.3X6
Tenoglicin	T48.4X1	T48.4X2	T48.4X3	T48.4X4	T48.4X5	T48.4X6
Tenonitrozole	T37.3X1	T37.3X2	T37.3X3	T37.3X4	T37.3X5	T37.3X6
Tenoxicam	T39.391	T39.392	T39.393	T39.394	T39.395	T39.396
TEPA	T45.1X1	T45.1X2	T45.1X3	T45.1X4	T45.1X5	T45.1X6
TEPP	T60.0X1	T60.0X2	T60.0X3	T60.0X4	—	—
Teprotide	T46.5X1	T46.5X2	T46.5X3	T46.5X4	T46.5X5	T46.5X6
Terazosin	T44.6X1	T44.6X2	T44.6X3	T44.6X4	T44.6X5	T44.6X6
Terbufos	T60.0X1	T60.0X2	T60.0X3	T60.0X4	—	—
Terbutaline	T48.6X1	T48.6X2	T48.6X3	T48.6X4	T48.6X5	T48.6X6
Terconazole	T49.0X1	T49.0X2	T49.0X3	T49.0X4	T49.0X5	T49.0X6
Terfenadine	T45.0X1	T45.0X2	T45.0X3	T45.0X4	T45.0X5	T45.0X6
Teriparatide (acetate)	T50.991	T50.992	T50.993	T50.994	T50.995	T50.996
Terizidone	T37.1X1	T37.1X2	T37.1X3	T37.1X4	T37.1X5	T37.1X6
Terlipressin	T38.891	T38.892	T38.893	T38.894	T38.895	T38.896
Terodiline	T46.3X1	T46.3X2	T46.3X3	T46.3X4	T46.3X5	T46.3X6
Teroxalene	T37.4X1	T37.4X2	T37.4X3	T37.4X4	T37.4X5	T37.4X6
Terpin (cis) hydrate	T48.4X1	T48.4X2	T48.4X3	T48.4X4	T48.4X5	T48.4X6
Terramycin	T36.4X1	T36.4X2	T36.4X3	T36.4X4	T36.4X5	T36.4X6
Tertatolol	T44.7X1	T44.7X2	T44.7X3	T44.7X4	T44.7X5	T44.7X6
Tessalon	T48.3X1	T48.3X2	T48.3X3	T48.3X4	T48.3X5	T48.3X6
Testolactone	T38.7X1	T38.7X2	T38.7X3	T38.7X4	T38.7X5	T38.7X6
Testosterone	T38.7X1	T38.7X2	T38.7X3	T38.7X4	T38.7X5	T38.7X6
Tetanus toxoid or vaccine	T50.A91	T50.A92	T50.A93	T50.A94	T50.A95	T50.A96
antitoxin	T50.Z11	T50.Z12	T50.Z13	T50.Z14	T50.Z15	T50.Z16
immune globulin (human)	T50.Z11	T50.Z12	T50.Z13	T50.Z14	T50.Z15	T50.Z16
toxoid	T50.A91	T50.A92	T50.A93	T50.A94	T50.A95	T50.A96
with diphtheria toxoid	T50.A21	T50.A22	T50.A23	T50.A24	T50.A25	T50.A26
with pertussis	T50.A11	T50.A12	T50.A13	T50.A14	T50.A15	T50.A16
Tetrabenazine	T43.591	T43.592	T43.593	T43.594	T43.595	T43.596
Tetracaine	T41.3X1	T41.3X2	T41.3X3	T41.3X4	T41.3X5	T41.3X6
nerve block (peripheral) (plexus)	T41.3X1	T41.3X2	T41.3X3	T41.3X4	T41.3X5	T41.3X6
regional	T41.3X1	T41.3X2	T41.3X3	T41.3X4	T41.3X5	T41.3X6
spinal	T41.3X1	T41.3X2	T41.3X3	T41.3X4	T41.3X5	T41.3X6
Tetrachlorethylene—*see Tetrachloroethylene*						
Tetrachlormethiazide	T50.2X1	T50.2X2	T50.2X3	T50.2X4	T50.2X5	T50.2X6
2,3,7,8-Tetrachlorod-ibenzo-p-dioxin	T53.7X1	T53.7X2	T53.7X3	T53.7X4	—	—
Tetrachloroethane	T53.6X1	T53.6X2	T53.6X3	T53.6X4	—	—
vapor	T53.6X1	T53.6X2	T53.6X3	T53.6X4	—	—
paint or varnish	T53.6X1	T53.6X2	T53.6X3	T53.6X4	—	—
Tetrachloroethylene (liquid)	T53.3X1	T53.3X2	T53.3X3	T53.3X4	—	—
medicinal	T37.4X1	T37.4X2	T37.4X3	T37.4X4	T37.4X5	T37.4X6
vapor	T53.3X1	T53.3X2	T53.3X3	T53.3X4	—	—
Tetrachloromethane—*see Carbon tetrachloride*						
Tetracosactide	T38.811	T38.812	T38.813	T38.814	T38.815	T38.816

Substance	Poisoning, Accidental (unintentional)	Poisoning, Intentional self-harm	Poisoning, Assault	Poisoning, Undetermined	Adverse effect	Underdosing
Tetracosactrin	T38.811	T38.812	T38.813	T38.814	T38.815	T38.816
Tetracycline	T36.4X1	T36.4X2	T36.4X3	T36.4X4	T36.4X5	T36.4X6
ophthalmic preparation	T49.5X1	T49.5X2	T49.5X3	T49.5X4	T49.5X5	T49.5X6
topical NEC	T49.0X1	T49.0X2	T49.0X3	T49.0X4	T49.0X5	T49.0X6
Tetradifon	T60.8X1	T60.8X2	T60.8X3	T60.8X4	—	—
Tetradotoxin	T61.771	T61.772	T61.773	T61.774	—	—
Tetraethyl						
lead	T56.0X1	T56.0X2	T56.0X3	T56.0X4	—	—
pyrophosphate	T60.0X1	T60.0X2	T60.0X3	T60.0X4	—	—
Tetraethylammonium chloride	T44.2X1	T44.2X2	T44.2X3	T44.2X4	T44.2X5	T44.2X6
Tetraethylthiuram disulfide	T50.6X1	T50.6X2	T50.6X3	T50.6X4	T50.6X5	T50.6X6
Tetrahydroaminoacri-dine	T44.0X1	T44.0X2	T44.0X3	T44.0X4	T44.0X5	T44.0X6
Tetrahydrocannabinol	T40.7X1	T40.7X2	T40.7X3	T40.7X4	T40.7X5	T40.7X6
Tetrahydrofuran	T52.8X1	T52.8X2	T52.8X3	T52.8X4	—	—
Tetrahydronaphthalene	T52.8X1	T52.8X2	T52.8X3	T52.8X4	—	—
Tetrahydrozoline	T49.5X1	T49.5X2	T49.5X3	T49.5X4	T49.5X5	T49.5X6
Tetralin	T52.8X1	T52.8X2	T52.8X3	T52.8X4	—	—
Tetramethrin	T60.2X1	T60.2X2	T60.2X3	T60.2X4	—	—
Tetramethylthiuram (disulfide) NEC	T60.3X1	T60.3X2	T60.3X3	T60.3X4	—	—
medicinal	T49.0X1	T49.0X2	T49.0X3	T49.0X4	T49.0X5	T49.0X6
Tetramisole	T37.4X1	T37.4X2	T37.4X3	T37.4X4	T37.4X5	T37.4X6
Tetranicotinoyl fructose	T46.7X1	T46.7X2	T46.7X3	T46.7X4	T46.7X5	T46.7X6
Tetrazepam	T42.4X1	T42.4X2	T42.4X3	T42.4X4	T42.4X5	T42.4X6
Tetronal	T42.6X1	T42.6X2	T42.6X3	T42.6X4	T42.6X5	T42.6X6
Tetryl	T65.3X1	T65.3X2	T65.3X3	T65.3X4	—	—
Tetrylammonium chloride	T44.2X1	T44.2X2	T44.2X3	T44.2X4	T44.2X5	T44.2X6
Tetryzoline	T49.5X1	T49.5X2	T49.5X3	T49.5X4	T49.5X5	T49.5X6
Thalidomide	T45.1X1	T45.1X2	T45.1X3	T45.1X4	T45.1X5	T45.1X6
Thallium (compounds) (dust) NEC	T56.811	T56.812	T56.813	T56.814	—	—
pesticide	T60.4X1	T60.4X2	T60.4X3	T60.4X4	—	—
THC	T40.7X1	T40.7X2	T40.7X3	T40.7X4	T40.7X5	T40.7X6
Thebacon	T48.3X1	T48.3X2	T48.3X3	T48.3X4	T48.3X5	T48.3X6
Thebaine	T40.2X1	T40.2X2	T40.2X3	T40.2X4	T40.2X5	T40.2X6
Thenoic acid	T49.6X1	T49.6X2	T49.6X3	T49.6X4	T49.6X5	T49.6X6
Thenyldiamine	T45.0X1	T45.0X2	T45.0X3	T45.0X4	T45.0X5	T45.0X6
Theobromine (calcium salicylate)	T48.6X1	T48.6X2	T48.6X3	T48.6X4	T48.6X5	T48.6X6
sodium salicylate	T48.6X1	T48.6X2	T48.6X3	T48.6X4	T48.6X5	T48.6X6
Theophyllamine	T48.6X1	T48.6X2	T48.6X3	T48.6X4	T48.6X5	T48.6X6
Theophylline	T48.6X1	T48.6X2	T48.6X3	T48.6X4	T48.6X5	T48.6X6
aminobenzoic acid	T48.6X1	T48.6X2	T48.6X3	T48.6X4	T48.6X5	T48.6X6
ethylenediamine	T48.6X1	T48.6X2	T48.6X3	T48.6X4	T48.6X5	T48.6X6
piperazine p-amino-benzoate	T48.6X1	T48.6X2	T48.6X3	T48.6X4	T48.6X5	T48.6X6
Thiabendazole	T37.4X1	T37.4X2	T37.4X3	T37.4X4	T37.4X5	T37.4X6
Thialbarbital	T41.1X1	T41.1X2	T41.1X3	T41.1X4	T41.1X5	T41.1X6
Thiamazole	T38.2X1	T38.2X2	T38.2X3	T38.2X4	T38.2X5	T38.2X6
Thiambutosine	T37.1X1	T37.1X2	T37.1X3	T37.1X4	T37.1X5	T37.1X6
Thiamine	T45.2X1	T45.2X2	T45.2X3	T45.2X4	T45.2X5	T45.2X6
Thiamphenicol	T36.2X1	T36.2X2	T36.2X3	T36.2X4	T36.2X5	T36.2X6
Thiamylal	T41.1X1	T41.1X2	T41.1X3	T41.1X4	T41.1X5	T41.1X6
sodium	T41.1X1	T41.1X2	T41.1X3	T41.1X4	T41.1X5	T41.1X6
Thiazesim	T43.291	T43.292	T43.293	T43.294	T43.295	T43.296
Thiazides (diuretics)	T50.2X1	T50.2X2	T50.2X3	T50.2X4	T50.2X5	T50.2X6
Thiazinamium metilsulfate	T43.3X1	T43.3X2	T43.3X3	T43.3X4	T43.3X5	T43.3X6
Thiethylperazine	T43.3X1	T43.3X2	T43.3X3	T43.3X4	T43.3X5	T43.3X6
Thimerosal	T49.0X1	T49.0X2	T49.0X3	T49.0X4	T49.0X5	T49.0X6
ophthalmic preparation	T49.5X1	T49.5X2	T49.5X3	T49.5X4	T49.5X5	T49.5X6
Thioacetazone	T37.1X1	T37.1X2	T37.1X3	T37.1X4	T37.1X5	T37.1X6
with isoniazid	T37.1X1	T37.1X2	T37.1X3	T37.1X4	T37.1X5	T37.1X6
Thiobarbital sodium	T41.1X1	T41.1X2	T41.1X3	T41.1X4	T41.1X5	T41.1X6
Thiobarbiturate anesthetic	T41.1X1	T41.1X2	T41.1X3	T41.1X4	T41.1X5	T41.1X6
Thiobismol	T37.8X1	T37.8X2	T37.8X3	T37.8X4	T37.8X5	T37.8X6
Thiobutabarbital sodium	T41.1X1	T41.1X2	T41.1X3	T41.1X4	T41.1X5	T41.1X6
Thiocarbamate (insecticide)	T60.0X1	T60.0X2	T60.0X3	T60.0X4	—	—
Thiocarbamide	T38.2X1	T38.2X2	T38.2X3	T38.2X4	T38.2X5	T38.2X6
Thiocarbarsone	T37.8X1	T37.8X2	T37.8X3	T37.8X4	T37.8X5	T37.8X6
Thiocarlide	T37.1X1	T37.1X2	T37.1X3	T37.1X4	T37.1X5	T37.1X6
Thioctamide	T50.991	T50.992	T50.993	T50.994	T50.995	T50.996
Thioctic acid	T50.991	T50.992	T50.993	T50.994	T50.995	T50.996
Thiofos	T60.0X1	T60.0X2	T60.0X3	T60.0X4	—	—
Thioglycolate	T49.4X1	T49.4X2	T49.4X3	T49.4X4	T49.4X5	T49.4X6
Thioglycolic acid	T65.891	T65.892	T65.893	T65.894	—	—
Thioguanine	T45.1X1	T45.1X2	T45.1X3	T45.1X4	T45.1X5	T45.1X6
Thiomercaptomerin	T50.2X1	T50.2X2	T50.2X3	T50.2X4	T50.2X5	T50.2X6
Thiomerin	T50.2X1	T50.2X2	T50.2X3	T50.2X4	T50.2X5	T50.2X6
Thiomersal	T49.0X1	T49.0X2	T49.0X3	T49.0X4	T49.0X5	T49.0X6
Thionazin	T60.0X1	T60.0X2	T60.0X3	T60.0X4	—	—
Thiopental (sodium)	T41.1X1	T41.1X2	T41.1X3	T41.1X4	T41.1X5	T41.1X6
Thiopentone (sodium)	T41.1X1	T41.1X2	T41.1X3	T41.1X4	T41.1X5	T41.1X6
Thiopropazate	T43.3X1	T43.3X2	T43.3X3	T43.3X4	T43.3X5	T43.3X6
Thioproperazine	T43.3X1	T43.3X2	T43.3X3	T43.3X4	T43.3X5	T43.3X6
Thioridazine	T43.3X1	T43.3X2	T43.3X3	T43.3X4	T43.3X5	T43.3X6
Thiosinamine	T49.3X1	T49.3X2	T49.3X3	T49.3X4	T49.3X5	T49.3X6
Thiotepa	T45.1X1	T45.1X2	T45.1X3	T45.1X4	T45.1X5	T45.1X6
Thiothixene	T43.4X1	T43.4X2	T43.4X3	T43.4X4	T43.4X5	T43.4X6
Thiouracil (benzyl) (methyl) (propyl)	T38.2X1	T38.2X2	T38.2X3	T38.2X4	T38.2X5	T38.2X6
Thiourea	T38.2X1	T38.2X2	T38.2X3	T38.2X4	T38.2X5	T38.2X6
Thiphenamil	T44.3X1	T44.3X2	T44.3X3	T44.3X4	T44.3X5	T44.3X6
Thiram	T60.3X1	T60.3X2	T60.3X3	T60.3X4	—	—
medicinal	T49.2X1	T49.2X2	T49.2X3	T49.2X4	T49.2X5	T49.2X6
Thonzylamine (systemic)	T45.0X1	T45.0X2	T45.0X3	T45.0X4	T45.0X5	T45.0X6
mucosal decongestant	T48.5X1	T48.5X2	T48.5X3	T48.5X4	T48.5X5	T48.5X6
Thorazine	T43.3X1	T43.3X2	T43.3X3	T43.3X4	T43.3X5	T43.3X6
Thorium dioxide suspension	T50.8X1	T50.8X2	T50.8X3	T50.8X4	T50.8X5	T50.8X6
Thornapple	T62.2X1	T62.2X2	T62.2X3	T62.2X4	—	—
Throat drug NEC	T49.6X1	T49.6X2	T49.6X3	T49.6X4	T49.6X5	T49.6X6
Thrombin	T45.7X1	T45.7X2	T45.7X3	T45.7X4	T45.7X5	T45.7X6
Thrombolysin	T45.611	T45.612	T45.613	T45.614	T45.615	T45.616
Thromboplastin	T45.7X1	T45.7X2	T45.7X3	T45.7X4	T45.7X5	T45.7X6
Thurfyl nicotinate	T46.7X1	T46.7X2	T46.7X3	T46.7X4	T46.7X5	T46.7X6
Thymol	T49.0X1	T49.0X2	T49.0X3	T49.0X4	T49.0X5	T49.0X6
Thymopentin	T37.5X1	T37.5X2	T37.5X3	T37.5X4	T37.5X5	T37.5X6
Thymoxamine	T46.7X1	T46.7X2	T46.7X3	T46.7X4	T46.7X5	T46.7X6
Thymus extract	T38.891	T38.892	T38.893	T38.894	T38.895	T38.896
Thyreotrophic hormone	T38.811	T38.812	T38.813	T38.814	T38.815	T38.816
Thyroglobulin	T38.1X1	T38.1X2	T38.1X3	T38.1X4	T38.1X5	T38.1X6
Thyroid (hormone)	T38.1X1	T38.1X2	T38.1X3	T38.1X4	T38.1X5	T38.1X6
Thyrolar	T38.1X1	T38.1X2	T38.1X3	T38.1X4	T38.1X5	T38.1X6
Thyrotrophin	T38.811	T38.812	T38.813	T38.814	T38.815	T38.816

Substance	Poisoning, Accidental (unintentional)	Poisoning, Intentional self-harm	Poisoning, Assault	Poisoning, Undetermined	Adverse effect	Underdosing
Thyrotropic hormone	T38.811	T38.812	T38.813	T38.814	T38.815	T38.816
Thyroxine	T38.1X1	T38.1X2	T38.1X3	T38.1X4	T38.1X5	T38.1X6
Tiabendazole	T37.4X1	T37.4X2	T37.4X3	T37.4X4	T37.4X5	T37.4X6
Tiamizide	T50.2X1	T50.2X2	T50.2X3	T50.2X4	T50.2X5	T50.2X6
Tianeptine	T43.291	T43.292	T43.293	T43.294	T43.295	T43.296
Tiapamil	T46.1X1	T46.1X2	T46.1X3	T46.1X4	T46.1X5	T46.1X6
Tiapride	T43.591	T43.592	T43.593	T43.594	T43.595	T43.596
Tiaprofenic acid	T39.311	T39.312	T39.313	T39.314	T39.315	T39.316
Tiaramide	T39.8X1	T39.8X2	T39.8X3	T39.8X4	T39.8X5	T39.8X6
Ticarcillin	T36.0X1	T36.0X2	T36.0X3	T36.0X4	T36.0X5	T36.0X6
Ticlatone	T49.0X1	T49.0X2	T49.0X3	T49.0X4	T49.0X5	T49.0X6
Ticlopidine	T45.521	T45.522	T45.523	T45.524	T45.525	T45.526
Ticrynafen	T50.1X1	T50.1X2	T50.1X3	T50.1X4	T50.1X5	T50.1X6
Tidiacic	T50.991	T50.992	T50.993	T50.994	T50.995	T50.996
Tiemonium	T44.3X1	T44.3X2	T44.3X3	T44.3X4	T44.3X5	T44.3X6
iodide	T44.3X1	T44.3X2	T44.3X3	T44.3X4	T44.3X5	T44.3X6
Tienilic acid	T50.1X1	T50.1X2	T50.1X3	T50.1X4	T50.1X5	T50.1X6
Tifenamil	T44.3X1	T44.3X2	T44.3X3	T44.3X4	T44.3X5	T44.3X6
Tigan	T45.0X1	T45.0X2	T45.0X3	T45.0X4	T45.0X5	T45.0X6
Tigloidine	T44.3X1	T44.3X2	T44.3X3	T44.3X4	T44.3X5	T44.3X6
Tilactase	T47.5X1	T47.5X2	T47.5X3	T47.5X4	T47.5X5	T47.5X6
Tiletamine	T41.291	T41.292	T41.293	T41.294	T41.295	T41.296
Tilidine	T40.4X1	T40.4X2	T40.4X3	T40.4X4	—	—
Timepidium bromide	T44.3X1	T44.3X2	T44.3X3	T44.3X4	T44.3X5	T44.3X6
Timiperone	T43.4X1	T43.4X2	T43.4X3	T43.4X4	T43.4X5	T43.4X6
Timolol	T44.7X1	T44.7X2	T44.7X3	T44.7X4	T44.7X5	T44.7X6
Tin (chloride) (dust) (oxide) NEC	T56.6X1	T56.6X2	T56.6X3	T56.6X4	—	—
anti-infectives	T37.8X1	T37.8X2	T37.8X3	T37.8X4	T37.8X5	T37.8X6
Tincture, iodine—see Iodine						
Tindal	T43.3X1	T43.3X2	T43.3X3	T43.3X4	T43.3X5	T43.3X6
Tinidazole	T37.3X1	T37.3X2	T37.3X3	T37.3X4	T37.3X5	T37.3X6
Tinoridine	T39.8X1	T39.8X2	T39.8X3	T39.8X4	T39.8X5	T39.8X6
Tiocarlide	T37.1X1	T37.1X2	T37.1X3	T37.1X4	T37.1X5	T37.1X6
Tioclomarol	T45.511	T45.512	T45.513	T45.514	T45.515	T45.516
Tioconazole	T49.0X1	T49.0X2	T49.0X3	T49.0X4	T49.0X5	T49.0X6
Tioguanine	T45.1X1	T45.1X2	T45.1X3	T45.1X4	T45.1X5	T45.1X6
Tiopronin	T50.991	T50.992	T50.993	T50.994	T50.995	T50.996
Tiotixene	T43.4X1	T43.4X2	T43.4X3	T43.4X4	T43.4X5	T43.4X6
Tioxolone	T49.4X1	T49.4X2	T49.4X3	T49.4X4	T49.4X5	T49.4X6
Tipepidine	T48.3X1	T48.3X2	T48.3X3	T48.3X4	T48.3X5	T48.3X6
Tiquizium bromide	T44.3X1	T44.3X2	T44.3X3	T44.3X4	T44.3X5	T44.3X6
Tiratricol	T38.1X1	T38.1X2	T38.1X3	T38.1X4	T38.1X5	T38.1X6
Tisopurine	T50.4X1	T50.4X2	T50.4X3	T50.4X4	T50.4X5	T50.4X6
Titanium (compounds) (vapor)	T56.891	T56.892	T56.893	T56.894	—	—
dioxide	T49.3X1	T49.3X2	T49.3X3	T49.3X4	T49.3X5	T49.3X6
ointment	T49.3X1	T49.3X2	T49.3X3	T49.3X4	T49.3X5	T49.3X6
oxide	T49.3X1	T49.3X2	T49.3X3	T49.3X4	T49.3X5	T49.3X6
tetrachloride	T56.891	T56.892	T56.893	T56.894	—	—
Titanocene	T56.891	T56.892	T56.893	T56.894	—	—
Titroid	T38.1X1	T38.1X2	T38.1X3	T38.1X4	T38.1X5	T38.1X6
Tizanidine	T42.8X1	T42.8X2	T42.8X3	T42.8X4	T42.8X5	T42.8X6
TMTD	T60.3X1	T60.3X2	T60.3X3	T60.3X4	—	—
TNT (fumes)	T65.3X1	T65.3X2	T65.3X3	T65.3X4	—	—
Toadstool	T62.0X1	T62.0X2	T62.0X3	T62.0X4	—	—
Tobacco NEC	T65.291	T65.292	T65.293	T65.294	—	—
cigarettes	T65.221	T65.222	T65.223	T65.224	—	—
Indian	T62.2X1	T62.2X2	T62.2X3	T62.2X4	—	—
smoke, second-hand	T65.221	T65.222	T65.223	T65.224	—	—

Substance	Poisoning, Accidental (unintentional)	Poisoning, Intentional self-harm	Poisoning, Assault	Poisoning, Undetermined	Adverse effect	Underdosing
Tobramycin	T36.5X1	T36.5X2	T36.5X3	T36.5X4	T36.5X5	T36.5X6
Tocainide	T46.2X1	T46.2X2	T46.2X3	T46.2X4	T46.2X5	T46.2X6
Tocoferol	T45.2X1	T45.2X2	T45.2X3	T45.2X4	T45.2X5	T45.2X6
Tocopherol	T45.2X1	T45.2X2	T45.2X3	T45.2X4	T45.2X5	T45.2X6
acetate	T45.2X1	T45.2X2	T45.2X3	T45.2X4	T45.2X5	T45.2X6
Tocosamine	T48.0X1	T48.0X2	T48.0X3	T48.0X4	T48.0X5	T48.0X6
Todralazine	T46.5X1	T46.5X2	T46.5X3	T46.5X4	T46.5X5	T46.5X6
Tofisopam	T42.4X1	T42.4X2	T42.4X3	T42.4X4	T42.4X5	T42.4X6
Tofranil	T43.011	T43.012	T43.013	T43.014	T43.015	T43.016
Toilet deodorizer	T65.891	T65.892	T65.893	T65.894	—	—
Tolamolol	T44.7X1	T44.7X2	T44.7X3	T44.7X4	T44.7X5	T44.7X6
Tolazamide	T38.3X1	T38.3X2	T38.3X3	T38.3X4	T38.3X5	T38.3X6
Tolazoline	T46.7X1	T46.7X2	T46.7X3	T46.7X4	T46.7X5	T46.7X6
Tolbutamide (sodium)	T38.3X1	T38.3X2	T38.3X3	T38.3X4	T38.3X5	T38.3X6
Tolciclate	T49.0X1	T49.0X2	T49.0X3	T49.0X4	T49.0X5	T49.0X6
Tolmetin	T39.391	T39.392	T39.393	T39.394	T39.395	T39.396
Tolnaftate	T49.0X1	T49.0X2	T49.0X3	T49.0X4	T49.0X5	T49.0X6
Tolonidine	T46.5X1	T46.5X2	T46.5X3	T46.5X4	T46.5X5	T46.5X6
Toloxatone	T42.6X1	T42.6X2	T42.6X3	T42.6X4	T42.6X5	T42.6X6
Tolperisone	T44.3X1	T44.3X2	T44.3X3	T44.3X4	T44.3X5	T44.3X6
Tolserol	T42.8X1	T42.8X2	T42.8X3	T42.8X4	T42.8X5	T42.8X6
Toluene (liquid)	T52.2X1	T52.2X2	T52.2X3	T52.2X4	—	—
diisocyanate	T65.0X1	T65.0X2	T65.0X3	T65.0X4	—	—
Toluidine	T65.891	T65.892	T65.893	T65.894	—	—
vapor	T59.891	T59.892	T59.893	T59.894	—	—
Toluol (liquid)	T52.2X1	T52.2X2	T52.2X3	T52.2X4	—	—
vapor	T52.2X1	T52.2X2	T52.2X3	T52.2X4	—	—
Toluylenediamine	T65.3X1	T65.3X2	T65.3X3	T65.3X4	—	—
Tolylene-2,4-diisocyanate	T65.0X1	T65.0X2	T65.0X3	T65.0X4	—	—
Tonic NEC	T50.901	T50.902	T50.903	T50.904	T50.905	T50.906
Topical action drug NEC	T49.91	T49.92	T49.93	T49.94	T49.95	T49.96
ear, nose or throat	T49.6X1	T49.6X2	T49.6X3	T49.6X4	T49.6X5	T49.6X6
eye	T49.5X1	T49.5X2	T49.5X3	T49.5X4	T49.5X5	T49.5X6
skin	T49.91	T49.92	T49.93	T49.94	T49.95	T49.96
specified NEC	T49.8X1	T49.8X2	T49.8X3	T49.8X4	T49.8X5	T49.8X6
Toquizine	T44.3X1	T44.3X2	T44.3X3	T44.3X4	T44.3X5	T44.3X6
Toremifene	T38.6X1	T38.6X2	T38.6X3	T38.6X4	T38.6X5	T38.6X6
Tosylchloramide sodium	T49.8X1	T49.8X2	T49.8X3	T49.8X4	T49.8X5	T49.8X6
Toxaphene (dust) (spray)	T60.1X1	T60.1X2	T60.1X3	T60.1X4	—	—
Toxin, diphtheria (Schick Test)	T50.8X1	T50.8X2	T50.8X3	T50.8X4	T50.8X5	T50.8X6
Toxoid						
combined	T50.A21	T50.A22	T50.A23	T50.A24	T50.A25	T50.A26
diphtheria	T50.A91	T50.A92	T50.A93	T50.A94	T50.A95	T50.A96
tetanus	T50.A91	T50.A92	T50.A93	T50.A94	T50.A95	T50.A96
Trace element NEC	T45.8X1	T45.8X2	T45.8X3	T45.8X4	T45.8X5	T45.8X6
Tractor fuel NEC	T52.0X1	T52.0X2	T52.0X3	T52.0X4	—	—
Tragacanth	T50.991	T50.992	T50.993	T50.994	T50.995	T50.996
Tramadol	T40.4X1	T40.4X2	T40.4X3	T40.4X4	T40.4X5	T40.4X6
Tramazoline	T48.5X1	T48.5X2	T48.5X3	T48.5X4	T48.5X5	T48.5X6
Tranexamic acid	T45.621	T45.622	T45.623	T45.624	T45.625	T45.626
Tranilast	T45.0X1	T45.0X2	T45.0X3	T45.0X4	T45.0X5	T45.0X6
Tranquilizer NEC	T43.501	T43.502	T43.503	T43.504	T43.505	T43.506
with hypnotic or sedative	T42.6X1	T42.6X2	T42.6X3	T42.6X4	T42.6X5	T42.6X6
benzodiazepine NEC	T42.4X1	T42.4X2	T42.4X3	T42.4X4	T42.4X5	T42.4X6
butyrophenone NEC	T43.4X1	T43.4X2	T43.4X3	T43.4X4	T43.4X5	T43.4X6
carbamate	T43.591	T43.592	T43.593	T43.594	T43.595	T43.596
dimethylamine	T43.3X1	T43.3X2	T43.3X3	T43.3X4	T43.3X5	T43.3X6
ethylamine	T43.3X1	T43.3X2	T43.3X3	T43.3X4	T43.3X5	T43.3X6

Substance	Poisoning, Accidental (unintentional)	Poisoning, Intentional self-harm	Poisoning, Assault	Poisoning, Undetermined	Adverse effect	Underdosing
Tranquilizer NEC — *continued*						
hydroxyzine	T43.591	T43.592	T43.593	T43.594	T43.595	T43.596
major NEC	T43.501	T43.502	T43.503	T43.504	T43.505	T43.506
penothiazine NEC	T43.3X1	T43.3X2	T43.3X3	T43.3X4	T43.3X5	T43.3X6
phenothiazine-based	T43.3X1	T43.3X2	T43.3X3	T43.3X4	T43.3X5	T43.3X6
piperazine NEC	T43.3X1	T43.3X2	T43.3X3	T43.3X4	T43.3X5	T43.3X6
piperidine	T43.3X1	T43.3X2	T43.3X3	T43.3X4	T43.3X5	T43.3X6
propylamine	T43.3X1	T43.3X2	T43.3X3	T43.3X4	T43.3X5	T43.3X6
specified NEC	T43.591	T43.592	T43.593	T43.594	T43.595	T43.596
thioxanthene NEC	T43.591	T43.592	T43.593	T43.594	T43.595	T43.596
Tranxene	T42.4X1	T42.4X2	T42.4X3	T42.4X4	T42.4X5	T42.4X6
Tranylcypromine	T43.1X1	T43.1X2	T43.1X3	T43.1X4	T43.1X5	T43.1X6
Trapidil	T46.3X1	T46.3X2	T46.3X3	T46.3X4	T46.3X5	T46.3X6
Trasentine	T44.3X1	T44.3X2	T44.3X3	T44.3X4	T44.3X5	T44.3X6
Travert	T50.3X1	T50.3X2	T50.3X3	T50.3X4	T50.3X5	T50.3X6
Trazodone	T43.211	T43.212	T43.213	T43.214	T43.215	T43.216
Trecator	T37.1X1	T37.1X2	T37.1X3	T37.1X4	T37.1X5	T37.1X6
Treosulfan	T45.1X1	T45.1X2	T45.1X3	T45.1X4	T45.1X5	T45.1X6
Tretamine	T45.1X1	T45.1X2	T45.1X3	T45.1X4	T45.1X5	T45.1X6
Tretinoin	T49.0X1	T49.0X2	T49.0X3	T49.0X4	T49.0X5	T49.0X6
Tretoquinol	T48.6X1	T48.6X2	T48.6X3	T48.6X4	T48.6X5	T48.6X6
Triacetin	T49.0X1	T49.0X2	T49.0X3	T49.0X4	T49.0X5	T49.0X6
Triacetoxyanthracene	T49.4X1	T49.4X2	T49.4X3	T49.4X4	T49.4X5	T49.4X6
Triacetyloleandomycin	T36.3X1	T36.3X2	T36.3X3	T36.3X4	T36.3X5	T36.3X6
Triamcinolone	T49.0X1	T49.0X2	T49.0X3	T49.0X4	T49.0X5	T49.0X6
ENT agent	T49.6X1	T49.6X2	T49.6X3	T49.6X4	T49.6X5	T49.6X6
hexacetonide	T49.0X1	T49.0X2	T49.0X3	T49.0X4	T49.0X5	T49.0X6
ophthalmic preparation	T49.5X1	T49.5X2	T49.5X3	T49.5X4	T49.5X5	T49.5X6
topical NEC	T49.0X1	T49.0X2	T49.0X3	T49.0X4	T49.0X5	T49.0X6
Triampyzine	T44.3X1	T44.3X2	T44.3X3	T44.3X4	T44.3X5	T44.3X6
Triamterene	T50.2X1	T50.2X2	T50.2X3	T50.2X4	T50.2X5	T50.2X6
Triazine (herbicide)	T60.3X1	T60.3X2	T60.3X3	T60.3X4	—	—
Triaziquone	T45.1X1	T45.1X2	T45.1X3	T45.1X4	T45.1X5	T45.1X6
Triazolam	T42.4X1	T42.4X2	T42.4X3	T42.4X4	T42.4X5	T42.4X6
Triazole (herbicide)	T60.3X1	T60.3X2	T60.3X3	T60.3X4	—	—
Tribenoside	T46.991	T46.992	T46.993	T46.994	T46.995	T46.996
Tribromacetaldehyde	T42.6X1	T42.6X2	T42.6X3	T42.6X4	T42.6X5	T42.6X6
Tribromoethanol, rectal	T41.291	T41.292	T41.293	T41.294	T41.295	T41.296
Tribromomethane	T42.6X1	T42.6X2	T42.6X3	T42.6X4	T42.6X5	T42.6X6
Trichlorethane	T53.2X1	T53.2X2	T53.2X3	T53.2X4	—	—
Trichlorethylene	T53.2X1	T53.2X2	T53.2X3	T53.2X4	—	—
Trichlorfon	T60.0X1	T60.0X2	T60.0X3	T60.0X4	—	—
Trichlormethiazide	T50.2X1	T50.2X2	T50.2X3	T50.2X4	T50.2X5	T50.2X6
Trichlormethine	T45.1X1	T45.1X2	T45.1X3	T45.1X4	T45.1X5	T45.1X6
Trichloroacetic acid, Trichloracetic acid	T54.2X1	T54.2X2	T54.2X3	T54.2X4	—	—
medicinal	T49.4X1	T49.4X2	T49.4X3	T49.4X4	T49.4X5	T49.4X6
Trichloroethane	T53.2X1	T53.2X2	T53.2X3	T53.2X4	—	—
Trichloroethanol	T42.6X1	T42.6X2	T42.6X3	T42.6X4	T42.6X5	T42.6X6
Trichloroethyl phosphate	T42.6X1	T42.6X2	T42.6X3	T42.6X4	T42.6X5	T42.6X6
Trichloroethylene (liquid) (vapor)	T53.2X1	T53.2X2	T53.2X3	T53.2X4	—	—
anesthetic (gas)	T41.0X1	T41.0X2	T41.0X3	T41.0X4	T41.0X5	T41.0X6
vapor NEC	T53.2X1	T53.2X2	T53.2X3	T53.2X4	—	—
Trichlorofluoromethane NEC	T53.5X1	T53.5X2	T53.5X3	T53.5X4	—	—
Trichloronate	T60.0X1	T60.0X2	T60.0X3	T60.0X4	—	—
2,4,5-Trichlorophenoxyacetic acid	T60.3X1	T60.3X2	T60.3X3	T60.3X4	—	—
Trichloropropane	T53.6X1	T53.6X2	T53.6X3	T53.6X4	—	—
Trichlorotriethylamine	T45.1X1	T45.1X2	T45.1X3	T45.1X4	T45.1X5	T45.1X6
Trichomonacides NEC	T37.3X1	T37.3X2	T37.3X3	T37.3X4	T37.3X5	T37.3X6
Trichomycin	T36.7X1	T36.7X2	T36.7X3	T36.7X4	T36.7X5	T36.7X6
Triclobisonium chloride	T49.0X1	T49.0X2	T49.0X3	T49.0X4	T49.0X5	T49.0X6
Triclocarban	T49.0X1	T49.0X2	T49.0X3	T49.0X4	T49.0X5	T49.0X6
Triclofos	T42.6X1	T42.6X2	T42.6X3	T42.6X4	T42.6X5	T42.6X6
Triclosan	T49.0X1	T49.0X2	T49.0X3	T49.0X4	T49.0X5	T49.0X6
Tricresyl phosphate	T65.891	T65.892	T65.893	T65.894	—	—
solvent	T52.91	T52.92	T52.93	T52.94	—	—
Tricyclamol chloride	T44.3X1	T44.3X2	T44.3X3	T44.3X4	T44.3X5	T44.3X6
Tridesilon	T49.0X1	T49.0X2	T49.0X3	T49.0X4	T49.0X5	T49.0X6
Tridihexethyl iodide	T44.3X1	T44.3X2	T44.3X3	T44.3X4	T44.3X5	T44.3X6
Tridione	T42.2X1	T42.2X2	T42.2X3	T42.2X4	T42.2X5	T42.2X6
Trientine	T45.8X1	T45.8X2	T45.8X3	T45.8X4	T45.8X5	T45.8X6
Triethanolamine NEC	T54.3X1	T54.3X2	T54.3X3	T54.3X4	—	—
detergent	T54.3X1	T54.3X2	T54.3X3	T54.3X4	—	—
trinitrate (biphosphate)	T46.3X1	T46.3X2	T46.3X3	T46.3X4	T46.3X5	T46.3X6
Triethanomelamine	T45.1X1	T45.1X2	T45.1X3	T45.1X4	T45.1X5	T45.1X6
Triethylenemelamine	T45.1X1	T45.1X2	T45.1X3	T45.1X4	T45.1X5	T45.1X6
Triethylenephosphora-mide	T45.1X1	T45.1X2	T45.1X3	T45.1X4	T45.1X5	T45.1X6
Triethylenethiophos-phoramide	T45.1X1	T45.1X2	T45.1X3	T45.1X4	T45.1X5	T45.1X6
Trifluoperazine	T43.3X1	T43.3X2	T43.3X3	T43.3X4	T43.3X5	T43.3X6
Trifluoroethyl vinyl ether	T41.0X1	T41.0X2	T41.0X3	T41.0X4	T41.0X5	T41.0X6
Trifluperidol	T43.4X1	T43.4X2	T43.4X3	T43.4X4	T43.4X5	T43.4X6
Triflupromazine	T43.3X1	T43.3X2	T43.3X3	T43.3X4	T43.3X5	T43.3X6
Trifluridine	T37.5X1	T37.5X2	T37.5X3	T37.5X4	T37.5X5	T37.5X6
Triflusal	T45.521	T45.522	T45.523	T45.524	T45.525	T45.526
Trihexyphenidyl	T44.3X1	T44.3X2	T44.3X3	T44.3X4	T44.3X5	T44.3X6
Triiodothyronine	T38.1X1	T38.1X2	T38.1X3	T38.1X4	T38.1X5	T38.1X6
Trilene	T41.0X1	T41.0X2	T41.0X3	T41.0X4	T41.0X5	T41.0X6
Trilostane	T38.991	T38.992	T38.993	T38.994	T38.995	T38.996
Trimebutine	T44.3X1	T44.3X2	T44.3X3	T44.3X4	T44.3X5	T44.3X6
Trimecaine	T41.3X1	T41.3X2	T41.3X3	T41.3X4	T41.3X5	T41.3X6
Trimeprazine (tartrate)	T44.3X1	T44.3X2	T44.3X3	T44.3X4	T44.3X5	T44.3X6
Trimetaphan camsilate	T44.2X1	T44.2X2	T44.2X3	T44.2X4	T44.2X5	T44.2X6
Trimetazidine	T46.7X1	T46.7X2	T46.7X3	T46.7X4	T46.7X5	T46.7X6
Trimethadione	T42.2X1	T42.2X2	T42.2X3	T42.2X4	T42.2X5	T42.2X6
Trimethaphan	T44.2X1	T44.2X2	T44.2X3	T44.2X4	T44.2X5	T44.2X6
Trimethidinium	T44.2X1	T44.2X2	T44.2X3	T44.2X4	T44.2X5	T44.2X6
Trimethobenzamide	T45.0X1	T45.0X2	T45.0X3	T45.0X4	T45.0X5	T45.0X6
Trimethoprim	T37.8X1	T37.8X2	T37.8X3	T37.8X4	T37.8X5	T37.8X6
with sulfamethoxazole	T36.8X1	T36.8X2	T36.8X3	T36.8X4	T36.8X5	T36.8X6
Trimethylcarbinol	T51.3X1	T51.3X2	T51.3X3	T51.3X4	—	—
Trimethylpsoralen	T49.3X1	T49.3X2	T49.3X3	T49.3X4	T49.3X5	T49.3X6
Trimeton	T45.0X1	T45.0X2	T45.0X3	T45.0X4	T45.0X5	T45.0X6
Trimetrexate	T45.1X1	T45.1X2	T45.1X3	T45.1X4	T45.1X5	T45.1X6
Trimipramine	T43.011	T43.012	T43.013	T43.014	T43.015	T43.016
Trimustine	T45.1X1	T45.1X2	T45.1X3	T45.1X4	T45.1X5	T45.1X6
Trinitrine	T46.3X1	T46.3X2	T46.3X3	T46.3X4	T46.3X5	T46.3X6
Trinitrobenzol	T65.3X1	T65.3X2	T65.3X3	T65.3X4	—	—
Trinitrophenol	T65.3X1	T65.3X2	T65.3X3	T65.3X4	—	—
Trinitrotoluene (fumes)	T65.3X1	T65.3X2	T65.3X3	T65.3X4	—	—
Trional	T42.6X1	T42.6X2	T42.6X3	T42.6X4	T42.6X5	T42.6X6
Triorthocresyl phosphate	T65.891	T65.892	T65.893	T65.894	—	—
Trioxide of arsenic	T57.0X1	T57.0X2	T57.0X3	T57.0X4	—	—
Trioxysalen	T49.4X1	T49.4X2	T49.4X3	T49.4X4	T49.4X5	T49.4X6
Tripamide	T50.2X1	T50.2X2	T50.2X3	T50.2X4	T50.2X5	T50.2X6

Triparanol - Vaccine NEC

Substance	Poisoning, Accidental (unintentional)	Poisoning, Intentional self-harm	Poisoning, Assault	Poisoning, Undetermined	Adverse effect	Underdosing
Triparanol	T46.6X1	T46.6X2	T46.6X3	T46.6X4	T46.6X5	T46.6X6
Tripelennamine	T45.0X1	T45.0X2	T45.0X3	T45.0X4	T45.0X5	T45.0X6
Triperiden	T44.3X1	T44.3X2	T44.3X3	T44.3X4	T44.3X5	T44.3X6
Triperidol	T43.4X1	T43.4X2	T43.4X3	T43.4X4	T43.4X5	T43.4X6
Triphenylphosphate	T65.891	T65.892	T65.893	T65.894	—	—
Triple						
bromides	T42.6X1	T42.6X2	T42.6X3	T42.6X4	T42.6X5	T42.6X6
carbonate	T47.1X1	T47.1X2	T47.1X3	T47.1X4	T47.1X5	T47.1X6
vaccine						
DPT	T50.A11	T50.A12	T50.A13	T50.A14	T50.A15	T50.A16
including pertussis	T50.A11	T50.A12	T50.A13	T50.A14	T50.A15	T50.A16
MMR	T50.B91	T50.B92	T50.B93	T50.B94	T50.B95	T50.B96
Triprolidine	T45.0X1	T45.0X2	T45.0X3	T45.0X4	T45.0X5	T45.0X6
Trisodium hydrogen edetate	T50.6X1	T50.6X2	T50.6X3	T50.6X4	T50.6X5	T50.6X6
Trisoralen	T49.3X1	T49.3X2	T49.3X3	T49.3X4	T49.3X5	T49.3X6
Trisulfapyrimidines	T37.0X1	T37.0X2	T37.0X3	T37.0X4	T37.0X5	T37.0X6
Trithiozine	T44.3X1	T44.3X2	T44.3X3	T44.3X4	T44.3X5	T44.3X6
Tritiozine	T44.3X1	T44.3X2	T44.3X3	T44.3X4	T44.3X5	T44.3X6
Tritoqualine	T45.0X1	T45.0X2	T45.0X3	T45.0X4	T45.0X5	T45.0X6
Trofosfamide	T45.1X1	T45.1X2	T45.1X3	T45.1X4	T45.1X5	T45.1X6
Troleandomycin	T36.3X1	T36.3X2	T36.3X3	T36.3X4	T36.3X5	T36.3X6
Trolnitrate (phosphate)	T46.3X1	T46.3X2	T46.3X3	T46.3X4	T46.3X5	T46.3X6
Tromantadine	T37.5X1	T37.5X2	T37.5X3	T37.5X4	T37.5X5	T37.5X6
Trometamol	T50.2X1	T50.2X2	T50.2X3	T50.2X4	T50.2X5	T50.2X6
Tromethamine	T50.2X1	T50.2X2	T50.2X3	T50.2X4	T50.2X5	T50.2X6
Tronothane	T41.3X1	T41.3X2	T41.3X3	T41.3X4	T41.3X5	T41.3X6
Tropacine	T44.3X1	T44.3X2	T44.3X3	T44.3X4	T44.3X5	T44.3X6
Tropatepine	T44.3X1	T44.3X2	T44.3X3	T44.3X4	T44.3X5	T44.3X6
Tropicamide	T44.3X1	T44.3X2	T44.3X3	T44.3X4	T44.3X5	T44.3X6
Trospium chloride	T44.3X1	T44.3X2	T44.3X3	T44.3X4	T44.3X5	T44.3X6
Troxerutin	T46.991	T46.992	T46.993	T46.994	T46.995	T46.996
Troxidone	T42.2X1	T42.2X2	T42.2X3	T42.2X4	T42.2X5	T42.2X6
Tryparsamide	T37.3X1	T37.3X2	T37.3X3	T37.3X4	T37.3X5	T37.3X6
Trypsin	T45.3X1	T45.3X2	T45.3X3	T45.3X4	T45.3X5	T45.3X6
Tryptizol	T43.011	T43.012	T43.013	T43.014	T43.015	T43.016
TSH	T38.811	T38.812	T38.813	T38.814	T38.815	T38.816
Tuaminoheptane	T48.5X1	T48.5X2	T48.5X3	T48.5X4	T48.5X5	T48.5X6
Tuberculin, purified protein derivative (PPD)	T50.8X1	T50.8X2	T50.8X3	T50.8X4	T50.8X5	T50.8X6
Tubocurare	T48.1X1	T48.1X2	T48.1X3	T48.1X4	T48.1X5	T48.1X6
Tubocurarine (chloride)	T48.1X1	T48.1X2	T48.1X3	T48.1X4	T48.1X5	T48.1X6
Tulobuterol	T48.6X1	T48.6X2	T48.6X3	T48.6X4	T48.6X5	T48.6X6
Turpentine (spirits of)	T52.8X1	T52.8X2	T52.8X3	T52.8X4	—	—
vapor	T52.8X1	T52.8X2	T52.8X3	T52.8X4	—	—
Tybamate	T43.591	T43.592	T43.593	T43.594	T43.595	T43.596
Tyloxapol	T48.4X1	T48.4X2	T48.4X3	T48.4X4	T48.4X5	T48.4X6
Tymazoline	T48.5X1	T48.5X2	T48.5X3	T48.5X4	T48.5X5	T48.5X6
Typhoid-paratyphoid vaccine	T50.A91	T50.A92	T50.A93	T50.A94	T50.A95	T50.A96
Typhus vaccine	T50.A91	T50.A92	T50.A93	T50.A94	T50.A95	T50.A96
Tyropanoate	T50.8X1	T50.8X2	T50.8X3	T50.8X4	T50.8X5	T50.8X6
Tyrothricin	T49.6X1	T49.6X2	T49.6X3	T49.6X4	T49.6X5	T49.6X6
ENT agent	T49.6X1	T49.6X2	T49.6X3	T49.6X4	T49.6X5	T49.6X6
ophthalmic preparation	T49.5X1	T49.5X2	T49.5X3	T49.5X4	T49.5X5	T49.5X6
U						
Ufenamate	T39.391	T39.392	T39.393	T39.394	T39.395	T39.396
Ultraviolet light protectant	T49.3X1	T49.3X2	T49.3X3	T49.3X4	T49.3X5	T49.3X6

Substance	Poisoning, Accidental (unintentional)	Poisoning, Intentional self-harm	Poisoning, Assault	Poisoning, Undetermined	Adverse effect	Underdosing
Undecenoic acid	T49.0X1	T49.0X2	T49.0X3	T49.0X4	T49.0X5	T49.0X6
Undecoylium	T49.0X1	T49.0X2	T49.0X3	T49.0X4	T49.0X5	T49.0X6
Undecylenic acid (derivatives)	T49.0X1	T49.0X2	T49.0X3	T49.0X4	T49.0X5	T49.0X6
Unna's boot	T49.3X1	T49.3X2	T49.3X3	T49.3X4	T49.3X5	T49.3X6
Unsaturated fatty acid	T46.6X1	T46.6X2	T46.6X3	T46.6X4	T46.6X5	T46.6X6
Uracil mustard	T45.1X1	T45.1X2	T45.1X3	T45.1X4	T45.1X5	T45.1X6
Uramustine	T45.1X1	T45.1X2	T45.1X3	T45.1X4	T45.1X5	T45.1X6
Urapidil	T46.5X1	T46.5X2	T46.5X3	T46.5X4	T46.5X5	T46.5X6
Urari	T48.1X1	T48.1X2	T48.1X3	T48.1X4	T48.1X5	T48.1X6
Urate oxidase	T50.4X1	T50.4X2	T50.4X3	T50.4X4	T50.4X5	T50.4X6
Urea	T47.3X1	T47.3X2	T47.3X3	T47.3X4	T47.3X5	T47.3X6
peroxide	T49.0X1	T49.0X2	T49.0X3	T49.0X4	T49.0X5	T49.0X6
stibamine	T37.4X1	T37.4X2	T37.4X3	T37.4X4	T37.4X5	T37.4X6
topical	T49.8X1	T49.8X2	T49.8X3	T49.8X4	T49.8X5	T49.8X6
Urethane	T45.1X1	T45.1X2	T45.1X3	T45.1X4	T45.1X5	T45.1X6
Urginea (maritima) (scilla)—see Squill						
Uric acid metabolism drug NEC	T50.4X1	T50.4X2	T50.4X3	T50.4X4	T50.4X5	T50.4X6
Uricosuric agent	T50.4X1	T50.4X2	T50.4X3	T50.4X4	T50.4X5	T50.4X6
Urinary anti-infective	T37.8X1	T37.8X2	T37.8X3	T37.8X4	T37.8X5	T37.8X6
Urofollitropin	T38.811	T38.812	T38.813	T38.814	T38.815	T38.816
Urokinase	T45.611	T45.612	T45.613	T45.614	T45.615	T45.616
Urokon	T50.8X1	T50.8X2	T50.8X3	T50.8X4	T50.8X5	T50.8X6
Ursodeoxycholic acid	T50.991	T50.992	T50.993	T50.994	T50.995	T50.996
Ursodiol	T50.991	T50.992	T50.993	T50.994	T50.995	T50.996
Urtica	T62.2X1	T62.2X2	T62.2X3	T62.2X4	—	—
Utility gas—see Gas, utility						
V						
Vaccine NEC	T50.Z91	T50.Z92	T50.Z93	T50.Z94	T50.Z95	T50.Z96
antineoplastic	T50.Z91	T50.Z92	T50.Z93	T50.Z94	T50.Z95	T50.Z96
bacterial NEC	T50.A91	T50.A92	T50.A93	T50.A94	T50.A95	T50.A96
with						
other bacterial component	T50.A21	T50.A22	T50.A23	T50.A24	T50.A25	T50.A26
pertussis component	T50.A11	T50.A12	T50.A13	T50.A14	T50.A15	T50.A16
viral-rickettsial component	T50.A21	T50.A22	T50.A23	T50.A24	T50.A25	T50.A26
mixed NEC	T50.A21	T50.A22	T50.A23	T50.A24	T50.A25	T50.A26
BCG	T50.A91	T50.A92	T50.A93	T50.A94	T50.A95	T50.A96
cholera	T50.A91	T50.A92	T50.A93	T50.A94	T50.A95	T50.A96
diphtheria	T50.A91	T50.A92	T50.A93	T50.A94	T50.A95	T50.A96
with tetanus	T50.A21	T50.A22	T50.A23	T50.A24	T50.A25	T50.A26
and pertussis	T50.A11	T50.A12	T50.A13	T50.A14	T50.A15	T50.A16
influenza	T50.B91	T50.B92	T50.B93	T50.B94	T50.B95	T50.B96
measles	T50.B91	T50.B92	T50.B93	T50.B94	T50.B95	T50.B96
with mumps and rubella	T50.B91	T50.B92	T50.B93	T50.B94	T50.B95	T50.B96
meningococcal	T50.A91	T50.A92	T50.A93	T50.A94	T50.A95	T50.A96
mumps	T50.B91	T50.B92	T50.B93	T50.B94	T50.B95	T50.B96
paratyphoid	T50.A91	T50.A92	T50.A93	T50.A94	T50.A95	T50.A96
pertussis	T50.A11	T50.A12	T50.A13	T50.A14	T50.A15	T50.A16
with diphtheria	T50.A11	T50.A12	T50.A13	T50.A14	T50.A15	T50.A16
and tetanus	T50.A11	T50.A12	T50.A13	T50.A14	T50.A15	T50.A16
with other component	T50.A11	T50.A12	T50.A13	T50.A14	T50.A15	T50.A16
plague	T50.A91	T50.A92	T50.A93	T50.A94	T50.A95	T50.A96
poliomyelitis	T50.B91	T50.B92	T50.B93	T50.B94	T50.B95	T50.B96
poliovirus	T50.B91	T50.B92	T50.B93	T50.B94	T50.B95	T50.B96

Substance	Poisoning, Accidental (unintentional)	Poisoning, Intentional self-harm	Poisoning, Assault	Poisoning, Undetermined	Adverse effect	Underdosing
Vitamin NEC — *continued*						
rabies	T50.B91	T50.B92	T50.B93	T50.B94	T50.B95	T50.B96
respiratory syncytial virus	T50.B91	T50.B92	T50.B93	T50.B94	T50.B95	T50.B96
rickettsial NEC	T50.A91	T50.A92	T50.A93	T50.A94	T50.A95	T50.A96
with						
bacterial component	T50.A21	T50.A22	T50.A23	T50.A24	T50.A25	T50.A26
Rocky Mountain spotted fever	T50.A91	T50.A92	T50.A93	T50.A94	T50.A95	T50.A96
rubella	T50.B91	T50.B92	T50.B93	T50.B94	T50.B95	T50.B96
sabin oral	T50.B91	T50.B92	T50.B93	T50.B94	T50.B95	T50.B96
smallpox	T50.B11	T50.B12	T50.B13	T50.B14	T50.B15	T50.B16
TAB	T50.A91	T50.A92	T50.A93	T50.A94	T50.A95	T50.A96
tetanus	T50.A91	T50.A92	T50.A93	T50.A94	T50.A95	T50.A96
typhoid	T50.A91	T50.A92	T50.A93	T50.A94	T50.A95	T50.A96
typhus	T50.A91	T50.A92	T50.A93	T50.A94	T50.A95	T50.A96
viral NEC	T50.B91	T50.B92	T50.B93	T50.B94	T50.B95	T50.B96
yellow fever	T50.B91	T50.B92	T50.B93	T50.B94	T50.B95	T50.B96
Vaccinia immune globulin	T50.Z11	T50.Z12	T50.Z13	T50.Z14	T50.Z15	T50.Z16
Vaginal contraceptives	T49.8X1	T49.8X2	T49.8X3	T49.8X4	T49.8X5	T49.8X6
Valerian						
root	T42.6X1	T42.6X2	T42.6X3	T42.6X4	T42.6X5	T42.6X6
tincture	T42.6X1	T42.6X2	T42.6X3	T42.6X4	T42.6X5	T42.6X6
Valethamate bromide	T44.3X1	T44.3X2	T44.3X3	T44.3X4	T44.3X5	T44.3X6
Valisone	T49.0X1	T49.0X2	T49.0X3	T49.0X4	T49.0X5	T49.0X6
Valium	T42.4X1	T42.4X2	T42.4X3	T42.4X4	T42.4X5	T42.4X6
Valmid	T42.6X1	T42.6X2	T42.6X3	T42.6X4	T42.6X5	T42.6X6
Valnoctamide	T42.6X1	T42.6X2	T42.6X3	T42.6X4	T42.6X5	T42.6X6
Valproate (sodium)	T42.6X1	T42.6X2	T42.6X3	T42.6X4	T42.6X5	T42.6X6
Valproic acid	T42.6X1	T42.6X2	T42.6X3	T42.6X4	T42.6X5	T42.6X6
Valpromide	T42.6X1	T42.6X2	T42.6X3	T42.6X4	T42.6X5	T42.6X6
Vanadium	T56.891	T56.892	T56.893	T56.894	—	—
Vancomycin	T36.8X1	T36.8X2	T36.8X3	T36.8X4	T36.8X5	T36.8X6
Vapor—*see also Gas*	T59.91	T59.92	T59.93	T59.94	—	—
kiln (carbon monoxide)	T58.8X1	T58.8X2	T58.8X3	T58.8X4		
lead—*see lead*						
specified source NEC	T59.891	T59.892	T59.893	T59.894	—	—
Vardenafil	T46.7X1	T46.7X2	T46.7X3	T46.7X4	T46.7X5	T46.7X6
Varicose reduction drug	T46.8X1	T46.8X2	T46.8X3	T46.8X4	T46.8X5	T46.8X6
Varnish	T65.4X1	T65.4X2	T65.4X3	T65.4X4	—	—
cleaner	T52.91	T52.92	T52.93	T52.94	—	—
Vaseline	T49.3X1	T49.3X2	T49.3X3	T49.3X4	T49.3X5	T49.3X6
Vasodilan	T46.7X1	T46.7X2	T46.7X3	T46.7X4	T46.7X5	T46.7X6
Vasodilator						
coronary NEC	T46.3X1	T46.3X2	T46.3X3	T46.3X4	T46.3X5	T46.3X6
peripheral NEC	T46.7X1	T46.7X2	T46.7X3	T46.7X4	T46.7X5	T46.7X6
Vasopressin	T38.891	T38.892	T38.893	T38.894	T38.895	T38.896
Vasopressor drugs	T38.891	T38.892	T38.893	T38.894	T38.895	T38.896
Vecuronium bromide	T48.1X1	T48.1X2	T48.1X3	T48.1X4	T48.1X5	T48.1X6
Vegetable extract, astringent	T49.2X1	T49.2X2	T49.2X3	T49.2X4	T49.2X5	T49.2X6
Venlafaxine	T43.211	T43.212	T43.213	T43.214	T43.215	T43.216
Venom, venomous (bite) (sting)	T63.91	T63.92	T63.93	T63.94	—	—
amphibian NEC	T63.831	T63.832	T63.833	T63.834	—	—
animal NEC	T63.891	T63.892	T63.893	T63.894	—	—
ant	T63.421	T63.422	T63.423	T63.424	—	—
arthropod NEC	T63.481	T63.482	T63.483	T63.484	—	—
bee	T63.441	T63.442	T63.443	T63.444	—	—

Substance	Poisoning, Accidental (unintentional)	Poisoning, Intentional self-harm	Poisoning, Assault	Poisoning, Undetermined	Adverse effect	Underdosing
Venom, venomous (bite) (sting) — *continued*						
centipede	T63.411	T63.412	T63.413	T63.414	—	—
fish	T63.591	T63.592	T63.593	T63.594	—	—
frog	T63.811	T63.812	T63.813	T63.814	—	—
hornet	T63.451	T63.452	T63.453	T63.454	—	—
insect NEC	T63.481	T63.482	T63.483	T63.484	—	—
lizard	T63.121	T63.122	T63.123	T63.124	—	—
marine						
animals	T63.691	T63.692	T63.693	T63.694	—	—
bluebottle	T63.611	T63.612	T63.613	T63.614	—	—
jellyfish NEC	T63.621	T63.622	T63.623	T63.624	—	—
Portugese Man-o-war	T63.611	T63.612	T63.613	T63.614	—	—
sea anemone	T63.631	T63.632	T63.633	T63.634	—	—
specified NEC	T63.691	T63.692	T63.693	T63.694	—	—
fish	T63.591	T63.592	T63.593	T63.594	—	—
plants	T63.711	T63.712	T63.713	T63.714	—	—
sting ray	T63.511	T63.512	T63.513	T63.514	—	—
millipede (tropical)	T63.411	T63.412	T63.413	T63.414	—	—
plant NEC	T63.791	T63.792	T63.793	T63.794	—	—
marine	T63.711	T63.712	T63.713	T63.714	—	—
reptile	T63.191	T63.192	T63.193	T63.194	—	—
gila monster	T63.111	T63.112	T63.113	T63.114	—	—
lizard NEC	T63.121	T63.122	T63.123	T63.124	—	—
scorpion	T63.2X1	T63.2X2	T63.2X3	T63.2X4	—	—
snake	T63.001	T63.002	T63.003	T63.004	—	—
African NEC	T63.081	T63.082	T63.083	T63.084	—	—
American (North) (South) NEC	T63.061	T63.062	T63.063	T63.064	—	—
Asian	T63.081	T63.082	T63.083	T63.084	—	—
Australian	T63.071	T63.072	T63.073	T63.074	—	—
cobra	T63.041	T63.042	T63.043	T63.044	—	—
coral snake	T63.021	T63.022	T63.023	T63.024	—	—
rattlesnake	T63.011	T63.012	T63.013	T63.014	—	—
specified NEC	T63.091	T63.092	T63.093	T63.094	—	—
taipan	T63.031	T63.032	T63.033	T63.034	—	—
specified NEC	T63.891	T63.892	T63.893	T63.894	—	—
spider	T63.301	T63.302	T63.303	T63.304	—	—
black widow	T63.311	T63.312	T63.313	T63.314	—	—
brown recluse	T63.331	T63.332	T63.333	T63.334	—	—
specified NEC	T63.391	T63.392	T63.393	T63.394	—	—
tarantula	T63.321	T63.322	T63.323	T63.324	—	—
sting ray	T63.511	T63.512	T63.513	T63.514	—	—
toad	T63.821	T63.822	T63.823	T63.824	—	—
wasp	T63.461	T63.462	T63.463	T63.464	—	—
Venous sclerosing drug NEC	T46.8X1	T46.8X2	T46.8X3	T46.8X4	T46.8X5	T46.8X6
Ventolin—*see Albuterol*						
Veramon	T42.3X1	T42.3X2	T42.3X3	T42.3X4	T42.3X5	T42.3X6
Verapamil	T46.1X1	T46.1X2	T46.1X3	T46.1X4	T46.1X5	T46.1X6
Veratrine	T46.5X1	T46.5X2	T46.5X3	T46.5X4	T46.5X5	T46.5X6
Veratrum						
album	T62.2X1	T62.2X2	T62.2X3	T62.2X4	—	—
alkaloids	T46.5X1	T46.5X2	T46.5X3	T46.5X4	T46.5X5	T46.5X6
viride	T62.2X1	T62.2X2	T62.2X3	T62.2X4	—	—
Verdigris	T60.3X1	T60.3X2	T60.3X3	T60.3X4	—	—
Veronal	T42.3X1	T42.3X2	T42.3X3	T42.3X4	T42.3X5	T42.3X6
Veroxil	T37.4X1	T37.4X2	T37.4X3	T37.4X4	T37.4X5	T37.4X6
Versenate	T50.6X1	T50.6X2	T50.6X3	T50.6X4	T50.6X5	T50.6X6
Versidyne	T39.8X1	T39.8X2	T39.8X3	T39.8X4	T39.8X5	T39.8X6

Substance	Poisoning, Accidental (unintentional)	Poisoning, Intentional self-harm	Poisoning, Assault	Poisoning, Undetermined	Adverse effect	Underdosing
Vetrabutine	T48.0X1	T48.0X2	T48.0X3	T48.0X4	T48.0X5	T48.0X6
Vidarabine	T37.5X1	T37.5X2	T37.5X3	T37.5X4	T37.5X5	T37.5X6
Vienna						
green	T57.0X1	T57.0X2	T57.0X3	T57.0X4	—	—
insecticide	T60.2X1	T60.2X2	T60.2X3	T60.2X4	—	—
red	T57.0X1	T57.0X2	T57.0X3	T57.0X4	—	—
pharmaceutical dye	T50.991	T50.992	T50.993	T50.994	T50.995	T50.996
Vigabatrin	T42.6X1	T42.6X2	T42.6X3	T42.6X4	T42.6X5	T42.6X6
Viloxazine	T43.291	T43.292	T43.293	T43.294	T43.295	T43.296
Viminol	T39.8X1	T39.8X2	T39.8X3	T39.8X4	T39.8X5	T39.8X6
Vinbarbital, vinbarbitone	T42.3X1	T42.3X2	T42.3X3	T42.3X4	T42.3X5	T42.3X6
Vinblastine	T45.1X1	T45.1X2	T45.1X3	T45.1X4	T45.1X5	T45.1X6
Vinburnine	T46.7X1	T46.7X2	T46.7X3	T46.7X4	T46.7X5	T46.7X6
Vincamine	T45.1X1	T45.1X2	T45.1X3	T45.1X4	T45.1X5	T45.1X6
Vincristine	T45.1X1	T45.1X2	T45.1X3	T45.1X4	T45.1X5	T45.1X6
Vindesine	T45.1X1	T45.1X2	T45.1X3	T45.1X4	T45.1X5	T45.1X6
Vinesthene, vinethene	T41.0X1	T41.0X2	T41.0X3	T41.0X4	T41.0X5	T41.0X6
Vinorelbine tartrate	T45.1X1	T45.1X2	T45.1X3	T45.1X4	T45.1X5	T45.1X6
Vinpocetine	T46.7X1	T46.7X2	T46.7X3	T46.7X4	T46.7X5	T46.7X6
Vinyl						
acetate	T65.891	T65.892	T65.893	T65.894	—	—
bital	T42.3X1	T42.3X2	T42.3X3	T42.3X4	T42.3X5	T42.3X6
bromide	T65.891	T65.892	T65.893	T65.894	—	—
chloride	T59.891	T59.892	T59.893	T59.894	—	—
ether	T41.0X1	T41.0X2	T41.0X3	T41.0X4	T41.0X5	T41.0X6
Vinylbital	T42.3X1	T42.3X2	T42.3X3	T42.3X4	T42.3X5	T42.3X6
Vinylidene chloride	T65.891	T65.892	T65.893	T65.894	—	—
Vioform	T37.8X1	T37.8X2	T37.8X3	T37.8X4	T37.8X5	T37.8X6
topical	T49.0X1	T49.0X2	T49.0X3	T49.0X4	T49.0X5	T49.0X6
Viomycin	T36.8X1	T36.8X2	T36.8X3	T36.8X4	T36.8X5	T36.8X6
Viosterol	T45.2X1	T45.2X2	T45.2X3	T45.2X4	T45.2X5	T45.2X6
Viper (venom)	T63.091	T63.092	T63.093	T63.094	—	—
Viprynium	T37.4X1	T37.4X2	T37.4X3	T37.4X4	T37.4X5	T37.4X6
Viquidil	T46.7X1	T46.7X2	T46.7X3	T46.7X4	T46.7X5	T46.7X6
Viral vaccine NEC	T50.B91	T50.B92	T50.B93	T50.B94	T50.B95	T50.B96
Virginiamycin	T36.8X1	T36.8X2	T36.8X3	T36.8X4	T36.8X5	T36.8X6
Virugon	T37.5X1	T37.5X2	T37.5X3	T37.5X4	T37.5X5	T37.5X6
Viscous agent	T50.901	T50.902	T50.903	T50.904	T50.905	T50.906
Visine	T49.5X1	T49.5X2	T49.5X3	T49.5X4	T49.5X5	T49.5X6
Visnadine	T46.3X1	T46.3X2	T46.3X3	T46.3X4	T46.3X5	T46.3X6
Vitamin NEC	T45.2X1	T45.2X2	T45.2X3	T45.2X4	T45.2X5	T45.2X6
A	T45.2X1	T45.2X2	T45.2X3	T45.2X4	T45.2X5	T45.2X6
B NEC	T45.2X1	T45.2X2	T45.2X3	T45.2X4	T45.2X5	T45.2X6
nicotinic acid	T46.7X1	T46.7X2	T46.7X3	T46.7X4	T46.7X5	T46.7X6
B1	T45.2X1	T45.2X2	T45.2X3	T45.2X4	T45.2X5	T45.2X6
B2	T45.2X1	T45.2X2	T45.2X3	T45.2X4	T45.2X5	T45.2X6
B6	T45.2X1	T45.2X2	T45.2X3	T45.2X4	T45.2X5	T45.2X6
B12	T45.2X1	T45.2X2	T45.2X3	T45.2X4	T45.2X5	T45.2X6
B15	T45.2X1	T45.2X2	T45.2X3	T45.2X4	T45.2X5	T45.2X6
C	T45.2X1	T45.2X2	T45.2X3	T45.2X4	T45.2X5	T45.2X6
D	T45.2X1	T45.2X2	T45.2X3	T45.2X4	T45.2X5	T45.2X6
D2	T45.2X1	T45.2X2	T45.2X3	T45.2X4	T45.2X5	T45.2X6
D3	T45.2X1	T45.2X2	T45.2X3	T45.2X4	T45.2X5	T45.2X6
E	T45.2X1	T45.2X2	T45.2X3	T45.2X4	T45.2X5	T45.2X6
E acetate	T45.2X1	T45.2X2	T45.2X3	T45.2X4	T45.2X5	T45.2X6
hematopoietic	T45.8X1	T45.8X2	T45.8X3	T45.8X4	T45.8X5	T45.8X6
K NEC	T45.7X1	T45.7X2	T45.7X3	T45.7X4	T45.7X5	T45.7X6
K1	T45.7X1	T45.7X2	T45.7X3	T45.7X4	T45.7X5	T45.7X6
K2	T45.7X1	T45.7X2	T45.7X3	T45.7X4	T45.7X5	T45.7X6

Substance	Poisoning, Accidental (unintentional)	Poisoning, Intentional self-harm	Poisoning, Assault	Poisoning, Undetermined	Adverse effect	Underdosing
Vitamin NEC — *continued*						
PP	T45.2X1	T45.2X2	T45.2X3	T45.2X4	T45.2X5	T45.2X6
ulceroprotectant	T47.1X1	T47.1X2	T47.1X3	T47.1X4	T47.1X5	T47.1X6
Vleminckx's solution	T49.4X1	T49.4X2	T49.4X3	T49.4X4	T49.4X5	T49.4X6
Voltaren—*see Diclofenac sodium*						
W						
Warfarin	T45.511	T45.512	T45.513	T45.514	T45.515	T45.516
rodenticide	T60.4X1	T60.4X2	T60.4X3	T60.4X4	—	—
sodium	T60.4X1	T60.4X2	T60.4X3	T60.4X4	—	—
Wasp (sting)	T63.461	T63.462	T63.463	T63.464	—	—
Water						
balance drug	T50.3X1	T50.3X2	T50.3X3	T50.3X4	T50.3X5	T50.3X6
distilled	T50.3X1	T50.3X2	T50.3X3	T50.3X4	T50.3X5	T50.3X6
gas—*see Gas, water*						
incomplete combustion of —*see Carbon, monoxide, fuel, utility*						
hemlock	T62.2X1	T62.2X2	T62.2X3	T62.2X4	—	—
moccasin (venom)	T63.061	T63.062	T63.063	T63.064	—	—
purified	T50.3X1	T50.3X2	T50.3X3	T50.3X4	T50.3X5	T50.3X6
Wax (paraffin) (petroleum)	T52.0X1	T52.0X2	T52.0X3	T52.0X4	—	—
automobile	T65.891	T65.892	T65.893	T65.894	—	—
floor	T52.0X1	T52.0X2	T52.0X3	T52.0X4	—	—
Weed killers NEC	T60.3X1	T60.3X2	T60.3X3	T60.3X4	—	—
Welldorm	T42.6X1	T42.6X2	T42.6X3	T42.6X4	T42.6X5	T42.6X6
White						
arsenic	T57.0X1	T57.0X2	T57.0X3	T57.0X4	—	—
hellebore	T62.2X1	T62.2X2	T62.2X3	T62.2X4	—	—
lotion (keratolytic)	T49.4X1	T49.4X2	T49.4X3	T49.4X4	T49.4X5	T49.4X6
spirit	T52.0X1	T52.0X2	T52.0X3	T52.0X4	—	—
Whitewash	T65.891	T65.892	T65.893	T65.894	—	—
Whole blood (human)	T45.8X1	T45.8X2	T45.8X3	T45.8X4	T45.8X5	T45.8X6
Wild						
black cherry	T62.2X1	T62.2X2	T62.2X3	T62.2X4	—	—
poisonous plants NEC	T62.2X1	T62.2X2	T62.2X3	T62.2X4	—	—
Window cleaning fluid	T65.891	T65.892	T65.893	T65.894	—	—
Wintergreen (oil)	T49.3X1	T49.3X2	T49.3X3	T49.3X4	T49.3X5	T49.3X6
Wisterine	T62.2X1	T62.2X2	T62.2X3	T62.2X4	—	—
Witch hazel	T49.2X1	T49.2X2	T49.2X3	T49.2X4	T49.2X5	T49.2X6
Wood alcohol or spirit	T51.1X1	T51.1X2	T51.1X3	T51.1X4	—	—
Wool fat (hydrous)	T49.3X1	T49.3X2	T49.3X3	T49.3X4	T49.3X5	T49.3X6
Woorali	T48.1X1	T48.1X2	T48.1X3	T48.1X4	T48.1X5	T48.1X6
Wormseed, American	T37.4X1	T37.4X2	T37.4X3	T37.4X4	T37.4X5	T37.4X6
X						
Xamoterol	T44.5X1	T44.5X2	T44.5X3	T44.5X4	T44.5X5	T44.5X6
Xanthine diuretics	T50.2X1	T50.2X2	T50.2X3	T50.2X4	T50.2X5	T50.2X6
Xanthinol nicotinate	T46.7X1	T46.7X2	T46.7X3	T46.7X4	T46.7X5	T46.7X6
Xanthotoxin	T49.3X1	T49.3X2	T49.3X3	T49.3X4	T49.3X5	T49.3X6
Xantinol nicotinate	T46.7X1	T46.7X2	T46.7X3	T46.7X4	T46.7X5	T46.7X6
Xantocillin	T36.0X1	T36.0X2	T36.0X3	T36.0X4	T36.0X5	T36.0X6
Xenon (127Xe) (133Xe)	T50.8X1	T50.8X2	T50.8X3	T50.8X4	T50.8X5	T50.8X6
Xenysalate	T49.4X1	T49.4X2	T49.4X3	T49.4X4	T49.4X5	T49.4X6
Xibornol	T37.8X1	T37.8X2	T37.8X3	T37.8X4	T37.8X5	T37.8X6
Xigris	T45.511	T45.512	T45.513	T45.514	T45.515	T45.516
Xipamide	T50.2X1	T50.2X2	T50.2X3	T50.2X4	T50.2X5	T50.2X6
Xylene (vapor)	T52.2X1	T52.2X2	T52.2X3	T52.2X4	—	—

Xylocaine (infiltration) (topical)	T41.3X1	T41.3X2	T41.3X3	T41.3X4	T41.3X5	T41.3X6
nerve block (peripheral) (plexus)	T41.3X1	T41.3X2	T41.3X3	T41.3X4	T41.3X5	T41.3X6
spinal	T41.3X1	T41.3X2	T41.3X3	T41.3X4	T41.3X5	T41.3X6
Xylol (vapor)	T52.2X1	T52.2X2	T52.2X3	T52.2X4	—	—
Xylometazoline	T48.5X1	T48.5X2	T48.5X3	T48.5X4	T48.5X5	T48.5X6
Y						
Yeast	T45.2X1	T45.2X2	T45.2X3	T45.2X4	T45.2X5	T45.2X6
dried	T45.2X1	T45.2X2	T45.2X3	T45.2X4	T45.2X5	T45.2X6
Yellow						
fever vaccine	T50.B91	T50.B92	T50.B93	T50.B94	T50.B95	T50.B96
jasmine	T62.2X1	T62.2X2	T62.2X3	T62.2X4	—	—
phenolphthalein	T47.2X1	T47.2X2	T47.2X3	T47.2X4	T47.2X5	T47.2X6
Yew	T62.2X1	T62.2X2	T62.2X3	T62.2X4	—	—
Yohimbic acid	T40.991	T40.992	T40.993	T40.994	T40.995	T40.996
Z						
Zactane	T39.8X1	T39.8X2	T39.8X3	T39.8X4	T39.8X5	T39.8X6
Zalcitabine	T37.5X1	T37.5X2	T37.5X3	T37.5X4	T37.5X5	T37.5X6
Zaroxolyn	T50.2X1	T50.2X2	T50.2X3	T50.2X4	T50.2X5	T50.2X6
Zephiran (topical)	T49.0X1	T49.0X2	T49.0X3	T49.0X4	T49.0X5	T49.0X6
ophthalmic preparation	T49.5X1	T49.5X2	T49.5X3	T49.5X4	T49.5X5	T49.5X6
Zeranol	T38.7X1	T38.7X2	T38.7X3	T38.7X4	T38.7X5	T38.7X6
Zerone	T51.1X1	T51.1X2	T51.1X3	T51.1X4	—	—
Zidovudine	T37.5X1	T37.5X2	T37.5X3	T37.5X4	T37.5X5	T37.5X6
Zimeldine	T43.221	T43.222	T43.223	T43.224	T43.225	T43.226
Zinc (compounds) (fumes) (vapor) NEC	T56.5X1	T56.5X2	T56.5X3	T56.5X4	—	—
anti-infectives	T49.0X1	T49.0X2	T49.0X3	T49.0X4	T49.0X5	T49.0X6
antivaricose	T46.8X1	T46.8X2	T46.8X3	T46.8X4	T46.8X5	T46.8X6
bacitracin	T49.0X1	T49.0X2	T49.0X3	T49.0X4	T49.0X5	T49.0X6
chloride (mouthwash)	T49.6X1	T49.6X2	T49.6X3	T49.6X4	T49.6X5	T49.6X6
chromate	T56.5X1	T56.5X2	T56.5X3	T56.5X4	—	—
gelatin	T49.3X1	T49.3X2	T49.3X3	T49.3X4	T49.3X5	T49.3X6
oxide	T49.3X1	T49.3X2	T49.3X3	T49.3X4	T49.3X5	T49.3X6
plaster	T49.3X1	T49.3X2	T49.3X3	T49.3X4	T49.3X5	T49.3X6
peroxide	T49.0X1	T49.0X2	T49.0X3	T49.0X4	T49.0X5	T49.0X6
pesticides	T56.5X1	T56.5X2	T56.5X3	T56.5X4	—	—
phosphide	T60.4X1	T60.4X2	T60.4X3	T60.4X4	—	—
pyrithionate	T49.4X1	T49.4X2	T49.4X3	T49.4X4	T49.4X5	T49.4X6
stearate	T49.3X1	T49.3X2	T49.3X3	T49.3X4	T49.3X5	T49.3X6
sulfate	T49.5X1	T49.5X2	T49.5X3	T49.5X4	T49.5X5	T49.5X6
ENT agent	T49.6X1	T49.6X2	T49.6X3	T49.6X4	T49.6X5	T49.6X6
ophthalmic solution	T49.5X1	T49.5X2	T49.5X3	T49.5X4	T49.5X5	T49.5X6
topical NEC	T49.0X1	T49.0X2	T49.0X3	T49.0X4	T49.0X5	T49.0X6
undecylenate	T49.0X1	T49.0X2	T49.0X3	T49.0X4	T49.0X5	T49.0X6
Zineb	T60.0X1	T60.0X2	T60.0X3	T60.0X4	—	—
Zinostatin	T45.1X1	T45.1X2	T45.1X3	T45.1X4	T45.1X5	T45.1X6
Zipeprol	T48.3X1	T48.3X2	T48.3X3	T48.3X4	T48.3X5	T48.3X6
Zofenopril	T46.4X1	T46.4X2	T46.4X3	T46.4X4	T46.4X5	T46.4X6
Zolpidem	T42.6X1	T42.6X2	T42.6X3	T42.6X4	T42.6X5	T42.6X6
Zomepirac	T39.391	T39.392	T39.393	T39.394	T39.395	T39.396
Zopiclone	T42.6X1	T42.6X2	T42.6X3	T42.6X4	T42.6X5	T42.6X6
Zorubicin	T45.1X1	T45.1X2	T45.1X3	T45.1X4	T45.1X5	T45.1X6
Zotepine	T43.591	T43.592	T43.593	T43.594	T43.595	T43.596
Zovant	T45.511	T45.512	T45.513	T45.514	T45.515	T45.516
Zoxazolamine	T42.8X1	T42.8X2	T42.8X3	T42.8X4	T42.8X5	T42.8X6
Zuclopenthixol	T43.4X1	T43.4X2	T43.4X3	T43.4X4	T43.4X5	T43.4X6
Zygadenus (venenosus)	T62.2X1	T62.2X2	T62.2X3	T62.2X4	—	—
Zyprexa	T43.591	T43.592	T43.593	T43.594	T43.595	T43.596

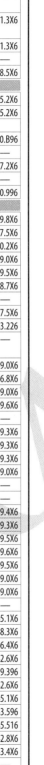

A

Abandonment (causing exposure to weather conditions) (with intent to injure or kill) NEC X58 ☑
Abuse (adult) (child) (mental) (physical) (sexual) X58 ☑
Accident (to) X58 ☑
  aircraft (in transit) (powered) (*see also* Accident, transport, aircraft)
    due to, caused by cataclysm — *see* Forces of nature, by type
  animal-rider — *see* Accident, transport, animal-rider
  animal-drawn vehicle — *see* Accident, transport, animal-drawn vehicle occupant
  automobile — *see* Accident, transport, car occupant
  bare foot water skiier V94.4 ☑
  boat, boating (*see also* Accident, watercraft)
    striking swimmer
      powered V94.11 ☑
      unpowered V94.12 ☑
  bus — *see* Accident, transport, bus occupant
  cable car, not on rails V98.0 ☑
    on rails — *see* Accident, transport, streetcar occupant
  car — *see* Accident, transport, car occupant
  caused by, due to
    animal NEC W64 ☑
    chain hoist W24.0 ☑
    cold (excessive) — *see* Exposure, cold
    corrosive liquid, substance — *see* Table of Drugs and Chemicals
    cutting or piercing instrument — *see* Contact, with, by type of instrument
    drive belt W24.0 ☑
    electric
      current — *see* Exposure, electric current
      motor (*see also* Contact, with, by type of machine) W31.3 ☑
      current (of) W86.8 ☑
    environmental factor NEC X58 ☑
    explosive material — *see* Explosion
    fire, flames — *see* Exposure, fire
    firearm missile — *see* Discharge, firearm by type
    heat (excessive) — *see* Heat
    hot — *see* Contact, with, hot
    ignition — *see* Ignition
    lifting device W24.0 ☑
    lightning T75.0
      causing fire — *see* Exposure, fire
    machine, machinery — *see* Contact, with, by type of machine
    natural factor NEC X58 ☑
    pulley (block) W24.0 ☑
    radiation — *see* Radiation
    steam X13.1 ☑
      inhalation X13.0 ☑
      pipe X16 ☑
    thunderbolt T75.0
      causing fire — *see* Exposure, fire
    transmission device W24.1 ☑
  coach — *see* Accident, transport, bus occupant
  coal car — *see* Accident, transport, industrial vehicle occupant
  diving (*see also* Fall, into, water)
    with
      drowning or submersion — *see* Drowning
  forklift — *see* Accident, transport, industrial vehicle occupant
  heavy transport vehicle NOS — *see* Accident, transport, truck occupant
  ice yacht V98.2 ☑
  in
    medical, surgical procedure
      as, or due to misadventure — *see* Misadventure
      causing an abnormal reaction or later complication without mention of misadventure (*see also* Complication of or following, by type of procedure) Y84.9
  land yacht V98.1 ☑
  late effect of — *see* W00-X58 with 7th character S
  logging car — *see* Accident, transport, industrial vehicle occupant
  machine, machinery (*see also* Contact, with, by type of machine)
    on board watercraft V93.69 ☑
      explosion — *see* Explosion, in, watercraft
      fire — *see* Burn, on board watercraft
      powered craft V93.63 ☑

Accident — *continued*
    ferry boat V93.61 ☑
    fishing boat V93.62 ☑
    jetskis V93.63 ☑
    liner V93.61 ☑
    merchant ship V93.60 ☑
    passenger ship V93.61 ☑
    sailboat V93.64 ☑
  mine tram — *see* Accident, transport, industrial vehicle occupant
  mobility scooter (motorized) — *see* Accident, transport, pedestrian, conveyance, specified type NEC
  motor scooter — *see* Accident, transport, motorcyclist
  motor vehicle NOS (traffic) (*see also* Accident, transport) V89.2 ☑
    nontraffic V89.0 ☑
    three-wheeled NOS — *see* Accident, transport, three-wheeled motor vehicle occupant
  motorcycle NOS — *see* Accident, transport, motorcyclist
  nonmotor vehicle NOS (nontraffic) (*see also* Accident, transport) V89.1 ☑
    traffic NOS V89.3 ☑
  nontraffic (victim's mode of transport NOS) V88.9 ☑
    collision (between) V88.7 ☑
      bus and truck V88.5 ☑
      car and:
        bus V88.3 ☑
        pickup V88.2 ☑
        three-wheeled motor vehicle V88.0 ☑
        train V88.6 ☑
        truck V88.4 ☑
        two-wheeled motor vehicle V88.0 ☑
        van V88.2 ☑
      specified vehicle NEC and:
        three-wheeled motor vehicle V88.1 ☑
        two-wheeled motor vehicle V88.1 ☑
    known mode of transport — *see* Accident, transport, by type of vehicle
    noncollision V88.8 ☑
  on board watercraft V93.89 ☑
    powered craft V93.83 ☑
      ferry boat V93.81 ☑
      fishing boat V93.82 ☑
      jetskis V93.83 ☑
      liner V93.81 ☑
      merchant ship V93.80 ☑
      passenger ship V93.81 ☑
    unpowered craft V93.88 ☑
      canoe V93.85 ☑
      inflatable V93.86 ☑
        in tow
          recreational V94.31 ☑
          specified NEC V94.32 ☑
      kayak V93.85 ☑
      sailboat V93.84 ☑
      surf-board V93.88 ☑
      water skis V93.87 ☑
      windsurfer V93.88 ☑
  parachutist V97.29 ☑
    entangled in object V97.21 ☑
    injured on landing V97.22 ☑
  pedal cycle — *see* Accident, transport, pedal cyclist
  pedestrian (on foot)
    with
      another pedestrian W51 ☑
        with fall W03 ☑
          due to ice or snow W00.0 ☑
        on pedestrian conveyance NEC V00.09 ☑
      roller skater (in-line) V00.01 ☑
      skate boarder V00.02 ☑
      transport vehicle — *see* Accident, transport
    on pedestrian conveyance — *see* Accident, transport, pedestrian, conveyance
  pick-up truck or van — *see* Accident, transport, pickup truck occupant
  quarry truck — *see* Accident, transport, industrial vehicle occupant
  railway vehicle (any) (in motion) — *see* Accident, transport, railway vehicle occupant
    due to cataclysm — *see* Forces of nature, by type
  scooter (non-motorized) — *see* Accident, transport, pedestrian, conveyance, scooter
  sequelae of — *see* W00-X58 with 7th character S
  skateboard — *see* Accident, transport, pedestrian, conveyance, skateboard

Accident — *continued*
    ski (ing) — *see* Accident, transport, pedestrian, conveyance
    lift V98.3 ☑
  specified cause NEC X58 ☑
  streetcar — *see* Accident, transport, streetcar occupant
  traffic (victim's mode of transport NOS) V87.9 ☑
    collision (between) V87.7 ☑
      bus and truck V87.5 ☑
      car and:
        bus V87.3 ☑
        pickup V87.2 ☑
        three-wheeled motor vehicle V87.0 ☑
        train V87.6 ☑
        truck V87.4 ☑
        two-wheeled motor vehicle V87.0 ☑
        van V87.2 ☑
      specified vehicle NEC and:
        three-wheeled motor vehicle V87.1 ☑
        two-wheeled motor vehicle V87.1 ☑
    known mode of transport — *see* Accident, transport, by type of vehicle
    noncollision V87.8 ☑
  transport (involving injury to) V99 ☑
    18 wheeler — *see* Accident, transport, truck occupant
    agricultural vehicle occupant (nontraffic) V84.9 ☑
      driver V84.5 ☑
      hanger-on V84.7 ☑
      passenger V84.6 ☑
      traffic V84.3 ☑
        driver V84.0 ☑
        hanger-on V84.2 ☑
        passenger V84.1 ☑
      while boarding or alighting V84.4 ☑
    aircraft NEC V97.89 ☑
      military NEC V97.818 ☑
        with civlian aircraft V97.810 ☑
        civilian injured by V97.811 ☑
      occupant injured (in)
        nonpowered craft accident V96.9 ☑
          balloon V96.00 ☑
            collision V96.03 ☑
            crash V96.01 ☑
            explosion V96.05 ☑
            fire V96.04 ☑
            forced landing V96.02 ☑
            specified type NEC V96.09 ☑
          glider V96.20 ☑
            collision V96.23 ☑
            crash V96.21 ☑
            explosion V96.25 ☑
            fire V96.24 ☑
            forced landing V96.22 ☑
            specified type NEC V96.29 ☑
          hang glider V96.10 ☑
            collision V96.13 ☑
            crash V96.11 ☑
            explosion V96.15 ☑
            fire V96.14 ☑
            forced landing V96.12 ☑
            specified type NEC V96.19 ☑
          specified craft NEC V96.8 ☑
        powered craft accident V95.9 ☑
          fixed wing NEC
            commercial V95.30 ☑
              collision V95.33 ☑
              crash V95.31 ☑
              explosion V95.35 ☑
              fire V95.34 ☑
              forced landing V95.32 ☑
              specified type NEC V95.39 ☑
            private V95.20 ☑
              collision V95.23 ☑
              crash V95.21 ☑
              explosion V95.25 ☑
              fire V95.24 ☑
              forced landing V95.22 ☑
              specified type NEC V95.29 ☑
          glider V95.10 ☑
            collision V95.13 ☑
            crash V95.11 ☑
            explosion V95.15 ☑
            fire V95.14 ☑
            forced landing V95.12 ☑
            specified type NEC V95.19 ☑
          helicopter V95.00 ☑
            collision V95.03 ☑
            crash V95.01 ☑
            explosion V95.05 ☑

Accident

Accident — *continued*
- two wheeled motor vehicle (traffic) V72.6 ☑
  - nontraffic V72.1 ☑
- van (traffic) V73.6 ☑
  - nontraffic V73.1 ☑
- noncollision accident (traffic) V78.6 ☑
  - nontraffic V78.1 ☑
- specified type NEC V79.88 ☑
- military vehicle V79.81 ☑
- cable car, not on rails V98.0 ☑
  - on rails — *see* Accident, transport, streetcar occupant
- car occupant V49.9 ☑
  - ambulance occupant — *see* Accident, transport, ambulance occupant
  - collision (with)
    - animal (traffic) V40.9 ☑
      - being ridden (traffic) V46.9 ☑
        - nontraffic V46.3 ☑
        - while boarding or alighting V46.4 ☑
      - nontraffic V40.3 ☑
      - while boarding or alighting V40.4 ☑
    - animal-drawn vehicle (traffic) V46.9 ☑
      - nontraffic V46.3 ☑
      - while boarding or alighting V46.4 ☑
    - bus (traffic) V44.9 ☑
      - nontraffic V44.3 ☑
      - while boarding or alighting V44.4 ☑
    - car (traffic) V43.92 ☑
      - nontraffic V43.32 ☑
      - while boarding or alighting V43.42 ☑
    - motor vehicle NOS (traffic) V49.60 ☑
      - nontraffic V49.20 ☑
      - specified type NEC (traffic) V49.69 ☑
        - nontraffic V49.29 ☑
    - pedal cycle (traffic) V41.9 ☑
      - nontraffic V41.3 ☑
      - while boarding or alighting V41.4 ☑
    - pickup truck (traffic) V43.93 ☑
      - nontraffic V43.33 ☑
      - while boarding or alighting V43.43 ☑
    - railway vehicle (traffic) V45.9 ☑
      - nontraffic V45.3 ☑
      - while boarding or alighting V45.4 ☑
    - specified vehicle NEC (traffic) V46.9 ☑
      - nontraffic V46.3 ☑
      - while boarding or alighting V46.4 ☑
    - sport utility vehicle (traffic) V43.91 ☑
      - nontraffic V43.31 ☑
      - while boarding or alighting V43.41 ☑
    - stationary object (traffic) V47.92 ☑
      - nontraffic V47.32 ☑
      - while boarding or alighting V47.4 ☑
    - streetcar (traffic) V46.9 ☑
      - nontraffic V46.3 ☑
      - while boarding or alighting V46.4 ☑
    - three wheeled motor vehicle (traffic) V42.9 ☑
      - nontraffic V42.3 ☑
      - while boarding or alighting V42.4 ☑
    - truck (traffic) V44.9 ☑
      - nontraffic V44.3 ☑
      - while boarding or alighting V44.4 ☑
    - two wheeled motor vehicle (traffic) V42.9 ☑
      - nontraffic V42.3 ☑
      - while boarding or alighting V42.4 ☑
    - van (traffic) V43.94 ☑
      - nontraffic V43.34 ☑
      - while boarding or alighting V43.44 ☑
  - driver
    - collision (with)
      - animal (traffic) V40.5 ☑
        - being ridden (traffic) V46.5 ☑
          - nontraffic V46.0 ☑
        - nontraffic V40.0 ☑
      - animal-drawn vehicle (traffic) V46.5 ☑
        - nontraffic V46.0 ☑
      - bus (traffic) V44.5 ☑
        - nontraffic V44.0 ☑
      - car (traffic) V43.52 ☑
        - nontraffic V43.02 ☑
      - motor vehicle NOS (traffic) V49.40 ☑
        - nontraffic V49.00 ☑
        - specified type NEC (traffic) V49.49 ☑
          - nontraffic V49.09 ☑
      - pedal cycle (traffic) V41.5 ☑
        - nontraffic V41.0 ☑
      - pickup truck (traffic) V43.53 ☑
        - nontraffic V43.03 ☑
      - railway vehicle (traffic) V45.5 ☑

- nontraffic V45.0 ☑
- specified vehicle NEC (traffic) V46.5 ☑
  - nontraffic V46.0 ☑
- sport utility vehicle (traffic) V43.51 ☑
  - nontraffic V43.01 ☑
- stationary object (traffic) V47.52 ☑
  - nontraffic V47.02 ☑
- streetcar (traffic) V46.5 ☑
  - nontraffic V46.0 ☑
- three wheeled motor vehicle (traffic) V42.5 ☑
  - nontraffic V42.0 ☑
- truck (traffic) V44.5 ☑
  - nontraffic V44.0 ☑
- two wheeled motor vehicle (traffic) V42.5 ☑
  - nontraffic V42.0 ☑
- van (traffic) V43.54 ☑
  - nontraffic V43.04 ☑
- noncollision accident (traffic) V48.5 ☑
  - nontraffic V48.0 ☑
- noncollision accident (traffic) V48.9 ☑
  - nontraffic V48.3 ☑
  - while boarding or alighting V48.4 ☑
- nontraffic V49.3 ☑
- hanger-on
  - collision (with)
    - animal (traffic) V40.7 ☑
      - being ridden (traffic) V46.7 ☑
        - nontraffic V46.2 ☑
      - nontraffic V40.2 ☑
    - animal-drawn vehicle (traffic) V46.7 ☑
      - nontraffic V46.2 ☑
    - bus (traffic) V44.7 ☑
      - nontraffic V44.2 ☑
    - car (traffic) V43.72 ☑
      - nontraffic V43.22 ☑
    - pedal cycle (traffic) V41.7 ☑
      - nontraffic V41.2 ☑
    - pickup truck (traffic) V43.73 ☑
      - nontraffic V43.23 ☑
    - railway vehicle (traffic) V45.7 ☑
      - nontraffic V45.2 ☑
    - specified vehicle NEC (traffic) V46.7 ☑
      - nontraffic V46.2 ☑
    - sport utility vehicle (traffic) V43.71 ☑
      - nontraffic V43.21 ☑
    - stationary object (traffic) V47.7 ☑
      - nontraffic V47.2 ☑
    - streetcar (traffic) V46.7 ☑
      - nontraffic V46.2 ☑
    - three wheeled motor vehicle (traffic) V42.7 ☑
      - nontraffic V42.2 ☑
    - truck (traffic) V44.7 ☑
      - nontraffic V44.2 ☑
    - two wheeled motor vehicle (traffic) V42.7 ☑
      - nontraffic V42.2 ☑
    - van (traffic) V43.74 ☑
      - nontraffic V43.24 ☑
  - noncollision accident (traffic) V48.7 ☑
    - nontraffic V48.2 ☑
- passenger
  - collision (with)
    - animal (traffic) V40.6 ☑
      - being ridden (traffic) V46.6 ☑
        - nontraffic V46.1 ☑
      - nontraffic V40.1 ☑
    - animal-drawn vehicle (traffic) V46.6 ☑
      - nontraffic V46.1 ☑
    - bus (traffic) V44.6 ☑
      - nontraffic V44.1 ☑
    - car (traffic) V43.62 ☑
      - nontraffic V43.12 ☑
    - motor vehicle NOS (traffic) V49.50 ☑
      - nontraffic V49.10 ☑
      - specified type NEC (traffic) V49.59 ☑
        - nontraffic V49.19 ☑
    - pedal cycle (traffic) V41.6 ☑
      - nontraffic V41.1 ☑
    - pickup truck (traffic) V43.63 ☑
      - nontraffic V43.13 ☑
    - railway vehicle (traffic) V45.6 ☑
      - nontraffic V45.1 ☑
    - specified vehicle NEC (traffic) V46.6 ☑
      - nontraffic V46.1 ☑
    - sport utility vehicle (traffic) V43.61 ☑
      - nontraffic V43.11 ☑
    - stationary object (traffic) V47.62 ☑
      - nontraffic V47.12 ☑

- streetcar (traffic) V46.6 ☑
  - nontraffic V46.1 ☑
- three wheeled motor vehicle (traffic) V42.6 ☑
  - nontraffic V42.1 ☑
- truck (traffic) V44.6 ☑
  - nontraffic V44.1 ☑
- two wheeled motor vehicle (traffic) V42.6 ☑
  - nontraffic V42.1 ☑
- van (traffic) V43.64 ☑
  - nontraffic V43.14 ☑
- noncollision accident (traffic) V48.6 ☑
  - nontraffic V48.1 ☑
- specified type NEC V49.88 ☑
- military vehicle V49.81 ☑
- coal car — *see* Accident, transport, industrial vehicle occupant
- construction vehicle occupant (nontraffic) V85.9 ☑
  - driver V85.5 ☑
  - hanger-on V85.7 ☑
  - passenger V85.6 ☑
  - traffic V85.3 ☑
    - driver V85.0 ☑
    - hanger-on V85.2 ☑
    - passenger V85.1 ☑
  - while boarding or alighting V85.4 ☑
- dirt bike rider — *see* Accident, transport, all-terrain vehicle occupant
- due to cataclysm — *see* Forces of nature, by type
- dune buggy occupant (nontraffic) V86.93 ☑
  - driver V86.53 ☑
  - hanger-on V86.73 ☑
  - passenger V86.63 ☑
  - traffic V86.33 ☑
    - driver V86.03 ☑
    - hanger-on V86.23 ☑
    - passenger V86.13 ☑
  - while boarding or alighting V86.43 ☑
- forklift — *see* Accident, transport, industrial vehicle occupant
- go cart — *see* Accident, transport, all-terrain vehicle occupant
- golf cart — *see* Accident, transport, all-terrain vehicle occupant
- heavy transport vehicle occupant — *see* Accident, transport, truck occupant
- ice yacht V98.2 ☑
- industrial vehicle occupant (nontraffic) V83.9 ☑
  - driver V83.5 ☑
  - hanger-on V83.7 ☑
  - passenger V83.6 ☑
  - traffic V83.3 ☑
    - driver V83.0 ☑
    - hanger-on V83.2 ☑
    - passenger V83.1 ☑
  - while boarding or alighting V83.4 ☑
- interurban electric car — *see* Accident, transport, streetcar
- land yacht V98.1 ☑
- logging car — *see* Accident, transport, industrial vehicle occupant
- military vehicle occupant (traffic) V86.34 ☑
  - driver V86.04 ☑
  - hanger-on V86.24 ☑
  - nontraffic V86.94 ☑
    - driver V86.54 ☑
    - hanger-on V86.74 ☑
    - passenger V86.64 ☑
  - passenger V86.14 ☑
  - while boarding or alighting V86.44 ☑
- mine tram — *see* Accident, transport, industrial vehicle occupant
- motorcoach — *see* Accident, transport, bus occupant
- motorcyclist V29.9 ☑
  - collision (with)
    - animal (traffic) V20.9 ☑
      - being ridden (traffic) V26.9 ☑
        - nontraffic V26.2 ☑
        - while boarding or alighting V26.3 ☑
      - nontraffic V20.2 ☑
      - while boarding or alighting V20.3 ☑
    - animal-drawn vehicle (traffic) V26.9 ☑
      - nontraffic V26.2 ☑
      - while boarding or alighting V26.3 ☑
    - bus (traffic) V24.9 ☑
      - nontraffic V24.2 ☑
      - while boarding or alighting V24.3 ☑

Accident

Accident — *continued*
- car (traffic) V23.9 ☑
  - nontraffic V23.2 ☑
  - while boarding or alighting V23.3 ☑
- motor vehicle NOS (traffic) V29.60 ☑
  - nontraffic V29.20 ☑
  - specified type NEC (traffic) V29.69 ☑
    - nontraffic V29.29 ☑
- pedal cycle (traffic) V21.9 ☑
  - nontraffic V21.2 ☑
  - while boarding or alighting V21.3 ☑
- pickup truck (traffic) V23.9 ☑
  - nontraffic V23.2 ☑
  - while boarding or alighting V23.3 ☑
- railway vehicle (traffic) V25.9 ☑
  - nontraffic V25.2 ☑
  - while boarding or alighting V25.3 ☑
- specified vehicle NEC (traffic) V26.9 ☑
  - nontraffic V26.2 ☑
  - while boarding or alighting V26.3 ☑
- stationary object (traffic) V27.9 ☑
  - nontraffic V27.2 ☑
  - while boarding or alighting V27.3 ☑
- streetcar (traffic) V26.9 ☑
  - nontraffic V26.2 ☑
  - while boarding or alighting V26.3 ☑
- three wheeled motor vehicle (traffic) V22.9 ☑
  - nontraffic V22.2 ☑
  - while boarding or alighting V22.3 ☑
- truck (traffic) V24.9 ☑
  - nontraffic V24.2 ☑
  - while boarding or alighting V24.3 ☑
- two wheeled motor vehicle (traffic) V22.9 ☑
  - nontraffic V22.2 ☑
  - while boarding or alighting V22.3 ☑
- van (traffic) V23.9 ☑
  - nontraffic V23.2 ☑
  - while boarding or alighting V23.3 ☑
- driver
  - collision (with)
    - animal (traffic) V20.4 ☑
      - being ridden (traffic) V26.4 ☑
        - nontraffic V26.0 ☑
      - nontraffic V20.0 ☑
    - animal-drawn vehicle (traffic) V26.4 ☑
      - nontraffic V26.0 ☑
    - bus (traffic) V24.4 ☑
      - nontraffic V24.0 ☑
    - car (traffic) V23.4 ☑
      - nontraffic V23.0 ☑
    - motor vehicle NOS (traffic) V29.40 ☑
      - nontraffic V29.00 ☑
      - specified type NEC (traffic) V29.49 ☑
        - nontraffic V29.09 ☑
    - pedal cycle (traffic) V21.4 ☑
      - nontraffic V21.0 ☑
    - pickup truck (traffic) V23.4 ☑
      - nontraffic V23.0 ☑
    - railway vehicle (traffic) V25.4 ☑
      - nontraffic V25.0 ☑
    - specified vehicle NEC (traffic) V26.4 ☑
      - nontraffic V26.0 ☑
    - stationary object (traffic) V27.4 ☑
      - nontraffic V27.0 ☑
    - streetcar (traffic) V26.4 ☑
      - nontraffic V26.0 ☑
    - three wheeled motor vehicle (traffic) V22.4 ☑
      - nontraffic V22.0 ☑
    - truck (traffic) V24.4 ☑
      - nontraffic V24.0 ☑
    - two wheeled motor vehicle (traffic) V22.4 ☑
      - nontraffic V22.0 ☑
    - van (traffic) V23.4 ☑
      - nontraffic V23.0 ☑
  - noncollision accident (traffic) V28.4 ☑
    - nontraffic V28.0 ☑
  - noncollision accident (traffic) V28.9 ☑
    - nontraffic V28.2 ☑
    - while boarding or alighting V28.3 ☑
  - nontraffic V29.3 ☑
- passenger
  - collision (with)
    - animal (traffic) V20.5 ☑
      - being ridden (traffic) V26.5 ☑
        - nontraffic V26.1 ☑
      - nontraffic V20.1 ☑
    - animal-drawn vehicle (traffic) V26.5 ☑
      - nontraffic V26.1 ☑

Accident — *continued*
- bus (traffic) V24.5 ☑
  - nontraffic V24.1 ☑
- car (traffic) V23.5 ☑
  - nontraffic V23.1 ☑
- motor vehicle NOS (traffic) V29.50 ☑
  - nontraffic V29.10 ☑
  - specified type NEC (traffic) V29.59 ☑
    - nontraffic V29.19 ☑
- pedal cycle (traffic) V21.5 ☑
  - nontraffic V21.1 ☑
- pickup truck (traffic) V23.5 ☑
  - nontraffic V23.1 ☑
- railway vehicle (traffic) V25.5 ☑
  - nontraffic V25.1 ☑
- specified vehicle NEC (traffic) V26.5 ☑
  - nontraffic V26.1 ☑
- stationary object (traffic) V27.5 ☑
  - nontraffic V27.1 ☑
- streetcar (traffic) V26.5 ☑
  - nontraffic V26.1 ☑
- three wheeled motor vehicle (traffic) V22.5 ☑
  - nontraffic V22.1 ☑
- truck (traffic) V24.5 ☑
  - nontraffic V24.1 ☑
- two wheeled motor vehicle (traffic) V22.5 ☑
  - nontraffic V22.1 ☑
- van (traffic) V23.5 ☑
  - nontraffic V23.1 ☑
- noncollision accident (traffic) V28.5 ☑
  - nontraffic V28.1 ☑
- specified type NEC V29.88 ☑
  - military vehicle V29.81 ☑
- motor vehicle NEC occupant (traffic) V86.39 ☑
  - driver V86.09 ☑
  - hanger-on V86.29 ☑
  - nontraffic V86.99 ☑
    - driver V86.59 ☑
    - hanger-on V86.79 ☑
    - passenger V86.69 ☑
  - passenger V86.19 ☑
  - while boarding or alighting V86.49 ☑
- occupant (of)
  - aircraft (powered) V95.9 ☑
    - fixed wing
      - commercial — *see* Accident, transport, aircraft, occupant, powered, fixed wing, commercial
      - private — *see* Accident, transport, aircraft, occupant, powered, fixed wing, private
    - nonpowered V96.9 ☑
    - specified NEC V95.8 ☑
  - airport battery-powered vehicle — *see* Accident, transport, industrial vehicle occupant
  - all-terrain vehicle (ATV) — *see* Accident, transport, all-terrain vehicle occupant
  - animal-drawn vehicle — *see* Accident, transport, animal-drawn vehicle occupant
  - automobile — *see* Accident, transport, car occupant
  - balloon V96.00 ☑
  - battery-powered vehicle — *see* Accident, transport, industrial vehicle occupant
  - bicycle — *see* Accident, transport, pedal cyclist
    - motorized — *see* Accident, transport, motorcycle rider
  - boat NEC — *see* Accident, watercraft
  - bulldozer — *see* Accident, transport, construction vehicle occupant
  - bus — *see* Accident, transport, bus occupant
  - cable car (on rails) (*see also* Accident, transport, streetcar occupant)
    - not on rails V98.0 ☑
  - car (*see also* Accident, transport, car occupant)
    - cable (on rails) (*see also* Accident, transport, streetcar occupant)
      - not on rails V98.0 ☑
  - coach — *see* Accident, transport, bus occupant
  - coal-car — *see* Accident, transport, industrial vehicle occupant
  - digger — *see* Accident, transport, construction vehicle occupant
  - dump truck — *see* Accident, transport, construction vehicle occupant

Accident — *continued*
- earth-leveler — *see* Accident, transport, construction vehicle occupant
- farm machinery (self-propelled) — *see* Accident, transport, agricultural vehicle occupant
- forklift — *see* Accident, transport, industrial vehicle occupant
- glider (unpowered) V96.20 ☑
  - hang V96.10 ☑
  - powered (microlight) (ultralight) — *see* Accident, transport, aircraft, occupant, powered, glider
- glider (unpowered) NEC V96.20 ☑
- hang-glider V96.10 ☑
- harvester — *see* Accident, transport, agricultural vehicle occupant
- heavy (transport) vehicle — *see* Accident, transport, truck occupant
- helicopter — *see* Accident, transport, aircraft, occupant, helicopter
- ice-yacht V98.2 ☑
- kite (carrying person) V96.8 ☑
- land-yacht V98.1 ☑
- logging car — *see* Accident, transport, industrial vehicle occupant
- mechanical shovel — *see* Accident, transport, construction vehicle occupant
- microlight — *see* Accident, transport, aircraft, occupant, powered, glider
- minibus — *see* Accident, transport, car occupant
- minivan — *see* Accident, transport, car occupant
- moped — *see* Accident, transport, motorcycle
- motor scooter — *see* Accident, transport, motorcycle
- motorcycle (with sidecar) — *see* Accident, transport, motorcycle
- pedal cycle (*see also* Accident, transport, pedal cyclist)
- pick-up (truck) — *see* Accident, transport, pickup truck occupant
- railway (train) (vehicle) (subterranean) (elevated) — *see* Accident, transport, railway vehicle occupant
- rickshaw — *see* Accident, transport, pedal cycle
  - motorized — *see* Accident, transport, three-wheeled motor vehicle
  - pedal driven — *see* Accident, transport, pedal cyclist
- road-roller — *see* Accident, transport, construction vehicle occupant
- ship NOS V94.9 ☑
- ski-lift (chair) (gondola) V98.3 ☑
- snowmobile — *see* Accident, transport, snowmobile occupant
- spacecraft, spaceship — *see* Accident, transport, aircraft, occupant, spacecraft
- sport utility vehicle — *see* Accident, transport, car occupant
- streetcar (interurban) (operating on public street or highway) — *see* Accident, transport, streetcar occupant
- SUV — *see* Accident, transport, car occupant
- téléférique V98.0 ☑
- three-wheeled vehicle (motorized) (*see also* Accident, transport, three-wheeled motor vehicle occupant)
  - nonmotorized — *see* Accident, transport, pedal cycle
- tractor (farm) (and trailer) — *see* Accident, transport, agricultural vehicle occupant
- train — *see* Accident, transport, railway vehicle occupant
- tram — *see* Accident, transport, streetcar occupant
  - in mine or quarry — *see* Accident, transport, industrial vehicle occupant
- tricycle — *see* Accident, transport, pedal cycle
  - motorized — *see* Accident, transport, three-wheeled motor vehicle
- trolley — *see* Accident, transport, streetcar occupant
  - in mine or quarry — *see* Accident, transport, industrial vehicle occupant
- tub, in mine or quarry — *see* Accident, transport, industrial vehicle occupant

☑ **Additional character required**

Accident — *continued*

- ultralight — *see* Accident, transport, aircraft, occupant, powered, glider
- van — *see* Accident, transport, van occupant
- vehicle NEC V89.9 ☑
  - heavy transport — *see* Accident, transport, truck occupant
  - motor (traffic) NEC V89.2 ☑
  - nontraffic NEC V89.0 ☑
- watercraft NOS V94.9 ☑
  - causing drowning — *see* Drowning, resulting from accident to boat
- parachutist V97.29 ☑
  - after accident to aircraft — *see* Accident, transport, aircraft
  - entangled in object V97.21 ☑
  - injured on landing V97.22 ☑
- pedal cyclist V19.9 ☑
  - collision (with)
    - animal (traffic) V10.9 ☑
      - being ridden (traffic) V16.9 ☑
        - nontraffic V16.2 ☑
        - while boarding or alighting V16.3 ☑
      - nontraffic V10.2 ☑
      - while boarding or alighting V10.3 ☑
    - animal-drawn vehicle (traffic) V16.9 ☑
      - nontraffic V16.2 ☑
      - while boarding or alighting V16.3 ☑
    - bus (traffic) V14.9 ☑
      - nontraffic V14.2 ☑
      - while boarding or alighting V14.3 ☑
    - car (traffic) V13.9 ☑
      - nontraffic V13.2 ☑
      - while boarding or alighting V13.3 ☑
    - motor vehicle NOS (traffic) V19.60 ☑
      - nontraffic V19.20 ☑
    - specified type NEC (traffic) V19.69 ☑
      - nontraffic V19.29 ☑
    - pedal cycle (traffic) V11.9 ☑
      - nontraffic V11.2 ☑
      - while boarding or alighting V11.3 ☑
    - pickup truck (traffic) V13.9 ☑
      - nontraffic V13.2 ☑
      - while boarding or alighting V13.3 ☑
    - railway vehicle (traffic) V15.9 ☑
      - nontraffic V15.2 ☑
      - while boarding or alighting V15.3 ☑
    - specified vehicle NEC (traffic) V16.9 ☑
      - nontraffic V16.2 ☑
      - while boarding or alighting V16.3 ☑
    - stationary object (traffic) V17.9 ☑
      - nontraffic V17.2 ☑
      - while boarding or alighting V17.3 ☑
    - streetcar (traffic) V16.9 ☑
      - nontraffic V16.2 ☑
      - while boarding or alighting V16.3 ☑
    - three wheeled motor vehicle (traffic) V12.9 ☑
      - nontraffic V12.2 ☑
      - while boarding or alighting V12.3 ☑
    - truck (traffic) V14.9 ☑
      - nontraffic V14.2 ☑
      - while boarding or alighting V14.3 ☑
    - two wheeled motor vehicle (traffic) V12.9 ☑
      - nontraffic V12.2 ☑
      - while boarding or alighting V12.3 ☑
    - van (traffic) V13.9 ☑
      - nontraffic V13.2 ☑
      - while boarding or alighting V13.3 ☑
  - driver
    - collision (with)
      - animal (traffic) V10.4 ☑
        - being ridden (traffic) V16.4 ☑
          - nontraffic V16.0 ☑
        - nontraffic V10.0 ☑
      - animal-drawn vehicle (traffic) V16.4 ☑
        - nontraffic V16.0 ☑
      - bus (traffic) V14.4 ☑
        - nontraffic V14.0 ☑
      - car (traffic) V13.4 ☑
        - nontraffic V13.0 ☑
      - motor vehicle NOS (traffic) V19.40 ☑
        - nontraffic V19.00 ☑
      - specified type NEC (traffic) V19.49 ☑
        - nontraffic V19.09 ☑
      - pedal cycle (traffic) V11.4 ☑
        - nontraffic V11.0 ☑
      - pickup truck (traffic) V13.4 ☑
        - nontraffic V13.0 ☑
      - railway vehicle (traffic) V15.4 ☑
        - nontraffic V15.0 ☑

Accident — *continued*

- specified vehicle NEC (traffic) V16.4 ☑
  - nontraffic V16.0 ☑
- stationary object (traffic) V17.4 ☑
  - nontraffic V17.0 ☑
- streetcar (traffic) V16.4 ☑
  - nontraffic V16.0 ☑
- three wheeled motor vehicle (traffic) V12.4 ☑
  - nontraffic V12.0 ☑
- truck (traffic) V14.4 ☑
  - nontraffic V14.0 ☑
- two wheeled motor vehicle (traffic) V12.4 ☑
  - nontraffic V12.0 ☑
- van (traffic) V13.4 ☑
  - nontraffic V13.0 ☑
- noncollision accident (traffic) V18.4 ☑
  - nontraffic V18.0 ☑
- noncollision accident (traffic) V18.9 ☑
  - nontraffic V18.2 ☑
  - while boarding or alighting V18.3 ☑
- nontraffic V19.3 ☑
- passenger
  - collision (with)
    - animal (traffic) V10.5 ☑
      - being ridden (traffic) V16.5 ☑
        - nontraffic V16.1 ☑
      - nontraffic V10.1 ☑
    - animal-drawn vehicle (traffic) V16.5 ☑
      - nontraffic V16.1 ☑
    - bus (traffic) V14.5 ☑
      - nontraffic V14.1 ☑
    - car (traffic) V13.5 ☑
      - nontraffic V13.1 ☑
    - motor vehicle NOS (traffic) V19.50 ☑
      - nontraffic V19.10 ☑
      - specified type NEC (traffic) V19.59 ☑
        - nontraffic V19.19 ☑
    - pedal cycle (traffic) V11.5 ☑
      - nontraffic V11.1 ☑
    - pickup truck (traffic) V13.5 ☑
      - nontraffic V13.1 ☑
    - railway vehicle (traffic) V15.5 ☑
      - nontraffic V15.1 ☑
    - specified vehicle NEC (traffic) V16.5 ☑
      - nontraffic V16.1 ☑
    - stationary object (traffic) V17.5 ☑
      - nontraffic V17.1 ☑
    - streetcar (traffic) V16.5 ☑
      - nontraffic V16.1 ☑
    - three wheeled motor vehicle (traffic) V12.5 ☑
      - nontraffic V12.1 ☑
    - truck (traffic) V14.5 ☑
      - nontraffic V14.1 ☑
    - two wheeled motor vehicle (traffic) V12.5 ☑
      - nontraffic V12.1 ☑
    - van (traffic) V13.5 ☑
      - nontraffic V13.1 ☑
  - noncollision accident (traffic) V18.5 ☑
    - nontraffic V18.1 ☑
  - specified type NEC V19.88 ☑
  - military vehicle V19.81 ☑
- pedestrian
  - conveyance (occupant) V09.9 ☑
    - babystroller V00.828 ☑
      - collision (with) V09.9 ☑
        - animal being ridden or animal drawn vehicle V06.99 ☑
          - nontraffic V06.09 ☑
          - traffic V06.19 ☑
        - bus or heavy transport V04.99 ☑
          - nontraffic V04.09 ☑
          - traffic V04.19 ☑
        - car V03.99 ☑
          - nontraffic V03.09 ☑
          - traffic V03.19 ☑
        - pedal cycle V01.99 ☑
          - nontraffic V01.09 ☑
          - traffic V01.19 ☑
        - pick-up truck or van V03.99 ☑
          - nontraffic V03.09 ☑
          - traffic V03.19 ☑
        - railway (train) (vehicle) V05.99 ☑
          - nontraffic V05.09 ☑
          - traffic V05.19 ☑
        - streetcar V06.99 ☑
          - nontraffic V06.09 ☑
          - traffic V06.19 ☑
        - stationary object V00.822 ☑

Accident — *continued*

- two- or three-wheeled motor vehicle V02.99 ☑
  - nontraffic V02.09 ☑
  - traffic V02.19 ☑
- vehicle V09.9 ☑
  - animal-drawn V06.99 ☑
    - nontraffic V06.09 ☑
    - traffic V06.19 ☑
  - motor
    - nontraffic V09.00 ☑
    - traffic V09.20 ☑
- fall V00.821 ☑
- nontraffic V09.1 ☑
  - involving motor vehicle NEC V09.00 ☑
- traffic V09.3 ☑
  - involving motor vehicle NEC V09.20 ☑
- flat-bottomed NEC V00.388 ☑
  - collision (with) V09.9 ☑
    - animal being ridden or animal drawn vehicle V06.99 ☑
      - nontraffic V06.09 ☑
      - traffic V06.19 ☑
    - bus or heavy transport V04.99 ☑
      - nontraffic V04.09 ☑
      - traffic V04.19 ☑
    - car V03.99 ☑
      - nontraffic V03.09 ☑
    - pedal cycle V01.99 ☑
      - nontraffic V01.09 ☑
      - traffic V01.19 ☑
    - pick-up truck or van V03.99 ☑
      - nontraffic V03.09 ☑
      - traffic V03.19 ☑
    - railway (train) (vehicle) V05.99 ☑
      - nontraffic V05.09 ☑
      - traffic V05.19 ☑
    - stationary object V00.382 ☑
    - streetcar V06.99 ☑
      - nontraffic V06.09 ☑
      - traffic V06.19 ☑
    - two- or three-wheeled motor vehicle V02.99 ☑
      - nontraffic V02.09 ☑
      - traffic V02.19 ☑
    - vehicle V09.9 ☑
      - animal-drawn V06.99 ☑
        - nontraffic V06.09 ☑
        - traffic V06.19 ☑
      - motor
        - nontraffic V09.00 ☑
        - traffic V09.20 ☑
  - fall V00.381 ☑
  - nontraffic V09.1 ☑
    - involving motor vehicle NEC V09.00 ☑
  - snow
    - board — *see* Accident, transport, pedestrian, conveyance, snow board
    - ski- — *see* Accident, transport, pedestrian, conveyance, skis (snow)
  - traffic V09.3 ☑
    - involving motor vehicle NEC V09.20 ☑
- gliding type NEC V00.288 ☑
  - collision (with) V09.9 ☑
    - animal being ridden or animal drawn vehicle V06.99 ☑
      - nontraffic V06.09 ☑
      - traffic V06.19 ☑
    - bus or heavy transport V04.99 ☑
      - nontraffic V04.09 ☑
      - traffic V04.19 ☑
    - car V03.99 ☑
      - nontraffic V03.09 ☑
      - traffic V03.19 ☑
    - pedal cycle V01.99 ☑
      - nontraffic V01.09 ☑
      - traffic V01.19 ☑
    - pick-up truck or van V03.99 ☑
      - nontraffic V03.09 ☑
      - traffic V03.19 ☑
    - railway (train) (vehicle) V05.99 ☑
      - nontraffic V05.09 ☑
      - traffic V05.19 ☑
    - stationary object V00.282 ☑
    - streetcar V06.99 ☑
      - nontraffic V06.09 ☑
      - traffic V06.19 ☑
    - two- or three-wheeled motor vehicle V02.99 ☑

☑ **Additional character required**

Accident

Accident — *continued*

nontraffic V02.09 ☑
traffic V02.19 ☑
vehicle V09.9 ☑
animal-drawn V06.99 ☑
nontraffic V06.09 ☑
traffic V06.19 ☑
motor
nontraffic V09.00 ☑
traffic V09.20 ☑
fall V00.281 ☑
heelies — *see* Accident, transport,
pedestrian, conveyance, heelies
ice skate — *see* Accident, transport,
pedestrian, conveyance, ice skate
nontraffic V09.1 ☑
involving motor vehicle NEC V09.00 ☑
sled — *see* Accident, transport,
pedestrian, conveyance, sled
traffic V09.3 ☑
involving motor vehicle NEC V09.20 ☑
wheelies — *see* Accident, transport,
pedestrian, conveyance, heelies
heelies V00.158 ☑
colliding with stationary object V00.152 ☑
fall V00.151 ☑
ice skates V00.218 ☑
collision (with) V09.9 ☑
animal being ridden or animal drawn
vehicle V06.99 ☑
nontraffic V06.09 ☑
traffic V06.19 ☑
bus or heavy transport V04.99 ☑
nontraffic V04.09 ☑
traffic V04.19 ☑
car V03.99 ☑
nontraffic V03.09 ☑
traffic V03.19 ☑
pedal cycle V01.99 ☑
nontraffic V01.09 ☑
traffic V01.19 ☑
pick-up truck or van V03.99 ☑
nontraffic V03.09 ☑
traffic V03.19 ☑
railway (train) (vehicle) V05.99 ☑
nontraffic V05.09 ☑
traffic V05.19 ☑
streetcar V06.99 ☑
nontraffic V06.09 ☑
traffic V06.19 ☑
stationary object V00.212 ☑
two- or three-wheeled motor vehicle
V02.99 ☑
nontraffic V02.09 ☑
traffic V02.19 ☑
vehicle V09.9 ☑
animal-drawn V06.99 ☑
nontraffic V06.09 ☑
traffic V06.19 ☑
motor
nontraffic V09.00 ☑
traffic V09.20 ☑
fall V00.211 ☑
nontraffic V09.1 ☑
involving motor vehicle NEC V09.00 ☑
traffic V09.3 ☑
involving motor vehicle NEC V09.20 ☑
motorized mobility scooter V00.838 ☑
collision with stationary object V00.832 ☑
fall from V00.831 ☑
nontraffic V09.1 ☑
involving motor vehicle V09.00 ☑
military V09.01 ☑
specified type NEC V09.09 ☑
roller skates (non in-line) V00.128 ☑
collision (with) V09.9 ☑
animal being ridden or animal drawn
vehicle V06.91 ☑
nontraffic V06.01 ☑
traffic V06.11 ☑
bus or heavy transport V04.91 ☑
nontraffic V04.01 ☑
traffic V04.11 ☑
car V03.91 ☑
nontraffic V03.01 ☑
traffic V03.11 ☑
pedal cycle V01.91 ☑
nontraffic V01.01 ☑
traffic V01.11 ☑
pick-up truck or van V03.91 ☑

Accident — *continued*

nontraffic V03.01 ☑
traffic V03.11 ☑
railway (train) (vehicle) V05.91 ☑
nontraffic V05.01 ☑
traffic V05.11 ☑
streetcar V06.91 ☑
nontraffic V06.01 ☑
traffic V06.11 ☑
stationary object V00.122 ☑
two- or three-wheeled motor vehicle
V02.91 ☑
nontraffic V02.01 ☑
traffic V02.11 ☑
vehicle V09.9 ☑
animal-drawn V06.91 ☑
nontraffic V06.01 ☑
traffic V06.11 ☑
motor
nontraffic V09.00 ☑
traffic V09.20 ☑
fall V00.121 ☑
in-line V00.118 ☑
collision- — *see also* Accident,
transport, pedestrian, conveyance
occupant, roller skates, collision
with stationary object V00.112 ☑
fall V00.111 ☑
nontraffic V09.1 ☑
involving motor vehicle NEC V09.00 ☑
traffic V09.3 ☑
involving motor vehicle NEC V09.20 ☑
rolling shoes V00.158 ☑
colliding with stationary object V00.152 ☑
fall V00.151 ☑
rolling type NEC V00.188 ☑
collision (with) V09.9 ☑
animal being ridden or animal drawn
vehicle V06.99 ☑
nontraffic V06.09 ☑
traffic V06.19 ☑
bus or heavy transport V04.99 ☑
nontraffic V04.09 ☑
traffic V04.19 ☑
car V03.99 ☑
nontraffic V03.09 ☑
traffic V03.19 ☑
pedal cycle V01.99 ☑
nontraffic V01.09 ☑
traffic V01.19 ☑
pick-up truck or van V03.99 ☑
nontraffic V03.09 ☑
traffic V03.19 ☑
railway (train) (vehicle) V05.99 ☑
nontraffic V05.09 ☑
traffic V05.19 ☑
stationary object V00.182 ☑
streetcar V06.99 ☑
nontraffic V06.09 ☑
traffic V06.19 ☑
two- or three-wheeled motor vehicle
V02.99 ☑
nontraffic V02.09 ☑
traffic V02.19 ☑
vehicle V09.9 ☑
animal-drawn V06.99 ☑
nontraffic V06.09 ☑
traffic V06.19 ☑
motor
nontraffic V09.00 ☑
traffic V09.20 ☑
fall V00.181 ☑
in-line roller skate — *see* Accident,
transport, pedestrian, conveyance,
roller skate, in-line
nontraffic V09.1 ☑
involving motor vehicle NEC V09.00 ☑
roller skate — *see* Accident, transport,
pedestrian, conveyance, roller skate
scooter (non-motorized) — *see* Accident,
transport, pedestrian, conveyance,
scooter
skateboard — *see* Accident, transport,
pedestrian, conveyance, skateboard
traffic V09.3 ☑
involving motor vehicle NEC V09.20 ☑
scooter (non-motorized) V00.148 ☑
collision (with) V09.9 ☑
animal being ridden or animal drawn
vehicle V06.99 ☑
nontraffic V06.09 ☑

Accident — *continued*

traffic V06.19 ☑
bus or heavy transport V04.99 ☑
nontraffic V04.09 ☑
traffic V04.19 ☑
car V03.99 ☑
nontraffic V03.09 ☑
traffic V03.19 ☑
pedal cycle V01.99 ☑
nontraffic V01.09 ☑
traffic V01.19 ☑
pick-up truck or van V03.99 ☑
nontraffic V03.09 ☑
traffic V03.19 ☑
railway (train) (vehicle) V05.99 ☑
nontraffic V05.09 ☑
traffic V05.19 ☑
streetcar V06.99 ☑
nontraffic V06.09 ☑
traffic V06.19 ☑
stationary object V00.142 ☑
two- or three-wheeled motor vehicle
V02.99 ☑
nontraffic V02.09 ☑
traffic V02.19 ☑
vehicle V09.9 ☑
animal-drawn V06.99 ☑
nontraffic V06.09 ☑
traffic V06.19 ☑
motor
nontraffic V09.00 ☑
traffic V09.20 ☑
fall V00.141 ☑
nontraffic V09.1 ☑
involving motor vehicle NEC V09.00 ☑
traffic V09.3 ☑
involving motor vehicle NEC V09.20 ☑
skate board V00.138 ☑
collision (with) V09.9 ☑
animal being ridden or animal drawn
vehicle V06.92 ☑
nontraffic V06.02 ☑
traffic V06.12 ☑
bus or heavy transport V04.92 ☑
nontraffic V04.02 ☑
traffic V04.12 ☑
car V03.92 ☑
nontraffic V03.02 ☑
traffic V03.12 ☑
pedal cycle V01.92 ☑
nontraffic V01.02 ☑
traffic V01.12 ☑
pick-up truck or van V03.92 ☑
nontraffic V03.02 ☑
traffic V03.12 ☑
railway (train) (vehicle) V05.92 ☑
nontraffic V05.02 ☑
traffic V05.12 ☑
streetcar V06.92 ☑
nontraffic V06.02 ☑
traffic V06.12 ☑
stationary object V00.132 ☑
two- or three-wheeled motor vehicle
V02.92 ☑
nontraffic V02.02 ☑
traffic V02.12 ☑
vehicle V09.9 ☑
animal-drawn V06.92 ☑
nontraffic V06.02 ☑
traffic V06.12 ☑
motor
nontraffic V09.00 ☑
traffic V09.20 ☑
fall V00.131 ☑
nontraffic V09.1 ☑
involving motor vehicle NEC V09.00 ☑
traffic V09.3 ☑
involving motor vehicle NEC V09.20 ☑
sled V00.228 ☑
collision (with) V09.9 ☑
animal being ridden or animal drawn
vehicle V06.99 ☑
nontraffic V06.09 ☑
traffic V06.19 ☑
bus or heavy transport V04.99 ☑
nontraffic V04.09 ☑
traffic V04.19 ☑
car V03.99 ☑
nontraffic V03.09 ☑
traffic V03.19 ☑
pedal cycle V01.99 ☑
nontraffic V01.09 ☑

☑ **Additional character required**

Accident — *continued*
    traffic V01.19 ☑
   pick-up truck or van V03.99 ☑
    nontraffic V03.09 ☑
    traffic V03.19 ☑
   railway (train) (vehicle) V05.99 ☑
    nontraffic V05.09 ☑
    traffic V05.19 ☑
   streetcar V06.99 ☑
    nontraffic V06.09 ☑
    traffic V06.19 ☑
   stationary object V00.222 ☑
   two- or three-wheeled motor vehicle
    V02.99 ☑
    nontraffic V02.09 ☑
    traffic V02.19 ☑
   vehicle V09.9 ☑
    animal-drawn V06.99 ☑
     nontraffic V06.09 ☑
     traffic V06.19 ☑
    motor
     nontraffic V09.00 ☑
     traffic V09.20 ☑
  fall V00.221 ☑
  nontraffic V09.1 ☑
   involving motor vehicle NEC V09.00 ☑
  traffic V09.3 ☑
   involving motor vehicle NEC V09.20 ☑
 skis (snow) V00.328 ☑
  collision (with) V09.9 ☑
   animal being ridden or animal drawn
    vehicle V06.99 ☑
    nontraffic V06.09 ☑
    traffic V06.19 ☑
   bus or heavy transport V04.99 ☑
    nontraffic V04.09 ☑
    traffic V04.19 ☑
   car V03.99 ☑
    nontraffic V03.09 ☑
    traffic V03.19 ☑
   pedal cycle V01.99 ☑
    nontraffic V01.09 ☑
    traffic V01.19 ☑
   pick-up truck or van V03.99 ☑
    nontraffic V03.09 ☑
    traffic V03.19 ☑
   railway (train) (vehicle) V05.99 ☑
    nontraffic V05.09 ☑
    traffic V05.19 ☑
   streetcar V06.99 ☑
    nontraffic V06.09 ☑
    traffic V06.19 ☑
   stationary object V00.322 ☑
   two- or three-wheeled motor vehicle
    V02.99 ☑
    nontraffic V02.09 ☑
    traffic V02.19 ☑
   vehicle V09.9 ☑
    animal-drawn V06.99 ☑
     nontraffic V06.09 ☑
     traffic V06.19 ☑
    motor
     nontraffic V09.00 ☑
     traffic V09.20 ☑
  fall V00.321 ☑
  nontraffic V09.1 ☑
   involving motor vehicle NEC V09.00 ☑
  traffic V09.3 ☑
   involving motor vehicle NEC V09.20 ☑
 snow board V00.318 ☑
  collision (with) V09.9 ☑
   animal being ridden or animal drawn
    vehicle V06.99 ☑
    nontraffic V06.09 ☑
    traffic V06.19 ☑
   bus or heavy transport V04.99 ☑
    nontraffic V04.09 ☑
    traffic V04.19 ☑
   car V03.99 ☑
    nontraffic V03.09 ☑
    traffic V03.19 ☑
   pedal cycle V01.99 ☑
    nontraffic V01.09 ☑
    traffic V01.19 ☑
   pick-up truck or van V03.99 ☑
    nontraffic V03.09 ☑
    traffic V03.19 ☑
   railway (train) (vehicle) V05.99 ☑
    nontraffic V05.09 ☑
    traffic V05.19 ☑
   streetcar V06.99 ☑
    nontraffic V06.09 ☑

Accident — *continued*
    traffic V06.19 ☑
   stationary object V00.312 ☑
   two- or three-wheeled motor vehicle
    V02.99 ☑
    nontraffic V02.09 ☑
    traffic V02.19 ☑
   vehicle V09.9 ☑
    animal-drawn V06.99 ☑
     nontraffic V06.09 ☑
     traffic V06.19 ☑
    motor
     nontraffic V09.00 ☑
     traffic V09.20 ☑
  fall V00.311 ☑
  nontraffic V09.1 ☑
   involving motor vehicle NEC V09.00 ☑
  traffic V09.3 ☑
   involving motor vehicle NEC V09.20 ☑
 specified type NEC V00.898 ☑
  collision (with) V09.9 ☑
   animal being ridden or animal drawn
    vehicle V06.99 ☑
    nontraffic V06.09 ☑
    traffic V06.19 ☑
   bus or heavy transport V04.99 ☑
    nontraffic V04.09 ☑
    traffic V04.19 ☑
   car V03.99 ☑
    nontraffic V03.09 ☑
    traffic V03.19 ☑
   pedal cycle V01.99 ☑
    nontraffic V01.09 ☑
    traffic V01.19 ☑
   pick-up truck or van V03.99 ☑
    nontraffic V03.09 ☑
    traffic V03.19 ☑
   railway (train) (vehicle) V05.99 ☑
    nontraffic V05.09 ☑
    traffic V05.19 ☑
   streetcar V06.99 ☑
    nontraffic V06.09 ☑
    traffic V06.19 ☑
   stationary object V00.892 ☑
   two- or three-wheeled motor vehicle
    V02.99 ☑
    nontraffic V02.09 ☑
    traffic V02.19 ☑
   vehicle V09.9 ☑
    animal-drawn V06.99 ☑
     nontraffic V06.09 ☑
     traffic V06.19 ☑
    motor
     nontraffic V09.00 ☑
     traffic V09.20 ☑
  fall V00.891 ☑
  nontraffic V09.1 ☑
   involving motor vehicle NEC V09.00 ☑
  traffic V09.3 ☑
   involving motor vehicle NEC V09.20 ☑
  traffic V09.3 ☑
   involving motor vehicle V09.20 ☑
    military V09.21 ☑
    specified type NEC V09.29 ☑
 wheelchair (powered) V00.818 ☑
  collision (with) V09.9 ☑
   animal being ridden or animal drawn
    vehicle V06.99 ☑
    nontraffic V06.09 ☑
    traffic V06.19 ☑
   bus or heavy transport V04.99 ☑
    nontraffic V04.09 ☑
    traffic V04.19 ☑
   car V03.99 ☑
    nontraffic V03.09 ☑
    traffic V03.19 ☑
   pedal cycle V01.99 ☑
    nontraffic V01.09 ☑
    traffic V01.19 ☑
   pick-up truck or van V03.99 ☑
    nontraffic V03.09 ☑
    traffic V03.19 ☑
   railway (train) (vehicle) V05.99 ☑
    nontraffic V05.09 ☑
    traffic V05.19 ☑
   streetcar V06.99 ☑
    nontraffic V06.09 ☑
    traffic V06.19 ☑
   stationary object V00.812 ☑
   two- or three-wheeled motor vehicle
    V02.99 ☑
    nontraffic V02.09 ☑

Accident — *continued*
    traffic V02.19 ☑
   vehicle V09.9 ☑
    animal-drawn V06.99 ☑
     nontraffic V06.09 ☑
     traffic V06.19 ☑
    motor
     nontraffic V09.00 ☑
     traffic V09.20 ☑
  fall V00.811 ☑
  nontraffic V09.1 ☑
   involving motor vehicle NEC V09.00 ☑
  traffic V09.3 ☑
   involving motor vehicle NEC V09.20 ☑
 wheeled shoe V00.158 ☑
  colliding with stationary object
   V00.152 ☑
  fall V00.151 ☑
 on foot (*see also* Accident, pedestrian)
  collision (with)
   animal being ridden or animal drawn
    vehicle V06.90 ☑
    nontraffic V06.00 ☑
    traffic V06.10 ☑
   bus or heavy transport V04.90 ☑
    nontraffic V04.00 ☑
    traffic V04.10 ☑
   car V03.90 ☑
    nontraffic V03.00 ☑
    traffic V03.10 ☑
   pedal cycle V01.90 ☑
    nontraffic V01.00 ☑
    traffic V01.10 ☑
   pick-up truck or van V03.90 ☑
    nontraffic V03.00 ☑
    traffic V03.10 ☑
   railway (train) (vehicle) V05.90 ☑
    nontraffic V05.00 ☑
    traffic V05.10 ☑
   streetcar V06.90 ☑
    nontraffic V06.00 ☑
    traffic V06.10 ☑
   two- or three-wheeled motor vehicle
    V02.90 ☑
    nontraffic V02.00 ☑
    traffic V02.10 ☑
   vehicle V09.9 ☑
    animal-drawn V06.90 ☑
     nontraffic V06.00 ☑
     traffic V06.10 ☑
    motor
     nontraffic V09.00 ☑
     traffic V09.20 ☑
  nontraffic V09.1 ☑
   involving motor vehicle V09.00 ☑
    military V09.01 ☑
    specified type NEC V09.09 ☑
  traffic V09.3 ☑
   involving motor vehicle V09.20 ☑
    military V09.21 ☑
    specified type NEC V09.29 ☑
 person NEC (unknown way or transportation)
  V99 ☑
  collision (between)
   bus (with)
    heavy transport vehicle (traffic) V87.5 ☑
    nontraffic V88.5 ☑
   car (with)
    nontraffic V88.5 ☑
    bus (traffic) V87.3 ☑
    nontraffic V88.3 ☑
    heavy transport vehicle (traffic) V87.4 ☑
    nontraffic V88.4 ☑
    pick-up truck or van (traffic) V87.2 ☑
    nontraffic V88.2 ☑
    train or railway vehicle (traffic) V87.6 ☑
    nontraffic V88.6 ☑
    two-or three-wheeled motor vehicle
     (traffic) V87.0 ☑
     nontraffic V88.0 ☑
   motor vehicle (traffic) NEC V87.7 ☑
    nontraffic V88.7 ☑
   two-or three-wheeled vehicle (with)
    (traffic)
    motor vehicle NEC V87.1 ☑
    nontraffic V88.1 ☑
   nonmotor vehicle (collision) (noncollision)
    (traffic) V87.9 ☑
    nontraffic V88.9 ☑
 pickup truck occupant V59.9 ☑
  collision (with)
   animal (traffic) V50.9 ☑

Accident — *continued*
  being ridden (traffic) V56.9 ☑
    nontraffic V56.3 ☑
      while boarding or alighting V56.4 ☑
    nontraffic V50.3 ☑
    while boarding or alighting V50.4 ☑
  animal-drawn vehicle (traffic) V56.9 ☑
    nontraffic V56.3 ☑
    while boarding or alighting V56.4 ☑
  bus (traffic) V54.9 ☑
    nontraffic V54.3 ☑
    while boarding or alighting V54.4 ☑
  car (traffic) V53.9 ☑
    nontraffic V53.3 ☑
    while boarding or alighting V53.4 ☑
  motor vehicle NOS (traffic) V59.60 ☑
    nontraffic V59.20 ☑
    specified type NEC (traffic) V59.69 ☑
      nontraffic V59.29 ☑
  pedal cycle (traffic) V51.9 ☑
    nontraffic V51.3 ☑
    while boarding or alighting V51.4 ☑
  pickup truck (traffic) V53.9 ☑
    nontraffic V53.3 ☑
    while boarding or alighting V53.4 ☑
  railway vehicle (traffic) V55.9 ☑
    nontraffic V55.3 ☑
    while boarding or alighting V55.4 ☑
  specified vehicle NEC (traffic) V56.9 ☑
    nontraffic V56.3 ☑
    while boarding or alighting V56.4 ☑
  stationary object (traffic) V57.9 ☑
    nontraffic V57.3 ☑
    while boarding or alighting V57.4 ☑
  streetcar (traffic) V56.9 ☑
    nontraffic V56.3 ☑
    while boarding or alighting V56.4 ☑
  three wheeled motor vehicle (traffic)
      V52.9 ☑
    nontraffic V52.3 ☑
    while boarding or alighting V52.4 ☑
  truck (traffic) V54.9 ☑
    nontraffic V54.3 ☑
    while boarding or alighting V54.4 ☑
  two wheeled motor vehicle (traffic) V52.9
      ☑
    nontraffic V52.3 ☑
    while boarding or alighting V52.4 ☑
  van (traffic) V53.9 ☑
    nontraffic V53.3 ☑
    while boarding or alighting V53.4 ☑
  driver
    collision (with)
      animal (traffic) V50.5 ☑
        being ridden (traffic) V56.5 ☑
          nontraffic V56.0 ☑
        nontraffic V50.0 ☑
      animal-drawn vehicle (traffic) V56.5 ☑
        nontraffic V56.0 ☑
      bus (traffic) V54.5 ☑
        nontraffic V54.0 ☑
      car (traffic) V53.5 ☑
        nontraffic V53.0 ☑
      motor vehicle NOS (traffic) V59.40 ☑
        nontraffic V59.00 ☑
        specified type NEC (traffic) V59.49 ☑
          nontraffic V59.09 ☑
      pedal cycle (traffic) V51.5 ☑
        nontraffic V51.0 ☑
      pickup truck (traffic) V53.5 ☑
        nontraffic V53.0 ☑
      railway vehicle (traffic) V55.5 ☑
        nontraffic V55.0 ☑
      specified vehicle NEC (traffic) V56.5 ☑
        nontraffic V56.0 ☑
      stationary object (traffic) V57.5 ☑
        nontraffic V57.0 ☑
      streetcar (traffic) V56.5 ☑
        nontraffic V56.0 ☑
      three wheeled motor vehicle (traffic)
          V52.5 ☑
        nontraffic V52.0 ☑
      truck (traffic) V54.5 ☑
        nontraffic V54.0 ☑
      two wheeled motor vehicle (traffic)
          V52.5 ☑
        nontraffic V52.0 ☑
      van (traffic) V53.5 ☑
        nontraffic V53.0 ☑
    noncollision accident (traffic) V58.5 ☑
      nontraffic V58.0 ☑
  noncollision accident (traffic) V58.9 ☑

Accident — *continued*
    nontraffic V58.3 ☑
    while boarding or alighting V58.4 ☑
  nontraffic V59.3 ☑
  hanger-on
    collision (with)
      animal (traffic) V50.7 ☑
        being ridden (traffic) V56.7 ☑
          nontraffic V56.2 ☑
        nontraffic V50.2 ☑
      animal-drawn vehicle (traffic) V56.7 ☑
        nontraffic V56.2 ☑
      bus (traffic) V54.7 ☑
        nontraffic V54.2 ☑
      car (traffic) V53.7 ☑
        nontraffic V53.2 ☑
      pedal cycle (traffic) V51.7 ☑
        nontraffic V51.2 ☑
      pickup truck (traffic) V53.7 ☑
        nontraffic V53.2 ☑
      railway vehicle (traffic) V55.7 ☑
        nontraffic V55.2 ☑
      specified vehicle NEC (traffic) V56.7 ☑
        nontraffic V56.2 ☑
      stationary object (traffic) V57.7 ☑
        nontraffic V57.2 ☑
      streetcar (traffic) V56.7 ☑
        nontraffic V56.2 ☑
      three wheeled motor vehicle (traffic)
          V52.7 ☑
        nontraffic V52.2 ☑
      truck (traffic) V54.7 ☑
        nontraffic V54.2 ☑
      two wheeled motor vehicle (traffic)
          V52.7 ☑
        nontraffic V52.2 ☑
      van (traffic) V53.7 ☑
        nontraffic V53.2 ☑
    noncollision accident (traffic) V58.7 ☑
      nontraffic V58.2 ☑
  passenger
    collision (with)
      animal (traffic) V50.6 ☑
        being ridden (traffic) V56.6 ☑
          nontraffic V56.1 ☑
        nontraffic V50.1 ☑
      animal-drawn vehicle (traffic) V56.6 ☑
        nontraffic V56.1 ☑
      bus (traffic) V54.6 ☑
        nontraffic V54.1 ☑
      car (traffic) V53.6 ☑
        nontraffic V53.1 ☑
      motor vehicle NOS (traffic) V59.50 ☑
        nontraffic V59.10 ☑
        specified type NEC (traffic) V59.59 ☑
          nontraffic V59.19 ☑
      pedal cycle (traffic) V51.6 ☑
        nontraffic V51.1 ☑
      pickup truck (traffic) V53.6 ☑
        nontraffic V53.1 ☑
      railway vehicle (traffic) V55.6 ☑
        nontraffic V55.1 ☑
      specified vehicle NEC (traffic) V56.6 ☑
        nontraffic V56.1 ☑
      stationary object (traffic) V57.6 ☑
        nontraffic V57.1 ☑
      streetcar (traffic) V56.6 ☑
        nontraffic V56.1 ☑
      three wheeled motor vehicle (traffic)
          V52.6 ☑
        nontraffic V52.1 ☑
      truck (traffic) V54.6 ☑
        nontraffic V54.1 ☑
      two wheeled motor vehicle (traffic)
          V52.6 ☑
        nontraffic V52.1 ☑
      van (traffic) V53.6 ☑
        nontraffic V53.1 ☑
    noncollision accident (traffic) V58.6 ☑
      nontraffic V58.1 ☑
    specified type NEC V59.88 ☑
    military vehicle V59.81 ☑
  quarry truck — *see* Accident, transport,
      industrial vehicle occupant
  race car — *see* Accident, transport, motor
      vehicle NEC occupant
  railway vehicle occupant V81.9 ☑
    collision (with) V81.3 ☑
      motor vehicle (non-military) (traffic) V81.1
          ☑
        military V81.83 ☑
      nontraffic V81.0 ☑

Accident — *continued*
      rolling stock V81.2 ☑
      specified object NEC V81.3 ☑
    during derailment V81.7 ☑
      with antecedent collision — *see* Accident,
          transport, railway vehicle occupant,
          collision
    explosion V81.81 ☑
    fall (in railway vehicle) V81.5 ☑
      during derailment V81.7 ☑
        with antecedent collision — *see* Accident,
            transport, railway vehicle occupant,
            collision
      from railway vehicle V81.6 ☑
        during derailment V81.7 ☑
          with antecedent collision — *see*
              Accident, transport, railway vehicle
              occupant, collision
      while boarding or alighting V81.4 ☑
    fire V81.81 ☑
    object falling onto train V81.82 ☑
    specified type NEC V81.89 ☑
    while boarding or alighting V81.4 ☑
  ski lift V98.3 ☑
  snowmobile occupant (nontraffic) V86.92 ☑
    driver V86.52 ☑
    hanger-on V86.72 ☑
    passenger V86.62 ☑
    traffic V86.32 ☑
      driver V86.02 ☑
      hanger-on V86.22 ☑
      passenger V86.12 ☑
    while boarding or alighting V86.42 ☑
    specified NEC V98.8 ☑
  sport utility vehicle occupant (*see also*
      Accident, transport, car occupant)
    collision (with)
      stationary object (traffic) V47.91 ☑
        nontraffic V47.31 ☑
    driver
      collision (with)
        stationary object (traffic) V47.51 ☑
          nontraffic V47.01 ☑
    passenger
      collision (with)
        stationary object (traffic) V47.61 ☑
          nontraffic V47.11 ☑
  streetcar occupant V82.9 ☑
    collision (with) V82.3 ☑
      motor vehicle (traffic) V82.1 ☑
        nontraffic V82.0 ☑
      rolling stock V82.2 ☑
    during derailment V82.7 ☑
      with antecedent collision — *see* Accident,
          transport, streetcar occupant, collision
    fall (in streetcar) V82.5 ☑
      during derailment V82.7 ☑
        with antecedent collision — *see* Accident,
            transport, streetcar occupant,
            collision
      from streetcar V82.6 ☑
        during derailment V82.7 ☑
          with antecedent collision — *see*
              Accident, transport, streetcar
              occupant, collision
      while boarding or alighting V82.4 ☑
    while boarding or alighting V82.4 ☑
    specified type NEC V82.8 ☑
    while boarding or alighting V82.4 ☑
  three-wheeled motor vehicle occupant V39.9
      ☑
    collision (with)
      animal (traffic) V30.9 ☑
        being ridden (traffic) V36.9 ☑
          nontraffic V36.3 ☑
          while boarding or alighting V36.4 ☑
        nontraffic V30.3 ☑
        while boarding or alighting V30.4 ☑
      animal-drawn vehicle (traffic) V36.9 ☑
        nontraffic V36.3 ☑
        while boarding or alighting V36.4 ☑
      bus (traffic) V34.9 ☑
        nontraffic V34.3 ☑
        while boarding or alighting V34.4 ☑
      car (traffic) V33.9 ☑
        nontraffic V33.3 ☑
        while boarding or alighting V33.4 ☑
      motor vehicle NOS (traffic) V39.60 ☑
        nontraffic V39.20 ☑
        specified type NEC (traffic) V39.69 ☑
          nontraffic V39.29 ☑
      pedal cycle (traffic) V31.9 ☑

☑ **Additional character required**

Accident

Accident — *continued*
  nontraffic V31.3 ☑
  while boarding or alighting V31.4 ☑
  pickup truck (traffic) V33.9 ☑
    nontraffic V33.3 ☑
    while boarding or alighting V33.4 ☑
  railway vehicle (traffic) V35.9 ☑
    nontraffic V35.3 ☑
    while boarding or alighting V35.4 ☑
  specified vehicle NEC (traffic) V36.9 ☑
    nontraffic V36.3 ☑
    while boarding or alighting V36.4 ☑
  stationary object (traffic) V37.9 ☑
    nontraffic V37.3 ☑
    while boarding or alighting V37.4 ☑
  streetcar (traffic) V36.9 ☑
    nontraffic V36.3 ☑
    while boarding or alighting V36.4 ☑
  three wheeled motor vehicle (traffic) V32.9 ☑
    nontraffic V32.3 ☑
    while boarding or alighting V32.4 ☑
  truck (traffic) V34.9 ☑
    nontraffic V34.3 ☑
    while boarding or alighting V34.4 ☑
  two wheeled motor vehicle (traffic) V32.9 ☑
    nontraffic V32.3 ☑
    while boarding or alighting V32.4 ☑
  van (traffic) V33.9 ☑
    nontraffic V33.3 ☑
    while boarding or alighting V33.4 ☑
 driver
  collision (with)
    animal (traffic) V30.5 ☑
     being ridden (traffic) V36.5 ☑
      nontraffic V36.0 ☑
     nontraffic V30.0 ☑
    animal-drawn vehicle (traffic) V36.5 ☑
     nontraffic V36.0 ☑
    bus (traffic) V34.5 ☑
     nontraffic V34.0 ☑
    car (traffic) V33.5 ☑
     nontraffic V33.0 ☑
    motor vehicle NOS (traffic) V39.40 ☑
     nontraffic V39.00 ☑
     specified type NEC (traffic) V39.49 ☑
      nontraffic V39.09 ☑
    pedal cycle (traffic) V31.5 ☑
     nontraffic V31.0 ☑
    pickup truck (traffic) V33.5 ☑
     nontraffic V33.0 ☑
    railway vehicle (traffic) V35.5 ☑
     nontraffic V35.0 ☑
    specified vehicle NEC (traffic) V36.5 ☑
     nontraffic V36.0 ☑
    stationary object (traffic) V37.5 ☑
     nontraffic V37.0 ☑
    streetcar (traffic) V36.5 ☑
     nontraffic V36.0 ☑
    three wheeled motor vehicle (traffic) V32.5 ☑
     nontraffic V32.0 ☑
    truck (traffic) V34.5 ☑
     nontraffic V34.0 ☑
    two wheeled motor vehicle (traffic) V32.5 ☑
     nontraffic V32.0 ☑
    van (traffic) V33.5 ☑
     nontraffic V33.0 ☑
    noncollision accident (traffic) V38.5 ☑
     nontraffic V38.0 ☑
  noncollision accident (traffic) V38.9 ☑
    nontraffic V38.3 ☑
    while boarding or alighting V38.4 ☑
  nontraffic V39.3 ☑
 hanger-on
  collision (with)
    animal (traffic) V30.7 ☑
     being ridden (traffic) V36.7 ☑
      nontraffic V36.2 ☑
     nontraffic V30.2 ☑
    animal-drawn vehicle (traffic) V36.7 ☑
     nontraffic V36.2 ☑
    bus (traffic) V34.7 ☑
     nontraffic V34.2 ☑
    car (traffic) V33.7 ☑
     nontraffic V33.2 ☑
    pedal cycle (traffic) V31.7 ☑
     nontraffic V31.2 ☑
    pickup truck (traffic) V33.7 ☑
     nontraffic V33.2 ☑

  railway vehicle (traffic) V35.7 ☑
    nontraffic V35.2 ☑
  specified vehicle NEC (traffic) V36.7 ☑
    nontraffic V36.2 ☑
  stationary object (traffic) V37.7 ☑
    nontraffic V37.2 ☑
  streetcar (traffic) V36.7 ☑
    nontraffic V36.2 ☑
  three wheeled motor vehicle (traffic) V32.7 ☑
    nontraffic V32.2 ☑
  truck (traffic) V34.7 ☑
    nontraffic V34.2 ☑
  two wheeled motor vehicle (traffic) V32.7 ☑
    nontraffic V32.2 ☑
  van (traffic) V33.7 ☑
    nontraffic V33.2 ☑
 noncollision accident (traffic) V38.7 ☑
  nontraffic V38.2 ☑
 passenger
  collision (with)
    animal (traffic) V30.6 ☑
     being ridden (traffic) V36.6 ☑
      nontraffic V36.1 ☑
     nontraffic V30.1 ☑
    animal-drawn vehicle (traffic) V36.6 ☑
     nontraffic V36.1 ☑
    bus (traffic) V34.6 ☑
     nontraffic V34.1 ☑
    car (traffic) V33.6 ☑
     nontraffic V33.1 ☑
    motor vehicle NOS (traffic) V39.50 ☑
     nontraffic V39.10 ☑
     specified type NEC (traffic) V39.59 ☑
      nontraffic V39.19 ☑
    pedal cycle (traffic) V31.6 ☑
     nontraffic V31.1 ☑
    pickup truck (traffic) V33.6 ☑
     nontraffic V33.1 ☑
    railway vehicle (traffic) V35.6 ☑
     nontraffic V35.1 ☑
    specified vehicle NEC (traffic) V36.6 ☑
     nontraffic V36.1 ☑
    stationary object (traffic) V37.6 ☑
     nontraffic V37.1 ☑
    streetcar (traffic) V36.6 ☑
     nontraffic V36.1 ☑
    three wheeled motor vehicle (traffic) V32.6 ☑
     nontraffic V32.1 ☑
    truck (traffic) V34.6 ☑
     nontraffic V34.1 ☑
    two wheeled motor vehicle (traffic) V32.6 ☑
     nontraffic V32.1 ☑
    van (traffic) V33.6 ☑
     nontraffic V33.1 ☑
    noncollision accident (traffic) V38.6 ☑
     nontraffic V38.1 ☑
  specified type NEC V39.89 ☑
    military vehicle V39.81 ☑
 tractor (farm) (and trailer) — *see* Accident, transport, agricultural vehicle occupant
 tram — *see* Accident, transport, streetcar
  in mine or quarry — *see* Accident, transport, industrial vehicle occupant
 trolley — *see* Accident, transport, streetcar
  in mine or quarry — *see* Accident, transport, industrial vehicle occupant
 truck (heavy) occupant V69.9 ☑
  collision (with)
    animal (traffic) V60.9 ☑
     being ridden (traffic) V66.9 ☑
      nontraffic V66.3 ☑
      while boarding or alighting V66.4 ☑
     nontraffic V60.3 ☑
     while boarding or alighting V60.4 ☑
    animal-drawn vehicle (traffic) V66.9 ☑
     nontraffic V66.3 ☑
     while boarding or alighting V66.4 ☑
    bus (traffic) V64.9 ☑
     nontraffic V64.3 ☑
     while boarding or alighting V64.4 ☑
    car (traffic) V63.9 ☑
     nontraffic V63.3 ☑
     while boarding or alighting V63.4 ☑
    motor vehicle NOS (traffic) V69.60 ☑
     nontraffic V69.20 ☑
     specified type NEC (traffic) V69.69 ☑
      nontraffic V69.29 ☑

  pedal cycle (traffic) V61.9 ☑
    nontraffic V61.3 ☑
    while boarding or alighting V61.4 ☑
  pickup truck (traffic) V63.9 ☑
    nontraffic V63.3 ☑
    while boarding or alighting V63.4 ☑
  railway vehicle (traffic) V65.9 ☑
    nontraffic V65.3 ☑
    while boarding or alighting V65.4 ☑
  specified vehicle NEC (traffic) V66.9 ☑
    nontraffic V66.3 ☑
    while boarding or alighting V66.4 ☑
  stationary object (traffic) V67.9 ☑
    nontraffic V67.3 ☑
    while boarding or alighting V67.4 ☑
  streetcar (traffic) V66.9 ☑
    nontraffic V66.3 ☑
    while boarding or alighting V66.4 ☑
  three wheeled motor vehicle (traffic) V62.9 ☑
    nontraffic V62.3 ☑
    while boarding or alighting V62.4 ☑
  truck (traffic) V64.9 ☑
    nontraffic V64.3 ☑
    while boarding or alighting V64.4 ☑
  two wheeled motor vehicle (traffic) V62.9 ☑
    nontraffic V62.3 ☑
    while boarding or alighting V62.4 ☑
  van (traffic) V63.9 ☑
    nontraffic V63.3 ☑
    while boarding or alighting V63.4 ☑
 driver
  collision (with)
    animal (traffic) V60.5 ☑
     being ridden (traffic) V66.5 ☑
      nontraffic V66.0 ☑
     nontraffic V60.0 ☑
    animal-drawn vehicle (traffic) V66.5 ☑
     nontraffic V66.0 ☑
    bus (traffic) V64.5 ☑
     nontraffic V64.0 ☑
    car (traffic) V63.5 ☑
     nontraffic V63.0 ☑
    motor vehicle NOS (traffic) V69.40 ☑
     nontraffic V69.00 ☑
     specified type NEC (traffic) V69.49 ☑
      nontraffic V69.09 ☑
    pedal cycle (traffic) V61.5 ☑
     nontraffic V61.0 ☑
    pickup truck (traffic) V63.5 ☑
     nontraffic V63.0 ☑
    railway vehicle (traffic) V65.5 ☑
     nontraffic V65.0 ☑
    specified vehicle NEC (traffic) V66.5 ☑
     nontraffic V66.0 ☑
    stationary object (traffic) V67.5 ☑
     nontraffic V67.0 ☑
    streetcar (traffic) V66.5 ☑
     nontraffic V66.0 ☑
    three wheeled motor vehicle (traffic) V62.5 ☑
     nontraffic V62.0 ☑
    truck (traffic) V64.5 ☑
     nontraffic V64.0 ☑
    two wheeled motor vehicle (traffic) V62.5 ☑
     nontraffic V62.0 ☑
    van (traffic) V63.5 ☑
     nontraffic V63.0 ☑
    noncollision accident (traffic) V68.5 ☑
     nontraffic V68.0 ☑
 dump — *see* Accident, transport, construction vehicle occupant
 hanger-on
  collision (with)
    animal (traffic) V60.7 ☑
     being ridden (traffic) V66.7 ☑
      nontraffic V66.2 ☑
     nontraffic V60.2 ☑
    animal-drawn vehicle (traffic) V66.7 ☑
     nontraffic V66.2 ☑
    bus (traffic) V64.7 ☑
     nontraffic V64.2 ☑
    car (traffic) V63.7 ☑
     nontraffic V63.2 ☑
    pedal cycle (traffic) V61.7 ☑
     nontraffic V61.2 ☑
    pickup truck (traffic) V63.7 ☑
     nontraffic V63.2 ☑
    railway vehicle (traffic) V65.7 ☑

☑ **Additional character required**

405

Accident

Accident — *continued*
- nontraffic V65.2 ☑
- specified vehicle NEC (traffic) V66.7 ☑
  - nontraffic V66.2 ☑
- stationary object (traffic) V67.7 ☑
  - nontraffic V67.2 ☑
- streetcar (traffic) V66.7 ☑
  - nontraffic V66.2 ☑
- three wheeled motor vehicle (traffic) V62.7 ☑
  - nontraffic V62.2 ☑
- truck (traffic) V64.7 ☑
  - nontraffic V64.2 ☑
- two wheeled motor vehicle (traffic) V62.7 ☑
  - nontraffic V62.2 ☑
- van (traffic) V63.7 ☑
  - nontraffic V63.2 ☑
- noncollision accident (traffic) V68.7 ☑
  - nontraffic V68.2 ☑
- noncollision accident (traffic) V68.9 ☑
  - nontraffic V68.3 ☑
  - while boarding or alighting V68.4 ☑
- nontraffic V69.3 ☑
- passenger
  - collision (with)
    - animal (traffic) V60.6 ☑
      - being ridden (traffic) V66.6 ☑
        - nontraffic V66.1 ☑
      - nontraffic V60.1 ☑
    - animal-drawn vehicle (traffic) V66.6 ☑
      - nontraffic V66.1 ☑
    - bus (traffic) V64.6 ☑
      - nontraffic V64.1 ☑
    - car (traffic) V63.6 ☑
      - nontraffic V63.1 ☑
    - motor vehicle NOS (traffic) V69.50 ☑
      - nontraffic V69.10 ☑
      - specified type NEC (traffic) V69.59 ☑
        - nontraffic V69.19 ☑
    - pedal cycle (traffic) V61.6 ☑
      - nontraffic V61.1 ☑
    - pickup truck (traffic) V63.6 ☑
      - nontraffic V63.1 ☑
    - railway vehicle (traffic) V65.6 ☑
      - nontraffic V65.1 ☑
    - specified vehicle NEC (traffic) V66.6 ☑
      - nontraffic V66.1 ☑
    - stationary object (traffic) V67.6 ☑
      - nontraffic V67.1 ☑
    - streetcar (traffic) V66.6 ☑
      - nontraffic V66.1 ☑
    - three wheeled motor vehicle (traffic) V62.6 ☑
      - nontraffic V62.1 ☑
    - truck (traffic) V64.6 ☑
      - nontraffic V64.1 ☑
    - two wheeled motor vehicle (traffic) V62.6 ☑
      - nontraffic V62.1 ☑
    - van (traffic) V63.6 ☑
      - nontraffic V63.1 ☑
  - noncollision accident (traffic) V68.6 ☑
    - nontraffic V68.1 ☑
- pickup — *see* Accident, transport, pickup truck occupant
- specified type NEC V69.88 ☑
- military vehicle V69.81 ☑
- van occupant V59.9 ☑
  - collision (with)
    - animal (traffic) V50.9 ☑
      - being ridden (traffic) V56.9 ☑
        - nontraffic V56.3 ☑
        - while boarding or alighting V56.4 ☑
      - nontraffic V50.3 ☑
      - while boarding or alighting V50.4 ☑
    - animal-drawn vehicle (traffic) V56.9 ☑
      - nontraffic V56.3 ☑
      - while boarding or alighting V56.4 ☑
    - bus (traffic) V54.9 ☑
      - nontraffic V54.3 ☑
      - while boarding or alighting V54.4 ☑
    - car (traffic) V53.9 ☑
      - nontraffic V53.3 ☑
      - while boarding or alighting V53.4 ☑
    - motor vehicle NOS (traffic) V59.60 ☑
      - nontraffic V59.20 ☑
      - specified type NEC (traffic) V59.69 ☑
        - nontraffic V59.29 ☑
    - pedal cycle (traffic) V51.9 ☑
      - nontraffic V51.3 ☑
      - while boarding or alighting V51.4 ☑

Accident — *continued*
- pickup truck (traffic) V53.9 ☑
  - nontraffic V53.3 ☑
  - while boarding or alighting V53.4 ☑
- railway vehicle (traffic) V55.9 ☑
  - nontraffic V55.3 ☑
  - while boarding or alighting V55.4 ☑
- specified vehicle NEC (traffic) V56.9 ☑
  - nontraffic V56.3 ☑
  - while boarding or alighting V56.4 ☑
- stationary object (traffic) V57.9 ☑
  - nontraffic V57.3 ☑
  - while boarding or alighting V57.4 ☑
- streetcar (traffic) V56.9 ☑
  - nontraffic V56.3 ☑
  - while boarding or alighting V56.4 ☑
- three wheeled motor vehicle (traffic) V52.9 ☑
  - nontraffic V52.3 ☑
  - while boarding or alighting V52.4 ☑
- truck (traffic) V54.9 ☑
  - nontraffic V54.3 ☑
  - while boarding or alighting V54.4 ☑
- two wheeled motor vehicle (traffic) V52.9 ☑
  - nontraffic V52.3 ☑
  - while boarding or alighting V52.4 ☑
- van (traffic) V53.9 ☑
  - nontraffic V53.3 ☑
  - while boarding or alighting V53.4 ☑
- driver
  - collision (with)
    - animal (traffic) V50.5 ☑
      - being ridden (traffic) V56.5 ☑
        - nontraffic V56.0 ☑
      - nontraffic V50.0 ☑
    - animal-drawn vehicle (traffic) V56.5 ☑
      - nontraffic V56.0 ☑
    - bus (traffic) V54.5 ☑
      - nontraffic V54.0 ☑
    - car (traffic) V53.5 ☑
      - nontraffic V53.0 ☑
    - motor vehicle NOS (traffic) V59.40 ☑
      - nontraffic V59.00 ☑
      - specified type NEC (traffic) V59.49 ☑
        - nontraffic V59.09 ☑
    - pedal cycle (traffic) V51.5 ☑
      - nontraffic V51.0 ☑
    - pickup truck (traffic) V53.5 ☑
      - nontraffic V53.0 ☑
    - railway vehicle (traffic) V55.5 ☑
      - nontraffic V55.0 ☑
    - specified vehicle NEC (traffic) V56.5 ☑
      - nontraffic V56.0 ☑
    - stationary object (traffic) V57.5 ☑
      - nontraffic V57.0 ☑
    - streetcar (traffic) V56.5 ☑
      - nontraffic V56.0 ☑
    - three wheeled motor vehicle (traffic) V52.5 ☑
      - nontraffic V52.0 ☑
    - truck (traffic) V54.5 ☑
      - nontraffic V54.0 ☑
    - two wheeled motor vehicle (traffic) V52.5 ☑
      - nontraffic V52.0 ☑
    - van (traffic) V53.5 ☑
      - nontraffic V53.0 ☑
  - noncollision accident (traffic) V58.5 ☑
    - nontraffic V58.0 ☑
- noncollision accident (traffic) V58.9 ☑
  - nontraffic V58.3 ☑
  - while boarding or alighting V58.4 ☑
- nontraffic V59.3 ☑
- hanger-on
  - collision (with)
    - animal (traffic) V50.7 ☑
      - being ridden (traffic) V56.7 ☑
        - nontraffic V56.2 ☑
      - nontraffic V50.2 ☑
    - animal-drawn vehicle (traffic) V56.7 ☑
      - nontraffic V56.2 ☑
    - bus (traffic) V54.7 ☑
      - nontraffic V54.2 ☑
    - car (traffic) V53.7 ☑
      - nontraffic V53.2 ☑
    - pedal cycle (traffic) V51.7 ☑
      - nontraffic V51.2 ☑
    - pickup truck (traffic) V53.7 ☑
      - nontraffic V53.2 ☑
    - railway vehicle (traffic) V55.7 ☑
      - nontraffic V55.2 ☑

Accident — *continued*
- specified vehicle NEC (traffic) V56.7 ☑
  - nontraffic V56.2 ☑
- stationary object (traffic) V57.7 ☑
  - nontraffic V57.2 ☑
- streetcar (traffic) V56.7 ☑
  - nontraffic V56.2 ☑
- three wheeled motor vehicle (traffic) V52.7 ☑
  - nontraffic V52.2 ☑
- truck (traffic) V54.7 ☑
  - nontraffic V54.2 ☑
- two wheeled motor vehicle (traffic) V52.7 ☑
  - nontraffic V52.2 ☑
- van (traffic) V53.7 ☑
  - nontraffic V53.2 ☑
- noncollision accident (traffic) V58.7 ☑
  - nontraffic V58.2 ☑
- passenger
  - collision (with)
    - animal (traffic) V50.6 ☑
      - being ridden (traffic) V56.6 ☑
        - nontraffic V56.1 ☑
      - nontraffic V50.1 ☑
    - animal-drawn vehicle (traffic) V56.6 ☑
      - nontraffic V56.1 ☑
    - bus (traffic) V54.6 ☑
      - nontraffic V54.1 ☑
    - car (traffic) V53.6 ☑
      - nontraffic V53.1 ☑
    - motor vehicle NOS (traffic) V59.50 ☑
      - nontraffic V59.10 ☑
      - specified type NEC (traffic) V59.59 ☑
        - nontraffic V59.19 ☑
    - pedal cycle (traffic) V51.6 ☑
      - nontraffic V51.1 ☑
    - pickup truck (traffic) V53.6 ☑
      - nontraffic V53.1 ☑
    - railway vehicle (traffic) V55.6 ☑
      - nontraffic V55.1 ☑
    - specified vehicle NEC (traffic) V56.6 ☑
      - nontraffic V56.1 ☑
    - stationary object (traffic) V57.6 ☑
      - nontraffic V57.1 ☑
    - streetcar (traffic) V56.6 ☑
      - nontraffic V56.1 ☑
    - three wheeled motor vehicle (traffic) V52.6 ☑
      - nontraffic V52.1 ☑
    - truck (traffic) V54.6 ☑
      - nontraffic V54.1 ☑
    - two wheeled motor vehicle (traffic) V52.6 ☑
      - nontraffic V52.1 ☑
    - van (traffic) V53.6 ☑
      - nontraffic V53.1 ☑
  - noncollision accident (traffic) V58.6 ☑
    - nontraffic V58.1 ☑
- specified type NEC V59.88 ☑
- military vehicle V59.81 ☑
- watercraft occupant — *see* Accident, watercraft
- vehicle NEC V89.9 ☑
  - animal-drawn NEC — *see* Accident, transport, animal-drawn vehicle occupant
  - special
    - agricultural — *see* Accident, transport, agricultural vehicle occupant
    - construction — *see* Accident, transport, construction vehicle occupant
    - industrial — *see* Accident, transport, industrial vehicle occupant
  - three-wheeled NEC (motorized) — *see* Accident, transport, three-wheeled motor vehicle occupant
- watercraft V94.9 ☑
  - causing
    - drowning — *see* Drowning, due to, accident to, watercraft
    - injury NEC V91.89 ☑
      - crushed between craft and object V91.19 ☑
        - powered craft V91.13 ☑
          - ferry boat V91.11 ☑
          - fishing boat V91.12 ☑
          - jetskis V91.13 ☑
          - liner V91.11 ☑
          - merchant ship V91.10 ☑
          - passenger ship V91.11 ☑
        - unpowered craft V91.18 ☑
          - canoe V91.15 ☑
          - inflatable V91.16 ☑

☑ **Additional character required**

Accident — continued
kayak V91.15 ☑
sailboat V91.14 ☑
surf-board V91.18 ☑
windsurfer V91.18 ☑
fall on board V91.29 ☑
powered craft V91.23 ☑
ferry boat V91.21 ☑
fishing boat V91.22 ☑
jetskis V91.23 ☑
liner V91.21 ☑
merchant ship V91.20 ☑
passenger ship V91.21 ☑
unpowered craft
canoe V91.25 ☑
inflatable V91.26 ☑
kayak V91.25 ☑
sailboat V91.24 ☑
fire on board causing burn V91.09 ☑
powered craft V91.03 ☑
ferry boat V91.01 ☑
fishing boat V91.02 ☑
jetskis V91.03 ☑
liner V91.01 ☑
merchant ship V91.00 ☑
passenger ship V91.01 ☑
unpowered craft V91.08 ☑
canoe V91.05 ☑
inflatable V91.06 ☑
kayak V91.05 ☑
sailboat V91.04 ☑
surf-board V91.08 ☑
water skis V91.07 ☑
windsurfer V91.08 ☑
hit by falling object V91.39 ☑
powered craft V91.33 ☑
ferry boat V91.31 ☑
fishing boat V91.32 ☑
jetskis V91.33 ☑
liner V91.31 ☑
merchant ship V91.30 ☑
passenger ship V91.31 ☑
unpowered craft V91.38 ☑
canoe V91.35 ☑
inflatable V91.36 ☑
kayak V91.35 ☑
sailboat V91.34 ☑
surf-board V91.38 ☑
water skis V91.37 ☑
windsurfer V91.38 ☑
specified type NEC V91.89 ☑
powered craft V91.83 ☑
ferry boat V91.81 ☑
fishing boat V91.82 ☑
jetskis V91.83 ☑
liner V91.81 ☑
merchant ship V91.80 ☑
passenger ship V91.81 ☑
unpowered craft V91.88 ☑
canoe V91.85 ☑
inflatable V91.86 ☑
kayak V91.85 ☑
sailboat V91.84 ☑
surf-board V91.88 ☑
water skis V91.87 ☑
windsurfer V91.88 ☑
due to, caused by cataclysm — see Forces of
nature, by type
military NEC V94.818 ☑
with civilian watercraft V94.810 ☑
civilian in water injured by V94.811 ☑
nonpowered, struck by
nonpowered vessel V94.22 ☑
powered vessel V94.21 ☑
specified type NEC V94.89 ☑
striking swimmer
powered V94.11 ☑
unpowered V94.12 ☑
Acid throwing (assault) Y08.89 ☑
Activity (involving) (of victim at time of event) Y93.9
aerobic and step exercise (class) Y93.A3
alpine skiing Y93.23
animal care NEC Y93.K9
arts and handcrafts NEC Y93.D9
athletics NEC Y93.79
athletics played as a team or group NEC Y93.69
athletics played individually NEC Y93.59
baking Y93.G3
ballet Y93.41
barbells Y93.B3
BASE (Building, Antenna, Span, Earth) jumping
Y93.33

Activity — continued
baseball Y93.64
basketball Y93.67
bathing (personal) Y93.E1
beach volleyball Y93.68
bike riding Y93.55
boogie boarding Y93.18
bowling Y93.54
boxing Y93.71
brass instrument playing Y93.J4
building construction Y93.H3
bungee jumping Y93.34
calisthenics Y93.A2
canoeing (in calm and turbulent water) Y93.16
capture the flag Y93.6A
cardiorespiratory exercise NEC Y93.A9
caregiving (providing) NEC Y93.F9
bathing Y93.F1
lifting Y93.F2
cellular
communication device Y93.C2
telephone Y93.C2
challenge course Y93.A5
cheerleading Y93.45
circuit training Y93.A4
cleaning
floor Y93.E5
climbing NEC Y93.39
mountain Y93.31
rock Y93.31
wall Y93.31
clothing care and maintenance NEC Y93.E9
combatives Y93.75
computer
keyboarding Y93.C1
technology NEC Y93.C9
confidence course Y93.A5
construction (building) Y93.H3
cooking and baking Y93.G3
cool down exercises Y93.A2
cricket Y93.69
crocheting Y93.D1
cross country skiing Y93.24
dancing (all types) Y93.41
digging
dirt Y93.H1
dirt digging Y93.H1
dishwashing Y93.G1
diving (platform) (springboard) Y93.12
underwater Y93.15
dodge ball Y93.6A
downhill skiing Y93.23
drum playing Y93.J2
dumbbells Y93.B3
electronic
devices NEC Y93.C9
hand held interactive Y93.C2
game playing (using) (with)
interactive device Y93.C2
keyboard or other stationary device Y93.C1
elliptical machine Y93.A1
exercise (s)
machines ((primarily) for)
cardiorespiratory conditioning Y93.A1
muscle strengthening Y93.B1
muscle strengthening (non-machine) NEC
Y93.B9
external motion NEC Y93.I9
rollercoaster Y93.I1
field hockey Y93.65
figure skating (pairs) (singles) Y93.21
flag football Y93.62
floor mopping and cleaning Y93.E5
food preparation and clean up Y93.G1
football (American) NOS Y93.61
flag Y93.62
tackle Y93.61
touch Y93.62
four square Y93.6A
free weights Y93.B3
frisbee (ultimate) Y93.74
furniture
building Y93.D3
finishing Y93.D3
repair Y93.D3
game playing (electronic)
using keyboard or other stationary device
Y93.C1
using interactive device Y93.C2
gardening Y93.H2
golf Y93.53
grass drills Y93.A6

Activity — continued
grilling and smoking food Y93.G2
grooming and shearing an animal Y93.K3
guerilla drills Y93.A6
gymnastics (rhythmic) Y93.43
handball Y93.73
handcrafts NEC Y93.D9
hand held interactive electronic device Y93.C2
hang gliding Y93.35
hiking (on level or elevated terrain) Y93.01
hockey (ice) Y93.22
field Y93.65
horseback riding Y93.52
household (interior) maintenance NEC Y93.E9
ice NEC Y93.29
dancing Y93.21
hockey Y93.22
skating Y93.21
inline roller skating Y93.51
ironing Y93.E4
judo Y93.75
jumping (off) NEC Y93.39
BASE (Building, Antenna, Span, Earth) Y93.33
bungee Y93.34
jacks Y93.A2
rope Y93.56
jumping jacks Y93.A2
jumping rope Y93.56
karate Y93.75
kayaking (in calm and turbulent water) Y93.16
keyboarding (computer) Y93.C1
kickball Y93.6A
knitting Y93.D1
lacrosse Y93.65
land maintenance NEC Y93.H9
landscaping Y93.H2
laundry Y93.E2
machines (exercise)
primarily for cardiorespiratory conditioning
Y93.A1
primarily for muscle strengthening Y93.B1
maintenance
exterior building NEC Y93.H9
household (interior) NEC Y93.E9
land Y93.H9
property Y93.H9
marching (on level or elevated terrain) Y93.01
martial arts Y93.75
microwave oven Y93.G3
milking an animal Y93.K2
mopping (floor) Y93.E5
mountain climbing Y93.31
muscle strengthening
exercises (non-machine) NEC Y93.B9
machines Y93.B1
musical keyboard (electronic) playing Y93.J1
nordic skiing Y93.24
obstacle course Y93.A5
oven (microwave) Y93.G3
packing up and unpacking in moving to a new
residence Y93.E6
parasailing Y93.19
percussion instrument playing NEC Y93.J2
personal
bathing and showering Y93.E1
hygiene NEC Y93.E8
showering Y93.E1
physical games generally associated with school
recess, summer camp and children Y93.6A
physical training NEC Y93.A9
piano playing Y93.J1
pilates Y93.B4
platform diving Y93.12
playing musical instrument
brass instrument Y93.J4
drum Y93.J2
musical keyboard (electronic) Y93.J1
percussion instrument NEC Y93.J2
piano Y93.J1
string instrument Y93.J3
winds instrument Y93.J4
property maintenance
exterior NEC Y93.H9
interior NEC Y93.E9
pruning (garden and lawn) Y93.H2
pull-ups Y93.B2
push-ups Y93.B2
racquetball Y93.73
rafting (in calm and turbulent water) Y93.16
raking (leaves) Y93.H1
rappelling Y93.32
refereeing a sports activity Y93.81

☑ **Additional character required**

B

Barotitis, barodontalgia, barosinusitis, barotrauma (otitic) (sinus) - — *see* Air, pressure
Battered (baby) (child) (person) (syndrome) X58 ☑
Bayonet wound W26.1 ☑
  in
    legal intervention — *see* Legal, intervention, sharp object, bayonet
    war operations — *see* War operations, combat
  stated as undetermined whether accidental or intentional Y28.8 ☑
  suicide (attempt) X78.2 ☑
Bean in nose — *see* categories T17 and T18 ☑
Bed set on fire NEC — *see* Exposure, fire, uncontrolled, building, bed
Beheading (by guillotine)
  homicide X99.9 ☑
  legal execution — *see* Legal, intervention
Bending, injury in Y93
Bends - — *see* Air, pressure, change
Bite, bitten by
  alligator W58.01 ☑
  arthropod (nonvenomous) NEC W57 ☑
  bull W55.21 ☑
  cat W55.01 ☑
  cow W55.21 ☑
  crocodile W58.11 ☑
  dog W54.0 ☑
  goat W55.31 ☑
  hoof stock NEC W55.31 ☑
  horse W55.11 ☑
  human being (accidentally) W50.3 ☑
    with intent to injure or kill Y04.1 ☑
    as, or caused by, a crowd or human stampede (with fall) W52 ☑
    assault Y04.1 ☑
    homicide (attempt) Y04.1 ☑
    in
      fight Y04.1 ☑
  insect (nonvenomous) W57 ☑
  lizard (nonvenomous) W59.01 ☑
  mammal NEC W55.81 ☑
    marine W56.31 ☑
  marine animal (nonvenomous) W56.81 ☑
  millipede W57 ☑
  moray eel W56.51 ☑
  mouse W53.01 ☑
  person (s) (accidentally) W50.3 ☑
    with intent to injure or kill Y04.1 ☑
    as, or caused by, a crowd or human stampede (with fall) W52 ☑
    assault Y04.1 ☑
    homicide (attempt) Y04.1 ☑
    in
      fight Y04.1 ☑
  pig W55.41 ☑
  raccoon W55.51 ☑
  rat W53.11 ☑
  reptile W59.81 ☑
    lizard W59.01 ☑
    snake W59.11 ☑
    turtle W59.21 ☑
    terrestrial W59.81 ☑
  rodent W53.81 ☑
    mouse W53.01 ☑
    rat W53.11 ☑
    specified NEC W53.81 ☑
    squirrel W53.21 ☑
  shark W56.41 ☑
  sheep W55.31 ☑
  snake (nonvenomous) W59.11 ☑
  spider (nonvenomous) W57 ☑
  squirrel W53.21 ☑
Blast (air) in war operations — *see* War operations, blast
Blizzard X37.2 ☑
Blood alcohol level Y90.9
  less than 20mg/100ml Y90.0
  presence in blood, level not specified Y90.9
  20-39mg/100ml Y90.1
  40-59mg/100ml Y90.2
  60-79mg/100ml Y90.3
  80-99mg/100ml Y90.4
  100-119mg/100ml Y90.5
  120-199mg/100ml Y90.6
  200-239mg/100ml Y90.7
Blow X58 ☑
  by law-enforcing agent, police (on duty) — *see* Legal, intervention, manhandling

Blow — *continued*
  blunt object — *see* Legal, intervention, blunt object
Blowing up — *see* Explosion
Brawl (hand) (fists) (foot) Y04.0 ☑
Breakage (accidental) (part of)
  ladder (causing fall) W11 ☑
  scaffolding (causing fall) W12 ☑
Broken
  glass, contact with — *see* Contact, with, glass
  power line (causing electric shock) W85 ☑
Bumping against, into (accidentally)
  object NEC W22.8 ☑
    with fall — *see* Fall, due to, bumping against, object
    caused by crowd or human stampede (with fall) W52 ☑
    sports equipment W21.9 ☑
  person (s) W51 ☑
    with fall W03 ☑
      due to ice or snow W00.0 ☑
    assault Y04.2 ☑
    caused by, a crowd or human stampede (with fall) W52 ☑
    homicide (attempt) Y04.2 ☑
  sports equipment W21.9 ☑
Burn, burned, burning (accidental) (by) (from) (on)
  acid NEC — *see* Table of Drugs and Chemicals
  bed linen — *see* Exposure, fire, uncontrolled, in building, bed
  blowtorch X08.8 ☑
    with ignition of clothing NEC X06.2 ☑
      nightwear X05 ☑
  bonfire, campfire (controlled) (*see also* Exposure, fire, controlled, not in building)
    uncontrolled — *see* Exposure, fire, uncontrolled, not in building
  candle X08.8 ☑
    with ignition of clothing NEC X06.2 ☑
      nightwear X05 ☑
  caustic liquid, substance (external) (internal) NEC — *see* Table of Drugs and Chemicals
  chemical (external) (internal) (*see also* Table of Drugs and Chemicals)
    in war operations — *see* War operations. fire
  cigar (s) or cigarette(s) X08.8 ☑
    with ignition of clothing NEC X06.2 ☑
      nightwear X05 ☑
  clothes, clothing NEC (from controlled fire) X06.2 ☑
    with conflagration — *see* Exposure, fire, uncontrolled, building
    not in building or structure — *see* Exposure, fire, uncontrolled, not in building
  cooker (hot) X15.8 ☑
    stated as undetermined whether accidental or intentional Y27.3 ☑
    suicide (attempt) X77.3 ☑
  electric blanket X16 ☑
  engine (hot) X17 ☑
  fire, flames — *see* Exposure, fire
  flare, Very pistol — *see* Discharge, firearm NEC
  heat
    from appliance (electrical) (household) X15.8 ☑
      cooker X15.8 ☑
      hotplate X15.2 ☑
      kettle X15.8 ☑
      light bulb X15.8 ☑
      saucepan X15.3 ☑
      skillet X15.3 ☑
      stove X15.0 ☑
      stated as undetermined whether accidental or intentional Y27.3 ☑
      suicide (attempt) X77.3 ☑
      toaster X15.1 ☑
    in local application or packing during medical or surgical procedure Y63.5
  heating
    appliance, radiator or pipe X16 ☑
  homicide (attempt) — *see* Assault, burning
  hot
    air X14.1 ☑
    cooker X15.8 ☑
    drink X10.0 ☑
    engine X17 ☑
    fat X10.2 ☑
    fluid NEC X12 ☑
    food X10.1 ☑
    gases X14.1 ☑
    heating appliance X16 ☑
    household appliance NEC X15.8 ☑
    kettle X15.8 ☑

Burn — *continued*
  liquid NEC X12 ☑
  machinery X17 ☑
  metal (molten) (liquid) NEC X18 ☑
  object (not producing fire or flames) NEC X19 ☑
  oil (cooking) X10.2 ☑
  pipe (s) X16 ☑
  radiator X16 ☑
  saucepan (glass) (metal) X15.3 ☑
  stove (kitchen) X15.0 ☑
  substance NEC X19 ☑
    caustic or corrosive NEC — *see* Table of Drugs and Chemicals
  toaster X15.1 ☑
  tool X17 ☑
  vapor X13.1 ☑
  water (tap) — *see* Contact, with, hot, tap water
  hotplate X15.2 ☑
    suicide (attempt) X77.3 ☑
  ignition — *see* Ignition
  in war operations — *see* War operations, fire
  inflicted by other person X97 ☑
    by hot objects, hot vapor, and steam — *see* Assault, burning, hot object
  internal, from swallowed caustic, corrosive liquid, substance — *see* Table of Drugs and Chemicals
  iron (hot) X15.8 ☑
    stated as undetermined whether accidental or intentional Y27.3 ☑
    suicide (attempt) X77.3 ☑
  kettle (hot) X15.8 ☑
    stated as undetermined whether accidental or intentional Y27.3 ☑
    suicide (attempt) X77.3 ☑
  lamp (flame) X08.8 ☑
    with ignition of clothing NEC X06.2 ☑
      nightwear X05 ☑
  lighter (cigar) (cigarette) X08.8 ☑
    with ignition of clothing NEC X06.2 ☑
      nightwear X05 ☑
  lightning T75.0
    causing fire — *see* Exposure, fire
  liquid (boiling) (hot) NEC X12 ☑
    stated as undetermined whether accidental or intentional Y27.2 ☑
    suicide (attempt) X77.2 ☑
  local application of externally applied substance in medical or surgical care Y63.5
  on board watercraft
    due to
      accident to watercraft V91.09 ☑
        powered craft V91.03 ☑
          ferry boat V91.01 ☑
          fishing boat V91.02 ☑
          jetskis V91.03 ☑
          liner V91.01 ☑
          merchant ship V91.00 ☑
          passenger ship V91.01 ☑
        unpowered craft V91.08 ☑
          canoe V91.05 ☑
          inflatable V91.06 ☑
          kayak V91.05 ☑
          sailboat V91.04 ☑
          surf-board V91.08 ☑
          water skis V91.07 ☑
          windsurfer V91.08 ☑
      fire on board V93.09 ☑
        ferry boat V93.01 ☑
        fishing boat V93.02 ☑
        jetskis V93.03 ☑
        liner V93.01 ☑
        merchant ship V93.00 ☑
        passenger ship V93.01 ☑
        powered craft NEC V93.03 ☑
        sailboat V93.04 ☑
      specified heat source NEC on board V93.19 ☑
        ferry boat V93.11 ☑
        fishing boat V93.12 ☑
        jetskis V93.13 ☑
        liner V93.11 ☑
        merchant ship V93.10 ☑
        passenger ship V93.11 ☑
        powered craft NEC V93.13 ☑
        sailboat V93.14 ☑
  machinery (hot) X08.8 ☑
  matches X08.8 ☑
    with ignition of clothing NEC X06.2 ☑
      nightwear X05 ☑
  mattress — *see* Exposure, fire, uncontrolled, building, bed

Burn — *continued*
  medicament, externally applied Y63.5
  metal (hot) (liquid) (molten) NEC X18 ☑
  nightwear (nightclothes, nightdress, gown, pajamas, robe) X05 ☑
  object (hot) NEC X19 ☑
  pipe (hot) X16 ☑
    smoking X08.8 ☑
      with ignition of clothing NEC X06.2 ☑
        nightwear X05 ☑
  powder — *see* Powder burn
  radiator (hot) X16 ☑
  saucepan (hot) (glass) (metal) X15.3 ☑
    stated as undetermined whether accidental or intentional Y27.3 ☑
    suicide (attempt) X77.3 ☑
  self-inflicted X76 ☑
    stated as undetermined whether accidental or intentional Y26 ☑
  steam X13.1 ☑
    pipe X16 ☑
      stated as undetermined whether accidental or intentional Y27.8 ☑
    stated as undetermined whether accidental or intentional Y27.0 ☑
    suicide (attempt) X77.0 ☑
  stove (hot) (kitchen) X15.0 ☑
    stated as undetermined whether accidental or intentional Y27.3 ☑
    suicide (attempt) X77.3 ☑
  substance (hot) NEC X19 ☑
    boiling X12 ☑
      stated as undetermined whether accidental or intentional Y27.2 ☑
      suicide (attempt) X77.2 ☑
    molten (metal) X18 ☑
  suicide (attempt) NEC X76 ☑
    hot
      household appliance X77.3 ☑
      object X77.9 ☑
  stated as undetermined whether accidental or intentional Y27.0 ☑
  therapeutic misadventure
    heat in local application or packing during medical or surgical procedure Y63.5
    overdose of radiation Y63.2
  toaster (hot) X15.1 ☑
    stated as undetermined whether accidental or intentional Y27.3 ☑
    suicide (attempt) X77.3 ☑
  tool (hot) X17 ☑
  torch, welding X08.8 ☑
    with ignition of clothing NEC X06.2 ☑
      nightwear X05 ☑
  trash fire (controlled) — *see* Exposure, fire, controlled, not in building
    uncontrolled — *see* Exposure, fire, uncontrolled, not in building
  vapor (hot) X13.1 ☑
    stated as undetermined whether accidental or intentional Y27.0 ☑
    suicide (attempt) X77.0 ☑
  Very pistol — *see* Discharge, firearm NEC
Butted by animal W55.82 ☑
  bull W55.22 ☑
  cow W55.22 ☑
  goat W55.32 ☑
  horse W55.12 ☑
  pig W55.42 ☑
  sheep W55.32 ☑

C

Caisson disease - — *see* Air, pressure, change
Campfire (exposure to) (controlled) (*see also* Exposure, fire, controlled, not in building)
  uncontrolled — *see* Exposure, fire, uncontrolled, not in building
Capital punishment (any means) — *see* Legal, intervention
Car sickness T75.3 ☑
Casualty (not due to war) NEC X58 ☑
  war — *see* War operations
Cat
  bite W55.01 ☑
  scratch W55.03 ☑
Cataclysm, cataclysmic (any injury) NEC — *see* Forces of nature
Catching fire — *see* Exposure, fire

Caught
  between
    folding object W23.0 ☑
    objects (moving) (stationary and moving) W23.0 ☑
      and machinery — *see* Contact, with, by type of machine
      stationary W23.1 ☑
    sliding door and door frame W23.0 ☑
  by, in
    machinery (moving parts of) — *see* Contact, with, by type of machine
    washing-machine wringer W23.0 ☑
    under packing crate (due to losing grip) W23.1 ☑
Cave-in caused by cataclysmic earth surface movement or eruption — *see* Landslide
Change (s) in air pressure - — *see* Air, pressure, change
Choked, choking (on) (any object except food or vomitus)
  food (bone) (seed) — *see* categories T17 and T18 ☑
  vomitus T17.81- ☑
Civil insurrection — *see* War operations
Cloudburst (any injury) X37.8 ☑
Cold, exposure to (accidental) (excessive) (extreme) (natural) (place) NEC — *see* Exposure, cold
Collapse
  building W20.1 ☑
    burning (uncontrolled fire) X00.2 ☑
  dam or man-made structure (causing earth movement) X36.0 ☑
  machinery — *see* Contact, with, by type of machine
  structure W20.1 ☑
    burning (uncontrolled fire) X00.2 ☑
Collision (accidental) NEC (*see also* Accident, transport) V89.9 ☑
  pedestrian W51 ☑
    with fall W03 ☑
      due to ice or snow W00.0 ☑
      involving pedestrian conveyance — *see* Accident, transport, pedestrian, conveyance
    and
      crowd or human stampede (with fall) W52 ☑
      object W22.8 ☑
        with fall — *see* Fall, due to, bumping against, object
  person (s) — *see* Collision, pedestrian
  transport vehicle NEC V89.9 ☑
    and
      avalanche, fallen or not moving — *see* Accident, transport
        falling or moving — *see* Landslide
      landslide, fallen or not moving — *see* Accident, transport
        falling or moving — *see* Landslide
    due to cataclysm — *see* Forces of nature, by type
  intentional, purposeful suicide (attempt) — *see* Suicide, collision
Combustion, spontaneous — *see* Ignition
Complication (delayed) of or following (medical or surgical procedure) Y84.9
  with misadventure — *see* Misadventure
  amputation of limb (s) Y83.5
  anastomosis (arteriovenous) (blood vessel) (gastrojejunal) (tendon) (natural or artificial material) Y83.2
  aspiration (of fluid) Y84.4
    tissue Y84.8
  biopsy Y84.8
  blood
    sampling Y84.7
    transfusion
      procedure Y84.8
  bypass Y83.2
  catheterization (urinary) Y84.6
    cardiac Y84.0
  colostomy Y83.3
  cystostomy Y83.3
  dialysis (kidney) Y84.1
  drug — *see* Table of Drugs and Chemicals
    due to misadventure — *see* Misadventure
  duodenostomy Y83.3
  electroshock therapy Y84.3
  external stoma, creation of Y83.3
  formation of external stoma Y83.3
  gastrostomy Y83.3
  graft Y83.2
  hypothermia (medically-induced) Y84.8

Complication — *continued*
  implant, implantation (of)
    artificial
      internal device (cardiac pacemaker) (electrodes in brain) (heart valve prosthesis) (orthopedic) Y83.1
      material or tissue (for anastomosis or bypass) Y83.2
        with creation of external stoma Y83.3
      natural tissues (for anastomosis or bypass) Y83.2
        with creation of external stoma Y83.3
  infusion
    procedure Y84.8
  injection — *see* Table of Drugs and Chemicals
    procedure Y84.8
  insertion of gastric or duodenal sound Y84.5
  insulin-shock therapy Y84.3
  paracentesis (abdominal) (thoracic) (aspirative) Y84.4
  procedures other than surgical operation — *see* Complication of or following, by type of procedure
  radiological procedure or therapy Y84.2
  removal of organ (partial) (total) NEC Y83.6
  sampling
    blood Y84.7
    fluid NEC Y84.4
    tissue Y84.8
  shock therapy Y84.3
  surgical operation NEC (*see also* Complication of or following, by type of operation) Y83.9
    reconstructive NEC Y83.4
      with
        anastomosis, bypass or graft Y83.2
        formation of external stoma Y83.3
    specified NEC Y83.8
  transfusion (*see also* Table of Drugs and Chemicals)
    procedure Y84.8
  transplant, transplantation (heart) (kidney) (liver) (whole organ, any) Y83.0
    partial organ Y83.4
  ureterostomy Y83.3
  vaccination (*see also* Table of Drugs and Chemicals)
    procedure Y84.8
Compression
  divers' squeeze - — *see* Air, pressure, change
  trachea by
    food (lodged in esophagus) — *see* categories T17 and T18 ☑
    vomitus (lodged in esophagus) T17.81- ☑
Conflagration — *see* Exposure, fire, uncontrolled
Constriction (external)
  hair W49.01 ☑
  jewelry W49.04 ☑
  ring W49.04 ☑
  rubber band W49.03 ☑
  specified item NEC W49.09 ☑
  string W49.02 ☑
  thread W49.02 ☑
Contact (accidental)
  with
    abrasive wheel (metalworking) W31.1 ☑
    alligator W58.09 ☑
      bite W58.01 ☑
      crushing W58.03 ☑
      strike W58.02 ☑
    amphibian W62.9 ☑
      frog W62.0 ☑
      toad W62.1 ☑
    animal (nonvenomous) NEC W64 ☑
      marine W56.89 ☑
        bite W56.81 ☑
        dolphin — *see* Contact, with, dolphin
        fish NEC — *see* Contact, with, fish
        mammal — *see* Contact, with, mammal, marine
        orca — *see* Contact, with, orca
        sea lion — *see* Contact, with, sea lion
        shark — *see* Contact, with, shark
        strike W56.82 ☑
    animate mechanical force NEC W64 ☑
    arrow W21.89 ☑
      not thrown, projected or falling W45.8 ☑
    arthropods (nonvenomous) W57 ☑
    axe W27.0 ☑
    band-saw (industrial) W31.2 ☑
    bayonet — *see* Bayonet wound
    bee (s) X58 ☑
    bench-saw (industrial) W31.2 ☑

☑ **Additional character required**

Contact — *continued*
- bird W61.99 ☑
  - bite W61.91 ☑
    - chicken — *see* Contact, with, chicken
    - duck — *see* Contact, with, duck
    - goose — *see* Contact, with, goose
    - macaw — *see* Contact, with, macaw
    - parrot — *see* Contact, with, parrot
    - psittacine — *see* Contact, with, psittacine
  - strike W61.92 ☑
    - turkey — *see* Contact, with, turkey
- blender W29.0 ☑
- boiling water X12 ☑
  - stated as undetermined whether accidental or intentional Y27.2 ☑
  - suicide (attempt) X77.2 ☑
- bore, earth-drilling or mining (land) (seabed) W31.0 ☑
- buffalo — *see* Contact, with, hoof stock NEC
- bull W55.29 ☑
  - bite W55.21 ☑
  - gored W55.22 ☑
  - strike W55.22 ☑
- bumper cars W31.81 ☑
- camel — *see* Contact, with, hoof stock NEC
- can
  - lid W45.2 ☑
  - opener W27.4 ☑
    - powered W29.0 ☑
- cat W55.09 ☑
  - bite W55.01 ☑
  - scratch W55.03 ☑
- caterpillar (venomous) X58 ☑
- centipede (venomous) X58 ☑
- chain
  - hoist W24.0 ☑
    - agricultural operations W30.89 ☑
  - saw W29.3 ☑
- chicken W61.39 ☑
  - peck W61.33 ☑
  - strike W61.32 ☑
- chisel W27.0 ☑
- circular saw W31.2 ☑
- cobra X58 ☑
- combine (harvester) W30.0 ☑
- conveyer belt W24.1 ☑
- cooker (hot) X15.8 ☑
  - stated as undetermined whether accidental or intentional Y27.3 ☑
  - suicide (attempt) X77.3 ☑
- coral X58 ☑
- cotton gin W31.82 ☑
- cow W55.29 ☑
  - bite W55.21 ☑
  - strike W55.22 ☑
- crane W24.0 ☑
  - agricultural operations W30.89 ☑
- crocodile W58.19 ☑
  - bite W58.11 ☑
  - crushing W58.13 ☑
  - strike W58.12 ☑
- dagger W26.1 ☑
  - stated as undetermined whether accidental or intentional Y28.2 ☑
  - suicide (attempt) X78.2 ☑
- dairy equipment W31.82 ☑
- dart W21.89 ☑
  - not thrown, projected or falling W45.8 ☑
- deer — *see* Contact, with, hoof stock NEC
- derrick W24.0 ☑
  - agricultural operations W30.89 ☑
    - hay W30.2 ☑
- dog W54.8 ☑
  - bite W54.0 ☑
  - strike W54.1 ☑
- dolphin W56.09 ☑
  - bite W56.01 ☑
  - strike W56.02 ☑
- donkey — *see* Contact, with, hoof stock NEC
- drill (powered) W29.8 ☑
  - earth (land) (seabed) W31.0 ☑
  - nonpowered W27.8 ☑
- drive belt W24.0 ☑
  - agricultural operations W30.89 ☑
- dry ice — *see* Exposure, cold, man-made
- dryer (clothes) (powered) (spin) W29.2 ☑
- duck W61.69 ☑
  - bite W61.61 ☑
  - strike W61.62 ☑
- earth (-)
  - drilling machine (industrial) W31.0 ☑
  - scraping machine in stationary use W31.83 ☑

Contact — *continued*
- edge of stiff paper W45.1 ☑
- electric
  - beater W29.0 ☑
  - blanket X16 ☑
  - fan W29.2 ☑
    - commercial W31.82 ☑
  - knife W29.1 ☑
  - mixer W29.0 ☑
- elevator (building) W24.0 ☑
  - agricultural operations W30.89 ☑
    - grain W30.3 ☑
- engine (s), hot NEC X17 ☑
- excavating machine W31.0 ☑
- farm machine W30.9 ☑
- feces — *see* Contact, with, by type of animal
- fer de lance X58 ☑
- fish W56.59 ☑
  - bite W56.51 ☑
  - shark — *see* Contact, with, shark
  - strike W56.52 ☑
- flying horses W31.81 ☑
- forging (metalworking) machine W31.1 ☑
- fork W27.4 ☑
- forklift (truck) W24.0 ☑
  - agricultural operations W30.89 ☑
- frog W62.0 ☑
- garden
  - cultivator (powered) W29.3 ☑
    - riding W30.89 ☑
  - fork W27.1 ☑
- gas turbine W31.3 ☑
- Gila monster X58 ☑
- giraffe — *see* Contact, with, hoof stock NEC
- glass (sharp) (broken) W25 ☑
  - with subsequent fall W18.02 ☑
  - assault X99.0 ☑
  - due to fall — *see* Fall, by type
  - stated as undetermined whether accidental or intentional Y28.0 ☑
  - suicide (attempt) X78.0 ☑
- goat W55.39 ☑
  - bite W55.31 ☑
  - strike W55.32 ☑
- goose W61.59 ☑
  - bite W61.51 ☑
  - strike W61.52 ☑
- hand
  - saw W27.0 ☑
  - tool (not powered) NEC W27.8 ☑
    - powered W29.8 ☑
- harvester W30.0 ☑
- hay-derrick W30.2 ☑
- heat NEC X19 ☑
  - from appliance (electrical) (household) — *see* Contact, with, hot, household appliance
  - heating appliance X16 ☑
- heating
  - appliance (hot) X16 ☑
  - pad (electric) X16 ☑
- hedge-trimmer (powered) W29.3 ☑
- hoe W27.1 ☑
- hoist (chain) (shaft) NEC W24.0 ☑
  - agricultural W30.89 ☑
- hoof stock NEC W55.39 ☑
  - bite W55.31 ☑
  - strike W55.32 ☑
- hornet (s) X58 ☑
- horse W55.19 ☑
  - bite W55.11 ☑
  - strike W55.12 ☑
- hot
  - air X14.1 ☑
    - inhalation X14.0 ☑
  - cooker X15.8 ☑
  - drinks X10.0 ☑
  - engine X17 ☑
  - fats X10.2 ☑
  - fluids NEC X12 ☑
    - assault X98.2 ☑
    - suicide (attempt) X77.2 ☑
    - undetermined whether accidental or intentional Y27.2 ☑
  - food X10.1 ☑
  - gases X14.1 ☑
    - inhalation X14.0 ☑
  - heating appliance X16 ☑
  - household appliance X15.8 ☑
    - assault X98.3 ☑
    - cooker X15.8 ☑
    - hotplate X15.2 ☑
    - kettle X15.8 ☑

Contact — *continued*
- light bulb X15.8 ☑
- object NEC X19 ☑
  - assault X98.8 ☑
  - stated as undetermined whether accidental or intentional Y27.9 ☑
  - suicide (attempt) X77.8 ☑
- saucepan X15.3 ☑
- skillet X15.3 ☑
- stove X15.0 ☑
  - stated as undetermined whether accidental or intentional Y27.3 ☑
  - suicide (attempt) X77.3 ☑
- toaster X15.1 ☑
- kettle X15.8 ☑
- light bulb X15.8 ☑
- liquid NEC (*see also* Burn) X12 ☑
  - drinks X10.0 ☑
  - stated as undetermined whether accidental or intentional Y27.2 ☑
  - suicide (attempt) X77.2 ☑
  - tap water X11.8 ☑
    - stated as undetermined whether accidental or intentional Y27.1 ☑
    - suicide (attempt) X77.1 ☑
- machinery X17 ☑
- metal (molten) (liquid) NEC X18 ☑
- object (not producing fire or flames) NEC X19 ☑
- oil (cooking) X10.2 ☑
- pipe X16 ☑
- plate X15.2 ☑
- radiator X16 ☑
- saucepan (glass) (metal) X15.3 ☑
- skillet X15.3 ☑
- stove (kitchen) X15.0 ☑
- substance NEC X19 ☑
- tap-water X11.8 ☑
  - assault X98.1 ☑
  - heated on stove X12 ☑
    - stated as undetermined whether accidental or intentional Y27.2 ☑
    - suicide (attempt) X77.2 ☑
  - in bathtub X11.0 ☑
  - running X11.1 ☑
    - stated as undetermined whether accidental or intentional Y27.1 ☑
    - suicide (attempt) X77.1 ☑
- toaster X15.1 ☑
- tool X17 ☑
- vapors X13.1 ☑
  - inhalation X13.0 ☑
- water (tap) X11.8 ☑
  - boiling X12 ☑
    - stated as undetermined whether accidental or intentional Y27.2 ☑
    - suicide (attempt) X77.2 ☑
  - heated on stove X12 ☑
    - stated as undetermined whether accidental or intentional Y27.2 ☑
    - suicide (attempt) X77.2 ☑
  - in bathtub X11.0 ☑
  - running X11.1 ☑
    - stated as undetermined whether accidental or intentional Y27.1 ☑
    - suicide (attempt) X77.1 ☑
- hotplate X15.2 ☑
- ice-pick W27.4 ☑
- insect (nonvenomous) NEC W57 ☑
- kettle (hot) X15.8 ☑
- knife W26.0 ☑
  - assault X99.1 ☑
  - electric W29.1 ☑
  - stated as undetermined whether accidental or intentional Y28.1 ☑
  - suicide (attempt) X78.1 ☑
- lathe (metalworking) W31.1 ☑
  - turnings W45.8 ☑
  - woodworking W31.2 ☑
- lawnmower (powered) (ridden) W28 ☑
  - causing electrocution W86.8 ☑
  - suicide (attempt) X83.1 ☑
  - unpowered W27.1 ☑
- lift, lifting (devices) W24.0 ☑
  - agricultural operations W30.89 ☑
  - shaft W24.0 ☑
- liquefied gas — *see* Exposure, cold, man-made
- liquid air, hydrogen, nitrogen — *see* Exposure, cold, man-made
- lizard (nonvenomous) W59.09 ☑
  - bite W59.01 ☑
  - strike W59.02 ☑

Contact

Contact — *continued*
- llama — *see* Contact, with, hoof stock NEC
- macaw W61.19 ☑
  - bite W61.11 ☑
  - strike W61.12 ☑
- machine, machinery W31.9 ☑
  - abrasive wheel W31.1 ☑
  - agricultural including animal-powered W30.9 ☑
    - combine harvester W30.0 ☑
    - grain storage elevator W30.3 ☑
    - hay derrick W30.2 ☑
    - power take-off device W30.1 ☑
    - reaper W30.0 ☑
    - specified NEC W30.89 ☑
    - thresher W30.0 ☑
    - transport vehicle, stationary W30.81 ☑
  - band saw W31.2 ☑
  - bench saw W31.2 ☑
  - circular saw W31.2 ☑
  - commercial NEC W31.82 ☑
  - drilling, metal (industrial) W31.1 ☑
  - earth-drilling W31.0 ☑
  - earthmoving or scraping W31.89 ☑
  - excavating W31.89 ☑
  - forging machine W31.1 ☑
  - gas turbine W31.3 ☑
  - hot X17 ☑
  - internal combustion engine W31.3 ☑
  - land drill W31.0 ☑
  - lathe W31.1 ☑
  - lifting (devices) W24.0 ☑
  - metal drill W31.1 ☑
  - metalworking (industrial) W31.1 ☑
  - milling, metal W31.1 ☑
  - mining W31.0 ☑
  - molding W31.2 ☑
  - overhead plane W31.2 ☑
  - power press, metal W31.1 ☑
  - prime mover W31.3 ☑
  - printing W31.89 ☑
  - radial saw W31.2 ☑
  - recreational W31.81 ☑
  - roller-coaster W31.81 ☑
  - rolling mill, metal W31.1 ☑
  - sander W31.2 ☑
  - seabed drill W31.0 ☑
  - shaft
    - hoist W31.0 ☑
    - lift W31.0 ☑
  - specified NEC W31.89 ☑
  - spinning W31.89 ☑
  - steam engine W31.3 ☑
  - transmission W24.1 ☑
  - undercutter W31.0 ☑
  - water driven turbine W31.3 ☑
  - weaving W31.89 ☑
  - woodworking or forming (industrial) W31.2 ☑
- mammal (feces) (urine) W55.89 ☑
  - bull — *see* Contact, with, bull
  - cat — *see* Contact, with, cat
  - cow — *see* Contact, with, cow
  - goat — *see* Contact, with, goat
  - hoof stock — *see* Contact, with, hoof stock
  - horse — *see* Contact, with, horse
  - marine W56.39 ☑
    - dolphin — *see* Contact, with, dolphin
    - orca — *see* Contact, with, orca
    - sea lion — *see* Contact, with, sea lion
    - specified NEC W56.39 ☑
      - bite W56.31 ☑
      - strike W56.32 ☑
  - pig — *see* Contact, with, pig
  - raccoon — *see* Contact, with, raccoon
  - rodent — *see* Contact, with, rodent
  - sheep — *see* Contact, with, sheep
  - specified NEC W55.89 ☑
    - bite W55.81 ☑
    - strike W55.82 ☑
- marine
  - animal W56.89 ☑
    - bite W56.81 ☑
    - dolphin — *see* Contact, with, dolphin
    - fish NEC — *see* Contact, with, fish
    - mammal — *see* Contact, with, mammal, marine
    - orca — *see* Contact, with, orca
    - sea lion — *see* Contact, with, sea lion
    - shark — *see* Contact, with, shark
    - strike W56.82 ☑
- meat

Contact — *continued*
- grinder (domestic) W29.0 ☑
  - industrial W31.82 ☑
  - nonpowered W27.4 ☑
- slicer (domestic) W29.0 ☑
  - industrial W31.82 ☑
- merry go round W31.81 ☑
- metal, hot (liquid) (molten) NEC X18 ☑
- millipede W57 ☑
- nail W45.0 ☑
  - gun W29.4 ☑
- needle (sewing) W27.3 ☑
  - hypodermic W46.0 ☑
    - contaminated W46.1 ☑
- object (blunt) NEC
  - hot NEC X19 ☑
  - legal intervention — *see* Legal, intervention, blunt object
  - sharp NEC W45.8 ☑
    - inflicted by other person NEC W45.8 ☑
      - stated as
        - intentional homicide (attempt) — *see* Assault, cutting or piercing instrument
    - legal intervention — *see* Legal, intervention, sharp object
    - self-inflicted X78.9 ☑
- orca W56.29 ☑
  - bite W56.21 ☑
  - strike W56.22 ☑
- overhead plane W31.2 ☑
- paper (as sharp object) W45.1 ☑
- paper-cutter W27.5 ☑
- parrot W61.09 ☑
  - bite W61.01 ☑
  - strike W61.02 ☑
- pig W55.49 ☑
  - bite W55.41 ☑
  - strike W55.42 ☑
- pipe, hot X16 ☑
- pitchfork W27.1 ☑
- plane (metal) (wood) W27.0 ☑
  - overhead W31.2 ☑
- plant thorns, spines, sharp leaves or other mechanisms W60 ☑
- powered
  - garden cultivator W29.3 ☑
  - household appliance, implement, or machine W29.8 ☑
  - saw (industrial) W31.2 ☑
    - hand W29.8 ☑
- printing machine W31.89 ☑
- psittacine bird W61.29 ☑
  - bite W61.21 ☑
  - macaw — *see* Contact, with, macaw
  - parrot — *see* Contact, with, parrot
  - strike W61.22 ☑
- pulley (block) (transmission) W24.0 ☑
  - agricultural operations W30.89 ☑
- raccoon W55.59 ☑
  - bite W55.51 ☑
  - strike W55.52 ☑
- radial-saw (industrial) W31.2 ☑
- radiator (hot) X16 ☑
- rake W27.1 ☑
- rattlesnake X58 ☑
- reaper W30.0 ☑
- reptile W59.89 ☑
  - lizard — *see* Contact, with, lizard
  - snake — *see* Contact, with, snake
  - specified NEC W59.89 ☑
    - bite W59.81 ☑
    - crushing W59.83 ☑
    - strike W59.82 ☑
  - turtle — *see* Contact, with, turtle
- rivet gun (powered) W29.4 ☑
- road scraper — *see* Accident, transport, construction vehicle
- rodent (feces) (urine) W53.89 ☑
  - bite W53.81 ☑
  - mouse W53.09 ☑
    - bite W53.01 ☑
  - rat W53.19 ☑
    - bite W53.11 ☑
  - specified NEC W53.89 ☑
    - bite W53.81 ☑
  - squirrel W53.29 ☑
    - bite W53.21 ☑
- roller coaster W31.81 ☑
- rope NEC W24.0 ☑
  - agricultural operations W30.89 ☑
- saliva — *see* Contact, with, by type of animal

Contact — *continued*
- sander W29.8 ☑
  - industrial W31.2 ☑
- saucepan (hot) (glass) (metal) X15.3 ☑
- saw W27.0 ☑
  - band (industrial) W31.2 ☑
  - bench (industrial) W31.2 ☑
  - chain W29.3 ☑
  - hand W27.0 ☑
- sawing machine, metal W31.1 ☑
- scissors W27.2 ☑
- scorpion X58 ☑
- screwdriver W27.0 ☑
  - powered W29.8 ☑
- sea
  - anemone, cucumber or urchin (spine) X58 ☑
  - lion W56.19 ☑
    - bite W56.11 ☑
    - strike W56.12 ☑
- serpent — *see* Contact, with, snake, by type
- sewing-machine (electric) (powered) W29.2 ☑
  - not powered W27.8 ☑
- shaft (hoist) (lift) (transmission) NEC W24.0 ☑
  - agricultural W30.89 ☑
- shark W56.49 ☑
  - bite W56.41 ☑
  - strike W56.42 ☑
- shears (hand) W27.2 ☑
  - powered (industrial) W31.1 ☑
    - domestic W29.2 ☑
- sheep W55.39 ☑
  - bite W55.31 ☑
  - strike W55.32 ☑
- shovel W27.8 ☑
  - steam — *see* Accident, transport, construction vehicle
- snake (nonvenomous) W59.19 ☑
  - bite W59.11 ☑
  - crushing W59.13 ☑
  - strike W59.12 ☑
- spade W27.1 ☑
- spider (venomous) X58 ☑
- spin-drier W29.2 ☑
- spinning machine W31.89 ☑
- splinter W45.8 ☑
- sports equipment W21.9 ☑
- staple gun (powered) W29.8 ☑
- steam X13.1 ☑
  - engine W31.3 ☑
  - inhalation X13.0 ☑
  - pipe X16 ☑
  - shovel W31.89 ☑
- stove (hot) (kitchen) X15.0 ☑
- substance, hot NEC X19 ☑
  - molten (metal) X18 ☑
- sword W26.1 ☑
  - assault X99.2 ☑
  - stated as undetermined whether accidental or intentional Y28.2 ☑
  - suicide (attempt) X78.2 ☑
- tarantula X58 ☑
- thresher W30.0 ☑
- tin can lid W45.2 ☑
- toad W62.1 ☑
- toaster (hot) X15.1 ☑
- tool W27.8 ☑
  - hand (not powered) W27.8 ☑
    - auger W27.0 ☑
    - axe W27.0 ☑
    - can opener W27.4 ☑
    - chisel W27.0 ☑
    - fork W27.4 ☑
    - garden W27.1 ☑
    - handsaw W27.0 ☑
    - hoe W27.1 ☑
    - ice-pick W27.4 ☑
    - kitchen utensil W27.4 ☑
    - manual
      - lawn mower W27.1 ☑
      - sewing machine W27.8 ☑
    - meat grinder W27.4 ☑
    - needle (sewing) W27.3 ☑
      - hypodermic W46.0 ☑
        - contaminated W46.1 ☑
    - paper cutter W27.5 ☑
    - pitchfork W27.1 ☑
    - rake W27.1 ☑
    - scissors W27.2 ☑
    - screwdriver W27.0 ☑
    - specified NEC W27.8 ☑
    - workbench W27.0 ☑
  - hot X17 ☑

☑ **Additional character required**

Contact — *continued*
- powered W29.8 ☑
  - blender W29.0 ☑
    - commercial W31.82 ☑
  - can opener W29.0 ☑
    - commercial W31.82 ☑
  - chainsaw W29.3 ☑
  - clothes dryer W29.2 ☑
    - commercial W31.82 ☑
  - dishwasher W29.2 ☑
    - commercial W31.82 ☑
  - edger W29.3 ☑
  - electric fan W29.2 ☑
    - commercial W31.82 ☑
  - electric knife W29.1 ☑
  - food processor W29.0 ☑
    - commercial W31.82 ☑
  - garbage disposal W29.0 ☑
    - commercial W31.82 ☑
  - garden tool W29.3 ☑
  - hedge trimmer W29.3 ☑
  - ice maker W29.0 ☑
    - commercial W31.82 ☑
  - kitchen appliance W29.0 ☑
    - commercial W31.82 ☑
  - lawn mower W28 ☑
  - meat grinder W29.0 ☑
    - commercial W31.82 ☑
  - mixer W29.0 ☑
    - commercial W31.82 ☑
  - rototiller W29.3 ☑
  - sewing machine W29.2 ☑
    - commercial W31.82 ☑
  - washing machine W29.2 ☑
    - commercial W31.82 ☑
- transmission device (belt, cable, chain, gear, pinion, shaft) W24.1 ☑
  - agricultural operations W30.89 ☑
- turbine (gas) (water-driven) W31.3 ☑
- turkey W61.49 ☑
  - peck W61.43 ☑
  - strike W61.42 ☑
- turtle (nonvenomous) W59.29 ☑
  - bite W59.21 ☑
  - strike W59.22 ☑
  - terrestrial W59.89 ☑
    - bite W59.81 ☑
    - crushing W59.83 ☑
    - strike W59.82 ☑
- under-cutter W31.0 ☑
- urine — *see* Contact, with, by type of animal
- vehicle
  - agricultural use (transport) — *see* Accident, transport, agricultural vehicle
    - not on public highway W30.81 ☑
  - industrial use (transport) — *see* Accident, transport, industrial vehicle
    - not on public highway W31.83 ☑
  - off-road use (transport) — *see* Accident, transport, all-terrain or off-road vehicle
    - not on public highway W31.83 ☑
  - special construction use (transport) — *see* Accident, transport, construction vehicle
    - not on public highway W31.83 ☑
- venomous
  - animal X58 ☑
  - arthropods X58 ☑
  - lizard X58 ☑
  - marine animal NEC X58 ☑
  - marine plant NEC X58 ☑
  - millipedes (tropical) X58 ☑
  - plant (s) X58 ☑
  - snake X58 ☑
  - spider X58 ☑
  - viper X58 ☑
- washing-machine (powered) W29.2 ☑
- wasp X58 ☑
- weaving-machine W31.89 ☑
- winch W24.0 ☑
  - agricultural operations W30.89 ☑
- wire NEC W24.0 ☑
  - agricultural operations W30.89 ☑
- wood slivers W45.8 ☑
- yellow jacket X58 ☑
- zebra — *see* Contact, with, hoof stock NEC

Coup de soleil X32 ☑

Crash
- aircraft (in transit) (powered) V95.9 ☑
  - balloon V96.01 ☑
  - fixed wing NEC (private) V95.21 ☑
    - commercial V95.31 ☑
  - glider V96.21 ☑

Crash — *continued*
- hang V96.11 ☑
  - powered V95.11 ☑
- helicopter V95.01 ☑
- in war operations — *see* War operations, destruction of aircraft
- microlight V95.11 ☑
- nonpowered V96.9 ☑
  - specified NEC V96.8 ☑
- powered NEC V95.8 ☑
- stated as
  - homicide (attempt) Y08.81 ☑
  - suicide (attempt) X83.0 ☑
- ultralight V95.11 ☑
- spacecraft V95.41 ☑
- transport vehicle NEC (*see also* Accident, transport) V89.9 ☑
  - homicide (attempt) Y03.8 ☑
  - motor NEC (traffic) V89.2 ☑
    - homicide (attempt) Y03.8 ☑
  - suicide (attempt) — *see* Suicide, collision

Cruelty (mental) (physical) (sexual) X58 ☑

Crushed (accidentally) X58 ☑
- between objects (moving) (stationary and moving) W23.0 ☑
  - stationary W23.1 ☑
- by
  - alligator W58.03 ☑
  - avalanche NEC — *see* Landslide
  - cave-in W20.0 ☑
    - caused by cataclysmic earth surface movement — *see* Landslide
  - crocodile W58.13 ☑
  - crowd or human stampede W52 ☑
  - falling
    - aircraft V97.39 ☑
      - in war operations — *see* War operations, destruction of aircraft
    - earth, material W20.0 ☑
      - caused by cataclysmic earth surface movement — *see* Landslide
    - object NEC W20.8 ☑
  - landslide NEC — *see* Landslide
  - lizard (nonvenomous) W59.09 ☑
  - machinery — *see* Contact, with, by type of machine
  - reptile NEC W59.89 ☑
  - snake (nonvenomous) W59.13 ☑
- in
  - machinery — *see* Contact, with, by type of machine

Cut, cutting (any part of body) (accidental) (*see also* Contact, with, by object or machine)
- during medical or surgical treatment as misadventure — *see* Index to Diseases and Injuries, Complications
- homicide (attempt) — *see* Assault, cutting or piercing instrument
- inflicted by other person — *see* Assault, cutting or piercing instrument
- legal
  - execution — *see* Legal, intervention
  - intervention — *see* Legal, intervention, sharp object
- machine NEC (*see also* Contact, with, by type of machine) W31.9 ☑
- self-inflicted — *see* Suicide, cutting or piercing instrument
- suicide (attempt) — *see* Suicide, cutting or piercing instrument

Cyclone (any injury) X37.1 ☑

D

Decapitation (accidental circumstances) NEC X58 ☑
- homicide X99.9 ☑
- legal execution — *see* Legal, intervention

Dehydration from lack of water X58 ☑

Deprivation X58 ☑

Derailment (accidental)
- railway (rolling stock) (train) (vehicle) (without antecedent collision) V81.7 ☑
  - with antecedent collision — *see* Accident, transport, railway vehicle occupant
- streetcar (without antecedent collision) V82.7 ☑
  - with antecedent collision — *see* Accident, transport, streetcar occupant

Descent
- parachute (voluntary) (without accident to aircraft) V97.29 ☑

Descent — *continued*
- due to accident to aircraft — *see* Accident, transport, aircraft

Desertion X58 ☑

Destitution X58 ☑

Disability, late effect or sequela of injury — *see* Sequelae

Discharge (accidental)
- airgun W34.010 ☑
  - assault X95.01 ☑
  - homicide (attempt) X95.01 ☑
  - stated as undetermined whether accidental or intentional Y24.0 ☑
  - suicide (attempt) X74.01 ☑
- BB gun — *see* Discharge, airgun
- firearm (accidental) W34.00 ☑
  - assault X95.9 ☑
  - handgun (pistol) (revolver) W32.0 ☑
    - assault X93 ☑
    - homicide (attempt) X93 ☑
    - legal intervention — *see* Legal, intervention, firearm, handgun
    - stated as undetermined whether accidental or intentional Y22 ☑
    - suicide (attempt) X72 ☑
  - homicide (attempt) X95.9 ☑
  - hunting rifle W33.02 ☑
    - assault X94.1 ☑
    - homicide (attempt) X94.1 ☑
    - legal intervention
      - injuring
        - bystander Y35.032 ☑
        - law enforcement personnel Y35.031 ☑
        - suspect Y35.033 ☑
    - stated as undetermined whether accidental or intentional Y23.1 ☑
    - suicide (attempt) X73.1 ☑
  - larger W33.00 ☑
    - assault X94.9 ☑
    - homicide (attempt) X94.9 ☑
    - hunting rifle — *see* Discharge, firearm, hunting rifle
    - legal intervention — *see* Legal, intervention, firearm by type of firearm
    - machine gun — *see* Discharge, firearm, machine gun
    - shotgun — *see* Discharge, firearm, shotgun
    - specified NEC W33.09 ☑
      - assault X94.8 ☑
      - homicide (attempt) X94.8 ☑
      - legal intervention
        - injuring
          - bystander Y35.092 ☑
          - law enforcement personnel Y35.091 ☑
          - suspect Y35.093 ☑
      - stated as undetermined whether accidental or intentional Y23.8 ☑
      - suicide (attempt) X73.8 ☑
    - stated as undetermined whether accidental or intentional Y23.9 ☑
    - suicide (attempt) X73.9 ☑
  - legal intervention
    - injuring
      - bystander Y35.002 ☑
      - law enforcement personnel Y35.001 ☑
      - suspect Y35.03 ☑
    - using rubber bullet
      - injuring
        - bystander Y35.042 ☑
        - law enforcement personnel Y35.041 ☑
        - suspect Y35.043 ☑
  - machine gun W33.03 ☑
    - assault X94.2 ☑
    - homicide (attempt) X94.2 ☑
    - legal intervention — *see* Legal, intervention, firearm, machine gun
    - stated as undetermined whether accidental or intentional Y23.3 ☑
    - suicide (attempt) X73.2 ☑
  - pellet gun — *see* Discharge, airgun
  - shotgun W33.01 ☑
    - assault X94.0 ☑
    - homicide (attempt) X94.0 ☑
    - legal intervention — *see* Legal, intervention, firearm, specified NEC
    - stated as undetermined whether accidental or intentional Y23.0 ☑
    - suicide (attempt) X73.0 ☑
  - specified NEC W34.09 ☑
    - assault X95.8 ☑
    - homicide (attempt) X95.8 ☑

Discharge — *continued*
　　legal intervention — *see* Legal, intervention, firearm, specified NEC
　　　stated as undetermined whether accidental or intentional Y24.8 ☑
　　　suicide (attempt) X74.8 ☑
　　stated as undetermined whether accidental or intentional Y24.9 ☑
　　suicide (attempt) X74.9 ☑
　　Very pistol W34.09 ☑
　　　assault X95.8 ☑
　　　homicide (attempt) X95.8 ☑
　　　stated as undetermined whether accidental or intentional Y24.8 ☑
　　　suicide (attempt) X74.8 ☑
　　firework (s) W39 ☑
　　　stated as undetermined whether accidental or intentional Y25 ☑
　　gas-operated gun NEC W34.018 ☑
　　　airgun — *see* Discharge, airgun
　　　assault X95.09 ☑
　　　homicide (attempt) X95.09 ☑
　　　paintball gun — *see* Discharge, paintball gun
　　　stated as undetermined whether accidental or intentional Y24.8 ☑
　　　suicide (attempt) X74.09 ☑
　　gun NEC (*see also* Discharge, firearm NEC)
　　　air — *see* Discharge, airgun
　　　BB — *see* Discharge, airgun
　　　for single hand use — *see* Discharge, firearm, handgun
　　　hand — *see* Discharge, firearm, handgun
　　　machine — *see* Discharge, firearm, machine gun
　　　other specified — *see* Discharge, firearm NEC
　　　paintball — *see* Discharge, paintball gun
　　　pellet — *see* Discharge, airgun
　　handgun — *see* Discharge, firearm, handgun
　　machine gun — *see* Discharge, firearm, machine gun
　　paintball gun W34.011 ☑
　　　assault X95.02 ☑
　　　homicide (attempt) X95.02 ☑
　　　stated as undetermined whether accidental or intentional Y24.8 ☑
　　　suicide (attempt) X74.02 ☑
　　pistol — *see* Discharge, firearm, handgun
　　　flare — *see* Discharge, firearm, Very pistol
　　　pellet — *see* Discharge, airgun
　　　Very — *see* Discharge, firearm, Very pistol
　　revolver — *see* Discharge, firearm, handgun
　　rifle (hunting) — *see* Discharge, firearm, hunting rifle
　　shotgun — *see* Discharge, firearm, shotgun
　　spring-operated gun NEC W34.018 ☑
　　　assault X95.09 ☑
　　　homicide (attempt) X95.09 ☑
　　　stated as undetermined whether accidental or intentional Y24.8 ☑
　　　suicide (attempt) X74.09 ☑
Disease
　　Andes W94.11 ☑
　　aviator's - — *see* Air, pressure
　　range W94.11 ☑
Diver's disease, palsy, paralysis, squeeze - — *see* Air, pressure
Diving (into water) — *see* Accident, diving
Dog bite W54.0 ☑
Dragged by transport vehicle NEC (*see also* Accident, transport) V09.9 ☑
Drinking poison (accidental) — *see* Table of Drugs and Chemicals
Dropped (accidentally) while being carried or supported by other person W04 ☑
Drowning (accidental) W74 ☑
　　assault X92.9 ☑
　　due to
　　　accident (to)
　　　　machinery — *see* Contact, with, by type of machine
　　　　watercraft V90.89 ☑
　　　　　burning V90.29 ☑
　　　　　　powered V90.23 ☑
　　　　　　　merchant ship V90.20 ☑
　　　　　　　passenger ship V90.21 ☑
　　　　　　　fishing boat V90.22 ☑
　　　　　　　jetskis V90.23 ☑
　　　　　　unpowered V90.28 ☑
　　　　　　　canoe V90.25 ☑
　　　　　　　inflatable V90.26 ☑
　　　　　　　kayak V90.25 ☑
　　　　　　　sailboat V90.24 ☑

Drowning — *continued*
　　　　　　water skis V90.27 ☑
　　　　　crushed V90.39 ☑
　　　　　　powered V90.33 ☑
　　　　　　　merchant ship V90.30 ☑
　　　　　　　passenger ship V90.31 ☑
　　　　　　　fishing boat V90.32 ☑
　　　　　　　jetskis V90.33 ☑
　　　　　　unpowered V90.38 ☑
　　　　　　　canoe V90.35 ☑
　　　　　　　inflatable V90.36 ☑
　　　　　　　kayak V90.35 ☑
　　　　　　　sailboat V90.34 ☑
　　　　　　　water skis V90.37 ☑
　　　　　overturning V90.09 ☑
　　　　　　powered V90.03 ☑
　　　　　　　merchant ship V90.00 ☑
　　　　　　　passenger ship V90.01 ☑
　　　　　　　fishing boat V90.02 ☑
　　　　　　　jetskis V90.03 ☑
　　　　　　unpowered V90.08 ☑
　　　　　　　canoe V90.05 ☑
　　　　　　　inflatable V90.06 ☑
　　　　　　　kayak V90.05 ☑
　　　　　　　sailboat V90.04 ☑
　　　　　sinking V90.19 ☑
　　　　　　powered V90.13 ☑
　　　　　　　merchant ship V90.10 ☑
　　　　　　　passenger ship V90.11 ☑
　　　　　　　fishing boat V90.12 ☑
　　　　　　　jetskis V90.13 ☑
　　　　　　unpowered V90.18 ☑
　　　　　　　canoe V90.15 ☑
　　　　　　　inflatable V90.16 ☑
　　　　　　　kayak V90.15 ☑
　　　　　　　sailboat V90.14 ☑
　　　　　specified type NEC V90.89 ☑
　　　　　　powered V90.83 ☑
　　　　　　　merchant ship V90.80 ☑
　　　　　　　passenger ship V90.81 ☑
　　　　　　　fishing boat V90.82 ☑
　　　　　　　jetskis V90.83 ☑
　　　　　　unpowered V90.88 ☑
　　　　　　　canoe V90.85 ☑
　　　　　　　inflatable V90.86 ☑
　　　　　　　kayak V90.85 ☑
　　　　　　　sailboat V90.84 ☑
　　　　　　　water skis V90.87 ☑
　　　avalanche — *see* Landslide
　　　cataclysmic
　　　　earth surface movement NEC — *see* Forces of nature, earth movement
　　　　storm — *see* Forces of nature, cataclysmic storm
　　　cloudburst X37.8 ☑
　　　cyclone X37.1 ☑
　　　fall overboard (from) V92.09 ☑
　　　　powered craft V92.03 ☑
　　　　　ferry boat V92.01 ☑
　　　　　liner V92.01 ☑
　　　　　merchant ship V92.00 ☑
　　　　　passenger ship V92.01 ☑
　　　　　fishing boat V92.02 ☑
　　　　　jetskis V92.03 ☑
　　　　unpowered craft V92.08 ☑
　　　　　canoe V92.05 ☑
　　　　　inflatable V92.06 ☑
　　　　　kayak V92.05 ☑
　　　　　sailboat V92.04 ☑
　　　　　surf-board V92.08 ☑
　　　　　water skis V92.07 ☑
　　　　　windsurfer V92.08 ☑
　　　resulting from
　　　　accident to watercraft — *see* Drowning, due to, accident to, watercraft
　　　　being washed overboard (from) V92.29 ☑
　　　　　powered craft V92.23 ☑
　　　　　　ferry boat V92.21 ☑
　　　　　　liner V92.21 ☑
　　　　　　merchant ship V92.20 ☑
　　　　　　passenger ship V92.21 ☑
　　　　　　fishing boat V92.22 ☑
　　　　　　jetskis V92.23 ☑
　　　　　unpowered craft V92.28 ☑
　　　　　　canoe V92.25 ☑
　　　　　　inflatable V92.26 ☑
　　　　　　kayak V92.25 ☑
　　　　　　sailboat V92.24 ☑
　　　　　　surf-board V92.28 ☑
　　　　　　water skis V92.27 ☑
　　　　　　windsurfer V92.28 ☑
　　　　motion of watercraft V92.19 ☑

Drowning — *continued*
　　　　　powered craft V92.13 ☑
　　　　　　ferry boat V92.11 ☑
　　　　　　liner V92.11 ☑
　　　　　　merchant ship V92.10 ☑
　　　　　　passenger ship V92.11 ☑
　　　　　　fishing boat V92.12 ☑
　　　　　　jetskis V92.13 ☑
　　　　　unpowered craft
　　　　　　canoe V92.15 ☑
　　　　　　inflatable V92.16 ☑
　　　　　　kayak V92.15 ☑
　　　　　　sailboat V92.14 ☑
　　　hurricane X37.0 ☑
　　　jumping into water from watercraft (involved in accident) (*see also* Drowning, due to, accident to, watercraft)
　　　　without accident to or on watercraft W16.711 ☑
　　　tidal wave NEC — *see* Forces of nature, tidal wave
　　　torrential rain X37.8 ☑
　　following
　　　fall
　　　　into
　　　　　bathtub W16.211 ☑
　　　　　bucket W16.221 ☑
　　　　　fountain — *see* Drowning, following, fall, into, water, specified NEC
　　　　　quarry — *see* Drowning, following, fall, into, water, specified NEC
　　　　　reservoir — *see* Drowning, following, fall, into, water, specified NEC
　　　　　swimming-pool W16.011 ☑
　　　　　　striking
　　　　　　　bottom W16.021 ☑
　　　　　　　wall W16.031 ☑
　　　　　　stated as undetermined whether accidental or intentional Y21.3 ☑
　　　　　　suicide (attempt) X71.2 ☑
　　　　　water NOS W16.41 ☑
　　　　　　natural (lake) (open sea) (river) (stream) (pond) W16.111 ☑
　　　　　　　striking
　　　　　　　　bottom W16.121 ☑
　　　　　　　　side W16.131 ☑
　　　　　　specified NEC W16.311 ☑
　　　　　　　striking
　　　　　　　　bottom W16.321 ☑
　　　　　　　　wall W16.331 ☑
　　　overboard NEC — *see* Drowning, due to, fall overboard
　　jump or dive
　　　from boat W16.711 ☑
　　　　striking bottom W16.721 ☑
　　　into
　　　　fountain — *see* Drowning, following, jump or dive, into, water, specified NEC
　　　　quarry — *see* Drowning, following, jump or dive, into, water, specified NEC
　　　　reservoir — *see* Drowning, following, jump or dive, into, water, specified NEC
　　　　swimming-pool W16.511 ☑
　　　　　striking
　　　　　　bottom W16.521 ☑
　　　　　　wall W16.531 ☑
　　　　　suicide (attempt) X71.2 ☑
　　　　water NOS W16.91 ☑
　　　　　natural (lake) (open sea) (river) (stream) (pond) W16.611 ☑
　　　　　specified NEC W16.811 ☑
　　　　　　striking
　　　　　　　bottom W16.821 ☑
　　　　　　　wall W16.831 ☑
　　　　　striking bottom W16.621 ☑
　　homicide (attempt) X92.9 ☑
　　in
　　　bathtub (accidental) W65 ☑
　　　　assault X92.0 ☑
　　　　following fall W16.211 ☑
　　　　stated as undetermined whether accidental or intentional Y21.1 ☑
　　　　stated as undetermined whether accidental or intentional Y21.0 ☑
　　　　suicide (attempt) X71.0 ☑
　　　lake — *see* Drowning, in, natural water
　　　natural water (lake) (open sea) (river) (stream) (pond) W69 ☑
　　　　assault X92.3 ☑
　　　　following
　　　　　dive or jump W16.611 ☑
　　　　　　striking bottom W16.621 ☑

☑ **Additional character required**

Drowning — *continued*
    fall W16.111 ☑
      striking
        bottom W16.121 ☑
        side W16.131 ☑
    stated as undetermined whether accidental
      or intentional Y21.4 ☑
    suicide (attempt) X71.3 ☑
    quarry — *see* Drowning, in, specified place NEC
    quenching tank — *see* Drowning, in, specified
      place NEC
    reservoir — *see* Drowning, in, specified place
      NEC
    river — *see* Drowning, in, natural water
    sea — *see* Drowning, in, natural water
    specified place NEC W73 ☑
      assault X92.8 ☑
      following
        dive or jump W16.811 ☑
          striking
            bottom W16.821 ☑
            wall W16.831 ☑
        fall W16.311 ☑
          striking
            bottom W16.321 ☑
            wall W16.331 ☑
      stated as undetermined whether accidental
        or intentional Y21.8 ☑
      suicide (attempt) X71.8 ☑
    stream — *see* Drowning, in, natural water
    swimming-pool W67 ☑
      assault X92.1 ☑
        following fall X92.2 ☑
      following
        dive or jump W16.511 ☑
          striking
            bottom W16.521 ☑
            wall W16.531 ☑
        fall W16.011 ☑
          striking
            bottom W16.021 ☑
            wall W16.031 ☑
      stated as undetermined whether accidental
        or intentional Y21.2 ☑
        following fall Y21.3 ☑
      suicide (attempt) X71.1 ☑
        following fall X71.2 ☑
    war operations — *see* War operations,
      restriction of airway
    resulting from accident to watercraftsee
      Drowning, due to, accident, watercraft
    self-inflicted X71.9 ☑
    stated as undetermined whether accidental or
      intentional Y21.9 ☑
    suicide (attempt) X71.9 ☑

E

Earth (surface) movement NEC — *see* Forces of
  nature, earth movement
Earth falling (on) W20.0 ☑
  caused by cataclysmic earth surface movement
    or eruption — *see* Landslide
Earthquake (any injury) X34 ☑
Effect (s) (adverse) of
  air pressure (any) - — *see* Air, pressure
  cold, excessive (exposure to) — *see* Exposure,
    cold
  heat (excessive) — *see* Heat
  hot place (weather) — *see* Heat
  insolation X30 ☑
  late — *see* Sequelae
  motion — *see* Motion
  nuclear explosion or weapon in war operations
    — *see* War operations, nuclear weapon
  radiation — *see* Radiation
  travel — *see* Travel
Electric shock (accidental) (by) (in) — *see* Exposure,
  electric current
Electrocution (accidental) — *see* Exposure, electric
  current
Endotracheal tube wrongly placed during
  anesthetic procedure
Entanglement
  in
    bed linen, causing suffocationT71
    wheel of pedal cycle V19.88 ☑
Entry of foreign body or material — *see* Foreign
  body

Environmental pollution related condition- see
  Z57 ☑
Execution, legal (any method) — *see* Legal,
  intervention
Exhaustion
  cold — *see* Exposure, cold
  due to excessive exertionY93
  heat — *see* Heat
Explosion (accidental) (of) (with secondary fire)
  W40.9 ☑
  acetylene W40.1 ☑
  aerosol can W36.1 ☑
  air tank (compressed) (in machinery) W36.2 ☑
  aircraft (in transit) (powered) NEC V95.9 ☑
    balloon V96.05 ☑
    fixed wing NEC (private) V95.25 ☑
      commercial V95.35 ☑
    glider V96.25 ☑
      hang V96.15 ☑
      powered V95.15 ☑
    helicopter V95.05 ☑
    in war operations — *see* War operations,
      destruction of aircraft
    microlight V95.15 ☑
    nonpowered V96.9 ☑
      specified NEC V96.8 ☑
    powered NEC V95.8 ☑
    stated as
      homicide (attempt) Y03.8 ☑
      suicide (attempt) X83.0 ☑
    ultralight V95.15 ☑
  anesthetic gas in operating room W40.1 ☑
  antipersonnel bomb W40.8 ☑
    assault X96.0 ☑
    homicide (attempt) X96.0 ☑
    suicide (attempt) X75 ☑
  assault X96.9 ☑
  bicycle tire W37.0 ☑
  blasting (cap) (materials) W40.0 ☑
  boiler (machinery), not on transport vehicle
    W35 ☑
    on watercraft — *see* Explosion, in, watercraft
  butane W40.1 ☑
  caused by other person X96.9 ☑
  coal gas W40.1 ☑
  detonator W40.0 ☑
  dump (munitions) W40.8 ☑
  dynamite W40.0 ☑
    in
      assault X96.8 ☑
      homicide (attempt) X96.8 ☑
      legal intervention
        injuring
          bystander Y35.112 ☑
          law enforcement personnel Y35.111 ☑
          suspect Y35.113 ☑
      suicide (attempt) X75 ☑
  explosive (material) W40.9 ☑
    gas W40.1 ☑
    in blasting operation W40.0 ☑
    specified NEC W40.8 ☑
      in
        assault X96.8 ☑
        homicide (attempt) X96.8 ☑
        legal intervention
          injuring
            bystander Y35.192 ☑
            law enforcement personnel Y35.191 ☑
            suspect Y35.193 ☑
        suicide (attempt) X75 ☑
  factory (munitions) W40.8 ☑
  fertilizer bomb W40.8 ☑
    assault X96.3 ☑
    homicide (attempt) X96.3 ☑
    suicide (attempt) X75 ☑
  firearm (parts) NEC W34.19 ☑
    airgun W34.110 ☑
    BB gun W34.110 ☑
    gas, air or spring-operated gun NEC W34.118 ☑
    hangun W32.1 ☑
    hunting rifle W33.12 ☑
    larger firearm W33.10 ☑
      specified NEC W33.19 ☑
    machine gun W33.13 ☑
    paintball gun W34.111 ☑
    pellet gun W34.110 ☑
    shotgun W33.11 ☑
    Very pistol [flare] W34.19 ☑
  fire-damp W40.1 ☑
  fireworks W39 ☑
  gas (coal) (explosive) W40.1 ☑
    cylinder W36.9 ☑

Explosion — *continued*
  aerosol can W36.1 ☑
  air tank W36.2 ☑
    pressurized W36.3 ☑
    specified NEC W36.8 ☑
  gasoline (fumes) (tank) not in moving motor
    vehicle W40.1 ☑
    bomb W40.8 ☑
      assault X96.1 ☑
      homicide (attempt) X96.1 ☑
      suicide (attempt) X75 ☑
    in motor vehicle — *see* Accident, transport, by
      type of vehicle
  grain store W40.8 ☑
  grenade W40.8 ☑
    in
      assault X96.8 ☑
      homicide (attempt) X96.8 ☑
      legal intervention
        injuring
          bystander Y35.192 ☑
          law enforcement personnel Y35.191 ☑
          suspect Y35.193 ☑
      suicide (attempt) X75 ☑
  handgun (parts) — *see* Explosion, firearm,
    hangun (parts)
  homicide (attempt) X96.9 ☑
    antipersonnel bomb — *see* Explosion,
      antipersonnel bomb
    fertilizer bomb — *see* Explosion, fertilizer bomb
    gasoline bomb — *see* Explosion, gasoline
      bomb
    letter bomb — *see* Explosion, letter bomb
    pipe bomb — *see* Explosion, pipe bomb
    specified NEC X96.8 ☑
  hose, pressurized W37.8 ☑
  hot water heater, tank (in machinery) W35 ☑
    on watercraft — *see* Explosion, in, watercraft
  in, on
    dump W40.8 ☑
    factory W40.8 ☑
    mine (of explosive gases) NEC W40.1 ☑
    watercraft V93.59 ☑
      powered craft V93.53 ☑
        ferry boat V93.51 ☑
        fishing boat V93.52 ☑
        jetskis V93.53 ☑
        liner V93.51 ☑
        merchant ship V93.50 ☑
        passenger ship V93.51 ☑
        sailboat V93.54 ☑
  letter bomb W40.8 ☑
    assault X96.2 ☑
    homicide (attempt) X96.2 ☑
    suicide (attempt) X75 ☑
  machinery (*see also* Contact, with, by type of
    machine)
    on board watercraft — *see* Explosion, in,
      watercraft
    pressure vessel — *see* Explosion, by type of
      vessel
  methane W40.1 ☑
  mine W40.1 ☑
  missile NEC W40.8 ☑
  mortar bomb W40.8 ☑
    in
      assault X96.8 ☑
      homicide (attempt) X96.8 ☑
      legal intervention
        injuring
          bystander Y35.192 ☑
          law enforcement personnel Y35.191 ☑
          suspect Y35.193 ☑
      suicide (attempt) X75 ☑
  munitions (dump) (factory) W40.8 ☑
  pipe, pressurized W37.8 ☑
    bomb W40.8 ☑
      assault X96.4 ☑
      homicide (attempt) X96.4 ☑
      suicide (attempt) X75 ☑
  pressure, pressurized
    cooker W38 ☑
    gas tank (in machinery) W36.3 ☑
    hose W37.8 ☑
    pipe W37.8 ☑
    specified device NEC W38 ☑
    tire W37.8 ☑
      bicycle W37.0 ☑
    vessel (in machinery) W38 ☑
  propane W40.1 ☑
  self inflicted X75 ☑
  shell (artillery) NEC W40.8 ☑

Explosion — *continued*
  during war operations — *see* War operations, explosion
  in
    legal intervention
      injuring
        bystander Y35.122 ☑
        law enforcement personnel Y35.121 ☑
        suspect Y35.123 ☑
      war — *see* War operations, explosion
  spacecraft V95.45 ☑
  steam or water lines (in machinery) W37.8 ☑
  stove W40.9 ☑
  stated as undetermined whether accidental or intentional Y25 ☑
  suicide (attempt) X75 ☑
  tire, pressurized W37.8 ☑
    bicycle W37.0 ☑
  undetermined whether accidental or intentional Y25 ☑
  vehicle tire NEC W37.8 ☑
    bicycle W37.0 ☑
  war operations — *see* War operations, explosion
Exposure (to) X58 ☑
  air pressure change — *see* Air, pressure
  cold (accidental) (excessive) (extreme) (natural) (place) X31 ☑
    assault Y08.89 ☑
    due to
      man-made conditions W93.8 ☑
        dry ice (contact) W93.01 ☑
          inhalation W93.02 ☑
        liquid air (contact) (hydrogen) (nitrogen) W93.11 ☑
          inhalation W93.12 ☑
        refrigeration unit (deep freeze) W93.2 ☑
        suicide (attempt) X83.2 ☑
      weather (conditions) X31 ☑
    homicide (attempt) Y08.89 ☑
    self-inflicted X83.2 ☑
  due to abandonment or neglect X58 ☑
  electric current W86.8 ☑
    appliance (faulty) W86.8 ☑
      domestic W86.0 ☑
    caused by other person Y08.89 ☑
    conductor (faulty) W86.1 ☑
    control apparatus (faulty) W86.1 ☑
    electric power generating plant, distribution station W86.1 ☑
    electroshock gun — *see* Exposure, electric current, taser
    high-voltage cable W85 ☑
    homicide (attempt) Y08.89 ☑
    legal execution — *see* Legal, intervention, specified means NEC
    lightning T75.0
    live rail W86.8 ☑
    misadventure in medical or surgical procedure in electroshock therapy Y63.4
    motor (electric) (faulty) W86.8 ☑
      domestic W86.0 ☑
    self-inflicted X83.1 ☑
    specified NEC W86.8 ☑
      domestic W86.0 ☑
    stun gun — *see* Exposure, electric current, taser
    suicide (attempt) X83.1 ☑
    taser W86.8 ☑
      assault Y08.89 ☑
      legal intervention Y35
      self-harm (intentional) X83.8 ☑
      undetermined intent Y33 ☑
    third rail W86.8 ☑
    transformer (faulty) W86.1 ☑
    transmission lines W85 ☑
  environmental tobacco smoke X58 ☑
  excessive
    cold — *see* Exposure, cold
    heat (natural) NEC X30 ☑
      man-made W92 ☑
  factor (s) NOS X58 ☑
    environmental NEC X58 ☑
      man-made NEC W99 ☑
      natural NEC — *see* Forces of nature
    specified NEC X58 ☑
  fire, flames (accidental) X08.8 ☑
    assault X97 ☑
    campfire — *see* Exposure, fire, controlled, not in building
    controlled (in)
      with ignition (of) clothing (*see also* Ignition, clothes) X06.2 ☑
        nightwear X05 ☑

Exposure — *continued*
  bonfire — *see* Exposure, fire, controlled, not in building
  brazier (in building or structure) (*see also* Exposure, fire, controlled, building)
    not in building or structure — *see* Exposure, fire, controlled, not in building
  building or structure X02.0 ☑
    with
      fall from building X02.3 ☑
      injury due to building collapse X02.2 ☑
      from building X02.5 ☑
      smoke inhalation X02.1 ☑
    hit by object from building X02.4 ☑
    specified mode of injury NEC X02.8 ☑
  fireplace, furnace or stove — *see* Exposure, fire, controlled, building
  not in building or structure X03.0 ☑
    with
      fall X03.3 ☑
      smoke inhalation X03.1 ☑
    hit by object X03.4 ☑
    specified mode of injury NEC X03.8 ☑
  trash — *see* Exposure, fire, controlled, not in building
  fireplace — *see* Exposure, fire, controlled, building
  fittings or furniture (in building or structure) (uncontrolled) — *see* Exposure, fire, uncontrolled, building
  forest (uncontrolled) — *see* Exposure, fire, uncontrolled, not in building
  grass (uncontrolled) — *see* Exposure, fire, uncontrolled, not in building
  hay (uncontrolled) — *see* Exposure, fire, uncontrolled, not in building
  homicide (attempt) X97 ☑
  ignition of highly flammable material X04 ☑
  in, of, on, starting in
    machinery — *see* Contact, with, by type of machine
    motor vehicle (in motion) (*see also* Accident, transport, occupant by type of vehicle) V87.8 ☑
      with collision — *see* Collision
    railway rolling stock, train, vehicle V81.81 ☑
      with collision — *see* Accident, transport, railway vehicle occupant
    street car (in motion) V82.8 ☑
      with collision — *see* Accident, transport, streetcar occupant
    transport vehicle NEC (*see also* Accident, transport)
      with collision — *see* Collision
    war operations (*see also* War operations, fire)
      from nuclear explosion — *see* War operations, nuclear weapons
  watercraft (in transit) (not in transit) V91.09 ☑
    localized — *see* Burn, on board watercraft, due to, fire on board
    powered craft V91.03 ☑
      ferry boat V91.01 ☑
      fishing boat V91.02 ☑
      jet skis V91.03 ☑
      liner V91.01 ☑
      merchant ship V91.00 ☑
      passenger ship V91.01 ☑
    unpowered craft V91.08 ☑
      canoe V91.05 ☑
      inflatable V91.06 ☑
      kayak V91.05 ☑
      sailboat V91.04 ☑
      surf-board V91.08 ☑
      waterskis V91.07 ☑
      windsurfer V91.08 ☑
  lumber (uncontrolled) — *see* Exposure, fire, uncontrolled, not in building
  mine (uncontrolled) — *see* Exposure, fire, uncontrolled, not in building
  prairie (uncontrolled) — *see* Exposure, fire, uncontrolled, not in building
  resulting from
    explosion — *see* Explosion
    lightning X08.8 ☑
  self-inflicted X76 ☑
  specified NEC X08.8 ☑
  started by other person X97 ☑
  stove — *see* Exposure, fire, controlled, building
  stated as undetermined whether accidental or intentional Y26 ☑
  suicide (attempt) X76 ☑

Exposure — *continued*
  tunnel (uncontrolled) — *see* Exposure, fire, uncontrolled, not in building
  uncontrolled
    in building or structure X00.0 ☑
      with
        fall from building X00.3 ☑
        injury due to building collapse X00.2 ☑
        jump from building X00.5 ☑
        smoke inhalation X00.1 ☑
      bed X08.00 ☑
        due to
          cigarette X08.01 ☑
          specified material NEC X08.09 ☑
      furniture NEC X08.20 ☑
        due to
          cigarette X08.21 ☑
          specified material NEC X08.29 ☑
      hit by object from building X00.4 ☑
      sofa X08.10 ☑
        due to
          cigarette X08.11 ☑
          specified material NEC X08.19 ☑
      specified mode of injury NEC X00.8 ☑
    not in building or structure (any) X01.0 ☑
      with
        fall X01.3 ☑
        smoke inhalation X01.1 ☑
      hit by object X01.4 ☑
      specified mode of injury NEC X01.8 ☑
  undetermined whether accidental or intentional Y26 ☑
  forces of nature NEC — *see* Forces of nature
  G-forces (abnormal) W49.9 ☑
  gravitational forces (abnormal) W49.9 ☑
  heat (natural) NEC — *see* Heat
  high-pressure jet (hydraulic) (pneumatic) W49.9 ☑
  hydraulic jet W49.9 ☑
  inanimate mechanical force W49.9 ☑
  jet, high-pressure (hydraulic) (pneumatic) W49.9 ☑
  lightning T75.0
    causing fire — *see* Exposure, fire
  mechanical forces NEC W49.9 ☑
    animate NEC W64 ☑
    inanimate NEC W49.9 ☑
  noise W42.9 ☑
    supersonic W42.0 ☑
  noxious substance — *see* Table of Drugs and Chemicals
  pneumatic jet W49.9 ☑
  prolonged in deep-freeze unit or refrigerator W93.2 ☑
  radiation — *see* Radiation
  smoke (*see also* Exposure, fire)
    tobacco, second hand Z77.22
  specified factors NEC X58 ☑
  sunlight X32 ☑
    man-made (sun lamp) W89.8 ☑
      tanning bed W89.1 ☑
  supersonic waves W42.0 ☑
  transmission line (s), electric W85 ☑
  vibration W49.9 ☑
  waves
    infrasound W49.9 ☑
    sound W42.9 ☑
    supersonic W42.0 ☑
  weather NEC — *see* Forces of nature
External cause status Y99.9
  child assisting in compensated work for family Y99.8
  civilian activity done for financial or other compensation Y99.0
  civilian activity done for income or pay Y99.0
  family member assisting in compensated work for other family member Y99.8
  hobby not done for income Y99.8
  leisure activity Y99.8
  military activity Y99.1
  off-duty activity of military personnel Y99.8
  recreation or sport not for income or while a student Y99.8
  specified NEC Y99.8
  student activity Y99.8
  volunteer activity Y99.2

☑ **Additional character required**

F

Factors, supplemental
  alcohol
    blood level
      less than 20mg/100ml Y90.0
      presence in blood, level not specified Y90.9
      20-39mg/100ml Y90.1
      40-59mg/100ml Y90.2
      60-79mg/100ml Y90.3
      80-99mg/100ml Y90.4
      100-119mg/100ml Y90.5
      120-199mg/100ml Y90.6
      200-239mg/100ml Y90.7
      240mg/100ml or more Y90.8
    presence in blood, but level not specified Y90.9
  environmental-pollution-related condition- see
    Z57 ☑
  nosocomial condition Y95
  work-related condition Y99.0
Failure
  in suture or ligature during surgical procedure
    Y65.2
  mechanical, of instrument or apparatus (any)
    (during any medical or surgical procedure)
    Y65.8
  sterile precautions (during medical and surgical
    care) — see Misadventure, failure, sterile
    precautions, by type of procedure
  to
    introduce tube or instrument Y65.4
      endotracheal tube during anesthesia Y65.3
    make curve (transport vehicle) NEC — see
      Accident, transport
    remove tube or instrument Y65.4
Fall, falling (accidental) W19 ☑
  building W20.1 ☑
    burning (uncontrolled fire) X00.3 ☑
  down
    embankment W17.81 ☑
    escalator W10.0 ☑
    hill W17.81 ☑
    ladder W11 ☑
    ramp W10.2 ☑
    stairs, steps W10.9 ☑
  due to
    bumping against
      object W18.00 ☑
        sharp glass W18.02 ☑
        specified NEC W18.09 ☑
        sports equipment W18.01 ☑
      person W03 ☑
        due to ice or snow W00.0 ☑
          on pedestrian conveyance — see Accident,
            transport, pedestrian, conveyance
    collision with another person W03 ☑
      due to ice or snow W00.0 ☑
      involving pedestrian conveyance — see
        Accident, transport, pedestrian,
        conveyance
    grocery cart tipping over W17.82 ☑
    ice or snow W00.9 ☑
      from one level to another W00.2 ☑
      on stairs or steps W00.1 ☑
      involving pedestrian conveyance — see
        Accident, transport, pedestrian,
        conveyance
      on same level W00.0 ☑
    slipping (on moving sidewalk) W01.0 ☑
      with subsequent striking against object
        W01.10 ☑
        furniture W01.190 ☑
        sharp object W01.119 ☑
          glass W01.110 ☑
          power tool or machine W01.111 ☑
          specified NEC W01.118 ☑
        specified NEC W01.198 ☑
    striking against
      object W18.00 ☑
        sharp glass W18.02 ☑
        specified NEC W18.09 ☑
        sports equipment W18.01 ☑
      person W03 ☑
        due to ice or snow W00.0 ☑
          on pedestrian conveyance — see Accident,
            transport, pedestrian, conveyance
  earth (with asphyxia or suffocation (by pressure))
    — see Earth, falling
  from, off, out of
    aircraft NEC (with accident to aircraft NEC)
      V97.0 ☑

Fall — continued
    while boarding or alighting V97.1 ☑
  balcony W13.0 ☑
  bed W06 ☑
  boat, ship, watercraft NEC (with drowning or
    submersion) — see Drowning, due to, fall
    overboard
    with hitting bottom or object V94.0 ☑
  bridge W13.1 ☑
  building W13.9 ☑
    burning (uncontrolled fire) X00.3 ☑
  cavity W17.2 ☑
  chair W07 ☑
  cherry picker W17.89 ☑
  cliff W15 ☑
  dock W17.4 ☑
  embankment W17.81 ☑
  escalator W10.0 ☑
  flagpole W13.8 ☑
  furniture NEC W08 ☑
  grocery cart W17.82 ☑
  haystack W17.89 ☑
  high place NEC W17.89 ☑
    stated as undetermined whether accidental
      or intentional Y30 ☑
  hole W17.2 ☑
  incline W10.2 ☑
  ladder W11 ☑
  lifting device W17.89 ☑
  machine, machinery (see also Contact, with, by
    type of machine)
    not in operation W17.89 ☑
  manhole W17.1 ☑
  mobile elevated work platform [MEWP] W17.89
    ☑
  motorized mobility scooter W05.2 ☑
  one level to another NEC W17.89 ☑
    intentional, purposeful, suicide (attempt)
      X80 ☑
    stated as undetermined whether accidental
      or intentional Y30 ☑
  pit W17.2 ☑
  playground equipment W09.8 ☑
    jungle gym W09.2 ☑
    slide W09.0 ☑
    swing W09.1 ☑
  quarry W17.89 ☑
  railing W13.9 ☑
  ramp W10.2 ☑
  roof W13.2 ☑
  scaffolding W12 ☑
  scooter (nonmotorized) W05.1 ☑
    motorized mobility W05.2 ☑
  sky lift W17.89 ☑
  stairs, steps W10.9 ☑
    curb W10.1 ☑
    due to ice or snow W00.1 ☑
    escalator W10.0 ☑
    incline W10.2 ☑
    ramp W10.2 ☑
    sidewalk curb W10.1 ☑
    specified NEC W10.8 ☑
  stepladder W11 ☑
  storm drain W17.1 ☑
  streetcar NEC V82.6 ☑
    with antecedent collision — see Accident,
      transport, streetcar occupant
    while boarding or alighting V82.4 ☑
  structure NEC W13.8 ☑
    burning (uncontrolled fire) X00.3 ☑
  table W08 ☑
  toilet W18.11 ☑
    with subsequent striking against object
      W18.12 ☑
  train NEC V81.6 ☑
    during derailment (without antecedent
      collision) V81.7 ☑
    with antecedent collision — see Accident,
      transport, railway vehicle occupant
    while boarding or alighting V81.4 ☑
  transport vehicle after collision — see Accident,
    transport, by type of vehicle, collision
  tree W14 ☑
  vehicle (in motion) NEC (see also Accident,
    transport) V89.9 ☑
    motor NEC (see also Accident, transport,
      occupant, by type of vehicle) V87.8 ☑
      stationary W17.89 ☑
        while boarding or alighting — see
          Accident, transport, by type of vehicle,
          while boarding or alighting
  viaduct W13.8 ☑

Fall — continued
  wall W13.8 ☑
  watercraft (see also Drowning, due to, fall
    overboard)
    with hitting bottom or object V94.0 ☑
  well W17.0 ☑
  wheelchair, non-moving W05.0 ☑
    powered — see Accident, transport,
      pedestrian, conveyance occupant,
      specified type NEC
  window W13.4 ☑
  in, on
    aircraft NEC V97.0 ☑
      with accident to aircraft V97.0 ☑
      while boarding or alighting V97.1 ☑
    bathtub (empty) W18.2 ☑
      filled W16.212 ☑
        causing drowning W16.211 ☑
    escalator W10.0 ☑
    incline W10.2 ☑
    ladder W11 ☑
    machine, machinery — see Contact, with, by
      type of machine
    object, edged, pointed or sharp (with cut) —
      see Fall, by type
    playground equipment W09.8 ☑
      jungle gym W09.2 ☑
      slide W09.0 ☑
      swing W09.1 ☑
    ramp W10.2 ☑
    scaffolding W12 ☑
    shower W18.2 ☑
      causing drowning W16.211 ☑
    staircase, stairs, steps W10.9 ☑
      curb W10.1 ☑
      due to ice or snow W00.1 ☑
      escalator W10.0 ☑
      incline W10.2 ☑
      specified NEC W10.8 ☑
    streetcar (without antecedent collision)
      V82.5 ☑
      with antecedent collision — see Accident,
        transport, streetcar occupant
      while boarding or alighting V82.4 ☑
    train (without antecedent collision) V81.5 ☑
      with antecedent collision — see Accident,
        transport, railway vehicle occupant
      during derailment (without antecedent
        collision) V81.7 ☑
      with antecedent collision — see Accident,
        transport, railway vehicle occupant
      while boarding or alighting V81.4 ☑
    transport vehicle after collision — see Accident,
      transport, by type of vehicle, collision
    watercraft V93.39 ☑
      due to
        accident to craft V91.29 ☑
          powered craft V91.23 ☑
            ferry boat V91.21 ☑
            fishing boat V91.22 ☑
            jetskis V91.23 ☑
            liner V91.21 ☑
            merchant ship V91.20 ☑
            passenger ship V91.21 ☑
          unpowered craft
            canoe V91.25 ☑
            inflatable V91.26 ☑
            kayak V91.25 ☑
            sailboat V91.24 ☑
        powered craft V93.33 ☑
          ferry boat V93.31 ☑
          fishing boat V93.32 ☑
          jetskis V93.33 ☑
          liner V93.31 ☑
          merchant ship V93.30 ☑
          passenger ship V93.31 ☑
        unpowered craft V93.38 ☑
          canoe V93.35 ☑
          inflatable V93.36 ☑
          kayak V93.35 ☑
          sailboat V93.34 ☑
          surf-board V93.38 ☑
          windsurfer V93.38 ☑
  into
    cavity W17.2 ☑
    dock W17.4 ☑
    fire — see Exposure, fire, by type
    haystack W17.89 ☑
    hole W17.2 ☑
    lake — see Fall, into, water
    manhole W17.1 ☑

Fall — continued
  moving part of machinery — *see* Contact, with, by type of machine
  ocean — *see* Fall, into, water
  opening in surface NEC W17.89 ☑
  pit W17.2 ☑
  pond — *see* Fall, into, water
  quarry W17.89 ☑
  river — *see* Fall, into, water
  shaft W17.89 ☑
  storm drain W17.1 ☑
  stream — *see* Fall, into, water
  swimming pool (*see also* Fall, into, water, in, swimming pool)
    empty W17.3 ☑
  tank W17.89 ☑
  water W16.42 ☑
    causing drowning W16.41 ☑
    from watercraft — *see* Drowning, due to, fall overboard
    hitting diving board W21.4 ☑
    in
      bathtub W16.212 ☑
        causing drowning W16.211 ☑
      bucket W16.222 ☑
        causing drowning W16.221 ☑
      natural body of water W16.112 ☑
        causing drowning W16.111 ☑
        striking
          bottom W16.122 ☑
            causing drowning W16.121 ☑
          side W16.132 ☑
            causing drowning W16.131 ☑
      specified water NEC W16.312 ☑
        causing drowning W16.311 ☑
        striking
          bottom W16.322 ☑
            causing drowning W16.321 ☑
          wall W16.332 ☑
            causing drowning W16.331 ☑
      swimming pool W16.012 ☑
        causing drowning W16.011 ☑
        striking
          bottom W16.022 ☑
            causing drowning W16.021 ☑
          wall W16.032 ☑
            causing drowning W16.031 ☑
      utility bucket W16.222 ☑
        causing drowning W16.221 ☑
  well W17.0 ☑
  involving
    bed W06 ☑
    chair W07 ☑
    furniture NEC W08 ☑
    glass — *see* Fall, by type
    playground equipment W09.8 ☑
      jungle gym W09.2 ☑
      slide W09.0 ☑
      swing W09.1 ☑
    roller blades — *see* Accident, transport, pedestrian, conveyance
    skateboard (s) — *see* Accident, transport, pedestrian, conveyance
    skates (ice) (in line) (roller) — *see* Accident, transport, pedestrian, conveyance
    skis — *see* Accident, transport, pedestrian, conveyance
    table W08 ☑
    wheelchair, non-moving W05.0 ☑
      powered — *see* Accident, transport, pedestrian, conveyance, specified type NEC
  object — *see* Struck by, object, falling
  off
    toilet W18.11 ☑
      with subsequent striking against object W18.12 ☑
  on same level W18.30 ☑
    due to
      specified NEC W18.39 ☑
      stepping on an object W18.31 ☑
  out of
    bed W06 ☑
    building NEC W13.8 ☑
    chair W07 ☑
    furniture NEC W08 ☑
    wheelchair, non-moving W05.0 ☑
      powered — *see* Accident, transport, pedestrian, conveyance, specified type NEC
    window W13.4 ☑
  over

Fall — continued
  animal W01.0 ☑
  cliff W15 ☑
  embankment W17.81 ☑
  small object W01.0 ☑
  rock W20.8 ☑
  same level W18.30 ☑
    from
      being crushed, pushed, or stepped on by a crowd or human stampede W52 ☑
      collision, pushing, shoving, by or with other person W03 ☑
      slipping, stumbling, tripping W01.0 ☑
    involving ice or snow W00.0 ☑
      involving skates (ice) (roller), skateboard, skis — *see* Accident, transport, pedestrian, conveyance
  snowslide (avalanche) — *see* Landslide
  stone W20.8 ☑
  structure W20.1 ☑
    burning (uncontrolled fire) X00.3 ☑
  through
    bridge W13.1 ☑
    floor W13.3 ☑
    roof W13.2 ☑
    wall W13.8 ☑
    window W13.4 ☑
  timber W20.8 ☑
  tree (caused by lightning) W20.8 ☑
  while being carried or supported by other person(s) W04 ☑
Fallen on by
  animal (not being ridden) NEC W55.89 ☑
Felo-de-se — *see* Suicide
Fight (hand) (fists) (foot) — *see* Assault, fight
Fire (accidental) — *see* Exposure, fire
Firearm discharge — *see* Discharge, firearm
Fireball effects from nuclear explosion in war operations — *see* War operations, nuclear weapons
Fireworks (explosion) W39 ☑
Flash burns from explosion — *see* Explosion
Flood (any injury) (caused by) X38 ☑
  collapse of man-made structure causing earth movement X36.0 ☑
  tidal wave — *see* Forces of nature, tidal wave
Food (any type) in
  air passages (with asphyxia, obstruction, or suffocation) — *see* categories T17 and T18 ☑
  alimentary tract causing asphyxia (due to compression of trachea) — *see* categories T17 and T18 ☑
Forces of nature X39.8 ☑
  avalanche X36.1 ☑
    causing transport accident — *see* Accident, transport, by type of vehicle
  blizzard X37.2 ☑
  cataclysmic storm X37.9 ☑
    with flood X38 ☑
    blizzard X37.2 ☑
    cloudburst X37.8 ☑
    cyclone X37.1 ☑
    dust storm X37.3 ☑
    hurricane X37.0 ☑
    specified storm NEC X37.8 ☑
    storm surge X37.0 ☑
    tornado X37.1 ☑
    twister X37.1 ☑
    typhoon X37.0 ☑
  cloudburst X37.8 ☑
  cold (natural) X31 ☑
  cyclone X37.1 ☑
  dam collapse causing earth movement X36.0 ☑
  dust storm X37.3 ☑
  earth movement X36.1 ☑
    earthquake X34 ☑
    caused by dam or structure collapse X36.0 ☑
  earthquake X34 ☑
  flood (caused by) X38 ☑
    dam collapse X36.0 ☑
    tidal wave — *see* Forces of nature, tidal wave
  heat (natural) X30 ☑
  hurricane X37.0 ☑
  landslide X36.1 ☑
    causing transport accident — *see* Accident, transport, by type of vehicle
  lightning T75.0
    causing fire — *see* Exposure, fire
  mudslide X36.1 ☑
    causing transport accident — *see* Accident, transport, by type of vehicle
  radiation (natural) X39.08 ☑
    radon X39.01 ☑

Forces — continued
  radon X39.01 ☑
  specified force NEC X39.8 ☑
  storm surge X37.0 ☑
  structure collapse causing earth movement X36.0 ☑
  sunlight X32 ☑
  tidal wave X37.41 ☑
    due to
      earthquake X37.41 ☑
      landslide X37.43 ☑
      storm X37.42 ☑
      volcanic eruption X37.41 ☑
  tornado X37.1 ☑
  tsunami X37.41 ☑
  twister X37.1 ☑
  typhoon X37.0 ☑
  volcanic eruption X35 ☑
Foreign body
  aspiration — *see* Index to Diseases and Injuries, Foreign body, respiratory tract
  entering through skin W45.8 ☑
    can lid W45.2 ☑
    nail W45.0 ☑
    paper W45.1 ☑
    specified NEC W45.8 ☑
    splinter W45.8 ☑
Forest fire (exposure to) — *see* Exposure, fire, uncontrolled, not in building
Found injured X58 ☑
  from exposure (to) — *see* Exposure
  on
    highway, road (way), street V89.9 ☑
    railway right of way V81.9 ☑
Fracture (circumstances unknown or unspecified) X58 ☑
  due to specified cause NEC X58 ☑
Freezing — *see* Exposure, cold
Frostbite X31 ☑
  due to man-made conditions — *see* Exposure, cold, man-made
Frozen — *see* Exposure, cold

G

Gored by bull W55.22 ☑
Gunshot wound W34.00 ☑

H

Hailstones, injured by X39.8 ☑
Hanged herself or himself — *see* Hanging, self-inflicted
Hanging (accidental) (*see also* category) T71 ☑
  legal execution — *see* Legal, intervention, specified means NEC
Heat (effects of) (excessive) X30 ☑
  due to
    man-made conditions W92 ☑
      on board watercraft V93.29 ☑
        fishing boat V93.22 ☑
        merchant ship V93.20 ☑
        passenger ship V93.21 ☑
        sailboat V93.24 ☑
        specified powered craft NEC V93.23 ☑
    weather (conditions) X30 ☑
  from
    electric heating apparatus causing burning X16 ☑
    nuclear explosion in war operations — *see* War operations, nuclear weapons
    inappropriate in local application or packing in medical or surgical procedure Y63.5
Hemorrhage
  delayed following medical or surgical treatment without mention of misadventure — *see* Index to Diseases and Injuries, Complication(s)
  during medical or surgical treatment as misadventure — *see* Index to Diseases and Injuries, Complication(s)
High
  altitude (effects) - — *see* Air, pressure, low
  level of radioactivity, effects — *see* Radiation
  pressure (effects) - — *see* Air, pressure, high
  temperature, effects — *see* Heat
Hit, hitting (accidental) by — *see* Struck by
Hitting against — *see* Striking against

☑ **Additional character required**

Homicide (attempt) (justifiable) — *see* Assault
Hot
  place, effects (*see also* Heat)
  weather, effects X30 ☑
House fire (uncontrolled) — *see* Exposure, fire,
  uncontrolled, building
Humidity, causing problem X39.8 ☑
Hunger X58 ☑
Hurricane (any injury) X37.0 ☑
Hypobarism, hypobaropathy - — *see* Air, pressure,
  low

I

Ictus
  caloris (*see also* Heat)
  solaris X30 ☑
Ignition (accidental) (*see also* Exposure, fire) X08.8 ☑
  anesthetic gas in operating room W40.1 ☑
  apparel X06.2 ☑
    from highly flammable material X04 ☑
    nightwear X05 ☑
  bed linen (sheets) (spreads) (pillows) (mattress)
    — *see* Exposure, fire, uncontrolled, building,
    bed
  benzine X04 ☑
  clothes, clothing NEC (from controlled fire) X06.2
    ☑
    from
      highly flammable material X04 ☑
  ether X04 ☑
    in operating room W40.1 ☑
  explosive material — *see* Explosion
  gasoline X04 ☑
  jewelry (plastic) (any) X06.0 ☑
  kerosene X04 ☑
  material
    explosive — *see* Explosion
    highly flammable with secondary explosion
      X04 ☑
  nightwear X05 ☑
  paraffin X04 ☑
  petrol X04 ☑
Immersion (accidental) (*see also* Drowning)
  hand or foot due to cold (excessive) X31 ☑
Implantation of quills of porcupine W55.89 ☑
Inanition (from) (hunger) X58 ☑
  thirst X58 ☑
Inappropriate operation performed
  correct operation on wrong side or body part
    (wrong side) (wrong site) Y65.53
  operation intended for another patient done on
    wrong patient Y65.52
  wrong operation performed on correct patient
    Y65.51
Inattention after, at birth (homicidal intent)
  (infanticidal intent) X58 ☑
Incident, adverse
  device
    anesthesiology Y70.8
      accessory Y70.2
      diagnostic Y70.0
      miscellaneous Y70.8
      monitoring Y70.0
      prosthetic Y70.2
      rehabilitative Y70.1
      surgical Y70.3
      therapeutic Y70.1
    cardiovascular Y71.8
      accessory Y71.2
      diagnostic Y71.0
      miscellaneous Y71.8
      monitoring Y71.0
      prosthetic Y71.2
      rehabilitative Y71.1
      surgical Y71.3
      therapeutic Y71.1
    gastroenterology Y73.8
      accessory Y73.2
      diagnostic Y73.0
      miscellaneous Y73.8
      monitoring Y73.0
      prosthetic Y73.2
      rehabilitative Y73.1
      surgical Y73.3
      therapeutic Y73.1
    general
      hospital Y74.8
        accessory Y74.2
        diagnostic Y74.0

Incident — *continued*
    miscellaneous Y74.8
    monitoring Y74.0
    prosthetic Y74.2
    rehabilitative Y74.1
    surgical Y74.3
    therapeutic Y74.1
  surgical Y81.8
    accessory Y81.2
    diagnostic Y81.0
    miscellaneous Y81.8
    monitoring Y81.0
    prosthetic Y81.2
    rehabilitative Y81.1
    surgical Y81.3
    therapeutic Y81.1
  gynecological Y76.8
    accessory Y76.2
    diagnostic Y76.0
    miscellaneous Y76.8
    monitoring Y76.0
    prosthetic Y76.2
    rehabilitative Y76.1
    surgical Y76.3
    therapeutic Y76.1
  medical Y82.9
    specified type NEC Y82.8
  neurological Y75.8
    accessory Y75.2
    diagnostic Y75.0
    miscellaneous Y75.8
    monitoring Y75.0
    prosthetic Y75.2
    rehabilitative Y75.1
    surgical Y75.3
    therapeutic Y75.1
  obstetrical Y76.8
    accessory Y76.2
    diagnostic Y76.0
    miscellaneous Y76.8
    monitoring Y76.0
    prosthetic Y76.2
    rehabilitative Y76.1
    surgical Y76.3
    therapeutic Y76.1
  ophthalmic Y77.8
    accessory Y77.2
    diagnostic Y77.0
    miscellaneous Y77.8
    monitoring Y77.0
    prosthetic Y77.2
    rehabilitative Y77.1
    surgical Y77.3
    therapeutic Y77.1
  orthopedic Y79.8
    accessory Y79.2
    diagnostic Y79.0
    miscellaneous Y79.8
    monitoring Y79.0
    prosthetic Y79.2
    rehabilitative Y79.1
    surgical Y79.3
    therapeutic Y79.1
  otorhinolaryngological Y72.8
    accessory Y72.2
    diagnostic Y72.0
    miscellaneous Y72.8
    monitoring Y72.0
    prosthetic Y72.2
    rehabilitative Y72.1
    surgical Y72.3
    therapeutic Y72.1
  personal use Y74.8
    accessory Y74.2
    diagnostic Y74.0
    miscellaneous Y74.8
    monitoring Y74.0
    prosthetic Y74.2
    rehabilitative Y74.1
    surgical Y74.3
    therapeutic Y74.1
  physical medicine Y80.8
    accessory Y80.2
    diagnostic Y80.0
    miscellaneous Y80.8
    monitoring Y80.0
    prosthetic Y80.2
    rehabilitative Y80.1
    surgical Y80.3
    therapeutic Y80.1
  plastic surgical Y81.8
    accessory Y81.2

Incident — *continued*
    diagnostic Y81.0
    miscellaneous Y81.8
    monitoring Y81.0
    prosthetic Y81.2
    rehabilitative Y81.1
    surgical Y81.3
    therapeutic Y81.1
  radiological Y78.8
    accessory Y78.2
    diagnostic Y78.0
    miscellaneous Y78.8
    monitoring Y78.0
    prosthetic Y78.2
    rehabilitative Y78.1
    surgical Y78.3
    therapeutic Y78.1
  urology Y73.8
    accessory Y73.2
    diagnostic Y73.0
    miscellaneous Y73.8
    monitoring Y73.0
    prosthetic Y73.2
    rehabilitative Y73.1
    surgical Y73.3
    therapeutic Y73.1
Incineration (accidental) — *see* Exposure, fire
Infanticide — *see* Assault
Infrasound waves (causing injury) W49.9 ☑
Ingestion
  foreign body (causing injury) (with obstruction)
    — *see* Foreign body, alimentary canal
  poisonous
    plant (s) X58 ☑
    substance NEC — *see* Table of Drugs and
      Chemicals
Inhalation
  excessively cold substance, man-made — *see*
    Exposure, cold, man-made
  food (any type) (into respiratory tract) (with
    asphyxia, obstruction respiratory tract,
    suffocation) — *see* categories T17 and T18 ☑
  foreign body — *see* Foreign body, aspiration
  gastric contents (with asphyxia, obstruction
    respiratory passage, suffocation) T17.81- ☑
  hot air or gases X14.0 ☑
  liquid air, hydrogen, nitrogen W93.12 ☑
    suicide (attempt) X83.2 ☑
  steam X13.0 ☑
    assault X98.0 ☑
    stated as undetermined whether accidental or
      intentional Y27.0 ☑
    suicide (attempt) X77.0 ☑
  toxic gas — *see* Table of Drugs and Chemicals
  vomitus (with asphyxia, obstruction respiratory
    passage, suffocation) T17.81- ☑
Injury, injured (accidental(ly)) NOS X58 ☑
  by, caused by, from
    assault — *see* Assault
    law-enforcing agent, police, in course of legal
      intervention — *see* Legal intervention
    suicide (attempt) X83.8 ☑
  due to, in
    civil insurrection — *see* War operations
    fight (*see also* Assault, fight) Y04.0 ☑
    war operations — *see* War operations
  homicide (*see also* Assault) Y09
  inflicted (by)
    in course of arrest (attempted), suppression of
      disturbance, maintenance of order, by law-
      enforcing agents — *see* Legal intervention
    other person
      stated as
        accidental X58 ☑
        intentional, homicide (attempt) — *see*
          Assault
        undetermined whether accidental or
          intentional Y33 ☑
    purposely (inflicted) by other person(s) — *see*
      Assault
  self-inflicted X83.8 ☑
    stated as accidental X58 ☑
  specified cause NEC X58 ☑
  undetermined whether accidental or intentional
    Y33 ☑
Insolation, effects X30 ☑
Insufficient nourishment X58 ☑
Interruption of respiration (by)
  food (lodged in esophagus) — *see* categories T17
    and T18 ☑
  vomitus (lodged in esophagus) T17.81- ☑
Intervention, legal — *see* Legal intervention

Intoxication
    drug — *see* Table of Drugs and Chemicals
    poison — *see* Table of Drugs and Chemicals

J

Jammed (accidentally)
    between objects (moving) (stationary and
        moving) W23.0 ☑
    stationary W23.1 ☑
Jumped, jumping
    before moving object NEC X81.8 ☑
        motor vehicle X81.0 ☑
        subway train X81.1 ☑
        train X81.1 ☑
        undetermined whether accidental or
            intentional Y31 ☑
    from
        boat (into water) voluntarily, without accident
            (to or on boat) W16.712 ☑
            with
                accident to or on boat — *see* Accident,
                    watercraft
                drowning or submersion W16.711 ☑
                    suicide (attempt) X71.3 ☑
                striking bottom W16.722 ☑
                    causing drowning W16.721 ☑
        building (*see also* Jumped, from, high place)
            W13.9 ☑
        burning (uncontrolled fire) X00.5 ☑
        high place NEC W17.89 ☑
            suicide (attempt) X80 ☑
            undetermined whether accidental or
                intentional Y30 ☑
        structure (*see also* Jumped, from, high place)
            W13.9 ☑
        burning (uncontrolled fire) X00.5 ☑
    into water W16.92 ☑
        causing drowning W16.91 ☑
        from, off watercraft — *see* Jumped, from, boat
        in
            natural body W16.612 ☑
                causing drowning W16.611 ☑
                striking bottom W16.622 ☑
                    causing drowning W16.621 ☑
            specified place NEC W16.812 ☑
                causing drowning W16.811 ☑
                striking
                    bottom W16.822 ☑
                        causing drowning W16.821 ☑
                    wall W16.832 ☑
                        causing drowning W16.831 ☑
            swimming pool W16.512 ☑
                causing drowning W16.511 ☑
                striking
                    bottom W16.522 ☑
                        causing drowning W16.521 ☑
                    wall W16.532 ☑
                        causing drowning W16.531 ☑
    suicide (attempt) X71.3 ☑

K

Kicked by
    animal NEC W55.82 ☑
    person (s) (accidentally) W50.1 ☑
        with intent to injure or kill Y04.0 ☑
        as, or caused by, a crowd or human stampede
            (with fall) W52 ☑
        assault Y04.0 ☑
        homicide (attempt) Y04.0 ☑
        in
            fight Y04.0 ☑
            legal intervention
                injuring
                    bystander Y35.812 ☑
                    law enforcement personnel Y35.811 ☑
                    suspect Y35.813 ☑
Kicking against
    object W22.8 ☑
        sports equipment W21.9 ☑
    stationary wW22.09
        sports equipment W21.89 ☑
    person — *see* Striking against, person
        sports equipment W21.9 ☑
Killed, killing (accidentally) NOS (*see also* Injury)
    X58 ☑
    in

Killed — *continued*
    action — *see* War operations
    brawl, fight (hand) (fists) (foot) Y04.0 ☑
        by weapon (*see also* Assault)
            cutting, piercing — *see* Assault, cutting or
                piercing instrument
            firearm — *see* Discharge, firearm, by type,
                homicide
    self
        stated as
            accident NOS X58 ☑
            suicide — *see* Suicide
            undetermined whether accidental or
                intentional Y33 ☑
Knocked down (accidentally) (by) NOS X58 ☑
    animal (not being ridden) NEC (*see also* Struck by,
        by type of animal)
    crowd or human stampede W52 ☑
    person W51 ☑
        in brawl, fight Y04.0 ☑
    transport vehicle NEC (*see also* Accident,
        transport) V09.9 ☑

L

Laceration NEC — *see* Injury
Lack of
    care (helpless person) (infant) (newborn) X58 ☑
    food except as result of abandonment or neglect
        X58 ☑
        due to abandonment or neglect X58 ☑
    water except as result of transport accident X58
        ☑
        due to transport accident — *see* Accident,
            transport, by type
    helpless person, infant, newborn X58 ☑
Landslide (falling on transport vehicle) X36.1 ☑
    caused by collapse of man-made structure X36.0
        ☑
Late effect — *see* Sequelae
Legal
    execution (any method) — *see* Legal, intervention
    intervention (by)
        baton — *see* Legal, intervention, blunt object,
            baton
        bayonet — *see* Legal, intervention, sharp
            object, bayonet
        blow — *see* Legal, intervention, manhandling
        blunt object
            baton
                injuring
                    bystander Y35.312 ☑
                    law enforcement personnel Y35.311 ☑
                    suspect Y35.313 ☑
            injuring
                bystander Y35.302 ☑
                law enforcement personnel Y35.301 ☑
                suspect Y35.303 ☑
            specified NEC
                injuring
                    bystander Y35.392 ☑
                    law enforcement personnel Y35.391 ☑
                    suspect Y35.393 ☑
            stave
                injuring
                    bystander Y35.392 ☑
                    law enforcement personnel Y35.391 ☑
                    suspect Y35.393 ☑
        bomb — *see* Legal, intervention, explosive
        cutting or piercing instrument — *see* Legal,
            intervention, sharp object
        dynamite — *see* Legal, intervention, explosive,
            dynamite
        explosive (s)
            dynamite
                injuring
                    bystander Y35.112 ☑
                    law enforcement personnel Y35.111 ☑
                    suspect Y35.113 ☑
            grenade
                injuring
                    bystander Y35.192 ☑
                    law enforcement personnel Y35.191 ☑
                    suspect Y35.193 ☑
            injuring
                bystander Y35.102 ☑
                law enforcement personnel Y35.101 ☑
                suspect Y35.103 ☑
            mortar bomb
                injuring

Legal — *continued*
                bystander Y35.192 ☑
                law enforcement personnel Y35.191 ☑
                suspect Y35.193 ☑
            shell
                injuring
                    bystander Y35.122 ☑
                    law enforcement personnel Y35.121 ☑
                    suspect Y35.123 ☑
            specified NEC
                injuring
                    bystander Y35.192 ☑
                    law enforcement personnel Y35.191 ☑
                    suspect Y35.193 ☑
        firearm (s) (discharge)
            handgun
                injuring
                    bystander Y35.022 ☑
                    law enforcement personnel Y35.021 ☑
                    suspect Y35.023 ☑
            injuring
                bystander Y35.002 ☑
                law enforcement personnel Y35.001 ☑
                suspect Y35.003 ☑
            machine gun
                injuring
                    bystander Y35.012 ☑
                    law enforcement personnel Y35.011 ☑
                    suspect Y35.013 ☑
            rifle pellet
                injuring
                    bystander Y35.032 ☑
                    law enforcement personnel Y35.031 ☑
                    suspect Y35.033 ☑
            rubber bullet
                injuring
                    bystander Y35.042 ☑
                    law enforcement personnel Y35.041 ☑
                    suspect Y35.043 ☑
            shotgun — *see* Legal, intervention, firearm,
                specified NEC
            specified NEC
                injuring
                    bystander Y35.092 ☑
                    law enforcement personnel Y35.091 ☑
                    suspect Y35.093 ☑
        gas (asphyxiation) (poisoning)
            injuring
                bystander Y35.202 ☑
                law enforcement personnel Y35.201 ☑
                suspect Y35.203 ☑
            specified NEC
                injuring
                    bystander Y35.292 ☑
                    law enforcement personnel Y35.291 ☑
                    suspect Y35.293 ☑
            tear gas
                injuring
                    bystander Y35.212 ☑
                    law enforcement personnel Y35.211 ☑
                    suspect Y35.213 ☑
        grenade — *see* Legal, intervention, explosive,
            grenade
        injuring
            bystander Y35.92 ☑
            law enforcement personnel Y35.91 ☑
            suspect Y35.93 ☑
        late effect (of) — *see* with 7th character S Y35
            ☑
        manhandling
            injuring
                bystander Y35.812 ☑
                law enforcement personnel Y35.811 ☑
                suspect Y35.813 ☑
        sequelae (of) — *see* with 7th character S Y35 ☑
        sharp objects
            bayonet
                injuring
                    bystander Y35.412 ☑
                    law enforcement personnel Y35.411 ☑
                    suspect Y35.413 ☑
            injuring
                bystander Y35.402 ☑
                law enforcement personnel Y35.401 ☑
                suspect Y35.403 ☑
            specified NEC
                injuring
                    bystander Y35.492 ☑
                    law enforcement personnel Y35.491 ☑
                    suspect Y35.493 ☑
        specified means NEC
            injuring

☑ **Additional character required**

Legal — *continued*
bystander Y35.892 ☑
law enforcement personnel Y35.891 ☑
suspect Y35.893 ☑
stabbing — *see* Legal, intervention, sharp object
stave — *see* Legal, intervention, blunt object, stave
tear gas — *see* Legal, intervention, gas, tear gas
truncheon — *see* Legal, intervention, blunt object, stave
Lightning (shock) (stroke) (struck by)T75.0
causing fire — *see* Exposure, fire
Loss of control (transport vehicle) NEC — *see* Accident, transport
Lost at sea NOS — *see* Drowning, due to, fall overboard
Low
pressure (effects) - — *see* Air, pressure, low
temperature (effects) — *see* Exposure, cold
Lying before train, vehicle or other moving object X81.8 ☑
subway train X81.1 ☑
train X81.1 ☑
undetermined whether accidental or intentional Y31 ☑
Lynching — *see* Assault

M

Malfunction (mechanism or component) (of)
firearm W34.10 ☑
airgun W34.110 ☑
BB gun W34.110 ☑
gas, air or spring-operated gun NEC W34.118 ☑
handgun W32.1 ☑
hunting rifle W33.12 ☑
larger firearm W33.10 ☑
specified NEC W33.19 ☑
machine gun W33.13 ☑
paintball gun W34.111 ☑
pellet gun W34.110 ☑
shotgun W33.11 ☑
specified NEC W34.19 ☑
Very pistol [flare] W34.19 ☑
handgun — *see* Malfunction, firearm, handgun
Maltreatment — *see* Perpetrator
Mangled (accidentally) NOS X58 ☑
Manhandling (in brawl, fight) Y04.0 ☑
legal intervention — *see* Legal, intervention, manhandling
Manslaughter (nonaccidental) — *see* Assault
Mauled by animal NEC W55.89 ☑
Medical procedure, complication of (delayed or as an abnormal reaction without mention of misadventure) — *see* Complication of or following, by specified type of procedure
due to or as a result of misadventure — *see* Misadventure
Melting (due to fire) (*see also* Exposure, fire)
apparel NEC X06.3 ☑
clothes, clothing NEC X06.3 ☑
nightwear X05 ☑
fittings or furniture (burning building) (uncontrolled fire) X00.8 ☑
nightwear X05 ☑
plastic jewelry X06.1 ☑
Mental cruelty X58 ☑
Military operations (injuries to military and civilians occuring during peacetime on military property and during routine military exercises and operations) (by) (from) (involving) Y37.90- ☑
air blast Y37.20- ☑
aircraft
destruction — *see* Military operations, destruction of aircraft
airway restriction — *see* Military operations, restriction of airways
asphyxiation — *see* Military operations, restriction of airways
biological weapons Y37.6X- ☑
blast Y37.20- ☑
blast fragments Y37.20- ☑
blast wave Y37.20- ☑
blast wind Y37.20- ☑
bomb Y37.20- ☑
dirty Y37.50- ☑
gasoline Y37.31- ☑
incendiary Y37.31- ☑
petrol Y37.31- ☑

Military — *continued*
bullet Y37.43- ☑
incendiary Y37.32- ☑
rubber Y37.41- ☑
chemical weapons Y37.7X- ☑
combat
hand to hand (unarmed) combat Y37.44- ☑
using blunt or piercing object Y37.45- ☑
conflagration — *see* Military operations, fire
conventional warfare NEC Y37.49- ☑
depth-charge Y37.01- ☑
destruction of aircraft Y37.10- ☑
due to
air to air missile Y37.11- ☑
collision with other aircraft Y37.12- ☑
detonation (accidental) of onboard munitions and explosives Y37.14- ☑
enemy fire or explosives Y37.11- ☑
explosive placed on aircraft Y37.11- ☑
onboard fire Y37.13- ☑
rocket propelled grenade [RPG] Y37.11- ☑
small arms fire Y37.11- ☑
surface to air missile Y37.11- ☑
specified NEC Y37.19- ☑
detonation (accidental) of
onboard marine weapons Y37.05- ☑
own munitions or munitions launch device Y37.24- ☑
dirty bomb Y37.50- ☑
explosion (of) Y37.20- ☑
aerial bomb Y37.21- ☑
bomb NOS (*see also* Military operations, bomb(s)) Y37.20- ☑
own munitions or munitions launch device (accidental) Y37.24- ☑
fragments Y37.20- ☑
grenade Y37.29- ☑
guided missile Y37.22- ☑
improvised explosive device [IED] (person-borne) (roadside) (vehicle-borne) Y37.23- ☑
land mine Y37.29- ☑
marine mine (at sea) (in harbor) Y37.02- ☑
marine weapon Y37.00- ☑
specified NEC Y37.09- ☑
sea-based artillery shell Y37.03- ☑
specified NEC Y37.29- ☑
torpedo Y37.04- ☑
fire Y37.30- ☑
specified NEC Y37.39- ☑
firearms
discharge Y37.43- ☑
pellets Y37.42- ☑
flamethrower Y37.33- ☑
fragments (from) (of)
improvised explosive device [IED] (person-borne) (roadside) (vehicle-borne) Y37.26- ☑
munitions Y37.25- ☑
specified NEC Y37.29- ☑
weapons Y37.27- ☑
friendly fire Y37.92- ☑
hand to hand (unarmed) combat Y37.44- ☑
hot substances — *see* Military operations, fire
incendiary bullet Y37.32- ☑
nuclear weapon (effects of) Y37.50- ☑
acute radiation exposure Y37.54- ☑
blast pressure Y37.51- ☑
direct blast Y37.51- ☑
direct heat Y37.53- ☑
fallout exposure Y37.54- ☑
fireball Y37.53- ☑
indirect blast (struck or crushed by blast debris) (being thrown by blast) Y37.52- ☑
ionizing radiation (immediate exposure) Y37.54- ☑
nuclear radiation Y37.54- ☑
radiation
ionizing (immediate exposure) Y37.54- ☑
nuclear Y37.54- ☑
thermal Y37.53- ☑
specified NEC Y37.59- ☑
secondary effects Y37.54- ☑
thermal radiation Y37.53- ☑
restriction of air (airway)
intentional Y37.46- ☑
unintentional Y37.47- ☑
rubber bullets Y37.41- ☑
shrapnel NOS Y37.29- ☑
suffocation — *see* Military operations, restriction of airways
unconventional warfare NEC Y37.7X- ☑

Military — *continued*
underwater blast NOS Y37.00- ☑
warfare
conventional NEC Y37.49- ☑
unconventional NEC Y37.7X- ☑
weapons
biological weapons Y37.6X- ☑
chemical Y37.7X- ☑
nuclear (effects of) Y37.50- ☑
acute radiation exposure Y37.54- ☑
blast pressure Y37.51- ☑
direct blast Y37.51- ☑
direct heat Y37.53- ☑
fallout exposure Y37.54- ☑
fireball Y37.53- ☑
indirect blast (struck or crushed by blast debris) (being thrown by blast) Y37.52- ☑
radiation
ionizing (immediate exposure) Y37.54- ☑
nuclear Y37.54- ☑
thermal Y37.53- ☑
secondary effects Y37.54- ☑
specified NEC Y37.59- ☑
of mass destruction [WMD] Y37.91- ☑
weapon of mass destruction [WMD] Y37.91- ☑
Misadventure (s) to patient(s) during surgical or medical care Y69
contaminated medical or biological substance (blood, drug, fluid) Y64.9
administered (by) NEC Y64.9
immunization Y64.1
infusion Y64.0
injection Y64.1
specified means NEC Y64.8
transfusion Y64.0
vaccination Y64.1
excessive amount of blood or other fluid during transfusion or infusion Y63.0
failure
in dosage Y63.9
electroshock therapy Y63.4
inappropriate temperature (too hot or too cold) in local application and packing Y63.5
infusion
excessive amount of fluid Y63.0
incorrect dilution of fluid Y63.1
insulin-shock therapy Y63.4
nonadministration of necessary drug or biological substance Y63.6
overdose — *see* Table of Drugs and Chemicals
radiation, in therapy Y63.2
radiation
overdose Y63.2
specified procedure NEC Y63.8
transfusion
excessive amount of blood Y63.0
mechanical, of instrument or apparatus (any) (during any procedure) Y65.8
sterile precautions (during procedure) Y62.9
aspiration of fluid or tissue (by puncture or catheterization, except heart) Y62.6
biopsy (except needle aspiration) Y62.8
needle (aspirating) Y62.6
blood sampling Y62.6
catheterization Y62.6
heart Y62.5
dialysis (kidney) Y62.2
endoscopic examination Y62.4
enema Y62.8
immunization Y62.3
infusion Y62.1
injection Y62.3
needle biopsy Y62.6
paracentesis (abdominal) (thoracic) Y62.6
perfusion Y62.2
puncture (lumbar) Y62.6
removal of catheter or packing Y62.8
specified procedure NEC Y62.8
surgical operation Y62.0
transfusion Y62.1
vaccination Y62.3
suture or ligature during surgical procedure Y65.2
to introduce or to remove tube or instrument — *see* Failure, to
hemorrhage — *see* Index to Diseases and Injuries, Complication(s)
inadvertent exposure of patient to radiation Y63.3
inappropriate

Misadventure — *continued*
  operation performed — *see* Inappropriate operation performed
  temperature (too hot or too cold) in local application or packing Y63.5
  infusion (*see also* Misadventure, by type, infusion) Y69
    excessive amount of fluid Y63.0
    incorrect dilution of fluid Y63.1
    wrong fluid Y65.1
  mismatched blood in transfusion Y65.0
  nonadministration of necessary drug or biological substance Y63.6
  overdose — *see* Table of Drugs and Chemicals
    radiation (in therapy) Y63.2
  perforation — *see* Index to Diseases and Injuries, Complication(s)
  performance of inappropriate operation — *see* Inappropriate operation performed
  puncture — *see* Index to Diseases and Injuries, Complication(s)
  specified type NEC Y65.8
    failure
      suture or ligature during surgical operation Y65.2
      to introduce or to remove tube or instrument — *see* Failure, to
    infusion of wrong fluid Y65.1
    performance of inappropriate operation — *see* Inappropriate operation performed
    transfusion of mismatched blood Y65.0
    wrong
      fluid in infusion Y65.1
      placement of endotracheal tube during anesthetic procedure Y65.3
  transfusion — *see* Misadventure, by type, transfusion
    excessive amount of blood Y63.0
    mismatched blood Y65.0
  wrong
    drug given in error — *see* Table of Drugs and Chemicals
    fluid in infusion Y65.1
    placement of endotracheal tube during anesthetic procedure Y65.3
Mismatched blood in transfusion Y65.0
Motion sickness T75.3 ☑
Mountain sickness W94.11 ☑
Mudslide (of cataclysmic nature) — *see* Landslide
Murder (attempt) — *see* Assault

N

Nail, contact with W45.0 ☑
  gun W29.4 ☑
Neglect (criminal) (homicidal intent) X58 ☑
Noise (causing injury) (pollution) W42.9 ☑
  supersonic W42.0 ☑
Nonadministration (of)
  drug or biological substance (necessary) Y63.6
  surgical and medical care Y66
Nosocomial condition Y95

O

Object
  falling
    from, in, on, hitting
      machinery — *see* Contact, with, by type of machine
  set in motion by
    accidental explosion or rupture of pressure vessel W38 ☑
    firearm — *see* Discharge, firearm, by type
    machine (ry) — *see* Contact, with, by type of machine
Overdose (drug) — *see* Table of Drugs and Chemicals
  radiation Y63.2
Overexertion Y93
Overexposure (accidental) (to)
  cold (*see also* Exposure, cold) X31 ☑
    due to man-made conditions — *see* Exposure, cold, man-made
  heat (*see also* Heat) X30 ☑
  radiation — *see* Radiation
  radioactivity W88.0 ☑
  sun (sunburn) X32 ☑

Overexposure — *continued*
  weather NEC — *see* Forces of nature
  wind NEC — *see* Forces of nature
Overheated — *see* Heat
Overturning (accidental)
  machinery — *see* Contact, with, by type of machine
  transport vehicle NEC (*see also* Accident, transport) V89.9 ☑
  watercraft (causing drowning, submersion) (*see also* Drowning, due to, accident to, watercraft, overturning)
    causing injury except drowning or submersion — *see* Accident, watercraft, causing, injury NEC

P

Parachute descent (voluntary) (without accident to aircraft) V97.29 ☑
  due to accident to aircraft — *see* Accident, transport, aircraft
Pecked by bird W61.99 ☑
Perforation during medical or surgical treatment as misadventure — *see* Index to Diseases and Injuries, Complication(s)
Perpetrator, perpetration, of assault, maltreatment and neglect (by) Y07.9
  boyfriend Y07.03
  brother Y07.410
    stepbrother Y07.435
  coach Y07.53
  cousin
    female Y07.491
    male Y07.490
  daycare provider Y07.519
    at-home
      adult care Y07.512
      childcare Y07.510
    care center
      adult care Y07.513
      childcare Y07.511
  family member NEC Y07.499
  father Y07.11
    adoptive Y07.13
    foster Y07.420
    stepfather Y07.430
  foster father Y07.420
  foster mother Y07.421
  girl friend Y07.04
  healthcare provider Y07.529
    mental health Y07.521
    specified NEC Y07.528
  husband Y07.01
  instructor Y07.53
  mother Y07.12
    adoptive Y07.14
    foster Y07.421
    stepmother Y07.433
  nonfamily member Y07.50
    specified NEC Y07.59
  nurse Y07.528
  occupational therapist Y07.528
  partner of parent
    female Y07.434
    male Y07.432
  physical therapist Y07.528
  sister Y07.411
  speech therapist Y07.528
  stepbrother Y07.435
  stepfather Y07.430
  stepmother Y07.433
  stepsister Y07.436
  teacher Y07.53
  wife Y07.02
Piercing — *see* Contact, with, by type of object or machine
Pinched
  between objects (moving) (stationary and moving) W23.0 ☑
  stationary W23.1 ☑
Pinned under machine (ry) — *see* Contact, with, by type of machine
Place of occurrence Y92.9
  abandoned house Y92.89
  airplane Y92.813
  airport Y92.520
  ambulatory health services establishment NEC Y92.538
  ambulatory surgery center Y92.530

Place — *continued*
  amusement park Y92.831
  apartment (co-op) — *see* Place of occurrence, residence, apartment
  assembly hall Y92.29
  bank Y92.510
  barn Y92.71
  baseball field Y92.320
  basketball court Y92.310
  beach Y92.832
  boarding house — *see* Place of occurrence, residence, boarding house
  boat Y92.814
  bowling alley Y92.39
  bridge Y92.89
  building under construction Y92.61
  bus Y92.811
    station Y92.521
  cafe Y92.511
  campsite Y92.833
  campus — *see* Place of occurrence, school
  canal Y92.89
  car Y92.810
  casino Y92.59
  children's home — *see* Place of occurrence, residence, institutional, orphanage
  church Y92.22
  cinema Y92.26
  clubhouse Y92.29
  coal pit Y92.64
  college (community) Y92.214
  condominium — *see* Place of occurrence, residence, apartment
  construction area — *see* Place of occurrence, industrial and construction area
  convalescent home — *see* Place of occurrence, residence, institutional, nursing home
  court-house Y92.240
  cricket ground Y92.328
  cultural building Y92.258
    art gallery Y92.250
    museum Y92.251
    music hall Y92.252
    opera house Y92.253
    specified NEC Y92.258
    theater Y92.254
  dancehall Y92.252
  day nursery Y92.210
  dentist office Y92.531
  derelict house Y92.89
  desert Y92.820
  dock NOS Y92.89
  dockyard Y92.62
  doctor's office Y92.531
  dormitory — *see* Place of occurrence, residence, institutional, school dormitory
  dry dock Y92.62
  factory (building) (premises) Y92.63
  farm (land under cultivation) (outbuildings) Y92.79
    barn Y92.71
    chicken coop Y92.72
    field Y92.73
    hen house Y92.72
    house — *see* Place of occurrence, residence, house
    orchard Y92.74
    specified NEC Y92.79
  football field Y92.321
  forest Y92.821
  freeway Y92.411
  gallery Y92.250
  garage (commercial) Y92.59
    boarding house Y92.044
    military base Y92.135
    mobile home Y92.025
    nursing home Y92.124
    orphanage Y92.114
    private house Y92.015
    reform school Y92.155
  gas station Y92.524
  gasworks Y92.69
  golf course Y92.39
  gravel pit Y92.64
  grocery Y92.512
  gymnasium Y92.39
  handball court Y92.318
  harbor Y92.89
  harness racing course Y92.39
  healthcare provider office Y92.531
  highway (interstate) Y92.411
  hill Y92.828

☑ **Additional character required**

Place — *continued*
- hockey rink Y92.330
- home — *see* Place of occurrence, residence
- hospice — *see* Place of occurrence, residence, institutional, nursing home
- hospital Y92.239
  - cafeteria Y92.233
  - corridor Y92.232
  - operating room Y92.234
  - patient
    - bathroom Y92.231
    - room Y92.230
  - specified NEC Y92.238
- hotel Y92.59
- house (*see also* Place of occurrence, residence)
  - abandoned Y92.89
  - under construction Y92.61
- industrial and construction area (yard) Y92.69
  - building under construction Y92.61
  - dock Y92.62
  - dry dock Y92.62
  - factory Y92.63
  - gasworks Y92.69
  - mine Y92.64
  - oil rig Y92.65
  - pit Y92.64
  - power station Y92.69
  - shipyard Y92.62
  - specified NEC Y92.69
  - tunnel under construction Y92.69
  - workshop Y92.69
- kindergarten Y92.211
- lacrosse field Y92.328
- lake Y92.828
- library Y92.241
- mall Y92.59
- market Y92.512
- marsh Y92.828
- military
  - base — *see* Place of occurrence, residence, institutional, military base
  - training ground Y92.84
- mine Y92.64
- mosque Y92.22
- motel Y92.59
- motorway (interstate) Y92.411
- mountain Y92.828
- movie-house Y92.26
- museum Y92.251
- music-hall Y92.252
- not applicable Y92.9
- nuclear power station Y92.69
- nursing home — *see* Place of occurrence, residence, institutional, nursing home
- office building Y92.59
- offshore installation Y92.65
- oil rig Y92.65
- old people's home — *see* Place of occurrence, residence, institutional, specified NEC
- opera-house Y92.253
- orphanage — *see* Place of occurrence, residence, institutional, orphanage
- outpatient surgery center Y92.530
- park (public) Y92.830
  - amusement Y92.831
- parking garage Y92.89
  - lot Y92.481
- pavement Y92.480
- physician office Y92.531
- polo field Y92.328
- pond Y92.828
- post office Y92.242
- power station Y92.69
- prairie Y92.828
- prison — *see* Place of occurrence, residence, institutional, prison
- public
  - administration building Y92.248
    - city hall Y92.243
    - courthouse Y92.240
    - library Y92.241
    - post office Y92.242
    - specified NEC Y92.248
  - building NEC Y92.29
  - hall Y92.29
  - place NOS Y92.89
- race course Y92.39
- radio station Y92.59
- railway line (bridge) Y92.85
- ranch (outbuildings) — *see* Place of occurrence, farm
- recreation area Y92.838

Place — *continued*
- amusement park Y92.831
- beach Y92.832
- campsite Y92.833
- park (public) Y92.830
- seashore Y92.832
- specified NEC Y92.838
- religious institution Y92.22
- reform school - — *see* Place of occurrence, residence, institutional, reform school
- residence (non-institutional) (private) Y92.009
  - apartment Y92.039
    - bathroom Y92.031
    - bedroom Y92.032
    - kitchen Y92.030
    - specified NEC Y92.038
  - bathroom Y92.002
  - bedroom Y92.003
  - boarding house Y92.049
    - bathroom Y92.041
    - bedroom Y92.042
    - driveway Y92.043
    - garage Y92.044
    - garden Y92.046
    - kitchen Y92.040
    - specified NEC Y92.048
    - swimming pool Y92.045
    - yard Y92.046
  - dining room Y92.001
  - garden Y92.007
  - home Y92.009
  - house, single family Y92.019
    - bathroom Y92.012
    - bedroom Y92.013
    - dining room Y92.011
    - driveway Y92.014
    - garage Y92.015
    - garden Y92.017
    - kitchen Y92.010
    - specified NEC Y92.018
    - swimming pool Y92.016
    - yard Y92.017
  - institutional Y92.10
    - children's home — *see* Place of occurrence, residence, institutional, orphanage
    - hospice — *see* Place of occurrence, residence, institutional, nursing home
    - military base Y92.139
      - barracks Y92.133
      - garage Y92.135
      - garden Y92.137
      - kitchen Y92.130
      - mess hall Y92.131
      - specified NEC Y92.138
      - swimming pool Y92.136
      - yard Y92.137
    - nursing home Y92.129
      - bathroom Y92.121
      - bedroom Y92.122
      - driveway Y92.123
      - garage Y92.124
      - garden Y92.126
      - kitchen Y92.120
      - specified NEC Y92.128
      - swimming pool Y92.125
      - yard Y92.126
    - orphanage Y92.119
      - bathroom Y92.111
      - bedroom Y92.112
      - driveway Y92.113
      - garage Y92.114
      - garden Y92.116
      - kitchen Y92.110
      - specified NEC Y92.118
      - swimming pool Y92.115
      - yard Y92.116
    - prison Y92.149
      - bathroom Y92.142
      - cell Y92.143
      - courtyard Y92.147
      - dining room Y92.141
      - kitchen Y92.140
      - specified NEC Y92.148
      - swimming pool Y92.146
    - reform school Y92.159
      - bathroom Y92.152
      - bedroom Y92.153
      - dining room Y92.151
      - driveway Y92.154
      - garage Y92.155
      - garden Y92.157
      - kitchen Y92.150

Place — *continued*
- specified NEC Y92.158
- swimming pool Y92.156
- yard Y92.157
- school dormitory Y92.169
  - bathroom Y92.162
  - bedroom Y92.163
  - dining room Y92.161
  - kitchen Y92.160
  - specified NEC Y92.168
- specified NEC Y92.199
  - bathroom Y92.192
  - bedroom Y92.193
  - dining room Y92.191
  - driveway Y92.194
  - garage Y92.195
  - garden Y92.197
  - kitchen Y92.190
  - specified NEC Y92.198
  - swimming pool Y92.196
  - yard Y92.197
- kitchen Y92.000
- mobile home Y92.029
  - bathroom Y92.022
  - bedroom Y92.023
  - dining room Y92.021
  - driveway Y92.024
  - garage Y92.025
  - garden Y92.027
  - kitchen Y92.020
  - specified NEC Y92.028
  - swimming pool Y92.026
  - yard Y92.027
- specified place in residence NEC Y92.008
- specified residence type NEC Y92.099
  - bathroom Y92.091
  - bedroom Y92.092
  - driveway Y92.093
  - garage Y92.094
  - garden Y92.096
  - kitchen Y92.090
  - specified NEC Y92.098
  - swimming pool Y92.095
  - yard Y92.096
- restaurant Y92.511
- riding school Y92.39
- river Y92.828
- road Y92.488
- rodeo ring Y92.39
- rugby field Y92.328
- same day surgery center Y92.530
- sand pit Y92.64
- school (private) (public) (state) Y92.219
  - college Y92.214
  - daycare center Y92.210
  - elementary school Y92.211
  - high school Y92.213
  - kindergarten Y92.211
  - middle school Y92.212
  - specified NEC Y92.218
  - trace school Y92.215
  - university Y92.214
  - vocational school Y92.215
- sea (shore) Y92.832
- senior citizen center Y92.29
- service area
  - airport Y92.520
  - bus station Y92.521
  - gas station Y92.524
  - highway rest stop Y92.523
  - railway station Y92.522
- shipyard Y92.62
- shop (commercial) Y92.513
- sidewalk Y92.480
- silo Y92.79
- skating rink (roller) Y92.331
  - ice Y92.330
- slaughter house Y92.86
- soccer field Y92.322
- specified place NEC Y92.89
- sports area Y92.39
  - athletic
    - court Y92.318
      - basketball Y92.310
      - specified NEC Y92.318
      - squash Y92.311
      - tennis Y92.312
    - field Y92.328
      - baseball Y92.320
      - cricket ground Y92.328
      - football Y92.321
      - hockey Y92.328

Place — *continued*
  soccer Y92.322
  specified NEC Y92.328
  golf course Y92.39
  gymnasium Y92.39
  riding school Y92.39
  skating rink (roller) Y92.331
  ice Y92.330
  stadium Y92.39
  swimming pool Y92.34
squash court Y92.311
stadium Y92.39
steeplechasing course Y92.39
store Y92.512
stream Y92.828
street and highway Y92.410
  bike path Y92.482
  freeway Y92.411
  highway ramp Y92.415
  interstate highway Y92.411
  local residential or business street Y92.414
  motorway Y92.411
  parkway Y92.412
  parking lot Y92.481
  sidewalk Y92.480
  specified NEC Y92.488
  state road Y92.413
subway car Y92.816
supermarket Y92.512
swamp Y92.828
swimming pool (public) Y92.34
  private (at) Y92.095
    boarding house Y92.045
    military base Y92.136
    mobile home Y92.026
    nursing home Y92.125
    orphanage Y92.115
    prison Y92.146
    reform school Y92.156
    single family residence Y92.016
synagogue Y92.22
television station Y92.59
tennis court Y92.312
theater Y92.254
trade area Y92.59
  bank Y92.510
  cafe Y92.511
  casino Y92.59
  garage Y92.59
  hotel Y92.59
  market Y92.512
  office building Y92.59
  radio station Y92.59
  restaurant Y92.511
  shop Y92.513
  shopping mall Y92.59
  store Y92.512
  supermarket Y92.512
  television station Y92.59
  warehouse Y92.59
trailer park, residential — *see* Place of occurrence, residence, mobile home
trailer site NOS Y92.89
train Y92.815
  station Y92.522
truck Y92.812
tunnel under construction Y92.69
urgent (health) care center Y92.532
university Y92.214
vehicle (transport) Y92.818
  airplane Y92.813
  boat Y92.814
  bus Y92.811
  car Y92.810
  specified NEC Y92.818
  subway car Y92.816
  train Y92.815
  truck Y92.812
warehouse Y92.59
water reservoir Y92.89
wilderness area Y92.828
  desert Y92.820
  forest Y92.821
  marsh Y92.828
  mountain Y92.828
  prairie Y92.828
  specified NEC Y92.828
  swamp Y92.828
workshop Y92.69
yard, private Y92.096
  boarding house Y92.046
  single family house Y92.017

Place — *continued*
  mobile home Y92.027
  youth center Y92.29
  zoo (zoological garden) Y92.834
Plumbism — *see* Table of Drugs and Chemicals, lead
Poisoning (accidental) (by) (*see also* Table of Drugs and Chemicals)
  by plant, thorns, spines, sharp leaves or other mechanisms NEC X58 ☑
  carbon monoxide
    generated by
      motor vehicle — *see* Accident, transport
      watercraft (in transit) (not in transit) V93.89 ☑
        ferry boat V93.81 ☑
        fishing boat V93.82 ☑
        jet skis V93.83 ☑
        liner V93.81 ☑
        merchant ship V93.80 ☑
        passenger ship V93.81 ☑
        powered craft NEC V93.83 ☑
  caused by injection of poisons into skin by plant thorns, spines, sharp leaves X58 ☑
  marine or sea plants (venomous) X58 ☑
  exhaust gas
    generated by
      motor vehicle — *see* Accident, transport
      watercraft (in transit) (not in transit) V93.89 ☑
        ferry boat V93.81 ☑
        fishing boat V93.82 ☑
        jet skis V93.83 ☑
        liner V93.81 ☑
        merchant ship V93.80 ☑
        passenger ship V93.81 ☑
        powered craft NEC V93.83 ☑
  fumes or smoke due to
    explosion (*see also* Explosion) W40.9 ☑
    fire — *see* Exposure, fire
    ignition — *see* Ignition
  gas
    in legal intervention — *see* Legal, intervention, gas
    legal execution — *see* Legal, intervention, gas
    in war operations — *see* War operations
  legal
    execution — *see* Legal, intervention, gas
    intervention
      by gas — *see* Legal, intervention, gas
      other specified means — *see* Legal, intervention, specified means NEC
Powder burn (by) (from)
  airgun W34.110 ☑
  BB gun W34.110 ☑
  firearm NEC W34.19 ☑
  gas, air or spring-operated gun NEC W34.118 ☑
  handgun W32.1 ☑
  hunting rifle W33.12 ☑
  larger firearm W33.10 ☑
    specified NEC W33.19 ☑
  machine gun W33.13 ☑
  paintball gun W34.111 ☑
  pellet gun W34.110 ☑
  shotgun W33.11 ☑
  Very pistol [flare] W34.19 ☑
Premature cessation (of) surgical and medical care Y66
Privation (food) (water) X58 ☑
Procedure (operation)
  correct, on wrong side or body part (wrong side) (wrong site) Y65.53
  intended for another patient done on wrong patient Y65.52
  performed on patient not scheduled for surgery Y65.52
  performed on wrong patient Y65.52
  wrong, performed on correct patient Y65.51
Prolonged
  sitting in transport vehicle — *see* Travel, by type of vehicle
  stay in
    high altitude as cause of anoxia, barodontalgia, barotitis or hypoxia W94.11 ☑
    weightless environment X52 ☑
Pulling, excessive Y93
Puncture, puncturing (*see also* Contact, with, by type of object or machine)
  by
    plant thorns, spines, sharp leaves or other mechanisms NEC W60 ☑
    during medical or surgical treatment as misadventure — *see* Index to Diseases and Injuries, Complication(s)

Pushed, pushing (accidental) (injury in) (overexertion) Y93
  by other person (s) (accidental) W51 ☑
    with fall W03 ☑
      due to ice or snow W00.0 ☑
    as, or caused by, a crowd or human stampede (with fall) W52 ☑
    before moving object NEC Y02.8 ☑
      motor vehicle Y02.0 ☑
      subway train Y02.1 ☑
      train Y02.1 ☑
  from
    high place NEC
      in accidental circumstances W17.89 ☑
      stated as
        intentional, homicide (attempt) Y01 ☑
        undetermined whether accidental or intentional Y30 ☑
    transport vehicle NEC (*see also* Accident, transport) V89.9 ☑
      stated as
        intentional, homicide (attempt) Y08.89 ☑

R

Radiation (exposure to)
  arc lamps W89.0 ☑
  atomic power plant (malfunction) NEC W88.1 ☑
  complication of or abnormal reaction to medical radiotherapy Y84.2
  electromagnetic, ionizing W88.0 ☑
  gamma rays W88.1 ☑
  in
    war operations (from or following nuclear explosion) — *see* War operations
  inadvertent exposure of patient (receiving test or therapy) Y63.3
  infrared (heaters and lamps) W90.1 ☑
    excessive heat from W92 ☑
  ionized, ionizing (particles, artificially accelerated) radioisotopes W88.1 ☑
    specified NEC W88.8 ☑
    x-rays W88.0 ☑
  isotopes, radioactive — *see* Radiation, radioactive isotopes
  laser (s) W90.2 ☑
    in war operations — *see* War operations
    misadventure in medical care Y63.2
  light sources (man-made visible and ultraviolet) W89.9 ☑
    natural X32 ☑
    specified NEC W89.8 ☑
    tanning bed W89.1 ☑
    welding light W89.0 ☑
  man-made visible light W89.9 ☑
    specified NEC W89.8 ☑
    tanning bed W89.1 ☑
    welding light W89.0 ☑
  microwave W90.8 ☑
  misadventure in medical or surgical procedure Y63.2
  natural NEC X39.08 ☑
    radon X39.01 ☑
  overdose (in medical or surgical procedure) Y63.2
  radar W90.0 ☑
  radioactive isotopes (any) W88.1 ☑
    atomic power plant malfunction W88.1 ☑
    misadventure in medical or surgical treatment Y63.2
  radiofrequency W90.0 ☑
  radium NEC W88.1 ☑
  sun X32 ☑
  ultraviolet (light) (man-made) W89.9 ☑
    natural X32 ☑
    specified NEC W89.8 ☑
    tanning bed W89.1 ☑
    welding light W89.0 ☑
  welding arc, torch, or light W89.0 ☑
    excessive heat from W92 ☑
  x-rays (hard) (soft) W88.0 ☑
Range disease W94.11 ☑
Rape (attempted) T74.2- ☑
Rat bite W53.11 ☑
Reaction, abnormal to medical procedure (*see also* Complication of or following, by type of procedure) Y84.9
  with misadventure — *see* Misadventure
  biologicals — *see* Table of Drugs and Chemicals
  drugs — *see* Table of Drugs and Chemicals
  vaccine — *see* Table of Drugs and Chemicals

☑ **Additional character required**

Recoil
  airgun W34.110 ☑
  BB gun W34.110 ☑
  firearm NEC W34.19 ☑
  gas, air or spring-operated gun NEC W34.118 ☑
  handgun W32.1 ☑
  hunting rifle W33.12 ☑
  larger firearm W33.10 ☑
    specified NEC W33.19 ☑
  machine gun W33.13 ☑
  paintball gun W34.111 ☑
  pellet W34.110 ☑
  shotgun W33.11 ☑
  Very pistol [flare] W34.19 ☑
Reduction in
  atmospheric pressure - — see Air, pressure, change
Rock falling on or hitting (accidentally) (person) W20.8 ☑
  in cave-in W20.0 ☑
Run over (accidentally) (by)
  animal (not being ridden) NEC W55.89 ☑
  machinery — see Contact, with, by specified type of machine
  transport vehicle NEC (see also Accident, transport) V09.9 ☑
    intentional homicide (attempt) Y03.0 ☑
    motor NEC V09.20 ☑
      intentional homicide (attempt) Y03.0 ☑
Running
  before moving object X81.8 ☑
    motor vehicle X81.0 ☑
Running off, away
  animal (being ridden) (see also Accident, transport) V80.918 ☑
    not being ridden W55.89 ☑
  animal-drawn vehicle NEC (see also Accident, transport) V80.928 ☑
  highway, road (way), street
    transport vehicle NEC (see also Accident, transport) V89.9 ☑
Rupture pressurized devices — see Explosion, by type of device

S

Saturnism — see Table of Drugs and Chemicals, lead
Scald, scalding (accidental) (by) (from) (in) X19 ☑
  air (hot) X14.1 ☑
  gases (hot) X14.1 ☑
  homicide (attempt) — see Assault, burning, hot object
  inflicted by other person
    stated as intentional, homicide (attempt) — see Assault, burning, hot object
  liquid (boiling) (hot) NEC X12 ☑
    stated as undetermined whether accidental or intentional Y27.2 ☑
    suicide (attempt) X77.2 ☑
  local application of externally applied substance in medical or surgical care Y63.5
  metal (molten) (liquid) (hot) NEC X18 ☑
  self-inflicted X77.9 ☑
    stated as undetermined whether accidental or intentional Y27.8 ☑
  steam X13.1 ☑
    assault X98.0 ☑
    stated as undetermined whether accidental or intentional Y27.0 ☑
    suicide (attempt) X77.0 ☑
  suicide (attempt) X77.9 ☑
  vapor (hot) X13.1 ☑
    assault X98.0 ☑
    stated as undetermined whether accidental or intentional Y27.0 ☑
    suicide (attempt) X77.0 ☑
Scratched by
  cat W55.03 ☑
  person (s) (accidentally) W50.4 ☑
    with intent to injure or kill Y04.0 ☑
    as, or caused by, a crowd or human stampede (with fall) W52 ☑
    assault Y04.0 ☑
    homicide (attempt) Y04.0 ☑
    in
      fight Y04.0 ☑
      legal intervention
        injuring
          bystander Y35.892 ☑
          law enforcement personnel Y35.891 ☑

Scratched — continued
        suspect Y35.893 ☑
Seasickness T75.3 ☑
Self-harm NEC (see also External cause by type, undetermined whether accidental or intentional)
  intentional — see Suicide
  poisoning NEC — see Table of drugs and biologicals, accident
Self-inflicted (injury) NEC (see also External cause by type, undetermined whether accidental or intentional)
  intentional — see Suicide
  poisoning NEC — see Table of drugs and biologicals, accident
Sequelae (of)
  accident NEC — see W00-X58 with 7th character S
  assault (homicidal) (any means) — see X92-Y08 with 7th character S
  homicide, attempt (any means) — see X92-Y08 with 7th character S
  injury undetermined whether accidentally or purposely inflicted — see Y21-Y33 with 7th character S
  intentional self-harm (classifiable to X71-X83) — see X71-X83 with 7th character S
  legal intervention — see with 7th character S Y35
  motor vehicle accident — see V00-V99 with 7th character S
  suicide, attempt (any means) — see X71-X83 with 7th character S
  transport accident — see V00-V99 with 7th character S
  war operations — see War operations
Shock
  electric — see Exposure, electric current
  from electric appliance (any) (faulty) W86.8 ☑
    domestic W86.0 ☑
    suicide (attempt) X83.1 ☑
Shooting, shot (accidental(ly)) (see also Discharge, firearm, by type)
  herself or himself — see Discharge, firearm by type, self-inflicted
  homicide (attempt) — see Discharge, firearm by type, homicide
  in war operations — see War operations
  inflicted by other person — see Discharge, firearm by type, homicide
    accidental — see Discharge, firearm, by type of firearm
  legal
    execution — see Legal, intervention, firearm
    intervention — see Legal, intervention, firearm
  self-inflicted — see Discharge, firearm by type, suicide
    accidental — see Discharge, firearm, by type of firearm
  suicide (attempt) — see Discharge, firearm by type, suicide
Shoving (accidentally) by other person — see Pushed, by other person
Sickness
  alpine W94.11 ☑
  motion — see Motion
  mountain W94.11 ☑
Sinking (accidental)
  watercraft (causing drowning, submersion) (see also Drowning, due to, accident to, watercraft, sinking)
  causing injury except drowning or submersion — see Accident, watercraft, causing, injury NEC
Siriasis X32 ☑
Slashed wrists — see Cut, self-inflicted
Slipping (accidental) (on same level) (with fall) W01.0 ☑
  on
    ice W00.0 ☑
      with skates — see Accident, transport, pedestrian, conveyance
    mud W01.0 ☑
    oil W01.0 ☑
    snow W00.0 ☑
      with skis — see Accident, transport, pedestrian, conveyance
    surface (slippery) (wet) NEC W01.0 ☑
  without fall W18.40 ☑
    due to
      specified NEC W18.49 ☑
      stepping from one level to another W10.43 ☑
      stepping into hole or opening W18.42 ☑
      stepping on object W18.41 ☑

Sliver, wood, contact with W45.8 ☑
Smoldering (due to fire) — see Exposure, fire
Sodomy (attempted) by force T74.2- ☑
Sound waves (causing injury) W42.9 ☑
  supersonic W42.0 ☑
Splinter, contact with W45.8 ☑
Stab, stabbing — see Cut
Starvation X58 ☑
Status of external cause Y99.9
  child assisting in compensated work for family Y99.8
  civilian activity done for financial or other compensation Y99.0
  civilian activity done for income or pay Y99.0
  family member assisting in compensated work for other family member Y99.8
  hobby not done for income Y99.8
  leisure activity Y99.8
  military activity Y99.1
  off-duty activity of military personnel Y99.8
  recreation or sport not for income or while a student Y99.8
  specified NEC Y99.8
  student activity Y99.8
  volunteer activity Y99.2
Stepped on
  by
    animal (not being ridden) NEC W55.89 ☑
    crowd or human stampede W52 ☑
    person W50.0 ☑
Stepping on
  object W22.8 ☑
    with fall W18.31 ☑
    sports equipment W21.9 ☑
    stationary W22.09 ☑
      sports equipment W21.89 ☑
  person W51 ☑
    by crowd or human stampede W52 ☑
  sports equipment W21.9 ☑
Sting
  arthropod, nonvenomous W57 ☑
  insect, nonvenomous W57 ☑
Storm (cataclysmic) — see Forces of nature, cataclysmic storm
Straining, excessive Y93
Strangling — see Strangulation
Strangulation (accidental) T71
Strenuous movements Y93
Striking against
  airbag (automobile) W22.10 ☑
    driver side W22.11 ☑
    front passenger side W22.12 ☑
    specified NEC W22.19 ☑
  bottom when
    diving or jumping into water (in) W16.822 ☑
      causing drowning W16.821 ☑
      from boat W16.722 ☑
        causing drowning W16.721 ☑
      natural body W16.622 ☑
        causing drowning W16.821 ☑
      swimming pool W16.522 ☑
        causing drowning W16.521 ☑
    falling into water (in) W16.322 ☑
      causing drowning W16.321 ☑
    fountain — see Striking against, bottom when, falling into water, specified NEC
    natural body W16.122 ☑
      causing drowning W16.121 ☑
    reservoir — see Striking against, bottom when, falling into water, specified NEC
    specified NEC W16.322 ☑
      causing drowning W16.321 ☑
    swimming pool W16.022 ☑
      causing drowning W16.021 ☑
  diving board (swimming-pool) W21.4 ☑
  object W22.8 ☑
    with
      drowning or submersion — see Drowning
      fall — see Fall, due to, bumping against, object
    caused by crowd or human stampede (with fall) W52 ☑
    furniture W22.03 ☑
    lamppost W22.02 ☑
    sports equipment W21.9 ☑
    stationary W22.09 ☑
      sports equipment W21.89 ☑
    wall W22.01 ☑
  person (s) W51 ☑
    with fall W03 ☑
      due to ice or snow W00.0 ☑

Striking - Stumbling

Striking — *continued*
  as, or caused by, a crowd or human stampede
    (with fall) W52 ☑
    assault Y04.2 ☑
    homicide (attempt) Y04.2 ☑
  sports equipment W21.9 ☑
  wall (when) W22.01 ☑
    diving or jumping into water (in) W16.832 ☑
      causing drowning W16.831 ☑
      swimming pool W16.532 ☑
        causing drowning W16.531 ☑
    falling into water (in) W16.332 ☑
      causing drowning W16.331 ☑
      fountain — *see* Striking against, wall when,
        falling into water, specified NEC
      natural body W16.132 ☑
        causing drowning W16.131 ☑
      reservoir — *see* Striking against, wall when,
        falling into water, specified NEC
      specified NEC W16.332 ☑
        causing drowning W16.331 ☑
      swimming pool W16.032 ☑
        causing drowning W16.031 ☑
    swimming pool (when) W22.042 ☑
      causing drowning W22.041 ☑
      diving or jumping into water W16.532 ☑
        causing drowning W16.531 ☑
      falling into water W16.032 ☑
        causing drowning W16.031 ☑

Struck (accidentally) by
  airbag (automobile) W22.10 ☑
    driver side W22.11 ☑
    front passenger side W22.12 ☑
    specified NEC W22.19 ☑
  alligator W58.02 ☑
  animal (not being ridden) NEC W55.89 ☑
  avalanche — *see* Landslide
  ball (hit) (thrown) W21.00 ☑
    assault Y08.09 ☑
    baseball W21.03 ☑
    basketball W21.05 ☑
    golf ball W21.04 ☑
    football W21.01 ☑
    soccer W21.02 ☑
    softball W21.07 ☑
    specified NEC W21.09 ☑
    volleyball W21.06 ☑
  bat or racquet
    baseball bat W21.11 ☑
      assault Y08.02 ☑
    golf club W21.13 ☑
      assault Y08.09 ☑
    specified NEC W21.19 ☑
      assault Y08.09 ☑
    tennis racquet W21.12 ☑
      assault Y08.09 ☑
  bullet (*see also* Discharge, firearm by type)
    in war operations — *see* War operations
  crocodile W58.12 ☑
  dog W54.1 ☑
  flare, Very pistol — *see* Discharge, firearm NEC
  hailstones X39.8 ☑
  hockey (ice)
    field
      puck W21.221 ☑
      stick W21.211 ☑
    puck W21.220 ☑
    stick W21.210 ☑
      assault Y08.01 ☑
  landslide — *see* Landslide
  law-enforcement agent (on duty) — *see* Legal,
    intervention, manhandling
    with blunt object — *see* Legal, intervention,
      blunt object
  lightning T75.0
    causing fire — *see* Exposure, fire
  machine — *see* Contact, with, by type of machine
  mammal NEC W55.89 ☑
    marine W56.32 ☑
  marine animal W56.82 ☑
  missile
    firearm — *see* Discharge, firearm by type
    in war operations — *see* War operations, missile
  object W22.8 ☑
    blunt W22.8 ☑
      assault Y00 ☑
      suicide (attempt) X79 ☑
      undetermined whether accidental or
        intentional Y29 ☑
    falling W20.8 ☑
      from, in, on
        building W20.1 ☑

Struck — *continued*
  burning (uncontrolled fire) X00.4 ☑
  cataclysmic
    earth surface movement NEC — *see*
      Landslide
    storm — *see* Forces of nature, cataclysmic
      storm
  cave-in W20.0 ☑
  earthquake X34 ☑
  machine (in operation) — *see* Contact,
    with, by type of machine
  structure W20.1 ☑
    burning X00.4 ☑
  transport vehicle (in motion) — *see*
    Accident, transport, by type of vehicle
  watercraft W93.49 ☑
    due to
      accident to craft V91.39 ☑
        powered craft V91.33 ☑
          ferry boat V91.31 ☑
          fishing boat V91.32 ☑
          jetskis V91.33 ☑
          liner V91.31 ☑
          merchant ship V91.30 ☑
          passenger ship V91.31 ☑
        unpowered craft V91.38 ☑
          canoe V91.35 ☑
          inflatable V91.36 ☑
          kayak V91.35 ☑
          sailboat V91.34 ☑
          surf-board V91.38 ☑
          windsurfer V91.38 ☑
      powered craft V93.43 ☑
        ferry boat V93.41 ☑
        fishing boat V93.42 ☑
        jetskis V93.43 ☑
        liner V93.41 ☑
        merchant ship V93.40 ☑
        passenger ship V93.41 ☑
      unpowered craft V93.48 ☑
        sailboat V93.44 ☑
        surf-board V93.48 ☑
        windsurfer V93.48 ☑
  moving NEC W20.8 ☑
  projected W20.8 ☑
    assault Y00 ☑
    in sports W21.9 ☑
      assault Y08.09 ☑
    ball W21.00 ☑
      baseball W21.03 ☑
      basketball W21.05 ☑
      football W21.01 ☑
      golf ball W21.04 ☑
      soccer W21.02 ☑
      softball W21.07 ☑
      specified NEC W21.09 ☑
      volleyball W21.06 ☑
    bat or racquet
      baseball bat W21.11 ☑
        assault Y08.02 ☑
      golf club W21.13 ☑
        assault Y08.09 ☑
      specified NEC W21.19 ☑
        assault Y08.09 ☑
      tennis racquet W21.12 ☑
        assault Y08.09 ☑
    hockey (ice)
      field
        puck W21.221 ☑
        stick W21.211 ☑
      puck W21.220 ☑
      stick W21.210 ☑
        assault Y08.01 ☑
    specified NEC W21.89 ☑
  set in motion by explosion — *see* Explosion
  thrown W20.8 ☑
    assault Y00 ☑
    in sports W21.9 ☑
      assault Y08.09 ☑
    ball W21.00 ☑
      baseball W21.03 ☑
      basketball W21.05 ☑
      football W21.01 ☑
      golf ball W21.04 ☑
      soccer W21.02 ☑
      soft ball W21.07 ☑
      specified NEC W21.09 ☑
      volleyball W21.06 ☑
    bat or racquet
      baseball bat W21.11 ☑
        assault Y08.02 ☑
      golf club W21.13 ☑

Struck — *continued*
      assault Y08.09 ☑
      specified NEC W21.19 ☑
        assault Y08.09 ☑
      tennis racquet W21.12 ☑
        assault Y08.09 ☑
    hockey (ice)
      field
        puck W21.221 ☑
        stick W21.211 ☑
      puck W21.220 ☑
      stick W21.210 ☑
        assault Y08.01 ☑
    specified NEC W21.89 ☑
  other person (s) W50.0 ☑
    with
      blunt object W22.8 ☑
        intentional, homicide (attempt) Y00 ☑
        sports equipment W21.9 ☑
        undetermined whether accidental or
          intentional Y29 ☑
      fall W03 ☑
        due to ice or snow W00.0 ☑
    as, or caused by, a crowd or human stampede
      (with fall) W52 ☑
    assault Y04.2 ☑
    homicide (attempt) Y04.2 ☑
    in legal intervention
      injuring
        bystander Y35.812 ☑
        law enforcement personnel Y35.811 ☑
        suspect Y35.813 ☑
    sports equipment W21.9 ☑
  police (on duty) — *see* Legal, intervention,
    manhandling
    with blunt object — *see* Legal, intervention,
      blunt object
  sports equipment W21.9 ☑
    assault Y08.09 ☑
    ball W21.00 ☑
      baseball W21.03 ☑
      basketball W21.05 ☑
      football W21.01 ☑
      golf ball W21.04 ☑
      soccer W21.02 ☑
      soft ball W21.07 ☑
      specified NEC W21.09 ☑
      volleyball W21.06 ☑
    bat or racquet
      baseball bat W21.11 ☑
        assault Y08.02 ☑
      golf club W21.13 ☑
        assault Y08.09 ☑
      specified NEC W21.19 ☑
      tennis racquet W21.12 ☑
        assault Y08.09 ☑
    cleats (shoe) W21.31 ☑
    foot wear NEC W21.39 ☑
    football helmet W21.81 ☑
    hockey (ice)
      field
        puck W21.221 ☑
        stick W21.211 ☑
      puck W21.220 ☑
      stick W21.210 ☑
        assault Y08.01 ☑
    skate blades W21.32 ☑
    specified NEC W21.89 ☑
      assault Y08.09 ☑
  thunderbolt T75.0
    causing fire — *see* Exposure, fire
  transport vehicle NEC (*see also* Accident,
    transport) V09.9 ☑
    intentional, homicide (attempt) Y03.0 ☑
    motor NEC (*see also* Accident, transport) V09.20
      ☑
      homicide Y03.0 ☑
  vehicle (transport) NEC — *see* Accident, transport,
    by type of vehicle
    stationary (falling from jack, hydraulic lift,
      ramp) W20.8 ☑

Stumbling
  over
    animal NEC W01.0 ☑
      with fall W18.09 ☑
    carpet, rug or (small) object W22.8 ☑
      with fall W18.09 ☑
    person W51 ☑
      with fall W03 ☑
        due to ice or snow W00.0 ☑
  without fall W18.40 ☑
    due to

☑ **Additional character required**

Stumbling — *continued*
    specified NEC W18.49 ☑
    stepping from one level to another W18.43 ☑
    stepping into hole or opening W18.42 ☑
    stepping on object W18.41 ☑
Submersion (accidental) — *see* Drowning
Suffocation (accidental) (by external means) (by pressure) (mechanical) (*see also* category) T71 ☑
    due to, by
        avalanche — *see* Landslide
        explosion — *see* Explosion
        fire — *see* Exposure, fire
        food, any type (aspiration) (ingestion) (inhalation) — *see* categories T17 and T18 ☑
        ignition — *see* Ignition
        landslide — *see* Landslide
        machine (ry) — *see* Contact, with, by type of machine
        vomitus (aspiration) (inhalation) T17.81- ☑
    in
        burning building X00.8 ☑
Suicide, suicidal (attempted) (by) X83.8 ☑
    blunt object X79 ☑
    burning, burns X76 ☑
        hot object X77.9 ☑
            fluid NEC X77.2 ☑
            household appliance X77.3 ☑
            specified NEC X77.8 ☑
            steam X77.0 ☑
            tap water X77.1 ☑
            vapors X77.0 ☑
    caustic substance — *see* Table of Drugs and Chemicals
    cold, extreme X83.2 ☑
    collision of motor vehicle with
        motor vehicle X82.0 ☑
        specified NEC X82.8 ☑
        train X82.1 ☑
        tree X82.2 ☑
    crashing of aircraft X83.0 ☑
    cut (any part of body) X78.9 ☑
    cutting or piercing instrument X78.9 ☑
        dagger X78.2 ☑
        glass X78.0 ☑
        knife X78.1 ☑
        specified NEC X78.8 ☑
        sword X78.2 ☑
    drowning (in) X71.9 ☑
        bathtub X71.0 ☑
        natural water X71.3 ☑
        specified NEC X71.8 ☑
        swimming pool X71.1 ☑
            following fall X71.2 ☑
    electrocution X83.1 ☑
    explosive (s) (material) X75 ☑
    fire, flames X76 ☑
    firearm X74.9 ☑
        airgun X74.01 ☑
        handgun X72 ☑
        hunting rifle X73.1 ☑
        larger X73.9 ☑
            specified NEC X73.8 ☑
        machine gun X73.2 ☑
        shotgun X73.0 ☑
        specified NEC X74.8 ☑
    hanging X83.8 ☑
    hot object — *see* Suicide, burning, hot object
    jumping
        before moving object X81.8 ☑
            motor vehicle X81.0 ☑
            subway train X81.1 ☑
            train X81.1 ☑
        from high place X80 ☑
    late effect of attempt — *see* X71-X83 with 7th character S
    lying before moving object, train, vehicle X81.8 ☑
    poisoning — *see* Table of Drugs and Chemicals
    puncture (any part of body) — *see* Suicide, cutting or piercing instrument
    scald — *see* Suicide, burning, hot object
    sequelae of attempt — *see* X71-X83 with 7th character S
    sharp object (any) — *see* Suicide, cutting or piercing instrument
    shooting — *see* Suicide, firearm
    specified means NEC X83.8 ☑
    stab (any part of body) — *see* Suicide, cutting or piercing instrument
    steam, hot vapors X77.0 ☑
    strangulation X83.8 ☑
    submersion — *see* Suicide, drowning

Suicide — *continued*
    suffocation X83.8 ☑
    wound NEC X83.8 ☑
Sunstroke X32 ☑
Supersonic waves (causing injury) W42.0 ☑
Surgical procedure, complication of (delayed or as an abnormal reaction without mention of misadventure) (*see also* Complication of or following, by type of procedure)
    due to or as a result of misadventure — *see* Misadventure
Swallowed, swallowing
    foreign body — *see* Foreign body, alimentary canal
    poison — *see* Table of Drugs and Chemicals
    substance
        caustic or corrosive — *see* Table of Drugs and Chemicals
        poisonous — *see* Table of Drugs and Chemicals

T

Tackle in sport W03 ☑
Terrorism (involving) Y38.80 ☑
    biological weapons Y38.6X- ☑
    chemical weapons Y38.7X- ☑
    conflagration Y38.3X- ☑
    drowning and submersion Y38.89- ☑
    explosion Y38.2X- ☑
        destruction of aircraft Y38.1X- ☑
        marine weapons Y38.0X- ☑
    fire Y38.3X- ☑
    firearms Y38.4X- ☑
    hot substances Y38.5X- ☑
    lasers Y38.89- ☑
    nuclear weapons Y38.5X- ☑
    piercing or stabbing instruments Y38.89- ☑
    secondary effects Y38.9X- ☑
    specified method NEC Y38.89- ☑
    suicide bomber Y38.81- ☑
Thirst X58 ☑
Threat to breathing
    aspiration — *see* Aspiration
    due to cave-in, falling earth or substance NEC T71 ☑
Thrown (accidentally)
    against part (any) of or object in transport vehicle (in motion) NEC (*see also* Accident, transport)
    from
        high place, homicide (attempt) Y01 ☑
        machinery — *see* Contact, with, by type of machine
        transport vehicle NEC (*see also* Accident, transport) V89.9 ☑
    off — *see* Thrown, from
Thunderbolt T75.0
    causing fire — *see* Exposure, fire
Tidal wave (any injury) NEC — *see* Forces of nature, tidal wave
Took
    overdose (drug) — *see* Table of Drugs and Chemicals
    poison — *see* Table of Drugs and Chemicals
Tornado (any injury) X37.1 ☑
Torrential rain (any injury) X37.8 ☑
Torture X58 ☑
Trampled by animal NEC W55.89 ☑
Trapped (accidentally)
    between objects (moving) (stationary and moving) — *see* Caught
    by part (any) of
        motorcycle V29.88 ☑
        pedal cycle V19.88 ☑
        transport vehicle NEC (*see also* Accident, transport) V89.9 ☑
Travel (effects) (sickness) T75.3 ☑
Tree falling on or hitting (accidentally) (person) W20.8 ☑
Tripping
    over
        animal W01.0 ☑
            with fall W01.0 ☑
        carpet, rug or (small) object W22.8 ☑
            with fall W18.09 ☑
        person W51 ☑
            with fall W03 ☑
                due to ice or snow W00.0 ☑
    without fall W18.40 ☑
        due to
            specified NEC W18.49 ☑
            stepping from one level to another W18.43 ☑

Tripping — *continued*
    stepping into hole or opening W18.42 ☑
    stepping on object W18.41 ☑
Twisted by person (s) (accidentally) W50.2 ☑
    with intent to injure or kill Y04.0 ☑
    as, or caused by, a crowd or human stampede (with fall) W52 ☑
    assault Y04.0 ☑
    homicide (attempt) Y04.0 ☑
    in
        fight Y04.0 ☑
        legal intervention — *see* Legal, intervention, manhandling
Twisting, excessive Y93

U

Underdosing of necessary drugs, medicaments or biological substances Y63.6
Undetermined intent (contact) (exposure)
    automobile collision Y32 ☑
    blunt object Y29 ☑
    drowning (submersion) (in) Y21.9 ☑
        bathtub Y21.0 ☑
            after fall Y21.1 ☑
        natural water (lake) (ocean) (pond) (river) (stream) Y21.4 ☑
        specified place NEC Y21.8 ☑
        swimming pool Y21.2 ☑
            after fall Y21.3 ☑
    explosive material Y25 ☑
    fall, jump or push from high place Y30 ☑
    falling, lying or running before moving object Y31 ☑
    fire Y26 ☑
    firearm discharge Y24.9 ☑
        airgun (BB) (pellet) Y24.0 ☑
        handgun (pistol) (revolver) Y22 ☑
        hunting rifle Y23.1 ☑
        larger Y23.9 ☑
            hunting rifle Y23.1 ☑
            machine gun Y23.3 ☑
            military Y23.2 ☑
            shotgun Y23.0 ☑
            specified type NEC Y23.8 ☑
        machine gun Y23.3 ☑
        military Y23.2 ☑
        shotgun Y23.0 ☑
        specified type NEC Y24.8 ☑
        Very pistol Y24.8 ☑
    hot object Y27.9 ☑
        fluid NEC Y27.2 ☑
        household appliance Y27.3 ☑
        specified object NEC Y27.8 ☑
        steam Y27.0 ☑
        tap water Y27.1 ☑
        vapor Y27.0 ☑
    jump, fall or push from high place Y30 ☑
    lying, falling or running before moving object Y31 ☑
    motor vehicle crash Y32 ☑
    push, fall or jump from high place Y30 ☑
    running, falling or lying before moving object Y31 ☑
    sharp object Y28.9 ☑
        dagger Y28.2 ☑
        glass Y28.0 ☑
        knife Y28.1 ☑
        specified object NEC Y28.8 ☑
        sword Y28.2 ☑
    smoke Y26 ☑
    specified event NEC Y33 ☑

V

Vibration (causing injury) W49.9 ☑
Victim (of)
    avalanche — *see* Landslide
    earth movements NEC — *see* Forces of nature, earth movement
    earthquake X34 ☑
    flood — *see* Flood
    landslide — *see* Landslide
    lightning T75.0
        causing fire — *see* Exposure, fire
    storm (cataclysmic) NEC — *see* Forces of nature, cataclysmic storm
    volcanic eruption X35 ☑

Volcanic eruption (any injury) X35 ☑
Vomitus, gastric contents in air passages (with asphyxia, obstruction or suffocation) T17.81- ☑

W

Walked into stationary object (any) W22.09 ☑
  furniture W22.03 ☑
  lamppost W22.02 ☑
  wall W22.01 ☑
War operations (injuries to military personnel and civilians during war, civil insurrection and peacekeeping missions) (by) (from) (involving) Y36.90 ☑
  after cessation of hostilities Y36.89- ☑
    explosion (of)
      bomb placed during war operations Y36.82- ☑
      mine placed during war operations Y36.81- ☑
    specified NEC Y36.88- ☑
  air blast Y36.20- ☑
  aircraft
    destruction — see War operations, destruction of aircraft
    airway restriction — see War operations, restriction of airways
  asphyxiation — see War operations, restriction of airways
  biological weapons Y36.6X- ☑
  blast Y36.20- ☑
  blast fragments Y36.20- ☑
  blast wave Y36.20- ☑
  blast wind Y36.20- ☑
  bomb Y36.20- ☑
    dirty Y36.50- ☑
    gasoline Y36.31- ☑
    incendiary Y36.31- ☑
    petrol Y36.31- ☑
  bullet Y36.43- ☑
    incendiary Y36.32- ☑
    rubber Y36.41- ☑
  chemical weapons Y36.7X- ☑
  combat
    hand to hand (unarmed) combat Y36.44- ☑
    using blunt or piercing object Y36.45- ☑
  conflagration — see War operations, fire
  conventional warfare NEC Y36.49- ☑
  depth-charge Y36.01- ☑
  destruction of aircraft Y36.10- ☑
    due to
      air to air missile Y36.11- ☑
      collision with other aircraft Y36.12- ☑
      detonation (accidental) of onboard munitions and explosives Y36.14- ☑
      enemy fire or explosives Y36.11- ☑
      explosive placed on aircraft Y36.11- ☑
      onboard fire Y36.13- ☑
      rocket propelled grenade [RPG] Y36.11- ☑

War — continued
    small arms fire Y36.11- ☑
    surface to air missile Y36.11- ☑
    specified NEC Y36.19- ☑
  detonation (accidental) of
    onboard marine weapons Y36.05- ☑
    own munitions or munitions launch device Y36.24- ☑
  dirty bomb Y36.50- ☑
  explosion (of) Y36.20- ☑
    after cessation of hostilities
      bomb placed during war operations Y36.82- ☑
      mine placed during war operations Y36.81- ☑
    aerial bomb Y36.21- ☑
    bomb NOS (see also War operations, bomb(s)) Y36.20- ☑
    own munitions or munitions launch device (accidental) Y36.24- ☑
    fragments Y36.20- ☑
    grenade Y36.29- ☑
    guided missile Y36.22- ☑
    improvised explosive device [IED] (person-borne) (roadside) (vehicle-borne) Y36.23- ☑
    land mine Y36.29- ☑
    marine mine (at sea) (in harbor) Y36.02- ☑
    marine weapon Y36.00- ☑
      specified NEC Y36.09- ☑
    sea-based artillery shell Y36.03- ☑
    specified NEC Y36.29- ☑
    torpedo Y36.04- ☑
  fire Y36.30- ☑
    specified NEC Y36.39- ☑
  firearms
    discharge Y36.43- ☑
    pellets Y36.42- ☑
  flamethrower Y36.33- ☑
  fragments (from) (of)
    improvised explosive device [IED] (person-borne) (roadside) (vehicle-borne) Y36.26- ☑
    munitions Y36.25- ☑
    specified NEC Y36.29- ☑
    weapons Y36.27- ☑
  friendly fire Y36.92 ☑
  hand to hand (unarmed) combat Y36.44- ☑
  hot substances — see War operations, fire
  incendiary bullet Y36.32- ☑
  nuclear weapon (effects of) Y36.50- ☑
    acute radiation exposure Y36.54- ☑
    blast pressure Y36.51- ☑
    direct blast Y36.51- ☑
    direct heat Y36.53- ☑
    fallout exposure Y36.54- ☑
    fireball Y36.53- ☑
    indirect blast (struck or crushed by blast debris) (being thrown by blast) Y36.52- ☑
    ionizing radiation (immediate exposure) Y36.54- ☑

War — continued
  nuclear radiation Y36.54- ☑
  radiation
    ionizing (immediate exposure) Y36.54- ☑
    nuclear Y36.54- ☑
    thermal Y36.53- ☑
    specified NEC Y36.59- ☑
    secondary effects Y36.54- ☑
    thermal radiation Y36.53- ☑
  restriction of air (airway)
    intentional Y36.46- ☑
    unintentional Y36.47- ☑
  rubber bullets Y36.41- ☑
  shrapnel NOS Y36.29- ☑
  suffocation — see War operations, restriction of airways
  unconventional warfare NEC Y36.7X- ☑
  underwater blast NOS Y36.00- ☑
  warfare
    conventional NEC Y36.49- ☑
    unconventional NEC Y36.7X- ☑
  weapons
    biological weapons Y36.6X- ☑
    chemical Y36.7X- ☑
    nuclear (effects of) Y36.50- ☑
      acute radiation exposure Y36.54- ☑
      blast pressure Y36.51- ☑
      direct blast Y36.51- ☑
      direct heat Y36.53- ☑
      fallout exposure Y36.54- ☑
      fireball Y36.53- ☑
      indirect blast (struck or crushed by blast debris) (being thrown by blast) Y36.52- ☑
      radiation
        ionizing (immediate exposure) Y36.54- ☑
        nuclear Y36.54- ☑
        thermal Y36.53- ☑
      secondary effects Y36.54- ☑
      specified NEC Y36.59- ☑
    of mass destruction [WMD] Y36.91 ☑
  weapon of mass destruction [WMD] Y36.91 ☑
Washed
  away by flood — see Flood
  off road by storm (transport vehicle) — see Forces of nature, cataclysmic storm
Weather exposure NEC — see Forces of nature
Weightlessness (causing injury) (effects of) (in spacecraft, real or simulated) X52 ☑
Work related condition Y99.0
Wound (accidental) NEC (see also Injury) X58 ☑
  battle (see also War operations) Y36.90 ☑
  gunshot — see Discharge, firearm by type
Wreck transport vehicle NEC (see also Accident, transport) V89.9 ☑
Wrong
  device implanted into correct surgical site Y65.51
  fluid in infusion Y65.1
  procedure (operation) on correct patient Y65.51
  patient, procedure performed on Y65.52

☑ **Additional character required**

Chapter 1: Certain Infectious and Parasitic Diseases (A00-B99)

Chapter Specific Coding Guidelines

a. **Human Immunodeficiency Virus (HIV) Infections**
   1) **Code only confirmed cases**

   Code only confirmed cases of HIV infection/illness. This is an exception to the hospital inpatient guideline Section II, H.

   In this context, "confirmation" does not require documentation of positive serology or culture for HIV; the provider's diagnostic statement that the patient is HIV positive, or has an HIV-related illness is sufficient.

   2) **Selection and sequencing of HIV codes**
      (a) **Patient admitted for HIV-related condition**

      If a patient is admitted for an HIV-related condition, the principal diagnosis should be B20, Human immunodeficiency virus [HIV] disease followed by additional diagnosis codes for all reported HIV-related conditions.

      (b) **Patient with HIV disease admitted for unrelated condition**

      If a patient with HIV disease is admitted for an unrelated condition (such as a traumatic injury), the code for the unrelated condition (e.g., the nature of injury code) should be the principal diagnosis. Other diagnoses would be B20 followed by additional diagnosis codes for all reported HIV-related conditions.

      (c) **Whether the patient is newly diagnosed**

      Whether the patient is newly diagnosed or has had previous admissions/encounters for HIV conditions is irrelevant to the sequencing decision.

      (d) **Asymptomatic human immunodeficiency virus**

      Z21, Asymptomatic human immunodeficiency virus [HIV] infection status, is to be applied when the patient without any documentation of symptoms is listed as being "HIV positive," "known HIV," "HIV test positive," or similar terminology. Do not use this code if the term "AIDS" is used or if the patient is treated for any HIV-related illness or is described as having any condition(s) resulting from his/her HIV positive status; use B20 in these cases.

      (e) **Patients with inconclusive HIV serology**

      Patients with inconclusive HIV serology, but no definitive diagnosis or manifestations of the illness, may be assigned code R75, Inconclusive laboratory evidence of human immunodeficiency virus [HIV].

      (f) **Previously diagnosed HIV-related illness**

      Patients with any known prior diagnosis of an HIV-related illness should be coded to B20. Once a patient has developed an HIV-related illness, the patient should always be assigned code B20 on every subsequent admission/encounter. Patients previously diagnosed with any HIV illness (B20) should never be assigned to R75 or Z21, Asymptomatic human immunodeficiency virus [HIV] infection status.

      (g) **HIV Infection in pregnancy, childbirth and the puerperium**

      During pregnancy, childbirth or the puerperium, a patient admitted (or presenting for a health care encounter) because of an HIV-related illness should receive a principal diagnosis code of O98.7-, Human immunodeficiency [HIV] disease complicating pregnancy, childbirth and the puerperium, followed by B20 and the code(s) for the HIV-related illness(es). Codes from Chapter 15 always take sequencing priority.

      Patients with asymptomatic HIV infection status admitted (or presenting for a health care encounter) during pregnancy, childbirth, or the puerperium should receive codes of O98.7- and Z21.

      (h) **Encounters for testing for HIV**

      If a patient is being seen to determine his/her HIV status, use code Z11.4, Encounter for screening for human immunodeficiency virus [HIV]. Use additional codes for any associated high risk behavior.

      If a patient with signs or symptoms is being seen for HIV testing, code the signs and symptoms. An additional counseling code Z71.7, Human immunodeficiency virus [HIV] counseling, may be used if counseling is provided during the encounter for the test.

      When a patient returns to be informed of his/her HIV test results and the test result is negative, use code Z71.7, Human immunodeficiency virus [HIV] counseling.

      If the results are positive, see previous guidelines and assign codes as appropriate.

b. **Infectious Agents as the Cause of Diseases Classified to Other Chapters**

   Certain infections are classified in chapters other than Chapter 1 and no organism is identified as part of the infection code. In these instances, it is necessary to use an additional code from Chapter 1 to identify the organism. A code from category B95, Streptococcus, Staphylococcus, and Enterococcus as the cause of diseases classified to other chapters, B96, Other bacterial agents as the cause of diseases classified to other chapters, or B97, Viral agents as the cause of diseases classified to other chapters, is to be used as an additional code to identify the organism. An instructional note will be found at the infection code advising that an additional organism code is required.

c. **Infections Resistant to Antibiotics**

   Many bacterial infections are resistant to current antibiotics. It is necessary to identify all infections documented as antibiotic resistant. Assign a code from category Z16, Resistance to antimicrobial drugs, following the infection code only if the infection code does not identify drug resistance.

d. **Sepsis, Severe Sepsis, and Septic Shock**
   1) **Coding of Sepsis and Severe Sepsis**
      (a) **Sepsis**

      For a diagnosis of sepsis, assign the appropriate code for the underlying systemic infection. If the type of infection or causal organism is not further specified, assign code A41.9, Sepsis, unspecified organism.

      A code from subcategory R65.2, Severe sepsis, should not be assigned unless severe sepsis or an associated acute organ dysfunction is documented.

      (i) Negative or inconclusive blood cultures and sepsis

      Negative or inconclusive blood cultures do not preclude a diagnosis of sepsis in patients with clinical evidence of the condition, however, the provider should be queried.

      (ii) Urosepsis

      The term urosepsis is a nonspecific term. It is not to be considered synonymous with sepsis. It has no default code in the Alphabetic Index. Should a provider use this term, he/she must be queried for clarification.

      (iii) Sepsis with organ dysfunction

      If a patient has sepsis and associated acute organ dysfunction or multiple organ dysfunction (MOD), follow the instructions for coding severe sepsis.

      (iv) Acute organ dysfunction that is not clearly associated with the sepsis

If a patient has sepsis and an acute organ dysfunction, but the medical record documentation indicates that the acute organ dysfunction is related to a medical condition other than the sepsis, do not assign a code from subcategory R65.2, Severe sepsis. An acute organ dysfunction must be associated with the sepsis in order to assign the severe sepsis code. If the documentation is not clear as to whether an acute organ dysfunction is related to the sepsis or another medical condition, query the provider.

(b) **Severe sepsis**

The coding of severe sepsis requires a minimum of 2 codes: first a code for the underlying systemic infection, followed by a code from subcategory R65.2, Severe sepsis. If the causal organism is not documented, assign code A41.9, Sepsis, unspecified organism, for the infection. Additional code(s) for the associated acute organ dysfunction are also required.

Due to the complex nature of severe sepsis, some cases may require querying the provider prior to assignment of the codes.

2) **Septic Shock**
(a) Septic shock generally refers to circulatory failure associated with severe sepsis, and therefore, it represents a type of acute organ dysfunction.

For cases of septic shock, the code for the systemic infection should be sequenced first, followed by code R65.21, Severe sepsis with septic shock or code T81.12, Postprocedural septic shock. Any additional codes for the other acute organ dysfunctions should also be assigned. As noted in the sequencing instructions in the Tabular List, the code for septic shock cannot be assigned as a principal diagnosis.

3) **Sequencing of Severe Sepsis**
If severe sepsis is present on admission, and meets the definition of principal diagnosis, the underlying systemic infection should be assigned as principal diagnosis followed by the appropriate code from subcategory R65.2 as required by the sequencing rules in the Tabular List. A code from subcategory R65.2 can never be assigned as a principal diagnosis.

When severe sepsis develops during an encounter (it was not present on admission) the underlying systemic infection and the appropriate code from subcategory R65.2 should be assigned as secondary diagnoses.

Severe sepsis may be present on admission but the diagnosis may not be confirmed until sometime after admission. If the documentation is not clear whether severe sepsis was present on admission, the provider should be queried.

4) **Sepsis and Severe Sepsis with a Localized Infection**
If the reason for admission is both sepsis or severe sepsis and a localized infection, such as pneumonia or cellulitis, a code(s) for the underlying systemic infection should be assigned first and the code for the localized infection should be assigned as a secondary diagnosis. If the patient has severe sepsis, a code from subcategory R65.2 should also be assigned as a secondary diagnosis. If the patient is admitted with a localized infection, such as pneumonia, and sepsis/severe sepsis doesn't develop until after admission, the localized infection should be assigned first, followed by the appropriate sepsis/severe sepsis codes.

5) **Sepsis Due to a Postprocedural Infection**
(a) **Documentation of causal relationship**

As with all postprocedural complications, code assignment is based on the provider's documentation of the relationship between the infection and the procedure.

(b) **Sepsis due to a postprocedural infection**

For such cases, the postprocedural infection code, such as, T80.2, Infections following infusion, transfusion, and therapeutic injection, T81.4, Infection following a procedure, T88.0, Infection following immunization, or O86.0, Infection of obstetric surgical wound, should be coded first, followed by the code for the specific infection. If the patient has severe sepsis the appropriate code from subcategory R65.2 should also be assigned with the additional code(s) for any acute organ dysfunction.

(c) **Postprocedural infection and postprocedural septic shock**

In cases where a postprocedural infection has occurred and has resulted in severe sepsis and postprocedural septic shock, the code for the precipitating complication such as code T81.4, Infection following a procedure, or O86.0, Infection of obstetrical surgical wound should be coded first followed by code R65.21, Severe sepsis with septic shock and a code for the systemic infection.

6) **Sepsis and severe sepsis associated with a noninfectious process (condition)**
In some cases a noninfectious process (condition), such as trauma, may lead to an infection which can result in sepsis or severe sepsis. If sepsis or severe sepsis is documented as associated with a noninfectious condition, such as a burn or serious injury, and this condition meets the definition for principal diagnosis, the code for the noninfectious condition should be sequenced first, followed by the code for the resulting infection. If severe sepsis, is present a code from subcategory R65.2 should also be assigned with any associated organ dysfunction(s) codes. It is not necessary to assign a code from subcategory R65.1, Systemic inflammatory response syndrome (SIRS) of non-infectious origin, for these cases.

If the infection meets the definition of principal diagnosis it should be sequenced before the non-infectious condition. When both the associated non-infectious condition and the infection meet the definition of principal diagnosis either may be assigned as principal diagnosis.

Only one code from category R65, Symptoms and signs specifically associated with systemic inflammation and infection, should be assigned. Therefore, when a non-infectious condition leads to an infection resulting in severe sepsis, assign the appropriate code from subcategory R65.2, Severe sepsis. Do not additionally assign a code from subcategory R65.1, Systemic inflammatory response syndrome (SIRS) of non-infectious origin.

See Section I.C.18. SIRS due to non-infectious process

7) **Sepsis and septic shock complicating abortion, pregnancy, childbirth, and the puerperium**
See Section I.C.15. Sepsis and septic shock complicating abortion, pregnancy, childbirth and the puerperium

8) **Newborn sepsis**
See Section I.C.16. f. Bacterial sepsis of Newborn

e. **Methicillin Resistant Staphylococcus aureus (MRSA) Conditions**
1) **Selection and sequencing of MRSA codes**
(a) **Combination codes for MRSA infection**

When a patient is diagnosed with an infection that is due to methicillin resistant *Staphylococcus aureus* (MRSA), and that infection has a combination code that includes the causal organism (e.g., sepsis, pneumonia) assign the appropriate combination code for the condition (e.g., code A41.02, Sepsis due to Methicillin resistant Staphylococcus aureus or code J15.212, Pneumonia due to Methicillin resistant Staphylococcus aureus). Do not assign code B95.62, Methicillin resistant Staphylococcus aureus infection as the cause of diseases classified elsewhere, as an additional code because the combination code includes the type of infection and the MRSA organism. Do not assign a code from subcategory Z16.11, Resistance to penicillins, as an additional diagnosis.

See Section C.1. for instructions on coding and sequencing of sepsis and severe sepsis.

(b) **Other codes for MRSA infection**

When there is documentation of a current infection (e.g., wound infection, stitch abscess, urinary tract infection) due to MRSA, and that infection does not have a combination code that includes the causal organism, assign the appropriate code to identify the condition along with code B95.62, Methicillin resistant Staphylococcus aureus infection as the cause of diseases classified elsewhere for the MRSA infection. Do not assign a code from subcategory Z16.11, Resistance to penicillins.

(c) **Methicillin susceptible Staphylococcus aureus (MSSA) and MRSA colonization**

The condition or state of being colonized or carrying MSSA or MRSA is called colonization or carriage, while an individual person is described as being colonized or being a carrier. Colonization means that MSSA or MSRA is present on or in the body without necessarily causing illness. A positive MRSA colonization test might be documented by the provider as "MRSA screen positive" or "MRSA nasal swab positive".

Assign code Z22.322, Carrier or suspected carrier of Methicillin resistant Staphylococcus aureus, for patients documented as having MRSA colonization. Assign code Z22.321, Carrier or suspected carrier of Methicillin susceptible Staphylococcus aureus, for patient documented as having MSSA colonization. Colonization is not necessarily indicative of a disease process or as the cause of a specific condition the patient may have unless documented as such by the provider.

(d) **MRSA colonization and infection**

If a patient is documented as having both MRSA colonization and infection during a hospital admission, code Z22.322, Carrier or suspected carrier of Methicillin resistant Staphylococcus aureus, and a code for the MRSA infection may both be assigned.

This page intentionally left blank

Certain infectious and parasitic diseases (A00-B99)

[INCLUDES] *diseases generally recognized as communicable or transmissible*

Use additional code to identify resistance to antimicrobial drugs (Z16.-)

[EXCLUDES1] *certain localized infections - see body system-related chapters*

[EXCLUDES2] *carrier or suspected carrier of infectious disease (Z22.-)*
infectious and parasitic diseases complicating pregnancy, childbirth and the puerperium (O98.-)
infectious and parasitic diseases specific to the perinatal period (P35-P39)
influenza and other acute respiratory infections (J00-J22)

Intestinal infectious diseases (A00-A09)

[4] **A00 Cholera**
- **A00.0 Cholera due to Vibrio cholerae 01, biovar cholerae**
  Classical cholera
- **A00.1 Cholera due to Vibrio cholerae 01, biovar eltor**
  Cholera eltor
- **A00.9 Cholera, unspecified**

[4] **A01 Typhoid and paratyphoid fevers**
- [5] **A01.0 Typhoid fever**
  Infection due to Salmonella typhi
  - **A01.00 Typhoid fever, unspecified**
  - **A01.01 Typhoid meningitis**
  - **A01.02 Typhoid fever with heart involvement**
    Typhoid endocarditis
    Typhoid myocarditis
  - **A01.03 Typhoid pneumonia**
  - **A01.04 Typhoid arthritis**
  - **A01.05 Typhoid osteomyelitis**
  - **A01.09 Typhoid fever with other complications**
- **A01.1 Paratyphoid fever A**
- **A01.2 Paratyphoid fever B**
- **A01.3 Paratyphoid fever C**
- **A01.4 Paratyphoid fever, unspecified**
  Infection due to Salmonella paratyphi NOS

[4] **A02 Other salmonella infections**

[INCLUDES] *infection or foodborne intoxication due to any Salmonella species other than S. typhi and S. paratyphi*

- **A02.0 Salmonella enteritis**
  Salmonellosis
- **A02.1 Salmonella sepsis**
- [5] **A02.2 Localized salmonella infections**
  - **A02.20 Localized salmonella infection, unspecified**
  - **A02.21 Salmonella meningitis**
  - **A02.22 Salmonella pneumonia**
  - **A02.23 Salmonella arthritis**
  - **A02.24 Salmonella osteomyelitis**
  - **A02.25 Salmonella pyelonephritis**
    Salmonella tubulo-interstitial nephropathy
  - **A02.29 Salmonella with other localized infection**
- **A02.8 Other specified salmonella infections**
- **A02.9 Salmonella infection, unspecified**

[4] **A03 Shigellosis**
- **A03.0 Shigellosis due to Shigella dysenteriae**
  Group A shigellosis [Shiga-Kruse dysentery]
- **A03.1 Shigellosis due to Shigella flexneri**
  Group B shigellosis
- **A03.2 Shigellosis due to Shigella boydii**
  Group C shigellosis
- **A03.3 Shigellosis due to Shigella sonnei**
  Group D shigellosis
- **A03.8 Other shigellosis**
- **A03.9 Shigellosis, unspecified**
  Bacillary dysentery NOS

[4] **A04 Other bacterial intestinal infections**

[EXCLUDES1] *bacterial foodborne intoxications, NEC (A05.-)*
tuberculous enteritis (A18.32)

- **A04.0 Enteropathogenic Escherichia coli infection**
- **A04.1 Enterotoxigenic Escherichia coli infection**
- **A04.2 Enteroinvasive Escherichia coli infection**
- **A04.3 Enterohemorrhagic Escherichia coli infection**
- **A04.4 Other intestinal Escherichia coli infections**
  Escherichia coli enteritis NOS
- **A04.5 Campylobacter enteritis**
- **A04.6 Enteritis due to Yersinia enterocolitica**
  [EXCLUDES1] *extraintestinal yersiniosis (A28.2)*
- **A04.7 Enterocolitis due to Clostridium difficile**
  Foodborne intoxication by Clostridium difficile
  Pseudomembraneous colitis
- **A04.8 Other specified bacterial intestinal infections**
- **A04.9 Bacterial intestinal infection, unspecified**
  Bacterial enteritis NOS

[4] **A05 Other bacterial foodborne intoxications, not elsewhere classified**

[EXCLUDES1] *Clostridium difficile foodborne intoxication and infection (A04.7)*
Escherichia coli infection (A04.0-A04.4)
listeriosis (A32.-)
salmonella foodborne intoxication and infection (A02.-)
toxic effect of noxious foodstuffs (T61-T62)

- **A05.0 Foodborne staphylococcal intoxication**
- **A05.1 Botulism food poisoning**
  Botulism NOS
  Classical foodborne intoxication due to Clostridium botulinum
  [EXCLUDES1] *infant botulism (A48.51)*
  wound botulism (A48.52)
- **A05.2 Foodborne Clostridium perfringens [Clostridium welchii] intoxication**
  Enteritis necroticans
  Pig-bel
- **A05.3 Foodborne Vibrio parahaemolyticus intoxication**
- **A05.4 Foodborne Bacillus cereus intoxication**
- **A05.5 Foodborne Vibrio vulnificus intoxication**
- **A05.8 Other specified bacterial foodborne intoxications**
- **A05.9 Bacterial foodborne intoxication, unspecified**

[4] **A06 Amebiasis**

[INCLUDES] *infection due to Entamoeba histolytica*

[EXCLUDES1] *other protozoal intestinal diseases (A07.-)*

[EXCLUDES2] *acanthamebiasis (B60.1-)*
Naegleriasis (B60.2)

- **A06.0 Acute amebic dysentery**
  Acute amebiasis
  Intestinal amebiasis NOS
- **A06.1 Chronic intestinal amebiasis**
- **A06.2 Amebic nondysenteric colitis**
- **A06.3 Ameboma of intestine**
  Ameboma NOS
- **A06.4 Amebic liver abscess**
  Hepatic amebiasis
- **A06.5 Amebic lung abscess**
  Amebic abscess of lung (and liver)
- **A06.6 Amebic brain abscess**
  Amebic abscess of brain (and liver) (and lung)
- **A06.7 Cutaneous amebiasis**

Unspecified Code | Other Specified Code | [N] Newborn Age: 0 | [P] Pediatric Age: 0-17 | [M] Maternity Age: 12-55
[A] Adult Age: 15-124 | ♂ Male | ♀ Female | ● New Code | ▲ Revised Code Title | ►◄ Revised Text

[5] **A06.8 Amebic infection of other sites**

A06.81 Amebic cystitis

A06.82 Other amebic genitourinary infections

Amebic balanitis
Amebic vesiculitis
Amebic vulvovaginitis

A06.89 Other amebic infections

Amebic appendicitis
Amebic splenic abscess

A06.9 Amebiasis, unspecified

[4] **A07 Other protozoal intestinal diseases**

A07.0 Balantidiasis

Balantidial dysentery

A07.1 Giardiasis [lambliasis]

A07.2 Cryptosporidiosis

A07.3 Isosporiasis

Infection due to Isospora belli and Isospora hominis
Intestinal coccidiosis
Isosporosis

A07.4 Cyclosporiasis

A07.8 Other specified protozoal intestinal diseases

Intestinal microsporidiosis
Intestinal trichomoniasis
Sarcocystosis
Sarcosporidiosis

A07.9 Protozoal intestinal disease, unspecified

Flagellate diarrhea
Protozoal colitis
Protozoal diarrhea
Protozoal dysentery

[4] **A08 Viral and other specified intestinal infections**

[EXCLUDES1] *influenza with involvement of gastrointestinal tract (J09.X3, J10.2, J11.2)*

A08.0 Rotaviral enteritis

[5] **A08.1 Acute gastroenteropathy due to Norwalk agent and other small round viruses**

A08.11 Acute gastroenteropathy due to Norwalk agent

Acute gastroenteropathy due to Norovirus
Acute gastroenteropathy due to Norwalk-like agent

A08.19 Acute gastroenteropathy due to other small round viruses

Acute gastroenteropathy due to small round virus [SRV] NOS

A08.2 Adenoviral enteritis

[5] **A08.3 Other viral enteritis**

A08.31 Calicivirus enteritis

A08.32 Astrovirus enteritis

A08.39 Other viral enteritis

Coxsackie virus enteritis
Echovirus enteritis
Enterovirus enteritis NEC
Torovirus enteritis

A08.4 Viral intestinal infection, unspecified

Viral enteritis NOS
Viral gastroenteritis NOS
Viral gastroenteropathy NOS

A08.8 Other specified intestinal infections

A09 Infectious gastroenteritis and colitis, unspecified

Infectious colitis NOS
Infectious enteritis NOS
Infectious gastroenteritis NOS

[EXCLUDES1] *colitis NOS (K52.9)*
diarrhea NOS (R19.7)
enteritis NOS (K52.9)
gastroenteritis NOS (K52.9)
noninfective gastroenteritis and colitis, unspecified (K52.9)

Tuberculosis (A15-A19)

[INCLUDES] *infections due to Mycobacterium tuberculosis and Mycobacterium bovis*

[EXCLUDES1] *congenital tuberculosis (P37.0)*
nonspecific reaction to test for tuberculosis without active tuberculosis (R76.1-)
pneumoconiosis associated with tuberculosis, any type in A15 (J65)
positive PPD (R76.11)
positive tuberculin skin test without active tuberculosis (R76.11)
sequelae of tuberculosis (B90.-)
silicotuberculosis (J65)

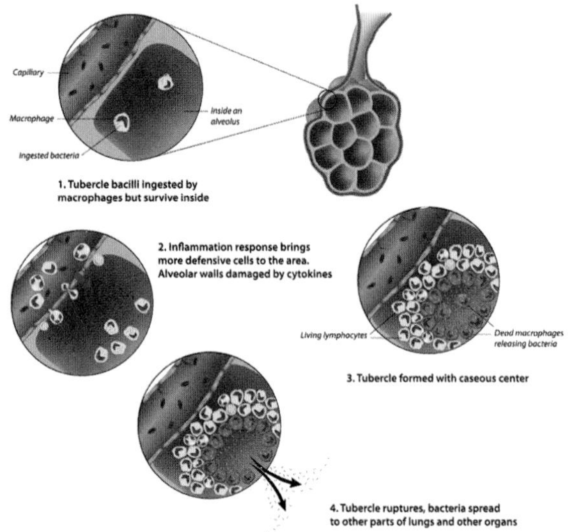

Figure 1.1 Progression of Tuberculosis

[4] **A15 Respiratory tuberculosis**

A15.0 Tuberculosis of lung

Tuberculous bronchiectasis
Tuberculous fibrosis of lung
Tuberculous pneumonia
Tuberculous pneumothorax

A15.4 Tuberculosis of intrathoracic lymph nodes

Tuberculosis of hilar lymph nodes
Tuberculosis of mediastinal lymph nodes
Tuberculosis of tracheobronchial lymph nodes

[EXCLUDES1] *tuberculosis specified as primary (A15.7)*

A15.5 Tuberculosis of larynx, trachea and bronchus

Tuberculosis of bronchus
Tuberculosis of glottis
Tuberculosis of larynx
Tuberculosis of trachea

A15.6 Tuberculous pleurisy

Tuberculosis of pleura Tuberculous empyema

[EXCLUDES1] *primary respiratory tuberculosis (A15.7)*

A15.7 Primary respiratory tuberculosis

A15.8 Other respiratory tuberculosis

Mediastinal tuberculosis
Nasopharyngeal tuberculosis
Tuberculosis of nose
Tuberculosis of sinus [any nasal]

A15.9 Respiratory tuberculosis unspecified

[4] **A17 Tuberculosis of nervous system**

A17.0 Tuberculous meningitis

Tuberculosis of meninges (cerebral)(spinal)
Tuberculous leptomeningitis

[4] 4th character required [5] 5th character required [6] 6th character required [7] 7th character required [X] Extension 'X' Alert
[EXCLUDES1] Not coded here [EXCLUDES2] Not included here [PDx] Primary Diagnosis Only Manifestation Code

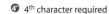

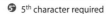

[EXCLUDES1] *tuberculous meningoencephalitis (A17.82)*

A17.1 Meningeal **tuberculoma**

Tuberculoma of meninges (cerebral) (spinal)

[EXCLUDES2] *tuberculoma of brain and spinal cord (A17.81)*

[5] A17.8 Other **tuberculosis of** nervous system

A17.81 **Tuberculoma of** brain and spinal cord

Tuberculous abscess of brain and spinal cord

A17.82 **Tuberculous** meningoencephalitis

Tuberculous myelitis

A17.83 **Tuberculous** neuritis

Tuberculous mononeuropathy

A17.89 **Other tuberculosis of nervous system**

Tuberculous polyneuropathy

A17.9 **Tuberculosis of nervous system, unspecified**

[4] A18 **Tuberculosis of** other organs

[5] A18.0 **Tuberculosis of** bones **and** joints

A18.01 **Tuberculosis of** spine

Pott's disease or curvature of spine
Tuberculous arthritis
Tuberculous osteomyelitis of spine
Tuberculous spondylitis

A18.02 **Tuberculous** arthritis of other joints

Tuberculosis of hip (joint)
Tuberculosis of knee (joint)

A18.03 **Tuberculosis of** other bones

Tuberculous mastoiditis
Tuberculous osteomyelitis

A18.09 **Other musculoskeletal tuberculosis**

Tuberculous myositis
Tuberculous synovitis
Tuberculous tenosynovitis

[5] A18.1 **Tuberculosis of** genitourinary **system**

A18.10 **Tuberculosis of genitourinary system, unspecified**

A18.11 **Tuberculosis of** kidney and ureter

A18.12 **Tuberculosis of** bladder

A18.13 **Tuberculosis of** other urinary **organs**

Tuberculous urethritis

A18.14 **Tuberculosis of** prostate [A] ♂

A18.15 **Tuberculosis of other male genital organs** ♂

A18.16 **Tuberculosis of** cervix ♀

A18.17 **Tuberculous** female pelvic inflammatory disease

Tuberculous endometritis
Tuberculous oophoritis and salpingitis ♀

A18.18 **Tuberculosis of other female genital organs**

Tuberculous ulceration of vulva ♀

A18.2 **Tuberculous** peripheral lymphadenopathy

Tuberculous adenitis

[EXCLUDES2] *tuberculosis of bronchial and mediastinal lymph nodes (A15.4)*
tuberculosis of mesenteric and retroperitoneal lymph nodes (A18.39)
tuberculous tracheobronchial adenopathy (A15.4)

[5] A18.3 **Tuberculosis of** intestines, peritoneum and mesenteric glands

A18.31 **Tuberculous** peritonitis

Tuberculous ascites

A18.32 **Tuberculous** enteritis

Tuberculosis of anus and rectum
Tuberculosis of intestine (large) (small)

A18.39 Retroperitoneal **tuberculosis**

Tuberculosis of mesenteric glands
Tuberculosis of retroperitoneal (lymph glands)

A18.4 **Tuberculosis of** skin and subcutaneous tissue

Erythema induratum, tuberculous
Lupus excedens
Lupus vulgaris NOS
Lupus vulgaris of eyelid
Scrofuloderma
Tuberculosis of external ear

[EXCLUDES2] *lupus erythematosus (L93.-)*
lupus NOS (M32.9)
systemic (M32.-)

[5] A18.5 **Tuberculosis of** eye

[EXCLUDES2] *lupus vulgaris of eyelid (A18.4)*

A18.50 **Tuberculosis of eye, unspecified**

A18.51 **Tuberculous** episcleritis

A18.52 **Tuberculous** keratitis

Tuberculous interstitial keratitis
Tuberculous keratoconjunctivitis (interstitial) (phlyctenular)

A18.53 **Tuberculous** chorioretinitis

A18.54 **Tuberculous** iridocyclitis

A18.59 **Other tuberculosis of eye**

Tuberculous conjunctivitis

A18.6 **Tuberculosis of** (inner) (middle) ear

Tuberculous otitis media

[EXCLUDES2] *tuberculosis of external ear (A18.4)*
tuberculous mastoiditis (A18.03)

A18.7 **Tuberculosis of** adrenal glands

Tuberculous Addison's disease

[5] A18.8 **Tuberculosis of other** specified organs

A18.81 **Tuberculosis of** thyroid gland

A18.82 **Tuberculosis of other endocrine glands**

Tuberculosis of pituitary gland
Tuberculosis of thymus gland

A18.83 **Tuberculosis of digestive tract organs, not elsewhere classified**

[EXCLUDES1] *tuberculosis of intestine (A18.32)*

A18.84 **Tuberculosis of** heart

Tuberculous cardiomyopathy
Tuberculous endocarditis
Tuberculous myocarditis
Tuberculous pericarditis

A18.85 **Tuberculosis of** spleen

A18.89 **Tuberculosis of other sites**

Tuberculosis of muscle
Tuberculous cerebral arteritis

[4] A19 Miliary **tuberculosis**

[INCLUDES] *disseminated tuberculosis*
generalized tuberculosis
tuberculous polyserositis

A19.0 **Acute miliary tuberculosis of a** single specified site

A19.1 **Acute miliary tuberculosis of** multiple sites

A19.2 **Acute miliary tuberculosis, unspecified**

A19.8 **Other miliary tuberculosis**

A19.9 **Miliary tuberculosis, unspecified**

Certain zoonotic bacterial diseases (A20-A28)

[4] A20 Plague

[INCLUDES] *infection due to Yersinia pestis*

A20.0 Bubonic **plague**

A20.1 Cellulocutaneous **plague**

A20.2 Pneumonic **plague**

A20.3 **Plague** meningitis

A20.7 Septicemic **plague**

A20.8 **Other forms of plague**

Abortive plague
Asymptomatic plague
Pestis minor

A20.9 **Plague, unspecified**

Unspecified Code | Other Specified Code | [N] Newborn Age: 0 | [P] Pediatric Age: 0-17 | [M] Maternity Age: 12-55
[A] Adult Age: 15-124 | ♂ Male | ♀ Female | ● New Code | ▲ Revised Code Title | ►◄ Revised Text

A21 Tularemia

    INCLUDES   *deer-fly fever*
           infection due to Francisella tularensis
           rabbit fever

  A21.0 Ulceroglandular **tularemia**

  A21.1 Oculoglandular **tularemia**

      Ophthalmic tularemia

  A21.2 Pulmonary **tularemia**

  A21.3 Gastrointestinal **tularemia**

      Abdominal tularemia

  A21.7 Generalized **tularemia**

  A21.8 Other forms of tularemia

  A21.9 Tularemia, unspecified

A22 Anthrax

    INCLUDES   *infection due to Bacillus anthracis*

  A22.0 Cutaneous **anthrax**

      Malignant carbuncle
      Malignant pustule

  A22.1 Pulmonary **anthrax**

      Inhalation anthrax
      Ragpicker's disease
      Woolsorter's disease

  A22.2 Gastrointestinal **anthrax**

  A22.7 **Anthrax** sepsis

  A22.8 Other forms of anthrax

      Anthrax meningitis

  A22.9 Anthrax, unspecified

A23 Brucellosis

    INCLUDES   *Malta fever*
           Mediterranean fever
           undulant fever

  A23.0 **Brucellosis due to Brucella** melitensis

  A23.1 **Brucellosis due to Brucella** abortus

  A23.2 **Brucellosis due to Brucella** suis

  A23.3 **Brucellosis due to Brucella** canis

  A23.8 Other brucellosis

  A23.9 Brucellosis, unspecified

A24 Glanders and melioidosis

  A24.0 Glanders

      Infection due to Pseudomonas mallei
      Malleus

  A24.1 Acute and fulminating **melioidosis**

      Melioidosis pneumonia
      Melioidosis sepsis

  A24.2 Subacute and chronic **melioidosis**

  A24.3 Other melioidosis

  A24.9 Melioidosis, unspecified

      Infection due to Pseudomonas pseudomallei NOS
      Whitmore's disease

A25 Rat-bite fevers

  A25.0 Spirillosis

      Sodoku

  A25.1 Streptobacillosis

      Epidemic arthritic erythema
      Haverhill fever
      Streptobacillary rat-bite fever

  A25.9 Rat-bite fever, unspecified

A26 Erysipeloid

  A26.0 Cutaneous **erysipeloid**

      Erythema migrans

  A26.7 Erysipelothrix **sepsis**

  A26.8 Other forms of erysipeloid

  A26.9 Erysipeloid, unspecified

A27 Leptospirosis

  A27.0 **Leptospirosis** icterohemorrhagica

      Leptospiral or spirochetal jaundice (hemorrhagic)
      Weil's disease

  A27.8 Other forms **of leptospirosis**

    A27.81 Aseptic meningitis in leptospirosis

    A27.89 Other forms of leptospirosis

  A27.9 Leptospirosis, unspecified

A28 Other zoonotic bacterial diseases, not elsewhere classified

  A28.0 Pasteurellosis

  A28.1 Cat-scratch disease

      Cat-scratch fever

  A28.2 Extraintestinal yersiniosis

    EXCLUDES1 *enteritis due to Yersinia enterocolitica (A04.6)*
          plague (A20.-)

  A28.8 Other specified zoonotic bacterial diseases, not elsewhere classified

  A28.9 Zoonotic bacterial disease, unspecified

Other bacterial diseases (A30-A49)

A30 Leprosy [Hansen's disease]

    INCLUDES   *infection due to Mycobacterium leprae*
    EXCLUDES1 *sequelae of leprosy (B92)*

  A30.0 Indeterminate **leprosy**

      I leprosy

  A30.1 Tuberculoid **leprosy**

      TT leprosy

  A30.2 Borderline tuberculoid **leprosy**

      BT leprosy

  A30.3 Borderline **leprosy**

      BB leprosy

  A30.4 Borderline lepromatous **leprosy**

      BL leprosy

  A30.5 Lepromatous **leprosy**

      LL leprosy

  A30.8 Other forms of leprosy

  A30.9 Leprosy, unspecified

A31 Infection due to other mycobacteria

    EXCLUDES2 *leprosy (A30.-)*
          tuberculosis (A15-A19)

  A31.0 Pulmonary **mycobacterial infection**

      Infection due to Mycobacterium avium
      Infection due to Mycobacterium intracellulare [Battey bacillus]
      Infection due to Mycobacterium kansasii

  A31.1 Cutaneous **mycobacterial infection**

      Buruli ulcer
      Infection due to Mycobacterium marinum
      Infection due to Mycobacterium ulcerans

  A31.2 Disseminated **mycobacterium avium-intracellulare complex (DMAC)**

      MAC sepsis

  A31.8 Other mycobacterial infections

  A31.9 Mycobacterial infection, unspecified

      Atypical mycobacterial infection NOS
      Mycobacteriosis NOS

A32 Listeriosis

    INCLUDES   *listerial foodborne infection*
    EXCLUDES1 *neonatal (disseminated) listeriosis (P37.2)*

  A32.0 Cutaneous **listeriosis**

  A32.1 Listerial meningitis and meningoencephalitis

    A32.11 Listerial meningitis

    A32.12 Listerial meningoencephalitis

  A32.7 Listerial sepsis

  A32.8 Other forms of listeriosis

    A32.81 Oculoglandular **listeriosis**

    A32.82 Listerial endocarditis

4th character required *5th* character required *6th* character required *7th* character required Extension 'X' Alert		
EXCLUDES1 Not coded here EXCLUDES2 Not included here PDX Primary Diagnosis Only Manifestation Code		

A32.89 Other forms of listeriosis
Listerial cerebral arteritis
A32.9 Listeriosis, unspecified
A33 Tetanus neonatorum
A34 Obstetrical tetanus ♀
A35 Other tetanus
Tetanus NOS
[EXCLUDES1] *obstetrical tetanus (A34)*
tetanus neonatorum (A33)
[4th] A36 Diphtheria
A36.0 Pharyngeal diphtheria
Diphtheritic membranous angina
Tonsillar diphtheria
A36.1 Nasopharyngeal diphtheria
A36.2 Laryngeal diphtheria
Diphtheritic laryngotracheitis
A36.3 Cutaneous diphtheria
[EXCLUDES2] *erythrasma (L08.1)*
[5th] A36.8 Other diphtheria
A36.81 Diphtheritic cardiomyopathy
Diphtheritic myocarditis
A36.82 Diphtheritic radiculomyelitis
A36.83 Diphtheritic polyneuritis
A36.84 Diphtheritic tubulo-interstitial nephropathy
A36.85 Diphtheritic cystitis
A36.86 Diphtheritic conjunctivitis
A36.89 Other diphtheritic complications
Diphtheritic peritonitis
A36.9 Diphtheria, unspecified
[4th] A37 Whooping cough
[5th] A37.0 Whooping cough due to Bordetella pertussis
A37.00 Whooping cough due to Bordetella pertussis without pneumonia
A37.01 Whooping cough due to Bordetella pertussis with pneumonia
[5th] A37.1 Whooping cough due to Bordetella parapertussis
A37.10 Whooping cough due to Bordetella parapertussis without pneumonia
A37.11 Whooping cough due to Bordetella parapertussis with pneumonia
[5th] A37.8 Whooping cough due to other Bordetella species
A37.80 Whooping cough due to other Bordetella species without pneumonia
A37.81 Whooping cough due to other Bordetella species with pneumonia
[5th] A37.9 Whooping cough, unspecified species
A37.90 Whooping cough, unspecified species without pneumonia
A37.91 Whooping cough, unspecified species with pneumonia
[4th] A38 Scarlet fever
[INCLUDES] *scarlatina*
[EXCLUDES2] *streptococcal sore throat (J02.0)*
A38.0 Scarlet fever with otitis media
A38.1 Scarlet fever with myocarditis
A38.8 Scarlet fever with other complications
A38.9 Scarlet fever, uncomplicated
Scarlet fever, NOS
[4th] A39 Meningococcal infection
A39.0 Meningococcal meningitis
A39.1 Waterhouse-Friderichsen syndrome
Meningococcal hemorrhagic adrenalitis
Meningococcic adrenal syndrome
A39.2 Acute meningococcemia
A39.3 Chronic meningococcemia
A39.4 Meningococcemia, unspecified
[5th] A39.5 Meningococcal heart disease
A39.50 Meningococcal carditis, unspecified
A39.51 Meningococcal endocarditis
A39.52 Meningococcal myocarditis
A39.53 Meningococcal pericarditis
[5th] A39.8 Other meningococcal infections
A39.81 Meningococcal encephalitis
A39.82 Meningococcal retrobulbar neuritis
A39.83 Meningococcal arthritis
A39.84 Postmeningococcal arthritis
A39.89 Other meningococcal infections
Meningococcal conjunctivitis
A39.9 Meningococcal infection, unspecified
Meningococcal disease NOS
[4th] A40 Streptococcal sepsis
Code first postprocedural streptococcal sepsis (T81.4)
streptococcal sepsis during labor (O75.3)
streptococcal sepsis following abortion or ectopic or molar pregnancy (O03-O07, O08.0)
streptococcal sepsis following immunization (T88.0)
streptococcal sepsis following infusion, transfusion or therapeutic injection (T80.2-)
[EXCLUDES1] *neonatal (P36.0-P36.1)*
puerperal sepsis (O85)
sepsis due to Streptococcus, group D (A41.81)
A40.0 Sepsis due to streptococcus, group A
A40.1 Sepsis due to streptococcus, group B
A40.3 Sepsis due to Streptococcus pneumoniae
Pneumococcal sepsis
A40.8 Other streptococcal sepsis
A40.9 Streptococcal sepsis, unspecified
[4th] A41 Other sepsis
Code first postprocedural sepsis (T81.4)
sepsis during labor (O75.3)
sepsis following abortion, ectopic or molar pregnancy (O03-O07, O08.0)
sepsis following immunization (T88.0)
sepsis following infusion, transfusion or therapeutic injection (T80.2-)
[EXCLUDES1] *bacteremia NOS (R78.81)*
neonatal (P36.-)
puerperal sepsis (O85)
sepsis NOS (A41.9)
streptococcal sepsis (A40.-)
[EXCLUDES2] *sepsis (due to) (in) actinomycotic (A42.7)*
sepsis (due to) (in) anthrax (A22.7)
sepsis (due to) (in) candidal (B37.7)
sepsis (due to) (in) Erysipelothrix (A26.7)
sepsis (due to) (in) extraintestinal yersiniosis (A28.2)
sepsis (due to) (in) gonococcal (A54.86)
sepsis (due to) (in) herpesviral (B00.7)
sepsis (due to) (in) listerial (A32.7)
sepsis (due to) (in) melioidosis (A24.1)
sepsis (due to) (in) meningococcal (A39.2-A39.4)
sepsis (due to) (in) plague (A20.7)
sepsis (due to) (in) tularemia (A21.7)
toxic shock syndrome (A48.3)
[5th] A41.0 Sepsis due to Staphylococcus aureus
A41.01 Sepsis due to Methicillin susceptible Staphylococcus aureus
MSSA sepsis
Staphylococcus aureus sepsis NOS
A41.02 Sepsis due to Methicillin resistant Staphylococcus aureus
A41.1 Sepsis due to other specified staphylococcus
Coagulase negative staphylococcus sepsis
A41.2 Sepsis due to unspecified staphylococcus
A41.3 Sepsis due to Hemophilus influenzae

Unspecified Code | Other Specified Code | [N] Newborn Age: 0 | [P] Pediatric Age: 0-17 | [M] Maternity Age: 12-55
[A] Adult Age: 15-124 | ♂ Male | ♀ Female | ● New Code | ▲ Revised Code Title | ►◄ Revised Text

A41.4 Sepsis due to anaerobes
[EXCLUDES1] *gas gangrene (A48.0)*

[5] A41.5 Sepsis due to other Gram-negative organisms
A41.50 Gram-negative sepsis, unspecified
Gram-negative sepsis NOS
A41.51 Sepsis due to Escherichia coli [E. coli]
A41.52 Sepsis due to Pseudomonas
Pseudomonas aeroginosa
A41.53 Sepsis due to Serratia
A41.59 Other Gram-negative sepsis

[5] A41.8 Other specified sepsis
A41.81 Sepsis due to Enterococcus
A41.89 Other specified sepsis

A41.9 Sepsis, unspecified organism
Septicemia NOS

[4] A42 Actinomycosis
[EXCLUDES1] *actinomycetoma (B47.1)*
A42.0 Pulmonary actinomycosis
A42.1 Abdominal actinomycosis
A42.2 Cervicofacial actinomycosis
A42.7 Actinomycotic sepsis
[5] A42.8 Other forms of actinomycosis
A42.81 Actinomycotic meningitis
A42.82 Actinomycotic encephalitis
A42.89 Other forms of actinomycosis
A42.9 Actinomycosis, unspecified

[4] A43 Nocardiosis
A43.0 Pulmonary nocardiosis
A43.1 Cutaneous nocardiosis
A43.8 Other forms of nocardiosis
A43.9 Nocardiosis, unspecified

[4] A44 Bartonellosis
A44.0 Systemic bartonellosis
Oroya fever
A44.1 Cutaneous and mucocutaneous bartonellosis
Verruga peruana
A44.8 Other forms of bartonellosis
A44.9 Bartonellosis, unspecified

A46 Erysipelas
[EXCLUDES1] *postpartum or puerperal erysipelas (O86.89)*

[4] A48 Other bacterial diseases, not elsewhere classified
[EXCLUDES1] *actinomycetoma (B47.1)*
A48.0 Gas gangrene
Clostridial cellulitis
Clostridial myonecrosis
A48.1 Legionnaires' disease
A48.2 Nonpneumonic Legionnaires' disease [Pontiac fever]
A48.3 Toxic shock syndrome
Use additional code to identify the organism (B95, B96)
[EXCLUDES1] *endotoxic shock NOS (R57.8)*
sepsis NOS (A41.9)
A48.4 Brazilian purpuric fever
Systemic Hemophilus aegyptius infection
[5] A48.5 Other specified botulism
Non-foodborne intoxication due to toxins of Clostridium botulinum [C. botulinum]
[EXCLUDES1] *food poisoning due to toxins of Clostridium botulinum (A05.1)*
A48.51 Infant botulism [P]
A48.52 Wound botulism
Non-foodborne botulism NOS
Use additional code for associated wound
A48.8 Other specified bacterial diseases

[4] A49 Bacterial infection of unspecified site
[EXCLUDES1] *bacterial agents as the cause of diseases classified elsewhere (B95-B96)*
chlamydial infection NOS (A74.9)
meningococcal infection NOS (A39.9)
rickettsial infection NOS (A79.9)
spirochetal infection NOS (A69.9)
[5] A49.0 Staphylococcal infection, unspecified site
A49.01 Methicillin susceptible Staphylococcus aureus infection, unspecified site
Methicillin susceptible Staphylococcus aureus (MSSA) infection
Staphylococcus aureus infection NOS
A49.02 Methicillin resistant Staphylococcus aureus infection, unspecified site
Methicillin resistant Staphylococcus aureus (MRSA) infection
A49.1 Streptococcal infection, unspecified site
A49.2 Hemophilus influenzae infection, unspecified site
A49.3 Mycoplasma infection, unspecified site
A49.8 Other bacterial infections of unspecified site
A49.9 Bacterial infection, unspecified
[EXCLUDES1] *bacteremia NOS (R78.81)*

Infections with a predominantly sexual mode of transmission (A50-A64)

[EXCLUDES1] *human immunodeficiency virus [HIV] disease (B20)*
nonspecific and nongonococcal urethritis (N34.1)
Reiter's disease (M02.3-)

[4] A50 Congenital syphilis
[5] A50.0 Early congenital syphilis, symptomatic
Any congenital syphilitic condition specified as early or manifest less than two years after birth.
A50.01 Early congenital syphilitic oculopathy
A50.02 Early congenital ~~syphilitic osteochondropathy~~
A50.03 Early congenital syphilitic pharyngitis
Early congenital syphilitic laryngitis
A50.04 Early congenital syphilitic pneumonia
A50.05 Early congenital syphilitic rhinitis
A50.06 Early cutaneous congenital syphilis
A50.07 Early mucocutaneous congenital syphilis
A50.08 Early visceral congenital syphilis
A50.09 Other early congenital syphilis, symptomatic
A50.1 Early congenital syphilis, latent
Congenital syphilis without clinical manifestations, with positive serological reaction and negative spinal fluid test, less than two years after birth.
A50.2 Early congenital syphilis, unspecified
Congenital syphilis NOS less than two years after birth.
[5] A50.3 Late congenital syphilitic oculopathy
[EXCLUDES1] *Hutchinson's triad (A50.53)*
A50.30 Late congenital syphilitic oculopathy, unspecified
A50.31 Late congenital syphilitic interstitial keratitis
A50.32 Late congenital syphilitic chorioretinitis
A50.39 Other late congenital syphilitic oculopathy
[5] A50.4 Late congenital neurosyphilis [juvenile neurosyphilis]
Use additional code to identify any associated mental disorder
[EXCLUDES1] *Hutchinson's triad (A50.53)*
A50.40 Late congenital neurosyphilis, unspecified
Juvenile neurosyphilis NOS
A50.41 Late congenital syphilitic meningitis
A50.42 Late congenital syphilitic encephalitis
A50.43 Late congenital syphilitic polyneuropathy
A50.44 Late congenital syphilitic optic nerve atrophy
A50.45 Juvenile general paresis
Dementia paralytica juvenilis
Juvenile tabetoparetic neurosyphilis

[4] 4th character required [5] 5th character required [6] 6th character required [7] 7th character required [X] Extension 'X' Alert
[EXCLUDES1] Not coded here [EXCLUDES2] Not included here [PDx] Primary Diagnosis Only Manifestation Code

A50.49 **Other late congenital neurosyphilis**
Juvenile tabes dorsalis

⑤ A50.5 Other late **congenital syphilis,** symptomatic
Any congenital syphilitic condition specified as late or manifest two years or more after birth.

A50.51 Clutton's joints
A50.52 Hutchinson's teeth
A50.53 Hutchinson's triad
A50.54 **Late congenital** cardiovascular syphilis
A50.55 **Late congenital** syphilitic arthropathy
A50.56 **Late congenital** syphilitic osteochondropathy
A50.57 **Syphilitic saddle nose**
A50.59 **Other late congenital syphilis, symptomatic**

A50.6 Late **congenital syphilis,** latent
Congenital syphilis without clinical manifestations, with positive serological reaction and negative spinal fluid test, two years or more after birth.

A50.7 **Late congenital syphilis, unspecified**
Congenital syphilis NOS two years or more after birth.

A50.9 **Congenital syphilis, unspecified**

④ A51 Early **syphilis**

A51.0 Primary genital **syphilis**
Syphilitic chancre NOS

A51.1 Primary anal **syphilis**
A51.2 **Primary syphilis of other sites**

⑤ A51.3 Secondary **syphilis of** skin and mucous membranes

A51.31 **Condyloma latum**
A51.32 **Syphilitic alopecia**
A51.39 **Other secondary syphilis of skin**
Syphilitic leukoderma
Syphilitic mucous patch
EXCLUDES1 *late syphilitic leukoderma (A52.79)*

⑤ A51.4 Other secondary **syphilis**

A51.41 **Secondary syphilitic** meningitis
A51.42 **Secondary syphilitic** female pelvic disease   ♀
A51.43 **Secondary syphilitic** oculopathy
Secondary syphilitic chorioretinitis
Secondary syphilitic iridocyclitis, iritis
Secondary syphilitic uveitis
A51.44 **Secondary syphilitic** nephritis
A51.45 **Secondary syphilitic** hepatitis
A51.46 **Secondary syphilitic** osteopathy
A51.49 **Other secondary syphilitic conditions**
Secondary syphilitic lymphadenopathy
Secondary syphilitic myositis

A51.5 Early **syphilis,** latent
Syphilis (acquired) without clinical manifestations, with positive serological reaction and negative spinal fluid test, less than two years after infection.

A51.9 **Early syphilis, unspecified**

④ A52 Late **syphilis**

⑤ A52.0 Cardiovascular and cerebrovascular **syphilis**

A52.00 **Cardiovascular syphilis, unspecified**
A52.01 **Syphilitic** aneurysm of aorta
A52.02 **Syphilitic** aortitis
A52.03 **Syphilitic** endocarditis
Syphilitic aortic valve incompetence or stenosis
Syphilitic mitral valve stenosis
Syphilitic pulmonary valve regurgitation
A52.04 **Syphilitic** cerebral arteritis
A52.05 **Other cerebrovascular syphilis**
Syphilitic cerebral aneurysm (ruptured) (non-ruptured)
Syphilitic cerebral thrombosis
A52.06 **Other syphilitic heart involvement**
Syphilitic coronary artery disease
Syphilitic myocarditis
Syphilitic pericarditis

A52.09 **Other cardiovascular syphilis**

⑤ A52.1 Symptomatic **neurosyphilis**

A52.10 **Symptomatic neurosyphilis, unspecified**
A52.11 **Tabes dorsalis**
Locomotor ataxia (progressive)
Tabetic neurosyphilis
A52.12 **Other cerebrospinal syphilis**
A52.13 **Late syphilitic** meningitis
A52.14 **Late syphilitic** encephalitis
A52.15 **Late syphilitic** neuropathy
Late syphilitic acoustic neuritis
Late syphilitic optic (nerve) atrophy
Late syphilitic polyneuropathy
Late syphilitic retrobulbar neuritis
A52.16 **Charcôt's arthropathy (tabetic)**
A52.17 **General paresis**
Dementia paralytica
A52.19 **Other symptomatic neurosyphilis**
Syphilitic parkinsonism

A52.2 Asymptomatic **neurosyphilis**
A52.3 **Neurosyphilis, unspecified**
Gumma (syphilitic)
Syphilis (late)
Syphiloma

⑤ A52.7 Other symptomatic **late syphilis**

A52.71 **Late syphilitic** oculopathy
Late syphilitic chorioretinitis
Late syphilitic episcleritis
A52.72 **Syphilis of** lung and bronchus
A52.73 **Symptomatic late syphilis of other respiratory organs**
A52.74 **Syphilis of** liver and other viscera
Late syphilitic peritonitis
A52.75 **Syphilis of** kidney and ureter
Syphilitic glomerular disease
A52.76 Other genitourinary **symptomatic late syphilis**
Late syphilitic female pelvic inflammatory disease
A52.77 **Syphilis of** bone and joint
A52.78 **Syphilis of** other musculoskeletal tissue
Late syphilitic bursitis
Syphilis [stage unspecified] of bursa
Syphilis [stage unspecified] of muscle
Syphilis [stage unspecified] of synovium
Syphilis [stage unspecified] of tendon
A52.79 **Other symptomatic late syphilis**
Late syphilitic leukoderma
Syphilis of adrenal gland
Syphilis of pituitary gland
Syphilis of thyroid gland
Syphilitic splenomegaly
EXCLUDES1 *syphilitic leukoderma (secondary) (A51.39)*

A52.8 **Late syphilis,** latent
Syphilis (acquired) without clinical manifestations, with positive serological reaction and negative spinal fluid test, two years or more after infection

A52.9 **Late syphilis, unspecified**

④ A53 **Other and unspecified syphilis**

A53.0 **Latent syphilis, unspecified as early or late**
Latent syphilis NOS
Positive serological reaction for syphilis

A53.9 **Syphilis, unspecified**
Infection due to Treponema pallidum NOS
Syphilis (acquired) NOS
EXCLUDES1 *syphilis NOS under two years of age (A50.2)*

Unspecified Code	Other Specified Code	N Newborn Age: 0	P Pediatric Age: 0-17	M Maternity Age: 12-55	
A Adult Age: 15-124	♂ Male	♀ Female	● New Code	▲ Revised Code Title	►◄ Revised Text

[4] **A54 Gonococcal infection**

- [5] **A54.0 Gonococcal infection of lower genitourinary tract without periurethral or accessory gland abscess**
  - [EXCLUDES1] *gonococcal infection with genitourinary gland abscess (A54.1)*
  - *gonococcal infection with periurethral abscess (A54.1)*
  - **A54.00 Gonococcal infection of lower genitourinary tract, unspecified**
  - **A54.01 Gonococcal cystitis and urethritis, unspecified**
  - **A54.02 Gonococcal vulvovaginitis, unspecified** ♀
  - **A54.03 Gonococcal cervicitis, unspecified** ♀
  - **A54.09 Other gonococcal infection of lower genitourinary tract**
- **A54.1 Gonococcal infection of lower genitourinary tract with periurethral and accessory gland abscess**
  - Gonococcal Bartholin's gland abscess
- [5] **A54.2 Gonococcal pelviperitonitis and other gonococcal genitourinary infection**
  - **A54.21 Gonococcal infection of kidney and ureter**
  - **A54.22 Gonococcal prostatitis** ♂
  - **A54.23 Gonococcal infection of other male genital organs**
    - Gonococcal epididymitis
    - Gonococcal orchitis ♂
  - **A54.24 Gonococcal female pelvic inflammatory disease**
    - Gonococcal pelviperitonitis
    - [EXCLUDES1] *gonococcal peritonitis (A54.85)* ♀
  - **A54.29 Other gonococcal genitourinary infections**
- [5] **A54.3 Gonococcal infection of eye**
  - **A54.30 Gonococcal infection of eye, unspecified**
  - **A54.31 Gonococcal conjunctivitis**
    - Ophthalmia neonatorum due to gonococcus
  - **A54.32 Gonococcal iridocyclitis**
  - **A54.33 Gonococcal keratitis**
  - **A54.39 Other gonococcal eye infection**
    - Gonococcal endophthalmia
- [5] **A54.4 Gonococcal infection of musculoskeletal system**
  - **A54.40 Gonococcal infection of musculoskeletal system, unspecified**
  - **A54.41 Gonococcal spondylopathy**
  - **A54.42 Gonococcal arthritis**
    - [EXCLUDES2] *gonococcal infection of spine (A54.41)*
  - **A54.43 Gonococcal osteomyelitis**
    - [EXCLUDES2] *gonococcal infection of spine (A54.41)*
  - **A54.49 Gonococcal infection of other musculoskeletal tissue**
    - Gonococcal bursitis
    - Gonococcal myositis
    - Gonococcal synovitis
    - Gonococcal tenosynovitis
- **A54.5 Gonococcal pharyngitis**
- **A54.6 Gonococcal infection of anus and rectum**
- [5] **A54.8 Other gonococcal infections**
  - **A54.81 Gonococcal meningitis**
  - **A54.82 Gonococcal brain abscess**
  - **A54.83 Gonococcal heart infection**
    - Gonococcal endocarditis
    - Gonococcal myocarditis
    - Gonococcal pericarditis
  - **A54.84 Gonococcal pneumonia**
  - **A54.85 Gonococcal peritonitis**
    - [EXCLUDES1] *gonococcal pelviperitonitis (A54.24)*
  - **A54.86 Gonococcal sepsis**
  - **A54.89 Other gonococcal infections**
    - Gonococcal keratoderma
    - Gonococcal lymphadenitis
- **A54.9 Gonococcal infection, unspecified**

A55 Chlamydial lymphogranuloma (venereum)

- Climatic or tropical bubo
- Durand-Nicolas-Favre disease
- Esthiomene
- Lymphogranuloma inguinale

[4] **A56 Other sexually transmitted chlamydial diseases**

- [INCLUDES] *sexually transmitted diseases due to Chlamydia trachomatis*
- [EXCLUDES1] *neonatal chlamydial conjunctivitis (P39.1)*
  neonatal chlamydial pneumonia (P23.1)
- [EXCLUDES2] *chlamydial lymphogranuloma (A55)*
  conditions classified to A74.-
- [5] **A56.0 Chlamydial infection of lower genitourinary tract**
  - **A56.00 Chlamydial infection of lower genitourinary tract, unspecified**
  - **A56.01 Chlamydial cystitis and urethritis**
  - **A56.02 Chlamydial vulvovaginitis** ♀
  - **A56.09 Other chlamydial infection of lower genitourinary tract**
    - Chlamydial cervicitis
- [5] **A56.1 Chlamydial infection of pelviperitoneum and other genitourinary organs**
  - **A56.11 Chlamydial female pelvic inflammatory disease** ♀
  - **A56.19 Other chlamydial genitourinary infection**
    - Chlamydial epididymitis
    - Chlamydial orchitis
- **A56.2 Chlamydial infection of genitourinary tract, unspecified**
- **A56.3 Chlamydial infection of anus and rectum**
- **A56.4 Chlamydial infection of pharynx**
- **A56.8 Sexually transmitted chlamydial infection of other sites**

A57 Chancroid

- Ulcus molle

A58 Granuloma inguinale

- Donovanosis

[4] **A59 Trichomoniasis**

- [EXCLUDES2] *intestinal trichomoniasis (A07.8)*
- [5] **A59.0 Urogenital trichomoniasis**
  - **A59.00 Urogenital trichomoniasis, unspecified**
    - Fluor (vaginalis) due to Trichomonas
    - Leukorrhea (vaginalis) due to Trichomonas
  - **A59.01 Trichomonal vulvovaginitis** ♀
  - **A59.02 Trichomonal prostatitis** ♂
  - **A59.03 Trichomonal cystitis and urethritis**
  - **A59.09 Other urogenital trichomoniasis**
    - Trichomonas cervicitis
- **A59.8 Trichomoniasis of other sites**
- **A59.9 Trichomoniasis, unspecified**

[4] **A60 Anogenital herpesviral [herpes simplex] infections**

- [5] **A60.0 Herpesviral infection of genitalia and urogenital tract**
  - **A60.00 Herpesviral infection of urogenital system, unspecified**
  - **A60.01 Herpesviral infection of penis** ♂
  - **A60.02 Herpesviral infection of other male genital organs** ♂
  - **A60.03 Herpesviral cervicitis** ♀
  - **A60.04 Herpesviral vulvovaginitis**
    - Herpesviral [herpes simplex] ulceration
    - Herpesviral [herpes simplex] vaginitis
    - Herpesviral [herpes simplex] vulvitis ♀
  - **A60.09 Herpesviral infection of other urogenital tract**
- **A60.1 Herpesviral infection of perianal skin and rectum**

[4] 4th character required [5] 5th character required [6] 6th character required [7] 7th character required [X] Extension 'X' Alert
[EXCLUDES1] Not coded here [EXCLUDES2] Not included here [PDx] Primary Diagnosis Only Manifestation Code

A60.9 Anogenital herpesviral infection, unspecified

⊕ A63 Other predominantly sexually transmitted diseases, not elsewhere classified

EXCLUDES2 *molluscum contagiosum (B08.1)*
papilloma of cervix (D26.0)

A63.0 Anogenital (venereal) warts

Anogenital warts due to (human) papillomavirus [HPV]
Condyloma acuminatum

A63.8 Other specified predominantly sexually transmitted diseases

A64 Unspecified sexually transmitted disease

Other spirochetal diseases (A65-A69)

EXCLUDES2 *leptospirosis (A27.-)*
syphilis (A50-A53)

A65 Nonvenereal syphilis

Bejel
Endemic syphilis
Njovera

⊕ A66 Yaws

INCLUDES *bouba*
frambesia (tropica)
pian

A66.0 Initial lesions of yaws

Chancre of yaws
Frambesia, initial or primary
Initial frambesial ulcer
Mother yaw

A66.1 Multiple papillomata and wet crab yaws

Frambesioma
Pianoma
Plantar or palmar papilloma of yaws

A66.2 Other early skin lesions of yaws

Cutaneous yaws, less than five years after infection
Early yaws (cutaneous)(macular)(maculopapular)(microp apular)(papular)
Frambeside of early yaws

A66.3 Hyperkeratosis of yaws

Ghoul hand
Hyperkeratosis, palmar or plantar (early) (late) due to yaws
Worm-eaten soles

A66.4 Gummata and ulcers of yaws

Gummatous frambeside
Nodular late yaws (ulcerated)

A66.5 Gangosa

Rhinopharyngitis mutilans

A66.6 Bone and joint lesions of yaws

Yaws ganglion
Yaws goundou
Yaws gumma, bone
Yaws gummatous osteitis or periostitis
Yaws hydrarthrosis
Yaws osteitis
Yaws periostitis (hypertrophic)

A66.7 Other manifestations of yaws

Juxta-articular nodules of yaws
Mucosal yaws

A66.8 Latent yaws

Yaws without clinical manifestations, with positive serology

A66.9 Yaws, unspecified

⊕ A67 Pinta [carate]

A67.0 Primary lesions of pinta

Chancre (primary) of pinta
Papule (primary) of pinta

A67.1 Intermediate lesions of pinta

Erythematous plaques of pinta
Hyperchromic lesions of pinta
Hyperkeratosis of pinta
Pintids

A67.2 Late lesions of pinta

Achromic skin lesions of pinta
Cicatricial skin lesions of pinta
Dyschromic skin lesions of pinta

A67.3 Mixed lesions of pinta

Achromic with hyperchromic skin lesions of pinta [carate]

A67.9 Pinta, unspecified

⊕ A68 Relapsing fevers

INCLUDES *recurrent fever*
EXCLUDES2 *Lyme disease (A69.2-)*

A68.0 Louse-borne relapsing fever

Relapsing fever due to Borrelia recurrentis

A68.1 Tick-borne relapsing fever

Relapsing fever due to any Borrelia species other than Borrelia recurrentis

A68.9 Relapsing fever, unspecified

⊕ A69 Other spirochetal infections

A69.0 Necrotizing ulcerative stomatitis

Cancrum oris
Fusospirochetal gangrene
Noma
Stomatitis gangrenosa

A69.1 Other Vincent's infections

Fusospirochetal pharyngitis
Necrotizing ulcerative (acute) gingivitis
Necrotizing ulcerative (acute) gingivostomatitis
Spirochetal stomatitis
Trench mouth
Vincent's angina
Vincent's gingivitis

⑤ A69.2 Lyme disease

Erythema chronicum migrans due to Borrelia burgdorferi

A69.20 Lyme disease, unspecified

A69.21 Meningitis due to Lyme disease

A69.22 Other neurologic disorders in Lyme disease

Cranial neuritis
Meningoencephalitis
Polyneuropathy

A69.23 Arthritis due to Lyme disease

A69.29 Other conditions associated with Lyme disease

Myopericarditis due to Lyme disease

A69.8 Other specified spirochetal infections

A69.9 Spirochetal infection, unspecified

Unspecified Code	Other Specified Code	N Newborn Age: 0	P Pediatric Age: 0-17	M Maternity Age: 12-55
A Adult Age: 15-124	♂ Male	♀ Female	● New Code	▲ Revised Code Title	►◄ Revised Text

Other diseases caused by chlamydiae (A70-A74)

[EXCLUDES1] *sexually transmitted chlamydial diseases (A55-A56)*

A70 Chlamydia psittaci infections

Ornithosis
Parrot fever
Psittacosis

[4th] **A71 Trachoma**

[EXCLUDES1] *sequelae of trachoma (B94.0)*

A71.0 Initial stage of trachoma

Trachoma dubium

A71.1 Active stage of trachoma

Granular conjunctivitis (trachomatous)
Trachomatous follicular conjunctivitis
Trachomatous pannus

A71.9 Trachoma, unspecified

[4th] **A74 Other diseases caused by chlamydiae**

[EXCLUDES1] *neonatal chlamydial conjunctivitis (P39.1)*
neonatal chlamydial pneumonia (P23.1)
Reiter's disease (M02.3-)
sexually transmitted chlamydial diseases (A55-A56)

[EXCLUDES2] *chlamydial pneumonia (J16.0)*

A74.0 Chlamydial conjunctivitis

Paratrachoma

[5th] **A74.8 Other chlamydial diseases**

A74.81 Chlamydial peritonitis

A74.89 Other chlamydial diseases

A74.9 Chlamydial infection, unspecified

Chlamydiosis NOS

Rickettsioses (A75-A79)

[4th] **A75 Typhus fever**

[EXCLUDES1] *rickettsiosis due to Ehrlichia sennetsu (A79.81)*

A75.0 Epidemic louse-borne typhus fever due to Rickettsia prowazekii

Classical typhus (fever)
Epidemic (louse-borne) typhus

A75.1 Recrudescent typhus [Brill's disease]

Brill-Zinsser disease

A75.2 Typhus fever due to Rickettsia typhi

Murine (flea-borne) typhus

A75.3 Typhus fever due to Rickettsia tsutsugamushi

Scrub (mite-borne) typhus
Tsutsugamushi fever

A75.9 Typhus fever, unspecified

Typhus (fever) NOS

[4th] **A77 Spotted fever [tick-borne rickettsioses]**

A77.0 Spotted fever due to Rickettsia rickettsii

Rocky Mountain spotted fever
Sao Paulo fever

A77.1 Spotted fever due to Rickettsia conorii

African tick typhus
Boutonneuse fever
India tick typhus
Kenya tick typhus
Marseilles fever
Mediterranean tick fever

A77.2 Spotted fever due to Rickettsia siberica

North Asian tick fever
Siberian tick typhus

A77.3 Spotted fever due to Rickettsia australis

Queensland tick typhus

[5th] **A77.4 Ehrlichiosis**

[EXCLUDES1] *Rickettsiosis due to Ehrlichia sennetsu (A79.81)*

A77.40 Ehrlichiosis, unspecified

A77.41 Ehrlichiosis chafeensis [E. chafeensis]

A77.49 Other ehrlichiosis

A77.8 Other spotted fevers

A77.9 Spotted fever, unspecified

Tick-borne typhus NOS

A78 Q fever

Infection due to Coxiella burnetii
Nine Mile fever
Quadrilateral fever

[4th] **A79 Other rickettsioses**

A79.0 Trench fever

Quintan fever
Wolhynian fever

A79.1 Rickettsialpox due to Rickettsia akari

Kew Garden fever
Vesicular rickettsiosis

[5th] **A79.8 Other specified rickettsioses**

A79.81 Rickettsiosis due to Ehrlichia sennetsu

A79.89 Other specified rickettsioses

A79.9 Rickettsiosis, unspecified

Rickettsial infection NOS

Viral and prion infections of the central nervous system (A80-A89)

[EXCLUDES1] *postpolio syndrome (G14)*
sequelae of poliomyelitis (B91)
sequelae of viral encephalitis (B94.1)

[4th] **A80 Acute poliomyelitis**

A80.0 Acute paralytic poliomyelitis, vaccine-associated

A80.1 Acute paralytic poliomyelitis, wild virus, imported

A80.2 Acute paralytic poliomyelitis, wild virus, indigenous

[5th] **A80.3 Acute paralytic poliomyelitis, other and unspecified**

A80.30 Acute paralytic poliomyelitis, unspecified

A80.39 Other acute paralytic poliomyelitis

A80.4 Acute nonparalytic poliomyelitis

A80.9 Acute poliomyelitis, unspecified

[4th] **A81 Atypical virus infections of central nervous system**

[INCLUDES] *diseases of the central nervous system caused by prions*

Use additional code to identify:
dementia with behavioral disturbance (F02.81)
dementia without behavioral disturbance (F02.80)

[5th] **A81.0 Creutzfeldt-Jakob disease**

A81.00 Creutzfeldt-Jakob disease, unspecified

Jakob-Creutzfeldt disease, unspecified

A81.01 Variant Creutzfeldt-Jakob disease

vCJD

A81.09 Other Creutzfeldt-Jakob disease

CJD
Familial Creutzfeldt-Jakob disease
Iatrogenic Creutzfeldt-Jakob disease
Sporadic Creutzfeldt-Jakob disease
Subacute spongiform encephalopathy (with dementia)

A81.1 Subacute sclerosing panencephalitis

Dawson's inclusion body encephalitis
Van Bogaert's sclerosing leukoencephalopathy

A81.2 Progressive multifocal leukoencephalopathy

Multifocal leukoencephalopathy NOS

[5th] **A81.8 Other atypical virus infections of central nervous system**

A81.81 Kuru

A81.82 Gerstmann-Sträussler-Scheinker syndrome

GSS syndrome

A81.83 Fatal familial insomnia

FFI

[4th] 4th character required [5th] 5th character required [6th] 6th character required [7th] 7th character required [X] Extension 'X' Alert
[EXCLUDES1] Not coded here [EXCLUDES2] Not included here [PDx] Primary Diagnosis Only Manifestation Code

A81.89 Other atypical virus infections of central nervous system

A81.9 Atypical virus infection of central nervous system, unspecified

Prion diseases of the central nervous system NOS

🔄 A82 Rabies

A82.0 Sylvatic rabies

A82.1 Urban rabies

A82.9 Rabies, unspecified

🔄 A83 Mosquito-borne viral encephalitis

INCLUDES   mosquito-borne viral meningoencephalitis

EXCLUDES2   Venezuelan equine encephalitis (A92.2)
West Nile fever (A92.3-)
West Nile virus (A92.3-)

A83.0 Japanese encephalitis

A83.1 Western equine encephalitis

A83.2 Eastern equine encephalitis

A83.3 St Louis encephalitis

A83.4 Australian encephalitis

Kunjin virus disease

A83.5 California encephalitis

California meningoencephalitis

La Crosse encephalitis

A83.6 Rocio virus disease

A83.8 Other mosquito-borne viral encephalitis

A83.9 Mosquito-borne viral encephalitis, unspecified

🔄 A84 Tick-borne viral encephalitis

INCLUDES   tick-borne viral meningoencephalitis

A84.0 Far Eastern tick-borne encephalitis [Russian spring-summer encephalitis]

A84.1 Central European tick-borne encephalitis

A84.8 Other tick-borne viral encephalitis

Louping ill

Powassan virus disease

A84.9 Tick-borne viral encephalitis, unspecified

🔄 A85 Other viral encephalitis, not elsewhere classified

INCLUDES   specified viral encephalomyelitis NEC
specified viral meningoencephalitis NEC

EXCLUDES1   benign myalgic encephalomyelitis (G93.3)
encephalitis due to cytomegalovirus (B25.8)
encephalitis due to herpesvirus NEC (B10.0-)
encephalitis due to herpesvirus [herpes simplex] (B00.4)
encephalitis due to measles virus (B05.0)
encephalitis due to mumps virus (B26.2)
encephalitis due to poliomyelitis virus (A80.-)
encephalitis due to zoster (B02.0)
lymphocytic choriomeningitis (A87.2)

A85.0 Enteroviral encephalitis

Enteroviral encephalomyelitis

A85.1 Adenoviral encephalitis

Adenoviral meningoencephalitis

A85.2 Arthropod-borne viral encephalitis, unspecified

EXCLUDES1   West nile virus with encephalitis (A92.31)

A85.8 Other specified viral encephalitis

Encephalitis lethargica

Von Economo-Cruchet disease

A86 Unspecified viral encephalitis

Viral encephalomyelitis NOS

Viral meningoencephalitis NOS

🔄 A87 Viral meningitis

EXCLUDES1   meningitis due to herpesvirus [herpes simplex] (B00.3)
meningitis due to herpesvirus [herpes simplex] (B00.3)
meningitis due to measles virus (B05.1)
meningitis due to mumps virus (B26.1)

meningitis due to poliomyelitis virus (A80.-)
meningitis due to zoster (B02.1)

A87.0 Enteroviral meningitis

Coxsackievirus meningitis

Echovirus meningitis

A87.1 Adenoviral meningitis

A87.2 Lymphocytic choriomeningitis

Lymphocytic meningoencephalitis

A87.8 Other viral meningitis

A87.9 Viral meningitis, unspecified

🔄 A88 Other viral infections of central nervous system, not elsewhere classified

EXCLUDES1   viral encephalitis NOS (A86)
viral meningitis NOS (A87.9)

A88.0 Enteroviral exanthematous fever [Boston exanthem]

A88.1 Epidemic vertigo

A88.8 Other specified viral infections of central nervous system

A89 Unspecified viral infection of central nervous system

Arthropod-borne viral fevers and viral hemorrhagic fevers (A90-A99)

A90 Dengue fever [classical dengue]

EXCLUDES1   dengue hemorrhagic fever (A91)

A91 Dengue hemorrhagic fever

🔄 A92 Other mosquito-borne viral fevers

EXCLUDES1   Ross River disease (B33.1)

A92.0 Chikungunya virus disease

Chikungunya (hemorrhagic) fever

A92.1 O'nyong-nyong fever

A92.2 Venezuelan equine fever

Venezuelan equine encephalitis

Venezuelan equine encephalomyelitis virus disease

5️⃣ A92.3 West Nile virus infection

West Nile fever

A92.30 West Nile virus infection, unspecified

West Nile fever NOS

West Nile fever without complications

West Nile virus NOS

A92.31 West Nile virus infection with encephalitis

West Nile encephalitis

West Nile encephalomyelitis

A92.32 West Nile virus infection with other neurologic manifestation

Use additional code to specify the neurologic manifestation

A92.39 West Nile virus infection with other complications

Use additional code to specify the other conditions

A92.4 Rift Valley fever

A92.8 Other specified mosquito-borne viral fevers

A92.9 Mosquito-borne viral fever, unspecified

🔄 A93 Other arthropod-borne viral fevers, not elsewhere classified

A93.0 Oropouche virus disease

Oropouche fever

A93.1 Sandfly fever

Pappataci fever

Phlebotomus fever

A93.2 Colorado tick fever

A93.8 Other specified arthropod-borne viral fevers

Piry virus disease

Vesicular stomatitis virus disease [Indiana fever]

Unspecified Code	Other Specified Code	N Newborn Age: 0	P Pediatric Age: 0-17	M Maternity Age: 12-55
A Adult Age: 15-124	♂ Male	♀ Female	● New Code	▲ Revised Code Title	▶◀ Revised Text

A94 Unspecified arthropod-borne viral fever
Arboviral fever NOS
Arbovirus infection NOS

[4] **A95 Yellow fever**
A95.0 Sylvatic **yellow fever**
Jungle yellow fever
A95.1 Urban **yellow fever**
A95.9 Yellow fever, unspecified

[4] **A96 Arenaviral** ~~hemorrhagic fever~~
A96.0 Junin **hemorrhagic fever**
Argentinian hemorrhagic fever
A96.1 Machupo **hemorrhagic fever**
Bolivian hemorrhagic fever
A96.2 Lassa **fever**
A96.8 Other arenaviral hemorrhagic fevers
A96.9 Arenaviral hemorrhagic fever, unspecified

[4] **A98 Other viral hemorrhagic fevers, not elsewhere classified**
[EXCLUDES1] *chikungunya hemorrhagic fever (A92.0)*
dengue hemorrhagic fever (A91)
A98.0 Crimean-Congo **hemorrhagic fever**
Central Asian hemorrhagic fever
A98.1 Omsk **hemorrhagic fever**
A98.2 Kyasanur Forest **disease**
A98.3 Marburg virus **disease**
A98.4 Ebola virus **disease**
A98.5 Hemorrhagic fever with renal syndrome
Epidemic hemorrhagic fever
Korean hemorrhagic fever
Russian hemorrhagic fever
Hantaan virus disease
Hantavirus disease with renal manifestations
Nephropathia epidemica
Songo fever
[EXCLUDES1] *hantavirus (cardio)-pulmonary syndrome (B33.4)*
A98.8 Other specified viral hemorrhagic fevers

A99 Unspecified viral hemorrhagic fever

Viral infections characterized by skin and mucous membrane lesions (B00-B09)

[4] **B00 Herpesviral [herpes simplex] infections**
[EXCLUDES1] *congenital herpesviral infections (P35.2)*
[EXCLUDES2] *anogenital herpesviral infection (A60.-)*
gammaherpesviral mononucleosis (B27.0-)
herpangina (B08.5)
B00.0 Eczema herpeticum
Kaposi's varicelliform eruption
B00.1 Herpesviral vesicular dermatitis
Herpes simplex facialis
Herpes simplex labialis
Herpes simplex otitis externa
Vesicular dermatitis of ear
Vesicular dermatitis of lip
B00.2 Herpesviral gingivostomatitis and pharyngotonsillitis
Herpesviral pharyngitis
B00.3 Herpesviral meningitis
B00.4 Herpesviral encephalitis
Herpesviral meningoencephalitis
Simian B disease
[EXCLUDES1] *herpesviral encephalitis due to herpesvirus 6 and 7 (B10.01, B10.09)*
non-simplex herpesviral encephalitis (B10.0-)
[5] **B00.5 Herpesviral ocular disease**
B00.50 Herpesviral ocular disease, unspecified
B00.51 Herpesviral iridocyclitis
Herpesviral iritis
Herpesviral uveitis, anterior
B00.52 Herpesviral keratitis
Herpesviral keratoconjunctivitis
B00.53 Herpesviral conjunctivitis
B00.59 Other herpesviral disease of eye
Herpesviral dermatitis of eyelid
B00.7 Disseminated herpesviral disease
Herpesviral sepsis
[5] **B00.8 Other forms of herpesviral infections**
B00.81 Herpesviral hepatitis
B00.82 Herpes simplex myelitis
B00.89 Other herpesviral infection
Herpesviral whitlow
B00.9 Herpesviral infection, unspecified
Herpes simplex infection NOS

[4] **B01 Varicella [chickenpox]**
B01.0 Varicella meningitis
[5] **B01.1 Varicella encephalitis, myelitis and encephalomyelitis**
Postchickenpox encephalitis, myelitis and encephalomyelitis
B01.11 Varicella encephalitis and encephalomyelitis
Postchickenpox encephalitis and encephalomyelitis
B01.12 Varicella myelitis
Postchickenpox myelitis
B01.2 Varicella pneumonia
[5] **B01.8 Varicella with other complications**
B01.81 Varicella keratitis
B01.89 Other varicella complications
B01.9 Varicella without complication
Varicella NOS

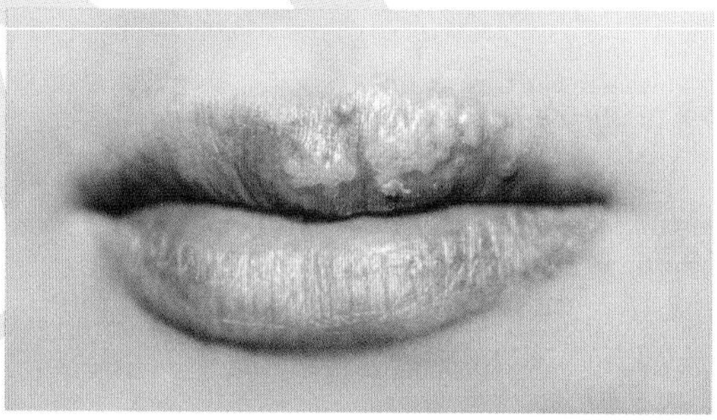

Figure 2.1 Oral Herpes

[4] **B02 Zoster [herpes zoster]**
[INCLUDES] *shingles*
zona
B02.0 Zoster encephalitis
Zoster meningoencephalitis
B02.1 Zoster meningitis
[5] **B02.2 Zoster with** other nervous system involvement
B02.21 Postherpetic geniculate ganglionitis
B02.22 Postherpetic trigeminal neuralgia
B02.23 Postherpetic polyneuropathy
B02.24 Postherpetic myelitis
Herpes zoster myelitis
B02.29 Other postherpetic nervous system involvement
Postherpetic radiculopathy
[5] **B02.3 Zoster** ocular **disease**
B02.30 Zoster ocular disease, unspecified
B02.31 Zoster conjunctivitis
B02.32 Zoster iridocyclitis
B02.33 Zoster keratitis
Herpes zoster keratoconjunctivitis
B02.34 Zoster scleritis
B02.39 Other herpes zoster eye disease

[4] 4th character required [5] 5th character required [6] 6th character required [7] 7th character required [7] Extension 'X' Alert
[EXCLUDES1] Not coded here [EXCLUDES2] Not included here [PDx] Primary Diagnosis Only Manifestation Code

Zoster blepharitis

B02.7 Disseminated zoster

B02.8 Zoster with other complications

Herpes zoster otitis externa

B02.9 Zoster without complications

Zoster NOS

B03 **Smallpox**

NOTES   In 1980 the 33rd World Health Assembly declared that smallpox had been eradicated.
The classification is maintained for surveillance purposes.

B04 **Monkeypox**

🔹 B05 **Measles**

INCLUDES   morbilli

EXCLUDES1   subacute sclerosing panencephalitis (A81.1)

B05.0 Measles complicated by encephalitis

Postmeasles encephalitis

B05.1 Measles complicated by meningitis

Postmeasles meningitis

B05.2 Measles complicated by pneumonia

Postmeasles pneumonia

B05.3 Measles complicated by otitis media

Postmeasles otitis media

B05.4 Measles with intestinal complications

🔹 **B05.8 Measles with other complications**

B05.81 Measles keratitis and keratoconjunctivitis

B05.89 Other measles complications

B05.9 Measles without complication

Measles NOS

🔹 B06 **Rubella [German measles]**

EXCLUDES1   congenital rubella (P35.0)

🔹 **B06.0 Rubella with** neurological complications

B06.00 Rubella with neurological complication, unspecified

B06.01 Rubella encephalitis

Rubella meningoencephalitis

B06.02 Rubella meningitis

B06.09 Other neurological complications of rubella

🔹 **B06.8 Rubella with** other complications

B06.81 Rubella pneumonia

B06.82 Rubella arthritis

B06.89 Other rubella complications

B06.9 Rubella without complication

Rubella NOS

🔹 B07 **Viral warts**

INCLUDES   verruca simplex
verruca vulgaris
viral warts due to human papillomavirus

EXCLUDES2   anogenital (venereal) warts (A63.0)
papilloma of bladder (D41.4)
papilloma of cervix (D26.0)
papilloma of larynx (D14.1)

B07.0 Plantar wart

Verruca plantaris

B07.8 Other viral warts

Common wart

Flat wart

Verruca plana

B07.9 Viral wart, unspecified

🔹 B08 **Other viral infections characterized by skin and mucous membrane lesions, not elsewhere classified**

EXCLUDES1   vesicular stomatitis virus disease (A93.8)

🔹 **B08.0 Other orthopoxvirus infections**

EXCLUDES2   monkeypox (B04)

🔹 **B08.01 Cowpox and vaccinia not from vaccine**

B08.010 Cowpox

B08.011 Vaccinia not from vaccine

EXCLUDES1   vaccinia (from vaccination) (generalized) (T88.1)

B08.02 Orf virus disease

Contagious pustular dermatitis

Ecthyma contagiosum

B08.03 Pseudocowpox [milker's node]

B08.04 Paravaccinia, unspecified

B08.09 Other orthopoxvirus infections

Orthopoxvirus infection NOS

B08.1 Molluscum contagiosum

🔹 **B08.2 Exanthema** subitum [sixth disease]

Roseola infantum

B08.20 Exanthema subitum [sixth disease], unspecified

Roseola infantum, unspecified   P

B08.21 Exanthema subitum [sixth disease] due to human herpesvirus 6

Roseola infantum due to human herpesvirus 6   P

B08.22 Exanthema subitum [sixth disease] due to human herpesvirus 7

Roseola infantum due to human herpesvirus 7   P

B08.3 Erythema infectiosum [fifth disease]

B08.4 Enteroviral vesicular stomatitis with exanthem

Hand, foot and mouth disease

B08.5 Enteroviral vesicular pharyngitis

Herpangina

🔹 **B08.6 Parapoxvirus** infections

B08.60 Parapoxvirus infection, unspecified

B08.61 Bovine stomatitis

B08.62 Sealpox

B08.69 Other parapoxvirus infections

🔹 **B08.7 Yatapoxvirus** infections

B08.70 Yatapoxvirus infection, unspecified

B08.71 Tanapox virus disease

B08.72 Yaba pox virus disease

Yaba monkey tumor disease

B08.79 Other yatapoxvirus infections

B08.8 Other specified viral infections characterized by skin and mucous membrane lesions

Enteroviral lymphonodular pharyngitis

Foot-and-mouth disease

Poxvirus NEC

B09 **Unspecified viral infection characterized by skin and mucous membrane lesions**

Viral enanthema NOS

Viral exanthema NOS

Other human herpesviruses (B10)

🔹 B10 **Other human herpesviruses**

EXCLUDES2   cytomegalovirus (B25.9)
Epstein-Barr virus (B27.0-)
herpes NOS (B00.9)
herpes simplex (B00.-)
herpes zoster (B02.-)
human herpesvirus NOS (B00.-)
human herpesvirus 1 and 2 (B00.-)
human herpesvirus 3 (B01.-, B02.-)
human herpesvirus 4 (B27.0-)
human herpesvirus 5 (B25.-)
varicella (B01.-)
zoster (B02.-)

🔹 **B10.0 Other human herpesvirus** encephalitis

EXCLUDES2   herpes encephalitis NOS (B00.4)
herpes simplex encephalitis (B00.4)
human herpesvirus encephalitis (B00.4)
simian B herpes virus encephalitis (B00.4)

B10.01 Human herpesvirus 6 encephalitis

B10.09 Other human herpesvirus encephalitis

Human herpesvirus 7 encephalitis

Unspecified Code	Other Specified Code	N Newborn Age: 0 P Pediatric Age: 0-17 M Maternity Age: 12-55
A Adult Age: 15-124 ♂ Male ♀ Female ● New Code ▲ Revised Code Title ►◄ Revised Text		

⑤ **B10.8 Other human herpesvirus infection**
  B10.81 Human herpesvirus 6 **infection**
  B10.82 Human herpesvirus 7 **infection**
  B10.89 Other human herpesvirus infection
    Human herpesvirus 8 infection
    Kaposi's sarcoma-associated herpesvirus infection

Viral hepatitis (B15-B19)

> EXCLUDES1 sequelae of viral hepatitis (B94.2)
> EXCLUDES2 cytomegaloviral hepatitis (B25.1)
>   herpesviral [herpes simplex] hepatitis (B00.81)

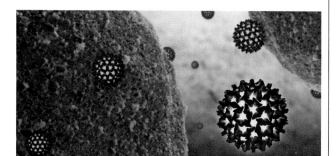

Figure 2.2 Hepatitis B virus

④ **B15 Acute** hepatitis A
  B15.0 Hepatitis A with hepatic coma
  B15.9 Hepatitis A without hepatic coma
    Hepatitis A (acute)(viral) NOS
④ **B16 Acute** hepatitis B
  B16.0 Acute hepatitis B with delta-agent with hepatic coma
  B16.1 Acute hepatitis B with delta-agent without hepatic coma
  B16.2 Acute hepatitis B without delta-agent **with hepatic coma**
  B16.9 Acute hepatitis B without delta-agent and without hepatic coma
    Hepatitis B (acute) (viral) NOS
④ **B17 Other acute viral hepatitis**
  B17.0 Acute delta-(super) infection of hepatitis B carrier
  ⑤ **B17.1 Acute** hepatitis C
    B17.10 Acute hepatitis C without hepatic coma
      Acute hepatitis C NOS
    B17.11 Acute hepatitis C with hepatic coma
  B17.2 Acute hepatitis E
  B17.8 Other specified acute viral hepatitis
    Hepatitis non-A non-B (acute) (viral) NEC
  B17.9 Acute viral hepatitis, unspecified
    Acute hepatitis NOS
④ **B18** Chronic **viral hepatitis**
  B18.0 Chronic viral hepatitis B with **delta-agent**
  B18.1 Chronic viral hepatitis B without **delta-agent**
    Chronic (viral) hepatitis B
  B18.2 Chronic viral hepatitis C
  B18.8 Other chronic viral hepatitis
  B18.9 Chronic viral hepatitis, unspecified
④ **B19 Unspecified viral hepatitis**
  B19.0 Unspecified viral hepatitis with hepatic coma
  ⑤ **B19.1 Unspecified viral** hepatitis B
    B19.10 Unspecified viral hepatitis B without hepatic coma
      Unspecified viral hepatitis B NOS
    B19.11 Unspecified viral hepatitis B with hepatic coma
  ⑤ **B19.2 Unspecified viral** hepatitis C

B19.20 Unspecified viral hepatitis C without hepatic coma
    Viral hepatitis C NOS
  B19.21 Unspecified viral hepatitis C with hepatic coma
B19.9 Unspecified viral hepatitis without hepatic coma
    Viral hepatitis NOS

Human immunodeficiency virus [HIV] disease (B20)

B20 Human immunodeficiency virus [HIV] disease

> INCLUDES acquired immune deficiency syndrome [AIDS]
>   AIDS-related complex [ARC]
>   HIV infection, symptomatic

Code first Human immunodeficiency virus [HIV] disease complicating pregnancy, childbirth and the puerperium, if applicable (O98.7-)
Use additional code(s) to identify all manifestations of HIV infection

> EXCLUDES1 asymptomatic human immunodeficiency virus [HIV] infection status (Z21)
>   exposure to HIV virus (Z20.6)
>   inconclusive serologic evidence of HIV (R75)

Other viral diseases (B25-B34)

④ **B25 Cytomegaloviral disease**

> EXCLUDES1 congenital cytomegalovirus infection (P35.1)
>   cytomegaloviral mononucleosis (B27.1-)

  B25.0 Cytomegaloviral pneumonitis
  B25.1 Cytomegaloviral hepatitis
  B25.2 Cytomegaloviral pancreatitis
  B25.8 Other cytomegaloviral diseases
    Cytomegaloviral encephalitis
  B25.9 Cytomegaloviral disease, unspecified
④ **B26 Mumps**

> INCLUDES epidemic parotitis
>   infectious parotitis

  B26.0 Mumps orchitis   ♂
  B26.1 Mumps meningitis
  B26.2 Mumps encephalitis
  B26.3 Mumps pancreatitis
  ⑤ **B26.8 Mumps with other complications**
    B26.81 Mumps hepatitis
    B26.82 Mumps myocarditis
    B26.83 Mumps nephritis
    B26.84 Mumps polyneuropathy
    B26.85 Mumps arthritis
    B26.89 Other mumps complications
  B26.9 Mumps without complication
    Mumps NOS
    Mumps parotitis NOS
④ **B27 Infectious** mononucleosis

> INCLUDES glandular fever
>   monocytic angina
>   Pfeiffer's disease

  ⑤ **B27.0** Gammaherpesviral **mononucleosis**
    Mononucleosis due to Epstein-Barr virus
    B27.00 Gammaherpesviral mononucleosis without complication
    B27.01 Gammaherpesviral mononucleosis with polyneuropathy
    B27.02 Gammaherpesviral mononucleosis with meningitis
    B27.09 Gammaherpesviral mononucleosis with other complications
      Hepatomegaly in gammaherpesviral mononucleosis
  ⑤ **B27.1** Cytomegaloviral **mononucleosis**
    B27.10 Cytomegaloviral mononucleosis without complications

---

④ 4th character required   ⑤ 5th character required   ⑥ 6th character required   ⑦ 7th character required   ⑩ Extension 'X' Alert
EXCLUDES 1 Not coded here   EXCLUDES 2 Not included here   PDx Primary Diagnosis Only   Manifestation Code

B27.11 **Cytomegaloviral mononucleosis** with polyneuropathy

B27.12 **Cytomegaloviral mononucleosis** with meningitis

B27.19 **Cytomegaloviral mononucleosis with other complication**

Hepatomegaly in cytomegaloviral mononucleosis

🔄 B27.8 Other **infectious mononucleosis**

B27.80 **Other infectious mononucleosis** without complication

B27.81 **Other infectious mononucleosis** with polyneuropathy

B27.82 **Other infectious mononucleosis** with meningitis

B27.89 **Other infectious mononucleosis with other complication**

Hepatomegaly in other infectious mononucleosis

Infectious Mononucleosis

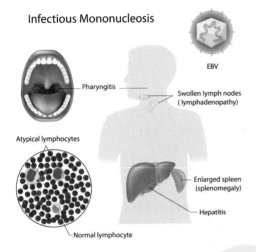

EBV

Pharyngitis

Swollen lymph nodes (lymphadenopathy)

Atypical lymphocytes

Enlarged spleen (splenomegaly)

Hepatitis

Normal lymphocyte

Figure 2.3 Infectious Mononucleosis

🔄 B27.9 **Infectious mononucleosis,** unspecified

B27.90 **Infectious mononucleosis, unspecified** without complication

B27.91 **Infectious mononucleosis, unspecified** with polyneuropathy

B27.92 **Infectious mononucleosis, unspecified** with meningitis

B27.99 **Infectious mononucleosis, unspecified** with other complication

Hepatomegaly in unspecified infectious mononucleosis

🔄 B30 **Viral conjunctivitis**

EXCLUDES1 *herpesviral [herpes simplex] ocular disease (B00.5)*
ocular zoster (B02.3)

B30.0 Keratoconjunctivitis **due to adenovirus**

Epidemic keratoconjunctivitis
Shipyard eye

B30.1 Conjunctivitis **due to adenovirus**

Acute adenoviral follicular conjunctivitis
Swimming-pool conjunctivitis

B30.2 **Viral** pharyngoconjunctivitis

B30.3 **Acute epidemic hemorrhagic conjunctivitis (enteroviral)**

Conjunctivitis due to coxsackievirus 24
Conjunctivitis due to enterovirus 70
Hemorrhagic conjunctivitis (acute)(epidemic)

B30.8 **Other viral conjunctivitis**

Newcastle conjunctivitis

B30.9 **Viral conjunctivitis, unspecified**

🔄 B33 **Other viral diseases, not elsewhere classified**

B33.0 **Epidemic myalgia**

Bornholm disease

B33.1 **Ross River disease**

Epidemic polyarthritis and exanthema
Ross River fever

🔄 B33.2 **Viral** carditis

Coxsackie (virus) carditis

B33.20 **Viral carditis, unspecified**

B33.21 **Viral** endocarditis

B33.22 **Viral** myocarditis

B33.23 **Viral** pericarditis

B33.24 **Viral** cardiomyopathy

B33.3 **Retrovirus infections, not elsewhere classified**

Retrovirus infection NOS

B33.4 **Hantavirus (cardio)-pulmonary syndrome [HPS] [HCPS]**

Hantavirus disease with pulmonary manifestations
Sin nombre virus disease
Use additional code to identify any associated acute kidney failure (N17.9)

EXCLUDES1 *hantavirus disease with renal manifestations (A98.5)*
hemorrhagic fever with renal manifestations (A98.5)

B33.8 **Other specified viral diseases**

EXCLUDES1 *anogenital human papillomavirus infection (A63.0)*
viral warts due to human papillomavirus infection (B07)

🔄 B34 **Viral infection of** unspecified site

EXCLUDES1 *anogenital human papillomavirus infection (A63.0)*
cytomegaloviral disease NOS (B25.9)
herpesvirus [herpes simplex] infection NOS (B00.9)
retrovirus infection NOS (B33.3)
viral agents as the cause of diseases classified elsewhere (B97.-)
viral warts due to human papillomavirus infection (B07)

B34.0 Adenovirus **infection, unspecified**

B34.1 Enterovirus **infection, unspecified**

Coxsackievirus infection NOS
Echovirus infection NOS

B34.2 Coronavirus **infection, unspecified**

EXCLUDES1 *pneumonia due to SARS-associated coronavirus (J12.81)*

B34.3 Parvovirus **infection, unspecified**

B34.4 Papovavirus **infection, unspecified**

B34.8 Other viral **infections of unspecified site**

B34.9 Viral **infection, unspecified**

Viremia NOS

Mycoses (B35-B49)

EXCLUDES2 *hypersensitivity pneumonitis due to organic dust (J67.-)*
mycosis fungoides (C84.0-)

🔄 B35 **Dermatophytosis**

INCLUDES *favus*
infections due to species of Epidermophyton, Micro-sporum and Trichophyton
tinea, any type except those in B36.-

B35.0 **Tinea** barbae **and tinea** capitis

Beard ringworm
Kerion
Scalp ringworm
Sycosis, mycotic

Unspecified Code	Other Specified Code	N Newborn Age: 0	P Pediatric Age: 0-17	M Maternity Age: 12-55
A Adult Age: 15-124	♂ Male	♀ Female	● New Code	▲ Revised Code Title	►◄ Revised Text

B35.1 **Tinea** unguium

Dermatophytic onychia

Dermatophytosis of nail

Onychomycosis

Ringworm of nails

B35.2 **Tinea** manuum

Dermatophytosis of hand

Hand ringworm

B35.3 **Tinea** pedis

Athlete's foot

Dermatophytosis of foot

Foot ringworm

B35.4 **Tinea** corporis

Ringworm of the body

B35.5 **Tinea** imbricata

Tokelau

B35.6 **Tinea** cruris

Dhobi itch

Groin ringworm

Jock itch

B35.8 **Other dermatophytoses**

Disseminated dermatophytosis

Granulomatous dermatophytosis

B35.9 **Dermatophytosis, unspecified**

Ringworm NOS

④ B36 **Other superficial mycoses**

B36.0 **Pityriasis versicolor**

Tinea flava

Tinea versicolor

B36.1 **Tinea nigra**

Keratomycosis nigricans palmaris

Microsporosis nigra

Pityriasis nigra

B36.2 **White piedra**

Tinea blanca

B36.3 **Black piedra**

B36.8 **Other specified superficial mycoses**

B36.9 **Superficial mycosis, unspecified**

④ B37 **Candidiasis**

> INCLUDES candidosis
> moniliasis
> EXCLUDES1 neonatal candidiasis (P37.5)

B37.0 **Candidal** stomatitis

Oral thrush

B37.1 Pulmonary **candidiasis**

Candidal bronchitis

Candidal pneumonia

B37.2 **Candidiasis of** skin and nail

Candidal onychia

Candidal paronychia

> EXCLUDES2 diaper dermatitis (L22)

B37.3 **Candidiasis of** vulva and vagina

Candidal vulvovaginitis

Monilial vulvovaginitis

Vaginal thrush   ♀

⑤ B37.4 **Candidiasis of** other urogenital sites

B37.41 **Candidal** cystitis and urethritis

B37.42 **Candidal** balanitis

B37.49 **Other urogenital candidiasis**

Candidal pyelonephritis

B37.5 **Candidal** meningitis

B37.6 **Candidal** endocarditis

B37.7 **Candidal** sepsis

Disseminated candidiasis

Systemic candidiasis

⑤ B37.8 **Candidiasis of** other sites

B37.81 **Candidal** esophagitis

B37.82 **Candidal** enteritis

Candidal proctitis

B37.83 **Candidal** cheilitis

B37.84 **Candidal** otitis externa

B37.89 **Other sites of candidiasis**

Candidal osteomyelitis

B37.9 **Candidiasis, unspecified**

Thrush NOS

④ B38 **Coccidioidomycosis**

B38.0 Acute pulmonary **coccidioidomycosis**

B38.1 Chronic pulmonary **coccidioidomycosis**

B38.2 Pulmonary **coccidioidomycosis,** unspecified

B38.3 Cutaneous **coccidioidomycosis**

B38.4 Coccidioidomycosis **meningitis**

B38.7 Disseminated **coccidioidomycosis**

Generalized coccidioidomycosis

⑤ B38.8 Other forms **of coccidioidomycosis**

B38.81 Prostatic **coccidioidomycosis**   ♂

B38.89 **Other forms of coccidioidomycosis**

B38.9 **Coccidioidomycosis, unspecified**

④ B39 **Histoplasmosis**

Code first associated AIDS (B20)

Use additional code for any associated manifestations, such as:

endocarditis (I39)

meningitis (G02)

pericarditis (I32)

retinitits (H32)

B39.0 Acute pulmonary **histoplasmosis capsulati**

B39.1 Chronic pulmonary **histoplasmosis capsulati**

B39.2 Pulmonary **histoplasmosis capsulati,** unspecified

B39.3 Disseminated **histoplasmosis capsulati**

Generalized histoplasmosis capsulati

B39.4 **Histoplasmosis capsulati, unspecified**

American histoplasmosis

B39.5 **Histoplasmosis** duboisii

African histoplasmosis

B39.9 **Histoplasmosis, unspecified**

④ B40 **Blastomycosis**

> EXCLUDES1 Brazilian blastomycosis (B41.-)
> keloidal blastomycosis (B48.0)

B40.0 Acute pulmonary **blastomycosis**

B40.1 Chronic pulmonary **blastomycosis**

B40.2 Pulmonary **blastomycosis,** unspecified

B40.3 Cutaneous **blastomycosis**

B40.7 Disseminated **blastomycosis**

Generalized blastomycosis

⑤ B40.8 Other forms **of blastomycosis**

B40.81 **Blastomycotic meningoencephalitis**

Meningomyelitis due to blastomycosis

B40.89 **Other forms of blastomycosis**

B40.9 **Blastomycosis, unspecified**

④ B41 **Paracoccidioidomycosis**

> INCLUDES Brazilian blastomycosis
> Lutz' disease

B41.0 Pulmonary **paracoccidioidomycosis**

B41.7 Disseminated **paracoccidioidomycosis**

Generalized paracoccidioidomycosis

B41.8 Other forms **of paracoccidioidomycosis**

B41.9 **Paracoccidioidomycosis, unspecified**

④ B42 **Sporotrichosis**

B42.0 Pulmonary **sporotrichosis**

B42.1 Lymphocutaneous **sporotrichosis**

B42.7 Disseminated **sporotrichosis**

Generalized sporotrichosis

---

④ 4th character required ⑤ 5th character required ⑥ 6th character required ⑦ 7th character required ⑩ Extension 'X' Alert

EXCLUDES1 Not coded here EXCLUDES2 Not included here PDx Primary Diagnosis Only Manifestation Code

[5] **B42.8 Other forms of sporotrichosis**
- **B42.81** Cerebral **sporotrichosis**
  - Meningitis due to sporotrichosis
- **B42.82 Sporotrichosis** arthritis
- **B42.89 Other forms of sporotrichosis**

B42.9 Sporotrichosis, unspecified

[4] **B43 Chromomycosis and pheomycotic abscess**
- **B43.0** Cutaneous **chromomycosis**
  - Dermatitis verrucosa
- **B43.1 Pheomycotic** brain abscess
  - Cerebral chromomycosis
- **B43.2** Subcutaneous **pheomycotic abscess and cyst**
- **B43.8 Other forms of chromomycosis**
- **B43.9 Chromomycosis, unspecified**

[4] **B44 Aspergillosis**
- INCLUDES *aspergilloma*
- **B44.0 Invasive** pulmonary **aspergillosis**
- **B44.1 Other** pulmonary **aspergillosis**
- **B44.2** Tonsillar **aspergillosis**
- **B44.7** Disseminated **aspergillosis**
  - Generalized aspergillosis

[5] **B44.8** Other forms **of aspergillosis**
- **B44.81 Allergic bronchopulmonary aspergillosis**
- **B44.89 Other forms of aspergillosis**

B44.9 Aspergillosis, unspecified

[4] **B45 Cryptococcosis**
- **B45.0** Pulmonary **cryptococcosis**
- **B45.1** Cerebral **cryptococcosis**
  - Cryptococcal meningitis
  - Cryptococcosis meningocerebralis
- **B45.2** Cutaneous **cryptococcosis**
- **B45.3** Osseous **cryptococcosis**
- **B45.7** Disseminated **cryptococcosis**
  - Generalized cryptococcosis
- **B45.8 Other forms of cryptococcosis**
- **B45.9 Cryptococcosis, unspecified**

[4] **B46 Zygomycosis**
- **B46.0** Pulmonary **mucormycosis**
- **B46.1** Rhinocerebral **mucormycosis**
- **B46.2** Gastrointestinal **mucormycosis**
- **B46.3** Cutaneous **mucormycosis**
  - Subcutaneous mucormycosis
- **B46.4** Disseminated **mucormycosis**
  - Generalized mucormycosis
- **B46.5 Mucormycosis, unspecified**
- **B46.8 Other zygomycoses**
  - Entomophthoromycosis
- **B46.9 Zygomycosis, unspecified**
  - Phycomycosis NOS

[4] **B47 Mycetoma**
- **B47.0 Eumycetoma**
  - Madura foot, mycotic
  - Maduromycosis
- **B47.1 Actinomycetoma**
- **B47.9 Mycetoma, unspecified**
  - Madura foot NOS

[4] **B48 Other mycoses, not elsewhere classified**
- **B48.0 Lobomycosis**
  - Keloidal blastomycosis
  - Lobo's disease
- **B48.1 Rhinosporidiosis**
- **B48.2 Allescheriasis**
  - Infection due to Pseudallescheria boydii
  - [EXCLUDES1] *eumycetoma (B47.0)*
- **B48.3 Geotrichosis**
  - Geotrichum stomatitis
- **B48.4 Penicillosis**
- **B48.8 Other specified mycoses**
  - Adiaspiromycosis
  - Infection of tissue and organs by Alternaria
  - Infection of tissue and organs by Drechslera
  - Infection of tissue and organs by Fusarium
  - Infection of tissue and organs by saprophytic fungi NEC

B49 Unspecified mycosis
- Fungemia NOS

Protozoal diseases (B50-B64)

[EXCLUDES1] *amebiasis (A06.-)*
other protozoal intestinal diseases (A07.-)

[4] **B50 Plasmodium** falciparum **malaria**
- INCLUDES *mixed infections of Plasmodium falciparum with any other Plasmodium species*
- **B50.0 Plasmodium falciparum malaria** with cerebral complications
  - Cerebral malaria NOS
- **B50.8 Other severe and complicated Plasmodium falciparum malaria**
  - Severe or complicated Plasmodium falciparum malaria NOS
- **B50.9 Plasmodium falciparum malaria, unspecified**

[4] **B51 Plasmodium** vivax **malaria**
- INCLUDES *mixed infections of Plasmodium vivax with other Plasmodium species, except Plasmodium falciparum*
- [EXCLUDES1] *plasmodium vivav with Plasmodium falciparum (B50.-)*
- **B51.0 Plasmodium vivax malaria** with rupture of spleen
- **B51.8 Plasmodium vivax malaria** with other complications
- **B51.9 Plasmodium vivax malaria** without complication
  - Plasmodium vivax malaria NOS

[4] **B52 Plasmodium** malariae **malaria**
- INCLUDES *mixed infections of Plasmodium malariae with other Plasmodium species, except Plasmodium falciparum and Plasmodium vivax*
- [EXCLUDES1] *Plasmodium falciparum (B50.-)*
  Plasmodium vivax (B51.-)
- **B52.0 Plasmodium malariae malaria** with nephropathy
- **B52.8 Plasmodium malariae malaria** with other complications
- **B52.9 Plasmodium malariae malaria** without complication
  - Plasmodium malariae malaria NOS

[4] **B53** Other specified **malaria**
- **B53.0 Plasmodium** ovale **malaria**
  - [EXCLUDES1] *Plasmodium ovale with Plasmodium falciparum (B50.-)*
    Plasmodium ovale with Plasmodium malariae (B52.-)
    Plasmodium ovale with Plasmodium vivax (B51.-)
- **B53.1 Malaria due to** simian plasmodia
  - [EXCLUDES1] *Malaria due to simian plasmodia with Plasmodium falciparum (B50.-)*
    Malaria due to simian plasmodia with Plasmodium malariae (B52.-)
    Malaria due to simian plasmodia with Plasmodium ovale (B53.0)
    Malaria due to simian plasmodia with Plasmodium vivax (B51.-)
- **B53.8 Other malaria, not elsewhere classified**

B54 Unspecified **malaria**

[4] **B55 Leishmaniasis**
- **B55.0** Visceral **leishmaniasis**
  - Kala-azar
  - Post-kala-azar dermal leishmaniasis

Unspecified Code | Other Specified Code | [N] Newborn Age: 0 | [P] Pediatric Age: 0-17 | [M] Maternity Age: 12-55 | [A] Adult Age: 15-124 | ♂ Male | ♀ Female | ● New Code | ▲ Revised Code Title | ►◄ Revised Text

B55.1 Cutaneous **leishmaniasis**
B55.2 Mucocutaneous **leishmaniasis**
B55.9 **Leishmaniasis, unspecified**
🔵 B56 African trypanosomiasis
B56.0 Gambiense **trypanosomiasis**
Infection due to Trypanosoma brucei gambiense
West African sleeping sickness
B56.1 Rhodesiense **trypanosomiasis**
East African sleeping sickness
Infection due to Trypanosoma brucei rhodesiense
B56.9 **African trypanosomiasis, unspecified**
Sleeping sickness NOS
🔵 B57 Chagas' disease
INCLUDES   *American trypanosomiasis*
infection due to Trypanosoma cruzi
B57.0 Acute **Chagas' disease** with heart involvement
Acute Chagas' disease with myocarditis
B57.1 Acute **Chagas' disease** without heart involvement
Acute Chagas' disease NOS
B57.2 **Chagas' disease** (chronic) **with heart involvement**
American trypanosomiasis NOS
Chagas' disease (chronic) NOS
Chagas' disease (chronic) with myocarditis
Trypanosomiasis NOS
🔵 B57.3 **Chagas' disease** (chronic) with digestive system involvement
B57.30 **Chagas' disease with digestive system involvement, unspecified**
B57.31 Megaesophagus in Chagas' disease
B57.32 Megacolon in Chagas' disease
B57.39 **Other digestive system involvement in Chagas' disease**
🔵 B57.4 **Chagas' disease** (chronic) with nervous system involvement
B57.40 **Chagas' disease with nervous system involvement, unspecified**
B57.41 Meningitis in Chagas' disease
B57.42 Meningoencephalitis in Chagas' disease
B57.49 **Other nervous system involvement in Chagas' disease**
🔵 B57.5 **Chagas' disease (chronic) with other organ involvement**
🔵 B58 Toxoplasmosis
INCLUDES   *infection due to Toxoplasma gondii*
EXCLUDES1   *congenital toxoplasmosis (P37.1)*
🔵 B58.0 **Toxoplasma** oculopathy
B58.00 **Toxoplasma oculopathy,** unspecified
B58.01 **Toxoplasma** chorioretinitis
B58.09 Other **toxoplasma oculopathy**
Toxoplasma uveitis
B58.1 **Toxoplasma** hepatitis
B58.2 **Toxoplasma** meningoencephalitis
B58.3 Pulmonary **toxoplasmosis**
🔵 B58.8 **Toxoplasmosis** with other organ involvement
B58.81 **Toxoplasma** myocarditis
B58.82 **Toxoplasma** myositis
B58.83 **Toxoplasma** tubulo-interstitial nephropathy
Toxoplasma pyelonephritis
B58.89 **Toxoplasmosis with other organ involvement**
B58.9 **Toxoplasmosis, unspecified**
B59 Pneumocystosis
Pneumonia due to Pneumocystis carinii
Pneumonia due to Pneumocystis jiroveci
🔵 B60 **Other protozoal diseases, not elsewhere classified**
EXCLUDES1   *cryptosporidiosis (A07.2)*
intestinal microsporidiosis (A07.8)
isosporiasis (A07.3)

B60.0 **Babesiosis**
Piroplasmosis
🔵 B60.1 **Acanthamebiasis**
B60.10 **Acanthamebiasis, unspecified**
B60.11 Meningoencephalitis **due to Acanthamoeba (culbertsoni)**
B60.12 Conjunctivitis **due to Acanthamoeba**
B60.13 Keratoconjunctivitis **due to Acanthamoeba**
B60.19 **Other acanthamebic disease**
B60.2 **Naegleriasis**
Primary amebic meningoencephalitis
B60.8 **Other specified protozoal diseases**
Microsporidiosis
B64 **Unspecified protozoal disease**

Helminthiases (B65-B83)

🔵 B65 Schistosomiasis [bilharziasis]
INCLUDES   *snail fever*
B65.0 **Schistosomiasis due to Schistosoma** haematobium **[urinary schistosomiasis]**
B65.1 **Schistosomiasis due to Schistosoma** mansoni **[intestinal schistosomiasis]**
B65.2 **Schistosomiasis due to Schistosoma** japonicum
Asiatic schistosomiasis
B65.3 **Cercarial dermatitis**
Swimmer's itch
B65.8 **Other schistosomiasis**
Infection due to Schistosoma intercalatum
Infection due to Schistosoma mattheei
Infection due to Schistosoma mekongi
B65.9 **Schistosomiasis, unspecified**
🔵 B66 **Other fluke infections**
B66.0 **Opisthorchiasis**
Infection due to cat liver fluke
Infection due to Opisthorchis (felineus)(viverrini)
B66.1 **Clonorchiasis**
Chinese liver fluke disease
Infection due to Clonorchis sinensis
Oriental liver fluke disease
B66.2 **Dicroceliasis**
Infection due to Dicrocoelium dendriticum
Lancet fluke infection
B66.3 **Fascioliasis**
Infection due to Fasciola gigantica
Infection due to Fasciola hepatica
Infection due to Fasciola indica
Sheep liver fluke disease
B66.4 **Paragonimiasis**
Infection due to Paragonimus species
Lung fluke disease
Pulmonary distomiasis
B66.5 **Fasciolopsiasis**
Infection due to Fasciolopsis buski
Intestinal distomiasis
B66.8 **Other specified fluke infections**
Echinostomiasis
Heterophyiasis
Metagonimiasis
Nanophyetiasis
Watsoniasis
B66.9 **Fluke infection, unspecified**
🔵 B67 Echinococcosis
INCLUDES   *hydatidosis*
B67.0 **Echinococcus** granulosus **infection of** liver
B67.1 **Echinococcus** granulosus **infection of** lung
B67.2 **Echinococcus** granulosus **infection of** bone

🔵 4th character required	🔵 5th character required	🔵 6th character required	🔵 7th character required	🔵 Extension 'X' Alert

EXCLUDES 1 Not coded here   **EXCLUDES 2** Not included here   PDx Primary Diagnosis Only   Manifestation Code

[5] **B67.3 Echinococcus granulosus infection, other and multiple sites**

B67.31 Echinococcus granulosus infection, thyroid gland

B67.32 Echinococcus granulosus infection, multiple sites

B67.39 Echinococcus granulosus infection, other sites

B67.4 Echinococcus granulosus infection, unspecified

Dog tapeworm (infection)

B67.5 Echinococcus multilocularis infection of liver

[5] **B67.6 Echinococcus multilocularis infection, other and multiple sites**

B67.61 Echinococcus multilocularis infection, multiple sites

B67.69 Echinococcus multilocularis infection, other sites

B67.7 Echinococcus multilocularis infection, unspecified

B67.8 Echinococcosis, unspecified, of liver

[5] **B67.9 Echinococcosis, other and unspecified**

B67.90 Echinococcosis, unspecified

Echinococcosis NOS

B67.99 Other echinococcosis

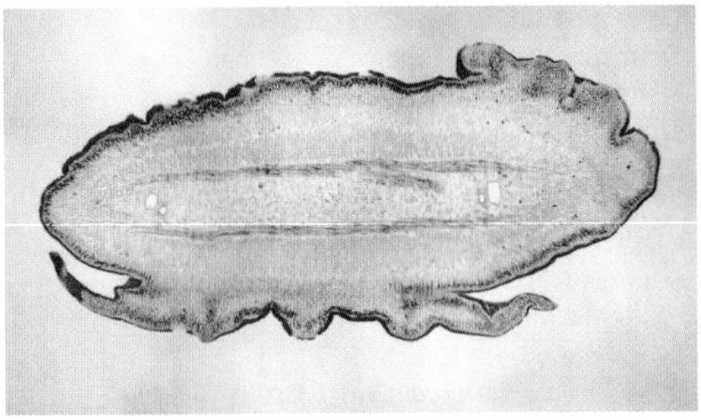

Figure 2.4 Taeniasis

[4] **B68 Taeniasis**

[EXCLUDES1] *cysticercosis (B69.-)*

B68.0 Taenia solium taeniasis

Pork tapeworm (infection)

B68.1 Taenia saginata taeniasis

Beef tapeworm (infection)
Infection due to adult tapeworm Taenia saginata

B68.9 Taeniasis, unspecified

[4] **B69 Cysticercosis**

[INCLUDES] *cysticerciasis infection due to larval form of Taenia solium*

B69.0 Cysticercosis of central nervous system

B69.1 Cysticercosis of eye

[5] **B69.8 Cysticercosis of other sites**

B69.81 Myositis in cysticercosis

B69.89 Cysticercosis of other sites

B69.9 Cysticercosis, unspecified

[4] **B70 Diphyllobothriasis and sparganosis**

B70.0 Diphyllobothriasis

Diphyllobothrium (adult) (latum) (pacificum) infection
Fish tapeworm (infection)

[EXCLUDES2] *larval diphyllobothriasis (B70.1)*

B70.1 Sparganosis

Infection due to Sparganum (mansoni) (proliferum)
Infection due to Spirometra larva
Larval diphyllobothriasis
Spirometrosis

[4] **B71 Other cestode infections**

B71.0 Hymenolepiasis

Dwarf tapeworm infection
Rat tapeworm (infection)

B71.1 Dipylidiasis

B71.8 Other specified cestode infections

Coenurosis

B71.9 Cestode infection, unspecified

Tapeworm (infection) NOS

B72 Dracunculiasis

[INCLUDES] *guinea worm infection*
infection due to Dracunculus medinensis

[4] **B73 Onchocerciasis**

[INCLUDES] *onchocerca volvulus infection*
onchocercosis
river blindness

[5] **B73.0 Onchocerciasis with eye disease**

B73.00 Onchocerciasis with eye involvement, unspecified

B73.01 Onchocerciasis with endophthalmitis

B73.02 Onchocerciasis with glaucoma

B73.09 Onchocerciasis with other eye involvement

Infestation of eyelid due to onchocerciasis

B73.1 Onchocerciasis without eye disease

[4] **B74 Filariasis**

[EXCLUDES2] *onchocerciasis (B73)*
tropical (pulmonary) eosinophilia NOS (J82)

B74.0 Filariasis due to Wuchereria bancrofti

Bancroftian elephantiasis
Bancroftian filariasis

B74.1 Filariasis due to Brugia malayi

B74.2 Filariasis due to Brugia timori

B74.3 Loiasis

Calabar swelling
Eyeworm disease of Africa
Loa loa infection

B74.4 Mansonelliasis

Infection due to Mansonella ozzardi
Infection due to Mansonella perstans
Infection due to Mansonella streptocerca

B74.8 Other filariases

Dirofilariasis

B74.9 Filariasis, unspecified

B75 Trichinellosis

[INCLUDES] *infection due to Trichinella species*
trichiniasis

[4] **B76 Hookworm diseases**

[INCLUDES] *uncinariasis*

B76.0 Ancylostomiasis

Infection due to Ancylostoma species

B76.1 Necatoriasis

Infection due to Necator americanus

B76.8 Other hookworm diseases

B76.9 Hookworm disease, unspecified

Cutaneous larva migrans NOS

[4] **B77 Ascariasis**

[INCLUDES] *ascaridiasis*
roundworm infection

B77.0 Ascariasis with intestinal complications

[5] **B77.8 Ascariasis with other complications**

B77.81 Ascariasis pneumonia

B77.89 Ascariasis with other complications

B77.9 Ascariasis, unspecified

[4] **B78 Strongyloidiasis**

[EXCLUDES1] *trichostrongyliasis (B81.2)*

B78.0 Intestinal strongyloidiasis

B78.1 Cutaneous strongyloidiasis

B78.7 Disseminated strongyloidiasis

B78.9 Strongyloidiasis, unspecified

B79 Trichuriasis

[INCLUDES] *trichocephaliasis*
whipworm (disease)(infection)

Unspecified Code | Other Specified Code | [N] Newborn Age: 0 | [P] Pediatric Age: 0-17 | [M] Maternity Age: 12-55
[A] Adult Age: 15-124 | ♂ Male | ♀ Female | ● New Code | ▲ Revised Code Title | ►◄ Revised Text

B80 Enterobiasis

[INCLUDES] *oxyuriasis*
pinworm infection
threadworm infection

[4] **B81 Other intestinal helminthiases, not elsewhere classified**

[EXCLUDES1] *angiostrongyliasis due to Parastrongylus cantonensis (B83.2)*

B81.0 Anisakiasis

Infection due to Anisakis larva

B81.1 Intestinal capillariasis

Capillariasis NOS
Infection due to Capillaria philippinensis
[EXCLUDES2] *hepatic capillariasis (B83.8)*

B81.2 Trichostrongyliasis

B81.3 Intestinal angiostrongyliasis

Angiostrongyliasis due to Parastrongylus costaricensis

B81.4 Mixed intestinal helminthiases

Infection due to intestinal helminths classified to more than one of the categories B65.0-B81.3 and B81.8
Mixed helminthiasis NOS

B81.8 Other specified intestinal helminthiases

Infection due to Oesophagostomum species [esophagostomiasis]
Infection due to Ternidens diminutus [ternidensiasis]

[4] **B82 Unspecified intestinal parasitism**

B82.0 Intestinal helminthiasis, unspecified

B82.9 Intestinal parasitism, unspecified

[4] **B83 Other helminthiases**

[EXCLUDES1] *capillariasis NOS (B81.1)*
[EXCLUDES2] *intestinal capillariasis (B81.1)*

B83.0 Visceral larva migrans

Toxocariasis

B83.1 Gnathostomiasis

Wandering swelling

B83.2 Angiostrongyliasis due to Parastrongylus cantonensis

Eosinophilic meningoencephalitis due to Parastrongylus cantonensis
[EXCLUDES2] *intestinal angiostrongyliasis (B81.3)*

B83.3 Syngamiasis

Syngamosis

B83.4 Internal hirudiniasis

[EXCLUDES2] *external hirudiniasis (B88.3)*

B83.8 Other specified helminthiases

Acanthocephaliasis
Gongylonemiasis
Hepatic capillariasis
Metastrongyliasis
Thelaziasis

B83.9 Helminthiasis, unspecified

Worms NOS
[EXCLUDES1] *intestinal helminthiasis NOS (B82.0)*

Pediculosis, acariasis and other infestations (B85-B89)

[4] **B85 Pediculosis and phthiriasis**

B85.0 Pediculosis due to Pediculus humanus capitis

Head-louse infestation

B85.1 Pediculosis due to Pediculus humanus corporis

Body-louse infestation

B85.2 Pediculosis, unspecified

B85.3 Phthiriasis

Infestation by crab-louse
Infestation by Phthirus pubis

B85.4 Mixed pediculosis and phthiriasis

Infestation classifiable to more than one of the categories B85.0-B85.3

B86 Scabies

Sarcoptic itch

[4] **B87 Myiasis**

[INCLUDES] *infestation by larva of flies*

B87.0 Cutaneous myiasis

Creeping myiasis

B87.1 Wound myiasis

Traumatic myiasis

B87.2 Ocular myiasis

B87.3 Nasopharyngeal myiasis

Laryngeal myiasis

B87.4 Aural myiasis

[5] **B87.8 Myiasis of other sites**

B87.81 Genitourinary myiasis

B87.82 Intestinal myiasis

B87.89 Myiasis of other sites

B87.9 Myiasis, unspecified

[4] **B88 Other infestations**

B88.0 Other acariasis

Acarine dermatitis
Dermatitis due to Demodex species
Dermatitis due to Dermanyssus gallinae
Dermatitis due to Liponyssoides sanguineus
Trombiculosis
[EXCLUDES2] *scabies (B86)*

B88.1 Tungiasis [sandflea infestation]

B88.2 Other arthropod infestations

Scarabiasis

B88.3 External hirudiniasis

Leech infestation NOS
[EXCLUDES2] *internal hirudiniasis (B83.4)*

B88.8 Other specified infestations

Ichthyoparasitism due to Vandellia cirrhosa
Linguatulosis
Porocephaliasis

B88.9 Infestation, unspecified

Infestation (skin) NOS
Infestation by mites NOS
Skin parasites NOS

B89 Unspecified parasitic disease

Sequelae of infectious and parasitic diseases (B90-B94)

Code first condition resulting from (sequela) the infectious or parasitic disease

[NOTES] Categories B90-B94 are to be used to indicate conditions in categories A00-B89 as the cause of sequelae, which are themselves classified elsewhere. The 'sequelae' include conditions specified as such; they also include residuals of diseases classifiable to the above categories if there is evidence that the disease itself is no longer present. Codes from these categories are not to be used for chronic infections. Code chronic current infections to active infectious disease as appropriate.

[4] **B90 Sequelae of tuberculosis**

B90.0 Sequelae of central nervous system tuberculosis

B90.1 Sequelae of genitourinary tuberculosis

B90.2 Sequelae of tuberculosis of bones and joints

B90.8 Sequelae of tuberculosis of other organs

[EXCLUDES2] *sequelae of respiratory tuberculosis (B90.9)*

B90.9 Sequelae of respiratory and unspecified tuberculosis

Sequelae of tuberculosis NOS

B91 Sequelae of poliomyelitis

[EXCLUDES1] *postpolio syndrome (G14)*

B92 Sequelae of leprosy

[4] B94 Sequelae of other and unspecified infectious and parasitic diseases
B94.0 Sequelae of trachoma
B94.1 Sequelae of viral encephalitis
B94.2 Sequelae of viral hepatitis
B94.8 Sequelae of other specified infectious and parasitic diseases
B94.9 Sequelae of unspecified infectious and parasitic disease

Bacterial and viral infectious agents (B95-B97)

[NOTES] These categories are provided for use as supplementary or additional codes to identify the infectious agent(s) in diseases classified elsewhere.

[4] B95 Streptococcus, Staphylococcus, and Enterococcus as the cause of diseases classified elsewhere
B95.0 Streptococcus, group A, as the cause of diseases classified elsewhere
B95.1 Streptococcus, group B, as the cause of diseases classified elsewhere
B95.2 Enterococcus as the cause of diseases classified elsewhere
B95.3 Streptococcus pneumoniae as the cause of diseases classified elsewhere
B95.4 Other streptococcus as the cause of diseases classified elsewhere
B95.5 Unspecified streptococcus as the cause of diseases classified elsewhere
[5] B95.6 Staphylococcus aureus as the cause of diseases classified elsewhere
B95.61 Methicillin susceptible Staphylococcus aureus infection as the cause of diseases classified elsewhere
Methicillin susceptible Staphylococcus aureus (MSSA) infection as the cause of diseases classified elsewhere
Staphylococcus aureus infection NOS as the cause of diseases classified elsewhere
B95.62 Methicillin resistant Staphylococcus aureus infection as the cause of diseases classified elsewhere
Methicillin resistant staphylococcus aureus (MRSA) infection as the cause of diseases classified elsewhere
B95.7 Other staphylococcus as the cause of diseases classified elsewhere
B95.8 Unspecified staphylococcus as the cause of diseases classified elsewhere

[4] B96 Other bacterial agents as the cause of diseases classified elsewhere
B96.0 Mycoplasma pneumoniae [M. pneumoniae] as the cause of diseases classified elsewhere
Pleuro-pneumonia-like-organism [PPLO]
B96.1 Klebsiella pneumoniae [K. pneumoniae] as the cause of diseases classified elsewhere
[5] B96.2 Escherichia coli [E. coli] as the cause of diseases classified elsewhere
B96.20 Unspecified Escherichia coli [E. coli] as the cause of diseases classified elsewhere
Escherichia coli [E. coli] NOS
B96.21 Shiga toxin-producing Escherichia coli [E. coli] (STEC) O157 as the cause of diseases classified elsewhere
E. coli O157:H- (nonmotile) with confirmation of Shiga toxin
E. coli O157 with confirmation of Shiga toxin when H antigen is unknown, or is not H7
O157:H7 Escherichia coli [E.coli] with or without confirmation of Shiga toxin-production
Shiga toxin-producing Escherichia coli [E.coli] O157:H7 with or without confirmation of Shiga toxin-production
STEC O157:H7 with or without confirmation of Shiga toxin-production
B96.22 Other specified Shiga toxin-producing Escherichia coli [E. coli] (STEC) as the cause of diseases classified elsewhere
Non-O157 Shiga toxin-producing Escherichia coli [E.coli]
Non-O157 Shiga toxin-producing Escherichia coli [E.coli] with known O group
B96.23 Unspecified Shiga toxin-producing Escherichia coli [E. coli] (STEC) as the cause of diseases classified elsewhere
Shiga toxin-producing Escherichia coli [E. coli] with unspecified O group
STEC NOS
B96.29 Other Escherichia coli [E. coli] as the cause of diseases classified elsewhere
Non-Shiga toxin-producing E. coli
B96.3 Hemophilus influenzae [H. influenzae] as the cause of diseases classified elsewhere
B96.4 Proteus (mirabilis) (morganii) as the cause of diseases classified elsewhere
B96.5 Pseudomonas (aeruginosa) (mallei) (pseudomallei) as the cause of diseases classified elsewhere
B96.6 Bacteroides fragilis [B. fragilis] as the cause of diseases classified elsewhere
B96.7 Clostridium perfringens [C. perfringens] as the cause of diseases classified elsewhere
[5] B96.8 Other specified bacterial agents as the cause of diseases classified elsewhere
B96.81 Helicobacter pylori [H. pylori] as the cause of diseases classified elsewhere
B96.82 Vibrio vulnificus as the cause of diseases classified elsewhere
B96.89 Other specified bacterial agents as the cause of diseases classified elsewhere

[4] B97 Viral agents as the cause of diseases classified elsewhere
B97.0 Adenovirus as the cause of diseases classified elsewhere
[5] B97.1 Enterovirus as the cause of diseases classified elsewhere
B97.10 Unspecified enterovirus as the cause of diseases classified elsewhere
B97.11 Coxsackievirus as the cause of diseases classified elsewhere
B97.12 Echovirus as the cause of diseases classified elsewhere
B97.19 Other enterovirus as the cause of diseases classified elsewhere
[5] B97.2 Coronavirus as the cause of diseases classified elsewhere
B97.21 SARS-associated coronavirus as the cause of diseases classified elsewhere
[EXCLUDES1] *pneumonia due to SARS-associated coronavirus (J12.81)*
B97.29 Other coronavirus as the cause of diseases classified elsewhere
[5] B97.3 Retrovirus as the cause of diseases classified elsewhere
[EXCLUDES1] *Human immunodeficiency virus [HIV] disease (B20)*
B97.30 Unspecified retrovirus as the cause of diseases classified elsewhere
B97.31 Lentivirus as the cause of diseases classified elsewhere

Unspecified Code | Other Specified Code | [N] Newborn Age: 0 | [P] Pediatric Age: 0-17 | [M] Maternity Age: 12-55
[A] Adult Age: 15-124 | ♂ Male | ♀ Female | ● New Code | ▲ Revised Code Title | ►◄ Revised Text

B97.32 Oncovirus as the cause of diseases classified elsewhere

B97.33 Human T-cell lymphotrophic virus, type I [HTLV-I] as the cause of diseases classified elsewhere

B97.34 Human T-cell lymphotrophic virus, type II [HTLV-II] as the cause of diseases classified elsewhere

B97.35 Human immunodeficiency virus, type 2 [HIV 2] as the cause of diseases classified elsewhere

B97.39 Other retrovirus as the cause of diseases classified elsewhere

B97.4 Respiratory syncytial virus as the cause of diseases classified elsewhere

B97.5 Reovirus as the cause of diseases classified elsewhere

B97.6 Parvovirus as the cause of diseases classified elsewhere

B97.7 Papillomavirus as the cause of diseases classified elsewhere

[5th] B97.8 Other viral agents as the cause of diseases classified elsewhere

B97.81 Human metapneumovirus as the cause of diseases classified elsewhere

B97.89 Other viral agents as the cause of diseases classified elsewhere

Other infectious diseases (B99)

[4th] B99 Other and unspecified infectious diseases

B99.8 Other infectious disease

B99.9 Unspecified infectious disease

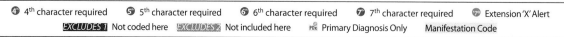

Chapter 2: Neoplasms (C00-D49)

Chapter Specific Coding Guidelines

General Guidelines

Chapter 2 of the ICD-10-CM contains the codes for most benign and all malignant neoplasms. Certain benign neoplasms, such as prostatic adenomas, may be found in the specific body system chapters. To properly code a neoplasm it is necessary to determine from the record if the neoplasm is benign, in-situ, malignant, or of uncertain histologic behavior. If malignant, any secondary (metastatic) sites should also be determined.

Primary malignant neoplasms overlapping site boundaries

A primary malignant neoplasm that overlaps two or more contiguous (next to each other) sites should be classified to the subcategory/code .8 ('overlapping lesion'), unless the combination is specifically indexed elsewhere. For multiple neoplasms of the same site that are not contiguous such as tumors in different quadrants of the same breast, codes for each site should be assigned.

Malignant neoplasm of ectopic tissue

Malignant neoplasms of ectopic tissue are to be coded to the site of origin mentioned, e.g., ectopic pancreatic malignant neoplasms involving the stomach are coded to pancreas, unspecified (C25.9).

The neoplasm table in the Alphabetic Index should be referenced first. However, if the histological term is documented, that term should be referenced first, rather than going immediately to the Neoplasm Table, in order to determine which column in the Neoplasm Table is appropriate. For example, if the documentation indicates "adenoma," refer to the term in the Alphabetic Index to review the entries under this term and the instructional note to "see also neoplasm, by site, benign." The table provides the proper code based on the type of neoplasm and the site. It is important to select the proper column in the table that corresponds to the type of neoplasm. The Tabular List should then be referenced to verify that the correct code has been selected from the table and that a more specific site code does not exist.

See Section I.C.21. Factors influencing health status and contact with health services, Status, for information regarding Z15.0, codes for genetic susceptibility to cancer.

a. Treatment directed at the malignancy

If the treatment is directed at the malignancy, designate the malignancy as the principal diagnosis.

The only exception to this guideline is if a patient admission/encounter is solely for the administration of chemotherapy, immunotherapy or radiation therapy, assign the appropriate Z51.-- code as the first-listed or principal diagnosis, and the diagnosis or problem for which the service is being performed as a secondary diagnosis.

b. Treatment of secondary site

When a patient is admitted because of a primary neoplasm with metastasis and treatment is directed toward the secondary site only, the secondary neoplasm is designated as the principal diagnosis even though the primary malignancy is still present.

c. Coding and sequencing of complications

Coding and sequencing of complications associated with the malignancies or with the therapy thereof are subject to the following guidelines:

1) **Anemia associated with malignancy**
When admission/encounter is for management of an anemia associated with the malignancy, and the treatment is only for anemia, the appropriate code for the malignancy is sequenced as the principal or first-listed diagnosis followed by the appropriate code for the anemia (such as code D63.0, Anemia in neoplastic disease).

2) **Anemia associated with chemotherapy, immunotherapy and radiation therapy**
When the admission/encounter is for management of an anemia associated with an adverse effect of the administration of chemotherapy or immunotherapy and the only treatment is for the anemia, the anemia code is sequenced first followed by the appropriate codes for the neoplasm and the adverse effect (T45.1X5, Adverse effect of antineoplastic and immunosuppressive drugs).

When the admission/encounter is for management of an anemia associated with an adverse effect of radiotherapy, the anemia code should be sequenced first, followed by the appropriate neoplasm code and code Y84.2, Radiological procedure and radiotherapy as the cause of abnormal reaction of the patient, or of later complication, without mention of misadventure at the time of the procedure.

3) **Management of dehydration due to the malignancy**
When the admission/encounter is for management of dehydration due to the malignancy and only the dehydration is being treated (intravenous rehydration), the dehydration is sequenced first, followed by the code(s) for the malignancy.

4) **Treatment of a complication resulting from a surgical procedure**
When the admission/encounter is for treatment of a complication resulting from a surgical procedure, designate the complication as the principal or first-listed diagnosis if treatment is directed at resolving the complication.

d. Primary malignancy previously excised

When a primary malignancy has been previously excised or eradicated from its site and there is no further treatment directed to that site and there is no evidence of any existing primary malignancy, a code from category Z85, Personal history of malignant neoplasm, should be used to indicate the former site of the malignancy. Any mention of extension, invasion, or metastasis to another site is coded as a secondary malignant neoplasm to that site. The secondary site may be the principal or first-listed with the Z85 code used as a secondary code.

e. Admissions/Encounters involving chemotherapy, immunotherapy and radiation therapy

1) **Episode of care involves surgical removal of neoplasm**
When an episode of care involves the surgical removal of a neoplasm, primary or secondary site, followed by adjunct chemotherapy or radiation treatment during the same episode of care, the code for the neoplasm should be assigned as principal or first-listed diagnosis.

2) **Patient admission/encounter solely for administration of chemotherapy, immunotherapy and radiation therapy**
If a patient admission/encounter is solely for the administration of chemotherapy, immunotherapy or radiation therapy assign code Z51.0, Encounter for antineoplastic radiation therapy, or Z51.11, Encounter for antineoplastic chemotherapy, or Z51.12, Encounter for antineoplastic immunotherapy as the first-listed or principal diagnosis. If a patient receives more than one of these therapies during the same admission more than one of these codes may be assigned, in any sequence.

The malignancy for which the therapy is being administered should be assigned as a secondary diagnosis.

3) **Patient admitted for radiation therapy, chemotherapy or immunotherapy and develops complications**
When a patient is admitted for the purpose of radiotherapy, immunotherapy or chemotherapy and develops complications such as uncontrolled nausea and vomiting or dehydration, the principal or first-listed diagnosis is Z51.0, Encounter for antineoplastic radiation therapy, or Z51.11,

Encounter for antineoplastic chemotherapy, or Z51.12, Encounter for antineoplastic immunotherapy followed by any codes for the complications.

f. **Admission/encounter to determine extent of malignancy**
When the reason for admission/encounter is to determine the extent of the malignancy, or for a procedure such as paracentesis or thoracentesis, the primary malignancy or appropriate metastatic site is designated as the principal or first-listed diagnosis, even though chemotherapy or radiotherapy is administered.

g. **Symptoms, signs, and abnormal findings listed in Chapter 18 associated with neoplasms**
Symptoms, signs, and ill-defined conditions listed in Chapter 18 characteristic of, or associated with, an existing primary or secondary site malignancy cannot be used to replace the malignancy as principal or first-listed diagnosis, regardless of the number of admissions or encounters for treatment and care of the neoplasm.

See section I.C.21. Factors Influencing Health Status and Contact with Health Services, Encounter for Prophylactic Organ Removal.

h. **Admission/encounter for pain control/management**
See Section I.C.6. for information on coding admission/encounter for pain control/management.

i. **Malignancy in two or more noncontiguous sites**
A patient may have more than one malignant tumor in the same organ. These tumors may represent different primaries or metastatic disease, depending on the site. Should the documentation be unclear, the provider should be queried as to the status of each tumor so that the correct codes can be assigned.

j. **Disseminated malignant neoplasm, unspecified**
Code C80.0, Disseminated malignant neoplasm, unspecified, is for use only in those cases where the patient has advanced metastatic disease and no known primary or secondary sites are specified. It should not be used in place of assigning codes for the primary site and all known secondary sites.

k. **Malignant neoplasm without specification of site**
Code C80.1, Malignant (primary) neoplasm, unspecified, equates to Cancer, unspecified. This code should only be used when no determination can be made as to the primary site of a malignancy. This code should rarely be used in the inpatient setting.

l. **Sequencing of neoplasm codes**
1) **Encounter for treatment of primary malignancy**
If the reason for the encounter is for treatment of a primary malignancy, assign the malignancy as the principal/first-listed diagnosis. The primary site is to be sequenced first, followed by any metastatic sites.

2) **Encounter for treatment of secondary malignancy**
When an encounter is for a primary malignancy with metastasis and treatment is directed toward the metastatic (secondary) site(s) only, the metastatic site(s) is designated as the principal/first-listed diagnosis. The primary malignancy is coded as an additional code.

3) **Malignant neoplasm in a pregnant patient**
When a pregnant woman has a malignant neoplasm, a code from subcategory O9A.1-, Malignant neoplasm complicating pregnancy, childbirth, and the puerperium, should be sequenced first, followed by the appropriate code from Chapter 2 to indicate the type of neoplasm.

4) **Encounter for complication associated with a neoplasm**
When an encounter is for management of a complication associated with a neoplasm, such as dehydration, and the treatment is only for the complication, the complication is coded first, followed by the appropriate code(s) for the neoplasm.

The exception to this guideline is anemia. When the admission/encounter is for management of an anemia associated with the malignancy, and the treatment is only for anemia, the appropriate code for the malignancy is sequenced as the principal or first-listed diagnosis followed by code D63.0, Anemia in neoplastic disease.

5) **Complication from surgical procedure for treatment of a neoplasm**
When an encounter is for treatment of a complication resulting from a surgical procedure performed for the treatment of the neoplasm, designate the complication as the principal/first-listed diagnosis. See guideline regarding the coding of a current malignancy versus personal history to determine if the code for the neoplasm should also be assigned.

6) **Pathologic fracture due to a neoplasm**
When an encounter is for a pathological fracture due to a neoplasm, and the focus of treatment is the fracture, a code from subcategory M84.5, Pathological fracture in neoplastic disease, should be sequenced first, followed by the code for the neoplasm.

If the focus of treatment is the neoplasm with an associated pathological fracture, the neoplasm code should be sequenced first, followed by a code from M84.5 for the pathological fracture.

m. **Current malignancy versus personal history of malignancy**
When a primary malignancy has been excised but further treatment, such as an additional surgery for the malignancy, radiation therapy or chemotherapy is directed to that site, the primary malignancy code should be used until treatment is completed.

When a primary malignancy has been previously excised or eradicated from its site, there is no further treatment (of the malignancy) directed to that site, and there is no evidence of any existing primary malignancy, a code from category Z85, Personal history of malignant neoplasm, should be used to indicate the former site of the malignancy.

See Section I.C.21. Factors influencing health status and contact with health services, History (of)

n. **Leukemia, Multiple Myeloma, and Malignant Plasma Cell Neoplasms in remission versus personal history**
The categories for leukemia, and category C90, Multiple myeloma and malignant plasma cell neoplasms, have codes indicating whether or not the leukemia has achieved remission. There are also codes Z85.6, Personal history of leukemia, and Z85.79, Personal history of other malignant neoplasms of lymphoid, hematopoietic and related tissues. If the documentation is unclear, as to whether the leukemia has achieved remission, the provider should be queried.

See Section I.C.21. Factors influencing health status and contact with health services, History (of)

o. **Aftercare following surgery for neoplasm**
See Section I.C.21. Factors influencing health status and contact with health services, Aftercare

p. **Follow-up care for completed treatment of a malignancy**
See Section I.C.21. Factors influencing health status and contact with health services, Follow-up

q. **Prophylactic organ removal for prevention of malignancy**
See Section I.C. 21, Factors influencing health status and contact with health services, Prophylactic organ removal

r. **Malignant neoplasm associated with transplanted organ**
A malignant neoplasm of a transplanted organ should be coded as a transplant complication. Assign first the appropriate code from category T86.-, Complications of transplanted organs and tissue, followed by code C80.2, Malignant neoplasm associated with transplanted organ. Use an additional code for the specific malignancy.

Neoplasms (C00-D49)

NOTES Functional activity

All neoplasms are classified in this chapter, whether they are functionally active or not. An additional code from Chapter 4 may be used, to identify functional activity associated with any neoplasm.

Morphology [Histology]

Chapter 2 classifies neoplasms primarily by site (topography), with broad groupings for behavior, malignant, in situ, benign, etc. The Table of Neoplasms should be used to identify the correct topography code. In a few cases, such as for malignant melanoma and certain neuroendocrine tumors, the morphology (histologic type) is included in the category and codes.

Primary malignant neoplasms overlapping site boundaries

A primary malignant neoplasm that overlaps two or more contiguous (next to each other) sites should be classified to the subcategory/code .8 ('overlapping lesion'), unless the combination is specifically indexed elsewhere.

For multiple neoplasms of the same site that are not contiguous, such as tumors in different quadrants of the same breast, codes for each site should be assigned.

Malignant neoplasm of ectopic tissue

Malignant neoplasms of ectopic tissue are to be coded to the site mentioned, e.g., ectopic pancreatic malignant neoplasms are coded to pancreas, unspecified (C25.9).

Malignant neoplasms (C00-C96)

Malignant neoplasms of lip, oral cavity and pharynx (C00-C14)

C00 Malignant neoplasm of lip

    Use additional code to identify:

    alcohol abuse and dependence (F10.-)

    history of tobacco use (Z87.891)

    tobacco dependence (F17.-)

    tobacco use (Z72.0)

    EXCLUDES1 *malignant melanoma of lip (C43.0)*

              Merkel cell carcinoma of lip (C4A.0)

              other and unspecified malignant neoplasm of skin of lip (C44.0-)

C00.0 Malignant neoplasm of external upper lip

    Malignant neoplasm of lipstick area of upper lip

    Malignant neoplasm of upper lip NOS

    Malignant neoplasm of vermilion border of upper lip

C00.1 Malignant neoplasm of external lower lip

    Malignant neoplasm of lower lip NOS

    Malignant neoplasm of lipstick area of lower lip

    Malignant neoplasm of vermilion border of lower lip

C00.2 Malignant neoplasm of external lip, unspecified

    Malignant neoplasm of vermilion border of lip NOS

C00.3 Malignant neoplasm of upper lip, inner aspect

    Malignant neoplasm of buccal aspect of upper lip

    Malignant neoplasm of frenulum of upper lip

    Malignant neoplasm of mucosa of upper lip

    Malignant neoplasm of oral aspect of upper lip

C00.4 Malignant neoplasm of lower lip, inner aspect

    Malignant neoplasm of buccal aspect of lower lip

    Malignant neoplasm of frenulum of lower lip

    Malignant neoplasm of mucosa of lower lip

    Malignant neoplasm of oral aspect of lower lip

C00.5 Malignant neoplasm of lip, unspecified, inner aspect

    Malignant neoplasm of buccal aspect of lip, unspecified

    Malignant neoplasm of frenulum of lip, unspecified

    Malignant neoplasm of mucosa of lip, unspecified

    Malignant neoplasm of oral aspect of lip, unspecified

C00.6 Malignant neoplasm of commissure of lip, **unspecified**

C00.8 Malignant neoplasm of overlapping sites **of lip**

C00.9 Malignant neoplasm of lip, unspecified

C01 Malignant neoplasm of base of tongue

    Malignant neoplasm of dorsal surface of base of tongue

    Malignant neoplasm of fixed part of tongue NOS

    Malignant neoplasm of posterior third of tongue

    Use additional code to identify:

    alcohol abuse and dependence (F10.-)

    history of tobacco use (Z87.891)

    tobacco dependence (F17.-)

    tobacco use (Z72.0)

C02 Malignant neoplasm of other and unspecified parts of tongue

    Use additional code to identify:

    alcohol abuse and dependence (F10.-)

    history of tobacco use (Z87.891)

    tobacco dependence (F17.-)

    tobacco use (Z72.0)

C02.0 Malignant neoplasm of dorsal surface **of tongue**

    Malignant neoplasm of anterior two-thirds of tongue, dorsal surface

    EXCLUDES2 *malignant neoplasm of dorsal surface of base of tongue (C01)*

C02.1 Malignant neoplasm of border **of tongue**

    Malignant neoplasm of tip of tongue

C02.2 Malignant neoplasm of ventral surface **of tongue**

    Malignant neoplasm of anterior two-thirds of tongue, ventral surface

    Malignant neoplasm of frenulum linguae

C02.3 Malignant neoplasm of anterior two-thirds **of tongue, part unspecified**

    Malignant neoplasm of middle third of tongue NOS

    Malignant neoplasm of mobile part of tongue NOS

C02.4 Malignant neoplasm of lingual tonsil

    EXCLUDES2 *malignant neoplasm of tonsil NOS (C09.9)*

C02.8 Malignant neoplasm of overlapping sites **of tongue**

    Malignant neoplasm of two or more contiguous sites of tongue

C02.9 Malignant neoplasm of tongue, unspecified

C03 Malignant neoplasm of gum

    INCLUDES *malignant neoplasm of alveolar (ridge) mucosa*

              malignant neoplasm of gingiva

    Use additional code to identify:

    alcohol abuse and dependence (F10.-)

    history of tobacco use (Z87.891)

    tobacco dependence (F17.-)

    tobacco use (Z72.0)

    EXCLUDES2 *malignant odontogenic neoplasms (C41.0-C41.1)*

C03.0 Malignant neoplasm of upper gum

C03.1 Malignant neoplasm of lower gum

C03.9 Malignant neoplasm of gum, unspecified

C04 Malignant neoplasm of floor of mouth

    Use additional code to identify:

    alcohol abuse and dependence (F10.-)

    history of tobacco use (Z87.891)

    tobacco dependence (F17.-)

    tobacco use (Z72.0)

C04.0 Malignant neoplasm of anterior floor **of mouth**

    Malignant neoplasm of anterior to the premolar-canine junction

C04.1 Malignant neoplasm of lateral floor **of mouth**

C04.8 Malignant neoplasm of overlapping sites **of floor of mouth**

C04.9 Malignant neoplasm of floor of mouth, unspecified

C05 Malignant neoplasm of palate

    Use additional code to identify:

    alcohol abuse and dependence (F10.-)

    history of tobacco use (Z87.891)

    tobacco dependence (F17.-)

    tobacco use (Z72.0)

    EXCLUDES1 *Kaposi's sarcoma of palate (C46.2)*

Unspecified Code	Other Specified Code	N Newborn Age: 0	P Pediatric Age: 0-17	M Maternity Age: 12-55
A Adult Age: 15-124	♂ Male	♀ Female	● New Code	▲ Revised Code Title ►◄ Revised Text

C05.0 **Malignant neoplasm of** hard **palate**
C05.1 **Malignant neoplasm of** soft **palate**

> EXCLUDES2 *malignant neoplasm of nasopharyngeal surface of soft palate (C11.3)*

C05.2 **Malignant neoplasm of** uvula
C05.8 **Malignant neoplasm of** overlapping sites **of palate**
C05.9 **Malignant neoplasm of palate, unspecified**

Malignant neoplasm of roof of mouth

④ C06 **Malignant neoplasm of other and unspecified parts of** mouth

Use additional code to identify:
alcohol abuse and dependence (F10.-)
history of tobacco use (Z87.891)
tobacco dependence (F17.-)
tobacco use (Z72.0)

C06.0 **Malignant neoplasm of** cheek mucosa

Malignant neoplasm of buccal mucosa NOS
Malignant neoplasm of internal cheek

C06.1 **Malignant neoplasm of** vestibule **of mouth**

Malignant neoplasm of buccal sulcus (upper) (lower)
Malignant neoplasm of labial sulcus (upper) (lower)

C06.2 **Malignant neoplasm of** retromolar area

⑤ C06.8 **Malignant neoplasm of** overlapping sites **of other and unspecified parts of mouth**

C06.80 **Malignant neoplasm of overlapping sites of unspecified parts of mouth**
C06.89 **Malignant neoplasm of overlapping sites of other parts of mouth**

'book leaf' neoplasm [ventral surface of tongue and floor of mouth]

C06.9 **Malignant neoplasm of mouth, unspecified**

Malignant neoplasm of minor salivary gland, unspecified site
Malignant neoplasm of oral cavity NOS

C07 **Malignant neoplasm of** parotid gland

Use additional code to identify:
alcohol abuse and dependence (F10.-)
exposure to environmental tobacco smoke (Z77.22)
exposure to tobacco smoke in the perinatal period (P96.81)
history of tobacco use (Z87.891)
occupational exposure to environmental tobacco smoke (Z57.31)
tobacco dependence (F17.-)
tobacco use (Z72.0)

④ C08 **Malignant neoplasm of other and unspecified** major salivary glands

> INCLUDES *malignant neoplasm of salivary ducts*

Use additional code to identify:
alcohol abuse and dependence (F10.-)
exposure to environmental tobacco smoke (Z77.22)
exposure to tobacco smoke in the perinatal period (P96.81)
history of tobacco use (Z87.891)
occupational exposure to environmental tobacco smoke (Z57.31)
tobacco dependence (F17.-)
tobacco use (Z72.0)

> EXCLUDES1 *malignant neoplasms of specified minor salivary glands which are classified according to their anatomical location*
> EXCLUDES2 *malignant neoplasms of minor salivary glands NOS (C06.9)*
> *malignant neoplasm of parotid gland (C07)*

C08.0 **Malignant neoplasm of** submandibular gland

Malignant neoplasm of submaxillary gland

C08.1 **Malignant neoplasm of** sublingual gland
C08.9 **Malignant neoplasm of major salivary gland, unspecified**

Malignant neoplasm of salivary gland (major) NOS

④ C09 **Malignant neoplasm of** tonsil

Use additional code to identify:
alcohol abuse and dependence (F10.-)
exposure to environmental tobacco smoke (Z77.22)
exposure to tobacco smoke in the perinatal period (P96.81)
history of tobacco use (Z87.891)
occupational exposure to environmental tobacco smoke (Z57.31)
tobacco dependence (F17.-)
tobacco use (Z72.0)

> EXCLUDES2 *malignant neoplasm of lingual tonsil (C02.4)*
> *malignant neoplasm of pharyngeal tonsil (C11.1)*

C09.0 **Malignant neoplasm of** tonsillar fossa
C09.1 **Malignant neoplasm of** tonsillar pillar (anterior) (posterior)
C09.8 **Malignant neoplasm of** overlapping sites **of tonsil**
C09.9 **Malignant neoplasm of tonsil, unspecified**

Malignant neoplasm of tonsil NOS
Malignant neoplasm of faucial tonsils
Malignant neoplasm of palatine tonsils

④ C10 **Malignant neoplasm of** oropharynx

Use additional code to identify:
alcohol abuse and dependence (F10.-)
exposure to environmental tobacco smoke (Z77.22)
exposure to tobacco smoke in the perinatal period (P96.81)
history of tobacco use (Z87.891)
occupational exposure to environmental tobacco smoke (Z57.31)
tobacco dependence (F17.-)
tobacco use (Z72.0)

> EXCLUDES2 *malignant neoplasm of tonsil (C09.-)*

C10.0 **Malignant neoplasm of** vallecula
C10.1 **Malignant neoplasm of** anterior surface of epiglottis

Malignant neoplasm of epiglottis, free border [margin]
Malignant neoplasm of glossoepiglottic fold(s)

> EXCLUDES2 *malignant neoplasm of epiglottis (suprahyoid portion) NOS (C32.1)*

C10.2 **Malignant neoplasm of** lateral wall **of oropharynx**
C10.3 **Malignant neoplasm of** posterior wall **of oropharynx**
C10.4 **Malignant neoplasm of** branchial cleft

Malignant neoplasm of branchial cyst [site of neoplasm]

C10.8 **Malignant neoplasm of** overlapping sites **of oropharynx**

Malignant neoplasm of junctional region of oropharynx

C10.9 **Malignant neoplasm of oropharynx, unspecified**

④ C11 **Malignant neoplasm of** nasopharynx

Use additional code to identify:
exposure to environmental tobacco smoke (Z77.22)
exposure to tobacco smoke in the perinatal period (P96.81)
history of tobacco use (Z87.891)
occupational exposure to environmental tobacco smoke (Z57.31)
tobacco dependence (F17.-)
tobacco use (Z72.0)

C11.0 **Malignant neoplasm of** superior wall **of nasopharynx**

Malignant neoplasm of roof of nasopharynx

C11.1 **Malignant neoplasm of** posterior wall **of nasopharynx**

Malignant neoplasm of adenoid
Malignant neoplasm of pharyngeal tonsil

C11.2 **Malignant neoplasm of** lateral wall **of nasopharynx**

Malignant neoplasm of fossa of Rosenmüller
Malignant neoplasm of opening of auditory tube
Malignant neoplasm of pharyngeal recess

C11.3 **Malignant neoplasm of** anterior wall **of nasopharynx**

---

④ 4th character required   ⑤ 5th character required   ⑥ 6th character required   ⑦ 7th character required   ⑩ Extension 'X' Alert

EXCLUDES 1 Not coded here   EXCLUDES 2 Not included here   PDx Primary Diagnosis Only   Manifestation Code

Malignant neoplasm of floor of nasopharynx
Malignant neoplasm of nasopharyngeal (anterior) (posterior) surface of soft palate
Malignant neoplasm of posterior margin of nasal choana
Malignant neoplasm of posterior margin of nasal septum

C11.8 Malignant neoplasm of overlapping sites **of nasopharynx**

C11.9 Malignant neoplasm of nasopharynx, unspecified

Malignant neoplasm of nasopharyngeal wall NOS

C12 Malignant neoplasm of pyriform sinus

Malignant neoplasm of pyriform fossa
Use additional code to identify:
exposure to environmental tobacco smoke (Z77.22)
exposure to tobacco smoke in the perinatal period (P96.81)
history of tobacco use (Z87.891)
occupational exposure to environmental tobacco smoke (Z57.31)
tobacco dependence (F17.-)
tobacco use (Z72.0)

C13 Malignant neoplasm of hypopharynx

Use additional code to identify:
exposure to environmental tobacco smoke (Z77.22)
exposure to tobacco smoke in the perinatal period (P96.81)
history of tobacco use (Z87.891)
occupational exposure to environmental tobacco smoke (Z57.31)
tobacco dependence (F17.-)
tobacco use (Z72.0)

EXCLUDES2 *malignant neoplasm of pyriform sinus (C12)*

C13.0 Malignant neoplasm of postcricoid region

C13.1 Malignant neoplasm of aryepiglottic fold, hypopharyngeal aspect

Malignant neoplasm of aryepiglottic fold, marginal zone
Malignant neoplasm of aryepiglottic fold NOS
Malignant neoplasm of interarytenoid fold, marginal zone
Malignant neoplasm of interarytenoid fold NOS

EXCLUDES2 *malignant neoplasm of aryepiglottic fold or interarytenoid fold, laryngeal aspect (C32.1)*

C13.2 Malignant neoplasm of posterior wall of **hypopharynx**

C13.8 Malignant neoplasm of overlapping sites **of hypopharynx**

C13.9 Malignant neoplasm of hypopharynx, unspecified

Malignant neoplasm of hypopharyngeal wall NOS

C14 Malignant neoplasm of other and ill-defined sites in the lip, oral cavity and pharynx

Use additional code to identify:
alcohol abuse and dependence (F10.-)
exposure to environmental tobacco smoke (Z77.22)
exposure to tobacco smoke in the perinatal period (P96.81)
history of tobacco use (Z87.891)
occupational exposure to environmental tobacco smoke (Z57.31)
tobacco dependence (F17.-)
tobacco use (Z72.0)

EXCLUDES1 *malignant neoplasm of oral cavity NOS (C06.9)*

C14.0 Malignant neoplasm of pharynx, unspecified

C14.2 Malignant neoplasm of Waldeyer's ring

C14.8 Malignant neoplasm of overlapping sites of lip, oral cavity and pharynx

Primary malignant neoplasm of two or more contiguous sites of lip, oral cavity and pharynx

EXCLUDES1 *'book leaf' neoplasm [ventral surface of tongue and floor of mouth] (C06.89)*

Malignant neoplasms of digestive organs (C15-C26)

EXCLUDES1 *Kaposi's sarcoma of gastrointestinal sites (C46.4)*

C15 Malignant neoplasm of esophagus

Use additional code to identify:
alcohol abuse and dependence (F10.-)

C15.3 Malignant neoplasm of upper third **of esophagus**

C15.4 Malignant neoplasm of middle third **of esophagus**

C15.5 Malignant neoplasm of lower third **of esophagus**

EXCLUDES1 *malignant neoplasm of cardio-esophageal junction (C16.0)*

C15.8 Malignant neoplasm of overlapping sites **of esophagus**

C15.9 Malignant neoplasm of esophagus, unspecified

C16 Malignant neoplasm of stomach

Use additional code to identify:
alcohol abuse and dependence (F10.-)

EXCLUDES2 *malignant carcinoid tumor of the stomach (C7A.092)*

C16.0 Malignant neoplasm of cardia

Malignant neoplasm of cardiac orifice
Malignant neoplasm of cardio-esophageal junction
Malignant neoplasm of esophagus and stomach
Malignant neoplasm of gastro-esophageal junction

C16.1 Malignant neoplasm of fundus **of stomach**

C16.2 Malignant neoplasm of body **of stomach**

C16.3 Malignant neoplasm of pyloric antrum

Malignant neoplasm of gastric antrum

C16.4 Malignant neoplasm of pylorus

Malignant neoplasm of prepylorus
Malignant neoplasm of pyloric canal

C16.5 Malignant neoplasm of lesser curvature **of stomach, unspecified**

Malignant neoplasm of lesser curvature of stomach, not classifiable to C16.1-C16.4

C16.6 Malignant neoplasm of greater curvature **of stomach, unspecified**

Malignant neoplasm of greater curvature of stomach, not classifiable to C16.0-C16.4

C16.8 Malignant neoplasm of overlapping sites **of stomach**

C16.9 Malignant neoplasm of stomach, unspecified

Gastric cancer NOS

C17 Malignant neoplasm of small intestine

EXCLUDES1 *malignant carcinoid tumors of the small intestine (C7A.01)*

C17.0 Malignant neoplasm of duodenum

C17.1 Malignant neoplasm of jejunum

C17.2 Malignant neoplasm of ileum

EXCLUDES1 *malignant neoplasm of ileocecal valve (C18.0)*

C17.3 Meckel's diverticulum, **malignant**

EXCLUDES1 *Meckel's diverticulum, congenital (Q43.0)*

C17.8 Malignant neoplasm of overlapping sites **of small intestine**

C17.9 Malignant neoplasm of small intestine, unspecified

C18 Malignant neoplasm of colon

EXCLUDES1 *malignant carcinoid tumors of the colon (C7A.02-)*

C18.0 Malignant neoplasm of cecum

Malignant neoplasm of ileocecal valve

C18.1 Malignant neoplasm of appendix

C18.2 Malignant neoplasm of ascending colon

C18.3 Malignant neoplasm of hepatic flexure

C18.4 Malignant neoplasm of transverse colon

C18.5 Malignant neoplasm of splenic flexure

C18.6 Malignant neoplasm of descending colon

C18.7 Malignant neoplasm of sigmoid colon

Malignant neoplasm of sigmoid (flexure)

EXCLUDES1 *malignant neoplasm of rectosigmoid junction (C19)*

Unspecified Code   Other Specified Code   N Newborn Age: 0   P Pediatric Age: 0-17   M Maternity Age: 12-55
A Adult Age: 15-124   ♂ Male   ♀ Female   ● New Code   ▲ Revised Code Title   ►◄ Revised Text

C18.8 **Malignant neoplasm of overlapping sites of colon**
C18.9 **Malignant neoplasm of colon, unspecified**
Malignant neoplasm of large intestine NOS

C19 Malignant neoplasm of rectosigmoid junction
Malignant neoplasm of colon with rectum
Malignant neoplasm of rectosigmoid (colon)
[EXCLUDES1] *malignant carcinoid tumors of the colon (C7A.02-)*

C20 Malignant neoplasm of rectum
Malignant neoplasm of rectal ampulla
[EXCLUDES1] *malignant carcinoid tumor of the rectum (C7A.026)*

[4th] **C21 Malignant neoplasm of anus and anal canal**
[EXCLUDES2] *malignant carcinoid tumors of the colon (C7A.02-)*
malignant melanoma of anal margin (C43.51)
malignant melanoma of anal skin (C43.51)
malignant melanoma of perianal skin (C43.51)
other and unspecified malignant neoplasm of anal margin (C44.500, C44.510, C44.520, C44.590)
other and unspecified malignant neoplasm of anal skin (C44.500, C44.510, C44.520, C44.590)
other and unspecified malignant neoplasm of perianal skin (C44.500, C44.510, C44.520, C44.590)

C21.0 **Malignant neoplasm of anus, unspecified**
C21.1 **Malignant neoplasm of anal canal**
Malignant neoplasm of anal sphincter
C21.2 **Malignant neoplasm of cloacogenic zone**
C21.8 **Malignant neoplasm of overlapping sites of rectum, anus and anal canal**
Malignant neoplasm of anorectal junction
Malignant neoplasm of anorectum
Primary malignant neoplasm of two or more contiguous sites of rectum, anus and anal canal

[4th] **C22 Malignant neoplasm of liver and intrahepatic bile ducts**
[EXCLUDES1] *malignant neoplasm of biliary tract NOS (C24.9)*
secondary malignant neoplasm of liver and intrahepatic bile duct (C78.7)
Use additional code to identify:
alcohol abuse and dependence (F10.-)
hepatitis B (B16.-, B18.0-B18.1)
hepatitis C (B17.1-, B18.2)

C22.0 **Liver cell carcinoma**
Hepatocellular carcinoma
Hepatoma
C22.1 **Intrahepatic bile duct carcinoma**
Cholangiocarcinoma
[EXCLUDES1] *malignant neoplasm of hepatic duct (C24.0)*
C22.2 **Hepatoblastoma**
C22.3 **Angiosarcoma of liver**
Kupffer cell sarcoma
C22.4 **Other sarcomas of liver**
C22.7 **Other specified carcinomas of liver**
C22.8 **Malignant neoplasm of liver, primary, unspecified as to type**
C22.9 **Malignant neoplasm of liver, not specified as primary or secondary**

C23 Malignant neoplasm of gallbladder

[4th] **C24 Malignant neoplasm of other and unspecified parts of biliary tract**
[EXCLUDES1] *malignant neoplasm of intrahepatic bile duct (C22.1)*

C24.0 **Malignant neoplasm of extrahepatic bile duct**
Malignant neoplasm of biliary duct or passage NOS
Malignant neoplasm of common bile duct
Malignant neoplasm of cystic duct
Malignant neoplasm of hepatic duct
C24.1 **Malignant neoplasm of ampulla of Vater**
C24.8 **Malignant neoplasm of overlapping sites of biliary tract**
Malignant neoplasm involving both intrahepatic and extrahepatic bile ducts
Primary malignant neoplasm of two or more contiguous sites of biliary tract
C24.9 **Malignant neoplasm of biliary tract, unspecified**

[4th] **C25 Malignant neoplasm of pancreas**
Use additional code to identify:
alcohol abuse and dependence (F10.-)

C25.0 **Malignant neoplasm of head of pancreas**
C25.1 **Malignant neoplasm of body of pancreas**
C25.2 **Malignant neoplasm of tail of pancreas**
C25.3 **Malignant neoplasm of pancreatic duct**
C25.4 **Malignant neoplasm of endocrine pancreas**
Malignant neoplasm of islets of Langerhans
Use additional code to identify any functional activity.
C25.7 **Malignant neoplasm of other parts of pancreas**
Malignant neoplasm of neck of pancreas
C25.8 **Malignant neoplasm of overlapping sites of pancreas**
C25.9 **Malignant neoplasm of pancreas, unspecified**

[4th] **C26 Malignant neoplasm of other and ill-defined digestive organs**
[EXCLUDES1] *malignant neoplasm of peritoneum and retroperitoneum (C48.-)*

C26.0 **Malignant neoplasm of intestinal tract, part unspecified**
Malignant neoplasm of intestine NOS
C26.1 **Malignant neoplasm of spleen**
[EXCLUDES1] *Hodgkin lymphoma (C81.-)*
non-Hodgkin lymphoma (C82-C85)
C26.9 **Malignant neoplasm of ill-defined sites within the digestive system**
Malignant neoplasm of alimentary canal or tract NOS
Malignant neoplasm of gastrointestinal tract NOS
[EXCLUDES1] *malignant neoplasm of abdominal NOS (C76.2)*
malignant neoplasm of intra-abdominal NOS (C76.2)

Malignant neoplasms of respiratory and intrathoracic organs (C30-C39)

[INCLUDES] *malignant neoplasm of middle ear*
[EXCLUDES1] *mesothelioma (C45.-)*

[4th] **C30 Malignant neoplasm of nasal cavity and middle ear**
C30.0 **Malignant neoplasm of nasal cavity**
Malignant neoplasm of cartilage of nose
Malignant neoplasm of nasal concha
Malignant neoplasm of internal nose
Malignant neoplasm of septum of nose
Malignant neoplasm of vestibule of nose
[EXCLUDES1] *malignant neoplasm of nasal bone (C41.0)*
malignant neoplasm of nose NOS (C76.0)
malignant neoplasm of olfactory bulb (C72.2-)
malignant neoplasm of posterior margin of nasal septum and choana (C11.3)
malignant melanoma of skin of nose (C43.31)
malignant neoplasm of turbinates (C41.0)
other and unspecified malignant neoplasm of skin of nose C44.301, C44.311, C44.321, C44.391)
C30.1 **Malignant neoplasm of middle ear**
Malignant neoplasm of antrum tympanicum
Malignant neoplasm of auditory tube
Malignant neoplasm of eustachian tube
Malignant neoplasm of inner ear
Malignant neoplasm of mastoid air cells
Malignant neoplasm of tympanic cavity

[4th] 4th character required [5th] 5th character required [6th] 6th character required [7th] 7th character required [X] Extension 'X' Alert
[EXCLUDES1] Not coded here [EXCLUDES2] Not included here [PDx] Primary Diagnosis Only Manifestation Code

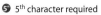

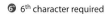

[EXCLUDES1] *malignant neoplasm of auricular canal (external) (C43.2-,C44.2-)*
malignant neoplasm of bone of ear (meatus) (C41.0)
malignant neoplasm of cartilage of ear (C49.0)
malignant melanoma of skin of (external) ear (C43.2-)
other and unspecified malignant neoplasm of skin of (external) ear (C44.2-)

[4th] **C31 Malignant neoplasm of accessory sinuses**
C31.0 Malignant neoplasm of maxillary sinus
Malignant neoplasm of antrum (Highmore) (maxillary)
C31.1 Malignant neoplasm of ethmoidal sinus
C31.2 Malignant neoplasm of frontal sinus
C31.3 Malignant neoplasm of sphenoid sinus
C31.8 Malignant neoplasm of overlapping sites of accessory sinuses
C31.9 Malignant neoplasm of accessory sinus, unspecified

[4th] **C32 Malignant neoplasm of larynx**
Use additional code to identify:
alcohol abuse and dependence (F10.-)
exposure to environmental tobacco smoke (Z77.22)
exposure to tobacco smoke in the perinatal period (P96.81)
history of tobacco use (Z87.891)
occupational exposure to environmental tobacco smoke (Z57.31)
tobacco dependence (F17.-)
tobacco use (Z72.0)
C32.0 Malignant neoplasm of glottis
Malignant neoplasm of intrinsic larynx
Malignant neoplasm of laryngeal commissure (anterior)(posterior)
Malignant neoplasm of vocal cord (true) NOS
C32.1 Malignant neoplasm of supraglottis
Malignant neoplasm of aryepiglottic fold or interarytenoid fold, laryngeal aspect
Malignant neoplasm of epiglottis (suprahyoid portion) NOS
Malignant neoplasm of extrinsic larynx
Malignant neoplasm of false vocal cord
Malignant neoplasm of posterior (laryngeal) surface of epiglottis
Malignant neoplasm of ventricular bands
[EXCLUDES2] *malignant neoplasm of anterior surface of epiglottis (C10.1)*
malignant neoplasm of aryepiglottic fold or interarytenoid fold, hypopharyngeal aspect (C13.1)
malignant neoplasm of aryepiglottic fold or interarytenoid fold, marginal zone (C13.1)
malignant neoplasm of aryepiglottic fold or interarytenoid fold NOS (C13.1)
C32.2 Malignant neoplasm of subglottis
C32.3 Malignant neoplasm of laryngeal cartilage
C32.8 Malignant neoplasm of overlapping sites of larynx
C32.9 Malignant neoplasm of larynx, unspecified

C33 Malignant neoplasm of trachea
Use additional code to identify:
exposure to environmental tobacco smoke (Z77.22)
exposure to tobacco smoke in the perinatal period (P96.81)
history of tobacco use (Z87.891)
occupational exposure to environmental tobacco smoke (Z57.31)
tobacco dependence (F17.-)
tobacco use (Z72.0)

[4th] **C34 Malignant neoplasm of bronchus and lung**
Use additional code to identify:
exposure to environmental tobacco smoke (Z77.22)
exposure to tobacco smoke in the perinatal period (P96.81)
history of tobacco use (Z87.891)
occupational exposure to environmental tobacco smoke (Z57.31)
tobacco dependence (F17.-)
tobacco use (Z72.0)
[EXCLUDES1] *Kaposi's sarcoma of lung (C46.5-)*
malignant carcinoid tumor of the bronchus and lung (C7A.090)

[5th] **C34.0 Malignant neoplasm of main bronchus**
Malignant neoplasm of carina
Malignant neoplasm of hilus (of lung)
C34.00 Malignant neoplasm of unspecified main bronchus
C34.01 Malignant neoplasm of right main bronchus
C34.02 Malignant neoplasm of left main bronchus
[5th] **C34.1 Malignant neoplasm of upper lobe, bronchus or lung**
C34.10 Malignant neoplasm of upper lobe, unspecified bronchus or lung
C34.11 Malignant neoplasm of upper lobe, right bronchus or lung
C34.12 Malignant neoplasm of upper lobe, left bronchus or lung
C34.2 Malignant neoplasm of middle lobe, bronchus or lung
[5th] **C34.3 Malignant neoplasm of lower lobe, bronchus or lung**
C34.30 Malignant neoplasm of lower lobe, unspecified bronchus or lung
C34.31 Malignant neoplasm of lower lobe, right bronchus or lung
C34.32 Malignant neoplasm of lower lobe, left bronchus or lung
[5th] **C34.8 Malignant neoplasm of overlapping sites of bronchus and lung**
C34.80 Malignant neoplasm of overlapping sites of unspecified bronchus and lung
C34.81 Malignant neoplasm of overlapping sites of right bronchus and lung
C34.82 Malignant neoplasm of overlapping sites of left bronchus and lung
[5th] **C34.9 Malignant neoplasm of unspecified part of bronchus or lung**
C34.90 Malignant neoplasm of unspecified part of unspecified bronchus or lung
Lung cancer NOS
C34.91 Malignant neoplasm of unspecified part of right bronchus or lung
C34.92 Malignant neoplasm of unspecified part of left bronchus or lung

C37 Malignant neoplasm of thymus
[EXCLUDES1] *malignant carcinoid tumor of the thymus (C7A.091)*

[4th] **C38 Malignant neoplasm of heart, mediastinum and pleura**
[EXCLUDES1] *mesothelioma (C45.-)*
C38.0 Malignant neoplasm of heart
Malignant neoplasm of pericardium
[EXCLUDES1] *malignant neoplasm of great vessels (C49.3)*
C38.1 Malignant neoplasm of anterior mediastinum
C38.2 Malignant neoplasm of posterior mediastinum
C38.3 Malignant neoplasm of mediastinum, part unspecified
C38.4 Malignant neoplasm of pleura
C38.8 Malignant neoplasm of overlapping sites of heart, mediastinum and pleura

Unspecified Code | Other Specified Code | [N] Newborn Age: 0 | [P] Pediatric Age: 0-17 | [M] Maternity Age: 12-55
[A] Adult Age: 15-124 | ♂ Male | ♀ Female | ● New Code | ▲ Revised Code Title | ►◄ Revised Text

④ **C39** **Malignant neoplasm of** other and ill-defined sites in the respiratory system and intrathoracic organs

Use additional code to identify:
exposure to environmental tobacco smoke (Z77.22)
exposure to tobacco smoke in the perinatal period (P96.81)
history of tobacco use (Z87.891)
occupational exposure to environmental tobacco smoke (Z57.31)
tobacco dependence (F17.-)
tobacco use (Z72.0)

EXCLUDES1 intrathoracic malignant neoplasm NOS (C76.1)
thoracic malignant neoplasm NOS (C76.1)

C39.0 **Malignant neoplasm of** upper **respiratory tract, part unspecified**

C39.9 **Malignant neoplasm of** lower **respiratory tract, part unspecified**

Malignant neoplasm of respiratory tract NOS

Malignant neoplasms of bone and articular cartilage (C40-C41)

INCLUDES malignant neoplasm of cartilage (articular) (joint)
malignant neoplasm of periosteum

EXCLUDES1 malignant neoplasm of bone marrow NOS (C96.9)
malignant neoplasm of synovia (C49.-)

④ **C40** **Malignant neoplasm of** bone and articular cartilage of limbs

Use additional code to identify major osseous defect, if applicable (M89.7-)

⑤ **C40.0** **Malignant neoplasm of** scapula and long bones of upper limb

C40.00 **Malignant neoplasm of scapula and long bones of unspecified upper limb**

C40.01 **Malignant neoplasm of scapula and long bones of** right **upper limb**

C40.02 **Malignant neoplasm of scapula and long bones of** left **upper limb**

⑤ **C40.1** **Malignant neoplasm of** short bones of upper limb

C40.10 **Malignant neoplasm of short bones of unspecified upper limb**

C40.11 **Malignant neoplasm of short bones of** right **upper limb**

C40.12 **Malignant neoplasm of short bones of** left **upper limb**

⑤ **C40.2** **Malignant neoplasm of** long bones of lower limb

C40.20 **Malignant neoplasm of long bones of unspecified lower limb**

C40.21 **Malignant neoplasm of long bones of** right **lower limb**

C40.22 **Malignant neoplasm of long bones of** left **lower limb**

⑤ **C40.3** **Malignant neoplasm of** short bones of lower limb

C40.30 **Malignant neoplasm of short bones of unspecified lower limb**

C40.31 **Malignant neoplasm of short bones of** right **lower limb**

C40.32 **Malignant neoplasm of short bones of** left **lower limb**

⑤ **C40.8** **Malignant neoplasm of** overlapping sites **of bone and articular cartilage of limb**

C40.80 **Malignant neoplasm of overlapping sites of bone and articular cartilage of unspecified limb**

C40.81 **Malignant neoplasm of overlapping sites of bone and articular cartilage of** right **limb**

C40.82 **Malignant neoplasm of overlapping sites of bone and articular cartilage of** left **limb**

⑤ **C40.9** **Malignant neoplasm of** unspecified bones **and articular cartilage of limb**

C40.90 **Malignant neoplasm of unspecified bones and articular cartilage of unspecified limb**

C40.91 **Malignant neoplasm of unspecified bones and articular cartilage of** right **limb**

C40.92 **Malignant neoplasm of unspecified bones and articular cartilage of** left **limb**

④ **C41** **Malignant neoplasm of bone and articular cartilage of other and unspecified sites**

EXCLUDES1 malignant neoplasm of bones of limbs (C40.-)
malignant neoplasm of cartilage of ear (C49.0)
malignant neoplasm of cartilage of eyelid (C49.0)
malignant neoplasm of cartilage of larynx (C32.3)
malignant neoplasm of cartilage of limbs (C40.-)
malignant neoplasm of cartilage of nose (C30.0)

C41.0 **Malignant neoplasm of bones of** skull and face

Malignant neoplasm of maxilla (superior)
Malignant neoplasm of orbital bone

EXCLUDES2 carcinoma, any type except intraosseous or odontogenic of:
maxillary sinus (C31.0)
upper jaw (C03.0)
malignant neoplasm of jaw bone (lower) (C41.1)

C41.1 **Malignant neoplasm of** mandible

Malignant neoplasm of inferior maxilla
Malignant neoplasm of lower jaw bone

EXCLUDES2 carcinoma, any type except intraosseous or odontogenic of:
jaw NOS (C03.9)
lower (C03.1)
malignant neoplasm of upper jaw bone (C41.0)

C41.2 **Malignant neoplasm of** vertebral column

EXCLUDES1 malignant neoplasm of sacrum and coccyx (C41.4)

C41.3 **Malignant neoplasm of** ribs, sternum and clavicle

C41.4 **Malignant neoplasm of** pelvic bones, sacrum and coccyx

C41.9 **Malignant neoplasm of** bone and articular cartilage, **unspecified**

Melanoma and other malignant neoplasms of skin (C43-C44)

④ **C43** **Malignant melanoma of** skin

EXCLUDES1 melanoma in situ (D03.-)

EXCLUDES2 malignant melanoma of skin of genital organs (C51-C52, C60.-, C63.-)
Merkel cell carcinoma (C4A.-)
sites other than skin-code to malignant neoplasm of the site

C43.0 **Malignant melanoma of** lip

EXCLUDES1 malignant neoplasm of vermilion border of lip (C00.0-C00.2)

⑤ **C43.1** **Malignant melanoma of** eyelid, including canthus

C43.10 **Malignant melanoma of unspecified eyelid, including canthus**

C43.11 **Malignant melanoma of** right **eyelid, including canthus**

C43.12 **Malignant melanoma of** left **eyelid, including canthus**

⑤ **C43.2** **Malignant melanoma of** ear and external auricular canal

C43.20 **Malignant melanoma of unspecified ear and external auricular canal**

C43.21 **Malignant melanoma of** right **ear and external auricular canal**

C43.22 **Malignant melanoma of** left **ear and external auricular canal**

⑤ **C43.3** **Malignant melanoma of other and unspecified** parts of face

---

④ 4th character required	⑤ 5th character required	⑥ 6th character required	⑦ 7th character required	⑦ Extension 'X' Alert

EXCLUDES1 Not coded here   EXCLUDES2 Not included here   PDx Primary Diagnosis Only   Manifestation Code

ICD-10-CM 2015

C43.30 **Malignant melanoma of unspecified part of face**
C43.31 **Malignant melanoma of nose**
C43.39 **Malignant melanoma of other parts of face**
C43.4 **Malignant melanoma of scalp and neck**
[5th] C43.5 **Malignant melanoma of trunk**
[EXCLUDES2] *malignant neoplasm of anus NOS (C21.0)*
malignant neoplasm of scrotum (C63.2)
C43.51 **Malignant melanoma of anal skin**
Malignant melanoma of anal margin
Malignant melanoma of perianal skin
C43.52 **Malignant melanoma of skin of breast**
C43.59 **Malignant melanoma of other part of trunk**
[5th] C43.6 **Malignant melanoma of upper limb, including shoulder**
C43.60 **Malignant melanoma of unspecified upper limb, including shoulder**
C43.61 **Malignant melanoma of right upper limb, including shoulder**
C43.62 **Malignant melanoma of left upper limb, including shoulder**
[5th] C43.7 **Malignant melanoma of lower limb, including hip**
C43.70 **Malignant melanoma of unspecified lower limb, including hip**
C43.71 **Malignant melanoma of right lower limb, including hip**
C43.72 **Malignant melanoma of left lower limb, including hip**
C43.8 **Malignant melanoma of overlapping sites of skin**
C43.9 **Malignant melanoma of skin, unspecified**
Malignant melanoma of unspecified site of skin
Melanoma (malignant) NOS
[4th] C4A **Merkel cell carcinoma**
C4A.0 **Merkel cell carcinoma of lip**
[EXCLUDES1] *malignant neoplasm of vermilion border of lip (C00.0-C00.2)*
[5th] C4A.1 **Merkel cell carcinoma of eyelid, including canthus**
C4A.10 **Merkel cell carcinoma of unspecified eyelid, including canthus**
C4A.11 **Merkel cell carcinoma of right eyelid, including canthus**
C4A.12 **Merkel cell carcinoma of left eyelid, including canthus**
[5th] C4A.2 **Merkel cell carcinoma of ear and external auricular canal**
C4A.20 **Merkel cell carcinoma of unspecified ear and external auricular canal**
C4A.21 **Merkel cell carcinoma of right ear and external auricular canal**
C4A.22 **Merkel cell carcinoma of left ear and external auricular canal**
[5th] C4A.3 **Merkel cell carcinoma of other and unspecified parts of face**
C4A.30 **Merkel cell carcinoma of unspecified part of face**
C4A.31 **Merkel cell carcinoma of nose**
C4A.39 **Merkel cell carcinoma of other parts of face**
C4A.4 **Merkel cell carcinoma of scalp and neck**
[5th] C4A.5 **Merkel cell carcinoma of trunk**
[EXCLUDES2] *malignant neoplasm of anus NOS (C21.0)*
malignant neoplasm of scrotum (C63.2)
C4A.51 **Merkel cell carcinoma of anal skin**
Merkel cell carcinoma of anal margin
Merkel cell carcinoma of perianal skin
C4A.52 **Merkel cell carcinoma of skin of breast**
C4A.59 **Merkel cell carcinoma of other part of trunk**
[5th] C4A.6 **Merkel cell carcinoma of upper limb, including shoulder**
C4A.60 **Merkel cell carcinoma of unspecified upper limb, including shoulder**
C4A.61 **Merkel cell carcinoma of right upper limb, including shoulder**
C4A.62 **Merkel cell carcinoma of left upper limb, including shoulder**
[5th] C4A.7 **Merkel cell carcinoma of lower limb, including hip**
C4A.70 **Merkel cell carcinoma of unspecified lower limb, including hip**
C4A.71 **Merkel cell carcinoma of right lower limb, including hip**
C4A.72 **Merkel cell carcinoma of left lower limb, including hip**
C4A.8 **Merkel cell carcinoma of overlapping sites**
C4A.9 **Merkel cell carcinoma, unspecified**
Merkel cell carcinoma of unspecified site
Merkel cell carcinoma NOS

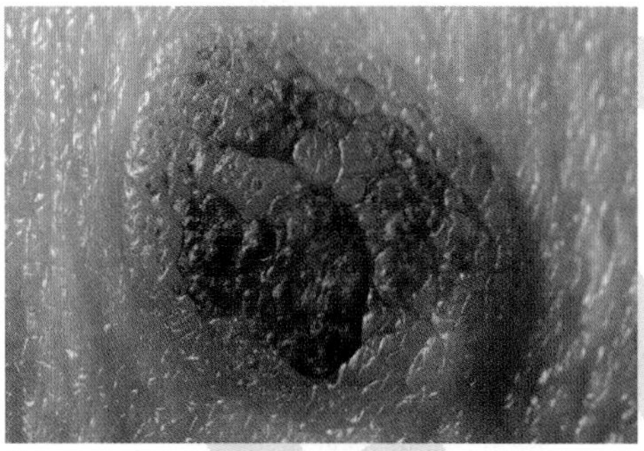

Figure 3.1 Malignant Neoplasm of Skin

[4th] C44 **Other and unspecified malignant neoplasm of skin**
[INCLUDES] *malignant neoplasm of sebaceous glands*
malignant neoplasm of sweat glands
[EXCLUDES1] *Kaposi's sarcoma of skin (C46.0)*
malignant melanoma of skin (C43.-)
malignant neoplasm of skin of genital organs (C51-C52, C60.-, C63.2)
Merkel cell carcinoma (C4A.-)
[5th] C44.0 **Other and unspecified malignant neoplasm of skin of lip**
[EXCLUDES1] *malignant neoplasm of lip (C00.-)*
C44.00 **Unspecified malignant neoplasm of skin of lip**
C44.01 **Basal cell carcinoma of skin of lip**
C44.02 **Squamous cell carcinoma of skin of lip**
C44.09 **Other specified malignant neoplasm of skin of lip**
[5th] C44.1 **Other and unspecified malignant neoplasm of skin of eyelid, including canthus**
[EXCLUDES1] *connective tissue of eyelid (C49.0)*
[6th] C44.10 **Unspecified malignant neoplasm of skin of eyelid, including canthus**
C44.101 **Unspecified malignant neoplasm of skin of unspecified eyelid, including canthus**
C44.102 **Unspecified malignant neoplasm of skin of right eyelid, including canthus**
C44.109 **Unspecified malignant neoplasm of skin of left eyelid, including canthus**
[6th] C44.11 **Basal cell carcinoma of skin of eyelid, including canthus**
C44.111 **Basal cell carcinoma of skin of unspecified eyelid, including canthus**
C44.112 **Basal cell carcinoma of skin of right eyelid, including canthus**
C44.119 **Basal cell carcinoma of skin of left eyelid, including canthus**
[6th] C44.12 **Squamous cell carcinoma of skin of eyelid, including canthus**
C44.121 **Squamous cell carcinoma of skin of unspecified eyelid, including canthus**

C44.122 Squamous cell carcinoma of skin of right eyelid, including canthus

C44.129 Squamous cell carcinoma of skin of left eyelid, including canthus

[6] C44.19 Other specified malignant neoplasm of skin of eyelid, including canthus

C44.191 Other specified malignant neoplasm of skin of unspecified eyelid, including canthus

C44.192 Other specified malignant neoplasm of skin of right eyelid, including canthus

C44.199 Other specified malignant neoplasm of skin of left eyelid, including canthus

[5] C44.2 Other and unspecified malignant neoplasm of skin of ear and external auricular canal

[EXCLUDES1] *connective tissue of ear (C49.0)*

[6] C44.20 Unspecified malignant neoplasm of skin of ear and external auricular canal

C44.201 Unspecified malignant neoplasm of skin of unspecified ear and external auricular canal

C44.202 Unspecified malignant neoplasm of skin of right ear and external auricular canal

C44.209 Unspecified malignant neoplasm of skin of left ear and external auricular canal

[6] C44.21 Basal cell carcinoma of skin of ear and external auricular canal

C44.211 Basal cell carcinoma of skin of unspecified ear and external auricular canal

C44.212 Basal cell carcinoma of skin of right ear and external auricular canal

C44.219 Basal cell carcinoma of skin of left ear and external auricular canal

[6] C44.22 Squamous cell carcinoma of skin of ear and external auricular canal

C44.221 Squamous cell carcinoma of skin of unspecified ear and external auricular canal

C44.222 Squamous cell carcinoma of skin of right ear and external auricular canal

C44.229 Squamous cell carcinoma of skin of left ear and external auricular canal

[6] C44.29 Other specified malignant neoplasm of skin of ear and external auricular canal

C44.291 Other specified malignant neoplasm of skin of unspecified ear and external auricular canal

C44.292 Other specified malignant neoplasm of skin of right ear and external auricular canal

C44.299 Other specified malignant neoplasm of skin of left ear and external auricular canal

[5] C44.3 Other and unspecified malignant neoplasm of skin of other and unspecified parts of face

[6] C44.30 Unspecified malignant neoplasm of skin of other and unspecified parts of face

C44.300 Unspecified malignant neoplasm of skin of unspecified part of face

C44.301 Unspecified malignant neoplasm of skin of nose

C44.309 Unspecified malignant neoplasm of skin of other parts of face

[6] C44.31 Basal cell carcinoma of skin of other and unspecified parts of face

C44.310 Basal cell carcinoma of skin of unspecified parts of face

C44.311 Basal cell carcinoma of skin of nose

C44.319 Basal cell carcinoma of skin of other parts of face

[6] C44.32 Squamous cell carcinoma of skin of other and unspecified parts of face

C44.320 Squamous cell carcinoma of skin of unspecified parts of face

C44.321 Squamous cell carcinoma of skin of nose

C44.329 Squamous cell carcinoma of skin of other parts of face

[6] C44.39 Other specified malignant neoplasm of skin of other and unspecified parts of face

C44.390 Other specified malignant neoplasm of skin of unspecified parts of face

C44.391 Other specified malignant neoplasm of skin of nose

C44.399 Other specified malignant neoplasm of skin of other parts of face

[5] C44.4 Other and unspecified malignant neoplasm of skin of scalp and neck

C44.40 Unspecified malignant neoplasm of skin of scalp and neck

C44.41 Basal cell carcinoma of skin of scalp and neck

C44.42 Squamous cell carcinoma of skin of scalp and neck

C44.49 Other specified malignant neoplasm of skin of scalp and neck

[5] C44.5 Other and unspecified malignant neoplasm of skin of trunk

[EXCLUDES1] *anus NOS (C21.0)*
scrotum (C63.2)

[6] C44.50 Unspecified malignant neoplasm of skin of trunk

C44.500 Unspecified malignant neoplasm of anal skin

Unspecified malignant neoplasm of anal margin
Unspecified malignant neoplasm of perianal skin

C44.501 Unspecified malignant neoplasm of skin of breast

C44.509 Unspecified malignant neoplasm of skin of other part of trunk

[6] C44.51 Basal cell carcinoma of skin of trunk

C44.510 Basal cell carcinoma of anal skin

Basal cell carcinoma of anal margin
Basal cell carcinoma of perianal skin

C44.511 Basal cell carcinoma of skin of breast

C44.519 Basal cell carcinoma of skin of other part of trunk

[6] C44.52 Squamous cell carcinoma of skin of trunk

C44.520 Squamous cell carcinoma of anal skin

Squamous cell carcinoma of anal margin
Squamous cell carcinoma of perianal skin

C44.521 Squamous cell carcinoma of skin of breast

C44.529 Squamous cell carcinoma of skin of other part of trunk

[6] C44.59 Other specified malignant neoplasm of skin of trunk

C44.590 Other specified malignant neoplasm of anal skin

Other specified malignant neoplasm of anal margin
Other specified malignant neoplasm of perianal skin

C44.591 Other specified malignant neoplasm of skin of breast

C44.599 Other specified malignant neoplasm of skin of other part of trunk

[5] C44.6 Other and unspecified malignant neoplasm of skin of upper limb, including shoulder

[6] C44.60 Unspecified malignant neoplasm of skin of upper limb, including shoulder

C44.601 Unspecified malignant neoplasm of skin of unspecified upper limb, including shoulder

C44.602 Unspecified malignant neoplasm of skin of right upper limb, including shoulder

C44.609 Unspecified malignant neoplasm of skin of left upper limb, including shoulder

[4] 4th character required [5] 5th character required [6] 6th character required [7] 7th character required [7X] Extension 'X' Alert
[EXCLUDES1] Not coded here [EXCLUDES2] Not included here [PDx] Primary Diagnosis Only Manifestation Code

Ⓖ C44.61 Basal cell carcinoma of skin of upper limb, including shoulder

    C44.611 **Basal cell carcinoma of skin of unspecified upper limb, including shoulder**

    C44.612 **Basal cell carcinoma of skin of** right **upper limb, including shoulder**

    C44.619 **Basal cell carcinoma of skin of** left **upper limb, including shoulder**

Ⓖ C44.62 Squamous cell carcinoma of skin of upper limb, including shoulder

    C44.621 **Squamous cell carcinoma of skin of unspecified upper limb, including shoulder**

    C44.622 **Squamous cell carcinoma of skin of** right **upper limb, including shoulder**

    C44.629 **Squamous cell carcinoma of skin of** left **upper limb, including shoulder**

Ⓖ C44.69 **Other specified malignant neoplasm of skin of upper limb, including shoulder**

    C44.691 **Other specified malignant neoplasm of skin of unspecified upper limb, including shoulder**

    C44.692 **Other specified malignant neoplasm of skin of** right **upper limb, including shoulder**

    C44.699 **Other specified malignant neoplasm of skin of** left **upper limb, including shoulder**

Ⓢ C44.7 **Other and unspecified malignant neoplasm of skin of** lower limb, including hip

Ⓖ C44.70 Unspecified **malignant neoplasm of skin of lower limb, including hip**

    C44.701 **Unspecified malignant neoplasm of skin of unspecified lower limb, including hip**

    C44.702 **Unspecified malignant neoplasm of skin of** right **lower limb, including hip**

    C44.709 **Unspecified malignant neoplasm of skin of** left **lower limb, including hip**

Ⓖ C44.71 Basal cell carcinoma **of skin of lower limb, including hip**

    C44.711 **Basal cell carcinoma of skin of unspecified lower limb, including hip**

    C44.712 **Basal cell carcinoma of skin of** right **lower limb, including hip**

    C44.719 **Basal cell carcinoma of skin of** left **lower limb, including hip**

Ⓖ C44.72 Squamous cell carcinoma **of skin of lower limb, including hip**

    C44.721 **Squamous cell carcinoma of skin of unspecified lower limb, including hip**

    C44.722 **Squamous cell carcinoma of skin of** right **lower limb, including hip**

    C44.729 **Squamous cell carcinoma of skin of** left **lower limb, including hip**

Ⓖ C44.79 Other specified **malignant neoplasm of skin of lower limb, including hip**

    C44.791 **Other specified malignant neoplasm of skin of unspecified lower limb, including hip**

    C44.792 **Other specified malignant neoplasm of skin of** right **lower limb, including hip**

    C44.799 **Other specified malignant neoplasm of skin of** left **lower limb, including hip**

Ⓢ C44.8 **Other and unspecified malignant neoplasm of** overlapping sites of skin

    C44.80 **Unspecified malignant neoplasm of overlapping sites of skin**

    C44.81 Basal cell carcinoma **of overlapping sites of skin**

    C44.82 Squamous cell carcinoma **of overlapping sites of skin**

    C44.89 **Other specified malignant neoplasm of overlapping sites of skin**

Ⓢ C44.9 **Other and unspecified malignant neoplasm of skin,** unspecified

    C44.90 **Unspecified malignant neoplasm of skin, unspecified**

    Malignant neoplasm of unspecified site of skin

    C44.91 Basal cell carcinoma **of skin, unspecified**

    C44.92 Squamous cell carcinoma **of skin, unspecified**

    C44.99 **Other specified malignant neoplasm of skin, unspecified**

Malignant neoplasms of mesothelial and soft tissue (C45-C49)

Ⓖ C45 **Mesothelioma**

    C45.0 **Mesothelioma of** pleura

        EXCLUDES1 *other malignant neoplasm of pleura (C38.4)*

    C45.1 **Mesothelioma of** peritoneum

        Mesothelioma of cul-de-sac

        Mesothelioma of mesentery

        Mesothelioma of mesocolon

        Mesothelioma of omentum

        Mesothelioma of peritoneum (parietal) (pelvic)

        EXCLUDES1 *other malignant neoplasm of soft tissue of peritoneum (C48.-)*

    C45.2 **Mesothelioma of** pericardium

        EXCLUDES1 *other malignant neoplasm of pericardium (C38.0)*

    C45.7 **Mesothelioma of other sites**

    C45.9 **Mesothelioma, unspecified**

Ⓖ C46 **Kaposi's sarcoma**

    Code first any human immunodeficiency virus [HIV] disease (B20)

    C46.0 **Kaposi's sarcoma of** skin

    C46.1 **Kaposi's sarcoma of** soft tissue

        Kaposi's sarcoma of blood vessel

        Kaposi's sarcoma of connective tissue

        Kaposi's sarcoma of fascia

        Kaposi's sarcoma of ligament

        Kaposi's sarcoma of lymphatic(s) NEC

        Kaposi's sarcoma of muscle

        EXCLUDES2 *Kaposi's sarcoma of lymph glands and nodes (C46.3)*

    C46.2 **Kaposi's sarcoma of** palate

    C46.3 **Kaposi's sarcoma of** lymph nodes

    C46.4 **Kaposi's sarcoma of** gastrointestinal sites

Ⓢ C46.5 **Kaposi's sarcoma of** lung

    C46.50 **Kaposi's sarcoma of unspecified lung**

    C46.51 **Kaposi's sarcoma of** right **lung**

    C46.52 **Kaposi's sarcoma of** left **lung**

    C46.7 **Kaposi's sarcoma of other sites**

    C46.9 **Kaposi's sarcoma, unspecified**

    Kaposi's sarcoma of unspecified site

Ⓖ C47 **Malignant neoplasm of** peripheral nerves and autonomic nervous system

    INCLUDES *malignant neoplasm of sympathetic and parasympathetic nerves and ganglia*

    EXCLUDES1 *Kaposi's sarcoma of soft tissue (C46.1)*

    C47.0 **Malignant neoplasm of peripheral nerves of** head, face and neck

        EXCLUDES1 *malignant neoplasm of peripheral nerves of orbit (C69.6-)*

Ⓢ C47.1 **Malignant neoplasm of peripheral nerves of** upper limb, including shoulder

    C47.10 **Malignant neoplasm of peripheral nerves of unspecified upper limb, including shoulder**

    C47.11 **Malignant neoplasm of peripheral nerves of** right **upper limb, including shoulder**

Unspecified Code   Other Specified Code   Ⓝ Newborn Age: 0   Ⓟ Pediatric Age: 0-17   Ⓜ Maternity Age: 12-55

Ⓐ Adult Age: 15-124   ♂ Male   ♀ Female   ● New Code   ▲ Revised Code Title   ►◄ Revised Text

C47.12 **Malignant neoplasm of peripheral nerves of left upper limb, including shoulder**

[5] C47.2 **Malignant neoplasm of peripheral nerves of lower limb, including hip**

C47.20 **Malignant neoplasm of peripheral nerves of unspecified lower limb, including hip**

C47.21 **Malignant neoplasm of peripheral nerves of right lower limb, including hip**

C47.22 **Malignant neoplasm of peripheral nerves of left lower limb, including hip**

C47.3 **Malignant neoplasm of peripheral nerves of thorax**

C47.4 **Malignant neoplasm of peripheral nerves of abdomen**

C47.5 **Malignant neoplasm of peripheral nerves of pelvis**

C47.6 **Malignant neoplasm of peripheral nerves of trunk, unspecified**

Malignant neoplasm of peripheral nerves of unspecified part of trunk

C47.8 **Malignant neoplasm of overlapping sites of peripheral nerves and autonomic nervous system**

C47.9 **Malignant neoplasm of peripheral nerves and autonomic nervous system, unspecified**

Malignant neoplasm of unspecified site of peripheral nerves and autonomic nervous system

[4] C48 **Malignant neoplasm of retroperitoneum and peritoneum**

EXCLUDES1 *Kaposi's sarcoma of connective tissue (C46.1)*
mesothelioma (C45.-)

C48.0 **Malignant neoplasm of retroperitoneum**

C48.1 **Malignant neoplasm of specified parts of peritoneum**

Malignant neoplasm of cul-de-sac
Malignant neoplasm of mesentery
Malignant neoplasm of mesocolon
Malignant neoplasm of omentum
Malignant neoplasm of parietal peritoneum
Malignant neoplasm of pelvic peritoneum

C48.2 **Malignant neoplasm of peritoneum, unspecified**

C48.8 **Malignant neoplasm of overlapping sites of retroperitoneum and peritoneum**

[4] C49 **Malignant neoplasm of other connective and soft tissue**

INCLUDES *malignant neoplasm of blood vessel*
malignant neoplasm of bursa
malignant neoplasm of cartilage
malignant neoplasm of fascia
malignant neoplasm of fat
malignant neoplasm of ligament, except uterine
malignant neoplasm of lymphatic vessel
malignant neoplasm of muscle
malignant neoplasm of synovia
malignant neoplasm of tendon (sheath)

EXCLUDES1 *malignant neoplasm of cartilage (of):*
articular (C40-C41)
larynx (C32.3)
nose (C30.0)
malignant neoplasm of connective tissue of breast (C50.-)

EXCLUDES2 *Kaposi's sarcoma of soft tissue (C46.1)*
malignant neoplasm of heart (C38.0)
malignant neoplasm of peripheral nerves and autonomic nervous system (C47.-)
malignant neoplasm of peritoneum (C48.2)
malignant neoplasm of retroperitoneum (C48.0)
malignant neoplasm of uterine ligament (C57.3)
mesothelioma (C45.-)

C49.0 **Malignant neoplasm of connective and soft tissue of head, face and neck**

Malignant neoplasm of connective tissue of ear
Malignant neoplasm of connective tissue of eyelid

EXCLUDES1 *connective tissue of orbit (C69.6-)*

[5] C49.1 **Malignant neoplasm of connective and soft tissue of upper limb, including shoulder**

C49.10 **Malignant neoplasm of connective and soft tissue of unspecified upper limb, including shoulder**

C49.11 **Malignant neoplasm of connective and soft tissue of right upper limb, including shoulder**

C49.12 **Malignant neoplasm of connective and soft tissue of left upper limb, including shoulder**

[5] C49.2 **Malignant neoplasm of connective and soft tissue of lower limb, including hip**

C49.20 **Malignant neoplasm of connective and soft tissue of unspecified lower limb, including hip**

C49.21 **Malignant neoplasm of connective and soft tissue of right lower limb, including hip**

C49.22 **Malignant neoplasm of connective and soft tissue of left lower limb, including hip**

C49.3 **Malignant neoplasm of connective and soft tissue of thorax**

Malignant neoplasm of axilla
Malignant neoplasm of diaphragm
Malignant neoplasm of great vessels

EXCLUDES1 *malignant neoplasm of breast (C50.-)*
malignant neoplasm of heart (C38.0)
malignant neoplasm of mediastinum (C38.1-C38.3)
malignant neoplasm of thymus (C37)

C49.4 **Malignant neoplasm of connective and soft tissue of abdomen**

Malignant neoplasm of abdominal wall
Malignant neoplasm of hypochondrium

C49.5 **Malignant neoplasm of connective and soft tissue of pelvis**

Malignant neoplasm of buttock
Malignant neoplasm of groin
Malignant neoplasm of perineum

C49.6 **Malignant neoplasm of connective and soft tissue of trunk, unspecified**

Malignant neoplasm of back NOS

C49.8 **Malignant neoplasm of overlapping sites of connective and soft tissue**

Primary malignant neoplasm of two or more contiguous sites of connective and soft tissue

C49.9 **Malignant neoplasm of connective and soft tissue, unspecified**

Malignant neoplasms of breast (C50)

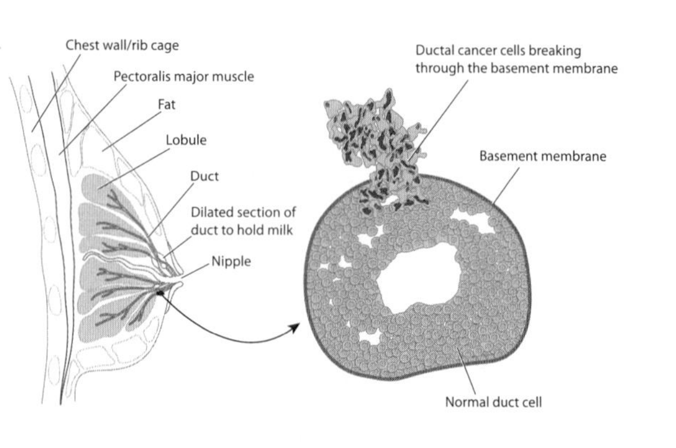

Figure 3.2 Breast Cancer Cells

[4] C50 **Malignant neoplasm of breast**

[4] 4th character required [5] 5th character required [6] 6th character required [7] 7th character required [X] Extension 'X' Alert
EXCLUDES1 Not coded here EXCLUDES2 Not included here PDx Primary Diagnosis Only Manifestation Code

[INCLUDES] *connective tissue of breast*
Paget's disease of breast
Paget's disease of nipple

Use additional code to identify estrogen receptor status (Z17.0, Z17.1)

[EXCLUDES1] *skin of breast (C44.501, C44.511, C44.521, C44.591)*

[5] **C50.0 Malignant neoplasm of nipple and areola**
- [6] **C50.01 Malignant neoplasm of nipple and areola, female**
  - **C50.011 Malignant neoplasm of nipple and areola, right female breast** ♀
  - **C50.012 Malignant neoplasm of nipple and areola, left female breast** ♀
  - **C50.019 Malignant neoplasm of nipple and areola, unspecified female breast** ♀
- [6] **C50.02 Malignant neoplasm of nipple and areola, male**
  - **C50.021 Malignant neoplasm of nipple and areola, right male breast** ♂
  - **C50.022 Malignant neoplasm of nipple and areola, left male breast** ♂
  - **C50.029 Malignant neoplasm of nipple and areola, unspecified male breast** ♂

[5] **C50.1 Malignant neoplasm of central portion of breast**
- [6] **C50.11 Malignant neoplasm of central portion of breast, female**
  - **C50.111 Malignant neoplasm of central portion of right female breast** ♀
  - **C50.112 Malignant neoplasm of central portion of left female breast** ♀
  - **C50.119 Malignant neoplasm of central portion of unspecified female breast** ♀
- [6] **C50.12 Malignant neoplasm of central portion of breast, male**
  - **C50.121 Malignant neoplasm of central portion of right male breast** ♂
  - **C50.122 Malignant neoplasm of central portion of left male breast** ♂
  - **C50.129 Malignant neoplasm of central portion of unspecified male breast** ♂

[5] **C50.2 Malignant neoplasm of upper-inner quadrant of breast**
- [6] **C50.21 Malignant neoplasm of upper-inner quadrant of breast, female**
  - **C50.211 Malignant neoplasm of upper-inner quadrant of right female breast** ♀
  - **C50.212 Malignant neoplasm of upper-inner quadrant of left female breast** ♀
  - **C50.219 Malignant neoplasm of upper-inner quadrant of unspecified female breast** ♀
- [6] **C50.22 Malignant neoplasm of upper-inner quadrant of breast, male**
  - **C50.221 Malignant neoplasm of upper-inner quadrant of right male breast** ♂
  - **C50.222 Malignant neoplasm of upper-inner quadrant of left male breast** ♂
  - **C50.229 Malignant neoplasm of upper-inner quadrant of unspecified male breast** ♂

[5] **C50.3 Malignant neoplasm of lower-inner quadrant of breast**
- [6] **C50.31 Malignant neoplasm of lower-inner quadrant of breast, female**
  - **C50.311 Malignant neoplasm of lower-inner quadrant of right female breast** ♀
  - **C50.312 Malignant neoplasm of lower-inner quadrant of left female breast** ♀
  - **C50.319 Malignant neoplasm of lower-inner quadrant of unspecified female breast** ♀
- [6] **C50.32 Malignant neoplasm of lower-inner quadrant of breast, male**
  - **C50.321 Malignant neoplasm of lower-inner quadrant of right male breast** ♂
  - **C50.322 Malignant neoplasm of lower-inner quadrant of left male breast** ♂
  - **C50.329 Malignant neoplasm of lower-inner quadrant of unspecified male breast** ♂

[5] **C50.4 Malignant neoplasm of upper-outer quadrant of breast**
- [6] **C50.41 Malignant neoplasm of upper-outer quadrant of breast, female**
  - **C50.411 Malignant neoplasm of upper-outer quadrant of right female breast** ♀
  - **C50.412 Malignant neoplasm of upper-outer quadrant of left female breast** ♀
  - **C50.419 Malignant neoplasm of upper-outer quadrant of unspecified female breast** ♀
- [6] **C50.42 Malignant neoplasm of upper-outer quadrant of breast, male**
  - **C50.421 Malignant neoplasm of upper-outer quadrant of right male breast** ♂
  - **C50.422 Malignant neoplasm of upper-outer quadrant of left male breast** ♂
  - **C50.429 Malignant neoplasm of upper-outer quadrant of unspecified male breast** ♂

[5] **C50.5 Malignant neoplasm of lower-outer quadrant of breast**
- [6] **C50.51 Malignant neoplasm of lower-outer quadrant of breast, female**
  - **C50.511 Malignant neoplasm of lower-outer quadrant of right female breast** ♀
  - **C50.512 Malignant neoplasm of lower-outer quadrant of left female breast** ♀
  - **C50.519 Malignant neoplasm of lower-outer quadrant of unspecified female breast** ♀
- [6] **C50.52 Malignant neoplasm of lower-outer quadrant of breast, male**
  - **C50.521 Malignant neoplasm of lower-outer quadrant of right male breast** ♂
  - **C50.522 Malignant neoplasm of lower-outer quadrant of left male breast** ♂
  - **C50.529 Malignant neoplasm of lower-outer quadrant of unspecified male breast** ♂

[5] **C50.6 Malignant neoplasm of axillary tail of breast**
- [6] **C50.61 Malignant neoplasm of axillary tail of breast, female**
  - **C50.611 Malignant neoplasm of axillary tail of right female breast** ♀
  - **C50.612 Malignant neoplasm of axillary tail of left female breast** ♀
  - **C50.619 Malignant neoplasm of axillary tail of unspecified female breast** ♀
- [6] **C50.62 Malignant neoplasm of axillary tail of breast, male**
  - **C50.621 Malignant neoplasm of axillary tail of right male breast** ♂
  - **C50.622 Malignant neoplasm of axillary tail of left male breast** ♂
  - **C50.629 Malignant neoplasm of axillary tail of unspecified male breast** ♂

[5] **C50.8 Malignant neoplasm of overlapping sites of breast**
- [6] **C50.81 Malignant neoplasm of overlapping sites of breast, female**
  - **C50.811 Malignant neoplasm of overlapping sites of right female breast** ♀
  - **C50.812 Malignant neoplasm of overlapping sites of left female breast** ♀
  - **C50.819 Malignant neoplasm of overlapping sites of unspecified female breast** ♀

Unspecified Code | Other Specified Code | [N] Newborn Age: 0 | [P] Pediatric Age: 0-17 | [M] Maternity Age: 12-55
[A] Adult Age: 15-124 | ♂ Male | ♀ Female | ● New Code | ▲ Revised Code Title | ►◄ Revised Text

C50.82 Malignant neoplasm of overlapping sites of breast, male
    C50.821 Malignant neoplasm of overlapping sites of right male breast ♂
    C50.822 Malignant neoplasm of overlapping sites of left male breast ♂
    C50.829 Malignant neoplasm of overlapping sites of unspecified male breast ♂

C50.9 Malignant neoplasm of breast of unspecified site
  C50.91 Malignant neoplasm of breast of unspecified site, female
    C50.911 Malignant neoplasm of unspecified site of right female breast ♀
    C50.912 Malignant neoplasm of unspecified site of left female breast ♀
    C50.919 Malignant neoplasm of unspecified site of unspecified female breast ♀
  C50.92 Malignant neoplasm of breast of unspecified site, male
    C50.921 Malignant neoplasm of unspecified site of right male breast ♂
    C50.922 Malignant neoplasm of unspecified site of left male breast ♂
    C50.929 Malignant neoplasm of unspecified site of unspecified male breast ♂

Malignant neoplasms of female genital organs (C51-C58)

    INCLUDES   *malignant neoplasm of skin of female genital organs*

C51 Malignant neoplasm of vulva
    EXCLUDES1   *carcinoma in situ of vulva (D07.1)*
  C51.0 Malignant neoplasm of labium majus
    Malignant neoplasm of Bartholin's [greater vestibular] gland ♀
  C51.1 Malignant neoplasm of labium minus ♀
  C51.2 Malignant neoplasm of clitoris ♀
  C51.8 Malignant neoplasm of overlapping sites of vulva ♀
  C51.9 Malignant neoplasm of vulva, unspecified
    Malignant neoplasm of external female genitalia NOS
    Malignant neoplasm of pudendum ♀

C52 Malignant neoplasm of vagina
    EXCLUDES1   *carcinoma in situ of vagina (D07.2)*

C53 Malignant neoplasm of cervix uteri
    EXCLUDES1   *carcinoma in situ of cervix uteri (D06.-)*
  C53.0 Malignant neoplasm of endocervix ♀
  C53.1 Malignant neoplasm of exocervix ♀
  C53.8 Malignant neoplasm of overlapping sites of cervix uteri ♀
  C53.9 Malignant neoplasm of cervix uteri, unspecified ♀

C54 Malignant neoplasm of corpus uteri
  C54.0 Malignant neoplasm of isthmus uteri
    Malignant neoplasm of lower uterine segment ♀
  C54.1 Malignant neoplasm of endometrium ♀
  C54.2 Malignant neoplasm of myometrium ♀
  C54.3 Malignant neoplasm of fundus uteri ♀
  C54.8 Malignant neoplasm of overlapping sites of corpus uteri ♀
  C54.9 Malignant neoplasm of corpus uteri, unspecified ♀

C55 Malignant neoplasm of uterus, part unspecified ♀

C56 Malignant neoplasm of ovary
    Use additional code to identify any functional activity
  C56.1 Malignant neoplasm of right ovary ♀
  C56.2 Malignant neoplasm of left ovary ♀
  C56.9 Malignant neoplasm of unspecified ovary ♀

C57 Malignant neoplasm of other and unspecified female genital organs
  C57.0 Malignant neoplasm of fallopian tube
    Malignant neoplasm of oviduct
    Malignant neoplasm of uterine tube

    C57.00 Malignant neoplasm of unspecified fallopian tube ♀
    C57.01 Malignant neoplasm of right fallopian tube ♀
    C57.02 Malignant neoplasm of left fallopian tube ♀
  C57.1 Malignant neoplasm of broad ligament
    C57.10 Malignant neoplasm of unspecified broad ligament ♀
    C57.11 Malignant neoplasm of right broad ligament ♀
    C57.12 Malignant neoplasm of left broad ligament ♀
  C57.2 Malignant neoplasm of round ligament
    C57.20 Malignant neoplasm of unspecified round ligament ♀
    C57.21 Malignant neoplasm of right round ligament ♀
    C57.22 Malignant neoplasm of left round ligament ♀
  C57.3 Malignant neoplasm of parametrium
    Malignant neoplasm of uterine ligament NOS ♀
  C57.4 Malignant neoplasm of uterine adnexa, unspecified ♀
  C57.7 Malignant neoplasm of other specified female genital organs
    Malignant neoplasm of wolffian body or duct ♀
  C57.8 Malignant neoplasm of overlapping sites of female genital organs
    Primary malignant neoplasm of two or more contiguous sites of the female genital organs whose point of origin cannot be determined
    Primary tubo-ovarian malignant neoplasm whose point of origin cannot be determined
    Primary utero-ovarian malignant neoplasm whose point of origin cannot be determined ♀
  C57.9 Malignant neoplasm of female genital organ, unspecified
    Malignant neoplasm of female genitourinary tract NOS ♀

C58 Malignant neoplasm of placenta
    INCLUDES   *choriocarcinoma NOS*
        chorionepithelioma NOS
    EXCLUDES1   *chorioadenoma (destruens) (D39.2)*
        hydatidiform mole NOS (O01.9)
        invasive hydatidiform mole (D39.2)
        male choriocarcinoma NOS (C62.9-)
        malignant hydatidiform mole (D39.2) ♀

Malignant neoplasms of male genital organs (C60-C63)

    INCLUDES   *malignant neoplasm of skin of male genital organs*

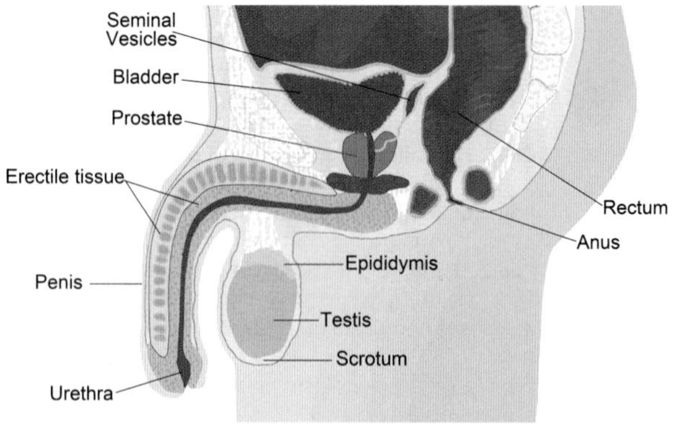

Seminal Vesicles
Bladder
Prostate
Erectile tissue
Penis
Urethra
Rectum
Anus
Epididymis
Testis
Scrotum

Figure 3.3 Male Reproductive Tract

C60 Malignant neoplasm of penis
  C60.0 Malignant neoplasm of prepuce
    Malignant neoplasm of foreskin ♂
  C60.1 Malignant neoplasm of glans penis ♂

---

❹ 4th character required   ❺ 5th character required   ❻ 6th character required   ❼ 7th character required   ⊕ Extension 'X' Alert

EXCLUDES 1 Not coded here   *EXCLUDES 2* Not included here   PDx Primary Diagnosis Only   Manifestation Code

C60.2 Malignant neoplasm of body of penis

Malignant neoplasm of corpus cavernosum ♂

C60.8 Malignant neoplasm of overlapping sites of penis ♂

C60.9 Malignant neoplasm of penis, unspecified

Malignant neoplasm of skin of penis NOS ♂

C61 Malignant neoplasm of prostate

EXCLUDES1 malignant neoplasm of seminal vesicle (C63.7) ♂

C62 Malignant neoplasm of testis

Use additional code to identify any functional activity

C62.0 Malignant neoplasm of undescended testis

Malignant neoplasm of ectopic testis
Malignant neoplasm of retained testis

C62.00 Malignant neoplasm of unspecified undescended testis ♂

C62.01 Malignant neoplasm of undescended right testis ♂

C62.02 Malignant neoplasm of undescended left testis ♂

C62.1 Malignant neoplasm of descended testis

Malignant neoplasm of scrotal testis

C62.10 Malignant neoplasm of unspecified descended testis ♂

C62.11 Malignant neoplasm of descended right testis ♂

C62.12 Malignant neoplasm of descended left testis ♂

C62.9 Malignant neoplasm of testis, unspecified whether descended or undescended

C62.90 Malignant neoplasm of unspecified testis, unspecified whether descended or undescended

Malignant neoplasm of testis NOS ♂

C62.91 Malignant neoplasm of right testis, unspecified whether descended or undescended ♂

C62.92 Malignant neoplasm of left testis, unspecified whether descended or undescended ♂

C63 Malignant neoplasm of other and unspecified male genital organs

C63.0 Malignant neoplasm of epididymis

C63.00 Malignant neoplasm of unspecified epididymis ♂

C63.01 Malignant neoplasm of right epididymis ♂

C63.02 Malignant neoplasm of left epididymis ♂

C63.1 Malignant neoplasm of spermatic cord

C63.10 Malignant neoplasm of unspecified spermatic cord ♂

C63.11 Malignant neoplasm of right spermatic cord ♂

C63.12 Malignant neoplasm of left spermatic cord ♂

C63.2 Malignant neoplasm of scrotum

Malignant neoplasm of skin of scrotum ♂

C63.7 Malignant neoplasm of other specified male genital organs

Malignant neoplasm of seminal vesicle
Malignant neoplasm of tunica vaginalis ♂

C63.8 Malignant neoplasm of overlapping sites of male genital organs

Primary malignant neoplasm of two or more contiguous sites of male genital organs whose point of origin cannot be determined ♂

C63.9 Malignant neoplasm of male genital organ, unspecified

Malignant neoplasm of male genitourinary tract NOS ♂

Malignant neoplasms of urinary tract (C64-C68)

C64 Malignant neoplasm of kidney, except renal pelvis

EXCLUDES1 malignant carcinoid tumor of the kidney (C7A.093)
malignant neoplasm of renal calyces (C65.-)
malignant neoplasm of renal pelvis (C65.-)

C64.1 Malignant neoplasm of right kidney, except renal pelvis

C64.2 Malignant neoplasm of left kidney, except renal pelvis

C64.9 Malignant neoplasm of unspecified kidney, except renal pelvis

C65 Malignant neoplasm of renal pelvis

INCLUDES malignant neoplasm of pelviureteric junction
malignant neoplasm of renal calyces

C65.1 Malignant neoplasm of right renal pelvis

C65.2 Malignant neoplasm of left renal pelvis

C65.9 Malignant neoplasm of unspecified renal pelvis

C66 Malignant neoplasm of ureter

EXCLUDES1 malignant neoplasm of ureteric orifice of bladder (C67.6)

C66.1 Malignant neoplasm of right ureter

C66.2 Malignant neoplasm of left ureter

C66.9 Malignant neoplasm of unspecified ureter

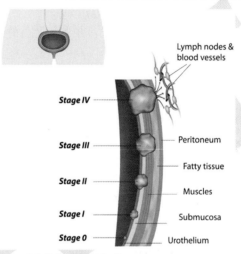

Lymph nodes & blood vessels

Stage IV

Stage III — Peritoneum

— Fatty tissue

Stage II — Muscles

Stage I — Submucosa

Stage 0 — Urothelium

Figure 3.4 Urinary Bladder Cancer

C67 Malignant neoplasm of bladder

C67.0 Malignant neoplasm of trigone of bladder

C67.1 Malignant neoplasm of dome of bladder

C67.2 Malignant neoplasm of lateral wall of bladder

C67.3 Malignant neoplasm of anterior wall of bladder

C67.4 Malignant neoplasm of posterior wall of bladder

C67.5 Malignant neoplasm of bladder neck

Malignant neoplasm of internal urethral orifice

C67.6 Malignant neoplasm of ureteric orifice

C67.7 Malignant neoplasm of urachus

C67.8 Malignant neoplasm of overlapping sites of bladder

C67.9 Malignant neoplasm of bladder, unspecified

C68 Malignant neoplasm of other and unspecified urinary organs

EXCLUDES1 malignant neoplasm of female genitourinary tract NOS (C57.9)
malignant neoplasm of male genitourinary tract NOS (C63.9)

C68.0 Malignant neoplasm of urethra

EXCLUDES1 malignant neoplasm of urethral orifice of bladder (C67.5)

C68.1 Malignant neoplasm of paraurethral glands

C68.8 Malignant neoplasm of overlapping sites of urinary organs

Primary malignant neoplasm of two or more contiguous sites of urinary organs whose point of origin cannot be determined

C68.9 Malignant neoplasm of urinary organ, unspecified

Malignant neoplasm of urinary system NOS

Unspecified Code	Other Specified Code	N Newborn Age: 0	P Pediatric Age: 0-17	M Maternity Age: 12-55
A Adult Age: 15-124	♂ Male	♀ Female	● New Code	▲ Revised Code Title	►◄ Revised Text

Malignant neoplasms of eye, brain and other parts of central nervous system (C69-C72)

[4] **C69 Malignant neoplasm of eye and adnexa**

[EXCLUDES1] *malignant neoplasm of connective tissue of eyelid (C49.0)*
malignant neoplasm of eyelid (skin) (C43.1-, C44.1-)
malignant neoplasm of optic nerve (C72.3)

[5] **C69.0 Malignant neoplasm of conjunctiva**
C69.00 Malignant neoplasm of unspecified conjunctiva
C69.01 Malignant neoplasm of right conjunctiva
C69.02 Malignant neoplasm of left conjunctiva

[5] **C69.1 Malignant neoplasm of cornea**
C69.10 Malignant neoplasm of unspecified cornea
C69.11 Malignant neoplasm of right cornea
C69.12 Malignant neoplasm of left cornea

[5] **C69.2 Malignant neoplasm of retina**

[EXCLUDES1] *dark area on retina (D49.81)*
neoplasm of unspecified behavior of retina and choroid (D49.81)
retinal freckle (D49.81)

C69.20 Malignant neoplasm of unspecified retina
C69.21 Malignant neoplasm of right retina
C69.22 Malignant neoplasm of left retina

[5] **C69.3 Malignant neoplasm of choroid**
C69.30 Malignant neoplasm of unspecified choroid
C69.31 Malignant neoplasm of right choroid
C69.32 Malignant neoplasm of left choroid

[5] **C69.4 Malignant neoplasm of ciliary body**
C69.40 Malignant neoplasm of unspecified ciliary body
C69.41 Malignant neoplasm of right ciliary body
C69.42 Malignant neoplasm of left ciliary body

[5] **C69.5 Malignant neoplasm of lacrimal gland and duct**

Malignant neoplasm of lacrimal sac
Malignant neoplasm of nasolacrimal duct

C69.50 Malignant neoplasm of unspecified lacrimal gland and duct
C69.51 Malignant neoplasm of right lacrimal gland and duct
C69.52 Malignant neoplasm of left lacrimal gland and duct

[5] **C69.6 Malignant neoplasm of orbit**

Malignant neoplasm of connective tissue of orbit
Malignant neoplasm of extraocular muscle
Malignant neoplasm of peripheral nerves of orbit
Malignant neoplasm of retrobulbar tissue
Malignant neoplasm of retro-ocular tissue

[EXCLUDES1] *malignant neoplasm of orbital bone (C41.0)*

C69.60 Malignant neoplasm of unspecified orbit
C69.61 Malignant neoplasm of right orbit
C69.62 Malignant neoplasm of left orbit

[5] **C69.8 Malignant neoplasm of overlapping sites of eye and adnexa**
C69.80 Malignant neoplasm of overlapping sites of unspecified eye and adnexa
C69.81 Malignant neoplasm of overlapping sites of right eye and adnexa
C69.82 Malignant neoplasm of overlapping sites of left eye and adnexa

[5] **C69.9 Malignant neoplasm of unspecified site of eye**

Malignant neoplasm of eyeball

C69.90 Malignant neoplasm of unspecified site of unspecified eye
C69.91 Malignant neoplasm of unspecified site of right eye
C69.92 Malignant neoplasm of unspecified site of left eye

[4] **C70 Malignant neoplasm of meninges**
C70.0 Malignant neoplasm of cerebral meninges
C70.1 Malignant neoplasm of spinal meninges
C70.9 Malignant neoplasm of meninges, unspecified

[4] **C71 Malignant neoplasm of brain**

[EXCLUDES1] *malignant neoplasm of cranial nerves (C72.2-C72.5)*
retrobulbar malignant neoplasm (C69.6-)

C71.0 Malignant neoplasm of ~~cerebrum, except lobes and ventricles~~

Malignant neoplasm of supratentorial NOS

C71.1 Malignant neoplasm of frontal lobe
C71.2 Malignant neoplasm of temporal lobe
C71.3 Malignant neoplasm of parietal lobe
C71.4 Malignant neoplasm of occipital lobe
C71.5 Malignant neoplasm of cerebral ventricle

[EXCLUDES1] *malignant neoplasm of fourth cerebral ventricle (C71.7)*

C71.6 Malignant neoplasm of cerebellum
C71.7 Malignant neoplasm of brain stem

Malignant neoplasm of fourth cerebral ventricle
Infratentorial malignant neoplasm NOS

C71.8 Malignant neoplasm of overlapping sites of brain
C71.9 Malignant neoplasm of brain, unspecified

[4] **C72 Malignant neoplasm of spinal cord, cranial nerves and other parts of central nervous system**

[EXCLUDES1] *malignant neoplasm of meninges (C70.-)*
malignant neoplasm of peripheral nerves and autonomic nervous system (C47.-)

C72.0 Malignant neoplasm of spinal cord
C72.1 Malignant neoplasm of cauda equina

[5] **C72.2 Malignant neoplasm of olfactory nerve**

Malignant neoplasm of olfactory bulb

C72.20 Malignant neoplasm of unspecified olfactory nerve
C72.21 Malignant neoplasm of right olfactory nerve
C72.22 Malignant neoplasm of left olfactory nerve

[5] **C72.3 Malignant neoplasm of optic nerve**
C72.30 Malignant neoplasm of unspecified optic nerve
C72.31 Malignant neoplasm of right optic nerve
C72.32 Malignant neoplasm of left optic nerve

[5] **C72.4 Malignant neoplasm of acoustic nerve**
C72.40 Malignant neoplasm of unspecified acoustic nerve
C72.41 Malignant neoplasm of right acoustic nerve
C72.42 Malignant neoplasm of left acoustic nerve

[5] **C72.5 Malignant neoplasm of other and unspecified cranial nerves**
C72.50 Malignant neoplasm of unspecified cranial nerve

Malignant neoplasm of cranial nerve NOS

C72.59 Malignant neoplasm of other cranial nerves
C72.9 Malignant neoplasm of central nervous system, unspecified

Malignant neoplasm of unspecified site of central nervous system
Malignant neoplasm of nervous system NOS

Malignant neoplasms of thyroid and other endocrine glands (C73-C75)

C73 Malignant neoplasm of thyroid gland

Use additional code to identify any functional activity

[4] **C74 Malignant neoplasm of adrenal gland**

[5] **C74.0 Malignant neoplasm of cortex of adrenal gland**
C74.00 Malignant neoplasm of cortex of unspecified adrenal gland

[4] 4th character required [5] 5th character required [6] 6th character required [7] 7th character required [X] Extension 'X' Alert
[EXCLUDES1] Not coded here [EXCLUDES2] Not included here [PDx] Primary Diagnosis Only Manifestation Code

C74.01 Malignant neoplasm of cortex of right adrenal gland

C74.02 Malignant neoplasm of cortex of left adrenal gland

🄯 **C74.1** Malignant neoplasm of medulla of adrenal gland

C74.10 Malignant neoplasm of medulla of unspecified adrenal gland

C74.11 Malignant neoplasm of medulla of right adrenal gland

C74.12 Malignant neoplasm of medulla of left adrenal gland

🄯 **C74.9** Malignant neoplasm of unspecified part of adrenal gland

C74.90 Malignant neoplasm of unspecified part of unspecified adrenal gland

C74.91 Malignant neoplasm of unspecified part of right adrenal gland

C74.92 Malignant neoplasm of unspecified part of left adrenal gland

🄯 **C75** Malignant neoplasm of other endocrine glands and related structures

> EXCLUDES1 *malignant carcinoid tumors (C7A.0-)*
> *malignant neoplasm of adrenal gland (C74.-)*
> *malignant neoplasm of endocrine pancreas (C25.4)*
> *malignant neoplasm of islets of Langerhans (C25.4)*
> *malignant neoplasm of ovary (C56.-)*
> *malignant neoplasm of testis (C62.-)*
> *malignant neoplasm of thymus (C37)*
> *malignant neoplasm of thyroid gland (C73)*
> *malignant neuroendocrine tumors (C7A.-)*

C75.0 Malignant neoplasm of parathyroid gland

C75.1 Malignant neoplasm of pituitary gland

C75.2 Malignant neoplasm of craniopharyngeal duct

C75.3 Malignant neoplasm of pineal gland

C75.4 Malignant neoplasm of carotid body

C75.5 Malignant neoplasm of aortic body and other paraganglia

C75.8 Malignant neoplasm with pluriglandular involvement, unspecified

C75.9 Malignant neoplasm of endocrine gland, unspecified

Malignant neuroendocrine tumors (C7A)

🄯 **C7A** Malignant neuroendocrine tumors

> Code also any associated multiple endocrine neoplasia [MEN] syndromes (E31.2-)
> Use additional code to identify any associated endocrine syndrome, such as:
> carcinoid syndrome (E34.0)

> EXCLUDES2 *malignant pancreatic islet cell tumors (C25.4)*
> *Merkel cell carcinoma (C4A.-)*

🄯 **C7A.0** Malignant carcinoid tumors

C7A.00 Malignant carcinoid tumor of unspecified site

🄯 **C7A.01** Malignant carcinoid tumors of the small intestine

C7A.010 Malignant carcinoid tumor of the duodenum

C7A.011 Malignant carcinoid tumor of the jejunum

C7A.012 Malignant carcinoid tumor of the ileum

C7A.019 Malignant carcinoid tumor of the small intestine, unspecified portion

🄯 **C7A.02** Malignant carcinoid tumors of the appendix, large intestine, and rectum

C7A.020 Malignant carcinoid tumor of the appendix

C7A.021 Malignant carcinoid tumor of the cecum

C7A.022 Malignant carcinoid tumor of the ascending colon

C7A.023 Malignant carcinoid tumor of the transverse colon

C7A.024 Malignant carcinoid tumor of the descending colon

C7A.025 Malignant carcinoid tumor of the sigmoid colon

C7A.026 Malignant carcinoid tumor of the rectum

C7A.029 Malignant carcinoid tumor of the large intestine, unspecified portion

> Malignant carcinoid tumor of the colon NOS

🄯 **C7A.09** Malignant carcinoid tumors of other sites

C7A.090 Malignant carcinoid tumor of the bronchus and lung

C7A.091 Malignant carcinoid tumor of the thymus

C7A.092 Malignant carcinoid tumor of the stomach

C7A.093 Malignant carcinoid tumor of the kidney

C7A.094 Malignant carcinoid tumor of the foregut NOS

C7A.095 Malignant carcinoid tumor of the midgut NOS

C7A.096 Malignant carcinoid tumor of the hindgut NOS

C7A.098 Malignant carcinoid tumors of other sites

C7A.1 Malignant poorly differentiated neuroendocrine tumors

> Malignant poorly differentiated neuroendocrine tumor NOS
> Malignant poorly differentiated neuroendocrine carcinoma, any site
> High grade neuroendocrine carcinoma, any site

C7A.8 Other malignant neuroendocrine tumors

Secondary neuroendocrine tumors (C7B)

🄯 **C7B** Secondary neuroendocrine tumors

> Use additional code to identify any functional activity

🄯 **C7B.0** Secondary carcinoid tumors

C7B.00 Secondary carcinoid tumors, unspecified site

C7B.01 Secondary carcinoid tumors of distant lymph nodes

C7B.02 Secondary carcinoid tumors of liver

C7B.03 Secondary carcinoid tumors of bone

C7B.04 Secondary carcinoid tumors of peritoneum

> Mesentary metastasis of carcinoid tumor

C7B.09 Secondary carcinoid tumors of other sites

C7B.1 Secondary Merkel cell carcinoma

> Merkel cell carcinoma nodal presentation
> Merkel cell carcinoma visceral metastatic presentation

C7B.8 Other secondary neuroendocrine tumors

Malignant neoplasms of ill-defined, other secondary and unspecified sites (C76-C80)

🄯 **C76** Malignant neoplasm of other and ill-defined sites

> EXCLUDES1 *malignant neoplasm of female genitourinary tract NOS (C57.9)*
> *malignant neoplasm of male genitourinary tract NOS (C63.9)*
> *malignant neoplasm of lymphoid, hematopoietic and related tissue (C81-C96)*
> *malignant neoplasm of skin (C44.-)*
> *malignant neoplasm of unspecified site NOS (C80.1)*

C76.0 Malignant neoplasm of head, face and neck

> Malignant neoplasm of cheek NOS
> Malignant neoplasm of nose NOS

C76.1 Malignant neoplasm of thorax

> Intrathoracic malignant neoplasm NOS
> Malignant neoplasm of axilla NOS
> Thoracic malignant neoplasm NOS

C76.2 Malignant neoplasm of abdomen

Unspecified Code	Other Specified Code	Ⓝ Newborn Age: 0	Ⓟ Pediatric Age: 0-17	Ⓜ Maternity Age: 12-55
Ⓐ Adult Age: 15-124	♂ Male	♀ Female	● New Code	▲ Revised Code Title	►◄ Revised Text

C76.3 **Malignant neoplasm of pelvis**
Malignant neoplasm of groin NOS
Malignant neoplasm of sites overlapping systems within the pelvis
Rectovaginal (septum) malignant neoplasm
Rectovesical (septum) malignant neoplasm
[5] C76.4 **Malignant neoplasm of upper limb**
C76.40 **Malignant neoplasm of unspecified upper limb**
C76.41 **Malignant neoplasm of right upper limb**
C76.42 **Malignant neoplasm of left upper limb**
[5] C76.5 **Malignant neoplasm of lower limb**
C76.50 **Malignant neoplasm of unspecified lower limb**
C76.51 **Malignant neoplasm of right lower limb**
C76.52 **Malignant neoplasm of left lower limb**
C76.8 **Malignant neoplasm of other specified ill-defined sites**
Malignant neoplasm of overlapping ill-defined sites
[4] C77 **Secondary and unspecified malignant neoplasm of lymph nodes**
[EXCLUDES1] *malignant neoplasm of lymph nodes, specified as primary (C81-C86, C88, C96.-)*
mesentary metastasis of carcinoid tumor (C7B.04)
secondary carcinoid tumors of distant lymph nodes (C7B.01)
C77.0 **Secondary and unspecified malignant neoplasm of lymph nodes of head, face and neck**
Secondary and unspecified malignant neoplasm of supraclavicular lymph nodes
C77.1 **Secondary and unspecified malignant neoplasm of intrathoracic lymph nodes**
C77.2 **Secondary and unspecified malignant neoplasm of intra-abdominal lymph nodes**
C77.3 **Secondary and unspecified malignant neoplasm of axilla and upper limb lymph nodes**
Secondary and unspecified malignant neoplasm of pectoral lymph nodes
C77.4 **Secondary and unspecified malignant neoplasm of inguinal and lower limb lymph nodes**
C77.5 **Secondary and unspecified malignant neoplasm of intrapelvic lymph nodes**
C77.8 **Secondary and unspecified malignant neoplasm of lymph nodes of multiple regions**
C77.9 **Secondary and unspecified malignant neoplasm of lymph node, unspecified**
[4] C78 **Secondary malignant neoplasm of respiratory and digestive organs**
[EXCLUDES1] *lymph node metastases (C77.0)*
secondary carcinoid tumors of liver (C7B.02)
secondary carcinoid tumors of peritoneum (C7B.04)
[5] C78.0 **Secondary malignant neoplasm of lung**
C78.00 **Secondary malignant neoplasm of unspecified lung**
C78.01 **Secondary malignant neoplasm of right lung**
C78.02 **Secondary malignant neoplasm of left lung**
C78.1 **Secondary malignant neoplasm of mediastinum**
C78.2 **Secondary malignant neoplasm of pleura**
[5] C78.3 **Secondary malignant neoplasm of other and unspecified respiratory organs**
C78.30 **Secondary malignant neoplasm of unspecified respiratory organ**
C78.39 **Secondary malignant neoplasm of other respiratory organs**
C78.4 **Secondary malignant neoplasm of small intestine**
C78.5 **Secondary malignant neoplasm of large intestine and rectum**
C78.6 **Secondary malignant neoplasm of retroperitoneum and peritoneum**
C78.7 **Secondary malignant neoplasm of liver and intrahepatic bile duct**
[5] C78.8 **Secondary malignant neoplasm of other and unspecified digestive organs**
C78.80 **Secondary malignant neoplasm of unspecified digestive organ**
C78.89 **Secondary malignant neoplasm of other digestive organs**
[4] C79 **Secondary malignant neoplasm of other and unspecified sites**
[EXCLUDES1] *lymph node metastases (C77.0)*
secondary carcinoid tumors (C7B.-)
secondary neuroendocrine tumors (C7B.-)
[5] C79.0 **Secondary malignant neoplasm of kidney and renal pelvis**
C79.00 **Secondary malignant neoplasm of unspecified kidney and renal pelvis**
C79.01 **Secondary malignant neoplasm of right kidney and renal pelvis**
C79.02 **Secondary malignant neoplasm of left kidney and renal pelvis**
[5] C79.1 **Secondary malignant neoplasm of bladder and other and unspecified urinary organs**
C79.10 **Secondary malignant neoplasm of unspecified urinary organs**
C79.11 **Secondary malignant neoplasm of bladder**
C79.19 **Secondary malignant neoplasm of other urinary organs**
C79.2 **Secondary malignant neoplasm of skin**
[EXCLUDES1] *secondary Merkel cell carcinoma (C7B.1)*
[5] C79.3 **Secondary malignant neoplasm of brain and cerebral meninges**
C79.31 **Secondary malignant neoplasm of brain**
C79.32 **Secondary malignant neoplasm of cerebral meninges**
[5] C79.4 **Secondary malignant neoplasm of other and unspecified parts of nervous system**
C79.40 **Secondary malignant neoplasm of unspecified part of nervous system**
C79.49 **Secondary malignant neoplasm of other parts of nervous system**
[5] C79.5 **Secondary malignant neoplasm of bone and bone marrow**
[EXCLUDES1] *secondary carcinoid tumors of bone (C7B.03)*
C79.51 **Secondary malignant neoplasm of bone**
C79.52 **Secondary malignant neoplasm of bone marrow**
[5] C79.6 **Secondary malignant neoplasm of ovary**
C79.60 **Secondary malignant neoplasm of unspecified ovary** ♀
C79.61 **Secondary malignant neoplasm of right ovary** ♀
C79.62 **Secondary malignant neoplasm of left ovary** ♀
[5] C79.7 **Secondary malignant neoplasm of adrenal gland**
C79.70 **Secondary malignant neoplasm of unspecified adrenal gland**
C79.71 **Secondary malignant neoplasm of right adrenal gland**
C79.72 **Secondary malignant neoplasm of left adrenal gland**
[5] C79.8 **Secondary malignant neoplasm of other specified sites**
C79.81 **Secondary malignant neoplasm of breast**
C79.82 **Secondary malignant neoplasm of genital organs**
C79.89 **Secondary malignant neoplasm of other specified sites**

[4] 4th character required [5] 5th character required [6] 6th character required [7] 7th character required [X] Extension 'X' Alert
[EXCLUDES 1] Not coded here [EXCLUDES 2] Not included here [PDX] Primary Diagnosis Only Manifestation Code

C79.9 **Secondary malignant neoplasm of unspecified site**

Metastatic cancer NOS

Metastatic disease NOS

EXCLUDES1 *carcinomatosis NOS (C80.0)*
generalized cancer NOS (C80.0)
malignant (primary) neoplasm of unspecified site (C80.1)

C80 **Malignant neoplasm** without specification of site

EXCLUDES1 *malignant carcinoid tumor of unspecified site (C7A.00)*
malignant neoplasm of specified multiple sites- code to each site

C80.0 **Disseminated malignant neoplasm, unspecified**

Carcinomatosis NOS

Generalized cancer, unspecified site (primary) (secondary)

Generalized malignancy, unspecified site (primary) (secondary)

C80.1 **Malignant (primary) neoplasm, unspecified**

Cancer NOS

Cancer unspecified site (primary)

Carcinoma unspecified site (primary)

Malignancy unspecified site (primary)

EXCLUDES1 *secondary malignant neoplasm of unspecified site (C79.9)*

C80.2 **Malignant neoplasm** associated with transplanted organ

Code first complication of transplanted organ (T86.-)

Use additional code to identify the specific malignancy

Malignant neoplasms of lymphoid, hematopoietic and related tissue (C81-C96)

EXCLUDES2 *Kaposi's sarcoma of lymph nodes (C46.3)*
secondary and unspecified neoplasm of lymph nodes (C77.-)
secondary neoplasm of bone marrow (C79.52)
secondary neoplasm of spleen (C78.89)

C81 **Hodgkin lymphoma**

EXCLUDES1 *personal history of Hodgkin lymphoma (Z85.71)*

C81.0 Nodular lymphocyte predominant **Hodgkin lymphoma**

C81.00 **Nodular lymphocyte predominant Hodgkin lymphoma, unspecified site**

C81.01 **Nodular lymphocyte predominant Hodgkin lymphoma, lymph nodes of** head, face, and neck

C81.02 **Nodular lymphocyte predominant Hodgkin lymphoma,** intrathoracic **lymph nodes**

C81.03 **Nodular lymphocyte predominant Hodgkin lymphoma,** intra-abdominal **lymph nodes**

C81.04 **Nodular lymphocyte predominant Hodgkin lymphoma, lymph nodes of** axilla and upper limb

C81.05 **Nodular lymphocyte predominant Hodgkin lymphoma, lymph nodes of** inguinal region and lower limb

C81.06 **Nodular lymphocyte predominant Hodgkin lymphoma,** intrapelvic **lymph nodes**

C81.07 **Nodular lymphocyte predominant Hodgkin lymphoma,** spleen

C81.08 **Nodular lymphocyte predominant Hodgkin lymphoma, lymph nodes of** multiple sites

C81.09 **Nodular lymphocyte predominant Hodgkin lymphoma,** extranodal and solid organ sites

C81.1 Nodular sclerosis classical **Hodgkin lymphoma**

C81.10 **Nodular sclerosis classical Hodgkin lymphoma, unspecified site**

C81.11 **Nodular sclerosis classical Hodgkin lymphoma, lymph nodes of** head, face, and neck

C81.12 **Nodular sclerosis classical Hodgkin lymphoma,** intrathoracic **lymph nodes**

C81.13 **Nodular sclerosis classical Hodgkin lymphoma,** intra-abdominal **lymph nodes**

C81.14 **Nodular sclerosis classical Hodgkin lymphoma, lymph nodes of** axilla and upper limb

C81.15 **Nodular sclerosis classical Hodgkin lymphoma, lymph nodes of** inguinal region and lower limb

C81.16 **Nodular sclerosis classical Hodgkin lymphoma,** intrapelvic **lymph nodes**

C81.17 **Nodular sclerosis classical Hodgkin lymphoma,** spleen

C81.18 **Nodular sclerosis classical Hodgkin lymphoma, lymph nodes of** multiple sites

C81.19 **Nodular sclerosis classical Hodgkin lymphoma,** extranodal and solid organ sites

C81.2 Mixed cellularity classical **Hodgkin lymphoma**

C81.20 **Mixed cellularity classical Hodgkin lymphoma, unspecified site**

C81.21 **Mixed cellularity classical Hodgkin lymphoma, lymph nodes of** head, face, and neck

C81.22 **Mixed cellularity classical Hodgkin lymphoma,** intrathoracic **lymph nodes**

C81.23 **Mixed cellularity classical Hodgkin lymphoma,** intra-abdominal **lymph nodes**

C81.24 **Mixed cellularity classical Hodgkin lymphoma, lymph nodes of** axilla and upper limb

C81.25 **Mixed cellularity classical Hodgkin lymphoma, lymph nodes of** inguinal region and lower limb

C81.26 **Mixed cellularity classical Hodgkin lymphoma,** intrapelvic **lymph nodes**

C81.27 **Mixed cellularity classical Hodgkin lymphoma,** spleen

C81.28 **Mixed cellularity classical Hodgkin lymphoma, lymph nodes of** multiple sites

C81.29 **Mixed cellularity classical Hodgkin lymphoma,** extranodal and solid organ sites

C81.3 Lymphocyte depleted classical **Hodgkin lymphoma**

C81.30 **Lymphocyte depleted classical Hodgkin lymphoma, unspecified site**

C81.31 **Lymphocyte depleted classical Hodgkin lymphoma, lymph nodes of** head, face, and neck

C81.32 **Lymphocyte depleted classical Hodgkin lymphoma,** intrathoracic **lymph nodes**

C81.33 **Lymphocyte depleted classical Hodgkin lymphoma,** intra-abdominal **lymph nodes**

C81.34 **Lymphocyte depleted classical Hodgkin lymphoma, lymph nodes of** axilla and upper limb

C81.35 **Lymphocyte depleted classical Hodgkin lymphoma, lymph nodes of** inguinal region and lower limb

C81.36 **Lymphocyte depleted classical Hodgkin lymphoma,** intrapelvic **lymph nodes**

C81.37 **Lymphocyte depleted classical Hodgkin lymphoma,** spleen

C81.38 **Lymphocyte depleted classical Hodgkin lymphoma, lymph nodes of** multiple sites

C81.39 **Lymphocyte depleted classical Hodgkin lymphoma,** extranodal and solid organ sites

C81.4 Lymphocyte-rich classical **Hodgkin lymphoma**

EXCLUDES1 *nodular lymphocyte predominant Hodgkin lymphoma (C81.0-)*

C81.40 **Lymphocyte-rich classical Hodgkin lymphoma, unspecified site**

C81.41 **Lymphocyte-rich classical Hodgkin lymphoma, lymph nodes of** head, face, and neck

C81.42 **Lymphocyte-rich classical Hodgkin lymphoma,** intrathoracic **lymph nodes**

Unspecified Code   Other Specified Code   N Newborn Age: 0   P Pediatric Age: 0-17   M Maternity Age: 12-55

A Adult Age: 15-124   ♂ Male   ♀ Female   ● New Code   ▲ Revised Code Title   ►◄ Revised Text

C81.43 Lymphocyte-rich classical Hodgkin lymphoma, intra-abdominal lymph nodes

C81.44 Lymphocyte-rich classical Hodgkin lymphoma, lymph nodes of axilla and upper limb

C81.45 Lymphocyte-rich classical Hodgkin lymphoma, lymph nodes of inguinal region and lower limb

C81.46 Lymphocyte-rich classical Hodgkin lymphoma, intrapelvic lymph nodes

C81.47 Lymphocyte-rich classical Hodgkin lymphoma, spleen

C81.48 Lymphocyte-rich classical Hodgkin lymphoma, lymph nodes of multiple sites

C81.49 Lymphocyte-rich classical Hodgkin lymphoma, extranodal and solid organ sites

⑤ C81.7 Other classical Hodgkin lymphoma

Classical Hodgkin lymphoma NOS

C81.70 Other classical Hodgkin lymphoma, unspecified site

C81.71 Other classical Hodgkin lymphoma, lymph nodes of head, face, and neck

C81.72 Other classical Hodgkin lymphoma, intrathoracic lymph nodes

C81.73 Other classical Hodgkin lymphoma, intra-abdominal lymph nodes

C81.74 Other classical Hodgkin lymphoma, lymph nodes of axilla and upper limb

C81.75 Other classical Hodgkin lymphoma, lymph nodes of inguinal region and lower limb

C81.76 Other classical Hodgkin lymphoma, intrapelvic lymph nodes

C81.77 Other classical Hodgkin lymphoma, spleen

C81.78 Other classical Hodgkin lymphoma, lymph nodes of multiple sites

C81.79 Other classical Hodgkin lymphoma, extranodal and solid organ sites

⑤ C81.9 Hodgkin lymphoma, unspecified

C81.90 Hodgkin lymphoma, unspecified, unspecified site

C81.91 Hodgkin lymphoma, unspecified, lymph nodes of head, face, and neck

C81.92 Hodgkin lymphoma, unspecified, intrathoracic lymph nodes

C81.93 Hodgkin lymphoma, unspecified, intra-abdominal lymph nodes

C81.94 Hodgkin lymphoma, unspecified, lymph nodes of axilla and upper limb

C81.95 Hodgkin lymphoma, unspecified, lymph nodes of inguinal region and lower limb

C81.96 Hodgkin lymphoma, unspecified, intrapelvic lymph nodes

C81.97 Hodgkin lymphoma, unspecified, spleen

C81.98 Hodgkin lymphoma, unspecified, lymph nodes of multiple sites

C81.99 Hodgkin lymphoma, unspecified, extranodal and solid organ sites

④ C82 Follicular lymphoma

INCLUDES follicular lymphoma with or without diffuse areas

EXCLUDES1 mature T/NK-cell lymphomas (C84.-)
personal history of non-Hodgkin lymphoma (Z85.72)

⑤ C82.0 Follicular lymphoma grade I

C82.00 Follicular lymphoma grade I, unspecified site

C82.01 Follicular lymphoma grade I, lymph nodes of head, face, and neck

C82.02 Follicular lymphoma grade I, intrathoracic lymph nodes

C82.03 Follicular lymphoma grade I, intra-abdominal lymph nodes

C82.04 Follicular lymphoma grade I, lymph nodes of axilla and upper limb

C82.05 Follicular lymphoma grade I, lymph nodes of inguinal region and lower limb

C82.06 Follicular lymphoma grade I, intrapelvic lymph nodes

C82.07 Follicular lymphoma grade I, spleen

C82.08 Follicular lymphoma grade I, lymph nodes of multiple sites

C82.09 Follicular lymphoma grade I, extranodal and solid organ sites

⑤ C82.1 Follicular lymphoma grade II

C82.10 Follicular lymphoma grade II, unspecified site

C82.11 Follicular lymphoma grade II, lymph nodes of head, face, and neck

C82.12 Follicular lymphoma grade II, intrathoracic lymph nodes

C82.13 Follicular lymphoma grade II, intra-abdominal lymph nodes

C82.14 Follicular lymphoma grade II, lymph nodes of axilla and upper limb

C82.15 Follicular lymphoma grade II, lymph nodes of inguinal region and lower limb

C82.16 Follicular lymphoma grade II, intrapelvic lymph nodes

C82.17 Follicular lymphoma grade II, spleen

C82.18 Follicular lymphoma grade II, lymph nodes of multiple sites

C82.19 Follicular lymphoma grade II, extranodal and solid organ sites

⑤ C82.2 Follicular lymphoma grade III, unspecified

C82.20 Follicular lymphoma grade III, unspecified, unspecified site

C82.21 Follicular lymphoma grade III, unspecified, lymph nodes of head, face, and neck

C82.22 Follicular lymphoma grade III, unspecified, intrathoracic lymph nodes

C82.23 Follicular lymphoma grade III, unspecified, intra-abdominal lymph nodes

C82.24 Follicular lymphoma grade III, unspecified, lymph nodes of axilla and upper limb

C82.25 Follicular lymphoma grade III, unspecified, lymph nodes of inguinal region and lower limb

C82.26 Follicular lymphoma grade III, unspecified, intrapelvic lymph nodes

C82.27 Follicular lymphoma grade III, unspecified, spleen

C82.28 Follicular lymphoma grade III, unspecified, lymph nodes of multiple sites

C82.29 Follicular lymphoma grade III, unspecified, extranodal and solid organ sites

⑤ C82.3 Follicular lymphoma grade IIIa

C82.30 Follicular lymphoma grade IIIa, unspecified site

C82.31 Follicular lymphoma grade IIIa, lymph nodes of head, face, and neck

C82.32 Follicular lymphoma grade IIIa, intrathoracic lymph nodes

C82.33 Follicular lymphoma grade IIIa, intra-abdominal lymph nodes

C82.34 Follicular lymphoma grade IIIa, lymph nodes of axilla and upper limb

C82.35 Follicular lymphoma grade IIIa, lymph nodes of inguinal region and lower limb

C82.36 Follicular lymphoma grade IIIa, intrapelvic lymph nodes

C82.37 Follicular lymphoma grade IIIa, spleen

C82.38 Follicular lymphoma grade IIIa, lymph nodes of multiple sites

---

④ 4th character required ⑤ 5th character required ⑥ 6th character required ⑦ 7th character required ⑩ Extension 'X' Alert

EXCLUDES 1 Not coded here EXCLUDES 2 Not included here PDx Primary Diagnosis Only Manifestation Code

C82.39 Follicular lymphoma grade IIIa, extranodal and solid organ sites

🔁 C82.4 Follicular lymphoma grade IIIb

C82.40 Follicular lymphoma grade IIIb, unspecified site

C82.41 Follicular lymphoma grade IIIb, lymph nodes of head, face, and neck

C82.42 Follicular lymphoma grade IIIb, intrathoracic lymph nodes

C82.43 Follicular lymphoma grade IIIb, intra-abdominal lymph nodes

C82.44 Follicular lymphoma grade IIIb, lymph nodes of axilla and upper limb

C82.45 Follicular lymphoma grade IIIb, lymph nodes of inguinal region and lower limb

C82.46 Follicular lymphoma grade IIIb, intrapelvic lymph nodes

C82.47 Follicular lymphoma grade IIIb, spleen

C82.48 Follicular lymphoma grade IIIb, lymph nodes of multiple sites

C82.49 Follicular lymphoma grade IIIb, extranodal and solid organ sites

🔁 C82.5 Diffuse follicle center lymphoma

C82.50 Diffuse follicle center lymphoma, unspecified site

C82.51 Diffuse follicle center lymphoma, lymph nodes of head, face, and neck

C82.52 Diffuse follicle center lymphoma, intrathoracic lymph nodes

C82.53 Diffuse follicle center lymphoma, intra-abdominal lymph nodes

C82.54 Diffuse follicle center lymphoma, lymph nodes of axilla and upper limb

C82.55 Diffuse follicle center lymphoma, lymph nodes of inguinal region and lower limb

C82.56 Diffuse follicle center lymphoma, intrapelvic lymph nodes

C82.57 Diffuse follicle center lymphoma, spleen

C82.58 Diffuse follicle center lymphoma, lymph nodes of multiple sites

C82.59 Diffuse follicle center lymphoma, extranodal and solid organ sites

🔁 C82.6 Cutaneous follicle center lymphoma

C82.60 Cutaneous follicle center lymphoma, unspecified site

C82.61 Cutaneous follicle center lymphoma, lymph nodes of head, face, and neck

C82.62 Cutaneous follicle center lymphoma, intrathoracic lymph nodes

C82.63 Cutaneous follicle center lymphoma, intra-abdominal lymph nodes

C82.64 Cutaneous follicle center lymphoma, lymph nodes of axilla and upper limb

C82.65 Cutaneous follicle center lymphoma, lymph nodes of inguinal region and lower limb

C82.66 Cutaneous follicle center lymphoma, intrapelvic lymph nodes

C82.67 Cutaneous follicle center lymphoma, spleen

C82.68 Cutaneous follicle center lymphoma, lymph nodes of multiple sites

C82.69 Cutaneous follicle center lymphoma, extranodal and solid organ sites

🔁 C82.8 Other types of follicular lymphoma

C82.80 Other types of follicular lymphoma, unspecified site

C82.81 Other types of follicular lymphoma, lymph nodes of head, face, and neck

C82.82 Other types of follicular lymphoma, intrathoracic lymph nodes

C82.83 Other types of follicular lymphoma, intra-abdominal lymph nodes

C82.84 Other types of follicular lymphoma, lymph nodes of axilla and upper limb

C82.85 Other types of follicular lymphoma, lymph nodes of inguinal region and lower limb

C82.86 Other types of follicular lymphoma, intrapelvic lymph nodes

C82.87 Other types of follicular lymphoma, spleen

C82.88 Other types of follicular lymphoma, lymph nodes of multiple sites

C82.89 Other types of follicular lymphoma, extranodal and solid organ sites

🔁 C82.9 Follicular lymphoma, unspecified

C82.90 Follicular lymphoma, unspecified, unspecified site

C82.91 Follicular lymphoma, unspecified, lymph nodes of head, face, and neck

C82.92 Follicular lymphoma, unspecified, intrathoracic lymph nodes

C82.93 Follicular lymphoma, unspecified, intra-abdominal lymph nodes

C82.94 Follicular lymphoma, unspecified, lymph nodes of axilla and upper limb

C82.95 Follicular lymphoma, unspecified, lymph nodes of inguinal region and lower limb

C82.96 Follicular lymphoma, unspecified, intrapelvic lymph nodes

C82.97 Follicular lymphoma, unspecified, spleen

C82.98 Follicular lymphoma, unspecified, lymph nodes of multiple sites

C82.99 Follicular lymphoma, unspecified, extranodal and solid organ sites

❹ C83 Non-follicular lymphoma

EXCLUDES1 personal history of non-Hodgkin lymphoma (Z85.72)

🔁 C83.0 Small cell B-cell lymphoma

Lymphoplasmacytic lymphoma
Nodal marginal zone lymphoma
Non-leukemic variant of B-CLL
Splenic marginal zone lymphoma

EXCLUDES1 chronic lymphocytic leukemia (C91.1)
mature T/NK-cell lymphomas (C84.-)
Waldenström macroglobulinemia (C88.0)

C83.00 Small cell B-cell lymphoma, unspecified site

C83.01 Small cell B-cell lymphoma, lymph nodes of head, face, and neck

C83.02 Small cell B-cell lymphoma, intrathoracic lymph nodes

C83.03 Small cell B-cell lymphoma, intra-abdominal lymph nodes

C83.04 Small cell B-cell lymphoma, lymph nodes of axilla and upper limb

C83.05 Small cell B-cell lymphoma, lymph nodes of inguinal region and lower limb

C83.06 Small cell B-cell lymphoma, intrapelvic lymph nodes

C83.07 Small cell B-cell lymphoma, spleen

C83.08 Small cell B-cell lymphoma, lymph nodes of multiple sites

C83.09 Small cell B-cell lymphoma, extranodal and solid organ sites

🔁 C83.1 Mantle cell lymphoma

Centrocytic lymphoma
Malignant lymphomatous polyposis

C83.10 Mantle cell lymphoma, unspecified site

C83.11 Mantle cell lymphoma, lymph nodes of head, face, and neck

C83.12 Mantle cell lymphoma, intrathoracic lymph nodes
C83.13 Mantle cell lymphoma, intra-abdominal lymph nodes
C83.14 Mantle cell lymphoma, lymph nodes of axilla and upper limb
C83.15 Mantle cell lymphoma, lymph nodes of inguinal region and lower limb
C83.16 Mantle cell lymphoma, intrapelvic lymph nodes
C83.17 Mantle cell lymphoma, spleen
C83.18 Mantle cell lymphoma, lymph nodes of multiple sites
C83.19 Mantle cell lymphoma, extranodal and solid organ sites

[5] **C83.3 Diffuse large B-cell lymphoma**

Anaplastic diffuse large B-cell lymphoma
CD30-positive diffuse large B-cell lymphoma
Centroblastic diffuse large B-cell lymphoma
Diffuse large B-cell lymphoma, subtype not specified
Immunoblastic diffuse large B-cell lymphoma
Plasmablastic diffuse large B-cell lymphoma
Diffuse large B-cell lymphoma, subtype not specified
T-cell rich diffuse large B-cell lymphoma

[EXCLUDES1] *mediastinal (thymic) large B-cell lymphoma (C85.2-)*
mature T/NK-cell lymphomas (C84.-)

C83.30 Diffuse large B-cell lymphoma, unspecified site
C83.31 Diffuse large B-cell lymphoma, lymph nodes of head, face, and neck
C83.32 Diffuse large B-cell lymphoma, intrathoracic lymph nodes
C83.33 Diffuse large B-cell lymphoma, intra-abdominal lymph nodes
C83.34 Diffuse large B-cell lymphoma, lymph nodes of axilla and upper limb
C83.35 Diffuse large B-cell lymphoma, lymph nodes of inguinal region and lower limb
C83.36 Diffuse large B-cell lymphoma, intrapelvic lymph nodes
C83.37 Diffuse large B-cell lymphoma, spleen
C83.38 Diffuse large B-cell lymphoma, lymph nodes of multiple sites
C83.39 Diffuse large B-cell lymphoma, extranodal and solid organ sites

[5] **C83.5 Lymphoblastic (diffuse) lymphoma**

B-precursor lymphoma
Lymphoblastic B-cell lymphoma
Lymphoblastic lymphoma NOS
Lymphoblastic T-cell lymphoma
T-precursor lymphoma

C83.50 Lymphoblastic (diffuse) lymphoma, unspecified site
C83.51 Lymphoblastic (diffuse) lymphoma, lymph nodes of head, face, and neck
C83.52 Lymphoblastic (diffuse) lymphoma, intrathoracic lymph nodes
C83.53 Lymphoblastic (diffuse) lymphoma, intra-abdominal lymph nodes
C83.54 Lymphoblastic (diffuse) lymphoma, lymph nodes of axilla and upper limb
C83.55 Lymphoblastic (diffuse) lymphoma, lymph nodes of inguinal region and lower limb
C83.56 Lymphoblastic (diffuse) lymphoma, intrapelvic lymph nodes
C83.57 Lymphoblastic (diffuse) lymphoma, spleen
C83.58 Lymphoblastic (diffuse) lymphoma, lymph nodes of multiple sites
C83.59 Lymphoblastic (diffuse) lymphoma, extranodal and solid organ sites

[5] **C83.7 Burkitt lymphoma**

Atypical Burkitt lymphoma
Burkitt-like lymphoma

[EXCLUDES1] *mature B-cell leukemia Burkitt type (C91.A-)*

C83.70 Burkitt lymphoma, unspecified site
C83.71 Burkitt lymphoma, lymph nodes of head, face, and neck
C83.72 Burkitt lymphoma, intrathoracic lymph nodes
C83.73 Burkitt lymphoma, intra-abdominal lymph nodes
C83.74 Burkitt lymphoma, lymph nodes of axilla and upper limb
C83.75 Burkitt lymphoma, lymph nodes of inguinal region and lower limb
C83.76 Burkitt lymphoma, intrapelvic lymph nodes
C83.77 Burkitt lymphoma, spleen
C83.78 Burkitt lymphoma, lymph nodes of multiple sites
C83.79 Burkitt lymphoma, extranodal and solid organ sites

[5] **C83.8 Other non-follicular lymphoma**

Intravascular large B-cell lymphoma
Lymphoid granulomatosis
Primary effusion B-cell lymphoma

[EXCLUDES1] *mediastinal (thymic) large B-cell lymphoma (C85.2-)*
T-cell rich B-cell lymphoma (C83.3-)

C83.80 Other non-follicular lymphoma, unspecified site
C83.81 Other non-follicular lymphoma, lymph nodes of head, face, and neck
C83.82 Other non-follicular lymphoma, intrathoracic lymph nodes
C83.83 Other non-follicular lymphoma, intra-abdominal lymph nodes
C83.84 Other non-follicular lymphoma, lymph nodes of axilla and upper limb
C83.85 Other non-follicular lymphoma, lymph nodes of inguinal region and lower limb
C83.86 Other non-follicular lymphoma, intrapelvic lymph nodes
C83.87 Other non-follicular lymphoma, spleen
C83.88 Other non-follicular lymphoma, lymph nodes of multiple sites
C83.89 Other non-follicular lymphoma, extranodal and solid organ sites

[5] **C83.9 Non-follicular (diffuse) lymphoma, unspecified**

C83.90 Non-follicular (diffuse) lymphoma, unspecified, unspecified site
C83.91 Non-follicular (diffuse) lymphoma, unspecified, lymph nodes of head, face, and neck
C83.92 Non-follicular (diffuse) lymphoma, unspecified, intrathoracic lymph nodes
C83.93 Non-follicular (diffuse) lymphoma, unspecified, intra-abdominal lymph nodes
C83.94 Non-follicular (diffuse) lymphoma, unspecified, lymph nodes of axilla and upper limb
C83.95 Non-follicular (diffuse) lymphoma, unspecified, lymph nodes of inguinal region and lower limb
C83.96 Non-follicular (diffuse) lymphoma, unspecified, intrapelvic lymph nodes
C83.97 Non-follicular (diffuse) lymphoma, unspecified, spleen
C83.98 Non-follicular (diffuse) lymphoma, unspecified, lymph nodes of multiple sites
C83.99 Non-follicular (diffuse) lymphoma, unspecified, extranodal and solid organ sites

[4] 4th character required [5] 5th character required [6] 6th character required [7] 7th character required [X] Extension 'X' Alert
[EXCLUDES1] Not coded here [EXCLUDES2] Not included here [PDx] Primary Diagnosis Only Manifestation Code

[4] C84 Mature T/NK-cell lymphomas
[EXCLUDES1] *personal history of non-Hodgkin lymphoma (Z85.72)*

[5] C84.0 Mycosis fungoides
[EXCLUDES1] *peripheral T-cell lymphoma, not classified (C84.4-)*

C84.00 Mycosis fungoides, unspecified site
C84.01 Mycosis fungoides, lymph nodes of head, face, and neck
C84.02 Mycosis fungoides, intrathoracic lymph nodes
C84.03 Mycosis fungoides, intra-abdominal lymph nodes
C84.04 Mycosis fungoides, lymph nodes of axilla and upper limb
C84.05 Mycosis fungoides, lymph nodes of inguinal region and lower limb
C84.06 Mycosis fungoides, intrapelvic lymph nodes
C84.07 Mycosis fungoides, spleen
C84.08 Mycosis fungoides, lymph nodes of multiple sites
C84.09 Mycosis fungoides, extranodal and solid organ sites

[5] C84.1 Sézary disease
C84.10 Sézary disease, unspecified site
C84.11 Sézary disease, lymph nodes of head, face, and neck
C84.12 Sézary disease, intrathoracic lymph nodes
C84.13 Sézary disease, intra-abdominal lymph nodes
C84.14 Sézary disease, lymph nodes of axilla and upper limb
C84.15 Sézary disease, lymph nodes of inguinal region and lower limb
C84.16 Sézary disease, intrapelvic lymph nodes
C84.17 Sézary disease, spleen
C84.18 Sézary disease, lymph nodes of multiple sites
C84.19 Sézary disease, extranodal and solid organ sites

[5] C84.4 Peripheral T-cell lymphoma, not classified
Lennert's lymphoma
Lymphoepithelioid lymphoma
Mature T-cell lymphoma, not elsewhere classified

C84.40 Peripheral T-cell lymphoma, not classified, unspecified site
C84.41 Peripheral T-cell lymphoma, not classified, lymph nodes of head, face, and neck
C84.42 Peripheral T-cell lymphoma, not classified, intrathoracic lymph nodes
C84.43 Peripheral T-cell lymphoma, not classified, intra-abdominal lymph nodes
C84.44 Peripheral T-cell lymphoma, not classified, lymph nodes of axilla and upper limb
C84.45 Peripheral T-cell lymphoma, not classified, lymph nodes of inguinal region and lower limb
C84.46 Peripheral T-cell lymphoma, not classified, intrapelvic lymph nodes
C84.47 Peripheral T-cell lymphoma, not classified, spleen
C84.48 Peripheral T-cell lymphoma, not classified, lymph nodes of multiple sites
C84.49 Peripheral T-cell lymphoma, not classified, extranodal and solid organ sites

[5] C84.6 Anaplastic large cell lymphoma, ALK-positive
Anaplastic large cell lymphoma, CD30-positive

C84.60 Anaplastic large cell lymphoma, ALK-positive, unspecified site
C84.61 Anaplastic large cell lymphoma, ALK-positive, lymph nodes of head, face, and neck
C84.62 Anaplastic large cell lymphoma, ALK-positive, intrathoracic lymph nodes
C84.63 Anaplastic large cell lymphoma, ALK-positive, intra-abdominal lymph nodes
C84.64 Anaplastic large cell lymphoma, ALK-positive, lymph nodes of axilla and upper limb
C84.65 Anaplastic large cell lymphoma, ALK-positive, lymph nodes of inguinal region and lower limb
C84.66 Anaplastic large cell lymphoma, ALK-positive, intrapelvic lymph nodes
C84.67 Anaplastic large cell lymphoma, ALK-positive, spleen
C84.68 Anaplastic large cell lymphoma, ALK-positive, lymph nodes of multiple sites
C84.69 Anaplastic large cell lymphoma, ALK-positive, extranodal and solid organ sites

[5] C84.7 Anaplastic large cell lymphoma, ALK-negative
[EXCLUDES1] *primary cutaneous CD30-positive T-cell proliferations (C86.6-)*

C84.70 Anaplastic large cell lymphoma, ALK-negative, unspecified site
C84.71 Anaplastic large cell lymphoma, ALK-negative, lymph nodes of head, face, and neck
C84.72 Anaplastic large cell lymphoma, ALK-negative, intrathoracic lymph nodes
C84.73 Anaplastic large cell lymphoma, ALK-negative, intra-abdominal lymph nodes
C84.74 Anaplastic large cell lymphoma, ALK-negative, lymph nodes of axilla and upper limb
C84.75 Anaplastic large cell lymphoma, ALK-negative, lymph nodes of inguinal region and lower limb
C84.76 Anaplastic large cell lymphoma, ALK-negative, intrapelvic lymph nodes
C84.77 Anaplastic large cell lymphoma, ALK-negative, spleen
C84.78 Anaplastic large cell lymphoma, ALK-negative, lymph nodes of multiple sites
C84.79 Anaplastic large cell lymphoma, ALK-negative, extranodal and solid organ sites

[5] C84.A Cutaneous T-cell lymphoma, unspecified
C84.A0 Cutaneous T-cell lymphoma, unspecified, unspecified site
C84.A1 Cutaneous T-cell lymphoma, unspecified lymph nodes of head, face, and neck
C84.A2 Cutaneous T-cell lymphoma, unspecified, intrathoracic lymph nodes
C84.A3 Cutaneous T-cell lymphoma, unspecified, intra-abdominal lymph nodes
C84.A4 Cutaneous T-cell lymphoma, unspecified, lymph nodes of axilla and upper limb
C84.A5 Cutaneous T-cell lymphoma, unspecified, lymph nodes of inguinal region and lower limb
C84.A6 Cutaneous T-cell lymphoma, unspecified, intrapelvic lymph nodes
C84.A7 Cutaneous T-cell lymphoma, unspecified, spleen
C84.A8 Cutaneous T-cell lymphoma, unspecified, lymph nodes of multiple sites
C84.A9 Cutaneous T-cell lymphoma, unspecified, extranodal and solid organ sites

[5] C84.Z Other mature T/NK-cell lymphomas
[NOTES] If T-cell lineage or involvement is mentioned in conjunction with a specific lymphoma, code to the more specific description.
[EXCLUDES1] *angioimmunoblastic T-cell lymphoma (C86.5)*
blastic NK-cell lymphoma (C86.4)
enteropathy-type T-cell lymphoma (C86.2)
extranodal NK-cell lymphoma, nasal type (C86.0)
hepatosplenic T-cell lymphoma (C86.1)
primary cutaneous CD30-positive T-cell proliferations (C86.6)
subcutaneous panniculitis-like T-cell lymphoma (C86.3)
T-cell leukemia (C91.1-)

C84.Z0 Other mature T/NK-cell lymphomas, unspecified site

Unspecified Code | Other Specified Code | [N] Newborn Age: 0 | [P] Pediatric Age: 0-17 | [M] Maternity Age: 12-55
[A] Adult Age: 15-124 | ♂ Male | ♀ Female | ● New Code | ▲ Revised Code Title | ►◄ Revised Text

C84.Z1 Other mature T/NK-cell lymphomas, lymph nodes of head, face, and neck
C84.Z2 Other mature T/NK-cell lymphomas, intrathoracic lymph nodes
C84.Z3 Other mature T/NK-cell lymphomas, intra-abdominal lymph nodes
C84.Z4 Other mature T/NK-cell lymphomas, lymph nodes of axilla and upper limb
C84.Z5 Other mature T/NK-cell lymphomas, lymph nodes of inguinal region and lower limb
C84.Z6 Other mature T/NK-cell lymphomas, intrapelvic lymph nodes
C84.Z7 Other mature T/NK-cell lymphomas, spleen
C84.Z8 Other mature T/NK-cell lymphomas, lymph nodes of multiple sites
C84.Z9 Other mature T/NK-cell lymphomas, extranodal and solid organ sites

[5] **C84.9 Mature T/NK-cell lymphomas, unspecified**
NK/T cell lymphoma NOS
[EXCLUDES1] *mature T-cell lymphoma, not elsewhere classified (C84.4-)*
C84.90 Mature T/NK-cell lymphomas, unspecified, unspecified site
C84.91 Mature T/NK-cell lymphomas, unspecified, lymph nodes of head, face, and neck
C84.92 Mature T/NK-cell lymphomas, unspecified, intrathoracic lymph nodes
C84.93 Mature T/NK-cell lymphomas, unspecified, intra-abdominal lymph nodes
C84.94 Mature T/NK-cell lymphomas, unspecified, lymph nodes of axilla and upper limb
C84.95 Mature T/NK-cell lymphomas, unspecified, lymph nodes of inguinal region and lower limb
C84.96 Mature T/NK-cell lymphomas, unspecified, intrapelvic lymph nodes
C84.97 Mature T/NK-cell lymphomas, unspecified, spleen
C84.98 Mature T/NK-cell lymphomas, unspecified, lymph nodes of multiple sites
C84.99 Mature T/NK-cell lymphomas, unspecified, extranodal and solid organ sites

[4] **C85 Other specified and unspecified types of non-Hodgkin lymphoma**
[EXCLUDES1] *other specified types of T/NK-cell lymphoma (C86.-)*
personal history of non-Hodgkin lymphoma (Z85.72)

[5] **C85.1 Unspecified B-cell lymphoma**
[NOTES] If B-cell lineage or involvement is mentioned in conjunction with a specific lymphoma, code to the more specific description.
C85.10 Unspecified B-cell lymphoma, unspecified site
C85.11 Unspecified B-cell lymphoma, lymph nodes of head, face, and neck
C85.12 Unspecified B-cell lymphoma, intrathoracic lymph nodes
C85.13 Unspecified B-cell lymphoma, intra-abdominal lymph nodes
C85.14 Unspecified B-cell lymphoma, lymph nodes of axilla and upper limb
C85.15 Unspecified B-cell lymphoma, lymph nodes of inguinal region and lower limb
C85.16 Unspecified B-cell lymphoma, intrapelvic lymph nodes
C85.17 Unspecified B-cell lymphoma, spleen
C85.18 Unspecified B-cell lymphoma, lymph nodes of multiple sites
C85.19 Unspecified B-cell lymphoma, extranodal and solid organ sites

[5] **C85.2 Mediastinal (thymic) large B-cell lymphoma**
C85.20 Mediastinal (thymic) large B-cell lymphoma, unspecified site
C85.21 Mediastinal (thymic) large B-cell lymphoma, lymph nodes of head, face, and neck
C85.22 Mediastinal (thymic) large B-cell lymphoma, intrathoracic lymph nodes
C85.23 Mediastinal (thymic) large B-cell lymphoma, intra-abdominal lymph nodes
C85.24 Mediastinal (thymic) large B-cell lymphoma, lymph nodes of axilla and upper limb
C85.25 Mediastinal (thymic) large B-cell lymphoma, lymph nodes of inguinal region and lower limb
C85.26 Mediastinal (thymic) large B-cell lymphoma, intrapelvic lymph nodes
C85.27 Mediastinal (thymic) large B-cell lymphoma, spleen
C85.28 Mediastinal (thymic) large B-cell lymphoma, lymph nodes of multiple sites
C85.29 Mediastinal (thymic) large B-cell lymphoma, extranodal and solid organ sites

[5] **C85.8 Other specified types of non-Hodgkin lymphoma**
C85.80 Other specified types of non-Hodgkin lymphoma, unspecified site
C85.81 Other specified types of non-Hodgkin lymphoma, lymph nodes of head, face, and neck
C85.82 Other specified types of non-Hodgkin lymphoma, intrathoracic lymph nodes
C85.83 Other specified types of non-Hodgkin lymphoma, intra-abdominal lymph nodes
C85.84 Other specified types of non-Hodgkin lymphoma, lymph nodes of axilla and upper limb
C85.85 Other specified types of non-Hodgkin lymphoma, lymph nodes of inguinal region and lower limb
C85.86 Other specified types of non-Hodgkin lymphoma, intrapelvic lymph nodes
C85.87 Other specified types of non-Hodgkin lymphoma, spleen
C85.88 Other specified types of non-Hodgkin lymphoma, lymph nodes of multiple sites
C85.89 Other specified types of non-Hodgkin lymphoma, extranodal and solid organ sites

[5] **C85.9 Non-Hodgkin lymphoma, unspecified**
Lymphoma NOS
Malignant lymphoma NOS
Non-Hodgkin lymphoma NOS
C85.90 Non-Hodgkin lymphoma, unspecified, unspecified site
C85.91 Non-Hodgkin lymphoma, unspecified, lymph nodes of head, face, and neck
C85.92 Non-Hodgkin lymphoma, unspecified, intrathoracic lymph nodes
C85.93 Non-Hodgkin lymphoma, unspecified, intra-abdominal lymph nodes
C85.94 Non-Hodgkin lymphoma, unspecified, lymph nodes of axilla and upper limb
C85.95 Non-Hodgkin lymphoma, unspecified, lymph nodes of inguinal region and lower limb
C85.96 Non-Hodgkin lymphoma, unspecified, intrapelvic lymph nodes
C85.97 Non-Hodgkin lymphoma, unspecified, spleen
C85.98 Non-Hodgkin lymphoma, unspecified, lymph nodes of multiple sites
C85.99 Non-Hodgkin lymphoma, unspecified, extranodal and solid organ sites

[4] **C86 Other specified types of T/NK-cell lymphoma**

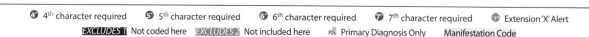

[4] 4th character required [5] 5th character required [6] 6th character required [7] 7th character required [x] Extension 'X' Alert
[EXCLUDES1] Not coded here [EXCLUDES2] Not included here [PDx] Primary Diagnosis Only Manifestation Code

[EXCLUDES1] *anaplastic large cell lymphoma, ALK negative (C84.7-)*
anaplastic large cell lymphoma, ALK positive (C84.6-)
mature T/NK-cell lymphomas (C84.-)
other specified types of non-Hodgkin lymphoma (C85.8-)

C86.0 Extranodal NK/T-cell lymphoma, nasal type

C86.1 Hepatosplenic T-cell lymphoma
Alpha-beta and gamma delta types

C86.2 Enteropathy-type (intestinal) T-cell lymphoma
Enteropathy associated T-cell lymphoma

C86.3 Subcutaneous panniculitis-like T-cell lymphoma

C86.4 Blastic NK-cell lymphoma

C86.5 Angioimmunoblastic T-cell lymphoma
Angioimmunoblastic lymphadenopathy with dysproteinemia (AILD)

C86.6 Primary cutaneous CD30-positive T-cell proliferations
Lymphomatoid papulosis
Primary cutaneous anaplastic large cell lymphoma
Primary cutaneous CD30-positive large T-cell lymphoma

[4] **C88 Malignant immunoproliferative diseases and certain other B-cell lymphomas**
[EXCLUDES1] *B-cell lymphoma, unspecified (C85.1-)*
personal history of other malignant neoplasms of lymphoid, hematopoietic and related tissues (Z85.79)

C88.0 Waldenström macroglobulinemia
Lymphoplasmacytic lymphoma with IgM-production
Macroglobulinemia (idiopathic) (primary)
[EXCLUDES1] *small cell B-cell lymphoma (C83.0)*

C88.2 Heavy chain disease
Franklin disease
Gamma heavy chain disease
Mu heavy chain disease

C88.3 Immunoproliferative small intestinal disease
Alpha heavy chain disease
Mediterranean lymphoma

C88.4 Extranodal marginal zone B-cell lymphoma of mucosa-associated lymphoid tissue [MALT-lymphoma]
Lymphoma of skin-associated lymphoid tissue [SALT-lymphoma]
Lymphoma of bronchial-associated lymphoid tissue [BALT-lymphoma]
[EXCLUDES1] *high malignant (diffuse large B-cell) lymphoma (C83.3-)*

C88.8 Other malignant immunoproliferative diseases

C88.9 Malignant immunoproliferative disease, unspecified
Immunoproliferative disease NOS

[4] **C90 Multiple myeloma and malignant plasma cell neoplasms**
[EXCLUDES1] *personal history of other malignant neoplasms of lymphoid, hematopoietic and related tissues (Z85.79)*

[5] **C90.0 Multiple myeloma**
Kahler's disease
Medullary plasmacytoma
Myelomatosis
Plasma cell myeloma
[EXCLUDES1] *solitary myeloma (C90.3-)*
solitary plasmactyoma (C90.3-)

C90.00 Multiple myeloma not having achieved remission
Multiple myeloma with failed remission
Multiple myeloma NOS

C90.01 Multiple myeloma in remission

C90.02 Multiple myeloma in relapse

[5] **C90.1 Plasma cell leukemia**
Plasmacytic leukemia

C90.10 Plasma cell leukemia not having achieved remission
Plasma cell leukemia with failed remission
Plasma cell leukemia NOS

C90.11 Plasma cell leukemia in remission

C90.12 Plasma cell leukemia in relapse

[5] **C90.2 Extramedullary plasmacytoma**

C90.20 Extramedullary plasmacytoma not having achieved remission
Extramedullary plasmacytoma with failed remission
Extramedullary plasmacytoma NOS

C90.21 Extramedullary plasmacytoma in remission

C90.22 Extramedullary plasmacytoma in relapse

[5] **C90.3 Solitary plasmacytoma**
Localized malignant plasma cell tumor NOS
Plasmacytoma NOS
Solitary myeloma

C90.30 Solitary plasmacytoma not having achieved remission
Solitary plasmacytoma with failed remission
Solitary plasmacytoma NOS

C90.31 Solitary plasmacytoma in remission

C90.32 Solitary plasmacytoma in relapse

[4] **C91 Lymphoid leukemia**
[EXCLUDES1] *personal history of leukemia (Z85.6)*

[5] **C91.0 Acute lymphoblastic leukemia [ALL]**
[NOTES] Code C91.0 should only be used for T-cell and B-cell precursor leukemia

C91.00 Acute lymphoblastic leukemia not having achieved remission
Acute lymphoblastic leukemia with failed remission
Acute lymphoblastic leukemia NOS

C91.01 Acute lymphoblastic leukemia, in remission

C91.02 Acute lymphoblastic leukemia, in relapse

[5] **C91.1 Chronic lymphocytic leukemia of B-cell type**
Lymphoplasmacytic leukemia
Richter syndrome
[EXCLUDES1] *lymphoplasmacytic lymphoma (C83.0-)*

C91.10 Chronic lymphocytic leukemia of B-cell type not having achieved remission
Chronic lymphocytic leukemia of B-cell type with failed remission
Chronic lymphocytic leukemia of B-cell type NOS

C91.11 Chronic lymphocytic leukemia of B-cell type in remission

C91.12 Chronic lymphocytic leukemia of B-cell type in relapse

[5] **C91.3 Prolymphocytic leukemia of B-cell type**

C91.30 Prolymphocytic leukemia of B-cell type not having achieved remission
Prolymphocytic leukemia of B-cell type with failed remission
Prolymphocytic leukemia of B-cell type NOS

C91.31 Prolymphocytic leukemia of B-cell type, in remission

C91.32 Prolymphocytic leukemia of B-cell type, in relapse

[5] **C91.4 Hairy cell leukemia**
Leukemic reticuloendotheliosis

C91.40 Hairy cell leukemia not having achieved remission
Hairy cell leukemia with failed remission
Hairy cell leukemia NOS

C91.41 Hairy cell leukemia, in remission

C91.42 Hairy cell leukemia, in relapse

Unspecified Code | Other Specified Code | [N] Newborn Age: 0 | [P] Pediatric Age: 0-17 | [M] Maternity Age: 12-55
[A] Adult Age: 15-124 | ♂ Male | ♀ Female | ● New Code | ▲ Revised Code Title | ►◄ Revised Text

[5] **C91.5 Adult T-cell lymphoma/leukemia (HTLV-1-associated)**
Acute variant of adult T-cell lymphoma/leukemia (HTLV-1-associated)
Chronic variant of adult T-cell lymphoma/leukemia (HTLV-1-associated)
Lymphomatoid variant of adult T-cell lymphoma/leukemia (HTLV-1-associated)
Smouldering variant of adult T-cell lymphoma/leukemia (HTLV-1-associated)
C91.50 Adult T-cell lymphoma/leukemia (HTLV-1-associated) not having achieved remission
Adult T-cell lymphoma/leukemia (HTLV-1-associated) with failed remission
Adult T-cell lymphoma/leukemia (HTLV-1-associated) NOS [A]
C91.51 Adult T-cell lymphoma/leukemia (HTLV-1-associated), in remission [A]
C91.52 Adult T-cell lymphoma/leukemia (HTLV-1-associated), in relapse [A]
[5] **C91.6 Prolymphocytic leukemia of T-cell type**
C91.60 Prolymphocytic leukemia of T-cell type not having achieved remission
Prolymphocytic leukemia of T-cell type with failed remission
Prolymphocytic leukemia of T-cell type NOS
C91.61 Prolymphocytic leukemia of T-cell type, in remission
C91.62 Prolymphocytic leukemia of T-cell type, in relapse
[5] **C91.A Mature B-cell leukemia Burkitt-type**
[EXCLUDES1] *Burkitt lymphoma (C83.7-)*
C91.A0 Mature B-cell leukemia Burkitt-type not having achieved remission
Mature B-cell leukemia Burkitt-type with failed remission
Mature B-cell leukemia Burkitt-type NOS
C91.A1 Mature B-cell leukemia Burkitt-type, in remission
C91.A2 Mature B-cell leukemia Burkitt-type, in relapse
[5] **C91.Z Other lymphoid leukemia**
T-cell large granular lymphocytic leukemia (associated with rheumatoid arthritis)
C91.Z0 Other lymphoid leukemia not having achieved remission
Other lymphoid leukemia with failed remission
Other lymphoid leukemia NOS
C91.Z1 Other lymphoid leukemia, in remission
C91.Z2 Other lymphoid leukemia, in relapse
[5] **C91.9 Lymphoid leukemia,** unspecified
C91.90 Lymphoid leukemia, unspecified not having achieved remission
Lymphoid leukemia with failed remission
Lymphoid leukemia NOS
C91.91 Lymphoid leukemia, unspecified, in remission
C91.92 Lymphoid leukemia, unspecified, in relapse

[4] **C92 Myeloid leukemia**
[INCLUDES] *granulocytic leukemia*
myelogenous leukemia
[EXCLUDES1] *personal history of leukemia (Z85.6)*
[5] **C92.0 Acute myeloblastic leukemia**
Acute myeloblastic leukemia, minimal differentiation
Acute myeloblastic leukemia (with maturation)
Acute myeloblastic leukemia 1/ETO
Acute myeloblastic leukemia M0
Acute myeloblastic leukemia M1
Acute myeloblastic leukemia M2
Acute myeloblastic leukemia with t(8;21)
Acute myeloblastic leukemia (without a FAB classification) NOS
Refractory anemia with excess blasts in transformation [RAEB T]
[EXCLUDES1] *acute exacerbation of chronic myeloid leukemia (C92.10)*
refractory anemia with excess of blasts not in transformation (D46.2-)
C92.00 Acute myeloblastic leukemia, not having achieved remission
Acute myeloblastic leukemia with failed remission
Acute myeloblastic leukemia NOS
C92.01 Acute myeloblastic leukemia, in remission
C92.02 Acute myeloblastic leukemia, in relapse
[5] **C92.1 Chronic myeloid leukemia, BCR/ABL-positive**
Chronic myelogenous leukemia, Philadelphia chromosome (Ph1) positive
Chronic myelogenous leukemia, t(9;22) (q34;q11)
Chronic myelogenous leukemia with crisis of blast cells
[EXCLUDES1] *atypical chronic myeloid leukemia BCR/ABL-negative (C92.2-)*
chronic myelomonocytic leukemia (C93.1-)
chronic myeloproliferative disease (D47.1)
C92.10 Chronic myeloid leukemia, BCR/ABL-positive, not having achieved remission
Chronic myeloid leukemia, BCR/ABL-positive with failed remission
Chronic myeloid leukemia, BCR/ABL-positive NOS
C92.11 Chronic myeloid leukemia, BCR/ABL-positive, in remission
C92.12 Chronic myeloid leukemia, BCR/ABL-positive, in relapse
[5] **C92.2 Atypical chronic myeloid leukemia, BCR/ABL-negative**
C92.20 Atypical chronic myeloid leukemia, BCR/ABL-negative, not having achieved remission
Atypical chronic myeloid leukemia, BCR/ABL-negative with failed remission
Atypical chronic myeloid leukemia, BCR/ABL-negative NOS
C92.21 Atypical chronic myeloid leukemia, BCR/ABL-negative, in remission
C92.22 Atypical chronic myeloid leukemia, BCR/ABL-negative, in relapse
[5] **C92.3 Myeloid sarcoma**
A malignant tumor of immature myeloid cells
Chloroma
Granulocytic sarcoma
C92.30 Myeloid sarcoma, not having achieved remission
Myeloid sarcoma with failed remission
Myeloid sarcoma NOS
C92.31 Myeloid sarcoma, in remission
C92.32 Myeloid sarcoma, in relapse
[5] **C92.4 Acute promyelocytic leukemia**
AML M3
AML Me with t(15;17) and variants
C92.40 Acute promyelocytic leukemia, not having achieved remission
Acute promyelocytic leukemia with failed remission
Acute promyelocytic leukemia NOS
C92.41 Acute promyelocytic leukemia, in remission
C92.42 Acute promyelocytic leukemia, in relapse
[5] **C92.5 Acute myelomonocytic leukemia**
AML M4
AML M4 Eo with inv(16) or t(16;16)
C92.50 Acute myelomonocytic leukemia, not having achieved remission
Acute myelomonocytic leukemia with failed remission
Acute myelomonocytic leukemia NOS

C92.51 **Acute myelomonocytic leukemia,** in remission
C92.52 **Acute myelomonocytic leukemia,** in relapse

[5] C92.6 Acute myeloid **leukemia with** 11q23-abnormality
Acute myeloid leukemia with variation of MLL-gene
C92.60 **Acute myeloid leukemia with 11q23-abnormality** not having achieved remission
Acute myeloid leukemia with 11q23-abnormality with failed remission
Acute myeloid leukemia with 11q23-abnormality NOS
C92.61 **Acute myeloid leukemia with 11q23-abnormality** in remission
C92.62 **Acute myeloid leukemia with 11q23-abnormality** in relapse

[5] C92.A Acute myeloid **leukemia with** multilineage dysplasia
Acute myeloid leukemia with dysplasia of remaining hematopoesis and/or myelodysplastic disease in its history
C92.A0 **Acute myeloid leukemia with multilineage dysplasia,** not having achieved remission
Acute myeloid leukemia with multilineage dysplasia with failed remission
Acute myeloid leukemia with multilineage dysplasia NOS
C92.A1 **Acute myeloid leukemia with multilineage dysplasia,** in remission
C92.A2 **Acute myeloid leukemia with multilineage dysplasia,** in relapse

[5] C92.Z Other **myeloid leukemia**
C92.Z0 **Other myeloid leukemia** not having achieved remission
Myeloid leukemia NEC with failed remission
Myeloid leukemia NEC
C92.Z1 **Other myeloid leukemia,** in remission
C92.Z2 **Other myeloid leukemia,** in relapse

[5] C92.9 **Myeloid leukemia,** unspecified
C92.90 **Myeloid leukemia, unspecified,** not having achieved remission
Myeloid leukemia, unspecified with failed remission
Myeloid leukemia, unspecified NOS
C92.91 **Myeloid leukemia, unspecified** in remission
C92.92 **Myeloid leukemia, unspecified** in relapse

[4] C93 **Monocytic leukemia**
INCLUDES *monocytoid leukemia*
EXCLUDES1 *personal history of leukemia (Z85.6)*

[5] C93.0 Acute **monoblastic/monocytic leukemia**
AML M5
AML M5a
AML M5b
C93.00 **Acute monoblastic/monocytic leukemia,** not having achieved remission
Acute monoblastic/monocytic leukemia with failed remission
Acute monoblastic/monocytic leukemia NOS
C93.01 **Acute monoblastic/monocytic leukemia,** in remission
C93.02 **Acute monoblastic/monocytic leukemia,** in relapse

[5] C93.1 Chronic **myelomonocytic leukemia**
Chronic monocytic leukemia
CMML-1
CMML-2
CMML with eosinophilia
C93.10 **Chronic myelomonocytic leukemia** not having achieved remission
Chronic myelomonocytic leukemia with failed remission
Chronic myelomonocytic leukemia NOS
C93.11 **Chronic myelomonocytic leukemia,** in remission
C93.12 **Chronic myelomonocytic leukemia,** in relapse

[5] C93.3 Juvenile **myelomonocytic leukemia**
C93.30 **Juvenile myelomonocytic leukemia,** not having achieved remission
Juvenile myelomonocytic leukemia with failed remission
Juvenile myelomonocytic leukemia NOS [P]
C93.31 **Juvenile myelomonocytic leukemia,** in remission [P]
C93.32 **Juvenile myelomonocytic leukemia,** in relapse [P]

[5] C93.Z Other **monocytic leukemia**
C93.Z0 **Other monocytic leukemia,** not having achieved remission
Other monocytic leukemia NOS
C93.Z1 **Other monocytic leukemia,** in remission
C93.Z2 **Other monocytic leukemia,** in relapse

[5] C93.9 **Monocytic leukemia,** unspecified
C93.90 **Monocytic leukemia, unspecified,** not having achieved remission
Monocytic leukemia, unspecified with failed remission
Monocytic leukemia, unspecified NOS
C93.91 **Monocytic leukemia, unspecified** in remission
C93.92 **Monocytic leukemia, unspecified** in relapse

[4] C94 Other **leukemias of** specified cell type
EXCLUDES1 *leukemic reticuloendotheliosis (C91.4-)*
myelodysplastic syndromes (D46.-)
personal history of leukemia (Z85.6)
plasma cell leukemia (C90.1-)

[5] C94.0 Acute erythroid **leukemia**
Acute myeloid leukemia M6(a)(b)
Erythroleukemia
C94.00 **Acute erythroid leukemia,** not having achieved remission
Acute erythroid leukemia with failed remission
Acute erythroid leukemia NOS
C94.01 **Acute erythroid leukemia,** in remission
C94.02 **Acute erythroid leukemia,** in relapse

[5] C94.2 Acute megakaryoblastic **leukemia**
Acute myeloid leukemia M7
Acute megakaryocytic leukemia
C94.20 **Acute megakaryoblastic leukemia** not having achieved remission
Acute megakaryoblastic leukemia with failied remission
Acute megakaryoblastic leukemia NOS
C94.21 **Acute megakaryoblastic leukemia,** in remission
C94.22 **Acute megakaryoblastic leukemia,** in relapse

[5] C94.3 Mast cell **leukemia**
C94.30 **Mast cell leukemia** not having achieved remission
Mast cell leukemia with failed remission
Mast cell leukemia NOS
C94.31 **Mast cell leukemia,** in remission
C94.32 **Mast cell leukemia,** in relapse

[5] C94.4 Acute panmyelosis **with** myelofibrosis
Acute myelofibrosis
EXCLUDES1 *myelofibrosis NOS (D75.81)*
secondary myelofibrosis NOS (D75.81)
C94.40 **Acute panmyelosis with myelofibrosis** not having achieved remission
Acute myelofibrosis NOS
Acute panmyelosis with myelofibrosis with failed remission
Acute panmyelosis NOS
C94.41 **Acute panmyelosis with myelofibrosis,** in remission
C94.42 **Acute panmyelosis with myelofibrosis,** in relapse

C94.6 **Myelodysplastic disease, not classified**
Myeloproliferative disease, not classified

⑤ **C94.8 Other specified leukemias**

Aggressive NK-cell leukemia

Acute basophilic leukemia

C94.80 Other specified leukemias not having achieved remission

Other specified leukemia with failed remission

Other specified leukemias NOS

C94.81 Other specified leukemias, in remission

C94.82 Other specified leukemias, in relapse

④ **C95 Leukemia of** unspecified cell type

EXCLUDES1 *personal history of leukemia (Z85.6)*

⑤ **C95.0 Acute leukemia of** unspecified cell type

Acute bilineal leukemia

Acute mixed lineage leukemia

Biphenotypic acute leukemia

Stem cell leukemia of unclear lineage

EXCLUDES1 *acute exacerbation of unspecified chronic leukemia (C95.10)*

C95.00 Acute leukemia of unspecified cell type not having achieved remission

Acute leukemia of unspecified cell type with failed remission

Acute leukemia NOS

C95.01 Acute leukemia of unspecified cell type, in remission

C95.02 Acute leukemia of unspecified cell type, in relapse

⑤ **C95.1 Chronic leukemia of** unspecified cell type

C95.10 Chronic leukemia of unspecified cell type not having achieved remission

Chronic leukemia of unspecified cell type with failed remission

Chronic leukemia NOS

C95.11 Chronic leukemia of unspecified cell type, in remission

C95.12 Chronic leukemia of unspecified cell type, in relapse

⑤ **C95.9 Leukemia,** unspecified

C95.90 Leukemia, unspecified not having achieved remission

Leukemia, unspecified with failed remission

Leukemia NOS

C95.91 Leukemia, unspecified, in remission

C95.92 Leukemia, unspecified, in relapse

④ **C96 Other and unspecified malignant neoplasms of lymphoid, hematopoietic and related tissue**

EXCLUDES1 *personal history of other malignant neoplasms of lymphoid, hematopoietic and related tissues (Z85.79)*

C96.0 Multifocal and multisystemic (disseminated) Langerhans-cell histiocytosis

Histiocytosis X, multisystemic

Letterer-Siwe disease

EXCLUDES1 *adult pulmonary Langerhans cell histiocytosis (J84.82)*
multifocal and unisystemic Langerhans-cell histiocytosis (C96.5)
unifocal Langerhans-cell histiocytosis (C96.6)

C96.2 Malignant mast cell tumor

Aggressive systemic mastocytosis

Mast cell sarcoma

EXCLUDES1 *indolent mastocytosis (D47.0)*
mast cell leukemia (C94.30)
mastocytosis (congenital) (cutaneous) (Q82.2)

C96.4 Sarcoma of dendritic cells (accessory cells)

Follicular dendritic cell sarcoma

Interdigitating dendritic cell sarcoma

Langerhans cell sarcoma

C96.5 Multifocal and unisystemic Langerhans-cell histiocytosis

Hand-Schüller-Christian Disease

Histiocytosis X, multifocal

EXCLUDES1 *multifocal and multisystemic (disseminated) Langerhans-cell histiocytosis (C96.0)*
unifocal Langerhans-cell histiocytosis (C96.6)

C96.6 Unifocal Langerhans-cell histiocytosis

Eosinophilic granuloma

Histiocytosis X, unifocal

Histiocytosis X NOS

Langerhans-cell histiocytosis NOS

EXCLUDES1 *multifocal and multisysemic (disseminated) Langerhans-cell histiocytosis (C96.0)*
multifocal and unisystemic Langerhans-cell histiocytosis (C96.5)

C96.A Histiocytic sarcoma

Malignant histiocytosis

C96.Z Other specified malignant neoplasms of lymphoid, hematopoietic and related tissue

C96.9 Malignant neoplasm of lymphoid, hematopoietic and related tissue, unspecified

In situ neoplasms (D00-D09)

INCLUDES *Bowen's disease*
erythroplasia
grade III intraepithelial neoplasia
Queyrat's erythroplasia

④ **D00 Carcinoma in situ of** oral cavity, esophagus and stomach

EXCLUDES1 *melanoma in situ (D03.-)*

⑤ **D00.0 Carcinoma in situ of** lip, oral cavity and pharynx

Use additional code to identify:

exposure to environmental tobacco smoke (Z77.22)

exposure to tobacco smoke in the perinatal period (P96.81)

history of tobacco use (Z87.891)

occupational exposure to environmental tobacco smoke (Z57.31)

tobacco dependence (F17.-)

tobacco use (Z72.0)

EXCLUDES1 *carcinoma in situ of aryepiglottic fold or interarytenoid fold, laryngeal aspect (D02.0)*
carcinoma in situ of epiglottis NOS (D02.0)
carcinoma in situ of epiglottis suprahyoid portion (D02.0)
carcinoma in situ of skin of lip (D03.0, D04.0)

D00.00 Carcinoma in situ of oral cavity, unspecified site

D00.01 Carcinoma in situ of labial mucosa and vermilion border

D00.02 Carcinoma in situ of buccal mucosa

D00.03 Carcinoma in situ of gingiva and edentulous alveolar ridge

D00.04 Carcinoma in situ of soft palate

D00.05 Carcinoma in situ of hard palate

D00.06 Carcinoma in situ of floor of mouth

D00.07 Carcinoma in situ of tongue

D00.08 Carcinoma in situ of pharynx

Carcinoma in situ of aryepiglottic fold NOS

Carcinoma in situ of hypopharyngeal aspect of aryepiglottic fold

Carcinoma in situ of marginal zone of aryepiglottic fold

D00.1 Carcinoma in situ of esophagus

D00.2 Carcinoma in situ of stomach

---

❹ 4th character required ❺ 5th character required ❻ 6th character required ❼ 7th character required ⑩ Extension 'X' Alert

EXCLUDES 1 Not coded here *EXCLUDES 2* Not included here PDx Primary Diagnosis Only Manifestation Code

[4] D01 Carcinoma in situ of other and unspecified digestive organs
EXCLUDES1 *melanoma in situ (D03.-)*
D01.0 Carcinoma in situ of colon
EXCLUDES1 *carcinoma in situ of rectosigmoid junction (D01.1)*
D01.1 Carcinoma in situ of rectosigmoid junction
D01.2 Carcinoma in situ of rectum
D01.3 Carcinoma in situ of anus and anal canal
EXCLUDES1 *carcinoma in situ of anal margin (D04.5)*
carcinoma in situ of anal skin (D04.5)
carcinoma in situ of perianal skin (D04.5)
[5] D01.4 Carcinoma in situ of other and unspecified parts of intestine
EXCLUDES1 *carcinoma in situ of ampulla of Vater (D01.5)*
D01.40 Carcinoma in situ of unspecified part of intestine
D01.49 Carcinoma in situ of other parts of intestine
D01.5 Carcinoma in situ of liver, gallbladder and bile ducts
Carcinoma in situ of ampulla of Vater
D01.7 Carcinoma in situ of other specified digestive organs
Carcinoma in situ of pancreas
D01.9 Carcinoma in situ of digestive organ, unspecified
[4] D02 Carcinoma in situ of middle ear and respiratory system
Use additional code to identify:
exposure to environmental tobacco smoke (Z77.22)
exposure to tobacco smoke in the perinatal period (P96.81)
history of tobacco use (Z87.891)
occupational exposure to environmental tobacco smoke (Z57.31)
tobacco dependence (F17.-)
tobacco use (Z72.0)
EXCLUDES1 *melanoma in situ (D03.-)*
D02.0 Carcinoma in situ of larynx
Carcinoma in situ of aryepiglottic fold or interarytenoid fold, laryngeal aspect
Carcinoma in situ of epiglottis (suprahyoid portion)
EXCLUDES1 *carcinoma in situ of aryepiglottic fold or interarytenoid fold NOS (D00.08)*
carcinoma in situ of hypopharyngeal aspect (D00.08)
carcinoma in situ of marginal zone (D00.08)
D02.1 Carcinoma in situ of trachea
[5] D02.2 Carcinoma in situ of bronchus and lung
D02.20 Carcinoma in situ of unspecified bronchus and lung
D02.21 Carcinoma in situ of right bronchus and lung
D02.22 Carcinoma in situ of left bronchus and lung
D02.3 Carcinoma in situ of other parts of respiratory system
Carcinoma in situ of accessory sinuses
Carcinoma in situ of middle ear
Carcinoma in situ of nasal cavities
EXCLUDES1 *carcinoma in situ of ear (external) (skin) (D04.2-)*
carcinoma in situ of nose NOS D09.8
carcinoma in situ of skin of nose (D04.3)
D02.4 Carcinoma in situ of respiratory system, unspecified
[4] D03 Melanoma in situ
D03.0 Melanoma in situ of lip
[5] D03.1 Melanoma in situ of eyelid, including canthus
D03.10 Melanoma in situ of unspecified eyelid, including canthus
D03.11 Melanoma in situ of right eyelid, including canthus
D03.12 Melanoma in situ of left eyelid, including canthus
[5] D03.2 Melanoma in situ of ear and external auricular canal
D03.20 Melanoma in situ of unspecified ear and external auricular canal
D03.21 Melanoma in situ of right ear and external auricular canal
D03.22 Melanoma in situ of left ear and external auricular canal
[5] D03.3 Melanoma in situ of other and unspecified parts of face
D03.30 Melanoma in situ of unspecified part of face
D03.39 Melanoma in situ of other parts of face
D03.4 Melanoma in situ of scalp and neck
[5] D03.5 Melanoma in situ of trunk
D03.51 Melanoma in situ of anal skin
Melanoma in situ of anal margin
Melanoma in situ of perianal skin
D03.52 Melanoma in situ of breast (skin) (soft tissue)
D03.59 Melanoma in situ of other part of trunk
[5] D03.6 Melanoma in situ of upper limb, including shoulder
D03.60 Melanoma in situ of unspecified upper limb, including shoulder
D03.61 Melanoma in situ of right upper limb, including shoulder
D03.62 Melanoma in situ of left upper limb, including shoulder
[5] D03.7 Melanoma in situ of lower limb, including hip
D03.70 Melanoma in situ of unspecified lower limb, including hip
D03.71 Melanoma in situ of right lower limb, including hip
D03.72 Melanoma in situ of left lower limb, including hip
D03.8 Melanoma in situ of other sites
Melanoma in situ of scrotum
EXCLUDES1 *carcinoma in situ of scrotum (D07.61)*
D03.9 Melanoma in situ, unspecified
[4] D04 Carcinoma in situ of skin
EXCLUDES1 *erythroplasia of Queyrat (penis) NOS (D07.4)*
melanoma in situ (D03.-)
D04.0 Carcinoma in situ of skin of lip
EXCLUDES1 *carcinoma in situ of vermilion border of lip (D00.01)*
[5] D04.1 Carcinoma in situ of skin of eyelid, including canthus
D04.10 Carcinoma in situ of skin of unspecified eyelid, including canthus
D04.11 Carcinoma in situ of skin of right eyelid, including canthus
D04.12 Carcinoma in situ of skin of left eyelid, including canthus
[5] D04.2 Carcinoma in situ of skin of ear and external auricular canal
D04.20 Carcinoma in situ of skin of unspecified ear and external auricular canal
D04.21 Carcinoma in situ of skin of right ear and external auricular canal
D04.22 Carcinoma in situ of skin of left ear and external auricular canal
[5] D04.3 Carcinoma in situ of skin of other and unspecified parts of face
D04.30 Carcinoma in situ of skin of unspecified part of face
D04.39 Carcinoma in situ of skin of other parts of face
D04.4 Carcinoma in situ of skin of scalp and neck
D04.5 Carcinoma in situ of skin of trunk
Carcinoma in situ of anal margin
Carcinoma in situ of anal skin
Carcinoma in situ of perianal skin
Carcinoma in situ of skin of breast
EXCLUDES1 *carcinoma in situ of anus NOS (D01.3)*
carcinoma in situ of scrotum (D07.61)
carcinoma in situ of skin of genital organs (D07.-)

Unspecified Code | Other Specified Code | [N] Newborn Age: 0 | [P] Pediatric Age: 0-17 | [M] Maternity Age: 12-55
[A] Adult Age: 15-124 | ♂ Male | ♀ Female | ● New Code | ▲ Revised Code Title | ►◄ Revised Text

[5] D04.6 Carcinoma in situ of skin of upper limb, including shoulder
D04.60 Carcinoma in situ of skin of unspecified upper limb, including shoulder
D04.61 Carcinoma in situ of skin of right upper limb, including shoulder
D04.62 Carcinoma in situ of skin of left upper limb, including shoulder
[5] D04.7 Carcinoma in situ of skin of lower limb, including hip
D04.70 Carcinoma in situ of skin of unspecified lower limb, including hip
D04.71 Carcinoma in situ of skin of right lower limb, including hip
D04.72 Carcinoma in situ of skin of left lower limb, including hip
D04.8 Carcinoma in situ of skin of other sites
D04.9 Carcinoma in situ of skin, unspecified
[4] D05 Carcinoma in situ of breast
[EXCLUDES1] *carcinoma in situ of skin of breast (D04.5)*
melanoma in situ of breast (skin) (D03.5)
Paget's disease of breast or nipple (C50.-)
[5] D05.0 Lobular carcinoma in situ of breast
D05.00 Lobular carcinoma in situ of unspecified breast
D05.01 Lobular carcinoma in situ of right breast
D05.02 Lobular carcinoma in situ of left breast
[5] D05.1 Intraductal carcinoma in situ of breast
D05.10 Intraductal carcinoma in situ of unspecified breast
D05.11 Intraductal carcinoma in situ of right breast
D05.12 Intraductal carcinoma in situ of left breast
[5] D05.8 Other specified type of carcinoma in situ of breast
D05.80 Other specified type of carcinoma in situ of unspecified breast
D05.81 Other specified type of carcinoma in situ of right breast
D05.82 Other specified type of carcinoma in situ of left breast
[5] D05.9 Unspecified type of carcinoma in situ of breast
D05.90 Unspecified type of carcinoma in situ of unspecified breast
D05.91 Unspecified type of carcinoma in situ of right breast
D05.92 Unspecified type of carcinoma in situ of left breast
[4] D06 Carcinoma in situ of cervix uteri
INCLUDES *cervical adenocarcinoma in situ*
cervical intraepithelial glandular neoplasia
cervical intraepithelial neoplasia III [CIN III]
severe dysplasia of cervix uteri
[EXCLUDES1] *cervical intraepithelial neoplasia II [CIN II] (N87.1)*
cytologic evidence of malignancy of cervix without histologic confirmation (R87.614)
high grade squamous intraepithelial lesion (HGSIL) of cervix (R87.613)
melanoma in situ of cervix (D03.5)
moderate cervical dysplasia (N87.1)
D06.0 Carcinoma in situ of endocervix ♀
D06.1 Carcinoma in situ of exocervix ♀
D06.7 Carcinoma in situ of other parts of cervix ♀
D06.9 Carcinoma in situ of cervix, unspecified ♀

[4] D07 Carcinoma in situ of other and unspecified genital organs
[EXCLUDES1] *melanoma in situ of trunk (D03.5)*
D07.0 Carcinoma in situ of endometrium ♀
D07.1 Carcinoma in situ of vulva
Severe dysplasia of vulva
Vulvar intraepithelial neoplasia III [VIN III]
[EXCLUDES1] *moderate dysplasia of vulva (N90.1)*
vulvar intraepithelial neoplasia II [VIN II] (N90.1) ♀
D07.2 Carcinoma in situ of vagina
Severe dysplasia of vagina
Vaginal intraepithelial neoplasia III [VAIN III]
[EXCLUDES1] *moderate dysplasia of vagina (N89.1)*
vaginal intraepithelial neoplasia II [VIN II] (N89.1) ♀
[5] D07.3 Carcinoma in situ of other and unspecified female genital organs
D07.30 Carcinoma in situ of unspecified female genital organs ♀
D07.39 Carcinoma in situ of other female genital organs ♀
D07.4 Carcinoma in situ of penis
Erythroplasia of Queyrat NOS ♂
D07.5 Carcinoma in situ of prostate
Prostatic intraepithelial neoplasia III (PIN III)
Severe dysplasia of prostate
[EXCLUDES1] *dysplasia (mild) (moderate) of prostate (N42.3)* ♂
[5] D07.6 Carcinoma in situ of other and unspecified male genital organs
D07.60 Carcinoma in situ of unspecified male genital organs ♂
D07.61 Carcinoma in situ of scrotum ♂
D07.69 Carcinoma in situ of other male genital organs ♂
[4] D09 Carcinoma in situ of other and unspecified sites
[EXCLUDES1] *melanoma in situ (D03.-)*
D09.0 Carcinoma in situ of bladder
[5] D09.1 Carcinoma in situ of other and unspecified urinary organs
D09.10 Carcinoma in situ of unspecified urinary organ
D09.19 Carcinoma in situ of other urinary organs
[5] D09.2 Carcinoma in situ of eye
[EXCLUDES1] *carcinoma in situ of skin of eyelid (D04.1-)*
D09.20 Carcinoma in situ of unspecified eye
D09.21 Carcinoma in situ of right eye
D09.22 Carcinoma in situ of left eye
D09.3 Carcinoma in situ of thyroid and other endocrine glands
[EXCLUDES1] *carcinoma in situ of endocrine pancreas (D01.7)*
carcinoma in situ of ovary (D07.39)
carcinoma in situ of testis (D07.69)
D09.8 Carcinoma in situ of other specified sites
D09.9 Carcinoma in situ, unspecified

Benign neoplasms, except benign neuroendocrine tumors (D10-D36)

[4] D10 Benign neoplasm of mouth and pharynx
D10.0 Benign neoplasm of lip
Benign neoplasm of lip (frenulum) (inner aspect) (mucosa) (vermilion border)
[EXCLUDES1] *benign neoplasm of skin of lip (D22.0, D23.0)*
D10.1 Benign neoplasm of tongue
Benign neoplasm of lingual tonsil
D10.2 Benign neoplasm of floor of mouth
[5] D10.3 Other and unspecified parts of mouth
D10.30 Benign neoplasm of unspecified part of mouth
D10.39 Benign neoplasm of other parts of mouth

[4] 4th character required [5] 5th character required [6] 6th character required [7] 7th character required [7x] Extension 'X' Alert
[EXCLUDES 1] Not coded here [EXCLUDES 2] Not included here [PDx] Primary Diagnosis Only Manifestation Code

Benign neoplasm of minor salivary gland NOS
[EXCLUDES1] *benign odontogenic neoplasms (D16.4-D16.5)*
benign neoplasm of mucosa of lip (D10.0)
benign neoplasm of nasopharyngeal surface of soft palate (D10.6)

D10.4 Benign neoplasm of tonsil
Benign neoplasm of tonsil (faucial) (palatine)
[EXCLUDES1] *benign neoplasm of lingual tonsil (D10.1)*
benign neoplasm of pharyngeal tonsil (D10.6)
benign neoplasm of tonsillar fossa (D10.5)
benign neoplasm of tonsillar pillars (D10.5)

D10.5 Benign neoplasm of other parts of oropharynx
Benign neoplasm of epiglottis, anterior aspect
Benign neoplasm of tonsillar fossa
Benign neoplasm of tonsillar pillars
Benign neoplasm of vallecula
[EXCLUDES1] *benign neoplasm of epiglottis NOS (D14.1)*
benign neoplasm of epiglottis, suprahyoid portion (D14.1)

D10.6 Benign neoplasm of nasopharynx
Benign neoplasm of pharyngeal tonsil
Benign neoplasm of posterior margin of septum and choanae

D10.7 Benign neoplasm of hypopharynx

D10.9 Benign neoplasm of pharynx, unspecified

[4] **D11 Benign neoplasm of major salivary glands**
[EXCLUDES1] *benign neoplasms of specified minor salivary glands which are classified according to their anatomical location*
benign neoplasms of minor salivary glands NOS (D10.39)

D11.0 Benign neoplasm of parotid gland

D11.7 Benign neoplasm of other major salivary glands
Benign neoplasm of sublingual salivary gland
Benign neoplasm of submandibular salivary gland

D11.9 Benign neoplasm of major salivary gland, unspecified

[4] **D12 Benign neoplasm of colon, rectum, anus and anal canal**
[EXCLUDES1] *benign carcinoid tumors of the large intestine, and rectum (D3A.02-)*

D12.0 Benign neoplasm of cecum
Benign neoplasm of ileocecal valve

D12.1 Benign neoplasm of appendix
[EXCLUDES1] *benign carcinoid tumor of the appendix (D3A.020)*

D12.2 Benign neoplasm of ascending colon

D12.3 Benign neoplasm of transverse colon
Benign neoplasm of hepatic flexure
Benign neoplasm of splenic flexure

D12.4 Benign neoplasm of descending colon

D12.5 Benign neoplasm of sigmoid colon

D12.6 Benign neoplasm of colon, unspecified
Adenomatosis of colon
Benign neoplasm of large intestine NOS
Polyposis (hereditary) of colon
[EXCLUDES1] *inflammatory polyp of colon (K51.4-)*
polyp of colon NOS (K63.5)

D12.7 Benign neoplasm of rectosigmoid junction

D12.8 Benign neoplasm of rectum
[EXCLUDES1] *benign carcinoid tumor of the rectum (D3A.026)*

D12.9 Benign neoplasm of anus and anal canal
Benign neoplasm of anus NOS
[EXCLUDES1] *benign neoplasm of anal margin (D22.5, D23.5)*
benign neoplasm of anal skin (D22.5, D23.5)
benign neoplasm of perianal skin (D22.5, D23.5)

[4] **D13 Benign neoplasm of other and ill-defined parts of digestive system**
[EXCLUDES1] *benign stromal tumors of digestive system (D21.4)*

D13.0 Benign neoplasm of esophagus

D13.1 Benign neoplasm of stomach
[EXCLUDES1] *benign carcinoid tumor of the stomach (D3A.092)*

D13.2 Benign neoplasm of duodenum
[EXCLUDES1] *benign carcinoid tumor of the duodenum (D3A.010)*

[5] **D13.3 Benign neoplasm of other and unspecified parts of small intestine**
[EXCLUDES1] *benign carcinoid tumors of the small intestine(D3A.01-)*
benign neoplasm of ileocecal valve (D12.0)

D13.30 Benign neoplasm of unspecified part of small intestine

D13.39 Benign neoplasm of other parts of small intestine

D13.4 Benign neoplasm of liver
Benign neoplasm of intrahepatic bile ducts

D13.5 Benign neoplasm of extrahepatic bile ducts

D13.6 Benign neoplasm of pancreas
[EXCLUDES1] *benign neoplasm of endocrine pancreas (D13.7)*

D13.7 Benign neoplasm of endocrine pancreas
Islet cell tumor
Benign neoplasm of islets of Langerhans
Use additional code to identify any functional activity.

D13.9 Benign neoplasm of ill-defined sites within the digestive system
Benign neoplasm of digestive system NOS
Benign neoplasm of intestine NOS
Benign neoplasm of spleen

[4] **D14 Benign neoplasm of middle ear and respiratory system**

D14.0 Benign neoplasm of middle ear, nasal cavity and accessory sinuses
Benign neoplasm of cartilage of nose
[EXCLUDES1] *benign neoplasm of auricular canal (external) (D22.2-, D23.2-)*
benign neoplasm of bone of ear (D16.4)
benign neoplasm of bone of nose (D16.4)
benign neoplasm of cartilage of ear (D21.0)
benign neoplasm of ear (external)(skin) (D22.2-, D23.2-)
benign neoplasm of nose NOS (D36.7)
benign neoplasm of skin of nose (D22.39, D23.39)
benign neoplasm of olfactory bulb (D33.3)
benign neoplasm of posterior margin of septum and choanae (D10.6)
polyp of accessory sinus (J33.8)
polyp of ear (middle) (H74.4)
polyp of nasal (cavity) (J33.-)

D14.1 Benign neoplasm of larynx
Adenomatous polyp of larynx
Benign neoplasm of epiglottis (suprahyoid portion)
[EXCLUDES1] *benign neoplasm of epiglottis, anterior aspect (D10.5)*
polyp (nonadenomatous) of vocal cord or larynx (J38.1)

D14.2 Benign neoplasm of trachea

[5] **D14.3 Benign neoplasm of bronchus and lung**
[EXCLUDES1] *benign carcinoid tumor of the bronchus and lung (D3A.090)*

D14.30 Benign neoplasm of unspecified bronchus and lung

D14.31 Benign neoplasm of right bronchus and lung

D14.32 Benign neoplasm of left bronchus and lung

D14.4 Benign neoplasm of respiratory system, unspecified

Unspecified Code | Other Specified Code | [N] Newborn Age: 0 | [P] Pediatric Age: 0-17 | [M] Maternity Age: 12-55
[A] Adult Age: 15-124 | ♂ Male | ♀ Female | ● New Code | ▲ Revised Code Title | ►◄ Revised Text

④ **D15 Benign neoplasm of** other and unspecified intrathoracic organs

> *EXCLUDES1* *benign neoplasm of mesothelial tissue (D19.-)*

D15.0 Benign neoplasm of thymus

> *EXCLUDES1* *benign carcinoid tumor of the thymus (D3A.091)*

D15.1 Benign neoplasm of heart

> *EXCLUDES1* *benign neoplasm of great vessels (D21.3)*

D15.2 Benign neoplasm of mediastinum

D15.7 Benign neoplasm of other specified **intrathoracic organs**

D15.9 Benign neoplasm of intrathoracic organ, unspecified

④ **D16 Benign neoplasm of** bone and articular cartilage

> *EXCLUDES1* *benign neoplasm of connective tissue of ear (D21.0)*
> *benign neoplasm of connective tissue of eyelid (D21.0)*
> *benign neoplasm of connective tissue of larynx (D14.1)*
> *benign neoplasm of connective tissue of nose (D14.0)*
> *benign neoplasm of synovia (D21.-)*

⑤ **D16.0 Benign neoplasm of** scapula and long bones of upper limb

D16.00 Benign neoplasm of scapula and long bones of unspecified upper limb

D16.01 Benign neoplasm of scapula and long bones of right **upper limb**

D16.02 Benign neoplasm of scapula and long bones of left **upper limb**

⑤ **D16.1 Benign neoplasm of** short bones of upper limb

D16.10 Benign neoplasm of short bones of unspecified upper limb

D16.11 Benign neoplasm of short bones of right **upper limb**

D16.12 Benign neoplasm of short bones of left **upper limb**

⑤ **D16.2 Benign neoplasm of** long bones of lower limb

D16.20 Benign neoplasm of long bones of unspecified lower limb

D16.21 Benign neoplasm of long bones of right **lower limb**

D16.22 Benign neoplasm of long bones of left **lower limb**

⑤ **D16.3 Benign neoplasm of** short bones of lower limb

D16.30 Benign neoplasm of short bones of unspecified lower limb

D16.31 Benign neoplasm of short bones of right **lower limb**

D16.32 Benign neoplasm of short bones of left **lower limb**

D16.4 Benign neoplasm of bones of skull and face

Benign neoplasm of maxilla (superior)
Benign neoplasm of orbital bone
Keratocyst of maxilla
Keratocystic odontogenic tumor of maxilla

> *EXCLUDES1* *benign neoplasm of lower jaw bone (D16.5)*

D16.5 Benign neoplasm of lower jaw bone

Keratocyst of mandible
Keratocystic odontogenic tumor of mandible

D16.6 Benign neoplasm of vertebral column

> *EXCLUDES1* *benign neoplasm of sacrum and coccyx (D16.8)*

D16.7 Benign neoplasm of ribs, sternum and clavicle

D16.8 Benign neoplasm of pelvic bones, sacrum and coccyx

D16.9 Benign neoplasm of bone and articular cartilage, unspecified

④ **D17** Benign lipomatous **neoplasm**

D17.0 Benign lipomatous neoplasm of skin and subcutaneous tissue of head, face and neck

D17.1 Benign lipomatous neoplasm of skin and subcutaneous tissue of trunk

⑤ **D17.2 Benign lipomatous neoplasm of** skin and subcutaneous tissue of limb

D17.20 Benign lipomatous neoplasm of skin and subcutaneous tissue of unspecified limb

D17.21 Benign lipomatous neoplasm of skin and subcutaneous tissue of right **arm**

D17.22 Benign lipomatous neoplasm of skin and subcutaneous tissue of left **arm**

D17.23 Benign lipomatous neoplasm of skin and subcutaneous tissue of right **leg**

D17.24 Benign lipomatous neoplasm of skin and subcutaneous tissue of left **leg**

⑤ **D17.3 Benign lipomatous neoplasm of skin and subcutaneous tissue of** other and unspecified sites

D17.30 Benign lipomatous neoplasm of skin and subcutaneous tissue of unspecified sites

D17.39 Benign lipomatous neoplasm of skin and subcutaneous tissue of other sites

D17.4 Benign lipomatous neoplasm of intrathoracic organs

D17.5 Benign lipomatous neoplasm of intra-abdominal organs

> *EXCLUDES1* *benign lipomatous neoplasm of peritoneum and retroperitoneum (D17.79)*

D17.6 Benign lipomatous neoplasm of spermatic cord ♂

⑤ **D17.7 Benign lipomatous neoplasm of** other sites

D17.71 Benign lipomatous neoplasm of kidney

D17.72 Benign lipomatous neoplasm of other genitourinary organ

D17.79 Benign lipomatous neoplasm of other sites

Benign lipomatous neoplasm of peritoneum
Benign lipomatous neoplasm of retroperitoneum

D17.9 Benign lipomatous neoplasm, unspecified

Lipoma NOS

④ **D18 Hemangioma and lymphangioma, any site**

> *EXCLUDES1* *benign neoplasm of glomus jugulare (D35.6)*
> *blue or pigmented nevus (D22.-)*
> *nevus NOS (D22.-)*
> *vascular nevus (Q82.5)*

⑤ **D18.0 Hemangioma**

Angioma NOS
Cavernous nevus

D18.00 Hemangioma unspecified site

D18.01 Hemangioma of skin and subcutaneous tissue

D18.02 Hemangioma of intracranial structures

D18.03 Hemangioma of intra-abdominal structures

D18.09 Hemangioma of other sites

D18.1 Lymphangioma, any site

④ **D19 Benign neoplasm of** mesothelial tissue

D19.0 Benign neoplasm of mesothelial tissue of pleura

D19.1 Benign neoplasm of mesothelial tissue of peritoneum

D19.7 Benign neoplasm of mesothelial tissue of other sites

D19.9 Benign neoplasm of mesothelial tissue, unspecified

Benign mesothelioma NOS

④ **D20 Benign neoplasm of** soft tissue of retroperitoneum and peritoneum

> *EXCLUDES1* *benign lipomatous neoplasm of peritoneum and retroperitoneum (D17.79)*
> *benign neoplasm of mesothelial tissue (D19.-)*

D20.0 Benign neoplasm of soft tissue of retroperitoneum

D20.1 Benign neoplasm of soft tissue of peritoneum

④ **D21 Other benign neoplasms of** connective and other soft tissue

> *INCLUDES* *benign neoplasm of blood vessel*
> *benign neoplasm of bursa*
> *benign neoplasm of cartilage*
> *benign neoplasm of fascia*

---

④ 4ᵗʰ character required   ⑤ 5ᵗʰ character required   ⑥ 6ᵗʰ character required   ⑦ 7ᵗʰ character required   ⑦ₓ Extension 'X' Alert

EXCLUDES1 Not coded here   *EXCLUDES2* Not included here   PDx Primary Diagnosis Only   Manifestation Code

benign neoplasm of fat
benign neoplasm of ligament, except uterine
benign neoplasm of lymphatic channel
benign neoplasm of muscle
benign neoplasm of synovia
benign neoplasm of tendon (sheath)
benign stromal tumors

[EXCLUDES1] *benign neoplasm of articular cartilage (D16.-)*
benign neoplasm of cartilage of larynx (D14.1)
benign neoplasm of cartilage of nose (D14.0)
benign neoplasm of connective tissue of breast (D24.-)
benign neoplasm of peripheral nerves and autonomic nervous system (D36.1-)
benign neoplasm of peritoneum (D20.1)
benign neoplasm of retroperitoneum (D20.0)
benign neoplasm of uterine ligament, any (D28.2)
benign neoplasm of vascular tissue (D18.-)
hemangioma (D18.0-)
lipomatous neoplasm (D17.-)
lymphangioma (D18.1)
uterine leiomyoma (D25.-)

D21.0 **Benign neoplasm of connective and other soft tissue of head, face and neck**

Benign neoplasm of connective tissue of ear
Benign neoplasm of connective tissue of eyelid

[EXCLUDES1] *benign neoplasm of connective tissue of orbit (D31.6-)*

[5] D21.1 Benign neoplasm of connective and other soft tissue of upper limb, including shoulder

D21.10 **Benign neoplasm of connective and other soft tissue of unspecified upper limb, including shoulder**

D21.11 **Benign neoplasm of connective and other soft tissue of right upper limb, including shoulder**

D21.12 **Benign neoplasm of connective and other soft tissue of left upper limb, including shoulder**

[5] D21.2 Benign neoplasm of connective and other soft tissue of lower limb, including hip

D21.20 **Benign neoplasm of connective and other soft tissue of unspecified lower limb, including hip**

D21.21 **Benign neoplasm of connective and other soft tissue of right lower limb, including hip**

D21.22 **Benign neoplasm of connective and other soft tissue of left lower limb, including hip**

D21.3 **Benign neoplasm of connective and other soft tissue of thorax**

Benign neoplasm of axilla
Benign neoplasm of diaphragm
Benign neoplasm of great vessels

[EXCLUDES1] *benign neoplasm of heart (D15.1)*
benign neoplasm of mediastinum (D15.2)
benign neoplasm of thymus (D15.0)

D21.4 **Benign neoplasm of connective and other soft tissue of abdomen**

Benign stromal tumors of abdomen

D21.5 **Benign neoplasm of connective and other soft tissue of pelvis**

[EXCLUDES1] *benign neoplasm of any uterine ligament (D28.2)*
uterine leiomyoma (D25.-)

D21.6 **Benign neoplasm of connective and other soft tissue of trunk, unspecified**

Benign neoplasm of back NOS

D21.9 **Benign neoplasm of connective and other soft tissue, unspecified**

[4] D22 Melanocytic nevi

[INCLUDES] *atypical nevus*
blue hairy pigmented nevus
nevus NOS

D22.0 **Melanocytic nevi of lip**

[5] D22.1 Melanocytic nevi of eyelid, including canthus

D22.10 **Melanocytic nevi of unspecified eyelid, including canthus**

D22.11 **Melanocytic nevi of right eyelid, including canthus**

D22.12 **Melanocytic nevi of left eyelid, including canthus**

[5] D22.2 Melanocytic nevi of ear and external auricular canal

D22.20 **Melanocytic nevi of unspecified ear and external auricular canal**

D22.21 **Melanocytic nevi of right ear and external auricular canal**

D22.22 **Melanocytic nevi of left ear and external auricular canal**

[5] D22.3 Melanocytic nevi of other and unspecified parts of face

D22.30 **Melanocytic nevi of unspecified part of face**

D22.39 **Melanocytic nevi of other parts of face**

D22.4 **Melanocytic nevi of scalp and neck**

D22.5 **Melanocytic nevi of trunk**

Melanocytic nevi of anal margin
Melanocytic nevi of anal skin
Melanocytic nevi of perianal skin
Melanocytic nevi of skin of breast

[5] D22.6 Melanocytic nevi of upper limb, including shoulder

D22.60 **Melanocytic nevi of unspecified upper limb, including shoulder**

D22.61 **Melanocytic nevi of right upper limb, including shoulder**

D22.62 **Melanocytic nevi of left upper limb, including shoulder**

[5] D22.7 Melanocytic nevi of lower limb, including hip

D22.70 **Melanocytic nevi of unspecified lower limb, including hip**

D22.71 **Melanocytic nevi of right lower limb, including hip**

D22.72 **Melanocytic nevi of left lower limb, including hip**

D22.9 **Melanocytic nevi, unspecified**

[4] D23 Other benign neoplasms of skin

[INCLUDES] *benign neoplasm of hair follicles*
benign neoplasm of sebaceous glands
benign neoplasm of sweat glands

[EXCLUDES1] *benign lipomatous neoplasms of skin (D17.0-D17.3)*
melanocytic nevi (D22.-)

D23.0 **Other benign neoplasm of skin of lip**

[EXCLUDES1] *benign neoplasm of vermilion border of lip (D10.0)*

[5] D23.1 Other benign neoplasm of skin of eyelid, including canthus

D23.10 **Other benign neoplasm of skin of unspecified eyelid, including canthus**

D23.11 **Other benign neoplasm of skin of right eyelid, including canthus**

D23.12 **Other benign neoplasm of skin of left eyelid, including canthus**

[5] D23.2 Other benign neoplasm of skin of ear and external auricular canal

D23.20 **Other benign neoplasm of skin of unspecified ear and external auricular canal**

D23.21 **Other benign neoplasm of skin of right ear and external auricular canal**

D23.22 **Other benign neoplasm of skin of left ear and external auricular canal**

[5] D23.3 Other benign neoplasm of skin of other and unspecified parts of face

Unspecified Code | Other Specified Code | [N] Newborn Age: 0 | [P] Pediatric Age: 0-17 | [M] Maternity Age: 12-55
[A] Adult Age: 15-124 | ♂ Male | ♀ Female | ● New Code | ▲ Revised Code Title | ►◄ Revised Text

D23.30 **Other benign neoplasm of skin of unspecified part of face**
D23.39 **Other benign neoplasm of skin of other parts of face**
D23.4 **Other benign neoplasm of skin of scalp and neck**
D23.5 **Other benign neoplasm of skin of trunk**
Other benign neoplasm of anal margin
Other benign neoplasm of anal skin
Other benign neoplasm of perianal skin
Other benign neoplasm of skin of breast
EXCLUDES1 *benign neoplasm of anus NOS (D12.9)*
[5] D23.6 **Other benign neoplasm of skin of upper limb, including shoulder**
D23.60 **Other benign neoplasm of skin of unspecified upper limb, including shoulder**
D23.61 **Other benign neoplasm of skin of right upper limb, including shoulder**
D23.62 **Other benign neoplasm of skin of left upper limb, including shoulder**
[5] D23.7 **Other benign neoplasm of skin of lower limb, including hip**
D23.70 **Other benign neoplasm of skin of unspecified lower limb, including hip**
D23.71 **Other benign neoplasm of skin of right lower limb, including hip**
D23.72 **Other benign neoplasm of skin of left lower limb, including hip**
D23.9 **Other benign neoplasm of skin, unspecified**
[4] D24 **Benign neoplasm of breast**
INCLUDES *benign neoplasm of connective tissue of breast*
benign neoplasm of soft parts of breast
fibroadenoma of breast
EXCLUDES2 *adenofibrosis of breast (N60.2)*
benign cyst of breast (N60.-)
benign mammary dysplasia (N60.-)
benign neoplasm of skin of breast (D22.5, D23.5)
fibrocystic disease of breast (N60.-)
D24.1 **Benign neoplasm of right breast**
D24.2 **Benign neoplasm of left breast**
D24.9 **Benign neoplasm of unspecified breast**

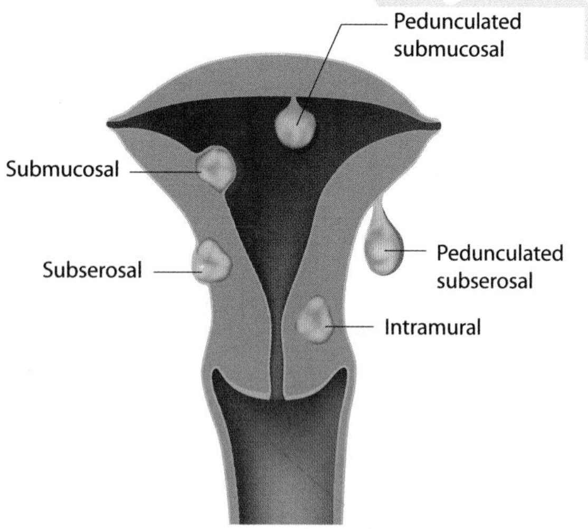
Pedunculated submucosal
Submucosal
Subserosal
Pedunculated subserosal
Intramural

Figure 4.1 Uterine Fibroids

[4] D25 **Leiomyoma of uterus**
INCLUDES *uterine fibroid*
uterine fibromyoma
uterine myoma
D25.0 **Submucous leiomyoma of uterus** ♀
D25.1 **Intramural leiomyoma of uterus**
Interstitial leiomyoma of uterus ♀
D25.2 **Subserosal leiomyoma of uterus**
Subperitoneal leiomyoma of uterus ♀
D25.9 **Leiomyoma of uterus, unspecified** ♀
[4] D26 **Other benign neoplasms of uterus**
D26.0 **Other benign neoplasm of cervix uteri** ♀
D26.1 **Other benign neoplasm of corpus uteri** ♀
D26.7 **Other benign neoplasm of other parts of uterus** ♀
D26.9 **Other benign neoplasm of uterus, unspecified** ♀
[4] D27 **Benign neoplasm of ovary**
Use additional code to identify any functional activity.
EXCLUDES2 *corpus albicans cyst (N83.2)*
corpus luteum cyst (N83.1)
endometrial cyst (N80.1)
follicular (atretic) cyst (N83.0)
graafian follicle cyst (N83.0)
ovarian cyst NEC (N83.2)
ovarian retention cyst (N83.2)
D27.0 **Benign neoplasm of right ovary** ♀
D27.1 **Benign neoplasm of left ovary** ♀
D27.9 **Benign neoplasm of unspecified ovary** ♀
[4] D28 **Benign neoplasm of other and unspecified female genital organs**
INCLUDES *adenomatous polyp*
benign neoplasm of skin of female genital organs
benign teratoma
EXCLUDES1 *epoophoron cyst (Q50.5)*
fimbrial cyst (Q50.4)
Gartner's duct cyst (Q52.4)
parovarian cyst (Q50.5)
D28.0 **Benign neoplasm of vulva** ♀
D28.1 **Benign neoplasm of vagina** ♀
D28.2 **Benign neoplasm of uterine tubes and ligaments**
Benign neoplasm of fallopian tube
Benign neoplasm of uterine ligament (broad) (round) ♀
D28.7 **Benign neoplasm of other specified female genital organs** ♀
D28.9 **Benign neoplasm of female genital organ, unspecified** ♀
[4] D29 **Benign neoplasm of male genital organs**
INCLUDES *benign neoplasm of skin of male genital organs*
D29.0 **Benign neoplasm of penis** ♂
D29.1 **Benign neoplasm of prostate**
EXCLUDES1 *enlarged prostate (N40.-)* ♂
[5] D29.2 **Benign neoplasm of testis**
Use additional code to identify any functional activity.
D29.20 **Benign neoplasm of unspecified testis** ♂
D29.21 **Benign neoplasm of right testis** ♂
D29.22 **Benign neoplasm of left testis** ♂
[5] D29.3 **Benign neoplasm of epididymis**
D29.30 **Benign neoplasm of unspecified epididymis** ♂
D29.31 **Benign neoplasm of right epididymis** ♂
D29.32 **Benign neoplasm of left epididymis** ♂
D29.4 **Benign neoplasm of scrotum**
Benign neoplasm of skin of scrotum ♂
D29.8 **Benign neoplasm of other specified male genital organs**
Benign neoplasm of seminal vesicle
Benign neoplasm of spermatic cord
Benign neoplasm of tunica vaginalis ♂
D29.9 **Benign neoplasm of male genital organ, unspecified** ♂
[4] D30 **Benign neoplasm of urinary organs**
[5] D30.0 **Benign neoplasm of kidney**
EXCLUDES1 *benign carcinoid tumor of the kidney (D3A.093)*
benign neoplasm of renal calyces (D30.1-)
benign neoplasm of renal pelvis (D30.1-)

D30.00 **Benign neoplasm of unspecified kidney**
D30.01 **Benign neoplasm of right kidney**
D30.02 **Benign neoplasm of left kidney**
[5] D30.1 Benign neoplasm of renal pelvis
D30.10 **Benign neoplasm of unspecified renal pelvis**
D30.11 **Benign neoplasm of right renal pelvis**
D30.12 **Benign neoplasm of left renal pelvis**
[5] D30.2 Benign neoplasm of ureter
[EXCLUDES1] *benign neoplasm of ureteric orifice of bladder (D30.3)*
D30.20 **Benign neoplasm of unspecified ureter**
D30.21 **Benign neoplasm of right ureter**
D30.22 **Benign neoplasm of left ureter**
D30.3 **Benign neoplasm of bladder**
Benign neoplasm of ureteric orifice of bladder
Benign neoplasm of urethral orifice of bladder
D30.4 **Benign neoplasm of urethra**
[EXCLUDES1] *benign neoplasm of urethral orifice of bladder (D30.3)*
D30.8 **Benign neoplasm of other specified urinary organs**
Benign neoplasm of paraurethral glands
D30.9 **Benign neoplasm of urinary organ, unspecified**
Benign neoplasm of urinary system NOS
[4] D31 Benign neoplasm of eye and adnexa
[EXCLUDES1] *benign neoplasm of connective tissue of eyelid (D21.0)*
benign neoplasm of optic nerve (D33.3)
benign neoplasm of skin of eyelid (D22.1-, D23.1-)
[5] D31.0 Benign neoplasm of conjunctiva
D31.00 **Benign neoplasm of unspecified conjunctiva**
D31.01 **Benign neoplasm of right conjunctiva**
D31.02 **Benign neoplasm of left conjunctiva**
[5] D31.1 Benign neoplasm of cornea
D31.10 **Benign neoplasm of unspecified cornea**
D31.11 **Benign neoplasm of right cornea**
D31.12 **Benign neoplasm of left cornea**
[5] D31.2 Benign neoplasm of retina
[EXCLUDES1] *dark area on retina (D49.81)*
hemangioma of retina (D49.81)
neoplasm of unspecified behavior of retina and choroid (D49.81)
retinal freckle (D49.81)
D31.20 **Benign neoplasm of unspecified retina**
D31.21 **Benign neoplasm of right retina**
D31.22 **Benign neoplasm of left retina**
[5] D31.3 Benign neoplasm of choroid
D31.30 **Benign neoplasm of unspecified choroid**
D31.31 **Benign neoplasm of right choroid**
D31.32 **Benign neoplasm of left choroid**
[5] D31.4 Benign neoplasm of ciliary body
D31.40 **Benign neoplasm of unspecified ciliary body**
D31.41 **Benign neoplasm of right ciliary body**
D31.42 **Benign neoplasm of left ciliary body**
[5] D31.5 Benign neoplasm of lacrimal gland and duct
Benign neoplasm of lacrimal sac
Benign neoplasm of nasolacrimal duct
D31.50 **Benign neoplasm of unspecified lacrimal gland and duct**
D31.51 **Benign neoplasm of right lacrimal gland and duct**
D31.52 **Benign neoplasm of left lacrimal gland and duct**
[5] D31.6 Benign neoplasm of unspecified site of orbit
Benign neoplasm of connective tissue of orbit
Benign neoplasm of extraocular muscle
Benign neoplasm of peripheral nerves of orbit
Benign neoplasm of retrobulbar tissue
Benign neoplasm of retro-ocular tissue
[EXCLUDES1] *benign neoplasm of orbital bone (D16.4)*
D31.60 **Benign neoplasm of unspecified site of unspecified orbit**
D31.61 **Benign neoplasm of unspecified site of right orbit**
D31.62 **Benign neoplasm of unspecified site of left orbit**
[5] D31.9 Benign neoplasm of unspecified part of eye
Benign neoplasm of eyeball
D31.90 **Benign neoplasm of unspecified part of unspecified eye**
D31.91 **Benign neoplasm of unspecified part of right eye**
D31.92 **Benign neoplasm of unspecified part of left eye**
[4] D32 Benign neoplasm of meninges
D32.0 **Benign neoplasm of cerebral meninges**
D32.1 **Benign neoplasm of spinal meninges**
D32.9 **Benign neoplasm of meninges, unspecified**
Meningioma NOS

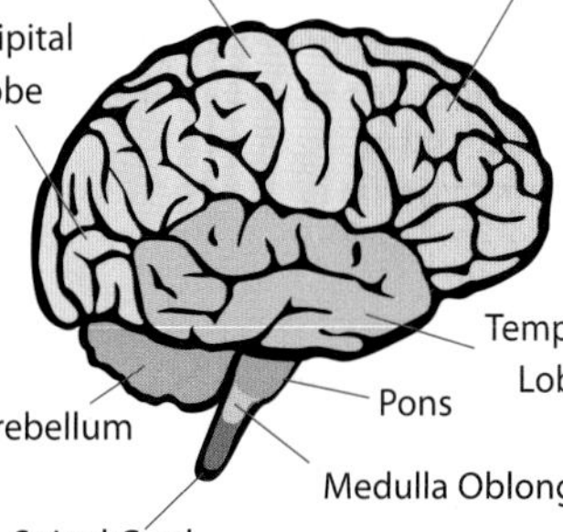

Figure 4.2 Brain lobes

[4] D33 Benign neoplasm of brain and other parts of central nervous system
[EXCLUDES1] *angioma (D18.0-)*
benign neoplasm of meninges (D32.-)
benign neoplasm of peripheral nerves and autonomic nervous system (D36.1-)
hemangioma (D18.0-)
neurofibromatosis (Q85.0-)
retro-ocular benign neoplasm (D31.6-)
D33.0 **Benign neoplasm of brain, supratentorial**
Benign neoplasm of cerebral ventricle
Benign neoplasm of cerebrum
Benign neoplasm of frontal lobe
Benign neoplasm of occipital lobe
Benign neoplasm of parietal lobe
Benign neoplasm of temporal lobe
[EXCLUDES1] *benign neoplasm of fourth ventricle (D33.1)*
D33.1 **Benign neoplasm of brain, infratentorial**
Benign neoplasm of brain stem
Benign neoplasm of cerebellum
Benign neoplasm of fourth ventricle
D33.2 **Benign neoplasm of brain, unspecified**
D33.3 **Benign neoplasm of cranial nerves**
Benign neoplasm of olfactory bulb
D33.4 **Benign neoplasm of spinal cord**
D33.7 **Benign neoplasm of other specified parts of central nervous system**
D33.9 **Benign neoplasm of central nervous system, unspecified**
Benign neoplasm of nervous system (central) NOS

Unspecified Code | Other Specified Code | [N] Newborn Age: 0 | [P] Pediatric Age: 0-17 | [M] Maternity Age: 12-55
[A] Adult Age: 15-124 | ♂ Male | ♀ Female | ● New Code | ▲ Revised Code Title | ►◄ Revised Text

D34 Benign neoplasm of thyroid gland
Use additional code to identify any functional activity

[4] D35 Benign neoplasm of other and unspecified endocrine glands
Use additional code to identify any functional activity
[EXCLUDES1] *benign neoplasm of endocrine pancreas (D13.7)*
benign neoplasm of ovary (D27.-)
benign neoplasm of testis (D29.2.-)
benign neoplasm of thymus (D15.0)

[5] D35.0 Benign neoplasm of adrenal gland
D35.00 **Benign neoplasm of unspecified adrenal gland**
D35.01 **Benign neoplasm of right adrenal gland**
D35.02 **Benign neoplasm of left adrenal gland**
D35.1 **Benign neoplasm of parathyroid gland**
D35.2 **Benign neoplasm of pituitary gland**
D35.3 **Benign neoplasm of craniopharyngeal duct**
D35.4 **Benign neoplasm of pineal gland**
D35.5 **Benign neoplasm of carotid body**
D35.6 **Benign neoplasm of aortic body and other paraganglia**
Benign tumor of glomus jugulare
D35.7 **Benign neoplasm of other specified endocrine glands**
D35.9 **Benign neoplasm of endocrine gland, unspecified**
Benign neoplasm of unspecified endocrine gland

[4] D36 Benign neoplasm of other and unspecified sites
D36.0 **Benign neoplasm of lymph nodes**
[EXCLUDES1] *lymphangioma (D18.1)*

[5] D36.1 Benign neoplasm of peripheral nerves and autonomic nervous system
[EXCLUDES1] *benign neoplasm of peripheral nerves of orbit (D31.6-)*
neurofibromatosis (Q85.0-)
D36.10 **Benign neoplasm of peripheral nerves and autonomic nervous system, unspecified**
D36.11 **Benign neoplasm of peripheral nerves and autonomic nervous system of face, head, and neck**
D36.12 **Benign neoplasm of peripheral nerves and autonomic nervous system, upper limb, including shoulder**
D36.13 **Benign neoplasm of peripheral nerves and autonomic nervous system of lower limb, including hip**
D36.14 **Benign neoplasm of peripheral nerves and autonomic nervous system of thorax**
D36.15 **Benign neoplasm of peripheral nerves and autonomic nervous system of abdomen**
D36.16 **Benign neoplasm of peripheral nerves and autonomic nervous system of pelvis**
D36.17 **Benign neoplasm of peripheral nerves and autonomic nervous system of trunk, unspecified**
D36.7 **Benign neoplasm of other specified sites**
Benign neoplasm of nose NOS
D36.9 **Benign neoplasm, unspecified site**

Benign neuroendocrine tumors (D3A)

[4] D3A Benign neuroendocrine tumors
Code also any associated multiple endocrine neoplasia [MEN] syndromes (E31.2-)
Use additional code to identify any associated endocrine syndrome, such as:
carcinoid syndrome (E34.0)
[EXCLUDES2] *benign pancreatic islet cell tumors (D13.7)*

[5] D3A.0 Benign carcinoid tumors
D3A.00 **Benign carcinoid tumor of unspecified site**
Carcinoid tumor NOS

[6] D3A.01 Benign carcinoid tumors of the small intestine
D3A.010 **Benign carcinoid tumor of the duodenum**
D3A.011 **Benign carcinoid tumor of the jejunum**
D3A.012 **Benign carcinoid tumor of the ileum**
D3A.019 **Benign carcinoid tumor of the small intestine, unspecified portion**

[6] D3A.02 Benign carcinoid tumors of the appendix, large intestine, and rectum
D3A.020 **Benign carcinoid tumor of the appendix**
D3A.021 **Benign carcinoid tumor of the cecum**
D3A.022 **Benign carcinoid tumor of the ascending colon**
D3A.023 **Benign carcinoid tumor of the transverse colon**
D3A.024 **Benign carcinoid tumor of the descending colon**
D3A.025 **Benign carcinoid tumor of the sigmoid colon**
D3A.026 **Benign carcinoid tumor of the rectum**
D3A.029 **Benign carcinoid tumor of the large intestine, unspecified portion**
Benign carcinoid tumor of the colon NOS

[6] D3A.09 Benign carcinoid tumors of other sites
D3A.090 **Benign carcinoid tumor of the bronchus and lung**
D3A.091 **Benign carcinoid tumor of the thymus**
D3A.092 **Benign carcinoid tumor of the stomach**
D3A.093 **Benign carcinoid tumor of the kidney**
D3A.094 **Benign carcinoid tumor of the foregut NOS**
D3A.095 **Benign carcinoid tumor of the midgut NOS**
D3A.096 **Benign carcinoid tumor of the hindgut NOS**
D3A.098 **Benign carcinoid tumors of other sites**
D3A.8 **Other benign neuroendocrine tumors**
Neuroendocrine tumor NOS

Neoplasms of uncertain behavior, polycythemia vera and myelodysplastic syndromes (D37-D48)

[NOTES] Categories D37-D44, and D48 classify by site neoplasms of uncertain behavior, i.e., histologic confirmation whether the neoplasm is malignant or benign cannot be made.
[EXCLUDES1] *neoplasms of unspecified behavior (D49.-)*

[4] D37 Neoplasm of uncertain behavior of oral cavity and digestive organs
[EXCLUDES1] *stromal tumors of uncertain behavior of digestive system (D48.1)*

[5] D37.0 Neoplasm of uncertain behavior of lip, oral cavity and pharynx
[EXCLUDES1] *neoplasm of uncertain behavior of aryepiglottic fold or interarytenoid fold, laryngeal aspect (D38.0)*
neoplasm of uncertain behavior of epiglottis NOS (D38.0)
neoplasm of uncertain behavior of skin of lip (D48.5)
neoplasm of uncertain behavior of suprahyoid portion of epiglottis (D38.0)
D37.01 **Neoplasm of uncertain behavior of lip**
Neoplasm of uncertain behavior of vermilion border of lip
D37.02 **Neoplasm of uncertain behavior of tongue**

[6] D37.03 Neoplasm of uncertain behavior of the major salivary glands
D37.030 **Neoplasm of uncertain behavior of the parotid salivary glands**
D37.031 **Neoplasm of uncertain behavior of the sublingual salivary glands**
D37.032 **Neoplasm of uncertain behavior of the submandibular salivary glands**

[4] 4th character required [5] 5th character required [6] 6th character required [7] 7th character required [X] Extension 'X' Alert
[EXCLUDES1] Not coded here [EXCLUDES2] Not included here [PDx] Primary Diagnosis Only Manifestation Code

D37.039 Neoplasm of uncertain behavior of the major salivary glands, unspecified

D37.04 Neoplasm of uncertain behavior of the minor salivary glands

Neoplasm of uncertain behavior of submucosal salivary glands of lip
Neoplasm of uncertain behavior of submucosal salivary glands of cheek
Neoplasm of uncertain behavior of submucosal salivary glands of hard palate
Neoplasm of uncertain behavior of submucosal salivary glands of soft palate

D37.05 Neoplasm of uncertain behavior of pharynx

Neoplasm of uncertain behavior of aryepiglottic fold of pharynx NOS
Neoplasm of uncertain behavior of hypopharyngeal aspect of aryepiglottic fold of pharynx
Neoplasm of uncertain behavior of marginal zone of aryepiglottic fold of pharynx

D37.09 Neoplasm of uncertain behavior of other specified sites of the oral cavity

D37.1 Neoplasm of uncertain behavior of stomach

D37.2 Neoplasm of uncertain behavior of small intestine

D37.3 Neoplasm of uncertain behavior of appendix

D37.4 Neoplasm of uncertain behavior of colon

D37.5 Neoplasm of uncertain behavior of rectum

Neoplasm of uncertain behavior of rectosigmoid junction

D37.6 Neoplasm of uncertain behavior of liver, gallbladder and bile ducts

Neoplasm of uncertain behavior of ampulla of Vater

D37.8 Neoplasm of uncertain behavior of other specified digestive organs

Neoplasm of uncertain behavior of anal canal
Neoplasm of uncertain behavior of anal sphincter
Neoplasm of uncertain behavior of anus NOS
Neoplasm of uncertain behavior of esophagus
Neoplasm of uncertain behavior of intestine NOS
Neoplasm of uncertain behavior of pancreas

[EXCLUDES1] *neoplasm of uncertain behavior of anal margin (D48.5)*
neoplasm of uncertain behavior of anal skin (D48.5)
neoplasm of uncertain behavior of perianal skin (D48.5)

D37.9 Neoplasm of uncertain behavior of digestive organ, unspecified

[4th] **D38 Neoplasm of uncertain behavior of middle ear and respiratory and intrathoracic organs**

[EXCLUDES1] *neoplasm of uncertain behavior of heart (D48.7)*

D38.0 Neoplasm of uncertain behavior of larynx

Neoplasm of uncertain behavior of aryepiglottic fold or interarytenoid fold, laryngeal aspect
Neoplasm of uncertain behavior of epiglottis (suprahyoid portion)

[EXCLUDES1] *neoplasm of uncertain behavior of aryepiglottic fold or interarytenoid fold NOS (D37.05)*
neoplasm of uncertain behavior of hypopharyngeal aspect of aryepiglottic fold (D37.05)
neoplasm of uncertain behavior of marginal zone of aryepiglottic fold (D37.05)

D38.1 Neoplasm of uncertain behavior of trachea, bronchus and lung

D38.2 Neoplasm of uncertain behavior of pleura

D38.3 Neoplasm of uncertain behavior of mediastinum

D38.4 Neoplasm of uncertain behavior of thymus

D38.5 Neoplasm of uncertain behavior of other respiratory organs

Neoplasm of uncertain behavior of accessory sinuses
Neoplasm of uncertain behavior of cartilage of nose
Neoplasm of uncertain behavior of middle ear
Neoplasm of uncertain behavior of nasal cavities

[EXCLUDES1] *neoplasm of uncertain behavior of ear (external) (skin) (D48.5)*
neoplasm of uncertain behavior of nose NOS (D48.7)
neoplasm of uncertain behavior of skin of nose (D48.5)

D38.6 Neoplasm of uncertain behavior of respiratory organ, unspecified

[4th] **D39 Neoplasm of uncertain behavior of female genital organs**

D39.0 Neoplasm of uncertain behavior of uterus ♀

[5th] **D39.1 Neoplasm of uncertain behavior of ovary**

Use additional code to identify any functional activity.

D39.10 Neoplasm of uncertain behavior of unspecified ovary ♀

D39.11 Neoplasm of uncertain behavior of right ovary ♀

D39.12 Neoplasm of uncertain behavior of left ovary ♀

D39.2 Neoplasm of uncertain behavior of placenta

Chorioadenoma destruens
Invasive hydatidiform mole
Malignant hydatidiform mole

[EXCLUDES1] *hydatidiform mole NOS (O01.9)* ♀

D39.8 Neoplasm of uncertain behavior of other specified female genital organs

Neoplasm of uncertain behavior of skin of female genital organs ♀

D39.9 Neoplasm of uncertain behavior of female genital organ, unspecified ♀

[4th] **D40 Neoplasm of uncertain behavior of male genital organs**

D40.0 Neoplasm of uncertain behavior of prostate ♂

[5th] **D40.1 Neoplasm of uncertain behavior of testis**

D40.10 Neoplasm of uncertain behavior of unspecified testis ♂

D40.11 Neoplasm of uncertain behavior of right testis ♂

D40.12 Neoplasm of uncertain behavior of left testis ♂

D40.8 Neoplasm of uncertain behavior of other specified male genital organs

Neoplasm of uncertain behavior of skin of male genital organs ♂

D40.9 Neoplasm of uncertain behavior of male genital organ, unspecified ♂

[4th] **D41 Neoplasm of uncertain behavior of urinary organs**

[5th] **D41.0 Neoplasm of uncertain behavior of kidney**

[EXCLUDES1] *neoplasm of uncertain behavior of renal pelvis (D41.1-)*

D41.00 Neoplasm of uncertain behavior of unspecified kidney

D41.01 Neoplasm of uncertain behavior of right kidney

D41.02 Neoplasm of uncertain behavior of left kidney

[5th] **D41.1 Neoplasm of uncertain behavior of renal pelvis**

D41.10 Neoplasm of uncertain behavior of unspecified renal pelvis

D41.11 Neoplasm of uncertain behavior of right renal pelvis

D41.12 Neoplasm of uncertain behavior of left renal pelvis

[5th] **D41.2 Neoplasm of uncertain behavior of ureter**

D41.20 Neoplasm of uncertain behavior of unspecified ureter

D41.21 Neoplasm of uncertain behavior of right ureter

D41.22 Neoplasm of uncertain behavior of left ureter

D41.3 Neoplasm of uncertain behavior of urethra

D41.4 Neoplasm of uncertain behavior of bladder

Unspecified Code | Other Specified Code | [N] Newborn Age: 0 | [P] Pediatric Age: 0-17 | [M] Maternity Age: 12-55
[A] Adult Age: 15-124 | ♂ Male | ♀ Female | ● New Code | ▲ Revised Code Title | ►◄ Revised Text

D41.8 Neoplasm of uncertain behavior of other specified urinary organs
D41.9 Neoplasm of uncertain behavior of unspecified urinary organ
[4] D42 Neoplasm of uncertain behavior of meninges
D42.0 Neoplasm of uncertain behavior of cerebral meninges
D42.1 Neoplasm of uncertain behavior of spinal meninges
D42.9 Neoplasm of uncertain behavior of meninges, unspecified
[4] D43 Neoplasm of uncertain behavior of brain and central nervous system
[EXCLUDES1] *neoplasm of uncertain behavior of peripheral nerves and autonomic nervous system (D48.2)*
D43.0 Neoplasm of uncertain behavior of brain, supratentorial
Neoplasm of uncertain behavior of cerebral ventricle
Neoplasm of uncertain behavior of cerebrum
Neoplasm of uncertain behavior of frontal lobe
Neoplasm of uncertain behavior of occipital lobe
Neoplasm of uncertain behavior of parietal lobe
Neoplasm of uncertain behavior of temporal lobe
[EXCLUDES1] *neoplasm of uncertain behavior of fourth ventricle (D43.1)*
D43.1 Neoplasm of uncertain behavior of brain, infratentorial
Neoplasm of uncertain behavior of brain stem
Neoplasm of uncertain behavior of cerebellum
Neoplasm of uncertain behavior of fourth ventricle
D43.2 Neoplasm of uncertain behavior of brain, unspecified
D43.3 Neoplasm of uncertain behavior of cranial nerves
D43.4 Neoplasm of uncertain behavior of spinal cord
D43.8 Neoplasm of uncertain behavior of other specified parts of central nervous system
D43.9 Neoplasm of uncertain behavior of central nervous system, unspecified
Neoplasm of uncertain behavior of nervous system (central) NOS
[4] D44 Neoplasm of uncertain behavior of endocrine glands
[EXCLUDES1] *multiple endocrine adenomatosis (E31.2-)*
multiple endocrine neoplasia (E31.2-)
neoplasm of uncertain behavior of endocrine pancreas (D37.8)
neoplasm of uncertain behavior of ovary (D39.1-)
neoplasm of uncertain behavior of testis (D40.1-)
neoplasm of uncertain behavior of thymus (D38.4)
D44.0 Neoplasm of uncertain behavior of thyroid gland
[5] D44.1 Neoplasm of uncertain behavior of adrenal gland
Use additional code to identify any functional activity.
D44.10 Neoplasm of uncertain behavior of unspecified adrenal gland
D44.11 Neoplasm of uncertain behavior of right adrenal gland
D44.12 Neoplasm of uncertain behavior of left adrenal gland
D44.2 Neoplasm of uncertain behavior of parathyroid gland
D44.3 Neoplasm of uncertain behavior of pituitary gland
Use additional code to identify any functional activity.
D44.4 Neoplasm of uncertain behavior of craniopharyngeal duct
D44.5 Neoplasm of uncertain behavior of pineal gland
D44.6 Neoplasm of uncertain behavior of carotid body
D44.7 Neoplasm of uncertain behavior of aortic body and other paraganglia
D44.9 Neoplasm of uncertain behavior of unspecified endocrine gland
D45 Polycythemia vera
[EXCLUDES1] *familial polycythemia (D75.0)*
secondary polycythemia (D75.1)
[4] D46 Myelodysplastic syndromes
Use additional code for adverse effect, if applicable, to identify drug (T36-T50 with fifth or sixth character 5)
[EXCLUDES2] *drug-induced aplastic anemia (D61.1)*
D46.0 Refractory anemia without ring sideroblasts, so stated
Refractory anemia without sideroblasts, without excess of blasts
D46.1 Refractory anemia with ring sideroblasts
RARS
[5] D46.2 Refractory anemia with excess of blasts
D46.20 Refractory anemia with excess of blasts, unspecified
RAEB NOS
D46.21 Refractory anemia with excess of blasts 1
RAEB 1
D46.22 Refractory anemia with excess of blasts 2
RAEB 2
D46.A Refractory cytopenia with multilineage dysplasia
D46.B Refractory cytopenia with multilineage dysplasia and ring sideroblasts
RCMD RS
D46.C Myelodysplastic syndrome with isolated del(5q) chromosomal abnormality
Myelodysplastic syndrome with 5q deletion
5q minus syndrome NOS
D46.4 Refractory anemia, unspecified
D46.Z Other myelodysplastic syndromes
[EXCLUDES1] *chronic myelomonocytic leukemia (C93.1-)*
D46.9 Myelodysplastic syndrome, unspecified
Myelodysplasia NOS
[4] D47 Other neoplasms of uncertain behavior of lymphoid, hematopoietic and related tissue
D47.0 Histiocytic and mast cell tumors of uncertain behavior
Indolent systemic mastocytosis
Mast cell tumor NOS
Mastocytoma NOS
[EXCLUDES1] *malignant mast cell tumor (C96.2)*
mastocytosis (congenital) (cutaneous) (Q82.2)
D47.1 Chronic myeloproliferative disease
Chronic neutrophilic leukemia
Myeloproliferative disease, unspecified
[EXCLUDES1] *atypical chronic myeloid leukemia BCR/ABL-negative (C92.2-)*
chronic myeloid leukemia BCR/ABL-positive (C92.1-)
myelofibrosis NOS (D75.81)
myelophthisic anemia (D61.82)
myelophthisis (D61.82)
secondary myelofibrosis NOS (D75.81)
D47.2 Monoclonal gammopathy
Monoclonal gammopathy of undetermined significance [MGUS]
D47.3 Essential (hemorrhagic) thrombocythemia
Essential thrombocytosis
Idiopathic hemorrhagic thrombocythemia

[4] 4th character required [5] 5th character required [6] 6th character required [7] 7th character required [x] Extension 'X' Alert
[EXCLUDES1] Not coded here [EXCLUDES2] Not included here [PDx] Primary Diagnosis Only Manifestation Code

D47.4 **Osteomyelofibrosis**

Chronic idiopathic myelofibrosis

Myelofibrosis (idiopathic) (with myeloid metaplasia)

Myelosclerosis (megakaryocytic) with myeloid metaplasia

Secondary myelofibrosis in myeloproliferative disease

EXCLUDES1 *acute myelofibrosis (C94.4-)*

⑤ D47.Z **Other specified neoplasms of uncertain behavior of lymphoid, hematopoietic and related tissue**

D47.Z1 **Post-transplant lymphoproliferative disorder (PTLD)**

Code first complications of transplanted organs and tissue (T86.-)

D47.Z9 **Other specified neoplasms of uncertain behavior of lymphoid, hematopoietic and related tissue**

Histiocytic tumors of uncertain behavior

D47.9 **Neoplasm of uncertain behavior of lymphoid, hematopoietic and related tissue, unspecified**

Lymphoproliferative disease NOS

④ D48 **Neoplasm of uncertain behavior of other and unspecified sites**

EXCLUDES1 *neurofibromatosis (nonmalignant) (Q85.0-)*

D48.0 **Neoplasm of uncertain behavior of bone and articular cartilage**

EXCLUDES1 *neoplasm of uncertain behavior of cartilage of ear (D48.1)*

neoplasm of uncertain behavior of cartilage of larynx (D38.0)

neoplasm of uncertain behavior of cartilage of nose (D38.5)

neoplasm of uncertain behavior of connective tissue of eyelid (D48.1)

neoplasm of uncertain behavior of synovia (D48.1)

D48.1 **Neoplasm of uncertain behavior of connective and other soft tissue**

Neoplasm of uncertain behavior of connective tissue of ear

Neoplasm of uncertain behavior of connective tissue of eyelid

Stromal tumors of uncertain behavior of digestive system

EXCLUDES1 *neoplasm of uncertain behavior of articular cartilage (D48.0)*

neoplasm of uncertain behavior of cartilage of larynx (D38.0)

neoplasm of uncertain behavior of cartilage of nose (D38.5)

neoplasm of uncertain behavior of connective tissue of breast (D48.6-)

D48.2 **Neoplasm of uncertain behavior of peripheral nerves and autonomic nervous system**

EXCLUDES1 *neoplasm of uncertain behavior of peripheral nerves of orbit (D48.7)*

D48.3 **Neoplasm of uncertain behavior of retroperitoneum**

D48.4 **Neoplasm of uncertain behavior of peritoneum**

D48.5 **Neoplasm of uncertain behavior of skin**

Neoplasm of uncertain behavior of anal margin

Neoplasm of uncertain behavior of anal skin

Neoplasm of uncertain behavior of perianal skin

Neoplasm of uncertain behavior of skin of breast

EXCLUDES1 *neoplasm of uncertain behavior of anus NOS (D37.8)*

neoplasm of uncertain behavior of skin of genital organs (D39.8, D40.8)

neoplasm of uncertain behavior of vermilion border of lip (D37.0)

⑤ D48.6 **Neoplasm of uncertain behavior of breast**

Neoplasm of uncertain behavior of connective tissue of breast

Cystosarcoma phyllodes

EXCLUDES1 *neoplasm of uncertain behavior of skin of breast (D48.5)*

D48.60 **Neoplasm of uncertain behavior of unspecified breast**

D48.61 **Neoplasm of uncertain behavior of right breast**

D48.62 **Neoplasm of uncertain behavior of left breast**

D48.7 **Neoplasm of uncertain behavior of other specified sites**

Neoplasm of uncertain behavior of eye

Neoplasm of uncertain behavior of heart

Neoplasm of uncertain behavior of peripheral nerves of orbit

EXCLUDES1 *neoplasm of uncertain behavior of connective tissue (D48.1)*

neoplasm of uncertain behavior of skin of eyelid (D48.5)

D48.9 **Neoplasm of uncertain behavior, unspecified**

Neoplasms of unspecified behavior (D49)

④ D49 **Neoplasms of unspecified behavior**

NOTES Category D49 classifies by site neoplasms of unspecified morphology and behavior. The term 'mass', unless otherwise stated, is not to be regarded as a neoplastic growth.

INCLUDES *'growth' NOS*

neoplasm NOS

new growth NOS

tumor NOS

EXCLUDES1 *neoplasms of uncertain behavior (D37-D44, D48)*

D49.0 **Neoplasm of unspecified behavior of digestive system**

EXCLUDES1 *neoplasm of unspecified behavior of margin of anus (D49.2)*

neoplasm of unspecified behavior of perianal skin (D49.2)

neoplasm of unspecified behavior of skin of anus (D49.2)

D49.1 **Neoplasm of unspecified behavior of respiratory system**

D49.2 **Neoplasm of unspecified behavior of bone, soft tissue, and skin**

EXCLUDES1 *neoplasm of unspecified behavior of anal canal (D49.0)*

neoplasm of unspecified behavior of anus NOS (D49.0)

neoplasm of unspecified behavior of bone marrow (D49.89)

neoplasm of unspecified behavior of cartilage of larynx (D49.1)

neoplasm of unspecified behavior of cartilage of nose (D49.1)

neoplasm of unspecified behavior of connective tissue of breast (D49.3)

neoplasm of unspecified behavior of skin of genital organs (D49.5)

neoplasm of unspecified behavior of vermilion border of lip (D49.0)

D49.3 **Neoplasm of unspecified behavior of breast**

EXCLUDES1 *neoplasm of unspecified behavior of skin of breast (D49.2)*

D49.4 **Neoplasm of unspecified behavior of bladder**

D49.5 **Neoplasm of unspecified behavior of other genitourinary organs**

Unspecified Code | Other Specified Code | N Newborn Age: 0 | P Pediatric Age: 0-17 | M Maternity Age: 12-55
A Adult Age: 15-124 | ♂ Male | ♀ Female | ● New Code | ▲ Revised Code Title | ►◄ Revised Text

D49.6 Neoplasm of unspecified behavior of brain

> *EXCLUDES1* *neoplasm of unspecified behavior of cerebral meninges (D49.7)*
> *neoplasm of unspecified behavior of cranial nerves (D49.7)*

D49.7 Neoplasm of unspecified behavior of endocrine glands and other parts of nervous system

> *EXCLUDES1* *neoplasm of unspecified behavior of peripheral, sympathetic, and parasympathetic nerves and ganglia (D49.2)*

🔵 **D49.8 Neoplasm of unspecified behavior of** other specified sites

> *EXCLUDES1* *neoplasm of unspecified behavior of eyelid (skin) (D49.2)*
> *neoplasm of unspecified behavior of eyelid cartilage (D49.2)*
> *neoplasm of unspecified behavior of great vessels (D49.2)*
> *neoplasm of unspecified behavior of optic nerve (D49.7)*

D49.81 Neoplasm of unspecified behavior of retina and choroid

Dark area on retina

Retinal freckle

D49.89 Neoplasm of unspecified behavior of other specified sites

D49.9 Neoplasm of unspecified behavior of unspecified site

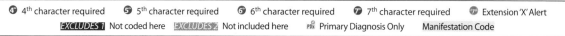

🔵 4th character required   🔵 5th character required   🔵 6th character required   🔵 7th character required   🔵 Extension 'X' Alert

EXCLUDES 1 Not coded here   *EXCLUDES 2* Not included here   Pᴅx Primary Diagnosis Only   Manifestation Code

66   **ICD-10-CM 2015**

Chapter 3: Disease of the Blood and Blood-Forming Organs and Certain Disorders Involving the Immune Mechanism (D50-D89)

EXCLUDES2   *autoimmune disease (systemic) NOS (M35.9)*
certain conditions originating in the perinatal period (P00-P96)
complications of pregnancy, childbirth and the puerperium (O00-O9A)
congenital malformations, deformations and chromosomal abnormalities (Q00-Q99)
endocrine, nutritional and metabolic diseases (E00-E88)
human immunodeficiency virus [HIV] disease (B20)
injury, poisoning and certain other consequences of external causes (S00-T88)
neoplasms (C00-D49)
symptoms, signs and abnormal clinical and laboratory findings, not elsewhere classified (R00-R94)

Nutritional anemias (D50-D53)

🔵 **D50** Iron deficiency anemia

INCLUDES   asiderotic anemia
hypochromic anemia

D50.0 Iron deficiency anemia secondary to blood loss (chronic)

Posthemorrhagic anemia (chronic)

EXCLUDES1   *acute posthemorrhagic anemia (D62)*
congenital anemia from fetal blood loss (P61.3)

D50.1 Sideropenic dysphagia

Kelly-Paterson syndrome

Plummer-Vinson syndrome

D50.8 Other iron deficiency anemias

Iron deficiency anemia due to inadequate dietary iron intake

D50.9 Iron deficiency anemia, unspecified

🔵 **D51** Vitamin B12 deficiency anemia

EXCLUDES1   *vitamin B12 deficiency (E53.8)*

D51.0 Vitamin B12 deficiency anemia due to intrinsic factor deficiency

Addison anemia

Biermer anemia

Pernicious (congenital) anemia

Congenital intrinsic factor deficiency

D51.1 Vitamin B12 deficiency anemia due to selective vitamin B12 malabsorption with proteinuria

Imerslund (Gräsbeck) syndrome

Megaloblastic hereditary anemia

D51.2 Transcobalamin II **deficiency**

D51.3 Other dietary vitamin B12 deficiency anemia

Vegan anemia

D51.8 Other vitamin B12 deficiency anemias

D51.9 Vitamin B12 deficiency anemia, unspecified

🔵 **D52** Folate deficiency anemia

EXCLUDES1   *folate deficiency without anemia (E53.8)*

D52.0 Dietary **folate deficiency anemia**

Nutritional megaloblastic anemia

D52.1 Drug-induced **folate deficiency anemia**

Use additional code for adverse effect, if applicable, to identify drug (T36-T50 with fifth or sixth character 5)

D52.8 Other folate deficiency anemias

D52.9 Folate deficiency anemia, unspecified

Folic acid deficiency anemia NOS

🔵 **D53** Other nutritional anemias

INCLUDES   megaloblastic anemia unresponsive to vitamin B12 or folate therapy

D53.0 Protein **deficiency anemia**

Amino-acid deficiency anemia

Orotaciduric anemia

EXCLUDES1   *Lesch-Nyhan syndrome (E79.1)*

D53.1 Other megaloblastic **anemias, not elsewhere classified**

Megaloblastic anemia NOS

EXCLUDES1   *Di Guglielmo's disease (C94.0)*

D53.2 Scorbutic **anemia**

EXCLUDES1   *scurvy (E54)*

D53.8 Other specified nutritional anemias

Anemia associated with deficiency of copper

Anemia associated with deficiency of molybdenum

Anemia associated with deficiency of zinc

EXCLUDES1   *nutritional deficiencies without anemia, such as:*
copper deficiency NOS (E61.0)
molybdenum deficiency NOS (E61.5)
zinc deficiency NOS (E60)

D53.9 Nutritional anemia, unspecified

Simple chronic anemia

EXCLUDES1   *anemia NOS (D64.9)*

Hemolytic anemias (D55-D59)

🔵 **D55** Anemia due to enzyme disorders

EXCLUDES1   *drug-induced enzyme deficiency anemia (D59.2)*

D55.0 Anemia due to glucose-6-phosphate dehydrogenase **[G6PD] deficiency**

Favism

G6PD deficiency anemia

D55.1 Anemia due to other disorders of glutathione metabolism

Anemia (due to) enzyme deficiencies, except G6PD, related to the hexose monophosphate [HMP] shunt pathway

Anemia (due to) hemolytic nonspherocytic (hereditary), type I

D55.2 Anemia due to disorders of glycolytic enzymes

Hemolytic nonspherocytic (hereditary) anemia, type II

Hexokinase deficiency anemia

Pyruvate kinase [PK] deficiency anemia

Triose-phosphate isomerase deficiency anemia

EXCLUDES1   *disorders of glycolysis not associated with anemia (E74.8)*

D55.3 Anemia due to disorders of nucleotide metabolism

D55.8 Other anemias due to enzyme disorders

D55.9 Anemia due to enzyme disorder, unspecified

🔵 **D56** Thalassemia

EXCLUDES1   *sickle-cell thalassemia (D57.4-)*

D56.0 Alpha **thalassemia**

Alpha thalassemia major

Hemoglobin H Constant Spring

Hemoglobin H disease

Hydrops fetalis due to alpha thalassemia

Severe alpha thalassemia

Triple gene defect alpha thalassemia

Use additional code, if applicable, for hydrops fetalis due to alpha thalassemia (P56.99)

EXCLUDES1   *alpha thalassemia trait or minor (D56.3)*
asymptomatic alpha thalassemia (D56.3)
hydrops fetalis due to isoimmunization (P56.0)
hydrops fetalis not due to immune hemolysis (P83.2)

Unspecified Code	Other Specified Code	Ⓝ Newborn Age: 0	Ⓟ Pediatric Age: 0-17	Ⓜ Maternity Age: 12-55
Ⓐ Adult Age: 15-124	♂ Male	♀ Female	● New Code	▲ Revised Code Title ►◄ Revised Text

D56.1 Beta **thalassemia**
Beta thalassemia major
Cooley's anemia
Homozygous beta thalassemia
Severe beta thalassemia
Thalassemia intermedia
Thalassemia major
EXCLUDES1 *beta thalassemia minor (D56.3)*
beta thalassemia trait (D56.3)
delta-beta thalassemia (D56.2)
hemoglobin E-beta thalassemia (D56.5)
sickle-cell beta thalassemia (D57.4-)

D56.2 Delta-beta **thalassemia**
Homozygous delta-beta thalassemia
EXCLUDES1 *delta-beta thalassemia minor (D56.3)*
delta-beta thalassemia trait (D56.3)

D56.3 **Thalassemia** minor
Alpha thalassemia minor
Alpha thalassemia silent carrier
Alpha thalassemia trait
Beta thalassemia minor
Beta thalassemia trait
Delta-beta thalassemia minor
Delta-beta thalassemia trait
Thalassemia trait NOS
EXCLUDES1 *alpha thalassemia (D56.0)*
beta thalassemia (D56.1)
delta-beta thalassemia (D56.2)
hemoglobin E-beta thalassemia (D56.5)
sickle-cell trait (D57.3)

D56.4 Hereditary persistence of fetal hemoglobin **[HPFH]**

D56.5 Hemoglobin E-beta **thalassemia**
EXCLUDES1 *beta thalassemia (D56.1)*
beta thalassemia minor (D56.3)
beta thalassemia trait (D56.3)
delta-beta thalassemia (D56.2)
delta-beta thalassemia trait (D56.3)
hemoglobin E disease (D58.2)
other hemoglobinopathies (D58.2)
sickle-cell beta thalassemia (D57.4-)

D56.8 **Other thalassemias**
Dominant thalassemia
Hemoglobin C thalassemia
Mixed thalassemia
Thalassemia with other hemoglobinopathy
EXCLUDES1 *hemoglobin C disease (D58.2)*
hemoglobin E disease (D58.2)
other hemoglobinopathies (D58.2)
sickle-cell anemia (D57.-)
sickle-cell thalassemia (D57.4)

D56.9 **Thalassemia, unspecified**
Mediterranean anemia (with other hemoglobinopathy)

④ D57 **Sickle-cell disorders**
Use additional code for any associated fever (R50.81)
EXCLUDES1 *other hemoglobinopathies (D58.-)*

⑤ D57.0 Hb-SS **disease** with crisis
Sickle-cell disease NOS with crisis
Hb-SS disease with vasoocclusive pain
D57.00 **Hb-SS disease with crisis, unspecified**
D57.01 **Hb-SS disease with** acute chest syndrome
D57.02 **Hb-SS disease with** splenic sequestration

D57.1 **Sickle-cell disease** without crisis
Hb-SS disease without crisis
Sickle-cell anemia NOS
Sickle-cell disease NOS
Sickle-cell disorder NOS

⑤ D57.2 **Sickle-cell/**Hb-C **disease**

Hb-SC disease
Hb-S/Hb-C disease
D57.20 **Sickle-cell/Hb-C disease** without crisis
⑥ D57.21 **Sickle-cell/Hb-C disease** with crisis
D57.211 **Sickle-cell/Hb-C disease with** acute chest syndrome
D57.212 **Sickle-cell/Hb-C disease with** splenic sequestration
D57.219 **Sickle-cell/Hb-C disease with crisis, unspecified**
Sickle-cell/Hb-C disease with crisis NOS

D57.3 **Sickle-cell** trait
Hb-S trait
Heterozygous hemoglobin S

⑤ D57.4 **Sickle-cell** thalassemia
Sickle-cell beta thalassemia
Thalassemia Hb-S disease
D57.40 **Sickle-cell thalassemia** without crisis
Microdrepanocytosis
Sickle-cell thalassemia NOS
⑥ D57.41 **Sickle-cell thalassemia** with crisis
Sickle-cell thalassemia with vasoocclusive pain
D57.411 **Sickle-cell thalassemia with** acute chest syndrome
D57.412 **Sickle-cell thalassemia with** splenic sequestration
D57.419 **Sickle-cell thalassemia with crisis, unspecified**
Sickle-cell thalassemia with crisis NOS

⑤ D57.8 **Other sickle-cell disorders**
Hb-SD disease
Hb-SE disease
D57.80 **Other sickle-cell disorders** without crisis
⑥ D57.81 **Other sickle-cell disorders** with crisis
D57.811 **Other sickle-cell disorders with** acute chest syndrome
D57.812 **Other sickle-cell disorders with** splenic sequestration
D57.819 **Other sickle-cell disorders with crisis, unspecified**
Other sickle-cell disorders with crisis NOS

④ D58 Other hereditary **hemolytic anemias**
EXCLUDES1 *hemolytic anemia of the newborn (P55.-)*

D58.0 **Hereditary** spherocytosis
Acholuric (familial) jaundice
Congenital (spherocytic) hemolytic icterus
Minkowski-Chauffard syndrome

D58.1 **Hereditary** elliptocytosis
Elliptocytosis (congenital)
Ovalocytosis (congenital) (hereditary)

D58.2 **Other** hemoglobinopathies
Abnormal hemoglobin NOS
Congenital Heinz body anemia
Hb-C disease
Hb-D disease
Hb-E disease
Hemoglobinopathy NOS
Unstable hemoglobin hemolytic disease
EXCLUDES1 *familial polycythemia (D75.0)*
Hb-M disease (D74.0)
hemoglobin E-beta thalassemia (D56.5)
hereditary persistence of fetal hemoglobin [HPFH] (D56.4)
high-altitude polycythemia (D75.1)
methemoglobinemia (D74.-)
other hemoglobinopathies with thalassemia (D56.8)

---

④ 4th character required	⑤ 5th character required	⑥ 6th character required	⑦ 7th character required	⑩ Extension 'X' Alert
	EXCLUDES 1 Not coded here	EXCLUDES 2 Not included here	PDx Primary Diagnosis Only	Manifestation Code

D58.8 Other specified hereditary hemolytic anemias
Stomatocytosis
D58.9 Hereditary hemolytic anemia, unspecified

[4] D59 Acquired hemolytic anemia
D59.0 Drug-induced autoimmune hemolytic anemia
Use additional code for adverse effect, if applicable, to identify drug (T36-T50 with fifth or sixth character 5)
D59.1 Other autoimmune hemolytic anemias
Autoimmune hemolytic disease (cold type) (warm type)
Chronic cold hemagglutinin disease
Cold agglutinin disease
Cold agglutinin hemoglobinuria
Cold type (secondary) (symptomatic) hemolytic anemia
Warm type (secondary) (symptomatic) hemolytic anemia
[EXCLUDES1] *Evans syndrome (D69.41)*
hemolytic disease of newborn (P55.-)
paroxysmal cold hemoglobinuria (D59.6)
D59.2 Drug-induced nonautoimmune hemolytic anemia
Drug-induced enzyme deficiency anemia
Use additional code for adverse effect, if applicable, to identify drug (T36-T50 with fifth or sixth character 5)
D59.3 Hemolytic-uremic syndrome
Use additional code to identify associated:
E. coli infection (B96.2-)
Pneumococcal pneumonia (J13)
Shigella dysenteriae (A03.9)
D59.4 Other nonautoimmune hemolytic anemias
Mechanical hemolytic anemia
Microangiopathic hemolytic anemia
Toxic hemolytic anemia
D59.5 Paroxysmal nocturnal hemoglobinuria [Marchiafava-Micheli]
[EXCLUDES1] *hemoglobinuria NOS (R82.3)*
D59.6 Hemoglobinuria due to hemolysis from other external causes
Hemoglobinuria from exertion
March hemoglobinuria
Paroxysmal cold hemoglobinuria
Use additional code (Chapter 20) to identify external cause
[EXCLUDES1] *hemoglobinuria NOS (R82.3)*
D59.8 Other acquired hemolytic anemias
D59.9 Acquired hemolytic anemia, unspecified
Idiopathic hemolytic anemia, chronic

Aplastic and other anemias and other bone marrow failure syndromes (D60-D64)

[4] D60 Acquired pure red cell aplasia [erythroblastopenia]
[INCLUDES] *red cell aplasia (acquired) (adult) (with thymoma)*
[EXCLUDES1] *congenital red cell aplasia (D61.01)*
D60.0 Chronic acquired pure red cell aplasia
D60.1 Transient acquired pure red cell aplasia
D60.8 Other acquired pure red cell aplasias
D60.9 Acquired pure red cell aplasia, unspecified

[4] D61 Other aplastic anemias and other bone marrow failure syndromes
[EXCLUDES1] *neutropenia (D70.-)*
[5] D61.0 Constitutional aplastic anemia
D61.01 Constitutional (pure) red blood cell aplasia
Blackfan-Diamond syndrome
Congenital (pure) red cell aplasia
Familial hypoplastic anemia
Primary (pure) red cell aplasia
Red cell (pure) aplasia of infants
[EXCLUDES1] *acquired red cell aplasia (D60.9)*
D61.09 Other constitutional aplastic anemia
Fanconi's anemia
Pancytopenia with malformations
D61.1 Drug-induced aplastic anemia
Use additional code for adverse effect, if applicable, to identify drug (T36-T50 with fifth or sixth character 5)
D61.2 Aplastic anemia due to other external agents
Code first , if applicable, toxic effects of substances chiefly nonmedicinal as to source (T51-T65)
D61.3 Idiopathic aplastic anemia
[5] D61.8 Other specified aplastic anemias and other bone marrow failure syndromes
[6] D61.81 Pancytopenia
[EXCLUDES1] *pancytopenia (due to) (with) aplastic anemia (D61.9)*
pancytopenia (due to) (with) bone marrow infiltration (D61.82)
pancytopenia (due to) (with) congenital (pure) red cell aplasia (D61.01)
pancytopenia (due to) (with) hairy cell leukemia (C91.4-)
pancytopenia (due to) (with) human immunodeficiency virus disease (B20.-)
pancytopenia (due to) (with) leukoerythroblastic anemia (D61.82)
pancytopenia (due to) (with) myelodysplastic syndromes (D46.-)
pancytopenia (due to) (with) myeloproliferative disease (D47.1)
D61.810 Antineoplastic chemotherapy induced pancytopenia
[EXCLUDES2] *aplastic anemia due to antineoplastic chemotherapy (D61.1)*
D61.811 Other drug-induced pancytopenia
[EXCLUDES2] *aplastic anemia due to drugs (D61.1)*
D61.818 Other pancytopenia
D61.82 Myelophthisis
Leukoerythroblastic anemia
Myelophthisic anemia
Panmyelophthisis
Code also the underlying disorder, such as:
malignant neoplasm of breast (C50.-)
tuberculosis (A15.-)
[EXCLUDES1] *idiopathic myelofibrosis (D47.1)*
myelofibrosis NOS (D75.81)
myelofibrosis with myeloid metaplasia (D47.4)
primary myelofibrosis (D47.1)
secondary myelofibrosis (D75.81)
D61.89 Other specified aplastic anemias and other bone marrow failure syndromes
D61.9 Aplastic anemia, unspecified
Hypoplastic anemia NOS
Medullary hypoplasia

D62 Acute posthemorrhagic anemia
[EXCLUDES1] *anemia due to chronic blood loss (D50.0)*
blood loss anemia NOS (D50.0)
congenital anemia from fetal blood loss (P61.3)

[4] D63 Anemia in chronic diseases classified elsewhere
D63.0 Anemia in neoplastic disease
Code first neoplasm (C00-D49)
[EXCLUDES1] *anemia due to antineoplastic chemotherapy (D64.81)*
aplastic anemia due to antineoplastic chemotherapy (D61.1)
D63.1 Anemia in chronic kidney disease
Erythropoietin resistant anemia (EPO resistant anemia)
Code first underlying chronic kidney disease (CKD) (N18.-)

Unspecified Code | Other Specified Code | [N] Newborn Age: 0 | [P] Pediatric Age: 0-17 | [M] Maternity Age: 12-55
[A] Adult Age: 15-124 | ♂ Male | ♀ Female | ● New Code | ▲ Revised Code Title | ►◄ Revised Text

D63.8 Anemia in other chronic diseases classified elsewhere

Code first underlying disease, such as:
diphyllobothriasis (B70.0)
hookworm disease (B76.0-B76.9)
hypothyroidism (E00.0-E03.9)
malaria (B50.0-B54)
symptomatic late syphilis (A52.79)
tuberculosis (A18.89)

[4] **D64 Other anemias**

[EXCLUDES1] *refractory anemia (D46.-)*
refractory anemia with excess blasts in transformation [RAEB T] (C92.0-)

D64.0 Hereditary sideroblastic anemia

Sex-linked hypochromic sideroblastic anemia

D64.1 Secondary sideroblastic anemia due to disease

Code first underlying disease

D64.2 Secondary sideroblastic anemia due to drugs and toxins

Code first poisoning due to drug or toxin, if applicable (T36-T65 with fifth or sixth character 1-4 or 6)
Use additional code for adverse effect, if applicable, to identify drug (T36-T50 with fifth or sixth character 5)

D64.3 Other sideroblastic anemias

Sideroblastic anemia NOS
Pyridoxine-responsive sideroblastic anemia NEC

D64.4 Congenital dyserythropoietic anemia

Dyshematopoietic anemia (congenital)

[EXCLUDES1] *Blackfan-Diamond syndrome (D61.01)*
Di Guglielmo's disease (C94.0)

[5] **D64.8 Other specified anemias**

D64.81 Anemia due to antineoplastic chemotherapy

Antineoplastic chemotherapy induced anemia

[EXCLUDES1] *anemia in neoplastic disease (D63.0)*
aplastic anemia due to antineoplastic chemotherapy (D61.1)

D64.89 Other specified anemias

Infantile pseudoleukemia

D64.9 Anemia, unspecified

Coagulation defects, purpura and other hemorrhagic conditions (D65-D69)

D65 Disseminated intravascular coagulation [defibrination syndrome]

Afibrinogenemia, acquired
Consumption coagulopathy
Diffuse or disseminated intravascular coagulation [DIC]
Fibrinolytic hemorrhage, acquired
Fibrinolytic purpura
Purpura fulminans

[EXCLUDES1] *disseminated intravascular coagulation (complicating):*
abortion or ectopic or molar pregnancy (O00-O07, O08.1)
in newborn (P60)
pregnancy, childbirth and the puerperium (O45.0, O46.0, O67.0, O72.3)

D66 Hereditary factor VIII deficiency

Classical hemophilia
Deficiency factor VIII (with functional defect)
Hemophilia NOS
Hemophilia A

[EXCLUDES1] *factor VIII deficiency with vascular defect (D68.0)*

D67 Hereditary factor IX deficiency

Christmas disease
Factor IX deficiency (with functional defect)
Hemophilia B
Plasma thromboplastin component [PTC] deficiency

[4] **D68 Other coagulation defects**

[EXCLUDES1] *abnormal coagulation profile (R79.1)*
coagulation defects complicating abortion or ectopic or molar pregnancy (O00-O07, O08.1)
coagulation defects complicating pregnancy, childbirth and the puerperium (O45.0, O46.0, O67.0, O72.3)

D68.0 Von Willebrand's disease

Angiohemophilia
Factor VIII deficiency with vascular defect
Vascular hemophilia

[EXCLUDES1] *capillary fragility (hereditary) (D69.8)*
factor VIII deficiency NOS (D66)
factor VIII deficiency with functional defect (D66)

D68.1 Hereditary factor XI deficiency

Hemophilia C
Plasma thromboplastin antecedent [PTA] deficiency
Rosenthal's disease

D68.2 Hereditary deficiency of other clotting factors

AC globulin deficiency
Congenital afibrinogenemia
Deficiency of factor I [fibrinogen]
Deficiency of factor II [prothrombin]
Deficiency of factor V [labile]
Deficiency of factor VII [stable]
Deficiency of factor X [Stuart-Prower]
Deficiency of factor XII [Hageman]
Deficiency of factor XIII [fibrin stabilizing]
Dysfibrinogenemia (congenital)
Hypoproconvertinemia
Owren's disease
Proaccelerin deficiency

[5] **D68.3 Hemorrhagic disorder due to circulating anticoagulants**

[6] **D68.31 Hemorrhagic disorder due to intrinsic circulating anticoagulants, antibodies, or inhibitors**

D68.311 Acquired hemophilia

Autoimmune hemophilia
Autoimmune inhibitors to clotting factors
Secondary hemophilia

D68.312 Antiphospholipid antibody with hemorrhagic disorder

Lupus anticoagulant (LAC) with hemorrhagic disorder
Systemic lupus erythematosus [SLE] inhibitor with hemorrhagic disorder

[EXCLUDES1] *antiphospholipid antibody, finding without diagnosis (R76.0)*
antiphospholipid antibody syndrome (D68.61)
antiphospholipid antibody with hypercoagulable state (D68.61)
lupus anticoagulant (LAC) finding without diagnosis (R76.0)
lupus anticoagulant (LAC) with hypercoagulable state (D68.62)
systemic lupus erythematosus [SLE] inhibitor finding without diagnosis (R76.0)
systemic lupus erythematosus [SLE] inhibitor with hypercoagulable state (D68.62)

D68.318 Other hemorrhagic disorder due to intrinsic circulating anticoagulants, antibodies, or inhibitors

Antithromboplastinemia
Antithromboplastinogenemia
Hemorrhagic disorder due to intrinsic increase in antithrombin
Hemorrhagic disorder due to intrinsic

increase in anti-VIIIa
Hemorrhagic disorder due to intrinsic increase in anti-IXa
Hemorrhagic disorder due to intrinsic increase in anti-XIa

D68.32 Hemorrhagic disorder due to extrinsic circulating anticoagulants
Drug-induced hemorrhagic disorder
Hemorrhagic disorder due to increase in anti-IIa
Hemorrhagic disorder due to increase in anti-Xa
Hyperheparinemia
Use additional code for adverse effect, if applicable, to identify drug (T45.515, T45.525)

D68.4 Acquired coagulation factor deficiency
Deficiency of coagulation factor due to liver disease
Deficiency of coagulation factor due to vitamin K deficiency
EXCLUDES1 *vitamin K deficiency of newborn (P53)*

[5] **D68.5 Primary thrombophilia**
Primary hypercoagulable states
EXCLUDES1 *antiphospholipid syndrome (D68.61)*
lupus anticoagulant (D68.62)
secondary activated protein C resistance (D68.69)
secondary antiphospholipid antibody syndrome (D68.69)
secondary lupus anticoagulant with hypercoagulable state (D68.69)
secondary systemic lupus erythematosus [SLE] inhibitor with hypercoagulable state (D68.69)
systemic lupus erythematosus [SLE] inhibitor finding without diagnosis (R76.0)
systemic lupus erythematosus [SLE] inhibitor with hemorrhagic disorder (D68.312)
thrombotic thrombocytopenic purpura (M31.1)

D68.51 Activated protein C resistance
Factor V Leiden mutation

D68.52 Prothrombin gene mutation

D68.59 Other primary thrombophilia
Antithrombin III deficiency
Hypercoagulable state NOS
Primary hypercoagulable state NEC
Primary thrombophilia NEC
Protein C deficiency
Protein S deficiency
Thrombophilia NOS

[5] **D68.6 Other thrombophilia**
Other hypercoagulable states
EXCLUDES1 *diffuse or disseminated intravascular coagulation [DIC] (D65)*
heparin induced thrombocytopenia (HIT) (D75.82)
hyperhomocysteinemia (E72.11)

D68.61 Antiphospholipid syndrome
Anticardiolipin syndrome
Antiphospholipid antibody syndrome
EXCLUDES1 *anti-phospholipid antibody, finding without diagnosis (R76.0)*
anti-phospholipid antibody with hemorrhagic disorder (D68.312)
lupus anticoagulant syndrome (D68.62)

D68.62 Lupus anticoagulant syndrome
Lupus anticoagulant
Presence of systemic lupus erythematosus [SLE] inhibitor
EXCLUDES1 *anticardiolipin syndrome (D68.61)*
antiphospholipid syndrome (D68.61)
lupus anticoagulant (LAC) finding without diagnosis (R79.0)
lupus anticoagulant (LAC) with hemorrhagic disorder (D68.312)

D68.69 Other thrombophilia
Hypercoagulable states NEC
Secondary hypercoagulable state NOS

D68.8 Other specified coagulation defects
EXCLUDES1 *hemorrhagic disease of newborn (P53)*

D68.9 Coagulation defect, unspecified

[4] **D69 Purpura and other hemorrhagic conditions**
EXCLUDES1 *benign hypergammaglobulinemic purpura (D89.0)*
cryoglobulinemic purpura (D89.1)
essential (hemorrhagic) thrombocythemia (D47.3)
hemorrhagic thrombocythemia (D47.3)
purpura fulminans (D65)
thrombotic thrombocytopenic purpura (M31.1)
Waldenström hypergammaglobulinemic purpura (D89.0)

D69.0 Allergic purpura
Allergic vasculitis
Nonthrombocytopenic hemorrhagic purpura
Nonthrombocytopenic idiopathic purpura
Purpura anaphylactoid
Purpura Henoch(-Schönlein)
Purpura rheumatica
Vascular purpura
EXCLUDES1 *thrombocytopenic hemorrhagic purpura (D69.3)*

D69.1 Qualitative platelet defects
Bernard-Soulier [giant platelet] syndrome
Glanzmann's disease
Grey platelet syndrome
Thromboasthenia (hemorrhagic) (hereditary)
Thrombocytopathy
EXCLUDES1 *von Willebrand's disease (D68.0)*

D69.2 Other nonthrombocytopenic purpura
Purpura NOS
Purpura simplex
Senile purpura

D69.3 Immune thrombocytopenic purpura
Hemorrhagic (thrombocytopenic) purpura
Idiopathic thrombocytopenic purpura
Tidal platelet dysgenesis

[5] **D69.4 Other primary thrombocytopenia**
EXCLUDES1 *transient neonatal thrombocytopenia (P61.0)*
Wiskott-Aldrich syndrome (D82.0)

D69.41 Evans syndrome

D69.42 Congenital and hereditary thrombocytopenia purpura
Congenital thrombocytopenia
Hereditary thrombocytopenia
Code first congenital or hereditary disorder, such as: thrombocytopenia with absent radius (TAR syndrome) (Q87.2)

D69.49 Other primary thrombocytopenia
Megakaryocytic hypoplasia
Primary thrombocytopenia NOS

[5] **D69.5 Secondary thrombocytopenia**
EXCLUDES1 *heparin induced thrombocytopenia (HIT) (D75.82)*
transient thrombocytopenia of newborn (P61.0)

D69.51 Posttransfusion purpura
Posttransfusion purpura from whole blood (fresh) or blood products
PTP

D69.59 Other secondary thrombocytopenia

D69.6 Thrombocytopenia, unspecified

Unspecified Code | Other Specified Code | [N] Newborn Age: 0 | [P] Pediatric Age: 0-17 | [M] Maternity Age: 12-55
[A] Adult Age: 15-124 | ♂ Male | ♀ Female | ● New Code | ▲ Revised Code Title | ►◄ Revised Text

D69.8 Other specified hemorrhagic conditions
Capillary fragility (hereditary)
Vascular pseudohemophilia
D69.9 Hemorrhagic condition, unspecified

Other disorders of blood and blood-forming organs (D70-D77)

[4] **D70 Neutropenia**
INCLUDES *agranulocytosis*
decreased absolute neurophile count (ANC)
Use additional code for any associated:
fever (R50.81)
mucositis (J34.81, K12.3-, K92.81, N76.81)
EXCLUDES1 *neutropenic splenomegaly (D73.81)*
transient neonatal neutropenia (P61.5)
D70.0 Congenital agranulocytosis
Congenital neutropenia
Infantile genetic agranulocytosis
Kostmann's disease
D70.1 Agranulocytosis secondary to cancer chemotherapy
Use additional code for adverse effect, if applicable, to identify drug (T45.1X5)
Code also underlying neoplasm
D70.2 Other drug-induced agranulocytosis
Use additional code for adverse effect, if applicable, to identify drug (T36-T50 with fifth or sixth character 5)
D70.3 Neutropenia due to infection
D70.4 Cyclic neutropenia
Cyclic hematopoiesis
Periodic neutropenia
D70.8 Other neutropenia
D70.9 Neutropenia, unspecified
D71 Functional disorders of polymorphonuclear neutrophils
Cell membrane receptor complex [CR3] defect
Chronic (childhood) granulomatous disease
Congenital dysphagocytosis
Progressive septic granulomatosis
[4] **D72 Other disorders of white blood cells**
EXCLUDES1 *basophilia (D72.824)*
immunity disorders (D80-D89)
neutropenia (D70)
preleukemia (syndrome) (D46.9)
D72.0 Genetic anomalies of leukocytes
Alder (granulation) (granulocyte) anomaly
Alder syndrome
Hereditary leukocytic hypersegmentation
Hereditary leukocytic hyposegmentation
Hereditary leukomelanopathy
May-Hegglin (granulation) (granulocyte) anomaly
May-Hegglin syndrome
Pelger-Huët (granulation) (granulocyte) anomaly
Pelger-Huët syndrome
EXCLUDES1 *Chédiak (-Steinbrinck)-Higashi syndrome (E70.330)*
D72.1 Eosinophilia
Allergic eosinophilia
Hereditary eosinophilia
EXCLUDES1 *Löffler's syndrome (J82)*
pulmonary eosinophilia (J82)
[5] **D72.8 Other specified disorders of white blood cells**
EXCLUDES1 *leukemia (C91-C95)*
[6] **D72.81 Decreased white blood cell count**
EXCLUDES1 *neutropenia (D70.-)*
D72.810 Lymphocytopenia
Decreased lymphocytes
D72.818 Other decreased white blood cell count
Basophilic leukopenia
Eosinophilic leukopenia
Monocytopenia
Other decreased leukocytes
Plasmacytopenia
D72.819 Decreased white blood cell count, unspecified
Decreased leukocytes, unspecified
Leukocytopenia, unspecified
Leukopenia
EXCLUDES1 *malignant leukopenia (D70.9)*
[6] **D72.82 Elevated white blood cell count**
EXCLUDES1 *eosinophilia (D72.1)*
D72.820 Lymphocytosis (symptomatic)
Elevated lymphocytes
D72.821 Monocytosis (symptomatic)
EXCLUDES1 *infectious mononucleosis (B27.-)*
D72.822 Plasmacytosis
D72.823 Leukemoid reaction
Basophilic leukemoid reaction
Leukemoid reaction NOS
Lymphocytic leukemoid reaction
Monocytic leukemoid reaction
Myelocytic leukemoid reaction
Neutrophilic leukemoid reaction
D72.824 Basophilia
D72.825 Bandemia
Bandemia without diagnosis of specific infection
EXCLUDES1 *confirmed infection - code to infection*
leukemia (C91.-, C92.-, C93.-, C94.-, C95.-)
D72.828 Other elevated white blood cell count
D72.829 Elevated white blood cell count, unspecified
Elevated leukocytes, unspecified
Leukocytosis, unspecified
D72.89 Other specified disorders of white blood cells
Abnormality of white blood cells NEC
D72.9 Disorder of white blood cells, unspecified
Abnormal leukocyte differential NOS
[4] **D73 Diseases of spleen**
D73.0 Hyposplenism
Atrophy of spleen
EXCLUDES1 *asplenia (congenital) (Q89.01)*
postsurgical absence of spleen (Z90.81)
D73.1 Hypersplenism
EXCLUDES1 *neutropenic splenomegaly (D73.81)*
primary splenic neutropenia (D73.81)
splenitis, splenomegaly in late syphilis (A52.79)
splenitis, splenomegaly in tuberculosis (A18.85)
splenomegaly NOS (R16.1)
splenomegaly congenital (Q89.0)
D73.2 Chronic congestive splenomegaly
D73.3 Abscess of spleen
D73.4 Cyst of spleen
D73.5 Infarction of spleen
Splenic rupture, nontraumatic
Torsion of spleen
EXCLUDES1 *rupture of spleen due to Plasmodium vivax malaria (B51.0)*
traumatic rupture of spleen (S36.03-)
[5] **D73.8 Other diseases of spleen**
D73.81 Neutropenic splenomegaly
Werner-Schultz disease
D73.89 Other diseases of spleen

Fibrosis of spleen NOS
Perisplenitis
Splenitis NOS

D73.9 Disease of spleen, unspecified

[4] **D74 Methemoglobinemia**

D74.0 Congenital methemoglobinemia
Congenital NADH-methemoglobin reductase deficiency
Hemoglobin-M [Hb-M] disease
Methemoglobinemia, hereditary

D74.8 Other methemoglobinemias
Acquired methemoglobinemia (with sulfhemoglobinemia)
Toxic methemoglobinemia

D74.9 Methemoglobinemia, unspecified

[4] **D75 Other and unspecified diseases of blood and blood-forming organs**

[EXCLUDES2] *acute lymphadenitis (L04.-)*
chronic lymphadenitis (I88.1)
enlarged lymph nodes (R59.-)
hypergammaglobulinemia NOS (D89.2)
lymphadenitis NOS (I88.9)
mesenteric lymphadenitis (acute) (chronic) (I88.0)

D75.0 Familial erythrocytosis
Benign polycythemia
Familial polycythemia
[EXCLUDES1] *hereditary ovalocytosis (D58.1)*

D75.1 Secondary polycythemia
Acquired polycythemia
Emotional polycythemia
Erythrocytosis NOS
Hypoxemic polycythemia
Nephrogenous polycythemia
Polycythemia due to erythropoietin
Polycythemia due to fall in plasma volume
Polycythemia due to high altitude
Polycythemia due to stress
Polycythemia NOS
Relative polycythemia
[EXCLUDES1] *polycythemia neonatorum (P61.1)*
polycythemia vera (D45)

[5] **D75.8 Other specified diseases of blood and blood-forming organs**

D75.81 Myelofibrosis
Myelofibrosis NOS
Secondary myelofibrosis NOS
Code first the underlying disorder, such as:
malignant neoplasm of breast (C50.-)
Use additional code, if applicable, for associated therapy-related myelodysplastic syndrome (D46.-)
code for adverse effect, if applicable, to identify drug (T45.1X5)
[EXCLUDES1] *acute myelofibrosis (C94.4-)*
idiopathic myelofibrosis (D47.1)
leukoerythroblastic anemia (D61.82)
myelofibrosis with myeloid metaplasia (D47.4)
myelophthisic anemia (D61.82)
myelophthisis (D61.82)
primary myelofibrosis (D47.1)

D75.82 Heparin induced thrombocytopenia (HIT)

D75.89 Other specified diseases of blood and blood-forming organs

D75.9 Disease of blood and blood-forming organs, unspecified

[4] **D76 Other specified diseases with participation of lymphoreticular and reticulohistiocytic tissue**

[EXCLUDES1] *(Abt-) Letterer-Siwe disease (C96.0)*
eosinophilic granuloma (C96.6)
Hand-Schüller-Christian disease (C96.5)
histiocytic sarcoma (C96.A)
histiocytosis X, multifocal (C96.5)
histiocytosis X, unifocal (C96.6)
malignant histiocytosis (C96.A)
Langerhans-cell histiocytosis, multifocal (C96.5)
Langerhans-cell histiocytosis NOS (C96.6)
Langerhans-cell histiocytosis, unifocal (C96.6)
leukemic reticuloendotheliosis or reticulosis (C91.4-)
lipomelanotic reticuloendotheliosis or reticulosis (I89.8)

D76.1 Hemophagocytic lymphohistiocytosis
Familial hemophagocytic reticulosis
Histiocytoses of mononuclear phagocytes

D76.2 Hemophagocytic syndrome, infection-associated
Use additional code to identify infectious agent or disease.

D76.3 Other histiocytosis syndromes
Reticulohistiocytoma (giant-cell)
Sinus histiocytosis with massive lymphadenopathy
Xanthogranuloma

D77 Other disorders of blood and blood-forming organs in diseases classified elsewhere
Code first underlying disease, such as:
amyloidosis (E85.-)
congenital early syphilis (A50.0)
echinococcosis (B67.0-B67.9)
malaria (B50.0-B54)
schistosomiasis [bilharziasis] (B65.0-B65.9)
vitamin C deficiency (E54)
[EXCLUDES1] *rupture of spleen due to Plasmodium vivax malaria (B51.0)*
splenitis, splenomegaly in late syphilis (A52.79)
splenitis, splenomegaly in tuberculosis (A18.85)

Intraoperative and postprocedural complications of the spleen (D78)

[4] **D78 Intraoperative and postprocedural complications of the spleen**

[5] **D78.0 Intraoperative hemorrhage and hematoma of the spleen complicating a procedure**
[EXCLUDES1] *intraoperative hemorrhage and hematoma of the spleen due to accidental puncture or laceration during a procedure (D78.1-)*

D78.01 Intraoperative hemorrhage and hematoma of the spleen complicating a procedure on the spleen

D78.02 Intraoperative hemorrhage and hematoma of the spleen complicating other procedure

[5] **D78.1 Accidental puncture and laceration of the spleen during a procedure**

D78.11 Accidental puncture and laceration of the spleen during a procedure on the spleen

D78.12 Accidental puncture and laceration of the spleen during other procedure

[5] **D78.2 Postprocedural hemorrhage and hematoma of the spleen following a procedure**

D78.21 Postprocedural hemorrhage and hematoma of the spleen following a procedure on the spleen

D78.22 Postprocedural hemorrhage and hematoma of the spleen following other procedure

[5] **D78.8 Other intraoperative and postprocedural complications of the spleen**
Use additional code, if applicable, to further specify disorder

D78.81 Other intraoperative complications of the spleen

D78.89 Other postprocedural complications of the spleen

Unspecified Code | Other Specified Code | [N] Newborn Age: 0 | [P] Pediatric Age: 0-17 | [M] Maternity Age: 12-55
[A] Adult Age: 15-124 | ♂ Male | ♀ Female | ● New Code | ▲ Revised Code Title | ►◄ Revised Text

Certain disorders involving the immune mechanism (D80-D89)

[INCLUDES] *defects in the complement system*
immunodeficiency disorders, except human immunodeficiency virus [HIV] disease
sarcoidosis

[EXCLUDES1] *autoimmune disease (systemic) NOS (M35.9)*
functional disorders of polymorphonuclear neutrophils (D71)
human immunodeficiency virus [HIV] disease (B20)

[4] **D80 Immunodeficiency with predominantly antibody defects**

D80.0 Hereditary hypogammaglobulinemia
Autosomal recessive agammaglobulinemia (Swiss type)
X-linked agammaglobulinemia [Bruton] (with growth hormone deficiency)

D80.1 Nonfamilial hypogammaglobulinemia
Agammaglobulinemia with immunoglobulin-bearing B-lymphocytes
Common variable agammaglobulinemia [CVAgamma]
Hypogammaglobulinemia NOS

D80.2 Selective deficiency of immunoglobulin A [IgA]

D80.3 Selective deficiency of immunoglobulin G [IgG] subclasses

D80.4 Selective deficiency of immunoglobulin M [IgM]

D80.5 Immunodeficiency with increased immunoglobulin M [IgM]

D80.6 Antibody deficiency with near-normal immunoglobulins or with hyperimmunoglobulinemia

D80.7 Transient hypogammaglobulinemia of infancy [N]

D80.8 Other immunodeficiencies with predominantly antibody defects
Kappa light chain deficiency

D80.9 Immunodeficiency with predominantly antibody defects, unspecified

[4] **D81 Combined immunodeficiencies**

[EXCLUDES1] *autosomal recessive agammaglobulinemia (Swiss type) (D80.0)*

D81.0 Severe combined immunodeficiency [SCID] with reticular dysgenesis

D81.1 Severe combined immunodeficiency [SCID] with low T- and B-cell numbers

D81.2 Severe combined immunodeficiency [SCID] with low or normal B-cell numbers

D81.3 Adenosine deaminase [ADA] deficiency

D81.4 Nezelof's syndrome

D81.5 Purine nucleoside phosphorylase [PNP] deficiency

D81.6 Major histocompatibility complex class I deficiency
Bare lymphocyte syndrome

D81.7 Major histocompatibility complex class II deficiency

[5] **D81.8 Other combined immunodeficiencies**

[6] **D81.81 Biotin-dependent carboxylase deficiency**
Multiple carboxylase deficiency

[EXCLUDES1] *biotin-dependent carboxylase deficiency due to dietary deficiency of biotin (E53.8)*

D81.810 Biotinidase deficiency

D81.818 Other biotin-dependent carboxylase deficiency
Holocarboxylase synthetase deficiency
Other multiple carboxylase deficiency

D81.819 Biotin-dependent carboxylase deficiency, unspecified
Multiple carboxylase deficiency, unspecified

D81.89 Other combined immunodeficiencies

D81.9 Combined immunodeficiency, unspecified
Severe combined immunodeficiency disorder [SCID] NOS

[4] **D82 Immunodeficiency associated with other major defects**

[EXCLUDES1] *ataxia telangiectasia [Louis-Bar] (G11.3)*

D82.0 Wiskott-Aldrich syndrome
Immunodeficiency with thrombocytopenia and eczema

D82.1 Di George's syndrome
Pharyngeal pouch syndrome
Thymic alymphoplasia
Thymic aplasia or hypoplasia with immunodeficiency

D82.2 Immunodeficiency with short-limbed stature

D82.3 Immunodeficiency following hereditary defective response to Epstein-Barr virus
X-linked lymphoproliferative disease

D82.4 Hyperimmunoglobulin E [IgE] syndrome

D82.8 Immunodeficiency associated with other specified major defects

D82.9 Immunodeficiency associated with major defect, unspecified

[4] **D83 Common variable immunodeficiency**

D83.0 Common variable immunodeficiency with predominant abnormalities of B-cell numbers and function

D83.1 Common variable immunodeficiency with predominant immunoregulatory T-cell disorders

D83.2 Common variable immunodeficiency with autoantibodies to B- or T-cells

D83.8 Other common variable immunodeficiencies

D83.9 Common variable immunodeficiency, unspecified

[4] **D84 Other immunodeficiencies**

D84.0 Lymphocyte function antigen-1 [LFA-1] defect

D84.1 Defects in the complement system
C1 esterase inhibitor [C1-INH] deficiency

D84.8 Other specified immunodeficiencies

D84.9 Immunodeficiency, unspecified

[4] **D86 Sarcoidosis**

D86.0 Sarcoidosis of lung

D86.1 Sarcoidosis of lymph nodes

D86.2 Sarcoidosis of lung with sarcoidosis of lymph nodes

D86.3 Sarcoidosis of skin

[5] **D86.8 Sarcoidosis of other sites**

D86.81 Sarcoid meningitis

D86.82 Multiple cranial nerve palsies in sarcoidosis

D86.83 Sarcoid iridocyclitis

D86.84 Sarcoid pyelonephritis
Tubulo-interstitial nephropathy in sarcoidosis

D86.85 Sarcoid myocarditis

D86.86 Sarcoid arthropathy
Polyarthritis in sarcoidosis

D86.87 Sarcoid myositis

D86.89 Sarcoidosis of other sites
Hepatic granuloma
Uveoparotid fever [Heerfordt]

D86.9 Sarcoidosis, unspecified

[4] **D89 Other disorders involving the immune mechanism, not elsewhere classified**

[EXCLUDES1] *hyperglobulinemia NOS (R77.1)*
monoclonal gammopathy (of undetermined significance) (D47.2)

[EXCLUDES2] *transplant failure and rejection (T86.-)*

D89.0 Polyclonal hypergammaglobulinemia
Benign hypergammaglobulinemic purpura
Polyclonal gammopathy NOS

D89.1 Cryoglobulinemia
Cryoglobulinemic purpura
Cryoglobulinemic vasculitis
Essential cryoglobulinemia

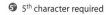

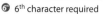

Idiopathic cryoglobulinemia
Mixed cryoglobulinemia
Primary cryoglobulinemia
Secondary cryoglobulinemia

D89.2 **Hypergammaglobulinemia, unspecified**

D89.3 **Immune reconstitution syndrome**

Immune reconstitution inflammatory syndrome [IRIS]
Use additional code for adverse effect, if applicable, to identify drug (T36-T50 with fifth or sixth character 5)

⑤ **D89.8** **Other specified disorders involving the immune mechanism, not elsewhere classified**

⑥ **D89.81** **Graft-versus-host disease**

Code first underlying cause, such as:
complications of transplanted organs and tissue (T86.-)
complications of blood transfusion (T80.89)
Use additional code to identify associated manifestations, such as:
desquamative dermatitis (L30.8)
diarrhea (R19.7)
elevated bilirubin (R17)
hair loss (L65.9)

D89.810 Acute **graft-versus-host disease**

D89.811 Chronic **graft-versus-host disease**

D89.812 Acute on chronic **graft-versus-host disease**

D89.813 **Graft-versus-host disease, unspecified**

D89.82 Autoimmune lymphoproliferative syndrome [ALPS]

D89.89 Other specified disorders involving the immune mechanism, not elsewhere classified

EXCLUDES1 *human immunodeficiency virus disease (B20)*

D89.9 **Disorder involving the immune mechanism, unspecified**

Immune disease NOS

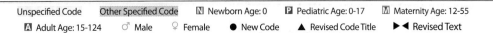

| Unspecified Code | Other Specified Code | Ⓝ Newborn Age: 0 | Ⓟ Pediatric Age: 0-17 | Ⓜ Maternity Age: 12-55 |
| Ⓐ Adult Age: 15-124 | ♂ Male | ♀ Female | ● New Code | ▲ Revised Code Title | ▶◀ Revised Text |

ICD-10-CM 2015

75

This page intentionally left blank

Chapter 4: Endocrine, Nutritional, and Metabolic Diseases (E00-E89)

Chapter Specific Coding Guidelines

a. Diabetes mellitus

The diabetes mellitus codes are combination codes that include the type of diabetes mellitus, the body system affected, and the complications affecting that body system. As many codes within a particular category as are necessary to describe all of the complications of the disease may be used. They should be sequenced based on the reason for a particular encounter. Assign as many codes from categories E08 – E13 as needed to identify all of the associated conditions that the patient has.

1) Type of diabetes

The age of a patient is not the sole determining factor, though most type 1 diabetics develop the condition before reaching puberty. For this reason, type 1 diabetes mellitus is also referred to as juvenile diabetes.

2) Type of diabetes mellitus not documented

If the type of diabetes mellitus is not documented in the medical record the default is E11.-, Type 2 diabetes mellitus.

3) Diabetes mellitus and the use of insulin

If the documentation in a medical record does not indicate the type of diabetes but does indicate that the patient uses insulin, code E11, Type 2 diabetes mellitus, should be assigned. Code Z79.4, Long-term (current) use of insulin, should also be assigned to indicate that the patient uses insulin. Code Z79.4 should not be assigned if insulin is given temporarily to bring a type 2 patient's blood sugar under control during an encounter.

4) Diabetes mellitus in pregnancy and gestational diabetes

See Section I.C.15. Diabetes mellitus in pregnancy.

See Section I.C.15. Gestational (pregnancy induced) diabetes

5) Complications due to insulin pump malfunction

(a) Underdose of insulin due to insulin pump failure

An underdose of insulin due to an insulin pump failure should be assigned to a code from subcategory T85.6, Mechanical complication of other specified internal and external prosthetic devices, implants and grafts, that specifies the type of pump malfunction, as the principal or first-listed code, followed by code T38.3x6-, Underdosing of insulin and oral hypoglycemic [antidiabetic] drugs. Additional codes for the type of diabetes mellitus and any associated complications due to the underdosing should also be assigned.

(b) Overdose of insulin due to insulin pump failure

The principal or first-listed code for an encounter due to an insulin pump malfunction resulting in an overdose of insulin, should also be T85.6-, Mechanical complication of other specified internal and external prosthetic devices, implants and grafts, followed by code T38.3x1-, Poisoning by insulin and oral hypoglycemic [antidiabetic] drugs, accidental (unintentional).

6) Secondary diabetes mellitus

Codes under categories E08, Diabetes mellitus due to underlying condition, E09, Drug or chemical induced diabetes mellitus, and E13, Other specified diabetes mellitus, identify complications/manifestations associated with secondary diabetes mellitus. Secondary diabetes is always caused by another condition or event (e.g., cystic fibrosis, malignant neoplasm of pancreas, pancreatectomy, adverse effect of drug, or poisoning).

(a) Secondary diabetes mellitus and the use of insulin

For patients who routinely use insulin, code Z79.4, Long-term (current) use of insulin, should also be assigned. Code Z79.4 should not be assigned if insulin is given temporarily to bring a patient's blood sugar under control during an encounter.

(b) Assigning and sequencing secondary diabetes codes and its causes

The sequencing of the secondary diabetes codes in relationship to codes for the cause of the diabetes is based on the Tabular List instructions for categories E08, E09 and E13.

(i) Secondary diabetes mellitus due to pancreatectomy

For postpancreatectomy diabetes mellitus (lack of insulin due to the surgical removal of all or part of the pancreas), assign code E89.1, Postprocedural hypoinsulinemia. Assign a code from category E13 and a code from subcategory Z90.41-, Acquired absence of pancreas, as additional codes.

(ii) Secondary diabetes due to drugs

Secondary diabetes may be caused by an adverse effect of correctly administered medications, poisoning or sequela of poisoning.

See section I.C.19.e for coding of adverse effects and poisoning, and section I.C.20 for external cause code reporting.

Anatomy of the Endocrine System

1. **An Outline of the Endocrine System**
    a) The endocrine system is primarily responsible for maintaining the body's homeostasis through various hormones.
    b) The endocrine system is based on the ductless endocrine glands that secrete their hormones directly into the blood stream. These hormones are further carried to the target organs through the blood stream.
    c) The pituitary gland (or hypophysis) is regarded as the master gland of the endocrine system. This gland is monitored and controlled by the hypothalamus of the brain.

The Endocrine System

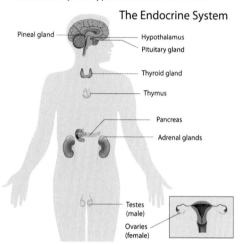

2. **The Endocrine Hormones**
    a) The names of various endocrine hormones of the body are as follows:
        i)   epinephrine
        ii)   norepinephrine
        iii) oxytosin
        iv)   vasopressin
        v)   insulin
        vi)   growth hormone
        vii) cortisol
        viii) estrogen
        ix)   testosterone
    b) The hormones monitor and control the processes of cellular respiration, growth, reproduction and electrolyte balances of the body. They also regulate the reproductive cycles, growth and the secretion of other hormones.

3. **The Hypothalamus (of the Brain)**
    a) The hypothalamus controls the secretions of pituitary gland.
    b) The hypothalamus controls and monitors the secretions of the endocrine system.
    c) The endocrine system can influence the functions of the hypothalamus via negative feedback mechanisms.

4. **The Major Endocrine Glands**
    a) The names of the major endocrine glands are as follows:
        i)   anterior pituitary gland
        ii)   posterior pituitary gland
        iii) pineal gland
        iv)   thyroid gland
        v)   parathyroid gland
        vi)   thymus
        vii) adrenal gland
        viii) pancreatic Islets
        ix)   ovaries
        x)   testes

5. **The Anatomy of the Anterior Pituitary Gland**
    The anterior pituitary gland is constituted by the glandular epithelium and generates the following hormones, which are listed below:
    a) Growth Hormone

    The growth hormone stimulates cell metabolism and growth of bones and muscles.
    b) Thyroid Stimulating Hormone (TSH)

    The TSH stimulates the thyroid gland for the production of T3, T4 and calcitonin hormones.
    c) Adrenocorticoid Hormone (ACTH)

    The ACTH stimulates the adrenal cortex for the secretion of the hormone cortisol.
    d) Melanocyte Stimulating Hormone (MSH)

    The MSH stimulates melanocytes for the production of melanin, which causes darkening of the skin.
    e) Luteinizing Hormone (LH)

    The LH stimulates the production of testosterone in males and progesterone in females.
    f) Prolactin

    The Prolactin provides stimulation for milk production in the mammary glands of female, after child birth.

6. **The Anatomy of the Posterior Pituitary Gland**
    The posterior pituitary gland is also known as neurohypophysis. It is made up of the posterior lobe of the pituitary gland. The hormones of the posterior pituitary gland are listed below:
    a) Antidiuretic Hormone (ADH)/Vasopressin

    Function of vasopressin is to enhance water re-absorption in the kidney tubules. Deficiency of vasopressin can cause Diabetes insipidus.
    b) Oxytosin

    Oxytosin facilitates the childbirth by causing the contraction of uterine smooth muscles. It also facilitates lactation by causing constriction of the mammary glands during breastfeeding.

7. **The Anatomy of the Thyroid Gland**
    a) The thyroid gland is located below the thyroid cartilage in the neck region. It is one of the largest endocrine glands in the body.
    b) The overactive thyroid gland causes excessive secretion of thyroid hormone or hyperthyroidism.
    c) The underactive thyroid gland causes a condition of lack of thyroid hormone, which is known as the hypothyroidism.
    d) The hormone calcitonin is secreted by the extrafollicular cells of the thyroid gland. It causes an increased excretion of the calcium and phosphate ions via the kidneys.

8. **The Anatomy of the Parathyroid Glands**
    a) The parathyroid glands are four in number and remain embedded in the posterior surface of the thyroid gland in the neck region. These glands secrete parathyroid hormone or parathormone (PTH).
    b) PTH stimulates the bone cells to release calcium and phosphate into the blood stream.
    c) A deficiency of PTH causes hypoparathyroidism.
    d) The high levels of PTH can result in the condition of hyperparathyroidism.

9. **The Anatomy of Adrenal Glands**
    a) The adrenal (or suprarenal) glands are located on top of each kidney.

b) The adrenal gland is divided into the following components:

   i)   adrenal medulla (or the inner portion)

   ii) adrenal cortex (or the outer portion)

c) The hormones epinephrine (or adrenalin) and norepinephrine (or noradrenalin) are produced by the adrenal medulla.

d) The adrenal cortex is divided into the following three layers:

   i)   outer layer of adrenal cortex secretes aldosterone, which is a mineralocorticoid hormone and regulates sodium reabsorption and potassium excretion by the kidney.

   ii) hormone cortisol (or hydrocortisone) is secreted by the middle layer of adrenal cortex. It stimulates the liver to manufacture glucose from the circulating amino acids. The cortisol also possesses anti-inflammatory proterties.

   iii) adrenal male sex hormones (or androgens) are produced by the inner layer of the adrenal cortex. These hormones enhance the male sex characteristics. The androgens are also the precursors of all estrogens (or the female sex hormones) and stimulate the female sex drive. The testosterone is the primary and most well-known androgen.

e) deficit of adrenal cortex hormones causes Addison's disease.

f) an increased secretion of adrenal cortex causes Cushing's syndrome.

10. The Anatomy of the Pancreas

a) The pancreas is a glandular organ of both digestive and endocrine systems.

b) The islets of Langerhans of pancreas constitute its endocrine portion, and produce insulin and glucagon hormones for the regulation of blood glucose levels.

c) The blood glucose concentration is regulated by the negative feedback mechanism.

d) The clinical abnormality of diabetes mellitus is caused by the insufficient production of insulin.

11. The Anatomy of the Testes and Ovaries

a) Each of the two testes is the component of the reproductive and endocrine systems and produces the male sex hormone, testosterone.

b) Testosterone is responsible for the development of secondary male sex characteristics, which include facial and chest hairs, narrow hips, broad shoulders and deep voice.

c) Each of the two ovaries is an ovum producing reproductive organ and secretes the estrogen and progesterone, which are the female sex hormones.

d) Estrogen and progesterone are responsible for the development of the female reproductive organs and the development of secondary female sex characteristics, which include the fat deposition on thighs, hips and legs, high pitched voice, broad hips and breast enlargement.

12. The Anatomy of the Thymus Gland

a) The thymus gland is regarded as a specialized organ of the immune system that produces the hormone thymosin.

b) Thymosin stimulates the production of the T-lymphocyte white blood cells (or T cells) that are critical cells of the adaptive immune system and protect the body against the invasion of foreign microbes.

13. The Anatomy of the Pineal Gland

a) The pineal gland is also known as the pineal body, epiphysis cerebri or epiphysis. It is a small endocrine gland located near the thalamus inside the human brain.

b) The pineal gland secretes the following hormones:

   i)   melatonin, which regulates the body rhythms (wake and sleep patterns) and inhibits the functions of the reproductive system.

   ii) serotonin, which acts as a neurotransmitter and vasoconstrictor.

Common Pathologies

Adrenal Insufficiency
This is a condition in which the production of steroid hormones such as cortisol and aldosterone becomes low. Symptoms include fatigue, stomach upset, dehydration, and skin changes. Addison's disease is a type of adrenal insufficiency.

Cushing's Syndrome
This is a condition in which overproduction of a pituitary gland hormone(ACTH) leads to an overactive adrenal gland. A similar condition called Cushing's disease may occur in people, particularly children, who take high doses of corticosteroid medications.

Gigantism (acromegaly) and other growth hormone problems
This is a condition in which, if the pituitary gland produces too much growth hormone, a child's bones and body parts may grow abnormally fast. If growth hormone levels are too low, a child can stop growing in height.

Hyperthyroidism
This is a condition in which, the thyroid gland produces too much thyroid hormone, leading to weight loss, fast heart rate, sweating, and nervousness. The most common cause for an overactive thyroid is an autoimmune disorder called Grave's disease.

Hypothyroidism
This is a condition in which, the thyroid gland does not produce enough thyroid hormone, leading to fatigue, constipation, dry skin, and depression. The underactive gland can cause slowed development in children. Some types of hypothyroidism are present at birth.

Hypopituitarism
This is a condition in which, the pituitary gland releases little or no hormones. It may be caused by a number of different diseases. Women with this condition may stop getting their periods.

Polycystic Ovary Syndrome (PCOS)
This is a condition in which, overproduction of androgens interfere with the development of eggs and their release from the female ovaries. PCOS is a leading cause of infertility.

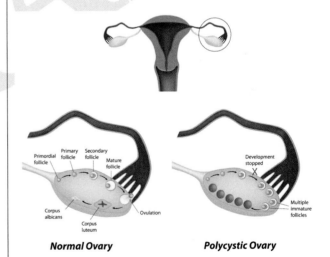

Normal Ovary   *Polycystic Ovary*

Precocious Puberty
This is a condition in which abnormally early puberty occurs when glands tell the body to release sex hormones too soon in life.

This page intentionally left blank

Endocrine, nutritional and metabolic diseases (E00-E89)

NOTES All neoplasms, whether functionally active or not, are classified in Chapter 2. Appropriate codes in this chapter (i.e. E05.8, E07.0, E16-E31, E34.-) may be used as additional codes to indicate either functional activity by neoplasms and ectopic endocrine tissue or hyperfunction and hypofunction of endocrine glands associated with neoplasms and other conditions classified elsewhere.

EXCLUDES1 *transitory endocrine and metabolic disorders specific to newborn (P70-P74)*

Disorders of thyroid gland (E00-E07)

E00 Congenital iodine-deficiency syndrome

Use additional code (F70-F79) to identify associated intellectual disabilities.

EXCLUDES1 *subclinical iodine-deficiency hypothyroidism (E02)*

E00.0 Congenital iodine-deficiency syndrome, neurological type

Endemic cretinism, neurological type

E00.1 Congenital iodine-deficiency syndrome, myxedematous type

Endemic hypothyroid cretinism

Endemic cretinism, myxedematous type

E00.2 Congenital iodine-deficiency syndrome, mixed type

Endemic cretinism, mixed type

E00.9 Congenital iodine-deficiency syndrome, unspecified

Congenital iodine-deficiency hypothyroidism NOS

Endemic cretinism NOS

E01 Iodine-deficiency related thyroid disorders and allied conditions

EXCLUDES1 *congenital iodine-deficiency syndrome (E00.-) subclinical iodine-deficiency hypothyroidism (E02)*

E01.0 Iodine-deficiency related diffuse (endemic) goiter

E01.1 Iodine-deficiency related multinodular (endemic) goiter

Iodine-deficiency related nodular goiter

E01.2 Iodine-deficiency related (endemic) goiter, unspecified

Endemic goiter NOS

E01.8 Other iodine-deficiency related thyroid disorders and allied conditions

Acquired iodine-deficiency hypothyroidism NOS

E02 Subclinical iodine-deficiency hypothyroidism

E03 Other hypothyroidism

EXCLUDES1 *iodine-deficiency related hypothyroidism (E00-E02) postprocedural hypothyroidism (E89.0)*

E03.0 Congenital hypothyroidism with diffuse goiter

Congenital parenchymatous goiter (nontoxic)

Congenital goiter (nontoxic) NOS

EXCLUDES1 *transitory congenital goiter with normal function (P72.0)*

E03.1 Congenital hypothyroidism without goiter

Aplasia of thyroid (with myxedema)

Congenital atrophy of thyroid

Congenital hypothyroidism NOS

E03.2 Hypothyroidism due to medicaments and other exogenous substances

Code first poisoning due to drug or toxin, if applicable (T36-T65 with fifth or sixth character 1-4 or 6)

Use additional code for adverse effect, if applicable, to identify drug (T36-T50 with fifth or sixth character 5)

E03.3 Postinfectious hypothyroidism

E03.4 Atrophy of thyroid (acquired)

EXCLUDES1 *congenital atrophy of thyroid (E03.1)*

E03.5 Myxedema coma

E03.8 Other specified hypothyroidism

E03.9 Hypothyroidism, unspecified

Myxedema NOS

E04 Other nontoxic goiter

EXCLUDES1 *congenital goiter (NOS) (diffuse) (parenchymatous) (E03.0) iodine-deficiency related goiter (E00-E02)*

E04.0 Nontoxic diffuse goiter

Diffuse (colloid) nontoxic goiter

Simple nontoxic goiter

E04.1 Nontoxic single thyroid nodule

Colloid nodule (cystic) (thyroid)

Nontoxic uninodular goiter

Thyroid (cystic) nodule NOS

E04.2 Nontoxic multinodular goiter

Cystic goiter NOS

Multinodular (cystic) goiter NOS

E04.8 Other specified nontoxic goiter

E04.9 Nontoxic goiter, unspecified

Goiter NOS

Nodular goiter (nontoxic) NOS

E05 Thyrotoxicosis [hyperthyroidism]

EXCLUDES1 *chronic thyroiditis with transient thyrotoxicosis (E06.2) neonatal thyrotoxicosis (P72.1)*

E05.0 Thyrotoxicosis with diffuse goiter

Exophthalmic or toxic goiter NOS

Graves' disease

Toxic diffuse goiter

E05.00 Thyrotoxicosis with diffuse goiter without thyrotoxic crisis or storm

E05.01 Thyrotoxicosis with diffuse goiter with thyrotoxic crisis or storm

E05.1 Thyrotoxicosis with toxic single thyroid nodule

Thyrotoxicosis with toxic uninodular goiter

E05.10 Thyrotoxicosis with toxic single thyroid nodule without thyrotoxic crisis or storm

E05.11 Thyrotoxicosis with toxic single thyroid nodule with thyrotoxic crisis or storm

E05.2 Thyrotoxicosis with toxic multinodular goiter

Toxic nodular goiter NOS

E05.20 Thyrotoxicosis with toxic multinodular goiter without thyrotoxic crisis or storm

E05.21 Thyrotoxicosis with toxic multinodular goiter with thyrotoxic crisis or storm

E05.3 Thyrotoxicosis from ectopic thyroid tissue

E05.30 Thyrotoxicosis from ectopic thyroid tissue without thyrotoxic crisis or storm

E05.31 Thyrotoxicosis from ectopic thyroid tissue with thyrotoxic crisis or storm

E05.4 Thyrotoxicosis factitia

E05.40 Thyrotoxicosis factitia without thyrotoxic crisis or storm

E05.41 Thyrotoxicosis factitia with thyrotoxic crisis or storm

E05.8 Other thyrotoxicosis

Overproduction of thyroid-stimulating hormone

E05.80 Other thyrotoxicosis without thyrotoxic crisis or storm

E05.81 Other thyrotoxicosis with thyrotoxic crisis or storm

E05.9 Thyrotoxicosis, unspecified

Hyperthyroidism NOS

E05.90 Thyrotoxicosis, unspecified without thyrotoxic crisis or storm

E05.91 Thyrotoxicosis, unspecified with thyrotoxic crisis or storm

Unspecified Code	Other Specified Code	N Newborn Age: 0	P Pediatric Age: 0-17	M Maternity Age: 12-55	
A Adult Age: 15-124	♂ Male	♀ Female	● New Code	▲ Revised Code Title	►◄ Revised Text

④ **E06 Thyroiditis**

EXCLUDES1 *postpartum thyroiditis (O90.5)*

E06.0 Acute thyroiditis

Abscess of thyroid

Pyogenic thyroiditis

Suppurative thyroiditis

Use additional code (B95-B97) to identify infectious agent.

E06.1 Subacute thyroiditis

de Quervain thyroiditis

Giant-cell thyroiditis

Granulomatous thyroiditis

Nonsuppurative thyroiditis

Viral thyroiditis

EXCLUDES1 *autoimmune thyroiditis (E06.3)*

E06.2 Chronic thyroiditis with transient thyrotoxicosis

EXCLUDES1 *autoimmune thyroiditis (E06.3)*

E06.3 Autoimmune thyroiditis

Hashimoto's thyroiditis

Hashitoxicosis (transient)

Lymphadenoid goiter

Lymphocytic thyroiditis

Struma lymphomatosa

E06.4 Drug-induced thyroiditis

Use additional code for adverse effect, if applicable, to identify drug (T36-T50 with fifth or sixth character 5)

E06.5 Other chronic thyroiditis

Chronic fibrous thyroiditis

Chronic thyroiditis NOS

Ligneous thyroiditis

Riedel thyroiditis

E06.9 Thyroiditis, unspecified

④ **E07 Other disorders of thyroid**

E07.0 Hypersecretion of calcitonin

C-cell hyperplasia of thyroid

Hypersecretion of thyrocalcitonin

E07.1 Dyshormogenetic goiter

Familial dyshormogenetic goiter

Pendred's syndrome

EXCLUDES1 *transitory congenital goiter with normal function (P72.0)*

⑤ **E07.8 Other specified disorders of thyroid**

E07.81 Sick-euthyroid syndrome

Euthyroid sick-syndrome

E07.89 Other specified disorders of thyroid

Abnormality of thyroid-binding globulin

Hemorrhage of thyroid

Infarction of thyroid

E07.9 Disorder of thyroid, unspecified

Diabetes mellitus (E08-E13)

④ **E08 Diabetes mellitus due to underlying condition**

Code first the underlying condition, such as:

congenital rubella (P35.0)

Cushing's syndrome (E24.-)

cystic fibrosis (E84.-)

malignant neoplasm (C00-C96)

malnutrition (E40-E46)

pancreatitis and other diseases of the pancreas (K85-K86.-)

Use additional code to identify any insulin use (Z79.4)

EXCLUDES1 *drug or chemical induced diabetes mellitus (E09.-)*

gestational diabetes (O24.4-)

neonatal diabetes mellitus (P70.2)

postpancreatectomy diabetes mellitus (E13.-)

postprocedural diabetes mellitus (E13.-)

secondary diabetes mellitus NEC (E13.-)

type 1 diabetes mellitus (E10.-)

type 2 diabetes mellitus (E11.-)

⑤ **E08.0 Diabetes mellitus due to underlying condition with hyperosmolarity**

E08.00 Diabetes mellitus due to underlying condition with hyperosmolarity without nonketotic hyperglycemic-hyperosmolar coma (NKHHC)

E08.01 Diabetes mellitus due to underlying condition with hyperosmolarity with coma

⑤ **E08.1 Diabetes mellitus due to underlying condition with ketoacidosis**

E08.10 Diabetes mellitus due to underlying condition with ketoacidosis without coma

E08.11 Diabetes mellitus due to underlying condition with ketoacidosis with coma

⑤ **E08.2 Diabetes mellitus due to underlying condition with kidney complications**

E08.21 Diabetes mellitus due to underlying condition with diabetic nephropathy

Diabetes mellitus due to underlying condition with intercapillary glomerulosclerosis

Diabetes mellitus due to underlying condition with intracapillary glomerulonephrosis

Diabetes mellitus due to underlying condition with Kimmelstiel-Wilson disease

E08.22 Diabetes mellitus due to underlying condition with diabetic chronic kidney disease

Use additional code to identify stage of chronic kidney disease (N18.1-N18.6)

E08.29 Diabetes mellitus due to underlying condition with other diabetic kidney complication

Renal tubular degeneration in diabetes mellitus due to underlying condition

Normal

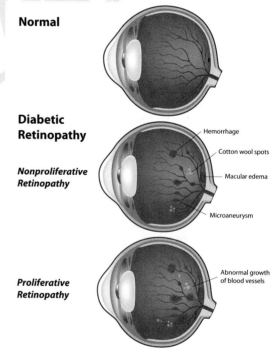

Diabetic Retinopathy

Nonproliferative Retinopathy

Hemorrhage

Cotton wool spots

Macular edema

Microaneurysm

Proliferative Retinopathy

Abnormal growth of blood vessels

Figure 5.1 Diabetic retinopathy

⑤ **E08.3 Diabetes mellitus due to underlying condition with ophthalmic complications**

⑥ **E08.31 Diabetes mellitus due to underlying condition with unspecified diabetic retinopathy**

④ 4th character required   ⑤ 5th character required   ⑥ 6th character required   ⑦ 7th character required   ⑦ Extension 'X' Alert

EXCLUDES 1 Not coded here   EXCLUDES 2 Not included here   PDx Primary Diagnosis Only   Manifestation Code

E08.311 Diabetes mellitus due to underlying condition with unspecified diabetic retinopathy with macular edema
E08.319 Diabetes mellitus due to underlying condition with unspecified diabetic retinopathy without macular edema
[6] E08.32 Diabetes mellitus due to underlying condition with mild nonproliferative diabetic retinopathy
Diabetes mellitus due to underlying condition with nonproliferative diabetic retinopathy NOS
E08.321 Diabetes mellitus due to underlying condition with mild nonproliferative diabetic retinopathy with macular edema
E08.329 Diabetes mellitus due to underlying condition with mild nonproliferative diabetic retinopathy without macular edema
[6] E08.33 Diabetes mellitus due to underlying condition with moderate nonproliferative diabetic retinopathy
E08.331 Diabetes mellitus due to underlying condition with moderate nonproliferative diabetic retinopathy with macular edema
E08.339 Diabetes mellitus due to underlying condition with moderate nonproliferative diabetic retinopathy without macular edema
[6] E08.34 Diabetes mellitus due to underlying condition with severe nonproliferative diabetic retinopathy
E08.341 Diabetes mellitus due to underlying condition with severe nonproliferative diabetic retinopathy with macular edema
E08.349 Diabetes mellitus due to underlying condition with severe nonproliferative diabetic retinopathy without macular edema
[6] E08.35 Diabetes mellitus due to underlying condition with proliferative diabetic retinopathy
E08.351 Diabetes mellitus due to underlying condition with proliferative diabetic retinopathy with macular edema
E08.359 Diabetes mellitus due to underlying condition with proliferative diabetic retinopathy without macular edema
E08.36 Diabetes mellitus due to underlying condition with diabetic cataract
E08.39 Diabetes mellitus due to underlying condition with other diabetic ophthalmic complication
Use additional code to identify manifestation, such as: diabetic glaucoma (H40-H42)
[5] E08.4 Diabetes mellitus due to underlying condition with neurological complications
E08.40 Diabetes mellitus due to underlying condition with diabetic neuropathy, unspecified
E08.41 Diabetes mellitus due to underlying condition with diabetic mononeuropathy
E08.42 Diabetes mellitus due to underlying condition with diabetic polyneuropathy
Diabetes mellitus due to underlying condition with diabetic neuralgia
E08.43 Diabetes mellitus due to underlying condition with diabetic autonomic (poly)neuropathy
Diabetes mellitus due to underlying condition with diabetic gastroparesis
E08.44 Diabetes mellitus due to underlying condition with diabetic amyotrophy
E08.49 Diabetes mellitus due to underlying condition with other diabetic neurological complication
[5] E08.5 Diabetes mellitus due to underlying condition with circulatory complications
E08.51 Diabetes mellitus due to underlying condition with diabetic peripheral angiopathy without gangrene
E08.52 Diabetes mellitus due to underlying condition with diabetic peripheral angiopathy with gangrene
Diabetes mellitus due to underlying condition with diabetic gangrene
E08.59 Diabetes mellitus due to underlying condition with other circulatory complications
[5] E08.6 Diabetes mellitus due to underlying condition with other specified complications
[6] E08.61 Diabetes mellitus due to underlying condition with diabetic arthropathy
E08.610 Diabetes mellitus due to underlying condition with diabetic neuropathic arthropathy
Diabetes mellitus due to underlying condition with Charcôt's joints
E08.618 Diabetes mellitus due to underlying condition with other diabetic arthropathy
[6] E08.62 Diabetes mellitus due to underlying condition with skin complications
E08.620 Diabetes mellitus due to underlying condition with diabetic dermatitis
Diabetes mellitus due to underlying condition with diabetic necrobiosis lipoidica
E08.621 Diabetes mellitus due to underlying condition with foot ulcer
Use additional code to identify site of ulcer (L97.4-, L97.5-)
E08.622 Diabetes mellitus due to underlying condition with other skin ulcer
Use additional code to identify site of ulcer (L97.1-L97.9, L98.41-L98.49)
E08.628 Diabetes mellitus due to underlying condition with other skin complications
[6] E08.63 Diabetes mellitus due to underlying condition with oral complications
E08.630 Diabetes mellitus due to underlying condition with periodontal disease
E08.638 Diabetes mellitus due to underlying condition with other oral complications
[6] E08.64 Diabetes mellitus due to underlying condition with hypoglycemia
E08.641 Diabetes mellitus due to underlying condition with hypoglycemia with coma
E08.649 Diabetes mellitus due to underlying condition with hypoglycemia without coma
E08.65 Diabetes mellitus due to underlying condition with hyperglycemia
E08.69 Diabetes mellitus due to underlying condition with other specified complication
Use additional code to identify complication
E08.8 Diabetes mellitus due to underlying condition with unspecified complications
E08.9 Diabetes mellitus due to underlying condition without complications
[4] E09 Drug or chemical induced diabetes mellitus
Code first poisoning due to drug or toxin, if applicable (T36-T65 with fifth or sixth character 1-4 or 6)
Use additional code for adverse effect, if applicable, to identify drug (T36-T50 with fifth or sixth character 5)
code to identify any insulin use (Z79.4)
[EXCLUDES1] *diabetes mellitus due to underlying condition (E08.-)*
gestational diabetes (O24.4-)
neonatal diabetes mellitus (P70.2)
postpancreatectomy diabetes mellitus (E13.-)
postprocedural diabetes mellitus (E13.-)
secondary diabetes mellitus NEC (E13.-)
type 1 diabetes mellitus (E10.-)
type 2 diabetes mellitus (E11.-)
[5] E09.0 Drug or chemical induced diabetes mellitus with hyperosmolarity

Unspecified Code | Other Specified Code | [N] Newborn Age: 0 | [P] Pediatric Age: 0-17 | [M] Maternity Age: 12-55
[A] Adult Age: 15-124 | ♂ Male | ♀ Female | ● New Code | ▲ Revised Code Title | ►◄ Revised Text

E09.00 Drug or chemical induced diabetes mellitus with hyperosmolarity without nonketotic hyperglycemic-hyperosmolar coma (NKHHC)

E09.01 Drug or chemical induced diabetes mellitus with hyperosmolarity with coma

[5] E09.1 Drug or chemical induced diabetes mellitus with ketoacidosis

E09.10 Drug or chemical induced diabetes mellitus with ketoacidosis without coma

E09.11 Drug or chemical induced diabetes mellitus with ketoacidosis with coma

[5] E09.2 Drug or chemical induced diabetes mellitus with kidney complications

E09.21 Drug or chemical induced diabetes mellitus with diabetic nephropathy

Drug or chemical induced diabetes mellitus with intercapillary glomerulosclerosis

Drug or chemical induced diabetes mellitus with intracapillary glomerulonephrosis

Drug or chemical induced diabetes mellitus with Kimmelstiel-Wilson disease

E09.22 Drug or chemical induced diabetes mellitus with diabetic chronic kidney disease

Use additional code to identify stage of chronic kidney disease (N18.1-N18.6)

E09.29 Drug or chemical induced diabetes mellitus with other diabetic kidney complication

Drug or chemical induced diabetes mellitus with renal tubular degeneration

[5] E09.3 Drug or chemical induced diabetes mellitus with ophthalmic complications

[6] E09.31 Drug or chemical induced diabetes mellitus with unspecified diabetic retinopathy

E09.311 Drug or chemical induced diabetes mellitus with unspecified diabetic retinopathy with macular edema

E09.319 Drug or chemical induced diabetes mellitus with unspecified diabetic retinopathy without macular edema

[6] E09.32 Drug or chemical induced diabetes mellitus with mild nonproliferative diabetic retinopathy

Drug or chemical induced diabetes mellitus with nonproliferative diabetic retinopathy NOS

E09.321 Drug or chemical induced diabetes mellitus with mild nonproliferative diabetic retinopathy with macular edema

E09.329 Drug or chemical induced diabetes mellitus with mild nonproliferative diabetic retinopathy without macular edema

[6] E09.33 Drug or chemical induced diabetes mellitus with moderate nonproliferative diabetic retinopathy

E09.331 Drug or chemical induced diabetes mellitus with moderate nonproliferative diabetic retinopathy with macular edema

E09.339 Drug or chemical induced diabetes mellitus with moderate nonproliferative diabetic retinopathy without macular edema

[6] E09.34 Drug or chemical induced diabetes mellitus with severe nonproliferative diabetic retinopathy

E09.341 Drug or chemical induced diabetes mellitus with severe nonproliferative diabetic retinopathy with macular edema

E09.349 Drug or chemical induced diabetes mellitus with severe nonproliferative diabetic retinopathy without macular edema

[6] E09.35 Drug or chemical induced diabetes mellitus with proliferative diabetic retinopathy

E09.351 Drug or chemical induced diabetes mellitus with proliferative diabetic retinopathy with macular edema

E09.359 Drug or chemical induced diabetes mellitus with proliferative diabetic retinopathy without macular edema

E09.36 Drug or chemical induced diabetes mellitus with diabetic cataract

E09.39 Drug or chemical induced diabetes mellitus with other diabetic ophthalmic complication

Use additional code to identify manifestation, such as: diabetic glaucoma (H40-H42)

[5] E09.4 Drug or chemical induced diabetes mellitus with neurological complications

E09.40 Drug or chemical induced diabetes mellitus with neurological complications with diabetic neuropathy, unspecified

E09.41 Drug or chemical induced diabetes mellitus with neurological complications with diabetic mononeuropathy

E09.42 Drug or chemical induced diabetes mellitus with neurological complications with diabetic polyneuropathy

Drug or chemical induced diabetes mellitus with diabetic neuralgia

E09.43 Drug or chemical induced diabetes mellitus with neurological complications with diabetic autonomic (poly)neuropathy

Drug or chemical induced diabetes mellitus with diabetic gastroparesis

E09.44 Drug or chemical induced diabetes mellitus with neurological complications with diabetic amyotrophy

E09.49 Drug or chemical induced diabetes mellitus with neurological complications with other diabetic neurological complication

[5] E09.5 Drug or chemical induced diabetes mellitus with circulatory complications

E09.51 Drug or chemical induced diabetes mellitus with diabetic peripheral angiopathy without gangrene

E09.52 Drug or chemical induced diabetes mellitus with diabetic peripheral angiopathy with gangrene

Drug or chemical induced diabetes mellitus with diabetic gangrene

E09.59 Drug or chemical induced diabetes mellitus with other circulatory complications

[5] E09.6 Drug or chemical induced diabetes mellitus with other specified complications

[6] E09.61 Drug or chemical induced diabetes mellitus with diabetic arthropathy

E09.610 Drug or chemical induced diabetes mellitus with diabetic neuropathic arthropathy

Drug or chemical induced diabetes mellitus with Charcôt's joints

E09.618 Drug or chemical induced diabetes mellitus with other diabetic arthropathy

[6] E09.62 Drug or chemical induced diabetes mellitus with skin complications

E09.620 Drug or chemical induced diabetes mellitus with diabetic dermatitis

Drug or chemical induced diabetes mellitus with diabetic necrobiosis lipoidica

E09.621 Drug or chemical induced diabetes mellitus with foot ulcer

Use additional code to identify site of ulcer (L97.4-, L97.5-)

E09.622 Drug or chemical induced diabetes mellitus with other skin ulcer

[4] 4th character required [5] 5th character required [6] 6th character required [7] 7th character required [7x] Extension 'X' Alert
EXCLUDES 1 Not coded here EXCLUDES 2 Not included here [PDx] Primary Diagnosis Only Manifestation Code

Use additional code to identify site of ulcer (L97.1-L97.9, L98.41-L98.49)

E09.628 Drug or chemical induced diabetes mellitus with other skin complications

[6] E09.63 Drug or chemical induced diabetes mellitus with oral complications

E09.630 Drug or chemical induced diabetes mellitus with periodontal disease

E09.638 Drug or chemical induced diabetes mellitus with other oral complications

[6] E09.64 Drug or chemical induced diabetes mellitus with hypoglycemia

E09.641 Drug or chemical induced diabetes mellitus with hypoglycemia with coma

E09.649 Drug or chemical induced diabetes mellitus with hypoglycemia without coma

E09.65 Drug or chemical induced diabetes mellitus with hyperglycemia

E09.69 Drug or chemical induced diabetes mellitus with other specified complication

Use additional code to identify complication

E09.8 Drug or chemical induced diabetes mellitus with unspecified complications

E09.9 Drug or chemical induced diabetes mellitus without complications

[4] **E10 Type 1 diabetes mellitus**

[INCLUDES] *brittle diabetes (mellitus)*
diabetes (mellitus) due to autoimmune process
diabetes (mellitus) due to immune mediated pancreatic islet beta-cell destruction
idiopathic diabetes (mellitus)
juvenile onset diabetes (mellitus)
ketosis-prone diabetes (mellitus)

[EXCLUDES1] *diabetes mellitus due to underlying condition (E08.-)*
drug or chemical induced diabetes mellitus (E09.-)
gestational diabetes (O24.4-)
hyperglycemia NOS (R73.9)
neonatal diabetes mellitus (P70.2)
postpancreatectomy diabetes mellitus (E13.-)
postprocedural diabetes mellitus (E13.-)
secondary diabetes mellitus NEC (E13.-)
type 2 diabetes mellitus (E11.-)

[5] E10.1 Type 1 diabetes mellitus with ketoacidosis

E10.10 Type 1 diabetes mellitus with ketoacidosis without coma

E10.11 Type 1 diabetes mellitus with ketoacidosis with coma

[5] E10.2 Type 1 diabetes mellitus with kidney complications

E10.21 Type 1 diabetes mellitus with diabetic nephropathy

Type 1 diabetes mellitus with intercapillary glomerulosclerosis
Type 1 diabetes mellitus with intracapillary glomerulonephrosis
Type 1 diabetes mellitus with Kimmelstiel-Wilson disease

E10.22 Type 1 diabetes mellitus with diabetic chronic kidney disease

Use additional code to identify stage of chronic kidney disease (N18.1-N18.6)

E10.29 Type 1 diabetes mellitus with other diabetic kidney complication

Type 1 diabetes mellitus with renal tubular degeneration

[5] E10.3 Type 1 diabetes mellitus with ophthalmic complications

[6] E10.31 Type 1 diabetes mellitus with unspecified diabetic retinopathy

E10.311 Type 1 diabetes mellitus with unspecified diabetic retinopathy with macular edema

E10.319 Type 1 diabetes mellitus with unspecified diabetic retinopathy without macular edema

[6] E10.32 Type 1 diabetes mellitus with mild nonproliferative diabetic retinopathy

Type 1 diabetes mellitus with nonproliferative diabetic retinopathy NOS

E10.321 Type 1 diabetes mellitus with mild nonproliferative diabetic retinopathy with macular edema

E10.329 Type 1 diabetes mellitus with mild nonproliferative diabetic retinopathy without macular edema

[6] E10.33 Type 1 diabetes mellitus with moderate nonproliferative diabetic retinopathy

E10.331 Type 1 diabetes mellitus with moderate nonproliferative diabetic retinopathy with macular edema

E10.339 Type 1 diabetes mellitus with moderate nonproliferative diabetic retinopathy without macular edema

[6] E10.34 Type 1 diabetes mellitus with severe nonproliferative diabetic retinopathy

E10.341 Type 1 diabetes mellitus with severe nonproliferative diabetic retinopathy with macular edema

E10.349 Type 1 diabetes mellitus with severe nonproliferative diabetic retinopathy without macular edema

[6] E10.35 Type 1 diabetes mellitus with proliferative diabetic retinopathy

E10.351 Type 1 diabetes mellitus with proliferative diabetic retinopathy with macular edema

E10.359 Type 1 diabetes mellitus with proliferative diabetic retinopathy without macular edema

E10.36 Type 1 diabetes mellitus with diabetic cataract

E10.39 Type 1 diabetes mellitus with other diabetic ophthalmic complication

Use additional code to identify manifestation, such as:
diabetic glaucoma (H40-H42)

[5] E10.4 Type 1 diabetes mellitus with neurological complications

E10.40 Type 1 diabetes mellitus with diabetic neuropathy, unspecified

E10.41 Type 1 diabetes mellitus with diabetic mononeuropathy

E10.42 Type 1 diabetes mellitus with diabetic polyneuropathy

Type 1 diabetes mellitus with diabetic neuralgia

E10.43 Type 1 diabetes mellitus with diabetic autonomic (poly)neuropathy

Type 1 diabetes mellitus with diabetic gastroparesis

E10.44 Type 1 diabetes mellitus with diabetic amyotrophy

E10.49 Type 1 diabetes mellitus with other diabetic neurological complication

[5] E10.5 Type 1 diabetes mellitus with circulatory complications

E10.51 Type 1 diabetes mellitus with diabetic peripheral angiopathy without gangrene

E10.52 Type 1 diabetes mellitus with diabetic peripheral angiopathy with gangrene

Type 1 diabetes mellitus with diabetic gangrene

E10.59 Type 1 diabetes mellitus with other circulatory complications

[5] E10.6 Type 1 diabetes mellitus with other specified complications

Unspecified Code | Other Specified Code | [N] Newborn Age: 0 | [P] Pediatric Age: 0-17 | [M] Maternity Age: 12-55
[A] Adult Age: 15-124 | ♂ Male | ♀ Female | ● New Code | ▲ Revised Code Title | ►◄ Revised Text

⑥ E10.61 Type 1 diabetes mellitus with diabetic arthropathy

E10.610 Type 1 diabetes mellitus with diabetic neuropathic **arthropathy**

Type 1 diabetes mellitus with Charcôt's joints

E10.618 Type 1 diabetes mellitus with other diabetic arthropathy

⑥ E10.62 Type 1 diabetes mellitus with skin complications

E10.620 Type 1 diabetes mellitus with diabetic dermatitis

Type 1 diabetes mellitus with diabetic necrobiosis lipoidica

E10.621 Type 1 diabetes mellitus with foot ulcer

Use additional code to identify site of ulcer (L97.4-, L97.5-)

E10.622 Type 1 diabetes mellitus with other skin ulcer

Use additional code to identify site of ulcer (L97.1-L97.9, L98.41-L98.49)

E10.628 Type 1 diabetes mellitus with other skin complications

⑥ E10.63 Type 1 diabetes mellitus with oral complications

E10.630 Type 1 diabetes mellitus with periodontal disease

E10.638 Type 1 diabetes mellitus with other oral complications

⑥ E10.64 Type 1 diabetes mellitus with hypoglycemia

E10.641 Type 1 diabetes mellitus with hypoglycemia with coma

E10.649 Type 1 diabetes mellitus with hypoglycemia without coma

E10.65 Type 1 diabetes mellitus with hyperglycemia

E10.69 Type 1 diabetes mellitus with other specified complication

Use additional code to identify complication

E10.8 Type 1 diabetes mellitus with unspecified complications

E10.9 Type 1 diabetes mellitus without complications

④ E11 Type 2 diabetes mellitus

INCLUDES   diabetes (mellitus) due to insulin secretory defect
diabetes NOS
insulin resistant diabetes (mellitus)

Use additional code to identify any insulin use (Z79.4)

EXCLUDES1   diabetes mellitus due to underlying condition (E08.-)
drug or chemical induced diabetes mellitus (E09.-)
gestational diabetes (O24.4-)
neonatal diabetes mellitus (P70.2)
postpancreatectomy diabetes mellitus (E13.-)
postprocedural diabetes mellitus (E13.-)
secondary diabetes mellitus NEC (E13.-)
type 1 diabetes mellitus (E10.-)

⑤ E11.0 Type 2 diabetes mellitus with hyperosmolarity

E11.00 Type 2 diabetes mellitus with hyperosmolarity without nonketotic hyperglycemic-hyperosmolar coma (NKHHC)

E11.01 Type 2 diabetes mellitus with hyperosmolarity with coma

⑤ E11.2 Type 2 diabetes mellitus with kidney complications

E11.21 Type 2 diabetes mellitus with diabetic nephropathy

Type 2 diabetes mellitus with intercapillary glomerulosclerosis

Type 2 diabetes mellitus with intracapillary glomerulonephrosis

Type 2 diabetes mellitus with Kimmelstiel-Wilson disease

E11.22 Type 2 diabetes mellitus with diabetic chronic kidney disease

Use additional code to identify stage of chronic kidney disease (N18.1-N18.6)

E11.29 Type 2 diabetes mellitus with other diabetic kidney complication

Type 2 diabetes mellitus with renal tubular degeneration

⑤ E11.3 Type 2 diabetes mellitus with ophthalmic complications

⑥ E11.31 Type 2 diabetes mellitus with unspecified diabetic retinopathy

E11.311 Type 2 diabetes mellitus with unspecified diabetic retinopathy with macular edema

E11.319 Type 2 diabetes mellitus with unspecified diabetic retinopathy without macular edema

⑥ E11.32 Type 2 diabetes mellitus with mild nonproliferative diabetic retinopathy

Type 2 diabetes mellitus with nonproliferative diabetic retinopathy NOS

E11.321 Type 2 diabetes mellitus with mild nonproliferative diabetic retinopathy with macular edema

E11.329 Type 2 diabetes mellitus with mild nonproliferative diabetic retinopathy without macular edema

⑥ E11.33 Type 2 diabetes mellitus with moderate nonproliferative diabetic retinopathy

E11.331 Type 2 diabetes mellitus with moderate nonproliferative diabetic retinopathy with macular edema

E11.339 Type 2 diabetes mellitus with moderate nonproliferative diabetic retinopathy without macular edema

⑥ E11.34 Type 2 diabetes mellitus with severe nonproliferative diabetic retinopathy

E11.341 Type 2 diabetes mellitus with severe nonproliferative diabetic retinopathy with macular edema

E11.349 Type 2 diabetes mellitus with severe nonproliferative diabetic retinopathy without macular edema

⑥ E11.35 Type 2 diabetes mellitus with proliferative diabetic retinopathy

E11.351 Type 2 diabetes mellitus with proliferative diabetic retinopathy with macular edema

E11.359 Type 2 diabetes mellitus with proliferative diabetic retinopathy without macular edema

E11.36 Type 2 diabetes mellitus with diabetic cataract

E11.39 Type 2 diabetes mellitus with other diabetic ophthalmic complication

Use additional code to identify manifestation, such as: diabetic glaucoma (H40-H42)

⑤ E11.4 Type 2 diabetes mellitus with neurological complications

E11.40 Type 2 diabetes mellitus with diabetic neuropathy, unspecified

E11.41 Type 2 diabetes mellitus with diabetic mononeuropathy

E11.42 Type 2 diabetes mellitus with diabetic polyneuropathy

Type 2 diabetes mellitus with diabetic neuralgia

E11.43 Type 2 diabetes mellitus with diabetic autonomic (poly)neuropathy

Type 2 diabetes mellitus with diabetic gastroparesis

E11.44 Type 2 diabetes mellitus with diabetic amyotrophy

E11.49 Type 2 diabetes mellitus with other diabetic neurological complication

---

④ 4th character required   ⑤ 5th character required   ⑥ 6th character required   ⑦ 7th character required   ⑦Ⓧ Extension 'X' Alert

EXCLUDES 1 Not coded here   EXCLUDES 2 Not included here   PDx Primary Diagnosis Only   Manifestation Code

[5] E11.5 Type 2 diabetes mellitus with circulatory complications
E11.51 Type 2 diabetes mellitus with diabetic peripheral angiopathy without gangrene
E11.52 Type 2 diabetes mellitus with diabetic peripheral angiopathy with gangrene
Type 2 diabetes mellitus with diabetic gangrene
E11.59 Type 2 diabetes mellitus with other circulatory complications
[5] E11.6 Type 2 diabetes mellitus with other specified complications
[6] E11.61 Type 2 diabetes mellitus with diabetic arthropathy
E11.610 Type 2 diabetes mellitus with diabetic neuropathic arthropathy
Type 2 diabetes mellitus with Charcôt's joints
E11.618 Type 2 diabetes mellitus with other diabetic arthropathy
[6] E11.62 Type 2 diabetes mellitus with skin complications
E11.620 Type 2 diabetes mellitus with diabetic dermatitis
Type 2 diabetes mellitus with diabetic necrobiosis lipoidica
E11.621 Type 2 diabetes mellitus with foot ulcer
Use additional code to identify site of ulcer (L97.4-, L97.5-)
E11.622 Type 2 diabetes mellitus with other skin ulcer
Use additional code to identify site of ulcer (L97.1-L97.9, L98.41-L98.49)
E11.628 Type 2 diabetes mellitus with other skin complications
[6] E11.63 Type 2 diabetes mellitus with oral complications
E11.630 Type 2 diabetes mellitus with periodontal disease
E11.638 Type 2 diabetes mellitus with other oral complications
[6] E11.64 Type 2 diabetes mellitus with hypoglycemia
E11.641 Type 2 diabetes mellitus with hypoglycemia with coma
E11.649 Type 2 diabetes mellitus with hypoglycemia without coma
E11.65 Type 2 diabetes mellitus with hyperglycemia
E11.69 Type 2 diabetes mellitus with other specified complication
Use additional code to identify complication
E11.8 Type 2 diabetes mellitus with unspecified complications
E11.9 Type 2 diabetes mellitus without complications

[4] E13 Other specified diabetes mellitus

INCLUDES *diabetes mellitus due to genetic defects of beta-cell function*
diabetes mellitus due to genetic defects in insulin action
postpancreatectomy diabetes mellitus
postprocedural diabetes mellitus
secondary diabetes mellitus NEC

Use additional code to identify any insulin use (Z79.4)

EXCLUDES1 *diabetes (mellitus) due to autoimmune process (E10.-)*
diabetes (mellitus) due to immune mediated pancreatic islet beta-cell destruction (E10.-)
diabetes mellitus due to underlying condition (E08.-)
drug or chemical induced diabetes mellitus (E09.-)
gestational diabetes (O24.4-)
neonatal diabetes mellitus (P70.2)
type 2 diabetes mellitus (E11.-)

[5] E13.0 Other specified diabetes mellitus with hyperosmolarity
E13.00 Other specified diabetes mellitus with hyperosmolarity without nonketotic hyperglycemic-hyperosmolar coma (NKHHC)
E13.01 Other specified diabetes mellitus with hyperosmolarity with coma
[5] E13.1 Other specified diabetes mellitus with ketoacidosis
E13.10 Other specified diabetes mellitus with ketoacidosis without coma
E13.11 Other specified diabetes mellitus with ketoacidosis with coma
[5] E13.2 Other specified diabetes mellitus with kidney complications
E13.21 Other specified diabetes mellitus with diabetic nephropathy
Other specified diabetes mellitus with intercapillary glomerulosclerosis
Other specified diabetes mellitus with intracapillary glomerulonephrosis
Other specified diabetes mellitus with Kimmelstiel-Wilson disease
E13.22 Other specified diabetes mellitus with diabetic chronic kidney disease
Use additional code to identify stage of chronic kidney disease (N18.1-N18.6)
E13.29 Other specified diabetes mellitus with other diabetic kidney complication
Other specified diabetes mellitus with renal tubular degeneration
[5] E13.3 Other specified diabetes mellitus with ophthalmic complications
[6] E13.31 Other specified diabetes mellitus with unspecified diabetic retinopathy
E13.311 Other specified diabetes mellitus with unspecified diabetic retinopathy with macular edema
E13.319 Other specified diabetes mellitus with unspecified diabetic retinopathy without macular edema
[6] E13.32 Other specified diabetes mellitus with mild nonproliferative diabetic retinopathy
Other specified diabetes mellitus with nonproliferative diabetic retinopathy NOS
E13.321 Other specified diabetes mellitus with mild nonproliferative diabetic retinopathy with macular edema
E13.329 Other specified diabetes mellitus with mild nonproliferative diabetic retinopathy without macular edema
[6] E13.33 Other specified diabetes mellitus with moderate nonproliferative diabetic retinopathy
E13.331 Other specified diabetes mellitus with moderate nonproliferative diabetic retinopathy with macular edema
E13.339 Other specified diabetes mellitus with moderate nonproliferative diabetic retinopathy without macular edema
[6] E13.34 Other specified diabetes mellitus with severe nonproliferative diabetic retinopathy
E13.341 Other specified diabetes mellitus with severe nonproliferative diabetic retinopathy with macular edema
E13.349 Other specified diabetes mellitus with severe nonproliferative diabetic retinopathy without macular edema
[6] E13.35 Other specified diabetes mellitus with proliferative diabetic retinopathy

Unspecified Code | Other Specified Code | [N] Newborn Age: 0 | [P] Pediatric Age: 0-17 | [M] Maternity Age: 12-55
[A] Adult Age: 15-124 | ♂ Male | ♀ Female | ● New Code | ▲ Revised Code Title | ►◄ Revised Text

E13.351 Other specified diabetes mellitus with proliferative diabetic retinopathy with macular edema

E13.359 Other specified diabetes mellitus with proliferative diabetic retinopathy without macular edema

E13.36 Other specified diabetes mellitus with diabetic cataract

E13.39 Other specified diabetes mellitus with other diabetic ophthalmic complication
Use additional code to identify manifestation, such as:
diabetic glaucoma (H40-H42)

[5] E13.4 Other specified diabetes mellitus with neurological complications

E13.40 Other specified diabetes mellitus with diabetic neuropathy, unspecified

E13.41 Other specified diabetes mellitus with diabetic mononeuropathy

E13.42 Other specified diabetes mellitus with diabetic polyneuropathy
Other specified diabetes mellitus with diabetic neuralgia

E13.43 Other specified diabetes mellitus with diabetic autonomic (poly)neuropathy
Other specified diabetes mellitus with diabetic gastroparesis

E13.44 Other specified diabetes mellitus with diabetic amyotrophy

E13.49 Other specified diabetes mellitus with other diabetic neurological complication

[5] E13.5 Other specified diabetes mellitus with circulatory complications

E13.51 Other specified diabetes mellitus with diabetic peripheral angiopathy without gangrene

E13.52 Other specified diabetes mellitus with diabetic peripheral angiopathy with gangrene
Other specified diabetes mellitus with diabetic gangrene

E13.59 Other specified diabetes mellitus with other circulatory complications

[5] E13.6 Other specified diabetes mellitus with other specified complications

[6] E13.61 Other specified diabetes mellitus with diabetic arthropathy

E13.610 Other specified diabetes mellitus with diabetic neuropathic arthropathy
Other specified diabetes mellitus with Charcôt's joints

E13.618 Other specified diabetes mellitus with other diabetic arthropathy

[6] E13.62 Other specified diabetes mellitus with skin complications

E13.620 Other specified diabetes mellitus with diabetic dermatitis
Other specified diabetes mellitus with diabetic necrobiosis lipoidica

E13.621 Other specified diabetes mellitus with foot ulcer
Use additional code to identify site of ulcer (L97.4-, L97.5-)

E13.622 Other specified diabetes mellitus with other skin ulcer
Use additional code to identify site of ulcer (L97.1-L97.9, L98.41-L98.49)

E13.628 Other specified diabetes mellitus with other skin complications

[6] E13.63 Other specified diabetes mellitus with oral complications

E13.630 Other specified diabetes mellitus with periodontal disease

E13.638 Other specified diabetes mellitus with other oral complications

[6] E13.64 Other specified diabetes mellitus with hypoglycemia

E13.641 Other specified diabetes mellitus with hypoglycemia with coma

E13.649 Other specified diabetes mellitus with hypoglycemia without coma

E13.65 Other specified diabetes mellitus with hyperglycemia

E13.69 Other specified diabetes mellitus with other specified complication
Use additional code to identify complication

E13.8 Other specified diabetes mellitus with unspecified complications

E13.9 Other specified diabetes mellitus without complications

Other disorders of glucose regulation and pancreatic internal secretion (E15-E16)

E15 Nondiabetic hypoglycemic coma
[INCLUDES] *drug-induced insulin coma in nondiabetic*
hyperinsulinism with hypoglycemic coma
hypoglycemic coma NOS

[4] E16 Other disorders of pancreatic internal secretion

E16.0 Drug-induced hypoglycemia without coma
Use additional code for adverse effect, if applicable, to identify drug (T36-T50 with fifth or sixth character 5)

E16.1 Other hypoglycemia
Functional hyperinsulinism
Functional nonhyperinsulinemic hypoglycemia
Hyperinsulinism NOS
Hyperplasia of pancreatic islet beta cells NOS
[EXCLUDES1] *hypoglycemia in infant of diabetic mother (P70.1)*
neonatal hypoglycemia (P70.4)

E16.2 Hypoglycemia, unspecified

E16.3 Increased secretion of glucagon
Hyperplasia of pancreatic endocrine cells with glucagon excess

E16.4 Increased secretion of gastrin
Hypergastrinemia
Hyperplasia of pancreatic endocrine cells with gastrin excess
Zollinger-Ellison syndrome

E16.8 Other specified disorders of pancreatic internal secretion
Increased secretion from endocrine pancreas of growth hormone-releasing hormone
Increased secretion from endocrine pancreas of pancreatic polypeptide
Increased secretion from endocrine pancreas of somatostatin
Increased secretion from endocrine pancreas of vasoactive-intestinal polypeptide

E16.9 Disorder of pancreatic internal secretion, unspecified
Islet-cell hyperplasia NOS
Pancreatic endocrine cell hyperplasia NOS

Disorders of other endocrine glands (E20-E35)

[EXCLUDES1] *galactorrhea (N64.3)*
gynecomastia (N62)

[4] E20 Hypoparathyroidism
[EXCLUDES1] *Di George's syndrome (D82.1)*
postprocedural hypoparathyroidism (E89.2)
tetany NOS (R29.0)
transitory neonatal hypoparathyroidism (P71.4)

[4] 4th character required [5] 5th character required [6] 6th character required [7] 7th character required [7x] Extension 'X' Alert
[EXCLUDES1] Not coded here [EXCLUDES2] Not included here [PDx] Primary Diagnosis Only Manifestation Code

E20.0 Idiopathic hypoparathyroidism
E20.1 Pseudohypoparathyroidism
E20.8 Other hypoparathyroidism
E20.9 Hypoparathyroidism, unspecified
Parathyroid tetany

[4th] **E21 Hyperparathyroidism and other disorders of parathyroid gland**

EXCLUDES1 *adult osteomalacia (M83.-)*
ectopic hyperparathyroidism (E34.2)
familial hypocalciuric hypercalcemia (E83.52)
hungry bone syndrome (E83.81)
infantile and juvenile osteomalacia (E55.0)

E21.0 Primary hyperparathyroidism
Hyperplasia of parathyroid
Osteitis fibrosa cystica generalisata [von Recklinghausen's disease of bone]
E21.1 Secondary hyperparathyroidism, not elsewhere classified
EXCLUDES1 *secondary hyperparathyroidism of renal origin (N25.81)*
E21.2 Other hyperparathyroidism
Tertiary hyperparathyroidism
EXCLUDES1 *familial hypocalciuric hypercalcemia (E83.52)*
E21.3 Hyperparathyroidism, unspecified
E21.4 Other specified disorders of parathyroid gland
E21.5 Disorder of parathyroid gland, unspecified

[4th] **E22 Hyperfunction of pituitary gland**

EXCLUDES1 *Cushing's syndrome (E24.-)*
Nelson's syndrome (E24.1)
overproduction of ACTH not associated with Cushing's disease (E27.0)
overproduction of pituitary ACTH (E24.0)
overproduction of thyroid-stimulating hormone (E05.8-)

E22.0 Acromegaly and pituitary gigantism
Overproduction of growth hormone
EXCLUDES1 *constitutional gigantism (E34.4)*
constitutional tall stature (E34.4)
increased secretion from endocrine pancreas of growth hormone-releasing hormone (E16.8)
E22.1 Hyperprolactinemia
Use additional code for adverse effect, if applicable, to identify drug (T36-T50 with fifth or sixth character 5)
E22.2 Syndrome of inappropriate secretion of antidiuretic hormone
E22.8 Other hyperfunction of pituitary gland
Central precocious puberty
E22.9 Hyperfunction of pituitary gland, unspecified

[4th] **E23 Hypofunction and other disorders of the pituitary gland**

INCLUDES *the listed conditions whether the disorder is in the pituitary or the hypothalamus*
EXCLUDES1 *postprocedural hypopituitarism (E89.3)*

E23.0 Hypopituitarism
Fertile eunuch syndrome
Hypogonadotropic hypogonadism
Idiopathic growth hormone deficiency
Isolated deficiency of gonadotropin
Isolated deficiency of growth hormone
Isolated deficiency of pituitary hormone
Kallmann's syndrome
Lorain-Levi short stature
Necrosis of pituitary gland (postpartum)
Panhypopituitarism
Pituitary cachexia
Pituitary insufficiency NOS
Pituitary short stature
Sheehan's syndrome
Simmonds' disease
E23.1 Drug-induced hypopituitarism
Use additional code for adverse effect, if applicable, to identify drug (T36-T50 with fifth or sixth character 5)
E23.2 Diabetes insipidus
EXCLUDES1 *nephrogenic diabetes insipidus (N25.1)*
E23.3 Hypothalamic dysfunction, not elsewhere classified
EXCLUDES1 *Prader-Willi syndrome (Q87.1)*
Russell-Silver syndrome (Q87.1)
E23.6 Other disorders of pituitary gland
Abscess of pituitary
Adiposogenital dystrophy
E23.7 Disorder of pituitary gland, unspecified

[4th] **E24 Cushing's syndrome**

EXCLUDES1 *congenital adrenal hyperplasia (E25.0)*

E24.0 Pituitary-dependent Cushing's disease
Overproduction of pituitary ACTH
Pituitary-dependent hypercorticalism
E24.1 Nelson's syndrome
E24.2 Drug-induced Cushing's syndrome
Use additional code for adverse effect, if applicable, to identify drug (T36-T50 with fifth or sixth character 5)
E24.3 Ectopic ACTH syndrome
E24.4 Alcohol-induced pseudo-Cushing's syndrome
E24.8 Other Cushing's syndrome
E24.9 Cushing's syndrome, unspecified

[4th] **E25 Adrenogenital disorders**

INCLUDES *adrenogenital syndromes, virilizing or feminizing, whether acquired or due to adrenal hyperplasia consequent on inborn enzyme defects in hormone synthesis*
Female adrenal pseudohermaphroditism
Female heterosexual precocious pseudopuberty
Male isosexual precocious pseudopuberty
Male macrogenitosomia praecox
Male sexual precocity with adrenal hyperplasia
Male virilization (female)
EXCLUDES1 *indeterminate sex and pseudohermaphroditism (Q56)*
chromosomal abnormalities (Q90-Q99)

E25.0 Congenital adrenogenital disorders associated with enzyme deficiency
Congenital adrenal hyperplasia
21-Hydroxylase deficiency
Salt-losing congenital adrenal hyperplasia
E25.8 Other adrenogenital disorders
Idiopathic adrenogenital disorder
Use additional code for adverse effect, if applicable, to identify drug (T36-T50 with fifth or sixth character 5)
E25.9 Adrenogenital disorder, unspecified
Adrenogenital syndrome NOS

[4th] **E26 Hyperaldosteronism**

[5th] E26.0 Primary hyperaldosteronism
E26.01 Conn's syndrome
Code also adrenal adenoma (D35.0-)
E26.02 Glucocorticoid-remediable aldosteronism
Familial aldosteronism type I
E26.09 Other primary hyperaldosteronism
Primary aldosteronism due to adrenal hyperplasia (bilateral)
E26.1 Secondary hyperaldosteronism
[5th] E26.8 Other hyperaldosteronism
E26.81 Bartter's syndrome
E26.89 Other hyperaldosteronism
E26.9 Hyperaldosteronism, unspecified
Aldosteronism NOS
Hyperaldosteronism NOS

[4th] **E27 Other disorders of adrenal gland**

Unspecified Code | Other Specified Code | [N] Newborn Age: 0 | [P] Pediatric Age: 0-17 | [M] Maternity Age: 12-55 | [A] Adult Age: 15-124 | ♂ Male | ♀ Female | ● New Code | ▲ Revised Code Title | ►◄ Revised Text

E27.0 Other adrenocortical overactivity
Overproduction of ACTH, not associated with Cushing's disease
Premature adrenarche
[EXCLUDES1] *Cushing's syndrome (E24.-)*

E27.1 Primary adrenocortical insufficiency
Addison's disease
Autoimmune adrenalitis
[EXCLUDES1] *Addison only phenotype adrenoleukodystrophy (E71.528)*
amyloidosis (E85.-)
tuberculous Addison's disease (A18.7)
Waterhouse-Friderichsen syndrome (A39.1)

E27.2 Addisonian crisis
Adrenal crisis
Adrenocortical crisis

E27.3 Drug-induced adrenocortical insufficiency
Use additional code for adverse effect, if applicable, to identify drug (T36-T50 with fifth or sixth character 5)

[5] **E27.4 Other and unspecified adrenocortical insufficiency**
[EXCLUDES1] *adrenoleukodystrophy [Addison-Schilder] (E71.528)*
Waterhouse-Friderichsen syndrome (A39.1)

E27.40 Unspecified adrenocortical insufficiency
Adrenocortical insufficiency NOS
Hypoaldosteronism

E27.49 Other adrenocortical insufficiency
Adrenal hemorrhage
Adrenal infarction

E27.5 Adrenomedullary hyperfunction
Adrenomedullary hyperplasia
Catecholamine hypersecretion

E27.8 Other specified disorders of adrenal gland
Abnormality of cortisol-binding globulin

E27.9 Disorder of adrenal gland, unspecified

[4] **E28 Ovarian dysfunction**
[EXCLUDES1] *isolated gonadotropin deficiency (E23.0)*
postprocedural ovarian failure (E89.4-)

E28.0 Estrogen excess
Use additional code for adverse effect, if applicable, to identify drug (T36-T50 with fifth or sixth character 5) ♀

E28.1 Androgen excess
Hypersecretion of ovarian androgens
Use additional code for adverse effect, if applicable, to identify drug (T36-T50 with fifth or sixth character 5) ♀

E28.2 Polycystic ovarian syndrome
Sclerocystic ovary syndrome
Stein-Leventhal syndrome ♀

[5] **E28.3 Primary ovarian failure**
[EXCLUDES1] *pure gonadal dysgenesis (Q99.1)*
Turner's syndrome (Q96.-)

[6] **E28.31 Premature menopause**

E28.310 Symptomatic premature menopause
Symptoms such as flushing, sleeplessness, headache, lack of concentration, associated with premature menopause [A] ♀

E28.319 Asymptomatic premature menopause
Premature menopause NOS [A] ♀

E28.39 Other primary ovarian failure
Decreased estrogen
Resistant ovary syndrome ♀

E28.8 Other ovarian dysfunction
Ovarian hyperfunction NOS
[EXCLUDES1] *postprocedural ovarian failure (E89.4-)* ♀

E28.9 Ovarian dysfunction, unspecified ♀

[4] **E29 Testicular dysfunction**
[EXCLUDES1] *androgen insensitivity syndrome (E34.5-)*
azoospermia or oligospermia NOS (N46.0-N46.1)
isolated gonadotropin deficiency (E23.0)
Klinefelter's syndrome (Q98.0-Q98.2, Q98.4)

E29.0 Testicular hyperfunction
Hypersecretion of testicular hormones ♂

E29.1 Testicular hypofunction
Defective biosynthesis of testicular androgen NOS
5-delta-Reductase deficiency (with male pseudohermaphroditism)
Testicular hypogonadism NOS
Use additional code for adverse effect, if applicable, to identify drug (T36-T50 with fifth or sixth character 5)
[EXCLUDES1] *postprocedural testicular hypofunction (E89.5)* ♂

E29.8 Other testicular dysfunction ♂

E29.9 Testicular dysfunction, unspecified ♂

[4] **E30 Disorders of puberty, not elsewhere classified**

E30.0 Delayed puberty
Constitutional delay of puberty
Delayed sexual development

E30.1 Precocious puberty
Precocious menstruation
[EXCLUDES1] *Albright (-McCune) (-Sternberg) syndrome (Q78.1)*
central precocious puberty (E22.8)
congenital adrenal hyperplasia (E25.0)
female heterosexual precocious pseudopuberty (E25.-)
male isosexual precocious pseudopuberty (E25.-) [P]

E30.8 Other disorders of puberty
Premature thelarche [P]

E30.9 Disorder of puberty, unspecified

[4] **E31 Polyglandular dysfunction**
[EXCLUDES1] *ataxia telangiectasia [Louis-Bar] (G11.3)*
dystrophia myotonica [Steinert] (G71.11)
pseudohypoparathyroidism (E20.1)

E31.0 Autoimmune polyglandular failure
Schmidt's syndrome

E31.1 Polyglandular hyperfunction
[EXCLUDES1] *multiple endocrine adenomatosis (E31.2-)*
multiple endocrine neoplasia (E31.2-)

[5] **E31.2 Multiple endocrine neoplasia [MEN] syndromes**
Multiple endocrine adenomatosis
Code also any associated malignancies and other conditions associated with the syndromes

E31.20 Multiple endocrine neoplasia [MEN] syndrome, unspecified
Multiple endocrine adenomatosis NOS
Multiple endocrine neoplasia [MEN] syndrome NOS

E31.21 Multiple endocrine neoplasia [MEN] type I
Wermer's syndrome

E31.22 Multiple endocrine neoplasia [MEN] type IIA
Sipple's syndrome

E31.23 Multiple endocrine neoplasia [MEN] type IIB

E31.8 Other polyglandular dysfunction

E31.9 Polyglandular dysfunction, unspecified

[4] **E32 Diseases of thymus**
[EXCLUDES1] *aplasia or hypoplasia of thymus with immunodeficiency (D82.1)*
myasthenia gravis (G70.0)

E32.0 Persistent hyperplasia of thymus
Hypertrophy of thymus

E32.1 Abscess of thymus

E32.8 Other diseases of thymus
[EXCLUDES1] *aplasia or hypoplasia with immunodeficiency (D82.1)*
thymoma (D15.0)

E32.9 Disease of thymus, unspecified

[4] 4th character required [5] 5th character required [6] 6th character required [7] 7th character required [7th] Extension 'X' Alert
[EXCLUDES1] Not coded here [EXCLUDES2] Not included here [PDx] Primary Diagnosis Only Manifestation Code

⊕ **E34 Other endocrine disorders**

EXCLUDES1 *pseudohypoparathyroidism (E20.1)*

E34.0 Carcinoid syndrome

NOTES May be used as an additional code to identify functional activity associated with a carcinoid tumor.

E34.1 Other hypersecretion of intestinal hormones

E34.2 Ectopic hormone secretion, not elsewhere classified

EXCLUDES1 *ectopic ACTH syndrome (E24.3)*

E34.3 Short stature due to endocrine disorder

Constitutional short stature

Laron-type short stature

EXCLUDES1 *achondroplastic short stature (Q77.4)*
hypochondroplastic short stature (Q77.4)
nutritional short stature (E45)
pituitary short stature (E23.0)
progeria (E34.8)
renal short stature (N25.0)
Russell-Silver syndrome (Q87.1)
short-limbed stature with immunodeficiency (D82.2)
short stature in specific dysmorphic syndromes - code to syndrome - see Alphabetical Index
short stature NOS (R62.52)

E34.4 Constitutional tall stature

Constitutional gigantism

⑤ **E34.5 Androgen insensitivity syndrome**

E34.50 Androgen insensitivity syndrome, unspecified

Androgen insensitivity NOS

E34.51 Complete androgen insensitivity syndrome

Complete androgen insensitivity

de Quervain syndrome

Goldberg-Maxwell syndrome

E34.52 Partial androgen insensitivity syndrome

Partial androgen insensitivity

Reifenstein syndrome

E34.8 Other specified endocrine disorders

Pineal gland dysfunction

Progeria

EXCLUDES2 *pseudohypoparathyroidism (E20.1)*

E34.9 Endocrine disorder, unspecified

Endocrine disturbance NOS

Hormone disturbance NOS

E35 Disorders of endocrine glands in diseases classified elsewhere

Code first underlying disease, such as:
late congenital syphilis of thymus gland [Dubois disease] (A50.5)

EXCLUDES1 *Echinococcus granulosus infection of thyroid gland (B67.3)*
meningococcal hemorrhagic adrenalitis (A39.1)
syphilis of endocrine gland (A52.79)
tuberculosis of adrenal gland, except calcification (A18.7)
tuberculosis of endocrine gland NEC (A18.82)
tuberculosis of thyroid gland (A18.81)
Waterhouse-Friderichsen syndrome (A39.1)

Use additional code , if applicable, to identify:
sequelae of tuberculosis of other organs (B90.8)

Intraoperative complications of endocrine system (E36)

⊕ **E36 Intraoperative complications of endocrine system**

EXCLUDES2 *postprocedural endocrine and metabolic complications and disorders, not elsewhere classified (E89.-)*

⑤ **E36.0 Intraoperative hemorrhage and hematoma of an endocrine system organ or structure complicating a procedure**

EXCLUDES1 *intraoperative hemorrhage and hematoma of an endocrine system organ or structure due to accidental puncture or laceration during a procedure (E36.1-)*

E36.01 Intraoperative hemorrhage and hematoma of an endocrine system organ or structure complicating an endocrine system procedure

E36.02 Intraoperative hemorrhage and hematoma of an endocrine system organ or structure complicating other procedure

⑤ **E36.1 Accidental puncture and laceration of an endocrine system organ or structure during a procedure**

E36.11 Accidental puncture and laceration of an endocrine system organ or structure during an endocrine system procedure

E36.12 Accidental puncture and laceration of an endocrine system organ or structure during other procedure

E36.8 Other intraoperative complications of endocrine system

Use additional code, if applicable, to further specify disorder

Malnutrition (E40-E46)

EXCLUDES1 *intestinal malabsorption (K90.-)*
sequelae of protein-calorie malnutrition (E64.0)

EXCLUDES2 *nutritional anemias (D50-D53)*
starvation (T73.0)

E40 Kwashiorkor

Severe malnutrition with nutritional edema with dyspigmentation of skin and hair

EXCLUDES1 *marasmic kwashiorkor (E42)*

E41 Nutritional marasmus

Severe malnutrition with marasmus

EXCLUDES1 *marasmic kwashiorkor (E42)*

E42 Marasmic kwashiorkor

Intermediate form severe protein-calorie malnutrition

Severe protein-calorie malnutrition with signs of both kwashiorkor and marasmus

E43 Unspecified severe protein-calorie malnutrition

Starvation edema

⊕ **E44 Protein-calorie malnutrition of moderate and mild degree**

E44.0 Moderate protein-calorie malnutrition

E44.1 Mild protein-calorie malnutrition

E45 Retarded development following protein-calorie malnutrition

Nutritional short stature

Nutritional stunting

Physical retardation due to malnutrition

E46 Unspecified protein-calorie malnutrition

Malnutrition NOS

Protein-calorie imbalance NOS

EXCLUDES1 *nutritional deficiency NOS (E63.9)*

Other nutritional deficiencies (E50-E64)

EXCLUDES2 *nutritional anemias (D50-D53)*

⊕ **E50 Vitamin A deficiency**

EXCLUDES1 *sequelae of vitamin A deficiency (E64.1)*

E50.0 Vitamin A deficiency with conjunctival xerosis

E50.1 Vitamin A deficiency with Bitot's spot and conjunctival xerosis

Bitot's spot in the young child

E50.2 Vitamin A deficiency with corneal xerosis

E50.3 Vitamin A deficiency with corneal ulceration and xerosis

E50.4 Vitamin A deficiency with keratomalacia

E50.5 Vitamin A deficiency with night blindness

E50.6 Vitamin A deficiency with xerophthalmic scars of cornea

E50.7 Other ocular manifestations of vitamin A deficiency

Xerophthalmia NOS

Unspecified Code	Other Specified Code	N Newborn Age: 0	P Pediatric Age: 0-17	M Maternity Age: 12-55

A Adult Age: 15-124 ♂ Male ♀ Female ● New Code ▲ Revised Code Title ►◄ Revised Text

E50.8 Other manifestations of vitamin A deficiency
Follicular keratosis
Xeroderma
E50.9 Vitamin A deficiency, unspecified
Hypovitaminosis A NOS

[4] E51 Thiamine deficiency
[EXCLUDES1] *sequelae of thiamine deficiency (E64.8)*

[5] E51.1 Beriberi
E51.11 Dry beriberi
Beriberi NOS
Beriberi with polyneuropathy
E51.12 Wet beriberi
Beriberi with cardiovascular manifestations
Cardiovascular beriberi
Shoshin disease
E51.2 Wernicke's encephalopathy
E51.8 Other manifestations of thiamine deficiency
E51.9 Thiamine deficiency, unspecified

E52 Niacin deficiency [pellagra]
Niacin (-tryptophan) deficiency
Nicotinamide deficiency
Pellagra (alcoholic)
[EXCLUDES1] *sequelae of niacin deficiency (E64.8)*

[4] E53 Deficiency of other B group vitamins
[EXCLUDES1] *sequelae of vitamin B deficiency (E64.8)*
E53.0 Riboflavin deficiency
Ariboflavinosis
Vitamin B2 deficiency
E53.1 Pyridoxine deficiency
Vitamin B6 deficiency
[EXCLUDES1] *pyridoxine-responsive sideroblastic anemia (D64.3)*
E53.8 Deficiency of other specified B group vitamins
Biotin deficiency
Cyanocobalamin deficiency
Folate deficiency
Folic acid deficiency
Pantothenic acid deficiency
Vitamin B12 deficiency
[EXCLUDES1] *folate deficiency anemia (D52.-)*
vitamin B12 deficiency anemia (D51.-)
E53.9 Vitamin B deficiency, unspecified

E54 Ascorbic acid deficiency
Deficiency of vitamin C
Scurvy
[EXCLUDES1] *scorbutic anemia (D53.2)*
sequelae of vitamin C deficiency (E64.2)

[4] E55 Vitamin D deficiency
[EXCLUDES1] *adult osteomalacia (M83.-)*
osteoporosis (M80.-)
sequelae of rickets (E64.3)
E55.0 Rickets, active
Infantile osteomalacia
Juvenile osteomalacia
[EXCLUDES1] *celiac rickets (K90.0)*
Crohn's rickets (K50.-)
hereditary vitamin D-dependent rickets (E83.32)
inactive rickets (E64.3)
renal rickets (N25.0)
sequelae of rickets (E64.3)
vitamin D-resistant rickets (E83.31)
E55.9 Vitamin D deficiency, unspecified
Avitaminosis D

[4] E56 Other vitamin deficiencies
[EXCLUDES1] *sequelae of other vitamin deficiencies (E64.8)*
E56.0 Deficiency of vitamin E
E56.1 Deficiency of vitamin K
[EXCLUDES1] *deficiency of coagulation factor due to vitamin K deficiency (D68.4)*
vitamin K deficiency of newborn (P53)
E56.8 Deficiency of other vitamins
E56.9 Vitamin deficiency, unspecified

E58 Dietary calcium deficiency
[EXCLUDES1] *disorders of calcium metabolism (E83.5-)*
sequelae of calcium deficiency (E64.8)

E59 Dietary selenium deficiency
Keshan disease
[EXCLUDES1] *sequelae of selenium deficiency (E64.8)*

E60 Dietary zinc deficiency

[4] E61 Deficiency of other nutrient elements
Use additional code for adverse effect, if applicable, to identify drug (T36-T50 with fifth or sixth character 5)
[EXCLUDES1] *disorders of mineral metabolism (E83.-)*
iodine deficiency related thyroid disorders (E00-E02)
sequelae of malnutrition and other nutritional deficiencies (E64.-)
E61.0 Copper deficiency
E61.1 Iron deficiency
[EXCLUDES1] *iron deficiency anemia (D50.-)*
E61.2 Magnesium deficiency
E61.3 Manganese deficiency
E61.4 Chromium deficiency
E61.5 Molybdenum deficiency
E61.6 Vanadium deficiency
E61.7 Deficiency of multiple nutrient elements
E61.8 Deficiency of other specified nutrient elements
E61.9 Deficiency of nutrient element, unspecified

[4] E63 Other nutritional deficiencies
[EXCLUDES1] *dehydration (E86.0)*
failure to thrive, adult (R62.7)
failure to thrive, child (R62.51)
feeding problems in newborn (P92.-)
sequelae of malnutrition and other nutritional deficiencies (E64.-)
E63.0 Essential fatty acid [EFA] deficiency
E63.1 Imbalance of constituents of food intake
E63.8 Other specified nutritional deficiencies
E63.9 Nutritional deficiency, unspecified

[4] E64 Sequelae of malnutrition and other nutritional deficiencies
[NOTES] This category is to be used to indicate conditions in categories E43, E44, E46, E50-E63 as the cause of sequelae, which are themselves classified elsewhere. The 'sequelae' include conditions specified as such; they also include the late effects of diseases classifiable to the above categories if the disease itself is no longer present
Code first condition resulting from (sequela) of malnutrition and other nutritional deficiencies
E64.0 Sequelae of protein-calorie malnutrition
[EXCLUDES2] *retarded development following protein-calorie malnutrition (E45)*
E64.1 Sequelae of vitamin A deficiency
E64.2 Sequelae of vitamin C deficiency
E64.3 Sequelae of rickets
E64.8 Sequelae of other nutritional deficiencies
E64.9 Sequelae of unspecified nutritional deficiency

Overweight, obesity and other hyperalimentation (E65-E68)

E65 Localized adiposity
Fat pad

[4] E66 Overweight and obesity
Code first obesity complicating pregnancy, childbirth and the puerperium, if applicable (O99.21-)

[4] 4th character required [5] 5th character required [6] 6th character required [7] 7th character required [X] Extension 'X' Alert
[EXCLUDES1] Not coded here [EXCLUDES2] Not included here [PDx] Primary Diagnosis Only Manifestation Code

Use additional code to identify body mass index (BMI), if known (Z68.-)

[EXCLUDES1] *adiposogenital dystrophy (E23.6)*
lipomatosis NOS (E88.2)
lipomatosis dolorosa [Dercum] (E88.2)
Prader-Willi syndrome (Q87.1)

[5] **E66.0 Obesity due to excess calories**

E66.01 Morbid (severe) obesity due to excess calories

[EXCLUDES1] *morbid (severe) obesity with alveolar hypoventilation (E66.2)*

E66.09 Other obesity due to excess calories

E66.1 Drug-induced obesity

Use additional code for adverse effect, if applicable, to identify drug (T36-T50 with fifth or sixth character 5)

E66.2 Morbid (severe) obesity with alveolar hypoventilation

Pickwickian syndrome

E66.3 Overweight

E66.8 Other obesity

E66.9 Obesity, unspecified

Obesity NOS

[4] **E67 Other hyperalimentation**

[EXCLUDES1] *hyperalimentation NOS (R63.2)*
sequelae of hyperalimentation (E68)

E67.0 Hypervitaminosis A

E67.1 Hypercarotinemia

E67.2 Megavitamin-B6 syndrome

E67.3 Hypervitaminosis D

E67.8 Other specified hyperalimentation

E68 Sequelae of hyperalimentation

Code first condition resulting from (sequela) of hyperalimentation

Metabolic disorders (E70-E88)

[EXCLUDES1] *androgen insensitivity syndrome (E34.5-)*
congenital adrenal hyperplasia (E25.0)
Ehlers-Danlos syndrome (Q79.6)
hemolytic anemias attributable to enzyme disorders (D55.-)
Marfan's syndrome (Q87.4)
5-alpha-reductase deficiency (E29.1)

[4] **E70 Disorders of aromatic amino-acid metabolism**

E70.0 Classical phenylketonuria

E70.1 Other hyperphenylalaninemias

[5] **E70.2 Disorders of tyrosine metabolism**

[EXCLUDES1] *transitory tyrosinemia of newborn (P74.5)*

E70.20 Disorder of tyrosine metabolism, unspecified

E70.21 Tyrosinemia

Hypertyrosinemia

E70.29 Other disorders of tyrosine metabolism

Alkaptonuria
Ochronosis

[5] **E70.3 Albinism**

E70.30 Albinism, unspecified

[6] **E70.31 Ocular albinism**

E70.310 X-linked ocular albinism

E70.311 Autosomal recessive ocular albinism

E70.318 Other ocular albinism

E70.319 Ocular albinism, unspecified

[6] **E70.32 Oculocutaneous albinism**

[EXCLUDES1] *Chediak-Higashi syndrome (E70.330)*
Hermansky-Pudlak syndrome (E70.331)

E70.320 Tyrosinase negative oculocutaneous albinism

Albinism I
Oculocutaneous albinism ty-neg

E70.321 Tyrosinase positive oculocutaneous albinism

Albinism II
Oculocutaneous albinism ty-pos

E70.328 Other oculocutaneous albinism

Cross syndrome

E70.329 Oculocutaneous albinism, unspecified

[6] **E70.33 Albinism with hematologic abnormality**

E70.330 Chediak-Higashi syndrome

E70.331 Hermansky-Pudlak syndrome

E70.338 Other albinism with hematologic abnormality

E70.339 Albinism with hematologic abnormality, unspecified

E70.39 Other specified albinism

Piebaldism

[5] **E70.4 Disorders of histidine metabolism**

E70.40 Disorders of histidine metabolism, unspecified

E70.41 Histidinemia

E70.49 Other disorders of histidine metabolism

E70.5 Disorders of tryptophan metabolism

E70.8 Other disorders of aromatic amino-acid metabolism

E70.9 Disorder of aromatic amino-acid metabolism, unspecified

[4] **E71 Disorders of branched-chain amino-acid metabolism and fatty-acid metabolism**

E71.0 Maple-syrup-urine disease

[5] **E71.1 Other disorders of branched-chain amino-acid metabolism**

[6] **E71.11 Branched-chain organic acidurias**

E71.110 Isovaleric acidemia

E71.111 3-methylglutaconic aciduria

E71.118 Other branched-chain organic acidurias

[6] **E71.12 Disorders of propionate metabolism**

E71.120 Methylmalonic acidemia

E71.121 Propionic acidemia

E71.128 Other disorders of propionate metabolism

E71.19 Other disorders of branched-chain amino-acid metabolism

Hyperleucine-isoleucinemia
Hypervalinemia

E71.2 Disorder of branched-chain amino-acid metabolism, unspecified

[5] **E71.3 Disorders of fatty-acid metabolism**

[EXCLUDES1] *peroxisomal disorders (E71.5)*
Refsum's disease (G60.1)
Schilder's disease (G37.0)

[EXCLUDES2] *carnitine deficiency due to inborn error of metabolism (E71.42)*

E71.30 Disorder of fatty-acid metabolism, unspecified

[6] **E71.31 Disorders of fatty-acid oxidation**

E71.310 Long chain/very long chain acyl CoA dehydrogenase deficiency

LCAD
VLCAD

E71.311 Medium chain acyl CoA dehydrogenase deficiency

MCAD

E71.312 Short chain acyl CoA dehydrogenase deficiency

SCAD

E71.313 Glutaric aciduria type II

Glutaric aciduria type II A
Glutaric aciduria type II B
Glutaric aciduria type II C

[EXCLUDES1] *glutaric aciduria (type 1) NOS (E72.3)*

E71.314 Muscle carnitine palmitoyltransferase deficiency

E71.318 Other disorders of fatty-acid oxidation

E71.32 Disorders of ketone metabolism

E71.39 Other disorders of fatty-acid metabolism

Unspecified Code | Other Specified Code | [N] Newborn Age: 0 | [P] Pediatric Age: 0-17 | [M] Maternity Age: 12-55
[A] Adult Age: 15-124 | ♂ Male | ♀ Female | ● New Code | ▲ Revised Code Title | ►◄ Revised Text

⑤ **E71.4 Disorders of carnitine metabolism**
  EXCLUDES1 *Muscle carnitine palmitoyltransferase deficiency (E71.314)*
  E71.40 Disorder of carnitine metabolism, unspecified
  E71.41 Primary carnitine deficiency
  E71.42 Carnitine deficiency due to inborn errors of metabolism
    Code also associated inborn error or metabolism
  E71.43 Iatrogenic carnitine deficiency
    Carnitine deficiency due to hemodialysis
    Carnitine deficiency due to Valproic acid therapy
  ⑥ **E71.44 Other secondary carnitine deficiency**
    E71.440 Ruvalcaba-Myhre-Smith syndrome
    E71.448 Other secondary carnitine deficiency
⑤ **E71.5 Peroxisomal disorders**
  EXCLUDES1 *Schilder's disease (G37.0)*
  E71.50 Peroxisomal disorder, unspecified
  ⑥ **E71.51 Disorders of peroxisome biogenesis**
    Group 1 peroxisomal disorders
    EXCLUDES1 *Refsum's disease (G60.1)*
    E71.510 Zellweger syndrome
    E71.511 Neonatal adrenoleukodystrophy
    EXCLUDES1 *X-linked adrenoleukodystrophy (E71.42-)* Ⓝ
    E71.518 Other disorders of peroxisome biogenesis
  ⑥ **E71.52 X-linked adrenoleukodystrophy**
    E71.520 Childhood cerebral X-linked adrenoleukodystrophy
    E71.521 Adolescent X-linked adrenoleukodystrophy
    E71.522 Adrenomyeloneuropathy
    E71.528 Other X-linked adrenoleukodystrophy
      Addison only phenotype adrenoleukodystrophy
      Addison-Schilder adrenoleukodystrophy
    E71.529 X-linked adrenoleukodystrophy, unspecified type
    E71.53 Other group 2 peroxisomal disorders
  ⑥ **E71.54 Other peroxisomal disorders**
    E71.540 Rhizomelic chondrodysplasia punctata
    EXCLUDES1 *chondrodysplasia punctata NOS (Q77.3)*
    E71.541 Zellweger-like syndrome
    E71.542 Other group 3 peroxisomal disorders
    E71.548 Other peroxisomal disorders
④ **E72 Other disorders of amino-acid metabolism**
  EXCLUDES1 *disorders of:*
    aromatic amino-acid metabolism (E70.-)
    branched-chain amino-acid metabolism (E71.0-E71.2)
    fatty-acid metabolism (E71.3)
    purine and pyrimidine metabolism (E79.-)
    gout (M1A.-, M10.-)
⑤ **E72.0 Disorders of amino-acid transport**
  EXCLUDES1 *disorders of tryptophan metabolism (E70.5)*
  E72.00 Disorders of amino-acid transport, unspecified
  E72.01 Cystinuria
  E72.02 Hartnup's disease
  E72.03 Lowe's syndrome
    Use additional code for associated glaucoma (H42)
  E72.04 Cystinosis
    Fanconi (-de Toni) (-Debré) syndrome with cystinosis
    EXCLUDES1 *Fanconi (-de Toni) (-Debré) syndrome without cystinosis (E72.09)*
  E72.09 Other disorders of amino-acid transport
    Fanconi (-de Toni) (-Debré) syndrome, unspecified
⑤ **E72.1 Disorders of sulfur-bearing amino-acid metabolism**

  EXCLUDES1 *cystinosis (E72.04)*
    cystinuria (E72.01)
    transcobalamin II deficiency (D51.2)
  E72.10 Disorders of sulfur-bearing amino-acid metabolism, unspecified
  E72.11 Homocystinuria
    Cystathionine synthase deficiency
  E72.12 Methylenetetrahydrofolate reductase deficiency
  E72.19 Other disorders of sulfur-bearing amino-acid metabolism
    Cystathioninuria
    Methioninemia
    Sulfite oxidase deficiency
⑤ **E72.2 Disorders of urea cycle metabolism**
  EXCLUDES1 *disorders of ornithine metabolism (E72.4)*
  E72.20 Disorder of urea cycle metabolism, unspecified
    Hyperammonemia
    EXCLUDES1 *hyperammonemia-hyperornithinemia-homocitrullinemia syndrome E72.4*
      transient hyperammonemia of newborn (P74.6)
  E72.21 Argininemia
  E72.22 Arginosuccinic aciduria
  E72.23 Citrullinemia
  E72.29 Other disorders of urea cycle metabolism
  E72.3 Disorders of lysine and hydroxylysine metabolism
    Glutaric aciduria NOS
    Glutaric aciduria (type I)
    Hydroxylysinemia
    Hyperlysinemia
    EXCLUDES1 *glutaric aciduria type II (E71.313)*
      Refsum's disease (G60.1)
      Zellweger syndrome (E71.510)
  E72.4 Disorders of ornithine metabolism
    Hyperammonemia-Hyperornithinemia-Homocitrullinemia syndrome
    Ornithinemia (types I, II)
    Ornithine transcarbamylase deficiency
    EXCLUDES1 *hereditary choroidal dystrophy (H31.2-)*
⑤ **E72.5 Disorders of glycine metabolism**
  E72.50 Disorder of glycine metabolism, unspecified
  E72.51 Non-ketotic hyperglycinemia
  E72.52 Trimethylaminuria
  E72.53 Hyperoxaluria
    Oxalosis
    Oxaluria
  E72.59 Other disorders of glycine metabolism
    D-glycericacidemia
    Hyperhydroxyprolinemia
    Hyperprolinemia (types I, II)
    Sarcosinemia
  E72.8 Other specified disorders of amino-acid metabolism
    Disorders of beta-amino-acid metabolism
    Disorders of gamma-glutamyl cycle
  E72.9 Disorder of amino-acid metabolism, unspecified
④ **E73 Lactose intolerance**
  E73.0 Congenital lactase deficiency
  E73.1 Secondary lactase deficiency
  E73.8 Other lactose intolerance
  E73.9 Lactose intolerance, unspecified
④ **E74 Other disorders of carbohydrate metabolism**
  EXCLUDES1 *diabetes mellitus (E08-E13)*
    hypoglycemia NOS (E16.2)
    increased secretion of glucagon (E16.3)
    mucopolysaccharidosis (E76.0-E76.3)
⑤ **E74.0 Glycogen storage disease**
  E74.00 Glycogen storage disease, unspecified
  E74.01 von Gierke disease
    Type I glycogen storage disease

---

④ 4th character required ⑤ 5th character required ⑥ 6th character required ⑦ 7th character required ⑩ Extension 'X' Alert

EXCLUDES 1 Not coded here EXCLUDES 2 Not included here PDx Primary Diagnosis Only Manifestation Code

E74.02 Pompe disease
Cardiac glycogenosis
Type II glycogen storage disease
E74.03 Cori disease
Forbes disease
Type III glycogen storage disease
E74.04 McArdle disease
Type V glycogen storage disease
E74.09 Other glycogen storage disease
Andersen disease
Hers disease
Tauri disease
Glycogen storage disease, types 0, IV, VI-XI
Liver phosphorylase deficiency
Muscle phosphofructokinase deficiency
[5] E74.1 Disorders of fructose metabolism
[EXCLUDES1] *muscle phosphofructokinase deficiency (E74.09)*
E74.10 Disorder of fructose metabolism, unspecified
E74.11 Essential fructosuria
Fructokinase deficiency
E74.12 Hereditary fructose intolerance
Fructosemia
E74.19 Other disorders of fructose metabolism
Fructose-1, 6-diphosphatase deficiency
[5] E74.2 Disorders of galactose metabolism
E74.20 Disorders of galactose metabolism, unspecified
E74.21 Galactosemia
E74.29 Other disorders of galactose metabolism
Galactokinase deficiency
[5] E74.3 Other disorders of intestinal carbohydrate absorption
[EXCLUDES2] *lactose intolerance (E73.-)*
E74.31 Sucrase-isomaltase deficiency
E74.39 Other disorders of intestinal carbohydrate absorption
Disorder of intestinal carbohydrate absorption NOS
Glucose-galactose malabsorption
Sucrase deficiency
E74.4 Disorders of pyruvate metabolism and gluconeogenesis
Deficiency of phosphoenolpyruvate carboxykinase
Deficiency of pyruvate carboxylase
Deficiency of pyruvate dehydrogenase
[EXCLUDES1] *disorders of pyruvate metabolism and gluconeogenesis with anemia (D55.-)*
Leigh's syndrome (G31.82)
E74.8 Other specified disorders of carbohydrate metabolism
Essential pentosuria
Renal glycosuria
E74.9 Disorder of carbohydrate metabolism, unspecified
[4] E75 Disorders of sphingolipid metabolism and other lipid storage disorders
[EXCLUDES1] *mucolipidosis, types I-III (E77.0-E77.1)*
Refsum's disease (G60.1)
[5] E75.0 GM2 gangliosidosis
E75.00 GM2 gangliosidosis, unspecified
E75.01 Sandhoff disease
E75.02 Tay-Sachs disease
E75.09 Other GM2 gangliosidosis
Adult GM2 gangliosidosis
Juvenile GM2 gangliosidosis
[5] E75.1 Other and unspecified gangliosidosis
E75.10 Unspecified gangliosidosis
Gangliosidosis NOS
E75.11 Mucolipidosis IV
E75.19 Other gangliosidosis
GM1 gangliosidosis
GM3 gangliosidosis
[5] E75.2 Other sphingolipidosis
[EXCLUDES1] *adrenoleukodystrophy [Addison-Schilder] (E71.528)*
E75.21 Fabry (-Anderson) disease
E75.22 Gaucher disease
E75.23 Krabbe disease
[6] E75.24 Niemann-Pick disease
E75.240 Niemann-Pick disease type A
E75.241 Niemann-Pick disease type B
E75.242 Niemann-Pick disease type C
E75.243 Niemann-Pick disease type D
E75.248 Other Niemann-Pick disease
E75.249 Niemann-Pick disease, unspecified
E75.25 Metachromatic leukodystrophy
E75.29 Other sphingolipidosis
Farber's syndrome
Sulfatase deficiency
Sulfatide lipidosis
E75.3 Sphingolipidosis, unspecified
E75.4 Neuronal ceroid lipofuscinosis
Batten disease
Bielschowsky-Jansky disease
Kufs disease
Spielmeyer-Vogt disease
E75.5 Other lipid storage disorders
Cerebrotendinous cholesterosis [van Bogaert-Scherer-Epstein]
Wolman's disease
E75.6 Lipid storage disorder, unspecified
[4] E76 Disorders of glycosaminoglycan metabolism
[5] E76.0 Mucopolysaccharidosis, type I
E76.01 Hurler's syndrome
E76.02 Hurler-Scheie syndrome
E76.03 Scheie's syndrome
E76.1 Mucopolysaccharidosis, type II
Hunter's syndrome
[5] E76.2 Other mucopolysaccharidoses
[6] E76.21 Morquio mucopolysaccharidoses
E76.210 Morquio A mucopolysaccharidoses
Classic Morquio syndrome
Morquio syndrome A
Mucopolysaccharidosis, type IVA
E76.211 Morquio B mucopolysaccharidoses
Morquio-like mucopolysaccharidoses
Morquio-like syndrome
Morquio syndrome B
Mucopolysaccharidosis, type IVB
E76.219 Morquio mucopolysaccharidoses, unspecified
Morquio syndrome
Mucopolysaccharidosis, type IV
E76.22 Sanfilippo mucopolysaccharidoses
Mucopolysaccharidosis, type III (A) (B) (C) (D)
Sanfilippo A syndrome
Sanfilippo B syndrome
Sanfilippo C syndrome
Sanfilippo D syndrome
E76.29 Other mucopolysaccharidoses
beta-Glucuronidase deficiency
Maroteaux-Lamy (mild) (severe) syndrome
Mucopolysaccharidosis, types VI, VII
E76.3 Mucopolysaccharidosis, unspecified
E76.8 Other disorders of glucosaminoglycan metabolism
E76.9 Glucosaminoglycan metabolism disorder, unspecified

Unspecified Code Other Specified Code [N] Newborn Age: 0 [P] Pediatric Age: 0-17 [M] Maternity Age: 12-55
[A] Adult Age: 15-124 ♂ Male ♀ Female ● New Code ▲ Revised Code Title ►◄ Revised Text

[4] E77 Disorders of glycoprotein metabolism

E77.0 Defects in post-translational modification of lysosomal enzymes
- Mucolipidosis II [I-cell disease]
- Mucolipidosis III [pseudo-Hurler polydystrophy]

E77.1 Defects in glycoprotein degradation
- Aspartylglucosaminuria
- Fucosidosis
- Mannosidosis
- Sialidosis [mucolipidosis I]

E77.8 Other disorders of glycoprotein metabolism

E77.9 Disorder of glycoprotein metabolism, unspecified

[4] E78 Disorders of lipoprotein metabolism and other lipidemias

[EXCLUDES1] *sphingolipidosis (E75.0-E75.3)*

E78.0 Pure hypercholesterolemia
- Familial hypercholesterolemia
- Fredrickson's hyperlipoproteinemia, type IIa
- Hyperbetalipoproteinemia
- Hyperlipidemia, Group A
- Low-density-lipoprotein-type [LDL] hyperlipoproteinemia

E78.1 Pure hyperglyceridemia
- Elevated fasting triglycerides
- Endogenous hyperglyceridemia
- Fredrickson's hyperlipoproteinemia, type IV
- Hyperlipidemia, group B
- Hyperprebetalipoproteinemia
- Very-low-density-lipoprotein-type [VLDL] hyperlipoproteinemia

E78.2 Mixed hyperlipidemia
- Broad- or floating-betalipoproteinemia
- Combined hyperlipidemia NOS
- Elevated cholesterol with elevated triglycerides NEC
- Fredrickson's hyperlipoproteinemia, type IIb or III
- Hyperbetalipoproteinemia with prebetalipoproteinemia
- Hypercholesteremia with endogenous hyperglyceridemia
- Hyperlipidemia, group C
- Tubo-eruptive xanthoma
- Xanthoma tuberosum

[EXCLUDES1] *cerebrotendinous cholesterosis [van Bogaert-Scherer- Epstein] (E75.5)*
familial combined hyperlipidemia (E78.4)

E78.3 Hyperchylomicronemia
- Chylomicron retention disease
- Fredrickson's hyperlipoproteinemia, type I or V
- Hyperlipidemia, group D
- Mixed hyperglyceridemia

E78.4 Other hyperlipidemia
- Familial combined hyperlipidemia

E78.5 Hyperlipidemia, unspecified

E78.6 Lipoprotein deficiency
- Abetalipoproteinemia
- Depressed HDL cholesterol
- High-density lipoprotein deficiency
- Hypoalphalipoproteinemia
- Hypobetalipoproteinemia (familial)
- Lecithin cholesterol acyltransferase deficiency
- Tangier disease

[5] E78.7 Disorders of bile acid and cholesterol metabolism

[EXCLUDES1] *Niemann-Pick disease type C (E75.242)*

E78.70 Disorder of bile acid and cholesterol metabolism, unspecified

E78.71 Barth syndrome

E78.72 Smith-Lemli-Opitz syndrome

E78.79 Other disorders of bile acid and cholesterol metabolism

[5] **E78.8 Other disorders of lipoprotein metabolism**

E78.81 Lipoid dermatoarthritis

E78.89 Other lipoprotein metabolism disorders

E78.9 Disorder of lipoprotein metabolism, unspecified

[4] E79 Disorders of purine and pyrimidine metabolism

[EXCLUDES1] *Ataxia-telangiectasia (Q87.1)*
Bloom's syndrome (Q82.8)
Cockayne's syndrome (Q87.1)
calculus of kidney (N20.0)
combined immunodeficiency disorders (D81.-)
Fanconi's anemia (D61.09)
gout (M1A.-, M10.-)
orotaciduric anemia (D53.0)
progeria (E34.8)
Werner's syndrome (E34.8)
xeroderma pigmentosum (Q82.1)

E79.0 Hyperuricemia without signs of inflammatory arthritis and tophaceous disease
- Asymptomatic hyperuricemia

E79.1 Lesch-Nyhan syndrome
- HGPRT deficiency

E79.2 Myoadenylate deaminase deficiency

E79.8 Other disorders of purine and pyrimidine metabolism
- Hereditary xanthinuria

E79.9 Disorder of purine and pyrimidine metabolism, unspecified

[4] E80 Disorders of porphyrin and bilirubin metabolism

INCLUDES *defects of catalase and peroxidase*

E80.0 Hereditary erythropoietic porphyria
- Congenital erythropoietic porphyria
- Erythropoietic protoporphyria

E80.1 Porphyria cutanea tarda

[5] **E80.2 Other and unspecified porphyria**

E80.20 Unspecified porphyria
- Porphyria NOS

E80.21 Acute intermittent **(hepatic) porphyria**

E80.29 Other porphyria
- Hereditary coproporphyria

E80.3 Defects of catalase and peroxidase
- Acatalasia [Takahara]

E80.4 Gilbert syndrome

E80.5 Crigler-Najjar syndrome

E80.6 Other disorders of bilirubin metabolism
- Dubin-Johnson syndrome
- Rotor's syndrome

E80.7 Disorder of bilirubin metabolism, unspecified

[4] E83 Disorders of mineral metabolism

[EXCLUDES1] *dietary mineral deficiency (E58-E61)*
parathyroid disorders (E20-E21)
vitamin D deficiency (E55.-)

[5] E83.0 Disorders of copper metabolism

E83.00 Disorder of copper metabolism, unspecified

E83.01 Wilson's disease
- Code also associated Kayser Fleischer ring (H18.04-)

E83.09 Other disorders of copper metabolism
- Menkes' (kinky hair) (steely hair) disease

[5] E83.1 Disorders of iron metabolism

[EXCLUDES1] *iron deficiency anemia (D50.-)*
sideroblastic anemia (D64.0-D64.3)

E83.10 Disorder of iron metabolism, unspecified

[6] **E83.11 Hemochromatosis**

E83.110 Hereditary **hemochromatosis**
- Bronzed diabetes
- Pigmentary cirrhosis (of liver)
- Primary (hereditary) hemochromatosis

E83.111 **Hemochromatosis** due to repeated red blood cell transfusions

Iron overload due to repeated red blood cell transfusions

Transfusion (red blood cell) associated hemochromatosis

E83.118 **Other hemochromatosis**

E83.119 **Hemochromatosis, unspecified**

E83.19 **Other disorders of iron metabolism**

Use additional code, if applicable, for idiopathic pulmonary hemosiderosis (J84.03)

E83.2 **Disorders of** zinc **metabolism**

Acrodermatitis enteropathica

⑤ E83.3 **Disorders of** phosphorus **metabolism and phosphatases**

EXCLUDES1 *adult osteomalacia (M83.-)*
osteoporosis (M80.-)

E83.30 **Disorder of phosphorus metabolism, unspecified**

E83.31 **Familial hypophosphatemia**

Vitamin D-resistant osteomalacia

Vitamin D-resistant rickets

EXCLUDES1 *vitamin D-deficiency rickets (E55.0)*

E83.32 **Hereditary vitamin D-dependent rickets (type 1) (type 2)**

25-hydroxyvitamin D 1-alpha-hydroxylase deficiency

Pseudovitamin D deficiency

Vitamin D receptor defect

E83.39 **Other disorders of phosphorus metabolism**

Acid phosphatase deficiency

Hypophosphatasia

⑤ E83.4 **Disorders of** magnesium **metabolism**

E83.40 **Disorders of magnesium metabolism, unspecified**

E83.41 **Hypermagnesemia**

E83.42 **Hypomagnesemia**

E83.49 **Other disorders of magnesium metabolism**

⑤ E83.5 **Disorders of** calcium **metabolism**

EXCLUDES1 *chondrocalcinosis (M11.1-M11.2)*
hungry bone syndrome (E83.81)
hyperparathyroidism (E21.0-E21.3)

E83.50 **Unspecified disorder of calcium metabolism**

E83.51 **Hypocalcemia**

E83.52 **Hypercalcemia**

Familial hypocalciuric hypercalcemia

E83.59 **Other disorders of calcium metabolism**

Idiopathic hypercalciuria

⑤ E83.8 **Other disorders of** mineral **metabolism**

E83.81 **Hungry bone syndrome**

E83.89 **Other disorders of mineral metabolism**

E83.9 **Disorder of mineral metabolism, unspecified**

④ E84 **Cystic fibrosis**

INCLUDES *mucoviscidosis*

E84.0 **Cystic fibrosis with** pulmonary manifestations

Use additional code to identify any infectious organism present, such as:

Pseudomonas (B96.5)

⑤ E84.1 **Cystic fibrosis with** intestinal manifestations

E84.11 **Meconium ileus** in cystic fibrosis

EXCLUDES1 *meconium ileus not due to cystic fibrosis (P76.0)*N

E84.19 **Cystic fibrosis with** other intestinal manifestations

Distal intestinal obstruction syndrome

E84.8 **Cystic fibrosis with other** manifestations

E84.9 **Cystic fibrosis, unspecified**

④ E85 **Amyloidosis**

EXCLUDES1 *Alzheimer's disease (G30.0-)*

E85.0 **Non-neuropathic heredofamilial amyloidosis**

Familial Mediterranean fever

Hereditary amyloid nephropathy

E85.1 **Neuropathic heredofamilial amyloidosis**

Amyloid polyneuropathy (Portuguese)

E85.2 **Heredofamilial amyloidosis, unspecified**

E85.3 **Secondary systemic amyloidosis**

Hemodialysis-associated amyloidosis

E85.4 **Organ-limited amyloidosis**

Localized amyloidosis

E85.8 **Other amyloidosis**

E85.9 **Amyloidosis, unspecified**

④ E86 **Volume depletion**

EXCLUDES1 *dehydration of newborn (P74.1)*
hypovolemic shock NOS (R57.1)
postprocedural hypovolemic shock (T81.19)
traumatic hypovolemic shock (T79.4)

E86.0 **Dehydration**

E86.1 **Hypovolemia**

Depletion of volume of plasma

E86.9 **Volume depletion, unspecified**

④ E87 **Other disorders of** fluid, electrolyte and acid-base balance

EXCLUDES1 *diabetes insipidus (E23.2)*
electrolyte imbalance associated with hyperemesis gravidarum (O21.1)
electrolyte imbalance following ectopic or molar pregnancy (O08.5)
familial periodic paralysis (G72.3)

E87.0 **Hyperosmolality and hypernatremia**

Sodium [Na] excess

Sodium [Na] overload

E87.1 **Hypo-osmolality and hyponatremia**

Sodium [Na] deficiency

EXCLUDES1 *syndrome of inappropriate secretion of antidiuretic hormone (E22.2)*

E87.2 **Acidosis**

Acidosis NOS

Lactic acidosis

Metabolic acidosis

Respiratory acidosis

EXCLUDES1 *diabetic acidosis - see categories E08-E10, E13 with ketoacidosis*

E87.3 **Alkalosis**

Alkalosis NOS

Metabolic alkalosis

Respiratory alkalosis

E87.4 **Mixed disorder of acid-base balance**

E87.5 **Hyperkalemia**

Potassium [K] excess

Potassium [K] overload

E87.6 **Hypokalemia**

Potassium [K] deficiency

⑤ E87.7 **Fluid overload**

EXCLUDES1 *edema NOS (R60.9)*
fluid retention (R60.9)

E87.70 **Fluid overload, unspecified**

E87.71 **Transfusion associated circulatory overload**

Fluid overload due to transfusion (blood) (blood components)

TACO

E87.79 **Other fluid overload**

E87.8 **Other disorders of electrolyte and fluid balance, not elsewhere classified**

Electrolyte imbalance NOS

Hyperchloremia

Hypochloremia

Unspecified Code   Other Specified Code   N Newborn Age: 0   P Pediatric Age: 0-17   M Maternity Age: 12-55
A Adult Age: 15-124   ♂ Male   ♀ Female   ● New Code   ▲ Revised Code Title   ►◄ Revised Text

④ *E88* **Other and unspecified metabolic disorders**

Use additional codes for associated conditions

EXCLUDES1 *histiocytosis X (chronic) (C96.6)*

⑤ **E88.0 Disorders of plasma-protein metabolism, not elsewhere classified**

EXCLUDES1 *disorder of lipoprotein metabolism (E78.-)*
monoclonal gammopathy (of undetermined significance) (D47.2)
polyclonal hypergammaglobulinemia (D89.0)
Waldenström macroglobulinemia (C88.0)

E88.01 Alpha-1-antitrypsin deficiency

AAT deficiency

E88.09 Other disorders of plasma-protein metabolism, not elsewhere classified

Bisalbuminemia

E88.1 Lipodystrophy, not elsewhere classified

Lipodystrophy NOS

EXCLUDES1 *Whipple's disease (K90.81)*

E88.2 Lipomatosis, not elsewhere classified

Lipomatosis NOS
Lipomatosis (Check) dolorosa [Dercum]

E88.3 Tumor lysis syndrome

Tumor lysis syndrome (spontaneous)
Tumor lysis syndrome following antineoplastic drug chemotherapy
Use additional code for adverse effect, if applicable, to identify drug (T45.1X5)

⑤ **E88.4 Mitochondrial metabolism disorders**

EXCLUDES1 *disorders of pyruvate metabolism (E74.4)*
Kearns-Sayre syndrome (H49.81)
Leber's disease (H47.22)
Leigh's encephalopathy (G31.82)
Mitochondrial myopathy, NEC (G71.3)
Reye's syndrome (G93.7)

E88.40 Mitochondrial metabolism disorder, unspecified

E88.41 MELAS syndrome

Mitochondrial myopathy, encephalopathy, lactic acidosis and stroke-like episodes

E88.42 MERRF syndrome

Myoclonic epilepsy associated with ragged-red fibers
Code also myoclonic epilepsy (G40.3-)

E88.49 Other mitochondrial metabolism disorders

⑤ **E88.8 Other specified metabolic disorders**

E88.81 Metabolic syndrome

Dysmetabolic syndrome X
Use additional codes for associated manifestations, such as:
obesity (E66.-)

E88.89 Other specified metabolic disorders

Launois-Bensaude adenolipomatosis

EXCLUDES1 *adult pulmonary Langerhans cell histiocytosis (J84.82)*

E88.9 Metabolic disorder, unspecified

Postprocedural endocrine and metabolic complications and disorders, not elsewhere classified (E89)

④ **E89 Postprocedural endocrine and metabolic complications and disorders, not elsewhere classified**

EXCLUDES2 *intraoperative complications of endocrine system organ or structure (E36.0-, E36.1-, E36.8)*

E89.0 Postprocedural hypothyroidism

Postirradiation hypothyroidism
Postsurgical hypothyroidism

E89.1 Postprocedural hypoinsulinemia

Postpancreatectomy hyperglycemia
Postsurgical hypoinsulinemia
Use additional code, if applicable, to identify:
acquired absence of pancreas (Z90.41-)
diabetes mellitus (postpancreatectomy) (postprocedural) (E13.-)
insulin use (Z79.4)

EXCLUDES1 *transient postprocedural hyperglycemia (R73.9)*
transient postprocedural hypoglycemia (E16.2)

E89.2 Postprocedural hypoparathyroidism

Parathyroprival tetany

E89.3 Postprocedural hypopituitarism

Postirradiation hypopituitarism

⑤ **E89.4 Postprocedural ovarian failure**

E89.40 Asymptomatic postprocedural ovarian failure

Postprocedural ovarian failure NOS ♀

E89.41 Symptomatic postprocedural ovarian failure

Symptoms such as flushing, sleeplessness, headache, lack of concentration, associated with postprocedural menopause ♀

E89.5 Postprocedural testicular hypofunction ♂

E89.6 Postprocedural adrenocortical (-medullary) hypofunction

⑤ **E89.8 Other postprocedural endocrine and metabolic complications and disorders**

⑥ **E89.81 Postprocedural hemorrhage and hematoma of an endocrine system organ or structure following a procedure**

E89.810 Postprocedural hemorrhage and hematoma of an endocrine system organ or structure following an endocrine system procedure

E89.811 Postprocedural hemorrhage and hematoma of an endocrine system organ or structure following other procedure

E89.89 Other postprocedural endocrine and metabolic complications and disorders

Use additional code, if applicable, to further specify disorder

---

④ 4th character required　⑤ 5th character required　⑥ 6th character required　⑦ 7th character required　⑦ₓ Extension 'X' Alert

EXCLUDES1 Not coded here　EXCLUDES2 Not included here　PDx Primary Diagnosis Only　Manifestation Code

Chapter 5: Mental, Behavioral and Neurodevelopmental Disorders (F01 – F99)

Chapter Specific Coding Guidelines

a. **Pain disorders related to psychological factors**

   Assign code F45.41, for pain that is exclusively related to psychological disorders. As indicated by the Excludes 1 note under category G89, a code from category G89 should not be assigned with code F45.41

   Code F45.42, Pain disorders with related psychological factors, should be used with a code from category G89, Pain, not elsewhere classified, if there is documentation of a psychological component for a patient with acute or chronic pain.

   See Section I.C.6. Pain

b. **Mental and behavioral disorders due to psychoactive substance use**

   1) **In Remission**

      Selection of codes for "in remission" for categories F10-F19, Mental and behavioral disorders due to psychoactive substance use (categories F10-F19 with -.21) requires the provider's clinical judgment. The appropriate codes for "in remission" are assigned only on the basis of provider documentation (as defined in the Official Guidelines for Coding and Reporting).

   2) **Psychoactive Substance Use, Abuse And Dependence**

      When the provider documentation refers to use, abuse and dependence of the same substance (e.g. alcohol, opioid, cannabis, etc.), only one code should be assigned to identify the pattern of use based on the following hierarchy:

      - If both use and abuse are documented, assign only the code for abuse
      - If both abuse and dependence are documented, assign only the code for dependence
      - If use, abuse and dependence are all documented, assign only the code for dependence
      - If both use and dependence are documented, assign only the code for dependence.

   3) **Psychoactive Substance Use**

      As with all other diagnoses, the codes for psychoactive substance use (F10.9-, F11.9-, F12.9-, F13.9-, F14.9-, F15.9-, F16.9-) should only be assigned based on provider documentation and when they meet the definition of a reportable diagnosis (see Section III, Reporting Additional Diagnoses). The codes are to be used only when the psychoactive substance use is associated with a mental or behavioral disorder, and such a relationship is documented by the provider.

This page intentionally left blank

Mental, Behavioral and Neurodevelopmental disorders (F01-F99)

> INCLUDES *disorders of psychological development*
>
> EXCLUDES2 *symptoms, signs and abnormal clinical laboratory findings, not elsewhere classified (R00-R99)*

Mental disorders due to known physiological conditions (F01-F09)

> NOTES This block comprises a range of mental disorders grouped together on the basis of their having in common a demonstrable etiology in cerebral disease, brain injury, or other insult leading to cerebral dysfunction. The dysfunction may be primary, as in diseases, injuries, and insults that affect the brain directly and selectively; or secondary, as in systemic diseases and disorders that attack the brain only as one of the multiple organs or systems of the body that are involved.

🄬 **F01 Vascular dementia**

Vascular dementia as a result of infarction of the brain due to vascular disease, including hypertensive cerebrovascular disease.

> INCLUDES *arteriosclerotic dementia*

Code first the underlying physiological condition or sequelae of cerebrovascular disease.

🄮 **F01.5 Vascular dementia**

F01.50 Vascular dementia without behavioral disturbance 🄰

F01.51 Vascular dementia with behavioral disturbance

Vascular dementia with aggressive behavior

Vascular dementia with combative behavior

Vascular dementia with violent behavior

Use additional code, if applicable, to identify wandering in vascular dementia (Z91.83) 🄰

🄬 **F02 Dementia in other diseases classified elsewhere**

Code first the underlying physiological condition, such as:

Alzheimer's (G30.-)

cerebral lipidosis (E75.4)

Creutzfeldt-Jakob disease (A81.0-)

dementia with Lewy bodies (G31.83)

epilepsy and recurrent seizures (G40.-)

frontotemporal dementia (G31.09)

hepatolenticular degeneration (E83.0)

human immunodeficiency virus [HIV] disease (B20)

hypercalcemia (E83.52)

hypothyroidism, acquired (E00-E03.-)

intoxications (T36-T65)

Jakob-Creutzfeldt disease (A81.0-)

multiple sclerosis (G35)

neurosyphilis (A52.17)

niacin deficiency [pellagra] (E52)

Parkinson's disease (G20)

Pick's disease (G31.01)

polyarteritis nodosa (M30.0)

systemic lupus erythematosus (M32.-)

trypanosomiasis (B56.-, B57.-)

vitamin B deficiency (E53.8)

> EXCLUDES1 *dementia with Parkinsonism (G31.83)*
>
> EXCLUDES2 *dementia in alcohol and psychoactive substance disorders (F10-F19, with .17, .27, .97)*
> *vascular dementia (F01.5-)*

🄮 **F02.8 Dementia in other diseases classified elsewhere**

F02.80 Dementia in other diseases classified elsewhere without behavioral disturbance

Dementia in other diseases classified elsewhere NOS

F02.81 Dementia in other diseases classified elsewhere with behavioral disturbance

Dementia in other diseases classified elsewhere with aggressive behavior

Dementia in other diseases classified elsewhere with combative behavior

Dementia in other diseases classified elsewhere with violent behavior

Use additional code, if applicable, to identify wandering in dementia in conditions classified elsewhere (Z91.83)

🄬 **F03 Unspecified dementia**

Presenile dementia NOS

Presenile psychosis NOS

Primary degenerative dementia NOS

Senile dementia NOS

Senile dementia depressed or paranoid type

Senile psychosis NOS

> EXCLUDES1 *senility NOS (R41.81)*
>
> EXCLUDES2 *mild memory disturbance due to known physiological condition (F06.8)*
> *senile dementia with delirium or acute confusional state (F05)*

🄮 **F03.9 Unspecified dementia**

F03.90 Unspecified dementia without behavioral disturbance

Dementia NOS 🄰

F03.91 Unspecified dementia with behavioral disturbance

Unspecified dementia with aggressive behavior

Unspecified dementia with combative behavior

Unspecified dementia with violent behavior

Use additional code, if applicable, to identify wandering in unspecified dementia (Z91.83) 🄰

F04 Amnestic disorder due to known physiological condition

Korsakov's psychosis or syndrome, nonalcoholic

Code first the underlying physiological condition

> EXCLUDES1 *amnesia NOS (R41.3)*
> *anterograde amnesia (R41.1)*
> *dissociative amnesia (F44.0)*
> *retrograde amnesia (R41.2)*
>
> EXCLUDES2 *alcohol-induced or unspecified Korsakov's syndrome (F10.26, F10.96)*
> *Korsakov's syndrome induced by other psychoactive substances (F13.26, F13.96, F19.16, F19.26, F19.96)*

F05 Delirium due to known physiological condition

Acute or subacute brain syndrome

Acute or subacute confusional state (nonalcoholic)

Acute or subacute infective psychosis

Acute or subacute organic reaction

Acute or subacute psycho-organic syndrome

Delirium of mixed etiology

Delirium superimposed on dementia

Sundowning

Code first the underlying physiological condition

> EXCLUDES1 *delirium NOS (R41.0)*
>
> EXCLUDES2 *delirium tremens alcohol-induced or unspecified (F10.231, F10.921)*

🄬 **F06 Other mental disorders due to known physiological condition**

> INCLUDES *mental disorders due to endocrine disorder*
> *mental disorders due to exogenous hormone*
> *mental disorders due to exogenous toxic substance*
> *mental disorders due to primary cerebral disease*
> *mental disorders due to somatic illness*
> *mental disorders due to systemic disease affecting the brain*

Code first the underlying physiological condition

> EXCLUDES1 *unspecified dementia (F03)*
>
> EXCLUDES2 *delirium due to known physiological condition (F05)*
> *dementia as classified in F01-F02*
> *other mental disorders associated with alcohol and other psychoactive substances (F10-F19)*

Unspecified Code	Other Specified Code	🄽 Newborn Age: 0	🄿 Pediatric Age: 0-17	🄼 Maternity Age: 12-55

🄰 Adult Age: 15-124   ♂ Male   ♀ Female   ● New Code   ▲ Revised Code Title   ►◄ Revised Text

F06.0 Psychotic disorder with hallucinations due to known physiological condition

Organic hallucinatory state (nonalcoholic)

EXCLUDES2 *hallucinations and perceptual disturbance induced by alcohol and other psychoactive substances (F10-F19 with .151, .251, .951)*
schizophrenia (F20.-)

F06.1 Catatonic disorder due to known physiological condition

EXCLUDES1 *catatonic stupor (R40.1)*
stupor NOS (R40.1)

EXCLUDES2 *catatonic schizophrenia (F20.2)*
dissociative stupor (F44.2)

F06.2 Psychotic disorder with delusions due to known physiological condition

Paranoid and paranoid-hallucinatory organic states
Schizophrenia-like psychosis in epilepsy

EXCLUDES2 *alcohol and drug-induced psychotic disorder (F10-F19 with .150, .250, .950)*
brief psychotic disorder (F23)
delusional disorder (F22)
schizophrenia (F20.-)

⑤ **F06.3** Mood disorder due to known physiological condition

EXCLUDES2 *mood disorders due to alcohol and other psychoactive substances (F10-F19 with .14, .24, .94)*
mood disorders, not due to known physiological condition or unspecified (F30-F39)

F06.30 Mood disorder due to known physiological condition, unspecified

F06.31 Mood disorder due to known physiological condition with depressive features

F06.32 Mood disorder due to known physiological condition with major depressive-like episode

F06.33 Mood disorder due to known physiological condition with manic features

F06.34 Mood disorder due to known physiological condition with mixed features

F06.4 Anxiety disorder due to known physiological condition

EXCLUDES2 *anxiety disorders due to alcohol and other psychoactive substances (F10-F19 with .180, .280, .980)*
anxiety disorders, not due to known physiological condition or unspecified (F40.-, F41.-)

F06.8 Other specified mental disorders due to known physiological condition

Epileptic psychosis NOS
Organic dissociative disorder
Organic emotionally labile [asthenic] disorder

④ **F07** Personality and behavioral disorders due to known physiological condition

Code first the underlying physiological condition

F07.0 Personality change due to known physiological condition

Frontal lobe syndrome
Limbic epilepsy personality syndrome
Lobotomy syndrome
Organic personality disorder
Organic pseudopsychopathic personality
Organic pseudoretarded personality
Postleucotomy syndrome
Code first underlying physiological condition

EXCLUDES1 *mild cognitive impairment (G31.84)*
postconcussional syndrome (F07.81)
postencephalitic syndrome (F07.89)
signs and symptoms involving emotional state (R45.-)

EXCLUDES2 *specific personality disorder (F60.-)*

⑤ **F07.8** Other personality and behavioral disorders due to known physiological condition

F07.81 Postconcussional syndrome

Postcontusional syndrome (encephalopathy)
Post-traumatic brain syndrome, nonpsychotic
Use additional code to identify associated post-traumatic headache, if applicable (G44.3-)

EXCLUDES1 *current concussion (brain) (S06.0-)*
postencephalitic syndrome (F07.89)

F07.89 Other personality and behavioral disorders due to known physiological condition

Postencephalitic syndrome
Right hemispheric organic affective disorder

F07.9 Unspecified personality and behavioral disorder due to known physiological condition

Organic psychosyndrome

F09 Unspecified mental disorder due to known physiological condition

Mental disorder NOS due to known physiological condition
Organic brain syndrome NOS
Organic mental disorder NOS
Organic psychosis NOS
Symptomatic psychosis NOS
Code first the underlying physiological condition

EXCLUDES1 *psychosis NOS (F29)*

Mental and behavioral disorders due to psychoactive substance use (F10-F19)

④ **F10** Alcohol related disorders

Use additional code for blood alcohol level, if applicable (Y90.-)

⑤ **F10.1** Alcohol abuse

EXCLUDES1 *alcohol dependence (F10.2-)*
alcohol use, unspecified (F10.9-)

F10.10 Alcohol abuse, uncomplicated

⑥ **F10.12** Alcohol abuse with intoxication

F10.120 Alcohol abuse with intoxication, uncomplicated

F10.121 Alcohol abuse with intoxication delirium

F10.129 Alcohol abuse with intoxication, unspecified

F10.14 Alcohol abuse with alcohol-induced mood disorder

⑥ **F10.15** Alcohol abuse with alcohol-induced psychotic disorder

F10.150 Alcohol abuse with alcohol-induced psychotic disorder with delusions

F10.151 Alcohol abuse with alcohol-induced psychotic disorder with hallucinations

F10.159 Alcohol abuse with alcohol-induced psychotic disorder, unspecified

⑥ **F10.18** Alcohol abuse with other alcohol-induced disorders

F10.180 Alcohol abuse with alcohol-induced anxiety disorder

F10.181 Alcohol abuse with alcohol-induced sexual dysfunction

F10.182 Alcohol abuse with alcohol-induced sleep disorder

F10.188 Alcohol abuse with other alcohol-induced disorder

F10.19 Alcohol abuse with unspecified alcohol-induced disorder

⑤ **F10.2** Alcohol dependence

EXCLUDES1 *alcohol abuse (F10.1-)*
alcohol use, unspecified (F10.9-)

EXCLUDES2 *toxic effect of alcohol (T51.0-)*

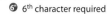

④ 4ᵗʰ character required   ⑤ 5ᵗʰ character required   ⑥ 6ᵗʰ character required   ⑦ 7ᵗʰ character required   ⑦ᵡ Extension 'X' Alert

EXCLUDES 1 Not coded here   EXCLUDES 2 Not included here   PDx Primary Diagnosis Only   Manifestation Code

F10.20 Alcohol dependence, uncomplicated

F10.21 Alcohol dependence, in remission

F10.22 Alcohol dependence with intoxication

Acute drunkenness (in alcoholism)

EXCLUDES1 alcohol dependence with withdrawal (F10.23-)

F10.220 Alcohol dependence with intoxication, uncomplicated

F10.221 Alcohol dependence with intoxication delirium

F10.229 Alcohol dependence with intoxication, unspecified

F10.23 Alcohol dependence with withdrawal

EXCLUDES1 Alcohol dependence with intoxication (F10.22-)

F10.230 Alcohol dependence with withdrawal, uncomplicated

F10.231 Alcohol dependence with withdrawal delirium

F10.232 Alcohol dependence with withdrawal with perceptual disturbance

F10.239 Alcohol dependence with withdrawal, unspecified

F10.24 Alcohol dependence with alcohol-induced mood disorder

F10.25 Alcohol dependence with alcohol-induced psychotic disorder

F10.250 Alcohol dependence with alcohol-induced psychotic disorder with delusions

F10.251 Alcohol dependence with alcohol-induced psychotic disorder with hallucinations

F10.259 Alcohol dependence with alcohol-induced psychotic disorder, unspecified

F10.26 Alcohol dependence with alcohol-induced persisting amnestic disorder

F10.27 Alcohol dependence with alcohol-induced persisting dementia

F10.28 Alcohol dependence with other alcohol-induced disorders

F10.280 Alcohol dependence with alcohol-induced anxiety disorder

F10.281 Alcohol dependence with alcohol-induced sexual dysfunction

F10.282 Alcohol dependence with alcohol-induced sleep disorder

F10.288 Alcohol dependence with other alcohol-induced disorder

F10.29 Alcohol dependence with unspecified alcohol-induced disorder

F10.9 Alcohol use, unspecified

EXCLUDES1 alcohol abuse (F10.1-)
alcohol dependence (F10.2-)

F10.92 Alcohol use, unspecified with intoxication

F10.920 Alcohol use, unspecified with intoxication, uncomplicated

F10.921 Alcohol use, unspecified with intoxication delirium

F10.929 Alcohol use, unspecified with intoxication, unspecified

F10.94 Alcohol use, unspecified with alcohol-induced mood disorder

F10.95 Alcohol use, unspecified with alcohol-induced psychotic disorder

F10.950 Alcohol use, unspecified with alcohol-induced psychotic disorder with delusions

F10.951 Alcohol use, unspecified with alcohol-induced psychotic disorder with hallucinations

F10.959 Alcohol use, unspecified with alcohol-induced psychotic disorder, unspecified

F10.96 Alcohol use, unspecified with alcohol-induced persisting amnestic disorder

F10.97 Alcohol use, unspecified with alcohol-induced persisting dementia

F10.98 Alcohol use, unspecified with other alcohol-induced disorders

F10.980 Alcohol use, unspecified with alcohol-induced anxiety disorder

F10.981 Alcohol use, unspecified with alcohol-induced sexual dysfunction

F10.982 Alcohol use, unspecified with alcohol-induced sleep disorder

F10.988 Alcohol use, unspecified with other alcohol-induced disorder

F10.99 Alcohol use, unspecified with unspecified alcohol-induced disorder

F11 Opioid related disorders

F11.1 Opioid abuse

EXCLUDES1 opioid dependence (F11.2-)
opioid use, unspecified (F11.9-)

F11.10 Opioid abuse, uncomplicated

F11.12 Opioid abuse with intoxication

F11.120 Opioid abuse with intoxication, uncomplicated

F11.121 Opioid abuse with intoxication delirium

F11.122 Opioid abuse with intoxication with perceptual disturbance

F11.129 Opioid abuse with intoxication, unspecified

F11.14 Opioid abuse with opioid-induced mood disorder

F11.15 Opioid abuse with opioid-induced psychotic disorder

F11.150 Opioid abuse with opioid-induced psychotic disorder with delusions

F11.151 Opioid abuse with opioid-induced psychotic disorder with hallucinations

F11.159 Opioid abuse with opioid-induced psychotic disorder, unspecified

F11.18 Opioid abuse with other opioid-induced disorder

F11.181 Opioid abuse with opioid-induced sexual dysfunction

F11.182 Opioid abuse with opioid-induced sleep disorder

F11.188 Opioid abuse with other opioid-induced disorder

F11.19 Opioid abuse with unspecified opioid-induced disorder

F11.2 Opioid dependence

EXCLUDES1 opioid abuse (F11.1-)
opioid use, unspecified (F11.9-)

EXCLUDES2 opioid poisoning (T40.0-T40.2-)

F11.20 Opioid dependence, uncomplicated

F11.21 Opioid dependence, in remission

F11.22 Opioid dependence with intoxication

EXCLUDES1 opioid dependence with withdrawal (F11.23)

F11.220 Opioid dependence with intoxication, uncomplicated

F11.221 Opioid dependence with intoxication delirium

F11.222 Opioid dependence with intoxication with perceptual disturbance

F11.229 Opioid dependence with intoxication, unspecified

F11.23 Opioid dependence with withdrawal

EXCLUDES1 opioid dependence with intoxication (F11.22-)

F11.24 Opioid dependence with opioid-induced mood disorder

Unspecified Code   Other Specified Code   N Newborn Age: 0   P Pediatric Age: 0-17   M Maternity Age: 12-55
A Adult Age: 15-124   ♂ Male   ♀ Female   ● New Code   ▲ Revised Code Title   ►◄ Revised Text

ⓢ **F11.25 Opioid dependence with opioid-induced** psychotic disorder
　　F11.250 Opioid dependence with opioid-induced psychotic disorder with delusions
　　F11.251 Opioid dependence with opioid-induced psychotic disorder with hallucinations
　　F11.259 Opioid dependence with opioid-induced psychotic disorder, unspecified

ⓢ **F11.28 Opioid dependence with** other opioid-induced disorder
　　F11.281 Opioid dependence with opioid-induced sexual dysfunction
　　F11.282 Opioid dependence with opioid-induced sleep disorder
　　F11.288 Opioid dependence with other opioid-induced disorder
　　F11.29 Opioid dependence with unspecified opioid-induced disorder

ⓢ **F11.9 Opioid** use, unspecified
　　EXCLUDES1 opioid abuse (F11.1-)
　　　　　　 opioid dependence (F11.2-)
　　F11.90 Opioid use, unspecified, uncomplicated

ⓢ **F11.92 Opioid use, unspecified** with intoxication
　　EXCLUDES1 opioid use, unspecified with withdrawal (F11.93)
　　F11.920 Opioid use, unspecified with intoxication, uncomplicated
　　F11.921 Opioid use, unspecified with intoxication delirium
　　F11.922 Opioid use, unspecified with intoxication with perceptual disturbance
　　F11.929 Opioid use, unspecified with intoxication, unspecified
　　F11.93 Opioid use, unspecified with withdrawal
　　EXCLUDES1 opioid use, unspecified with intoxication (F11.92-)
　　F11.94 Opioid use, unspecified with opioid-induced mood disorder

ⓢ **F11.95 Opioid use, unspecified with opioid-induced** psychotic disorder
　　F11.950 Opioid use, unspecified with opioid-induced psychotic disorder with delusions
　　F11.951 Opioid use, unspecified with opioid-induced psychotic disorder with hallucinations
　　F11.959 Opioid use, unspecified with opioid-induced psychotic disorder, unspecified

ⓢ **F11.98 Opioid use, unspecified with** other specified opioid-induced disorder
　　F11.981 Opioid use, unspecified with opioid-induced sexual dysfunction
　　F11.982 Opioid use, unspecified with opioid-induced sleep disorder
　　F11.988 Opioid use, unspecified with other opioid-induced disorder
　　F11.99 Opioid use, unspecified with unspecified opioid-induced disorder

④ **F12** Cannabis related disorders
　　INCLUDES marijuana

ⓢ **F12.1 Cannabis** abuse
　　EXCLUDES1 cannabis dependence (F12.2-)
　　　　　　 cannabis use, unspecified (F12.9-)
　　F12.10 Cannabis abuse, uncomplicated

ⓢ **F12.12 Cannabis abuse** with intoxication
　　F12.120 Cannabis abuse with intoxication, uncomplicated
　　F12.121 Cannabis abuse with intoxication delirium
　　F12.122 Cannabis abuse with intoxication with perceptual disturbance

　　F12.129 Cannabis abuse with intoxication, unspecified

ⓢ **F12.15 Cannabis abuse with psychotic disorder**
　　F12.150 Cannabis abuse with psychotic disorder with delusions
　　F12.151 Cannabis abuse with psychotic disorder with hallucinations
　　F12.159 Cannabis abuse with psychotic disorder, unspecified

ⓢ **F12.18 Cannabis abuse with** other cannabis-induced disorder
　　F12.180 Cannabis abuse with cannabis-induced anxiety disorder
　　F12.188 Cannabis abuse with other cannabis-induced disorder
　　F12.19 Cannabis abuse with unspecified cannabis-induced disorder

ⓢ **F12.2 Cannabis** dependence
　　EXCLUDES1 cannabis abuse (F12.1-)
　　　　　　 cannabis use, unspecified (F12.9-)
　　EXCLUDES2 cannabis poisoning (T40.7-)
　　F12.20 Cannabis dependence, uncomplicated
　　F12.21 Cannabis dependence, in remission

ⓢ **F12.22 Cannabis dependence** with intoxication
　　F12.220 Cannabis dependence with intoxication, uncomplicated
　　F12.221 Cannabis dependence with intoxication delirium
　　F12.222 Cannabis dependence with intoxication with perceptual disturbance
　　F12.229 Cannabis dependence with intoxication, unspecified

ⓢ **F12.25 Cannabis dependence** with psychotic disorder
　　F12.250 Cannabis dependence with psychotic disorder with delusions
　　F12.251 Cannabis dependence with psychotic disorder with hallucinations
　　F12.259 Cannabis dependence with psychotic disorder, unspecified

ⓢ **F12.28 Cannabis dependence with** other cannabis-induced disorder
　　F12.280 Cannabis dependence with cannabis-induced anxiety disorder
　　F12.288 Cannabis dependence with other cannabis-induced disorder
　　F12.29 Cannabis dependence with unspecified cannabis-induced disorder

ⓢ **F12.9 Cannabis** use, unspecified
　　EXCLUDES1 cannabis abuse (F12.1-)
　　　　　　 cannabis dependence (F12.2-)
　　F12.90 Cannabis use, unspecified, uncomplicated

ⓢ **F12.92 Cannabis use, unspecified** with intoxication
　　F12.920 Cannabis use, unspecified with intoxication, uncomplicated
　　F12.921 Cannabis use, unspecified with intoxication delirium
　　F12.922 Cannabis use, unspecified with intoxication with perceptual disturbance
　　F12.929 Cannabis use, unspecified with intoxication, unspecified

ⓢ **F12.95 Cannabis use, unspecified with** psychotic disorder
　　F12.950 Cannabis use, unspecified with psychotic disorder with delusions
　　F12.951 Cannabis use, unspecified with psychotic disorder with hallucinations
　　F12.959 Cannabis use, unspecified with psychotic disorder, unspecified

---

④ 4th character required　　ⓢ 5th character required　　ⓢ 6th character required　　ⓢ 7th character required　　Ⓧ Extension 'X' Alert

EXCLUDES 1 Not coded here　　EXCLUDES 2 Not included here　　ⓟⓓⓧ Primary Diagnosis Only　　Manifestation Code

[6] F12.98 Cannabis use, unspecified with other cannabis-induced disorder
F12.980 Cannabis use, unspecified with anxiety disorder
F12.988 Cannabis use, unspecified with other cannabis-induced disorder
F12.99 Cannabis use, unspecified with unspecified cannabis-induced disorder

[4] F13 Sedative, hypnotic, or anxiolytic related disorders

[5] F13.1 Sedative, hypnotic or anxiolytic-related abuse
[EXCLUDES1] *sedative, hypnotic or anxiolytic-related dependence (F13.2-)*
sedative, hypnotic, or anxiolytic use, unspecified (F13.9-)
F13.10 Sedative, hypnotic or anxiolytic abuse, uncomplicated
[6] F13.12 Sedative, hypnotic or anxiolytic abuse with intoxication
F13.120 Sedative, hypnotic or anxiolytic abuse with intoxication, uncomplicated
F13.121 Sedative, hypnotic or anxiolytic abuse with intoxication delirium
F13.129 Sedative, hypnotic or anxiolytic abuse with intoxication, unspecified
F13.14 Sedative, hypnotic or anxiolytic abuse with sedative, hypnotic or anxiolytic-induced mood disorder
[6] F13.15 Sedative, hypnotic or anxiolytic abuse with sedative, hypnotic or anxiolytic-induced psychotic disorder
F13.150 Sedative, hypnotic or anxiolytic abuse with sedative, hypnotic or anxiolytic-induced psychotic disorder with delusions
F13.151 Sedative, hypnotic or anxiolytic abuse with sedative, hypnotic or anxiolytic-induced psychotic disorder with hallucinations
F13.159 Sedative, hypnotic or anxiolytic abuse with sedative, hypnotic or anxiolytic-induced psychotic disorder, unspecified
[6] F13.18 Sedative, hypnotic or anxiolytic abuse with other sedative, hypnotic or anxiolytic-induced disorders
F13.180 Sedative, hypnotic or anxiolytic abuse with sedative, hypnotic or anxiolytic-induced anxiety disorder
F13.181 Sedative, hypnotic or anxiolytic abuse with sedative, hypnotic or anxiolytic-induced sexual dysfunction
F13.182 Sedative, hypnotic or anxiolytic abuse with sedative, hypnotic or anxiolytic-induced sleep disorder
F13.188 Sedative, hypnotic or anxiolytic abuse with other sedative, hypnotic or anxiolytic-induced disorder
F13.19 Sedative, hypnotic or anxiolytic abuse with unspecified sedative, hypnotic or anxiolytic-induced disorder

[5] F13.2 Sedative, hypnotic or anxiolytic-related dependence
[EXCLUDES1] *sedative, hypnotic or anxiolytic-related abuse (F13.1-)*
sedative, hypnotic, or anxiolytic use, unspecified (F13.9-)
[EXCLUDES2] *sedative, hypnotic, or anxiolytic poisoning (T42.-)*
F13.20 Sedative, hypnotic or anxiolytic dependence, uncomplicated
F13.21 Sedative, hypnotic or anxiolytic dependence, in remission
[6] F13.22 Sedative, hypnotic or anxiolytic dependence with intoxication
[EXCLUDES1] *sedative, hypnotic or anxiolytic dependence with withdrawal (F13.23-)*
F13.220 Sedative, hypnotic or anxiolytic dependence with intoxication, uncomplicated
F13.221 Sedative, hypnotic or anxiolytic dependence with intoxication delirium
F13.229 Sedative, hypnotic or anxiolytic dependence with intoxication, unspecified
[6] F13.23 Sedative, hypnotic or anxiolytic dependence with withdrawal
[EXCLUDES1] *sedative, hypnotic or anxiolytic dependence with intoxication (F13.22-)*
F13.230 Sedative, hypnotic or anxiolytic dependence with withdrawal, uncomplicated
F13.231 Sedative, hypnotic or anxiolytic dependence with withdrawal delirium
F13.232 Sedative, hypnotic or anxiolytic dependence with withdrawal with perceptual disturbance
F13.239 Sedative, hypnotic or anxiolytic dependence with withdrawal, unspecified
F13.24 Sedative, hypnotic or anxiolytic dependence with sedative, hypnotic or anxiolytic-induced mood disorder
[6] F13.25 Sedative, hypnotic or anxiolytic dependence with sedative, hypnotic or anxiolytic-induced psychotic disorder
F13.250 Sedative, hypnotic or anxiolytic dependence with sedative, hypnotic or anxiolytic-induced psychotic disorder with delusions
F13.251 Sedative, hypnotic or anxiolytic dependence with sedative, hypnotic or anxiolytic-induced psychotic disorder with hallucinations
F13.259 Sedative, hypnotic or anxiolytic dependence with sedative, hypnotic or anxiolytic-induced psychotic disorder, unspecified
F13.26 Sedative, hypnotic or anxiolytic dependence with sedative, hypnotic or anxiolytic-induced persisting amnestic disorder
F13.27 Sedative, hypnotic or anxiolytic dependence with sedative, hypnotic or anxiolytic-induced persisting dementia
[6] F13.28 Sedative, hypnotic or anxiolytic dependence with other sedative, hypnotic or anxiolytic-induced disorders
F13.280 Sedative, hypnotic or anxiolytic dependence with sedative, hypnotic or anxiolytic-induced anxiety disorder
F13.281 Sedative, hypnotic or anxiolytic dependence with sedative, hypnotic or anxiolytic-induced sexual dysfunction
F13.282 Sedative, hypnotic or anxiolytic dependence with sedative, hypnotic or anxiolytic-induced sleep disorder
F13.288 Sedative, hypnotic or anxiolytic dependence with other sedative, hypnotic or anxiolytic-induced disorder
F13.29 Sedative, hypnotic or anxiolytic dependence with unspecified sedative, hypnotic or anxiolytic-induced disorder

[5] F13.9 Sedative, hypnotic or anxiolytic-related use, unspecified
[EXCLUDES1] *sedative, hypnotic or anxiolytic-related abuse (F13.1-)*
sedative, hypnotic or anxiolytic-related dependence (F13.2-)

Unspecified Code | Other Specified Code | [N] Newborn Age: 0 | [P] Pediatric Age: 0-17 | [M] Maternity Age: 12-55
[A] Adult Age: 15-124 | ♂ Male | ♀ Female | ● New Code | ▲ Revised Code Title | ►◄ Revised Text

F13.90 Sedative, hypnotic, or anxiolytic use, unspecified, uncomplicated

⑥ F13.92 Sedative, hypnotic or anxiolytic use, unspecified with intoxication

> EXCLUDES1 *sedative, hypnotic or anxiolytic use, unspecified with withdrawal (F13.93-)*

F13.920 Sedative, hypnotic or anxiolytic use, unspecified with intoxication, uncomplicated

F13.921 Sedative, hypnotic or anxiolytic use, unspecified with intoxication delirium

F13.929 Sedative, hypnotic or anxiolytic use, unspecified with intoxication, unspecified

⑥ F13.93 Sedative, hypnotic or anxiolytic use, unspecified with withdrawal

> EXCLUDES1 *sedative, hypnotic or anxiolytic use, unspecified with intoxication (F13.92-)*

F13.930 Sedative, hypnotic or anxiolytic use, unspecified with withdrawal, uncomplicated

F13.931 Sedative, hypnotic or anxiolytic use, unspecified with withdrawal delirium

F13.932 Sedative, hypnotic or anxiolytic use, unspecified with withdrawal with perceptual disturbances

F13.939 Sedative, hypnotic or anxiolytic use, unspecified with withdrawal, unspecified

F13.94 Sedative, hypnotic or anxiolytic use, unspecified with sedative, hypnotic or anxiolytic-induced mood disorder

⑥ F13.95 Sedative, hypnotic or anxiolytic use, unspecified with sedative, hypnotic or anxiolytic-induced psychotic disorder

F13.950 Sedative, hypnotic or anxiolytic use, unspecified with sedative, hypnotic or anxiolytic-induced psychotic disorder with delusions

F13.951 Sedative, hypnotic or anxiolytic use, unspecified with sedative, hypnotic or anxiolytic-induced psychotic disorder with hallucinations

F13.959 Sedative, hypnotic or anxiolytic use, unspecified with sedative, hypnotic or anxiolytic-induced psychotic disorder, unspecified

F13.96 Sedative, hypnotic or anxiolytic use, unspecified with sedative, hypnotic or anxiolytic-induced persisting amnestic disorder

F13.97 Sedative, hypnotic or anxiolytic use, unspecified with sedative, hypnotic or anxiolytic-induced persisting dementia

⑥ F13.98 Sedative, hypnotic or anxiolytic use, unspecified with other sedative, hypnotic or anxiolytic-induced disorders

F13.980 Sedative, hypnotic or anxiolytic use, unspecified with sedative, hypnotic or anxiolytic-induced anxiety disorder

F13.981 Sedative, hypnotic or anxiolytic use, unspecified with sedative, hypnotic or anxiolytic-induced sexual dysfunction

F13.982 Sedative, hypnotic or anxiolytic use, unspecified with sedative, hypnotic or anxiolytic-induced sleep disorder

F13.988 Sedative, hypnotic or anxiolytic use, unspecified with other sedative, hypnotic or anxiolytic-induced disorder

F13.99 Sedative, hypnotic or anxiolytic use, unspecified with unspecified sedative, hypnotic or anxiolytic-induced disorder

④ F14 Cocaine related disorders

> EXCLUDES2 *other stimulant-related disorders (F15.-)*

⑤ F14.1 Cocaine abuse

> EXCLUDES1 *cocaine dependence (F14.2-)*
> *cocaine use, unspecified (F14.9-)*

F14.10 Cocaine abuse, uncomplicated

⑥ F14.12 Cocaine abuse with intoxication

F14.120 Cocaine abuse with intoxication, uncomplicated

F14.121 Cocaine abuse with intoxication with delirium

F14.122 Cocaine abuse with intoxication with perceptual disturbance

F14.129 Cocaine abuse with intoxication, unspecified

F14.14 Cocaine abuse with cocaine-induced mood disorder

⑥ F14.15 Cocaine abuse with cocaine-induced psychotic disorder

F14.150 Cocaine abuse with cocaine-induced psychotic disorder with delusions

F14.151 Cocaine abuse with cocaine-induced psychotic disorder with hallucinations

F14.159 Cocaine abuse with cocaine-induced psychotic disorder, unspecified

⑥ F14.18 Cocaine abuse with other cocaine-induced disorder

F14.180 Cocaine abuse with cocaine-induced anxiety disorder

F14.181 Cocaine abuse with cocaine-induced sexual dysfunction

F14.182 Cocaine abuse with cocaine-induced sleep disorder

F14.188 Cocaine abuse with other cocaine-induced disorder

F14.19 Cocaine abuse with unspecified cocaine-induced disorder

⑤ F14.2 Cocaine dependence

> EXCLUDES1 *cocaine abuse (F14.1-)*
> *cocaine use, unspecified (F14.9-)*

> EXCLUDES2 *cocaine poisoning (T40.5-)*

F14.20 Cocaine dependence, uncomplicated

F14.21 Cocaine dependence, in remission

⑥ F14.22 Cocaine dependence with intoxication

> EXCLUDES1 *cocaine dependence with withdrawal (F14.23)*

F14.220 Cocaine dependence with intoxication, uncomplicated

F14.221 Cocaine dependence with intoxication delirium

F14.222 Cocaine dependence with intoxication with perceptual disturbance

F14.229 Cocaine dependence with intoxication, unspecified

---

④ 4th character required   ⑤ 5th character required   ⑥ 6th character required   ⑦ 7th character required   ⑦ Extension 'X' Alert

EXCLUDES 1 Not coded here   EXCLUDES 2 Not included here   PDx Primary Diagnosis Only   Manifestation Code

F14.23 Cocaine dependence with withdrawal
[EXCLUDES1] *cocaine dependence with intoxication (F14.22-)*
F14.24 Cocaine dependence with cocaine-induced mood disorder
[6] F14.25 Cocaine dependence with cocaine-induced psychotic disorder
F14.250 Cocaine dependence with cocaine-induced psychotic disorder with delusions
F14.251 Cocaine dependence with cocaine-induced psychotic disorder with hallucinations
F14.259 Cocaine dependence with cocaine-induced psychotic disorder, unspecified
[6] F14.28 Cocaine dependence with other cocaine-induced disorder
F14.280 Cocaine dependence with cocaine-induced anxiety disorder
F14.281 Cocaine dependence with cocaine-induced sexual dysfunction
F14.282 Cocaine dependence with cocaine-induced sleep disorder
F14.288 Cocaine dependence with other cocaine-induced disorder
F14.29 Cocaine dependence with unspecified cocaine-induced disorder
[5] F14.9 Cocaine use, unspecified
[EXCLUDES1] *cocaine abuse (F14.1-)*
cocaine dependence (F14.2-)
F14.90 Cocaine use, unspecified, uncomplicated
[6] F14.92 Cocaine use, unspecified with intoxication
F14.920 Cocaine use, unspecified with intoxication, uncomplicated
F14.921 Cocaine use, unspecified with intoxication delirium
F14.922 Cocaine use, unspecified with intoxication with perceptual disturbance
F14.929 Cocaine use, unspecified with intoxication, unspecified
F14.94 Cocaine use, unspecified with cocaine-induced mood disorder
[6] F14.95 Cocaine use, unspecified with cocaine-induced psychotic disorder
F14.950 Cocaine use, unspecified with cocaine-induced psychotic disorder with delusions
F14.951 Cocaine use, unspecified with cocaine-induced psychotic disorder with hallucinations
F14.959 Cocaine use, unspecified with cocaine-induced psychotic disorder, unspecified
[6] F14.98 Cocaine use, unspecified with other specified cocaine-induced disorder
F14.980 Cocaine use, unspecified with cocaine-induced anxiety disorder
F14.981 Cocaine use, unspecified with cocaine-induced sexual dysfunction
F14.982 Cocaine use, unspecified with cocaine-induced sleep disorder
F14.988 Cocaine use, unspecified with other cocaine-induced disorder
F14.99 Cocaine use, unspecified with unspecified cocaine-induced disorder
[4] F15 Other stimulant related disorders
[INCLUDES] *amphetamine-related disorders*
caffeine
[EXCLUDES2] *cocaine-related disorders (F14.-)*
[5] F15.1 Other stimulant abuse
[EXCLUDES1] *other stimulant dependence (F15.2-)*
other stimulant use, unspecified (F15.9-)
F15.10 Other stimulant abuse, uncomplicated

[6] F15.12 Other stimulant abuse with intoxication
F15.120 Other stimulant abuse with intoxication, uncomplicated
F15.121 Other stimulant abuse with intoxication delirium
F15.122 Other stimulant abuse with intoxication with perceptual disturbance
F15.129 Other stimulant abuse with intoxication, unspecified
F15.14 Other stimulant abuse with stimulant-induced mood disorder
[6] F15.15 Other stimulant abuse with stimulant-induced psychotic disorder
F15.150 Other stimulant abuse with stimulant-induced psychotic disorder with delusions
F15.151 Other stimulant abuse with stimulant-induced psychotic disorder with hallucinations
F15.159 Other stimulant abuse with stimulant-induced psychotic disorder, unspecified
[6] F15.18 Other stimulant abuse with other stimulant-induced disorder
F15.180 Other stimulant abuse with stimulant-induced anxiety disorder
F15.181 Other stimulant abuse with stimulant-induced sexual dysfunction
F15.182 Other stimulant abuse with stimulant-induced sleep disorder
F15.188 Other stimulant abuse with other stimulant-induced disorder
F15.19 Other stimulant abuse with unspecified stimulant-induced disorder
[5] F15.2 Other stimulant dependence
[EXCLUDES1] *other stimulant abuse (F15.1-)*
other stimulant use, unspecified (F15.9-)
F15.20 Other stimulant dependence, uncomplicated
F15.21 Other stimulant dependence, in remission
[6] F15.22 Other stimulant dependence with intoxication
[EXCLUDES1] *other stimulant dependence with withdrawal (F15.23)*
F15.220 Other stimulant dependence with intoxication, uncomplicated
F15.221 Other stimulant dependence with intoxication delirium
F15.222 Other stimulant dependence with intoxication with perceptual disturbance
F15.229 Other stimulant dependence with intoxication, unspecified
F15.23 Other stimulant dependence with withdrawal
[EXCLUDES1] *other stimulant dependence with intoxication (F15.22-)*
F15.24 Other stimulant dependence with stimulant-induced mood disorder
[6] F15.25 Other stimulant dependence with stimulant-induced psychotic disorder
F15.250 Other stimulant dependence with stimulant-induced psychotic disorder with delusions
F15.251 Other stimulant dependence with stimulant-induced psychotic disorder with hallucinations
F15.259 Other stimulant dependence with stimulant-induced psychotic disorder, unspecified
[6] F15.28 Other stimulant dependence with other stimulant-induced disorder
F15.280 Other stimulant dependence with stimulant-induced anxiety disorder

Unspecified Code | Other Specified Code | [N] Newborn Age: 0 | [P] Pediatric Age: 0-17 | [M] Maternity Age: 12-55
[A] Adult Age: 15-124 | ♂ Male | ♀ Female | ● New Code | ▲ Revised Code Title | ►◄ Revised Text

F15.281 Other stimulant dependence with stimulant-induced sexual dysfunction

F15.282 Other stimulant dependence with stimulant-induced sleep disorder

F15.288 Other stimulant dependence with other stimulant-induced disorder

F15.29 Other stimulant dependence with unspecified stimulant-induced disorder

[5] F15.9 Other stimulant use, unspecified

EXCLUDES1 *other stimulant abuse (F15.1-)*
other stimulant dependence (F15.2-)

F15.90 Other stimulant use, unspecified, uncomplicated

[6] F15.92 Other stimulant use, unspecified with intoxication

EXCLUDES1 *other stimulant use, unspecified with withdrawal (F15.93)*

F15.920 Other stimulant use, unspecified with intoxication, uncomplicated

F15.921 Other stimulant use, unspecified with intoxication delirium

F15.922 Other stimulant use, unspecified with intoxication with perceptual disturbance

F15.929 Other stimulant use, unspecified with intoxication, unspecified

F15.93 Other stimulant use, unspecified with withdrawal

EXCLUDES1 *other stimulant use, unspecified with intoxication (F15.92-)*

F15.94 Other stimulant use, unspecified with stimulant-induced mood disorder

[6] F15.95 Other stimulant use, unspecified with stimulant-induced psychotic disorder

F15.950 Other stimulant use, unspecified with stimulant-induced psychotic disorder with delusions

F15.951 Other stimulant use, unspecified with stimulant-induced psychotic disorder with hallucinations

F15.959 Other stimulant use, unspecified with stimulant-induced psychotic disorder, unspecified

[6] F15.98 Other stimulant use, unspecified with other stimulant-induced disorder

F15.980 Other stimulant use, unspecified with stimulant-induced anxiety disorder

F15.981 Other stimulant use, unspecified with stimulant-induced sexual dysfunction

F15.982 Other stimulant use, unspecified with stimulant-induced sleep disorder

F15.988 Other stimulant use, unspecified with other stimulant-induced disorder

F15.99 Other stimulant use, unspecified with unspecified stimulant-induced disorder

[4] F16 Hallucinogen related disorders

INCLUDES *ecstasy*
PCP
phencyclidine

[5] F16.1 Hallucinogen abuse

EXCLUDES1 *hallucinogen dependence (F16.2-)*
hallucinogen use, unspecified (F16.9-)

F16.10 Hallucinogen abuse, uncomplicated

[6] F16.12 Hallucinogen abuse with intoxication

F16.120 Hallucinogen abuse with intoxication, uncomplicated

F16.121 Hallucinogen abuse with intoxication with delirium

F16.122 Hallucinogen abuse with intoxication with perceptual disturbance

F16.129 Hallucinogen abuse with intoxication, unspecified

F16.14 Hallucinogen abuse with hallucinogen-induced mood disorder

[6] F16.15 Hallucinogen abuse with hallucinogen-induced psychotic disorder

F16.150 Hallucinogen abuse with hallucinogen-induced psychotic disorder with delusions

F16.151 Hallucinogen abuse with hallucinogen-induced psychotic disorder with hallucinations

F16.159 Hallucinogen abuse with hallucinogen-induced psychotic disorder, unspecified

[6] F16.18 Hallucinogen abuse with other hallucinogen-induced disorder

F16.180 Hallucinogen abuse with hallucinogen-induced anxiety disorder

F16.183 Hallucinogen abuse with hallucinogen persisting perception disorder (flashbacks)

F16.188 Hallucinogen abuse with other hallucinogen-induced disorder

F16.19 Hallucinogen abuse with unspecified hallucinogen-induced disorder

[5] F16.2 Hallucinogen dependence

EXCLUDES1 *hallucinogen abuse (F16.1-)*
hallucinogen use, unspecified (F16.9-)

F16.20 Hallucinogen dependence, uncomplicated

F16.21 Hallucinogen dependence, in remission

[6] F16.22 Hallucinogen dependence with intoxication

F16.220 Hallucinogen dependence with intoxication, uncomplicated

F16.221 Hallucinogen dependence with intoxication with delirium

F16.229 Hallucinogen dependence with intoxication, unspecified

F16.24 Hallucinogen dependence with hallucinogen-induced mood disorder

[6] F16.25 Hallucinogen dependence with hallucinogen-induced psychotic disorder

F16.250 Hallucinogen dependence with hallucinogen-induced psychotic disorder with delusions

F16.251 Hallucinogen dependence with hallucinogen-induced psychotic disorder with hallucinations

F16.259 Hallucinogen dependence with hallucinogen-induced psychotic disorder, unspecified

[6] F16.28 Hallucinogen dependence with other hallucinogen-induced disorder

F16.280 Hallucinogen dependence with hallucinogen-induced anxiety disorder

F16.283 Hallucinogen dependence with hallucinogen persisting perception disorder (flashbacks)

F16.288 Hallucinogen dependence with other hallucinogen-induced disorder

F16.29 Hallucinogen dependence with unspecified hallucinogen-induced disorder

[5] F16.9 Hallucinogen use, unspecified

EXCLUDES1 *hallucinogen abuse (F16.1-)*
hallucinogen dependence (F16.2-)

F16.90 Hallucinogen use, unspecified, uncomplicated

[6] F16.92 Hallucinogen use, unspecified with intoxication

F16.920 Hallucinogen use, unspecified with intoxication, uncomplicated

F16.921 Hallucinogen use, unspecified with intoxication with delirium

[4] 4th character required [5] 5th character required [6] 6th character required [7] 7th character required [x7] Extension 'X' Alert
EXCLUDES1 Not coded here EXCLUDES2 Not included here [PDx] Primary Diagnosis Only Manifestation Code

F16.929 Hallucinogen use, unspecified with intoxication, unspecified
F16.94 Hallucinogen use, unspecified with hallucinogen-induced mood disorder
[6] F16.95 Hallucinogen use, unspecified with hallucinogen-induced psychotic disorder
F16.950 Hallucinogen use, unspecified with hallucinogen-induced psychotic disorder with delusions
F16.951 Hallucinogen use, unspecified with hallucinogen-induced psychotic disorder with hallucinations
F16.959 Hallucinogen use, unspecified with hallucinogen-induced psychotic disorder, unspecified
[6] F16.98 Hallucinogen use, unspecified with other specified hallucinogen-induced disorder
F16.980 Hallucinogen use, unspecified with hallucinogen-induced anxiety disorder
F16.983 Hallucinogen use, unspecified with hallucinogen persisting perception disorder (flashbacks)
F16.988 Hallucinogen use, unspecified with other hallucinogen-induced disorder
F16.99 Hallucinogen use, unspecified with unspecified hallucinogen-induced disorder

[4] F17 Nicotine dependence
[EXCLUDES1] *history of tobacco dependence (Z87.891)*
tobacco use NOS (Z72.0)
[EXCLUDES2] *tobacco use (smoking) during pregnancy, childbirth and the puerperium (O99.33-)*
toxic effect of nicotine (T65.2-)
[5] F17.2 Nicotine dependence
[6] F17.20 Nicotine dependence, unspecified
F17.200 Nicotine dependence, unspecified, uncomplicated
F17.201 Nicotine dependence, unspecified, in remission
F17.203 Nicotine dependence unspecified, with withdrawal
F17.208 Nicotine dependence, unspecified, with other nicotine-induced disorders
F17.209 Nicotine dependence, unspecified, with unspecified nicotine-induced disorders
[6] F17.21 Nicotine dependence, cigarettes
F17.210 Nicotine dependence, cigarettes, uncomplicated
F17.211 Nicotine dependence, cigarettes, in remission
F17.213 Nicotine dependence, cigarettes, with withdrawal
F17.218 Nicotine dependence, cigarettes, with other nicotine-induced disorders
F17.219 Nicotine dependence, cigarettes, with unspecified nicotine-induced disorders
[6] F17.22 Nicotine dependence, chewing tobacco
F17.220 Nicotine dependence, chewing tobacco, uncomplicated
F17.221 Nicotine dependence, chewing tobacco, in remission
F17.223 Nicotine dependence, chewing tobacco, with withdrawal
F17.228 Nicotine dependence, chewing tobacco, with other nicotine-induced disorders
F17.229 Nicotine dependence, chewing tobacco, with unspecified nicotine-induced disorders
[6] F17.29 Nicotine dependence, other tobacco product
F17.290 Nicotine dependence, other tobacco product, uncomplicated
F17.291 Nicotine dependence, other tobacco product, in remission
F17.293 Nicotine dependence, other tobacco product, with withdrawal
F17.298 Nicotine dependence, other tobacco product, with other nicotine-induced disorders
F17.299 Nicotine dependence, other tobacco product, with unspecified nicotine-induced disorders

[4] F18 Inhalant related disorders
[INCLUDES] *volatile solvents*
[5] F18.1 Inhalant abuse
[EXCLUDES1] *inhalant dependence (F18.2-)*
inhalant use, unspecified (F18.9-)
F18.10 Inhalant abuse, uncomplicated
[6] F18.12 Inhalant abuse with intoxication
F18.120 Inhalant abuse with intoxication, uncomplicated
F18.121 Inhalant abuse with intoxication delirium
F18.129 Inhalant abuse with intoxication, unspecified
F18.14 Inhalant abuse with inhalant-induced mood disorder
[6] F18.15 Inhalant abuse with inhalant-induced psychotic disorder
F18.150 Inhalant abuse with inhalant-induced psychotic disorder with delusions
F18.151 Inhalant abuse with inhalant-induced psychotic disorder with hallucinations
F18.159 Inhalant abuse with inhalant-induced psychotic disorder, unspecified
F18.17 Inhalant abuse with inhalant-induced dementia
[6] F18.18 Inhalant abuse with other inhalant-induced disorders
F18.180 Inhalant abuse with inhalant-induced anxiety disorder
F18.188 Inhalant abuse with other inhalant-induced disorder
F18.19 Inhalant abuse with unspecified inhalant-induced disorder
[5] F18.2 Inhalant dependence
[EXCLUDES1] *inhalant abuse (F18.1-)*
inhalant use, unspecified (F18.9-)
F18.20 Inhalant dependence, uncomplicated
F18.21 Inhalant dependence, in remission
[6] F18.22 Inhalant dependence with intoxication
F18.220 Inhalant dependence with intoxication, uncomplicated
F18.221 Inhalant dependence with intoxication delirium
F18.229 Inhalant dependence with intoxication, unspecified
F18.24 Inhalant dependence with inhalant-induced mood disorder
[6] F18.25 Inhalant dependence with inhalant-induced psychotic disorder
F18.250 Inhalant dependence with inhalant-induced psychotic disorder with delusions
F18.251 Inhalant dependence with inhalant-induced psychotic disorder with hallucinations
F18.259 Inhalant dependence with inhalant-induced psychotic disorder, unspecified
F18.27 Inhalant dependence with inhalant-induced dementia
[6] F18.28 Inhalant dependence with other inhalant-induced disorders
F18.280 Inhalant dependence with inhalant-induced anxiety disorder

Unspecified Code | Other Specified Code | [N] Newborn Age: 0 | [P] Pediatric Age: 0-17 | [M] Maternity Age: 12-55
[A] Adult Age: 15-124 | ♂ Male | ♀ Female | ● New Code | ▲ Revised Code Title | ►◄ Revised Text

F18.288 Inhalant dependence with other inhalant-induced disorder

F18.29 Inhalant dependence with unspecified inhalant-induced disorder

[5] F18.9 Inhalant use, unspecified

[EXCLUDES1] *inhalant abuse (F18.1-)*
inhalant dependence (F18.2-)

F18.90 Inhalant use, unspecified, uncomplicated

[6] F18.92 Inhalant use, unspecified with intoxication

F18.920 Inhalant use, unspecified with intoxication, uncomplicated

F18.921 Inhalant use, unspecified with intoxication with delirium

F18.929 Inhalant use, unspecified with intoxication, unspecified

F18.94 Inhalant use, unspecified with inhalant-induced mood disorder

[6] F18.95 Inhalant use, unspecified with inhalant-induced psychotic disorder

F18.950 Inhalant use, unspecified with inhalant-induced psychotic disorder with delusions

F18.951 Inhalant use, unspecified with inhalant-induced psychotic disorder with hallucinations

F18.959 Inhalant use, unspecified with inhalant-induced psychotic disorder, unspecified

F18.97 Inhalant use, unspecified with inhalant-induced persisting dementia

[6] F18.98 Inhalant use, unspecified with other inhalant-induced disorders

F18.980 Inhalant use, unspecified with inhalant-induced anxiety disorder

F18.988 Inhalant use, unspecified with other inhalant-induced disorder

F18.99 Inhalant use, unspecified with unspecified inhalant-induced disorder

[4] F19 Other psychoactive substance related disorders

INCLUDES *polysubstance drug use (indiscriminate drug use)*

[5] F19.1 Other psychoactive substance abuse

[EXCLUDES1] *other psychoactive substance dependence (F19.2-)*
other psychoactive substance use, unspecified (F19.9-)

F19.10 Other psychoactive substance abuse, uncomplicated

[6] F19.12 Other psychoactive substance abuse with intoxication

F19.120 Other psychoactive substance abuse with intoxication, uncomplicated

F19.121 Other psychoactive substance abuse with intoxication delirium

F19.122 Other psychoactive substance abuse with intoxication with perceptual disturbances

F19.129 Other psychoactive substance abuse with intoxication, unspecified

F19.14 Other psychoactive substance abuse with psychoactive substance-induced mood disorder

[6] F19.15 Other psychoactive substance abuse with psychoactive substance-induced psychotic disorder

F19.150 Other psychoactive substance abuse with psychoactive substance-induced psychotic disorder with delusions

F19.151 Other psychoactive substance abuse with psychoactive substance-induced psychotic disorder with hallucinations

F19.159 Other psychoactive substance abuse with psychoactive substance-induced psychotic disorder, unspecified

F19.16 Other psychoactive substance abuse with psychoactive substance-induced persisting amnestic disorder

F19.17 Other psychoactive substance abuse with psychoactive substance-induced persisting dementia

[6] F19.18 Other psychoactive substance abuse with other psychoactive substance-induced disorders

F19.180 Other psychoactive substance abuse with psychoactive substance-induced anxiety disorder

F19.181 Other psychoactive substance abuse with psychoactive substance-induced sexual dysfunction

F19.182 Other psychoactive substance abuse with psychoactive substance-induced sleep disorder

F19.188 Other psychoactive substance abuse with other psychoactive substance-induced disorder

F19.19 Other psychoactive substance abuse with unspecified psychoactive substance-induced disorder

[5] F19.2 Other psychoactive substance dependence

[EXCLUDES1] *other psychoactive substance abuse (F19.1-)*
other psychoactive substance use, unspecified (F19.9-)

F19.20 Other psychoactive substance dependence, uncomplicated

F19.21 Other psychoactive substance dependence, in remission

[6] F19.22 Other psychoactive substance dependence with intoxication

[EXCLUDES1] *other psychoactive substance dependence with withdrawal (F19.23-)*

F19.220 Other psychoactive substance dependence with intoxication, uncomplicated

F19.221 Other psychoactive substance dependence with intoxication delirium

F19.222 Other psychoactive substance dependence with intoxication with perceptual disturbance

F19.229 Other psychoactive substance dependence with intoxication, unspecified

[6] F19.23 Other psychoactive substance dependence with withdrawal

[EXCLUDES1] *other psychoactive substance dependence with intoxication (F19.22-)*

F19.230 Other psychoactive substance dependence with withdrawal, uncomplicated

F19.231 Other psychoactive substance dependence with withdrawal delirium

F19.232 Other psychoactive substance dependence with withdrawal with perceptual disturbance

F19.239 Other psychoactive substance dependence with withdrawal, unspecified

F19.24 Other psychoactive substance dependence with psychoactive substance-induced mood disorder

[6] F19.25 Other psychoactive substance dependence with psychoactive substance-induced psychotic disorder

F19.250 Other psychoactive substance dependence with psychoactive substance-induced psychotic disorder with delusions

F19.251 Other psychoactive substance dependence with psychoactive substance-induced psychotic disorder with hallucinations

F19.259 Other psychoactive substance dependence with psychoactive substance-induced psychotic disorder, unspecified

F19.26 Other psychoactive substance dependence with psychoactive substance-induced persisting amnestic disorder

F19.27 Other psychoactive substance dependence with psychoactive substance-induced persisting dementia

[6] F19.28 Other psychoactive substance dependence with other psychoactive substance-induced disorders

F19.280 Other psychoactive substance dependence with psychoactive substance-induced anxiety disorder

F19.281 Other psychoactive substance dependence with psychoactive substance-induced sexual dysfunction

F19.282 Other psychoactive substance dependence with psychoactive substance-induced sleep disorder

F19.288 Other psychoactive substance dependence with other psychoactive substance-induced disorder

F19.29 Other psychoactive substance dependence with unspecified psychoactive substance-induced disorder

[5] F19.9 Other psychoactive substance use, unspecified

[EXCLUDES1] *other psychoactive substance abuse (F19.1-)*
other psychoactive substance dependence (F19.2-)

F19.90 Other psychoactive substance use, unspecified, uncomplicated

[6] F19.92 Other psychoactive substance use, unspecified with intoxication

[EXCLUDES1] *other psychoactive substance use, unspecified with withdrawal (F19.93)*

F19.920 Other psychoactive substance use, unspecified with intoxication, uncomplicated

F19.921 Other psychoactive substance use, unspecified with intoxication with delirium

F19.922 Other psychoactive substance use, unspecified with intoxication with perceptual disturbance

F19.929 Other psychoactive substance use, unspecified with intoxication, unspecified

[6] F19.93 Other psychoactive substance use, unspecified with withdrawal

[EXCLUDES1] *other psychoactive substance use, unspecified with intoxication (F19.92-)*

F19.930 Other psychoactive substance use, unspecified with withdrawal, uncomplicated

F19.931 Other psychoactive substance use, unspecified with withdrawal delirium

F19.932 Other psychoactive substance use, unspecified with withdrawal with perceptual disturbance

F19.939 Other psychoactive substance use, unspecified with withdrawal, unspecified

F19.94 Other psychoactive substance use, unspecified with psychoactive substance-induced mood disorder

[6] F19.95 Other psychoactive substance use, unspecified with psychoactive substance-induced psychotic disorder

F19.950 Other psychoactive substance use, unspecified with psychoactive substance-induced psychotic disorder with delusions

F19.951 Other psychoactive substance use, unspecified with psychoactive substance-induced psychotic disorder with hallucinations

F19.959 Other psychoactive substance use, unspecified with psychoactive substance-induced psychotic disorder, unspecified

F19.96 Other psychoactive substance use, unspecified with psychoactive substance-induced persisting amnestic disorder

F19.97 Other psychoactive substance use, unspecified with psychoactive substance-induced persisting dementia

[6] F19.98 Other psychoactive substance use, unspecified with other psychoactive substance-induced disorders

F19.980 Other psychoactive substance use, unspecified with psychoactive substance-induced anxiety disorder

F19.981 Other psychoactive substance use, unspecified with psychoactive substance-induced sexual dysfunction

F19.982 Other psychoactive substance use, unspecified with psychoactive substance-induced sleep disorder

F19.988 Other psychoactive substance use, unspecified with other psychoactive substance-induced disorder

F19.99 Other psychoactive substance use, unspecified with unspecified psychoactive substance-induced disorder

Schizophrenia, schizotypal, delusional, and other non-mood psychotic disorders (F20-F29)

[4] F20 Schizophrenia

[EXCLUDES1] *brief psychotic disorder (F23)*
cyclic schizophrenia (F25.0)
mood [affective] disorders with psychotic symptoms (F30.2, F31.2, F31.5, F31.64, F32.3, F33.3)
schizoaffective disorder (F25.-)
schizophrenic reaction NOS (F23)

[EXCLUDES2] *schizophrenic reaction in:*
alcoholism (F10.15-, F10.25-, F10.95-)
brain disease (F06.2)
epilepsy (F06.2)
psychoactive drug use (F11-F19 with .15. .25, .95)
schizotypal disorder (F21)

F20.0 Paranoid schizophrenia

Paraphrenic schizophrenia

[EXCLUDES1] *involutional paranoid state (F22)*
paranoia (F22)

F20.1 Disorganized schizophrenia

Hebephrenic schizophrenia
Hebephrenia

F20.2 Catatonic schizophrenia

Schizophrenic catalepsy
Schizophrenic catatonia
Schizophrenic flexibilitas cerea

[EXCLUDES1] *catatonic stupor (R40.1)*

F20.3 Undifferentiated schizophrenia

Atypical schizophrenia

[EXCLUDES1] *acute schizophrenia-like psychotic disorder (F23)*

[EXCLUDES2] *post-schizophrenic depression (F32.8)*

F20.5 Residual schizophrenia

Restzustand (schizophrenic)
Schizophrenic residual state

Unspecified Code | Other Specified Code | [N] Newborn Age: 0 | [P] Pediatric Age: 0-17 | [M] Maternity Age: 12-55
[A] Adult Age: 15-124 | ♂ Male | ♀ Female | ● New Code | ▲ Revised Code Title | ►◄ Revised Text

[5] **F20.8 Other schizophrenia**
F20.81 Schizophreniform disorder
Schizophreniform psychosis NOS
F20.89 Other schizophrenia
Cenesthopathic schizophrenia
Simple schizophrenia
F20.9 Schizophrenia, unspecified

F21 Schizotypal disorder
Borderline schizophrenia
Latent schizophrenia
Latent schizophrenic reaction
Prepsychotic schizophrenia
Prodromal schizophrenia
Pseudoneurotic schizophrenia
Pseudopsychopathic schizophrenia
Schizotypal personality disorder
[EXCLUDES2] *Asperger's syndrome (F84.5)*
schizoid personality disorder (F60.1)

F22 Delusional disorders
Delusional dysmorphophobia
Involutional paranoid state
Paranoia
Paranoia querulans
Paranoid psychosis
Paranoid state
Paraphrenia (late)
Sensitiver Beziehungswahn
[EXCLUDES1] *mood [affective] disorders with psychotic symptoms (F30.2, F31.2, F31.5, F31.64, F32.3, F33.3)*
paranoid schizophrenia (F20.0)
[EXCLUDES2] *paranoid personality disorder (F60.0)*
paranoid psychosis, psychogenic (F23)
paranoid reaction (F23)

F23 Brief psychotic disorder
Paranoid reaction
Psychogenic paranoid psychosis
[EXCLUDES2] *mood [affective] disorders with psychotic symptoms (F30.2, F31.2, F31.5, F31.64, F32.3, F33.3)*

F24 Shared psychotic disorder
Folie á deux
Induced paranoid disorder
Induced psychotic disorder

[4] **F25 Schizoaffective disorders**
[EXCLUDES1] *mood [affective] disorders with psychotic symptoms (F30.2, F31.2, F31.5, F31.64, F32.3, F33.3)*
schizophrenia (F20.-)
F25.0 Schizoaffective disorder, bipolar type
Cyclic schizophrenia
Schizoaffective disorder, manic type
Schizoaffective disorder, mixed type
Schizoaffective psychosis, bipolar type
Schizophreniform psychosis, manic type
F25.1 Schizoaffective disorder, depressive type
Schizoaffective psychosis, depressive type
Schizophreniform psychosis, depressive type
F25.8 Other schizoaffective disorders
F25.9 Schizoaffective disorder, unspecified
Schizoaffective psychosis NOS

F28 Other psychotic disorder not due to a substance or known physiological condition
Chronic hallucinatory psychosis

F29 Unspecified psychosis not due to a substance or known physiological condition
Psychosis NOS

[EXCLUDES1] *mental disorder NOS (F99)*
unspecified mental disorder due to known physiological condition (F09)

Mood [affective] disorders (F30-F39)

[4] **F30 Manic episode**
[INCLUDES] *bipolar disorder, single manic episode*
mixed affective episode
[EXCLUDES1] *bipolar disorder (F31.-)*
major depressive disorder, single episode (F32.-)
major depressive disorder, recurrent (F33.-)
[5] **F30.1 Manic episode without psychotic symptoms**
F30.10 Manic episode without psychotic symptoms, unspecified
F30.11 Manic episode without psychotic symptoms, mild
F30.12 Manic episode without psychotic symptoms, moderate
F30.13 Manic episode, severe, without psychotic symptoms
F30.2 Manic episode, severe with psychotic symptoms
Manic stupor
Mania with mood-congruent psychotic symptoms
Mania with mood-incongruent psychotic symptoms
F30.3 Manic episode in partial remission
F30.4 Manic episode in full remission
F30.8 Other manic episodes
Hypomania
F30.9 Manic episode, unspecified
Mania NOS

[4] **F31 Bipolar disorder**
[INCLUDES] *manic-depressive illness*
manic-depressive psychosis
manic-depressive reaction
[EXCLUDES1] *bipolar disorder, single manic episode (F30.-)*
major depressive disorder, single episode (F32.-)
major depressive disorder, recurrent (F33.-)
[EXCLUDES2] *cyclothymia (F34.0)*
F31.0 Bipolar disorder, current episode hypomanic
[5] **F31.1 Bipolar disorder, current episode manic without psychotic features**
F31.10 Bipolar disorder, current episode manic without psychotic features, unspecified
F31.11 Bipolar disorder, current episode manic without psychotic features, mild
F31.12 Bipolar disorder, current episode manic without psychotic features, moderate
F31.13 Bipolar disorder, current episode manic without psychotic features, severe
F31.2 Bipolar disorder, current episode manic severe with psychotic features
Bipolar disorder, current episode manic with mood-congruent psychotic symptoms
Bipolar disorder, current episode manic with mood-incongruent psychotic symptoms
[5] **F31.3 Bipolar disorder, current episode depressed, mild or moderate severity**
F31.30 Bipolar disorder, current episode depressed, mild or moderate severity, unspecified
F31.31 Bipolar disorder, current episode depressed, mild
F31.32 Bipolar disorder, current episode depressed, moderate
F31.4 Bipolar disorder, current episode depressed, severe, without psychotic features
F31.5 Bipolar disorder, current episode depressed, severe, with psychotic features

[4] 4th character required [5] 5th character required [6] 6th character required [7] 7th character required [X] Extension 'X' Alert
[EXCLUDES 1] Not coded here [EXCLUDES 2] Not included here [PDx] Primary Diagnosis Only Manifestation Code

Bipolar disorder, current episode depressed with mood-incongruent psychotic symptoms

Bipolar disorder, current episode depressed with mood-congruent psychotic symptoms

⑤ **F31.6 Bipolar disorder, current episode** mixed

F31.60 Bipolar disorder, current episode mixed, unspecified

F31.61 Bipolar disorder, current episode mixed, mild

F31.62 Bipolar disorder, current episode mixed, moderate

F31.63 Bipolar disorder, current episode mixed, severe, without psychotic features

F31.64 Bipolar disorder, current episode mixed, severe, with psychotic features

Bipolar disorder, current episode mixed with mood-congruent psychotic symptoms

Bipolar disorder, current episode mixed with mood-incongruent psychotic symptoms

⑤ **F31.7 Bipolar disorder, currently** in remission

F31.70 Bipolar disorder, currently in remission, most recent episode unspecified

F31.71 Bipolar disorder, in partial remission, **most recent episode** hypomanic

F31.72 Bipolar disorder, in full remission, **most recent episode** hypomanic

F31.73 Bipolar disorder, in partial remission, **most recent episode** manic

F31.74 Bipolar disorder, in full remission, **most recent episode** manic

F31.75 Bipolar disorder, in partial remission, **most recent episode** depressed

F31.76 Bipolar disorder, in full remission, **most recent episode** depressed

F31.77 Bipolar disorder, in partial remission, **most recent episode** mixed

F31.78 Bipolar disorder, in full remission, **most recent episode** mixed

⑤ **F31.8** Other **bipolar disorders**

F31.81 Bipolar II disorder

F31.89 Other bipolar disorder

Recurrent manic episodes NOS

F31.9 Bipolar disorder, unspecified

④ **F32 Major depressive disorder,** single episode

INCLUDES   single episode of agitated depression
single episode of depressive reaction
single episode of major depression
single episode of psychogenic depression
single episode of reactive depression
single episode of vital depression

EXCLUDES1   bipolar disorder (F31.-)
manic episode (F30.-)
recurrent depressive disorder (F33.-)

EXCLUDES2   adjustment disorder (F43.2)

F32.0 Major depressive disorder, single episode, mild

F32.1 Major depressive disorder, single episode, moderate

F32.2 Major depressive disorder, single episode, severe **without psychotic features**

F32.3 Major depressive disorder, single episode, severe with psychotic features

Single episode of major depression with mood-congruent psychotic symptoms

Single episode of major depression with mood-incongruent psychotic symptoms

Single episode of major depression with psychotic symptoms

Single episode of psychogenic depressive psychosis

Single episode of psychotic depression

Single episode of reactive depressive psychosis

F32.4 Major depressive disorder, single episode, in partial remission

F32.5 Major depressive disorder, single episode, in full remission

F32.8 Other depressive episodes

Atypical depression

Post-schizophrenic depression

Single episode of 'masked' depression NOS

F32.9 Major depressive disorder, single episode, unspecified

Depression NOS

Depressive disorder NOS

Major depression NOS

④ **F33 Major depressive disorder,** recurrent

INCLUDES   recurrent episodes of depressive reaction
recurrent episodes of endogenous depression
recurrent episodes of major depression
recurrent episodes of psychogenic depression
recurrent episodes of reactive depression
recurrent episodes of seasonal depressive disorder
recurrent episodes of vital depression

EXCLUDES1   bipolar disorder (F31.-)
manic episode (F30.-)

F33.0 Major depressive disorder, recurrent, mild

F33.1 Major depressive disorder, recurrent, moderate

F33.2 Major depressive disorder, recurrent severe **without psychotic features**

F33.3 Major depressive disorder, recurrent, severe with psychotic symptoms

Endogenous depression with psychotic symptoms

Recurrent severe episodes of major depression with mood-congruent psychotic symptoms

Recurrent severe episodes of major depression with mood-incongruent psychotic symptoms

Recurrent severe episodes of major depression with psychotic symptoms

Recurrent severe episodes of psychogenic depressive psychosis

Recurrent severe episodes of psychotic depression

Recurrent severe episodes of reactive depressive psychosis

⑤ **F33.4 Major depressive disorder, recurrent,** in remission

F33.40 Major depressive disorder, recurrent, in remission, unspecified

F33.41 Major depressive disorder, recurrent, in partial remission

F33.42 Major depressive disorder, recurrent, in full remission

F33.8 Other recurrent depressive disorders

Recurrent brief depressive episodes

F33.9 Major depressive disorder, recurrent, unspecified

Monopolar depression NOS

④ **F34 Persistent mood [affective] disorders**

F34.0 Cyclothymic **disorder**

Affective personality disorder

Cycloid personality

Cyclothymia

Cyclothymic personality

F34.1 Dysthymic **disorder**

Depressive neurosis

Depressive personality disorder

Dysthymia

Neurotic depression

Persistent anxiety depression

EXCLUDES2   anxiety depression (mild or not persistent) (F41.8)

F34.8 Other persistent mood [affective] disorders

Unspecified Code	Other Specified Code	N Newborn Age: 0	P Pediatric Age: 0-17	M Maternity Age: 12-55	
A Adult Age: 15-124	♂ Male	♀ Female	● New Code	▲ Revised Code Title	►◄ Revised Text

F34.9 Persistent mood [affective] disorder, unspecified

F39 Unspecified mood [affective] disorder

Affective psychosis NOS

Anxiety, dissociative, stress-related, somatoform and other nonpsychotic mental disorders (F40-F48)

[4] **F40 Phobic anxiety disorders**

[5] **F40.0 Agoraphobia**

F40.00 Agoraphobia, unspecified

F40.01 Agoraphobia with panic disorder

Panic disorder with agoraphobia

[EXCLUDES1] *panic disorder without agoraphobia (F41.0)*

F40.02 Agoraphobia without panic disorder

[5] **F40.1 Social phobias**

Anthropophobia
Social anxiety disorder of childhood
Social neurosis

F40.10 Social phobia, unspecified

F40.11 Social phobia, generalized

[5] **F40.2 Specific (isolated) phobias**

[EXCLUDES2] *dysmorphophobia (nondelusional) (F45.22)*
nosophobia (F45.22)

[6] **F40.21 Animal type phobia**

F40.210 Arachnophobia

Fear of spiders

F40.218 Other animal type phobia

[6] **F40.22 Natural environment type phobia**

F40.220 Fear of thunderstorms

F40.228 Other natural environment type phobia

[6] **F40.23 Blood, injection, injury type phobia**

F40.230 Fear of blood

F40.231 Fear of injections and transfusions

F40.232 Fear of other medical care

F40.233 Fear of injury

[6] **F40.24 Situational type phobia**

F40.240 Claustrophobia

F40.241 Acrophobia

F40.242 Fear of bridges

F40.243 Fear of flying

F40.248 Other situational type phobia

[6] **F40.29 Other specified phobia**

F40.290 Androphobia

Fear of men

F40.291 Gynephobia

Fear of women

F40.298 Other specified phobia

F40.8 Other phobic anxiety disorders

Phobic anxiety disorder of childhood

F40.9 Phobic anxiety disorder, unspecified

Phobia NOS
Phobic state NOS

[4] **F41 Other anxiety disorders**

[EXCLUDES2] *anxiety in:*
acute stress reaction (F43.0)
transient adjustment reaction (F43.2)
neurasthenia (F48.8)
psychophysiologic disorders (F45.-)
separation anxiety (F93.0)

F41.0 Panic disorder [episodic paroxysmal anxiety] without agoraphobia

Panic attack
Panic state

[EXCLUDES1] *panic disorder with agoraphobia (F40.01)*

F41.1 Generalized anxiety disorder

Anxiety neurosis
Anxiety reaction
Anxiety state
Overanxious disorder

[EXCLUDES2] *neurasthenia (F48.8)*

F41.3 Other mixed anxiety disorders

F41.8 Other specified anxiety disorders

Anxiety depression (mild or not persistent)
Anxiety hysteria
Mixed anxiety and depressive disorder

F41.9 Anxiety disorder, unspecified

Anxiety NOS

F42 Obsessive-compulsive disorder

Anancastic neurosis
Obsessive-compulsive neurosis

[EXCLUDES2] *obsessive-compulsive personality (disorder) (F60.5)*
obsessive-compulsive symptoms occurring in depression (F32-F33)
obsessive-compulsive symptoms occurring in schizophrenia (F20.-)

[4] **F43 Reaction to severe stress, and adjustment disorders**

F43.0 Acute stress reaction

Acute crisis reaction
Acute reaction to stress
Combat and operational stress reaction
Combat fatigue
Crisis state
Psychic shock

[5] **F43.1 Post-traumatic stress disorder (PTSD)**

Traumatic neurosis

F43.10 Post-traumatic stress disorder, unspecified

F43.11 Post-traumatic stress disorder, acute

F43.12 Post-traumatic stress disorder, chronic

[5] **F43.2 Adjustment disorders**

Culture shock
Grief reaction
Hospitalism in children

[EXCLUDES2] *separation anxiety disorder of childhood (F93.0)*

F43.20 Adjustment disorder, unspecified

F43.21 Adjustment disorder with depressed mood

F43.22 Adjustment disorder with anxiety

F43.23 Adjustment disorder with mixed anxiety and depressed mood

F43.24 Adjustment disorder with disturbance of conduct

F43.25 Adjustment disorder with mixed disturbance of emotions and conduct

F43.29 Adjustment disorder with other symptoms

F43.8 Other reactions to severe stress

F43.9 Reaction to severe stress, unspecified

[4] **F44 Dissociative and conversion disorders**

[INCLUDES] *conversion hysteria*
conversion reaction
hysteria
hysterical psychosis

[EXCLUDES2] *malingering [conscious simulation] (Z76.5)*

F44.0 Dissociative amnesia

[EXCLUDES1] *amnesia NOS (R41.3)*
anterograde amnesia (R41.1)
retrograde amnesia (R41.2)

[EXCLUDES2] *alcohol-or other psychoactive substance-induced amnestic disorder (F10, F13, F19 with .26, .96)*
amnestic disorder due to known physiological condition (F04)
postictal amnesia in epilepsy (G40.-)

F44.1 Dissociative fugue

[EXCLUDES2] *postictal fugue in epilepsy (G40.-)*

F44.2 Dissociative stupor

[EXCLUDES1] *catatonic stupor (R40.1)*
stupor NOS (R40.1)

[4] 4th character required [5] 5th character required [6] 6th character required [7] 7th character required [X] Extension 'X' Alert
[EXCLUDES1] Not coded here [EXCLUDES2] Not included here [PDx] Primary Diagnosis Only Manifestation Code

[EXCLUDES2] *catatonic disorder due to known physiological condition (F06.1)*
depressive stupor (F32, F33)
manic stupor (F30, F31)

F44.4 Conversion disorder with motor symptom or deficit
Dissociative motor disorders
Psychogenic aphonia
Psychogenic dysphonia

F44.5 Conversion disorder with seizures or convulsions
Dissociative convulsions

F44.6 Conversion disorder with sensory symptom or deficit
Dissociative anesthesia and sensory loss
Psychogenic deafness

F44.7 Conversion disorder with mixed symptom presentation

[5] **F44.8 Other dissociative and conversion disorders**

F44.81 Dissociative identity disorder
Multiple personality disorder

F44.89 Other dissociative and conversion disorders
Ganser's syndrome
Psychogenic confusion
Psychogenic twilight state
Trance and possession disorders

F44.9 Dissociative and conversion disorder, unspecified
Dissociative disorder NOS

[4] **F45 Somatoform disorders**

[EXCLUDES2] *dissociative and conversion disorders (F44.-)*
factitious disorders (F68.1-)
hair-plucking (F63.3)
lalling (F80.0)
lisping (F80.0)
malingering [conscious simulation] (Z76.5)
nail-biting (F98.8)
psychological or behavioral factors associated with disorders or diseases classified elsewhere (F54)
sexual dysfunction, not due to a substance or known physiological condition (F52.-)
thumb-sucking (F98.8)
tic disorders (in childhood and adolescence) (F95.-)
Tourette's syndrome (F95.2)
trichotillomania (F63.3)

F45.0 Somatization disorder
Briquet's disorder
Multiple psychosomatic disorder

F45.1 Undifferentiated somatoform disorder
Undifferentiated psychosomatic disorder

[5] **F45.2 Hypochondriacal disorders**

[EXCLUDES2] *delusional dysmorphophobia (F22)*
fixed delusions about bodily functions or shape (F22)

F45.20 Hypochondriacal disorder, unspecified

F45.21 Hypochondriasis
Hypochondriacal neurosis

F45.22 Body dysmorphic disorder
Dysmorphophobia (nondelusional)
Nosophobia

F45.29 Other hypochondriacal disorders

[5] **F45.4 Pain disorders related to psychological factors**

[EXCLUDES1] *pain NOS (R52)*

F45.41 Pain disorder exclusively related to psychological factors
Somatoform pain disorder (persistent)

F45.42 Pain disorder with related psychological factors
Code also associated acute or chronic pain (G89.-)

F45.8 Other somatoform disorders
Psychogenic dysmenorrhea
Psychogenic dysphagia, including 'globus hystericus'
Psychogenic pruritus
Psychogenic torticollis
Somatoform autonomic dysfunction
Teeth grinding

[EXCLUDES1] *sleep related teeth grinding (G47.63)*

F45.9 Somatoform disorder, unspecified
Psychosomatic disorder NOS

[4] **F48 Other nonpsychotic mental disorders**

F48.1 Depersonalization-derealization syndrome

F48.2 Pseudobulbar affect
Involuntary emotional expression disorder
Code first underlying cause, if known, such as:
amyotrophic lateral sclerosis (G12.21)
multiple sclerosis (G35)
sequelae of cerebrovascular disease (I69.-)
sequelae of traumatic intracranial injury (S06.-)

F48.8 Other specified nonpsychotic mental disorders
Dhat syndrome
Neurasthenia
Occupational neurosis, including writer's cramp
Psychasthenia
Psychasthenic neurosis
Psychogenic syncope

F48.9 Nonpsychotic mental disorder, unspecified
Neurosis NOS

Behavioral syndromes associated with physiological disturbances and physical factors (F50-F59)

[4] **F50 Eating disorders**

[EXCLUDES1] *anorexia NOS (R63.0)*
feeding difficulties (R63.3)
polyphagia (R63.2)

[EXCLUDES2] *feeding disorder in infancy or childhood (F98.2-)*

[5] **F50.0 Anorexia nervosa**

[EXCLUDES1] *loss of appetite (R63.0)*
psychogenic loss of appetite (F50.8)

F50.00 Anorexia nervosa, unspecified

F50.01 Anorexia nervosa, restricting type

F50.02 Anorexia nervosa, binge eating/purging type

[EXCLUDES1] *bulimia nervosa (F50.2)*

F50.2 Bulimia nervosa
Bulimia NOS
Hyperorexia nervosa

[EXCLUDES1] *anorexia nervosa, binge eating/purging type (F50.02)*

F50.8 Other eating disorders
Pica in adults
Psychogenic loss of appetite

[EXCLUDES2] *pica of infancy and childhood (F98.3)*

F50.9 Eating disorder, unspecified
Atypical anorexia nervosa
Atypical bulimia nervosa

[4] **F51 Sleep disorders not due to a substance or known physiological condition**

[EXCLUDES2] *organic sleep disorders (G47.-)*

[5] **F51.0 Insomnia not due to a substance or known physiological condition**

[EXCLUDES2] *alcohol related insomnia (F10.182, F10.282, F10.982)*
drug-related insomnia (F11.182, F11.282, F11.982, F13.182, F13.282, F13.982, F14.182, F14.282, F14.982, F15.182, F15.282, F15.982, F19.182, F19.282, F19.982)
insomnia NOS (G47.0-)
insomnia due to known physiological condition (G47.0-)
organic insomnia (G47.0-)
sleep deprivation (Z72.820)

F51.01 Primary insomnia
Idiopathic insomnia

Unspecified Code | Other Specified Code | [N] Newborn Age: 0 | [P] Pediatric Age: 0-17 | [M] Maternity Age: 12-55
[A] Adult Age: 15-124 | ♂ Male | ♀ Female | ● New Code | ▲ Revised Code Title | ►◄ Revised Text

F51.02 Adjustment **insomnia**

F51.03 Paradoxical **insomnia**

F51.04 Psychophysiologic **insomnia**

F51.05 Insomnia due to other mental disorder

Code also associated mental disorder

F51.09 Other insomnia not due to a substance or known physiological condition

[5] **F51.1** Hypersomnia **not due to a substance or known physiological condition**

[EXCLUDES2] *alcohol related hypersomnia (F10.182, F10.282, F10.982)*
drug-related hypersomnia (F11.182, F11.282, F11.982, F13.182, F13.282, F13.982, F14.182, F14.282, F14.982, F15.182, F15.282, F15.982, F19.182, F19.282, F19.982)
hypersomnia NOS (G47.10)
hypersomnia due to known physiological condition (G47.10)
idiopathic hypersomnia (G47.11, G47.12)
narcolepsy (G47.4-)

F51.11 Primary **hypersomnia**

F51.12 Insufficient sleep syndrome

[EXCLUDES1] *sleep deprivation (Z72.820)*

F51.13 Hypersomnia due to other mental disorder

Code also associated mental disorder

F51.19 Other hypersomnia not due to a substance or known physiological condition

F51.3 Sleepwalking [somnambulism]

F51.4 Sleep terrors [night terrors]

F51.5 Nightmare disorder

Dream anxiety disorder

F51.8 Other sleep disorders not due to a substance or known physiological condition

F51.9 Sleep disorder not due to a substance or known physiological condition, unspecified

Emotional sleep disorder NOS

[4] **F52** Sexual dysfunction **not due to a substance or known physiological condition**

[EXCLUDES2] *Dhat syndrome (F48.8)*

F52.0 Hypoactive sexual desire **disorder**

Anhedonia (sexual)
Lack or loss of sexual desire

[EXCLUDES1] *decreased libido (R68.82)*

F52.1 Sexual aversion **disorder**

Sexual aversion and lack of sexual enjoyment

[5] **F52.2 Sexual arousal disorders**

Failure of genital response

F52.21 Male **erectile disorder**

Psychogenic impotence

[EXCLUDES1] *impotence of organic origin (N52.-)*
impotence NOS (N52.-) ♂

F52.22 Female **sexual arousal disorder**

Frigidity ♀

[5] **F52.3** Orgasmic **disorder**

Inhibited orgasm
Psychogenic anorgasmy

F52.31 Female **orgasmic disorder** ♀

F52.32 Male **orgasmic disorder** ♂

F52.4 Premature ejaculation ♂

F52.5 Vaginismus not due to a substance or known physiological condition

Psychogenic vaginismus

[EXCLUDES2] *vaginismus (due to a known physiological condition) (N94.2)* ♀

F52.6 Dyspareunia not due to a substance or known physiological condition

Psychogenic dyspareunia

[EXCLUDES2] *dyspareunia (due to a known physiological condition) (N94.1)* ♀

F52.8 Other sexual dysfunction not due to a substance or known physiological condition

Excessive sexual drive
Nymphomania
Satyriasis

F52.9 Unspecified sexual dysfunction not due to a substance or known physiological condition

Sexual dysfunction NOS

F53 Puerperal psychosis

Postpartum depression

[EXCLUDES1] *mood disorders with psychotic features (F30.2, F31.2, F31.5, F31.64, F32.3, F33.3)*
postpartum dysphoria (O90.6)
psychosis in schizophrenia, schizotypal, delusional, and other psychotic disorders (F20-F29) ♀

F54 Psychological and behavioral factors associated with disorders or diseases classified elsewhere

Psychological factors affecting physical conditions

Code first the associated physical disorder, such as:
asthma (J45.-)
dermatitis (L23-L25)
gastric ulcer (K25.-)
mucous colitis (K58.-)
ulcerative colitis (K51.-)
urticaria (L50.-)

[EXCLUDES2] *tension-type headache (G44.2)*

[4] **F55 Abuse of non-psychoactive substances**

[EXCLUDES2] *abuse of psychoactive substances (F10-F19)*

F55.0 Abuse of antacids

F55.1 Abuse of herbal or folk remedies

F55.2 Abuse of laxatives

F55.3 Abuse of steroids or hormones

F55.4 Abuse of vitamins

F55.8 Abuse of other non-psychoactive substances

F59 Unspecified behavioral syndromes associated with physiological disturbances and physical factors

Psychogenic physiological dysfunction NOS

Disorders of adult personality and behavior (F60-F69)

[4] **F60 Specific personality disorders**

F60.0 Paranoid **personality disorder**

Expansive paranoid personality (disorder)
Fanatic personality (disorder)
Querulant personality (disorder)
Paranoid personality (disorder)
Sensitive paranoid personality (disorder)

[EXCLUDES2] *paranoia (F22)*
paranoia querulans (F22)
paranoid psychosis (F22)
paranoid schizophrenia (F20.0)
paranoid state (F22)

F60.1 Schizoid **personality disorder**

[EXCLUDES2] *Asperger's syndrome (F84.5)*
delusional disorder (F22)
schizoid disorder of childhood (F84.5)
schizophrenia (F20.-)
schizotypal disorder (F21)

F60.2 Antisocial **personality disorder**

Amoral personality (disorder)
Asocial personality (disorder)
Dissocial personality disorder
Psychopathic personality (disorder)
Sociopathic personality (disorder)

[EXCLUDES1] *conduct disorders (F91.-)*

[EXCLUDES2] *borderline personality disorder (F60.3)*

F60.3 Borderline personality disorder
Aggressive personality (disorder)
Emotionally unstable personality disorder
Explosive personality (disorder)
[EXCLUDES2] *antisocial personality disorder (F60.2)*

F60.4 Histrionic personality disorder
Hysterical personality (disorder)
Psychoinfantile personality (disorder)

F60.5 Obsessive-compulsive personality disorder
Anankastic personality (disorder)
Compulsive personality (disorder)
Obsessional personality (disorder)
[EXCLUDES2] *obsessive-compulsive disorder (F42)*

F60.6 Avoidant personality disorder
Anxious personality disorder

F60.7 Dependent personality disorder
Asthenic personality (disorder)
Inadequate personality (disorder)
Passive personality (disorder)

[5] **F60.8 Other specific personality disorders**

F60.81 Narcissistic personality disorder

F60.89 Other specific personality disorders
Eccentric personality disorder
'Haltlose' type personality disorder
Immature personality disorder
Passive-aggressive personality disorder
Psychoneurotic personality disorder
Self-defeating personality disorder

F60.9 Personality disorder, unspecified
Character disorder NOS
Character neurosis NOS
Pathological personality NOS

[4] **F63 Impulse disorders**
[EXCLUDES2] *habitual excessive use of alcohol or psychoactive substances (F10-F19)*
impulse disorders involving sexual behavior (F65.-)

F63.0 Pathological gambling
Compulsive gambling
[EXCLUDES1] *gambling and betting NOS (Z72.6)*
[EXCLUDES2] *excessive gambling by manic patients (F30, F31)*
gambling in antisocial personality disorder (F60.2)

F63.1 Pyromania
Pathological fire-setting
[EXCLUDES2] *fire-setting (by) (in):*
adult with antisocial personality disorder (F60.2)
alcohol or psychoactive substance intoxication (F10-F19)
conduct disorders (F91.-)
mental disorders due to known physiological condition (F01-F09)
schizophrenia (F20.-)

F63.2 Kleptomania
Pathological stealing
[EXCLUDES1] *shoplifting as the reason for observation for suspected mental disorder (Z03.8)*
[EXCLUDES2] *depressive disorder with stealing (F31-F33)*
stealing due to underlying mental condition-code to mental condition
stealing in mental disorders due to known physiological condition (F01-F09)

F63.3 Trichotillomania
Hair plucking
[EXCLUDES2] *other stereotyped movement disorder (F98.4)*

[5] **F63.8 Other impulse disorders**

F63.81 Intermittent explosive disorder

F63.89 Other impulse disorders

F63.9 Impulse disorder, unspecified
Impulse control disorder NOS

[4] **F64 Gender identity disorders**

F64.1 Gender identity disorder in adolescence and adulthood
Dual role transvestism
Transsexualism
Use additional code to identify sex reassignment status (Z87.890)
[EXCLUDES1] *gender identity disorder in childhood (F64.2)*
[EXCLUDES2] *fetishistic transvestism (F65.1)*

F64.2 Gender identity disorder of childhood
[EXCLUDES1] *gender identity disorder in adolescence and adulthood (F64.1)*
[EXCLUDES2] *sexual maturation disorder (F66)* [P]

F64.8 Other gender identity disorders

F64.9 Gender identity disorder, unspecified
Gender-role disorder NOS

[4] **F65 Paraphilias**

F65.0 Fetishism

F65.1 Transvestic fetishism
Fetishistic transvestism

F65.2 Exhibitionism

F65.3 Voyeurism

F65.4 Pedophilia

[5] **F65.5 Sadomasochism**

F65.50 Sadomasochism, unspecified

F65.51 Sexual masochism

F65.52 Sexual sadism

[5] **F65.8 Other paraphilias**

F65.81 Frotteurism

F65.89 Other paraphilias
Necrophilia

F65.9 Paraphilia, unspecified
Sexual deviation NOS

F66 Other sexual disorders
Sexual maturation disorder
Sexual relationship disorder

[4] **F68 Other disorders of adult personality and behavior**

[5] **F68.1 Factitious disorder**
Compensation neurosis
Elaboration of physical symptoms for psychological reasons
Hospital hopper syndrome
Münchausen's syndrome
Peregrinating patient
[EXCLUDES2] *factitial dermatitis (L98.1)*
person feigning illness (with obvious motivation) (Z76.5)

F68.10 Factitious disorder, unspecified

F68.11 Factitious disorder with predominantly psychological signs and symptoms

F68.12 Factitious disorder with predominantly physical signs and symptoms

F68.13 Factitious disorder with combined psychological and physical signs and symptoms

F68.8 Other specified disorders of adult personality and behavior

F69 Unspecified disorder of adult personality and behavior [A]

Unspecified Code | Other Specified Code | [N] Newborn Age: 0 | [P] Pediatric Age: 0-17 | [M] Maternity Age: 12-55
[A] Adult Age: 15-124 | ♂ Male | ♀ Female | ● New Code | ▲ Revised Code Title | ►◄ Revised Text

Intellectual Disabilities (F70-F79)

Code first any associated physical or developmental disorders

[EXCLUDES1] *borderline intellectual functioning, IQ above 70 to 84 (R41.83)*

F70 Mild intellectual disabilities

IQ level 50-55 to approximately 70
Mild mental subnormality

F71 Moderate intellectual disabilities

IQ level 35-40 to 50-55
Moderate mental subnormality

F72 Severe intellectual disabilities

IQ 20-25 to 35-40
Severe mental subnormality

F73 Profound intellectual disabilities

IQ level below 20-25
Profound mental subnormality

F78 Other intellectual disabilities

F79 Unspecified intellectual disabilities

Mental deficiency NOS
Mental subnormality NOS

Pervasive and specific developmental disorders (F80-F89)

[4] F80 Specific developmental disorders of speech and language

F80.0 Phonological disorder

Dyslalia
Functional speech articulation disorder
Lalling
Lisping
Phonological developmental disorder
Speech articulation developmental disorder

[EXCLUDES1] *speech articulation impairment due to aphasia NOS (R47.01)*
speech articulation impairment due to apraxia (R48.2)

[EXCLUDES2] *speech articulation impairment due to hearing loss (F80.4)*
speech articulation impairment due to intellectual disabilities (F70-F79)
speech articulation impairment with expressive language developmental disorder (F80.1)
speech articulation impairment with mixed receptive expressive language developmental disorder (F80.2)

F80.1 Expressive language disorder

Developmental dysphasia or aphasia, expressive type

[EXCLUDES1] *mixed receptive-expressive language disorder (F80.2)*
dysphasia and aphasia NOS (R47.-)

[EXCLUDES2] *acquired aphasia with epilepsy [Landau-Kleffner] (G40.80-)*
selective mutism (F94.0)
intellectual disabilities (F70-F79)
pervasive developmental disorders (F84.-)

F80.2 Mixed receptive-expressive language disorder

Developmental dysphasia or aphasia, receptive type
Developmental Wernicke's aphasia

[EXCLUDES1] *central auditory processing disorder (H93.25)*
dysphasia or aphasia NOS (R47.-)
expressive language disorder (F80.1)
expressive type dysphasia or aphasia (F80.1)
word deafness (H93.25)

[EXCLUDES2] *acquired aphasia with epilepsy [Landau-Kleffner] (G40.80-)*
pervasive developmental disorders (F84.-)
selective mutism (F94.0)
intellectual disabilities (F70-F79)

F80.4 Speech and language development delay due to hearing loss

Code also type of hearing loss (H90.-, H91.-)

[5] F80.8 Other developmental disorders of speech and language

F80.81 Childhood onset fluency disorder

Cluttering NOS
Stuttering NOS

[EXCLUDES1] *adult onset fluency disorder (F98.5)*
fluency disorder in conditions classified elsewhere (R47.82)
fluency disorder (stuttering) following cerebrovascular disease (I69. with final characters -23)

F80.89 Other developmental disorders of speech and language

F80.9 Developmental disorder of speech and language, unspecified

Communication disorder NOS
Language disorder NOS

[4] F81 Specific developmental disorders of scholastic skills

F81.0 Specific reading disorder

'Backward reading'
Developmental dyslexia
Specific reading retardation

[EXCLUDES1] *alexia NOS (R48.0)*
dyslexia NOS (R48.0)

F81.2 Mathematics disorder

Developmental acalculia
Developmental arithmetical disorder
Developmental Gerstmann's syndrome

[EXCLUDES1] *acalculia NOS (R48.8)*

[EXCLUDES2] *arithmetical difficulties associated with a reading disorder (F81.0)*
arithmetical difficulties associated with a spelling disorder (F81.81)
arithmetical difficulties due to inadequate teaching (Z55.8)

[5] F81.8 Other developmental disorders of scholastic skills

F81.81 Disorder of written expression

Specific spelling disorder

F81.89 Other developmental disorders of scholastic skills

F81.9 Developmental disorder of scholastic skills, unspecified

Knowledge acquisition disability NOS
Learning disability NOS
Learning disorder NOS

F82 Specific developmental disorder of motor function

Clumsy child syndrome
Developmental coordination disorder
Developmental dyspraxia

[EXCLUDES1] *abnormalities of gait and mobility (R26.-)*
lack of coordination (R27.-)

[EXCLUDES2] *lack of coordination secondary to intellectual disabilities (F70-F79)*

[4] F84 Pervasive developmental disorders

Use additional code to identify any associated medical condition and intellectual disabilities.

F84.0 Autistic disorder

Infantile autism
Infantile psychosis
Kanner's syndrome

[EXCLUDES1] *Asperger's syndrome (F84.5)*

F84.2 Rett's syndrome

[EXCLUDES1] *Asperger's syndrome (F84.5)*
Autistic disorder (F84.0)
Other childhood disintegrative disorder (F84.3)

[4] 4th character required [5] 5th character required [6] 6th character required [7] 7th character required [X] Extension 'X' Alert
[EXCLUDES1] Not coded here [EXCLUDES2] Not included here [PDx] Primary Diagnosis Only Manifestation Code

F84.3 **Other childhood disintegrative disorder**

Dementia infantilis

Disintegrative psychosis

Heller's syndrome

Symbiotic psychosis

Use additional code to identify any associated neurological condition.

> EXCLUDES1 Asperger's syndrome (F84.5)
> Autistic disorder (F84.0)
> Rett's syndrome (F84.2) P

F84.5 Asperger's syndrome

Asperger's disorder

Autistic psychopathy

Schizoid disorder of childhood

F84.8 **Other pervasive developmental disorders**

Overactive disorder associated with intellectual disabilities and stereotyped movements

F84.9 **Pervasive developmental disorder, unspecified**

Atypical autism

F88 **Other disorders of psychological development**

Developmental agnosia

F89 **Unspecified disorder of psychological development**

Developmental disorder NOS

Behavioral and emotional disorders with onset usually occurring in childhood and adolescence (F90-F98)

> NOTES Codes within categories F90-F98 may be used regardless of the age of a patient. These disorders generally have onset within the childhood or adolescent years, but may continue throughout life or not be diagnosed until adulthood

F90 **Attention-deficit hyperactivity disorders**

> INCLUDES attention deficit disorder with hyperactivity
> attention deficit syndrome with hyperactivity

> EXCLUDES2 anxiety disorders (F40.-, F41.-)
> mood [affective] disorders (F30-F39)
> pervasive developmental disorders (F84.-)
> schizophrenia (F20.-)

F90.0 **Attention-deficit hyperactivity disorder, predominantly inattentive type**

F90.1 **Attention-deficit hyperactivity disorder, predominantly hyperactive type**

F90.2 **Attention-deficit hyperactivity disorder, combined type**

F90.8 **Attention-deficit hyperactivity disorder, other type**

F90.9 **Attention-deficit hyperactivity disorder, unspecified type**

Attention-deficit hyperactivity disorder of childhood or adolescence NOS

Attention-deficit hyperactivity disorder NOS

F91 **Conduct disorders**

> EXCLUDES1 antisocial behavior (Z72.81-)
> antisocial personality disorder (F60.2)

> EXCLUDES2 conduct problems associated with attention-deficit hyperactivity disorder (F90.-)
> mood [affective] disorders (F30-F39)
> pervasive developmental disorders (F84.-)
> schizophrenia (F20.-)

F91.0 **Conduct disorder** confined to family context

F91.1 **Conduct disorder,** childhood-onset type

Unsocialized conduct disorder

Conduct disorder, solitary aggressive type

Unsocialized aggressive disorder

F91.2 **Conduct disorder,** adolescent-onset type

Socialized conduct disorder

Conduct disorder, group type

F91.3 Oppositional defiant **disorder**

F91.8 **Other conduct disorders**

F91.9 **Conduct disorder, unspecified**

Behavioral disorder NOS

Conduct disorder NOS

Disruptive behavior disorder NOS

F93 **Emotional disorders with onset specific to childhood**

F93.0 **Separation anxiety disorder of childhood**

> EXCLUDES2 mood [affective] disorders (F30-F39)
> nonpsychotic mental disorders (F40-F48)
> phobic anxiety disorder of childhood (F40.8)
> social phobia (F40.1) P

F93.8 **Other childhood emotional disorders**

Identity disorder

> EXCLUDES2 gender identity disorder of childhood (F64.2) P

F93.9 **Childhood emotional disorder, unspecified** P

F94 **Disorders of social functioning with onset specific to childhood and adolescence**

F94.0 Selective **mutism**

Elective mutism

> EXCLUDES2 pervasive developmental disorders (F84.-)
> schizophrenia (F20.-)
> specific developmental disorders of speech and language (F80.-)
> transient mutism as part of separation anxiety in young children (F93.0)

F94.1 Reactive **attachment disorder of childhood**

Use additional code to identify any associated failure to thrive or growth retardation

> EXCLUDES1 disinhibited attachment disorder of childhood (F94.2)
> normal variation in pattern of selective attachment

> EXCLUDES2 Asperger's syndrome (F84.5)
> maltreatment syndromes (T74.-)
> sexual or physical abuse in childhood, resulting in psychosocial problems (Z62.81-) P

F94.2 Disinhibited **attachment disorder of childhood**

Affectionless psychopathy

Institutional syndrome

> EXCLUDES1 reactive attachment disorder of childhood (F94.1)

> EXCLUDES2 Asperger's syndrome (F84.5)
> attention-deficit hyperactivity disorders (F90.-)
> hospitalism in children (F43.2-) P

F94.8 **Other childhood disorders of social functioning** P

F94.9 **Childhood disorder of social functioning, unspecified** P

F95 **Tic disorder**

F95.0 Transient **tic disorder**

F95.1 Chronic motor or vocal **tic disorder**

F95.2 Tourette's **disorder**

Combined vocal and multiple motor tic disorder [de la Tourette]

Tourette's syndrome

F95.8 **Other tic disorders**

F95.9 **Tic disorder, unspecified**

Tic NOS

F98 **Other behavioral and emotional disorders with onset usually occurring in childhood and adolescence**

> EXCLUDES2 breath-holding spells (R06.89)
> gender identity disorder of childhood (F64.2)
> Kleine-Levin syndrome (G47.13)
> obsessive-compulsive disorder (F42)
> sleep disorders not due to a substance or known physiological condition (F51.-)

Unspecified Code	Other Specified Code	N Newborn Age: 0	P Pediatric Age: 0-17	M Maternity Age: 12-55
A Adult Age: 15-124	♂ Male	♀ Female	● New Code	▲ Revised Code Title	►◄ Revised Text

F98.0 Enuresis not due to a substance or known physiological condition

Enuresis (primary) (secondary) of nonorganic origin
Functional enuresis
Psychogenic enuresis
Urinary incontinence of nonorganic origin

[EXCLUDES1] *enuresis NOS (R32)*

F98.1 Encopresis not due to a substance or known physiological condition

Functional encopresis
Incontinence of feces of nonorganic origin
Psychogenic encopresis

Use additional code to identify the cause of any coexisting constipation.

[EXCLUDES1] *encopresis NOS (R15.-)*

[5] **F98.2 Other feeding disorders of infancy and childhood**

[EXCLUDES1] *feeding difficulties (R63.3)*

[EXCLUDES2] *anorexia nervosa and other eating disorders (F50.-)*
feeding problems of newborn (P92.-)
pica of infancy or childhood (F98.3)

F98.21 Rumination disorder of infancy [P]

F98.29 Other feeding disorders of infancy and early childhood [P]

F98.3 Pica of infancy and childhood [P]

F98.4 Stereotyped movement disorders

Stereotype/habit disorder

[EXCLUDES1] *abnormal involuntary movements (R25.-)*

[EXCLUDES2] *compulsions in obsessive-compulsive disorder (F42)*
hair plucking (F63.3)
movement disorders of organic origin (G20-G25)
nail-biting (F98.8)
nose-picking (F98.8)
stereotypies that are part of a broader psychiatric condition (F01-F95)
thumb-sucking (F98.8)
tic disorders (F95.-)
trichotillomania (F63.3)

F98.5 Adult onset fluency disorder

[EXCLUDES1] *childhood onset fluency disorder (F80.81)*
dysphasia (R47.02)
fluency disorder in conditions classified elsewhere (R47.82)
fluency disorder (stuttering) following cerebrovascular disease (I69. with final characters -23)
tic disorders (F95.-)

F98.8 Other specified behavioral and emotional disorders with onset usually occurring in childhood and adolescence

Excessive masturbation
Nail-biting
Nose-picking
Thumb-sucking [P]

F98.9 Unspecified behavioral and emotional disorders with onset usually occurring in childhood and adolescence [P]

Unspecified mental disorder (F99)

F99 Mental disorder, not otherwise specified

Mental illness NOS

[EXCLUDES1] *unspecified mental disorder due to known physiological condition (F09)*

[4] 4th character required [5] 5th character required [6] 6th character required [7] 7th character required [7th] Extension 'X' Alert
[EXCLUDES1] Not coded here [EXCLUDES2] Not included here [PDx] Primary Diagnosis Only Manifestation Code

Chapter 6: Diseases of the Nervous System (G00-G99)

Chapter Specific Coding Guidelines

a. Dominant/nondominant side

Codes from category G81, Hemiplegia and hemiparesis, and subcategories, G83.1, Monoplegia of lower limb, G83.2, Monoplegia of upper limb, and G83.3, Monoplegia, unspecified, identify whether the dominant or nondominant side is affected. Should the affected side be documented, but not specified as dominant or nondominant, and the classification system does not indicate a default, code selection is as follows:

- For ambidextrous patients, the default should be dominant.
- If the left side is affected, the default is non-dominant.
- If the right side is affected, the default is dominant.

b. Pain - Category G89

1) General coding information

Codes in category G89, Pain, not elsewhere classified, may be used in conjunction with codes from other categories and chapters to provide more detail about acute or chronic pain and neoplasm-related pain, unless otherwise indicated below.

If the pain is not specified as acute or chronic, post-thoracotomy, postprocedural, or neoplasm-related, do not assign codes from category G89.

A code from category G89 should not be assigned if the underlying (definitive) diagnosis is known, unless the reason for the encounter is pain control/ management and not management of the underlying condition.

When an admission or encounter is for a procedure aimed at treating the underlying condition (e.g., spinal fusion, kyphoplasty), a code for the underlying condition (e.g., vertebral fracture, spinal stenosis) should be assigned as the principal diagnosis. No code from category G89 should be assigned.

(a) Category G89 codes as principal or first-listed diagnosis

Category G89 codes are acceptable as principal diagnosis or the first-listed code:

- When pain control or pain management is the reason for the admission/encounter (e.g., a patient with displaced intervertebral disc, nerve impingement and severe back pain presents for injection of steroid into the spinal canal). The underlying cause of the pain should be reported as an additional diagnosis, if known.
- When a patient is admitted for the insertion of a neurostimulator for pain control, assign the appropriate pain code as the principal or first-listed diagnosis. When an admission or encounter is for a procedure aimed at treating the underlying condition and a neurostimulator is inserted for pain control during the same admission/encounter, a code for the underlying condition should be assigned as the principal diagnosis and the appropriate pain code should be assigned as a secondary diagnosis.

(b) Use of category G89 codes in conjunction with site specific pain codes

(i) Assigning category G89 and site-specific pain codes

Codes from category G89 may be used in conjunction with codes that identify the site of pain (including codes from chapter 18) if the category G89 code provides additional information. For example, if the code describes the site of the pain, but does not fully describe whether the pain is acute or chronic, then both codes should be assigned.

(ii) Sequencing of category G89 codes with site-specific pain codes

The sequencing of category G89 codes with site-specific pain codes (including chapter 18 codes), is dependent on the circumstances of the encounter/admission as follows:

- If the encounter is for pain control or pain management, assign the code from category G89 followed by the code identifying the specific site of pain (e.g., encounter for pain management for acute neck pain from trauma is assigned code G89.11, Acute pain due to trauma, followed by code M54.2, Cervicalgia, to identify the site of pain).
- If the encounter is for any other reason except pain control or pain management, and a related definitive diagnosis has not been established (confirmed) by the provider, assign the code for the specific site of pain first, followed by the appropriate code from category G89.

2) Pain due to devices, implants and grafts

See Section I.C.19. Pain due to medical devices

3) Postoperative Pain

The provider's documentation should be used to guide the coding of postoperative pain, as well as *Section III. Reporting Additional Diagnoses* and *Section IV. Diagnostic Coding and Reporting in the Outpatient Setting.*

The default for post-thoracotomy and other postoperative pain not specified as acute or chronic is the code for the acute form.

Routine or expected postoperative pain immediately after surgery should not be coded.

(a) Postoperative pain not associated with specific postoperative complication

Postoperative pain not associated with a specific postoperative complication is assigned to the appropriate postoperative pain code in category G89.

(b) Postoperative pain associated with specific postoperative complication

Postoperative pain associated with a specific postoperative complication (such as painful wire sutures) is assigned to the appropriate code(s) found in Chapter 19, Injury, poisoning, and certain other consequences of external causes. If appropriate, use additional code(s) from category G89 to identify acute or chronic pain (G89.18 or G89.28).

4) Chronic pain

Chronic pain is classified to subcategory G89.2. There is no time frame defining when pain becomes chronic pain. The provider's documentation should be used to guide use of these codes.

5) Neoplasm Related Pain

Code G89.3 is assigned to pain documented as being related, associated or due to cancer, primary or secondary malignancy, or tumor. This code is assigned regardless of whether the pain is acute or chronic.

This code may be assigned as the principal or first-listed code when the stated reason for the admission/encounter is documented as pain control/pain management. The underlying neoplasm should be reported as an additional diagnosis.

When the reason for the admission/encounter is management of the neoplasm and the pain associated with the neoplasm is also documented, code G89.3 may be assigned as an additional diagnosis. It is not necessary to assign an additional code for the site of the pain.

See Section I.C.2 for instructions on the sequencing of neoplasms for all other stated reasons for the admission/ encounter (except for pain control/pain management).

6) **Chronic pain syndrome**
Central pain syndrome (G89.0) and chronic pain syndrome (G89.4) are different than the term "chronic pain," and therefore codes should only be used when the provider has specifically documented this condition.

See Section I.C.5. Pain disorders related to psychological factors

Anatomy of the Nervous System

The nervous system constitutes the body's control center and the communication network and directs the functions of multiple body organs and systems. It helps the individual to interpret the external environmental events and respond to various environmental stimuli. The nervous system includes the following types and components:

1. **The Central Nervous System (CNS)**

   The central nervous system is regarded as the control center of the entire nervous system. It is composed of the brain and the spinal cord. The CNS receives the body's sensations and information about the external environmental changes via receptors and sense organs, and directs the body to act accordingly in response to these external environmental stimuli.

Human Nervous System

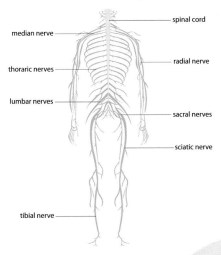

2. **The Peripheral Nervous System (PNS)**

   The peripheral nervous system is composed of the nerves that connect the brain and spinal cord with the glands, muscles and sensory receptors. The PNS can be further divided into the following subcategories:

   a) The Afferent Peripheral System

   The afferent peripheral system is composed of sensory (or afferent) neurons that transfer information to the brain and spinal cord via peripheral receptors.

   b) The Efferent Peripheral System

   The efferent peripheral system consists of the motor (or efferent) neurons that form a communication channel (for information transfer) between the brain, spinal cord, muscles and glands. This system of neurons is further divided into the following subcategories:

   i) Somatic Nervous System

   The somatic nervous system helps the individual to respond to the changes in the external environment by conducting the impulses from the brain and spinal cord to the skeletal muscle.

   ii) Autonomic Nervous System

   The autonomic nervous system is an involuntary system of nerves that conduct impulses from the brain and spinal cord to the smooth muscles of the intestine, the cardiac muscles of the heart, and the endocrine glands. The organs of this particular system receive nerve fibers from the following divisions of the ANS:

   iii) Sympathetic Division

   The sympathetic division acts to mobilize the body's resources and induce the fight-or-flight response. This

system uses norepinephrine as a neurotransmitter to speed up it's activity through energy expenditure.

   iv) Parasympathetic Division

   The parasympathetic division facilitates the vegetative activities of human body (like digestion, urination and defecation).

3. **The Spinal Cord (or Medulla Spinalis)**

   The spinal cord initiates as a continuation of the medulla oblongata of the brainstem. Its length varies between 16 to 18 inches and is made up of a series of 31 segments, each of which gives rise to a pair of spinal nerves. The human spinal cord is further protected by a series of connective tissue membranes that are known as the spinal meninges.

4. **The Brain or Encephalon**

   The brain is regarded as one of the largest organs of the body and weighs about 3 pounds in an average adult. The major parts of the human brain are described as follows:

   a) The Brainstem

   The brainstem is regarded as the posterior portion of the brain, which is structurally continuous with the spinal cord. It is composed of the medulla oblongata, the pons Varolii, and the midbrain.

   b) The Diencephalon

   The diencephalon is located between the two cerebral hemispheres, and superiorly to the midbrain. It surrounds the third ventricle of the brain and consists of the thalamus and hypothalamus regions.

   c) The Cerebrum (or Telencephalon)

   The cerebrum constitutes the bulk of the brain and composed of the gray matter (or cerebral cortex), longitudinal fissure, and the right and left cerebral hemispheres. It is further subdivided into the frontal, parietal, occipital and temporal lobes.

   d) The Cerebellum

   The cerebellum is regarded as the second largest portion of the brain. It is located under the occipital lobes of the cerebrum, and behind the pons and medulla oblongata of brainstem. The two partially separated hemispheres of the cerebellum are connected together by a centrally constricted structure, which is known as the vermis. The cerebellum is constituted primarily by the white matter and a thin layer of gray matter on its surface, which is known as the cerebellar cortex. The cerebrospinal fluid (CSF) is a colorless fluid that fills up the subarachnoid space (or interval between the arachnoid membrane and pia mater) and the ventricular system inside and around the spinal cord and brain.

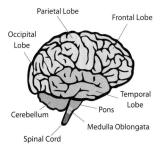

5. **The Cranial Nerves**

   The cranial nerves are based on 12 pairs that remain attached to the brain and leave the skull through various foramina in the cranial base. The names of the various cranial nerves are listed below:

   a) Olfactory (1st cranial nerve)

   b) Optic (2nd cranial nerve)

c) Oculomotor (3rd cranial nerve)

d) Trochlear (4th cranial nerve)

e) Trigeminal (5th cranial nerve)

f) Abducens (6th cranial nerve)

g) The Facial (7th cranial nerve)

h) Acoustic (8th cranial nerve)

i) Glossopharyngeal (9th cranial nerve)

j) Vagus/Pneumogastric (10th cranial nerve)

k) Accessory (11th cranial nerve)

l) Hypoglossal (12th cranial nerve)

The Cranial Nerves

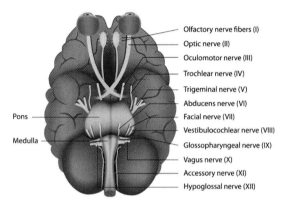

Olfactory nerve fibers (I)
Optic nerve (II)
Oculomotor nerve (III)
Trochlear nerve (IV)
Trigeminal nerve (V)
Abducens nerve (VI)
Facial nerve (VII)
Vestibulocochlear nerve (VIII)
Glossopharyngeal nerve (IX)
Vagus nerve (X)
Accessory nerve (XI)
Hypoglossal nerve (XII)

Pons
Medulla

6. **The Spinal Nerves**

The 31 pairs of spinal nerves originate from the integration of the dorsal and ventral roots of the spinal nerves. These nerves carry the motor, sensory and the autonomic signals between the spinal cord and the body. They are also called mixed nerves as they consist of both motor and sensory fibres. The spinal nerves exit the vertebral column between the adjacent vertebrae. The naming convention of the spinal nerves is based on the region and level of the spinal cord from which these nerves arise. The division of the spinal nerves is documented below:

a) 8 pairs of cervical nerves (C1-C8)

b) 12 pairs of thoracic nerves (T1-T12)

c) 5 pairs of lumbar nerves (L1-L5)

d) 5 pairs of sacral nerves (S1-S5)

e) 1 pair of coccygeal nerves (Cx)

7. **The Sympathetic Nerves**

The sympathetic nerves are a part of the sympathetic nervous system, which innervates the striated muscles of the heart, the smooth muscles, and multiple glands of the body. The sympathetic nervous system is that division of the autonomic nervous system which prepares the body for stressful conditions requiring energy expenditure. The nerve fibers of this system originate from the thoracic and lumbar regions of the spinal cord. The axons of these nerves leave the spinal cord via the anterior root. They further pass near the spinal ganglion and integrate with the anterior rami of the spinal nerves.

Common Pathologies

Muscular dystrophy (MD)

This is characterized by progressive muscle weakness, abnormal muscle protein, and death of muscle tissues and cells.

Spina Bifida

This is a type of birth defect of the brain, spine, or spinal cord, also

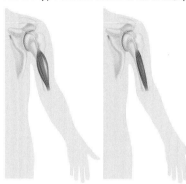

Normal biceps   Muscular dystrophy

known as the neural tube defect. It happens if the spinal column of the fetus doesn't close completely during the first month of pregnancy.

Parkinson's Disease (PD)

This is a progressive disorder of the nervous system which affects the movement and is known as a movement disorder.

Alzheimer's Disease (AD)

This is a brain disorder that seriously affects a person's ability to carry out daily activities. Alzheimer's disease is the most common form of dementia.

Strokes

This is a condition in which, due to lack of oxygen, the sudden death of brain cells occurs and can be caused by an obstruction in the blood flow to the brain. The more common kind, called ischemic stroke, is caused by a blood clot that blocks or plugs a blood vessel in the brain. The other kind, called hemorrhagic stroke, is caused by a blood vessel that breaks and bleeds into the brain. "Mini-strokes" or transient ischemic attacks (TIAs), occur when the blood supply to the brain is briefly interrupted.

Hemorrhagic Stroke

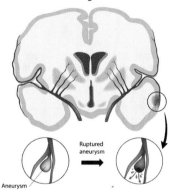

Ruptured
aneurysm

Aneurysm

Malignant Brain Tumor

Cancer of the brain is usually called a malignant brain tumor.

Meningitis

The inflammation of the thin tissue that surrounds the brain and spinal cord, called the meninges, is known as Meningitis.

Epilepsy

This is a neurological condition which affects the nervous system. Epilepsy is also known as a seizure disorder that causes people to have recurring seizures.

Bell's Palsy

This condition occurs due to compression of a facial nerve.

Diseases of the nervous system (G00-G99)

[EXCLUDES2] *certain conditions originating in the perinatal period (P04-P96)*
certain infectious and parasitic diseases (A00-B99)
complications of pregnancy, childbirth and the puerperium (O00-O9A)
congenital malformations, deformations, and chromosomal abnormalities (Q00-Q99)
endocrine, nutritional and metabolic diseases (E00-E88)
injury, poisoning and certain other consequences of external causes (S00-T88)
neoplasms (C00-D49)
symptoms, signs and abnormal clinical and laboratory findings, not elsewhere classified (R00-R94)

Inflammatory diseases of the central nervous system (G00-G09)

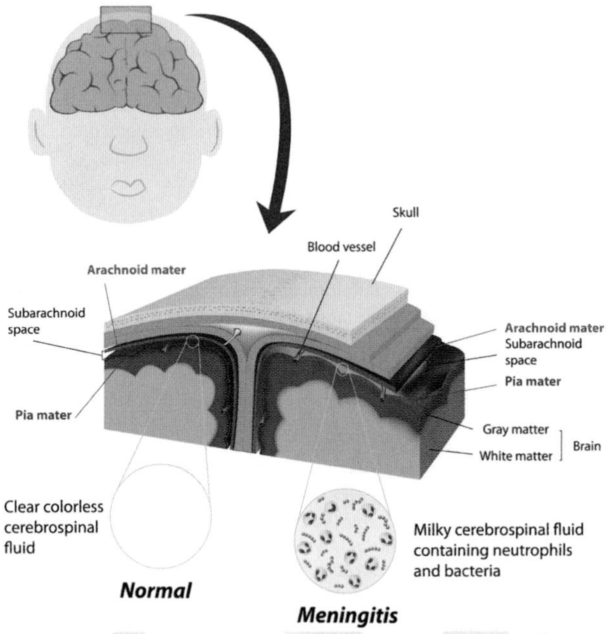
Skull
Blood vessel
Arachnoid mater
Subarachnoid space
Pia mater
Arachnoid mater
Subarachnoid space
Pia mater
Gray matter
White matter
Brain
Clear colorless cerebrospinal fluid
Milky cerebrospinal fluid containing neutrophils and bacteria
Normal
Meningitis

Figure 6.1 Meningitis

[4] **G00 Bacterial meningitis, not elsewhere classified**

[INCLUDES] *bacterial arachnoiditis*
bacterial leptomeningitis
bacterial meningitis
bacterial pachymeningitis

[EXCLUDES1] *bacterial:*
meningoencephalitis (G04.2)
meningomyelitis (G04.2)

G00.0 Hemophilus meningitis

Meningitis due to Hemophilus influenzae

G00.1 Pneumococcal meningitis

G00.2 Streptococcal meningitis

Use additional code to further identify organism (B95.0-B95.5)

G00.3 Staphylococcal meningitis

Use additional code to further identify organism (B95.61-B95.8)

G00.8 Other bacterial meningitis

Meningitis due to Escherichia coli
Meningitis due to Friedländer's bacillus
Meningitis due to Klebsiella
Use additional code to further identify organism (B96.-)

G00.9 Bacterial meningitis, unspecified

Meningitis due to gram-negative bacteria, unspecified
Purulent meningitis NOS
Pyogenic meningitis NOS
Suppurative meningitis NOS

G01 Meningitis in bacterial diseases classified elsewhere

Code first underlying disease

[EXCLUDES1] *meningitis (in):*
gonococcal (A54.81)
leptospirosis (A27.81)
listeriosis (A32.11)
Lyme disease (A69.21)
meningococcal (A39.0)
neurosyphilis (A52.13)
tuberculosis (A17.0)
meningoencephalitis and meningomyelitis in bacterial diseases classified elsewhere (G05)

G02 Meningitis in other infectious and parasitic diseases classified elsewhere

Code first underlying disease, such as:
African trypanosomiasis (B56.-)
poliovirus infection (A80.-)

[EXCLUDES1] *candidal meningitis (B37.5)*
coccidioidomycosis meningitis (B38.4)
cryptococcal meningitis (B45.1)
herpesviral [herpes simplex] meningitis (B00.3)
infectious mononucleosis complicated by meningitis (B27.- with fourth character 2)
measles complicated by meningitis (B05.1)
meningoencephalitis and meningomyelitis in other infectious and parasitic diseases classified elsewhere (G05)
mumps meningitis (B26.1)
rubella meningitis (B06.02)
varicella [chickenpox] meningitis (B01.0)
zoster meningitis (B02.1)

[4] **G03 Meningitis due to other and unspecified causes**

[INCLUDES] *arachnoiditis NOS*
leptomeningitis NOS
meningitis NOS
pachymeningitis NOS

[EXCLUDES1] *meningoencephalitis (G04.-)*
meningomyelitis (G04.-)

G03.0 Nonpyogenic meningitis

Aseptic meningitis
Nonbacterial meningitis

G03.1 Chronic meningitis

G03.2 Benign recurrent meningitis [Mollaret]

G03.8 Meningitis due to other specified causes

G03.9 Meningitis, unspecified

Arachnoiditis (spinal) NOS

[4] **G04 Encephalitis, myelitis and encephalomyelitis**

[INCLUDES] *acute ascending myelitis*
meningoencephalitis
meningomyelitis

[EXCLUDES1] *encephalopathy NOS (G93.40)*

[EXCLUDES2] *acute transverse myelitis (G37.3-)*
alcoholic encephalopathy (G31.2)
benign myalgic encephalomyelitis (G93.3)
multiple sclerosis (G35)
subacute necrotizing myelitis (G37.4)
toxic encephalitis (G92)
toxic encephalopathy (G92)

[5] **G04.0 Acute disseminated encephalitis and encephalomyelitis (ADEM)**

[EXCLUDES1] *acute necrotizing hemorrhagic encephalopathy (G04.3-)*
other noninfectious acute disseminated encephalomyelitis (noninfectious ADEM) (G04.81)

Unspecified Code | Other Specified Code | [N] Newborn Age: 0 | [P] Pediatric Age: 0-17 | [M] Maternity Age: 12-55
[A] Adult Age: 15-124 | ♂ Male | ♀ Female | ● New Code | ▲ Revised Code Title | ►◄ Revised Text

G04.00 **Acute disseminated encephalitis and encephalomyelitis, unspecified**

G04.01 Postinfectious **acute disseminated encephalitis and encephalomyelitis (postinfectious ADEM)**

[EXCLUDES1] *post chickenpox encephalitis (B01.1)*
post measles encephalitis (B05.0)
post measles myelitis (B05.1)

G04.02 Postimmunization **acute disseminated encephalitis, myelitis and encephalomyelitis**

Encephalitis, post immunization
Encephalomyelitis, post immunization
Use additional code to identify the vaccine (T50.A-, T50.B-, T50.Z-)

G04.1 **Tropical spastic paraplegia**

G04.2 **Bacterial meningoencephalitis and meningomyelitis, not elsewhere classified**

[5] G04.3 **Acute necrotizing hemorrhagic encephalopathy**

[EXCLUDES1] *acute disseminated encephalitis and encephalomyelitis (G04.0-)*

G04.30 **Acute necrotizing hemorrhagic encephalopathy, unspecified**

G04.31 Postinfectious **acute necrotizing hemorrhagic encephalopathy**

G04.32 Postimmunization **acute necrotizing hemorrhagic encephalopathy**

Use additional code to identify the vaccine (T50.A-, T50.B-, T50.Z-)

G04.39 **Other acute necrotizing hemorrhagic encephalopathy**

Code also underlying etiology, if applicable

[5] G04.8 Other **encephalitis, myelitis and encephalomyelitis**

Code also any associated seizure (G40.-, R56.9)

G04.81 **Other encephalitis and encephalomyelitis**

Noninfectious acute disseminated encephalomyelitis (noninfectious ADEM)

G04.89 **Other myelitis**

[5] G04.9 **Encephalitis, myelitis and encephalomyelitis, unspecified**

G04.90 **Encephalitis and encephalomyelitis, unspecified**

Ventriculitis (cerebral) NOS

G04.91 **Myelitis, unspecified**

[4] G05 **Encephalitis, myelitis and encephalomyelitis in diseases classified elsewhere**

Code first underlying disease, such as:
human immunodeficiency virus [HIV] disease (B20)
poliovirus (A80.-)
suppurative otitis media (H66.01-H66.4)
trichinellosis (B75)

[EXCLUDES1] *adenoviral encephalitis, myelitis and encephalomyelitis (A85.1)*
congenital toxoplasmosis encephalitis, myelitis and encephalomyelitis (P37.1)
cytomegaloviral encephalitis, myelitis and encephalomyelitis (B25.8)
encephalitis, myelitis and encephalomyelitis (in) measles (B05.0)
encephalitis, myelitis and encephalomyelitis (in) systemic lupus erythematosus (M32.19)
enteroviral encephalitis, myelitis and encephalomyelitis (A85.0)
eosinophilic meningoencephalitis (B83.2)
herpesviral [herpes simplex] encephalitis, myelitis and encephalomyelitis (B00.4)
listerial encephalitis, myelitis and encephalomyelitis (A32.12)
meningococcal encephalitis, myelitis and encephalomyelitis (A39.81)
mumps encephalitis, myelitis and encephalomyelitis (B26.2)
postchickenpox encephalitis, myelitis and encephalomyelitis (B01.1-)
rubella encephalitis, myelitis and encephalomyelitis (B06.01)
toxoplasmosis encephalitis, myelitis and encephalomyelitis (B58.2)
zoster encephalitis, myelitis and encephalomyelitis (B02.0)

G05.3 **Encephalitis and encephalomyelitis in diseases classified elsewhere**

Meningoencephalitis in diseases classified elsewhere

G05.4 **Myelitis in diseases classified elsewhere**

Meningomyelitis in diseases classified elsewhere

[4] G06 **Intracranial and intraspinal** abscess and granuloma

Use additional code (B95-B97) to identify infectious agent.

G06.0 Intracranial **abscess and granuloma**

Brain [any part] abscess (embolic)
Cerebellar abscess (embolic)
Cerebral abscess (embolic)
Intracranial epidural abscess or granuloma
Intracranial extradural abscess or granuloma
Intracranial subdural abscess or granuloma
Otogenic abscess (embolic)

[EXCLUDES1] *tuberculous intracranial abscess and granuloma (A17.81)*

G06.1 Intraspinal **abscess and granuloma**

Abscess (embolic) of spinal cord [any part]
Intraspinal epidural abscess or granuloma
Intraspinal extradural abscess or granuloma
Intraspinal subdural abscess or granuloma

[EXCLUDES1] *tuberculous intraspinal abscess and granuloma (A17.81)*

G06.2 **Extradural and subdural abscess, unspecified**

G07 **Intracranial and intraspinal abscess and granuloma in diseases classified elsewhere**

Code first underlying disease, such as:
schistosomiasis granuloma of brain (B65.-)

[EXCLUDES1] *abscess of brain:*
amebic (A06.6)
chromomycotic (B43.1)
gonococcal (A54.82)
tuberculous (A17.81)
tuberculoma of meninges (A17.1)

G08 **Intracranial and intraspinal** phlebitis and thrombophlebitis

Septic embolism of intracranial or intraspinal venous sinuses and veins
Septic endophlebitis of intracranial or intraspinal venous sinuses and veins
Septic phlebitis of intracranial or intraspinal venous sinuses and veins
Septic thrombophlebitis of intracranial or intraspinal venous sinuses and veins
Septic thrombosis of intracranial or intraspinal venous sinuses and veins

[EXCLUDES1] *intracranial phlebitis and thrombophlebitis complicating:*
abortion, ectopic or molar pregnancy (O00-O07, O08.7)
pregnancy, childbirth and the puerperium (O22.5, O87.3)
nonpyogenic intracranial phlebitis and thrombophlebitis (I67.6)

[EXCLUDES2] *intracranial phlebitis and thrombophlebitis complicating nonpyogenic intraspinal phlebitis andthrombophlebitis (G95.1)*

[4] 4th character required [5] 5th character required [6] 6th character required [7] 7th character required [x7] Extension 'X' Alert
[EXCLUDES1] Not coded here [EXCLUDES2] Not included here [PDx] Primary Diagnosis Only Manifestation Code

G09 Sequelae of inflammatory diseases of central nervous system

> **NOTES** Category G09 is to be used to indicate conditions whose primary classification is to G00-G08 as the cause of sequelae, themselves classifiable elsewhere. The 'sequelae' include conditions specified as residuals. Code first condition resulting from (sequela) of inflammatory diseases of central nervous system

Systemic atrophies primarily affecting the central nervous system (G10-G14)

G10 Huntington's disease

> Huntington's chorea
> Huntington's dementia

④ G11 Hereditary ataxia

> **EXCLUDES2** cerebral palsy (G80.-)
> hereditary and idiopathic neuropathy (G60.-)
> metabolic disorders (E70-E88)

> **G11.0 Congenital nonprogressive ataxia**
> **G11.1 Early-onset cerebellar ataxia**
>> Early-onset cerebellar ataxia with essential tremor
>> Early-onset cerebellar ataxia with myoclonus [Hunt's ataxia]
>> Early-onset cerebellar ataxia with retained tendon reflexes
>> Friedreich's ataxia (autosomal recessive)
>> X-linked recessive spinocerebellar ataxia
> **G11.2 Late-onset cerebellar ataxia** 🅐
> **G11.3 Cerebellar ataxia with defective DNA repair**
>> Ataxia telangiectasia [Louis-Bar]
>> **EXCLUDES2** Cockayne's syndrome (Q87.1)
>> other disorders of purine and pyrimidine metabolism (E79.-)
>> xeroderma pigmentosum (Q82.1)
> **G11.4 Hereditary spastic paraplegia**
> **G11.8 Other hereditary ataxias**
> **G11.9 Hereditary ataxia, unspecified**
>> Hereditary cerebellar ataxia NOS
>> Hereditary cerebellar degeneration
>> Hereditary cerebellar disease
>> Hereditary cerebellar syndrome

④ G12 Spinal muscular atrophy and related syndromes

> **G12.0 Infantile spinal muscular atrophy, type I [Werdnig-Hoffman]**
> **G12.1 Other inherited spinal muscular atrophy**
>> Adult form spinal muscular atrophy
>> Childhood form, type II spinal muscular atrophy
>> Distal spinal muscular atrophy
>> Juvenile form, type III spinal muscular atrophy [Kugelberg-Welander]
>> Progressive bulbar palsy of childhood [Fazio-Londe]
>> Scapuloperoneal form spinal muscular atrophy
> **⑤ G12.2 Motor neuron disease**
>> **G12.20 Motor neuron disease, unspecified**
>> **G12.21 Amyotrophic lateral sclerosis**
>>> Progressive spinal muscle atrophy 🅐
>> **G12.22 Progressive bulbar palsy**
>> **G12.29 Other motor neuron disease**
>>> Familial motor neuron disease
>>> Primary lateral sclerosis
> **G12.8 Other spinal muscular atrophies and related syndromes**
> **G12.9 Spinal muscular atrophy, unspecified**

④ G13 Systemic atrophies primarily affecting central nervous system in diseases classified elsewhere

> **G13.0 Paraneoplastic neuromyopathy and neuropathy**
>> Carcinomatous neuromyopathy
>> Sensorial paraneoplastic neuropathy [Denny Brown]
>> Code first underlying neoplasm (C00-D49)
> **G13.1 Other systemic atrophy primarily affecting central nervous system in neoplastic disease**
>> Paraneoplastic limbic encephalopathy
>> Code first underlying neoplasm (C00-D49)
> **G13.2 Systemic atrophy primarily affecting the central nervous system in myxedema**
>> Code first underlying disease, such as:
>> hypothyroidism (E03.-)
>> myxedematous congenital iodine deficiency (E00.1)
> **G13.8 Systemic atrophy primarily affecting central nervous system in other diseases classified elsewhere**
>> Code first underlying disease

G14 Postpolio syndrome

> **INCLUDES** postpolio myelitic syndrome
> **EXCLUDES1** sequelae of poliomyelitis (B91)

Extrapyramidal and movement disorders (G20-G26)

G20 Parkinson's disease

> Hemiparkinsonism
> Idiopathic Parkinsonism or Parkinson's disease
> Paralysis agitans
> Parkinsonism or Parkinson's disease NOS
> Primary Parkinsonism or Parkinson's disease
> **EXCLUDES1** dementia with Parkinsonism (G31.83)

④ G21 Secondary parkinsonism

> **EXCLUDES1** dementia with Parkinsonism (G31.83)
> Huntington's disease (G10)
> Shy-Drager syndrome (G90.3)
> syphilitic Parkinsonism (A52.19)

> **G21.0 Malignant neuroleptic syndrome**
>> Use additional code for adverse effect, if applicable, to identify drug (T43.3X5, T43.4X5, T43.505, T43.595)
>> **EXCLUDES1** neuroleptic induced parkinsonism (G21.11)
> **⑤ G21.1 Other drug-induced secondary parkinsonism**
>> **G21.11 Neuroleptic induced parkinsonism**
>>> Use additional code for adverse effect, if applicable, to identify drug (T43.3X5, T43.4X5, T43.505, T43.595)
>>> **EXCLUDES1** malignant neuroleptic syndrome (G21.0)
>> **G21.19 Other drug induced secondary parkinsonism**
>>> Use additional code for adverse effect, if applicable, to identify drug (T36-T50 with fifth or sixth character 5)
> **G21.2 Secondary parkinsonism due to other external agents**
>> Code first (T51-T65) to identify external agent
> **G21.3 Postencephalitic parkinsonism**
> **G21.4 Vascular parkinsonism**
> **G21.8 Other secondary parkinsonism**
> **G21.9 Secondary parkinsonism, unspecified**

④ G23 Other degenerative diseases of basal ganglia

> **EXCLUDES2** multi-system degeneration of the autonomic nervous system (G90.3)

> **G23.0 Hallervorden-Spatz disease**
>> Pigmentary pallidal degeneration
> **G23.1 Progressive supranuclear ophthalmoplegia [Steele-Richardson-Olszewski]**
>> Progressive supranuclear palsy
> **G23.2 Striatonigral degeneration**
> **G23.8 Other specified degenerative diseases of basal ganglia**
>> Calcification of basal ganglia
> **G23.9 Degenerative disease of basal ganglia, unspecified**

④ G24 Dystonia

> **INCLUDES** dyskinesia
> **EXCLUDES2** athetoid cerebral palsy (G80.3)

> **⑤ G24.0 Drug induced dystonia**
>> Use additional code code for adverse effect, if applicable, to identify drug (T36-T50 with fifth or sixth character 5)

Unspecified Code	Other Specified Code	**N** Newborn Age: 0 **P** Pediatric Age: 0-17 **M** Maternity Age: 12-55

🅐 Adult Age: 15-124   ♂ Male   ♀ Female   ● New Code   ▲ Revised Code Title   ►◄ Revised Text

G24.01 **Drug induced** subacute dyskinesia

Drug induced blepharospasm

Drug induced orofacial dyskinesia

Neuroleptic induced tardive dyskinesia

Tardive dyskinesia

G24.02 **Drug induced** acute dystonia

Acute dystonic reaction to drugs

Neuroleptic induced acute dystonia

G24.09 Other drug induced dystonia

G24.1 Genetic torsion **dystonia**

Dystonia deformans progressiva

Dystonia musculorum deformans

Familial torsion dystonia

Idiopathic familial dystonia

Idiopathic (torsion) dystonia NOS

(Schwalbe-) Ziehen-Oppenheim disease

G24.2 Idiopathic nonfamilial **dystonia**

G24.3 Spasmodic torticollis

EXCLUDES1 *congenital torticollis (Q68.0)*
hysterical torticollis (F44.4)
ocular torticollis (R29.891)
psychogenic torticollis (F45.8)
torticollis NOS (M43.6)
traumatic recurrent torticollis (S13.4)

G24.4 Idiopathic orofacial **dystonia**

Orofacial dyskinesia

EXCLUDES1 *drug induced orofacial dyskinesia (G24.01)*

G24.5 Blepharospasm

EXCLUDES1 *drug induced blepharospasm (G24.01)*

G24.8 **Other dystonia**

Acquired torsion dystonia NOS

G24.9 **Dystonia, unspecified**

Dyskinesia NOS

🄬 G25 Other extrapyramidal and movement disorders

EXCLUDES2 *sleep related movement disorders (G47.6-)*

G25.0 Essential **tremor**

Familial tremor

EXCLUDES1 *tremor NOS (R25.1)*

G25.1 Drug-induced **tremor**

Use additional code for adverse effect, if applicable, to identify drug (T36-T50 with fifth or sixth character 5)

G25.2 Other specified forms of tremor

Intention tremor

G25.3 Myoclonus

Drug-induced myoclonus

Palatal myoclonus

Use additional code for adverse effect, if applicable, to identify drug (T36-T50 with fifth or sixth character 5)

EXCLUDES1 *facial myokymia (G51.4)*
myoclonic epilepsy (G40.-)

G25.4 Drug-induced chorea

Use additional code for adverse effect, if applicable, to identify drug (T36-T50 with fifth or sixth character 5)

G25.5 **Other chorea**

Chorea NOS

EXCLUDES1 *chorea NOS with heart involvement (I02.0)*
Huntington's chorea (G10)
rheumatic chorea (I02.-)
Sydenham's chorea (I02.-)

🄬 G25.6 Drug induced tics and other tics of organic origin

G25.61 Drug induced tics

Use additional code for adverse effect, if applicable, to identify drug (T36-T50 with fifth or sixth character 5)

G25.69 Other tics of organic origin

EXCLUDES1 *habit spasm (F95.9)*
tic NOS (F95.9)
Tourette's syndrome (F95.2)

🄬 G25.7 Other and unspecified drug induced movement disorders

Use additional code for adverse effect, if applicable, to identify drug (T36-T50 with fifth or sixth character 5)

G25.70 **Drug induced movement disorder, unspecified**

G25.71 Drug induced **akathisia**

Drug induced acathisia

Neuroleptic induced acute akathisia

G25.79 Other drug induced movement disorders

🄬 G25.8 Other specified extrapyramidal and movement disorders

G25.81 Restless legs **syndrome**

G25.82 Stiff-man **syndrome**

G25.83 Benign shuddering attacks

G25.89 Other specified extrapyramidal and movement disorders

G25.9 Extrapyramidal and movement disorder, unspecified

G26 Extrapyramidal and movement disorders in diseases classified elsewhere

Code first underlying disease

Other degenerative diseases of the nervous system (G30-G32)

🄬 G30 Alzheimer's disease

INCLUDES *Alzheimer's dementia senile and presenile forms*

Use additional code to identify:

delirium, if applicable (F05)

dementia with behavioral disturbance (F02.81)

dementia without behavioral disturbance (F02.80)

EXCLUDES1 *senile degeneration of brain NEC (G31.1)*
senile dementia NOS (F03)
senility NOS (R41.81)

G30.0 Alzheimer's disease with early onset

G30.1 Alzheimer's disease with late onset 🄰

G30.8 **Other Alzheimer's disease**

G30.9 **Alzheimer's disease, unspecified**

🄬 G31 Other degenerative diseases of nervous system, not elsewhere classified

Use additional code to identify:

dementia with behavioral disturbance (F02.81)

dementia without behavioral disturbance (F02.80)

EXCLUDES2 *Reye's syndrome (G93.7)*

🄬 G31.0 Frontotemporal dementia

G31.01 **Pick's disease**

Primary progressive aphasia

Progressive isolated aphasia

G31.09 Other frontotemporal dementia

Frontal dementia

G31.1 **Senile degeneration of brain, not elsewhere classified**

EXCLUDES1 *Alzheimer's disease (G30.-)*
senility NOS (R41.81)

G31.2 **Degeneration of nervous system due to alcohol**

Alcoholic cerebellar ataxia

Alcoholic cerebellar degeneration

Alcoholic cerebral degeneration

Alcoholic encephalopathy

Dysfunction of the autonomic nervous system due to alcohol

Code also associated alcoholism (F10.-)

🄬 G31.8 Other specified degenerative diseases of nervous system

G31.81 **Alpers disease**

Grey-matter degeneration

G31.82 **Leigh's disease**

Subacute necrotizing encephalopathy

🄬 4th character required   🄬 5th character required   🄬 6th character required   🄬 7th character required   🄬 Extension 'X' Alert

EXCLUDES 1 Not coded here   EXCLUDES 2 Not included here   PDx Primary Diagnosis Only   Manifestation Code

G31.83 Dementia with Lewy bodies

Dementia with Parkinsonism

Lewy body dementia

Lewy body disease

G31.84 Mild cognitive impairment, so stated

EXCLUDES1 *age related cognitive decline (R41.81)*
altered mental status (R41.82)
cerebral degeneration (G31.9)
change in mental status (R41.82)
cognitive deficits following (sequelae of) cerebral hemorrhage or infarction (I69.01, I69.11, I69.21, I69.31, I69.81, I69.91)
cognitive impairment due to intracranial or head injury (S06.-)
dementia (F01.-, F02.-, F03)
mild memory disturbance (F06.8)
neurologic neglect syndrome (R41.4)
personality change, nonpsychotic (F68.8)

G31.85 Corticobasal degeneration

G31.89 Other specified degenerative diseases of nervous system

G31.9 Degenerative disease of nervous system, unspecified

🔄 **G32 Other degenerative disorders of nervous system in diseases classified elsewhere**

G32.0 Subacute combined degeneration of spinal cord in diseases classified elsewhere

Dana-Putnam syndrome

Sclerosis of spinal cord (combined) (dorsolateral) (posterolateral)

Code first underlying disease, such as:

vitamin B12 deficiency (E53.8)

anemia (D51.9)

dietary (D51.3)

pernicious (D51.0)

EXCLUDES1 *syphilitic combined degeneration of spinal cord (A52.11)*

🔄 **G32.8 Other specified degenerative disorders of nervous system in diseases classified elsewhere**

Code first underlying disease, such as:

amyloidosis cerebral degeneration (E85.-)

cerebral degeneration (due to) hypothyroidism (E00.0-E03.9)

cerebral degeneration (due to) neoplasm (C00-D49)

cerebral degeneration (due to) vitamin B deficiency, except thiamine (E52-E53.-)

EXCLUDES1 *superior hemorrhagic polioencephalitis [Wernicke's encephalopathy] (E51.2)*

G32.81 Cerebellar ataxia in diseases classified elsewhere

Code first underlying disease, such as:

celiac disease (with gluten ataxia) (K90.0)

cerebellar ataxia (in) neoplastic disease (paraneoplastic cerebellar degeneration) (C00-D49)

non-celiac gluten ataxia (M35.9)

EXCLUDES1 *systemic atrophy primarily affecting the central nervous system in alcoholic cerebellar ataxia (G31.2)*
systemic atrophy primarily affecting the central nervous system in myxedema (G13.2)

G32.89 Other specified degenerative disorders of nervous system in diseases classified elsewhere

Degenerative encephalopathy in diseases classified elsewhere

Demyelinating diseases of the central nervous system (G35-G37)

G35 Multiple sclerosis

Disseminated multiple sclerosis

Generalized multiple sclerosis

Multiple sclerosis NOS

Multiple sclerosis of brain stem

Multiple sclerosis of cord

🔄 **G36 Other acute disseminated demyelination**

EXCLUDES1 *postinfectious encephalitis and encephalomyelitis NOS (G04.01)*

G36.0 Neuromyelitis optica [Devic]

Demyelination in optic neuritis

EXCLUDES1 *optic neuritis NOS (H46)*

G36.1 Acute and subacute hemorrhagic leukoencephalitis [Hurst]

G36.8 Other specified acute disseminated demyelination

G36.9 Acute disseminated demyelination, unspecified

🔄 **G37 Other demyelinating diseases of central nervous system**

G37.0 Diffuse sclerosis of central nervous system

Periaxial encephalitis

Schilder's disease

EXCLUDES1 *X linked adrenoleukodystrophy (E71.52-)*

G37.1 Central demyelination of corpus callosum

G37.2 Central pontine myelinolysis

G37.3 Acute transverse myelitis in demyelinating disease of central nervous system

Acute transverse myelitis NOS

Acute transverse myelopathy

EXCLUDES1 *multiple sclerosis (G35)*
neuromyelitis optica [Devic] (G36.0)

G37.4 Subacute necrotizing myelitis of central nervous system

G37.5 Concentric sclerosis [Balo] of central nervous system

G37.8 Other specified demyelinating diseases of central nervous system

G37.9 Demyelinating disease of central nervous system, unspecified

Episodic and paroxysmal disorders (G40-G47)

🔄 **G40 Epilepsy and recurrent seizures**

NOTES the following terms are to be considered equivalent to intractable: pharmacoresistant (pharmacologically resistant), treatment resistant, refractory (medically) and poorly controlled

EXCLUDES1 *conversion disorder with seizures (F44.5)*
convulsions NOS (R56.9)
hippocampal sclerosis (G93.81)
mesial temporal sclerosis (G93.81)
post traumatic seizures (R56.1)
seizure (convulsive) NOS (R56.9)
seizure of newborn (P90)
temporal sclerosis (G93.81)
Todd's paralysis (G83.8)

🔄 **G40.0 Localization-related (focal) (partial) idiopathic epilepsy and epileptic syndromes** with seizures of localized onset

Benign childhood epilepsy with centrotemporal EEG spikes

Childhood epilepsy with occipital EEG paroxysms

EXCLUDES1 *adult onset localization-related epilepsy (G40.1-, G40.2-)*

🔄 **G40.00 Localization-related (focal) (partial) idiopathic epilepsy and epileptic syndromes with seizures of localized onset,** not intractable

Localization-related (focal) (partial) idiopathic epilepsy and epileptic syndromes with seizures of localized onset without intractability

Unspecified Code	Other Specified Code	N Newborn Age: 0 P Pediatric Age: 0-17 M Maternity Age: 12-55
A Adult Age: 15-124	♂ Male ♀ Female	● New Code ▲ Revised Code Title ▶◀ Revised Text

G40.001 Localization-related (focal) (partial) idiopathic epilepsy and epileptic syndromes with seizures of localized onset, not intractable, with status epilepticus

G40.009 Localization-related (focal) (partial) idiopathic epilepsy and epileptic syndromes with seizures of localized onset, not intractable, without status epilepticus

Localization-related (focal) (partial) idiopathic epilepsy and epileptic syndromes with seizures of localized onset NOS

[6] **G40.01 Localization-related (focal) (partial) idiopathic epilepsy and epileptic syndromes with seizures of localized onset,** intractable

G40.011 Localization-related (focal) (partial) idiopathic epilepsy and epileptic syndromes with seizures of localized onset, intractable, with status epilepticus

G40.019 Localization-related (focal) (partial) idiopathic epilepsy and epileptic syndromes with seizures of localized onset, intractable, without status epilepticus

[5] **G40.1 Localization-related (focal) (partial) symptomatic epilepsy and epileptic syndromes** with simple partial seizures

Attacks without alteration of consciousness
Epilepsia partialis continua [Kozhevnikof]
Simple partial seizures developing into secondarily generalized seizures

[6] **G40.10 Localization-related (focal) (partial) symptomatic epilepsy and epileptic syndromes with simple partial seizures,** not intractable

Localization-related (focal) (partial) symptomatic epilepsy and epileptic syndromes with simple partial seizures without intractability

G40.101 Localization-related (focal) (partial) symptomatic epilepsy and epileptic syndromes with simple partial seizures, not intractable, with status epilepticus

G40.109 Localization-related (focal) (partial) symptomatic epilepsy and epileptic syndromes with simple partial seizures, not intractable, without status epilepticus

Localization-related (focal) (partial) symptomatic epilepsy and epileptic syndromes with simple partial seizures NOS

[6] **G40.11 Localization-related (focal) (partial) symptomatic epilepsy and epileptic syndromes with simple partial seizures,** intractable

G40.111 Localization-related (focal) (partial) symptomatic epilepsy and epileptic syndromes with simple partial seizures, intractable, with status epilepticus

G40.119 Localization-related (focal) (partial) symptomatic epilepsy and epileptic syndromes with simple partial seizures, intractable, without status epilepticus

[5] **G40.2 Localization-related (focal) (partial) symptomatic epilepsy and epileptic syndromes** with complex partial seizures

Attacks with alteration of consciousness, often with automatisms
Complex partial seizures developing into secondarily generalized seizures

[6] **G40.20 Localization-related (focal) (partial) symptomatic epilepsy and epileptic syndromes with complex partial seizures,** not intractable

Localization-related (focal) (partial) symptomatic epilepsy and epileptic syndromes with complex partial seizures without intractability

G40.201 Localization-related (focal) (partial) symptomatic epilepsy and epileptic syndromes with complex partial seizures, not intractable, with status epilepticus

G40.209 Localization-related (focal) (partial) symptomatic epilepsy and epileptic syndromes with complex partial seizures, not intractable, without status epilepticus

Localization-related (focal) (partial) symptomatic epilepsy and epileptic syndromes with complex partial seizures NOS

[6] **G40.21 Localization-related (focal) (partial) symptomatic epilepsy and epileptic syndromes with complex partial seizures,** intractable

G40.211 Localization-related (focal) (partial) symptomatic epilepsy and epileptic syndromes with complex partial seizures, intractable, with status epilepticus

G40.219 Localization-related (focal) (partial) symptomatic epilepsy and epileptic syndromes with complex partial seizures, intractable, without status epilepticus

[5] **G40.3** Generalized **idiopathic epilepsy and epileptic syndromes**

Code also MERRF syndrome, if applicable (E88.42)

[6] **G40.30 Generalized idiopathic epilepsy and epileptic syndromes,** not intractable

Generalized idiopathic epilepsy and epileptic syndromes without intractability

G40.301 Generalized idiopathic epilepsy and epileptic syndromes, not intractable, with status epilepticus

G40.309 Generalized idiopathic epilepsy and epileptic syndromes, not intractable, without status epilepticus

Generalized idiopathic epilepsy and epileptic syndromes NOS

[6] **G40.31 Generalized idiopathic epilepsy and epileptic syndromes,** intractable

G40.311 Generalized idiopathic epilepsy and epileptic syndromes, intractable, with status epilepticus

G40.319 Generalized idiopathic epilepsy and epileptic syndromes, intractable, without status epilepticus

[5] **G40.A** Absence **epileptic syndrome**

Childhood absence epilepsy [pyknolepsy]
Juvenile absence epilepsy
Absence epileptic syndrome, NOS

[6] **G40.A0 Absence epileptic syndrome,** not intractable

G40.A01 Absence epileptic syndrome, not intractable, with status epilepticus

G40.A09 Absence epileptic syndrome, not intractable, without status epilepticus

[6] **G40.A1 Absence epileptic syndrome,** intractable

G40.A11 Absence epileptic syndrome, intractable, with status epilepticus

G40.A19 Absence epileptic syndrome, intractable, without status epilepticus

[5] **G40.B** Juvenile myoclonic **epilepsy [impulsive petit mal]**

[6] **G40.B0 Juvenile myoclonic epilepsy,** not intractable

G40.B01 Juvenile myoclonic epilepsy, not intractable, with status epilepticus

G40.B09 Juvenile myoclonic epilepsy, not intractable, without status epilepticus

[6] **G40.B1 Juvenile myoclonic epilepsy,** intractable

G40.B11 Juvenile myoclonic epilepsy, intractable, with status epilepticus

G40.B19 Juvenile myoclonic epilepsy, intractable, without status epilepticus

[5] **G40.4 Other generalized epilepsy and epileptic syndromes**

Epilepsy with grand mal seizures on awakening
Epilepsy with myoclonic absences
Epilepsy with myoclonic-astatic seizures
Grand mal seizure NOS
Nonspecific atonic epileptic seizures
Nonspecific clonic epileptic seizures
Nonspecific myoclonic epileptic seizures
Nonspecific tonic epileptic seizures
Nonspecific tonic-clonic epileptic seizures
Symptomatic early myoclonic encephalopathy

[6] **G40.40 Other generalized epilepsy and epileptic syndromes, not intractable**

Other generalized epilepsy and epileptic syndromes without intractability
Other generalized epilepsy and epileptic syndromes NOS

G40.401 Other generalized epilepsy and epileptic syndromes, not intractable, with status epilepticus

G40.409 Other generalized epilepsy and epileptic syndromes, not intractable, without status epilepticus

[6] **G40.41 Other generalized epilepsy and epileptic syndromes, intractable**

G40.411 Other generalized epilepsy and epileptic syndromes, intractable, with status epilepticus

G40.419 Other generalized epilepsy and epileptic syndromes, intractable, without status epilepticus

[5] **G40.5 Epileptic seizures related to external causes**

Epileptic seizures related to alcohol
Epileptic seizures related to drugs
Epileptic seizures related to hormonal changes
Epileptic seizures related to sleep deprivation
Epileptic seizures related to stress

Use additional code for adverse effect, if applicable, to identify drug (T36-T50 with fifth or sixth character 5)

Code also , if applicable, associated epilepsy and recurrent seizures (G40.-)

[6] **G40.50 Epileptic seizures related to external causes, not intractable**

G40.501 Epileptic seizures related to external causes, not intractable, with status epilepticus

G40.509 Epileptic seizures related to external causes, not intractable, without status epilepticus

Epileptic seizures related to external causes, NOS

[5] **G40.8 Other epilepsy and recurrent seizures**

Epilepsies and epileptic syndromes undetermined as to whether they are focal or generalized
Landau-Kleffner syndrome

[6] **G40.80 Other epilepsy**

G40.801 Other epilepsy, not intractable, with status epilepticus

Other epilepsy without intractability with status epilepticus

G40.802 Other epilepsy, not intractable, without status epilepticus

Other epilepsy NOS
Other epilepsy without intractability without status epilepticus

G40.803 Other epilepsy, intractable, with status epilepticus

G40.804 Other epilepsy, intractable, without status epilepticus

[6] **G40.81 Lennox-Gastaut syndrome**

G40.811 Lennox-Gastaut syndrome, not intractable, with status epilepticus

G40.812 Lennox-Gastaut syndrome, not intractable, without status epilepticus

G40.813 Lennox-Gastaut syndrome, intractable, with status epilepticus

G40.814 Lennox-Gastaut syndrome, intractable, without status epilepticus

[6] **G40.82 Epileptic spasms**

Infantile spasms
Salaam attacks
West's syndrome

G40.821 Epileptic spasms, not intractable, with status epilepticus

G40.822 Epileptic spasms, not intractable, without status epilepticus

G40.823 Epileptic spasms, intractable, with status epilepticus

G40.824 Epileptic spasms, intractable, without status epilepticus

G40.89 Other seizures

[EXCLUDES1] *post traumatic seizures (R56.1)*
recurrent seizures NOS (G40.909)
seizure NOS (R56.9)

[5] **G40.9 Epilepsy, unspecified**

[6] **G40.90 Epilepsy, unspecified, not intractable**

Epilepsy, unspecified, without intractability

G40.901 Epilepsy, unspecified, not intractable, with status epilepticus

G40.909 Epilepsy, unspecified, not intractable, without status epilepticus

Epilepsy NOS
Epileptic convulsions NOS
Epileptic fits NOS
Epileptic seizures NOS
Recurrent seizures NOS
Seizure disorder NOS

[6] **G40.91 Epilepsy, unspecified, intractable**

Intractable seizure disorder NOS

G40.911 Epilepsy, unspecified, intractable, with status epilepticus

G40.919 Epilepsy, unspecified, intractable, without status epilepticus

[4] **G43 Migraine**

[NOTES] the following terms are to be considered equivalent to intractable: pharmacoresistant (pharmacologically resistant), treatment resistant, refractory (medically) and poorly controlled

Use additional code for adverse effect, if applicable, to identify drug (T36-T50 with fifth or sixth character 5)

[EXCLUDES1] *headache NOS (R51)*
lower half migraine (G44.00)

[EXCLUDES2] *headache syndromes (G44.-)*

[5] **G43.0 Migraine without aura**

Common migraine

[EXCLUDES1] *chronic migraine without aura (G43.7-)*

[6] **G43.00 Migraine without aura, not intractable**

Migraine without aura without mention of refractory migraine

G43.001 Migraine without aura, not intractable, with status migrainosus

G43.009 Migraine without aura, not intractable, without status migrainosus

Migraine without aura NOS

Unspecified Code | Other Specified Code | [N] Newborn Age: 0 | [P] Pediatric Age: 0-17 | [M] Maternity Age: 12-55
[A] Adult Age: 15-124 | ♂ Male | ♀ Female | ● New Code | ▲ Revised Code Title | ►◄ Revised Text

⑥ **G43.01 Migraine without aura,** intractable

Migraine without aura with refractory migraine

G43.011 Migraine without aura, intractable, with status migrainosus

G43.019 Migraine without aura, intractable, without status migrainosus

⑤ **G43.1 Migraine** with aura

Basilar migraine

Classical migraine

Migraine equivalents

Migraine preceded or accompanied by transient focal neurological phenomena

Migraine triggered seizures

Migraine with acute-onset aura

Migraine with aura without headache (migraine equivalents)

Migraine with prolonged aura

Migraine with typical aura

Retinal migraine

Code also any associated seizure (G40.-, R56.9)

EXCLUDES1 persistent migraine aura (G43.5-, G43.6-)

⑥ **G43.10 Migraine with aura,** not intractable

Migraine with aura without mention of refractory migraine

G43.101 Migraine with aura, not intractable, with status migrainosus

G43.109 Migraine with aura, not intractable, without status migrainosus

Migraine with aura NOS

⑥ **G43.11 Migraine with aura,** intractable

Migraine with aura with refractory migraine

G43.111 Migraine with aura, intractable, with status migrainosus

G43.119 Migraine with aura, intractable, without status migrainosus

⑤ **G43.4 Hemiplegic migraine**

Familial migraine

Sporadic migraine

⑥ **G43.40 Hemiplegic migraine,** not intractable

Hemiplegic migraine without refractory migraine

G43.401 Hemiplegic migraine, not intractable, with status migrainosus

G43.409 Hemiplegic migraine, not intractable, without status migrainosus

Hemiplegic migraine NOS

⑥ **G43.41 Hemiplegic migraine,** intractable

Hemiplegic migraine with refractory migraine

G43.411 Hemiplegic migraine, intractable, with status migrainosus

G43.419 Hemiplegic migraine, intractable, without status migrainosus

⑤ **G43.5 Persistent migraine aura** without cerebral infarction

⑥ **G43.50 Persistent migraine aura without cerebral infarction,** not intractable

Persistent migraine aura without cerebral infarction, without refractory migraine

G43.501 Persistent migraine aura without cerebral infarction, not intractable, with status migrainosus

G43.509 Persistent migraine aura without cerebral infarction, not intractable, without status migrainosus

Persistent migraine aura NOS

⑥ **G43.51 Persistent migraine aura without cerebral infarction,** intractable

Persistent migraine aura without cerebral infarction, with refractory migraine

G43.511 Persistent migraine aura without cerebral infarction, intractable, with status migrainosus

G43.519 Persistent migraine aura without cerebral infarction, intractable, without status migrainosus

⑤ **G43.6 Persistent migraine aura** with cerebral infarction

Code also the type of cerebral infarction (I63.-)

⑥ **G43.60 Persistent migraine aura with cerebral infarction,** not intractable

Persistent migraine aura with cerebral infarction, without refractory migraine

G43.601 Persistent migraine aura with cerebral infarction, not intractable, with status migrainosus

G43.609 Persistent migraine aura with cerebral infarction, not intractable, without status migrainosus

⑥ **G43.61 Persistent migraine aura with cerebral infarction,** intractable

Persistent migraine aura with cerebral infarction, with refractory migraine

G43.611 Persistent migraine aura with cerebral infarction, intractable, with status migrainosus

G43.619 Persistent migraine aura with cerebral infarction, intractable, without status migrainosus

⑤ **G43.7 Chronic migraine** without aura

Transformed migraine

EXCLUDES1 migraine without aura (G43.0-)

⑥ **G43.70 Chronic migraine without aura,** not intractable

Chronic migraine without aura, without refractory migraine

G43.701 Chronic migraine without aura, not intractable, with status migrainosus

G43.709 Chronic migraine without aura, not intractable, without status migrainosus

Chronic migraine without aura NOS

⑥ **G43.71 Chronic migraine without aura,** intractable

Chronic migraine without aura, with refractory migraine

G43.711 Chronic migraine without aura, intractable, with status migrainosus

G43.719 Chronic migraine without aura, intractable, without status migrainosus

⑤ **G43.A Cyclical vomiting**

G43.A0 Cyclical vomiting, not intractable

Cyclical vomiting, without refractory migraine

G43.A1 Cyclical vomiting, intractable

Cyclical vomiting, with refractory migraine

⑤ **G43.B Ophthalmoplegic migraine**

G43.B0 Ophthalmoplegic migraine, not intractable

Ophthalmoplegic migraine, without refractory migraine

G43.B1 Ophthalmoplegic migraine, intractable

Ophthalmoplegic migraine, with refractory migraine

⑤ **G43.C Periodic headache syndromes in** child or adult

G43.C0 Periodic headache syndromes in child or adult, not intractable

Periodic headache syndromes in child or adult, without refractory migraine

G43.C1 Periodic headache syndromes in child or adult, intractable

Periodic headache syndromes in child or adult, with refractory migraine

⑤ **G43.D Abdominal migraine**

---

④ 4th character required　　⑤ 5th character required　　⑥ 6th character required　　⑦ 7th character required　　⑦ Extension 'X' Alert

EXCLUDES1 Not coded here　　EXCLUDES2 Not included here　　℞ Primary Diagnosis Only　　Manifestation Code

G43.D0 Abdominal migraine, not intractable
Abdominal migraine, without refractory migraine

G43.D1 Abdominal migraine, intractable
Abdominal migraine, with refractory migraine

[5] **G43.8 Other migraine**

[6] **G43.80 Other migraine, not intractable**
Other migraine, without refractory migraine

G43.801 Other migraine, not intractable, with status migrainosus

G43.809 Other migraine, not intractable, without status migrainosus

[6] **G43.81 Other migraine, intractable**
Other migraine, with refractory migraine

G43.811 Other migraine, intractable, with status migrainosus

G43.819 Other migraine, intractable, without status migrainosus

[6] **G43.82 Menstrual migraine, not intractable**
Menstrual headache, not intractable
Menstrual migraine, without refractory migraine
Menstrually related migraine, not intractable
Pre-menstrual headache, not intractable
Pre-menstrual migraine, not intractable
Pure menstrual migraine, not intractable
Code also associated premenstrual tension syndrome (N94.3)

G43.821 Menstrual migraine, not intractable, with status migrainosus ♀

G43.829 Menstrual migraine, not intractable, without status migrainosus ♀
Menstrual migraine NOS

[6] **G43.83 Menstrual migraine, intractable**
Menstrual headache, intractable
Menstrual migraine, with refractory migraine
Menstrually related migraine, intractable
Pre-menstrual headache, intractable
Pre-menstrual migraine, intractable
Pure menstrual migraine, intractable
Code also associated premenstrual tension syndrome (N94.3)

G43.831 Menstrual migraine, intractable, with status migrainosus ♀

G43.839 Menstrual migraine, intractable, without status migrainosus ♀

[5] **G43.9 Migraine, unspecified**

[6] **G43.90 Migraine, unspecified, not intractable**
Migraine, unspecified, without refractory migraine

G43.901 Migraine, unspecified, not intractable, with status migrainosus
Status migrainosus NOS

G43.909 Migraine, unspecified, not intractable, without status migrainosus
Migraine NOS

[6] **G43.91 Migraine, unspecified, intractable**
Migraine, unspecified, with refractory migraine

G43.911 Migraine, unspecified, intractable, with status migrainosus

G43.919 Migraine, unspecified, intractable, without status migrainosus

[4] **G44 Other headache syndromes**

[EXCLUDES1] *headache NOS (R51)*

[EXCLUDES2] *atypical facial pain (G50.1)*
headache due to lumbar puncture (G97.1)
migraines (G43.-)
trigeminal neuralgia (G50.0)

[5] **G44.0 Cluster headaches and other trigeminal autonomic cephalgias (TAC)**

[6] **G44.00 Cluster headache syndrome, unspecified**
Ciliary neuralgia
Cluster headache NOS
Histamine cephalgia
Lower half migraine
Migrainous neuralgia

G44.001 Cluster headache syndrome, unspecified, intractable

G44.009 Cluster headache syndrome, unspecified, not intractable
Cluster headache syndrome NOS

[6] **G44.01 Episodic cluster headache**

G44.011 Episodic cluster headache, intractable

G44.019 Episodic cluster headache, not intractable
Episodic cluster headache NOS

[6] **G44.02 Chronic cluster headache**

G44.021 Chronic cluster headache, intractable

G44.029 Chronic cluster headache, not intractable
Chronic cluster headache NOS

[6] **G44.03 Episodic paroxysmal hemicrania**
Paroxysmal hemicrania NOS

G44.031 Episodic paroxysmal hemicrania, intractable

G44.039 Episodic paroxysmal hemicrania, not intractable
Episodic paroxysmal hemicrania NOS

[6] **G44.04 Chronic paroxysmal hemicrania**

G44.041 Chronic paroxysmal hemicrania, intractable

G44.049 Chronic paroxysmal hemicrania, not intractable
Chronic paroxysmal hemicrania NOS

[6] **G44.05 Short lasting unilateral neuralgiform headache with conjunctival injection and tearing (SUNCT)**

G44.051 Short lasting unilateral neuralgiform headache with conjunctival injection and tearing (SUNCT), intractable

G44.059 Short lasting unilateral neuralgiform headache with conjunctival injection and tearing (SUNCT), not intractable
Short lasting unilateral neuralgiform headache with conjunctival injection and tearing (SUNCT) NOS

[6] **G44.09 Other trigeminal autonomic cephalgias (TAC)**

G44.091 Other trigeminal autonomic cephalgias (TAC), intractable

G44.099 Other trigeminal autonomic cephalgias (TAC), not intractable

G44.1 Vascular headache, not elsewhere classified

[EXCLUDES2] *cluster headache (G44.0)*
complicated headache syndromes (G44.5-)
drug-induced headache (G44.4-)
migraine (G43.-)
other specified headache syndromes (G44.8-)
post-traumatic headache (G44.3-)
tension-type headache (G44.2-)

[5] **G44.2 Tension-type headache**

[6] **G44.20 Tension-type headache, unspecified**

G44.201 Tension-type headache, unspecified, intractable

G44.209 Tension-type headache, unspecified, not intractable
Tension headache NOS

[6] **G44.21 Episodic tension-type headache**

G44.211 Episodic tension-type headache, intractable

G44.219 Episodic tension-type headache, not intractable
Episodic tension-type headache NOS

Unspecified Code | Other Specified Code | [N] Newborn Age: 0 | [P] Pediatric Age: 0-17 | [M] Maternity Age: 12-55
[A] Adult Age: 15-124 | ♂ Male | ♀ Female | ● New Code | ▲ Revised Code Title | ►◄ Revised Text

⑥ **G44.22** Chronic tension-type **headache**
    G44.221 Chronic tension-type headache, intractable
    G44.229 Chronic tension-type headache, not intractable
        Chronic tension-type headache NOS

⑤ **G44.3** Post-traumatic **headache**
  ⑥ **G44.30** Post-traumatic headache, unspecified
    G44.301 Post-traumatic headache, unspecified, intractable
    G44.309 Post-traumatic headache, unspecified, not intractable
        Post-traumatic headache NOS
  ⑥ **G44.31** Acute post-traumatic **headache**
    G44.311 Acute post-traumatic headache, intractable
    G44.319 Acute post-traumatic headache, not intractable
        Acute post-traumatic headache NOS
  ⑥ **G44.32** Chronic post-traumatic **headache**
    G44.321 Chronic post-traumatic headache, intractable
    G44.329 Chronic post-traumatic headache, not intractable
        Chronic post-traumatic headache NOS

⑤ **G44.4** Drug-induced **headache,** not elsewhere classified
    Medication overuse headache
    Use additional code for adverse effect, if applicable, to identify drug (T36-T50 with fifth or sixth character 5)
    G44.40 Drug-induced headache, not elsewhere classified, not intractable
    G44.41 Drug-induced headache, not elsewhere classified, intractable

⑤ **G44.5** Complicated **headache syndromes**
    G44.51 Hemicrania continua
    G44.52 New daily persistent **headache (NDPH)**
    G44.53 Primary thunderclap **headache**
    G44.59 Other complicated **headache syndrome**

⑤ **G44.8** Other specified **headache syndromes**
    G44.81 Hypnic **headache**
    G44.82 Headache associated with sexual activity
        Orgasmic headache
        Preorgasmic headache
    G44.83 Primary cough **headache**
    G44.84 Primary exertional **headache**
    G44.85 Primary stabbing **headache**
    G44.89 Other **headache syndrome**

④ **G45** Transient cerebral ischemic attacks and related syndromes
    EXCLUDES1 neonatal cerebral ischemia (P91.0)
            transient retinal artery occlusion (H34.0-)
    G45.0 Vertebro-basilar artery **syndrome**
    G45.1 Carotid artery **syndrome (hemispheric)**
    G45.2 Multiple and bilateral precerebral artery **syndromes**
    G45.3 Amaurosis fugax
    G45.4 Transient global amnesia
        EXCLUDES1 amnesia NOS (R41.3)
    G45.8 Other transient cerebral ischemic attacks and related syndromes
    G45.9 Transient cerebral ischemic attack, unspecified
        Spasm of cerebral artery
        TIA
        Transient cerebral ischemia NOS

④ **G46** Vascular syndromes of brain in cerebrovascular diseases
    Code first underlying cerebrovascular disease (I60-I69)
    G46.0 Middle **cerebral artery syndrome**
    G46.1 Anterior **cerebral artery syndrome**
    G46.2 Posterior **cerebral artery syndrome**
    G46.3 Brain stem stroke **syndrome**

        Benedikt syndrome
        Claude syndrome
        Foville syndrome
        Millard-Gubler syndrome
        Wallenberg syndrome
        Weber syndrome
    G46.4 Cerebellar stroke **syndrome**
    G46.5 Pure motor lacunar **syndrome**
    G46.6 Pure sensory lacunar **syndrome**
    G46.7 Other lacunar **syndromes**
    G46.8 Other vascular syndromes of brain in cerebrovascular diseases

④ **G47** Sleep disorders
    EXCLUDES2 nightmares (F51.5)
            nonorganic sleep disorders (F51.-)
            sleep terrors (F51.4)
            sleepwalking (F51.3)

  ⑤ **G47.0** Insomnia
    EXCLUDES2 alcohol related insomnia (F10.182, F10.282, F10.982)
            drug-related insomnia (F11.182, F11.282, F11.982, F13.182, F13.282, F13.982, F14.182,F14.282, F14.982, F15.182, F15.282, F15.982, F19.182, F19.282, F19.982)
            idiopathic insomnia (F51.01)
            insomnia due to a mental disorder (F51.05)
            insomnia not due to a substance or known physiological condition (F51.0-)
            nonorganic insomnia (F51.0-)
            primary insomnia (F51.01)
            sleep apnea (G47.3-)
    G47.00 Insomnia, unspecified
        Insomnia NOS
    G47.01 Insomnia due to medical condition
        Code also associated medical condition
    G47.09 Other insomnia

  ⑤ **G47.1** Hypersomnia
    EXCLUDES2 alcohol-related hypersomnia (F10.182, F10.282, F10.982)
            drug-related hypersomnia (F11.182, F11.282, F11.982, F13.182, F13.282, F13.982, F14.182,F14.282, F14.982, F15.182, F15.282, F15.982, F19.182, F19.282, F19.982)
            hypersomnia due to a mental disorder (F51.13)
            hypersomnia not due to a substance or known physiological condition (F51.1-)
            primary hypersomnia (F51.11)
            sleep apnea (G47.3-)
    G47.10 Hypersomnia, unspecified
        Hypersomnia NOS
    G47.11 Idiopathic hypersomnia with long sleep time
        Idiopathic hypersomnia NOS
    G47.12 Idiopathic hypersomnia without long sleep time
    G47.13 Recurrent hypersomnia
        Kleine-Levin syndrome
        Menstrual related hypersomnia
    G47.14 Hypersomnia due to medical condition
        Code also associated medical condition
    G47.19 Other hypersomnia

  ⑤ **G47.2** Circadian rhythm sleep disorders
    Disorders of the sleep wake schedule
    Inversion of nyctohemeral rhythm
    Inversion of sleep rhythm
    G47.20 Circadian rhythm sleep disorder, unspecified type
        Sleep wake schedule disorder NOS
    G47.21 Circadian rhythm sleep disorder, delayed sleep phase type
        Delayed sleep phase syndrome

---

④ 4ᵗʰ character required   ⑤ 5ᵗʰ character required   ⑥ 6ᵗʰ character required   ⑦ 7ᵗʰ character required   ⑳ Extension 'X' Alert

EXCLUDES 1 Not coded here   **EXCLUDES 2** Not included here   PDx Primary Diagnosis Only   Manifestation Code

G47.22 **Circadian rhythm sleep disorder, advanced sleep phase type**
G47.23 **Circadian rhythm sleep disorder, irregular sleep wake type**
Irregular sleep-wake pattern
G47.24 **Circadian rhythm sleep disorder, free running type**
G47.25 **Circadian rhythm sleep disorder, jet lag type**
G47.26 **Circadian rhythm sleep disorder, shift work type**
G47.27 **Circadian rhythm sleep disorder in conditions classified elsewhere**
Code first underlying condition
G47.29 **Other circadian rhythm sleep disorder**

[5] G47.3 **Sleep apnea**
Code also any associated underlying condition
[EXCLUDES1] *apnea NOS (R06.81)*
Cheyne-Stokes breathing (R06.3)
pickwickian syndrome (E66.2)
sleep apnea of newborn (P28.3)
G47.30 **Sleep apnea, unspecified**
Sleep apnea NOS
G47.31 **Primary central sleep apnea**
G47.32 **High altitude periodic breathing**
G47.33 **Obstructive sleep apnea (adult) (pediatric)**
[EXCLUDES1] *obstructive sleep apnea of newborn (P28.3)*
G47.34 **Idiopathic sleep related nonobstructive alveolar hypoventilation**
Sleep related hypoxia
G47.35 **Congenital central alveolar hypoventilation syndrome**
G47.36 **Sleep related hypoventilation in conditions classified elsewhere**
Sleep related hypoxemia in conditions classified elsewhere
Code first underlying condition
G47.37 **Central sleep apnea in conditions classified elsewhere**
Code first underlying condition
G47.39 **Other sleep apnea**

[5] G47.4 **Narcolepsy and cataplexy**
[6] G47.41 **Narcolepsy**
G47.411 **Narcolepsy with cataplexy**
G47.419 **Narcolepsy without cataplexy**
Narcolepsy NOS
[6] G47.42 **Narcolepsy in conditions classified elsewhere**
Code first underlying condition
G47.421 **Narcolepsy in conditions classified elsewhere with cataplexy**
G47.429 **Narcolepsy in conditions classified elsewhere without cataplexy**

[5] G47.5 **Parasomnia**
[EXCLUDES1] *alcohol induced parasomnia (F10.182, F10.282, F10.982)*
drug induced parasomnia (F11.182, F11.282, F11.982, F13.182, F13.282, F13.982, F14.182, F14.282, F14.982, F15.182, F15.282, F15.982, F19.182, F19.282, F19.982)
parasomnia not due to a substance or known physiological condition (F51.8)
G47.50 **Parasomnia, unspecified**
Parasomnia NOS
G47.51 **Confusional arousals**
G47.52 **REM sleep behavior disorder**
G47.53 **Recurrent isolated sleep paralysis**
G47.54 **Parasomnia in conditions classified elsewhere**
Code first underlying condition
G47.59 **Other parasomnia**

[5] G47.6 **Sleep related movement disorders**
[EXCLUDES2] *restless legs syndrome (G25.81)*
G47.61 **Periodic limb movement disorder**
Periodic limb movement disorder
G47.62 **Sleep related leg cramps**
G47.63 **Sleep related bruxism**
[EXCLUDES1] *psychogenic bruxism (F45.8)*
G47.69 **Other sleep related movement disorders**
G47.8 **Other sleep disorders**
G47.9 **Sleep disorder, unspecified**
Sleep disorder NOS

Nerve, nerve root and plexus disorders (G50-G59)

[EXCLUDES1] *current traumatic nerve, nerve root and plexus disorders - see Injury, nerve by body region*
neuralgia NOS (M79.2)
neuritis NOS (M79.2)
peripheral neuritis in pregnancy (O26.82-)
radiculitis NOS (M54.1-)

[4] G50 **Disorders of trigeminal nerve**
[INCLUDES] *disorders of 5th cranial nerve*
G50.0 **Trigeminal neuralgia**
Syndrome of paroxysmal facial pain
Tic douloureux
G50.1 **Atypical facial pain**
G50.8 **Other disorders of trigeminal nerve**
G50.9 **Disorder of trigeminal nerve, unspecified**

[4] G51 **Facial nerve disorders**
[INCLUDES] *disorders of 7th cranial nerve*
G51.0 **Bell's palsy**
Facial palsy
G51.1 **Geniculate ganglionitis**
[EXCLUDES1] *postherpetic geniculate ganglionitis (B02.21)*
G51.2 **Melkersson's syndrome**
Melkersson-Rosenthal syndrome
G51.3 **Clonic hemifacial spasm**
G51.4 **Facial myokymia**
G51.8 **Other disorders of facial nerve**
G51.9 **Disorder of facial nerve, unspecified**

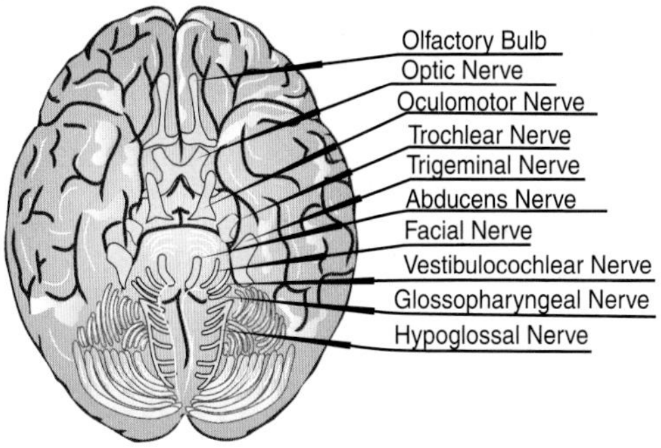
Olfactory Bulb
Optic Nerve
Oculomotor Nerve
Trochlear Nerve
Trigeminal Nerve
Abducens Nerve
Facial Nerve
Vestibulocochlear Nerve
Glossopharyngeal Nerve
Hypoglossal Nerve

Figure 6.2 The Cranial Nerves

[4] G52 **Disorders of other cranial nerves**
[EXCLUDES2] *disorders of acoustic [8th] nerve (H93.3)*
disorders of optic [2nd] nerve (H46, H47.0)
paralytic strabismus due to nerve palsy (H49.0-H49.2)
G52.0 **Disorders of olfactory nerve**
Disorders of 1st cranial nerve
G52.1 **Disorders of glossopharyngeal nerve**
Disorder of 9th cranial nerve
Glossopharyngeal neuralgia
G52.2 **Disorders of vagus nerve**
Disorders of pneumogastric [10th] nerve

Unspecified Code | Other Specified Code | [N] Newborn Age: 0 | [P] Pediatric Age: 0-17 | [M] Maternity Age: 12-55 | [A] Adult Age: 15-124 | ♂ Male | ♀ Female | ● New Code | ▲ Revised Code Title | ►◄ Revised Text

G52.3 Disorders of hypoglossal nerve
Disorders of 12th cranial nerve
G52.7 Disorders of multiple cranial nerves
Polyneuritis cranialis
G52.8 Disorders of other specified cranial nerves
G52.9 Cranial nerve disorder, unspecified

G53 Cranial nerve disorders in diseases classified elsewhere
Code first underlying disease, such as:
neoplasm (C00-D49)

[EXCLUDES1] *multiple cranial nerve palsy in sarcoidosis (D86.82)*
multiple cranial nerve palsy in syphilis (A52.15)
postherpetic geniculate ganglionitis (B02.21)
postherpetic trigeminal neuralgia (B02.22)

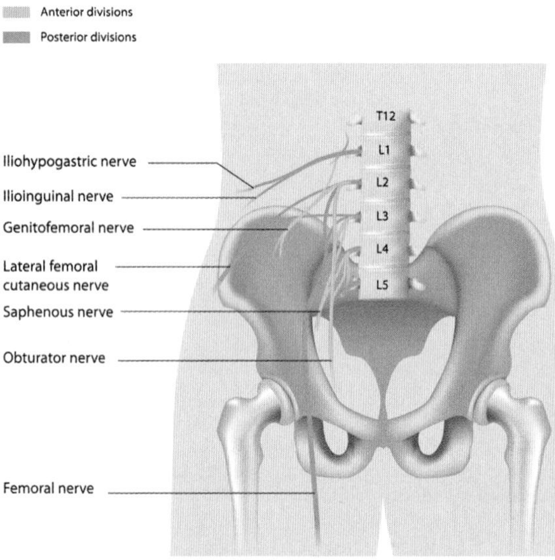
Anterior divisions
Posterior divisions
T12
L1
L2
L3
L4
L5
Iliohypogastric nerve
Ilioinguinal nerve
Genitofemoral nerve
Lateral femoral cutaneous nerve
Saphenous nerve
Obturator nerve
Femoral nerve

Figure 6.3 The lumbar Plexus

[4] **G54 Nerve root and plexus disorders**

[EXCLUDES1] *current traumatic nerve root and plexus disorders - see nerve injury by body region*
intervertebral disc disorders (M50-M51)
neuralgia or neuritis NOS (M79.2)
neuritis or radiculitis brachial NOS (M54.13)
neuritis or radiculitis lumbar NOS (M54.16)
neuritis or radiculitis lumbosacral NOS (M54.17)
neuritis or radiculitis thoracic NOS (M54.14)
radiculitis NOS (M54.10)
radiculopathy NOS (M54.10)
spondylosis (M47.-)

G54.0 Brachial plexus disorders
Thoracic outlet syndrome
G54.1 Lumbosacral plexus disorders
G54.2 Cervical root disorders, not elsewhere classified
G54.3 Thoracic root disorders, not elsewhere classified
G54.4 Lumbosacral root disorders, not elsewhere classified
G54.5 Neuralgic amyotrophy
Parsonage-Aldren-Turner syndrome
Shoulder-girdle neuritis

[EXCLUDES1] *neuralgic amyotrophy in diabetes mellitus (E08-E13 with .44)*

G54.6 Phantom limb syndrome with pain
G54.7 Phantom limb syndrome without pain
Phantom limb syndrome NOS
G54.8 Other nerve root and plexus disorders
G54.9 Nerve root and plexus disorder, unspecified

G55 Nerve root and plexus compressions in diseases classified elsewhere
Code first underlying disease, such as:
neoplasm (C00-D49)

[EXCLUDES1] *nerve root compression (due to) (in) ankylosing spondylitis (M45.-)*
nerve root compression (due to) (in) dorsopathies (M53.-, M54.-)
nerve root compression (due to) (in) intervertebral disc disorders (M50.1.-, M51.1.-)
nerve root compression (due to) (in) spondylopathies (M46.-, M48.-)
nerve root compression (due to) (in) spondylosis (M47.0-M47.2.-)

[4] **G56 Mononeuropathies of upper limb**

[EXCLUDES1] *current traumatic nerve disorder - see nerve injury by body region*

[5] **G56.0 Carpal tunnel syndrome**
G56.00 Carpal tunnel syndrome, unspecified upper limb
G56.01 Carpal tunnel syndrome, right upper limb
G56.02 Carpal tunnel syndrome, left upper limb

[5] **G56.1 Other lesions of median nerve**
G56.10 Other lesions of median nerve, unspecified upper limb
G56.11 Other lesions of median nerve, right upper limb
G56.12 Other lesions of median nerve, left upper limb

[5] **G56.2 Lesion of ulnar nerve**
Tardy ulnar nerve palsy
G56.20 Lesion of ulnar nerve, unspecified upper limb
G56.21 Lesion of ulnar nerve, right upper limb
G56.22 Lesion of ulnar nerve, left upper limb

[5] **G56.3 Lesion of radial nerve**
G56.30 Lesion of radial nerve, unspecified upper limb
G56.31 Lesion of radial nerve, right upper limb
G56.32 Lesion of radial nerve, left upper limb

[5] **G56.4 Causalgia of upper limb**
Complex regional pain syndrome II of upper limb

[EXCLUDES1] *complex regional pain syndrome I of lower limb (G90.52-)*
complex regional pain syndrome I of upper limb (G90.51-)
complex regional pain syndrome II of lower limb (G57.7-)
reflex sympathetic dystrophy of lower limb (G90.52-)
reflex sympathetic dystrophy of upper limb (G90.51-)

G56.40 Causalgia of unspecified upper limb
G56.41 Causalgia of right upper limb
G56.42 Causalgia of left upper limb

[5] **G56.8 Other specified mononeuropathies of upper limb**
Interdigital neuroma of upper limb
G56.80 Other specified mononeuropathies of unspecified upper limb
G56.81 Other specified mononeuropathies of right upper limb
G56.82 Other specified mononeuropathies of left upper limb

[5] **G56.9 Unspecified mononeuropathy of upper limb**
G56.90 Unspecified mononeuropathy of unspecified upper limb
G56.91 Unspecified mononeuropathy of right upper limb
G56.92 Unspecified mononeuropathy of left upper limb

[4] **G57 Mononeuropathies of lower limb**

[EXCLUDES1] *current traumatic nerve disorder - see nerve injury by body region*

[4] 4th character required [5] 5th character required [6] 6th character required [7] 7th character required [X] Extension 'X' Alert
[EXCLUDES1] Not coded here [EXCLUDES2] Not included here [PDx] Primary Diagnosis Only Manifestation Code

[5] G57.0 Lesion of sciatic nerve
[EXCLUDES1] *sciatica NOS (M54.3-)*
[EXCLUDES2] *sciatica attributed to intervertebral disc disorder (M51.1.-)*
G57.00 Lesion of sciatic nerve, unspecified lower limb
G57.01 Lesion of sciatic nerve, right lower limb
G57.02 Lesion of sciatic nerve, left lower limb

[5] G57.1 Meralgia paresthetica
Lateral cutaneous nerve of thigh syndrome
G57.10 Meralgia paresthetica, unspecified lower limb
G57.11 Meralgia paresthetica, right lower limb
G57.12 Meralgia paresthetica, left lower limb

[5] G57.2 Lesion of femoral nerve
G57.20 Lesion of femoral nerve, unspecified lower limb
G57.21 Lesion of femoral nerve, right lower limb
G57.22 Lesion of femoral nerve, left lower limb

[5] G57.3 Lesion of lateral popliteal nerve
Peroneal nerve palsy
G57.30 Lesion of lateral popliteal nerve, unspecified lower limb
G57.31 Lesion of lateral popliteal nerve, right lower limb
G57.32 Lesion of lateral popliteal nerve, left lower limb

[5] G57.4 Lesion of medial popliteal nerve
G57.40 Lesion of medial popliteal nerve, unspecified lower limb
G57.41 Lesion of medial popliteal nerve, right lower limb
G57.42 Lesion of medial popliteal nerve, left lower limb

[5] G57.5 Tarsal tunnel syndrome
G57.50 Tarsal tunnel syndrome, unspecified lower limb
G57.51 Tarsal tunnel syndrome, right lower limb
G57.52 Tarsal tunnel syndrome, left lower limb

[5] G57.6 Lesion of plantar nerve
Morton's metatarsalgia
G57.60 Lesion of plantar nerve, unspecified lower limb
G57.61 Lesion of plantar nerve, right lower limb
G57.62 Lesion of plantar nerve, left lower limb

[5] G57.7 Causalgia of lower limb
Complex regional pain syndrome II of lower limb
[EXCLUDES1] *complex regional pain syndrome I of lower limb (G90.52-)*
complex regional pain syndrome I of upper limb (G90.51-)
complex regional pain syndrome II of upper limb (G56.4-)
reflex sympathetic dystrophy of lower limb (G90.52-)
reflex sympathetic dystrophy of upper limb (G90.51-)
G57.70 Causalgia of unspecified lower limb
G57.71 Causalgia of right lower limb
G57.72 Causalgia of left lower limb

[5] G57.8 Other specified mononeuropathies of lower limb
Interdigital neuroma of lower limb
G57.80 Other specified mononeuropathies of unspecified lower limb
G57.81 Other specified mononeuropathies of right lower limb
G57.82 Other specified mononeuropathies of left lower limb

[5] G57.9 Unspecified mononeuropathy of lower limb
G57.90 Unspecified mononeuropathy of unspecified lower limb
G57.91 Unspecified mononeuropathy of right lower limb
G57.92 Unspecified mononeuropathy of left lower limb

[4] G58 Other mononeuropathies
G58.0 Intercostal neuropathy
G58.7 Mononeuritis multiplex
G58.8 Other specified mononeuropathies
G58.9 Mononeuropathy, unspecified

G59 Mononeuropathy in diseases classified elsewhere
Code first underlying disease
[EXCLUDES1] *diabetic mononeuropathy (E09-E14 with .41)*
syphilitic nerve paralysis (A52.19)
syphilitic neuritis (A52.15)
tuberculous mononeuropathy (A17.83)

Polyneuropathies and other disorders of the peripheral nervous system (G60-G65)

[EXCLUDES1] *neuralgia NOS (M79.2)*
neuritis NOS (M79.2)
peripheral neuritis in pregnancy (O26.82-)
radiculitis NOS (M54.10)

[4] G60 Hereditary and idiopathic neuropathy
G60.0 Hereditary motor and sensory neuropathy
Charcot-Marie-Tooth disease
Déjérine-Sottas disease
Hereditary motor and sensory neuropathy, types I-IV
Hypertrophic neuropathy of infancy
Peroneal muscular atrophy (axonal type) (hypertrophic type)
Roussy-Levy syndrome
G60.1 Refsum's disease
Infantile Refsum disease
G60.2 Neuropathy in association with hereditary ataxia
G60.3 Idiopathic progressive neuropathy
G60.8 Other hereditary and idiopathic neuropathies
Dominantly inherited sensory neuropathy
Morvan's disease
Nelaton's syndrome
Recessively inherited sensory neuropathy
G60.9 Hereditary and idiopathic neuropathy, unspecified

[4] G61 Inflammatory polyneuropathy
G61.0 Guillain-Barre syndrome
Acute (post-)infective polyneuritis
Miller Fisher Syndrome
G61.1 Serum neuropathy
Use additional code for adverse effect, if applicable, to identify serum (T50.-)
[5] G61.8 Other inflammatory polyneuropathies
G61.81 Chronic inflammatory demyelinating polyneuritis
G61.89 Other inflammatory polyneuropathies
G61.9 Inflammatory polyneuropathy, unspecified

[4] G62 Other and unspecified polyneuropathies
G62.0 Drug-induced polyneuropathy
Use additional code for adverse effect, if applicable, to identify drug (T36-T50 with fifth or sixth character 5)
G62.1 Alcoholic polyneuropathy
G62.2 Polyneuropathy due to other toxic agents
Code first (T51-T65) to identify toxic agent
[5] G62.8 Other specified polyneuropathies
G62.81 Critical illness polyneuropathy
Acute motor neuropathy
G62.82 Radiation-induced polyneuropathy
Use additional external cause code (W88-W90, X39.0-) to identify cause
G62.89 Other specified polyneuropathies
G62.9 Polyneuropathy, unspecified
Neuropathy NOS

Unspecified Code | Other Specified Code | [N] Newborn Age: 0 | [P] Pediatric Age: 0-17 | [M] Maternity Age: 12-55
[A] Adult Age: 15-124 | ♂ Male | ♀ Female | ● New Code | ▲ Revised Code Title | ►◄ Revised Text

G63 **Polyneuropathy in diseases classified elsewhere**
Code first underlying disease, such as:
amyloidosis (E85.-)
endocrine disease, except diabetes (E00-E07, E15-E16, E20-E34)
metabolic diseases (E70-E88)
neoplasm (C00-D49)
nutritional deficiency (E40-E64)
[EXCLUDES1] *polyneuropathy (in):*
diabetes mellitus (E08-E13 with .42)
diphtheria (A36.83)
infectious mononucleosis (B27.0-B27.9 with 1)
Lyme disease (A69.22)
mumps (B26.84)
postherpetic (B02.23)
rheumatoid arthritis (M05.33)
scleroderma (M34.83)
systemic lupus erythematosus (M32.19)

G64 **Other disorders of peripheral nervous system**
Disorder of peripheral nervous system NOS

[4] G65 **Sequelae of inflammatory and toxic polyneuropathies**
Code first condition resulting from (sequela) of inflammatory and toxic polyneuropathies
G65.0 **Sequelae of Guillain-Barré syndrome**
G65.1 **Sequelae of other inflammatory polyneuropathy**
G65.2 **Sequelae of toxic polyneuropathy**

Diseases of myoneural junction and muscle (G70-G73)

[4] G70 **Myasthenia gravis and other myoneural disorders**
[EXCLUDES1] *botulism (A05.1, A48.51-A48.52)*
transient neonatal myasthenia gravis (P94.0)
[5] G70.0 **Myasthenia gravis**
G70.00 **Myasthenia gravis without (acute) exacerbation**
Myasthenia gravis NOS
G70.01 **Myasthenia gravis with (acute) exacerbation**
Myasthenia gravis in crisis
G70.1 **Toxic myoneural disorders**
Code first (T51-T65) to identify toxic agent
G70.2 **Congenital and developmental myasthenia**
[5] G70.8 **Other specified myoneural disorders**
G70.80 **Lambert-Eaton syndrome, unspecified**
Lambert-Eaton syndrome NOS
G70.81 **Lambert-Eaton syndrome in disease classified elsewhere**
Code first underlying disease
[EXCLUDES1] *Lambert-Eaton syndrome in neoplastic disease (G73.1)*
G70.89 **Other specified myoneural disorders**
G70.9 **Myoneural disorder, unspecified**

[4] G71 **Primary disorders of muscles**
[EXCLUDES2] *arthrogryposis multiplex congenita (Q74.3)*
metabolic disorders (E70-E88)
myositis (M60.-)
G71.0 **Muscular dystrophy**
Autosomal recessive, childhood type, muscular dystrophy resembling Duchenne or Becker muscular dystrophy
Benign [Becker] muscular dystrophy
Benign scapuloperoneal muscular dystrophy with early contractures [Emery-Dreifuss]
Congenital muscular dystrophy NOS
Congenital muscular dystrophy with specific morphological abnormalities of the muscle fiber
Distal muscular dystrophy
Facioscapulohumeral muscular dystrophy
Limb-girdle muscular dystrophy
Ocular muscular dystrophy
Oculopharyngeal muscular dystrophy
Scapuloperoneal muscular dystrophy
Severe [Duchenne] muscular dystrophy
[5] G71.1 **Myotonic disorders**
G71.11 **Myotonic muscular dystrophy**
Dystrophia myotonica [Steinert]
Myotonia atrophica
Myotonic dystrophy
Proximal myotonic myopathy (PROMM)
Steinert disease
G71.12 **Myotonia congenita**
Acetazolamide responsive myotonia congenita
Dominant myotonia congenita [Thomsen disease]
Myotonia levior
Recessive myotonia congenita [Becker disease]
G71.13 **Myotonic chondrodystrophy**
Chondrodystrophic myotonia
Congenital myotonic chondrodystrophy
Schwartz-Jampel disease
G71.14 **Drug induced myotonia**
Use additional code for adverse effect, if applicable, to identify drug (T36-T50 with fifth or sixth character 5)
G71.19 **Other specified myotonic disorders**
Myotonia fluctuans
Myotonia permanens
Neuromyotonia [Isaacs]
Paramyotonia congenita (of von Eulenburg)
Pseudomyotonia
Symptomatic myotonia
G71.2 **Congenital myopathies**
Central core disease
Fiber-type disproportion
Minicore disease
Multicore disease
Myotubular (centronuclear) myopathy
Nemaline myopathy
[EXCLUDES1] *arthrogryposis multiplex congenita (Q74.3)*
G71.3 **Mitochondrial myopathy, not elsewhere classified**
[EXCLUDES1] *Kearns-Sayre syndrome (H49.81)*
Leber's disease (H47.21)
Leigh's encephalopathy (G31.82)
mitochondrial metabolism disorders (E88.4.-)
Reye's syndrome (G93.7)
G71.8 **Other primary disorders of muscles**
G71.9 **Primary disorder of muscle, unspecified**
Hereditary myopathy NOS

[4] G72 **Other and unspecified myopathies**
[EXCLUDES1] *arthrogryposis multiplex congenita (Q74.3)*
dermatopolymyositis (M33.-)
ischemic infarction of muscle (M62.2-)
myositis (M60.-)
polymyositis (M33.2.-)
G72.0 **Drug-induced myopathy**
Use additional code for adverse effect, if applicable, to identify drug (T36-T50 with fifth or sixth character 5)
G72.1 **Alcoholic myopathy**
Use additional code to identify alcoholism (F10.-)
G72.2 **Myopathy due to other toxic agents**
Code first (T51-T65) to identify toxic agent
G72.3 **Periodic paralysis**
Familial periodic paralysis
Hyperkalemic periodic paralysis (familial)
Hypokalemic periodic paralysis (familial)
Myotonic periodic paralysis (familial)
Normokalemic paralysis (familial)
Potassium sensitive periodic paralysis
[EXCLUDES1] *paramyotonia congenita (of von Eulenburg) (G71.19)*

[4] 4th character required [5] 5th character required [6] 6th character required [7] 7th character required [X] Extension 'X' Alert
[EXCLUDES1] Not coded here [EXCLUDES2] Not included here [PDx] Primary Diagnosis Only Manifestation Code

[5] G72.4 Inflammatory and immune myopathies, not elsewhere classified
G72.41 Inclusion body myositis [IBM]
G72.49 Other inflammatory and immune myopathies, not elsewhere classified
Inflammatory myopathy NOS
[5] G72.8 Other specified myopathies
G72.81 Critical illness myopathy
Acute necrotizing myopathy
Acute quadriplegic myopathy
Intensive care (ICU) myopathy
Myopathy of critical illness
G72.89 Other specified myopathies
G72.9 Myopathy, unspecified
[4] G73 Disorders of myoneural junction and muscle in diseases classified elsewhere
G73.1 Lambert-Eaton syndrome in neoplastic disease
Code first underlying neoplasm (C00-D49)
[EXCLUDES1] *Lambert-Eaton syndrome not associated with neoplasm (G70.80-G70.81)*
G73.3 Myasthenic syndromes in other diseases classified elsewhere
Code first underlying disease, such as:
neoplasm (C00-D49)
thyrotoxicosis (E05.-)
G73.7 Myopathy in diseases classified elsewhere
Code first underlying disease, such as:
hyperparathyroidism (E21.0, E21.3)
hypoparathyroidism (E20.-)
glycogen storage disease (E74.0)
lipid storage disorders (E75.-)
[EXCLUDES1] *myopathy in:*
rheumatoid arthritis (M05.32)
sarcoidosis (D86.87)
scleroderma (M34.82)
sicca syndrome [Sjögren] (M35.03)
systemic lupus erythematosus (M32.19)

Cerebral palsy and other paralytic syndromes (G80-G83)

[4] G80 Cerebral palsy
[EXCLUDES1] *hereditary spastic paraplegia (G11.4)*
G80.0 Spastic quadriplegic cerebral palsy
Congenital spastic paralysis (cerebral)
G80.1 Spastic diplegic cerebral palsy
Spastic cerebral palsy NOS
G80.2 Spastic hemiplegic cerebral palsy
G80.3 Athetoid cerebral palsy
Double athetosis (syndrome)
Dyskinetic cerebral palsy
Dystonic cerebral palsy
Vogt disease
G80.4 Ataxic cerebral palsy
G80.8 Other cerebral palsy
Mixed cerebral palsy syndromes
G80.9 Cerebral palsy, unspecified
Cerebral palsy NOS
[4] G81 Hemiplegia and hemiparesis
[NOTES] This category is to be used only when hemiplegia (complete)(incomplete) is reported without further specification, or is stated to be old or longstanding but of unspecified cause. The category is also for use in multiple coding to identify these types of hemiplegia resulting from any cause.
[EXCLUDES1] *congenital cerebral palsy (G80.-)*
hemiplegia and hemiparesis due to sequela of cerebrovascular disease (I69.05-, I69.15-, I69.25-, I69.35-, I69.85-, I69.95-)
[5] G81.0 Flaccid hemiplegia
G81.00 Flaccid hemiplegia affecting unspecified side
G81.01 Flaccid hemiplegia affecting right dominant side
G81.02 Flaccid hemiplegia affecting left dominant side
G81.03 Flaccid hemiplegia affecting right nondominant side
G81.04 Flaccid hemiplegia affecting left nondominant side
[5] G81.1 Spastic hemiplegia
G81.10 Spastic hemiplegia affecting unspecified side
G81.11 Spastic hemiplegia affecting right dominant side
G81.12 Spastic hemiplegia affecting left dominant side
G81.13 Spastic hemiplegia affecting right nondominant side
G81.14 Spastic hemiplegia affecting left nondominant side
[5] G81.9 Hemiplegia, unspecified
G81.90 Hemiplegia, unspecified affecting unspecified side
G81.91 Hemiplegia, unspecified affecting right dominant side
G81.92 Hemiplegia, unspecified affecting left dominant side
G81.93 Hemiplegia, unspecified affecting right nondominant side
G81.94 Hemiplegia, unspecified affecting left nondominant side
[4] G82 Paraplegia (paraparesis) and quadriplegia (quadriparesis)
[NOTES] This category is to be used only when the listed conditions are reported without further specification, or are stated to be old or longstanding but of unspecified cause. The category is also for use in multiple coding to identify these conditions resulting from any cause
[EXCLUDES1] *congenital cerebral palsy (G80.-)*
functional quadriplegia (R53.2)
hysterical paralysis (F44.4)
[5] G82.2 Paraplegia
Paralysis of both lower limbs NOS
Paraparesis (lower) NOS
Paraplegia (lower) NOS
G82.20 Paraplegia, unspecified
G82.21 Paraplegia, complete
G82.22 Paraplegia, incomplete
[5] G82.5 Quadriplegia
G82.50 Quadriplegia, unspecified
G82.51 Quadriplegia, C1-C4 complete
G82.52 Quadriplegia, C1-C4 incomplete
G82.53 Quadriplegia, C5-C7 complete
G82.54 Quadriplegia, C5-C7 incomplete
[4] G83 Other paralytic syndromes
[NOTES] This category is to be used only when the listed conditions are reported without further specification, or are stated to be old or longstanding but of unspecified cause. The category is also for use in multiple coding to identify these conditions resulting from any cause.
INCLUDES *paralysis (complete) (incomplete), except as in G80-G82*
G83.0 Diplegia of upper limbs
Diplegia (upper)
Paralysis of both upper limbs
[5] G83.1 Monoplegia of lower limb
Paralysis of lower limb
[EXCLUDES1] *monoplegia of lower limbs due to sequela of cerebrovascular disease (I69.04-, I69.14-, I69.24-, I69.34-, I69.84-, I69.94-)*
G83.10 Monoplegia of lower limb affecting unspecified side

Unspecified Code | Other Specified Code | [N] Newborn Age: 0 | [P] Pediatric Age: 0-17 | [M] Maternity Age: 12-55
[A] Adult Age: 15-124 | ♂ Male | ♀ Female | ● New Code | ▲ Revised Code Title | ►◄ Revised Text

G83.11 Monoplegia of lower limb affecting right dominant side

G83.12 Monoplegia of lower limb affecting left dominant side

G83.13 Monoplegia of lower limb affecting right nondominant side

G83.14 Monoplegia of lower limb affecting left nondominant side

⑤ G83.2 Monoplegia of upper limb

Paralysis of upper limb

EXCLUDES1 *monoplegia of upper limbs due to sequela of cerebrovascular disease (I69.03-, I69.13-, I69.23-, I69.33-, I69.83-, I69.93-)*

G83.20 Monoplegia of upper limb affecting unspecified side

G83.21 Monoplegia of upper limb affecting right dominant side

G83.22 Monoplegia of upper limb affecting left dominant side

G83.23 Monoplegia of upper limb affecting right nondominant side

G83.24 Monoplegia of upper limb affecting left nondominant side

⑤ G83.3 Monoplegia, unspecified

G83.30 Monoplegia, unspecified affecting unspecified side

G83.31 Monoplegia, unspecified affecting right dominant side

G83.32 Monoplegia, unspecified affecting left dominant side

G83.33 Monoplegia, unspecified affecting right nondominant side

G83.34 Monoplegia, unspecified affecting left nondominant side

G83.4 Cauda equina syndrome

Neurogenic bladder due to cauda equina syndrome

EXCLUDES1 *cord bladder NOS (G95.89)*
neurogenic bladder NOS (N31.9)

G83.5 Locked-in state

⑤ G83.8 Other specified paralytic syndromes

EXCLUDES1 *paralytic syndromes due to current spinal cord injury-code to spinal cord injury (S14, S24, S34)*

G83.81 Brown-Séquard syndrome

G83.82 Anterior cord syndrome

G83.83 Posterior cord syndrome

G83.84 Todd's paralysis (postepileptic)

G83.89 Other specified paralytic syndromes

G83.9 Paralytic syndrome, unspecified

Other disorders of the nervous system (G89-G99)

④ G89 Pain, not elsewhere classified

Code also related psychological factors associated with pain (F45.42)

EXCLUDES1 *generalized pain NOS (R52)*
pain disorders exclusively related to psychological factors (F45.41)
pain NOS (R52)

EXCLUDES2 *atypical face pain (G50.1)*
headache syndromes (G44.-)
localized pain, unspecified type - code to pain by site, such as:
abdomen pain (R10.-)
back pain (M54.9)
breast pain (N64.4)
chest pain (R07.1-R07.9)
ear pain (H92.0-)
eye pain (H57.1)
headache (R51)

joint pain (M25.5-)
limb pain (M79.6-)
lumbar region pain (M54.5)
painful urination (R30.9)
pelvic and perineal pain (R10.2)
shoulder pain (M25.51-)
spine pain (M54.-)
throat pain (R07.0)
tongue pain (K14.6)
tooth pain (K08.8)
renal colic (N23)
migraines (G43.-)
myalgia (M79.1)
pain from prosthetic devices, implants, and grafts (T82.84, T83.84, T84.84, T85.84)
phantom limb syndrome with pain (G54.6)
vulvar vestibulitis (N94.810)
vulvodynia (N94.81-)

G89.0 Central pain syndrome

Déjérine-Roussy syndrome

Myelopathic pain syndrome

Thalamic pain syndrome (hyperesthetic)

⑤ G89.1 Acute pain, not elsewhere classified

G89.11 Acute pain due to trauma

G89.12 Acute post-thoracotomy pain

Post-thoracotomy pain NOS

G89.18 Other acute postprocedural pain

Postoperative pain NOS

Postprocedural pain NOS

⑤ G89.2 Chronic pain, not elsewhere classified

EXCLUDES1 *causalgia, lower limb (G57.7-)*
causalgia, upper limb (G56.4-)
central pain syndrome (G89.0)
chronic pain syndrome (G89.4)
complex regional pain syndrome II, lower limb (G57.7-)
complex regional pain syndrome II, upper limb (G56.4-)
neoplasm related chronic pain (G89.3)
reflex sympathetic dystrophy (G90.5-)

G89.21 Chronic pain due to trauma

G89.22 Chronic post-thoracotomy pain

G89.28 Other chronic postprocedural pain

Other chronic postoperative pain

G89.29 Other chronic pain

G89.3 Neoplasm related pain (acute) (chronic)

Cancer associated pain

Pain due to malignancy (primary) (secondary)

Tumor associated pain

G89.4 Chronic pain syndrome

Chronic pain associated with significant psychosocial dysfunction

④ G90 Disorders of autonomic nervous system

EXCLUDES1 *dysfunction of the autonomic nervous system due to alcohol (G31.2)*

⑤ G90.0 Idiopathic peripheral autonomic neuropathy

G90.01 Carotid sinus syncope

Carotid sinus syndrome

G90.09 Other idiopathic peripheral autonomic neuropathy

Idiopathic peripheral autonomic neuropathy NOS

G90.1 Familial dysautonomia [Riley-Day]

G90.2 Horner's syndrome

Bernard(-Horner) syndrome

Cervical sympathetic dystrophy or paralysis

G90.3 Multi-system degeneration of the autonomic nervous system

Neurogenic orthostatic hypotension [Shy-Drager]

EXCLUDES1 *orthostatic hypotension NOS (I95.1)*

---

④ 4th character required   ⑤ 5th character required   ⑥ 6th character required   ⑦ 7th character required   ⑩ Extension 'X' Alert

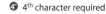 *EXCLUDES1* Not coded here   *EXCLUDES2* Not included here   PDx Primary Diagnosis Only   Manifestation Code

G90.4 Autonomic dysreflexia
Use additional code to identify the cause, such as:
fecal impaction (K56.41)
pressure ulcer (pressure area) (L89.-)
urinary tract infection (N39.0)

[5] G90.5 Complex regional pain syndrome I (CRPS I)
Reflex sympathetic dystrophy
EXCLUDES1 *causalgia of lower limb (G57.7-)*
causalgia of upper limb (G56.4-)
complex regional pain syndrome II of lower limb (G57.7-)
complex regional pain syndrome II of upper limb (G56.4-)

G90.50 Complex regional pain syndrome I, unspecified

[6] G90.51 Complex regional pain syndrome I of upper limb
G90.511 Complex regional pain syndrome I of right upper limb
G90.512 Complex regional pain syndrome I of left upper limb
G90.513 Complex regional pain syndrome I of upper limb, bilateral
G90.519 Complex regional pain syndrome I of unspecified upper limb

[6] G90.52 Complex regional pain syndrome I of lower limb
G90.521 Complex regional pain syndrome I of right lower limb
G90.522 Complex regional pain syndrome I of left lower limb
G90.523 Complex regional pain syndrome I of lower limb, bilateral
G90.529 Complex regional pain syndrome I of unspecified lower limb

G90.59 Complex regional pain syndrome I of other specified site

G90.8 Other disorders of autonomic nervous system
G90.9 Disorder of the autonomic nervous system, unspecified

[4] G91 Hydrocephalus
INCLUDES *acquired hydrocephalus*
EXCLUDES1 *Arnold-Chiari syndrome with hydrocephalus (Q07.-)*
congenital hydrocephalus (Q03.-)
spina bifida with hydrocephalus (Q05.-)

G91.0 Communicating hydrocephalus
Secondary normal pressure hydrocephalus
G91.1 Obstructive hydrocephalus
G91.2 (Idiopathic) normal pressure hydrocephalus
Normal pressure hydrocephalus NOS
G91.3 Post-traumatic hydrocephalus, unspecified
G91.4 Hydrocephalus in diseases classified elsewhere
Code first underlying condition, such as:
congenital syphilis (A50.4-)
neoplasm (C00-D49)
EXCLUDES1 *hydrocephalus due to congenital toxoplasmosis (P37.1)*
G91.8 Other hydrocephalus
G91.9 Hydrocephalus, unspecified

G92 Toxic encephalopathy
Toxic encephalitis
Toxic metabolic encephalopathy
Code first (T51-T65) to identify toxic agent

[4] G93 Other disorders of brain
G93.0 Cerebral cysts
Arachnoid cyst
Porencephalic cyst, acquired
EXCLUDES1 *acquired periventricular cysts of newborn (P91.1)*
congenital cerebral cysts (Q04.6)

G93.1 Anoxic brain damage, not elsewhere classified
EXCLUDES1 *cerebral anoxia due to anesthesia during labor and delivery (O74.3)*
cerebral anoxia due to anesthesia during the puerperium (O89.2)
neonatal anoxia (P84)

G93.2 Benign intracranial hypertension
EXCLUDES1 *hypertensive encephalopathy (I67.4)*

G93.3 Postviral fatigue syndrome
Benign myalgic encephalomyelitis
EXCLUDES1 *chronic fatigue syndrome NOS (R53.82)*

[5] G93.4 Other and unspecified encephalopathy
EXCLUDES1 *alcoholic encephalopathy (G31.2)*
encephalopathy in diseases classified elsewhere (G94)
hypertensive encephalopathy (I67.4)
toxic (metabolic) encephalopathy (G92)

G93.40 Encephalopathy, unspecified
G93.41 Metabolic encephalopathy
Septic encephalopathy
G93.49 Other encephalopathy
Encephalopathy NEC

G93.5 Compression of brain
Arnold-Chiari type 1 compression of brain
Compression of brain (stem)
Herniation of brain (stem)
EXCLUDES1 *diffuse traumatic compression of brain (S06.2-)*
focal traumatic compression of brain (S06.3-)

G93.6 Cerebral edema
EXCLUDES1 *cerebral edema due to birth injury (P11.0)*
traumatic cerebral edema (S06.1-)

G93.7 Reye's syndrome
Code first (T39.0-), if salicylates-induced [P]

[5] G93.8 Other specified disorders of brain
G93.81 Temporal sclerosis
Hippocampal sclerosis
Mesial temporal sclerosis
G93.82 Brain death
G93.89 Other specified disorders of brain
Postradiation encephalopathy

G93.9 Disorder of brain, unspecified

G94 Other disorders of brain in diseases classified elsewhere
Code first underlying disease
EXCLUDES1 *encephalopathy in congenital syphilis (A50.49)*
encephalopathy in influenza (J09.X9, J10.81, J11.81)
encephalopathy in syphilis (A52.19)
hydrocephalus in diseases classified elsewhere (G91.4)

[4] G95 Other and unspecified diseases of spinal cord
EXCLUDES2 *myelitis (G04.-)*

G95.0 Syringomyelia and syringobulbia

[5] G95.1 Vascular myelopathies
EXCLUDES2 *intraspinal phlebitis and thrombophlebitis, except non-pyogenic (G08)*
G95.11 Acute infarction of spinal cord (embolic) (nonembolic)
Anoxia of spinal cord
Arterial thrombosis of spinal cord
G95.19 Other vascular myelopathies
Edema of spinal cord
Hematomyelia
Nonpyogenic intraspinal phlebitis and thrombophlebitis
Subacute necrotic myelopathy

[5] G95.2 Other and unspecified cord compression
G95.20 Unspecified cord compression
G95.29 Other cord compression

Unspecified Code | Other Specified Code | [N] Newborn Age: 0 | [P] Pediatric Age: 0-17 | [M] Maternity Age: 12-55
[A] Adult Age: 15-124 | ♂ Male | ♀ Female | ● New Code | ▲ Revised Code Title | ►◄ Revised Text

⑤ **G95.8** Other specified diseases of spinal cord

> EXCLUDES1 *neurogenic bladder NOS (N31.9)*
> *neurogenic bladder due to cauda equina*
> *syndrome (G83.4)*
> *neuromuscular dysfunction of bladder without*
> *spinal cord lesion (N31.-)*

G95.81 Conus medullaris **syndrome**

G95.89 Other specified **diseases of spinal cord**

Cord bladder NOS

Drug-induced myelopathy

Radiation-induced myelopathy

> EXCLUDES1 *myelopathy NOS (G95.9)*

G95.9 Disease of spinal cord, unspecified

Myelopathy NOS

④ **G96** Other disorders of central nervous system

G96.0 Cerebrospinal fluid leak

> EXCLUDES1 *cerebrospinal fluid leak from spinal puncture*
> *(G97.0)*

⑤ **G96.1** Disorders of meninges, not elsewhere classified

G96.11 Dural tear

> EXCLUDES1 *accidental puncture or laceration of dura during*
> *a procedure (G97.41)*

G96.12 Meningeal adhesions (cerebral) (spinal)

G96.19 Other disorders of meninges, not elsewhere
classified

G96.8 Other specified disorders of central nervous system

G96.9 Disorder of central nervous system, unspecified

④ **G97** Intraoperative and postprocedural complications **and
disorders of nervous system, not elsewhere classified**

> EXCLUDES2 *intraoperative and postprocedural*
> *cerebrovascular infarction (I97.81-, I97.82-)*

G97.0 Cerebrospinal fluid leak **from spinal puncture**

G97.1 Other reaction **to spinal and lumbar puncture**

Headache due to lumbar puncture

G97.2 Intracranial hypotension **following ventricular
shunting**

⑤ **G97.3** Intraoperative hemorrhage and hematoma **of a
nervous system organ or structure complicating a
procedure**

> EXCLUDES1 *intraoperative hemorrhage and hematoma*
> *of a nervous system organ or structure due to*
> *accidental puncture and laceration during a*
> *procedure (G97.4-)*

G97.31 Intraoperative hemorrhage and hematoma of a
nervous system organ or structure complicating
a nervous system procedure

G97.32 Intraoperative hemorrhage and hematoma of a
nervous system organ or structure complicating
other procedure

⑤ **G97.4** Accidental puncture and laceration **of a nervous
system organ or structure during a procedure**

G97.41 Accidental puncture or laceration of dura during
a procedure

Incidental (inadvertent) durotomy

G97.48 Accidental puncture and laceration of other
nervous system organ or structure during a
nervous system procedure

G97.49 Accidental puncture and laceration of other
nervous system organ or structure during other
procedure

⑤ **G97.5** Postprocedural hemorrhage and hematoma **of
a nervous system organ or structure following a
procedure**

G97.51 Postprocedural hemorrhage and hematoma of
a nervous system organ or structure following a
nervous system procedure

G97.52 Postprocedural hemorrhage and hematoma of
a nervous system organ or structure following
other procedure

⑤ **G97.8** Other intraoperative and postprocedural
complications **and disorders of nervous system**
Use additional code to further specify disorder

G97.81 Other intraoperative **complications of nervous
system**

G97.82 Other postprocedural **complications and
disorders of nervous system**

④ **G98** Other disorders of nervous system not elsewhere classified

> INCLUDES *nervous system disorder NOS*

G98.0 Neurogenic arthritis, **not elsewhere classified**

Nonsyphilitic neurogenic arthropathy NEC

Nonsyphilitic neurogenic spondylopathy NEC

> EXCLUDES1 *spondylopathy (in):*
> *syringomyelia and syringobulbia (G95.0)*
> *tabes dorsalis (A52.11)*

G98.8 Other **disorders of nervous system**

Nervous system disorder NOS

④ **G99** Other disorders of nervous system in diseases classified
elsewhere

G99.0 Autonomic neuropathy **in diseases classified
elsewhere**
Code first underlying disease, such as:
amyloidosis (E85.-)
gout (M1A.-, M10.-)
hyperthyroidism (E05.-)

> EXCLUDES1 *diabetic autonomic neuropathy (E09-14 with .43)*

G99.2 Myelopathy **in diseases classified elsewhere**
Code first underlying disease, such as:
neoplasm (C00-D49)

> EXCLUDES1 *myelopathy in:*
> *intervertebral disease (M50.0-, M51.0-)*
> *spondylosis (M47.0-, M47.1-)*

G99.8 Other specified **disorders of nervous system in
diseases classified elsewhere**
Code first underlying disorder, such as:
amyloidosis (E85.-)
avitaminosis (E56.9)

> EXCLUDES1 *nervous system involvement in:*
> *cysticercosis (B69.0)*
> *rubella (B06.0-)*
> *syphilis (A52.1-)*

---

④ 4ᵗʰ character required   ⑤ 5ᵗʰ character required   ⑥ 6ᵗʰ character required   ⑦ 7ᵗʰ character required   ⑰ Extension 'X' Alert

EXCLUDES 1 Not coded here   EXCLUDES 2 Not included here   PDx Primary Diagnosis Only   Manifestation Code

Chapter 7: Diseases of the Eye and Adnexa (H00-H59)

Chapter Specific Coding Guidelines

a. **Glaucoma**

   1) **Assigning Glaucoma Codes**

      Assign as many codes from category H40, Glaucoma, as needed to identify the type of glaucoma, the affected eye, and the glaucoma stage.

   2) **Bilateral glaucoma with same type and stage**

      When a patient has bilateral glaucoma and both eyes are documented as being the same type and stage, and there is a code for bilateral glaucoma, report only the code for the type of glaucoma, bilateral, with the seventh character for the stage.

      When a patient has bilateral glaucoma and both eyes are documented as being the same type and stage, and the classification does not provide a code for bilateral glaucoma (i.e. subcategories H40.10, H40.11 and H40.20) report only one code for the type of glaucoma with the appropriate seventh character for the stage.

   3) **Bilateral glaucoma stage with different types or stages**

      When a patient has bilateral glaucoma and each eye is documented as having a different type or stage, and the classification distinguishes laterality, assign the appropriate code for each eye rather than the code for bilateral glaucoma.

   When a patient has bilateral glaucoma and each eye is documented as having a different type, and the classification does not distinguish laterality (i.e. subcategories H40.10, H40.11 and H40.20), assign one code for each type of glaucoma with the appropriate seventh character for the stage.

   When a patient has bilateral glaucoma and each eye is documented as having the same type, but different stage, and the classification does not distinguish laterality (i.e. subcategories H40.10, H40.11 and H40.20), assign a code for the type of glaucoma for each eye with the seventh character for the specific glaucoma stage documented for each eye.

   4) **Patient admitted with glaucoma and stage evolves during the admission**

      If a patient is admitted with glaucoma and the stage progresses during the admission, assign the code for highest stage documented.

   5) **Indeterminate stage glaucoma**

      Assignment of the seventh character "4" for "indeterminate stage" should be based on the clinical documentation. The seventh character "4" is used for glaucomas whose stage cannot be clinically determined. This seventh character should not be confused with the seventh character "0", unspecified, which should be assigned when there is no documentation regarding the stage of the glaucoma.

This page intentionally left blank

Anatomy of the Ocular System

1. The Organ of Sight

Eyes are regarded as the organs of sight. They are located in the orbits of the skull. The eyelids and eyelashes serve to protect the eyes from the foreign objects. Blinking of the eyelids lubricates the surface of the eye by spreading tears that are produced by the lacrimal gland. A typical human eye is in the form of a sphere a filled with the following two fluids:

a) Aqueous Humor

The frontal portion of the lens of the eye is known as the anterior compartment that remains filled with fluid, which is called the aqueous humor.

b) Vitreous Humor

The portion behind the lens of the eye is known as the posterior compartment that is filled with a fluid called the vitreous humor.

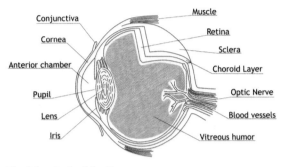

2. The Other Parts of the Eye:

a) **Ciliary Body and Muscle:** This is a ring of striated smooth muscle in the middle layer eye (vascular layer). It is triangular in the horizontal section and is coated by a double layer, the ciliary epithelium. The inner layer is transparent and covers the vitreous body and is continuation of neural tissue of the retina. The outer layer is a continuous with the retinal pigment epithelium and constitutes the cells of the dilator muscle.

b) **Suspensory Ligament:** A series of fibers that connect the ciliary body of the eye with the lens, holding it in place. Suspensory ligaments are thin fibers that connect the ciliary body of the lens with the receptors. It is a thickening of Tenon's capsule, the dense connective tissue capsule surrounding the globe and separating it from orbital fat. Suspensory ligaments in the eye lens allow easy focusing.

c) **Iris:** A thin, circular structure in the eye which covers the sclera. It is responsible for controlling the diameter and size of the pupils and thus the amount of light reaching the retina. In response to the amount of light entering the eye, muscles attached to the iris expand or contract the aperture at the center of the iris, known as the pupil.

d) **Pupil:** The dark center opening in the middle of the iris is called the pupil. The pupil is a hole located in the center of the iris of the eye that allows light to enter the retina. The pupil changes size to adjust for the amount of light available.

e) **Cornea:** The cornea is transparent and comprises the front part of the eye that covers the iris, pupil and anterior chamber. Together with the lens, the cornea refracts light accounting for approximately two-thirds of the eye's total optical power.

f) **Lens:** The crystalline lens is a biconvex structure and is suspended behind the colored iris. The lens is behind the covering known as the cornea. The lens is more flat on its anterior side than on its posterior side.

g) **Retina:** The vertebrate retina is 0.5 mm thick and lines the back of the eye. It is a light-sensitive layer of tissue, lining the inner surface of the eye. The optic nerve contains the ganglion cell axons running to the brain.

h) **Retinal Arteries and Veins:** The retinal arteries and veins emerge from the nasal side of the optic disc. Vessels directed temporally have an arching course; those directed nasally have a radial course. Arteries are brighter red and narrower than veins.

i) **Fovea Centralis:** The fovea is the depression in the inner retinal surface, about 1.5 mm wide and is specialized for maximum visual acuity. This is the thickest part of the retina. This part has the highest density of cones in the eye.

j) **Optic Nerve:** The optic nerve is the second of twelve paired cranial nerves, but is considered to be part of the central nervous system as it is derived from an out-pouching of the diencephalon during embryonic development. It consists mainly of fibers derived from the ganglionic cells of the retina. Its fibers are covered with myelin produced by oligodendrocytes rather than Schwann cells.

k) **Choroid Coat:** The choroid, also known as the choroidea or choroid coat, is the vascular layer of the eye containing connective tissue and lies between the retina and the sclera. It contains the retinal pigmented epithelial cells and provides oxygen and nourishment to the retina.

l) **Sclera:** The posterior five-sixths of the connective tissue coat of the ocular globe is formed by sclera. It maintains the shape of the globe and provides an attachment for the extraocular muscle insertions. The sclera is perforated by many nerves and vessels passing through the posterior scleral foramen, the hole that is formed by the optic nerve. The inner layer of the sclera (lamina fusca) blends with the suprachoroidal and supraciliary lamellae of the uveal tract.

m) **Blind Spot:** This is a small portion of the visual field of each eye where the optic nerve and blood vessels pass through to connect to the back of the eye and is also called as optic disk. There are no photoreceptors in the optic disk, therefore there is no image detection in this area. The blind spot of the right eye is located to the right of the centre of vision and vice versa in the left eye.

n) **Hyaloid Canal (or Cloquet's/Stilling's Canal):** This is a small transparent canal running through the vitreous body from the optical nerve disc to the lens. It is formed by pouch of the hyaloid membrane which encloses the vitreous body. It is filled with lymph.

Common Pathologies

Cataract

Cataracts are an eye disorder in which clouding of the lens occurs which leads to blurry vision. It is an ageing disorder. This disoder leads to dimness in eye vision, and if not treated can lead to blindness.

Cataract Surgery

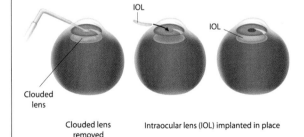

Clouded lens

Clouded lens removed

Intraocular lens (IOL) implanted in place

Glaucoma

In this disease, damage occurs to optic nerves due to increased intraocular pressure and leads to blindness.

Development of Glaucoma

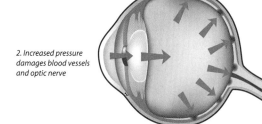

Healthy eye

Flow of aqueous humour

Vitreous body

Drainage canal

Glaucoma

1. Drainage canal blocked; build-up of fluid

2. Increased pressure damages blood vessels and optic nerve

Strabismus

A condition of eye in which there is non-alignment between both eyes. This condition is commonly called squint.

Strabismus

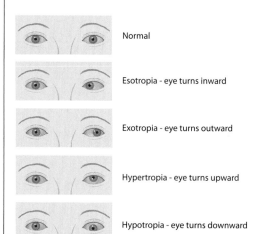

Normal

Esotropia - eye turns inward

Exotropia - eye turns outward

Hypertropia - eye turns upward

Hypotropia - eye turns downward

Macular Degeneration

The condition because of degeneration in macula of eye due to ageing and leads to blurry vision. It is a disease that destroys sharp, central vision. Central vision is required to see objects clearly and to do tasks such as reading and driving.

Conjunctivitis

An infection in eye. The conjuctiva in the eye gets exposed to bacteria and other allergic irritants which can lead to inflammation and infection. It is also known as red eye.

Optic Neuritis

This disorder occurs due to inflammation of the optic nerve. Pain and temporary vision loss are common

Diseases of the eye and adnexa (H00-H59)

[NOTES] Use an external cause code following the code for the eye condition, if applicable, to identify the cause of the eye condition

[EXCLUDES2] *certain conditions originating in the perinatal period (P04-P96)*
certain infectious and parasitic diseases (A00-B99)
complications of pregnancy, childbirth and the puerperium (O00-O9A)
congenital malformations, deformations, and chromosomal abnormalities (Q00-Q99)
diabetes mellitus related eye conditions (E09.3-, E10.3-, E11.3-, E13.3-)
endocrine, nutritional and metabolic diseases (E00-E88)
injury (trauma) of eye and orbit (S05.-)
injury, poisoning and certain other consequences of external causes (S00-T88)
neoplasms (C00-D49)
symptoms, signs and abnormal clinical and laboratory findings, not elsewhere classified (R00-R94)
syphilis related eye disorders (A50.01, A50.3-, A51.43, A52.71)

Disorders of eyelid, lacrimal system and orbit (H00-H05)

[EXCLUDES2] *open wound of eyelid (S01.1-)*
superficial injury of eyelid (S00.1-, S00.2-)

[4] **H00 Hordeolum and chalazion**

[5] **H00.0 Hordeolum (externum) (internum) of eyelid**

[6] **H00.01 Hordeolum externum**

Hordeolum NOS
Stye

- **H00.011 Hordeolum externum right upper eyelid**
- **H00.012 Hordeolum externum right lower eyelid**
- **H00.013 Hordeolum externum right eye, unspecified eyelid**
- **H00.014 Hordeolum externum left upper eyelid**
- **H00.015 Hordeolum externum left lower eyelid**
- **H00.016 Hordeolum externum left eye, unspecified eyelid**
- **H00.019 Hordeolum externum unspecified eye, unspecified eyelid**

[6] **H00.02 Hordeolum internum**

Infection of meibomian gland

- **H00.021 Hordeolum internum right upper eyelid**
- **H00.022 Hordeolum internum right lower eyelid**
- **H00.023 Hordeolum internum right eye, unspecified eyelid**
- **H00.024 Hordeolum internum left upper eyelid**
- **H00.025 Hordeolum internum left lower eyelid**
- **H00.026 Hordeolum internum left eye, unspecified eyelid**
- **H00.029 Hordeolum internum unspecified eye, unspecified eyelid**

[6] **H00.03 Abscess of eyelid**

Furuncle of eyelid

- **H00.031 Abscess of right upper eyelid**
- **H00.032 Abscess of right lower eyelid**
- **H00.033 Abscess of eyelid right eye, unspecified eyelid**
- **H00.034 Abscess of left upper eyelid**
- **H00.035 Abscess of left lower eyelid**
- **H00.036 Abscess of eyelid left eye, unspecified eyelid**
- **H00.039 Abscess of eyelid unspecified eye, unspecified eyelid**

[5] **H00.1 Chalazion**

Meibomian (gland) cyst

[EXCLUDES2] *infected meibomian gland (H00.02-)*

- **H00.11 Chalazion right upper eyelid**
- **H00.12 Chalazion right lower eyelid**
- **H00.13 Chalazion right eye, unspecified eyelid**
- **H00.14 Chalazion left upper eyelid**
- **H00.15 Chalazion left lower eyelid**
- **H00.16 Chalazion left eye, unspecified eyelid**
- **H00.19 Chalazion unspecified eye, unspecified eyelid**

[4] **H01 Other inflammation of eyelid**

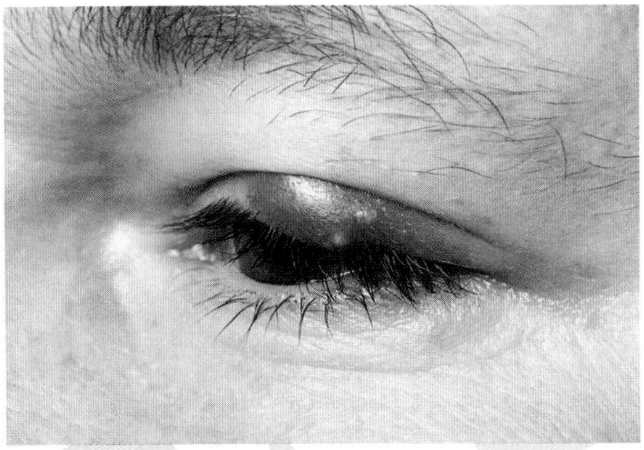

Figure 7.1 Blepharitis

[5] **H01.0 Blepharitis**

[EXCLUDES1] *blepharoconjunctivitis (H10.5-)*

[6] **H01.00 Unspecified blepharitis**

- **H01.001 Unspecified blepharitis right upper eyelid**
- **H01.002 Unspecified blepharitis right lower eyelid**
- **H01.003 Unspecified blepharitis right eye, unspecified eyelid**
- **H01.004 Unspecified blepharitis left upper eyelid**
- **H01.005 Unspecified blepharitis left lower eyelid**
- **H01.006 Unspecified blepharitis left eye, unspecified eyelid**
- **H01.009 Unspecified blepharitis unspecified eye, unspecified eyelid**

[6] **H01.01 Ulcerative blepharitis**

- **H01.011 Ulcerative blepharitis right upper eyelid**
- **H01.012 Ulcerative blepharitis right lower eyelid**
- **H01.013 Ulcerative blepharitis right eye, unspecified eyelid**
- **H01.014 Ulcerative blepharitis left upper eyelid**
- **H01.015 Ulcerative blepharitis left lower eyelid**
- **H01.016 Ulcerative blepharitis left eye, unspecified eyelid**
- **H01.019 Ulcerative blepharitis unspecified eye, unspecified eyelid**

[6] **H01.02 Squamous blepharitis**

- **H01.021 Squamous blepharitis right upper eyelid**
- **H01.022 Squamous blepharitis right lower eyelid**
- **H01.023 Squamous blepharitis right eye, unspecified eyelid**
- **H01.024 Squamous blepharitis left upper eyelid**
- **H01.025 Squamous blepharitis left lower eyelid**
- **H01.026 Squamous blepharitis left eye, unspecified eyelid**
- **H01.029 Squamous blepharitis unspecified eye, unspecified eyelid**

[5] **H01.1 Noninfectious dermatoses of eyelid**

[6] **H01.11 Allergic dermatitis of eyelid**

Contact dermatitis of eyelid

- **H01.111 Allergic dermatitis of right upper eyelid**

Unspecified Code | Other Specified Code | [N] Newborn Age: 0 | [P] Pediatric Age: 0-17 | [M] Maternity Age: 12-55
[A] Adult Age: 15-124 | ♂ Male | ♀ Female | ● New Code | ▲ Revised Code Title | ►◄ Revised Text

H01.112 Allergic dermatitis of right lower eyelid
H01.113 Allergic dermatitis of right eye, unspecified eyelid
H01.114 Allergic dermatitis of left upper eyelid
H01.115 Allergic dermatitis of left lower eyelid
H01.116 Allergic dermatitis of left eye, unspecified eyelid
H01.119 Allergic dermatitis of unspecified eye, unspecified eyelid

[6] H01.12 Discoid lupus erythematosus of eyelid
H01.121 Discoid lupus erythematosus of right upper eyelid
H01.122 Discoid lupus erythematosus of right lower eyelid
H01.123 Discoid lupus erythematosus of right eye, unspecified eyelid
H01.124 Discoid lupus erythematosus of left upper eyelid
H01.125 Discoid lupus erythematosus of left lower eyelid
H01.126 Discoid lupus erythematosus of left eye, unspecified eyelid
H01.129 Discoid lupus erythematosus of unspecified eye, unspecified eyelid

[6] H01.13 Eczematous dermatitis of eyelid
H01.131 Eczematous dermatitis of right upper eyelid
H01.132 Eczematous dermatitis of right lower eyelid
H01.133 Eczematous dermatitis of right eye, unspecified eyelid
H01.134 Eczematous dermatitis of left upper eyelid
H01.135 Eczematous dermatitis of left lower eyelid
H01.136 Eczematous dermatitis of left eye, unspecified eyelid
H01.139 Eczematous dermatitis of unspecified eye, unspecified eyelid

[6] H01.14 Xeroderma of eyelid
H01.141 Xeroderma of right upper eyelid
H01.142 Xeroderma of right lower eyelid
H01.143 Xeroderma of right eye, unspecified eyelid
H01.144 Xeroderma of left upper eyelid
H01.145 Xeroderma of left lower eyelid
H01.146 Xeroderma of left eye, unspecified eyelid
H01.149 Xeroderma of unspecified eye, unspecified eyelid

H01.8 Other specified inflammations of eyelid
H01.9 Unspecified inflammation of eyelid
Inflammation of eyelid NOS

[4] H02 Other disorders of eyelid
[EXCLUDES1] *congenital malformations of eyelid (Q10.0-Q10.3)*

[5] H02.0 Entropion and trichiasis of eyelid

[6] H02.00 Unspecified entropion of eyelid
H02.001 Unspecified entropion of right upper eyelid
H02.002 Unspecified entropion of right lower eyelid
H02.003 Unspecified entropion of right eye, unspecified eyelid
H02.004 Unspecified entropion of left upper eyelid
H02.005 Unspecified entropion of left lower eyelid
H02.006 Unspecified entropion of left eye, unspecified eyelid
H02.009 Unspecified entropion of unspecified eye, unspecified eyelid

[6] H02.01 Cicatricial entropion of eyelid
H02.011 Cicatricial entropion of right upper eyelid
H02.012 Cicatricial entropion of right lower eyelid
H02.013 Cicatricial entropion of right eye, unspecified eyelid
H02.014 Cicatricial entropion of left upper eyelid
H02.015 Cicatricial entropion of left lower eyelid
H02.016 Cicatricial entropion of left eye, unspecified eyelid
H02.019 Cicatricial entropion of unspecified eye, unspecified eyelid

[6] H02.02 Mechanical entropion of eyelid
H02.021 Mechanical entropion of right upper eyelid
H02.022 Mechanical entropion of right lower eyelid
H02.023 Mechanical entropion of right eye, unspecified eyelid
H02.024 Mechanical entropion of left upper eyelid
H02.025 Mechanical entropion of left lower eyelid
H02.026 Mechanical entropion of left eye, unspecified eyelid
H02.029 Mechanical entropion of unspecified eye, unspecified eyelid

[6] H02.03 Senile entropion of eyelid
H02.031 Senile entropion of right upper eyelid [A]
H02.032 Senile entropion of right lower eyelid [A]
H02.033 Senile entropion of right eye, unspecified eyelid [A]
H02.034 Senile entropion of left upper eyelid [A]
H02.035 Senile entropion of left lower eyelid [A]
H02.036 Senile entropion of left eye, unspecified eyelid [A]
H02.039 Senile entropion of unspecified eye, unspecified eyelid [A]

[6] H02.04 Spastic entropion of eyelid
H02.041 Spastic entropion of right upper eyelid
H02.042 Spastic entropion of right lower eyelid
H02.043 Spastic entropion of right eye, unspecified eyelid
H02.044 Spastic entropion of left upper eyelid
H02.045 Spastic entropion of left lower eyelid
H02.046 Spastic entropion of left eye, unspecified eyelid
H02.049 Spastic entropion of unspecified eye, unspecified eyelid

[6] H02.05 Trichiasis without entropian
H02.051 Trichiasis without entropian right upper eyelid
H02.052 Trichiasis without entropian right lower eyelid
H02.053 Trichiasis without entropian right eye, unspecified eyelid
H02.054 Trichiasis without entropian left upper eyelid
H02.055 Trichiasis without entropian left lower eyelid
H02.056 Trichiasis without entropian left eye, unspecified eyelid
H02.059 Trichiasis without entropian unspecified eye, unspecified eyelid

[5] H02.1 Ectropion of eyelid

[6] H02.10 Unspecified ectropion of eyelid
H02.101 Unspecified ectropion of right upper eyelid
H02.102 Unspecified ectropion of right lower eyelid
H02.103 Unspecified ectropion of right eye, unspecified eyelid
H02.104 Unspecified ectropion of left upper eyelid
H02.105 Unspecified ectropion of left lower eyelid
H02.106 Unspecified ectropion of left eye, unspecified eyelid
H02.109 Unspecified ectropion of unspecified eye, unspecified eyelid

[6] H02.11 Cicatricial ectropion of eyelid
H02.111 Cicatricial ectropion of right upper eyelid

[4] 4th character required [5] 5th character required [6] 6th character required [7] 7th character required [X] Extension 'X' Alert
[EXCLUDES 1] Not coded here [EXCLUDES 2] Not included here [PDx] Primary Diagnosis Only Manifestation Code

H02.112 Cicatricial ectropion of right lower eyelid
H02.113 Cicatricial ectropion of right eye, unspecified eyelid
H02.114 Cicatricial ectropion of left upper eyelid
H02.115 Cicatricial ectropion of left lower eyelid
H02.116 Cicatricial ectropion of left eye, unspecified eyelid
H02.119 Cicatricial ectropion of unspecified eye, unspecified eyelid

🄶 H02.12 Mechanical ectropion of eyelid
H02.121 Mechanical ectropion of right upper eyelid
H02.122 Mechanical ectropion of right lower eyelid
H02.123 Mechanical ectropion of right eye, unspecified eyelid
H02.124 Mechanical ectropion of left upper eyelid
H02.125 Mechanical ectropion of left lower eyelid
H02.126 Mechanical ectropion of left eye, unspecified eyelid
H02.129 Mechanical ectropion of unspecified eye, unspecified eyelid

🄶 H02.13 Senile ectropion of eyelid
H02.131 Senile ectropion of right upper eyelid Ⓐ
H02.132 Senile ectropion of right lower eyelid Ⓐ
H02.133 Senile ectropion of right eye, unspecified eyelid Ⓐ
H02.134 Senile ectropion of left upper eyelid Ⓐ
H02.135 Senile ectropion of left lower eyelid Ⓐ
H02.136 Senile ectropion of left eye, unspecified eyelid Ⓐ
H02.139 Senile ectropion of unspecified eye, unspecified eyelid Ⓐ

🄶 H02.14 Spastic ectropion of eyelid
H02.141 Spastic ectropion of right upper eyelid
H02.142 Spastic ectropion of right lower eyelid
H02.143 Spastic ectropion of right eye, unspecified eyelid
H02.144 Spastic ectropion of left upper eyelid
H02.145 Spastic ectropion of left lower eyelid
H02.146 Spastic ectropion of left eye, unspecified eyelid
H02.149 Spastic ectropion of unspecified eye, unspecified eyelid

🄢 H02.2 Lagophthalmos
🄶 H02.20 Unspecified lagophthalmos
H02.201 Unspecified lagophthalmos right upper eyelid
H02.202 Unspecified lagophthalmos right lower eyelid
H02.203 Unspecified lagophthalmos right eye, unspecified eyelid
H02.204 Unspecified lagophthalmos left upper eyelid
H02.205 Unspecified lagophthalmos left lower eyelid
H02.206 Unspecified lagophthalmos left eye, unspecified eyelid
H02.209 Unspecified lagophthalmos unspecified eye, unspecified eyelid

🄶 H02.21 Cicatricial lagophthalmos
H02.211 Cicatricial lagophthalmos right upper eyelid
H02.212 Cicatricial lagophthalmos right lower eyelid
H02.213 Cicatricial lagophthalmos right eye, unspecified eyelid
H02.214 Cicatricial lagophthalmos left upper eyelid
H02.215 Cicatricial lagophthalmos left lower eyelid
H02.216 Cicatricial lagophthalmos left eye, unspecified eyelid

H02.219 Cicatricial lagophthalmos unspecified eye, unspecified eyelid
🄶 H02.22 Mechanical lagophthalmos
H02.221 Mechanical lagophthalmos right upper eyelid
H02.222 Mechanical lagophthalmos right lower eyelid
H02.223 Mechanical lagophthalmos right eye, unspecified eyelid
H02.224 Mechanical lagophthalmos left upper eyelid
H02.225 Mechanical lagophthalmos left lower eyelid
H02.226 Mechanical lagophthalmos left eye, unspecified eyelid
H02.229 Mechanical lagophthalmos unspecified eye, unspecified eyelid

🄶 H02.23 Paralytic lagophthalmos
H02.231 Paralytic lagophthalmos right upper eyelid
H02.232 Paralytic lagophthalmos right lower eyelid
H02.233 Paralytic lagophthalmos right eye, unspecified eyelid
H02.234 Paralytic lagophthalmos left upper eyelid
H02.235 Paralytic lagophthalmos left lower eyelid
H02.236 Paralytic lagophthalmos left eye, unspecified eyelid
H02.239 Paralytic lagophthalmos unspecified eye, unspecified eyelid

🄢 H02.3 Blepharochalasis
Pseudoptosis
H02.30 Blepharochalasis unspecified eye, unspecified eyelid
H02.31 Blepharochalasis right upper eyelid
H02.32 Blepharochalasis right lower eyelid
H02.33 Blepharochalasis right eye, unspecified eyelid
H02.34 Blepharochalasis left upper eyelid
H02.35 Blepharochalasis left lower eyelid
H02.36 Blepharochalasis left eye, unspecified eyelid

🄢 H02.4 Ptosis of eyelid
🄶 H02.40 Unspecified ptosis of eyelid
H02.401 Unspecified ptosis of right eyelid
H02.402 Unspecified ptosis of left eyelid
H02.403 Unspecified ptosis of bilateral eyelids
H02.409 Unspecified ptosis of unspecified eyelid
🄶 H02.41 Mechanical ptosis of eyelid
H02.411 Mechanical ptosis of right eyelid
H02.412 Mechanical ptosis of left eyelid
H02.413 Mechanical ptosis of bilateral eyelids
H02.419 Mechanical ptosis of unspecified eyelid
🄶 H02.42 Myogenic ptosis of eyelid
H02.421 Myogenic ptosis of right eyelid
H02.422 Myogenic ptosis of left eyelid
H02.423 Myogenic ptosis of bilateral eyelids
H02.429 Myogenic ptosis of unspecified eyelid
🄶 H02.43 Paralytic ptosis of eyelid
Neurogenic ptosis of eyelid
H02.431 Paralytic ptosis of right eyelid
H02.432 Paralytic ptosis of left eyelid
H02.433 Paralytic ptosis of bilateral eyelids
H02.439 Paralytic ptosis unspecified eyelid
🄢 H02.5 Other disorders affecting eyelid function
EXCLUDES2 blepharospasm (G24.5)
organic tic (G25.69)
psychogenic tic (F95.-)
🄶 H02.51 Abnormal innervation syndrome
H02.511 Abnormal innervation syndrome right upper eyelid

Unspecified Code Other Specified Code Ⓝ Newborn Age: 0 Ⓟ Pediatric Age: 0-17 Ⓜ Maternity Age: 12-55
Ⓐ Adult Age: 15-124 ♂ Male ♀ Female ● New Code ▲ Revised Code Title ►◄ Revised Text

H02.512 Abnormal innervation syndrome right lower eyelid
H02.513 Abnormal innervation syndrome right eye, unspecified eyelid
H02.514 Abnormal innervation syndrome left upper eyelid
H02.515 Abnormal innervation syndrome left lower eyelid
H02.516 Abnormal innervation syndrome left eye, unspecified eyelid
H02.519 Abnormal innervation syndrome unspecified eye, unspecified eyelid

[6] H02.52 Blepharophimosis
Ankyloblepharon
H02.521 Blepharophimosis right upper eyelid
H02.522 Blepharophimosis right lower eyelid
H02.523 Blepharophimosis right eye, unspecified eyelid
H02.524 Blepharophimosis left upper eyelid
H02.525 Blepharophimosis left lower eyelid
H02.526 Blepharophimosis left eye, unspecified eyelid
H02.529 Blepharophimosis unspecified eye, unspecified lid

[6] H02.53 Eyelid retraction
Eyelid lag
H02.531 Eyelid retraction right upper eyelid
H02.532 Eyelid retraction right lower eyelid
H02.533 Eyelid retraction right eye, unspecified eyelid
H02.534 Eyelid retraction left upper eyelid
H02.535 Eyelid retraction left lower eyelid
H02.536 Eyelid retraction left eye, unspecified eyelid
H02.539 Eyelid retraction unspecified eye, unspecified lid

H02.59 Other disorders affecting eyelid function
Deficient blink reflex
Sensory disorders

[5] H02.6 Xanthelasma of eyelid
H02.60 Xanthelasma of unspecified eye, unspecified eyelid
H02.61 Xanthelasma of right upper eyelid
H02.62 Xanthelasma of right lower eyelid
H02.63 Xanthelasma of right eye, unspecified eyelid
H02.64 Xanthelasma of left upper eyelid
H02.65 Xanthelasma of left lower eyelid
H02.66 Xanthelasma of left eye, unspecified eyelid

[5] H02.7 Other and unspecified degenerative disorders of eyelid and periocular area
H02.70 Unspecified degenerative disorders of eyelid and periocular area

[6] H02.71 Chloasma of eyelid and periocular area
Dyspigmentation of eyelid
Hyperpigmentation of eyelid
H02.711 Chloasma of right upper eyelid and periocular area
H02.712 Chloasma of right lower eyelid and periocular area
H02.713 Chloasma of right eye, unspecified eyelid and periocular area
H02.714 Chloasma of left upper eyelid and periocular area
H02.715 Chloasma of left lower eyelid and periocular area
H02.716 Chloasma of left eye, unspecified eyelid and periocular area
H02.719 Chloasma of unspecified eye, unspecified eyelid and periocular area

[6] H02.72 Madarosis of eyelid and periocular area
Hypotrichosis of eyelid
H02.721 Madarosis of right upper eyelid and periocular area
H02.722 Madarosis of right lower eyelid and periocular area
H02.723 Madarosis of right eye, unspecified eyelid and periocular area
H02.724 Madarosis of left upper eyelid and periocular area
H02.725 Madarosis of left lower eyelid and periocular area
H02.726 Madarosis of left eye, unspecified eyelid and periocular area
H02.729 Madarosis of unspecified eye, unspecified eyelid and periocular area

[6] H02.73 Vitiligo of eyelid and periocular area
Hypopigmentation of eyelid
H02.731 Vitiligo of right upper eyelid and periocular area
H02.732 Vitiligo of right lower eyelid and periocular area
H02.733 Vitiligo of right eye, unspecified eyelid and periocular area
H02.734 Vitiligo of left upper eyelid and periocular area
H02.735 Vitiligo of left lower eyelid and periocular area
H02.736 Vitiligo of left eye, unspecified eyelid and periocular area
H02.739 Vitiligo of unspecified eye, unspecified eyelid and periocular area

H02.79 Other degenerative disorders of eyelid and periocular area

[5] H02.8 Other specified disorders of eyelid

[6] H02.81 Retained foreign body in eyelid
Use additional code to identify the type of retained foreign body (Z18.-)
EXCLUDES1 *laceration of eyelid with foreign body (S01.12-)*
retained intraocular foreign body (H44.6-, H44.7-)
superficial foreign body of eyelid and periocular area (S00.25-)
H02.811 Retained foreign body in right upper eyelid
H02.812 Retained foreign body in right lower eyelid
H02.813 Retained foreign body in right eye, unspecified eyelid
H02.814 Retained foreign body in left upper eyelid
H02.815 Retained foreign body in left lower eyelid
H02.816 Retained foreign body in left eye, unspecified eyelid
H02.819 Retained foreign body in unspecified eye, unspecified eyelid

[6] H02.82 Cysts of eyelid
Sebaceous cyst of eyelid
H02.821 Cysts of right upper eyelid
H02.822 Cysts of right lower eyelid
H02.823 Cysts of right eye, unspecified eyelid
H02.824 Cysts of left upper eyelid
H02.825 Cysts of left lower eyelid
H02.826 Cysts of left eye, unspecified eyelid
H02.829 Cysts of unspecified eye, unspecified eyelid

[6] H02.83 Dermatochalasis of eyelid
H02.831 Dermatochalasis of right upper eyelid
H02.832 Dermatochalasis of right lower eyelid
H02.833 Dermatochalasis of right eye, unspecified eyelid
H02.834 Dermatochalasis of left upper eyelid
H02.835 Dermatochalasis of left lower eyelid

[4] 4th character required [5] 5th character required [6] 6th character required [7] 7th character required [x] Extension 'X' Alert
EXCLUDES 1 Not coded here EXCLUDES 2 Not included here PDx Primary Diagnosis Only Manifestation Code

H02.836 Dermatochalasis of left eye, unspecified eyelid
H02.839 Dermatochalasis of unspecified eye, unspecified eyelid

[6] H02.84 Edema of eyelid
Hyperemia of eyelid
H02.841 Edema of right upper eyelid
H02.842 Edema of right lower eyelid
H02.843 Edema of right eye, unspecified eyelid
H02.844 Edema of left upper eyelid
H02.845 Edema of left lower eyelid
H02.846 Edema of left eye, unspecified eyelid
H02.849 Edema of unspecified eye, unspecified eyelid

[6] H02.85 Elephantiasis of eyelid
H02.851 Elephantiasis of right upper eyelid
H02.852 Elephantiasis of right lower eyelid
H02.853 Elephantiasis of right eye, unspecified eyelid
H02.854 Elephantiasis of left upper eyelid
H02.855 Elephantiasis of left lower eyelid
H02.856 Elephantiasis of left eye, unspecified eyelid
H02.859 Elephantiasis of unspecified eye, unspecified eyelid

[6] H02.86 Hypertrichosis of eyelid
H02.861 Hypertrichosis of right upper eyelid
H02.862 Hypertrichosis of right lower eyelid
H02.863 Hypertrichosis of right eye, unspecified eyelid
H02.864 Hypertrichosis of left upper eyelid
H02.865 Hypertrichosis of left lower eyelid
H02.866 Hypertrichosis of left eye, unspecified eyelid
H02.869 Hypertrichosis of unspecified eye, unspecified eyelid

[6] H02.87 Vascular anomalies of eyelid
H02.871 Vascular anomalies of right upper eyelid
H02.872 Vascular anomalies of right lower eyelid
H02.873 Vascular anomalies of right eye, unspecified eyelid
H02.874 Vascular anomalies of left upper eyelid
H02.875 Vascular anomalies of left lower eyelid
H02.876 Vascular anomalies of left eye, unspecified eyelid
H02.879 Vascular anomalies of unspecified eye, unspecified eyelid

H02.89 Other specified disorders of eyelid
Hemorrhage of eyelid

H02.9 Unspecified disorder of eyelid
Disorder of eyelid NOS

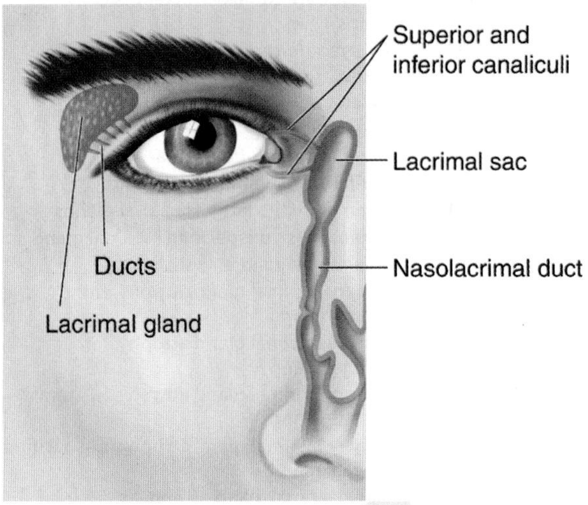

Figure 7.2 lacrimal system

[4] H04 Disorders of lacrimal system
[EXCLUDES1] *congenital malformations of lacrimal system (Q10.4-Q10.6)*

[5] H04.0 Dacryoadenitis

[6] H04.00 Unspecified dacryoadenitis
H04.001 Unspecified dacryoadenitis, right lacrimal gland
H04.002 Unspecified dacryoadenitis, left lacrimal gland
H04.003 Unspecified dacryoadenitis, bilateral lacrimal glands
H04.009 Unspecified dacryoadenitis, unspecified lacrimal gland

[6] H04.01 Acute dacryoadenitis
H04.011 Acute dacryoadenitis, right lacrimal gland
H04.012 Acute dacryoadenitis, left lacrimal gland
H04.013 Acute dacryoadenitis, bilateral lacrimal glands
H04.019 Acute dacryoadenitis, unspecified lacrimal gland

[6] H04.02 Chronic dacryoadenitis
H04.021 Chronic dacryoadenitis, right lacrimal gland
H04.022 Chronic dacryoadenitis, left lacrimal gland
H04.023 Chronic dacryoadenitis, bilateral lacrimal gland
H04.029 Chronic dacryoadenitis, unspecified lacrimal gland

[6] H04.03 Chronic enlargement of lacrimal gland
H04.031 Chronic enlargement of right lacrimal gland
H04.032 Chronic enlargement of left lacrimal gland
H04.033 Chronic enlargement of bilateral lacrimal glands
H04.039 Chronic enlargement of unspecified lacrimal gland

[5] H04.1 Other disorders of lacrimal gland

[6] H04.11 Dacryops
H04.111 Dacryops of right lacrimal gland
H04.112 Dacryops of left lacrimal gland
H04.113 Dacryops of bilateral lacrimal glands
H04.119 Dacryops of unspecified lacrimal gland

[6] H04.12 Dry eye syndrome
Tear film insufficiency, NOS
H04.121 Dry eye syndrome of right lacrimal gland
H04.122 Dry eye syndrome of left lacrimal gland

Unspecified Code | Other Specified Code | [N] Newborn Age: 0 | [P] Pediatric Age: 0-17 | [M] Maternity Age: 12-55
[A] Adult Age: 15-124 | ♂ Male | ♀ Female | ● New Code | ▲ Revised Code Title | ►◄ Revised Text

H04.123 Dry eye syndrome of bilateral lacrimal glands
H04.129 Dry eye syndrome of unspecified lacrimal gland
⑥ H04.13 Lacrimal cyst
  Lacrimal cystic degeneration
  H04.131 Lacrimal cyst, right lacrimal gland
  H04.132 Lacrimal cyst, left lacrimal gland
  H04.133 Lacrimal cyst, bilateral lacrimal glands
  H04.139 Lacrimal cyst, unspecified lacrimal gland
⑥ H04.14 Primary lacrimal gland atrophy
  H04.141 Primary lacrimal gland atrophy, right lacrimal gland
  H04.142 Primary lacrimal gland atrophy, left lacrimal gland
  H04.143 Primary lacrimal gland atrophy, bilateral lacrimal glands
  H04.149 Primary lacrimal gland atrophy, unspecified lacrimal gland
⑥ H04.15 Secondary lacrimal gland atrophy
  H04.151 Secondary lacrimal gland atrophy, right lacrimal gland
  H04.152 Secondary lacrimal gland atrophy, left lacrimal gland
  H04.153 Secondary lacrimal gland atrophy, bilateral lacrimal glands
  H04.159 Secondary lacrimal gland atrophy, unspecified lacrimal gland
⑥ H04.16 Lacrimal gland dislocation
  H04.161 Lacrimal gland dislocation, right lacrimal gland
  H04.162 Lacrimal gland dislocation, left lacrimal gland
  H04.163 Lacrimal gland dislocation, bilateral lacrimal glands
  H04.169 Lacrimal gland dislocation, unspecified lacrimal gland
  H04.19 Other specified disorders of lacrimal gland
⑤ H04.2 Epiphora
⑥ H04.20 Unspecified epiphora
  H04.201 Unspecified epiphora, right lacrimal gland
  H04.202 Unspecified epiphora, left lacrimal gland
  H04.203 Unspecified epiphora, bilateral lacrimal glands
  H04.209 Unspecified epiphora, unspecified lacrimal gland
⑥ H04.21 Epiphora due to excess lacrimation
  H04.211 Epiphora due to excess lacrimation, right lacrimal gland
  H04.212 Epiphora due to excess lacrimation, left lacrimal gland
  H04.213 Epiphora due to excess lacrimation, bilateral lacrimal glands
  H04.219 Epiphora due to excess lacrimation, unspecified lacrimal gland
⑥ H04.22 Epiphora due to insufficient drainage
  H04.221 Epiphora due to insufficient drainage, right lacrimal gland
  H04.222 Epiphora due to insufficient drainage, left lacrimal gland
  H04.223 Epiphora due to insufficient drainage, bilateral lacrimal glands
  H04.229 Epiphora due to insufficient drainage, unspecified lacrimal gland
⑤ H04.3 Acute and unspecified inflammation of lacrimal passages
  EXCLUDES1 neonatal dacryocystitis (P39.1)
⑥ H04.30 Unspecified dacryocystitis

H04.301 Unspecified dacryocystitis of right lacrimal passage
H04.302 Unspecified dacryocystitis of left lacrimal passage
H04.303 Unspecified dacryocystitis of bilateral lacrimal passages
H04.309 Unspecified dacryocystitis of unspecified lacrimal passage
⑥ H04.31 Phlegmonous dacryocystitis
  H04.311 Phlegmonous dacryocystitis of right lacrimal passage
  H04.312 Phlegmonous dacryocystitis of left lacrimal passage
  H04.313 Phlegmonous dacryocystitis of bilateral lacrimal passages
  H04.319 Phlegmonous dacryocystitis of unspecified lacrimal passage
⑥ H04.32 Acute dacryocystitis
  Acute dacryopericystitis
  H04.321 Acute dacryocystitis of right lacrimal passage
  H04.322 Acute dacryocystitis of left lacrimal passage
  H04.323 Acute dacryocystitis of bilateral lacrimal passages
  H04.329 Acute dacryocystitis of unspecified lacrimal passage
⑥ H04.33 Acute lacrimal canaliculitis
  H04.331 Acute lacrimal canaliculitis of right lacrimal passage
  H04.332 Acute lacrimal canaliculitis of left lacrimal passage
  H04.333 Acute lacrimal canaliculitis of bilateral lacrimal passages
  H04.339 Acute lacrimal canaliculitis of unspecified lacrimal passage
⑤ H04.4 Chronic inflammation of lacrimal passages
⑥ H04.41 Chronic dacryocystitis
  H04.411 Chronic dacryocystitis of right lacrimal passage
  H04.412 Chronic dacryocystitis of left lacrimal passage
  H04.413 Chronic dacryocystitis of bilateral lacrimal passages
  H04.419 Chronic dacryocystitis of unspecified lacrimal passage
⑥ H04.42 Chronic lacrimal canaliculitis
  H04.421 Chronic lacrimal canaliculitis of right lacrimal passage
  H04.422 Chronic lacrimal canaliculitis of left lacrimal passage
  H04.423 Chronic lacrimal canaliculitis of bilateral lacrimal passages
  H04.429 Chronic lacrimal canaliculitis of unspecified lacrimal passage
⑥ H04.43 Chronic lacrimal mucocele
  H04.431 Chronic lacrimal mucocele of right lacrimal passage
  H04.432 Chronic lacrimal mucocele of left lacrimal passage
  H04.433 Chronic lacrimal mucocele of bilateral lacrimal passages
  H04.439 Chronic lacrimal mucocele of unspecified lacrimal passage
⑤ H04.5 Stenosis and insufficiency of lacrimal passages
⑥ H04.51 Dacryolith
  H04.511 Dacryolith of right lacrimal passage
  H04.512 Dacryolith of left lacrimal passage
  H04.513 Dacryolith of bilateral lacrimal passages
  H04.519 Dacryolith of unspecified lacrimal passage

---

④ 4th character required   ⑤ 5th character required   ⑥ 6th character required   ⑦ 7th character required   ⑦ₓ Extension 'X' Alert

EXCLUDES 1 Not coded here   EXCLUDES 2 Not included here   PDx Primary Diagnosis Only   Manifestation Code

[6] H04.52 Eversion of lacrimal punctum
H04.521 Eversion of right lacrimal punctum
H04.522 Eversion of left lacrimal punctum
H04.523 Eversion of bilateral lacrimal punctum
H04.529 Eversion of unspecified lacrimal punctum
[6] H04.53 Neonatal obstruction of nasolacrimal duct
[EXCLUDES1] *congenital stenosis and stricture of lacrimal duct (Q10.5)*
H04.531 Neonatal obstruction of right nasolacrimal duct [N]
H04.532 Neonatal obstruction of left nasolacrimal duct [N]
H04.533 Neonatal obstruction of bilateral nasolacrimal duct [N]
H04.539 Neonatal obstruction of unspecified nasolacrimal duct [N]
[6] H04.54 Stenosis of lacrimal canaliculi
H04.541 Stenosis of right lacrimal canaliculi
H04.542 Stenosis of left lacrimal canaliculi
H04.543 Stenosis of bilateral lacrimal canaliculi
H04.549 Stenosis of unspecified lacrimal canaliculi
[6] H04.55 Acquired stenosis of nasolacrimal duct
H04.551 Acquired stenosis of right nasolacrimal duct
H04.552 Acquired stenosis of left nasolacrimal duct
H04.553 Acquired stenosis of bilateral nasolacrimal duct
H04.559 Acquired stenosis of unspecified nasolacrimal duct
[6] H04.56 Stenosis of lacrimal punctum
H04.561 Stenosis of right lacrimal punctum
H04.562 Stenosis of left lacrimal punctum
H04.563 Stenosis of bilateral lacrimal punctum
H04.569 Stenosis of unspecified lacrimal punctum
[6] H04.57 Stenosis of lacrimal sac
H04.571 Stenosis of right lacrimal sac
H04.572 Stenosis of left lacrimal sac
H04.573 Stenosis of bilateral lacrimal sac
H04.579 Stenosis of unspecified lacrimal sac
[5] H04.6 Other changes of lacrimal passages
[6] H04.61 Lacrimal fistula
H04.611 Lacrimal fistula right lacrimal passage
H04.612 Lacrimal fistula left lacrimal passage
H04.613 Lacrimal fistula bilateral lacrimal passages
H04.619 Lacrimal fistula unspecified lacrimal passage
H04.69 Other changes of lacrimal passages
[5] H04.8 Other disorders of lacrimal system
[6] H04.81 Granuloma of lacrimal passages
H04.811 Granuloma of right lacrimal passage
H04.812 Granuloma of left lacrimal passage
H04.813 Granuloma of bilateral lacrimal passages
H04.819 Granuloma of unspecified lacrimal passage
H04.89 Other disorders of lacrimal system
H04.9 Disorder of lacrimal system, unspecified
[4] H05 Disorders of orbit
[EXCLUDES1] *congenital malformation of orbit (Q10.7)*
[5] H05.0 Acute inflammation of orbit
H05.00 Unspecified acute inflammation of orbit
[6] H05.01 Cellulitis of orbit
Abscess of orbit
H05.011 Cellulitis of right orbit
H05.012 Cellulitis of left orbit
H05.013 Cellulitis of bilateral orbits
H05.019 Cellulitis of unspecified orbit
[6] H05.02 Osteomyelitis of orbit
H05.021 Osteomyelitis of right orbit
H05.022 Osteomyelitis of left orbit
H05.023 Osteomyelitis of bilateral orbits
H05.029 Osteomyelitis of unspecified orbit
[6] H05.03 Periostitis of orbit
H05.031 Periostitis of right orbit
H05.032 Periostitis of left orbit
H05.033 Periostitis of bilateral orbits
H05.039 Periostitis of unspecified orbit
[6] H05.04 Tenonitis of orbit
H05.041 Tenonitis of right orbit
H05.042 Tenonitis of left orbit
H05.043 Tenonitis of bilateral orbits
H05.049 Tenonitis of unspecified orbit
[5] H05.1 Chronic inflammatory disorders of orbit
H05.10 Unspecified chronic inflammatory disorders of orbit
[6] H05.11 Granuloma of orbit
Pseudotumor (inflammatory) of orbit
H05.111 Granuloma of right orbit
H05.112 Granuloma of left orbit
H05.113 Granuloma of bilateral orbits
H05.119 Granuloma of unspecified orbit
[6] H05.12 Orbital myositis
H05.121 Orbital myositis, right orbit
H05.122 Orbital myositis, left orbit
H05.123 Orbital myositis, bilateral
H05.129 Orbital myositis, unspecified orbit
[5] H05.2 Exophthalmic conditions
H05.20 Unspecified exophthalmos
[6] H05.21 Displacement (lateral) of globe
H05.211 Displacement (lateral) of globe, right eye
H05.212 Displacement (lateral) of globe, left eye
H05.213 Displacement (lateral) of globe, bilateral
H05.219 Displacement (lateral) of globe, unspecified eye
[6] H05.22 Edema of orbit
Orbital congestion
H05.221 Edema of right orbit
H05.222 Edema of left orbit
H05.223 Edema of bilateral orbit
H05.229 Edema of unspecified orbit
[6] H05.23 Hemorrhage of orbit
H05.231 Hemorrhage of right orbit
H05.232 Hemorrhage of left orbit
H05.233 Hemorrhage of bilateral orbit
H05.239 Hemorrhage of unspecified orbit
[6] H05.24 Constant exophthalmos
H05.241 Constant exophthalmos, right eye
H05.242 Constant exophthalmos, left eye
H05.243 Constant exophthalmos, bilateral
H05.249 Constant exophthalmos, unspecified eye
[6] H05.25 Intermittent exophthalmos
H05.251 Intermittent exophthalmos, right eye
H05.252 Intermittent exophthalmos, left eye
H05.253 Intermittent exophthalmos, bilateral
H05.259 Intermittent exophthalmos, unspecified eye
[6] H05.26 Pulsating exophthalmos
H05.261 Pulsating exophthalmos, right eye
H05.262 Pulsating exophthalmos, left eye
H05.263 Pulsating exophthalmos, bilateral
H05.269 Pulsating exophthalmos, unspecified eye
[5] H05.3 Deformity of orbit
[EXCLUDES1] *congenital deformity of orbit (Q10.7)*
hypertelorism (Q75.2)
H05.30 Unspecified deformity of orbit

Unspecified Code | Other Specified Code | [N] Newborn Age: 0 | [P] Pediatric Age: 0-17 | [M] Maternity Age: 12-55
[A] Adult Age: 15-124 | ♂ Male | ♀ Female | ● New Code | ▲ Revised Code Title | ▶◀ Revised Text

[6] H05.31 Atrophy of orbit
H05.311 Atrophy of right orbit
H05.312 Atrophy of left orbit
H05.313 Atrophy of bilateral orbit
H05.319 Atrophy of unspecified orbit
[6] H05.32 Deformity of orbit due to bone disease
Code also associated bone disease
H05.321 Deformity of right orbit due to bone disease
H05.322 Deformity of left orbit due to bone disease
H05.323 Deformity of bilateral orbits due to bone disease
H05.329 Deformity of unspecified orbit due to bone disease
[6] H05.33 Deformity of orbit due to trauma or surgery
H05.331 Deformity of right orbit due to trauma or surgery
H05.332 Deformity of left orbit due to trauma or surgery
H05.333 Deformity of bilateral orbits due to trauma or surgery
H05.339 Deformity of unspecified orbit due to trauma or surgery
[6] H05.34 Enlargement of orbit
H05.341 Enlargement of right orbit
H05.342 Enlargement of left orbit
H05.343 Enlargement of bilateral orbits
H05.349 Enlargement of unspecified orbit
[6] H05.35 Exostosis of orbit
H05.351 Exostosis of right orbit
H05.352 Exostosis of left orbit
H05.353 Exostosis of bilateral orbits
H05.359 Exostosis of unspecified orbit
[5] H05.4 Enophthalmos
[6] H05.40 Unspecified enophthalmos
H05.401 Unspecified enophthalmos, right eye
H05.402 Unspecified enophthalmos, left eye
H05.403 Unspecified enophthalmos, bilateral
H05.409 Unspecified enophthalmos, unspecified eye
[6] H05.41 Enophthalmos due to atrophy of orbital tissue
H05.411 Enophthalmos due to atrophy of orbital tissue, right eye
H05.412 Enophthalmos due to atrophy of orbital tissue, left eye
H05.413 Enophthalmos due to atrophy of orbital tissue, bilateral
H05.419 Enophthalmos due to atrophy of orbital tissue, unspecified eye
[6] H05.42 Enophthalmos due to trauma or surgery
H05.421 Enophthalmos due to trauma or surgery, right eye
H05.422 Enophthalmos due to trauma or surgery, left eye
H05.423 Enophthalmos due to trauma or surgery, bilateral
H05.429 Enophthalmos due to trauma or surgery, unspecified eye
[5] H05.5 Retained (old) foreign body following penetrating wound of orbit
Retrobulbar foreign body
Use additional code to identify the type of retained foreign body (Z18.-)
[EXCLUDES1] *current penetrating wound of orbit (S05.4-)*
[EXCLUDES2] *retained foreign body of eyelid (H02.81-)*
retained intraocular foreign body (H44.6-, H44.7-)
H05.50 Retained (old) foreign body following penetrating wound of unspecified orbit
H05.51 Retained (old) foreign body following penetrating wound of right orbit
H05.52 Retained (old) foreign body following penetrating wound of left orbit
H05.53 Retained (old) foreign body following penetrating wound of bilateral orbits
[5] H05.8 Other disorders of orbit
[6] H05.81 Cyst of orbit
Encephalocele of orbit
H05.811 Cyst of right orbit
H05.812 Cyst of left orbit
H05.813 Cyst of bilateral orbits
H05.819 Cyst of unspecified orbit
[6] H05.82 Myopathy of extraocular muscles
H05.821 Myopathy of extraocular muscles, right orbit
H05.822 Myopathy of extraocular muscles, left orbit
H05.823 Myopathy of extraocular muscles, bilateral
H05.829 Myopathy of extraocular muscles, unspecified orbit
H05.89 Other disorders of orbit
H05.9 Unspecified disorder of orbit

Disorders of conjunctiva (H10-H11)

[4] H10 Conjunctivitis
[EXCLUDES1] *keratoconjunctivitis (H16.2-)*
[5] H10.0 Mucopurulent conjunctivitis
[6] H10.01 Acute follicular conjunctivitis
H10.011 Acute follicular conjunctivitis, right eye
H10.012 Acute follicular conjunctivitis, left eye
H10.013 Acute follicular conjunctivitis, bilateral
H10.019 Acute follicular conjunctivitis, unspecified eye
[6] H10.02 Other mucopurulent conjunctivitis
H10.021 Other mucopurulent conjunctivitis, right eye
H10.022 Other mucopurulent conjunctivitis, left eye
H10.023 Other mucopurulent conjunctivitis, bilateral
H10.029 Other mucopurulent conjunctivitis, unspecified eye
[5] H10.1 Acute atopic conjunctivitis
Acute papillary conjunctivitis
H10.10 Acute atopic conjunctivitis, unspecified eye
H10.11 Acute atopic conjunctivitis, right eye
H10.12 Acute atopic conjunctivitis, left eye
H10.13 Acute atopic conjunctivitis, bilateral
[5] H10.2 Other acute conjunctivitis
[6] H10.21 Acute toxic conjunctivitis
Acute chemical conjunctivitis
Code first (T51-T65) to identify chemical and intent
[EXCLUDES1] *burn and corrosion of eye and adnexa (T26.-)*
H10.211 Acute toxic conjunctivitis, right eye
H10.212 Acute toxic conjunctivitis, left eye
H10.213 Acute toxic conjunctivitis, bilateral
H10.219 Acute toxic conjunctivitis, unspecified eye
[6] H10.22 Pseudomembranous conjunctivitis
H10.221 Pseudomembranous conjunctivitis, right eye
H10.222 Pseudomembranous conjunctivitis, left eye
H10.223 Pseudomembranous conjunctivitis, bilateral
H10.229 Pseudomembranous conjunctivitis, unspecified eye
[6] H10.23 Serous conjunctivitis, except viral
[EXCLUDES1] *viral conjunctivitis (B30.-)*
H10.231 Serous conjunctivitis, except viral, right eye
H10.232 Serous conjunctivitis, except viral, left eye

[4] 4th character required [5] 5th character required [6] 6th character required [7] 7th character required [7th] Extension 'X' Alert
[EXCLUDES1] Not coded here [EXCLUDES2] Not included here [PDx] Primary Diagnosis Only Manifestation Code

H10.233 Serous conjunctivitis, except viral, bilateral
H10.239 Serous conjunctivitis, except viral, unspecified eye

[5] H10.3 Unspecified acute conjunctivitis

EXCLUDES1 *ophthalmia neonatorum NOS (P39.1)*

H10.30 Unspecified acute conjunctivitis, unspecified eye
H10.31 Unspecified acute conjunctivitis, right eye
H10.32 Unspecified acute conjunctivitis, left eye
H10.33 Unspecified acute conjunctivitis, bilateral

[5] H10.4 Chronic conjunctivitis

[6] H10.40 Unspecified chronic conjunctivitis
H10.401 Unspecified chronic conjunctivitis, right eye
H10.402 Unspecified chronic conjunctivitis, left eye
H10.403 Unspecified chronic conjunctivitis, bilateral
H10.409 Unspecified chronic conjunctivitis, unspecified eye

[6] H10.41 Chronic giant papillary conjunctivitis
H10.411 Chronic giant papillary conjunctivitis, right eye
H10.412 Chronic giant papillary conjunctivitis, left eye
H10.413 Chronic giant papillary conjunctivitis, bilateral
H10.419 Chronic giant papillary conjunctivitis, unspecified eye

[6] H10.42 Simple chronic conjunctivitis
H10.421 Simple chronic conjunctivitis, right eye
H10.422 Simple chronic conjunctivitis, left eye
H10.423 Simple chronic conjunctivitis, bilateral
H10.429 Simple chronic conjunctivitis, unspecified eye

[6] H10.43 Chronic follicular conjunctivitis
H10.431 Chronic follicular conjunctivitis, right eye
H10.432 Chronic follicular conjunctivitis, left eye
H10.433 Chronic follicular conjunctivitis, bilateral
H10.439 Chronic follicular conjunctivitis, unspecified eye

H10.44 Vernal conjunctivitis

EXCLUDES1 *vernal keratoconjunctivitis with limbar and corneal involvement (H16.26-)*

H10.45 Other chronic allergic conjunctivitis

[5] H10.5 Blepharoconjunctivitis

[6] H10.50 Unspecified blepharoconjunctivitis
H10.501 Unspecified blepharoconjunctivitis, right eye
H10.502 Unspecified blepharoconjunctivitis, left eye
H10.503 Unspecified blepharoconjunctivitis, bilateral
H10.509 Unspecified blepharoconjunctivitis, unspecified eye

[6] H10.51 Ligneous conjunctivitis
H10.511 Ligneous conjunctivitis, right eye
H10.512 Ligneous conjunctivitis, left eye
H10.513 Ligneous conjunctivitis, bilateral
H10.519 Ligneous conjunctivitis, unspecified eye

[6] H10.52 Angular blepharoconjunctivitis
H10.521 Angular blepharoconjunctivitis, right eye
H10.522 Angular blepharoconjunctivitis, left eye
H10.523 Angular blepharoconjunctivitis, bilateral
H10.529 Angular blepharoconjunctivitis, unspecified eye

[6] H10.53 Contact blepharoconjunctivitis
H10.531 Contact blepharoconjunctivitis, right eye
H10.532 Contact blepharoconjunctivitis, left eye
H10.533 Contact blepharoconjunctivitis, bilateral
H10.539 Contact blepharoconjunctivitis, unspecified eye

[5] H10.8 Other conjunctivitis

[6] H10.81 Pingueculitis

EXCLUDES1 *pinguecula (H11.15-)*

H10.811 Pingueculitis, right eye
H10.812 Pingueculitis, left eye
H10.813 Pingueculitis, bilateral
H10.819 Pingueculitis, unspecified eye

H10.89 Other conjunctivitis

H10.9 Unspecified conjunctivitis

[4] H11 Other disorders of conjunctiva

EXCLUDES1 *keratoconjunctivitis (H16.2-)*

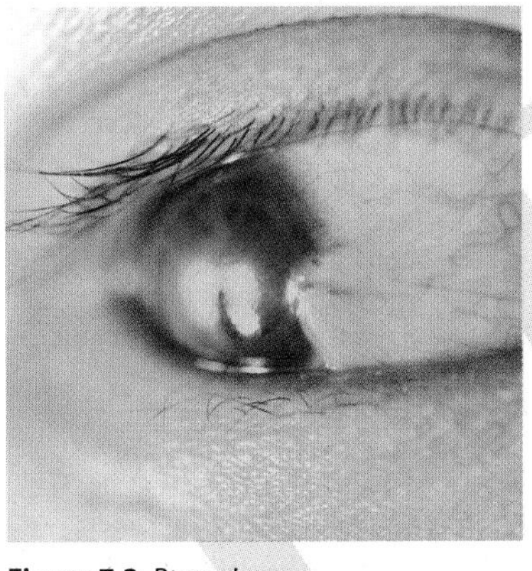

Figure 7.3 Pterygium

[5] H11.0 Pterygium of eye

EXCLUDES1 *pseudopterygium (H11.81-)*

[6] H11.00 Unspecified pterygium of eye
H11.001 Unspecified pterygium of right eye
H11.002 Unspecified pterygium of left eye
H11.003 Unspecified pterygium of eye, bilateral
H11.009 Unspecified pterygium of unspecified eye

[6] H11.01 Amyloid pterygium
H11.011 Amyloid pterygium of right eye
H11.012 Amyloid pterygium of left eye
H11.013 Amyloid pterygium of eye, bilateral
H11.019 Amyloid pterygium of unspecified eye

[6] H11.02 Central pterygium of eye
H11.021 Central pterygium of right eye
H11.022 Central pterygium of left eye
H11.023 Central pterygium of eye, bilateral
H11.029 Central pterygium of unspecified eye

[6] H11.03 Double pterygium of eye
H11.031 Double pterygium of right eye
H11.032 Double pterygium of left eye
H11.033 Double pterygium of eye, bilateral
H11.039 Double pterygium of unspecified eye

[6] H11.04 Peripheral pterygium of eye, stationary
H11.041 Peripheral pterygium, stationary, right eye
H11.042 Peripheral pterygium, stationary, left eye
H11.043 Peripheral pterygium, stationary, bilateral
H11.049 Peripheral pterygium, stationary, unspecified eye

[6] H11.05 Peripheral pterygium of eye, progressive
H11.051 Peripheral pterygium, progressive, right eye
H11.052 Peripheral pterygium, progressive, left eye
H11.053 Peripheral pterygium, progressive, bilateral
H11.059 Peripheral pterygium, progressive, unspecified eye

Unspecified Code | Other Specified Code | [N] Newborn Age: 0 | [P] Pediatric Age: 0-17 | [M] Maternity Age: 12-55
[A] Adult Age: 15-124 | ♂ Male | ♀ Female | ● New Code | ▲ Revised Code Title | ►◄ Revised Text

[6] H11.06 Recurrent pterygium of eye
H11.061 Recurrent pterygium of right eye
H11.062 Recurrent pterygium of left eye
H11.063 Recurrent pterygium of eye, bilateral
H11.069 Recurrent pterygium of unspecified eye

[5] H11.1 Conjunctival degenerations and deposits
EXCLUDES2 *pseudopterygium (H11.81)*
H11.10 Unspecified conjunctival degenerations

[6] H11.11 Conjunctival deposits
H11.111 Conjunctival deposits, right eye
H11.112 Conjunctival deposits, left eye
H11.113 Conjunctival deposits, bilateral
H11.119 Conjunctival deposits, unspecified eye

[6] H11.12 Conjunctival concretions
H11.121 Conjunctival concretions, right eye
H11.122 Conjunctival concretions, left eye
H11.123 Conjunctival concretions, bilateral
H11.129 Conjunctival concretions, unspecified eye

[6] H11.13 Conjunctival pigmentations
Conjunctival argyrosis [argyria]
H11.131 Conjunctival pigmentations, right eye
H11.132 Conjunctival pigmentations, left eye
H11.133 Conjunctival pigmentations, bilateral
H11.139 Conjunctival pigmentations, unspecified eye

[6] H11.14 Conjunctival xerosis, unspecified
EXCLUDES1 *xerosis of conjunctiva due to vitamin A deficiency (E50.0, E50.1)*
H11.141 Conjunctival xerosis, unspecified, right eye
H11.142 Conjunctival xerosis, unspecified, left eye
H11.143 Conjunctival xerosis, unspecified, bilateral
H11.149 Conjunctival xerosis, unspecified, unspecified eye

[6] H11.15 Pinguecula
EXCLUDES1 *pingueculitis (H10.81-)*
H11.151 Pinguecula, right eye
H11.152 Pinguecula, left eye
H11.153 Pinguecula, bilateral
H11.159 Pinguecula, unspecified eye

[5] H11.2 Conjunctival scars

[6] H11.21 Conjunctival adhesions and strands (localized)
H11.211 Conjunctival adhesions and strands (localized), right eye
H11.212 Conjunctival adhesions and strands (localized), left eye
H11.213 Conjunctival adhesions and strands (localized), bilateral
H11.219 Conjunctival adhesions and strands (localized), unspecified eye

[6] H11.22 Conjunctival granuloma
H11.221 Conjunctival granuloma, right eye
H11.222 Conjunctival granuloma, left eye
H11.223 Conjunctival granuloma, bilateral
H11.229 Conjunctival granuloma, unspecified

[6] H11.23 Symblepharon
H11.231 Symblepharon, right eye
H11.232 Symblepharon, left eye
H11.233 Symblepharon, bilateral
H11.239 Symblepharon, unspecified eye

[6] H11.24 Scarring of conjunctiva
H11.241 Scarring of conjunctiva, right eye
H11.242 Scarring of conjunctiva, left eye
H11.243 Scarring of conjunctiva, bilateral
H11.249 Scarring of conjunctiva, unspecified eye

[5] H11.3 Conjunctival hemorrhage
Subconjunctival hemorrhage
H11.30 Conjunctival hemorrhage, unspecified eye
H11.31 Conjunctival hemorrhage, right eye
H11.32 Conjunctival hemorrhage, left eye
H11.33 Conjunctival hemorrhage, bilateral

[5] H11.4 Other conjunctival vascular disorders and cysts

[6] H11.41 Vascular abnormalities of conjunctiva
Conjunctival aneurysm
H11.411 Vascular abnormalities of conjunctiva, right eye
H11.412 Vascular abnormalities of conjunctiva, left eye
H11.413 Vascular abnormalities of conjunctiva, bilateral
H11.419 Vascular abnormalities of conjunctiva, unspecified eye

[6] H11.42 Conjunctival edema
H11.421 Conjunctival edema, right eye
H11.422 Conjunctival edema, left eye
H11.423 Conjunctival edema, bilateral
H11.429 Conjunctival edema, unspecified eye

[6] H11.43 Conjunctival hyperemia
H11.431 Conjunctival hyperemia, right eye
H11.432 Conjunctival hyperemia, left eye
H11.433 Conjunctival hyperemia, bilateral
H11.439 Conjunctival hyperemia, unspecified eye

[6] H11.44 Conjunctival cysts
H11.441 Conjunctival cysts, right eye
H11.442 Conjunctival cysts, left eye
H11.443 Conjunctival cysts, bilateral
H11.449 Conjunctival cysts, unspecified eye

[5] H11.8 Other specified disorders of conjunctiva

[6] H11.81 Pseudopterygium of conjunctiva
H11.811 Pseudopterygium of conjunctiva, right eye
H11.812 Pseudopterygium of conjunctiva, left eye
H11.813 Pseudopterygium of conjunctiva, bilateral
H11.819 Pseudopterygium of conjunctiva, unspecified eye

[6] H11.82 Conjunctivochalasis
H11.821 Conjunctivochalasis, right eye
H11.822 Conjunctivochalasis, left eye
H11.823 Conjunctivochalasis, bilateral
H11.829 Conjunctivochalasis, unspecified eye
H11.89 Other specified disorders of conjunctiva
H11.9 Unspecified disorder of conjunctiva

Disorders of sclera, cornea, iris and ciliary body (H15-H22)

[4] H15 Disorders of sclera

[5] H15.0 Scleritis

[6] H15.00 Unspecified scleritis
H15.001 Unspecified scleritis, right eye
H15.002 Unspecified scleritis, left eye
H15.003 Unspecified scleritis, bilateral
H15.009 Unspecified scleritis, unspecified eye

[6] H15.01 Anterior scleritis
H15.011 Anterior scleritis, right eye
H15.012 Anterior scleritis, left eye
H15.013 Anterior scleritis, bilateral
H15.019 Anterior scleritis, unspecified eye

[6] H15.02 Brawny scleritis
H15.021 Brawny scleritis, right eye
H15.022 Brawny scleritis, left eye
H15.023 Brawny scleritis, bilateral
H15.029 Brawny scleritis, unspecified eye

[6] H15.03 Posterior scleritis
Sclerotenonitis

[4] 4th character required [5] 5th character required [6] 6th character required [7] 7th character required [X] Extension 'X' Alert
EXCLUDES1 Not coded here EXCLUDES2 Not included here [PDx] Primary Diagnosis Only Manifestation Code

H15.031 Posterior scleritis, right eye
H15.032 Posterior scleritis, left eye
H15.033 Posterior scleritis, bilateral
H15.039 Posterior scleritis, unspecified eye
[6] H15.04 Scleritis with corneal involvement
H15.041 Scleritis with corneal involvement, right eye
H15.042 Scleritis with corneal involvement, left eye
H15.043 Scleritis with corneal involvement, bilateral
H15.049 Scleritis with corneal involvement, unspecified eye
[6] H15.05 Scleromalacia perforans
H15.051 Scleromalacia perforans, right eye
H15.052 Scleromalacia perforans, left eye
H15.053 Scleromalacia perforans, bilateral
H15.059 Scleromalacia perforans, unspecified eye
[6] H15.09 Other scleritis
Scleral abscess
H15.091 Other scleritis, right eye
H15.092 Other scleritis, left eye
H15.093 Other scleritis, bilateral
H15.099 Other scleritis, unspecified eye
[5] H15.1 Episcleritis
[6] H15.10 Unspecified episcleritis
H15.101 Unspecified episcleritis, right eye
H15.102 Unspecified episcleritis, left eye
H15.103 Unspecified episcleritis, bilateral
H15.109 Unspecified episcleritis, unspecified eye
[6] H15.11 Episcleritis periodica fugax
H15.111 Episcleritis periodica fugax, right eye
H15.112 Episcleritis periodica fugax, left eye
H15.113 Episcleritis periodica fugax, bilateral
H15.119 Episcleritis periodica fugax, unspecified eye
[6] H15.12 Nodular episcleritis
H15.121 Nodular episcleritis, right eye
H15.122 Nodular episcleritis, left eye
H15.123 Nodular episcleritis, bilateral
H15.129 Nodular episcleritis, unspecified eye
[5] H15.8 Other disorders of sclera
[EXCLUDES2] *blue sclera (Q13.5)*
degenerative myopia (H44.2-)
[6] H15.81 Equatorial staphyloma
H15.811 Equatorial staphyloma, right eye
H15.812 Equatorial staphyloma, left eye
H15.813 Equatorial staphyloma, bilateral
H15.819 Equatorial staphyloma, unspecified eye
[6] H15.82 Localized anterior staphyloma
H15.821 Localized anterior staphyloma, right eye
H15.822 Localized anterior staphyloma, left eye
H15.823 Localized anterior staphyloma, bilateral
H15.829 Localized anterior staphyloma, unspecified eye
[6] H15.83 Staphyloma posticum
H15.831 Staphyloma posticum, right eye
H15.832 Staphyloma posticum, left eye
H15.833 Staphyloma posticum, bilateral
H15.839 Staphyloma posticum, unspecified eye
[6] H15.84 Scleral ectasia
H15.841 Scleral ectasia, right eye
H15.842 Scleral ectasia, left eye
H15.843 Scleral ectasia, bilateral
H15.849 Scleral ectasia, unspecified eye
[6] H15.85 Ring staphyloma
H15.851 Ring staphyloma, right eye
H15.852 Ring staphyloma, left eye
H15.853 Ring staphyloma, bilateral
H15.859 Ring staphyloma, unspecified eye
H15.89 Other disorders of sclera
H15.9 Unspecified disorder of sclera
[4] H16 Keratitis
[5] H16.0 Corneal ulcer
[6] H16.00 Unspecified corneal ulcer
H16.001 Unspecified corneal ulcer, right eye
H16.002 Unspecified corneal ulcer, left eye
H16.003 Unspecified corneal ulcer, bilateral
H16.009 Unspecified corneal ulcer, unspecified eye
[6] H16.01 Central corneal ulcer
H16.011 Central corneal ulcer, right eye
H16.012 Central corneal ulcer, left eye
H16.013 Central corneal ulcer, bilateral
H16.019 Central corneal ulcer, unspecified eye
[6] H16.02 Ring corneal ulcer
H16.021 Ring corneal ulcer, right eye
H16.022 Ring corneal ulcer, left eye
H16.023 Ring corneal ulcer, bilateral
H16.029 Ring corneal ulcer, unspecified eye
[6] H16.03 Corneal ulcer with hypopyon
H16.031 Corneal ulcer with hypopyon, right eye
H16.032 Corneal ulcer with hypopyon, left eye
H16.033 Corneal ulcer with hypopyon, bilateral
H16.039 Corneal ulcer with hypopyon, unspecified eye
[6] H16.04 Marginal corneal ulcer
H16.041 Marginal corneal ulcer, right eye
H16.042 Marginal corneal ulcer, left eye
H16.043 Marginal corneal ulcer, bilateral
H16.049 Marginal corneal ulcer, unspecified eye
[6] H16.05 Mooren's corneal ulcer
H16.051 Mooren's corneal ulcer, right eye
H16.052 Mooren's corneal ulcer, left eye
H16.053 Mooren's corneal ulcer, bilateral
H16.059 Mooren's corneal ulcer, unspecified eye
[6] H16.06 Mycotic corneal ulcer
H16.061 Mycotic corneal ulcer, right eye
H16.062 Mycotic corneal ulcer, left eye
H16.063 Mycotic corneal ulcer, bilateral
H16.069 Mycotic corneal ulcer, unspecified eye
[6] H16.07 Perforated corneal ulcer
H16.071 Perforated corneal ulcer, right eye
H16.072 Perforated corneal ulcer, left eye
H16.073 Perforated corneal ulcer, bilateral
H16.079 Perforated corneal ulcer, unspecified eye
[5] H16.1 Other and unspecified superficial keratitis without conjunctivitis
[6] H16.10 Unspecified superficial keratitis
H16.101 Unspecified superficial keratitis, right eye
H16.102 Unspecified superficial keratitis, left eye
H16.103 Unspecified superficial keratitis, bilateral
H16.109 Unspecified superficial keratitis, unspecified eye
[6] H16.11 Macular keratitis
Areolar keratitis
Nummular keratitis
Stellate keratitis
Striate keratitis
H16.111 Macular keratitis, right eye
H16.112 Macular keratitis, left eye
H16.113 Macular keratitis, bilateral
H16.119 Macular keratitis, unspecified eye
[6] H16.12 Filamentary keratitis
H16.121 Filamentary keratitis, right eye
H16.122 Filamentary keratitis, left eye

Unspecified Code | Other Specified Code | [N] Newborn Age: 0 | [P] Pediatric Age: 0-17 | [M] Maternity Age: 12-55
[A] Adult Age: 15-124 | ♂ Male | ♀ Female | ● New Code | ▲ Revised Code Title | ►◄ Revised Text

⑥ H16.123 Filamentary keratitis, bilateral
H16.129 Filamentary keratitis, unspecified eye
⑥ H16.13 Photokeratitis
Snow blindness
Welders keratitis
H16.131 Photokeratitis, right eye
H16.132 Photokeratitis, left eye
H16.133 Photokeratitis, bilateral
H16.139 Photokeratitis, unspecified eye
⑥ H16.14 Punctate keratitis
H16.141 Punctate keratitis, right eye
H16.142 Punctate keratitis, left eye
H16.143 Punctate keratitis, bilateral
H16.149 Punctate keratitis, unspecified eye
⑤ H16.2 Keratoconjunctivitis
⑥ H16.20 Unspecified keratoconjunctivitis
Superficial keratitis with conjunctivitis NOS
H16.201 Unspecified keratoconjunctivitis, right eye
H16.202 Unspecified keratoconjunctivitis, left eye
H16.203 Unspecified keratoconjunctivitis, bilateral
H16.209 Unspecified keratoconjunctivitis, unspecified eye
⑥ H16.21 Exposure keratoconjunctivitis
H16.211 Exposure keratoconjunctivitis, right eye
H16.212 Exposure keratoconjunctivitis, left eye
H16.213 Exposure keratoconjunctivitis, bilateral
H16.219 Exposure keratoconjunctivitis, unspecified eye
⑥ H16.22 Keratoconjunctivitis sicca, not specified as Sjögren's
EXCLUDES1 Sjögren's syndrome (M35.01)
H16.221 Keratoconjunctivitis sicca, not specified as Sjögren's, right eye
H16.222 Keratoconjunctivitis sicca, not specified as Sjögren's, left eye
H16.223 Keratoconjunctivitis sicca, not specified as Sjögren's, bilateral
H16.229 Keratoconjunctivitis sicca, not specified as Sjögren's, unspecified eye
⑥ H16.23 Neurotrophic keratoconjunctivitis
H16.231 Neurotrophic keratoconjunctivitis, right eye
H16.232 Neurotrophic keratoconjunctivitis, left eye
H16.233 Neurotrophic keratoconjunctivitis, bilateral
H16.239 Neurotrophic keratoconjunctivitis, unspecified eye
⑥ H16.24 Ophthalmia nodosa
H16.241 Ophthalmia nodosa, right eye
H16.242 Ophthalmia nodosa, left eye
H16.243 Ophthalmia nodosa, bilateral
H16.249 Ophthalmia nodosa, unspecified eye
⑥ H16.25 Phlyctenular keratoconjunctivitis
H16.251 Phlyctenular keratoconjunctivitis, right eye
H16.252 Phlyctenular keratoconjunctivitis, left eye
H16.253 Phlyctenular keratoconjunctivitis, bilateral
H16.259 Phlyctenular keratoconjunctivitis, unspecified eye
⑥ H16.26 Vernal keratoconjunctivitis, with limbar and corneal involvement
EXCLUDES1 vernal conjunctivitis without limbar and corneal involvement (H10.44)
H16.261 Vernal keratoconjunctivitis, with limbar and corneal involvement, right eye
H16.262 Vernal keratoconjunctivitis, with limbar and corneal involvement, left eye
H16.263 Vernal keratoconjunctivitis, with limbar and corneal involvement, bilateral

H16.269 Vernal keratoconjunctivitis, with limbar and corneal involvement, unspecified eye
⑥ H16.29 Other keratoconjunctivitis
H16.291 Other keratoconjunctivitis, right eye
H16.292 Other keratoconjunctivitis, left eye
H16.293 Other keratoconjunctivitis, bilateral
H16.299 Other keratoconjunctivitis, unspecified eye
⑤ H16.3 Interstitial and deep keratitis
⑥ H16.30 Unspecified interstitial keratitis
H16.301 Unspecified interstitial keratitis, right eye
H16.302 Unspecified interstitial keratitis, left eye
H16.303 Unspecified interstitial keratitis, bilateral
H16.309 Unspecified interstitial keratitis, unspecified eye
⑥ H16.31 Corneal abscess
H16.311 Corneal abscess, right eye
H16.312 Corneal abscess, left eye
H16.313 Corneal abscess, bilateral
H16.319 Corneal abscess, unspecified eye
⑥ H16.32 Diffuse interstitial keratitis
Cogan's syndrome
H16.321 Diffuse interstitial keratitis, right eye
H16.322 Diffuse interstitial keratitis, left eye
H16.323 Diffuse interstitial keratitis, bilateral
H16.329 Diffuse interstitial keratitis, unspecified eye
⑥ H16.33 Sclerosing keratitis
H16.331 Sclerosing keratitis, right eye
H16.332 Sclerosing keratitis, left eye
H16.333 Sclerosing keratitis, bilateral
H16.339 Sclerosing keratitis, unspecified eye
⑥ H16.39 Other interstitial and deep keratitis
H16.391 Other interstitial and deep keratitis, right eye
H16.392 Other interstitial and deep keratitis, left eye
H16.393 Other interstitial and deep keratitis, bilateral
H16.399 Other interstitial and deep keratitis, unspecified eye
⑤ H16.4 Corneal neovascularization
⑥ H16.40 Unspecified corneal neovascularization
H16.401 Unspecified corneal neovascularization, right eye
H16.402 Unspecified corneal neovascularization, left eye
H16.403 Unspecified corneal neovascularization, bilateral
H16.409 Unspecified corneal neovascularization, unspecified eye
⑥ H16.41 Ghost vessels (corneal)
H16.411 Ghost vessels (corneal), right eye
H16.412 Ghost vessels (corneal), left eye
H16.413 Ghost vessels (corneal), bilateral
H16.419 Ghost vessels (corneal), unspecified eye
⑥ H16.42 Pannus (corneal)
H16.421 Pannus (corneal), right eye
H16.422 Pannus (corneal), left eye
H16.423 Pannus (corneal), bilateral
H16.429 Pannus (corneal), unspecified eye
⑥ H16.43 Localized vascularization of cornea
H16.431 Localized vascularization of cornea, right eye
H16.432 Localized vascularization of cornea, left eye
H16.433 Localized vascularization of cornea, bilateral
H16.439 Localized vascularization of cornea, unspecified eye
⑥ H16.44 Deep vascularization of cornea

---

④ 4th character required   ⑤ 5th character required   ⑥ 6th character required   ⑦ 7th character required   ⑰ Extension 'X' Alert

EXCLUDES 1 Not coded here   EXCLUDES 2 Not included here   PDx Primary Diagnosis Only   Manifestation Code

H16.441 Deep vascularization of cornea, right eye
H16.442 Deep vascularization of cornea, left eye
H16.443 Deep vascularization of cornea, bilateral
H16.449 Deep vascularization of cornea, unspecified eye
H16.8 Other keratitis
H16.9 Unspecified keratitis

[4] H17 Corneal scars and opacities
[5] H17.0 Adherent leukoma
H17.00 Adherent leukoma, unspecified eye
H17.01 Adherent leukoma, right eye
H17.02 Adherent leukoma, left eye
H17.03 Adherent leukoma, bilateral
[5] H17.1 Central corneal opacity
H17.10 Central corneal opacity, unspecified eye
H17.11 Central corneal opacity, right eye
H17.12 Central corneal opacity, left eye
H17.13 Central corneal opacity, bilateral
[5] H17.8 Other corneal scars and opacities
[6] H17.81 Minor opacity of cornea
Corneal nebula
H17.811 Minor opacity of cornea, right eye
H17.812 Minor opacity of cornea, left eye
H17.813 Minor opacity of cornea, bilateral
H17.819 Minor opacity of cornea, unspecified eye
[6] H17.82 Peripheral opacity of cornea
H17.821 Peripheral opacity of cornea, right eye
H17.822 Peripheral opacity of cornea, left eye
H17.823 Peripheral opacity of cornea, bilateral
H17.829 Peripheral opacity of cornea, unspecified eye
H17.89 Other corneal scars and opacities
H17.9 Unspecified corneal scar and opacity

[4] H18 Other disorders of cornea
[5] H18.0 Corneal pigmentations and deposits
[6] H18.00 Unspecified corneal deposit
H18.001 Unspecified corneal deposit, right eye
H18.002 Unspecified corneal deposit, left eye
H18.003 Unspecified corneal deposit, bilateral
H18.009 Unspecified corneal deposit, unspecified eye
[6] H18.01 Anterior corneal pigmentations
Staehli's line
H18.011 Anterior corneal pigmentations, right eye
H18.012 Anterior corneal pigmentations, left eye
H18.013 Anterior corneal pigmentations, bilateral
H18.019 Anterior corneal pigmentations, unspecified eye
[6] H18.02 Argentous corneal deposits
H18.021 Argentous corneal deposits, right eye
H18.022 Argentous corneal deposits, left eye
H18.023 Argentous corneal deposits, bilateral
H18.029 Argentous corneal deposits, unspecified eye
[6] H18.03 Corneal deposits in metabolic disorders
Code also associated metabolic disorder
H18.031 Corneal deposits in metabolic disorders, right eye
H18.032 Corneal deposits in metabolic disorders, left eye
H18.033 Corneal deposits in metabolic disorders, bilateral
H18.039 Corneal deposits in metabolic disorders, unspecified eye
[6] H18.04 Kayser-Fleischer ring
Code also associated Wilson's disease (E83.01)
H18.041 Kayser-Fleischer ring, right eye
H18.042 Kayser-Fleischer ring, left eye
H18.043 Kayser-Fleischer ring, bilateral
H18.049 Kayser-Fleischer ring, unspecified eye
[6] H18.05 Posterior corneal pigmentations
Krukenberg's spindle
H18.051 Posterior corneal pigmentations, right eye
H18.052 Posterior corneal pigmentations, left eye
H18.053 Posterior corneal pigmentations, bilateral
H18.059 Posterior corneal pigmentations, unspecified eye
[6] H18.06 Stromal corneal pigmentations
Hematocornea
H18.061 Stromal corneal pigmentations, right eye
H18.062 Stromal corneal pigmentations, left eye
H18.063 Stromal corneal pigmentations, bilateral
H18.069 Stromal corneal pigmentations, unspecified eye
[5] H18.1 Bullous keratopathy
H18.10 Bullous keratopathy, unspecified eye
H18.11 Bullous keratopathy, right eye
H18.12 Bullous keratopathy, left eye
H18.13 Bullous keratopathy, bilateral
[5] H18.2 Other and unspecified corneal edema
H18.20 Unspecified corneal edema
[6] H18.21 Corneal edema secondary to contact lens
[EXCLUDES2] *other corneal disorders due to contact lens (H18.82-)*
H18.211 Corneal edema secondary to contact lens, right eye
H18.212 Corneal edema secondary to contact lens, left eye
H18.213 Corneal edema secondary to contact lens, bilateral
H18.219 Corneal edema secondary to contact lens, unspecified eye
[6] H18.22 Idiopathic corneal edema
H18.221 Idiopathic corneal edema, right eye
H18.222 Idiopathic corneal edema, left eye
H18.223 Idiopathic corneal edema, bilateral
H18.229 Idiopathic corneal edema, unspecified eye
[6] H18.23 Secondary corneal edema
H18.231 Secondary corneal edema, right eye
H18.232 Secondary corneal edema, left eye
H18.233 Secondary corneal edema, bilateral
H18.239 Secondary corneal edema, unspecified eye
[5] H18.3 Changes of corneal membranes
H18.30 Unspecified corneal membrane change
[6] H18.31 Folds and rupture in Bowman's membrane
H18.311 Folds and rupture in Bowman's membrane, right eye
H18.312 Folds and rupture in Bowman's membrane, left eye
H18.313 Folds and rupture in Bowman's membrane, bilateral
H18.319 Folds and rupture in Bowman's membrane, unspecified eye
[6] H18.32 Folds in Descemet's membrane
H18.321 Folds in Descemet's membrane, right eye
H18.322 Folds in Descemet's membrane, left eye
H18.323 Folds in Descemet's membrane, bilateral
H18.329 Folds in Descemet's membrane, unspecified eye
[6] H18.33 Rupture in Descemet's membrane
H18.331 Rupture in Descemet's membrane, right eye
H18.332 Rupture in Descemet's membrane, left eye
H18.333 Rupture in Descemet's membrane, bilateral

Unspecified Code | Other Specified Code | [N] Newborn Age: 0 | [P] Pediatric Age: 0-17 | [M] Maternity Age: 12-55
[A] Adult Age: 15-124 | ♂ Male | ♀ Female | ● New Code | ▲ Revised Code Title | ►◄ Revised Text

H18.339 Rupture in Descemet's membrane, unspecified eye

[5] H18.4 Corneal degeneration

[EXCLUDES1] *Mooren's ulcer (H16.0-)*
recurrent erosion of cornea (H18.83-)

H18.40 Unspecified corneal degeneration

[6] H18.41 Arcus senilis

Senile corneal changes

H18.411 Arcus senilis, right eye
H18.412 Arcus senilis, left eye
H18.413 Arcus senilis, bilateral
H18.419 Arcus senilis, unspecified eye

[6] H18.42 Band keratopathy

H18.421 Band keratopathy, right eye
H18.422 Band keratopathy, left eye
H18.423 Band keratopathy, bilateral
H18.429 Band keratopathy, unspecified eye

H18.43 Other calcerous corneal degeneration

[6] H18.44 Keratomalacia

[EXCLUDES1] *keratomalacia due to vitamin A deficiency (E50.4)*

H18.441 Keratomalacia, right eye
H18.442 Keratomalacia, left eye
H18.443 Keratomalacia, bilateral
H18.449 Keratomalacia, unspecified eye

[6] H18.45 Nodular corneal degeneration

H18.451 Nodular corneal degeneration, right eye
H18.452 Nodular corneal degeneration, left eye
H18.453 Nodular corneal degeneration, bilateral
H18.459 Nodular corneal degeneration, unspecified eye

[6] H18.46 Peripheral corneal degeneration

H18.461 Peripheral corneal degeneration, right eye
H18.462 Peripheral corneal degeneration, left eye
H18.463 Peripheral corneal degeneration, bilateral
H18.469 Peripheral corneal degeneration, unspecified eye

H18.49 Other corneal degeneration

[5] H18.5 Hereditary corneal dystrophies

H18.50 Unspecified hereditary corneal dystrophies
H18.51 Endothelial corneal dystrophy

Fuchs' dystrophy

H18.52 Epithelial (juvenile) corneal dystrophy
H18.53 Granular corneal dystrophy
H18.54 Lattice corneal dystrophy
H18.55 Macular corneal dystrophy
H18.59 Other hereditary corneal dystrophies

[5] H18.6 Keratoconus

[6] H18.60 Keratoconus, unspecified

H18.601 Keratoconus, unspecified, right eye
H18.602 Keratoconus, unspecified, left eye
H18.603 Keratoconus, unspecified, bilateral
H18.609 Keratoconus, unspecified, unspecified eye

[6] H18.61 Keratoconus, stable

H18.611 Keratoconus, stable, right eye
H18.612 Keratoconus, stable, left eye
H18.613 Keratoconus, stable, bilateral
H18.619 Keratoconus, stable, unspecified eye

[6] H18.62 Keratoconus, unstable

Acute hydrops

H18.621 Keratoconus, unstable, right eye
H18.622 Keratoconus, unstable, left eye
H18.623 Keratoconus, unstable, bilateral
H18.629 Keratoconus, unstable, unspecified eye

[5] H18.7 Other and unspecified corneal deformities

[EXCLUDES1] *congenital malformations of cornea (Q13.3-Q13.4)*

H18.70 Unspecified corneal deformity

[6] H18.71 Corneal ectasia

H18.711 Corneal ectasia, right eye
H18.712 Corneal ectasia, left eye
H18.713 Corneal ectasia, bilateral
H18.719 Corneal ectasia, unspecified eye

[6] H18.72 Corneal staphyloma

H18.721 Corneal staphyloma, right eye
H18.722 Corneal staphyloma, left eye
H18.723 Corneal staphyloma, bilateral
H18.729 Corneal staphyloma, unspecified eye

[6] H18.73 Descemetocele

H18.731 Descemetocele, right eye
H18.732 Descemetocele, left eye
H18.733 Descemetocele, bilateral
H18.739 Descemetocele, unspecified eye

[6] H18.79 Other corneal deformities

H18.791 Other corneal deformities, right eye
H18.792 Other corneal deformities, left eye
H18.793 Other corneal deformities, bilateral
H18.799 Other corneal deformities, unspecified eye

[5] H18.8 Other specified disorders of cornea

[6] H18.81 Anesthesia and hypoesthesia of cornea

H18.811 Anesthesia and hypoesthesia of cornea, right eye
H18.812 Anesthesia and hypoesthesia of cornea, left eye
H18.813 Anesthesia and hypoesthesia of cornea, bilateral
H18.819 Anesthesia and hypoesthesia of cornea, unspecified eye

[6] H18.82 Corneal disorder due to contact lens

[EXCLUDES2] *corneal edema due to contact lens (H18.21-)*

H18.821 Corneal disorder due to contact lens, right eye
H18.822 Corneal disorder due to contact lens, left eye
H18.823 Corneal disorder due to contact lens, bilateral
H18.829 Corneal disorder due to contact lens, unspecified eye

[6] H18.83 Recurrent erosion of cornea

H18.831 Recurrent erosion of cornea, right eye
H18.832 Recurrent erosion of cornea, left eye
H18.833 Recurrent erosion of cornea, bilateral
H18.839 Recurrent erosion of cornea, unspecified eye

[6] H18.89 Other specified disorders of cornea

H18.891 Other specified disorders of cornea, right eye
H18.892 Other specified disorders of cornea, left eye
H18.893 Other specified disorders of cornea, bilateral
H18.899 Other specified disorders of cornea, unspecified eye

H18.9 Unspecified disorder of cornea

[4] H20 Iridocyclitis

[5] H20.0 Acute and subacute iridocyclitis

Acute anterior uveitis
Acute cyclitis

[4] 4th character required [5] 5th character required [6] 6th character required [7] 7th character required [7] Extension 'X' Alert
[EXCLUDES1] Not coded here [EXCLUDES2] Not included here [PDx] Primary Diagnosis Only Manifestation Code

Acute iritis

Subacute anterior uveitis

Subacute cyclitis

Subacute iritis

EXCLUDES1 *iridocyclitis, iritis, uveitis (due to) (in) diabetes mellitus (E08-E13 with .39)*

iridocyclitis, iritis, uveitis (due to) (in) diphtheria (A36.89)

iridocyclitis, iritis, uveitis (due to) (in) gonococcal (A54.32)

iridocyclitis, iritis, uveitis (due to) (in) herpes (simplex) (B00.51)

iridocyclitis, iritis, uveitis (due to) (in) herpes zoster (B02.32)

iridocyclitis, iritis, uveitis (due to) (in) late congenital syphilis (A50.39)

iridocyclitis, iritis, uveitis (due to) (in) late syphilis (A52.71)

iridocyclitis, iritis, uveitis (due to) (in) sarcoidosis (D86.83)

iridocyclitis, iritis, uveitis (due to) (in) syphilis (A51.43)

iridocyclitis, iritis, uveitis (due to) (in) toxoplasmosis (B58.09)

iridocyclitis, iritis, uveitis (due to) (in) tuberculosis (A18.54)

    H20.00 Unspecified acute and subacute iridocyclitis

6️⃣ **H20.01 Primary iridocyclitis**

    H20.011 Primary iridocyclitis, right **eye**

    H20.012 Primary iridocyclitis, left **eye**

    H20.013 Primary iridocyclitis, bilateral

    H20.019 Primary iridocyclitis, unspecified eye

6️⃣ **H20.02 Recurrent acute iridocyclitis**

    H20.021 Recurrent acute iridocyclitis, right **eye**

    H20.022 Recurrent acute iridocyclitis, left **eye**

    H20.023 Recurrent acute iridocyclitis, bilateral

    H20.029 Recurrent acute iridocyclitis, unspecified eye

6️⃣ **H20.03 Secondary infectious iridocyclitis**

    H20.031 Secondary infectious iridocyclitis, right **eye**

    H20.032 Secondary infectious iridocyclitis, left **eye**

    H20.033 Secondary infectious iridocyclitis, bilateral

    H20.039 Secondary infectious iridocyclitis, unspecified eye

6️⃣ **H20.04 Secondary noninfectious iridocyclitis**

    H20.041 Secondary noninfectious iridocyclitis, right **eye**

    H20.042 Secondary noninfectious iridocyclitis, left **eye**

    H20.043 Secondary noninfectious iridocyclitis, bilateral

    H20.049 Secondary noninfectious iridocyclitis, unspecified eye

6️⃣ **H20.05 Hypopyon**

    H20.051 Hypopyon, right **eye**

    H20.052 Hypopyon, left **eye**

    H20.053 Hypopyon, bilateral

    H20.059 Hypopyon, unspecified eye

5️⃣ **H20.1 Chronic iridocyclitis**

    Use additional code for any associated cataract (H26.21-)

    EXCLUDES2 *posterior cyclitis (H30.2-)*

    H20.10 Chronic iridocyclitis, unspecified eye

    H20.11 Chronic iridocyclitis, right **eye**

    H20.12 Chronic iridocyclitis, left **eye**

    H20.13 Chronic iridocyclitis, bilateral

5️⃣ **H20.2 Lens-induced iridocyclitis**

    H20.20 Lens-induced iridocyclitis, unspecified eye

    H20.21 Lens-induced iridocyclitis, right **eye**

    H20.22 Lens-induced iridocyclitis, left **eye**

    H20.23 Lens-induced iridocyclitis, bilateral

5️⃣ **H20.8 Other iridocyclitis**

    EXCLUDES2 *glaucomatocyclitis crises (H40.4-)*

posterior cyclitis (H30.2-)

sympathetic uveitis (H44.13-)

6️⃣ **H20.81 Fuchs' heterochromic cyclitis**

    H20.811 Fuchs' heterochromic cyclitis, right **eye**

    H20.812 Fuchs' heterochromic cyclitis, left **eye**

    H20.813 Fuchs' heterochromic cyclitis, bilateral

    H20.819 Fuchs' heterochromic cyclitis, unspecified eye

6️⃣ **H20.82 Vogt-Koyanagi syndrome**

    H20.821 Vogt-Koyanagi syndrome, right **eye**

    H20.822 Vogt-Koyanagi syndrome, left **eye**

    H20.823 Vogt-Koyanagi syndrome, bilateral

    H20.829 Vogt-Koyanagi syndrome, unspecified eye

H20.9 Unspecified iridocyclitis

    Uveitis NOS

4️⃣ **H21 Other disorders of iris and ciliary body**

    EXCLUDES2 *sympathetic uveitis (H44.1-)*

5️⃣ **H21.0 Hyphema**

    EXCLUDES1 *traumatic hyphema (S05.1-)*

    H21.00 Hyphema, unspecified eye

    H21.01 Hyphema, right **eye**

    H21.02 Hyphema, left **eye**

    H21.03 Hyphema, bilateral

5️⃣ **H21.1 Other vascular disorders of iris and ciliary body**

    Neovascularization of iris or ciliary body

    Rubeosis iridis

    Rubeosis of iris

6️⃣ **H21.1X Other vascular disorders of iris and ciliary body**

    H21.1X1 Other vascular disorders of iris and ciliary body, right **eye**

    H21.1X2 Other vascular disorders of iris and ciliary body, left **eye**

    H21.1X3 Other vascular disorders of iris and ciliary body, bilateral

    H21.1X9 Other vascular disorders of iris and ciliary body, unspecified eye

5️⃣ **H21.2 Degeneration of iris and ciliary body**

6️⃣ **H21.21 Degeneration of chamber angle**

    H21.211 Degeneration of chamber angle, right **eye**

    H21.212 Degeneration of chamber angle, left **eye**

    H21.213 Degeneration of chamber angle, bilateral

    H21.219 Degeneration of chamber angle, unspecified eye

6️⃣ **H21.22 Degeneration of ciliary body**

    H21.221 Degeneration of ciliary body, right **eye**

    H21.222 Degeneration of ciliary body, left **eye**

    H21.223 Degeneration of ciliary body, bilateral

    H21.229 Degeneration of ciliary body, unspecified eye

6️⃣ **H21.23 Degeneration of iris (pigmentary)**

    Translucency of iris

    H21.231 Degeneration of iris (pigmentary), right **eye**

    H21.232 Degeneration of iris (pigmentary), left **eye**

    H21.233 Degeneration of iris (pigmentary), bilateral

    H21.239 Degeneration of iris (pigmentary), unspecified eye

6️⃣ **H21.24 Degeneration of pupillary margin**

    H21.241 Degeneration of pupillary margin, right **eye**

    H21.242 Degeneration of pupillary margin, left **eye**

    H21.243 Degeneration of pupillary margin, bilateral

    H21.249 Degeneration of pupillary margin, unspecified eye

6️⃣ **H21.25 Iridoschisis**

Unspecified Code	Other Specified Code	N Newborn Age: 0	P Pediatric Age: 0-17	M Maternity Age: 12-55
A Adult Age: 15-124	♂ Male	♀ Female	● New Code	▲ Revised Code Title	▶◀ Revised Text

H21.251 Iridoschisis, right eye
H21.252 Iridoschisis, left eye
H21.253 Iridoschisis, bilateral
H21.259 Iridoschisis, unspecified eye

[6] H21.26 Iris atrophy (essential) (progressive)
H21.261 Iris atrophy (essential) (progressive), right eye
H21.262 Iris atrophy (essential) (progressive), left eye
H21.263 Iris atrophy (essential) (progressive), bilateral
H21.269 Iris atrophy (essential) (progressive), unspecified eye

[6] H21.27 Miotic pupillary cyst
H21.271 Miotic pupillary cyst, right eye
H21.272 Miotic pupillary cyst, left eye
H21.273 Miotic pupillary cyst, bilateral
H21.279 Miotic pupillary cyst, unspecified eye

H21.29 Other iris atrophy

[5] H21.3 Cyst of iris, ciliary body and anterior chamber

EXCLUDES2 *miotic pupillary cyst (H21.27-)*

[6] H21.30 Idiopathic cysts of iris, ciliary body or anterior chamber

Cyst of iris, ciliary body or anterior chamber NOS

H21.301 Idiopathic cysts of iris, ciliary body or anterior chamber, right eye
H21.302 Idiopathic cysts of iris, ciliary body or anterior chamber, left eye
H21.303 Idiopathic cysts of iris, ciliary body or anterior chamber, bilateral
H21.309 Idiopathic cysts of iris, ciliary body or anterior chamber, unspecified eye

[6] H21.31 Exudative cysts of iris or anterior chamber
H21.311 Exudative cysts of iris or anterior chamber, right eye
H21.312 Exudative cysts of iris or anterior chamber, left eye
H21.313 Exudative cysts of iris or anterior chamber, bilateral
H21.319 Exudative cysts of iris or anterior chamber, unspecified eye

[6] H21.32 Implantation cysts of iris, ciliary body or anterior chamber
H21.321 Implantation cysts of iris, ciliary body or anterior chamber, right eye
H21.322 Implantation cysts of iris, ciliary body or anterior chamber, left eye
H21.323 Implantation cysts of iris, ciliary body or anterior chamber, bilateral
H21.329 Implantation cysts of iris, ciliary body or anterior chamber, unspecified eye

[6] H21.33 Parasitic cyst of iris, ciliary body or anterior chamber
H21.331 Parasitic cyst of iris, ciliary body or anterior chamber, right eye
H21.332 Parasitic cyst of iris, ciliary body or anterior chamber, left eye
H21.333 Parasitic cyst of iris, ciliary body or anterior chamber, bilateral
H21.339 Parasitic cyst of iris, ciliary body or anterior chamber, unspecified eye

[6] H21.34 Primary cyst of pars plana
H21.341 Primary cyst of pars plana, right eye
H21.342 Primary cyst of pars plana, left eye
H21.343 Primary cyst of pars plana, bilateral
H21.349 Primary cyst of pars plana, unspecified eye

[6] H21.35 Exudative cyst of pars plana
H21.351 Exudative cyst of pars plana, right eye
H21.352 Exudative cyst of pars plana, left eye
H21.353 Exudative cyst of pars plana, bilateral
H21.359 Exudative cyst of pars plana, unspecified eye

[5] H21.4 Pupillary membranes

Iris bombé
Pupillary occlusion
Pupillary seclusion

EXCLUDES1 *congenital pupillary membranes (Q13.8)*

H21.40 Pupillary membranes, unspecified eye
H21.41 Pupillary membranes, right eye
H21.42 Pupillary membranes, left eye
H21.43 Pupillary membranes, bilateral

[5] H21.5 Other and unspecified adhesions and disruptions of iris and ciliary body

EXCLUDES1 *corectopia (Q13.2)*

[6] H21.50 Unspecified adhesions of iris

Synechia (iris) NOS

H21.501 Unspecified adhesions of iris, right eye
H21.502 Unspecified adhesions of iris, left eye
H21.503 Unspecified adhesions of iris, bilateral
H21.509 Unspecified adhesions of iris and ciliary body, unspecified eye

[6] H21.51 Anterior synechiae (iris)
H21.511 Anterior synechiae (iris), right eye
H21.512 Anterior synechiae (iris), left eye
H21.513 Anterior synechiae (iris), bilateral
H21.519 Anterior synechiae (iris), unspecified eye

[6] H21.52 Goniosynechiae
H21.521 Goniosynechiae, right eye
H21.522 Goniosynechiae, left eye
H21.523 Goniosynechiae, bilateral
H21.529 Goniosynechiae, unspecified eye

[6] H21.53 Iridodialysis
H21.531 Iridodialysis, right eye
H21.532 Iridodialysis, left eye
H21.533 Iridodialysis, bilateral
H21.539 Iridodialysis, unspecified eye

[6] H21.54 Posterior synechiae (iris)
H21.541 Posterior synechiae (iris), right eye
H21.542 Posterior synechiae (iris), left eye
H21.543 Posterior synechiae (iris), bilateral
H21.549 Posterior synechiae (iris), unspecified eye

[6] H21.55 Recession of chamber angle
H21.551 Recession of chamber angle, right eye
H21.552 Recession of chamber angle, left eye
H21.553 Recession of chamber angle, bilateral
H21.559 Recession of chamber angle, unspecified eye

[6] H21.56 Pupillary abnormalities

Deformed pupil
Ectopic pupil
Rupture of sphincter, pupil

EXCLUDES1 *congenital deformity of pupil (Q13.2-)*

H21.561 Pupillary abnormality, right eye
H21.562 Pupillary abnormality, left eye
H21.563 Pupillary abnormality, bilateral
H21.569 Pupillary abnormality, unspecified eye

[5] H21.8 Other specified disorders of iris and ciliary body
H21.81 Floppy iris syndrome

Intraoperative floppy iris syndrome (IFIS)
Use additional code for adverse effect, if applicable, to identify drug (T36-T50 with fifth or sixth character 5)

[4] 4th character required [5] 5th character required [6] 6th character required [7] 7th character required [x7] Extension 'X' Alert
EXCLUDES1 Not coded here EXCLUDES2 Not included here [PDx] Primary Diagnosis Only Manifestation Code

H21.82 Plateau iris syndrome (post-iridectomy) (postprocedural)
H21.89 Other specified disorders of iris and ciliary body
H21.9 Unspecified disorder of iris and ciliary body
H22 Disorders of iris and ciliary body in diseases classified elsewhere
Code first underlying disease, such as:
gout (M1A.-, M10.-)
leprosy (A30.-)
parasitic disease (B89)

Disorders of lens (H25-H28)

[4] H25 Age-related cataract
Senile cataract
[EXCLUDES2] *capsular glaucoma with pseudoexfoliation of lens (H40.1-)*
[5] H25.0 Age-related incipient cataract
[6] H25.01 Cortical age-related cataract
H25.011 Cortical age-related cataract, right eye [A]
H25.012 Cortical age-related cataract, left eye [A]
H25.013 Cortical age-related cataract, bilateral [A]
H25.019 Cortical age-related cataract, unspecified eye [A]
[6] H25.03 Anterior subcapsular polar age-related cataract
H25.031 Anterior subcapsular polar age-related cataract, right eye [A]
H25.032 Anterior subcapsular polar age-related cataract, left eye [A]
H25.033 Anterior subcapsular polar age-related cataract, bilateral [A]
H25.039 Anterior subcapsular polar age-related cataract, unspecified eye [A]
[6] H25.04 Posterior subcapsular polar age-related cataract
H25.041 Posterior subcapsular polar age-related cataract, right eye [A]
H25.042 Posterior subcapsular polar age-related cataract, left eye [A]
H25.043 Posterior subcapsular polar age-related cataract, bilateral [A]
H25.049 Posterior subcapsular polar age-related cataract, unspecified eye [A]
[6] H25.09 Other age-related incipient cataract
Coronary age-related cataract
Punctate age-related cataract
Water clefts
H25.091 Other age-related incipient cataract, right eye [A]
H25.092 Other age-related incipient cataract, left eye [A]
H25.093 Other age-related incipient cataract, bilateral [A]
H25.099 Other age-related incipient cataract, unspecified eye [A]
[5] H25.1 Age-related nuclear cataract
Cataracta brunescens
Nuclear sclerosis cataract
H25.10 Age-related nuclear cataract, unspecified eye [A]
H25.11 Age-related nuclear cataract, right eye [A]
H25.12 Age-related nuclear cataract, left eye [A]
H25.13 Age-related nuclear cataract, bilateral [A]
[5] H25.2 Age-related cataract, morgagnian type
Age-related hypermature cataract
H25.20 Age-related cataract, morgagnian type, unspecified eye [A]
H25.21 Age-related cataract, morgagnian type, right eye [A]
H25.22 Age-related cataract, morgagnian type, left eye [A]
H25.23 Age-related cataract, morgagnian type, bilateral [A]
[5] H25.8 Other age-related cataract
[6] H25.81 Combined forms of age-related cataract
H25.811 Combined forms of age-related cataract, right eye [A]
H25.812 Combined forms of age-related cataract, left eye [A]
H25.813 Combined forms of age-related cataract, bilateral [A]
H25.819 Combined forms of age-related cataract, unspecified eye [A]
H25.89 Other age-related cataract [A]
H25.9 Unspecified age-related cataract [A]
[4] H26 Other cataract
[EXCLUDES1] *congenital cataract (Q12.0)*
[5] H26.0 Infantile and juvenile cataract
[6] H26.00 Unspecified infantile and juvenile cataract
H26.001 Unspecified infantile and juvenile cataract, right eye [P]
H26.002 Unspecified infantile and juvenile cataract, left eye [P]
H26.003 Unspecified infantile and juvenile cataract, bilateral [P]
H26.009 Unspecified infantile and juvenile cataract, unspecified eye [P]
[6] H26.01 Infantile and juvenile cortical, lamellar, or zonular cataract
H26.011 Infantile and juvenile cortical, lamellar, or zonular cataract, right eye [P]
H26.012 Infantile and juvenile cortical, lamellar, or zonular cataract, left eye [P]
H26.013 Infantile and juvenile cortical, lamellar, or zonular cataract, bilateral [P]
H26.019 Infantile and juvenile cortical, lamellar, or zonular cataract, unspecified eye [P]
[6] H26.03 Infantile and juvenile nuclear cataract
H26.031 Infantile and juvenile nuclear cataract, right eye [P]
H26.032 Infantile and juvenile nuclear cataract, left eye [P]
H26.033 Infantile and juvenile nuclear cataract, bilateral [P]
H26.039 Infantile and juvenile nuclear cataract, unspecified eye [P]
[6] H26.04 Anterior subcapsular polar infantile and juvenile cataract
H26.041 Anterior subcapsular polar infantile and juvenile cataract, right eye [P]
H26.042 Anterior subcapsular polar infantile and juvenile cataract, left eye [P]
H26.043 Anterior subcapsular polar infantile and juvenile cataract, bilateral [P]
H26.049 Anterior subcapsular polar infantile and juvenile cataract, unspecified eye [P]
[6] H26.05 Posterior subcapsular polar infantile and juvenile cataract
H26.051 Posterior subcapsular polar infantile and juvenile cataract, right eye [P]
H26.052 Posterior subcapsular polar infantile and juvenile cataract, left eye [P]
H26.053 Posterior subcapsular polar infantile and juvenile cataract, bilateral [P]
H26.059 Posterior subcapsular polar infantile and juvenile cataract, unspecified eye [P]
[6] H26.06 Combined forms of infantile and juvenile cataract
H26.061 Combined forms of infantile and juvenile cataract, right eye [P]

Unspecified Code   Other Specified Code   [N] Newborn Age: 0   [P] Pediatric Age: 0-17   [M] Maternity Age: 12-55
[A] Adult Age: 15-124   ♂ Male   ♀ Female   ● New Code   ▲ Revised Code Title   ►◄ Revised Text

H26.062 Combined forms of infantile and juvenile cataract, left eye 🄿
H26.063 Combined forms of infantile and juvenile cataract, bilateral 🄿
H26.069 Combined forms of infantile and juvenile cataract, unspecified eye 🄿
H26.09 Other infantile and juvenile cataract 🄿
⑤ H26.1 Traumatic cataract
Use additional code (Chapter 20) to identify external cause
⑥ H26.10 Unspecified traumatic cataract
H26.101 Unspecified traumatic cataract, right eye
H26.102 Unspecified traumatic cataract, left eye
H26.103 Unspecified traumatic cataract, bilateral
H26.109 Unspecified traumatic cataract, unspecified eye
⑥ H26.11 Localized traumatic opacities
H26.111 Localized traumatic opacities, right eye
H26.112 Localized traumatic opacities, left eye
H26.113 Localized traumatic opacities, bilateral
H26.119 Localized traumatic opacities, unspecified eye
⑥ H26.12 Partially resolved traumatic cataract
H26.121 Partially resolved traumatic cataract, right eye
H26.122 Partially resolved traumatic cataract, left eye
H26.123 Partially resolved traumatic cataract, bilateral
H26.129 Partially resolved traumatic cataract, unspecified eye
⑥ H26.13 Total traumatic cataract
H26.131 Total traumatic cataract, right eye
H26.132 Total traumatic cataract, left eye
H26.133 Total traumatic cataract, bilateral
H26.139 Total traumatic cataract, unspecified eye
⑤ H26.2 Complicated cataract
H26.20 Unspecified complicated cataract
Cataracta complicata NOS
⑥ H26.21 Cataract with neovascularization
Code also associated condition, such as: chronic iridocyclitis (H20.1-)
H26.211 Cataract with neovascularization, right eye
H26.212 Cataract with neovascularization, left eye
H26.213 Cataract with neovascularization, bilateral
H26.219 Cataract with neovascularization, unspecified eye
⑥ H26.22 Cataract secondary to ocular disorders (degenerative) (inflammatory)
Code also associated ocular disorder
H26.221 Cataract secondary to ocular disorders (degenerative) (inflammatory), right eye
H26.222 Cataract secondary to ocular disorders (degenerative) (inflammatory), left eye
H26.223 Cataract secondary to ocular disorders (degenerative) (inflammatory), bilateral
H26.229 Cataract secondary to ocular disorders (degenerative) (inflammatory), unspecified eye
⑥ H26.23 Glaucomatous flecks (subcapsular)
Code first underlying glaucoma (H40-H42)
H26.231 Glaucomatous flecks (subcapsular), right eye
H26.232 Glaucomatous flecks (subcapsular), left eye
H26.233 Glaucomatous flecks (subcapsular), bilateral
H26.239 Glaucomatous flecks (subcapsular), unspecified eye

⑤ H26.3 Drug-induced cataract
Toxic cataract
Use additional code for adverse effect, if applicable, to identify drug (T36-T50 with fifth or sixth character 5)
H26.30 Drug-induced cataract, unspecified eye
H26.31 Drug-induced cataract, right eye
H26.32 Drug-induced cataract, left eye
H26.33 Drug-induced cataract, bilateral
⑤ H26.4 Secondary cataract
H26.40 Unspecified secondary cataract
⑥ H26.41 Soemmering's ring
H26.411 Soemmering's ring, right eye
H26.412 Soemmering's ring, left eye
H26.413 Soemmering's ring, bilateral
H26.419 Soemmering's ring, unspecified eye
⑥ H26.49 Other secondary cataract
H26.491 Other secondary cataract, right eye
H26.492 Other secondary cataract, left eye
H26.493 Other secondary cataract, bilateral
H26.499 Other secondary cataract, unspecified eye
H26.8 Other specified cataract
H26.9 Unspecified cataract
④ H27 Other disorders of lens
EXCLUDES1 congenital lens malformations (Q12.-)
mechanical complications of intraocular lens implant (T85.2)
pseudophakia (Z96.1)
⑤ H27.0 Aphakia
Acquired absence of lens
Acquired aphakia
Aphakia due to trauma
EXCLUDES1 cataract extraction status (Z98.4-)
congenital absence of lens (Q12.3)
congenital aphakia (Q12.3)
H27.00 Aphakia, unspecified eye
H27.01 Aphakia, right eye
H27.02 Aphakia, left eye
H27.03 Aphakia, bilateral
⑤ H27.1 Dislocation of lens
H27.10 Unspecified dislocation of lens
⑥ H27.11 Subluxation of lens
H27.111 Subluxation of lens, right eye
H27.112 Subluxation of lens, left eye
H27.113 Subluxation of lens, bilateral
H27.119 Subluxation of lens, unspecified eye
⑥ H27.12 Anterior dislocation of lens
H27.121 Anterior dislocation of lens, right eye
H27.122 Anterior dislocation of lens, left eye
H27.123 Anterior dislocation of lens, bilateral
H27.129 Anterior dislocation of lens, unspecified eye
⑥ H27.13 Posterior dislocation of lens
H27.131 Posterior dislocation of lens, right eye
H27.132 Posterior dislocation of lens, left eye
H27.133 Posterior dislocation of lens, bilateral
H27.139 Posterior dislocation of lens, unspecified eye
H27.8 Other specified disorders of lens
H27.9 Unspecified disorder of lens

H28 Cataract in diseases classified elsewhere
Code first underlying disease, such as:
hypoparathyroidism (E20.-)
myotonia (G71.1-)
myxedema (E03.-)
protein-calorie malnutrition (E40-E46)

---

④ 4th character required   ⑤ 5th character required   ⑥ 6th character required   ⑦ 7th character required   ⑩ Extension 'X' Alert
EXCLUDES 1 Not coded here   EXCLUDES 2 Not included here   🄿 Primary Diagnosis Only   Manifestation Code

[EXCLUDES1] *cataract in diabetes mellitus (E08.36, E09.36, E10.36, E11.36, E13.36)*

Disorders of choroid and retina (H30-H36)

[4th] **H30 Chorioretinal inflammation**

[5th] **H30.0 Focal chorioretinal inflammation**

Focal chorioretinitis
Focal choroiditis
Focal retinitis
Focal retinochoroiditis

[6th] **H30.00 Unspecified focal chorioretinal inflammation**

Focal chorioretinitis NOS
Focal choroiditis NOS
Focal retinitis NOS
Focal retinochoroiditis NOS

H30.001 Unspecified focal chorioretinal inflammation, right eye
H30.002 Unspecified focal chorioretinal inflammation, left eye
H30.003 Unspecified focal chorioretinal inflammation, bilateral
H30.009 Unspecified focal chorioretinal inflammation, unspecified eye

[6th] **H30.01 Focal chorioretinal inflammation, juxtapapillary**

H30.011 Focal chorioretinal inflammation, juxtapapillary, right eye
H30.012 Focal chorioretinal inflammation, juxtapapillary, left eye
H30.013 Focal chorioretinal inflammation, juxtapapillary, bilateral
H30.019 Focal chorioretinal inflammation, juxtapapillary, unspecified eye

[6th] **H30.02 Focal chorioretinal inflammation of posterior pole**

H30.021 Focal chorioretinal inflammation of posterior pole, right eye
H30.022 Focal chorioretinal inflammation of posterior pole, left eye
H30.023 Focal chorioretinal inflammation of posterior pole, bilateral
H30.029 Focal chorioretinal inflammation of posterior pole, unspecified eye

[6th] **H30.03 Focal chorioretinal inflammation, peripheral**

H30.031 Focal chorioretinal inflammation, peripheral, right eye
H30.032 Focal chorioretinal inflammation, peripheral, left eye
H30.033 Focal chorioretinal inflammation, peripheral, bilateral
H30.039 Focal chorioretinal inflammation, peripheral, unspecified eye

[6th] **H30.04 Focal chorioretinal inflammation, macular or paramacular**

H30.041 Focal chorioretinal inflammation, macular or paramacular, right eye
H30.042 Focal chorioretinal inflammation, macular or paramacular, left eye
H30.043 Focal chorioretinal inflammation, macular or paramacular, bilateral
H30.049 Focal chorioretinal inflammation, macular or paramacular, unspecified eye

[5th] **H30.1 Disseminated chorioretinal inflammation**

Disseminated chorioretinitis
Disseminated choroiditis
Disseminated retinitis
Disseminated retinochoroiditis

[EXCLUDES2] *exudative retinopathy (H35.02-)*

[6th] **H30.10 Unspecified disseminated chorioretinal inflammation**

Disseminated chorioretinitis NOS
Disseminated choroiditis NOS
Disseminated retinitis NOS
Disseminated retinochoroiditis NOS

H30.101 Unspecified disseminated chorioretinal inflammation, right eye
H30.102 Unspecified disseminated chorioretinal inflammation, left eye
H30.103 Unspecified disseminated chorioretinal inflammation, bilateral
H30.109 Unspecified disseminated chorioretinal inflammation, unspecified eye

[6th] **H30.11 Disseminated chorioretinal inflammation of posterior pole**

H30.111 Disseminated chorioretinal inflammation of posterior pole, right eye
H30.112 Disseminated chorioretinal inflammation of posterior pole, left eye
H30.113 Disseminated chorioretinal inflammation of posterior pole, bilateral
H30.119 Disseminated chorioretinal inflammation of posterior pole, unspecified eye

[6th] **H30.12 Disseminated chorioretinal inflammation, peripheral**

H30.121 Disseminated chorioretinal inflammation, peripheral right eye
H30.122 Disseminated chorioretinal inflammation, peripheral, left eye
H30.123 Disseminated chorioretinal inflammation, peripheral, bilateral
H30.129 Disseminated chorioretinal inflammation, peripheral, unspecified eye

[6th] **H30.13 Disseminated chorioretinal inflammation, generalized**

H30.131 Disseminated chorioretinal inflammation, generalized, right eye
H30.132 Disseminated chorioretinal inflammation, generalized, left eye
H30.133 Disseminated chorioretinal inflammation, generalized, bilateral
H30.139 Disseminated chorioretinal inflammation, generalized, unspecified eye

[6th] **H30.14 Acute posterior multifocal placoid pigment epitheliopathy**

H30.141 Acute posterior multifocal placoid pigment epitheliopathy, right eye
H30.142 Acute posterior multifocal placoid pigment epitheliopathy, left eye
H30.143 Acute posterior multifocal placoid pigment epitheliopathy, bilateral
H30.149 Acute posterior multifocal placoid pigment epitheliopathy, unspecified eye

[5th] **H30.2 Posterior cyclitis**

Pars planitis

H30.20 Posterior cyclitis, unspecified eye
H30.21 Posterior cyclitis, right eye
H30.22 Posterior cyclitis, left eye
H30.23 Posterior cyclitis, bilateral

[5th] **H30.8 Other chorioretinal inflammations**

[6th] **H30.81 Harada's disease**

H30.811 Harada's disease, right eye
H30.812 Harada's disease, left eye
H30.813 Harada's disease, bilateral
H30.819 Harada's disease, unspecified eye

[6th] **H30.89 Other chorioretinal inflammations**

H30.891 Other chorioretinal inflammations, right eye
H30.892 Other chorioretinal inflammations, left eye
H30.893 Other chorioretinal inflammations, bilateral

Unspecified Code | Other Specified Code | [N] Newborn Age: 0 | [P] Pediatric Age: 0-17 | [M] Maternity Age: 12-55
[A] Adult Age: 15-124 | ♂ Male | ♀ Female | ● New Code | ▲ Revised Code Title | ►◄ Revised Text

H30.899 Other chorioretinal inflammations, unspecified eye

[5] H30.9 Unspecified chorioretinal inflammation
Chorioretinitis NOS
Choroiditis NOS
Neuroretinitis NOS
Retinitis NOS
Retinochoroiditis NOS
H30.90 Unspecified chorioretinal inflammation, unspecified eye
H30.91 Unspecified chorioretinal inflammation, right eye
H30.92 Unspecified chorioretinal inflammation, left eye
H30.93 Unspecified chorioretinal inflammation, bilateral

[4] H31 Other disorders of choroid

[5] H31.0 Chorioretinal scars
EXCLUDES2 *postsurgical chorioretinal scars (H59.81-)*
[6] H31.00 Unspecified chorioretinal scars
H31.001 Unspecified chorioretinal scars, right eye
H31.002 Unspecified chorioretinal scars, left eye
H31.003 Unspecified chorioretinal scars, bilateral
H31.009 Unspecified chorioretinal scars, unspecified eye
[6] H31.01 Macula scars of posterior pole (postinflammatory) (post-traumatic)
EXCLUDES1 *postprocedural chorioretinal scar (H59.81-)*
H31.011 Macula scars of posterior pole (postinflammatory) (post-traumatic), right eye
H31.012 Macula scars of posterior pole (postinflammatory) (post-traumatic), left eye
H31.013 Macula scars of posterior pole (postinflammatory) (post-traumatic), bilateral
H31.019 Macula scars of posterior pole (postinflammatory) (post-traumatic), unspecified eye
[6] H31.02 Solar retinopathy
H31.021 Solar retinopathy, right eye
H31.022 Solar retinopathy, left eye
H31.023 Solar retinopathy, bilateral
H31.029 Solar retinopathy, unspecified eye
[6] H31.09 Other chorioretinal scars
H31.091 Other chorioretinal scars, right eye
H31.092 Other chorioretinal scars, left eye
H31.093 Other chorioretinal scars, bilateral
H31.099 Other chorioretinal scars, unspecified eye

[5] H31.1 Choroidal degeneration
EXCLUDES2 *angioid streaks of macula (H35.33)*
[6] H31.10 Unspecified choroidal degeneration
Choroidal sclerosis NOS
H31.101 Choroidal degeneration, unspecified, right eye
H31.102 Choroidal degeneration, unspecified, left eye
H31.103 Choroidal degeneration, unspecified, bilateral
H31.109 Choroidal degeneration, unspecified, unspecified eye
[6] H31.11 Age-related choroidal atrophy
H31.111 Age-related choroidal atrophy, right eye [A]
H31.112 Age-related choroidal atrophy, left eye [A]
H31.113 Age-related choroidal atrophy, bilateral [A]
H31.119 Age-related choroidal atrophy, unspecified eye [A]
[6] H31.12 Diffuse secondary atrophy of choroid
H31.121 Diffuse secondary atrophy of choroid, right eye
H31.122 Diffuse secondary atrophy of choroid, left eye
H31.123 Diffuse secondary atrophy of choroid, bilateral
H31.129 Diffuse secondary atrophy of choroid, unspecified eye

[5] H31.2 Hereditary choroidal dystrophy
EXCLUDES2 *hyperornithinemia (E72.4)*
ornithinemia (E72.4)
H31.20 Hereditary choroidal dystrophy, unspecified
H31.21 Choroideremia
H31.22 Choroidal dystrophy (central areolar) (generalized) (peripapillary)
H31.23 Gyrate atrophy, choroid
H31.29 Other hereditary choroidal dystrophy

[5] H31.3 Choroidal hemorrhage and rupture
[6] H31.30 Unspecified choroidal hemorrhage
H31.301 Unspecified choroidal hemorrhage, right eye
H31.302 Unspecified choroidal hemorrhage, left eye
H31.303 Unspecified choroidal hemorrhage, bilateral
H31.309 Unspecified choroidal hemorrhage, unspecified eye
[6] H31.31 Expulsive choroidal hemorrhage
H31.311 Expulsive choroidal hemorrhage, right eye
H31.312 Expulsive choroidal hemorrhage, left eye
H31.313 Expulsive choroidal hemorrhage, bilateral
H31.319 Expulsive choroidal hemorrhage, unspecified eye
[6] H31.32 Choroidal rupture
H31.321 Choroidal rupture, right eye
H31.322 Choroidal rupture, left eye
H31.323 Choroidal rupture, bilateral
H31.329 Choroidal rupture, unspecified eye

[5] H31.4 Choroidal detachment
[6] H31.40 Unspecified choroidal detachment
H31.401 Unspecified choroidal detachment, right eye
H31.402 Unspecified choroidal detachment, left eye
H31.403 Unspecified choroidal detachment, bilateral
H31.409 Unspecified choroidal detachment, unspecified eye
[6] H31.41 Hemorrhagic choroidal detachment
H31.411 Hemorrhagic choroidal detachment, right eye
H31.412 Hemorrhagic choroidal detachment, left eye
H31.413 Hemorrhagic choroidal detachment, bilateral
H31.419 Hemorrhagic choroidal detachment, unspecified eye
[6] H31.42 Serous choroidal detachment
H31.421 Serous choroidal detachment, right eye
H31.422 Serous choroidal detachment, left eye
H31.423 Serous choroidal detachment, bilateral
H31.429 Serous choroidal detachment, unspecified eye

H31.8 Other specified disorders of choroid

H31.9 Unspecified disorder of choroid

H32 Chorioretinal disorders in diseases classified elsewhere
Code first underlying disease, such as:
congenital toxoplasmosis (P37.1)
histoplasmosis (B39.-)
leprosy (A30.-)

[4] 4th character required [5] 5th character required [6] 6th character required [7] 7th character required [x7] Extension 'X' Alert
EXCLUDES1 Not coded here EXCLUDES2 Not included here [PDx] Primary Diagnosis Only Manifestation Code

[EXCLUDES1] *chorioretinitis (in):*
toxoplasmosis (acquired) (B58.01)
tuberculosis (A18.53)

[4] **H33 Retinal detachments and breaks**

[EXCLUDES1] *detachment of retinal pigment epithelium (H35.72-, H35.73-)*

[5] **H33.0 Retinal detachment with retinal break**

Rhegmatogenous retinal detachment

[EXCLUDES1] *serous retinal detachment (without retinal break) (H33.2-)*

[6] **H33.00 Unspecified retinal detachment with retinal break**
- **H33.001 Unspecified retinal detachment with retinal break, right eye**
- **H33.002 Unspecified retinal detachment with retinal break, left eye**
- **H33.003 Unspecified retinal detachment with retinal break, bilateral**
- **H33.009 Unspecified retinal detachment with retinal break, unspecified eye**

[6] **H33.01 Retinal detachment with single break**
- **H33.011 Retinal detachment with single break, right eye**
- **H33.012 Retinal detachment with single break, left eye**
- **H33.013 Retinal detachment with single break, bilateral**
- **H33.019 Retinal detachment with single break, unspecified eye**

[6] **H33.02 Retinal detachment with multiple breaks**
- **H33.021 Retinal detachment with multiple breaks, right eye**
- **H33.022 Retinal detachment with multiple breaks, left eye**
- **H33.023 Retinal detachment with multiple breaks, bilateral**
- **H33.029 Retinal detachment with multiple breaks, unspecified eye**

[6] **H33.03 Retinal detachment with giant retinal tear**
- **H33.031 Retinal detachment with giant retinal tear, right eye**
- **H33.032 Retinal detachment with giant retinal tear, left eye**
- **H33.033 Retinal detachment with giant retinal tear, bilateral**
- **H33.039 Retinal detachment with giant retinal tear, unspecified eye**

[6] **H33.04 Retinal detachment with retinal dialysis**
- **H33.041 Retinal detachment with retinal dialysis, right eye**
- **H33.042 Retinal detachment with retinal dialysis, left eye**
- **H33.043 Retinal detachment with retinal dialysis, bilateral**
- **H33.049 Retinal detachment with retinal dialysis, unspecified eye**

[6] **H33.05 Total retinal detachment**
- **H33.051 Total retinal detachment, right eye**
- **H33.052 Total retinal detachment, left eye**
- **H33.053 Total retinal detachment, bilateral**
- **H33.059 Total retinal detachment, unspecified eye**

[5] **H33.1 Retinoschisis and retinal cysts**

[EXCLUDES1] *congenital retinoschisis (Q14.1)*
microcystoid degeneration of retina (H35.42-)

[6] **H33.10 Unspecified retinoschisis**
- **H33.101 Unspecified retinoschisis, right eye**
- **H33.102 Unspecified retinoschisis, left eye**
- **H33.103 Unspecified retinoschisis, bilateral**
- **H33.109 Unspecified retinoschisis, unspecified eye**

[6] **H33.11 Cyst of ora serrata**
- **H33.111 Cyst of ora serrata, right eye**
- **H33.112 Cyst of ora serrata, left eye**
- **H33.113 Cyst of ora serrata, bilateral**
- **H33.119 Cyst of ora serrata, unspecified eye**

[6] **H33.12 Parasitic cyst of retina**
- **H33.121 Parasitic cyst of retina, right eye**
- **H33.122 Parasitic cyst of retina, left eye**
- **H33.123 Parasitic cyst of retina, bilateral**
- **H33.129 Parasitic cyst of retina, unspecified eye**

[6] **H33.19 Other retinoschisis and retinal cysts**

Pseudocyst of retina
- **H33.191 Other retinoschisis and retinal cysts, right eye**
- **H33.192 Other retinoschisis and retinal cysts, left eye**
- **H33.193 Other retinoschisis and retinal cysts, bilateral**
- **H33.199 Other retinoschisis and retinal cysts, unspecified eye**

[5] **H33.2 Serous retinal detachment**

Retinal detachment NOS
Retinal detachment without retinal break

[EXCLUDES1] *central serous chorioretinopathy (H35.71-)*
- **H33.20 Serous retinal detachment, unspecified eye**
- **H33.21 Serous retinal detachment, right eye**
- **H33.22 Serous retinal detachment, left eye**
- **H33.23 Serous retinal detachment, bilateral**

[5] **H33.3 Retinal breaks without detachment**

[EXCLUDES1] *chorioretinal scars after surgery for detachment (H59.81-)*
peripheral retinal degeneration without break (H35.4-)

[6] **H33.30 Unspecified retinal break**
- **H33.301 Unspecified retinal break, right eye**
- **H33.302 Unspecified retinal break, left eye**
- **H33.303 Unspecified retinal break, bilateral**
- **H33.309 Unspecified retinal break, unspecified eye**

[6] **H33.31 Horseshoe tear of retina without detachment**

Operculum of retina without detachment
- **H33.311 Horseshoe tear of retina without detachment, right eye**
- **H33.312 Horseshoe tear of retina without detachment, left eye**
- **H33.313 Horseshoe tear of retina without detachment, bilateral**
- **H33.319 Horseshoe tear of retina without detachment, unspecified eye**

[6] **H33.32 Round hole of retina without detachment**
- **H33.321 Round hole, right eye**
- **H33.322 Round hole, left eye**
- **H33.323 Round hole, bilateral**
- **H33.329 Round hole, unspecified eye**

[6] **H33.33 Multiple defects of retina without detachment**
- **H33.331 Multiple defects of retina without detachment, right eye**
- **H33.332 Multiple defects of retina without detachment, left eye**
- **H33.333 Multiple defects of retina without detachment, bilateral**
- **H33.339 Multiple defects of retina without detachment, unspecified eye**

[5] **H33.4 Traction detachment of retina**

Proliferative vitreo-retinopathy with retinal detachment

Unspecified Code | Other Specified Code | [N] Newborn Age: 0 | [P] Pediatric Age: 0-17 | [M] Maternity Age: 12-55
[A] Adult Age: 15-124 | ♂ Male | ♀ Female | ● New Code | ▲ Revised Code Title | ►◄ Revised Text

H33.40 Traction detachment of retina, unspecified eye
H33.41 Traction detachment of retina, right eye
H33.42 Traction detachment of retina, left eye
H33.43 Traction detachment of retina, bilateral
H33.8 Other retinal detachments

[4] **H34 Retinal vascular occlusions**
EXCLUDES1 *amaurosis fugax (G45.3)*

[5] H34.0 Transient retinal artery occlusion
H34.00 Transient retinal artery occlusion, unspecified eye
H34.01 Transient retinal artery occlusion, right eye
H34.02 Transient retinal artery occlusion, left eye
H34.03 Transient retinal artery occlusion, bilateral

[5] H34.1 Central retinal artery occlusion
H34.10 Central retinal artery occlusion, unspecified eye
H34.11 Central retinal artery occlusion, right eye
H34.12 Central retinal artery occlusion, left eye
H34.13 Central retinal artery occlusion, bilateral

[5] H34.2 Other retinal artery occlusions

[6] H34.21 Partial retinal artery occlusion
Hollenhorst's plaque
Retinal microembolism
H34.211 Partial retinal artery occlusion, right eye
H34.212 Partial retinal artery occlusion, left eye
H34.213 Partial retinal artery occlusion, bilateral
H34.219 Partial retinal artery occlusion, unspecified eye

[6] H34.23 Retinal artery branch occlusion
H34.231 Retinal artery branch occlusion, right eye
H34.232 Retinal artery branch occlusion, left eye
H34.233 Retinal artery branch occlusion, bilateral
H34.239 Retinal artery branch occlusion, unspecified eye

[5] H34.8 Other retinal vascular occlusions

[6] H34.81 Central retinal vein occlusion
H34.811 Central retinal vein occlusion, right eye
H34.812 Central retinal vein occlusion, left eye
H34.813 Central retinal vein occlusion, bilateral
H34.819 Central retinal vein occlusion, unspecified eye

[6] H34.82 Venous engorgement
Incipient retinal vein occlusion
Partial retinal vein occlusion
H34.821 Venous engorgement, right eye
H34.822 Venous engorgement, left eye
H34.823 Venous engorgement, bilateral
H34.829 Venous engorgement, unspecified eye

[6] H34.83 Tributary (branch) retinal vein occlusion
H34.831 Tributary (branch) retinal vein occlusion, right eye
H34.832 Tributary (branch) retinal vein occlusion, left eye
H34.833 Tributary (branch) retinal vein occlusion, bilateral
H34.839 Tributary (branch) retinal vein occlusion, unspecified eye

H34.9 Unspecified retinal vascular occlusion

[4] **H35 Other retinal disorders**
EXCLUDES2 *diabetic retinal disorders (E08.311-E08.359, E09.311-E09.359, E10.311-E10.359, E11.311-E11.359,E13.311-E13.359)*

[5] H35.0 Background retinopathy and retinal vascular changes
Code also any associated hypertension (I10.-)
H35.00 Unspecified background retinopathy

[6] H35.01 Changes in retinal vascular appearance
Retinal vascular sheathing
H35.011 Changes in retinal vascular appearance, right eye
H35.012 Changes in retinal vascular appearance, left eye
H35.013 Changes in retinal vascular appearance, bilateral
H35.019 Changes in retinal vascular appearance, unspecified eye

[6] H35.02 Exudative retinopathy
Coats retinopathy
H35.021 Exudative retinopathy, right eye
H35.022 Exudative retinopathy, left eye
H35.023 Exudative retinopathy, bilateral
H35.029 Exudative retinopathy, unspecified eye

[6] H35.03 Hypertensive retinopathy
H35.031 Hypertensive retinopathy, right eye
H35.032 Hypertensive retinopathy, left eye
H35.033 Hypertensive retinopathy, bilateral
H35.039 Hypertensive retinopathy, unspecified eye

[6] H35.04 Retinal micro-aneurysms, unspecified
H35.041 Retinal micro-aneurysms, unspecified, right eye
H35.042 Retinal micro-aneurysms, unspecified, left eye
H35.043 Retinal micro-aneurysms, unspecified, bilateral
H35.049 Retinal micro-aneurysms, unspecified, unspecified eye

[6] H35.05 Retinal neovascularization, unspecified
H35.051 Retinal neovascularization, unspecified, right eye
H35.052 Retinal neovascularization, unspecified, left eye
H35.053 Retinal neovascularization, unspecified, bilateral
H35.059 Retinal neovascularization, unspecified, unspecified eye

[6] H35.06 Retinal vasculitis
Eales disease
Retinal perivasculitis
H35.061 Retinal vasculitis, right eye
H35.062 Retinal vasculitis, left eye
H35.063 Retinal vasculitis, bilateral
H35.069 Retinal vasculitis, unspecified eye

[6] H35.07 Retinal telangiectasis
H35.071 Retinal telangiectasis, right eye
H35.072 Retinal telangiectasis, left eye
H35.073 Retinal telangiectasis, bilateral
H35.079 Retinal telangiectasis, unspecified eye

H35.09 Other intraretinal microvascular abnormalities
Retinal varices

[5] H35.1 Retinopathy of prematurity

[6] H35.10 Retinopathy of prematurity, unspecified
Retinopathy of prematurity NOS
H35.101 Retinopathy of prematurity, unspecified, right eye
H35.102 Retinopathy of prematurity, unspecified, left eye
H35.103 Retinopathy of prematurity, unspecified, bilateral
H35.109 Retinopathy of prematurity, unspecified, unspecified eye

[6] H35.11 Retinopathy of prematurity, stage 0
H35.111 Retinopathy of prematurity, stage 0, right eye
H35.112 Retinopathy of prematurity, stage 0, left eye

[4] 4th character required [5] 5th character required [6] 6th character required [7] 7th character required [7] Extension 'X' Alert
EXCLUDES1 Not coded here EXCLUDES2 Not included here PDx Primary Diagnosis Only Manifestation Code

H35.113 Retinopathy of prematurity, stage 0, bilateral
H35.119 Retinopathy of prematurity, stage 0, unspecified eye
[6] H35.12 Retinopathy of prematurity, stage 1
H35.121 Retinopathy of prematurity, stage 1, right eye
H35.122 Retinopathy of prematurity, stage 1, left eye
H35.123 Retinopathy of prematurity, stage 1, bilateral
H35.129 Retinopathy of prematurity, stage 1, unspecified eye
[6] H35.13 Retinopathy of prematurity, stage 2
H35.131 Retinopathy of prematurity, stage 2, right eye
H35.132 Retinopathy of prematurity, stage 2, left eye
H35.133 Retinopathy of prematurity, stage 2, bilateral
H35.139 Retinopathy of prematurity, stage 2, unspecified eye
[6] H35.14 Retinopathy of prematurity, stage 3
H35.141 Retinopathy of prematurity, stage 3, right eye
H35.142 Retinopathy of prematurity, stage 3, left eye
H35.143 Retinopathy of prematurity, stage 3, bilateral
H35.149 Retinopathy of prematurity, stage 3, unspecified eye
[6] H35.15 Retinopathy of prematurity, stage 4
H35.151 Retinopathy of prematurity, stage 4, right eye
H35.152 Retinopathy of prematurity, stage 4, left eye
H35.153 Retinopathy of prematurity, stage 4, bilateral
H35.159 Retinopathy of prematurity, stage 4, unspecified eye
[6] H35.16 Retinopathy of prematurity, stage 5
H35.161 Retinopathy of prematurity, stage 5, right eye
H35.162 Retinopathy of prematurity, stage 5, left eye
H35.163 Retinopathy of prematurity, stage 5, bilateral
H35.169 Retinopathy of prematurity, stage 5, unspecified eye
[6] H35.17 Retrolental fibroplasia
H35.171 Retrolental fibroplasia, right eye
H35.172 Retrolental fibroplasia, left eye
H35.173 Retrolental fibroplasia, bilateral
H35.179 Retrolental fibroplasia, unspecified eye
[5] H35.2 Other non-diabetic proliferative retinopathy
Proliferative vitreo-retinopathy
[EXCLUDES1] *proliferative vitreo-retinopathy with retinal detachment (H33.4-)*
H35.20 Other non-diabetic proliferative retinopathy, unspecified eye
H35.21 Other non-diabetic proliferative retinopathy, right eye
H35.22 Other non-diabetic proliferative retinopathy, left eye
H35.23 Other non-diabetic proliferative retinopathy, bilateral
[5] H35.3 Degeneration of macula and posterior pole
H35.30 Unspecified macular degeneration
Age-related macular degeneration [A]
H35.31 Nonexudative age-related macular degeneration
Atrophic age-related macular degeneration [A]
H35.32 Exudative age-related macular degeneration [A]
H35.33 Angioid streaks of macula
[6] H35.34 Macular cyst, hole, or pseudohole
H35.341 Macular cyst, hole, or pseudohole, right eye
H35.342 Macular cyst, hole, or pseudohole, left eye
H35.343 Macular cyst, hole, or pseudohole, bilateral
H35.349 Macular cyst, hole, or pseudohole, unspecified eye
[6] H35.35 Cystoid macular degeneration
[EXCLUDES1] *cystoid macular edema following cataract surgery (H59.03-)*
H35.351 Cystoid macular degeneration, right eye
H35.352 Cystoid macular degeneration, left eye
H35.353 Cystoid macular degeneration, bilateral
H35.359 Cystoid macular degeneration, unspecified eye
[6] H35.36 Drusen (degenerative) of macula
H35.361 Drusen (degenerative) of macula, right eye
H35.362 Drusen (degenerative) of macula, left eye
H35.363 Drusen (degenerative) of macula, bilateral
H35.369 Drusen (degenerative) of macula, unspecified eye
[6] H35.37 Puckering of macula
H35.371 Puckering of macula, right eye
H35.372 Puckering of macula, left eye
H35.373 Puckering of macula, bilateral
H35.379 Puckering of macula, unspecified eye
[6] H35.38 Toxic maculopathy
Code first poisoning due to drug or toxin, if applicable (T36-T65 with fifth or sixth character 1-4 or 6)
Use additional code for adverse effect, if applicable, to identify drug (T36-T50 with fifth or sixth character 5)
H35.381 Toxic maculopathy, right eye
H35.382 Toxic maculopathy, left eye
H35.383 Toxic maculopathy, bilateral
H35.389 Toxic maculopathy, unspecified eye
[5] H35.4 Peripheral retinal degeneration
[EXCLUDES1] *hereditary retinal degeneration (dystrophy) (H35.5-)*
peripheral retinal degeneration with retinal break (H33.3-)
H35.40 Unspecified peripheral retinal degeneration
[6] H35.41 Lattice degeneration of retina
Palisade degeneration of retina
H35.411 Lattice degeneration of retina, right eye
H35.412 Lattice degeneration of retina, left eye
H35.413 Lattice degeneration of retina, bilateral
H35.419 Lattice degeneration of retina, unspecified eye
[6] H35.42 Microcystoid degeneration of retina
H35.421 Microcystoid degeneration of retina, right eye
H35.422 Microcystoid degeneration of retina, left eye
H35.423 Microcystoid degeneration of retina, bilateral
H35.429 Microcystoid degeneration of retina, unspecified eye
[6] H35.43 Paving stone degeneration of retina
H35.431 Paving stone degeneration of retina, right eye
H35.432 Paving stone degeneration of retina, left eye

Unspecified Code | Other Specified Code | [N] Newborn Age: 0 | [P] Pediatric Age: 0-17 | [M] Maternity Age: 12-55
[A] Adult Age: 15-124 | ♂ Male | ♀ Female | ● New Code | ▲ Revised Code Title | ►◄ Revised Text

H35.433 Paving stone degeneration of retina, bilateral

H35.439 Paving stone degeneration of retina, unspecified eye

⑥ H35.44 Age-related reticular degeneration of retina

H35.441 Age-related reticular degeneration of retina, right eye Ⓐ

H35.442 Age-related reticular degeneration of retina, left eye Ⓐ

H35.443 Age-related reticular degeneration of retina, bilateral Ⓐ

H35.449 Age-related reticular degeneration of retina, unspecified eye Ⓐ

⑥ H35.45 Secondary pigmentary degeneration

H35.451 Secondary pigmentary degeneration, right eye

H35.452 Secondary pigmentary degeneration, left eye

H35.453 Secondary pigmentary degeneration, bilateral

H35.459 Secondary pigmentary degeneration, unspecified eye

⑥ H35.46 Secondary vitreoretinal degeneration

H35.461 Secondary vitreoretinal degeneration, right eye

H35.462 Secondary vitreoretinal degeneration, left eye

H35.463 Secondary vitreoretinal degeneration, bilateral

H35.469 Secondary vitreoretinal degeneration, unspecified eye

⑤ H35.5 Hereditary retinal dystrophy

EXCLUDES1 dystrophies primarily involving Bruch's membrane (H31.1-)

H35.50 Unspecified hereditary retinal dystrophy

H35.51 Vitreoretinal dystrophy

H35.52 Pigmentary retinal dystrophy

Albipunctate retinal dystrophy
Retinitis pigmentosa
Tapetoretinal dystrophy

H35.53 Other dystrophies primarily involving the sensory retina

Stargardt's disease

H35.54 Dystrophies primarily involving the retinal pigment epithelium

Vitelliform retinal dystrophy

⑤ H35.6 Retinal hemorrhage

H35.60 Retinal hemorrhage, unspecified eye
H35.61 Retinal hemorrhage, right eye
H35.62 Retinal hemorrhage, left eye
H35.63 Retinal hemorrhage, bilateral

⑤ H35.7 Separation of retinal layers

EXCLUDES1 retinal detachment (serous) (H33.2-)
rhegmatogenous retinal detachment (H33.0-)

H35.70 Unspecified separation of retinal layers

⑥ H35.71 Central serous chorioretinopathy

H35.711 Central serous chorioretinopathy, right eye
H35.712 Central serous chorioretinopathy, left eye
H35.713 Central serous chorioretinopathy, bilateral
H35.719 Central serous chorioretinopathy, unspecified eye

⑥ H35.72 Serous detachment of retinal pigment epithelium

H35.721 Serous detachment of retinal pigment epithelium, right eye
H35.722 Serous detachment of retinal pigment epithelium, left eye

H35.723 Serous detachment of retinal pigment epithelium, bilateral

H35.729 Serous detachment of retinal pigment epithelium, unspecified eye

⑥ H35.73 Hemorrhagic detachment of retinal pigment epithelium

H35.731 Hemorrhagic detachment of retinal pigment epithelium, right eye

H35.732 Hemorrhagic detachment of retinal pigment epithelium, left eye

H35.733 Hemorrhagic detachment of retinal pigment epithelium, bilateral

H35.739 Hemorrhagic detachment of retinal pigment epithelium, unspecified eye

⑤ H35.8 Other specified retinal disorders

EXCLUDES2 retinal hemorrhage (H35.6-)

H35.81 Retinal edema

Retinal cotton wool spots

H35.82 Retinal ischemia

H35.89 Other specified retinal disorders

H35.9 Unspecified retinal disorder

H36 Retinal disorders in diseases classified elsewhere

Code first underlying disease, such as:
lipid storage disorders (E75.-)
sickle-cell disorders (D57.-)

EXCLUDES1 arteriosclerotic retinopathy (H35.0-)
diabetic retinopathy (E08.3-, E09.3-, E10.3-, E11.3-, E13.3-)

---

⑥ 4th character required ⑤ 5th character required ⑥ 6th character required ⑦ 7th character required Ⓧ Extension 'X' Alert

EXCLUDES 1 Not coded here EXCLUDES 2 Not included here PDX Primary Diagnosis Only Manifestation Code

Glaucoma (H40-H42)

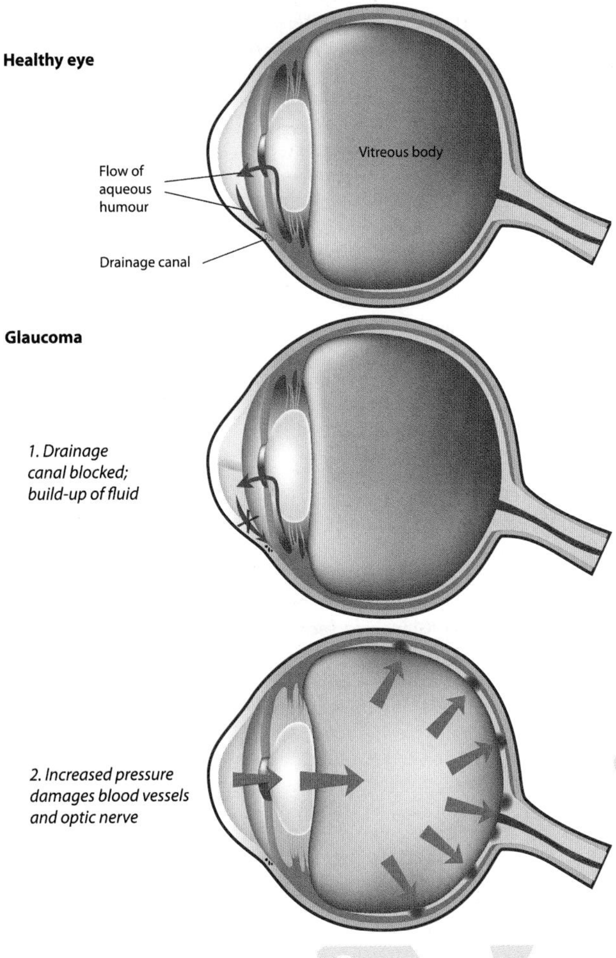
Healthy eye
Vitreous body
Flow of aqueous humour
Drainage canal
Glaucoma
1. Drainage canal blocked; build-up of fluid
2. Increased pressure damages blood vessels and optic nerve

Figure 7.4 Development of Glaucoma

[4] **H40 Glaucoma**

[EXCLUDES1] *absolute glaucoma (H44.51-)*
congenital glaucoma (Q15.0)
traumatic glaucoma due to birth injury (P15.3)

[5] **H40.0 Glaucoma suspect**

[6] **H40.00 Preglaucoma, unspecified**
- **H40.001 Preglaucoma, unspecified, right eye**
- **H40.002 Preglaucoma, unspecified, left eye**
- **H40.003 Preglaucoma, unspecified, bilateral**
- **H40.009 Preglaucoma, unspecified, unspecified eye**

[6] **H40.01 Open angle with borderline findings, low risk**
Open angle, low risk
- **H40.011 Open angle with borderline findings, low risk, right eye**
- **H40.012 Open angle with borderline findings, low risk, left eye**
- **H40.013 Open angle with borderline findings, low risk, bilateral**
- **H40.019 Open angle with borderline findings, low risk, unspecified eye**

[6] **H40.02 Open angle with borderline findings, high risk**
Open angle, high risk
- **H40.021 Open angle with borderline findings, high risk, right eye**
- **H40.022 Open angle with borderline findings, high risk, left eye**
- **H40.023 Open angle with borderline findings, high risk, bilateral**
- **H40.029 Open angle with borderline findings, high risk, unspecified eye**

[6] **H40.03 Anatomical narrow angle**
Primary angle closure suspect
- **H40.031 Anatomical narrow angle, right eye**
- **H40.032 Anatomical narrow angle, left eye**
- **H40.033 Anatomical narrow angle, bilateral**
- **H40.039 Anatomical narrow angle, unspecified eye**

[6] **H40.04 Steroid responder**
- **H40.041 Steroid responder, right eye**
- **H40.042 Steroid responder, left eye**
- **H40.043 Steroid responder, bilateral**
- **H40.049 Steroid responder, unspecified eye**

[6] **H40.05 Ocular hypertension**
- **H40.051 Ocular hypertension, right eye**
- **H40.052 Ocular hypertension, left eye**
- **H40.053 Ocular hypertension, bilateral**
- **H40.059 Ocular hypertension, unspecified eye**

[6] **H40.06 Primary angle closure without glaucoma damage**
- **H40.061 Primary angle closure without glaucoma damage, right eye**
- **H40.062 Primary angle closure without glaucoma damage, left eye**
- **H40.063 Primary angle closure without glaucoma damage, bilateral**
- **H40.069 Primary angle closure without glaucoma damage, unspecified eye**

[5] **H40.1 Open-angle glaucoma**

[7th] **H40.10 Unspecified open-angle glaucoma**
One of the following 7th characters is to be assigned to code H40.10 to designate the stage of glaucoma
0 = stage unspecified
1 = mild stage
2 = moderate stage
3 = severe stage
4 = indeterminate stage

[7th] **H40.11 Primary open-angle glaucoma**
Chronic simple glaucoma
One of the following 7th characters is to be assigned to code H40.11 to designate the stage of glaucoma
0 = stage unspecified
1 = mild stage
2 = moderate stage
3 = severe stage
4 = indeterminate stage

[6] **H40.12 Low-tension glaucoma**
One of the following 7th characters is to be assigned to each code in subcategory H40.12 to designate the stage of glaucoma
0 = stage unspecified
1 = mild stage
2 = moderate stage
3 = severe stage
4 = indeterminate stage
- [7] **H40.121 Low-tension glaucoma, right eye**
- [7] **H40.122 Low-tension glaucoma, left eye**
- [7] **H40.123 Low-tension glaucoma, bilateral**
- [7] **H40.129 Low-tension glaucoma, unspecified eye**

[6] **H40.13 Pigmentary glaucoma**
One of the following 7th characters is to be assigned to each code in subcategory H40.13 to designate the stage of glaucoma
0 = stage unspecified
1 = mild stage
2 = moderate stage
3 = severe stage
4 = indeterminate stage
- [7] **H40.131 Pigmentary glaucoma, right eye**

[7] H40.132 Pigmentary glaucoma, left eye
[7] H40.133 Pigmentary glaucoma, bilateral
[7] H40.139 Pigmentary glaucoma, unspecified eye
[6] H40.14 Capsular glaucoma with pseudoexfoliation of lens
One of the following 7th characters is to be assigned to each code in subcategory H40.14 to designate the stage of glaucoma
0 = stage unspecified
1 = mild stage
2 = moderate stage
3 = severe stage
4 = indeterminate stage
[7] H40.141 Capsular glaucoma with pseudoexfoliation of lens, right eye
[7] H40.142 Capsular glaucoma with pseudoexfoliation of lens, left eye
[7] H40.143 Capsular glaucoma with pseudoexfoliation of lens, bilateral
[7] H40.149 Capsular glaucoma with pseudoexfoliation of lens, unspecified eye
[6] H40.15 Residual stage of open-angle glaucoma
H40.151 Residual stage of open-angle glaucoma, right eye
H40.152 Residual stage of open-angle glaucoma, left eye
H40.153 Residual stage of open-angle glaucoma, bilateral
H40.159 Residual stage of open-angle glaucoma, unspecified eye
[5] H40.2 Primary angle-closure glaucoma
[EXCLUDES1] *aqueous misdirection (H40.83-)*
malignant glaucoma (H40.83-)
[7th] H40.20 Unspecified primary angle-closure glaucoma
One of the following 7th characters is to be assigned to code H40.20 to designate the stage of glaucoma
0 = stage unspecified
1 = mild stage
2 = moderate stage
3 = severe stage
4 = indeterminate stage
[6] H40.21 Acute angle-closure glaucoma
Acute angle-closure glaucoma attack
Acute angle-closure glaucoma crisis
H40.211 Acute angle-closure glaucoma, right eye
H40.212 Acute angle-closure glaucoma, left eye
H40.213 Acute angle-closure glaucoma, bilateral
H40.219 Acute angle-closure glaucoma, unspecified eye
[6] H40.22 Chronic angle-closure glaucoma
Chronic primary angle closure glaucoma
One of the following 7th characters is to be assigned to each code in subcategory H40.22 to designate the stage of glaucoma
0 = stage unspecified
1 = mild stage
2 = moderate stage
3 = severe stage
4 = indeterminate stage
[7] H40.221 Chronic angle-closure glaucoma, right eye
[7] H40.222 Chronic angle-closure glaucoma, left eye
[7] H40.223 Chronic angle-closure glaucoma, bilateral
[7] H40.229 Chronic angle-closure glaucoma, unspecified eye
[6] H40.23 Intermittent angle-closure glaucoma
H40.231 Intermittent angle-closure glaucoma, right eye
H40.232 Intermittent angle-closure glaucoma, left eye
H40.233 Intermittent angle-closure glaucoma, bilateral
H40.239 Intermittent angle-closure glaucoma, unspecified eye
[6] H40.24 Residual stage of angle-closure glaucoma
H40.241 Residual stage of angle-closure glaucoma, right eye
H40.242 Residual stage of angle-closure glaucoma, left eye
H40.243 Residual stage of angle-closure glaucoma, bilateral
H40.249 Residual stage of angle-closure glaucoma, unspecified eye
[5] H40.3 Glaucoma secondary to eye trauma
Code also underlying condition
One of the following 7th characters is to be assigned to each code in subcategory H40.3 to designate the stage of glaucoma
0 = stage unspecified
1 = mild stage
2 = moderate stage
3 = severe stage
4 = indeterminate stage
[7th] H40.30 Glaucoma secondary to eye trauma, unspecified eye
[7th] H40.31 Glaucoma secondary to eye trauma, right eye
[7th] H40.32 Glaucoma secondary to eye trauma, left eye
[7th] H40.33 Glaucoma secondary to eye trauma, bilateral
[5] H40.4 Glaucoma secondary to eye inflammation
Code also underlying condition
One of the following 7th characters is to be assigned to each code in subcategory H40.4 to designate the stage of glaucoma
0 = stage unspecified
1 = mild stage
2 = moderate stage
3 = severe stage
4 = indeterminate stage
[7th] H40.40 Glaucoma secondary to eye inflammation, unspecified eye
[7th] H40.41 Glaucoma secondary to eye inflammation, right eye
[7th] H40.42 Glaucoma secondary to eye inflammation, left eye
[7th] H40.43 Glaucoma secondary to eye inflammation, bilateral
[5] H40.5 Glaucoma secondary to other eye disorders
Code also underlying eye disorder
One of the following 7th characters is to be assigned to each code in subcategory H40.5 to designate the stage of glaucoma
0 = stage unspecified
1 = mild stage
2 = moderate stage
3 = severe stage
4 = indeterminate stage
[7th] H40.50 Glaucoma secondary to other eye disorders, unspecified eye
[7th] H40.51 Glaucoma secondary to other eye disorders, right eye
[7th] H40.52 Glaucoma secondary to other eye disorders, left eye
[7th] H40.53 Glaucoma secondary to other eye disorders, bilateral
[5] H40.6 Glaucoma secondary to drugs
Use additional code for adverse effect, if applicable, to identify drug (T36-T50 with fifth or sixth character 5)
One of the following 7th characters is to be assigned to each code in subcategory H40.6 to designate the stage of glaucoma

[4] 4th character required [5] 5th character required [6] 6th character required [7] 7th character required [7th] Extension 'X' Alert
[EXCLUDES 1] Not coded here [EXCLUDES 2] Not included here [PDx] Primary Diagnosis Only Manifestation Code

0 = stage unspecified
1 = mild stage
2 = moderate stage
3 = severe stage
4 = indeterminate stage

[7th] H40.60 Glaucoma secondary to drugs, unspecified eye
[7th] H40.61 Glaucoma secondary to drugs, right eye
[7th] H40.62 Glaucoma secondary to drugs, left eye
[7th] H40.63 Glaucoma secondary to drugs, bilateral

[5] H40.8 Other glaucoma
[6] H40.81 Glaucoma with increased episcleral venous pressure
H40.811 Glaucoma with increased episcleral venous pressure, right eye
H40.812 Glaucoma with increased episcleral venous pressure, left eye
H40.813 Glaucoma with increased episcleral venous pressure, bilateral
H40.819 Glaucoma with increased episcleral venous pressure, unspecified eye

[6] H40.82 Hypersecretion glaucoma
H40.821 Hypersecretion glaucoma, right eye
H40.822 Hypersecretion glaucoma, left eye
H40.823 Hypersecretion glaucoma, bilateral
H40.829 Hypersecretion glaucoma, unspecified eye

[6] H40.83 Aqueous misdirection
Malignant glaucoma
H40.831 Aqueous misdirection, right eye
H40.832 Aqueous misdirection, left eye
H40.833 Aqueous misdirection, bilateral
H40.839 Aqueous misdirection, unspecified eye

H40.89 Other specified glaucoma
H40.9 Unspecified glaucoma

H42 Glaucoma in diseases classified elsewhere
Code first underlying condition, such as:
amyloidosis (E85.-)
aniridia (Q13.1)
Lowe's syndrome (E72.03)
Reiger's anomaly (Q13.81)
specified metabolic disorder (E70-E88)

EXCLUDES1 *glaucoma (in):*
diabetes mellitus (E08.39, E09.39, E10.39, E11.39, E13.39)
onchocerciasis (B73.02)
syphilis (A52.71)
tuberculous (A18.59)

Disorders of vitreous body and globe (H43-H44)

[4] H43 Disorders of vitreous body
[5] H43.0 Vitreous prolapse
EXCLUDES1 *vitreous syndrome following cataract surgery (H59.0-)*
traumatic vitreous prolapse (S05.2-)
H43.00 Vitreous prolapse, unspecified eye
H43.01 Vitreous prolapse, right eye
H43.02 Vitreous prolapse, left eye
H43.03 Vitreous prolapse, bilateral

[5] H43.1 Vitreous hemorrhage
H43.10 Vitreous hemorrhage, unspecified eye
H43.11 Vitreous hemorrhage, right eye
H43.12 Vitreous hemorrhage, left eye
H43.13 Vitreous hemorrhage, bilateral

[5] H43.2 Crystalline deposits in vitreous body
H43.20 Crystalline deposits in vitreous body, unspecified eye
H43.21 Crystalline deposits in vitreous body, right eye
H43.22 Crystalline deposits in vitreous body, left eye
H43.23 Crystalline deposits in vitreous body, bilateral

[5] H43.3 Other vitreous opacities
[6] H43.31 Vitreous membranes and strands
H43.311 Vitreous membranes and strands, right eye
H43.312 Vitreous membranes and strands, left eye
H43.313 Vitreous membranes and strands, bilateral
H43.319 Vitreous membranes and strands, unspecified eye

[6] H43.39 Other vitreous opacities
Vitreous floaters
H43.391 Other vitreous opacities, right eye
H43.392 Other vitreous opacities, left eye
H43.393 Other vitreous opacities, bilateral
H43.399 Other vitreous opacities, unspecified eye

[5] H43.8 Other disorders of vitreous body
EXCLUDES1 *proliferative vitreo-retinopathy with retinal detachment (H33.4-)*
EXCLUDES2 *vitreous abscess (H44.02-)*

[6] H43.81 Vitreous degeneration
Vitreous detachment
H43.811 Vitreous degeneration, right eye
H43.812 Vitreous degeneration, left eye
H43.813 Vitreous degeneration, bilateral
H43.819 Vitreous degeneration, unspecified eye

[6] H43.82 Vitreomacular adhesion
Vitreomacular traction
H43.821 Vitreomacular adhesion, right eye [A]
H43.822 Vitreomacular adhesion, left eye [A]
H43.823 Vitreomacular adhesion, bilateral [A]
H43.829 Vitreomacular adhesion, unspecified eye [A]

H43.89 Other disorders of vitreous body
H43.9 Unspecified disorder of vitreous body

[4] H44 Disorders of globe
INCLUDES *disorders affecting multiple structures of eye*

[5] H44.0 Purulent endophthalmitis
Use additional code to identify organism
EXCLUDES1 *bleb associated endophthalmitis (H59.4-)*

[6] H44.00 Unspecified purulent endophthalmitis
H44.001 Unspecified purulent endophthalmitis, right eye
H44.002 Unspecified purulent endophthalmitis, left eye
H44.003 Unspecified purulent endophthalmitis, bilateral
H44.009 Unspecified purulent endophthalmitis, unspecified eye

[6] H44.01 Panophthalmitis (acute)
H44.011 Panophthalmitis (acute), right eye
H44.012 Panophthalmitis (acute), left eye
H44.013 Panophthalmitis (acute), bilateral
H44.019 Panophthalmitis (acute), unspecified eye

[6] H44.02 Vitreous abscess (chronic)
H44.021 Vitreous abscess (chronic), right eye
H44.022 Vitreous abscess (chronic), left eye
H44.023 Vitreous abscess (chronic), bilateral
H44.029 Vitreous abscess (chronic), unspecified eye

[5] H44.1 Other endophthalmitis
EXCLUDES1 *bleb associated endophthalmitis (H59.4-)*
EXCLUDES2 *ophthalmia nodosa (H16.2-)*

[6] H44.11 Panuveitis
H44.111 Panuveitis, right eye
H44.112 Panuveitis, left eye
H44.113 Panuveitis, bilateral
H44.119 Panuveitis, unspecified eye

[6] H44.12 Parasitic endophthalmitis, unspecified
H44.121 Parasitic endophthalmitis, unspecified, right eye
H44.122 Parasitic endophthalmitis, unspecified, left eye

H44.123 Parasitic endophthalmitis, unspecified, bilateral
H44.129 Parasitic endophthalmitis, unspecified, unspecified eye

[6] H44.13 Sympathetic uveitis
H44.131 Sympathetic uveitis, right eye
H44.132 Sympathetic uveitis, left eye
H44.133 Sympathetic uveitis, bilateral
H44.139 Sympathetic uveitis, unspecified eye

H44.19 Other endophthalmitis

[5] H44.2 Degenerative myopia
Malignant myopia
H44.20 Degenerative myopia, unspecified eye
H44.21 Degenerative myopia, right eye
H44.22 Degenerative myopia, left eye
H44.23 Degenerative myopia, bilateral

[5] H44.3 Other and unspecified degenerative disorders of globe
H44.30 Unspecified degenerative disorder of globe

[6] H44.31 Chalcosis
H44.311 Chalcosis, right eye
H44.312 Chalcosis, left eye
H44.313 Chalcosis, bilateral
H44.319 Chalcosis, unspecified eye

[6] H44.32 Siderosis of eye
H44.321 Siderosis of eye, right eye
H44.322 Siderosis of eye, left eye
H44.323 Siderosis of eye, bilateral
H44.329 Siderosis of eye, unspecified eye

[6] H44.39 Other degenerative disorders of globe
H44.391 Other degenerative disorders of globe, right eye
H44.392 Other degenerative disorders of globe, left eye
H44.393 Other degenerative disorders of globe, bilateral
H44.399 Other degenerative disorders of globe, unspecified eye

[5] H44.4 Hypotony of eye
H44.40 Unspecified hypotony of eye

[6] H44.41 Flat anterior chamber hypotony of eye
H44.411 Flat anterior chamber hypotony of right eye
H44.412 Flat anterior chamber hypotony of left eye
H44.413 Flat anterior chamber hypotony of eye, bilateral
H44.419 Flat anterior chamber hypotony of unspecified eye

[6] H44.42 Hypotony of eye due to ocular fistula
H44.421 Hypotony of right eye due to ocular fistula
H44.422 Hypotony of left eye due to ocular fistula
H44.423 Hypotony of eye due to ocular fistula, bilateral
H44.429 Hypotony of unspecified eye due to ocular fistula

[6] H44.43 Hypotony of eye due to other ocular disorders
H44.431 Hypotony of eye due to other ocular disorders, right eye
H44.432 Hypotony of eye due to other ocular disorders, left eye
H44.433 Hypotony of eye due to other ocular disorders, bilateral
H44.439 Hypotony of eye due to other ocular disorders, unspecified eye

[6] H44.44 Primary hypotony of eye
H44.441 Primary hypotony of right eye
H44.442 Primary hypotony of left eye
H44.443 Primary hypotony of eye, bilateral
H44.449 Primary hypotony of unspecified eye

[5] H44.5 Degenerated conditions of globe
H44.50 Unspecified degenerated conditions of globe

[6] H44.51 Absolute glaucoma
H44.511 Absolute glaucoma, right eye
H44.512 Absolute glaucoma, left eye
H44.513 Absolute glaucoma, bilateral
H44.519 Absolute glaucoma, unspecified eye

[6] H44.52 Atrophy of globe
Phthisis bulbi
H44.521 Atrophy of globe, right eye
H44.522 Atrophy of globe, left eye
H44.523 Atrophy of globe, bilateral
H44.529 Atrophy of globe, unspecified eye

[6] H44.53 Leucocoria
H44.531 Leucocoria, right eye
H44.532 Leucocoria, left eye
H44.533 Leucocoria, bilateral
H44.539 Leucocoria, unspecified eye

[5] H44.6 Retained (old) intraocular foreign body, magnetic
Use additional code to identify magnetic foreign body (Z18.11)

[EXCLUDES1] *current intraocular foreign body (S05.-)*

[EXCLUDES2] *retained foreign body in eyelid (H02.81-)*
retained (old) foreign body following penetrating wound of orbit (H05.5-)
retained (old) intraocular foreign body, nonmagnetic (H44.7-)

[6] H44.60 Unspecified retained (old) intraocular foreign body, magnetic
H44.601 Unspecified retained (old) intraocular foreign body, magnetic, right eye
H44.602 Unspecified retained (old) intraocular foreign body, magnetic, left eye
H44.603 Unspecified retained (old) intraocular foreign body, magnetic, bilateral
H44.609 Unspecified retained (old) intraocular foreign body, magnetic, unspecified eye

[6] H44.61 Retained (old) magnetic foreign body in anterior chamber
H44.611 Retained (old) magnetic foreign body in anterior chamber, right eye
H44.612 Retained (old) magnetic foreign body in anterior chamber, left eye
H44.613 Retained (old) magnetic foreign body in anterior chamber, bilateral
H44.619 Retained (old) magnetic foreign body in anterior chamber, unspecified eye

[6] H44.62 Retained (old) magnetic foreign body in iris or ciliary body
H44.621 Retained (old) magnetic foreign body in iris or ciliary body, right eye
H44.622 Retained (old) magnetic foreign body in iris or ciliary body, left eye
H44.623 Retained (old) magnetic foreign body in iris or ciliary body, bilateral
H44.629 Retained (old) magnetic foreign body in iris or ciliary body, unspecified eye

[6] H44.63 Retained (old) magnetic foreign body in lens
H44.631 Retained (old) magnetic foreign body in lens, right eye
H44.632 Retained (old) magnetic foreign body in lens, left eye
H44.633 Retained (old) magnetic foreign body in lens, bilateral
H44.639 Retained (old) magnetic foreign body in lens, unspecified eye

[6] H44.64 Retained (old) magnetic foreign body in posterior wall of globe

[4] 4th character required [5] 5th character required [6] 6th character required [7] 7th character required [7] Extension 'X' Alert
[EXCLUDES 1] Not coded here [EXCLUDES 2] Not included here [PDx] Primary Diagnosis Only Manifestation Code

H44.641 Retained (old) magnetic foreign body in posterior wall of globe, right eye

H44.642 Retained (old) magnetic foreign body in posterior wall of globe, left eye

H44.643 Retained (old) magnetic foreign body in posterior wall of globe, bilateral

H44.649 Retained (old) magnetic foreign body in posterior wall of globe, unspecified eye

H44.65 Retained (old) magnetic foreign body in vitreous body

H44.651 Retained (old) magnetic foreign body in vitreous body, right eye

H44.652 Retained (old) magnetic foreign body in vitreous body, left eye

H44.653 Retained (old) magnetic foreign body in vitreous body, bilateral

H44.659 Retained (old) magnetic foreign body in vitreous body, unspecified eye

H44.69 Retained (old) intraocular foreign body, magnetic, in other or multiple sites

H44.691 Retained (old) intraocular foreign body, magnetic, in other or multiple sites, right eye

H44.692 Retained (old) intraocular foreign body, magnetic, in other or multiple sites, left eye

H44.693 Retained (old) intraocular foreign body, magnetic, in other or multiple sites, bilateral

H44.699 Retained (old) intraocular foreign body, magnetic, in other or multiple sites, unspecified eye

H44.7 Retained (old) intraocular foreign body, nonmagnetic
Use additional code to identify nonmagnetic foreign body (Z18.01-Z18.10, Z18.12, Z18.2-Z18.9)
EXCLUDES1 current intraocular foreign body (S05.-)
EXCLUDES2 retained foreign body in eyelid (H02.81-)
retained (old) foreign body following penetrating wound of orbit (H05.5-)
retained (old) intraocular foreign body, magnetic (H44.6-)

H44.70 Unspecified retained (old) intraocular foreign body, nonmagnetic

H44.701 Unspecified retained (old) intraocular foreign body, nonmagnetic, right eye

H44.702 Unspecified retained (old) intraocular foreign body, nonmagnetic, left eye

H44.703 Unspecified retained (old) intraocular foreign body, nonmagnetic, bilateral

H44.709 Unspecified retained (old) intraocular foreign body, nonmagnetic, unspecified eye
Retained (old) intraocular foreign body NOS

H44.71 Retained (nonmagnetic) (old) foreign body in anterior chamber

H44.711 Retained (nonmagnetic) (old) foreign body in anterior chamber, right eye

H44.712 Retained (nonmagnetic) (old) foreign body in anterior chamber, left eye

H44.713 Retained (nonmagnetic) (old) foreign body in anterior chamber, bilateral

H44.719 Retained (nonmagnetic) (old) foreign body in anterior chamber, unspecified eye

H44.72 Retained (nonmagnetic) (old) foreign body in iris or ciliary body

H44.721 Retained (nonmagnetic) (old) foreign body in iris or ciliary body, right eye

H44.722 Retained (nonmagnetic) (old) foreign body in iris or ciliary body, left eye

H44.723 Retained (nonmagnetic) (old) foreign body in iris or ciliary body, bilateral

H44.729 Retained (nonmagnetic) (old) foreign body in iris or ciliary body, unspecified eye

H44.73 Retained (nonmagnetic) (old) foreign body in lens

H44.731 Retained (nonmagnetic) (old) foreign body in lens, right eye

H44.732 Retained (nonmagnetic) (old) foreign body in lens, left eye

H44.733 Retained (nonmagnetic) (old) foreign body in lens, bilateral

H44.739 Retained (nonmagnetic) (old) foreign body in lens, unspecified eye

H44.74 Retained (nonmagnetic) (old) foreign body in posterior wall of globe

H44.741 Retained (nonmagnetic) (old) foreign body in posterior wall of globe, right eye

H44.742 Retained (nonmagnetic) (old) foreign body in posterior wall of globe, left eye

H44.743 Retained (nonmagnetic) (old) foreign body in posterior wall of globe, bilateral

H44.749 Retained (nonmagnetic) (old) foreign body in posterior wall of globe, unspecified eye

H44.75 Retained (nonmagnetic) (old) foreign body in vitreous body

H44.751 Retained (nonmagnetic) (old) foreign body in vitreous body, right eye

H44.752 Retained (nonmagnetic) (old) foreign body in vitreous body, left eye

H44.753 Retained (nonmagnetic) (old) foreign body in vitreous body, bilateral

H44.759 Retained (nonmagnetic) (old) foreign body in vitreous body, unspecified eye

H44.79 Retained (old) intraocular foreign body, nonmagnetic, in other or multiple sites

H44.791 Retained (old) intraocular foreign body, nonmagnetic, in other or multiple sites, right eye

H44.792 Retained (old) intraocular foreign body, nonmagnetic, in other or multiple sites, left eye

H44.793 Retained (old) intraocular foreign body, nonmagnetic, in other or multiple sites, bilateral

H44.799 Retained (old) intraocular foreign body, nonmagnetic, in other or multiple sites, unspecified eye

H44.8 Other disorders of globe

H44.81 Hemophthalmos

H44.811 Hemophthalmos, right eye

H44.812 Hemophthalmos, left eye

H44.813 Hemophthalmos, bilateral

H44.819 Hemophthalmos, unspecified eye

H44.82 Luxation of globe

H44.821 Luxation of globe, right eye

H44.822 Luxation of globe, left eye

H44.823 Luxation of globe, bilateral

H44.829 Luxation of globe, unspecified eye

H44.89 Other disorders of globe

H44.9 Unspecified disorder of globe

Disorders of optic nerve and visual pathways (H46-H47)

[4] H46 Optic neuritis
[EXCLUDES2] *ischemic optic neuropathy (H47.01-)*
neuromyelitis optica [Devic] (G36.0)
[5] H46.0 Optic papillitis
H46.00 Optic papillitis, unspecified eye
H46.01 Optic papillitis, right eye
H46.02 Optic papillitis, left eye
H46.03 Optic papillitis, bilateral
[5] H46.1 Retrobulbar neuritis
Retrobulbar neuritis NOS
[EXCLUDES1] *syphilitic retrobulbar neuritis (A52.15)*
H46.10 Retrobulbar neuritis, unspecified eye
H46.11 Retrobulbar neuritis, right eye
H46.12 Retrobulbar neuritis, left eye
H46.13 Retrobulbar neuritis, bilateral
H46.2 Nutritional optic neuropathy
H46.3 Toxic optic neuropathy
Code first (T51-T65) to identify cause
H46.8 Other optic neuritis
H46.9 Unspecified optic neuritis
[4] H47 Other disorders of optic [2nd] nerve and visual pathways
[5] H47.0 Disorders of optic nerve, not elsewhere classified
[6] H47.01 Ischemic optic neuropathy
H47.011 Ischemic optic neuropathy, right eye
H47.012 Ischemic optic neuropathy, left eye
H47.013 Ischemic optic neuropathy, bilateral
H47.019 Ischemic optic neuropathy, unspecified eye
[6] H47.02 Hemorrhage in optic nerve sheath
H47.021 Hemorrhage in optic nerve sheath, right eye
H47.022 Hemorrhage in optic nerve sheath, left eye
H47.023 Hemorrhage in optic nerve sheath, bilateral
H47.029 Hemorrhage in optic nerve sheath, unspecified eye
[6] H47.03 Optic nerve hypoplasia
H47.031 Optic nerve hypoplasia, right eye
H47.032 Optic nerve hypoplasia, left eye
H47.033 Optic nerve hypoplasia, bilateral
H47.039 Optic nerve hypoplasia, unspecified eye
[6] H47.09 Other disorders of optic nerve, not elsewhere classified
Compression of optic nerve
H47.091 Other disorders of optic nerve, not elsewhere classified, right eye
H47.092 Other disorders of optic nerve, not elsewhere classified, left eye
H47.093 Other disorders of optic nerve, not elsewhere classified, bilateral
H47.099 Other disorders of optic nerve, not elsewhere classified, unspecified eye
[5] H47.1 Papilledema
H47.10 Unspecified papilledema
H47.11 Papilledema associated with increased intracranial pressure
H47.12 Papilledema associated with decreased ocular pressure
H47.13 Papilledema associated with retinal disorder
[6] H47.14 Foster-Kennedy syndrome
H47.141 Foster-Kennedy syndrome, right eye
H47.142 Foster-Kennedy syndrome, left eye
H47.143 Foster-Kennedy syndrome, bilateral
H47.149 Foster-Kennedy syndrome, unspecified eye
[5] H47.2 Optic atrophy
H47.20 Unspecified optic atrophy
[6] H47.21 Primary optic atrophy
H47.211 Primary optic atrophy, right eye
H47.212 Primary optic atrophy, left eye
H47.213 Primary optic atrophy, bilateral
H47.219 Primary optic atrophy, unspecified eye
H47.22 Hereditary optic atrophy
Leber's optic atrophy
[6] H47.23 Glaucomatous optic atrophy
H47.231 Glaucomatous optic atrophy, right eye
H47.232 Glaucomatous optic atrophy, left eye
H47.233 Glaucomatous optic atrophy, bilateral
H47.239 Glaucomatous optic atrophy, unspecified eye
[6] H47.29 Other optic atrophy
Temporal pallor of optic disc
H47.291 Other optic atrophy, right eye
H47.292 Other optic atrophy, left eye
H47.293 Other optic atrophy, bilateral
H47.299 Other optic atrophy, unspecified eye
[5] H47.3 Other disorders of optic disc
[6] H47.31 Coloboma of optic disc
H47.311 Coloboma of optic disc, right eye
H47.312 Coloboma of optic disc, left eye
H47.313 Coloboma of optic disc, bilateral
H47.319 Coloboma of optic disc, unspecified eye
[6] H47.32 Drusen of optic disc
H47.321 Drusen of optic disc, right eye
H47.322 Drusen of optic disc, left eye
H47.323 Drusen of optic disc, bilateral
H47.329 Drusen of optic disc, unspecified eye
[6] H47.33 Pseudopapilledema of optic disc
H47.331 Pseudopapilledema of optic disc, right eye
H47.332 Pseudopapilledema of optic disc, left eye
H47.333 Pseudopapilledema of optic disc, bilateral
H47.339 Pseudopapilledema of optic disc, unspecified eye
[6] H47.39 Other disorders of optic disc
H47.391 Other disorders of optic disc, right eye
H47.392 Other disorders of optic disc, left eye
H47.393 Other disorders of optic disc, bilateral
H47.399 Other disorders of optic disc, unspecified eye
[5] H47.4 Disorders of optic chiasm
Code also underlying condition
H47.41 Disorders of optic chiasm in (due to) inflammatory disorders
H47.42 Disorders of optic chiasm in (due to) neoplasm
H47.43 Disorders of optic chiasm in (due to) vascular disorders
H47.49 Disorders of optic chiasm in (due to) other disorders
[5] H47.5 Disorders of other visual pathways
Disorders of optic tracts, geniculate nuclei and optic radiations
Code also underlying condition
[6] H47.51 Disorders of visual pathways in (due to) inflammatory disorders
H47.511 Disorders of visual pathways in (due to) inflammatory disorders, right side
H47.512 Disorders of visual pathways in (due to) inflammatory disorders, left side
H47.519 Disorders of visual pathways in (due to) inflammatory disorders, unspecified side
[6] H47.52 Disorders of visual pathways in (due to) neoplasm
H47.521 Disorders of visual pathways in (due to) neoplasm, right side

[4] 4th character required [5] 5th character required [6] 6th character required [7] 7th character required [x7] Extension 'X' Alert
[EXCLUDES1] Not coded here [EXCLUDES2] Not included here [PDx] Primary Diagnosis Only Manifestation Code

H47.522 Disorders of visual pathways in (due to) neoplasm, left side
H47.529 Disorders of visual pathways in (due to) neoplasm, unspecified side
[6] H47.53 Disorders of visual pathways in (due to) vascular disorders
H47.531 Disorders of visual pathways in (due to) vascular disorders, right side
H47.532 Disorders of visual pathways in (due to) vascular disorders, left side
H47.539 Disorders of visual pathways in (due to) vascular disorders, unspecified side
[5] H47.6 Disorders of visual cortex
Code also underlying condition
[EXCLUDES1] *injury to visual cortex S04.04*
[6] H47.61 Cortical blindness
H47.611 Cortical blindness, right side of brain
H47.612 Cortical blindness, left side of brain
H47.619 Cortical blindness, unspecified side of brain
[6] H47.62 Disorders of visual cortex in (due to) inflammatory disorders
H47.621 Disorders of visual cortex in (due to) inflammatory disorders, right side of brain
H47.622 Disorders of visual cortex in (due to) inflammatory disorders, left side of brain
H47.629 Disorders of visual cortex in (due to) inflammatory disorders, unspecified side of brain
[6] H47.63 Disorders of visual cortex in (due to) neoplasm
H47.631 Disorders of visual cortex in (due to) neoplasm, right side of brain
H47.632 Disorders of visual cortex in (due to) neoplasm, left side of brain
H47.639 Disorders of visual cortex in (due to) neoplasm, unspecified side of brain
[6] H47.64 Disorders of visual cortex in (due to) vascular disorders
H47.641 Disorders of visual cortex in (due to) vascular disorders, right side of brain
H47.642 Disorders of visual cortex in (due to) vascular disorders, left side of brain
H47.649 Disorders of visual cortex in (due to) vascular disorders, unspecified side of brain
H47.9 Unspecified disorder of visual pathways

Disorders of ocular muscles, binocular movement, accommodation and refraction (H49-H52)

[EXCLUDES2] *nystagmus and other irregular eye movements (H55)*

[4] H49 Paralytic strabismus
[EXCLUDES2] *internal ophthalmoplegia (H52.51-)*
internuclear ophthalmoplegia (H51.2-)
progressive supranuclear ophthalmoplegia (G23.1)
[5] H49.0 Third [oculomotor] nerve palsy
H49.00 Third [oculomotor] nerve palsy, unspecified eye
H49.01 Third [oculomotor] nerve palsy, right eye
H49.02 Third [oculomotor] nerve palsy, left eye
H49.03 Third [oculomotor] nerve palsy, bilateral
[5] H49.1 Fourth [trochlear] nerve palsy
H49.10 Fourth [trochlear] nerve palsy, unspecified eye
H49.11 Fourth [trochlear] nerve palsy, right eye
H49.12 Fourth [trochlear] nerve palsy, left eye
H49.13 Fourth [trochlear] nerve palsy, bilateral
[5] H49.2 Sixth [abducent] nerve palsy
H49.20 Sixth [abducent] nerve palsy, unspecified eye
H49.21 Sixth [abducent] nerve palsy, right eye
H49.22 Sixth [abducent] nerve palsy, left eye
H49.23 Sixth [abducent] nerve palsy, bilateral
[5] H49.3 Total (external) ophthalmoplegia
H49.30 Total (external) ophthalmoplegia, unspecified eye
H49.31 Total (external) ophthalmoplegia, right eye
H49.32 Total (external) ophthalmoplegia, left eye
H49.33 Total (external) ophthalmoplegia, bilateral
[5] H49.4 Progressive external ophthalmoplegia
[EXCLUDES1] *Kearns-Sayre syndrome (H49.81-)*
H49.40 Progressive external ophthalmoplegia, unspecified eye
H49.41 Progressive external ophthalmoplegia, right eye
H49.42 Progressive external ophthalmoplegia, left eye
H49.43 Progressive external ophthalmoplegia, bilateral
[5] H49.8 Other paralytic strabismus
[6] H49.81 Kearns-Sayre syndrome
Progressive external ophthalmoplegia with pigmentary retinopathy
Use additional code for other manifestation, such as: heart block (I45.9)
H49.811 Kearns-Sayre syndrome, right eye
H49.812 Kearns-Sayre syndrome, left eye
H49.813 Kearns-Sayre syndrome, bilateral
H49.819 Kearns-Sayre syndrome, unspecified eye
[6] H49.88 Other paralytic strabismus
External ophthalmoplegia NOS
H49.881 Other paralytic strabismus, right eye
H49.882 Other paralytic strabismus, left eye
H49.883 Other paralytic strabismus, bilateral
H49.889 Other paralytic strabismus, unspecified eye
H49.9 Unspecified paralytic strabismus

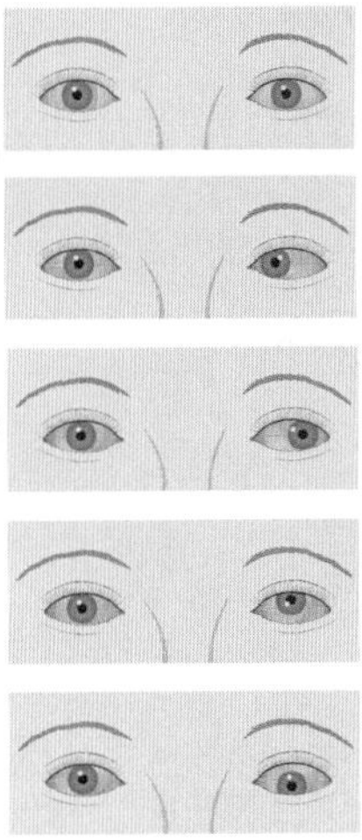
Normal
Esotropia - eye turns inward
Exotropia - eye turns outward
Hypertropia - eye turns upward
Hypotropia - eye turns downward

Figure 7.5 Types of Strabismus

[4] H50 Other strabismus
[5] H50.0 Esotropia
Convergent concomitant strabismus
[EXCLUDES1] *intermittent esotropia (H50.31-, H50.32)*
H50.00 Unspecified esotropia
[6] H50.01 Monocular esotropia
H50.011 Monocular esotropia, right eye
H50.012 Monocular esotropia, left eye
[6] H50.02 Monocular esotropia with A pattern
H50.021 Monocular esotropia with A pattern, right eye
H50.022 Monocular esotropia with A pattern, left eye
[6] H50.03 Monocular esotropia with V pattern

Unspecified Code | Other Specified Code | [N] Newborn Age: 0 | [P] Pediatric Age: 0-17 | [M] Maternity Age: 12-55
[A] Adult Age: 15-124 | ♂ Male | ♀ Female | ● New Code | ▲ Revised Code Title | ►◄ Revised Text

H50.031 Monocular esotropia with V pattern, right eye

H50.032 Monocular esotropia with V pattern, left eye

H50.04 Monocular esotropia with other noncomitancies

H50.041 Monocular esotropia with other noncomitancies, right eye

H50.042 Monocular esotropia with other noncomitancies, left eye

H50.05 Alternating esotropia

H50.06 Alternating esotropia with A pattern

H50.07 Alternating esotropia with V pattern

H50.08 Alternating esotropia with other noncomitancies

H50.1 Exotropia

Divergent concomitant strabismus

EXCLUDES1 intermittent exotropia (H50.33-, H50.34)

H50.10 Unspecified exotropia

H50.11 Monocular exotropia

H50.111 Monocular exotropia, right eye

H50.112 Monocular exotropia, left eye

H50.12 Monocular exotropia with A pattern

H50.121 Monocular exotropia with A pattern, right eye

H50.122 Monocular exotropia with A pattern, left eye

H50.13 Monocular exotropia with V pattern

H50.131 Monocular exotropia with V pattern, right eye

H50.132 Monocular exotropia with V pattern, left eye

H50.14 Monocular exotropia with other noncomitancies

H50.141 Monocular exotropia with other noncomitancies, right eye

H50.142 Monocular exotropia with other noncomitancies, left eye

H50.15 Alternating exotropia

H50.16 Alternating exotropia with A pattern

H50.17 Alternating exotropia with V pattern

H50.18 Alternating exotropia with other noncomitancies

H50.2 Vertical strabismus

Hypertropia

H50.21 Vertical strabismus, right eye

H50.22 Vertical strabismus, left eye

H50.3 Intermittent heterotropia

H50.30 Unspecified intermittent heterotropia

H50.31 Intermittent monocular esotropia

H50.311 Intermittent monocular esotropia, right eye

H50.312 Intermittent monocular esotropia, left eye

H50.32 Intermittent alternating esotropia

H50.33 Intermittent monocular exotropia

H50.331 Intermittent monocular exotropia, right eye

H50.332 Intermittent monocular exotropia, left eye

H50.34 Intermittent alternating exotropia

H50.4 Other and unspecified heterotropia

H50.40 Unspecified heterotropia

H50.41 Cyclotropia

H50.411 Cyclotropia, right eye

H50.412 Cyclotropia, left eye

H50.42 Monofixation syndrome

H50.43 Accommodative component in esotropia

H50.5 Heterophoria

H50.50 Unspecified heterophoria

H50.51 Esophoria

H50.52 Exophoria

H50.53 Vertical heterophoria

H50.54 Cyclophoria

H50.55 Alternating heterophoria

H50.6 Mechanical strabismus

H50.60 Mechanical strabismus, unspecified

H50.61 Brown's sheath syndrome

H50.611 Brown's sheath syndrome, right eye

H50.612 Brown's sheath syndrome, left eye

H50.69 Other mechanical strabismus

Strabismus due to adhesions

Traumatic limitation of duction of eye muscle

H50.8 Other specified strabismus

H50.81 Duane's syndrome

H50.811 Duane's syndrome, right eye

H50.812 Duane's syndrome, left eye

H50.89 Other specified strabismus

H50.9 Unspecified strabismus

H51 Other disorders of binocular movement

H51.0 Palsy (spasm) of conjugate gaze

H51.1 Convergence insufficiency and excess

H51.11 Convergence insufficiency

H51.12 Convergence excess

H51.2 Internuclear ophthalmoplegia

H51.20 Internuclear ophthalmoplegia, unspecified eye

H51.21 Internuclear ophthalmoplegia, right eye

H51.22 Internuclear ophthalmoplegia, left eye

H51.23 Internuclear ophthalmoplegia, bilateral

H51.8 Other specified disorders of binocular movement

H51.9 Unspecified disorder of binocular movement

H52 Disorders of refraction and accommodation

H52.0 Hypermetropia

H52.00 Hypermetropia, unspecified eye

H52.01 Hypermetropia, right eye

H52.02 Hypermetropia, left eye

H52.03 Hypermetropia, bilateral

H52.1 Myopia

EXCLUDES1 degenerative myopia (H44.2-)

H52.10 Myopia, unspecified eye

H52.11 Myopia, right eye

H52.12 Myopia, left eye

H52.13 Myopia, bilateral

H52.2 Astigmatism

H52.20 Unspecified astigmatism

H52.201 Unspecified astigmatism, right eye

H52.202 Unspecified astigmatism, left eye

H52.203 Unspecified astigmatism, bilateral

H52.209 Unspecified astigmatism, unspecified eye

H52.21 Irregular astigmatism

H52.211 Irregular astigmatism, right eye

H52.212 Irregular astigmatism, left eye

H52.213 Irregular astigmatism, bilateral

H52.219 Irregular astigmatism, unspecified eye

H52.22 Regular astigmatism

H52.221 Regular astigmatism, right eye

H52.222 Regular astigmatism, left eye

H52.223 Regular astigmatism, bilateral

H52.229 Regular astigmatism, unspecified eye

H52.3 Anisometropia and aniseikonia

H52.31 Anisometropia

H52.32 Aniseikonia

H52.4 Presbyopia

H52.5 Disorders of accommodation

H52.51 Internal ophthalmoplegia (complete) (total)

H52.511 Internal ophthalmoplegia (complete) (total), right eye

---

4th character required   5th character required   6th character required   7th character required   Extension 'X' Alert

EXCLUDES1 Not coded here   EXCLUDES2 Not included here   Primary Diagnosis Only   Manifestation Code

H52.512 Internal ophthalmoplegia (complete) (total), left eye
H52.513 Internal ophthalmoplegia (complete) (total), bilateral
H52.519 Internal ophthalmoplegia (complete) (total), unspecified eye
H52.52 Paresis of accommodation
  H52.521 Paresis of accommodation, right eye
  H52.522 Paresis of accommodation, left eye
  H52.523 Paresis of accommodation, bilateral
  H52.529 Paresis of accommodation, unspecified eye
H52.53 Spasm of accommodation
  H52.531 Spasm of accommodation, right eye
  H52.532 Spasm of accommodation, left eye
  H52.533 Spasm of accommodation, bilateral
  H52.539 Spasm of accommodation, unspecified eye
H52.6 Other disorders of refraction
H52.7 Unspecified disorder of refraction

Visual disturbances and blindness (H53-H54)

H53 Visual disturbances
H53.0 Amblyopia ex anopsia
  EXCLUDES1 amblyopia due to vitamin A deficiency (E50.5)
H53.00 Unspecified amblyopia
  H53.001 Unspecified amblyopia, right eye
  H53.002 Unspecified amblyopia, left eye
  H53.003 Unspecified amblyopia, bilateral
  H53.009 Unspecified amblyopia, unspecified eye
H53.01 Deprivation amblyopia
  H53.011 Deprivation amblyopia, right eye
  H53.012 Deprivation amblyopia, left eye
  H53.013 Deprivation amblyopia, bilateral
  H53.019 Deprivation amblyopia, unspecified eye
H53.02 Refractive amblyopia
  H53.021 Refractive amblyopia, right eye
  H53.022 Refractive amblyopia, left eye
  H53.023 Refractive amblyopia, bilateral
  H53.029 Refractive amblyopia, unspecified eye
H53.03 Strabismic amblyopia
  EXCLUDES1 strabismus (H50.-)
  H53.031 Strabismic amblyopia, right eye
  H53.032 Strabismic amblyopia, left eye
  H53.033 Strabismic amblyopia, bilateral
  H53.039 Strabismic amblyopia, unspecified eye
H53.1 Subjective visual disturbances
  EXCLUDES1 subjective visual disturbances due to vitamin A deficiency (E50.5)
    visual hallucinations (R44.1)
H53.10 Unspecified subjective visual disturbances
H53.11 Day blindness
  Hemeralopia
H53.12 Transient visual loss
  Scintillating scotoma
  EXCLUDES1 amaurosis fugax (G45.3-)
    transient retinal artery occlusion (H34.0-)
  H53.121 Transient visual loss, right eye
  H53.122 Transient visual loss, left eye
  H53.123 Transient visual loss, bilateral
  H53.129 Transient visual loss, unspecified eye
H53.13 Sudden visual loss
  H53.131 Sudden visual loss, right eye
  H53.132 Sudden visual loss, left eye
  H53.133 Sudden visual loss, bilateral
  H53.139 Sudden visual loss, unspecified eye
H53.14 Visual discomfort
  Asthenopia
  Photophobia

H53.141 Visual discomfort, right eye
H53.142 Visual discomfort, left eye
H53.143 Visual discomfort, bilateral
H53.149 Visual discomfort, unspecified
H53.15 Visual distortions of shape and size
  Metamorphopsia
H53.16 Psychophysical visual disturbances
H53.19 Other subjective visual disturbances
  Visual halos
H53.2 Diplopia
  Double vision
H53.3 Other and unspecified disorders of binocular vision
H53.30 Unspecified disorder of binocular vision
H53.31 Abnormal retinal correspondence
H53.32 Fusion with defective stereopsis
H53.33 Simultaneous visual perception without fusion
H53.34 Suppression of binocular vision
H53.4 Visual field defects
H53.40 Unspecified visual field defects
H53.41 Scotoma involving central area
  Central scotoma
  H53.411 Scotoma involving central area, right eye
  H53.412 Scotoma involving central area, left eye
  H53.413 Scotoma involving central area, bilateral
  H53.419 Scotoma involving central area, unspecified eye
H53.42 Scotoma of blind spot area
  Enlarged blind spot
  H53.421 Scotoma of blind spot area, right eye
  H53.422 Scotoma of blind spot area, left eye
  H53.423 Scotoma of blind spot area, bilateral
  H53.429 Scotoma of blind spot area, unspecified eye
H53.43 Sector or arcuate defects
  Arcuate scotoma
  Bjerrum scotoma
  H53.431 Sector or arcuate defects, right eye
  H53.432 Sector or arcuate defects, left eye
  H53.433 Sector or arcuate defects, bilateral
  H53.439 Sector or arcuate defects, unspecified eye
H53.45 Other localized visual field defect
  Peripheral visual field defect
  Ring scotoma NOS
  Scotoma NOS
  H53.451 Other localized visual field defect, right eye
  H53.452 Other localized visual field defect, left eye
  H53.453 Other localized visual field defect, bilateral
  H53.459 Other localized visual field defect, unspecified eye
H53.46 Homonymous bilateral field defects
  Homonymous hemianopia
  Homonymous hemianopsia
  Quadrant anopia
  Quadrant anopsia
  H53.461 Homonymous bilateral field defects, right side
  H53.462 Homonymous bilateral field defects, left side
  H53.469 Homonymous bilateral field defects, unspecified side
    Homonymous bilateral field defects NOS
H53.47 Heteronymous bilateral field defects
  Heteronymous hemianop(s)ia
H53.48 Generalized contraction of visual field
  H53.481 Generalized contraction of visual field, right eye
  H53.482 Generalized contraction of visual field, left eye

Unspecified Code | Other Specified Code | N Newborn Age: 0 | P Pediatric Age: 0-17 | M Maternity Age: 12-55 | A Adult Age: 15-124 | ♂ Male | ♀ Female | ● New Code | ▲ Revised Code Title | ▶◀ Revised Text

H53.483 **Generalized contraction of visual field, bilateral**

H53.489 **Generalized contraction of visual field, unspecified eye**

[5th] **H53.5 Color vision deficiencies**

Color blindness

EXCLUDES2 *day blindness (H53.11)*

H53.50 **Unspecified color vision deficiencies**

Color blindness NOS

H53.51 **Achromatopsia**

H53.52 **Acquired color vision deficiency**

H53.53 **Deuteranomaly**

Deuteranopia

H53.54 **Protanomaly**

Protanopia

H53.55 **Tritanomaly**

Tritanopia

H53.59 **Other color vision deficiencies**

[5th] **H53.6 Night blindness**

EXCLUDES1 *night blindness due to vitamin A deficiency (E50.5)*

H53.60 **Unspecified night blindness**

H53.61 **Abnormal dark adaptation curve**

H53.62 **Acquired night blindness**

H53.63 **Congenital night blindness**

H53.69 **Other night blindness**

[5th] **H53.7 Vision sensitivity deficiencies**

H53.71 **Glare sensitivity**

H53.72 **Impaired contrast sensitivity**

H53.8 Other visual disturbances

H53.9 Unspecified visual disturbance

[4th] **H54 Blindness and low vision**

NOTES For definition of visual impairment categories see table below

Code first any associated underlying cause of the blindness

EXCLUDES1 *amaurosis fugax (G45.3)*

H54.0 Blindness, both eyes

Visual impairment categories 3, 4, 5 in both eyes.

[5th] **H54.1 Blindness, one eye, low vision other eye**

Visual impairment categories 3, 4, 5 in one eye, with categories 1 or 2 in the other eye.

H54.10 **Blindness, one eye, low vision other eye, unspecified eyes**

H54.11 **Blindness, right eye, low vision left eye**

H54.12 **Blindness, left eye, low vision right eye**

H54.2 Low vision, both eyes

Visual impairment categories 1 or 2 in both eyes.

H54.3 Unqualified visual loss, both eyes

Visual impairment category 9 in both eyes.

[5th] **H54.4 Blindness, one eye**

Visual impairment categories 3, 4, 5 in one eye [normal vision in other eye]

H54.40 **Blindness, one eye, unspecified eye**

H54.41 **Blindness, right eye, normal vision left eye**

H54.42 **Blindness, left eye, normal vision right eye**

[5th] **H54.5 Low vision, one eye**

Visual impairment categories 1 or 2 in one eye [normal vision in other eye].

H54.50 **Low vision, one eye, unspecified eye**

H54.51 **Low vision, right eye, normal vision left eye**

H54.52 **Low vision, left eye, normal vision right eye**

[5th] **H54.6 Unqualified visual loss, one eye**

Visual impairment category 9 in one eye [normal vision in other eye].

H54.60 **Unqualified visual loss, one eye, unspecified**

H54.61 **Unqualified visual loss, right eye, normal vision left eye**

H54.62 **Unqualified visual loss, left eye, normal vision right eye**

H54.7 Unspecified visual loss

Visual impairment category 9 NOS

H54.8 Legal blindness, as defined in USA

Blindness NOS according to USA definition

EXCLUDES1 *legal blindness with specification of impairment level (H54.0-H54.7)*

NOTES The table below gives a classification of severity of visual impairment recommended by a WHO Study Group on the Prevention of Blindness, Geneva, 6-10 November 1972.
The term 'low vision' in category H54 comprises categories 1 and 2 of the table, the term 'blindness' categories 3, 4 and 5, and the term 'unqualified visual loss' category 9.
If the extent of the visual field is taken into account, patients with a field no greater than 10 but greater than 5 around central fixation should be placed in category 3 and patients with a field no greater than 5 around central fixation should be placed in category 4, even if the central acuity is not impaired.

Category of visual impairment	Visual acuity with best possible correction	
	Maximum less than:	Minimum equal to or better than:
	6/18	6/60
3/10(0.3)	1/10(0.1)	
20/70	20/200	
	6/60	3/60
1/10(0.1)	1/20(0.05)	
20/200	20/400	
	3/60	1/60 (finger counting at one meter)
1/20(0.05)	1/50(0.02)	
20/400	5/300(20/1200)	
	1/60 (finger counting at one meter)	Light perception
1/50(0.02)		
5/300		
	No light perception	
	Undetermined or unspecified	

Other disorders of eye and adnexa (H55-H57)

[4th] **H55 Nystagmus and other irregular eye movements**

[5th] **H55.0 Nystagmus**

H55.00 **Unspecified nystagmus**

H55.01 **Congenital nystagmus**

H55.02 **Latent nystagmus**

H55.03 **Visual deprivation nystagmus**

H55.04 **Dissociated nystagmus**

H55.09 **Other forms of nystagmus**

[5th] **H55.8 Other irregular eye movements**

H55.81 **Saccadic eye movements**

H55.89 **Other irregular eye movements**

[4th] **H57 Other disorders of eye and adnexa**

[5th] **H57.0 Anomalies of pupillary function**

H57.00 **Unspecified anomaly of pupillary function**

H57.01 **Argyll Robertson pupil, atypical**

EXCLUDES1 *syphilitic Argyll Robertson pupil (A52.19)*

H57.02 **Anisocoria**

H57.03 **Miosis**

H57.04 **Mydriasis**

[6th] H57.05 **Tonic pupil**

H57.051 **Tonic pupil, right eye**

H57.052 **Tonic pupil, left eye**

H57.053 **Tonic pupil, bilateral**

H57.059 **Tonic pupil, unspecified eye**

H57.09 **Other anomalies of pupillary function**

[5th] **H57.1 Ocular pain**

H57.10 **Ocular pain, unspecified eye**

[4th] 4th character required [5th] 5th character required [6th] 6th character required [7th] 7th character required [X] Extension 'X' Alert
EXCLUDES1 Not coded here EXCLUDES2 Not included here [Pdx] Primary Diagnosis Only Manifestation Code

H57.11 Ocular pain, right eye
H57.12 Ocular pain, left eye
H57.13 Ocular pain, bilateral
H57.8 Other specified disorders of eye and adnexa
H57.9 Unspecified disorder of eye and adnexa

Intraoperative and postprocedural complications and disorders of eye and adnexa, not elsewhere classified (H59)

[4] **H59 Intraoperative and postprocedural complications and disorders of eye and adnexa, not elsewhere classified**

[EXCLUDES1] *mechanical complication of intraocular lens (T85.2)*
mechanical complication of other ocular prosthetic devices, implants and grafts (T85.3)
pseudophakia (Z96.1)
secondary cataracts (H26.4-)

[5] H59.0 Disorders of the eye following cataract surgery

[6] H59.01 Keratopathy (bullous aphakic) following cataract surgery
Vitreal corneal syndrome
Vitreous (touch) syndrome
H59.011 Keratopathy (bullous aphakic) following cataract surgery, right eye
H59.012 Keratopathy (bullous aphakic) following cataract surgery, left eye
H59.013 Keratopathy (bullous aphakic) following cataract surgery, bilateral
H59.019 Keratopathy (bullous aphakic) following cataract surgery, unspecified eye

[6] H59.02 Cataract (lens) fragments in eye following cataract surgery
H59.021 Cataract (lens) fragments in eye following cataract surgery, right eye
H59.022 Cataract (lens) fragments in eye following cataract surgery, left eye
H59.023 Cataract (lens) fragments in eye following cataract surgery, bilateral
H59.029 Cataract (lens) fragments in eye following cataract surgery, unspecified eye

[6] H59.03 Cystoid macular edema following cataract surgery
H59.031 Cystoid macular edema following cataract surgery, right eye
H59.032 Cystoid macular edema following cataract surgery, left eye
H59.033 Cystoid macular edema following cataract surgery, bilateral
H59.039 Cystoid macular edema following cataract surgery, unspecified eye

[6] H59.09 Other disorders of the eye following cataract surgery
H59.091 Other disorders of the right eye following cataract surgery
H59.092 Other disorders of the left eye following cataract surgery
H59.093 Other disorders of the eye following cataract surgery, bilateral
H59.099 Other disorders of unspecified eye following cataract surgery

[5] H59.1 Intraoperative hemorrhage and hematoma of eye and adnexa complicating a procedure

[EXCLUDES1] *intraoperative hemorrhage and hematoma of eye and adnexa due to accidental puncture or laceration during a procedure (H59.2-)*

[6] H59.11 Intraoperative hemorrhage and hematoma of eye and adnexa complicating an ophthalmic procedure
H59.111 Intraoperative hemorrhage and hematoma of right eye and adnexa complicating an ophthalmic procedure
H59.112 Intraoperative hemorrhage and hematoma of left eye and adnexa complicating an ophthalmic procedure
H59.113 Intraoperative hemorrhage and hematoma of eye and adnexa complicating an ophthalmic procedure, bilateral
H59.119 Intraoperative hemorrhage and hematoma of unspecified eye and adnexa complicating an ophthalmic procedure

[6] H59.12 Intraoperative hemorrhage and hematoma of eye and adnexa complicating other procedure
H59.121 Intraoperative hemorrhage and hematoma of right eye and adnexa complicating other procedure
H59.122 Intraoperative hemorrhage and hematoma of left eye and adnexa complicating other procedure
H59.123 Intraoperative hemorrhage and hematoma of eye and adnexa complicating other procedure, bilateral
H59.129 Intraoperative hemorrhage and hematoma of unspecified eye and adnexa complicating other procedure

[5] H59.2 Accidental puncture and laceration of eye and adnexa during a procedure

[6] H59.21 Accidental puncture and laceration of eye and adnexa during an ophthalmic procedure
H59.211 Accidental puncture and laceration of right eye and adnexa during an ophthalmic procedure
H59.212 Accidental puncture and laceration of left eye and adnexa during an ophthalmic procedure
H59.213 Accidental puncture and laceration of eye and adnexa during an ophthalmic procedure, bilateral
H59.219 Accidental puncture and laceration of unspecified eye and adnexa during an ophthalmic procedure

[6] H59.22 Accidental puncture and laceration of eye and adnexa during other procedure
H59.221 Accidental puncture and laceration of right eye and adnexa during other procedure
H59.222 Accidental puncture and laceration of left eye and adnexa during other procedure
H59.223 Accidental puncture and laceration of eye and adnexa during other procedure, bilateral
H59.229 Accidental puncture and laceration of unspecified eye and adnexa during other procedure

[5] H59.3 Postprocedural hemorrhage and hematoma of eye and adnexa following a procedure

[6] H59.31 Postprocedural hemorrhage and hematoma of eye and adnexa following an ophthalmic procedure
H59.311 Postprocedural hemorrhage and hematoma of right eye and adnexa following an ophthalmic procedure
H59.312 Postprocedural hemorrhage and hematoma of left eye and adnexa following an ophthalmic procedure
H59.313 Postprocedural hemorrhage and hematoma of eye and adnexa following an ophthalmic procedure, bilateral

Unspecified Code | Other Specified Code | [N] Newborn Age: 0 | [P] Pediatric Age: 0-17 | [M] Maternity Age: 12-55
[A] Adult Age: 15-124 | ♂ Male | ♀ Female | ● New Code | ▲ Revised Code Title | ►◄ Revised Text

H59.319 Postprocedural hemorrhage and hematoma of unspecified eye and adnexa following an ophthalmic procedure

[6] H59.32 Postprocedural hemorrhage and hematoma of eye and adnexa following other procedure

H59.321 Postprocedural hemorrhage and hematoma of right eye and adnexa following other procedure

H59.322 Postprocedural hemorrhage and hematoma of left eye and adnexa following other procedure

H59.323 Postprocedural hemorrhage and hematoma of eye and adnexa following other procedure, bilateral

H59.329 Postprocedural hemorrhage and hematoma of unspecified eye and adnexa following other procedure

[5] H59.4 Inflammation (infection) of postprocedural bleb

Postprocedural blebitis

[EXCLUDES1] *filtering (vitreous) bleb after glaucoma surgery status (Z98.83)*

H59.40 Inflammation (infection) of postprocedural bleb, unspecified

H59.41 Inflammation (infection) of postprocedural bleb, stage 1

H59.42 Inflammation (infection) of postprocedural bleb, stage 2

H59.43 Inflammation (infection) of postprocedural bleb, stage 3

Bleb endophthalmitis

[5] H59.8 Other intraoperative and postprocedural complications and disorders of eye and adnexa, not elsewhere classified

[6] H59.81 Chorioretinal scars after surgery for detachment

H59.811 Chorioretinal scars after surgery for detachment, right eye

H59.812 Chorioretinal scars after surgery for detachment, left eye

H59.813 Chorioretinal scars after surgery for detachment, bilateral

H59.819 Chorioretinal scars after surgery for detachment, unspecified eye

H59.88 Other intraoperative complications of eye and adnexa, not elsewhere classified

H59.89 Other postprocedural complications and disorders of eye and adnexa, not elsewhere classified

Chapter 8: Diseases of the Ear and Mastoid Process (H60-H95)

Anatomy of the Sense Organ (Ear)

The Organ of Hearing

The external, inner and middle ear contain the organs of hearing and balance. The external ear extends from outside of the head to the eardrum. The middle ear is the air filled chamber and located medially to the eardrum. It contains the auditory ossciles (the malleus, incus, and stapes). The external and middle ears are primarily involved in the process of hearing. The inner ear comprises of fluid filled chambers which serve to maintain balance (or equilibrium) and hearing. The various organs of a typical human ear are listed below:

1. **The External Ear**
   a) Auricle (or Pinna)
   b) External Auditory (or Auricular) Canal (or Ear Canal/External Auditory Meatus/External Acoustic Meatus)
   c) Surface of Ear Drum

2. **The Middle Ear**
   a) Malleus
   b) Incus
   c) Stapes
   d) Tympanic Membrane (or Ear Drum)
   e) Auditory/Eustachian Tube (or Pharyngotympanic Tube)

3. **The Inner Ear**
   a) Cochlea
   b) Vestibule
   c) Semicircular Canals

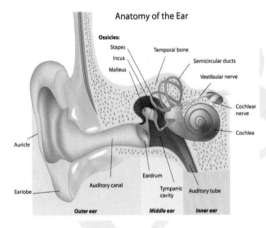

Anatomy of the Ear

Common Pathologies

Swimmer's ear
Swimmer's ear is an inflammation, irritation, or infection of the outer ear and ear canal. The medical term for swimmer's ear is otitis externa. Acute external otitis is commonly a bacterial infection caused by streptococcus, staphylococcus, or pseudomonas types of bacteria.

Otitis media
Otitis media is the medical term for middle ear infection. Symptom of acute otitis media is ear pain; other possible symptoms include fever, and irritability (in infants) often with drainage of purulent material. After an acute infection, fluid (an effusion) may remain behind the ear drum (tympanic membrane) leading to otitis media with effusion chronic suppurative otitis media.

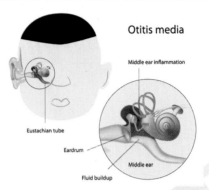

Meniere's disease
Meniere's disease is a disorder of the inner ear that can affect hearing. It causes severe dizziness and feeling of ear pressure or pain. It is characterized by episodes of vertigo low-pitched tinnitus and hearing loss. It usually affects just one ear. It may occur when the pressure of the fluid in part of the inner ear gets too high. The inner ear contains fluid-filled tubes called semicircular canals. These canals help to maintain position and balance.

Vestibular neuritis
Vestibular neuritis is a disorder resulting from an acute infection of nerves of inner ear. This disrupts transmission of sensory information. Its main symptom is vertigo which appears suddenly, often with nausea and vomiting. This can be made worse by head movement. Vertigo usually lasts for several days or weeks. In rare cases it can take months to go away entirely. Vestibular neuritis does not lead to loss of hearing.

Cholesteatoma
Cholesteatoma can be congenital, but it more commonly occurs as a complication of chronic ear infection. An abnormal skin growth in the middle ear behind the eardrum is called cholesteatoma. Poor function in the eustachian tube leads to negative pressure in the middle ear. Over time, the cholesteatoma can increase in size and destroy the surrounding delicate bones of the middle ear leading to hearing loss.

Otosclerosis
Otosclerosis is an abnormal bone growth in the middle ear that causes hearing loss. This bone prevents structures within the ear from working properly and causes hearing loss. It is a condition that mainly affects the stapes, one of the tiny bony ossicles in the middle ear. It significantly involves the bone which surrounds the inner ear, called the otic capsule, a sensory type hearing loss occurs.

Acoustic Neuroma
An acoustic neuroma is a benign tumor of the nerve that connects the ear to the brain. This nerve is called the vestibular cochlear nerve. It is also called as vestibular schwannoma. The cause is generally unknown. If an acoustic tumor becomes large it will push on the surface of the brainstem but not really grow into brain tissue. Symptoms of acoustic neuroma are loss of hearing on one side, ringing in ears, dizziness and balance problems

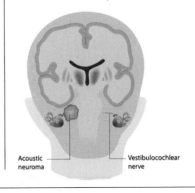

This page intentionally left blank

Diseases of the ear and mastoid process (H60-H95)

NOTES Use an external cause code following the code for the ear condition, if applicable, to identify the cause of the ear condition

EXCLUDES2 certain conditions originating in the perinatal period (P04-P96)
certain infectious and parasitic diseases (A00-B99)
complications of pregnancy, childbirth and the puerperium (O00-O9A)
congenital malformations, deformations and chromosomal abnormalities (Q00-Q99)
endocrine, nutritional and metabolic diseases (E00-E88)
injury, poisoning and certain other consequences of external causes (S00-T88)
neoplasms (C00-D49)
symptoms, signs and abnormal clinical and laboratory findings, not elsewhere classified (R00-R94)

Diseases of external ear (H60-H62)

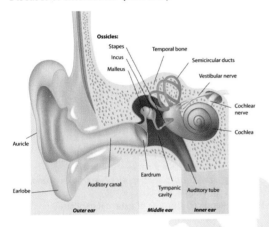

Figure 7.6 Anatomy of the Ear

4 H60 Otitis externa
  5 H60.0 Abscess of external ear
    Boil of external ear
    Carbuncle of auricle or external auditory canal
    Furuncle of external ear
    H60.00 Abscess of external ear, unspecified ear
    H60.01 Abscess of right external ear
    H60.02 Abscess of left external ear
    H60.03 Abscess of external ear, bilateral
  5 H60.1 Cellulitis of external ear
    Cellulitis of auricle
    Cellulitis of external auditory canal
    H60.10 Cellulitis of external ear, unspecified ear
    H60.11 Cellulitis of right external ear
    H60.12 Cellulitis of left external ear
    H60.13 Cellulitis of external ear, bilateral
  5 H60.2 Malignant otitis externa
    H60.20 Malignant otitis externa, unspecified ear
    H60.21 Malignant otitis externa, right ear
    H60.22 Malignant otitis externa, left ear
    H60.23 Malignant otitis externa, bilateral
  5 H60.3 Other infective otitis externa
    6 H60.31 Diffuse otitis externa
      H60.311 Diffuse otitis externa, right ear
      H60.312 Diffuse otitis externa, left ear
      H60.313 Diffuse otitis externa, bilateral
      H60.319 Diffuse otitis externa, unspecified ear

6 H60.32 Hemorrhagic otitis externa
  H60.321 Hemorrhagic otitis externa, right ear
  H60.322 Hemorrhagic otitis externa, left ear
  H60.323 Hemorrhagic otitis externa, bilateral
  H60.329 Hemorrhagic otitis externa, unspecified ear
6 H60.33 Swimmer's ear
  H60.331 Swimmer's ear, right ear
  H60.332 Swimmer's ear, left ear
  H60.333 Swimmer's ear, bilateral
  H60.339 Swimmer's ear, unspecified ear
6 H60.39 Other infective otitis externa
  H60.391 Other infective otitis externa, right ear
  H60.392 Other infective otitis externa, left ear
  H60.393 Other infective otitis externa, bilateral
  H60.399 Other infective otitis externa, unspecified ear
5 H60.4 Cholesteatoma of external ear
  Keratosis obturans of external ear (canal)
  EXCLUDES2 cholesteatoma of middle ear (H71.-)
    recurrent cholesteatoma of postmastoidectomy cavity (H95.0-)
  H60.40 Cholesteatoma of external ear, unspecified ear
  H60.41 Cholesteatoma of right external ear
  H60.42 Cholesteatoma of left external ear
  H60.43 Cholesteatoma of external ear, bilateral
5 H60.5 Acute noninfective otitis externa
  6 H60.50 Unspecified acute noninfective otitis externa
    Acute otitis externa NOS
    H60.501 Unspecified acute noninfective otitis externa, right ear
    H60.502 Unspecified acute noninfective otitis externa, left ear
    H60.503 Unspecified acute noninfective otitis externa, bilateral
    H60.509 Unspecified acute noninfective otitis externa, unspecified ear
  6 H60.51 Acute actinic otitis externa
    H60.511 Acute actinic otitis externa, right ear
    H60.512 Acute actinic otitis externa, left ear
    H60.513 Acute actinic otitis externa, bilateral
    H60.519 Acute actinic otitis externa, unspecified ear
  6 H60.52 Acute chemical otitis externa
    H60.521 Acute chemical otitis externa, right ear
    H60.522 Acute chemical otitis externa, left ear
    H60.523 Acute chemical otitis externa, bilateral
    H60.529 Acute chemical otitis externa, unspecified ear
  6 H60.53 Acute contact otitis externa
    H60.531 Acute contact otitis externa, right ear
    H60.532 Acute contact otitis externa, left ear
    H60.533 Acute contact otitis externa, bilateral
    H60.539 Acute contact otitis externa, unspecified ear
  6 H60.54 Acute eczematoid otitis externa
    H60.541 Acute eczematoid otitis externa, right ear
    H60.542 Acute eczematoid otitis externa, left ear
    H60.543 Acute eczematoid otitis externa, bilateral
    H60.549 Acute eczematoid otitis externa, unspecified ear
  6 H60.55 Acute reactive otitis externa
    H60.551 Acute reactive otitis externa, right ear
    H60.552 Acute reactive otitis externa, left ear
    H60.553 Acute reactive otitis externa, bilateral
    H60.559 Acute reactive otitis externa, unspecified ear
  6 H60.59 Other noninfective acute otitis externa

Unspecified Code	Other Specified Code	N Newborn Age: 0	P Pediatric Age: 0-17	M Maternity Age: 12-55
A Adult Age: 15-124	♂ Male	♀ Female	● New Code	▲ Revised Code Title	◄ Revised Text

H60.591 Other noninfective acute otitis externa, right ear
H60.592 Other noninfective acute otitis externa, left ear
H60.593 Other noninfective acute otitis externa, bilateral
H60.599 Other noninfective acute otitis externa, unspecified ear

[5] H60.6 Unspecified chronic otitis externa
H60.60 Unspecified chronic otitis externa, unspecified ear
H60.61 Unspecified chronic otitis externa, right ear
H60.62 Unspecified chronic otitis externa, left ear
H60.63 Unspecified chronic otitis externa, bilateral

[5] H60.8 Other otitis externa
[6] H60.8X Other otitis externa
H60.8X1 Other otitis externa, right ear
H60.8X2 Other otitis externa, left ear
H60.8X3 Other otitis externa, bilateral
H60.8X9 Other otitis externa, unspecified ear

[5] H60.9 Unspecified otitis externa
H60.90 Unspecified otitis externa, unspecified ear
H60.91 Unspecified otitis externa, right ear
H60.92 Unspecified otitis externa, left ear
H60.93 Unspecified otitis externa, bilateral

[4] H61 Other disorders of external ear

[5] H61.0 Chondritis and perichondritis of external ear
Chondrodermatitis nodularis chronica helicis
Perichondritis of auricle
Perichondritis of pinna
[6] H61.00 Unspecified perichondritis of external ear
H61.001 Unspecified perichondritis of right external ear
H61.002 Unspecified perichondritis of left external ear
H61.003 Unspecified perichondritis of external ear, bilateral
H61.009 Unspecified perichondritis of external ear, unspecified ear
[6] H61.01 Acute perichondritis of external ear
H61.011 Acute perichondritis of right external ear
H61.012 Acute perichondritis of left external ear
H61.013 Acute perichondritis of external ear, bilateral
H61.019 Acute perichondritis of external ear, unspecified ear
[6] H61.02 Chronic perichondritis of external ear
H61.021 Chronic perichondritis of right external ear
H61.022 Chronic perichondritis of left external ear
H61.023 Chronic perichondritis of external ear, bilateral
H61.029 Chronic perichondritis of external ear, unspecified ear
[6] H61.03 Chondritis of external ear
Chondritis of auricle
Chondritis of pinna
H61.031 Chondritis of right external ear
H61.032 Chondritis of left external ear
H61.033 Chondritis of external ear, bilateral
H61.039 Chondritis of external ear, unspecified ear

[5] H61.1 Noninfective disorders of pinna
[EXCLUDES2] *cauliflower ear (M95.1-)*
gouty tophi of ear (M1A.-)
[6] H61.10 Unspecified noninfective disorders of pinna
Disorder of pinna NOS
H61.101 Unspecified noninfective disorders of pinna, right ear
H61.102 Unspecified noninfective disorders of pinna, left ear
H61.103 Unspecified noninfective disorders of pinna, bilateral
H61.109 Unspecified noninfective disorders of pinna, unspecified ear
[6] H61.11 Acquired deformity of pinna
Acquired deformity of auricle
[EXCLUDES2] *cauliflower ear (M95.1-)*
H61.111 Acquired deformity of pinna, right ear
H61.112 Acquired deformity of pinna, left ear
H61.113 Acquired deformity of pinna, bilateral
H61.119 Acquired deformity of pinna, unspecified ear
[6] H61.12 Hematoma of pinna
Hematoma of auricle
H61.121 Hematoma of pinna, right ear
H61.122 Hematoma of pinna, left ear
H61.123 Hematoma of pinna, bilateral
H61.129 Hematoma of pinna, unspecified ear
[6] H61.19 Other noninfective disorders of pinna
H61.191 Noninfective disorders of pinna, right ear
H61.192 Noninfective disorders of pinna, left ear
H61.193 Noninfective disorders of pinna, bilateral
H61.199 Noninfective disorders of pinna, unspecified ear

[5] H61.2 Impacted cerumen
Wax in ear
H61.20 Impacted cerumen, unspecified ear
H61.21 Impacted cerumen, right ear
H61.22 Impacted cerumen, left ear
H61.23 Impacted cerumen, bilateral

[5] H61.3 Acquired stenosis of external ear canal
Collapse of external ear canal
[EXCLUDES1] *postprocedural stenosis of external ear canal (H95.81-)*
[6] H61.30 Acquired stenosis of external ear canal, unspecified
H61.301 Acquired stenosis of right external ear canal, unspecified
H61.302 Acquired stenosis of left external ear canal, unspecified
H61.303 Acquired stenosis of external ear canal, unspecified, bilateral
H61.309 Acquired stenosis of external ear canal, unspecified, unspecified ear
[6] H61.31 Acquired stenosis of external ear canal secondary to trauma
H61.311 Acquired stenosis of right external ear canal secondary to trauma
H61.312 Acquired stenosis of left external ear canal secondary to trauma
H61.313 Acquired stenosis of external ear canal secondary to trauma, bilateral
H61.319 Acquired stenosis of external ear canal secondary to trauma, unspecified ear
[6] H61.32 Acquired stenosis of external ear canal secondary to inflammation and infection
H61.321 Acquired stenosis of right external ear canal secondary to inflammation and infection
H61.322 Acquired stenosis of left external ear canal secondary to inflammation and infection
H61.323 Acquired stenosis of external ear canal secondary to inflammation and infection, bilateral

[4] 4th character required [5] 5th character required [6] 6th character required [7] 7th character required [7x] Extension 'X' Alert
[EXCLUDES1] Not coded here [EXCLUDES2] Not included here [PDx] Primary Diagnosis Only Manifestation Code

H61.329 Acquired stenosis of external ear canal secondary to inflammation and infection, unspecified ear

H61.39 Other acquired stenosis of external ear canal

H61.391 Other acquired stenosis of right external ear canal

H61.392 Other acquired stenosis of left external ear canal

H61.393 Other acquired stenosis of external ear canal, bilateral

H61.399 Other acquired stenosis of external ear canal, unspecified ear

H61.8 Other specified disorders of external ear

H61.81 Exostosis of external canal

H61.811 Exostosis of right external canal

H61.812 Exostosis of left external canal

H61.813 Exostosis of external canal, bilateral

H61.819 Exostosis of external canal, unspecified ear

H61.89 Other specified disorders of external ear

H61.891 Other specified disorders of right external ear

H61.892 Other specified disorders of left external ear

H61.893 Other specified disorders of external ear, bilateral

H61.899 Other specified disorders of external ear, unspecified ear

H61.9 Disorder of external ear, unspecified

H61.90 Disorder of external ear, unspecified, unspecified ear

H61.91 Disorder of right external ear, unspecified

H61.92 Disorder of left external ear, unspecified

H61.93 Disorder of external ear, unspecified, bilateral

H62 Disorders of external ear in diseases classified elsewhere

H62.4 Otitis externa in other diseases classified elsewhere

Code first underlying disease, such as:
erysipelas (A46)
impetigo (L01.0)

EXCLUDES1 otitis externa (in):
candidiasis (B37.84)
herpes viral [herpes simplex] (B00.1)
herpes zoster (B02.8)

H62.40 Otitis externa in other diseases classified elsewhere, unspecified ear

H62.41 Otitis externa in other diseases classified elsewhere, right ear

H62.42 Otitis externa in other diseases classified elsewhere, left ear

H62.43 Otitis externa in other diseases classified elsewhere, bilateral

H62.8 Other disorders of external ear in diseases classified elsewhere

Code first underlying disease, such as:
gout (M1A.-, M10.-)

H62.8X Other disorders of external ear in diseases classified elsewhere

H62.8X1 Other disorders of right external ear in diseases classified elsewhere

H62.8X2 Other disorders of left external ear in diseases classified elsewhere

H62.8X3 Other disorders of external ear in diseases classified elsewhere, bilateral

H62.8X9 Other disorders of external ear in diseases classified elsewhere, unspecified ear

Diseases of middle ear and mastoid (H65-H75)

H65 Nonsuppurative otitis media

INCLUDES nonsuppurative otitis media with myringitis
Use additional code for any associated perforated tympanic membrane (H72.-)
code to identify:
exposure to environmental tobacco smoke (Z77.22)
exposure to tobacco smoke in the perinatal period (P96.81)
history of tobacco use (Z87.891)
occupational exposure to environmental tobacco smoke (Z57.31)
tobacco dependence (F17.-)
tobacco use (Z72.0)

H65.0 Acute serous otitis media

Acute and subacute secretory otitis

H65.00 Acute serous otitis media, unspecified ear

H65.01 Acute serous otitis media, right ear

H65.02 Acute serous otitis media, left ear

H65.03 Acute serous otitis media, bilateral

H65.04 Acute serous otitis media, recurrent, right ear

H65.05 Acute serous otitis media, recurrent, left ear

H65.06 Acute serous otitis media, recurrent, bilateral

H65.07 Acute serous otitis media, recurrent, unspecified ear

H65.1 Other acute nonsuppurative otitis media

EXCLUDES1 otitic barotrauma (T70.0)
otitis media (acute) NOS (H66.9)

H65.11 Acute and subacute allergic otitis media (mucoid) (sanguinous) (serous)

H65.111 Acute and subacute allergic otitis media (mucoid) (sanguinous) (serous), right ear

H65.112 Acute and subacute allergic otitis media (mucoid) (sanguinous) (serous), left ear

H65.113 Acute and subacute allergic otitis media (mucoid) (sanguinous) (serous), bilateral

H65.114 Acute and subacute allergic otitis media (mucoid) (sanguinous) (serous), recurrent, right ear

H65.115 Acute and subacute allergic otitis media (mucoid) (sanguinous) (serous), recurrent, left ear

H65.116 Acute and subacute allergic otitis media (mucoid) (sanguinous) (serous), recurrent, bilateral

H65.117 Acute and subacute allergic otitis media (mucoid) (sanguinous) (serous), recurrent, unspecified ear

H65.119 Acute and subacute allergic otitis media (mucoid) (sanguinous) (serous), unspecified ear

H65.19 Other acute nonsuppurative otitis media

Acute and subacute mucoid otitis media
Acute and subacute nonsuppurative otitis media NOS
Acute and subacute sanguinous otitis media
Acute and subacute seromucinous otitis media

H65.191 Other acute nonsuppurative otitis media, right ear

H65.192 Other acute nonsuppurative otitis media, left ear

H65.193 Other acute nonsuppurative otitis media, bilateral

H65.194 Other acute nonsuppurative otitis media, recurrent, right ear

H65.195 Other acute nonsuppurative otitis media, recurrent, left ear

H65.196 Other acute nonsuppurative otitis media, recurrent, bilateral

H65.197 Other acute nonsuppurative otitis media recurrent, unspecified ear
H65.199 Other acute nonsuppurative otitis media, unspecified ear

[5] H65.2 Chronic serous otitis media
Chronic tubotympanal catarrh
H65.20 Chronic serous otitis media, unspecified ear
H65.21 Chronic serous otitis media, right ear
H65.22 Chronic serous otitis media, left ear
H65.23 Chronic serous otitis media, bilateral

[5] H65.3 Chronic mucoid otitis media
Chronic mucinous otitis media
Chronic secretory otitis media
Chronic transudative otitis media
Glue ear
[EXCLUDES1] *adhesive middle ear disease (H74.1)*
H65.30 Chronic mucoid otitis media, unspecified ear
H65.31 Chronic mucoid otitis media, right ear
H65.32 Chronic mucoid otitis media, left ear
H65.33 Chronic mucoid otitis media, bilateral

[5] H65.4 Other chronic nonsuppurative otitis media
[6] H65.41 Chronic allergic otitis media
H65.411 Chronic allergic otitis media, right ear
H65.412 Chronic allergic otitis media, left ear
H65.413 Chronic allergic otitis media, bilateral
H65.419 Chronic allergic otitis media, unspecified ear
[6] H65.49 Other chronic nonsuppurative otitis media
Chronic exudative otitis media
Chronic nonsuppurative otitis media NOS
Chronic otitis media with effusion (nonpurulent)
Chronic seromucinous otitis media
H65.491 Other chronic nonsuppurative otitis media, right ear
H65.492 Other chronic nonsuppurative otitis media, left ear
H65.493 Other chronic nonsuppurative otitis media, bilateral
H65.499 Other chronic nonsuppurative otitis media, unspecified ear

[5] H65.9 Unspecified nonsuppurative otitis media
Allergic otitis media NOS
Catarrhal otitis media NOS
Exudative otitis media NOS
Mucoid otitis media NOS
Otitis media with effusion (nonpurulent) NOS
Secretory otitis media NOS
Seromucinous otitis media NOS
Serous otitis media NOS
Transudative otitis media NOS
H65.90 Unspecified nonsuppurative otitis media, unspecified ear
H65.91 Unspecified nonsuppurative otitis media, right ear
H65.92 Unspecified nonsuppurative otitis media, left ear
H65.93 Unspecified nonsuppurative otitis media, bilateral

[4] H66 Suppurative and unspecified otitis media
[INCLUDES] *suppurative and unspecified otitis media with myringitis*
Use additional code to identify:
exposure to environmental tobacco smoke (Z77.22)
exposure to tobacco smoke in the perinatal period (P96.81)
history of tobacco use (Z87.891)
occupational exposure to environmental tobacco smoke (Z57.31)
tobacco dependence (F17.-)
tobacco use (Z72.0)

[5] H66.0 Acute suppurative otitis media
[6] H66.00 Acute suppurative otitis media without spontaneous rupture of ear drum
H66.001 Acute suppurative otitis media without spontaneous rupture of ear drum, right ear
H66.002 Acute suppurative otitis media without spontaneous rupture of ear drum, left ear
H66.003 Acute suppurative otitis media without spontaneous rupture of ear drum, bilateral
H66.004 Acute suppurative otitis media without spontaneous rupture of ear drum, recurrent, right ear
H66.005 Acute suppurative otitis media without spontaneous rupture of ear drum, recurrent, left ear
H66.006 Acute suppurative otitis media without spontaneous rupture of ear drum, recurrent, bilateral
H66.007 Acute suppurative otitis media without spontaneous rupture of ear drum, recurrent, unspecified ear
H66.009 Acute suppurative otitis media without spontaneous rupture of ear drum, unspecified ear
[6] H66.01 Acute suppurative otitis media with spontaneous rupture of ear drum
H66.011 Acute suppurative otitis media with spontaneous rupture of ear drum, right ear
H66.012 Acute suppurative otitis media with spontaneous rupture of ear drum, left ear
H66.013 Acute suppurative otitis media with spontaneous rupture of ear drum, bilateral
H66.014 Acute suppurative otitis media with spontaneous rupture of ear drum, recurrent, right ear
H66.015 Acute suppurative otitis media with spontaneous rupture of ear drum, recurrent, left ear
H66.016 Acute suppurative otitis media with spontaneous rupture of ear drum, recurrent, bilateral
H66.017 Acute suppurative otitis media with spontaneous rupture of ear drum, recurrent, unspecified ear
H66.019 Acute suppurative otitis media with spontaneous rupture of ear drum, unspecified ear

[5] H66.1 Chronic tubotympanic suppurative otitis media
Benign chronic suppurative otitis media
Chronic tubotympanic disease
Use additional code for any associated perforated tympanic membrane (H72.-)
H66.10 Chronic tubotympanic suppurative otitis media, unspecified
H66.11 Chronic tubotympanic suppurative otitis media, right ear
H66.12 Chronic tubotympanic suppurative otitis media, left ear
H66.13 Chronic tubotympanic suppurative otitis media, bilateral

[5] H66.2 Chronic atticoantral suppurative otitis media
Chronic atticoantral disease
Use additional code for any associated perforated tympanic membrane (H72.-)
H66.20 Chronic atticoantral suppurative otitis media, unspecified ear
H66.21 Chronic atticoantral suppurative otitis media, right ear
H66.22 Chronic atticoantral suppurative otitis media, left ear

[4] 4th character required [5] 5th character required [6] 6th character required [7] 7th character required [X] Extension 'X' Alert
[EXCLUDES1] Not coded here [EXCLUDES2] Not included here [PDx] Primary Diagnosis Only Manifestation Code

H66.23 Chronic atticoantral suppurative otitis media, bilateral

[5] H66.3 Other chronic suppurative otitis media
Chronic suppurative otitis media NOS
[EXCLUDES1] *tuberculous otitis media (A18.6)*
Use additional code for any associated perforated tympanic membrane (H72.-)

[6] H66.3X Other chronic suppurative otitis media
H66.3X1 **Other chronic suppurative otitis media, right ear**
H66.3X2 **Other chronic suppurative otitis media, left ear**
H66.3X3 **Other chronic suppurative otitis media, bilateral**
H66.3X9 **Other chronic suppurative otitis media, unspecified ear**

[5] H66.4 Suppurative otitis media, unspecified
Purulent otitis media NOS
Use additional code for any associated perforated tympanic membrane (H72.-)
H66.40 **Suppurative otitis media, unspecified, unspecified ear**
H66.41 **Suppurative otitis media, unspecified, right ear**
H66.42 **Suppurative otitis media, unspecified, left ear**
H66.43 **Suppurative otitis media, unspecified, bilateral**

[5] H66.9 Otitis media, unspecified
Otitis media NOS
Acute otitis media NOS
Chronic otitis media NOS
Use additional code for any associated perforated tympanic membrane (H72.-)
H66.90 **Otitis media, unspecified, unspecified ear**
H66.91 **Otitis media, unspecified, right ear**
H66.92 **Otitis media, unspecified, left ear**
H66.93 **Otitis media, unspecified, bilateral**

[4] H67 Otitis media in diseases classified elsewhere
Code first underlying disease, such as:
viral disease NEC (B00-B34)
Use additional code for any associated perforated tympanic membrane (H72.-)
[EXCLUDES1] *otitis media in:*
influenza (J09.X9, J10.83, J11.83)
measles (B05.3)
scarlet fever (A38.0)
tuberculosis (A18.6)
H67.1 **Otitis media in diseases classified elsewhere, right ear**
H67.2 **Otitis media in diseases classified elsewhere, left ear**
H67.3 **Otitis media in diseases classified elsewhere, bilateral**
H67.9 **Otitis media in diseases classified elsewhere, unspecified ear**

[4] H68 Eustachian salpingitis and obstruction
[5] H68.0 Eustachian salpingitis
[6] H68.00 Unspecified Eustachian salpingitis
H68.001 **Unspecified Eustachian salpingitis, right ear**
H68.002 **Unspecified Eustachian salpingitis, left ear**
H68.003 **Unspecified Eustachian salpingitis, bilateral**
H68.009 **Unspecified Eustachian salpingitis, unspecified ear**
[6] H68.01 Acute Eustachian salpingitis
H68.011 **Acute Eustachian salpingitis, right ear**
H68.012 **Acute Eustachian salpingitis, left ear**
H68.013 **Acute Eustachian salpingitis, bilateral**
H68.019 **Acute Eustachian salpingitis, unspecified ear**
[6] H68.02 Chronic Eustachian salpingitis
H68.021 **Chronic Eustachian salpingitis, right ear**
H68.022 **Chronic Eustachian salpingitis, left ear**
H68.023 **Chronic Eustachian salpingitis, bilateral**
H68.029 **Chronic Eustachian salpingitis, unspecified ear**

[5] H68.1 Obstruction of Eustachian tube
Stenosis of Eustachian tube
Stricture of Eustachian tube
[6] H68.10 Unspecified obstruction of Eustachian tube
H68.101 **Unspecified obstruction of Eustachian tube, right ear**
H68.102 **Unspecified obstruction of Eustachian tube, left ear**
H68.103 **Unspecified obstruction of Eustachian tube, bilateral**
H68.109 **Unspecified obstruction of Eustachian tube, unspecified ear**
[6] H68.11 Osseous obstruction of Eustachian tube
H68.111 **Osseous obstruction of Eustachian tube, right ear**
H68.112 **Osseous obstruction of Eustachian tube, left ear**
H68.113 **Osseous obstruction of Eustachian tube, bilateral**
H68.119 **Osseous obstruction of Eustachian tube, unspecified ear**
[6] H68.12 Intrinsic cartilagenous obstruction of Eustachian tube
H68.121 **Intrinsic cartilagenous obstruction of Eustachian tube, right ear**
H68.122 **Intrinsic cartilagenous obstruction of Eustachian tube, left ear**
H68.123 **Intrinsic cartilagenous obstruction of Eustachian tube, bilateral**
H68.129 **Intrinsic cartilagenous obstruction of Eustachian tube, unspecified ear**
[6] H68.13 Extrinsic cartilagenous obstruction of Eustachian tube
Compression of Eustachian tube
H68.131 **Extrinsic cartilagenous obstruction of Eustachian tube, right ear**
H68.132 **Extrinsic cartilagenous obstruction of Eustachian tube, left ear**
H68.133 **Extrinsic cartilagenous obstruction of Eustachian tube, bilateral**
H68.139 **Extrinsic cartilagenous obstruction of Eustachian tube, unspecified ear**

[4] H69 Other and unspecified disorders of Eustachian tube
[5] H69.0 Patulous Eustachian tube
H69.00 **Patulous Eustachian tube, unspecified ear**
H69.01 **Patulous Eustachian tube, right ear**
H69.02 **Patulous Eustachian tube, left ear**
H69.03 **Patulous Eustachian tube, bilateral**
[5] H69.8 Other specified disorders of Eustachian tube
H69.80 **Other specified disorders of Eustachian tube, unspecified ear**
H69.81 **Other specified disorders of Eustachian tube, right ear**
H69.82 **Other specified disorders of Eustachian tube, left ear**
H69.83 **Other specified disorders of Eustachian tube, bilateral**
[5] H69.9 Unspecified Eustachian tube disorder
H69.90 **Unspecified Eustachian tube disorder, unspecified ear**
H69.91 **Unspecified Eustachian tube disorder, right ear**
H69.92 **Unspecified Eustachian tube disorder, left ear**
H69.93 **Unspecified Eustachian tube disorder, bilateral**

Unspecified Code | Other Specified Code | [N] Newborn Age: 0 | [P] Pediatric Age: 0-17 | [M] Maternity Age: 12-55
[A] Adult Age: 15-124 | ♂ Male | ♀ Female | ● New Code | ▲ Revised Code Title | ►◄ Revised Text

[4] H70 Mastoiditis and related conditions

[5] H70.0 Acute mastoiditis
Abscess of mastoid
Empyema of mastoid

[6] H70.00 Acute mastoiditis without complications
H70.001 Acute mastoiditis without complications, right ear
H70.002 Acute mastoiditis without complications, left ear
H70.003 Acute mastoiditis without complications, bilateral
H70.009 Acute mastoiditis without complications, unspecified ear

[6] H70.01 Subperiosteal abscess of mastoid
H70.011 Subperiosteal abscess of mastoid, right ear
H70.012 Subperiosteal abscess of mastoid, left ear
H70.013 Subperiosteal abscess of mastoid, bilateral
H70.019 Subperiosteal abscess of mastoid, unspecified ear

[6] H70.09 Acute mastoiditis with other complications
H70.091 Acute mastoiditis with other complications, right ear
H70.092 Acute mastoiditis with other complications, left ear
H70.093 Acute mastoiditis with other complications, bilateral
H70.099 Acute mastoiditis with other complications, unspecified ear

[5] H70.1 Chronic mastoiditis
Caries of mastoid
Fistula of mastoid
[EXCLUDES1] *tuberculous mastoiditis (A18.03)*
H70.10 Chronic mastoiditis, unspecified ear
H70.11 Chronic mastoiditis, right ear
H70.12 Chronic mastoiditis, left ear
H70.13 Chronic mastoiditis, bilateral

[5] H70.2 Petrositis
Inflammation of petrous bone

[6] H70.20 Unspecified petrositis
H70.201 Unspecified petrositis, right ear
H70.202 Unspecified petrositis, left ear
H70.203 Unspecified petrositis, bilateral
H70.209 Unspecified petrositis, unspecified ear

[6] H70.21 Acute petrositis
H70.211 Acute petrositis, right ear
H70.212 Acute petrositis, left ear
H70.213 Acute petrositis, bilateral
H70.219 Acute petrositis, unspecified ear

[6] H70.22 Chronic petrositis
H70.221 Chronic petrositis, right ear
H70.222 Chronic petrositis, left ear
H70.223 Chronic petrositis, bilateral
H70.229 Chronic petrositis, unspecified ear

[5] H70.8 Other mastoiditis and related conditions
[EXCLUDES1] *preauricular sinus and cyst (Q18.1)*
sinus, fistula, and cyst of branchial cleft (Q18.0)

[6] H70.81 Postauricular fistula
H70.811 Postauricular fistula, right ear
H70.812 Postauricular fistula, left ear
H70.813 Postauricular fistula, bilateral
H70.819 Postauricular fistula, unspecified ear

[6] H70.89 Other mastoiditis and related conditions
H70.891 Other mastoiditis and related conditions, right ear
H70.892 Other mastoiditis and related conditions, left ear
H70.893 Other mastoiditis and related conditions, bilateral
H70.899 Other mastoiditis and related conditions, unspecified ear

[5] H70.9 Unspecified mastoiditis
H70.90 Unspecified mastoiditis, unspecified ear
H70.91 Unspecified mastoiditis, right ear
H70.92 Unspecified mastoiditis, left ear
H70.93 Unspecified mastoiditis, bilateral

[4] H71 Cholesteatoma of middle ear
[EXCLUDES2] *cholesteatoma of external ear (H60.4-)*
recurrent cholesteatoma of postmastoidectomy cavity (H95.0-)

[5] H71.0 Cholesteatoma of attic
H71.00 Cholesteatoma of attic, unspecified ear
H71.01 Cholesteatoma of attic, right ear
H71.02 Cholesteatoma of attic, left ear
H71.03 Cholesteatoma of attic, bilateral

[5] H71.1 Cholesteatoma of tympanum
H71.10 Cholesteatoma of tympanum, unspecified ear
H71.11 Cholesteatoma of tympanum, right ear
H71.12 Cholesteatoma of tympanum, left ear
H71.13 Cholesteatoma of tympanum, bilateral

[5] H71.2 Cholesteatoma of mastoid
H71.20 Cholesteatoma of mastoid, unspecified ear
H71.21 Cholesteatoma of mastoid, right ear
H71.22 Cholesteatoma of mastoid, left ear
H71.23 Cholesteatoma of mastoid, bilateral

[5] H71.3 Diffuse cholesteatosis
H71.30 Diffuse cholesteatosis, unspecified ear
H71.31 Diffuse cholesteatosis, right ear
H71.32 Diffuse cholesteatosis, left ear
H71.33 Diffuse cholesteatosis, bilateral

[5] H71.9 Unspecified cholesteatoma
H71.90 Unspecified cholesteatoma, unspecified ear
H71.91 Unspecified cholesteatoma, right ear
H71.92 Unspecified cholesteatoma, left ear
H71.93 Unspecified cholesteatoma, bilateral

[4] H72 Perforation of tympanic membrane
[INCLUDES] *persistent post-traumatic perforation of ear drum*
postinflammatory perforation of ear drum
Code first any associated otitis media (H65.-, H66.1-, H66.2-, H66.3-, H66.4-, H66.9-, H67.-)
[EXCLUDES1] *acute suppurative otitis media with rupture of the tympanic membrane (H66.01-)*
traumatic rupture of ear drum (S09.2-)

[5] H72.0 Central perforation of tympanic membrane
H72.00 Central perforation of tympanic membrane, unspecified ear
H72.01 Central perforation of tympanic membrane, right ear
H72.02 Central perforation of tympanic membrane, left ear
H72.03 Central perforation of tympanic membrane, bilateral

[5] H72.1 Attic perforation of tympanic membrane
Perforation of pars flaccida
H72.10 Attic perforation of tympanic membrane, unspecified ear
H72.11 Attic perforation of tympanic membrane, right ear
H72.12 Attic perforation of tympanic membrane, left ear
H72.13 Attic perforation of tympanic membrane, bilateral

[5] H72.2 Other marginal perforations of tympanic membrane

[4] 4th character required [5] 5th character required [6] 6th character required [7] 7th character required [X] Extension 'X' Alert
[EXCLUDES1] Not coded here [EXCLUDES2] Not included here [PDx] Primary Diagnosis Only Manifestation Code

ⓖ H72.2X Other marginal perforations of tympanic membrane

H72.2X1 Other marginal perforations of tympanic membrane, right ear

H72.2X2 Other marginal perforations of tympanic membrane, left ear

H72.2X3 Other marginal perforations of tympanic membrane, bilateral

H72.2X9 Other marginal perforations of tympanic membrane, unspecified ear

ⓔ H72.8 Other perforations of tympanic membrane

ⓖ H72.81 Multiple perforations of tympanic membrane

H72.811 Multiple perforations of tympanic membrane, right ear

H72.812 Multiple perforations of tympanic membrane, left ear

H72.813 Multiple perforations of tympanic membrane, bilateral

H72.819 Multiple perforations of tympanic membrane, unspecified ear

ⓖ H72.82 Total perforations of tympanic membrane

H72.821 Total perforations of tympanic membrane, right ear

H72.822 Total perforations of tympanic membrane, left ear

H72.823 Total perforations of tympanic membrane, bilateral

H72.829 Total perforations of tympanic membrane, unspecified ear

ⓔ H72.9 Unspecified perforation of tympanic membrane

H72.90 Unspecified perforation of tympanic membrane, unspecified ear

H72.91 Unspecified perforation of tympanic membrane, right ear

H72.92 Unspecified perforation of tympanic membrane, left ear

H72.93 Unspecified perforation of tympanic membrane, bilateral

ⓓ H73 Other disorders of tympanic membrane

ⓔ H73.0 Acute myringitis

EXCLUDES1 acute myringitis with otitis media (H65, H66)

ⓖ H73.00 Unspecified acute myringitis

Acute tympanitis NOS

H73.001 Acute myringitis, right ear

H73.002 Acute myringitis, left ear

H73.003 Acute myringitis, bilateral

H73.009 Acute myringitis, unspecified ear

ⓖ H73.01 Bullous myringitis

H73.011 Bullous myringitis, right ear

H73.012 Bullous myringitis, left ear

H73.013 Bullous myringitis, bilateral

H73.019 Bullous myringitis, unspecified ear

ⓖ H73.09 Other acute myringitis

H73.091 Other acute myringitis, right ear

H73.092 Other acute myringitis, left ear

H73.093 Other acute myringitis, bilateral

H73.099 Other acute myringitis, unspecified ear

ⓔ H73.1 Chronic myringitis

Chronic tympanitis

EXCLUDES1 chronic myringitis with otitis media (H65, H66)

H73.10 Chronic myringitis, unspecified ear

H73.11 Chronic myringitis, right ear

H73.12 Chronic myringitis, left ear

H73.13 Chronic myringitis, bilateral

ⓔ H73.2 Unspecified myringitis

H73.20 Unspecified myringitis, unspecified ear

H73.21 Unspecified myringitis, right ear

H73.22 Unspecified myringitis, left ear

H73.23 Unspecified myringitis, bilateral

ⓔ H73.8 Other specified disorders of tympanic membrane

ⓖ H73.81 Atrophic flaccid tympanic membrane

H73.811 Atrophic flaccid tympanic membrane, right ear

H73.812 Atrophic flaccid tympanic membrane, left ear

H73.813 Atrophic flaccid tympanic membrane, bilateral

H73.819 Atrophic flaccid tympanic membrane, unspecified ear

ⓖ H73.82 Atrophic nonflaccid tympanic membrane

H73.821 Atrophic nonflaccid tympanic membrane, right ear

H73.822 Atrophic nonflaccid tympanic membrane, left ear

H73.823 Atrophic nonflaccid tympanic membrane, bilateral

H73.829 Atrophic nonflaccid tympanic membrane, unspecified ear

ⓖ H73.89 Other specified disorders of tympanic membrane

H73.891 Other specified disorders of tympanic membrane, right ear

H73.892 Other specified disorders of tympanic membrane, left ear

H73.893 Other specified disorders of tympanic membrane, bilateral

H73.899 Other specified disorders of tympanic membrane, unspecified ear

ⓔ H73.9 Unspecified disorder of tympanic membrane

H73.90 Unspecified disorder of tympanic membrane, unspecified ear

H73.91 Unspecified disorder of tympanic membrane, right ear

H73.92 Unspecified disorder of tympanic membrane, left ear

H73.93 Unspecified disorder of tympanic membrane, bilateral

ⓓ H74 Other disorders of middle ear mastoid

EXCLUDES2 mastoiditis (H70.-)

ⓔ H74.0 Tympanosclerosis

H74.01 Tympanosclerosis, right ear

H74.02 Tympanosclerosis, left ear

H74.03 Tympanosclerosis, bilateral

H74.09 Tympanosclerosis, unspecified ear

ⓔ H74.1 Adhesive middle ear disease

Adhesive otitis

EXCLUDES1 glue ear (H65.3-)

H74.11 Adhesive right middle ear disease

H74.12 Adhesive left middle ear disease

H74.13 Adhesive middle ear disease, bilateral

H74.19 Adhesive middle ear disease, unspecified ear

ⓔ H74.2 Discontinuity and dislocation of ear ossicles

H74.20 Discontinuity and dislocation of ear ossicles, unspecified ear

H74.21 Discontinuity and dislocation of right ear ossicles

H74.22 Discontinuity and dislocation of left ear ossicles

H74.23 Discontinuity and dislocation of ear ossicles, bilateral

ⓔ H74.3 Other acquired abnormalities of ear ossicles

ⓖ H74.31 Ankylosis of ear ossicles

H74.311 Ankylosis of ear ossicles, right ear

H74.312 Ankylosis of ear ossicles, left ear

H74.313 Ankylosis of ear ossicles, bilateral

H74.319 Ankylosis of ear ossicles, unspecified ear

Unspecified Code	Other Specified Code	Ⓝ Newborn Age: 0	Ⓟ Pediatric Age: 0-17	Ⓜ Maternity Age: 12-55

Ⓐ Adult Age: 15-124   ♂ Male   ♀ Female   ● New Code   ▲ Revised Code Title   ►◄ Revised Text

[6] H74.32 Partial loss of ear ossicles
H74.321 Partial loss of ear ossicles, right ear
H74.322 Partial loss of ear ossicles, left ear
H74.323 Partial loss of ear ossicles, bilateral
H74.329 Partial loss of ear ossicles, unspecified ear
[6] H74.39 Other acquired abnormalities of ear ossicles
H74.391 Other acquired abnormalities of right ear ossicles
H74.392 Other acquired abnormalities of left ear ossicles
H74.393 Other acquired abnormalities of ear ossicles, bilateral
H74.399 Other acquired abnormalities of ear ossicles, unspecified ear
[5] H74.4 Polyp of middle ear
H74.40 Polyp of middle ear, unspecified ear
H74.41 Polyp of right middle ear
H74.42 Polyp of left middle ear
H74.43 Polyp of middle ear, bilateral
[5] H74.8 Other specified disorders of middle ear and mastoid
[6] H74.8X Other specified disorders of middle ear and mastoid
H74.8X1 Other specified disorders of right middle ear and mastoid
H74.8X2 Other specified disorders of left middle ear and mastoid
H74.8X3 Other specified disorders of middle ear and mastoid, bilateral
H74.8X9 Other specified disorders of middle ear and mastoid, unspecified ear
[5] H74.9 Unspecified disorder of middle ear and mastoid
H74.90 Unspecified disorder of middle ear and mastoid, unspecified ear
H74.91 Unspecified disorder of right middle ear and mastoid
H74.92 Unspecified disorder of left middle ear and mastoid
H74.93 Unspecified disorder of middle ear and mastoid, bilateral
[4] H75 Other disorders of middle ear and mastoid in diseases classified elsewhere
Code first underlying disease
[5] H75.0 Mastoiditis in infectious and parasitic diseases classified elsewhere
[EXCLUDES1] *mastoiditis (in):*
syphilis (A52.77)
tuberculosis (A18.03)
H75.00 Mastoiditis in infectious and parasitic diseases classified elsewhere, unspecified ear
H75.01 Mastoiditis in infectious and parasitic diseases classified elsewhere, right ear
H75.02 Mastoiditis in infectious and parasitic diseases classified elsewhere, left ear
H75.03 Mastoiditis in infectious and parasitic diseases classified elsewhere, bilateral
[5] H75.8 Other specified disorders of middle ear and mastoid in diseases classified elsewhere
H75.80 Other specified disorders of middle ear and mastoid in diseases classified elsewhere, unspecified ear
H75.81 Other specified disorders of right middle ear and mastoid in diseases classified elsewhere
H75.82 Other specified disorders of left middle ear and mastoid in diseases classified elsewhere
H75.83 Other specified disorders of middle ear and mastoid in diseases classified elsewhere, bilateral

Diseases of inner ear (H80-H83)

[4] H80 Otosclerosis
[INCLUDES] *Otospongiosis*
[5] H80.0 Otosclerosis involving oval window, nonobliterative
H80.00 Otosclerosis involving oval window, nonobliterative, unspecified ear
H80.01 Otosclerosis involving oval window, nonobliterative, right ear
H80.02 Otosclerosis involving oval window, nonobliterative, left ear
H80.03 Otosclerosis involving oval window, nonobliterative, bilateral
[5] H80.1 Otosclerosis involving oval window, obliterative
H80.10 Otosclerosis involving oval window, obliterative, unspecified ear
H80.11 Otosclerosis involving oval window, obliterative, right ear
H80.12 Otosclerosis involving oval window, obliterative, left ear
H80.13 Otosclerosis involving oval window, obliterative, bilateral
[5] H80.2 Cochlear otosclerosis
Otosclerosis involving otic capsule
Otosclerosis involving round window
H80.20 Cochlear otosclerosis, unspecified ear
H80.21 Cochlear otosclerosis, right ear
H80.22 Cochlear otosclerosis, left ear
H80.23 Cochlear otosclerosis, bilateral
[5] H80.8 Other otosclerosis
H80.80 Other otosclerosis, unspecified ear
H80.81 Other otosclerosis, right ear
H80.82 Other otosclerosis, left ear
H80.83 Other otosclerosis, bilateral
[5] H80.9 Unspecified otosclerosis
H80.90 Unspecified otosclerosis, unspecified ear
H80.91 Unspecified otosclerosis, right ear
H80.92 Unspecified otosclerosis, left ear
H80.93 Unspecified otosclerosis, bilateral
[4] H81 Disorders of vestibular function
[EXCLUDES1] *epidemic vertigo (A88.1)*
vertigo NOS (R42)
[5] H81.0 Ménière's disease
Labyrinthine hydrops
Ménière's syndrome or vertigo
H81.01 Ménière's disease, right ear
H81.02 Ménière's disease, left ear
H81.03 Ménière's disease, bilateral
H81.09 Ménière's disease, unspecified ear
[5] H81.1 Benign paroxysmal vertigo
H81.10 Benign paroxysmal vertigo, unspecified ear
H81.11 Benign paroxysmal vertigo, right ear
H81.12 Benign paroxysmal vertigo, left ear
H81.13 Benign paroxysmal vertigo, bilateral
[5] H81.2 Vestibular neuronitis
H81.20 Vestibular neuronitis, unspecified ear
H81.21 Vestibular neuronitis, right ear
H81.22 Vestibular neuronitis, left ear
H81.23 Vestibular neuronitis, bilateral
[5] H81.3 Other peripheral vertigo
[6] H81.31 Aural vertigo
H81.311 Aural vertigo, right ear
H81.312 Aural vertigo, left ear
H81.313 Aural vertigo, bilateral
H81.319 Aural vertigo, unspecified ear
[6] H81.39 Other peripheral vertigo

[4] 4th character required [5] 5th character required [6] 6th character required [7] 7th character required [7th] Extension 'X' Alert
[EXCLUDES1] Not coded here [EXCLUDES2] Not included here [PDx] Primary Diagnosis Only Manifestation Code

Lermoyez' syndrome
Otogenic vertigo
Peripheral vertigo NOS

H81.391 Other peripheral vertigo, right ear
H81.392 Other peripheral vertigo, left ear
H81.393 Other peripheral vertigo, bilateral
H81.399 Other peripheral vertigo, unspecified ear

[5] H81.4 Vertigo of central origin

Central positional nystagmus

H81.41 Vertigo of central origin, right ear
H81.42 Vertigo of central origin, left ear
H81.43 Vertigo of central origin, bilateral
H81.49 Vertigo of central origin, unspecified ear

[5] H81.8 Other disorders of vestibular function

[6] H81.8X Other disorders of vestibular function

H81.8X1 Other disorders of vestibular function, right ear
H81.8X2 Other disorders of vestibular function, left ear
H81.8X3 Other disorders of vestibular function, bilateral
H81.8X9 Other disorders of vestibular function, unspecified ear

[5] H81.9 Unspecified disorder of vestibular function

Vertiginous syndrome NOS

H81.90 Unspecified disorder of vestibular function, unspecified ear
H81.91 Unspecified disorder of vestibular function, right ear
H81.92 Unspecified disorder of vestibular function, left ear
H81.93 Unspecified disorder of vestibular function, bilateral

[4] H82 Vertiginous syndromes in diseases classified elsewhere

Code first underlying disease

[EXCLUDES1] *epidemic vertigo (A88.1)*

H82.1 Vertiginous syndromes in diseases classified elsewhere, right ear
H82.2 Vertiginous syndromes in diseases classified elsewhere, left ear
H82.3 Vertiginous syndromes in diseases classified elsewhere, bilateral
H82.9 Vertiginous syndromes in diseases classified elsewhere, unspecified ear

[4] H83 Other diseases of inner ear

[5] H83.0 Labyrinthitis

H83.01 Labyrinthitis, right ear
H83.02 Labyrinthitis, left ear
H83.03 Labyrinthitis, bilateral
H83.09 Labyrinthitis, unspecified ear

[5] H83.1 Labyrinthine fistula

H83.11 Labyrinthine fistula, right ear
H83.12 Labyrinthine fistula, left ear
H83.13 Labyrinthine fistula, bilateral
H83.19 Labyrinthine fistula, unspecified ear

[5] H83.2 Labyrinthine dysfunction

Labyrinthine hypersensitivity
Labyrinthine hypofunction
Labyrinthine loss of function

[6] H83.2X Labyrinthine dysfunction

H83.2X1 Labyrinthine dysfunction, right ear
H83.2X2 Labyrinthine dysfunction, left ear
H83.2X3 Labyrinthine dysfunction, bilateral
H83.2X9 Labyrinthine dysfunction, unspecified ear

[5] H83.3 Noise effects on inner ear

Acoustic trauma of inner ear
Noise-induced hearing loss of inner ear

[6] H83.3X Noise effects on inner ear

H83.3X1 Noise effects on right inner ear
H83.3X2 Noise effects on left inner ear
H83.3X3 Noise effects on inner ear, bilateral
H83.3X9 Noise effects on inner ear, unspecified ear

[5] H83.8 Other specified diseases of inner ear

[6] H83.8X Other specified diseases of inner ear

H83.8X1 Other specified diseases of right inner ear
H83.8X2 Other specified diseases of left inner ear
H83.8X3 Other specified diseases of inner ear, bilateral
H83.8X9 Other specified diseases of inner ear, unspecified ear

[5] H83.9 Unspecified disease of inner ear

H83.90 Unspecified disease of inner ear, unspecified ear
H83.91 Unspecified disease of right inner ear
H83.92 Unspecified disease of left inner ear
H83.93 Unspecified disease of inner ear, bilateral

Other disorders of ear (H90-H94)

[4] H90 Conductive and sensorineural hearing loss

[EXCLUDES1] *deaf nonspeaking NEC (H91.3)*
deafness NOS (H91.9-)
hearing loss NOS (H91.9-)
noise-induced hearing loss (H83.3-)
ototoxic hearing loss (H91.0-)
sudden (idiopathic) hearing loss (H91.2-)

H90.0 Conductive hearing loss, bilateral

[5] H90.1 Conductive hearing loss, unilateral with unrestricted hearing on the contralateral side

H90.11 Conductive hearing loss, unilateral, right ear, with unrestricted hearing on the contralateral side
H90.12 Conductive hearing loss, unilateral, left ear, with unrestricted hearing on the contralateral side

H90.2 Conductive hearing loss, unspecified

Conductive deafness NOS

H90.3 Sensorineural hearing loss, bilateral

[5] H90.4 Sensorineural hearing loss, unilateral with unrestricted hearing on the contralateral side

H90.41 Sensorineural hearing loss, unilateral, right ear, with unrestricted hearing on the contralateral side
H90.42 Sensorineural hearing loss, unilateral, left ear, with unrestricted hearing on the contralateral side

H90.5 Unspecified sensorineural hearing loss

Central hearing loss NOS
Congenital deafness NOS
Neural hearing loss NOS
Perceptive hearing loss NOS
Sensorineural deafness NOS
Sensory hearing loss NOS

[EXCLUDES1] *abnormal auditory perception (H93.2-)*
psychogenic deafness (F44.6)

H90.6 Mixed conductive and sensorineural hearing loss, bilateral

[5] H90.7 Mixed conductive and sensorineural hearing loss, unilateral with unrestricted hearing on the contralateral side

H90.71 Mixed conductive and sensorineural hearing loss, unilateral, right ear, with unrestricted hearing on the contralateral side
H90.72 Mixed conductive and sensorineural hearing loss, unilateral, left ear, with unrestricted hearing on the contralateral side

H90.8 Mixed conductive and sensorineural hearing loss, unspecified

Unspecified Code | Other Specified Code | [N] Newborn Age: 0 | [P] Pediatric Age: 0-17 | [M] Maternity Age: 12-55
[A] Adult Age: 15-124 | ♂ Male | ♀ Female | ● New Code | ▲ Revised Code Title | ►◄ Revised Text

H91 Other and unspecified **hearing loss**

> EXCLUDES1 *abnormal auditory perception (H93.2-)*
> *hearing loss as classified in H90.-*
> *impacted cerumen (H61.2-)*
> *noise-induced hearing loss (H83.3-)*
> *psychogenic deafness (F44.6)*
> *transient ischemic deafness (H93.01-)*

H91.0 Ototoxic **hearing loss**

> Code first poisoning due to drug or toxin, if applicable (T36-T65 with fifth or sixth character 1-4 or 6)
> Use additional code for adverse effect, if applicable, to identify drug (T36-T50 with fifth or sixth character 5)

H91.01 Ototoxic hearing loss, right ear
H91.02 Ototoxic hearing loss, left ear
H91.03 Ototoxic hearing loss, bilateral
H91.09 Ototoxic hearing loss, unspecified ear

H91.1 Presbycusis

> Presbyacusia

H91.10 Presbycusis, unspecified ear
H91.11 Presbycusis, right ear
H91.12 Presbycusis, left ear
H91.13 Presbycusis, bilateral

H91.2 Sudden idiopathic **hearing loss**

> Sudden hearing loss NOS

H91.20 Sudden idiopathic hearing loss, unspecified ear
H91.21 Sudden idiopathic hearing loss, right ear
H91.22 Sudden idiopathic hearing loss, left ear
H91.23 Sudden idiopathic hearing loss, bilateral
H91.3 Deaf nonspeaking, not elsewhere classified

H91.8 Other specified **hearing loss**

H91.8X Other specified hearing loss

H91.8X1 Other specified hearing loss, right ear
H91.8X2 Other specified hearing loss, left ear
H91.8X3 Other specified hearing loss, bilateral
H91.8X9 Other specified hearing loss, unspecified ear

H91.9 Unspecified **hearing loss**

> Deafness NOS
> High frequency deafness
> Low frequency deafness

H91.90 Unspecified hearing loss, unspecified ear
H91.91 Unspecified hearing loss, right ear
H91.92 Unspecified hearing loss, left ear
H91.93 Unspecified hearing loss, bilateral

H92 Otalgia and effusion of ear

H92.0 Otalgia

H92.01 Otalgia, right ear
H92.02 Otalgia, left ear
H92.03 Otalgia, bilateral
H92.09 Otalgia, unspecified ear

H92.1 Otorrhea

> EXCLUDES1 *leakage of cerebrospinal fluid through ear (G96.0)*

H92.10 Otorrhea, unspecified ear
H92.11 Otorrhea, right ear
H92.12 Otorrhea, left ear
H92.13 Otorrhea, bilateral

H92.2 Otorrhagia

> EXCLUDES1 *traumatic otorrhagia - code to injury*

H92.20 Otorrhagia, unspecified ear
H92.21 Otorrhagia, right ear
H92.22 Otorrhagia, left ear
H92.23 Otorrhagia, bilateral

H93 Other disorders of ear, not elsewhere classified

H93.0 Degenerative and vascular disorders of ear

> EXCLUDES1 *presbycusis (H91.1)*

H93.01 Transient ischemic deafness

H93.011 Transient ischemic deafness, right ear
H93.012 Transient ischemic deafness, left ear
H93.013 Transient ischemic deafness, bilateral
H93.019 Transient ischemic deafness, unspecified ear

H93.09 Unspecified degenerative and vascular disorders of ear

H93.091 Unspecified degenerative and vascular disorders of right ear
H93.092 Unspecified degenerative and vascular disorders of left ear
H93.093 Unspecified degenerative and vascular disorders of ear, bilateral
H93.099 Unspecified degenerative and vascular disorders of unspecified ear

H93.1 Tinnitus

H93.11 Tinnitus, right ear
H93.12 Tinnitus, left ear
H93.13 Tinnitus, bilateral
H93.19 Tinnitus, unspecified ear

H93.2 Other abnormal auditory perceptions

> EXCLUDES2 *auditory hallucinations (R44.0)*

H93.21 Auditory recruitment

H93.211 Auditory recruitment, right ear
H93.212 Auditory recruitment, left ear
H93.213 Auditory recruitment, bilateral
H93.219 Auditory recruitment, unspecified ear

H93.22 Diplacusis

H93.221 Diplacusis, right ear
H93.222 Diplacusis, left ear
H93.223 Diplacusis, bilateral
H93.229 Diplacusis, unspecified ear

H93.23 Hyperacusis

H93.231 Hyperacusis, right ear
H93.232 Hyperacusis, left ear
H93.233 Hyperacusis, bilateral
H93.239 Hyperacusis, unspecified ear

H93.24 Temporary auditory threshold shift

H93.241 Temporary auditory threshold shift, right ear
H93.242 Temporary auditory threshold shift, left ear
H93.243 Temporary auditory threshold shift, bilateral
H93.249 Temporary auditory threshold shift, unspecified ear

H93.25 Central auditory processing disorder

> Congenital auditory imperception
> Word deafness
> EXCLUDES1 *mixed receptive-expressive language disorder (F80.2)*

H93.29 Other abnormal auditory perceptions

H93.291 Other abnormal auditory perceptions, right ear
H93.292 Other abnormal auditory perceptions, left ear
H93.293 Other abnormal auditory perceptions, bilateral
H93.299 Other abnormal auditory perceptions, unspecified ear

H93.3 Disorders of acoustic nerve

> Disorder of 8th cranial nerve
> EXCLUDES1 *acoustic neuroma (D33.3)*
> *syphilitic acoustic neuritis (A52.15)*

H93.3X Disorders of acoustic nerve

H93.3X1 Disorders of right acoustic nerve
H93.3X2 Disorders of left acoustic nerve
H93.3X3 Disorders of bilateral acoustic nerves

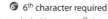

4th character required   5th character required   6th character required   7th character required   Extension 'X' Alert

EXCLUDES 1 Not coded here   EXCLUDES 2 Not included here   PDx Primary Diagnosis Only   Manifestation Code

H93.3X9 Disorders of unspecified acoustic nerve
- H93.8 Other specified disorders of ear
  - H93.8X Other specified disorders of ear
    - H93.8X1 Other specified disorders of right ear
    - H93.8X2 Other specified disorders of left ear
    - H93.8X3 Other specified disorders of ear, bilateral
    - H93.8X9 Other specified disorders of ear, unspecified ear
- H93.9 Unspecified disorder of ear
  - H93.90 Unspecified disorder of ear, unspecified ear
  - H93.91 Unspecified disorder of right ear
  - H93.92 Unspecified disorder of left ear
  - H93.93 Unspecified disorder of ear, bilateral
- H94 Other disorders of ear in diseases classified elsewhere
  - H94.0 Acoustic neuritis in infectious and parasitic diseases classified elsewhere
    Code first underlying disease, such as:
    parasitic disease (B65-B89)
    EXCLUDES1 acoustic neuritis (in):
    herpes zoster (B02.29)
    syphilis (A52.15)
    - H94.00 Acoustic neuritis in infectious and parasitic diseases classified elsewhere, unspecified ear
    - H94.01 Acoustic neuritis in infectious and parasitic diseases classified elsewhere, right ear
    - H94.02 Acoustic neuritis in infectious and parasitic diseases classified elsewhere, left ear
    - H94.03 Acoustic neuritis in infectious and parasitic diseases classified elsewhere, bilateral
  - H94.8 Other specified disorders of ear in diseases classified elsewhere
    Code first underlying disease, such as:
    congenital syphilis (A50.0)
    EXCLUDES1 aural myiasis (B87.4)
    syphilitic labyrinthitis (A52.79)
    - H94.80 Other specified disorders of ear in diseases classified elsewhere, unspecified ear
    - H94.81 Other specified disorders of right ear in diseases classified elsewhere
    - H94.82 Other specified disorders of left ear in diseases classified elsewhere
    - H94.83 Other specified disorders of ear in diseases classified elsewhere, bilateral

Intraoperative and postprocedural complications and disorders of ear and mastoid process, not elsewhere classified (H95)

- H95 Intraoperative and postprocedural complications and disorders of ear and mastoid process, not elsewhere classified
  - H95.0 Recurrent cholesteatoma of postmastoidectomy cavity
    - H95.00 Recurrent cholesteatoma of postmastoidectomy cavity, unspecified ear
    - H95.01 Recurrent cholesteatoma of postmastoidectomy cavity, right ear
    - H95.02 Recurrent cholesteatoma of postmastoidectomy cavity, left ear
    - H95.03 Recurrent cholesteatoma of postmastoidectomy cavity, bilateral ears
  - H95.1 Other disorders of ear and mastoid process following mastoidectomy
    - H95.11 Chronic inflammation of postmastoidectomy cavity
      - H95.111 Chronic inflammation of postmastoidectomy cavity, right ear
      - H95.112 Chronic inflammation of postmastoidectomy cavity, left ear
      - H95.113 Chronic inflammation of postmastoidectomy cavity, bilateral ears
      - H95.119 Chronic inflammation of postmastoidectomy cavity, unspecified ear
    - H95.12 Granulation of postmastoidectomy cavity
      - H95.121 Granulation of postmastoidectomy cavity, right ear
      - H95.122 Granulation of postmastoidectomy cavity, left ear
      - H95.123 Granulation of postmastoidectomy cavity, bilateral ears
      - H95.129 Granulation of postmastoidectomy cavity, unspecified ear
    - H95.13 Mucosal cyst of postmastoidectomy cavity
      - H95.131 Mucosal cyst of postmastoidectomy cavity, right ear
      - H95.132 Mucosal cyst of postmastoidectomy cavity, left ear
      - H95.133 Mucosal cyst of postmastoidectomy cavity, bilateral ears
      - H95.139 Mucosal cyst of postmastoidectomy cavity, unspecified ear
    - H95.19 Other disorders following mastoidectomy
      - H95.191 Other disorders following mastoidectomy, right ear
      - H95.192 Other disorders following mastoidectomy, left ear
      - H95.193 Other disorders following mastoidectomy, bilateral ears
      - H95.199 Other disorders following mastoidectomy, unspecified ear
  - H95.2 Intraoperative hemorrhage and hematoma of ear and mastoid process complicating a procedure
    EXCLUDES1 intraoperative hemorrhage and hematoma of ear and mastoid process due to accidental puncture or laceration during a procedure (H95.3-)
    - H95.21 Intraoperative hemorrhage and hematoma of ear and mastoid process complicating a procedure on the ear and mastoid process
    - H95.22 Intraoperative hemorrhage and hematoma of ear and mastoid process complicating other procedure
  - H95.3 Accidental puncture and laceration of ear and mastoid process during a procedure

Unspecified Code	Other Specified Code	N Newborn Age: 0	P Pediatric Age: 0-17	M Maternity Age: 12-55	
A Adult Age: 15-124	♂ Male	♀ Female	● New Code	▲ Revised Code Title	▶◀ Revised Text

H95.31 Accidental puncture and laceration of the ear and mastoid process during a procedure on the ear and mastoid process

H95.32 Accidental puncture and laceration of the ear and mastoid process during other procedure

[5] H95.4 Postprocedural hemorrhage and hematoma of ear and mastoid process following a procedure

H95.41 Postprocedural hemorrhage and hematoma of ear and mastoid process following a procedure on the ear and mastoid process

H95.42 Postprocedural hemorrhage and hematoma of ear and mastoid process following other procedure

[5] H95.8 Other intraoperative and postprocedural complications and disorders of the ear and mastoid process, not elsewhere classified

[EXCLUDES2] *postprocedural complications and disorders following mastoidectomy (H95.0-, H95.1-)*

[6] H95.81 Postprocedural stenosis of external ear canal

H95.811 Postprocedural stenosis of right external ear canal

H95.812 Postprocedural stenosis of left external ear canal

H95.813 Postprocedural stenosis of external ear canal, bilateral

H95.819 Postprocedural stenosis of unspecified external ear canal

H95.88 Other intraoperative complications and disorders of the ear and mastoid process, not elsewhere classified

Use additional code , if applicable, to further specify disorder

H95.89 Other postprocedural complications and disorders of the ear and mastoid process, not elsewhere classified

Use additional code, if applicable, to further specify disorder

[4] 4th character required [5] 5th character required [6] 6th character required [7] 7th character required [7x] Extension 'X' Alert
[EXCLUDES1] Not coded here [EXCLUDES2] Not included here [PDx] Primary Diagnosis Only Manifestation Code

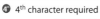

Chapter 9: Diseases of the Circulatory System (I00-I99)

Chapter Specific Coding Guidelines

a. Hypertension

1) Hypertension with Heart Disease
Heart conditions classified to I50.- or I51.4-I51.9, are assigned to, a code from category I11, Hypertensive heart disease, when a causal relationship is stated (due to hypertension) or implied (hypertensive). Use an additional code from category I50, Heart failure, to identify the type of heart failure in those patients with heart failure.

The same heart conditions (I50.-, I51.4-I51.9) with hypertension, but without a stated causal relationship, are coded separately. Sequence according to the circumstances of the admission/encounter.

2) Hypertensive Chronic Kidney Disease
Assign codes from category I12, Hypertensive chronic kidney disease, when both hypertension and a condition classifiable to category N18, Chronic kidney disease (CKD), are present. Unlike hypertension with heart disease, ICD-10-CM presumes a cause-and-effect relationship and classifies chronic kidney disease with hypertension as hypertensive chronic kidney disease.

The appropriate code from category N18 should be used as a secondary code with a code from category I12 to identify the stage of chronic kidney disease.

See Section I.C.14. Chronic kidney disease.

If a patient has hypertensive chronic kidney disease and acute renal failure, an additional code for the acute renal failure is required.

3) Hypertensive Heart and Chronic Kidney Disease
Assign codes from combination category I13, Hypertensive heart and chronic kidney disease, when both hypertensive kidney disease and hypertensive heart disease are stated in the diagnosis. Assume a relationship between the hypertension and the chronic kidney disease, whether or not the condition is so designated. If heart failure is present, assign an additional code from category I50 to identify the type of heart failure.

The appropriate code from category N18, Chronic kidney disease, should be used as a secondary code with a code from category I13 to identify the stage of chronic kidney disease.

See Section I.C.14. Chronic kidney disease.

The codes in category I13, Hypertensive heart and chronic kidney disease, are combination codes that include hypertension, heart disease and chronic kidney disease. The Includes note at I13 specifies that the conditions included at I11 and I12 are included together in I13. If a patient has hypertension, heart disease and chronic kidney disease then a code from I13 should be used, not individual codes for hypertension, heart disease and chronic kidney disease, or codes from I11 or I12.

For patients with both acute renal failure and chronic kidney disease an additional code for acute renal failure is required.

4) Hypertensive Cerebrovascular Disease
For hypertensive cerebrovascular disease, first assign the appropriate code from categories I60-I69, followed by the appropriate hypertension code.

5) Hypertensive Retinopathy
Subcategory H35.0, Background retinopathy and retinal vascular changes, should be used with a code from category I10 – I15, Hypertensive disease to include the systemic hypertension. The sequencing is based on the reason for the encounter.

6) Hypertension, Secondary
Secondary hypertension is due to an underlying condition. Two codes are required: one to identify the underlying etiology and one from category I15 to identify the hypertension. Sequencing of codes is determined by the reason for admission/encounter.

7) Hypertension, Transient
Assign code R03.0, Elevated blood pressure reading without diagnosis of hypertension, unless patient has an established diagnosis of hypertension. Assign code O13.-, Gestational [pregnancy-induced] hypertension without significant proteinuria, or O14.-, Pre-eclampsia, for transient hypertension of pregnancy.

8) Hypertension, Controlled
This diagnostic statement usually refers to an existing state of hypertension under control by therapy. Assign the appropriate code from categories I10-I15, Hypertensive diseases.

9) Hypertension, Uncontrolled
Uncontrolled hypertension may refer to untreated hypertension or hypertension not responding to current therapeutic regimen. In either case, assign the appropriate code from categories I10-I15, Hypertensive diseases.

b. Atherosclerotic Coronary Artery Disease and Angina
ICD-10-CM has combination codes for atherosclerotic heart disease with angina pectoris. The subcategories for these codes are I25.11, Atherosclerotic heart disease of native coronary artery with angina pectoris and I25.7, Atherosclerosis of coronary artery bypass graft(s) and coronary artery of transplanted heart with angina pectoris.

When using one of these combination codes it is not necessary to use an additional code for angina pectoris. A causal relationship can be assumed in a patient with both atherosclerosis and angina pectoris, unless the documentation indicates the angina is due to something other than the atherosclerosis.

If a patient with coronary artery disease is admitted due to an acute myocardial infarction (AMI), the AMI should be sequenced before the coronary artery disease.

See Section I.C.9. Acute myocardial infarction (AMI)

c. Intraoperative and Postprocedural Cerebrovascular Accident

Medical record documentation should clearly specify the cause-and-effect relationship between the medical intervention and the cerebrovascular accident in order to assign a code for intraoperative or postprocedural cerebrovascular accident.

Proper code assignment depends on whether it was an infarction or hemorrhage and whether it occurred intraoperatively or postoperatively. If it was a cerebral hemorrhage, code assignment depends on the type of procedure performed.

d. Sequelae of Cerebrovascular Disease

1) Category I69, Sequelae of Cerebrovascular disease
Category I69 is used to indicate conditions classifiable to categories I60-I67 as the causes of sequela (neurologic deficits), themselves classified elsewhere. These "late effects" include neurologic deficits that persist after initial onset of conditions classifiable to categories I60-I67. The neurologic deficits caused by cerebrovascular disease may be present from the onset or may arise at any time after the onset of the condition classifiable to categories I60-I67.

Codes from category I69, Sequelae of cerebrovascular disease, that specify hemiplegia, hemiparesis and monoplegia identify whether the dominant or nondominant side is affected. Should the affected side be documented, but not specified as dominant or nondominant, and the classification system does not indicate a default, code selection is as follows:

- For ambidextrous patients, the default should be dominant.
- If the left side is affected, the default is non-dominant.
- If the right side is affected, the default is dominant.

2) **Codes from category I69 with codes from I60-I67**
Codes from category I69 may be assigned on a health care record with codes from I60-I67, if the patient has a current cerebrovascular disease and deficits from an old cerebrovascular disease.

3) **Codes from category I69 and Personal history of transient ischemic attack (TIA) and cerebral infarction (Z86.73)**
Codes from category I69 should not be assigned if the patient does not have neurologic deficits.

See Section I.C.21. 4. History (of) for use of personal history codes

e. **Acute Myocardial Infarction (AMI)**
1) **ST elevation myocardial infarction (STEMI) and non ST elevation myocardial infarction (NSTEMI)**
The ICD-10-CM codes for acute myocardial infarction (AMI) identify the site, such as anterolateral wall or true posterior wall. Subcategories I21.0-I21.2 and code I21.3 are used for ST elevation myocardial infarction (STEMI). Code I21.4, Non-ST elevation (NSTEMI) myocardial infarction, is used for non ST elevation myocardial infarction (NSTEMI) and nontransmural MIs.

If NSTEMI evolves to STEMI, assign the STEMI code. If STEMI converts to NSTEMI due to thrombolytic therapy, it is still coded as STEMI.

For encounters occurring while the myocardial infarction is equal to, or less than, four weeks old, including transfers to another acute setting or a postacute setting, and the patient requires continued care for the myocardial infarction, codes from category I21 may continue to be reported. For encounters after the 4 week time frame and the patient is still receiving care related to the myocardial infarction, the appropriate aftercare code should be assigned, rather than a code from category I21. For old or healed myocardial infarctions not requiring further care, code I25.2, Old myocardial infarction, may be assigned.

2) **Acute myocardial infarction, unspecified**
Code I21.3, ST elevation (STEMI) myocardial infarction of unspecified site, is the default for unspecified acute myocardial infarction. If only STEMI or transmural MI without the site is documented, assign code I21.3.

3) **AMI documented as nontransmural or subendocardial but site provided**
If an AMI is documented as nontransmural or subendocardial, but the site is provided, it is still coded as a subendocardial AMI.

See Section I.C.21.3 for information on coding status post administration of tPA in a different facility within the last 24 hours.

4) **Subsequent acute myocardial infarction**
A code from category I22, Subsequent ST elevation (STEMI) and non ST elevation (NSTEMI) myocardial infarction, is to be used when a patient who has suffered an AMI has a new AMI within the 4 week time frame of the initial AMI. A code from category I22 must be used in conjunction with a code from category I21. The sequencing of the I22 and I21 codes depends on the circumstances of the encounter.

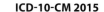

Anatomy of the Cardiovascular System

Introduction

The human vascular system comprises a series of tubes (which are known as vessels) that travel in almost all parts of the human body. It is categorized into the following two classes:

1. **Blood Vascular System**

    The blood vascular system includes the heart and blood vessels required to facilitate the circulation of the colored fluid (blood) inside the body.

    a) The Structure of Arteries

    The arteries possess stronger and thicker walls than the corresponding veins and are based on the following components:

    i)   Tunica Intima

    ii) Tunica Media

    iii) Tunica Externa

    b. The Structure of Veins

    The veins have a similar structure as that of the arteries. The components of a typical vein are described below:

    i)   Tunica Intima

    ii) Tunica Media

    iii) Tunica Externa

    c. The Blood

    The blood is considered as a uniquely specialized connective tissue that is composed of the formed elements (or the blood cells) and the fluid portion (or plasma). The formed elements of blood are based on the red blood cells (RBCs or erythrocytes), the white blood cells (WBCs or leukocytes) and the platelets (or thrombocytes). The blood contributes to about 8% of total body weight. The quantity of blood in an average human varies between 5 to 6 litres. The elements of blood are categorized below:

    d. Erythrocytes or Red Blood Cells: The red blood cells are the most common type of blood cells that contribute to about 95% of the blood cell volume.

    e. Leukocytes or White Blood Cells: The white blood cells can be divided into the following subcategories:

    f. Granular Leukocytes- The granular leukocytes contain granules in their cytoplasm and can be further classified into the following three types:

    i)   neutrophils constitute about 60% to 70% of the white blood cells.

    ii) eosinophils constitute about 2% to 4% of the white blood cells.

    iii) basophils constitute about 0.5% to 1% of the white blood cells.

    g. Agranular Leukocytes: The agranular leukocytes do not contain granules in their cytoplasm and can be further classified into the following two types:

    i)   monocytes constitute about 3% to 8% of the white blood cells.

    ii) lymphocytes constitute about 20% to 25% of the white blood cells.

    h. Thrombocytes or Platelets: The platelets are small cell fragments that do not contain nucleus in their cytoplasm.

    i. Blood Plasma

    The plasma is the fluid component of blood in which the blood cells usually remain suspended. The blood plasma is composed of 91% water, 7% proteins, and 2% solutes.

2. **Lymph Vascular System**

    The lymph vascular system includes the lymph glands and lymphatic vessels for circulating the colourless fluid (lymph) throughout the human body. Both of the blood vascular and the lymph vascular systems work in close association with each other for sustaining the human life cycle.

Circulation of Blood Through the Heart

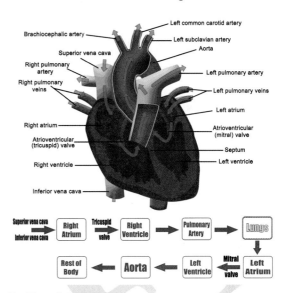

3. **The Thoracic Cavity**

    The thoracic cavity is enclosed by the thoracic wall and primarily contains the structures of the cardiovascular and respiratory systems.

    a) The Pericardium

    The heart and the roots of the great vessels are contained within the conical and fibro-serous sac, which is known as the pericardium. It is composed of two closely connected sacs, which are known as the fibrous pericardium (or the outer sac) and the serous pericardium (the inner sac).

    b) The Heart

    The heart is a hollow muscular organ which remains enclosed in the fibro-serous sac (or the pericardium) and regarded as the central organ of the cardiovascular system. It lies between the lungs in the middle mediastinum and receives blood from the veins.

4. **The Chambers of Heart**

    The human heart is based on the following four chambers:

    a) The Right Atrium: The right border of human heart is formed by the right atrium. The superior vena cava, inferior vena cava and coronary sinus provide venous blood supply to the right atrium of heart.

    The right atrium contains the following elements inside it:

    i)   Sinus Venarum

    ii)   Pectinate Muscles

    iii) Opening of Superior Vena Cava

    iv)   Opening of Inferior Vena Cava

    v)   Opening of Coronary Sinus

    vi)   The Right Atrioventricular Orifice

    vii) Interatrial Septum

    b) The Right Ventricle: The inferior border of the human heart is constituted by the right ventricle.

    c) The Left Atrium: The left atrium chiefly constitutes the base of the heart and utilizes the mitral valve to pump the oxygenated blood received from the pulmonary veins into the left ventricle of heart. The interior of the left atrium is based on the following components:

i) Two superior and two inferior pulmonary veins that enter the posterior wall of the left atrium.

ii) A posteriorly directed interatrial septum that separates the right atrium from the left atrium of the heart.

iii) A smooth walled portion and a muscular auricle containing pectinate muscles.

iv) A comparatively thicker wall than the corresponding right atrium.

v) A left atrioventricular orifice that facilitates the discharge of oxygenated blood into the left ventricle.

d) The Left Ventricle: The left ventricle pumps the oxygenated blood (through the aortic valve) to the whole body by aorta. The interior of the left ventricle is based on the following elements:

i) a double-leaflet/dual-flap mitral (bicuspid or left atrioventricular) valve, which is located between the left atrium and ventricle for guarding the left atrioventricular orifice.

ii) walls of the left ventricle, which are comparatively thicker than the corresponding right ventricle.

iii) conical cavity of the left ventricle that is comparatively longer than the corresponding right ventricle.

iv) anterior and posterior left ventricular papillary muscles that get attached to the cusps of the mitral valve through the tendinous cords (or the chordae tendineae).

v) aortic vestibule, which is a smooth-walled, non-muscular, superoanterior outflow portion of the left ventricle that lies inferior to the aortic orifice and possesses fibrous walls.

vi) aortic orifice (or opening) is an opening of the left ventricle into the aorta. This valve is usually tricuspid (with three leaflets) and located posterior to the left side of the sternum at the level of the third intercostal space.

vii) inner surface of the left ventricle gives rise to the irregular, rounded and thick muscular ridges that are termed as the trabeculae carneae.

5. **The Cardiac Cycle:**
The cardiac cycle is based on the synchronous pumping of the right and left chambers of the heart.

a) The Arterial Supply of the Heart

The heart is supplied by the following arteries:

i) right coronary artery (RCA)

ii) sinu-atrial nodal artery

iii) right marginal artery

iv) posterior interventricular artery

v) atrio-ventricular nodal artery

vi) left coronary artery

vii) anterior interventricular artery (or Left Anterior Descending Artery)

viii) circumflex artery

ix) left marginal artery

x) posterior interventricular artery

b) The Arteries

The major types of arteries are described below:

i) pulmonary arteries- pulmonary arteries carry the oxygen deficient blood from the heart to the lungs for attaining oxygen.

ii) systemic arteries- systemic arteries transport the oxygenated blood to the rest of the body.

c) The Aorta

The aorta is divided into the following components:

i) ascending aorta

ii) arch of aorta

iii) descending aorta

d) Thoracic Aorta

i) aortic intercostal arteries (nine pairs)

ii) left bronchial arteries (two in number)

iii) posterior mediastinal arteries

iv) pericardial arteries

v) superior phrenic arteries

e) The Abdominal Aorta

Circulatory System

6. **The Arteries of the Head and Neck**
The major arteries that supply blood to the head and neck regions are the two common carotid arteries. These arteries travel through the neck and each one of them gets divided into the following branches:

a) External Carotid Arteries

b) Ascending Pharyngeal Artery

c) Occipital Artery

i) muscular branches

ii) sternocleidomastoid branch/sternocleidomastoid artery

iii) auricular branch

iv) meningeal or dural branch

v) descending branch

d) Posterior Auricular Artery

i) stylomastoid branch/stylomastoid artery

ii) auricular branch

iii) occipital branch

e) Superior Thyroid Artery

i) hyoid branch

ii) sternocleidomastoid branch/sternocleidomastoid artery

iii) superior laryngeal branch/superior laryngeal artery

iv) cricothyroid branch

f) Lingual Artery

i) hyoid branch

ii) dorsal lingual branches

iii) sublingual branch/sublingual artery

iv) deep lingual branch/deep lingual artery

g) Facial (or External Maxillary) Artery

Cervical Branches		Facial Branches	
i)	ascending palatine artery	i)	inferior labial artery
ii)	tonsillar branch	ii)	superior labial artery
iii)	glandular branches	iii)	lateral nasal branch
iv)	submental artery	iv)	angular artery
v)	muscular branches	v)	muscular branches

7. **The Internal Carotid Arteries:** The internal carotid arteries are the direct continuation of the common carotid arteries. However, the other portions of these arteries extend into the following arterial branches:

   a) The petrous portion of the internal carotid arteries gives rise to the following branches:
      i) caroticotympanic artery
      ii) artery of the pterygoid canal (or vidian artery)

   b) The cavernous portion of the internal carotid arteries gives rise to the following branches:
      i) cavernous artery
      ii) hypophyseal artery
      iii) semilunar arterial branches
      iv) anterior meningeal artery
      v) ophthalmic artery

   c) Anterior Cerebral Artery
      i) antero-medial ganglionic branches
      ii) inferior branches
      iii) anterior branches
      iv) middle branches
      v) posterior branches

   d) The Middle Cerebral Artery
      i) antero-lateral ganglionic branches
      ii) inferior lateral frontal branch
      iii) ascending frontal branch
      iv) ascending parietal branch
      v) parietotemporal branch
      vi) temporal branches

   e) Posterior Communicating Artery

   f) Anterior Choroidal Artery (or Choroid Artery)

8. **The Arteries of the Upper Extremity:** Subclavian Artery divides in to following branches:

   a) Vertebral Artery: The vertebral artery is divided into the following branches:

Cervical Branches	Cranial Branches
i) spinal branches	i) posterior meningeal branch
ii) muscular branches	ii) posterior/dorsal spinal artery
	iii) anterior/ventral spinal artery
	iv) posterior inferior cerebellar artery
	v) medullary arteries

   b) Internal Thoracic (or Internal Mammary) Artery
      i) pericardiacophrenic artery
      ii) anterior mediastinal arteries
      iii) pericardial branches
      iv) sternal branches
      v) anterior intercostal arteries
      vi) perforating branches
      vii) musculophrenic artery
      viii) superior epigastric artery

   c) Thyrocervical trunk (or Thyroid Axis)
      i) inferior thyroid artery
      ii) inferior laryngeal artery
      iii) esophageal branches
      iv) tracheal artery
      v) ascending cervical artery
      vi) muscular branches

   d) Suprascapular (or Transverse Scapular) Artery
      i) suprasternal branch
      ii) acromial branch

   e) Transverse Cervical Artery (or Transverse Artery of Neck)
      i) ascending branch
      ii) descending branch

   f) Costocervical trunk is the highest intercostal artery (superior intercostal artery)
      i) first posterior intercostal artery
      ii) second posterior intercostal artery
      iii) deep cervical artery
      iv) third arterialPart

   g) Axillary Artery
      i) first part
      ii) second part
      iii) third part

   h) Brachial Artery
      i) muscular branches
      ii) human nutrient artery
      iii) profunda brachii artery (deep artery of the arm/superior profunda artery)
      iv) superior ulnar collateral artery (or inferior profunda artery)
      v) inferior ulnar collateral artery (or anastomotica magna artery)

   i) Radial Artery

Branches of the Radial Artery in Forearm	Branches of the Radial Artery in Wrist	Branches of the Radial Artery in Hand
The Radial Recurrent Artery	The Posterior Radial Carpal Artery (The Dorsal Carpal Branch)	The Princeps Pollicis Artery
The Muscular (Arterial) Branches	The First Dorsal Metacarpal Artery	The Radialis Indicis Artery
The Anterior Radial Carpal Artery (The Volar Carpal Branch)		The Deep Palmar/Volar Arch
The Superficial Volar Artery (The Superficial Palmar Branch of Radial Artery)		The Palmar Interosseous (or Volar Metacarpal) Arteries
		The Perforating (Arterial) Branches
		The Recurrent (Arterial) Branches

   j) Ulnar Artery- ulnar artery originates from the brachial artery and runs along the medial aspect (or ulnar side) of forearm. A tabular representation of the arterial branches of ulnar artery is provided below:

Branches of the Ulnar Artery in Forearm	Branches of the Ulnar Artery in Wrist	Branches of the Ulnar Artery in Hand
The Anterior Ulnar Recurrent Artery	The Volar Carpal Branch (or Anterior Ulnar Carpal Artery)	The Deep Volar Branch (or Profunda Branch)

The Posterior Ulnar Recurrent Artery	The Dorsal Carpal Branch (or Posterior Ulnar Carpal Artery)	The Superficial Volar Arch (or Superficial Palmar Arch)
The Common Interosseous Artery (divides into the following two branches) ➲ The Volar Interosseous Artery (or Anterior Interosseous Artery) ➲ The Dorsal Interosseous Artery (or Posterior Interosseous Artery)		
The Muscular (Arterial) Branches		

9. **Arteries of the Trunk**
   Arteries of the trunk are based on the following arteries:
   a) The Descending Aorta
      i) thoracic aorta
      ii) abdominal aorta
   b) The Common Iliac Arteries
   c) internal iliac (or Hypogastric) artery

The Anterior Trunk	The Posterior Trunk
The Superior Vesical Artery	The Iliolumbar Artery-with the following branches: - The Lumbar (Arterial) Branch - The Iliac (Arterial) Branch
The Middle Vesical Artery	
The Inferior Vesical Artery	
The Middle Hemorrhoidal Artery	The Superior and Inferior Lateral Sacral Arteries
The Uterine Artery (In Female)	
The Vaginal Artery (In Female)	The Superior Gluteal Artery (or Gluteal Artery)-with the following branches: - The Superficial (Arterial) Branch - The Deep (Arterial) Branch
The Obturator Artery	
The Internal Pudendal Artery (Internal Pudic Artery)-with the following branches: The Muscular (Arterial) Branches The Inferior Hemorrhoidal Artery The Perineal (or Superficial Perineal)Artery The Artery of the Urethral Bulb The Urethral Artery The Deep Artery of the Penis (or Artery to the Corpus Cavernosum) The Dorsal Artery of the Penis	
The Inferior Gluteal Artery (Sciatic Artery)-with the following branches: The Muscular (Arterial) Branches The Coccygeal (Arterial) Branches The Arteria Comitans Nervi Ischiadici The Anastomotic (Arterial) Branch The Articular (Arterial) Branch The Cutaneous (Arterial) Branches	

   d) External Iliac Artery divides in to inferior epigastric artery
      i) muscular branches
      ii) cutaneous branches
      iii) external spermatic branch (in males) and artery of round ligament of uterus (in females)
      iv) pubic branch
   e) Deep Iliac Circumflex Artery
      i) muscular branch
      ii) cutaneous branch

18. **The Arteries of the Lower Extremity**
    a) Femoral Artery- The branches of the femoral artery are presented below in a tabular format:

The Branches of the Femoral Artery		
The Superficial Epigastric Artery		
The Superficial Iliac Circumflex Artery		
The Superficial External Pudendal Artery (or Superficial External Pudic Artery)		
The Deep External Pudendal Artery (or Deep External Pudic Artery)		
The Muscular (Arterial) Branches		
The Profunda Femoris Artery (or Deep Femoral Artery)		
Branches and Subordinate Branches of the Profunda Femoris Artery	The Lateral Femoral Circumflex Artery	
	Sub-Branches	The Ascending (Arterial) Branch
		The Descending (Arterial) Branch
		The Transverse (Arterial) Branch
	The Medial Femoral Circumflex Artery (or Internal Circumflex Artery)	
	Sub-Branches	The Superficial (Arterial) Branch
		The Deep (Arterial) Branch
		The Acetabular (Arterial) Branch
	The Perforating Arteries	
	Sub-Branches	The First Perforating Artery
		The Second Perforating Artery
		The Third Perforating Artery
	The Muscular (Arterial) Branches	
The Highest Genicular Artery (or Anastomotica Magna Artery)		
Branches of the Highest Genicular Artery	The Saphenous (Arterial) Branch	
	The Musculo-articular (Arterial) Branch	

    b) Popliteal Artery- A tabular presentation of the branches of the popliteal artery is given below:

Branches of the Popliteal Artery	
The Superior Muscular Branches	
The Sural Arteries (or Inferior Muscular Arteries)	
The Cutaneous Branches	
The Superior Genicular Arteries (or Superior Articular Arteries)	
Branches of the Superior Genicular Arteries	The Medial Superior Genicular Artery
	The Lateral Superior Genicular Artery
The Middle Genicular Artery (or Azygos Articular Artery)	
The Inferior Genicular Arteries (or Inferior Articular Arteries)	
Branches of the Inferior Genicular Arteries	The Medial Inferior Genicular Artery
	The Lateral Inferior Genicular Artery

c) Anterior Tibial Artery
   a. Posterior Tibial Recurrent Artery
   b. Fibular Artery
   c. Anterior Tibial Recurrent Artery
   d. Muscular (Arterial) Branches
   e. Anterior Medial Malleolar Artery (or Internal Malleolar Artery)
   f. Anterior Lateral Malleolar Artery (or External Malleolar Artery)

d) Dorsalis Pedis Artery (or Dorsal Artery of Foot)- A tabular presentation of the branches of dorsalis pedis artery is given below:

Branches of the Dorsalis Pedis Artery	
The lateral Tarsal Artery (or Tarsal Artery)	
The Medial Tarsal Arteries	
The Arcuate Artery (or Metatarsal Artery)	
Branches of Arcuate Artery	The Second Dorsal Metatarsal Artery
	The Third Dorsal Metatarsal Artery
	The Fourth Dorsal Metatarsal Artery
The First Dorsal Metatarsal Artery	
The Deep Plantar Artery (or Communicating Artery)	

e) Posterior Tibial Artery- The branching tree of the posterior tibial artery is presented below:

Branches of the Posterior Tibial Artery	
The Peroneal Artery	
Branches of Peroneal Artery	The Muscular (Arterial) Branches
	The Nutrient Artery of Fibula
	The Perforating Branch (or Anterior Peroneal Artery)
	The Communicating Branch of Peroneal Artery
	The Lateral Calcaneal Arteries (or External Calcaneal Arteries)
The Nutrient Artery of Tibia	
The Muscular Branches of the Posterior Tibial Artery	
The Posterior Medial Malleolar Artery (or Internal Malleolar Artery)	
The Communicating Branch of Posterior Tibial Artery	
The Medial Calcaneal Arteries (or Internal Calcaneal Arteries)	
The Medial Plantar Artery (or Internal Plantar Artery)	
The Lateral Plantar Artery (or External Plantar Artery)	

19. The Veins

The veins are the blood vessels that carry deoxygenated blood from the body tissues towards the heart via capillaries. The veins can be categorized into the following classes:

a) Pulmonary Veins: The pulmonary veins carry oxygenated blood from the lungs to the left atrium of the heart. The pulmonary veins are of the following types:
   i) right inferior pulmonary vein
   ii) right superior pulmonary vein
   iii) left inferior pulmonary vein
   iv) left superior pulmonary vein

b) Systemic Veins: The systemic veins deliver deoxygenated blood from the body tissues to the right atrium of human heart.

c) Superficial (or Cutaneous) Veins: The superficial veins are found immediately beneath the skin between the layers of the superficial fascia.

d) Deep Veins: The deep veins are located under the deep fascia with their corresponding arteries.

e) Systemic Veins

The systemic veins are divided into the following groups:
   i) veins of the heart
   ii) veins of the head and neck
   iii) veins of the upper extremity and thorax
   iv) veins of the lower extremity, abdomen, and pelvis

f) Veins of the Heart
   i) great cardiac vein
   ii) small cardiac vein
   iii) middle cardiac vein
   iv) posterior vein of the left ventricle
   v) oblique vein of the left atrium

g) Veins of the Head and Neck
   i) frontal vein (or supratrochlear vein)
   ii) supraorbital vein
   iii) angular vein
   iv) anterior facial vein (or facial vein)
   v) superficial temporal vein
   vi) parotid veins
   vii) articular veins (from temporomandibular joint)
   viii) anterior auricular veins
   ix) transverse facial veins
   x) internal maxillary vein
   xi) posterior facial vein (or temporomaxillary vein)
   xii) posterior auricular vein
   xiii) occipital vein

h) Veins of the Neck
   i) external jugular vein
   ii) posterior external jugular vein
   iii) anterior jugular vein
   iv) internal jugular vein
   v) vertebral vein
   i) Diploic Veins
   i) frontal diploic vein
   ii) anterior temporal diploic vein
   iii) posterior temporal diploic vein
   iv) occipital diploic vein

20. Veins of the Brain

a) External Cerebral Veins
   i) superior cerebral veins
   ii) middle cerebral vein (or superficial sylvian vein)
   iii) inferior cerebral veins

b) Internal Cerebral Veins (or deep cerebral veins)

c) Terminal Vein

d) Great Cerebral Veins (or Great Vein of Galen)

e) Cerebellar Veins
   i) superior cerebellar veins
   ii) inferior cerebellar veins

f) Ophthalmic and Emissary Veins
   i) ophthalmic veins are the veins that serve to perform the venous drainage of the orbit and pass through the superior orbital fissure to enter into the cavernous sinus.
   ii) superior ophthalmic veins
   iii) inferior opthalmic veins
   iv) emissary veins are those valveless veins which connect the dural venous sinuses with veins outside the cranium.

g) Sinuses of the Dura Mater
   i) posterosuperior sinuses
   ii) superior sagittal sinus (or superior longitudinal sinus)
   iii) inferior sagittal sinus (or inferior sagittal sinus)
   iv) straight sinus (or tentorial sinus)
   v) transverse sinuses (or lateral sinuses)
h) Occipital Sinuses
   i) anteroinferior sinuses
   ii) cavernous sinuses
   iii) intercavernous sinuses
   iv) superior petrosal sinuses
   v) inferior petrosal sinuses
   vi) basilar plexus (or transverse/basilar sinus)

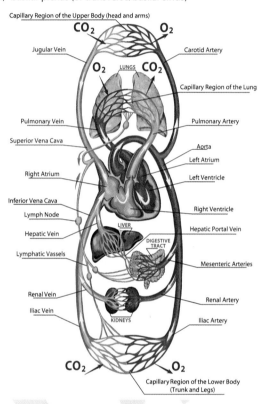

21. **Veins of the Upper Extremity, Thorax and Vertebral Column**
    The veins of the upper extremity are divided into the following two major groups:
    a) Superficial Veins of the Upper Extremity
       i) cephalic vein (or antecubital vein)
       ii) accessory cephalic vein
       iii) median cubital vein (or median basilic vein/antecubital vein)
       iv) basilic vein
       v) median antebrachial vein
       vi) dorsal venous network of the hand
       vii) intercapitular veins
       viii) dorsal metacarpal veins
       ix) dorsal digital veins
    b) Deep Veins of the Upper Extremity
       i) radial veins
       ii) ulnar veins
       iii) brachial veins
       iv) axillary veins

v) subclavian veins
vi) deep palmar venous arch
c) Veins of the thorax
   i) innominate veins (or brachiocephalic veins)
   ii) internal mammary veins (or internal thoracic veins)
   iii) inferior thyroid veins
   iv) highest intercostal vein (or superior intercostal vein)
   v) right superior intercostal vein
   vi) left superior intercostal vein
   vii) superior vena cava
   viii) azygos vein
   ix) hemiazygos vein
   x) accessory hemiazygous vein (or vena azygous minor superior)
   xi) bronchial veins
d) Veins of the vertebral column
   i) external vertebral venous plexuses (or extraspinal veins)
   ii) anterior external vertebral plexuses
   iii) posterior external vertebral plexuses
   iv) internal vertebral venous plexus (or intraspinal veins)
   v) basivertebral veins
   vi) intervertebral veins
   vii) veins of the medulla spinalis (or veins of spinal cord)

22. **Veins of the Lower Extremity, Abdomen, and Pelvis**
    The veins of the lower extremity are arranged into the following groups:
    a. Superficial Veins of the Lower Extremity
       i) great saphenous vein
       ii) small saphenous vein (or lesser saphenous vein)
    b. Deep Veins of the Lower Extremity
       a) posterior tibial veins
       b) peroneal veins
       c) tibioperoneal trunk
       d) anterior tibial veins
       e) popliteal vein
       f) femoral vein
       g) deep femoral vein (or profunda femoris vein)
       h) common femoral vein
       i) external iliac vein
    b) Major Veins of Abdomen and Pelvis:
       i) ascending lumbar vein
       ii) left gastric vein
       iii) right gastric vein
       iv) left gastro-omental vein
       v) right gastro-omental vein
       vi) left hepatic vein
       vii) middle hepatic vein
       viii) right hepatic vein
       ix) superior mesenteric vein
       x) inferior phrenic veins
       xi) inferior vena cava
       xii) left renal vein
       xiii) right renal vein
       xiv) splenic vein
       xv) suprarenal veins
       xvi) deep dorsal vein of clitoris

xvii)　deep dorsal vein of penis

xviii)　external pudendal veins

xix)　internal pudendal vein

xx)　ovarian vein

xxi)　pampiniform venous plexus

xxii)　prostatic venous plexus

xxiii)　rectal venous plexus

xxiv)　uterine venous plexus

xxv)　vaginal venous plexus

xxvi)　common iliac veins

xxvii)　middle sacral veins

xxviii)　vesical venous plexus

23. **The Portal System of Veins**

The hepatic portal system of the veins is responsible for the portal circulation, which denotes the passage of blood from the gastrointestinal tract and spleen through the portal vein to the liver.

The tributaries and sub-tributaries of the portal vein are presented below:

The Tributaries and Sub-Tributaries of the Portal Vein			
The Lienal Vein			
The Tributaries of Lienal Vein	The Short Gastric Veins		
	The Left Gastroepiploic Vein		
	The Pancreatic Veins		
	The Inferior Mesenteric Vein		
	The Tributaries of Inferior Mesenteric Vein	The Sigmoid Veins	
		The Left Colic Vein	
The Superior Mesenteric Vein			
The Tributaries of Superior Mesenteric Vein	The Right Gastroepiploic Vein		
	The Pancreaticoduodenal Veins		
The Coronary Vein			
The Pyloric Vein			
The Cystic Vein			
The Parumbilical Veins			

Common Pathologies

Angina pectoris
Commonly known as angina, angina pectoris chest pain due to ischemia of the heart muscle, generally due to obstruction or spasm of the coronary arteries. The main cause of angina pectoris is coronary artery disease, due to atherosclerosis of the arteries feeding the heart

Cardiomyopathy
Cardiomyopathy is a chronic disease of the heart muscle, in which the muscle is abnormally enlarged, thickened, and/or stiffened. The weakened heart muscle loses the ability to pump blood effectively, resulting in irregular heartbeats (arrhythmias) and possibly even heart failure.

Rheumatic Heart Disease
Rheumatic heart disease is a condition in which permanent damage to heart valves is caused by rheumatic fever. The heart valve is damaged by a disease process that generally begins with a strep throat caused by bacteria called Streptococcus, and may eventually cause rheumatic fever.

Arrhythmia
An arrhythmia is an abnormal rate or rhythm of the heart beat. It can beat too fast, too slow, or with an irregular rhythm. If the heart beat is fast it is called as tachycardia and if is too slow, it is referred to as bradycardia.

Congenital Heart Defects
Congenital heart defects are abnormalities in the morphological or physiological functioning of the heart that are present at the time of birth. The primary cause is the incomplete or abnormal development of the fetal heart during the early weeks of pregnancy

Hypertension
Hypertension, also referred to as high blood pressure, is a condition in which the arteries have persistently elevated blood pressure. Every time the human heart beats, it pumps blood to the whole body through the arteries. The pumping through the narrowed vessel consistently increases the systolic and diastolic pressure above normal reference range.

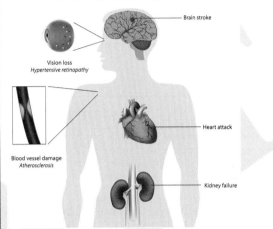

Main complications of hypertension

Aortic Aneurysm
An aneurysm is an abnormal bulging or swelling of a portion of a blood vessel. The aorta, which can develop these abnormal bulges, is the large blood vessel that carries oxygen-rich blood away from the heart to the rest of the body.

Atherosclerosis
Atherosclerosis is a disease of the arterial blood vessels (arteries), in which the walls of the blood vessels become thickened and hardened by "plaques." The plaques are composed of cholesterol and other lipids, inflammatory cells, and calcium deposits.

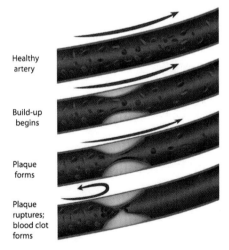

STAGES OF ATHEROSCLEROSIS

Deep Vein Thrombosis
Deep vein thrombosis (DVT) is a blood clot in a major vein that usually develops in the legs and/or pelvis.

Coronary Artery Disease
Coronary artery disease (CAD) is one of the common vascular diseases marked by accumulation of atherosclerotic plaque in the coronary blood vessels. As the plaque thickens, secondary changes may take place like enlargement of size and calcification that may lead to complete occlusion of the lumen of the coronary artery, resulting in inadequate supply of oxygen to the heart muscle

Peripheral Vascular Disease
Peripheral vascular disease is a narrowing of blood vessels that restricts blood flow. It mostly occurs in the legs, but is sometimes seen in the arms.

Hypercholesterolemia
Hypercholesterolemia is the presence of high levels of cholesterol in the blood. It is a form of "hyperlipidemia" (elevated levels of lipids in the blood) and "hyperlipoproteinemia" (elevated levels of lipoproteins in the blood).

Lymphedema
A condition in which excess fluid collects in tissue and causes swelling. Lymphedema may occur in the arm or leg after lymph vessels or lymph nodes in the underarm or groin are removed.

Hodgkin's Lymphoma
This is a type of cancer of the lymphatic system. It can start almost anywhere in the body. It's believed to be caused by HIV, Epstein-Barr Syndrome, age, and family history.

Non-Hodgkin's Lymphoma
Non-Hodgkin's lymphoma is a cancer of the lymphoid system. It is divided into three types: high-grade, intermediate-grade and low-grade.

Lymphangitis
Lymphangitis is an inflammation of the lymphatics (lymph channels) due to an infection by a microbe or some chemical irritant. It occurs when an infection or inflammation occurs somewhere else and the microbe or the irritant is transported along with lymph fluid through the lymphatics.

Splenomegaly
Splenomegaly is a condition in which the spleen becomes enlarged, tender and painful. It can occur due to a number of reasons, ranging from certain infections to cancers.

Anatomy of the Lymphatic System

1. **Introduction**
   The human lymphatic system is closely linked with the blood and the vascular system. Both of these systems work in an intimate association with each other and transport vital fluids throughout the body via a system of vessels. The lymph capillaries and lymphatics are the special vessels that serve to transport a fluid (called lymph). The human lymphatic system consists of the below mentioned components:

   a) The Lymph
   b) The Lymph Vessels
   c) The Lymph Nodes
   d) The Tonsils, Spleen, Thymus Gland and Peyer's Patches

   The most important function of the lymphatic system is to drain the protein containing fluid from the tissue spaces. The entire lymphatics of the body converge into one of the following major channels:

   i) thoracic duct (or the main collecting channel)
   ii) right lymphatic duct

   e) The lymph nodes (or lymph glands) are oval structures that are found along the length of lymphatics at various intervals. The lymph trunk is a specific lymph vessel containing lymph. The various types of lymph trunks are documented below:

   i) jugular lymph trunk
   ii) subclavian lymph trunk
   iii) bronchomediastinal lymph trunk
   iv) lumbar lymph trunk
   v) intestinal lymph trunk

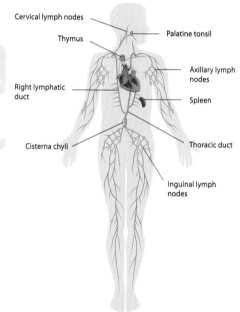
The Lymphatic System

2. **Thoracic Duct**
   The thoracic duct is the largest lymphatic vessel in the body and constitutes an essential part of the lymphatic system. It is also called the alimentary duct, chyliferous duct, left lymphatic duct or Van Hoorne's canal.

3. **Lymphatics of the Head, Face and Neck**
   The entire lymph glands of the head are mostly extra-cranial, and arranged in the following groups:

   a) Occipital Lymph Glands: The occipital lymph glands are two or three in number and located on the back of the head.
   b) Posterior Auricular Lymph Glands (or Mastoid Glands): The posterior auricular lymph glands are two in number and exist on the upper part of the sternomastoid muscle and mastoid portion of the temporal bone.

c) Anterior Auricular Lymph Glands (or Superficial Parotid/Preauricular Glands): The superficial parotid glands are present on the lateral surface of the parotid gland.

d) Parotid Lymph Glands (or Deep Parotid Glands): The parotid lymph glands remain embedded in the deeper portions of the parotid gland.

e) Superficial Facial Lymph Glands: The superficial facial lymph glands are based on several lymph glands in the region of face. However, the major ones are described below:

　i) Infraorbital Lymph Glands (or Maxillary Glands): The infraorbital lymph glands remain scattered along the angle between the nose and cheek, and below the margin of the orbit.

　ii) Buccinator Lymph Glands: The buccinator lymph glands are found on the superficial surface of the anterior part of buccinator muscle, opposite to the angle of the mouth.

　iii) Supramandibular Lymph Glands: The supramandibular lymph glands lie on the outer surface of the mandible at the anterior border of the masseter muscle, between the external maxillary artery and the anterior facial vein.

f) The Deep Facial Lymph Glands (or Internal Maxillary Glands): The deep facial lymph glands are found in association with the internal maxillary artery, on the outer surface of the external pterygoid muscle.

g) The Lingual Lymph Glands: The lingual lymph glands are based on two or three small nodules that exist on the lateral surfaces of the hypo-glossi and genio-glossi muscles.

h) The Retropharyngeal Glands: The retropharyngeal glands are located in the buccopharyngeal fascia behind the upper part of pharynx.

4. **The Lymph Glands of the Neck:** The lymph glands of the neck are divided into the following major groups:

a) The Submaxillary Glands: The submaxillary glands are a pair of salivary glands located on each side under the body of mandible.

b) The Submental (or Suprahyoid Glands): The submental glands are located beneath the chin, and between the anterior bellies of the two digastric muscles.

c) The Superficial Cervical Glands: The superficial cervical glands remain embedded in the deep fascia along the course of the external jugular vein, and superficial to the sternomastoid muscle.

5. **The Anterior Cervical Glands:** The lymph glands of the anterior neck region are divisible into the following two groups:

a) Superficial Anterior Cervical Lymph Glands- The superficial anterior cervical lymph glands exist in association with the anterior jugular veins.

b) Deep Anterior Cervical Lymph Glands: The deep anterior cervical lymph glands are divisible into the following groups/types:

　i) infrahyoid glands obtain lymph fluid from the region of epiglottis and transport it to the deep cervical glands.

　ii) prelaryngeal gland obtains lymph from the anterior portion of the larynx, the isthmus, and the portions of the right and left lobes of thyroid gland.

　iii) pretracheal lymph glands are the numerous small nodules that follow the course of the inferior thyroid veins.

　iv) paratracheal lymph glands lie in association with the branches of the superior and inferior thyroid arteries and the recurrent nerves.

c) Deep Cervical Glands: The deep cervical glands are the intercommunicating lymph vessels that remain positioned in the anterior and posterior triangles of the neck, and under the cover of sterno-mastoid muscle. These glands are divisible into the following groups:

　i) superior deep cervical glands are located under the cover of sterno-mastoid muscle, and lie in close association with the accessory nerve and internal jugular vein.

　ii) inferior deep cervical glands are located below the level of omo-hyoid muscle.

d) Lymphatic vessels of the scalp are distributed in the soft tissue envelope of the frontal, temporoparietal and the occipital regions of the cranium.

e) Lymphatic Vessels of the Ear divide in to upper and lateral portion of the auricle terminate into the anterior auricular glands.

f) Lymphatic vessels of the face are more widely distributed than the scalp vessels, and can be divided into the following groups:

6. **Lymphatic Vessels of the Eyelids and Conjunctiva:** The lymphatic vessels of the eyelids and conjunctiva form the following two groups:

a) Medial Lymph Vessels: The medial lymph vessels travel from the medial portions of the superior and inferior eyelids, and terminate to the submaxillary lymph glands.

b) Lateral Lymph Vessels: The lateral lymph vessels arise from the lateral parts of the eyelids, and terminate into the anterior auricular and the parotid lymph glands.

c) Lymphatic Vessels of the Cheeks: The superficial and deep lymphatic vessels of the cheeks usually communicate with the submaxillary glands.

d) Lymphatic Vessels of the Lips: The lymphatic vessels of the lips drain lymph fluid to the submental and submaxillary glands.

e) Lymphatic Vessels of the Nose: The lymphatic vessels from the external part of the nose drain lymph fluid to the anterior auricular and submaxillary glands.

f) Lymphatic Vessels of the Nasal Cavities: The lymphatic vessels from the anterior and posterior portions of the nasal cavities drain lymph fluid to the submaxillary, the retropharyngeal, and the superior deep cervical glands.

g) Lymphatic Vessels of the Mouth: The lymphatic vessels of the mouth can be divided into the following groups:

h) Lymphatic Vessels of the Palatine Tonsil: The lymphatic vessels of the palatine tonsil arise from the buccopharyngeal fascia and constrictor pharyngis superior and meet with the superior deep cervical glands.

i) Lymphatic Vessels of the Tongue: The lymphatic vessels of the tongue are divided into the following three groups:

　i) anterior lymph vessels of the tongue drain lymph fluid from the tip and lower surface of tongue to the submental glands.

　ii) middle lymph vessels of the tongue drain lymph fluid from the anterior two third portion of the tongue to the submaxillary and medial superior deep cervical glands.

　iii) posterior lymph vessels of the tongue drain lymph fluid from the portion of tongue which lies in the anterior wall of pharynx.

j) Lymphatic Vessels of the Gums: The lymph vessels of the anterior portion of mandibular gum drain lymph fluid to the submandibular gland. The lymph vessels from the inner portion of the mandibular gum also drain lymph fluid to the submaxillary glands.

k) Lymphatic Vessels of the Teeth: The lymph vessels of the teeth of mandible transport lymph fluid to the sub maxillary or the superior deep cervical glands.

7. **The Lymphatics of the Upper Extremity:** The lymph glands of the upper extremity are divisible into the following two groups:

a) The Superficial Lymph Glands- The superficial lymph glands of the upper extremity are of the following types:

　i) supratrochlear lymph glands are situated above the medial epicondyle of humerus, and drain lymph fluid from the middle, ring and little fingers, and the portions of the hand and forearm.

ii) deltoideopectoral lymph glands are located in the groove between the pectoralis major and deltoid muscles.

b) The Deep Lymph Glands: The deep lymph glands are chiefly found in the axillary region, where they constitute several constant as well as variable groups.

   i) lateral group of axillary lymph glands lies along the line of the great axillary vessels. These glands drain lymph fluid from the greater part of the upper extremity to the central and inferior deep cervical glands.

   ii) anterior group of axillary lymph glands travels from third to sixth intercostal space, along the line of the lateral thoracic artery.

   iii) posterior Group of axillary lymph glands lies along the posterior wall of axilla, and follow the course of the subscapular vessels.

   iv) central group of axillary lymph glands are located in the central part of the axilla, and along the line of the intercosto-brachial nerve.

   v) infra-clavicular Group of axillary lymph glands is found between the upper border of the pectoralis minor muscle and the clavicle, along the medial side of the axillary artery.

c) The Lymphatic Vessels of the Upper Extremity: The lymphatic vessels of the upper extremity are divisible into the following two groups:

   i) superficial lymph vessels of the upper extremity are located in the skin and subcutaneous tissues, and commence in the cutaneous plexuses on the volar aspects of the fingers and hand.

   ii) deep lymph vessels of the upper extremity follow the course of the deeper blood vessels in the regions of the forearm and hand.

8. **Lymphatics of the Lower Extremity:** The lymph glands of the lower extremity are divisible into the following groups:

   a) The Superficial Lymph Glands- superficial lymph glands are found in the superficial fascia in subinguinal and inguinal regions. These glands are separable into the following groups:

      i) inguinal lymph glands are located above the level of the inguinal ligament.

      ii) superficial sublingual lymph glands are divisible into the proximal and distal groups.

   b) Deep Lymph Glands: The deep lymph glands of the inferior extremity are divided into the following two groups:

      i) popliteal lymph glands are located in the popliteal fossa.

      ii) deep sublingual lymph glands are located in the femoral trigone.

   c) Lymphatic Vessels of the Lower Extremity: The lymphatic vessels of the lower extremity are based on the following two groups:

      i) superficial lymphatic vessels are located in the superficial fascia and divided in to vessels of the medial group arises on the tibial side and dorsum of the foot, and terminates in the distal group of superficial subinguinal glands and vessels of the lateral group commences from the fibular side of the foot.

      ii) deep lymphatic vessels of the lower extremity follow the course of the deep blood vessels, and terminate into the deep subinguinal and hypogastric glands.

9. **The Lymphatics of the Abdomen and Pelvis:** The lymph glands of the abdomen and pelvis are divisible into parietal lymph glands and visceral lymph glands.

   a) External Iliac Glands: The external iliac group of glands pertains to the pelvic region, located along the course of the external iliac vessels, and constitutes the lateral, intermediate and medial chains.

   b) Common Iliac Glands: The common iliac glands of the pelvis are located on the sides of the common iliac artery and below the bifurcation of aorta.

c) Epigastric Glands: The epigastric glands of the anterior abdominal wall are divisible into the following types:

   i) superior epigastric gland is located in the superficial fascia of the median part of the epigastric region.

   ii) inferior epigastric glands are located along the course of the inferior epigastric artery.

d) Circumflex Iliac Glands: The circumflex iliac glands of the anterior abdominal wall follow the course of the deep circumflex iliac artery in the lateral aspect of groin.

e) Hypogastric Glands: The hypogastric glands of the pelvis are located along the course of the hypogastric vessels.

   i) gluteal lymph glands

   ii) pubo-gluteal lymph glands

   iii) middle haemorrhoidal gland

   iv) inter-iliac glands

   v) obturator gland

f) Sacral Glands: The sacral lymph glands of the pelvis are located along the anterior aspect of sacrum, between the anterior sacral foramina.

g) Lumbar Glands: The lumbar lymph glands are located behind the peritoneum of the posterior wall of abdomen. The lumbar lymph glands are further separable into the following groups:

   i) right lateral aortic glands

   ii) left lateral aortic glands

   iii) preaortic glands

   iv) retroaortic glands

h) Superior Gastric Glands: The superior gastric glands exist in association with the left gastric artery and constitute the following subdivisions:

   i) anterior left gastric glands (or lower coronary glands)

   ii) right paracardial glands

   iii) left paracardial glands

   iv) posterior paracardial glands

   v) posterior left gastric glands (or upper coronary glands)

   vi) right gastric gland (or pyloric gland)

   vii) left suprapancreatic glands

   viii) right suprapancreatic glands

   ix) subpyloric glands

   x) biliary lymph glands

i) Inferior Gastric Glands (or Right Gastroepiploic Glands): The inferior gastric glands are associated with the greater curvature of stomach and follow the course of the right gastroepiploic artery.

j) Hepatic Glands: The hepatic lymph glands exist in the region of porta hepatis (or transverse fissure of the liver), between the layers of the lesser omentum.

k) Pancreaticolienal Glands (or Splenic Glands): The pancreaticolienal glands are positioned in relation to the posterior surface and upper border of pancreas, and follow the course of the lienal (or splenic) artery.

l) Mesenteric Glands: The mesenteric lymph glands are located between the layers of the mesentery.

m) Ileocolic glands: The ileocolic glands are located around the ileocolic artery and form the following major groups:

   i) ileal glands

   ii) anterior ileocolic glands

   iii) posterior ileocolic glands

   iv) right colic glands

n) Mesocolic Glands: The mesocolic glands exist in close association with the transverse colon.

o) Inferior Mesenteric Glands- The inferior mesenteric glands are located on the branches of the left colic and sigmoid arteries, the superior hemorrhoidal artery, and the muscular coat of the rectum.

10. **The Lymphatic Vessels of the Abdominal Viscera and the Superior and Posterior Walls of the Abdomen**
    a) Lymphatic Vessels of the Abdominal Part of the Alimentary Canal
    b) Lymphatic Vessels of the Stomach
    c) Lymphatic Vessels of the Duodenum
    d) Lymphatic Vessels of the Jejunum and Ileum (or the Lacteals)
    e) Lymphatic Vessels of the Cecum, Vermiform Process, and the Ascending colon
    f) Lymphatic Vessels of the Right Colic Flexure and the Transverse colon
    g) Lymphatic Vessels of the Left Colic Flexure, Descending Colon, Iliac Colon, and Pelvic Colon
    h) Lymphatic Vessels of the Liver
    i) Lymphatic Vessels of the Gall Bladder
    j) Lymphatic Vessels of the Pancreas
    k) Lymphatic Vessels of the Spleen
    l) Lymphatic Vessels of the Kidneys
    m) Lymphatic Vessels of the Ureters
    n) Lymphatic Vessels of the Suprarenal Glands
    o) Lymphatic Vessels of the Diaphragm

11. **The Lymphatic Vessels of the Pelvic Viscera**
    a) lymphatic Vessels of the Male Urethra
    b) Lymphatic Vessels of the Prostate
    c) Lymphatic Vessels of the Female Urethra
    d) Lymphatic Vessels of the Seminal Vesicle
    e) Lymphatic Vessels of the of the Ductus Deferens
    f) Lymphatic Vessels of the Urinary Bladder
    g) Lymphatic Vessels of the Ureter
    h) Lymphatic Vessels of the Vagina
    i) Lymphatic Vessels of the Uterus
    j) Lymphatic Vessels of the Uterine Tube
    k) Lymphatic Vessels of the Ovaries
    l) Lymphatic Vessels of the Testis and Epididymis
    m) Lymphatic Vessels of the Anus, Anal Canal and Rectum

12. **The Lymphatics of the Thorax**
    The Lymph Glands of the thorax are separable into the following groups:
    a) Sternal Lymph Glands- The sternal lymph glands are located at the margins of the sternum along the side of the internal mammary artery.
    b) Intercostal Lymph Glands- The intercostal lymph glands are situated in the posterior portions of the intercostal spaces (in relation to the intercostal vessels), and in front of the heads of the ribs.
    c) Anterior Mediastinal Lymph Glands- The anterior mediastinal lymph glands are located in the lower portion of the anterior mediastinum, and the anterior part of the superior mediastinal cavity.
    d) Posterior Mediastinal Lymph Glands- The posterior mediastinal lymph glands exist along the thoracic part of the esophagus and the descending thoracic aorta.
    e) Bronchial Lymph Glands- The bronchial lymph glands lie along the walls of the intrathoracic part of trachea, the bronchi and their intrapulmonary branches. These glands are further categorized into the following groups:
       i) tracheo-bronchial lymph glands

       ii) lymph glands of the bifurcation (or intertracheo-bronchial lymph glands)
       iii) broncho-pulmonary lymph glands
       iv) pulmonary lymph glands

13. **The Lymphatic Vessels of the Thorax**
    These vessels are divisible into the following groups:
    a) Intercostal Lymph Vessels
    b) Lymph Vessels of the Diaphragm
    c) Lymphatic Vessels of the Contents of the Thorax: The lymphatic vessels of the contents of the thorax are divisible into the following groups:
       i) lymph vessels of the heart
       ii) lymph vessels of the pericardium
       iii) lymph vessels of the thymus
       iv) lymph vessels of the thoracic part of esophagus
       v) lymph vessels of the pleura
       vi) lymph vessels of the lungs

This page intentionally left blank

Diseases of the circulatory system (I00-I99)

EXCLUDES2 *certain conditions originating in the perinatal period (P04-P96)*
certain infectious and parasitic diseases (A00-B99)
complications of pregnancy, childbirth and the puerperium (O00-O9A)
congenital malformations, deformations, and chromosomal abnormalities (Q00-Q99)
endocrine, nutritional and metabolic diseases (E00-E88)
injury, poisoning and certain other consequences of external causes (S00-T88)
neoplasms (C00-D49)
symptoms, signs and abnormal clinical and laboratory findings, not elsewhere classified (R00-R94)
systemic connective tissue disorders (M30-M36)
transient cerebral ischemic attacks and related syndromes (G45.-)

Acute rheumatic fever (I00-I02)

I00 Rheumatic fever without heart involvement

INCLUDES *arthritis, rheumatic, acute or subacute*
EXCLUDES1 *rheumatic fever with heart involvement (I01.0 -I01.9)*

I01 Rheumatic fever with heart involvement

EXCLUDES1 *chronic diseases of rheumatic origin (I05-I09) unless rheumatic fever is also present or there is evidence of reactivation or activity of the rheumatic process.*

I01.0 Acute rheumatic pericarditis

Any condition in I00 with pericarditis
Rheumatic pericarditis (acute)

EXCLUDES1 *acute pericarditis not specified as rheumatic (I30.-)*

I01.1 Acute rheumatic endocarditis

Any condition in I00 with endocarditis or valvulitis
Acute rheumatic valvulitis

I01.2 Acute rheumatic myocarditis

Any condition in I00 with myocarditis

I01.8 Other acute rheumatic heart disease

Any condition in I00 with other or multiple types of heart involvement
Acute rheumatic pancarditis

I01.9 Acute rheumatic heart disease, unspecified

Any condition in I00 with unspecified type of heart involvement
Rheumatic carditis, acute
Rheumatic heart disease, active or acute

I02 Rheumatic chorea

INCLUDES *Sydenham's chorea*
EXCLUDES1 *chorea NOS (G25.5)*
Huntington's chorea (G10)

I02.0 Rheumatic chorea with heart involvement

Chorea NOS with heart involvement
Rheumatic chorea with heart involvement of any type classifiable under I01.-

I02.9 Rheumatic chorea without heart involvement

Rheumatic chorea NOS

Chronic rheumatic heart diseases (I05-I09)

I05 Rheumatic mitral valve **diseases**

INCLUDES *conditions classifiable to both I05.0 and I05.2-I05.9, whether specified as rheumatic or not*

EXCLUDES1 *mitral valve disease specified as nonrheumatic (I34.-)*
mitral valve disease with aortic and/or tricuspid valve involvement (I08.-)

I05.0 Rheumatic mitral stenosis

Mitral (valve) obstruction (rheumatic)

I05.1 Rheumatic mitral insufficiency

Rheumatic mitral incompetence
Rheumatic mitral regurgitation

EXCLUDES1 *mitral insufficiency not specified as rheumatic (I34.0)*

I05.2 Rheumatic mitral stenosis with insufficiency

Rheumatic mitral stenosis with incompetence or regurgitation

I05.8 Other rheumatic mitral valve diseases

Rheumatic mitral (valve) failure

I05.9 Rheumatic mitral valve disease, unspecified

Rheumatic mitral (valve) disorder (chronic) NOS

I06 Rheumatic aortic valve **diseases**

EXCLUDES1 *aortic valve disease not specified as rheumatic (I35.-)*
aortic valve disease with mitral and/or tricuspid valve involvement (I08.-)

I06.0 Rheumatic aortic stenosis

Rheumatic aortic (valve) obstruction

I06.1 Rheumatic aortic insufficiency

Rheumatic aortic incompetence
Rheumatic aortic regurgitation

I06.2 Rheumatic aortic stenosis with insufficiency

Rheumatic aortic stenosis with incompetence or regurgitation

I06.8 Other rheumatic aortic valve diseases

I06.9 Rheumatic aortic valve disease, unspecified

Rheumatic aortic (valve) disease NOS

I07 Rheumatic tricuspid valve **diseases**

INCLUDES *rheumatic tricuspid valve diseases specified as rheumatic or unspecified*

EXCLUDES1 *tricuspid valve disease specified as nonrheumatic (I36.-)*
tricuspid valve disease with aortic and/or mitral valve involvement (I08.-)

I07.0 Rheumatic tricuspid stenosis

Tricuspid (valve) stenosis (rheumatic)

I07.1 Rheumatic tricuspid insufficiency

Tricuspid (valve) insufficiency (rheumatic)

I07.2 Rheumatic tricuspid stenosis and insufficiency

I07.8 Other rheumatic tricuspid valve diseases

I07.9 Rheumatic tricuspid valve disease, unspecified

Rheumatic tricuspid valve disorder NOS

I08 Multiple valve diseases

INCLUDES *multiple valve diseases specified as rheumatic or unspecified*

EXCLUDES1 *endocarditis, valve unspecified (I38)*
multiple valve disease specified a nonrheumatic (I34.-, I35.-, I36.-, I37.-, I38.-, Q22.-, Q23.-, Q24.8-)
rheumatic valve disease NOS (I09.1)

I08.0 Rheumatic disorders of both mitral **and** aortic **valves**

Involvement of both mitral and aortic valves specified as rheumatic or unspecified

I08.1 Rheumatic disorders of both mitral **and** tricuspid **valves**

I08.2 Rheumatic disorders of both aortic **and** tricuspid **valves**

I08.3 Combined rheumatic disorders of mitral, aortic **and** tricuspid **valves**

I08.8 Other rheumatic multiple valve diseases

I08.9 Rheumatic multiple valve disease, unspecified

Unspecified Code	Other Specified Code	N Newborn Age: 0	P Pediatric Age: 0-17	M Maternity Age: 12-55
A Adult Age: 15-124	♂ Male	♀ Female	● New Code	▲ Revised Code Title	►◄ Revised Text

[4] **I09 Other rheumatic heart diseases**

I09.0 Rheumatic myocarditis

EXCLUDES1 *myocarditis not specified as rheumatic (I51.4)*

I09.1 Rheumatic diseases of endocardium, valve unspecified

Rheumatic endocarditis (chronic)
Rheumatic valvulitis (chronic)

EXCLUDES1 *endocarditis, valve unspecified (I38)*

I09.2 Chronic rheumatic pericarditis

Adherent pericardium, rheumatic
Chronic rheumatic mediastinopericarditis
Chronic rheumatic myopericarditis

EXCLUDES1 *chronic pericarditis not specified as rheumatic (I31.-)*

[5] **I09.8 Other specified rheumatic heart diseases**

I09.81 Rheumatic heart failure

Use additional code to identify type of heart failure (I50.-)

I09.89 Other specified rheumatic heart diseases

Rheumatic disease of pulmonary valve

I09.9 Rheumatic heart disease, unspecified

Rheumatic carditis

EXCLUDES1 *rheumatoid carditis (M05.31)*

Hypertensive diseases (I10-I15)

Use additional code to identify:
exposure to environmental tobacco smoke (Z77.22)
history of tobacco use (Z87.891)
occupational exposure to environmental tobacco smoke (Z57.31)
tobacco dependence (F17.-)
tobacco use (Z72.0)

EXCLUDES1 *hypertensive disease complicating pregnancy, childbirth and the puerperium (O10-O11, O13-O16)*
neonatal hypertension (P29.2)
primary pulmonary hypertension (I27.0)

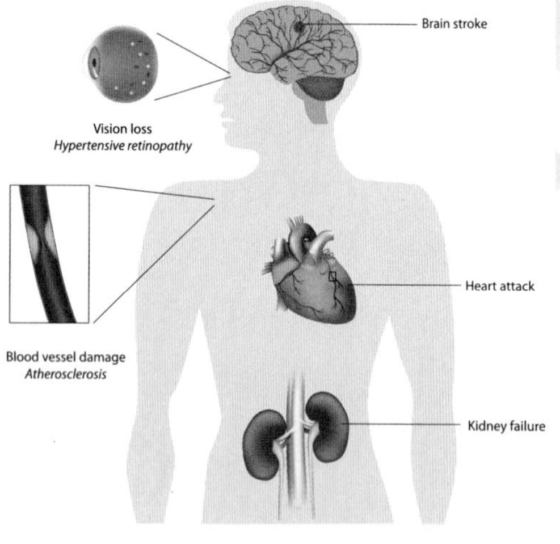

Figure 8.1 Main complications of Hypertension

I10 Essential (primary) hypertension

INCLUDES *high blood pressure*
hypertension (arterial) (benign) (essential) (malignant) (primary) (systemic)

EXCLUDES1 *hypertensive disease complicating pregnancy, childbirth and the puerperium (O10-O11, O13-O16)*

EXCLUDES2 *essential (primary) hypertension involving vessels of brain (I60-I69)*
essential (primary) hypertension involving vessels of eye (H35.0-)

[4] **I11 Hypertensive heart disease**

INCLUDES *any condition in I51.4-I51.9 due to hypertension*

I11.0 Hypertensive heart disease with heart failure

Hypertensive heart failure
Use additional code to identify type of heart failure (I50.-)

I11.9 Hypertensive heart disease without heart failure

Hypertensive heart disease NOS

[4] **I12 Hypertensive chronic kidney disease**

INCLUDES *any condition in N18 and N26 - due to hypertension*
arteriosclerosis of kidney
arteriosclerotic nephritis (chronic) (interstitial)
hypertensive nephropathy
nephrosclerosis

EXCLUDES1 *hypertension due to kidney disease (I15.0, I15.1)*
renovascular hypertension (I15.0)
secondary hypertension (I15.-)

EXCLUDES2 *acute kidney failure (N17.-)*

I12.0 Hypertensive chronic kidney disease with stage 5 chronic kidney disease or end stage renal disease

Use additional code to identify the stage of chronic kidney disease (N18.5, N18.6)

I12.9 Hypertensive chronic kidney disease with stage 1 through stage 4 chronic kidney disease, or unspecified chronic kidney disease

Hypertensive chronic kidney disease NOS
Hypertensive renal disease NOS
Use additional code to identify the stage of chronic kidney disease (N18.1-N18.4, N18.9)

[4] **I13 Hypertensive heart and chronic kidney disease**

INCLUDES *any condition in I11.- with any condition in I12.-*
cardiorenal disease
cardiovascular renal disease

I13.0 Hypertensive heart and chronic kidney disease with heart failure and stage 1 through stage 4 chronic kidney disease, or unspecified chronic kidney disease

Use additional code to identify type of heart failure (I50.-)
code to identify stage of chronic kidney disease (N18.1-N18.4, N18.9)

[5] **I13.1 Hypertensive heart and chronic kidney disease without heart failure**

I13.10 Hypertensive heart and chronic kidney disease without heart failure, with stage 1 through stage 4 chronic kidney disease, or unspecified chronic kidney disease

Hypertensive heart disease and hypertensive chronic kidney disease NOS
Use additional code to identify the stage of chronic kidney disease (N18.1-N18.4, N18.9)

I13.11 Hypertensive heart and chronic kidney disease without heart failure, with stage 5 chronic kidney disease, or end stage renal disease

Use additional code to identify the stage of chronic kidney disease (N18.5, N18.6)

I13.2 Hypertensive heart and chronic kidney disease with heart failure and with stage 5 chronic kidney disease, or end stage renal disease

Use additional code to identify type of heart failure (I50.-)
code to identify the stage of chronic kidney disease (N18.5, N18.6)

[4] **I15 Secondary hypertension**

Code also underlying condition

EXCLUDES1 *postprocedural hypertension (I97.3)*

[EXCLUDES2] *secondary hypertension involving vessels of brain (I60-I69)*
secondary hypertension involving vessels of eye (H35.0-)

I15.0 Renovascular hypertension

I15.1 Hypertension secondary to other renal disorders

I15.2 Hypertension secondary to endocrine disorders

I15.8 Other secondary hypertension

I15.9 Secondary hypertension, unspecified

Ischemic heart diseases (I20-I25)

Use additional code to identify presence of hypertension (I10-I15)

[4] I20 Angina pectoris

Use additional code to identify:
exposure to environmental tobacco smoke (Z77.22)
history of tobacco use (Z87.891)
occupational exposure to environmental tobacco smoke (Z57.31)
tobacco dependence (F17.-)
tobacco use (Z72.0)

[EXCLUDES1] *angina pectoris with atherosclerotic heart disease of native coronary arteries (I25.1-)*
atherosclerosis of coronary artery bypass graft(s) and coronary artery of transplanted heart with angina pectoris (I25.7-)
postinfarction angina (I23.7)

I20.0 Unstable angina

Accelerated angina
Crescendo angina
De novo effort angina
Intermediate coronary syndrome
Preinfarction syndrome
Worsening effort angina

I20.1 Angina pectoris with documented spasm

Angiospastic angina
Prinzmetal angina
Spasm-induced angina
Variant angina

I20.8 Other forms of angina pectoris

Angina equivalent
Angina of effort
Coronary slow flow syndrome
Stenocardia
Use additional code(s) for symptoms associated with angina equivalent

I20.9 Angina pectoris, unspecified

Angina NOS
Anginal syndrome
Cardiac angina
Ischemic chest pain

[4] I21 ST elevation (STEMI) and non-ST elevation (NSTEMI) myocardial infarction

[INCLUDES] *cardiac infarction*
coronary (artery) embolism
coronary (artery) occlusion
coronary (artery) rupture
coronary (artery) thrombosis
infarction of heart, myocardium, or ventricle
myocardial infarction specified as acute or with a stated duration of 4 weeks (28 days) or less from onset

Use additional code, if applicable, to identify:
exposure to environmental tobacco smoke (Z77.22)
history of tobacco use (Z87.891)
occupational exposure to environmental tobacco smoke (Z57.31)
status post administration of tPA (rtPA) in a different facility within the last 24 hours prior to admission to current facility (Z92.82)
tobacco dependence (F17.-)
tobacco use (Z72.0)

[EXCLUDES2] *old myocardial infarction (I25.2)*
postmyocardial infarction syndrome (I24.1)
subsequent myocardial infarction (I22.-)

[5] I21.0 ST elevation (STEMI) myocardial infarction of anterior wall

I21.01 ST elevation (STEMI) myocardial infarction involving left main coronary artery

I21.02 ST elevation (STEMI) myocardial infarction involving left anterior descending coronary artery

ST elevation (STEMI) myocardial infarction involving diagonal coronary artery

I21.09 ST elevation (STEMI) myocardial infarction involving other coronary artery of anterior wall

Acute transmural myocardial infarction of anterior wall
Anteroapical transmural (Q wave) infarction (acute)
Anterolateral transmural (Q wave) infarction (acute)
Anteroseptal transmural (Q wave) infarction (acute)
Transmural (Q wave) infarction (acute) (of) anterior (wall) NOS

[5] I21.1 ST elevation (STEMI) myocardial infarction of inferior wall

I21.11 ST elevation (STEMI) myocardial infarction involving right coronary artery

Inferoposterior transmural (Q wave) infarction (acute)

I21.19 ST elevation (STEMI) myocardial infarction involving other coronary artery of inferior wall

Acute transmural myocardial infarction of inferior wall
Inferolateral transmural (Q wave) infarction (acute)
Transmural (Q wave) infarction (acute) (of) diaphragmatic wall
Transmural (Q wave) infarction (acute) (of) inferior (wall) NOS

[EXCLUDES2] *ST elevation (STEMI) myocardial infarction involving left circumflex coronary artery (I21.21)*

[5] I21.2 ST elevation (STEMI) myocardial infarction of other sites

I21.21 ST elevation (STEMI) myocardial infarction involving left circumflex coronary artery

ST elevation (STEMI) myocardial infarction involving oblique marginal coronary artery

I21.29 ST elevation (STEMI) myocardial infarction involving other sites

Acute transmural myocardial infarction of other sites
Apical-lateral transmural (Q wave) infarction (acute)
Basal-lateral transmural (Q wave) infarction (acute)
High lateral transmural (Q wave) infarction (acute)
Lateral (wall) NOS transmural (Q wave) infarction (acute)
Posterior (true) transmural (Q wave) infarction (acute)
Posterobasal transmural (Q wave) infarction (acute)
Posterolateral transmural (Q wave) infarction (acute)
Posteroseptal transmural (Q wave) infarction (acute)
Septal transmural (Q wave) infarction (acute) NOS

I21.3 ST elevation (STEMI) myocardial infarction of unspecified site

Acute transmural myocardial infarction of unspecified site
Myocardial infarction (acute) NOS
Transmural (Q wave) myocardial infarction NOS

I21.4 Non-ST elevation (NSTEMI) myocardial infarction

Acute subendocardial myocardial infarction
Non-Q wave myocardial infarction NOS
Nontransmural myocardial infarction NOS

Unspecified Code   Other Specified Code   [N] Newborn Age: 0   [P] Pediatric Age: 0-17   [M] Maternity Age: 12-55
[A] Adult Age: 15-124   ♂ Male   ♀ Female   ● New Code   ▲ Revised Code Title   ►◄ Revised Text

[4] **I22 Subsequent ST elevation (STEMI) and non-ST elevation (NSTEMI) myocardial infarction**

[INCLUDES] *acute myocardial infarction occurring within four weeks (28 days) of a previous acute myocardial infarction, regardless of site*
cardiac infarction
coronary (artery) embolism
coronary (artery) occlusion
coronary (artery) rupture
coronary (artery) thrombosis
infarction of heart, myocardium, or ventricle
recurrent myocardial infarction
reinfarction of myocardium
rupture of heart, myocardium, or ventricle

Use additional code, if applicable, to identify:
exposure to environmental tobacco smoke (Z77.22)
history of tobacco use (Z87.891)
occupational exposure to environmental tobacco smoke (Z57.31)
status post administration of tPA (rtPA) in a different facility within the last 24 hours prior to admission to current facility (Z92.82)
tobacco dependence (F17.-)
tobacco use (Z72.0)

I22.0 Subsequent ST elevation (STEMI) myocardial infarction of anterior wall
Subsequent acute transmural myocardial infarction of anterior wall
Subsequent transmural (Q wave) infarction (acute)(of) anterior (wall) NOS
Subsequent anteroapical transmural (Q wave) infarction (acute)
Subsequent anterolateral transmural (Q wave) infarction (acute)
Subsequent anteroseptal transmural (Q wave) infarction (acute)

I22.1 Subsequent ST elevation (STEMI) myocardial infarction of inferior wall
Subsequent acute transmural myocardial infarction of inferior wall
Subsequent transmural (Q wave) infarction (acute)(of) diaphragmatic wall
Subsequent transmural (Q wave) infarction (acute)(of) inferior (wall) NOS
Subsequent inferolateral transmural (Q wave) infarction (acute)
Subsequent inferoposterior transmural (Q wave) infarction (acute)

I22.2 Subsequent non-ST elevation (NSTEMI) myocardial infarction
Subsequent acute subendocardial myocardial infarction
Subsequent non-Q wave myocardial infarction NOS
Subsequent nontransmural myocardial infarction NOS

I22.8 Subsequent ST elevation (STEMI) myocardial infarction of other sites
Subsequent acute transmural myocardial infarction of other sites
Subsequent apical-lateral transmural (Q wave) myocardial infarction (acute)
Subsequent basal-lateral transmural (Q wave) myocardial infarction (acute)
Subsequent high lateral transmural (Q wave) myocardial infarction (acute)
Subsequent transmural (Q wave) myocardial infarction (acute)(of) lateral (wall) NOS
Subsequent posterior (true)transmural (Q wave) myocardial infarction (acute)
Subsequent posterobasal transmural (Q wave) myocardial infarction (acute)
Subsequent posterolateral transmural (Q wave) myocardial infarction (acute)
Subsequent posteroseptal transmural (Q wave) myocardial infarction (acute)
Subsequent septal NOS transmural (Q wave) myocardial infarction (acute)

I22.9 Subsequent ST elevation (STEMI) myocardial infarction of unspecified site
Subsequent acute myocardial infarction of unspecified site
Subsequent myocardial infarction (acute) NOS

[4] **I23 Certain current complications following ST elevation (STEMI) and non-ST elevation (NSTEMI) myocardial infarction (within the 28 day period)**

I23.0 Hemopericardium as current complication following acute myocardial infarction
[EXCLUDES1] *hemopericardium not specified as current complication following acute myocardial infarction (I31.2)* [A]

I23.1 Atrial septal defect as current complication following acute myocardial infarction
[EXCLUDES1] *acquired atrial septal defect not specified as current complication following acute myocardial infarction (I51.0)* [A]

I23.2 Ventricular septal defect as current complication following acute myocardial infarction
[EXCLUDES1] *acquired ventricular septal defect not specified as current complication following acute myocardial infarction (I51.0)* [A]

I23.3 Rupture of cardiac wall without hemopericardium as current complication following acute myocardial infarction [A]

I23.4 Rupture of chordae tendineae as current complication following acute myocardial infarction
[EXCLUDES1] *rupture of chordae tendineae not specified as current complication following acute myocardial infarction (I51.1)*

I23.5 Rupture of papillary muscle as current complication following acute myocardial infarction
[EXCLUDES1] *rupture of papillary muscle not specified as current complication following acute myocardial infarction (I51.2)*

I23.6 Thrombosis of atrium, auricular appendage, and ventricle as current complications following acute myocardial infarction
[EXCLUDES1] *thrombosis of atrium, auricular appendage, and ventricle not specified as current complication following acute myocardial infarction (I51.3)* [A]

I23.7 Postinfarction angina [A]

I23.8 Other current complications following acute myocardial infarction [A]

[4] **I24 Other acute ischemic heart diseases**
[EXCLUDES1] *angina pectoris (I20.-)*
transient myocardial ischemia in newborn (P29.4)

I24.0 Acute coronary thrombosis not resulting in myocardial infarction
Acute coronary (artery) (vein) embolism not resulting in myocardial infarction
Acute coronary (artery) (vein) occlusion not resulting in myocardial infarction
Acute coronary (artery) (vein) thromboembolism not resulting in myocardial infarction
[EXCLUDES1] *atherosclerotic heart disease (I25.1-)*

I24.1 Dressler's syndrome
Postmyocardial infarction syndrome
[EXCLUDES1] *postinfarction angina (I23.7)*

[4] 4th character required [5] 5th character required [6] 6th character required [7] 7th character required [X] Extension 'X' Alert
[EXCLUDES1] Not coded here [EXCLUDES2] Not included here [PDx] Primary Diagnosis Only Manifestation Code

I24.8 Other forms of acute ischemic heart disease

I24.9 Acute ischemic heart disease, unspecified

[EXCLUDES1] *ischemic heart disease (chronic) NOS (I25.9)*

[4] **I25 Chronic ischemic heart disease**

Use additional code to identify:
chronic total occlusion of coronary artery (I25.82)
exposure to environmental tobacco smoke (Z77.22)
history of tobacco use (Z87.891)
occupational exposure to environmental tobacco smoke (Z57.31)
tobacco dependence (F17.-)
tobacco use (Z72.0)

[5] **I25.1 Atherosclerotic heart disease of native coronary artery**

Atherosclerotic cardiovascular disease
Coronary (artery) atheroma
Coronary (artery) atherosclerosis
Coronary (artery) disease
Coronary (artery) sclerosis
Use additional code, if applicable, to identify:
coronary atherosclerosis due to calcified coronary lesion (I25.84)
coronary atherosclerosis due to lipid rich plaque (I25.83)

[EXCLUDES2] *atheroembolism (I75.-)*
atherosclerosis of coronary artery bypass graft(s) and transplanted heart (I25.7-)

I25.10 Atherosclerotic heart disease of native coronary artery without angina pectoris

Atherosclerotic heart disease NOS [A]

[6] **I25.11 Atherosclerotic heart disease of native coronary artery with angina pectoris**

I25.110 Atherosclerotic heart disease of native coronary artery with unstable angina pectoris

[EXCLUDES1] *unstable angina without atherosclerotic heart disease (I20.0)* [A]

I25.111 Atherosclerotic heart disease of native coronary artery with angina pectoris with documented spasm

[EXCLUDES1] *angina pectoris with documented spasm without atherosclerotic heart disease (I20.1)* [A]

I25.118 Atherosclerotic heart disease of native coronary artery with other forms of angina pectoris

[EXCLUDES1] *other forms of angina pectoris without atherosclerotic heart disease (I20.8)* [A]

I25.119 Atherosclerotic heart disease of native coronary artery with unspecified angina pectoris

Atherosclerotic heart disease with angina NOS
Atherosclerotic heart disease with ischemic chest pain

[EXCLUDES1] *unspecified angina pectoris without atherosclerotic heart disease (I20.9)* [A]

I25.2 Old myocardial infarction

Healed myocardial infarction
Past myocardial infarction diagnosed by ECG or other investigation, but currently presenting no symptoms

I25.3 Aneurysm of heart

Mural aneurysm
Ventricular aneurysm

[5] **I25.4 Coronary artery aneurysm and dissection**

I25.41 Coronary artery aneurysm

Coronary arteriovenous fistula, acquired

[EXCLUDES1] *congenital coronary (artery) aneurysm (Q24.5)*

I25.42 Coronary artery dissection

I25.5 Ischemic cardiomyopathy

[EXCLUDES2] *coronary atherosclerosis (I25.1-, I25.7-)*

I25.6 Silent myocardial ischemia

[5] **I25.7 Atherosclerosis of coronary artery bypass graft(s) and coronary artery of transplanted heart with angina pectoris**

Use additional code, if applicable, to identify:
coronary atherosclerosis due to calcified coronary lesion (I25.84)
coronary atherosclerosis due to lipid rich plaque (I25.83)

[EXCLUDES1] *atherosclerosis of bypass graft(s) of transplanted heart without angina pectoris (I25.812)*
atherosclerosis of coronary artery bypass graft(s) without angina pectoris (I25.810)
atherosclerosis of native coronary artery of transplanted heart without angina pectoris (I25.811)
embolism or thrombus of coronary artery bypass graft(s) (T82.8-)

[6] **I25.70 Atherosclerosis of coronary artery bypass graft(s), unspecified, with angina pectoris**

I25.700 Atherosclerosis of coronary artery bypass graft(s), unspecified, with unstable angina pectoris

[EXCLUDES1] *unstable angina pectoris without atherosclerosis of coronary artery bypass graft (I20.0)* [A]

I25.701 Atherosclerosis of coronary artery bypass graft(s), unspecified, with angina pectoris with documented spasm

[EXCLUDES1] *angina pectoris with documented spasm without atherosclerosis of coronary artery bypass graft (I20.1)* [A]

I25.708 Atherosclerosis of coronary artery bypass graft(s), unspecified, with other forms of angina pectoris

[EXCLUDES1] *other forms of angina pectoris without atherosclerosis of coronary artery bypass graft (I20.8)* [A]

I25.709 Atherosclerosis of coronary artery bypass graft(s), unspecified, with unspecified angina pectoris

[EXCLUDES1] *unspecified angina pectoris without atherosclerosis of coronary artery bypass graft (I20.9)* [A]

[6] **I25.71 Atherosclerosis of autologous vein coronary artery bypass graft(s) with angina pectoris**

I25.710 Atherosclerosis of autologous vein coronary artery bypass graft(s) with unstable angina pectoris

[EXCLUDES1] *unstable angina without atherosclerosis of autologous vein coronary artery bypass graft(s) (I20.0)* [A]

I25.711 Atherosclerosis of autologous vein coronary artery bypass graft(s) with angina pectoris with documented spasm

[EXCLUDES1] *angina pectoris with documented spasm without atherosclerosis of autologous vein coronary artery bypass graft(s) (I20.1)* [A]

I25.718 Atherosclerosis of autologous vein coronary artery bypass graft(s) with other forms of angina pectoris

[EXCLUDES1] *other forms of angina pectoris without atherosclerosis of autologous vein coronary artery bypass graft(s) (I20.8)* [A]

I25.719 Atherosclerosis of autologous vein coronary artery bypass graft(s) with unspecified angina pectoris

[EXCLUDES1] *unspecified angina pectoris without atherosclerosis of autologous vein coronary artery bypass graft(s) (I20.9)* [A]

Unspecified Code | Other Specified Code | [N] Newborn Age: 0 | [P] Pediatric Age: 0-17 | [M] Maternity Age: 12-55
[A] Adult Age: 15-124 | ♂ Male | ♀ Female | ● New Code | ▲ Revised Code Title | ►◄ Revised Text

[6] **I25.72 Atherosclerosis of autologous artery coronary artery bypass graft(s) with angina pectoris**
Atherosclerosis of internal mammary artery graft with angina pectoris

I25.720 Atherosclerosis of autologous artery coronary artery bypass graft(s) with unstable angina pectoris
[EXCLUDES1] *unstable angina without atherosclerosis of autologous artery coronary artery bypass graft(s) (I20.0)* [A]

I25.721 Atherosclerosis of autologous artery coronary artery bypass graft(s) with angina pectoris with documented spasm
[EXCLUDES1] *angina pectoris with documented spasm without atherosclerosis of autologous artery coronary artery bypass graft(s) (I20.1)* [A]

I25.728 Atherosclerosis of autologous artery coronary artery bypass graft(s) with other forms of angina pectoris
[EXCLUDES1] *other forms of angina pectoris without atherosclerosis of autologous artery coronary artery bypass graft(s) (I20.8)* [A]

I25.729 Atherosclerosis of autologous artery coronary artery bypass graft(s) with unspecified angina pectoris
[EXCLUDES1] *unspecified angina pectoris without atherosclerosis of autologous artery coronary artery bypass graft(s) (I20.9)* [A]

[6] **I25.73 Atherosclerosis of nonautologous biological coronary artery bypass graft(s) with angina pectoris**

I25.730 Atherosclerosis of nonautologous biological coronary artery bypass graft(s) with unstable angina pectoris
[EXCLUDES1] *unstable angina without atherosclerosis of nonautologous biological coronary artery bypass graft(s) (I20.0)* [A]

I25.731 Atherosclerosis of nonautologous biological coronary artery bypass graft(s) with angina pectoris with documented spasm
[EXCLUDES1] *angina pectoris with documented spasm without atherosclerosis of nonautologous biological coronary artery bypass graft(s) (I20.1)* [A]

I25.738 Atherosclerosis of nonautologous biological coronary artery bypass graft(s) with other forms of angina pectoris
[EXCLUDES1] *other forms of angina pectoris without atherosclerosis of nonautologous biological coronary artery bypass graft(s) (I20.8)* [A]

I25.739 Atherosclerosis of nonautologous biological coronary artery bypass graft(s) with unspecified angina pectoris
[EXCLUDES1] *unspecified angina pectoris without atherosclerosis of nonautologous biological coronary artery bypass graft(s) (I20.9)* [A]

[6] **I25.75 Atherosclerosis of native coronary artery of transplanted heart with angina pectoris**
[EXCLUDES1] *atherosclerosis of native coronary artery of transplanted heart without angina pectoris (I25.811)*

I25.750 Atherosclerosis of native coronary artery of transplanted heart with unstable angina

I25.751 Atherosclerosis of native coronary artery of transplanted heart with angina pectoris with documented spasm

I25.758 Atherosclerosis of native coronary artery of transplanted heart with other forms of angina pectoris

I25.759 Atherosclerosis of native coronary artery of transplanted heart with unspecified angina pectoris

[6] **I25.76 Atherosclerosis of bypass graft of coronary artery of transplanted heart with angina pectoris**
[EXCLUDES1] *atherosclerosis of bypass graft of coronary artery of transplanted heart without angina pectoris (I25.812)*

I25.760 Atherosclerosis of bypass graft of coronary artery of transplanted heart with unstable angina [A]

I25.761 Atherosclerosis of bypass graft of coronary artery of transplanted heart with angina pectoris with documented spasm [A]

I25.768 Atherosclerosis of bypass graft of coronary artery of transplanted heart with other forms of angina pectoris [A]

I25.769 Atherosclerosis of bypass graft of coronary artery of transplanted heart with unspecified angina pectoris [A]

[6] **I25.79 Atherosclerosis of other coronary artery bypass graft(s) with angina pectoris**

I25.790 Atherosclerosis of other coronary artery bypass graft(s) with unstable angina pectoris
[EXCLUDES1] *unstable angina without atherosclerosis of other coronary artery bypass graft(s) (I20.0)* [A]

I25.791 Atherosclerosis of other coronary artery bypass graft(s) with angina pectoris with documented spasm
[EXCLUDES1] *angina pectoris with documented spasm without atherosclerosis of other coronary artery bypass graft(s) (I20.1)* [A]

I25.798 Atherosclerosis of other coronary artery bypass graft(s) with other forms of angina pectoris
[EXCLUDES1] *other forms of angina pectoris without atherosclerosis of other coronary artery bypass graft(s) (I20.8)* [A]

I25.799 Atherosclerosis of other coronary artery bypass graft(s) with unspecified angina pectoris
[EXCLUDES1] *unspecified angina pectoris without atherosclerosis of other coronary artery bypass graft(s) (I20.9)* [A]

[5] **I25.8 Other forms of chronic ischemic heart disease**

[6] **I25.81 Atherosclerosis of other coronary vessels without angina pectoris**
Use additional code, if applicable, to identify:
coronary atherosclerosis due to calcified coronary lesion (I25.84)
coronary atherosclerosis due to lipid rich plaque (I25.83)
[EXCLUDES1] *atherosclerotic heart disease of native coronary artery without angina pectoris (I25.10)*

I25.810 Atherosclerosis of coronary artery bypass graft(s) without angina pectoris
Atherosclerosis of coronary artery bypass graft NOS
[EXCLUDES1] *atherosclerosis of coronary bypass graft(s) with angina pectoris (I25.70-I25.73-, I25.79-)* [A]

I25.811 Atherosclerosis of native coronary artery of transplanted heart without angina pectoris
Atherosclerosis of native coronary artery of transplanted heart NOS
[EXCLUDES1] *atherosclerosis of native coronary artery of transplanted heart with angina pectoris (I25.75-)*

I25.812 Atherosclerosis of bypass graft of coronary artery of transplanted heart without angina pectoris

[4] 4th character required [5] 5th character required [6] 6th character required [7] 7th character required [7th] Extension 'X' Alert
[EXCLUDES 1] Not coded here [EXCLUDES 2] Not included here [PDx] Primary Diagnosis Only Manifestation Code

Atherosclerosis of bypass graft of transplanted heart NOS

[EXCLUDES1] *atherosclerosis of bypass graft of transplanted heart with angina pectoris (I25.76)* [A]

I25.82 Chronic total occlusion of coronary artery

Complete occlusion of coronary artery

Total occlusion of coronary artery

Code first coronary atherosclerosis (I25.1-, I25.7-, I25.81-)

[EXCLUDES1] *acute coronary occulsion with myocardial infarction (I21.-, I22.-)*
acute coronary occulsion without myocardial infarction (I24.0)

I25.83 Coronary atherosclerosis due to lipid rich plaque

Code first coronary atherosclerosis (I25.1-, I25.7-, I25.81-) [A]

I25.84 Coronary atherosclerosis due to calcified coronary lesion

Coronary atherosclerosis due to severely calcified coronary lesion

Code first coronary atherosclerosis (I25.1-, I25.7-, I25.81-)

I25.89 Other forms of chronic ischemic heart disease

I25.9 Chronic ischemic heart disease, unspecified

Ischemic heart disease (chronic) NOS

Pulmonary heart disease and diseases of pulmonary circulation (I26-I28)

[4] **I26 Pulmonary embolism**

[INCLUDES] *pulmonary (acute) (artery)(vein) infarction*
pulmonary (acute) (artery)(vein) thromboembolism
pulmonary (acute) (artery)(vein) thrombosis

[EXCLUDES2] *chronic pulmonary embolism (I27.82)*
personal history of pulmonary embolism (Z86.711)
pulmonary embolism complicating abortion, ectopic or molar pregnancy (O00-O07, O08.2)
pulmonary embolism complicating pregnancy, childbirth and the puerperium (O88.-)
pulmonary embolism due to trauma (T79.0, T79.1)
pulmonary embolism due to complications of surgical and medical care (T80.0, T81.7-, T82.8-)
septic (non-pulmonary) arterial embolism (I76)

[5] **I26.0 Pulmonary embolism with acute cor pulmonale**

I26.01 Septic pulmonary embolism with acute cor pulmonale

Code first underlying infection

I26.02 Saddle embolus of pulmonary artery with acute cor pulmonale

I26.09 Other pulmonary embolism with acute cor pulmonale

Acute cor pulmonale NOS

[5] **I26.9 Pulmonary embolism without acute cor pulmonale**

I26.90 Septic pulmonary embolism without acute cor pulmonale

Code first underlying infection

I26.92 Saddle embolus of pulmonary artery without acute cor pulmonale

I26.99 Other pulmonary embolism without acute cor pulmonale

Acute pulmonary embolism NOS

Pulmonary embolism NOS

[4] **I27 Other pulmonary heart diseases**

I27.0 Primary pulmonary hypertension

[EXCLUDES1] *pulmonary hypertension NOS (I27.2)*
secondary pulmonary hypertension (I27.2)

I27.1 Kyphoscoliotic heart disease

I27.2 Other secondary pulmonary hypertension

Pulmonary hypertension NOS

Code also associated underlying condition

[5] **I27.8 Other specified pulmonary heart diseases**

I27.81 Cor pulmonale (chronic)

Cor pulmonale NOS

[EXCLUDES1] *acute cor pulmonale (I26.0-)*

I27.82 Chronic pulmonary embolism

Use additional code, if applicable, for associated long-term (current) use of anticoagulants (Z79.01)

[EXCLUDES1] *personal history of pulmonary embolism (Z86.711)*

I27.89 Other specified pulmonary heart diseases

Eisenmenger's complex

Eisenmenger's syndrome

[EXCLUDES1] *Eisenmenger's defect (Q21.8)*

I27.9 Pulmonary heart disease, unspecified

Chronic cardiopulmonary disease

[4] **I28 Other diseases of pulmonary vessels**

I28.0 Arteriovenous fistula of pulmonary vessels

[EXCLUDES1] *congenital arteriovenous fistula (Q25.72)*

I28.1 Aneurysm of pulmonary artery

[EXCLUDES1] *congenital aneurysm (Q25.79)*
congenital arteriovenous aneurysm (Q25.72)

I28.8 Other diseases of pulmonary vessels

Pulmonary arteritis

Pulmonary endarteritis

Rupture of pulmonary vessels

Stenosis of pulmonary vessels

Stricture of pulmonary vessels

I28.9 Disease of pulmonary vessels, unspecified

Other forms of heart disease (I30-I52)

[4] **I30 Acute pericarditis**

[INCLUDES] *acute mediastinopericarditis*
acute myopericarditis
acute pericardial effusion
acute pleuropericarditis
acute pneumopericarditis

[EXCLUDES1] *Dressler's syndrome (I24.1)*
rheumatic pericarditis (acute) (I01.0)

I30.0 Acute nonspecific idiopathic pericarditis

I30.1 Infective pericarditis

Pneumococcal pericarditis

Pneumopyopericardium

Purulent pericarditis

Pyopericarditis

Pyopericardium

Pyopneumopericardium

Staphylococcal pericarditis

Streptococcal pericarditis

Suppurative pericarditis

Viral pericarditis

Use additional code (B95-B97) to identify infectious agent

I30.8 Other forms of acute pericarditis

I30.9 Acute pericarditis, unspecified

[4] **I31 Other diseases of pericardium**

[EXCLUDES1] *diseases of pericardium specified as rheumatic (I09.2)*
postcardiotomy syndrome (I97.0)
traumatic injury to pericardium (S26.-)

I31.0 Chronic adhesive pericarditis

Accretio cordis

Adherent pericardium

Adhesive mediastinopericarditis

Unspecified Code | Other Specified Code | [N] Newborn Age: 0 | [P] Pediatric Age: 0-17 | [M] Maternity Age: 12-55
[A] Adult Age: 15-124 | ♂ Male | ♀ Female | ● New Code | ▲ Revised Code Title | ►◄ Revised Text

I31.1 **Chronic constrictive pericarditis**
Concretio cordis
Pericardial calcification

I31.2 **Hemopericardium, not elsewhere classified**
[EXCLUDES1] *hemopericardium as current complication following acute myocardial infarction (I23.0)*

I31.3 **Pericardial effusion (noninflammatory)**
Chylopericardium
[EXCLUDES1] *acute pericardial effusion (I30.9)*

I31.4 **Cardiac tamponade**
Code first underlying cause

I31.8 **Other specified diseases of pericardium**
Epicardial plaques
Focal pericardial adhesions

I31.9 **Disease of pericardium, unspecified**
Pericarditis (chronic) NOS

I32 **Pericarditis in diseases classified elsewhere**
Code first underlying disease
[EXCLUDES1] *pericarditis (in):*
coxsackie (virus) (B33.23)
gonococcal (A54.83)
meningococcal (A39.53)
rheumatoid (arthritis) (M05.31)
syphilitic (A52.06)
systemic lupus erythematosus (M32.12)
tuberculosis (A18.84)

[4] I33 **Acute and subacute endocarditis**
[EXCLUDES1] *acute rheumatic endocarditis (I01.1)*
endocarditis NOS (I38)

I33.0 **Acute and subacute infective endocarditis**
Bacterial endocarditis (acute) (subacute)
Infective endocarditis (acute) (subacute) NOS
Endocarditis lenta (acute) (subacute)
Malignant endocarditis (acute) (subacute)
Purulent endocarditis (acute) (subacute)
Septic endocarditis (acute) (subacute)
Ulcerative endocarditis (acute) (subacute)
Vegetative endocarditis (acute) (subacute)
Use additional code (B95-B97) to identify infectious agent

I33.9 **Acute and subacute endocarditis, unspecified**
Acute endocarditis NOS
Acute myoendocarditis NOS
Acute periendocarditis NOS
Subacute endocarditis NOS
Subacute myoendocarditis NOS
Subacute periendocarditis NOS

[4] I34 **Nonrheumatic mitral valve disorders**
[EXCLUDES1] *mitral valve disease (I05.9)*
mitral valve failure (I05.8)
mitral valve stenosis (I05.0)
mitral valve disorder of unspecified cause with diseases of aortic and/or tricuspid valve(s) (I08.-)
mitral valve disorder of unspecified cause with mitral stenosis or obstruction (I05.0)
mitral valve disorder specified as congenital (Q23.2, Q23.3)
mitral valve disorder specified as rheumatic (I05.-)

I34.0 **Nonrheumatic mitral (valve) insufficiency**
Nonrheumatic mitral (valve) incompetence NOS
Nonrheumatic mitral (valve) regurgitation NOS

I34.1 **Nonrheumatic mitral (valve) prolapse**
Floppy nonrheumatic mitral valve syndrome
[EXCLUDES1] *Marfan's syndrome (Q87.4-)*

I34.2 **Nonrheumatic mitral (valve) stenosis**

I34.8 **Other nonrheumatic mitral valve disorders**

I34.9 **Nonrheumatic mitral valve disorder, unspecified**

[4] I35 **Nonrheumatic aortic valve disorders**
[EXCLUDES1] *aortic valve disorder of unspecified cause but with diseases of mitral and/or tricuspid valve(s) (I08.-)*
aortic valve disorder specified as congenital (Q23.0, Q23.1)
aortic valve disorder specified as rheumatic (I06.-)
hypertrophic subaortic stenosis (I42.1)

I35.0 **Nonrheumatic aortic (valve) stenosis**

I35.1 **Nonrheumatic aortic (valve) insufficiency**
Nonrheumatic aortic (valve) incompetence NOS
Nonrheumatic aortic (valve) regurgitation NOS

I35.2 **Nonrheumatic aortic (valve) stenosis with insufficiency**

I35.8 **Other nonrheumatic aortic valve disorders**

I35.9 **Nonrheumatic aortic valve disorder, unspecified**

[4] I36 **Nonrheumatic tricuspid valve disorders**
[EXCLUDES1] *tricuspid valve disorders of unspecified cause (I07.-)*
tricuspid valve disorders specified as congenital (Q22.4, Q22.8, Q22.9)
tricuspid valve disorders specified as rheumatic (I07.-)
tricuspid valve disorders with aortic and/or mitral valve involvement (I08.-)

I36.0 **Nonrheumatic tricuspid (valve) stenosis**

I36.1 **Nonrheumatic tricuspid (valve) insufficiency**
Nonrheumatic tricuspid (valve) incompetence
Nonrheumatic tricuspid (valve) regurgitation

I36.2 **Nonrheumatic tricuspid (valve) stenosis with insufficiency**

I36.8 **Other nonrheumatic tricuspid valve disorders**

I36.9 **Nonrheumatic tricuspid valve disorder, unspecified**

[4] I37 **Nonrheumatic pulmonary valve disorders**
[EXCLUDES1] *pulmonary valve disorder specified as congenital (Q22.1, Q22.2, Q22.3)*
pulmonary valve disorder specified as rheumatic (I09.89)

I37.0 **Nonrheumatic pulmonary valve stenosis**

I37.1 **Nonrheumatic pulmonary valve insufficiency**
Nonrheumatic pulmonary valve incompetence
Nonrheumatic pulmonary valve regurgitation

I37.2 **Nonrheumatic pulmonary valve stenosis with insufficiency**

I37.8 **Other nonrheumatic pulmonary valve disorders**

I37.9 **Nonrheumatic pulmonary valve disorder, unspecified**

I38 **Endocarditis, valve unspecified**
[INCLUDES] *endocarditis (chronic) NOS*
valvular incompetence NOS
valvular insufficiency NOS
valvular regurgitation NOS
valvular stenosis NOS
valvulitis (chronic) NOS
[EXCLUDES1] *congenital insufficiency of cardiac valve NOS (Q24.8)*
congenital stenosis of cardiac valve NOS (Q24.8)
endocardial fibroelastosis (I42.4)
endocarditis specified as rheumatic (I09.1)

I39 Endocarditis and heart valve disorders in diseases classified elsewhere

Code first underlying disease, such as:
Q fever (A78)

EXCLUDES1 *endocardial involvement in:*
candidiasis (B37.6)
gonococcal infection (A54.83)
Libman-Sacks disease (M32.11)
listerosis (A32.82)
meningococcal infection (A39.51)
rheumatoid arthritis (M05.31)
syphilis (A52.03)
tuberculosis (A18.84)
typhoid fever (A01.02)

I40 Acute myocarditis

INCLUDES *subacute myocarditis*

EXCLUDES1 *acute rheumatic myocarditis (I01.2)*

I40.0 Infective myocarditis

Septic myocarditis
Use additional code (B95-B97) to identify infectious agent

I40.1 Isolated myocarditis

Fiedler's myocarditis
Giant cell myocarditis
Idiopathic myocarditis

I40.8 Other acute myocarditis

I40.9 Acute myocarditis, unspecified

I41 Myocarditis in diseases classified elsewhere

Code first underlying disease, such as:
typhus (A75.0-A75.9)

EXCLUDES1 *myocarditis (in):*
Chagas' disease (chronic) (B57.2)
acute (B57.0)
coxsackie (virus) infection (B33.22)
diphtheritic (A36.81)
gonococcal (A54.83)
influenzal (J09.X9, J10.82, J11.82)
meningococcal (A39.52)
mumps (B26.82)
rheumatoid arthritis (M05.31)
sarcoid (D86.85)
syphilis (A52.06)
toxoplasmosis (B58.81)
tuberculous (A18.84)

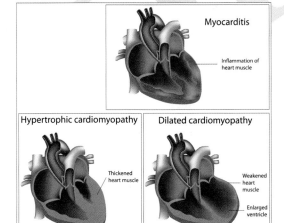

Figure 8.2 Heart Muscle Disease

I42 Cardiomyopathy

INCLUDES *myocardiopathy*

Code first pre-existing cardiomyopathy complicating pregnancy and puerperium (O99.4)

EXCLUDES1 *ischemic cardiomyopathy (I25.5)*
peripartum cardiomyopathy (O90.3)
EXCLUDES2 *ventricular hypertrophy (I51.7)*

I42.0 Dilated cardiomyopathy

Congestive cardiomyopathy

I42.1 Obstructive hypertrophic cardiomyopathy

Hypertrophic subaortic stenosis (idiopathic)

I42.2 Other hypertrophic cardiomyopathy

Nonobstructive hypertrophic cardiomyopathy

I42.3 Endomyocardial (eosinophilic) disease

Endomyocardial (tropical) fibrosis
Löffler's endocarditis

I42.4 Endocardial fibroelastosis

Congenital cardiomyopathy
Elastomyofibrosis

I42.5 Other restrictive cardiomyopathy

Constrictive cardiomyopathy NOS

I42.6 Alcoholic cardiomyopathy

Code also presence of alcoholism (F10.-)

I42.7 Cardiomyopathy due to drug and external agent

Code first poisoning due to drug or toxin, if applicable (T36-T65 with fifth or sixth character 1-4 or 6)
Use additional code for adverse effect, if applicable, to identify drug (T36-T50 with fifth or sixth character 5)

I42.8 Other cardiomyopathies

I42.9 Cardiomyopathy, unspecified

Cardiomyopathy (primary) (secondary) NOS

I43 Cardiomyopathy in diseases classified elsewhere

Code first underlying disease, such as:
amyloidosis (E85.-)
glycogen storage disease (E74.0)
gout (M10.0-)
thyrotoxicosis (E05.0-E05.9-)

EXCLUDES1 *cardiomyopathy (in):*
coxsackie (virus) (B33.24)
diphtheria (A36.81)
sarcoidosis (D86.85)
tuberculosis (A18.84)

I44 Atrioventricular and left bundle-branch block

I44.0 Atrioventricular block, first degree

I44.1 Atrioventricular block, second degree

Atrioventricular block, type I and II
Möbitz block block, type I and II
Second degree block, type I and II
Wenckebach's block

I44.2 Atrioventricular block, complete

Complete heart block NOS
Third degree block

I44.3 Other and unspecified atrioventricular block

Atrioventricular block NOS

I44.30 Unspecified atrioventricular block

I44.39 Other atrioventricular block

I44.4 Left anterior fascicular block

I44.5 Left posterior fascicular block

I44.6 Other and unspecified fascicular block

I44.60 Unspecified fascicular block

Left bundle-branch hemiblock NOS

I44.69 Other fascicular block

I44.7 Left bundle-branch block, unspecified

I45 Other conduction disorders

I45.0 Right fascicular block

I45.1 Other and unspecified right bundle-branch block

I45.10 Unspecified right bundle-branch block

Right bundle-branch block NOS

I45.19 Other right bundle-branch block

I45.2 Bifascicular block

I45.3 Trifascicular block

| Unspecified Code | Other Specified Code | Ⓝ Newborn Age: 0 | Ⓟ Pediatric Age: 0-17 | Ⓜ Maternity Age: 12-55 |
| Ⓐ Adult Age: 15-124 | ♂ Male | ♀ Female | ● New Code | ▲ Revised Code Title | ►◄ Revised Text |

I45.4 Nonspecific intraventricular block
Bundle-branch block NOS
I45.5 Other specified heart block
Sinoatrial block
Sinoauricular block
[EXCLUDES1] *heart block NOS (I45.9)*
I45.6 Pre-excitation syndrome
Accelerated atrioventricular conduction
Accessory atrioventricular conduction
Anomalous atrioventricular excitation
Lown-Ganong-Levine syndrome
Pre-excitation atrioventricular conduction
Wolff-Parkinson-White syndrome
[5] I45.8 Other specified conduction disorders
I45.81 Long QT syndrome
I45.89 Other specified conduction disorders
Atrioventricular [AV] dissociation
Interference dissociation
Isorhythmic dissociation
Nonparoxysmal AV nodal tachycardia
I45.9 Conduction disorder, unspecified
Heart block NOS
Stokes-Adams syndrome
[4] I46 Cardiac arrest
[EXCLUDES1] *cardiogenic shock (R57.0)*
I46.2 Cardiac arrest due to underlying cardiac condition
Code first underlying cardiac condition
I46.8 Cardiac arrest due to other underlying condition
Code first underlying condition
I46.9 Cardiac arrest, cause unspecified
[4] I47 Paroxysmal tachycardia
Code first tachycardia complicating:
abortion or ectopic or molar pregnancy (O00-O07, O08.8)
obstetric surgery and procedures (O75.4)
[EXCLUDES1] *tachycardia NOS (R00.0)*
sinoauricular tachycardia NOS (R00.0)
sinus [sinusal] tachycardia NOS (R00.0)
I47.0 Re-entry ventricular arrhythmia
I47.1 Supraventricular tachycardia
Atrial (paroxysmal) tachycardia
Atrioventricular [AV] (paroxysmal) tachycardia
Atrioventricular re-entrant (nodal) tachycardia [AVNRT] [AVRT]
Junctional (paroxysmal) tachycardia
Nodal (paroxysmal) tachycardia
I47.2 Ventricular tachycardia
I47.9 Paroxysmal tachycardia, unspecified
Bouveret (-Hoffman) syndrome
[4] I48 Atrial fibrillation and flutter
I48.0 Paroxysmal atrial fibrillation
I48.1 Persistent atrial fibrillation
I48.2 Chronic atrial fibrillation
Permanent atrial fibrillation
I48.3 Typical atrial flutter
Type I atrial flutter
I48.4 Atypical atrial flutter
Type II atrial flutter
[5] I48.9 Unspecified atrial fibrillation and atrial flutter
I48.91 Unspecified atrial fibrillation
I48.92 Unspecified atrial flutter
[4] I49 Other cardiac arrhythmias
Code first cardiac arrhythmia complicating:
abortion or ectopic or molar pregnancy (O00-O07, O08.8)
obstetric surgery and procedures (O75.4)
[EXCLUDES1] *bradycardia NOS (R00.1)*
neonatal dysrhythmia (P29.1-)
sinoatrial bradycardia (R00.1)
sinus bradycardia (R00.1)
vagal bradycardia (R00.1)
[5] I49.0 Ventricular fibrillation and flutter
I49.01 Ventricular fibrillation
I49.02 Ventricular flutter
I49.1 Atrial premature depolarization
Atrial premature beats
I49.2 Junctional premature depolarization
I49.3 Ventricular premature depolarization
[5] I49.4 Other and unspecified premature depolarization
I49.40 Unspecified premature depolarization
Premature beats NOS
I49.49 Other premature depolarization
Ectopic beats
Extrasystoles
Extrasystolic arrhythmias
Premature contractions
I49.5 Sick sinus syndrome
Tachycardia-bradycardia syndrome
I49.8 Other specified cardiac arrhythmias
Coronary sinus rhythm disorder
Ectopic rhythm disorder
Nodal rhythm disorder
I49.9 Cardiac arrhythmia, unspecified
Arrhythmia (cardiac) NOS
[4] I50 Heart failure
Code first:
heart failure complicating abortion or ectopic or molar pregnancy (O00-O07, O08.8)
heart failure following surgery (I97.13-)
heart failure due to hypertension (I11.0)
heart failure due to hypertension with chronic kidney disease (I13.-)
obstetric surgery and procedures (O75.4)
rheumatic heart failure (I09.81)
[EXCLUDES1] *cardiac arrest (I46.-)*
neonatal cardiac failure (P29.0)
I50.1 Left ventricular failure
Cardiac asthma
Edema of lung with heart disease NOS
Edema of lung with heart failure
Left heart failure
Pulmonary edema with heart disease NOS
Pulmonary edema with heart failure
[EXCLUDES1] *edema of lung without heart disease or heart failure (J81.-)*
pulmonary edema without heart disease or failure (J81.-)
[5] I50.2 Systolic (congestive) heart failure
[EXCLUDES1] *combined systolic (congestive) and diastolic (congestive) heart failure (I50.4-)*
I50.20 Unspecified systolic (congestive) heart failure
I50.21 Acute systolic (congestive) heart failure
I50.22 Chronic systolic (congestive) heart failure
I50.23 Acute on chronic systolic (congestive) heart failure
[5] I50.3 Diastolic (congestive) heart failure
[EXCLUDES1] *combined systolic (congestive) and diastolic (congestive) heart failure (I50.4-)*
I50.30 Unspecified diastolic (congestive) heart failure
I50.31 Acute diastolic (congestive) heart failure
I50.32 Chronic diastolic (congestive) heart failure
I50.33 Acute on chronic diastolic (congestive) heart failure
[5] I50.4 Combined systolic (congestive) and diastolic (congestive) heart failure

[4] 4th character required [5] 5th character required [6] 6th character required [7] 7th character required [7x] Extension 'X' Alert
[EXCLUDES1] Not coded here [EXCLUDES2] Not included here [PDx] Primary Diagnosis Only Manifestation Code

I50.40 **Unspecified combined systolic (congestive) and diastolic (congestive) heart failure**

I50.41 Acute **combined systolic (congestive) and diastolic (congestive) heart failure**

I50.42 Chronic **combined systolic (congestive) and diastolic (congestive) heart failure**

I50.43 Acute on chronic **combined systolic (congestive) and diastolic (congestive) heart failure**

I50.9 **Heart failure, unspecified**

Biventricular (heart) failure NOS

Cardiac, heart or myocardial failure NOS

Congestive heart disease

Congestive heart failure NOS

Right ventricular failure (secondary to left heart failure)

EXCLUDES1 *fluid overload (E87.70)*

I51 **Complications and ill-defined descriptions of heart disease**

EXCLUDES1 *any condition in I51.4-I51.9 due to hypertension (I11.-)*
any condition in I51.4-I51.9 due to hypertension and chronic kidney disease (I13.-)
heart disease specified as rheumatic (I00-I09)

I51.0 **Cardiac septal defect, acquired**

Acquired septal atrial defect (old)

Acquired septal auricular defect (old)

Acquired septal ventricular defect (old)

EXCLUDES1 *cardiac septal defect as current complication following acute myocardial infarction (I23.1, I23.2)* 🅰

I51.1 **Rupture of chordae tendineae, not elsewhere classified**

EXCLUDES1 *rupture of chordae tendineae as current complication following acute myocardial infarction (I23.4)*

I51.2 **Rupture of papillary muscle, not elsewhere classified**

EXCLUDES1 *rupture of papillary muscle as current complication following acute myocardial infarction (I23.5)*

I51.3 **Intracardiac thrombosis, not elsewhere classified**

Apical thrombosis (old)

Atrial thrombosis (old)

Auricular thrombosis (old)

Mural thrombosis (old)

Ventricular thrombosis (old)

EXCLUDES1 *intracardiac thrombosis as current complication following acute myocardial infarction (I23.6)* 🅰

I51.4 **Myocarditis, unspecified**

Chronic (interstitial) myocarditis

Myocardial fibrosis

Myocarditis NOS

EXCLUDES1 *acute or subacute myocarditis (I40.-)*

I51.5 **Myocardial degeneration**

Fatty degeneration of heart or myocardium

Myocardial disease

Senile degeneration of heart or myocardium

I51.7 **Cardiomegaly**

Cardiac dilatation

Cardiac hypertrophy

Ventricular dilatation

I51.8 **Other ill-defined heart diseases**

I51.81 **Takotsubo syndrome**

Reversible left ventricular dysfunction following sudden emotional stress

Stress induced cardiomyopathy

Takotsubo cardiomyopathy

Transient left ventricular apical ballooning syndrome

I51.89 Other ill-defined heart diseases

Carditis (acute)(chronic)

Pancarditis (acute)(chronic)

I51.9 **Heart disease, unspecified**

I52 **Other heart disorders in diseases classified elsewhere**

Code first underlying disease, such as:

congenital syphilis (A50.5)

mucopolysaccharidosis (E76.3)

schistosomiasis (B65.0-B65.9)

EXCLUDES1 *heart disease (in):*
gonococcal infection (A54.83)
meningococcal infection (A39.50)
rheumatoid arthritis (M05.31)
syphilis (A52.06)

Cerebrovascular diseases (I60-I69)

Use additional code to identify presence of:

alcohol abuse and dependence (F10.-)

exposure to environmental tobacco smoke (Z77.22)

history of tobacco use (Z87.891)

hypertension (I10-I15)

occupational exposure to environmental tobacco smoke (Z57.31)

tobacco dependence (F17.-)

tobacco use (Z72.0)

EXCLUDES1 *transient cerebral ischemic attacks and related syndromes (G45.-)*
traumatic intracranial hemorrhage (S06.-)

I60 **Nontraumatic** subarachnoid **hemorrhage**

INCLUDES *ruptured cerebral aneurysm*

EXCLUDES1 *sequelae of subarachnoid hemorrhage (I69.0-)*
syphilitic ruptured cerebral aneurysm (A52.05)

I60.0 **Nontraumatic subarachnoid hemorrhage from** carotid siphon and bifurcation

I60.00 **Nontraumatic subarachnoid hemorrhage from** unspecified **carotid siphon and bifurcation**

I60.01 **Nontraumatic subarachnoid hemorrhage from** right **carotid siphon and bifurcation**

I60.02 **Nontraumatic subarachnoid hemorrhage from** left **carotid siphon and bifurcation**

I60.1 **Nontraumatic subarachnoid hemorrhage from** middle cerebral artery

I60.10 **Nontraumatic subarachnoid hemorrhage from** unspecified **middle cerebral artery**

I60.11 **Nontraumatic subarachnoid hemorrhage from** right **middle cerebral artery**

I60.12 **Nontraumatic subarachnoid hemorrhage from** left **middle cerebral artery**

I60.2 **Nontraumatic subarachnoid hemorrhage** from anterior communicating artery

I60.20 **Nontraumatic subarachnoid hemorrhage from** unspecified **anterior communicating artery**

I60.21 **Nontraumatic subarachnoid hemorrhage from** right **anterior communicating artery**

I60.22 **Nontraumatic subarachnoid hemorrhage from** left **anterior communicating artery**

I60.3 **Nontraumatic subarachnoid hemorrhage from** posterior communicating artery

I60.30 **Nontraumatic subarachnoid hemorrhage from** unspecified **posterior communicating artery**

I60.31 **Nontraumatic subarachnoid hemorrhage from** right **posterior communicating artery**

I60.32 **Nontraumatic subarachnoid hemorrhage from** left **posterior communicating artery**

I60.4 **Nontraumatic subarachnoid hemorrhage from basilar artery**

I60.5 **Nontraumatic subarachnoid hemorrhage from** vertebral artery

I60.50 **Nontraumatic subarachnoid hemorrhage from** unspecified **vertebral artery**

Unspecified Code   Other Specified Code   🅝 Newborn Age: 0   🅟 Pediatric Age: 0-17   🅜 Maternity Age: 12-55

🅰 Adult Age: 15-124   ♂ Male   ♀ Female   ● New Code   ▲ Revised Code Title   ►◄ Revised Text

I60.51 Nontraumatic subarachnoid hemorrhage from right vertebral artery

I60.52 Nontraumatic subarachnoid hemorrhage from left vertebral artery

I60.6 Nontraumatic subarachnoid hemorrhage from other intracranial arteries

I60.7 Nontraumatic subarachnoid hemorrhage from unspecified intracranial artery

Ruptured (congenital) berry aneurysm

Ruptured (congenital) cerebral aneurysm

Subarachnoid hemorrhage (nontraumatic) from cerebral artery NOS

Subarachnoid hemorrhage (nontraumatic) from communicating artery NOS

EXCLUDES1 berry aneurysm, nonruptured (I67.1)

I60.8 Other nontraumatic subarachnoid hemorrhage

Meningeal hemorrhage

Rupture of cerebral arteriovenous malformation

I60.9 Nontraumatic subarachnoid hemorrhage, unspecified

④ I61 Nontraumatic intracerebral hemorrhage

EXCLUDES1 sequelae of intracerebral hemorrhage (I69.1-)

I61.0 Nontraumatic intracerebral hemorrhage in hemisphere, subcortical

Deep intracerebral hemorrhage (nontraumatic)

I61.1 Nontraumatic intracerebral hemorrhage in hemisphere, cortical

Cerebral lobe hemorrhage (nontraumatic)

Superficial intracerebral hemorrhage (nontraumatic)

I61.2 Nontraumatic intracerebral hemorrhage in hemisphere, unspecified

I61.3 Nontraumatic intracerebral hemorrhage in brain stem

I61.4 Nontraumatic intracerebral hemorrhage in cerebellum

I61.5 Nontraumatic intracerebral hemorrhage, intraventricular

I61.6 Nontraumatic intracerebral hemorrhage, multiple localized

I61.8 Other nontraumatic intracerebral hemorrhage

I61.9 Nontraumatic intracerebral hemorrhage, unspecified

④ I62 Other and unspecified nontraumatic intracranial hemorrhage

EXCLUDES1 sequelae of intracranial hemorrhage (I69.2)

⑤ I62.0 Nontraumatic subdural hemorrhage

I62.00 Nontraumatic subdural hemorrhage, unspecified

I62.01 Nontraumatic acute subdural hemorrhage

I62.02 Nontraumatic subacute subdural hemorrhage

I62.03 Nontraumatic chronic subdural hemorrhage

I62.1 Nontraumatic extradural hemorrhage

Nontraumatic epidural hemorrhage

I62.9 Nontraumatic intracranial hemorrhage, unspecified

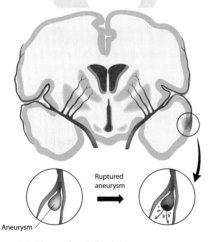

Ruptured aneurysm

Aneurysm

Figure 8.3 Hemorrhagic Stroke

④ I63 Cerebral infarction

INCLUDES occlusion and stenosis of cerebral and precerebral arteries, resulting in cerebral infarction

Use additional code, if applicable, to identify status post administration of tPA (rtPA) in a different facility within the last 24 hours prior to admission to current facility (Z92.82)

EXCLUDES1 sequelae of cerebral infarction (I69.3-)

⑤ I63.0 Cerebral infarction due to thrombosis of precerebral arteries

I63.00 Cerebral infarction due to thrombosis of unspecified precerebral artery

⑥ I63.01 Cerebral infarction due to thrombosis of vertebral artery

I63.011 Cerebral infarction due to thrombosis of right vertebral artery

I63.012 Cerebral infarction due to thrombosis of left vertebral artery

I63.019 Cerebral infarction due to thrombosis of unspecified vertebral artery

I63.02 Cerebral infarction due to thrombosis of basilar artery

⑥ I63.03 Cerebral infarction due to thrombosis of carotid artery

I63.031 Cerebral infarction due to thrombosis of right carotid artery

I63.032 Cerebral infarction due to thrombosis of left carotid artery

I63.039 Cerebral infarction due to thrombosis of unspecified carotid artery

I63.09 Cerebral infarction due to thrombosis of other precerebral artery

⑤ I63.1 Cerebral infarction due to embolism of precerebral arteries

I63.10 Cerebral infarction due to embolism of unspecified precerebral artery

⑥ I63.11 Cerebral infarction due to embolism of vertebral artery

I63.111 Cerebral infarction due to embolism of right vertebral artery

I63.112 Cerebral infarction due to embolism of left vertebral artery

I63.119 Cerebral infarction due to embolism of unspecified vertebral artery

I63.12 Cerebral infarction due to embolism of basilar artery

⑥ I63.13 Cerebral infarction due to embolism of carotid artery

I63.131 Cerebral infarction due to embolism of right carotid artery

I63.132 Cerebral infarction due to embolism of left carotid artery

I63.139 Cerebral infarction due to embolism of unspecified carotid artery

I63.19 Cerebral infarction due to embolism of other precerebral artery

⑤ I63.2 Cerebral infarction due to unspecified occlusion or stenosis of precerebral arteries

I63.20 Cerebral infarction due to unspecified occlusion or stenosis of unspecified precerebral arteries

⑥ I63.21 Cerebral infarction due to unspecified occlusion or stenosis of vertebral arteries

I63.211 Cerebral infarction due to unspecified occlusion or stenosis of right vertebral arteries

I63.212 Cerebral infarction due to unspecified occlusion or stenosis of left vertebral arteries

---

④ 4th character required ⑤ 5th character required ⑥ 6th character required ⑦ 7th character required ⑦ₓ Extension 'X' Alert

EXCLUDES 1 Not coded here EXCLUDES 2 Not included here PDx Primary Diagnosis Only Manifestation Code

I63.219 Cerebral infarction due to unspecified occlusion or stenosis of unspecified vertebral arteries

I63.22 Cerebral infarction due to unspecified occlusion or stenosis of basilar arteries

[6] I63.23 Cerebral infarction due to unspecified occlusion or stenosis of carotid arteries

I63.231 Cerebral infarction due to unspecified occlusion or stenosis of right carotid arteries

I63.232 Cerebral infarction due to unspecified occlusion or stenosis of left carotid arteries

I63.239 Cerebral infarction due to unspecified occlusion or stenosis of unspecified carotid arteries

I63.29 Cerebral infarction due to unspecified occlusion or stenosis of other precerebral arteries

[5] I63.3 Cerebral infarction due to thrombosis of cerebral arteries

I63.30 Cerebral infarction due to thrombosis of unspecified cerebral artery

[6] I63.31 Cerebral infarction due to thrombosis of middle cerebral artery

I63.311 Cerebral infarction due to thrombosis of right middle cerebral artery

I63.312 Cerebral infarction due to thrombosis of left middle cerebral artery

I63.319 Cerebral infarction due to thrombosis of unspecified middle cerebral artery

[6] I63.32 Cerebral infarction due to thrombosis of anterior cerebral artery

I63.321 Cerebral infarction due to thrombosis of right anterior cerebral artery

I63.322 Cerebral infarction due to thrombosis of left anterior cerebral artery

I63.329 Cerebral infarction due to thrombosis of unspecified anterior cerebral artery

[6] I63.33 Cerebral infarction due to thrombosis of posterior cerebral artery

I63.331 Cerebral infarction due to thrombosis of right posterior cerebral artery

I63.332 Cerebral infarction due to thrombosis of left posterior cerebral artery

I63.339 Cerebral infarction due to thrombosis of unspecified posterior cerebral artery

[6] I63.34 Cerebral infarction due to thrombosis of cerebellar artery

I63.341 Cerebral infarction due to thrombosis of right cerebellar artery

I63.342 Cerebral infarction due to thrombosis of left cerebellar artery

I63.349 Cerebral infarction due to thrombosis of unspecified cerebellar artery

I63.39 Cerebral infarction due to thrombosis of other cerebral artery

[5] I63.4 Cerebral infarction due to embolism of cerebral arteries

I63.40 Cerebral infarction due to embolism of unspecified cerebral artery

[6] I63.41 Cerebral infarction due to embolism of middle cerebral artery

I63.411 Cerebral infarction due to embolism of right middle cerebral artery

I63.412 Cerebral infarction due to embolism of left middle cerebral artery

I63.419 Cerebral infarction due to embolism of unspecified middle cerebral artery

[6] I63.42 Cerebral infarction due to embolism of anterior cerebral artery

I63.421 Cerebral infarction due to embolism of right anterior cerebral artery

I63.422 Cerebral infarction due to embolism of left anterior cerebral artery

I63.429 Cerebral infarction due to embolism of unspecified anterior cerebral artery

[6] I63.43 Cerebral infarction due to embolism of posterior cerebral artery

I63.431 Cerebral infarction due to embolism of right posterior cerebral artery

I63.432 Cerebral infarction due to embolism of left posterior cerebral artery

I63.439 Cerebral infarction due to embolism of unspecified posterior cerebral artery

[6] I63.44 Cerebral infarction due to embolism of cerebellar artery

I63.441 Cerebral infarction due to embolism of right cerebellar artery

I63.442 Cerebral infarction due to embolism of left cerebellar artery

I63.449 Cerebral infarction due to embolism of unspecified cerebellar artery

I63.49 Cerebral infarction due to embolism of other cerebral artery

[5] I63.5 Cerebral infarction due to unspecified occlusion or stenosis of cerebral arteries

I63.50 Cerebral infarction due to unspecified occlusion or stenosis of unspecified cerebral artery

[6] I63.51 Cerebral infarction due to unspecified occlusion or stenosis of middle cerebral artery

I63.511 Cerebral infarction due to unspecified occlusion or stenosis of right middle cerebral artery

I63.512 Cerebral infarction due to unspecified occlusion or stenosis of left middle cerebral artery

I63.519 Cerebral infarction due to unspecified occlusion or stenosis of unspecified middle cerebral artery

[6] I63.52 Cerebral infarction due to unspecified occlusion or stenosis of anterior cerebral artery

I63.521 Cerebral infarction due to unspecified occlusion or stenosis of right anterior cerebral artery

I63.522 Cerebral infarction due to unspecified occlusion or stenosis of left anterior cerebral artery

I63.529 Cerebral infarction due to unspecified occlusion or stenosis of unspecified anterior cerebral artery

[6] I63.53 Cerebral infarction due to unspecified occlusion or stenosis of posterior cerebral artery

I63.531 Cerebral infarction due to unspecified occlusion or stenosis of right posterior cerebral artery

I63.532 Cerebral infarction due to unspecified occlusion or stenosis of left posterior cerebral artery

I63.539 Cerebral infarction due to unspecified occlusion or stenosis of unspecified posterior cerebral artery

[6] I63.54 Cerebral infarction due to unspecified occlusion or stenosis of cerebellar artery

I63.541 Cerebral infarction due to unspecified occlusion or stenosis of right cerebellar artery

I63.542 Cerebral infarction due to unspecified occlusion or stenosis of left cerebellar artery

I63.549 Cerebral infarction due to unspecified occlusion or stenosis of unspecified cerebellar artery

Unspecified Code | Other Specified Code | [N] Newborn Age: 0 | [P] Pediatric Age: 0-17 | [M] Maternity Age: 12-55
[A] Adult Age: 15-124 | ♂ Male | ♀ Female | ● New Code | ▲ Revised Code Title | ►◄ Revised Text

I63.59 Cerebral infarction due to unspecified occlusion or stenosis of other cerebral artery

I63.6 Cerebral infarction due to cerebral venous thrombosis, nonpyogenic

I63.8 Other cerebral infarction

I63.9 Cerebral infarction, unspecified

Stroke NOS

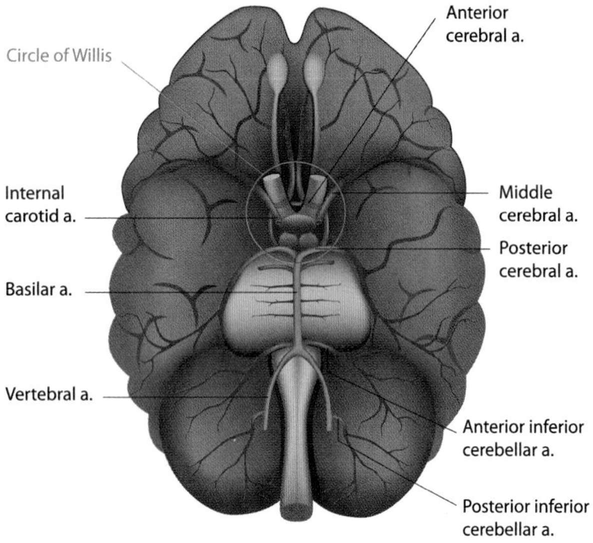
Circle of Willis
Anterior cerebral a.
Internal carotid a.
Middle cerebral a.
Posterior cerebral a.
Basilar a.
Vertebral a.
Anterior inferior cerebellar a.
Posterior inferior cerebellar a.

Figure 8.4 Blood Supply of the Brain

[4] I65 Occlusion and stenosis of precerebral arteries, not resulting in cerebral infarction

INCLUDES *embolism of precerebral artery*
narrowing of precerebral artery
obstruction (complete) (partial) of precerebral artery
thrombosis of precerebral artery

EXCLUDES1 *insufficiency, NOS, of precerebral artery (G45.-)*
insufficiency of precerebral arteries causing cerebral infarction (I63.0-I63.2)

[5] I65.0 Occlusion and stenosis of vertebral artery

I65.01 Occlusion and stenosis of right vertebral artery

I65.02 Occlusion and stenosis of left vertebral artery

I65.03 Occlusion and stenosis of bilateral vertebral arteries

I65.09 Occlusion and stenosis of unspecified vertebral artery

I65.1 Occlusion and stenosis of basilar artery

[5] I65.2 Occlusion and stenosis of carotid artery

I65.21 Occlusion and stenosis of right carotid artery

I65.22 Occlusion and stenosis of left carotid artery

I65.23 Occlusion and stenosis of bilateral carotid arteries

I65.29 Occlusion and stenosis of unspecified carotid artery

I65.8 Occlusion and stenosis of other precerebral arteries

I65.9 Occlusion and stenosis of unspecified precerebral artery

Occlusion and stenosis of precerebral artery NOS

[4] I66 Occlusion and stenosis of cerebral arteries, not resulting in cerebral infarction

INCLUDES *embolism of cerebral artery*
narrowing of cerebral artery
obstruction (complete) (partial) of cerebral artery
thrombosis of cerebral artery

EXCLUDES1 *Occlusion and stenosis of cerebral artery causing cerebral infarction (I63.3-I63.5)*

[5] I66.0 Occlusion and stenosis of middle cerebral artery

I66.01 Occlusion and stenosis of right middle cerebral artery

I66.02 Occlusion and stenosis of left middle cerebral artery

I66.03 Occlusion and stenosis of bilateral middle cerebral arteries

I66.09 Occlusion and stenosis of unspecified middle cerebral artery

[5] I66.1 Occlusion and stenosis of anterior cerebral artery

I66.11 Occlusion and stenosis of right anterior cerebral artery

I66.12 Occlusion and stenosis of left anterior cerebral artery

I66.13 Occlusion and stenosis of bilateral anterior cerebral arteries

I66.19 Occlusion and stenosis of unspecified anterior cerebral artery

[5] I66.2 Occlusion and stenosis of posterior cerebral artery

I66.21 Occlusion and stenosis of right posterior cerebral artery

I66.22 Occlusion and stenosis of left posterior cerebral artery

I66.23 Occlusion and stenosis of bilateral posterior cerebral arteries

I66.29 Occlusion and stenosis of unspecified posterior cerebral artery

I66.3 Occlusion and stenosis of cerebellar arteries

I66.8 Occlusion and stenosis of other cerebral arteries

Occlusion and stenosis of perforating arteries

I66.9 Occlusion and stenosis of unspecified cerebral artery

[4] I67 Other cerebrovascular diseases

EXCLUDES1 *sequelae of the listed conditions (I69.8)*

I67.0 Dissection of cerebral arteries, nonruptured

EXCLUDES1 *ruptured cerebral arteries (I60.7)*

I67.1 Cerebral aneurysm, nonruptured

Cerebral aneurysm NOS
Cerebral arteriovenous fistula, acquired
Internal carotid artery aneurysm, intracranial portion
Internal carotid artery aneurysm, NOS

EXCLUDES1 *congenital cerebral aneurysm, nonruptured (Q28.-)*
ruptured cerebral aneurysm (I60.7)

I67.2 Cerebral atherosclerosis

Atheroma of cerebral and precerebral arteries [A]

I67.3 Progressive vascular leukoencephalopathy

Binswanger's disease

I67.4 Hypertensive encephalopathy

I67.5 Moyamoya disease

I67.6 Nonpyogenic thrombosis of intracranial venous system

Nonpyogenic thrombosis of cerebral vein
Nonpyogenic thrombosis of intracranial venous sinus

EXCLUDES1 *nonpyogenic thrombosis of intracranial venous system causing infarction (I63.6)*

I67.7 Cerebral arteritis, not elsewhere classified

Granulomatous angiitis of the nervous system

EXCLUDES1 *allergic granulomatous angiitis (M30.1)*

[5] I67.8 Other specified cerebrovascular diseases

I67.81 Acute cerebrovascular insufficiency

Acute cerebrovascular insufficiency unspecified as to location or reversibility

I67.82 Cerebral ischemia

Chronic cerebral ischemia

I67.83 Posterior reversible encephalopathy syndrome

PRES

[4] 4th character required [5] 5th character required [6] 6th character required [7] 7th character required [x7] Extension 'X' Alert
EXCLUDES1 Not coded here EXCLUDES2 Not included here PDx Primary Diagnosis Only Manifestation Code

[6] I67.84 Cerebral vasospasm and vasoconstriction
I67.841 Reversible cerebrovascular vasoconstriction syndrome
Call-Fleming syndrome
Code first underlying condition, if applicable, such as eclampsia (O15.00-O15.9)
I67.848 Other cerebrovascular vasospasm and vasoconstriction
I67.89 Other cerebrovascular disease
I67.9 Cerebrovascular disease, unspecified
[4] I68 Cerebrovascular disorders in diseases classified elsewhere
I68.0 Cerebral amyloid angiopathy
Code first underlying amyloidosis (E85.-)
I68.2 Cerebral arteritis in other diseases classified elsewhere
Code first underlying disease
[EXCLUDES1] *cerebral arteritis (in):*
listerosis (A32.89)
systemic lupus erythematosus (M32.19)
syphilis (A52.04)
tuberculosis (A18.89)
I68.8 Other cerebrovascular disorders in diseases classified elsewhere
Code first underlying disease
[EXCLUDES1] *syphilitic cerebral aneurysm (A52.05)*
[4] I69 Sequelae of cerebrovascular disease
[NOTES] Category I69 is to be used to indicate conditions in I60-I67 as the cause of sequelae. The 'sequelae' include conditions specified as such or as residuals which may occur at any time after the onset of the causal condition
[EXCLUDES1] *personal history of cerebral infarction without residual deficit (Z86.73)*
personal history of prolonged reversible ischemic neurologic deficit (PRIND) (Z86.73)
personal history of reversible ischemic neurologcial deficit (RIND) (Z86.73)
sequelae of traumatic intracranial injury (S06.-)
transient ischemic attack (TIA) (G45.9)
[5] I69.0 Sequelae of nontraumatic subarachnoid hemorrhage
I69.00 Unspecified sequelae of nontraumatic subarachnoid hemorrhage
I69.01 Cognitive deficits following nontraumatic subarachnoid hemorrhage
[6] I69.02 Speech and language deficits following nontraumatic subarachnoid hemorrhage
I69.020 Aphasia following nontraumatic subarachnoid hemorrhage
I69.021 Dysphasia following nontraumatic subarachnoid hemorrhage
I69.022 Dysarthria following nontraumatic subarachnoid hemorrhage
I69.023 Fluency disorder following nontraumatic subarachnoid hemorrhage
Stuttering following nontraumatic subarachnoid hemorrhage
I69.028 Other speech and language deficits following nontraumatic subarachnoid hemorrhage
[6] I69.03 Monoplegia of upper limb following nontraumatic subarachnoid hemorrhage
I69.031 Monoplegia of upper limb following nontraumatic subarachnoid hemorrhage affecting right dominant side
I69.032 Monoplegia of upper limb following nontraumatic subarachnoid hemorrhage affecting left dominant side
I69.033 Monoplegia of upper limb following nontraumatic subarachnoid hemorrhage affecting right non-dominant side
I69.034 Monoplegia of upper limb following nontraumatic subarachnoid hemorrhage affecting left non-dominant side
I69.039 Monoplegia of upper limb following nontraumatic subarachnoid hemorrhage affecting unspecified side
[6] I69.04 Monoplegia of lower limb following nontraumatic subarachnoid hemorrhage
I69.041 Monoplegia of lower limb following nontraumatic subarachnoid hemorrhage affecting right dominant side
I69.042 Monoplegia of lower limb following nontraumatic subarachnoid hemorrhage affecting left dominant side
I69.043 Monoplegia of lower limb following nontraumatic subarachnoid hemorrhage affecting right non-dominant side
I69.044 Monoplegia of lower limb following nontraumatic subarachnoid hemorrhage affecting left non-dominant side
I69.049 Monoplegia of lower limb following nontraumatic subarachnoid hemorrhage affecting unspecified side
[6] I69.05 Hemiplegia and hemiparesis following nontraumatic subarachnoid hemorrhage
I69.051 Hemiplegia and hemiparesis following nontraumatic subarachnoid hemorrhage affecting right dominant side
I69.052 Hemiplegia and hemiparesis following nontraumatic subarachnoid hemorrhage affecting left dominant side
I69.053 Hemiplegia and hemiparesis following nontraumatic subarachnoid hemorrhage affecting right non-dominant side
I69.054 Hemiplegia and hemiparesis following nontraumatic subarachnoid hemorrhage affecting left non-dominant side
I69.059 Hemiplegia and hemiparesis following nontraumatic subarachnoid hemorrhage affecting unspecified side
[6] I69.06 Other paralytic syndrome following nontraumatic subarachnoid hemorrhage
Use additional code to identify type of paralytic syndrome, such as:
locked-in state (G83.5)
quadriplegia (G82.5-)
[EXCLUDES1] *hemiplegia/hemiparesis following nontraumatic subarachnoid hemorrhage (I69.05-)*
monoplegia of lower limb following nontraumatic subarachnoid hemorrhage (I69.04-)
monoplegia of upper limb following nontraumatic subarachnoid hemorrhage (I69.03-)
I69.061 Other paralytic syndrome following nontraumatic subarachnoid hemorrhage affecting right dominant side
I69.062 Other paralytic syndrome following nontraumatic subarachnoid hemorrhage affecting left dominant side
I69.063 Other paralytic syndrome following nontraumatic subarachnoid hemorrhage affecting right non-dominant side
I69.064 Other paralytic syndrome following nontraumatic subarachnoid hemorrhage affecting left non-dominant side

Unspecified Code | Other Specified Code | [N] Newborn Age: 0 | [P] Pediatric Age: 0-17 | [M] Maternity Age: 12-55
[A] Adult Age: 15-124 | ♂ Male | ♀ Female | ● New Code | ▲ Revised Code Title | ►◄ Revised Text

I69.065　Other paralytic syndrome following nontraumatic subarachnoid hemorrhage, bilateral

I69.069　Other paralytic syndrome following nontraumatic subarachnoid hemorrhage affecting unspecified side

⑤ I69.09　Other sequelae of nontraumatic subarachnoid hemorrhage

I69.090　Apraxia following nontraumatic subarachnoid hemorrhage

I69.091　Dysphagia following nontraumatic subarachnoid hemorrhage

Use additional code to identify the type of dysphagia, if known (R13.1-)

I69.092　Facial weakness following nontraumatic subarachnoid hemorrhage

Facial droop following nontraumatic subarachnoid hemorrhage

I69.093　Ataxia following nontraumatic subarachnoid hemorrhage

I69.098　Other sequelae following nontraumatic subarachnoid hemorrhage

Alterations of sensation following nontraumatic subarachnoid hemorrhage

Disturbance of vision following nontraumatic subarachnoid hemorrhage

Use additional code to identify the sequelae

⑤ I69.1　Sequelae of nontraumatic intracerebral hemorrhage

I69.10　Unspecified sequelae of nontraumatic intracerebral hemorrhage

I69.11　Cognitive deficits following nontraumatic intracerebral hemorrhage

⑥ I69.12　Speech and language deficits following nontraumatic intracerebral hemorrhage

I69.120　Aphasia following nontraumatic intracerebral hemorrhage

I69.121　Dysphasia following nontraumatic intracerebral hemorrhage

I69.122　Dysarthria following nontraumatic intracerebral hemorrhage

I69.123　Fluency disorder following nontraumatic intracerebral hemorrhage

Stuttering following nontraumatic subarachnoid hemorrhage

I69.128　Other speech and language deficits following nontraumatic intracerebral hemorrhage

⑥ I69.13　Monoplegia of upper limb following nontraumatic intracerebral hemorrhage

I69.131　Monoplegia of upper limb following nontraumatic intracerebral hemorrhage affecting right dominant side

I69.132　Monoplegia of upper limb following nontraumatic intracerebral hemorrhage affecting left dominant side

I69.133　Monoplegia of upper limb following nontraumatic intracerebral hemorrhage affecting right non-dominant side

I69.134　Monoplegia of upper limb following nontraumatic intracerebral hemorrhage affecting left non-dominant side

I69.139　Monoplegia of upper limb following nontraumatic intracerebral hemorrhage affecting unspecified side

⑥ I69.14　Monoplegia of lower limb following nontraumatic intracerebral hemorrhage

I69.141　Monoplegia of lower limb following nontraumatic intracerebral hemorrhage affecting right dominant side

I69.142　Monoplegia of lower limb following nontraumatic intracerebral hemorrhage affecting left dominant side

I69.143　Monoplegia of lower limb following nontraumatic intracerebral hemorrhage affecting right non-dominant side

I69.144　Monoplegia of lower limb following nontraumatic intracerebral hemorrhage affecting left non-dominant side

I69.149　Monoplegia of lower limb following nontraumatic intracerebral hemorrhage affecting unspecified side

⑥ I69.15　Hemiplegia and hemiparesis following nontraumatic intracerebral hemorrhage

I69.151　Hemiplegia and hemiparesis following nontraumatic intracerebral hemorrhage affecting right dominant side

I69.152　Hemiplegia and hemiparesis following nontraumatic intracerebral hemorrhage affecting left dominant side

I69.153　Hemiplegia and hemiparesis following nontraumatic intracerebral hemorrhage affecting right non-dominant side

I69.154　Hemiplegia and hemiparesis following nontraumatic intracerebral hemorrhage affecting left non-dominant side

I69.159　Hemiplegia and hemiparesis following nontraumatic intracerebral hemorrhage affecting unspecified side

⑥ I69.16　Other paralytic syndrome following nontraumatic intracerebral hemorrhage

Use additional code to identify type of paralytic syndrome, such as:
locked-in state (G83.5)
quadriplegia (G82.5-)

EXCLUDES1　hemiplegia/hemiparesis following nontraumatic intracerebral hemorrhage (I69.15-)
monoplegia of lower limb following nontraumatic intracerebral hemorrhage (I69.14-)
monoplegia of upper limb following nontraumatic intracerebral hemorrhage (I69.13-)

I69.161　Other paralytic syndrome following nontraumatic intracerebral hemorrhage affecting right dominant side

I69.162　Other paralytic syndrome following nontraumatic intracerebral hemorrhage affecting left dominant side

I69.163　Other paralytic syndrome following nontraumatic intracerebral hemorrhage affecting right non-dominant side

I69.164　Other paralytic syndrome following nontraumatic intracerebral hemorrhage affecting left non-dominant side

I69.165　Other paralytic syndrome following nontraumatic intracerebral hemorrhage, bilateral

I69.169　Other paralytic syndrome following nontraumatic intracerebral hemorrhage affecting unspecified side

⑥ I69.19　Other sequelae of nontraumatic intracerebral hemorrhage

I69.190　Apraxia following nontraumatic intracerebral hemorrhage

I69.191　Dysphagia following nontraumatic intracerebral hemorrhage

Use additional code to identify the type of dysphagia, if known (R13.1-)

---

④ 4th character required　　⑤ 5th character required　　⑥ 6th character required　　⑦ 7th character required　　⑦ˣ Extension 'X' Alert

EXCLUDES 1 Not coded here　　EXCLUDES 2 Not included here　　PDx Primary Diagnosis Only　　Manifestation Code

I69.192 Facial weakness following nontraumatic intracerebral hemorrhage
Facial droop following nontraumatic intracerebral hemorrhage

I69.193 Ataxia following nontraumatic intracerebral hemorrhage

I69.198 Other sequelae of nontraumatic intracerebral hemorrhage
Alteration of sensations following nontraumatic intracerebral hemorrhage
Disturbance of vision following nontraumatic intracerebral hemorrhage
Use additional code to identify the sequelae

[5] I69.2 Sequelae of other nontraumatic intracranial hemorrhage

I69.20 Unspecified sequelae of other nontraumatic intracranial hemorrhage

I69.21 Cognitive deficits following other nontraumatic intracranial hemorrhage

[6] I69.22 Speech and language deficits following other nontraumatic intracranial hemorrhage

I69.220 Aphasia following other nontraumatic intracranial hemorrhage

I69.221 Dysphasia following other nontraumatic intracranial hemorrhage

I69.222 Dysarthria following other nontraumatic intracranial hemorrhage

I69.223 Fluency disorder following other nontraumatic intracranial hemorrhage
Stuttering following nontraumatic subarachnoid hemorrhage

I69.228 Other speech and language deficits following other nontraumatic intracranial hemorrhage

[6] I69.23 Monoplegia of upper limb following other nontraumatic intracranial hemorrhage

I69.231 Monoplegia of upper limb following other nontraumatic intracranial hemorrhage affecting right dominant side

I69.232 Monoplegia of upper limb following other nontraumatic intracranial hemorrhage affecting left dominant side

I69.233 Monoplegia of upper limb following other nontraumatic intracranial hemorrhage affecting right non-dominant side

I69.234 Monoplegia of upper limb following other nontraumatic intracranial hemorrhage affecting left non-dominant side

I69.239 Monoplegia of upper limb following other nontraumatic intracranial hemorrhage affecting unspecified side

[6] I69.24 Monoplegia of lower limb following other nontraumatic intracranial hemorrhage

I69.241 Monoplegia of lower limb following other nontraumatic intracranial hemorrhage affecting right dominant side

I69.242 Monoplegia of lower limb following other nontraumatic intracranial hemorrhage affecting left dominant side

I69.243 Monoplegia of lower limb following other nontraumatic intracranial hemorrhage affecting right non-dominant side

I69.244 Monoplegia of lower limb following other nontraumatic intracranial hemorrhage affecting left non-dominant side

I69.249 Monoplegia of lower limb following other nontraumatic intracranial hemorrhage affecting unspecified side

[6] I69.25 Hemiplegia and hemiparesis following other nontraumatic intracranial hemorrhage

I69.251 Hemiplegia and hemiparesis following other nontraumatic intracranial hemorrhage affecting right dominant side

I69.252 Hemiplegia and hemiparesis following other nontraumatic intracranial hemorrhage affecting left dominant side

I69.253 Hemiplegia and hemiparesis following other nontraumatic intracranial hemorrhage affecting right non-dominant side

I69.254 Hemiplegia and hemiparesis following other nontraumatic intracranial hemorrhage affecting left non-dominant side

I69.259 Hemiplegia and hemiparesis following other nontraumatic intracranial hemorrhage affecting unspecified side

[6] I69.26 Other paralytic syndrome following other nontraumatic intracranial hemorrhage
Use additional code to identify type of paralytic syndrome, such as:
locked-in state (G83.5)
quadriplegia (G82.5-)

[EXCLUDES1] *hemiplegia/hemiparesis following other nontraumatic intracranial hemorrhage (I69.25-)*
monoplegia of lower limb following other nontraumatic intracranial hemorrhage (I69.24-)
monoplegia of upper limb following other nontraumatic intracranial hemorrhage (I69.23-)

I69.261 Other paralytic syndrome following other nontraumatic intracranial hemorrhage affecting right dominant side

I69.262 Other paralytic syndrome following other nontraumatic intracranial hemorrhage affecting left dominant side

I69.263 Other paralytic syndrome following other nontraumatic intracranial hemorrhage affecting right non-dominant side

I69.264 Other paralytic syndrome following other nontraumatic intracranial hemorrhage affecting left non-dominant side

I69.265 Other paralytic syndrome following other nontraumatic intracranial hemorrhage, bilateral

I69.269 Other paralytic syndrome following other nontraumatic intracranial hemorrhage affecting unspecified side

[6] I69.29 Other sequelae of other nontraumatic intracranial hemorrhage

I69.290 Apraxia following other nontraumatic intracranial hemorrhage

I69.291 Dysphagia following other nontraumatic intracranial hemorrhage
Use additional code to identify the type of dysphagia, if known (R13.1-)

I69.292 Facial weakness following other nontraumatic intracranial hemorrhage
Facial droop following other nontraumatic intracranial hemorrhage

I69.293 Ataxia following other nontraumatic intracranial hemorrhage

I69.298 Other sequelae of other nontraumatic intracranial hemorrhage
Alteration of sensation following other nontraumatic intracranial hemorrhage
Disturbance of vision following other nontraumatic intracranial hemorrhage
Use additional code to identify the sequelae

⑤ **I69.3 Sequelae of** cerebral infarction

Sequelae of stroke NOS

I69.30 Unspecified sequelae of cerebral infarction

I69.31 Cognitive deficits **following cerebral infarction**

⑥ **I69.32** Speech and language deficits **following cerebral infarction**

I69.320 Aphasia **following cerebral infarction**

I69.321 Dysphasia **following cerebral infarction**

I69.322 Dysarthria **following cerebral infarction**

I69.323 Fluency disorder **following cerebral infarction**

Stuttering following nontraumatic subarachnoid hemorrhage

I69.328 Other speech and language deficits following cerebral infarction

⑥ **I69.33** Monoplegia of upper limb **following cerebral infarction**

I69.331 Monoplegia of upper limb following cerebral infarction affecting right dominant side

I69.332 Monoplegia of upper limb following cerebral infarction affecting left dominant side

I69.333 Monoplegia of upper limb following cerebral infarction affecting right non-dominant side

I69.334 Monoplegia of upper limb following cerebral infarction affecting left non-dominant side

I69.339 Monoplegia of upper limb following cerebral infarction affecting unspecified side

⑥ **I69.34** Monoplegia of lower limb **following cerebral infarction**

I69.341 Monoplegia of lower limb following cerebral infarction affecting right dominant side

I69.342 Monoplegia of lower limb following cerebral infarction affecting left dominant side

I69.343 Monoplegia of lower limb following cerebral infarction affecting right non-dominant side

I69.344 Monoplegia of lower limb following cerebral infarction affecting left non-dominant side

I69.349 Monoplegia of lower limb following cerebral infarction affecting unspecified side

⑥ **I69.35** Hemiplegia and hemiparesis **following cerebral infarction**

I69.351 Hemiplegia and hemiparesis following cerebral infarction affecting right dominant side

I69.352 Hemiplegia and hemiparesis following cerebral infarction affecting left dominant side

I69.353 Hemiplegia and hemiparesis following cerebral infarction affecting right non-dominant side

I69.354 Hemiplegia and hemiparesis following cerebral infarction affecting left non-dominant side

I69.359 Hemiplegia and hemiparesis following cerebral infarction affecting unspecified side

⑥ **I69.36** Other paralytic syndrome **following cerebral infarction**

Use additional code to identify type of paralytic syndrome, such as:

locked-in state (G83.5)

quadriplegia (G82.5-)

EXCLUDES1 *hemiplegia/hemiparesis following cerebral infarction (I69.35-)*

monoplegia of lower limb following cerebral infarction (I69.34-)

monoplegia of upper limb following cerebral infarction (I69.33-)

I69.361 Other paralytic syndrome following cerebral infarction affecting right dominant side

I69.362 Other paralytic syndrome following cerebral infarction affecting left dominant side

I69.363 Other paralytic syndrome following cerebral infarction affecting right non-dominant side

I69.364 Other paralytic syndrome following cerebral infarction affecting left non-dominant side

I69.365 Other paralytic syndrome following cerebral infarction, bilateral

I69.369 Other paralytic syndrome following cerebral infarction affecting unspecified side

⑥ **I69.39** Other sequelae of cerebral infarction

I69.390 Apraxia **following cerebral infarction**

I69.391 Dysphagia **following cerebral infarction**

Use additional code to identify the type of dysphagia, if known (R13.1-)

I69.392 Facial weakness **following cerebral infarction**

Facial droop following cerebral infarction

I69.393 Ataxia **following cerebral infarction**

I69.398 Other sequelae of cerebral infarction

Alteration of sensation following cerebral infarction

Disturbance of vision following cerebral infarction

Use additional code to identify the sequelae

⑤ **I69.8 Sequelae of** other cerebrovascular diseases

EXCLUDES1 *sequelae of traumatic intracranial injury (S06.-)*

I69.80 Unspecified sequelae of other cerebrovascular disease

I69.81 Cognitive deficits following other cerebrovascular disease

⑥ **I69.82** Speech and language deficits **following other cerebrovascular disease**

I69.820 Aphasia **following other cerebrovascular disease**

I69.821 Dysphasia **following other cerebrovascular disease**

I69.822 Dysarthria **following other cerebrovascular disease**

I69.823 Fluency disorder **following other cerebrovascular disease**

Stuttering following nontraumatic subarachnoid hemorrhage

I69.828 Other speech and language deficits following other cerebrovascular disease

⑥ **I69.83** Monoplegia of upper limb **following other cerebrovascular disease**

I69.831 Monoplegia of upper limb following other cerebrovascular disease affecting right dominant side

I69.832 Monoplegia of upper limb following other cerebrovascular disease affecting left dominant side

I69.833 Monoplegia of upper limb following other cerebrovascular disease affecting right non-dominant side

I69.834 Monoplegia of upper limb following other cerebrovascular disease affecting left non-dominant side

I69.839 Monoplegia of upper limb following other cerebrovascular disease affecting unspecified side

⑥ **I69.84** Monoplegia of lower limb **following other cerebrovascular disease**

---

④ 4ᵗʰ character required   ⑤ 5ᵗʰ character required   ⑥ 6ᵗʰ character required   ⑦ 7ᵗʰ character required   ⑦ˣ Extension 'X' Alert

EXCLUDES 1 Not coded here   *EXCLUDES 2* Not included here   ᴾᴰˣ Primary Diagnosis Only   Manifestation Code

228

ICD-10-CM 2015

I69.841 Monoplegia of lower limb following other cerebrovascular disease affecting right dominant side
I69.842 Monoplegia of lower limb following other cerebrovascular disease affecting left dominant side
I69.843 Monoplegia of lower limb following other cerebrovascular disease affecting right non-dominant side
I69.844 Monoplegia of lower limb following other cerebrovascular disease affecting left non-dominant side
I69.849 Monoplegia of lower limb following other cerebrovascular disease affecting unspecified side

[6] I69.85 Hemiplegia and hemiparesis following other cerebrovascular disease
I69.851 Hemiplegia and hemiparesis following other cerebrovascular disease affecting right dominant side
I69.852 Hemiplegia and hemiparesis following other cerebrovascular disease affecting left dominant side
I69.853 Hemiplegia and hemiparesis following other cerebrovascular disease affecting right non-dominant side
I69.854 Hemiplegia and hemiparesis following other cerebrovascular disease affecting left non-dominant side
I69.859 Hemiplegia and hemiparesis following other cerebrovascular disease affecting unspecified side

[6] I69.86 Other paralytic syndrome following other cerebrovascular disease
Use additional code to identify type of paralytic syndrome, such as:
locked-in state (G83.5)
quadriplegia (G82.5-)
[EXCLUDES1] *hemiplegia/hemiparesis following other cerebrovascular disease (I69.85-)*
monoplegia of lower limb following other cerebrovascular disease (I69.84-)
monoplegia of upper limb following other cerebrovascular disease (I69.83-)
I69.861 Other paralytic syndrome following other cerebrovascular disease affecting right dominant side
I69.862 Other paralytic syndrome following other cerebrovascular disease affecting left dominant side
I69.863 Other paralytic syndrome following other cerebrovascular disease affecting right non-dominant side
I69.864 Other paralytic syndrome following other cerebrovascular disease affecting left non-dominant side
I69.865 Other paralytic syndrome following other cerebrovascular disease, bilateral
I69.869 Other paralytic syndrome following other cerebrovascular disease affecting unspecified side

[6] I69.89 Other sequelae of other cerebrovascular disease
I69.890 Apraxia following other cerebrovascular disease
I69.891 Dysphagia following other cerebrovascular disease
Use additional code to identify the type of dysphagia, if known (R13.1-)
I69.892 Facial weakness following other cerebrovascular disease
Facial droop following other cerebrovascular disease
I69.893 Ataxia following other cerebrovascular disease
I69.898 Other sequelae of other cerebrovascular disease
Alteration of sensation following other cerebrovascular disease
Disturbance of vision following other cerebrovascular disease
Use additional code to identify the sequelae

[5] I69.9 Sequelae of unspecified cerebrovascular diseases
[EXCLUDES1] *sequelae of stroke (I69.3)*
sequelae of traumatic intracranial injury (S06.-)
I69.90 Unspecified sequelae of unspecified cerebrovascular disease
I69.91 Cognitive deficits following unspecified cerebrovascular disease

[6] I69.92 Speech and language deficits following unspecified cerebrovascular disease
I69.920 Aphasia following unspecified cerebrovascular disease
I69.921 Dysphasia following unspecified cerebrovascular disease
I69.922 Dysarthria following unspecified cerebrovascular disease
I69.923 Fluency disorder following unspecified cerebrovascular disease
Stuttering following nontraumatic subarachnoid hemorrhage
I69.928 Other speech and language deficits following unspecified cerebrovascular disease

[6] I69.93 Monoplegia of upper limb following unspecified cerebrovascular disease
I69.931 Monoplegia of upper limb following unspecified cerebrovascular disease affecting right dominant side
I69.932 Monoplegia of upper limb following unspecified cerebrovascular disease affecting left dominant side
I69.933 Monoplegia of upper limb following unspecified cerebrovascular disease affecting right non-dominant side
I69.934 Monoplegia of upper limb following unspecified cerebrovascular disease affecting left non-dominant side
I69.939 Monoplegia of upper limb following unspecified cerebrovascular disease affecting unspecified side

[6] I69.94 Monoplegia of lower limb following unspecified cerebrovascular disease
I69.941 Monoplegia of lower limb following unspecified cerebrovascular disease affecting right dominant side
I69.942 Monoplegia of lower limb following unspecified cerebrovascular disease affecting left dominant side
I69.943 Monoplegia of lower limb following unspecified cerebrovascular disease affecting right non-dominant side
I69.944 Monoplegia of lower limb following unspecified cerebrovascular disease affecting left non-dominant side
I69.949 Monoplegia of lower limb following unspecified cerebrovascular disease affecting unspecified side

Unspecified Code | Other Specified Code | [N] Newborn Age: 0 | [P] Pediatric Age: 0-17 | [M] Maternity Age: 12-55
[A] Adult Age: 15-124 | ♂ Male | ♀ Female | ● New Code | ▲ Revised Code Title | ►◄ Revised Text

[6] **I69.95 Hemiplegia and hemiparesis following unspecified cerebrovascular disease**

I69.951 Hemiplegia and hemiparesis following unspecified cerebrovascular disease affecting right dominant side

I69.952 Hemiplegia and hemiparesis following unspecified cerebrovascular disease affecting left dominant side

I69.953 Hemiplegia and hemiparesis following unspecified cerebrovascular disease affecting right non-dominant side

I69.954 Hemiplegia and hemiparesis following unspecified cerebrovascular disease affecting left non-dominant side

I69.959 Hemiplegia and hemiparesis following unspecified cerebrovascular disease affecting unspecified side

[6] **I69.96 Other paralytic syndrome following unspecified cerebrovascular disease**

Use additional code to identify type of paralytic syndrome, such as:
locked-in state (G83.5)
quadriplegia (G82.5-)

[EXCLUDES1] *hemiplegia/hemiparesis following unspecified cerebrovascular disease (I69.95-)*
monoplegia of lower limb following unspecified cerebrovascular disease (I69.94-)
monoplegia of upper limb following unspecified cerebrovascular disease (I69.93-)

I69.961 Other paralytic syndrome following unspecified cerebrovascular disease affecting right dominant side

I69.962 Other paralytic syndrome following unspecified cerebrovascular disease affecting left dominant side

I69.963 Other paralytic syndrome following unspecified cerebrovascular disease affecting right non-dominant side

I69.964 Other paralytic syndrome following unspecified cerebrovascular disease affecting left non-dominant side

I69.965 Other paralytic syndrome following unspecified cerebrovascular disease, bilateral

I69.969 Other paralytic syndrome following unspecified cerebrovascular disease affecting unspecified side

[6] **I69.99 Other sequelae of unspecified cerebrovascular disease**

I69.990 Apraxia following unspecified cerebrovascular disease

I69.991 Dysphagia following unspecified cerebrovascular disease

Use additional code to identify the type of dysphagia, if known (R13.1-)

I69.992 Facial weakness following unspecified cerebrovascular disease

Facial droop following unspecified cerebrovascular disease

I69.993 Ataxia following unspecified cerebrovascular disease

I69.998 Other sequelae following unspecified cerebrovascular disease

Alteration in sensation following unspecified cerebrovascular disease
Disturbance of vision following unspecified cerebrovascular disease

Use additional code to identify the sequelae

Diseases of arteries, arterioles and capillaries (I70-I79)

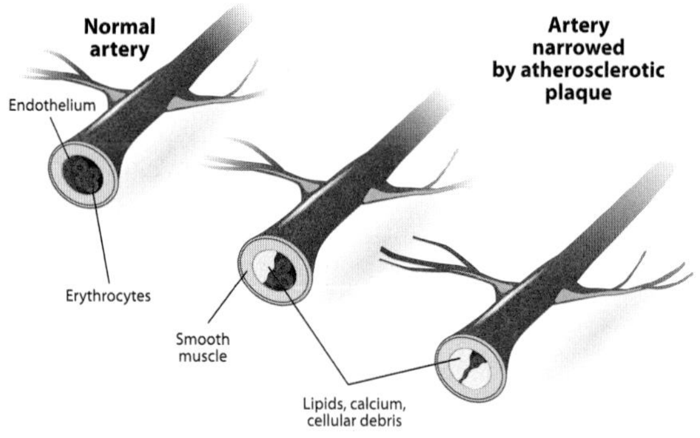

Figure 8.5 Atherosclerosis

[4] **I70 Atherosclerosis**

[INCLUDES] *arteriolosclerosis*
arterial degeneration
arteriosclerosis
arteriosclerotic vascular disease
arteriovascular degeneration
atheroma
endarteritis deformans or obliterans
senile arteritis
senile endarteritis
vascular degeneration

Use additional code to identify:
exposure to environmental tobacco smoke (Z77.22)
history of tobacco use (Z87.891)
occupational exposure to environmental tobacco smoke (Z57.31)
tobacco dependence (F17.-)
tobacco use (Z72.0)

[EXCLUDES2] *arteriosclerotic cardiovascular disease (I25.1-)*
arteriosclerotic heart disease (I25.1-)
atheroembolism (I75.-)
cerebral atherosclerosis (I67.2)
coronary atherosclerosis (I25.1-)
mesenteric atherosclerosis (K55.1)
precerebral atherosclerosis (I67.2)
primary pulmonary atherosclerosis (I27.0)

I70.0 Atherosclerosis of aorta [A]

I70.1 Atherosclerosis of renal artery

Goldblatt's kidney

[EXCLUDES2] *atherosclerosis of renal arterioles (I12.-)* [A]

[5] **I70.2 Atherosclerosis of native arteries of the extremities**

Mönckeberg's (medial) sclerosis
Use additional code, if applicable, to identify chronic total occlusion of artery of extremity (I70.92)

[EXCLUDES2] *atherosclerosis of bypass graft of extremities (I70.30-I70.79)*

[6] **I70.20 Unspecified atherosclerosis of native arteries of extremities**

I70.201 Unspecified atherosclerosis of native arteries of extremities, right leg [A]

I70.202 Unspecified atherosclerosis of native arteries of extremities, left leg [A]

I70.203 Unspecified atherosclerosis of native arteries of extremities, bilateral legs [A]

I70.208 Unspecified atherosclerosis of native arteries of extremities, other extremity [A]

I70.209 Unspecified atherosclerosis of native arteries of extremities, unspecified extremity [A]

[6] **I70.21 Atherosclerosis of native arteries of extremities with intermittent claudication**

[4] 4th character required [5] 5th character required [6] 6th character required [7] 7th character required [X] Extension 'X' Alert
[EXCLUDES 1] Not coded here [EXCLUDES 2] Not included here [PDX] Primary Diagnosis Only Manifestation Code

I70.211 Atherosclerosis of native arteries of extremities with intermittent claudication, right leg [A]

I70.212 Atherosclerosis of native arteries of extremities with intermittent claudication, left leg [A]

I70.213 Atherosclerosis of native arteries of extremities with intermittent claudication, bilateral legs [A]

I70.218 Atherosclerosis of native arteries of extremities with intermittent claudication, other extremity [A]

I70.219 Atherosclerosis of native arteries of extremities with intermittent claudication, unspecified extremity [A]

[6] I70.22 Atherosclerosis of native arteries of extremities with rest pain

INCLUDES *any condition classifiable to I70.21-*

I70.221 Atherosclerosis of native arteries of extremities with rest pain, right leg [A]

I70.222 Atherosclerosis of native arteries of extremities with rest pain, left leg [A]

I70.223 Atherosclerosis of native arteries of extremities with rest pain, bilateral legs [A]

I70.228 Atherosclerosis of native arteries of extremities with rest pain, other extremity [A]

I70.229 Atherosclerosis of native arteries of extremities with rest pain, unspecified extremity [A]

[6] I70.23 Atherosclerosis of native arteries of right leg with ulceration

INCLUDES *any condition classifiable to I70.211 and I70.221*

Use additional code to identify severity of ulcer (L97.-)

I70.231 Atherosclerosis of native arteries of right leg with ulceration of thigh [A]

I70.232 Atherosclerosis of native arteries of right leg with ulceration of calf [A]

I70.233 Atherosclerosis of native arteries of right leg with ulceration of ankle [A]

I70.234 Atherosclerosis of native arteries of right leg with ulceration of heel and midfoot

Atherosclerosis of native arteries of right leg with ulceration of plantar surface of midfoot [A]

I70.235 Atherosclerosis of native arteries of right leg with ulceration of other part of foot

Atherosclerosis of native arteries of right leg extremities with ulceration of toe [A]

I70.238 Atherosclerosis of native arteries of right leg with ulceration of other part of lower right leg [A]

I70.239 Atherosclerosis of native arteries of right leg with ulceration of unspecified site [A]

[6] I70.24 Atherosclerosis of native arteries of left leg with ulceration

INCLUDES *any condition classifiable to I70.212 and I70.222*

Use additional code to identify severity of ulcer (L97.-)

I70.241 Atherosclerosis of native arteries of left leg with ulceration of thigh [A]

I70.242 Atherosclerosis of native arteries of left leg with ulceration of calf [A]

I70.243 Atherosclerosis of native arteries of left leg with ulceration of ankle [A]

I70.244 Atherosclerosis of native arteries of left leg with ulceration of heel and midfoot

Atherosclerosis of native arteries of left leg with ulceration of plantar surface of midfoot [A]

I70.245 Atherosclerosis of native arteries of left leg with ulceration of other part of foot

Atherosclerosis of native arteries of left leg extremities with ulceration of toe [A]

I70.248 Atherosclerosis of native arteries of left leg with ulceration of other part of lower left leg [A]

I70.249 Atherosclerosis of native arteries of left leg with ulceration of unspecified site [A]

I70.25 Atherosclerosis of native arteries of other extremities with ulceration

INCLUDES *any condition classifiable to I70.218 and I70.228*

Use additional code to identify the severity of the ulcer (L98.49-) [A]

[6] I70.26 Atherosclerosis of native arteries of extremities with gangrene

INCLUDES *any condition classifiable to I70.21-, I70.22-, I70.23-, I70.24-, and I70.25-*

Use additional code to identify the severity of any ulcer (L97.-, L98.49-), if applicable

I70.261 Atherosclerosis of native arteries of extremities with gangrene, right leg [A]

I70.262 Atherosclerosis of native arteries of extremities with gangrene, left leg [A]

I70.263 Atherosclerosis of native arteries of extremities with gangrene, bilateral legs [A]

I70.268 Atherosclerosis of native arteries of extremities with gangrene, other extremity [A]

I70.269 Atherosclerosis of native arteries of extremities with gangrene, unspecified extremity [A]

[6] I70.29 Other atherosclerosis of native arteries of extremities

I70.291 Other atherosclerosis of native arteries of extremities, right leg [A]

I70.292 Other atherosclerosis of native arteries of extremities, left leg [A]

I70.293 Other atherosclerosis of native arteries of extremities, bilateral legs [A]

I70.298 Other atherosclerosis of native arteries of extremities, other extremity [A]

I70.299 Other atherosclerosis of native arteries of extremities, unspecified extremity [A]

[5] I70.3 Atherosclerosis of unspecified type of bypass graft(s) of the extremities

Use additional code, if applicable, to identify chronic total occlusion of artery of extremity (I70.92)

EXCLUDES1 *embolism or thrombus of bypass graft(s) of extremities (T82.8-)*

[6] I70.30 Unspecified atherosclerosis of unspecified type of bypass graft(s) of the extremities

I70.301 Unspecified atherosclerosis of unspecified type of bypass graft(s) of the extremities, right leg [A]

I70.302 Unspecified atherosclerosis of unspecified type of bypass graft(s) of the extremities, left leg [A]

I70.303 Unspecified atherosclerosis of unspecified type of bypass graft(s) of the extremities, bilateral legs [A]

I70.308 Unspecified atherosclerosis of unspecified type of bypass graft(s) of the extremities, other extremity [A]

I70.309 Unspecified atherosclerosis of unspecified type of bypass graft(s) of the extremities, unspecified extremity [A]

[6] I70.31 Atherosclerosis of unspecified type of bypass graft(s) of the extremities with intermittent claudication

Unspecified Code | Other Specified Code | [N] Newborn Age: 0 | [P] Pediatric Age: 0-17 | [M] Maternity Age: 12-55
[A] Adult Age: 15-124 | ♂ Male | ♀ Female | ● New Code | ▲ Revised Code Title | ►◄ Revised Text

I70.311 Atherosclerosis of unspecified type of bypass graft(s) of the extremities with intermittent claudication, right leg [A]
I70.312 Atherosclerosis of unspecified type of bypass graft(s) of the extremities with intermittent claudication, left leg [A]
I70.313 Atherosclerosis of unspecified type of bypass graft(s) of the extremities with intermittent claudication, bilateral legs [A]
I70.318 Atherosclerosis of unspecified type of bypass graft(s) of the extremities with intermittent claudication, other extremity [A]
I70.319 Atherosclerosis of unspecified type of bypass graft(s) of the extremities with intermittent claudication, unspecified extremity [A]

[6] I70.32 Atherosclerosis of unspecified type of bypass graft(s) of the extremities with rest pain

INCLUDES *any condition classifiable to I70.31-*

I70.321 Atherosclerosis of unspecified type of bypass graft(s) of the extremities with rest pain, right leg [A]
I70.322 Atherosclerosis of unspecified type of bypass graft(s) of the extremities with rest pain, left leg [A]
I70.323 Atherosclerosis of unspecified type of bypass graft(s) of the extremities with rest pain, bilateral legs [A]
I70.328 Atherosclerosis of unspecified type of bypass graft(s) of the extremities with rest pain, other extremity [A]
I70.329 Atherosclerosis of unspecified type of bypass graft(s) of the extremities with rest pain, unspecified extremity [A]

[6] I70.33 Atherosclerosis of unspecified type of bypass graft(s) of the right leg with ulceration

INCLUDES *any condition classifiable to I70.311 and I70.321*

Use additional code to identify severity of ulcer (L97.-)

I70.331 Atherosclerosis of unspecified type of bypass graft(s) of the right leg with ulceration of thigh [A]
I70.332 Atherosclerosis of unspecified type of bypass graft(s) of the right leg with ulceration of calf [A]
I70.333 Atherosclerosis of unspecified type of bypass graft(s) of the right leg with ulceration of ankle [A]
I70.334 Atherosclerosis of unspecified type of bypass graft(s) of the right leg with ulceration of heel and midfoot

Atherosclerosis of unspecified type of bypass graft(s) of right leg with ulceration of plantar surface of midfoot [A]

I70.335 Atherosclerosis of unspecified type of bypass graft(s) of the right leg with ulceration of other part of foot

Atherosclerosis of unspecified type of bypass graft(s) of the right leg with ulceration of toe [A]

I70.338 Atherosclerosis of unspecified type of bypass graft(s) of the right leg with ulceration of other part of lower leg [A]
I70.339 Atherosclerosis of unspecified type of bypass graft(s) of the right leg with ulceration of unspecified site [A]

[6] I70.34 Atherosclerosis of unspecified type of bypass graft(s) of the left leg with ulceration

INCLUDES *any condition classifiable to I70.312 and I70.322*

Use additional code to identify severity of ulcer (L97.-)

I70.341 Atherosclerosis of unspecified type of bypass graft(s) of the left leg with ulceration of thigh [A]
I70.342 Atherosclerosis of unspecified type of bypass graft(s) of the left leg with ulceration of calf [A]
I70.343 Atherosclerosis of unspecified type of bypass graft(s) of the left leg with ulceration of ankle [A]
I70.344 Atherosclerosis of unspecified type of bypass graft(s) of the left leg with ulceration of heel and midfoot

Atherosclerosis of unspecified type of bypass graft(s) of left leg with ulceration of plantar surface of midfoot [A]

I70.345 Atherosclerosis of unspecified type of bypass graft(s) of the left leg with ulceration of other part of foot

Atherosclerosis of unspecified type of bypass graft(s) of the left leg with ulceration of toe [A]

I70.348 Atherosclerosis of unspecified type of bypass graft(s) of the left leg with ulceration of other part of lower leg [A]
I70.349 Atherosclerosis of unspecified type of bypass graft(s) of the left leg with ulceration of unspecified site [A]

I70.35 Atherosclerosis of unspecified type of bypass graft(s) of other extremity with ulceration

INCLUDES *any condition classifiable to I70.318 and I70.328*

Use additional code to identify severity of ulcer (L98.49-) [A]

[6] I70.36 Atherosclerosis of unspecified type of bypass graft(s) of the extremities with gangrene

INCLUDES *any condition classifiable to I70.31-, I70.32-, I70.33-, I70.34-, I70.35*

Use additional code to identify the severity of any ulcer (L97.-, L98.49-), if applicable

I70.361 Atherosclerosis of unspecified type of bypass graft(s) of the extremities with gangrene, right leg [A]
I70.362 Atherosclerosis of unspecified type of bypass graft(s) of the extremities with gangrene, left leg [A]
I70.363 Atherosclerosis of unspecified type of bypass graft(s) of the extremities with gangrene, bilateral legs [A]
I70.368 Atherosclerosis of unspecified type of bypass graft(s) of the extremities with gangrene, other extremity [A]
I70.369 Atherosclerosis of unspecified type of bypass graft(s) of the extremities with gangrene, unspecified extremity [A]

[6] I70.39 Other atherosclerosis of unspecified type of bypass graft(s) of the extremities

I70.391 Other atherosclerosis of unspecified type of bypass graft(s) of the extremities, right leg [A]
I70.392 Other atherosclerosis of unspecified type of bypass graft(s) of the extremities, left leg [A]
I70.393 Other atherosclerosis of unspecified type of bypass graft(s) of the extremities, bilateral legs [A]
I70.398 Other atherosclerosis of unspecified type of bypass graft(s) of the extremities, other extremity [A]
I70.399 Other atherosclerosis of unspecified type of bypass graft(s) of the extremities, unspecified extremity [A]

[5] I70.4 Atherosclerosis of autologous vein bypass graft(s) of the extremities

Use additional code, if applicable, to identify chronic total occlusion of artery of extremity (I70.92)

[6] I70.40 Unspecified atherosclerosis of autologous vein bypass graft(s) of the extremities

[4] 4th character required [5] 5th character required [6] 6th character required [7] 7th character required [X] Extension 'X' Alert
EXCLUDES 1 Not coded here EXCLUDES 2 Not included here PDX Primary Diagnosis Only Manifestation Code

I70.401 Unspecified atherosclerosis of autologous vein bypass graft(s) of the extremities, right leg 🄰

I70.402 Unspecified atherosclerosis of autologous vein bypass graft(s) of the extremities, left leg 🄰

I70.403 Unspecified atherosclerosis of autologous vein bypass graft(s) of the extremities, bilateral legs 🄰

I70.408 Unspecified atherosclerosis of autologous vein bypass graft(s) of the extremities, other extremity 🄰

I70.409 Unspecified atherosclerosis of autologous vein bypass graft(s) of the extremities, unspecified extremity 🄰

⑥ I70.41 Atherosclerosis of autologous vein bypass graft(s) of the extremities with intermittent claudication

I70.411 Atherosclerosis of autologous vein bypass graft(s) of the extremities with intermittent claudication, right leg 🄰

I70.412 Atherosclerosis of autologous vein bypass graft(s) of the extremities with intermittent claudication, left leg 🄰

I70.413 Atherosclerosis of autologous vein bypass graft(s) of the extremities with intermittent claudication, bilateral legs 🄰

I70.418 Atherosclerosis of autologous vein bypass graft(s) of the extremities with intermittent claudication, other extremity 🄰

I70.419 Atherosclerosis of autologous vein bypass graft(s) of the extremities with intermittent claudication, unspecified extremity 🄰

⑥ I70.42 Atherosclerosis of autologous vein bypass graft(s) of the extremities with rest pain

INCLUDES any condition classifiable to I70.41-

I70.421 Atherosclerosis of autologous vein bypass graft(s) of the extremities with rest pain, right leg 🄰

I70.422 Atherosclerosis of autologous vein bypass graft(s) of the extremities with rest pain, left leg 🄰

I70.423 Atherosclerosis of autologous vein bypass graft(s) of the extremities with rest pain, bilateral legs 🄰

I70.428 Atherosclerosis of autologous vein bypass graft(s) of the extremities with rest pain, other extremity 🄰

I70.429 Atherosclerosis of autologous vein bypass graft(s) of the extremities with rest pain, unspecified extremity 🄰

⑥ I70.43 Atherosclerosis of autologous vein bypass graft(s) of the right leg with ulceration

INCLUDES any condition classifiable to I70.411 and I70.421
Use additional code to identify severity of ulcer (L97.-)

I70.431 Atherosclerosis of autologous vein bypass graft(s) of the right leg with ulceration of thigh 🄰

I70.432 Atherosclerosis of autologous vein bypass graft(s) of the right leg with ulceration of calf 🄰

I70.433 Atherosclerosis of autologous vein bypass graft(s) of the right leg with ulceration of ankle 🄰

I70.434 Atherosclerosis of autologous vein bypass graft(s) of the right leg with ulceration of heel and midfoot
Atherosclerosis of autologous vein bypass graft(s) of right leg with ulceration of plantar surface of midfoot 🄰

I70.435 Atherosclerosis of autologous vein bypass graft(s) of the right leg with ulceration of other part of foot
Atherosclerosis of autologous vein bypass graft(s) of right leg with ulceration of toe 🄰

I70.438 Atherosclerosis of autologous vein bypass graft(s) of the right leg with ulceration of other part of lower leg 🄰

I70.439 Atherosclerosis of autologous vein bypass graft(s) of the right leg with ulceration of unspecified site 🄰

⑥ I70.44 Atherosclerosis of autologous vein bypass graft(s) of the left leg with ulceration

INCLUDES any condition classifiable to I70.412 and I70.422
Use additional code to identify severity of ulcer (L97.-)

I70.441 Atherosclerosis of autologous vein bypass graft(s) of the left leg with ulceration of thigh 🄰

I70.442 Atherosclerosis of autologous vein bypass graft(s) of the left leg with ulceration of calf 🄰

I70.443 Atherosclerosis of autologous vein bypass graft(s) of the left leg with ulceration of ankle 🄰

I70.444 Atherosclerosis of autologous vein bypass graft(s) of the left leg with ulceration of heel and midfoot
Atherosclerosis of autologous vein bypass graft(s) of left leg with ulceration of plantar surface of midfoot 🄰

I70.445 Atherosclerosis of autologous vein bypass graft(s) of the left leg with ulceration of other part of foot
Atherosclerosis of autologous vein bypass graft(s) of left leg with ulceration of toe 🄰

I70.448 Atherosclerosis of autologous vein bypass graft(s) of the left leg with ulceration of other part of lower leg 🄰

I70.449 Atherosclerosis of autologous vein bypass graft(s) of the left leg with ulceration of unspecified site 🄰

I70.45 Atherosclerosis of autologous vein bypass graft(s) of other extremity with ulceration

INCLUDES any condition classifiable to I70.418, I70.428, and I70.438
Use additional code to identify severity of ulcer (L98.49) 🄰

⑥ I70.46 Atherosclerosis of autologous vein bypass graft(s) of the extremities with gangrene

INCLUDES any condition classifiable to I70.41-, I70.42-, and I70.43-, I70.44-, I70.45
Use additional code to identify the severity of any ulcer (L97.-, L98.49-), if applicable

I70.461 Atherosclerosis of autologous vein bypass graft(s) of the extremities with gangrene, right leg 🄰

I70.462 Atherosclerosis of autologous vein bypass graft(s) of the extremities with gangrene, left leg 🄰

I70.463 Atherosclerosis of autologous vein bypass graft(s) of the extremities with gangrene, bilateral legs 🄰

I70.468 Atherosclerosis of autologous vein bypass graft(s) of the extremities with gangrene, other extremity 🄰

I70.469 Atherosclerosis of autologous vein bypass graft(s) of the extremities with gangrene, unspecified extremity 🄰

Unspecified Code   Other Specified Code   🄽 Newborn Age: 0   🄿 Pediatric Age: 0-17   🄼 Maternity Age: 12-55
🄰 Adult Age: 15-124   ♂ Male   ♀ Female   ● New Code   ▲ Revised Code Title   ►◄ Revised Text

CHAPTER 9: DISEASES OF THE CIRCULATORY SYSTEM (I00-I99)

I70.49 - I70.55

⑥ I70.49 Other atherosclerosis of autologous vein bypass graft(s) of the extremities
- I70.491 Other atherosclerosis of autologous vein bypass graft(s) of the extremities, right leg Ⓐ
- I70.492 Other atherosclerosis of autologous vein bypass graft(s) of the extremities, left leg Ⓐ
- I70.493 Other atherosclerosis of autologous vein bypass graft(s) of the extremities, bilateral legs Ⓐ
- I70.498 Other atherosclerosis of autologous vein bypass graft(s) of the extremities, other extremity Ⓐ
- I70.499 Other atherosclerosis of autologous vein bypass graft(s) of the extremities, unspecified extremity Ⓐ

⑤ I70.5 Atherosclerosis of nonautologous biological bypass graft(s) of the extremities

Use additional code, if applicable, to identify chronic total occlusion of artery of extremity (I70.92)

⑥ I70.50 Unspecified atherosclerosis of nonautologous biological bypass graft(s) of the extremities
- I70.501 Unspecified atherosclerosis of nonautologous biological bypass graft(s) of the extremities, right leg Ⓐ
- I70.502 Unspecified atherosclerosis of nonautologous biological bypass graft(s) of the extremities, left leg Ⓐ
- I70.503 Unspecified atherosclerosis of nonautologous biological bypass graft(s) of the extremities, bilateral legs Ⓐ
- I70.508 Unspecified atherosclerosis of nonautologous biological bypass graft(s) of the extremities, other extremity Ⓐ
- I70.509 Unspecified atherosclerosis of nonautologous biological bypass graft(s) of the extremities, unspecified extremity Ⓐ

⑥ I70.51 Atherosclerosis of nonautologous biological bypass graft(s) of the extremities with intermittent claudication
- I70.511 Atherosclerosis of nonautologous biological bypass graft(s) of the extremities with intermittent claudication, right leg Ⓐ
- I70.512 Atherosclerosis of nonautologous biological bypass graft(s) of the extremities with intermittent claudication, left leg Ⓐ
- I70.513 Atherosclerosis of nonautologous biological bypass graft(s) of the extremities with intermittent claudication, bilateral legs Ⓐ
- I70.518 Atherosclerosis of nonautologous biological bypass graft(s) of the extremities with intermittent claudication, other extremity Ⓐ
- I70.519 Atherosclerosis of nonautologous biological bypass graft(s) of the extremities with intermittent claudication, unspecified extremity Ⓐ

⑥ I70.52 Atherosclerosis of nonautologous biological bypass graft(s) of the extremities with rest pain
  INCLUDES   any condition classifiable to I70.51-
- I70.521 Atherosclerosis of nonautologous biological bypass graft(s) of the extremities with rest pain, right leg Ⓐ
- I70.522 Atherosclerosis of nonautologous biological bypass graft(s) of the extremities with rest pain, left leg Ⓐ
- I70.523 Atherosclerosis of nonautologous biological bypass graft(s) of the extremities with rest pain, bilateral legs Ⓐ
- I70.528 Atherosclerosis of nonautologous biological bypass graft(s) of the extremities with rest pain, other extremity Ⓐ

- I70.529 Atherosclerosis of nonautologous biological bypass graft(s) of the extremities with rest pain, unspecified extremity Ⓐ

⑥ I70.53 Atherosclerosis of nonautologous biological bypass graft(s) of the right leg with ulceration
  INCLUDES   any condition classifiable to I70.511 and I70.521
  Use additional code to identify severity of ulcer (L97.-)
- I70.531 Atherosclerosis of nonautologous biological bypass graft(s) of the right leg with ulceration of thigh Ⓐ
- I70.532 Atherosclerosis of nonautologous biological bypass graft(s) of the right leg with ulceration of calf Ⓐ
- I70.533 Atherosclerosis of nonautologous biological bypass graft(s) of the right leg with ulceration of ankle Ⓐ
- I70.534 Atherosclerosis of nonautologous biological bypass graft(s) of the right leg with ulceration of heel and midfoot

  Atherosclerosis of nonautologous biological bypass graft(s) of right leg with ulceration of plantar surface of midfoot Ⓐ
- I70.535 Atherosclerosis of nonautologous biological bypass graft(s) of the right leg with ulceration of other part of foot

  Atherosclerosis of nonautologous biological bypass graft(s) of the right leg with ulceration of toe Ⓐ
- I70.538 Atherosclerosis of nonautologous biological bypass graft(s) of the right leg with ulceration of other part of lower leg Ⓐ
- I70.539 Atherosclerosis of nonautologous biological bypass graft(s) of the right leg with ulceration of unspecified site Ⓐ

⑥ I70.54 Atherosclerosis of nonautologous biological bypass graft(s) of the left leg with ulceration
  INCLUDES   any condition classifiable to I70.512 and I70.522
  Use additional code to identify severity of ulcer (L97.-)
- I70.541 Atherosclerosis of nonautologous biological bypass graft(s) of the left leg with ulceration of thigh Ⓐ
- I70.542 Atherosclerosis of nonautologous biological bypass graft(s) of the left leg with ulceration of calf Ⓐ
- I70.543 Atherosclerosis of nonautologous biological bypass graft(s) of the left leg with ulceration of ankle Ⓐ
- I70.544 Atherosclerosis of nonautologous biological bypass graft(s) of the left leg with ulceration of heel and midfoot

  Atherosclerosis of nonautologous biological bypass graft(s) of left leg with ulceration of plantar surface of midfoot Ⓐ
- I70.545 Atherosclerosis of nonautologous biological bypass graft(s) of the left leg with ulceration of other part of foot

  Atherosclerosis of nonautologous biological bypass graft(s) of the left leg with ulceration of toe Ⓐ
- I70.548 Atherosclerosis of nonautologous biological bypass graft(s) of the left leg with ulceration of other part of lower leg Ⓐ
- I70.549 Atherosclerosis of nonautologous biological bypass graft(s) of the left leg with ulceration of unspecified site Ⓐ

I70.55 Atherosclerosis of nonautologous biological bypass graft(s) of other extremity with ulceration
  INCLUDES   any condition classifiable to I70.518, I70.528, and I70.538
  Use additional code to identify severity of ulcer (L98.49) Ⓐ

---

④ 4ᵗʰ character required   ⑤ 5ᵗʰ character required   ⑥ 6ᵗʰ character required   ⑦ 7ᵗʰ character required   ⑩ Extension 'X' Alert

EXCLUDES 1 Not coded here   **EXCLUDES 2** Not included here   PDx Primary Diagnosis Only   Manifestation Code

[6] I70.56 Atherosclerosis of nonautologous biological bypass graft(s) of the extremities with gangrene
[INCLUDES] *any condition classifiable to I70.51-, I70.52-, and I70.53-, I70.54-, I70.55*
Use additional code to identify the severity of any ulcer (L97.-, L98.49-), if applicable
I70.561 Atherosclerosis of nonautologous biological bypass graft(s) of the extremities with gangrene, right leg [A]
I70.562 Atherosclerosis of nonautologous biological bypass graft(s) of the extremities with gangrene, left leg [A]
I70.563 Atherosclerosis of nonautologous biological bypass graft(s) of the extremities with gangrene, bilateral legs [A]
I70.568 Atherosclerosis of nonautologous biological bypass graft(s) of the extremities with gangrene, other extremity [A]
I70.569 Atherosclerosis of nonautologous biological bypass graft(s) of the extremities with gangrene, unspecified extremity [A]
[6] I70.59 Other atherosclerosis of nonautologous biological bypass graft(s) of the extremities
I70.591 Other atherosclerosis of nonautologous biological bypass graft(s) of the extremities, right leg [A]
I70.592 Other atherosclerosis of nonautologous biological bypass graft(s) of the extremities, left leg [A]
I70.593 Other atherosclerosis of nonautologous biological bypass graft(s) of the extremities, bilateral legs [A]
I70.598 Other atherosclerosis of nonautologous biological bypass graft(s) of the extremities, other extremity [A]
I70.599 Other atherosclerosis of nonautologous biological bypass graft(s) of the extremities, unspecified extremity [A]
[5] I70.6 Atherosclerosis of nonbiological bypass graft(s) of the extremities
Use additional code, if applicable, to identify chronic total occlusion of artery of extremity (I70.92)
[6] I70.60 Unspecified atherosclerosis of nonbiological bypass graft(s) of the extremities
I70.601 Unspecified atherosclerosis of nonbiological bypass graft(s) of the extremities, right leg [A]
I70.602 Unspecified atherosclerosis of nonbiological bypass graft(s) of the extremities, left leg [A]
I70.603 Unspecified atherosclerosis of nonbiological bypass graft(s) of the extremities, bilateral legs [A]
I70.608 Unspecified atherosclerosis of nonbiological bypass graft(s) of the extremities, other extremity [A]
I70.609 Unspecified atherosclerosis of nonbiological bypass graft(s) of the extremities, unspecified extremity [A]
[6] I70.61 Atherosclerosis of nonbiological bypass graft(s) of the extremities with intermittent claudication
I70.611 Atherosclerosis of nonbiological bypass graft(s) of the extremities with intermittent claudication, right leg [A]
I70.612 Atherosclerosis of nonbiological bypass graft(s) of the extremities with intermittent claudication, left leg [A]
I70.613 Atherosclerosis of nonbiological bypass graft(s) of the extremities with intermittent claudication, bilateral legs [A]
I70.618 Atherosclerosis of nonbiological bypass graft(s) of the extremities with intermittent claudication, other extremity [A]
I70.619 Atherosclerosis of nonbiological bypass graft(s) of the extremities with intermittent claudication, unspecified extremity [A]
[6] I70.62 Atherosclerosis of nonbiological bypass graft(s) of the extremities with rest pain
[INCLUDES] *any condition classifiable to I70.61-*
I70.621 Atherosclerosis of nonbiological bypass graft(s) of the extremities with rest pain, right leg [A]
I70.622 Atherosclerosis of nonbiological bypass graft(s) of the extremities with rest pain, left leg [A]
I70.623 Atherosclerosis of nonbiological bypass graft(s) of the extremities with rest pain, bilateral legs [A]
I70.628 Atherosclerosis of nonbiological bypass graft(s) of the extremities with rest pain, other extremity [A]
I70.629 Atherosclerosis of nonbiological bypass graft(s) of the extremities with rest pain, unspecified extremity [A]
[6] I70.63 Atherosclerosis of nonbiological bypass graft(s) of the right leg with ulceration
[INCLUDES] *any condition classifiable to I70.611 and I70.621*
Use additional code to identify severity of ulcer (L97.-)
I70.631 Atherosclerosis of nonbiological bypass graft(s) of the right leg with ulceration of thigh [A]
I70.632 Atherosclerosis of nonbiological bypass graft(s) of the right leg with ulceration of calf [A]
I70.633 Atherosclerosis of nonbiological bypass graft(s) of the right leg with ulceration of ankle [A]
I70.634 Atherosclerosis of nonbiological bypass graft(s) of the right leg with ulceration of heel and midfoot
Atherosclerosis of nonbiological bypass graft(s) of right leg with ulceration of plantar surface of midfoot [A]
I70.635 Atherosclerosis of nonbiological bypass graft(s) of the right leg with ulceration of other part of foot
Atherosclerosis of nonbiological bypass graft(s) of the right leg with ulceration of toe [A]
I70.638 Atherosclerosis of nonbiological bypass graft(s) of the right leg with ulceration of other part of lower leg [A]
I70.639 Atherosclerosis of nonbiological bypass graft(s) of the right leg with ulceration of unspecified site [A]
[6] I70.64 Atherosclerosis of nonbiological bypass graft(s) of the left leg with ulceration
[INCLUDES] *any condition classifiable to I70.612 and I70.622*
Use additional code to identify severity of ulcer (L97.-)
I70.641 Atherosclerosis of nonbiological bypass graft(s) of the left leg with ulceration of thigh [A]
I70.642 Atherosclerosis of nonbiological bypass graft(s) of the left leg with ulceration of calf [A]
I70.643 Atherosclerosis of nonbiological bypass graft(s) of the left leg with ulceration of ankle [A]
I70.644 Atherosclerosis of nonbiological bypass graft(s) of the left leg with ulceration of heel and midfoot
Atherosclerosis of nonbiological bypass graft(s) of left leg with ulceration of plantar surface of midfoot [A]

Unspecified Code | Other Specified Code | [N] Newborn Age: 0 | [P] Pediatric Age: 0-17 | [M] Maternity Age: 12-55
[A] Adult Age: 15-124 | ♂ Male | ♀ Female | ● New Code | ▲ Revised Code Title | ►◄ Revised Text

I70.645 Atherosclerosis of nonbiological bypass graft(s) of the left leg with ulceration of other part of foot

Atherosclerosis of nonbiological bypass graft(s) of the left leg with ulceration of toe Ⓐ

I70.648 Atherosclerosis of nonbiological bypass graft(s) of the left leg with ulceration of other part of lower leg Ⓐ

I70.649 Atherosclerosis of nonbiological bypass graft(s) of the left leg with ulceration of unspecified site Ⓐ

I70.65 Atherosclerosis of nonbiological bypass graft(s) of other extremity with ulceration

INCLUDES any condition classifiable to I70.618 and I70.628

Use additional code to identify severity of ulcer (L98.49) Ⓐ

Ⓖ **I70.66** Atherosclerosis of nonbiological bypass graft(s) of the extremities with gangrene

INCLUDES any condition classifiable to I70.61-, I70.62-, I70.63-, I70.64-, I70.65

Use additional code to identify the severity of any ulcer (L97.-, L98.49-), if applicable

I70.661 Atherosclerosis of nonbiological bypass graft(s) of the extremities with gangrene, right leg Ⓐ

I70.662 Atherosclerosis of nonbiological bypass graft(s) of the extremities with gangrene, left leg Ⓐ

I70.663 Atherosclerosis of nonbiological bypass graft(s) of the extremities with gangrene, bilateral legs Ⓐ

I70.668 Atherosclerosis of nonbiological bypass graft(s) of the extremities with gangrene, other extremity Ⓐ

I70.669 Atherosclerosis of nonbiological bypass graft(s) of the extremities with gangrene, unspecified extremity Ⓐ

Ⓖ **I70.69** Other atherosclerosis of nonbiological bypass graft(s) of the extremities

I70.691 Other atherosclerosis of nonbiological bypass graft(s) of the extremities, right leg Ⓐ

I70.692 Other atherosclerosis of nonbiological bypass graft(s) of the extremities, left leg Ⓐ

I70.693 Other atherosclerosis of nonbiological bypass graft(s) of the extremities, bilateral legs Ⓐ

I70.698 Other atherosclerosis of nonbiological bypass graft(s) of the extremities, other extremity Ⓐ

I70.699 Other atherosclerosis of nonbiological bypass graft(s) of the extremities, unspecified extremity Ⓐ

Ⓢ **I70.7** Atherosclerosis of other type of bypass graft(s) of the extremities

Use additional code, if applicable, to identify chronic total occlusion of artery of extremity (I70.92)

Ⓖ **I70.70** Unspecified atherosclerosis of other type of bypass graft(s) of the extremities

I70.701 Unspecified atherosclerosis of other type of bypass graft(s) of the extremities, right leg Ⓐ

I70.702 Unspecified atherosclerosis of other type of bypass graft(s) of the extremities, left leg Ⓐ

I70.703 Unspecified atherosclerosis of other type of bypass graft(s) of the extremities, bilateral legs Ⓐ

I70.708 Unspecified atherosclerosis of other type of bypass graft(s) of the extremities, other extremity Ⓐ

I70.709 Unspecified atherosclerosis of other type of bypass graft(s) of the extremities, unspecified extremity Ⓐ

Ⓖ **I70.71** Atherosclerosis of other type of bypass graft(s) of the extremities with intermittent claudication

I70.711 Atherosclerosis of other type of bypass graft(s) of the extremities with intermittent claudication, right leg Ⓐ

I70.712 Atherosclerosis of other type of bypass graft(s) of the extremities with intermittent claudication, left leg Ⓐ

I70.713 Atherosclerosis of other type of bypass graft(s) of the extremities with intermittent claudication, bilateral legs Ⓐ

I70.718 Atherosclerosis of other type of bypass graft(s) of the extremities with intermittent claudication, other extremity Ⓐ

I70.719 Atherosclerosis of other type of bypass graft(s) of the extremities with intermittent claudication, unspecified extremity Ⓐ

Ⓖ **I70.72** Atherosclerosis of other type of bypass graft(s) of the extremities with rest pain

INCLUDES any condition classifiable to I70.71-

I70.721 Atherosclerosis of other type of bypass graft(s) of the extremities with rest pain, right leg Ⓐ

I70.722 Atherosclerosis of other type of bypass graft(s) of the extremities with rest pain, left leg Ⓐ

I70.723 Atherosclerosis of other type of bypass graft(s) of the extremities with rest pain, bilateral legs Ⓐ

I70.728 Atherosclerosis of other type of bypass graft(s) of the extremities with rest pain, other extremity Ⓐ

I70.729 Atherosclerosis of other type of bypass graft(s) of the extremities with rest pain, unspecified extremity Ⓐ

Ⓖ **I70.73** Atherosclerosis of other type of bypass graft(s) of the right leg with ulceration

INCLUDES any condition classifiable to I70.711 and I70.721

Use additional code to identify severity of ulcer (L97.-)

I70.731 Atherosclerosis of other type of bypass graft(s) of the right leg with ulceration of thigh Ⓐ

I70.732 Atherosclerosis of other type of bypass graft(s) of the right leg with ulceration of calf Ⓐ

I70.733 Atherosclerosis of other type of bypass graft(s) of the right leg with ulceration of ankle Ⓐ

I70.734 Atherosclerosis of other type of bypass graft(s) of the right leg with ulceration of heel and midfoot

Atherosclerosis of other type of bypass graft(s) of right leg with ulceration of plantar surface of midfoot Ⓐ

I70.735 Atherosclerosis of other type of bypass graft(s) of the right leg with ulceration of other part of foot

Atherosclerosis of other type of bypass graft(s) of right leg with ulceration of toe Ⓐ

I70.738 Atherosclerosis of other type of bypass graft(s) of the right leg with ulceration of other part of lower leg Ⓐ

I70.739 Atherosclerosis of other type of bypass graft(s) of the right leg with ulceration of unspecified site Ⓐ

Ⓐ 4ᵗʰ character required   Ⓢ 5ᵗʰ character required   Ⓖ 6ᵗʰ character required   Ⓐ 7ᵗʰ character required   Ⓐ Extension 'X' Alert

EXCLUDES 1 Not coded here   **EXCLUDES 2** Not included here   ℞ Primary Diagnosis Only   Manifestation Code

[6] I70.74 Atherosclerosis of other type of bypass graft(s) of the left leg with ulceration

INCLUDES *any condition classifiable to I70.712 and I70.722*

Use additional code to identify severity of ulcer (L97.-)

I70.741 Atherosclerosis of other type of bypass graft(s) of the left leg with ulceration of thigh [A]

I70.742 Atherosclerosis of other type of bypass graft(s) of the left leg with ulceration of calf [A]

I70.743 Atherosclerosis of other type of bypass graft(s) of the left leg with ulceration of ankle [A]

I70.744 Atherosclerosis of other type of bypass graft(s) of the left leg with ulceration of heel and midfoot

Atherosclerosis of other type of bypass graft(s) of left leg with ulceration of plantar surface of midfoot [A]

I70.745 Atherosclerosis of other type of bypass graft(s) of the left leg with ulceration of other part of foot

Atherosclerosis of other type of bypass graft(s) of left leg with ulceration of toe [A]

I70.748 Atherosclerosis of other type of bypass graft(s) of the left leg with ulceration of other part of lower leg [A]

I70.749 Atherosclerosis of other type of bypass graft(s) of the left leg with ulceration of unspecified site [A]

I70.75 Atherosclerosis of other type of bypass graft(s) of other extremity with ulceration

INCLUDES *any condition classifiable to I70.718 and I70.728*

Use additional code to identify severity of ulcer (L98.49) [A]

[6] I70.76 Atherosclerosis of other type of bypass graft(s) of the extremities with gangrene

INCLUDES *any condition classifiable to I70.71-, I70.72-, I70.73-, I70.74-, I70.75*

Use additional code to identify the severity of any ulcer (L97.-, L98.49-), if applicable

I70.761 Atherosclerosis of other type of bypass graft(s) of the extremities with gangrene, right leg [A]

I70.762 Atherosclerosis of other type of bypass graft(s) of the extremities with gangrene, left leg [A]

I70.763 Atherosclerosis of other type of bypass graft(s) of the extremities with gangrene, bilateral legs [A]

I70.768 Atherosclerosis of other type of bypass graft(s) of the extremities with gangrene, other extremity [A]

I70.769 Atherosclerosis of other type of bypass graft(s) of the extremities with gangrene, unspecified extremity [A]

[6] I70.79 Other atherosclerosis of other type of bypass graft(s) of the extremities

I70.791 Other atherosclerosis of other type of bypass graft(s) of the extremities, right leg [A]

I70.792 Other atherosclerosis of other type of bypass graft(s) of the extremities, left leg [A]

I70.793 Other atherosclerosis of other type of bypass graft(s) of the extremities, bilateral legs [A]

I70.798 Other atherosclerosis of other type of bypass graft(s) of the extremities, other extremity [A]

I70.799 Other atherosclerosis of other type of bypass graft(s) of the extremities, unspecified extremity [A]

I70.8 Atherosclerosis of other arteries [A]

[5] I70.9 Other and unspecified atherosclerosis

I70.90 Unspecified atherosclerosis [A]

I70.91 Generalized atherosclerosis [A]

I70.92 Chronic total occlusion of artery of the extremities

Complete occlusion of artery of the extremities

Total occlusion of artery of the extremities

Code first atherosclerosis of arteries of the extremities (I70.2-, I70.3-, I70.4-, I70.5-, I70.6-, I70.7-) [A]

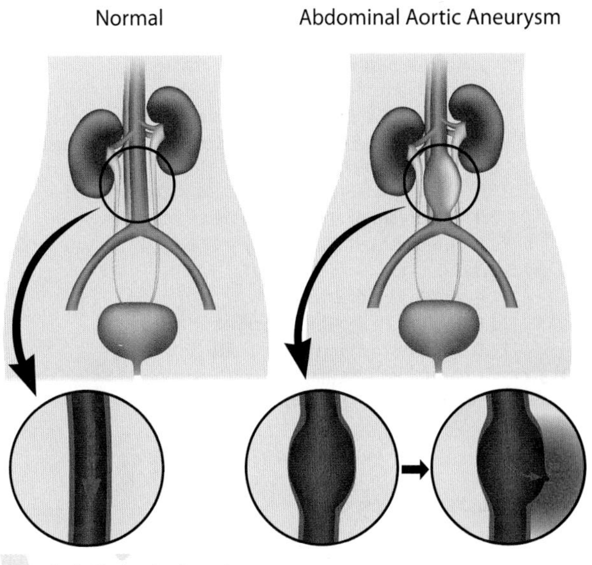

Figure 8.6 Abdominal aortic aneurysm

[4] I71 Aortic aneurysm and dissection

EXCLUDES1 *aortic ectasia (I77.81-)*
syphilitic aortic aneurysm (A52.01)
traumatic aortic aneurysm (S25.09, S35.09)

[5] I71.0 Dissection of aorta

I71.00 Dissection of unspecified site of aorta

I71.01 Dissection of thoracic aorta

I71.02 Dissection of abdominal aorta

I71.03 Dissection of thoracoabdominal aorta

I71.1 Thoracic aortic aneurysm, ruptured

I71.2 Thoracic aortic aneurysm, without rupture

I71.3 Abdominal aortic aneurysm, ruptured

I71.4 Abdominal aortic aneurysm, without rupture

I71.5 Thoracoabdominal aortic aneurysm, ruptured

I71.6 Thoracoabdominal aortic aneurysm, without rupture

I71.8 Aortic aneurysm of unspecified site, ruptured

Rupture of aorta NOS

I71.9 Aortic aneurysm of unspecified site, without rupture

Aneurysm of aorta

Dilatation of aorta

Hyaline necrosis of aorta

Unspecified Code | Other Specified Code | [N] Newborn Age: 0 | [P] Pediatric Age: 0-17 | [M] Maternity Age: 12-55
[A] Adult Age: 15-124 | ♂ Male | ♀ Female | ● New Code | ▲ Revised Code Title | ►◄ Revised Text

[4] I72 Other aneurysm

INCLUDES *aneurysm (cirsoid) (false) (ruptured)*

EXCLUDES2 *acquired aneurysm (I77.0)*
aneurysm (of) aorta (I71.-)
aneurysm (of) arteriovenous NOS (Q27.3-)
carotid artery dissection (I77.71)
cerebral (nonruptured) aneurysm (I67.1)
coronary aneurysm (I25.4)
coronary artery dissection (I25.42)
dissection of artery NEC (I77.79)
heart aneurysm (I25.3)
iliac artery dissection (I77.72)
pulmonary artery aneurysm (I28.1)
renal artery dissection (I77.73)
retinal aneurysm (H35.0)
ruptured cerebral aneurysm (I60.7)
varicose aneurysm (I77.0)
vertebral artery dissection (I77.74)

I72.0 Aneurysm of carotid artery
Aneurysm of common carotid artery
Aneurysm of external carotid artery
Aneurysm of internal carotid artery, extracranial portion
EXCLUDES1 *aneurysm of internal carotid artery, intracranial portion (I67.1)*
aneurysm of internal carotid artery NOS (I67.1)

I72.1 Aneurysm of artery of upper extremity
I72.2 Aneurysm of renal artery
I72.3 Aneurysm of iliac artery
I72.4 Aneurysm of artery of lower extremity
I72.8 Aneurysm of other specified arteries
I72.9 Aneurysm of unspecified site

[4] I73 Other peripheral vascular diseases

EXCLUDES2 *chilblains (T69.1)*
frostbite (T33-T34)
immersion hand or foot (T69.0-)
spasm of cerebral artery (G45.9)

[5] **I73.0 Raynaud's syndrome**
Raynaud's disease
Raynaud's phenomenon (secondary)
I73.00 Raynaud's syndrome without gangrene
I73.01 Raynaud's syndrome with gangrene

I73.1 Thromboangiitis obliterans [Buerger's disease]

[5] **I73.8 Other specified peripheral vascular diseases**
EXCLUDES1 *diabetic (peripheral) angiopathy (E08-E13 with .51-.52)*
I73.81 Erythromelalgia
I73.89 Other specified peripheral vascular diseases
Acrocyanosis
Erythrocyanosis
Simple acroparesthesia [Schultze's type]
Vasomotor acroparesthesia [Nothnagel's type]

I73.9 Peripheral vascular disease, unspecified
Intermittent claudication
Peripheral angiopathy NOS
Spasm of artery
EXCLUDES1 *atherosclerosis of the extremities (I70.2--I70.7-)*

[4] I74 Arterial embolism and thrombosis

INCLUDES *embolic infarction*
embolic occlusion
thrombotic infarction
thrombotic occlusion

Code first embolism and thrombosis complicating abortion or ectopic or molar pregnancy (O00-O07, O08.2)
embolism and thrombosis complicating pregnancy, childbirth and the puerperium (O88.-)

EXCLUDES2 *atheroembolism (I75.-)*
basilar embolism and thrombosis (I63.0-I63.2, I65.1)
carotid embolism and thrombosis (I63.0-I63.2, I65.2)
cerebral embolism and thrombosis (I63.3-I63.5, I66.-)
coronary embolism and thrombosis (I21-I25)
mesenteric embolism and thrombosis (K55.0)
ophthalmic embolism and thrombosis (H34.-)
precerebral embolism and thrombosis NOS (I63.0-I63.2, I65.9)
pulmonary embolism and thrombosis (I26.-)
renal embolism and thrombosis (N28.0)
retinal embolism and thrombosis (H34.-)
septic embolism and thrombosis (I76)
vertebral embolism and thrombosis (I63.0-I63.2, I65.0)

[5] **I74.0 Embolism and thrombosis of abdominal aorta**
I74.01 Saddle embolus of abdominal aorta
I74.09 Other arterial embolism and thrombosis of abdominal aorta
Aortic bifurcation syndrome
Aortoiliac obstruction
Leriche's syndrome

[5] **I74.1 Embolism and thrombosis of other and unspecified parts of aorta**
I74.10 Embolism and thrombosis of unspecified parts of aorta
I74.11 Embolism and thrombosis of thoracic aorta
I74.19 Embolism and thrombosis of other parts of aorta

I74.2 Embolism and thrombosis of arteries of the upper extremities
I74.3 Embolism and thrombosis of arteries of the lower extremities
I74.4 Embolism and thrombosis of arteries of extremities, unspecified
Peripheral arterial embolism NOS
I74.5 Embolism and thrombosis of iliac artery
I74.8 Embolism and thrombosis of other arteries
I74.9 Embolism and thrombosis of unspecified artery

[4] I75 Atheroembolism

INCLUDES *atherothrombotic microembolism*
cholesterol embolism

[5] **I75.0 Atheroembolism of extremities**
[6] **I75.01 Atheroembolism of upper extremity**
I75.011 Atheroembolism of right upper extremity
I75.012 Atheroembolism of left upper extremity
I75.013 Atheroembolism of bilateral upper extremities
I75.019 Atheroembolism of unspecified upper extremity
[6] **I75.02 Atheroembolism of lower extremity**
I75.021 Atheroembolism of right lower extremity
I75.022 Atheroembolism of left lower extremity
I75.023 Atheroembolism of bilateral lower extremities
I75.029 Atheroembolism of unspecified lower extremity

[5] **I75.8 Atheroembolism of other sites**
I75.81 Atheroembolism of kidney
Use additional code for any associated acute kidney failure and chronic kidney disease (N17.-, N18.-)
I75.89 Atheroembolism of other site

I76 Septic arterial embolism

Code first underlying infection, such as:
infective endocarditis (I33.0)
lung abscess (J85.-)
Use additional code to identify the site of the embolism (I74.-)

EXCLUDES2 *septic pulmonary embolism (I26.01, I26.90)*

[4] 4th character required [5] 5th character required [6] 6th character required [7] 7th character required [X] Extension 'X' Alert
EXCLUDES1 Not coded here EXCLUDES2 Not included here [PDx] Primary Diagnosis Only Manifestation Code

[4] I77 Other disorders of arteries and arterioles
EXCLUDES2 *collagen (vascular) diseases (M30-M36)*
hypersensitivity angiitis (M31.0)
pulmonary artery (I28.-)

I77.0 Arteriovenous fistula, acquired
Aneurysmal varix
Arteriovenous aneurysm, acquired
EXCLUDES1 *arteriovenous aneurysm NOS (Q27.3-)*
presence of arteriovenous shunt (fistula) for dialysis (Z99.2)
traumatic - see injury of blood vessel by body region
EXCLUDES2 *cerebral (I67.1)*
coronary (I25.4)

I77.1 Stricture of artery
Narrowing of artery

I77.2 Rupture of artery
Erosion of artery
Fistula of artery
Ulcer of artery
EXCLUDES1 *traumatic rupture of artery - see injury of blood vessel by body region*

I77.3 Arterial fibromuscular dysplasia
Fibromuscular hyperplasia (of) carotid artery
Fibromuscular hyperplasia (of) renal artery

I77.4 Celiac artery compression syndrome

I77.5 Necrosis of artery

I77.6 Arteritis, unspecified
Aortitis NOS
Endarteritis NOS
EXCLUDES1 *arteritis or endarteritis:*
aortic arch (M31.4)
cerebral NEC (I67.7)
coronary (I25.89)
deformans (I70.-)
giant cell (M31.5., M31.6)
obliterans (I70.-)
senile (I70.-)

[5] I77.7 Other arterial dissection
EXCLUDES2 *dissection of aorta (I71.0-)*
dissection of coronary artery (I25.42)

I77.71 Dissection of carotid artery
I77.72 Dissection of iliac artery
I77.73 Dissection of renal artery
I77.74 Dissection of vertebral artery
I77.79 Dissection of other artery

[5] I77.8 Other specified disorders of arteries and arterioles

[6] I77.81 Aortic ectasia
Ectasis aorta
EXCLUDES1 *aortic aneurysm and dissection (I71.0-)*

I77.810 Thoracic aortic ectasia
I77.811 Abdominal aortic ectasia
I77.812 Thoracoabdominal aortic ectasia
I77.819 Aortic ectasia, unspecified site

I77.89 Other specified disorders of arteries and arterioles

I77.9 Disorder of arteries and arterioles, unspecified

[4] I78 Diseases of capillaries

I78.0 Hereditary hemorrhagic telangiectasia
Rendu-Osler-Weber disease

I78.1 Nevus, non-neoplastic
Araneus nevus
Senile nevus
Spider nevus
Stellar nevus
EXCLUDES1 *nevus NOS (D22.-)*
vascular NOS (Q82.5)
EXCLUDES2 *blue nevus (D22.-)*
flammeus nevus (Q82.5)
hairy nevus (D22.-)
melanocytic nevus (D22.-)
pigmented nevus (D22.-)
portwine nevus (Q82.5)
sanguineous nevus (Q82.5)
strawberry nevus (Q82.5)
verrucous nevus (Q82.5)

I78.8 Other diseases of capillaries

I78.9 Disease of capillaries, unspecified

[4] I79 Disorders of arteries, arterioles and capillaries in diseases classified elsewhere

I79.0 Aneurysm of aorta in diseases classified elsewhere
Code first underlying disease
EXCLUDES1 *syphilitic aneurysm (A52.01)*

I79.1 Aortitis in diseases classified elsewhere
Code first underlying disease
EXCLUDES1 *syphilitic aortitis (A52.02)*

I79.8 Other disorders of arteries, arterioles and capillaries in diseases classified elsewhere
Code first underlying disease, such as:
amyloidosis (E85.-)
EXCLUDES1 *diabetic (peripheral) angiopathy (E08-E13 with .51-.52)*
syphilitic endarteritis (A52.09)
tuberculous endarteritis (A18.89)

Diseases of veins, lymphatic vessels and lymph nodes, not elsewhere classified (I80-I89)

[4] I80 Phlebitis and thrombophlebitis
INCLUDES *endophlebitis*
inflammation, vein
periphlebitis
suppurative phlebitis
Code first phlebitis and thrombophlebitis complicating abortion, ectopic or molar pregnancy (O00-O07, O08.7)
phlebitis and thrombophlebitis complicating pregnancy, childbirth and the puerperium (O22.-, O87.-)
EXCLUDES1 *venous embolism and thrombosis of lower extremities (I82.4-, I82.5-, I82.81-)*

[5] I80.0 Phlebitis and thrombophlebitis of superficial vessels of lower extremities
Phlebitis and thrombophlebitis of femoropopliteal vein

I80.00 Phlebitis and thrombophlebitis of superficial vessels of unspecified lower extremity
I80.01 Phlebitis and thrombophlebitis of superficial vessels of right lower extremity
I80.02 Phlebitis and thrombophlebitis of superficial vessels of left lower extremity
I80.03 Phlebitis and thrombophlebitis of superficial vessels of lower extremities, bilateral

[5] I80.1 Phlebitis and thrombophlebitis of femoral vein

I80.10 Phlebitis and thrombophlebitis of unspecified femoral vein
I80.11 Phlebitis and thrombophlebitis of right femoral vein
I80.12 Phlebitis and thrombophlebitis of left femoral vein
I80.13 Phlebitis and thrombophlebitis of femoral vein, bilateral

[5] I80.2 Phlebitis and thrombophlebitis of other and unspecified deep vessels of lower extremities

[6] I80.20 Phlebitis and thrombophlebitis of unspecified deep vessels of lower extremities

Unspecified Code | Other Specified Code | [N] Newborn Age: 0 | [P] Pediatric Age: 0-17 | [M] Maternity Age: 12-55
[A] Adult Age: 15-124 | ♂ Male | ♀ Female | ● New Code | ▲ Revised Code Title | ►◄ Revised Text

I80.201 Phlebitis and thrombophlebitis of unspecified deep vessels of right lower extremity

I80.202 Phlebitis and thrombophlebitis of unspecified deep vessels of left lower extremity

I80.203 Phlebitis and thrombophlebitis of unspecified deep vessels of lower extremities, bilateral

I80.209 Phlebitis and thrombophlebitis of unspecified deep vessels of unspecified lower extremity

⑥ I80.21 Phlebitis and thrombophlebitis of iliac vein

I80.211 Phlebitis and thrombophlebitis of right iliac vein

I80.212 Phlebitis and thrombophlebitis of left iliac vein

I80.213 Phlebitis and thrombophlebitis of iliac vein, bilateral

I80.219 Phlebitis and thrombophlebitis of unspecified iliac vein

⑥ I80.22 Phlebitis and thrombophlebitis of popliteal vein

I80.221 Phlebitis and thrombophlebitis of right popliteal vein

I80.222 Phlebitis and thrombophlebitis of left popliteal vein

I80.223 Phlebitis and thrombophlebitis of popliteal vein, bilateral

I80.229 Phlebitis and thrombophlebitis of unspecified popliteal vein

⑥ I80.23 Phlebitis and thrombophlebitis of tibial vein

I80.231 Phlebitis and thrombophlebitis of right tibial vein

I80.232 Phlebitis and thrombophlebitis of left tibial vein

I80.233 Phlebitis and thrombophlebitis of tibial vein, bilateral

I80.239 Phlebitis and thrombophlebitis of unspecified tibial vein

⑥ I80.29 Phlebitis and thrombophlebitis of other deep vessels of lower extremities

I80.291 Phlebitis and thrombophlebitis of other deep vessels of right lower extremity

I80.292 Phlebitis and thrombophlebitis of other deep vessels of left lower extremity

I80.293 Phlebitis and thrombophlebitis of other deep vessels of lower extremity, bilateral

I80.299 Phlebitis and thrombophlebitis of other deep vessels of unspecified lower extremity

I80.3 Phlebitis and thrombophlebitis of lower extremities, unspecified

I80.8 Phlebitis and thrombophlebitis of other sites

I80.9 Phlebitis and thrombophlebitis of unspecified site

I81 Portal vein thrombosis

Portal (vein) obstruction

EXCLUDES2 hepatic vein thrombosis (I82.0)
phlebitis of portal vein (K75.1)

④ I82 Other venous embolism and thrombosis

Code first venous embolism and thrombosis complicating:
abortion, ectopic or molar pregnancy (O00-O07, O08.7)
pregnancy, childbirth and the puerperium (O22.-, O87.-)

EXCLUDES2 venous embolism and thrombosis (of):
cerebral (I63.6, I67.6)
coronary (I21-I25)
intracranial and intraspinal, septic or NOS (G08)
intracranial, nonpyogenic (I67.6)
intraspinal, nonpyogenic (G95.1)
mesenteric (K55.0)
portal (I81)
pulmonary (I26.-)

I82.0 Budd-Chiari syndrome

Hepatic vein thrombosis

I82.1 Thrombophlebitis migrans

⑤ I82.2 Embolism and thrombosis of vena cava and other thoracic veins

⑥ I82.21 Embolism and thrombosis of superior vena cava

I82.210 Acute embolism and thrombosis of superior vena cava

Embolism and thrombosis of superior vena cava NOS

I82.211 Chronic embolism and thrombosis of superior vena cava

⑥ I82.22 Embolism and thrombosis of inferior vena cava

I82.220 Acute embolism and thrombosis of inferior vena cava

Embolism and thrombosis of inferior vena cava NOS

I82.221 Chronic embolism and thrombosis of inferior vena cava

⑥ I82.29 Embolism and thrombosis of other thoracic veins

Embolism and thrombosis of brachiocephalic (innominate) vein

I82.290 Acute embolism and thrombosis of other thoracic veins

I82.291 Chronic embolism and thrombosis of other thoracic veins

I82.3 Embolism and thrombosis of renal vein

⑤ I82.4 Acute embolism and thrombosis of deep veins of lower extremity

⑥ I82.40 Acute embolism and thrombosis of unspecified deep veins of lower extremity

Deep vein thrombosis NOS
DVT NOS

EXCLUDES1 acute embolism and thrombosis of unspecified deep veins of distal lower extremity (I82.4Z-)
acute embolism and thrombosis of unspecified deep veins of proximal lower extremity (I82.4Y-)

I82.401 Acute embolism and thrombosis of unspecified deep veins of right lower extremity

I82.402 Acute embolism and thrombosis of unspecified deep veins of left lower extremity

I82.403 Acute embolism and thrombosis of unspecified deep veins of lower extremity, bilateral

I82.409 Acute embolism and thrombosis of unspecified deep veins of unspecified lower extremity

⑥ I82.41 Acute embolism and thrombosis of femoral vein

I82.411 Acute embolism and thrombosis of right femoral vein

I82.412 Acute embolism and thrombosis of left femoral vein

④ 4th character required   ⑤ 5th character required   ⑥ 6th character required   ⑦ 7th character required   Ⓧ Extension 'X' Alert

EXCLUDES 1 Not coded here   EXCLUDES 2 Not included here   PDx Primary Diagnosis Only   Manifestation Code

240

ICD-10-CM 2015

I82.413 Acute embolism and thrombosis of femoral vein, bilateral

I82.419 Acute embolism and thrombosis of unspecified femoral vein

[6] I82.42 Acute embolism and thrombosis of iliac vein

I82.421 Acute embolism and thrombosis of right iliac vein

I82.422 Acute embolism and thrombosis of left iliac vein

I82.423 Acute embolism and thrombosis of iliac vein, bilateral

I82.429 Acute embolism and thrombosis of unspecified iliac vein

[6] I82.43 Acute embolism and thrombosis of popliteal vein

I82.431 Acute embolism and thrombosis of right popliteal vein

I82.432 Acute embolism and thrombosis of left popliteal vein

I82.433 Acute embolism and thrombosis of popliteal vein, bilateral

I82.439 Acute embolism and thrombosis of unspecified popliteal vein

[6] I82.44 Acute embolism and thrombosis of tibial vein

I82.441 Acute embolism and thrombosis of right tibial vein

I82.442 Acute embolism and thrombosis of left tibial vein

I82.443 Acute embolism and thrombosis of tibial vein, bilateral

I82.449 Acute embolism and thrombosis of unspecified tibial vein

[6] I82.49 Acute embolism and thrombosis of other specified deep vein of lower extremity

I82.491 Acute embolism and thrombosis of other specified deep vein of right lower extremity

I82.492 Acute embolism and thrombosis of other specified deep vein of left lower extremity

I82.493 Acute embolism and thrombosis of other specified deep vein of lower extremity, bilateral

I82.499 Acute embolism and thrombosis of other specified deep vein of unspecified lower extremity

[6] I82.4Y Acute embolism and thrombosis of unspecified deep veins of proximal lower extremity

Acute embolism and thrombosis of deep vein of thigh NOS

Acute embolism and thrombosis of deep vein of upper leg NOS

I82.4Y1 Acute embolism and thrombosis of unspecified deep veins of right proximal lower extremity

I82.4Y2 Acute embolism and thrombosis of unspecified deep veins of left proximal lower extremity

I82.4Y3 Acute embolism and thrombosis of unspecified deep veins of proximal lower extremity, bilateral

I82.4Y9 Acute embolism and thrombosis of unspecified deep veins of unspecified proximal lower extremity

[6] I82.4Z Acute embolism and thrombosis of unspecified deep veins of distal lower extremity

Acute embolism and thrombosis of deep vein of calf NOS

Acute embolism and thrombosis of deep vein of lower leg NOS

I82.4Z1 Acute embolism and thrombosis of unspecified deep veins of right distal lower extremity

I82.4Z2 Acute embolism and thrombosis of unspecified deep veins of left distal lower extremity

I82.4Z3 Acute embolism and thrombosis of unspecified deep veins of distal lower extremity, bilateral

I82.4Z9 Acute embolism and thrombosis of unspecified deep veins of unspecified distal lower extremity

[5] I82.5 Chronic embolism and thrombosis of deep veins of lower extremity

Use additional code, if applicable, for associated long-term (current) use of anticoagulants (Z79.01)

[EXCLUDES1] *personal history of venous embolism and thrombosis (Z86.718)*

[6] I82.50 Chronic embolism and thrombosis of unspecified deep veins of lower extremity

[EXCLUDES1] *chronic embolism and thrombosis of unspecified deep veins of distal lower extremity (I82.5Z-)*
chronic embolism and thrombosis of unspecified deep veins of proximal lower extremity (I82.5Y-)

I82.501 Chronic embolism and thrombosis of unspecified deep veins of right lower extremity

I82.502 Chronic embolism and thrombosis of unspecified deep veins of left lower extremity

I82.503 Chronic embolism and thrombosis of unspecified deep veins of lower extremity, bilateral

I82.509 Chronic embolism and thrombosis of unspecified deep veins of unspecified lower extremity

[6] I82.51 Chronic embolism and thrombosis of femoral vein

I82.511 Chronic embolism and thrombosis of right femoral vein

I82.512 Chronic embolism and thrombosis of left femoral vein

I82.513 Chronic embolism and thrombosis of femoral vein, bilateral

I82.519 Chronic embolism and thrombosis of unspecified femoral vein

[6] I82.52 Chronic embolism and thrombosis of iliac vein

I82.521 Chronic embolism and thrombosis of right iliac vein

I82.522 Chronic embolism and thrombosis of left iliac vein

I82.523 Chronic embolism and thrombosis of iliac vein, bilateral

I82.529 Chronic embolism and thrombosis of unspecified iliac vein

[6] I82.53 Chronic embolism and thrombosis of popliteal vein

I82.531 Chronic embolism and thrombosis of right popliteal vein

I82.532 Chronic embolism and thrombosis of left popliteal vein

I82.533 Chronic embolism and thrombosis of popliteal vein, bilateral

I82.539 Chronic embolism and thrombosis of unspecified popliteal vein

[6] I82.54 Chronic embolism and thrombosis of tibial vein

I82.541 Chronic embolism and thrombosis of right tibial vein

I82.542 Chronic embolism and thrombosis of left tibial vein

I82.543 Chronic embolism and thrombosis of tibial vein, bilateral

I82.549 Chronic embolism and thrombosis of unspecified tibial vein

⑥ I82.59 Chronic embolism and thrombosis of other specified deep vein of lower extremity

I82.591 Chronic embolism and thrombosis of other specified deep vein of right lower extremity

I82.592 Chronic embolism and thrombosis of other specified deep vein of left lower extremity

I82.593 Chronic embolism and thrombosis of other specified deep vein of lower extremity, bilateral

I82.599 Chronic embolism and thrombosis of other specified deep vein of unspecified lower extremity

⑥ I82.5Y Chronic embolism and thrombosis of unspecified deep veins of proximal lower extremity

Chronic embolism and thrombosis of deep veins of thigh NOS
Chronic embolism and thrombosis of deep veins of upper leg NOS

I82.5Y1 Chronic embolism and thrombosis of unspecified deep veins of right proximal lower extremity

I82.5Y2 Chronic embolism and thrombosis of unspecified deep veins of left proximal lower extremity

I82.5Y3 Chronic embolism and thrombosis of unspecified deep veins of proximal lower extremity, bilateral

I82.5Y9 Chronic embolism and thrombosis of unspecified deep veins of unspecified proximal lower extremity

⑥ I82.5Z Chronic embolism and thrombosis of unspecified deep veins of distal lower extremity

Chronic embolism and thrombosis of deep veins of calf NOS
Chronic embolism and thrombosis of deep veins of lower leg NOS

I82.5Z1 Chronic embolism and thrombosis of unspecified deep veins of right distal lower extremity

I82.5Z2 Chronic embolism and thrombosis of unspecified deep veins of left distal lower extremity

I82.5Z3 Chronic embolism and thrombosis of unspecified deep veins of distal lower extremity, bilateral

I82.5Z9 Chronic embolism and thrombosis of unspecified deep veins of unspecified distal lower extremity

⑤ I82.6 Acute embolism and thrombosis of veins of upper extremity

⑥ I82.60 Acute embolism and thrombosis of unspecified veins of upper extremity

I82.601 Acute embolism and thrombosis of unspecified veins of right upper extremity

I82.602 Acute embolism and thrombosis of unspecified veins of left upper extremity

I82.603 Acute embolism and thrombosis of unspecified veins of upper extremity, bilateral

I82.609 Acute embolism and thrombosis of unspecified veins of unspecified upper extremity

⑥ I82.61 Acute embolism and thrombosis of superficial veins of upper extremity

Acute embolism and thrombosis of antecubital vein
Acute embolism and thrombosis of basilic vein
Acute embolism and thrombosis of cephalic vein

I82.611 Acute embolism and thrombosis of superficial veins of right upper extremity

I82.612 Acute embolism and thrombosis of superficial veins of left upper extremity

I82.613 Acute embolism and thrombosis of superficial veins of upper extremity, bilateral

I82.619 Acute embolism and thrombosis of superficial veins of unspecified upper extremity

⑥ I82.62 Acute embolism and thrombosis of deep veins of upper extremity

Acute embolism and thrombosis of brachial vein
Acute embolism and thrombosis of radial vein
Acute embolism and thrombosis of ulnar vein

I82.621 Acute embolism and thrombosis of deep veins of right upper extremity

I82.622 Acute embolism and thrombosis of deep veins of left upper extremity

I82.623 Acute embolism and thrombosis of deep veins of upper extremity, bilateral

I82.629 Acute embolism and thrombosis of deep veins of unspecified upper extremity

⑤ I82.7 Chronic embolism and thrombosis of veins of upper extremity

Use additional code, if applicable, for associated long-term (current) use of anticoagulants (Z79.01)

EXCLUDES1 personal history of venous embolism and thrombosis (Z86.718)

⑥ I82.70 Chronic embolism and thrombosis of unspecified veins of upper extremity

I82.701 Chronic embolism and thrombosis of unspecified veins of right upper extremity

I82.702 Chronic embolism and thrombosis of unspecified veins of left upper extremity

I82.703 Chronic embolism and thrombosis of unspecified veins of upper extremity, bilateral

I82.709 Chronic embolism and thrombosis of unspecified veins of unspecified upper extremity

⑥ I82.71 Chronic embolism and thrombosis of superficial veins of upper extremity

Chronic embolism and thrombosis of antecubital vein
Chronic embolism and thrombosis of basilic vein
Chronic embolism and thrombosis of cephalic vein

I82.711 Chronic embolism and thrombosis of superficial veins of right upper extremity

I82.712 Chronic embolism and thrombosis of superficial veins of left upper extremity

I82.713 Chronic embolism and thrombosis of superficial veins of upper extremity, bilateral

I82.719 Chronic embolism and thrombosis of superficial veins of unspecified upper extremity

⑥ I82.72 Chronic embolism and thrombosis of deep veins of upper extremity

Chronic embolism and thrombosis of brachial vein
Chronic embolism and thrombosis of radial vein
Chronic embolism and thrombosis of ulnar vein

I82.721 Chronic embolism and thrombosis of deep veins of right upper extremity

④ 4th character required   ⑤ 5th character required   ⑥ 6th character required   ⑦ 7th character required   ⑦ Extension 'X' Alert
EXCLUDES 1 Not coded here   EXCLUDES 2 Not included here   Primary Diagnosis Only   Manifestation Code

242

ICD-10-CM 2015

I82.722 Chronic embolism and thrombosis of deep veins of left upper extremity

I82.723 Chronic embolism and thrombosis of deep veins of upper extremity, bilateral

I82.729 Chronic embolism and thrombosis of deep veins of unspecified upper extremity

I82.A Embolism and thrombosis of axillary vein

  I82.A1 Acute embolism and thrombosis of axillary vein

    I82.A11 Acute embolism and thrombosis of right axillary vein

    I82.A12 Acute embolism and thrombosis of left axillary vein

    I82.A13 Acute embolism and thrombosis of axillary vein, bilateral

    I82.A19 Acute embolism and thrombosis of unspecified axillary vein

  I82.A2 Chronic embolism and thrombosis of axillary vein

    I82.A21 Chronic embolism and thrombosis of right axillary vein

    I82.A22 Chronic embolism and thrombosis of left axillary vein

    I82.A23 Chronic embolism and thrombosis of axillary vein, bilateral

    I82.A29 Chronic embolism and thrombosis of unspecified axillary vein

I82.B Embolism and thrombosis of subclavian vein

  I82.B1 Acute embolism and thrombosis of subclavian vein

    I82.B11 Acute embolism and thrombosis of right subclavian vein

    I82.B12 Acute embolism and thrombosis of left subclavian vein

    I82.B13 Acute embolism and thrombosis of subclavian vein, bilateral

    I82.B19 Acute embolism and thrombosis of unspecified subclavian vein

  I82.B2 Chronic embolism and thrombosis of subclavian vein

    I82.B21 Chronic embolism and thrombosis of right subclavian vein

    I82.B22 Chronic embolism and thrombosis of left subclavian vein

    I82.B23 Chronic embolism and thrombosis of subclavian vein, bilateral

    I82.B29 Chronic embolism and thrombosis of unspecified subclavian vein

I82.C Embolism and thrombosis of internal jugular vein

  I82.C1 Acute embolism and thrombosis of internal jugular vein

    I82.C11 Acute embolism and thrombosis of right internal jugular vein

    I82.C12 Acute embolism and thrombosis of left internal jugular vein

    I82.C13 Acute embolism and thrombosis of internal jugular vein, bilateral

    I82.C19 Acute embolism and thrombosis of unspecified internal jugular vein

  I82.C2 Chronic embolism and thrombosis of internal jugular vein

    I82.C21 Chronic embolism and thrombosis of right internal jugular vein

    I82.C22 Chronic embolism and thrombosis of left internal jugular vein

    I82.C23 Chronic embolism and thrombosis of internal jugular vein, bilateral

    I82.C29 Chronic embolism and thrombosis of unspecified internal jugular vein

I82.8 Embolism and thrombosis of other specified veins
Use additional code, if applicable, for associated long-term (current) use of anticoagulants (Z79.01)

  I82.81 Embolism and thrombosis of superficial veins of lower extremities

    Embolism and thrombosis of saphenous vein (greater) (lesser)

    I82.811 Embolism and thrombosis of superficial veins of right lower extremities

    I82.812 Embolism and thrombosis of superficial veins of left lower extremities

    I82.813 Embolism and thrombosis of superficial veins of lower extremities, bilateral

    I82.819 Embolism and thrombosis of superficial veins of unspecified lower extremities

  I82.89 Embolism and thrombosis of other specified veins

    I82.890 Acute embolism and thrombosis of other specified veins

    I82.891 Chronic embolism and thrombosis of other specified veins

I82.9 Embolism and thrombosis of unspecified vein

  I82.90 Acute embolism and thrombosis of unspecified vein

    Embolism of vein NOS
    Thrombosis (vein) NOS

  I82.91 Chronic embolism and thrombosis of unspecified vein

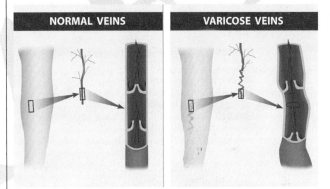

Figure 8.7 Illustration showing Normal and Varicose Veins

I83 Varicose veins of lower extremities

    EXCLUDES1 varicose veins complicating pregnancy (O22.0-)
    varicose veins complicating the puerperium (O87.4)

I83.0 Varicose veins of lower extremities with ulcer
Use additional code to identify severity of ulcer (L97.-)

  I83.00 Varicose veins of unspecified lower extremity with ulcer

    I83.001 Varicose veins of unspecified lower extremity with ulcer of thigh   🅰

    I83.002 Varicose veins of unspecified lower extremity with ulcer of calf   🅰

    I83.003 Varicose veins of unspecified lower extremity with ulcer of ankle   🅰

    I83.004 Varicose veins of unspecified lower extremity with ulcer of heel and midfoot
      Varicose veins of unspecified lower extremity with ulcer of plantar surface of midfoot   🅰

    I83.005 Varicose veins of unspecified lower extremity with ulcer other part of foot
      Varicose veins of unspecified lower extremity with ulcer of toe   🅰

    I83.008 Varicose veins of unspecified lower extremity with ulcer other part of lower leg   🅰

Unspecified Code	Other Specified Code	N Newborn Age: 0	P Pediatric Age: 0-17	M Maternity Age: 12-55
	🅰 Adult Age: 15-124	♂ Male	♀ Female	● New Code	▲ Revised Code Title	►◄ Revised Text

I83.009 Varicose veins of unspecified lower extremity with ulcer of unspecified site [A]

[6] I83.01 Varicose veins of right lower extremity with ulcer

I83.011 Varicose veins of right lower extremity with ulcer of thigh [A]

I83.012 Varicose veins of right lower extremity with ulcer of calf [A]

I83.013 Varicose veins of right lower extremity with ulcer of ankle [A]

I83.014 Varicose veins of right lower extremity with ulcer of heel and midfoot

Varicose veins of right lower extremity with ulcer of plantar surface of midfoot [A]

I83.015 Varicose veins of right lower extremity with ulcer other part of foot

Varicose veins of right lower extremity with ulcer of toe [A]

I83.018 Varicose veins of right lower extremity with ulcer other part of lower leg [A]

I83.019 Varicose veins of right lower extremity with ulcer of unspecified site [A]

[6] I83.02 Varicose veins of left lower extremity with ulcer

I83.021 Varicose veins of left lower extremity with ulcer of thigh [A]

I83.022 Varicose veins of left lower extremity wlth ulcer of calf [A]

I83.023 Varicose veins of left lower extremity with ulcer of ankle [A]

I83.024 Varicose veins of left lower extremity with ulcer of heel and midfoot

Varicose veins of left lower extremity with ulcer of plantar surface of midfoot [A]

I83.025 Varicose veins of left lower extremity with ulcer other part of foot

Varicose veins of left lower extremity with ulcer of toe [A]

I83.028 Varicose veins of left lower extremity with ulcer other part of lower leg [A]

I83.029 Varicose veins of left lower extremity with ulcer of unspecified site [A]

[5] I83.1 Varicose veins of lower extremities with inflammation

Stasis dermatitis

I83.10 Varicose veins of unspecified lower extremity with inflammation [A]

I83.11 Varicose veins of right lower extremity with inflammation [A]

I83.12 Varicose veins of left lower extremity with inflammation [A]

[5] I83.2 Varicose veins of lower extremities with both ulcer and inflammation

Use additional code to identify severity of ulcer (L97.-)

[6] I83.20 Varicose veins of unspecified lower extremity with both ulcer and inflammation

I83.201 Varicose veins of unspecified lower extremity with both ulcer of thigh and inflammation [A]

I83.202 Varicose veins of unspecified lower extremity with both ulcer of calf and inflammation [A]

I83.203 Varicose veins of unspecified lower extremity with both ulcer of ankle and inflammation [A]

I83.204 Varicose veins of unspecified lower extremity with both ulcer of heel and midfoot and inflammation

Varicose veins of unspecified lower extremity with both ulcer of plantar surface of midfoot and inflammation [A]

I83.205 Varicose veins of unspecified lower extremity with both ulcer other part of foot and inflammation

Varicose veins of unspecified lower extremity with both ulcer of toe and inflammation [A]

I83.208 Varicose veins of unspecified lower extremity with both ulcer of other part of lower extremity and inflammation [A]

I83.209 Varicose veins of unspecified lower extremity with both ulcer of unspecified site and inflammation [A]

[6] I83.21 Varicose veins of right lower extremity with both ulcer and inflammation

I83.211 Varicose veins of right lower extremity with both ulcer of thigh and inflammation [A]

I83.212 Varicose veins of right lower extremity with both ulcer of calf and inflammation [A]

I83.213 Varicose veins of right lower extremity with both ulcer of ankle and inflammation [A]

I83.214 Varicose veins of right lower extremity with both ulcer of heel and midfoot and inflammation

Varicose veins of right lower extremity with both ulcer of plantar surface of midfoot and inflammation [A]

I83.215 Varicose veins of right lower extremity with both ulcer other part of foot and inflammation

Varicose veins of right lower extremity with both ulcer of toe and inflammation [A]

I83.218 Varicose veins of right lower extremity with both ulcer of other part of lower extremity and inflammation [A]

I83.219 Varicose veins of right lower extremity with both ulcer of unspecified site and inflammation [A]

[6] I83.22 Varicose veins of left lower extremity with both ulcer and inflammation

I83.221 Varicose veins of left lower extremity with both ulcer of thigh and inflammation [A]

I83.222 Varicose veins of left lower extremity with both ulcer of calf and inflammation [A]

I83.223 Varicose veins of left lower extremity with both ulcer of ankle and inflammation [A]

I83.224 Varicose veins of left lower extremity with both ulcer of heel and midfoot and inflammation

Varicose veins of left lower extremity with both ulcer of plantar surface of midfoot and inflammation [A]

I83.225 Varicose veins of left lower extremity with both ulcer other part of foot and inflammation

Varicose veins of left lower extremity with both ulcer of toe and inflammation [A]

I83.228 Varicose veins of left lower extremity with both ulcer of other part of lower extremity and inflammation [A]

I83.229 Varicose veins of left lower extremity with both ulcer of unspecified site and inflammation [A]

[5] I83.8 Varicose veins of lower extremities with other complications

[6] I83.81 Varicose veins of lower extremities with pain

I83.811 Varicose veins of right lower extremities with pain [A]

I83.812 Varicose veins of left lower extremities with pain [A]

I83.813 Varicose veins of bilateral lower extremities with pain [A]

[4] 4th character required [5] 5th character required [6] 6th character required [7] 7th character required Extension 'X' Alert
EXCLUDES 1 Not coded here EXCLUDES 2 Not included here PDx Primary Diagnosis Only Manifestation Code

I83.819 Varicose veins of unspecified lower extremities with pain [A]

[6] I83.89 Varicose veins of lower extremities with other complications

Varicose veins of lower extremities with edema
Varicose veins of lower extremities with swelling

I83.891 Varicose veins of right lower extremities with other complications [A]

I83.892 Varicose veins of left lower extremities with other complications [A]

I83.893 Varicose veins of bilateral lower extremities with other complications [A]

I83.899 Varicose veins of unspecified lower extremities with other complications [A]

[5] I83.9 Asymptomatic varicose veins of lower extremities

Phlebectasia of lower extremities
Varicose veins of lower extremities
Varix of lower extremities

I83.90 Asymptomatic varicose veins of unspecified lower extremity

Varicose veins NOS [A]

I83.91 Asymptomatic varicose veins of right lower extremity [A]

I83.92 Asymptomatic varicose veins of left lower extremity [A]

I83.93 Asymptomatic varicose veins of bilateral lower extremities [A]

[4] I85 Esophageal varices

Use additional code to identify:
alcohol abuse and dependence (F10.-)

[5] I85.0 Esophageal varices

Idiopathic esophageal varices
Primary esophageal varices

I85.00 Esophageal varices without bleeding

Esophageal varices NOS

I85.01 Esophageal varices with bleeding

[5] I85.1 Secondary esophageal varices

Esophageal varices secondary to alcoholic liver disease
Esophageal varices secondary to cirrhosis of liver
Esophageal varices secondary to schistosomiasis
Esophageal varices secondary to toxic liver disease
Code first underlying disease

I85.10 Secondary esophageal varices without bleeding

I85.11 Secondary esophageal varices with bleeding

[4] I86 Varicose veins of other sites

[EXCLUDES1] *varicose veins of unspecified site (I83.9-)*
[EXCLUDES2] *retinal varices (H35.0-)*

I86.0 Sublingual varices

I86.1 Scrotal varices

Varicocele ♂

I86.2 Pelvic varices

I86.3 Vulval varices

[EXCLUDES1] *vulval varices complicating childbirth and the puerperium (O87.8)*
vulval varices complicating pregnancy (O22.1-) ♀

I86.4 Gastric varices

I86.8 Varicose veins of other specified sites

Varicose ulcer of nasal septum [A]

[4] I87 Other disorders of veins

[5] I87.0 Postthrombotic syndrome

Chronic venous hypertension due to deep vein thrombosis
Postphlebitic syndrome
[EXCLUDES1] *chronic venous hypertension without deep vein thrombosis (I87.3-)*

[6] I87.00 Postthrombotic syndrome without complications

Asymptomatic Postthrombotic syndrome

I87.001 Postthrombotic syndrome without complications of right lower extremity

I87.002 Postthrombotic syndrome without complications of left lower extremity

I87.003 Postthrombotic syndrome without complications of bilateral lower extremity

I87.009 Postthrombotic syndrome without complications of unspecified extremity

Postthrombotic syndrome NOS

[6] I87.01 Postthrombotic syndrome with ulcer

Use additional code to specify site and severity of ulcer (L97.-)

I87.011 Postthrombotic syndrome with ulcer of right lower extremity

I87.012 Postthrombotic syndrome with ulcer of left lower extremity

I87.013 Postthrombotic syndrome with ulcer of bilateral lower extremity

I87.019 Postthrombotic syndrome with ulcer of unspecified lower extremity

[6] I87.02 Postthrombotic syndrome with inflammation

I87.021 Postthrombotic syndrome with inflammation of right lower extremity

I87.022 Postthrombotic syndrome with inflammation of left lower extremity

I87.023 Postthrombotic syndrome with inflammation of bilateral lower extremity

I87.029 Postthrombotic syndrome with inflammation of unspecified lower extremity

[6] I87.03 Postthrombotic syndrome with ulcer and inflammation

Use additional code to specify site and severity of ulcer (L97.-)

I87.031 Postthrombotic syndrome with ulcer and inflammation of right lower extremity

I87.032 Postthrombotic syndrome with ulcer and inflammation of left lower extremity

I87.033 Postthrombotic syndrome with ulcer and inflammation of bilateral lower extremity

I87.039 Postthrombotic syndrome with ulcer and inflammation of unspecified lower extremity

[6] I87.09 Postthrombotic syndrome with other complications

I87.091 Postthrombotic syndrome with other complications of right lower extremity

I87.092 Postthrombotic syndrome with other complications of left lower extremity

I87.093 Postthrombotic syndrome with other complications of bilateral lower extremity

I87.099 Postthrombotic syndrome with other complications of unspecified lower extremity

I87.1 Compression of vein

Stricture of vein
Vena cava syndrome (inferior) (superior)
[EXCLUDES2] *compression of pulmonary vein (I28.8)*

I87.2 Venous insufficiency (chronic) (peripheral)

[5] I87.3 Chronic venous hypertension (idiopathic)

Stasis edema
[EXCLUDES1] *chronic venous hypertension due to deep vein thrombosis (I87.0-)*
varicose veins of lower extremities (I83.-)

[6] I87.30 Chronic venous hypertension (idiopathic) without complications

Asymptomatic chronic venous hypertension (idiopathic)

I87.301 Chronic venous hypertension (idiopathic) without complications of right lower extremity

Unspecified Code | Other Specified Code | [N] Newborn Age: 0 | [P] Pediatric Age: 0-17 | [M] Maternity Age: 12-55
[A] Adult Age: 15-124 | ♂ Male | ♀ Female | ● New Code | ▲ Revised Code Title | ►◄ Revised Text

I87.302 Chronic venous hypertension (idiopathic) without complications of left lower extremity

I87.303 Chronic venous hypertension (idiopathic) without complications of bilateral lower extremity

I87.309 Chronic venous hypertension (idiopathic) without complications of unspecified lower extremity

Chronic venous hypertension NOS

[6] **I87.31 Chronic venous hypertension (idiopathic) with ulcer**

Use additional code to specify site and severity of ulcer (L97.-)

I87.311 Chronic venous hypertension (idiopathic) with ulcer of right lower extremity

I87.312 Chronic venous hypertension (idiopathic) with ulcer of left lower extremity

I87.313 Chronic venous hypertension (idiopathic) with ulcer of bilateral lower extremity

I87.319 Chronic venous hypertension (idiopathic) with ulcer of unspecified lower extremity

[6] **I87.32 Chronic venous hypertension (idiopathic) with inflammation**

I87.321 Chronic venous hypertension (idiopathic) with inflammation of right lower extremity

I87.322 Chronic venous hypertension (idiopathic) with inflammation of left lower extremity

I87.323 Chronic venous hypertension (idiopathic) with inflammation of bilateral lower extremity

I87.329 Chronic venous hypertension (idiopathic) with inflammation of unspecified lower extremity

[6] **I87.33 Chronic venous hypertension (idiopathic) with ulcer and inflammation**

Use additional code to specify site and severity of ulcer (L97.-)

I87.331 Chronic venous hypertension (idiopathic) with ulcer and inflammation of right lower extremity

I87.332 Chronic venous hypertension (idiopathic) with ulcer and inflammation of left lower extremity

I87.333 Chronic venous hypertension (idiopathic) with ulcer and inflammation of bilateral lower extremity

I87.339 Chronic venous hypertension (idiopathic) with ulcer and inflammation of unspecified lower extremity

[6] **I87.39 Chronic venous hypertension (idiopathic) with other complications**

I87.391 Chronic venous hypertension (idiopathic) with other complications of right lower extremity

I87.392 Chronic venous hypertension (idiopathic) with other complications of left lower extremity

I87.393 Chronic venous hypertension (idiopathic) with other complications of bilateral lower extremity

I87.399 Chronic venous hypertension (idiopathic) with other complications of unspecified lower extremity

I87.8 Other specified disorders of veins

Phlebosclerosis
Venofibrosis

I87.9 Disorder of vein, unspecified

[4] **I88 Nonspecific lymphadenitis**

[EXCLUDES1] *acute lymphadenitis, except mesenteric (L04.-)*
enlarged lymph nodes NOS (R59.-)
human immunodeficiency virus [HIV] disease resulting in generalized lymphadenopathy (B20)

I88.0 Nonspecific mesenteric lymphadenitis

Mesenteric lymphadenitis (acute)(chronic)

I88.1 Chronic lymphadenitis, except mesenteric

Adenitis
Lymphadenitis

I88.8 Other nonspecific lymphadenitis

I88.9 Nonspecific lymphadenitis, unspecified

Lymphadenitis NOS

[4] **I89 Other noninfective disorders of lymphatic vessels and lymph nodes**

[EXCLUDES1] *chylocele, tunica vaginalis (nonfilarial) NOS (N50.8)*
enlarged lymph nodes NOS (R59.-)
filarial chylocele (B74.-)
hereditary lymphedema (Q82.0)

I89.0 Lymphedema, not elsewhere classified

Elephantiasis (nonfilarial) NOS
Lymphangiectasis
Obliteration, lymphatic vessel
Praecox lymphedema
Secondary lymphedema

[EXCLUDES1] *postmastectomy lymphedema (I97.2)*

I89.1 Lymphangitis

Chronic lymphangitis
Lymphangitis NOS
Subacute lymphangitis

[EXCLUDES1] *acute lymphangitis (L03.-)*

I89.8 Other specified noninfective disorders of lymphatic vessels and lymph nodes

Chylocele (nonfilarial)
Chylous ascites
Chylous cyst
Lipomelanotic reticulosis
Lymph node or vessel fistula
Lymph node or vessel infarction
Lymph node or vessel rupture

I89.9 Noninfective disorder of lymphatic vessels and lymph nodes, unspecified

Disease of lymphatic vessels NOS

Other and unspecified disorders of the circulatory system (I95-I99)

[4] **I95 Hypotension**

[EXCLUDES1] *cardiovascular collapse (R57.9)*
maternal hypotension syndrome (O26.5-)
nonspecific low blood pressure reading NOS (R03.1)

I95.0 Idiopathic hypotension

I95.1 Orthostatic hypotension

Hypotension, postural

[EXCLUDES1] *neurogenic orthostatic hypotension [Shy-Drager] (G90.3)*
orthostatic hypotension due to drugs (I95.2)

I95.2 Hypotension due to drugs

Orthostatic hypotension due to drugs
Use additional code for adverse effect, if applicable, to identify drug (T36-T50 with fifth or sixth character 5)

I95.3 Hypotension of hemodialysis

Intra-dialytic hypotension

[5] **I95.8 Other hypotension**

I95.81 Postprocedural hypotension

I95.89 Other hypotension

Chronic hypotension

I95.9 Hypotension, unspecified

I96 Gangrene, not elsewhere classified

Gangrenous cellulitis

[EXCLUDES1] *gangrene in atherosclerosis of native arteries of the extremities (I70.26)*
gangrene in diabetes mellitus (E08-E13)
gangrene in hernia (K40.1, K40.4, K41.1, K41.4, K42.1, K43.1-, K44.1, K45.1, K46.1)
gangrene in other peripheral vascular diseases (I73.-)
gangrene of certain specified sites - see Alphabetical Index
gas gangrene (A48.0)
pyoderma gangrenosum (L88)

[4] **I97 Intraoperative and postprocedural complications and disorders of circulatory system, not elsewhere classified**

[EXCLUDES2] *postprocedural shock (T81.1-)*

I97.0 Postcardiotomy syndrome

[5] **I97.1 Other postprocedural cardiac functional disturbances**

[EXCLUDES2] *acute pulmonary insufficiency following thoracic surgery (J95.1)*
intraoperative cardiac functional disturbances (I97.7-)

[6] **I97.11 Postprocedural cardiac insufficiency**

I97.110 Postprocedural cardiac insufficiency following cardiac surgery

I97.111 Postprocedural cardiac insufficiency following other surgery

[6] **I97.12 Postprocedural cardiac arrest**

I97.120 Postprocedural cardiac arrest following cardiac surgery

I97.121 Postprocedural cardiac arrest following other surgery

[6] **I97.13 Postprocedural heart failure**

Use additional code to identify the heart failure (I50.-)

I97.130 Postprocedural heart failure following cardiac surgery

I97.131 Postprocedural heart failure following other surgery

[6] **I97.19 Other postprocedural cardiac functional disturbances**

Use additional code, if applicable, to further specify disorder

I97.190 Other postprocedural cardiac functional disturbances following cardiac surgery

I97.191 Other postprocedural cardiac functional disturbances following other surgery

I97.2 Postmastectomy lymphedema syndrome

Elephantiasis due to mastectomy
Obliteration of lymphatic vessels [A]

I97.3 Postprocedural hypertension

[5] **I97.4 Intraoperative hemorrhage and hematoma of a circulatory system organ or structure complicating a procedure**

[EXCLUDES1] *intraoperative hemorrhage and hematoma of a circulatory system organ or structure due to accidental puncture and laceration during a procedure (I97.5-)*

[EXCLUDES2] *intraoperative cerebrovascular hemorrhage complicating a procedure (G97.3-)*

[6] **I97.41 Intraoperative hemorrhage and hematoma of a circulatory system organ or structure complicating a circulatory system procedure**

I97.410 Intraoperative hemorrhage and hematoma of a circulatory system organ or structure complicating a cardiac catheterization

I97.411 Intraoperative hemorrhage and hematoma of a circulatory system organ or structure complicating a cardiac bypass

I97.418 Intraoperative hemorrhage and hematoma of a circulatory system organ or structure complicating other circulatory system procedure

I97.42 Intraoperative hemorrhage and hematoma of a circulatory system organ or structure complicating other procedure

[5] **I97.5 Accidental puncture and laceration of a circulatory system organ or structure during a procedure**

[EXCLUDES2] *accidental puncture and laceration of brain during a procedure (G97.4-)*

I97.51 Accidental puncture and laceration of a circulatory system organ or structure during a circulatory system procedure

I97.52 Accidental puncture and laceration of a circulatory system organ or structure during other procedure

[5] **I97.6 Postprocedural hemorrhage and hematoma of a circulatory system organ or structure following a procedure**

[EXCLUDES2] *postprocedural cerebrovascular hemorrhage complicating a procedure (G97.5-)*

[6] **I97.61 Postprocedural hemorrhage and hematoma of a circulatory system organ or structure following a circulatory system procedure**

I97.610 Postprocedural hemorrhage and hematoma of a circulatory system organ or structure following a cardiac catheterization

I97.611 Postprocedural hemorrhage and hematoma of a circulatory system organ or structure following cardiac bypass

I97.618 Postprocedural hemorrhage and hematoma of a circulatory system organ or structure following other circulatory system procedure

I97.62 Postprocedural hemorrhage and hematoma of a circulatory system organ or structure following other procedure

[5] **I97.7 Intraoperative cardiac functional disturbances**

[EXCLUDES2] *acute pulmonary insufficiency following thoracic surgery (J95.1)*
postprocedural cardiac functional disturbances (I97.1-)

[6] **I97.71 Intraoperative cardiac arrest**

I97.710 Intraoperative cardiac arrest during cardiac surgery

Unspecified Code | Other Specified Code | [N] Newborn Age: 0 | [P] Pediatric Age: 0-17 | [M] Maternity Age: 12-55
[A] Adult Age: 15-124 | ♂ Male | ♀ Female | ● New Code | ▲ Revised Code Title | ►◄ Revised Text

I97.711 Intraoperative cardiac arrest during other surgery

[6th] I97.79 Other intraoperative cardiac functional disturbances

Use additional code, if applicable, to further specify disorder

I97.790 Other intraoperative cardiac functional disturbances during cardiac surgery

I97.791 Other intraoperative cardiac functional disturbances during other surgery

[5th] I97.8 Other intraoperative and postprocedural complications and disorders of the circulatory system, not elsewhere classified

Use additional code, if applicable, to further specify disorder

[6th] I97.81 Intraoperative cerebrovascular infarction

I97.810 Intraoperative cerebrovascular infarction during cardiac surgery

I97.811 Intraoperative cerebrovascular infarction during other surgery

[6th] I97.82 Postprocedural cerebrovascular infarction

I97.820 Postprocedural cerebrovascular infarction during cardiac surgery

I97.821 Postprocedural cerebrovascular infarction during other surgery

I97.88 Other intraoperative complications of the circulatory system, not elsewhere classified

I97.89 Other postprocedural complications and disorders of the circulatory system, not elsewhere classified

[4th] I99 Other and unspecified disorders of circulatory system

I99.8 Other disorder of circulatory system

I99.9 Unspecified disorder of circulatory system

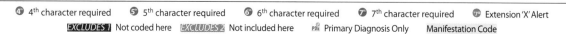

Chapter 10: Diseases of the Respiratory System (J00-J99)

Chapter Specific Coding Guidelines

a. Chronic Obstructive Pulmonary Disease [COPD] and Asthma
1) Acute exacerbation of chronic obstructive bronchitis and asthma
The codes in categories J44 and J45 distinguish between uncomplicated cases and those in acute exacerbation. An acute exacerbation is a worsening or a decompensation of a chronic condition. An acute exacerbation is not equivalent to an infection superimposed on a chronic condition, though an exacerbation may be triggered by an infection.

b. Acute Respiratory Failure
1) Acute respiratory failure as principal diagnosis
A code from subcategory J96.0, Acute respiratory failure, or subcategory J96.2, Acute and chronic respiratory failure, may be assigned as a principal diagnosis when it is the condition established after study to be chiefly responsible for occasioning the admission to the hospital, and the selection is supported by the Alphabetic Index and Tabular List. However, chapter-specific coding guidelines (such as obstetrics, poisoning, HIV, newborn) that provide sequencing direction take precedence.

2) Acute respiratory failure as secondary diagnosis
Respiratory failure may be listed as a secondary diagnosis if it occurs after admission, or if it is present on admission, but does not meet the definition of principal diagnosis.

3) Sequencing of acute respiratory failure and another acute condition
When a patient is admitted with respiratory failure and another acute condition, (e.g., myocardial infarction, cerebrovascular accident, aspiration pneumonia), the principal diagnosis will not be the same in every situation. This applies whether the other acute condition is a respiratory or nonrespiratory condition. Selection of the principal diagnosis will be dependent on the circumstances of admission. If both the respiratory failure and the other acute condition are equally responsible for occasioning the admission to the hospital, and there are no chapter-specific sequencing rules, the guideline regarding two or more diagnoses that equally meet the definition for principal diagnosis (Section II, C.) may be applied in these situations.

If the documentation is not clear as to whether acute respiratory failure and another condition are equally responsible for occasioning the admission, query the provider for clarification.

c. Influenza due to certain identified influenza viruses
Code only confirmed cases of influenza due to certain identified influenza viruses (category J09), and due to other identified influenza virus (category J10). This is an exception to the hospital inpatient guideline Section II, H. (Uncertain Diagnosis).

In this context, "confirmation" does not require documentation of positive laboratory testing specific for avian or other novel influenza A or other identified influenza virus. However, coding should be based on the provider's diagnostic statement that the patient has avian influenza, or other novel influenza A, for category J09, or has another particular identified strain of influenza, such as H1N1 or H3N2, but not identified as novel or variant, for category J10.

If the provider records "suspected" or "possible" or "probable" avian influenza, or novel influenza, or other identified influenza, then the appropriate influenza code from category J11, Influenza due to unidentified influenza virus, should be assigned. A code from category J09, Influenza due to certain identified influenza viruses, should not be assigned nor should a code from category J10, Influenza due to other identified influenza virus.

d. Ventilator-associated Pneumonia
1) Documentation of Ventilator-associated Pneumonia
As with all procedural or postprocedural complications, code assignment is based on the provider's documentation of the relationship between the condition and the procedure.

Code J95.851, Ventilator associated pneumonia, should be assigned only when the provider has documented ventilator associated pneumonia (VAP). An additional code to identify the organism (e.g., Pseudomonas aeruginosa, code B96.5) should also be assigned. Do not assign an additional code from categories J12-J18 to identify the type of pneumonia.

Code J95.851 should not be assigned for cases where the patient has pneumonia and is on a mechanical ventilator and the provider has not specifically stated that the pneumonia is ventilator-associated pneumonia. If the documentation is unclear as to whether the patient has a pneumonia that is a complication attributable to the mechanical ventilator, query the provider.

2) Ventilator-associated Pneumonia Develops after Admission
A patient may be admitted with one type of pneumonia (e.g., code J13, Pneumonia due to Streptococcus pneumonia) and subsequently develop VAP. In this instance, the principal diagnosis would be the appropriate code from categories J12-J18 for the pneumonia diagnosed at the time of admission. Code J95.851, Ventilator associated pneumonia, would be assigned as an additional diagnosis when the provider has also documented the presence of ventilator associated pneumonia.

This page intentionally left blank

Anatomy of the Respiratory System

1. **An Outline of the Respiratory System**
   a) The human respiratory system is based on the following organs:
      i) nose
      ii) pharynx
      iii) larynx
      iv) trachea
      v) bronchi
      vi) lungs
   b) The process of respiration involves the exchange of oxygen and carbon dioxide between the atmosphere, blood and cells.

The Respiratory System

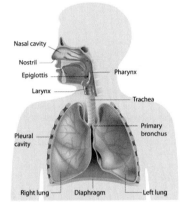

Nasal cavity
Nostril
Epiglottis
Larynx
Pharynx
Trachea
Primary bronchus
Pleural cavity
Right lung
Diaphragm
Left lung

2. **The Anatomy of Nose**
   a) The nostrils or external nares are openings into the external nose.
   b) The internal nares serve to connect the internal nose with the throat or pharynx.
   c) The nasal septum divides the nose into the right and left nasal cavities.
   d) The internal nose contains three turbinate bones (superior, middle and inferior meatus).
   e) The olfactory receptors are located in the superior meatus.

3. **The Anatomy of the Pharynx**
   a) The pharynx is a resonating chamber for speech sounds and also provides a passage to both air and food.
   b) The nasopharynx, oropharynx and laryngopharynx are the parts of the pharynx.
   c) The nasopharynx surrounds the pharyngeal tonsils. It contains two internal nares and the openings of the eustachian tubes.
   d) The oropharynx surrounds the palatine and lingual tonsils and it's opening (or fauces) provides connection to the mouth.
   e) The laryngopharynx gets connected with the larynx on anterior aspect and the esophagus posteriorly.

4. **The Anatomy of the Larynx**
   a) The larynx is also known as the voice box.
   b) The skeleton of the larynx is made up of nine cartilages. Three of them are single (thyroid, cricoid, and epiglottis) and the remaining three (arytenoid, corniculate, and cuneiform) are paired cartilages.
   c) The thyroid cartilage is also known as Adam's apple. It is the largest single cartilage of the laryngeal skeleton.
   d) The cricoid cartilage connects with the first tracheal ring and is made up of a single ring of cartilage.
   e) The epiglottis is a large and single leaf-shaped flap of elastic cartilage. It is lined with the mucous membrane and remains

attached to the entrance of larynx. It pulls down over the glottis during the process of swallowing to obstruct the entrance of the fluids and food in the trachea.
   f) The arytenoid cartilages are formed by a pair of three ladle shaped pyraminds that remain attached to the laryngeal muscles and the vocal cords.
   g) The corniculate cartilages are based on two cone shaped nodules of yellow elastic cartilage.
   h) The cuneiform cartilages are also known as the cartilages of Wrisberg. They are based on two rod shaped pieces of yellow elastic cartilage.
   i) The mucous membrane of the larynx is divided into two pairs of folds. The vestibular folds (or false vocal cords) constitute the upper pair, while the vocal folds (or true vocal cords) form the lower pair of fold.
   j) The opening over the true vocal cords is known as the glottis.

5. **The Anatomy of Trachea**
   a) The trachea is also known as the windpipe and located anteriorly to the esophagus.
   b) It begins at the larynx and gets divided into primary bronchi at the level of T4/T5 vertebrae.
   c) The trachea is lined by the respiratory epithelium and consists of a series of incomplete C-shaped cartilaginous rings.

6. **The Anatomy of the Bronchial Tree**
   a) The bronchial tree is based on right and left primary bronchi, secondary and tertiary bronchi, and the bronchioles.
   b) The right and left primary bronchi emanate from the trachea and merge with the right and left lungs.
   c) The primary bronchi further get branched into the secondary (or lobar) bronchi that penetrate into the lobes of the lungs.
   d) The secondary bronchi further get divided into the tertiary or segmental bronchi that penetrate into the segments of the lobes of lungs.
   e) The bronchioles are the branches that emanate from the tertiary bronchi.

7. **The Anatomy of the Lungs**
   a) The lungs are the human organs of respiration.
   b) The right and left lungs are based on multiple lobes. The right lung contains three lobes, while the left lung is based on two lobes.
   c) The lungs are protected by the pleural membrane. The pleural membrane is further made up of two layers of serous membranes. The outer layer is known as the parietal pleura, while the inner layer is termed as the visceral pleura.
   d) The bronchopulmonary segment is a segment of lung tissue which is supplied by each of the tertiary bronchi. It is divided into multiple lobules that remain covered with the elastic connective tissue.
   e) A terminal bronchiole exists at the end of the conducting zone of the respiratory system.
   f) The microscopic respiratory bronchioles are the subdivisions of the terminal bronchioles. The atria or the alveolar ducts emanate from these respiratory bronchioles.
   g) The alveoli and alveolar sacs lie around the circumference of the alveolar ducts.
   h) The alveolar sac is made up of two or more alveoli with a common opening.
   i) The respiratory (or the alveolar capillary) membrane is a membrane which provides a medium for the movement of respiratory gases.

8. **The Process of Respiration**
   a) The respiration in humans is based on the following stages:

i)　ventilation is also known as the breathing, which involves the movement of the ambient air into the alveoli of the lungs.

ii)　The process of pulmonary gas exchange is based on the exchange of respiratory gases between the alveoli and the pulmonary capillaries.

iii)　gas process involves the transport of respiratory gases from the pulmonary capillaries to the peripheral capillaries in the organs via circulation.

iv)　peripheral gas exchange is the process of exchange of respiratory gases between the tissue capillaries and the cells and mitochondria.

b)　The nasal breathing in the process of respiration that involves the inhalation and exhalation of the respiratory gases through the nose.

Common Pathologies

Sinusitis
Inflammation of mucous membrane lining that lines the paranasal sinuses- sinuses dry out, humidifiers used - can also cause dizziness and difficulty breathing.

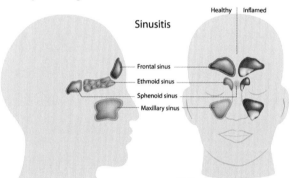

Epiglottitis
Inflammation of the epiglottis caused by H. Influenzae type B; characterized by fever and a severe sore throat and difficulty in swallowing.

Laryngitis
Inflammation of larynx and vocal cords resulting in hoarseness of the voice (Dysphonia), and difficulty in swallowing (Dysphagia).

Pharyngitis
Inflammation of the pharynx, usually causing a sore throat. Acute Pharyngitis is a sudden, severe inflammation of the pharynx. Chronic Pharyngitis is a persistent throat inflammation that may be associated with the lymphoid granules in the pharyngeal mucosa.

Acute Bronchitis
Inflammation of the mucous membrane lining the bronchus, involves the trachea resulting in tracheobrochitis, chest tightness, fever, cough that progresses from nonproductive to productive.

Chronic Bronchitis
Inflammation of the bronchial mucous membrane characterized by cough, hyper-secretion of mucus, and expectoration of sputum over a long period of time and associated with increased vulnerability to bronchial infection.

Influenza
Influenza is a highly infectious respiratory disease. The disease is caused by certain strains of the influenza virus.

Pneumonia
Pneumonia is an infection of the lung that can be caused by nearly any class of organism known to cause human infections. These include bacteria, amoebae, viruses, fungi, and parasites.

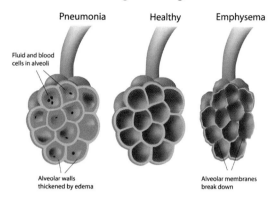

Pulmonary Abscess
Lung abscess that is a collection of infectious material contained within a capsule in the lung which results into coughing of bloody or foul-smelling sputum (breath foul-smelling). The most important preventative measure to avoid pulmonary abscess is to prevent aspiration.

Pulmonary TB
Pulmonary tuberculosis is an infection (inflammation) caused by mycobacterium tuberculosis.
Pathologic changes depend on the type of infection or "exposure." given below:
Primary pulmonary TB (Primary Exposure), Secondary pulmonary TB(Reactivation) and Progressive pulmonary TB.

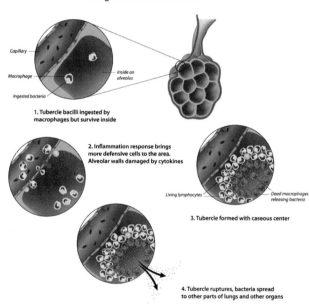

Asthma
Asthma is a common chronic inflammatory disease of the airways characterized by variable and recurring symptoms, reversible airflow obstruction, and bronchospasm. Common symptoms include wheezing, coughing, chest tightness, and shortness of breath.

Pathology of Asthma

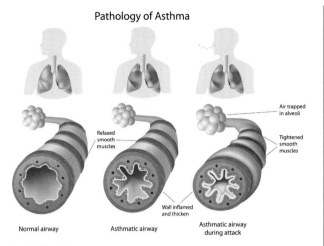

Normal airway　　Asthmatic airway　　Asthmatic airway during attack

Cystic Fibrosis
Cystic Fibrosis is an autosomal recessive genetic disorder that affects most critically the lungs, and also the pancreas, liver, and intestine. It is characterized by abnormal transport of chloride and sodium across an epithelium, leading to thick, viscous secretions.

Cystic Fibrosis

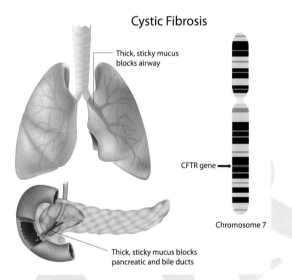

Chronic Obstructive Pulmonary Disease (COPD)
Chronic obstructive pulmonary disease (COPD) is a lung disease characterized by chronic obstruction of lung airflow that interferes with normal breathing and is not fully reversible. The more familiar terms 'chronic bronchitis' and 'emphysema' are no longer used, but are now included within the COPD diagnosis.

Emphysema
Emphysema is a chronic lung disease caused by damage to the alveoli, the tiny air sacs in the lung where exchange of oxygen and carbon dioxide takes place. With emphysema, damage to the alveoli results in air becoming trapped, causing them to expand and rupture.

Bronchiectasis
Bronchiectasis is a disease state defined by localized, irreversible dilation of part of the bronchial tree caused by destruction of the muscle and elastic tissue. It is classified as an obstructive lung disease, along with emphysema, bronchitis, asthma, and cystic fibrosis.

This page intentionally left blank

Diseases of the respiratory system (J00-J99)

[NOTES] When a respiratory condition is described as occurring in more than one site and is not specifically indexed, it should be classified to the lower anatomic site (e.g. tracheobronchitis to bronchitis in J40).

Use additional code, where applicable, to identify:
exposure to environmental tobacco smoke (Z77.22)
exposure to tobacco smoke in the perinatal period (P96.81)
history of tobacco use (Z87.891)
occupational exposure to environmental tobacco smoke (Z57.31)
tobacco dependence (F17.-)
tobacco use (Z72.0)

[EXCLUDES2] *certain conditions originating in the perinatal period (P04-P96)*
certain infectious and parasitic diseases (A00-B99)
complications of pregnancy, childbirth and the puerperium (O00-O9A)
congenital malformations, deformations and chromosomal abnormalities (Q00-Q99)
endocrine, nutritional and metabolic diseases (E00-E88)
injury, poisoning and certain other consequences of external causes (S00-T88)
neoplasms (C00-D49)
smoke inhalation (T59.81-)
symptoms, signs and abnormal clinical and laboratory findings, not elsewhere classified (R00-R94)

Acute upper respiratory infections (J00-J06)

[EXCLUDES1] *chronic obstructive pulmonary disease with acute lower respiratory infection (J44.0)*
influenza virus with other respiratory manifestations (J09.X2, J10.1, J11.1)

J00 Acute nasopharyngitis [common cold]
Acute rhinitis
Coryza (acute)
Infective nasopharyngitis NOS
Infective rhinitis
Nasal catarrh, acute
Nasopharyngitis NOS
[EXCLUDES1] *acute pharyngitis (J02.-)*
acute sore throat NOS (J02.9)
pharyngitis NOS (J02.9)
rhinitis NOS (J31.0)
sore throat NOS (J02.9)
[EXCLUDES2] *allergic rhinitis (J30.1-J30.9)*
chronic pharyngitis (J31.2)
chronic rhinitis (J31.0)
chronic sore throat (J31.2)
nasopharyngitis, chronic (J31.1)
vasomotor rhinitis (J30.0)

[4] **J01 Acute sinusitis**
[INCLUDES] *acute abscess of sinus*
acute empyema of sinus
acute infection of sinus
acute inflammation of sinus
acute suppuration of sinus
Use additional code (B95-B97) to identify infectious agent.
[EXCLUDES1] *sinusitis NOS (J32.9)*
[EXCLUDES2] *chronic sinusitis (J32.0-J32.8)*

[5] **J01.0 Acute maxillary sinusitis**
Acute antritis
J01.00 Acute maxillary sinusitis, unspecified
J01.01 Acute recurrent maxillary sinusitis

[5] **J01.1 Acute frontal sinusitis**
J01.10 Acute frontal sinusitis, unspecified
J01.11 Acute recurrent frontal sinusitis

[5] **J01.2 Acute ethmoidal sinusitis**
J01.20 Acute ethmoidal sinusitis, unspecified
J01.21 Acute recurrent ethmoidal sinusitis

[5] **J01.3 Acute sphenoidal sinusitis**
J01.30 Acute sphenoidal sinusitis, unspecified
J01.31 Acute recurrent sphenoidal sinusitis

[5] **J01.4 Acute pansinusitis**
J01.40 Acute pansinusitis, unspecified
J01.41 Acute recurrent pansinusitis

[5] **J01.8 Other acute sinusitis**
J01.80 Other acute sinusitis
Acute sinusitis involving more than one sinus but not pansinusitis
J01.81 Other acute recurrent sinusitis
Acute recurrent sinusitis involving more than one sinus but not pansinusitis

[5] **J01.9 Acute sinusitis, unspecified**
J01.90 Acute sinusitis, unspecified
J01.91 Acute recurrent sinusitis, unspecified

[4] **J02 Acute pharyngitis**
[INCLUDES] *acute sore throat*
[EXCLUDES1] *acute laryngopharyngitis (J06.0)*
peritonsillar abscess (J36)
pharyngeal abscess (J39.1)
retropharyngeal abscess (J39.0)
[EXCLUDES2] *chronic pharyngitis (J31.2)*

J02.0 Streptococcal pharyngitis
Septic pharyngitis
Streptococcal sore throat
[EXCLUDES2] *scarlet fever (A38.-)*

J02.8 Acute pharyngitis due to other specified organisms
Use additional code (B95-B97) to identify infectious agent
[EXCLUDES1] *acute pharyngitis due to coxsackie virus (B08.5)*
acute pharyngitis due to gonococcus (A54.5)
acute pharyngitis due to herpes [simplex] virus (B00.2)
acute pharyngitis due to infectious mononucleosis (B27.-)
enteroviral vesicular pharyngitis (B08.5)

J02.9 Acute pharyngitis, unspecified
Gangrenous pharyngitis (acute)
Infective pharyngitis (acute) NOS
Pharyngitis (acute) NOS
Sore throat (acute) NOS
Suppurative pharyngitis (acute)
Ulcerative pharyngitis (acute)

[4] **J03 Acute tonsillitis**
[EXCLUDES1] *acute sore throat (J02.-)*
hypertrophy of tonsils (J35.1)
peritonsillar abscess (J36)
sore throat NOS (J02.9)
streptococcal sore throat (J02.0)
[EXCLUDES2] *chronic tonsillitis (J35.0)*

[5] **J03.0 Streptococcal tonsillitis**
J03.00 Acute streptococcal tonsillitis, unspecified
J03.01 Acute recurrent streptococcal tonsillitis

[5] **J03.8 Acute tonsillitis due to other specified organisms**
Use additional code (B95-B97) to identify infectious agent.
[EXCLUDES1] *diphtheritic tonsillitis (A36.0)*
herpesviral pharyngotonsillitis (B00.2)
streptococcal tonsillitis (J03.0)
tuberculous tonsillitis (A15.8)
Vincent's tonsillitis (A69.1)

Unspecified Code | Other Specified Code | [N] Newborn Age: 0 | [P] Pediatric Age: 0-17 | [M] Maternity Age: 12-55
[A] Adult Age: 15-124 | ♂ Male | ♀ Female | ● New Code | ▲ Revised Code Title | ▶◀ Revised Text

J03.80 Acute tonsillitis due to other specified organisms
J03.81 Acute recurrent tonsillitis due to other specified organisms

[5] J03.9 Acute tonsillitis, unspecified
- Follicular tonsillitis (acute)
- Gangrenous tonsillitis (acute)
- Infective tonsillitis (acute)
- Tonsillitis (acute) NOS
- Ulcerative tonsillitis (acute)

J03.90 Acute tonsillitis, unspecified
J03.91 Acute recurrent tonsillitis, unspecified

[4] J04 Acute laryngitis and tracheitis
Use additional code (B95-B97) to identify infectious agent.
EXCLUDES1 *acute obstructive laryngitis [croup] and epiglottitis (J05.-)*
EXCLUDES2 *laryngismus (stridulus) (J38.5)*

J04.0 Acute laryngitis
- Edematous laryngitis (acute)
- Laryngitis (acute) NOS
- Subglottic laryngitis (acute)
- Suppurative laryngitis (acute)
- Ulcerative laryngitis (acute)

EXCLUDES1 *acute obstructive laryngitis (J05.0)*
EXCLUDES2 *chronic laryngitis (J37.0)*

[5] J04.1 Acute tracheitis
- Acute viral tracheitis
- Catarrhal tracheitis (acute)
- Tracheitis (acute) NOS

EXCLUDES2 *chronic tracheitis (J42)*

J04.10 Acute tracheitis without obstruction
J04.11 Acute tracheitis with obstruction

J04.2 Acute laryngotracheitis
- Laryngotracheitis NOS
- Tracheitis (acute) with laryngitis (acute)

EXCLUDES1 *acute obstructive laryngotracheitis (J05.0)*
EXCLUDES2 *chronic laryngotracheitis (J37.1)*

[5] J04.3 Supraglottitis, unspecified
J04.30 Supraglottitis, unspecified, without obstruction
J04.31 Supraglottitis, unspecified, with obstruction

[4] J05 Acute obstructive laryngitis [croup] and epiglottitis
Use additional code (B95-B97) to identify infectious agent.

J05.0 Acute obstructive laryngitis [croup]
- Obstructive laryngitis (acute) NOS
- Obstructive laryngotracheitis NOS

[5] J05.1 Acute epiglottitis
EXCLUDES2 *epiglottitis, chronic (J37.0)*

J05.10 Acute epiglottitis without obstruction
- Epiglottitis NOS

J05.11 Acute epiglottitis with obstruction

[4] J06 Acute upper respiratory infections of multiple and unspecified sites
EXCLUDES1 *acute respiratory infection NOS (J22)*
streptococcal pharyngitis (J02.0)

J06.0 Acute laryngopharyngitis
J06.9 Acute upper respiratory infection, unspecified
- Upper respiratory disease, acute
- Upper respiratory infection NOS

Influenza and pneumonia (J09-J18)

EXCLUDES2 *allergic or eosinophilic pneumonia (J82)*
aspiration pneumonia NOS (J69.0)
meconium pneumonia (P24.01)
neonatal aspiration pneumonia (P24.-)
pneumonia due to solids and liquids (J69.-)
congenital pneumonia (P23.9)
lipid pneumonia (J69.1)
rheumatic pneumonia (I00)
ventilator associated pneumonia (J95.851)

[4] J09 Influenza due to certain identified influenza viruses
EXCLUDES1 *influenza due to other identified influenza virus (J10.-)*
influenza due to unidentified influenza virus (J11.-)
seasonal influenza due to other identified influenza virus (J10.-)
seasonal influenza due to unidentified influenza virus (J11.-)

[5] J09.X Influenza due to identified novel influenza A virus

J09.X1 Influenza due to identified novel influenza A virus with pneumonia
Code also , if applicable, associated:
lung abscess (J85.1)
other specified type of pneumonia

J09.X2 Influenza due to identified novel influenza A virus with other respiratory manifestations
- Influenza due to identified novel influenza A virus NOS
- Influenza due to identified novel influenza A virus with laryngitis
- Influenza due to identified novel influenza A virus with pharyngitis
- Influenza due to identified novel influenza A virus with upper respiratory symptoms

Use additional code, if applicable, for associated:
pleural effusion (J91.8)
sinusitis (J01.-)

J09.X3 Influenza due to identified novel influenza A virus with gastrointestinal manifestations
- Influenza due to identified novel influenza A virus gastroenteritis

EXCLUDES1 *'intestinal flu' [viral gastroenteritis] (A08.-)*

J09.X9 Influenza due to identified novel influenza A virus with other manifestations
- Influenza due to identified novel influenza A virus with encephalopathy
- Influenza due to identified novel influenza A virus with myocarditis
- Influenza due to identified novel influenza A virus with otitis media

Use additional code to identify manifestation

[4] J10 Influenza due to other identified influenza virus
EXCLUDES1 *influenza due to avian influenza virus (J09.X-)*
influenza due to swine flu (J09.X-)
influenza due to unidentifed influenza virus (J11.-)

[5] J10.0 Influenza due to other identified influenza virus with pneumonia
Code also associated lung abscess, if applicable (J85.1)

J10.00 Influenza due to other identified influenza virus with unspecified type of pneumonia
J10.01 Influenza due to other identified influenza virus with the same other identified influenza virus pneumonia
J10.08 Influenza due to other identified influenza virus with other specified pneumonia
Code also other specified type of pneumonia

[4] 4th character required [5] 5th character required [6] 6th character required [7] 7th character required [X] Extension 'X' Alert
EXCLUDES1 Not coded here EXCLUDES2 Not included here [PDx] Primary Diagnosis Only Manifestation Code

J10.1 Influenza due to other identified influenza virus with other respiratory manifestations
Influenza due to other identified influenza virus NOS
Influenza due to other identified influenza virus with laryngitis
Influenza due to other identified influenza virus with pharyngitis
Influenza due to other identified influenza virus with upper respiratory symptoms
Use additional code for associated pleural effusion, if applicable (J91.8)
code for associated sinusitis, if applicable (J01.-)

J10.2 Influenza due to other identified influenza virus with gastrointestinal manifestations
Influenza due to other identified influenza virus gastroenteritis
[EXCLUDES1] *'intestinal flu' [viral gastroenteritis] (A08.-)*

[5] **J10.8 Influenza due to other identified influenza virus with other manifestations**

J10.81 Influenza due to other identified influenza virus with encephalopathy

J10.82 Influenza due to other identified influenza virus with myocarditis

J10.83 Influenza due to other identified influenza virus with otitis media
Use additional code for any associated perforated tympanic membrane (H72.-)

J10.89 Influenza due to other identified influenza virus with other manifestations
Use additional codes to identify the manifestations

[4] **J11 Influenza due to unidentified influenza virus**

[5] **J11.0 Influenza due to unidentified influenza virus with pneumonia**
Code also associated lung abscess, if applicable (J85.1)

J11.00 Influenza due to unidentified influenza virus with unspecified type of pneumonia
Influenza with pneumonia NOS

J11.08 Influenza due to unidentified influenza virus with specified pneumonia
Code also other specified type of pneumonia

J11.1 Influenza due to unidentified influenza virus with other respiratory manifestations
Influenza NOS
Influenzal laryngitis NOS
Influenzal pharyngitis NOS
Influenza with upper respiratory symptoms NOS
Use additional code for associated pleural effusion, if applicable (J91.8)
code for associated sinusitis, if applicable (J01.-)

J11.2 Influenza due to unidentified influenza virus with gastrointestinal manifestations
Influenza gastroenteritis NOS
[EXCLUDES1] *'intestinal flu' [viral gastroenteritis] (A08.-)*

[5] **J11.8 Influenza due to unidentified influenza virus with other manifestations**

J11.81 Influenza due to unidentified influenza virus with encephalopathy
Influenzal encephalopathy NOS

J11.82 Influenza due to unidentified influenza virus with myocarditis
Influenzal myocarditis NOS

J11.83 Influenza due to unidentified influenza virus with otitis media
Influenzal otitis media NOS
Use additional code for any associated perforated tympanic membrane (H72.-)

J11.89 Influenza due to unidentified influenza virus with other manifestations
Use additional codes to identify the manifestations

[4] **J12 Viral pneumonia, not elsewhere classified**
[INCLUDES] *bronchopneumonia due to viruses other than influenza viruses*
Code first associated influenza, if applicable (J09.X1, J10.0-, J11.0-)
Code also associated abscess, if applicable (J85.1)
[EXCLUDES1] *aspiration pneumonia due to anesthesia during labor and delivery (O74.0)*
aspiration pneumonia due to anesthesia during pregnancy (O29)
aspiration pneumonia due to anesthesia during puerperium (O89.0)
aspiration pneumonia due to solids and liquids (J69.-)
aspiration pneumonia NOS (J69.0)
congenital pneumonia (P23.0)
congenital rubella pneumonitis (P35.0)
interstitial pneumonia NOS (J84.9)
lipid pneumonia (J69.1)
neonatal aspiration pneumonia (P24.-)

J12.0 Adenoviral pneumonia

J12.1 Respiratory syncytial virus pneumonia

J12.2 Parainfluenza virus pneumonia

J12.3 Human metapneumovirus pneumonia

[5] **J12.8 Other viral pneumonia**

J12.81 Pneumonia due to SARS-associated coronavirus
Severe acute respiratory syndrome NOS

J12.89 Other viral pneumonia

J12.9 Viral pneumonia, unspecified

J13 Pneumonia due to Streptococcus pneumoniae
Bronchopneumonia due to S. pneumoniae
Code first associated influenza, if applicable (J09.X1, J10.0-, J11.0-)
Code also associated abscess, if applicable (J85.1)
[EXCLUDES1] *congenital pneumonia due to S. pneumoniae (P23.6)*
lobar pneumonia, unspecified organism (J18.1)
pneumonia due to other streptococci (J15.3-J15.4)

J14 Pneumonia due to Hemophilus influenzae
Bronchopneumonia due to H. influenzae
Code first associated influenza, if applicable (J09.X1, J10.0-, J11.0-)
Code also associated abscess, if applicable (J85.1)
[EXCLUDES1] *congenital pneumonia due to H. influenzae (P23.6)*

[4] **J15 Bacterial pneumonia, not elsewhere classified**
[INCLUDES] *bronchopneumonia due to bacteria other than S. pneumoniae and H. influenzae*
Code first associated influenza, if applicable (J09.X1, J10.0-, J11.0-)
Code also associated abscess, if applicable (J85.1)
[EXCLUDES1] *chlamydial pneumonia (J16.0)*
congenital pneumonia (P23.-)
Legionnaires' disease (A48.1)
spirochetal pneumonia (A69.8)

J15.0 Pneumonia due to Klebsiella pneumoniae

J15.1 Pneumonia due to Pseudomonas

[5] **J15.2 Pneumonia due to staphylococcus**

J15.20 Pneumonia due to staphylococcus, unspecified

[6] **J15.21 Pneumonia due to staphylococcus aureus**

J15.211 Pneumonia due to Methicillin susceptible Staphylococcus aureus
MSSA pneumonia
Pneumonia due to Staphylococcus aureus NOS

J15.212 Pneumonia due to Methicillin resistant Staphylococcus aureus

J15.29 Pneumonia due to other staphylococcus

Unspecified Code | Other Specified Code | [N] Newborn Age: 0 | [P] Pediatric Age: 0-17 | [M] Maternity Age: 12-55
[A] Adult Age: 15-124 | ♂ Male | ♀ Female | ● New Code | ▲ Revised Code Title | ►◄ Revised Text

J15.3 Pneumonia due to streptococcus, group B
J15.4 Pneumonia due to other streptococci

EXCLUDES1 pneumonia due to streptococcus, group B (J15.3)
pneumonia due to Streptococcus pneumoniae (J13)

J15.5 Pneumonia due to Escherichia coli
J15.6 Pneumonia due to other aerobic Gram-negative bacteria

Pneumonia due to Serratia marcescens

J15.7 Pneumonia due to Mycoplasma pneumoniae
J15.8 Pneumonia due to other specified bacteria
J15.9 Unspecified bacterial pneumonia

Pneumonia due to gram-positive bacteria

④ J16 Pneumonia due to other infectious organisms, not elsewhere classified

Code first associated influenza, if applicable (J09.X1, J10.0-, J11.0-)

Code also associated abscess, if applicable (J85.1)

EXCLUDES1 congenital pneumonia (P23.-)
ornithosis (A70)
pneumocystosis (B59)
pneumonia NOS (J18.9)

J16.0 Chlamydial pneumonia
J16.8 Pneumonia due to other specified infectious organisms

J17 Pneumonia in diseases classified elsewhere

Code first underlying disease, such as:
Q fever (A78)
rheumatic fever (I00)
schistosomiasis (B65.0-B65.9)

EXCLUDES1 candidial pneumonia (B37.1)
chlamydial pneumonia (J16.0)
gonorrheal pneumonia (A54.84)
histoplasmosis pneumonia (B39.0-B39.2)
measles pneumonia (B05.2)
nocardiosis pneumonia (A43.0)
pneumocystosis (B59)
pneumonia due to Pneumocystis carinii (B59)
pneumonia due to Pneumocystis jiroveci (B59)
pneumonia in actinomycosis (A42.0)
pneumonia in anthrax (A22.1)
pneumonia in ascariasis (B77.81)
pneumonia in aspergillosis (B44.0-B44.1)
pneumonia in coccidioidomycosis (B38.0-B38.2)
pneumonia in cytomegalovirus disease (B25.0)
pneumonia in toxoplasmosis (B58.3)
rubella pneumonia (B06.81)
salmonella pneumonia (A02.22)
spirochetal infection NEC with pneumonia (A69.8)
tularemia pneumonia (A21.2)
typhoid fever with pneumonia (A01.03)
varicella pneumonia (B01.2)
whooping cough with pneumonia (A37 with fifth-character 1)

④ J18 Pneumonia, unspecified organism

Code first associated influenza, if applicable (J09.X1, J10.0-, J11.0-)

EXCLUDES1 abscess of lung with pneumonia (J85.1)
aspiration pneumonia due to anesthesia during labor and delivery (O74.0)
aspiration pneumonia due to anesthesia during pregnancy (O29)
aspiration pneumonia due to anesthesia during puerperium (O89.0)
aspiration pneumonia due to solids and liquids (J69.-)
aspiration pneumonia NOS (J69.0)
congenital pneumonia (P23.0)
drug-induced interstitial lung disorder (J70.2-

J70.4)
interstitial pneumonia NOS (J84.9)
lipid pneumonia (J69.1)
neonatal aspiration pneumonia (P24.-)
pneumonitis due to external agents (J67-J70)
pneumonitis due to fumes and vapors (J68.0)
usual interstitial pneumonia (J84.17)

J18.0 Bronchopneumonia, unspecified organism

EXCLUDES1 hypostatic bronchopneumonia (J18.2)
lipid pneumonia (J69.1)

EXCLUDES2 acute bronchiolitis (J21.-)
chronic bronchiolitis (J44.9)

J18.1 Lobar pneumonia, unspecified organism
J18.2 Hypostatic pneumonia, unspecified organism

Hypostatic bronchopneumonia
Passive pneumonia

J18.8 Other pneumonia, unspecified organism
J18.9 Pneumonia, unspecified organism

Other acute lower respiratory infections (J20-J22)

EXCLUDES2 chronic obstructive pulmonary disease with acute lower respiratory infection (J44.0)

④ J20 Acute bronchitis

INCLUDES acute and subacute bronchitis (with) bronchospasm
acute and subacute bronchitis (with) tracheitis
acute and subacute bronchitis (with) tracheobronchitis, acute
acute and subacute fibrinous bronchitis
acute and subacute membranous bronchitis
acute and subacute purulent bronchitis
acute and subacute septic bronchitis

EXCLUDES2 acute bronchitis with bronchiectasis (J47.0)
acute bronchitis with chronic obstructive asthma (J44.0)
acute bronchitis with chronic obstructive pulmonary disease (J44.0)
allergic bronchitis NOS (J45.909-)
bronchitis due to chemicals, fumes and vapors (J68.0)
chronic bronchitis NOS (J42)
chronic mucopurulent bronchitis (J41.1)
chronic obstructive bronchitis (J44.-)
chronic obstructive tracheobronchitis (J44.-)
chronic simple bronchitis (J41.0)
chronic tracheobronchitis (J42)

EXCLUDES1 bronchitis NOS (J40)
tracheobronchitis NOS (J40)

J20.0 Acute bronchitis due to Mycoplasma pneumoniae
J20.1 Acute bronchitis due to Hemophilus influenzae
J20.2 Acute bronchitis due to streptococcus
J20.3 Acute bronchitis due to coxsackievirus
J20.4 Acute bronchitis due to parainfluenza virus
J20.5 Acute bronchitis due to respiratory syncytial virus
J20.6 Acute bronchitis due to rhinovirus
J20.7 Acute bronchitis due to echovirus
J20.8 Acute bronchitis due to other specified organisms
J20.9 Acute bronchitis, unspecified

④ J21 Acute bronchiolitis

INCLUDES acute bronchiolitis with bronchospasm

EXCLUDES2 respiratory bronchiolitis interstitial lung disease (J84.115)

J21.0 Acute bronchiolitis due to respiratory syncytial virus
J21.1 Acute bronchiolitis due to human metapneumovirus
J21.8 Acute bronchiolitis due to other specified organisms
J21.9 Acute bronchiolitis, unspecified

Bronchiolitis (acute)

EXCLUDES1 chronic bronchiolitis (J44.-)

J22 Unspecified acute lower respiratory infection

Acute (lower) respiratory (tract) infection NOS

EXCLUDES1 upper respiratory infection (acute) (J06.9)

---

④ 4th character required   ⑤ 5th character required   ⑥ 6th character required   ⑦ 7th character required   ⑦ˣ Extension 'X' Alert

EXCLUDES 1 Not coded here   EXCLUDES 2 Not included here   ᴾᴰˣ Primary Diagnosis Only   Manifestation Code

Other diseases of upper respiratory tract (J30-J39)

⊕ **J30 Vasomotor and allergic rhinitis**

INCLUDES spasmodic rhinorrhea

EXCLUDES1 allergic rhinitis with asthma (bronchial) (J45.909)
rhinitis NOS (J31.0)

J30.0 Vasomotor rhinitis

J30.1 Allergic rhinitis due to pollen

Allergy NOS due to pollen

Hay fever

Pollinosis

J30.2 Other seasonal allergic rhinitis

J30.5 Allergic rhinitis due to food

⑤ **J30.8 Other allergic rhinitis**

J30.81 Allergic rhinitis due to animal (cat) (dog) hair and dander

J30.89 Other allergic rhinitis

Perennial allergic rhinitis

J30.9 Allergic rhinitis, unspecified

⊕ **J31 Chronic rhinitis, nasopharyngitis and pharyngitis**

Use additional code to identify:

exposure to environmental tobacco smoke (Z77.22)

exposure to tobacco smoke in the perinatal period (P96.81)

history of tobacco use (Z87.891)

occupational exposure to environmental tobacco smoke (Z57.31)

tobacco dependence (F17.-)

tobacco use (Z72.0)

J31.0 Chronic rhinitis

Atrophic rhinitis (chronic)

Granulomatous rhinitis (chronic)

Hypertrophic rhinitis (chronic)

Obstructive rhinitis (chronic)

Ozena

Purulent rhinitis (chronic)

Rhinitis (chronic) NOS

Ulcerative rhinitis (chronic)

EXCLUDES1 allergic rhinitis (J30.1-J30.9)
vasomotor rhinitis (J30.0)

J31.1 Chronic nasopharyngitis

EXCLUDES2 acute nasopharyngitis (J00)

J31.2 Chronic pharyngitis

Chronic sore throat

Atrophic pharyngitis (chronic)

Granular pharyngitis (chronic)

Hypertrophic pharyngitis (chronic)

EXCLUDES2 acute pharyngitis (J02.9)

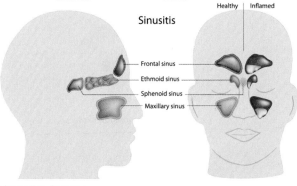

Figure 9.1 Sinusitis

⊕ **J32 Chronic sinusitis**

INCLUDES sinus abscess
sinus empyema
sinus infection
sinus suppuration

Use additional code to identify:

exposure to environmental tobacco smoke (Z77.22)

exposure to tobacco smoke in the perinatal period (P96.81)

history of tobacco use (Z87.891)

infectious agent (B95-B97)

occupational exposure to environmental tobacco smoke (Z57.31)

tobacco dependence (F17.-)

tobacco use (Z72.0)

EXCLUDES2 acute sinusitis (J01.-)

J32.0 Chronic maxillary sinusitis

Antritis (chronic)

Maxillary sinusitis NOS

J32.1 Chronic frontal sinusitis

Frontal sinusitis NOS

J32.2 Chronic ethmoidal sinusitis

Ethmoidal sinusitis NOS

EXCLUDES1 Woakes' ethmoiditis (J33.1)

J32.3 Chronic sphenoidal sinusitis

Sphenoidal sinusitis NOS

J32.4 Chronic pansinusitis

Pansinusitis NOS

J32.8 Other chronic sinusitis

Sinusitis (chronic) involving more than one sinus but not pansinusitis

J32.9 Chronic sinusitis, unspecified

Sinusitis (chronic) NOS

⊕ **J33 Nasal polyp**

Use additional code to identify:

exposure to environmental tobacco smoke (Z77.22)

exposure to tobacco smoke in the perinatal period (P96.81)

history of tobacco use (Z87.891)

occupational exposure to environmental tobacco smoke (Z57.31)

tobacco dependence (F17.-)

tobacco use (Z72.0)

EXCLUDES1 adenomatous polyps (D14.0)

J33.0 Polyp of nasal cavity

Choanal polyp

Nasopharyngeal polyp

J33.1 Polypoid sinus degeneration

Woakes' syndrome or ethmoiditis

J33.8 Other polyp of sinus

Accessory polyp of sinus

Ethmoidal polyp of sinus

Maxillary polyp of sinus

Sphenoidal polyp of sinus

J33.9 Nasal polyp, unspecified

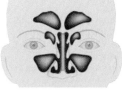

Normal

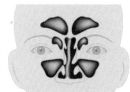

Deviated Septum

Figure 9.2 Deviated nasal septum

Unspecified Code	Other Specified Code	N Newborn Age: 0	P Pediatric Age: 0-17	M Maternity Age: 12-55
A Adult Age: 15-124	♂ Male	♀ Female	● New Code	▲ Revised Code Title ►◄ Revised Text

J34 Other and unspecified disorders of nose and nasal sinuses

> *EXCLUDES2 varicose ulcer of nasal septum (I86.8)*

J34.0 Abscess, furuncle and carbuncle of nose

Cellulitis of nose
Necrosis of nose
Ulceration of nose

J34.1 Cyst and mucocele of nose and nasal sinus

J34.2 Deviated nasal septum

Deflection or deviation of septum (nasal) (acquired)

> *EXCLUDES1 congenital deviated nasal septum (Q67.4)*

J34.3 Hypertrophy of nasal turbinates

J34.8 Other specified disorders of nose and nasal sinuses

J34.81 Nasal mucositis (ulcerative)

Code also type of associated therapy, such as:
antineoplastic and immunosuppressive drugs (T45.1X-)
radiological procedure and radiotherapy (Y84.2)

> *EXCLUDES2 gastrointestinal mucositis (ulcerative) (K92.81)*
> *mucositis (ulcerative) of vagina and vulva (N76.81)*
> *oral mucositis (ulcerative) (K12.3-)*

J34.89 Other specified disorders of nose and nasal sinuses

Perforation of nasal septum NOS
Rhinolith

J34.9 Unspecified disorder of nose and nasal sinuses

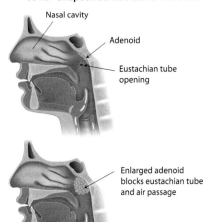

Figure 9.3 Adenoid hypertrophy

J35 Chronic diseases of tonsils and adenoids

Use additional code to identify:
exposure to environmental tobacco smoke (Z77.22)
exposure to tobacco smoke in the perinatal period (P96.81)
history of tobacco use (Z87.891)
occupational exposure to environmental tobacco smoke (Z57.31)
tobacco dependence (F17.-)
tobacco use (Z72.0)

J35.0 Chronic tonsillitis and adenoiditis

> *EXCLUDES2 acute tonsillitis (J03.-)*

J35.01 Chronic tonsillitis
J35.02 Chronic adenoiditis
J35.03 Chronic tonsillitis and adenoiditis

J35.1 Hypertrophy of tonsils

Enlargement of tonsils

> *EXCLUDES1 hypertrophy of tonsils with tonsillitis (J35.0-)*

J35.2 Hypertrophy of adenoids

Enlargement of adenoids

> *EXCLUDES1 hypertrophy of adenoids with adenoiditis (J35.0-)*

J35.3 Hypertrophy of tonsils with hypertrophy of adenoids

> *EXCLUDES1 hypertrophy of tonsils and adenoids with tonsillitis and adenoiditis (J35.03)*

J35.8 Other chronic diseases of tonsils and adenoids

Adenoid vegetations
Amygdalolith
Calculus, tonsil
Cicatrix of tonsil (and adenoid)
Tonsillar tag
Ulcer of tonsil

J35.9 Chronic disease of tonsils and adenoids, unspecified

Disease (chronic) of tonsils and adenoids NOS

J36 Peritonsillar abscess

> *INCLUDES abscess of tonsil*
> *peritonsillar cellulitis*
> *quinsy*

Use additional code (B95-B97) to identify infectious agent.

> *EXCLUDES1 acute tonsillitis (J03.-)*
> *chronic tonsillitis (J35.0)*
> *retropharyngeal abscess (J39.0)*
> *tonsillitis NOS (J03.9-)*

J37 Chronic laryngitis and laryngotracheitis

Use additional code to identify:
exposure to environmental tobacco smoke (Z77.22)
exposure to tobacco smoke in the perinatal period (P96.81)
history of tobacco use (Z87.891)
infectious agent (B95-B97)
occupational exposure to environmental tobacco smoke (Z57.31)
tobacco dependence (F17.-)
tobacco use (Z72.0)

J37.0 Chronic laryngitis

Catarrhal laryngitis
Hypertrophic laryngitis
Sicca laryngitis

> *EXCLUDES2 acute laryngitis (J04.0)*
> *obstructive (acute) laryngitis (J05.0)*

J37.1 Chronic laryngotracheitis

Laryngitis, chronic, with tracheitis (chronic)
Tracheitis, chronic, with laryngitis

> *EXCLUDES1 chronic tracheitis (J42)*

> *EXCLUDES2 acute laryngotracheitis (J04.2)*
> *acute tracheitis (J04.1)*

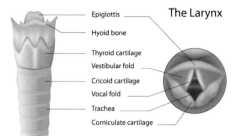

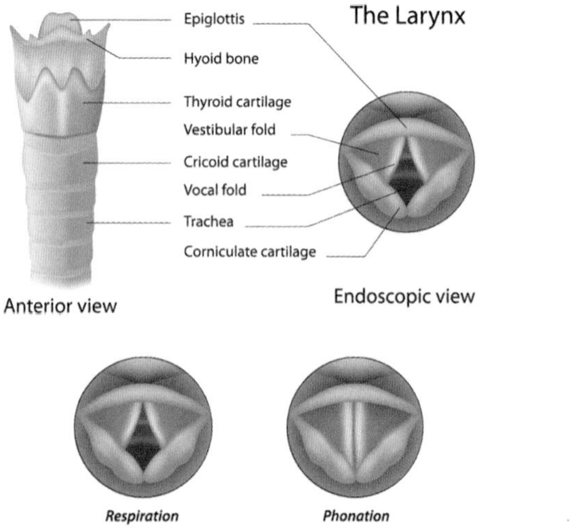

Figure 9.4 The Larynx

| ④ 4th character required | ⑤ 5th character required | ⑥ 6th character required | ⑦ 7th character required | ⑦ Extension 'X' Alert |

EXCLUDES 1 Not coded here   *EXCLUDES 2* Not included here   PDx Primary Diagnosis Only   Manifestation Code

260   ICD-10-CM 2015

J38 Diseases of vocal cords and larynx, not elsewhere classified
>Use additional code to identify:
>exposure to environmental tobacco smoke (Z77.22)
>exposure to tobacco smoke in the perinatal period (P96.81)
>history of tobacco use (Z87.891)
>occupational exposure to environmental tobacco smoke (Z57.31)
>tobacco dependence (F17.-)
>tobacco use (Z72.0)
>
>> *EXCLUDES1* *congenital laryngeal stridor (P28.89)*
>> *obstructive laryngitis (acute) (J05.0)*
>> *postprocedural subglottic stenosis (J95.5)*
>> *stridor (R06.1)*
>> *ulcerative laryngitis (J04.0)*

J38.0 Paralysis of vocal cords and larynx
>Laryngoplegia
>Paralysis of glottis
>
>J38.00 Paralysis of vocal cords and larynx, unspecified
>J38.01 Paralysis of vocal cords and larynx, unilateral
>J38.02 Paralysis of vocal cords and larynx, bilateral

J38.1 Polyp of vocal cord and larynx
>> *EXCLUDES1* *adenomatous polyps (D14.1)*

J38.2 Nodules of vocal cords
>Chorditis (fibrinous)(nodosa)(tuberosa)
>Singer's nodes
>Teacher's nodes

J38.3 Other diseases of vocal cords
>Abscess of vocal cords
>Cellulitis of vocal cords
>Granuloma of vocal cords
>Leukokeratosis of vocal cords
>Leukoplakia of vocal cords

J38.4 Edema of larynx
>Edema (of) glottis
>Subglottic edema
>Supraglottic edema
>
>> *EXCLUDES1* *acute obstructive laryngitis [croup] (J05.0)*
>> *edematous laryngitis (J04.0)*

J38.5 Laryngeal spasm
>Laryngismus (stridulus)

J38.6 Stenosis of larynx

J38.7 Other diseases of larynx
>Abscess of larynx
>Cellulitis of larynx
>Disease of larynx NOS
>Necrosis of larynx
>Pachyderma of larynx
>Perichondritis of larynx
>Ulcer of larynx

J39 Other diseases of upper respiratory tract
>> *EXCLUDES1* *acute respiratory infection NOS (J22)*
>> *acute upper respiratory infection (J06.9)*
>> *upper respiratory inflammation due to chemicals, gases, fumes or vapors (J68.2)*

J39.0 Retropharyngeal and parapharyngeal abscess
>Peripharyngeal abscess
>
>> *EXCLUDES1* *peritonsillar abscess (J36)*

J39.1 Other abscess of pharynx
>Cellulitis of pharynx
>Nasopharyngeal abscess

J39.2 Other diseases of pharynx
>Cyst of pharynx
>Edema of pharynx
>
>> *EXCLUDES2* *chronic pharyngitis (J31.2)*
>> *ulcerative pharyngitis (J02.9)*

J39.3 Upper respiratory tract hypersensitivity reaction, site unspecified
>> *EXCLUDES1* *hypersensitivity reaction of upper respiratory tract, such as:*
>> *extrinsic allergic alveolitis (J67.9)*
>> *pneumoconiosis (J60-J67.9)*

J39.8 Other specified diseases of upper respiratory tract
J39.9 Disease of upper respiratory tract, unspecified

Chronic lower respiratory diseases (J40-J47)

>> *EXCLUDES1* *bronchitis due to chemicals, gases, fumes and vapors (J68.0)*
>> *EXCLUDES2* *cystic fibrosis (E84.-)*

J40 Bronchitis, not specified as acute or chronic
>Bronchitis NOS
>Bronchitis with tracheitis NOS
>Catarrhal bronchitis
>Tracheobronchitis NOS
>Use additional code to identify:
>exposure to environmental tobacco smoke (Z77.22)
>exposure to tobacco smoke in the perinatal period (P96.81)
>history of tobacco use (Z87.891)
>occupational exposure to environmental tobacco smoke (Z57.31)
>tobacco dependence (F17.-)
>tobacco use (Z72.0)
>
>> *EXCLUDES1* *acute bronchitis (J20.-)*
>> *allergic bronchitis NOS (J45.909-)*
>> *asthmatic bronchitis NOS (J45.9-)*
>> *bronchitis due to chemicals, gases, fumes and vapors (J68.0)*

J41 Simple and mucopurulent chronic bronchitis
>Use additional code to identify:
>exposure to environmental tobacco smoke (Z77.22)
>exposure to tobacco smoke in the perinatal period (P96.81)
>history of tobacco use (Z87.891)
>occupational exposure to environmental tobacco smoke (Z57.31)
>tobacco dependence (F17.-)
>tobacco use (Z72.0)
>
>> *EXCLUDES1* *chronic bronchitis NOS (J42)*
>> *chronic obstructive bronchitis (J44.-)*

>J41.0 Simple chronic bronchitis
>J41.1 Mucopurulent chronic bronchitis
>J41.8 Mixed simple and mucopurulent chronic bronchitis

J42 Unspecified chronic bronchitis
>Chronic bronchitis NOS
>Chronic tracheitis
>Chronic tracheobronchitis
>Use additional code to identify:
>exposure to environmental tobacco smoke (Z77.22)
>exposure to tobacco smoke in the perinatal period (P96.81)
>history of tobacco use (Z87.891)
>occupational exposure to environmental tobacco smoke (Z57.31)
>tobacco dependence (F17.-)
>tobacco use (Z72.0)
>
>> *EXCLUDES1* *chronic asthmatic bronchitis (J44.-)*
>> *chronic bronchitis with airways obstruction (J44.-)*
>> *chronic emphysematous bronchitis (J44.-)*
>> *chronic obstructive pulmonary disease NOS (J44.9)*
>> *simple and mucopurulent chronic bronchitis (J41.-)*

Unspecified Code	Other Specified Code	N Newborn Age: 0 P Pediatric Age: 0-17 M Maternity Age: 12-55
A Adult Age: 15-124 ♂ Male ♀ Female ● New Code ▲ Revised Code Title ►◄ Revised Text	

[4] **J43 Emphysema**

Use additional code to identify:
exposure to environmental tobacco smoke (Z77.22)
history of tobacco use (Z87.891)
occupational exposure to environmental tobacco smoke (Z57.31)
tobacco dependence (F17.-)
tobacco use (Z72.0)

[EXCLUDES1] *compensatory emphysema (J98.3)*
emphysema due to inhalation of chemicals, gases, fumes or vapors (J68.4)
emphysema with chronic (obstructive) bronchitis (J44.-)
emphysematous (obstructive) bronchitis (J44.-)
interstitial emphysema (J98.2)
mediastinal emphysema (J98.2)
neonatal interstitial emphysema (P25.0)
surgical (subcutaneous) emphysema (T81.82)
traumatic subcutaneous emphysema (T79.7)

J43.0 Unilateral pulmonary emphysema [MacLeod's syndrome]
Swyer-James syndrome
Unilateral emphysema
Unilateral hyperlucent lung
Unilateral pulmonary artery functional hypoplasia
Unilateral transparency of lung

J43.1 Panlobular emphysema
Panacinar emphysema

J43.2 Centrilobular emphysema

J43.8 Other emphysema

J43.9 Emphysema, unspecified
Bullous emphysema (lung)(pulmonary)
Emphysema (lung)(pulmonary) NOS
Emphysematous bleb
Vesicular emphysema (lung)(pulmonary)

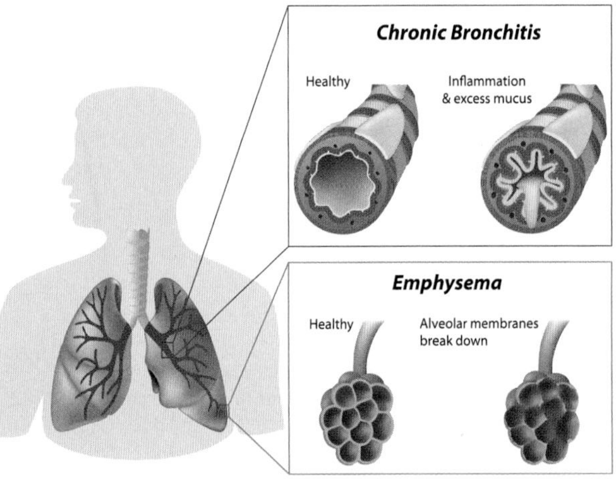
Chronic Bronchitis
Healthy
Inflammation
& excess mucus
Emphysema
Healthy
Alveolar membranes
break down

Figure 9.5 Chronic Obstructive Pulmonary Disease (COPD): Chronic Bronchitis and Emphysema

[4] **J44 Other chronic obstructive pulmonary disease**

[INCLUDES] *asthma with chronic obstructive pulmonary disease*
chronic asthmatic (obstructive) bronchitis
chronic bronchitis with airways obstruction
chronic bronchitis with emphysema
chronic emphysematous bronchitis
chronic obstructive asthma
chronic obstructive bronchitis
chronic obstructive tracheobronchitis

Code also type of asthma, if applicable (J45.-)
Use additional code to identify:
exposure to environmental tobacco smoke (Z77.22)
history of tobacco use (Z87.891)
occupational exposure to environmental tobacco smoke (Z57.31)
tobacco dependence (F17.-)
tobacco use (Z72.0)

[EXCLUDES1] *bronchiectasis (J47.-)*
chronic bronchitis NOS (J42)
chronic simple and mucopurulent bronchitis (J41.-)
chronic tracheitis (J42)
chronic tracheobronchitis (J42)
emphysema without chronic bronchitis (J43.-)
lung diseases due to external agents (J60-J70)

J44.0 Chronic obstructive pulmonary disease with acute lower respiratory infection
Use additional code to identify the infection

J44.1 Chronic obstructive pulmonary disease with (acute) exacerbation
Decompensated COPD
Decompensated COPD with (acute) exacerbation
[EXCLUDES2] *chronic obstructive pulmonary disease [COPD] with acute bronchitis (J44.0)*

J44.9 Chronic obstructive pulmonary disease, unspecified
Chronic obstructive airway disease NOS
Chronic obstructive lung disease NOS

[4] **J45 Asthma**

[INCLUDES] *allergic (predominantly) asthma*
allergic bronchitis NOS
allergic rhinitis with asthma
atopic asthma
extrinsic allergic asthma
hay fever with asthma
idiosyncratic asthma
intrinsic nonallergic asthma
nonallergic asthma

Use additional code to identify:
exposure to environmental tobacco smoke (Z77.22)
exposure to tobacco smoke in the perinatal period (P96.81)
history of tobacco use (Z87.891)
occupational exposure to environmental tobacco smoke (Z57.31)
tobacco dependence (F17.-)
tobacco use (Z72.0)

[EXCLUDES1] *detergent asthma (J69.8)*
eosinophilic asthma (J82)
lung diseases due to external agents (J60-J70)
miner's asthma (J60)
wheezing NOS (R06.2)
wood asthma (J67.8)

[EXCLUDES2] *asthma with chronic obstructive pulmonary disease (J44.9)*
chronic asthmatic (obstructive) bronchitis (J44.9)
chronic obstructive asthma (J44.9)

[5] **J45.2 Mild intermittent asthma**
J45.20 Mild intermittent asthma, uncomplicated
Mild intermittent asthma NOS
J45.21 Mild intermittent asthma with (acute) exacerbation
J45.22 Mild intermittent asthma with status asthmaticus

[5] **J45.3 Mild persistent asthma**
J45.30 Mild persistent asthma, uncomplicated
Mild persistent asthma NOS
J45.31 Mild persistent asthma with (acute) exacerbation
J45.32 Mild persistent asthma with status asthmaticus

[5] **J45.4 Moderate persistent asthma**
J45.40 Moderate persistent asthma, uncomplicated
Moderate persistent asthma NOS

[4] 4th character required [5] 5th character required [6] 6th character required [7] 7th character required [x7th] Extension 'X' Alert
[EXCLUDES1] Not coded here [EXCLUDES2] Not included here [PDx] Primary Diagnosis Only Manifestation Code

K05.30 Chronic periodontitis, unspecified
K05.31 Chronic periodontitis, localized
K05.32 Chronic periodontitis, generalized
K05.4 Periodontosis
Juvenile periodontosis
K05.5 Other periodontal diseases
[EXCLUDES2] *leukoplakia of gingiva (K13.21)*
K05.6 Periodontal disease, unspecified

[4] K06 Other disorders of gingiva and edentulous alveolar ridge
[EXCLUDES2] *acute gingivitis (K05.0)*
atrophy of edentulous alveolar ridge (K08.2)
chronic gingivitis (K05.1)
gingivitis NOS (K05.1)
K06.0 Gingival recession
Gingival recession (generalized) (localized) (postinfective) (postprocedural)
K06.1 Gingival enlargement
Gingival fibromatosis
K06.2 Gingival and edentulous alveolar ridge lesions associated with trauma
Irritative hyperplasia of edentulous ridge [denture hyperplasia]
Use additional code (Chapter 20) to identify external cause or denture status (Z97.2)
K06.8 Other specified disorders of gingiva and edentulous alveolar ridge
Fibrous epulis
Flabby alveolar ridge
Giant cell epulis
Peripheral giant cell granuloma of gingiva
Pyogenic granuloma of gingiva
[EXCLUDES2] *gingival cyst (K09.0)*
K06.9 Disorder of gingiva and edentulous alveolar ridge, unspecified

[4] K08 Other disorders of teeth and supporting structures
[EXCLUDES2] *dentofacial anomalies [including malocclusion] (M26.-)*
disorders of jaw (M27.-)
K08.0 Exfoliation of teeth due to systemic causes
Code also underlying systemic condition
[5] K08.1 Complete loss of teeth
Acquired loss of teeth, complete
[EXCLUDES1] *congenital absence of teeth (K00.0)*
exfoliation of teeth due to systemic causes (K08.0)
partial loss of teeth (K08.4-)
[6] K08.10 Complete loss of teeth, unspecified cause
K08.101 Complete loss of teeth, unspecified cause, class I
K08.102 Complete loss of teeth, unspecified cause, class II
K08.103 Complete loss of teeth, unspecified cause, class III
K08.104 Complete loss of teeth, unspecified cause, class IV
K08.109 Complete loss of teeth, unspecified cause, unspecified class
Edentulism NOS
[6] K08.11 Complete loss of teeth due to trauma
K08.111 Complete loss of teeth due to trauma, class I
K08.112 Complete loss of teeth due to trauma, class II
K08.113 Complete loss of teeth due to trauma, class III
K08.114 Complete loss of teeth due to trauma, class IV
K08.119 Complete loss of teeth due to trauma, unspecified class
[6] K08.12 Complete loss of teeth due to periodontal diseases
K08.121 Complete loss of teeth due to periodontal diseases, class I
K08.122 Complete loss of teeth due to periodontal diseases, class II
K08.123 Complete loss of teeth due to periodontal diseases, class III
K08.124 Complete loss of teeth due to periodontal diseases, class IV
K08.129 Complete loss of teeth due to periodontal diseases, unspecified class
[6] K08.13 Complete loss of teeth due to caries
K08.131 Complete loss of teeth due to caries, class I
K08.132 Complete loss of teeth due to caries, class II
K08.133 Complete loss of teeth due to caries, class III
K08.134 Complete loss of teeth due to caries, class IV
K08.139 Complete loss of teeth due to caries, unspecified class
[6] K08.19 Complete loss of teeth due to other specified cause
K08.191 Complete loss of teeth due to other specified cause, class I
K08.192 Complete loss of teeth due to other specified cause, class II
K08.193 Complete loss of teeth due to other specified cause, class III
K08.194 Complete loss of teeth due to other specified cause, class IV
K08.199 Complete loss of teeth due to other specified cause, unspecified class
[5] K08.2 Atrophy of edentulous alveolar ridge
K08.20 Unspecified atrophy of edentulous alveolar ridge
Atrophy of the mandible NOS
Atrophy of the maxilla NOS
K08.21 Minimal atrophy of the mandible
Minimal atrophy of the edentulous mandible
K08.22 Moderate atrophy of the mandible
Moderate atrophy of the edentulous mandible
K08.23 Severe atrophy of the mandible
Severe atrophy of the edentulous mandible
K08.24 Minimal atrophy of maxilla
Minimal atrophy of the edentulous maxilla
K08.25 Moderate atrophy of the maxilla
Moderate atrophy of the edentulous maxilla
K08.26 Severe atrophy of the maxilla
Severe atrophy of the edentulous maxilla
K08.3 Retained dental root
[5] K08.4 Partial loss of teeth
Acquired loss of teeth, partial
[EXCLUDES1] *complete loss of teeth (K08.1-)*
congenital absence of teeth (K00.0)
[EXCLUDES2] *exfoliation of teeth due to systemic causes (K08.0)*
[6] K08.40 Partial loss of teeth, unspecified cause
K08.401 Partial loss of teeth, unspecified cause, class I
K08.402 Partial loss of teeth, unspecified cause, class II
K08.403 Partial loss of teeth, unspecified cause, class III
K08.404 Partial loss of teeth, unspecified cause, class IV
K08.409 Partial loss of teeth, unspecified cause, unspecified class
Tooth extraction status NOS
[6] K08.41 Partial loss of teeth due to trauma
K08.411 Partial loss of teeth due to trauma, class I
K08.412 Partial loss of teeth due to trauma, class II
K08.413 Partial loss of teeth due to trauma, class III
K08.414 Partial loss of teeth due to trauma, class IV
K08.419 Partial loss of teeth due to trauma, unspecified class

Unspecified Code | Other Specified Code | [N] Newborn Age: 0 | [P] Pediatric Age: 0-17 | [M] Maternity Age: 12-55
[A] Adult Age: 15-124 | ♂ Male | ♀ Female | ● New Code | ▲ Revised Code Title | ▶◀ Revised Text

[6] K08.42 Partial loss of teeth due to periodontal diseases
- **K08.421 Partial loss of teeth due to periodontal diseases,** class I
- **K08.422 Partial loss of teeth due to periodontal diseases,** class II
- **K08.423 Partial loss of teeth due to periodontal diseases,** class III
- **K08.424 Partial loss of teeth due to periodontal diseases,** class IV
- **K08.429 Partial loss of teeth due to periodontal diseases, unspecified class**

[6] K08.43 Partial loss of teeth due to caries
- **K08.431 Partial loss of teeth due to caries,** class I
- **K08.432 Partial loss of teeth due to caries,** class II
- **K08.433 Partial loss of teeth due to caries,** class III
- **K08.434 Partial loss of teeth due to caries,** class IV
- **K08.439 Partial loss of teeth due to caries, unspecified class**

[6] K08.49 Partial loss of teeth due to other specified cause
- **K08.491 Partial loss of teeth due to other specified cause,** class I
- **K08.492 Partial loss of teeth due to other specified cause,** class II
- **K08.493 Partial loss of teeth due to other specified cause,** class III
- **K08.494 Partial loss of teeth due to other specified cause,** class IV
- **K08.499 Partial loss of teeth due to other specified cause, unspecified class**

[5] K08.5 Unsatisfactory restoration of tooth

Defective bridge, crown, filling
Defective dental restoration

[EXCLUDES1] *dental restoration status (Z98.811)*

[EXCLUDES2] *endosseous dental implant failure (M27.6-)*
unsatisfactory endodontic treatment (M27.5-)

K08.50 Unsatisfactory restoration of tooth, unspecified
Defective dental restoration NOS

K08.51 Open **restoration margins of tooth**
Dental restoration failure of marginal integrity
Open margin on tooth restoration
Poor gingival margin to tooth restoration

K08.52 Unrepairable overhanging of dental restorative materials
Overhanging of tooth restoration

[6] K08.53 Fractured dental restorative material

[EXCLUDES1] *cracked tooth (K03.81)*
traumatic fracture of tooth (S02.5)

- **K08.530 Fractured dental restorative material** without loss of material
- **K08.531 Fractured dental restorative material** with loss of material
- **K08.539 Fractured dental restorative material, unspecified**

K08.54 Contour of existing restoration of tooth biologically incompatible with oral health
Dental restoration failure of periodontal anatomical integrity
Unacceptable contours of existing restoration of tooth
Unacceptable morphology of existing restoration of tooth

K08.55 Allergy to existing dental restorative material
Use additional code to identify the specific type of allergy

K08.56 Poor aesthetic of existing restoration of tooth
Dental restoration aesthetically inadequate or displeasing

K08.59 Other unsatisfactory restoration of tooth
Other defective dental restoration

K08.8 Other specified disorders of teeth and supporting structures
Enlargement of alveolar ridge NOS
Irregular alveolar process
Toothache NOS

K08.9 Disorder of teeth and supporting structures, unspecified

[4] K09 Cysts of oral region, not elsewhere classified

[INCLUDES] *lesions showing histological features both of aneurysmal cyst and of another fibro-osseous lesion*

[EXCLUDES2] *cysts of jaw (M27.0-, M27.4-)*
radicular cyst (K04.8)

K09.0 Developmental odontogenic **cysts**
Dentigerous cyst
Eruption cyst
Follicular cyst
Gingival cyst
Lateral periodontal cyst
Primordial cyst

[EXCLUDES2] *keratocysts (D16.4, D16.5)*
odontogenic keratocystic tumors (D16.4, D16.5)

K09.1 Developmental (nonodontogenic) **cysts of oral region**
Cyst (of) incisive canal
Cyst (of) palatine of papilla
Globulomaxillary cyst
Median palatal cyst
Nasoalveolar cyst
Nasolabial cyst
Nasopalatine duct cyst

K09.8 Other cysts of oral region, not elsewhere classified
Dermoid cyst
Epidermoid cyst
Lymphoepithelial cyst
Epstein's pearl

K09.9 Cyst of oral region, unspecified

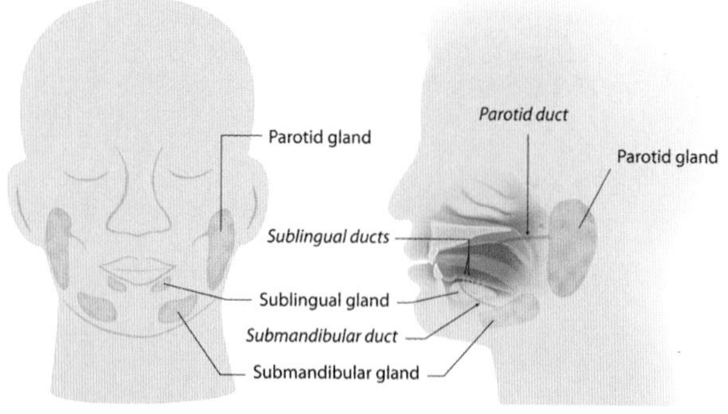

Figure 10.2 The Salivary Glands

[4] K11 Diseases of salivary glands

Use additional code to identify:
alcohol abuse and dependence (F10.-)
exposure to environmental tobacco smoke (Z77.22)
exposure to tobacco smoke in the perinatal period (P96.81)
history of tobacco use (Z87.891)
occupational exposure to environmental tobacco smoke (Z57.31)
tobacco dependence (F17.-)
tobacco use (Z72.0)

K11.0 Atrophy **of salivary gland**

K11.1 Hypertrophy **of salivary gland**

[4] 4th character required [5] 5th character required [6] 6th character required [7] 7th character required [X] Extension 'X' Alert
[EXCLUDES1] Not coded here [EXCLUDES2] Not included here [PDx] Primary Diagnosis Only Manifestation Code

[5] K11.2 Sialoadenitis
Parotitis
[EXCLUDES1] *epidemic parotitis (B26.-)*
mumps (B26.-)
uveoparotid fever [Heerfordt] (D86.89)
K11.20 Sialoadenitis, unspecified
K11.21 Acute sialoadenitis
[EXCLUDES1] *acute recurrent sialoadenitis (K11.22)*
K11.22 Acute recurrent sialoadenitis
K11.23 Chronic sialoadenitis
K11.3 Abscess of salivary gland
K11.4 Fistula of salivary gland
[EXCLUDES1] *congenital fistula of salivary gland (Q38.4)*
K11.5 Sialolithiasis
Calculus of salivary gland or duct
Stone of salivary gland or duct
K11.6 Mucocele of salivary gland
Mucous extravasation cyst of salivary gland
Mucous retention cyst of salivary gland
Ranula
K11.7 Disturbances of salivary secretion
Hypoptyalism
Ptyalism
Xerostomia
[EXCLUDES2] *dry mouth NOS (R68.2)*
K11.8 Other diseases of salivary glands
Benign lymphoepithelial lesion of salivary gland
Mikulicz' disease
Necrotizing sialometaplasia
Sialectasia
Stenosis of salivary duct
Stricture of salivary duct
[EXCLUDES1] *sicca syndrome [Sjögren] (M35.0-)*
K11.9 Disease of salivary gland, unspecified
Sialoadenopathy NOS
[4] **K12 Stomatitis and related lesions**
Use additional code to identify:
alcohol abuse and dependence (F10.-)
exposure to environmental tobacco smoke (Z77.22)
exposure to tobacco smoke in the perinatal period (P96.81)
history of tobacco use (Z87.891)
occupational exposure to environmental tobacco smoke (Z57.31)
tobacco dependence (F17.-)
tobacco use (Z72.0)
[EXCLUDES1] *cancrum oris (A69.0)*
cheilitis (K13.0)
gangrenous stomatitis (A69.0)
herpesviral [herpes simplex] gingivostomatitis (B00.2)
noma (A69.0)
K12.0 Recurrent oral aphthae
Aphthous stomatitis (major) (minor)
Bednar's aphthae
Periadenitis mucosa necrotica recurrens
Recurrent aphthous ulcer
Stomatitis herpetiformis
K12.1 Other forms of stomatitis
Stomatitis NOS
Denture stomatitis
Ulcerative stomatitis
Vesicular stomatitis
[EXCLUDES1] *acute necrotizing ulcerative stomatitis (A69.1)*
Vincent's stomatitis (A69.1)
K12.2 Cellulitis and abscess of mouth
Cellulitis of mouth (floor)
Submandibular abscess
[EXCLUDES2] *abscess of salivary gland (K11.3)*
abscess of tongue (K14.0)
periapical abscess (K04.6-K04.7)
periodontal abscess (K05.21)
peritonsillar abscess (J36)
[5] **K12.3 Oral mucositis (ulcerative)**
Mucositis (oral) (oropharyneal)
[EXCLUDES2] *gastrointestinal mucositis (ulcerative) (K92.81)*
mucositis (ulcerative) of vagina and vulva (N76.81)
nasal mucositis (ulcerative) (J34.81)
K12.30 Oral mucositis (ulcerative), unspecified
K12.31 Oral mucositis (ulcerative) due to antineoplastic therapy
Use additional code for adverse effect, if applicable, to identify antineoplastic and immunosuppressive drugs (T45.1X5)
code for other antineoplastic therapy, such as: radiological procedure and radiotherapy (Y84.2)
K12.32 Oral mucositis (ulcerative) due to other drugs
Use additional code for adverse effect, if applicable, to identify drug (T36-T50 with fifth or sixth character 5)
K12.33 Oral mucositis (ulcerative) due to radiation
Use additional external cause code (W88-W90, X39.0-) to identify cause
K12.39 Other oral mucositis (ulcerative)
Viral oral mucositis (ulcerative)
[4] **K13 Other diseases of lip and oral mucosa**
INCLUDES *epithelial disturbances of tongue*
Use additional code to identify:
alcohol abuse and dependence (F10.-)
exposure to environmental tobacco smoke (Z77.22)
exposure to tobacco smoke in the perinatal period (P96.81)
history of tobacco use (Z87.891)
occupational exposure to environmental tobacco smoke (Z57.31)
tobacco dependence (F17.-)
tobacco use (Z72.0)
[EXCLUDES2] *certain disorders of gingiva and edentulous alveolar ridge (K05-K06)*
cysts of oral region (K09.-)
diseases of tongue (K14.-)
stomatitis and related lesions (K12.-)
K13.0 Diseases of lips
Abscess of lips
Angular cheilitis
Cellulitis of lips
Cheilitis NOS
Cheilodynia
Cheilosis
Exfoliative cheilitis
Fistula of lips
Glandular cheilitis
Hypertrophy of lips
Perlèche NEC
[EXCLUDES1] *ariboflavinosis (E53.0)*
cheilitis due to radiation-related disorders (L55-L59)
congenital fistula of lips (Q38.0)
congenital hypertrophy of lips (Q18.6)
Perlèche due to candidiasis (B37.83)
Perlèche due to riboflavin deficiency (E53.0)
K13.1 Cheek and lip biting

Unspecified Code | Other Specified Code | [N] Newborn Age: 0 | [P] Pediatric Age: 0-17 | [M] Maternity Age: 12-55
[A] Adult Age: 15-124 | ♂ Male | ♀ Female | ● New Code | ▲ Revised Code Title | ►◄ Revised Text

[5] **K13.2 Leukoplakia and other disturbances of oral epithelium, including tongue**

[EXCLUDES1] *carcinoma in situ of oral epithelium (D00.0-)*
hairy leukoplakia (K13.3)

K13.21 Leukoplakia of oral mucosa, including tongue

Leukokeratosis of oral mucosa
Leukoplakia of gingiva, lips, tongue

[EXCLUDES1] *hairy leukoplakia (K13.3)*
leukokeratosis nicotina palati (K13.24)

K13.22 Minimal keratinized residual ridge mucosa

Minimal keratinization of alveolar ridge mucosa

K13.23 Excessive keratinized residual ridge mucosa

Excessive keratinization of alveolar ridge mucosa

K13.24 Leukokeratosis nicotina palati

Smoker's palate

K13.29 Other disturbances of oral epithelium, including tongue

Erythroplakia of mouth or tongue
Focal epithelial hyperplasia of mouth or tongue
Leukoedema of mouth or tongue
Other oral epithelium disturbances

K13.3 Hairy leukoplakia

K13.4 Granuloma and granuloma-like lesions of oral mucosa

Eosinophilic granuloma
Granuloma pyogenicum
Verrucous xanthoma

K13.5 Oral submucous fibrosis

Submucous fibrosis of tongue

K13.6 Irritative hyperplasia of oral mucosa

[EXCLUDES2] *irritative hyperplasia of edentulous ridge [denture hyperplasia] (K06.2)*

[5] **K13.7 Other and unspecified lesions of oral mucosa**

K13.70 Unspecified lesions of oral mucosa

K13.79 Other lesions of oral mucosa

Focal oral mucinosis

[4] **K14 Diseases of tongue**

Use additional code to identify:
alcohol abuse and dependence (F10.-)
exposure to environmental tobacco smoke (Z77.22)
history of tobacco use (Z87.891)
occupational exposure to environmental tobacco smoke (Z57.31)
tobacco dependence (F17.-)
tobacco use (Z72.0)

[EXCLUDES2] *erythroplakia (K13.29)*
focal epithelial hyperplasia (K13.29)
leukedema of tongue (K13.29)
leukoplakia of tongue (K13.21)
hairy leukoplakia (K13.3)
macroglossia (congenital) (Q38.2)
submucous fibrosis of tongue (K13.5)

K14.0 Glossitis

Abscess of tongue
Ulceration (traumatic) of tongue

[EXCLUDES1] *atrophic glossitis (K14.4)*

K14.1 Geographic tongue

Benign migratory glossitis
Glossitis areata exfoliativa

K14.2 Median rhomboid glossitis

K14.3 Hypertrophy of tongue papillae

Black hairy tongue
Coated tongue
Hypertrophy of foliate papillae
Lingua villosa nigra

K14.4 Atrophy of tongue papillae

Atrophic glossitis

K14.5 Plicated tongue

Fissured tongue
Furrowed tongue
Scrotal tongue

[EXCLUDES1] *fissured tongue, congenital (Q38.3)*

K14.6 Glossodynia

Glossopyrosis
Painful tongue

K14.8 Other diseases of tongue

Atrophy of tongue
Crenated tongue
Enlargement of tongue
Glossocele
Glossoptosis
Hypertrophy of tongue

K14.9 Disease of tongue, unspecified

Glossopathy NOS

Diseases of esophagus, stomach and duodenum (K20-K31)

[EXCLUDES2] *hiatus hernia (K44.-)*

[4] **K20 Esophagitis**

Use additional code to identify:
alcohol abuse and dependence (F10.-)

[EXCLUDES1] *erosion of esophagus (K22.1-)*
esophagitis with gastro-esophageal reflux disease (K21.0)
reflux esophagitis (K21.0)
ulcerative esophagitis (K22.1-)

[EXCLUDES2] *eosinophilic gastritis or gastroenteritis (K52.81)*

K20.0 Eosinophilic esophagitis

K20.8 Other esophagitis

Abscess of esophagus

K20.9 Esophagitis, unspecified

Esophagitis NOS

[4] **K21 Gastro-esophageal reflux disease**

[EXCLUDES1] *newborn esophageal reflux (P78.83)*

K21.0 Gastro-esophageal reflux disease with esophagitis

Reflux esophagitis

K21.9 Gastro-esophageal reflux disease without esophagitis

Esophageal reflux NOS

[4] **K22 Other diseases of esophagus**

[EXCLUDES2] *esophageal varices (I85.-)*

K22.0 Achalasia of cardia

Achalasia NOS
Cardiospasm

[EXCLUDES1] *congenital cardiospasm (Q39.5)*

[5] **K22.1 Ulcer of esophagus**

Barrett's ulcer
Erosion of esophagus
Fungal ulcer of esophagus
Peptic ulcer of esophagus
Ulcer of esophagus due to ingestion of chemicals
Ulcer of esophagus due to ingestion of drugs and medicaments
Ulcerative esophagitis

Code first poisoning due to drug or toxin, if applicable (T36-T65 with fifth or sixth character 1-4 or 6)

Use additional code for adverse effect, if applicable, to identify drug (T36-T50 with fifth or sixth character 5)

[EXCLUDES1] *Barrett's esophagus (K22.7-)*

K22.10 Ulcer of esophagus without bleeding

Ulcer of esophagus NOS

K22.11 Ulcer of esophagus with bleeding

[EXCLUDES2] *bleeding esophageal varices (I85.01, I85.11)*

[4] 4th character required [5] 5th character required [6] 6th character required [7] 7th character required [X] Extension 'X' Alert
[EXCLUDES1] Not coded here [EXCLUDES2] Not included here [PDx] Primary Diagnosis Only Manifestation Code

K22.2 Esophageal obstruction
- Compression of esophagus
- Constriction of esophagus
- Stenosis of esophagus
- Stricture of esophagus

[EXCLUDES1] *congenital stenosis or stricture of esophagus (Q39.3)*

K22.3 Perforation of esophagus
- Rupture of esophagus

[EXCLUDES1] *traumatic perforation of (thoracic) esophagus (S27.8-)*

K22.4 Dyskinesia of esophagus
- Corkscrew esophagus
- Diffuse esophageal spasm
- Spasm of esophagus

[EXCLUDES1] *cardiospasm (K22.0)*

K22.5 Diverticulum of esophagus, acquired
- Esophageal pouch, acquired

[EXCLUDES1] *diverticulum of esophagus (congenital) (Q39.6)*

K22.6 Gastro-esophageal laceration-hemorrhage syndrome
- Mallory-Weiss syndrome

[5] K22.7 Barrett's esophagus
- Barrett's disease
- Barrett's syndrome

[EXCLUDES1] *Barrett's ulcer (K22.1)*
malignant neoplasm of esophagus (C15.-)

K22.70 Barrett's esophagus without dysplasia
- Barrett's esophagus NOS

[6] K22.71 Barrett's esophagus with dysplasia

K22.710 Barrett's esophagus with low grade dysplasia

K22.711 Barrett's esophagus with high grade dysplasia

K22.719 Barrett's esophagus with dysplasia, unspecified

K22.8 Other specified diseases of esophagus
- Hemorrhage of esophagus NOS

[EXCLUDES2] *esophageal varices (I85.-)*
Paterson-Kelly syndrome (D50.1)

K22.9 Disease of esophagus, unspecified

K23 Disorders of esophagus in diseases classified elsewhere

Code first underlying disease, such as:
congenital syphilis (A50.5)

[EXCLUDES1] *late syphilis (A52.79)*
megaesophagus due to Chagas' disease (B57.31)
tuberculosis (A18.83)

[4] **K25 Gastric ulcer**

[INCLUDES] *erosion (acute) of stomach*
pylorus ulcer (peptic)
stomach ulcer (peptic)

Use additional code to identify:
alcohol abuse and dependence (F10.-)

[EXCLUDES1] *acute gastritis (K29.0-)*
peptic ulcer NOS (K27.-)

K25.0 Acute gastric ulcer with hemorrhage

K25.1 Acute gastric ulcer with perforation

K25.2 Acute gastric ulcer with both hemorrhage and perforation

K25.3 Acute gastric ulcer without hemorrhage or perforation

K25.4 Chronic or unspecified gastric ulcer with hemorrhage

K25.5 Chronic or unspecified gastric ulcer with perforation

K25.6 Chronic or unspecified gastric ulcer with both hemorrhage and perforation

K25.7 Chronic gastric ulcer without hemorrhage or perforation

K25.9 Gastric ulcer, unspecified as acute or chronic, without hemorrhage or perforation

[4] **K26 Duodenal ulcer**

[INCLUDES] *erosion (acute) of duodenum*
duodenum ulcer (peptic)
postpyloric ulcer (peptic)

Use additional code to identify:
alcohol abuse and dependence (F10.-)

[EXCLUDES1] *peptic ulcer NOS (K27.-)*

K26.0 Acute duodenal ulcer with hemorrhage

K26.1 Acute duodenal ulcer with perforation

K26.2 Acute duodenal ulcer with both hemorrhage and perforation

K26.3 Acute duodenal ulcer without hemorrhage or perforation

K26.4 Chronic or unspecified duodenal ulcer with hemorrhage

K26.5 Chronic or unspecified duodenal ulcer with perforation

K26.6 Chronic or unspecified duodenal ulcer with both hemorrhage and perforation

K26.7 Chronic duodenal ulcer without hemorrhage or perforation

K26.9 Duodenal ulcer, unspecified as acute or chronic, without hemorrhage or perforation

[4] **K27 Peptic ulcer, site unspecified**

[INCLUDES] *gastroduodenal ulcer NOS*
peptic ulcer NOS

Use additional code to identify:
alcohol abuse and dependence (F10.-)

[EXCLUDES1] *peptic ulcer of newborn (P78.82)*

K27.0 Acute peptic ulcer, site unspecified, with hemorrhage

K27.1 Acute peptic ulcer, site unspecified, with perforation

K27.2 Acute peptic ulcer, site unspecified, with both hemorrhage and perforation

K27.3 Acute peptic ulcer, site unspecified, without hemorrhage or perforation

K27.4 Chronic or unspecified peptic ulcer, site unspecified, with hemorrhage

K27.5 Chronic or unspecified peptic ulcer, site unspecified, with perforation

K27.6 Chronic or unspecified peptic ulcer, site unspecified, with both hemorrhage and perforation

K27.7 Chronic peptic ulcer, site unspecified, without hemorrhage or perforation

K27.9 Peptic ulcer, site unspecified, unspecified as acute or chronic, without hemorrhage or perforation

[4] **K28 Gastrojejunal ulcer**

[INCLUDES] *anastomotic ulcer (peptic) or erosion*
gastrocolic ulcer (peptic) or erosion
gastrointestinal ulcer (peptic) or erosion
gastrojejunal ulcer (peptic) or erosion
jejunal ulcer (peptic) or erosion
marginal ulcer (peptic) or erosion
stomal ulcer (peptic) or erosion

Use additional code to identify:
alcohol abuse and dependence (F10.-)

[EXCLUDES1] *primary ulcer of small intestine (K63.3)*

K28.0 Acute gastrojejunal ulcer with hemorrhage

K28.1 Acute gastrojejunal ulcer with perforation

K28.2 Acute gastrojejunal ulcer with both hemorrhage and perforation

K28.3 Acute gastrojejunal ulcer without hemorrhage or perforation

K28.4 Chronic or unspecified gastrojejunal ulcer with hemorrhage

K28.5 Chronic or unspecified gastrojejunal ulcer with perforation

K28.6 Chronic or unspecified gastrojejunal ulcer with both hemorrhage and perforation

K28.7 Chronic gastrojejunal ulcer without hemorrhage or perforation

K28.9 Gastrojejunal ulcer, unspecified as acute or chronic, without hemorrhage or perforation

[4] **K29 Gastritis and duodenitis**

[EXCLUDES1] *eosinophilic gastritis or gastroenteritis (K52.81)*
Zollinger-Ellison syndrome (E16.4)

[5] K29.0 Acute gastritis
Use additional code to identify:
alcohol abuse and dependence (F10.-)
[EXCLUDES1] *erosion (acute) of stomach (K25.-)*

K29.00 Acute gastritis without bleeding
K29.01 Acute gastritis with bleeding

[5] K29.2 Alcoholic gastritis
Use additional code to identify:
alcohol abuse and dependence (F10.-)

K29.20 Alcoholic gastritis without bleeding
K29.21 Alcoholic gastritis with bleeding

[5] K29.3 Chronic superficial gastritis
K29.30 Chronic superficial gastritis without bleeding
K29.31 Chronic superficial gastritis with bleeding

[5] K29.4 Chronic atrophic gastritis
Gastric atrophy
K29.40 Chronic atrophic gastritis without bleeding
K29.41 Chronic atrophic gastritis with bleeding

[5] K29.5 Unspecified chronic gastritis
Chronic antral gastritis
Chronic fundal gastritis
K29.50 Unspecified chronic gastritis without bleeding
K29.51 Unspecified chronic gastritis with bleeding

[5] K29.6 Other gastritis
Giant hypertrophic gastritis
Granulomatous gastritis
Ménétrier's disease
K29.60 Other gastritis without bleeding
K29.61 Other gastritis with bleeding

[5] K29.7 Gastritis, unspecified
K29.70 Gastritis, unspecified, without bleeding
K29.71 Gastritis, unspecified, with bleeding

[5] K29.8 Duodenitis
K29.80 Duodenitis without bleeding
K29.81 Duodenitis with bleeding

[5] K29.9 Gastroduodenitis, unspecified
K29.90 Gastroduodenitis, unspecified, without bleeding
K29.91 Gastroduodenitis, unspecified, with bleeding

K30 Functional dyspepsia
Indigestion
[EXCLUDES1] *dyspepsia NOS (R10.13)*
heartburn (R12)
nervous dyspepsia (F45.8)
neurotic dyspepsia (F45.8)
psychogenic dyspepsia (F45.8)

[4] **K31 Other diseases of stomach and duodenum**
[INCLUDES] *functional disorders of stomach*
[EXCLUDES2] *diabetic gastroparesis (E08.43, E09.43, E10.43, E11.43, E13.43)*
diverticulum of duodenum (K57.00-K57.13)

K31.0 Acute dilatation of stomach
Acute distention of stomach

K31.1 Adult hypertrophic pyloric stenosis
Pyloric stenosis NOS
[EXCLUDES1] *congenital or infantile pyloric stenosis (Q40.0)* [A]

K31.2 Hourglass stricture and stenosis of stomach
[EXCLUDES1] *congenital hourglass stomach (Q40.2)*
hourglass contraction of stomach (K31.89)

K31.3 Pylorospasm, not elsewhere classified
[EXCLUDES1] *congenital or infantile pylorospasm (Q40.0)*
neurotic pylorospasm (F45.8)
psychogenic pylorospasm (F45.8)

K31.4 Gastric diverticulum
[EXCLUDES1] *congenital diverticulum of stomach (Q40.2)*

K31.5 Obstruction of duodenum
Constriction of duodenum
Duodenal ileus (chronic)
Stenosis of duodenum
Stricture of duodenum
Volvulus of duodenum
[EXCLUDES1] *congenital stenosis of duodenum (Q41.0)*

K31.6 Fistula of stomach and duodenum
Gastrocolic fistula
Gastrojejunocolic fistula

K31.7 Polyp of stomach and duodenum
[EXCLUDES1] *adenomatous polyp of stomach (D13.1)*

[5] K31.8 Other specified diseases of stomach and duodenum

[6] K31.81 Angiodysplasia of stomach and duodenum
K31.811 Angiodysplasia of stomach and duodenum with bleeding
K31.819 Angiodysplasia of stomach and duodenum without bleeding
Angiodysplasia of stomach and duodenum NOS

K31.82 Dieulafoy lesion (hemorrhagic) of stomach and duodenum
[EXCLUDES2] *Dieulafoy lesion of intestine (K63.81)*

K31.83 Achlorhydria

K31.84 Gastroparesis
Gastroparalysis
Code first underlying disease, if known, such as:
anorexia nervosa (F50.0-)
diabetes mellitus (E08.43, E09.43, E10.43, E11.43, E13.43)
scleroderma (M34.-)

K31.89 Other diseases of stomach and duodenum

K31.9 Disease of stomach and duodenum, unspecified

Diseases of appendix (K35-K38)

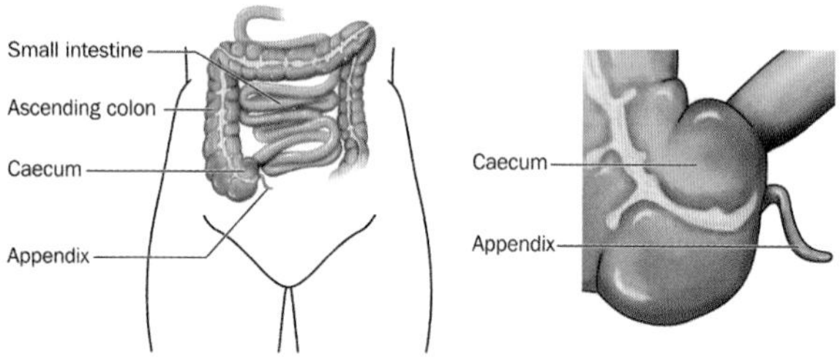
Small intestine
Ascending colon
Caecum
Appendix
Caecum
Appendix

Figure 10.3 Vermiform appendix

[4] **K35 Acute appendicitis**

K35.2 Acute appendicitis with generalized peritonitis
Appendicitis (acute) with generalized (diffuse) peritonitis following rupture or perforation of appendix
Perforated appendix NOS
Ruptured appendix NOS

K35.3 Acute appendicitis with localized peritonitis
Acute appendicitis with or without perforation or rupture NOS
Acute appendicitis with or without perforation or rupture with localized peritonitis
Acute appendicitis with peritoneal abscess

[5] K35.8 Other and unspecified acute appendicitis

[4] 4th character required [5] 5th character required [6] 6th character required [7] 7th character required [7x] Extension 'X' Alert
[EXCLUDES1] Not coded here [EXCLUDES2] Not included here [PDx] Primary Diagnosis Only Manifestation Code

K35.80 **Unspecified acute appendicitis**
Acute appendicitis NOS
Acute appendicitis without (localized) (generalized) peritonitis

K35.89 **Other acute appendicitis**

K36 **Other appendicitis**
Chronic appendicitis
Recurrent appendicitis

K37 **Unspecified appendicitis**
[EXCLUDES1] *-unspecified appendicitis with peritonitis (K35.2-K35.3)*

[4th] K38 **Other diseases of appendix**

K38.0 **Hyperplasia of appendix**

K38.1 **Appendicular concretions**
Fecalith of appendix
Stercolith of appendix

K38.2 **Diverticulum of appendix**

K38.3 **Fistula of appendix**

K38.8 **Other specified diseases of appendix**
Intussusception of appendix

K38.9 **Disease of appendix, unspecified**

Hernia (K40-K46)

[NOTES] Hernia with both gangrene and obstruction is classified to hernia with gangrene.

[INCLUDES] *acquired hernia*
congenital [except diaphragmatic or hiatus] hernia
recurrent hernia

[4th] K40 Inguinal **hernia**

[INCLUDES] *bubonocele*
direct inguinal hernia
double inguinal hernia
indirect inguinal hernia
inguinal hernia NOS
oblique inguinal hernia
scrotal hernia

[5th] K40.0 Bilateral **inguinal hernia,** with obstruction, without gangrene
Inguinal hernia (bilateral) causing obstruction without gangrene
Incarcerated inguinal hernia (bilateral) without gangrene
Irreducible inguinal hernia (bilateral) without gangrene
Strangulated inguinal hernia (bilateral) without gangrene

K40.00 **Bilateral inguinal hernia, with obstruction, without gangrene,** not specified as recurrent
Bilateral inguinal hernia, with obstruction, without gangrene NOS

K40.01 **Bilateral inguinal hernia, with obstruction, without gangrene,** recurrent

[5th] K40.1 Bilateral **inguinal hernia,** with gangrene

K40.10 **Bilateral inguinal hernia, with gangrene,** not specified as recurrent
Bilateral inguinal hernia, with gangrene NOS

K40.11 **Bilateral inguinal hernia, with gangrene,** recurrent

[5th] K40.2 Bilateral **inguinal hernia,** without obstruction or gangrene

K40.20 **Bilateral inguinal hernia, without obstruction or gangrene,** not specified as recurrent
Bilateral inguinal hernia NOS

K40.21 **Bilateral inguinal hernia, without obstruction or gangrene,** recurrent

[5th] K40.3 Unilateral **inguinal hernia,** with obstruction, without gangrene
Inguinal hernia (unilateral) causing obstruction without gangrene
Incarcerated inguinal hernia (unilateral) without gangrene
Irreducible inguinal hernia (unilateral) without gangrene
Strangulated inguinal hernia (unilateral) without gangrene

K40.30 **Unilateral inguinal hernia, with obstruction, without gangrene,** not specified as recurrent
Inguinal hernia, with obstruction NOS
Unilateral inguinal hernia, with obstruction, without gangrene NOS

K40.31 **Unilateral inguinal hernia, with obstruction, without gangrene, recurrent**

[5th] K40.4 **Unilateral inguinal hernia, with gangrene**

K40.40 **Unilateral inguinal hernia, with gangrene, not specified as** recurrent
Inguinal hernia with gangrene NOS
Unilateral inguinal hernia with gangrene NOS

K40.41 **Unilateral inguinal hernia, with gangrene,** recurrent

[5th] K40.9 Unilateral **inguinal hernia,** without obstruction or gangrene

K40.90 **Unilateral inguinal hernia, without obstruction or gangrene,** not specified as recurrent
Inguinal hernia NOS
Unilateral inguinal hernia NOS

K40.91 **Unilateral inguinal hernia, without obstruction or gangrene,** recurrent

[4th] K41 Femoral **hernia**

[5th] K41.0 Bilateral **femoral hernia,** with obstruction, without gangrene
Femoral hernia (bilateral) causing obstruction, without gangrene
Incarcerated femoral hernia (bilateral), without gangrene
Irreducible femoral hernia (bilateral), without gangrene
Strangulated femoral hernia (bilateral), without gangrene

K41.00 **Bilateral femoral hernia, with obstruction, without gangrene,** not specified as recurrent
Bilateral femoral hernia, with obstruction, without gangrene NOS

K41.01 **Bilateral femoral hernia, with obstruction, without gangrene,** recurrent

[5th] K41.1 Bilateral **femoral hernia,** with gangrene

K41.10 **Bilateral femoral hernia, with gangrene,** not specified as recurrent
Bilateral femoral hernia, with gangrene NOS

K41.11 **Bilateral femoral hernia, with gangrene,** recurrent

[5th] K41.2 Bilateral **femoral hernia,** without obstruction or gangrene

K41.20 **Bilateral femoral hernia, without obstruction or gangrene,** not specified as recurrent
Bilateral femoral hernia NOS

K41.21 **Bilateral femoral hernia, without obstruction or gangrene,** recurrent

[5th] K41.3 Unilateral **femoral hernia,** with obstruction, without gangrene
Femoral hernia (unilateral) causing obstruction, without gangrene
Incarcerated femoral hernia (unilateral), without gangrene
Irreducible femoral hernia (unilateral), without gangrene
Strangulated femoral hernia (unilateral), without gangrene

K41.30 **Unilateral femoral hernia, with obstruction, without gangrene,** not specified as recurrent
Femoral hernia, with obstruction NOS
Unilateral femoral hernia, with obstruction NOS

K41.31 Unilateral femoral hernia, with obstruction, without gangrene, recurrent

[5] **K41.4** Unilateral **femoral hernia,** with gangrene

K41.40 Unilateral femoral hernia, with gangrene, not specified as recurrent

Femoral hernia, with gangrene NOS
Unilateral femoral hernia, with gangrene NOS

K41.41 Unilateral femoral hernia, with gangrene, recurrent

[5] **K41.9** Unilateral **femoral hernia,** without obstruction or gangrene

K41.90 Unilateral femoral hernia, without obstruction or gangrene, not specified as recurrent

Femoral hernia NOS
Unilateral femoral hernia NOS

K41.91 Unilateral femoral hernia, without obstruction or gangrene, recurrent

[4] **K42** Umbilical **hernia**

INCLUDES *paraumbilical hernia*

EXCLUDES1 *omphalocele (Q79.2)*

K42.0 Umbilical hernia with obstruction, without gangrene

Umbilical hernia causing obstruction, without gangrene
Incarcerated umbilical hernia, without gangrene
Irreducible umbilical hernia, without gangrene
Strangulated umbilical hernia, without gangrene

K42.1 Umbilical hernia with gangrene

Gangrenous umbilical hernia

K42.9 Umbilical hernia without obstruction or gangrene

Umbilical hernia NOS

[4] **K43** Ventral **hernia**

K43.0 Incisional **hernia with obstruction,** without gangrene

Incisional hernia causing obstruction, without gangrene
Incarcerated incisional hernia, without gangrene
Irreducible incisional hernia, without gangrene
Strangulated incisional hernia, without gangrene

K43.1 Incisional **hernia** with gangrene

Gangrenous incisional hernia

K43.2 Incisional **hernia** without obstruction or gangrene

Incisional hernia NOS

K43.3 Parastomal **hernia with obstruction, w**ithout gangrene

Incarcerated parastomal hernia, without gangrene
Irreducible parastomal hernia, without gangrene
Parastomal hernia causing obstruction, without gangrene
Strangulated parastomal hernia, without gangrene

K43.4 Parastomal **hernia** with gangrene

Gangrenous parastomal hernia

K43.5 Parastomal **hernia** without obstruction or gangrene

Parastomal hernia NOS

K43.6 Other and unspecified ventral hernia with obstruction, without gangrene

Epigastric hernia causing obstruction, without gangrene
Hypogastric hernia causing obstruction, without gangrene
Incarcerated epigastric hernia without gangrene
Incarcerated hypogastric hernia without gangrene
Incarcerated midline hernia without gangrene
Incarcerated spigelian hernia without gangrene
Incarcerated subxiphoid hernia without gangrene
Irreducible epigastric hernia without gangrene
Irreducible hypogastric hernia without gangrene
Irreducible midline hernia without gangrene
Irreducible spigelian hernia without gangrene
Irreducible subxiphoid hernia without gangrene
Midline hernia causing obstruction, without gangrene
Spigelian hernia causing obstruction, without gangrene
Strangulated epigastric hernia without gangrene
Strangulated hypogastric hernia without gangrene
Strangulated midline hernia without gangrene
Strangulated spigelian hernia without gangrene
Strangulated subxiphoid hernia without gangrene
Subxiphoid hernia causing obstruction, without gangrene

K43.7 Other and unspecified ventral hernia with gangrene

Any condition listed under K43.6 specified as gangrenous

K43.9 Ventral hernia without obstruction or gangrene

Epigastric hernia
Ventral hernia NOS

[4] **K44** Diaphragmatic **hernia**

INCLUDES *hiatus hernia (esophageal) (sliding)*
paraesophageal hernia

EXCLUDES1 *congenital diaphragmatic hernia (Q79.0)*
congenital hiatus hernia (Q40.1)

K44.0 Diaphragmatic hernia with obstruction, without gangrene

Diaphragmatic hernia causing obstruction
Incarcerated diaphragmatic hernia
Irreducible diaphragmatic hernia
Strangulated diaphragmatic hernia

K44.1 Diaphragmatic hernia with gangrene

Gangrenous diaphragmatic hernia

K44.9 Diaphragmatic hernia without obstruction or gangrene

Diaphragmatic hernia NOS

[4] **K45** Other abdominal **hernia**

INCLUDES *abdominal hernia, specified site NEC*
lumbar hernia
obturator hernia
pudendal hernia
retroperitoneal hernia
sciatic hernia

K45.0 Other specified abdominal hernia with obstruction, without gangrene

Other specified abdominal hernia causing obstruction
Other specified incarcerated abdominal hernia
Other specified irreducible abdominal hernia
Other specified strangulated abdominal hernia

K45.1 Other specified abdominal hernia with gangrene

Any condition listed under K45 specified as gangrenous

K45.8 Other specified abdominal hernia without obstruction or gangrene

[4] **K46 Unspecified** abdominal hernia

INCLUDES *enterocele*
epiplocele
hernia NOS
interstitial hernia
intestinal hernia
intra-abdominal hernia

EXCLUDES1 *vaginal enterocele (N81.5)*

K46.0 Unspecified abdominal hernia with obstruction, without gangrene

Unspecified abdominal hernia causing obstruction
Unspecified incarcerated abdominal hernia
Unspecified irreducible abdominal hernia
Unspecified strangulated abdominal hernia

K46.1 Unspecified abdominal hernia with gangrene

Any condition listed under K46 specified as gangrenous

K46.9 Unspecified abdominal hernia without obstruction or gangrene

Abdominal hernia NOS

[4] 4th character required [5] 5th character required [6] 6th character required [7] 7th character required [7x] Extension 'X' Alert
EXCLUDES 1 Not coded here EXCLUDES 2 Not included here PDx Primary Diagnosis Only Manifestation Code

Noninfective enteritis and colitis (K50-K52)

> INCLUDES   *noninfective inflammatory bowel disease*
> EXCLUDES1   *irritable bowel syndrome (K58.-)*
>   *megacolon (K59.3)*

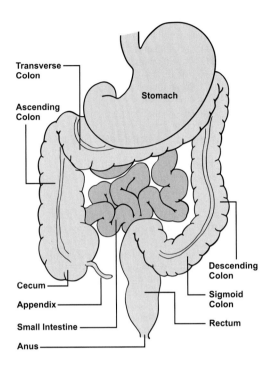

Figure 10.4 Large and Small Intestine

🟢 **K50 Crohn's disease [regional enteritis]**

> INCLUDES   *granulomatous enteritis*
> Use additional code to identify manifestations, such as:
> pyoderma gangrenosum (L88)
> EXCLUDES1   *ulcerative colitis (K51.-)*

🟢 **K50.0 Crohn's disease of** small intestine

> Crohn's disease [regional enteritis] of duodenum
> Crohn's disease [regional enteritis] of ileum
> Crohn's disease [regional enteritis] of jejunum
> Regional ileitis
> Terminal ileitis
> EXCLUDES1   *Crohn's disease of both small and large intestine (K50.8-)*

  K50.00 Crohn's disease of small intestine without complications

🟢 **K50.01 Crohn's disease of small intestine** with complications

    K50.011 Crohn's disease of small intestine with rectal bleeding

    K50.012 Crohn's disease of small intestine with intestinal obstruction

    K50.013 Crohn's disease of small intestine with fistula

    K50.014 Crohn's disease of small intestine with abscess

    K50.018 Crohn's disease of small intestine with other complication

    K50.019 Crohn's disease of small intestine with unspecified complications

🟢 **K50.1 Crohn's disease of** large intestine

> Crohn's disease [regional enteritis] of colon
> Crohn's disease [regional enteritis] of large bowel
> Crohn's disease [regional enteritis] of rectum
> Granulomatous colitis
> Regional colitis
> EXCLUDES1   *Crohn's disease of both small and large intestine (K50.8)*

  K50.10 Crohn's disease of large intestine without complications

🟢 **K50.11 Crohn's disease of large intestine** with complications

    K50.111 Crohn's disease of large intestine with rectal bleeding

    K50.112 Crohn's disease of large intestine with intestinal obstruction

    K50.113 Crohn's disease of large intestine with fistula

    K50.114 Crohn's disease of large intestine with abscess

    K50.118 Crohn's disease of large intestine with other complication

    K50.119 Crohn's disease of large intestine with unspecified complications

🟢 **K50.8 Crohn's disease of** both small and large intestine

  K50.80 Crohn's disease of both small and large intestine without complications

🟢 **K50.81 Crohn's disease of both small and large intestine with complications**

    K50.811 Crohn's disease of both small and large intestine with rectal bleeding

    K50.812 Crohn's disease of both small and large intestine with intestinal obstruction

    K50.813 Crohn's disease of both small and large intestine with fistula

    K50.814 Crohn's disease of both small and large intestine with abscess

    K50.818 Crohn's disease of both small and large intestine with other complication

    K50.819 Crohn's disease of both small and large intestine with unspecified complications

🟢 **K50.9 Crohn's disease, unspecified**

  K50.90 Crohn's disease, unspecified, without complications

> Crohn's disease NOS
> Regional enteritis NOS

🟢 **K50.91 Crohn's disease, unspecified, with complications**

    K50.911 Crohn's disease, unspecified, with rectal bleeding

    K50.912 Crohn's disease, unspecified, with intestinal obstruction

    K50.913 Crohn's disease, unspecified, with fistula

    K50.914 Crohn's disease, unspecified, with abscess

    K50.918 Crohn's disease, unspecified, with other complication

    K50.919 Crohn's disease, unspecified, with unspecified complications

🟢 **K51 Ulcerative colitis**

> Use additional code to identify manifestations, such as:
> pyoderma gangrenosum (L88)
> EXCLUDES1   *Crohn's disease [regional enteritis] (K50.-)*

🟢 **K51.0 Ulcerative (chronic)** pancolitis

> Backwash ileitis

  K51.00 Ulcerative (chronic) pancolitis without complications

> Ulcerative (chronic) pancolitis NOS

🟢 **K51.01 Ulcerative (chronic) pancolitis** with complications

---

Unspecified Code	Other Specified Code	🅽 Newborn Age: 0	🅿 Pediatric Age: 0-17	🅼 Maternity Age: 12-55
🅰 Adult Age: 15-124	♂ Male	♀ Female	● New Code	▲ Revised Code Title ►◄ Revised Text

K51.011 Ulcerative (chronic) pancolitis with rectal bleeding
K51.012 Ulcerative (chronic) pancolitis with intestinal obstruction
K51.013 Ulcerative (chronic) pancolitis with fistula
K51.014 Ulcerative (chronic) pancolitis with abscess
K51.018 Ulcerative (chronic) pancolitis with other complication
K51.019 Ulcerative (chronic) pancolitis with unspecified complications
⑤ K51.2 Ulcerative (chronic) proctitis
K51.20 Ulcerative (chronic) proctitis without complications
Ulcerative (chronic) proctitis NOS
⑥ K51.21 Ulcerative (chronic) proctitis with complications
K51.211 Ulcerative (chronic) proctitis with rectal bleeding
K51.212 Ulcerative (chronic) proctitis with intestinal obstruction
K51.213 Ulcerative (chronic) proctitis with fistula
K51.214 Ulcerative (chronic) proctitis with abscess
K51.218 Ulcerative (chronic) proctitis with other complication
K51.219 Ulcerative (chronic) proctitis with unspecified complications
⑤ K51.3 Ulcerative (chronic) rectosigmoiditis
K51.30 Ulcerative (chronic) rectosigmoiditis without complications
Ulcerative (chronic) rectosigmoiditis NOS
⑥ K51.31 Ulcerative (chronic) rectosigmoiditis with complications
K51.311 Ulcerative (chronic) rectosigmoiditis with rectal bleeding
K51.312 Ulcerative (chronic) rectosigmoiditis with intestinal obstruction
K51.313 Ulcerative (chronic) rectosigmoiditis with fistula
K51.314 Ulcerative (chronic) rectosigmoiditis with abscess
K51.318 Ulcerative (chronic) rectosigmoiditis with other complication
K51.319 Ulcerative (chronic) rectosigmoiditis with unspecified complications
⑤ K51.4 Inflammatory polyps of colon
EXCLUDES1 adenomatous polyp of colon (D12.6)
polyposis of colon (D12.6)
polyps of colon NOS (K63.5)
K51.40 Inflammatory polyps of colon without complications
Inflammatory polyps of colon NOS
⑥ K51.41 Inflammatory polyps of colon with complications
K51.411 Inflammatory polyps of colon with rectal bleeding
K51.412 Inflammatory polyps of colon with intestinal obstruction
K51.413 Inflammatory polyps of colon with fistula
K51.414 Inflammatory polyps of colon with abscess
K51.418 Inflammatory polyps of colon with other complication
K51.419 Inflammatory polyps of colon with unspecified complications
⑤ K51.5 Left sided colitis
Left hemicolitis
K51.50 Left sided colitis without complications
Left sided colitis NOS
⑥ K51.51 Left sided colitis with complications
K51.511 Left sided colitis with rectal bleeding
K51.512 Left sided colitis with intestinal obstruction

K51.513 Left sided colitis with fistula
K51.514 Left sided colitis with abscess
K51.518 Left sided colitis with other complication
K51.519 Left sided colitis with unspecified complications
⑤ K51.8 Other ulcerative colitis
K51.80 Other ulcerative colitis without complications
⑥ K51.81 Other ulcerative colitis with complications
K51.811 Other ulcerative colitis with rectal bleeding
K51.812 Other ulcerative colitis with intestinal obstruction
K51.813 Other ulcerative colitis with fistula
K51.814 Other ulcerative colitis with abscess
K51.818 Other ulcerative colitis with other complication
K51.819 Other ulcerative colitis with unspecified complications
⑤ K51.9 Ulcerative colitis, unspecified
K51.90 Ulcerative colitis, unspecified, without complications
⑥ K51.91 Ulcerative colitis, unspecified, with complications
K51.911 Ulcerative colitis, unspecified with rectal bleeding
K51.912 Ulcerative colitis, unspecified with intestinal obstruction
K51.913 Ulcerative colitis, unspecified with fistula
K51.914 Ulcerative colitis, unspecified with abscess
K51.918 Ulcerative colitis, unspecified with other complication
K51.919 Ulcerative colitis, unspecified with unspecified complications
④ K52 Other and unspecified noninfective gastroenteritis and colitis
K52.0 Gastroenteritis and colitis due to radiation
K52.1 Toxic gastroenteritis and colitis
Drug-induced gastroenteritis and colitis
Code first (T51-T65) to identify toxic agent
Use additional code for adverse effect, if applicable, to identify drug (T36-T50 with fifth or sixth character 5)
K52.2 Allergic and dietetic gastroenteritis and colitis
Food hypersensitivity gastroenteritis or colitis
Use additional code to identify type of food allergy (Z91.01-, Z91.02-)
⑤ K52.8 Other specified noninfective gastroenteritis and colitis
K52.81 Eosinophilic gastritis or gastroenteritis
Eosinophilic enteritis
EXCLUDES1 eosinophilic esophagitis (K20.0)
K52.82 Eosinophilic colitis
K52.89 Other specified noninfective gastroenteritis and colitis
Collagenous colitis
Lymphocytic colitis
Microscopic colitis (collagenous or lymphocytic)
K52.9 Noninfective gastroenteritis and colitis, unspecified
Colitis NOS
Enteritis NOS
Gastroenteritis NOS
Ileitis NOS
Jejunitis NOS
Sigmoiditis NOS
EXCLUDES1 diarrhea NOS (R19.7)
functional diarrhea (K59.1)
infectious gastroenteritis and colitis NOS (A09)
neonatal diarrhea (noninfective) (P78.3)
psychogenic diarrhea (F45.8)

④ 4th character required   ⑤ 5th character required   ⑥ 6th character required   ⑦ 7th character required   ⑩ Extension 'X' Alert

EXCLUDES1 Not coded here   EXCLUDES2 Not included here   PDx Primary Diagnosis Only   Manifestation Code

284

ICD-10-CM 2015

Other diseases of intestines (K55-K64)

K55 Vascular disorders of intestine
> *EXCLUDES1* necrotizing enterocolitis of newborn (P77.-)

K55.0 Acute **vascular disorders of intestine**
Acute fulminant ischemic colitis
Acute intestinal infarction
Acute small intestine ischemia
Infarction of appendices epiploicae
Mesenteric (artery) (vein) embolism
Mesenteric (artery) (vein) infarction
Mesenteric (artery) (vein) thrombosis
Necrosis of intestine
Subacute ischemic colitis

K55.1 Chronic **vascular disorders of intestine**
Chronic ischemic colitis
Chronic ischemic enteritis
Chronic ischemic enterocolitis
Ischemic stricture of intestine
Mesenteric atherosclerosis
Mesenteric vascular insufficiency

K55.2 Angiodysplasia **of colon**
K55.20 Angiodysplasia of colon without hemorrhage
K55.21 Angiodysplasia of colon with hemorrhage

K55.8 Other vascular disorders of intestine

K55.9 Vascular disorder of intestine, unspecified
Ischemic colitis
Ischemic enteritis
Ischemic enterocolitis

K56 Paralytic ileus and intestinal obstruction without hernia
> *EXCLUDES1* congenital stricture or stenosis of intestine (Q41-Q42)
> cystic fibrosis with meconium ileus (E84.11)
> ischemic stricture of intestine (K55.1)
> meconium ileus NOS (P76.0)
> neonatal intestinal obstructions classifiable to P76.-
> obstruction of duodenum (K31.5)
> postprocedural intestinal obstruction (K91.3)
> stenosis of anus or rectum (K62.4)
> intestinal obstruction with hernia (K40-K46)

K56.0 Paralytic ileus
Paralysis of bowel
Paralysis of colon
Paralysis of intestine
> *EXCLUDES1* gallstone ileus (K56.3)
> ileus NOS (K56.7)
> obstructive ileus NOS (K56.69)

K56.1 Intussusception
Intussusception or invagination of bowel
Intussusception or invagination of colon
Intussusception or invagination of intestine
Intussusception or invagination of rectum
> *EXCLUDES2* intussusception of appendix (K38.8)

K56.2 Volvulus
Strangulation of colon or intestine
Torsion of colon or intestine
Twist of colon or intestine
> *EXCLUDES2* volvulus of duodenum (K31.5)

K56.3 Gallstone ileus
Obstruction of intestine by gallstone

K56.4 Other impaction of intestine
K56.41 Fecal impaction
> *EXCLUDES1* constipation (K59.0-)
> incomplete defecation (R15.0)
K56.49 Other impaction of intestine

K56.5 Intestinal adhesions [bands] with obstruction (postprocedural) (postinfection)
Abdominal hernia due to adhesions with obstruction
Peritoneal adhesions [bands] with intestinal obstruction (postprocedural) (postinfection)

K56.6 Other and unspecified intestinal obstruction
K56.60 Unspecified intestinal obstruction
Intestinal obstruction NOS
> *EXCLUDES1* intestinal obstruction due to specified condition-code to condition
K56.69 Other intestinal obstruction
Enterostenosis NOS
Obstructive ileus NOS
Occlusion of colon or intestine NOS
Stenosis of colon or intestine NOS
Stricture of colon or intestine NOS
> *EXCLUDES1* intestinal obstruction due to specified condition-code to condition

K56.7 Ileus, unspecified
> *EXCLUDES1* obstructive ileus (K56.69)

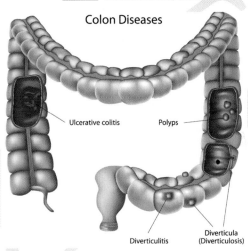

Figure 10.6 Diverticulosis

K57 Diverticular disease of intestine
> *EXCLUDES1* congenital diverticulum of intestine (Q43.8)
> Meckel's diverticulum (Q43.0)
> *EXCLUDES2* diverticulum of appendix (K38.2)

K57.0 Diverticulitis of small intestine with perforation and abscess
Diverticulitis of small intestine with peritonitis
> *EXCLUDES1* diverticulitis of both small and large intestine with perforation and abscess (K57.4-)
K57.00 Diverticulitis of small intestine with perforation and abscess without bleeding
K57.01 Diverticulitis of small intestine with perforation and abscess with bleeding

K57.1 Diverticular disease of small intestine without perforation or abscess
> *EXCLUDES1* diverticular disease of both small and large intestine without perforation or abscess (K57.5-)
K57.10 Diverticulosis of small intestine without perforation or abscess without bleeding
Diverticular disease of small intestine NOS
K57.11 Diverticulosis of small intestine without perforation or abscess with bleeding
K57.12 Diverticulitis of small intestine without perforation or abscess without bleeding
K57.13 Diverticulitis of small intestine without perforation or abscess with bleeding

⑤ **K57.2 Diverticulitis of** large intestine with perforation and abscess

Diverticulitis of colon with peritonitis

EXCLUDES1 *diverticulitis of both small and large intestine with perforation and abscess (K57.4-)*

K57.20 Diverticulitis of large intestine with perforation and abscess without bleeding

K57.21 Diverticulitis of large intestine with perforation and abscess with bleeding

⑤ **K57.3 Diverticular disease of** large intestine without perforation or abscess

EXCLUDES1 *diverticular disease of both small and large intestine without perforation or abscess (K57.5-)*

K57.30 Diverticulosis **of large intestine without perforation or abscess** without bleeding

Diverticular disease of colon NOS

K57.31 Diverticulosis **of large intestine without perforation or abscess** with bleeding

K57.32 Diverticulitis **of large intestine without perforation or abscess** without bleeding

K57.33 Diverticulitis **of large intestine without perforation or abscess** with bleeding

⑤ **K57.4 Diverticulitis of both** small and large intestine with perforation and abscess

Diverticulitis of both small and large intestine with peritonitis

K57.40 Diverticulitis of both small and large intestine with perforation and abscess without bleeding

K57.41 Diverticulitis of both small and large intestine with perforation and abscess with bleeding

⑤ **K57.5 Diverticular disease of** both small and large intestine without perforation or abscess

K57.50 Diverticulosis of both small and large intestine without perforation or abscess without bleeding

Diverticular disease of both small and large intestine NOS

K57.51 Diverticulosis **of both small and large intestine without perforation or abscess** with bleeding

K57.52 Diverticulitis **of both small and large intestine without perforation or abscess** without bleeding

K57.53 Diverticulitis **of both small and large intestine without perforation or abscess** with bleeding

⑤ **K57.8 Diverticulitis of intestine, part unspecified, with perforation and abscess**

Diverticulitis of intestine NOS with peritonitis

K57.80 Diverticulitis of intestine, part unspecified, with perforation and abscess without bleeding

K57.81 Diverticulitis of intestine, part unspecified, with perforation and abscess with bleeding

⑤ **K57.9 Diverticular disease of intestine, part unspecified, without perforation or abscess**

K57.90 Diverticulosis of intestine, part unspecified, without perforation or abscess without bleeding

Diverticular disease of intestine NOS

K57.91 Diverticulosis of intestine, part unspecified, without perforation or abscess with bleeding

K57.92 Diverticulitis of intestine, part unspecified, without perforation or abscess without bleeding

K57.93 Diverticulitis of intestine, part unspecified, without perforation or abscess with bleeding

④ **K58 Irritable bowel syndrome**

INCLUDES *irritable colon*
spastic colon

K58.0 Irritable bowel syndrome with diarrhea

K58.9 Irritable bowel syndrome without diarrhea

Irritable bowel syndrome NOS

④ **K59 Other functional intestinal disorders**

EXCLUDES1 *change in bowel habit NOS (R19.4)*
intestinal malabsorption (K90.-)
psychogenic intestinal disorders (F45.8)

EXCLUDES2 *functional disorders of stomach (K31.-)*

⑤ **K59.0 Constipation**

EXCLUDES1 *fecal impaction (K56.41)*
incomplete defecation (R15.0)

K59.00 Constipation, unspecified

K59.01 Slow transit **constipation**

K59.02 Outlet dysfunction **constipation**

K59.09 Other constipation

K59.1 Functional diarrhea

EXCLUDES1 *diarrhea NOS (R19.7)*
irritable bowel syndrome with diarrhea (K58.0)

K59.2 Neurogenic bowel, not elsewhere classified

K59.3 Megacolon, not elsewhere classified

Dilatation of colon

Toxic megacolon

Code first (T51-T65) to identify toxic agent

EXCLUDES1 *congenital megacolon (aganglionic) (Q43.1)*
megacolon (due to) (in) Chagas' disease (B57.32)
megacolon (due to) (in) Clostridium difficile (A04.7)
megacolon (due to) (in) Hirschsprung's disease (Q43.1)

K59.4 Anal spasm

Proctalgia fugax

K59.8 Other specified functional intestinal disorders

Atony of colon

Pseudo-obstruction (acute) (chronic) of intestine

K59.9 Functional intestinal disorder, unspecified

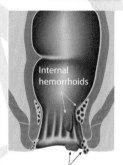 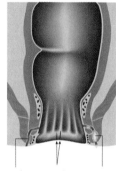

Internal hemorrhoids

External hemorrhoids

Anal fistula

Anal fissures

Anal abscess

Figure 10.7 Anal Disorders

④ **K60 Fissure and fistula of anal and rectal regions**

EXCLUDES1 *fissure and fistula of anal and rectal regions with abscess or cellulitis (K61.-)*

EXCLUDES2 *anal sphincter tear (healed) (nontraumatic) (old) (K62.81)*

K60.0 Acute **anal fissure**

K60.1 Chronic **anal fissure**

K60.2 Anal fissure, unspecified

K60.3 Anal **fistula**

K60.4 Rectal **fistula**

Fistula of rectum to skin

EXCLUDES1 *rectovaginal fistula (N82.3)*
vesicorectal fistual (N32.1)

K60.5 Anorectal **fistula**

④ **K61 Abscess of anal and rectal regions**

INCLUDES *abscess of anal and rectal regions*
cellulitis of anal and rectal regions

K61.0 Anal **abscess**

Perianal abscess

EXCLUDES1 *intrasphincteric abscess (K61.4)*

---

④ 4th character required ⑤ 5th character required ⑥ 6th character required ⑦ 7th character required ⑦ˣ Extension 'X' Alert

EXCLUDES 1 Not coded here   *EXCLUDES 2* Not included here   ᴾᴰˣ Primary Diagnosis Only   Manifestation Code

K61.1 Rectal **abscess**

Perirectal abscess

EXCLUDES1 *ischiorectal abscess (K61.3)*

K61.2 Anorectal **abscess**

K61.3 Ischiorectal **abscess**

Abscess of ischiorectal fossa

K61.4 Intrasphincteric **abscess**

🍀 K62 Other diseases of anus and rectum

INCLUDES *anal canal*

EXCLUDES2 *colostomy and enterostomy malfunction (K94.0-, K94.1-)*

fecal incontinence (R15.-)

hemorrhoids (K64.-)

K62.0 Anal polyp

K62.1 Rectal polyp

EXCLUDES1 *adenomatous polyp (D12.8)*

K62.2 Anal prolapse

Prolapse of anal canal

K62.3 Rectal prolapse

Prolapse of rectal mucosa

K62.4 Stenosis of anus and rectum

Stricture of anus (sphincter)

K62.5 Hemorrhage of anus and rectum

EXCLUDES1 *gastrointestinal bleeding NOS (K92.2)*

melena (K92.1)

neonatal rectal hemorrhage (P54.2)

K62.6 Ulcer of anus and rectum

Solitary ulcer of anus and rectum

Stercoral ulcer of anus and rectum

EXCLUDES1 *fissure and fistula of anus and rectum (K60.-)*

ulcerative colitis (K51.-)

K62.7 Radiation proctitis

Use additional code to identify the type of radiation (W90.-)

🍵 K62.8 Other specified diseases of anus and rectum

EXCLUDES2 *ulcerative proctitis (K51.2)*

K62.81 Anal sphincter tear (healed) (nontraumatic) (old)

Tear of anus, nontraumatic

Use additional code for any associated fecal incontinence (R15.-)

EXCLUDES2 *anal fissure (K60.-)*

anal sphincter tear (healed) (old) complicating delivery (O34.7-)

traumatic tear of anal sphincter (S31.831)

K62.82 Dysplasia of anus

Anal intraepithelial neoplasia I and II (AIN I and II) (histologically confirmed)

Dysplasia of anus NOS

Mild and moderate dysplasia of anus (histologically confirmed)

EXCLUDES1 *abnormal results from anal cytologic examination without histologic confirmation (R85.61-)*

anal intraepithelial neoplasia III (D01.3)

carcinoma in situ of anus (D01.3)

HGSIL of anus (R85.613)

severe dysplasia of anus (D01.3)

K62.89 Other specified diseases of anus and rectum

Proctitis NOS

Use additional code for any associated fecal incontinence (R15.-)

K62.9 Disease of anus and rectum, unspecified

🍀 K63 Other diseases of intestine

K63.0 Abscess of intestine

EXCLUDES1 *abscess of intestine with Crohn's disease (K50.014, K50.114, K50.814, K50.914,)*

abscess of intestine with diverticular disease (K57.0, K57.2, K57.4, K57.8)

abscess of intestine with ulcerative colitis (K51.014, K51.214, K51.314, K51.414, K51.514,K51.814, K51.914)

EXCLUDES2 *abscess of anal and rectal regions (K61.-)*

abscess of appendix (K35.3)

K63.1 Perforation of intestine (nontraumatic)

Perforation (nontraumatic) of rectum

EXCLUDES1 *perforation (nontraumatic) of duodenum (K26.-)*

perforation (nontraumatic) of intestine with diverticular disease (K57.0, K57.2, K57.4, K57.8)

EXCLUDES2 *perforation (nontraumatic) of appendix (K35.2, K35.3)*

K63.2 Fistula of intestine

EXCLUDES1 *fistula of duodenum (K31.6)*

fistula of intestine with Crohn's disease (K50.013, K50.113, K50.813, K50.913,)

fistula of intestine with ulcerative colitis (K51.013, K51.213, K51.313, K51.413, K51.513, K51.813,K51.913)

EXCLUDES2 *fistula of anal and rectal regions (K60.-)*

fistula of appendix (K38.3)

intestinal-genital fistula, female (N82.2-N82.4)

vesicointestinal fistula (N32.1)

K63.3 Ulcer of intestine

Primary ulcer of small intestine

EXCLUDES1 *duodenal ulcer (K26.-)*

gastrointestinal ulcer (K28.-)

gastrojejunal ulcer (K28.-)

jejunal ulcer (K28.-)

peptic ulcer, site unspecified (K27.-)

ulcer of intestine with perforation (K63.1)

ulcer of anus or rectum (K62.6)

ulcerative colitis (K51.-)

K63.4 Enteroptosis

K63.5 Polyp of colon

EXCLUDES1 *adenomatous polyp of colon (D12.6)*

inflammatory polyp of colon (K51.4-)

polyposis of colon (D12.6)

🍵 K63.8 Other specified diseases of intestine

K63.81 Dieulafoy lesion of intestine

EXCLUDES2 *Dieulafoy lesion of stomach and duodenum (K31.82)*

K63.89 Other specified diseases of intestine

K63.9 Disease of intestine, unspecified

🍀 K64 Hemorrhoids and perianal venous thrombosis

INCLUDES *piles*

EXCLUDES1 *hemorrhoids complicating childbirth and the puerperium (O87.2)*

hemorrhoids complicating pregnancy (O22.4)

K64.0 First degree hemorrhoids

Grade/stage I hemorrhoids

Hemorrhoids (bleeding) without prolapse outside of anal canal

K64.1 Second degree hemorrhoids

Grade/stage II hemorrhoids

Hemorrhoids (bleeding) that prolapse with straining, but retract spontaneously

K64.2 Third degree hemorrhoids

Grade/stage III hemorrhoids

Hemorrhoids (bleeding) that prolapse with straining and require manual replacement back inside anal canal

Unspecified Code	Other Specified Code	N Newborn Age: 0	P Pediatric Age: 0-17	M Maternity Age: 12-55
A Adult Age: 15-124	♂ Male	♀ Female	● New Code	▲ Revised Code Title	►◄ Revised Text

K64.3 Fourth degree hemorrhoids

Grade/stage IV hemorrhoids

Hemorrhoids (bleeding) with prolapsed tissue that cannot be manually replaced

K64.4 Residual hemorrhoidal skin tags

External hemorrhoids, NOS

Skin tags of anus

K64.5 Perianal venous thrombosis

External hemorrhoids with thrombosis

Perianal hematoma

Thrombosed hemorrhoids NOS

K64.8 Other hemorrhoids

Internal hemorrhoids, without mention of degree

Prolapsed hemorrhoids, degree not specified

K64.9 Unspecified hemorrhoids

Hemorrhoids (bleeding) NOS

Hemorrhoids (bleeding) without mention of degree

Diseases of peritoneum and retroperitoneum (K65-K68)

🔵 K65 Peritonitis

Use additional code (B95-B97), to identify infectious agent

EXCLUDES1 acute appendicitis with generalized peritonitis (K35.2)

aseptic peritonitis (T81.6)

benign paroxysmal peritonitis (E85.0)

chemical peritonitis (T81.6)

diverticulitis of both small and large intestine with peritonitis (K57.4-)

diverticulitis of colon with peritonitis (K57.2-)

diverticulitis of intestine, NOS, with peritonitis (K57.8-)

diverticulitis of small intestine with peritonitis (K57.0-)

gonococcal peritonitis (A54.85)

neonatal peritonitis (P78.0-P78.1)

pelvic peritonitis, female (N73.3-N73.5)

periodic familial peritonitis (E85.0)

peritonitis due to talc or other foreign substance (T81.6)

peritonitis in chlamydia (A74.81)

peritonitis in diphtheria (A36.89)

peritonitis in syphilis (late) (A52.74)

peritonitis in tuberculosis (A18.31)

peritonitis with or following abortion or ectopic or molar pregnancy (O00-O07, O08.0)

peritonitis with or following appendicitis (K35.-)

peritonitis with or following diverticular disease of intestine (K57.-)

puerperal peritonitis (O85)

retroperitoneal infections (K68.-)

K65.0 Generalized (acute) peritonitis

Pelvic peritonitis (acute), male

Subphrenic peritonitis (acute)

Suppurative peritonitis (acute)

K65.1 Peritoneal abscess

Abdominopelvic abscess

Abscess (of) omentum

Abscess (of) peritoneum

Mesenteric abscess

Retrocecal abscess

Subdiaphragmatic abscess

Subhepatic abscess

Subphrenic abscess

K65.2 Spontaneous bacterial peritonitis

EXCLUDES1 bacterial peritonitis NOS (K65.9)

K65.3 Choleperitonitis

Peritonitis due to bile

K65.4 Sclerosing mesenteritis

Fat necrosis of peritoneum

(Idiopathic) sclerosing mesenteric fibrosis

Mesenteric lipodystrophy

Mesenteric panniculitis

Retractile mesenteritis

K65.8 Other peritonitis

Chronic proliferative peritonitis

Peritonitis due to urine

K65.9 Peritonitis, unspecified

Bacterial peritonitis NOS

🔵 K66 Other disorders of peritoneum

EXCLUDES2 ascites (R18.-)

peritoneal effusion (chronic) (R18.8)

K66.0 Peritoneal adhesions (postprocedural) (postinfection)

Adhesions (of) abdominal (wall)

Adhesions (of) diaphragm

Adhesions (of) intestine

Adhesions (of) male pelvis

Adhesions (of) omentum

Adhesions (of) stomach

Adhesive bands

Mesenteric adhesions

EXCLUDES1 female pelvic adhesions [bands] (N73.6)

peritoneal adhesions with intestinal obstruction (K56.5)

K66.1 Hemoperitoneum

EXCLUDES1 traumatic hemoperitoneum (S36.8-)

K66.8 Other specified disorders of peritoneum

K66.9 Disorder of peritoneum, unspecified

K67 Disorders of peritoneum in infectious diseases classified elsewhere

Code first underlying disease, such as :

congenital syphilis (A50.0)

helminthiasis (B65.0 -B83.9)

EXCLUDES1 peritonitis in chlamydia (A74.81)

peritonitis in diphtheria (A36.89)

peritonitis in gonococcal (A54.85)

peritonitis in syphilis (late) (A52.74)

peritonitis in tuberculosis (A18.31)

🔵 K68 Disorders of retroperitoneum

🔵 K68.1 Retroperitoneal abscess

K68.11 Postprocedural retroperitoneal abscess

K68.12 Psoas muscle abscess

K68.19 Other retroperitoneal abscess

K68.9 Other disorders of retroperitoneum

🔵 4th character required   🔵 5th character required   🔵 6th character required   🔵 7th character required   🔵 Extension 'X' Alert

EXCLUDES 1 Not coded here   EXCLUDES 2 Not included here   🔵 Primary Diagnosis Only   Manifestation Code

ICD-10-CM 2015

Diseases of liver (K70-K77)

[EXCLUDES1] *jaundice NOS (R17)*
[EXCLUDES2] *hemochromatosis (E83.11-)*
Reye's syndrome (G93.7)
viral hepatitis (B15-B19)
Wilson's disease (E83.0)

[4] **K70 Alcoholic liver disease**
Use additional code to identify:
alcohol abuse and dependence (F10.-)
K70.0 Alcoholic fatty liver [A]
[5] **K70.1 Alcoholic** hepatitis
K70.10 Alcoholic hepatitis without ascites [A]
K70.11 Alcoholic hepatitis with ascites [A]
K70.2 Alcoholic fibrosis and sclerosis **of liver** [A]
[5] **K70.3 Alcoholic** cirrhosis **of liver**
Alcoholic cirrhosis NOS
K70.30 Alcoholic cirrhosis of liver without ascites [A]
K70.31 Alcoholic cirrhosis of liver with ascites [A]
[5] **K70.4 Alcoholic** hepatic failure
Acute alcoholic hepatic failure
Alcoholic hepatic failure NOS
Chronic alcoholic hepatic failure
Subacute alcoholic hepatic failure
K70.40 Alcoholic hepatic failure without coma [A]
K70.41 Alcoholic hepatic failure with coma [A]
K70.9 Alcoholic liver disease, unspecified [A]

[4] **K71 Toxic liver disease**
[INCLUDES] *drug-induced idiosyncratic (unpredictable) liver disease*
drug-induced toxic (predictable) liver disease
Code first poisoning due to drug or toxin, if applicable (T36-T65 with fifth or sixth character 1-4 or 6)
Use additional code for adverse effect, if applicable, to identify drug (T36-T50 with fifth or sixth character 5)
[EXCLUDES2] *alcoholic liver disease (K70.-)*
Budd-Chiari syndrome (I82.0)
K71.0 Toxic liver disease with cholestasis
Cholestasis with hepatocyte injury
'Pure' cholestasis
[5] **K71.1 Toxic liver disease with** hepatic necrosis
Hepatic failure (acute) (chronic) due to drugs
K71.10 Toxic liver disease with hepatic necrosis, without coma
K71.11 Toxic liver disease with hepatic necrosis, with coma
K71.2 Toxic liver disease with acute hepatitis
K71.3 Toxic liver disease with chronic persistent hepatitis
K71.4 Toxic liver disease with chronic lobular hepatitis
[5] **K71.5 Toxic liver disease with** chronic active hepatitis
Toxic liver disease with lupoid hepatitis
K71.50 Toxic liver disease with chronic active hepatitis without ascites
K71.51 Toxic liver disease with chronic active hepatitis with ascites
K71.6 Toxic liver disease with hepatitis, not elsewhere classified
K71.7 Toxic liver disease with fibrosis and cirrhosis **of liver**
K71.8 Toxic liver disease with other disorders of liver
Toxic liver disease with focal nodular hyperplasia
Toxic liver disease with hepatic granulomas
Toxic liver disease with peliosis hepatis
Toxic liver disease with veno-occlusive disease of liver
K71.9 Toxic liver disease, unspecified

[4] **K72 Hepatic failure, not elsewhere classified**
[INCLUDES] *acute hepatitis NEC, with hepatic failure*
fulminant hepatitis NEC, with hepatic failure
hepatic encephalopathy NOS
liver (cell) necrosis with hepatic failure
malignant hepatitis NEC, with hepatic failure
yellow liver atrophy or dystrophy
[EXCLUDES1] *alcoholic hepatic failure (K70.4)*
hepatic failure with toxic liver disease (K71.1-)
icterus of newborn (P55-P59)
postprocedural hepatic failure (K91.82)
viral hepatitis with hepatic coma (B15-B19)
[EXCLUDES2] *hepatic failure complicating abortion or ectopic or molar pregnancy (O00-O07, O08.8)*
hepatic failure complicating pregnancy, childbirth and the puerperium (O26.6-)
[5] **K72.0** Acute and subacute **hepatic failure**
K72.00 Acute and subacute hepatic failure without coma
K72.01 Acute and subacute hepatic failure with coma
[5] **K72.1** Chronic **hepatic failure**
K72.10 Chronic hepatic failure without coma
K72.11 Chronic hepatic failure with coma
[5] **K72.9 Hepatic failure, unspecified**
K72.90 Hepatic failure, unspecified without coma
K72.91 Hepatic failure, unspecified with coma
Hepatic coma NOS

[4] **K73 Chronic hepatitis, not elsewhere classified**
[EXCLUDES1] *alcoholic hepatitis (chronic) (K70.1-)*
drug-induced hepatitis (chronic) (K71.-)
granulomatous hepatitis (chronic) NEC (K75.3)
reactive, nonspecific hepatitis (chronic) (K75.2)
viral hepatitis (chronic) (B15-B19)
K73.0 Chronic persistent **hepatitis, not elsewhere classified**
K73.1 Chronic lobular **hepatitis, not elsewhere classified**
K73.2 Chronic active **hepatitis, not elsewhere classified**
K73.8 Other chronic hepatitis, not elsewhere classified
K73.9 Chronic hepatitis, unspecified

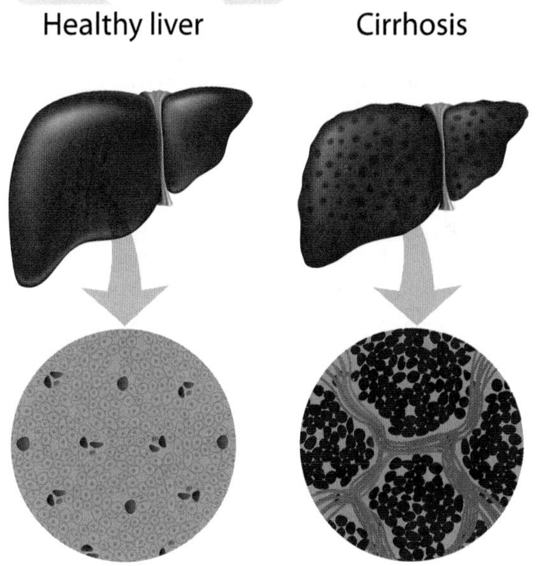

Figure 10.8 Cirrhosis of the Liver

[4] **K74 Fibrosis and cirrhosis of liver**
Code also , if applicable, viral hepatitis (acute) (chronic) (B15-B19)
[EXCLUDES1] *alcoholic cirrhosis (of liver) (K70.3)*
alcoholic fibrosis of liver (K70.2)
cardiac sclerosis of liver (K76.1)
cirrhosis (of liver) with toxic liver disease (K71.7)
congenital cirrhosis (of liver) (P78.81)
pigmentary cirrhosis (of liver) (E83.110)
K74.0 Hepatic fibrosis

Unspecified Code | Other Specified Code | [N] Newborn Age: 0 | [P] Pediatric Age: 0-17 | [M] Maternity Age: 12-55
[A] Adult Age: 15-124 | ♂ Male | ♀ Female | ● New Code | ▲ Revised Code Title | ►◄ Revised Text

K74.1 **Hepatic** sclerosis
K74.2 **Hepatic** fibrosis with hepatic sclerosis
K74.3 Primary **biliary cirrhosis**
Chronic nonsuppurative destructive cholangitis
K74.4 Secondary **biliary cirrhosis**
K74.5 Biliary cirrhosis, unspecified
[5] **K74.6 Other and unspecified cirrhosis of liver**
K74.60 Unspecified cirrhosis of liver
Cirrhosis (of liver) NOS
K74.69 Other cirrhosis of liver
Cryptogenic cirrhosis (of liver)
Macronodular cirrhosis (of liver)
Micronodular cirrhosis (of liver)
Mixed type cirrhosis (of liver)
Portal cirrhosis (of liver)
Postnecrotic cirrhosis (of liver)

[4] **K75 Other inflammatory liver diseases**
[EXCLUDES2] *toxic liver disease (K71.-)*
K75.0 Abscess of liver
Cholangitic hepatic abscess
Hematogenic hepatic abscess
Hepatic abscess NOS
Lymphogenic hepatic abscess
Pylephlebitic hepatic abscess
[EXCLUDES1] *amebic liver abscess (A06.4)*
cholangitis without liver abscess (K83.0)
pylephlebitis without liver abscess (K75.1)
K75.1 Phlebitis of portal vein
Pylephlebitis
[EXCLUDES1] *pylephlebitic liver abscess (K75.0)*
K75.2 Nonspecific reactive hepatitis
[EXCLUDES1] *acute or subacute hepatitis (K72.0-)*
chronic hepatitis NEC (K73.-)
viral hepatitis (B15-B19)
K75.3 Granulomatous hepatitis, not elsewhere classified
[EXCLUDES1] *acute or subacute hepatitis (K72.0-)*
chronic hepatitis NEC (K73.-)
viral hepatitis (B15-B19)
K75.4 Autoimmune hepatitis
Lupoid hepatitis NEC
[5] **K75.8 Other specified inflammatory liver diseases**
K75.81 Nonalcoholic steatohepatitis (NASH)
K75.89 Other specified inflammatory liver diseases
K75.9 Inflammatory liver disease, unspecified
Hepatitis NOS
[EXCLUDES1] *acute or subacute hepatitis (K72.0-)*
chronic hepatitis NEC (K73.-)
viral hepatitis (B15-B19)

[4] **K76 Other diseases of liver**
[EXCLUDES2] *alcoholic liver disease (K70.-)*
amyloid degeneration of liver (E85.-)
cystic disease of liver (congenital) (Q44.6)
hepatic vein thrombosis (I82.0)
hepatomegaly NOS (R16.0)
pigmentary cirrhosis (of liver) (E83.110)
portal vein thrombosis (I81)
toxic liver disease (K71.-)
K76.0 Fatty (change of) liver, not elsewhere classified
Nonalcoholic fatty liver disease (NAFLD)
[EXCLUDES1] *nonalcoholic steatohepatitis (NASH) (K75.81)*
K76.1 Chronic passive congestion of liver
Cardiac cirrhosis
Cardiac sclerosis
K76.2 Central hemorrhagic necrosis of liver
[EXCLUDES1] *liver necrosis with hepatic failure (K72.-)*
K76.3 Infarction of liver
K76.4 Peliosis hepatis
Hepatic angiomatosis
K76.5 Hepatic veno-occlusive disease
[EXCLUDES1] *Budd-Chiari syndrome (I82.0)*
K76.6 Portal hypertension
Use additional code for any associated complications, such as:
portal hypertensive gastropathy (K31.89)
K76.7 Hepatorenal syndrome
[EXCLUDES1] *hepatorenal syndrome following labor and delivery (O90.4)*
postprocedural hepatorenal syndrome (K91.82)
[5] **K76.8 Other specified diseases of liver**
K76.81 Hepatopulmonary syndrome
Code first underlying liver disease, such as:
alcoholic cirrhosis of liver (K70.3-)
cirrhosis of liver without mention of alcohol (K74.6-)
K76.89 Other specified diseases of liver
Cyst (simple) of liver
Focal nodular hyperplasia of liver
Hepatoptosis
K76.9 Liver disease, unspecified

K77 Liver disorders in diseases classified elsewhere
Code first underlying disease, such as:
amyloidosis (E85.-)
congenital syphilis (A50.0, A50.5)
congenital toxoplasmosis (P37.1)
schistosomiasis (B65.0-B65.9)
[EXCLUDES1] *alcoholic hepatitis (K70.1-)*
alcoholic liver disease (K70.-)
cytomegaloviral hepatitis (B25.1)
herpesviral [herpes simplex] hepatitis (B00.81)
infectious mononucleosis with liver disease (B27.0-B27.9 with .9)
mumps hepatitis (B26.81)
sarcoidosis with liver disease (D86.89)
secondary syphilis with liver disease (A51.45)
syphilis (late) with liver disease (A52.74)
toxoplasmosis (acquired) hepatitis (B58.1)
tuberculosis with liver disease (A18.83)

Disorders of gallbladder, biliary tract and pancreas (K80-K87)

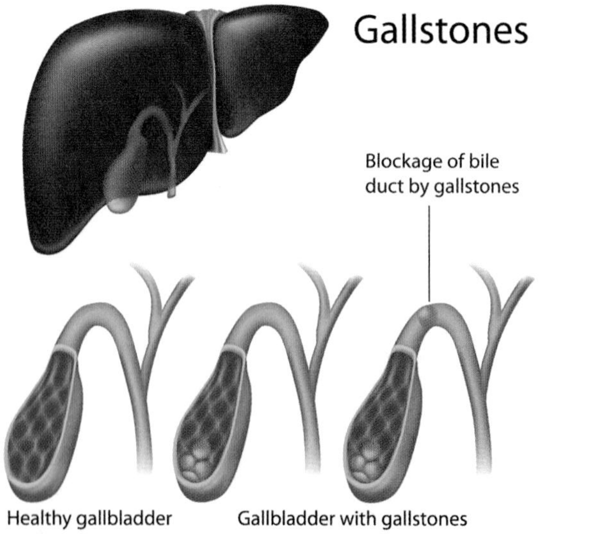
Gallstones
Blockage of bile duct by gallstones
Healthy gallbladder
Gallbladder with gallstones

Figure 10.9 Illustration showing normal and obstructed gall bladder

[4] **K80 Cholelithiasis**
[EXCLUDES1] *retained cholelithiasis following cholecystectomy (K91.86)*

[5] **K80.0 Calculus of gallbladder with acute cholecystitis**
Any condition listed in K80.2 with acute cholecystitis
K80.00 Calculus of gallbladder with acute cholecystitis without obstruction
K80.01 Calculus of gallbladder with acute cholecystitis with obstruction

[5] **K80.1 Calculus of gallbladder with other cholecystitis**
K80.10 Calculus of gallbladder with chronic cholecystitis without obstruction
Cholelithiasis with cholecystitis NOS
K80.11 Calculus of gallbladder with chronic cholecystitis with obstruction
K80.12 Calculus of gallbladder with acute and chronic cholecystitis without obstruction
K80.13 Calculus of gallbladder with acute and chronic cholecystitis with obstruction
K80.18 Calculus of gallbladder with other cholecystitis without obstruction
K80.19 Calculus of gallbladder with other cholecystitis with obstruction

[5] **K80.2 Calculus of gallbladder without cholecystitis**
Cholecystolithiasis without cholecystitis
Cholelithiasis (without cholecystitis)
Colic (recurrent) of gallbladder (without cholecystitis)
Gallstone (impacted) of cystic duct (without cholecystitis)
Gallstone (impacted) of gallbladder (without cholecystitis)
K80.20 Calculus of gallbladder without cholecystitis without obstruction
K80.21 Calculus of gallbladder without cholecystitis with obstruction

[5] **K80.3 Calculus of bile duct with cholangitis**
Any condition listed in K80.5 with cholangitis
K80.30 Calculus of bile duct with cholangitis, unspecified, without obstruction
K80.31 Calculus of bile duct with cholangitis, unspecified, with obstruction
K80.32 Calculus of bile duct with acute cholangitis without obstruction
K80.33 Calculus of bile duct with acute cholangitis with obstruction
K80.34 Calculus of bile duct with chronic cholangitis without obstruction
K80.35 Calculus of bile duct with chronic cholangitis with obstruction
K80.36 Calculus of bile duct with acute and chronic cholangitis without obstruction
K80.37 Calculus of bile duct with acute and chronic cholangitis with obstruction

[5] **K80.4 Calculus of bile duct with cholecystitis**
Any condition listed in K80.5 with cholecystitis (with cholangitis)
K80.40 Calculus of bile duct with cholecystitis, unspecified, without obstruction
K80.41 Calculus of bile duct with cholecystitis, unspecified, with obstruction
K80.42 Calculus of bile duct with acute cholecystitis without obstruction
K80.43 Calculus of bile duct with acute cholecystitis with obstruction
K80.44 Calculus of bile duct with chronic cholecystitis without obstruction
K80.45 Calculus of bile duct with chronic cholecystitis with obstruction
K80.46 Calculus of bile duct with acute and chronic cholecystitis without obstruction
K80.47 Calculus of bile duct with acute and chronic cholecystitis with obstruction

[5] **K80.5 Calculus of bile duct without cholangitis or cholecystitis**
Choledocholithiasis (without cholangitis or cholecystitis)
Gallstone (impacted) of bile duct NOS (without cholangitis or cholecystitis)
Gallstone (impacted) of common duct (without cholangitis or cholecystitis)
Gallstone (impacted) of hepatic duct (without cholangitis or cholecystitis)
Hepatic cholelithiasis (without cholangitis or cholecystitis)
Hepatic colic (recurrent) (without cholangitis or cholecystitis)
K80.50 Calculus of bile duct without cholangitis or cholecystitis without obstruction
K80.51 Calculus of bile duct without cholangitis or cholecystitis with obstruction

[5] **K80.6 Calculus of gallbladder and bile duct with cholecystitis**
K80.60 Calculus of gallbladder and bile duct with cholecystitis, unspecified, without obstruction
K80.61 Calculus of gallbladder and bile duct with cholecystitis, unspecified, with obstruction
K80.62 Calculus of gallbladder and bile duct with acute cholecystitis without obstruction
K80.63 Calculus of gallbladder and bile duct with acute cholecystitis with obstruction
K80.64 Calculus of gallbladder and bile duct with chronic cholecystitis without obstruction
K80.65 Calculus of gallbladder and bile duct with chronic cholecystitis with obstruction
K80.66 Calculus of gallbladder and bile duct with acute and chronic cholecystitis without obstruction
K80.67 Calculus of gallbladder and bile duct with acute and chronic cholecystitis with obstruction

[5] **K80.7 Calculus of gallbladder and bile duct without cholecystitis**
K80.70 Calculus of gallbladder and bile duct without cholecystitis without obstruction
K80.71 Calculus of gallbladder and bile duct without cholecystitis with obstruction

[5] **K80.8 Other cholelithiasis**
K80.80 Other cholelithiasis without obstruction
K80.81 Other cholelithiasis with obstruction

[4] **K81 Cholecystitis**
[EXCLUDES1] *cholecystitis with cholelithiasis (K80.-)*
K81.0 Acute cholecystitis
Abscess of gallbladder
Angiocholecystitis
Emphysematous (acute) cholecystitis
Empyema of gallbladder
Gangrene of gallbladder
Gangrenous cholecystitis
Suppurative cholecystitis
K81.1 Chronic cholecystitis
K81.2 Acute cholecystitis with chronic cholecystitis
K81.9 Cholecystitis, unspecified

[4] **K82 Other diseases of gallbladder**
[EXCLUDES1] *nonvisualization of gallbladder (R93.2)*
postcholecystectomy syndrome (K91.5)
K82.0 Obstruction of gallbladder
Occlusion of cystic duct or gallbladder without cholelithiasis
Stenosis of cystic duct or gallbladder without cholelithiasis
Stricture of cystic duct or gallbladder without cholelithiasis
[EXCLUDES1] *obstruction of gallbladder with cholelithiasis (K80.-)*

Unspecified Code | Other Specified Code | [N] Newborn Age: 0 | [P] Pediatric Age: 0-17 | [M] Maternity Age: 12-55
[A] Adult Age: 15-124 | ♂ Male | ♀ Female | ● New Code | ▲ Revised Code Title | ►◄ Revised Text

K82.1 **Hydrops of gallbladder**
Mucocele of gallbladder
K82.2 **Perforation of gallbladder**
Rupture of cystic duct or gallbladder
K82.3 **Fistula of gallbladder**
Cholecystocolic fistula
Cholecystoduodenal fistula
K82.4 **Cholesterolosis of gallbladder**
Strawberry gallbladder
EXCLUDES1 *cholesterolosis of gallbladder with cholecystitis*
(K81.-)
cholesterolosis of gallbladder with cholelithiasis
(K80.-)
K82.8 **Other specified diseases of gallbladder**
Adhesions of cystic duct or gallbladder
Atrophy of cystic duct or gallbladder
Cyst of cystic duct or gallbladder
Dyskinesia of cystic duct or gallbladder
Hypertrophy of cystic duct or gallbladder
Nonfunctioning of cystic duct or gallbladder
Ulcer of cystic duct or gallbladder
K82.9 **Disease of gallbladder, unspecified**
④ K83 **Other diseases of biliary tract**
EXCLUDES1 *postcholecystectomy syndrome (K91.5)*
EXCLUDES2 *conditions involving the gallbladder (K81-K82)*
conditions involving the cystic duct (K81-K82)
K83.0 **Cholangitis**
Ascending cholangitis
Cholangitis NOS
Primary cholangitis
Recurrent cholangitis
Sclerosing cholangitis
Secondary cholangitis
Stenosing cholangitis
Suppurative cholangitis
EXCLUDES1 *cholangitic liver abscess (K75.0)*
cholangitis with choledocholithiasis (K80.3-,
K80.4-)
chronic nonsuppurative destructive cholangitis
(K74.3)
K83.1 **Obstruction of bile duct**
Occlusion of bile duct without cholelithiasis
Stenosis of bile duct without cholelithiasis
Stricture of bile duct without cholelithiasis
EXCLUDES1 *congenital obstruction of bile duct (Q44.3)*
obstruction of bile duct with cholelithiasis (K80.-)
K83.2 **Perforation of bile duct**
Rupture of bile duct
K83.3 **Fistula of bile duct**
Choledochoduodenal fistula
K83.4 **Spasm of sphincter of Oddi**
K83.5 **Biliary cyst**
K83.8 **Other specified diseases of biliary tract**
Adhesions of biliary tract
Atrophy of biliary tract
Hypertrophy of biliary tract
Ulcer of biliary tract
K83.9 **Disease of biliary tract, unspecified**

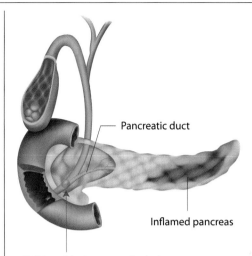

Gallstone blocks pancreatic duct

Figure 10.10 Acute Pancreatitis

④ K85 **Acute pancreatitis**
INCLUDES *abscess of pancreas*
acute necrosis of pancreas
acute (recurrent) pancreatitis
gangrene of (gangrenous) pancreas
hemorrhagic pancreatitis
infective necrosis of pancreas
subacute pancreatitis
suppurative pancreatitis
K85.0 **Idiopathic acute pancreatitis**
K85.1 **Biliary acute pancreatitis**
Gallstone pancreatitis
K85.2 **Alcohol induced acute pancreatitis**
EXCLUDES2 *alcohol induced chronic pancreatitis (K86.0)*
K85.3 **Drug induced acute pancreatitis**
Use additional code for adverse effect, if applicable, to
identify drug (T36-T50 with fifth or sixth character 5)
code to identify drug abuse and dependence (F11.-
F17.-)
K85.8 **Other acute pancreatitis**
K85.9 **Acute pancreatitis, unspecified**
Pancreatitis NOS
④ K86 **Other diseases of pancreas**
EXCLUDES2 *fibrocystic disease of pancreas (E84.-)*
islet cell tumor (of pancreas) (D13.7)
pancreatic steatorrhea (K90.3)
K86.0 **Alcohol-induced chronic pancreatitis**
Use additional code to identify:
alcohol abuse and dependence (F10.-)
EXCLUDES2 *alcohol induced acute pancreatitis (K85.2)*
K86.1 **Other chronic pancreatitis**
Chronic pancreatitis NOS
Infectious chronic pancreatitis
Recurrent chronic pancreatitis
Relapsing chronic pancreatitis
K86.2 **Cyst of pancreas**
K86.3 **Pseudocyst of pancreas**
K86.8 **Other specified diseases of pancreas**
Aseptic pancreatic necrosis
Atrophy of pancreas
Calculus of pancreas
Cirrhosis of pancreas
Fibrosis of pancreas
Pancreatic fat necrosis
Pancreatic infantilism
Pancreatic necrosis NOS
K86.9 **Disease of pancreas, unspecified**

---

④ 4th character required   ⑤ 5th character required   ⑥ 6th character required   ⑦ 7th character required   Ⓧ Extension 'X' Alert

EXCLUDES 1 Not coded here   *EXCLUDES 2* Not included here   PDx Primary Diagnosis Only   Manifestation Code

K87 Disorders of gallbladder, biliary tract and pancreas in diseases classified elsewhere

Code first underlying disease

[EXCLUDES1] *cytomegaloviral pancreatitis(B25.2)*
mumps pancreatitis (B26.3)
syphilitic gallbladder (A52.74)
syphilitic pancreas (A52.74)
tuberculosis of gallbladder (A18.83)
tuberculosis of pancreas (A18.83)

Other diseases of the digestive system (K90-K95)

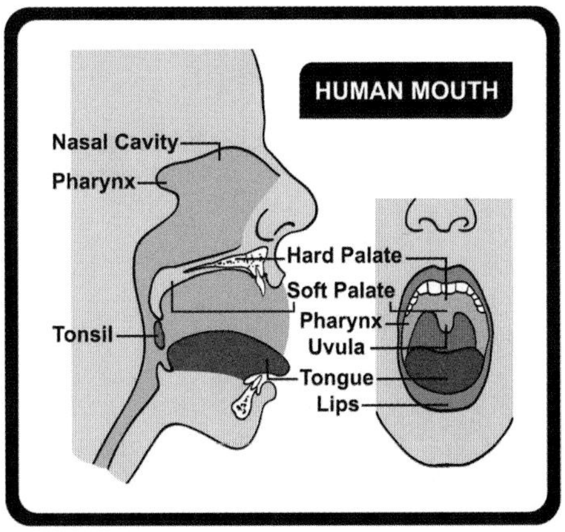

Figure 10.11 Human mouth

[4] **K90 Intestinal malabsorption**

[EXCLUDES1] *intestinal malabsorption following gastrointestinal surgery (K91.2)*

K90.0 Celiac disease

Gluten-sensitive enteropathy
Idiopathic steatorrhea
Nontropical sprue
Use additional code for associated disorders including:
dermatitis herpetiformis (L13.0)
gluten ataxia (G32.81)

K90.1 Tropical sprue

Sprue NOS
Tropical steatorrhea

K90.2 Blind loop syndrome, not elsewhere classified

Blind loop syndrome NOS

[EXCLUDES1] *congenital blind loop syndrome (Q43.8)*
postsurgical blind loop syndrome (K91.2)

K90.3 Pancreatic steatorrhea

K90.4 Malabsorption due to intolerance, not elsewhere classified

Malabsorption due to intolerance to carbohydrate
Malabsorption due to intolerance to fat
Malabsorption due to intolerance to protein
Malabsorption due to intolerance to starch

[EXCLUDES2] *gluten-sensitive enteropathy (K90.0)*
lactose intolerance (E73.-)

[5] **K90.8 Other intestinal malabsorption**

K90.81 Whipple's disease

K90.89 Other intestinal malabsorption

K90.9 Intestinal malabsorption, unspecified

[4] **K91 Intraoperative and postprocedural complications and disorders of digestive system, not elsewhere classified**

[EXCLUDES2] *complications of artificial opening of digestive system (K94.-)*
complications of bariatric procedures (K95.-)
gastrojejunal ulcer (K28.-)
postprocedural (radiation) retroperitoneal abscess (K68.11)
radiation colitis (K52.0)
radiation gastroenteritis (K52.0)
radiation proctitis (K62.7)

K91.0 Vomiting following gastrointestinal surgery

K91.1 Postgastric surgery syndromes

Dumping syndrome
Postgastrectomy syndrome
Postvagotomy syndrome

K91.2 Postsurgical malabsorption, not elsewhere classified

Postsurgical blind loop syndrome

[EXCLUDES1] *malabsorption osteomalacia in adults (M83.2)*
malabsorption osteoporosis, postsurgical (M80.8-, M81.8)

K91.3 Postprocedural intestinal obstruction

K91.5 Postcholecystectomy syndrome

[5] **K91.6 Intraoperative hemorrhage and hematoma of a digestive system organ or structure complicating a procedure**

[EXCLUDES1] *intraoperative hemorrhage and hematoma of a digestive system organ or structure due to accidental puncture and laceration during a procedure (K91.7-)*

K91.61 Intraoperative hemorrhage and hematoma of a digestive system organ or structure complicating a digestive sytem procedure

K91.62 Intraoperative hemorrhage and hematoma of a digestive system organ or structure complicating other procedure

[5] **K91.7 Accidental puncture and laceration of a digestive system organ or structure during a procedure**

K91.71 Accidental puncture and laceration of a digestive system organ or structure during a digestive system procedure

K91.72 Accidental puncture and laceration of a digestive system organ or structure during other procedure

[5] **K91.8 Other intraoperative and postprocedural complications and disorders of digestive system**

K91.81 Other intraoperative complications of digestive system

K91.82 Postprocedural hepatic failure

K91.83 Postprocedural hepatorenal syndrome

[6] **K91.84 Postprocedural hemorrhage and hematoma of a digestive system organ or structure following a procedure**

K91.840 Postprocedural hemorrhage and hematoma of a digestive system organ or structure following a digestive system procedure

K91.841 Postprocedural hemorrhage and hematoma of a digestive system organ or structure following other procedure

[6] **K91.85 Complications of intestinal pouch**

K91.850 Pouchitis

Inflammation of internal ileoanal pouch

K91.858 Other complications of intestinal pouch

K91.86 Retained cholelithiasis following cholecystectomy

K91.89 Other postprocedural complications and disorders of digestive system

Use additional code, if applicable, to further specify disorder

[EXCLUDES2] *postprocedural retroperitoneal abscess (K68.11)*

[4] **K92 Other diseases of digestive system**

[EXCLUDES1] *neonatal gastrointestinal hemorrhage (P54.0-P54.3)*

K92.0 Hematemesis

Unspecified Code Other Specified Code [N] Newborn Age: 0 [P] Pediatric Age: 0-17 [M] Maternity Age: 12-55
[A] Adult Age: 15-124 ♂ Male ♀ Female ● New Code ▲ Revised Code Title ►◄ Revised Text

K92.1 **Melena**
> EXCLUDES1 *occult blood in feces (R19.5)*

K92.2 **Gastrointestinal hemorrhage, unspecified**
> Gastric hemorrhage NOS
> Intestinal hemorrhage NOS
> EXCLUDES1 *acute hemorrhagic gastritis (K29.01)*
> *hemorrhage of anus and rectum (K62.5)*
> *angiodysplasia of stomach with hemorrhage (K31.811)*
> *diverticular disease with hemorrhage (K57.-)*
> *gastritis and duodenitis with hemorrhage (K29.-)*
> *peptic ulcer with hemorrhage (K25-K28)*

⑤ K92.8 **Other specified diseases of the digestive system**

K92.81 **Gastrointestinal mucositis (ulcerative)**
> Code also type of associated therapy, such as:
> antineoplastic and immunosuppressive drugs (T45.1X-)
> radiological procedure and radiotherapy (Y84.2)
> EXCLUDES2 *mucositis (ulcerative) of vagina and vulva (N76.81)*
> *nasal mucositis (ulcerative) (J34.81)*
> *oral mucositis (ulcerative) (K12.3-)*

K92.89 **Other specified diseases of the digestive system**

K92.9 **Disease of digestive system, unspecified**

④ K94 **Complications of artificial openings of the digestive system**

⑤ K94.0 **Colostomy complications**

K94.00 **Colostomy complication, unspecified**

K94.01 **Colostomy hemorrhage**

K94.02 **Colostomy infection**
> Use additional code to specify type of infection, such as:
> cellulitis of abdominal wall (L03.311)
> sepsis (A40.-, A41.-)

K94.03 **Colostomy malfunction**
> Mechanical complication of colostomy

K94.09 **Other complications of colostomy**

⑤ K94.1 **Enterostomy complications**

K94.10 **Enterostomy complication, unspecified**

K94.11 **Enterostomy hemorrhage**

K94.12 **Enterostomy infection**
> Use additional code to specify type of infection, such as:
> cellulitis of abdominal wall (L03.311)
> sepsis (A40.-, A41.-)

K94.13 **Enterostomy malfunction**
> Mechanical complication of enterostomy

K94.19 **Other complications of enterostomy**

⑤ K94.2 **Gastrostomy complications**

K94.20 **Gastrostomy complication, unspecified**

K94.21 **Gastrostomy hemorrhage**

K94.22 **Gastrostomy infection**
> Use additional code to specify type of infection, such as:
> cellulitis of abdominal wall (L03.311)
> sepsis (A40.-, A41.-)

K94.23 **Gastrostomy malfunction**
> Mechanical complication of gastrostomy

K94.29 **Other complications of gastrostomy**

⑤ K94.3 **Esophagostomy complications**

K94.30 **Esophagostomy complications, unspecified**

K94.31 **Esophagostomy hemorrhage**

K94.32 **Esophagostomy infection**
> Use additional code to identify the infection

K94.33 **Esophagostomy malfunction**
> Mechanical complication of esophagostomy

K94.39 **Other complications of esophagostomy**

④ K95 **Complications of bariatric procedures**

⑤ K95.0 **Complications of gastric band procedure**

K95.01 **Infection due to gastric band procedure**

> Use additional code to specify type of infection or organism, such as:
> bacterial and viral infectious agents (B95.-, B96.-)
> cellulitis of abdominal wall (L03.311)
> sepsis (A40.-, A41.-)

K95.09 **Other complications of gastric band procedure**
> Use additional code, if applicable, to further specify complication

⑤ K95.8 **Complications of other bariatric procedure**
> EXCLUDES1 *complications of gastric band surgery (K95.0-)*

K95.81 **Infection due to other bariatric procedure**
> Use additional code to specify type of infection or organism, such as:
> bacterial and viral infectious agents(B95-, B96-)
> cellulitis of abdominal wall (L03.311)
> sepsis (A40.-, A41.-)

K95.89 **Other complications of other bariatric procedure**
> Use additional code, if applicable, to further specify complication

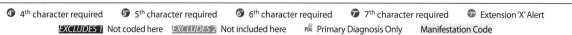

④ 4ᵗʰ character required   ⑤ 5ᵗʰ character required   ⑥ 6ᵗʰ character required   ⑦ 7ᵗʰ character required   ⑰ Extension 'X' Alert

EXCLUDES1 Not coded here   EXCLUDES2 Not included here   PDx Primary Diagnosis Only   Manifestation Code

Chapter 12: Diseases of the Skin and Subcutaneous Tissue (L00-L99)

Chapter Specific Coding Guidelines

a. Pressure ulcer stage codes

1) Pressure ulcer stages

Codes from category L89, Pressure ulcer, are combination codes that identify the site of the pressure ulcer as well as the stage of the ulcer.

The ICD-10-CM classifies pressure ulcer stages based on severity, which is designated by stages 1-4, unspecified stage and unstageable.

Assign as many codes from category L89 as needed to identify all the pressure ulcers the patient has, if applicable.

2) Unstageable pressure ulcers

Assignment of the code for unstageable pressure ulcer (L89.--0) should be based on the clinical documentation. These codes are used for pressure ulcers whose stage cannot be clinically determined (e.g., the ulcer is covered by eschar or has been treated with a skin or muscle graft) and pressure ulcers that are documented as deep tissue injury but not documented as due to trauma. This code should not be confused with the codes for unspecified stage (L89.--9). When there is no documentation regarding the stage of the pressure ulcer, assign the appropriate code for unspecified stage (L89.--9).

3) Documented pressure ulcer stage

Assignment of the pressure ulcer stage code should be guided by clinical documentation of the stage or documentation of the terms found in the Alphabetic Index. For clinical terms describing the stage that are not found in the Alphabetic Index, and there is no documentation of the stage, the provider should be queried.

4) Patients admitted with pressure ulcers documented as healed

No code is assigned if the documentation states that the pressure ulcer is completely healed.

5) Patients admitted with pressure ulcers documented as healing

Pressure ulcers described as healing should be assigned the appropriate pressure ulcer stage code based on the documentation in the medical record. If the documentation does not provide information about the stage of the healing pressure ulcer, assign the appropriate code for unspecified stage.

If the documentation is unclear as to whether the patient has a current (new) pressure ulcer or if the patient is being treated for a healing pressure ulcer, query the provider.

6) Patient admitted with pressure ulcer evolving into another stage during the admission

If a patient is admitted with a pressure ulcer at one stage and it progresses to a higher stage, assign the code for the highest stage reported for that site.

This page intentionally left blank

Anatomy of the Integumentary System

The Common Integument

The integumentary system is composed of the common integument (or skin) and it's appendages. The skin covers the body and proves to be an affective barrier to most harmful chemicals that can cause damage to our internal body system. It contains the peripheral endings of various sensory nerves and plays an important role in the regulation of our body temperature. The various layers/components of the skin (from outside to inside) are listed below:

1. **The Epidermis**
   a) Stratum Corneum
   b) Stratum Lucidum
   c) Stratum Granulosum
   d) Stratum Spinosum
   e) Stratum Germinativum (or Basal Layer/Stratum Basale)
2. **The Dermis (or Corium)**
   a) Papillary Layer of Dermis
   b) Reticular Layer of Dermis
3. **The Subcutaneous Tissue/Superficial Fascia (or Hypodermis)**
4. **The Appendages of the Skin**
   a) Hair (for protection and sensation)
   b) Nails (for protection)
   c) Sebaceous Glands (or the glands that secrete sebum onto hair follicle)
   d) Sweat Glands (or the glands that secrete sweat) and ducts
      i) eccrine sweat glands (or the glands secreting sweet with faint odor)
      ii) apocrine sweat glands (or the glands secreting sweet with strong odor)
   e) Arrector Pilli (or smooth muscles that pull hairs straight)

Common Pathologies

Cellulitis
It is a noncontiguous inflammation of the skin and deeper tissues. It is a diffuse inflammation of connective tissue with severe inflammation of dermal and subcutaneous layers of the skin. Skin in the infected area will become red, hot, irritated and painful. Group A strep (streptococcal) bacteria are the most common cause of cellulitis.

Impetigo
Impetigo is a highly contagious skin infection which causes sores and blisters. This contagious superficial skin infection is generally caused by one of two bacteria; Staphylococcus aureus or Streptococcus pyogenes. Symptoms start with red or pimple-like sores surrounded by red skin.

Folliculitis
It is the infection and inflammation of one or more hair follicles. It usually is caused by bacteria. It can occur anywhere on the skin. Numerous smooth little red bumps form around hair follicles and are most common seen on the chest, back, buttocks and legs.

Acne
Acne vulgaris is a common human skin disease. Human skin has pores which connect to oil glands located under the skin. A small hair grows through the follicle out of the skin. Pimples grow when these follicles get blocked. Pimples form when hair follicles under the skin clog up. Acne lesions heal slowly, and when one begins to resolve, others seem to crop up.

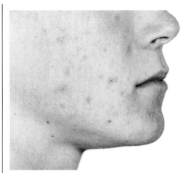

Herpes simplex
Herpes is an infection that is caused by a herpes simplex virus (HSV). Oral herpes is the most common form of infection followed by genital herpes. Main symptoms of herpes are tingling, itching and burning.

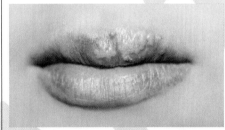

Chicken pox
Chicken pox is a viral infection in which extremely itchy blisters develops all over the body. It is a highly contagious disease caused by primary infection with varicella zoster virus. The classic symptoms of this disease are an uncomfortable itchy rash, fever, headache, tiredness and loss of appetite. The rash turns into fluid-filled blisters and eventually into scabs. It usually shows up on the face, chest, and back and then spread to the rest of the body. If the virus becomes active again, it can cause a painful infection called shingles.

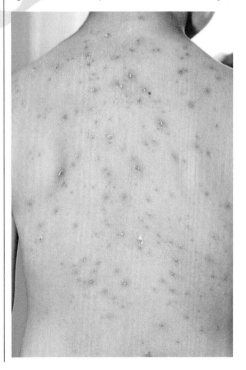

Verrucae

A verruca is simply a wart that is found on the soles of your feet, though they can also appear around the toes. Warts are rough lumps that often develop on the skin of the hands and feet. It is a small growth on the sole of the foot often with tiny black dots on the surface.

Scabies

Scabies is a contagious and itchy skin infection caused by the mite Sarcoptes scabiei. The mite is a tiny and usually not directly visible parasite which burrows under the patients, skin, causing intense allergic itching. Direct skin-to-skin contact is the mode of transmission. Scabies can also be spread by sharing towels, bed sheets, and other personal belongings. Scabies causes severe itching that is usually worse at night and a rash with tiny blisters. It spreads quickly in crowded conditions.

Psoriasis

Psoriasis is a chronic skin problem that causes skin cells to grow too quickly, resulting in thick, white, silvery patches of skin. This occurs when the immune system mistakenly attacks and destroys healthy body tissue. Bacteria or viral infections, stress, dry air, injury to the skin and some medicines may trigger the condition. It is a non-contagious skin condition that produces red papules that merge together into plaques of thickened scaling skin. Psoriasis commonly affects the skin of the elbows, knees, and scalp. Psoriasis symptoms improve or can go into remission.

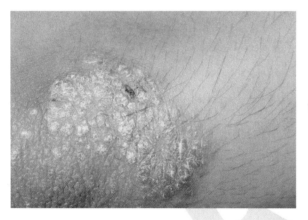

Ringworm

Ringworm is a type of fungal skin infection which is caused by fungi called tinea. It grows and multiplies on the skin. It is a common highly contagious. Skin infection causes a ring-like red rash on the skin. The rash can appear almost anywhere on the body, with the scalp, feet and groin being most common sites.

Diseases of the skin and subcutaneous tissue (L00-L99)

> EXCLUDES2 certain conditions originating in the perinatal period (P04-P96)
> certain infectious and parasitic diseases (A00-B99)
> complications of pregnancy, childbirth and the puerperium (O00-O9A)
> congenital malformations, deformations, and chromosomal abnormalities (Q00-Q99)
> endocrine, nutritional and metabolic diseases (E00-E88)
> lipomelanotic reticulosis (I89.8)
> neoplasms (C00-D49)
> symptoms, signs and abnormal clinical and laboratory findings, not elsewhere classified (R00-R94)
> systemic connective tissue disorders (M30-M36)
> viral warts (B07.-)

Infections of the skin and subcutaneous tissue (L00-L08)

> EXCLUDES2 hordeolum (H00.0)
> infective dermatitis (L30.3)
> local infections of skin classified in Chapter 1
> lupus panniculitis (L93.2)
> panniculitis NOS (M79.3)
> panniculitis of neck and back (M54.0-)
> Perlèche NOS (K13.0)
> Perlèche due to candidiasis (B37.0)
> Perlèche due to riboflavin deficiency (E53.0)
> pyogenic granuloma (L98.0)
> relapsing panniculitis [Weber-Christian] (M35.6)
> viral warts (B07.-)
> zoster (B02.-)

L00 Staphylococcal scalded skin syndrome

Ritter's disease
Use additional code to identify percentage of skin exfoliation (L49.-)

> EXCLUDES1 bullous impetigo (L01.03)
> pemphigus neonatorum (L01.03)
> toxic epidermal necrolysis [Lyell] (L51.2)

L01 Impetigo

> EXCLUDES1 impetigo herpetiformis (L40.1)

L01.0 Impetigo

Impetigo contagiosa
Impetigo vulgaris

L01.00 Impetigo, unspecified

Impetigo NOS

L01.01 Non-bullous impetigo

L01.02 Bockhart's impetigo

Impetigo follicularis
Perifolliculitis NOS
Superficial pustular perifolliculitis

L01.03 Bullous impetigo

Impetigo neonatorum
Pemphigus neonatorum

L01.09 Other impetigo

Ulcerative impetigo

L01.1 Impetiginization of other dermatoses

L02 Cutaneous abscess, furuncle and carbuncle

Use additional code to identify organism (B95-B96)

> EXCLUDES2 abscess of anus and rectal regions (K61.-)
> abscess of female genital organs (external) (N76.4)
> abscess of male genital organs (external) (N48.2, N49.-)

L02.0 Cutaneous abscess, furuncle and carbuncle of face

> EXCLUDES2 abscess of ear, external (H60.0)
> abscess of eyelid (H00.0)
> abscess of head [any part, except face] (L02.8)
> abscess of lacrimal gland (H04.0)
> abscess of lacrimal passages (H04.3)
> abscess of mouth (K12.2)
> abscess of nose (J34.0)
> abscess of orbit (H05.0)
> submandibular abscess (K12.2)

L02.01 Cutaneous abscess of face

L02.02 Furuncle of face

Boil of face
Folliculitis of face

L02.03 Carbuncle of face

L02.1 Cutaneous abscess, furuncle and carbuncle of neck

L02.11 Cutaneous abscess of neck

L02.12 Furuncle of neck

Boil of neck
Folliculitis of neck

L02.13 Carbuncle of neck

L02.2 Cutaneous abscess, furuncle and carbuncle of trunk

> EXCLUDES1 non-newborn omphalitis (L08.82)
> omphalitis of newborn (P38.-)

> EXCLUDES2 abscess of breast (N61)
> abscess of buttocks (L02.3)
> abscess of female external genital organs (N76.4)
> abscess of male external genital organs (N48.2, N49.-)
> abscess of hip (L02.4)

L02.21 Cutaneous abscess of trunk

L02.211 Cutaneous abscess of abdominal wall

L02.212 Cutaneous abscess of back [any part, except buttock]

L02.213 Cutaneous abscess of chest wall

L02.214 Cutaneous abscess of groin

L02.215 Cutaneous abscess of perineum

L02.216 Cutaneous abscess of umbilicus

L02.219 Cutaneous abscess of trunk, unspecified

L02.22 Furuncle of trunk

Boil of trunk
Folliculitis of trunk

L02.221 Furuncle of abdominal wall

L02.222 Furuncle of back [any part, except buttock]

L02.223 Furuncle of chest wall

L02.224 Furuncle of groin

L02.225 Furuncle of perineum

L02.226 Furuncle of umbilicus

L02.229 Furuncle of trunk, unspecified

L02.23 Carbuncle of trunk

L02.231 Carbuncle of abdominal wall

L02.232 Carbuncle of back [any part, except buttock]

L02.233 Carbuncle of chest wall

L02.234 Carbuncle of groin

L02.235 Carbuncle of perineum

L02.236 Carbuncle of umbilicus

L02.239 Carbuncle of trunk, unspecified

L02.3 Cutaneous abscess, furuncle and carbuncle of buttock

> EXCLUDES1 pilonidal cyst with abscess (L05.01)

L02.31 Cutaneous abscess of buttock

Cutaneous abscess of gluteal region

L02.32 Furuncle of buttock

Boil of buttock
Folliculitis of buttock
Furuncle of gluteal region

L02.33 Carbuncle of buttock

Carbuncle of gluteal region

Unspecified Code	Other Specified Code	N Newborn Age: 0	P Pediatric Age: 0-17	M Maternity Age: 12-55	
A Adult Age: 15-124	♂ Male	♀ Female	● New Code	▲ Revised Code Title	►◄ Revised Text

[5] L02.4 Cutaneous abscess, furuncle and carbuncle of limb

[EXCLUDES2] *Cutaneous abscess, furuncle and carbuncle of groin (L02.214, L02.224, L02.234)*
Cutaneous abscess, furuncle and carbuncle of hand (L02.5-)
Cutaneous abscess, furuncle and carbuncle of foot (L02.6-)

[6] L02.41 Cutaneous abscess of limb
- L02.411 Cutaneous abscess of right axilla
- L02.412 Cutaneous abscess of left axilla
- L02.413 Cutaneous abscess of right upper limb
- L02.414 Cutaneous abscess of left upper limb
- L02.415 Cutaneous abscess of right lower limb
- L02.416 Cutaneous abscess of left lower limb
- L02.419 Cutaneous abscess of limb, unspecified

[6] L02.42 Furuncle of limb

Boil of limb
Folliculitis of limb
- L02.421 Furuncle of right axilla
- L02.422 Furuncle of left axilla
- L02.423 Furuncle of right upper limb
- L02.424 Furuncle of left upper limb
- L02.425 Furuncle of right lower limb
- L02.426 Furuncle of left lower limb
- L02.429 Furuncle of limb, unspecified

[6] L02.43 Carbuncle of limb
- L02.431 Carbuncle of right axilla
- L02.432 Carbuncle of left axilla
- L02.433 Carbuncle of right upper limb
- L02.434 Carbuncle of left upper limb
- L02.435 Carbuncle of right lower limb
- L02.436 Carbuncle of left lower limb
- L02.439 Carbuncle of limb, unspecified

[5] L02.5 Cutaneous abscess, furuncle and carbuncle of hand

[6] L02.51 Cutaneous abscess of hand
- L02.511 Cutaneous abscess of right hand
- L02.512 Cutaneous abscess of left hand
- L02.519 Cutaneous abscess of unspecified hand

[6] L02.52 Furuncle hand

Boil of hand
Folliculitis of hand
- L02.521 Furuncle right hand
- L02.522 Furuncle left hand
- L02.529 Furuncle unspecified hand

[6] L02.53 Carbuncle of hand
- L02.531 Carbuncle of right hand
- L02.532 Carbuncle of left hand
- L02.539 Carbuncle of unspecified hand

[5] L02.6 Cutaneous abscess, furuncle and carbuncle of foot

[6] L02.61 Cutaneous abscess of foot
- L02.611 Cutaneous abscess of right foot
- L02.612 Cutaneous abscess of left foot
- L02.619 Cutaneous abscess of unspecified foot

[6] L02.62 Furuncle of foot

Boil of foot
Folliculitis of foot
- L02.621 Furuncle of right foot
- L02.622 Furuncle of left foot
- L02.629 Furuncle of unspecified foot

[6] L02.63 Carbuncle of foot
- L02.631 Carbuncle of right foot
- L02.632 Carbuncle of left foot
- L02.639 Carbuncle of unspecified foot

[5] L02.8 Cutaneous abscess, furuncle and carbuncle of other sites

[6] L02.81 Cutaneous abscess of other sites
- L02.811 Cutaneous abscess of head [any part, except face]
- L02.818 Cutaneous abscess of other sites

[6] L02.82 Furuncle of other sites

Boil of other sites
Folliculitis of other sites
- L02.821 Furuncle of head [any part, except face]
- L02.828 Furuncle of other sites

[6] L02.83 Carbuncle of other sites
- L02.831 Carbuncle of head [any part, except face]
- L02.838 Carbuncle of other sites

[5] L02.9 Cutaneous abscess, furuncle and carbuncle, unspecified
- L02.91 Cutaneous abscess, unspecified
- L02.92 Furuncle, unspecified

  Boil NOS
  Furunculosis NOS
- L02.93 Carbuncle, unspecified

[4] L03 Cellulitis and acute lymphangitis

[EXCLUDES2] *cellulitis of anal and rectal region (K61.-)*
cellulitis of external auditory canal (H60.1)
cellulitis of eyelid (H00.0)
cellulitis of female external genital organs (N76.4)
cellulitis of lacrimal apparatus (H04.3)
cellulitis of male external genital organs (N48.2, N49.-)
cellulitis of mouth (K12.2)
cellulitis of nose (J34.0)
eosinophilic cellulitis [Wells] (L98.3)
febrile neutrophilic dermatosis [Sweet] (L98.2)
lymphangitis (chronic) (subacute) (I89.1)

[5] L03.0 Cellulitis and acute lymphangitis of finger and toe

Infection of nail
Onychia
Paronychia
Perionychia

[6] L03.01 Cellulitis of finger

Felon
Whitlow

[EXCLUDES1] *herpetic whitlow (B00.89)*
- L03.011 Cellulitis of right finger
- L03.012 Cellulitis of left finger
- L03.019 Cellulitis of unspecified finger

[6] L03.02 Acute lymphangitis of finger

Hangnail with lymphangitis of finger
- L03.021 Acute lymphangitis of right finger
- L03.022 Acute lymphangitis of left finger
- L03.029 Acute lymphangitis of unspecified finger

[6] L03.03 Cellulitis of toe
- L03.031 Cellulitis of right toe
- L03.032 Cellulitis of left toe
- L03.039 Cellulitis of unspecified toe

[6] L03.04 Acute lymphangitis of toe

Hangnail with lymphangitis of toe
- L03.041 Acute lymphangitis of right toe
- L03.042 Acute lymphangitis of left toe
- L03.049 Acute lymphangitis of unspecified toe

[5] L03.1 Cellulitis and acute lymphangitis of other parts of limb

[6] L03.11 Cellulitis of other parts of limb

[EXCLUDES2] *cellulitis of fingers (L03.01-)*
cellulitis of toes (L03.03-)
groin (L03.314)
- L03.111 Cellulitis of right axilla
- L03.112 Cellulitis of left axilla
- L03.113 Cellulitis of right upper limb
- L03.114 Cellulitis of left upper limb

[4] 4th character required [5] 5th character required [6] 6th character required [7] 7th character required [7] Extension 'X' Alert
[EXCLUDES1] Not coded here [EXCLUDES2] Not included here [PDx] Primary Diagnosis Only Manifestation Code

L03.115 Cellulitis of right lower limb
L03.116 Cellulitis of left lower limb
L03.119 Cellulitis of unspecified part of limb
[6] L03.12 Acute lymphangitis of other parts of limb
[EXCLUDES2] *acute lymphangitis of fingers (L03.2-)*
acute lymphangitis of toes (L03.0-)
acute lymphangitis of groin (L03.324)
L03.121 Acute lymphangitis of right axilla
L03.122 Acute lymphangitis of left axilla
L03.123 Acute lymphangitis of right upper limb
L03.124 Acute lymphangitis of left upper limb
L03.125 Acute lymphangitis of right lower limb
L03.126 Acute lymphangitis of left lower limb
L03.129 Acute lymphangitis of unspecified part of limb
[5] L03.2 Cellulitis and acute lymphangitis of face and neck
[6] L03.21 Cellulitis and acute lymphangitis of face
L03.211 Cellulitis of face
[EXCLUDES2] *cellulitis of ear (H60.1-)*
cellulitis of eyelid (H00.0-)
cellulitis of head (L03.81)
cellulitis of lacrimal apparatus (H04.3)
cellulitis of lip (K13.0)
cellulitis of mouth (K12.2)
cellulitis of nose (internal) (J34.0)
cellulitis of orbit (H05.0)
cellulitis of scalp (L03.81)
L03.212 Acute lymphangitis of face
[6] L03.22 Cellulitis and acute lymphangitis of neck
L03.221 Cellulitis of neck
L03.222 Acute lymphangitis of neck
[5] L03.3 Cellulitis and acute lymphangitis of trunk
[6] L03.31 Cellulitis of trunk
[EXCLUDES2] *cellulitis of anal and rectal regions (K61.-)*
cellulitis of breast NOS (N61)
cellulitis of female external genital organs (N76.4)
cellulitis of male external genital organs (N48.2, N49.-)
omphalitis of newborn (P38.-)
puerperal cellulitis of breast (O91.2)
L03.311 Cellulitis of abdominal wall
[EXCLUDES2] *cellulitis of umbilicus (L03.316)*
cellulitis of groin (L03.314)
L03.312 Cellulitis of back [any part except buttock]
L03.313 Cellulitis of chest wall
L03.314 Cellulitis of groin
L03.315 Cellulitis of perineum
L03.316 Cellulitis of umbilicus
L03.317 Cellulitis of buttock
L03.319 Cellulitis of trunk, unspecified
[6] L03.32 Acute lymphangitis of trunk
L03.321 Acute lymphangitis of abdominal wall
L03.322 Acute lymphangitis of back [any part except buttock]
L03.323 Acute lymphangitis of chest wall
L03.324 Acute lymphangitis of groin
L03.325 Acute lymphangitis of perineum
L03.326 Acute lymphangitis of umbilicus
L03.327 Acute lymphangitis of buttock
L03.329 Acute lymphangitis of trunk, unspecified
[5] L03.8 Cellulitis and acute lymphangitis of other sites
[6] L03.81 Cellulitis of other sites
L03.811 Cellulitis of head [any part, except face]
Cellulitis of scalp
[EXCLUDES2] *cellulitis of face (L03.211)*
L03.818 Cellulitis of other sites
[6] L03.89 Acute lymphangitis of other sites
L03.891 Acute lymphangitis of head [any part, except face]
L03.898 Acute lymphangitis of other sites
[5] L03.9 Cellulitis and acute lymphangitis, unspecified
L03.90 Cellulitis, unspecified
L03.91 Acute lymphangitis, unspecified
[EXCLUDES1] *lymphangitis NOS (I89.1)*
[4] L04 Acute lymphadenitis
[INCLUDES] *abscess (acute) of lymph nodes, except mesenteric*
acute lymphadenitis, except mesenteric
[EXCLUDES1] *chronic or subacute lymphadenitis, except mesenteric (I88.1)*
enlarged lymph nodes (R59.-)
human immunodeficiency virus [HIV] disease resulting in generalized lymphadenopathy (B20)
lymphadenitis NOS (I88.9)
nonspecific mesenteric lymphadenitis (I88.0)
L04.0 Acute lymphadenitis of face, head and neck
L04.1 Acute lymphadenitis of trunk
L04.2 Acute lymphadenitis of upper limb
Acute lymphadenitis of axilla
Acute lymphadenitis of shoulder
L04.3 Acute lymphadenitis of lower limb
Acute lymphadenitis of hip
[EXCLUDES2] *acute lymphadenitis of groin (L04.1)*
L04.8 Acute lymphadenitis of other sites
L04.9 Acute lymphadenitis, unspecified
[4] L05 Pilonidal cyst and sinus
[5] L05.0 Pilonidal cyst and sinus with abscess
L05.01 Pilonidal cyst with abscess
Parasacral dimple with abscess
Pilonidal abscess
Pilonidal dimple with abscess
Postanal dimple with abscess
L05.02 Pilonidal sinus with abscess
Coccygeal fistula with abscess
Coccygeal sinus with abscess
Pilonidal fistula with abscess
[5] L05.9 Pilonidal cyst and sinus without abscess
L05.91 Pilonidal cyst without abscess
Parasacral dimple
Pilonidal dimple
Postanal dimple
Pilonidal cyst NOS
L05.92 Pilonidal sinus without abscess
Coccygeal fistula
Coccygeal sinus without abscess
Pilonidal fistula
[4] L08 Other local infections of skin and subcutaneous tissue
L08.0 Pyoderma
Dermatitis gangrenosa
Purulent dermatitis
Septic dermatitis
Suppurative dermatitis
[EXCLUDES1] *pyoderma gangrenosum (L88)*
pyoderma vegetans (L08.81)
L08.1 Erythrasma
[5] L08.8 Other specified local infections of the skin and subcutaneous tissue
L08.81 Pyoderma vegetans
[EXCLUDES1] *pyoderma gangrenosum (L88)*
pyoderma NOS (L08.0)
L08.82 Omphalitis not of newborn
[EXCLUDES1] *omphalitis of newborn (P38.-)*
L08.89 Other specified local infections of the skin and subcutaneous tissue
L08.9 Local infection of the skin and subcutaneous tissue, unspecified

Unspecified Code | Other Specified Code | [N] Newborn Age: 0 | [P] Pediatric Age: 0-17 | [M] Maternity Age: 12-55
[A] Adult Age: 15-124 | ♂ Male | ♀ Female | ● New Code | ▲ Revised Code Title | ►◄ Revised Text

Bullous disorders (L10-L14)

[EXCLUDES1] *benign familial pemphigus [Hailey-Hailey] (Q82.8)*
staphylococcal scalded skin syndrome (L00)
toxic epidermal necrolysis [Lyell] (L51.2)

[4] **L10 Pemphigus**

[EXCLUDES1] *pemphigus neonatorum (L01.03)*

L10.0 Pemphigus vulgaris
L10.1 Pemphigus vegetans
L10.2 Pemphigus foliaceous
L10.3 Brazilian **pemphigus [fogo selvagem]**
L10.4 Pemphigus erythematosus

Senear-Usher syndrome

L10.5 Drug-induced **pemphigus**

Use additional code for adverse effect, if applicable, to identify drug (T36-T50 with fifth or sixth character 5)

[5] **L10.8** Other **pemphigus**

L10.81 Paraneoplastic **pemphigus**
L10.89 Other pemphigus

L10.9 Pemphigus, unspecified

[4] **L11** Other **acantholytic disorders**

L11.0 Acquired keratosis follicularis

[EXCLUDES1] *keratosis follicularis (congenital) [Darier-White] (Q82.8)*

L11.1 Transient acantholytic dermatosis [Grover]
L11.8 Other specified acantholytic disorders
L11.9 Acantholytic disorder, unspecified

[4] **L12 Pemphigoid**

[EXCLUDES1] *herpes gestationis (O26.4-)*
impetigo herpetiformis (L40.1)

L12.0 Bullous **pemphigoid**
L12.1 Cicatricial **pemphigoid**

Benign mucous membrane pemphigoid

L12.2 Chronic bullous disease of childhood

Juvenile dermatitis herpetiformis [P]

[5] **L12.3** Acquired epidermolysis **bullosa**

[EXCLUDES1] *epidermolysis bullosa (congenital) (Q81.-)*

L12.30 Acquired epidermolysis bullosa, unspecified
L12.31 Epidermolysis bullosa due to drug

Use additional code for adverse effect, if applicable, to identify drug (T36-T50 with fifth or sixth character 5)

L12.35 Other acquired epidermolysis bullosa

L12.8 Other pemphigoid
L12.9 Pemphigoid, unspecified

[4] **L13** Other **bullous disorders**

L13.0 Dermatitis herpetiformis

Duhring's disease
Hydroa herpetiformis

[EXCLUDES1] *juvenile dermatitis herpetiformis (L12.2)*
senile dermatitis herpetiformis (L12.0)

L13.1 Subcorneal pustular **dermatitis**

Sneddon-Wilkinson disease

L13.8 Other specified bullous disorders
L13.9 Bullous disorder, unspecified

L14 Bullous disorders in diseases classified elsewhere

Code first underlying disease

Dermatitis and eczema (L20-L30)

[NOTES] In this block the terms dermatitis and eczema are used synonymously and interchangeably.

[EXCLUDES2] *chronic (childhood) granulomatous disease (D71)*
dermatitis gangrenosa (L08.0)
dermatitis herpetiformis (L13.0)
dry skin dermatitis (L85.3)
factitial dermatitis (L98.1)
perioral dermatitis (L71.0)
radiation-related disorders of the skin and subcutaneous tissue (L55-L59)
stasis dermatitis (I83.1-I83.2)

[4] **L20** Atopic **dermatitis**

L20.0 Besnier's prurigo

[5] **L20.8 Other atopic dermatitis**

[EXCLUDES2] *circumscribed neurodermatitis (L28.0)*

L20.81 Atopic neurodermatitis

Diffuse neurodermatitis

L20.82 Flexural **eczema**
L20.83 Infantile (acute) (chronic) **eczema** [P]
L20.84 Intrinsic (allergic) **eczema**
L20.89 Other atopic dermatitis

L20.9 Atopic dermatitis, unspecified

[4] **L21** Seborrheic **dermatitis**

[EXCLUDES2] *infective dermatitis (L30.3)*
seborrheic keratosis (L82.-)

L21.0 Seborrhea capitis

Cradle cap [P]

L21.1 Seborrheic infantile dermatitis [P]
L21.8 Other seborrheic dermatitis
L21.9 Seborrheic dermatitis, unspecified

Seborrhea NOS

L22 Diaper **dermatitis**

Diaper erythema
Diaper rash
Psoriasiform diaper rash

[4] **L23** Allergic contact **dermatitis**

[EXCLUDES1] *allergy NOS (T78.40)*
contact dermatitis NOS (L25.9)
dermatitis NOS (L30.9)

[EXCLUDES2] *dermatitis due to substances taken internally (L27.-)*
dermatitis of eyelid (H01.1-)
diaper dermatitis (L22)
eczema of external ear (H60.5-)
irritant contact dermatitis (L24.-)
perioral dermatitis (L71.0)
radiation-related disorders of the skin and subcutaneous tissue (L55-L59)

L23.0 Allergic contact dermatitis due to metals

Allergic contact dermatitis due to chromium
Allergic contact dermatitis due to nickel

L23.1 Allergic contact dermatitis due to adhesives
L23.2 Allergic contact dermatitis due to cosmetics
L23.3 Allergic contact dermatitis due to drugs in contact with skin

Use additional code for adverse effect, if applicable, to identify drug (T36-T50 with fifth or sixth character 5)

[EXCLUDES2] *dermatitis due to ingested drugs and medicaments (L27.0-L27.1)*

L23.4 Allergic contact dermatitis due to dyes
L23.5 Allergic contact dermatitis due to other chemical products

Allergic contact dermatitis due to cement
Allergic contact dermatitis due to insecticide
Allergic contact dermatitis due to plastic
Allergic contact dermatitis due to rubber

L23.6 Allergic contact dermatitis due to food in contact with the skin

[EXCLUDES2] *dermatitis due to ingested food (L27.2)*

L23.7 Allergic contact dermatitis due to plants, except food

[EXCLUDES2] *allergy NOS due to pollen (J30.1)*

[5] **L23.8 Allergic contact dermatitis** due to other agents

L23.81 Allergic contact dermatitis due to animal (cat) (dog) dander

Allergic contact dermatitis due to animal (cat) (dog) hair

L23.89 Allergic contact dermatitis due to other agents

L23.9 Allergic contact dermatitis, unspecified cause
Allergic contact eczema NOS

[4] **L24 Irritant contact dermatitis**

[EXCLUDES1] *allergy NOS (T78.40)*
contact dermatitis NOS (L25.9)
dermatitis NOS (L30.9)

[EXCLUDES2] *allergic contact dermatitis (L23.-)*
dermatitis due to substances taken internally (L27.-)
dermatitis of eyelid (H01.1-)
diaper dermatitis (L22)
eczema of external ear (H60.5-)
perioral dermatitis (L71.0)
radiation-related disorders of the skin and subcutaneous tissue (L55-L59)

L24.0 Irritant contact dermatitis due to detergents

L24.1 Irritant contact dermatitis due to oils and greases

L24.2 Irritant contact dermatitis due to solvents
Irritant contact dermatitis due to chlorocompound
Irritant contact dermatitis due to cyclohexane
Irritant contact dermatitis due to ester
Irritant contact dermatitis due to glycol
Irritant contact dermatitis due to hydrocarbon
Irritant contact dermatitis due to ketone

L24.3 Irritant contact dermatitis due to cosmetics

L24.4 Irritant contact dermatitis due to drugs in contact with skin
Use additional code for adverse effect, if applicable, to identify drug (T36-T50 with fifth or sixth character 5)

L24.5 Irritant contact dermatitis due to other chemical products
Irritant contact dermatitis due to cement
Irritant contact dermatitis due to insecticide
Irritant contact dermatitis due to plastic
Irritant contact dermatitis due to rubber

L24.6 Irritant contact dermatitis due to food in contact with skin

[EXCLUDES2] *dermatitis due to ingested food (L27.2)*

L24.7 Irritant contact dermatitis due to plants, except food

[EXCLUDES2] *allergy NOS to pollen (J30.1)*

[5] **L24.8 Irritant contact dermatitis** due to other agents

L24.81 Irritant contact dermatitis due to metals
Irritant contact dermatitis due to chromium
Irritant contact dermatitis due to nickel

L24.89 Irritant contact dermatitis due to other agents
Irritant contact dermatitis due to dyes

L24.9 Irritant contact dermatitis, unspecified cause
Irritant contact eczema NOS

[4] **L25 Unspecified contact dermatitis**

[EXCLUDES1] *allergic contact dermatitis (L23.-)*
allergy NOS (T78.40)
dermatitis NOS (L30.9)
irritant contact dermatitis (L24.-)

[EXCLUDES2] *dermatitis due to ingested substances (L27.-)*
dermatitis of eyelid (H01.1-)
eczema of external ear (H60.5-)
perioral dermatitis (L71.0)
radiation-related disorders of the skin and subcutaneous tissue (L55-L59)

L25.0 Unspecified contact dermatitis due to cosmetics

L25.1 Unspecified contact dermatitis due to drugs in contact with skin
Use additional code for adverse effect, if applicable, to identify drug (T36-T50 with fifth or sixth character 5)

[EXCLUDES2] *dermatitis due to ingested drugs and medicaments (L27.0-L27.1)*

L25.2 Unspecified contact dermatitis due to dyes

L25.3 Unspecified contact dermatitis due to other chemical products
Unspecified contact dermatitis due to cement
Unspecified contact dermatitis due to insecticide

L25.4 Unspecified contact dermatitis due to food in contact with skin

[EXCLUDES2] *dermatitis due to ingested food (L27.2)*

L25.5 Unspecified contact dermatitis due to plants, except food

[EXCLUDES1] *nettle rash (L50.9)*

[EXCLUDES2] *allergy NOS due to pollen (J30.1)*

L25.8 Unspecified contact dermatitis due to other agents

L25.9 Unspecified contact dermatitis, unspecified cause
Contact dermatitis (occupational) NOS
Contact eczema (occupational) NOS

L26 Exfoliative dermatitis
Hebra's pityriasis

[EXCLUDES1] *Ritter's disease (L00)*

[4] **L27 Dermatitis due to** substances taken internally

[EXCLUDES1] *allergy NOS (T78.40)*

[EXCLUDES2] *adverse food reaction, except dermatitis (T78.0-T78.1)*
contact dermatitis (L23-L25)
drug photoallergic response (L56.1)
drug phototoxic response (L56.0)
urticaria (L50.-)

L27.0 Generalized skin eruption **due to drugs and medicaments taken internally**
Use additional code for adverse effect, if applicable, to identify drug (T36-T50 with fifth or sixth character 5)

L27.1 Localized skin eruption **due to drugs and medicaments taken internally**
Use additional code for adverse effect, if applicable, to identify drug (T36-T50 with fifth or sixth character 5)

L27.2 Dermatitis **due to ingested food**

[EXCLUDES2] *dermatitis due to food in contact with skin (L23.6, L24.6, L25.4)*

L27.8 Dermatitis due to other substances taken internally

L27.9 Dermatitis due to unspecified substance taken internally

[4] **L28 Lichen simplex chronicus and prurigo**

L28.0 Lichen simplex chronicus
Circumscribed neurodermatitis
Lichen NOS

L28.1 Prurigo nodularis

L28.2 Other prurigo
Prurigo NOS
Prurigo Hebra
Prurigo mitis
Urticaria papulosa

[4] **L29 Pruritus**

[EXCLUDES1] *neurotic excoriation (L98.1)*
psychogenic pruritus (F45.8)

L29.0 Pruritus ani

L29.1 Pruritus scroti ♂

L29.2 Pruritus vulvae ♀

L29.3 Anogenital **pruritus, unspecified**

L29.8 Other pruritus

L29.9 Pruritus, unspecified
Itch NOS

[4] **L30** Other and unspecified **dermatitis**

[EXCLUDES2] *contact dermatitis (L23-L25)*
dry skin dermatitis (L85.3)
small plaque parapsoriasis (L41.3)
stasis dermatitis (I83.1-.2)

L30.0 Nummular **dermatitis**

L30.1 Dyshidrosis [pompholyx]

L30.2 Cutaneous autosensitization
Candidid [levurid]
Dermatophytid
Eczematid
L30.3 Infective dermatitis
Infectious eczematoid dermatitis
L30.4 Erythema intertrigo
L30.5 Pityriasis alba
L30.8 Other specified dermatitis
L30.9 Dermatitis, unspecified
Eczema NOS

Papulosquamous disorders (L40-L45)

L40 Psoriasis
L40.0 Psoriasis vulgaris
Nummular psoriasis
Plaque psoriasis
L40.1 Generalized pustular psoriasis
Impetigo herpetiformis
Von Zumbusch's disease
L40.2 Acrodermatitis continua
L40.3 Pustulosis palmaris et plantaris
L40.4 Guttate psoriasis
L40.5 Arthropathic psoriasis
L40.50 Arthropathic psoriasis, unspecified
L40.51 Distal interphalangeal psoriatic arthropathy
L40.52 Psoriatic arthritis mutilans
L40.53 Psoriatic spondylitis
L40.54 Psoriatic juvenile arthropathy
L40.59 Other psoriatic arthropathy
L40.8 Other psoriasis
Flexural psoriasis
L40.9 Psoriasis, unspecified
L41 Parapsoriasis
EXCLUDES1 poikiloderma vasculare atrophicans (L94.5)
L41.0 Pityriasis lichenoides et varioliformis acuta
Mucha-Habermann disease
L41.1 Pityriasis lichenoides chronica
L41.3 Small plaque parapsoriasis
L41.4 Large plaque parapsoriasis
L41.5 Retiform parapsoriasis
L41.8 Other parapsoriasis
L41.9 Parapsoriasis, unspecified
L42 Pityriasis rosea
L43 Lichen planus
EXCLUDES1 lichen planopilaris (L66.1)
L43.0 Hypertrophic lichen planus
L43.1 Bullous lichen planus
L43.2 Lichenoid drug reaction
Use additional code for adverse effect, if applicable, to identify drug (T36-T50 with fifth or sixth character 5)
L43.3 Subacute (active) lichen planus
Lichen planus tropicus
L43.8 Other lichen planus
L43.9 Lichen planus, unspecified
L44 Other papulosquamous disorders
L44.0 Pityriasis rubra pilaris
L44.1 Lichen nitidus
L44.2 Lichen striatus
L44.3 Lichen ruber moniliformis
L44.4 Infantile papular acrodermatitis [Gianotti-Crosti] P
L44.8 Other specified papulosquamous disorders
L44.9 Papulosquamous disorder, unspecified
L45 Papulosquamous disorders in diseases classified elsewhere
Code first underlying disease.

Urticaria and erythema (L49-L54)

EXCLUDES1 Lyme disease (A69.2-)
rosacea (L71.-)
L49 Exfoliation due to erythematous conditions according to extent of body surface involved
Code first erythematous condition causing exfoliation, such as:
Ritter's disease (L00)
(Staphylococcal) scalded skin syndrom (L00)
Stevens-Johnson syndrome (L51.1)
Stevens-Johnson syndrome-toxic epidermal necrolysis overlap syndrome (L51.3)
Toxic epidermal necrolysis (L51.2)
L49.0 Exfoliation due to erythematous condition involving less than 10 percent of body surface
Exfoliation due to erythematous condition NOS
L49.1 Exfoliation due to erythematous condition involving 10-19 percent of body surface
L49.2 Exfoliation due to erythematous condition involving 20-29 percent of body surface
L49.3 Exfoliation due to erythematous condition involving 30-39 percent of body surface
L49.4 Exfoliation due to erythematous condition involving 40-49 percent of body surface
L49.5 Exfoliation due to erythematous condition involving 50-59 percent of body surface
L49.6 Exfoliation due to erythematous condition involving 60-69 percent of body surface
L49.7 Exfoliation due to erythematous condition involving 70-79 percent of body surface
L49.8 Exfoliation due to erythematous condition involving 80-89 percent of body surface
L49.9 Exfoliation due to erythematous condition involving 90 or more percent of body surface

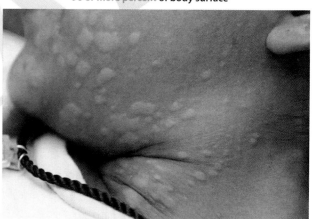

Figure 11.1 Urticaria

L50 Urticaria
EXCLUDES1 allergic contact dermatitis (L23.-)
angioneurotic edema (T78.3)
giant urticaria (T78.3)
hereditary angio-edema (D84.1)
Quincke's edema (T78.3)
serum urticaria (T80.6-)
solar urticaria (L56.3)
urticaria neonatorum (P83.8)
urticaria papulosa (L28.2)
urticaria pigmentosa (Q82.2)
L50.0 Allergic urticaria
L50.1 Idiopathic urticaria
L50.2 Urticaria due to cold and heat
L50.3 Dermatographic urticaria
L50.4 Vibratory urticaria

4th character required   5th character required   6th character required   7th character required   Extension 'X' Alert

EXCLUDES1 Not coded here   EXCLUDES2 Not included here   PDx Primary Diagnosis Only   Manifestation Code

L50.5 Cholinergic **urticaria**

L50.6 Contact **urticaria**

L50.8 Other urticaria

Chronic urticaria

Recurrent periodic urticaria

L50.9 **Urticaria, unspecified**

④ L51 **Erythema multiforme**

Use additional code for adverse effect, if applicable, to identify drug (T36-T50 with fifth or sixth character 5) code to identify associated manifestations, such as: arthropathy associated with dermatological disorders (M14.8-)

conjunctival edema (H11.42)

conjunctivitis (H10.22-)

corneal scars and opacities (H17.-)

corneal ulcer (H16.0-)

edema of eyelid (H02.84)

inflammation of eyelid (H01.8)

keratoconjunctivitis sicca (H16.22-)

mechanical lagophthalmos (H02.22-)

stomatitis (K12.-)

symblepharon (H11.23-)

code to identify percentage of skin exfoliation (L49.-)

EXCLUDES1 *staphylococcal scalded skin syndrome (L00) Ritter's disease (L00)*

L51.0 **Nonbullous erythema multiforme**

L51.1 **Stevens-Johnson syndrome**

L51.2 **Toxic epidermal necrolysis [Lyell]**

L51.3 **Stevens-Johnson syndrome-toxic epidermal necrolysis overlap syndrome**

SJS-TEN overlap syndrome

L51.8 Other erythema multiforme

L51.9 **Erythema multiforme, unspecified**

Erythema iris

Erythema multiforme major NOS

Erythema multiforme minor NOS

Herpes iris

L52 **Erythema nodosum**

EXCLUDES1 *tuberculous erythema nodosum (A18.4)*

④ L53 Other erythematous **conditions**

EXCLUDES1 *erythema ab igne (L59.0) erythema due to external agents in contact with skin (L23-L25) erythema intertrigo (L30.4)*

L53.0 Toxic **erythema**

Code first poisoning due to drug or toxin, if applicable (T36-T65 with fifth or sixth character 1-4 or 6)

Use additional code for adverse effect, if applicable, to identify drug (T36-T50 with fifth or sixth character 5)

EXCLUDES1 *neonatal erythema toxicum (P83.1)*

L53.1 **Erythema** annulare centrifugum

L53.2 **Erythema** marginatum

L53.3 Other chronic figurate erythema

L53.8 Other specified erythematous conditions

L53.9 **Erythematous condition, unspecified**

Erythema NOS

Erythroderma NOS

L54 **Erythema in diseases classified elsewhere**

Code first underlying disease.

Radiation-related disorders of the skin and subcutaneous tissue (L55-L59)

④ L55 **Sunburn**

L55.0 **Sunburn of** first **degree**

L55.1 **Sunburn of** second **degree**

L55.2 **Sunburn of** third **degree**

L55.9 **Sunburn, unspecified**

④ L56 **Other acute skin changes due to ultraviolet radiation**

Use additional code to identify the source of the ultraviolet radiation (W89, X32)

L56.0 **Drug phototoxic response**

Use additional code for adverse effect, if applicable, to identify drug (T36-T50 with fifth or sixth character 5)

L56.1 **Drug photoallergic response**

Use additional code for adverse effect, if applicable, to identify drug (T36-T50 with fifth or sixth character 5)

L56.2 **Photocontact dermatitis [berloque dermatitis]**

L56.3 **Solar urticaria**

L56.4 **Polymorphous light eruption**

L56.5 **Disseminated superficial actinic porokeratosis (DSAP)**

L56.8 Other specified acute skin changes due to ultraviolet radiation

L56.9 **Acute skin change due to ultraviolet radiation, unspecified**

④ L57 **Skin changes due to chronic exposure to nonionizing radiation**

Use additional code to identify the source of the ultraviolet radiation (W89, X32)

L57.0 **Actinic keratosis**

Keratosis NOS

Senile keratosis

Solar keratosis

L57.1 **Actinic reticuloid**

L57.2 **Cutis rhomboidalis nuchae**

L57.3 **Poikiloderma of Civatte**

L57.4 **Cutis laxa senilis**

Elastosis senilis

L57.5 **Actinic granuloma**

L57.8 Other skin changes due to chronic exposure to nonionizing radiation

Farmer's skin

Sailor's skin

Solar dermatitis

L57.9 **Skin changes due to chronic exposure to nonionizing radiation, unspecified**

④ L58 **Radiodermatitis**

Use additional code to identify the source of the radiation (W88, W90)

L58.0 Acute **radiodermatitis**

L58.1 Chronic **radiodermatitis**

L58.9 **Radiodermatitis, unspecified**

④ L59 **Other disorders of skin and subcutaneous tissue related to radiation**

L59.0 **Erythema ab igne [dermatitis ab igne]**

L59.8 Other specified disorders of the skin and subcutaneous tissue related to radiation

L59.9 **Disorder of the skin and subcutaneous tissue related to radiation, unspecified**

Disorders of skin appendages (L60-L75)

EXCLUDES1 *congenital malformations of integument (Q84.-)*

④ L60 **Nail disorders**

EXCLUDES2 *clubbing of nails (R68.3) onychia and paronychia (L03.0-)*

L60.0 **Ingrowing nail**

L60.1 **Onycholysis**

Unspecified Code	Other Specified Code	N Newborn Age: 0	P Pediatric Age: 0 17	M Maternity Age: 12-55	
A Adult Age: 15-124	♂ Male	♀ Female	● New Code	▲ Revised Code Title	►◄ Revised Text

L60.2 Onychogryphosis
L60.3 Nail dystrophy
L60.4 Beau's lines
L60.5 Yellow nail syndrome
L60.8 Other nail disorders
L60.9 Nail disorder, unspecified

L62 Nail disorders in diseases classified elsewhere

Code first underlying disease, such as:
pachydermoperiostosis (M89.4-)

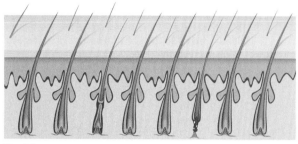

Healthy

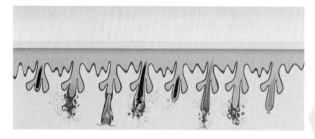

Figure 11.2 Alopecia areata

❹ L63 Alopecia areata
L63.0 Alopecia (capitis) totalis
L63.1 Alopecia universalis
L63.2 Ophiasis
L63.8 Other alopecia areata
L63.9 Alopecia areata, unspecified

❹ L64 Androgenic alopecia

INCLUDES   male-pattern baldness

L64.0 Drug-induced androgenic alopecia

Use additional code for adverse effect, if applicable, to
identify drug (T36-T50 with fifth or sixth character 5)

L64.8 Other androgenic alopecia
L64.9 Androgenic alopecia, unspecified

❹ L65 Other nonscarring hair loss

Use additional code for adverse effect, if applicable, to
identify drug (T36-T50 with fifth or sixth character 5)

EXCLUDES1   trichotillomania (F63.3)

L65.0 Telogen effluvium
L65.1 Anagen effluvium
L65.2 Alopecia mucinosa
L65.8 Other specified nonscarring hair loss
L65.9 Nonscarring hair loss, unspecified

Alopecia NOS

❹ L66 Cicatricial alopecia [scarring hair loss]
L66.0 Pseudopelade
L66.1 Lichen planopilaris

Follicular lichen planus

L66.2 Folliculitis decalvans
L66.3 Perifolliculitis capitis abscedens
L66.4 Folliculitis ulerythematosa reticulata
L66.8 Other cicatricial alopecia
L66.9 Cicatricial alopecia, unspecified

❹ L67 Hair color and hair shaft abnormalities

EXCLUDES1   monilethrix (Q84.1)
pili annulati (Q84.1)
telogen effluvium (L65.0)

L67.0 Trichorrhexis nodosa
L67.1 Variations in hair color

Canities
Greyness, hair (premature)
Heterochromia of hair
Poliosis circumscripta, acquired
Poliosis NOS

L67.8 Other hair color and hair shaft abnormalities

Fragilitas crinium

L67.9 Hair color and hair shaft abnormality, unspecified

❹ L68 Hypertrichosis

INCLUDES   excess hair

EXCLUDES1   congenital hypertrichosis (Q84.2)
persistent lanugo (Q84.2)

L68.0 Hirsutism
L68.1 Acquired hypertrichosis lanuginosa
L68.2 Localized hypertrichosis
L68.3 Polytrichia
L68.8 Other hypertrichosis
L68.9 Hypertrichosis, unspecified

❹ L70 Acne

EXCLUDES2   acne keloid (L73.0)

L70.0 Acne vulgaris
L70.1 Acne conglobata
L70.2 Acne varioliformis

Acne necrotica miliaris

L70.3 Acne tropica
L70.4 Infantile acne   ℗
L70.5 Acné excoriée des jeunes filles   ▲

Picker's acne

L70.8 Other acne
L70.9 Acne, unspecified

❹ L71 Rosacea

Use additional code for adverse effect, if applicable, to
identify drug (T36-T50 with fifth or sixth character 5)

L71.0 Perioral dermatitis
L71.1 Rhinophyma
L71.8 Other rosacea
L71.9 Rosacea, unspecified

❹ L72 Follicular cysts of skin and subcutaneous tissue
L72.0 Epidermal cyst
❺ L72.1 Pilar and trichodermal cyst
L72.11 Pilar cyst
L72.12 Trichodermal cyst

Trichilemmal (proliferating) cyst

L72.2 Steatocystoma multiplex
L72.3 Sebaceous cyst

EXCLUDES2   pilar cyst (L72.11)
trichilemmal (proliferating) cyst (L72.12)

L72.8 Other follicular cysts of the skin and subcutaneous
tissue

L72.9 Follicular cyst of the skin and subcutaneous tissue,
unspecified

❹ L73 Other follicular disorders
L73.0 Acne keloid
L73.1 Pseudofolliculitis barbae
L73.2 Hidradenitis suppurativa
L73.8 Other specified follicular disorders

Sycosis barbae

L73.9 Follicular disorder, unspecified

❹ L74 Eccrine sweat disorders

EXCLUDES2   generalized hyperhidrosis (R61)

---

❹ 4th character required   ❺ 5th character required   ❻ 6th character required   ❼ 7th character required   ⓔ Extension 'X' Alert

EXCLUDES1 Not coded here   EXCLUDES2 Not included here   ℗ Primary Diagnosis Only   Manifestation Code

L74.0 Miliaria rubra
L74.1 Miliaria crystallina
L74.2 Miliaria profunda
Miliaria tropicalis
L74.3 Miliaria, unspecified
L74.4 Anhidrosis
Hypohidrosis
[5] L74.5 Focal hyperhidrosis
[6] L74.51 Primary focal hyperhidrosis
L74.510 Primary focal hyperhidrosis, axilla
L74.511 Primary focal hyperhidrosis, face
L74.512 Primary focal hyperhidrosis, palms
L74.513 Primary focal hyperhidrosis, soles
L74.519 Primary focal hyperhidrosis, unspecified
L74.52 Secondary focal hyperhidrosis
Frey's syndrome
L74.8 Other eccrine sweat disorders
L74.9 Eccrine sweat disorder, unspecified
Sweat gland disorder NOS
[4] L75 Apocrine sweat disorders
[EXCLUDES1] *dyshidrosis (L30.1)*
hidradenitis suppurativa (L73.2)
L75.0 Bromhidrosis
L75.1 Chromhidrosis
L75.2 Apocrine miliaria
Fox-Fordyce disease
L75.8 Other apocrine sweat disorders
L75.9 Apocrine sweat disorder, unspecified

Intraoperative and postprocedural complications of skin and subcutaneous tissue (L76)

[4] L76 Intraoperative and postprocedural complications of skin and subcutaneous tissue
[5] L76.0 Intraoperative hemorrhage and hematoma of skin and subcutaneous tissue complicating a procedure
[EXCLUDES1] *intraoperative hemorrhage and hematoma of skin and subcutaneous tissue due to accidental puncture and laceration during a procedure (L76.1-)*
L76.01 Intraoperative hemorrhage and hematoma of skin and subcutaneous tissue complicating a dermatologic procedure
L76.02 Intraoperative hemorrhage and hematoma of skin and subcutaneous tissue complicating other procedure
[5] L76.1 Accidental puncture and laceration of skin and subcutaneous tissue during a procedure
L76.11 Accidental puncture and laceration of skin and subcutaneous tissue during a dermatologic procedure
L76.12 Accidental puncture and laceration of skin and subcutaneous tissue during other procedure
[5] L76.2 Postprocedural hemorrhage and hematoma of skin and subcutaneous tissue following a procedure
L76.21 Postprocedural hemorrhage and hematoma of skin and subcutaneous tissue following a dermatologic procedure
L76.22 Postprocedural hemorrhage and hematoma of skin and subcutaneous tissue following other procedure
[5] L76.8 Other intraoperative and postprocedural complications of skin and subcutaneous tissue
Use additional code, if applicable, to further specify disorder
L76.81 Other intraoperative complications of skin and subcutaneous tissue
L76.82 Other postprocedural complications of skin and subcutaneous tissue

Other disorders of the skin and subcutaneous tissue (L80-L99)

L80 Vitiligo
[EXCLUDES2] *vitiligo of eyelids (H02.73-)*
vitiligo of vulva (N90.89)
[4] L81 Other disorders of pigmentation
[EXCLUDES1] *birthmark NOS (Q82.5)*
Peutz-Jeghers syndrome (Q85.8)
[EXCLUDES2] *nevus - see Alphabetical Index*
L81.0 Postinflammatory hyperpigmentation
L81.1 Chloasma
L81.2 Freckles
L81.3 Café au lait spots
L81.4 Other melanin hyperpigmentation
Lentigo
L81.5 Leukoderma, not elsewhere classified
L81.6 Other disorders of diminished melanin formation
L81.7 Pigmented purpuric dermatosis
Angioma serpiginosum
L81.8 Other specified disorders of pigmentation
Iron pigmentation
Tattoo pigmentation
L81.9 Disorder of pigmentation, unspecified
[4] L82 Seborrheic keratosis
[INCLUDES] *dermatosis papulosa nigra*
Leser-Trélat disease
[EXCLUDES2] *seborrheic dermatitis (L21.-)*
L82.0 Inflamed seborrheic keratosis
L82.1 Other seborrheic keratosis
Seborrheic keratosis NOS
L83 Acanthosis nigricans
Confluent and reticulated papillomatosis
L84 Corns and callosities
Callus
Clavus
[4] L85 Other epidermal thickening
[EXCLUDES2] *hypertrophic disorders of the skin (L91.-)*
L85.0 Acquired ichthyosis
[EXCLUDES1] *congenital ichthyosis (Q80.-)*
L85.1 Acquired keratosis [keratoderma] palmaris et plantaris
[EXCLUDES1] *inherited keratosis palmaris et plantaris (Q82.8)*
L85.2 Keratosis punctata (palmaris et plantaris)
L85.3 Xerosis cutis
Dry skin dermatitis
L85.8 Other specified epidermal thickening
Cutaneous horn
L85.9 Epidermal thickening, unspecified
L86 Keratoderma in diseases classified elsewhere
Code first underlying disease, such as:
Reiter's disease (M02.3-)
[EXCLUDES1] *gonococcal keratoderma (A54.89)*
gonococcal keratosis (A54.89)
keratoderma due to vitamin A deficiency (E50.8)
keratosis due to vitamin A deficiency (E50.8)
xeroderma due to vitamin A deficiency (E50.8)
[4] L87 Transepidermal elimination disorders
[EXCLUDES1] *granuloma annulare (perforating) (L92.0)*
L87.0 Keratosis follicularis et parafollicularis in cutem penetrans
Kyrle disease
Hyperkeratosis follicularis penetrans
L87.1 Reactive perforating collagenosis
L87.2 Elastosis perforans serpiginosa
L87.8 Other transepidermal elimination disorders
L87.9 Transepidermal elimination disorder, unspecified

Unspecified Code | Other Specified Code | [N] Newborn Age: 0 | [P] Pediatric Age: 0-17 | [M] Maternity Age: 12-55
[A] Adult Age: 15-124 | ♂ Male | ♀ Female | ● New Code | ▲ Revised Code Title | ►◄ Revised Text

L88 Pyoderma gangrenosum
Phagedenic pyoderma
[EXCLUDES1] *dermatitis gangrenosa (L08.0)*

[4] **L89 Pressure ulcer**
[INCLUDES] *bed sore*
decubitus ulcer
plaster ulcer
pressure area
pressure sore
Code first any associated gangrene (I96)
[EXCLUDES2] *decubitus (trophic) ulcer of cervix (uteri) (N86)*
diabetic ulcers (E08.621, E08.622, E09.621, E09.622, E10.621, E10.622, E11.621, E11.622, E13.621, E13.622)
non-pressure chronic ulcer of skin (L97.-)
skin infections (L00-L08)
varicose ulcer (I83.0, I83.2)

[5] **L89.0 Pressure ulcer of elbow**

[6] **L89.00 Pressure ulcer of unspecified elbow**

L89.000 Pressure ulcer of unspecified elbow, unstageable

L89.001 Pressure ulcer of unspecified elbow, stage 1
Healing pressure ulcer of unspecified elbow, stage 1
Pressure pre-ulcer skin changes limited to persistent focal edema, unspecified elbow

L89.002 Pressure ulcer of unspecified elbow, stage 2
Healing pressure ulcer of unspecified elbow, stage 2
Pressure ulcer with abrasion, blister, partial thickness skin loss involving epidermis and/ or dermis, unspecified elbow

L89.003 Pressure ulcer of unspecified elbow, stage 3
Healing pressure ulcer of unspecified elbow, stage 3
Pressure ulcer with full thickness skin loss involving damage or necrosis of subcutaneous tissue, unspecified elbow

L89.004 Pressure ulcer of unspecified elbow, stage 4
Healing pressure ulcer of unspecified elbow, stage 4
Pressure ulcer with necrosis of soft tissues through to underlying muscle, tendon, or bone, unspecified elbow

L89.009 Pressure ulcer of unspecified elbow, unspecified stage
Healing pressure ulcer of elbow NOS
Healing pressure ulcer of unspecified elbow, unspecified stage

[6] **L89.01 Pressure ulcer of right elbow**

L89.010 Pressure ulcer of right elbow, unstageable

L89.011 Pressure ulcer of right elbow, stage 1
Healing pressure ulcer of right elbow, stage 1
Pressure pre-ulcer skin changes limited to persistent focal edema, right elbow

L89.012 Pressure ulcer of right elbow, stage 2
Healing pressure ulcer of right elbow, stage 2
Pressure ulcer with abrasion, blister, partial thickness skin loss involving epidermis and/ or dermis, right elbow

L89.013 Pressure ulcer of right elbow, stage 3
Healing pressure ulcer of right elbow, stage 3
Pressure ulcer with full thickness skin loss involving damage or necrosis of subcutaneous tissue, right elbow

L89.014 Pressure ulcer of right elbow, stage 4
Healing pressure ulcer of right elbow, stage 4
Pressure ulcer with necrosis of soft tissues through to underlying muscle, tendon, or bone, right elbow

L89.019 Pressure ulcer of right elbow, unspecified stage
Healing pressure right of elbow NOS
Healing pressure ulcer of unspecified elbow, unspecified stage

[6] **L89.02 Pressure ulcer of left elbow**

L89.020 Pressure ulcer of left elbow, unstageable

L89.021 Pressure ulcer of left elbow, stage 1
Healing pressure ulcer of left elbow, stage 1
Pressure pre-ulcer skin changes limited to persistent focal edema, left elbow

L89.022 Pressure ulcer of left elbow, stage 2
Healing pressure ulcer of left elbow, stage 2
Pressure ulcer with abrasion, blister, partial thickness skin loss involving epidermis and/ or dermis, left elbow

L89.023 Pressure ulcer of left elbow, stage 3
Healing pressure ulcer of left elbow, stage 3
Pressure ulcer with full thickness skin loss involving damage or necrosis of subcutaneous tissue, left elbow

L89.024 Pressure ulcer of left elbow, stage 4
Healing pressure ulcer of left elbow, stage 4
Pressure ulcer with necrosis of soft tissues through to underlying muscle, tendon, or bone, left elbow

L89.029 Pressure ulcer of left elbow, unspecified stage
Healing pressure ulcer of left of elbow NOS
Healing pressure ulcer of unspecified elbow, unspecified stage

[5] **L89.1 Pressure ulcer of back**

[6] **L89.10 Pressure ulcer of unspecified part of back**

L89.100 Pressure ulcer of unspecified part of back, unstageable

L89.101 Pressure ulcer of unspecified part of back, stage 1
Healing pressure ulcer of unspecified part of back, stage 1
Pressure pre-ulcer skin changes limited to persistent focal edema, unspecified part of back

L89.102 Pressure ulcer of unspecified part of back, stage 2
Healing pressure ulcer of unspecified part of back, stage 2
Pressure ulcer with abrasion, blister, partial thickness skin loss involving epidermis and/ or dermis, unspecified part of back

L89.103 Pressure ulcer of unspecified part of back, stage 3
Healing pressure ulcer of unspecified part of back, stage 3
Pressure ulcer with full thickness skin loss involving damage or necrosis of subcutaneous tissue, unspecified part of back

L89.104 Pressure ulcer of unspecified part of back, stage 4
Healing pressure ulcer of unspecified part of back, stage 4
Pressure ulcer with necrosis of soft tissues through to underlying muscle, tendon, or bone, unspecified part of back

L89.109 Pressure ulcer of unspecified part of back, unspecified stage

Healing pressure ulcer of unspecified part of back NOS
Healing pressure ulcer of unspecified part of back, unspecified stage

⑥ **L89.11 Pressure ulcer of** right upper back
Pressure ulcer of right shoulder blade

    L89.110 Pressure ulcer of right upper back, unstageable

    L89.111 Pressure ulcer of right upper back, stage 1
Healing pressure ulcer of right upper back, stage 1
Pressure pre-ulcer skin changes limited to persistent focal edema, right upper back

    L89.112 Pressure ulcer of right upper back, stage 2
Healing pressure ulcer of right upper back, stage 2
Pressure ulcer with abrasion, blister, partial thickness skin loss involving epidermis and/or dermis, right upper back

    L89.113 Pressure ulcer of right upper back, stage 3
Healing pressure ulcer of right upper back, stage 3
Pressure ulcer with full thickness skin loss involving damage or necrosis of subcutaneous tissue, right upper back

    L89.114 Pressure ulcer of right upper back, stage 4
Healing pressure ulcer of right upper back, stage 4
Pressure ulcer with necrosis of soft tissues through to underlying muscle, tendon, or bone, right upper back

    L89.119 Pressure ulcer of right upper back, unspecified stage
Healing pressure ulcer of right upper back NOS
Healing pressure ulcer of right upper back, unspecified stage

⑥ **L89.12 Pressure ulcer of** left upper back
Pressure ulcer of left shoulder blade

    L89.120 Pressure ulcer of left upper back, unstageable

    L89.121 Pressure ulcer of left upper back, stage 1
Healing pressure ulcer of left upper back, stage 1
Pressure pre-ulcer skin changes limited to persistent focal edema, left upper back

    L89.122 Pressure ulcer of left upper back, stage 2
Healing pressure ulcer of left upper back, stage 2
Pressure ulcer with abrasion, blister, partial thickness skin loss involving epidermis and/or dermis, left upper back

    L89.123 Pressure ulcer of left upper back, stage 3
Healing pressure ulcer of left upper back, stage 3
Pressure ulcer with full thickness skin loss involving damage or necrosis of subcutaneous tissue, left upper back

    L89.124 Pressure ulcer of left upper back, stage 4
Healing pressure ulcer of left upper back, stage 4
Pressure ulcer with necrosis of soft tissues through to underlying muscle, tendon, or bone, left upper back

    L89.129 Pressure ulcer of left upper back, unspecified stage
Healing pressure ulcer of left upper back NOS
Healing pressure ulcer of left upper back, unspecified stage

⑥ **L89.13 Pressure ulcer of** right lower back

    L89.130 Pressure ulcer of right lower back, unstageable

    L89.131 Pressure ulcer of right lower back, stage 1
Healing pressure ulcer of right lower back, stage 1
Pressure pre-ulcer skin changes limited to persistent focal edema, right lower back

    L89.132 Pressure ulcer of right lower back, stage 2
Healing pressure ulcer of right lower back, stage 2
Pressure ulcer with abrasion, blister, partial thickness skin loss involving epidermis and/or dermis, right lower back

    L89.133 Pressure ulcer of right lower back, stage 3
Healing pressure ulcer of right lower back, stage 3
Pressure ulcer with full thickness skin loss involving damage or necrosis of subcutaneous tissue, right lower back

    L89.134 Pressure ulcer of right lower back, stage 4
Healing pressure ulcer of right lower back, stage 4
Pressure ulcer with necrosis of soft tissues through to underlying muscle, tendon, or bone, right lower back

    L89.139 Pressure ulcer of right lower back, unspecified stage
Healing pressure ulcer of right lower back NOS
Healing pressure ulcer of right lower back, unspecified stage

⑥ **L89.14 Pressure ulcer of** left lower back

    L89.140 Pressure ulcer of left lower back, unstageable

    L89.141 Pressure ulcer of left lower back, stage 1
Healing pressure ulcer of left lower back, stage 1
Pressure pre-ulcer skin changes limited to persistent focal edema, left lower back

    L89.142 Pressure ulcer of left lower back, stage 2
Healing pressure ulcer of left lower back, stage 2
Pressure ulcer with abrasion, blister, partial thickness skin loss involving epidermis and/or dermis, left lower back

    L89.143 Pressure ulcer of left lower back, stage 3
Healing pressure ulcer of left lower back, stage 3
Pressure ulcer with full thickness skin loss involving damage or necrosis of subcutaneous tissue, left lower back

    L89.144 Pressure ulcer of left lower back, stage 4
Healing pressure ulcer of left lower back, stage 4
Pressure ulcer with necrosis of soft tissues through to underlying muscle, tendon, or bone, left lower back

    L89.149 Pressure ulcer of left lower back, unspecified stage
Healing pressure ulcer of left lower back NOS
Healing pressure ulcer of left lower back, unspecified stage

⑥ **L89.15 Pressure ulcer of** sacral region
Pressure ulcer of coccyx
Pressure ulcer of tailbone

    L89.150 Pressure ulcer of sacral region, unstageable

    L89.151 Pressure ulcer of sacral region, stage 1
Healing pressure ulcer of sacral region, stage 1
Pressure pre-ulcer skin changes limited to persistent focal edema, sacral region

    L89.152 Pressure ulcer of sacral region, stage 2
Healing pressure ulcer of sacral region, stage 2
Pressure ulcer with abrasion, blister, partial thickness skin loss involving epidermis and/or dermis, sacral region

    L89.153 Pressure ulcer of sacral region, stage 3
Healing pressure ulcer of sacral region, stage 3
Pressure ulcer with full thickness skin loss involving damage or necrosis of subcutaneous tissue, sacral region

---

Unspecified Code	Other Specified Code	N Newborn Age: 0	P Pediatric Age: 0 17	M Maternity Age: 12-55	
A Adult Age: 15-124	♂ Male	♀ Female	● New Code	▲ Revised Code Title	►◄ Revised Text

L89.154 **Pressure ulcer of sacral region,** stage 4
Healing pressure ulcer of sacral region, stage 4
Pressure ulcer with necrosis of soft tissues through to underlying muscle, tendon, or bone, sacral region

L89.159 **Pressure ulcer of sacral region,** unspecified stage
Healing pressure ulcer of sacral region NOS
Healing pressure ulcer of sacral region, unspecified stage

[5] L89.2 **Pressure ulcer of** hip

[6] L89.20 **Pressure ulcer of** unspecified **hip**

L89.200 **Pressure ulcer of unspecified hip,** unstageable

L89.201 **Pressure ulcer of unspecified hip,** stage 1
Healing pressure ulcer of unspecified hip back, stage 1
Pressure pre-ulcer skin changes limited to persistent focal edema, unspecified hip

L89.202 **Pressure ulcer of unspecified hip,** stage 2
Healing pressure ulcer of unspecified hip, stage 2
Pressure ulcer with abrasion, blister, partial thickness skin loss involving epidermis and/or dermis, unspecified hip

L89.203 **Pressure ulcer of unspecified hip,** stage 3
Healing pressure ulcer of unspecified hip, stage 3
Pressure ulcer with full thickness skin loss involving damage or necrosis of subcutaneous tissue, unspecified hip

L89.204 **Pressure ulcer of unspecified hip,** stage 4
Healing pressure ulcer of unspecified hip, stage 4
Pressure ulcer with necrosis of soft tissues through to underlying muscle, tendon, or bone, unspecified hip

L89.209 **Pressure ulcer of unspecified hip,** unspecified stage
Healing pressure ulcer of unspecified hip NOS
Healing pressure ulcer of unspecified hip, unspecified stage

[6] L89.21 **Pressure ulcer of** right hip

L89.210 **Pressure ulcer of right hip,** unstageable

L89.211 **Pressure ulcer of right hip,** stage 1
Healing pressure ulcer of right hip back, stage 1
Pressure pre-ulcer skin changes limited to persistent focal edema, right hip

L89.212 **Pressure ulcer of right hip,** stage 2
Healing pressure ulcer of right hip, stage 2
Pressure ulcer with abrasion, blister, partial thickness skin loss involving epidermis and/or dermis, right hip

L89.213 **Pressure ulcer of right hip,** stage 3
Healing pressure ulcer of right hip, stage 3
Pressure ulcer with full thickness skin loss involving damage or necrosis of subcutaneous tissue, right hip

L89.214 **Pressure ulcer of right hip,** stage 4
Healing pressure ulcer of right hip, stage 4
Pressure ulcer with necrosis of soft tissues through to underlying muscle, tendon, or bone, right hip

L89.219 **Pressure ulcer of right hip,** unspecified stage
Healing pressure ulcer of right hip NOS
Healing pressure ulcer of right hip, unspecified stage

[6] L89.22 **Pressure ulcer of** left hip

L89.220 **Pressure ulcer of left hip,** unstageable

L89.221 **Pressure ulcer of left hip,** stage 1
Healing pressure ulcer of left hip back, stage 1
Pressure pre-ulcer skin changes limited to persistent focal edema, left hip

L89.222 **Pressure ulcer of left hip,** stage 2
Healing pressure ulcer of left hip, stage 2
Pressure ulcer with abrasion, blister, partial thickness skin loss involving epidermis and/or dermis, left hip

L89.223 **Pressure ulcer of left hip,** stage 3
Healing pressure ulcer of left hip, stage 3
Pressure ulcer with full thickness skin loss involving damage or necrosis of subcutaneous tissue, left hip

L89.224 **Pressure ulcer of left hip,** stage 4
Healing pressure ulcer of left hip, stage 4
Pressure ulcer with necrosis of soft tissues through to underlying muscle, tendon, or bone, left hip

L89.229 **Pressure ulcer of left hip,** unspecified stage
Healing pressure ulcer of left hip NOS
Healing pressure ulcer of left hip, unspecified stage

[5] L89.3 **Pressure ulcer of** buttock

[6] L89.30 **Pressure ulcer of** unspecified **buttock**

L89.300 **Pressure ulcer of unspecified buttock,** unstageable

L89.301 **Pressure ulcer of unspecified buttock,** stage 1
Healing pressure ulcer of unspecified buttock, stage 1
Pressure pre-ulcer skin changes limited to persistent focal edema, unspecified buttock

L89.302 **Pressure ulcer of unspecified buttock,** stage 2
Healing pressure ulcer of unspecified buttock, stage 2
Pressure ulcer with abrasion, blister, partial thickness skin loss involving epidermis and/or dermis, unspecified buttock

L89.303 **Pressure ulcer of unspecified buttock,** stage 3
Healing pressure ulcer of unspecified buttock, stage 3
Pressure ulcer with full thickness skin loss involving damage or necrosis of subcutaneous tissue, unspecified buttock

L89.304 **Pressure ulcer of unspecified buttock,** stage 4
Healing pressure ulcer of unspecified buttock, stage 4
Pressure ulcer with necrosis of soft tissues through to underlying muscle, tendon, or bone, unspecified buttock

L89.309 **Pressure ulcer of unspecified buttock,** unspecified stage
Healing pressure ulcer of unspecified buttock NOS
Healing pressure ulcer of unspecified buttock, unspecified stage

[6] L89.31 **Pressure ulcer of** right buttock

L89.310 **Pressure ulcer of right buttock,** unstageable

L89.311 **Pressure ulcer of right buttock,** stage 1
Healing pressure ulcer of right buttock, stage 1
Pressure pre-ulcer skin changes limited to persistent focal edema, right buttock

L89.312 **Pressure ulcer of right buttock,** stage 2
Healing pressure ulcer of right buttock, stage 2
Pressure ulcer with abrasion, blister, partial thickness skin loss involving epidermis and/or dermis, right buttock

L89.313 **Pressure ulcer of right buttock,** stage 3
Healing pressure ulcer of right buttock, stage 3
Pressure ulcer with full thickness skin loss involving damage or necrosis of subcutaneous tissue, right buttock

L89.314 **Pressure ulcer of right buttock,** stage 4
Healing pressure ulcer of right buttock, stage 4
Pressure ulcer with necrosis of soft tissues through to underlying muscle, tendon, or bone, right buttock

L89.319 **Pressure ulcer of right buttock,** unspecified stage
Healing pressure ulcer of right buttock NOS
Healing pressure ulcer of right buttock, unspecified stage

[6] L89.32 **Pressure ulcer of** left buttock

L89.320 **Pressure ulcer of left buttock,** unstageable

L89.321 **Pressure ulcer of left buttock,** stage 1
Healing pressure ulcer of left buttock, stage 1
Pressure pre-ulcer skin changes limited to persistent focal edema, left buttock

L89.322 **Pressure ulcer of left buttock,** stage 2
Healing pressure ulcer of left buttock, stage 2
Pressure ulcer with abrasion, blister, partial thickness skin loss involving epidermis and/ or dermis, left buttock

L89.323 **Pressure ulcer of left buttock,** stage 3
Healing pressure ulcer of left buttock, stage 3
Pressure ulcer with full thickness skin loss involving damage or necrosis of subcutaneous tissue, left buttock

L89.324 **Pressure ulcer of left buttock,** stage 4
Healing pressure ulcer of left buttock, stage 4
Pressure ulcer with necrosis of soft tissues through to underlying muscle, tendon, or bone, left buttock

L89.329 **Pressure ulcer of left buttock,** unspecified stage
Healing pressure ulcer of left buttock NOS
Healing pressure ulcer of left buttock, unspecified stage

[5] L89.4 **Pressure ulcer of** contiguous site of back, buttock and hip

L89.40 **Pressure ulcer of contiguous site of back, buttock and hip,** unspecified stage
Healing pressure ulcer of contiguous site of back, buttock and hip NOS
Healing pressure ulcer of contiguous site of back, buttock and hip, unspecified stage

L89.41 **Pressure ulcer of contiguous site of back, buttock and hip,** stage 1
Healing pressure ulcer of contiguous site of back, buttock and hip, stage 1
Pressure pre-ulcer skin changes limited to persistent focal edema, contiguous site of back, buttock and hip

L89.42 **Pressure ulcer of contiguous site of back, buttock and hip,** stage 2
Healing pressure ulcer of contiguous site of back, buttock and hip, stage 2
Pressure ulcer with abrasion, blister, partial thickness skin loss involving epidermis and/or dermis, contiguous site of back, buttock and hip

L89.43 **Pressure ulcer of contiguous site of back, buttock and hip,** stage 3
Healing pressure ulcer of contiguous site of back, buttock and hip, stage 3
Pressure ulcer with full thickness skin loss involving damage or necrosis of subcutaneous tissue, contiguous site of back, buttock and hip

L89.44 **Pressure ulcer of contiguous site of back, buttock and hip,** stage 4
Healing pressure ulcer of contiguous site of back, buttock and hip, stage 4
Pressure ulcer with necrosis of soft tissues through to underlying muscle, tendon, or bone, contiguous site of back, buttock and hip

L89.45 **Pressure ulcer of contiguous site of back, buttock and hip,** unstageable

[5] L89.5 **Pressure ulcer of** ankle

[6] L89.50 **Pressure ulcer of** unspecified **ankle**

L89.500 **Pressure ulcer of unspecified ankle,** unstageable

L89.501 **Pressure ulcer of unspecified ankle,** stage 1
Healing pressure ulcer of unspecified ankle, stage 1
Pressure pre-ulcer skin changes limited to persistent focal edema, unspecified ankle

L89.502 **Pressure ulcer of unspecified ankle,** stage 2
Healing pressure ulcer of unspecified ankle, stage 2
Pressure ulcer with abrasion, blister, partial thickness skin loss involving epidermis and/ or dermis, unspecified ankle

L89.503 **Pressure ulcer of unspecified ankle,** stage 3
Healing pressure ulcer of unspecified ankle, stage 3
Pressure ulcer with full thickness skin loss involving damage or necrosis of subcutaneous tissue, unspecified ankle

L89.504 **Pressure ulcer of unspecified ankle,** stage 4
Healing pressure ulcer of unspecified ankle, stage 4
Pressure ulcer with necrosis of soft tissues through to underlying muscle, tendon, or bone, unspecified ankle

L89.509 **Pressure ulcer of unspecified ankle,** unspecified stage
Healing pressure ulcer of unspecified ankle NOS
Healing pressure ulcer of unspecified ankle, unspecified stage

[6] L89.51 **Pressure ulcer of** right ankle

L89.510 **Pressure ulcer of right ankle,** unstageable

L89.511 **Pressure ulcer of right ankle,** stage 1
Healing pressure ulcer of right ankle, stage 1
Pressure pre-ulcer skin changes limited to persistent focal edema, right ankle

L89.512 **Pressure ulcer of right ankle,** stage 2
Healing pressure ulcer of right ankle, stage 2
Pressure ulcer with abrasion, blister, partial thickness skin loss involving epidermis and/ or dermis, right ankle

L89.513 **Pressure ulcer of right ankle,** stage 3
Healing pressure ulcer of right ankle, stage 3
Pressure ulcer with full thickness skin loss involving damage or necrosis of subcutaneous tissue, right ankle

L89.514 **Pressure ulcer of right ankle,** stage 4
Healing pressure ulcer of right ankle, stage 4
Pressure ulcer with necrosis of soft tissues through to underlying muscle, tendon, or bone, right ankle

L89.519 **Pressure ulcer of right ankle,** unspecified stage
Healing pressure ulcer of right ankle NOS
Healing pressure ulcer of right ankle, unspecified stage

[6] L89.52 Pressure ulcer of left ankle
L89.520 **Pressure ulcer of left ankle,** unstageable
L89.521 **Pressure ulcer of left ankle,** stage 1
Healing pressure ulcer of left ankle, stage 1
Pressure pre-ulcer skin changes limited to persistnt focal edema, left ankle
L89.522 **Pressure ulcer of left ankle,** stage 2
Healing pressure ulcer of left ankle, stage 2
Pressure ulcer with abrasion, blister, partial thickness skin loss involving epidermis and/or dermis, left ankle
L89.523 **Pressure ulcer of left ankle,** stage 3
Healing pressure ulcer of left ankle, stage 3
Pressure ulcer with full thickness skin loss involving damage or necrosis of subcutaneous tissue, left ankle
L89.524 **Pressure ulcer of left ankle,** stage 4
Healing pressure ulcer of left ankle, stage 4
Pressure ulcer with necrosis of soft tissues through to underlying muscle, tendon, or bone, left ankle
L89.529 **Pressure ulcer of left ankle,** unspecified stage
Healing pressure ulcer of left ankle NOS
Healing pressure ulcer of left ankle, unspecified stage

[5] L89.6 Pressure ulcer of heel

[6] L89.60 Pressure ulcer of unspecified heel
L89.600 **Pressure ulcer of unspecified heel,** unstageable
L89.601 **Pressure ulcer of unspecified heel,** stage 1
Healing pressure ulcer of unspecified heel, stage 1
Pressure pre-ulcer skin changes limited to persistent focal edema, unspecified heel
L89.602 **Pressure ulcer of unspecified heel,** stage 2
Healing pressure ulcer of unspecified heel, stage 2
Pressure ulcer with abrasion, blister, partial thickness skin loss involving epidermis and/or dermis, unspecified heel
L89.603 **Pressure ulcer of unspecified heel,** stage 3
Healing pressure ulcer of unspecified heel, stage 3
Pressure ulcer with full thickness skin loss involving damage or necrosis of subcutaneous tissue, unspecified heel
L89.604 **Pressure ulcer of unspecified heel,** stage 4
Healing pressure ulcer of unspecified heel, stage 4
Pressure ulcer with necrosis of soft tissues through to underlying muscle, tendon, or bone, unspecified heel
L89.609 **Pressure ulcer of unspecified heel,** unspecified stage
Healing pressure ulcer of unspecified heel NOS
Healing pressure ulcer of unspecified heel, unspecified stage

[6] L89.61 Pressure ulcer of right heel
L89.610 **Pressure ulcer of right heel,** unstageable
L89.611 **Pressure ulcer of right heel,** stage 1
Healing pressure ulcer of right heel, stage 1
Pressure pre-ulcer skin changes limited to persistent focal edema, right heel
L89.612 **Pressure ulcer of right heel,** stage 2
Healing pressure ulcer of right heel, stage 2
Pressure ulcer with abrasion, blister, partial thickness skin loss involving epidermis and/or dermis, right heel
L89.613 **Pressure ulcer of right heel,** stage 3
Healing pressure ulcer of right heel, stage 3
Pressure ulcer with full thickness skin loss involving damage or necrosis of subcutaneous tissue, right heel
L89.614 **Pressure ulcer of right heel,** stage 4
Healing pressure ulcer of right heel, stage 4
Pressure ulcer with necrosis of soft tissues through to underlying muscle, tendon, or bone, right heel
L89.619 **Pressure ulcer of right heel,** unspecified stage
Healing pressure ulcer of right heel NOS
Healing pressure ulcer of unspecified heel, right stage

[6] L89.62 Pressure ulcer of left heel
L89.620 **Pressure ulcer of left heel,** unstageable
L89.621 **Pressure ulcer of left heel,** stage 1
Healing pressure ulcer of left heel, stage 1
Pressure pre-ulcer skin changes limited to persistent focal edema, left heel
L89.622 **Pressure ulcer of left heel,** stage 2
Healing pressure ulcer of left heel, stage 2
Pressure ulcer with abrasion, blister, partial thickness skin loss involving epidermis and/or dermis, left heel
L89.623 **Pressure ulcer of left heel,** stage 3
Healing pressure ulcer of left heel, stage 3
Pressure ulcer with full thickness skin loss involving damage or necrosis of subcutaneous tissue, left heel
L89.624 **Pressure ulcer of left heel,** stage 4
Healing pressure ulcer of left heel, stage 4
Pressure ulcer with necrosis of soft tissues through to underlying muscle, tendon, or bone, left heel
L89.629 **Pressure ulcer of left heel,** unspecified stage
Healing pressure ulcer of left heel NOS
Healing pressure ulcer of left heel, unspecified stage

[5] L89.8 Pressure ulcer of other site

[6] L89.81 Pressure ulcer of head
Pressure ulcer of face
L89.810 **Pressure ulcer of head,** unstageable
L89.811 **Pressure ulcer of head,** stage 1
Healing pressure ulcer of head, stage 1
Pressure pre-ulcer skin changes limited to persistent focal edema, head
L89.812 **Pressure ulcer of head,** stage 2
Healing pressure ulcer of head, stage 2
Pressure ulcer with abrasion, blister, partial thickness skin loss involving epidermis and/or dermis, head
L89.813 **Pressure ulcer of head,** stage 3
Healing pressure ulcer of head, stage 3
Pressure ulcer with full thickness skin loss involving damage or necrosis of subcutaneous tissue, head
L89.814 **Pressure ulcer of head,** stage 4
Healing pressure ulcer of head, stage 4
Pressure ulcer with necrosis of soft tissues through to underlying muscle, tendon, or bone, head
L89.819 **Pressure ulcer of head, unspecified stage**
Healing pressure ulcer of head NOS
Healing pressure ulcer of head, unspecified stage

[6] L89.89 Pressure ulcer of other site

[4] 4th character required [5] 5th character required [6] 6th character required [7] 7th character required [7x] Extension 'X' Alert
EXCLUDES 1 Not coded here EXCLUDES 2 Not included here PDx Primary Diagnosis Only Manifestation Code

L89.890 Pressure ulcer of other site, unstageable
L89.891 Pressure ulcer of other site, stage 1
Healing pressure ulcer of other site, stage 1
Pressure pre-ulcer skin changes limited to persistent focal edema, other site
L89.892 Pressure ulcer of other site, stage 2
Healing pressure ulcer of other site, stage 2
Pressure ulcer with abrasion, blister, partial thickness skin loss involving epidermis and/or dermis, other site
L89.893 Pressure ulcer of other site, stage 3
Healing pressure ulcer of other site, stage 3
Pressure ulcer with full thickness skin loss involving damage or necrosis of subcutaneous tissue, other site
L89.894 Pressure ulcer of other site, stage 4
Healing pressure ulcer of other site, stage 4
Pressure ulcer with necrosis of soft tissues through to underlying muscle, tendon, or bone, other site
L89.899 Pressure ulcer of other site, unspecified stage
Healing pressure ulcer of other site NOS
Healing pressure ulcer of other site, unspecified stage

[5] L89.9 Pressure ulcer of unspecified site
L89.90 Pressure ulcer of unspecified site, unspecified stage
Healing pressure ulcer of unspecified site NOS
Healing pressure ulcer of unspecified site, unspecified stage
L89.91 Pressure ulcer of unspecified site, stage 1
Healing pressure ulcer of unspecified site, stage 1
Pressure pre-ulcer skin changes limited to persistent focal edema, unspecified site
L89.92 Pressure ulcer of unspecified site, stage 2
Healing pressure ulcer of unspecified site, stage 2
Pressure ulcer with abrasion, blister, partial thickness skin loss involving epidermis and/or dermis, unspecified site
L89.93 Pressure ulcer of unspecified site, stage 3
Healing pressure ulcer of unspecified site, stage 3
Pressure ulcer with full thickness skin loss involving damage or necrosis of subcutaneous tissue, unspecified site
L89.94 Pressure ulcer of unspecified site, stage 4
Healing pressure ulcer of unspecified site, stage 4
Pressure ulcer with necrosis of soft tissues through to underlying muscle, tendon, or bone, unspecified site
L89.95 Pressure ulcer of unspecified site, unstageable

[4] L90 Atrophic disorders of skin
L90.0 Lichen sclerosus et atrophicus
[EXCLUDES2] *lichen sclerosus of external female genital organs (N90.4)*
lichen sclerosus of external male genital organs (N48.0)
L90.1 Anetoderma of Schweninger-Buzzi
L90.2 Anetoderma of Jadassohn-Pellizzari
L90.3 Atrophoderma of Pasini and Pierini
L90.4 Acrodermatitis chronica atrophicans
L90.5 Scar conditions and fibrosis of skin
Adherent scar (skin)
Cicatrix
Disfigurement of skin due to scar
Fibrosis of skin NOS
Scar NOS
[EXCLUDES2] *hypertrophic scar (L91.0)*
keloid scar (L91.0)
L90.6 Striae atrophicae
L90.8 Other atrophic disorders of skin
L90.9 Atrophic disorder of skin, unspecified

[4] L91 Hypertrophic disorders of skin
L91.0 Hypertrophic scar
Keloid
Keloid scar
[EXCLUDES2] *acne keloid (L73.0)*
scar NOS (L90.5)
L91.8 Other hypertrophic disorders of the skin
L91.9 Hypertrophic disorder of the skin, unspecified

[4] L92 Granulomatous disorders of skin and subcutaneous tissue
[EXCLUDES2] *actinic granuloma (L57.5)*
L92.0 Granuloma annulare
Perforating granuloma annulare
L92.1 Necrobiosis lipoidica, not elsewhere classified
[EXCLUDES1] *necrobiosis lipoidica associated with diabetes mellitus (E08-E13 with .620)*
L92.2 Granuloma faciale [eosinophilic granuloma of skin]
L92.3 Foreign body granuloma of the skin and subcutaneous tissue
Use additional code to identify the type of retained foreign body (Z18.-)
L92.8 Other granulomatous disorders of the skin and subcutaneous tissue
L92.9 Granulomatous disorder of the skin and subcutaneous tissue, unspecified

[4] L93 Lupus erythematosus
Use additional code for adverse effect, if applicable, to identify drug (T36-T50 with fifth or sixth character 5)
[EXCLUDES1] *lupus exedens (A18.4)*
lupus vulgaris (A18.4)
scleroderma (M34.-)
systemic lupus erythematosus (M32.-)
L93.0 Discoid lupus erythematosus
Lupus erythematosus NOS
L93.1 Subacute cutaneous lupus erythematosus
L93.2 Other local lupus erythematosus
Lupus erythematosus profundus
Lupus panniculitis

[4] L94 Other localized connective tissue disorders
[EXCLUDES1] *systemic connective tissue disorders (M30-M36)*
L94.0 Localized scleroderma [morphea]
Circumscribed scleroderma
L94.1 Linear scleroderma
En coup de sabre lesion
L94.2 Calcinosis cutis
L94.3 Sclerodactyly
L94.4 Gottron's papules
L94.5 Poikiloderma vasculare atrophicans
L94.6 Ainhum
L94.8 Other specified localized connective tissue disorders
L94.9 Localized connective tissue disorder, unspecified

[4] L95 Vasculitis limited to skin, not elsewhere classified
[EXCLUDES1] *angioma serpiginosum (L81.7)*
Henoch(-Schönlein) purpura (D69.0)
hypersensitivity angiitis (M31.0)
lupus panniculitis (L93.2)
panniculitis NOS (M79.3)
panniculitis of neck and back (M54.0-)
polyarteritis nodosa (M30.0)
relapsing panniculitis (M35.6)
rheumatoid vasculitis (M05.2)
serum sickness (T80.6-)
urticaria (L50.-)
Wegener's granulomatosis (M31.3-)

Unspecified Code | Other Specified Code | [N] Newborn Age: 0 | [P] Pediatric Age: 0-17 | [M] Maternity Age: 12-55
[A] Adult Age: 15-124 | ♂ Male | ♀ Female | ● New Code | ▲ Revised Code Title | ►◄ Revised Text

L95.0 Livedoid vasculitis
Atrophie blanche (en plaque)
L95.1 Erythema elevatum diutinum
L95.8 Other vasculitis limited to the skin
L95.9 Vasculitis limited to the skin, unspecified

[4] L97 Non-pressure chronic ulcer of lower limb, not elsewhere classified

INCLUDES *chronic ulcer of skin of lower limb NOS*
non-healing ulcer of skin
non-infected sinus of skin
trophic ulcer NOS
tropical ulcer NOS
ulcer of skin of lower limb NOS

Code first any associated underlying condition, such as:
any associated gangrene (I96)
atherosclerosis of the lower extremities (I70.23-, I70.24-, I70.33-, I70.34-, I70.43-, I70.44-, I70.53-, I70.54-, I70.63-, I70.64-, I70.73-, I70.74-)
chronic venous hypertension (I87.31-, I87.33-)
diabetic ulcers (E08.621, E08.622, E09.621, E09.622, E10.621, E10.622, E11.621, E11.622, E13.621, E13.622)
postphlebitic syndrome (I87.01-, I87.03-)
postthrombotic syndrome (I87.01-, I87.03-)
varicose ulcer (I83.0-, I83.2-)

EXCLUDES2 *pressure ulcer (pressure area) (L89.-)*
skin infections (L00-L08)
specific infections classified to A00-B99

[5] L97.1 Non-pressure chronic ulcer of thigh

[6] L97.10 Non-pressure chronic ulcer of unspecified thigh
L97.101 Non-pressure chronic ulcer of unspecified thigh limited to breakdown of skin
L97.102 Non-pressure chronic ulcer of unspecified thigh with fat layer exposed
L97.103 Non-pressure chronic ulcer of unspecified thigh with necrosis of muscle
L97.104 Non-pressure chronic ulcer of unspecified thigh with necrosis of bone
L97.109 Non-pressure chronic ulcer of unspecified thigh with unspecified severity

[6] L97.11 Non-pressure chronic ulcer of right thigh
L97.111 Non-pressure chronic ulcer of right thigh limited to breakdown of skin
L97.112 Non-pressure chronic ulcer of right thigh with fat layer exposed
L97.113 Non-pressure chronic ulcer of right thigh with necrosis of muscle
L97.114 Non-pressure chronic ulcer of right thigh with necrosis of bone
L97.119 Non-pressure chronic ulcer of right thigh with unspecified severity

[6] L97.12 Non-pressure chronic ulcer of left thigh
L97.121 Non-pressure chronic ulcer of left thigh limited to breakdown of skin
L97.122 Non-pressure chronic ulcer of left thigh with fat layer exposed
L97.123 Non-pressure chronic ulcer of left thigh with necrosis of muscle
L97.124 Non-pressure chronic ulcer of left thigh with necrosis of bone
L97.129 Non-pressure chronic ulcer of left thigh with unspecified severity

[5] L97.2 Non-pressure chronic ulcer of calf

[6] L97.20 Non-pressure chronic ulcer of unspecified calf
L97.201 Non-pressure chronic ulcer of unspecified calf limited to breakdown of skin
L97.202 Non-pressure chronic ulcer of unspecified calf with fat layer exposed
L97.203 Non-pressure chronic ulcer of unspecified calf with necrosis of muscle
L97.204 Non-pressure chronic ulcer of unspecified calf with necrosis of bone
L97.209 Non-pressure chronic ulcer of unspecified calf with unspecified severity

[6] L97.21 Non-pressure chronic ulcer of right calf
L97.211 Non-pressure chronic ulcer of right calf limited to breakdown of skin
L97.212 Non-pressure chronic ulcer of right calf with fat layer exposed
L97.213 Non-pressure chronic ulcer of right calf with necrosis of muscle
L97.214 Non-pressure chronic ulcer of right calf with necrosis of bone
L97.219 Non-pressure chronic ulcer of right calf with unspecified severity

[6] L97.22 Non-pressure chronic ulcer of left calf
L97.221 Non-pressure chronic ulcer of left calf limited to breakdown of skin
L97.222 Non-pressure chronic ulcer of left calf with fat layer exposed
L97.223 Non-pressure chronic ulcer of left calf with necrosis of muscle
L97.224 Non-pressure chronic ulcer of left calf with necrosis of bone
L97.229 Non-pressure chronic ulcer of left calf with unspecified severity

[5] L97.3 Non-pressure chronic ulcer of ankle

[6] L97.30 Non-pressure chronic ulcer of unspecified ankle
L97.301 Non-pressure chronic ulcer of unspecified ankle limited to breakdown of skin
L97.302 Non-pressure chronic ulcer of unspecified ankle with fat layer exposed
L97.303 Non-pressure chronic ulcer of unspecified ankle with necrosis of muscle
L97.304 Non-pressure chronic ulcer of unspecified ankle with necrosis of bone
L97.309 Non-pressure chronic ulcer of unspecified ankle with unspecified severity

[6] L97.31 Non-pressure chronic ulcer of right ankle
L97.311 Non-pressure chronic ulcer of right ankle limited to breakdown of skin
L97.312 Non-pressure chronic ulcer of right ankle with fat layer exposed
L97.313 Non-pressure chronic ulcer of right ankle with necrosis of muscle
L97.314 Non-pressure chronic ulcer of right ankle with necrosis of bone
L97.319 Non-pressure chronic ulcer of right ankle with unspecified severity

[6] L97.32 Non-pressure chronic ulcer of left ankle
L97.321 Non-pressure chronic ulcer of left ankle limited to breakdown of skin
L97.322 Non-pressure chronic ulcer of left ankle with fat layer exposed
L97.323 Non-pressure chronic ulcer of left ankle with necrosis of muscle
L97.324 Non-pressure chronic ulcer of left ankle with necrosis of bone
L97.329 Non-pressure chronic ulcer of left ankle with unspecified severity

[5] L97.4 Non-pressure chronic ulcer of heel and midfoot
Non-pressure chronic ulcer of plantar surface of midfoot

[6] L97.40 Non-pressure chronic ulcer of unspecified heel and midfoot
L97.401 Non-pressure chronic ulcer of unspecified heel and midfoot limited to breakdown of skin
L97.402 Non-pressure chronic ulcer of unspecified heel and midfoot with fat layer exposed

[4] 4th character required [5] 5th character required [6] 6th character required [7] 7th character required [7X] Extension 'X' Alert
EXCLUDES1 Not coded here EXCLUDES2 Not included here [PDx] Primary Diagnosis Only Manifestation Code

L97.403 Non-pressure chronic ulcer of unspecified heel and midfoot with necrosis of muscle
L97.404 Non-pressure chronic ulcer of unspecified heel and midfoot with necrosis of bone
L97.409 Non-pressure chronic ulcer of unspecified heel and midfoot with unspecified severity

[6] L97.41 Non-pressure chronic ulcer of right heel and midfoot
L97.411 Non-pressure chronic ulcer of right heel and midfoot limited to breakdown of skin
L97.412 Non-pressure chronic ulcer of right heel and midfoot with fat layer exposed
L97.413 Non-pressure chronic ulcer of right heel and midfoot with necrosis of muscle
L97.414 Non-pressure chronic ulcer of right heel and midfoot with necrosis of bone
L97.419 Non-pressure chronic ulcer of right heel and midfoot with unspecified severity

[6] L97.42 Non-pressure chronic ulcer of left heel and midfoot
L97.421 Non-pressure chronic ulcer of left heel and midfoot limited to breakdown of skin
L97.422 Non-pressure chronic ulcer of left heel and midfoot with fat layer exposed
L97.423 Non-pressure chronic ulcer of left heel and midfoot with necrosis of muscle
L97.424 Non-pressure chronic ulcer of left heel and midfoot with necrosis of bone
L97.429 Non-pressure chronic ulcer of left heel and midfoot with unspecified severity

[5] L97.5 Non-pressure chronic ulcer of other part of foot
Non-pressure chronic ulcer of toe

[6] L97.50 Non-pressure chronic ulcer of other part of unspecified foot
L97.501 Non-pressure chronic ulcer of other part of unspecified foot limited to breakdown of skin
L97.502 Non-pressure chronic ulcer of other part of unspecified foot with fat layer exposed
L97.503 Non-pressure chronic ulcer of other part of unspecified foot with necrosis of muscle
L97.504 Non-pressure chronic ulcer of other part of unspecified foot with necrosis of bone
L97.509 Non-pressure chronic ulcer of other part of unspecified foot with unspecified severity

[6] L97.51 Non-pressure chronic ulcer of other part of right foot
L97.511 Non-pressure chronic ulcer of other part of right foot limited to breakdown of skin
L97.512 Non-pressure chronic ulcer of other part of right foot with fat layer exposed
L97.513 Non-pressure chronic ulcer of other part of right foot with necrosis of muscle
L97.514 Non-pressure chronic ulcer of other part of right foot with necrosis of bone
L97.519 Non-pressure chronic ulcer of other part of right foot with unspecified severity

[6] L97.52 Non-pressure chronic ulcer of other part of left foot
L97.521 Non-pressure chronic ulcer of other part of left foot limited to breakdown of skin
L97.522 Non-pressure chronic ulcer of other part of left foot with fat layer exposed
L97.523 Non-pressure chronic ulcer of other part of left foot with necrosis of muscle
L97.524 Non-pressure chronic ulcer of other part of left foot with necrosis of bone
L97.529 Non-pressure chronic ulcer of other part of left foot with unspecified severity

[5] L97.8 Non-pressure chronic ulcer of other part of lower leg

[6] L97.80 Non-pressure chronic ulcer of other part of unspecified lower leg
L97.801 Non-pressure chronic ulcer of other part of unspecified lower leg limited to breakdown of skin
L97.802 Non-pressure chronic ulcer of other part of unspecified lower leg with fat layer exposed
L97.803 Non-pressure chronic ulcer of other part of unspecified lower leg with necrosis of muscle
L97.804 Non-pressure chronic ulcer of other part of unspecified lower leg with necrosis of bone
L97.809 Non-pressure chronic ulcer of other part of unspecified lower leg with unspecified severity

[6] L97.81 Non-pressure chronic ulcer of other part of right lower leg
L97.811 Non-pressure chronic ulcer of other part of right lower leg limited to breakdown of skin
L97.812 Non-pressure chronic ulcer of other part of right lower leg with fat layer exposed
L97.813 Non-pressure chronic ulcer of other part of right lower leg with necrosis of muscle
L97.814 Non-pressure chronic ulcer of other part of right lower leg with necrosis of bone
L97.819 Non-pressure chronic ulcer of other part of right lower leg with unspecified severity

[6] L97.82 Non-pressure chronic ulcer of other part of left lower leg
L97.821 Non-pressure chronic ulcer of other part of left lower leg limited to breakdown of skin
L97.822 Non-pressure chronic ulcer of other part of left lower leg with fat layer exposed
L97.823 Non-pressure chronic ulcer of other part of left lower leg with necrosis of muscle
L97.824 Non-pressure chronic ulcer of other part of left lower leg with necrosis of bone
L97.829 Non-pressure chronic ulcer of other part of left lower leg with unspecified severity

[5] L97.9 Non-pressure chronic ulcer of unspecified part of lower leg

[6] L97.90 Non-pressure chronic ulcer of unspecified part of unspecified lower leg
L97.901 Non-pressure chronic ulcer of unspecified part of unspecified lower leg limited to breakdown of skin
L97.902 Non-pressure chronic ulcer of unspecified part of unspecified lower leg with fat layer exposed
L97.903 Non-pressure chronic ulcer of unspecified part of unspecified lower leg with necrosis of muscle
L97.904 Non-pressure chronic ulcer of unspecified part of unspecified lower leg with necrosis of bone
L97.909 Non-pressure chronic ulcer of unspecified part of unspecified lower leg with unspecified severity

[6] L97.91 Non-pressure chronic ulcer of unspecified part of right lower leg
L97.911 Non-pressure chronic ulcer of unspecified part of right lower leg limited to breakdown of skin
L97.912 Non-pressure chronic ulcer of unspecified part of right lower leg with fat layer exposed
L97.913 Non-pressure chronic ulcer of unspecified part of right lower leg with necrosis of muscle

Unspecified Code | Other Specified Code | [N] Newborn Age: 0 | [P] Pediatric Age: 0-17 | [M] Maternity Age: 12-55
[A] Adult Age: 15-124 | ♂ Male | ♀ Female | ● New Code | ▲ Revised Code Title | ►◄ Revised Text

L97.914 **Non-pressure chronic ulcer of unspecified part of right lower leg** with necrosis of bone

L97.919 **Non-pressure chronic ulcer of unspecified part of right lower leg** with unspecified severity

⑥ L97.92 **Non-pressure chronic ulcer of** unspecified part of left lower leg

L97.921 **Non-pressure chronic ulcer of unspecified part of left lower leg** limited to breakdown of skin

L97.922 **Non-pressure chronic ulcer of unspecified part of left lower leg** with fat layer exposed

L97.923 **Non-pressure chronic ulcer of unspecified part of left lower leg** with necrosis of muscle

L97.924 **Non-pressure chronic ulcer of unspecified part of left lower leg** with necrosis of bone

L97.929 **Non-pressure chronic ulcer of unspecified part of left lower leg** with unspecified severity

④ L98 **Other disorders of skin and subcutaneous tissue, not elsewhere classified**

L98.0 **Pyogenic granuloma**

EXCLUDES2 *pyogenic granuloma of gingiva (K06.8)*
pyogenic granuloma of maxillary alveolar ridge (K04.5)
pyogenic granuloma of oral mucosa (K13.4)

L98.1 **Factitial dermatitis**

Neurotic excoriation

L98.2 **Febrile neutrophilic dermatosis [Sweet]**

L98.3 **Eosinophilic cellulitis [Wells]**

⑤ L98.4 **Non-pressure chronic ulcer of skin, not elsewhere classified**

Chronic ulcer of skin NOS
Tropical ulcer NOS
Ulcer of skin NOS

EXCLUDES2 *pressure ulcer (pressure area) (L89.-)*
gangrene (I96)
skin infections (L00-L08)
specific infections classified to A00-B99
ulcer of lower limb NEC (L97.-)
varicose ulcer (I83.0-I82.2)

⑥ L98.41 **Non-pressure chronic ulcer of** buttock

L98.411 **Non-pressure chronic ulcer of buttock** limited to breakdown of skin

L98.412 **Non-pressure chronic ulcer of buttock** with fat layer exposed

L98.413 **Non-pressure chronic ulcer of buttock** with necrosis of muscle

L98.414 **Non-pressure chronic ulcer of buttock** with necrosis of bone

L98.419 **Non-pressure chronic ulcer of buttock** with unspecified severity

⑥ L98.42 **Non-pressure chronic ulcer of** back

L98.421 **Non-pressure chronic ulcer of back** limited to breakdown of skin

L98.422 **Non-pressure chronic ulcer of back** with fat layer exposed

L98.423 **Non-pressure chronic ulcer of back** with necrosis of muscle

L98.424 **Non-pressure chronic ulcer of back** with necrosis of bone

L98.429 **Non-pressure chronic ulcer of back** with unspecified severity

⑥ L98.49 **Non-pressure chronic ulcer of skin of** other sites

Non-pressure chronic ulcer of skin NOS

L98.491 **Non-pressure chronic ulcer of skin of other sites** limited to breakdown of skin

L98.492 **Non-pressure chronic ulcer of skin of other sites** with fat layer exposed

L98.493 **Non-pressure chronic ulcer of skin of other sites** with necrosis of muscle

L98.494 **Non-pressure chronic ulcer of skin of other sites** with necrosis of bone

L98.499 **Non-pressure chronic ulcer of skin of other sites** with unspecified severity

L98.5 **Mucinosis of the skin**

Focal mucinosis
Lichen myxedematosus

EXCLUDES1 *focal oral mucinosis (K13.79)*
myxedema (E03.9)

Reticular erythematous mucinosis

L98.6 **Other infiltrative disorders of the skin and subcutaneous tissue**

EXCLUDES1 *hyalinosis cutis et mucosae (E78.89)*

L98.8 **Other specified disorders of the skin and subcutaneous tissue**

L98.9 **Disorder of the skin and subcutaneous tissue, unspecified**

L99 **Other disorders of skin and subcutaneous tissue in diseases classified elsewhere**

Code first underlying disease, such as:
amyloidosis (E85.-)

EXCLUDES1 *skin disorders in diabetes (E08-E13 with .62)*
skin disorders in gonorrhea (A54.89)
skin disorders in syphilis (A51.31, A52.79)

---

④ 4th character required   ⑤ 5th character required   ⑥ 6th character required   ⑦ 7th character required   ⑩ Extension 'X' Alert

EXCLUDES 1 Not coded here   *EXCLUDES 2* Not included here   PDx Primary Diagnosis Only   Manifestation Code

ICD-10-CM 2015

Chapter 13: Diseases of the Musculoskeletal System and Connective Tissue (M00-M99)

Chapter Specific Coding Guidelines

a. **Site and Laterality**

Most of the codes within Chapter 13 have site and laterality designations. The site represents the bone, joint or the muscle involved. For some conditions where more than one bone, joint or muscle is usually involved, such as osteoarthritis, there is a "multiple sites" code available. For categories where no multiple site code is provided and more than one bone, joint or muscle is involved, multiple codes should be used to indicate the different sites involved.

1) **Bone versus joint**

For certain conditions, the bone may be affected at the upper or lower end, (e.g., avascular necrosis of bone, M87, Osteoporosis, M80, M81). Though the portion of the bone affected may be at the joint, the site designation will be the bone, not the joint.

b. **Acute Traumatic Versus Chronic or Recurrent Musculoskeletal Conditions**

Many musculoskeletal conditions are a result of previous injury or trauma to a site, or are recurrent conditions. Bone, joint or muscle conditions that are the result of a healed injury are usually found in chapter 13. Recurrent bone, joint or muscle conditions are also usually found in chapter 13. Any current, acute injury should be coded to the appropriate injury code from chapter 19. Chronic or recurrent conditions should generally be coded with a code from chapter 13. If it is difficult to determine from the documentation in the record which code is best to describe a condition, query the provider.

c. **Coding of Pathologic Fractures**

7th character A is for use as long as the patient is receiving active treatment for the fracture. Examples of active treatment are: surgical treatment, emergency department encounter, evaluation and treatment by a new physician. 7th character, D is to be used for encounters after the patient has completed active treatment. The other 7th characters, listed under each subcategory in the Tabular List, are to be used for subsequent encounters for treatment of problems associated with the healing, such as malunions, nonunions, and sequelae.

Care for complications of surgical treatment for fracture repairs during the healing or recovery phase should be coded with the appropriate complication codes.

See Section I.C.19. Coding of traumatic fractures.

d. **Osteoporosis**

Osteoporosis is a systemic condition, meaning that all bones of the musculoskeletal system are affected. Therefore, site is not a component of the codes under category M81, Osteoporosis without current pathological fracture. The site codes under category M80, Osteoporosis with current pathological fracture, identify the site of the fracture, not the osteoporosis.

1) **Osteoporosis without pathological fracture**

Category M81, Osteoporosis without current pathological fracture, is for use for patients with osteoporosis who do not currently have a pathologic fracture due to the osteoporosis, even if they have had a fracture in the past. For patients with a history of osteoporosis fractures, status code Z87.310, Personal history of (healed) osteoporosis fracture, should follow the code from M81.

2) **Osteoporosis with current pathological fracture**

Category M80, Osteoporosis with current pathological fracture, is for patients who have a current pathologic fracture at the time of an encounter. The codes under M80 identify the site of the fracture. A code from category M80, not a traumatic fracture code, should be used for any patient with known osteoporosis who suffers a fracture, even if the patient had a minor fall or trauma, if that fall or trauma would not usually break a normal, healthy bone.

This page intentionally left blank

Anatomy of the Musculoskeletal System

Introduction

Osteology (Osteo: bone; logy: study) is the branch of anatomy that deals with the detailed analysis of structure, function and diseases of the skeletal elements. It constitutes the bony framework of the body. Human bony skeleton is composed of the below mentioned components (and is derived from the mesoderm, which is the primary germ cell layer).

Skeletal Region	Body Structure	Quantity of bones
Axial Skeleton (The trunk)	Skull	22
	Hyoid Bone	1
	Ribs & Sternum	25
	Vertebral Column	26
Appendicular Skeleton (The limbs)	Upper Extremities	64
	Lower Extremities	62
Auditory Ossicles		6

1. **Structure of a Normal Human Bone:** Bone comprises of a rigid structure, which is based on dense connective tissue. A normal human bone is made up of the following essential macro and micro elements:
   a) Periosteum
   b) Medullary Membrane
   c) Marrow
   d) Blood Vessels and Nerves of Bone
   e) Haversian Canals (Canals of Havers)
   f) Lamellae
   g) Lacunae
   h) Canaliculi
   i) Perichondrium
   j) Osteoblasts
   k) Osteoclasts
   l) Medullary spaces
   m) Epiphysis
   n) Diaphysis
   o) Metaphysis

2. **The Vertebral Column**
   a) Anatomical Detail: The vertebral column is composed of a continuous series of compact bones that articulate with each other via intervertebral discs, and are called as vertebrae. The structure forms the dorsal aspect of the trunk. The vertebral column is also called as spine. The spinal cord traverses through the spinal canal of the vertebral column. The individual vertebrae remain connected together by intervertebral discs. The cervical, thoracic and lumbar vertebrae are termed as true vertebrae. However, sacral and coccygeal ones are false vertebrae. The concept behind considering them as true or false is based on mobility of the individual vertebrae through intervertebral discs. Cervical, thoracic and lumbar vertebrae are moveable to some extent and therefore, termed as true vertebral bodies. In contrast, sacral-coccygeal section is rather fixed and thus, not categorized as true vertebrae. Each vertebral segment is associated with a portion of spinal cord, which travels the entire vertebral column, and each spinal cord segment has specific physiology and functions. The vertebral bodies communicate with each other through the pads of elastic fibro-cartilage. These flexible pads constitute the intervertebral discs, which help in the movement of vertebral

bodies and provide protection from trauma or shocks. However, the length of the adult vertebral column ranges from 60-70 cm. The entire vertebral column is based on a total of 33 vertebrae that are categorized (below) in accordance with the occupied region.

   i) neck or the cervical region is composed of seven cervical vertebrae.
   ii) back or thorax region contains twelve thoracic vertebrae.
   iii) loin or lumbar region is based on five lumbar vertebrae.
   iv) sacrum forms five (fused) sacral vertebrae.
   v) coccyx (tail) has usually four (fused) coccygeal vertebrae.

   b) Cervical Vertebrae

   These are small and delicate bones, which are marked by the existence of a foramen in every transverse process. The cervical region is based on the seven cervical bones (C1-C7). However, the first cervical vertebra is known as Atlas and the second one is Axis.

   c) Thoracic Vertebrae

   Thoracic vertebrae are 12 in quantity (T1–T12), and communicate with the head (tubercles) of ribs in the thoracic region through articular facets of the transverse processes. Their body structure is similar to the shape of the heart, with nearly circular vertebral foramina.

   d) Lumbar Vertebrae

   These are 5 vertebrae (L1-L5), with kidney shaped body. Lumbar vertebrae are in fact, the most toughest and robust in configuration. These are enlarged in size and marked by the absence of transverse process foramen and vertebral facets. They are true vertebrae, thereby allowing flexion and extension movements via flexible intervertebral discs. Their broad lamellae, large bodies, long transverse processes and strong pedicles make them suitable to support additional body weight as compared to other similar vertebrae.

   e) Sacral Vertebrae

   These are composed of 5 vertebral bodies (S1-S5), which constitute a portion of the pelvic cavity. Sacral vertebral bodies consist of 5 separate segments that get fused together at maturity. As a matter of fact, these vertebrae lack intervertebral discs, which restrict their mobility and put them into the category of false vertebrae.

   f) Coccygeal Vertebrae

   The 4 coccygeal vertebrae constitute the human vestigial tail bone, in which vertebral bodies are fused together without the existence of any intervertebral disc. Movement of the individual vertebral bodies is restricted due to their interfusion. Hence, these are considered as false vertebrae. The number of bones in the coccygeal region may rarely vary between three to five vertebrae, in few individuals.

3. **Thorax; Anatomical Detail**
   The part of the trunk situated between neck and abdomen constitutes the thorax. Thoracic cavity is bounded by ribs, sternum, costal cartilages and the thoracic vertebrae. Thorax is also known as the chest region. The osseocartilagenous cage of the thorax covers and protects the prime organs of circulation and respiration. Furthermore, this osseocartilagenous cage is composed mainly of the ribcage, shoulder girdle and spine.

   The twelve thoracic vertebrae and certain component of the ribs constitute the posterior (back) wall of the thoracic cavity. However, the anterior (front) region is composed of sternum and the costal cartilages. The entire human chest (thorax) region contains multiple organs, muscles, bones, vasculature, internal and external structures. These contents include heart, lungs, thymus, pectoral muscles, scapula, sternum, ribs, aorta, trachea, diaphragm and mammary glands etc.

4. **Sternum (Chest or Breast Bone)**
   a) Sternum: It is a flat and long bone situated in the center of the thorax and forms the midline of anterior thoracic cage. It articulates with both clavicles (collar bones) through its upper ends It is composed of the following three (interfused) components:
      i)   manubrium
      ii) body (gladiolus/corpus sterni)
      iii) xiphoid process (processus xiphoideus/ensiform or xiphoid appendix) ribs.
   b) Ribs are the elongated, flattened, lightweight, resilient and twisted bones that are the essential constituent of thoracic skeleton. The total number of ribs in human body is 24 (12 on each side). The ribs can be classified as follows:
      i)   True Ribs-These are also called as vertebro-sternal ribs. True ribs comprise of the first seven ribs that communicate (to the dorsum) with the vertebral column as well as sternum (in front) via costal cartilages.
      ii) False Ribs-These are also called as vertebro-chondral ribs. False ribs comprise of 8, 9, and10 ribs that are indirectly attached to the sternum through costal cartilages. The individual cartilages of each of these ribs are connected to the cartilage of the rib lying just above them.
      iii) Floating Ribs-These are also termed as vertebral ribs. These ribs include 11th and 12th ribs that are free at their anterior extremities (without any attachment with the sternum) and are connected to the vertebral bodies on their dorsal ends.

5. **The Skull**
   The human skull is based on the skeleton of the head. Several bones of the skull integrate together to form the cranium (or the skull). The skull can be categorized as follows:
   a) The Brain Box or Brain Case (The Calvaria). It constitute the upper cranium and contain the brain.
   b) The Facial Skeleton comprises of the portion of skull (other than the brain box) and includes the mandible bone of face.

The Composition of Human Skull

The Calvaria			
Paired Bones		**Unpaired Bones**	
i)	Parietal	i)	Frontal
ii)	Temporal	ii)	Occipital
		iii)	Sphenoid
		iv)	Ethmoid
The Facial Skeleton			
Paired Bones		**Unpaired Bones**	
iii)	Maxilla	v)	Mandible
iv)	Zygomatic	vi)	Vomer
v)	Nasal		
vi)	Lacrimal		
vii)	Palatine		
viii)	Inferior Nasal Concha		

   c) The Facial Bones- The facial skeleton comprises of the lower and anterior portion of human skull and includes the following bones:
      i)   nasal bones
      ii) maxillae (upper jaw)
      iii) lacrimal bone
      iv) zygomatic bone
      v)   palatine bone
      vi) inferior nasal concha
      vii) vomer
      viii) mandible (lower jaw)
      ix) hyoid bone

6. **The Bones of the Upper Extremity**
   a. Clavicle

      The clavicle is also called as the collar bone that forms the anterior portion of the shoulder girdle. The clavicles are 2 in number and called as the right and left clavicles.

   b. Scapula

      The scapula is also called as shoulder blade and constitutes the back portion of the shoulder girdle. It is a flat bone that articulates with the clavicle and humerus. It also contains a triangular process that projects laterally and is called as the acromion. Additionally, the upper part of the neck of the scapula contains a curved process, which is known as the coracoid process. The scapulae are 2 in number (right and left scapula).

   c. Humerus

      The humerus is the long bone of the arm that begins from shoulder and ends up at elbow. It is the largest bone of the upper extremity and consists of the following major components:
      i)   greater tubercle (greater tuberosity)
      ii)   lesser tubercle (lesser tuberosity)
      iii) body or shaft (corpus humeri)
      iv)   anterior, lateral and medial borders
      v)   medial and lateral epicondyles
      vi)   radial sulcus (musculospiral groove)
      vii) lateral and medial supracondylar ridges
      viii) deltoid tuberosity.

   d. Ulna

      The ulna is one of the two long and prismatic bones of the forearm that extends parallel with the radius. The ulna possesses a body and two extremities. The proximal or upper extremity contains olecranon and coronoid processes, and the semilunar and radial notches respectively. The body or shaft of ulna is also known as corpus ulnae. The lower or distal extremity comprises of an articular eminence (the head of the ulna) and a non-articular eminence (the styloid process).

   e. Radius

      The radius is one of the two long bones of the foerarm that extends laterally with ulna. Its lower end participates in the formation of the wrist joint and upper end helps to create the elbow joint. The upper or proximal extremity comprises of a head, neck, and tuberosity. The body or shaft is also known as corpus radii. The lateral surface of the lower extremity contains a conical projection, which is known as the styloid process.

   f. Carpus

      The carpus region of hand contains the carpal bones, which are based on a total of 8 bones positioned in proximal and distal rows to facilitate uninterrupted movement of the wrist joint. The carpal bones of the proximal row are: navicular, lunate, triangular, and pisiform. The bones of the distal row are: greater multangular, lesser multangular, capitate, and hamate.

   g. Metacarpus

      The metacarpus region of hand is based on cylindrical (metacarpal) bones that are five in number and constitute the intermediary portion of the bony skeleton of hand. The first till fifth metacarpal bones belong to the thumb, index, middle, ring and little fingers respectively.

   h. Phalanges of the Hand

      The phalanges (finger bones) of the hand constitute the fingers. These are 14 in number. Each finger comprises of 3 phalanges. However, the thumb is based on only two phalanges. A single finger bone has a body, with 2 extremities. The finger bones serve to facilitate the basic functions of hand, like-effective grasping of objects and writing etc.

7. **The Bones of the Lower Extremity**
    a. Hip Bone

    The hip bone is also known as the coxal bone. It's based on three components-ilium: ischium, and pubis. The ilium holds the flank and it's the broad portion situated on top of the large cup-shaped articular cavity, the acetabulum. The ischium forms the lower back part of the hip bone that facilitates sitting. It's located downward from the acetabulum and is the strongest component of the hip bone containing an enlarged opening, the obturator foramen. The pubis is the lower frontal portion of the hip bone, which is located medially below the acetabulum. It supports the external organs of generation. The angle across the pubic symphysis is known as the pubic arch.

    b. Pelvis

    The pelvis comprises of a bony ring that provides a connecting medium between the vertebral column and femurs. It is based on the following 4 bones:

    i)   The hip bones-2 in number.
    ii) The sacrum-The fused vertebrae that are 5 in number, and connected to the hip bones.
    iii) The coccyx-The fused vertebrae that are 4 in number, and constitute the tailbone.

    The space surrounded by the pelvic girdle is known as the pelvic cavity. The pelvic girdle bears the entire weight of the trunk and upper body while sitting, and transfers this weight to the lower limbs during standing, walking or running.

    c. Femur

    The femur is one of the two largest, longest and strongest bones in the human skeleton that bears the load of the upper body via pelvis in standing, walking or running. It also participates in the formation of the hip and knee joints. The components of a normal femur bone are as follows:

    The Upper (Proximal) Extremity comprises of the following elements:

    i)   Head
    ii) Neck
    iii) Greater Trochanter
    iv) Lesser Trochanter

    The Body or Shaft-The body is cylindrical in shape, lies between the upper and   lower extremities, and is also known as corpus femoris.

    The Lower (Distal) Extremity -The distal extremity is based on two projections (the lateral and medial condyles). These projections (condyles) are separated in front by an articular depression, known as the patellar surface. The same condyles are further interrupted from behind by a deep pit, which is termed as the intercondyloid fossa.

    d. Patella

    The knee cap (patella) is a flat, thick, circular-triangular and dense cancellous articular bone that is situated on the frontal portion of the knee joint. The superior border is thick and forms the base of patella. The patella is further marked by medial and lateral borders. The apex of patella is a pointed region that provides attachment to the patellar ligament. The patella articulates with the femur through patellofemoral joint.

    e. Tibia

    The tibia (shin bone) is located medially in the lower leg and is regarded as the largest and strongest bone of the skeleton after femur. It also participates in the formation of the knee and ankle joints. The tibia is composed of the following elements:

    i)   upper (proximal) end – The proximal extremity is composed of the projections, which are known as the medial and lateral condyles. The condylar surfaces further merge to form an eminence on the frontal side, which is known as the tibial tuberosity.

    ii) body or shaft of tibia – The shaft of tibia is also known as corpus tibiae and contains the anterior crest (or border), the medial border and the interosseous crest (or lateral border).

    iii) lower (distal) end – The distal extremity contains the inferior articular surface, the anterior surface, the posterior surface, the lateral surface and the medial surface. However, the medial surface extends medially to form a pyrimidal process, which is termed as the medial malleolus.

    f. Fibula

    The fibula (calf bone) is located laterally in the lower leg and runs laterally with the adjacent shin bone (tibia). It's a thin and slender bone which is composed of a body with upper and lower extremities. The lower or distal extremity constitutes the lateral malleolus, which is also known as the external malleolus or malleolus lateralis.

    g. Tarsus

    The tarsus region of foot is based on the following seven tarsal bones:

    i)   calcaneus
    ii) talus
    iii) cuboid
    iv) navicular
    v)   three cuneiforms the metatarsus

    h. Phalanges of the Foot

    The phalanges of the foot constitute the region of forefoot. These are also known as the toe bones. The great toe (hallux) contains 2 phalanges (proximal and distal). The proximal and distal phalangeal bones of the great toe articulate with each other to form the first interphalangeal joint. The proximal phalanges of the other 4 toes articulate with their respective metatarsal heads to form the metatarsophalangeal joints.

8. **Introduction of Syndesmology (The Articulations or Joints)**
    Syndesmology is defined as the branch of anatomy that deals with the joints and their components (including ligaments). The junctions of bones, where multiple parts of the individual bones connect together are called as articulations or joints. These articulations are further supported by sheets of tough fibrous tissue that connect the joint bones together, and are termed as the ligaments. Various components of the joints are listed below:

    a) Bones
    b) Cartilages

    The cartilages are flexible non-vascluar structures composed of connective tissue and found mainly in joints. A cartilage can be categorized into the following elements:

    c) Hyaline cartilage
    d) White fibrocartilage

    The white fibrocartilage can further be categorized into four subcategories:

    i)   interarticular fibrocartilage
    ii) connecting fibrocartilage
    iii) circumferential fibrocartilage
    iv) stratiform fibrocartilage

    e) Yellow or elastic fibrocartilage
    f) Articular Capsule

    The articular capsule is also known as the joint capsule that completely covers and protects the freely movable (synovial) joints.

    g) Mucous Sheaths

    The mucous sheaths cover a part of the fibroosseous canals and surface of the tendons that glide upon these canals, to facilitate the movement of these tendons on their respective canals.

9. **Classification of Joints**
   The joints can be classified into the following three classes:
   a) Synarthroses (Immovable Joints)
   b) Amphiarthroses (Slightly Movable Joints)
   c) Diarthroses (Freely Movable Joints)

10. **Joints of the Trunk**
   a) Joints between Vertebral Bodies

   The articulations between the individual vertebral bodies are based on the amphiarthrodial (slightly movable) intervertebral joints that possess only a very slight degree of mobility.

   b) Joints between Vertebral Arches

   The articulations between the individual vertebral arches are carried out through the two pairs of articular processes. The articular processes of a typical vertebral arch connect together with the articular processes of the adjacent vertebral arch to form true diarthrosis of arthrodial variety.

   c) Joints of the Atlas with the Axis

   The atlas forms three diarthroses with the axis. Moreover, the articulations of the axis with the atlas are known as the Atlantoaxial articulations.

   d) Joints of the Vertebral Column with the Cranium

   The atlas forms two articulations (known as diarthrosis) with the occipital bone. The occipital condyles interact with the articular surfaces of the atlas to constitute diarthoses. The synovial stratum covers the articular capsules around the condyles of the occipital bone.

   e) Joints of the Mandible

   The temporomandibular articulation forms an arthrodial diarthrosis. The temporal mandibular fossa and mandibular condyle interact together to constitute the temporomandibular articulation.

   f) Joints of the Ribs with the Vertebrae

   The head and tubercle of a typical rib articulates with the vertebral column to form a costovertebral articulation.

   g) Joints of the Vertebral Column with the Pelvis

   The fifth lumbar vertebra connects with the sacrum to form the lumbosacral articulation. The inner lip of the iliac crest connects with the transverse processes of the fifth lumbar vertebra through iliolumbar ligament.

   h) Joints of the Pelvis

   The articulations of the pelvis are mainly based on the following types of joints:

   i) symphysis pubis

   The two pubic bones articulate with each other to constitute a joint, which is known as the symphysis pubis.

   ii) sacroiliac articulation

   The auricular surfaces of sacrum and ilium connect with each other to form an amphiarthrodial joint, which is termed as the sacroiliac articulation.

   iii) sacrococcygeal symphysis

   The apex of the sacrum and base of the coccyx articulate with each other to form an amphiarthrodial joint, which is known as the sacrococcygeal symphysis.

11. **Joints of Upper Extremity**
   a) The Acromioclavicular Joint

   The medial aspect of the acromion (of the scapula) connects with the acromial end of the clavicle to constitute the acromioclavicular articulation. However, this type of joint is categorized as an arthrodial diarthrosis.

   b) The Shoulder Joint

   The humeral articulation constitutes the shoulder joint, which is an enarthrodial (ball and socket) joint and considered as the largest joint of the upper limb. The shoulder joint offers an extended range of movement and is composed of the articular head of humerus and the shallow glenoid cavity of the scapula. The ligaments of the shoulder joint include the articular capsule (capsular ligament), glenoid labrum (glenoid ligament) as well as the glenohumeral, coracohumeral and transverse humeral ligaments.

   c) The Elbow Joint

   The elbow articulation falls under the category of hinge joint (ginglymus diarthrosis). The elbow joint performs the flexion and extension movements around a transversely placed single axis. The elbow joint comprises of the humerus, ulna and radius bones. An elbow joint is formed when the trochlea of humerus connects with the semilunar notch of ulna and the capitulum of humerus interacts with the cup (shallow-depression or fovea) on the proximal aspect of the head of radius. The articular surfaces of the elbow joint are enclosed by and interact with each other through a well defined articular capsule.

   d) The Radioulnar Joint

   The radioulnar joint is based on two articulations positioned at the proximal and distal ends of the radius and ulna. These articulations facilitate the rotational movements of the radius around its longitudnal axis to constitute a uniaxial diarthrosis, which is known as lateral ginglymus.

   e) The Radiocarpal Joint

   The radiocarpal articulation is also known as the wrist joint, which is a type of condyloid articulation. The distal (lower) end of radius, discus articularis (the articular disc), proximal articular surfaces of navicular, lunate and triquetral bones (including their interosseous ligaments) together constitute the wrist articulation. Moreover, the wrist joint is completely encapsulated by the articular capsule.

   f) The Intercarpal Joint

   The carpal joints are based on the articulations between the carpal bones with limited range of movement. These joints comprise of the arthrodial diarthroses, and are therefore known as the gliding joints. The carpal bone articulations are characterized as follows:

   i) Proximal Row (Carpal) Joint
   ii) Distal Row (Carpal) Joint
   iii) Transverse (Carpal) Joint

   g) The Carpometacarpal joint

   The Carpometacarpal (CMC) joints are based on the interaction between the carpal and metacarpal bones. However, the carpometacarpal articulation of the thumb region differs from the articulations of the other four metacarpal bones with the carpus. Therefore, the carpometacarpal articulations can be categorized as follows:

   h) The Joints of the other Four Metacarpal Bones with the Carpus

   These types of carpometacarpal articulations are formed by the connections between the bases of the second, third, fourth, and fifth medial metacarpal bones and the four bones of the distal carpal row.

   i) The Intermetacarpal Joints

   The four medial metacarpal bones articulate with each other to form the arthrodial diarthroses, which are known as the intermetacarpal joints.

   j) The Metacarpophalangeal Joints

   With the exception of the thumb, the spherical head of each metacarpal bone articulates with the shallow oval cavity on the base of the first phalanx to constitute the metacarpophalangeal joints. The metacarpophalangeal articulations facilitate flexion, extension, adduction, abduction, and circumduction type of joint movements.

   k) The Joints of the Digits

   The interphalangeal joints are categorized as hinge joints that are two in number for each finger and only one for the thumb.

The interphalangeal joints can perform movements like flexion and extension.

12. Joints of the Lower Extremity

a) The Hip Joint

The coxal articulation constitutes the hip joint, which is a type of enarthrodial diarthrosis (ball and socket joint). The articular surfaces of the hip joint comprise of the head of the femur and a cup shaped cavity (acetabulum) that connect together to constitute the coxal articulation. The hip joint can perform multi-axial movements like rotation, flexion, extension, abduction and adduction. The hip joint cavity is completely encapsulated by an articular capsule or the capsular ligament. Other ligaments of the hip joint are described below:

i) iliofemoral ligament (ligamentum iliofemorale/Y-ligament/ligament of Bigelow)

ii) pubocapsular ligament (ligamentum pubocapsulare/pubofemoral ligament)

iii) ischiocapsular ligament (ligamentum ischiocapsulare/ischiocapsular band/ligament of Bertin)

iv) ligamentum teres femoris

v) glenoidal labrum (labrum glenoidale/cotyloid ligament)

vi) transverse acetabular ligament (ligamentum transversum acetabuli/transverse ligament)

b) The Knee Joint

The knee articulation/joint is considered as the largest articulation in the human body and related to the ginglymus (hinge) variety of diarthroses. However, its structure is much elaborate and complicated. The articular surfaces of the knee joint pertain to specific portions of the femur, tibia and patella bones. The ligaments associated with the knee joint are as follows:

i) articular capsule (capsula articularis/capsular ligament)

ii) ligamentum patellae (anterior ligament)

iii) oblique popliteal ligament (ligamentum popliteum obliquum/posterior ligament)

iv) tibial collateral ligament (ligamentum collaterale tibiale/internal lateral ligament)

v) fibular collateral ligament (ligamentum collaterale fibulare/external lateral or long external lateral ligament)

vi) anterior cruciate ligament (ligamentum cruciatum anterius/external crucial ligament)

vii) posterior cruciate ligament (ligamentum cruciatum posterius/internal crucial ligament)

viii) medial meniscus (meniscus medialis/internal semilunar fibrocartilage)

ix) lateral meniscus (meniscus lateralis/external semilunar fibrocartilage)

x) transverse ligament (ligamentum transversum genu)

xi) coronary ligaments

xii) synovial membrane encapsulates the upper border of the patella and the lower portion of the front of femur. The movements associated with the knee joint are flexion, extension, internal and external rotation.

c) The Joints between Tibia and Fibula

The articulations between the tibia and fibula constitute the tibiofibular joints. The fibula articulates with the tibia through its proximal and distal ends. The proximal tibiofibular joint is an arthrodial articulation between head of fibula and lateral condyle of tibia. The interosseous membrane acts as an accessory ligament to bind the shafts of tibia and fibula together. However, the tibiofibular syndesmosis constitutes the distal tibiofibular joint, which presents a series of ligaments that are accessory to the ankle joint.

d) The Talocrural Joint

The talocrural articulation constitutes the ankle joint, which is a ginglymus variety of diarthrosis. In other words, ankle joint is a type of hinge joint. The ankle joint facilitates the movements like dorsiflexion and extension.

e) The Intertarsal Joints

The intertarsal articulations (joints) are diarthroses that facilitate the gliding movements of the foot. These joints can be categorized in the following manner:

i) talocalcaneal joint

ii) talocalcaneonavicular joint

iii) calcaneocuboid joint

iv) cuneonavicular joint

v) cuboideonavicular joint

vi) intercuneiform and cuneocuboid joint

f) The Tarsometatarsal Joint

The tarsometatarsal joints include the articular surfaces of the cuneiform, the cuboid and the metatarsal bones. The articular facets of the three cuneiform and cuboid bones connect with the bases of the five metatarsal bones to constitute the tarsometatarsal articulations.

g) The Intermetatarsal Joint

The articular facets on the bases of the four metatarsal bones connect with each other via dorsal, plantar and interosseous ligaments to form the intermetatarsal joints. However, no ligament acts to connect the first metatarsal base with the second one.

h) The Metatarsophalangeal Joint

The metatarsophalangeal joints are a type of modified ball and socket articulations, wherein globular heads of metatarsal bones articulate with the shallow cups upon the bases of the first phalanges via plantar and collateral ligaments. These joints are encapsulated by an articular capsule.

i) The Joints of the Digits

The articulations between the digits constitute the interphalangeal joints. The phalanges of the toes connect with each other to form the interphalangeal articulations. The great toe possesses only one interphalangeal joint. However, each other toe (except great toe) comprises of two interphalangeal joints.

13. Myology (The Muscular System)
Introduction

The muscle cells of the human body facilitate the movements of various body parts through their special function of contraction in response to a requisite external or internal stimulus. These muscle cells can be characterized under the below mentioned three different classes:

a) Striated Muscle Cells

The striated muscle cells are those voluntary muscle cells that constitute the skeletal muscular system.

b) Non Striated Muscle Cells

The non striated muscle cells are those involuntary muscle cells that occur in the vessel walls and hollow viscera.

c) Cardiac Muscle Cells

The cardiac muscle cells comprise of those striated cells that constitute the substance of the heart. However, these muscle cells are involuntary in nature.

14. The Muscles of the Trunk
The muscles of the back are based on the following group of muscles:

a) Splenius

The splenius muscles constitute the superficial layer of the intrinsic back muscles that occupy the back of neck and upper portion of the thoracic region. The splenius muscles overlap the vertical muscles like a bandage and have the following two types:

   i)   splenius capitis

   ii) splenius cervicis

b) Sacrospinalis (Erector Spinae)

The erector spinae muscles are positioned in a groove between the angle of ribs and spinal processes on each side of the vertebral column. The erector spinae is divided into the following three muscle columns:

c) Iliocostalis

The lateral column is further divided into the following muscle components:

   i)   iliocostalis lumborum (iliocostalis/sacrolumbalis muscle)

   ii) iliocostalis dorsi (musculus accessorius)

   iii) iliocostalis cervicis (cervicalis ascendens)

d) Longissimus

   i)   longissimus dorsi

   ii) longissimus cervicis (transversalis cervicis)

   iii) longissimus capitis (trachelomastoid muscle)

e) Spinalis

   i)   spinalis dorsi

   ii) spinalis cervicis (spinalis coli)

   iii) spinalis capitis (biventer cervicis)

f) Semispinalis

The semispinalis constitute the deeper layer of intrinsic back muscles. These muscles originate from half of the vertebral column and categorized into three distinct parts:

   i)   semispinalis dorsi

   ii) semispinalis cervicis (semispinalis colli)

   iii) semispinalis capitis (complexus)

g) Multifidus (Multifidus Spinae)

The multifundus comprises of short triangular muscular bundles that remain apparent from sacrum to the axis.

h) Rotatores (Rotatores Spinae)

It remain confined in the thoracic region.

   i)   Interspinales and Intertransversarii (Intertransversales) are best developed and most distinct in the cervical region, and considered as the smallest of the deep back muscles.

15. The Muscles of the Pelvis

The muscles of the pelvis include the following:

a) Obturator Internus

b) Piriformis

c) Levator Ani (Pubococcygeus and Iliococcygeus)

d) Coccygeus (Ischiococcygeus)

16. The Muscles of the Upper Extremity

a) The muscles that connect the upper extremity to the vertebral column are defined below:

   i)   trapezius

   ii) rhomboideus major

   iii) latissimus dorsi

   iv) rhomboideus minor

   v)   levator scapulae

b) The Muscles Connecting the Upper Extremity to the Anterior and Lateral Thoracic Walls

   i)   pectoralis major

   ii) subclavius

   iii) pectoralis minor

   iv) serratus anterior

c) The Muscles of the Shoulder

   i)   Deltoid muscle originates from the lateral third portion of clavicle, the acromion and the spine of scapula. However, it gets inserted into the deltoid tuberosity of humerus. This muscle facilitates the abduction and medial and lateral rotation of the arm.

   ii) Subscapularis muscle originates from the subscapular fossa that forms the ventral surface of scapula. However, it gets inserted into the lesser tubercle of humerus. The subscapularis helps to medially rotate and adduct the arm and fixes the humeral head in glenoid cavity (of the scapula).

   iii) Supraspinatus muscle originates from the supraspinatous fossa of scapula and gets inserted into the superior facet of greater tubercle of humerus. This muscle assists the deltoid in the abduction of arm.

   iv) Infraspinatus muscle arises from the infraspinatous fossa of scapula and gets inserted into the middle facet of greater tubercle of humerus. This muscle helps in the lateral rotation of arm and fixes the head of humerus into the glenoid cavity of scapula.

   v)   Teres Minor muscle originates from the middle portion of lateral border of scapula and gets inserted into the inferior facet of greater tubercle of humerus. Like infraspnatous, teres minor muscle also helps in the lateral rotation of arm and fixes the head of humerus into the glenoid cavity of scapula.

   vi) Teres Major muscle arises from the posterior surface of inferior angle of scapula and gets inserted into the medial lip of intertubercular groove of humerus. This muscle facilitates the adduction and medial rotation of the arm.

d) The Muscles of the Arm

   i)   coracobrachialis

   ii) biceps brachii

   iii) brachialis

   iv) triceps brachii

e) The Muscles of the Forearm: muscles of the Anterior Compartment of Forearm

The Muscles of the Superficial (First) Layer

   i)   pronator teres

   ii) flexor carpi radialis

   iii) the palmaris longus

   iv) flexor carpi ulnaris

The Muscle of the Intermediate (Second) Layer

   i)   flexor digitorum superficialis

The Muscles of the Deep (Third) Layer

   i)   flexor digitorum profundus

   ii) flexor pollicis longus

   iii) pronator quadrates

f) Muscles of the Posterior Compartment of Forearm: of the Superficial Layer

   i)   brachioradialis

   ii) extensor carpi radialis longus

   iii) extensor carpii radialis brevis

   iv) extensor digitorum

   v)   extensor digiti minimi

   vi) extensor carpi ulnaris

g) The Muscles of the Deep Layer

   i)   supinator

   ii) abductor pollicis longus

   iii) extensor pollicis longus

   iv) extensor pollicis brevis

   v)   extensor indicis

h) The Muscles of the Hand: thenar muscles
  i) opponens pollicis
  ii) abductor pollicis brevis
  iii) flexor pollicis brevis
  iv) adductor pollicis
  Hypothenar muscles
  i) abductor digiti minimi
  ii) flexor digiti minimi Brevis
  iii) opponens digiti minimi
i) The Short Muscles
  i) Lumbricals
  ii) Dorsal Interossei
  iii) Palmar Interossei

17. The Muscles of the Thigh : Anterior Thigh Muscles
  a) The below mentioned anterior thigh muscles are based on the anterior compartment of thigh:
    i) pectineus
    ii) iliopsoas
    iii) psoas major
    iv) iliacus
    v) femoris
    vi) vastus lateralis
    vii) vastus intermedius
    viii) vastus medialis
  b) Medial Thigh Muscles
    i) adductor longus
    ii) adductor brevis
    iii) adductor magnus
    iv) gracilis
    v) obturator externus
  c) Gluteal Region Muscles
    i) gluteus maximus
    ii) gluteus medius
    iii) gluteus minimus
    iv) tensor fasciae latae
    v) piriformis
    vi) obturator internus
    vii) superior and inferior gemelli
    viii) quadratus femoris
  d) Posterior Thigh Muscles
    i) semitendinosus
    ii) semimembranosus
    iii) biceps femoris (long head)
  e) The Muscles of the Leg: The Anterior Compartment Muscles
    i) tibialis anterior
    ii) extensor hallucis longus
    iii) extensor digitorum longus
    iv) fibularis tertius
  f) The Lateral Compartment Muscles
    i) fibularis longus
    ii) fibularis brevis
  g) The Posterior Compartment Muscles: Superficial Muscle Group
    i) gastrocnemius
    ii) soleus
    iii) plantaris

h) The Deep Muscle Group
  i) Popliteus
  ii) Flexor Hallucis Longus
  iii) Flexor Digitorum Longus
  iv) Tibialis Posterior
i) The Muscles of the Foot: First Layer Muscles
  i) abductor hallucis
  ii) flexor digitorum brevis
  iii) abductor digiti minimi
j) Second Layer Muscles
  i) quadratus plantae
  ii) lumbricals
k) The Third Layer Muscles
  i) flexor hallucis brevis
  ii) adductor hallucis
  iii) flexor digiti minimi brevis
l) The Fourth Layer Muscles
  i) plantar interossei (three muscles)
  ii) dorsal interossei (four muscles)
m) Muscles of Dorsum of Foot
  i) extensor digitorum brevis
  ii) extensor hallucis brevis

Common Pathologies

Rotator Cuff Tendinitis
Rotator cuff tendinitis, or impingement syndrome, is often associated with bursitis of the overlying subacromial bursa and is the cause of most non traumatic cases of shoulder pain. It refers to irritation of these tendons and inflammation of the bursa (a normally smooth layer) lining these tendons. Pain commonly causes local swelling and tenderness in the front of the shoulder. It results from inflammation, degeneration of the rotator cuff by mechanical impingement on the acromion and sometimes the acromioclavicular joint.

Frozen Shoulder
Frozen shoulder, also called adhesive capsulitis, causes pain and stiffness in the shoulder. It is characterized by progressive pain and global loss of motion in the shoulder. Movement of the shoulder is severely restricted. Pain is usually constant, worse at night. When the capsule becomes inflamed, the shoulder bones are unable to move freely in the joint. The pathophysiology of frozen shoulder is still unclear. As the condition progresses, the stiffness may continue to the point where range of motion can be severely limited.

De Quervain's Tenosynovitis
De Quervain's tenosynovitis is a painful condition affecting the tendons on the thumb side of wrist. Tendons include the extensor pollicis brevis and the abductor pollicis longus tendons. The swollen tendons and their coverings rub against the narrow tunnel through which they pass. The result is pain at the base of the thumb and extending into the lower arm. Pain is reproduced by stretching the tendons with the thumb inside a closed fist.

Carpal Tunnel Syndrome
Carpal tunnel syndrome is caused by compression of the median nerve at the wrist. Carpal tunnel is a narrow passageway of ligament and bones at the base of your hand. It contains nerve and tendons. The main symptom of carpal tunnel syndrome is intermittent numbness of the thumb, index, long and radial half of the ring finger. Symptoms are often worse at night or after use of vibrating tools or great force.

Dupuytren Contracture
Dupuytren's contracture is a thickening of the fibrous tissue layer underneath the skin of the palm and fingers. It involves the palmar

fascia of the hand. The finger affected by contracture cannot be straightened completely, which can complicate everyday activities. The ring finger is affected most often.

Osteoarthrosis

Osteoarthrosis is a noninflammatory degenerative join disease. The cause of osteoarthritis is unknown. Symptoms may include degeneration of the articular cartilage, hypertrophy of bone at the margins, changes in the synovial membrane, tenderness, stiffness, locking and sometimes an effusion. It may be present in many joints. Symptoms are usually evident in one or two joints at the most. The three main symptoms are pain, morning stiffness and a tendency for the affected joint to gel with immobility.

Osteoporosis

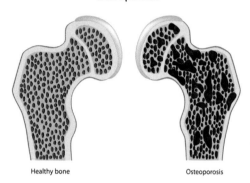

Healthy bone   Osteoporosis

Rheumatoid arthritis

Rheumatoid arthritis is a chronic progressive and disabling autoimmune disease that causes inflammation, swelling, and pain in the joints, the tissue around the joints, and other organs in the human body. The cause of rheumatoid arthritis is not known. It can affect any joint but is common in the wrist and fingers. It can be a disabling and painful condition, which can lead to substantial loss of functioning and mobility.

Common types of Arthritis

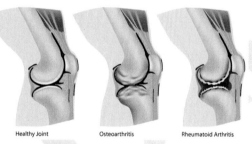

Healthy Joint   Osteoarthritis   Rheumatoid Arthritis

Stages of Rheumatoid Arthritis

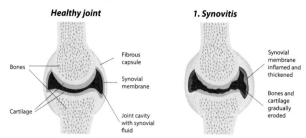

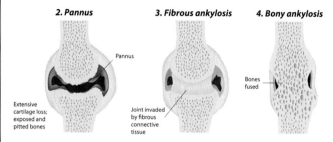

Osteoporosis

Osteoporosis is a systemic bone disease characterized as the diminishment of bone mass and damage of bone micro-structural. It is a silent disease. It causes bones to become weak and brittle. Its risk factors include aging, being female, low body weight, low sex hormones or menopause, smoking, and some medications. Osteoporosis related fractures most commonly occur in the hip, wrist or spine.

Septic Arthritis

Septic arthritis is the purulent invasion of a joint by an infectious agent which produces arthritis. Septic arthritis develops when bacteria or other tiny disease-causing microorganisms spread through the bloodstream to a joint. It is a sterile inflammatory process that usually results from an extra-articular infectious process. Bacteria are the most significant pathogens because of their rapidly destructive nature.

Meralgia Paresthetica

Meralgia paresthetica is a condition characterized by tingling, numbness and burning pain in the outer part of your thigh. Pain in the outer thigh is caused by injury to lateral cutaneous nerve of thigh. Entrapment occurs at the level of the anterosuperior iliac spine where the nerve passes through the lateral end of the inguinal ligament. It typically occurs in isolation

Diseases of the musculoskeletal system and connective tissue (M00-M99)

NOTES Use an external cause code following the code for the musculoskeletal condition, if applicable, to identify the cause of the musculoskeletal condition

EXCLUDES2 arthropathic psoriasis (L40.5-)
certain conditions originating in the perinatal period (P04-P96)
certain infectious and parasitic diseases (A00-B99)
compartment syndrome (traumatic) (T79.A-)
complications of pregnancy, childbirth and the puerperium (O00-O9A)
congenital malformations, deformations, and chromosomal abnormalities (Q00-Q99)
endocrine, nutritional and metabolic diseases (E00-E88)
injury, poisoning and certain other consequences of external causes (S00-T88)
neoplasms (C00-D49)
symptoms, signs and abnormal clinical and laboratory findings, not elsewhere classified (R00-R94)

Arthropathies (M00-M25)

INCLUDES Disorders affecting predominantly peripheral (limb) joints

Infectious arthropathies (M00-M02)

NOTES This block comprises arthropathies due to microbiological agents. Distinction is made between the following types of etiological relationship:
a) direct infection of joint, where organisms invade synovial tissue and microbial antigen is present in the joint;
b) indirect infection, which may be of two types: a reactive arthropathy, where microbial infection of the body is established but neither organisms nor antigens can be identified in the joint, and a postinfective arthropathy, where microbial antigen is present but recovery of an organism is inconstant and evidence of local multiplication is lacking.

M00 Pyogenic arthritis
M00.0 Staphylococcal arthritis and polyarthritis
Use additional code (B95.61-B95.8) to identify bacterial agent
EXCLUDES2 infection and inflammatory reaction due to internal joint prosthesis (T84.5-)
M00.00 Staphylococcal arthritis, unspecified joint
M00.01 Staphylococcal arthritis, shoulder
M00.011 Staphylococcal arthritis, right shoulder
M00.012 Staphylococcal arthritis, left shoulder
M00.019 Staphylococcal arthritis, unspecified shoulder
M00.02 Staphylococcal arthritis, elbow
M00.021 Staphylococcal arthritis, right elbow
M00.022 Staphylococcal arthritis, left elbow
M00.029 Staphylococcal arthritis, unspecified elbow
M00.03 Staphylococcal arthritis, wrist
Staphylococcal arthritis of carpal bones
M00.031 Staphylococcal arthritis, right wrist
M00.032 Staphylococcal arthritis, left wrist
M00.039 Staphylococcal arthritis, unspecified wrist
M00.04 Staphylococcal arthritis, hand
Staphylococcal arthritis of metacarpus and phalanges
M00.041 Staphylococcal arthritis, right hand
M00.042 Staphylococcal arthritis, left hand
M00.049 Staphylococcal arthritis, unspecified hand

M00.05 Staphylococcal arthritis, hip
M00.051 Staphylococcal arthritis, right hip
M00.052 Staphylococcal arthritis, left hip
M00.059 Staphylococcal arthritis, unspecified hip
M00.06 Staphylococcal arthritis, knee
M00.061 Staphylococcal arthritis, right knee
M00.062 Staphylococcal arthritis, left knee
M00.069 Staphylococcal arthritis, unspecified knee
M00.07 Staphylococcal arthritis, ankle and foot
Staphylococcal arthritis, tarsus, metatarsus and phalanges
M00.071 Staphylococcal arthritis, right ankle and foot
M00.072 Staphylococcal arthritis, left ankle and foot
M00.079 Staphylococcal arthritis, unspecified ankle and foot
M00.08 Staphylococcal arthritis, vertebrae
M00.09 Staphylococcal polyarthritis
M00.1 Pneumococcal arthritis and polyarthritis
M00.10 Pneumococcal arthritis, unspecified joint
M00.11 Pneumococcal arthritis, shoulder
M00.111 Pneumococcal arthritis, right shoulder
M00.112 Pneumococcal arthritis, left shoulder
M00.119 Pneumococcal arthritis, unspecified shoulder
M00.12 Pneumococcal arthritis, elbow
M00.121 Pneumococcal arthritis, right elbow
M00.122 Pneumococcal arthritis, left elbow
M00.129 Pneumococcal arthritis, unspecified elbow
M00.13 Pneumococcal arthritis, wrist
Pneumococcal arthritis of carpal bones
M00.131 Pneumococcal arthritis, right wrist
M00.132 Pneumococcal arthritis, left wrist
M00.139 Pneumococcal arthritis, unspecified wrist
M00.14 Pneumococcal arthritis, hand
Pneumococcal arthritis of metacarpus and phalanges
M00.141 Pneumococcal arthritis, right hand
M00.142 Pneumococcal arthritis, left hand
M00.149 Pneumococcal arthritis, unspecified hand
M00.15 Pneumococcal arthritis, hip
M00.151 Pneumococcal arthritis, right hip
M00.152 Pneumococcal arthritis, left hip
M00.159 Pneumococcal arthritis, unspecified hip
M00.16 Pneumococcal arthritis, knee
M00.161 Pneumococcal arthritis, right knee
M00.162 Pneumococcal arthritis, left knee
M00.169 Pneumococcal arthritis, unspecified knee
M00.17 Pneumococcal arthritis, ankle and foot
Pneumococcal arthritis, tarsus, metatarsus and phalanges
M00.171 Pneumococcal arthritis, right ankle and foot
M00.172 Pneumococcal arthritis, left ankle and foot
M00.179 Pneumococcal arthritis, unspecified ankle and foot
M00.18 Pneumococcal arthritis, vertebrae
M00.19 Pneumococcal polyarthritis
M00.2 Other streptococcal arthritis and polyarthritis
Use additional code (B95.0-B95.2, B95.4-B95.5) to identify bacterial agent
M00.20 Other streptococcal arthritis, unspecified joint
M00.21 Other streptococcal arthritis, shoulder
M00.211 Other streptococcal arthritis, right shoulder
M00.212 Other streptococcal arthritis, left shoulder
M00.219 Other streptococcal arthritis, unspecified shoulder

| Unspecified Code | Other Specified Code | N Newborn Age: 0 | P Pediatric Age: 0-17 | M Maternity Age: 12-55 |
| A Adult Age: 15-124 | ♂ Male | ♀ Female | ● New Code | ▲ Revised Code Title | ►◄ Revised Text |

[6] M00.22 Other streptococcal arthritis, elbow
- M00.221 Other streptococcal arthritis, right elbow
- M00.222 Other streptococcal arthritis, left elbow
- M00.229 Other streptococcal arthritis, unspecified elbow

[6] M00.23 Other streptococcal arthritis, wrist
Other streptococcal arthritis of carpal bones
- M00.231 Other streptococcal arthritis, right wrist
- M00.232 Other streptococcal arthritis, left wrist
- M00.239 Other streptococcal arthritis, unspecified wrist

[6] M00.24 Other streptococcal arthritis, hand
Other streptococcal arthritis metacarpus and phalanges
- M00.241 Other streptococcal arthritis, right hand
- M00.242 Other streptococcal arthritis, left hand
- M00.249 Other streptococcal arthritis, unspecified hand

[6] M00.25 Other streptococcal arthritis, hip
- M00.251 Other streptococcal arthritis, right hip
- M00.252 Other streptococcal arthritis, left hip
- M00.259 Other streptococcal arthritis, unspecified hip

[6] M00.26 Other streptococcal arthritis, knee
- M00.261 Other streptococcal arthritis, right knee
- M00.262 Other streptococcal arthritis, left knee
- M00.269 Other streptococcal arthritis, unspecified knee

[6] M00.27 Other streptococcal arthritis, ankle and foot
Other streptococcal arthritis, tarsus, metatarsus and phalanges
- M00.271 Other streptococcal arthritis, right ankle and foot
- M00.272 Other streptococcal arthritis, left ankle and foot
- M00.279 Other streptococcal arthritis, unspecified ankle and foot

M00.28 Other streptococcal arthritis, vertebrae
M00.29 Other streptococcal polyarthritis

[5] M00.8 Arthritis and polyarthritis due to other bacteria
Use additional code (B96) to identify bacteria

M00.80 Arthritis due to other bacteria, unspecified joint

[6] M00.81 Arthritis due to other bacteria, shoulder
- M00.811 Arthritis due to other bacteria, right shoulder
- M00.812 Arthritis due to other bacteria, left shoulder
- M00.819 Arthritis due to other bacteria, unspecified shoulder

[6] M00.82 Arthritis due to other bacteria, elbow
- M00.821 Arthritis due to other bacteria, right elbow
- M00.822 Arthritis due to other bacteria, left elbow
- M00.829 Arthritis due to other bacteria, unspecified elbow

[6] M00.83 Arthritis due to other bacteria, wrist
Arthritis due to other bacteria, carpal bones
- M00.831 Arthritis due to other bacteria, right wrist
- M00.832 Arthritis due to other bacteria, left wrist
- M00.839 Arthritis due to other bacteria, unspecified wrist

[6] M00.84 Arthritis due to other bacteria, hand
Arthritis due to other bacteria, metacarpus and phalanges
- M00.841 Arthritis due to other bacteria, right hand
- M00.842 Arthritis due to other bacteria, left hand
- M00.849 Arthritis due to other bacteria, unspecified hand

[6] M00.85 Arthritis due to other bacteria, hip
- M00.851 Arthritis due to other bacteria, right hip
- M00.852 Arthritis due to other bacteria, left hip
- M00.859 Arthritis due to other bacteria, unspecified hip

[6] M00.86 Arthritis due to other bacteria, knee
- M00.861 Arthritis due to other bacteria, right knee
- M00.862 Arthritis due to other bacteria, left knee
- M00.869 Arthritis due to other bacteria, unspecified knee

[6] M00.87 Arthritis due to other bacteria, ankle and foot
Arthritis due to other bacteria, tarsus, metatarsus, and phalanges
- M00.871 Arthritis due to other bacteria, right ankle and foot
- M00.872 Arthritis due to other bacteria, left ankle and foot
- M00.879 Arthritis due to other bacteria, unspecified ankle and foot

M00.88 Arthritis due to other bacteria, vertebrae
M00.89 Polyarthritis due to other bacteria

M00.9 Pyogenic arthritis, unspecified
Infective arthritis NOS

[4] M01 Direct infections of joint in infectious and parasitic diseases classified elsewhere
Code first underlying disease, such as:
leprosy [Hansen's disease] (A30.-)
mycoses (B35-B49)
O'nyong-nyong fever (A92.1)
paratyphoid fever (A01.1-A01.4)

[EXCLUDES1] *arthropathy in Lyme disease (A69.23)*
gonococcal arthritis (A54.42)
meningococcal arthritis (A39.83)
mumps arthritis (B26.85)
postinfective arthropathy (M02.-)
postmeningococcal arthritis (A39.84)
reactive arthritis (M02.3)
rubella arthritis (B06.82)
sarcoidosis arthritis (D86.86)
typhoid fever arthritis (A01.04)
tuberculosis arthritis (A18.01-A18.02)

[5] M01.X Direct infection of joint in infectious and parasitic diseases classified elsewhere

M01.X0 Direct infection of unspecified joint in infectious and parasitic diseases classified elsewhere

[6] M01.X1 Direct infection of shoulder joint in infectious and parasitic diseases classified elsewhere
- M01.X11 Direct infection of right shoulder in infectious and parasitic diseases classified elsewhere
- M01.X12 Direct infection of left shoulder in infectious and parasitic diseases classified elsewhere
- M01.X19 Direct infection of unspecified shoulder in infectious and parasitic diseases classified elsewhere

[6] M01.X2 Direct infection of elbow in infectious and parasitic diseases classified elsewhere
- M01.X21 Direct infection of right elbow in infectious and parasitic diseases classified elsewhere
- M01.X22 Direct infection of left elbow in infectious and parasitic diseases classified elsewhere
- M01.X29 Direct infection of unspecified elbow in infectious and parasitic diseases classified elsewhere

[6] M01.X3 Direct infection of wrist in infectious and parasitic diseases classified elsewhere
Direct infection of carpal bones in infectious and parasitic diseases classified elsewhere

M01.X31 Direct infection of right wrist in infectious and parasitic diseases classified elsewhere

M01.X32 Direct infection of left wrist in infectious and parasitic diseases classified elsewhere

M01.X39 Direct infection of unspecified wrist in infectious and parasitic diseases classified elsewhere

M01.X4 Direct infection of hand in infectious and parasitic diseases classified elsewhere

Direct infection of metacarpus and phalanges in infectious and parasitic diseases classified elsewhere

M01.X41 Direct infection of right hand in infectious and parasitic diseases classified elsewhere

M01.X42 Direct infection of left hand in infectious and parasitic diseases classified elsewhere

M01.X49 Direct infection of unspecified hand in infectious and parasitic diseases classified elsewhere

M01.X5 Direct infection of hip in infectious and parasitic diseases classified elsewhere

M01.X51 Direct infection of right hip in infectious and parasitic diseases classified elsewhere

M01.X52 Direct infection of left hip in infectious and parasitic diseases classified elsewhere

M01.X59 Direct infection of unspecified hip in infectious and parasitic diseases classified elsewhere

M01.X6 Direct infection of knee in infectious and parasitic diseases classified elsewhere

M01.X61 Direct infection of right knee in infectious and parasitic diseases classified elsewhere

M01.X62 Direct infection of left knee in infectious and parasitic diseases classified elsewhere

M01.X69 Direct infection of unspecified knee in infectious and parasitic diseases classified elsewhere

M01.X7 Direct infection of ankle and foot in infectious and parasitic diseases classified elsewhere

Direct infection of tarsus, metatarsus and phalanges in infectious and parasitic diseases classified elsewhere

M01.X71 Direct infection of right ankle and foot in infectious and parasitic diseases classified elsewhere

M01.X72 Direct infection of left ankle and foot in infectious and parasitic diseases classified elsewhere

M01.X79 Direct infection of unspecified ankle and foot in infectious and parasitic diseases classified elsewhere

M01.X8 Direct infection of vertebrae in infectious and parasitic diseases classified elsewhere

M01.X9 Direct infection of multiple joints in infectious and parasitic diseases classified elsewhere

M02 Postinfective and reactive arthropathies

Code first underlying disease, such as:
congenital syphilis [Clutton's joints] (A50.5)
enteritis due to Yersinia enterocolitica (A04.6)
infective endocarditis (I33.0)
viral hepatitis (B15-B19)

EXCLUDES1 Behçet's disease (M35.2)
direct infections of joint in infectious and parasitic diseases classified elsewhere (M01.-)
postmeningococcal arthritis (A39.84)
mumps arthritis (B26.85)
rubella arthritis (B06.82)
syphilis arthritis (late) (A52.77)
rheumatic fever (I00)
tabetic arthropathy [Charcôt's] (A52.16)

M02.0 Arthropathy following intestinal bypass

M02.00 Arthropathy following intestinal bypass, unspecified site

M02.01 Arthropathy following intestinal bypass, shoulder

M02.011 Arthropathy following intestinal bypass, right shoulder

M02.012 Arthropathy following intestinal bypass, left shoulder

M02.019 Arthropathy following intestinal bypass, unspecified shoulder

M02.02 Arthropathy following intestinal bypass, elbow

M02.021 Arthropathy following intestinal bypass, right elbow

M02.022 Arthropathy following intestinal bypass, left elbow

M02.029 Arthropathy following intestinal bypass, unspecified elbow

M02.03 Arthropathy following intestinal bypass, wrist

Arthropathy following intestinal bypass, carpal bones

M02.031 Arthropathy following intestinal bypass, right wrist

M02.032 Arthropathy following intestinal bypass, left wrist

M02.039 Arthropathy following intestinal bypass, unspecified wrist

M02.04 Arthropathy following intestinal bypass, hand

Arthropathy following intestinal bypass, metacarpals and phalanges

M02.041 Arthropathy following intestinal bypass, right hand

M02.042 Arthropathy following intestinal bypass, left hand

M02.049 Arthropathy following intestinal bypass, unspecified hand

M02.05 Arthropathy following intestinal bypass, hip

M02.051 Arthropathy following intestinal bypass, right hip

M02.052 Arthropathy following intestinal bypass, left hip

M02.059 Arthropathy following intestinal bypass, unspecified hip

M02.06 Arthropathy following intestinal bypass, knee

M02.061 Arthropathy following intestinal bypass, right knee

M02.062 Arthropathy following intestinal bypass, left knee

M02.069 Arthropathy following intestinal bypass, unspecified knee

M02.07 Arthropathy following intestinal bypass, ankle and foot

Arthropathy following intestinal bypass, tarsus, metatarsus and phalanges

M02.071 Arthropathy following intestinal bypass, right ankle and foot

M02.072 Arthropathy following intestinal bypass, left ankle and foot

M02.079 Arthropathy following intestinal bypass, unspecified ankle and foot

M02.08 Arthropathy following intestinal bypass, vertebrae

M02.09 Arthropathy following intestinal bypass, multiple sites

M02.1 Postdysenteric arthropathy

M02.10 Postdysenteric arthropathy, unspecified site

M02.11 Postdysenteric arthropathy, shoulder

M02.111 Postdysenteric arthropathy, right shoulder

M02.112 Postdysenteric arthropathy, left shoulder

M02.119 Postdysenteric arthropathy, unspecified shoulder

Unspecified Code	Other Specified Code	N Newborn Age: 0	P Pediatric Age: 0-17	M Maternity Age: 12-55
A Adult Age: 15-124	♂ Male	♀ Female	● New Code	▲ Revised Code Title	►◄ Revised Text

[6] M02.12 Postdysenteric arthropathy, elbow
M02.121 Postdysenteric arthropathy, right elbow
M02.122 Postdysenteric arthropathy, left elbow
M02.129 Postdysenteric arthropathy, unspecified elbow
[6] M02.13 Postdysenteric arthropathy, wrist
Postdysenteric arthropathy, carpal bones
M02.131 Postdysenteric arthropathy, right wrist
M02.132 Postdysenteric arthropathy, left wrist
M02.139 Postdysenteric arthropathy, unspecified wrist
[6] M02.14 Postdysenteric arthropathy, hand
Postdysenteric arthropathy, metacarpus and phalanges
M02.141 Postdysenteric arthropathy, right hand
M02.142 Postdysenteric arthropathy, left hand
M02.149 Postdysenteric arthropathy, unspecified hand
[6] M02.15 Postdysenteric arthropathy, hip
M02.151 Postdysenteric arthropathy, right hip
M02.152 Postdysenteric arthropathy, left hip
M02.159 Postdysenteric arthropathy, unspecified hip
[6] M02.16 Postdysenteric arthropathy, knee
M02.161 Postdysenteric arthropathy, right knee
M02.162 Postdysenteric arthropathy, left knee
M02.169 Postdysenteric arthropathy, unspecified knee
[6] M02.17 Postdysenteric arthropathy, ankle and foot
Postdysenteric arthropathy, tarsus, metatarsus and phalanges
M02.171 Postdysenteric arthropathy, right ankle and foot
M02.172 Postdysenteric arthropathy, left ankle and foot
M02.179 Postdysenteric arthropathy, unspecified ankle and foot
M02.18 Postdysenteric arthropathy, vertebrae
M02.19 Postdysenteric arthropathy, multiple sites
[5] M02.2 Postimmunization arthropathy
M02.20 Postimmunization arthropathy, unspecified site
[6] M02.21 Postimmunization arthropathy, shoulder
M02.211 Postimmunization arthropathy, right shoulder
M02.212 Postimmunization arthropathy, left shoulder
M02.219 Postimmunization arthropathy, unspecified shoulder
[6] M02.22 Postimmunization arthropathy, elbow
M02.221 Postimmunization arthropathy, right elbow
M02.222 Postimmunization arthropathy, left elbow
M02.229 Postimmunization arthropathy, unspecified elbow
[6] M02.23 Postimmunization arthropathy, wrist
Postimmunization arthropathy, carpal bones
M02.231 Postimmunization arthropathy, right wrist
M02.232 Postimmunization arthropathy, left wrist
M02.239 Postimmunization arthropathy, unspecified wrist
[6] M02.24 Postimmunization arthropathy, hand
Postimmunization arthropathy, metacarpus and phalanges
M02.241 Postimmunization arthropathy, right hand
M02.242 Postimmunization arthropathy, left hand
M02.249 Postimmunization arthropathy, unspecified hand
[6] M02.25 Postimmunization arthropathy, hip
M02.251 Postimmunization arthropathy, right hip
M02.252 Postimmunization arthropathy, left hip
M02.259 Postimmunization arthropathy, unspecified hip
[6] M02.26 Postimmunization arthropathy, knee
M02.261 Postimmunization arthropathy, right knee
M02.262 Postimmunization arthropathy, left knee
M02.269 Postimmunization arthropathy, unspecified knee
[6] M02.27 Postimmunization arthropathy, ankle and foot
Postimmunization arthropathy, tarsus, metatarsus and phalanges
M02.271 Postimmunization arthropathy, right ankle and foot
M02.272 Postimmunization arthropathy, left ankle and foot
M02.279 Postimmunization arthropathy, unspecified ankle and foot
M02.28 Postimmunization arthropathy, vertebrae
M02.29 Postimmunization arthropathy, multiple sites
[5] M02.3 Reiter's disease
Reactive arthritis
M02.30 Reiter's disease, unspecified site
[6] M02.31 Reiter's disease, shoulder
M02.311 Reiter's disease, right shoulder
M02.312 Reiter's disease, left shoulder
M02.319 Reiter's disease, unspecified shoulder
[6] M02.32 Reiter's disease, elbow
M02.321 Reiter's disease, right elbow
M02.322 Reiter's disease, left elbow
M02.329 Reiter's disease, unspecified elbow
[6] M02.33 Reiter's disease, wrist
Reiter's disease, carpal bones
M02.331 Reiter's disease, right wrist
M02.332 Reiter's disease, left wrist
M02.339 Reiter's disease, unspecified wrist
[6] M02.34 Reiter's disease, hand
Reiter's disease, metacarpus and phalanges
M02.341 Reiter's disease, right hand
M02.342 Reiter's disease, left hand
M02.349 Reiter's disease, unspecified hand
[6] M02.35 Reiter's disease, hip
M02.351 Reiter's disease, right hip
M02.352 Reiter's disease, left hip
M02.359 Reiter's disease, unspecified hip
[6] M02.36 Reiter's disease, knee
M02.361 Reiter's disease, right knee
M02.362 Reiter's disease, left knee
M02.369 Reiter's disease, unspecified knee
[6] M02.37 Reiter's disease, ankle and foot
Reiter's disease, tarsus, metatarsus and phalanges
M02.371 Reiter's disease, right ankle and foot
M02.372 Reiter's disease, left ankle and foot
M02.379 Reiter's disease, unspecified ankle and foot
M02.38 Reiter's disease, vertebrae
M02.39 Reiter's disease, multiple sites
[5] M02.8 Other reactive arthropathies
M02.80 Other reactive arthropathies, unspecified site
[6] M02.81 Other reactive arthropathies, shoulder
M02.811 Other reactive arthropathies, right shoulder
M02.812 Other reactive arthropathies, left shoulder
M02.819 Other reactive arthropathies, unspecified shoulder
[6] M02.82 Other reactive arthropathies, elbow
M02.821 Other reactive arthropathies, right elbow
M02.822 Other reactive arthropathies, left elbow

[4] 4th character required [5] 5th character required [6] 6th character required [7] 7th character required [x7] Extension 'X' Alert
[EXCLUDES 1] Not coded here [EXCLUDES 2] Not included here [PDx] Primary Diagnosis Only Manifestation Code

M02.829 Other reactive arthropathies, unspecified elbow
⑥ M02.83 Other reactive arthropathies, wrist
Other reactive arthropathies, carpal bones
M02.831 Other reactive arthropathies, right wrist
M02.832 Other reactive arthropathies, left wrist
M02.839 Other reactive arthropathies, unspecified wrist
⑥ M02.84 Other reactive arthropathies, hand
Other reactive arthropathies, metacarpus and phalanges
M02.841 Other reactive arthropathies, right hand
M02.842 Other reactive arthropathies, left hand
M02.849 Other reactive arthropathies, unspecified hand
⑥ M02.85 Other reactive arthropathies, hip
M02.851 Other reactive arthropathies, right hip
M02.852 Other reactive arthropathies, left hip
M02.859 Other reactive arthropathies, unspecified hip
⑥ M02.86 Other reactive arthropathies, knee
M02.861 Other reactive arthropathies, right knee
M02.862 Other reactive arthropathies, left knee
M02.869 Other reactive arthropathies, unspecified knee
⑥ M02.87 Other reactive arthropathies, ankle and foot
Other reactive arthropathies, tarsus, metatarsus and phalanges
M02.871 Other reactive arthropathies, right ankle and foot
M02.872 Other reactive arthropathies, left ankle and foot
M02.879 Other reactive arthropathies, unspecified ankle and foot
M02.88 Other reactive arthropathies, vertebrae
M02.89 Other reactive arthropathies, multiple sites
M02.9 Reactive arthropathy, unspecified

Inflammatory polyarthropathies (M05-M14)

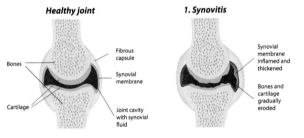

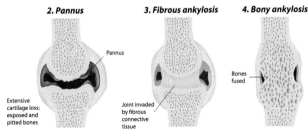

Figure 12.1 Stages of Rheumatoid Athritis

④ M05 Rheumatoid arthritis with rheumatoid factor
EXCLUDES1 rheumatic fever (I00)
juvenile rheumatoid arthritis (M08.-)
rheumatoid arthritis of spine (M45.-)

⑤ M05.0 Felty's syndrome
Rheumatoid arthritis with splenoadenomegaly and leukopenia
M05.00 Felty's syndrome, unspecified site
⑥ M05.01 Felty's syndrome, shoulder
M05.011 Felty's syndrome, right shoulder
M05.012 Felty's syndrome, left shoulder
M05.019 Felty's syndrome, unspecified shoulder
⑥ M05.02 Felty's syndrome, elbow
M05.021 Felty's syndrome, right elbow
M05.022 Felty's syndrome, left elbow
M05.029 Felty's syndrome, unspecified elbow
⑥ M05.03 Felty's syndrome, wrist
Felty's syndrome, carpal bones
M05.031 Felty's syndrome, right wrist
M05.032 Felty's syndrome, left wrist
M05.039 Felty's syndrome, unspecified wrist
⑥ M05.04 Felty's syndrome, hand
Felty's syndrome, metacarpus and phalanges
M05.041 Felty's syndrome, right hand
M05.042 Felty's syndrome, left hand
M05.049 Felty's syndrome, unspecified hand
⑥ M05.05 Felty's syndrome, hip
M05.051 Felty's syndrome, right hip
M05.052 Felty's syndrome, left hip
M05.059 Felty's syndrome, unspecified hip
⑥ M05.06 Felty's syndrome, knee
M05.061 Felty's syndrome, right knee
M05.062 Felty's syndrome, left knee
M05.069 Felty's syndrome, unspecified knee
⑥ M05.07 Felty's syndrome, ankle and foot
Felty's syndrome, tarsus, metatarsus and phalanges
M05.071 Felty's syndrome, right ankle and foot
M05.072 Felty's syndrome, left ankle and foot
M05.079 Felty's syndrome, unspecified ankle and foot
M05.09 Felty's syndrome, multiple sites
⑤ M05.1 Rheumatoid lung disease with rheumatoid arthritis
M05.10 Rheumatoid lung disease with rheumatoid arthritis of unspecified site
⑥ M05.11 Rheumatoid lung disease with rheumatoid arthritis of shoulder
M05.111 Rheumatoid lung disease with rheumatoid arthritis of right shoulder
M05.112 Rheumatoid lung disease with rheumatoid arthritis of left shoulder
M05.119 Rheumatoid lung disease with rheumatoid arthritis of unspecified shoulder
⑥ M05.12 Rheumatoid lung disease with rheumatoid arthritis of elbow
M05.121 Rheumatoid lung disease with rheumatoid arthritis of right elbow
M05.122 Rheumatoid lung disease with rheumatoid arthritis of left elbow
M05.129 Rheumatoid lung disease with rheumatoid arthritis of unspecified elbow
⑥ M05.13 Rheumatoid lung disease with rheumatoid arthritis of wrist
Rheumatoid lung disease with rheumatoid arthritis, carpal bones
M05.131 Rheumatoid lung disease with rheumatoid arthritis of right wrist
M05.132 Rheumatoid lung disease with rheumatoid arthritis of left wrist
M05.139 Rheumatoid lung disease with rheumatoid arthritis of unspecified wrist

| Unspecified Code | Other Specified Code | N Newborn Age: 0 | P Pediatric Age: 0-17 | M Maternity Age: 12-55 |

A Adult Age: 15-124   ♂ Male   ♀ Female   ● New Code   ▲ Revised Code Title   ►◄ Revised Text

[6] M05.14 Rheumatoid lung disease with rheumatoid arthritis of hand
Rheumatoid lung disease with rheumatoid arthritis, metacarpus and phalanges
M05.141 Rheumatoid lung disease with rheumatoid arthritis of right hand
M05.142 Rheumatoid lung disease with rheumatoid arthritis of left hand
M05.149 Rheumatoid lung disease with rheumatoid arthritis of unspecified hand
[6] M05.15 Rheumatoid lung disease with rheumatoid arthritis of hip
M05.151 Rheumatoid lung disease with rheumatoid arthritis of right hip
M05.152 Rheumatoid lung disease with rheumatoid arthritis of left hip
M05.159 Rheumatoid lung disease with rheumatoid arthritis of unspecified hip
[6] M05.16 Rheumatoid lung disease with rheumatoid arthritis of knee
M05.161 Rheumatoid lung disease with rheumatoid arthritis of right knee
M05.162 Rheumatoid lung disease with rheumatoid arthritis of left knee
M05.169 Rheumatoid lung disease with rheumatoid arthritis of unspecified knee
[6] M05.17 Rheumatoid lung disease with rheumatoid arthritis of ankle and foot
Rheumatoid lung disease with rheumatoid arthritis, tarsus, metatarsus and phalanges
M05.171 Rheumatoid lung disease with rheumatoid arthritis of right ankle and foot
M05.172 Rheumatoid lung disease with rheumatoid arthritis of left ankle and foot
M05.179 Rheumatoid lung disease with rheumatoid arthritis of unspecified ankle and foot
M05.19 Rheumatoid lung disease with rheumatoid arthritis of multiple sites
[5] M05.2 Rheumatoid vasculitis with rheumatoid arthritis
M05.20 Rheumatoid vasculitis with rheumatoid arthritis of unspecified site
[6] M05.21 Rheumatoid vasculitis with rheumatoid arthritis of shoulder
M05.211 Rheumatoid vasculitis with rheumatoid arthritis of right shoulder
M05.212 Rheumatoid vasculitis with rheumatoid arthritis of left shoulder
M05.219 Rheumatoid vasculitis with rheumatoid arthritis of unspecified shoulder
[6] M05.22 Rheumatoid vasculitis with rheumatoid arthritis of elbow
M05.221 Rheumatoid vasculitis with rheumatoid arthritis of right elbow
M05.222 Rheumatoid vasculitis with rheumatoid arthritis of left elbow
M05.229 Rheumatoid vasculitis with rheumatoid arthritis of unspecified elbow
[6] M05.23 Rheumatoid vasculitis with rheumatoid arthritis of wrist
Rheumatoid vasculitis with rheumatoid arthritis, carpal bones
M05.231 Rheumatoid vasculitis with rheumatoid arthritis of right wrist
M05.232 Rheumatoid vasculitis with rheumatoid arthritis of left wrist
M05.239 Rheumatoid vasculitis with rheumatoid arthritis of unspecified wrist
[6] M05.24 Rheumatoid vasculitis with rheumatoid arthritis of hand
Rheumatoid vasculitis with rheumatoid arthritis, metacarpus and phalanges
M05.241 Rheumatoid vasculitis with rheumatoid arthritis of right hand
M05.242 Rheumatoid vasculitis with rheumatoid arthritis of left hand
M05.249 Rheumatoid vasculitis with rheumatoid arthritis of unspecified hand
[6] M05.25 Rheumatoid vasculitis with rheumatoid arthritis of hip
M05.251 Rheumatoid vasculitis with rheumatoid arthritis of right hip
M05.252 Rheumatoid vasculitis with rheumatoid arthritis of left hip
M05.259 Rheumatoid vasculitis with rheumatoid arthritis of unspecified hip
[6] M05.26 Rheumatoid vasculitis with rheumatoid arthritis of knee
M05.261 Rheumatoid vasculitis with rheumatoid arthritis of right knee
M05.262 Rheumatoid vasculitis with rheumatoid arthritis of left knee
M05.269 Rheumatoid vasculitis with rheumatoid arthritis of unspecified knee
[6] M05.27 Rheumatoid vasculitis with rheumatoid arthritis of ankle and foot
Rheumatoid vasculitis with rheumatoid arthritis, tarsus, metatarsus and phalanges
M05.271 Rheumatoid vasculitis with rheumatoid arthritis of right ankle and foot
M05.272 Rheumatoid vasculitis with rheumatoid arthritis of left ankle and foot
M05.279 Rheumatoid vasculitis with rheumatoid arthritis of unspecified ankle and foot
M05.29 Rheumatoid vasculitis with rheumatoid arthritis of multiple sites
[5] M05.3 Rheumatoid heart disease with rheumatoid arthritis
Rheumatoid carditis
Rheumatoid endocarditis
Rheumatoid myocarditis
Rheumatoid pericarditis
M05.30 Rheumatoid heart disease with rheumatoid arthritis of unspecified site
[6] M05.31 Rheumatoid heart disease with rheumatoid arthritis of shoulder
M05.311 Rheumatoid heart disease with rheumatoid arthritis of right shoulder
M05.312 Rheumatoid heart disease with rheumatoid arthritis of left shoulder
M05.319 Rheumatoid heart disease with rheumatoid arthritis of unspecified shoulder
[6] M05.32 Rheumatoid heart disease with rheumatoid arthritis of elbow
M05.321 Rheumatoid heart disease with rheumatoid arthritis of right elbow
M05.322 Rheumatoid heart disease with rheumatoid arthritis of left elbow
M05.329 Rheumatoid heart disease with rheumatoid arthritis of unspecified elbow
[6] M05.33 Rheumatoid heart disease with rheumatoid arthritis of wrist
Rheumatoid heart disease with rheumatoid arthritis, carpal bones
M05.331 Rheumatoid heart disease with rheumatoid arthritis of right wrist
M05.332 Rheumatoid heart disease with rheumatoid arthritis of left wrist
M05.339 Rheumatoid heart disease with rheumatoid arthritis of unspecified wrist

[4] 4th character required [5] 5th character required [6] 6th character required [7] 7th character required [7th] Extension 'X' Alert
EXCLUDES 1 Not coded here EXCLUDES 2 Not included here PDx Primary Diagnosis Only Manifestation Code

[6] M05.34 Rheumatoid heart disease with rheumatoid arthritis of hand
Rheumatoid heart disease with rheumatoid arthritis, metacarpus and phalanges
M05.341 Rheumatoid heart disease with rheumatoid arthritis of right hand
M05.342 Rheumatoid heart disease with rheumatoid arthritis of left hand
M05.349 Rheumatoid heart disease with rheumatoid arthritis of unspecified hand
[6] M05.35 Rheumatoid heart disease with rheumatoid arthritis of hip
M05.351 Rheumatoid heart disease with rheumatoid arthritis of right hip
M05.352 Rheumatoid heart disease with rheumatoid arthritis of left hip
M05.359 Rheumatoid heart disease with rheumatoid arthritis of unspecified hip
[6] M05.36 Rheumatoid heart disease with rheumatoid arthritis of knee
M05.361 Rheumatoid heart disease with rheumatoid arthritis of right knee
M05.362 Rheumatoid heart disease with rheumatoid arthritis of left knee
M05.369 Rheumatoid heart disease with rheumatoid arthritis of unspecified knee
[6] M05.37 Rheumatoid heart disease with rheumatoid arthritis of ankle and foot
Rheumatoid heart disease with rheumatoid arthritis, tarsus, metatarsus and phalanges
M05.371 Rheumatoid heart disease with rheumatoid arthritis of right ankle and foot
M05.372 Rheumatoid heart disease with rheumatoid arthritis of left ankle and foot
M05.379 Rheumatoid heart disease with rheumatoid arthritis of unspecified ankle and foot
M05.39 Rheumatoid heart disease with rheumatoid arthritis of multiple sites
[5] M05.4 Rheumatoid myopathy with rheumatoid arthritis
M05.40 Rheumatoid myopathy with rheumatoid arthritis of unspecified site
[6] M05.41 Rheumatoid myopathy with rheumatoid arthritis of shoulder
M05.411 Rheumatoid myopathy with rheumatoid arthritis of right shoulder
M05.412 Rheumatoid myopathy with rheumatoid arthritis of left shoulder
M05.419 Rheumatoid myopathy with rheumatoid arthritis of unspecified shoulder
[6] M05.42 Rheumatoid myopathy with rheumatoid arthritis of elbow
M05.421 Rheumatoid myopathy with rheumatoid arthritis of right elbow
M05.422 Rheumatoid myopathy with rheumatoid arthritis of left elbow
M05.429 Rheumatoid myopathy with rheumatoid arthritis of unspecified elbow
[6] M05.43 Rheumatoid myopathy with rheumatoid arthritis of wrist
Rheumatoid myopathy with rheumatoid arthritis, carpal bones
M05.431 Rheumatoid myopathy with rheumatoid arthritis of right wrist
M05.432 Rheumatoid myopathy with rheumatoid arthritis of left wrist
M05.439 Rheumatoid myopathy with rheumatoid arthritis of unspecified wrist
[6] M05.44 Rheumatoid myopathy with rheumatoid arthritis of hand
Rheumatoid myopathy with rheumatoid arthritis, metacarpus and phalanges
M05.441 Rheumatoid myopathy with rheumatoid arthritis of right hand
M05.442 Rheumatoid myopathy with rheumatoid arthritis of left hand
M05.449 Rheumatoid myopathy with rheumatoid arthritis of unspecified hand
[6] M05.45 Rheumatoid myopathy with rheumatoid arthritis of hip
M05.451 Rheumatoid myopathy with rheumatoid arthritis of right hip
M05.452 Rheumatoid myopathy with rheumatoid arthritis of left hip
M05.459 Rheumatoid myopathy with rheumatoid arthritis of unspecified hip
[6] M05.46 Rheumatoid myopathy with rheumatoid arthritis of knee
M05.461 Rheumatoid myopathy with rheumatoid arthritis of right knee
M05.462 Rheumatoid myopathy with rheumatoid arthritis of left knee
M05.469 Rheumatoid myopathy with rheumatoid arthritis of unspecified knee
[6] M05.47 Rheumatoid myopathy with rheumatoid arthritis of ankle and foot
Rheumatoid myopathy with rheumatoid arthritis, tarsus, metatarsus and phalanges
M05.471 Rheumatoid myopathy with rheumatoid arthritis of right ankle and foot
M05.472 Rheumatoid myopathy with rheumatoid arthritis of left ankle and foot
M05.479 Rheumatoid myopathy with rheumatoid arthritis of unspecified ankle and foot
M05.49 Rheumatoid myopathy with rheumatoid arthritis of multiple sites
[5] M05.5 Rheumatoid polyneuropathy with rheumatoid arthritis
M05.50 Rheumatoid polyneuropathy with rheumatoid arthritis of unspecified site
[6] M05.51 Rheumatoid polyneuropathy with rheumatoid arthritis of shoulder
M05.511 Rheumatoid polyneuropathy with rheumatoid arthritis of right shoulder
M05.512 Rheumatoid polyneuropathy with rheumatoid arthritis of left shoulder
M05.519 Rheumatoid polyneuropathy with rheumatoid arthritis of unspecified shoulder
[6] M05.52 Rheumatoid polyneuropathy with rheumatoid arthritis of elbow
M05.521 Rheumatoid polyneuropathy with rheumatoid arthritis of right elbow
M05.522 Rheumatoid polyneuropathy with rheumatoid arthritis of left elbow
M05.529 Rheumatoid polyneuropathy with rheumatoid arthritis of unspecified elbow
[6] M05.53 Rheumatoid polyneuropathy with rheumatoid arthritis of wrist
Rheumatoid polyneuropathy with rheumatoid arthritis, carpal bones
M05.531 Rheumatoid polyneuropathy with rheumatoid arthritis of right wrist
M05.532 Rheumatoid polyneuropathy with rheumatoid arthritis of left wrist
M05.539 Rheumatoid polyneuropathy with rheumatoid arthritis of unspecified wrist

Unspecified Code | Other Specified Code | [N] Newborn Age: 0 | [P] Pediatric Age: 0-17 | [M] Maternity Age: 12-55
[A] Adult Age: 15-124 | ♂ Male | ♀ Female | ● New Code | ▲ Revised Code Title | ►◄ Revised Text

⑥ M05.54 Rheumatoid polyneuropathy with rheumatoid arthritis of hand
Rheumatoid polyneuropathy with rheumatoid arthritis, metacarpus and phalanges
M05.541 Rheumatoid polyneuropathy with rheumatoid arthritis of right hand
M05.542 Rheumatoid polyneuropathy with rheumatoid arthritis of left hand
M05.549 Rheumatoid polyneuropathy with rheumatoid arthritis of unspecified hand
⑥ M05.55 Rheumatoid polyneuropathy with rheumatoid arthritis of hip
M05.551 Rheumatoid polyneuropathy with rheumatoid arthritis of right hip
M05.552 Rheumatoid polyneuropathy with rheumatoid arthritis of left hip
M05.559 Rheumatoid polyneuropathy with rheumatoid arthritis of unspecified hip
⑥ M05.56 Rheumatoid polyneuropathy with rheumatoid arthritis of knee
M05.561 Rheumatoid polyneuropathy with rheumatoid arthritis of right knee
M05.562 Rheumatoid polyneuropathy with rheumatoid arthritis of left knee
M05.569 Rheumatoid polyneuropathy with rheumatoid arthritis of unspecified knee
⑥ M05.57 Rheumatoid polyneuropathy with rheumatoid arthritis of ankle and foot
Rheumatoid polyneuropathy with rheumatoid arthritis, tarsus, metatarsus and phalanges
M05.571 Rheumatoid polyneuropathy with rheumatoid arthritis of right ankle and foot
M05.572 Rheumatoid polyneuropathy with rheumatoid arthritis of left ankle and foot
M05.579 Rheumatoid polyneuropathy with rheumatoid arthritis of unspecified ankle and foot
M05.59 Rheumatoid polyneuropathy with rheumatoid arthritis of multiple sites
⑤ M05.6 Rheumatoid arthritis with involvement of other organs and systems
M05.60 Rheumatoid arthritis of unspecified site with involvement of other organs and systems
⑥ M05.61 Rheumatoid arthritis of shoulder with involvement of other organs and systems
M05.611 Rheumatoid arthritis of right shoulder with involvement of other organs and systems
M05.612 Rheumatoid arthritis of left shoulder with involvement of other organs and systems
M05.619 Rheumatoid arthritis of unspecified shoulder with involvement of other organs and systems
⑥ M05.62 Rheumatoid arthritis of elbow with involvement of other organs and systems
M05.621 Rheumatoid arthritis of right elbow with involvement of other organs and systems
M05.622 Rheumatoid arthritis of left elbow with involvement of other organs and systems
M05.629 Rheumatoid arthritis of unspecified elbow with involvement of other organs and systems
⑥ M05.63 Rheumatoid arthritis of wrist with involvement of other organs and systems
Rheumatoid arthritis of carpal bones with involvement of other organs and systems
M05.631 Rheumatoid arthritis of right wrist with involvement of other organs and systems
M05.632 Rheumatoid arthritis of left wrist with involvement of other organs and systems
M05.639 Rheumatoid arthritis of unspecified wrist with involvement of other organs and systems
⑥ M05.64 Rheumatoid arthritis of hand with involvement of other organs and systems
Rheumatoid arthritis of metacarpus and phalanges with involvement of other organs and systems
M05.641 Rheumatoid arthritis of right hand with involvement of other organs and systems
M05.642 Rheumatoid arthritis of left hand with involvement of other organs and systems
M05.649 Rheumatoid arthritis of unspecified hand with involvement of other organs and systems
⑥ M05.65 Rheumatoid arthritis of hip with involvement of other organs and systems
M05.651 Rheumatoid arthritis of right hip with involvement of other organs and systems
M05.652 Rheumatoid arthritis of left hip with involvement of other organs and systems
M05.659 Rheumatoid arthritis of unspecified hip with involvement of other organs and systems
⑥ M05.66 Rheumatoid arthritis of knee with involvement of other organs and systems
M05.661 Rheumatoid arthritis of right knee with involvement of other organs and systems
M05.662 Rheumatoid arthritis of left knee with involvement of other organs and systems
M05.669 Rheumatoid arthritis of unspecified knee with involvement of other organs and systems
⑥ M05.67 Rheumatoid arthritis of ankle and foot with involvement of other organs and systems
Rheumatoid arthritis of tarsus, metatarsus and phalanges with involvement of other organs and systems
M05.671 Rheumatoid arthritis of right ankle and foot with involvement of other organs and systems
M05.672 Rheumatoid arthritis of left ankle and foot with involvement of other organs and systems
M05.679 Rheumatoid arthritis of unspecified ankle and foot with involvement of other organs and systems
M05.69 Rheumatoid arthritis of multiple sites with involvement of other organs and systems
⑤ M05.7 Rheumatoid arthritis with rheumatoid factor without organ or systems involvement
M05.70 Rheumatoid arthritis with rheumatoid factor of unspecified site without organ or systems involvement
⑥ M05.71 Rheumatoid arthritis with rheumatoid factor of shoulder without organ or systems involvement
M05.711 Rheumatoid arthritis with rheumatoid factor of right shoulder without organ or systems involvement
M05.712 Rheumatoid arthritis with rheumatoid factor of left shoulder without organ or systems involvement
M05.719 Rheumatoid arthritis with rheumatoid factor of unspecified shoulder without organ or systems involvement
⑥ M05.72 Rheumatoid arthritis with rheumatoid factor of elbow without organ or systems involvement
M05.721 Rheumatoid arthritis with rheumatoid factor of right elbow without organ or systems involvement

M05.722 Rheumatoid arthritis with rheumatoid factor of left elbow without organ or systems involvement
M05.729 Rheumatoid arthritis with rheumatoid factor of unspecified elbow without organ or systems involvement
[6] M05.73 Rheumatoid arthritis with rheumatoid factor of wrist without organ or systems involvement
M05.731 Rheumatoid arthritis with rheumatoid factor of right wrist without organ or systems involvement
M05.732 Rheumatoid arthritis with rheumatoid factor of left wrist without organ or systems involvement
M05.739 Rheumatoid arthritis with rheumatoid factor of unspecified wrist without organ or systems involvement
[6] M05.74 Rheumatoid arthritis with rheumatoid factor of hand without organ or systems involvement
M05.741 Rheumatoid arthritis with rheumatoid factor of right hand without organ or systems involvement
M05.742 Rheumatoid arthritis with rheumatoid factor of left hand without organ or systems involvement
M05.749 Rheumatoid arthritis with rheumatoid factor of unspecified hand without organ or systems involvement
[6] M05.75 Rheumatoid arthritis with rheumatoid factor of hip without organ or systems involvement
M05.751 Rheumatoid arthritis with rheumatoid factor of right hip without organ or systems involvement
M05.752 Rheumatoid arthritis with rheumatoid factor of left hip without organ or systems involvement
M05.759 Rheumatoid arthritis with rheumatoid factor of unspecified hip without organ or systems involvement
[6] M05.76 Rheumatoid arthritis with rheumatoid factor of knee without organ or systems involvement
M05.761 Rheumatoid arthritis with rheumatoid factor of right knee without organ or systems involvement
M05.762 Rheumatoid arthritis with rheumatoid factor of left knee without organ or systems involvement
M05.769 Rheumatoid arthritis with rheumatoid factor of unspecified knee without organ or systems involvement
[6] M05.77 Rheumatoid arthritis with rheumatoid factor of ankle and foot without organ or systems involvement
M05.771 Rheumatoid arthritis with rheumatoid factor of right ankle and foot without organ or systems involvement
M05.772 Rheumatoid arthritis with rheumatoid factor of left ankle and foot without organ or systems involvement
M05.779 Rheumatoid arthritis with rheumatoid factor of unspecified ankle and foot without organ or systems involvement
M05.79 Rheumatoid arthritis with rheumatoid factor of multiple sites without organ or systems involvement
[5] M05.8 Other rheumatoid arthritis with rheumatoid factor
M05.80 Other rheumatoid arthritis with rheumatoid factor of unspecified site
[6] M05.81 Other rheumatoid arthritis with rheumatoid factor of shoulder
M05.811 Other rheumatoid arthritis with rheumatoid factor of right shoulder
M05.812 Other rheumatoid arthritis with rheumatoid factor of left shoulder
M05.819 Other rheumatoid arthritis with rheumatoid factor of unspecified shoulder
[6] M05.82 Other rheumatoid arthritis with rheumatoid factor of elbow
M05.821 Other rheumatoid arthritis with rheumatoid factor of right elbow
M05.822 Other rheumatoid arthritis with rheumatoid factor of left elbow
M05.829 Other rheumatoid arthritis with rheumatoid factor of unspecified elbow
[6] M05.83 Other rheumatoid arthritis with rheumatoid factor of wrist
M05.831 Other rheumatoid arthritis with rheumatoid factor of right wrist
M05.832 Other rheumatoid arthritis with rheumatoid factor of left wrist
M05.839 Other rheumatoid arthritis with rheumatoid factor of unspecified wrist
[6] M05.84 Other rheumatoid arthritis with rheumatoid factor of hand
M05.841 Other rheumatoid arthritis with rheumatoid factor of right hand
M05.842 Other rheumatoid arthritis with rheumatoid factor of left hand
M05.849 Other rheumatoid arthritis with rheumatoid factor of unspecified hand
[6] M05.85 Other rheumatoid arthritis with rheumatoid factor of hip
M05.851 Other rheumatoid arthritis with rheumatoid factor of right hip
M05.852 Other rheumatoid arthritis with rheumatoid factor of left hip
M05.859 Other rheumatoid arthritis with rheumatoid factor of unspecified hip
[6] M05.86 Other rheumatoid arthritis with rheumatoid factor of knee
M05.861 Other rheumatoid arthritis with rheumatoid factor of right knee
M05.862 Other rheumatoid arthritis with rheumatoid factor of left knee
M05.869 Other rheumatoid arthritis with rheumatoid factor of unspecified knee
[6] M05.87 Other rheumatoid arthritis with rheumatoid factor of ankle and foot
M05.871 Other rheumatoid arthritis with rheumatoid factor of right ankle and foot
M05.872 Other rheumatoid arthritis with rheumatoid factor of left ankle and foot
M05.879 Other rheumatoid arthritis with rheumatoid factor of unspecified ankle and foot
M05.89 Other rheumatoid arthritis with rheumatoid factor of multiple sites
M05.9 Rheumatoid arthritis with rheumatoid factor, unspecified
[4] M06 Other rheumatoid arthritis
[5] M06.0 Rheumatoid arthritis without rheumatoid factor
M06.00 Rheumatoid arthritis without rheumatoid factor, unspecified site
[6] M06.01 Rheumatoid arthritis without rheumatoid factor, shoulder
M06.011 Rheumatoid arthritis without rheumatoid factor, right shoulder
M06.012 Rheumatoid arthritis without rheumatoid factor, left shoulder

Unspecified Code | Other Specified Code | [N] Newborn Age: 0 | [P] Pediatric Age: 0-17 | [M] Maternity Age: 12-55
[A] Adult Age: 15-124 | ♂ Male | ♀ Female | ● New Code | ▲ Revised Code Title | ►◄ Revised Text

M06.019 Rheumatoid arthritis without rheumatoid factor, unspecified shoulder
[6] M06.02 Rheumatoid arthritis without rheumatoid factor, elbow
M06.021 Rheumatoid arthritis without rheumatoid factor, right elbow
M06.022 Rheumatoid arthritis without rheumatoid factor, left elbow
M06.029 Rheumatoid arthritis without rheumatoid factor, unspecified elbow
[6] M06.03 Rheumatoid arthritis without rheumatoid factor, wrist
M06.031 Rheumatoid arthritis without rheumatoid factor, right wrist
M06.032 Rheumatoid arthritis without rheumatoid factor, left wrist
M06.039 Rheumatoid arthritis without rheumatoid factor, unspecified wrist
[6] M06.04 Rheumatoid arthritis without rheumatoid factor, hand
M06.041 Rheumatoid arthritis without rheumatoid factor, right hand
M06.042 Rheumatoid arthritis without rheumatoid factor, left hand
M06.049 Rheumatoid arthritis without rheumatoid factor, unspecified hand
[6] M06.05 Rheumatoid arthritis without rheumatoid factor, hip
M06.051 Rheumatoid arthritis without rheumatoid factor, right hip
M06.052 Rheumatoid arthritis without rheumatoid factor, left hip
M06.059 Rheumatoid arthritis without rheumatoid factor, unspecified hip
[6] M06.06 Rheumatoid arthritis without rheumatoid factor, knee
M06.061 Rheumatoid arthritis without rheumatoid factor, right knee
M06.062 Rheumatoid arthritis without rheumatoid factor, left knee
M06.069 Rheumatoid arthritis without rheumatoid factor, unspecified knee
[6] M06.07 Rheumatoid arthritis without rheumatoid factor, ankle and foot
M06.071 Rheumatoid arthritis without rheumatoid factor, right ankle and foot
M06.072 Rheumatoid arthritis without rheumatoid factor, left ankle and foot
M06.079 Rheumatoid arthritis without rheumatoid factor, unspecified ankle and foot
M06.08 Rheumatoid arthritis without rheumatoid factor, vertebrae
M06.09 Rheumatoid arthritis without rheumatoid factor, multiple sites
M06.1 Adult-onset Still's disease
[EXCLUDES1] *Still's disease NOS (M08.2-)* [A]
[5] M06.2 Rheumatoid bursitis
M06.20 Rheumatoid bursitis, unspecified site
[6] M06.21 Rheumatoid bursitis, shoulder
M06.211 Rheumatoid bursitis, right shoulder
M06.212 Rheumatoid bursitis, left shoulder
M06.219 Rheumatoid bursitis, unspecified shoulder
[6] M06.22 Rheumatoid bursitis, elbow
M06.221 Rheumatoid bursitis, right elbow
M06.222 Rheumatoid bursitis, left elbow
M06.229 Rheumatoid bursitis, unspecified elbow
[6] M06.23 Rheumatoid bursitis, wrist
M06.231 Rheumatoid bursitis, right wrist
M06.232 Rheumatoid bursitis, left wrist
M06.239 Rheumatoid bursitis, unspecified wrist
[6] M06.24 Rheumatoid bursitis, hand
M06.241 Rheumatoid bursitis, right hand
M06.242 Rheumatoid bursitis, left hand
M06.249 Rheumatoid bursitis, unspecified hand
[6] M06.25 Rheumatoid bursitis, hip
M06.251 Rheumatoid bursitis, right hip
M06.252 Rheumatoid bursitis, left hip
M06.259 Rheumatoid bursitis, unspecified hip
[6] M06.26 Rheumatoid bursitis, knee
M06.261 Rheumatoid bursitis, right knee
M06.262 Rheumatoid bursitis, left knee
M06.269 Rheumatoid bursitis, unspecified knee
[6] M06.27 Rheumatoid bursitis, ankle and foot
M06.271 Rheumatoid bursitis, right ankle and foot
M06.272 Rheumatoid bursitis, left ankle and foot
M06.279 Rheumatoid bursitis, unspecified ankle and foot
M06.28 Rheumatoid bursitis, vertebrae
M06.29 Rheumatoid bursitis, multiple sites
[5] M06.3 Rheumatoid nodule
M06.30 Rheumatoid nodule, unspecified site
[6] M06.31 Rheumatoid nodule, shoulder
M06.311 Rheumatoid nodule, right shoulder
M06.312 Rheumatoid nodule, left shoulder
M06.319 Rheumatoid nodule, unspecified shoulder
[6] M06.32 Rheumatoid nodule, elbow
M06.321 Rheumatoid nodule, right elbow
M06.322 Rheumatoid nodule, left elbow
M06.329 Rheumatoid nodule, unspecified elbow
[6] M06.33 Rheumatoid nodule, wrist
M06.331 Rheumatoid nodule, right wrist
M06.332 Rheumatoid nodule, left wrist
M06.339 Rheumatoid nodule, unspecified wrist
[6] M06.34 Rheumatoid nodule, hand
M06.341 Rheumatoid nodule, right hand
M06.342 Rheumatoid nodule, left hand
M06.349 Rheumatoid nodule, unspecified hand
[6] M06.35 Rheumatoid nodule, hip
M06.351 Rheumatoid nodule, right hip
M06.352 Rheumatoid nodule, left hip
M06.359 Rheumatoid nodule, unspecified hip
[6] M06.36 Rheumatoid nodule, knee
M06.361 Rheumatoid nodule, right knee
M06.362 Rheumatoid nodule, left knee
M06.369 Rheumatoid nodule, unspecified knee
[6] M06.37 Rheumatoid nodule, ankle and foot
M06.371 Rheumatoid nodule, right ankle and foot
M06.372 Rheumatoid nodule, left ankle and foot
M06.379 Rheumatoid nodule, unspecified ankle and foot
M06.38 Rheumatoid nodule, vertebrae
M06.39 Rheumatoid nodule, multiple sites
M06.4 Inflammatory polyarthropathy
[EXCLUDES1] *polyarthritis NOS (M13.0)*
[5] M06.8 Other specified rheumatoid arthritis
M06.80 Other specified rheumatoid arthritis, unspecified site
[6] M06.81 Other specified rheumatoid arthritis, shoulder
M06.811 Other specified rheumatoid arthritis, right shoulder
M06.812 Other specified rheumatoid arthritis, left shoulder
M06.819 Other specified rheumatoid arthritis, unspecified shoulder
[6] M06.82 Other specified rheumatoid arthritis, elbow

[4] 4th character required [5] 5th character required [6] 6th character required [7] 7th character required [X] Extension 'X' Alert
[EXCLUDES1] Not coded here [EXCLUDES2] Not included here [PDx] Primary Diagnosis Only Manifestation Code

M06.821 Other specified rheumatoid arthritis, right elbow

M06.822 Other specified rheumatoid arthritis, left elbow

M06.829 Other specified rheumatoid arthritis, unspecified elbow

⑥ M06.83 Other specified rheumatoid arthritis, wrist

M06.831 Other specified rheumatoid arthritis, right wrist

M06.832 Other specified rheumatoid arthritis, left wrist

M06.839 Other specified rheumatoid arthritis, unspecified wrist

⑥ M06.84 Other specified rheumatoid arthritis, hand

M06.841 Other specified rheumatoid arthritis, right hand

M06.842 Other specified rheumatoid arthritis, left hand

M06.849 Other specified rheumatoid arthritis, unspecified hand

⑥ M06.85 Other specified rheumatoid arthritis, hip

M06.851 Other specified rheumatoid arthritis, right hip

M06.852 Other specified rheumatoid arthritis, left hip

M06.859 Other specified rheumatoid arthritis, unspecified hip

⑥ M06.86 Other specified rheumatoid arthritis, knee

M06.861 Other specified rheumatoid arthritis, right knee

M06.862 Other specified rheumatoid arthritis, left knee

M06.869 Other specified rheumatoid arthritis, unspecified knee

⑥ M06.87 Other specified rheumatoid arthritis, ankle and foot

M06.871 Other specified rheumatoid arthritis, right ankle and foot

M06.872 Other specified rheumatoid arthritis, left ankle and foot

M06.879 Other specified rheumatoid arthritis, unspecified ankle and foot

M06.88 Other specified rheumatoid arthritis, vertebrae

M06.89 Other specified rheumatoid arthritis, multiple sites

M06.9 Rheumatoid arthritis, unspecified

④ M07 Enteropathic arthropathies

Code also associated enteropathy, such as:
regional enteritis [Crohn's disease] (K50.-)
ulcerative colitis (K51.-)

EXCLUDES1 psoriatic arthropathies (L40.5-)

⑤ M07.6 Enteropathic arthropathies

M07.60 Enteropathic arthropathies, unspecified site

⑥ M07.61 Enteropathic arthropathies, shoulder

M07.611 Enteropathic arthropathies, right shoulder

M07.612 Enteropathic arthropathies, left shoulder

M07.619 Enteropathic arthropathies, unspecified shoulder

⑥ M07.62 Enteropathic arthropathies, elbow

M07.621 Enteropathic arthropathies, right elbow

M07.622 Enteropathic arthropathies, left elbow

M07.629 Enteropathic arthropathies, unspecified elbow

⑥ M07.63 Enteropathic arthropathies, wrist

M07.631 Enteropathic arthropathies, right wrist

M07.632 Enteropathic arthropathies, left wrist

M07.639 Enteropathic arthropathies, unspecified wrist

⑥ M07.64 Enteropathic arthropathies, hand

M07.641 Enteropathic arthropathies, right hand

M07.642 Enteropathic arthropathies, left hand

M07.649 Enteropathic arthropathies, unspecified hand

⑥ M07.65 Enteropathic arthropathies, hip

M07.651 Enteropathic arthropathies, right hip

M07.652 Enteropathic arthropathies, left hip

M07.659 Enteropathic arthropathies, unspecified hip

⑥ M07.66 Enteropathic arthropathies, knee

M07.661 Enteropathic arthropathies, right knee

M07.662 Enteropathic arthropathies, left knee

M07.669 Enteropathic arthropathies, unspecified knee

⑥ M07.67 Enteropathic arthropathies, ankle and foot

M07.671 Enteropathic arthropathies, right ankle and foot

M07.672 Enteropathic arthropathies, left ankle and foot

M07.679 Enteropathic arthropathies, unspecified ankle and foot

M07.68 Enteropathic arthropathies, vertebrae

M07.69 Enteropathic arthropathies, multiple sites

④ M08 Juvenile arthritis

Code also any associated underlying condition, such as:
regional enteritis [Crohn's disease] (K50.-)
ulcerative colitis (K51.-)

EXCLUDES1 arthropathy in Whipple's disease (M14.8)
Felty's syndrome (M05.0)
juvenile dermatomyositis (M33.0-)
psoriatic juvenile arthropathy (L40.54)

⑤ M08.0 Unspecified juvenile rheumatoid arthritis

Juvenile rheumatoid arthritis with or without rheumatoid factor

M08.00 Unspecified juvenile rheumatoid arthritis of unspecified site

⑥ M08.01 Unspecified juvenile rheumatoid arthritis, shoulder

M08.011 Unspecified juvenile rheumatoid arthritis, right shoulder

M08.012 Unspecified juvenile rheumatoid arthritis, left shoulder

M08.019 Unspecified juvenile rheumatoid arthritis, unspecified shoulder

⑥ M08.02 Unspecified juvenile rheumatoid arthritis of elbow

M08.021 Unspecified juvenile rheumatoid arthritis, right elbow

M08.022 Unspecified juvenile rheumatoid arthritis, left elbow

M08.029 Unspecified juvenile rheumatoid arthritis, unspecified elbow

⑥ M08.03 Unspecified juvenile rheumatoid arthritis, wrist

M08.031 Unspecified juvenile rheumatoid arthritis, right wrist

M08.032 Unspecified juvenile rheumatoid arthritis, left wrist

M08.039 Unspecified juvenile rheumatoid arthritis, unspecified wrist

⑥ M08.04 Unspecified juvenile rheumatoid arthritis, hand

M08.041 Unspecified juvenile rheumatoid arthritis, right hand

M08.042 Unspecified juvenile rheumatoid arthritis, left hand

M08.049 Unspecified juvenile rheumatoid arthritis, unspecified hand

---

Unspecified Code	Other Specified Code	Ⓝ Newborn Age: 0	Ⓟ Pediatric Age: 0-17	Ⓜ Maternity Age: 12-55
Ⓐ Adult Age: 15-124	♂ Male	♀ Female	● New Code	▲ Revised Code Title	►◄ Revised Text

[6] M08.05 Unspecified juvenile rheumatoid arthritis, hip
M08.051 Unspecified juvenile rheumatoid arthritis, right hip
M08.052 Unspecified juvenile rheumatoid arthritis, left hip
M08.059 Unspecified juvenile rheumatoid arthritis, unspecified hip
[6] M08.06 Unspecified juvenile rheumatoid arthritis, knee
M08.061 Unspecified juvenile rheumatoid arthritis, right knee
M08.062 Unspecified juvenile rheumatoid arthritis, left knee
M08.069 Unspecified juvenile rheumatoid arthritis, unspecified knee
[6] M08.07 Unspecified juvenile rheumatoid arthritis, ankle and foot
M08.071 Unspecified juvenile rheumatoid arthritis, right ankle and foot
M08.072 Unspecified juvenile rheumatoid arthritis, left ankle and foot
M08.079 Unspecified juvenile rheumatoid arthritis, unspecified ankle and foot
M08.08 Unspecified juvenile rheumatoid arthritis, vertebrae
M08.09 Unspecified juvenile rheumatoid arthritis, multiple sites
M08.1 Juvenile ankylosing spondylitis
[EXCLUDES1] *ankylosing spondylitis in adults (M45.0-)*
[5] M08.2 Juvenile rheumatoid arthritis with systemic onset
Still's disease NOS
[EXCLUDES1] *adult-onset Still's disease (M06.1-)*
M08.20 Juvenile rheumatoid arthritis with systemic onset, unspecified site
[6] M08.21 Juvenile rheumatoid arthritis with systemic onset, shoulder
M08.211 Juvenile rheumatoid arthritis with systemic onset, right shoulder
M08.212 Juvenile rheumatoid arthritis with systemic onset, left shoulder
M08.219 Juvenile rheumatoid arthritis with systemic onset, unspecified shoulder
[6] M08.22 Juvenile rheumatoid arthritis with systemic onset, elbow
M08.221 Juvenile rheumatoid arthritis with systemic onset, right elbow
M08.222 Juvenile rheumatoid arthritis with systemic onset, left elbow
M08.229 Juvenile rheumatoid arthritis with systemic onset, unspecified elbow
[6] M08.23 Juvenile rheumatoid arthritis with systemic onset, wrist
M08.231 Juvenile rheumatoid arthritis with systemic onset, right wrist
M08.232 Juvenile rheumatoid arthritis with systemic onset, left wrist
M08.239 Juvenile rheumatoid arthritis with systemic onset, unspecified wrist
[6] M08.24 Juvenile rheumatoid arthritis with systemic onset, hand
M08.241 Juvenile rheumatoid arthritis with systemic onset, right hand
M08.242 Juvenile rheumatoid arthritis with systemic onset, left hand
M08.249 Juvenile rheumatoid arthritis with systemic onset, unspecified hand
[6] M08.25 Juvenile rheumatoid arthritis with systemic onset, hip
M08.251 Juvenile rheumatoid arthritis with systemic onset, right hip
M08.252 Juvenile rheumatoid arthritis with systemic onset, left hip
M08.259 Juvenile rheumatoid arthritis with systemic onset, unspecified hip
[6] M08.26 Juvenile rheumatoid arthritis with systemic onset, knee
M08.261 Juvenile rheumatoid arthritis with systemic onset, right knee
M08.262 Juvenile rheumatoid arthritis with systemic onset, left knee
M08.269 Juvenile rheumatoid arthritis with systemic onset, unspecified knee
[6] M08.27 Juvenile rheumatoid arthritis with systemic onset, ankle and foot
M08.271 Juvenile rheumatoid arthritis with systemic onset, right ankle and foot
M08.272 Juvenile rheumatoid arthritis with systemic onset, left ankle and foot
M08.279 Juvenile rheumatoid arthritis with systemic onset, unspecified ankle and foot
M08.28 Juvenile rheumatoid arthritis with systemic onset, vertebrae
M08.29 Juvenile rheumatoid arthritis with systemic onset, multiple sites
M08.3 Juvenile rheumatoid polyarthritis (seronegative)
[5] M08.4 Pauciarticular juvenile rheumatoid arthritis
M08.40 Pauciarticular juvenile rheumatoid arthritis, unspecified site
[6] M08.41 Pauciarticular juvenile rheumatoid arthritis, shoulder
M08.411 Pauciarticular juvenile rheumatoid arthritis, right shoulder
M08.412 Pauciarticular juvenile rheumatoid arthritis, left shoulder
M08.419 Pauciarticular juvenile rheumatoid arthritis, unspecified shoulder
[6] M08.42 Pauciarticular juvenile rheumatoid arthritis, elbow
M08.421 Pauciarticular juvenile rheumatoid arthritis, right elbow
M08.422 Pauciarticular juvenile rheumatoid arthritis, left elbow
M08.429 Pauciarticular juvenile rheumatoid arthritis, unspecified elbow
[6] M08.43 Pauciarticular juvenile rheumatoid arthritis, wrist
M08.431 Pauciarticular juvenile rheumatoid arthritis, right wrist
M08.432 Pauciarticular juvenile rheumatoid arthritis, left wrist
M08.439 Pauciarticular juvenile rheumatoid arthritis, unspecified wrist
[6] M08.44 Pauciarticular juvenile rheumatoid arthritis, hand
M08.441 Pauciarticular juvenile rheumatoid arthritis, right hand
M08.442 Pauciarticular juvenile rheumatoid arthritis, left hand
M08.449 Pauciarticular juvenile rheumatoid arthritis, unspecified hand
[6] M08.45 Pauciarticular juvenile rheumatoid arthritis, hip
M08.451 Pauciarticular juvenile rheumatoid arthritis, right hip
M08.452 Pauciarticular juvenile rheumatoid arthritis, left hip
M08.459 Pauciarticular juvenile rheumatoid arthritis, unspecified hip
[6] M08.46 Pauciarticular juvenile rheumatoid arthritis, knee

[4] 4th character required [5] 5th character required [6] 6th character required [7] 7th character required [7x] Extension 'X' Alert
[EXCLUDES1] Not coded here [EXCLUDES2] Not included here [PDx] Primary Diagnosis Only Manifestation Code

M08.461 Pauciarticular juvenile rheumatoid arthritis, right knee
M08.462 Pauciarticular juvenile rheumatoid arthritis, left knee
M08.469 Pauciarticular juvenile rheumatoid arthritis, unspecified knee
[6] M08.47 Pauciarticular juvenile rheumatoid arthritis, ankle and foot
M08.471 Pauciarticular juvenile rheumatoid arthritis, right ankle and foot
M08.472 Pauciarticular juvenile rheumatoid arthritis, left ankle and foot
M08.479 Pauciarticular juvenile rheumatoid arthritis, unspecified ankle and foot
M08.48 Pauciarticular juvenile rheumatoid arthritis, vertebrae
[5] M08.8 Other juvenile arthritis
M08.80 Other juvenile arthritis, unspecified site
[6] M08.81 Other juvenile arthritis, shoulder
M08.811 Other juvenile arthritis, right shoulder
M08.812 Other juvenile arthritis, left shoulder
M08.819 Other juvenile arthritis, unspecified shoulder
[6] M08.82 Other juvenile arthritis, elbow
M08.821 Other juvenile arthritis, right elbow
M08.822 Other juvenile arthritis, left elbow
M08.829 Other juvenile arthritis, unspecified elbow
[6] M08.83 Other juvenile arthritis, wrist
M08.831 Other juvenile arthritis, right wrist
M08.832 Other juvenile arthritis, left wrist
M08.839 Other juvenile arthritis, unspecified wrist
[6] M08.84 Other juvenile arthritis, hand
M08.841 Other juvenile arthritis, right hand
M08.842 Other juvenile arthritis, left hand
M08.849 Other juvenile arthritis, unspecified hand
[6] M08.85 Other juvenile arthritis, hip
M08.851 Other juvenile arthritis, right hip
M08.852 Other juvenile arthritis, left hip
M08.859 Other juvenile arthritis, unspecified hip
[6] M08.86 Other juvenile arthritis, knee
M08.861 Other juvenile arthritis, right knee
M08.862 Other juvenile arthritis, left knee
M08.869 Other juvenile arthritis, unspecified knee
[6] M08.87 Other juvenile arthritis, ankle and foot
M08.871 Other juvenile arthritis, right ankle and foot
M08.872 Other juvenile arthritis, left ankle and foot
M08.879 Other juvenile arthritis, unspecified ankle and foot
M08.88 Other juvenile arthritis, other specified site ▲
Other juvenile arthritis, vertebrae
M08.89 Other juvenile arthritis, multiple sites
[5] M08.9 Juvenile arthritis, unspecified
[EXCLUDES1] *juvenile rheumatoid arthritis, unspecified (M08.0-)*
M08.90 Juvenile arthritis, unspecified, unspecified site
[6] M08.91 Juvenile arthritis, unspecified, shoulder
M08.911 Juvenile arthritis, unspecified, right shoulder
M08.912 Juvenile arthritis, unspecified, left shoulder
M08.919 Juvenile arthritis, unspecified, unspecified shoulder
[6] M08.92 Juvenile arthritis, unspecified, elbow
M08.921 Juvenile arthritis, unspecified, right elbow
M08.922 Juvenile arthritis, unspecified, left elbow
M08.929 Juvenile arthritis, unspecified, unspecified elbow
[6] M08.93 Juvenile arthritis, unspecified, wrist
M08.931 Juvenile arthritis, unspecified, right wrist
M08.932 Juvenile arthritis, unspecified, left wrist
M08.939 Juvenile arthritis, unspecified, unspecified wrist
[6] M08.94 Juvenile arthritis, unspecified, hand
M08.941 Juvenile arthritis, unspecified, right hand
M08.942 Juvenile arthritis, unspecified, left hand
M08.949 Juvenile arthritis, unspecified, unspecified hand
[6] M08.95 Juvenile arthritis, unspecified, hip
M08.951 Juvenile arthritis, unspecified, right hip
M08.952 Juvenile arthritis, unspecified, left hip
M08.959 Juvenile arthritis, unspecified, unspecified hip
[6] M08.96 Juvenile arthritis, unspecified, knee
M08.961 Juvenile arthritis, unspecified, right knee
M08.962 Juvenile arthritis, unspecified, left knee
M08.969 Juvenile arthritis, unspecified, unspecified knee
[6] M08.97 Juvenile arthritis, unspecified, ankle and foot
M08.971 Juvenile arthritis, unspecified, right ankle and foot
M08.972 Juvenile arthritis, unspecified, left ankle and foot
M08.979 Juvenile arthritis, unspecified, unspecified ankle and foot
M08.98 Juvenile arthritis, unspecified, vertebrae
M08.99 Juvenile arthritis, unspecified, multiple sites
[4] M1A Chronic gout
Use additional code to identify:
Autonomic neuropathy in diseases classified elsewhere (G99.0)
Calculus of urinary tract in diseases classified elsewhere (N22)
Cardiomyopathy in diseases classified elsewhere (I43)
Disorders of external ear in diseases classified elsewhere (H61.1-, H62.8-)
Disorders of iris and ciliary body in diseases classified elsewhere (H22)
Glomerular disorders in diseases classified elsewhere (N08)
[EXCLUDES1] *acute gout (M10.-)*
gout NOS (M10.-)

The appropriate 7th character is to be added to each code from category M1A
0 = without tophus (tophi)
1 = with tophus (tophi)

[5] M1A.0 Idiopathic chronic gout
Chronic gouty bursitis
Primary chronic gout
[7] M1A.00 Idiopathic chronic gout, unspecified site
[6] M1A.01 Idiopathic chronic gout, shoulder
[7] M1A.011 Idiopathic chronic gout, right shoulder
[7] M1A.012 Idiopathic chronic gout, left shoulder
[7] M1A.019 Idiopathic chronic gout, unspecified shoulder
[6] M1A.02 Idiopathic chronic gout, elbow
[7] M1A.021 Idiopathic chronic gout, right elbow
[7] M1A.022 Idiopathic chronic gout, left elbow
[7] M1A.029 Idiopathic chronic gout, unspecified elbow
[6] M1A.03 Idiopathic chronic gout, wrist
[7] M1A.031 Idiopathic chronic gout, right wrist
[7] M1A.032 Idiopathic chronic gout, left wrist
[7] M1A.039 Idiopathic chronic gout, unspecified wrist
[6] M1A.04 Idiopathic chronic gout, hand
[7] M1A.041 Idiopathic chronic gout, right hand
[7] M1A.042 Idiopathic chronic gout, left hand
[7] M1A.049 Idiopathic chronic gout, unspecified hand

Unspecified Code | Other Specified Code | [N] Newborn Age: 0 | [P] Pediatric Age: 0-17 | [M] Maternity Age: 12-55
[A] Adult Age: 15-124 | ♂ Male | ♀ Female | ● New Code | ▲ Revised Code Title | ►◄ Revised Text

[6th] M1A.05 Idiopathic chronic gout, hip
- [7th] M1A.051 Idiopathic chronic gout, right hip
- [7th] M1A.052 Idiopathic chronic gout, left hip
- [7th] M1A.059 Idiopathic chronic gout, unspecified hip

[6th] M1A.06 Idiopathic chronic gout, knee
- [7th] M1A.061 Idiopathic chronic gout, right knee
- [7th] M1A.062 Idiopathic chronic gout, left knee
- [7th] M1A.069 Idiopathic chronic gout, unspecified knee

[6th] M1A.07 Idiopathic chronic gout, ankle and foot
- [7th] M1A.071 Idiopathic chronic gout, right ankle and foot
- [7th] M1A.072 Idiopathic chronic gout, left ankle and foot
- [7th] M1A.079 Idiopathic chronic gout, unspecified ankle and foot

[X7th] M1A.08 Idiopathic chronic gout, vertebrae

[X7th] M1A.09 Idiopathic chronic gout, multiple sites

[5th] M1A.1 Lead-induced chronic gout

Code first toxic effects of lead and its compounds (T56.0-)

[X7th] M1A.10 Lead-induced chronic gout, unspecified site

[6th] M1A.11 Lead-induced chronic gout, shoulder
- [7th] M1A.111 Lead-induced chronic gout, right shoulder
- [7th] M1A.112 Lead-induced chronic gout, left shoulder
- [7th] M1A.119 Lead-induced chronic gout, unspecified shoulder

[6th] M1A.12 Lead-induced chronic gout, elbow
- [7th] M1A.121 Lead-induced chronic gout, right elbow
- [7th] M1A.122 Lead-induced chronic gout, left elbow
- [7th] M1A.129 Lead-induced chronic gout, unspecified elbow

[6th] M1A.13 Lead-induced chronic gout, wrist
- [7th] M1A.131 Lead-induced chronic gout, right wrist
- [7th] M1A.132 Lead-induced chronic gout, left wrist
- [7th] M1A.139 Lead-induced chronic gout, unspecified wrist

[6th] M1A.14 Lead-induced chronic gout, hand
- [7th] M1A.141 Lead-induced chronic gout, right hand
- [7th] M1A.142 Lead-induced chronic gout, left hand
- [7th] M1A.149 Lead-induced chronic gout, unspecified hand

[6th] M1A.15 Lead-induced chronic gout, hip
- [7th] M1A.151 Lead-induced chronic gout, right hip
- [7th] M1A.152 Lead-induced chronic gout, left hip
- [7th] M1A.159 Lead-induced chronic gout, unspecified hip

[6th] M1A.16 Lead-induced chronic gout, knee
- [7th] M1A.161 Lead-induced chronic gout, right knee
- [7th] M1A.162 Lead-induced chronic gout, left knee
- [7th] M1A.169 Lead-induced chronic gout, unspecified knee

[6th] M1A.17 Lead-induced chronic gout, ankle and foot
- [7th] M1A.171 Lead-induced chronic gout, right ankle and foot
- [7th] M1A.172 Lead-induced chronic gout, left ankle and foot
- [7th] M1A.179 Lead-induced chronic gout, unspecified ankle and foot

[X7th] M1A.18 Lead-induced chronic gout, vertebrae

[X7th] M1A.19 Lead-induced chronic gout, multiple sites

[5th] M1A.2 Drug-induced chronic gout

Use additional code for adverse effect, if applicable, to identify drug (T36-T50 with fifth or sixth character 5)

[X7th] M1A.20 Drug-induced chronic gout, unspecified site

[6th] M1A.21 Drug-induced chronic gout, shoulder
- [7th] M1A.211 Drug-induced chronic gout, right shoulder
- [7th] M1A.212 Drug-induced chronic gout, left shoulder
- [7th] M1A.219 Drug-induced chronic gout, unspecified shoulder

[6th] M1A.22 Drug-induced chronic gout, elbow
- [7th] M1A.221 Drug-induced chronic gout, right elbow
- [7th] M1A.222 Drug-induced chronic gout, left elbow
- [7th] M1A.229 Drug-induced chronic gout, unspecified elbow

[6th] M1A.23 Drug-induced chronic gout, wrist
- [7th] M1A.231 Drug-induced chronic gout, right wrist
- [7th] M1A.232 Drug-induced chronic gout, left wrist
- [7th] M1A.239 Drug-induced chronic gout, unspecified wrist

[6th] M1A.24 Drug-induced chronic gout, hand
- [7th] M1A.241 Drug-induced chronic gout, right hand
- [7th] M1A.242 Drug-induced chronic gout, left hand
- [7th] M1A.249 Drug-induced chronic gout, unspecified hand

[6th] M1A.25 Drug-induced chronic gout, hip
- [7th] M1A.251 Drug-induced chronic gout, right hip
- [7th] M1A.252 Drug-induced chronic gout, left hip
- [7th] M1A.259 Drug-induced chronic gout, unspecified hip

[6th] M1A.26 Drug-induced chronic gout, knee
- [7th] M1A.261 Drug-induced chronic gout, right knee
- [7th] M1A.262 Drug-induced chronic gout, left knee
- [7th] M1A.269 Drug-induced chronic gout, unspecified knee

[6th] M1A.27 Drug-induced chronic gout, ankle and foot
- [7th] M1A.271 Drug-induced chronic gout, right ankle and foot
- [7th] M1A.272 Drug-induced chronic gout, left ankle and foot
- [7th] M1A.279 Drug-induced chronic gout, unspecified ankle and foot

[X7th] M1A.28 Drug-induced chronic gout, vertebrae

[X7th] M1A.29 Drug-induced chronic gout, multiple sites

[5th] M1A.3 Chronic gout due to renal impairment

Code first associated renal disease

[X7th] M1A.30 Chronic gout due to renal impairment, unspecified site

[6th] M1A.31 Chronic gout due to renal impairment, shoulder
- [7th] M1A.311 Chronic gout due to renal impairment, right shoulder
- [7th] M1A.312 Chronic gout due to renal impairment, left shoulder
- [7th] M1A.319 Chronic gout due to renal impairment, unspecified shoulder

[6th] M1A.32 Chronic gout due to renal impairment, elbow
- [7th] M1A.321 Chronic gout due to renal impairment, right elbow
- [7th] M1A.322 Chronic gout due to renal impairment, left elbow
- [7th] M1A.329 Chronic gout due to renal impairment, unspecified elbow

[6th] M1A.33 Chronic gout due to renal impairment, wrist
- [7th] M1A.331 Chronic gout due to renal impairment, right wrist
- [7th] M1A.332 Chronic gout due to renal impairment, left wrist
- [7th] M1A.339 Chronic gout due to renal impairment, unspecified wrist

[6th] M1A.34 Chronic gout due to renal impairment, hand
- [7th] M1A.341 Chronic gout due to renal impairment, right hand
- [7th] M1A.342 Chronic gout due to renal impairment, left hand
- [7th] M1A.349 Chronic gout due to renal impairment, unspecified hand

[6th] M1A.35 Chronic gout due to renal impairment, hip

[4th] 4th character required [5th] 5th character required [6th] 6th character required [7th] 7th character required [X7th] Extension 'X' Alert
EXCLUDES 1 Not coded here EXCLUDES 2 Not included here PDx Primary Diagnosis Only Manifestation Code

⑦ M1A.351 Chronic gout due to renal impairment, right hip

⑦ M1A.352 Chronic gout due to renal impairment, left hip

⑦ M1A.359 Chronic gout due to renal impairment, unspecified hip

⑥ M1A.36 Chronic gout due to renal impairment, knee

⑦ M1A.361 Chronic gout due to renal impairment, right knee

⑦ M1A.362 Chronic gout due to renal impairment, left knee

⑦ M1A.369 Chronic gout due to renal impairment, unspecified knee

⑥ M1A.37 Chronic gout due to renal impairment, ankle and foot

⑦ M1A.371 Chronic gout due to renal impairment, right ankle and foot

⑦ M1A.372 Chronic gout due to renal impairment, left ankle and foot

⑦ M1A.379 Chronic gout due to renal impairment, unspecified ankle and foot

⑦ᵖ M1A.38 Chronic gout due to renal impairment, vertebrae

⑦ᵖ M1A.39 Chronic gout due to renal impairment, multiple sites

⑤ M1A.4 Other secondary chronic gout
Code first associated condition

⑦ᵖ M1A.40 Other secondary chronic gout, unspecified site

⑥ M1A.41 Other secondary chronic gout, shoulder

⑦ M1A.411 Other secondary chronic gout, right shoulder

⑦ M1A.412 Other secondary chronic gout, left shoulder

⑦ M1A.419 Other secondary chronic gout, unspecified shoulder

⑥ M1A.42 Other secondary chronic gout, elbow

⑦ M1A.421 Other secondary chronic gout, right elbow

⑦ M1A.422 Other secondary chronic gout, left elbow

⑦ M1A.429 Other secondary chronic gout, unspecified elbow

⑥ M1A.43 Other secondary chronic gout, wrist

⑦ M1A.431 Other secondary chronic gout, right wrist

⑦ M1A.432 Other secondary chronic gout, left wrist

⑦ M1A.439 Other secondary chronic gout, unspecified wrist

⑥ M1A.44 Other secondary chronic gout, hand

⑦ M1A.441 Other secondary chronic gout, right hand

⑦ M1A.442 Other secondary chronic gout, left hand

⑦ M1A.449 Other secondary chronic gout, unspecified hand

⑥ M1A.45 Other secondary chronic gout, hip

⑦ M1A.451 Other secondary chronic gout, right hip

⑦ M1A.452 Other secondary chronic gout, left hip

⑦ M1A.459 Other secondary chronic gout, unspecified hip

⑥ M1A.46 Other secondary chronic gout, knee

⑦ M1A.461 Other secondary chronic gout, right knee

⑦ M1A.462 Other secondary chronic gout, left knee

⑦ M1A.469 Other secondary chronic gout, unspecified knee

⑥ M1A.47 Other secondary chronic gout, ankle and foot

⑦ M1A.471 Other secondary chronic gout, right ankle and foot

⑦ M1A.472 Other secondary chronic gout, left ankle and foot

⑦ M1A.479 Other secondary chronic gout, unspecified ankle and foot

⑦ᵖ M1A.48 Other secondary chronic gout, vertebrae

⑦ᵖ M1A.49 Other secondary chronic gout, multiple sites

⑦ᵖ M1A.9 Chronic gout, unspecified

④ M10 Gout
Acute gout
Gout attack
Gout flare
Gout NOS
Podagra
Use additional code to identify:
Autonomic neuropathy in diseases classified elsewhere (G99.0)
Calculus of urinary tract in diseases classified elsewhere (N22)
Cardiomyopathy in diseases classified elsewhere (I43)
Disorders of external ear in diseases classified elsewhere (H61.1-, H62.8-)
Disorders of iris and ciliary body in diseases classified elsewhere (H22)
Glomerular disorders in diseases classified elsewhere (N08)

EXCLUDES1 chronic gout (M1A.-)

⑤ M10.0 Idiopathic gout
Gouty bursitis
Primary gout
M10.00 Idiopathic gout, unspecified site

⑥ M10.01 Idiopathic gout, shoulder
M10.011 Idiopathic gout, right shoulder
M10.012 Idiopathic gout, left shoulder
M10.019 Idiopathic gout, unspecified shoulder

⑥ M10.02 Idiopathic gout, elbow
M10.021 Idiopathic gout, right elbow
M10.022 Idiopathic gout, left elbow
M10.029 Idiopathic gout, unspecified elbow

⑥ M10.03 Idiopathic gout, wrist
M10.031 Idiopathic gout, right wrist
M10.032 Idiopathic gout, left wrist
M10.039 Idiopathic gout, unspecified wrist

⑥ M10.04 Idiopathic gout, hand
M10.041 Idiopathic gout, right hand
M10.042 Idiopathic gout, left hand
M10.049 Idiopathic gout, unspecified hand

⑥ M10.05 Idiopathic gout, hip
M10.051 Idiopathic gout, right hip
M10.052 Idiopathic gout, left hip
M10.059 Idiopathic gout, unspecified hip

⑥ M10.06 Idiopathic gout, knee
M10.061 Idiopathic gout, right knee
M10.062 Idiopathic gout, left knee
M10.069 Idiopathic gout, unspecified knee

⑥ M10.07 Idiopathic gout, ankle and foot
M10.071 Idiopathic gout, right ankle and foot
M10.072 Idiopathic gout, left ankle and foot
M10.079 Idiopathic gout, unspecified ankle and foot

M10.08 Idiopathic gout, vertebrae
M10.09 Idiopathic gout, multiple sites

⑤ M10.1 Lead-induced gout
Code first toxic effects of lead and its compounds (T56.0-)
M10.10 Lead-induced gout, unspecified site

⑥ M10.11 Lead-induced gout, shoulder
M10.111 Lead-induced gout, right shoulder
M10.112 Lead-induced gout, left shoulder
M10.119 Lead-induced gout, unspecified shoulder

⑥ M10.12 Lead-induced gout, elbow
M10.121 Lead-induced gout, right elbow
M10.122 Lead-induced gout, left elbow
M10.129 Lead-induced gout, unspecified elbow

Unspecified Code | Other Specified Code | Ⓝ Newborn Age: 0 | Ⓟ Pediatric Age: 0-17 | Ⓜ Maternity Age: 12-55
Ⓐ Adult Age: 15-124 | ♂ Male | ♀ Female | ● New Code | ▲ Revised Code Title | ►◄ Revised Text

[6] M10.13 Lead-induced gout, wrist
M10.131 Lead-induced gout, right wrist
M10.132 Lead-induced gout, left wrist
M10.139 Lead-induced gout, unspecified wrist
[6] M10.14 Lead-induced gout, hand
M10.141 Lead-induced gout, right hand
M10.142 Lead-induced gout, left hand
M10.149 Lead-induced gout, unspecified hand
[6] M10.15 Lead-induced gout, hip
M10.151 Lead-induced gout, right hip
M10.152 Lead-induced gout, left hip
M10.159 Lead-induced gout, unspecified hip
[6] M10.16 Lead-induced gout, knee
M10.161 Lead-induced gout, right knee
M10.162 Lead-induced gout, left knee
M10.169 Lead-induced gout, unspecified knee
[6] M10.17 Lead-induced gout, ankle and foot
M10.171 Lead-induced gout, right ankle and foot
M10.172 Lead-induced gout, left ankle and foot
M10.179 Lead-induced gout, unspecified ankle and foot
M10.18 Lead-induced gout, vertebrae
M10.19 Lead-induced gout, multiple sites
[5] M10.2 Drug-induced gout
Use additional code for adverse effect, if applicable, to identify drug (T36-T50 with fifth or sixth character 5)
M10.20 Drug-induced gout, unspecified site
[6] M10.21 Drug-induced gout, shoulder
M10.211 Drug-induced gout, right shoulder
M10.212 Drug-induced gout, left shoulder
M10.219 Drug-induced gout, unspecified shoulder
[6] M10.22 Drug-induced gout, elbow
M10.221 Drug-induced gout, right elbow
M10.222 Drug-induced gout, left elbow
M10.229 Drug-induced gout, unspecified elbow
[6] M10.23 Drug-induced gout, wrist
M10.231 Drug-induced gout, right wrist
M10.232 Drug-induced gout, left wrist
M10.239 Drug-induced gout, unspecified wrist
[6] M10.24 Drug-induced gout, hand
M10.241 Drug-induced gout, right hand
M10.242 Drug-induced gout, left hand
M10.249 Drug-induced gout, unspecified hand
[6] M10.25 Drug-induced gout, hip
M10.251 Drug-induced gout, right hip
M10.252 Drug-induced gout, left hip
M10.259 Drug-induced gout, unspecified hip
[6] M10.26 Drug-induced gout, knee
M10.261 Drug-induced gout, right knee
M10.262 Drug-induced gout, left knee
M10.269 Drug-induced gout, unspecified knee
[6] M10.27 Drug-induced gout, ankle and foot
M10.271 Drug-induced gout, right ankle and foot
M10.272 Drug-induced gout, left ankle and foot
M10.279 Drug-induced gout, unspecified ankle and foot
M10.28 Drug-induced gout, vertebrae
M10.29 Drug-induced gout, multiple sites
[5] M10.3 Gout due to renal impairment
Code first associated renal disease
M10.30 Gout due to renal impairment, unspecified site
[6] M10.31 Gout due to renal impairment, shoulder
M10.311 Gout due to renal impairment, right shoulder
M10.312 Gout due to renal impairment, left shoulder
M10.319 Gout due to renal impairment, unspecified shoulder
[6] M10.32 Gout due to renal impairment, elbow
M10.321 Gout due to renal impairment, right elbow
M10.322 Gout due to renal impairment, left elbow
M10.329 Gout due to renal impairment, unspecified elbow
[6] M10.33 Gout due to renal impairment, wrist
M10.331 Gout due to renal impairment, right wrist
M10.332 Gout due to renal impairment, left wrist
M10.339 Gout due to renal impairment, unspecified wrist
[6] M10.34 Gout due to renal impairment, hand
M10.341 Gout due to renal impairment, right hand
M10.342 Gout due to renal impairment, left hand
M10.349 Gout due to renal impairment, unspecified hand
[6] M10.35 Gout due to renal impairment, hip
M10.351 Gout due to renal impairment, right hip
M10.352 Gout due to renal impairment, left hip
M10.359 Gout due to renal impairment, unspecified hip
[6] M10.36 Gout due to renal impairment, knee
M10.361 Gout due to renal impairment, right knee
M10.362 Gout due to renal impairment, left knee
M10.369 Gout due to renal impairment, unspecified knee
[6] M10.37 Gout due to renal impairment, ankle and foot
M10.371 Gout due to renal impairment, right ankle and foot
M10.372 Gout due to renal impairment, left ankle and foot
M10.379 Gout due to renal impairment, unspecified ankle and foot
M10.38 Gout due to renal impairment, vertebrae
M10.39 Gout due to renal impairment, multiple sites
[5] M10.4 Other secondary gout
Code first associated condition
M10.40 Other secondary gout, unspecified site
[6] M10.41 Other secondary gout, shoulder
M10.411 Other secondary gout, right shoulder
M10.412 Other secondary gout, left shoulder
M10.419 Other secondary gout, unspecified shoulder
[6] M10.42 Other secondary gout, elbow
M10.421 Other secondary gout, right elbow
M10.422 Other secondary gout, left elbow
M10.429 Other secondary gout, unspecified elbow
[6] M10.43 Other secondary gout, wrist
M10.431 Other secondary gout, right wrist
M10.432 Other secondary gout, left wrist
M10.439 Other secondary gout, unspecified wrist
[6] M10.44 Other secondary gout, hand
M10.441 Other secondary gout, right hand
M10.442 Other secondary gout, left hand
M10.449 Other secondary gout, unspecified hand
[6] M10.45 Other secondary gout, hip
M10.451 Other secondary gout, right hip
M10.452 Other secondary gout, left hip
M10.459 Other secondary gout, unspecified hip
[6] M10.46 Other secondary gout, knee
M10.461 Other secondary gout, right knee
M10.462 Other secondary gout, left knee
M10.469 Other secondary gout, unspecified knee
[6] M10.47 Other secondary gout, ankle and foot
M10.471 Other secondary gout, right ankle and foot
M10.472 Other secondary gout, left ankle and foot

[4] 4th character required [5] 5th character required [6] 6th character required [7] 7th character required [X] Extension 'X' Alert
[EXCLUDES 1] Not coded here [EXCLUDES 2] Not included here [PDx] Primary Diagnosis Only Manifestation Code

M10.479 Other secondary gout, unspecified ankle and foot
M10.48 Other secondary gout, vertebrae
M10.49 Other secondary gout, multiple sites
M10.9 Gout, unspecified
Gout NOS

[4] M11 Other crystal arthropathies
[5] M11.0 Hydroxyapatite deposition disease
M11.00 Hydroxyapatite deposition disease, unspecified site
[6] M11.01 Hydroxyapatite deposition disease, shoulder
M11.011 Hydroxyapatite deposition disease, right shoulder
M11.012 Hydroxyapatite deposition disease, left shoulder
M11.019 Hydroxyapatite deposition disease, unspecified shoulder
[6] M11.02 Hydroxyapatite deposition disease, elbow
M11.021 Hydroxyapatite deposition disease, right elbow
M11.022 Hydroxyapatite deposition disease, left elbow
M11.029 Hydroxyapatite deposition disease, unspecified elbow
[6] M11.03 Hydroxyapatite deposition disease, wrist
M11.031 Hydroxyapatite deposition disease, right wrist
M11.032 Hydroxyapatite deposition disease, left wrist
M11.039 Hydroxyapatite deposition disease, unspecified wrist
[6] M11.04 Hydroxyapatite deposition disease, hand
M11.041 Hydroxyapatite deposition disease, right hand
M11.042 Hydroxyapatite deposition disease, left hand
M11.049 Hydroxyapatite deposition disease, unspecified hand
[6] M11.05 Hydroxyapatite deposition disease, hip
M11.051 Hydroxyapatite deposition disease, right hip
M11.052 Hydroxyapatite deposition disease, left hip
M11.059 Hydroxyapatite deposition disease, unspecified hip
[6] M11.06 Hydroxyapatite deposition disease, knee
M11.061 Hydroxyapatite deposition disease, right knee
M11.062 Hydroxyapatite deposition disease, left knee
M11.069 Hydroxyapatite deposition disease, unspecified knee
[6] M11.07 Hydroxyapatite deposition disease, ankle and foot
M11.071 Hydroxyapatite deposition disease, right ankle and foot
M11.072 Hydroxyapatite deposition disease, left ankle and foot
M11.079 Hydroxyapatite deposition disease, unspecified ankle and foot
M11.08 Hydroxyapatite deposition disease, vertebrae
M11.09 Hydroxyapatite deposition disease, multiple sites
[5] M11.1 Familial chondrocalcinosis
M11.10 Familial chondrocalcinosis, unspecified site
[6] M11.11 Familial chondrocalcinosis, shoulder
M11.111 Familial chondrocalcinosis, right shoulder
M11.112 Familial chondrocalcinosis, left shoulder
M11.119 Familial chondrocalcinosis, unspecified shoulder
[6] M11.12 Familial chondrocalcinosis, elbow
M11.121 Familial chondrocalcinosis, right elbow
M11.122 Familial chondrocalcinosis, left elbow
M11.129 Familial chondrocalcinosis, unspecified elbow
[6] M11.13 Familial chondrocalcinosis, wrist
M11.131 Familial chondrocalcinosis, right wrist
M11.132 Familial chondrocalcinosis, left wrist
M11.139 Familial chondrocalcinosis, unspecified wrist
[6] M11.14 Familial chondrocalcinosis, hand
M11.141 Familial chondrocalcinosis, right hand
M11.142 Familial chondrocalcinosis, left hand
M11.149 Familial chondrocalcinosis, unspecified hand
[6] M11.15 Familial chondrocalcinosis, hip
M11.151 Familial chondrocalcinosis, right hip
M11.152 Familial chondrocalcinosis, left hip
M11.159 Familial chondrocalcinosis, unspecified hip
[6] M11.16 Familial chondrocalcinosis, knee
M11.161 Familial chondrocalcinosis, right knee
M11.162 Familial chondrocalcinosis, left knee
M11.169 Familial chondrocalcinosis, unspecified knee
[6] M11.17 Familial chondrocalcinosis, ankle and foot
M11.171 Familial chondrocalcinosis, right ankle and foot
M11.172 Familial chondrocalcinosis, left ankle and foot
M11.179 Familial chondrocalcinosis, unspecified ankle and foot
M11.18 Familial chondrocalcinosis, vertebrae
M11.19 Familial chondrocalcinosis, multiple sites
[5] M11.2 Other chondrocalcinosis
Chondrocalcinosis NOS
M11.20 Other chondrocalcinosis, unspecified site
[6] M11.21 Other chondrocalcinosis, shoulder
M11.211 Other chondrocalcinosis, right shoulder
M11.212 Other chondrocalcinosis, left shoulder
M11.219 Other chondrocalcinosis, unspecified shoulder
[6] M11.22 Other chondrocalcinosis, elbow
M11.221 Other chondrocalcinosis, right elbow
M11.222 Other chondrocalcinosis, left elbow
M11.229 Other chondrocalcinosis, unspecified elbow
[6] M11.23 Other chondrocalcinosis, wrist
M11.231 Other chondrocalcinosis, right wrist
M11.232 Other chondrocalcinosis, left wrist
M11.239 Other chondrocalcinosis, unspecified wrist
[6] M11.24 Other chondrocalcinosis, hand
M11.241 Other chondrocalcinosis, right hand
M11.242 Other chondrocalcinosis, left hand
M11.249 Other chondrocalcinosis, unspecified hand
[6] M11.25 Other chondrocalcinosis, hip
M11.251 Other chondrocalcinosis, right hip
M11.252 Other chondrocalcinosis, left hip
M11.259 Other chondrocalcinosis, unspecified hip
[6] M11.26 Other chondrocalcinosis, knee
M11.261 Other chondrocalcinosis, right knee
M11.262 Other chondrocalcinosis, left knee
M11.269 Other chondrocalcinosis, unspecified knee
[6] M11.27 Other chondrocalcinosis, ankle and foot
M11.271 Other chondrocalcinosis, right ankle and foot

Unspecified Code | Other Specified Code | [N] Newborn Age: 0 | [P] Pediatric Age: 0-17 | [M] Maternity Age: 12-55
[A] Adult Age: 15-124 | ♂ Male | ♀ Female | ● New Code | ▲ Revised Code Title | ►◄ Revised Text

M11.272 Other chondrocalcinosis, left ankle and foot
M11.279 Other chondrocalcinosis, unspecified ankle and foot
M11.28 Other chondrocalcinosis, vertebrae
M11.29 Other chondrocalcinosis, multiple sites
[5] M11.8 Other specified crystal arthropathies
M11.80 Other specified crystal arthropathies, unspecified site
[6] M11.81 Other specified crystal arthropathies, shoulder
M11.811 Other specified crystal arthropathies, right shoulder
M11.812 Other specified crystal arthropathies, left shoulder
M11.819 Other specified crystal arthropathies, unspecified shoulder
[6] M11.82 Other specified crystal arthropathies, elbow
M11.821 Other specified crystal arthropathies, right elbow
M11.822 Other specified crystal arthropathies, left elbow
M11.829 Other specified crystal arthropathies, unspecified elbow
[6] M11.83 Other specified crystal arthropathies, wrist
M11.831 Other specified crystal arthropathies, right wrist
M11.832 Other specified crystal arthropathies, left wrist
M11.839 Other specified crystal arthropathies, unspecified wrist
[6] M11.84 Other specified crystal arthropathies, hand
M11.841 Other specified crystal arthropathies, right hand
M11.842 Other specified crystal arthropathies, left hand
M11.849 Other specified crystal arthropathies, unspecified hand
[6] M11.85 Other specified crystal arthropathies, hip
M11.851 Other specified crystal arthropathies, right hip
M11.852 Other specified crystal arthropathies, left hip
M11.859 Other specified crystal arthropathies, unspecified hip
[6] M11.86 Other specified crystal arthropathies, knee
M11.861 Other specified crystal arthropathies, right knee
M11.862 Other specified crystal arthropathies, left knee
M11.869 Other specified crystal arthropathies, unspecified knee
[6] M11.87 Other specified crystal arthropathies, ankle and foot
M11.871 Other specified crystal arthropathies, right ankle and foot
M11.872 Other specified crystal arthropathies, left ankle and foot
M11.879 Other specified crystal arthropathies, unspecified ankle and foot
M11.88 Other specified crystal arthropathies, vertebrae
M11.89 Other specified crystal arthropathies, multiple sites
M11.9 Crystal arthropathy, unspecified
[4] M12 Other and unspecified arthropathy
[EXCLUDES1] *arthrosis (M15-M19)*
cricoarytenoid arthropathy (J38.7)
[5] M12.0 Chronic postrheumatic arthropathy [Jaccoud]
M12.00 Chronic postrheumatic arthropathy [Jaccoud], unspecified site
[6] M12.01 Chronic postrheumatic arthropathy [Jaccoud], shoulder
M12.011 Chronic postrheumatic arthropathy [Jaccoud], right shoulder
M12.012 Chronic postrheumatic arthropathy [Jaccoud], left shoulder
M12.019 Chronic postrheumatic arthropathy [Jaccoud], unspecified shoulder
[6] M12.02 Chronic postrheumatic arthropathy [Jaccoud], elbow
M12.021 Chronic postrheumatic arthropathy [Jaccoud], right elbow
M12.022 Chronic postrheumatic arthropathy [Jaccoud], left elbow
M12.029 Chronic postrheumatic arthropathy [Jaccoud], unspecified elbow
[6] M12.03 Chronic postrheumatic arthropathy [Jaccoud], wrist
M12.031 Chronic postrheumatic arthropathy [Jaccoud], right wrist
M12.032 Chronic postrheumatic arthropathy [Jaccoud], left wrist
M12.039 Chronic postrheumatic arthropathy [Jaccoud], unspecified wrist
[6] M12.04 Chronic postrheumatic arthropathy [Jaccoud], hand
M12.041 Chronic postrheumatic arthropathy [Jaccoud], right hand
M12.042 Chronic postrheumatic arthropathy [Jaccoud], left hand
M12.049 Chronic postrheumatic arthropathy [Jaccoud], unspecified hand
[6] M12.05 Chronic postrheumatic arthropathy [Jaccoud], hip
M12.051 Chronic postrheumatic arthropathy [Jaccoud], right hip
M12.052 Chronic postrheumatic arthropathy [Jaccoud], left hip
M12.059 Chronic postrheumatic arthropathy [Jaccoud], unspecified hip
[6] M12.06 Chronic postrheumatic arthropathy [Jaccoud], knee
M12.061 Chronic postrheumatic arthropathy [Jaccoud], right knee
M12.062 Chronic postrheumatic arthropathy [Jaccoud], left knee
M12.069 Chronic postrheumatic arthropathy [Jaccoud], unspecified knee
[6] M12.07 Chronic postrheumatic arthropathy [Jaccoud], ankle and foot
M12.071 Chronic postrheumatic arthropathy [Jaccoud], right ankle and foot
M12.072 Chronic postrheumatic arthropathy [Jaccoud], left ankle and foot
M12.079 Chronic postrheumatic arthropathy [Jaccoud], unspecified ankle and foot
M12.08 Chronic postrheumatic arthropathy [Jaccoud], other specified site ▲
Chronic postrheumatic arthropathy [Jaccoud], vertebrae
M12.09 Chronic postrheumatic arthropathy [Jaccoud], multiple sites
[5] M12.1 Kaschin-Beck disease
Osteochondroarthrosis deformans endemica
M12.10 Kaschin-Beck disease, unspecified site
[6] M12.11 Kaschin-Beck disease, shoulder
M12.111 Kaschin-Beck disease, right shoulder
M12.112 Kaschin-Beck disease, left shoulder
M12.119 Kaschin-Beck disease, unspecified shoulder
[6] M12.12 Kaschin-Beck disease, elbow

[4] 4th character required [5] 5th character required [6] 6th character required [7] 7th character required [x7] Extension 'X' Alert
[EXCLUDES1] Not coded here [EXCLUDES2] Not included here [PDx] Primary Diagnosis Only Manifestation Code

M12.121 Kaschin-Beck disease, right elbow
M12.122 Kaschin-Beck disease, left elbow
M12.129 Kaschin-Beck disease, unspecified elbow
[6] M12.13 Kaschin-Beck disease, wrist
M12.131 Kaschin-Beck disease, right wrist
M12.132 Kaschin-Beck disease, left wrist
M12.139 Kaschin-Beck disease, unspecified wrist
[6] M12.14 Kaschin-Beck disease, hand
M12.141 Kaschin-Beck disease, right hand
M12.142 Kaschin-Beck disease, left hand
M12.149 Kaschin-Beck disease, unspecified hand
[6] M12.15 Kaschin-Beck disease, hip
M12.151 Kaschin-Beck disease, right hip
M12.152 Kaschin-Beck disease, left hip
M12.159 Kaschin-Beck disease, unspecified hip
[6] M12.16 Kaschin-Beck disease, knee
M12.161 Kaschin-Beck disease, right knee
M12.162 Kaschin-Beck disease, left knee
M12.169 Kaschin-Beck disease, unspecified knee
[6] M12.17 Kaschin-Beck disease, ankle and foot
M12.171 Kaschin-Beck disease, right ankle and foot
M12.172 Kaschin-Beck disease, left ankle and foot
M12.179 Kaschin-Beck disease, unspecified ankle and foot
M12.18 Kaschin-Beck disease, vertebrae
M12.19 Kaschin-Beck disease, multiple sites
[5] M12.2 Villonodular synovitis (pigmented)
M12.20 Villonodular synovitis (pigmented), unspecified site
[6] M12.21 Villonodular synovitis (pigmented), shoulder
M12.211 Villonodular synovitis (pigmented), right shoulder
M12.212 Villonodular synovitis (pigmented), left shoulder
M12.219 Villonodular synovitis (pigmented), unspecified shoulder
[6] M12.22 Villonodular synovitis (pigmented), elbow
M12.221 Villonodular synovitis (pigmented), right elbow
M12.222 Villonodular synovitis (pigmented), left elbow
M12.229 Villonodular synovitis (pigmented), unspecified elbow
[6] M12.23 Villonodular synovitis (pigmented), wrist
M12.231 Villonodular synovitis (pigmented), right wrist
M12.232 Villonodular synovitis (pigmented), left wrist
M12.239 Villonodular synovitis (pigmented), unspecified wrist
[6] M12.24 Villonodular synovitis (pigmented), hand
M12.241 Villonodular synovitis (pigmented), right hand
M12.242 Villonodular synovitis (pigmented), left hand
M12.249 Villonodular synovitis (pigmented), unspecified hand
[6] M12.25 Villonodular synovitis (pigmented), hip
M12.251 Villonodular synovitis (pigmented), right hip
M12.252 Villonodular synovitis (pigmented), left hip
M12.259 Villonodular synovitis (pigmented), unspecified hip
[6] M12.26 Villonodular synovitis (pigmented), knee
M12.261 Villonodular synovitis (pigmented), right knee
M12.262 Villonodular synovitis (pigmented), left knee
M12.269 Villonodular synovitis (pigmented), unspecified knee
[6] M12.27 Villonodular synovitis (pigmented), ankle and foot
M12.271 Villonodular synovitis (pigmented), right ankle and foot
M12.272 Villonodular synovitis (pigmented), left ankle and foot
M12.279 Villonodular synovitis (pigmented), unspecified ankle and foot
M12.28 Villonodular synovitis (pigmented), other specified site ▲
Villonodular synovitis (pigmented), vertebrae
M12.29 Villonodular synovitis (pigmented), multiple sites
[5] M12.3 Palindromic rheumatism
M12.30 Palindromic rheumatism, unspecified site
[6] M12.31 Palindromic rheumatism, shoulder
M12.311 Palindromic rheumatism, right shoulder
M12.312 Palindromic rheumatism, left shoulder
M12.319 Palindromic rheumatism, unspecified shoulder
[6] M12.32 Palindromic rheumatism, elbow
M12.321 Palindromic rheumatism, right elbow
M12.322 Palindromic rheumatism, left elbow
M12.329 Palindromic rheumatism, unspecified elbow
[6] M12.33 Palindromic rheumatism, wrist
M12.331 Palindromic rheumatism, right wrist
M12.332 Palindromic rheumatism, left wrist
M12.339 Palindromic rheumatism, unspecified wrist
[6] M12.34 Palindromic rheumatism, hand
M12.341 Palindromic rheumatism, right hand
M12.342 Palindromic rheumatism, left hand
M12.349 Palindromic rheumatism, unspecified hand
[6] M12.35 Palindromic rheumatism, hip
M12.351 Palindromic rheumatism, right hip
M12.352 Palindromic rheumatism, left hip
M12.359 Palindromic rheumatism, unspecified hip
[6] M12.36 Palindromic rheumatism, knee
M12.361 Palindromic rheumatism, right knee
M12.362 Palindromic rheumatism, left knee
M12.369 Palindromic rheumatism, unspecified knee
[6] M12.37 Palindromic rheumatism, ankle and foot
M12.371 Palindromic rheumatism, right ankle and foot
M12.372 Palindromic rheumatism, left ankle and foot
M12.379 Palindromic rheumatism, unspecified ankle and foot
M12.38 Palindromic rheumatism, other specified site ▲
Palindromic rheumatism, vertebrae
M12.39 Palindromic rheumatism, multiple sites
[5] M12.4 Intermittent hydrarthrosis
M12.40 Intermittent hydrarthrosis, unspecified site
[6] M12.41 Intermittent hydrarthrosis, shoulder
M12.411 Intermittent hydrarthrosis, right shoulder
M12.412 Intermittent hydrarthrosis, left shoulder
M12.419 Intermittent hydrarthrosis, unspecified shoulder
[6] M12.42 Intermittent hydrarthrosis, elbow
M12.421 Intermittent hydrarthrosis, right elbow
M12.422 Intermittent hydrarthrosis, left elbow
M12.429 Intermittent hydrarthrosis, unspecified elbow
[6] M12.43 Intermittent hydrarthrosis, wrist
M12.431 Intermittent hydrarthrosis, right wrist

Unspecified Code | Other Specified Code | [N] Newborn Age: 0 | [P] Pediatric Age: 0-17 | [M] Maternity Age: 12-55
[A] Adult Age: 15-124 | ♂ Male | ♀ Female | ● New Code | ▲ Revised Code Title | ►◄ Revised Text

M12.432 Intermittent hydrarthrosis, left wrist
M12.439 Intermittent hydrarthrosis, unspecified wrist
[6] M12.44 Intermittent hydrarthrosis, hand
M12.441 Intermittent hydrarthrosis, right hand
M12.442 Intermittent hydrarthrosis, left hand
M12.449 Intermittent hydrarthrosis, unspecified hand
[6] M12.45 Intermittent hydrarthrosis, hip
M12.451 Intermittent hydrarthrosis, right hip
M12.452 Intermittent hydrarthrosis, left hip
M12.459 Intermittent hydrarthrosis, unspecified hip
[6] M12.46 Intermittent hydrarthrosis, knee
M12.461 Intermittent hydrarthrosis, right knee
M12.462 Intermittent hydrarthrosis, left knee
M12.469 Intermittent hydrarthrosis, unspecified knee
[6] M12.47 Intermittent hydrarthrosis, ankle and foot
M12.471 Intermittent hydrarthrosis, right ankle and foot
M12.472 Intermittent hydrarthrosis, left ankle and foot
M12.479 Intermittent hydrarthrosis, unspecified ankle and foot
M12.48 Intermittent hydrarthrosis, other site
M12.49 Intermittent hydrarthrosis, multiple sites
[5] M12.5 Traumatic arthropathy

[EXCLUDES1] *current injury-see Alphabetic Index*
post-traumatic osteoarthritis of first carpometacarpal joint (M18.2-M18.3)
post-traumatic osteoarthritis of hip (M16.4-M16.5)
post-traumatic osteoarthritis of knee (M17.2-M17.3)
post-traumatic osteoarthritis NOS (M19.1-)
post-traumatic osteoarthritis of other single joints (M19.1-)

M12.50 Traumatic arthropathy, unspecified site
[6] M12.51 Traumatic arthropathy, shoulder
M12.511 Traumatic arthropathy, right shoulder
M12.512 Traumatic arthropathy, left shoulder
M12.519 Traumatic arthropathy, unspecified shoulder
[6] M12.52 Traumatic arthropathy, elbow
M12.521 Traumatic arthropathy, right elbow
M12.522 Traumatic arthropathy, left elbow
M12.529 Traumatic arthropathy, unspecified elbow
[6] M12.53 Traumatic arthropathy, wrist
M12.531 Traumatic arthropathy, right wrist
M12.532 Traumatic arthropathy, left wrist
M12.539 Traumatic arthropathy, unspecified wrist
[6] M12.54 Traumatic arthropathy, hand
M12.541 Traumatic arthropathy, right hand
M12.542 Traumatic arthropathy, left hand
M12.549 Traumatic arthropathy, unspecified hand
[6] M12.55 Traumatic arthropathy, hip
M12.551 Traumatic arthropathy, right hip
M12.552 Traumatic arthropathy, left hip
M12.559 Traumatic arthropathy, unspecified hip
[6] M12.56 Traumatic arthropathy, knee
M12.561 Traumatic arthropathy, right knee
M12.562 Traumatic arthropathy, left knee
M12.569 Traumatic arthropathy, unspecified knee
[6] M12.57 Traumatic arthropathy, ankle and foot
M12.571 Traumatic arthropathy, right ankle and foot
M12.572 Traumatic arthropathy, left ankle and foot
M12.579 Traumatic arthropathy, unspecified ankle and foot
M12.58 Traumatic arthropathy, other specified site ▲
Traumatic arthropathy, vertebrae
M12.59 Traumatic arthropathy, multiple sites
[5] M12.8 Other specific arthropathies, not elsewhere classified
Transient arthropathy
M12.80 Other specific arthropathies, not elsewhere classified, unspecified site
[6] M12.81 Other specific arthropathies, not elsewhere classified, shoulder
M12.811 Other specific arthropathies, not elsewhere classified, right shoulder
M12.812 Other specific arthropathies, not elsewhere classified, left shoulder
M12.819 Other specific arthropathies, not elsewhere classified, unspecified shoulder
[6] M12.82 Other specific arthropathies, not elsewhere classified, elbow
M12.821 Other specific arthropathies, not elsewhere classified, right elbow
M12.822 Other specific arthropathies, not elsewhere classified, left elbow
M12.829 Other specific arthropathies, not elsewhere classified, unspecified elbow
[6] M12.83 Other specific arthropathies, not elsewhere classified, wrist
M12.831 Other specific arthropathies, not elsewhere classified, right wrist
M12.832 Other specific arthropathies, not elsewhere classified, left wrist
M12.839 Other specific arthropathies, not elsewhere classified, unspecified wrist
[6] M12.84 Other specific arthropathies, not elsewhere classified, hand
M12.841 Other specific arthropathies, not elsewhere classified, right hand
M12.842 Other specific arthropathies, not elsewhere classified, left hand
M12.849 Other specific arthropathies, not elsewhere classified, unspecified hand
[6] M12.85 Other specific arthropathies, not elsewhere classified, hip
M12.851 Other specific arthropathies, not elsewhere classified, right hip
M12.852 Other specific arthropathies, not elsewhere classified, left hip
M12.859 Other specific arthropathies, not elsewhere classified, unspecified hip
[6] M12.86 Other specific arthropathies, not elsewhere classified, knee
M12.861 Other specific arthropathies, not elsewhere classified, right knee
M12.862 Other specific arthropathies, not elsewhere classified, left knee
M12.869 Other specific arthropathies, not elsewhere classified, unspecified knee
[6] M12.87 Other specific arthropathies, not elsewhere classified, ankle and foot
M12.871 Other specific arthropathies, not elsewhere classified, right ankle and foot
M12.872 Other specific arthropathies, not elsewhere classified, left ankle and foot
M12.879 Other specific arthropathies, not elsewhere classified, unspecified ankle and foot
M12.88 Other specific arthropathies, not elsewhere classified, other specified site ▲
Other specific arthropathies, not elsewhere classified, vertebrae
M12.89 Other specific arthropathies, not elsewhere classified, multiple sites

[4] 4th character required [5] 5th character required [6] 6th character required [7] 7th character required [x7] Extension 'X' Alert
[EXCLUDES1] Not coded here [EXCLUDES2] Not included here [PDx] Primary Diagnosis Only Manifestation Code

M12.9 Arthropathy, unspecified

[4] M13 Other arthritis

[EXCLUDES1] *arthrosis (M15-M19)*
osteoarthritis (M15-M19)

M13.0 Polyarthritis, unspecified

[5] M13.1 Monoarthritis, not elsewhere classified

M13.10 Monoarthritis, not elsewhere classified, unspecified site

[6] M13.11 Monoarthritis, not elsewhere classified, shoulder

M13.111 Monoarthritis, not elsewhere classified, right shoulder

M13.112 Monoarthritis, not elsewhere classified, left shoulder

M13.119 Monoarthritis, not elsewhere classified, unspecified shoulder

[6] M13.12 Monoarthritis, not elsewhere classified, elbow

M13.121 Monoarthritis, not elsewhere classified, right elbow

M13.122 Monoarthritis, not elsewhere classified, left elbow

M13.129 Monoarthritis, not elsewhere classified, unspecified elbow

[6] M13.13 Monoarthritis, not elsewhere classified, wrist

M13.131 Monoarthritis, not elsewhere classified, right wrist

M13.132 Monoarthritis, not elsewhere classified, left wrist

M13.139 Monoarthritis, not elsewhere classified, unspecified wrist

[6] M13.14 Monoarthritis, not elsewhere classified, hand

M13.141 Monoarthritis, not elsewhere classified, right hand

M13.142 Monoarthritis, not elsewhere classified, left hand

M13.149 Monoarthritis, not elsewhere classified, unspecified hand

[6] M13.15 Monoarthritis, not elsewhere classified, hip

M13.151 Monoarthritis, not elsewhere classified, right hip

M13.152 Monoarthritis, not elsewhere classified, left hip

M13.159 Monoarthritis, not elsewhere classified, unspecified hip

[6] M13.16 Monoarthritis, not elsewhere classified, knee

M13.161 Monoarthritis, not elsewhere classified, right knee

M13.162 Monoarthritis, not elsewhere classified, left knee

M13.169 Monoarthritis, not elsewhere classified, unspecified knee

[6] M13.17 Monoarthritis, not elsewhere classified, ankle and foot

M13.171 Monoarthritis, not elsewhere classified, right ankle and foot

M13.172 Monoarthritis, not elsewhere classified, left ankle and foot

M13.179 Monoarthritis, not elsewhere classified, unspecified ankle and foot

[5] M13.8 Other specified arthritis

Allergic arthritis

[EXCLUDES1] *osteoarthritis (M15-M19)*

M13.80 Other specified arthritis, unspecified site

[6] M13.81 Other specified arthritis, shoulder

M13.811 Other specified arthritis, right shoulder

M13.812 Other specified arthritis, left shoulder

M13.819 Other specified arthritis, unspecified shoulder

[6] M13.82 Other specified arthritis, elbow

M13.821 Other specified arthritis, right elbow

M13.822 Other specified arthritis, left elbow

M13.829 Other specified arthritis, unspecified elbow

[6] M13.83 Other specified arthritis, wrist

M13.831 Other specified arthritis, right wrist

M13.832 Other specified arthritis, left wrist

M13.839 Other specified arthritis, unspecified wrist

[6] M13.84 Other specified arthritis, hand

M13.841 Other specified arthritis, right hand

M13.842 Other specified arthritis, left hand

M13.849 Other specified arthritis, unspecified hand

[6] M13.85 Other specified arthritis, hip

M13.851 Other specified arthritis, right hip

M13.852 Other specified arthritis, left hip

M13.859 Other specified arthritis, unspecified hip

[6] M13.86 Other specified arthritis, knee

M13.861 Other specified arthritis, right knee

M13.862 Other specified arthritis, left knee

M13.869 Other specified arthritis, unspecified knee

[6] M13.87 Other specified arthritis, ankle and foot

M13.871 Other specified arthritis, right ankle and foot

M13.872 Other specified arthritis, left ankle and foot

M13.879 Other specified arthritis, unspecified ankle and foot

M13.88 Other specified arthritis, other site

M13.89 Other specified arthritis, multiple sites

[4] M14 Arthropathies in other diseases classified elsewhere

[EXCLUDES1] *arthropathy in:*
diabetes mellitus (E08-E13 with .61-)
hematological disorders (M36.2-M36.3)
hypersensitivity reactions (M36.4)
neoplastic disease (M36.1)
neurosyphillis (A52.16)
sarcoidosis (D86.86)
enteropathic arthropathies (M07.-)
juvenile psoriatic arthropathy (L40.54)
lipoid dermatoarthritis (E78.81)

[5] M14.6 Charcôt's joint

Neuropathic arthropathy

[EXCLUDES1] *Charcôt's joint in diabetes mellitus (E08-E13 with .610)*
Charcôt's joint in tabes dorsalis (A52.16)

M14.60 Charcôt's joint, unspecified site

[6] M14.61 Charcôt's joint, shoulder

M14.611 Charcôt's joint, right shoulder

M14.612 Charcôt's joint, left shoulder

M14.619 Charcôt's joint, unspecified shoulder

[6] M14.62 Charcôt's joint, elbow

M14.621 Charcôt's joint, right elbow

M14.622 Charcôt's joint, left elbow

M14.629 Charcôt's joint, unspecified elbow

[6] M14.63 Charcôt's joint, wrist

M14.631 Charcôt's joint, right wrist

M14.632 Charcôt's joint, left wrist

M14.639 Charcôt's joint, unspecified wrist

[6] M14.64 Charcôt's joint, hand

M14.641 Charcôt's joint, right hand

M14.642 Charcôt's joint, left hand

M14.649 Charcôt's joint, unspecified hand

[6] M14.65 Charcôt's joint, hip

M14.651 Charcôt's joint, right hip

M14.652 Charcôt's joint, left hip

M14.659 Charcôt's joint, unspecified hip

[6] M14.66 Charcôt's joint, knee

M14.661 Charcôt's joint, right knee

Unspecified Code | Other Specified Code | [N] Newborn Age: 0 | [P] Pediatric Age: 0-17 | [M] Maternity Age: 12-55
[A] Adult Age: 15-124 | ♂ Male | ♀ Female | ● New Code | ▲ Revised Code Title | ►◄ Revised Text

M14.662 Charcôt's joint, left knee
M14.669 Charcôt's joint, unspecified knee
⑥ M14.67 Charcôt's joint, ankle and foot
M14.671 Charcôt's joint, right ankle and foot
M14.672 Charcôt's joint, left ankle and foot
M14.679 Charcôt's joint, unspecified ankle and foot
M14.68 Charcôt's joint, vertebrae
M14.69 Charcôt's joint, multiple sites
⑤ M14.8 Arthropathies in other specified diseases classified elsewhere

Code first underlying disease, such as:
amyloidosis (E85.-)
erythema multiforme (L51.-)
erythema nodosum (L52)
hemochromatosis (E83.11-)
hyperparathyroidism (E21.-)
hypothyroidism (E00-E03)
sickle-cell disorders (D57.-)
thyrotoxicosis [hyperthyroidism] (E05.-)
Whipple's disease (K90.81)

M14.80 Arthropathies in other specified diseases classified elsewhere, unspecified site
⑤ M14.81 Arthropathies in other specified diseases classified elsewhere, shoulder
M14.811 Arthropathies in other specified diseases classified elsewhere, right shoulder
M14.812 Arthropathies in other specified diseases classified elsewhere, left shoulder
M14.819 Arthropathies in other specified diseases classified elsewhere, unspecified shoulder
⑥ M14.82 Arthropathies in other specified diseases classified elsewhere, elbow
M14.821 Arthropathies in other specified diseases classified elsewhere, right elbow
M14.822 Arthropathies in other specified diseases classified elsewhere, left elbow
M14.829 Arthropathies in other specified diseases classified elsewhere, unspecified elbow
⑥ M14.83 Arthropathies in other specified diseases classified elsewhere, wrist
M14.831 Arthropathies in other specified diseases classified elsewhere, right wrist
M14.832 Arthropathies in other specified diseases classified elsewhere, left wrist
M14.839 Arthropathies in other specified diseases classified elsewhere, unspecified wrist
⑥ M14.84 Arthropathies in other specified diseases classified elsewhere, hand
M14.841 Arthropathies in other specified diseases classified elsewhere, right hand
M14.842 Arthropathies in other specified diseases classified elsewhere, left hand
M14.849 Arthropathies in other specified diseases classified elsewhere, unspecified hand
⑥ M14.85 Arthropathies in other specified diseases classified elsewhere, hip
M14.851 Arthropathies in other specified diseases classified elsewhere, right hip
M14.852 Arthropathies in other specified diseases classified elsewhere, left hip
M14.859 Arthropathies in other specified diseases classified elsewhere, unspecified hip
⑥ M14.86 Arthropathies in other specified diseases classified elsewhere, knee
M14.861 Arthropathies in other specified diseases classified elsewhere, right knee
M14.862 Arthropathies in other specified diseases classified elsewhere, left knee

M14.869 Arthropathies in other specified diseases classified elsewhere, unspecified knee
⑥ M14.87 Arthropathies in other specified diseases classified elsewhere, ankle and foot
M14.871 Arthropathies in other specified diseases classified elsewhere, right ankle and foot
M14.872 Arthropathies in other specified diseases classified elsewhere, left ankle and foot
M14.879 Arthropathies in other specified diseases classified elsewhere, unspecified ankle and foot
M14.88 Arthropathies in other specified diseases classified elsewhere, vertebrae
M14.89 Arthropathies in other specified diseases classified elsewhere, multiple sites

Osteoarthritis (M15-M19)

EXCLUDES2 osteoarthritis of spine (M47.-)
④ M15 Polyosteoarthritis
INCLUDES arthritis of multiple sites
EXCLUDES1 bilateral involvement of single joint (M16-M19)
M15.0 Primary generalized (osteo)arthritis
M15.1 Heberden's nodes (with arthropathy)
Interphalangeal distal osteoarthritis
M15.2 Bouchard's nodes (with arthropathy)
Juxtaphalangeal distal osteoarthritis
M15.3 Secondary multiple arthritis
Post-traumatic polyosteoarthritis
M15.4 Erosive (osteo)arthritis
M15.8 Other polyosteoarthritis
M15.9 Polyosteoarthritis, unspecified
Generalized osteoarthritis NOS
④ M16 Osteoarthritis of hip
M16.0 Bilateral primary osteoarthritis of hip
⑤ M16.1 Unilateral primary osteoarthritis of hip
Primary osteoarthritis of hip NOS
M16.10 Unilateral primary osteoarthritis, unspecified hip
M16.11 Unilateral primary osteoarthritis, right hip
M16.12 Unilateral primary osteoarthritis, left hip
M16.2 Bilateral osteoarthritis resulting from hip dysplasia
⑤ M16.3 Unilateral osteoarthritis resulting from hip dysplasia
Dysplastic osteoarthritis of hip NOS
M16.30 Unilateral osteoarthritis resulting from hip dysplasia, unspecified hip
M16.31 Unilateral osteoarthritis resulting from hip dysplasia, right hip
M16.32 Unilateral osteoarthritis resulting from hip dysplasia, left hip
M16.4 Bilateral post-traumatic osteoarthritis of hip
⑤ M16.5 Unilateral post-traumatic osteoarthritis of hip
Post-traumatic osteoarthritis of hip NOS
M16.50 Unilateral post-traumatic osteoarthritis, unspecified hip
M16.51 Unilateral post-traumatic osteoarthritis, right hip
M16.52 Unilateral post-traumatic osteoarthritis, left hip
M16.6 Other bilateral secondary osteoarthritis of hip
M16.7 Other unilateral secondary osteoarthritis of hip
Secondary osteoarthritis of hip NOS
M16.9 Osteoarthritis of hip, unspecified
④ M17 Osteoarthritis of knee
M17.0 Bilateral primary osteoarthritis of knee
⑤ M17.1 Unilateral primary osteoarthritis of knee
Primary osteoarthritis of knee NOS
M17.10 Unilateral primary osteoarthritis, unspecified knee

---

④ 4th character required   ⑤ 5th character required   ⑥ 6th character required   ⑦ 7th character required   ⑦ Extension 'X' Alert

EXCLUDES 1 Not coded here   EXCLUDES 2 Not included here   PDx Primary Diagnosis Only   Manifestation Code

M17.11 Unilateral primary osteoarthritis, right knee
M17.12 Unilateral primary osteoarthritis, left knee
M17.2 Bilateral post-traumatic osteoarthritis of knee
[5] M17.3 Unilateral post-traumatic osteoarthritis of knee
Post-traumatic osteoarthritis of knee NOS
M17.30 Unilateral post-traumatic osteoarthritis, unspecified knee
M17.31 Unilateral post-traumatic osteoarthritis, right knee
M17.32 Unilateral post-traumatic osteoarthritis, left knee
M17.4 Other bilateral secondary osteoarthritis of knee
M17.5 Other unilateral secondary osteoarthritis of knee
Secondary osteoarthritis of knee NOS
M17.9 Osteoarthritis of knee, unspecified
[4] M18 Osteoarthritis of first carpometacarpal joint
M18.0 Bilateral primary osteoarthritis of first carpometacarpal joints
[5] M18.1 Unilateral primary osteoarthritis of first carpometacarpal joint
Primary osteoarthritis of first carpometacarpal joint NOS
M18.10 Unilateral primary osteoarthritis of first carpometacarpal joint, unspecified hand
M18.11 Unilateral primary osteoarthritis of first carpometacarpal joint, right hand
M18.12 Unilateral primary osteoarthritis of first carpometacarpal joint, left hand
M18.2 Bilateral post-traumatic osteoarthritis of first carpometacarpal joints
[5] M18.3 Unilateral post-traumatic osteoarthritis of first carpometacarpal joint
Post-traumatic osteoarthritis of first carpometacarpal joint NOS
M18.30 Unilateral post-traumatic osteoarthritis of first carpometacarpal joint, unspecified hand
M18.31 Unilateral post-traumatic osteoarthritis of first carpometacarpal joint, right hand
M18.32 Unilateral post-traumatic osteoarthritis of first carpometacarpal joint, left hand
M18.4 Other bilateral secondary osteoarthritis of first carpometacarpal joints
[5] M18.5 Other unilateral secondary osteoarthritis of first carpometacarpal joint
Secondary osteoarthritis of first carpometacarpal joint NOS
M18.50 Other unilateral secondary osteoarthritis of first carpometacarpal joint, unspecified hand
M18.51 Other unilateral secondary osteoarthritis of first carpometacarpal joint, right hand
M18.52 Other unilateral secondary osteoarthritis of first carpometacarpal joint, left hand
M18.9 Osteoarthritis of first carpometacarpal joint, unspecified
[4] M19 Other and unspecified osteoarthritis
EXCLUDES1 *polyarthritis (M15.-)*
EXCLUDES2 *arthrosis of spine (M47.-)*
hallux rigidus (M20.2)
osteoarthritis of spine (M47.-)
[5] M19.0 Primary osteoarthritis of other joints
[6] M19.01 Primary osteoarthritis, shoulder
M19.011 Primary osteoarthritis, right shoulder
M19.012 Primary osteoarthritis, left shoulder
M19.019 Primary osteoarthritis, unspecified shoulder
[6] M19.02 Primary osteoarthritis, elbow
M19.021 Primary osteoarthritis, right elbow
M19.022 Primary osteoarthritis, left elbow
M19.029 Primary osteoarthritis, unspecified elbow
[6] M19.03 Primary osteoarthritis, wrist
M19.031 Primary osteoarthritis, right wrist
M19.032 Primary osteoarthritis, left wrist
M19.039 Primary osteoarthritis, unspecified wrist
[6] M19.04 Primary osteoarthritis, hand
EXCLUDES2 *primary osteoarthritis of first carpometacarpal joint (M18.0-, M18.1-)*
M19.041 Primary osteoarthritis, right hand
M19.042 Primary osteoarthritis, left hand
M19.049 Primary osteoarthritis, unspecified hand
[6] M19.07 Primary osteoarthritis ankle and foot
M19.071 Primary osteoarthritis, right ankle and foot
M19.072 Primary osteoarthritis, left ankle and foot
M19.079 Primary osteoarthritis, unspecified ankle and foot
[5] M19.1 Post-traumatic osteoarthritis of other joints
[6] M19.11 Post-traumatic osteoarthritis, shoulder
M19.111 Post-traumatic osteoarthritis, right shoulder
M19.112 Post-traumatic osteoarthritis, left shoulder
M19.119 Post-traumatic osteoarthritis, unspecified shoulder
[6] M19.12 Post-traumatic osteoarthritis, elbow
M19.121 Post-traumatic osteoarthritis, right elbow
M19.122 Post-traumatic osteoarthritis, left elbow
M19.129 Post-traumatic osteoarthritis, unspecified elbow
[6] M19.13 Post-traumatic osteoarthritis, wrist
M19.131 Post-traumatic osteoarthritis, right wrist
M19.132 Post-traumatic osteoarthritis, left wrist
M19.139 Post-traumatic osteoarthritis, unspecified wrist
[6] M19.14 Post-traumatic osteoarthritis, hand
EXCLUDES2 *post-traumatic osteoarthritis of first carpometacarpal joint (M18.2-, M18.3-)*
M19.141 Post-traumatic osteoarthritis, right hand
M19.142 Post-traumatic osteoarthritis, left hand
M19.149 Post-traumatic osteoarthritis, unspecified hand
[6] M19.17 Post-traumatic osteoarthritis, ankle and foot
M19.171 Post-traumatic osteoarthritis, right ankle and foot
M19.172 Post-traumatic osteoarthritis, left ankle and foot
M19.179 Post-traumatic osteoarthritis, unspecified ankle and foot
[5] M19.2 Secondary osteoarthritis of other joints
[6] M19.21 Secondary osteoarthritis, shoulder
M19.211 Secondary osteoarthritis, right shoulder
M19.212 Secondary osteoarthritis, left shoulder
M19.219 Secondary osteoarthritis, unspecified shoulder
[6] M19.22 Secondary osteoarthritis, elbow
M19.221 Secondary osteoarthritis, right elbow
M19.222 Secondary osteoarthritis, left elbow
M19.229 Secondary osteoarthritis, unspecified elbow
[6] M19.23 Secondary osteoarthritis, wrist
M19.231 Secondary osteoarthritis, right wrist
M19.232 Secondary osteoarthritis, left wrist
M19.239 Secondary osteoarthritis, unspecified wrist
[6] M19.24 Secondary osteoarthritis, hand
M19.241 Secondary osteoarthritis, right hand
M19.242 Secondary osteoarthritis, left hand
M19.249 Secondary osteoarthritis, unspecified hand
[6] M19.27 Secondary osteoarthritis, ankle and foot

Unspecified Code | Other Specified Code | [N] Newborn Age: 0 | [P] Pediatric Age: 0-17 | [M] Maternity Age: 12-55
[A] Adult Age: 15-124 | ♂ Male | ♀ Female | ● New Code | ▲ Revised Code Title | ►◄ Revised Text

M19.271 Secondary osteoarthritis, right ankle and foot

M19.272 Secondary osteoarthritis, left ankle and foot

M19.279 Secondary osteoarthritis, unspecified ankle and foot

⑤ M19.9 Osteoarthritis, unspecified site

M19.90 Unspecified osteoarthritis, unspecified site

Arthrosis NOS

Arthritis NOS

Osteoarthritis NOS

M19.91 Primary osteoarthritis, unspecified site

Primary osteoarthritis NOS

M19.92 Post-traumatic osteoarthritis, unspecified site

Post-traumatic osteoarthritis NOS

M19.93 Secondary osteoarthritis, unspecified site

Secondary osteoarthritis NOS

Other joint disorders (M20-M25)

EXCLUDES2 joints of the spine (M40-M54)

④ M20 Acquired deformities of fingers and toes

EXCLUDES1 acquired absence of fingers and toes (Z89.-)
congenital absence of fingers and toes (Q71.3-, Q72.3-)
congenital deformities and malformations of fingers and toes (Q66.-, Q68-Q70, Q74.-)

⑤ M20.0 Deformity of finger(s)

EXCLUDES1 clubbing of fingers (R68.3)
palmar fascial fibromatosis [Dupuytren] (M72.0)
trigger finger (M65.3)

⑥ M20.00 Unspecified deformity of finger(s)

M20.001 Unspecified deformity of right finger(s)

M20.002 Unspecified deformity of left finger(s)

M20.009 Unspecified deformity of unspecified finger(s)

⑥ M20.01 Mallet finger

M20.011 Mallet finger of right finger(s)

M20.012 Mallet finger of left finger(s)

M20.019 Mallet finger of unspecified finger(s)

⑥ M20.02 Boutonniére deformity

M20.021 Boutonniére deformity of right finger(s)

M20.022 Boutonniére deformity of left finger(s)

M20.029 Boutonniére deformity of unspecified finger(s)

⑥ M20.03 Swan-neck deformity

M20.031 Swan-neck deformity of right finger(s)

M20.032 Swan-neck deformity of left finger(s)

M20.039 Swan-neck deformity of unspecified finger(s)

⑥ M20.09 Other deformity of finger(s)

M20.091 Other deformity of right finger(s)

M20.092 Other deformity of left finger(s)

M20.099 Other deformity of finger(s), unspecified finger(s)

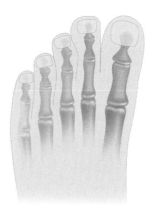 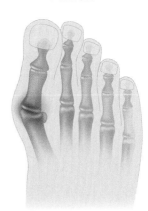

Normal   Bunion

Figure 12.2 Bunion

⑤ M20.1 Hallux valgus (acquired)

Bunion

M20.10 Hallux valgus (acquired), unspecified foot

M20.11 Hallux valgus (acquired), right foot

M20.12 Hallux valgus (acquired), left foot

⑤ M20.2 Hallux rigidus

M20.20 Hallux rigidus, unspecified foot

M20.21 Hallux rigidus, right foot

M20.22 Hallux rigidus, left foot

⑤ M20.3 Hallux varus (acquired)

M20.30 Hallux varus (acquired), unspecified foot

M20.31 Hallux varus (acquired), right foot

M20.32 Hallux varus (acquired), left foot

⑤ M20.4 Other hammer toe(s) (acquired)

M20.40 Other hammer toe(s) (acquired), unspecified foot

M20.41 Other hammer toe(s) (acquired), right foot

M20.42 Other hammer toe(s) (acquired), left foot

⑤ M20.5 Other deformities of toe(s) (acquired)

⑥ M20.5X Other deformities of toe(s) (acquired)

M20.5X1 Other deformities of toe(s) (acquired), right foot

M20.5X2 Other deformities of toe(s) (acquired), left foot

M20.5X9 Other deformities of toe(s) (acquired), unspecified foot

⑤ M20.6 Acquired deformities of toe(s), unspecified

M20.60 Acquired deformities of toe(s), unspecified, unspecified foot

M20.61 Acquired deformities of toe(s), unspecified, right foot

M20.62 Acquired deformities of toe(s), unspecified, left foot

④ M21 Other acquired deformities of limbs

EXCLUDES1 acquired absence of limb (Z89.-)
congenital absence of limbs (Q71-Q73)
congenital deformities and malformations of limbs (Q65-Q66, Q68-Q74)

EXCLUDES2 acquired deformities of fingers or toes (M20.-)
coxa plana (M91.2)

⑤ M21.0 Valgus deformity, not elsewhere classified

EXCLUDES1 metatarsus valgus (Q66.6)
talipes calcaneovalgus (Q66.4)

M21.00 Valgus deformity, not elsewhere classified, unspecified site

---

④ 4th character required   ⑤ 5th character required   ⑥ 6th character required   ⑦ 7th character required   ⑦ Extension 'X' Alert

EXCLUDES1 Not coded here   EXCLUDES2 Not included here   PDx Primary Diagnosis Only   Manifestation Code

[6] M21.02 Valgus deformity, not elsewhere classified, elbow
Cubitus valgus
M21.021 Valgus deformity, not elsewhere classified, right elbow
M21.022 Valgus deformity, not elsewhere classified, left elbow
M21.029 Valgus deformity, not elsewhere classified, unspecified elbow

[6] M21.05 Valgus deformity, not elsewhere classified, hip
M21.051 Valgus deformity, not elsewhere classified, right hip
M21.052 Valgus deformity, not elsewhere classified, left hip
M21.059 Valgus deformity, not elsewhere classified, unspecified hip

[6] M21.06 Valgus deformity, not elsewhere classified, knee
Genu valgum
Knock knee
M21.061 Valgus deformity, not elsewhere classified, right knee
M21.062 Valgus deformity, not elsewhere classified, left knee
M21.069 Valgus deformity, not elsewhere classified, unspecified knee

[6] M21.07 Valgus deformity, not elsewhere classified, ankle
M21.071 Valgus deformity, not elsewhere classified, right ankle
M21.072 Valgus deformity, not elsewhere classified, left ankle
M21.079 Valgus deformity, not elsewhere classified, unspecified ankle

[5] M21.1 Varus deformity, not elsewhere classified
[EXCLUDES1] *metatarsus varus (Q66.2)*
tibia vara (M92.5)
M21.10 Varus deformity, not elsewhere classified, unspecified site

[6] M21.12 Varus deformity, not elsewhere classified, elbow
Cubitus varus, elbow
M21.121 Varus deformity, not elsewhere classified, right elbow
M21.122 Varus deformity, not elsewhere classified, left elbow
M21.129 Varus deformity, not elsewhere classified, unspecified elbow

[6] M21.15 Varus deformity, not elsewhere classified, hip
M21.151 Varus deformity, not elsewhere classified, right hip
M21.152 Varus deformity, not elsewhere classified, left hip
M21.159 Varus deformity, not elsewhere classified, unspecified

[6] M21.16 Varus deformity, not elsewhere classified, knee
Bow leg
Genu varum
M21.161 Varus deformity, not elsewhere classified, right knee
M21.162 Varus deformity, not elsewhere classified, left knee
M21.169 Varus deformity, not elsewhere classified, unspecified knee

[6] M21.17 Varus deformity, not elsewhere classified, ankle
M21.171 Varus deformity, not elsewhere classified, right ankle
M21.172 Varus deformity, not elsewhere classified, left ankle
M21.179 Varus deformity, not elsewhere classified, unspecified ankle

[5] M21.2 Flexion deformity
M21.20 Flexion deformity, unspecified site

[6] M21.21 Flexion deformity, shoulder
M21.211 Flexion deformity, right shoulder
M21.212 Flexion deformity, left shoulder
M21.219 Flexion deformity, unspecified shoulder

[6] M21.22 Flexion deformity, elbow
M21.221 Flexion deformity, right elbow
M21.222 Flexion deformity, left elbow
M21.229 Flexion deformity, unspecified elbow

[6] M21.23 Flexion deformity, wrist
M21.231 Flexion deformity, right wrist
M21.232 Flexion deformity, left wrist
M21.239 Flexion deformity, unspecified wrist

[6] M21.24 Flexion deformity, finger joints
M21.241 Flexion deformity, right finger joints
M21.242 Flexion deformity, left finger joints
M21.249 Flexion deformity, unspecified finger joints

[6] M21.25 Flexion deformity, hip
M21.251 Flexion deformity, right hip
M21.252 Flexion deformity, left hip
M21.259 Flexion deformity, unspecified hip

[6] M21.26 Flexion deformity, knee
M21.261 Flexion deformity, right knee
M21.262 Flexion deformity, left knee
M21.269 Flexion deformity, unspecified knee

[6] M21.27 Flexion deformity, ankle and toes
M21.271 Flexion deformity, right ankle and toes
M21.272 Flexion deformity, left ankle and toes
M21.279 Flexion deformity, unspecified ankle and toes

[5] M21.3 Wrist or foot drop (acquired)

[6] M21.33 Wrist drop (acquired)
M21.331 Wrist drop, right wrist
M21.332 Wrist drop, left wrist
M21.339 Wrist drop, unspecified wrist

[6] M21.37 Foot drop (acquired)
M21.371 Foot drop, right foot
M21.372 Foot drop, left foot
M21.379 Foot drop, unspecified foot

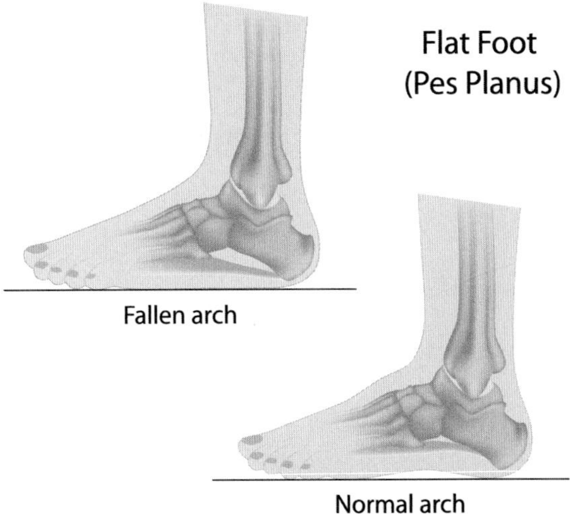

Figure 12.3 Illustration showing normal and Flat Foot

[5] M21.4 Flat foot [pes planus] (acquired)
[EXCLUDES1] *congenital pes planus (Q66.5-)*
M21.40 Flat foot [pes planus] (acquired), unspecified foot

Unspecified Code | Other Specified Code | [N] Newborn Age: 0 | [P] Pediatric Age: 0-17 | [M] Maternity Age: 12-55
[A] Adult Age: 15-124 | ♂ Male | ♀ Female | ● New Code | ▲ Revised Code Title | ►◄ Revised Text

M21.41 Flat foot [pes planus] (acquired), right foot
M21.42 Flat foot [pes planus] (acquired), left foot

[5] M21.5 Acquired clawhand, clubhand, clawfoot and clubfoot
[EXCLUDES1] *clubfoot, not specified as acquired (Q66.89)*

[6] M21.51 Acquired clawhand
M21.511 Acquired clawhand, right hand
M21.512 Acquired clawhand, left hand
M21.519 Acquired clawhand, unspecified hand

[6] M21.52 Acquired clubhand
M21.521 Acquired clubhand, right hand
M21.522 Acquired clubhand, left hand
M21.529 Acquired clubhand, unspecified hand

[6] M21.53 Acquired clawfoot
M21.531 Acquired clawfoot, right foot
M21.532 Acquired clawfoot, left foot
M21.539 Acquired clawfoot, unspecified foot

[6] M21.54 Acquired clubfoot
M21.541 Acquired clubfoot, right foot
M21.542 Acquired clubfoot, left foot
M21.549 Acquired clubfoot, unspecified foot

[5] M21.6 Other acquired deformities of foot
[EXCLUDES2] *deformities of toe (acquired) (M20.1-M20.6)*

[6] M21.6X Other acquired deformities of foot
M21.6X1 Other acquired deformities of right foot
M21.6X2 Other acquired deformities of left foot
M21.6X9 Other acquired deformities of unspecified foot

[5] M21.7 Unequal limb length (acquired)
[NOTES] The site used should correspond to the shorter limb
M21.70 Unequal limb length (acquired), unspecified site

[6] M21.72 Unequal limb length (acquired), humerus
M21.721 Unequal limb length (acquired), right humerus
M21.722 Unequal limb length (acquired), left humerus
M21.729 Unequal limb length (acquired), unspecified humerus

[6] M21.73 Unequal limb length (acquired), ulna and radius
M21.731 Unequal limb length (acquired), right ulna
M21.732 Unequal limb length (acquired), left ulna
M21.733 Unequal limb length (acquired), right radius
M21.734 Unequal limb length (acquired), left radius
M21.739 Unequal limb length (acquired), unspecified ulna and radius

[6] M21.75 Unequal limb length (acquired), femur
M21.751 Unequal limb length (acquired), right femur
M21.752 Unequal limb length (acquired), left femur
M21.759 Unequal limb length (acquired), unspecified femur

[6] M21.76 Unequal limb length (acquired), tibia and fibula
M21.761 Unequal limb length (acquired), right tibia
M21.762 Unequal limb length (acquired), left tibia
M21.763 Unequal limb length (acquired), right fibula
M21.764 Unequal limb length (acquired), left fibula
M21.769 Unequal limb length (acquired), unspecified tibia and fibula

[5] M21.8 Other specified acquired deformities of limbs
[EXCLUDES2] *coxa plana (M91.2)*
M21.80 Other specified acquired deformities of unspecified limb

[6] M21.82 Other specified acquired deformities of upper arm
M21.821 Other specified acquired deformities of right upper arm
M21.822 Other specified acquired deformities of left upper arm
M21.829 Other specified acquired deformities of unspecified upper arm

[6] M21.83 Other specified acquired deformities of forearm
M21.831 Other specified acquired deformities of right forearm
M21.832 Other specified acquired deformities of left forearm
M21.839 Other specified acquired deformities of unspecified forearm

[6] M21.85 Other specified acquired deformities of thigh
M21.851 Other specified acquired deformities of right thigh
M21.852 Other specified acquired deformities of left thigh
M21.859 Other specified acquired deformities of unspecified thigh

[6] M21.86 Other specified acquired deformities of lower leg
M21.861 Other specified acquired deformities of right lower leg
M21.862 Other specified acquired deformities of left lower leg
M21.869 Other specified acquired deformities of unspecified lower leg

[5] M21.9 Unspecified acquired deformity of limb and hand
M21.90 Unspecified acquired deformity of unspecified limb

[6] M21.92 Unspecified acquired deformity of upper arm
M21.921 Unspecified acquired deformity of right upper arm
M21.922 Unspecified acquired deformity of left upper arm
M21.929 Unspecified acquired deformity of unspecified upper arm

[6] M21.93 Unspecified acquired deformity of forearm
M21.931 Unspecified acquired deformity of right forearm
M21.932 Unspecified acquired deformity of left forearm
M21.939 Unspecified acquired deformity of unspecified forearm

[6] M21.94 Unspecified acquired deformity of hand
M21.941 Unspecified acquired deformity of hand, right hand
M21.942 Unspecified acquired deformity of hand, left hand
M21.949 Unspecified acquired deformity of hand, unspecified hand

[6] M21.95 Unspecified acquired deformity of thigh
M21.951 Unspecified acquired deformity of right thigh
M21.952 Unspecified acquired deformity of left thigh
M21.959 Unspecified acquired deformity of unspecified thigh

[6] M21.96 Unspecified acquired deformity of lower leg
M21.961 Unspecified acquired deformity of right lower leg
M21.962 Unspecified acquired deformity of left lower leg
M21.969 Unspecified acquired deformity of unspecified lower leg

[4] M22 Disorder of patella
[EXCLUDES1] *traumatic dislocation of patella (S83.0-)*

[5] M22.0 Recurrent dislocation of patella
M22.00 Recurrent dislocation of patella, unspecified knee

[4] 4th character required [5] 5th character required [6] 6th character required [7] 7th character required [7] Extension 'X' Alert
[EXCLUDES1] Not coded here [EXCLUDES2] Not included here [PDx] Primary Diagnosis Only Manifestation Code

M22.01 Recurrent dislocation of patella, right knee
M22.02 Recurrent dislocation of patella, left knee

[5] M22.1 Recurrent subluxation of patella
Incomplete dislocation of patella
M22.10 Recurrent subluxation of patella, unspecified knee
M22.11 Recurrent subluxation of patella, right knee
M22.12 Recurrent subluxation of patella, left knee

[5] M22.2 Patellofemoral disorders
[6] M22.2X Patellofemoral disorders
M22.2X1 Patellofemoral disorders, right knee
M22.2X2 Patellofemoral disorders, left knee
M22.2X9 Patellofemoral disorders, unspecified knee

[5] M22.3 Other derangements of patella
[6] M22.3X Other derangements of patella
M22.3X1 Other derangements of patella, right knee
M22.3X2 Other derangements of patella, left knee
M22.3X9 Other derangements of patella, unspecified knee

[5] M22.4 Chondromalacia patellae
M22.40 Chondromalacia patellae, unspecified knee
M22.41 Chondromalacia patellae, right knee
M22.42 Chondromalacia patellae, left knee

[5] M22.8 Other disorders of patella
[6] M22.8X Other disorders of patella
M22.8X1 Other disorders of patella, right knee
M22.8X2 Other disorders of patella, left knee
M22.8X9 Other disorders of patella, unspecified knee

[5] M22.9 Unspecified disorder of patella
M22.90 Unspecified disorder of patella, unspecified knee
M22.91 Unspecified disorder of patella, right knee
M22.92 Unspecified disorder of patella, left knee

[4] M23 Internal derangement of knee

[EXCLUDES1] *ankylosis (M24.66)*
current injury - see injury of knee and lower leg (S80-S89)
deformity of knee (M21.-)
osteochondritis dissecans (M93.2)
recurrent dislocation or subluxation of joints (M24.4)
recurrent dislocation or subluxation of patella (M22.0-M22.1)

[5] M23.0 Cystic meniscus
[6] M23.00 Cystic meniscus, unspecified meniscus
Cystic meniscus, unspecified lateral meniscus
Cystic meniscus, unspecified medial meniscus
M23.000 Cystic meniscus, unspecified lateral meniscus, right knee
M23.001 Cystic meniscus, unspecified lateral meniscus, left knee
M23.002 Cystic meniscus, unspecified lateral meniscus, unspecified knee
M23.003 Cystic meniscus, unspecified medial meniscus, right knee
M23.004 Cystic meniscus, unspecified medial meniscus, left knee
M23.005 Cystic meniscus, unspecified medial meniscus, unspecified knee
M23.006 Cystic meniscus, unspecified meniscus, right knee
M23.007 Cystic meniscus, unspecified meniscus, left knee
M23.009 Cystic meniscus, unspecified meniscus, unspecified knee

[6] M23.01 Cystic meniscus, anterior horn of medial meniscus
M23.011 Cystic meniscus, anterior horn of medial meniscus, right knee
M23.012 Cystic meniscus, anterior horn of medial meniscus, left knee
M23.019 Cystic meniscus, anterior horn of medial meniscus, unspecified knee

[6] M23.02 Cystic meniscus, posterior horn of medial meniscus
M23.021 Cystic meniscus, posterior horn of medial meniscus, right knee
M23.022 Cystic meniscus, posterior horn of medial meniscus, left knee
M23.029 Cystic meniscus, posterior horn of medial meniscus, unspecified knee

[6] M23.03 Cystic meniscus, other medial meniscus
M23.031 Cystic meniscus, other medial meniscus, right knee
M23.032 Cystic meniscus, other medial meniscus, left knee
M23.039 Cystic meniscus, other medial meniscus, unspecified knee

[6] M23.04 Cystic meniscus, anterior horn of lateral meniscus
M23.041 Cystic meniscus, anterior horn of lateral meniscus, right knee
M23.042 Cystic meniscus, anterior horn of lateral meniscus, left knee
M23.049 Cystic meniscus, anterior horn of lateral meniscus, unspecified knee

[6] M23.05 Cystic meniscus, posterior horn of lateral meniscus
M23.051 Cystic meniscus, posterior horn of lateral meniscus, right knee
M23.052 Cystic meniscus, posterior horn of lateral meniscus, left knee
M23.059 Cystic meniscus, posterior horn of lateral meniscus, unspecified knee

[6] M23.06 Cystic meniscus, other lateral meniscus
M23.061 Cystic meniscus, other lateral meniscus, right knee
M23.062 Cystic meniscus, other lateral meniscus, left knee
M23.069 Cystic meniscus, other lateral meniscus, unspecified knee

[5] M23.2 Derangement of meniscus due to old tear or injury
Old bucket-handle tear
[6] M23.20 Derangement of unspecified meniscus due to old tear or injury
Derangement of unspecified lateral meniscus due to old tear or injury
Derangement of unspecified medial meniscus due to old tear or injury
M23.200 Derangement of unspecified lateral meniscus due to old tear or injury, right knee
M23.201 Derangement of unspecified lateral meniscus due to old tear or injury, left knee
M23.202 Derangement of unspecified lateral meniscus due to old tear or injury, unspecified knee
M23.203 Derangement of unspecified medial meniscus due to old tear or injury, right knee
M23.204 Derangement of unspecified medial meniscus due to old tear or injury, left knee
M23.205 Derangement of unspecified medial meniscus due to old tear or injury, unspecified knee

Unspecified Code | Other Specified Code | [N] Newborn Age: 0 | [P] Pediatric Age: 0-17 | [M] Maternity Age: 12-55
[A] Adult Age: 15-124 | ♂ Male | ♀ Female | ● New Code | ▲ Revised Code Title | ►◄ Revised Text

M23.206 Derangement of unspecified meniscus due to old tear or injury, right knee
M23.207 Derangement of unspecified meniscus due to old tear or injury, left knee
M23.209 Derangement of unspecified meniscus due to old tear or injury, unspecified knee

⑥ M23.21 Derangement of anterior horn of medial meniscus due to old tear or injury
M23.211 Derangement of anterior horn of medial meniscus due to old tear or injury, right knee
M23.212 Derangement of anterior horn of medial meniscus due to old tear or injury, left knee
M23.219 Derangement of anterior horn of medial meniscus due to old tear or injury, unspecified knee

⑥ M23.22 Derangement of posterior horn of medial meniscus due to old tear or injury
M23.221 Derangement of posterior horn of medial meniscus due to old tear or injury, right knee
M23.222 Derangement of posterior horn of medial meniscus due to old tear or injury, left knee
M23.229 Derangement of posterior horn of medial meniscus due to old tear or injury, unspecified knee

⑥ M23.23 Derangement of other medial meniscus due to old tear or injury
M23.231 Derangement of other medial meniscus due to old tear or injury, right knee
M23.232 Derangement of other medial meniscus due to old tear or injury, left knee
M23.239 Derangement of other medial meniscus due to old tear or injury, unspecified knee

⑥ M23.24 Derangement of anterior horn of lateral meniscus due to old tear or injury
M23.241 Derangement of anterior horn of lateral meniscus due to old tear or injury, right knee
M23.242 Derangement of anterior horn of lateral meniscus due to old tear or injury, left knee
M23.249 Derangement of anterior horn of lateral meniscus due to old tear or injury, unspecified knee

⑥ M23.25 Derangement of posterior horn of lateral meniscus due to old tear or injury
M23.251 Derangement of posterior horn of lateral meniscus due to old tear or injury, right knee
M23.252 Derangement of posterior horn of lateral meniscus due to old tear or injury, left knee
M23.259 Derangement of posterior horn of lateral meniscus due to old tear or injury, unspecified knee

⑥ M23.26 Derangement of other lateral meniscus due to old tear or injury
M23.261 Derangement of other lateral meniscus due to old tear or injury, right knee
M23.262 Derangement of other lateral meniscus due to old tear or injury, left knee
M23.269 Derangement of other lateral meniscus due to old tear or injury, unspecified knee

⑤ M23.3 Other meniscus derangements
Degenerate meniscus
Detached meniscus
Retained meniscus

⑥ M23.30 Other meniscus derangements, unspecified meniscus
Other meniscus derangements, unspecified lateral meniscus
Other meniscus derangements, unspecified medial meniscus

M23.300 Other meniscus derangements, unspecified lateral meniscus, right knee
M23.301 Other meniscus derangements, unspecified lateral meniscus, left knee
M23.302 Other meniscus derangements, unspecified lateral meniscus, unspecified knee
M23.303 Other meniscus derangements, unspecified medial meniscus, right knee
M23.304 Other meniscus derangements, unspecified medial meniscus, left knee
M23.305 Other meniscus derangements, unspecified medial meniscus, unspecified knee
M23.306 Other meniscus derangements, unspecified meniscus, right knee
M23.307 Other meniscus derangements, unspecified meniscus, left knee
M23.309 Other meniscus derangements, unspecified meniscus, unspecified knee

⑥ M23.31 Other meniscus derangements, anterior horn of medial meniscus
M23.311 Other meniscus derangements, anterior horn of medial meniscus, right knee
M23.312 Other meniscus derangements, anterior horn of medial meniscus, left knee
M23.319 Other meniscus derangements, anterior horn of medial meniscus, unspecified knee

⑥ M23.32 Other meniscus derangements, posterior horn of medial meniscus
M23.321 Other meniscus derangements, posterior horn of medial meniscus, right knee
M23.322 Other meniscus derangements, posterior horn of medial meniscus, left knee
M23.329 Other meniscus derangements, posterior horn of medial meniscus, unspecified knee

⑥ M23.33 Other meniscus derangements, other medial meniscus
M23.331 Other meniscus derangements, other medial meniscus, right knee
M23.332 Other meniscus derangements, other medial meniscus, left knee
M23.339 Other meniscus derangements, other medial meniscus, unspecified knee

⑥ M23.34 Other meniscus derangements, anterior horn of lateral meniscus
M23.341 Other meniscus derangements, anterior horn of lateral meniscus, right knee
M23.342 Other meniscus derangements, anterior horn of lateral meniscus, left knee
M23.349 Other meniscus derangements, anterior horn of lateral meniscus, unspecified knee

⑥ M23.35 Other meniscus derangements, posterior horn of lateral meniscus
M23.351 Other meniscus derangements, posterior horn of lateral meniscus, right knee
M23.352 Other meniscus derangements, posterior horn of lateral meniscus, left knee
M23.359 Other meniscus derangements, posterior horn of lateral meniscus, unspecified knee

⑥ M23.36 Other meniscus derangements, other lateral meniscus
M23.361 Other meniscus derangements, other lateral meniscus, right knee
M23.362 Other meniscus derangements, other lateral meniscus, left knee
M23.369 Other meniscus derangements, other lateral meniscus, unspecified knee

⑤ M23.4 Loose body in knee

④ 4th character required   ⑤ 5th character required   ⑥ 6th character required   ⑦ 7th character required   ⑩ Extension 'X' Alert
EXCLUDES 1 Not coded here   EXCLUDES 2 Not included here   PDx Primary Diagnosis Only   Manifestation Code

354

ICD-10-CM 2015

M23.40 Loose body in knee, unspecified knee
M23.41 Loose body in knee, right knee
M23.42 Loose body in knee, left knee

[5] M23.5 Chronic instability of knee
M23.50 Chronic instability of knee, unspecified knee
M23.51 Chronic instability of knee, right knee
M23.52 Chronic instability of knee, left knee

[5] M23.6 Other spontaneous disruption of ligament(s) of knee
[6] M23.60 Other spontaneous disruption of unspecified ligament of knee
M23.601 Other spontaneous disruption of unspecified ligament of right knee
M23.602 Other spontaneous disruption of unspecified ligament of left knee
M23.609 Other spontaneous disruption of unspecified ligament of unspecified knee
[6] M23.61 Other spontaneous disruption of anterior cruciate ligament of knee
M23.611 Other spontaneous disruption of anterior cruciate ligament of right knee
M23.612 Other spontaneous disruption of anterior cruciate ligament of left knee
M23.619 Other spontaneous disruption of anterior cruciate ligament of unspecified knee
[6] M23.62 Other spontaneous disruption of posterior cruciate ligament of knee
M23.621 Other spontaneous disruption of posterior cruciate ligament of right knee
M23.622 Other spontaneous disruption of posterior cruciate ligament of left knee
M23.629 Other spontaneous disruption of posterior cruciate ligament of unspecified knee
[6] M23.63 Other spontaneous disruption of medial collateral ligament of knee
M23.631 Other spontaneous disruption of medial collateral ligament of right knee
M23.632 Other spontaneous disruption of medial collateral ligament of left knee
M23.639 Other spontaneous disruption of medial collateral ligament of unspecified knee
[6] M23.64 Other spontaneous disruption of lateral collateral ligament of knee
M23.641 Other spontaneous disruption of lateral collateral ligament of right knee
M23.642 Other spontaneous disruption of lateral collateral ligament of left knee
M23.649 Other spontaneous disruption of lateral collateral ligament of unspecified knee
[6] M23.67 Other spontaneous disruption of capsular ligament of knee
M23.671 Other spontaneous disruption of capsular ligament of right knee
M23.672 Other spontaneous disruption of capsular ligament of left knee
M23.679 Other spontaneous disruption of capsular ligament of unspecified knee

[5] M23.8 Other internal derangements of knee
Laxity of ligament of knee
Snapping knee
[6] M23.8X Other internal derangements of knee
M23.8X1 Other internal derangements of right knee
M23.8X2 Other internal derangements of left knee
M23.8X9 Other internal derangements of unspecified knee

[5] M23.9 Unspecified internal derangement of knee
M23.90 Unspecified internal derangement of unspecified knee
M23.91 Unspecified internal derangement of right knee
M23.92 Unspecified internal derangement of left knee

[4] M24 Other specific joint derangements
[EXCLUDES1] *current injury - see injury of joint by body region*
[EXCLUDES2] *ganglion (M67.4)*
snapping knee (M23.8-)
temporomandibular joint disorders (M26.6-)

[5] M24.0 Loose body in joint
[EXCLUDES2] *loose body in knee (M23.4)*
M24.00 Loose body in unspecified joint
[6] M24.01 Loose body in shoulder
M24.011 Loose body in right shoulder
M24.012 Loose body in left shoulder
M24.019 Loose body in unspecified shoulder
[6] M24.02 Loose body in elbow
M24.021 Loose body in right elbow
M24.022 Loose body in left elbow
M24.029 Loose body in unspecified elbow
[6] M24.03 Loose body in wrist
M24.031 Loose body in right wrist
M24.032 Loose body in left wrist
M24.039 Loose body in unspecified wrist
[6] M24.04 Loose body in finger joints
M24.041 Loose body in right finger joint(s)
M24.042 Loose body in left finger joint(s)
M24.049 Loose body in unspecified finger joint(s)
[6] M24.05 Loose body in hip
M24.051 Loose body in right hip
M24.052 Loose body in left hip
M24.059 Loose body in unspecified hip
[6] M24.07 Loose body in ankle and toe joints
M24.071 Loose body in right ankle
M24.072 Loose body in left ankle
M24.073 Loose body in unspecified ankle
M24.074 Loose body in right toe joint(s)
M24.075 Loose body in left toe joint(s)
M24.076 Loose body in unspecified toe joints
M24.08 Loose body, other site

[5] M24.1 Other articular cartilage disorders
[EXCLUDES2] *chondrocalcinosis (M11.1, M11.2-)*
internal derangement of knee (M23.-)
metastatic calcification (E83.5)
ochronosis (E70.2)
M24.10 Other articular cartilage disorders, unspecified site
[6] M24.11 Other articular cartilage disorders, shoulder
M24.111 Other articular cartilage disorders, right shoulder
M24.112 Other articular cartilage disorders, left shoulder
M24.119 Other articular cartilage disorders, unspecified shoulder
[6] M24.12 Other articular cartilage disorders, elbow
M24.121 Other articular cartilage disorders, right elbow
M24.122 Other articular cartilage disorders, left elbow
M24.129 Other articular cartilage disorders, unspecified elbow
[6] M24.13 Other articular cartilage disorders, wrist
M24.131 Other articular cartilage disorders, right wrist
M24.132 Other articular cartilage disorders, left wrist
M24.139 Other articular cartilage disorders, unspecified wrist
[6] M24.14 Other articular cartilage disorders, hand
M24.141 Other articular cartilage disorders, right hand

Unspecified Code | Other Specified Code | [N] Newborn Age: 0 | [P] Pediatric Age: 0-17 | [M] Maternity Age: 12-55
[A] Adult Age: 15-124 | ♂ Male | ♀ Female | ● New Code | ▲ Revised Code Title | ►◄ Revised Text

       M24.142 Other articular cartilage disorders, left hand

       M24.149 Other articular cartilage disorders, unspecified hand

⑥ M24.15 Other articular cartilage disorders, hip

       M24.151 Other articular cartilage disorders, right hip

       M24.152 Other articular cartilage disorders, left hip

       M24.159 Other articular cartilage disorders, unspecified hip

⑥ M24.17 Other articular cartilage disorders, ankle and foot

       M24.171 Other articular cartilage disorders, right ankle

       M24.172 Other articular cartilage disorders, left ankle

       M24.173 Other articular cartilage disorders, unspecified ankle

       M24.174 Other articular cartilage disorders, right foot

       M24.175 Other articular cartilage disorders, left foot

       M24.176 Other articular cartilage disorders, unspecified foot

⑤ M24.2 Disorder of ligament

       Instability secondary to old ligament injury

       Ligamentous laxity NOS

       EXCLUDES1 familial ligamentous laxity (M35.7)

       EXCLUDES2 internal derangement of knee (M23.5-M23.89)

       M24.20 Disorder of ligament, unspecified site

⑥ M24.21 Disorder of ligament, shoulder

       M24.211 Disorder of ligament, right shoulder

       M24.212 Disorder of ligament, left shoulder

       M24.219 Disorder of ligament, unspecified shoulder

⑥ M24.22 Disorder of ligament, elbow

       M24.221 Disorder of ligament, right elbow

       M24.222 Disorder of ligament, left elbow

       M24.229 Disorder of ligament, unspecified elbow

⑥ M24.23 Disorder of ligament, wrist

       M24.231 Disorder of ligament, right wrist

       M24.232 Disorder of ligament, left wrist

       M24.239 Disorder of ligament, unspecified wrist

⑥ M24.24 Disorder of ligament, hand

       M24.241 Disorder of ligament, right hand

       M24.242 Disorder of ligament, left hand

       M24.249 Disorder of ligament, unspecified hand

⑥ M24.25 Disorder of ligament, hip

       M24.251 Disorder of ligament, right hip

       M24.252 Disorder of ligament, left hip

       M24.259 Disorder of ligament, unspecified hip

⑥ M24.27 Disorder of ligament, ankle and foot

       M24.271 Disorder of ligament, right ankle

       M24.272 Disorder of ligament, left ankle

       M24.273 Disorder of ligament, unspecified ankle

       M24.274 Disorder of ligament, right foot

       M24.275 Disorder of ligament, left foot

       M24.276 Disorder of ligament, unspecified foot

       M24.28 Disorder of ligament, vertebrae

⑤ M24.3 Pathological dislocation of joint, not elsewhere classified

       EXCLUDES1 congenital dislocation or displacement of joint- see congenital malformations and deformations of the musculoskeletal system (Q65-Q79)
current injury - see injury of joints and ligaments by body region
recurrent dislocation of joint (M24.4-)

       M24.30 Pathological dislocation of unspecified joint, not elsewhere classified

⑥ M24.31 Pathological dislocation of shoulder, not elsewhere classified

       M24.311 Pathological dislocation of right shoulder, not elsewhere classified

       M24.312 Pathological dislocation of left shoulder, not elsewhere classified

       M24.319 Pathological dislocation of unspecified shoulder, not elsewhere classified

⑥ M24.32 Pathological dislocation of elbow, not elsewhere classified

       M24.321 Pathological dislocation of right elbow, not elsewhere classified

       M24.322 Pathological dislocation of left elbow, not elsewhere classified

       M24.329 Pathological dislocation of unspecified elbow, not elsewhere classified

⑥ M24.33 Pathological dislocation of wrist, not elsewhere classified

       M24.331 Pathological dislocation of right wrist, not elsewhere classified

       M24.332 Pathological dislocation of left wrist, not elsewhere classified

       M24.339 Pathological dislocation of unspecified wrist, not elsewhere classified

⑥ M24.34 Pathological dislocation of hand, not elsewhere classified

       M24.341 Pathological dislocation of right hand, not elsewhere classified

       M24.342 Pathological dislocation of left hand, not elsewhere classified

       M24.349 Pathological dislocation of unspecified hand, not elsewhere classified

⑥ M24.35 Pathological dislocation of hip, not elsewhere classified

       M24.351 Pathological dislocation of right hip, not elsewhere classified

       M24.352 Pathological dislocation of left hip, not elsewhere classified

       M24.359 Pathological dislocation of unspecified hip, not elsewhere classified

⑥ M24.36 Pathological dislocation of knee, not elsewhere classified

       M24.361 Pathological dislocation of right knee, not elsewhere classified

       M24.362 Pathological dislocation of left knee, not elsewhere classified

       M24.369 Pathological dislocation of unspecified knee, not elsewhere classified

⑥ M24.37 Pathological dislocation of ankle and foot, not elsewhere classified

       M24.371 Pathological dislocation of right ankle, not elsewhere classified

       M24.372 Pathological dislocation of left ankle, not elsewhere classified

       M24.373 Pathological dislocation of unspecified ankle, not elsewhere classified

       M24.374 Pathological dislocation of right foot, not elsewhere classified

---

④ 4th character required   ⑤ 5th character required   ⑥ 6th character required   ⑦ 7th character required   ⑰ Extension 'X' Alert

EXCLUDES1 Not coded here   EXCLUDES2 Not included here   PDx Primary Diagnosis Only   Manifestation Code

M24.375 Pathological dislocation of left foot, not elsewhere classified
M24.376 Pathological dislocation of unspecified foot, not elsewhere classified

[5] M24.4 Recurrent dislocation of joint
Recurrent subluxation of joint
[EXCLUDES2] *recurrent dislocation of patella (M22.0-M22.1)*
recurrent vertebral dislocation (M43.3-, M43.4, M43.5-)
M24.40 Recurrent dislocation, unspecified joint
[6] M24.41 Recurrent dislocation, shoulder
M24.411 Recurrent dislocation, right shoulder
M24.412 Recurrent dislocation, left shoulder
M24.419 Recurrent dislocation, unspecified shoulder
[6] M24.42 Recurrent dislocation, elbow
M24.421 Recurrent dislocation, right elbow
M24.422 Recurrent dislocation, left elbow
M24.429 Recurrent dislocation, unspecified elbow
[6] M24.43 Recurrent dislocation, wrist
M24.431 Recurrent dislocation, right wrist
M24.432 Recurrent dislocation, left wrist
M24.439 Recurrent dislocation, unspecified wrist
[6] M24.44 Recurrent dislocation, hand and finger(s)
M24.441 Recurrent dislocation, right hand
M24.442 Recurrent dislocation, left hand
M24.443 Recurrent dislocation, unspecified hand
M24.444 Recurrent dislocation, right finger
M24.445 Recurrent dislocation, left finger
M24.446 Recurrent dislocation, unspecified finger
[6] M24.45 Recurrent dislocation, hip
M24.451 Recurrent dislocation, right hip
M24.452 Recurrent dislocation, left hip
M24.459 Recurrent dislocation, unspecified hip
[6] M24.46 Recurrent dislocation, knee
M24.461 Recurrent dislocation, right knee
M24.462 Recurrent dislocation, left knee
M24.469 Recurrent dislocation, unspecified knee
[6] M24.47 Recurrent dislocation, ankle, foot and toes
M24.471 Recurrent dislocation, right ankle
M24.472 Recurrent dislocation, left ankle
M24.473 Recurrent dislocation, unspecified ankle
M24.474 Recurrent dislocation, right foot
M24.475 Recurrent dislocation, left foot
M24.476 Recurrent dislocation, unspecified foot
M24.477 Recurrent dislocation, right toe(s)
M24.478 Recurrent dislocation, left toe(s)
M24.479 Recurrent dislocation, unspecified toe(s)

[5] M24.5 Contracture of joint
[EXCLUDES1] *contracture of muscle without contracture of joint (M62.4-)*
contracture of tendon (sheath) without contracture of joint (M62.4-)
Dupuytren's contracture (M72.0)
[EXCLUDES2] *acquired deformities of limbs (M20-M21)*
M24.50 Contracture, unspecified joint
[6] M24.51 Contracture, shoulder
M24.511 Contracture, right shoulder
M24.512 Contracture, left shoulder
M24.519 Contracture, unspecified shoulder
[6] M24.52 Contracture, elbow
M24.521 Contracture, right elbow
M24.522 Contracture, left elbow
M24.529 Contracture, unspecified elbow
[6] M24.53 Contracture, wrist
M24.531 Contracture, right wrist
M24.532 Contracture, left wrist
M24.539 Contracture, unspecified wrist
[6] M24.54 Contracture, hand
M24.541 Contracture, right hand
M24.542 Contracture, left hand
M24.549 Contracture, unspecified hand
[6] M24.55 Contracture, hip
M24.551 Contracture, right hip
M24.552 Contracture, left hip
M24.559 Contracture, unspecified hip
[6] M24.56 Contracture, knee
M24.561 Contracture, right knee
M24.562 Contracture, left knee
M24.569 Contracture, unspecified knee
[6] M24.57 Contracture, ankle and foot
M24.571 Contracture, right ankle
M24.572 Contracture, left ankle
M24.573 Contracture, unspecified ankle
M24.574 Contracture, right foot
M24.575 Contracture, left foot
M24.576 Contracture, unspecified foot

[5] M24.6 Ankylosis of joint
[EXCLUDES1] *stiffness of joint without ankylosis (M25.6-)*
[EXCLUDES2] *spine (M43.2-)*
M24.60 Ankylosis, unspecified joint
[6] M24.61 Ankylosis, shoulder
M24.611 Ankylosis, right shoulder
M24.612 Ankylosis, left shoulder
M24.619 Ankylosis, unspecified shoulder
[6] M24.62 Ankylosis, elbow
M24.621 Ankylosis, right elbow
M24.622 Ankylosis, left elbow
M24.629 Ankylosis, unspecified elbow
[6] M24.63 Ankylosis, wrist
M24.631 Ankylosis, right wrist
M24.632 Ankylosis, left wrist
M24.639 Ankylosis, unspecified wrist
[6] M24.64 Ankylosis, hand
M24.641 Ankylosis, right hand
M24.642 Ankylosis, left hand
M24.649 Ankylosis, unspecified hand
[6] M24.65 Ankylosis, hip
M24.651 Ankylosis, right hip
M24.652 Ankylosis, left hip
M24.659 Ankylosis, unspecified hip
[6] M24.66 Ankylosis, knee
M24.661 Ankylosis, right knee
M24.662 Ankylosis, left knee
M24.669 Ankylosis, unspecified knee
[6] M24.67 Ankylosis, ankle and foot
M24.671 Ankylosis, right ankle
M24.672 Ankylosis, left ankle
M24.673 Ankylosis, unspecified ankle
M24.674 Ankylosis, right foot
M24.675 Ankylosis, left foot
M24.676 Ankylosis, unspecified foot

M24.7 Protrusio acetabuli

[5] M24.8 Other specific joint derangements, not elsewhere classified
[EXCLUDES2] *iliotibial band syndrome (M76.3)*
M24.80 Other specific joint derangements of unspecified joint, not elsewhere classified
[6] M24.81 Other specific joint derangements of shoulder, not elsewhere classified
M24.811 Other specific joint derangements of right shoulder, not elsewhere classified

Unspecified Code | Other Specified Code | [N] Newborn Age: 0 | [P] Pediatric Age: 0-17 | [M] Maternity Age: 12-55
[A] Adult Age: 15-124 | ♂ Male | ♀ Female | ● New Code | ▲ Revised Code Title | ►◄ Revised Text

M24.812 Other specific joint derangements of left shoulder, not elsewhere classified
M24.819 Other specific joint derangements of unspecified shoulder, not elsewhere classified
[6] M24.82 Other specific joint derangements of elbow, not elsewhere classified
M24.821 Other specific joint derangements of right elbow, not elsewhere classified
M24.822 Other specific joint derangements of left elbow, not elsewhere classified
M24.829 Other specific joint derangements of unspecified elbow, not elsewhere classified
[6] M24.83 Other specific joint derangements of wrist, not elsewhere classified
M24.831 Other specific joint derangements of right wrist, not elsewhere classified
M24.832 Other specific joint derangements of left wrist, not elsewhere classified
M24.839 Other specific joint derangements of unspecified wrist, not elsewhere classified
[6] M24.84 Other specific joint derangements of hand, not elsewhere classified
M24.841 Other specific joint derangements of right hand, not elsewhere classified
M24.842 Other specific joint derangements of left hand, not elsewhere classified
M24.849 Other specific joint derangements of unspecified hand, not elsewhere classified
[6] M24.85 Other specific joint derangements of hip, not elsewhere classified
Irritable hip
M24.851 Other specific joint derangements of right hip, not elsewhere classified
M24.852 Other specific joint derangements of left hip, not elsewhere classified
M24.859 Other specific joint derangements of unspecified hip, not elsewhere classified
[6] M24.87 Other specific joint derangements of ankle and foot, not elsewhere classified
M24.871 Other specific joint derangements of right ankle, not elsewhere classified
M24.872 Other specific joint derangements of left ankle, not elsewhere classified
M24.873 Other specific joint derangements of unspecified ankle, not elsewhere classified
M24.874 Other specific joint derangements of right foot, not elsewhere classified
M24.875 Other specific joint derangements left foot, not elsewhere classified
M24.876 Other specific joint derangements of unspecified foot, not elsewhere classified
M24.9 Joint derangement, unspecified

[4] M25 Other joint disorder, not elsewhere classified
[EXCLUDES2] *abnormality of gait and mobility (R26.-)*
acquired deformities of limb (M20-M21)
calcification of bursa (M71.4-)
calcification of shoulder (joint) (M75.3)
calcification of tendon (M65.2-)
difficulty in walking (R26.2)
temporomandibular joint disorder (M26.6-)
[5] M25.0 Hemarthrosis
[EXCLUDES1] *current injury - see injury of joint by body region*
hemophilic arthropathy (M36.2)
M25.00 Hemarthrosis, unspecified joint
[6] M25.01 Hemarthrosis, shoulder
M25.011 Hemarthrosis, right shoulder
M25.012 Hemarthrosis, left shoulder
M25.019 Hemarthrosis, unspecified shoulder
[6] M25.02 Hemarthrosis, elbow
M25.021 Hemarthrosis, right elbow
M25.022 Hemarthrosis, left elbow
M25.029 Hemarthrosis, unspecified elbow
[6] M25.03 Hemarthrosis, wrist
M25.031 Hemarthrosis, right wrist
M25.032 Hemarthrosis, left wrist
M25.039 Hemarthrosis, unspecified wrist
[6] M25.04 Hemarthrosis, hand
M25.041 Hemarthrosis, right hand
M25.042 Hemarthrosis, left hand
M25.049 Hemarthrosis, unspecified hand
[6] M25.05 Hemarthrosis, hip
M25.051 Hemarthrosis, right hip
M25.052 Hemarthrosis, left hip
M25.059 Hemarthrosis, unspecified hip
[6] M25.06 Hemarthrosis, knee
M25.061 Hemarthrosis, right knee
M25.062 Hemarthrosis, left knee
M25.069 Hemarthrosis, unspecified knee
[6] M25.07 Hemarthrosis, ankle and foot
M25.071 Hemarthrosis, right ankle
M25.072 Hemarthrosis, left ankle
M25.073 Hemarthrosis, unspecified ankle
M25.074 Hemarthrosis, right foot
M25.075 Hemarthrosis, left foot
M25.076 Hemarthrosis, unspecified foot
M25.08 Hemarthrosis, other specified site ▲
Hemarthrosis, vertebrae
[5] M25.1 Fistula of joint
M25.10 Fistula, unspecified joint
[6] M25.11 Fistula, shoulder
M25.111 Fistula, right shoulder
M25.112 Fistula, left shoulder
M25.119 Fistula, unspecified shoulder
[6] M25.12 Fistula, elbow
M25.121 Fistula, right elbow
M25.122 Fistula, left elbow
M25.129 Fistula, unspecified elbow
[6] M25.13 Fistula, wrist
M25.131 Fistula, right wrist
M25.132 Fistula, left wrist
M25.139 Fistula, unspecified wrist
[6] M25.14 Fistula, hand
M25.141 Fistula, right hand
M25.142 Fistula, left hand
M25.149 Fistula, unspecified hand
[6] M25.15 Fistula, hip
M25.151 Fistula, right hip
M25.152 Fistula, left hip

[4] 4th character required [5] 5th character required [6] 6th character required [7] 7th character required [7th] Extension 'X' Alert
[EXCLUDES1] Not coded here [EXCLUDES2] Not included here [PDx] Primary Diagnosis Only Manifestation Code

M25.159 Fistula, unspecified hip
🔟 M25.16 Fistula, knee
    M25.161 Fistula, right knee
    M25.162 Fistula, left knee
    M25.169 Fistula, unspecified knee
🔟 M25.17 Fistula, ankle and foot
    M25.171 Fistula, right ankle
    M25.172 Fistula, left ankle
    M25.173 Fistula, unspecified ankle
    M25.174 Fistula, right foot
    M25.175 Fistula, left foot
    M25.176 Fistula, unspecified foot
    M25.18 Fistula, other specified site ▲
      Fistula, vertebrae
5️⃣ M25.2 Flail joint
    M25.20 Flail joint, unspecified joint
🔟 M25.21 Flail joint, shoulder
    M25.211 Flail joint, right shoulder
    M25.212 Flail joint, left shoulder
    M25.219 Flail joint, unspecified shoulder
🔟 M25.22 Flail joint, elbow
    M25.221 Flail joint, right elbow
    M25.222 Flail joint, left elbow
    M25.229 Flail joint, unspecified elbow
🔟 M25.23 Flail joint, wrist
    M25.231 Flail joint, right wrist
    M25.232 Flail joint, left wrist
    M25.239 Flail joint, unspecified wrist
🔟 M25.24 Flail joint, hand
    M25.241 Flail joint, right hand
    M25.242 Flail joint, left hand
    M25.249 Flail joint, unspecified hand
🔟 M25.25 Flail joint, hip
    M25.251 Flail joint, right hip
    M25.252 Flail joint, left hip
    M25.259 Flail joint, unspecified hip
🔟 M25.26 Flail joint, knee
    M25.261 Flail joint, right knee
    M25.262 Flail joint, left knee
    M25.269 Flail joint, unspecified knee
🔟 M25.27 Flail joint, ankle and foot
    M25.271 Flail joint, right ankle and foot
    M25.272 Flail joint, left ankle and foot
    M25.279 Flail joint, unspecified ankle and foot
    M25.28 Flail joint, other site
5️⃣ M25.3 Other instability of joint
    EXCLUDES1 instability of joint secondary to old ligament
        injury (M24.2-)
        instability of joint secondary to removal of joint
        prosthesis (M96.8-)
    EXCLUDES2 spinal instabilities (M53.2-)
    M25.30 Other instability, unspecified joint
🔟 M25.31 Other instability, shoulder
    M25.311 Other instability, right shoulder
    M25.312 Other instability, left shoulder
    M25.319 Other instability, unspecified shoulder
🔟 M25.32 Other instability, elbow
    M25.321 Other instability, right elbow
    M25.322 Other instability, left elbow
    M25.329 Other instability, unspecified elbow
🔟 M25.33 Other instability, wrist
    M25.331 Other instability, right wrist
    M25.332 Other instability, left wrist
    M25.339 Other instability, unspecified wrist
🔟 M25.34 Other instability, hand
    M25.341 Other instability, right hand

    M25.342 Other instability, left hand
    M25.349 Other instability, unspecified hand
🔟 M25.35 Other instability, hip
    M25.351 Other instability, right hip
    M25.352 Other instability, left hip
    M25.359 Other instability, unspecified hip
🔟 M25.36 Other instability, knee
    M25.361 Other instability, right knee
    M25.362 Other instability, left knee
    M25.369 Other instability, unspecified knee
🔟 M25.37 Other instability, ankle and foot
    M25.371 Other instability, right ankle
    M25.372 Other instability, left ankle
    M25.373 Other instability, unspecified ankle
    M25.374 Other instability, right foot
    M25.375 Other instability, left foot
    M25.376 Other instability, unspecified foot
5️⃣ M25.4 Effusion of joint
    EXCLUDES1 hydrarthrosis in yaws (A66.6)
        intermittent hydrarthrosis (M12.4-)
        other infective (teno)synovitis (M65.1-)
    M25.40 Effusion, unspecified joint
🔟 M25.41 Effusion, shoulder
    M25.411 Effusion, right shoulder
    M25.412 Effusion, left shoulder
    M25.419 Effusion, unspecified shoulder
🔟 M25.42 Effusion, elbow
    M25.421 Effusion, right elbow
    M25.422 Effusion, left elbow
    M25.429 Effusion, unspecified elbow
🔟 M25.43 Effusion, wrist
    M25.431 Effusion, right wrist
    M25.432 Effusion, left wrist
    M25.439 Effusion, unspecified wrist
🔟 M25.44 Effusion, hand
    M25.441 Effusion, right hand
    M25.442 Effusion, left hand
    M25.449 Effusion, unspecified hand
🔟 M25.45 Effusion, hip
    M25.451 Effusion, right hip
    M25.452 Effusion, left hip
    M25.459 Effusion, unspecified hip
🔟 M25.46 Effusion, knee
    M25.461 Effusion, right knee
    M25.462 Effusion, left knee
    M25.469 Effusion, unspecified knee
🔟 M25.47 Effusion, ankle and foot
    M25.471 Effusion, right ankle
    M25.472 Effusion, left ankle
    M25.473 Effusion, unspecified ankle
    M25.474 Effusion, right foot
    M25.475 Effusion, left foot
    M25.476 Effusion, unspecified foot
    M25.48 Effusion, other site
5️⃣ M25.5 Pain in joint
    EXCLUDES2 pain in hand (M79.64-)
        pain in fingers (M79.64-)
        pain in foot (M79.67-)
        pain in limb (M79.6-)
        pain in toes (M79.67-)
    M25.50 Pain in unspecified joint
🔟 M25.51 Pain in shoulder
    M25.511 Pain in right shoulder
    M25.512 Pain in left shoulder
    M25.519 Pain in unspecified shoulder
🔟 M25.52 Pain in elbow

Unspecified Code   Other Specified Code   🅽 Newborn Age: 0   🅿 Pediatric Age: 0-17   🅼 Maternity Age: 12-55
🅰 Adult Age: 15-124   ♂ Male   ♀ Female   ● New Code   ▲ Revised Code Title   ►◄ Revised Text

M25.521 Pain in right elbow
M25.522 Pain in left elbow
M25.529 Pain in unspecified elbow
[6] M25.53 Pain in wrist
M25.531 Pain in right wrist
M25.532 Pain in left wrist
M25.539 Pain in unspecified wrist
[6] M25.55 Pain in hip
M25.551 Pain in right hip
M25.552 Pain in left hip
M25.559 Pain in unspecified hip
[6] M25.56 Pain in knee
M25.561 Pain in right knee
M25.562 Pain in left knee
M25.569 Pain in unspecified knee
[6] M25.57 Pain in ankle and joints of foot
M25.571 Pain in right ankle and joints of right foot
M25.572 Pain in left ankle and joints of left foot
M25.579 Pain in unspecified ankle and joints of unspecified foot
[5] M25.6 Stiffness of joint, not elsewhere classified
[EXCLUDES1] *ankylosis of joint (M24.6-)*
contracture of joint (M24.5-)
M25.60 Stiffness of unspecified joint, not elsewhere classified
[6] M25.61 Stiffness of shoulder, not elsewhere classified
M25.611 Stiffness of right shoulder, not elsewhere classified
M25.612 Stiffness of left shoulder, not elsewhere classified
M25.619 Stiffness of unspecified shoulder, not elsewhere classified
[6] M25.62 Stiffness of elbow, not elsewhere classified
M25.621 Stiffness of right elbow, not elsewhere classified
M25.622 Stiffness of left elbow, not elsewhere classified
M25.629 Stiffness of unspecified elbow, not elsewhere classified
[6] M25.63 Stiffness of wrist, not elsewhere classified
M25.631 Stiffness of right wrist, not elsewhere classified
M25.632 Stiffness of left wrist, not elsewhere classified
M25.639 Stiffness of unspecified wrist, not elsewhere classified
[6] M25.64 Stiffness of hand, not elsewhere classified
M25.641 Stiffness of right hand, not elsewhere classified
M25.642 Stiffness of left hand, not elsewhere classified
M25.649 Stiffness of unspecified hand, not elsewhere classified
[6] M25.65 Stiffness of hip, not elsewhere classified
M25.651 Stiffness of right hip, not elsewhere classified
M25.652 Stiffness of left hip, not elsewhere classified
M25.659 Stiffness of unspecified hip, not elsewhere classified
[6] M25.66 Stiffness of knee, not elsewhere classified
M25.661 Stiffness of right knee, not elsewhere classified
M25.662 Stiffness of left knee, not elsewhere classified
M25.669 Stiffness of unspecified knee, not elsewhere classified
[6] M25.67 Stiffness of ankle and foot, not elsewhere classified
M25.671 Stiffness of right ankle, not elsewhere classified
M25.672 Stiffness of left ankle, not elsewhere classified
M25.673 Stiffness of unspecified ankle, not elsewhere classified
M25.674 Stiffness of right foot, not elsewhere classified
M25.675 Stiffness of left foot, not elsewhere classified
M25.676 Stiffness of unspecified foot, not elsewhere classified
[5] M25.7 Osteophyte
M25.70 Osteophyte, unspecified joint
[6] M25.71 Osteophyte, shoulder
M25.711 Osteophyte, right shoulder
M25.712 Osteophyte, left shoulder
M25.719 Osteophyte, unspecified shoulder
[6] M25.72 Osteophyte, elbow
M25.721 Osteophyte, right elbow
M25.722 Osteophyte, left elbow
M25.729 Osteophyte, unspecified elbow
[6] M25.73 Osteophyte, wrist
M25.731 Osteophyte, right wrist
M25.732 Osteophyte, left wrist
M25.739 Osteophyte, unspecified wrist
[6] M25.74 Osteophyte, hand
M25.741 Osteophyte, right hand
M25.742 Osteophyte, left hand
M25.749 Osteophyte, unspecified hand
[6] M25.75 Osteophyte, hip
M25.751 Osteophyte, right hip
M25.752 Osteophyte, left hip
M25.759 Osteophyte, unspecified hip
[6] M25.76 Osteophyte, knee
M25.761 Osteophyte, right knee
M25.762 Osteophyte, left knee
M25.769 Osteophyte, unspecified knee
[6] M25.77 Osteophyte, ankle and foot
M25.771 Osteophyte, right ankle
M25.772 Osteophyte, left ankle
M25.773 Osteophyte, unspecified ankle
M25.774 Osteophyte, right foot
M25.775 Osteophyte, left foot
M25.776 Osteophyte, unspecified foot
M25.78 Osteophyte, vertebrae
[5] M25.8 Other specified joint disorders
M25.80 Other specified joint disorders, unspecified joint
[6] M25.81 Other specified joint disorders, shoulder
M25.811 Other specified joint disorders, right shoulder
M25.812 Other specified joint disorders, left shoulder
M25.819 Other specified joint disorders, unspecified shoulder
[6] M25.82 Other specified joint disorders, elbow
M25.821 Other specified joint disorders, right elbow
M25.822 Other specified joint disorders, left elbow
M25.829 Other specified joint disorders, unspecified elbow
[6] M25.83 Other specified joint disorders, wrist
M25.831 Other specified joint disorders, right wrist
M25.832 Other specified joint disorders, left wrist

M25.839 Other specified joint disorders, unspecified wrist
[6] M25.84 Other specified joint disorders, hand
M25.841 Other specified joint disorders, right hand
M25.842 Other specified joint disorders, left hand
M25.849 Other specified joint disorders, unspecified hand
[6] M25.85 Other specified joint disorders, hip
M25.851 Other specified joint disorders, right hip
M25.852 Other specified joint disorders, left hip
M25.859 Other specified joint disorders, unspecified hip
[6] M25.86 Other specified joint disorders, knee
M25.861 Other specified joint disorders, right knee
M25.862 Other specified joint disorders, left knee
M25.869 Other specified joint disorders, unspecified knee
[6] M25.87 Other specified joint disorders, ankle and foot
M25.871 Other specified joint disorders, right ankle and foot
M25.872 Other specified joint disorders, left ankle and foot
M25.879 Other specified joint disorders, unspecified ankle and foot
M25.9 Joint disorder, unspecified

Dentofacial anomalies [including malocclusion] and other disorders of jaw (M26-M27)

[EXCLUDES1] *hemifacial atrophy or hypertrophy (Q67.4)*
unilateral condylar hyperplasia or hypoplasia (M27.8)

[4] M26 Dentofacial anomalies [including malocclusion]
[5] M26.0 Major anomalies of jaw size
[EXCLUDES1] *acromegaly (E22.0)*
Robin's syndrome (Q87.0)
M26.00 Unspecified anomaly of jaw size
M26.01 Maxillary hyperplasia
M26.02 Maxillary hypoplasia
M26.03 Mandibular hyperplasia
M26.04 Mandibular hypoplasia
M26.05 Macrogenia
M26.06 Microgenia
M26.07 Excessive tuberosity of jaw
Entire maxillary tuberosity
M26.09 Other specified anomalies of jaw size
[5] M26.1 Anomalies of jaw-cranial base relationship
M26.10 Unspecified anomaly of jaw-cranial base relationship
M26.11 Maxillary asymmetry
M26.12 Other jaw asymmetry
M26.19 Other specified anomalies of jaw-cranial base relationship
[5] M26.2 Anomalies of dental arch relationship
M26.20 Unspecified anomaly of dental arch relationship
[6] M26.21 Malocclusion, Angle's class
M26.211 Malocclusion, Angle's class I
Neutro-occlusion
M26.212 Malocclusion, Angle's class II
Disto-occlusion Division I
Disto-occlusion Division II
M26.213 Malocclusion, Angle's class III
Mesio-occlusion
M26.219 Malocclusion, Angle's class, unspecified
[6] M26.22 Open occlusal relationship
M26.220 Open anterior occlusal relationship
Anterior openbite
M26.221 Open posterior occlusal relationship
Posterior openbite
M26.23 Excessive horizontal overlap
Excessive horizontal overjet
M26.24 Reverse articulation
Crossbite (anterior) (posterior)
M26.25 Anomalies of interarch distance
M26.29 Other anomalies of dental arch relationship
Midline deviation of dental arch
Overbite (excessive) deep
Overbite (excessive) horizontal
Overbite (excessive) vertical
Posterior lingual occlusion of mandibular teeth
[5] M26.3 Anomalies of tooth position of fully erupted tooth or teeth
[EXCLUDES2] *embedded and impacted teeth (K01.-)*
M26.30 Unspecified anomaly of tooth position of fully erupted tooth or teeth
Abnormal spacing of fully erupted tooth or teeth NOS
Displacement of fully erupted tooth or teeth NOS
Transposition of fully erupted tooth or teeth NOS
M26.31 Crowding of fully erupted teeth
M26.32 Excessive spacing of fully erupted teeth
Diastema of fully erupted tooth or teeth NOS
M26.33 Horizontal displacement of fully erupted tooth or teeth
Tipped tooth or teeth
Tipping of fully erupted tooth
M26.34 Vertical displacement of fully erupted tooth or teeth
Extruded tooth
Infraeruption of tooth or teeth
Supraeruption of tooth or teeth
M26.35 Rotation of fully erupted tooth or teeth
M26.36 Insufficient interocclusal distance of fully erupted teeth (ridge)
Lack of adequate intermaxillary vertical dimension of fully erupted teeth
M26.37 Excessive interocclusal distance of fully erupted teeth
Excessive intermaxillary vertical dimension of fully erupted teeth
Loss of occlusal vertical dimension of fully erupted teeth
M26.39 Other anomalies of tooth position of fully erupted tooth or teeth
M26.4 Malocclusion, unspecified
[5] M26.5 Dentofacial functional abnormalities
[EXCLUDES1] *bruxism (F45.8)*
teeth-grinding NOS (F45.8)
M26.50 Dentofacial functional abnormalities, unspecified
M26.51 Abnormal jaw closure
M26.52 Limited mandibular range of motion
M26.53 Deviation in opening and closing of the mandible
M26.54 Insufficient anterior guidance
Insufficient anterior occlusal guidance
M26.55 Centric occlusion maximum intercuspation discrepancy
[EXCLUDES1] *centric occlusion NOS (M26.59)*
M26.56 Non-working side interference
Balancing side interference
M26.57 Lack of posterior occlusal support
M26.59 Other dentofacial functional abnormalities
Centric occlusion (of teeth) NOS
Malocclusion due to abnormal swallowing
Malocclusion due to mouth breathing
Malocclusion due to tongue, lip or finger habits

Unspecified Code | Other Specified Code | [N] Newborn Age: 0 | [P] Pediatric Age: 0-17 | [M] Maternity Age: 12-55
[A] Adult Age: 15-124 | ♂ Male | ♀ Female | ● New Code | ▲ Revised Code Title | ►◄ Revised Text

[5] **M26.6 Temporomandibular joint disorders**

[EXCLUDES2] *current temporomandibular joint dislocation (S03.0)*
current temporomandibular joint sprain (S03.4)

M26.60 Temporomandibular joint disorder, unspecified
M26.61 Adhesions and ankylosis of temporomandibular joint
M26.62 Arthralgia of temporomandibular joint
M26.63 Articular disc disorder of temporomandibular joint
M26.69 Other specified disorders of temporomandibular joint

[5] **M26.7 Dental alveolar anomalies**

M26.70 Unspecified alveolar anomaly
M26.71 Alveolar maxillary hyperplasia
M26.72 Alveolar mandibular hyperplasia
M26.73 Alveolar maxillary hypoplasia
M26.74 Alveolar mandibular hypoplasia
M26.79 Other specified alveolar anomalies

[5] **M26.8 Other dentofacial anomalies**

M26.81 Anterior soft tissue impingement
Anterior soft tissue impingement on teeth
M26.82 Posterior soft tissue impingement
Posterior soft tissue impingement on teeth
M26.89 Other dentofacial anomalies

M26.9 Dentofacial anomaly, unspecified

[4] **M27 Other diseases of jaws**

M27.0 Developmental disorders of jaws
Latent bone cyst of jaw
Stafne's cyst
Torus mandibularis
Torus palatinus

M27.1 Giant cell granuloma, central
Giant cell granuloma NOS
[EXCLUDES1] *peripheral giant cell granuloma (K06.8)*

M27.2 Inflammatory conditions of jaws
Osteitis of jaw(s)
Osteomyelitis (neonatal) jaw(s)
Osteoradionecrosis jaw(s)
Periostitis jaw(s)
Sequestrum of jaw bone
Use additional code (W88-W90, X39.0) to identify radiation, if radiation-induced
[EXCLUDES2] *osteonecrosis of jaw due to drug (M87.180)*

M27.3 Alveolitis of jaws
Alveolar osteitis
Dry socket

[5] **M27.4 Other and unspecified cysts of jaw**

[EXCLUDES1] *cysts of oral region (K09.-)*
latent bone cyst of jaw (M27.0)
Stafne's cyst (M27.0)

M27.40 Unspecified cyst of jaw
Cyst of jaw NOS
M27.49 Other cysts of jaw
Aneurysmal cyst of jaw
Hemorrhagic cyst of jaw
Traumatic cyst of jaw

[5] **M27.5 Periradicular pathology associated with previous endodontic treatment**

M27.51 Perforation of root canal space due to endodontic treatment
M27.52 Endodontic overfill
M27.53 Endodontic underfill
M27.59 Other periradicular pathology associated with previous endodontic treatment

[5] **M27.6 Endosseous dental implant failure**

M27.61 Osseointegration failure of dental implant
Hemorrhagic complications of dental implant placement
Iatrogenic osseointegration failure of dental implant
Osseointegration failure of dental implant due to complications of systemic disease
Osseointegration failure of dental implant due to poor bone quality
Pre-integration failure of dental implant NOS
Pre-osseointegration failure of dental implant

M27.62 Post-osseointegration biological failure of dental implant
Failure of dental implant due to lack of attached gingiva
Failure of dental implant due to occlusal trauma (caused by poor prosthetic design)
Failure of dental implant due to parafunctional habits
Failure of dental implant due to periodontal infection (peri-implantitis)
Failure of dental implant due to poor oral hygiene
Iatrogenic post-osseointegration failure of dental implant
Post-osseointegration failure of dental implant due to complications of systemic disease

M27.63 Post-osseointegration mechanical failure of dental implant
Failure of dental prosthesis causing loss of dental implant
Fracture of dental implant
[EXCLUDES2] *cracked tooth (K03.81)*
fractured dental restorative material with loss of material (K08.531)
fractured dental restorative material without loss of material (K08.530)
fractured tooth (S02.5)

M27.69 Other endosseous dental implant failure
Dental implant failure NOS

M27.8 Other specified diseases of jaws
Cherubism
Exostosis
Fibrous dysplasia
Unilateral condylar hyperplasia
Unilateral condylar hypoplasia
[EXCLUDES1] *jaw pain (R68.84)*

M27.9 Disease of jaws, unspecified

Systemic connective tissue disorders (M30-M36)

[INCLUDES] *autoimmune disease NOS*
collagen (vascular) disease NOS
systemic autoimmune disease
systemic collagen (vascular) disease

[EXCLUDES1] *autoimmune disease, single organ or single cell-type -code to relevant condition category*

[4] **M30 Polyarteritis nodosa and related conditions**

[EXCLUDES1] *microscopic polyarteritis (M31.7)*

M30.0 Polyarteritis nodosa
M30.1 Polyarteritis with lung involvement [Churg-Strauss]
Allergic granulomatous angiitis
M30.2 Juvenile polyarteritis
M30.3 Mucocutaneous lymph node syndrome [Kawasaki]
M30.8 Other conditions related to polyarteritis nodosa
Polyangiitis overlap syndrome

[4] **M31 Other necrotizing vasculopathies**

CHAPTER 13: DISEASES OF THE MUSCULOSKELETAL SYSTEM AND CONNECTIVE TISSUE (M00-M99)
M26.6 - M31

M31.0 Hypersensitivity angiitis
Goodpasture's syndrome
M31.1 Thrombotic microangiopathy
Thrombotic thrombocytopenic purpura
M31.2 Lethal midline granuloma
[5] **M31.3 Wegener's granulomatosis**
Necrotizing respiratory granulomatosis
M31.30 Wegener's granulomatosis without renal involvement
Wegener's granulomatosis NOS
M31.31 Wegener's granulomatosis with renal involvement
M31.4 Aortic arch syndrome [Takayasu]
M31.5 Giant cell arteritis with polymyalgia rheumatica
M31.6 Other giant cell arteritis
M31.7 Microscopic polyangiitis
Microscopic polyarteritis
[EXCLUDES1] *polyarteritis nodosa (M30.0)*
M31.8 Other specified necrotizing vasculopathies
Hypocomplementemic vasculitis
Septic vasculitis
M31.9 Necrotizing vasculopathy, unspecified
[4] **M32 Systemic lupus erythematosus (SLE)**
[EXCLUDES1] *lupus erythematosus (discoid) (NOS) (L93.0)*
M32.0 Drug-induced systemic lupus erythematosus
Use additional code for adverse effect, if applicable, to identify drug (T36-T50 with fifth or sixth character 5)
[5] **M32.1 Systemic lupus erythematosus with organ or system involvement**
M32.10 Systemic lupus erythematosus, organ or system involvement unspecified
M32.11 Endocarditis in systemic lupus erythematosus
Libman-Sacks disease
M32.12 Pericarditis in systemic lupus erythematosus
Lupus pericarditis
M32.13 Lung involvement in systemic lupus erythematosus
Pleural effusion due to systemic lupus erythematosus
M32.14 Glomerular disease in systemic lupus erythematosus
Lupus renal disease NOS
M32.15 Tubulo-interstitial nephropathy in systemic lupus erythematosus
M32.19 Other organ or system involvement in systemic lupus erythematosus
M32.8 Other forms of systemic lupus erythematosus
M32.9 Systemic lupus erythematosus, unspecified
SLE NOS
Systemic lupus erythematosus NOS
Systemic lupus erythematosus without organ involvement
[4] **M33 Dermatopolymyositis**
[5] **M33.0 Juvenile dermatopolymyositis**
M33.00 Juvenile dermatopolymyositis, organ involvement unspecified
M33.01 Juvenile dermatopolymyositis with respiratory involvement
M33.02 Juvenile dermatopolymyositis with myopathy
M33.09 Juvenile dermatopolymyositis with other organ involvement
[5] **M33.1 Other dermatopolymyositis**
M33.10 Other dermatopolymyositis, organ involvement unspecified
M33.11 Other dermatopolymyositis with respiratory involvement
M33.12 Other dermatopolymyositis with myopathy
M33.19 Other dermatopolymyositis with other organ involvement
[5] **M33.2 Polymyositis**
M33.20 Polymyositis, organ involvement unspecified
M33.21 Polymyositis with respiratory involvement
M33.22 Polymyositis with myopathy
M33.29 Polymyositis with other organ involvement
[5] **M33.9 Dermatopolymyositis, unspecified**
M33.90 Dermatopolymyositis, unspecified, organ involvement unspecified
M33.91 Dermatopolymyositis, unspecified with respiratory involvement
M33.92 Dermatopolymyositis, unspecified with myopathy
M33.99 Dermatopolymyositis, unspecified with other organ involvement
[4] **M34 Systemic sclerosis [scleroderma]**
[EXCLUDES1] *circumscribed scleroderma (L94.0)*
neonatal scleroderma (P83.8)
M34.0 Progressive systemic sclerosis
M34.1 CR(E)ST syndrome
Combination of calcinosis, Raynaud's phenomenon, esophageal dysfunction, sclerodactyly, telangiectasia
M34.2 Systemic sclerosis induced by drug and chemical
Code first poisoning due to drug or toxin, if applicable (T36-T65 with fifth or sixth character 1-4 or 6)
Use additional code for adverse effect, if applicable, to identify drug (T36-T50 with fifth or sixth character 5)
[5] **M34.8 Other forms of systemic sclerosis**
M34.81 Systemic sclerosis with lung involvement
M34.82 Systemic sclerosis with myopathy
M34.83 Systemic sclerosis with polyneuropathy
M34.89 Other systemic sclerosis
M34.9 Systemic sclerosis, unspecified
[4] **M35 Other systemic involvement of connective tissue**
[EXCLUDES1] *reactive perforating collagenosis (L87.1)*
[5] **M35.0 Sicca syndrome [Sjögren]**
M35.00 Sicca syndrome, unspecified
M35.01 Sicca syndrome with keratoconjunctivitis
M35.02 Sicca syndrome with lung involvement
M35.03 Sicca syndrome with myopathy
M35.04 Sicca syndrome with tubulo-interstitial nephropathy
Renal tubular acidosis in sicca syndrome
M35.09 Sicca syndrome with other organ involvement
M35.1 Other overlap syndromes
Mixed connective tissue disease
[EXCLUDES1] *polyangiitis overlap syndrome (M30.8)*
M35.2 Behçet's disease
M35.3 Polymyalgia rheumatica
[EXCLUDES1] *polymyalgia rheumatica with giant cell arteritis (M31.5)*
M35.4 Diffuse (eosinophilic) fasciitis
M35.5 Multifocal fibrosclerosis
M35.6 Relapsing panniculitis [Weber-Christian]
[EXCLUDES1] *lupus panniculitis (L93.2)*
panniculitis NOS (M79.3-)
M35.7 Hypermobility syndrome
Familial ligamentous laxity
[EXCLUDES1] *Ehlers-Danlos syndrome (Q79.6)*
ligamentous laxity, NOS (M24.2-)
M35.8 Other specified systemic involvement of connective tissue
M35.9 Systemic involvement of connective tissue, unspecified
Autoimmune disease (systemic) NOS
Collagen (vascular) disease NOS

Unspecified Code | Other Specified Code | [N] Newborn Age: 0 | [P] Pediatric Age: 0-17 | [M] Maternity Age: 12-55
[A] Adult Age: 15-124 | ♂ Male | ♀ Female | ● New Code | ▲ Revised Code Title | ►◄ Revised Text

[4] **M36 Systemic disorders of connective tissue in diseases classified elsewhere**

[EXCLUDES2] *arthropathies in diseases classified elsewhere (M14.-)*

M36.0 Dermato(poly)myositis in neoplastic disease

Code first underlying neoplasm (C00-D49)

M36.1 Arthropathy in neoplastic disease

Code first underlying neoplasm, such as:
leukemia (C91-C95)
malignant histiocytosis (C96.A)
multiple myeloma (C90.0)

M36.2 Hemophilic arthropathy

Hemarthrosis in hemophilic arthropathy
Code first underlying disease, such as:
factor VIII deficiency (D66)
with vascular defect (D68.0)
factor IX deficiency (D67)
hemophilia (classical) (D66)
hemophilia B (D67)
hemophilia C (D68.1)

M36.3 Arthropathy in other blood disorders

M36.4 Arthropathy in hypersensitivity reactions classified elsewhere

Code first underlying disease, such as:
Henoch (-Schönlein) purpura (D69.0)
serum sickness (T80.6-)

M36.8 Systemic disorders of connective tissue in other diseases classified elsewhere

Code first underlying disease, such as:
alkaptonuria (E70.2)
hypogammaglobulinemia (D80.-)
ochronosis (E70.2)

Dorsopathies (M40-M54)

Deforming dorsopathies (M40-M43)

[4] **M40 Kyphosis and lordosis**

[EXCLUDES1] *congenital kyphosis and lordosis (Q76.4)*
kyphoscoliosis (M41.-)
postprocedural kyphosis and lordosis (M96.-)

[5] **M40.0 Postural kyphosis**

[EXCLUDES1] *osteochondrosis of spine (M42.-)*

M40.00 Postural kyphosis, site unspecified
M40.03 Postural kyphosis, cervicothoracic region
M40.04 Postural kyphosis, thoracic region
M40.05 Postural kyphosis, thoracolumbar region

[5] **M40.1 Other secondary kyphosis**

M40.10 Other secondary kyphosis, site unspecified
M40.12 Other secondary kyphosis, cervical region
M40.13 Other secondary kyphosis, cervicothoracic region
M40.14 Other secondary kyphosis, thoracic region
M40.15 Other secondary kyphosis, thoracolumbar region

[5] **M40.2 Other and unspecified kyphosis**

[6] **M40.20 Unspecified kyphosis**

M40.202 Unspecified kyphosis, cervical region
M40.203 Unspecified kyphosis, cervicothoracic region
M40.204 Unspecified kyphosis, thoracic region
M40.205 Unspecified kyphosis, thoracolumbar region
M40.209 Unspecified kyphosis, site unspecified

[6] **M40.29 Other kyphosis**

M40.292 Other kyphosis, cervical region
M40.293 Other kyphosis, cervicothoracic region
M40.294 Other kyphosis, thoracic region
M40.295 Other kyphosis, thoracolumbar region
M40.299 Other kyphosis, site unspecified

[5] **M40.3 Flatback syndrome**

M40.30 Flatback syndrome, site unspecified
M40.35 Flatback syndrome, thoracolumbar region
M40.36 Flatback syndrome, lumbar region
M40.37 Flatback syndrome, lumbosacral region

[5] **M40.4 Postural lordosis**

Acquired lordosis

M40.40 Postural lordosis, site unspecified
M40.45 Postural lordosis, thoracolumbar region
M40.46 Postural lordosis, lumbar region
M40.47 Postural lordosis, lumbosacral region

[5] **M40.5 Lordosis, unspecified**

M40.50 Lordosis, unspecified, site unspecified
M40.55 Lordosis, unspecified, thoracolumbar region
M40.56 Lordosis, unspecified, lumbar region
M40.57 Lordosis, unspecified, lumbosacral region

[4] **M41 Scoliosis**

[INCLUDES] *kyphoscoliosis*

[EXCLUDES1] *congenital scoliosis NOS (Q67.5)*
congenital scoliosis due to bony malformation (Q76.3)
postural congenital scoliosis (Q67.5)
kyphoscoliotic heart disease (I27.1)
postprocedural scoliosis (M96.-)

[5] **M41.0 Infantile idiopathic scoliosis**

M41.00 Infantile idiopathic scoliosis, site unspecified
M41.02 Infantile idiopathic scoliosis, cervical region
M41.03 Infantile idiopathic scoliosis, cervicothoracic region
M41.04 Infantile idiopathic scoliosis, thoracic region
M41.05 Infantile idiopathic scoliosis, thoracolumbar region
M41.06 Infantile idiopathic scoliosis, lumbar region
M41.07 Infantile idiopathic scoliosis, lumbosacral region
M41.08 Infantile idiopathic scoliosis, sacral and sacrococcygeal region

[5] **M41.1 Juvenile and adolescent idiopathic scoliosis**

[6] **M41.11 Juvenile idiopathic scoliosis**

M41.112 Juvenile idiopathic scoliosis, cervical region
M41.113 Juvenile idiopathic scoliosis, cervicothoracic region
M41.114 Juvenile idiopathic scoliosis, thoracic region
M41.115 Juvenile idiopathic scoliosis, thoracolumbar region
M41.116 Juvenile idiopathic scoliosis, lumbar region
M41.117 Juvenile idiopathic scoliosis, lumbosacral region
M41.119 Juvenile idiopathic scoliosis, site unspecified

[6] **M41.12 Adolescent scoliosis**

M41.122 Adolescent idiopathic scoliosis, cervical region
M41.123 Adolescent idiopathic scoliosis, cervicothoracic region
M41.124 Adolescent idiopathic scoliosis, thoracic region
M41.125 Adolescent idiopathic scoliosis, thoracolumbar region
M41.126 Adolescent idiopathic scoliosis, lumbar region
M41.127 Adolescent idiopathic scoliosis, lumbosacral region

M41.129 Adolescent idiopathic scoliosis, site unspecified

🔵 M41.2 Other idiopathic scoliosis
M41.20 Other idiopathic scoliosis, site unspecified
M41.22 Other idiopathic scoliosis, cervical region
M41.23 Other idiopathic scoliosis, cervicothoracic region
M41.24 Other idiopathic scoliosis, thoracic region
M41.25 Other idiopathic scoliosis, thoracolumbar region
M41.26 Other idiopathic scoliosis, lumbar region
M41.27 Other idiopathic scoliosis, lumbosacral region

🔵 M41.3 Thoracogenic scoliosis
M41.30 Thoracogenic scoliosis, site unspecified
M41.34 Thoracogenic scoliosis, thoracic region
M41.35 Thoracogenic scoliosis, thoracolumbar region

🔵 M41.4 Neuromuscular scoliosis
Scoliosis secondary to cerebral palsy, Friedreich's ataxia, poliomyelitis and other neuromuscular disorders
Code also underlying condition
M41.40 Neuromuscular scoliosis, site unspecified
M41.41 Neuromuscular scoliosis, occipito-atlanto-axial region
M41.42 Neuromuscular scoliosis, cervical region
M41.43 Neuromuscular scoliosis, cervicothoracic region
M41.44 Neuromuscular scoliosis, thoracic region
M41.45 Neuromuscular scoliosis, thoracolumbar region
M41.46 Neuromuscular scoliosis, lumbar region
M41.47 Neuromuscular scoliosis, lumbosacral region

🔵 M41.5 Other secondary scoliosis
M41.50 Other secondary scoliosis, site unspecified
M41.52 Other secondary scoliosis, cervical region
M41.53 Other secondary scoliosis, cervicothoracic region
M41.54 Other secondary scoliosis, thoracic region
M41.55 Other secondary scoliosis, thoracolumbar region
M41.56 Other secondary scoliosis, lumbar region
M41.57 Other secondary scoliosis, lumbosacral region

🔵 M41.8 Other forms of scoliosis
M41.80 Other forms of scoliosis, site unspecified
M41.82 Other forms of scoliosis, cervical region
M41.83 Other forms of scoliosis, cervicothoracic region
M41.84 Other forms of scoliosis, thoracic region
M41.85 Other forms of scoliosis, thoracolumbar region
M41.86 Other forms of scoliosis, lumbar region
M41.87 Other forms of scoliosis, lumbosacral region
M41.9 Scoliosis, unspecified

🔵 M42 Spinal osteochondrosis
🔵 M42.0 Juvenile osteochondrosis of spine
Calvé's disease
Scheuermann's disease
EXCLUDES1 postural kyphosis (M40.0)
M42.00 Juvenile osteochondrosis of spine, site unspecified
M42.01 Juvenile osteochondrosis of spine, occipito-atlanto-axial region
M42.02 Juvenile osteochondrosis of spine, cervical region
M42.03 Juvenile osteochondrosis of spine, cervicothoracic region
M42.04 Juvenile osteochondrosis of spine, thoracic region
M42.05 Juvenile osteochondrosis of spine, thoracolumbar region
M42.06 Juvenile osteochondrosis of spine, lumbar region
M42.07 Juvenile osteochondrosis of spine, lumbosacral region
M42.08 Juvenile osteochondrosis of spine, sacral and sacrococcygeal region
M42.09 Juvenile osteochondrosis of spine, multiple sites in spine

🔵 M42.1 Adult osteochondrosis of spine
M42.10 Adult osteochondrosis of spine, site unspecified 🅐
M42.11 Adult osteochondrosis of spine, occipito-atlanto-axial region 🅐
M42.12 Adult osteochondrosis of spine, cervical region 🅐
M42.13 Adult osteochondrosis of spine, cervicothoracic region 🅐
M42.14 Adult osteochondrosis of spine, thoracic region 🅐
M42.15 Adult osteochondrosis of spine, thoracolumbar region 🅐
M42.16 Adult osteochondrosis of spine, lumbar region 🅐
M42.17 Adult osteochondrosis of spine, lumbosacral region 🅐
M42.18 Adult osteochondrosis of spine, sacral and sacrococcygeal region 🅐
M42.19 Adult osteochondrosis of spine, multiple sites in spine 🅐
M42.9 Spinal osteochondrosis, unspecified

🔵 M43 Other deforming dorsopathies
EXCLUDES1 congenital spondylolysis and spondylolisthesis (Q76.2)
hemivertebra (Q76.3-Q76.4)
Klippel-Feil syndrome (Q76.1)
lumbarization and sacralization (Q76.4)
platyspondylisis (Q76.4)
spina bifida occulta (Q76.0)
spinal curvature in osteoporosis (M80.-)
spinal curvature in Paget's disease of bone [osteitis deformans] (M88.-)

🔵 M43.0 Spondylolysis
EXCLUDES1 congenital spondylolysis (Q76.2)
spondylolisthesis (M43.1)
M43.00 Spondylolysis, site unspecified
M43.01 Spondylolysis, occipito-atlanto-axial region
M43.02 Spondylolysis, cervical region
M43.03 Spondylolysis, cervicothoracic region
M43.04 Spondylolysis, thoracic region
M43.05 Spondylolysis, thoracolumbar region
M43.06 Spondylolysis, lumbar region
M43.07 Spondylolysis, lumbosacral region
M43.08 Spondylolysis, sacral and sacrococcygeal region
M43.09 Spondylolysis, multiple sites in spine

🔵 M43.1 Spondylolisthesis
EXCLUDES1 acute traumatic of lumbosacral region (S33.1)
acute traumatic of sites other than lumbosacral-code to Fracture, vertebra, by region
congenital spondylolisthesis (Q76.2)
M43.10 Spondylolisthesis, site unspecified
M43.11 Spondylolisthesis, occipito-atlanto-axial region
M43.12 Spondylolisthesis, cervical region
M43.13 Spondylolisthesis, cervicothoracic region
M43.14 Spondylolisthesis, thoracic region
M43.15 Spondylolisthesis, thoracolumbar region
M43.16 Spondylolisthesis, lumbar region
M43.17 Spondylolisthesis, lumbosacral region
M43.18 Spondylolisthesis, sacral and sacrococcygeal region
M43.19 Spondylolisthesis, multiple sites in spine

Unspecified Code   Other Specified Code   🅝 Newborn Age: 0   🅟 Pediatric Age: 0-17   🅜 Maternity Age: 12-55
🅐 Adult Age: 15-124   ♂ Male   ♀ Female   ● New Code   ▲ Revised Code Title   ►◄ Revised Text

[5] **M43.2 Fusion of spine**

Ankylosis of spinal joint

[EXCLUDES1] *ankylosing spondylitis (M45.0-)*
congenital fusion of spine (Q76.4)

[EXCLUDES2] *arthrodesis status (Z98.1)*
pseudoarthrosis after fusion or arthrodesis (M96.0)

M43.20 Fusion of spine, site unspecified
M43.21 Fusion of spine, occipito-atlanto-axial region
M43.22 Fusion of spine, cervical region
M43.23 Fusion of spine, cervicothoracic region
M43.24 Fusion of spine, thoracic region
M43.25 Fusion of spine, thoracolumbar region
M43.26 Fusion of spine, lumbar region
M43.27 Fusion of spine, lumbosacral region
M43.28 Fusion of spine, sacral and sacrococcygeal region

M43.3 Recurrent atlantoaxial dislocation with myelopathy

M43.4 Other recurrent atlantoaxial dislocation

[5] **M43.5 Other recurrent vertebral dislocation**

[EXCLUDES1] *biomechanical lesions NEC (M99.-)*

[6] **M43.5X Other recurrent vertebral dislocation**

M43.5X2 Other recurrent vertebral dislocation, cervical region
M43.5X3 Other recurrent vertebral dislocation, cervicothoracic region
M43.5X4 Other recurrent vertebral dislocation, thoracic region
M43.5X5 Other recurrent vertebral dislocation, thoracolumbar region
M43.5X6 Other recurrent vertebral dislocation, lumbar region
M43.5X7 Other recurrent vertebral dislocation, lumbosacral region
M43.5X8 Other recurrent vertebral dislocation, sacral and sacrococcygeal region
M43.5X9 Other recurrent vertebral dislocation, site unspecified

M43.6 Torticollis

[EXCLUDES1] *congenital (sternomastoid) torticollis (Q68.0)*
current injury - see Injury, of spine, by body region
ocular torticollis (R29.891)
psychogenic torticollis (F45.8)
spasmodic torticollis (G24.3)
torticollis due to birth injury (P15.2)

[5] **M43.8 Other specified deforming dorsopathies**

[EXCLUDES2] *kyphosis and lordosis (M40.-)*
scoliosis (M41.-)

[6] **M43.8X Other specified deforming dorsopathies**

M43.8X1 Other specified deforming dorsopathies, occipito-atlanto-axial region
M43.8X2 Other specified deforming dorsopathies, cervical region
M43.8X3 Other specified deforming dorsopathies, cervicothoracic region
M43.8X4 Other specified deforming dorsopathies, thoracic region
M43.8X5 Other specified deforming dorsopathies, thoracolumbar region
M43.8X6 Other specified deforming dorsopathies, lumbar region
M43.8X7 Other specified deforming dorsopathies, lumbosacral region
M43.8X8 Other specified deforming dorsopathies, sacral and sacrococcygeal region
M43.8X9 Other specified deforming dorsopathies, site unspecified

M43.9 Deforming dorsopathy, unspecified

Curvature of spine NOS

Spondylopathies (M45-M49)

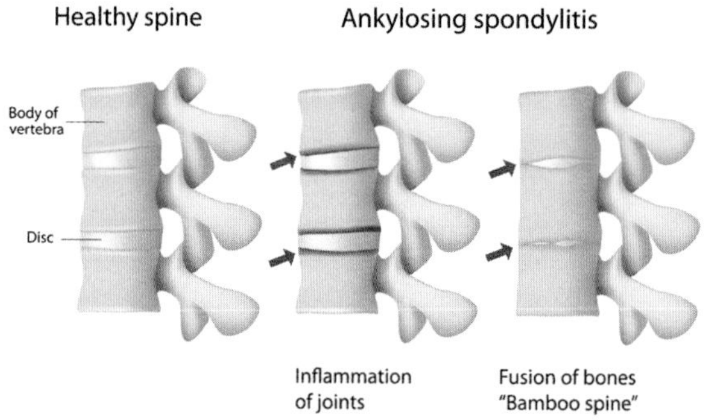
Healthy spine
Ankylosing spondylitis
Body of vertebra
Disc
Inflammation of joints
Fusion of bones "Bamboo spine"

Figure 12.4 Healthy spine changing in to Ankylosing Spondylitis

[4] **M45 Ankylosing spondylitis**

Rheumatoid arthritis of spine

[EXCLUDES1] *arthropathy in Reiter's disease (M02.3-)*
juvenile (ankylosing) spondylitis (M08.1)

[EXCLUDES2] *Behçet's disease (M35.2)*

M45.0 Ankylosing spondylitis of multiple sites in spine
M45.1 Ankylosing spondylitis of occipito-atlanto-axial region
M45.2 Ankylosing spondylitis of cervical region
M45.3 Ankylosing spondylitis of cervicothoracic region
M45.4 Ankylosing spondylitis of thoracic region
M45.5 Ankylosing spondylitis of thoracolumbar region
M45.6 Ankylosing spondylitis lumbar region
M45.7 Ankylosing spondylitis of lumbosacral region
M45.8 Ankylosing spondylitis sacral and sacrococcygeal region
M45.9 Ankylosing spondylitis of unspecified sites in spine

[4] **M46 Other inflammatory spondylopathies**

[5] **M46.0 Spinal enthesopathy**

Disorder of ligamentous or muscular attachments of spine

M46.00 Spinal enthesopathy, site unspecified
M46.01 Spinal enthesopathy, occipito-atlanto-axial region
M46.02 Spinal enthesopathy, cervical region
M46.03 Spinal enthesopathy, cervicothoracic region
M46.04 Spinal enthesopathy, thoracic region
M46.05 Spinal enthesopathy, thoracolumbar region
M46.06 Spinal enthesopathy, lumbar region
M46.07 Spinal enthesopathy, lumbosacral region
M46.08 Spinal enthesopathy, sacral and sacrococcygeal region
M46.09 Spinal enthesopathy, multiple sites in spine

M46.1 Sacroiliitis, not elsewhere classified

[5] **M46.2 Osteomyelitis of vertebra**

M46.20 Osteomyelitis of vertebra, site unspecified
M46.21 Osteomyelitis of vertebra, occipito-atlanto-axial region
M46.22 Osteomyelitis of vertebra, cervical region
M46.23 Osteomyelitis of vertebra, cervicothoracic region
M46.24 Osteomyelitis of vertebra, thoracic region
M46.25 Osteomyelitis of vertebra, thoracolumbar region
M46.26 Osteomyelitis of vertebra, lumbar region
M46.27 Osteomyelitis of vertebra, lumbosacral region
M46.28 Osteomyelitis of vertebra, sacral and sacrococcygeal region

[5] **M46.3 Infection of intervertebral disc (pyogenic)**

Use additional code (B95-B97) to identify infectious agent.

[4] 4th character required [5] 5th character required [6] 6th character required [7] 7th character required [7th] Extension 'X' Alert
[EXCLUDES1] Not coded here [EXCLUDES2] Not included here [PDx] Primary Diagnosis Only Manifestation Code

M46.30 Infection of intervertebral disc (pyogenic), site unspecified
M46.31 Infection of intervertebral disc (pyogenic), occipito-atlanto-axial region
M46.32 Infection of intervertebral disc (pyogenic), cervical region
M46.33 Infection of intervertebral disc (pyogenic), cervicothoracic region
M46.34 Infection of intervertebral disc (pyogenic), thoracic region
M46.35 Infection of intervertebral disc (pyogenic), thoracolumbar region
M46.36 Infection of intervertebral disc (pyogenic), lumbar region
M46.37 Infection of intervertebral disc (pyogenic), lumbosacral region
M46.38 Infection of intervertebral disc (pyogenic), sacral and sacrococcygeal region
M46.39 Infection of intervertebral disc (pyogenic), multiple sites in spine

[5] M46.4 Discitis, unspecified
M46.40 Discitis, unspecified, site unspecified
M46.41 Discitis, unspecified, occipito-atlanto-axial region
M46.42 Discitis, unspecified, cervical region
M46.43 Discitis, unspecified, cervicothoracic region
M46.44 Discitis, unspecified, thoracic region
M46.45 Discitis, unspecified, thoracolumbar region
M46.46 Discitis, unspecified, lumbar region
M46.47 Discitis, unspecified, lumbosacral region
M46.48 Discitis, unspecified, sacral and sacrococcygeal region
M46.49 Discitis, unspecified, multiple sites in spine

[5] M46.5 Other infective spondylopathies
M46.50 Other infective spondylopathies, site unspecified
M46.51 Other infective spondylopathies, occipito-atlanto-axial region
M46.52 Other infective spondylopathies, cervical region
M46.53 Other infective spondylopathies, cervicothoracic region
M46.54 Other infective spondylopathies, thoracic region
M46.55 Other infective spondylopathies, thoracolumbar region
M46.56 Other infective spondylopathies, lumbar region
M46.57 Other infective spondylopathies, lumbosacral region
M46.58 Other infective spondylopathies, sacral and sacrococcygeal region
M46.59 Other infective spondylopathies, multiple sites in spine

[5] M46.8 Other specified inflammatory spondylopathies
M46.80 Other specified inflammatory spondylopathies, site unspecified
M46.81 Other specified inflammatory spondylopathies, occipito-atlanto-axial region
M46.82 Other specified inflammatory spondylopathies, cervical region
M46.83 Other specified inflammatory spondylopathies, cervicothoracic region
M46.84 Other specified inflammatory spondylopathies, thoracic region
M46.85 Other specified inflammatory spondylopathies, thoracolumbar region
M46.86 Other specified inflammatory spondylopathies, lumbar region
M46.87 Other specified inflammatory spondylopathies, lumbosacral region
M46.88 Other specified inflammatory spondylopathies, sacral and sacrococcygeal region
M46.89 Other specified inflammatory spondylopathies, multiple sites in spine

[5] M46.9 Unspecified inflammatory spondylopathy
M46.90 Unspecified inflammatory spondylopathy, site unspecified
M46.91 Unspecified inflammatory spondylopathy, occipito-atlanto-axial region
M46.92 Unspecified inflammatory spondylopathy, cervical region
M46.93 Unspecified inflammatory spondylopathy, cervicothoracic region
M46.94 Unspecified inflammatory spondylopathy, thoracic region
M46.95 Unspecified inflammatory spondylopathy, thoracolumbar region
M46.96 Unspecified inflammatory spondylopathy, lumbar region
M46.97 Unspecified inflammatory spondylopathy, lumbosacral region
M46.98 Unspecified inflammatory spondylopathy, sacral and sacrococcygeal region
M46.99 Unspecified inflammatory spondylopathy, multiple sites in spine

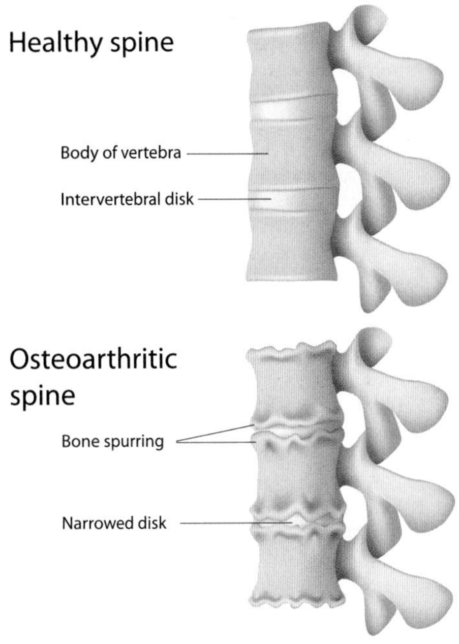
Healthy spine
Body of vertebra
Intervertebral disk
Osteoarthritic spine
Bone spurring
Narrowed disk

Figure 12.5 Remarkable changes in Healthy and Osteoarthritic spine

[4] M47 Spondylosis
[INCLUDES] *arthrosis or osteoarthritis of spine*
degeneration of facet joints

[5] M47.0 Anterior spinal and vertebral artery compression syndromes
[6] M47.01 Anterior spinal artery compression syndromes
M47.011 Anterior spinal artery compression syndromes, occipito-atlanto-axial region
M47.012 Anterior spinal artery compression syndromes, cervical region
M47.013 Anterior spinal artery compression syndromes, cervicothoracic region
M47.014 Anterior spinal artery compression syndromes, thoracic region
M47.015 Anterior spinal artery compression syndromes, thoracolumbar region

Unspecified Code | Other Specified Code | [N] Newborn Age: 0 | [P] Pediatric Age: 0-17 | [M] Maternity Age: 12-55
[A] Adult Age: 15-124 | ♂ Male | ♀ Female | ● New Code | ▲ Revised Code Title | ►◄ Revised Text

M47.016 Anterior spinal artery compression syndromes, lumbar region

M47.019 Anterior spinal artery compression syndromes, site unspecified

⑤ M47.02 Vertebral artery compression syndromes

M47.021 Vertebral artery compression syndromes, occipito-atlanto-axial region

M47.022 Vertebral artery compression syndromes, cervical region

M47.029 Vertebral artery compression syndromes, site unspecified

⑤ M47.1 Other spondylosis with myelopathy

Spondylogenic compression of spinal cord

EXCLUDES1 vertebral subluxation (M43.3-M43.59)

M47.10 Other spondylosis with myelopathy, site unspecified

M47.11 Other spondylosis with myelopathy, occipito-atlanto-axial region

M47.12 Other spondylosis with myelopathy, cervical region

M47.13 Other spondylosis with myelopathy, cervicothoracic region

M47.14 Other spondylosis with myelopathy, thoracic region

M47.15 Other spondylosis with myelopathy, thoracolumbar region

M47.16 Other spondylosis with myelopathy, lumbar region

⑤ M47.2 Other spondylosis with radiculopathy

M47.20 Other spondylosis with radiculopathy, site unspecified

M47.21 Other spondylosis with radiculopathy, occipito-atlanto-axial region

M47.22 Other spondylosis with radiculopathy, cervical region

M47.23 Other spondylosis with radiculopathy, cervicothoracic region

M47.24 Other spondylosis with radiculopathy, thoracic region

M47.25 Other spondylosis with radiculopathy, thoracolumbar region

M47.26 Other spondylosis with radiculopathy, lumbar region

M47.27 Other spondylosis with radiculopathy, lumbosacral region

M47.28 Other spondylosis with radiculopathy, sacral and sacrococcygeal region

⑤ M47.8 Other spondylosis

⑥ M47.81 Spondylosis without myelopathy or radiculopathy

M47.811 Spondylosis without myelopathy or radiculopathy, occipito-atlanto-axial region

M47.812 Spondylosis without myelopathy or radiculopathy, cervical region

M47.813 Spondylosis without myelopathy or radiculopathy, cervicothoracic region

M47.814 Spondylosis without myelopathy or radiculopathy, thoracic region

M47.815 Spondylosis without myelopathy or radiculopathy, thoracolumbar region

M47.816 Spondylosis without myelopathy or radiculopathy, lumbar region

M47.817 Spondylosis without myelopathy or radiculopathy, lumbosacral region

M47.818 Spondylosis without myelopathy or radiculopathy, sacral and sacrococcygeal region

M47.819 Spondylosis without myelopathy or radiculopathy, site unspecified

⑥ M47.89 Other spondylosis

M47.891 Other spondylosis, occipito-atlanto-axial region

M47.892 Other spondylosis, cervical region

M47.893 Other spondylosis, cervicothoracic region

M47.894 Other spondylosis, thoracic region

M47.895 Other spondylosis, thoracolumbar region

M47.896 Other spondylosis, lumbar region

M47.897 Other spondylosis, lumbosacral region

M47.898 Other spondylosis, sacral and sacrococcygeal region

M47.899 Other spondylosis, site unspecified

M47.9 Spondylosis, unspecified

④ M48 Other spondylopathies

⑤ M48.0 Spinal stenosis

Caudal stenosis

M48.00 Spinal stenosis, site unspecified

M48.01 Spinal stenosis, occipito-atlanto-axial region

M48.02 Spinal stenosis, cervical region

M48.03 Spinal stenosis, cervicothoracic region

M48.04 Spinal stenosis, thoracic region

M48.05 Spinal stenosis, thoracolumbar region

M48.06 Spinal stenosis, lumbar region

M48.07 Spinal stenosis, lumbosacral region

M48.08 Spinal stenosis, sacral and sacrococcygeal region

⑤ M48.1 Ankylosing hyperostosis [Forestier]

Diffuse idiopathic skeletal hyperostosis [DISH]

M48.10 Ankylosing hyperostosis [Forestier], site unspecified

M48.11 Ankylosing hyperostosis [Forestier], occipito-atlanto-axial region

M48.12 Ankylosing hyperostosis [Forestier], cervical region

M48.13 Ankylosing hyperostosis [Forestier], cervicothoracic region

M48.14 Ankylosing hyperostosis [Forestier], thoracic region

M48.15 Ankylosing hyperostosis [Forestier], thoracolumbar region

M48.16 Ankylosing hyperostosis [Forestier], lumbar region

M48.17 Ankylosing hyperostosis [Forestier], lumbosacral region

M48.18 Ankylosing hyperostosis [Forestier], sacral and sacrococcygeal region

M48.19 Ankylosing hyperostosis [Forestier], multiple sites in spine

⑤ M48.2 Kissing spine

M48.20 Kissing spine, site unspecified

M48.21 Kissing spine, occipito-atlanto-axial region

M48.22 Kissing spine, cervical region

M48.23 Kissing spine, cervicothoracic region

M48.24 Kissing spine, thoracic region

M48.25 Kissing spine, thoracolumbar region

M48.26 Kissing spine, lumbar region

M48.27 Kissing spine, lumbosacral region

⑤ M48.3 Traumatic spondylopathy

M48.30 Traumatic spondylopathy, site unspecified

M48.31 Traumatic spondylopathy, occipito-atlanto-axial region

M48.32 Traumatic spondylopathy, cervical region

M48.33 Traumatic spondylopathy, cervicothoracic region

M48.34 Traumatic spondylopathy, thoracic region

---

④ 4th character required   ⑤ 5th character required   ⑥ 6th character required   ⑦ 7th character required   Ⓧ Extension 'X' Alert

EXCLUDES1 Not coded here   EXCLUDES2 Not included here   PDx Primary Diagnosis Only   Manifestation Code

M48.35 Traumatic spondylopathy, thoracolumbar region

M48.36 Traumatic spondylopathy, lumbar region

M48.37 Traumatic spondylopathy, lumbosacral region

M48.38 Traumatic spondylopathy, sacral and sacrococcygeal region

⑤ M48.4 Fatigue fracture of vertebra

Stress fracture of vertebra

EXCLUDES1 *pathological fracture NOS (M84.4-)*
pathological fracture of vertebra due to neoplasm (M84.58)
pathological fracture of vertebra due to other diagnosis (M84.68)
pathological fracture of vertebra due to osteoporosis (M80.-)
traumatic fracture of vertebrae (S12.0-S12.3-, S22.0-, S32.0-)

The appropriate 7th character is to be added to each code from subcategory M48.4:
A = initial encounter for fracture
D = subsequent encounter for fracture with routine healing
G = subsequent encounter for fracture with delayed healing
S = sequela of fracture

⑦ M48.40 Fatigue fracture of vertebra, site unspecified

⑦ M48.41 Fatigue fracture of vertebra, occipito-atlanto-axial region

⑦ M48.42 Fatigue fracture of vertebra, cervical region

⑦ M48.43 Fatigue fracture of vertebra, cervicothoracic region

⑦ M48.44 Fatigue fracture of vertebra, thoracic region

⑦ M48.45 Fatigue fracture of vertebra, thoracolumbar region

⑦ M48.46 Fatigue fracture of vertebra, lumbar region

⑦ M48.47 Fatigue fracture of vertebra, lumbosacral region

⑦ M48.48 Fatigue fracture of vertebra, sacral and sacrococcygeal region

⑤ M48.5 Collapsed vertebra, not elsewhere classified

Collapsed vertebra NOS

Wedging of vertebra NOS

EXCLUDES1 *current injury - see Injury of spine, by body region*
fatigue fracture of vertebra (M48.4)
pathological fracture of vertebra due to neoplasm (M84.58)
pathological fracture of vertebra due to other diagnosis (M84.68)
pathological fracture of vertebra due to osteoporosis (M80.-)
pathological fracture NOS (M84.4-)
stress fracture of vertebra (M48.4-)
traumatic fracture of vertebra (S12.-, S22.-, S32.-)

The appropriate 7th character is to be added to each code from subcategory M48.5:
A = initial encounter for fracture
D = subsequent encounter for fracture with routine healing
G = subsequent encounter for fracture with delayed healing
S = sequela of fracture

⑦ M48.50 Collapsed vertebra, not elsewhere classified, site unspecified

⑦ M48.51 Collapsed vertebra, not elsewhere classified, occipito-atlanto-axial region

⑦ M48.52 Collapsed vertebra, not elsewhere classified, cervical region

⑦ M48.53 Collapsed vertebra, not elsewhere classified, cervicothoracic region

⑦ M48.54 Collapsed vertebra, not elsewhere classified, thoracic region

⑦ M48.55 Collapsed vertebra, not elsewhere classified, thoracolumbar region

⑦ M48.56 Collapsed vertebra, not elsewhere classified, lumbar region

⑦ M48.57 Collapsed vertebra, not elsewhere classified, lumbosacral region

⑦ M48.58 Collapsed vertebra, not elsewhere classified, sacral and sacrococcygeal region

⑤ M48.8 Other specified spondylopathies

Ossification of posterior longitudinal ligament

⑥ M48.8X Other specified spondylopathies

M48.8X1 Other specified spondylopathies, occipito-atlanto-axial region

M48.8X2 Other specified spondylopathies, cervical region

M48.8X3 Other specified spondylopathies, cervicothoracic region

M48.8X4 Other specified spondylopathies, thoracic region

M48.8X5 Other specified spondylopathies, thoracolumbar region

M48.8X6 Other specified spondylopathies, lumbar region

M48.8X7 Other specified spondylopathies, lumbosacral region

M48.8X8 Other specified spondylopathies, sacral and sacrococcygeal region

M48.8X9 Other specified spondylopathies, site unspecified

M48.9 Spondylopathy, unspecified

④ M49 Spondylopathies in diseases classified elsewhere

INCLUDES *curvature of spine in diseases classified elsewhere*
deformity of spine in diseases classified elsewhere
kyphosis in diseases classified elsewhere
scoliosis in diseases classified elsewhere
spondylopathy in diseases classified elsewhere

EXCLUDES1 *curvature of spine in tuberculosis [Pott's] (A18.01)*
enteropathic arthropathies (M07.-)
gonococcal spondylitis (A54.41)
neuropathic [tabes dorsalis] spondylitis (A52.11)
neuropathic spondylopathy in syringomyelia (G95.0)
neuropathic spondylopathy in tabes dorsalis (A52.11)
nonsyphilitic neuropathic spondylopathy NEC (G98.0)
spondylitis in syphilis (acquired) (A52.77)
tuberculous spondylitis (A18.01)
typhoid fever spondylitis (A01.05)

Code first underlying disease, such as:
brucellosis (A23.-)
Charcot-Marie-Tooth disease (G60.0)
enterobacterial infections (A01-A04)
osteitis fibrosa cystica (E21.0)

⑤ M49.8 Spondylopathy in diseases classified elsewhere

M49.80 Spondylopathy in diseases classified elsewhere, site unspecified

M49.81 Spondylopathy in diseases classified elsewhere, occipito-atlanto-axial region

M49.82 Spondylopathy in diseases classified elsewhere, cervical region

M49.83 Spondylopathy in diseases classified elsewhere, cervicothoracic region

M49.84 Spondylopathy in diseases classified elsewhere, thoracic region

M49.85 Spondylopathy in diseases classified elsewhere, thoracolumbar region

M49.86 Spondylopathy in diseases classified elsewhere, lumbar region

---

Unspecified Code   Other Specified Code   N Newborn Age: 0   P Pediatric Age: 0-17   M Maternity Age: 12-55

A Adult Age: 15-124   ♂ Male   ♀ Female   ● New Code   ▲ Revised Code Title   ►◄ Revised Text

M49.87 **Spondylopathy in diseases classified elsewhere, lumbosacral region**
M49.88 **Spondylopathy in diseases classified elsewhere, sacral and sacrococcygeal region**
M49.89 **Spondylopathy in diseases classified elsewhere, multiple sites in spine**

Other dorsopathies (M50-M54)

[EXCLUDES1] *current injury - see injury of spine by body region*
discitis NOS (M46.4-)

[4] **M50 Cervical disc disorders**
[NOTES] code to the most superior level of disorder
[INCLUDES] *cervicothoracic disc disorders with cervicalgia*
cervicothoracic disc disorders

[5] **M50.0 Cervical disc disorder with myelopathy**
M50.00 **Cervical disc disorder with myelopathy, unspecified cervical region**
M50.01 **Cervical disc disorder with myelopathy, high cervical region** ▲
C2-C3 disc disorder with myelopathy
C3-C4 disc disorder with myelopathy
M50.02 **Cervical disc disorder with myelopathy, mid-cervical region**
C4-C5 disc disorder with myelopathy
C5-C6 disc disorder with myelopathy
C6-C7 disc disorder with myelopathy
M50.03 **Cervical disc disorder with myelopathy, cervicothoracic region**
C7-T1 disc disorder with myelopathy

[5] **M50.1 Cervical disc disorder with radiculopathy**
[EXCLUDES2] *brachial radiculitis NOS (M54.13)*
M50.10 **Cervical disc disorder with radiculopathy, unspecified cervical region**
M50.11 **Cervical disc disorder with radiculopathy, high cervical region** ▲
C2-C3 disc disorder with radiculopathy
C3 radiculopathy due to disc disorder
C3-C4 disc disorder with radiculopathy
C4 radiculopathy due to disc disorder
M50.12 **Cervical disc disorder with radiculopathy, mid-cervical region**
C4-C5 disc disorder with radiculopathy
C5 radiculopathy due to disc disorder
C5-C6 disc disorder with radiculopathy
C6 radiculopathy due to disc disorder
C6-C7 disc disorder with radiculopathy
C7 radiculopathy due to disc disorder
M50.13 **Cervical disc disorder with radiculopathy, cervicothoracic region**
C7-T1 disc disorder with radiculopathy
C8 radiculopathy due to disc disorder

[5] **M50.2 Other cervical disc displacement**
M50.20 **Other cervical disc displacement, unspecified cervical region**
M50.21 **Other cervical disc displacement, high cervical region** ▲
Other C2-C3 cervical disc displacement
Other C3-C4 cervical disc displacement
M50.22 **Other cervical disc displacement, mid-cervical region**
Other C4-C5 cervical disc displacement
Other C5-C6 cervical disc displacement
Other C6-C7 cervical disc displacement
M50.23 **Other cervical disc displacement, cervicothoracic region**
Other C7-T1 cervical disc displacement

[5] **M50.3 Other cervical disc degeneration**
M50.30 **Other cervical disc degeneration, unspecified cervical region**
M50.31 **Other cervical disc degeneration, high cervical region** ▲
Other C2-C3 cervical disc degeneration
Other C3-C4 cervical disc degeneration
M50.32 **Other cervical disc degeneration, mid-cervical region**
Other C4-C5 cervical disc degeneration
Other C5-C6 cervical disc degeneration
Other C6-C7 cervical disc degeneration
M50.33 **Other cervical disc degeneration, cervicothoracic region**
Other C7-T1 cervical disc degeneration

[5] **M50.8 Other cervical disc disorders**
M50.80 **Other cervical disc disorders, unspecified cervical region**
M50.81 **Other cervical disc disorders, high cervical region** ▲
Other C2-C3 cervical disc disorders
Other C3-C4 cervical disc disorders
M50.82 **Other cervical disc disorders, mid-cervical region**
Other C4-C5 cervical disc disorders
Other C5-C6 cervical disc disorders
Other C6-C7 cervical disc disorders
M50.83 **Other cervical disc disorders, cervicothoracic region**
Other C7-T1 cervical disc disorders

[5] **M50.9 Cervical disc disorder, unspecified**
M50.90 **Cervical disc disorder, unspecified, unspecified cervical region**
M50.91 **Cervical disc disorder, unspecified, high cervical region** ▲
C2-C3 cervical disc disorder, unspecified
C3-C4 cervical disc disorder, unspecified
M50.92 **Cervical disc disorder, unspecified, mid-cervical region**
C4-C5 cervical disc disorder, unspecified
C5-C6 cervical disc disorder, unspecified
C6-C7 cervical disc disorder, unspecified
M50.93 **Cervical disc disorder, unspecified, cervicothoracic region**
C7-T1 cervical disc disorder, unspecified

[4] **M51 Thoracic, thoracolumbar, and lumbosacral intervertebral disc disorders**
[EXCLUDES2] *cervical and cervicothoracic disc disorders (M50.-)*
sacral and sacrococcygeal disorders (M53.3)

[5] **M51.0 Thoracic, thoracolumbar and lumbosacral intervertebral disc disorders with myelopathy**
M51.04 **Intervertebral disc disorders with myelopathy, thoracic region**
M51.05 **Intervertebral disc disorders with myelopathy, thoracolumbar region**
M51.06 **Intervertebral disc disorders with myelopathy, lumbar region**

[5] **M51.1 Thoracic, thoracolumbar and lumbosacral intervertebral disc disorders with radiculopathy**
Sciatica due to intervertebral disc disorder
[EXCLUDES1] *lumbar radiculitis NOS (M54.16)*
sciatica NOS (M54.3)
M51.14 **Intervertebral disc disorders with radiculopathy, thoracic region**
M51.15 **Intervertebral disc disorders with radiculopathy, thoracolumbar region**
M51.16 **Intervertebral disc disorders with radiculopathy, lumbar region**

[4] 4th character required [5] 5th character required [6] 6th character required [7] 7th character required [7x] Extension 'X' Alert
[EXCLUDES1] Not coded here [EXCLUDES2] Not included here [PDx] Primary Diagnosis Only Manifestation Code

M51.17 Intervertebral disc disorders with radiculopathy, lumbosacral region

[5] M51.2 Other thoracic, thoracolumbar and lumbosacral intervertebral disc displacement

Lumbago due to displacement of intervertebral disc

M51.24 Other intervertebral disc displacement, thoracic region

M51.25 Other intervertebral disc displacement, thoracolumbar region

M51.26 Other intervertebral disc displacement, lumbar region

M51.27 Other intervertebral disc displacement, lumbosacral region

[5] M51.3 Other thoracic, thoracolumbar and lumbosacral intervertebral disc degeneration

M51.34 Other intervertebral disc degeneration, thoracic region

M51.35 Other intervertebral disc degeneration, thoracolumbar region

M51.36 Other intervertebral disc degeneration, lumbar region

M51.37 Other intervertebral disc degeneration, lumbosacral region

[5] M51.4 Schmorl's nodes

M51.44 Schmorl's nodes, thoracic region

M51.45 Schmorl's nodes, thoracolumbar region

M51.46 Schmorl's nodes, lumbar region

M51.47 Schmorl's nodes, lumbosacral region

[5] M51.8 Other thoracic, thoracolumbar and lumbosacral intervertebral disc disorders

M51.84 Other intervertebral disc disorders, thoracic region

M51.85 Other intervertebral disc disorders, thoracolumbar region

M51.86 Other intervertebral disc disorders, lumbar region

M51.87 Other intervertebral disc disorders, lumbosacral region

M51.9 Unspecified thoracic, thoracolumbar and lumbosacral intervertebral disc disorder

[4] M53 Other and unspecified dorsopathies, not elsewhere classified

M53.0 Cervicocranial syndrome

Posterior cervical sympathetic syndrome

M53.1 Cervicobrachial syndrome

[EXCLUDES2] *cervical disc disorder (M50.-)*
thoracic outlet syndrome (G54.0)

[5] M53.2 Spinal instabilities

[6] M53.2X Spinal instabilities

M53.2X1 Spinal instabilities, occipito-atlanto-axial region

M53.2X2 Spinal instabilities, cervical region

M53.2X3 Spinal instabilities, cervicothoracic region

M53.2X4 Spinal instabilities, thoracic region

M53.2X5 Spinal instabilities, thoracolumbar region

M53.2X6 Spinal instabilities, lumbar region

M53.2X7 Spinal instabilities, lumbosacral region

M53.2X8 Spinal instabilities, sacral and sacrococcygeal region

M53.2X9 Spinal instabilities, site unspecified

M53.3 Sacrococcygeal disorders, not elsewhere classified

Coccygodynia

[5] M53.8 Other specified dorsopathies

M53.80 Other specified dorsopathies, site unspecified

M53.81 Other specified dorsopathies, occipito-atlanto-axial region

M53.82 Other specified dorsopathies, cervical region

M53.83 Other specified dorsopathies, cervicothoracic region

M53.84 Other specified dorsopathies, thoracic region

M53.85 Other specified dorsopathies, thoracolumbar region

M53.86 Other specified dorsopathies, lumbar region

M53.87 Other specified dorsopathies, lumbosacral region

M53.88 Other specified dorsopathies, sacral and sacrococcygeal region

M53.9 Dorsopathy, unspecified

[4] M54 Dorsalgia

[EXCLUDES1] *psychogenic dorsalgia (F45.41)*

[5] M54.0 Panniculitis affecting regions of neck and back

[EXCLUDES1] *lupus panniculitis (L93.2)*
panniculitis NOS (M79.3)
relapsing [Weber-Christian] panniculitis (M35.6)

M54.00 Panniculitis affecting regions of neck and back, site unspecified

M54.01 Panniculitis affecting regions of neck and back, occipito-atlanto-axial region

M54.02 Panniculitis affecting regions of neck and back, cervical region

M54.03 Panniculitis affecting regions of neck and back, cervicothoracic region

M54.04 Panniculitis affecting regions of neck and back, thoracic region

M54.05 Panniculitis affecting regions of neck and back, thoracolumbar region

M54.06 Panniculitis affecting regions of neck and back, lumbar region

M54.07 Panniculitis affecting regions of neck and back, lumbosacral region

M54.08 Panniculitis affecting regions of neck and back, sacral and sacrococcygeal region

M54.09 Panniculitis affecting regions, neck and back, multiple sites in spine

[5] M54.1 Radiculopathy

Brachial neuritis or radiculitis NOS
Lumbar neuritis or radiculitis NOS
Lumbosacral neuritis or radiculitis NOS
Thoracic neuritis or radiculitis NOS
Radiculitis NOS

[EXCLUDES1] *neuralgia and neuritis NOS (M79.2)*
radiculopathy with cervical disc disorder (M50.1)
radiculopathy with lumbar and other intervertebral disc disorder (M51.1-)
radiculopathy with spondylosis (M47.2-)

M54.10 Radiculopathy, site unspecified

M54.11 Radiculopathy, occipito-atlanto-axial region

M54.12 Radiculopathy, cervical region

M54.13 Radiculopathy, cervicothoracic region

M54.14 Radiculopathy, thoracic region

M54.15 Radiculopathy, thoracolumbar region

M54.16 Radiculopathy, lumbar region

M54.17 Radiculopathy, lumbosacral region

M54.18 Radiculopathy, sacral and sacrococcygeal region

M54.2 Cervicalgia

[EXCLUDES1] *cervicalgia due to intervertebral cervical disc disorder (M50.-)*

[5] M54.3 Sciatica

[EXCLUDES1] *lesion of sciatic nerve (G57.0)*
sciatica due to intervertebral disc disorder (M51.1-)
sciatica with lumbago (M54.4-)

M54.30 Sciatica, unspecified side

M54.31 Sciatica, right side

M54.32 Sciatica, left side

Unspecified Code Other Specified Code [N] Newborn Age: 0 [P] Pediatric Age: 0-17 [M] Maternity Age: 12-55
[A] Adult Age: 15-124 ♂ Male ♀ Female ● New Code ▲ Revised Code Title ►◄ Revised Text

[5] M54.4 Lumbago with sciatica

[EXCLUDES1] *lumbago with sciatica due to intervertebral disc disorder (M51.1-)*

M54.40 Lumbago with sciatica, unspecified side

M54.41 Lumbago with sciatica, right side

M54.42 Lumbago with sciatica, left side

M54.5 Low back pain

Loin pain

Lumbago NOS

[EXCLUDES1] *low back strain (S39.012)*
lumbago due to intervertebral disc displacement (M51.2-)
lumbago with sciatica (M54.4-)

M54.6 Pain in thoracic spine

[EXCLUDES1] *pain in thoracic spine due to intervertebral disc disorder (M51.-)*

[5] M54.8 Other dorsalgia

[EXCLUDES1] *dorsalgia in thoracic region (M54.6)*
low back pain (M54.5)

M54.81 Occipital neuralgia

M54.89 Other dorsalgia

M54.9 Dorsalgia, unspecified

Backache NOS

Back pain NOS

Soft tissue disorders (M60-M79)

Disorders of muscles (M60-M63)

[EXCLUDES1] *dermatopolymyositis (M33.-)*
muscular dystrophies and myopathies (G71-G72)
myopathy in amyloidosis (E85.-)
myopathy in polyarteritis nodosa (M30.0)
myopathy in rheumatoid arthritis (M05.32)
myopathy in scleroderma (M34.-)
myopathy in Sjögren's syndrome (M35.03)
myopathy in systemic lupus erythematosus (M32.-)

[4] M60 Myositis

[EXCLUDES2] *inclusion body myositis [IBM] (G72.41)*

[5] M60.0 Infective myositis

Tropical pyomyositis

Use additional code (B95-B97) to identify infectious agent

[6] M60.00 Infective myositis, unspecified site

M60.000 Infective myositis, unspecified right arm

Infective myositis, right upper limb NOS

M60.001 Infective myositis, unspecified left arm

Infective myositis, left upper limb NOS

M60.002 Infective myositis, unspecified arm

Infective myositis, upper limb NOS

M60.003 Infective myositis, unspecified right leg

Infective myositis, right lower limb NOS

M60.004 Infective myositis, unspecified left leg

Infective myositis, left lower limb NOS

M60.005 Infective myositis, unspecified leg

Infective myositis, lower limb NOS

M60.009 Infective myositis, unspecified site

[6] M60.01 Infective myositis, shoulder

M60.011 Infective myositis, right shoulder

M60.012 Infective myositis, left shoulder

M60.019 Infective myositis, unspecified shoulder

[6] M60.02 Infective myositis, upper arm

M60.021 Infective myositis, right upper arm

M60.022 Infective myositis, left upper arm

M60.029 Infective myositis, unspecified upper arm

[6] M60.03 Infective myositis, forearm

M60.031 Infective myositis, right forearm

M60.032 Infective myositis, left forearm

M60.039 Infective myositis, unspecified forearm

[6] M60.04 Infective myositis, hand and fingers

M60.041 Infective myositis, right hand

M60.042 Infective myositis, left hand

M60.043 Infective myositis, unspecified hand

M60.044 Infective myositis, right finger(s)

M60.045 Infective myositis, left finger(s)

M60.046 Infective myositis, unspecified finger(s)

[6] M60.05 Infective myositis, thigh

M60.051 Infective myositis, right thigh

M60.052 Infective myositis, left thigh

M60.059 Infective myositis, unspecified thigh

[6] M60.06 Infective myositis, lower leg

M60.061 Infective myositis, right lower leg

M60.062 Infective myositis, left lower leg

M60.069 Infective myositis, unspecified lower leg

[6] M60.07 Infective myositis, ankle, foot and toes

M60.070 Infective myositis, right ankle

M60.071 Infective myositis, left ankle

M60.072 Infective myositis, unspecified ankle

M60.073 Infective myositis, right foot

M60.074 Infective myositis, left foot

M60.075 Infective myositis, unspecified foot

M60.076 Infective myositis, right toe(s)

M60.077 Infective myositis, left toe(s)

M60.078 Infective myositis, unspecified toe(s)

M60.08 Infective myositis, other site

M60.09 Infective myositis, multiple sites

[5] M60.1 Interstitial myositis

M60.10 Interstitial myositis of unspecified site

[6] M60.11 Interstitial myositis, shoulder

M60.111 Interstitial myositis, right shoulder

M60.112 Interstitial myositis, left shoulder

M60.119 Interstitial myositis, unspecified shoulder

[6] M60.12 Interstitial myositis, upper arm

M60.121 Interstitial myositis, right upper arm

M60.122 Interstitial myositis, left upper arm

M60.129 Interstitial myositis, unspecified upper arm

[6] M60.13 Interstitial myositis, forearm

M60.131 Interstitial myositis, right forearm

M60.132 Interstitial myositis, left forearm

M60.139 Interstitial myositis, unspecified forearm

[6] M60.14 Interstitial myositis, hand

M60.141 Interstitial myositis, right hand

M60.142 Interstitial myositis, left hand

M60.149 Interstitial myositis, unspecified hand

[6] M60.15 Interstitial myositis, thigh

M60.151 Interstitial myositis, right thigh

M60.152 Interstitial myositis, left thigh

M60.159 Interstitial myositis, unspecified thigh

[6] M60.16 Interstitial myositis, lower leg

M60.161 Interstitial myositis, right lower leg

M60.162 Interstitial myositis, left lower leg

M60.169 Interstitial myositis, unspecified lower leg

[6] M60.17 Interstitial myositis, ankle and foot

M60.171 Interstitial myositis, right ankle and foot

M60.172 Interstitial myositis, left ankle and foot

M60.179 Interstitial myositis, unspecified ankle and foot

M60.18 Interstitial myositis, other site

M60.19 Interstitial myositis, multiple sites

[5] M60.2 Foreign body granuloma of soft tissue, not elsewhere classified
Use additional code to identify the type of retained foreign body (Z18.-)
[EXCLUDES1] *foreign body granuloma of skin and subcutaneous tissue (L92.3)*
M60.20 Foreign body granuloma of soft tissue, not elsewhere classified, unspecified site
[6] M60.21 Foreign body granuloma of soft tissue, not elsewhere classified, shoulder
M60.211 Foreign body granuloma of soft tissue, not elsewhere classified, right shoulder
M60.212 Foreign body granuloma of soft tissue, not elsewhere classified, left shoulder
M60.219 Foreign body granuloma of soft tissue, not elsewhere classified, unspecified shoulder
[6] M60.22 Foreign body granuloma of soft tissue, not elsewhere classified, upper arm
M60.221 Foreign body granuloma of soft tissue, not elsewhere classified, right upper arm
M60.222 Foreign body granuloma of soft tissue, not elsewhere classified, left upper arm
M60.229 Foreign body granuloma of soft tissue, not elsewhere classified, unspecified upper arm
[6] M60.23 Foreign body granuloma of soft tissue, not elsewhere classified, forearm
M60.231 Foreign body granuloma of soft tissue, not elsewhere classified, right forearm
M60.232 Foreign body granuloma of soft tissue, not elsewhere classified, left forearm
M60.239 Foreign body granuloma of soft tissue, not elsewhere classified, unspecified forearm
[6] M60.24 Foreign body granuloma of soft tissue, not elsewhere classified, hand
M60.241 Foreign body granuloma of soft tissue, not elsewhere classified, right hand
M60.242 Foreign body granuloma of soft tissue, not elsewhere classified, left hand
M60.249 Foreign body granuloma of soft tissue, not elsewhere classified, unspecified hand
[6] M60.25 Foreign body granuloma of soft tissue, not elsewhere classified, thigh
M60.251 Foreign body granuloma of soft tissue, not elsewhere classified, right thigh
M60.252 Foreign body granuloma of soft tissue, not elsewhere classified, left thigh
M60.259 Foreign body granuloma of soft tissue, not elsewhere classified, unspecified thigh
[6] M60.26 Foreign body granuloma of soft tissue, not elsewhere classified, lower leg
M60.261 Foreign body granuloma of soft tissue, not elsewhere classified, right lower leg
M60.262 Foreign body granuloma of soft tissue, not elsewhere classified, left lower leg
M60.269 Foreign body granuloma of soft tissue, not elsewhere classified, unspecified lower leg
[6] M60.27 Foreign body granuloma of soft tissue, not elsewhere classified, ankle and foot
M60.271 Foreign body granuloma of soft tissue, not elsewhere classified, right ankle and foot
M60.272 Foreign body granuloma of soft tissue, not elsewhere classified, left ankle and foot
M60.279 Foreign body granuloma of soft tissue, not elsewhere classified, unspecified ankle and foot
M60.28 Foreign body granuloma of soft tissue, not elsewhere classified, other site
[5] M60.8 Other myositis
M60.80 Other myositis, unspecified site
[6] M60.81 Other myositis shoulder
M60.811 Other myositis, right shoulder
M60.812 Other myositis, left shoulder
M60.819 Other myositis, unspecified shoulder
[6] M60.82 Other myositis, upper arm
M60.821 Other myositis, right upper arm
M60.822 Other myositis, left upper arm
M60.829 Other myositis, unspecified upper arm
[6] M60.83 Other myositis, forearm
M60.831 Other myositis, right forearm
M60.832 Other myositis, left forearm
M60.839 Other myositis, unspecified forearm
[6] M60.84 Other myositis, hand
M60.841 Other myositis, right hand
M60.842 Other myositis, left hand
M60.849 Other myositis, unspecified hand
[6] M60.85 Other myositis, thigh
M60.851 Other myositis, right thigh
M60.852 Other myositis, left thigh
M60.859 Other myositis, unspecified thigh
[6] M60.86 Other myositis, lower leg
M60.861 Other myositis, right lower leg
M60.862 Other myositis, left lower leg
M60.869 Other myositis, unspecified lower leg
[6] M60.87 Other myositis, ankle and foot
M60.871 Other myositis, right ankle and foot
M60.872 Other myositis, left ankle and foot
M60.879 Other myositis, unspecified ankle and foot
M60.88 Other myositis, other site
M60.89 Other myositis, multiple sites
M60.9 Myositis, unspecified
[4] M61 Calcification and ossification of muscle
[5] M61.0 Myositis ossificans traumatica
M61.00 Myositis ossificans traumatica, unspecified site
[6] M61.01 Myositis ossificans traumatica, shoulder
M61.011 Myositis ossificans traumatica, right shoulder
M61.012 Myositis ossificans traumatica, left shoulder
M61.019 Myositis ossificans traumatica, unspecified shoulder
[6] M61.02 Myositis ossificans traumatica, upper arm
M61.021 Myositis ossificans traumatica, right upper arm
M61.022 Myositis ossificans traumatica, left upper arm
M61.029 Myositis ossificans traumatica, unspecified upper arm
[6] M61.03 Myositis ossificans traumatica, forearm
M61.031 Myositis ossificans traumatica, right forearm
M61.032 Myositis ossificans traumatica, left forearm
M61.039 Myositis ossificans traumatica, unspecified forearm
[6] M61.04 Myositis ossificans traumatica, hand
M61.041 Myositis ossificans traumatica, right hand
M61.042 Myositis ossificans traumatica, left hand
M61.049 Myositis ossificans traumatica, unspecified hand
[6] M61.05 Myositis ossificans traumatica, thigh
M61.051 Myositis ossificans traumatica, right thigh
M61.052 Myositis ossificans traumatica, left thigh
M61.059 Myositis ossificans traumatica, unspecified thigh

Unspecified Code Other Specified Code [N] Newborn Age: 0 [P] Pediatric Age: 0-17 [M] Maternity Age: 12-55
[A] Adult Age: 15-124 ♂ Male ♀ Female ● New Code ▲ Revised Code Title ►◄ Revised Text

[6] M61.06 Myositis ossificans traumatica, lower leg
M61.061 Myositis ossificans traumatica, right lower leg
M61.062 Myositis ossificans traumatica, left lower leg
M61.069 Myositis ossificans traumatica, unspecified lower leg
[6] M61.07 Myositis ossificans traumatica, ankle and foot
M61.071 Myositis ossificans traumatica, right ankle and foot
M61.072 Myositis ossificans traumatica, left ankle and foot
M61.079 Myositis ossificans traumatica, unspecified ankle and foot
M61.08 Myositis ossificans traumatica, other site
M61.09 Myositis ossificans traumatica, multiple sites
[5] M61.1 Myositis ossificans progressiva
Fibrodysplasia ossificans progressiva
M61.10 Myositis ossificans progressiva, unspecified site
[6] M61.11 Myositis ossificans progressiva, shoulder
M61.111 Myositis ossificans progressiva, right shoulder
M61.112 Myositis ossificans progressiva, left shoulder
M61.119 Myositis ossificans progressiva, unspecified shoulder
[6] M61.12 Myositis ossificans progressiva, upper arm
M61.121 Myositis ossificans progressiva, right upper arm
M61.122 Myositis ossificans progressiva, left upper arm
M61.129 Myositis ossificans progressiva, unspecified arm
[6] M61.13 Myositis ossificans progressiva, forearm
M61.131 Myositis ossificans progressiva, right forearm
M61.132 Myositis ossificans progressiva, left forearm
M61.139 Myositis ossificans progressiva, unspecified forearm
[6] M61.14 Myositis ossificans progressiva, hand and finger(s)
M61.141 Myositis ossificans progressiva, right hand
M61.142 Myositis ossificans progressiva, left hand
M61.143 Myositis ossificans progressiva, unspecified hand
M61.144 Myositis ossificans progressiva, right finger(s)
M61.145 Myositis ossificans progressiva, left finger(s)
M61.146 Myositis ossificans progressiva, unspecified finger(s)
[6] M61.15 Myositis ossificans progressiva, thigh
M61.151 Myositis ossificans progressiva, right thigh
M61.152 Myositis ossificans progressiva, left thigh
M61.159 Myositis ossificans progressiva, unspecified thigh
[6] M61.16 Myositis ossificans progressiva, lower leg
M61.161 Myositis ossificans progressiva, right lower leg
M61.162 Myositis ossificans progressiva, left lower leg
M61.169 Myositis ossificans progressiva, unspecified lower leg
[6] M61.17 Myositis ossificans progressiva, ankle, foot and toe(s)
M61.171 Myositis ossificans progressiva, right ankle
M61.172 Myositis ossificans progressiva, left ankle
M61.173 Myositis ossificans progressiva, unspecified ankle
M61.174 Myositis ossificans progressiva, right foot
M61.175 Myositis ossificans progressiva, left foot
M61.176 Myositis ossificans progressiva, unspecified foot
M61.177 Myositis ossificans progressiva, right toe(s)
M61.178 Myositis ossificans progressiva, left toe(s)
M61.179 Myositis ossificans progressiva, unspecified toe(s)
M61.18 Myositis ossificans progressiva, other site
M61.19 Myositis ossificans progressiva, multiple sites
[5] M61.2 Paralytic calcification and ossification of muscle
Myositis ossificans associated with quadriplegia or paraplegia
M61.20 Paralytic calcification and ossification of muscle, unspecified site
[6] M61.21 Paralytic calcification and ossification of muscle, shoulder
M61.211 Paralytic calcification and ossification of muscle, right shoulder
M61.212 Paralytic calcification and ossification of muscle, left shoulder
M61.219 Paralytic calcification and ossification of muscle, unspecified shoulder
[6] M61.22 Paralytic calcification and ossification of muscle, upper arm
M61.221 Paralytic calcification and ossification of muscle, right upper arm
M61.222 Paralytic calcification and ossification of muscle, left upper arm
M61.229 Paralytic calcification and ossification of muscle, unspecified upper arm
[6] M61.23 Paralytic calcification and ossification of muscle, forearm
M61.231 Paralytic calcification and ossification of muscle, right forearm
M61.232 Paralytic calcification and ossification of muscle, left forearm
M61.239 Paralytic calcification and ossification of muscle, unspecified forearm
[6] M61.24 Paralytic calcification and ossification of muscle, hand
M61.241 Paralytic calcification and ossification of muscle, right hand
M61.242 Paralytic calcification and ossification of muscle, left hand
M61.249 Paralytic calcification and ossification of muscle, unspecified hand
[6] M61.25 Paralytic calcification and ossification of muscle, thigh
M61.251 Paralytic calcification and ossification of muscle, right thigh
M61.252 Paralytic calcification and ossification of muscle, left thigh
M61.259 Paralytic calcification and ossification of muscle, unspecified thigh
[6] M61.26 Paralytic calcification and ossification of muscle, lower leg
M61.261 Paralytic calcification and ossification of muscle, right lower leg
M61.262 Paralytic calcification and ossification of muscle, left lower leg
M61.269 Paralytic calcification and ossification of muscle, unspecified lower leg
[6] M61.27 Paralytic calcification and ossification of muscle, ankle and foot
M61.271 Paralytic calcification and ossification of muscle, right ankle and foot

M61.272 Paralytic calcification and ossification of muscle, left ankle and foot
M61.279 Paralytic calcification and ossification of muscle, unspecified ankle and foot
M61.28 Paralytic calcification and ossification of muscle, other site
M61.29 Paralytic calcification and ossification of muscle, multiple sites
[5] M61.3 Calcification and ossification of muscles associated with burns
Myositis ossificans associated with burns
M61.30 Calcification and ossification of muscles associated with burns, unspecified site
[6] M61.31 Calcification and ossification of muscles associated with burns, shoulder
M61.311 Calcification and ossification of muscles associated with burns, right shoulder
M61.312 Calcification and ossification of muscles associated with burns, left shoulder
M61.319 Calcification and ossification of muscles associated with burns, unspecified shoulder
[6] M61.32 Calcification and ossification of muscles associated with burns, upper arm
M61.321 Calcification and ossification of muscles associated with burns, right upper arm
M61.322 Calcification and ossification of muscles associated with burns, left upper arm
M61.329 Calcification and ossification of muscles associated with burns, unspecified upper arm
[6] M61.33 Calcification and ossification of muscles associated with burns, forearm
M61.331 Calcification and ossification of muscles associated with burns, right forearm
M61.332 Calcification and ossification of muscles associated with burns, left forearm
M61.339 Calcification and ossification of muscles associated with burns, unspecified forearm
[6] M61.34 Calcification and ossification of muscles associated with burns, hand
M61.341 Calcification and ossification of muscles associated with burns, right hand
M61.342 Calcification and ossification of muscles associated with burns, left hand
M61.349 Calcification and ossification of muscles associated with burns, unspecified hand
[6] M61.35 Calcification and ossification of muscles associated with burns, thigh
M61.351 Calcification and ossification of muscles associated with burns, right thigh
M61.352 Calcification and ossification of muscles associated with burns, left thigh
M61.359 Calcification and ossification of muscles associated with burns, unspecified thigh
[6] M61.36 Calcification and ossification of muscles associated with burns, lower leg
M61.361 Calcification and ossification of muscles associated with burns, right lower leg
M61.362 Calcification and ossification of muscles associated with burns, left lower leg
M61.369 Calcification and ossification of muscles associated with burns, unspecified lower leg
[6] M61.37 Calcification and ossification of muscles associated with burns, ankle and foot
M61.371 Calcification and ossification of muscles associated with burns, right ankle and foot
M61.372 Calcification and ossification of muscles associated with burns, left ankle and foot
M61.379 Calcification and ossification of muscles associated with burns, unspecified ankle and foot
M61.38 Calcification and ossification of muscles associated with burns, other site
M61.39 Calcification and ossification of muscles associated with burns, multiple sites
[5] M61.4 Other calcification of muscle
[EXCLUDES1] *calcific tendinitis NOS (M65.2-)*
calcific tendinitis of shoulder (M75.3)
M61.40 Other calcification of muscle, unspecified site
[6] M61.41 Other calcification of muscle, shoulder
M61.411 Other calcification of muscle, right shoulder
M61.412 Other calcification of muscle, left shoulder
M61.419 Other calcification of muscle, unspecified shoulder
[6] M61.42 Other calcification of muscle, upper arm
M61.421 Other calcification of muscle, right upper arm
M61.422 Other calcification of muscle, left upper arm
M61.429 Other calcification of muscle, unspecified upper arm
[6] M61.43 Other calcification of muscle, forearm
M61.431 Other calcification of muscle, right forearm
M61.432 Other calcification of muscle, left forearm
M61.439 Other calcification of muscle, unspecified forearm
[6] M61.44 Other calcification of muscle, hand
M61.441 Other calcification of muscle, right hand
M61.442 Other calcification of muscle, left hand
M61.449 Other calcification of muscle, unspecified hand
[6] M61.45 Other calcification of muscle, thigh
M61.451 Other calcification of muscle, right thigh
M61.452 Other calcification of muscle, left thigh
M61.459 Other calcification of muscle, unspecified thigh
[6] M61.46 Other calcification of muscle, lower leg
M61.461 Other calcification of muscle, right lower leg
M61.462 Other calcification of muscle, left lower leg
M61.469 Other calcification of muscle, unspecified lower leg
[6] M61.47 Other calcification of muscle, ankle and foot
M61.471 Other calcification of muscle, right ankle and foot
M61.472 Other calcification of muscle, left ankle and foot
M61.479 Other calcification of muscle, unspecified ankle and foot
M61.48 Other calcification of muscle, other site
M61.49 Other calcification of muscle, multiple sites
[5] M61.5 Other ossification of muscle
M61.50 Other ossification of muscle, unspecified site
[6] M61.51 Other ossification of muscle, shoulder
M61.511 Other ossification of muscle, right shoulder
M61.512 Other ossification of muscle, left shoulder
M61.519 Other ossification of muscle, unspecified shoulder
[6] M61.52 Other ossification of muscle, upper arm
M61.521 Other ossification of muscle, right upper arm
M61.522 Other ossification of muscle, left upper arm
M61.529 Other ossification of muscle, unspecified upper arm

Unspecified Code | Other Specified Code | [N] Newborn Age: 0 | [P] Pediatric Age: 0-17 | [M] Maternity Age: 12-55
[A] Adult Age: 15-124 | ♂ Male | ♀ Female | ● New Code | ▲ Revised Code Title | ►◄ Revised Text

⑥ M61.53 Other ossification of muscle, forearm
　　　M61.531 Other ossification of muscle, right forearm
　　　M61.532 Other ossification of muscle, left forearm
　　　M61.539 Other ossification of muscle, unspecified forearm
⑥ M61.54 Other ossification of muscle, hand
　　　M61.541 Other ossification of muscle, right hand
　　　M61.542 Other ossification of muscle, left hand
　　　M61.549 Other ossification of muscle, unspecified hand
⑥ M61.55 Other ossification of muscle, thigh
　　　M61.551 Other ossification of muscle, right thigh
　　　M61.552 Other ossification of muscle, left thigh
　　　M61.559 Other ossification of muscle, unspecified thigh
⑥ M61.56 Other ossification of muscle, lower leg
　　　M61.561 Other ossification of muscle, right lower leg
　　　M61.562 Other ossification of muscle, left lower leg
　　　M61.569 Other ossification of muscle, unspecified lower leg
⑥ M61.57 Other ossification of muscle, ankle and foot
　　　M61.571 Other ossification of muscle, right ankle and foot
　　　M61.572 Other ossification of muscle, left ankle and foot
　　　M61.579 Other ossification of muscle, unspecified ankle and foot
　　M61.58 Other ossification of muscle, other site
　　M61.59 Other ossification of muscle, multiple sites
　M61.9 Calcification and ossification of muscle, unspecified
④ M62 Other disorders of muscle
　　　EXCLUDES1 alcoholic myopathy (G72.1)
　　　　　　cramp and spasm (R25.2)
　　　　　　drug-induced myopathy (G72.0)
　　　　　　myalgia (M79.1)
　　　　　　stiff-man syndrome (G25.82)
　　　EXCLUDES2 nontraumatic hematoma of muscle (M79.81)
⑤ M62.0 Separation of muscle (nontraumatic)
　　　Diastasis of muscle
　　　EXCLUDES1 diastasis recti complicating pregnancy, labor and delivery (O71.8)
　　　　　　traumatic separation of muscle- see strain of muscle by body region
　　M62.00 Separation of muscle (nontraumatic), unspecified site
⑥ M62.01 Separation of muscle (nontraumatic), shoulder
　　　M62.011 Separation of muscle (nontraumatic), right shoulder
　　　M62.012 Separation of muscle (nontraumatic), left shoulder
　　　M62.019 Separation of muscle (nontraumatic), unspecified shoulder
⑥ M62.02 Separation of muscle (nontraumatic), upper arm
　　　M62.021 Separation of muscle (nontraumatic), right upper arm
　　　M62.022 Separation of muscle (nontraumatic), left upper arm
　　　M62.029 Separation of muscle (nontraumatic), unspecified upper arm
⑥ M62.03 Separation of muscle (nontraumatic), forearm
　　　M62.031 Separation of muscle (nontraumatic), right forearm
　　　M62.032 Separation of muscle (nontraumatic), left forearm
　　　M62.039 Separation of muscle (nontraumatic), unspecified forearm
⑥ M62.04 Separation of muscle (nontraumatic), hand

　　　M62.041 Separation of muscle (nontraumatic), right hand
　　　M62.042 Separation of muscle (nontraumatic), left hand
　　　M62.049 Separation of muscle (nontraumatic), unspecified hand
⑥ M62.05 Separation of muscle (nontraumatic), thigh
　　　M62.051 Separation of muscle (nontraumatic), right thigh
　　　M62.052 Separation of muscle (nontraumatic), left thigh
　　　M62.059 Separation of muscle (nontraumatic), unspecified thigh
⑥ M62.06 Separation of muscle (nontraumatic), lower leg
　　　M62.061 Separation of muscle (nontraumatic), right lower leg
　　　M62.062 Separation of muscle (nontraumatic), left lower leg
　　　M62.069 Separation of muscle (nontraumatic), unspecified lower leg
⑥ M62.07 Separation of muscle (nontraumatic), ankle and foot
　　　M62.071 Separation of muscle (nontraumatic), right ankle and foot
　　　M62.072 Separation of muscle (nontraumatic), left ankle and foot
　　　M62.079 Separation of muscle (nontraumatic), unspecified ankle and foot
　　M62.08 Separation of muscle (nontraumatic), other site
⑤ M62.1 Other rupture of muscle (nontraumatic)
　　　EXCLUDES1 traumatic rupture of muscle - see strain of muscle by body region
　　　EXCLUDES2 rupture of tendon (M66.-)
　　M62.10 Other rupture of muscle (nontraumatic), unspecified site
⑥ M62.11 Other rupture of muscle (nontraumatic), shoulder
　　　M62.111 Other rupture of muscle (nontraumatic), right shoulder
　　　M62.112 Other rupture of muscle (nontraumatic), left shoulder
　　　M62.119 Other rupture of muscle (nontraumatic), unspecified shoulder
⑥ M62.12 Other rupture of muscle (nontraumatic), upper arm
　　　M62.121 Other rupture of muscle (nontraumatic), right upper arm
　　　M62.122 Other rupture of muscle (nontraumatic), left upper arm
　　　M62.129 Other rupture of muscle (nontraumatic), unspecified upper arm
⑥ M62.13 Other rupture of muscle (nontraumatic), forearm
　　　M62.131 Other rupture of muscle (nontraumatic), right forearm
　　　M62.132 Other rupture of muscle (nontraumatic), left forearm
　　　M62.139 Other rupture of muscle (nontraumatic), unspecified forearm
⑥ M62.14 Other rupture of muscle (nontraumatic), hand
　　　M62.141 Other rupture of muscle (nontraumatic), right hand
　　　M62.142 Other rupture of muscle (nontraumatic), left hand
　　　M62.149 Other rupture of muscle (nontraumatic), unspecified hand
⑥ M62.15 Other rupture of muscle (nontraumatic), thigh
　　　M62.151 Other rupture of muscle (nontraumatic), right thigh

---

④ 4th character required   ⑤ 5th character required   ⑥ 6th character required   ⑦ 7th character required   ⑩ Extension 'X' Alert

EXCLUDES1 Not coded here   EXCLUDES2 Not included here   PDx Primary Diagnosis Only   Manifestation Code

M62.152 Other rupture of muscle (nontraumatic), left thigh
M62.159 Other rupture of muscle (nontraumatic), unspecified thigh
[6] M62.16 Other rupture of muscle (nontraumatic), lower leg
M62.161 Other rupture of muscle (nontraumatic), right lower leg
M62.162 Other rupture of muscle (nontraumatic), left lower leg
M62.169 Other rupture of muscle (nontraumatic), unspecified lower leg
[6] M62.17 Other rupture of muscle (nontraumatic), ankle and foot
M62.171 Other rupture of muscle (nontraumatic), right ankle and foot
M62.172 Other rupture of muscle (nontraumatic), left ankle and foot
M62.179 Other rupture of muscle (nontraumatic), unspecified ankle and foot
M62.18 Other rupture of muscle (nontraumatic), other site
[5] M62.2 Nontraumatic ischemic infarction of muscle
[EXCLUDES1] *compartment syndrome (traumatic) (T79.A-)*
nontraumatic compartment syndrome (M79.A-)
traumatic ischemia of muscle (T79.6)
rhabdomyolysis (M62.82)
Volkmann's ischemic contracture (T79.6)
M62.20 Nontraumatic ischemic infarction of muscle, unspecified site
[6] M62.21 Nontraumatic ischemic infarction of muscle, shoulder
M62.211 Nontraumatic ischemic infarction of muscle, right shoulder
M62.212 Nontraumatic ischemic infarction of muscle, left shoulder
M62.219 Nontraumatic ischemic infarction of muscle, unspecified shoulder
[6] M62.22 Nontraumatic ischemic infarction of muscle, upper arm
M62.221 Nontraumatic ischemic infarction of muscle, right upper arm
M62.222 Nontraumatic ischemic infarction of muscle, left upper arm
M62.229 Nontraumatic ischemic infarction of muscle, unspecified upper arm
[6] M62.23 Nontraumatic ischemic infarction of muscle, forearm
M62.231 Nontraumatic ischemic infarction of muscle, right forearm
M62.232 Nontraumatic ischemic infarction of muscle, left forearm
M62.239 Nontraumatic ischemic infarction of muscle, unspecified forearm
[6] M62.24 Nontraumatic ischemic infarction of muscle, hand
M62.241 Nontraumatic ischemic infarction of muscle, right hand
M62.242 Nontraumatic ischemic infarction of muscle, left hand
M62.249 Nontraumatic ischemic infarction of muscle, unspecified hand
[6] M62.25 Nontraumatic ischemic infarction of muscle, thigh
M62.251 Nontraumatic ischemic infarction of muscle, right thigh
M62.252 Nontraumatic ischemic infarction of muscle, left thigh
M62.259 Nontraumatic ischemic infarction of muscle, unspecified thigh
[6] M62.26 Nontraumatic ischemic infarction of muscle, lower leg
M62.261 Nontraumatic ischemic infarction of muscle, right lower leg
M62.262 Nontraumatic ischemic infarction of muscle, left lower leg
M62.269 Nontraumatic ischemic infarction of muscle, unspecified lower leg
[6] M62.27 Nontraumatic ischemic infarction of muscle, ankle and foot
M62.271 Nontraumatic ischemic infarction of muscle, right ankle and foot
M62.272 Nontraumatic ischemic infarction of muscle, left ankle and foot
M62.279 Nontraumatic ischemic infarction of muscle, unspecified ankle and foot
M62.28 Nontraumatic ischemic infarction of muscle, other site
M62.3 Immobility syndrome (paraplegic)
[5] M62.4 Contracture of muscle
Contracture of tendon (sheath)
[EXCLUDES1] *contracture of joint (M24.5-)*
M62.40 Contracture of muscle, unspecified site
[6] M62.41 Contracture of muscle, shoulder
M62.411 Contracture of muscle, right shoulder
M62.412 Contracture of muscle, left shoulder
M62.419 Contracture of muscle, unspecified shoulder
[6] M62.42 Contracture of muscle, upper arm
M62.421 Contracture of muscle, right upper arm
M62.422 Contracture of muscle, left upper arm
M62.429 Contracture of muscle, unspecified upper arm
[6] M62.43 Contracture of muscle, forearm
M62.431 Contracture of muscle, right forearm
M62.432 Contracture of muscle, left forearm
M62.439 Contracture of muscle, unspecified forearm
[6] M62.44 Contracture of muscle, hand
M62.441 Contracture of muscle, right hand
M62.442 Contracture of muscle, left hand
M62.449 Contracture of muscle, unspecified hand
[6] M62.45 Contracture of muscle, thigh
M62.451 Contracture of muscle, right thigh
M62.452 Contracture of muscle, left thigh
M62.459 Contracture of muscle, unspecified thigh
[6] M62.46 Contracture of muscle, lower leg
M62.461 Contracture of muscle, right lower leg
M62.462 Contracture of muscle, left lower leg
M62.469 Contracture of muscle, unspecified lower leg
[6] M62.47 Contracture of muscle, ankle and foot
M62.471 Contracture of muscle, right ankle and foot
M62.472 Contracture of muscle, left ankle and foot
M62.479 Contracture of muscle, unspecified ankle and foot
M62.48 Contracture of muscle, other site
M62.49 Contracture of muscle, multiple sites
[5] M62.5 Muscle wasting and atrophy, not elsewhere classified
Disuse atrophy NEC
[EXCLUDES1] *neuralgic amyotrophy (G54.5)*
progressive muscular atrophy (G12.29)
[EXCLUDES2] *pelvic muscle wasting (N81.84)*
M62.50 Muscle wasting and atrophy, not elsewhere classified, unspecified site

Unspecified Code | Other Specified Code | [N] Newborn Age: 0 | [P] Pediatric Age: 0-17 | [M] Maternity Age: 12-55
[A] Adult Age: 15-124 | ♂ Male | ♀ Female | ● New Code | ▲ Revised Code Title | ►◄ Revised Text

M62.51 Muscle wasting and atrophy, not elsewhere classified, shoulder
- M62.511 Muscle wasting and atrophy, not elsewhere classified, right shoulder
- M62.512 Muscle wasting and atrophy, not elsewhere classified, left shoulder
- M62.519 Muscle wasting and atrophy, not elsewhere classified, unspecified shoulder

M62.52 Muscle wasting and atrophy, not elsewhere classified, upper arm
- M62.521 Muscle wasting and atrophy, not elsewhere classified, right upper arm
- M62.522 Muscle wasting and atrophy, not elsewhere classified, left upper arm
- M62.529 Muscle wasting and atrophy, not elsewhere classified, unspecified upper arm

M62.53 Muscle wasting and atrophy, not elsewhere classified, forearm
- M62.531 Muscle wasting and atrophy, not elsewhere classified, right forearm
- M62.532 Muscle wasting and atrophy, not elsewhere classified, left forearm
- M62.539 Muscle wasting and atrophy, not elsewhere classified, unspecified forearm

M62.54 Muscle wasting and atrophy, not elsewhere classified, hand
- M62.541 Muscle wasting and atrophy, not elsewhere classified, right hand
- M62.542 Muscle wasting and atrophy, not elsewhere classified, left hand
- M62.549 Muscle wasting and atrophy, not elsewhere classified, unspecified hand

M62.55 Muscle wasting and atrophy, not elsewhere classified, thigh
- M62.551 Muscle wasting and atrophy, not elsewhere classified, right thigh
- M62.552 Muscle wasting and atrophy, not elsewhere classified, left thigh
- M62.559 Muscle wasting and atrophy, not elsewhere classified, unspecified thigh

M62.56 Muscle wasting and atrophy, not elsewhere classified, lower leg
- M62.561 Muscle wasting and atrophy, not elsewhere classified, right lower leg
- M62.562 Muscle wasting and atrophy, not elsewhere classified, left lower leg
- M62.569 Muscle wasting and atrophy, not elsewhere classified, unspecified lower leg

M62.57 Muscle wasting and atrophy, not elsewhere classified, ankle and foot
- M62.571 Muscle wasting and atrophy, not elsewhere classified, right ankle and foot
- M62.572 Muscle wasting and atrophy, not elsewhere classified, left ankle and foot
- M62.579 Muscle wasting and atrophy, not elsewhere classified, unspecified ankle and foot

M62.58 Muscle wasting and atrophy, not elsewhere classified, other site

M62.59 Muscle wasting and atrophy, not elsewhere classified, multiple sites

M62.8 Other specified disorders of muscle
- EXCLUDES2 nontraumatic hematoma of muscle (M79.81)
- M62.81 Muscle weakness (generalized)
- M62.82 Rhabdomyolysis
  - EXCLUDES1 traumatic rhabdomyolysis (T79.6)
- M62.83 Muscle spasm
  - M62.830 Muscle spasm of back
  - M62.831 Muscle spasm of calf
    - Charley-horse

- M62.838 Other muscle spasm
- M62.89 Other specified disorders of muscle
  - Muscle (sheath) hernia
- M62.9 Disorder of muscle, unspecified

M63 Disorders of muscle in diseases classified elsewhere
Code first underlying disease, such as:
leprosy (A30.-)
neoplasm (C49.-, C79.89, D21.-, D48.1)
schistosomiasis (B65.-)
trichinellosis (B75)
- EXCLUDES1 myopathy in cysticercosis (B69.81)
  - myopathy in endocrine diseases (G73.7)
  - myopathy in metabolic diseases (G73.7)
  - myopathy in sarcoidosis (D86.87)
  - myopathy in secondary syphilis (A51.49)
  - myopathy in syphilis (late) (A52.78)
  - myopathy in toxoplasmosis (B58.82)
  - myopathy in tuberculosis (A18.09)

M63.8 Disorders of muscle in diseases classified elsewhere
- M63.80 Disorders of muscle in diseases classified elsewhere, unspecified site
- M63.81 Disorders of muscle in diseases classified elsewhere, shoulder
  - M63.811 Disorders of muscle in diseases classified elsewhere, right shoulder
  - M63.812 Disorders of muscle in diseases classified elsewhere, left shoulder
  - M63.819 Disorders of muscle in diseases classified elsewhere, unspecified shoulder
- M63.82 Disorders of muscle in diseases classified elsewhere, upper arm
  - M63.821 Disorders of muscle in diseases classified elsewhere, right upper arm
  - M63.822 Disorders of muscle in diseases classified elsewhere, left upper arm
  - M63.829 Disorders of muscle in diseases classified elsewhere, unspecified upper arm
- M63.83 Disorders of muscle in diseases classified elsewhere, forearm
  - M63.831 Disorders of muscle in diseases classified elsewhere, right forearm
  - M63.832 Disorders of muscle in diseases classified elsewhere, left forearm
  - M63.839 Disorders of muscle in diseases classified elsewhere, unspecified forearm
- M63.84 Disorders of muscle in diseases classified elsewhere, hand
  - M63.841 Disorders of muscle in diseases classified elsewhere, right hand
  - M63.842 Disorders of muscle in diseases classified elsewhere, left hand
  - M63.849 Disorders of muscle in diseases classified elsewhere, unspecified hand
- M63.85 Disorders of muscle in diseases classified elsewhere, thigh
  - M63.851 Disorders of muscle in diseases classified elsewhere, right thigh
  - M63.852 Disorders of muscle in diseases classified elsewhere, left thigh
  - M63.859 Disorders of muscle in diseases classified elsewhere, unspecified thigh
- M63.86 Disorders of muscle in diseases classified elsewhere, lower leg
  - M63.861 Disorders of muscle in diseases classified elsewhere, right lower leg
  - M63.862 Disorders of muscle in diseases classified elsewhere, left lower leg
  - M63.869 Disorders of muscle in diseases classified elsewhere, unspecified lower leg

4th character required   5th character required   6th character required   7th character required   Extension 'X' Alert
EXCLUDES1 Not coded here   EXCLUDES2 Not included here   PDx Primary Diagnosis Only   Manifestation Code

[6] M63.87 Disorders of muscle in diseases classified elsewhere, ankle and foot
- M63.871 Disorders of muscle in diseases classified elsewhere, right ankle and foot
- M63.872 Disorders of muscle in diseases classified elsewhere, left ankle and foot
- M63.879 Disorders of muscle in diseases classified elsewhere, unspecified ankle and foot

M63.88 Disorders of muscle in diseases classified elsewhere, other site

M63.89 Disorders of muscle in diseases classified elsewhere, multiple sites

Disorders of synovium and tendon (M65-M67)

[4] M65 Synovitis and tenosynovitis

[EXCLUDES1] *chronic crepitant synovitis of hand and wrist (M70.0-)*
current injury - see injury of ligament or tendon by body region
soft tissue disorders related to use, overuse and pressure (M70.-)

[5] M65.0 Abscess of tendon sheath

Use additional code (B95-B96) to identify bacterial agent.

M65.00 Abscess of tendon sheath, unspecified site

[6] M65.01 Abscess of tendon sheath, shoulder
- M65.011 Abscess of tendon sheath, right shoulder
- M65.012 Abscess of tendon sheath, left shoulder
- M65.019 Abscess of tendon sheath, unspecified shoulder

[6] M65.02 Abscess of tendon sheath, upper arm
- M65.021 Abscess of tendon sheath, right upper arm
- M65.022 Abscess of tendon sheath, left upper arm
- M65.029 Abscess of tendon sheath, unspecified upper arm

[6] M65.03 Abscess of tendon sheath, forearm
- M65.031 Abscess of tendon sheath, right forearm
- M65.032 Abscess of tendon sheath, left forearm
- M65.039 Abscess of tendon sheath, unspecified forearm

[6] M65.04 Abscess of tendon sheath, hand
- M65.041 Abscess of tendon sheath, right hand
- M65.042 Abscess of tendon sheath, left hand
- M65.049 Abscess of tendon sheath, unspecified hand

[6] M65.05 Abscess of tendon sheath, thigh
- M65.051 Abscess of tendon sheath, right thigh
- M65.052 Abscess of tendon sheath, left thigh
- M65.059 Abscess of tendon sheath, unspecified thigh

[6] M65.06 Abscess of tendon sheath, lower leg
- M65.061 Abscess of tendon sheath, right lower leg
- M65.062 Abscess of tendon sheath, left lower leg
- M65.069 Abscess of tendon sheath, unspecified lower leg

[6] M65.07 Abscess of tendon sheath, ankle and foot
- M65.071 Abscess of tendon sheath, right ankle and foot
- M65.072 Abscess of tendon sheath, left ankle and foot
- M65.079 Abscess of tendon sheath, unspecified ankle and foot

M65.08 Abscess of tendon sheath, other site

[5] M65.1 Other infective (teno)synovitis

M65.10 Other infective (teno)synovitis, unspecified site

[6] M65.11 Other infective (teno)synovitis, shoulder
- M65.111 Other infective (teno)synovitis, right shoulder
- M65.112 Other infective (teno)synovitis, left shoulder
- M65.119 Other infective (teno)synovitis, unspecified shoulder

[6] M65.12 Other infective (teno)synovitis, elbow
- M65.121 Other infective (teno)synovitis, right elbow
- M65.122 Other infective (teno)synovitis, left elbow
- M65.129 Other infective (teno)synovitis, unspecified elbow

[6] M65.13 Other infective (teno)synovitis, wrist
- M65.131 Other infective (teno)synovitis, right wrist
- M65.132 Other infective (teno)synovitis, left wrist
- M65.139 Other infective (teno)synovitis, unspecified wrist

[6] M65.14 Other infective (teno)synovitis, hand
- M65.141 Other infective (teno)synovitis, right hand
- M65.142 Other infective (teno)synovitis, left hand
- M65.149 Other infective (teno)synovitis, unspecified hand

[6] M65.15 Other infective (teno)synovitis, hip
- M65.151 Other infective (teno)synovitis, right hip
- M65.152 Other infective (teno)synovitis, left hip
- M65.159 Other infective (teno)synovitis, unspecified hip

[6] M65.16 Other infective (teno)synovitis, knee
- M65.161 Other infective (teno)synovitis, right knee
- M65.162 Other infective (teno)synovitis, left knee
- M65.169 Other infective (teno)synovitis, unspecified knee

[6] M65.17 Other infective (teno)synovitis, ankle and foot
- M65.171 Other infective (teno)synovitis, right ankle and foot
- M65.172 Other infective (teno)synovitis, left ankle and foot
- M65.179 Other infective (teno)synovitis, unspecified ankle and foot

M65.18 Other infective (teno)synovitis, other site

M65.19 Other infective (teno)synovitis, multiple sites

[5] M65.2 Calcific tendinitis

[EXCLUDES1] *tendinitis as classified in M75-M77*
calcified tendinitis of shoulder (M75.3)

M65.20 Calcific tendinitis, unspecified site

[6] M65.22 Calcific tendinitis, upper arm
- M65.221 Calcific tendinitis, right upper arm
- M65.222 Calcific tendinitis, left upper arm
- M65.229 Calcific tendinitis, unspecified upper arm

[6] M65.23 Calcific tendinitis, forearm
- M65.231 Calcific tendinitis, right forearm
- M65.232 Calcific tendinitis, left forearm
- M65.239 Calcific tendinitis, unspecified forearm

[6] M65.24 Calcific tendinitis, hand
- M65.241 Calcific tendinitis, right hand
- M65.242 Calcific tendinitis, left hand
- M65.249 Calcific tendinitis, unspecified hand

[6] M65.25 Calcific tendinitis, thigh
- M65.251 Calcific tendinitis, right thigh
- M65.252 Calcific tendinitis, left thigh
- M65.259 Calcific tendinitis, unspecified thigh

[6] M65.26 Calcific tendinitis, lower leg
- M65.261 Calcific tendinitis, right lower leg
- M65.262 Calcific tendinitis, left lower leg
- M65.269 Calcific tendinitis, unspecified lower leg

[6] M65.27 Calcific tendinitis, ankle and foot
- M65.271 Calcific tendinitis, right ankle and foot
- M65.272 Calcific tendinitis, left ankle and foot

M65.279 Calcific tendinitis, unspecified ankle and foot
M65.28 Calcific tendinitis, other site
M65.29 Calcific tendinitis, multiple sites
[5] M65.3 Trigger finger
Nodular tendinous disease
M65.30 Trigger finger, unspecified finger
[6] M65.31 Trigger thumb
M65.311 Trigger thumb, right thumb
M65.312 Trigger thumb, left thumb
M65.319 Trigger thumb, unspecified thumb
[6] M65.32 Trigger finger, index finger
M65.321 Trigger finger, right index finger
M65.322 Trigger finger, left index finger
M65.329 Trigger finger, unspecified index finger
[6] M65.33 Trigger finger, middle finger
M65.331 Trigger finger, right middle finger
M65.332 Trigger finger, left middle finger
M65.339 Trigger finger, unspecified middle finger
[6] M65.34 Trigger finger, ring finger
M65.341 Trigger finger, right ring finger
M65.342 Trigger finger, left ring finger
M65.349 Trigger finger, unspecified ring finger
[6] M65.35 Trigger finger, little finger
M65.351 Trigger finger, right little finger
M65.352 Trigger finger, left little finger
M65.359 Trigger finger, unspecified little finger
M65.4 Radial styloid tenosynovitis [de Quervain]
[5] M65.8 Other synovitis and tenosynovitis
M65.80 Other synovitis and tenosynovitis, unspecified site
[6] M65.81 Other synovitis and tenosynovitis, shoulder
M65.811 Other synovitis and tenosynovitis, right shoulder
M65.812 Other synovitis and tenosynovitis, left shoulder
M65.819 Other synovitis and tenosynovitis, unspecified shoulder
[6] M65.82 Other synovitis and tenosynovitis, upper arm
M65.821 Other synovitis and tenosynovitis, right upper arm
M65.822 Other synovitis and tenosynovitis, left upper arm
M65.829 Other synovitis and tenosynovitis, unspecified upper arm
[6] M65.83 Other synovitis and tenosynovitis, forearm
M65.831 Other synovitis and tenosynovitis, right forearm
M65.832 Other synovitis and tenosynovitis, left forearm
M65.839 Other synovitis and tenosynovitis, unspecified forearm
[6] M65.84 Other synovitis and tenosynovitis, hand
M65.841 Other synovitis and tenosynovitis, right hand
M65.842 Other synovitis and tenosynovitis, left hand
M65.849 Other synovitis and tenosynovitis, unspecified hand
[6] M65.85 Other synovitis and tenosynovitis, thigh
M65.851 Other synovitis and tenosynovitis, right thigh
M65.852 Other synovitis and tenosynovitis, left thigh
M65.859 Other synovitis and tenosynovitis, unspecified thigh
[6] M65.86 Other synovitis and tenosynovitis, lower leg
M65.861 Other synovitis and tenosynovitis, right lower leg
M65.862 Other synovitis and tenosynovitis, left lower leg
M65.869 Other synovitis and tenosynovitis, unspecified lower leg
[6] M65.87 Other synovitis and tenosynovitis, ankle and foot
M65.871 Other synovitis and tenosynovitis, right ankle and foot
M65.872 Other synovitis and tenosynovitis, left ankle and foot
M65.879 Other synovitis and tenosynovitis, unspecified ankle and foot
M65.88 Other synovitis and tenosynovitis, other site
M65.89 Other synovitis and tenosynovitis, multiple sites
M65.9 Synovitis and tenosynovitis, unspecified
[4] M66 Spontaneous rupture of synovium and tendon
[INCLUDES] *rupture that occurs when a normal force is applied to tissues that are inferred to have less than normal strength*
[EXCLUDES2] *rotator cuff syndrome (M75.1-)*
rupture where an abnormal force is applied to normal tissue - see injury of tendon by body region
M66.0 Rupture of popliteal cyst
[5] M66.1 Rupture of synovium
Rupture of synovial cyst
[EXCLUDES2] *rupture of popliteal cyst (M66.0)*
M66.10 Rupture of synovium, unspecified joint
[6] M66.11 Rupture of synovium, shoulder
M66.111 Rupture of synovium, right shoulder
M66.112 Rupture of synovium, left shoulder
M66.119 Rupture of synovium, unspecified shoulder
[6] M66.12 Rupture of synovium, elbow
M66.121 Rupture of synovium, right elbow
M66.122 Rupture of synovium, left elbow
M66.129 Rupture of synovium, unspecified elbow
[6] M66.13 Rupture of synovium, wrist
M66.131 Rupture of synovium, right wrist
M66.132 Rupture of synovium, left wrist
M66.139 Rupture of synovium, unspecified wrist
[6] M66.14 Rupture of synovium, hand and fingers
M66.141 Rupture of synovium, right hand
M66.142 Rupture of synovium, left hand
M66.143 Rupture of synovium, unspecified hand
M66.144 Rupture of synovium, right finger(s)
M66.145 Rupture of synovium, left finger(s)
M66.146 Rupture of synovium, unspecified finger(s)
[6] M66.15 Rupture of synovium, hip
M66.151 Rupture of synovium, right hip
M66.152 Rupture of synovium, left hip
M66.159 Rupture of synovium, unspecified hip
[6] M66.17 Rupture of synovium, ankle, foot and toes
M66.171 Rupture of synovium, right ankle
M66.172 Rupture of synovium, left ankle
M66.173 Rupture of synovium, unspecified ankle
M66.174 Rupture of synovium, right foot
M66.175 Rupture of synovium, left foot
M66.176 Rupture of synovium, unspecified foot
M66.177 Rupture of synovium, right toe(s)
M66.178 Rupture of synovium, left toe(s)
M66.179 Rupture of synovium, unspecified toe(s)
M66.18 Rupture of synovium, other site
[5] M66.2 Spontaneous rupture of extensor tendons
M66.20 Spontaneous rupture of extensor tendons, unspecified site

M66.21 Spontaneous rupture of extensor tendons, shoulder
- M66.211 Spontaneous rupture of extensor tendons, right shoulder
- M66.212 Spontaneous rupture of extensor tendons, left shoulder
- M66.219 Spontaneous rupture of extensor tendons, unspecified shoulder

M66.22 Spontaneous rupture of extensor tendons, upper arm
- M66.221 Spontaneous rupture of extensor tendons, right upper arm
- M66.222 Spontaneous rupture of extensor tendons, left upper arm
- M66.229 Spontaneous rupture of extensor tendons, unspecified upper arm

M66.23 Spontaneous rupture of extensor tendons, forearm
- M66.231 Spontaneous rupture of extensor tendons, right forearm
- M66.232 Spontaneous rupture of extensor tendons, left forearm
- M66.239 Spontaneous rupture of extensor tendons, unspecified forearm

M66.24 Spontaneous rupture of extensor tendons, hand
- M66.241 Spontaneous rupture of extensor tendons, right hand
- M66.242 Spontaneous rupture of extensor tendons, left hand
- M66.249 Spontaneous rupture of extensor tendons, unspecified hand

M66.25 Spontaneous rupture of extensor tendons, thigh
- M66.251 Spontaneous rupture of extensor tendons, right thigh
- M66.252 Spontaneous rupture of extensor tendons, left thigh
- M66.259 Spontaneous rupture of extensor tendons, unspecified thigh

M66.26 Spontaneous rupture of extensor tendons, lower leg
- M66.261 Spontaneous rupture of extensor tendons, right lower leg
- M66.262 Spontaneous rupture of extensor tendons, left lower leg
- M66.269 Spontaneous rupture of extensor tendons, unspecified lower leg

M66.27 Spontaneous rupture of extensor tendons, ankle and foot
- M66.271 Spontaneous rupture of extensor tendons, right ankle and foot
- M66.272 Spontaneous rupture of extensor tendons, left ankle and foot
- M66.279 Spontaneous rupture of extensor tendons, unspecified ankle and foot

M66.28 Spontaneous rupture of extensor tendons, other site

M66.29 Spontaneous rupture of extensor tendons, multiple sites

M66.3 Spontaneous rupture of flexor tendons
- M66.30 Spontaneous rupture of flexor tendons, unspecified site
- M66.31 Spontaneous rupture of flexor tendons, shoulder
  - M66.311 Spontaneous rupture of flexor tendons, right shoulder
  - M66.312 Spontaneous rupture of flexor tendons, left shoulder
  - M66.319 Spontaneous rupture of flexor tendons, unspecified shoulder

M66.32 Spontaneous rupture of flexor tendons, upper arm
- M66.321 Spontaneous rupture of flexor tendons, right upper arm
- M66.322 Spontaneous rupture of flexor tendons, left upper arm
- M66.329 Spontaneous rupture of flexor tendons, unspecified upper arm

M66.33 Spontaneous rupture of flexor tendons, forearm
- M66.331 Spontaneous rupture of flexor tendons, right forearm
- M66.332 Spontaneous rupture of flexor tendons, left forearm
- M66.339 Spontaneous rupture of flexor tendons, unspecified forearm

M66.34 Spontaneous rupture of flexor tendons, hand
- M66.341 Spontaneous rupture of flexor tendons, right hand
- M66.342 Spontaneous rupture of flexor tendons, left hand
- M66.349 Spontaneous rupture of flexor tendons, unspecified hand

M66.35 Spontaneous rupture of flexor tendons, thigh
- M66.351 Spontaneous rupture of flexor tendons, right thigh
- M66.352 Spontaneous rupture of flexor tendons, left thigh
- M66.359 Spontaneous rupture of flexor tendons, unspecified thigh

M66.36 Spontaneous rupture of flexor tendons, lower leg
- M66.361 Spontaneous rupture of flexor tendons, right lower leg
- M66.362 Spontaneous rupture of flexor tendons, left lower leg
- M66.369 Spontaneous rupture of flexor tendons, unspecified lower leg

M66.37 Spontaneous rupture of flexor tendons, ankle and foot
- M66.371 Spontaneous rupture of flexor tendons, right ankle and foot
- M66.372 Spontaneous rupture of flexor tendons, left ankle and foot
- M66.379 Spontaneous rupture of flexor tendons, unspecified ankle and foot

M66.38 Spontaneous rupture of flexor tendons, other site

M66.39 Spontaneous rupture of flexor tendons, multiple sites

M66.8 Spontaneous rupture of other tendons
- M66.80 Spontaneous rupture of other tendons, unspecified site
- M66.81 Spontaneous rupture of other tendons, shoulder
  - M66.811 Spontaneous rupture of other tendons, right shoulder
  - M66.812 Spontaneous rupture of other tendons, left shoulder
  - M66.819 Spontaneous rupture of other tendons, unspecified shoulder
- M66.82 Spontaneous rupture of other tendons, upper arm
  - M66.821 Spontaneous rupture of other tendons, right upper arm
  - M66.822 Spontaneous rupture of other tendons, left upper arm
  - M66.829 Spontaneous rupture of other tendons, unspecified upper arm

[6] M66.83 Spontaneous rupture of other tendons, forearm
- M66.831 Spontaneous rupture of other tendons, right forearm
- M66.832 Spontaneous rupture of other tendons, left forearm
- M66.839 Spontaneous rupture of other tendons, unspecified forearm

[6] M66.84 Spontaneous rupture of other tendons, hand
- M66.841 Spontaneous rupture of other tendons, right hand
- M66.842 Spontaneous rupture of other tendons, left hand
- M66.849 Spontaneous rupture of other tendons, unspecified hand

[6] M66.85 Spontaneous rupture of other tendons, thigh
- M66.851 Spontaneous rupture of other tendons, right thigh
- M66.852 Spontaneous rupture of other tendons, left thigh
- M66.859 Spontaneous rupture of other tendons, unspecified thigh

[6] M66.86 Spontaneous rupture of other tendons, lower leg
- M66.861 Spontaneous rupture of other tendons, right lower leg
- M66.862 Spontaneous rupture of other tendons, left lower leg
- M66.869 Spontaneous rupture of other tendons, unspecified lower leg

[6] M66.87 Spontaneous rupture of other tendons, ankle and foot
- M66.871 Spontaneous rupture of other tendons, right ankle and foot
- M66.872 Spontaneous rupture of other tendons, left ankle and foot
- M66.879 Spontaneous rupture of other tendons, unspecified ankle and foot

M66.88 Spontaneous rupture of other tendons, other

M66.89 Spontaneous rupture of other tendons, multiple sites

M66.9 Spontaneous rupture of unspecified tendon

Rupture at musculotendinous junction, nontraumatic

[4] **M67 Other disorders of synovium and tendon**

[EXCLUDES1] *palmar fascial fibromatosis [Dupuytren] (M72.0)*
tendinitis NOS (M77.9-)
xanthomatosis localized to tendons (E78.2)

[5] M67.0 Short Achilles tendon (acquired)
- M67.00 Short Achilles tendon (acquired), unspecified ankle
- M67.01 Short Achilles tendon (acquired), right ankle
- M67.02 Short Achilles tendon (acquired), left ankle

[5] M67.2 Synovial hypertrophy, not elsewhere classified

[EXCLUDES1] *villonodular synovitis (pigmented) (M12.2-)*

M67.20 Synovial hypertrophy, not elsewhere classified, unspecified site

[6] M67.21 Synovial hypertrophy, not elsewhere classified, shoulder
- M67.211 Synovial hypertrophy, not elsewhere classified, right shoulder
- M67.212 Synovial hypertrophy, not elsewhere classified, left shoulder
- M67.219 Synovial hypertrophy, not elsewhere classified, unspecified shoulder

[6] M67.22 Synovial hypertrophy, not elsewhere classified, upper arm
- M67.221 Synovial hypertrophy, not elsewhere classified, right upper arm
- M67.222 Synovial hypertrophy, not elsewhere classified, left upper arm
- M67.229 Synovial hypertrophy, not elsewhere classified, unspecified upper arm

[6] M67.23 Synovial hypertrophy, not elsewhere classified, forearm
- M67.231 Synovial hypertrophy, not elsewhere classified, right forearm
- M67.232 Synovial hypertrophy, not elsewhere classified, left forearm
- M67.239 Synovial hypertrophy, not elsewhere classified, unspecified forearm

[6] M67.24 Synovial hypertrophy, not elsewhere classified, hand
- M67.241 Synovial hypertrophy, not elsewhere classified, right hand
- M67.242 Synovial hypertrophy, not elsewhere classified, left hand
- M67.249 Synovial hypertrophy, not elsewhere classified, unspecified hand

[6] M67.25 Synovial hypertrophy, not elsewhere classified, thigh
- M67.251 Synovial hypertrophy, not elsewhere classified, right thigh
- M67.252 Synovial hypertrophy, not elsewhere classified, left thigh
- M67.259 Synovial hypertrophy, not elsewhere classified, unspecified thigh

[6] M67.26 Synovial hypertrophy, not elsewhere classified, lower leg
- M67.261 Synovial hypertrophy, not elsewhere classified, right lower leg
- M67.262 Synovial hypertrophy, not elsewhere classified, left lower leg
- M67.269 Synovial hypertrophy, not elsewhere classified, unspecified lower leg

[6] M67.27 Synovial hypertrophy, not elsewhere classified, ankle and foot
- M67.271 Synovial hypertrophy, not elsewhere classified, right ankle and foot
- M67.272 Synovial hypertrophy, not elsewhere classified, left ankle and foot
- M67.279 Synovial hypertrophy, not elsewhere classified, unspecified ankle and foot

M67.28 Synovial hypertrophy, not elsewhere classified, other site

M67.29 Synovial hypertrophy, not elsewhere classified, multiple sites

[5] M67.3 Transient synovitis

Toxic synovitis

[EXCLUDES1] *palindromic rheumatism (M12.3-)*

M67.30 Transient synovitis, unspecified site

[6] M67.31 Transient synovitis, shoulder
- M67.311 Transient synovitis, right shoulder
- M67.312 Transient synovitis, left shoulder
- M67.319 Transient synovitis, unspecified shoulder

[6] M67.32 Transient synovitis, elbow
- M67.321 Transient synovitis, right elbow
- M67.322 Transient synovitis, left elbow
- M67.329 Transient synovitis, unspecified elbow

[6] M67.33 Transient synovitis, wrist
- M67.331 Transient synovitis, right wrist
- M67.332 Transient synovitis, left wrist
- M67.339 Transient synovitis, unspecified wrist

[6] M67.34 Transient synovitis, hand
- M67.341 Transient synovitis, right hand
- M67.342 Transient synovitis, left hand
- M67.349 Transient synovitis, unspecified hand

[6] M67.35 Transient synovitis, hip
- M67.351 Transient synovitis, right hip

[4] 4th character required [5] 5th character required [6] 6th character required [7] 7th character required [x7] Extension 'X' Alert
[EXCLUDES1] Not coded here [EXCLUDES2] Not included here [PDx] Primary Diagnosis Only Manifestation Code

M67.352 Transient synovitis, left hip
M67.359 Transient synovitis, unspecified hip
[6] M67.36 Transient synovitis, knee
M67.361 Transient synovitis, right knee
M67.362 Transient synovitis, left knee
M67.369 Transient synovitis, unspecified knee
[6] M67.37 Transient synovitis, ankle and foot
M67.371 Transient synovitis, right ankle and foot
M67.372 Transient synovitis, left ankle and foot
M67.379 Transient synovitis, unspecified ankle and foot
M67.38 Transient synovitis, other site
M67.39 Transient synovitis, multiple sites
[5] M67.4 Ganglion
Ganglion of joint or tendon (sheath)
[EXCLUDES1] *ganglion in yaws (A66.6)*
[EXCLUDES2] *cyst of bursa (M71.2-M71.3)*
cyst of synovium (M71.2-M71.3)
M67.40 Ganglion, unspecified site
[6] M67.41 Ganglion, shoulder
M67.411 Ganglion, right shoulder
M67.412 Ganglion, left shoulder
M67.419 Ganglion, unspecified shoulder
[6] M67.42 Ganglion, elbow
M67.421 Ganglion, right elbow
M67.422 Ganglion, left elbow
M67.429 Ganglion, unspecified elbow
[6] M67.43 Ganglion, wrist
M67.431 Ganglion, right wrist
M67.432 Ganglion, left wrist
M67.439 Ganglion, unspecified wrist
[6] M67.44 Ganglion, hand
M67.441 Ganglion, right hand
M67.442 Ganglion, left hand
M67.449 Ganglion, unspecified hand
[6] M67.45 Ganglion, hip
M67.451 Ganglion, right hip
M67.452 Ganglion, left hip
M67.459 Ganglion, unspecified hip
[6] M67.46 Ganglion, knee
M67.461 Ganglion, right knee
M67.462 Ganglion, left knee
M67.469 Ganglion, unspecified knee
[6] M67.47 Ganglion, ankle and foot
M67.471 Ganglion, right ankle and foot
M67.472 Ganglion, left ankle and foot
M67.479 Ganglion, unspecified ankle and foot
M67.48 Ganglion, other site
M67.49 Ganglion, multiple sites
[5] M67.5 Plica syndrome
Plica knee
M67.50 Plica syndrome, unspecified knee
M67.51 Plica syndrome, right knee
M67.52 Plica syndrome, left knee
[5] M67.8 Other specified disorders of synovium and tendon
M67.80 Other specified disorders of synovium and tendon, unspecified site
[6] M67.81 Other specified disorders of synovium and tendon, shoulder
M67.811 Other specified disorders of synovium, right shoulder
M67.812 Other specified disorders of synovium, left shoulder
M67.813 Other specified disorders of tendon, right shoulder
M67.814 Other specified disorders of tendon, left shoulder
M67.819 Other specified disorders of synovium and tendon, unspecified shoulder
[6] M67.82 Other specified disorders of synovium and tendon, elbow
M67.821 Other specified disorders of synovium, right elbow
M67.822 Other specified disorders of synovium, left elbow
M67.823 Other specified disorders of tendon, right elbow
M67.824 Other specified disorders of tendon, left elbow
M67.829 Other specified disorders of synovium and tendon, unspecified elbow
[6] M67.83 Other specified disorders of synovium and tendon, wrist
M67.831 Other specified disorders of synovium, right wrist
M67.832 Other specified disorders of synovium, left wrist
M67.833 Other specified disorders of tendon, right wrist
M67.834 Other specified disorders of tendon, left wrist
M67.839 Other specified disorders of synovium and tendon, unspecified forearm
[6] M67.84 Other specified disorders of synovium and tendon, hand
M67.841 Other specified disorders of synovium, right hand
M67.842 Other specified disorders of synovium, left hand
M67.843 Other specified disorders of tendon, right hand
M67.844 Other specified disorders of tendon, left hand
M67.849 Other specified disorders of synovium and tendon, unspecified hand
[6] M67.85 Other specified disorders of synovium and tendon, hip
M67.851 Other specified disorders of synovium, right hip
M67.852 Other specified disorders of synovium, left hip
M67.853 Other specified disorders of tendon, right hip
M67.854 Other specified disorders of tendon, left hip
M67.859 Other specified disorders of synovium and tendon, unspecified hip
[6] M67.86 Other specified disorders of synovium and tendon, knee
M67.861 Other specified disorders of synovium, right knee
M67.862 Other specified disorders of synovium, left knee
M67.863 Other specified disorders of tendon, right knee
M67.864 Other specified disorders of tendon, left knee
M67.869 Other specified disorders of synovium and tendon, unspecified knee
[6] M67.87 Other specified disorders of synovium and tendon, ankle and foot
M67.871 Other specified disorders of synovium, right ankle and foot
M67.872 Other specified disorders of synovium, left ankle and foot

Unspecified Code | Other Specified Code | [N] Newborn Age: 0 | [P] Pediatric Age: 0-17 | [M] Maternity Age: 12-55
[A] Adult Age: 15-124 | ♂ Male | ♀ Female | ● New Code | ▲ Revised Code Title | ►◄ Revised Text

M67.873 Other specified disorders of tendon, right ankle and foot
M67.874 Other specified disorders of tendon, left ankle and foot
M67.879 Other specified disorders of synovium and tendon, unspecified ankle and foot
M67.88 Other specified disorders of synovium and tendon, other site
M67.89 Other specified disorders of synovium and tendon, multiple sites
[5] M67.9 Unspecified disorder of synovium and tendon
M67.90 Unspecified disorder of synovium and tendon, unspecified site
[6] M67.91 Unspecified disorder of synovium and tendon, shoulder
M67.911 Unspecified disorder of synovium and tendon, right shoulder
M67.912 Unspecified disorder of synovium and tendon, left shoulder
M67.919 Unspecified disorder of synovium and tendon, unspecified shoulder
[6] M67.92 Unspecified disorder of synovium and tendon, upper arm
M67.921 Unspecified disorder of synovium and tendon, right upper arm
M67.922 Unspecified disorder of synovium and tendon, left upper arm
M67.929 Unspecified disorder of synovium and tendon, unspecified upper arm
[6] M67.93 Unspecified disorder of synovium and tendon, forearm
M67.931 Unspecified disorder of synovium and tendon, right forearm
M67.932 Unspecified disorder of synovium and tendon, left forearm
M67.939 Unspecified disorder of synovium and tendon, unspecified forearm
[6] M67.94 Unspecified disorder of synovium and tendon, hand
M67.941 Unspecified disorder of synovium and tendon, right hand
M67.942 Unspecified disorder of synovium and tendon, left hand
M67.949 Unspecified disorder of synovium and tendon, unspecified hand
[6] M67.95 Unspecified disorder of synovium and tendon, thigh
M67.951 Unspecified disorder of synovium and tendon, right thigh
M67.952 Unspecified disorder of synovium and tendon, left thigh
M67.959 Unspecified disorder of synovium and tendon, unspecified thigh
[6] M67.96 Unspecified disorder of synovium and tendon, lower leg
M67.961 Unspecified disorder of synovium and tendon, right lower leg
M67.962 Unspecified disorder of synovium and tendon, left lower leg
M67.969 Unspecified disorder of synovium and tendon, unspecified lower leg
[6] M67.97 Unspecified disorder of synovium and tendon, ankle and foot
M67.971 Unspecified disorder of synovium and tendon, right ankle and foot
M67.972 Unspecified disorder of synovium and tendon, left ankle and foot
M67.979 Unspecified disorder of synovium and tendon, unspecified ankle and foot
M67.98 Unspecified disorder of synovium and tendon, other site
M67.99 Unspecified disorder of synovium and tendon, multiple sites

Other soft tissue disorders (M70-M79)

[4] M70 Soft tissue disorders related to use, overuse and pressure
INCLUDES *soft tissue disorders of occupational origin*
Use additional external cause code to identify activity causing disorder (Y93.-)
EXCLUDES1 *bursitis NOS (M71.9-)*
EXCLUDES2 *bursitis of shoulder (M75.5)*
enthesopathies (M76-M77)
pressure ulcer (pressure area) (L89.-)
[5] M70.0 Crepitant synovitis (acute) (chronic) of hand and wrist
[6] M70.03 Crepitant synovitis (acute) (chronic), wrist
M70.031 Crepitant synovitis (acute) (chronic), right wrist
M70.032 Crepitant synovitis (acute) (chronic), left wrist
M70.039 Crepitant synovitis (acute) (chronic), unspecified wrist
[6] M70.04 Crepitant synovitis (acute) (chronic), hand
M70.041 Crepitant synovitis (acute) (chronic), right hand
M70.042 Crepitant synovitis (acute) (chronic), left hand
M70.049 Crepitant synovitis (acute) (chronic), unspecified hand
[5] M70.1 Bursitis of hand
M70.10 Bursitis, unspecified hand
M70.11 Bursitis, right hand
M70.12 Bursitis, left hand
[5] M70.2 Olecranon bursitis
M70.20 Olecranon bursitis, unspecified elbow
M70.21 Olecranon bursitis, right elbow
M70.22 Olecranon bursitis, left elbow
[5] M70.3 Other bursitis of elbow
M70.30 Other bursitis of elbow, unspecified elbow
M70.31 Other bursitis of elbow, right elbow
M70.32 Other bursitis of elbow, left elbow
[5] M70.4 Prepatellar bursitis
M70.40 Prepatellar bursitis, unspecified knee
M70.41 Prepatellar bursitis, right knee
M70.42 Prepatellar bursitis, left knee
[5] M70.5 Other bursitis of knee
M70.50 Other bursitis of knee, unspecified knee
M70.51 Other bursitis of knee, right knee
M70.52 Other bursitis of knee, left knee
[5] M70.6 Trochanteric bursitis
Trochanteric tendinitis
M70.60 Trochanteric bursitis, unspecified hip
M70.61 Trochanteric bursitis, right hip
M70.62 Trochanteric bursitis, left hip
[5] M70.7 Other bursitis of hip
Ischial bursitis
M70.70 Other bursitis of hip, unspecified hip
M70.71 Other bursitis of hip, right hip
M70.72 Other bursitis of hip, left hip
[5] M70.8 Other soft tissue disorders related to use, overuse and pressure
M70.80 Other soft tissue disorders related to use, overuse and pressure of unspecified site
[6] M70.81 Other soft tissue disorders related to use, overuse and pressure of shoulder

[4] 4th character required [5] 5th character required [6] 6th character required [7] 7th character required [7x] Extension 'X' Alert
EXCLUDES1 Not coded here EXCLUDES2 Not included here [PDx] Primary Diagnosis Only Manifestation Code

M70.811 Other soft tissue disorders related to use, overuse and pressure, right shoulder
M70.812 Other soft tissue disorders related to use, overuse and pressure, left shoulder
M70.819 Other soft tissue disorders related to use, overuse and pressure, unspecified shoulder

[6] M70.82 Other soft tissue disorders related to use, overuse and pressure of upper arm
M70.821 Other soft tissue disorders related to use, overuse and pressure, right upper arm
M70.822 Other soft tissue disorders related to use, overuse and pressure, left upper arm
M70.829 Other soft tissue disorders related to use, overuse and pressure, unspecified upper arms

[6] M70.83 Other soft tissue disorders related to use, overuse and pressure of forearm
M70.831 Other soft tissue disorders related to use, overuse and pressure, right forearm
M70.832 Other soft tissue disorders related to use, overuse and pressure, left forearm
M70.839 Other soft tissue disorders related to use, overuse and pressure, unspecified forearm

[6] M70.84 Other soft tissue disorders related to use, overuse and pressure of hand
M70.841 Other soft tissue disorders related to use, overuse and pressure, right hand
M70.842 Other soft tissue disorders related to use, overuse and pressure, left hand
M70.849 Other soft tissue disorders related to use, overuse and pressure, unspecified hand

[6] M70.85 Other soft tissue disorders related to use, overuse and pressure of thigh
M70.851 Other soft tissue disorders related to use, overuse and pressure, right thigh
M70.852 Other soft tissue disorders related to use, overuse and pressure, left thigh
M70.859 Other soft tissue disorders related to use, overuse and pressure, unspecified thigh

[6] M70.86 Other soft tissue disorders related to use, overuse and pressure lower leg
M70.861 Other soft tissue disorders related to use, overuse and pressure, right lower leg
M70.862 Other soft tissue disorders related to use, overuse and pressure, left lower leg
M70.869 Other soft tissue disorders related to use, overuse and pressure, unspecified leg

[6] M70.87 Other soft tissue disorders related to use, overuse and pressure of ankle and foot
M70.871 Other soft tissue disorders related to use, overuse and pressure, right ankle and foot
M70.872 Other soft tissue disorders related to use, overuse and pressure, left ankle and foot
M70.879 Other soft tissue disorders related to use, overuse and pressure, unspecified ankle and foot

M70.88 Other soft tissue disorders related to use, overuse and pressure other site
M70.89 Other soft tissue disorders related to use, overuse and pressure multiple sites

[5] M70.9 Unspecified soft tissue disorder related to use, overuse and pressure
M70.90 Unspecified soft tissue disorder related to use, overuse and pressure of unspecified site

[6] M70.91 Unspecified soft tissue disorder related to use, overuse and pressure of shoulder
M70.911 Unspecified soft tissue disorder related to use, overuse and pressure, right shoulder
M70.912 Unspecified soft tissue disorder related to use, overuse and pressure, left shoulder
M70.919 Unspecified soft tissue disorder related to use, overuse and pressure, unspecified shoulder

[6] M70.92 Unspecified soft tissue disorder related to use, overuse and pressure of upper arm
M70.921 Unspecified soft tissue disorder related to use, overuse and pressure, right upper arm
M70.922 Unspecified soft tissue disorder related to use, overuse and pressure, left upper arm
M70.929 Unspecified soft tissue disorder related to use, overuse and pressure, unspecified upper arm

[6] M70.93 Unspecified soft tissue disorder related to use, overuse and pressure of forearm
M70.931 Unspecified soft tissue disorder related to use, overuse and pressure, right forearm
M70.932 Unspecified soft tissue disorder related to use, overuse and pressure, left forearm
M70.939 Unspecified soft tissue disorder related to use, overuse and pressure, unspecified forearm

[6] M70.94 Unspecified soft tissue disorder related to use, overuse and pressure of hand
M70.941 Unspecified soft tissue disorder related to use, overuse and pressure, right hand
M70.942 Unspecified soft tissue disorder related to use, overuse and pressure, left hand
M70.949 Unspecified soft tissue disorder related to use, overuse and pressure, unspecified hand

[6] M70.95 Unspecified soft tissue disorder related to use, overuse and pressure of thigh
M70.951 Unspecified soft tissue disorder related to use, overuse and pressure, right thigh
M70.952 Unspecified soft tissue disorder related to use, overuse and pressure, left thigh
M70.959 Unspecified soft tissue disorder related to use, overuse and pressure, unspecified thigh

[6] M70.96 Unspecified soft tissue disorder related to use, overuse and pressure lower leg
M70.961 Unspecified soft tissue disorder related to use, overuse and pressure, right lower leg
M70.962 Unspecified soft tissue disorder related to use, overuse and pressure, left lower leg
M70.969 Unspecified soft tissue disorder related to use, overuse and pressure, unspecified lower leg

[6] M70.97 Unspecified soft tissue disorder related to use, overuse and pressure of ankle and foot
M70.971 Unspecified soft tissue disorder related to use, overuse and pressure, right ankle and foot
M70.972 Unspecified soft tissue disorder related to use, overuse and pressure, left ankle and foot
M70.979 Unspecified soft tissue disorder related to use, overuse and pressure, unspecified ankle and foot

M70.98 Unspecified soft tissue disorder related to use, overuse and pressure other
M70.99 Unspecified soft tissue disorder related to use, overuse and pressure multiple sites

Unspecified Code | Other Specified Code | [N] Newborn Age: 0 | [P] Pediatric Age: 0-17 | [M] Maternity Age: 12-55
[A] Adult Age: 15-124 | ♂ Male | ♀ Female | ● New Code | ▲ Revised Code Title | ►◄ Revised Text

M71 Other bursopathies

EXCLUDES1 bunion (M20.1)
bursitis related to use, overuse or pressure (M70.-)
enthesopathies (M76-M77)

M71.0 Abscess of bursa
Use additional code (B95.-, B96.-) to identify causative organism

M71.00 Abscess of bursa, unspecified site

M71.01 Abscess of bursa, shoulder
M71.011 Abscess of bursa, right shoulder
M71.012 Abscess of bursa, left shoulder
M71.019 Abscess of bursa, unspecified shoulder

M71.02 Abscess of bursa, elbow
M71.021 Abscess of bursa, right elbow
M71.022 Abscess of bursa, left elbow
M71.029 Abscess of bursa, unspecified elbow

M71.03 Abscess of bursa, wrist
M71.031 Abscess of bursa, right wrist
M71.032 Abscess of bursa, left wrist
M71.039 Abscess of bursa, unspecified wrist

M71.04 Abscess of bursa, hand
M71.041 Abscess of bursa, right hand
M71.042 Abscess of bursa, left hand
M71.049 Abscess of bursa, unspecified hand

M71.05 Abscess of bursa, hip
M71.051 Abscess of bursa, right hip
M71.052 Abscess of bursa, left hip
M71.059 Abscess of bursa, unspecified hip

M71.06 Abscess of bursa, knee
M71.061 Abscess of bursa, right knee
M71.062 Abscess of bursa, left knee
M71.069 Abscess of bursa, unspecified knee

M71.07 Abscess of bursa, ankle and foot
M71.071 Abscess of bursa, right ankle and foot
M71.072 Abscess of bursa, left ankle and foot
M71.079 Abscess of bursa, unspecified ankle and foot

M71.08 Abscess of bursa, other site
M71.09 Abscess of bursa, multiple sites

M71.1 Other infective bursitis
Use additional code (B95.-, B96.-) to identify causative organism

M71.10 Other infective bursitis, unspecified site

M71.11 Other infective bursitis, shoulder
M71.111 Other infective bursitis, right shoulder
M71.112 Other infective bursitis, left shoulder
M71.119 Other infective bursitis, unspecified shoulder

M71.12 Other infective bursitis, elbow
M71.121 Other infective bursitis, right elbow
M71.122 Other infective bursitis, left elbow
M71.129 Other infective bursitis, unspecified elbow

M71.13 Other infective bursitis, wrist
M71.131 Other infective bursitis, right wrist
M71.132 Other infective bursitis, left wrist
M71.139 Other infective bursitis, unspecified wrist

M71.14 Other infective bursitis, hand
M71.141 Other infective bursitis, right hand
M71.142 Other infective bursitis, left hand
M71.149 Other infective bursitis, unspecified hand

M71.15 Other infective bursitis, hip
M71.151 Other infective bursitis, right hip
M71.152 Other infective bursitis, left hip
M71.159 Other infective bursitis, unspecified hip

M71.16 Other infective bursitis, knee
M71.161 Other infective bursitis, right knee
M71.162 Other infective bursitis, left knee
M71.169 Other infective bursitis, unspecified knee

M71.17 Other infective bursitis, ankle and foot
M71.171 Other infective bursitis, right ankle and foot
M71.172 Other infective bursitis, left ankle and foot
M71.179 Other infective bursitis, unspecified ankle and foot

M71.18 Other infective bursitis, other site
M71.19 Other infective bursitis, multiple sites

M71.2 Synovial cyst of popliteal space [Baker]

EXCLUDES1 synovial cyst of popliteal space with rupture (M66.0)

M71.20 Synovial cyst of popliteal space [Baker], unspecified knee
M71.21 Synovial cyst of popliteal space [Baker], right knee
M71.22 Synovial cyst of popliteal space [Baker], left knee

M71.3 Other bursal cyst
Synovial cyst NOS

EXCLUDES1 synovial cyst with rupture (M66.1-)

M71.30 Other bursal cyst, unspecified site

M71.31 Other bursal cyst, shoulder
M71.311 Other bursal cyst, right shoulder
M71.312 Other bursal cyst, left shoulder
M71.319 Other bursal cyst, unspecified shoulder

M71.32 Other bursal cyst, elbow
M71.321 Other bursal cyst, right elbow
M71.322 Other bursal cyst, left elbow
M71.329 Other bursal cyst, unspecified elbow

M71.33 Other bursal cyst, wrist
M71.331 Other bursal cyst, right wrist
M71.332 Other bursal cyst, left wrist
M71.339 Other bursal cyst, unspecified wrist

M71.34 Other bursal cyst, hand
M71.341 Other bursal cyst, right hand
M71.342 Other bursal cyst, left hand
M71.349 Other bursal cyst, unspecified hand

M71.35 Other bursal cyst, hip
M71.351 Other bursal cyst, right hip
M71.352 Other bursal cyst, left hip
M71.359 Other bursal cyst, unspecified hip

M71.37 Other bursal cyst, ankle and foot
M71.371 Other bursal cyst, right ankle and foot
M71.372 Other bursal cyst, left ankle and foot
M71.379 Other bursal cyst, unspecified ankle and foot

M71.38 Other bursal cyst, other site
M71.39 Other bursal cyst, multiple sites

M71.4 Calcium deposit in bursa

EXCLUDES2 calcium deposit in bursa of shoulder (M75.3)

M71.40 Calcium deposit in bursa, unspecified site

M71.42 Calcium deposit in bursa, elbow
M71.421 Calcium deposit in bursa, right elbow
M71.422 Calcium deposit in bursa, left elbow
M71.429 Calcium deposit in bursa, unspecified elbow

M71.43 Calcium deposit in bursa, wrist
M71.431 Calcium deposit in bursa, right wrist
M71.432 Calcium deposit in bursa, left wrist
M71.439 Calcium deposit in bursa, unspecified wrist

M71.44 Calcium deposit in bursa, hand
M71.441 Calcium deposit in bursa, right hand
M71.442 Calcium deposit in bursa, left hand
M71.449 Calcium deposit in bursa, unspecified hand

4ᵗʰ character required 　5ᵗʰ character required 　6ᵗʰ character required 　7ᵗʰ character required 　Extension 'X' Alert

EXCLUDES 1 Not coded here 　EXCLUDES 2 Not included here 　PDx Primary Diagnosis Only 　Manifestation Code

[6] M71.45 Calcium deposit in bursa, hip
- M71.451 Calcium deposit in bursa, right hip
- M71.452 Calcium deposit in bursa, left hip
- M71.459 Calcium deposit in bursa, unspecified hip

[6] M71.46 Calcium deposit in bursa, knee
- M71.461 Calcium deposit in bursa, right knee
- M71.462 Calcium deposit in bursa, left knee
- M71.469 Calcium deposit in bursa, unspecified knee

[6] M71.47 Calcium deposit in bursa, ankle and foot
- M71.471 Calcium deposit in bursa, right ankle and foot
- M71.472 Calcium deposit in bursa, left ankle and foot
- M71.479 Calcium deposit in bursa, unspecified ankle and foot

M71.48 Calcium deposit in bursa, other site

M71.49 Calcium deposit in bursa, multiple sites

[5] M71.5 Other bursitis, not elsewhere classified

[EXCLUDES1] *bursitis NOS (M71.9-)*

[EXCLUDES2] *bursitis of shoulder (M75.5)*
bursitis of tibial collateral [Pellegrini-Stieda] (M76.4)

M71.50 Other bursitis, not elsewhere classified, unspecified site

[6] M71.52 Other bursitis, not elsewhere classified, elbow
- M71.521 Other bursitis, not elsewhere classified, right elbow
- M71.522 Other bursitis, not elsewhere classified, left elbow
- M71.529 Other bursitis, not elsewhere classified, unspecified elbow

[6] M71.53 Other bursitis, not elsewhere classified, wrist
- M71.531 Other bursitis, not elsewhere classified, right wrist
- M71.532 Other bursitis, not elsewhere classified, left wrist
- M71.539 Other bursitis, not elsewhere classified, unspecified wrist

[6] M71.54 Other bursitis, not elsewhere classified, hand
- M71.541 Other bursitis, not elsewhere classified, right hand
- M71.542 Other bursitis, not elsewhere classified, left hand
- M71.549 Other bursitis, not elsewhere classified, unspecified hand

[6] M71.55 Other bursitis, not elsewhere classified, hip
- M71.551 Other bursitis, not elsewhere classified, right hip
- M71.552 Other bursitis, not elsewhere classified, left hip
- M71.559 Other bursitis, not elsewhere classified, unspecified hip

[6] M71.56 Other bursitis, not elsewhere classified, knee
- M71.561 Other bursitis, not elsewhere classified, right knee
- M71.562 Other bursitis, not elsewhere classified, left knee
- M71.569 Other bursitis, not elsewhere classified, unspecified knee

[6] M71.57 Other bursitis, not elsewhere classified, ankle and foot
- M71.571 Other bursitis, not elsewhere classified, right ankle and foot
- M71.572 Other bursitis, not elsewhere classified, left ankle and foot
- M71.579 Other bursitis, not elsewhere classified, unspecified ankle and foot

M71.58 Other bursitis, not elsewhere classified, other site

[5] M71.8 Other specified bursopathies

M71.80 Other specified bursopathies, unspecified site

[6] M71.81 Other specified bursopathies, shoulder
- M71.811 Other specified bursopathies, right shoulder
- M71.812 Other specified bursopathies, left shoulder
- M71.819 Other specified bursopathies, unspecified shoulder

[6] M71.82 Other specified bursopathies, elbow
- M71.821 Other specified bursopathies, right elbow
- M71.822 Other specified bursopathies, left elbow
- M71.829 Other specified bursopathies, unspecified elbow

[6] M71.83 Other specified bursopathies, wrist
- M71.831 Other specified bursopathies, right wrist
- M71.832 Other specified bursopathies, left wrist
- M71.839 Other specified bursopathies, unspecified wrist

[6] M71.84 Other specified bursopathies, hand
- M71.841 Other specified bursopathies, right hand
- M71.842 Other specified bursopathies, left hand
- M71.849 Other specified bursopathies, unspecified hand

[6] M71.85 Other specified bursopathies, hip
- M71.851 Other specified bursopathies, right hip
- M71.852 Other specified bursopathies, left hip
- M71.859 Other specified bursopathies, unspecified hip

[6] M71.86 Other specified bursopathies, knee
- M71.861 Other specified bursopathies, right knee
- M71.862 Other specified bursopathies, left knee
- M71.869 Other specified bursopathies, unspecified knee

[6] M71.87 Other specified bursopathies, ankle and foot
- M71.871 Other specified bursopathies, right ankle and foot
- M71.872 Other specified bursopathies, left ankle and foot
- M71.879 Other specified bursopathies, unspecified ankle and foot

M71.88 Other specified bursopathies, other site

M71.89 Other specified bursopathies, multiple sites

M71.9 Bursopathy, unspecified
Bursitis NOS

[4] M72 Fibroblastic disorders

[EXCLUDES2] *retroperitoneal fibromatosis (D48.3)*

M72.0 Palmar fascial fibromatosis [Dupuytren] [A]

M72.1 Knuckle pads

M72.2 Plantar fascial fibromatosis
Plantar fasciitis

M72.4 Pseudosarcomatous fibromatosis
Nodular fasciitis

M72.6 Necrotizing fasciitis
Use additional code (B95.-, B96.-) to identify causative organism

M72.8 Other fibroblastic disorders
Abscess of fascia
Fasciitis NEC
Other infective fasciitis
Use additional code to (B95.-, B96.-) identify causative organism

[EXCLUDES1] *diffuse (eosinophilic) fasciitis (M35.4)*
necrotizing fasciitis (M72.6)
nodular fasciitis (M72.4)
perirenal fasciitis NOS (N13.5)
perirenal fasciitis with infection (N13.6)
plantar fasciitis (M72.2)

M72.9 Fibroblastic disorder, unspecified
Fasciitis NOS
Fibromatosis NOS

[4] **M75 Shoulder lesions**
[EXCLUDES2] *shoulder-hand syndrome (M89.0-)*

[5] **M75.0 Adhesive capsulitis of shoulder**
Frozen shoulder
Periarthritis of shoulder
M75.00 Adhesive capsulitis of unspecified shoulder
M75.01 Adhesive capsulitis of right shoulder
M75.02 Adhesive capsulitis of left shoulder

[5] **M75.1 Rotator cuff tear or rupture, not specified as traumatic**
Rotator cuff syndrome
Supraspinatus tear or rupture, not specified as traumatic
Supraspinatus syndrome
[EXCLUDES1] *tear of rotator cuff, traumatic (S46.01-)*

[6] **M75.10 Unspecified rotator cuff tear or rupture, not specified as traumatic**
M75.100 Unspecified rotator cuff tear or rupture of unspecified shoulder, not specified as traumatic
M75.101 Unspecified rotator cuff tear or rupture of right shoulder, not specified as traumatic
M75.102 Unspecified rotator cuff tear or rupture of left shoulder, not specified as traumatic

[6] **M75.11 Incomplete rotator cuff tear or rupture not specified as traumatic**
M75.110 Incomplete rotator cuff tear or rupture of unspecified shoulder, not specified as traumatic
M75.111 Incomplete rotator cuff tear or rupture of right shoulder, not specified as traumatic
M75.112 Incomplete rotator cuff tear or rupture of left shoulder, not specified as traumatic

[6] **M75.12 Complete rotator cuff tear or rupture not specified as traumatic**
M75.120 Complete rotator cuff tear or rupture of unspecified shoulder, not specified as traumatic
M75.121 Complete rotator cuff tear or rupture of right shoulder, not specified as traumatic
M75.122 Complete rotator cuff tear or rupture of left shoulder, not specified as traumatic

[5] **M75.2 Bicipital tendinitis**
M75.20 Bicipital tendinitis, unspecified shoulder
M75.21 Bicipital tendinitis, right shoulder
M75.22 Bicipital tendinitis, left shoulder

[5] **M75.3 Calcific tendinitis of shoulder**
Calcified bursa of shoulder
M75.30 Calcific tendinitis of unspecified shoulder
M75.31 Calcific tendinitis of right shoulder
M75.32 Calcific tendinitis of left shoulder

[5] **M75.4 Impingement syndrome of shoulder**
M75.40 Impingement syndrome of unspecified shoulder
M75.41 Impingement syndrome of right shoulder
M75.42 Impingement syndrome of left shoulder

[5] **M75.5 Bursitis of shoulder**
M75.50 Bursitis of unspecified shoulder
M75.51 Bursitis of right shoulder
M75.52 Bursitis of left shoulder

[5] **M75.8 Other shoulder lesions**
M75.80 Other shoulder lesions, unspecified shoulder
M75.81 Other shoulder lesions, right shoulder
M75.82 Other shoulder lesions, left shoulder

[5] **M75.9 Shoulder lesion, unspecified**
M75.90 Shoulder lesion, unspecified, unspecified shoulder
M75.91 Shoulder lesion, unspecified, right shoulder
M75.92 Shoulder lesion, unspecified, left shoulder

[4] **M76 Enthesopathies, lower limb, excluding foot**
[EXCLUDES2] *bursitis due to use, overuse and pressure (M70.-)*
enthesopathies of ankle and foot (M77.5-)

[5] **M76.0 Gluteal tendinitis**
M76.00 Gluteal tendinitis, unspecified hip
M76.01 Gluteal tendinitis, right hip
M76.02 Gluteal tendinitis, left hip

[5] **M76.1 Psoas tendinitis**
M76.10 Psoas tendinitis, unspecified hip
M76.11 Psoas tendinitis, right hip
M76.12 Psoas tendinitis, left hip

[5] **M76.2 Iliac crest spur**
M76.20 Iliac crest spur, unspecified hip
M76.21 Iliac crest spur, right hip
M76.22 Iliac crest spur, left hip

[5] **M76.3 Iliotibial band syndrome**
M76.30 Iliotibial band syndrome, unspecified leg
M76.31 Iliotibial band syndrome, right leg
M76.32 Iliotibial band syndrome, left leg

[5] **M76.4 Tibial collateral bursitis [Pellegrini-Stieda]**
M76.40 Tibial collateral bursitis [Pellegrini-Stieda], unspecified leg
M76.41 Tibial collateral bursitis [Pellegrini-Stieda], right leg
M76.42 Tibial collateral bursitis [Pellegrini-Stieda], left leg

[5] **M76.5 Patellar tendinitis**
M76.50 Patellar tendinitis, unspecified knee
M76.51 Patellar tendinitis, right knee
M76.52 Patellar tendinitis, left knee

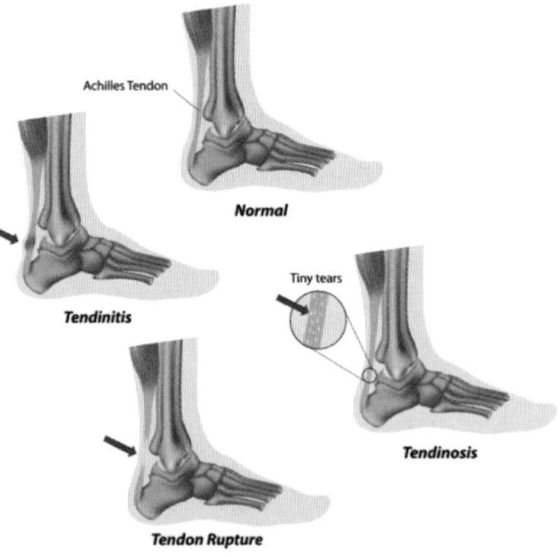

Figure 12.6 Achilles Tendon Problems

[5] **M76.6 Achilles tendinitis**
Achilles bursitis
M76.60 Achilles tendinitis, unspecified leg
M76.61 Achilles tendinitis, right leg
M76.62 Achilles tendinitis, left leg

[5] **M76.7 Peroneal tendinitis**
M76.70 Peroneal tendinitis, unspecified leg
M76.71 Peroneal tendinitis, right leg
M76.72 Peroneal tendinitis, left leg

[5] **M76.8 Other specified enthesopathies of lower limb, excluding foot**

[4] 4th character required [5] 5th character required [6] 6th character required [7] 7th character required Extension 'X' Alert
[EXCLUDES1] Not coded here [EXCLUDES2] Not included here [PDx] Primary Diagnosis Only Manifestation Code

[6] M76.81 Anterior tibial syndrome
M76.811 Anterior tibial syndrome, right leg
M76.812 Anterior tibial syndrome, left leg
M76.819 Anterior tibial syndrome, unspecified leg
[6] M76.82 Posterior tibial tendinitis
M76.821 Posterior tibial tendinitis, right leg
M76.822 Posterior tibial tendinitis, left leg
M76.829 Posterior tibial tendinitis, unspecified leg
[6] M76.89 Other specified enthesopathies of lower limb, excluding foot
M76.891 Other specified enthesopathies of right lower limb, excluding foot
M76.892 Other specified enthesopathies of left lower limb, excluding foot
M76.899 Other specified enthesopathies of unspecified lower limb, excluding foot
M76.9 Unspecified enthesopathy, lower limb, excluding foot

[4] M77 Other enthesopathies
[EXCLUDES1] *bursitis NOS (M71.9-)*
[EXCLUDES2] *bursitis due to use, overuse and pressure (M70.-)*
osteophyte (M25.7)
spinal enthesopathy (M46.0-)
[5] M77.0 Medial epicondylitis
M77.00 Medial epicondylitis, unspecified elbow
M77.01 Medial epicondylitis, right elbow
M77.02 Medial epicondylitis, left elbow
[5] M77.1 Lateral epicondylitis
Tennis elbow
M77.10 Lateral epicondylitis, unspecified elbow
M77.11 Lateral epicondylitis, right elbow
M77.12 Lateral epicondylitis, left elbow
[5] M77.2 Periarthritis of wrist
M77.20 Periarthritis, unspecified wrist
M77.21 Periarthritis, right wrist
M77.22 Periarthritis, left wrist
[5] M77.3 Calcaneal spur
M77.30 Calcaneal spur, unspecified foot
M77.31 Calcaneal spur, right foot
M77.32 Calcaneal spur, left foot
[5] M77.4 Metatarsalgia
[EXCLUDES1] *Morton's metatarsalgia (G57.6)*
M77.40 Metatarsalgia, unspecified foot
M77.41 Metatarsalgia, right foot
M77.42 Metatarsalgia, left foot
[5] M77.5 Other enthesopathy of foot
M77.50 Other enthesopathy of unspecified foot
M77.51 Other enthesopathy of right foot
M77.52 Other enthesopathy of left foot
M77.8 Other enthesopathies, not elsewhere classified
M77.9 Enthesopathy, unspecified
Bone spur NOS
Capsulitis NOS
Periarthritis NOS
Tendinitis NOS

[4] M79 Other and unspecified soft tissue disorders, not elsewhere classified
[EXCLUDES1] *psychogenic rheumatism (F45.8)*
soft tissue pain, psychogenic (F45.41)
M79.0 Rheumatism, unspecified
[EXCLUDES1] *fibromyalgia (M79.7)*
palindromic rheumatism (M12.3-)
M79.1 Myalgia
Myofascial pain syndrome
[EXCLUDES1] *fibromyalgia (M79.7)*
myositis (M60.-)
M79.2 Neuralgia and neuritis, unspecified
[EXCLUDES1] *brachial radiculitis NOS (M54.1)*
lumbosacral radiculitis NOS (M54.1)
mononeuropathies (G56-G58)
radiculitis NOS (M54.1)
sciatica (M54.3-M54.4)
M79.3 Panniculitis, unspecified
[EXCLUDES1] *lupus panniculitis (L93.2)*
neck and back panniculitis (M54.0-)
relapsing [Weber-Christian] panniculitis (M35.6)
M79.4 Hypertrophy of (infrapatellar) fat pad
M79.5 Residual foreign body in soft tissue
[EXCLUDES1] *foreign body granuloma of skin and subcutaneous tissue (L92.3)*
foreign body granuloma of soft tissue (M60.2-)
[5] M79.6 Pain in limb, hand, foot, fingers and toes
[EXCLUDES2] *pain in joint (M25.5-)*
[6] M79.60 Pain in limb, unspecified
M79.601 Pain in right arm
Pain in right upper limb NOS
M79.602 Pain in left arm
Pain in left upper limb NOS
M79.603 Pain in arm, unspecified
Pain in upper limb NOS
M79.604 Pain in right leg
Pain in right lower limb NOS
M79.605 Pain in left leg
Pain in left lower limb NOS
M79.606 Pain in leg, unspecified
Pain in lower limb NOS
M79.609 Pain in unspecified limb
Pain in limb NOS
[6] M79.62 Pain in upper arm
Pain in axillary region
M79.621 Pain in right upper arm
M79.622 Pain in left upper arm
M79.629 Pain in unspecified upper arm
[6] M79.63 Pain in forearm
M79.631 Pain in right forearm
M79.632 Pain in left forearm
M79.639 Pain in unspecified forearm
[6] M79.64 Pain in hand and fingers
M79.641 Pain in right hand
M79.642 Pain in left hand
M79.643 Pain in unspecified hand
M79.644 Pain in right finger(s)
M79.645 Pain in left finger(s)
M79.646 Pain in unspecified finger(s)
[6] M79.65 Pain in thigh
M79.651 Pain in right thigh
M79.652 Pain in left thigh
M79.659 Pain in unspecified thigh
[6] M79.66 Pain in lower leg
M79.661 Pain in right lower leg
M79.662 Pain in left lower leg
M79.669 Pain in unspecified lower leg
[6] M79.67 Pain in foot and toes
M79.671 Pain in right foot
M79.672 Pain in left foot
M79.673 Pain in unspecified foot
M79.674 Pain in right toe(s)
M79.675 Pain in left toe(s)
M79.676 Pain in unspecified toe(s)
M79.7 Fibromyalgia
Fibromyositis
Fibrositis
Myofibrositis

Unspecified Code | Other Specified Code | [N] Newborn Age: 0 | [P] Pediatric Age: 0-17 | [M] Maternity Age: 12-55
[A] Adult Age: 15-124 | ♂ Male | ♀ Female | ● New Code | ▲ Revised Code Title | ►◄ Revised Text

⑤ **M79.A** Nontraumatic compartment syndrome

Code first , if applicable, associated postprocedural complication

> EXCLUDES1 *compartment syndrome NOS (T79.A-)*
> *fibromyalgia (M79.7)*
> *nontraumatic ischemic infarction of muscle (M62.2-)*
> *traumatic compartment syndrome (T79.A-)*

⑥ **M79.A1** Nontraumatic compartment syndrome of upper extremity

Nontraumatic compartment syndrome of shoulder, arm, forearm, wrist, hand, and fingers

M79.A11 **Nontraumatic compartment syndrome of** right **upper extremity**

M79.A12 **Nontraumatic compartment syndrome of** left **upper extremity**

M79.A19 **Nontraumatic compartment syndrome of unspecified upper extremity**

⑥ **M79.A2** Nontraumatic compartment syndrome of lower extremity

Nontraumatic compartment syndrome of hip, buttock, thigh, leg, foot, and toes

M79.A21 **Nontraumatic compartment syndrome of** right **lower extremity**

M79.A22 **Nontraumatic compartment syndrome of** left **lower extremity**

M79.A29 **Nontraumatic compartment syndrome of unspecified lower extremity**

M79.A3 **Nontraumatic compartment syndrome of** abdomen

M79.A9 **Nontraumatic compartment syndrome of** other sites

⑤ **M79.8** Other specified soft tissue disorders

M79.81 **Nontraumatic hematoma of soft tissue**

Nontraumatic hematoma of muscle
Nontraumatic seroma of muscle and soft tissue

M79.89 **Other specified soft tissue disorders**

Polyalgia

M79.9 Soft tissue disorder, unspecified

Osteopathies and chondropathies (M80-M94)

Disorders of bone density and structure (M80-M85)

Osteoporosis

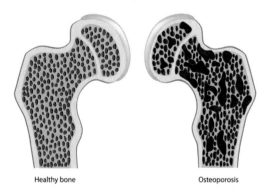

Healthy bone   Osteoporosis

Figure 12.7 Reduced Bone matrix in Osteoporosis

④ **M80** Osteoporosis with current pathological fracture

> INCLUDES *osteoporosis with current fragility fracture*
> Use additional code to identify major osseous defect, if applicable (M89.7-)

> EXCLUDES1 *collapsed vertebra NOS (M48.5)*
> *pathological fracture NOS (M84.4)*
> *wedging of vertebra NOS (M48.5)*
> EXCLUDES2 *personal history of (healed) osteoporosis fracture (Z87.310)*

The appropriate 7th character is to be added to each code from category M80:
A = initial encounter for fracture
D = subsequent encounter for fracture with routine healing
G = subsequent encounter for fracture with delayed healing
K = subsequent encounter for fracture with nonunion
P = subsequent encounter for fracture with malunion
S = sequela

⑤ **M80.0** Age-related osteoporosis with current pathological fracture

Involutional osteoporosis with current pathological fracture
Osteoporosis NOS with current pathological fracture
Postmenopausal osteoporosis with current pathological fracture
Senile osteoporosis with current pathological fracture

⑦ **M80.00** Age-related osteoporosis with current pathological fracture, unspecified site

⑥ **M80.01** Age-related osteoporosis with current pathological fracture, shoulder

⑦ **M80.011** Age-related osteoporosis with current pathological fracture, right shoulder

⑦ **M80.012** Age-related osteoporosis with current pathological fracture, left shoulder

⑦ **M80.019** Age-related osteoporosis with current pathological fracture, unspecified shoulder

⑥ **M80.02** Age-related osteoporosis with current pathological fracture, humerus

⑦ **M80.021** Age-related osteoporosis with current pathological fracture, right humerus

⑦ **M80.022** Age-related osteoporosis with current pathological fracture, left humerus

⑦ **M80.029** Age-related osteoporosis with current pathological fracture, unspecified humerus

⑥ **M80.03** Age-related osteoporosis with current pathological fracture, forearm

Age-related osteoporosis with current pathological fracture of wrist

⑦ **M80.031** Age-related osteoporosis with current pathological fracture, right forearm

⑦ **M80.032** Age-related osteoporosis with current pathological fracture, left forearm

⑦ **M80.039** Age-related osteoporosis with current pathological fracture, unspecified forearm

⑥ **M80.04** Age-related osteoporosis with current pathological fracture, hand

⑦ **M80.041** Age-related osteoporosis with current pathological fracture, right hand

⑦ **M80.042** Age-related osteoporosis with current pathological fracture, left hand

⑦ **M80.049** Age-related osteoporosis with current pathological fracture, unspecified hand

⑥ **M80.05** Age-related osteoporosis with current pathological fracture, femur

Age-related osteoporosis with current pathological fracture of hip

⑦ **M80.051** Age-related osteoporosis with current pathological fracture, right femur

⑦ **M80.052** Age-related osteoporosis with current pathological fracture, left femur

⑦ **M80.059** Age-related osteoporosis with current pathological fracture, unspecified femur

⑥ **M80.06** Age-related osteoporosis with current pathological fracture, lower leg

---

④ 4ᵗʰ character required   ⑤ 5ᵗʰ character required   ⑥ 6ᵗʰ character required   ⑦ 7ᵗʰ character required   ⓧ Extension 'X' Alert

EXCLUDES 1 Not coded here   EXCLUDES 2 Not included here   PDx Primary Diagnosis Only   Manifestation Code

⑦ M80.061 Age-related osteoporosis with current pathological fracture, right lower leg

⑦ M80.062 Age-related osteoporosis with current pathological fracture, left lower leg

⑦ M80.069 Age-related osteoporosis with current pathological fracture, unspecified lower leg

⑥ M80.07 Age-related osteoporosis with current pathological fracture, ankle and foot

⑦ M80.071 Age-related osteoporosis with current pathological fracture, right ankle and foot

⑦ M80.072 Age-related osteoporosis with current pathological fracture, left ankle and foot

⑦ M80.079 Age-related osteoporosis with current pathological fracture, unspecified ankle and foot

⑦ M80.08 Age-related osteoporosis with current pathological fracture, vertebra(e)

⑤ M80.8 Other osteoporosis with current pathological fracture

Drug-induced osteoporosis with current pathological fracture

Idiopathic osteoporosis with current pathological fracture

Osteoporosis of disuse with current pathological fracture

Postoophorectomy osteoporosis with current pathological fracture

Postsurgical malabsorption osteoporosis with current pathological fracture

Post-traumatic osteoporosis with current pathological fracture

Use additional code for adverse effect, if applicable, to identify drug (T36-T50 with fifth or sixth character 5)

⑦ M80.80 Other osteoporosis with current pathological fracture, unspecified site

⑥ M80.81 Other osteoporosis with pathological fracture, shoulder

⑦ M80.811 Other osteoporosis with current pathological fracture, right shoulder

⑦ M80.812 Other osteoporosis with current pathological fracture, left shoulder

⑦ M80.819 Other osteoporosis with current pathological fracture, unspecified shoulder

⑥ M80.82 Other osteoporosis with current pathological fracture, humerus

⑦ M80.821 Other osteoporosis with current pathological fracture, right humerus

⑦ M80.822 Other osteoporosis with current pathological fracture, left humerus

⑦ M80.829 Other osteoporosis with current pathological fracture, unspecified humerus

⑥ M80.83 Other osteoporosis with current pathological fracture, forearm

Other osteoporosis with current pathological fracture of wrist

⑦ M80.831 Other osteoporosis with current pathological fracture, right forearm

⑦ M80.832 Other osteoporosis with current pathological fracture, left forearm

⑦ M80.839 Other osteoporosis with current pathological fracture, unspecified forearm

⑥ M80.84 Other osteoporosis with current pathological fracture, hand

⑦ M80.841 Other osteoporosis with current pathological fracture, right hand

⑦ M80.842 Other osteoporosis with current pathological fracture, left hand

⑦ M80.849 Other osteoporosis with current pathological fracture, unspecified hand

⑥ M80.85 Other osteoporosis with current pathological fracture, femur

Other osteoporosis with current pathological fracture of hip

⑦ M80.851 Other osteoporosis with current pathological fracture, right femur

⑦ M80.852 Other osteoporosis with current pathological fracture, left femur

⑦ M80.859 Other osteoporosis with current pathological fracture, unspecified femur

⑥ M80.86 Other osteoporosis with current pathological fracture, lower leg

⑦ M80.861 Other osteoporosis with current pathological fracture, right lower leg

⑦ M80.862 Other osteoporosis with current pathological fracture, left lower leg

⑦ M80.869 Other osteoporosis with current pathological fracture, unspecified lower leg

⑥ M80.87 Other osteoporosis with current pathological fracture, ankle and foot

⑦ M80.871 Other osteoporosis with current pathological fracture, right ankle and foot

⑦ M80.872 Other osteoporosis with current pathological fracture, left ankle and foot

⑦ M80.879 Other osteoporosis with current pathological fracture, unspecified ankle and foot

⑦ M80.88 Other osteoporosis with current pathological fracture, vertebra(e)

④ M81 Osteoporosis without current pathological fracture

Use additional code to identify:
major osseous defect, if applicable (M89.7-)
personal history of (healed) osteoporosis fracture, if applicable (Z87.310)

EXCLUDES1 osteoporosis with current pathological fracture (M80.-)
Sudeck's atrophy (M89.0)

M81.0 Age-related osteoporosis without current pathological fracture

Involutional osteoporosis without current pathological fracture

Osteoporosis NOS

Postmenopausal osteoporosis without current pathological fracture

Senile osteoporosis without current pathological fracture Ⓐ

M81.6 Localized osteoporosis [Lequesne]

EXCLUDES1 Sudeck's atrophy (M89.0)

M81.8 Other osteoporosis without current pathological fracture

Drug-induced osteoporosis without current pathological fracture

Idiopathic osteoporosis without current pathological fracture

Osteoporosis of disuse without current pathological fracture

Postoophorectomy osteoporosis without current pathological fracture

Postsurgical malabsorption osteoporosis without current pathological fracture

Post-traumatic osteoporosis without current pathological fracture

Use additional code for adverse effect, if applicable, to identify drug (T36-T50 with fifth or sixth character 5)

Unspecified Code Other Specified Code Ⓝ Newborn Age: 0 Ⓟ Pediatric Age: 0-17 Ⓜ Maternity Age: 12-55
Ⓐ Adult Age: 15-124 ♂ Male ♀ Female ● New Code ▲ Revised Code Title ►◄ Revised Text

④ **M83** Adult osteomalacia

> EXCLUDES1 *infantile and juvenile osteomalacia (E55.0)*
> *renal osteodystrophy (N25.0)*
> *rickets (active) (E55.0)*
> *rickets (active) sequelae (E64.3)*
> *vitamin D-resistant osteomalacia (E83.3)*
> *vitamin D-resistant rickets (active) (E83.3)*

  M83.0 Puerperal osteomalacia   Ⓜ ♀
  M83.1 Senile osteomalacia   Ⓐ
  M83.2 Adult osteomalacia due to malabsorption
    Postsurgical malabsorption osteomalacia in adults   Ⓐ
  M83.3 Adult osteomalacia due to malnutrition   Ⓐ
  M83.4 Aluminum bone disease
  M83.5 Other drug-induced osteomalacia in adults
    Use additional code for adverse effect, if applicable, to
    identify drug (T36-T50 with fifth or sixth character 5) Ⓐ
  M83.8 Other adult osteomalacia   Ⓐ
  M83.9 Adult osteomalacia, unspecified   Ⓐ

④ **M84** Disorder of continuity of bone

> EXCLUDES2 *traumatic fracture of bone-see fracture, by site*

⑤ **M84.3** Stress fracture

    Fatigue fracture
    March fracture
    Stress fracture NOS
    Stress reaction
    Use additional external cause code(s) to identify the
    cause of the stress fracture

> EXCLUDES1 *pathological fracture NOS (M84.4.-)*
> *pathological fracture due to osteoporosis (M80.-)*
> *traumatic fracture (S12.-, S22.-, S32.-, S42.-, S52.-, S62.-, S72.-, S82.-, S92.-)*

> EXCLUDES2 *personal history of (healed) stress (fatigue) fracture (Z87.312)*
> *stress fracture of vertebra (M48.4-)*

The appropriate 7th character is to be added to each code from subcategory M84.3:
A = initial encounter for fracture
D = subsequent encounter for fracture with routine healing
G = subsequent encounter for fracture with delayed healing
K = subsequent encounter for fracture with nonunion
P = subsequent encounter for fracture with malunion
S = sequela

  ⑦ **M84.30** Stress fracture, unspecified site
  ⑥ **M84.31** Stress fracture, shoulder
    ⑦ M84.311 Stress fracture, right shoulder
    ⑦ M84.312 Stress fracture, left shoulder
    ⑦ M84.319 Stress fracture, unspecified shoulder
  ⑥ **M84.32** Stress fracture, humerus
    ⑦ M84.321 Stress fracture, right humerus
    ⑦ M84.322 Stress fracture, left humerus
    ⑦ M84.329 Stress fracture, unspecified humerus
  ⑥ **M84.33** Stress fracture, ulna and radius
    ⑦ M84.331 Stress fracture, right ulna
    ⑦ M84.332 Stress fracture, left ulna
    ⑦ M84.333 Stress fracture, right radius
    ⑦ M84.334 Stress fracture, left radius
    ⑦ M84.339 Stress fracture, unspecified ulna and radius
  ⑥ **M84.34** Stress fracture, hand and fingers
    ⑦ M84.341 Stress fracture, right hand
    ⑦ M84.342 Stress fracture, left hand
    ⑦ M84.343 Stress fracture, unspecified hand
    ⑦ M84.344 Stress fracture, right finger(s)
    ⑦ M84.345 Stress fracture, left finger(s)
    ⑦ M84.346 Stress fracture, unspecified finger(s)

⑥ **M84.35** Stress fracture, pelvis and femur
    Stress fracture, hip
    ⑦ M84.350 Stress fracture, pelvis
    ⑦ M84.351 Stress fracture, right femur
    ⑦ M84.352 Stress fracture, left femur
    ⑦ M84.353 Stress fracture, unspecified femur
    ⑦ M84.359 Stress fracture, hip, unspecified
  ⑥ **M84.36** Stress fracture, tibia and fibula
    ⑦ M84.361 Stress fracture, right tibia
    ⑦ M84.362 Stress fracture, left tibia
    ⑦ M84.363 Stress fracture, right fibula
    ⑦ M84.364 Stress fracture, left fibula
    ⑦ M84.369 Stress fracture, unspecified tibia and fibula
  ⑥ **M84.37** Stress fracture, ankle, foot and toes
    ⑦ M84.371 Stress fracture, right ankle
    ⑦ M84.372 Stress fracture, left ankle
    ⑦ M84.373 Stress fracture, unspecified ankle
    ⑦ M84.374 Stress fracture, right foot
    ⑦ M84.375 Stress fracture, left foot
    ⑦ M84.376 Stress fracture, unspecified foot
    ⑦ M84.377 Stress fracture, right toe(s)
    ⑦ M84.378 Stress fracture, left toe(s)
    ⑦ M84.379 Stress fracture, unspecified toe(s)
  ⑦ **M84.38** Stress fracture, other site

> EXCLUDES2 *stress fracture of vertebra (M48.4-)*

⑤ **M84.4** Pathological fracture, not elsewhere classified
    Chronic fracture
    Pathological fracture NOS

> EXCLUDES1 *collapsed vertebra NEC (M48.5)*
> *pathological fracture in neoplastic disease (M84.5-)*
> *pathological fracture in osteoporosis (M80.-)*
> *pathological fracture in other disease (M84.6-)*
> *stress fracture (M84.3-)*
> *traumatic fracture (S12.-, S22.-, S32.-, S42.-, S52.-, S62.-, S72.-, S82.-, S92.-)*

> EXCLUDES2 *personal history of (healed) pathological fracture (Z87.311)*

The appropriate 7th character is to be added to each code from subcategory M84.4:
A = initial encounter for fracture
D = subsequent encounter for fracture with routine healing
G = subsequent encounter for fracture with delayed healing
K = subsequent encounter for fracture with nonunion
P = subsequent encounter for fracture with malunion
S = sequela

  ⑦ **M84.40** Pathological fracture, unspecified site
  ⑥ **M84.41** Pathological fracture, shoulder
    ⑦ M84.411 Pathological fracture, right shoulder
    ⑦ M84.412 Pathological fracture, left shoulder
    ⑦ M84.419 Pathological fracture, unspecified shoulder
  ⑥ **M84.42** Pathological fracture, humerus
    ⑦ M84.421 Pathological fracture, right humerus
    ⑦ M84.422 Pathological fracture, left humerus
    ⑦ M84.429 Pathological fracture, unspecified humerus
  ⑥ **M84.43** Pathological fracture, ulna and radius
    ⑦ M84.431 Pathological fracture, right ulna
    ⑦ M84.432 Pathological fracture, left ulna
    ⑦ M84.433 Pathological fracture, right radius
    ⑦ M84.434 Pathological fracture, left radius
    ⑦ M84.439 Pathological fracture, unspecified ulna and radius
  ⑥ **M84.44** Pathological fracture, hand and fingers
    ⑦ M84.441 Pathological fracture, right hand
    ⑦ M84.442 Pathological fracture, left hand

---

④ 4th character required   ⑤ 5th character required   ⑥ 6th character required   ⑦ 7th character required   ⑦ Extension 'X' Alert

EXCLUDES 1 Not coded here   EXCLUDES 2 Not included here   PDx Primary Diagnosis Only   Manifestation Code

- [7] M84.443 Pathological fracture, unspecified hand
- [7] M84.444 Pathological fracture, right finger(s)
- [7] M84.445 Pathological fracture, left finger(s)
- [7] M84.446 Pathological fracture, unspecified finger(s)
- [6] M84.45 Pathological fracture, femur and pelvis
  - [7] M84.451 Pathological fracture, right femur
  - [7] M84.452 Pathological fracture, left femur
  - [7] M84.453 Pathological fracture, unspecified femur
  - [7] M84.454 Pathological fracture, pelvis
  - [7] M84.459 Pathological fracture, hip, unspecified
- [6] M84.46 Pathological fracture, tibia and fibula
  - [7] M84.461 Pathological fracture, right tibia
  - [7] M84.462 Pathological fracture, left tibia
  - [7] M84.463 Pathological fracture, right fibula
  - [7] M84.464 Pathological fracture, left fibula
  - [7] M84.469 Pathological fracture, unspecified tibia and fibula
- [6] M84.47 Pathological fracture, ankle, foot and toes
  - [7] M84.471 Pathological fracture, right ankle
  - [7] M84.472 Pathological fracture, left ankle
  - [7] M84.473 Pathological fracture, unspecified ankle
  - [7] M84.474 Pathological fracture, right foot
  - [7] M84.475 Pathological fracture, left foot
  - [7] M84.476 Pathological fracture, unspecified foot
  - [7] M84.477 Pathological fracture, right toe(s)
  - [7] M84.478 Pathological fracture, left toe(s)
  - [7] M84.479 Pathological fracture, unspecified toe(s)
- [7th] M84.48 Pathological fracture, other site

[5] M84.5 Pathological fracture in neoplastic disease

Code also underlying neoplasm

The appropriate 7th character is to be added to each code from subcategory M84.5:

A = initial encounter for fracture
D = subsequent encounter for fracture with routine healing
G = subsequent encounter for fracture with delayed healing
K = subsequent encounter for fracture with nonunion
P = subsequent encounter for fracture with malunion
S = sequela

- [7th] M84.50 Pathological fracture in neoplastic disease, unspecified site
- [6] M84.51 Pathological fracture in neoplastic disease, shoulder
  - [7] M84.511 Pathological fracture in neoplastic disease, right shoulder
  - [7] M84.512 Pathological fracture in neoplastic disease, left shoulder
  - [7] M84.519 Pathological fracture in neoplastic disease, unspecified shoulder
- [6] M84.52 Pathological fracture in neoplastic disease, humerus
  - [7] M84.521 Pathological fracture in neoplastic disease, right humerus
  - [7] M84.522 Pathological fracture in neoplastic disease, left humerus
  - [7] M84.529 Pathological fracture in neoplastic disease, unspecified humerus
- [6] M84.53 Pathological fracture in neoplastic disease, ulna and radius
  - [7] M84.531 Pathological fracture in neoplastic disease, right ulna
  - [7] M84.532 Pathological fracture in neoplastic disease, left ulna
  - [7] M84.533 Pathological fracture in neoplastic disease, right radius
  - [7] M84.534 Pathological fracture in neoplastic disease, left radius
  - [7] M84.539 Pathological fracture in neoplastic disease, unspecified ulna and radius
- [6] M84.54 Pathological fracture in neoplastic disease, hand
  - [7] M84.541 Pathological fracture in neoplastic disease, right hand
  - [7] M84.542 Pathological fracture in neoplastic disease, left hand
  - [7] M84.549 Pathological fracture in neoplastic disease, unspecified hand
- [6] M84.55 Pathological fracture in neoplastic disease, pelvis and femur
  - [7] M84.550 Pathological fracture in neoplastic disease, pelvis
  - [7] M84.551 Pathological fracture in neoplastic disease, right femur
  - [7] M84.552 Pathological fracture in neoplastic disease, left femur
  - [7] M84.553 Pathological fracture in neoplastic disease, unspecified femur
  - [7] M84.559 Pathological fracture in neoplastic disease, hip, unspecified
- [6] M84.56 Pathological fracture in neoplastic disease, tibia and fibula
  - [7] M84.561 Pathological fracture in neoplastic disease, right tibia
  - [7] M84.562 Pathological fracture in neoplastic disease, left tibia
  - [7] M84.563 Pathological fracture in neoplastic disease, right fibula
  - [7] M84.564 Pathological fracture in neoplastic disease, left fibula
  - [7] M84.569 Pathological fracture in neoplastic disease, unspecified tibia and fibula
- [6] M84.57 Pathological fracture in neoplastic disease, ankle and foot
  - [7] M84.571 Pathological fracture in neoplastic disease, right ankle
  - [7] M84.572 Pathological fracture in neoplastic disease, left ankle
  - [7] M84.573 Pathological fracture in neoplastic disease, unspecified ankle
  - [7] M84.574 Pathological fracture in neoplastic disease, right foot
  - [7] M84.575 Pathological fracture in neoplastic disease, left foot
  - [7] M84.576 Pathological fracture in neoplastic disease, unspecified foot
- [7th] M84.58 Pathological fracture in neoplastic disease, other specified site ▲

  Pathological fracture in neoplastic disease, vertebrae

[5] M84.6 Pathological fracture in other disease

Code also underlying condition

[EXCLUDES1] *pathological fracture in osteoporosis (M80.-)*

The appropriate 7th character is to be added to each code from subcategory M84.6:

A = initial encounter for fracture
D = subsequent encounter for fracture with routine healing
G = subsequent encounter for fracture with delayed healing
K = subsequent encounter for fracture with nonunion
P = subsequent encounter for fracture with malunion
S = sequela

- [7th] M84.60 Pathological fracture in other disease, unspecified site
- [6] M84.61 Pathological fracture in other disease, shoulder
  - [7] M84.611 Pathological fracture in other disease, right shoulder

Unspecified Code | Other Specified Code | [N] Newborn Age: 0 | [P] Pediatric Age: 0-17 | [M] Maternity Age: 12-55
[A] Adult Age: 15-124 | ♂ Male | ♀ Female | ● New Code | ▲ Revised Code Title | ►◄ Revised Text

[7] M84.612 Pathological fracture in other disease, left shoulder
[7] M84.619 Pathological fracture in other disease, unspecified shoulder
[6] M84.62 Pathological fracture in other disease, humerus
[7] M84.621 Pathological fracture in other disease, right humerus
[7] M84.622 Pathological fracture in other disease, left humerus
[7] M84.629 Pathological fracture in other disease, unspecified humerus
[6] M84.63 Pathological fracture in other disease, ulna and radius
[7] M84.631 Pathological fracture in other disease, right ulna
[7] M84.632 Pathological fracture in other disease, left ulna
[7] M84.633 Pathological fracture in other disease, right radius
[7] M84.634 Pathological fracture in other disease, left radius
[7] M84.639 Pathological fracture in other disease, unspecified ulna and radius
[6] M84.64 Pathological fracture in other disease, hand
[7] M84.641 Pathological fracture in other disease, right hand
[7] M84.642 Pathological fracture in other disease, left hand
[7] M84.649 Pathological fracture in other disease, unspecified hand
[6] M84.65 Pathological fracture in other disease, pelvis and femur
[7] M84.650 Pathological fracture in other disease, pelvis
[7] M84.651 Pathological fracture in other disease, right femur
[7] M84.652 Pathological fracture in other disease, left femur
[7] M84.653 Pathological fracture in other disease, unspecified femur
[7] M84.659 Pathological fracture in other disease, hip, unspecified
[6] M84.66 Pathological fracture in other disease, tibia and fibula
[7] M84.661 Pathological fracture in other disease, right tibia
[7] M84.662 Pathological fracture in other disease, left tibia
[7] M84.663 Pathological fracture in other disease, right fibula
[7] M84.664 Pathological fracture in other disease, left fibula
[7] M84.669 Pathological fracture in other disease, unspecified tibia and fibula
[6] M84.67 Pathological fracture in other disease, ankle and foot
[7] M84.671 Pathological fracture in other disease, right ankle
[7] M84.672 Pathological fracture in other disease, left ankle
[7] M84.673 Pathological fracture in other disease, unspecified ankle
[7] M84.674 Pathological fracture in other disease, right foot
[7] M84.675 Pathological fracture in other disease, left foot
[7] M84.676 Pathological fracture in other disease, unspecified foot
[7X] M84.68 Pathological fracture in other disease, other site

[5] M84.8 Other disorders of continuity of bone
M84.80 Other disorders of continuity of bone, unspecified site
[6] M84.81 Other disorders of continuity of bone, shoulder
M84.811 Other disorders of continuity of bone, right shoulder
M84.812 Other disorders of continuity of bone, left shoulder
M84.819 Other disorders of continuity of bone, unspecified shoulder
[6] M84.82 Other disorders of continuity of bone, humerus
M84.821 Other disorders of continuity of bone, right humerus
M84.822 Other disorders of continuity of bone, left humerus
M84.829 Other disorders of continuity of bone, unspecified humerus
[6] M84.83 Other disorders of continuity of bone, ulna and radius
M84.831 Other disorders of continuity of bone, right ulna
M84.832 Other disorders of continuity of bone, left ulna
M84.833 Other disorders of continuity of bone, right radius
M84.834 Other disorders of continuity of bone, left radius
M84.839 Other disorders of continuity of bone, unspecified ulna and radius
[6] M84.84 Other disorders of continuity of bone, hand
M84.841 Other disorders of continuity of bone, right hand
M84.842 Other disorders of continuity of bone, left hand
M84.849 Other disorders of continuity of bone, unspecified hand
[6] M84.85 Other disorders of continuity of bone, pelvic region and thigh
M84.851 Other disorders of continuity of bone, right pelvic region and thigh
M84.852 Other disorders of continuity of bone, left pelvic region and thigh
M84.859 Other disorders of continuity of bone, unspecified pelvic region and thigh
[6] M84.86 Other disorders of continuity of bone, tibia and fibula
M84.861 Other disorders of continuity of bone, right tibia
M84.862 Other disorders of continuity of bone, left tibia
M84.863 Other disorders of continuity of bone, right fibula
M84.864 Other disorders of continuity of bone, left fibula
M84.869 Other disorders of continuity of bone, unspecified tibia and fibula
[6] M84.87 Other disorders of continuity of bone, ankle and foot
M84.871 Other disorders of continuity of bone, right ankle and foot
M84.872 Other disorders of continuity of bone, left ankle and foot
M84.879 Other disorders of continuity of bone, unspecified ankle and foot
M84.88 Other disorders of continuity of bone, other site
M84.9 Disorder of continuity of bone, unspecified

[4] 4th character required [5] 5th character required [6] 6th character required [7] 7th character required [7X] Extension 'X' Alert
[EXCLUDES 1] Not coded here [EXCLUDES 2] Not included here [PDx] Primary Diagnosis Only Manifestation Code

M85 Other disorders of bone density and structure

> EXCLUDES1 osteogenesis imperfecta (Q78.0)
> osteopetrosis (Q78.2)
> osteopoikilosis (Q78.8)
> polyostotic fibrous dysplasia (Q78.1)

M85.0 Fibrous dysplasia (monostotic)

> EXCLUDES2 fibrous dysplasia of jaw (M27.8)

M85.00 Fibrous dysplasia (monostotic), unspecified site

M85.01 Fibrous dysplasia (monostotic), shoulder
M85.011 Fibrous dysplasia (monostotic), right shoulder
M85.012 Fibrous dysplasia (monostotic), left shoulder
M85.019 Fibrous dysplasia (monostotic), unspecified shoulder

M85.02 Fibrous dysplasia (monostotic), upper arm
M85.021 Fibrous dysplasia (monostotic), right upper arm
M85.022 Fibrous dysplasia (monostotic), left upper arm
M85.029 Fibrous dysplasia (monostotic), unspecified upper arm

M85.03 Fibrous dysplasia (monostotic), forearm
M85.031 Fibrous dysplasia (monostotic), right forearm
M85.032 Fibrous dysplasia (monostotic), left forearm
M85.039 Fibrous dysplasia (monostotic), unspecified forearm

M85.04 Fibrous dysplasia (monostotic), hand
M85.041 Fibrous dysplasia (monostotic), right hand
M85.042 Fibrous dysplasia (monostotic), left hand
M85.049 Fibrous dysplasia (monostotic), unspecified hand

M85.05 Fibrous dysplasia (monostotic), thigh
M85.051 Fibrous dysplasia (monostotic), right thigh
M85.052 Fibrous dysplasia (monostotic), left thigh
M85.059 Fibrous dysplasia (monostotic), unspecified thigh

M85.06 Fibrous dysplasia (monostotic), lower leg
M85.061 Fibrous dysplasia (monostotic), right lower leg
M85.062 Fibrous dysplasia (monostotic), left lower leg
M85.069 Fibrous dysplasia (monostotic), unspecified lower leg

M85.07 Fibrous dysplasia (monostotic), ankle and foot
M85.071 Fibrous dysplasia (monostotic), right ankle and foot
M85.072 Fibrous dysplasia (monostotic), left ankle and foot
M85.079 Fibrous dysplasia (monostotic), unspecified ankle and foot

M85.08 Fibrous dysplasia (monostotic), other site
M85.09 Fibrous dysplasia (monostotic), multiple sites

M85.1 Skeletal fluorosis
M85.10 Skeletal fluorosis, unspecified site

M85.11 Skeletal fluorosis, shoulder
M85.111 Skeletal fluorosis, right shoulder
M85.112 Skeletal fluorosis, left shoulder
M85.119 Skeletal fluorosis, unspecified shoulder

M85.12 Skeletal fluorosis, upper arm
M85.121 Skeletal fluorosis, right upper arm
M85.122 Skeletal fluorosis, left upper arm
M85.129 Skeletal fluorosis, unspecified upper arm

M85.13 Skeletal fluorosis, forearm
M85.131 Skeletal fluorosis, right forearm
M85.132 Skeletal fluorosis, left forearm

M85.139 Skeletal fluorosis, unspecified forearm

M85.14 Skeletal fluorosis, hand
M85.141 Skeletal fluorosis, right hand
M85.142 Skeletal fluorosis, left hand
M85.149 Skeletal fluorosis, unspecified hand

M85.15 Skeletal fluorosis, thigh
M85.151 Skeletal fluorosis, right thigh
M85.152 Skeletal fluorosis, left thigh
M85.159 Skeletal fluorosis, unspecified thigh

M85.16 Skeletal fluorosis, lower leg
M85.161 Skeletal fluorosis, right lower leg
M85.162 Skeletal fluorosis, left lower leg
M85.169 Skeletal fluorosis, unspecified lower leg

M85.17 Skeletal fluorosis, ankle and foot
M85.171 Skeletal fluorosis, right ankle and foot
M85.172 Skeletal fluorosis, left ankle and foot
M85.179 Skeletal fluorosis, unspecified ankle and foot

M85.18 Skeletal fluorosis, other site
M85.19 Skeletal fluorosis, multiple sites

M85.2 Hyperostosis of skull

M85.3 Osteitis condensans
M85.30 Osteitis condensans, unspecified site

M85.31 Osteitis condensans, shoulder
M85.311 Osteitis condensans, right shoulder
M85.312 Osteitis condensans, left shoulder
M85.319 Osteitis condensans, unspecified shoulder

M85.32 Osteitis condensans, upper arm
M85.321 Osteitis condensans, right upper arm
M85.322 Osteitis condensans, left upper arm
M85.329 Osteitis condensans, unspecified upper arm

M85.33 Osteitis condensans, forearm
M85.331 Osteitis condensans, right forearm
M85.332 Osteitis condensans, left forearm
M85.339 Osteitis condensans, unspecified forearm

M85.34 Osteitis condensans, hand
M85.341 Osteitis condensans, right hand
M85.342 Osteitis condensans, left hand
M85.349 Osteitis condensans, unspecified hand

M85.35 Osteitis condensans, thigh
M85.351 Osteitis condensans, right thigh
M85.352 Osteitis condensans, left thigh
M85.359 Osteitis condensans, unspecified thigh

M85.36 Osteitis condensans, lower leg
M85.361 Osteitis condensans, right lower leg
M85.362 Osteitis condensans, left lower leg
M85.369 Osteitis condensans, unspecified lower leg

M85.37 Osteitis condensans, ankle and foot
M85.371 Osteitis condensans, right ankle and foot
M85.372 Osteitis condensans, left ankle and foot
M85.379 Osteitis condensans, unspecified ankle and foot

M85.38 Osteitis condensans, other site
M85.39 Osteitis condensans, multiple sites

M85.4 Solitary bone cyst

> EXCLUDES2 solitary cyst of jaw (M27.4)

M85.40 Solitary bone cyst, unspecified site

M85.41 Solitary bone cyst, shoulder
M85.411 Solitary bone cyst, right shoulder
M85.412 Solitary bone cyst, left shoulder
M85.419 Solitary bone cyst, unspecified shoulder

M85.42 Solitary bone cyst, humerus
M85.421 Solitary bone cyst, right humerus
M85.422 Solitary bone cyst, left humerus
M85.429 Solitary bone cyst, unspecified humerus

Unspecified Code   Other Specified Code   N Newborn Age: 0   P Pediatric Age: 0-17   M Maternity Age: 12-55
A Adult Age: 15-124   ♂ Male   ♀ Female   ● New Code   ▲ Revised Code Title   ►◄ Revised Text

ICD-10-CM 2015   395

M85.43 Solitary bone cyst, ulna and radius
   M85.431 Solitary bone cyst, right ulna and radius
   M85.432 Solitary bone cyst, left ulna and radius
   M85.439 Solitary bone cyst, unspecified ulna and radius
M85.44 Solitary bone cyst, hand
   M85.441 Solitary bone cyst, right hand
   M85.442 Solitary bone cyst, left hand
   M85.449 Solitary bone cyst, unspecified hand
M85.45 Solitary bone cyst, pelvis
   M85.451 Solitary bone cyst, right pelvis
   M85.452 Solitary bone cyst, left pelvis
   M85.459 Solitary bone cyst, unspecified pelvis
M85.46 Solitary bone cyst, tibia and fibula
   M85.461 Solitary bone cyst, right tibia and fibula
   M85.462 Solitary bone cyst, left tibia and fibula
   M85.469 Solitary bone cyst, unspecified tibia and fibula
M85.47 Solitary bone cyst, ankle and foot
   M85.471 Solitary bone cyst, right ankle and foot
   M85.472 Solitary bone cyst, left ankle and foot
   M85.479 Solitary bone cyst, unspecified ankle and foot
M85.48 Solitary bone cyst, other site
M85.5 Aneurysmal bone cyst
   EXCLUDES2 aneurysmal cyst of jaw (M27.4)
M85.50 Aneurysmal bone cyst, unspecified site
M85.51 Aneurysmal bone cyst, shoulder
   M85.511 Aneurysmal bone cyst, right shoulder
   M85.512 Aneurysmal bone cyst, left shoulder
   M85.519 Aneurysmal bone cyst, unspecified shoulder
M85.52 Aneurysmal bone cyst, upper arm
   M85.521 Aneurysmal bone cyst, right upper arm
   M85.522 Aneurysmal bone cyst, left upper arm
   M85.529 Aneurysmal bone cyst, unspecified upper arm
M85.53 Aneurysmal bone cyst, forearm
   M85.531 Aneurysmal bone cyst, right forearm
   M85.532 Aneurysmal bone cyst, left forearm
   M85.539 Aneurysmal bone cyst, unspecified forearm
M85.54 Aneurysmal bone cyst, hand
   M85.541 Aneurysmal bone cyst, right hand
   M85.542 Aneurysmal bone cyst, left hand
   M85.549 Aneurysmal bone cyst, unspecified hand
M85.55 Aneurysmal bone cyst, thigh
   M85.551 Aneurysmal bone cyst, right thigh
   M85.552 Aneurysmal bone cyst, left thigh
   M85.559 Aneurysmal bone cyst, unspecified thigh
M85.56 Aneurysmal bone cyst, lower leg
   M85.561 Aneurysmal bone cyst, right lower leg
   M85.562 Aneurysmal bone cyst, left lower leg
   M85.569 Aneurysmal bone cyst, unspecified lower leg
M85.57 Aneurysmal bone cyst, ankle and foot
   M85.571 Aneurysmal bone cyst, right ankle and foot
   M85.572 Aneurysmal bone cyst, left ankle and foot
   M85.579 Aneurysmal bone cyst, unspecified ankle and foot
M85.58 Aneurysmal bone cyst, other site
M85.59 Aneurysmal bone cyst, multiple sites
M85.6 Other cyst of bone
   EXCLUDES1 cyst of jaw NEC (M27.4)
      osteitis fibrosa cystica generalisata [von Recklinghausen's disease of bone] (E21.0)
M85.60 Other cyst of bone, unspecified site
M85.61 Other cyst of bone, shoulder

M85.611 Other cyst of bone, right shoulder
M85.612 Other cyst of bone, left shoulder
M85.619 Other cyst of bone, unspecified shoulder
M85.62 Other cyst of bone, upper arm
   M85.621 Other cyst of bone, right upper arm
   M85.622 Other cyst of bone, left upper arm
   M85.629 Other cyst of bone, unspecified upper arm
M85.63 Other cyst of bone, forearm
   M85.631 Other cyst of bone, right forearm
   M85.632 Other cyst of bone, left forearm
   M85.639 Other cyst of bone, unspecified forearm
M85.64 Other cyst of bone, hand
   M85.641 Other cyst of bone, right hand
   M85.642 Other cyst of bone, left hand
   M85.649 Other cyst of bone, unspecified hand
M85.65 Other cyst of bone, thigh
   M85.651 Other cyst of bone, right thigh
   M85.652 Other cyst of bone, left thigh
   M85.659 Other cyst of bone, unspecified thigh
M85.66 Other cyst of bone, lower leg
   M85.661 Other cyst of bone, right lower leg
   M85.662 Other cyst of bone, left lower leg
   M85.669 Other cyst of bone, unspecified lower leg
M85.67 Other cyst of bone, ankle and foot
   M85.671 Other cyst of bone, right ankle and foot
   M85.672 Other cyst of bone, left ankle and foot
   M85.679 Other cyst of bone, unspecified ankle and foot
M85.68 Other cyst of bone, other site
M85.69 Other cyst of bone, multiple sites
M85.8 Other specified disorders of bone density and structure
   Hyperostosis of bones, except skull
   Osteosclerosis, acquired
   EXCLUDES1 diffuse idiopathic skeletal hyperostosis [DISH] (M48.1)
      osteosclerosis congenita (Q77.4)
      osteosclerosis fragilitas (generalista) (Q78.2)
      osteosclerosis myelofibrosis (D75.81)
M85.80 Other specified disorders of bone density and structure, unspecified site
M85.81 Other specified disorders of bone density and structure, shoulder
   M85.811 Other specified disorders of bone density and structure, right shoulder
   M85.812 Other specified disorders of bone density and structure, left shoulder
   M85.819 Other specified disorders of bone density and structure, unspecified shoulder
M85.82 Other specified disorders of bone density and structure, upper arm
   M85.821 Other specified disorders of bone density and structure, right upper arm
   M85.822 Other specified disorders of bone density and structure, left upper arm
   M85.829 Other specified disorders of bone density and structure, unspecified upper arm
M85.83 Other specified disorders of bone density and structure, forearm
   M85.831 Other specified disorders of bone density and structure, right forearm
   M85.832 Other specified disorders of bone density and structure, left forearm
   M85.839 Other specified disorders of bone density and structure, unspecified forearm
M85.84 Other specified disorders of bone density and structure, hand

---

4️⃣ 4th character required   5️⃣ 5th character required   6️⃣ 6th character required   7️⃣ 7th character required   🅧 Extension 'X' Alert

EXCLUDES 1 Not coded here   EXCLUDES 2 Not included here   PDx Primary Diagnosis Only   Manifestation Code

M85.841 Other specified disorders of bone density and structure, right hand
M85.842 Other specified disorders of bone density and structure, left hand
M85.849 Other specified disorders of bone density and structure, unspecified hand
[6] M85.85 Other specified disorders of bone density and structure, thigh
M85.851 Other specified disorders of bone density and structure, right thigh
M85.852 Other specified disorders of bone density and structure, left thigh
M85.859 Other specified disorders of bone density and structure, unspecified thigh
[6] M85.86 Other specified disorders of bone density and structure, lower leg
M85.861 Other specified disorders of bone density and structure, right lower leg
M85.862 Other specified disorders of bone density and structure, left lower leg
M85.869 Other specified disorders of bone density and structure, unspecified lower leg
[6] M85.87 Other specified disorders of bone density and structure, ankle and foot
M85.871 Other specified disorders of bone density and structure, right ankle and foot
M85.872 Other specified disorders of bone density and structure, left ankle and foot
M85.879 Other specified disorders of bone density and structure, unspecified ankle and foot
M85.88 Other specified disorders of bone density and structure, other site
M85.89 Other specified disorders of bone density and structure, multiple sites
M85.9 Disorder of bone density and structure, unspecified

Other osteopathies (M86-M90)

[EXCLUDES1] *postprocedural osteopathies (M96.-)*

[4] M86 Osteomyelitis
Use additional code (B95-B97) to identify infectious agent
code to identify major osseous defect, if applicable (M89.7-)
[EXCLUDES1] *osteomyelitis due to:*
echinococcus (B67.2)
gonococcus (A54.43)
salmonella (A02.24)
[EXCLUDES2] *ostemyelitis of:*
orbit (H05.0-)
petrous bone (H70.2-)
vertebra (M46.2-)
[5] M86.0 Acute hematogenous osteomyelitis
M86.00 Acute hematogenous osteomyelitis, unspecified site
[6] M86.01 Acute hematogenous osteomyelitis, shoulder
M86.011 Acute hematogenous osteomyelitis, right shoulder
M86.012 Acute hematogenous osteomyelitis, left shoulder
M86.019 Acute hematogenous osteomyelitis, unspecified shoulder
[6] M86.02 Acute hematogenous osteomyelitis, humerus
M86.021 Acute hematogenous osteomyelitis, right humerus
M86.022 Acute hematogenous osteomyelitis, left humerus
M86.029 Acute hematogenous osteomyelitis, unspecified humerus
[6] M86.03 Acute hematogenous osteomyelitis, radius and ulna
M86.031 Acute hematogenous osteomyelitis, right radius and ulna
M86.032 Acute hematogenous osteomyelitis, left radius and ulna
M86.039 Acute hematogenous osteomyelitis, unspecified radius and ulna
[6] M86.04 Acute hematogenous osteomyelitis, hand
M86.041 Acute hematogenous osteomyelitis, right hand
M86.042 Acute hematogenous osteomyelitis, left hand
M86.049 Acute hematogenous osteomyelitis, unspecified hand
[6] M86.05 Acute hematogenous osteomyelitis, femur
M86.051 Acute hematogenous osteomyelitis, right femur
M86.052 Acute hematogenous osteomyelitis, left femur
M86.059 Acute hematogenous osteomyelitis, unspecified femur
[6] M86.06 Acute hematogenous osteomyelitis, tibia and fibula
M86.061 Acute hematogenous osteomyelitis, right tibia and fibula
M86.062 Acute hematogenous osteomyelitis, left tibia and fibula
M86.069 Acute hematogenous osteomyelitis, unspecified tibia and fibula
[6] M86.07 Acute hematogenous osteomyelitis, ankle and foot
M86.071 Acute hematogenous osteomyelitis, right ankle and foot
M86.072 Acute hematogenous osteomyelitis, left ankle and foot
M86.079 Acute hematogenous osteomyelitis, unspecified ankle and foot
M86.08 Acute hematogenous osteomyelitis, other sites
M86.09 Acute hematogenous osteomyelitis, multiple sites
[5] M86.1 Other acute osteomyelitis
M86.10 Other acute osteomyelitis, unspecified site
[6] M86.11 Other acute osteomyelitis, shoulder
M86.111 Other acute osteomyelitis, right shoulder
M86.112 Other acute osteomyelitis, left shoulder
M86.119 Other acute osteomyelitis, unspecified shoulder
[6] M86.12 Other acute osteomyelitis, humerus
M86.121 Other acute osteomyelitis, right humerus
M86.122 Other acute osteomyelitis, left humerus
M86.129 Other acute osteomyelitis, unspecified humerus
[6] M86.13 Other acute osteomyelitis, radius and ulna
M86.131 Other acute osteomyelitis, right radius and ulna
M86.132 Other acute osteomyelitis, left radius and ulna
M86.139 Other acute osteomyelitis, unspecified radius and ulna
[6] M86.14 Other acute osteomyelitis, hand
M86.141 Other acute osteomyelitis, right hand
M86.142 Other acute osteomyelitis, left hand
M86.149 Other acute osteomyelitis, unspecified hand
[6] M86.15 Other acute osteomyelitis, femur
M86.151 Other acute osteomyelitis, right femur
M86.152 Other acute osteomyelitis, left femur

Unspecified Code | Other Specified Code | [N] Newborn Age: 0 | [P] Pediatric Age: 0-17 | [M] Maternity Age: 12-55
[A] Adult Age: 15-124 | ♂ Male | ♀ Female | ● New Code | ▲ Revised Code Title | ►◄ Revised Text

M86.159 Other acute osteomyelitis, unspecified femur
[6] M86.16 Other acute osteomyelitis, tibia and fibula
M86.161 Other acute osteomyelitis, right tibia and fibula
M86.162 Other acute osteomyelitis, left tibia and fibula
M86.169 Other acute osteomyelitis, unspecified tibia and fibula
[6] M86.17 Other acute osteomyelitis, ankle and foot
M86.171 Other acute osteomyelitis, right ankle and foot
M86.172 Other acute osteomyelitis, left ankle and foot
M86.179 Other acute osteomyelitis, unspecified ankle and foot
M86.18 Other acute osteomyelitis, other site
M86.19 Other acute osteomyelitis, multiple sites
[5] M86.2 Subacute osteomyelitis
M86.20 Subacute osteomyelitis, unspecified site
[6] M86.21 Subacute osteomyelitis, shoulder
M86.211 Subacute osteomyelitis, right shoulder
M86.212 Subacute osteomyelitis, left shoulder
M86.219 Subacute osteomyelitis, unspecified shoulder
[6] M86.22 Subacute osteomyelitis, humerus
M86.221 Subacute osteomyelitis, right humerus
M86.222 Subacute osteomyelitis, left humerus
M86.229 Subacute osteomyelitis, unspecified humerus
[6] M86.23 Subacute osteomyelitis, radius and ulna
M86.231 Subacute osteomyelitis, right radius and ulna
M86.232 Subacute osteomyelitis, left radius and ulna
M86.239 Subacute osteomyelitis, unspecified radius and ulna
[6] M86.24 Subacute osteomyelitis, hand
M86.241 Subacute osteomyelitis, right hand
M86.242 Subacute osteomyelitis, left hand
M86.249 Subacute osteomyelitis, unspecified hand
[6] M86.25 Subacute osteomyelitis, femur
M86.251 Subacute osteomyelitis, right femur
M86.252 Subacute osteomyelitis, left femur
M86.259 Subacute osteomyelitis, unspecified femur
[6] M86.26 Subacute osteomyelitis, tibia and fibula
M86.261 Subacute osteomyelitis, right tibia and fibula
M86.262 Subacute osteomyelitis, left tibia and fibula
M86.269 Subacute osteomyelitis, unspecified tibia and fibula
[6] M86.27 Subacute osteomyelitis, ankle and foot
M86.271 Subacute osteomyelitis, right ankle and foot
M86.272 Subacute osteomyelitis, left ankle and foot
M86.279 Subacute osteomyelitis, unspecified ankle and foot
M86.28 Subacute osteomyelitis, other site
M86.29 Subacute osteomyelitis, multiple sites
[5] M86.3 Chronic multifocal osteomyelitis
M86.30 Chronic multifocal osteomyelitis, unspecified site
[6] M86.31 Chronic multifocal osteomyelitis, shoulder
M86.311 Chronic multifocal osteomyelitis, right shoulder
M86.312 Chronic multifocal osteomyelitis, left shoulder
M86.319 Chronic multifocal osteomyelitis, unspecified shoulder
[6] M86.32 Chronic multifocal osteomyelitis, humerus
M86.321 Chronic multifocal osteomyelitis, right humerus
M86.322 Chronic multifocal osteomyelitis, left humerus
M86.329 Chronic multifocal osteomyelitis, unspecified humerus
[6] M86.33 Chronic multifocal osteomyelitis, radius and ulna
M86.331 Chronic multifocal osteomyelitis, right radius and ulna
M86.332 Chronic multifocal osteomyelitis, left radius and ulna
M86.339 Chronic multifocal osteomyelitis, unspecified radius and ulna
[6] M86.34 Chronic multifocal osteomyelitis, hand
M86.341 Chronic multifocal osteomyelitis, right hand
M86.342 Chronic multifocal osteomyelitis, left hand
M86.349 Chronic multifocal osteomyelitis, unspecified hand
[6] M86.35 Chronic multifocal osteomyelitis, femur
M86.351 Chronic multifocal osteomyelitis, right femur
M86.352 Chronic multifocal osteomyelitis, left femur
M86.359 Chronic multifocal osteomyelitis, unspecified femur
[6] M86.36 Chronic multifocal osteomyelitis, tibia and fibula
M86.361 Chronic multifocal osteomyelitis, right tibia and fibula
M86.362 Chronic multifocal osteomyelitis, left tibia and fibula
M86.369 Chronic multifocal osteomyelitis, unspecified tibia and fibula
[6] M86.37 Chronic multifocal osteomyelitis, ankle and foot
M86.371 Chronic multifocal osteomyelitis, right ankle and foot
M86.372 Chronic multifocal osteomyelitis, left ankle and foot
M86.379 Chronic multifocal osteomyelitis, unspecified ankle and foot
M86.38 Chronic multifocal osteomyelitis, other site
M86.39 Chronic multifocal osteomyelitis, multiple sites
[5] M86.4 Chronic osteomyelitis with draining sinus
M86.40 Chronic osteomyelitis with draining sinus, unspecified site
[6] M86.41 Chronic osteomyelitis with draining sinus, shoulder
M86.411 Chronic osteomyelitis with draining sinus, right shoulder
M86.412 Chronic osteomyelitis with draining sinus, left shoulder
M86.419 Chronic osteomyelitis with draining sinus, unspecified shoulder
[6] M86.42 Chronic osteomyelitis with draining sinus, humerus
M86.421 Chronic osteomyelitis with draining sinus, right humerus
M86.422 Chronic osteomyelitis with draining sinus, left humerus
M86.429 Chronic osteomyelitis with draining sinus, unspecified humerus
[6] M86.43 Chronic osteomyelitis with draining sinus, radius and ulna
M86.431 Chronic osteomyelitis with draining sinus, right radius and ulna

[4] 4th character required [5] 5th character required [6] 6th character required [7] 7th character required [7] Extension 'X' Alert
EXCLUDES 1 Not coded here EXCLUDES 2 Not included here PDx Primary Diagnosis Only Manifestation Code

M86.432 Chronic osteomyelitis with draining sinus, left radius and ulna

M86.439 Chronic osteomyelitis with draining sinus, unspecified radius and ulna

6⃝ M86.44 Chronic osteomyelitis with draining sinus, hand

M86.441 Chronic osteomyelitis with draining sinus, right hand

M86.442 Chronic osteomyelitis with draining sinus, left hand

M86.449 Chronic osteomyelitis with draining sinus, unspecified hand

6⃝ M86.45 Chronic osteomyelitis with draining sinus, femur

M86.451 Chronic osteomyelitis with draining sinus, right femur

M86.452 Chronic osteomyelitis with draining sinus, left femur

M86.459 Chronic osteomyelitis with draining sinus, unspecified femur

6⃝ M86.46 Chronic osteomyelitis with draining sinus, tibia and fibula

M86.461 Chronic osteomyelitis with draining sinus, right tibia and fibula

M86.462 Chronic osteomyelitis with draining sinus, left tibia and fibula

M86.469 Chronic osteomyelitis with draining sinus, unspecified tibia and fibula

6⃝ M86.47 Chronic osteomyelitis with draining sinus, ankle and foot

M86.471 Chronic osteomyelitis with draining sinus, right ankle and foot

M86.472 Chronic osteomyelitis with draining sinus, left ankle and foot

M86.479 Chronic osteomyelitis with draining sinus, unspecified ankle and foot

M86.48 Chronic osteomyelitis with draining sinus, other site

M86.49 Chronic osteomyelitis with draining sinus, multiple sites

5⃝ M86.5 Other chronic hematogenous osteomyelitis

M86.50 Other chronic hematogenous osteomyelitis, unspecified site

6⃝ M86.51 Other chronic hematogenous osteomyelitis, shoulder

M86.511 Other chronic hematogenous osteomyelitis, right shoulder

M86.512 Other chronic hematogenous osteomyelitis, left shoulder

M86.519 Other chronic hematogenous osteomyelitis, unspecified shoulder

6⃝ M86.52 Other chronic hematogenous osteomyelitis, humerus

M86.521 Other chronic hematogenous osteomyelitis, right humerus

M86.522 Other chronic hematogenous osteomyelitis, left humerus

M86.529 Other chronic hematogenous osteomyelitis, unspecified humerus

6⃝ M86.53 Other chronic hematogenous osteomyelitis, radius and ulna

M86.531 Other chronic hematogenous osteomyelitis, right radius and ulna

M86.532 Other chronic hematogenous osteomyelitis, left radius and ulna

M86.539 Other chronic hematogenous osteomyelitis, unspecified radius and ulna

6⃝ M86.54 Other chronic hematogenous osteomyelitis, hand

M86.541 Other chronic hematogenous osteomyelitis, right hand

M86.542 Other chronic hematogenous osteomyelitis, left hand

M86.549 Other chronic hematogenous osteomyelitis, unspecified hand

6⃝ M86.55 Other chronic hematogenous osteomyelitis, femur

M86.551 Other chronic hematogenous osteomyelitis, right femur

M86.552 Other chronic hematogenous osteomyelitis, left femur

M86.559 Other chronic hematogenous osteomyelitis, unspecified femur

6⃝ M86.56 Other chronic hematogenous osteomyelitis, tibia and fibula

M86.561 Other chronic hematogenous osteomyelitis, right tibia and fibula

M86.562 Other chronic hematogenous osteomyelitis, left tibia and fibula

M86.569 Other chronic hematogenous osteomyelitis, unspecified tibia and fibula

6⃝ M86.57 Other chronic hematogenous osteomyelitis, ankle and foot

M86.571 Other chronic hematogenous osteomyelitis, right ankle and foot

M86.572 Other chronic hematogenous osteomyelitis, left ankle and foot

M86.579 Other chronic hematogenous osteomyelitis, unspecified ankle and foot

M86.58 Other chronic hematogenous osteomyelitis, other site

M86.59 Other chronic hematogenous osteomyelitis, multiple sites

5⃝ M86.6 Other chronic osteomyelitis

M86.60 Other chronic osteomyelitis, unspecified site

6⃝ M86.61 Other chronic osteomyelitis, shoulder

M86.611 Other chronic osteomyelitis, right shoulder

M86.612 Other chronic osteomyelitis, left shoulder

M86.619 Other chronic osteomyelitis, unspecified shoulder

6⃝ M86.62 Other chronic osteomyelitis, humerus

M86.621 Other chronic osteomyelitis, right humerus

M86.622 Other chronic osteomyelitis, left humerus

M86.629 Other chronic osteomyelitis, unspecified humerus

6⃝ M86.63 Other chronic osteomyelitis, radius and ulna

M86.631 Other chronic osteomyelitis, right radius and ulna

M86.632 Other chronic osteomyelitis, left radius and ulna

M86.639 Other chronic osteomyelitis, unspecified radius and ulna

6⃝ M86.64 Other chronic osteomyelitis, hand

M86.641 Other chronic osteomyelitis, right hand

M86.642 Other chronic osteomyelitis, left hand

M86.649 Other chronic osteomyelitis, unspecified hand

6⃝ M86.65 Other chronic osteomyelitis, thigh

M86.651 Other chronic osteomyelitis, right thigh

M86.652 Other chronic osteomyelitis, left thigh

M86.659 Other chronic osteomyelitis, unspecified thigh

6⃝ M86.66 Other chronic osteomyelitis, tibia and fibula

M86.661 Other chronic osteomyelitis, right tibia and fibula

M86.662 Other chronic osteomyelitis, left tibia and fibula

M86.669 Other chronic osteomyelitis, unspecified tibia and fibula

| Unspecified Code | Other Specified Code | N Newborn Age: 0 | P Pediatric Age: 0-17 | M Maternity Age: 12-55 |
| A Adult Age: 15-124 | ♂ Male | ♀ Female | ● New Code | ▲ Revised Code Title | ►◄ Revised Text |

ICD-10-CM 2015

399

Ⓖ M86.67 Other chronic osteomyelitis, ankle and foot
  M86.671 Other chronic osteomyelitis, right ankle and foot
  M86.672 Other chronic osteomyelitis, left ankle and foot
  M86.679 Other chronic osteomyelitis, unspecified ankle and foot
M86.68 Other chronic osteomyelitis, other site
M86.69 Other chronic osteomyelitis, multiple sites
Ⓔ M86.8 Other osteomyelitis
  Brodie's abscess
  Ⓖ M86.8X Other osteomyelitis
    M86.8X0 Other osteomyelitis, multiple sites
    M86.8X1 Other osteomyelitis, shoulder
    M86.8X2 Other osteomyelitis, upper arm
    M86.8X3 Other osteomyelitis, forearm
    M86.8X4 Other osteomyelitis, hand
    M86.8X5 Other osteomyelitis, thigh
    M86.8X6 Other osteomyelitis, lower leg
    M86.8X7 Other osteomyelitis, ankle and foot
    M86.8X8 Other osteomyelitis, other site
    M86.8X9 Other osteomyelitis, unspecified sites
M86.9 Osteomyelitis, unspecified
  Infection of bone NOS
  Periostitis without osteomyelitis
Ⓓ M87 Osteonecrosis
  INCLUDES avascular necrosis of bone
  Use additional code to identify major osseous defect, if applicable (M89.7-)
  EXCLUDES1 juvenile osteonecrosis (M91-M92)
             osteochondropathies (M90-M93)
Ⓔ M87.0 Idiopathic aseptic necrosis of bone
  M87.00 Idiopathic aseptic necrosis of unspecified bone
  Ⓖ M87.01 Idiopathic aseptic necrosis of shoulder
    Idiopathic aseptic necrosis of clavicle and scapula
    M87.011 Idiopathic aseptic necrosis of right shoulder
    M87.012 Idiopathic aseptic necrosis of left shoulder
    M87.019 Idiopathic aseptic necrosis of unspecified shoulder
  Ⓖ M87.02 Idiopathic aseptic necrosis of humerus
    M87.021 Idiopathic aseptic necrosis of right humerus
    M87.022 Idiopathic aseptic necrosis of left humerus
    M87.029 Idiopathic aseptic necrosis of unspecified humerus
  Ⓖ M87.03 Idiopathic aseptic necrosis of radius, ulna and carpus
    M87.031 Idiopathic aseptic necrosis of right radius
    M87.032 Idiopathic aseptic necrosis of left radius
    M87.033 Idiopathic aseptic necrosis of unspecified radius
    M87.034 Idiopathic aseptic necrosis of right ulna
    M87.035 Idiopathic aseptic necrosis of left ulna
    M87.036 Idiopathic aseptic necrosis of unspecified ulna
    M87.037 Idiopathic aseptic necrosis of right carpus
    M87.038 Idiopathic aseptic necrosis of left carpus
    M87.039 Idiopathic aseptic necrosis of unspecified carpus
  Ⓖ M87.04 Idiopathic aseptic necrosis of hand and fingers
    Idiopathic aseptic necrosis of metacarpals and phalanges of hands
    M87.041 Idiopathic aseptic necrosis of right hand
    M87.042 Idiopathic aseptic necrosis of left hand
    M87.043 Idiopathic aseptic necrosis of unspecified hand

  M87.044 Idiopathic aseptic necrosis of right finger(s)
  M87.045 Idiopathic aseptic necrosis of left finger(s)
  M87.046 Idiopathic aseptic necrosis of unspecified finger(s)
Ⓖ M87.05 Idiopathic aseptic necrosis of pelvis and femur
  M87.050 Idiopathic aseptic necrosis of pelvis
  M87.051 Idiopathic aseptic necrosis of right femur
  M87.052 Idiopathic aseptic necrosis of left femur
  M87.059 Idiopathic aseptic necrosis of unspecified femur
  Idiopathic aseptic necrosis of hip NOS
Ⓖ M87.06 Idiopathic aseptic necrosis of tibia and fibula
  M87.061 Idiopathic aseptic necrosis of right tibia
  M87.062 Idiopathic aseptic necrosis of left tibia
  M87.063 Idiopathic aseptic necrosis of unspecified tibia
  M87.064 Idiopathic aseptic necrosis of right fibula
  M87.065 Idiopathic aseptic necrosis of left fibula
  M87.066 Idiopathic aseptic necrosis of unspecified fibula
Ⓖ M87.07 Idiopathic aseptic necrosis of ankle, foot and toes
  Idiopathic aseptic necrosis of metatarsus, tarsus, and phalanges of toes
  M87.071 Idiopathic aseptic necrosis of right ankle
  M87.072 Idiopathic aseptic necrosis of left ankle
  M87.073 Idiopathic aseptic necrosis of unspecified ankle
  M87.074 Idiopathic aseptic necrosis of right foot
  M87.075 Idiopathic aseptic necrosis of left foot
  M87.076 Idiopathic aseptic necrosis of unspecified foot
  M87.077 Idiopathic aseptic necrosis of right toe(s)
  M87.078 Idiopathic aseptic necrosis of left toe(s)
  M87.079 Idiopathic aseptic necrosis of unspecified toe(s)
M87.08 Idiopathic aseptic necrosis of bone, other site
M87.09 Idiopathic aseptic necrosis of bone, multiple sites
Ⓔ M87.1 Osteonecrosis due to drugs
  Use additional code for adverse effect, if applicable, to identify drug (T36-T50 with fifth or sixth character 5)
  M87.10 Osteonecrosis due to drugs, unspecified bone
Ⓖ M87.11 Osteonecrosis due to drugs, shoulder
  M87.111 Osteonecrosis due to drugs, right shoulder
  M87.112 Osteonecrosis due to drugs, left shoulder
  M87.119 Osteonecrosis due to drugs, unspecified shoulder
Ⓖ M87.12 Osteonecrosis due to drugs, humerus
  M87.121 Osteonecrosis due to drugs, right humerus
  M87.122 Osteonecrosis due to drugs, left humerus
  M87.129 Osteonecrosis due to drugs, unspecified humerus
Ⓖ M87.13 Osteonecrosis due to drugs of radius, ulna and carpus
  M87.131 Osteonecrosis due to drugs of right radius
  M87.132 Osteonecrosis due to drugs of left radius
  M87.133 Osteonecrosis due to drugs of unspecified radius
  M87.134 Osteonecrosis due to drugs of right ulna
  M87.135 Osteonecrosis due to drugs of left ulna
  M87.136 Osteonecrosis due to drugs of unspecified ulna
  M87.137 Osteonecrosis due to drugs of right carpus
  M87.138 Osteonecrosis due to drugs of left carpus
  M87.139 Osteonecrosis due to drugs of unspecified carpus
Ⓖ M87.14 Osteonecrosis due to drugs, hand and fingers

Ⓓ 4th character required   Ⓔ 5th character required   Ⓖ 6th character required   Ⓟ 7th character required   Ⓧ Extension 'X' Alert

EXCLUDES 1 Not coded here   EXCLUDES 2 Not included here   PDx Primary Diagnosis Only   Manifestation Code

M87.141 Osteonecrosis due to drugs, right hand
M87.142 Osteonecrosis due to drugs, left hand
M87.143 Osteonecrosis due to drugs, unspecified hand
M87.144 Osteonecrosis due to drugs, right finger(s)
M87.145 Osteonecrosis due to drugs, left finger(s)
M87.146 Osteonecrosis due to drugs, unspecified finger(s)

[6] M87.15 Osteonecrosis due to drugs, pelvis and femur
M87.150 Osteonecrosis due to drugs, pelvis
M87.151 Osteonecrosis due to drugs, right femur
M87.152 Osteonecrosis due to drugs, left femur
M87.159 Osteonecrosis due to drugs, unspecified femur

[6] M87.16 Osteonecrosis due to drugs, tibia and fibula
M87.161 Osteonecrosis due to drugs, right tibia
M87.162 Osteonecrosis due to drugs, left tibia
M87.163 Osteonecrosis due to drugs, unspecified tibia
M87.164 Osteonecrosis due to drugs, right fibula
M87.165 Osteonecrosis due to drugs, left fibula
M87.166 Osteonecrosis due to drugs, unspecified fibula

[6] M87.17 Osteonecrosis due to drugs, ankle, foot and toes
M87.171 Osteonecrosis due to drugs, right ankle
M87.172 Osteonecrosis due to drugs, left ankle
M87.173 Osteonecrosis due to drugs, unspecified ankle
M87.174 Osteonecrosis due to drugs, right foot
M87.175 Osteonecrosis due to drugs, left foot
M87.176 Osteonecrosis due to drugs, unspecified foot
M87.177 Osteonecrosis due to drugs, right toe(s)
M87.178 Osteonecrosis due to drugs, left toe(s)
M87.179 Osteonecrosis due to drugs, unspecified toe(s)

[6] M87.18 Osteonecrosis due to drugs, other site
M87.180 Osteonecrosis due to drugs, jaw
M87.188 Osteonecrosis due to drugs, other site

M87.19 Osteonecrosis due to drugs, multiple sites

[5] M87.2 Osteonecrosis due to previous trauma
M87.20 Osteonecrosis due to previous trauma, unspecified bone

[6] M87.21 Osteonecrosis due to previous trauma, shoulder
M87.211 Osteonecrosis due to previous trauma, right shoulder
M87.212 Osteonecrosis due to previous trauma, left shoulder
M87.219 Osteonecrosis due to previous trauma, unspecified shoulder

[6] M87.22 Osteonecrosis due to previous trauma, humerus
M87.221 Osteonecrosis due to previous trauma, right humerus
M87.222 Osteonecrosis due to previous trauma, left humerus
M87.229 Osteonecrosis due to previous trauma, unspecified humerus

[6] M87.23 Osteonecrosis due to previous trauma of radius, ulna and carpus
M87.231 Osteonecrosis due to previous trauma of right radius
M87.232 Osteonecrosis due to previous trauma of left radius
M87.233 Osteonecrosis due to previous trauma of unspecified radius
M87.234 Osteonecrosis due to previous trauma of right ulna
M87.235 Osteonecrosis due to previous trauma of left ulna
M87.236 Osteonecrosis due to previous trauma of unspecified ulna
M87.237 Osteonecrosis due to previous trauma of right carpus
M87.238 Osteonecrosis due to previous trauma of left carpus
M87.239 Osteonecrosis due to previous trauma of unspecified carpus

[6] M87.24 Osteonecrosis due to previous trauma, hand and fingers
M87.241 Osteonecrosis due to previous trauma, right hand
M87.242 Osteonecrosis due to previous trauma, left hand
M87.243 Osteonecrosis due to previous trauma, unspecified hand
M87.244 Osteonecrosis due to previous trauma, right finger(s)
M87.245 Osteonecrosis due to previous trauma, left finger(s)
M87.246 Osteonecrosis due to previous trauma, unspecified finger(s)

[6] M87.25 Osteonecrosis due to previous trauma, pelvis and femur
M87.250 Osteonecrosis due to previous trauma, pelvis
M87.251 Osteonecrosis due to previous trauma, right femur
M87.252 Osteonecrosis due to previous trauma, left femur
M87.256 Osteonecrosis due to previous trauma, unspecified femur

[6] M87.26 Osteonecrosis due to previous trauma, tibia and fibula
M87.261 Osteonecrosis due to previous trauma, right tibia
M87.262 Osteonecrosis due to previous trauma, left tibia
M87.263 Osteonecrosis due to previous trauma, unspecified tibia
M87.264 Osteonecrosis due to previous trauma, right fibula
M87.265 Osteonecrosis due to previous trauma, left fibula
M87.266 Osteonecrosis due to previous trauma, unspecified fibula

[6] M87.27 Osteonecrosis due to previous trauma, ankle, foot and toes
M87.271 Osteonecrosis due to previous trauma, right ankle
M87.272 Osteonecrosis due to previous trauma, left ankle
M87.273 Osteonecrosis due to previous trauma, unspecified ankle
M87.274 Osteonecrosis due to previous trauma, right foot
M87.275 Osteonecrosis due to previous trauma, left foot
M87.276 Osteonecrosis due to previous trauma, unspecified foot
M87.277 Osteonecrosis due to previous trauma, right toe(s)
M87.278 Osteonecrosis due to previous trauma, left toe(s)
M87.279 Osteonecrosis due to previous trauma, unspecified toe(s)

Unspecified Code | Other Specified Code | [N] Newborn Age: 0 | [P] Pediatric Age: 0-17 | [M] Maternity Age: 12-55
[A] Adult Age: 15-124 | ♂ Male | ♀ Female | ● New Code | ▲ Revised Code Title | ►◄ Revised Text

M87.28 Osteonecrosis due to previous trauma, other site
M87.29 Osteonecrosis due to previous trauma, multiple sites

[5] M87.3 Other secondary osteonecrosis
M87.30 Other secondary osteonecrosis, unspecified bone

[6] M87.31 Other secondary osteonecrosis, shoulder
M87.311 Other secondary osteonecrosis, right shoulder
M87.312 Other secondary osteonecrosis, left shoulder
M87.319 Other secondary osteonecrosis, unspecified shoulder

[6] M87.32 Other secondary osteonecrosis, humerus
M87.321 Other secondary osteonecrosis, right humerus
M87.322 Other secondary osteonecrosis, left humerus
M87.329 Other secondary osteonecrosis, unspecified humerus

[6] M87.33 Other secondary osteonecrosis of radius, ulna and carpus
M87.331 Other secondary osteonecrosis of right radius
M87.332 Other secondary osteonecrosis of left radius
M87.333 Other secondary osteonecrosis of unspecified radius
M87.334 Other secondary osteonecrosis of right ulna
M87.335 Other secondary osteonecrosis of left ulna
M87.336 Other secondary osteonecrosis of unspecified ulna
M87.337 Other secondary osteonecrosis of right carpus
M87.338 Other secondary osteonecrosis of left carpus
M87.339 Other secondary osteonecrosis of unspecified carpus

[6] M87.34 Other secondary osteonecrosis, hand and fingers
M87.341 Other secondary osteonecrosis, right hand
M87.342 Other secondary osteonecrosis, left hand
M87.343 Other secondary osteonecrosis, unspecified hand
M87.344 Other secondary osteonecrosis, right finger(s)
M87.345 Other secondary osteonecrosis, left finger(s)
M87.346 Other secondary osteonecrosis, unspecified finger(s)

[6] M87.35 Other secondary osteonecrosis, pelvis and femur
M87.350 Other secondary osteonecrosis, pelvis
M87.351 Other secondary osteonecrosis, right femur
M87.352 Other secondary osteonecrosis, left femur
M87.353 Other secondary osteonecrosis, unspecified femur

[6] M87.36 Other secondary osteonecrosis, tibia and fibula
M87.361 Other secondary osteonecrosis, right tibia
M87.362 Other secondary osteonecrosis, left tibia
M87.363 Other secondary osteonecrosis, unspecified tibia
M87.364 Other secondary osteonecrosis, right fibula
M87.365 Other secondary osteonecrosis, left fibula
M87.366 Other secondary osteonecrosis, unspecified fibula

[6] M87.37 Other secondary osteonecrosis, ankle and foot
M87.371 Other secondary osteonecrosis, right ankle
M87.372 Other secondary osteonecrosis, left ankle
M87.373 Other secondary osteonecrosis, unspecified ankle
M87.374 Other secondary osteonecrosis, right foot
M87.375 Other secondary osteonecrosis, left foot
M87.376 Other secondary osteonecrosis, unspecified foot
M87.377 Other secondary osteonecrosis, right toe(s)
M87.378 Other secondary osteonecrosis, left toe(s)
M87.379 Other secondary osteonecrosis, unspecified toe(s)

M87.38 Other secondary osteonecrosis, other site
M87.39 Other secondary osteonecrosis, multiple sites

[5] M87.8 Other osteonecrosis
M87.80 Other osteonecrosis, unspecified bone

[6] M87.81 Other osteonecrosis, shoulder
M87.811 Other osteonecrosis, right shoulder
M87.812 Other osteonecrosis, left shoulder
M87.819 Other osteonecrosis, unspecified shoulder

[6] M87.82 Other osteonecrosis, humerus
M87.821 Other osteonecrosis, right humerus
M87.822 Other osteonecrosis, left humerus
M87.829 Other osteonecrosis, unspecified humerus

[6] M87.83 Other osteonecrosis of radius, ulna and carpus
M87.831 Other osteonecrosis of right radius
M87.832 Other osteonecrosis of left radius
M87.833 Other osteonecrosis of unspecified radius
M87.834 Other osteonecrosis of right ulna
M87.835 Other osteonecrosis of left ulna
M87.836 Other osteonecrosis of unspecified ulna
M87.837 Other osteonecrosis of right carpus
M87.838 Other osteonecrosis of left carpus
M87.839 Other osteonecrosis of unspecified carpus

[6] M87.84 Other osteonecrosis, hand and fingers
M87.841 Other osteonecrosis, right hand
M87.842 Other osteonecrosis, left hand
M87.843 Other osteonecrosis, unspecified hand
M87.844 Other osteonecrosis, right finger(s)
M87.845 Other osteonecrosis, left finger(s)
M87.849 Other osteonecrosis, unspecified finger(s)

[6] M87.85 Other osteonecrosis, pelvis and femur
M87.850 Other osteonecrosis, pelvis
M87.851 Other osteonecrosis, right femur
M87.852 Other osteonecrosis, left femur
M87.859 Other osteonecrosis, unspecified femur

[6] M87.86 Other osteonecrosis, tibia and fibula
M87.861 Other osteonecrosis, right tibia
M87.862 Other osteonecrosis, left tibia
M87.863 Other osteonecrosis, unspecified tibia
M87.864 Other osteonecrosis, right fibula
M87.865 Other osteonecrosis, left fibula
M87.869 Other osteonecrosis, unspecified fibula

[6] M87.87 Other osteonecrosis, ankle, foot and toes
M87.871 Other osteonecrosis, right ankle
M87.872 Other osteonecrosis, left ankle
M87.873 Other osteonecrosis, unspecified ankle
M87.874 Other osteonecrosis, right foot
M87.875 Other osteonecrosis, left foot
M87.876 Other osteonecrosis, unspecified foot
M87.877 Other osteonecrosis, right toe(s)
M87.878 Other osteonecrosis, left toe(s)
M87.879 Other osteonecrosis, unspecified toe(s)

M87.88 Other osteonecrosis, other site
M87.89 Other osteonecrosis, multiple sites

M87.9 Osteonecrosis, unspecified
Necrosis of bone NOS

[4] M88 Osteitis deformans [Paget's disease of bone]
[EXCLUDES1] *osteitis deformans in neoplastic disease (M90.6)*
M88.0 Osteitis deformans of skull
M88.1 Osteitis deformans of vertebrae
[5] M88.8 Osteitis deformans of other bones
[6] M88.81 Osteitis deformans of shoulder
M88.811 Osteitis deformans of right shoulder
M88.812 Osteitis deformans of left shoulder
M88.819 Osteitis deformans of unspecified shoulder
[6] M88.82 Osteitis deformans of upper arm
M88.821 Osteitis deformans of right upper arm
M88.822 Osteitis deformans of left upper arm
M88.829 Osteitis deformans of unspecified upper arm
[6] M88.83 Osteitis deformans of forearm
M88.831 Osteitis deformans of right forearm
M88.832 Osteitis deformans of left forearm
M88.839 Osteitis deformans of unspecified forearm
[6] M88.84 Osteitis deformans of hand
M88.841 Osteitis deformans of right hand
M88.842 Osteitis deformans of left hand
M88.849 Osteitis deformans of unspecified hand
[6] M88.85 Osteitis deformans of thigh
M88.851 Osteitis deformans of right thigh
M88.852 Osteitis deformans of left thigh
M88.859 Osteitis deformans of unspecified thigh
[6] M88.86 Osteitis deformans of lower leg
M88.861 Osteitis deformans of right lower leg
M88.862 Osteitis deformans of left lower leg
M88.869 Osteitis deformans of unspecified lower leg
[6] M88.87 Osteitis deformans of ankle and foot
M88.871 Osteitis deformans of right ankle and foot
M88.872 Osteitis deformans of left ankle and foot
M88.879 Osteitis deformans of unspecified ankle and foot
M88.88 Osteitis deformans of other bones
[EXCLUDES2] *osteitis deformans of skull (M88.0)*
osteitis deformans of vertebrae (M88.1)
M88.89 Osteitis deformans of multiple sites
M88.9 Osteitis deformans of unspecified bone
[4] M89 Other disorders of bone
[5] M89.0 Algoneurodystrophy
Shoulder-hand syndrome
Sudeck's atrophy
[EXCLUDES1] *causalgia, lower limb (G57.7-)*
causalgia, upper limb (G56.4-)
complex regional pain syndrome II, lower limb (G57.7-)
complex regional pain syndrome II, upper limb (G56.4-)
reflex sympathetic dystrophy (G90.5-)
M89.00 Algoneurodystrophy, unspecified site
[6] M89.01 Algoneurodystrophy, shoulder
M89.011 Algoneurodystrophy, right shoulder
M89.012 Algoneurodystrophy, left shoulder
M89.019 Algoneurodystrophy, unspecified shoulder
[6] M89.02 Algoneurodystrophy, upper arm
M89.021 Algoneurodystrophy, right upper arm
M89.022 Algoneurodystrophy, left upper arm
M89.029 Algoneurodystrophy, unspecified upper arm
[6] M89.03 Algoneurodystrophy, forearm
M89.031 Algoneurodystrophy, right forearm
M89.032 Algoneurodystrophy, left forearm
M89.039 Algoneurodystrophy, unspecified forearm
[6] M89.04 Algoneurodystrophy, hand
M89.041 Algoneurodystrophy, right hand
M89.042 Algoneurodystrophy, left hand
M89.049 Algoneurodystrophy, unspecified hand
[6] M89.05 Algoneurodystrophy, thigh
M89.051 Algoneurodystrophy, right thigh
M89.052 Algoneurodystrophy, left thigh
M89.059 Algoneurodystrophy, unspecified thigh
[6] M89.06 Algoneurodystrophy, lower leg
M89.061 Algoneurodystrophy, right lower leg
M89.062 Algoneurodystrophy, left lower leg
M89.069 Algoneurodystrophy, unspecified lower leg
[6] M89.07 Algoneurodystrophy, ankle and foot
M89.071 Algoneurodystrophy, right ankle and foot
M89.072 Algoneurodystrophy, left ankle and foot
M89.079 Algoneurodystrophy, unspecified ankle and foot
M89.08 Algoneurodystrophy, other site
M89.09 Algoneurodystrophy, multiple sites
[5] M89.1 Physeal arrest
Arrest of growth plate
Epiphyseal arrest
Growth plate arrest
[6] M89.12 Physeal arrest, humerus
M89.121 Complete physeal arrest, right proximal humerus
M89.122 Complete physeal arrest, left proximal humerus
M89.123 Partial physeal arrest, right proximal humerus
M89.124 Partial physeal arrest, left proximal humerus
M89.125 Complete physeal arrest, right distal humerus
M89.126 Complete physeal arrest, left distal humerus
M89.127 Partial physeal arrest, right distal humerus
M89.128 Partial physeal arrest, left distal humerus
M89.129 Physeal arrest, humerus, unspecified
[6] M89.13 Physeal arrest, forearm
M89.131 Complete physeal arrest, right distal radius
M89.132 Complete physeal arrest, left distal radius
M89.133 Partial physeal arrest, right distal radius
M89.134 Partial physeal arrest, left distal radius
M89.138 Other physeal arrest of forearm
M89.139 Physeal arrest, forearm, unspecified
[6] M89.15 Physeal arrest, femur
M89.151 Complete physeal arrest, right proximal femur
M89.152 Complete physeal arrest, left proximal femur
M89.153 Partial physeal arrest, right proximal femur
M89.154 Partial physeal arrest, left proximal femur
M89.155 Complete physeal arrest, right distal femur
M89.156 Complete physeal arrest, left distal femur
M89.157 Partial physeal arrest, right distal femur
M89.158 Partial physeal arrest, left distal femur
M89.159 Physeal arrest, femur, unspecified
[6] M89.16 Physeal arrest, lower leg
M89.160 Complete physeal arrest, right proximal tibia
M89.161 Complete physeal arrest, left proximal tibia
M89.162 Partial physeal arrest, right proximal tibia
M89.163 Partial physeal arrest, left proximal tibia
M89.164 Complete physeal arrest, right distal tibia
M89.165 Complete physeal arrest, left distal tibia
M89.166 Partial physeal arrest, right distal tibia
M89.167 Partial physeal arrest, left distal tibia
M89.168 Other physeal arrest of lower leg
M89.169 Physeal arrest, lower leg, unspecified
M89.18 Physeal arrest, other site

Unspecified Code | Other Specified Code | [N] Newborn Age: 0 | [P] Pediatric Age: 0-17 | [M] Maternity Age: 12-55
[A] Adult Age: 15-124 | ♂ Male | ♀ Female | ● New Code | ▲ Revised Code Title | ►◄ Revised Text

⑤ **M89.2 Other disorders of bone development and growth**

M89.20 Other disorders of bone development and growth, unspecified site

⑥ M89.21 Other disorders of bone development and growth, shoulder

M89.211 **Other disorders of bone development and growth, right shoulder**

M89.212 **Other disorders of bone development and growth, left shoulder**

M89.219 Other disorders of bone development and growth, unspecified shoulder

⑥ M89.22 Other disorders of bone development and growth, humerus

M89.221 **Other disorders of bone development and growth, right humerus**

M89.222 **Other disorders of bone development and growth, left humerus**

M89.229 Other disorders of bone development and growth, unspecified humerus

⑥ M89.23 Other disorders of bone development and growth, ulna and radius

M89.231 **Other disorders of bone development and growth, right ulna**

M89.232 **Other disorders of bone development and growth, left ulna**

M89.233 **Other disorders of bone development and growth, right radius**

M89.234 **Other disorders of bone development and growth, left radius**

M89.239 Other disorders of bone development and growth, unspecified ulna and radius

⑥ M89.24 Other disorders of bone development and growth, hand

M89.241 **Other disorders of bone development and growth, right hand**

M89.242 **Other disorders of bone development and growth, left hand**

M89.249 Other disorders of bone development and growth, unspecified hand

⑥ M89.25 Other disorders of bone development and growth, femur

M89.251 **Other disorders of bone development and growth, right femur**

M89.252 **Other disorders of bone development and growth, left femur**

M89.259 Other disorders of bone development and growth, unspecified femur

⑥ M89.26 Other disorders of bone development and growth, tibia and fibula

M89.261 **Other disorders of bone development and growth, right tibia**

M89.262 **Other disorders of bone development and growth, left tibia**

M89.263 **Other disorders of bone development and growth, right fibula**

M89.264 **Other disorders of bone development and growth, left fibula**

M89.269 Other disorders of bone development and growth, unspecified lower leg

⑥ M89.27 Other disorders of bone development and growth, ankle and foot

M89.271 **Other disorders of bone development and growth, right ankle and foot**

M89.272 **Other disorders of bone development and growth, left ankle and foot**

M89.279 Other disorders of bone development and growth, unspecified ankle and foot

M89.28 **Other disorders of bone development and growth, other site**

M89.29 **Other disorders of bone development and growth, multiple sites**

⑤ M89.3 Hypertrophy of bone

M89.30 Hypertrophy of bone, unspecified site

⑥ M89.31 Hypertrophy of bone, shoulder

M89.311 Hypertrophy of bone, right shoulder

M89.312 Hypertrophy of bone, left shoulder

M89.319 Hypertrophy of bone, unspecified shoulder

⑥ M89.32 Hypertrophy of bone, humerus

M89.321 Hypertrophy of bone, right humerus

M89.322 Hypertrophy of bone, left humerus

M89.329 Hypertrophy of bone, unspecified humerus

⑥ M89.33 Hypertrophy of bone, ulna and radius

M89.331 Hypertrophy of bone, right ulna

M89.332 Hypertrophy of bone, left ulna

M89.333 Hypertrophy of bone, right radius

M89.334 Hypertrophy of bone, left radius

M89.339 Hypertrophy of bone, unspecified ulna and radius

⑥ M89.34 Hypertrophy of bone, hand

M89.341 Hypertrophy of bone, right hand

M89.342 Hypertrophy of bone, left hand

M89.349 Hypertrophy of bone, unspecified hand

⑥ M89.35 Hypertrophy of bone, femur

M89.351 Hypertrophy of bone, right femur

M89.352 Hypertrophy of bone, left femur

M89.359 Hypertrophy of bone, unspecified femur

⑥ M89.36 Hypertrophy of bone, tibia and fibula

M89.361 Hypertrophy of bone, right tibia

M89.362 Hypertrophy of bone, left tibia

M89.363 Hypertrophy of bone, right fibula

M89.364 Hypertrophy of bone, left fibula

M89.369 Hypertrophy of bone, unspecified tibia and fibula

⑥ M89.37 Hypertrophy of bone, ankle and foot

M89.371 Hypertrophy of bone, right ankle and foot

M89.372 Hypertrophy of bone, left ankle and foot

M89.379 Hypertrophy of bone, unspecified ankle and foot

M89.38 **Hypertrophy of bone, other site**

M89.39 Hypertrophy of bone, multiple sites

⑤ M89.4 Other hypertrophic osteoarthropathy

Marie-Bamberger disease

Pachydermoperiostosis

M89.40 Other hypertrophic osteoarthropathy, unspecified site

⑥ M89.41 Other hypertrophic osteoarthropathy, shoulder

M89.411 **Other hypertrophic osteoarthropathy, right shoulder**

M89.412 **Other hypertrophic osteoarthropathy, left shoulder**

M89.419 Other hypertrophic osteoarthropathy, unspecified shoulder

⑥ M89.42 Other hypertrophic osteoarthropathy, upper arm

M89.421 **Other hypertrophic osteoarthropathy, right upper arm**

M89.422 **Other hypertrophic osteoarthropathy, left upper arm**

M89.429 Other hypertrophic osteoarthropathy, unspecified upper arm

⑥ M89.43 Other hypertrophic osteoarthropathy, forearm

M89.431 **Other hypertrophic osteoarthropathy, right forearm**

M89.432 **Other hypertrophic osteoarthropathy, left forearm**

---

④ 4th character required   ⑤ 5th character required   ⑥ 6th character required   ⑦ 7th character required   ⑰ Extension 'X' Alert

EXCLUDES1 Not coded here   EXCLUDES2 Not included here   📠 Primary Diagnosis Only   Manifestation Code

M89.439 Other hypertrophic osteoarthropathy, unspecified forearm
[6] M89.44 Other hypertrophic osteoarthropathy, hand
M89.441 Other hypertrophic osteoarthropathy, right hand
M89.442 Other hypertrophic osteoarthropathy, left hand
M89.449 Other hypertrophic osteoarthropathy, unspecified hand
[6] M89.45 Other hypertrophic osteoarthropathy, thigh
M89.451 Other hypertrophic osteoarthropathy, right thigh
M89.452 Other hypertrophic osteoarthropathy, left thigh
M89.459 Other hypertrophic osteoarthropathy, unspecified thigh
[6] M89.46 Other hypertrophic osteoarthropathy, lower leg
M89.461 Other hypertrophic osteoarthropathy, right lower leg
M89.462 Other hypertrophic osteoarthropathy, left lower leg
M89.469 Other hypertrophic osteoarthropathy, unspecified lower leg
[6] M89.47 Other hypertrophic osteoarthropathy, ankle and foot
M89.471 Other hypertrophic osteoarthropathy, right ankle and foot
M89.472 Other hypertrophic osteoarthropathy, left ankle and foot
M89.479 Other hypertrophic osteoarthropathy, unspecified ankle and foot
M89.48 Other hypertrophic osteoarthropathy, other site
M89.49 Other hypertrophic osteoarthropathy, multiple sites
[5] M89.5 Osteolysis
Use additional code to identify major osseous defect, if applicable (M89.7-)
[EXCLUDES2] *periprosthetic osteolysis of internal prosthetic joint (T84.05-)*
M89.50 Osteolysis, unspecified site
[6] M89.51 Osteolysis, shoulder
M89.511 Osteolysis, right shoulder
M89.512 Osteolysis, left shoulder
M89.519 Osteolysis, unspecified shoulder
[6] M89.52 Osteolysis, upper arm
M89.521 Osteolysis, right upper arm
M89.522 Osteolysis, left upper arm
M89.529 Osteolysis, unspecified upper arm
[6] M89.53 Osteolysis, forearm
M89.531 Osteolysis, right forearm
M89.532 Osteolysis, left forearm
M89.539 Osteolysis, unspecified forearm
[6] M89.54 Osteolysis, hand
M89.541 Osteolysis, right hand
M89.542 Osteolysis, left hand
M89.549 Osteolysis, unspecified hand
[6] M89.55 Osteolysis, thigh
M89.551 Osteolysis, right thigh
M89.552 Osteolysis, left thigh
M89.559 Osteolysis, unspecified thigh
[6] M89.56 Osteolysis, lower leg
M89.561 Osteolysis, right lower leg
M89.562 Osteolysis, left lower leg
M89.569 Osteolysis, unspecified lower leg
[6] M89.57 Osteolysis, ankle and foot
M89.571 Osteolysis, right ankle and foot
M89.572 Osteolysis, left ankle and foot
M89.579 Osteolysis, unspecified ankle and foot
M89.58 Osteolysis, other site
M89.59 Osteolysis, multiple sites
[5] M89.6 Osteopathy after poliomyelitis
Use additional code (B91) to identify previous poliomyelitis
[EXCLUDES1] *postpolio syndrome (G14)*
M89.60 Osteopathy after poliomyelitis, unspecified site
[6] M89.61 Osteopathy after poliomyelitis, shoulder
M89.611 Osteopathy after poliomyelitis, right shoulder
M89.612 Osteopathy after poliomyelitis, left shoulder
M89.619 Osteopathy after poliomyelitis, unspecified shoulder
[6] M89.62 Osteopathy after poliomyelitis, upper arm
M89.621 Osteopathy after poliomyelitis, right upper arm
M89.622 Osteopathy after poliomyelitis, left upper arm
M89.629 Osteopathy after poliomyelitis, unspecified upper arm
[6] M89.63 Osteopathy after poliomyelitis, forearm
M89.631 Osteopathy after poliomyelitis, right forearm
M89.632 Osteopathy after poliomyelitis, left forearm
M89.639 Osteopathy after poliomyelitis, unspecified forearm
[6] M89.64 Osteopathy after poliomyelitis, hand
M89.641 Osteopathy after poliomyelitis, right hand
M89.642 Osteopathy after poliomyelitis, left hand
M89.649 Osteopathy after poliomyelitis, unspecified hand
[6] M89.65 Osteopathy after poliomyelitis, thigh
M89.651 Osteopathy after poliomyelitis, right thigh
M89.652 Osteopathy after poliomyelitis, left thigh
M89.659 Osteopathy after poliomyelitis, unspecified thigh
[6] M89.66 Osteopathy after poliomyelitis, lower leg
M89.661 Osteopathy after poliomyelitis, right lower leg
M89.662 Osteopathy after poliomyelitis, left lower leg
M89.669 Osteopathy after poliomyelitis, unspecified lower leg
[6] M89.67 Osteopathy after poliomyelitis, ankle and foot
M89.671 Osteopathy after poliomyelitis, right ankle and foot
M89.672 Osteopathy after poliomyelitis, left ankle and foot
M89.679 Osteopathy after poliomyelitis, unspecified ankle and foot
M89.68 Osteopathy after poliomyelitis, other site
M89.69 Osteopathy after poliomyelitis, multiple sites
[5] M89.7 Major osseous defect
Code first underlying disease, if known, such as:
aseptic necrosis of bone (M87.-)
malignant neoplasm of bone (C40.-)
osteolysis (M89.5)
osteomyelitis (M86.-)
osteonecrosis (M87.-)
osteoporosis (M80.-, M81.-)
periprosthetic osteolysis (T84.05-)
M89.70 Major osseous defect, unspecified site
[6] M89.71 Major osseous defect, shoulder region
Major osseous defect clavicle or scapula
M89.711 Major osseous defect, right shoulder region

Unspecified Code | Other Specified Code | [N] Newborn Age: 0 | [P] Pediatric Age: 0-17 | [M] Maternity Age: 12-55 | [A] Adult Age: 15-124 | ♂ Male | ♀ Female | ● New Code | ▲ Revised Code Title | ►◄ Revised Text

M89.712 Major osseous defect, left shoulder region
M89.719 Major osseous defect, unspecified shoulder region
[6] M89.72 Major osseous defect, humerus
M89.721 Major osseous defect, right humerus
M89.722 Major osseous defect, left humerus
M89.729 Major osseous defect, unspecified humerus
[6] M89.73 Major osseous defect, forearm
Major osseous defect of radius and ulna
M89.731 Major osseous defect, right forearm
M89.732 Major osseous defect, left forearm
M89.739 Major osseous defect, unspecified forearm
[6] M89.74 Major osseous defect, hand
Major osseous defect of carpus, fingers, metacarpus
M89.741 Major osseous defect, right hand
M89.742 Major osseous defect, left hand
M89.749 Major osseous defect, unspecified hand
[6] M89.75 Major osseous defect, pelvic region and thigh
Major osseous defect of femur and pelvis
M89.751 Major osseous defect, right pelvic region and thigh
M89.752 Major osseous defect, left pelvic region and thigh
M89.759 Major osseous defect, unspecified pelvic region and thigh
[6] M89.76 Major osseous defect, lower leg
Major osseous defect of fibula and tibia
M89.761 Major osseous defect, right lower leg
M89.762 Major osseous defect, left lower leg
M89.769 Major osseous defect, unspecified lower leg
[6] M89.77 Major osseous defect, ankle and foot
Major osseous defect of metatarsus, tarsus, toes
M89.771 Major osseous defect, right ankle and foot
M89.772 Major osseous defect, left ankle and foot
M89.779 Major osseous defect, unspecified ankle and foot
M89.78 Major osseous defect, other site
M89.79 Major osseous defect, multiple sites
[5] M89.8 Other specified disorders of bone
Infantile cortical hyperostoses
Post-traumatic subperiosteal ossification
[6] M89.8X Other specified disorders of bone
M89.8X0 Other specified disorders of bone, multiple sites
M89.8X1 Other specified disorders of bone, shoulder
M89.8X2 Other specified disorders of bone, upper arm
M89.8X3 Other specified disorders of bone, forearm
M89.8X4 Other specified disorders of bone, hand
M89.8X5 Other specified disorders of bone, thigh
M89.8X6 Other specified disorders of bone, lower leg
M89.8X7 Other specified disorders of bone, ankle and foot
M89.8X8 Other specified disorders of bone, other site
M89.8X9 Other specified disorders of bone, unspecified site
M89.9 Disorder of bone, unspecified

[4] M90 Osteopathies in diseases classified elsewhere
[EXCLUDES1] *osteochondritis, osteomyelitis, and osteopathy (in):*
cryptococcosis (B45.3)
diabetes mellitus (E08-E13 with .61-)
gonococcal (A54.43)
neurogenic syphilis (A52.11)
renal osteodystrophy (N25.0)
salmonellosis (A02.24)
secondary syphilis (A51.46)
syphilis (late) (A52.77)
[5] M90.5 Osteonecrosis in diseases classified elsewhere
Code first underlying disease, such as:
caisson disease (T70.3)
hemoglobinopathy (D50-D64)
M90.50 Osteonecrosis in diseases classified elsewhere, unspecified site
[6] M90.51 Osteonecrosis in diseases classified elsewhere, shoulder
M90.511 Osteonecrosis in diseases classified elsewhere, right shoulder
M90.512 Osteonecrosis in diseases classified elsewhere, left shoulder
M90.519 Osteonecrosis in diseases classified elsewhere, unspecified shoulder
[6] M90.52 Osteonecrosis in diseases classified elsewhere, upper arm
M90.521 Osteonecrosis in diseases classified elsewhere, right upper arm
M90.522 Osteonecrosis in diseases classified elsewhere, left upper arm
M90.529 Osteonecrosis in diseases classified elsewhere, unspecified upper arm
[6] M90.53 Osteonecrosis in diseases classified elsewhere, forearm
M90.531 Osteonecrosis in diseases classified elsewhere, right forearm
M90.532 Osteonecrosis in diseases classified elsewhere, left forearm
M90.539 Osteonecrosis in diseases classified elsewhere, unspecified forearm
[6] M90.54 Osteonecrosis in diseases classified elsewhere, hand
M90.541 Osteonecrosis in diseases classified elsewhere, right hand
M90.542 Osteonecrosis in diseases classified elsewhere, left hand
M90.549 Osteonecrosis in diseases classified elsewhere, unspecified hand
[6] M90.55 Osteonecrosis in diseases classified elsewhere, thigh
M90.551 Osteonecrosis in diseases classified elsewhere, right thigh
M90.552 Osteonecrosis in diseases classified elsewhere, left thigh
M90.559 Osteonecrosis in diseases classified elsewhere, unspecified thigh
[6] M90.56 Osteonecrosis in diseases classified elsewhere, lower leg
M90.561 Osteonecrosis in diseases classified elsewhere, right lower leg
M90.562 Osteonecrosis in diseases classified elsewhere, left lower leg
M90.569 Osteonecrosis in diseases classified elsewhere, unspecified lower leg
[6] M90.57 Osteonecrosis in diseases classified elsewhere, ankle and foot
M90.571 Osteonecrosis in diseases classified elsewhere, right ankle and foot

M90.572 Osteonecrosis in diseases classified elsewhere, left ankle and foot
M90.579 Osteonecrosis in diseases classified elsewhere, unspecified ankle and foot
M90.58 Osteonecrosis in diseases classified elsewhere, other site
M90.59 Osteonecrosis in diseases classified elsewhere, multiple sites

[5] M90.6 Osteitis deformans in neoplastic diseases
Osteitis deformans in malignant neoplasm of bone
Code first the neoplasm (C40.-, C41.-)
[EXCLUDES1] *osteitis deformans [Paget's disease of bone] (M88.-)*
M90.60 Osteitis deformans in neoplastic diseases, unspecified site
[6] M90.61 Osteitis deformans in neoplastic diseases, shoulder
M90.611 Osteitis deformans in neoplastic diseases, right shoulder
M90.612 Osteitis deformans in neoplastic diseases, left shoulder
M90.619 Osteitis deformans in neoplastic diseases, unspecified shoulder
[6] M90.62 Osteitis deformans in neoplastic diseases, upper arm
M90.621 Osteitis deformans in neoplastic diseases, right upper arm
M90.622 Osteitis deformans in neoplastic diseases, left upper arm
M90.629 Osteitis deformans in neoplastic diseases, unspecified upper arm
[6] M90.63 Osteitis deformans in neoplastic diseases, forearm
M90.631 Osteitis deformans in neoplastic diseases, right forearm
M90.632 Osteitis deformans in neoplastic diseases, left forearm
M90.639 Osteitis deformans in neoplastic diseases, unspecified forearm
[6] M90.64 Osteitis deformans in neoplastic diseases, hand
M90.641 Osteitis deformans in neoplastic diseases, right hand
M90.642 Osteitis deformans in neoplastic diseases, left hand
M90.649 Osteitis deformans in neoplastic diseases, unspecified hand
[6] M90.65 Osteitis deformans in neoplastic diseases, thigh
M90.651 Osteitis deformans in neoplastic diseases, right thigh
M90.652 Osteitis deformans in neoplastic diseases, left thigh
M90.659 Osteitis deformans in neoplastic diseases, unspecified thigh
[6] M90.66 Osteitis deformans in neoplastic diseases, lower leg
M90.661 Osteitis deformans in neoplastic diseases, right lower leg
M90.662 Osteitis deformans in neoplastic diseases, left lower leg
M90.669 Osteitis deformans in neoplastic diseases, unspecified lower leg
[6] M90.67 Osteitis deformans in neoplastic diseases, ankle and foot
M90.671 Osteitis deformans in neoplastic diseases, right ankle and foot
M90.672 Osteitis deformans in neoplastic diseases, left ankle and foot
M90.679 Osteitis deformans in neoplastic diseases, unspecified ankle and foot
M90.68 Osteitis deformans in neoplastic diseases, other site
M90.69 Osteitis deformans in neoplastic diseases, multiple sites

[5] M90.8 Osteopathy in diseases classified elsewhere
Code first underlying disease, such as:
rickets (E55.0)
vitamin-D-resistant rickets (E83.3)
M90.80 Osteopathy in diseases classified elsewhere, unspecified site
[6] M90.81 Osteopathy in diseases classified elsewhere, shoulder
M90.811 Osteopathy in diseases classified elsewhere, right shoulder
M90.812 Osteopathy in diseases classified elsewhere, left shoulder
M90.819 Osteopathy in diseases classified elsewhere, unspecified shoulder
[6] M90.82 Osteopathy in diseases classified elsewhere, upper arm
M90.821 Osteopathy in diseases classified elsewhere, right upper arm
M90.822 Osteopathy in diseases classified elsewhere, left upper arm
M90.829 Osteopathy in diseases classified elsewhere, unspecified upper arm
[6] M90.83 Osteopathy in diseases classified elsewhere, forearm
M90.831 Osteopathy in diseases classified elsewhere, right forearm
M90.832 Osteopathy in diseases classified elsewhere, left forearm
M90.839 Osteopathy in diseases classified elsewhere, unspecified forearm
[6] M90.84 Osteopathy in diseases classified elsewhere, hand
M90.841 Osteopathy in diseases classified elsewhere, right hand
M90.842 Osteopathy in diseases classified elsewhere, left hand
M90.849 Osteopathy in diseases classified elsewhere, unspecified hand
[6] M90.85 Osteopathy in diseases classified elsewhere, thigh
M90.851 Osteopathy in diseases classified elsewhere, right thigh
M90.852 Osteopathy in diseases classified elsewhere, left thigh
M90.859 Osteopathy in diseases classified elsewhere, unspecified thigh
[6] M90.86 Osteopathy in diseases classified elsewhere, lower leg
M90.861 Osteopathy in diseases classified elsewhere, right lower leg
M90.862 Osteopathy in diseases classified elsewhere, left lower leg
M90.869 Osteopathy in diseases classified elsewhere, unspecified lower leg
[6] M90.87 Osteopathy in diseases classified elsewhere, ankle and foot
M90.871 Osteopathy in diseases classified elsewhere, right ankle and foot
M90.872 Osteopathy in diseases classified elsewhere, left ankle and foot
M90.879 Osteopathy in diseases classified elsewhere, unspecified ankle and foot
M90.88 Osteopathy in diseases classified elsewhere, other site
M90.89 Osteopathy in diseases classified elsewhere, multiple sites

Unspecified Code | Other Specified Code | [N] Newborn Age: 0 | [P] Pediatric Age: 0-17 | [M] Maternity Age: 12-55
[A] Adult Age: 15-124 | ♂ Male | ♀ Female | ● New Code | ▲ Revised Code Title | ►◄ Revised Text

Chondropathies (M91-M94)

[EXCLUDES1] *postprocedural chondropathies (M96.-)*

[4] **M91 Juvenile osteochondrosis of hip and pelvis**

[EXCLUDES1] *slipped upper femoral epiphysis (nontraumatic) (M93.0)*

M91.0 Juvenile osteochondrosis of pelvis
Osteochondrosis (juvenile) of acetabulum
Osteochondrosis (juvenile) of iliac crest [Buchanan]
Osteochondrosis (juvenile) of ischiopubic synchondrosis [van Neck]
Osteochondrosis (juvenile) of symphysis pubis [Pierson]

[5] **M91.1 Juvenile osteochondrosis of head of femur [Legg-Calvé-Perthes]**
M91.10 Juvenile osteochondrosis of head of femur [Legg-Calvé-Perthes], unspecified leg
M91.11 Juvenile osteochondrosis of head of femur [Legg-Calvé-Perthes], right leg
M91.12 Juvenile osteochondrosis of head of femur [Legg-Calvé-Perthes], left leg

[5] **M91.2 Coxa plana**
Hip deformity due to previous juvenile osteochondrosis
M91.20 Coxa plana, unspecified hip
M91.21 Coxa plana, right hip
M91.22 Coxa plana, left hip

[5] **M91.3 Pseudocoxalgia**
M91.30 Pseudocoxalgia, unspecified hip
M91.31 Pseudocoxalgia, right hip
M91.32 Pseudocoxalgia, left hip

[5] **M91.4 Coxa magna**
M91.40 Coxa magna, unspecified hip
M91.41 Coxa magna, right hip
M91.42 Coxa magna, left hip

[5] **M91.8 Other juvenile osteochondrosis of hip and pelvis**
Juvenile osteochondrosis after reduction of congenital dislocation of hip
M91.80 Other juvenile osteochondrosis of hip and pelvis, unspecified leg
M91.81 Other juvenile osteochondrosis of hip and pelvis, right leg
M91.82 Other juvenile osteochondrosis of hip and pelvis, left leg

[5] **M91.9 Juvenile osteochondrosis of hip and pelvis, unspecified**
M91.90 Juvenile osteochondrosis of hip and pelvis, unspecified, unspecified leg
M91.91 Juvenile osteochondrosis of hip and pelvis, unspecified, right leg
M91.92 Juvenile osteochondrosis of hip and pelvis, unspecified, left leg

[4] **M92 Other juvenile osteochondrosis**

[5] **M92.0 Juvenile osteochondrosis of humerus**
Osteochondrosis (juvenile) of capitulum of humerus [Panner]
Osteochondrosis (juvenile) of head of humerus [Haas]
M92.00 Juvenile osteochondrosis of humerus, unspecified arm
M92.01 Juvenile osteochondrosis of humerus, right arm
M92.02 Juvenile osteochondrosis of humerus, left arm

[5] **M92.1 Juvenile osteochondrosis of radius and ulna**
Osteochondrosis (juvenile) of lower ulna [Burns]
Osteochondrosis (juvenile) of radial head [Brailsford]
M92.10 Juvenile osteochondrosis of radius and ulna, unspecified arm
M92.11 Juvenile osteochondrosis of radius and ulna, right arm
M92.12 Juvenile osteochondrosis of radius and ulna, left arm

[5] **M92.2 Juvenile osteochondrosis, hand**
[6] **M92.20 Unspecified juvenile osteochondrosis, hand**
M92.201 Unspecified juvenile osteochondrosis, right hand
M92.202 Unspecified juvenile osteochondrosis, left hand
M92.209 Unspecified juvenile osteochondrosis, unspecified hand
[6] **M92.21 Osteochondrosis (juvenile) of carpal lunate [Kienböck]**
M92.211 Osteochondrosis (juvenile) of carpal lunate [Kienböck], right hand
M92.212 Osteochondrosis (juvenile) of carpal lunate [Kienböck], left hand
M92.219 Osteochondrosis (juvenile) of carpal lunate [Kienböck], unspecified hand
[6] **M92.22 Osteochondrosis (juvenile) of metacarpal heads [Mauclaire]**
M92.221 Osteochondrosis (juvenile) of metacarpal heads [Mauclaire], right hand
M92.222 Osteochondrosis (juvenile) of metacarpal heads [Mauclaire], left hand
M92.229 Osteochondrosis (juvenile) of metacarpal heads [Mauclaire], unspecified hand
[6] **M92.29 Other juvenile osteochondrosis, hand**
M92.291 Other juvenile osteochondrosis, right hand
M92.292 Other juvenile osteochondrosis, left hand
M92.299 Other juvenile osteochondrosis, unspecified hand

[5] **M92.3 Other juvenile osteochondrosis, upper limb**
M92.30 Other juvenile osteochondrosis, unspecified upper limb
M92.31 Other juvenile osteochondrosis, right upper limb
M92.32 Other juvenile osteochondrosis, left upper limb

[5] **M92.4 Juvenile osteochondrosis of patella**
Osteochondrosis (juvenile) of primary patellar center [Köhler]
Osteochondrosis (juvenile) of secondary patellar centre [Sinding Larsen]
M92.40 Juvenile osteochondrosis of patella, unspecified knee
M92.41 Juvenile osteochondrosis of patella, right knee
M92.42 Juvenile osteochondrosis of patella, left knee

[5] **M92.5 Juvenile osteochondrosis of tibia and fibula**
Osteochondrosis (juvenile) of proximal tibia [Blount]
Osteochondrosis (juvenile) of tibial tubercle [Osgood-Schlatter]
Tibia vara
M92.50 Juvenile osteochondrosis of tibia and fibula, unspecified leg
M92.51 Juvenile osteochondrosis of tibia and fibula, right leg
M92.52 Juvenile osteochondrosis of tibia and fibula, left leg

[5] **M92.6 Juvenile osteochondrosis of tarsus**
Osteochondrosis (juvenile) of calcaneum [Sever]
Osteochondrosis (juvenile) of os tibiale externum [Haglund]
Osteochondrosis (juvenile) of talus [Diaz]
Osteochondrosis (juvenile) of tarsal navicular [Köhler]
M92.60 Juvenile osteochondrosis of tarsus, unspecified ankle
M92.61 Juvenile osteochondrosis of tarsus, right ankle
M92.62 Juvenile osteochondrosis of tarsus, left ankle

[5] **M92.7 Juvenile osteochondrosis of metatarsus**

[4] 4th character required [5] 5th character required [6] 6th character required [7] 7th character required [7] Extension 'X' Alert
[EXCLUDES 1] Not coded here [EXCLUDES 2] Not included here [PDx] Primary Diagnosis Only Manifestation Code

Osteochondrosis (juvenile) of fifth metatarsus [Iselin]

Osteochondrosis (juvenile) of second metatarsus [Freiberg]

M92.70 **Juvenile osteochondrosis of metatarsus, unspecified foot**

M92.71 **Juvenile osteochondrosis of metatarsus,** right **foot**

M92.72 **Juvenile osteochondrosis of metatarsus,** left **foot**

M92.8 Other specified juvenile osteochondrosis

Calcaneal apophysitis

M92.9 **Juvenile osteochondrosis, unspecified**

Juvenile apophysitis NOS

Juvenile epiphysitis NOS

Juvenile osteochondritis NOS

Juvenile osteochondrosis NOS

🜋 M93 **Other osteochondropathies**

EXCLUDES2 *osteochondrosis of spine (M42.-)*

🜊 M93.0 **Slipped upper femoral epiphysis (nontraumatic)**

Use additional code for associated chondrolysis (M94.3)

🜌 M93.00 Unspecified **slipped upper femoral epiphysis (nontraumatic)**

M93.001 **Unspecified slipped upper femoral epiphysis (nontraumatic),** right **hip**

M93.002 **Unspecified slipped upper femoral epiphysis (nontraumatic),** left **hip**

M93.003 **Unspecified slipped upper femoral epiphysis (nontraumatic), unspecified hip**

🜌 M93.01 Acute **slipped upper femoral epiphysis (nontraumatic)**

M93.011 **Acute slipped upper femoral epiphysis (nontraumatic),** right **hip**

M93.012 **Acute slipped upper femoral epiphysis (nontraumatic),** left **hip**

M93.013 **Acute slipped upper femoral epiphysis (nontraumatic), unspecified hip**

🜌 M93.02 Chronic **slipped upper femoral epiphysis (nontraumatic)**

M93.021 **Chronic slipped upper femoral epiphysis (nontraumatic),** right **hip**

M93.022 **Chronic slipped upper femoral epiphysis (nontraumatic),** left **hip**

M93.023 **Chronic slipped upper femoral epiphysis (nontraumatic), unspecified hip**

🜌 M93.03 Acute on chronic **slipped upper femoral epiphysis (nontraumatic)**

M93.031 **Acute on chronic slipped upper femoral epiphysis (nontraumatic),** right **hip**

M93.032 **Acute on chronic slipped upper femoral epiphysis (nontraumatic),** left **hip**

M93.033 **Acute on chronic slipped upper femoral epiphysis (nontraumatic), unspecified hip**

M93.1 **Kienböck's disease of adults**

Adult osteochondrosis of carpal lunates 🅰

🜊 M93.2 Osteochondritis dissecans

M93.20 **Osteochondritis dissecans of unspecified site**

🜌 M93.21 **Osteochondritis dissecans of** shoulder

M93.211 **Osteochondritis dissecans,** right **shoulder**

M93.212 **Osteochondritis dissecans,** left **shoulder**

M93.219 **Osteochondritis dissecans, unspecified shoulder**

🜌 M93.22 **Osteochondritis dissecans of** elbow

M93.221 **Osteochondritis dissecans,** right **elbow**

M93.222 **Osteochondritis dissecans,** left **elbow**

M93.229 **Osteochondritis dissecans, unspecified elbow**

🜌 M93.23 **Osteochondritis dissecans of** wrist

M93.231 **Osteochondritis dissecans,** right **wrist**

M93.232 **Osteochondritis dissecans,** left **wrist**

M93.239 **Osteochondritis dissecans, unspecified wrist**

🜌 M93.24 **Osteochondritis dissecans of** joints of hand

M93.241 **Osteochondritis dissecans, joints of** right **hand**

M93.242 **Osteochondritis dissecans, joints of** left **hand**

M93.249 **Osteochondritis dissecans, joints of unspecified hand**

🜌 M93.25 **Osteochondritis dissecans of** hip

M93.251 **Osteochondritis dissecans,** right **hip**

M93.252 **Osteochondritis dissecans,** left **hip**

M93.259 **Osteochondritis dissecans, unspecified hip**

🜌 M93.26 **Osteochondritis dissecans** knee

M93.261 **Osteochondritis dissecans,** right **knee**

M93.262 **Osteochondritis dissecans,** left **knee**

M93.269 **Osteochondritis dissecans, unspecified knee**

🜌 M93.27 **Osteochondritis dissecans of** ankle and joints of foot

M93.271 **Osteochondritis dissecans,** right ankle and **joints of** right foot

M93.272 **Osteochondritis dissecans,** left ankle and **joints of** left foot

M93.279 **Osteochondritis dissecans, unspecified ankle and joints of foot**

M93.28 Osteochondritis dissecans other site

M93.29 **Osteochondritis dissecans** multiple sites

🜊 M93.8 **Other specified osteochondropathies**

M93.80 **Other specified osteochondropathies of unspecified site**

🜌 M93.81 **Other specified osteochondropathies of** shoulder

M93.811 Other specified osteochondropathies, right shoulder

M93.812 Other specified osteochondropathies, left shoulder

M93.819 **Other specified osteochondropathies, unspecified shoulder**

🜌 M93.82 **Other specified osteochondropathies of upper** arm

M93.821 Other specified osteochondropathies, right upper arm

M93.822 Other specified osteochondropathies, left upper arm

M93.829 **Other specified osteochondropathies, unspecified upper arm**

🜌 M93.83 **Other specified osteochondropathies of** forearm

M93.831 Other specified osteochondropathies, right forearm

M93.832 Other specified osteochondropathies, left forearm

M93.839 **Other specified osteochondropathies, unspecified forearm**

🜌 M93.84 **Other specified osteochondropathies of** hand

M93.841 Other specified osteochondropathies, right hand

M93.842 Other specified osteochondropathies, left hand

M93.849 **Other specified osteochondropathies, unspecified hand**

🜌 M93.85 **Other specified osteochondropathies of** thigh

M93.851 Other specified osteochondropathies, right thigh

M93.852 Other specified osteochondropathies, left thigh

Unspecified Code	Other Specified Code	N Newborn Age: 0	P Pediatric Age: 0-17	M Maternity Age: 12-55	
A Adult Age: 15-124	♂ Male	♀ Female	● New Code	▲ Revised Code Title	►◄ Revised Text

M93.859 Other specified osteochondropathies, unspecified thigh

⑥ M93.86 Other specified osteochondropathies lower leg

M93.861 Other specified osteochondropathies, right lower leg

M93.862 Other specified osteochondropathies, left lower leg

M93.869 Other specified osteochondropathies, unspecified lower leg

⑥ M93.87 Other specified osteochondropathies of ankle and foot

M93.871 Other specified osteochondropathies, right ankle and foot

M93.872 Other specified osteochondropathies, left ankle and foot

M93.879 Other specified osteochondropathies, unspecified ankle and foot

M93.88 Other specified osteochondropathies other

M93.89 Other specified osteochondropathies multiple sites

⑤ M93.9 Osteochondropathy, unspecified

Apophysitis NOS

Epiphysitis NOS

Osteochondritis NOS

Osteochondrosis NOS

M93.90 Osteochondropathy, unspecified of unspecified site

⑥ M93.91 Osteochondropathy, unspecified of shoulder

M93.911 Osteochondropathy, unspecified, right shoulder

M93.912 Osteochondropathy, unspecified, left shoulder

M93.919 Osteochondropathy, unspecified, unspecified shoulder

⑥ M93.92 Osteochondropathy, unspecified of upper arm

M93.921 Osteochondropathy, unspecified, right upper arm

M93.922 Osteochondropathy, unspecified, left upper arm

M93.929 Osteochondropathy, unspecified, unspecified upper arm

⑥ M93.93 Osteochondropathy, unspecified of forearm

M93.931 Osteochondropathy, unspecified, right forearm

M93.932 Osteochondropathy, unspecified, left forearm

M93.939 Osteochondropathy, unspecified, unspecified forearm

⑥ M93.94 Osteochondropathy, unspecified of hand

M93.941 Osteochondropathy, unspecified, right hand

M93.942 Osteochondropathy, unspecified, left hand

M93.949 Osteochondropathy, unspecified, unspecified hand

⑥ M93.95 Osteochondropathy, unspecified of thigh

M93.951 Osteochondropathy, unspecified, right thigh

M93.952 Osteochondropathy, unspecified, left thigh

M93.959 Osteochondropathy, unspecified, unspecified thigh

⑥ M93.96 Osteochondropathy, unspecified lower leg

M93.961 Osteochondropathy, unspecified, right lower leg

M93.962 Osteochondropathy, unspecified, left lower leg

M93.969 Osteochondropathy, unspecified, unspecified lower leg

⑥ M93.97 Osteochondropathy, unspecified of ankle and foot

M93.971 Osteochondropathy, unspecified, right ankle and foot

M93.972 Osteochondropathy, unspecified, left ankle and foot

M93.979 Osteochondropathy, unspecified, unspecified ankle and foot

M93.98 Osteochondropathy, unspecified other

M93.99 Osteochondropathy, unspecified multiple sites

④ M94 Other disorders of cartilage

M94.0 Chondrocostal junction syndrome [Tietze]

Costochondritis

M94.1 Relapsing polychondritis

⑤ M94.2 Chondromalacia

EXCLUDES1 chondromalacia patellae (M22.4)

M94.20 Chondromalacia, unspecified site

⑥ M94.21 Chondromalacia, shoulder

M94.211 Chondromalacia, right shoulder

M94.212 Chondromalacia, left shoulder

M94.219 Chondromalacia, unspecified shoulder

⑥ M94.22 Chondromalacia, elbow

M94.221 Chondromalacia, right elbow

M94.222 Chondromalacia, left elbow

M94.229 Chondromalacia, unspecified elbow

⑥ M94.23 Chondromalacia, wrist

M94.231 Chondromalacia, right wrist

M94.232 Chondromalacia, left wrist

M94.239 Chondromalacia, unspecified wrist

⑥ M94.24 Chondromalacia, joints of hand

M94.241 Chondromalacia, joints of right hand

M94.242 Chondromalacia, joints of left hand

M94.249 Chondromalacia, joints of unspecified hand

⑥ M94.25 Chondromalacia, hip

M94.251 Chondromalacia, right hip

M94.252 Chondromalacia, left hip

M94.259 Chondromalacia, unspecified hip

⑥ M94.26 Chondromalacia, knee

M94.261 Chondromalacia, right knee

M94.262 Chondromalacia, left knee

M94.269 Chondromalacia, unspecified knee

⑥ M94.27 Chondromalacia, ankle and joints of foot

M94.271 Chondromalacia, right ankle and joints of right foot

M94.272 Chondromalacia, left ankle and joints of left foot

M94.279 Chondromalacia, unspecified ankle and joints of foot

M94.28 Chondromalacia, other site

M94.29 Chondromalacia, multiple sites

⑤ M94.3 Chondrolysis

Code first any associated slipped upper femoral epiphysis (nontraumatic) (M93.0-)

⑥ M94.35 Chondrolysis, hip

M94.351 Chondrolysis, right hip

M94.352 Chondrolysis, left hip

M94.359 Chondrolysis, unspecified hip

⑤ M94.8 Other specified disorders of cartilage

⑥ M94.8X Other specified disorders of cartilage

M94.8X0 Other specified disorders of cartilage, multiple sites

M94.8X1 Other specified disorders of cartilage, shoulder

M94.8X2 Other specified disorders of cartilage, upper arm

M94.8X3 Other specified disorders of cartilage, forearm

M94.8X4 Other specified disorders of cartilage, hand

---

④ 4th character required   ⑤ 5th character required   ⑥ 6th character required   ⑦ 7th character required   ⑦ₓ Extension 'X' Alert

EXCLUDES1 Not coded here   EXCLUDES2 Not included here   ℞ Primary Diagnosis Only   Manifestation Code

M94.8X5 Other specified disorders of cartilage, thigh

M94.8X6 Other specified disorders of cartilage, lower leg

M94.8X7 Other specified disorders of cartilage, ankle and foot

M94.8X8 Other specified disorders of cartilage, other site

M94.8X9 Other specified disorders of cartilage, unspecified sites

M94.9 Disorder of cartilage, unspecified

Other disorders of the musculoskeletal system and connective tissue (M95)

M95 Other acquired deformities of musculoskeletal system and connective tissue

EXCLUDES2 acquired absence of limbs and organs (Z89-Z90)
acquired deformities of limbs (M20-M21)
congenital malformations and deformations of the musculoskeletal system (Q65-Q79)
deforming dorsopathies (M40-M43)
dentofacial anomalies [including malocclusion] (M26.-)
postprocedural musculoskeletal disorders (M96.-)

M95.0 Acquired deformity of nose

EXCLUDES2 deviated nasal septum (J34.2)

M95.1 Cauliflower ear

EXCLUDES2 other acquired deformities of ear (H61.1)

M95.10 Cauliflower ear, unspecified ear

M95.11 Cauliflower ear, right ear

M95.12 Cauliflower ear, left ear

M95.2 Other acquired deformity of head

M95.3 Acquired deformity of neck

M95.4 Acquired deformity of chest and rib

M95.5 Acquired deformity of pelvis

EXCLUDES1 maternal care for known or suspected disproportion (O33.-)

M95.8 Other specified acquired deformities of musculoskeletal system

M95.9 Acquired deformity of musculoskeletal system, unspecified

Intraoperative and postprocedural complications and disorders of musculoskeletal system, not elsewhere classified (M96)

M96 Intraoperative and postprocedural complications and disorders of musculoskeletal system, not elsewhere classified

EXCLUDES2 arthropathy following intestinal bypass (M02.0-)
complications of internal orthopedic prosthetic devices, implants and grafts (T84.-)
disorders associated with osteoporosis (M80)
presence of functional implants and other devices (Z96-Z97)

M96.0 Pseudarthrosis after fusion or arthrodesis

M96.1 Postlaminectomy syndrome, not elsewhere classified

M96.2 Postradiation kyphosis

M96.3 Postlaminectomy kyphosis

M96.4 Postsurgical lordosis

M96.5 Postradiation scoliosis

M96.6 Fracture of bone following insertion of orthopedic implant, joint prosthesis, or bone plate

Intraoperative fracture of bone during insertion of orthopedic implant, joint prosthesis, or bone plate

EXCLUDES2 complication of internal orthopedic devices, implants or grafts (T84.-)

M96.62 Fracture of humerus following insertion of orthopedic implant, joint prosthesis, or bone plate

M96.621 Fracture of humerus following insertion of orthopedic implant, joint prosthesis, or bone plate, right arm

M96.622 Fracture of humerus following insertion of orthopedic implant, joint prosthesis, or bone plate, left arm

M96.629 Fracture of humerus following insertion of orthopedic implant, joint prosthesis, or bone plate, unspecified arm

M96.63 Fracture of radius or ulna following insertion of orthopedic implant, joint prosthesis, or bone plate

M96.631 Fracture of radius or ulna following insertion of orthopedic implant, joint prosthesis, or bone plate, right arm

M96.632 Fracture of radius or ulna following insertion of orthopedic implant, joint prosthesis, or bone plate, left arm

M96.639 Fracture of radius or ulna following insertion of orthopedic implant, joint prosthesis, or bone plate, unspecified arm

M96.65 Fracture of pelvis following insertion of orthopedic implant, joint prosthesis, or bone plate

M96.66 Fracture of femur following insertion of orthopedic implant, joint prosthesis, or bone plate

M96.661 Fracture of femur following insertion of orthopedic implant, joint prosthesis, or bone plate, right leg

M96.662 Fracture of femur following insertion of orthopedic implant, joint prosthesis, or bone plate, left leg

M96.669 Fracture of femur following insertion of orthopedic implant, joint prosthesis, or bone plate, unspecified leg

M96.67 Fracture of tibia or fibula following insertion of orthopedic implant, joint prosthesis, or bone plate

M96.671 Fracture of tibia or fibula following insertion of orthopedic implant, joint prosthesis, or bone plate, right leg

Unspecified Code	Other Specified Code	N Newborn Age: 0	P Pediatric Age: 0-17	M Maternity Age: 12-55
A Adult Age: 15-124	♂ Male	♀ Female	● New Code	▲ Revised Code Title	►◄ Revised Text

M96.672 Fracture of tibia or fibula following insertion of orthopedic implant, joint prosthesis, or bone plate, left leg

M96.679 Fracture of tibia or fibula following insertion of orthopedic implant, joint prosthesis, or bone plate, unspecified leg

M96.69 Fracture of other bone following insertion of orthopedic implant, joint prosthesis, or bone plate

[5] M96.8 Other intraoperative and postprocedural complications and disorders of musculoskeletal system, not elsewhere classified

[6] M96.81 Intraoperative hemorrhage and hematoma of a musculoskeletal structure complicating a procedure

[EXCLUDES1] *intraoperative hemorrhage and hematoma of a musculoskeletal structure due to accidental puncture and laceration during a procedure (M96.82-)*

M96.810 Intraoperative hemorrhage and hematoma of a musculoskeletal structure complicating a musculoskeletal system procedure

M96.811 Intraoperative hemorrhage and hematoma of a musculoskeletal structure complicating other procedure

[6] M96.82 Accidental puncture and laceration of a musculoskeletal structure during a procedure

M96.820 Accidental puncture and laceration of a musculoskeletal structure during a musculoskeletal system procedure

M96.821 Accidental puncture and laceration of a musculoskeletal structure during other procedure

[6] M96.83 Postprocedural hemorrhage and hematoma of a musculoskeletal structure following a procedure

M96.830 Postprocedural hemorrhage and hematoma of a musculoskeletal structure following a musculoskeletal system procedure

M96.831 Postprocedural hemorrhage and hematoma of a musculoskeletal structure following other procedure

M96.89 Other intraoperative and postprocedural complications and disorders of the musculoskeletal system

Instability of joint secondary to removal of joint prosthesis

Use additional code, if applicable, to further specify disorder

Biomechanical lesions, not elsewhere classified (M99)

[4] M99 Biomechanical lesions, not elsewhere classified

[NOTES] This category should not be used if the condition can be classified elsewhere.

[5] M99.0 Segmental and somatic dysfunction

M99.00 Segmental and somatic dysfunction of head region

M99.01 Segmental and somatic dysfunction of cervical region

M99.02 Segmental and somatic dysfunction of thoracic region

M99.03 Segmental and somatic dysfunction of lumbar region

M99.04 Segmental and somatic dysfunction of sacral region

M99.05 Segmental and somatic dysfunction of pelvic region

M99.06 Segmental and somatic dysfunction of lower extremity

M99.07 Segmental and somatic dysfunction of upper extremity

M99.08 Segmental and somatic dysfunction of rib cage

M99.09 Segmental and somatic dysfunction of abdomen and other regions

[5] M99.1 Subluxation complex (vertebral)

M99.10 Subluxation complex (vertebral) of head region

M99.11 Subluxation complex (vertebral) of cervical region

M99.12 Subluxation complex (vertebral) of thoracic region

M99.13 Subluxation complex (vertebral) of lumbar region

M99.14 Subluxation complex (vertebral) of sacral region

M99.15 Subluxation complex (vertebral) of pelvic region

M99.16 Subluxation complex (vertebral) of lower extremity

M99.17 Subluxation complex (vertebral) of upper extremity

M99.18 Subluxation complex (vertebral) of rib cage

M99.19 Subluxation complex (vertebral) of abdomen and other regions

[5] M99.2 Subluxation stenosis of neural canal

M99.20 Subluxation stenosis of neural canal of head region

M99.21 Subluxation stenosis of neural canal of cervical region

M99.22 Subluxation stenosis of neural canal of thoracic region

M99.23 Subluxation stenosis of neural canal of lumbar region

M99.24 Subluxation stenosis of neural canal of sacral region

M99.25 Subluxation stenosis of neural canal of pelvic region

M99.26 Subluxation stenosis of neural canal of lower extremity

M99.27 Subluxation stenosis of neural canal of upper extremity

M99.28 Subluxation stenosis of neural canal of rib cage

M99.29 Subluxation stenosis of neural canal of abdomen and other regions

[5] M99.3 Osseous stenosis of neural canal

M99.30 Osseous stenosis of neural canal of head region

M99.31 Osseous stenosis of neural canal of cervical region

M99.32 Osseous stenosis of neural canal of thoracic region

M99.33 Osseous stenosis of neural canal of lumbar region

M99.34 Osseous stenosis of neural canal of sacral region

M99.35 Osseous stenosis of neural canal of pelvic region

M99.36 Osseous stenosis of neural canal of lower extremity

M99.37 Osseous stenosis of neural canal of upper extremity

M99.38 Osseous stenosis of neural canal of rib cage

M99.39 Osseous stenosis of neural canal of abdomen and other regions

[5] M99.4 Connective tissue stenosis of neural canal

M99.40 Connective tissue stenosis of neural canal of head region

M99.41 Connective tissue stenosis of neural canal of cervical region

[4] 4th character required [5] 5th character required [6] 6th character required [7] 7th character required [X] Extension 'X' Alert
[EXCLUDES 1] Not coded here [EXCLUDES 2] Not included here [PDx] Primary Diagnosis Only Manifestation Code

M99.42 Connective tissue stenosis of neural canal of thoracic region
M99.43 Connective tissue stenosis of neural canal of lumbar region
M99.44 Connective tissue stenosis of neural canal of sacral region
M99.45 Connective tissue stenosis of neural canal of pelvic region
M99.46 Connective tissue stenosis of neural canal of lower extremity
M99.47 Connective tissue stenosis of neural canal of upper extremity
M99.48 Connective tissue stenosis of neural canal of rib cage
M99.49 Connective tissue stenosis of neural canal of abdomen and other regions

[5] M99.5 Intervertebral disc stenosis of neural canal
M99.50 Intervertebral disc stenosis of neural canal of head region
M99.51 Intervertebral disc stenosis of neural canal of cervical region
M99.52 Intervertebral disc stenosis of neural canal of thoracic region
M99.53 Intervertebral disc stenosis of neural canal of lumbar region
M99.54 Intervertebral disc stenosis of neural canal of sacral region
M99.55 Intervertebral disc stenosis of neural canal of pelvic region
M99.56 Intervertebral disc stenosis of neural canal of lower extremity
M99.57 Intervertebral disc stenosis of neural canal of upper extremity
M99.58 Intervertebral disc stenosis of neural canal of rib cage
M99.59 Intervertebral disc stenosis of neural canal of abdomen and other regions

[5] M99.6 Osseous and subluxation stenosis of intervertebral foramina
M99.60 Osseous and subluxation stenosis of intervertebral foramina of head region
M99.61 Osseous and subluxation stenosis of intervertebral foramina of cervical region
M99.62 Osseous and subluxation stenosis of intervertebral foramina of thoracic region
M99.63 Osseous and subluxation stenosis of intervertebral foramina of lumbar region
M99.64 Osseous and subluxation stenosis of intervertebral foramina of sacral region
M99.65 Osseous and subluxation stenosis of intervertebral foramina of pelvic region
M99.66 Osseous and subluxation stenosis of intervertebral foramina of lower extremity
M99.67 Osseous and subluxation stenosis of intervertebral foramina of upper extremity
M99.68 Osseous and subluxation stenosis of intervertebral foramina of rib cage
M99.69 Osseous and subluxation stenosis of intervertebral foramina of abdomen and other regions

[5] M99.7 Connective tissue and disc stenosis of intervertebral foramina
M99.70 Connective tissue and disc stenosis of intervertebral foramina of head region
M99.71 Connective tissue and disc stenosis of intervertebral foramina of cervical region
M99.72 Connective tissue and disc stenosis of intervertebral foramina of thoracic region
M99.73 Connective tissue and disc stenosis of intervertebral foramina of lumbar region
M99.74 Connective tissue and disc stenosis of intervertebral foramina of sacral region
M99.75 Connective tissue and disc stenosis of intervertebral foramina of pelvic region
M99.76 Connective tissue and disc stenosis of intervertebral foramina of lower extremity
M99.77 Connective tissue and disc stenosis of intervertebral foramina of upper extremity
M99.78 Connective tissue and disc stenosis of intervertebral foramina of rib cage
M99.79 Connective tissue and disc stenosis of intervertebral foramina of abdomen and other regions

[5] M99.8 Other biomechanical lesions
M99.80 Other biomechanical lesions of head region
M99.81 Other biomechanical lesions of cervical region
M99.82 Other biomechanical lesions of thoracic region
M99.83 Other biomechanical lesions of lumbar region
M99.84 Other biomechanical lesions of sacral region
M99.85 Other biomechanical lesions of pelvic region
M99.86 Other biomechanical lesions of lower extremity
M99.87 Other biomechanical lesions of upper extremity
M99.88 Other biomechanical lesions of rib cage
M99.89 Other biomechanical lesions of abdomen and other regions

M99.9 Biomechanical lesion, unspecified

Unspecified Code | Other Specified Code | [N] Newborn Age: 0 | [P] Pediatric Age: 0-17 | [M] Maternity Age: 12-55
[A] Adult Age: 15-124 | ♂ Male | ♀ Female | ● New Code | ▲ Revised Code Title | ►◄ Revised Text

This page intentionally left blank

Chapter Specific Coding Guidelines

a. **Chronic Kidney Disease**
   1) **Stages of chronic kidney disease (CKD)**
   The ICD-10-CM classifies CKD based on severity. The severity of CKD is designated by stages 1-5. Stage 2, code N18.2, equates to mild CKD; stage 3, code N18.3, equates to moderate CKD; and stage 4, code N18.4, equates to severe CKD. Code N18.6, End stage renal disease (ESRD), is assigned when the provider has documented end-stage-renal disease (ESRD).

   If both a stage of CKD and ESRD are documented, assign code N18.6 only.

   2) **Chronic kidney disease and kidney transplant status**
   Patients who have undergone kidney transplant may still have some form of chronic kidney disease (CKD) because the kidney transplant may not fully restore kidney function. Therefore, the presence of CKD alone does not constitute a transplant complication. Assign the appropriate N18 code for the patient's stage of CKD and code Z94.0, Kidney transplant status. If a transplant complication such as failure or rejection or other transplant complication is documented, see section I.C.19.g for information on coding complications of a kidney transplant. If the documentation is unclear as to whether the patient has a complication of the transplant, query the provider.

   3) **Chronic kidney disease with other conditions**
   Patients with CKD may also suffer from other serious conditions, most commonly diabetes mellitus and hypertension. The sequencing of the CKD code in relationship to codes for other contributing conditions is based on the conventions in the Tabular List.

   See I.C.9. Hypertensive chronic kidney disease.

   See I.C.19. Chronic kidney disease and kidney transplant complications.

This page intentionally left blank

Anatomy of the Male Reproductive System

1. **The male reproductive system includes the following:**
   a) The primary sex organs (or the Testes/Male Gonads) that produce sperms and the male sex hormones.
   b) The accessory organs (or the scrotum and ducts) that support the testes and transport the sperm.
   c) The accessory glands that produce secretions for constituting the semen.
   d) The penis, which acts as a transporting and supporting structure of the male reproductive system

2. **The anatomy of structures/components of the male reproductive system is further described below:**
   a) Scrotum
      i) It is an extension from the abdominal wall that supports the testes.
      ii) It is divided into two lateral pouches via a septum, and each pouch contains a single testis.
      iii) The scrotal sac serves to provide protection to the sperms from the changes in the external environment.
   b) The Testes
      i) The testes are covered by a capsule of connective tissue, which is known as the tunica albuginea.
      ii) The tunica albuginea travels inwards to constitute a series of compartments, which are known as lobules.
      iii) A single lobule carries convoluted seminiferous tubules for spermatogenesis.
      iv) Male sex hormone (testosterone) is produced by the interstitial cells of Leydig that remain located in the individual lobules.
   c) The Spermatozoa (or Mature Sperm Cell)
      i) A typical sperm cell is composed of a head, a middle piece, and a tail (or flagellum)
      ii) Spermatozoa can survive up to a period of 48 hours in the female reproductive tract. Approximately three hundred million spermatozoa are produced on a daily basis in a male.
   d) The Ducts of the Male Reproductive System
      i) Convoluted seminiferous tubules of the testis contain the mature sperm cells.
      ii) A tightly coiled structure (or epididymis) is positioned on the posterior border of the testis.
      iii) The straightened epididymis is known as the ductus deferens (or vas deferens).
      iv) The spermatic cord is a sheath that contains the vas deferens and empties into the ejaculatory duct.
      v) The urethra is regarded as the terminal duct of the male reproductive system. The ejaculatory duct ejects the spermatozoa into the urethra. Moreover, the urethra provides a common passage for both sperm and urine.
      vi) The urethra traverses through the prostate gland, urogenital diaphragm, and penis.
   e) The Accessory Glands
      i) Paired seminal vesicles generate the alkaline viscous part of the semen and transfer it to the ejaculatory duct.
      ii) Prostate gland produces the semen that provides a medium to the sperm cells for swimming.
      iii) Bulbourethral glands (or Cowper's glands) generate the viscous mucous that acts as a lubricant for sexual intercourse.
   f) Semen
      i) Semen is a milky fluid, which is a mixture of the matured sperm cells and secretions of the accessory glands.
      ii) It provides a transport medium for the sperm.
   g) The Penis
      i) It acts to transport the matured sperms to the female reproductive tract.
      ii) It is composed of a shaft, and the terminal point of the shaft is known as the glans penis (or head). The head of the penis is covered with loose skin, which is called as the prepuce or foreskin.

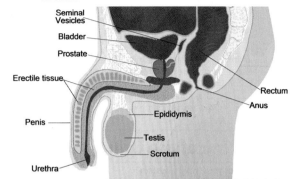

MALE REPRODUCTIVE TRACT

Common Pathologies

Benign Prostate Hypertrophy (BPH)
Benign prostatic hyperplasia (BPH) is a common urological condition caused by the non-cancerous enlargement of the prostate gland as men get older. As the prostate enlarges, it can squeeze down on the urethra. The symptoms associated with BPH are known as lower urinary tract symptoms. This can cause men to have trouble urinating and leads to symptoms of BPH. The symptoms associated with BPH are known as lower urinary tract symptoms (LUTS)

Benign Prostatic Hyperplasia

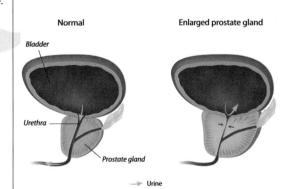

Gynaecomastia
Gynaecomastia is a common condition that causes boys' and men's breasts to swell and become larger than normal. It is most common in teenage boys and older men

Hypospadias
Hypospadias is an abnormality of anterior urethral and penile development in which the urethral opening is ectopically located on the ventrum of the penis proximal to the tip of the glans penis, which, in this condition, is splayed open. The urethral opening may be located as far down as in the scrotum or perineum.

Orchitis
Orchitis is an acute inflammatory reaction of the testis secondary to infection. Most cases are associated with a viral mumps infection; however, other viruses and bacteria can cause orchitis

Torsion of Testis

Testicular torsion, or testis torsion, occurs when the spermatic cord that provides blood flow to the testicle rotates and becomes twisted, usually due to an injury or medical condition. This cuts off the testicle's blood supply and causes sudden and severe pain and swelling.

Hydrocele

Accumulation of liquid in the scrotum between the visceral and parietal areas of the tunica vaginalis that in infants is usually the result of incomplete closure of the processus vaginalis. It may or may not be associated with inguinal hernia.

Phimosis

Phimosis is the inability to fully retract the foreskin (or prepuce) over the glans penis due to a narrow opening

Balanitis

Balanitis is an infection or inflammation of the skin on the head (glans) of the penis. In men who are not circumcised, this area is covered by a flap of skin known as the foreskin, or prepuce. Balanitis can occur in both circumcised and uncircumcised men, although it occurs more commonly in men who are not circumcised

Anatomy of the Urinary System

1. **An Outline of the Urinary System**
   a) Two Kidneys
   b) Two Ureters
   c) The Urinary Bladder
   d) The Urethra
   e) Urinary system maintains the state of homeostasis by regulating water and solutes in the human body.
   f) Kidneys produce the urine and function as the major filtering organs of the urinary system.
   g) Urine is composed of components like urea, water, ions and toxic wastes that need to be regulated in the human body by the entire urinary system.

2. **The Functions of Kidneys**
   a) Excretion
   b) Maintenance of blood volume and concentration
   c) pH regulation
   d) Maintenance of blood pressure
   e) Maintenance of erythrocyte concentration
   f) The conversion of vitamin D to its active form (or calciferol).

3. **The Anatomy of Kidneys**
   a) Kidneys are situated between the parietal peritoneum and posterior wall of abdomen.
   b) There is a notch (known as hilum) located in the concave center of each kidney. The ureter exits the kidney and blood vessels, lymph vessels and nerves enter and leave the kidney through the hilum.
   c) The kidney is surrounded by the following three layers:
      i) The innermost layer of the kidney is known as the renal capsule. It acts as a barrier against trauma and infection.
      ii) Adipose capsule is the middle layer of the kidney. It is made up of fatty tissue and protects the kidney from blows.
      iii) The renal fascia is the outermost layer of the kidney. It serves to attach the kidney to the abdominal wall.
   d) Cortex is the outer region of the kidney.
   e) Medulla is the inner area of the kidney.
   f) Renal pyramids are striated triangular structures that are found within the medulla. The bases of these pyramids face toward the cortex. However, their tips point to the center of the kidney and are known as the renal papillae.
   g) The renal columns constitute the cortical material that extends between the pyramids.

   h) The parenchyma of the kidney is formed by the cortex and renal pyramids.
   i) The parenchyma is further composed of the microscopic units or nephrons, which are the structural and functional units of the kidneys.
   j) The minor calyx is a funnel-shaped structure that surrounds the tip of each renal pyramid. The function of this minor calyx is to collect the urine from the ducts of the renal pyramids. The minor calyces integrate to constitute the major calyces.
   k) The renal pelvis is the large collecting funnel that is formed by a bunch of major calyces. The renal pelvis is further narrowed and extended to constitute the ureter.

4. **The Ureter**
   a) It is the extension of the renal pelvis of the kidney and communicates with the urinary bladder.
   b) They are two in number and carry urine from the renal pelvis to the urinary bladder.
   c) Urine is expelled from the bladder by the act of micturition.

5. **The Urethra**
   a) It is a thin walled tube that connects the floor of the urinary bladder to the genitals for the expulsion of fluids (urine, semen etc) out of the body.
   b) It is located in the wall of the vagina and above the vaginal opening in females. The female urethral orifice is the opening of the urethra and situated between the vaginal opening and clitoris.
   c) It lies below the bladder in males and travels through the prostate gland and penis.
   d) The opening at the tip of the male penis is known as the male urethral orifice.
   e) The external urethral sphincter is a striated muscle and provides voluntary control on urination.

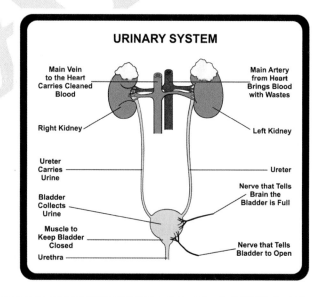

Common Pathologies

Glomerulonephritis

Glomerulonephritis is also known as glomerular nephritis (GN) or glomerular disease. It is a disease of the kidney, characterized by inflammation of the glomeruli. the individual filtering units of the kidney that produce urine. When the glomeruli become inflamed, the kidneys can't filter urine properly. This results in a buildup of excess fluid and toxins in the body. Glomerulonephritis can lead to chronic renal (kidney) failure.

Acute Renal Failure

Acute kidney failure occurs when your kidneys suddenly become unable to filter waste products from your blood. When your kidneys lose their filtering ability, dangerous levels of wastes may accumulate and your blood's chemical makeup may get out of balance.

Chronic Kidney Disease

Chronic kidney disease (CKD) is defined as the presence of kidney damage, or a decreased level of kidney function, for a period of three months or more. CKD can be divided into five stages, depending on how severe the damage is to the kidneys, or the level of decrease in kidney function.

Usually, kidney disease starts slowly and silently, and progresses over a number of years. Not everyone progresses from Stage 1 to Stage 5. Stage 5 is also known as End-Stage Renal Disease (ESRD). It may also be called end-stage renal failure. It is important to remember that end-stage refers to the end of your kidney function (your kidneys are working at less than 15% of normal), not the end of your life.

Bladder Cancer

Cancer that forms in tissues of the bladder (the organ that stores urine). Most bladder cancers are transitional cell carcinomas (cancer that begins in cells that normally make up the inner lining of the bladder). Other types include squamous cell carcinoma (cancer that begins in thin, flat cells) and adenocarcinoma (cancer that begins in cells that make and release mucus and other fluids). The cells that form squamous cell carcinoma and adenocarcinoma develop in the inner lining of the bladder as a result of chronic irritation and inflammation

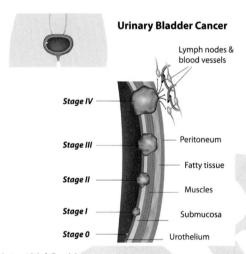

Urinary Bladder Cancer

Lymph nodes & blood vessels

Stage IV

Stage III — Peritoneum

— Fatty tissue

Stage II — Muscles

Stage I — Submucosa

Stage 0 — Urothelium

Interstitial Cystitis

Interstitial cystitis is a chronic inflammation of the bladder that causes chronic pain and discomfort. Symptoms often include a sense of urgency and increased frequency of urination.

Cystocele

Cystocele is a condition that is sometimes referred to as bladder hernia or a prolapsed bladder. This is a condition that affects women and is characterized by a protrusion of the urinary bladder into the vagina due to the stretching and relaxation of the tissues between the bladder and vagina.

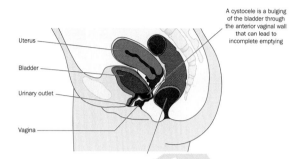

A cystocele is a bulging of the bladder through the anterior vaginal wall that can lead to incomplete emptying

Uterus

Bladder

Urinary outlet

Vagina

UTI

A urinary tract infection (UTI) is an infection in any part of urinary system (kidneys, ureters, bladder and urethra). Most infections involve the lower urinary tract the bladder and the urethra.

Kidney Stones

A kidney stone is a solid piece of material that forms in a kidney when substances that are normally found in the urine become highly concentrated. A stone may stay in the kidney or travel down the urinary tract. Kidney stones vary in size. A small stone may pass on its own, causing little or no pain. A larger stone may get stuck along the urinary tract and can block the flow of urine, causing severe pain or bleeding

Diseases of the genitourinary system (N00-N99)

> EXCLUDES2   *certain conditions originating in the perinatal period (P04-P96)*
> *certain infectious and parasitic diseases (A00-B99)*
> *complications of pregnancy, childbirth and the puerperium (O00-O9A)*
> *congenital malformations, deformations and chromosomal abnormalities (Q00-Q99)*
> *endocrine, nutritional and metabolic diseases (E00-E88)*
> *injury, poisoning and certain other consequences of external causes (S00-T88)*
> *neoplasms (C00-D49)*
> *symptoms, signs and abnormal clinical and laboratory findings, not elsewhere classified (R00-R94)*

Glomerular diseases (N00-N08)

Code also any associated kidney failure (N17-N19).

> EXCLUDES1   *hypertensive chronic kidney disease (I12.-)*

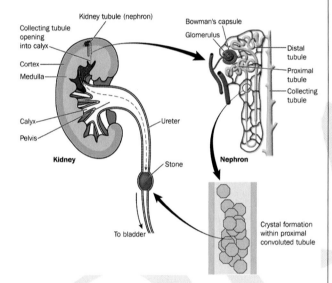

Figure 13.1 Kidney and Nephron

N00 Acute **nephritic syndrome**

> INCLUDES   *acute glomerular disease*
> *acute glomerulonephritis*
> *acute nephritis*
>
> EXCLUDES1   *acute tubulo-interstitial nephritis (N10)*
> *nephritic syndrome NOS (N05.-)*

N00.0 **Acute nephritic syndrome** with minor glomerular abnormality

Acute nephritic syndrome with minimal change lesion

N00.1 **Acute nephritic syndrome** with focal and segmental glomerular lesions

Acute nephritic syndrome with focal and segmental hyalinosis

Acute nephritic syndrome with focal and segmental sclerosis

Acute nephritic syndrome with focal glomerulonephritis

N00.2 **Acute nephritic syndrome** with diffuse membranous glomerulonephritis

N00.3 **Acute nephritic syndrome** with diffuse mesangial proliferative glomerulonephritis

N00.4 **Acute nephritic syndrome** with diffuse endocapillary proliferative glomerulonephritis

N00.5 Acute nephritic syndrome with diffuse mesangiocapillary glomerulonephritis

Acute nephritic syndrome with membranoproliferative glomerulonephritis, types 1 and 3, or NOS

N00.6 **Acute nephritic syndrome** with dense deposit disease

Acute nephritic syndrome with membranoproliferative glomerulonephritis, type 2

N00.7 **Acute nephritic syndrome** with diffuse crescentic glomerulonephritis

Acute nephritic syndrome with extracapillary glomerulonephritis

N00.8 Acute nephritic syndrome with other morphologic changes

Acute nephritic syndrome with proliferative glomerulonephritis NOS

N00.9 Acute nephritic syndrome with unspecified morphologic changes

N01 Rapidly progressive **nephritic syndrome**

> INCLUDES   *rapidly progressive glomerular disease*
> *rapidly progressive glomerulonephritis*
> *rapidly progressive nephritis*
>
> EXCLUDES1   *nephritic syndrome NOS (N05.-)*

N01.0 **Rapidly progressive nephritic syndrome** with minor glomerular abnormality

Rapidly progressive nephritic syndrome with minimal change lesion

N01.1 **Rapidly progressive nephritic syndrome** with focal and segmental glomerular lesions

Rapidly progressive nephritic syndrome with focal and segmental hyalinosis

Rapidly progressive nephritic syndrome with focal and segmental sclerosis

Rapidly progressive nephritic syndrome with focal glomerulonephritis

N01.2 **Rapidly progressive nephritic syndrome** with diffuse membranous glomerulonephritis

N01.3 **Rapidly progressive nephritic syndrome** with diffuse mesangial proliferative glomerulonephritis

N01.4 **Rapidly progressive nephritic syndrome** with diffuse endocapillary proliferative glomerulonephritis

N01.5 **Rapidly progressive nephritic syndrome** with diffuse mesangiocapillary glomerulonephritis

Rapidly progressive nephritic syndrome with membranoproliferative glomerulonephritis, types 1 and 3, or NOS

N01.6 **Rapidly progressive nephritic syndrome** with dense deposit disease

Rapidly progressive nephritic syndrome with membranoproliferative glomerulonephritis, type 2

N01.7 **Rapidly progressive nephritic syndrome** with diffuse crescentic glomerulonephritis

Rapidly progressive nephritic syndrome with extracapillary glomerulonephritis

N01.8 Rapidly progressive nephritic syndrome with other morphologic changes

Rapidly progressive nephritic syndrome with proliferative glomerulonephritis NOS

N01.9 **Rapidly progressive nephritic syndrome with unspecified morphologic changes**

N02 Recurrent and persistent hematuria

> EXCLUDES1   *acute cystitis with hematuria (N30.01)*
> *hematuria NOS (R31.9)*
> *hematuria not associated with specified morphologic lesions (R31.-)*

N02.0 Recurrent and persistent hematuria with minor glomerular abnormality

Recurrent and persistent hematuria with minimal change lesion

---

Unspecified Code   Other Specified Code   N Newborn Age: 0   P Pediatric Age: 0-17   M Maternity Age: 12-55

A Adult Age: 15-124   ♂ Male   ♀ Female   ● New Code   ▲ Revised Code Title   ►◄ Revised Text

N02.1 Recurrent and persistent hematuria with focal and segmental glomerular lesions

Recurrent and persistent hematuria with focal and segmental hyalinosis

Recurrent and persistent hematuria with focal and segmental sclerosis

Recurrent and persistent hematuria with focal glomerulonephritis

N02.2 Recurrent and persistent hematuria with diffuse membranous glomerulonephritis

N02.3 Recurrent and persistent hematuria with diffuse mesangial proliferative glomerulonephritis

N02.4 Recurrent and persistent hematuria with diffuse endocapillary proliferative glomerulonephritis

N02.5 Recurrent and persistent hematuria with diffuse mesangiocapillary glomerulonephritis

Recurrent and persistent hematuria with membranoproliferative glomerulonephritis, types 1 and 3, or NOS

N02.6 Recurrent and persistent hematuria with dense deposit disease

Recurrent and persistent hematuria with membranoproliferative glomerulonephritis, type 2

N02.7 Recurrent and persistent hematuria with diffuse crescentic glomerulonephritis

Recurrent and persistent hematuria with extracapillary glomerulonephritis

N02.8 Recurrent and persistent hematuria with other morphologic changes

Recurrent and persistent hematuria with proliferative glomerulonephritis NOS

N02.9 Recurrent and persistent hematuria with unspecified morphologic changes

④ **N03** Chronic nephritic syndrome

INCLUDES   chronic glomerular disease
chronic glomerulonephritis
chronic nephritis

EXCLUDES1   chronic tubulo-interstitial nephritis (N11.-)
diffuse sclerosing glomerulonephritis (N05.8-)
nephritic syndrome NOS (N05.-)

N03.0 Chronic nephritic syndrome with minor glomerular abnormality

Chronic nephritic syndrome with minimal change lesion

N03.1 Chronic nephritic syndrome with focal and segmental glomerular lesions

Chronic nephritic syndrome with focal and segmental hyalinosis

Chronic nephritic syndrome with focal and segmental sclerosis

Chronic nephritic syndrome with focal glomerulonephritis

N03.2 Chronic nephritic syndrome with diffuse membranous glomerulonephritis

N03.3 Chronic nephritic syndrome with diffuse mesangial proliferative glomerulonephritis

N03.4 Chronic nephritic syndrome with diffuse endocapillary proliferative glomerulonephritis

N03.5 Chronic nephritic syndrome with diffuse mesangiocapillary glomerulonephritis

Chronic nephritic syndrome with membranoproliferative glomerulonephritis, types 1 and 3, or NOS

N03.6 Chronic nephritic syndrome with dense deposit disease

Chronic nephritic syndrome with membranoproliferative glomerulonephritis, type 2

N03.7 Chronic nephritic syndrome with diffuse crescentic glomerulonephritis

Chronic nephritic syndrome with extracapillary glomerulonephritis

N03.8 Chronic nephritic syndrome with other morphologic changes

Chronic nephritic syndrome with proliferative glomerulonephritis NOS

N03.9 Chronic nephritic syndrome with unspecified morphologic changes

④ **N04** Nephrotic syndrome

INCLUDES   congenital nephrotic syndrome
lipoid nephrosis

N04.0 Nephrotic syndrome with minor glomerular abnormality

Nephrotic syndrome with minimal change lesion

N04.1 Nephrotic syndrome with focal and segmental glomerular lesions

Nephrotic syndrome with focal and segmental hyalinosis

Nephrotic syndrome with focal and segmental sclerosis

Nephrotic syndrome with focal glomerulonephritis

N04.2 Nephrotic syndrome with diffuse membranous glomerulonephritis

N04.3 Nephrotic syndrome with diffuse mesangial proliferative glomerulonephritis

N04.4 Nephrotic syndrome with diffuse endocapillary proliferative glomerulonephritis

N04.5 Nephrotic syndrome with diffuse mesangiocapillary glomerulonephritis

Nephrotic syndrome with membranoproliferative glomerulonephritis, types 1 and 3, or NOS

N04.6 Nephrotic syndrome with dense deposit disease

Nephrotic syndrome with membranoproliferative glomerulonephritis, type 2

N04.7 Nephrotic syndrome with diffuse crescentic glomerulonephritis

Nephrotic syndrome with extracapillary glomerulonephritis

N04.8 Nephrotic syndrome with other morphologic changes

Nephrotic syndrome with proliferative glomerulonephritis NOS

N04.9 Nephrotic syndrome with unspecified morphologic changes

④ **N05** Unspecified nephritic syndrome

INCLUDES   glomerular disease NOS
glomerulonephritis NOS
nephritis NOS
nephropathy NOS and renal disease NOS with morphological lesion specified in .0-.8

EXCLUDES1   nephropathy NOS with no stated morphological lesion (N28.9)
renal disease NOS with no stated morphological lesion (N28.9)
tubulo-interstitial nephritis NOS (N12)

N05.0 Unspecified nephritic syndrome with minor glomerular abnormality

Unspecified nephritic syndrome with minimal change lesion

N05.1 Unspecified nephritic syndrome with focal and segmental glomerular lesions

Unspecified nephritic syndrome with focal and segmental hyalinosis

Unspecified nephritic syndrome with focal and segmental sclerosis

Unspecified nephritic syndrome with focal glomerulonephritis

N05.2 Unspecified nephritic syndrome with diffuse membranous glomerulonephritis

N05.3 Unspecified nephritic syndrome with diffuse mesangial proliferative glomerulonephritis

---

④ 4ᵗʰ character required   ⑤ 5ᵗʰ character required   ⑥ 6ᵗʰ character required   ⑦ 7ᵗʰ character required   ⑩ Extension 'X' Alert

EXCLUDES 1 Not coded here   EXCLUDES 2 Not included here   Pᴅx Primary Diagnosis Only   Manifestation Code

N05.4 **Unspecified nephritic syndrome** with diffuse endocapillary proliferative glomerulonephritis

N05.5 **Unspecified nephritic syndrome** with diffuse mesangiocapillary glomerulonephritis

Unspecified nephritic syndrome with membranoproliferative glomerulonephritis, types 1 and 3, or NOS

N05.6 **Unspecified nephritic syndrome** with dense deposit disease

Unspecified nephritic syndrome with membranoproliferative glomerulonephritis, type 2

N05.7 **Unspecified nephritic syndrome** with diffuse crescentic glomerulonephritis

Unspecified nephritic syndrome with extracapillary glomerulonephritis

N05.8 **Unspecified nephritic syndrome** with other morphologic changes

Unspecified nephritic syndrome with proliferative glomerulonephritis NOS

N05.9 **Unspecified nephritic syndrome** with unspecified morphologic changes

🔵 **N06** **Isolated proteinuria with specified morphological lesion**

> EXCLUDES1 Proteinuria not associated with specific morphologic lesions (R80.0)

N06.0 **Isolated proteinuria** with minor glomerular abnormality

Isolated proteinuria with minimal change lesion

N06.1 **Isolated proteinuria** with focal and segmental glomerular lesions

Isolated proteinuria with focal and segmental hyalinosis
Isolated proteinuria with focal and segmental sclerosis
Isolated proteinuria with focal glomerulonephritis

N06.2 **Isolated proteinuria** with diffuse membranous glomerulonephritis

N06.3 **Isolated proteinuria** with diffuse mesangial proliferative glomerulonephritis

N06.4 **Isolated proteinuria** with diffuse endocapillary proliferative glomerulonephritis

N06.5 **Isolated proteinuria** with diffuse mesangiocapillary glomerulonephritis

Isolated proteinuria with membranoproliferative glomerulonephritis, types 1 and 3, or NOS

N06.6 **Isolated proteinuria** with dense deposit disease

Isolated proteinuria with membranoproliferative glomerulonephritis, type 2

N06.7 **Isolated proteinuria** with diffuse crescentic glomerulonephritis

Isolated proteinuria with extracapillary glomerulonephritis

N06.8 **Isolated proteinuria with other morphologic lesion**

Isolated proteinuria with proliferative glomerulonephritis NOS

N06.9 **Isolated proteinuria with unspecified morphologic lesion**

🔵 **N07** **Hereditary nephropathy, not elsewhere classified**

> EXCLUDES2 Alport's syndrome (Q87.81-)
> hereditary amyloid nephropathy (E85.-)
> nail patella syndrome (Q87.2)
> non-neuropathic heredofamilial amyloidosis (E85.-)

N07.0 **Hereditary nephropathy, not elsewhere classified** with minor glomerular abnormality

Hereditary nephropathy, not elsewhere classified with minimal change lesion

N07.1 **Hereditary nephropathy, not elsewhere classified** with focal and segmental glomerular lesions

Hereditary nephropathy, not elsewhere classified with focal and segmental hyalinosis

Hereditary nephropathy, not elsewhere classified with focal and segmental sclerosis

Hereditary nephropathy, not elsewhere classified with focal glomerulonephritis

N07.2 **Hereditary nephropathy, not elsewhere classified** with diffuse membranous glomerulonephritis

N07.3 **Hereditary nephropathy, not elsewhere classified** with diffuse mesangial proliferative glomerulonephritis

N07.4 **Hereditary nephropathy, not elsewhere classified** with diffuse endocapillary proliferative glomerulonephritis

N07.5 **Hereditary nephropathy, not elsewhere classified** with diffuse mesangiocapillary glomerulonephritis

Hereditary nephropathy, not elsewhere classified with membranoproliferative glomerulonephritis, types 1 and 3, or NOS

N07.6 **Hereditary nephropathy, not elsewhere classified** with dense deposit disease

Hereditary nephropathy, not elsewhere classified with membranoproliferative glomerulonephritis, type 2

N07.7 **Hereditary nephropathy, not elsewhere classified** with diffuse crescentic glomerulonephritis

Hereditary nephropathy, not elsewhere classified with extracapillary glomerulonephritis

N07.8 **Hereditary nephropathy, not elsewhere classified with other morphologic lesions**

Hereditary nephropathy, not elsewhere classified with proliferative glomerulonephritis NOS

N07.9 **Hereditary nephropathy, not elsewhere classified with unspecified morphologic lesions**

N08 **Glomerular disorders in diseases classified elsewhere**

Glomerulonephritis
Nephritis
Nephropathy
Code first underlying disease, such as:
amyloidosis (E85.-)
congenital syphilis (A50.5)
cryoglobulinemia (D89.1)
disseminated intravascular coagulation (D65)
gout (M1A.-, M10.-)
microscopic polyangiitis (M31.7)
multiple myeloma (C90.0-)
sepsis (A40.0-A41.9)
sickle-cell disease (D57.0-D57.8)

> EXCLUDES1 glomerulonephritis, nephritis and nephropathy (in):
> antiglomerular basement membrane disease (M31.0)
> diabetes (E08-E13 with .21)
> gonococcal (A54.21)
> Goodpasture's syndrome (M31.0)
> hemolytic-uremic syndrome (D59.3)
> lupus (M32.14)
> mumps (B26.83)
> syphilis (A52.75)
> systemic lupus erythematosus (M32.14)
> Wegener's granulomatosis (M31.31)
> pyelonephritis in diseases classified elsewhere (N16)
> renal tubulo-interstitial disorders classified elsewhere (N16)

Unspecified Code	Other Specified Code	N Newborn Age: 0	P Pediatric Age: 0-17	M Maternity Age: 12-55
	A Adult Age: 15-124	♂ Male	♀ Female	● New Code	▲ Revised Code Title	◄► Revised Text

Renal tubulo-interstitial diseases (N10-N16)

> INCLUDES   pyelonephritis
>
> EXCLUDES1   pyeloureteritis cystica (N28.85)

N10 Acute tubulo-interstitial nephritis

Acute infectious interstitial nephritis
Acute pyelitis
Acute pyelonephritis
Hemoglobin nephrosis
Myoglobin nephrosis
Use additional code (B95-B97), to identify infectious agent.

④ N11 Chronic tubulo-interstitial nephritis

> INCLUDES   chronic infectious interstitial nephritis
>   chronic pyelitis
>   chronic pyelonephritis

Use additional code (B95-B97), to identify infectious agent.

N11.0 Nonobstructive reflux-associated chronic pyelonephritis

Pyelonephritis (chronic) associated with (vesicoureteral) reflux

> EXCLUDES1   vesicoureteral reflux NOS (N13.70)

N11.1 Chronic obstructive pyelonephritis

Pyelonephritis (chronic) associated with anomaly of pelviureteric junction
Pyelonephritis (chronic) associated with anomaly of pyeloureteric junction
Pyelonephritis (chronic) associated with crossing of vessel
Pyelonephritis (chronic) associated with kinking of ureter
Pyelonephritis (chronic) associated with obstruction of ureter
Pyelonephritis (chronic) associated with stricture of pelviureteric junction
Pyelonephritis (chronic) associated with stricture of ureter

> EXCLUDES1   calculous pyelonephritis (N20.9)
>   obstructive uropathy (N13.-)

N11.8 Other chronic tubulo-interstitial nephritis

Nonobstructive chronic pyelonephritis NOS

N11.9 Chronic tubulo-interstitial nephritis, unspecified

Chronic interstitial nephritis NOS
Chronic pyelitis NOS
Chronic pyelonephritis NOS

N12 Tubulo-interstitial nephritis, not specified as acute or chronic

Interstitial nephritis NOS
Pyelitis NOS
Pyelonephritis NOS

> EXCLUDES1   calculous pyelonephritis (N20.9)

④ N13 Obstructive and reflux uropathy

> EXCLUDES2   calculus of kidney and ureter without
>   hydronephrosis (N20.-)
>   congenital obstructive defects of renal pelvis and
>   ureter (Q62.0-Q62.3)
>   hydronephrosis with ureteropelvic junction
>   obstruction (Q62.1)
>   obstructive pyelonephritis (N11.1)

N13.1 Hydronephrosis with ureteral stricture, not elsewhere classified

> EXCLUDES1   Hydronephrosis with ureteral stricture with
>   infection (N13.6)

N13.2 Hydronephrosis with renal and ureteral calculous obstruction

> EXCLUDES1   Hydronephrosis with renal and ureteral calculous
>   obstruction with infection (N13.6)

⑤ N13.3 Other and unspecified hydronephrosis

> EXCLUDES1   hydronephrosis with infection (N13.6)

N13.30 Unspecified hydronephrosis
N13.39 Other hydronephrosis

N13.4 Hydroureter

> EXCLUDES1   congenital hydroureter (Q62.3-)
>   hydroureter with infection (N13.6)
>   vesicoureteral-reflux with hydroureter (N13.73-)

N13.5 Crossing vessel and stricture of ureter without hydronephrosis

Kinking and stricture of ureter without hydronephrosis

> EXCLUDES1   Crossing vessel and stricture of ureter without
>   hydronephrosis with infection (N13.6)

N13.6 Pyonephrosis

Conditions in N13.1-N13.5 with infection
Obstructive uropathy with infection
Use additional code (B95-B97), to identify infectious agent.

⑤ N13.7 Vesicoureteral-reflux

> EXCLUDES1   reflux-associated pyelonephritis (N11.0)

N13.70 Vesicoureteral-reflux, unspecified

Vesicoureteral-reflux NOS

N13.71 Vesicoureteral-reflux without reflux nephropathy

⑥ N13.72 Vesicoureteral-reflux with reflux nephropathy without hydroureter

N13.721 Vesicoureteral-reflux with reflux nephropathy without hydroureter, unilateral

N13.722 Vesicoureteral-reflux with reflux nephropathy without hydroureter, bilateral

N13.729 Vesicoureteral-reflux with reflux nephropathy without hydroureter, unspecified

⑥ N13.73 Vesicoureteral-reflux with reflux nephropathy with hydroureter

N13.731 Vesicoureteral-reflux with reflux nephropathy with hydroureter, unilateral

N13.732 Vesicoureteral-reflux with reflux nephropathy with hydroureter, bilateral

N13.739 Vesicoureteral-reflux with reflux nephropathy with hydroureter, unspecified

N13.8 Other obstructive and reflux uropathy

Urinary tract obstruction due to specified cause
Code first, if applicable, any causal condition, such as: enlarged prostate (N40.1)

N13.9 Obstructive and reflux uropathy, unspecified

Urinary tract obstruction NOS

④ N14 Drug- and heavy-metal-induced tubulo-interstitial and tubular conditions

Code first poisoning due to drug or toxin, if applicable (T36-T65 with fifth or sixth character 1-4 or 6)
Use additional code for adverse effect, if applicable, to identify drug (T36-T50 with fifth or sixth character 5)

N14.0 Analgesic nephropathy

N14.1 Nephropathy induced by other drugs, medicaments and biological substances

N14.2 Nephropathy induced by unspecified drug, medicament or biological substance

N14.3 Nephropathy induced by heavy metals

N14.4 Toxic nephropathy, not elsewhere classified

④ N15 Other renal tubulo-interstitial diseases

N15.0 Balkan nephropathy

Balkan endemic nephropathy

N15.1 Renal and perinephric abscess

N15.8 Other specified renal tubulo-interstitial diseases

N15.9 Renal tubulo-interstitial disease, unspecified

Infection of kidney NOS

> EXCLUDES1   urinary tract infection NOS (N39.0)

---

④ 4th character required   ⑤ 5th character required   ⑥ 6th character required   ⑦ 7th character required   ⑩ Extension 'X' Alert

EXCLUDES 1 Not coded here   EXCLUDES 2 Not included here   PDx Primary Diagnosis Only   Manifestation Code

N16 Renal tubulo-interstitial disorders in diseases classified elsewhere

Pyelonephritis

Tubulo-interstitial nephritis

Code first underlying disease, such as:

brucellosis (A23.0-A23.9)

cryoglobulinemia (D89.1)

glycogen storage disease (E74.0)

leukemia (C91-C95)

lymphoma (C81.0-C85.9, C96.0-C96.9)

multiple myeloma (C90.0-)

sepsis (A40.0-A41.9)

Wilson's disease (E83.0)

EXCLUDES1 *diphtheritic pyelonephritis and tubulo-interstitial nephritis (A36.84)*

pyelonephritis and tubulo-interstitial nephritis in candidiasis (B37.49)

pyelonephritis and tubulo-interstitial nephritis in cystinosis (E72.04)

pyelonephritis and tubulo-interstitial nephritis in salmonella infection (A02.25)

pyelonephritis and tubulo-interstitial nephritis in sarcoidosis (D86.84)

pyelonephritis and tubulo-interstitial nephritis in sicca syndrome [Sjogren's] (M35.04)

pyelonephritis and tubulo-interstitial nephritis in systemic lupus erythematosus (M32.15)

pyelonephritis and tubulo-interstitial nephritis in toxoplasmosis (B58.83)

renal tubular degeneration in diabetes (E08-E13 with .29)

syphilitic pyelonephritis and tubulo-interstitial nephritis (A52.75)

Acute kidney failure and chronic kidney disease (N17-N19)

EXCLUDES2 *congenital renal failure (P96.0)*

drug- and heavy-metal-induced tubulo-interstitial and tubular conditions (N14.-)

extrarenal uremia (R39.2)

hemolytic-uremic syndrome (D59.3)

hepatorenal syndrome (K76.7)

postpartum hepatorenal syndrome (O90.4)

posttraumatic renal failure (T79.5)

prerenal uremia (R39.2)

renal failure complicating abortion or ectopic or molar pregnancy (O00-O07, O08.4)

renal failure following labor and delivery (O90.4)

renal failure postprocedural (N99.0)

⊕ **N17 Acute kidney failure**

Code also associated underlying condition

EXCLUDES1 *posttraumatic renal failure (T79.5)*

N17.0 Acute kidney failure with tubular necrosis

Acute tubular necrosis

Renal tubular necrosis

Tubular necrosis NOS

N17.1 Acute kidney failure with acute cortical necrosis

Acute cortical necrosis

Cortical necrosis NOS

Renal cortical necrosis

N17.2 Acute kidney failure with medullary necrosis

Medullary [papillary] necrosis NOS

Acute medullary [papillary] necrosis

Renal medullary [papillary] necrosis

N17.8 Other acute kidney failure

N17.9 Acute kidney failure, unspecified

Acute kidney injury (nontraumatic)

EXCLUDES2 *traumatic kidney injury (S37.0-)*

⊕ **N18 Chronic kidney disease (CKD)**

Code first any associated:

diabetic chronic kidney disease (E08.22, E09.22, E10.22, E11.22, E13.22)

hypertensive chronic kidney disease (I12.-, I13.-)

Use additional code to identify kidney transplant status, if applicable, (Z94.0)

N18.1 Chronic kidney disease, stage 1

N18.2 Chronic kidney disease, stage 2 (mild)

N18.3 Chronic kidney disease, stage 3 (moderate)

N18.4 Chronic kidney disease, stage 4 (severe)

N18.5 Chronic kidney disease, stage 5

EXCLUDES1 *chronic kidney disease, stage 5 requiring chronic dialysis (N18.6)*

N18.6 End stage renal disease

Chronic kidney disease requiring chronic dialysis

Use additional code to identify dialysis status (Z99.2)

N18.9 Chronic kidney disease, unspecified

Chronic renal failure NOS

Chronic renal insufficiency

Chronic uremia

N19 Unspecified kidney failure

Uremia NOS

EXCLUDES1 *acute kidney failure (N17.-)*

chronic kidney disease (N18.-)

chronic uremia (N18.9)

extrarenal uremia (R39.2)

prerenal uremia (R39.2)

renal insufficiency (acute) (N28.9)

uremia of newborn (P96.0)

Urolithiasis (N20-N23)

⊕ **N20 Calculus of kidney and ureter**

Calculous pyelonephritis

EXCLUDES1 *nephrocalcinosis (E83.5)*

that with hydronephrosis (N13.2)

N20.0 Calculus of kidney

Nephrolithiasis NOS

Renal calculus

Renal stone

Staghorn calculus

Stone in kidney

N20.1 Calculus of ureter

Ureteric stone

N20.2 Calculus of kidney with calculus of ureter

N20.9 Urinary calculus, unspecified

⊕ **N21 Calculus of lower urinary tract**

INCLUDES *calculus of lower urinary tract with cystitis and urethritis*

N21.0 Calculus in bladder

Calculus in diverticulum of bladder

Urinary bladder stone

EXCLUDES2 *staghorn calculus (N20.0)*

N21.1 Calculus in urethra

EXCLUDES2 *calculus of prostate (N42.0)*

N21.8 Other lower urinary tract calculus

N21.9 Calculus of lower urinary tract, unspecified

EXCLUDES1 *calculus of urinary tract NOS (N20.9)*

N22 Calculus of urinary tract in diseases classified elsewhere

Code first underlying disease, such as:

gout (M1A.-, M10.-)

schistosomiasis (B65.0-B65.9)

N23 Unspecified renal colic

Unspecified Code	Other Specified Code	N Newborn Age: 0	P Pediatric Age: 0-17	M Maternity Age: 12-55
A Adult Age: 15-124	♂ Male	♀ Female	● New Code	▲ Revised Code Title ►◄ Revised Text

Other disorders of kidney and ureter (N25-N29)

[EXCLUDES2] *disorders of kidney and ureter with urolithiasis (N20-N23)*

[4] **N25 Disorders resulting from impaired renal tubular function**

[EXCLUDES1] *metabolic disorders classifiable to E70-E88*

N25.0 Renal osteodystrophy

Azotemic osteodystrophy
Phosphate-losing tubular disorders
Renal rickets
Renal short stature

N25.1 Nephrogenic diabetes insipidus

[EXCLUDES1] *diabetes insipidus NOS (E23.2)*

[5] **N25.8 Other disorders resulting from impaired renal tubular function**

N25.81 Secondary hyperparathyroidism of renal origin

[EXCLUDES1] *secondary hyperparathyroidism, non-renal (E21.1)*

N25.89 Other disorders resulting from impaired renal tubular function

Hypokalemic nephropathy
Lightwood-Albright syndrome
Renal tubular acidosis NOS

N25.9 Disorder resulting from impaired renal tubular function, unspecified

[4] **N26 Unspecified contracted kidney**

[EXCLUDES1] *contracted kidney due to hypertension (I12.-)*
diffuse sclerosing glomerulonephritis (N05.8.-)
hypertensive nephrosclerosis (arteriolar) (arteriosclerotic) (I12.-)
small kidney of unknown cause (N27.-)

N26.1 Atrophy of kidney (terminal)

N26.2 Page kidney

N26.9 Renal sclerosis, unspecified

[4] **N27 Small kidney of unknown cause**

[INCLUDES] *oligonephronia*

N27.0 Small kidney, unilateral

N27.1 Small kidney, bilateral

N27.9 Small kidney, unspecified

[4] **N28 Other disorders of kidney and ureter, not elsewhere classified**

N28.0 Ischemia and infarction of kidney

Renal artery embolism
Renal artery obstruction
Renal artery occlusion
Renal artery thrombosis
Renal infarct

[EXCLUDES1] *atherosclerosis of renal artery (extrarenal part) (I70.1)*
congenital stenosis of renal artery (Q27.1)
Goldblatt's kidney (I70.1)

N28.1 Cyst of kidney, acquired

Cyst (multiple)(solitary) of kidney, acquired

[EXCLUDES1] *cystic kidney disease (congenital) (Q61.-)*

[5] **N28.8 Other specified disorders of kidney and ureter**

[EXCLUDES1] *hydroureter (N13.4)*
ureteric stricture with hydronephrosis (N13.1)
ureteric stricture without hydronephrosis (N13.5)

N28.81 Hypertrophy of kidney

N28.82 Megaloureter

N28.83 Nephroptosis

N28.84 Pyelitis cystica

N28.85 Pyeloureteritis cystica

N28.86 Ureteritis cystica

N28.89 Other specified disorders of kidney and ureter

N28.9 Disorder of kidney and ureter, unspecified

Nephropathy NOS
Renal disease (acute) NOS
Renal insufficiency (acute)

[EXCLUDES1] *chronic renal insufficiency (N18.9)*
unspecified nephritic syndrome (N05.-)

N29 Other disorders of kidney and ureter in diseases classified elsewhere

Code first underlying disease, such as:
amyloidosis (E85.-)
nephrocalcinosis (E83.5)
schistosomiasis (B65.0-B65.9)

[EXCLUDES1] *disorders of kidney and ureter in:*
cystinosis (E72.0)
gonorrhea (A54.21)
syphilis (A52.75)
tuberculosis (A18.11)

Other diseases of the urinary system (N30-N39)

[EXCLUDES1] *urinary infection (complicating):*
abortion or ectopic or molar pregnancy (O00-O07, O08.8)
pregnancy, childbirth and the puerperium (O23.-, O75.3, O86.2-)

[4] **N30 Cystitis**

Use additional code to identify infectious agent (B95-B97)

[EXCLUDES1] *prostatocystitis (N41.3)*

[5] **N30.0 Acute cystitis**

[EXCLUDES1] *irradiation cystitis (N30.4-)*
trigonitis (N30.3-)

N30.00 Acute cystitis without hematuria

N30.01 Acute cystitis with hematuria

[5] **N30.1 Interstitial cystitis (chronic)**

N30.10 Interstitial cystitis (chronic) without hematuria

N30.11 Interstitial cystitis (chronic) with hematuria

[5] **N30.2 Other chronic cystitis**

N30.20 Other chronic cystitis without hematuria

N30.21 Other chronic cystitis with hematuria

[5] **N30.3 Trigonitis**

Urethrotrigonitis

N30.30 Trigonitis without hematuria

N30.31 Trigonitis with hematuria

[5] **N30.4 Irradiation cystitis**

N30.40 Irradiation cystitis without hematuria

N30.41 Irradiation cystitis with hematuria

[5] **N30.8 Other cystitis**

Abscess of bladder

N30.80 Other cystitis without hematuria

N30.81 Other cystitis with hematuria

[5] **N30.9 Cystitis, unspecified**

N30.90 Cystitis, unspecified without hematuria

N30.91 Cystitis, unspecified with hematuria

[4] **N31 Neuromuscular dysfunction of bladder, not elsewhere classified**

Use additional code to identify any associated urinary incontinence (N39.3-N39.4-)

[EXCLUDES1] *cord bladder NOS (G95.89)*
neurogenic bladder due to cauda equina syndrome (G83.4)
neuromuscular dysfunction due to spinal cord lesion (G95.89)

N31.0 Uninhibited neuropathic bladder, not elsewhere classified

N31.1 Reflex neuropathic bladder, not elsewhere classified

N31.2 Flaccid neuropathic bladder, not elsewhere classified

Atonic (motor) (sensory) neuropathic bladder
Autonomous neuropathic bladder
Nonreflex neuropathic bladder

N31.8 Other neuromuscular dysfunction of bladder

[4] 4th character required [5] 5th character required [6] 6th character required [7] 7th character required [7] Extension 'X' Alert
[EXCLUDES1] Not coded here [EXCLUDES2] Not included here [PDx] Primary Diagnosis Only Manifestation Code

N31.9 Neuromuscular dysfunction of bladder, unspecified
Neurogenic bladder dysfunction NOS

[4] **N32 Other disorders of bladder**
[EXCLUDES2] *calculus of bladder (N21.0)*
cystocele (N81.1-)
hernia or prolapse of bladder, female (N81.1-)

N32.0 Bladder-neck obstruction
Bladder-neck stenosis (acquired)
[EXCLUDES1] *congenital bladder-neck obstruction (Q64.3-)*

N32.1 Vesicointestinal fistula
Vesicorectal fistula

N32.2 Vesical fistula, not elsewhere classified
[EXCLUDES1] *fistula between bladder and female genital tract (N82.0-N82.1)*

N32.3 Diverticulum of bladder
[EXCLUDES1] *congenital diverticulum of bladder (Q64.6)*
diverticulitis of bladder (N30.8-)

[5] **N32.8 Other specified disorders of bladder**
N32.81 Overactive bladder
Detrusor muscle hyperactivity
[EXCLUDES1] *frequent urination due to specified bladder condition- code to condition*

N32.89 Other specified disorders of bladder
Bladder hemorrhage
Bladder hypertrophy
Calcified bladder
Contracted bladder

N32.9 Bladder disorder, unspecified

N33 Bladder disorders in diseases classified elsewhere
Code first underlying disease, such as:
schistosomiasis (B65.0-B65.9)
[EXCLUDES1] *bladder disorder in syphilis (A52.76)*
bladder disorder in tuberculosis (A18.12)
candidal cystitis (B37.41)
chlamydial cystitis (A56.01)
cystitis in gonorrhea (A54.01)
cystitis in neurogenic bladder (N31.-)
diphtheritic cystitis (A36.85)
syphilitic cystitis (A52.76)
trichomonal cystitis (A59.03)

[4] **N34 Urethritis and urethral syndrome**
Use additional code (B95-B97), to identify infectious agent.
[EXCLUDES2] *Reiter's disease (M02.3-)*
urethritis in diseases with a predominantly sexual mode of transmission (A50-A64)
urethrotrigonitis (N30.3-)

N34.0 Urethral abscess
Abscess (of) Cowper's gland
Abscess (of) Littré's gland
Abscess (of) urethral (gland)
Periurethral abscess
[EXCLUDES1] *urethral caruncle (N36.2)*

N34.1 Nonspecific urethritis
Nongonococcal urethritis
Nonvenereal urethritis

N34.2 Other urethritis
Meatitis, urethral
Postmenopausal urethritis
Ulcer of urethra (meatus)
Urethritis NOS

N34.3 Urethral syndrome, unspecified

[4] **N35 Urethral stricture**
[EXCLUDES1] *congenital urethral stricture (Q64.3-)*
postprocedural urethral stricture (N99.1-)

[5] **N35.0 Post-traumatic urethral stricture**
Urethral stricture due to injury
[EXCLUDES1] *postprocedural urethral stricture (N99.1-)*

[6] **N35.01 Post-traumatic urethral stricture, male**
N35.010 Post-traumatic urethral stricture, male, meatal ♂
N35.011 Post-traumatic bulbous urethral stricture
N35.012 Post-traumatic membranous urethral stricture
N35.013 Post-traumatic anterior urethral stricture
N35.014 Post-traumatic urethral stricture, male, unspecified ♂

[6] **N35.02 Post-traumatic urethral stricture, female**
N35.021 Urethral stricture due to childbirth ♀
N35.028 Other post-traumatic urethral stricture, female ♀

[5] **N35.1 Postinfective urethral stricture, not elsewhere classified**
[EXCLUDES1] *urethral stricture associated with schistosomiasis (B65.-, N29)*
gonococcal urethral stricture (A54.01)
syphilitic urethral stricture (A52.76)

[6] **N35.11 Postinfective urethral stricture, not elsewhere classified, male**
N35.111 Postinfective urethral stricture, not elsewhere classified, male, meatal ♂
N35.112 Postinfective bulbous urethral stricture, not elsewhere classified
N35.113 Postinfective membranous urethral stricture, not elsewhere classified
N35.114 Postinfective anterior urethral stricture, not elsewhere classified
N35.119 Postinfective urethral stricture, not elsewhere classified, male, unspecified ♂

N35.12 Postinfective urethral stricture, not elsewhere classified, female ♀

N35.8 Other urethral stricture
[EXCLUDES1] *postprocedural urethral stricture (N99.1-)*

N35.9 Urethral stricture, unspecified

[4] **N36 Other disorders of urethra**
N36.0 Urethral fistula
Urethroperineal fistula
Urethrorectal fistula
Urinary fistula NOS
[EXCLUDES1] *urethroscrotal fistula (N50.8)*
urethrovaginal fistula (N82.1)
urethrovesicovaginal fistula (N82.1)

N36.1 Urethral diverticulum
N36.2 Urethral caruncle

[5] **N36.4 Urethral functional and muscular disorders**
Use additional code to identify associated urinary stress incontinence (N39.3)
N36.41 Hypermobility of urethra
N36.42 Intrinsic sphincter deficiency (ISD)
N36.43 Combined hypermobility of urethra and intrinsic sphincter deficiency
N36.44 Muscular disorders of urethra
Bladder sphincter dyssynergy

N36.5 Urethral false passage
N36.8 Other specified disorders of urethra
N36.9 Urethral disorder, unspecified

N37 Urethral disorders in diseases classified elsewhere
Code first underlying disease
[EXCLUDES1] *urethritis (in):*
candidal infection (B37.41)
chlamydial (A56.01)
gonorrhea (A54.01)
syphilis (A52.76)
trichomonal infection (A59.03)
tuberculosis (A18.13)

Unspecified Code	Other Specified Code	[N] Newborn Age: 0	[P] Pediatric Age: 0-17	[M] Maternity Age: 12-55
[A] Adult Age: 15-124	♂ Male	♀ Female	● New Code	▲ Revised Code Title ▶◀ Revised Text

N31.9 - N37
CHAPTER 14: DISEASES OF GENITOURINARY SYSTEM (N00-N99)

[4] **N39 Other disorders of urinary system**

[EXCLUDES2] *hematuria NOS (R31.-)*
recurrent or persistent hematuria (N02.-)
recurrent or persistent hematuria with specified morphological lesion (N02.-)
proteinuria NOS (R80.-)

N39.0 Urinary tract infection, site not specified

Use additional code (B95-B97), to identify infectious agent.

[EXCLUDES1] *candidiasis of urinary tract (B37.4-)*
neonatal urinary tract infection (P39.3)
urinary tract infection of specified site, such as:
cystitis (N30.-)
urethritis (N34.-)

N39.3 Stress incontinence (female) (male)

Code also any associated overactive bladder (N32.81)

[EXCLUDES1] *mixed incontinence (N39.46)*

[5] **N39.4 Other specified urinary incontinence**

Code also any associated overactive bladder (N32.81)

[EXCLUDES1] *enuresis NOS (R32)*
functional urinary incontinence (R39.81)
urinary incontinence associated with cognitive impairment (R39.81)
urinary incontinence NOS (R32)
urinary incontinence of nonorganic origin (F98.0)

N39.41 Urge incontinence

[EXCLUDES1] *mixed incontinence (N39.46)*

N39.42 Incontinence without sensory awareness

N39.43 Post-void dribbling

N39.44 Nocturnal enuresis

N39.45 Continuous leakage

N39.46 Mixed incontinence

Urge and stress incontinence

[6] **N39.49 Other specified urinary incontinence**

N39.490 Overflow incontinence

N39.498 Other specified urinary incontinence

Reflex incontinence
Total incontinence

N39.8 Other specified disorders of urinary system

N39.9 Disorder of urinary system, unspecified

Diseases of male genital organs (N40-N53)

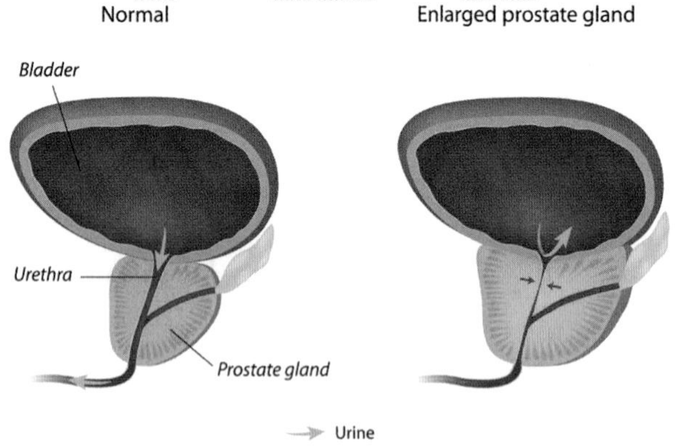

Figure 13.2 Benign prostatic hypertrophy

[4] **N40 Enlarged prostate**

[INCLUDES] *adenofibromatous hypertrophy of prostate*
benign hypertrophy of the prostate
benign prostatic hyperplasia
benign prostatic hypertrophy
BPH
nodular prostate
polyp of prostate

[EXCLUDES1] *benign neoplasms of prostate (adenoma, benign) (fibroadenoma) (fibroma) (myoma) (D29.1)*

[EXCLUDES2] *malignant neoplasm of prostate (C61)*

N40.0 Enlarged prostate without lower urinary tract symptoms

Enlarged prostate without LUTS
Enlarged prostate NOS [A] ♂

N40.1 Enlarged prostate with lower urinary tract symptoms

Enlarged prostate with LUTS
Use additional code for associated symptoms, when specified:
incomplete bladder emptying (R39.14)
nocturia (R35.1)
straining on urination (R39.16)
urinary frequency (R35.0)
urinary hesitancy (R39.11)
urinary incontinence (N39.4-)
urinary obstruction (N13.8)
urinary retention (R33.8)
urinary urgency (R39.15)
weak urinary stream (R39.12) [A] ♂

N40.2 Nodular prostate without lower urinary tract symptoms

Nodular prostate without LUTS [A] ♂

N40.3 Nodular prostate with lower urinary tract symptoms

Use additional code for associated symptoms, when specified:
incomplete bladder emptying (R39.14)
nocturia (R35.1)
straining on urination (R39.16)
urinary frequency (R35.0)
urinary hesitancy (R39.11)
urinary incontinence (N39.4-)
urinary obstruction (N13.8)
urinary retention (R33.8)
urinary urgency (R39.15)
weak urinary stream (R39.12) [A] ♂

[4] **N41 Inflammatory diseases of prostate**

Use additional code (B95-B97), to identify infectious agent.

N41.0 Acute prostatitis [A] ♂

N41.1 Chronic prostatitis [A] ♂

N41.2 Abscess of prostate [A] ♂

N41.3 Prostatocystitis [A] ♂

N41.4 Granulomatous prostatitis [A] ♂

N41.8 Other inflammatory diseases of prostate [A] ♂

N41.9 Inflammatory disease of prostate, unspecified

Prostatitis NOS [A] ♂

[4] **N42 Other and unspecified disorders of prostate**

N42.0 Calculus of prostate

Prostatic stone [A] ♂

N42.1 Congestion and hemorrhage of prostate

[EXCLUDES1] *enlarged prostate (N40.-)*
hematuria (R31.-)
hyperplasia of prostate (N40.-)
inflammatory diseases of prostate (N41.-) [A] ♂

N42.3 Dysplasia of prostate

Prostatic intraepithelial neoplasia I (PIN I)
Prostatic intraepithelial neoplasia II (PIN II)

[EXCLUDES1] *prostatic intraepithelial neoplasia III (PIN III) (D07.5)* ♂

[5] **N42.8 Other specified disorders of prostate**

N42.81 Prostatodynia syndrome

Painful prostate syndrome [A] ♂

N42.82 Prostatosis syndrome [A] ♂

N42.83 Cyst of prostate [A] ♂

N42.89 Other specified disorders of prostate [A] ♂

[4] 4th character required [5] 5th character required [6] 6th character required [7] 7th character required [X] Extension 'X' Alert
[EXCLUDES1] Not coded here [EXCLUDES2] Not included here [PDx] Primary Diagnosis Only Manifestation Code

N42.9 Disorder of prostate, unspecified [A] ♂

[4] **N43 Hydrocele and spermatocele**

INCLUDES hydrocele of spermatic cord, testis or tunica vaginalis

EXCLUDES1 congenital hydrocele (P83.5)

N43.0 Encysted hydrocele ♂

N43.1 Infected hydrocele
Use additional code (B95-B97), to identify infectious agent ♂

N43.2 Other hydrocele ♂

N43.3 Hydrocele, unspecified ♂

[5] N43.4 Spermatocele of epididymis
Spermatic cyst

N43.40 Spermatocele of epididymis, unspecified ♂

N43.41 Spermatocele of epididymis, single ♂

N43.42 Spermatocele of epididymis, multiple ♂

[4] **N44 Noninflammatory disorders of testis**

[5] N44.0 Torsion of testis

N44.00 Torsion of testis, unspecified ♂

N44.01 Extravaginal torsion of spermatic cord ♂

N44.02 Intravaginal torsion of spermatic cord
Torsion of spermatic cord NOS ♂

N44.03 Torsion of appendix testis ♂

N44.04 Torsion of appendix epididymis ♂

N44.1 Cyst of tunica albuginea testis ♂

N44.2 Benign cyst of testis ♂

N44.8 Other noninflammatory disorders of the testis ♂

[4] **N45 Orchitis and epididymitis**
Use additional code (B95-B97), to identify infectious agent.

N45.1 Epididymitis ♂

N45.2 Orchitis ♂

N45.3 Epididymo-orchitis ♂

N45.4 Abscess of epididymis or testis ♂

[4] **N46 Male infertility**

EXCLUDES1 vasectomy status (Z98.52)

[5] N46.0 Azoospermia
Absolute male infertility
Male infertility due to germinal (cell) aplasia
Male infertility due to spermatogenic arrest (complete)

N46.01 Organic azoospermia
Azoospermia NOS [A] ♂

[6] N46.02 Azoospermia due to extratesticular causes
Code also associated cause

N46.021 Azoospermia due to drug therapy [A] ♂

N46.022 Azoospermia due to infection [A] ♂

N46.023 Azoospermia due to obstruction of efferent ducts [A] ♂

N46.024 Azoospermia due to radiation [A] ♂

N46.025 Azoospermia due to systemic disease [A] ♂

N46.029 Azoospermia due to other extratesticular causes [A] ♂

[5] N46.1 Oligospermia
Male infertility due to germinal cell desquamation
Male infertility due to hypospermatogenesis
Male infertility due to incomplete spermatogenic arrest

N46.11 Organic oligospermia
Oligospermia NOS [A] ♂

[6] N46.12 Oligospermia due to extratesticular causes
Code also associated cause

N46.121 Oligospermia due to drug therapy [A] ♂

N46.122 Oligospermia due to infection [A] ♂

N46.123 Oligospermia due to obstruction of efferent ducts [A] ♂

N46.124 Oligospermia due to radiation [A] ♂

N46.125 Oligospermia due to systemic disease [A] ♂

N46.129 Oligospermia due to other extratesticular causes [A] ♂

N46.8 Other male infertility [A] ♂

N46.9 Male infertility, unspecified [A] ♂

[4] **N47 Disorders of prepuce**

N47.0 Adherent prepuce, newborn [N] ♂

N47.1 Phimosis ♂

N47.2 Paraphimosis ♂

N47.3 Deficient foreskin ♂

N47.4 Benign cyst of prepuce ♂

N47.5 Adhesions of prepuce and glans penis ♂

N47.6 Balanoposthitis
Use additional code (B95-B97), to identify infectious agent.

EXCLUDES1 balanitis (N48.1) ♂

N47.7 Other inflammatory diseases of prepuce
Use additional code (B95-B97), to identify infectious agent. ♂

N47.8 Other disorders of prepuce ♂

[4] **N48 Other disorders of penis**

N48.0 Leukoplakia of penis
Balanitis xerotica obliterans
Kraurosis of penis
Lichen sclerosus of external male genital organs

EXCLUDES1 carcinoma in situ of penis (D07.4) ♂

N48.1 Balanitis
Use additional code (B95-B97), to identify infectious agent

EXCLUDES1 amebic balanitis (A06.8)
balanitis xerotica obliterans (N48.0)
candidal balanitis (B37.42)
gonococcal balanitis (A54.23)
herpesviral [herpes simplex] balanitis (A60.01) ♂

[5] N48.2 Other inflammatory disorders of penis
Use additional code (B95-B97), to identify infectious agent.

EXCLUDES1 balanitis (N48.1)
balanitis xerotica obliterans (N48.0)
balanoposthitis (N47.6)

N48.21 Abscess of corpus cavernosum and penis ♂

N48.22 Cellulitis of corpus cavernosum and penis ♂

N48.29 Other inflammatory disorders of penis ♂

[5] N48.3 Priapism
Painful erection
Code first underlying cause

N48.30 Priapism, unspecified ♂

N48.31 Priapism due to trauma ♂

N48.32 Priapism due to disease classified elsewhere ♂

N48.33 Priapism, drug-induced ♂

N48.39 Other priapism ♂

N48.5 Ulcer of penis ♂

N48.6 Induration penis plastica
Peyronie's disease
Plastic induration of penis ♂

[5] N48.8 Other specified disorders of penis

N48.81 Thrombosis of superficial vein of penis ♂

N48.82 Acquired torsion of penis
Acquired torsion of penis NOS

EXCLUDES1 congenital torsion of penis (Q55.63) ♂

N48.83 Acquired buried penis

EXCLUDES1 congenital hidden penis (Q55.64) ♂

N48.89 Other specified disorders of penis ♂

N48.9 Disorder of penis, unspecified ♂

Unspecified Code | Other Specified Code | [N] Newborn Age: 0 | [P] Pediatric Age: 0-17 | [M] Maternity Age: 12-55
[A] Adult Age: 15-124 | ♂ Male | ♀ Female | ● New Code | ▲ Revised Code Title | ►◄ Revised Text

[4] *N49* **Inflammatory disorders of male genital organs, not elsewhere classified**
Use additional code (B95-B97), to identify infectious agent
[EXCLUDES1] *inflammation of penis (N48.1, N48.2-)*
orchitis and epididymitis (N45.-)
N49.0 **Inflammatory disorders of seminal vesicle**
Vesiculitis NOS ♂
N49.1 **Inflammatory disorders of spermatic cord, tunica vaginalis and vas deferens**
Vasitis ♂
N49.2 **Inflammatory disorders of scrotum** ♂
N49.3 **Fournier gangrene** ♂
N49.8 **Inflammatory disorders of other specified male genital organs**
Inflammation of multiple sites in male genital organs ♂
N49.9 **Inflammatory disorder of unspecified male genital organ**
Abscess of unspecified male genital organ
Boil of unspecified male genital organ
Carbuncle of unspecified male genital organ
Cellulitis of unspecified male genital organ ♂

[4] N50 **Other and unspecified disorders of male genital organs**
[EXCLUDES2] *torsion of testis (N44.0-)*
N50.0 **Atrophy of testis** ♂
N50.1 **Vascular disorders of male genital organs**
Hematocele, NOS, of male genital organs
Hemorrhage of male genital organs
Thrombosis of male genital organs ♂
N50.3 **Cyst of epididymis** ♂
N50.8 **Other specified disorders of male genital organs**
Atrophy of scrotum, seminal vesicle, spermatic cord, tunica vaginalis and vas deferens
Edema of scrotum, seminal vesicle, spermatic cord, testis, tunica vaginalis and vas deferens
Hypertrophy of scrotum, seminal vesicle, spermatic cord, testis, tunica vaginalis and vas deferens
Ulcer of scrotum, seminal vesicle, spermatic cord, testis, tunica vaginalis and vas deferens
Chylocele, tunica vaginalis (nonfilarial) NOS
Urethroscrotal fistula
Stricture of spermatic cord, tunica vaginalis, and vas deferens ♂
N50.9 **Disorder of male genital organs, unspecified** ♂

N51 **Disorders of male genital organs in diseases classified elsewhere**
Code first underlying disease, such as:
filariasis (B74.0-B74.9)
[EXCLUDES1] *amebic balanitis (A06.8)*
candidal balanitis (B37.42)
gonococcal balanitis (A54.23)
gonococcal prostatitis (A54.22)
herpesviral [herpes simplex] balanitis (A60.01)
trichomonal prostatitis (A59.02)
tuberculous prostatitis (A18.14) ♂

[4] N52 **Male erectile dysfunction**
[EXCLUDES1] *psychogenic impotence (F52.21)*
[5] N52.0 **Vasculogenic erectile dysfunction**
N52.01 **Erectile dysfunction due to arterial insufficiency** [A] ♂
N52.02 **Corporo-venous occlusive erectile dysfunction** [A] ♂
N52.03 **Combined arterial insufficiency and corporo-venous occlusive erectile dysfunction** [A] ♂
N52.1 **Erectile dysfunction due to diseases classified elsewhere**
Code first underlying disease [A] ♂
N52.2 **Drug-induced erectile dysfunction** [A] ♂
[5] N52.3 **Post-surgical erectile dysfunction**
N52.31 **Erectile dysfunction following radical prostatectomy** [A] ♂
N52.32 **Erectile dysfunction following radical cystectomy** [A] ♂
N52.33 **Erectile dysfunction following urethral surgery** [A] ♂
N52.34 **Erectile dysfunction following simple prostatectomy** [A] ♂
N52.39 **Other post-surgical erectile dysfunction** [A] ♂
N52.8 **Other male erectile dysfunction** [A] ♂
N52.9 **Male erectile dysfunction, unspecified**
Impotence NOS [A] ♂

[4] N53 **Other male sexual dysfunction**
[EXCLUDES1] *psychogenic sexual dysfunction (F52.-)*
[5] N53.1 **Ejaculatory dysfunction**
[EXCLUDES1] *premature ejaculation (F52.4)*
N53.11 **Retarded ejaculation** ♂
N53.12 **Painful ejaculation** ♂
N53.13 **Anejaculatory orgasm** ♂
N53.14 **Retrograde ejaculation** ♂
N53.19 **Other ejaculatory dysfunction**
Ejaculatory dysfunction NOS ♂
N53.8 **Other male sexual dysfunction** ♂
N53.9 **Unspecified male sexual dysfunction** ♂

Disorders of breast (N60-N65)

[EXCLUDES1] *disorders of breast associated with childbirth (O91-O92)*

[4] N60 **Benign mammary dysplasia**
INCLUDES *fibrocystic mastopathy*
[5] N60.0 **Solitary cyst of breast**
Cyst of breast
N60.01 **Solitary cyst of right breast**
N60.02 **Solitary cyst of left breast**
N60.09 **Solitary cyst of unspecified breast**
[5] N60.1 **Diffuse cystic mastopathy**
Cystic breast
Fibrocystic disease of breast
[EXCLUDES1] *diffuse cystic mastopathy with epithelial proliferation (N60.3-)*
N60.11 **Diffuse cystic mastopathy of right breast** [A]
N60.12 **Diffuse cystic mastopathy of left breast** [A]
N60.19 **Diffuse cystic mastopathy of unspecified breast** [A]
[5] N60.2 **Fibroadenosis of breast**
Adenofibrosis of breast
[EXCLUDES2] *fibroadenoma of breast (D24.-)*
N60.21 **Fibroadenosis of right breast**
N60.22 **Fibroadenosis of left breast**
N60.29 **Fibroadenosis of unspecified breast**
[5] N60.3 **Fibrosclerosis of breast**
Cystic mastopathy with epithelial proliferation
N60.31 **Fibrosclerosis of right breast**
N60.32 **Fibrosclerosis of left breast**
N60.39 **Fibrosclerosis of unspecified breast**
[5] N60.4 **Mammary duct ectasia**
N60.41 **Mammary duct ectasia of right breast**
N60.42 **Mammary duct ectasia of left breast**
N60.49 **Mammary duct ectasia of unspecified breast**
[5] N60.8 **Other benign mammary dysplasias**
N60.81 **Other benign mammary dysplasias of right breast**
N60.82 **Other benign mammary dysplasias of left breast**

[4] 4th character required [5] 5th character required [6] 6th character required [7] 7th character required [x7th] Extension 'X' Alert
[EXCLUDES1] Not coded here [EXCLUDES2] Not included here [PDx] Primary Diagnosis Only Manifestation Code

N60.89 Other benign mammary dysplasias of unspecified breast

⑤ N60.9 Unspecified benign mammary dysplasia

N60.91 Unspecified benign mammary dysplasia of right breast

N60.92 Unspecified benign mammary dysplasia of left breast

N60.99 Unspecified benign mammary dysplasia of unspecified breast

N61 Inflammatory disorders of breast

Abscess (acute) (chronic) (nonpuerperal) of areola
Abscess (acute) (chronic) (nonpuerperal) of breast
Carbuncle of breast
Infective mastitis (acute) (subacute) (nonpuerperal)
Mastitis (acute) (subacute) (nonpuerperal) NOS

EXCLUDES1 inflammatory carcinoma of breast (C50.9)
inflammatory disorder of breast associated with childbirth (O91.-)
neonatal infective mastitis (P39.0)
thrombophlebitis of breast [Mondor's disease] (I80.8)

N62 Hypertrophy of breast

Gynecomastia
Hypertrophy of breast NOS
Massive pubertal hypertrophy of breast

EXCLUDES1 breast engorgement of newborn (P83.4)
disproportion of reconstructed breast (N65.1)

N63 Unspecified lump in breast

Nodule(s) NOS in breast

④ N64 Other disorders of breast

EXCLUDES2 mechanical complication of breast prosthesis and implant (T85.4-)

N64.0 Fissure and fistula of nipple

N64.1 Fat necrosis of breast

Fat necrosis (segmental) of breast
Code first breast necrosis due to breast graft (T85.89)

N64.2 Atrophy of breast

N64.3 Galactorrhea not associated with childbirth

N64.4 Mastodynia

⑤ N64.5 Other signs and symptoms in breast

EXCLUDES2 abnormal findings on diagnostic imaging of breast (R92.-)

N64.51 Induration of breast

N64.52 Nipple discharge

EXCLUDES1 abnormal findings in nipple discharge (R89.-)

N64.53 Retraction of nipple

N64.59 Other signs and symptoms in breast

⑤ N64.8 Other specified disorders of breast

N64.81 Ptosis of breast

EXCLUDES1 ptosis of native breast in relation to reconstructed breast (N65.1) A

N64.82 Hypoplasia of breast

Micromastia

EXCLUDES1 congenital absence of breast (Q83.0)
hypoplasia of native breast in relation to reconstructed breast (N65.1) A

N64.89 Other specified disorders of breast

Galactocele
Subinvolution of breast (postlactational)

N64.9 Disorder of breast, unspecified

④ N65 Deformity and disproportion of reconstructed breast

N65.0 Deformity of reconstructed breast

Contour irregularity in reconstructed breast
Excess tissue in reconstructed breast
Misshapen reconstructed breast A

N65.1 Disproportion of reconstructed breast

Breast asymmetry between native breast and reconstructed breast
Disproportion between native breast and reconstructed breast A

Inflammatory diseases of female pelvic organs (N70-N77)

EXCLUDES1 inflammatory diseases of female pelvic organs complicating:
abortion or ectopic or molar pregnancy (O00-O07, O08.0)
pregnancy, childbirth and the puerperium (O23.-, O75.3, O85, O86.-)

④ N70 Salpingitis and oophoritis

INCLUDES abscess (of) fallopian tube
abscess (of) ovary
pyosalpinx
salpingo-oophoritis
tubo-ovarian abscess
tubo-ovarian inflammatory disease

Use additional code (B95-B97), to identify infectious agent

EXCLUDES1 gonococcal infection (A54.24)
tuberculous infection (A18.17)

⑤ N70.0 Acute salpingitis and oophoritis

N70.01 Acute salpingitis ♀
N70.02 Acute oophoritis ♀
N70.03 Acute salpingitis and oophoritis ♀

⑤ N70.1 Chronic salpingitis and oophoritis

Hydrosalpinx

N70.11 Chronic salpingitis ♀
N70.12 Chronic oophoritis ♀
N70.13 Chronic salpingitis and oophoritis ♀

⑤ N70.9 Salpingitis and oophoritis, unspecified

N70.91 Salpingitis, unspecified ♀
N70.92 Oophoritis, unspecified ♀
N70.93 Salpingitis and oophoritis, unspecified ♀

④ N71 Inflammatory disease of uterus, except cervix

INCLUDES endo (myo) metritis
metritis
myometritis
pyometra
uterine abscess

Use additional code (B95-B97), to identify infectious agent

EXCLUDES1 hyperplastic endometritis (N85.0-)
infection of uterus following delivery (O85, O86.-)

N71.0 Acute inflammatory disease of uterus ♀
N71.1 Chronic inflammatory disease of uterus ♀
N71.9 Inflammatory disease of uterus, unspecified ♀

N72 Inflammatory disease of cervix uteri

INCLUDES cervicitis (with or without erosion or ectropion)
endocervicitis (with or without erosion or ectropion)
exocervicitis (with or without erosion or ectropion)

Use additional code (B95-B97), to identify infectious agent

EXCLUDES1 erosion and ectropion of cervix without cervicitis (N86) ♀

④ N73 Other female pelvic inflammatory diseases

Use additional code (B95-B97), to identify infectious agent.

N73.0 Acute parametritis and pelvic cellulitis

Abscess of broad ligament
Abscess of parametrium
Pelvic cellulitis, female ♀

N73.1 Chronic parametritis and pelvic cellulitis

Any condition in N73.0 specified as chronic

EXCLUDES1 tuberculous parametritis and pelvic cellultis (A18.17) ♀

Unspecified Code   Other Specified Code   N Newborn Age: 0   P Pediatric Age: 0-17   M Maternity Age: 12-55
A Adult Age: 15-124   ♂ Male   ♀ Female   ● New Code   ▲ Revised Code Title   ▶◀ Revised Text

N73.2 **Unspecified parametritis and pelvic cellulitis**
Any condition in N73.0 unspecified whether acute or chronic ♀
N73.3 **Female acute pelvic peritonitis** ♀
N73.4 **Female chronic pelvic peritonitis**
[EXCLUDES1] *tuberculous pelvic (female) peritonitis (A18.17)* ♀
N73.5 **Female pelvic peritonitis, unspecified** ♀
N73.6 **Female pelvic peritoneal adhesions (postinfective)**
[EXCLUDES2] *postprocedural pelvic peritoneal adhesions (N99.4)* ♀
N73.8 **Other specified female pelvic inflammatory diseases** ♀
N73.9 **Female pelvic inflammatory disease, unspecified**
Female pelvic infection or inflammation NOS ♀

N74 **Female pelvic inflammatory disorders in diseases classified elsewhere**
Code first underlying disease
[EXCLUDES1] *chlamydial cervicitis (A56.02)*
chlamydial pelvic inflammatory disease (A56.11)
gonococcal cervicitis (A54.03)
gonococcal pelvic inflammatory disease (A54.24)
herpesviral [herpes simplex] cervicitis (A60.03)
herpesviral [herpes simplex] pelvic inflammatory disease (A60.09)
syphilitic cervicitis (A52.76)
syphilitic pelvic inflammatory disease (A52.76)
trichomonal cervicitis (A59.09)
tuberculous cervicitis (A18.16)
tuberculous pelvic inflammatory disease (A18.17) ♀

[4] N75 **Diseases of Bartholin's gland**
N75.0 **Cyst of Bartholin's gland** ♀
N75.1 **Abscess of Bartholin's gland** ♀
N75.8 **Other diseases of Bartholin's gland**
Bartholinitis ♀
N75.9 **Disease of Bartholin's gland, unspecified** ♀

[4] N76 **Other inflammation of vagina and vulva**
Use additional code (B95-B97), to identify infectious agent
[EXCLUDES2] *senile (atrophic) vaginitis (N95.2)*
vulvar vestibulitis (N94.810)
N76.0 **Acute vaginitis**
Acute vulvovaginitis
Vaginitis NOS
Vulvovaginitis NOS ♀
N76.1 **Subacute and chronic vaginitis**
Chronic vulvovaginitis
Subacute vulvovaginitis ♀
N76.2 **Acute vulvitis**
Vulvitis NOS ♀
N76.3 **Subacute and chronic vulvitis** ♀
N76.4 **Abscess of vulva**
Furuncle of vulva ♀
N76.5 **Ulceration of vagina** ♀
N76.6 **Ulceration of vulva** ♀
[5] N76.8 **Other specified inflammation of vagina and vulva**
N76.81 **Mucositis (ulcerative) of vagina and vulva**
Code also type of associated therapy, such as:
antineoplastic and immunosuppressive drugs (T45.1X-)
radiological procedure and radiotherapy (Y84.2)
[EXCLUDES2] *gastrointestinal mucositis (ulcerative) (K92.81)*
nasal mucositis (ulcerative) (J34.81)
oral mucositis (ulcerative) (K12.3-) ♀
N76.89 **Other specified inflammation of vagina and vulva** ♀

[4] N77 **Vulvovaginal ulceration and inflammation in diseases classified elsewhere**
N77.0 **Ulceration of vulva in diseases classified elsewhere**
Code first underlying disease, such as:
Behçet's disease (M35.2)
[EXCLUDES1] *ulceration of vulva in gonococcal infection (A54.02)*
ulceration of vulva in herpesviral [herpes simplex] infection (A60.04)
ulceration of vulva in syphilis (A51.0)
ulceration of vulva in tuberculosis (A18.18) ♀
N77.1 **Vaginitis, vulvitis and vulvovaginitis in diseases classified elsewhere**
Code first underlying disease, such as:
pinworm (B80)
[EXCLUDES1] *candidal vulvovaginitis (B37.3)*
chlamydial vulvovaginitis (A56.02)
gonococcal vulvovaginitis (A54.02)
herpesviral [herpes simplex] vulvovaginitis (A60.04)
trichomonal vulvovaginitis (A59.01)
tuberculous vulvovaginitis (A18.18)
vulvovaginitis in early syphilis (A51.0)
vulvovaginitis in late syphilis (A52.76) ♀

Noninflammatory disorders of female genital tract (N80-N98)

[4] N80 **Endometriosis**
N80.0 **Endometriosis of uterus**
Adenomyosis
[EXCLUDES1] *stromal endometriosis (D39.0)* ♀
N80.1 **Endometriosis of ovary** ♀
N80.2 **Endometriosis of fallopian tube** ♀
N80.3 **Endometriosis of pelvic peritoneum** ♀
N80.4 **Endometriosis of rectovaginal septum and vagina** ♀
N80.5 **Endometriosis of intestine** ♀
N80.6 **Endometriosis in cutaneous scar** ♀
N80.8 **Other endometriosis** ♀
N80.9 **Endometriosis, unspecified** ♀

[4] N81 **Female genital prolapse**
[EXCLUDES1] *genital prolapse complicating pregnancy, labor or delivery (O34.5-)*
prolapse and hernia of ovary and fallopian tube (N83.4)
prolapse of vaginal vault after hysterectomy (N99.3)
N81.0 **Urethrocele**
[EXCLUDES1] *urethrocele with cystocele (N81.1-)*
urethrocele with prolapse of uterus (N81.2-N81.4) ♀
[5] N81.1 **Cystocele**
Cystocele with urethrocele
Cystourethrocele
[EXCLUDES1] *cystocele with prolapse of uterus (N81.2-N81.4)*
N81.10 **Cystocele, unspecified**
Prolapse of (anterior) vaginal wall NOS ♀
N81.11 **Cystocele, midline** ♀
N81.12 **Cystocele, lateral**
Paravaginal cystocele ♀
N81.2 **Incomplete uterovaginal prolapse**
First degree uterine prolapse
Prolapse of cervix NOS
Second degree uterine prolapse
[EXCLUDES1] *cervical stump prolaspe (N81.85)* ♀
N81.3 **Complete uterovaginal prolapse**
Procidentia (uteri) NOS
Third degree uterine prolapse ♀
N81.4 **Uterovaginal prolapse, unspecified**
Prolapse of uterus NOS ♀

[4] 4th character required [5] 5th character required [6] 6th character required [7] 7th character required [7x] Extension 'X' Alert
[EXCLUDES 1] Not coded here [EXCLUDES 2] Not included here [PDx] Primary Diagnosis Only Manifestation Code

N81.5 Vaginal enterocele
[EXCLUDES1] *enterocele with prolapse of uterus (N81.2-N81.4)* ♀

N81.6 Rectocele
Prolapse of posterior vaginal wall
Use additional code for any associated fecal incontinence, if applicable (R15.-)
[EXCLUDES2] *perineocele (N81.81)*
rectal prolapse (K62.3)
rectocele with prolapse of uterus (N81.2-N81.4) ♀

[5] **N81.8 Other female genital prolapse**
N81.81 Perineocele ♀
N81.82 Incompetence or weakening of pubocervical tissue ♀
N81.83 Incompetence or weakening of rectovaginal tissue ♀
N81.84 Pelvic muscle wasting
Disuse atrophy of pelvic muscles and anal sphincter ♀
N81.85 Cervical stump prolapse ♀
N81.89 Other female genital prolapse
Deficient perineum
Old laceration of muscles of pelvic floor ♀

N81.9 Female genital prolapse, unspecified ♀

[4] **N82 Fistulae involving female genital tract**
[EXCLUDES1] *vesicointestinal fistulae (N32.1)*

N82.0 Vesicovaginal fistula ♀
N82.1 Other female urinary-genital tract fistulae
Cervicovesical fistula
Ureterovaginal fistula
Urethrovaginal fistula
Uteroureteric fistula
Uterovesical fistula ♀
N82.2 Fistula of vagina to small intestine ♀
N82.3 Fistula of vagina to large intestine
Rectovaginal fistula ♀
N82.4 Other female intestinal-genital tract fistulae
Intestinouterine fistula ♀
N82.5 Female genital tract-skin fistulae
Uterus to abdominal wall fistula
Vaginoperineal fistula ♀
N82.8 Other female genital tract fistulae ♀
N82.9 Female genital tract fistula, unspecified ♀

[4] **N83 Noninflammatory disorders of ovary, fallopian tube and broad ligament**
[EXCLUDES2] *hydrosalpinx (N70.1-)*

N83.0 Follicular cyst of ovary
Cyst of graafian follicle
Hemorrhagic follicular cyst (of ovary) ♀
N83.1 Corpus luteum cyst
Hemorrhagic corpus luteum cyst ♀
[5] **N83.2 Other and unspecified ovarian cysts**
[EXCLUDES1] *developmental ovarian cyst (Q50.1)*
neoplastic ovarian cyst (D27.-)
polycystic ovarian syndrome (E28.2)
Stein-Leventhal syndrome (E28.2)
N83.20 Unspecified ovarian cysts ♀
N83.29 Other ovarian cysts
Retention cyst of ovary
Simple cyst of ovary ♀
[5] **N83.3 Acquired atrophy of ovary and fallopian tube**
N83.31 Acquired atrophy of ovary ♀
N83.32 Acquired atrophy of fallopian tube ♀
N83.33 Acquired atrophy of ovary and fallopian tube ♀
N83.4 Prolapse and hernia of ovary and fallopian tube ♀
[5] **N83.5 Torsion of ovary, ovarian pedicle and fallopian tube**
Torsion of accessory tube
N83.51 Torsion of ovary and ovarian pedicle ♀
N83.52 Torsion of fallopian tube
Torsion of hydatid of Morgagni ♀
N83.53 Torsion of ovary, ovarian pedicle and fallopian tube ♀
N83.6 Hematosalpinx
[EXCLUDES1] *hematosalpinx (with) (in):*
hematocolpos (N89.7)
hematometra (N85.7)
tubal pregnancy (O00.1) ♀
N83.7 Hematoma of broad ligament ♀
N83.8 Other noninflammatory disorders of ovary, fallopian tube and broad ligament
Broad ligament laceration syndrome [Allen-Masters] ♀
N83.9 Noninflammatory disorder of ovary, fallopian tube and broad ligament, unspecified ♀

[4] **N84 Polyp of female genital tract**
[EXCLUDES1] *adenomatous polyp (D28.-)*
placental polyp (O90.89)

N84.0 Polyp of corpus uteri
Polyp of endometrium
Polyp of uterus NOS
[EXCLUDES1] *polypoid endometrial hyperplasia (N85.0-)* ♀
N84.1 Polyp of cervix uteri
Mucous polyp of cervix ♀
N84.2 Polyp of vagina ♀
N84.3 Polyp of vulva
Polyp of labia ♀
N84.8 Polyp of other parts of female genital tract ♀
N84.9 Polyp of female genital tract, unspecified ♀

[4] **N85 Other noninflammatory disorders of uterus, except cervix**
[EXCLUDES1] *endometriosis (N80.-)*
inflammatory diseases of uterus (N71.-)
noninflammatory disorders of cervix, except malposition (N86-N88)
polyp of corpus uteri (N84.0)
uterine prolapse (N81.-)

[5] **N85.0 Endometrial hyperplasia**
N85.00 Endometrial hyperplasia, unspecified
Hyperplasia (adenomatous) (cystic) (glandular) of endometrium
Hyperplastic endometritis ♀
N85.01 Benign endometrial hyperplasia
Endometrial hyperplasia (complex) (simple) without atypia ♀
N85.02 Endometrial intraepithelial neoplasia [EIN]
Endometrial hyperplasia with atypia
[EXCLUDES1] *malignant neoplasm of endometrium (with endometrial intraepithelial neoplasia [EIN]) (C54.1)* ♀
N85.2 Hypertrophy of uterus
Bulky or enlarged uterus
[EXCLUDES1] *puerperal hypertrophy of uterus (O90.89)* ♀
N85.3 Subinvolution of uterus
[EXCLUDES1] *puerperal subinvolution of uterus (O90.89)* ♀
N85.4 Malposition of uterus
Anteversion of uterus
Retroflexion of uterus
Retroversion of uterus
[EXCLUDES1] *malposition of uterus complicating pregnancy, labor or delivery (O34.5-, O65.5)* ♀
N85.5 Inversion of uterus
[EXCLUDES1] *current obstetric trauma (O71.2)*
postpartum inversion of uterus (O71.2) ♀
N85.6 Intrauterine synechiae ♀
N85.7 Hematometra
Hematosalpinx with hematometra
[EXCLUDES1] *hematometra with hematocolpos (N89.7)* ♀

Unspecified Code | Other Specified Code | [N] Newborn Age: 0 | [P] Pediatric Age: 0-17 | [M] Maternity Age: 12-55
[A] Adult Age: 15-124 | ♂ Male | ♀ Female | ● New Code | ▲ Revised Code Title | ►◄ Revised Text

N85.8 Other specified noninflammatory disorders of uterus
Atrophy of uterus, acquired
Fibrosis of uterus NOS ♀

N85.9 Noninflammatory disorder of uterus, unspecified
Disorder of uterus NOS ♀

N86 Erosion and ectropion of cervix uteri
Decubitus (trophic) ulcer of cervix
Eversion of cervix
[EXCLUDES1] *erosion and ectropion of cervix with cervicitis (N72)* ♀

[4] **N87 Dysplasia of cervix uteri**
[EXCLUDES1] *abnormal results from cervical cytologic examination without histologic confirmation (R87.61-)*
carcinoma in situ of cervix uteri (D06.-)
cervical intraepithelial neoplasia III [CIN III] (D06.-)
HGSIL of cervix (R87.613)
severe dysplasia of cervix uteri (D06.-)

N87.0 Mild cervical dysplasia
Cervical intraepithelial neoplasia I [CIN I] ♀

N87.1 Moderate cervical dysplasia
Cervical intraepithelial neoplasia II [CIN II] ♀

N87.9 Dysplasia of cervix uteri, unspecified
Anaplasia of cervix
Cervical atypism
Cervical dysplasia NOS ♀

[4] **N88 Other noninflammatory disorders of cervix uteri**
[EXCLUDES2] *inflammatory disease of cervix (N72)*
polyp of cervix (N84.1)

N88.0 Leukoplakia of cervix uteri ♀

N88.1 Old laceration of cervix uteri
Adhesions of cervix
[EXCLUDES1] *current obstetric trauma (O71.3)* ♀

N88.2 Stricture and stenosis of cervix uteri
[EXCLUDES1] *stricture and stenosis of cervix uteri complicating labor (O65.5)* ♀

N88.3 Incompetence of cervix uteri
Investigation and management of (suspected) cervical incompetence in a nonpregnant woman
[EXCLUDES1] *cervical incompetence complicating pregnancy (O34.3-)* ♀

N88.4 Hypertrophic elongation of cervix uteri ♀

N88.8 Other specified noninflammatory disorders of cervix uteri
[EXCLUDES1] *current obstetric trauma (O71.3)* ♀

N88.9 Noninflammatory disorder of cervix uteri, unspecified ♀

[4] **N89 Other noninflammatory disorders of vagina**
[EXCLUDES1] *abnormal results from vaginal cytologic examination without histologic confirmation (R87.62-)*
carcinoma in situ of vagina (D07.2)
HGSIL of vagina (R87.623)
inflammation of vagina (N76.-)
senile (atrophic) vaginitis (N95.2)
severe dysplasia of vagina (D07.2)
trichomonal leukorrhea (A59.00)
vaginal intraepithelial neoplasia [VAIN], grade III (D07.2)

N89.0 Mild vaginal dysplasia
Vaginal intraepithelial neoplasia [VAIN], grade I ♀

N89.1 Moderate vaginal dysplasia
Vaginal intraepithelial neoplasia [VAIN], grade II ♀

N89.3 Dysplasia of vagina, unspecified ♀

N89.4 Leukoplakia of vagina ♀

N89.5 Stricture and atresia of vagina
Vaginal adhesions
Vaginal stenosis
[EXCLUDES1] *congenital atresia or stricture (Q52.4)*
postprocedural adhesions of vagina (N99.2) ♀

N89.6 Tight hymenal ring
Rigid hymen
Tight introitus
[EXCLUDES1] *imperforate hymen (Q52.3)* ♀

N89.7 Hematocolpos
Hematocolpos with hematometra or hematosalpinx ♀

N89.8 Other specified noninflammatory disorders of vagina
Leukorrhea NOS
Old vaginal laceration
Pessary ulcer of vagina
[EXCLUDES1] *current obstetric trauma (O70.-, O71.4, O71.7-O71.8)*
old laceration involving muscles of pelvic floor (N81.8) ♀

N89.9 Noninflammatory disorder of vagina, unspecified ♀

[4] **N90 Other noninflammatory disorders of vulva and perineum**
[EXCLUDES1] *anogenital (venereal) warts (A63.0)*
carcinoma in situ of vulva (D07.1)
condyloma acuminatum (A63.0)
current obstetric trauma (O70.-, O71.7-O71.8)
inflammation of vulva (N76.-)
severe dysplasia of vulva (D07.1)
vulvar intraepithelial neoplasm III [VIN III] (D07.1)

N90.0 Mild vulvar dysplasia
Vulvar intraepithelial neoplasia [VIN], grade I ♀

N90.1 Moderate vulvar dysplasia
Vulvar intraepithelial neoplasia [VIN], grade II ♀

N90.3 Dysplasia of vulva, unspecified ♀

N90.4 Leukoplakia of vulva
Dystrophy of vulva
Kraurosis of vulva
Lichen sclerosus of external female genital organs ♀

N90.5 Atrophy of vulva
Stenosis of vulva ♀

N90.6 Hypertrophy of vulva
Hypertrophy of labia ♀

N90.7 Vulvar cyst ♀

[5] **N90.8 Other specified noninflammatory disorders of vulva and perineum**

[6] **N90.81 Female genital mutilation status**
Female genital cutting status

N90.810 Female genital mutilation status, unspecified
Female genital cutting status, unspecified
Female genital mutilation status NOS ♀

N90.811 Female genital mutilation Type I status
Clitorectomy status
Female genital cutting Type I status ♀

N90.812 Female genital mutilation Type II status
Clitorectomy with excision of labia minora status
Female genital cutting Type II status ♀

N90.813 Female genital mutilation Type III status
Female genital cutting Type III status
Infibulation status ♀

N90.818 Other female genital mutilation status
Female genital cutting Type IV status
Female genital mutilation Type IV status
Other female genital cutting status ♀

N90.89 Other specified noninflammatory disorders of vulva and perineum
Adhesions of vulva
Hypertrophy of clitoris ♀

[4] 4th character required [5] 5th character required [6] 6th character required [7] 7th character required [7] Extension 'X' Alert
[EXCLUDES1] Not coded here [EXCLUDES2] Not included here [PDx] Primary Diagnosis Only Manifestation Code

N90.9 Noninflammatory disorder of vulva and perineum, unspecified ♀

🔵 N91 Absent, scanty and rare menstruation

EXCLUDES1 ovarian dysfunction (E28.-)

N91.0 Primary amenorrhea ♀

N91.1 Secondary amenorrhea ♀

N91.2 Amenorrhea, unspecified ♀

N91.3 Primary oligomenorrhea ♀

N91.4 Secondary oligomenorrhea ♀

N91.5 Oligomenorrhea, unspecified

Hypomenorrhea NOS ♀

🔵 N92 Excessive, frequent and irregular menstruation

EXCLUDES1 postmenopausal bleeding (N95.0)
precocious puberty (menstruation) (E30.1)

N92.0 Excessive and frequent menstruation with regular cycle

Heavy periods NOS
Menorrhagia NOS
Polymenorrhea ♀

N92.1 Excessive and frequent menstruation with irregular cycle

Irregular intermenstrual bleeding
Irregular, shortened intervals between menstrual bleeding
Menometrorrhagia
Metrorrhagia ♀

N92.2 Excessive menstruation at puberty

Excessive bleeding associated with onset of menstrual periods
Pubertal menorrhagia
Puberty bleeding ℙ ♀

N92.3 Ovulation bleeding

Regular intermenstrual bleeding ♀

N92.4 Excessive bleeding in the premenopausal period

Climacteric menorrhagia or metrorrhagia
Menopausal menorrhagia or metrorrhagia
Preclimacteric menorrhagia or metrorrhagia
Premenopausal menorrhagia or metrorrhagia ♀

N92.5 Other specified irregular menstruation ♀

N92.6 Irregular menstruation, unspecified

Irregular bleeding NOS
Irregular periods NOS

EXCLUDES1 irregular menstruation with:
lengthened intervals or scanty bleeding (N91.3-N91.5)
shortened intervals or excessive bleeding (N92.1) ♀

🔵 N93 Other abnormal uterine and vaginal bleeding

EXCLUDES1 neonatal vaginal hemorrhage (P54.6)
precocious puberty (menstruation) (E30.1)
pseudomenses (P54.6)

N93.0 Postcoital and contact bleeding ♀

N93.8 Other specified abnormal uterine and vaginal bleeding

Dysfunctional or functional uterine or vaginal bleeding NOS ♀

N93.9 Abnormal uterine and vaginal bleeding, unspecified ♀

🔵 N94 Pain and other conditions associated with female genital organs and menstrual cycle

N94.0 Mittelschmerz ♀

N94.1 Dyspareunia

EXCLUDES1 psychogenic dyspareunia (F52.6) ♀

N94.2 Vaginismus

EXCLUDES1 psychogenic vaginismus (F52.5) ♀

N94.3 Premenstrual tension syndrome

Premenstrual dysphoric disorder
Code also associated menstrual migraine (G43.82-, G43.83-) ♀

N94.4 Primary dysmenorrhea ♀

N94.5 Secondary dysmenorrhea ♀

N94.6 Dysmenorrhea, unspecified ♀

EXCLUDES1 psychogenic dysmenorrhea (F45.8)

🔵 N94.8 Other specified conditions associated with female genital organs and menstrual cycle

🔵 N94.81 Vulvodynia

N94.810 Vulvar vestibulitis ♀

N94.818 Other vulvodynia ♀

N94.819 Vulvodynia, unspecified

Vulvodynia NOS ♀

N94.89 Other specified conditions associated with female genital organs and menstrual cycle ♀

N94.9 Unspecified condition associated with female genital organs and menstrual cycle ♀

🔵 N95 Menopausal and other perimenopausal disorders

Menopausal and other perimenopausal disorders due to naturally occurring (age-related) menopause and perimenopause

EXCLUDES1 excessive bleeding in the premenopausal period (N92.4)
menopausal and perimenopausal disorders due to artificial or premature menopause (E89.4-, E28.31-)
premature menopause (E28.31-)

EXCLUDES2 postmenopausal osteoporosis (M81.0-)
postmenopausal osteoporosis with current pathological fracture (M80.0-)
postmenopausal urethritis (N34.2)

N95.0 Postmenopausal bleeding ♀

N95.1 Menopausal and female climacteric states

Symptoms such as flushing, sleeplessness, headache, lack of concentration, associated with natural (age-related) menopause
Use additional code for associated symptoms

EXCLUDES1 asymptomatic menopausal state (Z78.0)
symptoms associated with artificial menopause (E89.41)
symptoms associated with premature menopause (E28.310) ♀

N95.2 Postmenopausal atrophic vaginitis

Senile (atrophic) vaginitis ♀

N95.8 Other specified menopausal and perimenopausal disorders ♀

N95.9 Unspecified menopausal and perimenopausal disorder ♀

N96 Recurrent pregnancy loss

Investigation or care in a nonpregnant woman with history of recurrent pregnancy loss

EXCLUDES1 recurrent pregnancy loss with current pregnancy (O26.2-) ♀

🔵 N97 Female infertility

INCLUDES inability to achieve a pregnancy
sterility, female NOS

EXCLUDES1 female infertility associated with:
hypopituitarism (E23.0)
Stein-Leventhal syndrome (E28.2)

EXCLUDES2 incompetence of cervix uteri (N88.3)

N97.0 Female infertility associated with anovulation ♀

N97.1 Female infertility of tubal origin

Female infertility associated with congenital anomaly of tube
Female infertility due to tubal block
Female infertility due to tubal occlusion
Female infertility due to tubal stenosis ♀

N97.2 Female infertility of uterine origin

Female infertility associated with congenital anomaly of uterus
Female infertility due to nonimplantation of ovum ♀

Unspecified Code	Other Specified Code	ℕ Newborn Age: 0	ℙ Pediatric Age: 0-17	𝕄 Maternity Age: 12-55
𝔸 Adult Age: 15-124	♂ Male	♀ Female	● New Code	▲ Revised Code Title	▶◀ Revised Text

N97.8 **Female infertility of other origin** ♀
N97.9 Female infertility, unspecified ♀
④ N98 Complications associated with artificial fertilization
N98.0 Infection associated with artificial insemination ♀
N98.1 Hyperstimulation of ovaries
Hyperstimulation of ovaries NOS
Hyperstimulation of ovaries associated with induced ovulation ♀
N98.2 Complications of attempted introduction of fertilized ovum following in vitro fertilization ♀
N98.3 Complications of attempted introduction of embryo in embryo transfer ♀
N98.8 **Other complications associated with artificial fertilization** ♀
N98.9 Complication associated with artificial fertilization, unspecified ♀

Intraoperative and postprocedural complications and disorders of genitourinary system, not elsewhere classified (N99)

④ N99 Intraoperative and postprocedural complications and disorders of genitourinary system, not elsewhere classified
EXCLUDES2 irradiation cystitis (N30.4-)
postoophorectomy osteoporosis with current pathological fracture (M80.8-)
postoophorectomy osteoporosis without current pathological fracture (M81.8)
N99.0 Postprocedural (acute) (chronic) kidney failure
Use additional code to type of kidney disease
⑤ N99.1 Postprocedural urethral stricture
Postcatheterization urethral stricture
⑥ N99.11 Postprocedural urethral stricture, male
N99.110 Postprocedural urethral stricture, male, meatal ♂
N99.111 Postprocedural bulbous urethral stricture
N99.112 Postprocedural membranous urethral stricture
N99.113 Postprocedural anterior urethral stricture
N99.114 Postprocedural urethral stricture, male, unspecified ♂
N99.12 Postprocedural urethral stricture, female ♀
N99.2 Postprocedural adhesions of vagina ♀
N99.3 Prolapse of vaginal vault after hysterectomy ♀
N99.4 Postprocedural pelvic peritoneal adhesions
EXCLUDES2 pelvic peritoneal adhesions NOS (N73.6)
postinfective pelvic peritoneal adhesions (N73.6)
⑤ N99.5 Complications of stoma of urinary tract
EXCLUDES2 mechanical complication of urinary (indwelling) catheter (T83.0-)
⑥ N99.51 Complication of cystostomy
N99.510 Cystostomy hemorrhage
N99.511 Cystostomy infection
N99.512 Cystostomy malfunction
N99.518 **Other cystostomy complication**
⑥ N99.52 Complication of other external stoma of urinary tract
N99.520 Hemorrhage of other external stoma of urinary tract
N99.521 Infection of other external stoma of urinary tract
N99.522 Malfunction of other external stoma of urinary tract
N99.528 **Other complication of other external stoma of urinary tract**
⑥ N99.53 Complication of other stoma of urinary tract
N99.530 Hemorrhage of other stoma of urinary tract
N99.531 Infection of other stoma of urinary tract
N99.532 Malfunction of other stoma of urinary tract

N99.538 **Other complication of other stoma of urinary tract**
⑤ N99.6 Intraoperative hemorrhage and hematoma of a genitourinary system organ or structure complicating a procedure
EXCLUDES1 intraoperative hemorrhage and hematoma of a genitourinary system organ or structure due to accidental puncture or laceration during a procedure (N99.7-)
N99.61 Intraoperative hemorrhage and hematoma of a genitourinary system organ or structure complicating a genitourinary system procedure
N99.62 Intraoperative hemorrhage and hematoma of a genitourinary system organ or structure complicating other procedure
⑤ N99.7 Accidental puncture and laceration of a genitourinary system organ or structure during a procedure
N99.71 Accidental puncture and laceration of a genitourinary system organ or structure during a genitourinary system procedure
N99.72 Accidental puncture and laceration of a genitourinary system organ or structure during other procedure
⑤ N99.8 Other intraoperative and postprocedural complications and disorders of genitourinary system
N99.81 Other intraoperative complications of genitourinary system
⑥ N99.82 Postprocedural hemorrhage and hematoma of a genitourinary system organ or structure following a procedure
N99.820 Postprocedural hemorrhage and hematoma of a genitourinary system organ or structure following a genitourinary system procedure
N99.821 Postprocedural hemorrhage and hematoma of a genitourinary system organ or structure following other procedure
N99.83 Residual ovary syndrome ♀
N99.89 **Other postprocedural complications and disorders of genitourinary system**

---

④ 4th character required   ⑤ 5th character required   ⑥ 6th character required   ⑦ 7th character required   ⑦ᵇ Extension 'X' Alert

EXCLUDES1 Not coded here   EXCLUDES2 Not included here   ᴾᴰˣ Primary Diagnosis Only   Manifestation Code

Chapter 15: Pregnancy, Childbirth, and the Puerperium (O00-O9A)

Chapter Specific Coding Guidelines

a. **General Rules for Obstetric Cases**

1) **Codes from chapter 15 and sequencing priority**
Obstetric cases require codes from chapter 15, codes in the range O00-O9A, Pregnancy, Childbirth, and the Puerperium. Chapter 15 codes have sequencing priority over codes from other chapters. Additional codes from other chapters may be used in conjunction with chapter 15 codes to further specify conditions. Should the provider document that the pregnancy is incidental to the encounter, then code Z33.1, Pregnant state, incidental, should be used in place of any chapter 15 codes. It is the provider's responsibility to state that the condition being treated is not affecting the pregnancy.

2) **Chapter 15 codes used only on the maternal record**
Chapter 15 codes are to be used only on the maternal record, never on the record of the newborn.

3) **Final character for trimester**
The majority of codes in Chapter 15 have a final character indicating the trimester of pregnancy. The timeframes for the trimesters are indicated at the beginning of the chapter. If trimester is not a component of a code it is because the condition always occurs in a specific trimester, or the concept of trimester of pregnancy is not applicable. Certain codes have characters for only certain trimesters because the condition does not occur in all trimesters, but it may occur in more than just one.

Assignment of the final character for trimester should be based on the provider's documentation of the trimester (or number of weeks) for the current admission/encounter. This applies to the assignment of trimester for pre-existing conditions as well as those that develop during or are due to the pregnancy. The provider's documentation of the number of weeks may be used to assign the appropriate code identifying the trimester.

Whenever delivery occurs during the current admission, and there is an "in childbirth" option for the obstetric complication being coded, the "in childbirth" code should be assigned.

4) **Selection of trimester for inpatient admissions that encompass more than one trimester**
In instances when a patient is admitted to a hospital for complications of pregnancy during one trimester and remains in the hospital into a subsequent trimester, the trimester character for the antepartum complication code should be assigned on the basis of the trimester when the complication developed, not the trimester of the discharge. If the condition developed prior to the current admission/encounter or represents a pre-existing condition, the trimester character for the trimester at the time of the admission/encounter should be assigned.

5) **Unspecified trimester**
Each category that includes codes for trimester has a code for "unspecified trimester." The "unspecified trimester" code should rarely be used, such as when the documentation in the record is insufficient to determine the trimester and it is not possible to obtain clarification.

6) **7th character for Fetus Identification**
Where applicable, a 7th character is to be assigned for certain categories (O31, O32, O33.3 - O33.6, O35, O36, O40, O41, O60.1, O60.2, O64, and O69) to identify the fetus for which the complication code applies.

Assign 7th character "0":
- For single gestations

- When the documentation in the record is insufficient to determine the fetus affected and it is not possible to obtain clarification.
- When it is not possible to clinically determine which fetus is affected.

b. **Selection of OB Principal or First-listed Diagnosis**

1) **Routine outpatient prenatal visits**
For routine outpatient prenatal visits when no complications are present, a code from category Z34, Encounter for supervision of normal pregnancy, should be used as the first-listed diagnosis. These codes should not be used in conjunction with chapter 15 codes.

2) **Prenatal outpatient visits for high-risk patients**
For routine prenatal outpatient visits for patients with high-risk pregnancies, a code from category O09, Supervision of high-risk pregnancy, should be used as the first-listed diagnosis. Secondary chapter 15 codes may be used in conjunction with these codes if appropriate.

3) **Episodes when no delivery occurs**
In episodes when no delivery occurs, the principal diagnosis should correspond to the principal complication of the pregnancy which necessitated the encounter. Should more than one complication exist, all of which are treated or monitored, any of the complications codes may be sequenced first.

4) **When a delivery occurs**
When a delivery occurs, the principal diagnosis should correspond to the main circumstances or complication of the delivery. In cases of cesarean delivery, the selection of the principal diagnosis should be the condition established after study that was responsible for the patient's admission. If the patient was admitted with a condition that resulted in the performance of a cesarean procedure, that condition should be selected as the principal diagnosis. If the reason for the admission/encounter was unrelated to the condition resulting in the cesarean delivery, the condition related to the reason for the admission/encounter should be selected as the principal diagnosis.

5) **Outcome of delivery**
A code from category Z37, Outcome of delivery, should be included on every maternal record when a delivery has occurred. These codes are not to be used on subsequent records or on the newborn record.

c. **Pre-existing conditions versus conditions due to the pregnancy**
Certain categories in Chapter 15 distinguish between conditions of the mother that existed prior to pregnancy (pre-existing) and those that are a direct result of pregnancy. When assigning codes from Chapter 15, it is important to assess if a condition was pre-existing prior to pregnancy or developed during or due to the pregnancy in order to assign the correct code.

Categories that do not distinguish between pre-existing and pregnancy-related conditions may be used for either. It is acceptable to use codes specifically for the puerperium with codes complicating pregnancy and childbirth if a condition arises postpartum during the delivery encounter.

d. **Pre-existing hypertension in pregnancy**
Category O10, Pre-existing hypertension complicating pregnancy, childbirth and the puerperium, includes codes for hypertensive heart and hypertensive chronic kidney disease. When assigning one of the O10 codes that includes hypertensive heart disease or hypertensive chronic kidney disease, it is necessary to add a secondary code from the appropriate hypertension category to specify the type of heart failure or chronic kidney disease.

See Section I.C.9. Hypertension.

e. **Fetal Conditions Affecting the Management of the Mother**
   1) **Codes from categories O35 and O36**
      Codes from categories O35, Maternal care for known or suspected fetal abnormality and damage, and O36, Maternal care for other fetal problems, are assigned only when the fetal condition is actually responsible for modifying the management of the mother, i.e., by requiring diagnostic studies, additional observation, special care, or termination of pregnancy. The fact that the fetal condition exists does not justify assigning a code from this series to the mother's record.

   2) **In utero surgery**
      In cases when surgery is performed on the fetus, a diagnosis code from category O35, Maternal care for known or suspected fetal abnormality and damage, should be assigned identifying the fetal condition. Assign the appropriate procedure code for the procedure performed.

      No code from Chapter 16, the perinatal codes, should be used on the mother's record to identify fetal conditions. Surgery performed in utero on a fetus is still to be coded as an obstetric encounter.

f. **HIV Infection in Pregnancy, Childbirth and the Puerperium**
   During pregnancy, childbirth or the puerperium, a patient admitted because of an HIV-related illness should receive a principal diagnosis from subcategory O98.7-, Human immunodeficiency [HIV] disease complicating pregnancy, childbirth and the puerperium, followed by the code(s) for the HIV-related illness(es).

   Patients with asymptomatic HIV infection status admitted during pregnancy, childbirth, or the puerperium should receive codes of O98.7- and Z21, Asymptomatic human immunodeficiency virus [HIV] infection status.

g. **Diabetes mellitus in pregnancy**
   Diabetes mellitus is a significant complicating factor in pregnancy. Pregnant women who are diabetic should be assigned a code from category O24, Diabetes mellitus in pregnancy, childbirth, and the puerperium, first, followed by the appropriate diabetes code(s) (E08-E13) from Chapter 4.

h. **Long term use of insulin**
   Code Z79.4, Long-term (current) use of insulin, should also be assigned if the diabetes mellitus is being treated with insulin.

i. **Gestational (pregnancy induced) diabetes**
   Gestational (pregnancy induced) diabetes can occur during the second and third trimester of pregnancy in women who were not diabetic prior to pregnancy. Gestational diabetes can cause complications in the pregnancy similar to those of pre-existing diabetes mellitus. It also puts the woman at greater risk of developing diabetes after the pregnancy. Codes for gestational diabetes are in subcategory O24.4, Gestational diabetes mellitus. No other code from category O24,

   Diabetes mellitus in pregnancy, childbirth, and the puerperium, should be used with a code from O24.4

   The codes under subcategory O24.4 include diet controlled and insulin controlled. If a patient with gestational diabetes is treated with both diet and insulin, only the code for insulin-controlled is required.

   Code Z79.4, Long-term (current) use of insulin, should not be assigned with codes from subcategory O24.4.

   An abnormal glucose tolerance in pregnancy is assigned a code from subcategory O99.81, Abnormal glucose complicating pregnancy, childbirth, and the puerperium.

j. **Sepsis and septic shock complicating abortion, pregnancy, childbirth and the puerperium**
   When assigning a chapter 15 code for sepsis complicating abortion, pregnancy, childbirth, and the puerperium, a code for the specific type of infection should be assigned as an additional diagnosis. If severe sepsis is present, a code from subcategory R65.2, Severe sepsis, and code(s) for associated organ dysfunction(s) should also be assigned as additional diagnoses.

k. **Puerperal sepsis**
   Code O85, Puerperal sepsis, should be assigned with a secondary code to identify the causal organism (e.g., for a bacterial infection, assign a code from category B95-B96, Bacterial infections in conditions classified elsewhere). A code from category A40, Streptococcal sepsis, or A41, Other sepsis, should not be used for puerperal sepsis. If applicable, use additional codes to identify severe sepsis (R65.2-) and any associated acute organ dysfunction.

l. **Alcohol and tobacco use during pregnancy, childbirth and the puerperium**
   1) **Alcohol use during pregnancy, childbirth and the puerperium**
      Codes under subcategory O99.31, Alcohol use complicating pregnancy, childbirth, and the puerperium, should be assigned for any pregnancy case when a mother uses alcohol during the pregnancy or postpartum. A secondary code from category F10, Alcohol related disorders, should also be assigned to identify manifestations of the alcohol use.

   2) **Tobacco use during pregnancy, childbirth and the puerperium**
      Codes under subcategory O99.33, Smoking (tobacco) complicating pregnancy, childbirth, and the puerperium, should be assigned for any pregnancy case when a mother uses any type of tobacco product during the pregnancy or postpartum. A secondary code from category F17, Nicotine dependence, should also be assigned to identify the type of nicotine dependence.

m. **Poisoning, toxic effects, adverse effects and underdosing in a pregnant patient**
   A code from subcategory O9A.2, Injury, poisoning and certain other consequences of external causes complicating pregnancy, childbirth, and the puerperium, should be sequenced first, followed by the appropriate injury, poisoning, toxic effect, adverse effect or underdosing code, and then the additional code(s) that specifies the condition caused by the poisoning, toxic effect, adverse effect or underdosing.

   See Section I.C.19. Adverse effects, poisoning, underdosing and toxic effects.

n. **Normal Delivery, Code O80**
   1) **Encounter for full term uncomplicated delivery**
      Code O80 should be assigned when a woman is admitted for a full-term normal delivery and delivers a single, healthy infant without any complications antepartum, during the delivery, or postpartum during the delivery episode. Code O80 is always a principal diagnosis. It is not to be used if any other code from chapter 15 is needed to describe a current complication of the antenatal, delivery, or perinatal period. Additional codes from other chapters may be used with code O80 if they are not related to or are in any way complicating the pregnancy.

   2) **Uncomplicated delivery with resolved antepartum complication**
      Code O80 may be used if the patient had a complication at some point during the pregnancy, but the complication is not present at the time of the admission for delivery.

   3) **Outcome of delivery for O80**
      Z37.0, Single live birth, is the only outcome of delivery code appropriate for use with O80.

o. **The Peripartum and Postpartum Periods**
   1) **Peripartum and Postpartum periods**
      The postpartum period begins immediately after delivery and   continues for six weeks following delivery. The peripartum period is defined as the last month of pregnancy to five months postpartum.

   2) **Peripartum and postpartum complication**
      A postpartum complication is any complication occurring within the six-week period.

3) **Pregnancy-related complications after 6 week period**
Chapter 15 codes may also be used to describe pregnancy-related complications after the peripartum or postpartum period if the provider documents that a condition is pregnancy related.

4) **Admission for routine postpartum care following delivery outside hospital**
When the mother delivers outside the hospital prior to admission and is admitted for routine postpartum care and no complications are noted, code Z39.0, Encounter for care and examination of mother immediately after delivery, should be assigned as the principal diagnosis.

5) **Pregnancy associated cardiomyopathy**
Pregnancy associated cardiomyopathy, code O90.3, is unique in that it may be diagnosed in the third trimester of pregnancy but may continue to progress months after delivery. For this reason, it is referred to as peripartum cardiomyopathy. Code O90.3 is only for use when the cardiomyopathy develops as a result of pregnancy in a woman who did not have pre-existing heart disease.

p. **Code O94, Sequelae of complication of pregnancy, childbirth, and the puerperium**
1) **Code O94**
Code O94, Sequelae of complication of pregnancy, childbirth, and the puerperium, is for use in those cases when an initial complication of a pregnancy develops a sequelae requiring care or treatment at a future date.

2) **After the initial postpartum period**
This code may be used at any time after the initial postpartum period.

3) **Sequencing of Code O94**
This code, like all sequela codes, is to be sequenced following the code describing the sequelae of the complication.

q. **Termination of Pregnancy and Spontaneous abortions**
1) **Abortion with Liveborn Fetus**
When an attempted termination of pregnancy results in a liveborn fetus, assign code Z33.2, Encounter for elective termination of pregnancy and a code from category Z37, Outcome of Delivery.

2) **Retained Products of Conception following an abortion**
Subsequent encounters for retained products of conception following a spontaneous abortion or elective termination of pregnancy are assigned the appropriate code from category O03, Spontaneous abortion, or codes O07.4, Failed attempted termination of pregnancy without complication and Z33.2, Encounter for elective termination of pregnancy. This advice is appropriate even when the patient was discharged previously with a discharge diagnosis of complete abortion.

3) **Complications leading to abortion**
Codes from Chapter 15 may be used as additional codes to identify any documented complications of the pregnancy in conjunction with codes in categories in O07 and O08.

r. **Abuse in a pregnant patient**
For suspected or confirmed cases of abuse of a pregnant patient, a code(s) from subcategories O9A.3, Physical abuse complicating pregnancy, childbirth, and the puerperium, O9A.4, Sexual abuse complicating pregnancy, childbirth, and the puerperium, and O9A.5, Psychological abuse complicating pregnancy, childbirth, and the puerperium, should be sequenced first, followed by the appropriate codes (if applicable) to identify any associated current injury due to physical abuse, sexual abuse, and the perpetrator of abuse.

See Section I.C.19. Adult and child abuse, neglect and other maltreatment.

This page intentionally left blank

Anatomy of the Female Reproductive System

1. **The female reproductive system includes the following:**
   a) The ovaries or female gonads are the primary sex organs of the female reproductive system.
   b) The uterine (or fallopian) tubes, uterus, vagina and external genitalia serve as the accessory organs of the female reproductive system.
   c) The accessory glands act to produce the mucus for providing lubrication during sexual intercourse.

2. **The anatomy of structures/components of the female reproductive system is further described below:**
   a) The Ovaries
      i) Ovaries are the paired glands in the upper pelvic cavity and remain located on each side of the uterus.
      ii) Capsule of the ovary is termed as the tunica albuginea. The outer region of the ovarian capsule is known as the cortex, which contains the ovarian follicles (or eggs).
      iii) Ovaries facilitate the discharge of eggs in ovulation and secrete the female sex hormones estrogen and progesterone.
   b) The Uterine (or Fallopian) Tubes
      i) Fallopian tubes are two in number and serve to transport the ova from the ovaries to the uterus.
      ii) The open end of the fallopian tube is of the shape of a funnel, and is known as the infundibulum. The infundibulum is surrounded by the fimbriae, which form a fringe of finger like projections.
   c) The Uterus
      i) The uterus is known as the site of menstruation and fetal development.
      ii) The uterus is a pear shaped organ. The dome shaped part of the uterus above the uterine tubes is known as the fundus. The major tapering portion of the uterus is called as the body. However, the narrow inferior part of the uterus is known as the cervix (or cervix uteri/neck of uterus).
      iii) The uterine cavity forms the interior of the body of uterus. The interior portion of the cervix is known as the cervical canal.
      iv) The internal os is the opening between the uterine cavity and the cervical canal. The external os is the opening between the cervical canal and the vagina.
      v) The endometrium is the innermost layer of the wall of uterus and forms the site of implantation of the fertilized egg.
      vi) The myometrium is the middle layer of the wall of uterus and composed of the smooth muscle.
      vii) The perimetrium (or visceral peritoneum) is the outermost layer of the wall of uterus.
   d) The Vagina
      i) Its provides a passage for the menstrual flow. It is the lower part of the birth canal and serves as a receptacle for the penis during sexual intercourse.
      ii) Its attachment to the cervix is surrounded by a recess, which is known as the fornix.
   e) The External Genitalia of the Female
      i) The external genitalia of the female are constituted by the vulva (or pudendum).
      ii) The mons pubis (or veneris) is a rounded eminence of adipose or fatty tissue upon the pubic symphysis.
      iii) The outer fatty folds of the vulva that extend from the mons pubis are known as the labia majora.
      iv) Inner and highly vascular connective tissue folds of the vulva are known as the labia minora. These folds lack hairs and are also known as the nymphae.

   v) The small mass of erectile tissue at the anterior junction of labia minora is known as the clitoris. The clitoris remains covered with a skin layer, which is known as the prepuce. The glans is the exposed part of the clitoris.
   vi) The vestibule is an opening between the folds of the labia minora. This opening contains a thin fold of tissue (or the hymen) that gets ruptured at the time of the first sexual intercourse.
   vii) The vestibule is further linked to the vaginal and urethral orifices.
   viii) Lesser vestibular or Skene's glands secrete mucous and the openings of their ducts lie on each side of the urethral orifice.
   ix) Bartholin's or greater vestibular glands generate mucous to facilitate the process of sexual intercourse. The openings of these glands lie on each side of the vaginal orifice.
   f) The Perineum
      i) The perineum is a region between the thighs and buttocks of both males and females. This area marks the boundary of the pelvic outlet and provides passage to the urogenital ducts and rectum.
      ii) The perineum is further divided into an anterior urogenital triangle containing the external genitalia, and a posterior anal triangle containing the anus.
   g) The Menstrual Cycle
      i) The menstrual cycle is also known by the names of menstruation or menses.
      ii) The menstrual cycle is divided into the menstrual, proliferative and secretory phases.
      iii) The shedding of the endometrial lining of uterus, blood and tissue fluid occurs during the menstrual phase of the menstrual cycle.
      iv) The proliferative phase of the menstrual cycle is also known as the follicular phase. The lining of the uterus grows and proliferates during this phase. The process of ovulation also starts in the follicular phase, wherein the egg ruptures from the Graafian follicle and the rising estrogen levels cause the endometrial lining of the uterus to thicken. The follicle eventually collapses and gets transformed to the corpus luteum.
      v) The estrogen and progesterone hormones are secreted during the secretory phase of the menstrual cycle. The fertilization and implantation process can occur in this stage after the hymen rupture during the first sexual intercourse. The corpus luteum degenerates and gets transformed to corpus albicans if the fertilization and implantation processes do not occur during this phase.
      vi) Following fertilization, the development of placenta is started. The placenta facilitates the secretion of estrogen and progesterone hormones to support the pregnancy and breast development for the production of milk inside the mammary glands.
   h) The Mammary Glands
      i) They serve to produce milk in females, and are found in both males and females.
      ii) The mammary ducts expand into milk storage sinuses (or ampullae) near the nipple.
      iii) The areola is a circular pigmented area around the nipple.
      iv) They facilitate the process of lactation (which includes milk production and it's ejection from the nipple).
   i) Pregnancy and Embryonic Development
      i) Pregnancy is initiated with the formation of a viable zygote (or fertilized egg) by the union of the male sperm and the female ovum (or fertilization).

ii) Fertilization occurs in the upper two third portion of the fallopian tube.

iii) The zygote travels down the uterine tube and forms the blastocyst or blastula through mitotic division.

iv) The tygote eventually gets transformed to the chorionic vesicle in the uterine cavity. This chorionic vesicle secretes the chorionic gonadotropin hormone that gets embedded in the endometrial lining and maintains it via hormones.

v) The ectoderm forms the outer layer of the germ cells and develops into skin and nervous system.

vi) The endoderm initially consists of the flattened cells that form the epithelial linings of the internal organs.

vii) The Mesoderm induces the formation of coelom (or the fluid-filled cavity within the mesoderm) and gives rise to muscles, bones, cartilages, connective tissues and other structures.

viii) The chorionic villi are the projections of the trophoblast (or the fluid-filled sphere of the blastocyst). These chorionic villi communicate with the uterine tissue to form the placenta.

ix) The amnion is the fluid filled sac that surrounds and protects the embryo as and when the placenta is formed.

x) The umbilical cord or birth cord is the stalk that connects the fetus (or embryo) to the placenta.

xi) The placenta serves to exchange oxygen, nutrients and wastes between the embryo and the mother.

xii) With the ongoing pregnancy, the uterus expands in the abdominal cavity for accommodating the growing fetus.

xiii) The childbirth (or parturition) is induced by the uterine contractions and this process is termed as the labor.

xiv) The dilation stage involves the complete dilation of the cervix by the head of the fetus. The amniotic fluid (or bag of waters) is also released during the rupture of the amnion.

xv) The expulsion stage child moves out through the cervix and vagina during the expulsion stage.

xvi) The placental stage (or afterbirth) is marked by the detachment of the placenta from the uterus following the birth.

Common Pathologies

Dysfunctional uterine bleeding (DUB)
Dysfunctional uterine bleeding (DUB) refers to uncategorized bleeding from the uterus; typically in the adolescent or perimenopausal period. DUB is broadly characterized clinically as ovulatory or anovulatory.

Dysmenorrhea
Dysmenorrhea refers to the symptom of painful menstruation. It can be divided into 2 broad categories: primary (occurring in the absence of pelvic pathology) and secondary (resulting from identifiable organic diseases).

Dyspareunia
Dyspareunia is pain that occurs only (or primarily) during sexual intercourse. It is not a disease, but rather a symptom of an underlying physical or psychological disorder. The pain, which can be mild or severe, may appear in the genitals, the pelvic region, or the lower back. The condition is much more common among women

Menorrhagia
Menorrhagia is an abnormally heavy and prolonged menstrual period at regular intervals. Menorrhagia can be caused by abnormal blood clotting, disruption of normal hormonal regulation of periods, or disorders of the endometrial lining of the uterus. Depending upon the cause, it may be associated with abnormally painful periods.

Endometriosis
Endometriosis is the abnormal growth of cells (endometrial cells) similar to those that form the inside of the uterus, but in a location outside of the uterus. Endometriosis is most commonly found on other organs of the pelvis.

Fibroids
Fibroids are non-cancerous (benign) tumors that grow from the muscle layers of the uterus (womb). They are also known as uterine fibroids, myomas, or fibromyomas. The singular of uterine fibroids is Uterine Fibroma. Fibroids are growths of smooth muscle and fibrous tissue. Fibroids can vary in size, from that of a bean to as large as a melon. There are four types of fibroids

Intramural
These are located in the wall of the uterus. These are the most common types of fibroids.

Subserosal
These are located outside the wall of the uterus. They can develop into pedunculated fibroids (stalks). Subserosal fibroids can become quite large.

Submucosal
These are located in the muscle beneath the lining of the uterus wall.

Cervical
These are located in the neck of the womb (the cervix).

Uterine fibroids

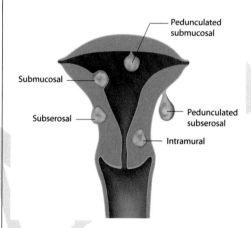

Gonorrhea
Gonorrhea is an infection caused by a sexually transmitted bacterium that can infect both males and females. Gonorrhea most often affects the urethra, rectum or throat. In females, gonorrhea can also infect the cervix.

Urinary Incontinence
Urinary incontinence (UI) is loss of bladder control. Symptoms can range from mild leaking to uncontrollable wetting. It can happen to anyone, but it becomes more common with age. Women experience UI twice as often as men. Most bladder control problems happen when muscles are too weak or too active. If the muscles that keep your bladder closed are weak, you may have accidents when you sneeze, laugh or lift a heavy object. This is stress incontinence. If bladder muscles become too active, you may feel a strong urge to go to the bathroom when you have little urine in your bladder. This is urge incontinence or overactive bladder. There are other causes of incontinence, such as prostate problems and nerve damage

Infertility
Infertility is fundamentally the inability to conceive a baby. Infertility also refers to the state of a woman who is unable to carry a pregnancy to full term. About 40 percent of the issues involved with infertility are due to the man, another 40 percent due to the woman, and 20 percent result from complications with both partners

Polycystic Ovarian Syndrome (PCOS)
Polycystic ovarian syndrome (PCOS), also known by the name Stein-Leventhal syndrome, is a hormonal problem that causes women to have a variety of symptoms. It should be noted that most women with the condition have a number of small cysts in the ovaries. However, women may have cysts in the ovaries for a number of reasons, and it is the characteristic constellation of symptoms, rather than the presence of the cysts themselves, that is important in establishing the diagnosis of PCOS.

Pregnancy, childbirth and the puerperium (O00-O9A)

NOTES CODES FROM THIS CHAPTER ARE FOR USE ONLY ON MATERNAL RECORDS, NEVER ON NEWBORN RECORDS
Codes from this chapter are for use for conditions related to or aggravated by the pregnancy, childbirth, or by the puerperium (maternal causes or obstetric causes)

Trimesters are counted from the first day of the last menstrual period. They are defined as follows:
1st trimester- less than 14 weeks 0 days
2nd trimester- 14 weeks 0 days to less than 28 weeks 0 days
3rd trimester- 28 weeks 0 days until delivery
Use additional code from category Z3A, Weeks of gestation, to identify the specific week of the pregnancy

EXCLUDES1 *supervision of normal pregnancy (Z34.-)*

EXCLUDES2 *mental and behavioral disorders associated with the puerperium (F53)*
obstetrical tetanus (A34)
postpartum necrosis of pituitary gland (E23.0)
puerperal osteomalacia (M83.0)

Pregnancy with abortive outcome (O00-O08)

EXCLUDES1 *continuing pregnancy in multiple gestation after abortion of one fetus or more (O31.1-, O31.3-)*

4️⃣ **O00 Ectopic pregnancy**
INCLUDES *ruptured ectopic pregnancy*
Use additional code from category O08 to identify any associated complication

O00.0 Abdominal pregnancy
EXCLUDES1 *maternal care for viable fetus in abdominal pregnancy (O36.7-)* Ⓜ ♀

O00.1 Tubal pregnancy
Fallopian pregnancy
Rupture of (fallopian) tube due to pregnancy
Tubal abortion Ⓜ ♀

O00.2 Ovarian pregnancy Ⓜ ♀

O00.8 Other ectopic pregnancy
Cervical pregnancy
Cornual pregnancy
Intraligamentous pregnancy
Mural pregnancy Ⓜ ♀

O00.9 Ectopic pregnancy, unspecified Ⓜ ♀

4️⃣ **O01 Hydatidiform mole**
Use additional code from category O08 to identify any associated complication.
EXCLUDES1 *chorioadenoma (destruens) (D39.2)*
malignant hydatidiform mole (D39.2)

O01.0 Classical hydatidiform mole
Complete hydatidiform mole Ⓜ ♀

O01.1 Incomplete and partial hydatidiform mole Ⓜ ♀

O01.9 Hydatidiform mole, unspecified
Trophoblastic disease NOS
Vesicular mole NOS Ⓜ ♀

4️⃣ **O02 Other abnormal products of conception**
Use additional code from category O08 to identify any associated complication.
EXCLUDES1 *papyraceous fetus (O31.0-)*

O02.0 Blighted ovum and nonhydatidiform mole
Carneous mole
Fleshy mole
Intrauterine mole NOS
Molar pregnancy NEC
Pathological ovum Ⓜ ♀

O02.1 Missed abortion
Early fetal death, before completion of 20 weeks of gestation, with retention of dead fetus

EXCLUDES1 *failed induced abortion (O07.-)*
fetal death (intrauterine) (late) (O36.4)
missed abortion with blighted ovum (O02.0)
missed abortion with hydatidiform mole (O01.-)
missed abortion with nonhydatidiform (O02.0)
missed abortion with other abnormal products of conception (O02.8-)
missed delivery (O36.4)
stillbirth (P95) Ⓜ ♀

5️⃣ **O02.8 Other specified abnormal products of conception**
EXCLUDES1 *abnormal products of conception with blighted ovum (O02.0)*
abnormal products of conception with hydatidiform mole (O01.-)
abnormal products of conception with nonhydatidiform mole (O02.0)

O02.81 Inappropriate change in quantitative human chorionic gonadotropin (hCG) in early pregnancy
Biochemical pregnancy
Chemical pregnancy
Inappropriate level of quantitative human chorionic gonadotropin (hCG) for gestational age in early pregnancy Ⓜ ♀

O02.89 Other abnormal products of conception Ⓜ ♀

O02.9 Abnormal product of conception, unspecified Ⓜ ♀

4️⃣ **O03 Spontaneous abortion**
NOTES Incomplete abortion includes retained products of conception following spontaneous abortion
INCLUDES *miscarriage*

O03.0 Genital tract and pelvic infection following incomplete spontaneous abortion
Endometritis following incomplete spontaneous abortion
Oophoritis following incomplete spontaneous abortion
Parametritis following incomplete spontaneous abortion
Pelvic peritonitis following incomplete spontaneous abortion
Salpingitis following incomplete spontaneous abortion
Salpingo-oophoritis following incomplete spontaneous abortion
EXCLUDES1 *sepsis following incomplete spontaneous abortion (O03.37)*
urinary tract infection following incomplete spontaneous abortion (O03.38) Ⓜ ♀

O03.1 Delayed or excessive hemorrhage following incomplete spontaneous abortion
Afibrinogenemia following incomplete spontaneous abortion
Defibrination syndrome following incomplete spontaneous abortion
Hemolysis following incomplete spontaneous abortion
Intravascular coagulation following incomplete spontaneous abortion Ⓜ ♀

O03.2 Embolism following incomplete spontaneous abortion
Air embolism following incomplete spontaneous abortion
Amniotic fluid embolism following incomplete spontaneous abortion
Blood-clot embolism following incomplete spontaneous abortion
Embolism NOS following incomplete spontaneous abortion
Fat embolism following incomplete spontaneous abortion
Pulmonary embolism following incomplete spontaneous abortion
Pyemic embolism following incomplete spontaneous abortion
Septic or septicopyemic embolism following incomplete spontaneous abortion
Soap embolism following incomplete spontaneous abortion Ⓜ ♀

Unspecified Code	Other Specified Code	Ⓝ Newborn Age: 0	Ⓟ Pediatric Age: 0-17	Ⓜ Maternity Age: 12-55	
Ⓐ Adult Age: 15-124	♂ Male	♀ Female	● New Code	▲ Revised Code Title	▶◀ Revised Text

[5] **O03.3 Other and unspecified complications following incomplete spontaneous abortion**

O03.30 Unspecified complication following incomplete spontaneous abortion [M] ♀

O03.31 Shock following incomplete spontaneous abortion

Circulatory collapse following incomplete spontaneous abortion
Shock (postprocedural) following incomplete spontaneous abortion

[EXCLUDES1] *shock due to infection following incomplete spontaneous abortion (O03.37)* [M] ♀

O03.32 Renal failure following incomplete spontaneous abortion

Kidney failure (acute) following incomplete spontaneous abortion
Oliguria following incomplete spontaneous abortion
Renal shutdown following incomplete spontaneous abortion
Renal tubular necrosis following incomplete spontaneous abortion
Uremia following incomplete spontaneous abortion [M] ♀

O03.33 Metabolic disorder following incomplete spontaneous abortion [M] ♀

O03.34 Damage to pelvic organs following incomplete spontaneous abortion

Laceration, perforation, tear or chemical damage of bladder following incomplete spontaneous abortion
Laceration, perforation, tear or chemical damage of bowel following incomplete spontaneous abortion
Laceration, perforation, tear or chemical damage of broad ligament following incomplete spontaneous abortion
Laceration, perforation, tear or chemical damage of cervix following incomplete spontaneous abortion
Laceration, perforation, tear or chemical damage of periurethral tissue following incomplete spontaneous abortion
Laceration, perforation, tear or chemical damage of uterus following incomplete spontaneous abortion
Laceration, perforation, tear or chemical damage of vagina following incomplete spontaneous abortion [M] ♀

O03.35 Other venous complications following incomplete spontaneous abortion [M] ♀

O03.36 Cardiac arrest following incomplete spontaneous abortion [M] ♀

O03.37 Sepsis following incomplete spontaneous abortion

Use additional code to identify infectious agent (B95-B97)
code to identify severe sepsis, if applicable (R65.2-)

[EXCLUDES1] *septic or septicopyemic embolism following incomplete spontaneous abortion (O03.2)* [M] ♀

O03.38 Urinary tract infection following incomplete spontaneous abortion

Cystitis following incomplete spontaneous abortion [M] ♀

O03.39 Incomplete spontaneous abortion with other complications [M] ♀

O03.4 Incomplete spontaneous abortion without complication [M] ♀

O03.5 Genital tract and pelvic infection following complete or unspecified spontaneous abortion

Endometritis following complete or unspecified spontaneous abortion
Oophoritis following complete or unspecified spontaneous abortion
Parametritis following complete or unspecified spontaneous abortion
Pelvic peritonitis following complete or unspecified spontaneous abortion
Salpingitis following complete or unspecified spontaneous abortion
Salpingo-oophoritis following complete or unspecified spontaneous abortion

[EXCLUDES1] *sepsis following complete or unspecified spontaneous abortion (O03.87)*
urinary tract infection following complete or unspecified spontaneous abortion (O03.88) [M] ♀

O03.6 Delayed or excessive hemorrhage following complete or unspecified spontaneous abortion

Afibrinogenemia following complete or unspecified spontaneous abortion
Defibrination syndrome following complete or unspecified spontaneous abortion
Hemolysis following complete or unspecified spontaneous abortion
Intravascular coagulation following complete or unspecified spontaneous abortion [M] ♀

O03.7 Embolism following complete or unspecified spontaneous abortion

Air embolism following complete or unspecified spontaneous abortion
Amniotic fluid embolism following complete or unspecified spontaneous abortion
Blood-clot embolism following complete or unspecified spontaneous abortion
Embolism NOS following complete or unspecified spontaneous abortion
Fat embolism following complete or unspecified spontaneous abortion
Pulmonary embolism following complete or unspecified spontaneous abortion
Pyemic embolism following complete or unspecified spontaneous abortion
Septic or septicopyemic embolism following complete or unspecified spontaneous abortion
Soap embolism following complete or unspecified spontaneous abortion [M] ♀

[5] **O03.8 Other and unspecified complications following complete or unspecified spontaneous abortion**

O03.80 Unspecified complication following complete or unspecified spontaneous abortion [M] ♀

O03.81 Shock following complete or unspecified spontaneous abortion

Circulatory collapse following complete or unspecified spontaneous abortion
Shock (postprocedural) following complete or unspecified spontaneous abortion

[EXCLUDES1] *shock due to infection following complete or unspecified spontaneous abortion (O03.87)* [M] ♀

O03.82 Renal failure following complete or unspecified spontaneous abortion

Kidney failure (acute) following complete or unspecified spontaneous abortion
Oliguria following complete or unspecified spontaneous abortion
Renal shutdown following complete or unspecified spontaneous abortion
Renal tubular necrosis following complete or unspecified spontaneous abortion
Uremia following complete or unspecified spontaneous abortion [M] ♀

[4] 4th character required [5] 5th character required [6] 6th character required [7] 7th character required [x7] Extension 'X' Alert
[EXCLUDES1] Not coded here [EXCLUDES2] Not included here [PDx] Primary Diagnosis Only Manifestation Code

O03.83 Metabolic disorder **following complete or unspecified spontaneous abortion** [M] ♀

O03.84 Damage to pelvic organs **following complete or unspecified spontaneous abortion**
Laceration, perforation, tear or chemical damage of bladder following complete or unspecified spontaneous abortion
Laceration, perforation, tear or chemical damage of bowel following complete or unspecified spontaneous abortion
Laceration, perforation, tear or chemical damage of broad ligament following complete or unspecified spontaneous abortion
Laceration, perforation, tear or chemical damage of cervix following complete or unspecified spontaneous abortion
Laceration, perforation, tear or chemical damage of periurethral tissue following complete or unspecified spontaneous abortion
Laceration, perforation, tear or chemical damage of uterus following complete or unspecified spontaneous abortion
Laceration, perforation, tear or chemical damage of vagina following complete or unspecified spontaneous abortion [M] ♀

O03.85 **Other venous complications following complete or unspecified spontaneous abortion** [M] ♀

O03.86 Cardiac arrest **following complete or unspecified spontaneous abortion** [M] ♀

O03.87 Sepsis **following complete or unspecified spontaneous abortion**
Use additional code to identify infectious agent (B95-B97)
code to identify severe sepsis, if applicable (R65.2-)
[EXCLUDES1] *septic or septicopyemic embolism following complete or unspecified spontaneous abortion (O03.7)* [M] ♀

O03.88 Urinary tract infection **following complete or unspecified spontaneous abortion**
Cystitis following complete or unspecified spontaneous abortion [M] ♀

O03.89 **Complete or unspecified spontaneous abortion with other complications** [M] ♀

O03.9 **Complete or unspecified spontaneous abortion** without complication
Miscarriage NOS
Spontaneous abortion NOS [M] ♀

[4] O04 Complications **following (induced)** termination of pregnancy
[INCLUDES] *complications following (induced) termination of pregnancy*
[EXCLUDES1] *encounter for elective termination of pregnancy, uncomplicated (Z33.2)*
failed attempted termination of pregnancy (O07.-)

O04.5 Genital tract and pelvic infection **following (induced) termination of pregnancy**
Endometritis following (induced) termination of pregnancy
Oophoritis following (induced) termination of pregnancy
Parametritis following (induced) termination of pregnancy
Pelvic peritonitis following (induced) termination of pregnancy
Salpingitis following (induced) termination of pregnancy
Salpingo-oophoritis following (induced) termination of pregnancy
[EXCLUDES1] *sepsis following (induced) termination of pregnancy (O04.87)*
urinary tract infection following (induced) termination of pregnancy (O04.88) [M] ♀

O04.6 Delayed or excessive hemorrhage **following (induced) termination of pregnancy**
Afibrinogenemia following (induced) termination of pregnancy
Defibrination syndrome following (induced) termination of pregnancy
Hemolysis following (induced) termination of pregnancy
Intravascular coagulation following (induced) termination of pregnancy [M] ♀

O04.7 Embolism **following (induced) termination of pregnancy**
Air embolism following (induced) termination of pregnancy
Amniotic fluid embolism following (induced) termination of pregnancy
Blood-clot embolism following (induced) termination of pregnancy
Embolism NOS following (induced) termination of pregnancy
Fat embolism following (induced) termination of pregnancy
Pulmonary embolism following (induced) termination of pregnancy
Pyemic embolism following (induced) termination of pregnancy
Septic or septicopyemic embolism following (induced) termination of pregnancy
Soap embolism following (induced) termination of pregnancy [M] ♀

[5] O04.8 **(Induced) termination of pregnancy with** other and unspecified **complications**

O04.80 **(Induced) termination of pregnancy with unspecified complications** [M] ♀

O04.81 Shock **following (induced) termination of pregnancy**
Circulatory collapse following (induced) termination of pregnancy
Shock (postprocedural) following (induced) termination of pregnancy
[EXCLUDES1] *shock due to infection following (induced) termination of pregnancy (O04.87)* [M] ♀

O04.82 Renal failure **following (induced) termination of pregnancy**
Kidney failure (acute) following (induced) termination of pregnancy
Oliguria following (induced) termination of pregnancy
Renal shutdown following (induced) termination of pregnancy
Renal tubular necrosis following (induced) termination of pregnancy
Uremia following (induced) termination of pregnancy [M] ♀

O04.83 Metabolic disorder **following (induced) termination of pregnancy** [M] ♀

O04.84 Damage to pelvic organs **following (induced) termination of pregnancy**
Laceration, perforation, tear or chemical damage of bladder following (induced) termination of pregnancy
Laceration, perforation, tear or chemical damage of bowel following (induced) termination of pregnancy
Laceration, perforation, tear or chemical damage of broad ligament following (induced) termination of pregnancy

Unspecified Code | Other Specified Code | [N] Newborn Age: 0 | [P] Pediatric Age: 0-17 | [M] Maternity Age: 12-55
[A] Adult Age: 15-124 | ♂ Male | ♀ Female | ● New Code | ▲ Revised Code Title | ►◄ Revised Text

Laceration, perforation, tear or chemical damage of cervix following (induced) termination of pregnancy

Laceration, perforation, tear or chemical damage of periurethral tissue following (induced) termination of pregnancy

Laceration, perforation, tear or chemical damage of uterus following (induced) termination of pregnancy

Laceration, perforation, tear or chemical damage of vagina following (induced) termination of pregnancy Ⓜ ♀

O04.85 Other venous complications following (induced) termination of pregnancy Ⓜ ♀

O04.86 Cardiac arrest following (induced) termination of pregnancy Ⓜ ♀

O04.87 Sepsis following (induced) termination of pregnancy

Use additional code to identify infectious agent (B95-B97)

code to identify severe sepsis, if applicable (R65.2-)

EXCLUDES1 septic or septicopyemic embolism following (induced) termination of pregnancy (O04.7) Ⓜ ♀

O04.88 Urinary tract infection following (induced) termination of pregnancy

Cystitis following (induced) termination of pregnancy Ⓜ ♀

O04.89 (Induced) termination of pregnancy with other complications Ⓜ ♀

❹ **O07 Failed attempted termination of pregnancy**

INCLUDES failure of attempted induction of termination of pregnancy

incomplete elective abortion

EXCLUDES1 incomplete spontaneous abortion (O03.0-)

O07.0 Genital tract and pelvic infection following failed attempted termination of pregnancy

Endometritis following failed attempted termination of pregnancy

Oophoritis following failed attempted termination of pregnancy

Parametritis following failed attempted termination of pregnancy

Pelvic peritonitis following failed attempted termination of pregnancy

Salpingitis following failed attempted termination of pregnancy

Salpingo-oophoritis following failed attempted termination of pregnancy

EXCLUDES1 sepsis following failed attempted termination of pregnancy (O07.37)

urinary tract infection following failed attempted termination of pregnancy (O07.38) Ⓜ ♀

O07.1 Delayed or excessive hemorrhage following failed attempted termination of pregnancy

Afibrinogenemia following failed attempted termination of pregnancy

Defibrination syndrome following failed attempted termination of pregnancy

Hemolysis following failed attempted termination of pregnancy

Intravascular coagulation following failed attempted termination of pregnancy Ⓜ ♀

O07.2 Embolism following failed attempted termination of pregnancy

Air embolism following failed attempted termination of pregnancy

Amniotic fluid embolism following failed attempted

termination of pregnancy

Blood-clot embolism following failed attempted termination of pregnancy

Embolism NOS following failed attempted termination of pregnancy

Fat embolism following failed attempted termination of pregnancy

Pulmonary embolism following failed attempted termination of pregnancy

Pyemic embolism following failed attempted termination of pregnancy

Septic or septicopyemic embolism following failed attempted termination of pregnancy

Soap embolism following failed attempted termination of pregnancy Ⓜ ♀

❺ **O07.3 Failed attempted termination of pregnancy with other and unspecified complications**

O07.30 Failed attempted termination of pregnancy with unspecified complications Ⓜ ♀

O07.31 Shock following failed attempted termination of pregnancy

Circulatory collapse following failed attempted termination of pregnancy

Shock (postprocedural) following failed attempted termination of pregnancy

EXCLUDES1 shock due to infection following failed attempted termination of pregnancy (O07.37) Ⓜ ♀

O07.32 Renal failure following failed attempted termination of pregnancy

Kidney failure (acute) following failed attempted termination of pregnancy

Oliguria following failed attempted termination of pregnancy

Renal shutdown following failed attempted termination of pregnancy

Renal tubular necrosis following failed attempted termination of pregnancy

Uremia following failed attempted termination of pregnancy Ⓜ ♀

O07.33 Metabolic disorder following failed attempted termination of pregnancy Ⓜ ♀

O07.34 Damage to pelvic organs following failed attempted termination of pregnancy

Laceration, perforation, tear or chemical damage of bladder following failed attempted termination of pregnancy

Laceration, perforation, tear or chemical damage of bowel following failed attempted termination of pregnancy

Laceration, perforation, tear or chemical damage of broad ligament following failed attempted termination of pregnancy

Laceration, perforation, tear or chemical damage of cervix following failed attempted termination of pregnancy

Laceration, perforation, tear or chemical damage of periurethral tissue following failed attempted termination of pregnancy

Laceration, perforation, tear or chemical damage of uterus following failed attempted termination of pregnancy

Laceration, perforation, tear or chemical damage of vagina following failed attempted termination of pregnancy Ⓜ ♀

O07.35 Other venous complications following failed attempted termination of pregnancy Ⓜ ♀

---

❹ 4th character required   ❺ 5th character required   ❻ 6th character required   ❼ 7th character required   ⓧ Extension 'X' Alert

EXCLUDES 1 Not coded here   *EXCLUDES 2* Not included here   ℞ Primary Diagnosis Only   Manifestation Code

O07.36 Cardiac arrest following failed attempted termination of pregnancy [M] ♀

O07.37 Sepsis following failed attempted termination of pregnancy
Use additional code (B95-B97), to identify infectious agent
code (R65.2-) to identify severe sepsis, if applicable
EXCLUDES1 *septic or septicopyemic embolism following failed attempted termination of pregnancy (O07.2)* [M] ♀

O07.38 Urinary tract infection following failed attempted termination of pregnancy
Cystitis following failed attempted termination of pregnancy [M] ♀

O07.39 Failed attempted termination of pregnancy with other complications [M] ♀

O07.4 Failed attempted termination of pregnancy without complication [M] ♀

④ O08 Complications following ectopic and molar pregnancy
This category is for use with categories O00-O02 to identify any associated complications

O08.0 Genital tract and pelvic infection following ectopic and molar pregnancy
Endometritis following ectopic and molar pregnancy
Oophoritis following ectopic and molar pregnancy
Parametritis following ectopic and molar pregnancy
Pelvic peritonitis following ectopic and molar pregnancy
Salpingitis following ectopic and molar pregnancy
Salpingo-oophoritis following ectopic and molar pregnancy
EXCLUDES1 *sepsis following ectopic and molar pregnancy (O08.82)*
urinary tract infection (O08.83) [M] ♀

O08.1 Delayed or excessive hemorrhage following ectopic and molar pregnancy
Afibrinogenemia following ectopic and molar pregnancy
Defibrination syndrome following ectopic and molar pregnancy
Hemolysis following ectopic and molar pregnancy
Intravascular coagulation following ectopic and molar pregnancy
EXCLUDES1 *delayed or excessive hemorrhage due to incomplete abortion (O03.1)* [M] ♀

O08.2 Embolism following ectopic and molar pregnancy
Air embolism following ectopic and molar pregnancy
Amniotic fluid embolism following ectopic and molar pregnancy
Blood-clot embolism following ectopic and molar pregnancy
Embolism NOS following ectopic and molar pregnancy
Fat embolism following ectopic and molar pregnancy
Pulmonary embolism following ectopic and molar pregnancy
Pyemic embolism following ectopic and molar pregnancy
Septic or septicopyemic embolism following ectopic and molar pregnancy
Soap embolism following ectopic and molar pregnancy [M] ♀

O08.3 Shock following ectopic and molar pregnancy
Circulatory collapse following ectopic and molar pregnancy
Shock (postprocedural) following ectopic and molar pregnancy
EXCLUDES1 *shock due to infection following ectopic and molar pregnancy (O08.82)* [M] ♀

O08.4 Renal failure following ectopic and molar pregnancy
Kidney failure (acute) following ectopic and molar pregnancy
Oliguria following ectopic and molar pregnancy
Renal shutdown following ectopic and molar pregnancy
Renal tubular necrosis following ectopic and molar pregnancy
Uremia following ectopic and molar pregnancy [M] ♀

O08.5 Metabolic disorders following an ectopic and molar pregnancy [M] ♀

O08.6 Damage to pelvic organs and tissues following an ectopic and molar pregnancy
Laceration, perforation, tear or chemical damage of bladder following an ectopic and molar pregnancy
Laceration, perforation, tear or chemical damage of bowel following an ectopic and molar pregnancy
Laceration, perforation, tear or chemical damage of broad ligament following an ectopic and molar pregnancy
Laceration, perforation, tear or chemical damage of cervix following an ectopic and molar pregnancy
Laceration, perforation, tear or chemical damage of periurethral tissue following an ectopic and molar pregnancy
Laceration, perforation, tear or chemical damage of uterus following an ectopic and molar pregnancy
Laceration, perforation, tear or chemical damage of vagina following an ectopic and molar pregnancy [M] ♀

O08.7 Other venous complications following an ectopic and molar pregnancy [M] ♀

⑤ O08.8 Other complications following an ectopic and molar pregnancy

O08.81 Cardiac arrest following an ectopic and molar pregnancy [M] ♀

O08.82 Sepsis following ectopic and molar pregnancy
Use additional code (B95-B97), to identify infectious agent
code (R65.2-) to identify severe sepsis, if applicable
EXCLUDES1 *septic or septicopyemic embolism following ectopic and molar pregnancy (O08.2)* [M] ♀

O08.83 Urinary tract infection following an ectopic and molar pregnancy
Cystitis following an ectopic and molar pregnancy [M] ♀

O08.89 Other complications following an ectopic and molar pregnancy [M] ♀

O08.9 Unspecified complication following an ectopic and molar pregnancy [M] ♀

Supervision of high risk pregnancy (O09)

④ O09 Supervision of high risk pregnancy

⑤ O09.0 Supervision of pregnancy with history of infertility

O09.00 Supervision of pregnancy with history of infertility, unspecified trimester [M] ♀

O09.01 Supervision of pregnancy with history of infertility, first trimester [M] ♀

O09.02 Supervision of pregnancy with history of infertility, second trimester [M] ♀

O09.03 Supervision of pregnancy with history of infertility, third trimester [M] ♀

⑤ O09.1 Supervision of pregnancy with history of ectopic or molar pregnancy

O09.10 Supervision of pregnancy with history of ectopic or molar pregnancy, unspecified trimester [M] ♀

O09.11 Supervision of pregnancy with history of ectopic or molar pregnancy, first trimester [M] ♀

O09.12 Supervision of pregnancy with history of ectopic or molar pregnancy, second trimester [M] ♀

Unspecified Code | Other Specified Code | [N] Newborn Age: 0 | [P] Pediatric Age: 0-17 | [M] Maternity Age: 12-55
[A] Adult Age: 15-124 | ♂ Male | ♀ Female | ● New Code | ▲ Revised Code Title | ►◄ Revised Text

O09.13 Supervision of pregnancy with history of ectopic or molar pregnancy, third trimester [M] ♀

[5] O09.2 Supervision of pregnancy with other poor reproductive or obstetric history

[EXCLUDES2] *pregnancy care for patient with history of recurrent pregnancy loss (O26.2-)*

[6] O09.21 Supervision of pregnancy with history of pre-term labor

O09.211 Supervision of pregnancy with history of pre-term labor, first trimester [M] ♀

O09.212 Supervision of pregnancy with history of pre-term labor, second trimester [M] ♀

O09.213 Supervision of pregnancy with history of pre-term labor, third trimester [M] ♀

O09.219 Supervision of pregnancy with history of pre-term labor, unspecified trimester [M] ♀

[6] O09.29 Supervision of pregnancy with other poor reproductive or obstetric history

Supervision of pregnancy with history of neonatal death
Supervision of pregnancy with history of stillbirth

O09.291 Supervision of pregnancy with other poor reproductive or obstetric history, first trimester [M] ♀

O09.292 Supervision of pregnancy with other poor reproductive or obstetric history, second trimester [M] ♀

O09.293 Supervision of pregnancy with other poor reproductive or obstetric history, third trimester [M] ♀

O09.299 Supervision of pregnancy with other poor reproductive or obstetric history, unspecified trimester [M] ♀

[5] O09.3 Supervision of pregnancy with insufficient antenatal care

Supervision of concealed pregnancy
Supervision of hidden pregnancy

O09.30 Supervision of pregnancy with insufficient antenatal care, unspecified trimester [M] ♀

O09.31 Supervision of pregnancy with insufficient antenatal care, first trimester [M] ♀

O09.32 Supervision of pregnancy with insufficient antenatal care, second trimester [M] ♀

O09.33 Supervision of pregnancy with insufficient antenatal care, third trimester [M] ♀

[5] O09.4 Supervision of pregnancy with grand multiparity

O09.40 Supervision of pregnancy with grand multiparity, unspecified trimester [M] ♀

O09.41 Supervision of pregnancy with grand multiparity, first trimester [M] ♀

O09.42 Supervision of pregnancy with grand multiparity, second trimester [M] ♀

O09.43 Supervision of pregnancy with grand multiparity, third trimester [M] ♀

[5] O09.5 Supervision of elderly primigravida and multigravida

Pregnancy for a female 35 years and older at expected date of delivery

[6] O09.51 Supervision of elderly primigravida

O09.511 Supervision of elderly primigravida, first trimester [M] ♀

O09.512 Supervision of elderly primigravida, second trimester [M] ♀

O09.513 Supervision of elderly primigravida, third trimester [M] ♀

O09.519 Supervision of elderly primigravida, unspecified trimester [M] ♀

[6] O09.52 Supervision of elderly multigravida

O09.521 Supervision of elderly multigravida, first trimester [M] ♀

O09.522 Supervision of elderly multigravida, second trimester [M] ♀

O09.523 Supervision of elderly multigravida, third trimester [M] ♀

O09.529 Supervision of elderly multigravida, unspecified trimester [M] ♀

[5] O09.6 Supervision of young primigravida and multigravida

Supervision of pregnancy for a female less than 16 years old at expected date of delivery

[6] O09.61 Supervision of young primigravida

O09.611 Supervision of young primigravida, first trimester [M] ♀

O09.612 Supervision of young primigravida, second trimester [M] ♀

O09.613 Supervision of young primigravida, third trimester [M] ♀

O09.619 Supervision of young primigravida, unspecified trimester [M] ♀

[6] O09.62 Supervision of young multigravida

O09.621 Supervision of young multigravida, first trimester [M] ♀

O09.622 Supervision of young multigravida, second trimester [M] ♀

O09.623 Supervision of young multigravida, third trimester [M] ♀

O09.629 Supervision of young multigravida, unspecified trimester [M] ♀

[5] O09.7 Supervision of high risk pregnancy due to social problems

O09.70 Supervision of high risk pregnancy due to social problems, unspecified trimester [M] ♀

O09.71 Supervision of high risk pregnancy due to social problems, first trimester [M] ♀

O09.72 Supervision of high risk pregnancy due to social problems, second trimester [M] ♀

O09.73 Supervision of high risk pregnancy due to social problems, third trimester [M] ♀

[5] O09.8 Supervision of other high risk pregnancies

[6] O09.81 Supervision of pregnancy resulting from assisted reproductive technology

Supervision of pregnancy resulting from in-vitro fertilization

O09.811 Supervision of pregnancy resulting from assisted reproductive technology, first trimester [M] ♀

O09.812 Supervision of pregnancy resulting from assisted reproductive technology, second trimester [M] ♀

O09.813 Supervision of pregnancy resulting from assisted reproductive technology, third trimester [M] ♀

O09.819 Supervision of pregnancy resulting from assisted reproductive technology, unspecified trimester [M] ♀

[6] O09.82 Supervision of pregnancy with history of in utero procedure during previous pregnancy

O09.821 Supervision of pregnancy with history of in utero procedure during previous pregnancy, first trimester [M] ♀

O09.822 Supervision of pregnancy with history of in utero procedure during previous pregnancy, second trimester [M] ♀

O09.823 Supervision of pregnancy with history of in utero procedure during previous pregnancy, third trimester [M] ♀

O09.829 Supervision of pregnancy with history of in utero procedure during previous pregnancy, unspecified trimester

[4] 4th character required [5] 5th character required [6] 6th character required [7] 7th character required [X] Extension 'X' Alert
[EXCLUDES1] Not coded here [EXCLUDES2] Not included here [PDx] Primary Diagnosis Only Manifestation Code

[EXCLUDES1] *supervision of pregnancy affected by in utero procedure during current pregnancy (O35.7)* [M] ♀

[6] O09.89 Supervision of other high risk pregnancies

- O09.891 Supervision of other high risk pregnancies, first trimester [M] ♀
- O09.892 Supervision of other high risk pregnancies, second trimester [M] ♀
- O09.893 Supervision of other high risk pregnancies, third trimester [M] ♀
- O09.899 Supervision of other high risk pregnancies, unspecified trimester [M] ♀

[5] O09.9 Supervision of high risk pregnancy, unspecified

- O09.90 Supervision of high risk pregnancy, unspecified, unspecified trimester [M] ♀
- O09.91 Supervision of high risk pregnancy, unspecified, first trimester [M] ♀
- O09.92 Supervision of high risk pregnancy, unspecified, second trimester [M] ♀
- O09.93 Supervision of high risk pregnancy, unspecified, third trimester [M] ♀

Edema, proteinuria and hypertensive disorders in pregnancy, childbirth and the puerperium (O10-O16)

[4] **O10 Pre-existing hypertension complicating pregnancy, childbirth and the puerperium**

[INCLUDES] *pre-existing hypertension with pre-existing proteinuria complicating pregnancy, childbirth and the puerperium*

[EXCLUDES2] *pre-existing hypertension with superimposed pre-eclampsia complicating pregnancy, childbirth and the puerperium (O11.-)*

[5] O10.0 Pre-existing essential hypertension complicating pregnancy, childbirth and the puerperium

Any condition in I10 specified as a reason for obstetric care during pregnancy, childbirth or the puerperium

[6] O10.01 Pre-existing essential hypertension complicating pregnancy,

- O10.011 Pre-existing essential hypertension complicating pregnancy, first trimester [M] ♀
- O10.012 Pre-existing essential hypertension complicating pregnancy, second trimester [M] ♀
- O10.013 Pre-existing essential hypertension complicating pregnancy, third trimester [M] ♀
- O10.019 Pre-existing essential hypertension complicating pregnancy, unspecified trimester [M] ♀

O10.02 Pre-existing essential hypertension complicating childbirth [M] ♀

O10.03 Pre-existing essential hypertension complicating the puerperium [M] ♀

[5] O10.1 Pre-existing hypertensive heart disease complicating pregnancy, childbirth and the puerperium

Any condition in I11 specified as a reason for obstetric care during pregnancy, childbirth or the puerperium

Use additional code from I11 to identify the type of hypertensive heart disease

[6] O10.11 Pre-existing hypertensive heart disease complicating pregnancy

- O10.111 Pre-existing hypertensive heart disease complicating pregnancy, first trimester [M] ♀
- O10.112 Pre-existing hypertensive heart disease complicating pregnancy, second trimester [M] ♀
- O10.113 Pre-existing hypertensive heart disease complicating pregnancy, third trimester [M] ♀
- O10.119 Pre-existing hypertensive heart disease complicating pregnancy, unspecified trimester [M] ♀

O10.12 Pre-existing hypertensive heart disease complicating childbirth [M] ♀

O10.13 Pre-existing hypertensive heart disease complicating the puerperium [M] ♀

[5] O10.2 Pre-existing hypertensive chronic kidney disease complicating pregnancy, childbirth and the puerperium

Any condition in I12 specified as a reason for obstetric care during pregnancy, childbirth or the puerperium

Use additional code from I12 to identify the type of hypertensive chronic kidney disease

[6] O10.21 Pre-existing hypertensive chronic kidney disease complicating pregnancy

- O10.211 Pre-existing hypertensive chronic kidney disease complicating pregnancy, first trimester [M] ♀
- O10.212 Pre-existing hypertensive chronic kidney disease complicating pregnancy, second trimester [M] ♀
- O10.213 Pre-existing hypertensive chronic kidney disease complicating pregnancy, third trimester [M] ♀
- O10.219 Pre-existing hypertensive chronic kidney disease complicating pregnancy, unspecified trimester [M] ♀

O10.22 Pre-existing hypertensive chronic kidney disease complicating childbirth [M] ♀

O10.23 Pre-existing hypertensive chronic kidney disease complicating the puerperium [M] ♀

[5] O10.3 Pre-existing hypertensive heart and chronic kidney disease complicating pregnancy, childbirth and the puerperium

Any condition in I13 specified as a reason for obstetric care during pregnancy, childbirth or the puerperium

Use additional code from I13 to identify the type of hypertensive heart and chronic kidney disease

[6] O10.31 Pre-existing hypertensive heart and chronic kidney disease complicating pregnancy

- O10.311 Pre-existing hypertensive heart and chronic kidney disease complicating pregnancy, first trimester [M] ♀
- O10.312 Pre-existing hypertensive heart and chronic kidney disease complicating pregnancy, second trimester [M] ♀
- O10.313 Pre-existing hypertensive heart and chronic kidney disease complicating pregnancy, third trimester [M] ♀
- O10.319 Pre-existing hypertensive heart and chronic kidney disease complicating pregnancy, unspecified trimester [M] ♀

O10.32 Pre-existing hypertensive heart and chronic kidney disease complicating childbirth [M] ♀

O10.33 Pre-existing hypertensive heart and chronic kidney disease complicating the puerperium [M] ♀

[5] O10.4 Pre-existing secondary hypertension complicating pregnancy, childbirth and the puerperium

Any condition in I15 specified as a reason for obstetric care during pregnancy, childbirth or the puerperium

Use additional code from I15 to identify the type of secondary hypertension

[6] O10.41 Pre-existing secondary hypertension complicating pregnancy

O10.411 Pre-existing secondary hypertension complicating pregnancy, first trimester   Ⓜ ♀

O10.412 Pre-existing secondary hypertension complicating pregnancy, second trimester   Ⓜ ♀

O10.413 Pre-existing secondary hypertension complicating pregnancy, third trimester   Ⓜ ♀

O10.419 Pre-existing secondary hypertension complicating pregnancy, unspecified trimester   Ⓜ ♀

O10.42 Pre-existing secondary hypertension complicating childbirth   Ⓜ ♀

O10.43 Pre-existing secondary hypertension complicating the puerperium   Ⓜ ♀

⑤ O10.9 Unspecified pre-existing hypertension complicating pregnancy, childbirth and the puerperium

⑥ O10.91 Unspecified pre-existing hypertension complicating pregnancy

O10.911 Unspecified pre-existing hypertension complicating pregnancy, first trimester   Ⓜ ♀

O10.912 Unspecified pre-existing hypertension complicating pregnancy, second trimester   Ⓜ ♀

O10.913 Unspecified pre-existing hypertension complicating pregnancy, third trimester   Ⓜ ♀

O10.919 Unspecified pre-existing hypertension complicating pregnancy, unspecified trimester   Ⓜ ♀

O10.92 Unspecified pre-existing hypertension complicating childbirth   Ⓜ ♀

O10.93 Unspecified pre-existing hypertension complicating the puerperium   Ⓜ ♀

④ O11 Pre-existing hypertension with pre-eclampsia

INCLUDES   conditions in O10 complicated by pre-eclampsia
pre-eclampsia superimposed pre-existing hypertension

Use additional code from O10 to identify the type of hypertension

O11.1 Pre-existing hypertension with pre-eclampsia, first trimester   Ⓜ ♀

O11.2 Pre-existing hypertension with pre-eclampsia, second trimester   Ⓜ ♀

O11.3 Pre-existing hypertension with pre-eclampsia, third trimester   Ⓜ ♀

O11.9 Pre-existing hypertension with pre-eclampsia, unspecified trimester   Ⓜ ♀

④ O12 Gestational [pregnancy-induced] edema and proteinuria without hypertension

⑤ O12.0 Gestational edema

O12.00 Gestational edema, unspecified trimester   Ⓜ ♀

O12.01 Gestational edema, first trimester   Ⓜ ♀

O12.02 Gestational edema, second trimester   Ⓜ ♀

O12.03 Gestational edema, third trimester   Ⓜ ♀

⑤ O12.1 Gestational proteinuria

O12.10 Gestational proteinuria, unspecified trimester   Ⓜ ♀

O12.11 Gestational proteinuria, first trimester   Ⓜ ♀

O12.12 Gestational proteinuria, second trimester   Ⓜ ♀

O12.13 Gestational proteinuria, third trimester   Ⓜ ♀

⑤ O12.2 Gestational edema with proteinuria

O12.20 Gestational edema with proteinuria, unspecified trimester   Ⓜ ♀

O12.21 Gestational edema with proteinuria, first trimester   Ⓜ ♀

O12.22 Gestational edema with proteinuria, second trimester   Ⓜ ♀

O12.23 Gestational edema with proteinuria, third trimester   Ⓜ ♀

④ O13 Gestational [pregnancy-induced] hypertension without significant proteinuria

INCLUDES   gestational hypertension NOS

O13.1 Gestational [pregnancy-induced] hypertension without significant proteinuria, first trimester   Ⓜ ♀

O13.2 Gestational [pregnancy-induced] hypertension without significant proteinuria, second trimester   Ⓜ ♀

O13.3 Gestational [pregnancy-induced] hypertension without significant proteinuria, third trimester   Ⓜ ♀

O13.9 Gestational [pregnancy-induced] hypertension without significant proteinuria, unspecified trimester   Ⓜ ♀

④ O14 Pre-eclampsia

EXCLUDES1   pre-existing hypertension with pre-eclampsia (O11)

⑤ O14.0 Mild to moderate pre-eclampsia

O14.00 Mild to moderate pre-eclampsia, unspecified trimester   Ⓜ ♀

O14.02 Mild to moderate pre-eclampsia, second trimester   Ⓜ ♀

O14.03 Mild to moderate pre-eclampsia, third trimester   Ⓜ ♀

⑤ O14.1 Severe pre-eclampsia

EXCLUDES1   HELLP syndrome (O14.2-)

O14.10 Severe pre-eclampsia, unspecified trimester   Ⓜ ♀

O14.12 Severe pre-eclampsia, second trimester   Ⓜ ♀

O14.13 Severe pre-eclampsia, third trimester   Ⓜ ♀

⑤ O14.2 HELLP syndrome

Severe pre-eclampsia with hemolysis, elevated liver enzymes and low platelet count (HELLP)

O14.20 HELLP syndrome (HELLP), unspecified trimester   Ⓜ ♀

O14.22 HELLP syndrome (HELLP), second trimester   Ⓜ ♀

O14.23 HELLP syndrome (HELLP), third trimester   Ⓜ ♀

⑤ O14.9 Unspecified pre-eclampsia

O14.90 Unspecified pre-eclampsia, unspecified trimester   Ⓜ ♀

O14.92 Unspecified pre-eclampsia, second trimester   Ⓜ ♀

O14.93 Unspecified pre-eclampsia, third trimester   Ⓜ ♀

④ O15 Eclampsia

INCLUDES   convulsions following conditions in O10-O14 and O16

⑤ O15.0 Eclampsia in pregnancy

O15.00 Eclampsia in pregnancy, unspecified trimester   Ⓜ ♀

O15.02 Eclampsia in pregnancy, second trimester   Ⓜ ♀

O15.03 Eclampsia in pregnancy, third trimester   Ⓜ ♀

O15.1 Eclampsia in labor   Ⓜ ♀

O15.2 Eclampsia in the puerperium   Ⓜ ♀

O15.9 Eclampsia, unspecified as to time period
Eclampsia NOS   Ⓜ ♀

④ O16 Unspecified maternal hypertension

O16.1 Unspecified maternal hypertension, first trimester   Ⓜ ♀

O16.2 Unspecified maternal hypertension, second trimester   Ⓜ ♀

O16.3 Unspecified maternal hypertension, third trimester   Ⓜ ♀

O16.9 Unspecified maternal hypertension, unspecified trimester   Ⓜ ♀

---

④ 4th character required   ⑤ 5th character required   ⑥ 6th character required   ⑦ 7th character required   ⑦ˣ Extension 'X' Alert

EXCLUDES1 Not coded here   EXCLUDES2 Not included here   PDx Primary Diagnosis Only   Manifestation Code

Other maternal disorders predominantly related to pregnancy (O20-O29)

[EXCLUDES2] *maternal care related to the fetus and amniotic cavity and possible delivery problems (O30-O48)*
maternal diseases classifiable elsewhere but complicating pregnancy, labor and delivery, and the puerperium (O98-O99)

[4] **O20 Hemorrhage in early pregnancy**

[INCLUDES] *hemorrhage before completion of 20 weeks gestation*

[EXCLUDES1] *pregnancy with abortive outcome (O00-O08)*

O20.0 Threatened abortion

Hemorrhage specified as due to threatened abortion [M] ♀

O20.8 Other hemorrhage in early pregnancy [M] ♀

O20.9 Hemorrhage in early pregnancy, unspecified [M] ♀

[4] **O21 Excessive vomiting in pregnancy**

O21.0 Mild hyperemesis gravidarum

Hyperemesis gravidarum, mild or unspecified, starting before the end of the 20th week of gestation [M] ♀

O21.1 Hyperemesis gravidarum with metabolic disturbance

Hyperemesis gravidarum, starting before the end of the 20th week of gestation, with metabolic disturbance such as carbohydrate depletion

Hyperemesis gravidarum, starting before the end of the 20th week of gestation, with metabolic disturbance such as dehydration

Hyperemesis gravidarum, starting before the end of the 20th week of gestation, with metabolic disturbance such as electrolyte imbalance [M] ♀

O21.2 Late vomiting of pregnancy

Excessive vomiting starting after 20 completed weeks of gestation [M] ♀

O21.8 Other vomiting complicating pregnancy

Vomiting due to diseases classified elsewhere, complicating pregnancy

Use additional code, to identify cause. [M] ♀

O21.9 Vomiting of pregnancy, unspecified [M] ♀

[4] **O22 Venous complications and hemorrhoids in pregnancy**

[EXCLUDES1] *venous complications of:*
abortion NOS (O03.9)
ectopic or molar pregnancy (O08.7)
failed attempted abortion (O07.35)
induced abortion (O04.85)
spontaneous abortion (O03.89)

[EXCLUDES2] *obstetric pulmonary embolism (O88.-)*
venous complications and hemorrhoids of childbirth and the puerperium (O87.-)

[5] **O22.0 Varicose veins of lower extremity in pregnancy**

Varicose veins NOS in pregnancy

O22.00 Varicose veins of lower extremity in pregnancy, unspecified trimester [M] ♀

O22.01 Varicose veins of lower extremity in pregnancy, first trimester [M] ♀

O22.02 Varicose veins of lower extremity in pregnancy, second trimester [M] ♀

O22.03 Varicose veins of lower extremity in pregnancy, third trimester [M] ♀

[5] **O22.1 Genital varices in pregnancy**

Perineal varices in pregnancy

Vaginal varices in pregnancy

Vulval varices in pregnancy

O22.10 Genital varices in pregnancy, unspecified trimester [M] ♀

O22.11 Genital varices in pregnancy, first trimester [M] ♀

O22.12 Genital varices in pregnancy, second trimester [M] ♀

O22.13 Genital varices in pregnancy, third trimester [M] ♀

[5] **O22.2 Superficial thrombophlebitis in pregnancy**

Phlebitis in pregnancy NOS

Thrombophlebitis of legs in pregnancy

Thrombosis in pregnancy NOS

Use additional code to identify the superficial thrombophlebitis (I80.0-)

O22.20 Superficial thrombophlebitis in pregnancy, unspecified trimester [M] ♀

O22.21 Superficial thrombophlebitis in pregnancy, first trimester [M] ♀

O22.22 Superficial thrombophlebitis in pregnancy, second trimester [M] ♀

O22.23 Superficial thrombophlebitis in pregnancy, third trimester [M] ♀

[5] **O22.3 Deep phlebothrombosis in pregnancy**

Deep vein thrombosis, antepartum

Use additional code to identify the deep vein thrombosis (I82.4-, I82.5-, I82.62-. I82.72-)

code, if applicable, for associated long-term (current) use of anticoagulants (Z79.01)

O22.30 Deep phlebothrombosis in pregnancy, unspecified trimester [M] ♀

O22.31 Deep phlebothrombosis in pregnancy, first trimester [M] ♀

O22.32 Deep phlebothrombosis in pregnancy, second trimester [M] ♀

O22.33 Deep phlebothrombosis in pregnancy, third trimester [M] ♀

[5] **O22.4 Hemorrhoids in pregnancy**

O22.40 Hemorrhoids in pregnancy, unspecified trimester [M] ♀

O22.41 Hemorrhoids in pregnancy, first trimester [M] ♀

O22.42 Hemorrhoids in pregnancy, second trimester [M] ♀

O22.43 Hemorrhoids in pregnancy, third trimester [M] ♀

[5] **O22.5 Cerebral venous thrombosis in pregnancy**

Cerebrovenous sinus thrombosis in pregnancy

O22.50 Cerebral venous thrombosis in pregnancy, unspecified trimester [M] ♀

O22.51 Cerebral venous thrombosis in pregnancy, first trimester [M] ♀

O22.52 Cerebral venous thrombosis in pregnancy, second trimester [M] ♀

O22.53 Cerebral venous thrombosis in pregnancy, third trimester [M] ♀

[5] **O22.8 Other venous complications in pregnancy**

[6] **O22.8X Other venous complications in pregnancy**

O22.8X1 Other venous complications in pregnancy, first trimester [M] ♀

O22.8X2 Other venous complications in pregnancy, second trimester [M] ♀

O22.8X3 Other venous complications in pregnancy, third trimester [M] ♀

O22.8X9 Other venous complications in pregnancy, unspecified trimester [M] ♀

[5] **O22.9 Venous complication in pregnancy, unspecified**

Gestational phlebitis NOS

Gestational phlebopathy NOS

Gestational thrombosis NOS

O22.90 Venous complication in pregnancy, unspecified, unspecified trimester [M] ♀

O22.91 Venous complication in pregnancy, unspecified, first trimester [M] ♀

O22.92 Venous complication in pregnancy, unspecified, second trimester [M] ♀

Unspecified Code | Other Specified Code | [N] Newborn Age: 0 | [P] Pediatric Age: 0-17 | [M] Maternity Age: 12-55
[A] Adult Age: 15-124 | ♂ Male | ♀ Female | ● New Code | ▲ Revised Code Title | ►◄ Revised Text

O22.93 Venous complication in pregnancy, unspecified, third trimester M ♀

❹ O23 Infections of genitourinary tract in pregnancy

Use additional code to identify organism (B95.-, B96.-)

EXCLUDES2 gonococcal infections complicating pregnancy, childbirth and the puerperium (O98.2)
infections with a predominantly sexual mode of transmission NOS complicating pregnancy, childbirth and the puerperium (O98.3)
syphilis complicating pregnancy, childbirth and the puerperium (O98.1)
tuberculosis of genitourinary system complicating pregnancy, childbirth and the puerperium (O98.0)
venereal disease NOS complicating pregnancy, childbirth and the puerperium (O98.3)

❺ O23.0 Infections of kidney in pregnancy

Pyelonephritis in pregnancy

O23.00 Infections of kidney in pregnancy, unspecified trimester M ♀
O23.01 Infections of kidney in pregnancy, first trimester M ♀
O23.02 Infections of kidney in pregnancy, second trimester M ♀
O23.03 Infections of kidney in pregnancy, third trimester M ♀

❺ O23.1 Infections of bladder in pregnancy

O23.10 Infections of bladder in pregnancy, unspecified trimester M ♀
O23.11 Infections of bladder in pregnancy, first trimester M ♀
O23.12 Infections of bladder in pregnancy, second trimester M ♀
O23.13 Infections of bladder in pregnancy, third trimester M ♀

❺ O23.2 Infections of urethra in pregnancy

O23.20 Infections of urethra in pregnancy, unspecified trimester M ♀
O23.21 Infections of urethra in pregnancy, first trimester M ♀
O23.22 Infections of urethra in pregnancy, second trimester M ♀
O23.23 Infections of urethra in pregnancy, third trimester M ♀

❺ O23.3 Infections of other parts of urinary tract in pregnancy

O23.30 Infections of other parts of urinary tract in pregnancy, unspecified trimester M ♀
O23.31 Infections of other parts of urinary tract in pregnancy, first trimester M ♀
O23.32 Infections of other parts of urinary tract in pregnancy, second trimester M ♀
O23.33 Infections of other parts of urinary tract in pregnancy, third trimester M ♀

❺ O23.4 Unspecified infection of urinary tract in pregnancy

O23.40 Unspecified infection of urinary tract in pregnancy, unspecified trimester M ♀
O23.41 Unspecified infection of urinary tract in pregnancy, first trimester M ♀
O23.42 Unspecified infection of urinary tract in pregnancy, second trimester M ♀
O23.43 Unspecified infection of urinary tract in pregnancy, third trimester M ♀

❺ O23.5 Infections of the genital tract in pregnancy

❻ O23.51 Infection of cervix in pregnancy

O23.511 Infections of cervix in pregnancy, first trimester M ♀
O23.512 Infections of cervix in pregnancy, second trimester M ♀
O23.513 Infections of cervix in pregnancy, third trimester M ♀
O23.519 Infections of cervix in pregnancy, unspecified trimester M ♀

❻ O23.52 Salpingo-oophoritis in pregnancy

Oophoritis in pregnancy
Salpingitis in pregnancy

O23.521 Salpingo-oophoritis in pregnancy, first trimester M ♀
O23.522 Salpingo-oophoritis in pregnancy, second trimester M ♀
O23.523 Salpingo-oophoritis in pregnancy, third trimester M ♀
O23.529 Salpingo-oophoritis in pregnancy, unspecified trimester M ♀

❻ O23.59 Infection of other part of genital tract in pregnancy

O23.591 Infection of other part of genital tract in pregnancy, first trimester M ♀
O23.592 Infection of other part of genital tract in pregnancy, second trimester M ♀
O23.593 Infection of other part of genital tract in pregnancy, third trimester M ♀
O23.599 Infection of other part of genital tract in pregnancy, unspecified trimester M ♀

❺ O23.9 Unspecified genitourinary tract infection in pregnancy

Genitourinary tract infection in pregnancy NOS

O23.90 Unspecified genitourinary tract infection in pregnancy, unspecified trimester M ♀
O23.91 Unspecified genitourinary tract infection in pregnancy, first trimester M ♀
O23.92 Unspecified genitourinary tract infection in pregnancy, second trimester M ♀
O23.93 Unspecified genitourinary tract infection in pregnancy, third trimester M ♀

❹ O24 Diabetes mellitus in pregnancy, childbirth, and the puerperium

❺ O24.0 Pre-existing diabetes mellitus, type 1, in pregnancy, childbirth and the puerperium

Juvenile onset diabetes mellitus, in pregnancy, childbirth and the puerperium
Ketosis-prone diabetes mellitus in pregnancy, childbirth and the puerperium
Use additional code from category E10 to further identify any manifestations

❻ O24.01 Pre-existing diabetes mellitus, type 1, in pregnancy

O24.011 Pre-existing diabetes mellitus, type 1, in pregnancy, first trimester M ♀
O24.012 Pre-existing diabetes mellitus, type 1, in pregnancy, second trimester M ♀
O24.013 Pre-existing diabetes mellitus, type 1, in pregnancy, third trimester M ♀
O24.019 Pre-existing diabetes mellitus, type 1, in pregnancy, unspecified trimester M ♀

O24.02 Pre-existing diabetes mellitus, type 1, in childbirth M ♀
O24.03 Pre-existing diabetes mellitus, type 1, in the puerperium M ♀

❺ O24.1 Pre-existing diabetes mellitus, type 2, in pregnancy, childbirth and the puerperium

Insulin-resistant diabetes mellitus in pregnancy, childbirth and the puerperium
Use additional code (for):
from category E11 to further identify any manifestations
long-term (current) use of insulin (Z79.4)

❹ 4th character required   ❺ 5th character required   ❻ 6th character required   ❼ 7th character required   Extension 'X' Alert
EXCLUDES 1 Not coded here   EXCLUDES 2 Not included here   PDx Primary Diagnosis Only   Manifestation Code

452

ICD-10-CM 2015

[6] O24.11 Pre-existing diabetes mellitus, type 2, in pregnancy
- O24.111 Pre-existing diabetes mellitus, type 2, in pregnancy, first trimester [M] ♀
- O24.112 Pre-existing diabetes mellitus, type 2, in pregnancy, second trimester [M] ♀
- O24.113 Pre-existing diabetes mellitus, type 2, in pregnancy, third trimester [M] ♀
- O24.119 Pre-existing diabetes mellitus, type 2, in pregnancy, unspecified trimester [M] ♀

O24.12 Pre-existing diabetes mellitus, type 2, in childbirth [M] ♀

O24.13 Pre-existing diabetes mellitus, type 2, in the puerperium [M] ♀

[5] O24.3 Unspecified pre-existing diabetes mellitus in pregnancy, childbirth and the puerperium

Use additional code (for):
from category E11 to further identify any manifestation
long-term (current) use of insulin (Z79.4)

[6] O24.31 Unspecified pre-existing diabetes mellitus in pregnancy
- O24.311 Unspecified pre-existing diabetes mellitus in pregnancy, first trimester [M] ♀
- O24.312 Unspecified pre-existing diabetes mellitus in pregnancy, second trimester [M] ♀
- O24.313 Unspecified pre-existing diabetes mellitus in pregnancy, third trimester [M] ♀
- O24.319 Unspecified pre-existing diabetes mellitus in pregnancy, unspecified trimester [M] ♀

O24.32 Unspecified pre-existing diabetes mellitus in childbirth [M] ♀

O24.33 Unspecified pre-existing diabetes mellitus in the puerperium [M] ♀

[5] O24.4 Gestational diabetes mellitus

Diabetes mellitus arising in pregnancy
Gestational diabetes mellitus NOS

[6] O24.41 Gestational diabetes mellitus in pregnancy
- O24.410 Gestational diabetes mellitus in pregnancy, diet controlled [M] ♀
- O24.414 Gestational diabetes mellitus in pregnancy, insulin controlled [M] ♀
- O24.419 Gestational diabetes mellitus in pregnancy, unspecified control [M] ♀

[6] O24.42 Gestational diabetes mellitus in childbirth
- O24.420 Gestational diabetes mellitus in childbirth, diet controlled [M] ♀
- O24.424 Gestational diabetes mellitus in childbirth, insulin controlled [M] ♀
- O24.429 Gestational diabetes mellitus in childbirth, unspecified control [M] ♀

[6] O24.43 Gestational diabetes mellitus in the puerperium
- O24.430 Gestational diabetes mellitus in the puerperium, diet controlled [M] ♀
- O24.434 Gestational diabetes mellitus in the puerperium, insulin controlled [M] ♀
- O24.439 Gestational diabetes mellitus in the puerperium, unspecified control [M] ♀

[5] O24.8 Other pre-existing diabetes mellitus in pregnancy, childbirth, and the puerperium

Use additional code (for):
from categories E08, E09 and E13 to further identify any manifestation
long-term (current) use of insulin (Z79.4)

[6] O24.81 Other pre-existing diabetes mellitus in pregnancy
- O24.811 Other pre-existing diabetes mellitus in pregnancy, first trimester [M] ♀
- O24.812 Other pre-existing diabetes mellitus in pregnancy, second trimester [M] ♀
- O24.813 Other pre-existing diabetes mellitus in pregnancy, third trimester [M] ♀
- O24.819 Other pre-existing diabetes mellitus in pregnancy, unspecified trimester [M] ♀

O24.82 Other pre-existing diabetes mellitus in childbirth [M] ♀

O24.83 Other pre-existing diabetes mellitus in the puerperium [M] ♀

[5] O24.9 Unspecified diabetes mellitus in pregnancy, childbirth and the puerperium

Use additional code for long-term (current) use of insulin (Z79.4)

[6] O24.91 Unspecified diabetes mellitus in pregnancy
- O24.911 Unspecified diabetes mellitus in pregnancy, first trimester [M] ♀
- O24.912 Unspecified diabetes mellitus in pregnancy, second trimester [M] ♀
- O24.913 Unspecified diabetes mellitus in pregnancy, third trimester [M] ♀
- O24.919 Unspecified diabetes mellitus in pregnancy, unspecified trimester [M] ♀

O24.92 Unspecified diabetes mellitus in childbirth [M] ♀

O24.93 Unspecified diabetes mellitus in the puerperium [M] ♀

[4] O25 Malnutrition in pregnancy, childbirth and the puerperium

[5] O25.1 Malnutrition in pregnancy
- O25.10 Malnutrition in pregnancy, unspecified trimester [M] ♀
- O25.11 Malnutrition in pregnancy, first trimester [M] ♀
- O25.12 Malnutrition in pregnancy, second trimester [M] ♀
- O25.13 Malnutrition in pregnancy, third trimester [M] ♀

O25.2 Malnutrition in childbirth [M] ♀

O25.3 Malnutrition in the puerperium [M] ♀

[4] O26 Maternal care for other conditions predominantly related to pregnancy

[5] O26.0 Excessive weight gain in pregnancy

[EXCLUDES2] *gestational edema (O12.0, O12.2)*

- O26.00 Excessive weight gain in pregnancy, unspecified trimester [M] ♀
- O26.01 Excessive weight gain in pregnancy, first trimester [M] ♀
- O26.02 Excessive weight gain in pregnancy, second trimester [M] ♀
- O26.03 Excessive weight gain in pregnancy, third trimester [M] ♀

[5] O26.1 Low weight gain in pregnancy
- O26.10 Low weight gain in pregnancy, unspecified trimester [M] ♀
- O26.11 Low weight gain in pregnancy, first trimester [M] ♀
- O26.12 Low weight gain in pregnancy, second trimester [M] ♀
- O26.13 Low weight gain in pregnancy, third trimester [M] ♀

[5] O26.2 Pregnancy care for patient with recurrent pregnancy loss
- O26.20 Pregnancy care for patient with recurrent pregnancy loss, unspecified trimester [M] ♀
- O26.21 Pregnancy care for patient with recurrent pregnancy loss, first trimester [M] ♀
- O26.22 Pregnancy care for patient with recurrent pregnancy loss, second trimester [M] ♀
- O26.23 Pregnancy care for patient with recurrent pregnancy loss, third trimester [M] ♀

Unspecified Code | Other Specified Code | [N] Newborn Age: 0 | [P] Pediatric Age: 0-17 | [M] Maternity Age: 12-55
[A] Adult Age: 15-124 | ♂ Male | ♀ Female | ● New Code | ▲ Revised Code Title | ►◄ Revised Text

Ⓢ **O26.3** Retained intrauterine contraceptive device in pregnancy

    O26.30 Retained intrauterine contraceptive device in pregnancy, unspecified trimester Ⓜ ♀

    O26.31 Retained intrauterine contraceptive device in pregnancy, first trimester Ⓜ ♀

    O26.32 Retained intrauterine contraceptive device in pregnancy, second trimester Ⓜ ♀

    O26.33 Retained intrauterine contraceptive device in pregnancy, third trimester Ⓜ ♀

Ⓢ **O26.4** Herpes gestationis

    O26.40 Herpes gestationis, unspecified trimester Ⓜ ♀

    O26.41 Herpes gestationis, first trimester Ⓜ ♀

    O26.42 Herpes gestationis, second trimester Ⓜ ♀

    O26.43 Herpes gestationis, third trimester Ⓜ ♀

Ⓢ **O26.5** Maternal hypotension syndrome

    Supine hypotensive syndrome

    O26.50 Maternal hypotension syndrome, unspecified trimester Ⓜ ♀

    O26.51 Maternal hypotension syndrome, first trimester Ⓜ ♀

    O26.52 Maternal hypotension syndrome, second trimester Ⓜ ♀

    O26.53 Maternal hypotension syndrome, third trimester Ⓜ ♀

Ⓢ **O26.6** Liver and biliary tract disorders in pregnancy, childbirth and the puerperium

    Use additional code to identify the specific disorder

    EXCLUDES2 *hepatorenal syndrome following labor and delivery (O90.4)*

    Ⓢ **O26.61** Liver and biliary tract disorders in pregnancy

        O26.611 Liver and biliary tract disorders in pregnancy, first trimester Ⓜ ♀

        O26.612 Liver and biliary tract disorders in pregnancy, second trimester Ⓜ ♀

        O26.613 Liver and biliary tract disorders in pregnancy, third trimester Ⓜ ♀

        O26.619 Liver and biliary tract disorders in pregnancy, unspecified trimester Ⓜ ♀

    O26.62 Liver and biliary tract disorders in childbirth Ⓜ ♀

    O26.63 Liver and biliary tract disorders in the puerperium Ⓜ ♀

Ⓢ **O26.7** Subluxation of symphysis (pubis) in pregnancy, childbirth and the puerperium

    EXCLUDES1 *traumatic separation of symphysis (pubis) during childbirth (O71.6)*

    Ⓢ **O26.71** Subluxation of symphysis (pubis) in pregnancy

        O26.711 Subluxation of symphysis (pubis) in pregnancy, first trimester Ⓜ ♀

        O26.712 Subluxation of symphysis (pubis) in pregnancy, second trimester Ⓜ ♀

        O26.713 Subluxation of symphysis (pubis) in pregnancy, third trimester Ⓜ ♀

        O26.719 Subluxation of symphysis (pubis) in pregnancy, unspecified trimester Ⓜ ♀

    O26.72 Subluxation of symphysis (pubis) in childbirth Ⓜ ♀

    O26.73 Subluxation of symphysis (pubis) in the puerperium Ⓜ ♀

Ⓢ **O26.8** Other specified pregnancy related conditions

    Ⓢ **O26.81** Pregnancy related exhaustion and fatigue

        O26.811 Pregnancy related exhaustion and fatigue, first trimester Ⓜ ♀

        O26.812 Pregnancy related exhaustion and fatigue, second trimester Ⓜ ♀

        O26.813 Pregnancy related exhaustion and fatigue, third trimester Ⓜ ♀

        O26.819 Pregnancy related exhaustion and fatigue, unspecified trimester Ⓜ ♀

    Ⓢ **O26.82** Pregnancy related peripheral neuritis

        O26.821 Pregnancy related peripheral neuritis, first trimester Ⓜ ♀

        O26.822 Pregnancy related peripheral neuritis, second trimester Ⓜ ♀

        O26.823 Pregnancy related peripheral neuritis, third trimester Ⓜ ♀

        O26.829 Pregnancy related peripheral neuritis, unspecified trimester Ⓜ ♀

    Ⓢ **O26.83** Pregnancy related renal disease

    Use additional code to identify the specific disorder

        O26.831 Pregnancy related renal disease, first trimester Ⓜ ♀

        O26.832 Pregnancy related renal disease, second trimester Ⓜ ♀

        O26.833 Pregnancy related renal disease, third trimester Ⓜ ♀

        O26.839 Pregnancy related renal disease, unspecified trimester Ⓜ ♀

    Ⓢ **O26.84** Uterine size-date discrepancy complicating pregnancy

    EXCLUDES1 *encounter for suspected problem with fetal growth ruled out (Z03.74)*

        O26.841 Uterine size-date discrepancy, first trimester Ⓜ ♀

        O26.842 Uterine size-date discrepancy, second trimester Ⓜ ♀

        O26.843 Uterine size-date discrepancy, third trimester Ⓜ ♀

        O26.849 Uterine size-date discrepancy, unspecified trimester Ⓜ ♀

    Ⓢ **O26.85** Spotting complicating pregnancy

        O26.851 Spotting complicating pregnancy, first trimester Ⓜ ♀

        O26.852 Spotting complicating pregnancy, second trimester Ⓜ ♀

        O26.853 Spotting complicating pregnancy, third trimester Ⓜ ♀

        O26.859 Spotting complicating pregnancy, unspecified trimester Ⓜ ♀

    O26.86 Pruritic urticarial papules and plaques of pregnancy (PUPPP)

    Polymorphic eruption of pregnancy Ⓜ ♀

    Ⓢ **O26.87** Cervical shortening

    EXCLUDES1 *encounter for suspected cervical shortening ruled out (Z03.75)*

        O26.872 Cervical shortening, second trimester Ⓜ ♀

        O26.873 Cervical shortening, third trimester Ⓜ ♀

        O26.879 Cervical shortening, unspecified trimester Ⓜ ♀

    Ⓢ **O26.89** Other specified pregnancy related conditions

        O26.891 Other specified pregnancy related conditions, first trimester Ⓜ ♀

        O26.892 Other specified pregnancy related conditions, second trimester Ⓜ ♀

        O26.893 Other specified pregnancy related conditions, third trimester Ⓜ ♀

        O26.899 Other specified pregnancy related conditions, unspecified trimester Ⓜ ♀

Ⓢ **O26.9** Pregnancy related conditions, unspecified

    O26.90 Pregnancy related conditions, unspecified, unspecified trimester Ⓜ ♀

    O26.91 Pregnancy related conditions, unspecified, first trimester Ⓜ ♀

    O26.92 Pregnancy related conditions, unspecified, second trimester Ⓜ ♀

Ⓐ 4th character required   Ⓢ 5th character required   Ⓖ 6th character required   Ⓖ 7th character required   Ⓧ Extension 'X' Alert

EXCLUDES 1 Not coded here   EXCLUDES 2 Not included here   Pᴅx Primary Diagnosis Only   Manifestation Code

O26.93 Pregnancy related conditions, unspecified, third trimester [M] ♀

[4] O28 Abnormal findings on antenatal screening of mother

[EXCLUDES1] *diagnostic findings classified elsewhere - see Alphabetical Index*

O28.0 Abnormal hematological finding on antenatal screening of mother [M] ♀

O28.1 Abnormal biochemical finding on antenatal screening of mother [M] ♀

O28.2 Abnormal cytological finding on antenatal screening of mother [M] ♀

O28.3 Abnormal ultrasonic finding on antenatal screening of mother [M] ♀

O28.4 Abnormal radiological finding on antenatal screening of mother [M] ♀

O28.5 Abnormal chromosomal and genetic finding on antenatal screening of mother [M] ♀

O28.8 Other abnormal findings on antenatal screening of mother [M] ♀

O28.9 Unspecified abnormal findings on antenatal screening of mother [M] ♀

[4] O29 Complications of anesthesia during pregnancy

[INCLUDES] *maternal complications arising from the administration of a general, regional or local anesthetic, analgesic or other sedation during pregnancy*

Use additional code, if necessary, to identify the complication

[EXCLUDES2] *complications of anesthesia during labor and delivery (O74.-)*
complications of anesthesia during the puerperium (O89.-)

[5] O29.0 Pulmonary complications of anesthesia during pregnancy

[6] O29.01 Aspiration pneumonitis due to anesthesia during pregnancy

Inhalation of stomach contents or secretions NOS due to anesthesia during pregnancy
Mendelson's syndrome due to anesthesia during pregnancy

O29.011 Aspiration pneumonitis due to anesthesia during pregnancy, first trimester [M] ♀

O29.012 Aspiration pneumonitis due to anesthesia during pregnancy, second trimester [M] ♀

O29.013 Aspiration pneumonitis due to anesthesia during pregnancy, third trimester [M] ♀

O29.019 Aspiration pneumonitis due to anesthesia during pregnancy, unspecified trimester [M] ♀

[6] O29.02 Pressure collapse of lung due to anesthesia during pregnancy

O29.021 Pressure collapse of lung due to anesthesia during pregnancy, first trimester [M] ♀

O29.022 Pressure collapse of lung due to anesthesia during pregnancy, second trimester [M] ♀

O29.023 Pressure collapse of lung due to anesthesia during pregnancy, third trimester [M] ♀

O29.029 Pressure collapse of lung due to anesthesia during pregnancy, unspecified trimester [M] ♀

[6] O29.09 Other pulmonary complications of anesthesia during pregnancy

O29.091 Other pulmonary complications of anesthesia during pregnancy, first trimester [M] ♀

O29.092 Other pulmonary complications of anesthesia during pregnancy, second trimester [M] ♀

O29.093 Other pulmonary complications of anesthesia during pregnancy, third trimester [M] ♀

O29.099 Other pulmonary complications of anesthesia during pregnancy, unspecified trimester [M] ♀

[5] O29.1 Cardiac complications of anesthesia during pregnancy

[6] O29.11 Cardiac arrest due to anesthesia during pregnancy

O29.111 Cardiac arrest due to anesthesia during pregnancy, first trimester [M] ♀

O29.112 Cardiac arrest due to anesthesia during pregnancy, second trimester [M] ♀

O29.113 Cardiac arrest due to anesthesia during pregnancy, third trimester [M] ♀

O29.119 Cardiac arrest due to anesthesia during pregnancy, unspecified trimester [M] ♀

[6] O29.12 Cardiac failure due to anesthesia during pregnancy

O29.121 Cardiac failure due to anesthesia during pregnancy, first trimester [M] ♀

O29.122 Cardiac failure due to anesthesia during pregnancy, second trimester [M] ♀

O29.123 Cardiac failure due to anesthesia during pregnancy, third trimester [M] ♀

O29.129 Cardiac failure due to anesthesia during pregnancy, unspecified trimester [M] ♀

[6] O29.19 Other cardiac complications of anesthesia during pregnancy

O29.191 Other cardiac complications of anesthesia during pregnancy, first trimester [M] ♀

O29.192 Other cardiac complications of anesthesia during pregnancy, second trimester [M] ♀

O29.193 Other cardiac complications of anesthesia during pregnancy, third trimester [M] ♀

O29.199 Other cardiac complications of anesthesia during pregnancy, unspecified trimester [M] ♀

[5] O29.2 Central nervous system complications of anesthesia during pregnancy

[6] O29.21 Cerebral anoxia due to anesthesia during pregnancy

O29.211 Cerebral anoxia due to anesthesia during pregnancy, first trimester [M] ♀

O29.212 Cerebral anoxia due to anesthesia during pregnancy, second trimester [M] ♀

O29.213 Cerebral anoxia due to anesthesia during pregnancy, third trimester [M] ♀

O29.219 Cerebral anoxia due to anesthesia during pregnancy, unspecified trimester [M] ♀

[6] O29.29 Other central nervous system complications of anesthesia during pregnancy

O29.291 Other central nervous system complications of anesthesia during pregnancy, first trimester [M] ♀

O29.292 Other central nervous system complications of anesthesia during pregnancy, second trimester [M] ♀

O29.293 Other central nervous system complications of anesthesia during pregnancy, third trimester [M] ♀

O29.299 Other central nervous system complications of anesthesia during pregnancy, unspecified trimester [M] ♀

[5] O29.3 Toxic reaction to local anesthesia during pregnancy

[6] O29.3X Toxic reaction to local anesthesia during pregnancy

O29.3X1 Toxic reaction to local anesthesia during pregnancy, first trimester [M] ♀

Unspecified Code | Other Specified Code | [N] Newborn Age: 0 | [P] Pediatric Age: 0-17 | [M] Maternity Age: 12-55
[A] Adult Age: 15-124 | ♂ Male | ♀ Female | ● New Code | ▲ Revised Code Title | ►◄ Revised Text

O29.3X2 Toxic reaction to local anesthesia during pregnancy, second trimester Ⓜ ♀

O29.3X3 Toxic reaction to local anesthesia during pregnancy, third trimester Ⓜ ♀

O29.3X9 Toxic reaction to local anesthesia during pregnancy, unspecified trimester Ⓜ ♀

⑤ O29.4 Spinal and epidural anesthesia induced headache during pregnancy

O29.40 Spinal and epidural anesthesia induced headache during pregnancy, unspecified trimester Ⓜ ♀

O29.41 Spinal and epidural anesthesia induced headache during pregnancy, first trimester Ⓜ ♀

O29.42 Spinal and epidural anesthesia induced headache during pregnancy, second trimester Ⓜ ♀

O29.43 Spinal and epidural anesthesia induced headache during pregnancy, third trimester Ⓜ ♀

⑤ O29.5 Other complications of spinal and epidural anesthesia during pregnancy

⑥ O29.5X Other complications of spinal and epidural anesthesia during pregnancy

O29.5X1 Other complications of spinal and epidural anesthesia during pregnancy, first trimester Ⓜ ♀

O29.5X2 Other complications of spinal and epidural anesthesia during pregnancy, second trimester Ⓜ ♀

O29.5X3 Other complications of spinal and epidural anesthesia during pregnancy, third trimester Ⓜ ♀

O29.5X9 Other complications of spinal and epidural anesthesia during pregnancy, unspecified trimester Ⓜ ♀

⑤ O29.6 Failed or difficult intubation for anesthesia during pregnancy

O29.60 Failed or difficult intubation for anesthesia during pregnancy, unspecified trimester Ⓜ ♀

O29.61 Failed or difficult intubation for anesthesia during pregnancy, first trimester Ⓜ ♀

O29.62 Failed or difficult intubation for anesthesia during pregnancy, second trimester Ⓜ ♀

O29.63 Failed or difficult intubation for anesthesia during pregnancy, third trimester Ⓜ ♀

⑤ O29.8 Other complications of anesthesia during pregnancy

⑥ O29.8X Other complications of anesthesia during pregnancy

O29.8X1 Other complications of anesthesia during pregnancy, first trimester Ⓜ ♀

O29.8X2 Other complications of anesthesia during pregnancy, second trimester Ⓜ ♀

O29.8X3 Other complications of anesthesia during pregnancy, third trimester Ⓜ ♀

O29.8X9 Other complications of anesthesia during pregnancy, unspecified trimester Ⓜ ♀

⑤ O29.9 Unspecified complication of anesthesia during pregnancy

O29.90 Unspecified complication of anesthesia during pregnancy, unspecified trimester Ⓜ ♀

O29.91 Unspecified complication of anesthesia during pregnancy, first trimester Ⓜ ♀

O29.92 Unspecified complication of anesthesia during pregnancy, second trimester Ⓜ ♀

O29.93 Unspecified complication of anesthesia during pregnancy, third trimester Ⓜ ♀

Maternal care related to the fetus and amniotic cavity and possible delivery problems (O30-O48)

④ O30 Multiple gestation

Code also any complications specific to multiple gestation

⑤ O30.0 Twin pregnancy

⑥ O30.00 Twin pregnancy, unspecified number of placenta and unspecified number of amniotic sacs

O30.001 Twin pregnancy, unspecified number of placenta and unspecified number of amniotic sacs, first trimester 1st Ⓜ ♀

O30.002 Twin pregnancy, unspecified number of placenta and unspecified number of amniotic sacs, second trimester 2nd Ⓜ ♀

O30.003 Twin pregnancy, unspecified number of placenta and unspecified number of amniotic sacs, third trimester 3rd Ⓜ ♀

O30.009 Twin pregnancy, unspecified number of placenta and unspecified number of amniotic sacs, unspecified trimester Ⓜ ♀

⑥ O30.01 Twin pregnancy, monochorionic/monoamniotic

Twin pregnancy, one placenta, one amniotic sac

EXCLUDES1 conjoined twins (O30.02-)

O30.011 Twin pregnancy, monochorionic/ monoamniotic, first trimester 1st Ⓜ ♀

O30.012 Twin pregnancy, monochorionic/ monoamniotic, second trimester 2nd Ⓜ ♀

O30.013 Twin pregnancy, monochorionic/ monoamniotic, third trimester 3rd Ⓜ ♀

O30.019 Twin pregnancy, monochorionic/ monoamniotic, unspecified trimester Ⓜ ♀

⑥ O30.02 Conjoined twin pregnancy

O30.021 Conjoined twin pregnancy, first trimester 1st Ⓜ ♀

O30.022 Conjoined twin pregnancy, second trimester 2nd Ⓜ ♀

O30.023 Conjoined twin pregnancy, third trimester 3rd Ⓜ ♀

O30.029 Conjoined twin pregnancy, unspecified trimester Ⓜ ♀

⑥ O30.03 Twin pregnancy, monochorionic/diamniotic

Twin pregnancy, one placenta, two amniotic sacs

O30.031 Twin pregnancy, monochorionic/ diamniotic, first trimester 1st Ⓜ ♀

O30.032 Twin pregnancy, monochorionic/ diamniotic, second trimester 2nd Ⓜ ♀

O30.033 Twin pregnancy, monochorionic/ diamniotic, third trimester 3rd Ⓜ ♀

O30.039 Twin pregnancy, monochorionic/ diamniotic, unspecified trimester Ⓜ ♀

⑥ O30.04 Twin pregnancy, dichorionic/diamniotic

Twin pregnancy, two placentae, two amniotic sacs

O30.041 Twin pregnancy, dichorionic/diamniotic, first trimester 1st Ⓜ ♀

O30.042 Twin pregnancy, dichorionic/diamniotic, second trimester 2nd Ⓜ ♀

O30.043 Twin pregnancy, dichorionic/diamniotic, third trimester 3rd Ⓜ ♀

O30.049 Twin pregnancy, dichorionic/diamniotic, unspecified trimester Ⓜ ♀

⑥ O30.09 Twin pregnancy, unable to determine number of placenta and number of amniotic sacs

O30.091 Twin pregnancy, unable to determine number of placenta and number of amniotic sacs, first trimester 1st Ⓜ ♀

O30.092 Twin pregnancy, unable to determine number of placenta and number of amniotic sacs, second trimester 2nd Ⓜ ♀

---

④ 4th character required   ⑤ 5th character required   ⑥ 6th character required   ⑦ 7th character required   ⑦ Extension 'X' Alert

EXCLUDES1 Not coded here   EXCLUDES2 Not included here   PDx Primary Diagnosis Only   Manifestation Code

O30.093 Twin pregnancy, unable to determine number of placenta and number of amniotic sacs, third trimester [3rd] [M] ♀

O30.099 Twin pregnancy, unable to determine number of placenta and number of amniotic sacs, unspecified trimester [M] ♀

[5] O30.1 Triplet pregnancy

[6] O30.10 Triplet pregnancy, unspecified number of placenta and unspecified number of amniotic sacs

O30.101 Triplet pregnancy, unspecified number of placenta and unspecified number of amniotic sacs, first trimester [1st] [M] ♀

O30.102 Triplet pregnancy, unspecified number of placenta and unspecified number of amniotic sacs, second trimester [2nd] [M] ♀

O30.103 Triplet pregnancy, unspecified number of placenta and unspecified number of amniotic sacs, third trimester [3rd] [M] ♀

O30.109 Triplet pregnancy, unspecified number of placenta and unspecified number of amniotic sacs, unspecified trimester [M] ♀

[6] O30.11 Triplet pregnancy with two or more monochorionic fetuses

O30.111 Triplet pregnancy with two or more monochorionic fetuses, first trimester [1st] [M] ♀

O30.112 Triplet pregnancy with two or more monochorionic fetuses, second trimester [2nd] [M] ♀

O30.113 Triplet pregnancy with two or more monochorionic fetuses, third trimester [3rd] [M] ♀

O30.119 Triplet pregnancy with two or more monochorionic fetuses, unspecified trimester [M] ♀

[6] O30.12 Triplet pregnancy with two or more monoamniotic fetuses

O30.121 Triplet pregnancy with two or more monoamniotic fetuses, first trimester [1st] [M] ♀

O30.122 Triplet pregnancy with two or more monoamniotic fetuses, second trimester [2nd] [M] ♀

O30.123 Triplet pregnancy with two or more monoamniotic fetuses, third trimester [3rd] [M] ♀

O30.129 Triplet pregnancy with two or more monoamniotic fetuses, unspecified trimester [M] ♀

[6] O30.19 Triplet pregnancy, unable to determine number of placenta and number of amniotic sacs

O30.191 Triplet pregnancy, unable to determine number of placenta and number of amniotic sacs, first trimester [1st] [M] ♀

O30.192 Triplet pregnancy, unable to determine number of placenta and number of amniotic sacs, second trimester [2nd] [M] ♀

O30.193 Triplet pregnancy, unable to determine number of placenta and number of amniotic sacs, third trimester [3rd] [M] ♀

O30.199 Triplet pregnancy, unable to determine number of placenta and number of amniotic sacs, unspecified trimester [M] ♀

[5] O30.2 Quadruplet pregnancy

[6] O30.20 Quadruplet pregnancy, unspecified number of placenta and unspecified number of amniotic sacs

O30.201 Quadruplet pregnancy, unspecified number of placenta and unspecified number of amniotic sacs, first trimester [1st] [M] ♀

O30.202 Quadruplet pregnancy, unspecified number of placenta and unspecified number of amniotic sacs, second trimester [2nd] [M] ♀

O30.203 Quadruplet pregnancy, unspecified number of placenta and unspecified number of amniotic sacs, third trimester [3rd] [M] ♀

O30.209 Quadruplet pregnancy, unspecified number of placenta and unspecified number of amniotic sacs, unspecified trimester [M] ♀

[6] O30.21 Quadruplet pregnancy with two or more monochorionic fetuses

O30.211 Quadruplet pregnancy with two or more monochorionic fetuses, first trimester [1st] [M] ♀

O30.212 Quadruplet pregnancy with two or more monochorionic fetuses, second trimester [2nd] [M] ♀

O30.213 Quadruplet pregnancy with two or more monochorionic fetuses, third trimester [3rd] [M] ♀

O30.219 Quadruplet pregnancy with two or more monochorionic fetuses, unspecified trimester [M] ♀

[6] O30.22 Quadruplet pregnancy with two or more monoamniotic fetuses

O30.221 Quadruplet pregnancy with two or more monoamniotic fetuses, first trimester [1st] [M] ♀

O30.222 Quadruplet pregnancy with two or more monoamniotic fetuses, second trimester [2nd] [M] ♀

O30.223 Quadruplet pregnancy with two or more monoamniotic fetuses, third trimester [3rd] [M] ♀

O30.229 Quadruplet pregnancy with two or more monoamniotic fetuses, unspecified trimester [M] ♀

[6] O30.29 Quadruplet pregnancy, unable to determine number of placenta and number of amniotic sacs

O30.291 Quadruplet pregnancy, unable to determine number of placenta and number of amniotic sacs, first trimester [1st] [M] ♀

O30.292 Quadruplet pregnancy, unable to determine number of placenta and number of amniotic sacs, second trimester [2nd] [M] ♀

O30.293 Quadruplet pregnancy, unable to determine number of placenta and number of amniotic sacs, third trimester [3rd] [M] ♀

O30.299 Quadruplet pregnancy, unable to determine number of placenta and number of amniotic sacs, unspecified trimester [M] ♀

[5] O30.8 Other specified multiple gestation

Multiple gestation pregnancy greater then quadruplets

[6] O30.80 Other specified multiple gestation, unspecified number of placenta and unspecified number of amniotic sacs

O30.801 Other specified multiple gestation, unspecified number of placenta and unspecified number of amniotic sacs, first trimester [1st] [M] ♀

Unspecified Code | Other Specified Code | [N] Newborn Age: 0 | [P] Pediatric Age: 0-17 | [M] Maternity Age: 12-55
[A] Adult Age: 15-124 | ♂ Male | ♀ Female | ● New Code | ▲ Revised Code Title | ►◄ Revised Text

O30.802 Other specified multiple gestation, unspecified number of placenta and unspecified number of amniotic sacs, second trimester [2nd] [M] ♀

O30.803 Other specified multiple gestation, unspecified number of placenta and unspecified number of amniotic sacs, third trimester [3rd] [M] ♀

O30.809 Other specified multiple gestation, unspecified number of placenta and unspecified number of amniotic sacs, unspecified trimester [M] ♀

[6] O30.81 Other specified multiple gestation with two or more monochorionic fetuses

O30.811 Other specified multiple gestation with two or more monochorionic fetuses, first trimester [1st] [M] ♀

O30.812 Other specified multiple gestation with two or more monochorionic fetuses, second trimester [2nd] [M] ♀

O30.813 Other specified multiple gestation with two or more monochorionic fetuses, third trimester [3rd] [M] ♀

O30.819 Other specified multiple gestation with two or more monochorionic fetuses, unspecified trimester [M] ♀

[6] O30.82 Other specified multiple gestation with two or more monoamniotic fetuses

O30.821 Other specified multiple gestation with two or more monoamniotic fetuses, first trimester [1st] [M] ♀

O30.822 Other specified multiple gestation with two or more monoamniotic fetuses, second trimester [2nd] [M] ♀

O30.823 Other specified multiple gestation with two or more monoamniotic fetuses, third trimester [3rd] [M] ♀

O30.829 Other specified multiple gestation with two or more monoamniotic fetuses, unspecified trimester [M] ♀

[6] O30.89 Other specified multiple gestation, unable to determine number of placenta and number of amniotic sacs

O30.891 Other specified multiple gestation, unable to determine number of placenta and number of amniotic sacs, first trimester [1st] [M] ♀

O30.892 Other specified multiple gestation, unable to determine number of placenta and number of amniotic sacs, second trimester [2nd] [M] ♀

O30.893 Other specified multiple gestation, unable to determine number of placenta and number of amniotic sacs, third trimester [3rd] [M] ♀

O30.899 Other specified multiple gestation, unable to determine number of placenta and number of amniotic sacs, unspecified trimester [M] ♀

[5] O30.9 Multiple gestation, unspecified

Multiple pregnancy NOS

O30.90 Multiple gestation, unspecified, unspecified trimester [M] ♀

O30.91 Multiple gestation, unspecified, first trimester [1st] [M] ♀

O30.92 Multiple gestation, unspecified, second trimester [2nd] [M] ♀

O30.93 Multiple gestation, unspecified, third trimester [3rd] [M] ♀

[4] O31 Complications specific to multiple gestation

[EXCLUDES2] *delayed delivery of second twin, triplet, etc. (O63.2)*
malpresentation of one fetus or more (O32.9)
placental transfusion syndromes (O43.0-)

One of the following 7th characters is to be assigned to each code under category O31. 7th character 0 is for single gestations and multiple gestations where the fetus is unspecified. 7th characters 1 through 9 are for cases of multiple gestations to identify the fetus for which the code applies. The appropriate code from category O30, Multiple gestation, must also be assigned when assigning a code from category O31 that has a 7th character of 1 through 9.

0 = not applicable or unspecified
1 = fetus 1
2 = fetus 2
3 = fetus 3
4 = fetus 4
5 = fetus 5
9 = other fetus

[5] O31.0 Papyraceous fetus

Fetus compressus

[7] O31.00 Papyraceous fetus, unspecified trimester

[7] O31.01 Papyraceous fetus, first trimester [1st]

[7] O31.02 Papyraceous fetus, second trimester [2nd]

[7] O31.03 Papyraceous fetus, third trimester [3rd]

[5] O31.1 Continuing pregnancy after spontaneous abortion of one fetus or more

[7] O31.10 Continuing pregnancy after spontaneous abortion of one fetus or more, unspecified trimester

[7] O31.11 Continuing pregnancy after spontaneous abortion of one fetus or more, first trimester [1st]

[7] O31.12 Continuing pregnancy after spontaneous abortion of one fetus or more, second trimester [2nd]

[7] O31.13 Continuing pregnancy after spontaneous abortion of one fetus or more, third trimester [3rd]

[5] O31.2 Continuing pregnancy after intrauterine death of one fetus or more

[7] O31.20 Continuing pregnancy after intrauterine death of one fetus or more, unspecified trimester

[7] O31.21 Continuing pregnancy after intrauterine death of one fetus or more, first trimester [1st]

[7] O31.22 Continuing pregnancy after intrauterine death of one fetus or more, second trimester [2nd]

[7] O31.23 Continuing pregnancy after intrauterine death of one fetus or more, third trimester [3rd]

[5] O31.3 Continuing pregnancy after elective fetal reduction of one fetus or more

Continuing pregnancy after selective termination of one fetus or more

[7] O31.30 Continuing pregnancy after elective fetal reduction of one fetus or more, unspecified trimester

[7] O31.31 Continuing pregnancy after elective fetal reduction of one fetus or more, first trimester [1st]

[7] O31.32 Continuing pregnancy after elective fetal reduction of one fetus or more, second trimester [2nd]

[7] O31.33 Continuing pregnancy after elective fetal reduction of one fetus or more, third trimester [3rd]

[5] O31.8 Other complications specific to multiple gestation

[6] O31.8X Other complications specific to multiple gestation

[7] O31.8X1 Other complications specific to multiple gestation, first trimester [1st]

[7] O31.8X2 Other complications specific to multiple gestation, second trimester [2nd]

[4] 4th character required [5] 5th character required [6] 6th character required [7] 7th character required [X] Extension 'X' Alert
[EXCLUDES1] Not coded here [EXCLUDES2] Not included here [PDx] Primary Diagnosis Only Manifestation Code

❼ **O31.8X3 Other complications specific to multiple gestation,** third trimester ▣3rd

❼ **O31.8X9 Other complications specific to multiple gestation, unspecified trimester**

❹ **O32 Maternal care for malpresentation of fetus**

> *INCLUDES* *the listed conditions as a reason for observation, hospitalization or other obstetric care of the mother, or for cesarean delivery before onset of labor*

> *EXCLUDES1* *malpresentation of fetus with obstructed labor (O64.-)*

One of the following 7th characters is to be assigned to each code under category O32. 7th character 0 is for single gestations and multiple gestations where the fetus is unspecified. 7th characters 1 through 9 are for cases of multiple gestations to identify the fetus for which the code applies. The appropriate code from category O30, Multiple gestation, must also be assigned when assigning a code from category O32 that has a 7th character of 1 through 9.

0 = not applicable or unspecified
1 = fetus 1
2 = fetus 2
3 = fetus 3
4 = fetus 4
5 = fetus 5
9 = other fetus

❼ **O32.0 Maternal care for** unstable lie

❼ **O32.1 Maternal care for** breech presentation

Maternal care for buttocks presentation
Maternal care for complete breech
Maternal care for frank breech
> *EXCLUDES1* *footling presentation (O32.8)*
> *incomplete breech (O32.8)*

❼ **O32.2 Maternal care for** transverse and oblique lie

Maternal care for oblique presentation
Maternal care for transverse presentation

❼ **O32.3 Maternal care for** face, brow and chin presentation

❼ **O32.4 Maternal care for** high head at term

Maternal care for failure of head to enter pelvic brim

❼ **O32.6 Maternal care for** compound presentation

❼ **O32.8 Maternal care for** other malpresentation of fetus

Maternal care for footling presentation
Maternal care for incomplete breech

❼ **O32.9 Maternal care for malpresentation of fetus, unspecified**

❹ **O33 Maternal care for** disproportion

> *INCLUDES* *the listed conditions as a reason for observation, hospitalization or other obstetric care of the mother, or for cesarean delivery before onset of labor*

> *EXCLUDES1* *disproportion with obstructed labor (O65-O66)*

O33.0 Maternal care for disproportion due to deformity of maternal pelvic bones

Maternal care for disproportion due to pelvic deformity causing disproportion NOS   Ⓜ ♀

O33.1 Maternal care for disproportion due to generally contracted pelvis

Maternal care for disproportion due to contracted pelvis NOS causing disproportion   Ⓜ ♀

O33.2 Maternal care for disproportion due to inlet contraction of pelvis

Maternal care for disproportion due to inlet contraction (pelvis) causing disproportion   Ⓜ ♀

❼ **O33.3 Maternal care for disproportion due to** outlet contraction of pelvis

Maternal care for disproportion due to mid-cavity contraction (pelvis)
Maternal care for disproportion due to outlet contraction (pelvis)

One of the following 7th characters is to be assigned to code O33.3. 7th character 0 is for single gestations and multiple gestations where the fetus is unspecified. 7th characters 1 through 9 are for cases of multiple gestations to identify the fetus for which the code applies. The appropriate code from category O30, Multiple gestation, must also be assigned when assigning code O33.3 with a 7th character of 1 through 9.
0 = not applicable or unspecified
1 = fetus 1
2 = fetus 2
3 = fetus 3
4 = fetus 4
5 = fetus 5
9 = other fetus

❼ **O33.4 Maternal care for disproportion of mixed maternal and fetal origin**

One of the following 7th characters is to be assigned to code O33.4. 7th character 0 is for single gestations and multiple gestations where the fetus is unspecified. 7th characters 1 through 9 are for cases of multiple gestations to identify the fetus for which the code applies. The appropriate code from category O30, Multiple gestation, must also be assigned when assigning code O33.4 with a 7th character of 1 through 9.
0 = not applicable or unspecified
1 = fetus 1
2 = fetus 2
3 = fetus 3
4 = fetus 4
5 = fetus 5
9 = other fetus

❼ **O33.5 Maternal care for disproportion due to unusually large fetus**

Maternal care for disproportion due to disproportion of fetal origin with normally formed fetus
Maternal care for disproportion due to fetal disproportion NOS

One of the following 7th characters is to be assigned to code O33.5. 7th character 0 is for single gestations and multiple gestations where the fetus is unspecified. 7th characters 1 through 9 are for cases of multiple gestations to identify the fetus for which the code applies. The appropriate code from category O30, Multiple gestation, must also be assigned when assigning code O33.5 with a 7th character of 1 through 9.
0 = not applicable or unspecified
1 = fetus 1
2 = fetus 2
3 = fetus 3
4 = fetus 4
5 = fetus 5
9 = other fetus

❼ **O33.6 Maternal care for disproportion due to hydrocephalic fetus**

One of the following 7th characters is to be assigned to code O33.6. 7th character 0 is for single gestations and multiple gestations where the fetus is unspecified. 7th characters 1 through 9 are for cases of multiple gestations to identify the fetus for which the code applies. The appropriate code from category O30, Multiple gestation, must also be assigned when assigning code O33.6 with a 7th character of 1 through 9.
0 = not applicable or unspecified
1 = fetus 1
2 = fetus 2
3 = fetus 3
4 = fetus 4
5 = fetus 5
9 = other fetus

Unspecified Code | Other Specified Code | Ⓝ Newborn Age: 0 | Ⓟ Pediatric Age: 0-17 | Ⓜ Maternity Age: 12-55
Ⓐ Adult Age: 15-124 | ♂ Male | ♀ Female | ● New Code | ▲ Revised Code Title | ►◄ Revised Text

O33.7 Maternal care for disproportion due to other fetal deformities

Maternal care for disproportion due to fetal ascites

Maternal care for disproportion due to fetal hydrops

Maternal care for disproportion due to fetal meningomyelocele

Maternal care for disproportion due to fetal sacral teratoma

Maternal care for disproportion due to fetal tumor

EXCLUDES1 obstructed labor due to other fetal deformities (O66.3) M ♀

O33.8 Maternal care for disproportion of other origin M ♀

O33.9 Maternal care for disproportion, unspecified

Maternal care for disproportion due to cephalopelvic disproportion NOS

Maternal care for disproportion due to fetopelvic disproportion NOS M ♀

🌕 O34 Maternal care for abnormality of pelvic organs

    INCLUDES the listed conditions as a reason for hospitalization or other obstetric care of the mother, or for cesarean delivery before onset of labor

Code first any associated obstructed labor (O65.5)

Use additional code for specific condition

🌕 O34.0 Maternal care for congenital malformation of uterus

    O34.00 Maternal care for unspecified congenital malformation of uterus, unspecified trimester M ♀

    O34.01 Maternal care for unspecified congenital malformation of uterus, first trimester M ♀

    O34.02 Maternal care for unspecified congenital malformation of uterus, second trimester M ♀

    O34.03 Maternal care for unspecified congenital malformation of uterus, third trimester M ♀

🌕 O34.1 Maternal care for benign tumor of corpus uteri

    EXCLUDES2 maternal care for benign tumor of cervix (O34.4-)

    maternal care for malignant neoplasm of uterus (O9A.1-)

    O34.10 Maternal care for benign tumor of corpus uteri, unspecified trimester M ♀

    O34.11 Maternal care for benign tumor of corpus uteri, first trimester M ♀

    O34.12 Maternal care for benign tumor of corpus uteri, second trimester M ♀

    O34.13 Maternal care for benign tumor of corpus uteri, third trimester M ♀

🌕 O34.2 Maternal care due to uterine scar from previous surgery

    O34.21 Maternal care for scar from previous cesarean delivery M ♀

    O34.29 Maternal care due to uterine scar from other previous surgery M ♀

🌕 O34.3 Maternal care for cervical incompetence

Maternal care for cerclage with or without cervical incompetence

Maternal care for Shirodkar suture with or without cervical incompetence

    O34.30 Maternal care for cervical incompetence, unspecified trimester M ♀

    O34.31 Maternal care for cervical incompetence, first trimester M ♀

    O34.32 Maternal care for cervical incompetence, second trimester M ♀

    O34.33 Maternal care for cervical incompetence, third trimester M ♀

🌕 O34.4 Maternal care for other abnormalities of cervix

    O34.40 Maternal care for other abnormalities of cervix, unspecified trimester M ♀

    O34.41 Maternal care for other abnormalities of cervix, first trimester M ♀

    O34.42 Maternal care for other abnormalities of cervix, second trimester M ♀

    O34.43 Maternal care for other abnormalities of cervix, third trimester M ♀

🌕 O34.5 Maternal care for other abnormalities of gravid uterus

    🌕 O34.51 Maternal care for incarceration of gravid uterus

        O34.511 Maternal care for incarceration of gravid uterus, first trimester M ♀

        O34.512 Maternal care for incarceration of gravid uterus, second trimester M ♀

        O34.513 Maternal care for incarceration of gravid uterus, third trimester M ♀

        O34.519 Maternal care for incarceration of gravid uterus, unspecified trimester M ♀

    🌕 O34.52 Maternal care for prolapse of gravid uterus

        O34.521 Maternal care for prolapse of gravid uterus, first trimester M ♀

        O34.522 Maternal care for prolapse of gravid uterus, second trimester M ♀

        O34.523 Maternal care for prolapse of gravid uterus, third trimester M ♀

        O34.529 Maternal care for prolapse of gravid uterus, unspecified trimester M ♀

    🌕 O34.53 Maternal care for retroversion of gravid uterus

        O34.531 Maternal care for retroversion of gravid uterus, first trimester M ♀

        O34.532 Maternal care for retroversion of gravid uterus, second trimester M ♀

        O34.533 Maternal care for retroversion of gravid uterus, third trimester M ♀

        O34.539 Maternal care for retroversion of gravid uterus, unspecified trimester M ♀

    🌕 O34.59 Maternal care for other abnormalities of gravid uterus

        O34.591 Maternal care for other abnormalities of gravid uterus, first trimester M ♀

        O34.592 Maternal care for other abnormalities of gravid uterus, second trimester M ♀

        O34.593 Maternal care for other abnormalities of gravid uterus, third trimester M ♀

        O34.599 Maternal care for other abnormalities of gravid uterus, unspecified trimester M ♀

🌕 O34.6 Maternal care for abnormality of vagina

    EXCLUDES2 maternal care for vaginal varices in pregnancy (O22.1-)

    O34.60 Maternal care for abnormality of vagina, unspecified trimester M ♀

    O34.61 Maternal care for abnormality of vagina, first trimester M ♀

    O34.62 Maternal care for abnormality of vagina, second trimester M ♀

    O34.63 Maternal care for abnormality of vagina, third trimester M ♀

🌕 O34.7 Maternal care for abnormality of vulva and perineum

    EXCLUDES2 maternal care for perineal and vulval varices in pregnancy (O22.1-)

    O34.70 Maternal care for abnormality of vulva and perineum, unspecified trimester M ♀

    O34.71 Maternal care for abnormality of vulva and perineum, first trimester M ♀

    O34.72 Maternal care for abnormality of vulva and perineum, second trimester M ♀

    O34.73 Maternal care for abnormality of vulva and perineum, third trimester M ♀

🌕 O34.8 Maternal care for other abnormalities of pelvic organs

O34.80 Maternal care for other abnormalities of pelvic organs, unspecified trimester [M] ♀
O34.81 Maternal care for other abnormalities of pelvic organs, first trimester [M] ♀
O34.82 Maternal care for other abnormalities of pelvic organs, second trimester [M] ♀
O34.83 Maternal care for other abnormalities of pelvic organs, third trimester [M] ♀

5 O34.9 Maternal care for abnormality of pelvic organ, unspecified
O34.90 Maternal care for abnormality of pelvic organ, unspecified, unspecified trimester [M] ♀
O34.91 Maternal care for abnormality of pelvic organ, unspecified, first trimester [M] ♀
O34.92 Maternal care for abnormality of pelvic organ, unspecified, second trimester [M] ♀
O34.93 Maternal care for abnormality of pelvic organ, unspecified, third trimester [M] ♀

4 O35 Maternal care for known or suspected fetal abnormality and damage

[INCLUDES] *the listed conditions in the fetus as a reason for hospitalization or other obstetric care to the mother, or for termination of pregnancy*

Code also any associated maternal condition

[EXCLUDES1] *encounter for suspected maternal and fetal conditions ruled out (Z03.7-)*

One of the following 7th characters is to be assigned to each code under category O35. 7th character 0 is for single gestations and multiple gestations where the fetus is unspecified. 7th characters 1 through 9 are for cases of multiple gestations to identify the fetus for which the code applies. The appropriate code from category O30, Multiple gestation, must also be assigned when assigning a code from category O35 that has a 7th character of 1 through 9.

0 = not applicable or unspecified
1 = fetus 1
2 = fetus 2
3 = fetus 3
4 = fetus 4
5 = fetus 5
9 = other fetus

7 O35.0 Maternal care for (suspected) central nervous system malformation in fetus
Maternal care for fetal anencephaly
Maternal care for fetal hydrocephalus
Maternal care for fetal spina bifida
[EXCLUDES2] *chromosomal abnormality in fetus (O35.1)*

7 O35.1 Maternal care for (suspected) chromosomal abnormality in fetus

7 O35.2 Maternal care for (suspected) hereditary disease in fetus
[EXCLUDES2] *chromosomal abnormality in fetus (O35.1)*

7 O35.3 Maternal care for (suspected) damage to fetus from viral disease in mother
Maternal care for damage to fetus from maternal cytomegalovirus infection
Maternal care for damage to fetus from maternal rubella

7 O35.4 Maternal care for (suspected) damage to fetus from alcohol

7 O35.5 Maternal care for (suspected) damage to fetus by drugs
Maternal care for damage to fetus from drug addiction

7 O35.6 Maternal care for (suspected) damage to fetus by radiation

7 O35.7 Maternal care for (suspected) damage to fetus by other medical procedures
Maternal care for damage to fetus by amniocentesis
Maternal care for damage to fetus by biopsy procedures
Maternal care for damage to fetus by hematological investigation
Maternal care for damage to fetus by intrauterine contraceptive device
Maternal care for damage to fetus by intrauterine surgery

7 O35.8 Maternal care for other (suspected) fetal abnormality and damage
Maternal care for damage to fetus from maternal listeriosis
Maternal care for damage to fetus from maternal toxoplasmosis

7 O35.9 Maternal care for (suspected) fetal abnormality and damage, unspecified

4 O36 Maternal care for other fetal problems

[INCLUDES] *the listed conditions in the fetus as a reason for hospitalization or other obstetric care of the mother, or for termination of pregnancy*

[EXCLUDES1] *encounter for suspected maternal and fetal conditions ruled out (Z03.7-)*
placental transfusion syndromes (O43.0-)

[EXCLUDES2] *labor and delivery complicated by fetal stress (O77.-)*

One of the following 7th characters is to be assigned to each code under category O36. 7th character 0 is for single gestations and multiple gestations where the fetus is unspecified. 7th characters 1 through 9 are for cases of multiple gestations to identify the fetus for which the code applies. The appropriate code from category O30, Multiple gestation, must also be assigned when assigning a code from category O36 that has a 7th character of 1 through 9.

0 = not applicable or unspecified
1 = fetus 1
2 = fetus 2
3 = fetus 3
4 = fetus 4
5 = fetus 5
9 = other fetus

5 O36.0 Maternal care for rhesus isoimmunization
Maternal care for Rh incompatibility (with hydrops fetalis)

6 O36.01 Maternal care for anti-D [Rh] antibodies
7 O36.011 Maternal care for anti-D [Rh] antibodies, first trimester
7 O36.012 Maternal care for anti-D [Rh] antibodies, second trimester
7 O36.013 Maternal care for anti-D [Rh] antibodies, third trimester
7 O36.019 Maternal care for anti-D [Rh] antibodies, unspecified trimester

6 O36.09 Maternal care for other rhesus isoimmunization
7 O36.091 Maternal care for other rhesus isoimmunization, first trimester
7 O36.092 Maternal care for other rhesus isoimmunization, second trimester
7 O36.093 Maternal care for other rhesus isoimmunization, third trimester
7 O36.099 Maternal care for other rhesus isoimmunization, unspecified trimester

5 O36.1 Maternal care for other isoimmunization
Maternal care for ABO isoimmunization

6 O36.11 Maternal care for Anti-A sensitization
Maternal care for isoimmunization NOS (with hydrops fetalis)
7 O36.111 Maternal care for Anti-A sensitization, first trimester
7 O36.112 Maternal care for Anti-A sensitization, second trimester
7 O36.113 Maternal care for Anti-A sensitization, third trimester
7 O36.119 Maternal care for Anti-A sensitization, unspecified trimester

Unspecified Code | Other Specified Code | [N] Newborn Age: 0 | [P] Pediatric Age: 0-17 | [M] Maternity Age: 12-55
[A] Adult Age: 15-124 | ♂ Male | ♀ Female | ● New Code | ▲ Revised Code Title | ▶◀ Revised Text

⑥ **O36.19** **Maternal care for** other isoimmunization

Maternal care for Anti-B sensitization

⑦ **O36.191** **Maternal care for other isoimmunization, first trimester**

⑦ **O36.192** **Maternal care for other isoimmunization, second trimester**

⑦ **O36.193** **Maternal care for other isoimmunization, third trimester**

⑦ **O36.199** **Maternal care for other isoimmunization, unspecified trimester**

⑤ **O36.2** **Maternal care for** hydrops fetalis

Maternal care for hydrops fetalis NOS

Maternal care for hydrops fetalis not associated with isoimmunization

> *EXCLUDES1* *hydrops fetalis associated with ABO isoimmunization (O36.1-)*
> *hydrops fetalis associated with rhesus isoimmunization (O36.0-)*

⑦ **O36.20** **Maternal care for hydrops fetalis, unspecified trimester**

⑦ **O36.21** **Maternal care for hydrops fetalis,** first trimester

⑦ **O36.22** **Maternal care for hydrops fetalis,** second trimester

⑦ **O36.23** **Maternal care for hydrops fetalis,** third trimester

⑦ **O36.4** **Maternal care for** intrauterine death

Maternal care for intrauterine fetal death NOS

Maternal care for intrauterine fetal death after completion of 20 weeks of gestation

Maternal care for late fetal death

Maternal care for missed delivery

> *EXCLUDES1* *missed abortion (O02.1)*
> *stillbirth (P95)*

⑤ **O36.5** **Maternal care for** known or suspected poor fetal growth

⑥ **O36.51** **Maternal care for known or suspected** placental insufficiency

⑦ **O36.511** **Maternal care for known or suspected placental insufficiency,** first trimester

⑦ **O36.512** **Maternal care for known or suspected placental insufficiency,** second trimester

⑦ **O36.513** **Maternal care for known or suspected placental insufficiency,** third trimester

⑦ **O36.519** **Maternal care for known or suspected placental insufficiency,** unspecified trimester

⑥ **O36.59** **Maternal care for** other **known or suspected poor fetal growth**

Maternal care for known or suspected light-for-dates NOS

Maternal care for known or suspected small-for-dates NOS

⑦ **O36.591** **Maternal care for other known or suspected poor fetal growth,** first trimester

⑦ **O36.592** **Maternal care for other known or suspected poor fetal growth,** second trimester

⑦ **O36.593** **Maternal care for other known or suspected poor fetal growth,** third trimester

⑦ **O36.599** **Maternal care for other known or suspected poor fetal growth,** unspecified trimester

⑤ **O36.6** **Maternal care for** excessive fetal growth

Maternal care for known or suspected large-for-dates

⑦ **O36.60** **Maternal care for excessive fetal growth, unspecified trimester**

⑦ **O36.61** **Maternal care for excessive fetal growth,** first trimester

⑦ **O36.62** **Maternal care for excessive fetal growth,** second trimester

⑦ **O36.63** **Maternal care for excessive fetal growth,** third trimester

⑤ **O36.7** **Maternal care for** viable fetus in abdominal pregnancy

⑦ **O36.70** **Maternal care for viable fetus in abdominal pregnancy, unspecified trimester**

⑦ **O36.71** **Maternal care for viable fetus in abdominal pregnancy,** first trimester

⑦ **O36.72** **Maternal care for viable fetus in abdominal pregnancy,** second trimester

⑦ **O36.73** **Maternal care for viable fetus in abdominal pregnancy,** third trimester

⑤ **O36.8** **Maternal care for** other specified **fetal problems**

⑦ **O36.80** **Pregnancy with inconclusive fetal viability**

Encounter to determine fetal viability of pregnancy

⑥ **O36.81** **Decreased fetal movements**

⑦ **O36.812** **Decreased fetal movements,** second trimester

⑦ **O36.813** **Decreased fetal movements,** third trimester

⑦ **O36.819** **Decreased fetal movements, unspecified trimester**

⑥ **O36.82** **Fetal anemia and thrombocytopenia**

⑦ **O36.821** **Fetal anemia and thrombocytopenia,** first trimester

⑦ **O36.822** **Fetal anemia and thrombocytopenia,** second trimester

⑦ **O36.823** **Fetal anemia and thrombocytopenia,** third trimester

⑦ **O36.829** **Fetal anemia and thrombocytopenia, unspecified trimester**

⑥ **O36.89** **Maternal care for other specified fetal problems**

⑦ **O36.891** **Maternal care for other specified fetal problems,** first trimester

⑦ **O36.892** **Maternal care for other specified fetal problems,** second trimester

⑦ **O36.893** **Maternal care for other specified fetal problems,** third trimester

⑦ **O36.899** **Maternal care for other specified fetal problems, unspecified trimester**

⑤ **O36.9** **Maternal care for fetal problem, unspecified**

⑦ **O36.90** **Maternal care for fetal problem, unspecified, unspecified trimester**

⑦ **O36.91** **Maternal care for fetal problem, unspecified,** first trimester

⑦ **O36.92** **Maternal care for fetal problem, unspecified,** second trimester

⑦ **O36.93** **Maternal care for fetal problem, unspecified,** third trimester

④ **O40** **Polyhydramnios**

> *INCLUDES* *hydramnios*
> *EXCLUDES1* *encounter for suspected maternal and fetal conditions ruled out (Z03.7-)*

One of the following 7th characters is to be assigned to each code under category O40. 7th character 0 is for single gestations and multiple gestations where the fetus is unspecified. 7th characters 1 through 9 are for cases of multiple gestations to identify the fetus for which the code applies. The appropriate code from category O30, Multiple gestation, must also be assigned when assigning a code from category O40 that has a 7th character of 1 through 9.

0 = not applicable or unspecified
1 = fetus 1
2 = fetus 2
3 = fetus 3
4 = fetus 4
5 = fetus 5
9 = other fetus

⑦ **O40.1** **Polyhydramnios,** first trimester

⑦ **O40.2** **Polyhydramnios,** second trimester

⑦ **O40.3** **Polyhydramnios,** third trimester

---

④ 4th character required	⑤ 5th character required	⑥ 6th character required	⑦ 7th character required	ⓧ Extension 'X' Alert

EXCLUDES 1 Not coded here   *EXCLUDES 2* Not included here   🔖 Primary Diagnosis Only   Manifestation Code

[7] O40.9 Polyhydramnios, unspecified trimester

[4] O41 Other disorders of amniotic fluid and membranes

[EXCLUDES1] *encounter for suspected maternal and fetal conditions ruled out (Z03.7-)*

One of the following 7th characters is to be assigned to each code under category O41. 7th character 0 is for single gestations and multiple gestations where the fetus is unspecified. 7th characters 1 through 9 are for cases of multiple gestations to identify the fetus for which the code applies. The appropriate code from category O30, Multiple gestation, must also be assigned when assigning a code from category O41 that has a 7th character of 1 through 9.

0 = not applicable or unspecified
1 = fetus 1
2 = fetus 2
3 = fetus 3
4 = fetus 4
5 = fetus 5
9 = other fetus

[5] O41.0 Oligohydramnios
Oligohydramnios without rupture of membranes
[7] O41.00 Oligohydramnios, unspecified trimester
[7] O41.01 Oligohydramnios, first trimester
[7] O41.02 Oligohydramnios, second trimester
[7] O41.03 Oligohydramnios, third trimester

[5] O41.1 Infection of amniotic sac and membranes
[6] O41.10 Infection of amniotic sac and membranes, unspecified
[7] O41.101 Infection of amniotic sac and membranes, unspecified, first trimester
[7] O41.102 Infection of amniotic sac and membranes, unspecified, second trimester
[7] O41.103 Infection of amniotic sac and membranes, unspecified, third trimester
[7] O41.109 Infection of amniotic sac and membranes, unspecified, unspecified trimester
[6] O41.12 Chorioamnionitis
[7] O41.121 Chorioamnionitis, first trimester
[7] O41.122 Chorioamnionitis, second trimester
[7] O41.123 Chorioamnionitis, third trimester
[7] O41.129 Chorioamnionitis, unspecified trimester
[6] O41.14 Placentitis
[7] O41.141 Placentitis, first trimester
[7] O41.142 Placentitis, second trimester
[7] O41.143 Placentitis, third trimester
[7] O41.149 Placentitis, unspecified trimester

[5] O41.8 Other specified disorders of amniotic fluid and membranes
[6] O41.8X Other specified disorders of amniotic fluid and membranes
[7] O41.8X1 Other specified disorders of amniotic fluid and membranes, first trimester
[7] O41.8X2 Other specified disorders of amniotic fluid and membranes, second trimester
[7] O41.8X3 Other specified disorders of amniotic fluid and membranes, third trimester
[7] O41.8X9 Other specified disorders of amniotic fluid and membranes, unspecified trimester

[5] O41.9 Disorder of amniotic fluid and membranes, unspecified
[7] O41.90 Disorder of amniotic fluid and membranes, unspecified, unspecified trimester
[7] O41.91 Disorder of amniotic fluid and membranes, unspecified, first trimester
[7] O41.92 Disorder of amniotic fluid and membranes, unspecified, second trimester
[7] O41.93 Disorder of amniotic fluid and membranes, unspecified, third trimester

[4] O42 Premature rupture of membranes
[5] O42.0 Premature rupture of membranes, onset of labor within 24 hours of rupture
O42.00 Premature rupture of membranes, onset of labor within 24 hours of rupture, unspecified weeks of gestation [M] ♀
[6] O42.01 Preterm premature rupture of membranes, onset of labor within 24 hours of rupture
Premature rupture of membranes before 37 completed weeks of gestation
O42.011 Preterm premature rupture of membranes, onset of labor within 24 hours of rupture, first trimester [M] ♀
O42.012 Preterm premature rupture of membranes, onset of labor within 24 hours of rupture, second trimester [M] ♀
O42.013 Preterm premature rupture of membranes, onset of labor within 24 hours of rupture, third trimester [M] ♀
O42.019 Preterm premature rupture of membranes, onset of labor within 24 hours of rupture, unspecified trimester [M] ♀
O42.02 Full-term premature rupture of membranes, onset of labor within 24 hours of rupture
Premature rupture of membranes after 37 completed weeks of gestation [M] ♀

[5] O42.1 Premature rupture of membranes, onset of labor more than 24 hours following rupture
O42.10 Premature rupture of membranes, onset of labor more than 24 hours following rupture, unspecified weeks of gestation [M] ♀
[6] O42.11 Preterm premature rupture of membranes, onset of labor more than 24 hours following rupture
Premature rupture of membranes before 37 completed weeks of gestation
O42.111 Preterm premature rupture of membranes, onset of labor more than 24 hours following rupture, first trimester [M] ♀
O42.112 Preterm premature rupture of membranes, onset of labor more than 24 hours following rupture, second trimester [M] ♀
O42.113 Preterm premature rupture of membranes, onset of labor more than 24 hours following rupture, third trimester [M] ♀
O42.119 Preterm premature rupture of membranes, onset of labor more than 24 hours following rupture, unspecified trimester [M] ♀
O42.12 Full-term premature rupture of membranes, onset of labor more than 24 hours following rupture
Premature rupture of membranes after 37 completed weeks of gestation [M] ♀

[5] O42.9 Premature rupture of membranes, unspecified as to length of time between rupture and onset of labor
O42.90 Premature rupture of membranes, unspecified as to length of time between rupture and onset of labor, unspecified weeks of gestation [M] ♀
[6] O42.91 Preterm premature rupture of membranes, unspecified as to length of time between rupture and onset of labor
Premature rupture of membranes before 37 completed weeks of gestation
O42.911 Preterm premature rupture of membranes, unspecified as to length of time between rupture and onset of labor, first trimester [M] ♀

Unspecified Code | Other Specified Code | [N] Newborn Age: 0 | [P] Pediatric Age: 0-17 | [M] Maternity Age: 12-55 | [A] Adult Age: 15-124 | ♂ Male | ♀ Female | ● New Code | ▲ Revised Code Title | ►◄ Revised Text

O42.912 Preterm premature rupture of membranes, unspecified as to length of time between rupture and onset of labor, second trimester M ♀

O42.913 Preterm premature rupture of membranes, unspecified as to length of time between rupture and onset of labor, third trimester M ♀

O42.919 Preterm premature rupture of membranes, unspecified as to length of time between rupture and onset of labor, unspecified trimester M ♀

O42.92 Full-term premature rupture of membranes, unspecified as to length of time between rupture and onset of labor

Premature rupture of membranes after 37 completed weeks of gestation M ♀

④ O43 **Placental disorders**

EXCLUDES2 maternal care for poor fetal growth due to placental insufficiency (O36.5-)
placenta previa (O44.-)
placental polyp (O90.89)
placentitis (O41.14-)
premature separation of placenta [abruptio placentae] (O45.-)

⑤ O43.0 **Placental transfusion syndromes**

⑥ O43.01 Fetomaternal placental transfusion syndrome

Maternofetal placental transfusion syndrome

O43.011 **Fetomaternal placental transfusion syndrome**, first trimester M ♀

O43.012 **Fetomaternal placental transfusion syndrome**, second trimester M ♀

O43.013 **Fetomaternal placental transfusion syndrome**, third trimester M ♀

O43.019 **Fetomaternal placental transfusion syndrome**, unspecified trimester M ♀

⑥ O43.02 Fetus-to-fetus placental transfusion syndrome

O43.021 **Fetus-to-fetus placental transfusion syndrome**, first trimester M ♀

O43.022 **Fetus-to-fetus placental transfusion syndrome**, second trimester M ♀

O43.023 **Fetus-to-fetus placental transfusion syndrome**, third trimester M ♀

O43.029 **Fetus-to-fetus placental transfusion syndrome**, unspecified trimester M ♀

⑤ O43.1 **Malformation of placenta**

⑥ O43.10 Malformation of placenta, unspecified

Abnormal placenta NOS

O43.101 **Malformation of placenta, unspecified**, first trimester M ♀

O43.102 **Malformation of placenta, unspecified**, second trimester M ♀

O43.103 **Malformation of placenta, unspecified**, third trimester M ♀

O43.109 **Malformation of placenta, unspecified**, unspecified trimester M ♀

⑥ O43.11 Circumvallate placenta

O43.111 **Circumvallate placenta**, first trimester M ♀

O43.112 **Circumvallate placenta**, second trimester M ♀

O43.113 **Circumvallate placenta**, third trimester M ♀

O43.119 **Circumvallate placenta**, unspecified trimester M ♀

⑥ O43.12 Velamentous insertion of umbilical cord

O43.121 **Velamentous insertion of umbilical cord**, first trimester M ♀

O43.122 **Velamentous insertion of umbilical cord**, second trimester M ♀

O43.123 **Velamentous insertion of umbilical cord**, third trimester M ♀

O43.129 **Velamentous insertion of umbilical cord**, unspecified trimester M ♀

⑥ O43.19 Other malformation of placenta

O43.191 **Other malformation of placenta**, first trimester M ♀

O43.192 **Other malformation of placenta**, second trimester M ♀

O43.193 **Other malformation of placenta**, third trimester M ♀

O43.199 **Other malformation of placenta**, unspecified trimester M ♀

⑤ O43.2 **Morbidly adherent placenta**

Code also associated third stage postpartum hemorrhage, if applicable (O72.0)

EXCLUDES1 retained placenta (O73.-)

⑥ O43.21 Placenta accreta

O43.211 **Placenta accreta**, first trimester M ♀

O43.212 **Placenta accreta**, second trimester M ♀

O43.213 **Placenta accreta**, third trimester M ♀

O43.219 **Placenta accreta**, unspecified trimester M ♀

⑥ O43.22 Placenta increta

O43.221 **Placenta increta**, first trimester M ♀

O43.222 **Placenta increta**, second trimester M ♀

O43.223 **Placenta increta**, third trimester M ♀

O43.229 **Placenta increta**, unspecified trimester M ♀

⑥ O43.23 Placenta percreta

O43.231 **Placenta percreta**, first trimester M ♀

O43.232 **Placenta percreta**, second trimester M ♀

O43.233 **Placenta percreta**, third trimester M ♀

O43.239 **Placenta percreta**, unspecified trimester M ♀

⑤ O43.8 **Other placental disorders**

⑥ O43.81 Placental infarction

O43.811 **Placental infarction**, first trimester M ♀

O43.812 **Placental infarction**, second trimester M ♀

O43.813 **Placental infarction**, third trimester M ♀

O43.819 **Placental infarction**, unspecified trimester M ♀

⑥ O43.89 Other placental disorders

Placental dysfunction

O43.891 **Other placental disorders**, first trimester M ♀

O43.892 **Other placental disorders**, second trimester M ♀

O43.893 **Other placental disorders**, third trimester M ♀

O43.899 **Other placental disorders**, unspecified trimester M ♀

⑤ O43.9 **Unspecified placental disorder**

O43.90 **Unspecified placental disorder**, unspecified trimester M ♀

O43.91 **Unspecified placental disorder**, first trimester M ♀

O43.92 **Unspecified placental disorder**, second trimester M ♀

O43.93 **Unspecified placental disorder**, third trimester M ♀

④ O44 **Placenta previa**

⑤ O44.0 **Placenta previa specified as** without hemorrhage

Low implantation of placenta specified as without hemorrhage

O44.00 **Placenta previa specified as without hemorrhage**, unspecified trimester M ♀

---

④ 4th character required ⑤ 5th character required ⑥ 6th character required ⑦ 7th character required ⑦ Extension 'X' Alert

EXCLUDES 1 Not coded here EXCLUDES 2 Not included here PDx Primary Diagnosis Only Manifestation Code

O44.01 **Placenta previa specified as without hemorrhage, first trimester** [M] ♀

O44.02 **Placenta previa specified as without hemorrhage, second trimester** [M] ♀

O44.03 **Placenta previa specified as without hemorrhage, third trimester** [M] ♀

[5] **O44.1 Placenta previa with hemorrhage**

Low implantation of placenta, NOS or with hemorrhage
Marginal placenta previa, NOS or with hemorrhage
Partial placenta previa, NOS or with hemorrhage
Total placenta previa, NOS or with hemorrhage

[EXCLUDES1] *labor and delivery complicated by hemorrhage from vasa previa (O69.4)*

O44.10 **Placenta previa with hemorrhage, unspecified trimester** [M] ♀

O44.11 **Placenta previa with hemorrhage, first trimester** [M] ♀

O44.12 **Placenta previa with hemorrhage, second trimester** [M] ♀

O44.13 **Placenta previa with hemorrhage, third trimester** [M] ♀

[4] **O45 Premature separation of placenta [abruptio placentae]**

[5] **O45.0 Premature separation of placenta with coagulation defect**

[6] **O45.00 Premature separation of placenta with coagulation defect, unspecified**

O45.001 **Premature separation of placenta with coagulation defect, unspecified, first trimester** [M] ♀

O45.002 **Premature separation of placenta with coagulation defect, unspecified, second trimester** [M] ♀

O45.003 **Premature separation of placenta with coagulation defect, unspecified, third trimester** [M] ♀

O45.009 **Premature separation of placenta with coagulation defect, unspecified, unspecified trimester** [M] ♀

[6] **O45.01 Premature separation of placenta with afibrinogenemia**

Premature separation of placenta with hypofibrinogenemia

O45.011 **Premature separation of placenta with afibrinogenemia, first trimester** [M] ♀

O45.012 **Premature separation of placenta with afibrinogenemia, second trimester** [M] ♀

O45.013 **Premature separation of placenta with afibrinogenemia, third trimester** [M] ♀

O45.019 **Premature separation of placenta with afibrinogenemia, unspecified trimester** [M] ♀

[6] **O45.02 Premature separation of placenta with disseminated intravascular coagulation**

O45.021 **Premature separation of placenta with disseminated intravascular coagulation, first trimester** [M] ♀

O45.022 **Premature separation of placenta with disseminated intravascular coagulation, second trimester** [M] ♀

O45.023 **Premature separation of placenta with disseminated intravascular coagulation, third trimester** [M] ♀

O45.029 **Premature separation of placenta with disseminated intravascular coagulation, unspecified trimester** [M] ♀

[6] **O45.09 Premature separation of placenta with other coagulation defect**

O45.091 **Premature separation of placenta with other coagulation defect, first trimester** [M] ♀

O45.092 **Premature separation of placenta with other coagulation defect, second trimester** [M] ♀

O45.093 **Premature separation of placenta with other coagulation defect, third trimester** [M] ♀

O45.099 **Premature separation of placenta with other coagulation defect, unspecified trimester** [M] ♀

[5] **O45.8 Other premature separation of placenta**

[6] **O45.8X Other premature separation of placenta**

O45.8X1 **Other premature separation of placenta, first trimester** [M] ♀

O45.8X2 **Other premature separation of placenta, second trimester** [M] ♀

O45.8X3 **Other premature separation of placenta, third trimester** [M] ♀

O45.8X9 **Other premature separation of placenta, unspecified trimester** [M] ♀

[5] **O45.9 Premature separation of placenta, unspecified**

Abruptio placentae NOS

O45.90 **Premature separation of placenta, unspecified, unspecified trimester** [M] ♀

O45.91 **Premature separation of placenta, unspecified, first trimester** [M] ♀

O45.92 **Premature separation of placenta, unspecified, second trimester** [M] ♀

O45.93 **Premature separation of placenta, unspecified, third trimester** [M] ♀

[4] **O46 Antepartum hemorrhage, not elsewhere classified**

[EXCLUDES1] *hemorrhage in early pregnancy (O20.-)*
intrapartum hemorrhage NEC (O67.-)
placenta previa (O44.-)
premature separation of placenta [abruptio placentae] (O45.-)

[5] **O46.0 Antepartum hemorrhage with coagulation defect**

[6] **O46.00 Antepartum hemorrhage with coagulation defect, unspecified**

O46.001 **Antepartum hemorrhage with coagulation defect, unspecified, first trimester** [M] ♀

O46.002 **Antepartum hemorrhage with coagulation defect, unspecified, second trimester** [M] ♀

O46.003 **Antepartum hemorrhage with coagulation defect, unspecified, third trimester** [M] ♀

O46.009 **Antepartum hemorrhage with coagulation defect, unspecified, unspecified trimester** [M] ♀

[6] **O46.01 Antepartum hemorrhage with afibrinogenemia**

Antepartum hemorrhage with hypofibrinogenemia

O46.011 **Antepartum hemorrhage with afibrinogenemia, first trimester** [M] ♀

O46.012 **Antepartum hemorrhage with afibrinogenemia, second trimester** [M] ♀

O46.013 **Antepartum hemorrhage with afibrinogenemia, third trimester** [M] ♀

O46.019 **Antepartum hemorrhage with afibrinogenemia, unspecified trimester** [M] ♀

[6] **O46.02 Antepartum hemorrhage with disseminated intravascular coagulation**

O46.021 **Antepartum hemorrhage with disseminated intravascular coagulation, first trimester** [M] ♀

O46.022 **Antepartum hemorrhage with disseminated intravascular coagulation, second trimester** [M] ♀

Unspecified Code | Other Specified Code | [N] Newborn Age: 0 | [P] Pediatric Age: 0-17 | [M] Maternity Age: 12-55
[A] Adult Age: 15-124 | ♂ Male | ♀ Female | ● New Code | ▲ Revised Code Title | ►◄ Revised Text

O46.023 Antepartum hemorrhage with disseminated intravascular coagulation, third trimester [M] ♀

O46.029 Antepartum hemorrhage with disseminated intravascular coagulation, unspecified trimester [M] ♀

[6] O46.09 Antepartum hemorrhage with other coagulation defect

O46.091 Antepartum hemorrhage with other coagulation defect, first trimester [M] ♀

O46.092 Antepartum hemorrhage with other coagulation defect, second trimester [M] ♀

O46.093 Antepartum hemorrhage with other coagulation defect, third trimester [M] ♀

O46.099 Antepartum hemorrhage with other coagulation defect, unspecified trimester [M] ♀

[5] O46.8 Other antepartum hemorrhage

[6] O46.8X Other antepartum hemorrhage

O46.8X1 Other antepartum hemorrhage, first trimester [M] ♀

O46.8X2 Other antepartum hemorrhage, second trimester [M] ♀

O46.8X3 Other antepartum hemorrhage, third trimester [M] ♀

O46.8X9 Other antepartum hemorrhage, unspecified trimester [M] ♀

[5] O46.9 Antepartum hemorrhage, unspecified

O46.90 Antepartum hemorrhage, unspecified, unspecified trimester [M] ♀

O46.91 Antepartum hemorrhage, unspecified, first trimester [M] ♀

O46.92 Antepartum hemorrhage, unspecified, second trimester [M] ♀

O46.93 Antepartum hemorrhage, unspecified, third trimester [M] ♀

[4] O47 False labor

[INCLUDES] *Braxton Hicks contractions*
threatened labor

[EXCLUDES1] *preterm labor (O60.-)*

[5] O47.0 False labor before 37 completed weeks of gestation

O47.00 False labor before 37 completed weeks of gestation, unspecified trimester [M] ♀

O47.02 False labor before 37 completed weeks of gestation, second trimester [M] ♀

O47.03 False labor before 37 completed weeks of gestation, third trimester [M] ♀

O47.1 False labor at or after 37 completed weeks of gestation [M] ♀

O47.9 False labor, unspecified [M] ♀

[4] O48 Late pregnancy

O48.0 Post-term pregnancy

Pregnancy over 40 completed weeks to 42 completed weeks gestation [M] ♀

O48.1 Prolonged pregnancy

Pregnancy which has advanced beyond 42 completed weeks gestation [M] ♀

Complications of labor and delivery (O60-O77)

[4] O60 Preterm labor

[INCLUDES] *onset (spontaneous) of labor before 37 completed weeks of gestation*

[EXCLUDES1] *false labor (O47.0-)*
threatened labor NOS (O47.0-)

[5] O60.0 Preterm labor without delivery

O60.00 Preterm labor without delivery, unspecified trimester [M] ♀

O60.02 Preterm labor without delivery, second trimester [M] ♀

O60.03 Preterm labor without delivery, third trimester [M] ♀

[5] O60.1 Preterm labor with preterm delivery

One of the following 7th characters is to be assigned to each code under subcategory O60.1. 7th character 0 is for single gestations and multiple gestations where the fetus is unspecified. 7th characters 1 through 9 are for cases of multiple gestations to identify the fetus for which the code applies. The appropriate code from category O30, Multiple gestation, must also be assigned when assigning a code from subcategory O60.1 that has a 7th character of 1 through 9.

0 = not applicable or unspecified
1 = fetus 1
2 = fetus 2
3 = fetus 3
4 = fetus 4
5 = fetus 5
9 = other fetus

[7] O60.10 Preterm labor with preterm delivery, unspecified trimester

Preterm labor with delivery NOS

[7] O60.12 Preterm labor second trimester with preterm delivery second trimester

[7] O60.13 Preterm labor second trimester with preterm delivery third trimester

[7] O60.14 Preterm labor third trimester with preterm delivery third trimester

[5] O60.2 Term delivery with preterm labor

One of the following 7th characters is to be assigned to each code under subcategory O60.2. 7th character 0 is for single gestations and multiple gestations where the fetus is unspecified. 7th characters 1 through 9 are for cases of multiple gestations to identify the fetus for which the code applies. The appropriate code from category O30, Multiple gestation, must also be assigned when assigning a code from subcategory O60.2 that has a 7th character of 1 through 9.

0 = not applicable or unspecified
1 = fetus 1
2 = fetus 2
3 = fetus 3
4 = fetus 4
5 = fetus 5
9 = other fetus

[7] O60.20 Term delivery with preterm labor, unspecified trimester

[7] O60.22 Term delivery with preterm labor, second trimester

[7] O60.23 Term delivery with preterm labor, third trimester

[4] O61 Failed induction of labor

O61.0 Failed medical induction of labor

Failed induction (of labor) by oxytocin
Failed induction (of labor) by prostaglandins [M] ♀

O61.1 Failed instrumental induction of labor

Failed mechanical induction (of labor)
Failed surgical induction (of labor) [M] ♀

O61.8 Other failed induction of labor [M] ♀

O61.9 Failed induction of labor, unspecified [M] ♀

[4] O62 Abnormalities of forces of labor

O62.0 Primary inadequate contractions

Failure of cervical dilatation
Primary hypotonic uterine dysfunction
Uterine inertia during latent phase of labor [M] ♀

O62.1 Secondary uterine inertia

Arrested active phase of labor
Secondary hypotonic uterine dysfunction [M] ♀

O62.2 Other uterine inertia
Atony of uterus without hemorrhage
Atony of uterus NOS
Desultory labor
Hypotonic uterine dysfunction NOS
Irregular labor
Poor contractions
Slow slope active phase of labor
Uterine inertia NOS
[EXCLUDES1] *atony of uterus with hemorrhage (postpartum) (O72.1)*
postpartum atony of uterus without hemorrhage (O75.89) [M] ♀

O62.3 Precipitate labor [M] ♀

O62.4 Hypertonic, incoordinate, and prolonged uterine contractions
Cervical spasm
Contraction ring dystocia
Dyscoordinate labor
Hour-glass contraction of uterus
Hypertonic uterine dysfunction
Incoordinate uterine action
Tetanic contractions
Uterine dystocia NOS
Uterine spasm
[EXCLUDES1] *dystocia (fetal) (maternal) NOS (O66.9)* [M] ♀

O62.8 Other abnormalities of forces of labor [M] ♀

O62.9 Abnormality of forces of labor, unspecified [M] ♀

[4th] **O63 Long labor**

O63.0 Prolonged first stage (of labor) [M] ♀

O63.1 Prolonged second stage (of labor) [M] ♀

O63.2 Delayed delivery of second twin, triplet, etc. [M] ♀

O63.9 Long labor, unspecified
Prolonged labor NOS [M] ♀

[4th] **O64 Obstructed labor due to malposition and malpresentation of fetus**

One of the following 7th characters is to be assigned to each code under category O64. 7th character 0 is for single gestations and multiple gestations where the fetus is unspecified. 7th characters 1 through 9 are for cases of multiple gestations to identify the fetus for which the code applies. The appropriate code from category O30, Multiple gestation, must also be assigned when assigning a code from category O64 that has a 7th character of 1 through 9.

0 = not applicable or unspecified
1 = fetus 1
2 = fetus 2
3 = fetus 3
4 = fetus 4
5 = fetus 5
9 = other fetus

[7th] **O64.0 Obstructed labor due to incomplete rotation of fetal head**
Deep transverse arrest
Obstructed labor due to persistent occipitoiliac (position)
Obstructed labor due to persistent occipitoposterior (position)
Obstructed labor due to persistent occipitosacral (position)
Obstructed labor due to persistent occipitotransverse (position)

[7th] **O64.1 Obstructed labor due to breech presentation**
Obstructed labor due to buttocks presentation
Obstructed labor due to complete breech presentation
Obstructed labor due to frank breech presentation

[7th] **O64.2 Obstructed labor due to face presentation**
Obstructed labor due to chin presentation

[7th] **O64.3 Obstructed labor due to brow presentation**

[7th] **O64.4 Obstructed labor due to shoulder presentation**
Prolapsed arm
[EXCLUDES1] *impacted shoulders (O66.0)*
shoulder dystocia (O66.0)

[7th] **O64.5 Obstructed labor due to compound presentation**

[7th] **O64.8 Obstructed labor due to other malposition and malpresentation**
Obstructed labor due to footling presentation
Obstructed labor due to incomplete breech presentation

[7th] **O64.9 Obstructed labor due to malposition and malpresentation, unspecified**

[4th] **O65 Obstructed labor due to maternal pelvic abnormality**

O65.0 Obstructed labor due to deformed pelvis [M] ♀

O65.1 Obstructed labor due to generally contracted pelvis [M] ♀

O65.2 Obstructed labor due to pelvic inlet contraction [M] ♀

O65.3 Obstructed labor due to pelvic outlet and mid-cavity contraction [M] ♀

O65.4 Obstructed labor due to fetopelvic disproportion, unspecified
[EXCLUDES1] *dystocia due to abnormality of fetus (O66.2-O66.3)* [M] ♀

O65.5 Obstructed labor due to abnormality of maternal pelvic organs
Obstructed labor due to conditions listed in O34.-
Use additional code to identify abnormality of pelvic organs O34.- [M] ♀

O65.8 Obstructed labor due to other maternal pelvic abnormalities [M] ♀

O65.9 Obstructed labor due to maternal pelvic abnormality, unspecified [M] ♀

[4th] **O66 Other obstructed labor**

O66.0 Obstructed labor due to shoulder dystocia
Impacted shoulders [M] ♀

O66.1 Obstructed labor due to locked twins [M] ♀

O66.2 Obstructed labor due to unusually large fetus [M] ♀

O66.3 Obstructed labor due to other abnormalities of fetus
Dystocia due to fetal ascites
Dystocia due to fetal hydrops
Dystocia due to fetal meningomyelocele
Dystocia due to fetal sacral teratoma
Dystocia due to fetal tumor
Dystocia due to hydrocephalic fetus
Use additional code to identify cause of obstruction [M] ♀

[5th] **O66.4 Failed trial of labor**

O66.40 Failed trial of labor, unspecified [M] ♀

O66.41 Failed attempted vaginal birth after previous cesarean delivery
Code first rupture of uterus, if applicable (O71.0-, O71.1) [M] ♀

O66.5 Attempted application of vacuum extractor and forceps
Attempted application of vacuum or forceps, with subsequent delivery by forceps or cesarean delivery [M] ♀

O66.6 Obstructed labor due to other multiple fetuses [M] ♀

O66.8 Other specified obstructed labor
Use additional code to identify cause of obstruction [M] ♀

O66.9 Obstructed labor, unspecified
Dystocia NOS
Fetal dystocia NOS
Maternal dystocia NOS [M] ♀

Unspecified Code | Other Specified Code | [N] Newborn Age: 0 | [P] Pediatric Age: 0-17 | [M] Maternity Age: 12-55
[A] Adult Age: 15-124 | ♂ Male | ♀ Female | ● New Code | ▲ Revised Code Title | ►◄ Revised Text

O67 Labor and delivery complicated by intrapartum hemorrhage, not elsewhere classified

> EXCLUDES1 antepartum hemorrhage NEC (O46.-)
> placenta previa (O44.-)
> premature separation of placenta [abruptio placentae] (O45.-)
>
> EXCLUDES2 postpartum hemorrhage (O72.-)

O67.0 Intrapartum hemorrhage with coagulation defect

Intrapartum hemorrhage (excessive) associated with afibrinogenemia

Intrapartum hemorrhage (excessive) associated with disseminated intravascular coagulation

Intrapartum hemorrhage (excessive) associated with hyperfibrinolysis

Intrapartum hemorrhage (excessive) associated with hypofibrinogenemia ♀

O67.8 Other intrapartum hemorrhage

Excessive intrapartum hemorrhage ♀

O67.9 Intrapartum hemorrhage, unspecified ♀

O68 Labor and delivery complicated by abnormality of fetal acid-base balance

Fetal acidemia complicating labor and delivery

Fetal acidosis complicating labor and delivery

Fetal alkalosis complicating labor and delivery

Fetal metabolic acidemia complicating labor and delivery

> EXCLUDES1 fetal stress NOS (O77.9)
> labor and delivery complicated by electrocardiographic evidence of fetal stress (O77.8)
> labor and delivery complicated by ultrasonic evidence of fetal stress (O77.8)
>
> EXCLUDES2 abnormality in fetal heart rate or rhythm (O76)
> labor and delivery complicated by meconium in amniotic fluid (O77.0) ♀

O69 Labor and delivery complicated by umbilical cord complications

One of the following 7th characters is to be assigned to each code under category O69. 7th character 0 is for single gestations and multiple gestations where the fetus is unspecified. 7th characters 1 through 9 are for cases of multiple gestations to identify the fetus for which the code applies. The appropriate code from category O30, Multiple gestation, must also be assigned when assigning a code from category O69 that has a 7th character of 1 through 9.

0 = not applicable or unspecified
1 = fetus 1
2 = fetus 2
3 = fetus 3
4 = fetus 4
5 = fetus 5
9 = other fetus

O69.0 Labor and delivery complicated by prolapse of cord

O69.1 Labor and delivery complicated by cord around neck, with compression

> EXCLUDES1 labor and delivery complicated by cord around neck, without compression (O69.81)

O69.2 Labor and delivery complicated by other cord entanglement, with compression

Labor and delivery complicated by compression of cord NOS

Labor and delivery complicated by entanglement of cords of twins in monoamniotic sac

Labor and delivery complicated by knot in cord

> EXCLUDES1 labor and delivery complicated by other cord entanglement, without compression (O69.82)

O69.3 Labor and delivery complicated by short cord

O69.4 Labor and delivery complicated by vasa previa

Labor and delivery complicated by hemorrhage from vasa previa

O69.5 Labor and delivery complicated by vascular lesion of cord

Labor and delivery complicated by cord bruising

Labor and delivery complicated by cord hematoma

Labor and delivery complicated by thrombosis of umbilical vessels

O69.8 Labor and delivery complicated by other cord complications

O69.81 Labor and delivery complicated by cord around neck, without compression

O69.82 Labor and delivery complicated by other cord entanglement, without compression

O69.89 Labor and delivery complicated by other cord complications

O69.9 Labor and delivery complicated by cord complication, unspecified

O70 Perineal laceration during delivery

> INCLUDES episiotomy extended by laceration
>
> EXCLUDES1 obstetric high vaginal laceration alone (O71.4)

O70.0 First degree perineal laceration during delivery

Perineal laceration, rupture or tear involving fourchette during delivery

Perineal laceration, rupture or tear involving labia during delivery

Perineal laceration, rupture or tear involving skin during delivery

Perineal laceration, rupture or tear involving vagina during delivery

Perineal laceration, rupture or tear involving vulva during delivery

Slight perineal laceration, rupture or tear during delivery ♀

O70.1 Second degree perineal laceration during delivery

Perineal laceration, rupture or tear during delivery as in O70.0, also involving pelvic floor

Perineal laceration, rupture or tear during delivery as in O70.0, also involving perineal muscles

Perineal laceration, rupture or tear during delivery as in O70.0, also involving vaginal muscles

> EXCLUDES1 perineal laceration involving anal sphincter (O70.2) ♀

O70.2 Third degree perineal laceration during delivery

Perineal laceration, rupture or tear during delivery as in O70.1, also involving anal sphincter

Perineal laceration, rupture or tear during delivery as in O70.1, also involving rectovaginal septum

Perineal laceration, rupture or tear during delivery as in O70.1, also involving sphincter NOS

> EXCLUDES1 anal sphincter tear during delivery without third degree perineal laceration (O70.4)
> perineal laceration involving anal or rectal mucosa (O70.3) ♀

O70.3 Fourth degree perineal laceration during delivery

Perineal laceration, rupture or tear during delivery as in O70.2, also involving anal mucosa

Perineal laceration, rupture or tear during delivery as in O70.2, also involving rectal mucosa ♀

O70.4 Anal sphincter tear complicating delivery, not associated with third degree laceration

> EXCLUDES1 anal sphincter tear with third degree perineal laceration (O70.2) ♀

O70.9 Perineal laceration during delivery, unspecified ♀

4th character required   5th character required   6th character required   7th character required   Extension 'X' Alert

EXCLUDES 1 Not coded here   EXCLUDES 2 Not included here   Primary Diagnosis Only   Manifestation Code

🔵 **O71 Other obstetric trauma**

INCLUDES *obstetric damage from instruments*

🔵 **O71.0 Rupture of uterus (spontaneous)** before onset of labor

EXCLUDES1 *disruption of (current) cesarean delivery wound (O90.0)*
laceration of uterus, NEC (O71.81)

O71.00 Rupture of uterus before onset of labor, unspecified trimester Ⓜ ♀

O71.02 Rupture of uterus before onset of labor, second trimester Ⓜ ♀

O71.03 Rupture of uterus before onset of labor, third trimester Ⓜ ♀

O71.1 Rupture of uterus during labor

Rupture of uterus not stated as occurring before onset of labor

EXCLUDES1 *disruption of cesarean delivery wound (O90.0)*
laceration of uterus, NEC (O71.81) Ⓜ ♀

O71.2 Postpartum inversion of uterus Ⓜ ♀

O71.3 Obstetric laceration of cervix

Annular detachment of cervix Ⓜ ♀

O71.4 Obstetric high vaginal laceration **alone**

Laceration of vaginal wall without perineal laceration

EXCLUDES1 *obstetric high vaginal laceration with perineal laceration (O70.-)* Ⓜ ♀

O71.5 Other obstetric injury to pelvic organs

Obstetric injury to bladder

Obstetric injury to urethra

EXCLUDES2 *obstetric periurethral trauma (O71.82)* Ⓜ ♀

O71.6 Obstetric damage to pelvic joints and ligaments

Obstetric avulsion of inner symphyseal cartilage

Obstetric damage to coccyx

Obstetric traumatic separation of symphysis (pubis) Ⓜ ♀

O71.7 Obstetric hematoma of pelvis

Obstetric hematoma of perineum

Obstetric hematoma of vagina

Obstetric hematoma of vulva Ⓜ ♀

🔵 **O71.8 Other specified obstetric trauma**

O71.81 Laceration of uterus, not elsewhere classified Ⓜ ♀

O71.82 Other specified trauma to perineum and vulva

Obstetric periurethral trauma Ⓜ ♀

O71.89 Other specified obstetric trauma Ⓜ ♀

O71.9 Obstetric trauma, unspecified Ⓜ ♀

🔵 **O72 Postpartum hemorrhage**

INCLUDES *hemorrhage after delivery of fetus or infant*

O72.0 Third-stage hemorrhage

Hemorrhage associated with retained, trapped or adherent placenta

Retained placenta NOS

Code also type of adherent placenta (O43.2-) Ⓜ ♀

O72.1 Other immediate postpartum hemorrhage

Hemorrhage following delivery of placenta

Postpartum hemorrhage (atonic) NOS

Uterine atony with hemorrhage

EXCLUDES1 *uterine atony NOS (O62.2)*
uterine atony without hemorrhage (O62.2)
postpartum atony of uterus without hemorrhage (O75.89) Ⓜ ♀

O72.2 Delayed and secondary postpartum hemorrhage

Hemorrhage associated with retained portions of placenta or membranes after the first 24 hours following delivery of placenta

Retained products of conception NOS, following delivery Ⓜ ♀

O72.3 Postpartum coagulation defects

Postpartum afibrinogenemia

Postpartum fibrinolysis Ⓜ ♀

🔵 **O73 Retained placenta and membranes, without hemorrhage**

EXCLUDES1 *placenta accreta (O43.21-)*
placenta increta (O43.22-)
placenta percreta (O43.23-)

O73.0 Retained placenta **without hemorrhage**

Adherent placenta, without hemorrhage

Trapped placenta without hemorrhage Ⓜ ♀

O73.1 Retained portions of placenta and membranes, **without hemorrhage**

Retained products of conception following delivery, without hemorrhage Ⓜ ♀

🔵 **O74 Complications of anesthesia during labor and delivery**

INCLUDES *maternal complications arising from the administration of a general, regional or local anesthetic, analgesic or other sedation during labor and delivery*

Use additional code, if applicable, to identify specific complication

O74.0 Aspiration pneumonitis due to anesthesia during labor and delivery

Inhalation of stomach contents or secretions NOS due to anesthesia during labor and delivery

Mendelson's syndrome due to anesthesia during labor and delivery Ⓜ ♀

O74.1 Other pulmonary complications of anesthesia during labor and delivery Ⓜ ♀

O74.2 Cardiac complications of anesthesia during labor and delivery Ⓜ ♀

O74.3 Central nervous system complications of anesthesia during labor and delivery Ⓜ ♀

O74.4 Toxic reaction to local anesthesia during labor and delivery Ⓜ ♀

O74.5 Spinal and epidural anesthesia-induced headache during labor and delivery Ⓜ ♀

O74.6 Other complications of spinal and epidural anesthesia **during labor and delivery** Ⓜ ♀

O74.7 Failed or difficult intubation for anesthesia during labor and delivery Ⓜ ♀

O74.8 Other complications of anesthesia during labor and delivery Ⓜ ♀

O74.9 Complication of anesthesia during labor and delivery, unspecified Ⓜ ♀

🔵 **O75 Other complications of labor and delivery, not elsewhere classified**

EXCLUDES2 *puerperal (postpartum) infection (O86.-)*
puerperal (postpartum) sepsis (O85)

O75.0 Maternal distress during labor and delivery Ⓜ ♀

O75.1 Shock during or following labor and delivery

Obstetric shock following labor and delivery Ⓜ ♀

O75.2 Pyrexia during labor, not elsewhere classified Ⓜ ♀

O75.3 Other infection during labor

Sepsis during labor

Use additional code (B95-B97), to identify infectious agent Ⓜ ♀

O75.4 Other complications of obstetric surgery and procedures

Cardiac arrest following obstetric surgery or procedures

Cardiac failure following obstetric surgery or procedures

Cerebral anoxia following obstetric surgery or procedures

Pulmonary edema following obstetric surgery or procedures

Use additional code to identify specific complication

EXCLUDES2 *complications of anesthesia during labor and delivery (O74.-)*
disruption of obstetrical (surgical) wound (O90.0-O90.1)
hematoma of obstetrical (surgical) wound (O90.2)
infection of obstetrical (surgical) wound (O86.0) Ⓜ ♀

Unspecified Code	Other Specified Code	Ⓝ Newborn Age: 0	Ⓟ Pediatric Age: 0-17	Ⓜ Maternity Age: 12-55
Ⓐ Adult Age: 15-124	♂ Male	♀ Female	● New Code	▲ Revised Code Title	►◄ Revised Text

O75.5 Delayed delivery after artificial rupture of membranes [M] ♀

[5] O75.8 Other specified complications of labor and delivery

O75.81 Maternal exhaustion complicating labor and delivery [M] ♀

O75.82 Onset (spontaneous) of labor after 37 completed weeks of gestation but before 39 completed weeks gestation, with delivery by (planned) cesarean section

Delivery by (planned) cesarean section occurring after 37 completed weeks of gestation but before 39 completed weeks gestation due to (spontaneous) onset of labor

Code first to specify reason for planned cesarean section such as: cephalopelvic disproportion (normally formed fetus) (O33.9) previous cesarean delivery (O34.21) [M] ♀

O75.89 Other specified complications of labor and delivery [M] ♀

O75.9 Complication of labor and delivery, unspecified [M] ♀

O76 Abnormality in fetal heart rate and rhythm complicating labor and delivery

Depressed fetal heart rate tones complicating labor and delivery

Fetal bradycardia complicating labor and delivery

Fetal heart rate decelerations complicating labor and delivery

Fetal heart rate irregularity complicating labor and delivery

Fetal heart rate abnormal variability complicating labor and delivery

Fetal tachycardia complicating labor and delivery

Non-reassuring fetal heart rate or rhythm complicating labor and delivery

[EXCLUDES1] *fetal stress NOS (O77.9)*
labor and delivery complicated by electrocardiographic evidence of fetal stress (O77.8)
labor and delivery complicated by ultrasonic evidence of fetal stress (O77.8)

[EXCLUDES2] *fetal metabolic acidemia (O68)*
other fetal stress (O77.0-O77.1) [M] ♀

[4] O77 Other fetal stress complicating labor and delivery

O77.0 Labor and delivery complicated by meconium in amniotic fluid [M] ♀

O77.1 Fetal stress in labor or delivery due to drug administration [M] ♀

O77.8 Labor and delivery complicated by other evidence of fetal stress

Labor and delivery complicated by electrocardiographic evidence of fetal stress

Labor and delivery complicated by ultrasonic evidence of fetal stress

[EXCLUDES1] *abnormality of fetal acid-base balance (O68)*
abnormality in fetal heart rate or rhythm (O76)
fetal metabolic acidemia (O68) [M] ♀

O77.9 Labor and delivery complicated by fetal stress, unspecified

[EXCLUDES1] *abnormality of fetal acid-base balance (O68)*
abnormality in fetal heart rate or rhythm (O76)
fetal metabolic acidemia (O68) [M] ♀

Encounter for delivery (O80, O82)

O80 Encounter for full-term uncomplicated delivery

Delivery requiring minimal or no assistance, with or without episiotomy, without fetal manipulation [e.g., rotation version] or instrumentation [forceps] of a spontaneous, cephalic, vaginal, full-term, single, live-born infant. This code is for use as a single diagnosis code and is not to be used with any other code from chapter 15.

Use additional code to indicate outcome of delivery (Z37.0) ♀

O82 Encounter for cesarean delivery without indication

Use additional code to indicate outcome of delivery (Z37.0) ♀

Complications predominantly related to the puerperium (O85-O92)

[EXCLUDES2] *mental and behavioral disorders associated with the puerperium (F53)*
obstetrical tetanus (A34)
puerperal osteomalacia (M83.0)

O85 Puerperal sepsis

Postpartum sepsis

Puerperal peritonitis

Puerperal pyemia

Use additional code (B95-B97), to identify infectious agent

code (R65.2-) to identify severe sepsis, if applicable

[EXCLUDES1] *fever of unknown origin following delivery (O86.4)*
genital tract infection following delivery (O86.1-)
obstetric pyemic and septic embolism (O88.3-)
puerperal septic thrombophlebitis (O86.81)
urinary tract infection following delivery (O86.2-)

[EXCLUDES2] *sepsis during labor (O75.3)* [M] ♀

[4] O86 Other puerperal infections

Use additional code (B95-B97), to identify infectious agent

[EXCLUDES2] *infection during labor (O75.3)*
obstetrical tetanus (A34)

O86.0 Infection of obstetric surgical wound

Infected cesarean delivery wound following delivery

Infected perineal repair following delivery [M] ♀

[5] O86.1 Other infection of genital tract following delivery

O86.11 Cervicitis following delivery [M] ♀

O86.12 Endometritis following delivery [M] ♀

O86.13 Vaginitis following delivery [M] ♀

O86.19 Other infection of genital tract following delivery [M] ♀

[5] O86.2 Urinary tract infection following delivery

O86.20 Urinary tract infection following delivery, unspecified

Puerperal urinary tract infection NOS [M] ♀

O86.21 Infection of kidney following delivery [M] ♀

O86.22 Infection of bladder following delivery

Infection of urethra following delivery [M] ♀

O86.29 Other urinary tract infection following delivery [M] ♀

O86.4 Pyrexia of unknown origin following delivery

Puerperal infection NOS following delivery

Puerperal pyrexia NOS following delivery

[EXCLUDES2] *pyrexia during labor (O75.2)* [M] ♀

[5] O86.8 Other specified puerperal infections

O86.81 Puerperal septic thrombophlebitis [M] ♀

O86.89 Other specified puerperal infections [M] ♀

[4] 4th character required [5] 5th character required [6] 6th character required [7] 7th character required [x7] Extension 'X' Alert
[EXCLUDES1] Not coded here [EXCLUDES2] Not included here [Pdx] Primary Diagnosis Only Manifestation Code

○ O87 Venous complications and hemorrhoids in the puerperium

INCLUDES venous complications in labor, delivery and the puerperium

EXCLUDES2 obstetric embolism (O88.-)
puerperal septic thrombophlebitis (O86.81)
venous complications in pregnancy (O22.-)

O87.0 Superficial thrombophlebitis in the puerperium
Puerperal phlebitis NOS
Puerperal thrombosis NOS Ⓜ ♀

O87.1 Deep phlebothrombosis in the puerperium
Deep vein thrombosis, postpartum
Pelvic thrombophlebitis, postpartum
Use additional code to identify the deep vein thrombosis (I82.4-, I82.5-, I82.62-. I82.72-)
code, if applicable, for associated long-term (current) use of anticoagulants (Z79.01) Ⓜ ♀

O87.2 Hemorrhoids in the puerperium Ⓜ ♀

O87.3 Cerebral venous thrombosis in the puerperium
Cerebrovenous sinus thrombosis in the puerperium Ⓜ ♀

O87.4 Varicose veins of lower extremity in the puerperium Ⓜ ♀

O87.8 Other venous complications in the puerperium
Genital varices in the puerperium Ⓜ ♀

O87.9 Venous complication in the puerperium, unspecified
Puerperal phlebopathy NOS Ⓜ ♀

○ O88 Obstetric embolism

EXCLUDES1 embolism complicating abortion NOS (O03.2)
embolism complicating ectopic or molar pregnancy (O08.2)
embolism complicating failed attempted abortion (O07.2)
embolism complicating induced abortion (O04.7)
embolism complicating spontaneous abortion (O03.2, O03.7)

○ O88.0 Obstetric air embolism
○ O88.01 Obstetric air embolism in pregnancy
O88.011 Air embolism in pregnancy, first trimester Ⓜ ♀
O88.012 Air embolism in pregnancy, second trimester Ⓜ ♀
O88.013 Air embolism in pregnancy, third trimester Ⓜ ♀
O88.019 Air embolism in pregnancy, unspecified trimester Ⓜ ♀
O88.02 Air embolism in childbirth Ⓜ ♀
O88.03 Air embolism in the puerperium Ⓜ ♀

○ O88.1 Amniotic fluid embolism
Anaphylactoid syndrome in pregnancy
○ O88.11 Amniotic fluid embolism in pregnancy
O88.111 Amniotic fluid embolism in pregnancy, first trimester Ⓜ ♀
O88.112 Amniotic fluid embolism in pregnancy, second trimester Ⓜ ♀
O88.113 Amniotic fluid embolism in pregnancy, third trimester Ⓜ ♀
O88.119 Amniotic fluid embolism in pregnancy, unspecified trimester Ⓜ ♀
O88.12 Amniotic fluid embolism in childbirth Ⓜ ♀
O88.13 Amniotic fluid embolism in the puerperium Ⓜ ♀

○ O88.2 Obstetric thromboembolism
○ O88.21 Thromboembolism in pregnancy
Obstetric (pulmonary) embolism NOS
O88.211 Thromboembolism in pregnancy, first trimester Ⓜ ♀
O88.212 Thromboembolism in pregnancy, second trimester ♀

O88.213 Thromboembolism in pregnancy, third trimester Ⓜ ♀
O88.219 Thromboembolism in pregnancy, unspecified trimester Ⓜ ♀
O88.22 Thromboembolism in childbirth Ⓜ ♀
O88.23 Thromboembolism in the puerperium
Puerperal (pulmonary) embolism NOS Ⓜ ♀

○ O88.3 Obstetric pyemic and septic embolism
○ O88.31 Pyemic and septic embolism in pregnancy
O88.311 Pyemic and septic embolism in pregnancy, first trimester Ⓜ ♀
O88.312 Pyemic and septic embolism in pregnancy, second trimester Ⓜ ♀
O88.313 Pyemic and septic embolism in pregnancy, third trimester Ⓜ ♀
O88.319 Pyemic and septic embolism in pregnancy, unspecified trimester Ⓜ ♀
O88.32 Pyemic and septic embolism in childbirth Ⓜ ♀
O88.33 Pyemic and septic embolism in the puerperium Ⓜ ♀

○ O88.8 Other obstetric embolism
Obstetric fat embolism
○ O88.81 Other embolism in pregnancy
O88.811 Other embolism in pregnancy, first trimester Ⓜ ♀
O88.812 Other embolism in pregnancy, second trimester Ⓜ ♀
O88.813 Other embolism in pregnancy, third trimester Ⓜ ♀
O88.819 Other embolism in pregnancy, unspecified trimester Ⓜ ♀
O88.82 Other embolism in childbirth Ⓜ ♀
O88.83 Other embolism in the puerperium Ⓜ ♀

○ O89 Complications of anesthesia during the puerperium

INCLUDES maternal complications arising from the administration of a general, regional or local anesthetic, analgesic or other sedation during the puerperium

Use additional code, if applicable, to identify specific complication

○ O89.0 Pulmonary complications of anesthesia during the puerperium
O89.01 Aspiration pneumonitis due to anesthesia during the puerperium
Inhalation of stomach contents or secretions NOS due to anesthesia during the puerperium
Mendelson's syndrome due to anesthesia during the puerperium Ⓜ ♀
O89.09 Other pulmonary complications of anesthesia during the puerperium Ⓜ ♀

O89.1 Cardiac complications of anesthesia during the puerperium Ⓜ ♀

O89.2 Central nervous system complications of anesthesia during the puerperium Ⓜ ♀

O89.3 Toxic reaction to local anesthesia during the puerperium Ⓜ ♀

O89.4 Spinal and epidural anesthesia-induced headache during the puerperium Ⓜ ♀

O89.5 Other complications of spinal and epidural anesthesia during the puerperium Ⓜ ♀

O89.6 Failed or difficult intubation for anesthesia during the puerperium Ⓜ ♀

O89.8 Other complications of anesthesia during the puerperium Ⓜ ♀

O89.9 Complication of anesthesia during the puerperium, unspecified Ⓜ ♀

Unspecified Code	Other Specified Code	Ⓝ Newborn Age: 0	Ⓟ Pediatric Age: 0-17	Ⓜ Maternity Age: 12-55
Ⓐ Adult Age: 15-124	♂ Male	♀ Female	● New Code	▲ Revised Code Title	►◄ Revised Text

[4] O90 Complications of the puerperium, not elsewhere classified
O90.0 Disruption of cesarean delivery wound
Dehiscence of cesarean delivery wound
EXCLUDES1 *rupture of uterus (spontaneous) before onset of labor (O71.0-)*
rupture of uterus during labor (O71.1) [M] ♀
O90.1 Disruption of perineal obstetric wound
Disruption of wound of episiotomy
Disruption of wound of perineal laceration
Secondary perineal tear [M] ♀
O90.2 Hematoma of obstetric wound [M] ♀
O90.3 Peripartum cardiomyopathy
Conditions in I42.- arising during pregnancy and the puerperium
EXCLUDES1 *pre-existing heart disease complicating pregnancy and the puerperium (O99.4-)* [M] ♀
O90.4 Postpartum acute kidney failure
Hepatorenal syndrome following labor and delivery [M] ♀
O90.5 Postpartum thyroiditis [M] ♀
O90.6 Postpartum mood disturbance
Postpartum blues
Postpartum dysphoria
Postpartum sadness
EXCLUDES1 *postpartum depression (F53)*
puerperal psychosis (F53) [M] ♀
[5] O90.8 Other complications of the puerperium, not elsewhere classified
O90.81 Anemia of the puerperium
Postpartum anemia NOS
EXCLUDES1 *pre-existing anemia complicating the puerperium (O99.03)* [M] ♀
O90.89 Other complications of the puerperium, not elsewhere classified
Placental polyp [M] ♀
O90.9 Complication of the puerperium, unspecified [M] ♀
[4] O91 Infections of breast associated with pregnancy, the puerperium and lactation
Use additional code to identify infection
[5] O91.0 Infection of nipple associated with pregnancy, the puerperium and lactation
[6] O91.01 Infection of nipple associated with pregnancy
Gestational abscess of nipple
O91.011 Infection of nipple associated with pregnancy, first trimester [M] ♀
O91.012 Infection of nipple associated with pregnancy, second trimester [M] ♀
O91.013 Infection of nipple associated with pregnancy, third trimester [M] ♀
O91.019 Infection of nipple associated with pregnancy, unspecified trimester [M] ♀
O91.02 Infection of nipple associated with the puerperium
Puerperal abscess of nipple [M] ♀
O91.03 Infection of nipple associated with lactation
Abscess of nipple associated with lactation [M] ♀
[5] O91.1 Abscess of breast associated with pregnancy, the puerperium and lactation
[6] O91.11 Abscess of breast associated with pregnancy
Gestational mammary abscess
Gestational purulent mastitis
Gestational subareolar abscess
O91.111 Abscess of breast associated with pregnancy, first trimester [M] ♀
O91.112 Abscess of breast associated with pregnancy, second trimester [M] ♀
O91.113 Abscess of breast associated with pregnancy, third trimester [M] ♀
O91.119 Abscess of breast associated with pregnancy, unspecified trimester [M] ♀
O91.12 Abscess of breast associated with the puerperium
Puerperal mammary abscess
Puerperal purulent mastitis
Puerperal subareolar abscess [M] ♀
O91.13 Abscess of breast associated with lactation
Mammary abscess associated with lactation
Purulent mastitis associated with lactation
Subareolar abscess associated with lactation [M] ♀
[5] O91.2 Nonpurulent mastitis associated with pregnancy, the puerperium and lactation
[6] O91.21 Nonpurulent mastitis associated with pregnancy
Gestational interstitial mastitis
Gestational lymphangitis of breast
Gestational mastitis NOS
Gestational parenchymatous mastitis
O91.211 Nonpurulent mastitis associated with pregnancy, first trimester [M] ♀
O91.212 Nonpurulent mastitis associated with pregnancy, second trimester [M] ♀
O91.213 Nonpurulent mastitis associated with pregnancy, third trimester [M] ♀
O91.219 Nonpurulent mastitis associated with pregnancy, unspecified trimester [M] ♀
O91.22 Nonpurulent mastitis associated with the puerperium
Puerperal interstitial mastitis
Puerperal lymphangitis of breast
Puerperal mastitis NOS
Puerperal parenchymatous mastitis [M] ♀
O91.23 Nonpurulent mastitis associated with lactation
Interstitial mastitis associated with lactation
Lymphangitis of breast associated with lactation
Mastitis NOS associated with lactation
Parenchymatous mastitis associated with lactation [M] ♀
[4] O92 Other disorders of breast and disorders of lactation associated with pregnancy and the puerperium
[5] O92.0 Retracted nipple associated with pregnancy, the puerperium, and lactation
[6] O92.01 Retracted nipple associated with pregnancy
O92.011 Retracted nipple associated with pregnancy, first trimester [M] ♀
O92.012 Retracted nipple associated with pregnancy, second trimester [M] ♀
O92.013 Retracted nipple associated with pregnancy, third trimester [M] ♀
O92.019 Retracted nipple associated with pregnancy, unspecified trimester [M] ♀
O92.02 Retracted nipple associated with the puerperium [M] ♀
O92.03 Retracted nipple associated with lactation [M] ♀
[5] O92.1 Cracked nipple associated with pregnancy, the puerperium, and lactation
Fissure of nipple, gestational or puerperal
[6] O92.11 Cracked nipple associated with pregnancy
O92.111 Cracked nipple associated with pregnancy, first trimester [M] ♀
O92.112 Cracked nipple associated with pregnancy, second trimester [M] ♀
O92.113 Cracked nipple associated with pregnancy, third trimester [M] ♀
O92.119 Cracked nipple associated with pregnancy, unspecified trimester [M] ♀
O92.12 Cracked nipple associated with the puerperium [M] ♀
O92.13 Cracked nipple associated with lactation [M] ♀

[4] 4th character required [5] 5th character required [6] 6th character required [7] 7th character required [7th] Extension 'X' Alert
EXCLUDES1 Not coded here EXCLUDES2 Not included here [PDx] Primary Diagnosis Only Manifestation Code

[5] O92.2 Other and unspecified disorders of breast associated with pregnancy and the puerperium
O92.20 Unspecified disorder of breast associated with pregnancy and the puerperium [M] ♀
O92.29 Other disorders of breast associated with pregnancy and the puerperium [M] ♀
O92.3 Agalactia
Primary agalactia
EXCLUDES1 *Elective agalactia (O92.5)*
Secondary agalactia (O92.5)
Therapeutic agalactia (O92.5) [M] ♀
O92.4 Hypogalactia [M] ♀
O92.5 Suppressed lactation
Elective agalactia
Secondary agalactia
Therapeutic agalactia
EXCLUDES1 *primary agalactia (O92.3)* [M] ♀
O92.6 Galactorrhea [M] ♀
[5] O92.7 Other and unspecified disorders of lactation
O92.70 Unspecified disorders of lactation [M] ♀
O92.79 Other disorders of lactation
Puerperal galactocele [M] ♀

Other obstetric conditions, not elsewhere classified (O94-O9A)

O94 Sequelae of complication of pregnancy, childbirth, and the puerperium
NOTES This category is to be used to indicate conditions in O00-O77.-, O85-O94 and O98-O9A.- as the cause of late effects. The sequelae include conditions specified as such, or as late effects, which may occur at any time after the puerperium
Code first condition resulting from (sequela) of complication of pregnancy, childbirth, and the puerperium [M] ♀
[4] O98 Maternal infectious and parasitic diseases classifiable elsewhere but complicating pregnancy, childbirth and the puerperium
INCLUDES *the listed conditions when complicating the pregnant state, when aggravated by the pregnancy, or as a reason for obstetric care*
Use additional code (Chapter 1), to identify specific infectious or parasitic disease
EXCLUDES2 *herpes gestationis (O26.4-)*
infectious carrier state (O99.82-, O99.83-)
obstetrical tetanus (A34)
puerperal infection (O86.-)
puerperal sepsis (O85)
when the reason for maternal care is that the disease is known or suspected to have affected the fetus (O35-O36)
[5] O98.0 Tuberculosis complicating pregnancy, childbirth and the puerperium
Conditions in A15-A19
[6] O98.01 Tuberculosis complicating pregnancy
O98.011 Tuberculosis complicating pregnancy, first trimester [M] ♀
O98.012 Tuberculosis complicating pregnancy, second trimester [M] ♀
O98.013 Tuberculosis complicating pregnancy, third trimester [M] ♀
O98.019 Tuberculosis complicating pregnancy, unspecified trimester [M] ♀
O98.02 Tuberculosis complicating childbirth [M] ♀
O98.03 Tuberculosis complicating the puerperium [M] ♀
[5] O98.1 Syphilis complicating pregnancy, childbirth and the puerperium
Conditions in A50-A53
[6] O98.11 Syphilis complicating pregnancy
O98.111 Syphilis complicating pregnancy, first trimester [M] ♀
O98.112 Syphilis complicating pregnancy, second trimester [M] ♀
O98.113 Syphilis complicating pregnancy, third trimester [M] ♀
O98.119 Syphilis complicating pregnancy, unspecified trimester [M] ♀
O98.12 Syphilis complicating childbirth [M] ♀
O98.13 Syphilis complicating the puerperium [M] ♀
[5] O98.2 Gonorrhea complicating pregnancy, childbirth and the puerperium
Conditions in A54.-
[6] O98.21 Gonorrhea complicating pregnancy
O98.211 Gonorrhea complicating pregnancy, first trimester [M] ♀
O98.212 Gonorrhea complicating pregnancy, second trimester [M] ♀
O98.213 Gonorrhea complicating pregnancy, third trimester [M] ♀
O98.219 Gonorrhea complicating pregnancy, unspecified trimester [M] ♀
O98.22 Gonorrhea complicating childbirth [M] ♀
O98.23 Gonorrhea complicating the puerperium [M] ♀
[5] O98.3 Other infections with a predominantly sexual mode of transmission complicating pregnancy, childbirth and the puerperium
Conditions in A55-A64
[6] O98.31 Other infections with a predominantly sexual mode of transmission complicating pregnancy
O98.311 Other infections with a predominantly sexual mode of transmission complicating pregnancy, first trimester [M] ♀
O98.312 Other infections with a predominantly sexual mode of transmission complicating pregnancy, second trimester [M] ♀
O98.313 Other infections with a predominantly sexual mode of transmission complicating pregnancy, third trimester [M] ♀
O98.319 Other infections with a predominantly sexual mode of transmission complicating pregnancy, unspecified trimester [M] ♀
O98.32 Other infections with a predominantly sexual mode of transmission complicating childbirth [M] ♀
O98.33 Other infections with a predominantly sexual mode of transmission complicating the puerperium [M] ♀
[5] O98.4 Viral hepatitis complicating pregnancy, childbirth and the puerperium
Conditions in B15-B19
[6] O98.41 Viral hepatitis complicating pregnancy
O98.411 Viral hepatitis complicating pregnancy, first trimester [M] ♀
O98.412 Viral hepatitis complicating pregnancy, second trimester [M] ♀
O98.413 Viral hepatitis complicating pregnancy, third trimester [M] ♀
O98.419 Viral hepatitis complicating pregnancy, unspecified trimester [M] ♀
O98.42 Viral hepatitis complicating childbirth [M] ♀
O98.43 Viral hepatitis complicating the puerperium [M] ♀
[5] O98.5 Other viral diseases complicating pregnancy, childbirth and the puerperium
Conditions in A80-B09, B25-B34, R87.81-, R87.82-
EXCLUDES1 *human immunodeficiency virus [HIV] disease complicating pregnancy, childbirth and the puerperium (O98.7-)*
[6] O98.51 Other viral diseases complicating pregnancy

Unspecified Code | Other Specified Code | [N] Newborn Age: 0 | [P] Pediatric Age: 0-17 | [M] Maternity Age: 12-55
[A] Adult Age: 15-124 | ♂ Male | ♀ Female | ● New Code | ▲ Revised Code Title | ►◄ Revised Text

O98.511 Other viral diseases complicating pregnancy, first trimester   M ♀

O98.512 Other viral diseases complicating pregnancy, second trimester   M ♀

O98.513 Other viral diseases complicating pregnancy, third trimester   M ♀

O98.519 Other viral diseases complicating pregnancy, unspecified trimester   M ♀

O98.52 Other viral diseases complicating childbirth   M ♀

O98.53 Other viral diseases complicating the puerperium   M ♀

⑤ O98.6 Protozoal diseases complicating pregnancy, childbirth and the puerperium

Conditions in B50-B64

⑥ O98.61 Protozoal diseases complicating pregnancy

O98.611 Protozoal diseases complicating pregnancy, first trimester   M ♀

O98.612 Protozoal diseases complicating pregnancy, second trimester   M ♀

O98.613 Protozoal diseases complicating pregnancy, third trimester   M ♀

O98.619 Protozoal diseases complicating pregnancy, unspecified trimester   M ♀

O98.62 Protozoal diseases complicating childbirth   M ♀

O98.63 Protozoal diseases complicating the puerperium   M ♀

⑤ O98.7 Human immunodeficiency virus [HIV] disease complicating pregnancy, childbirth and the puerperium

Use additional code to identify the type of HIV disease:
Acquired immune deficiency syndrome (AIDS) (B20)
Asymptomatic HIV status (Z21)
HIV positive NOS (Z21)
Symptomatic HIV disease (B20)

⑥ O98.71 Human immunodeficiency virus [HIV] disease complicating pregnancy

O98.711 Human immunodeficiency virus [HIV] disease complicating pregnancy, first trimester   M ♀

O98.712 Human immunodeficiency virus [HIV] disease complicating pregnancy, second trimester   M ♀

O98.713 Human immunodeficiency virus [HIV] disease complicating pregnancy, third trimester   M ♀

O98.719 Human immunodeficiency virus [HIV] disease complicating pregnancy, unspecified trimester   M ♀

O98.72 Human immunodeficiency virus [HIV] disease complicating childbirth   M ♀

O98.73 Human immunodeficiency virus [HIV] disease complicating the puerperium   M ♀

⑤ O98.8 Other maternal infectious and parasitic diseases complicating pregnancy, childbirth and the puerperium

⑥ O98.81 Other maternal infectious and parasitic diseases complicating pregnancy

O98.811 Other maternal infectious and parasitic diseases complicating pregnancy, first trimester   M ♀

O98.812 Other maternal infectious and parasitic diseases complicating pregnancy, second trimester   M ♀

O98.813 Other maternal infectious and parasitic diseases complicating pregnancy, third trimester   M ♀

O98.819 Other maternal infectious and parasitic diseases complicating pregnancy, unspecified trimester   M ♀

O98.82 Other maternal infectious and parasitic diseases complicating childbirth   M ♀

O98.83 Other maternal infectious and parasitic diseases complicating the puerperium   M ♀

⑤ O98.9 Unspecified maternal infectious and parasitic disease complicating pregnancy, childbirth and the puerperium

⑥ O98.91 Unspecified maternal infectious and parasitic disease complicating pregnancy

O98.911 Unspecified maternal infectious and parasitic disease complicating pregnancy, first trimester   M ♀

O98.912 Unspecified maternal infectious and parasitic disease complicating pregnancy, second trimester   M ♀

O98.913 Unspecified maternal infectious and parasitic disease complicating pregnancy, third trimester   M ♀

O98.919 Unspecified maternal infectious and parasitic disease complicating pregnancy, unspecified trimester   M ♀

O98.92 Unspecified maternal infectious and parasitic disease complicating childbirth   M ♀

O98.93 Unspecified maternal infectious and parasitic disease complicating the puerperium   M ♀

④ O99 Other maternal diseases classifiable elsewhere but complicating pregnancy, childbirth and the puerperium

INCLUDES   conditions which complicate the pregnant state, are aggravated by the pregnancy or are a main reason for obstetric care

Use additional code to identify specific condition

EXCLUDES2   when the reason for maternal care is that the condition is known or suspected to have affected the fetus (O35-O36)

⑤ O99.0 Anemia complicating pregnancy, childbirth and the puerperium

Conditions in D50-D64

EXCLUDES1   anemia arising in the puerperium (O90.81)
postpartum anemia NOS (O90.81)

⑥ O99.01 Anemia complicating pregnancy

O99.011 Anemia complicating pregnancy, first trimester   M ♀

O99.012 Anemia complicating pregnancy, second trimester   M ♀

O99.013 Anemia complicating pregnancy, third trimester   M ♀

O99.019 Anemia complicating pregnancy, unspecified trimester   M ♀

O99.02 Anemia complicating childbirth   M ♀

O99.03 Anemia complicating the puerperium

EXCLUDES1   postpartum anemia not pre-existing prior to delivery (O90.81)   M ♀

⑤ O99.1 Other diseases of the blood and blood-forming organs and certain disorders involving the immune mechanism complicating pregnancy, childbirth and the puerperium

Conditions in D65-D89

EXCLUDES2   hemorrhage with coagulation defects (O45.-, O46.0-, O67.0, O72.3)

⑥ O99.11 Other diseases of the blood and blood-forming organs and certain disorders involving the immune mechanism complicating pregnancy

O99.111 Other diseases of the blood and blood-forming organs and certain disorders involving the immune mechanism

---

④ 4th character required   ⑤ 5th character required   ⑥ 6th character required   ⑦ 7th character required   ⑩ Extension 'X' Alert

EXCLUDES 1 Not coded here   EXCLUDES 2 Not included here   PDx Primary Diagnosis Only   Manifestation Code

ICD-10-CM 2015

complicating pregnancy, first trimester [M] ♀

O99.112 Other diseases of the blood and blood-forming organs and certain disorders involving the immune mechanism complicating pregnancy, second trimester [M] ♀

O99.113 Other diseases of the blood and blood-forming organs and certain disorders involving the immune mechanism complicating pregnancy, third trimester [M] ♀

O99.119 Other diseases of the blood and blood-forming organs and certain disorders involving the immune mechanism complicating pregnancy, unspecified trimester [M] ♀

O99.12 Other diseases of the blood and blood-forming organs and certain disorders involving the immune mechanism complicating childbirth [M] ♀

O99.13 Other diseases of the blood and blood-forming organs and certain disorders involving the immune mechanism complicating the puerperium [M] ♀

[5] O99.2 Endocrine, nutritional and metabolic diseases complicating pregnancy, childbirth and the puerperium

Conditions in E00-E88

[EXCLUDES2] *diabetes mellitus (O24.-)*
malnutrition (O25.-)
postpartum thyroiditis (O90.5)

[6] O99.21 Obesity complicating pregnancy, childbirth, and the puerperium

Use additional code to identify the type of obesity (E66.-)

O99.210 Obesity complicating pregnancy, unspecified trimester [M] ♀

O99.211 Obesity complicating pregnancy, first trimester [M] ♀

O99.212 Obesity complicating pregnancy, second trimester [M] ♀

O99.213 Obesity complicating pregnancy, third trimester [M] ♀

O99.214 Obesity complicating childbirth [M] ♀

O99.215 Obesity complicating the puerperium [M] ♀

[6] O99.28 Other endocrine, nutritional and metabolic diseases complicating pregnancy, childbirth and the puerperium

O99.280 Endocrine, nutritional and metabolic diseases complicating pregnancy, unspecified trimester [M] ♀

O99.281 Endocrine, nutritional and metabolic diseases complicating pregnancy, first trimester [M] ♀

O99.282 Endocrine, nutritional and metabolic diseases complicating pregnancy, second trimester [M] ♀

O99.283 Endocrine, nutritional and metabolic diseases complicating pregnancy, third trimester [M] ♀

O99.284 Endocrine, nutritional and metabolic diseases complicating childbirth [M] ♀

O99.285 Endocrine, nutritional and metabolic diseases complicating the puerperium [M] ♀

[5] O99.3 Mental disorders and diseases of the nervous system complicating pregnancy, childbirth and the puerperium

[6] O99.31 Alcohol use complicating pregnancy, childbirth, and the puerperium

Use additional code(s) from F10 to identify manifestations of the alcohol use

O99.310 Alcohol use complicating pregnancy, unspecified trimester [M] ♀

O99.311 Alcohol use complicating pregnancy, first trimester [M] ♀

O99.312 Alcohol use complicating pregnancy, second trimester [M] ♀

O99.313 Alcohol use complicating pregnancy, third trimester [M] ♀

O99.314 Alcohol use complicating childbirth [M] ♀

O99.315 Alcohol use complicating the puerperium [M] ♀

[6] O99.32 Drug use complicating pregnancy, childbirth, and the puerperium

Use additional code(s) from F11-F16 and F18-F19 to identify manifestations of the drug use

O99.320 Drug use complicating pregnancy, unspecified trimester [M] ♀

O99.321 Drug use complicating pregnancy, first trimester [M] ♀

O99.322 Drug use complicating pregnancy, second trimester [M] ♀

O99.323 Drug use complicating pregnancy, third trimester [M] ♀

O99.324 Drug use complicating childbirth [M] ♀

O99.325 Drug use complicating the puerperium [M] ♀

[6] O99.33 Smoking (tobacco) complicating pregnancy, childbirth, and the puerperium

Use additional code from F17 to identify type of tobacco

O99.330 Smoking (tobacco) complicating pregnancy, unspecified trimester [M] ♀

O99.331 Smoking (tobacco) complicating pregnancy, first trimester [M] ♀

O99.332 Smoking (tobacco) complicating pregnancy, second trimester [M] ♀

O99.333 Smoking (tobacco) complicating pregnancy, third trimester [M] ♀

O99.334 Smoking (tobacco) complicating childbirth [M] ♀

O99.335 Smoking (tobacco) complicating the puerperium [M] ♀

[6] O99.34 Other mental disorders complicating pregnancy, childbirth, and the puerperium

Conditions in F01-F09 and F20-F99

[EXCLUDES2] *postpartum mood disturbance (O90.6)*
postnatal psychosis (F53)
puerperal psychosis (F53)

O99.340 Other mental disorders complicating pregnancy, unspecified trimester [M] ♀

O99.341 Other mental disorders complicating pregnancy, first trimester [M] ♀

O99.342 Other mental disorders complicating pregnancy, second trimester [M] ♀

O99.343 Other mental disorders complicating pregnancy, third trimester [M] ♀

O99.344 Other mental disorders complicating childbirth [M] ♀

O99.345 Other mental disorders complicating the puerperium [M] ♀

Unspecified Code | Other Specified Code | [N] Newborn Age: 0 | [P] Pediatric Age: 0-17 | [M] Maternity Age: 12-55
[A] Adult Age: 15-124 | ♂ Male | ♀ Female | ● New Code | ▲ Revised Code Title | ►◄ Revised Text

[6] **O99.35 Diseases of the nervous system complicating pregnancy, childbirth, and the puerperium**
Conditions in G00-G99
[EXCLUDES2] *pregnancy related peripheral neuritis (O26.8-)*
O99.350 Diseases of the nervous system complicating pregnancy, unspecified trimester [M] ♀
O99.351 Diseases of the nervous system complicating pregnancy, first trimester [M] ♀
O99.352 Diseases of the nervous system complicating pregnancy, second trimester [M] ♀
O99.353 Diseases of the nervous system complicating pregnancy, third trimester [M] ♀
O99.354 Diseases of the nervous system complicating childbirth [M] ♀
O99.355 Diseases of the nervous system complicating the puerperium [M] ♀

[5] **O99.4 Diseases of the circulatory system complicating pregnancy, childbirth and the puerperium**
Conditions in I00-I99
[EXCLUDES1] *peripartum cardiomyopathy (O90.3)*
[EXCLUDES2] *hypertensive disorders (O10-O16)*
obstetric embolism (O88.-)
venous complications and cerebrovenous sinus thrombosis in labor, childbirth and the puerperium (O87.-)
venous complications and cerebrovenous sinus thrombosis in pregnancy (O22.-)
[6] **O99.41 Diseases of the circulatory system complicating pregnancy**
O99.411 Diseases of the circulatory system complicating pregnancy, first trimester [M] ♀
O99.412 Diseases of the circulatory system complicating pregnancy, second trimester [M] ♀
O99.413 Diseases of the circulatory system complicating pregnancy, third trimester [M] ♀
O99.419 Diseases of the circulatory system complicating pregnancy, unspecified trimester [M] ♀
O99.42 Diseases of the circulatory system complicating childbirth [M] ♀
O99.43 Diseases of the circulatory system complicating the puerperium [M] ♀

[5] **O99.5 Diseases of the respiratory system complicating pregnancy, childbirth and the puerperium**
Conditions in J00-J99
[6] **O99.51 Diseases of the respiratory system complicating pregnancy**
O99.511 Diseases of the respiratory system complicating pregnancy, first trimester [M] ♀
O99.512 Diseases of the respiratory system complicating pregnancy, second trimester [M] ♀
O99.513 Diseases of the respiratory system complicating pregnancy, third trimester [M] ♀
O99.519 Diseases of the respiratory system complicating pregnancy, unspecified trimester [M] ♀
O99.52 Diseases of the respiratory system complicating childbirth [M] ♀
O99.53 Diseases of the respiratory system complicating the puerperium [M] ♀

[5] **O99.6 Diseases of the digestive system complicating pregnancy, childbirth and the puerperium**
Conditions in K00-K93
[EXCLUDES2] *liver and biliary tract disorders in pregnancy, childbirth and the puerperium (O26.6-)*
[6] **O99.61 Diseases of the digestive system complicating pregnancy**
O99.611 Diseases of the digestive system complicating pregnancy, first trimester [M] ♀
O99.612 Diseases of the digestive system complicating pregnancy, second trimester [M] ♀
O99.613 Diseases of the digestive system complicating pregnancy, third trimester [M] ♀
O99.619 Diseases of the digestive system complicating pregnancy, unspecified trimester [M] ♀
O99.62 Diseases of the digestive system complicating childbirth [M] ♀
O99.63 Diseases of the digestive system complicating the puerperium [M] ♀

[5] **O99.7 Diseases of the skin and subcutaneous tissue complicating pregnancy, childbirth and the puerperium**
Conditions in L00-L99
[EXCLUDES2] *herpes gestationis (O26.4)*
pruritic urticarial papules and plaques of pregnancy (PUPPP) (O26.86)
[6] **O99.71 Diseases of the skin and subcutaneous tissue complicating pregnancy**
O99.711 Diseases of the skin and subcutaneous tissue complicating pregnancy, first trimester [M] ♀
O99.712 Diseases of the skin and subcutaneous tissue complicating pregnancy, second trimester [M] ♀
O99.713 Diseases of the skin and subcutaneous tissue complicating pregnancy, third trimester [M] ♀
O99.719 Diseases of the skin and subcutaneous tissue complicating pregnancy, unspecified trimester [M] ♀
O99.72 Diseases of the skin and subcutaneous tissue complicating childbirth [M] ♀
O99.73 Diseases of the skin and subcutaneous tissue complicating the puerperium [M] ♀

[5] **O99.8 Other specified diseases and conditions complicating pregnancy, childbirth and the puerperium**
Conditions in D00-D48, H00-H95, M00-N99, and Q00-Q99
Use additional code to identify condition
[EXCLUDES2] *genitourinary infections in pregnancy (O23.-)*
infection of genitourinary tract following delivery (O86.1-O86.3)
malignant neoplasm complicating pregnancy, childbirth and the puerperium (O9A.1-)
maternal care for known or suspected abnormality of maternal pelvic organs (O34.-)
postpartum acute kidney failure (O90.4)
traumatic injuries in pregnancy (O9A.2-)
[6] **O99.81 Abnormal glucose complicating pregnancy, childbirth and the puerperium**
[EXCLUDES1] *gestational diabetes (O24.4-)*
O99.810 Abnormal glucose complicating pregnancy [M] ♀
O99.814 Abnormal glucose complicating childbirth [M] ♀

[4] 4th character required [5] 5th character required [6] 6th character required [7] 7th character required [7th] Extension 'X' Alert
[EXCLUDES1] Not coded here [EXCLUDES2] Not included here [PDx] Primary Diagnosis Only Manifestation Code

O99.815 Abnormal glucose complicating the puerperium [M] ♀

[6] O99.82 Streptococcus B carrier state complicating pregnancy, childbirth and the puerperium

O99.820 Streptococcus B carrier state complicating pregnancy [M] ♀

O99.824 Streptococcus B carrier state complicating childbirth [M] ♀

O99.825 Streptococcus B carrier state complicating the puerperium [M] ♀

[6] O99.83 Other infection carrier state complicating pregnancy, childbirth and the puerperium

Use additional code to identify the carrier state (Z22.-)

O99.830 Other infection carrier state complicating pregnancy [M] ♀

O99.834 Other infection carrier state complicating childbirth [M] ♀

O99.835 Other infection carrier state complicating the puerperium [M] ♀

[6] O99.84 Bariatric surgery status complicating pregnancy, childbirth and the puerperium

Gastric banding status complicating pregnancy, childbirth and the puerperium
Gastric bypass status for obesity complicating pregnancy, childbirth and the puerperium
Obesity surgery status complicating pregnancy, childbirth and the puerperium

O99.840 Bariatric surgery status complicating pregnancy, unspecified trimester [M] ♀

O99.841 Bariatric surgery status complicating pregnancy, first trimester [M] ♀

O99.842 Bariatric surgery status complicating pregnancy, second trimester [M] ♀

O99.843 Bariatric surgery status complicating pregnancy, third trimester [M] ♀

O99.844 Bariatric surgery status complicating childbirth [M] ♀

O99.845 Bariatric surgery status complicating the puerperium [M] ♀

O99.89 Other specified diseases and conditions complicating pregnancy, childbirth and the puerperium [M] ♀

[4] O9A Maternal malignant neoplasms, traumatic injuries and abuse classifiable elsewhere but complicating pregnancy, childbirth and the puerperium

[5] O9A.1 Malignant neoplasm complicating pregnancy, childbirth and the puerperium

Conditions in C00-C96
Use additional code to identify neoplasm

[EXCLUDES2] *maternal care for benign tumor of corpus uteri (O34.1-)*
maternal care for benign tumor of cervix (O34.4-)

[6] O9A.11 Malignant neoplasm complicating pregnancy

O9A.111 Malignant neoplasm complicating pregnancy, first trimester [M] ♀

O9A.112 Malignant neoplasm complicating pregnancy, second trimester [M] ♀

O9A.113 Malignant neoplasm complicating pregnancy, third trimester [M] ♀

O9A.119 Malignant neoplasm complicating pregnancy, unspecified trimester [M] ♀

O9A.12 Malignant neoplasm complicating childbirth [M] ♀

O9A.13 Malignant neoplasm complicating the puerperium [M] ♀

[5] O9A.2 Injury, poisoning and certain other consequences of external causes complicating pregnancy, childbirth and the puerperium

Conditions in S00-T88, except T74 and T76
Use additional code(s) to identify the injury or poisoning

[EXCLUDES2] *physical, sexual and psychological abuse complicating pregnancy, childbirth and the puerperium (O9A.3-, O9A.4-, O9A.5-)*

[6] O9A.21 Injury, poisoning and certain other consequences of external causes complicating pregnancy

O9A.211 Injury, poisoning and certain other consequences of external causes complicating pregnancy, first trimester [M] ♀

O9A.212 Injury, poisoning and certain other consequences of external causes complicating pregnancy, second trimester [M] ♀

O9A.213 Injury, poisoning and certain other consequences of external causes complicating pregnancy, third trimester [M] ♀

O9A.219 Injury, poisoning and certain other consequences of external causes complicating pregnancy, unspecified trimester [M] ♀

O9A.22 Injury, poisoning and certain other consequences of external causes complicating childbirth [M] ♀

O9A.23 Injury, poisoning and certain other consequences of external causes complicating the puerperium [M] ♀

[5] O9A.3 Physical abuse complicating pregnancy, childbirth and the puerperium

Conditions in T74.11 or T76.11
Use additional code (if applicable):
to identify any associated current injury due to physical abuse
to identify the perpetrator of abuse (Y07.-)

[EXCLUDES2] *sexual abuse complicating pregnancy, childbirth and the puerperium (O9A.4)*

[6] O9A.31 Physical abuse complicating pregnancy

O9A.311 Physical abuse complicating pregnancy, first trimester [M] ♀

O9A.312 Physical abuse complicating pregnancy, second trimester [M] ♀

O9A.313 Physical abuse complicating pregnancy, third trimester [M] ♀

O9A.319 Physical abuse complicating pregnancy, unspecified trimester [M] ♀

O9A.32 Physical abuse complicating childbirth [M] ♀

O9A.33 Physical abuse complicating the puerperium [M] ♀

[5] O9A.4 Sexual abuse complicating pregnancy, childbirth and the puerperium

Conditions in T74.21 or T76.21
Use additional code (if applicable):
to identify any associated current injury due to sexual abuse
to identify the perpetrator of abuse (Y07.-)

[6] O9A.41 Sexual abuse complicating pregnancy

O9A.411 Sexual abuse complicating pregnancy, first trimester [M] ♀

O9A.412 Sexual abuse complicating pregnancy, second trimester [M] ♀

O9A.413 Sexual abuse complicating pregnancy, third trimester [M] ♀

Unspecified Code | Other Specified Code | [N] Newborn Age: 0 | [P] Pediatric Age: 0-17 | [M] Maternity Age: 12-55
[A] Adult Age: 15-124 | ♂ Male | ♀ Female | ● New Code | ▲ Revised Code Title | ►◄ Revised Text

O9A.419 **Sexual abuse complicating pregnancy, unspecified trimester** Ⓜ ♀

O9A.42 **Sexual abuse complicating** childbirth Ⓜ ♀

O9A.43 **Sexual abuse complicating the** puerperium Ⓜ ♀

Ⓢ O9A.5 Psychological abuse **complicating pregnancy, childbirth and the puerperium**

Conditions in T74.31 or T76.31

Use additional code to identify the perpetrator of abuse (Y07.-)

Ⓖ O9A.51 **Psychological abuse complicating** pregnancy

O9A.511 **Psychological abuse complicating pregnancy,** first trimester Ⓜ ♀

O9A.512 **Psychological abuse complicating pregnancy,** second trimester Ⓜ ♀

O9A.513 **Psychological abuse complicating pregnancy,** third trimester Ⓜ ♀

O9A.519 **Psychological abuse complicating pregnancy, unspecified trimester** Ⓜ ♀

O9A.52 **Psychological abuse complicating** childbirth Ⓜ ♀

O9A.53 **Psychological abuse complicating the** puerperium Ⓜ ♀

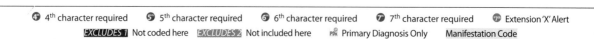

Ⓐ 4ᵗʰ character required   Ⓢ 5ᵗʰ character required   Ⓖ 6ᵗʰ character required   Ⓟ 7ᵗʰ character required   Ⓧ Extension 'X' Alert

EXCLUDES 1 Not coded here   EXCLUDES 2 Not included here   PDX Primary Diagnosis Only   Manifestation Code

Chapter 16: Certain Conditions Originating in the Perinatal Period (P00-P96)

Chapter Specific Coding Guidelines

For coding and reporting purposes the perinatal period is defined as before birth through the 28th day following birth. The following guidelines are provided for reporting purposes

a. **General Perinatal Rules**

1) **Use of Chapter 16 Codes**
   Codes in this chapter are never for use on the maternal record. Codes from Chapter 15, the obstetric chapter, are never permitted on the newborn record. Chapter 16 codes may be used throughout the life of the patient if the condition is still present.

2) **Principal Diagnosis for Birth Record**
   When coding the birth episode in a newborn record, assign a code from category Z38, Liveborn infants according to place of birth and type of delivery, as the principal diagnosis. A code from category Z38 is assigned only once, to a newborn at the time of birth. If a newborn is transferred to another institution, a code from category Z38 should not be used at the receiving hospital.

   A code from category Z38 is used only on the newborn record, not on the mother's record.

3) **Use of Codes from other Chapters with Codes from Chapter 16**
   Codes from other chapters may be used with codes from chapter 16 if the codes from the other chapters provide more specific detail. Codes for signs and symptoms may be assigned when a definitive diagnosis has not been established. If the reason for the encounter is a perinatal condition, the code from chapter 16 should be sequenced first.

4) **Use of Chapter 16 Codes after the Perinatal Period**
   Should a condition originate in the perinatal period, and continue throughout the life of the patient, the perinatal code should continue to be used regardless of the patient's age.

5) **Birth process or community acquired conditions**
   If a newborn has a condition that may be either due to the birth process or community acquired and the documentation does not indicate which it is, the default is due to the birth process and the code from Chapter 16 should be used. If the condition is community-acquired, a code from Chapter 16 should not be assigned.

6) **Code all clinically significant conditions**
   All clinically significant conditions noted on routine newborn examination should be coded. A condition is clinically significant if it requires:

   - clinical evaluation; or
   - therapeutic treatment; or
   - diagnostic procedures; or
   - extended length of hospital stay; or
   - increased nursing care and/or monitoring; or
   - has implications for future health care needs

     Note: The perinatal guidelines listed above are the same as the general coding guidelines for "additional diagnoses", except for the final point regarding implications for future health care needs. Codes should be assigned for conditions that have been specified by the provider as having implications for future health care needs.

b. **Observation and Evaluation of Newborns for Suspected Conditions not Found**
   Reserved for future expansion

c. **Coding Additional Perinatal Diagnoses**

1) **Assigning codes for conditions that require treatment**
   Assign codes for conditions that require treatment or further investigation, prolong the length of stay, or require resource utilization.

2) **Codes for conditions specified as having implications for future health care needs**
   Assign codes for conditions that have been specified by the provider as having implications for future health care needs.

   Note: This guideline should not be used for adult patients.

d. **Prematurity and Fetal Growth Retardation**
   Providers utilize different criteria in determining prematurity. A code for prematurity should not be assigned unless it is documented. Assignment of codes in categories P05, Disorders of newborn related to slow fetal growth and fetal malnutrition, and P07, Disorders of newborn related to short gestation and low birth weight, not elsewhere classified, should be based on the recorded birth weight and estimated gestational age. Codes from category P05 should not be assigned with codes from category P07.

   When both birth weight and gestational age are available, two codes from category P07 should be assigned, with the code for birth weight sequenced before the code for gestational age.

e. **Low birth weight and immaturity status**
   Codes from category P07, Disorders of newborn related to short gestation and low birth weight, not elsewhere classified, are for use for a child or adult who was premature or had a low birth weight as a newborn and this is affecting the patient's current health status.

   See Section I.C.21. Factors influencing health status and contact with health services, Status.

f. **Bacterial Sepsis of Newborn**
   Category P36, Bacterial sepsis of newborn, includes congenital sepsis. If a perinate is documented as having sepsis without documentation of congenital or community acquired, the default is congenital and a code from category P36 should be assigned. If the P36 code includes the causal organism, an additional code from category B95, Streptococcus, Staphylococcus, and Enterococcus as the cause of diseases classified elsewhere, or B96, Other bacterial agents as the cause of diseases classified elsewhere, should not be assigned. If the P36 code does not include the causal organism, assign an additional code from category B96. If applicable, use additional codes to identify severe sepsis (R65.2-) and any associated acute organ dysfunction.

g. **Stillbirth**
   Code P95, Stillbirth, is only for use in institutions that maintain separate records for stillbirths. No other code should be used with P95. Code P95 should not be used on the mother's record.

This page intentionally left blank

Certain conditions originating in the perinatal period (P00-P96)

[NOTES] Codes from this chapter are for use on newborn records only, never on maternal records

[INCLUDES] *conditions that have their origin in the fetal or perinatal period (before birth through the first 28 days after birth) even if morbidity occurs later*

[EXCLUDES2] *congenital malformations, deformations and chromosomal abnormalities (Q00-Q99)*
endocrine, nutritional and metabolic diseases (E00-E88)
injury, poisoning and certain other consequences of external causes (S00-T88)
neoplasms (C00-D49)
tetanus neonatorum (A33)

Newborn affected by maternal factors and by complications of pregnancy, labor, and delivery (P00-P04)

[NOTES] These codes are for use when the listed maternal conditions are specified as the cause of confirmed morbidity or potential morbidity which have their origin in the perinatal period (before birth through the first 28 days after birth). Codes from these categories are also for use for newborns who are suspected of having an abnormal condition resulting from exposure from the mother or the birth process, but without signs or symptoms, and, which after examination and observation, is found not to exist. These codes may be used even if treatment is begun for a suspected condition that is ruled out.

[4] **P00 Newborn (suspected to be) affected by maternal conditions that may be unrelated to present pregnancy**

Code first any current condition in newborn

[EXCLUDES2] *newborn (suspected to be) affected by maternal complications of pregnancy (P01.-)*
newborn affected by maternal endocrine and metabolic disorders (P70-P74)
newborn affected by noxious substances transmitted via placenta or breast milk (P04.-)

P00.0 Newborn (suspected to be) affected by maternal hypertensive disorders
Newborn (suspected to be) affected by maternal conditions classifiable to O10-O11, O13-O16 [N]

P00.1 Newborn (suspected to be) affected by maternal renal and urinary tract diseases
Newborn (suspected to be) affected by maternal conditions classifiable to N00-N39 [N]

P00.2 Newborn (suspected to be) affected by maternal infectious and parasitic diseases
Newborn (suspected to be) affected by maternal infectious disease classifiable to A00-B99, J09 and J10

[EXCLUDES1] *infections specific to the perinatal period (P35-P39)*
maternal genital tract or other localized infections (P00.8) [N]

P00.3 Newborn (suspected to be) affected by other maternal circulatory and respiratory diseases
Newborn (suspected to be) affected by maternal conditions classifiable to I00-I99, J00-J99, Q20-Q34 and not included in P00.0, P00.2 [N]

P00.4 Newborn (suspected to be) affected by maternal nutritional disorders
Newborn (suspected to be) affected by maternal disorders classifiable to E40-E64
Maternal malnutrition NOS [N]

P00.5 Newborn (suspected to be) affected by maternal injury
Newborn (suspected to be) affected by maternal conditions classifiable to O9A.2- [N]

P00.6 Newborn (suspected to be) affected by surgical procedure on mother
Newborn (suspected to be) affected by amniocentesis

[EXCLUDES1] *Cesarean delivery for present delivery (P03.4)*
damage to placenta from amniocentesis, Cesarean delivery or surgical induction (P02.1)
previous surgery to uterus or pelvic organs (P03.89)

[EXCLUDES2] *newborn affected by complication of (fetal) intrauterine procedure (P96.5)* [N]

P00.7 Newborn (suspected to be) affected by other medical procedures on mother, not elsewhere classified
Newborn (suspected to be) affected by radiation to mother

[EXCLUDES1] *damage to placenta from amniocentesis, cesarean delivery or surgical induction (P02.1)*
newborn affected by other complications of labor and delivery (P03.-) [N]

[5] **P00.8 Newborn (suspected to be) affected by other maternal conditions**

P00.81 Newborn (suspected to be) affected by periodontal disease in mother [N]

P00.89 Newborn (suspected to be) affected by other maternal conditions
Newborn (suspected to be) affected by conditions classifiable to T80-T88
Newborn (suspected to be) affected by maternal genital tract or other localized infections
Newborn (suspected to be) affected by maternal systemic lupus erythematosus [N]

P00.9 Newborn (suspected to be) affected by unspecified maternal condition [N]

[4] **P01 Newborn (suspected to be) affected by maternal complications of pregnancy**

Code first any current condition in newborn

P01.0 Newborn (suspected to be) affected by incompetent cervix [N]

P01.1 Newborn (suspected to be) affected by premature rupture of membranes [N]

P01.2 Newborn (suspected to be) affected by oligohydramnios

[EXCLUDES1] *oligohydramnios due to premature rupture of membranes (P01.1)* [N]

P01.3 Newborn (suspected to be) affected by polyhydramnios
Newborn (suspected to be) affected by hydramnios [N]

P01.4 Newborn (suspected to be) affected by ectopic pregnancy
Newborn (suspected to be) affected by abdominal pregnancy [N]

P01.5 Newborn (suspected to be) affected by multiple pregnancy
Newborn (suspected to be) affected by triplet (pregnancy)
Newborn (suspected to be) affected by twin (pregnancy) [N]

P01.6 Newborn (suspected to be) affected by maternal death [N]

P01.7 Newborn (suspected to be) affected by malpresentation before labor
Newborn (suspected to be) affected by breech presentation before labor
Newborn (suspected to be) affected by external version before labor
Newborn (suspected to be) affected by face presentation before labor
Newborn (suspected to be) affected by transverse lie before labor
Newborn (suspected to be) affected by unstable lie before labor [N]

Unspecified Code | Other Specified Code | [N] Newborn Age: 0 | [P] Pediatric Age: 0-17 | [M] Maternity Age: 12-55
[A] Adult Age: 15-124 | ♂ Male | ♀ Female | ● New Code | ▲ Revised Code Title | ►◄ Revised Text

P01.8 Newborn (suspected to be) affected by other maternal complications of pregnancy 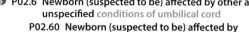 N

P01.9 Newborn (suspected to be) affected by maternal complication of pregnancy, unspecified N

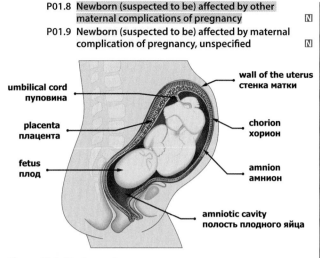

umbilical cord
пуповина

placenta
плацента

fetus
плод

wall of the uterus
стенка матки

chorion
хорион

amnion
амнион

amniotic cavity
полость плодного яйца

Figure 14.1 Uterine cavity

④ P02 Newborn (suspected to be) affected by complications of placenta, cord and membranes

Code first any current condition in newborn

P02.0 Newborn (suspected to be) affected by placenta previa N

P02.1 Newborn (suspected to be) affected by other forms of placental separation and hemorrhage

Newborn (suspected to be) affected by abruptio placenta

Newborn (suspected to be) affected by accidental hemorrhage

Newborn (suspected to be) affected by antepartum hemorrhage

Newborn (suspected to be) affected by damage to placenta from amniocentesis, cesarean delivery or surgical induction

Newborn (suspected to be) affected by maternal blood loss

Newborn (suspected to be) affected by premature separation of placenta N

⑤ P02.2 Newborn (suspected to be) affected by other and unspecified morphological and functional abnormalities of placenta

P02.20 Newborn (suspected to be) affected by unspecified morphological and functional abnormalities of placenta N

P02.29 Newborn (suspected to be) affected by other morphological and functional abnormalities of placenta

Newborn (suspected to be) affected by placental dysfunction

Newborn (suspected to be) affected by placental infarction

Newborn (suspected to be) affected by placental insufficiency N

P02.3 Newborn (suspected to be) affected by placental transfusion syndromes

Newborn (suspected to be) affected by placental and cord abnormalities resulting in twin-to-twin or other transplacental transfusion N

P02.4 Newborn (suspected to be) affected by prolapsed cord N

P02.5 Newborn (suspected to be) affected by other compression of umbilical cord

Newborn (suspected to be) affected by umbilical cord (tightly) around neck

Newborn (suspected to be) affected by entanglement of umbilical cord

Newborn (suspected to be) affected by knot in umbilical cord N

⑤ P02.6 Newborn (suspected to be) affected by other and unspecified conditions of umbilical cord

P02.60 Newborn (suspected to be) affected by unspecified conditions of umbilical cord N

P02.69 Newborn (suspected to be) affected by other conditions of umbilical cord

Newborn (suspected to be) affected by short umbilical cord

Newborn (suspected to be) affected by vasa previa

EXCLUDES1 newborn affected by single umbilical artery (Q27.0) N

P02.7 Newborn (suspected to be) affected by chorioamnionitis

Newborn (suspected to be) affected by amnionitis

Newborn (suspected to be) affected by membranitis

Newborn (suspected to be) affected by placentitis N

P02.8 Newborn (suspected to be) affected by other abnormalities of membranes N

P02.9 Newborn (suspected to be) affected by abnormality of membranes, unspecified N

④ P03 Newborn (suspected to be) affected by other complications of labor and delivery

Code first any current condition in newborn

P03.0 Newborn (suspected to be) affected by breech delivery and extraction N

P03.1 Newborn (suspected to be) affected by other malpresentation, malposition and disproportion during labor and delivery

Newborn (suspected to be) affected by contracted pelvis

Newborn (suspected to be) affected by conditions classifiable to O64-O66

Newborn (suspected to be) affected by persistent occipitoposterior

Newborn (suspected to be) affected by transverse lie N

P03.2 Newborn (suspected to be) affected by forceps delivery N

P03.3 Newborn (suspected to be) affected by delivery by vacuum extractor [ventouse] N

P03.4 Newborn (suspected to be) affected by Cesarean delivery N

P03.5 Newborn (suspected to be) affected by precipitate delivery

Newborn (suspected to be) affected by rapid second stage N

P03.6 Newborn (suspected to be) affected by abnormal uterine contractions

Newborn (suspected to be) affected by conditions classifiable to O62.-, except O62.3

Newborn (suspected to be) affected by hypertonic labor

Newborn (suspected to be) affected by uterine inertia N

⑤ P03.8 Newborn (suspected to be) affected by other specified complications of labor and delivery

⑥ P03.81 Newborn (suspected to be) affected by abnormality in fetal (intrauterine) heart rate or rhythm

EXCLUDES1 neonatal cardiac dysrhythmia (P29.1-)

P03.810 Newborn (suspected to be) affected by abnormality in fetal (intrauterine) heart rate or rhythm before the onset of labor N

---

④ 4ᵗʰ character required   ⑤ 5ᵗʰ character required   ⑥ 6ᵗʰ character required   ⑦ 7ᵗʰ character required   ⑦ˣ Extension 'X' Alert

EXCLUDES 1 Not coded here   EXCLUDES 2 Not included here   Pᴅx Primary Diagnosis Only   Manifestation Code

P03.811 Newborn (suspected to be) affected by abnormality in fetal (intrauterine) heart rate or rhythm during labor N

P03.819 Newborn (suspected to be) affected by abnormality in fetal (intrauterine) heart rate or rhythm, unspecified as to time of onset N

P03.82 Meconium passage during delivery

EXCLUDES1 meconium aspiration (P24.00, P24.01)
meconium staining (P96.83) N

P03.89 Newborn (suspected to be) affected by other specified complications of labor and delivery

Newborn (suspected to be) affected by abnormality of maternal soft tissues
Newborn (suspected to be) affected by conditions classifiable to O60-O75 and by procedures used in labor and delivery not included in P02.- and P03.0-P03.6
Newborn (suspected to be) affected by induction of labor N

P03.9 Newborn (suspected to be) affected by complication of labor and delivery, unspecified N

④ P04 Newborn (suspected to be) affected by noxious substances transmitted via placenta or breast milk

INCLUDES nonteratogenic effects of substances transmitted via placenta

EXCLUDES2 congenital malformations (Q00-Q99)
neonatal jaundice from excessive hemolysis due to drugs or toxins transmitted from mother (P58.4)
newborn in contact with and (suspected) exposures hazardous to health not transmitted via placenta or breast milk (Z77.-)

P04.0 Newborn (suspected to be) affected by maternal anesthesia and analgesia in pregnancy, labor and delivery

Newborn (suspected to be) affected by reactions and intoxications from maternal opiates and tranquilizers administered during labor and delivery N

P04.1 Newborn (suspected to be) affected by other maternal medication

Newborn (suspected to be) affected by cancer chemotherapy
Newborn (suspected to be) affected by cytotoxic drugs

EXCLUDES1 dysmorphism due to warfarin (Q86.2)
fetal hydantoin syndrome (Q86.1)
maternal use of drugs of addiction (P04.4-) N

P04.2 Newborn (suspected to be) affected by maternal use of tobacco

Newborn (suspected to be) affected by exposure in utero to tobacco smoke

EXCLUDES2 newborn exposure to environmental tobacco smoke (P96.81) N

P04.3 Newborn (suspected to be) affected by maternal use of alcohol

EXCLUDES1 fetal alcohol syndrome (Q86.0) N

⑤ P04.4 Newborn (suspected to be) affected by maternal use of drugs of addiction

P04.41 Newborn (suspected to be) affected by maternal use of cocaine

'Crack baby' N

P04.49 Newborn (suspected to be) affected by maternal use of other drugs of addiction

EXCLUDES2 newborn (suspected to be) affected by maternal anesthesia and analgesia (P04.0)
withdrawal symptoms from maternal use of drugs of addiction (P96.1) N

P04.5 Newborn (suspected to be) affected by maternal use of nutritional chemical substances N

P04.6 Newborn (suspected to be) affected by maternal exposure to environmental chemical substances N

P04.8 Newborn (suspected to be) affected by other maternal noxious substances N

P04.9 Newborn (suspected to be) affected by maternal noxious substance, unspecified N

Disorders of newborn related to length of gestation and fetal growth (P05-P08)

④ P05 Disorders of newborn related to slow fetal growth and fetal malnutrition

⑤ P05.0 Newborn light for gestational age

Newborn light-for-dates

P05.00 Newborn light for gestational age, unspecified weight N

P05.01 Newborn light for gestational age, less than 500 grams N

P05.02 Newborn light for gestational age, 500-749 grams N

P05.03 Newborn light for gestational age, 750-999 grams N

P05.04 Newborn light for gestational age, 1000-1249 grams N

P05.05 Newborn light for gestational age, 1250-1499 grams N

P05.06 Newborn light for gestational age, 1500-1749 grams N

P05.07 Newborn light for gestational age, 1750-1999 grams N

P05.08 Newborn light for gestational age, 2000-2499 grams N

⑤ P05.1 Newborn small for gestational age

Newborn small-and-light-for-dates
Newborn small-for-dates

P05.10 Newborn small for gestational age, unspecified weight N

P05.11 Newborn small for gestational age, less than 500 grams N

P05.12 Newborn small for gestational age, 500-749 grams N

P05.13 Newborn small for gestational age, 750-999 grams N

P05.14 Newborn small for gestational age, 1000-1249 grams N

P05.15 Newborn small for gestational age, 1250-1499 grams N

P05.16 Newborn small for gestational age, 1500-1749 grams N

P05.17 Newborn small for gestational age, 1750-1999 grams N

P05.18 Newborn small for gestational age, 2000-2499 grams N

P05.2 Newborn affected by fetal (intrauterine) malnutrition not light or small for gestational age

Infant, not light or small for gestational age, showing signs of fetal malnutrition, such as dry, peeling skin and loss of subcutaneous tissue

EXCLUDES1 newborn affected by fetal malnutrition with light for gestational age (P05.0-)
newborn affected by fetal malnutrition with small for gestational age (P05.1-) N

P05.9 Newborn affected by slow intrauterine growth, unspecified

Newborn affected by fetal growth retardation NOS N

| Unspecified Code | Other Specified Code | N Newborn Age: 0 | P Pediatric Age: 0-17 | M Maternity Age: 12-55 |
| A Adult Age: 15-124 | ♂ Male | ♀ Female | ● New Code | ▲ Revised Code Title | ►◄ Revised Text |

④ P07 Disorders of newborn related to short gestation and low birth weight, not elsewhere classified

NOTES   When both birth weight and gestational age of the newborn are available, both should be coded with birth weight sequenced before gestational age

INCLUDES   the listed conditions, without further specification, as the cause of morbidity or additional care, in newborn

EXCLUDES1   low birth weight due to slow fetal growth and fetal malnutrition (P05.-)

⑤ P07.0 Extremely low birth weight newborn

Newborn birth weight 999 g. or less

P07.00 Extremely low birth weight newborn, unspecified weight N

P07.01 Extremely low birth weight newborn, less than 500 grams N

P07.02 Extremely low birth weight newborn, 500-749 grams N

P07.03 Extremely low birth weight newborn, 750-999 grams N

⑤ P07.1 Other low birth weight newborn

Newborn birth weight 1000-2499 g.

P07.10 Other low birth weight newborn, unspecified weight N

P07.14 Other low birth weight newborn, 1000-1249 grams N

P07.15 Other low birth weight newborn, 1250-1499 grams N

P07.16 Other low birth weight newborn, 1500-1749 grams N

P07.17 Other low birth weight newborn, 1750-1999 grams N

P07.18 Other low birth weight newborn, 2000-2499 grams N

⑤ P07.2 Extreme immaturity of newborn

Less than 28 completed weeks (less than 196 completed days) of gestation.

P07.20 Extreme immaturity of newborn, unspecified weeks of gestation

Gestational age less than 28 completed weeks NOS N

P07.21 Extreme immaturity of newborn, gestational age less than 23 completed weeks

Extreme immaturity of newborn, gestational age less than 23 weeks, 0 days N

P07.22 Extreme immaturity of newborn, gestational age 23 completed weeks

Extreme immaturity of newborn, gestational age 23 weeks, 0 days through 23 weeks, 6 days N

P07.23 Extreme immaturity of newborn, gestational age 24 completed weeks

Extreme immaturity of newborn, gestational age 24 weeks, 0 days through 24 weeks, 6 days N

P07.24 Extreme immaturity of newborn, gestational age 25 completed weeks

Extreme immaturity of newborn, gestational age 25 weeks, 0 days through 25 weeks, 6 days N

P07.25 Extreme immaturity of newborn, gestational age 26 completed weeks

Extreme immaturity of newborn, gestational age 26 weeks, 0 days through 26 weeks, 6 days N

P07.26 Extreme immaturity of newborn, gestational age 27 completed weeks

Extreme immaturity of newborn, gestational age 27 weeks, 0 days through 27 weeks, 6 days N

⑤ P07.3 Preterm [premature] newborn [other]

28 completed weeks or more but less than 37 completed weeks (196 completed days but less than 259 completed days) of gestation.

Prematurity NOS

P07.30 Preterm newborn, unspecified weeks of gestation N

P07.31 Preterm newborn, gestational age 28 completed weeks

Preterm newborn, gestational age 28 weeks, 0 days through 28 weeks, 6 days N

P07.32 Preterm newborn, gestational age 29 completed weeks

Preterm newborn, gestational age 29 weeks, 0 days through 29 weeks, 6 days N

P07.33 Preterm newborn, gestational age 30 completed weeks

Preterm newborn, gestational age 30 weeks, 0 days through 30 weeks, 6 days N

P07.34 Preterm newborn, gestational age 31 completed weeks

Preterm newborn, gestational age 31 weeks, 0 days through 31 weeks, 6 days N

P07.35 Preterm newborn, gestational age 32 completed weeks

Preterm newborn, gestational age 32 weeks, 0 days through 32 weeks, 6 days N

P07.36 Preterm newborn, gestational age 33 completed weeks

Preterm newborn, gestational age 33 weeks, 0 days through 33 weeks, 6 days N

P07.37 Preterm newborn, gestational age 34 completed weeks

Preterm newborn, gestational age 34 weeks, 0 days through 34 weeks, 6 days N

P07.38 Preterm newborn, gestational age 35 completed weeks

Preterm newborn, gestational age 35 weeks, 0 days through 35 weeks, 6 days N

P07.39 Preterm newborn, gestational age 36 completed weeks

Preterm newborn, gestational age 36 weeks, 0 days through 36 weeks, 6 days N

④ P08 Disorders of newborn related to long gestation and high birth weight

NOTES   When both birth weight and gestational age of the newborn are available, priority of assignment should be given to birth weight

INCLUDES   the listed conditions, without further specification, as causes of morbidity or additional care, in newborn

P08.0 Exceptionally large newborn baby

Usually implies a birth weight of 4500 g. or more

EXCLUDES1   syndrome of infant of diabetic mother (P70.1)
syndrome of infant of mother with gestational diabetes (P70.0) N

P08.1 Other heavy for gestational age newborn

Other newborn heavy- or large-for-dates regardless of period of gestation

Usually implies a birth weight of 4000 g. to 4499 g.

EXCLUDES1   newborn with a birth weight of 4500 or more (P08.0)
syndrome of infant of diabetic mother (P70.1)
syndrome of infant of mother with gestational diabetes (P70.0). N

⑤ P08.2 Late newborn, not heavy for gestational age

④ 4th character required   ⑤ 5th character required   ⑥ 6th character required   ⑦ 7th character required   ⑦x Extension 'X' Alert

EXCLUDES 1 Not coded here   EXCLUDES 2 Not included here   PDx Primary Diagnosis Only   Manifestation Code

484   ICD-10-CM 2015

P08.21 **Post-term newborn**

Newborn with gestation period over 40 completed weeks to 42 completed weeks Ⓝ

P08.22 **Prolonged gestation of newborn**

Newborn with gestation period over 42 completed weeks (294 days or more), not heavy- or large-for-dates.

Postmaturity NOS Ⓝ

Abnormal findings on neonatal screening (P09)

P09 **Abnormal findings on neonatal screening**

Use additional code to identify signs, symptoms and conditions associated with the screening

EXCLUDES2 *nonspecific serologic evidence of human immunodeficiency virus [HIV] (R75)*

Birth trauma (P10-P15)

⊕ P10 Intracranial laceration and hemorrhage **due to birth injury**

EXCLUDES1 *intracranial hemorrhage of newborn NOS (P52.9)*
intracranial hemorrhage of newborn due to anoxia or hypoxia (P52.-)
nontraumatic intracranial hemorrhage of newborn (P52.-)

P10.0 Subdural hemorrhage **due to birth injury**

Subdural hematoma (localized) due to birth injury

EXCLUDES1 *subdural hemorrhage accompanying tentorial tear (P10.4)* Ⓝ

P10.1 Cerebral hemorrhage **due to birth injury** Ⓝ
P10.2 Intraventricular hemorrhage **due to birth injury** Ⓝ
P10.3 Subarachnoid hemorrhage **due to birth injury** Ⓝ
P10.4 Tentorial tear **due to birth injury** Ⓝ
P10.8 **Other intracranial lacerations and hemorrhages due to birth injury** Ⓝ
P10.9 **Unspecified intracranial laceration and hemorrhage due to birth injury** Ⓝ

⊕ P11 Other birth injuries to central nervous system

P11.0 Cerebral edema **due to birth injury** Ⓝ
P11.1 **Other specified brain damage due to birth injury** Ⓝ
P11.2 **Unspecified brain damage due to birth injury** Ⓝ
P11.3 **Birth injury to** facial nerve

Facial palsy due to birth injury Ⓝ

P11.4 **Birth injury to other** cranial nerves Ⓝ
P11.5 **Birth injury to** spine and spinal cord

Fracture of spine due to birth injury Ⓝ

P11.9 **Birth injury to central nervous system, unspecified** Ⓝ

⊕ P12 Birth injury to scalp

P12.0 Cephalhematoma **due to birth injury** Ⓝ
P12.1 Chignon (from vacuum extraction) **due to birth injury** Ⓝ
P12.2 Epicranial subaponeurotic hemorrhage **due to birth injury**

Subgaleal hemorrhage Ⓝ

P12.3 Bruising of scalp **due to birth injury** Ⓝ
P12.4 **Injury of scalp of newborn due to** monitoring equipment

Sampling incision of scalp of newborn
Scalp clip (electrode) injury of newborn Ⓝ

⊕ P12.8 **Other** birth injuries to scalp

P12.81 Caput succedaneum Ⓝ
P12.89 **Other birth injuries to scalp** Ⓝ

P12.9 **Birth injury to scalp, unspecified** Ⓝ

⊕ P13 Birth injury to skeleton

EXCLUDES2 *birth injury to spine (P11.5)*

P13.0 Fracture of skull **due to birth injury** Ⓝ
P13.1 **Other birth injuries to skull**

EXCLUDES1 *cephalhematoma (P12.0)* Ⓝ

P13.2 Birth injury to femur Ⓝ
P13.3 **Birth injury to other** long bones Ⓝ
P13.4 Fracture of clavicle **due to birth injury** Ⓝ
P13.8 **Birth injuries to other** parts **of skeleton** Ⓝ
P13.9 **Birth injury to skeleton, unspecified** Ⓝ

⊕ P14 **Birth injury to** peripheral nervous system

P14.0 Erb's paralysis **due to birth injury** Ⓝ
P14.1 Klumpke's paralysis **due to birth injury** Ⓝ
P14.2 Phrenic nerve paralysis **due to birth injury** Ⓝ
P14.3 **Other** brachial plexus **birth injuries** Ⓝ
P14.8 **Birth injuries to other parts of** peripheral nervous system Ⓝ
P14.9 **Birth injury to peripheral nervous system, unspecified** Ⓝ

⊕ P15 Other **birth injuries**

P15.0 **Birth injury to** liver

Rupture of liver due to birth injury Ⓝ

P15.1 **Birth injury to** spleen

Rupture of spleen due to birth injury Ⓝ

P15.2 Sternomastoid **injury due to birth injury** Ⓝ
P15.3 **Birth injury to** eye

Subconjunctival hemorrhage due to birth injury
Traumatic glaucoma due to birth injury Ⓝ

P15.4 **Birth injury to** face

Facial congestion due to birth injury Ⓝ

P15.5 **Birth injury to** external genitalia Ⓝ
P15.6 Subcutaneous fat necrosis **due to birth injury** Ⓝ
P15.8 **Other specified birth injuries** Ⓝ
P15.9 **Birth injury, unspecified** Ⓝ

Respiratory and cardiovascular disorders specific to the perinatal period (P19-P29)

⊕ P19 Metabolic acidemia in newborn

INCLUDES *metabolic acidemia in newborn*

P19.0 **Metabolic acidemia in newborn first noted** before onset of labor Ⓝ
P19.1 **Metabolic acidemia in newborn first noted** during labor Ⓝ
P19.2 **Metabolic acidemia noted** at birth Ⓝ
P19.9 **Metabolic acidemia, unspecified** Ⓝ

⊕ P22 Respiratory distress of newborn

EXCLUDES1 *respiratory arrest of newborn (P28.81)*
respiratory failure of newborn NOS (P28.5)

P22.0 **Respiratory distress syndrome of newborn**

Cardiorespiratory distress syndrome of newborn
Hyaline membrane disease
Idiopathic respiratory distress syndrome [IRDS or RDS] of newborn
Pulmonary hypoperfusion syndrome
Respiratory distress syndrome, type I Ⓝ

P22.1 **Transient tachypnea of newborn**

Idiopathic tachypnea of newborn
Respiratory distress syndrome, type II
Wet lung syndrome Ⓝ

P22.8 **Other respiratory distress of newborn** Ⓝ
P22.9 **Respiratory distress of newborn, unspecified** Ⓝ

⊕ P23 Congenital pneumonia

INCLUDES *infective pneumonia acquired in utero or during birth*

EXCLUDES1 *neonatal pneumonia resulting from aspiration (P24.-)*

P23.0 **Congenital pneumonia due to** viral agent

Use additional code (B97) to identify organism

EXCLUDES1 *congenital rubella pneumonitis (P35.0)* Ⓝ

P23.1 **Congenital pneumonia due to** Chlamydia Ⓝ
P23.2 **Congenital pneumonia due to** staphylococcus Ⓝ

Unspecified Code   Other Specified Code   Ⓝ Newborn Age: 0   Ⓟ Pediatric Age: 0-17   Ⓜ Maternity Age: 12-55
Ⓐ Adult Age: 15-124   ♂ Male   ♀ Female   ● New Code   ▲ Revised Code Title   ►◄ Revised Text

P23.3 **Congenital pneumonia due to** streptococcus, group B N

P23.4 **Congenital pneumonia due to** Escherichia coli N

P23.5 **Congenital pneumonia due to** Pseudomonas N

P23.6 **Congenital pneumonia due to other** bacterial agents N

    Congenital pneumonia due to Hemophilus influenzae

    Congenital pneumonia due to Klebsiella pneumoniae

    Congenital pneumonia due to Mycoplasma

    Congenital pneumonia due to Streptococcus, except group B

    Use additional code (B95-B96) to identify organism N

P23.8 **Congenital pneumonia due to other organisms** N

P23.9 **Congenital pneumonia, unspecified** N

④ P24 Neonatal aspiration

    INCLUDES aspiration in utero and during delivery

⑤ P24.0 Meconium aspiration

    EXCLUDES1 meconium passage (without aspiration) during delivery (P03.82)

    meconium staining (P96.83)

    P24.00 **Meconium aspiration** without respiratory symptoms

    Meconium aspiration NOS N

    P24.01 **Meconium aspiration** with respiratory symptoms

    Meconium aspiration pneumonia

    Meconium aspiration pneumonitis

    Meconium aspiration syndrome NOS

    Use additional code to identify any secondary pulmonary hypertension, if applicable (I27.2) N

⑤ P24.1 **Neonatal aspiration of (clear)** amniotic fluid and mucus

    Neonatal aspiration of liquor (amnii)

    P24.10 **Neonatal aspiration of (clear) amniotic fluid and mucus** without respiratory symptoms

    Neonatal aspiration of amniotic fluid and mucus NOS N

    P24.11 **Neonatal aspiration of (clear) amniotic fluid and mucus** with respiratory symptoms

        Neonatal aspiration of amniotic fluid and mucus with pneumonia

        Neonatal aspiration of amniotic fluid and mucus with pneumonitis

    Use additional code to identify any secondary pulmonary hypertension, if applicable (I27.2) N

⑤ P24.2 **Neonatal aspiration of** blood

    P24.20 **Neonatal aspiration of blood** without respiratory symptoms

        Neonatal aspiration of blood NOS N

    P24.21 **Neonatal aspiration of blood** with respiratory symptoms

        Neonatal aspiration of blood with pneumonia

        Neonatal aspiration of blood with pneumonitis

    Use additional code to identify any secondary pulmonary hypertension, if applicable (I27.2) N

⑤ P24.3 **Neonatal aspiration of** milk **and regurgitated** food

    Neonatal aspiration of stomach contents

    P24.30 **Neonatal aspiration of milk and regurgitated food** without respiratory symptoms

    Neonatal aspiration of milk and regurgitated food NOS N

    P24.31 **Neonatal aspiration of milk and regurgitated food** with respiratory symptoms

        Neonatal aspiration of milk and regurgitated food with pneumonia

        Neonatal aspiration of milk and regurgitated food with pneumonitis

    Use additional code to identify any secondary pulmonary hypertension, if applicable (I27.2) N

⑤ P24.8 **Other** neonatal aspiration

P24.80 **Other neonatal aspiration** without respiratory symptoms

    Neonatal aspiration NEC N

P24.81 **Other neonatal aspiration** with respiratory symptoms

    Neonatal aspiration pneumonia NEC

    Neonatal aspiration with pneumonitis NEC

    Neonatal aspiration with pneumonia NOS

    Neonatal aspiration with pneumonitis NOS

    Use additional code to identify any secondary pulmonary hypertension, if applicable (I27.2) N

P24.9 **Neonatal aspiration, unspecified** N

④ P25 Interstitial emphysema and related conditions originating in the perinatal period

P25.0 Interstitial emphysema **originating in the perinatal period** N

P25.1 Pneumothorax **originating in the perinatal period** N

P25.2 Pneumomediastinum **originating in the perinatal period** N

P25.3 Pneumopericardium **originating in the perinatal period** N

P25.8 **Other conditions related to interstitial emphysema originating in the perinatal period** N

④ P26 Pulmonary hemorrhage originating in the perinatal period

    EXCLUDES1 acute idiopathic hemorrhage in infants over 28 days old (R04.81)

P26.0 Tracheobronchial **hemorrhage originating in the perinatal period** N

P26.1 Massive pulmonary **hemorrhage originating in the perinatal period** N

P26.8 **Other pulmonary hemorrhages originating in the perinatal period** N

P26.9 **Unspecified pulmonary hemorrhage originating in the perinatal period** N

④ P27 Chronic respiratory disease originating in the perinatal period

    EXCLUDES1 respiratory distress of newborn (P22.0-P22.9)

P27.0 **Wilson-Mikity syndrome**

    Pulmonary dysmaturity

P27.1 **Bronchopulmonary dysplasia originating in the perinatal period**

P27.8 **Other chronic respiratory diseases originating in the perinatal period**

    Congenital pulmonary fibrosis

    Ventilator lung in newborn

P27.9 **Unspecified chronic respiratory disease originating in the perinatal period**

④ P28 Other respiratory conditions originating in the perinatal period

    EXCLUDES1 congenital malformations of the respiratory system (Q30-Q34)

P28.0 **Primary atelectasis of newborn**

    Primary failure to expand terminal respiratory units

    Pulmonary hypoplasia associated with short gestation

    Pulmonary immaturity NOS N

⑤ P28.1 **Other and unspecified atelectasis of newborn**

    P28.10 **Unspecified atelectasis of newborn**

    Atelectasis of newborn NOS N

    P28.11 **Resorption atelectasis without respiratory distress syndrome**

    EXCLUDES1 resorption atelectasis with respiratory distress syndrome (P22.0) N

    P28.19 **Other atelectasis of newborn**

    Partial atelectasis of newborn

    Secondary atelectasis of newborn N

P28.2 **Cyanotic attacks of newborn**

    EXCLUDES1 apnea of newborn (P28.3-P28.4) N

---

④ 4th character required   ⑤ 5th character required   ⑥ 6th character required   ⑦ 7th character required   Ⓧ Extension 'X' Alert

EXCLUDES 1 Not coded here   *EXCLUDES 2* Not included here   PDx Primary Diagnosis Only   Manifestation Code

P28.3 Primary sleep apnea of newborn
Central sleep apnea of newborn
Obstructive sleep apnea of newborn
Sleep apnea of newborn NOS [N]

P28.4 Other apnea of newborn
Apnea of prematurity
Obstructive apnea of newborn
[EXCLUDES1] *obstructive sleep apnea of newborn (P28.3)* [N]

P28.5 Respiratory failure of newborn
[EXCLUDES1] *respiratory arrest of newborn (P28.81)*
respiratory distress of newborn (P22.0-) [N]

[5th] **P28.8 Other specified respiratory conditions of newborn**
P28.81 Respiratory arrest of newborn [N]
P28.89 Other specified respiratory conditions of newborn
Congenital laryngeal stridor
Sniffles in newborn
Snuffles in newborn
[EXCLUDES1] *early congenital syphilitic rhinitis (A50.05)* [N]

P28.9 Respiratory condition of newborn, unspecified
Respiratory depression in newborn [N]

[4th] **P29 Cardiovascular disorders originating in the perinatal period**
[EXCLUDES1] *congenital malformations of the circulatory system (Q20-Q28)*

P29.0 Neonatal cardiac failure [N]
[5th] **P29.1 Neonatal cardiac dysrhythmia**
P29.11 Neonatal tachycardia [N]
P29.12 Neonatal bradycardia [N]
P29.2 Neonatal hypertension [N]
P29.3 Persistent fetal circulation
Delayed closure of ductus arteriosus
(Persistent) pulmonary hypertension of newborn [N]
P29.4 Transient myocardial ischemia in newborn [N]
[5th] **P29.8 Other cardiovascular disorders originating in the perinatal period**
P29.81 Cardiac arrest of newborn [N]
P29.89 Other cardiovascular disorders originating in the perinatal period [N]
P29.9 Cardiovascular disorder originating in the perinatal period, unspecified [N]

Infections specific to the perinatal period (P35-P39)

Infections acquired in utero, during birth via the umbilicus, or during the first 28 days after birth

[EXCLUDES2] *asymptomatic human immunodeficiency virus [HIV] infection status (Z21)*
congenital gonococcal infection (A54.-)
congenital pneumonia (P23.-)
congenital syphilis (A50.-)
human immunodeficiency virus [HIV] disease (B20)
infant botulism (A48.51)
infectious diseases not specific to the perinatal period (A00-B99, J09, J10.-)
intestinal infectious disease (A00-A09)
laboratory evidence of human immunodeficiency virus [HIV] (R75)
tetanus neonatorum (A33)

[4th] **P35 Congenital viral diseases**
[INCLUDES] *infections acquired in utero or during birth*

P35.0 Congenital rubella syndrome
Congenital rubella pneumonitis [N]
P35.1 Congenital cytomegalovirus infection [N]
P35.2 Congenital herpesviral [herpes simplex] infection [N]
P35.3 Congenital viral hepatitis [N]
P35.8 Other congenital viral diseases
Congenital varicella [chickenpox] [N]
P35.9 Congenital viral disease, unspecified [N]

[4th] **P36 Bacterial sepsis of newborn**
[INCLUDES] *congenital sepsis*
Use additional code(s), if applicable, to identify severe sepsis (R65.2-) and associated acute organ dysfunction(s)

P36.0 Sepsis of newborn due to streptococcus, group B [N]
[5th] **P36.1 Sepsis of newborn due to other and unspecified streptococci**
P36.10 Sepsis of newborn due to unspecified streptococci [N]
P36.19 Sepsis of newborn due to other streptococci [N]
P36.2 Sepsis of newborn due to Staphylococcus aureus [N]
[5th] **P36.3 Sepsis of newborn due to other and unspecified staphylococci**
P36.30 Sepsis of newborn due to unspecified staphylococci [N]
P36.39 Sepsis of newborn due to other staphylococci [N]
P36.4 Sepsis of newborn due to Escherichia coli [N]
P36.5 Sepsis of newborn due to anaerobes [N]
P36.8 Other bacterial sepsis of newborn
Use additional code from category B96 to identify organism [N]
P36.9 Bacterial sepsis of newborn, unspecified [N]

[4th] **P37 Other congenital infectious and parasitic diseases**
[EXCLUDES2] *congenital syphilis (A50.-)*
infectious neonatal diarrhea (A00-A09)
necrotizing enterocolitis in newborn (P77.-)
noninfectious neonatal diarrhea (P78.3)
ophthalmia neonatorum due to gonococcus (A54.31)
tetanus neonatorum (A33)

P37.0 Congenital tuberculosis [N]
P37.1 Congenital toxoplasmosis
Hydrocephalus due to congenital toxoplasmosis [N]
P37.2 Neonatal (disseminated) listeriosis [N]
P37.3 Congenital falciparum malaria [N]
P37.4 Other congenital malaria [N]
P37.5 Neonatal candidiasis [N]
P37.8 Other specified congenital infectious and parasitic diseases [N]
P37.9 Congenital infectious or parasitic disease, unspecified [N]

[4th] **P38 Omphalitis of newborn**
[EXCLUDES1] *omphalitis not of newborn (L08.82)*
tetanus omphalitis (A33)
umbilical hemorrhage of newborn (P51.-)

P38.1 Omphalitis with mild hemorrhage [N]
P38.9 Omphalitis without hemorrhage
Omphalitis of newborn NOS [N]

[4th] **P39 Other infections specific to the perinatal period**
Use additional code to identify organism or specific infection

P39.0 Neonatal infective mastitis
[EXCLUDES1] *breast engorgement of newborn (P83.4)*
noninfective mastitis of newborn (P83.4) [N]
P39.1 Neonatal conjunctivitis and dacryocystitis
Neonatal chlamydial conjunctivitis
Ophthalmia neonatorum NOS
[EXCLUDES1] *gonococcal conjunctivitis (A54.31)* [N]
P39.2 Intra-amniotic infection affecting newborn, not elsewhere classified [N]
P39.3 Neonatal urinary tract infection [N]
P39.4 Neonatal skin infection
Neonatal pyoderma
[EXCLUDES1] *pemphigus neonatorum (L00)*
staphylococcal scalded skin syndrome (L00) [N]
P39.8 Other specified infections specific to the perinatal period [N]
P39.9 Infection specific to the perinatal period, unspecified [N]

Unspecified Code | Other Specified Code | [N] Newborn Age: 0 | [P] Pediatric Age: 0-17 | [M] Maternity Age: 12-55
[A] Adult Age: 15-124 | ♂ Male | ♀ Female | ● New Code | ▲ Revised Code Title | ►◄ Revised Text

Hemorrhagic and hematological disorders of newborn (P50-P61)

[EXCLUDES1] *congenital stenosis and stricture of bile ducts (Q44.3)*
Crigler-Najjar syndrome (E80.5)
Dubin-Johnson syndrome (E80.6)
Gilbert syndrome (E80.4)
hereditary hemolytic anemias (D55-D58)

[4th] **P50 Newborn affected by intrauterine (fetal) blood loss**
[EXCLUDES1] *congenital anemia from intrauterine (fetal) blood loss (P61.3)*
P50.0 Newborn affected by intrauterine (fetal) blood loss from vasa previa [N]
P50.1 Newborn affected by intrauterine (fetal) blood loss from ruptured cord [N]
P50.2 Newborn affected by intrauterine (fetal) blood loss from placenta [N]
P50.3 Newborn affected by hemorrhage into co-twin [N]
P50.4 Newborn affected by hemorrhage into maternal circulation [N]
P50.5 Newborn affected by intrauterine (fetal) blood loss from cut end of co-twin's cord [N]
P50.8 Newborn affected by other intrauterine (fetal) blood loss [N]
P50.9 Newborn affected by intrauterine (fetal) blood loss, unspecified
Newborn affected by fetal hemorrhage NOS [N]

[4th] **P51 Umbilical hemorrhage of newborn**
[EXCLUDES1] *omphalitis with mild hemorrhage (P38.1)*
umbilical hemorrhage from cut end of co-twins cord (P50.5)
P51.0 Massive umbilical hemorrhage of newborn [N]
P51.8 Other umbilical hemorrhages of newborn
Slipped umbilical ligature NOS [N]
P51.9 Umbilical hemorrhage of newborn, unspecified [N]

[4th] **P52 Intracranial nontraumatic hemorrhage of newborn**
INCLUDES *intracranial hemorrhage due to anoxia or hypoxia*
[EXCLUDES1] *intracranial hemorrhage due to birth injury (P10.-)*
intracranial hemorrhage due to other injury (S06.-)
P52.0 Intraventricular (nontraumatic) hemorrhage, grade 1, of newborn
Subependymal hemorrhage (without intraventricular extension)
Bleeding into germinal matrix [N]
P52.1 Intraventricular (nontraumatic) hemorrhage, grade 2, of newborn
Subependymal hemorrhage with intraventricular extension
Bleeding into ventricle [N]
[5th] **P52.2 Intraventricular (nontraumatic) hemorrhage, grade 3 and grade 4, of newborn**
P52.21 Intraventricular (nontraumatic) hemorrhage, grade 3, of newborn
Subependymal hemorrhage with intraventricular extension with enlargement of ventricle [N]
P52.22 Intraventricular (nontraumatic) hemorrhage, grade 4, of newborn
Bleeding into cerebral cortex
Subependymal hemorrhage with intracerebral extension [N]
P52.3 Unspecified intraventricular (nontraumatic) hemorrhage of newborn [N]
P52.4 Intracerebral (nontraumatic) hemorrhage of newborn [N]
P52.5 Subarachnoid (nontraumatic) hemorrhage of newborn [N]
P52.6 Cerebellar (nontraumatic) and posterior fossa hemorrhage of newborn [N]
P52.8 Other intracranial (nontraumatic) hemorrhages of newborn [N]
P52.9 Intracranial (nontraumatic) hemorrhage of newborn, unspecified [N]

P53 Hemorrhagic disease of newborn
Vitamin K deficiency of newborn

[4th] **P54 Other neonatal hemorrhages**
[EXCLUDES1] *newborn affected by (intrauterine) blood loss (P50.-)*
pulmonary hemorrhage originating in the perinatal period (P26.-)
P54.0 Neonatal hematemesis
[EXCLUDES1] *neonatal hematemesis due to swallowed maternal blood (P78.2)* [N]
P54.1 Neonatal melena
[EXCLUDES1] *neonatal melena due to swallowed maternal blood (P78.2)* [N]
P54.2 Neonatal rectal hemorrhage [N]
P54.3 Other neonatal gastrointestinal hemorrhage [N]
P54.4 Neonatal adrenal hemorrhage [N]
P54.5 Neonatal cutaneous hemorrhage
Neonatal bruising
Neonatal ecchymoses
Neonatal petechiae
Neonatal superficial hematomata
[EXCLUDES2] *bruising of scalp due to birth injury (P12.3)*
cephalhematoma due to birth injury (P12.0) [N]
P54.6 Neonatal vaginal hemorrhage
Neonatal pseudomenses [N] ♀
P54.8 Other specified neonatal hemorrhages [N]
P54.9 Neonatal hemorrhage, unspecified [N]

[4th] **P55 Hemolytic disease of newborn**
P55.0 Rh isoimmunization of newborn [N]
P55.1 ABO isoimmunization of newborn [N]
P55.8 Other hemolytic diseases of newborn [N]
P55.9 Hemolytic disease of newborn, unspecified [N]

[4th] **P56 Hydrops fetalis due to hemolytic disease**
[EXCLUDES1] *hydrops fetalis NOS (P83.2)*
P56.0 Hydrops fetalis due to isoimmunization [N]
[5th] **P56.9 Hydrops fetalis due to other and unspecified hemolytic disease**
P56.90 Hydrops fetalis due to unspecified hemolytic disease [N]
P56.99 Hydrops fetalis due to other hemolytic disease [N]

[4th] **P57 Kernicterus**
P57.0 Kernicterus due to isoimmunization [N]
P57.8 Other specified kernicterus
[EXCLUDES1] *Crigler-Najjar syndrome (E80.5)* [N]
P57.9 Kernicterus, unspecified [N]

[4th] **P58 Neonatal jaundice due to other excessive hemolysis**
[EXCLUDES1] *jaundice due to isoimmunization (P55-P57)*
P58.0 Neonatal jaundice due to bruising [N]
P58.1 Neonatal jaundice due to bleeding [N]
P58.2 Neonatal jaundice due to infection [N]
P58.3 Neonatal jaundice due to polycythemia [N]
[5th] **P58.4 Neonatal jaundice due to drugs or toxins transmitted from mother or given to newborn**
Code first poisoning due to drug or toxin, if applicable (T36-T65 with fifth or sixth character 1-4 or 6)
Use additional code for adverse effect, if applicable, to identify drug (T36-T50 with fifth or sixth character 5)
P58.41 Neonatal jaundice due to drugs or toxins transmitted from mother [N]
P58.42 Neonatal jaundice due to drugs or toxins given to newborn [N]

[4th] 4th character required [5th] 5th character required [6th] 6th character required [7th] 7th character required [7th] Extension 'X' Alert
[EXCLUDES1] Not coded here [EXCLUDES2] Not included here [PDx] Primary Diagnosis Only Manifestation Code

P58.5 Neonatal jaundice due to swallowed maternal blood [N]
P58.8 Neonatal jaundice due to other specified excessive hemolysis [N]
P58.9 Neonatal jaundice due to excessive hemolysis, unspecified [N]

[4] P59 Neonatal jaundice from other and unspecified causes
EXCLUDES1 *jaundice due to inborn errors of metabolism (E70-E88)*
kernicterus (P57.-)

P59.0 Neonatal jaundice associated with preterm delivery
Hyperbilirubinemia of prematurity
Jaundice due to delayed conjugation associated with preterm delivery [N]
P59.1 Inspissated bile syndrome [N]
[5] P59.2 Neonatal jaundice from other and unspecified hepatocellular damage
EXCLUDES1 *congenital viral hepatitis (P35.3)*
P59.20 Neonatal jaundice from unspecified hepatocellular damage [N]
P59.29 Neonatal jaundice from other hepatocellular damage
Neonatal giant cell hepatitis
Neonatal (idiopathic) hepatitis [N]
P59.3 Neonatal jaundice from breast milk inhibitor [N]
P59.8 Neonatal jaundice from other specified causes [N]
P59.9 Neonatal jaundice, unspecified
Neonatal physiological jaundice (intense)(prolonged) NOS [N]

P60 Disseminated intravascular coagulation of newborn
Defibrination syndrome of newborn

[4] P61 Other perinatal hematological disorders
EXCLUDES1 *transient hypogammaglobulinemia of infancy (D80.7)*

P61.0 Transient neonatal thrombocytopenia
Neonatal thrombocytopenia due to exchange transfusion
Neonatal thrombocytopenia due to idiopathic maternal thrombocytopenia
Neonatal thrombocytopenia due to isoimmunization [N]
P61.1 Polycythemia neonatorum [N]
P61.2 Anemia of prematurity [N]
P61.3 Congenital anemia from fetal blood loss [N]
P61.4 Other congenital anemias, not elsewhere classified
Congenital anemia NOS [N]
P61.5 Transient neonatal neutropenia
EXCLUDES1 *congenital neutropenia (nontransient) (D70.0)* [N]
P61.6 Other transient neonatal disorders of coagulation [N]
P61.8 Other specified perinatal hematological disorders [N]
P61.9 Perinatal hematological disorder, unspecified [N]

Transitory endocrine and metabolic disorders specific to newborn (P70-P74)

INCLUDES *transitory endocrine and metabolic disturbances caused by the infant's response to maternal endocrine and metabolic factors, or its adjustment to extrauterine environment*

[4] P70 Transitory disorders of carbohydrate metabolism specific to newborn

P70.0 Syndrome of infant of mother with gestational diabetes
Newborn (with hypoglycemia) affected by maternal gestational diabetes
EXCLUDES1 *newborn (with hypoglycemia) affected by maternal (pre-existing) diabetes mellitus (P70.1)*
syndrome of infant of a diabetic mother (P70.1) [N]
P70.1 Syndrome of infant of a diabetic mother
Newborn (with hypoglycemia) affected by maternal (pre-existing) diabetes mellitus
EXCLUDES1 *newborn (with hypoglycemia) affected by maternal gestational diabetes (P70.0)*
syndrome of infant of mother with gestational diabetes (P70.0) [N]
P70.2 Neonatal diabetes mellitus [N]
P70.3 Iatrogenic neonatal hypoglycemia [N]
P70.4 Other neonatal hypoglycemia
Transitory neonatal hypoglycemia [N]
P70.8 Other transitory disorders of carbohydrate metabolism of newborn [N]
P70.9 Transitory disorder of carbohydrate metabolism of newborn, unspecified [N]

[4] P71 Transitory neonatal disorders of calcium and magnesium metabolism

P71.0 Cow's milk hypocalcemia in newborn [N]
P71.1 Other neonatal hypocalcemia
EXCLUDES1 *neonatal hypoparathyroidism (P71.4)* [N]
P71.2 Neonatal hypomagnesemia [N]
P71.3 Neonatal tetany without calcium or magnesium deficiency
Neonatal tetany NOS [N]
P71.4 Transitory neonatal hypoparathyroidism [N]
P71.8 Other transitory neonatal disorders of calcium and magnesium metabolism [N]
P71.9 Transitory neonatal disorder of calcium and magnesium metabolism, unspecified [N]

[4] P72 Other transitory neonatal endocrine disorders
EXCLUDES1 *congenital hypothyroidism with or without goiter (E03.0-E03.1)*
dyshormogenetic goiter (E07.1)
Pendred's syndrome (E07.1)

P72.0 Neonatal goiter, not elsewhere classified
Transitory congenital goiter with normal functioning [N]
P72.1 Transitory neonatal hyperthyroidism
Neonatal thyrotoxicosis [N]
P72.2 Other transitory neonatal disorders of thyroid function, not elsewhere classified
Transitory neonatal hypothyroidism [N]
P72.8 Other specified transitory neonatal endocrine disorders [N]
P72.9 Transitory neonatal endocrine disorder, unspecified [N]

[4] P74 Other transitory neonatal electrolyte and metabolic disturbances

P74.0 Late metabolic acidosis of newborn
EXCLUDES1 *(fetal) metabolic acidosis of newborn (P19)* [N]
P74.1 Dehydration of newborn [N]
P74.2 Disturbances of sodium balance of newborn [N]
P74.3 Disturbances of potassium balance of newborn [N]
P74.4 Other transitory electrolyte disturbances of newborn [N]
P74.5 Transitory tyrosinemia of newborn [N]
P74.6 Transitory hyperammonemia of newborn [N]
P74.8 Other transitory metabolic disturbances of newborn
Amino-acid metabolic disorders described as transitory [N]
P74.9 Transitory metabolic disturbance of newborn, unspecified [N]

Unspecified Code | Other Specified Code | [N] Newborn Age: 0 | [P] Pediatric Age: 0-17 | [M] Maternity Age: 12-55
[A] Adult Age: 15-124 | ♂ Male | ♀ Female | ● New Code | ▲ Revised Code Title | ►◄ Revised Text

Digestive system disorders of newborn (P76-P78)

④ P76 Other intestinal obstruction of newborn
P76.0 Meconium plug syndrome
Meconium ileus NOS
EXCLUDES1 *meconium ileus in cystic fibrosis (E84.11)* Ⓝ
P76.1 Transitory ileus of newborn
EXCLUDES1 *Hirschsprung's disease (Q43.1)* Ⓝ
P76.2 Intestinal obstruction due to inspissated milk Ⓝ
P76.8 Other specified intestinal obstruction of newborn
EXCLUDES1 *intestinal obstruction classifiable to K56.-* Ⓝ
P76.9 Intestinal obstruction of newborn, unspecified Ⓝ

④ P77 Necrotizing enterocolitis of newborn
P77.1 Stage 1 necrotizing enterocolitis in newborn
Necrotizing enterocolitis without pneumatosis, without perforation Ⓝ
P77.2 Stage 2 necrotizing enterocolitis in newborn
Necrotizing enterocolitis with pneumatosis, without perforation Ⓝ
P77.3 Stage 3 necrotizing enterocolitis in newborn
Necrotizing enterocolitis with perforation
Necrotizing enterocolitis with pneumatosis and perforation Ⓝ
P77.9 Necrotizing enterocolitis in newborn, unspecified
Necrotizing enterocolitis in newborn, NOS Ⓝ

④ P78 Other perinatal digestive system disorders
EXCLUDES1 *cystic fibrosis (E84.0-E84.9)*
neonatal gastrointestinal hemorrhages (P54.0-P54.3)
P78.0 Perinatal intestinal perforation
Meconium peritonitis Ⓝ
P78.1 Other neonatal peritonitis
Neonatal peritonitis NOS Ⓝ
P78.2 Neonatal hematemesis and melena due to swallowed maternal blood Ⓝ
P78.3 Noninfective neonatal diarrhea
Neonatal diarrhea NOS Ⓝ
⑤ P78.8 Other specified perinatal digestive system disorders
P78.81 Congenital cirrhosis (of liver) Ⓝ
P78.82 Peptic ulcer of newborn Ⓝ
P78.83 Newborn esophageal reflux
Neonatal esophageal reflux Ⓝ
P78.89 Other specified perinatal digestive system disorders Ⓝ
P78.9 Perinatal digestive system disorder, unspecified Ⓝ

Conditions involving the integument and temperature regulation of newborn (P80-P83)

④ P80 Hypothermia of newborn
P80.0 Cold injury syndrome
Severe and usually chronic hypothermia associated with a pink flushed appearance, edema and neurological and biochemical abnormalities.
EXCLUDES1 *mild hypothermia of newborn (P80.8)* Ⓝ
P80.8 Other hypothermia of newborn
Mild hypothermia of newborn Ⓝ
P80.9 Hypothermia of newborn, unspecified Ⓝ

④ P81 Other disturbances of temperature regulation of newborn
P81.0 Environmental hyperthermia of newborn Ⓝ
P81.8 Other specified disturbances of temperature regulation of newborn Ⓝ
P81.9 Disturbance of temperature regulation of newborn, unspecified
Fever of newborn NOS Ⓝ

④ P83 Other conditions of integument specific to newborn
EXCLUDES1 *congenital malformations of skin and integument (Q80-Q84)*
hydrops fetalis due to hemolytic disease (P56.-)
neonatal skin infection (P39.4)
staphylococcal scalded skin syndrome (L00)
EXCLUDES2 *cradle cap (L21.0)*
diaper [napkin] dermatitis (L22)
P83.0 Sclerema neonatorum Ⓝ
P83.1 Neonatal erythema toxicum Ⓝ
P83.2 Hydrops fetalis not due to hemolytic disease
Hydrops fetalis NOS Ⓝ
⑤ P83.3 Other and unspecified edema specific to newborn
P83.30 Unspecified edema specific to newborn Ⓝ
P83.39 Other edema specific to newborn Ⓝ
P83.4 Breast engorgement of newborn
Noninfective mastitis of newborn Ⓝ
P83.5 Congenital hydrocele ♂
P83.6 Umbilical polyp of newborn Ⓝ
P83.8 Other specified conditions of integument specific to newborn
Bronze baby syndrome
Neonatal scleroderma
Urticaria neonatorum Ⓝ
P83.9 Condition of the integument specific to newborn, unspecified Ⓝ

Other problems with newborn (P84)

P84 Other problems with newborn
Acidemia of newborn
Acidosis of newborn
Anoxia of newborn NOS
Asphyxia of newborn NOS
Hypercapnia of newborn
Hypoxemia of newborn
Hypoxia of newborn NOS
Mixed metabolic and respiratory acidosis of newborn
EXCLUDES1 *intracranial hemorrhage due to anoxia or hypoxia (P52.-)*
hypoxic ischemic encephalopathy [HIE] (P91.6-)
late metabolic acidosis of newborn (P74.0)

Other disorders originating in the perinatal period (P90-P96)

P90 Convulsions of newborn
EXCLUDES1 *benign myoclonic epilepsy in infancy (G40.3-)*
benign neonatal convulsions (familial) (G40.3-)
④ P91 Other disturbances of cerebral status of newborn
P91.0 Neonatal cerebral ischemia Ⓝ
P91.1 Acquired periventricular cysts of newborn Ⓝ
P91.2 Neonatal cerebral leukomalacia
Periventricular leukomalacia Ⓝ
P91.3 Neonatal cerebral irritability Ⓝ
P91.4 Neonatal cerebral depression Ⓝ
P91.5 Neonatal coma Ⓝ
⑤ P91.6 Hypoxic ischemic encephalopathy [HIE]
P91.60 Hypoxic ischemic encephalopathy [HIE], unspecified Ⓝ
P91.61 Mild hypoxic ischemic encephalopathy [HIE] Ⓝ
P91.62 Moderate hypoxic ischemic encephalopathy [HIE] Ⓝ
P91.63 Severe hypoxic ischemic encephalopathy [HIE] Ⓝ
P91.8 Other specified disturbances of cerebral status of newborn Ⓝ
P91.9 Disturbance of cerebral status of newborn, unspecified Ⓝ

④ 4th character required　⑤ 5th character required　⑥ 6th character required　⑦ 7th character required　⑩ Extension 'X' Alert
EXCLUDES 1 Not coded here　EXCLUDES 2 Not included here　PDx Primary Diagnosis Only　Manifestation Code

490

ICD-10-CM 2015

❹ **P92 Feeding problems of newborn**

> EXCLUDES1 *feeding problems in child over 28 days old (R63.3)*

❺ **P92.0 Vomiting of newborn**

> EXCLUDES1 *vomiting of child over 28 days old (R11.-)*

P92.01 Bilious vomiting of newborn

> EXCLUDES1 *bilious vomiting in child over 28 days old (R11.14)* Ⓝ

P92.09 Other vomiting of newborn

> EXCLUDES1 *regurgitation of food in newborn (P92.1)* Ⓝ

P92.1 Regurgitation and rumination of newborn Ⓝ

P92.2 Slow feeding of newborn Ⓝ

P92.3 Underfeeding of newborn Ⓝ

P92.4 Overfeeding of newborn Ⓝ

P92.5 Neonatal difficulty in feeding at breast Ⓝ

P92.6 Failure to thrive in newborn

> EXCLUDES1 *failure to thrive in child over 28 days old (R62.51)* Ⓝ

P92.8 Other feeding problems of newborn Ⓝ

P92.9 Feeding problem of newborn, unspecified Ⓝ

❹ **P93 Reactions and intoxications due to drugs administered to newborn**

> INCLUDES *reactions and intoxications due to drugs administered to fetus affecting newborn*

> EXCLUDES1 *jaundice due to drugs or toxins transmitted from mother or given to newborn (P58.4-)*
> *reactions and intoxications from maternal opiates, tranquilizers and other medication (P04.0-P04.1, P04.4)*
> *withdrawal symptoms from maternal use of drugs of addiction (P96.1)*
> *withdrawal symptoms from therapeutic use of drugs in newborn (P96.2)*

P93.0 Grey baby syndrome

Grey syndrome from chloramphenicol administration in newborn Ⓝ

P93.8 Other reactions and intoxications due to drugs administered to newborn

Use additional code for adverse effect, if applicable, to identify drug (T36-T50 with fifth or sixth character 5) Ⓝ

❹ **P94 Disorders of muscle tone of newborn**

P94.0 Transient neonatal myasthenia gravis

> EXCLUDES1 *myasthenia gravis (G70.0)* Ⓝ

P94.1 Congenital hypertonia Ⓝ

P94.2 Congenital hypotonia

Floppy baby syndrome, unspecified Ⓝ

P94.8 Other disorders of muscle tone of newborn Ⓝ

P94.9 Disorder of muscle tone of newborn, unspecified Ⓝ

P95 Stillbirth

Deadborn fetus NOS

Fetal death of unspecified cause

Stillbirth NOS

> EXCLUDES1 *maternal care for intrauterine death (O36.4)*
> *missed abortion (O02.1)*
> *outcome of delivery, stillbirth (Z37.1, Z37.3, Z37.4, Z37.7)*

❹ **P96 Other conditions originating in the perinatal period**

P96.0 Congenital renal failure

Uremia of newborn Ⓝ

P96.1 Neonatal withdrawal symptoms from maternal use of drugs of addiction

Drug withdrawal syndrome in infant of dependent mother

Neonatal abstinence syndrome

> EXCLUDES1 *reactions and intoxications from maternal opiates and tranquilizers administered during labor and delivery (P04.0)* Ⓝ

P96.2 Withdrawal symptoms from therapeutic use of drugs in newborn Ⓝ

P96.3 Wide cranial sutures of newborn

Neonatal craniotabes Ⓝ

P96.5 Complication to newborn due to (fetal) intrauterine procedure

> EXCLUDES2 *newborn (suspected to be) affected by amniocentesis (P00.6)* Ⓝ

❺ **P96.8 Other specified conditions originating in the perinatal period**

P96.81 Exposure to (parental) (environmental) tobacco smoke in the perinatal period

> EXCLUDES2 *newborn affected by in utero exposure to tobacco (P04.2)*
> *exposure to environmental tobacco smoke after the perinatal period (Z77.22)*

P96.82 Delayed separation of umbilical cord Ⓝ

P96.83 Meconium staining

> EXCLUDES1 *meconium aspiration (P24.00, P24.01)*
> *meconium passage during delivery (P03.82)* Ⓝ

P96.89 Other specified conditions originating in the perinatal period

Use additional code to specify condition Ⓝ

P96.9 Condition originating in the perinatal period, unspecified

Congenital debility NOS Ⓝ

Unspecified Code	Other Specified Code	Ⓝ Newborn Age: 0	Ⓟ Pediatric Age: 0-17	Ⓜ Maternity Age: 12-55
Ⓐ Adult Age: 15-124	♂ Male	♀ Female	● New Code	▲ Revised Code Title	▶◀ Revised Text

This page intentionally left blank

Chapter 17: Congenital Malformations, Deformations, and Chromosomal Abnormalities (Q00-Q99)

Chapter Specific Coding Guidelines

Assign an appropriate code(s) from categories Q00-Q99, Congenital malformations, deformations, and chromosomal abnormalities when a malformation/deformation or chromosomal abnormality is documented. A malformation/deformation/or chromosomal abnormality may be the principal/first-listed diagnosis on a record or a secondary diagnosis.

When a malformation/deformation/or chromosomal abnormality does not have a unique code assignment, assign additional code(s) for any manifestations that may be present.

When the code assignment specifically identifies the malformation/deformation/or chromosomal abnormality, manifestations that are an inherent component of the anomaly should not be coded separately. Additional codes should be assigned for manifestations that are not an inherent component.

Codes from Chapter 17 may be used throughout the life of the patient. If a congenital malformation or deformity has been corrected, a personal history code should be used to identify the history of the malformation or deformity. Although present at birth, malformation/deformation/or chromosomal abnormality may not be identified until later in life. Whenever the condition is diagnosed by the physician, it is appropriate to assign a code from codes Q00-Q99. For the birth admission, the appropriate code from category Z38, Liveborn infants, according to place of birth and type of delivery, should be sequenced as the principal diagnosis, followed by any congenital anomaly codes, Q00- Q99.

This page intentionally left blank

Congenital malformations, deformations and chromosomal abnormalities (Q00-Q99)

NOTES Codes from this chapter are not for use on maternal or fetal records

EXCLUDES2 *inborn errors of metabolism (E70-E88)*

Congenital malformations of the nervous system (Q00-Q07)

⊕ **Q00 Anencephaly and similar malformations**

Q00.0 Anencephaly

Acephaly

Acrania

Amyelencephaly

Hemianencephaly

Hemicephaly

Q00.1 Craniorachischisis

Q00.2 Iniencephaly

⊕ **Q01 Encephalocele**

INCLUDES *Arnold-Chiari syndrome, type III*
encephalocystocele
encephalomyelocele
hydroencephalocele
hydromeningocele, cranial
meningocele, cerebral
meningoencephalocele

EXCLUDES1 *Meckel-Gruber syndrome (Q61.9)*

Q01.0 Frontal encephalocele

Q01.1 Nasofrontal encephalocele

Q01.2 Occipital encephalocele

Q01.8 Encephalocele of other sites

Q01.9 Encephalocele, unspecified

Q02 Microcephaly

INCLUDES *hydromicrocephaly*
micrencephalon

EXCLUDES1 *Meckel-Gruber syndrome (Q61.9)*

⊕ **Q03 Congenital hydrocephalus**

INCLUDES *hydrocephalus in newborn*

EXCLUDES1 *Arnold-Chiari syndrome, type II (Q07.0-)*
acquired hydrocephalus (G91.-)
hydrocephalus due to congenital toxoplasmosis (P37.1)
hydrocephalus with spina bifida (Q05.0-Q05.4)

Q03.0 Malformations of aqueduct of Sylvius

Anomaly of aqueduct of Sylvius

Obstruction of aqueduct of Sylvius, congenital

Stenosis of aqueduct of Sylvius

Q03.1 Atresia of foramina of Magendie and Luschka

Dandy-Walker syndrome

Q03.8 Other congenital hydrocephalus

Q03.9 Congenital hydrocephalus, unspecified

⊕ **Q04 Other congenital malformations of brain**

EXCLUDES1 *cyclopia (Q87.0)*
macrocephaly (Q75.3)

Q04.0 Congenital malformations of corpus callosum

Agenesis of corpus callosum

Q04.1 Arhinencephaly

Q04.2 Holoprosencephaly

Q04.3 Other reduction deformities of brain

Absence of part of brain

Agenesis of part of brain

Agyria

Aplasia of part of brain

Hydranencephaly

Hypoplasia of part of brain

Lissencephaly

Microgyria

Pachygyria

EXCLUDES1 *congenital malformations of corpus callosum (Q04.0)*

Q04.4 Septo-optic dysplasia of brain

Q04.5 Megalencephaly

Q04.6 Congenital cerebral cysts

Porencephaly

Schizencephaly

EXCLUDES1 *acquired porencephalic cyst (G93.0)*

Q04.8 Other specified congenital malformations of brain

Arnold-Chiari syndrome, type IV

Macrogyria

Q04.9 Congenital malformation of brain, unspecified

Congenital anomaly NOS of brain

Congenital deformity NOS of brain

Congenital disease or lesion NOS of brain

Multiple anomalies NOS of brain, congenital

⊕ **Q05 Spina bifida**

INCLUDES *hydromeningocele (spinal)*
meningocele (spinal)
meningomyelocele
myelocele
myelomeningocele
rachischisis
spina bifida (aperta)(cystica)
syringomyelocele

Use additional code for any associated paraplegia (paraparesis) (G82.2-)

EXCLUDES1 *Arnold-Chiari syndrome, type II (Q07.0-)*
spina bifida occulta (Q76.0)

Q05.0 Cervical spina bifida with hydrocephalus

Q05.1 Thoracic spina bifida with hydrocephalus

Dorsal spina bifida with hydrocephalus

Thoracolumbar spina bifida with hydrocephalus

Q05.2 Lumbar spina bifida with hydrocephalus

Lumbosacral spina bifida with hydrocephalus

Q05.3 Sacral spina bifida with hydrocephalus

Q05.4 Unspecified spina bifida with hydrocephalus

Q05.5 Cervical spina bifida without hydrocephalus

Q05.6 Thoracic spina bifida without hydrocephalus

Dorsal spina bifida NOS

Thoracolumbar spina bifida NOS

Q05.7 Lumbar spina bifida without hydrocephalus

Lumbosacral spina bifida NOS

Q05.8 Sacral spina bifida without hydrocephalus

Q05.9 Spina bifida, unspecified

⊕ **Q06 Other congenital malformations of spinal cord**

Q06.0 Amyelia

Q06.1 Hypoplasia and dysplasia of spinal cord

Atelomyelia

Myelatelia

Myelodysplasia of spinal cord

Q06.2 Diastematomyelia

Q06.3 Other congenital cauda equina malformations

Q06.4 Hydromyelia

Hydrorachis

Q06.8 Other specified congenital malformations of spinal cord

Q06.9 Congenital malformation of spinal cord, unspecified

Congenital anomaly NOS of spinal cord

Congenital deformity NOS of spinal cord

Congenital disease or lesion NOS of spinal cord

⊕ **Q07 Other congenital malformations of nervous system**

EXCLUDES2 *congenital central alveolar hypoventilation syndrome (G47.35)*
familial dysautonomia [Riley-Day] (G90.1)
neurofibromatosis (nonmalignant) (Q85.0-)

Unspecified Code   Other Specified Code   N Newborn Age: 0   P Pediatric Age: 0-17   M Maternity Age: 12-55

A Adult Age: 15-124   ♂ Male   ♀ Female   ● New Code   ▲ Revised Code Title   ►◄ Revised Text

⑤ **Q07.0** **Arnold-Chiari syndrome**

Arnold-Chiari syndrome, type II

EXCLUDES1 Arnold-Chiari syndrome, type III (Q01.-)
Arnold-Chiari syndrome, type IV (Q04.8)

Q07.00 **Arnold-Chiari syndrome** without spina bifida or hydrocephalus

Q07.01 **Arnold-Chiari syndrome** with spina bifida

Q07.02 **Arnold-Chiari syndrome** with hydrocephalus

Q07.03 **Arnold-Chiari syndrome** with spina bifida and hydrocephalus

Q07.8 **Other specified congenital malformations of nervous system**

Agenesis of nerve

Displacement of brachial plexus

Jaw-winking syndrome

Marcus Gunn's syndrome

Q07.9 **Congenital malformation of nervous system, unspecified**

Congenital anomaly NOS of nervous system

Congenital deformity NOS of nervous system

Congenital disease or lesion NOS of nervous system

Congenital malformations of eye, ear, face and neck (Q10-Q18)

EXCLUDES2 cleft lip and cleft palate (Q35-Q37)
congenital malformation of cervical spine (Q05.0, Q05.5, Q67.5, Q76.0-Q76.4)
congenital malformation of larynx (Q31.-)
congenital malformation of lip NEC (Q38.0)
congenital malformation of nose (Q30.-)
congenital malformation of parathyroid gland (Q89.2)
congenital malformation of thyroid gland (Q89.2)

④ **Q10** **Congenital malformations of** eyelid, lacrimal apparatus and orbit

EXCLUDES1 cryptophthalmos NOS (Q11.2)
cryptophthalmos syndrome (Q87.0)

Q10.0 **Congenital** ptosis

Q10.1 **Congenital** ectropion

Q10.2 **Congenital** entropion

Q10.3 Other **congenital malformations of eyelid**

Ablepharon

Blepharophimosis, congenital

Coloboma of eyelid

Congenital absence or agenesis of cilia

Congenital absence or agenesis of eyelid

Congenital accessory eyelid

Congenital accessory eye muscle

Congenital malformation of eyelid NOS

Q10.4 **Absence and agenesis of lacrimal apparatus**

Congenital absence of punctum lacrimale

Q10.5 **Congenital** stenosis and stricture of lacrimal duct

Q10.6 Other **congenital malformations of lacrimal apparatus**

Congenital malformation of lacrimal apparatus NOS

Q10.7 **Congenital malformation of** orbit

④ **Q11** **Anophthalmos, microphthalmos and macrophthalmos**

Q11.0 **Cystic eyeball**

Q11.1 **Other anophthalmos**

Anophthalmos NOS

Agenesis of eye

Aplasia of eye

Q11.2 **Microphthalmos**

Cryptophthalmos NOS

Dysplasia of eye

Hypoplasia of eye

Rudimentary eye

EXCLUDES1 cryptophthalmos syndrome (Q87.0)

Q11.3 **Macrophthalmos**

EXCLUDES1 macrophthalmos in congenital glaucoma (Q15.0)

④ **Q12** **Congenital** lens malformations

Q12.0 **Congenital** cataract

Q12.1 **Congenital** displaced lens

Q12.2 Coloboma of lens

Q12.3 **Congenital** aphakia

Q12.4 **Spherophakia**

Q12.8 Other **congenital lens malformations**

Microphakia

Q12.9 **Congenital lens malformation, unspecified**

④ **Q13** **Congenital malformations of** anterior segment of eye

Q13.0 Coloboma **of iris**

Coloboma NOS

Q13.1 Absence **of iris**

Aniridia

Use additional code for associated glaucoma (H42)

Q13.2 Other **congenital malformations of iris**

Anisocoria, congenital

Atresia of pupil

Congenital malformation of iris NOS

Corectopia

Q13.3 **Congenital** corneal opacity

Q13.4 **Other congenital corneal malformations**

Congenital malformation of cornea NOS

Microcornea

Peter's anomaly

Q13.5 **Blue sclera**

⑤ **Q13.8** Other **congenital malformations of anterior segment of eye**

Q13.81 **Rieger's anomaly**

Use additional code for associated glaucoma (H42)

Q13.89 **Other congenital malformations of anterior segment of eye**

Q13.9 **Congenital malformation of anterior segment of eye, unspecified**

④ **Q14** **Congenital malformations of** posterior segment of eye

EXCLUDES2 optic nerve hypoplasia (H47.03-)

Q14.0 **Congenital malformation of** vitreous humor

Congenital vitreous opacity

Q14.1 **Congenital malformation of** retina

Congenital retinal aneurysm

Q14.2 **Congenital malformation of** optic disc

Coloboma of optic disc

Q14.3 **Congenital malformation of** choroid

Q14.8 Other **congenital malformations of posterior segment of eye**

Coloboma of the fundus

Q14.9 **Congenital malformation of posterior segment of eye, unspecified**

④ **Q15** Other **congenital malformations of** eye

EXCLUDES1 congenital nystagmus (H55.01)
ocular albinism (E70.31-)
optic nerve hypoplasia (H47.03-)
retinitis pigmentosa (H35.52)

Q15.0 **Congenital** glaucoma

Axenfeld's anomaly

Buphthalmos

Glaucoma of childhood

Glaucoma of newborn

Hydrophthalmos

Keratoglobus, congenital, with glaucoma

Macrocornea with glaucoma

Macrophthalmos in congenital glaucoma

Megalocornea with glaucoma

---

④ 4th character required	⑤ 5th character required	⑥ 6th character required	⑦ 7th character required	ⓧ Extension 'X' Alert
EXCLUDES 1 Not coded here	*EXCLUDES 2* Not included here	℞ₓ Primary Diagnosis Only	Manifestation Code	

Q15.8 Other specified congenital malformations of eye

Q15.9 Congenital malformation of eye, unspecified

Congenital anomaly of eye
Congenital deformity of eye

[4th] Q16 Congenital malformations of ear causing impairment of hearing

[EXCLUDES1] *congenital deafness (H90.-)*

Q16.0 Congenital absence of (ear) auricle

Q16.1 Congenital absence, atresia and stricture of auditory canal (external)

Congenital atresia or stricture of osseous meatus

Q16.2 Absence of eustachian tube

Q16.3 Congenital malformation of ear ossicles

Congenital fusion of ear ossicles

Q16.4 Other congenital malformations of middle ear

Congenital malformation of middle ear NOS

Q16.5 Congenital malformation of inner ear

Congenital anomaly of membranous labyrinth
Congenital anomaly of organ of Corti

Q16.9 Congenital malformation of ear causing impairment of hearing, unspecified

Congenital absence of ear NOS

[4th] Q17 Other congenital malformations of ear

[EXCLUDES1] *congenital malformations of ear with impairment of hearing (Q16.0-Q16.9)*
preauricular sinus (Q18.1)

Q17.0 Accessory auricle

Accessory tragus
Polyotia
Preauricular appendage or tag
Supernumerary ear
Supernumerary lobule

Q17.1 Macrotia

Q17.2 Microtia

Q17.3 Other misshapen ear

Pointed ear

Q17.4 Misplaced ear

Low-set ears

[EXCLUDES1] *cervical auricle (Q18.2)*

Q17.5 Prominent ear

Bat ear

Q17.8 Other specified congenital malformations of ear

Congenital absence of lobe of ear

Q17.9 Congenital malformation of ear, unspecified

Congenital anomaly of ear NOS

[4th] Q18 Other congenital malformations of face and neck

[EXCLUDES1] *cleft lip and cleft palate (Q35-Q37)*
conditions classified to Q67.0-Q67.4
congenital malformations of skull and face bones (Q75.-)
cyclopia (Q87.0)
dentofacial anomalies [including malocclusion] (M26.-)
malformation syndromes affecting facial appearance (Q87.0)
persistent thyroglossal duct (Q89.2)

Q18.0 Sinus, fistula and cyst of branchial cleft

Branchial vestige

Q18.1 Preauricular sinus and cyst

Fistula of auricle, congenital
Cervicoaural fistula

Q18.2 Other branchial cleft malformations

Branchial cleft malformation NOS
Cervical auricle
Otocephaly

Q18.3 Webbing of neck

Pterygium colli

Q18.4 Macrostomia

Q18.5 Microstomia

Q18.6 Macrocheilia

Hypertrophy of lip, congenital

Q18.7 Microcheilia

Q18.8 Other specified congenital malformations of face and neck

Medial cyst of face and neck
Medial fistula of face and neck
Medial sinus of face and neck

Q18.9 Congenital malformation of face and neck, unspecified

Congenital anomaly NOS of face and neck

Congenital malformations of the circulatory system (Q20-Q28)

[4th] Q20 Congenital malformations of cardiac chambers and connections

[EXCLUDES1] *dextrocardia with situs inversus (Q89.3)*
mirror-image atrial arrangement with situs inversus (Q89.3)

Q20.0 Common arterial trunk

Persistent truncus arteriosus

[EXCLUDES1] *aortic septal defect (Q21.4)*

Q20.1 Double outlet right ventricle

Taussig-Bing syndrome

Q20.2 Double outlet left ventricle

Q20.3 Discordant ventriculoarterial connection

Dextrotransposition of aorta
Transposition of great vessels (complete)

Q20.4 Double inlet ventricle

Common ventricle
Cor triloculare biatriatum
Single ventricle

Q20.5 Discordant atrioventricular connection

Corrected transposition
Levotransposition
Ventricular inversion

Q20.6 Isomerism of atrial appendages

Isomerism of atrial appendages with asplenia or polysplenia

Q20.8 Other congenital malformations of cardiac chambers and connections

Cor binoculare

Q20.9 Congenital malformation of cardiac chambers and connections, unspecified

[4th] Q21 Congenital malformations of cardiac septa

[EXCLUDES1] *acquired cardiac septal defect (I51.0)*

Q21.0 Ventricular septal defect

Roger's disease

Q21.1 Atrial septal defect

Coronary sinus defect
Patent or persistent foramen ovale
Patent or persistent ostium secundum defect (type II)
Patent or persistent sinus venosus defect

Q21.2 Atrioventricular septal defect

Common atrioventricular canal
Endocardial cushion defect
Ostium primum atrial septal defect (type I)

Q21.3 Tetralogy of Fallot

Ventricular septal defect with pulmonary stenosis or atresia, dextroposition of aorta and hypertrophy of right ventricle.

Q21.4 Aortopulmonary septal defect

Aortic septal defect
Aortopulmonary window

Unspecified Code | Other Specified Code | [N] Newborn Age: 0 | [P] Pediatric Age: 0-17 | [M] Maternity Age: 12-55
[A] Adult Age: 15-124 | ♂ Male | ♀ Female | ● New Code | ▲ Revised Code Title | ►◄ Revised Text

Q21.8 Other congenital malformations of cardiac septa
Eisenmenger's defect
Pentalogy of Fallot
[EXCLUDES1] *Eisenmenger's complex (I27.8)*
Eisenmenger's syndrome (I27.8)
Q21.9 **Congenital malformation of cardiac septum, unspecified**
Septal (heart) defect NOS

[4] Q22 **Congenital malformations of pulmonary and tricuspid valves**
Q22.0 **Pulmonary valve atresia**
Q22.1 **Congenital pulmonary valve stenosis**
Q22.2 **Congenital pulmonary valve insufficiency**
Congenital pulmonary valve regurgitation
Q22.3 **Other congenital malformations of pulmonary valve**
Congenital malformation of pulmonary valve NOS
Supernumerary cusps of pulmonary valve
Q22.4 **Congenital tricuspid stenosis**
Congenital tricuspid atresia
Q22.5 **Ebstein's anomaly**
Q22.6 **Hypoplastic right heart syndrome**
Q22.8 **Other congenital malformations of tricuspid valve**
Q22.9 **Congenital malformation of tricuspid valve, unspecified**

[4] Q23 **Congenital malformations of aortic and mitral valves**
Q23.0 **Congenital stenosis of aortic valve**
Congenital aortic atresia
Congenital aortic stenosis NOS
[EXCLUDES1] *congenital stenosis of aortic valve in hypoplastic left heart syndrome (Q23.4)*
congenital subaortic stenosis (Q24.4)
supravalvular aortic stenosis (congenital) (Q25.3)
Q23.1 **Congenital insufficiency of aortic valve**
Bicuspid aortic valve
Congenital aortic insufficiency
Q23.2 **Congenital mitral stenosis**
Congenital mitral atresia
Q23.3 **Congenital mitral insufficiency**
Q23.4 **Hypoplastic left heart syndrome**
Q23.8 **Other congenital malformations of aortic and mitral valves**
Q23.9 **Congenital malformation of aortic and mitral valves, unspecified**

[4] Q24 **Other congenital malformations of heart**
[EXCLUDES1] *endocardial fibroelastosis (I42.4)*
Q24.0 **Dextrocardia**
[EXCLUDES1] *dextrocardia with situs inversus (Q89.3)*
isomerism of atrial appendages (with asplenia or polysplenia) (Q20.6)
mirror-image atrial arrangement with situs inversus (Q89.3)
Q24.1 **Levocardia**
Q24.2 **Cor triatriatum**
Q24.3 **Pulmonary infundibular stenosis**
Subvalvular pulmonic stenosis
Q24.4 **Congenital subaortic stenosis**
Q24.5 **Malformation of coronary vessels**
Congenital coronary (artery) aneurysm
Q24.6 **Congenital heart block**
Q24.8 **Other specified congenital malformations of heart**
Congenital diverticulum of left ventricle
Congenital malformation of myocardium
Congenital malformation of pericardium
Malposition of heart
Uhl's disease
Q24.9 **Congenital malformation of heart, unspecified**
Congenital anomaly of heart
Congenital disease of heart

[4] Q25 **Congenital malformations of great arteries**
Q25.0 **Patent ductus arteriosus**
Patent ductus Botallo
Persistent ductus arteriosus
Q25.1 **Coarctation of aorta**
Coarctation of aorta (preductal) (postductal)
Q25.2 **Atresia of aorta**
Q25.3 **Supravalvular aortic stenosis**
[EXCLUDES1] *congenital aortic stenosis NOS (Q23.0)*
congenital stenosis of aortic valve (Q23.0)
Q25.4 **Other congenital malformations of aorta**
Absence of aorta
Aneurysm of sinus of Valsalva (ruptured)
Aplasia of aorta
Congenital aneurysm of aorta
Congenital malformations of aorta
Congenital dilatation of aorta
Double aortic arch [vascular ring of aorta]
Hypoplasia of aorta
Persistent convolutions of aortic arch
Persistent right aortic arch
[EXCLUDES1] *hypoplasia of aorta in hypoplastic left heart syndrome (Q23.4)*
Q25.5 **Atresia of pulmonary artery**
Q25.6 **Stenosis of pulmonary artery**
Supravalvular pulmonary stenosis
[5] Q25.7 **Other congenital malformations of pulmonary artery**
Q25.71 **Coarctation of pulmonary artery**
Q25.72 **Congenital pulmonary arteriovenous malformation**
Congenital pulmonary arteriovenous aneurysm
Q25.79 **Other congenital malformations of pulmonary artery**
Aberrant pulmonary artery
Agenesis of pulmonary artery
Congenital aneurysm of pulmonary artery
Congenital anomaly of pulmonary artery
Hypoplasia of pulmonary artery
Q25.8 **Other congenital malformations of other great arteries**
Q25.9 **Congenital malformation of great arteries, unspecified**

[4] Q26 **Congenital malformations of great veins**
Q26.0 **Congenital stenosis of vena cava**
Congenital stenosis of vena cava (inferior)(superior)
Q26.1 **Persistent left superior vena cava**
Q26.2 **Total anomalous pulmonary venous connection**
Total anomalous pulmonary venous return [TAPVR], subdiaphragmatic
Total anomalous pulmonary venous return [TAPVR], supradiaphragmatic
Q26.3 **Partial anomalous pulmonary venous connection**
Partial anomalous pulmonary venous return
Q26.4 **Anomalous pulmonary venous connection, unspecified**
Q26.5 **Anomalous portal venous connection**
Q26.6 **Portal vein-hepatic artery fistula**
Q26.8 **Other congenital malformations of great veins**
Absence of vena cava (inferior) (superior)
Azygos continuation of inferior vena cava
Persistent left posterior cardinal vein
Scimitar syndrome
Q26.9 **Congenital malformation of great vein, unspecified**
Congenital anomaly of vena cava (inferior) (superior) NOS

[4] 4th character required [5] 5th character required [6] 6th character required [7] 7th character required [7th] Extension 'X' Alert
[EXCLUDES1] Not coded here [EXCLUDES2] Not included here [PDx] Primary Diagnosis Only Manifestation Code

[4] **Q27 Other congenital malformations of peripheral vascular system**

[EXCLUDES2] *anomalies of cerebral and precerebral vessels (Q28.0-Q28.3)*
anomalies of coronary vessels (Q24.5)
anomalies of pulmonary artery (Q25.5-Q25.7)
congenital retinal aneurysm (Q14.1)
hemangioma and lymphangioma (D18.-)

Q27.0 Congenital absence and hypoplasia of umbilical artery
Single umbilical artery

Q27.1 Congenital renal artery stenosis

Q27.2 Other congenital malformations of renal artery
Congenital malformation of renal artery NOS
Multiple renal arteries

[5] **Q27.3 Arteriovenous malformation (peripheral)**
Arteriovenous aneurysm
[EXCLUDES1] *acquired arteriovenous aneurysm (I77.0)*
[EXCLUDES2] *arteriovenous malformation of cerebral vessels (Q28.2)*
arteriovenous malformation of precerebral vessels (Q28.0)

Q27.30 Arteriovenous malformation, site unspecified

Q27.31 Arteriovenous malformation of vessel of upper limb

Q27.32 Arteriovenous malformation of vessel of lower limb

Q27.33 Arteriovenous malformation of digestive system vessel

Q27.34 Arteriovenous malformation of renal vessel

Q27.39 Arteriovenous malformation, other site

Q27.4 Congenital phlebectasia

Q27.8 Other specified congenital malformations of peripheral vascular system
Absence of peripheral vascular system
Atresia of peripheral vascular system
Congenital aneurysm (peripheral)
Congenital stricture, artery
Congenital varix
[EXCLUDES1] *arteriovenous malformation (Q27.3-)*

Q27.9 Congenital malformation of peripheral vascular system, unspecified
Anomaly of artery or vein NOS

[4] **Q28 Other congenital malformations of circulatory system**

[EXCLUDES1] *congenital aneurysm NOS (Q27.8)*
congenital coronary aneurysm (Q24.5)
ruptured cerebral arteriovenous malformation (I60.8)
ruptured malformation of precerebral vessels (I72.0)
[EXCLUDES2] *congenital peripheral aneurysm (Q27.8)*
congenital pulmonary aneurysm (Q25.79)
congenital retinal aneurysm (Q14.1)

Q28.0 Arteriovenous malformation of precerebral vessels
Congenital arteriovenous precerebral aneurysm (nonruptured)

Q28.1 Other malformations of precerebral vessels
Congenital malformation of precerebral vessels NOS
Congenital precerebral aneurysm (nonruptured)

Q28.2 Arteriovenous malformation of cerebral vessels
Arteriovenous malformation of brain NOS
Congenital arteriovenous cerebral aneurysm (nonruptured)

Q28.3 Other malformations of cerebral vessels
Congenital cerebral aneurysm (nonruptured)
Congenital malformation of cerebral vessels NOS
Developmental venous anomaly

Q28.8 Other specified congenital malformations of circulatory system
Congenital aneurysm, specified site NEC
Spinal vessel anomaly

Q28.9 Congenital malformation of circulatory system, unspecified

Congenital malformations of the respiratory system (Q30-Q34)

[4] **Q30 Congenital malformations of nose**

[EXCLUDES1] *congenital deviation of nasal septum (Q67.4)*

Q30.0 Choanal atresia
Atresia of nares (anterior) (posterior)
Congenital stenosis of nares (anterior) (posterior)

Q30.1 Agenesis and underdevelopment of nose
Congenital absent of nose

Q30.2 Fissured, notched and cleft nose

Q30.3 Congenital perforated nasal septum

Q30.8 Other congenital malformations of nose
Accessory nose
Congenital anomaly of nasal sinus wall

Q30.9 Congenital malformation of nose, unspecified

[4] **Q31 Congenital malformations of larynx**

[EXCLUDES1] *congenital laryngeal stridor NOS (P28.89)*

Q31.0 Web of larynx
Glottic web of larynx
Subglottic web of larynx
Web of larynx NOS

Q31.1 Congenital subglottic stenosis

Q31.2 Laryngeal hypoplasia

Q31.3 Laryngocele

Q31.5 Congenital laryngomalacia

Q31.8 Other congenital malformations of larynx
Absence of larynx
Agenesis of larynx
Atresia of larynx
Congenital cleft thyroid cartilage
Congenital fissure of epiglottis
Congenital stenosis of larynx NEC
Posterior cleft of cricoid cartilage

Q31.9 Congenital malformation of larynx, unspecified

[4] **Q32 Congenital malformations of trachea and bronchus**

[EXCLUDES1] *congenital bronchiectasis (Q33.4)*

Q32.0 Congenital tracheomalacia

Q32.1 Other congenital malformations of trachea
Atresia of trachea
Congenital anomaly of tracheal cartilage
Congenital dilatation of trachea
Congenital malformation of trachea
Congenital stenosis of trachea
Congenital tracheocele

Q32.2 Congenital bronchomalacia

Q32.3 Congenital stenosis of bronchus

Q32.4 Other congenital malformations of bronchus
Absence of bronchus
Agenesis of bronchus
Atresia of bronchus
Congenital diverticulum of bronchus
Congenital malformation of bronchus NOS

[4] **Q33 Congenital malformations of lung**

Q33.0 Congenital cystic lung
Congenital cystic lung disease
Congenital honeycomb lung
Congenital polycystic lung disease
[EXCLUDES1] *cystic fibrosis (E84.0)*
cystic lung disease, acquired or unspecified (J98.4)

Unspecified Code | Other Specified Code | [N] Newborn Age: 0 | [P] Pediatric Age: 0-17 | [M] Maternity Age: 12-55
[A] Adult Age: 15-124 | ♂ Male | ♀ Female | ● New Code | ▲ Revised Code Title | ►◄ Revised Text

Q33.1 Accessory lobe of lung
Azygos lobe (fissured), lung
Q33.2 Sequestration of lung
Q33.3 Agenesis of lung
Congenital absence of lung (lobe)
Q33.4 Congenital bronchiectasis
Q33.5 Ectopic tissue in lung
Q33.6 Congenital hypoplasia and dysplasia of lung
[EXCLUDES1] *pulmonary hypoplasia associated with short gestation (P28.0)*
Q33.8 Other congenital malformations of lung
Q33.9 Congenital malformation of lung, unspecified
[4th] Q34 Other congenital malformations of respiratory system
[EXCLUDES2] *congenital central alveolar hypoventilation syndrome (G47.35)*
Q34.0 Anomaly of pleura
Q34.1 Congenital cyst of mediastinum
Q34.8 Other specified congenital malformations of respiratory system
Atresia of nasopharynx
Q34.9 Congenital malformation of respiratory system, unspecified
Congenital absence of respiratory system
Congenital anomaly of respiratory system NOS

Cleft lip and cleft palate (Q35-Q37)

Use additional code to identify associated malformation of the nose (Q30.2)
[EXCLUDES1] *Robin's syndrome (Q87.0)*
[4th] Q35 Cleft palate
[INCLUDES] *fissure of palate*
palatoschisis
[EXCLUDES1] *cleft palate with cleft lip (Q37.-)*
Q35.1 Cleft hard palate
Q35.3 Cleft soft palate
Q35.5 Cleft hard palate with cleft soft palate
Q35.7 Cleft uvula
Q35.9 Cleft palate, unspecified
Cleft palate NOS
[4th] Q36 Cleft lip
[INCLUDES] *cheiloschisis*
congenital fissure of lip
harelip
labium leporinum
[EXCLUDES1] *cleft lip with cleft palate (Q37.-)*
Q36.0 Cleft lip, bilateral
Q36.1 Cleft lip, median
Q36.9 Cleft lip, unilateral
Cleft lip NOS
[4th] Q37 Cleft palate with cleft lip
[INCLUDES] *cheilopalatoschisis*
Q37.0 Cleft hard palate with bilateral cleft lip
Q37.1 Cleft hard palate with unilateral cleft lip
Cleft hard palate with cleft lip NOS
Q37.2 Cleft soft palate with bilateral cleft lip
Q37.3 Cleft soft palate with unilateral cleft lip
Cleft soft palate with cleft lip NOS
Q37.4 Cleft hard and soft palate with bilateral cleft lip
Q37.5 Cleft hard and soft palate with unilateral cleft lip
Cleft hard and soft palate with cleft lip NOS
Q37.8 Unspecified cleft palate with bilateral cleft lip
Q37.9 Unspecified cleft palate with unilateral cleft lip
Cleft palate with cleft lip NOS

Other congenital malformations of the digestive system (Q38-Q45)

[4th] Q38 Other congenital malformations of tongue, mouth and pharynx
[EXCLUDES1] *dentofacial anomalies (M26.-)*
macrostomia (Q18.4)
microstomia (Q18.5)
Q38.0 Congenital malformations of lips, not elsewhere classified
Congenital fistula of lip
Congenital malformation of lip NOS
Van der Woude's syndrome
[EXCLUDES1] *cleft lip (Q36.-)*
cleft lip with cleft palate (Q37.-)
macrocheilia (Q18.6)
microcheilia (Q18.7)
Q38.1 Ankyloglossia
Tongue tie
Q38.2 Macroglossia
Congenital hypertrophy of tongue
Q38.3 Other congenital malformations of tongue
Aglossia
Bifid tongue
Congenital adhesion of tongue
Congenital fissure of tongue
Congenital malformation of tongue NOS
Double tongue
Hypoglossia
Hypoplasia of tongue
Microglossia
Q38.4 Congenital malformations of salivary glands and ducts
Atresia of salivary glands and ducts
Congenital absence of salivary glands and ducts
Congenital accessory salivary glands and ducts
Congenital fistula of salivary gland
Q38.5 Congenital malformations of palate, not elsewhere classified
Congenital absence of uvula
Congenital malformation of palate NOS
Congenital high arched palate
[EXCLUDES1] *cleft palate (Q35.-)*
cleft palate with cleft lip (Q37.-)
Q38.6 Other congenital malformations of mouth
Congenital malformation of mouth NOS
Q38.7 Congenital pharyngeal pouch
Congenital diverticulum of pharynx
[EXCLUDES1] *pharyngeal pouch syndrome (D82.1)*
Q38.8 Other congenital malformations of pharynx
Congenital malformation of pharynx NOS
Imperforate pharynx
[4th] Q39 Congenital malformations of esophagus
Q39.0 Atresia of esophagus without fistula
Atresia of esophagus NOS
Q39.1 Atresia of esophagus with tracheo-esophageal fistula
Atresia of esophagus with broncho-esophageal fistula
Q39.2 Congenital tracheo-esophageal fistula without atresia
Congenital tracheo-esophageal fistula NOS
Q39.3 Congenital stenosis and stricture of esophagus
Q39.4 Esophageal web
Q39.5 Congenital dilatation of esophagus
Congenital cardiospasm
Q39.6 Congenital diverticulum of esophagus
Congenital esophageal pouch

[4th] 4th character required [5th] 5th character required [6th] 6th character required [7th] 7th character required [X] Extension 'X' Alert
[EXCLUDES1] Not coded here [EXCLUDES2] Not included here [PDx] Primary Diagnosis Only Manifestation Code

Q39.8 **Other congenital** malformations **of** esophagus
  Congenital absence of esophagus
  Congenital displacement of esophagus
  Congenital duplication of esophagus
Q39.9 **Congenital malformation of esophagus, unspecified**

Q40 Other **congenital malformations of** upper alimentary tract

Q40.0 **Congenital** hypertrophic pyloric stenosis
  Congenital or infantile constriction
  Congenital or infantile hypertrophy
  Congenital or infantile spasm
  Congenital or infantile stenosis
  Congenital or infantile stricture
Q40.1 **Congenital** hiatus hernia
  Congenital displacement of cardia through esophageal hiatus
  EXCLUDES1 *congenital diaphragmatic hernia (Q79.0)*
Q40.2 **Other specified congenital malformations of** stomach
  Congenital displacement of stomach
  Congenital diverticulum of stomach
  Congenital hourglass stomach
  Congenital duplication of stomach
  Megalogastria
  Microgastria
Q40.3 **Congenital malformation of** stomach**, unspecified**
Q40.8 **Other specified congenital malformations of** upper alimentary tract
Q40.9 **Congenital malformation of** upper alimentary tract**, unspecified**
  Congenital anomaly of upper alimentary tract
  Congenital deformity of upper alimentary tract

Q41 **Congenital absence, atresia and stenosis of** small intestine
  INCLUDES *congenital obstruction, occlusion or stricture of small intestine or intestine NOS*
  EXCLUDES1 *cystic fibrosis with intestinal manifestation (E84.11)*
    meconium ileus NOS (without cystic fibrosis) (P76.0)
Q41.0 **Congenital absence, atresia and stenosis of** duodenum
Q41.1 **Congenital absence, atresia and stenosis of** jejunum
  Apple peel syndrome
  Imperforate jejunum
Q41.2 **Congenital absence, atresia and stenosis of** ileum
Q41.8 **Congenital absence, atresia and stenosis of** other specified parts of small intestine
Q41.9 **Congenital absence, atresia and stenosis of** small intestine, part unspecified
  Congenital absence, atresia and stenosis of intestine NOS

Q42 **Congenital absence, atresia and stenosis of** large intestine
  INCLUDES *congenital obstruction, occlusion and stricture of large intestine*
Q42.0 **Congenital absence, atresia and stenosis of** rectum with fistula
Q42.1 **Congenital absence, atresia and stenosis of** rectum without fistula
  Imperforate rectum
Q42.2 **Congenital absence, atresia and stenosis of** anus with fistula
Q42.3 **Congenital absence, atresia and stenosis of** anus without fistula
  Imperforate anus
Q42.8 **Congenital absence, atresia and stenosis of** other parts of large intestine
Q42.9 **Congenital absence, atresia and stenosis of** large intestine, part unspecified

Q43 Other **congenital malformations of** intestine
Q43.0 **Meckel's diverticulum (displaced) (hypertrophic)**
  Persistent omphalomesenteric duct
  Persistent vitelline duct
Q43.1 **Hirschsprung's disease**
  Aganglionosis
  Congenital (aganglionic) megacolon
Q43.2 **Other congenital functional disorders of** colon
  Congenital dilatation of colon
Q43.3 **Congenital malformations of** intestinal fixation
  Congenital omental, anomalous adhesions [bands]
  Congenital peritoneal adhesions [bands]
  Incomplete rotation of cecum and colon
  Insufficient rotation of cecum and colon
  Jackson's membrane
  Malrotation of colon
  Rotation failure of cecum and colon
  Universal mesentery
Q43.4 Duplication **of intestine**
Q43.5 **Ectopic anus**
Q43.6 **Congenital fistula of** rectum and anus
  EXCLUDES1 *congenital fistula of anus with absence, atresia and stenosis (Q42.2)*
    congenital fistula of rectum with absence, atresia and stenosis (Q42.0)
    congenital rectovaginal fistula (Q52.2)
    congenital urethrorectal fistula (Q64.73)
    pilonidal fistula or sinus (L05.-)
Q43.7 **Persistent** cloaca
  Cloaca NOS
Q43.8 **Other specified congenital malformations of** intestine
  Congenital blind loop syndrome
  Congenital diverticulitis, colon
  Congenital diverticulum, intestine
  Dolichocolon
  Megaloappendix
  Megaloduodenum
  Microcolon
  Transposition of appendix
  Transposition of colon
  Transposition of intestine
Q43.9 **Congenital malformation of intestine, unspecified**

Q44 **Congenital malformations of** gallbladder, bile ducts and liver
Q44.0 Agenesis, aplasia and hypoplasia **of gallbladder**
  Congenital absence of gallbladder
Q44.1 **Other congenital malformations of gallbladder**
  Congenital malformation of gallbladder NOS
  Intrahepatic gallbladder
Q44.2 Atresia **of** bile ducts
Q44.3 **Congenital** stenosis and stricture of bile ducts
Q44.4 Choledochal cyst
Q44.5 **Other congenital malformations of** bile ducts
  Accessory hepatic duct
  Biliary duct duplication
  Congenital malformation of bile duct NOS
  Cystic duct duplication
Q44.6 Cystic **disease of** liver
  Fibrocystic disease of liver
Q44.7 **Other congenital malformations of** liver
  Accessory liver
  Alagille's syndrome
  Congenital absence of liver
  Congenital hepatomegaly
  Congenital malformation of liver NOS

Unspecified Code Other Specified Code N Newborn Age: 0 P Pediatric Age: 0-17 M Maternity Age: 12-55
A Adult Age: 15-124 ♂ Male ♀ Female ● New Code ▲ Revised Code Title ►◄ Revised Text

[4] **Q45 Other congenital malformations of digestive system**

[EXCLUDES2] *congenital diaphragmatic hernia (Q79.0)*
congenital hiatus hernia (Q40.1)

Q45.0 Agenesis, aplasia and hypoplasia of pancreas
Congenital absence of pancreas

Q45.1 Annular pancreas

Q45.2 Congenital pancreatic cyst

Q45.3 Other congenital malformations of pancreas and pancreatic duct
Accessory pancreas
Congenital malformation of pancreas or pancreatic duct NOS
[EXCLUDES1] *congenital diabetes mellitus (E10.-)*
cystic fibrosis (E84.0-E84.9)
fibrocystic disease of pancreas (E84.-)
neonatal diabetes mellitus (P70.2)

Q45.8 Other specified congenital malformations of digestive system
Absence (complete) (partial) of alimentary tract NOS
Duplication of digestive system
Malposition, congenital of digestive system

Q45.9 Congenital malformation of digestive system, unspecified
Congenital anomaly of digestive system
Congenital deformity of digestive system

Congenital malformations of genital organs (Q50-Q56)

[EXCLUDES1] *androgen insensitivity syndrome (E34.5-)*
syndromes associated with anomalies in the number and form of chromosomes (Q90-Q99)

[4] **Q50 Congenital malformations of ovaries, fallopian tubes and broad ligaments**

[5] **Q50.0 Congenital absence of ovary**
[EXCLUDES1] *Turner's syndrome (Q96.-)*
Q50.01 Congenital absence of ovary, unilateral ♀
Q50.02 Congenital absence of ovary, bilateral ♀

Q50.1 Developmental ovarian cyst ♀

Q50.2 Congenital torsion of ovary ♀

[5] **Q50.3 Other congenital malformations of ovary**
Q50.31 Accessory ovary ♀
Q50.32 Ovarian streak
46, XX with streak gonads ♀
Q50.39 Other congenital malformation of ovary
Congenital malformation of ovary NOS ♀

Q50.4 Embryonic cyst of fallopian tube
Fimbrial cyst ♀

Q50.5 Embryonic cyst of broad ligament
Epoophoron cyst
Parovarian cyst ♀

Q50.6 Other congenital malformations of fallopian tube and broad ligament
Absence of fallopian tube and broad ligament
Accessory fallopian tube and broad ligament
Atresia of fallopian tube and broad ligament
Congenital malformation of fallopian tube or broad ligament NOS ♀

[4] **Q51 Congenital malformations of uterus and cervix**

Q51.0 Agenesis and aplasia of uterus
Congenital absence of uterus ♀

[5] **Q51.1 Doubling of uterus with doubling of cervix and vagina**
Q51.10 Doubling of uterus with doubling of cervix and vagina without obstruction
Doubling of uterus with doubling of cervix and vagina NOS ♀
Q51.11 Doubling of uterus with doubling of cervix and vagina with obstruction ♀

Q51.2 Other doubling of uterus
Doubling of uterus NOS
Septate uterus, complete or partial ♀

Q51.3 Bicornate uterus
Bicornate uterus, complete or partial ♀

Q51.4 Unicornate uterus
Unicornate uterus with or without a separate uterine horn
Uterus with only one functioning horn ♀

Q51.5 Agenesis and aplasia of cervix
Congenital absence of cervix ♀

Q51.6 Embryonic cyst of cervix ♀

Q51.7 Congenital fistulae between uterus and digestive and urinary tracts ♀

[5] **Q51.8 Other congenital malformations of uterus and cervix**
[6] **Q51.81 Other congenital malformations of uterus**
Q51.810 Arcuate uterus
Arcuatus uterus ♀
Q51.811 Hypoplasia of uterus ♀
Q51.818 Other congenital malformations of uterus
Müllerian anomaly of uterus NEC ♀
[6] **Q51.82 Other congenital malformations of cervix**
Q51.820 Cervical duplication ♀
Q51.821 Hypoplasia of cervix ♀
Q51.828 Other congenital malformations of cervix ♀

Q51.9 Congenital malformation of uterus and cervix, unspecified ♀

[4] **Q52 Other congenital malformations of female genitalia**

Q52.0 Congenital absence of vagina
Vaginal agenesis, total or partial ♀

[5] **Q52.1 Doubling of vagina**
[EXCLUDES1] *doubling of vagina with doubling of uterus and cervix (Q51.1-)*
Q52.10 Doubling of vagina, unspecified
Septate vagina NOS ♀
Q52.11 Transverse vaginal septum ♀
Q52.12 Longitudinal vaginal septum
Longitudinal vaginal septum with or without obstruction ♀

Q52.2 Congenital rectovaginal fistula
[EXCLUDES1] *cloaca (Q43.7)* ♀

Q52.3 Imperforate hymen ♀

Q52.4 Other congenital malformations of vagina
Canal of Nuck cyst, congenital
Congenital malformation of vagina NOS
Embryonic vaginal cyst
Gartner's duct cyst ♀

Q52.5 Fusion of labia ♀

Q52.6 Congenital malformation of clitoris ♀

[5] **Q52.7 Other and unspecified congenital malformations of vulva**
Q52.70 Unspecified congenital malformations of vulva
Congenital malformation of vulva NOS ♀
Q52.71 Congenital absence of vulva ♀
Q52.79 Other congenital malformations of vulva
Congenital cyst of vulva ♀

Q52.8 Other specified congenital malformations of female genitalia ♀

Q52.9 Congenital malformation of female genitalia, unspecified ♀

[4] **Q53 Undescended and ectopic testicle**

[5] **Q53.0 Ectopic testis**
Q53.00 Ectopic testis, unspecified ♂
Q53.01 Ectopic testis, unilateral ♂

[4] 4th character required [5] 5th character required [6] 6th character required [7] 7th character required [X] Extension 'X' Alert
[EXCLUDES1] Not coded here [EXCLUDES2] Not included here [PDx] Primary Diagnosis Only Manifestation Code

Q53.02 Ectopic testes, bilateral ♂
[5] Q53.1 Undescended testicle, unilateral
Q53.10 Unspecified undescended testicle, unilateral ♂
Q53.11 Abdominal testis, unilateral ♂
Q53.12 Ectopic perineal testis, unilateral ♂
[5] Q53.2 Undescended testicle, bilateral
Q53.20 Undescended testicle, unspecified, bilateral ♂
Q53.21 Abdominal testis, bilateral ♂
Q53.22 Ectopic perineal testis, bilateral ♂
Q53.9 Undescended testicle, unspecified
Cryptorchism NOS ♂

[4] Q54 Hypospadias
[EXCLUDES1] *epispadias (Q64.0)*
Q54.0 Hypospadias, balanic
Hypospadias, coronal
Hypospadias, glandular ♂
Q54.1 Hypospadias, penile ♂
Q54.2 Hypospadias, penoscrotal ♂
Q54.3 Hypospadias, perineal ♂
Q54.4 Congenital chordee
Chordee without hypospadias ♂
Q54.8 Other hypospadias
Hypospadias with intersex state ♂
Q54.9 Hypospadias, unspecified ♂

[4] Q55 Other congenital malformations of male genital organs
[EXCLUDES1] *congenital hydrocele (P83.5)*
hypospadias (Q54.-)
Q55.0 Absence and aplasia of testis
Monorchism ♂
Q55.1 Hypoplasia of testis and scrotum
Fusion of testes ♂
[5] Q55.2 Other and unspecified congenital malformations of testis and scrotum
Q55.20 Unspecified congenital malformations of testis and scrotum
Congenital malformation of testis or scrotum NOS ♂
Q55.21 Polyorchism ♂
Q55.22 Retractile testis ♂
Q55.23 Scrotal transposition ♂
Q55.29 Other congenital malformations of testis and scrotum ♂
Q55.3 Atresia of vas deferens
Code first any associated cystic fibrosis (E84.-) ♂
Q55.4 Other congenital malformations of vas deferens, epididymis, seminal vesicles and prostate
Absence or aplasia of prostate
Absence or aplasia of spermatic cord
Congenital malformation of vas deferens, epididymis, seminal vesicles or prostate NOS ♂
Q55.5 Congenital absence and aplasia of penis ♂
[5] Q55.6 Other congenital malformations of penis
Q55.61 Curvature of penis (lateral) ♂
Q55.62 Hypoplasia of penis
Micropenis ♂
Q55.63 Congenital torsion of penis
[EXCLUDES1] *acquired torsion of penis (N48.82)* ♂
Q55.64 Hidden penis
Buried penis
Concealed penis
[EXCLUDES1] *acquired buried penis (N48.83)* ♂
Q55.69 Other congenital malformation of penis
Congenital malformation of penis NOS ♂
Q55.7 Congenital vasocutaneous fistula ♂
Q55.8 Other specified congenital malformations of male genital organs ♂
Q55.9 Congenital malformation of male genital organ, unspecified
Congenital anomaly of male genital organ
Congenital deformity of male genital organ ♂

[4] Q56 Indeterminate sex and pseudohermaphroditism
[EXCLUDES1] *46,XX true hermaphrodite (Q99.1)*
androgen insensitivity syndrome (E34.5-)
chimera 46,XX/46,XY true hermaphrodite (Q99.0)
female pseudohermaphroditism with adrenocortical disorder (E25.-)
pseudohermaphroditism with specified chromosomal anomaly (Q96-Q99)
pure gonadal dysgenesis (Q99.1)
Q56.0 Hermaphroditism, not elsewhere classified
Ovotestis
Q56.1 Male pseudohermaphroditism, not elsewhere classified
46, XY with streak gonads
Male pseudohermaphroditism NOS ♂
Q56.2 Female pseudohermaphroditism, not elsewhere classified
Female pseudohermaphroditism NOS ♀
Q56.3 Pseudohermaphroditism, unspecified
Q56.4 Indeterminate sex, unspecified
Ambiguous genitalia

Congenital malformations of the urinary system (Q60-Q64)

[4] Q60 Renal agenesis and other reduction defects of kidney
[INCLUDES] *congenital absence of kidney*
congenital atrophy of kidney
infantile atrophy of kidney
Q60.0 Renal agenesis, unilateral
Q60.1 Renal agenesis, bilateral
Q60.2 Renal agenesis, unspecified
Q60.3 Renal hypoplasia, unilateral
Q60.4 Renal hypoplasia, bilateral
Q60.5 Renal hypoplasia, unspecified
Q60.6 Potter's syndrome

[4] Q61 Cystic kidney disease
[EXCLUDES1] *acquired cyst of kidney (N28.1)*
Potter's syndrome (Q60.6)
[5] Q61.0 Congenital renal cyst
Q61.00 Congenital renal cyst, unspecified
Cyst of kidney NOS (congenital)
Q61.01 Congenital single renal cyst
Q61.02 Congenital multiple renal cysts
[5] Q61.1 Polycystic kidney, infantile type
Polycystic kidney, autosomal recessive
Q61.11 Cystic dilatation of collecting ducts
Q61.19 Other polycystic kidney, infantile type
Q61.2 Polycystic kidney, adult type
Polycystic kidney, autosomal dominant
Q61.3 Polycystic kidney, unspecified
Q61.4 Renal dysplasia
Multicystic dysplastic kidney
Multicystic kidney (development)
Multicystic kidney disease
Multicystic renal dysplasia
[EXCLUDES1] *polycystic kidney disease (Q61.11-Q61.3)*
Q61.5 Medullary cystic kidney
Nephronopthisis
Sponge kidney NOS
Q61.8 Other cystic kidney diseases
Fibrocystic kidney
Fibrocystic renal degeneration or disease
Q61.9 Cystic kidney disease, unspecified
Meckel-Gruber syndrome

Unspecified Code | Other Specified Code | [N] Newborn Age: 0 | [P] Pediatric Age: 0-17 | [M] Maternity Age: 12-55
[A] Adult Age: 15-124 | ♂ Male | ♀ Female | ● New Code | ▲ Revised Code Title | ►◄ Revised Text

Q53.02 - Q61.9
CHAPTER 17: CONGENITAL MALFORMATIONS, DEFORMATIONS, AND CHROMOSOMAL ABNORMALITIES (Q00-Q99)

④ Q62 Congenital obstructive defects of renal pelvis and congenital malformations of ureter

   Q62.0 Congenital hydronephrosis

⑤ Q62.1 Congenital occlusion of ureter

   Atresia and stenosis of ureter

   Q62.10 Congenital occlusion of ureter, unspecified

   Q62.11 Congenital occlusion of ureteropelvic junction

   Q62.12 Congenital occlusion of ureterovesical orifice

   Q62.2 Congenital megaureter

   Congenital dilatation of ureter

⑤ Q62.3 Other obstructive defects of renal pelvis and ureter

   Q62.31 Congenital ureterocele, orthotopic

   Q62.32 Cecoureterocele

      Ectopic ureterocele

   Q62.39 Other obstructive defects of renal pelvis and ureter

      Ureteropelvic junction obstruction NOS

   Q62.4 Agenesis of ureter

      Congenital absence ureter

   Q62.5 Duplication of ureter

      Accessory ureter

      Double ureter

⑤ Q62.6 Malposition of ureter

   Q62.60 Malposition of ureter, unspecified

   Q62.61 Deviation of ureter

   Q62.62 Displacement of ureter

   Q62.63 Anomalous implantation of ureter

      Ectopia of ureter

      Ectopic ureter

   Q62.69 Other malposition of ureter

   Q62.7 Congenital vesico-uretero-renal reflux

   Q62.8 Other congenital malformations of ureter

      Anomaly of ureter NOS

④ Q63 Other congenital malformations of kidney

   EXCLUDES1 congenital nephrotic syndrome (N04.-)

   Q63.0 Accessory kidney

   Q63.1 Lobulated, fused and horseshoe kidney

   Q63.2 Ectopic kidney

      Congenital displaced kidney

      Malrotation of kidney

   Q63.3 Hyperplastic and giant kidney

      Compensatory hypertrophy of kidney

   Q63.8 Other specified congenital malformations of kidney

      Congenital renal calculi

   Q63.9 Congenital malformation of kidney, unspecified

④ Q64 Other congenital malformations of urinary system

   Q64.0 Epispadias

   EXCLUDES1 hypospadias (Q54.-) ♂

⑤ Q64.1 Exstrophy of urinary bladder

   Q64.10 Exstrophy of urinary bladder, unspecified

      Ectopia vesicae

   Q64.11 Supravesical fissure of urinary bladder

   Q64.12 Cloacal extrophy of urinary bladder

   Q64.19 Other exstrophy of urinary bladder

      Extroversion of bladder

   Q64.2 Congenital posterior urethral valves

⑤ Q64.3 Other atresia and stenosis of urethra and bladder neck

   Q64.31 Congenital bladder neck obstruction

      Congenital obstruction of vesicourethral orifice

   Q64.32 Congenital stricture of urethra

   Q64.33 Congenital stricture of urinary meatus

   Q64.39 Other atresia and stenosis of urethra and bladder neck

      Atresia and stenosis of urethra and bladder neck NOS

   Q64.4 Malformation of urachus

      Cyst of urachus

      Patent urachus

      Prolapse of urachus

   Q64.5 Congenital absence of bladder and urethra

   Q64.6 Congenital diverticulum of bladder

⑤ Q64.7 Other and unspecified congenital malformations of bladder and urethra

   EXCLUDES1 congenital prolapse of bladder (mucosa) (Q79.4)

   Q64.70 Unspecified congenital malformation of bladder and urethra

      Malformation of bladder or urethra NOS

   Q64.71 Congenital prolapse of urethra

   Q64.72 Congenital prolapse of urinary meatus

   Q64.73 Congenital urethrorectal fistula

   Q64.74 Double urethra

   Q64.75 Double urinary meatus

   Q64.79 Other congenital malformations of bladder and urethra

   Q64.8 Other specified congenital malformations of urinary system

   Q64.9 Congenital malformation of urinary system, unspecified

      Congenital anomaly NOS of urinary system

      Congenital deformity NOS of urinary system

Congenital malformations and deformations of the musculoskeletal system (Q65-Q79)

④ Q65 Congenital deformities of hip

   EXCLUDES1 clicking hip (R29.4)

⑤ Q65.0 Congenital dislocation of hip, unilateral

   Q65.00 Congenital dislocation of unspecified hip, unilateral

   Q65.01 Congenital dislocation of right hip, unilateral

   Q65.02 Congenital dislocation of left hip, unilateral

   Q65.1 Congenital dislocation of hip, bilateral

   Q65.2 Congenital dislocation of hip, unspecified

⑤ Q65.3 Congenital partial dislocation of hip, unilateral

   Q65.30 Congenital partial dislocation of unspecified hip, unilateral

   Q65.31 Congenital partial dislocation of right hip, unilateral

   Q65.32 Congenital partial dislocation of left hip, unilateral

   Q65.4 Congenital partial dislocation of hip, bilateral

   Q65.5 Congenital partial dislocation of hip, unspecified

   Q65.6 Congenital unstable hip

      Congenital dislocatable hip

⑤ Q65.8 Other congenital deformities of hip

   Q65.81 Congenital coxa valga

   Q65.82 Congenital coxa vara

   Q65.89 Other specified congenital deformities of hip

      Anteversion of femoral neck

      Congenital acetabular dysplasia

   Q65.9 Congenital deformity of hip, unspecified

④ Q66 Congenital deformities of feet

   EXCLUDES1 reduction defects of feet (Q72.-)
          valgus deformities (acquired) (M21.0-)
          varus deformities (acquired) (M21.1-)

   Q66.0 Congenital talipes equinovarus

   Q66.1 Congenital talipes calcaneovarus

   Q66.2 Congenital metatarsus (primus) varus

   Q66.3 Other congenital varus deformities of feet

      Hallux varus, congenital

   Q66.4 Congenital talipes calcaneovalgus

---

④ 4th character required   ⑤ 5th character required   ⑥ 6th character required   ⑦ 7th character required   Ⓧ Extension 'X' Alert

EXCLUDES1 Not coded here   EXCLUDES2 Not included here   𝓅𝓍 Primary Diagnosis Only   Manifestation Code

[5] **Q66.5 Congenital pes planus**
Congenital flat foot
Congenital rigid flat foot
Congenital spastic (everted) flat foot
[EXCLUDES1] *pes planus, acquired (M21.4)*
Q66.50 Congenital pes planus, unspecified foot
Q66.51 Congenital pes planus, right foot
Q66.52 Congenital pes planus, left foot
Q66.6 Other congenital valgus deformities of feet
Congenital metatarsus valgus
Q66.7 Congenital pes cavus
[5] **Q66.8 Other congenital deformities of feet**
Q66.80 Congenital vertical talus deformity, unspecified foot
Q66.81 Congenital vertical talus deformity, right foot
Q66.82 Congenital vertical talus deformity, left foot
Q66.89 Other specified congenital deformities of feet
Congenital asymmetric talipes
Congenital clubfoot NOS
Congenital talipes NOS
Congenital tarsal coalition
Hammer toe, congenital
Q66.9 Congenital deformity of feet, unspecified
[4] **Q67 Congenital musculoskeletal deformities of head, face, spine and chest**
[EXCLUDES1] *congenital malformation syndromes classified to Q87.-*
Potter's syndrome (Q60.6)
Q67.0 Congenital facial asymmetry
Q67.1 Congenital compression facies
Q67.2 Dolichocephaly
Q67.3 Plagiocephaly
Q67.4 Other congenital deformities of skull, face and jaw
Congenital depressions in skull
Congenital hemifacial atrophy or hypertrophy
Deviation of nasal septum, congenital
Squashed or bent nose, congenital
[EXCLUDES1] *dentofacial anomalies [including malocclusion] (M26.-)*
syphilitic saddle nose (A50.5)
Q67.5 Congenital deformity of spine
Congenital postural scoliosis
Congenital scoliosis NOS
[EXCLUDES1] *infantile idiopathic scoliosis (M41.0)*
scoliosis due to congenital bony malformation (Q76.3)
Q67.6 Pectus excavatum
Congenital funnel chest
Q67.7 Pectus carinatum
Congenital pigeon chest
Q67.8 Other congenital deformities of chest
Congenital deformity of chest wall NOS
[4] **Q68 Other congenital musculoskeletal deformities**
[EXCLUDES1] *reduction defects of limb(s) (Q71-Q73)*
[EXCLUDES2] *congenital myotonic chondrodystrophy (G71.13)*
Q68.0 Congenital deformity of sternocleidomastoid muscle
Congenital contracture of sternocleidomastoid (muscle)
Congenital (sternomastoid) torticollis
Sternomastoid tumor (congenital)
Q68.1 Congenital deformity of finger(s) and hand
Congenital clubfinger
Spade-like hand (congenital)
Q68.2 Congenital deformity of knee
Congenital dislocation of knee
Congenital genu recurvatum
Q68.3 Congenital bowing of femur
[EXCLUDES1] *anteversion of femur (neck) (Q65.89)*
Q68.4 Congenital bowing of tibia and fibula
Q68.5 Congenital bowing of long bones of leg, unspecified
Q68.6 Discoid meniscus
Q68.8 Other specified congenital musculoskeletal deformities
Congenital deformity of clavicle
Congenital deformity of elbow
Congenital deformity of forearm
Congenital deformity of scapula
Congenital deformity of wrist
Congenital dislocation of elbow
Congenital dislocation of shoulder
Congenital dislocation of wrist
[4] **Q69 Polydactyly**
Q69.0 Accessory finger(s)
Q69.1 Accessory thumb(s)
Q69.2 Accessory toe(s)
Accessory hallux
Q69.9 Polydactyly, unspecified
Supernumerary digit(s) NOS
[4] **Q70 Syndactyly**
[5] **Q70.0 Fused fingers**
Complex syndactyly of fingers with synostosis
Q70.00 Fused fingers, unspecified hand
Q70.01 Fused fingers, right hand
Q70.02 Fused fingers, left hand
Q70.03 Fused fingers, bilateral
[5] **Q70.1 Webbed fingers**
Simple syndactyly of fingers without synostosis
Q70.10 Webbed fingers, unspecified hand
Q70.11 Webbed fingers, right hand
Q70.12 Webbed fingers, left hand
Q70.13 Webbed fingers, bilateral
[5] **Q70.2 Fused toes**
Complex syndactyly of toes with synostosis
Q70.20 Fused toes, unspecified foot
Q70.21 Fused toes, right foot
Q70.22 Fused toes, left foot
Q70.23 Fused toes, bilateral
[5] **Q70.3 Webbed toes**
Simple syndactyly of toes without synostosis
Q70.30 Webbed toes, unspecified foot
Q70.31 Webbed toes, right foot
Q70.32 Webbed toes, left foot
Q70.33 Webbed toes, bilateral
Q70.4 Polysyndactyly, unspecified
[EXCLUDES1] *specified syndactyly of hand and feet - code to specified conditions (Q70.0- -Q70.3-)*
Q70.9 Syndactyly, unspecified
Symphalangy NOS
[4] **Q71 Reduction defects of upper limb**
[5] **Q71.0 Congenital complete absence of upper limb**
Q71.00 Congenital complete absence of unspecified upper limb
Q71.01 Congenital complete absence of right upper limb
Q71.02 Congenital complete absence of left upper limb
Q71.03 Congenital complete absence of upper limb, bilateral
[5] **Q71.1 Congenital absence of upper arm and forearm with hand present**
Q71.10 Congenital absence of unspecified upper arm and forearm with hand present
Q71.11 Congenital absence of right upper arm and forearm with hand present

Unspecified Code | Other Specified Code | [N] Newborn Age: 0 | [P] Pediatric Age: 0-17 | [M] Maternity Age: 12-55
[A] Adult Age: 15-124 | ♂ Male | ♀ Female | ● New Code | ▲ Revised Code Title | ►◄ Revised Text

Q71.12 Congenital absence of left upper arm and forearm with hand present
Q71.13 Congenital absence of upper arm and forearm with hand present, bilateral

[5] Q71.2 Congenital absence of both forearm and hand
Q71.20 Congenital absence of both forearm and hand, unspecified upper limb
Q71.21 Congenital absence of both forearm and hand, right upper limb
Q71.22 Congenital absence of both forearm and hand, left upper limb
Q71.23 Congenital absence of both forearm and hand, bilateral

[5] Q71.3 Congenital absence of hand and finger
Q71.30 Congenital absence of unspecified hand and finger
Q71.31 Congenital absence of right hand and finger
Q71.32 Congenital absence of left hand and finger
Q71.33 Congenital absence of hand and finger, bilateral

[5] Q71.4 Longitudinal reduction defect of radius
Clubhand (congenital)
Radial clubhand
Q71.40 Longitudinal reduction defect of unspecified radius
Q71.41 Longitudinal reduction defect of right radius
Q71.42 Longitudinal reduction defect of left radius
Q71.43 Longitudinal reduction defect of radius, bilateral

[5] Q71.5 Longitudinal reduction defect of ulna
Q71.50 Longitudinal reduction defect of unspecified ulna
Q71.51 Longitudinal reduction defect of right ulna
Q71.52 Longitudinal reduction defect of left ulna
Q71.53 Longitudinal reduction defect of ulna, bilateral

[5] Q71.6 Lobster-claw hand
Q71.60 Lobster-claw hand, unspecified hand
Q71.61 Lobster-claw right hand
Q71.62 Lobster-claw left hand
Q71.63 Lobster-claw hand, bilateral

[5] Q71.8 Other reduction defects of upper limb
[6] Q71.81 Congenital shortening of upper limb
Q71.811 Congenital shortening of right upper limb
Q71.812 Congenital shortening of left upper limb
Q71.813 Congenital shortening of upper limb, bilateral
Q71.819 Congenital shortening of unspecified upper limb
[6] Q71.89 Other reduction defects of upper limb
Q71.891 Other reduction defects of right upper limb
Q71.892 Other reduction defects of left upper limb
Q71.893 Other reduction defects of upper limb, bilateral
Q71.899 Other reduction defects of unspecified upper limb

[5] Q71.9 Unspecified reduction defect of upper limb
Q71.90 Unspecified reduction defect of unspecified upper limb
Q71.91 Unspecified reduction defect of right upper limb
Q71.92 Unspecified reduction defect of left upper limb
Q71.93 Unspecified reduction defect of upper limb, bilateral

[4] Q72 Reduction defects of lower limb

[5] Q72.0 Congenital complete absence of lower limb
Q72.00 Congenital complete absence of unspecified lower limb
Q72.01 Congenital complete absence of right lower limb
Q72.02 Congenital complete absence of left lower limb
Q72.03 Congenital complete absence of lower limb, bilateral

[5] Q72.1 Congenital absence of thigh and lower leg with foot present
Q72.10 Congenital absence of unspecified thigh and lower leg with foot present
Q72.11 Congenital absence of right thigh and lower leg with foot present
Q72.12 Congenital absence of left thigh and lower leg with foot present
Q72.13 Congenital absence of thigh and lower leg with foot present, bilateral

[5] Q72.2 Congenital absence of both lower leg and foot
Q72.20 Congenital absence of both lower leg and foot, unspecified lower limb
Q72.21 Congenital absence of both lower leg and foot, right lower limb
Q72.22 Congenital absence of both lower leg and foot, left lower limb
Q72.23 Congenital absence of both lower leg and foot, bilateral

[5] Q72.3 Congenital absence of foot and toe(s)
Q72.30 Congenital absence of unspecified foot and toe(s)
Q72.31 Congenital absence of right foot and toe(s)
Q72.32 Congenital absence of left foot and toe(s)
Q72.33 Congenital absence of foot and toe(s), bilateral

[5] Q72.4 Longitudinal reduction defect of femur
Proximal femoral focal deficiency
Q72.40 Longitudinal reduction defect of unspecified femur
Q72.41 Longitudinal reduction defect of right femur
Q72.42 Longitudinal reduction defect of left femur
Q72.43 Longitudinal reduction defect of femur, bilateral

[5] Q72.5 Longitudinal reduction defect of tibia
Q72.50 Longitudinal reduction defect of unspecified tibia
Q72.51 Longitudinal reduction defect of right tibia
Q72.52 Longitudinal reduction defect of left tibia
Q72.53 Longitudinal reduction defect of tibia, bilateral

[5] Q72.6 Longitudinal reduction defect of fibula
Q72.60 Longitudinal reduction defect of unspecified fibula
Q72.61 Longitudinal reduction defect of right fibula
Q72.62 Longitudinal reduction defect of left fibula
Q72.63 Longitudinal reduction defect of fibula, bilateral

[5] Q72.7 Split foot
Q72.70 Split foot, unspecified lower limb
Q72.71 Split foot, right lower limb
Q72.72 Split foot, left lower limb
Q72.73 Split foot, bilateral

[5] Q72.8 Other reduction defects of lower limb
[6] Q72.81 Congenital shortening of lower limb
Q72.811 Congenital shortening of right lower limb
Q72.812 Congenital shortening of left lower limb
Q72.813 Congenital shortening of lower limb, bilateral
Q72.819 Congenital shortening of unspecified lower limb
[6] Q72.89 Other reduction defects of lower limb
Q72.891 Other reduction defects of right lower limb
Q72.892 Other reduction defects of left lower limb
Q72.893 Other reduction defects of lower limb, bilateral
Q72.899 Other reduction defects of unspecified lower limb

[5] Q72.9 Unspecified reduction defect of lower limb

[4] 4th character required [5] 5th character required [6] 6th character required [7] 7th character required [X] Extension 'X' Alert
EXCLUDES 1 Not coded here EXCLUDES 2 Not included here PDx Primary Diagnosis Only Manifestation Code

Q72.90 **Unspecified reduction defect of unspecified lower limb**

Q72.91 **Unspecified reduction defect of** right **lower limb**

Q72.92 **Unspecified reduction defect of** left **lower limb**

Q72.93 **Unspecified reduction defect of lower limb, bilateral**

Q73 **Reduction defects of** unspecified limb

Q73.0 **Congenital absence of unspecified limb(s)**

Amelia NOS

Q73.1 Phocomelia, **unspecified limb(s)**

Phocomelia NOS

Q73.8 Other reduction defects **of unspecified limb(s)**

Longitudinal reduction deformity of unspecified limb(s)

Ectromelia of limb NOS

Hemimelia of limb NOS

Reduction defect of limb NOS

Q74 Other **congenital malformations of** limb(s)

> *EXCLUDES1* *polydactyly (Q69.-)*
> *reduction defect of limb (Q71-Q73)*
> *syndactyly (Q70.-)*

Q74.0 **Other congenital malformations of** upper limb(s), including shoulder girdle

Accessory carpal bones

Cleidocranial dysostosis

Congenital pseudarthrosis of clavicle

Macrodactylia (fingers)

Madelung's deformity

Radioulnar synostosis

Sprengel's deformity

Triphalangeal thumb

Q74.1 **Congenital malformation of** knee

Congenital absence of patella

Congenital dislocation of patella

Congenital genu valgum

Congenital genu varum

Rudimentary patella

> *EXCLUDES1* *congenital dislocation of knee (Q68.2)*
> *congenital genu recurvatum (Q68.2)*
> *nail patella syndrome (Q87.2)*

Q74.2 **Other congenital malformations of** lower limb(s), including pelvic girdle

Congenital fusion of sacroiliac joint

Congenital malformation of ankle joint

Congenital malformation of sacroiliac joint

> *EXCLUDES1* *anteversion of femur (neck) (Q65.89)*

Q74.3 **Arthrogryposis multiplex congenita**

Q74.8 **Other specified congenital malformations of limb(s)**

Q74.9 **Unspecified congenital malformation of limb(s)**

Congenital anomaly of limb(s) NOS

Q75 Other **congenital malformations of** skull and face bones

> *EXCLUDES1* *congenital malformation of face NOS (Q18.-)*
> *congenital malformation syndromes classified to Q87.-*
> *dentofacial anomalies [including malocclusion] (M26.-)*
> *musculoskeletal deformities of head and face (Q67.0-Q67.4)*
> *skull defects associated with congenital anomalies of brain such as:*
> *anencephaly (Q00.0)*
> *encephalocele (Q01.-)*
> *hydrocephalus (Q03.-)*
> *microcephaly (Q02)*

Q75.0 **Craniosynostosis**

Acrocephaly

Imperfect fusion of skull

Oxycephaly

Trigonocephaly

Q75.1 **Craniofacial dysostosis**

Crouzon's disease

Q75.2 **Hypertelorism**

Q75.3 **Macrocephaly**

Q75.4 **Mandibulofacial dysostosis**

Franceschetti syndrome

Treacher Collins syndrome

Q75.5 **Oculomandibular dysostosis**

Q75.8 **Other specified congenital malformations of skull and face bones**

Absence of skull bone, congenital

Congenital deformity of forehead

Platybasia

Q75.9 **Congenital malformation of skull and face bones, unspecified**

Congenital anomaly of face bones NOS

Congenital anomaly of skull NOS

Q76 Congenital malformations of spine and bony thorax

> *EXCLUDES1* *congenital musculoskeletal deformities of spine and chest (Q67.5-Q67.8)*

Q76.0 **Spina bifida occulta**

> *EXCLUDES1* *meningocele (spinal) (Q05.-)*
> *spina bifida (aperta) (cystica) (Q05.-)*

Q76.1 **Klippel-Feil syndrome**

Cervical fusion syndrome

Q76.2 **Congenital spondylolisthesis**

Congenital spondylolysis

> *EXCLUDES1* *spondylolisthesis (acquired) (M43.1-)*
> *spondylolysis (acquired) (M43.0-)*

Q76.3 **Congenital scoliosis due to congenital bony malformation**

Hemivertebra fusion or failure of segmentation with scoliosis

Q76.4 Other **congenital malformations of** spine, not associated with scoliosis

Q76.41 **Congenital** kyphosis

Q76.411 **Congenital kyphosis,** occipito-atlanto-axial **region**

Q76.412 **Congenital kyphosis,** cervical **region**

Q76.413 **Congenital kyphosis,** cervicothoracic **region**

Q76.414 **Congenital kyphosis,** thoracic **region**

Q76.415 **Congenital kyphosis,** thoracolumbar **region**

Q76.419 **Congenital kyphosis, unspecified region**

Q76.42 **Congenital** lordosis

Q76.425 **Congenital lordosis,** thoracolumbar **region**

Q76.426 **Congenital lordosis,** lumbar **region**

Q76.427 **Congenital lordosis,** lumbosacral **region**

Q76.428 **Congenital lordosis,** sacral and sacrococcygeal **region**

Q76.429 **Congenital lordosis, unspecified region**

Q76.49 **Other congenital malformations of spine, not associated with scoliosis**

Congenital absence of vertebra NOS

Congenital fusion of spine NOS

Congenital malformation of lumbosacral (joint) (region) NOS

Congenital malformation of spine NOS

Hemivertebra NOS

Malformation of spine NOS

Platyspondylisis NOS

Supernumerary vertebra NOS

Q76.5 Cervical rib

Supernumerary rib in cervical region

Q76.6 **Other congenital malformations of** ribs

Accessory rib

Congenital absence of rib

Congenital fusion of ribs

Congenital malformation of ribs NOS

> *EXCLUDES1* *short rib syndrome (Q77.2)*

Unspecified Code	Other Specified Code	N Newborn Age: 0	P Pediatric Age: 0-17	M Maternity Age: 12-55	
A Adult Age: 15-124	♂ Male	♀ Female	● New Code	▲ Revised Code Title	►◄ Revised Text

Q76.7 Congenital malformation of sternum
Congenital absence of sternum
Sternum bifidum
Q76.8 Other congenital malformations of bony thorax
Q76.9 Congenital malformation of bony thorax, unspecified

[4] **Q77 Osteochondrodysplasia with defects of growth of tubular bones and spine**
[EXCLUDES1] *mucopolysaccharidosis (E76.0-E76.3)*
[EXCLUDES2] *congenital myotonic chondrodystrophy (G71.13)*
Q77.0 Achondrogenesis
Hypochondrogenesis
Q77.1 Thanatophoric short stature
Q77.2 Short rib syndrome
Asphyxiating thoracic dysplasia [Jeune]
Q77.3 Chondrodysplasia punctata
[EXCLUDES1] *Rhizomelic chondrodysplasia punctata (E71.43)*
Q77.4 Achondroplasia
Hypochondroplasia
Osteosclerosis congenita
Q77.5 Diastrophic dysplasia
Q77.6 Chondroectodermal dysplasia
Ellis-van Creveld syndrome
Q77.7 Spondyloepiphyseal dysplasia
Q77.8 Other osteochondrodysplasia with defects of growth of tubular bones and spine
Q77.9 Osteochondrodysplasia with defects of growth of tubular bones and spine, unspecified

[4] **Q78 Other osteochondrodysplasias**
[EXCLUDES2] *congenital myotonic chondrodystrophy (G71.13)*
Q78.0 Osteogenesis imperfecta
Fragilitas ossium
Osteopsathyrosis
Q78.1 Polyostotic fibrous dysplasia
Albright(-McCune)(-Sternberg) syndrome
Q78.2 Osteopetrosis
Albers-Schönberg syndrome
Osteosclerosis NOS
Q78.3 Progressive diaphyseal dysplasia
Camurati-Engelmann syndrome
Q78.4 Enchondromatosis
Maffucci's syndrome
Ollier's disease
Q78.5 Metaphyseal dysplasia
Pyle's syndrome
Q78.6 Multiple congenital exostoses
Diaphyseal aclasis
Q78.8 Other specified osteochondrodysplasias
Osteopoikilosis
Q78.9 Osteochondrodysplasia, unspecified
Chondrodystrophy NOS
Osteodystrophy NOS

[4] **Q79 Congenital malformations of musculoskeletal system, not elsewhere classified**
[EXCLUDES2] *congenital (sternomastoid) torticollis (Q68.0)*
Q79.0 Congenital diaphragmatic hernia
[EXCLUDES1] *congenital hiatus hernia (Q40.1)*
Q79.1 Other congenital malformations of diaphragm
Absence of diaphragm
Congenital malformation of diaphragm NOS
Eventration of diaphragm
Q79.2 Exomphalos
Omphalocele
[EXCLUDES1] *umbilical hernia (K42.-)*
Q79.3 Gastroschisis
Q79.4 Prune belly syndrome
Congenital prolapse of bladder mucosa
Eagle-Barrett syndrome
[5] **Q79.5 Other congenital malformations of abdominal wall**
[EXCLUDES1] *umbilical hernia (K42.-)*
Q79.51 Congenital hernia of bladder
Q79.59 Other congenital malformations of abdominal wall
Q79.6 Ehlers-Danlos syndrome
Q79.8 Other congenital malformations of musculoskeletal system
Absence of muscle
Absence of tendon
Accessory muscle
Amyotrophia congenita
Congenital constricting bands
Congenital shortening of tendon
Poland syndrome
Q79.9 Congenital malformation of musculoskeletal system, unspecified
Congenital anomaly of musculoskeletal system NOS
Congenital deformity of musculoskeletal system NOS

Other congenital malformations (Q80-Q89)

[4] **Q80 Congenital ichthyosis**
[EXCLUDES1] *Refsum's disease (G60.1)*
Q80.0 Ichthyosis vulgaris
Q80.1 X-linked ichthyosis
Q80.2 Lamellar ichthyosis
Collodion baby
Q80.3 Congenital bullous ichthyosiform erythroderma
Q80.4 Harlequin fetus
Q80.8 Other congenital ichthyosis
Q80.9 Congenital ichthyosis, unspecified

[4] **Q81 Epidermolysis bullosa**
Q81.0 Epidermolysis bullosa simplex
[EXCLUDES1] *Cockayne's syndrome (Q87.1)*
Q81.1 Epidermolysis bullosa letalis
Herlitz' syndrome
Q81.2 Epidermolysis bullosa dystrophica
Q81.8 Other epidermolysis bullosa
Q81.9 Epidermolysis bullosa, unspecified

[4] **Q82 Other congenital malformations of skin**
[EXCLUDES1] *acrodermatitis enteropathica (E83.2)*
congenital erythropoietic porphyria (E80.0)
pilonidal cyst or sinus (L05.-)
Sturge-Weber (-Dimitri) syndrome (Q85.8)
Q82.0 Hereditary lymphedema
Q82.1 Xeroderma pigmentosum
Q82.2 Mastocytosis
Urticaria pigmentosa
[EXCLUDES1] *malignant mastocytosis (C96.2)*
Q82.3 Incontinentia pigmenti
Q82.4 Ectodermal dysplasia (anhidrotic)
[EXCLUDES1] *Ellis-van Creveld syndrome (Q77.6)*
Q82.5 Congenital non-neoplastic nevus
Birthmark NOS
Flammeus Nevus
Portwine Nevus
Sanguineous Nevus
Strawberry Nevus
Vascular Nevus NOS
Verrucous Nevus
[EXCLUDES2] *Café au lait spots (L81.3)*
lentigo (L81.4)
nevus NOS (D22.-)

araneus nevus (I78.1)
melanocytic nevus (D22.-)
pigmented nevus (D22.-)
spider nevus (I78.1)
stellar nevus (I78.1)

Q82.8 **Other specified congenital malformations of skin**

Abnormal palmar creases

Accessory skin tags

Benign familial pemphigus [Hailey-Hailey]

Congenital poikiloderma

Cutis laxa (hyperelastica)

Dermatoglyphic anomalies

Inherited keratosis palmaris et plantaris

Keratosis follicularis [Darier-White]

EXCLUDES1 *Ehlers-Danlos syndrome (Q79.6)*

Q82.9 **Congenital malformation of skin, unspecified**

Q83 **Congenital malformations of** breast

EXCLUDES2 *absence of pectoral muscle (Q79.8)*
hypoplasia of breast (N64.82)
micromastia (N64.82)

Q83.0 **Congenital** absence of breast **with** absent nipple

Q83.1 Accessory breast

Supernumerary breast

Q83.2 Absent nipple

Q83.3 Accessory nipple

Supernumerary nipple

Q83.8 **Other congenital malformations of breast**

Q83.9 **Congenital malformation of breast, unspecified**

Q84 Other **congenital malformations of** integument

Q84.0 **Congenital alopecia**

Congenital atrichosis

Q84.1 **Congenital morphological disturbances of** hair, **not elsewhere classified**

Beaded hair

Monilethrix

Pili annulati

EXCLUDES1 *Menkes' kinky hair syndrome (E83.0)*

Q84.2 **Other congenital malformations of** hair

Congenital hypertrichosis

Congenital malformation of hair NOS

Persistent lanugo

Q84.3 **Anonychia**

EXCLUDES1 *nail patella syndrome (Q87.2)*

Q84.4 **Congenital leukonychia**

Q84.5 **Enlarged and hypertrophic** nails

Congenital onychauxis

Pachyonychia

Q84.6 **Other congenital malformations of** nails

Congenital clubnail

Congenital koilonychia

Congenital malformation of nail NOS

Q84.8 **Other specified congenital malformations of** integument

Aplasia cutis congenita

Q84.9 **Congenital malformation of integument, unspecified**

Congenital anomaly of integument NOS

Congenital deformity of integument NOS

Q85 **Phakomatoses, not elsewhere classified**

EXCLUDES1 *ataxia telangiectasia [Louis-Bar] (G11.3)*
familial dysautonomia [Riley-Day] (G90.1)

Q85.0 **Neurofibromatosis (nonmalignant)**

Q85.00 **Neurofibromatosis, unspecified**

Q85.01 **Neurofibromatosis,** type 1

Von Recklinghausen disease

Q85.02 **Neurofibromatosis,** type 2

Acoustic neurofibromatosis

Q85.03 Schwannomatosis

Q85.09 Other neurofibromatosis

Q85.1 **Tuberous sclerosis**

Bourneville's disease

Epiloia

Q85.8 **Other phakomatoses, not elsewhere classified**

Peutz-Jeghers Syndrome

Sturge-Weber(-Dimitri) syndrome

von Hippel-Lindau syndrome

EXCLUDES1 *Meckel-Gruber syndrome (Q61.9)*

Q85.9 **Phakomatosis, unspecified**

Hamartosis NOS

Q86 **Congenital malformation syndromes** due to known exogenous causes, **not elsewhere classified**

EXCLUDES2 *iodine-deficiency-related hypothyroidism (E00-E02)*
nonteratogenic effects of substances transmitted via placenta or breast milk (P04.-)

Q86.0 **Fetal alcohol syndrome (dysmorphic)**

Q86.1 **Fetal hydantoin syndrome**

Meadow's syndrome   N

Q86.2 **Dysmorphism due to warfarin**

Q86.8 **Other congenital malformation syndromes due to known exogenous causes**

Q87 Other specified **congenital malformation syndromes** affecting multiple systems

Use additional code(s) to identify all associated manifestations

Q87.0 **Congenital malformation syndromes predominantly affecting** facial appearance

Acrocephalopolysyndactyly

Acrocephalosyndactyly [Apert]

Cryptophthalmos syndrome

Cyclopia

Goldenhar syndrome

Moebius syndrome

Oro-facial-digital syndrome

Robin syndrome

Whistling face

Q87.1 **Congenital malformation syndromes predominantly** associated with short stature

Aarskog syndrome

Cockayne syndrome

De Lange syndrome

Dubowitz syndrome

Noonan syndrome

Prader-Willi syndrome

Robinow-Silverman-Smith syndrome

Russell-Silver syndrome

Seckel syndrome

EXCLUDES1 *Ellis-van Creveld syndrome (Q77.6)*
Smith-Lemli-Opitz syndrome (E78.72)

Q87.2 **Congenital malformation syndromes predominantly** involving limbs

Holt-Oram syndrome

Klippel-Trenaunay-Weber syndrome

Nail patella syndrome

Rubinstein-Taybi syndrome

Sirenomelia syndrome

Thrombocytopenia with absent radius [TAR] syndrome

VATER syndrome

Q87.3 **Congenital malformation syndromes** involving early overgrowth

Beckwith-Wiedemann syndrome

Sotos syndrome

Weaver syndrome

Q87.4 **Marfan's syndrome**

Q87.40 **Marfan's syndrome, unspecified**

Unspecified Code	Other Specified Code	N Newborn Age: 0	P Pediatric Age: 0-17	M Maternity Age: 12-55	
A Adult Age: 15-124	♂ Male	♀ Female	● New Code	▲ Revised Code Title	►◄ Revised Text

[6] Q87.41 Marfan's syndrome with cardiovascular manifestations
Q87.410 Marfan's syndrome with aortic dilation
Q87.418 Marfan's syndrome with other cardiovascular manifestations
Q87.42 Marfan's syndrome with ocular manifestations
Q87.43 Marfan's syndrome with skeletal manifestation
Q87.5 Other congenital malformation syndromes with other skeletal changes
[5] Q87.8 Other specified congenital malformation syndromes, not elsewhere classified
[EXCLUDES1] *Zellweger syndrome (E71.510)*
Q87.81 Alport syndrome
Use additional code to identify stage of chronic kidney disease (N18.1-N18.6)
Q87.89 Other specified congenital malformation syndromes, not elsewhere classified
Laurence-Moon (-Bardet)-Biedl syndrome
[4] Q89 Other congenital malformations, not elsewhere classified
[5] Q89.0 Congenital absence and malformations of spleen
[EXCLUDES1] *isomerism of atrial appendages (with asplenia or polysplenia) (Q20.6)*
Q89.01 Asplenia (congenital)
Q89.09 Congenital malformations of spleen
Congenital splenomegaly
Q89.1 Congenital malformations of adrenal gland
[EXCLUDES1] *adrenogenital disorders (E25.-)*
congenital adrenal hyperplasia (E25.0)
Q89.2 Congenital malformations of other endocrine glands
Congenital malformation of parathyroid or thyroid gland
Persistent thyroglossal duct
Thyroglossal cyst
[EXCLUDES1] *congenital goiter (E03.0)*
congenital hypothyroidism (E03.1)
Q89.3 Situs inversus
Dextrocardia with situs inversus
Mirror-image atrial arrangement with situs inversus
Situs inversus or transversus abdominalis
Situs inversus or transversus thoracis
Transposition of abdominal viscera
Transposition of thoracic viscera
[EXCLUDES1] *dextrocardia NOS (Q24.0)*
Q89.4 Conjoined twins
Craniopagus
Dicephaly
Pygopagus
Thoracopagus
Q89.7 Multiple congenital malformations, not elsewhere classified
Multiple congenital anomalies NOS
Multiple congenital deformities NOS
[EXCLUDES1] *congenital malformation syndromes affecting multiple systems (Q87.-)*
Q89.8 Other specified congenital malformations
Use additional code(s) to identify all associated manifestations
Q89.9 Congenital malformation, unspecified
Congenital anomaly NOS
Congenital deformity NOS

Chromosomal abnormalities, not elsewhere classified (Q90-Q99)

[EXCLUDES2] *mitochondrial metabolic disorders (E88.4-)*
[4] Q90 Down syndrome
Use additional code(s) to identify any associated physical conditions and degree of intellectual disabilities (F70-F79)
Q90.0 Trisomy 21, nonmosaicism (meiotic nondisjunction)
Q90.1 Trisomy 21, mosaicism (mitotic nondisjunction)
Q90.2 Trisomy 21, translocation
Q90.9 Down syndrome, unspecified
Trisomy 21 NOS
[4] Q91 Trisomy 18 and Trisomy 13
Q91.0 Trisomy 18, nonmosaicism (meiotic nondisjunction)
Q91.1 Trisomy 18, mosaicism (mitotic nondisjunction)
Q91.2 Trisomy 18, translocation
Q91.3 Trisomy 18, unspecified
Q91.4 Trisomy 13, nonmosaicism (meiotic nondisjunction)
Q91.5 Trisomy 13, mosaicism (mitotic nondisjunction)
Q91.6 Trisomy 13, translocation
Q91.7 Trisomy 13, unspecified
[4] Q92 Other trisomies and partial trisomies of the autosomes, not elsewhere classified
[INCLUDES] *unbalanced translocations and insertions*
[EXCLUDES1] *trisomies of chromosomes 13, 18, 21 (Q90-Q91)*
Q92.0 Whole chromosome trisomy, nonmosaicism (meiotic nondisjunction)
Q92.1 Whole chromosome trisomy, mosaicism (mitotic nondisjunction)
Q92.2 Partial trisomy
Less than whole arm duplicated
Whole arm or more duplicated
[EXCLUDES1] *partial trisomy due to unbalanced translocation (Q92.5)*
Q92.5 Duplications with other complex rearrangements
Partial trisomy due to unbalanced translocations
Code also any associated deletions due to unbalanced translocations, inversions and insertions (Q93.7)
[5] Q92.6 Marker chromosomes
Trisomies due to dicentrics
Trisomies due to extra rings
Trisomies due to isochromosomes
Individual with marker heterochromatin
Q92.61 Marker chromosomes in normal individual
Q92.62 Marker chromosomes in abnormal individual
Q92.7 Triploidy and polyploidy
Q92.8 Other specified trisomies and partial trisomies of autosomes
Duplications identified by fluorescence in situ hybridization (FISH)
Duplications identified by in situ hybridization (ISH)
Duplications seen only at prometaphase
Q92.9 Trisomy and partial trisomy of autosomes, unspecified
[4] Q93 Monosomies and deletions from the autosomes, not elsewhere classified
Q93.0 Whole chromosome monosomy, nonmosaicism (meiotic nondisjunction)
Q93.1 Whole chromosome monosomy, mosaicism (mitotic nondisjunction)
Q93.2 Chromosome replaced with ring, dicentric or isochromosome
Q93.3 Deletion of short arm of chromosome 4
Wolff-Hirschorn syndrome
Q93.4 Deletion of short arm of chromosome 5
Cri-du-chat syndrome
Q93.5 Other deletions of part of a chromosome
Angelman syndrome
Q93.7 Deletions with other complex rearrangements
Deletions due to unbalanced translocations, inversions and insertions
Code also any associated duplications due to unbalanced translocations, inversions and insertions (Q92.5)

[4] 4th character required [5] 5th character required [6] 6th character required [7] 7th character required [x7] Extension 'X' Alert
[EXCLUDES1] Not coded here [EXCLUDES2] Not included here [PDx] Primary Diagnosis Only Manifestation Code

[5] **Q93.8 Other deletions from the autosomes**

Q93.81 Velo-cardio-facial syndrome

Deletion 22q11.2

Q93.88 Other microdeletions

Miller-Dieker syndrome
Smith-Magenis syndrome

Q93.89 Other deletions from the autosomes

Deletions identified by fluorescence in situ hybridization (FISH)
Deletions identified by in situ hybridization (ISH)
Deletions seen only at prometaphase

Q93.9 Deletion from autosomes, unspecified

[4] **Q95 Balanced rearrangements and structural markers, not elsewhere classified**

[INCLUDES] *Robertsonian and balanced reciprocal translocations and insertions*

Q95.0 Balanced translocation and insertion in normal individual

Q95.1 Chromosome inversion in normal individual

Q95.2 Balanced autosomal rearrangement in abnormal individual

Q95.3 Balanced sex/autosomal rearrangement in abnormal individual

Q95.5 Individual with autosomal fragile site

Q95.8 Other balanced rearrangements and structural markers

Q95.9 Balanced rearrangement and structural marker, unspecified

[4] **Q96 Turner's syndrome**

[EXCLUDES1] *Noonan syndrome (Q87.1)*

Q96.0 Karyotype 45, X ♀

Q96.1 Karyotype 46, X iso (Xq)

Karyotype 46, isochromosome Xq ♀

Q96.2 Karyotype 46, X with abnormal sex chromosome, except iso (Xq)

Karyotype 46, X with abnormal sex chromosome, except isochromosome Xq ♀

Q96.3 Mosaicism, 45, X/46, XX or XY ♀

Q96.4 Mosaicism, 45, X/other cell line(s) with abnormal sex chromosome ♀

Q96.8 Other variants of Turner's syndrome ♀

Q96.9 Turner's syndrome, unspecified ♀

[4] **Q97 Other sex chromosome abnormalities, female phenotype, not elsewhere classified**

[EXCLUDES1] *Turner's syndrome (Q96.-)*

Q97.0 Karyotype 47, XXX ♀

Q97.1 Female with more than three X chromosomes ♀

Q97.2 Mosaicism, lines with various numbers of X chromosomes ♀

Q97.3 Female with 46, XY karyotype ♀

Q97.8 Other specified sex chromosome abnormalities, female phenotype ♀

Q97.9 Sex chromosome abnormality, female phenotype, unspecified ♀

[4] **Q98 Other sex chromosome abnormalities, male phenotype, not elsewhere classified**

Q98.0 Klinefelter syndrome karyotype 47, XXY ♂

Q98.1 Klinefelter syndrome, male with more than two X chromosomes ♂

Q98.3 Other male with 46, XX karyotype ♂

Q98.4 Klinefelter syndrome, unspecified ♂

Q98.5 Karyotype 47, XYY

Q98.6 Male with structurally abnormal sex chromosome ♂

Q98.7 Male with sex chromosome mosaicism ♂

Q98.8 Other specified sex chromosome abnormalities, male phenotype ♂

Q98.9 Sex chromosome abnormality, male phenotype, unspecified ♂

[4] **Q99 Other chromosome abnormalities, not elsewhere classified**

Q99.0 Chimera 46, XX/46, XY

Chimera 46, XX/46, XY true hermaphrodite

Q99.1 46, XX true hermaphrodite

46, XX with streak gonads
46, XY with streak gonads
Pure gonadal dysgenesis

Q99.2 Fragile X chromosome

Fragile X syndrome

Q99.8 Other specified chromosome abnormalities

Q99.9 Chromosomal abnormality, unspecified

This page intentionally left blank

Chapter 18: Symptoms, Signs, and Abnormal Clinical and Laboratory Findings, Not Elsewhere Classified (R00-R99)

Chapter Specific Coding Guidelines

Chapter 18 includes symptoms, signs, abnormal results of clinical or other investigative procedures, and ill-defined conditions regarding which no diagnosis classifiable elsewhere is recorded. Signs and symptoms that point to a specific diagnosis have been assigned to a category in other chapters of the classification.

a. **Use of symptom codes**
Codes that describe symptoms and signs are acceptable for reporting purposes when a related definitive diagnosis has not been established (confirmed) by the provider.

b. **Use of a symptom code with a definitive diagnosis code**
Codes for signs and symptoms may be reported in addition to a related definitive diagnosis when the sign or symptom is not routinely associated with that diagnosis, such as the various signs and symptoms associated with complex syndromes. The definitive diagnosis code should be sequenced before the symptom code.

Signs or symptoms that are associated routinely with a disease process should not be assigned as additional codes, unless otherwise instructed by the classification.

c. **Combination codes that include symptoms**
ICD-10-CM contains a number of combination codes that identify both the definitive diagnosis and common symptoms of that diagnosis. When using one of these combination codes, an additional code should not be assigned for the symptom.

d. **Repeated falls**
Code R29.6, Repeated falls, is for use for encounters when a patient has recently fallen and the reason for the fall is being investigated.

Code Z91.81, History of falling, is for use when a patient has fallen in the past and is at risk for future falls. When appropriate, both codes R29.6 and Z91.81 may be assigned together.

e. **Coma scale**
The coma scale codes (R40.2-) can be used in conjunction with traumatic brain injury codes, acute cerebrovascular disease or sequelae of cerebrovascular disease codes. These codes are primarily for use by trauma registries, but they may be used in any setting where this information is collected. The coma scale codes should be sequenced after the diagnosis code(s).

These codes, one from each subcategory, are needed to complete the scale. The 7th character indicates when the scale was recorded. The 7th character should match for all three codes.

At a minimum, report the initial score documented on presentation at your facility. This may be a score from the emergency medicine technician (EMT) or in the emergency department. If desired, a facility may choose to capture multiple coma scale scores.

Assign code R40.24, Glasgow coma scale, total score, when only the total score is documented in the medical record and not the individual score(s).

f. **Functional quadriplegia**
Functional quadriplegia (code R53.2) is the lack of ability to use one's limbs or to ambulate due to extreme debility. It is not associated with neurologic deficit or injury, and code R53.2 should not be used for cases of neurologic quadriplegia. It should only be assigned if functional quadriplegia is specifically documented in the medical record.

g. **SIRS due to Non-Infectious Process**
The systemic inflammatory response syndrome (SIRS) can develop as a result of certain non-infectious disease processes, such as trauma, malignant neoplasm, or pancreatitis. When SIRS is documented with a noninfectious condition, and no subsequent infection is documented, the code for the underlying condition, such as an injury, should be assigned, followed by code R65.10, Systemic inflammatory response syndrome (SIRS) of non-infectious origin without acute organ dysfunction, or code R65.11, Systemic inflammatory response syndrome (SIRS) of non-infectious origin with acute organ dysfunction. If an associated acute organ dysfunction is documented, the appropriate code(s) for the specific type of organ dysfunction(s) should be assigned in addition to code R65.11. If acute organ dysfunction is documented, but it cannot be determined if the acute organ dysfunction is associated with SIRS or due to another condition (e.g., directly due to the trauma), the provider should be queried.

h. **Death NOS**
Code R99, Ill-defined and unknown cause of mortality, is only for use in the very limited circumstance when a patient who has already died is brought into an emergency department or other healthcare facility and is pronounced dead upon arrival. It does not represent the discharge disposition of death.

This page intentionally left blank

Symptoms, signs and abnormal clinical and laboratory findings, not elsewhere classified (R00-R99)

NOTES This chapter includes symptoms, signs, abnormal results of clinical or other investigative procedures, and ill-defined conditions regarding which no diagnosis classifiable elsewhere is recorded.

Signs and symptoms that point rather definitely to a given diagnosis have been assigned to a category in other chapters of the classification. In general, categories in this chapter include the less well-defined conditions and symptoms that, without the necessary study of the case to establish a final diagnosis, point perhaps equally to two or more diseases or to two or more systems of the body. Practically all categories in the chapter could be designated 'not otherwise specified', 'unknown etiology' or 'transient'. The Alphabetical Index should be consulted to determine which symptoms and signs are to be allocated here and which to other chapters. The residual subcategories, numbered .8, are generally provided for other relevant symptoms that cannot be allocated elsewhere in the classification.

The conditions and signs or symptoms included in categories R00-R94 consist of:

(a) cases for which no more specific diagnosis can be made even after all the facts bearing on the case have been investigated;
(b) signs or symptoms existing at the time of initial encounter that proved to be transient and whose causes could not be determined;
(c) provisional diagnosis in a patient who failed to return for further investigation or care;
(d) cases referred elsewhere for investigation or treatment before the diagnosis was made;
(e) cases in which a more precise diagnosis was not available for any other reason;
(f) certain symptoms, for which supplementary information is provided, that represent important problems in medical care in their own right.

EXCLUDES2 *abnormal findings on antenatal screening of mother (O28.-)*
certain conditions originating in the perinatal period (P04-P96)
signs and symptoms classified in the body system chapters
signs and symptoms of breast (N63, N64.5)

Symptoms and signs involving the circulatory and respiratory systems (R00-R09)

R00 Abnormalities of heart beat
EXCLUDES1 *abnormalities originating in the perinatal period (P29.1-)*
specified arrhythmias (I47-I49)

R00.0 Tachycardia, unspecified
Rapid heart beat
Sinoauricular tachycardia NOS
Sinus [sinusal] tachycardia NOS
EXCLUDES1 *neonatal tachycardia (P29.11)*
paroxysmal tachycardia (I47.-)

R00.1 Bradycardia, unspecified
Sinoatrial bradycardia
Sinus bradycardia
Slow heart beat
Vagal bradycardia
Use additional code for adverse effect, if applicable, to identify drug (T36-T50 with fifth or sixth character 5)
EXCLUDES1 *neonatal bradycardia (P29.12)*

R00.2 Palpitations
Awareness of heart beat

R00.8 Other abnormalities of heart beat

R00.9 Unspecified abnormalities of heart beat

R01 Cardiac murmurs and other cardiac sounds
EXCLUDES1 *cardiac murmurs and sounds originating in the perinatal period (P29.8)*

R01.0 Benign and innocent cardiac murmurs
Functional cardiac murmur

R01.1 Cardiac murmur, unspecified
Cardiac bruit NOS
Heart murmur NOS

R01.2 Other cardiac sounds
Cardiac dullness, increased or decreased
Precordial friction

R03 Abnormal blood-pressure reading, without diagnosis
R03.0 Elevated blood-pressure reading, without diagnosis of hypertension
NOTES This category is to be used to record an episode of elevated blood pressure in a patient in whom no formal diagnosis of hypertension has been made, or as an isolated incidental finding.

R03.1 Nonspecific low blood-pressure reading
EXCLUDES1 *hypotension (I95.-)*
maternal hypotension syndrome (O26.5-)
neurogenic orthostatic hypotension (G90.3)

R04 Hemorrhage from respiratory passages
R04.0 Epistaxis
Hemorrhage from nose
Nosebleed

R04.1 Hemorrhage from throat
EXCLUDES2 *hemoptysis (R04.2)*

R04.2 Hemoptysis
Blood-stained sputum
Cough with hemorrhage

R04.8 Hemorrhage from other sites in respiratory passages
R04.81 Acute idiopathic pulmonary hemorrhage in infants
AIPHI
Acute idiopathic hemorrhage in infants over 28 days old
EXCLUDES1 *perinatal pulmonary hemorrhage (P26.-)*
von Willebrand's disease (D68.0) **P**

R04.89 Hemorrhage from other sites in respiratory passages
Pulmonary hemorrhage NOS

R04.9 Hemorrhage from respiratory passages, unspecified

R05 Cough
EXCLUDES1 *cough with hemorrhage (R04.2)*
smoker's cough (J41.0)

R06 Abnormalities of breathing
EXCLUDES1 *acute respiratory distress syndrome (J80)*
respiratory arrest (R09.2)
respiratory arrest of newborn (P28.81)
respiratory distress syndrome of newborn (P22.-)
respiratory failure (J96.-)
respiratory failure of newborn (P28.5)

R06.0 Dyspnea
EXCLUDES1 *tachypnea NOS (R06.82)*
transient tachypnea of newborn (P22.1)

R06.00 Dyspnea, unspecified
R06.01 Orthopnea
R06.02 Shortness of breath
R06.09 Other forms of dyspnea

R06.1 Stridor
EXCLUDES1 *congenital laryngeal stridor (P28.89)*
laryngismus (stridulus) (J38.5)

R06.2 Wheezing
EXCLUDES1 *Asthma (J45.-)*

R06.3 Periodic breathing
Cheyne-Stokes breathing

Unspecified Code | Other Specified Code | **N** Newborn Age: 0 | **P** Pediatric Age: 0-17 | **M** Maternity Age: 12-55
A Adult Age: 15-124 | ♂ Male | ♀ Female | ● New Code | ▲ Revised Code Title | ►◄ Revised Text

R06.4 Hyperventilation
[EXCLUDES1] *psychogenic hyperventilation (F45.8)*

R06.5 Mouth breathing
[EXCLUDES2] *dry mouth NOS (R68.2)*

R06.6 Hiccough
[EXCLUDES1] *psychogenic hiccough (F45.8)*

R06.7 Sneezing

[5] **R06.8 Other abnormalities of breathing**

R06.81 Apnea, not elsewhere classified
Apnea NOS
[EXCLUDES1] *apnea (of) newborn (P28.4)*
sleep apnea (G47.3-)
sleep apnea of newborn (primary) (P28.3)

R06.82 Tachypnea, not elsewhere classified
Tachypnea NOS
[EXCLUDES1] *transitory tachypnea of newborn (P22.1)*

R06.83 Snoring

R06.89 Other abnormalities of breathing
Breath-holding (spells)
Sighing

R06.9 Unspecified abnormalities of breathing

[4] **R07 Pain in throat and chest**
[EXCLUDES1] *epidemic myalgia (B33.0)*
[EXCLUDES2] *jaw pain R68.84*
pain in breast (N64.4)

R07.0 Pain in throat
[EXCLUDES1] *chronic sore throat (J31.2)*
sore throat (acute) NOS (J02.9)
[EXCLUDES2] *dysphagia (R13.1-)*
pain in neck (M54.2)

R07.1 Chest pain on breathing
Painful respiration

R07.2 Precordial pain

[5] **R07.8 Other chest pain**

R07.81 Pleurodynia
Pleurodynia NOS
[EXCLUDES1] *epidemic pleurodynia (B33.0)*

R07.82 Intercostal pain

R07.89 Other chest pain
Anterior chest-wall pain NOS

R07.9 Chest pain, unspecified

[4] **R09 Other symptoms and signs involving the circulatory and respiratory system**
[EXCLUDES1] *acute respiratory distress syndrome (J80)*
respiratory arrest of newborn (P28.81)
respiratory distress syndrome of newborn (P22.0)
respiratory failure (J96.-)
respiratory failure of newborn (P28.5)

[5] **R09.0 Asphyxia and hypoxemia**
[EXCLUDES1] *asphyxia due to carbon monoxide (T58.-)*
asphyxia due to foreign body in respiratory tract (T17.-)
birth (intrauterine) asphyxia (P84)
hypercapnia (R06.4)
hyperventilation (R06.4)
traumatic asphyxia (T71.-)

R09.01 Asphyxia

R09.02 Hypoxemia

R09.1 Pleurisy
[EXCLUDES1] *pleurisy with effusion (J90)*

R09.2 Respiratory arrest
Cardiorespiratory failure
[EXCLUDES1] *cardiac arrest (I46.-)*
respiratory arrest of newborn (P28.81)
respiratory distress of newborn (P22.0)
respiratory failure (J96.-)
respiratory failure of newborn (P28.5)
respiratory insufficiency (R06.89)
respiratory insufficiency of newborn (P28.5)

R09.3 Abnormal sputum
Abnormal amount of sputum
Abnormal color of sputum
Abnormal odor of sputum
Excessive sputum
[EXCLUDES1] *blood-stained sputum (R04.2)*

[5] **R09.8 Other specified symptoms and signs involving the circulatory and respiratory systems**

R09.81 Nasal congestion

R09.82 Postnasal drip

R09.89 Other specified symptoms and signs involving the circulatory and respiratory systems
Bruit (arterial)
Abnormal chest percussion
Feeling of foreign body in throat
Friction sounds in chest
Chest tympany
Choking sensation
Rales
Weak pulse
[EXCLUDES2] *foreign body in throat (T17.2-)*
wheezing (R06.2)

Symptoms and signs involving the digestive system and abdomen (R10-R19)

[EXCLUDES1] *congenital or infantile pylorospasm (Q40.0)*
gastrointestinal hemorrhage (K92.0-K92.2)
intestinal obstruction (K56.-)
newborn gastrointestinal hemorrhage (P54.0-P54.3)
newborn intestinal obstruction (P76.-)
pylorospasm (K31.3)
signs and symptoms involving the urinary system (R30-R39)
symptoms referable to female genital organs (N94.-)
symptoms referable to male genital organs male (N48-N50)

[4] **R10 Abdominal and pelvic pain**
[EXCLUDES1] *renal colic (N23)*
[EXCLUDES2] *dorsalgia (M54.-)*
flatulence and related conditions (R14.-)

R10.0 Acute abdomen
Severe abdominal pain (generalized) (with abdominal rigidity)
[EXCLUDES1] *abdominal rigidity NOS (R19.3)*
generalized abdominal pain NOS (R10.84)
localized abdominal pain (R10.1-R10.3-)

[5] **R10.1 Pain localized to upper abdomen**

R10.10 Upper abdominal pain, unspecified

R10.11 Right upper quadrant pain

R10.12 Left upper quadrant pain

R10.13 Epigastric pain
Dyspepsia
[EXCLUDES1] *functional dyspepsia (K30)*

R10.2 Pelvic and perineal pain
[EXCLUDES1] *vulvodynia (N94.81)*

[5] **R10.3 Pain localized to other parts of lower abdomen**

R10.30 Lower abdominal pain, unspecified

R10.31 Right lower quadrant pain

R10.32 Left lower quadrant pain

R10.33 Periumbilical pain

[5] **R10.8 Other abdominal pain**

[6] **R10.81 Abdominal tenderness**
Abdominal tenderness NOS

R10.811 Right upper quadrant abdominal tenderness

R10.812 Left upper quadrant abdominal tenderness
R10.813 Right lower quadrant abdominal tenderness
R10.814 Left lower quadrant abdominal tenderness
R10.815 Periumbilic abdominal tenderness
R10.816 Epigastric abdominal tenderness
R10.817 Generalized abdominal tenderness
R10.819 Abdominal tenderness, unspecified site
R10.82 Rebound abdominal tenderness
R10.821 Right upper quadrant rebound abdominal tenderness
R10.822 Left upper quadrant rebound abdominal tenderness
R10.823 Right lower quadrant rebound abdominal tenderness
R10.824 Left lower quadrant rebound abdominal tenderness
R10.825 Periumbilic rebound abdominal tenderness
R10.826 Epigastric rebound abdominal tenderness
R10.827 Generalized rebound abdominal tenderness
R10.829 Rebound abdominal tenderness, unspecified site
R10.83 Colic
Colic NOS
Infantile colic
EXCLUDES1 colic in adult and child over 12 months old (R10.84)
R10.84 Generalized abdominal pain
EXCLUDES1 generalized abdominal pain associated with acute abdomen (R10.0)
R10.9 Unspecified abdominal pain
R11 Nausea and vomiting
EXCLUDES1 cyclical vomiting associated with migraine (G43.A-)
excessive vomiting in pregnancy (O21.-)
hematemesis (K92.0)
neonatal hematemesis (P54.0)
newborn vomiting (P92.0-)
psychogenic vomiting (F50.8)
vomiting associated with bulimia nervosa (F50.2)
vomiting following gastrointestinal surgery (K91.0)
R11.0 Nausea
Nausea NOS
Nausea without vomiting
R11.1 Vomiting
R11.10 Vomiting, unspecified
Vomiting NOS
R11.11 Vomiting without nausea
R11.12 Projectile vomiting
R11.13 Vomiting of fecal matter
R11.14 Bilious vomiting
Bilious emesis
R11.2 Nausea with vomiting, unspecified
Persistent nausea with vomiting NOS
R12 Heartburn
EXCLUDES1 dyspepsia NOS (R10.13)
functional dyspepsia (K30)
R13 Aphagia and dysphagia
R13.0 Aphagia
Inability to swallow
EXCLUDES1 psychogenic aphagia (F50.9)
R13.1 Dysphagia
Code first , if applicable, dysphagia following cerebrovascular disease (I69. with final characters -91)
EXCLUDES1 psychogenic dysphagia (F45.8)

R13.10 Dysphagia, unspecified
Difficulty in swallowing NOS
R13.11 Dysphagia, oral phase
R13.12 Dysphagia, oropharyngeal phase
R13.13 Dysphagia, pharyngeal phase
R13.14 Dysphagia, pharyngoesophageal phase
R13.19 Other dysphagia
Cervical dysphagia
Neurogenic dysphagia
R14 Flatulence and related conditions
EXCLUDES1 psychogenic aerophagy (F45.8)
R14.0 Abdominal distension (gaseous)
Bloating
Tympanites (abdominal) (intestinal)
R14.1 Gas pain
R14.2 Eructation
R14.3 Flatulence
R15 Fecal incontinence
INCLUDES encopresis NOS
EXCLUDES1 fecal incontinence of nonorganic origin (F98.1)
R15.0 Incomplete defecation
EXCLUDES1 constipation (K59.0-)
fecal impaction (K56.41)
R15.1 Fecal smearing
Fecal soiling
R15.2 Fecal urgency
R15.9 Full incontinence of feces
Fecal incontinence NOS
R16 Hepatomegaly and splenomegaly, not elsewhere classified
R16.0 Hepatomegaly, not elsewhere classified
Hepatomegaly NOS
R16.1 Splenomegaly, not elsewhere classified
Splenomegaly NOS
R16.2 Hepatomegaly with splenomegaly, not elsewhere classified
Hepatosplenomegaly NOS
R17 Unspecified jaundice
EXCLUDES1 neonatal jaundice (P55, P57-P59)
R18 Ascites
INCLUDES fluid in peritoneal cavity
EXCLUDES1 ascites in alcoholic cirrhosis (K70.31)
ascites in alcoholic hepatitis (K70.11)
ascites in toxic liver disease with chronic active hepatitis (K71.51)
R18.0 Malignant ascites
Code first malignancy, such as:
malignant neoplasm of ovary (C56.-)
secondary malignant neoplasm of retroperitoneum and peritoneum (C78.6)
R18.8 Other ascites
Ascites NOS
Peritoneal effusion (chronic)
R19 Other symptoms and signs involving the digestive system and abdomen
EXCLUDES1 acute abdomen (R10.0)
R19.0 Intra-abdominal and pelvic swelling, mass and lump
EXCLUDES1 abdominal distension (gaseous) (R14.-)
ascites (R18.-)
R19.00 Intra-abdominal and pelvic swelling, mass and lump, unspecified site
R19.01 Right upper quadrant abdominal swelling, mass and lump
R19.02 Left upper quadrant abdominal swelling, mass and lump
R19.03 Right lower quadrant abdominal swelling, mass and lump

Unspecified Code	Other Specified Code N Newborn Age: 0 P Pediatric Age: 0-17 M Maternity Age: 12-55
A Adult Age: 15-124 ♂ Male ♀ Female ● New Code ▲ Revised Code Title ►◄ Revised Text	

R19.04 Left lower quadrant abdominal swelling, mass and lump

R19.05 Periumbilic swelling, mass or lump

Diffuse or generalized umbilical swelling or mass

R19.06 Epigastric swelling, mass or lump

R19.07 Generalized intra-abdominal and pelvic swelling, mass and lump

Diffuse or generalized intra-abdominal swelling or mass NOS

Diffuse or generalized pelvic swelling or mass NOS

R19.09 Other intra-abdominal and pelvic swelling, mass and lump

[5] **R19.1 Abnormal bowel sounds**

R19.11 Absent bowel sounds

R19.12 Hyperactive bowel sounds

R19.15 Other abnormal bowel sounds

Abnormal bowel sounds NOS

R19.2 Visible peristalsis

Hyperperistalsis

[5] **R19.3 Abdominal rigidity**

EXCLUDES1 *abdominal rigidity with severe abdominal pain (R10.0)*

R19.30 Abdominal rigidity, unspecified site

R19.31 Right upper quadrant abdominal rigidity

R19.32 Left upper quadrant abdominal rigidity

R19.33 Right lower quadrant abdominal rigidity

R19.34 Left lower quadrant abdominal rigidity

R19.35 Periumbilic abdominal rigidity

R19.36 Epigastric abdominal rigidity

R19.37 Generalized abdominal rigidity

R19.4 Change in bowel habit

EXCLUDES1 *constipation (K59.0-)*
functional diarrhea (K59.1)

R19.5 Other fecal abnormalities

Abnormal stool color
Bulky stools
Mucus in stools
Occult blood in feces
Occult blood in stools

EXCLUDES1 *melena (K92.1)*
neonatal melena (P54.1)

R19.6 Halitosis

R19.7 Diarrhea, unspecified

Diarrhea NOS

EXCLUDES1 *functional diarrhea (K59.1)*
neonatal diarrhea (P78.3)
psychogenic diarrhea (F45.8)

R19.8 Other specified symptoms and signs involving the digestive system and abdomen

Symptoms and signs involving the skin and subcutaneous tissue (R20-R23)

EXCLUDES2 *symptoms relating to breast (N64.4-N64.5)*

[4] **R20 Disturbances of skin sensation**

EXCLUDES1 *dissociative anesthesia and sensory loss (F44.6)*
psychogenic disturbances (F45.8)

R20.0 Anesthesia of skin

R20.1 Hypoesthesia of skin

R20.2 Paresthesia of skin

Formication
Pins and needles
Tingling skin

EXCLUDES1 *acroparesthesia (I73.8)*

R20.3 Hyperesthesia

R20.8 Other disturbances of skin sensation

R20.9 Unspecified disturbances of skin sensation

R21 Rash and other nonspecific skin eruption

INCLUDES *rash NOS*

EXCLUDES1 *specified type of rash- code to condition*
vesicular eruption (R23.8)

[4] **R22 Localized swelling, mass and lump of skin and subcutaneous tissue**

INCLUDES *subcutaneous nodules (localized)(superficial)*

EXCLUDES1 *abnormal findings on diagnostic imaging (R90-R93)*
edema (R60.-)
enlarged lymph nodes (R59.-)
localized adiposity (E65)
swelling of joint (M25.4-)

R22.0 Localized swelling, mass and lump, head

R22.1 Localized swelling, mass and lump, neck

R22.2 Localized swelling, mass and lump, trunk

EXCLUDES1 *intra-abdominal or pelvic mass and lump (R19.0-)*
intra-abdominal or pelvic swelling (R19.0-)

EXCLUDES2 *breast mass and lump (N63)*

[5] **R22.3 Localized swelling, mass and lump, upper limb**

R22.30 Localized swelling, mass and lump, unspecified upper limb

R22.31 Localized swelling, mass and lump, right upper limb

R22.32 Localized swelling, mass and lump, left upper limb

R22.33 Localized swelling, mass and lump, upper limb, bilateral

[5] **R22.4 Localized swelling, mass and lump, lower limb**

R22.40 Localized swelling, mass and lump, unspecified lower limb

R22.41 Localized swelling, mass and lump, right lower limb

R22.42 Localized swelling, mass and lump, left lower limb

R22.43 Localized swelling, mass and lump, lower limb, bilateral

R22.9 Localized swelling, mass and lump, unspecified

[4] **R23 Other skin changes**

R23.0 Cyanosis

EXCLUDES1 *acrocyanosis (I73.8)*
cyanotic attacks of newborn (P28.2)

R23.1 Pallor

Clammy skin

R23.2 Flushing

Excessive blushing

Code first , if applicable, menopausal and female climacteric states (N95.1)

R23.3 Spontaneous ecchymoses

Petechiae

EXCLUDES1 *ecchymoses of newborn (P54.5)*
purpura (D69.-)

R23.4 Changes in skin texture

Desquamation of skin
Induration of skin
Scaling of skin

EXCLUDES1 *epidermal thickening NOS (L85.9)*

R23.8 Other skin changes

R23.9 Unspecified skin changes

Symptoms and signs involving the nervous and musculoskeletal systems (R25-R29)

◔ **R25 Abnormal involuntary movements**

   EXCLUDES1 specific movement disorders (G20-G26)
               stereotyped movement disorders (F98.4)
               tic disorders (F95.-)

   R25.0 Abnormal head movements
   R25.1 Tremor, unspecified

   EXCLUDES1 chorea NOS (G25.5)
               essential tremor (G25.0)
               hysterical tremor (F44.4)
               intention tremor (G25.2)

   R25.2 Cramp and spasm

   EXCLUDES2 carpopedal spasm (R29.0)
               charley-horse (M62.831)
               infantile spasms (G40.4-)
               muscle spasm of back (M62.830)
               muscle spasm of calf (M62.831)

   R25.3 Fasciculation

   Twitching NOS
   R25.8 Other abnormal involuntary movements
   R25.9 Unspecified abnormal involuntary movements

◑ **R26 Abnormalities of gait and mobility**

   EXCLUDES1 ataxia NOS (R27.0)
               hereditary ataxia (G11.-)
               locomotor (syphilitic) ataxia (A52.11)
               immobility syndrome (paraplegic) (M62.3)

   R26.0 Ataxic gait

   Staggering gait
   R26.1 Paralytic gait

   Spastic gait
   R26.2 Difficulty in walking, not elsewhere classified

   EXCLUDES1 falling (R29.6)
               unsteadiness on feet (R26.81)

◕ **R26.8 Other abnormalities of gait and mobility**
   R26.81 Unsteadiness on feet
   R26.89 Other abnormalities of gait and mobility
   R26.9 Unspecified abnormalities of gait and mobility

◔ **R27 Other lack of coordination**

   EXCLUDES1 ataxic gait (R26.0)
               hereditary ataxia (G11.-)
               vertigo NOS (R42)

   R27.0 Ataxia, unspecified

   EXCLUDES1 ataxia following cerebrovascular disease (I69. with final characters -93)

   R27.8 Other lack of coordination
   R27.9 Unspecified lack of coordination

◔ **R29 Other symptoms and signs involving the nervous and musculoskeletal systems**

   R29.0 Tetany

   Carpopedal spasm
   EXCLUDES1 hysterical tetany (F44.5)
               neonatal tetany (P71.3)
               parathyroid tetany (E20.9)
               post-thyroidectomy tetany (E89.2)

   R29.1 Meningismus
   R29.2 Abnormal reflex

   EXCLUDES2 abnormal pupillary reflex (H57.0)
               hyperactive gag reflex (J39.2)
               vasovagal reaction or syncope (R55)

   R29.3 Abnormal posture
   R29.4 Clicking hip

   EXCLUDES1 congenital deformities of hip (Q65.-)

   R29.5 Transient paralysis

   Code first any associated spinal cord injury (S14.0, S14.1-, S24.0, S24.1-, S34.0-, S34.1-)
   EXCLUDES1 transient ischemic attack (G45.9)

   R29.6 Repeated falls

   Falling
   Tendency to fall
   EXCLUDES2 at risk for falling (Z91.81)
               history of falling (Z91.81)

◕ **R29.8 Other symptoms and signs involving the nervous and musculoskeletal systems**

   ◕ **R29.81 Other symptoms and signs involving the nervous system**
      R29.810 Facial weakness

      Facial droop
      EXCLUDES1 Bell's palsy (G51.0)
                  facial weakness following cerebrovascular disease (I69. with final characters -92)
      R29.818 Other symptoms and signs involving the nervous system

   ◕ **R29.89 Other symptoms and signs involving the musculoskeletal system**

      EXCLUDES2 pain in limb (M79.6-)
      R29.890 Loss of height

      EXCLUDES1 osteoporosis (M80-M81)
      R29.891 Ocular torticollis

      EXCLUDES1 congenital (sternomastoid) torticollis Q68.0
                  psychogenic torticollis (F45.8)
                  spasmodic torticollis (G24.3)
                  torticollis due to birth injury (P15.8)
                  torticollis NOS M43.6
      R29.898 Other symptoms and signs involving the musculoskeletal system

◕ **R29.9 Unspecified symptoms and signs involving the nervous and musculoskeletal systems**
   R29.90 Unspecified symptoms and signs involving the nervous system
   R29.91 Unspecified symptoms and signs involving the musculoskeletal system

Symptoms and signs involving the genitourinary system (R30-R39)

◔ **R30 Pain associated with micturition**

   EXCLUDES1 psychogenic pain associated with micturition (F45.8)

   R30.0 Dysuria

   Strangury
   R30.1 Vesical tenesmus
   R30.9 Painful micturition, unspecified

   Painful urination NOS

◔ **R31 Hematuria**

   EXCLUDES1 hematuria included with underlying conditions, such as:
               acute cystitis with hematuria (N30.01)
               recurrent and persistent hematuria in glomerular diseases (N02.-)

   R31.0 Gross hematuria
   R31.1 Benign essential microscopic hematuria
   R31.2 Other microscopic hematuria
   R31.9 Hematuria, unspecified

R32 Unspecified urinary incontinence

   Enuresis NOS
   EXCLUDES1 functional urinary incontinence (R39.81)
               nonorganic enuresis (F98.0)
               stress incontinence and other specified urinary incontinence (N39.3-N39.4-)
               urinary incontinence associated with cognitive impairment (R39.81)

◔ **R33 Retention of urine**

   EXCLUDES1 psychogenic retention of urine (F45.8)
   R33.0 Drug induced retention of urine

   Use additional code for adverse effect, if applicable, to identify drug (T36-T50 with fifth or sixth character 5)

Unspecified Code	Other Specified Code	N Newborn Age: 0	P Pediatric Age: 0-17	M Maternity Age: 12-55
A Adult Age: 15-124	♂ Male	♀ Female	● New Code	▲ Revised Code Title ►◄ Revised Text

R33.8 **Other retention of urine**
Code first , if applicable, any causal condition, such as: enlarged prostate (N40.1)

R33.9 **Retention of urine, unspecified**

R34 **Anuria and oliguria**
> EXCLUDES1   anuria and oliguria complicating abortion or ectopic or molar pregnancy (O00-O07, O08.4)
> anuria and oliguria complicating pregnancy (O26.83-)
> anuria and oliguria complicating the puerperium (O90.4)

🔵 R35 **Polyuria**
Code first , if applicable, any causal condition, such as: enlarged prostate (N40.1)
> EXCLUDES1   psychogenic polyuria (F45.8)

R35.0 **Frequency of micturition**

R35.1 **Nocturia**

R35.8 **Other polyuria**
Polyuria NOS

🔵 R36 **Urethral discharge**

R36.0 **Urethral discharge without blood**

R36.1 **Hematospermia**   ♂

R36.9 **Urethral discharge, unspecified**
Penile discharge NOS
Urethrorrhea

R37 **Sexual dysfunction, unspecified**

🔵 R39 **Other and unspecified symptoms and signs involving the genitourinary system**

R39.0 **Extravasation of urine**

🔵 R39.1 **Other difficulties with micturition**
Code first , if applicable, any causal condition, such as: enlarged prostate (N40.1)

R39.11 **Hesitancy of micturition**

R39.12 **Poor urinary stream**
Weak urinary steam

R39.13 **Splitting of urinary stream**

R39.14 **Feeling of incomplete bladder emptying**

R39.15 **Urgency of urination**
> EXCLUDES1   urge incontinence (N39.41, N39.46)

R39.16 **Straining to void**

R39.19 **Other difficulties with micturition**

R39.2 **Extrarenal uremia**
Prerenal uremia
> EXCLUDES1   uremia NOS (N19)

🔵 R39.8 **Other symptoms and signs involving the genitourinary system**

R39.81 **Functional urinary incontinence**
Urinary incontinence due to cognitive impairment, or severe physical disability or immobility
> EXCLUDES1   stress incontinence and other specified urinary incontinence (N39.3-N39.4-)
> urinary incontinence NOS (R32)

R39.89 **Other symptoms and signs involving the genitourinary system**

R39.9 **Unspecified symptoms and signs involving the genitourinary system**

Symptoms and signs involving cognition, perception, emotional state and behavior (R40-R46)

> EXCLUDES1   symptoms and signs constituting part of a pattern of mental disorder (F01-F99)

🔵 R40 **Somnolence, stupor and coma**
> EXCLUDES1   neonatal coma (P91.5)
> somnolence, stupor and coma in diabetes (E08-E13)
> somnolence, stupor and coma in hepatic failure (K72.-)
> somnolence, stupor and coma in hypoglycemia (nondiabetic) (E15)

R40.0 **Somnolence**
Drowsiness
> EXCLUDES1   coma (R40.2-)

R40.1 **Stupor**
Catatonic stupor
Semicoma
> EXCLUDES1   catatonic schizophrenia (F20.2)
> coma (R40.2-)
> depressive stupor (F31-F33)
> dissociative stupor (F44.2)
> manic stupor (F30.2)

🔵 R40.2 **Coma**
Code first any associated:
fracture of skull (S02.-)
intracranial injury (S06.-)
The appropriate 7th character is to be added to each code from subcategory R40.21-, R40.22-, R40.23-:

NOTES   One code from subcategories R40.21-R40-23 is required to complete the coma scale

R40.20 **Unspecified coma**
Coma NOS
Unconsciousness NOS

🔵 R40.21 **Coma scale,** eyes open
0 = unspecified time
1 = in the field [EMT or ambulance]
2 = at arrival to emergency department
3 = at hospital admission
4 = 24 hours or more after hospital admission
The following appropriate 7th character is to be added to subcategory R40.21-:

🕖 R40.211 **Coma scale, eyes open,** never

🕖 R40.212 **Coma scale, eyes open,** to pain

🕖 R40.213 **Coma scale, eyes open,** to sound

🕖 R40.214 **Coma scale, eyes open,** spontaneous

🔵 R40.22 **Coma scale,** best verbal response
0 = unspecified time
1 = in the field [EMT or ambulance]
2 = at arrival to emergency department
3 = at hospital admission
4 = 24 hours or more after hospital admission
The following appropriate 7th character is to be added to subcategory R40.22-:

🕖 R40.221 **Coma scale, best verbal response,** none

🕖 R40.222 **Coma scale, best verbal response,** incomprehensible words

🕖 R40.223 **Coma scale, best verbal response,** inappropriate words

🕖 R40.224 **Coma scale, best verbal response,** confused conversation

🕖 R40.225 **Coma scale, best verbal response,** oriented

🔵 R40.23 **Coma scale,** best motor response
0 = unspecified time
1 = in the field [EMT or ambulance]
2 = at arrival to emergency department
3 = at hospital admission
4 = 24 hours or more after hospital admission

🔵 4th character required   🔵 5th character required   🔵 6th character required   🕖 7th character required   🔵 Extension 'X' Alert

EXCLUDES 1 Not coded here   **EXCLUDES 2** Not included here   PDx Primary Diagnosis Only   Manifestation Code

The following appropriate 7th character is to be added to subcategory R40.23-:

⑦ **R40.231 Coma scale, best motor response,** none
⑦ **R40.232 Coma scale, best motor response,** extension
⑦ **R40.233 Coma scale, best motor response,** abnormal
⑦ **R40.234 Coma scale, best motor response,** flexion withdrawal
⑦ **R40.235 Coma scale, best motor response,** localizes pain
⑦ **R40.236 Coma scale, best motor response,** obeys commands

⑥ **R40.24** Glasgow coma scale, **total score**

Use codes R40.21- through R40.23- only when the individual score(s) are documented

R40.241 Glasgow coma scale score 13-15
R40.242 Glasgow coma scale score 9-12
R40.243 Glasgow coma scale score 3-8
R40.244 Other coma, without documented Glasgow coma scale score, or with partial score reported

R40.3 Persistent vegetative state
R40.4 Transient alteration of awareness

④ **R41 Other symptoms and signs involving cognitive functions and awareness**

EXCLUDES1   *dissociative [conversion] disorders (F44.-)*
mild cognitive impairment, so stated (G31.84)

R41.0 Disorientation, unspecified

Confusion NOS
Delirium NOS

R41.1 Anterograde amnesia
R41.2 Retrograde amnesia
R41.3 Other amnesia

Amnesia NOS
Memory loss NOS

EXCLUDES1   *amnestic disorder due to known physiologic condition (F04)*
amnestic syndrome due to psychoactive substance use (F10-F19 with 5th character .6)
mild memory disturbance due to known physiological condition (F06.8)
transient global amnesia (G45.4)

R41.4 Neurologic neglect syndrome

Asomatognosia
Hemi-akinesia
Hemi-inattention
Hemispatial neglect
Left-sided neglect
Sensory neglect
Visuospatial neglect

EXCLUDES1   *visuospatial deficit (R41.842)*

⑤ **R41.8 Other symptoms and signs involving cognitive functions and awareness**

R41.81 Age-related **cognitive decline**

Senility NOS   Ⓐ

R41.82 Altered mental status, unspecified

Change in mental status NOS

EXCLUDES1   *altered level of consciousness (R40.-)*
altered mental status due to known condition - code to condition
delirium NOS (R41.0)

R41.83 Borderline intellectual **functioning**

IQ level 71 to 84

EXCLUDES1   *intellectual disabilities (F70-F79)*

⑥ **R41.84** Other **specified** cognitive deficit

R41.840 Attention **and** concentration **deficit**

EXCLUDES1   *attention-deficit hyperactivity disorders (F90.-)*

R41.841 Cognitive communication **deficit**

R41.842 Visuospatial **deficit**
R41.843 Psychomotor **deficit**
R41.844 Frontal lobe and executive function **deficit**

R41.89 Other symptoms and signs involving cognitive functions and awareness

Anosognosia

R41.9 Unspecified symptoms and signs involving cognitive functions and awareness

R42 Dizziness and giddiness

Light-headedness
Vertigo NOS

EXCLUDES1   *vertiginous syndromes (H81.-)*
vertigo from infrasound (T75.23)

④ **R43 Disturbances of smell and taste**

R43.0 Anosmia
R43.1 Parosmia
R43.2 Parageusia
R43.8 Other disturbances of smell and taste

Mixed disturbance of smell and taste

R43.9 Unspecified disturbances of smell and taste

④ **R44 Other symptoms and signs involving general sensations and perceptions**

EXCLUDES1   *alcoholic hallucinations (F1.5)*
hallucinations in drug psychosis (F11-F19 with .5)
hallucinations in mood disorders with psychotic symptoms (F30.2, F31.5, F32.3, F33.3)
hallucinations in schizophrenia, schizotypal and delusional disorders (F20-F29)

EXCLUDES2   *disturbances of skin sensation (R20.-)*

R44.0 Auditory hallucinations
R44.1 Visual hallucinations
R44.2 Other hallucinations
R44.3 Hallucinations, unspecified
R44.8 Other symptoms and signs involving general sensations and perceptions
R44.9 Unspecified symptoms and signs involving general sensations and perceptions

④ **R45 Symptoms and signs involving emotional state**

R45.0 Nervousness

Nervous tension

R45.1 Restlessness and agitation
R45.2 Unhappiness
R45.3 Demoralization and apathy

EXCLUDES1   *anhedonia (R45.84)*

R45.4 Irritability and anger
R45.5 Hostility
R45.6 Violent behavior
R45.7 State of emotional shock and stress, unspecified

⑤ **R45.8 Other symptoms and signs involving emotional state**

R45.81 Low self-esteem
R45.82 Worries
R45.83 Excessive crying of child, adolescent or adult

EXCLUDES1   *excessive crying of infant (baby) R68.11*

R45.84 Anhedonia
⑥ **R45.85 Homicidal and suicidal ideations**

EXCLUDES1   *suicide attempt (T14.91)*

R45.850 Homicidal **ideations**
R45.851 Suicidal **ideations**

R45.86 Emotional lability
R45.87 Impulsiveness
R45.89 Other symptoms and signs involving emotional state

④ **R46 Symptoms and signs involving appearance and behavior**

EXCLUDES1   *appearance and behavior in schizophrenia, schizotypal and delusional disorders (F20-F29)*
mental and behavioral disorders (F01-F99)

R46.0 Very low level of personal hygiene

Unspecified Code	Other Specified Code	Ⓝ Newborn Age: 0	Ⓟ Pediatric Age: 0-17	Ⓜ Maternity Age: 12-55
Ⓐ Adult Age: 15-124	♂ Male	♀ Female	● New Code	▲ Revised Code Title ►◄ Revised Text

R46.1   Bizarre personal appearance
R46.2   Strange and inexplicable behavior
R46.3   Overactivity
R46.4   Slowness and poor responsiveness
> EXCLUDES1 *stupor (R40.1)*

R46.5   Suspiciousness and marked evasiveness
R46.6   Undue concern and preoccupation with stressful events
R46.7   Verbosity and circumstantial detail obscuring reason for contact
R46.8   Other symptoms and signs involving appearance and behavior
   R46.81 Obsessive-compulsive behavior
   > EXCLUDES1 *obsessive-compulsive disorder (F42)*
   R46.89 Other symptoms and signs involving appearance and behavior

Symptoms and signs involving speech and voice (R47-R49)

R47   Speech disturbances, not elsewhere classified
   > EXCLUDES1 *autism (F84.0)*
   > *cluttering (F80.81)*
   > *specific developmental disorders of speech and language (F80.-)*
   > *stuttering (F80.81)*
   R47.0 Dysphasia and aphasia
      R47.01 Aphasia
      > EXCLUDES1 *aphasia following cerebrovascular disease (I69. with final characters -20)*
      > *progressive isolated aphasia (G31.01)*
      R47.02 Dysphasia
      > EXCLUDES1 *dysphasia following cerebrovascular disease (I69. with final characters -21)*
   R47.1 Dysarthria and anarthria
      > EXCLUDES1 *dysarthria following cerebrovascular disease (I69. with final characters -22)*
   R47.8 Other speech disturbances
      > EXCLUDES1 *dysarthria following cerebrovascular disease (I69. with final characters -28)*
      R47.81 Slurred speech
      R47.82 Fluency disorder in conditions classified elsewhere
         Stuttering in conditions classified elsewhere
         Code first underlying disease or condition, such as:
         Parkinson's disease (G20)
         > EXCLUDES1 *adult onset fluency disorder (F98.5)*
         > *childhood onset fluency disorder (F80.81)*
         > *fluency disorder (stuttering) following cerebrovascular disease (I69. with final characters -23)*
      R47.89 Other speech disturbances
   R47.9 Unspecified speech disturbances
R48   Dyslexia and other symbolic dysfunctions, not elsewhere classified
   > EXCLUDES1 *specific developmental disorders of scholastic skills (F81.-)*
   R48.0 Dyslexia and alexia
   R48.1 Agnosia
      Astereognosia (astereognosis)
      Autotopagnosia
      > EXCLUDES1 *visual object agnosia (R48.3)*
   R48.2 Apraxia
      > EXCLUDES1 *apraxia following cerebrovascular disease (I69. with final characters -90)*
   R48.3 Visual agnosia
      Prosopagnosia
      Simultanagnosia (asimultagnosia)
   R48.8 Other symbolic dysfunctions
      Acalculia
      Agraphia

R48.9   Unspecified symbolic dysfunctions
R49   Voice and resonance disorders
   > EXCLUDES1 *psychogenic voice and resonance disorders (F44.4)*
   R49.0 Dysphonia
      Hoarseness
   R49.1 Aphonia
      Loss of voice
   R49.2 Hypernasality and hyponasality
      R49.21 Hypernasality
      R49.22 Hyponasality
   R49.8 Other voice and resonance disorders
   R49.9 Unspecified voice and resonance disorder
      Change in voice NOS
      Resonance disorder NOS

General symptoms and signs (R50-R69)

R50   Fever of other and unknown origin
   > EXCLUDES1 *chills without fever (R68.83)*
   > *febrile convulsions (R56.0-)*
   > *fever of unknown origin during labor (O75.2)*
   > *fever of unknown origin in newborn (P81.9)*
   > *hypothermia due to illness (R68.0)*
   > *malignant hyperthermia due to anesthesia (T88.3)*
   > *puerperal pyrexia NOS (O86.4)*
   R50.2 Drug induced fever
      Use additional code for adverse effect, if applicable, to identify drug (T36-T50 with fifth or sixth character 5)
      > EXCLUDES1 *postvaccination (postimmunization) fever (R50.83)*
   R50.8 Other specified fever
      R50.81 Fever presenting with conditions classified elsewhere
         Code first underlying condition when associated fever is present, such as with:
         leukemia (C91-C95)
         neutropenia (D70.-)
         sickle-cell disease (D57.-)
      R50.82 Postprocedural fever
         > EXCLUDES1 *postprocedural infection (T81.4)*
         > *posttransfusion fever (R50.84)*
         > *postvaccination (postimmunization) fever (R50.83)*
      R50.83 Postvaccination fever
         Postimmunization fever
      R50.84 Febrile nonhemolytic transfusion reaction
         FNHTR
         Posttransfusion fever
   R50.9 Fever, unspecified
      Fever NOS
      Fever of unknown origin [FUO]
      Fever with chills
      Fever with rigors
      Hyperpyrexia NOS
      Persistent fever
      Pyrexia NOS
R51   Headache
      Facial pain NOS
      > EXCLUDES1 *atypical face pain (G50.1)*
      > *migraine and other headache syndromes (G43-G44)*
      > *trigeminal neuralgia (G50.0)*
R52   Pain, unspecified
      Acute pain NOS
      Generalized pain NOS
      Pain NOS

---

❹ 4ᵗʰ character required   ❺ 5ᵗʰ character required   ❻ 6ᵗʰ character required   ❼ 7ᵗʰ character required   Ⓧ Extension 'X' Alert
 EXCLUDES 1 Not coded here   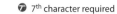 EXCLUDES 2 Not included here   PDx Primary Diagnosis Only   Manifestation Code

EXCLUDES1 acute and chronic pain, not elsewhere classified
(G89.-)
*localized pain, unspecified type - code to pain by
site, such as:*
abdomen pain (R10.-)
back pain (M54.9)
breast pain (N64.4)
chest pain (R07.1-R07.9)
ear pain (H92.0-)
eye pain (H57.1)
headache (R51)
joint pain (M25.5-)
limb pain (M79.6-)
lumbar region pain (M54.5)
pelvic and perineal pain (R10.2)
shoulder pain (M25.51-)
spine pain (M54.-)
throat pain (R07.0)
tongue pain (K14.6)
tooth pain (K08.8)
renal colic (N23)
*pain disorders exclusively related to
psychological factors (F45.41)*

R53 Malaise and fatigue

R53.0 Neoplastic (malignant) related fatigue

Code first associated neoplasm

R53.1 Weakness

Asthenia NOS

EXCLUDES1 age-related weakness (R54)
muscle weakness (M62.8-)
senile asthenia (R54)

R53.2 Functional quadriplegia

Complete immobility due to severe physical disability
or frailty

EXCLUDES1 frailty NOS (R54)
hysterical paralysis (F44.4)
immobility syndrome (M62.3)
neurologic quadriplegia (G82.5-)
quadriplegia (G82.50)

R53.8 Other malaise and fatigue

EXCLUDES1 combat exhaustion and fatigue (F43.0)
congenital debility (P96.9)
*exhaustion and fatigue due to depressive episode
(F32.-)*
*exhaustion and fatigue due to excessive exertion
(T73.3)*
exhaustion and fatigue due to exposure (T73.2)
exhaustion and fatigue due to heat (T67.-)
*exhaustion and fatigue due to pregnancy
(O26.8-)*
*exhaustion and fatigue due to recurrent
depressive episode (F33)*
*exhaustion and fatigue due to senile debility
(R54)*

R53.81 Other malaise

Chronic debility
Debility NOS
General physical deterioration
Malaise NOS
Nervous debility

EXCLUDES1 age-related physical debility (R54)

R53.82 Chronic fatigue, unspecified

Chronic fatigue syndrome NOS

EXCLUDES1 postviral fatigue syndrome (G93.3)

R53.83 Other fatigue

Fatigue NOS
Lack of energy
Lethargy
Tiredness

R54 Age-related physical debility

Frailty
Old age
Senescence
Senile asthenia
Senile debility

EXCLUDES1 age-related cognitive decline (R41.81)
senile psychosis (F03)
senility NOS (R41.81) 🅰

R55 Syncope and collapse

Blackout
Fainting
Vasovagal attack

EXCLUDES1 cardiogenic shock (R57.0)
carotid sinus syncope (G90.01)
heat syncope (T67.1)
neurocirculatory asthenia (F45.8)
neurogenic orthostatic hypotension (G90.3)
orthostatic hypotension (I95.1)
postprocedural shock (T81.1-)
psychogenic syncope (F48.8)
shock NOS (R57.9)
*shock complicating or following abortion or
ectopic or molar pregnancy (O00-O07, O08.3)*
*shock complicating or following labor and
delivery (O75.1)*
Stokes-Adams attack (I45.9)
unconsciousness NOS (R40.2-)

R56 Convulsions, not elsewhere classified

EXCLUDES1 dissociative convulsions and seizures (F44.5)
epileptic convulsions and seizures (G40.-)
newborn convulsions and seizures (P90)

R56.0 Febrile convulsions

R56.00 Simple febrile convulsions

Febrile convulsion NOS
Febrile seizure NOS

R56.01 Complex febrile convulsions

Atypical febrile seizure
Complex febrile seizure
Complicated febrile seizure

EXCLUDES1 status epilepticus (G40.901)

R56.1 Post traumatic seizures

EXCLUDES1 post traumatic epilepsy (G40.-)

R56.9 Unspecified convulsions

Convulsion disorder
Fit NOS
Recurrent convulsions
Seizure(s) (convulsive) NOS

R57 Shock, not elsewhere classified

EXCLUDES1 anaphylactic shock NOS (T78.2)
*anaphylactic reaction or shock due to adverse
food reaction (T78.0-)*
*anaphylactic shock due to adverse effect
of correct drug or medicament properly
administered (T88.6)*
anaphylactic shock due to serum (T80.5-)
anesthetic shock (T88.3)
electric shock (T75.4)
obstetric shock (O75.1)
postprocedural shock (T81.1-)
psychic shock (F43.0)
septic shock (R65.21)
*shock complicating or following ectopic or molar
pregnancy (O00-O07, O08.3)*
shock due to lightning (T75.01)
traumatic shock (T79.4)
toxic shock syndrome (A48.3)

R57.0 Cardiogenic shock

R57.1 Hypovolemic shock

Unspecified Code	Other Specified Code	N Newborn Age: 0	P Pediatric Age: 0-17	M Maternity Age: 12-55
🅰 Adult Age: 15-124	♂ Male	♀ Female	● New Code	▲ Revised Code Title	►◄ Revised Text

R57.8　**Other shock**

R57.9　**Shock, unspecified**

　　Failure of peripheral circulation NOS

R58　**Hemorrhage, not elsewhere classified**

　　Hemorrhage NOS

　　EXCLUDES1　*hemorrhage included with underlying conditions,*
　　　such as:
　　　acute duodenal ulcer with hemorrhage (K26.0)
　　　acute gastritis with bleeding (K29.01)
　　　ulcerative enterocolitis with rectal bleeding
　　　(K51.01)

❹ R59　**Enlarged lymph nodes**

　　INCLUDES　*swollen glands*

　　EXCLUDES1　*lymphadenitis NOS (I88.9)*
　　　acute lymphadenitis (L04.-)
　　　chronic lymphadenitis (I88.1)
　　　mesenteric (acute) (chronic) lymphadenitis (I88.0)

R59.0　Localized **enlarged lymph nodes**

R59.1　Generalized **enlarged lymph nodes**

　　Lymphadenopathy NOS

R59.9　**Enlarged lymph nodes, unspecified**

❹ R60　**Edema, not elsewhere classified**

　　EXCLUDES1　*angioneurotic edema (T78.3)*
　　　ascites (R18.-)
　　　cerebral edema (G93.6)
　　　cerebral edema due to birth injury (P11.0)
　　　edema of larynx (J38.4)
　　　edema of nasopharynx (J39.2)
　　　edema of pharynx (J39.2)
　　　gestational edema (O12.0-)
　　　hereditary edema (Q82.0)
　　　hydrops fetalis NOS (P83.2)
　　　hydrothorax (J94.8)
　　　nutritional edema (E40-E46)
　　　hydrops fetalis NOS (P83.2)
　　　newborn edema (P83.3)
　　　pulmonary edema (J81.-)

R60.0　Localized **edema**

R60.1　Generalized **edema**

R60.9　**Edema, unspecified**

　　Fluid retention NOS

R61　**Generalized hyperhidrosis**

　　Excessive sweating

　　Night sweats

　　Secondary hyperhidrosis

　　Code first , if applicable, menopausal and female
　　climacteric states (N95.1)

　　EXCLUDES1　*focal (primary) (secondary) hyperhidrosis (L74.5-)*
　　　Frey's syndrome (L74.52)
　　　localized (primary) (secondary) hyperhidrosis
　　　(L74.5-)

❹ R62　**Lack of expected normal physiological development in
　　childhood and adults**

　　EXCLUDES1　*delayed puberty (E30.0)*
　　　gonadal dysgenesis (Q99.1)
　　　hypopituitarism (E23.0)

R62.0　**Delayed milestone in childhood**

　　Delayed attainment of expected physiological
　　developmental stage

　　Late talker

　　Late walker　　　　　　　　　　　　　　　　　P

❺ R62.5　Other and unspecified **lack of expected normal
　　physiological development in childhood**

　　EXCLUDES1　*HIV disease resulting in failure to thrive (B20)*
　　　physical retardation due to malnutrition (E45)

R62.50　**Unspecified lack of expected normal
　　physiological development in childhood**

　　Infantilism NOS　　　　　　　　　　　　P

R62.51　**Failure to thrive (child)**

　　Failure to gain weight

　　EXCLUDES1　*failure to thrive in child under 28 days old
　　　(P92.6)*　　　　　　　　　　　　P

R62.52　**Short stature (child)**

　　Lack of growth

　　Physical retardation

　　Short stature NOS

　　EXCLUDES1　*short stature due to endocrine disorder (E34.3)*　P

R62.59　**Other lack of expected normal physiological
　　development in childhood**　　　　　　P

R62.7　**Adult failure to thrive**　　　　　　　　A

❹ R63　**Symptoms and signs concerning food and fluid intake**

　　EXCLUDES1　*bulimia NOS (F50.2)*
　　　eating disorders of nonorganic origin (F50.-)
　　　malnutrition (E40-E46)

R63.0　**Anorexia**

　　Loss of appetite

　　EXCLUDES1　*anorexia nervosa (F50.0-)*
　　　loss of appetite of nonorganic origin (F50.8)

R63.1　**Polydipsia**

　　Excessive thirst

R63.2　**Polyphagia**

　　Excessive eating

　　Hyperalimentation NOS

R63.3　**Feeding difficulties**

　　Feeding problem (elderly) (infant) NOS

　　EXCLUDES1　*feeding problems of newborn (P92.-)*
　　　*infant feeding disorder of nonorganic origin
　　　(F98.2-)*

R63.4　**Abnormal weight loss**

R63.5　**Abnormal weight gain**

　　EXCLUDES1　*excessive weight gain in pregnancy (O26.0-)*
　　　obesity (E66.-)

R63.6　**Underweight**

　　Use additional code to identify body mass index (BMI),
　　if known (Z68.-)

　　EXCLUDES1　*abnormal weight loss (R63.4)*
　　　anorexia nervosa (F50.0-)
　　　malnutrition (E40-E46)

R63.8　**Other symptoms and signs concerning food and fluid
　　intake**

R64　**Cachexia**

　　Wasting syndrome

　　Code first underlying condition, if known

　　EXCLUDES1　*abnormal weight loss (R63.4)*
　　　nutritional marasmus (E41)

❹ R65　**Symptoms and signs specifically associated with systemic
　　inflammation and infection**

❺ R65.1　**Systemic inflammatory response syndrome (SIRS) of**
　　non-infectious origin

　　Code first underlying condition, such as:
　　heatstroke (T67.0)
　　injury and trauma (S00-T88)

　　EXCLUDES1　*sepsis- code to infection
　　　severe sepsis (R65.2)*

R65.10　**Systemic inflammatory response syndrome
　　(SIRS) of non-infectious origin** without acute
　　organ dysfunction

　　Systemic inflammatory response syndrome (SIRS) NOS

R65.11　**Systemic inflammatory response syndrome
　　(SIRS) of non-infectious origin** with acute organ
　　dysfunction

　　Use additional code to identify specific acute organ
　　dysfunction, such as:
　　acute kidney failure (N17.-)
　　acute respiratory failure (J96.0-)

---

❹ 4th character required　　❺ 5th character required　　❻ 6th character required　　❼ 7th character required　　❼ Extension 'X' Alert

EXCLUDES1 Not coded here　　EXCLUDES2 Not included here　　PDX Primary Diagnosis Only　　Manifestation Code

critical illness myopathy (G72.81)
critical illness polyneuropathy (G62.81)
disseminated intravascular coagulopathy [DIC] (D65)
encephalopathy (metabolic) (septic) (G93.41)
hepatic failure (K72.0-)

[5] **R65.2 Severe sepsis**

Infection with associated acute organ dysfunction
Sepsis with acute organ dysfunction
Sepsis with multiple organ dysfunction
Systemic inflammatory response syndrome due to infectious process with acute organ dysfunction
Code first underlying infection, such as:
infection following a procedure (T81.4)
infections following infusion, transfusion and therapeutic injection (T80.2-)
puerperal sepsis (O85)
sepsis following complete or unspecified spontaneous abortion (O03.87)
sepsis following ectopic and molar pregnancy (O08.82)
sepsis following incomplete spontaneous abortion (O03.37)
sepsis following (induced) termination of pregnancy (O04.87)
sepsis NOS (A41.9)
Use additional code to identify specific acute organ dysfunction, such as:
acute kidney failure (N17.-)
acute respiratory failure (J96.0-)
critical illness myopathy (G72.81)
critical illness polyneuropathy (G62.81)
disseminated intravascular coagulopathy [DIC] (D65)
encephalopathy (metabolic) (septic) (G93.41)
hepatic failure (K72.0-)

R65.20 Severe sepsis without septic shock

Severe sepsis NOS

R65.21 Severe sepsis with septic shock

[4] **R68 Other general symptoms and signs**

R68.0 Hypothermia, not associated with low environmental temperature

EXCLUDES1 *hypothermia NOS (accidental) (T68)*
hypothermia due to anesthesia (T88.51)
hypothermia due to low environmental temperature (T68)
newborn hypothermia (P80.-)

[5] **R68.1 Nonspecific symptoms peculiar to infancy**

EXCLUDES1 *colic, infantile (R10.83)*
neonatal cerebral irritability (P91.3)
teething syndrome (K00.7)

R68.11 Excessive crying of infant (baby)

EXCLUDES1 *excessive crying of child, adolescent, or adult (R45.83)* [P]

R68.12 Fussy infant (baby)

Irritable infant [P]

R68.13 Apparent life threatening event in infant (ALTE)

Apparent life threatening event in newborn
Code first confirmed diagnosis, if known
Use additional code(s) for associated signs and symptoms if no confirmed diagnosis established, or if signs and symptoms are not associated routinely with confirmed diagnosis, or provide additional information for cause of ALTE [P]

R68.19 Other nonspecific symptoms peculiar to infancy [P]

R68.2 Dry mouth, unspecified

EXCLUDES1 *dry mouth due to dehydration (E86.0)*
dry mouth due to sicca syndrome [Sjögren] (M35.0-)
salivary gland hyposecretion (K11.7)

R68.3 Clubbing of fingers

Clubbing of nails

EXCLUDES1 *congenital clubfinger (Q68.1)*

[5] **R68.8 Other general symptoms and signs**

R68.81 Early satiety

R68.82 Decreased libido

Decreased sexual desire [A]

R68.83 Chills (without fever)

Chills NOS

EXCLUDES1 *chills with fever (R50.9)*

R68.84 Jaw pain

Mandibular pain
Maxilla pain

EXCLUDES1 *temporomandibular joint arthralgia (M26.62)*

R68.89 Other general symptoms and signs

R69 Illness, unspecified

Unknown and unspecified cases of morbidity

Abnormal findings on examination of blood, without diagnosis (R70-R79)

EXCLUDES1 *abnormalities (of)(on):*
abnormal findings on antenatal screening of mother (O28.-)
coagulation hemorrhagic disorders (D65-D68)
lipids (E78.-)
platelets and thrombocytes (D69.-)
white blood cells classified elsewhere (D70-D72)
diagnostic abnormal findings classified elsewhere - see Alphabetical Index
hemorrhagic and hematological disorders of newborn (P50-P61)

[4] **R70 Elevated erythrocyte sedimentation rate and abnormality of plasma viscosity**

R70.0 Elevated erythrocyte sedimentation rate

R70.1 Abnormal plasma viscosity

[4] **R71 Abnormality of red blood cells**

EXCLUDES1 *anemias (D50-D64)*
anemia of premature infant (P61.2)
benign (familial) polycythemia (D75.0)
congenital anemias (P61.2-P61.4)
newborn anemia due to isoimmunization (P55.-)
polycythemia neonatorum (P61.1)
polycythemia NOS (D75.1)
polycythemia vera (D45)
secondary polycythemia (D75.1)

R71.0 Precipitous drop in hematocrit

Drop (precipitous) in hemoglobin
Drop in hematocrit

R71.8 Other abnormality of red blood cells

Abnormal red-cell morphology NOS
Abnormal red-cell volume NOS
Anisocytosis
Poikilocytosis

[4] **R73 Elevated blood glucose level**

EXCLUDES1 *diabetes mellitus (E08-E13)*
diabetes mellitus in pregnancy, childbirth and the puerperium (O24.-)
neonatal disorders (P70.0-P70.2)
postsurgical hypoinsulinemia (E89.1)

[5] **R73.0 Abnormal glucose**

EXCLUDES1 *abnormal glucose in pregnancy (O99.81-)*
diabetes mellitus (E08-E13)
dysmetabolic syndrome X (E88.81)
gestational diabetes (O24.4-)
glycosuria (R81)
hypoglycemia (E16.2)

R73.01 Impaired fasting glucose

Elevated fasting glucose

Unspecified Code | Other Specified Code | [N] Newborn Age: 0 | [P] Pediatric Age: 0-17 | [M] Maternity Age: 12-55
[A] Adult Age: 15-124 | ♂ Male | ♀ Female | ● New Code | ▲ Revised Code Title | ►◄ Revised Text

R73.02 **Impaired glucose tolerance (oral)**

Elevated glucose tolerance

R73.09 Other abnormal glucose

Abnormal glucose NOS

Abnormal non-fasting glucose tolerance

Latent diabetes

Prediabetes

R73.9 **Hyperglycemia, unspecified**

R74 **Abnormal serum enzyme levels**

R74.0 **Nonspecific elevation of levels of transaminase and lactic acid dehydrogenase [LDH]**

R74.8 Abnormal levels of other serum enzymes

Abnormal level of acid phosphatase

Abnormal level of alkaline phosphatase

Abnormal level of amylase

Abnormal level of lipase [triacylglycerol lipase]

R74.9 **Abnormal serum enzyme level, unspecified**

R75 **Inconclusive laboratory evidence of human immunodeficiency virus [HIV]**

Nonconclusive HIV-test finding in infants

EXCLUDES1 *asymptomatic human immunodeficiency virus [HIV] infection status (Z21)*
human immunodeficiency virus [HIV] disease (B20)

R76 Other **abnormal immunological findings in serum**

R76.0 **Raised antibody titer**

EXCLUDES1 *isoimmunization in pregnancy (O36.0-O36.1)*
isoimmunization affecting newborn (P55.-)

R76.1 **Nonspecific reaction to test for tuberculosis**

R76.11 **Nonspecific reaction to** tuberculin skin test without active tuberculosis

Abnormal result of Mantoux test

PPD positive

Tuberculin (skin test) positive

Tuberculin (skin test) reactor

EXCLUDES1 *nonspecific reaction to cell mediated immunity measurement of gamma interferon antigen response without active tuberculosis (R76.12)*

R76.12 **Nonspecific reaction to** cell mediated immunity measurement of gamma interferon antigen response without active tuberculosis

Nonspecific reaction to QuantiFERON-TB test (QFT) without active tuberculosis

EXCLUDES1 *nonspecific reaction to tuberculin skin test without active tuberculosis (R76.11)*
positive tuberculin skin test (R76.11)

R76.8 Other specified abnormal immunological findings in serum

Raised level of immunoglobulins NOS

R76.9 **Abnormal immunological finding in serum, unspecified**

R77 Other **abnormalities of plasma proteins**

EXCLUDES1 *disorders of plasma-protein metabolism (E88.0)*

R77.0 **Abnormality of** albumin

R77.1 **Abnormality of** globulin

Hyperglobulinemia NOS

R77.2 **Abnormality of** alphafetoprotein

R77.8 Other specified abnormalities of plasma proteins

R77.9 **Abnormality of plasma protein, unspecified**

R78 **Findings of drugs and other substances, not normally found in blood**

Use additional code to identify the any retained foreign body, if applicable (Z18.-)

EXCLUDES1 *mental or behavioral disorders due to psychoactive substance use (F10-F19)*

R78.0 **Finding of** alcohol **in blood**

Use additional external cause code (Y90.-), for detail regarding alcohol level.

R78.1 **Finding of** opiate **drug in blood**

R78.2 **Finding of** cocaine **in blood**

R78.3 **Finding of** hallucinogen **in blood**

R78.4 Finding of other drugs of addictive potential in blood

R78.5 Finding of other psychotropic drug in blood

R78.6 **Finding of** steroid **agent in blood**

R78.7 **Finding of abnormal level of** heavy metals **in blood**

R78.71 **Abnormal** lead **level in blood**

EXCLUDES1 *lead poisoning (T56.0-)*

R78.79 **Finding of abnormal level of** heavy metals **in blood**

R78.8 **Finding of other specified substances, not normally found in blood**

R78.81 **Bacteremia**

EXCLUDES1 *sepsis-code to specified infection (A00-B99)*

R78.89 Finding of other specified substances, not normally found in blood

Finding of abnormal level of lithium in blood

R78.9 **Finding of unspecified substance, not normally found in blood**

R79 Other **abnormal findings of blood chemistry**

Use additional code to identify any retained foreign body, if applicable (Z18.-)

EXCLUDES1 *abnormality of fluid, electrolyte or acid-base balance (E86-E87)*
asymptomatic hyperuricemia (E79.0)
hyperglycemia NOS (R73.9)

hypoglycemia NOS (E16.2)
neonatal hypoglycemia (P70.3-P70.4)
specific findings indicating disorder of amino-acid metabolism (E70-E72)
specific findings indicating disorder of carbohydrate metabolism (E73-E74)
specific findings indicating disorder of lipid metabolism (E75.-)

R79.0 **Abnormal level of** blood mineral

Abnormal blood level of cobalt

Abnormal blood level of copper

Abnormal blood level of iron

Abnormal blood level of magnesium

Abnormal blood level of mineral NEC

Abnormal blood level of zinc

EXCLUDES1 *abnormal level of lithium (R78.89)*
disorders of mineral metabolism (E83.-)
neonatal hypomagnesemia (P71.2)
nutritional mineral deficiency (E58-E61)

R79.1 **Abnormal** coagulation profile

Abnormal or prolonged bleeding time

Abnormal or prolonged coagulation time

Abnormal or prolonged partial thromboplastin time [PTT]

Abnormal or prolonged prothrombin time [PT]

EXCLUDES1 *coagulation defects (D68.-)*

R79.8 Other specified **abnormal findings of blood chemistry**

R79.81 **Abnormal** blood-gas level

R79.82 Elevated C-reactive protein (CRP)

R79.89 Other specified abnormal findings of blood chemistry

R79.9 **Abnormal finding of blood chemistry, unspecified**

---

④ 4th character required ⑤ 5th character required ⑥ 6th character required ⑦ 7th character required ⑦ Extension 'X' Alert

EXCLUDES 1 Not coded here EXCLUDES 2 Not included here PDx Primary Diagnosis Only Manifestation Code

Abnormal findings on examination of urine, without diagnosis (R80-R82)

[EXCLUDES1] *abnormal findings on antenatal screening of mother (O28.-)*
diagnostic abnormal findings classified elsewhere - see Alphabetical Index
specific findings indicating disorder of amino-acid metabolism (E70-E72)
specific findings indicating disorder of carbohydrate metabolism (E73-E74)

[4] **R80 Proteinuria**

[EXCLUDES1] *gestational proteinuria (O12.1-)*

R80.0 Isolated proteinuria
Idiopathic proteinuria
[EXCLUDES1] *isolated proteinuria with specific morphological lesion (N06.-)*

R80.1 Persistent proteinuria, unspecified

R80.2 Orthostatic proteinuria, unspecified
Postural proteinuria

R80.3 Bence Jones proteinuria

R80.8 Other proteinuria

R80.9 Proteinuria, unspecified
Albuminuria NOS

R81 Glycosuria

[EXCLUDES1] *renal glycosuria (E74.8)*

[4] **R82 Other and unspecified abnormal findings in urine**

[INCLUDES] *chromoabnormalities in urine*
Use additional code to identify any retained foreign body, if applicable (Z18.-)
[EXCLUDES2] *hematuria (R31.-)*

R82.0 Chyluria
[EXCLUDES1] *filarial chyluria (B74.-)*

R82.1 Myoglobinuria

R82.2 Biliuria

R82.3 Hemoglobinuria
[EXCLUDES1] *hemoglobinuria due to hemolysis from external causes NEC (D59.6)*
hemoglobinuria due to paroxysmal nocturnal [Marchiafava-Micheli] (D59.5)

R82.4 Acetonuria
Ketonuria

R82.5 Elevated urine levels of drugs, medicaments and biological substances
Elevated urine levels of catecholamines
Elevated urine levels of indoleacetic acid
Elevated urine levels of 17-ketosteroids
Elevated urine levels of steroids

R82.6 Abnormal urine levels of substances chiefly nonmedicinal as to source
Abnormal urine level of heavy metals

R82.7 Abnormal findings on microbiological examination of urine
Positive culture findings of urine
[EXCLUDES1] *colonization status (Z22.-)*

R82.8 Abnormal findings on cytological and histological examination of urine

[5] **R82.9 Other and unspecified abnormal findings in urine**

R82.90 Unspecified abnormal findings in urine

R82.91 Other chromoabnormalities of urine
Chromoconversion (dipstick)
Idiopathic dipstick converts positive for blood with no cellular forms in sediment
[EXCLUDES1] *hemoglobinuria (R82.3)*
myoglobinuria (R82.1)

R82.99 Other abnormal findings in urine
Cells and casts in urine
Crystalluria
Melanuria

Abnormal findings on examination of other body fluids, substances and tissues, without diagnosis (R83-R89)

[EXCLUDES1] *abnormal findings on antenatal screening of mother (O28.-)*
diagnostic abnormal findings classified elsewhere - see Alphabetical Index
[EXCLUDES2] *abnormal findings on examination of blood, without diagnosis (R70-R79)*
abnormal findings on examination of urine, without diagnosis (R80-R82)
abnormal tumor markers (R97.-)

[4] **R83 Abnormal findings in cerebrospinal fluid**

R83.0 Abnormal level of enzymes in cerebrospinal fluid

R83.1 Abnormal level of hormones in cerebrospinal fluid

R83.2 Abnormal level of other drugs, medicaments and biological substances in cerebrospinal fluid

R83.3 Abnormal level of substances chiefly nonmedicinal as to source in cerebrospinal fluid

R83.4 Abnormal immunological findings in cerebrospinal fluid

R83.5 Abnormal microbiological findings in cerebrospinal fluid
Positive culture findings in cerebrospinal fluid
[EXCLUDES1] *colonization status (Z22.-)*

R83.6 Abnormal cytological findings in cerebrospinal fluid

R83.8 Other abnormal findings in cerebrospinal fluid
Abnormal chromosomal findings in cerebrospinal fluid

R83.9 Unspecified abnormal finding in cerebrospinal fluid

[4] **R84 Abnormal findings in specimens from respiratory organs and thorax**

[INCLUDES] *abnormal findings in bronchial washings*
abnormal findings in nasal secretions
abnormal findings in pleural fluid
abnormal findings in sputum
abnormal findings in throat scrapings
[EXCLUDES1] *blood-stained sputum (R04.2)*

R84.0 Abnormal level of enzymes in specimens from respiratory organs and thorax

R84.1 Abnormal level of hormones in specimens from respiratory organs and thorax

R84.2 Abnormal level of other drugs, medicaments and biological substances in specimens from respiratory organs and thorax

R84.3 Abnormal level of substances chiefly nonmedicinal as to source in specimens from respiratory organs and thorax

R84.4 Abnormal immunological findings in specimens from respiratory organs and thorax

R84.5 Abnormal microbiological findings in specimens from respiratory organs and thorax
Positive culture findings in specimens from respiratory organs and thorax
[EXCLUDES1] *colonization status (Z22.-)*

R84.6 Abnormal cytological findings in specimens from respiratory organs and thorax

R84.7 Abnormal histological findings in specimens from respiratory organs and thorax

R84.8 Other abnormal findings in specimens from respiratory organs and thorax
Abnormal chromosomal findings in specimens from respiratory organs and thorax

R84.9 Unspecified abnormal finding in specimens from respiratory organs and thorax

[4] **R85 Abnormal findings in specimens from digestive organs and abdominal cavity**

[INCLUDES] *abnormal findings in peritoneal fluid*
abnormal findings in saliva
[EXCLUDES1] *cloudy peritoneal dialysis effluent (R88.0)*
fecal abnormalities (R19.5)

Unspecified Code | Other Specified Code | [N] Newborn Age: 0 | [P] Pediatric Age: 0-17 | [M] Maternity Age: 12-55
[A] Adult Age: 15-124 | ♂ Male | ♀ Female | ● New Code | ▲ Revised Code Title | ▶◀ Revised Text

R85.0 Abnormal level of enzymes in specimens from digestive organs and abdominal cavity

R85.1 Abnormal level of hormones in specimens from digestive organs and abdominal cavity

R85.2 Abnormal level of other drugs, medicaments and biological substances in specimens from digestive organs and abdominal cavity

R85.3 Abnormal level of substances chiefly nonmedicinal as to source in specimens from digestive organs and abdominal cavity

R85.4 Abnormal immunological findings in specimens from digestive organs and abdominal cavity

R85.5 Abnormal microbiological findings in specimens from digestive organs and abdominal cavity

Positive culture findings in specimens from digestive organs and abdominal cavity

[EXCLUDES1] *colonization status (Z22.-)*

[5] R85.6 Abnormal cytological findings in specimens from digestive organs and abdominal cavity

[6] R85.61 Abnormal cytologic smear of anus

[EXCLUDES1] *abnormal cytological findings in specimens from other digestive organs and abdominal cavity (R85.69)*
carcinoma in situ of anus (histologically confirmed) (D01.3)
anal intraepithelial neoplasia I [AIN I] (K62.82)
anal intraepithelial neoplasia II [AIN II] (K62.82)
anal intraepithelial neoplasia III [AIN III] (D01.3)
dysplasia (mild) (moderate) of anus (histologically confirmed) (K62.82)
severe dysplasia of anus (histologically confirmed) (D01.3)

[EXCLUDES2] *anal high risk human papillomavirus (HPV) DNA test positive (R85.81)*
anal low risk human papillomavirus (HPV) DNA test positive (R85.82)

R85.610 Atypical squamous cells of undetermined significance on cytologic smear of anus (ASC-US)

R85.611 Atypical squamous cells cannot exclude high grade squamous intraepithelial lesion on cytologic smear of anus (ASC-H)

R85.612 Low grade squamous intraepithelial lesion on cytologic smear of anus (LGSIL)

R85.613 High grade squamous intraepithelial lesion on cytologic smear of anus (HGSIL)

R85.614 Cytologic evidence of malignancy on smear of anus

R85.615 Unsatisfactory cytologic smear of anus

Inadequate sample of cytologic smear of anus

R85.616 Satisfactory anal smear but lacking transformation zone

R85.618 Other abnormal cytological findings on specimens from anus

R85.619 Unspecified abnormal cytological findings in specimens from anus

Abnormal anal cytology NOS

Atypical glandular cells of anus NOS

R85.69 Abnormal cytological findings in specimens from other digestive organs and abdominal cavity

R85.7 Abnormal histological findings in specimens from digestive organs and abdominal cavity

[5] R85.8 Other abnormal findings in specimens from digestive organs and abdominal cavity

R85.81 Anal high risk human papillomavirus (HPV) DNA test positive

[EXCLUDES1] *anogenital warts due to human papillomavirus (HPV) (A63.0)*
condyloma acuminatum (A63.0)

R85.82 Anal low risk human papillomavirus (HPV) DNA test positive

Use additional code for associated human papillomavirus (B97.7)

R85.89 Other abnormal findings in specimens from digestive organs and abdominal cavity

Abnormal chromosomal findings in specimens from digestive organs and abdominal cavity

R85.9 Unspecified abnormal finding in specimens from digestive organs and abdominal cavity

[4] R86 Abnormal findings in specimens from male genital organs

[INCLUDES] *abnormal findings in prostatic secretions*
abnormal findings in semen, seminal fluid
abnormal spermatozoa

[EXCLUDES1] *azoospermia (N46.0-)*
oligospermia (N46.1-)

R86.0 Abnormal level of enzymes in specimens from male genital organs ♂

R86.1 Abnormal level of hormones in specimens from male genital organs ♂

R86.2 Abnormal level of other drugs, medicaments and biological substances in specimens from male genital organs ♂

R86.3 Abnormal level of substances chiefly nonmedicinal as to source in specimens from male genital organs ♂

R86.4 Abnormal immunological findings in specimens from male genital organs ♂

R86.5 Abnormal microbiological findings in specimens from male genital organs

Positive culture findings in specimens from male genital organs

[EXCLUDES1] *colonization status (Z22.-)* ♂

R86.6 Abnormal cytological findings in specimens from male genital organs ♂

R86.7 Abnormal histological findings in specimens from male genital organs ♂

R86.8 Other abnormal findings in specimens from male genital organs

Abnormal chromosomal findings in specimens from male genital organs ♂

R86.9 Unspecified abnormal finding in specimens from male genital organs ♂

[4] R87 Abnormal findings in specimens from female genital organs

[INCLUDES] *abnormal findings in secretion and smears from cervix uteri*
abnormal findings in secretion and smears from vagina
abnormal findings in secretion and smears from vulva

R87.0 Abnormal level of enzymes in specimens from female genital organs ♀

R87.1 Abnormal level of hormones in specimens from female genital organs ♀

R87.2 Abnormal level of other drugs, medicaments and biological substances in specimens from female genital organs ♀

R87.3 Abnormal level of substances chiefly nonmedicinal as to source in specimens from female genital organs ♀

R87.4 Abnormal immunological findings in specimens from female genital organs ♀

R87.5 Abnormal microbiological findings in specimens from female genital organs

Positive culture findings in specimens from female genital organs

[EXCLUDES1] *colonization status (Z22.-)* ♀

[5] R87.6 Abnormal cytological findings in specimens from female genital organs

[4] 4th character required [5] 5th character required [6] 6th character required [7] 7th character required [X] Extension 'X' Alert
[EXCLUDES1] Not coded here [EXCLUDES2] Not included here [PDx] Primary Diagnosis Only Manifestation Code

[6] R87.61 **Abnormal cytological findings in specimens from cervix uteri**

[EXCLUDES1] *abnormal cytological findings in specimens from other female genital organs (R87.69)*
abnormal cytological findings in specimens from vagina (R87.62-)
carcinoma in situ of cervix uteri (histologically confirmed) (D06.-)
cervical intraepithelial neoplasia I [CIN I] (N87.0)
cervical intraepithelial neoplasia II [CIN II] (N87.1)
cervical intraepithelial neoplasia III [CIN III] (D06.-)
dysplasia (mild) (moderate) of cervix uteri (histologically confirmed) (N87.-)
severe dysplasia of cervix uteri (histologically confirmed) (D06.-)

[EXCLUDES2] *cervical high risk human papillomavirus (HPV) DNA test positive (R87.810)*
cervical low risk human papillomavirus (HPV) DNA test positive (R87.820)

R87.610 **Atypical squamous cells of undetermined significance on cytologic smear of cervix (ASC-US)** ♀

R87.611 **Atypical squamous cells cannot exclude high grade squamous intraepithelial lesion on cytologic smear of cervix (ASC-H)** ♀

R87.612 **Low grade squamous intraepithelial lesion on cytologic smear of cervix (LGSIL)** ♀

R87.613 **High grade squamous intraepithelial lesion on cytologic smear of cervix (HGSIL)** ♀

R87.614 **Cytologic evidence of malignancy on smear of cervix** ♀

R87.615 **Unsatisfactory cytologic smear of cervix**

Inadequate sample of cytologic smear of cervix ♀

R87.616 **Satisfactory cervical smear but lacking transformation zone** ♀

R87.618 **Other abnormal cytological findings on specimens from cervix uteri** ♀

R87.619 **Unspecified abnormal cytological findings in specimens from cervix uteri**

Abnormal cervical cytology NOS
Abnormal Papanicolaou smear of cervix NOS
Abnormal thin preparation smear of cervix NOS
Atypical endocervial cells of cervix NOS
Atypical endometrial cells of cervix NOS
Atypical glandular cells of cervix NOS ♀

[6] R87.62 **Abnormal cytological findings in specimens from vagina**

Use additional code to identify acquired absence of uterus and cervix, if applicable (Z90.71-)

[EXCLUDES1] *abnormal cytological findings in specimens from cervix uteri (R87.61-)*
abnormal cytological findings in specimens from other female genital organs (R87.69)
carcinoma in situ of vagina (histologically confirmed) (D07.2)
vaginal intraepithelial neoplasia I [VAIN I] (N89.0)
vaginal intraepithelial neoplasia II [VAIN II] (N89.1)
vaginal intraepithelial neoplasia III [VAIN III] (D07.2)
dysplasia (mild) (moderate) of vagina (histologically confirmed) (N89.-)
severe dysplasia of vagina (histologically confirmed) (D07.2)

[EXCLUDES2] *vaginal high risk human papillomavirus (HPV) DNA test positive (R87.811)*
vaginal low risk human papillomavirus (HPV) DNA test positive (R87.821)

R87.620 **Atypical squamous cells of undetermined significance on cytologic smear of vagina (ASC-US)** ♀

R87.621 **Atypical squamous cells cannot exclude high grade squamous intraepithelial lesion on cytologic smear of vagina (ASC-H)** ♀

R87.622 **Low grade squamous intraepithelial lesion on cytologic smear of vagina (LGSIL)** ♀

R87.623 **High grade squamous intraepithelial lesion on cytologic smear of vagina (HGSIL)** ♀

R87.624 **Cytologic evidence of malignancy on smear of vagina** ♀

R87.625 **Unsatisfactory cytologic smear of vagina**

Inadequate sample of cytologic smear of vagina ♀

R87.628 **Other abnormal cytological findings on specimens from vagina** ♀

R87.629 **Unspecified abnormal cytological findings in specimens from vagina**

Abnormal Papanicolaou smear of vagina NOS
Abnormal thin preparation smear of vagina NOS
Abnormal vaginal cytology NOS
Atypical endocervical cells of vagina NOS
Atypical endometrial cells of vagina NOS
Atypical glandular cells of vagina NOS ♀

R87.69 **Abnormal cytological findings in specimens from other female genital organs**

Abnormal cytological findings in specimens from female genital organs NOS

[EXCLUDES1] *dysplasia of vulva (histologically confirmed) (N90.0-N90.3)* ♀

R87.7 **Abnormal histological findings in specimens from female genital organs**

[EXCLUDES1] *carcinoma in situ (histologically confirmed) of female genital organs (D06-D07.3)*
cervical intraepithelial neoplasia I [CIN I] (N87.0)
cervical intraepithelial neoplasia II [CIN II] (N87.1)
cervical intraepithelial neoplasia III [CIN III] (D06.-)
dysplasia (mild) (moderate) of cervix uteri (histologically confirmed) (N87.-)
dysplasia (mild) (moderate) of vagina (histologically confirmed) (N89.-)
vaginal intraepithelial neoplasia I [VAIN I] (N89.0)
vaginal intraepithelial neoplasia II [VAIN II] (N89.1)
vaginal intraepithelial neoplasia III [VAIN III] (D07.2)
severe dysplasia of cervix uteri (histologically confirmed) (D06.-)
severe dysplasia of vagina (histologically confirmed) (D07.2) ♀

[5] R87.8 **Other abnormal findings in specimens from female genital organs**

[6] R87.81 **High risk human papillomavirus (HPV) DNA test positive from female genital organs**

[EXCLUDES1] *anogenital warts due to human papillomavirus (HPV) (A63.0)*
condyloma acuminatum (A63.0)

R87.810 **Cervical high risk human papillomavirus (HPV) DNA test positive** ♀

R87.811 **Vaginal high risk human papillomavirus (HPV) DNA test positive** ♀

[6] R87.82 **Low risk human papillomavirus (HPV) DNA test positive from female genital organs**

Use additional code for associated human papillomavirus (B97.7)

R87.820 **Cervical low risk human papillomavirus (HPV) DNA test positive** ♀

R87.821 **Vaginal low risk human papillomavirus (HPV) DNA test positive** ♀

Unspecified Code | Other Specified Code | [N] Newborn Age: 0 | [P] Pediatric Age: 0-17 | [M] Maternity Age: 12-55 | [A] Adult Age: 15-124 | ♂ Male | ♀ Female | ● New Code | ▲ Revised Code Title | ▶◀ Revised Text

R87.89 Other abnormal findings in specimens from female genital organs

Abnormal chromosomal findings in specimens from female genital organs ♀

R87.9 Unspecified abnormal finding in specimens from female genital organs ♀

④ R88 Abnormal findings in other body fluids and substances

R88.0 Cloudy (hemodialysis) (peritoneal) dialysis effluent

R88.8 Abnormal findings in other body fluids and substances

④ R89 Abnormal findings in specimens from other organs, systems and tissues

INCLUDES abnormal findings in nipple discharge
abnormal findings in synovial fluid
abnormal findings in wound secretions

R89.0 Abnormal level of enzymes in specimens from other organs, systems and tissues

R89.1 Abnormal level of hormones in specimens from other organs, systems and tissues

R89.2 Abnormal level of other drugs, medicaments and biological substances in specimens from other organs, systems and tissues

R89.3 Abnormal level of substances chiefly nonmedicinal as to source in specimens from other organs, systems and tissues

R89.4 Abnormal immunological findings in specimens from other organs, systems and tissues

R89.5 Abnormal microbiological findings in specimens from other organs, systems and tissues

Positive culture findings in specimens from other organs, systems and tissues

EXCLUDES1 colonization status (Z22.-)

R89.6 Abnormal cytological findings in specimens from other organs, systems and tissues

R89.7 Abnormal histological findings in specimens from other organs, systems and tissues

R89.8 Other abnormal findings in specimens from other organs, systems and tissues

Abnormal chromosomal findings in specimens from other organs, systems and tissues

R89.9 Unspecified abnormal finding in specimens from other organs, systems and tissues

Abnormal findings on diagnostic imaging and in function studies, without diagnosis (R90-R94)

INCLUDES nonspecific abnormal findings on diagnostic imaging by computerized axial tomography [CAT scan]
nonspecific abnormal findings on diagnostic imaging by magnetic resonance imaging [MRI][NMR]
nonspecific abnormal findings on diagnostic imaging by positron emission tomography [PET scan]
nonspecific abnormal findings on diagnostic imaging by thermography
nonspecific abnormal findings on diagnostic imaging by ultrasound [echogram]
nonspecific abnormal findings on diagnostic imaging by X-ray examination

EXCLUDES1 abnormal findings on antenatal screening of mother (O28.-)
diagnostic abnormal findings classified elsewhere - see Alphabetical Index

④ R90 Abnormal findings on diagnostic imaging of central nervous system

R90.0 Intracranial space-occupying lesion found on diagnostic imaging of central nervous system

⑤ R90.8 Other abnormal findings on diagnostic imaging of central nervous system

R90.81 Abnormal echoencephalogram

R90.82 White matter disease, unspecified

R90.89 Other abnormal findings on diagnostic imaging of central nervous system

Other cerebrovascular abnormality found on diagnostic imaging of central nervous system

④ R91 Abnormal findings on diagnostic imaging of lung

R91.1 Solitary pulmonary nodule

Coin lesion lung

Solitary pulmonary nodule, subsegmental branch of the bronchial tree

R91.8 Other nonspecific abnormal finding of lung field

Lung mass NOS found on diagnostic imaging of lung

Pulmonary infiltrate NOS

Shadow, lung

④ R92 Abnormal and inconclusive findings on diagnostic imaging of breast

R92.0 Mammographic microcalcification found on diagnostic imaging of breast

EXCLUDES1 mammographic calcification (calculus) found on diagnostic imaging of breast (R92.1)

R92.1 Mammographic calcification found on diagnostic imaging of breast

Mammographic calculus found on diagnostic imaging of breast

R92.2 Inconclusive mammogram

Dense breasts NOS

Inconclusive mammogram NEC

Inconclusive mammography due to dense breasts

Inconclusive mammography NEC

R92.8 Other abnormal and inconclusive findings on diagnostic imaging of breast

④ R93 Abnormal findings on diagnostic imaging of other body structures

R93.0 Abnormal findings on diagnostic imaging of skull and head, not elsewhere classified

EXCLUDES1 intracranial space-occupying lesion found on diagnostic imaging (R90.0)

R93.1 Abnormal findings on diagnostic imaging of heart and coronary circulation

Abnormal echocardiogram NOS

Abnormal heart shadow

R93.2 Abnormal findings on diagnostic imaging of liver and biliary tract

Nonvisualization of gallbladder

R93.3 Abnormal findings on diagnostic imaging of other parts of digestive tract

R93.4 Abnormal findings on diagnostic imaging of urinary organs

Filling defect of bladder found on diagnostic imaging

Filling defect of kidney found on diagnostic imaging

Filling defect of ureter found on diagnostic imaging

EXCLUDES1 hypertrophy of kidney (N28.81)

R93.5 Abnormal findings on diagnostic imaging of other abdominal regions, including retroperitoneum

R93.6 Abnormal findings on diagnostic imaging of limbs

EXCLUDES2 abnormal finding in skin and subcutaneous tissue (R93.8)

R93.7 Abnormal findings on diagnostic imaging of other parts of musculoskeletal system

EXCLUDES2 abnormal findings on diagnostic imaging of skull (R93.0)

---

④ 4th character required ⑤ 5th character required ⑥ 6th character required ⑦ 7th character required ⑨ Extension 'X' Alert

EXCLUDES 1 Not coded here   EXCLUDES 2 Not included here   PDx Primary Diagnosis Only   Manifestation Code

530

ICD-10-CM 2015

R93.8 **Abnormal findings on diagnostic imaging of other specified body structures**

Abnormal finding by radioisotope localization of placenta

Abnormal radiological finding in skin and subcutaneous tissue

Mediastinal shift

R93.9 **Diagnostic imaging inconclusive due to** excess body fat of patient

R94 **Abnormal results of function studies**

> *INCLUDES* abnormal results of radionuclide [radioisotope] uptake studies
> abnormal results of scintigraphy

R94.0 **Abnormal results of function studies of** central nervous system

R94.01 **Abnormal** electroencephalogram **[EEG]**

R94.02 **Abnormal** brain scan

R94.09 **Abnormal results of other function studies of central nervous system**

R94.1 **Abnormal results of function studies of** peripheral nervous system and special senses

R94.11 **Abnormal results of function studies of** eye

R94.110 **Abnormal** electro-oculogram **[EOG]**

R94.111 **Abnormal** electroretinogram **[ERG]**

Abnormal retinal function study

R94.112 **Abnormal** visually evoked potential **[VEP]**

R94.113 **Abnormal** oculomotor **study**

R94.118 **Abnormal results of other function studies of eye**

R94.12 **Abnormal results of function studies of** ear and other special senses

R94.120 **Abnormal** auditory **function study**

R94.121 **Abnormal** vestibular **function study**

R94.128 **Abnormal results of other function studies of ear and other special senses**

R94.13 **Abnormal results of function studies of** peripheral nervous system

R94.130 **Abnormal response to nerve stimulation, unspecified**

R94.131 **Abnormal** electromyogram **[EMG]**

> *EXCLUDES1* electromyogram of eye (R94.113)

R94.138 **Abnormal results of other function studies of peripheral nervous system**

R94.2 **Abnormal results of** pulmonary function **studies**

Reduced ventilatory capacity

Reduced vital capacity

R94.3 **Abnormal results of** cardiovascular function **studies**

R94.30 **Abnormal result of cardiovascular function study, unspecified**

R94.31 **Abnormal** electrocardiogram **[ECG] [EKG]**

> *EXCLUDES1* long QT syndrome (I45.81)

R94.39 **Abnormal result of other cardiovascular function study**

Abnormal electrophysiological intracardiac studies

Abnormal phonocardiogram

Abnormal vectorcardiogram

R94.4 **Abnormal results of** kidney function **studies**

Abnormal renal function test

R94.5 **Abnormal results of** liver function **studies**

R94.6 **Abnormal results of** thyroid function **studies**

R94.7 **Abnormal results of other endocrine function studies**

> *EXCLUDES2* abnormal glucose (R73.0-)

R94.8 **Abnormal results of function studies of** other organs and systems

Abnormal basal metabolic rate [BMR]

Abnormal bladder function test

Abnormal splenic function test

Abnormal tumor markers (R97)

R97 **Abnormal tumor markers**

Elevated tumor associated antigens [TAA]

Elevated tumor specific antigens [TSA]

R97.0 **Elevated carcinoembryonic antigen [CEA]**

R97.1 **Elevated cancer antigen 125 [CA 125]**   ♀

R97.2 **Elevated prostate specific antigen [PSA]**   A ♂

R97.8 **Other abnormal tumor markers**

Ill-defined and unknown cause of mortality (R99)

R99 **Ill-defined and unknown cause of mortality**

Death (unexplained) NOS

Unspecified cause of mortality

Unspecified Code	Other Specified Code	N Newborn Age: 0	P Pediatric Age: 0-17	M Maternity Age: 12-55	
A Adult Age: 15-124	♂ Male	♀ Female	● New Code	▲ Revised Code Title	►◄ Revised Text

This page intentionally left blank

Chapter 19: Injury, Poisoning, and Certain Other Consequences of External Causes (S00-T88)

Chapter Specific Coding Guidelines

a. Application of 7th Characters in Chapter 19

Most categories in chapter 19 have a 7th character requirement for each applicable code. Most categories in this chapter have three 7th character values (with the exception of fractures): A, initial encounter, D, subsequent encounter and S, sequela. Categories for traumatic fractures have additional 7th character values.

7th character "A", initial encounter is used while the patient is receiving active treatment for the condition. Examples of active treatment are: surgical treatment, emergency department encounter, and evaluation and treatment by a new physician.

7th character "D" subsequent encounter is used for encounters after the patient has received active treatment of the condition and is receiving routine care for the condition during the healing or recovery phase. Examples of subsequent care are: cast change or removal, removal of external or internal fixation device, medication adjustment, other aftercare and follow up visits following treatment of the injury or condition.

The aftercare Z codes should not be used for aftercare for conditions such as injuries or poisonings, where 7th characters are provided to identify subsequent care. For example, for aftercare of an injury, assign the acute injury code with the 7th character "D" (subsequent encounter).

7th character "S", sequela, is for use for complications or conditions that arise as a direct result of a condition, such as scar formation after a burn. The scars are sequelae of the burn. When using 7th character "S", it is necessary to use both the injury code that precipitated the sequela and the code for the sequela itself. The "S" is added only to the injury code, not the sequela code. The 7th character "S" identifies the injury responsible for the sequela. The specific type of sequela (e.g. scar) is sequenced first, followed by the injury code.

b. Coding of Injuries

When coding injuries, assign separate codes for each injury unless a combination code is provided, in which case the combination code is assigned. Code T07, Unspecified multiple injuries should not be assigned in the inpatient setting unless information for a more specific code is not available. Traumatic injury codes (S00-T14.9) are not to be used for normal, healing surgical wounds or to identify complications of surgical wounds.

The code for the most serious injury, as determined by the provider and the focus of treatment, is sequenced first.

1) Superficial injuries

Superficial injuries such as abrasions or contusions are not coded when associated with more severe injuries of the same site.

2) Primary injury with damage to nerves/blood vessels

When a primary injury results in minor damage to peripheral nerves or blood vessels, the primary injury is sequenced first with additional code(s) for injuries to nerves and spinal cord (such as category S04), and/or injury to blood vessels (such as category S15). When the primary injury is to the blood vessels or nerves, that injury should be sequenced first.

c. Coding of Traumatic Fractures

The principles of multiple coding of injuries should be followed in coding fractures. Fractures of specified sites are coded individually by site in accordance with both the provisions within categories S02, S12, S22, S32, S42, S49, S52, S59, S62, S72, S79, S82, S89, S92 and the level of detail furnished by medical record content.

A fracture not indicated as open or closed should be coded to closed. A fracture not indicated whether displaced or not displaced should be coded to displaced.

More specific guidelines are as follows:

1) Initial vs. Subsequent Encounter for Fractures

Traumatic fractures are coded using the appropriate 7th character for initial encounter (A, B, C) while the patient is receiving active treatment for the fracture. Examples of active treatment are: surgical treatment, emergency department encounter, and evaluation and treatment by a new physician. The appropriate 7th character for initial encounter should also be assigned for a patient who delayed seeking treatment for the fracture or nonunion.

Fractures are coded using the appropriate 7th character for subsequent care for encounters after the patient has completed active treatment of the fracture and is receiving routine care for the fracture during the healing or recovery phase. Examples of fracture aftercare are: cast change or removal, removal of external or internal fixation device, medication adjustment, and follow-up visits following fracture treatment.

Care for complications of surgical treatment for fracture repairs during the healing or recovery phase should be coded with the appropriate complication codes.

Care of complications of fractures, such as malunion and nonunion, should be reported with the appropriate 7th character for subsequent care with nonunion (K, M, N,) or subsequent care with malunion (P, Q, R).

A code from category M80, not a traumatic fracture code, should be used for any patient with known osteoporosis who suffers a fracture, even if the patient had a minor fall or trauma, if that fall or trauma would not usually break a normal, healthy bone.

See Section I.C.13. Osteoporosis.

The aftercare Z codes should not be used for aftercare for traumatic fractures. For aftercare of a traumatic fracture, assign the acute fracture code with the appropriate 7th character.

2) Multiple fractures sequencing

Multiple fractures are sequenced in accordance with the severity of the fracture.

d. Coding of Burns and Corrosions

The ICD-10-CM makes a distinction between burns and corrosions. The burn codes are for thermal burns, except sunburns, that come from a heat source, such as a fire or hot appliance. The burn codes are also for burns resulting from electricity and radiation. Corrosions are burns due to chemicals. The guidelines are the same for burns and corrosions.

Current burns (T20-T25) are classified by depth, extent and by agent (X code). Burns are classified by depth as first degree (erythema), second degree (blistering), and third degree (full-thickness involvement). Burns of the eye and internal organs (T26-T28) are classified by site, but not by degree.

1) Sequencing of burn and related condition codes

Sequence first the code that reflects the highest degree of burn when more than one burn is present.

a. When the reason for the admission or encounter is for treatment of external multiple burns, sequence first the code that reflects the burn of the highest degree.

b. When a patient has both internal and external burns, the circumstances of admission govern the selection of the principal diagnosis or first-listed diagnosis.

c. When a patient is admitted for burn injuries and other related conditions such as smoke inhalation and/or respiratory failure, the circumstances of admission govern the selection of the principal or first-listed diagnosis.

2) **Burns of the same local site**
Classify burns of the same local site (three-character category level, T20-T28) but of different degrees to the subcategory identifying the highest degree recorded in the diagnosis.

3) **Non-healing burns**
Non-healing burns are coded as acute burns.

Necrosis of burned skin should be coded as a non-healed burn.

4) **Infected Burn**
For any documented infected burn site, use an additional code for the infection.

5) **Assign separate codes for each burn site**
When coding burns, assign separate codes for each burn site. Category T30, Burn and corrosion, body region unspecified is extremely vague and should rarely be used.

6) **Burns and Corrosions Classified According to Extent of Body Surface Involved**
Assign codes from category T31, Burns classified according to extent of body surface involved, or T32, Corrosions classified according to extent of body surface involved, when the site of the burn is not specified or when there is a need for additional data. It is advisable to use category T31 as additional coding when needed to provide data for evaluating burn mortality, such as that needed by burn units. It is also advisable to use category T31 as an additional code for reporting purposes when there is mention of a third-degree burn involving 20 percent or more of the body surface.

Categories T31 and T32 are based on the classic "rule of nines" in estimating body surface involved: head and neck are assigned nine percent, each arm nine percent, each leg 18 percent, the anterior trunk 18 percent, posterior trunk 18 percent, and genitalia one percent. Providers may change these percentage assignments where necessary to accommodate infants and children who have proportionately larger heads than adults, and patients who have large buttocks, thighs, or abdomen that involve burns.

7) **Encounters for treatment of sequela of burns**
Encounters for the treatment of the late effects of burns or corrosions (i.e., scars or joint contractures) should be coded with a burn or corrosion code with the 7th character "S" for sequela.

8) **Sequelae with a late effect code and current burn**
When appropriate, both a code for a current burn or corrosion with 7th character "A" or "D" and a burn or corrosion code with 7th character "S" may be assigned on the same record (when both a current burn and sequelae of an old burn exist). Burns and corrosions do not heal at the same rate and a current healing wound may still exist with sequela of a healed burn or corrosion.

9) **Use of an external cause code with burns and corrosions**
An external cause code should be used with burns and corrosions to identify the source and intent of the burn, as well as the place where it occurred.

e. **Adverse Effects, Poisoning, Underdosing and Toxic Effects**
Codes in categories T36-T65 are combination codes that include the substance that was taken as well as the intent. No additional external cause code is required for poisonings, toxic effects, adverse effects and underdosing codes.

1) **Do not code directly from the Table of Drugs**
Do not code directly from the Table of Drugs and Chemicals. Always refer back to the Tabular List.

2) **Use as many codes as necessary to describe**
Use as many codes as necessary to describe completely all drugs, medicinal or biological substances.

3) **If the same code would describe the causative agent**
If the same code would describe the causative agent for more than one adverse reaction, poisoning, toxic effect or underdosing, assign the code only once.

4) **If two or more drugs, medicinal or biological substances**
If two or more drugs, medicinal or biological substances are reported, code each individually unless a combination code is listed in the Table of Drugs and Chemicals.

5) **The occurrence of drug toxicity is classified in ICD-10-CM as follows:**
(a) **Adverse effect**

When coding an adverse effect of a drug that has been correctly prescribed and properly administered, assign the appropriate code for the nature of the adverse effect followed by the appropriate code for the adverse effect of the drug (T36-T50). The code for the drug should have a 5th or 6th character "5" (for example T36.0X5-) Examples of the nature of an adverse effect are tachycardia, delirium, gastrointestinal hemorrhaging, vomiting, hypokalemia, hepatitis, renal failure, or respiratory failure.

(b) **Poisoning**

When coding a poisoning or reaction to the improper use of a medication (e.g., overdose, wrong substance given or taken in error, wrong route of administration), first assign the appropriate code from categories T36-T50. The poisoning codes have an associated intent as their 5th or 6th character (accidental, intentional self-harm, assault and undetermined. Use additional code(s) for all manifestations of poisonings.

If there is also a diagnosis of abuse or dependence of the substance, the abuse or dependence is assigned as an additional code.

Examples of poisoning include:

(i) Error was made in drug prescription

Errors made in drug prescription or in the administration of the drug by provider, nurse, patient, or other person.

(ii) Overdose of a drug intentionally taken

If an overdose of a drug was intentionally taken or administered and resulted in drug toxicity, it would be coded as a poisoning.

(iii) Nonprescribed drug taken with correctly prescribed and properly administered drug

If a nonprescribed drug or medicinal agent was taken in combination with a correctly prescribed and properly administered drug, any drug toxicity or other reaction resulting from the interaction of the two drugs would be classified as a poisoning.

(iv) Interaction of drug(s) and alcohol

When a reaction results from the interaction of a drug(s) and alcohol, this would be classified as poisoning.

See Section I.C.4. if poisoning is the result of insulin pump malfunctions.

(c) **Underdosing**

Underdosing refers to taking less of a medication than is prescribed by a provider or a manufacturer's instruction. For underdosing, assign the code from categories T36-T50 (fifth or sixth character "6").

Codes for underdosing should never be assigned as principal or first-listed codes. If a patient has a relapse or exacerbation of the medical condition for which the drug is prescribed because of the reduction in dose, then the medical condition itself should be coded.

Noncompliance (Z91.12-, Z91.13-) or complication of care (Y63.6-Y63.9) codes are to be used with an underdosing code to indicate intent, if known.

(d) **Toxic Effects**

When a harmful substance is ingested or comes in contact with a person, this is classified as a toxic effect. The toxic effect codes are in categories T51-T65.

Toxic effect codes have an associated intent: accidental, intentional self-harm, assault and undetermined.

f. **Adult and child abuse, neglect and other maltreatment**
Sequence first the appropriate code from categories T74.- (Adult and child abuse, neglect and other maltreatment, confirmed) or T76.- (Adult and child abuse, neglect and other maltreatment, suspected) for abuse, neglect and other maltreatment, followed by any accompanying mental health or injury code(s).

If the documentation in the medical record states abuse or neglect it is coded as confirmed (T74.-). It is coded as suspected if it is documented as suspected (T76.-).

For cases of confirmed abuse or neglect an external cause code from the assault section (X92-Y08) should be added to identify the cause of any physical injuries. A perpetrator code (Y07) should be added when the perpetrator of the abuse is known. For suspected cases of abuse or neglect, do not report external cause or perpetrator code.

If a suspected case of abuse, neglect or mistreatment is ruled out during an encounter code Z04.71, Encounter for examination and observation following alleged physical adult abuse, ruled out, or code Z04.72, Encounter for examination and observation following alleged child physical abuse, ruled out, should be used, not a code from T76.

If a suspected case of alleged rape or sexual abuse is ruled out during an encounter code Z04.41, Encounter for examination and observation following alleged physical adult abuse, ruled out, or code Z04.42, Encounter for examination and observation following alleged rape or sexual abuse, ruled out, should be used, not a code from T76.

See Section I.C.15. Abuse in a pregnant patient.

g. **Complications of care**
1) **General guidelines for complications of care**
(a) **Documentation of complications of care**

See Section I.B.16. for information on documentation of complications of care.

2) **Pain due to medical devices**
Pain associated with devices, implants or grafts left in a surgical site (for example painful hip prosthesis) is assigned to the appropriate code(s) found in Chapter 19, Injury, poisoning, and certain other consequences of external causes. Specific codes for pain due to medical devices are found in the T code section of the ICD-10-CM. Use additional code(s) from category G89 to identify acute or chronic pain due to presence of the device, implant or graft (G89.18 or G89.28).

3) **Transplant complications**
(a) **Transplant complications other than kidney**

Codes under category T86, Complications of transplanted organs and tissues, are for use for both complications and rejection of transplanted organs. A transplant complication code is only assigned if the complication affects the function of the transplanted organ. Two codes are required to fully describe a transplant complication: the appropriate code from category T86 and a secondary code that identifies the complication.

Pre-existing conditions or conditions that develop after the transplant are not coded as complications unless they affect the function of the transplanted organs.

See I.C.21. for transplant organ removal status

See I.C.2. for malignant neoplasm associated with transplanted organ.

(b) **Kidney transplant complications**

Patients who have undergone kidney transplant may still have some form of chronic kidney disease (CKD) because the kidney transplant may not fully restore kidney function. Code T86.1- should be assigned for documented complications of a kidney transplant, such as transplant failure or rejection or other transplant complication. Code T86.1- should not be assigned for post kidney transplant patients who have chronic kidney (CKD) unless a transplant complication such as transplant failure or rejection is documented. If the documentation is unclear as to whether the patient has a complication of the transplant, query the provider.

Conditions that affect the function of the transplanted kidney, other than CKD, should be assigned a code from subcategory T86.1, Complications of transplanted organ, Kidney, and a secondary code that identifies the complication.

For patients with CKD following a kidney transplant, but who do not have a complication such as failure or rejection, *see section I.C.14. Chronic kidney disease and kidney transplant status.*

4) **Complication codes that include the external cause**
As with certain other T codes, some of the complications of care codes have the external cause included in the code. The code includes the nature of the complication as well as the type of procedure that caused the complication. No external cause code indicating the type of procedure is necessary for these codes.

5) **Complications of care codes within the body system chapters**
Intraoperative and postprocedural complication codes are found within the body system chapters with codes specific to the organs and structures of that body system. These codes should be sequenced first, followed by a code(s) for the specific complication, if applicable.

This page intentionally left blank

Injury, poisoning and certain other consequences of external causes (S00-T88)

NOTES Use secondary code(s) from Chapter 20, External causes of morbidity, to indicate cause of injury. Codes within the T section that include the external cause do not require an additional external cause code

NOTES The chapter uses the S-section for coding different types of injuries related to single body regions and the T-section to cover injuries to unspecified body regions as well as poisoning and certain other consequences of external causes.

Use additional code to identify any retained foreign body, if applicable (Z18.-)

EXCLUDES1 *birth trauma (P10-P15)*
obstetric trauma (O70-O71)

Injuries to the head (S00-S09)

INCLUDES *injuries of ear*
injuries of eye
injuries of face [any part]
injuries of gum
injuries of jaw
injuries of oral cavity
injuries of palate
injuries of periocular area
injuries of scalp
injuries of temporomandibular joint area
injuries of tongue
injuries of tooth

Code also for any associated infection

EXCLUDES2 *burns and corrosions (T20-T32)*
effects of foreign body in ear (T16)
effects of foreign body in larynx (T17.3)
effects of foreign body in mouth NOS (T18.0)
effects of foreign body in nose (T17.0-T17.1)
effects of foreign body in pharynx (T17.2)
effects of foreign body on external eye (T15.-)
frostbite (T33-T34)
insect bite or sting, venomous (T63.4)

● **S00** Superficial injury of head

EXCLUDES1 *diffuse cerebral contusion (S06.2-)*
focal cerebral contusion (S06.3-)
injury of eye and orbit (S05.-)
open wound of head (S01.-)

The appropriate 7th character is to be added to each code from category S00
A = initial encounter
D = subsequent encounter
S = sequela

● **S00.0** Superficial injury of scalp
  S00.00 Unspecified superficial injury of scalp
  S00.01 Abrasion of scalp
  S00.02 Blister (nonthermal) of scalp
  S00.03 Contusion of scalp
    Bruise of scalp
    Hematoma of scalp
  S00.04 External constriction of part of scalp
  S00.05 Superficial foreign body of scalp
    Splinter in the scalp
  S00.06 Insect bite (nonvenomous) of scalp
  S00.07 Other superficial bite of scalp
    EXCLUDES1 *open bite of scalp (S01.05)*
● **S00.1** Contusion of eyelid and periocular area
    Black eye
    EXCLUDES2 *contusion of eyeball and orbital tissues (S05.1)*
  S00.10 Contusion of unspecified eyelid and periocular area
  S00.11 Contusion of right eyelid and periocular area

  S00.12 Contusion of left eyelid and periocular area
● **S00.2** Other and unspecified superficial injuries of eyelid and periocular area
    EXCLUDES2 *superficial injury of conjunctiva and cornea (S05.0-)*
  ● **S00.20** Unspecified superficial injury of eyelid and periocular area
    S00.201 Unspecified superficial injury of right eyelid and periocular area
    S00.202 Unspecified superficial injury of left eyelid and periocular area
    S00.209 Unspecified superficial injury of unspecified eyelid and periocular area
  ● **S00.21** Abrasion of eyelid and periocular area
    S00.211 Abrasion of right eyelid and periocular area
    S00.212 Abrasion of left eyelid and periocular area
    S00.219 Abrasion of unspecified eyelid and periocular area
  ● **S00.22** Blister (nonthermal) of eyelid and periocular area
    S00.221 Blister (nonthermal) of right eyelid and periocular area
    S00.222 Blister (nonthermal) of left eyelid and periocular area
    S00.229 Blister (nonthermal) of unspecified eyelid and periocular area
  ● **S00.24** External constriction of eyelid and periocular area
    S00.241 External constriction of right eyelid and periocular area+
    S00.242 External constriction of left eyelid and periocular area
    S00.249 External constriction of unspecified eyelid and periocular area
  ● **S00.25** Superficial foreign body of eyelid and periocular area
    Splinter of eyelid and periocular area
    EXCLUDES2 *retained foreign body in eyelid (H02.81-)*
    S00.251 Superficial foreign body of right eyelid and periocular area
    S00.252 Superficial foreign body of left eyelid and periocular area
    S00.259 Superficial foreign body of unspecified eyelid and periocular area
  ● **S00.26** Insect bite (nonvenomous) of eyelid and periocular area
    S00.261 Insect bite (nonvenomous) of right eyelid and periocular area
    S00.262 Insect bite (nonvenomous) of left eyelid and periocular area
    S00.269 Insect bite (nonvenomous) of unspecified eyelid and periocular area
  ● **S00.27** Other superficial bite of eyelid and periocular area
    EXCLUDES1 *open bite of eyelid and periocular area (S01.15)*
    S00.271 Other superficial bite of right eyelid and periocular area
    S00.272 Other superficial bite of left eyelid and periocular area
    S00.279 Other superficial bite of unspecified eyelid and periocular area
● **S00.3** Superficial injury of nose
  S00.30 Unspecified superficial injury of nose
  S00.31 Abrasion of nose
  S00.32 Blister (nonthermal) of nose
  S00.33 Contusion of nose
    Bruise of nose
    Hematoma of nose
  S00.34 External constriction of nose

Unspecified Code	Other Specified Code	N Newborn Age: 0	P Pediatric Age: 0-17	M Maternity Age: 12-55	
A Adult Age: 15-124	♂ Male	♀ Female	● New Code	▲ Revised Code Title	►◄ Revised Text

🅗 S00.35 Superficial foreign body of nose
       Splinter in the nose
🅗 S00.36 Insect bite (nonvenomous) of nose
🅗 S00.37 Other superficial bite of nose
       EXCLUDES1 open bite of nose (S01.25)
🅢 S00.4 Superficial injury of ear
    🅖 S00.40 Unspecified superficial injury of ear
        🅗 S00.401 Unspecified superficial injury of right ear
        🅗 S00.402 Unspecified superficial injury of left ear
        🅗 S00.409 Unspecified superficial injury of unspecified ear
    🅖 S00.41 Abrasion of ear
        🅗 S00.411 Abrasion of right ear
        🅗 S00.412 Abrasion of left ear
        🅗 S00.419 Abrasion of unspecified ear
    🅖 S00.42 Blister (nonthermal) of ear
        🅗 S00.421 Blister (nonthermal) of right ear
        🅗 S00.422 Blister (nonthermal) of left ear
        🅗 S00.429 Blister (nonthermal) of unspecified ear
    🅖 S00.43 Contusion of ear
           Bruise of ear
           Hematoma of ear
        🅗 S00.431 Contusion of right ear
        🅗 S00.432 Contusion of left ear
        🅗 S00.439 Contusion of unspecified ear
    🅖 S00.44 External constriction of ear
        🅗 S00.441 External constriction of right ear
        🅗 S00.442 External constriction of left ear
        🅗 S00.449 External constriction of unspecified ear
    🅖 S00.45 Superficial foreign body of ear
           Splinter in the ear
        🅗 S00.451 Superficial foreign body of right ear
        🅗 S00.452 Superficial foreign body of left ear
        🅗 S00.459 Superficial foreign body of unspecified ear
    🅖 S00.46 Insect bite (nonvenomous) of ear
        🅗 S00.461 Insect bite (nonvenomous) of right ear
        🅗 S00.462 Insect bite (nonvenomous) of left ear
        🅗 S00.469 Insect bite (nonvenomous) of unspecified ear
    🅖 S00.47 Other superficial bite of ear
           EXCLUDES1 open bite of ear (S01.35)
        🅗 S00.471 Other superficial bite of right ear
        🅗 S00.472 Other superficial bite of left ear
        🅗 S00.479 Other superficial bite of unspecified ear
🅢 S00.5 Superficial injury of lip and oral cavity
    🅖 S00.50 Unspecified superficial injury of lip and oral cavity
        🅗 S00.501 Unspecified superficial injury of lip
        🅗 S00.502 Unspecified superficial injury of oral cavity
    🅖 S00.51 Abrasion of lip and oral cavity
        🅗 S00.511 Abrasion of lip
        🅗 S00.512 Abrasion of oral cavity
    🅖 S00.52 Blister (nonthermal) of lip and oral cavity
        🅗 S00.521 Blister (nonthermal) of lip
        🅗 S00.522 Blister (nonthermal) of oral cavity
    🅖 S00.53 Contusion of lip and oral cavity
        🅗 S00.531 Contusion of lip
               Bruise of lip
               Hematoma of oral cavity
        🅗 S00.532 Contusion of oral cavity
               Bruise of lip
               Hematoma of oral cavity
    🅖 S00.54 External constriction of lip and oral cavity
        🅗 S00.541 External constriction of lip
        🅗 S00.542 External constriction of oral cavity
    🅖 S00.55 Superficial foreign body of lip and oral cavity

        🅗 S00.551 Superficial foreign body of lip
               Splinter of lip and oral cavity
        🅗 S00.552 Superficial foreign body of oral cavity
               Splinter of lip and oral cavity
    🅖 S00.56 Insect bite (nonvenomous) of lip and oral cavity
        🅗 S00.561 Insect bite (nonvenomous) of lip
        🅗 S00.562 Insect bite (nonvenomous) of oral cavity
    🅖 S00.57 Other superficial bite of lip and oral cavity
        🅗 S00.571 Other superficial bite of lip
               EXCLUDES1 open bite of lip (S01.551)
        🅗 S00.572 Other superficial bite of oral cavity
               EXCLUDES1 open bite of oral cavity (S01.552)
🅢 S00.8 Superficial injury of other parts of head
    🅗 S00.80 Unspecified superficial injury of other part of head
    🅗 S00.81 Abrasion of other part of head
    🅗 S00.82 Blister (nonthermal) of other part of head
    🅗 S00.83 Contusion of other part of head
           Bruise of other part of head
           Hematoma of other part of head
    🅗 S00.84 External constriction of other part of head
    🅗 S00.85 Superficial foreign body of other part of head
           Splinter in other part of head
    🅗 S00.86 Insect bite (nonvenomous) of other part of head
    🅗 S00.87 Other superficial bite of other part of head
           EXCLUDES1 open bite of other part of head (S01.85)
🅢 S00.9 Superficial injury of unspecified part of head
    🅗 S00.90 Unspecified superficial injury of unspecified part of head
    🅗 S00.91 Abrasion of unspecified part of head
    🅗 S00.92 Blister (nonthermal) of unspecified part of head
    🅗 S00.93 Contusion of unspecified part of head
           Bruise of head
           Hematoma of head
    🅗 S00.94 External constriction of unspecified part of head
    🅗 S00.95 Superficial foreign body of unspecified part of head
           Splinter of head
    🅗 S00.96 Insect bite (nonvenomous) of unspecified part of head
    🅗 S00.97 Other superficial bite of unspecified part of head
           EXCLUDES1 open bite of head (S01.95)
🅓 S01 Open wound of head
       Code also any associated:
       injury of cranial nerve (S04.-)
       injury of muscle and tendon of head (S09.1-)
       intracranial injury (S06.-)
       wound infection
       EXCLUDES1 open skull fracture (S02.- with 7th character B)
       EXCLUDES2 injury of eye and orbit (S05.-)
                  traumatic amputation of part of head (S08.-)
       The appropriate 7th character is to be added to each code from category S01
       A = initial encounter
       D = subsequent encounter
       S = sequela
    🅢 S01.0 Open wound of scalp
           EXCLUDES1 avulsion of scalp (S08.0)
        🅗 S01.00 Unspecified open wound of scalp
        🅗 S01.01 Laceration without foreign body of scalp
        🅗 S01.02 Laceration with foreign body of scalp
        🅗 S01.03 Puncture wound without foreign body of scalp
        🅗 S01.04 Puncture wound with foreign body of scalp
        🅗 S01.05 Open bite of scalp
               Bite of scalp NOS
               EXCLUDES1 superficial bite of scalp (S00.06, S00.07-)

🅓 4th character required   🅢 5th character required   🅖 6th character required   🅗 7th character required   🅐 Extension 'X' Alert

EXCLUDES1 Not coded here   EXCLUDES2 Not included here   ᴾᴰˣ Primary Diagnosis Only   Manifestation Code

S01.1 Open wound of eyelid and periocular area

Open wound of eyelid and periocular area with or without involvement of lacrimal passages

S01.10 Unspecified open wound of eyelid and periocular area

S01.101 Unspecified open wound of right eyelid and periocular area

S01.102 Unspecified open wound of left eyelid and periocular area

S01.109 Unspecified open wound of unspecified eyelid and periocular area

S01.11 Laceration without foreign body of eyelid and periocular area

S01.111 Laceration without foreign body of right eyelid and periocular area

S01.112 Laceration without foreign body of left eyelid and periocular area

S01.119 Laceration without foreign body of unspecified eyelid and periocular area

S01.12 Laceration with foreign body of eyelid and periocular area

S01.121 Laceration with foreign body of right eyelid and periocular area

S01.122 Laceration with foreign body of left eyelid and periocular area

S01.129 Laceration with foreign body of unspecified eyelid and periocular area

S01.13 Puncture wound without foreign body of eyelid and periocular area

S01.131 Puncture wound without foreign body of right eyelid and periocular area

S01.132 Puncture wound without foreign body of left eyelid and periocular area

S01.139 Puncture wound without foreign body of unspecified eyelid and periocular area

S01.14 Puncture wound with foreign body of eyelid and periocular area

S01.141 Puncture wound with foreign body of right eyelid and periocular area

S01.142 Puncture wound with foreign body of left eyelid and periocular area

S01.149 Puncture wound with foreign body of unspecified eyelid and periocular area

S01.15 Open bite of eyelid and periocular area

Bite of eyelid and periocular area NOS

EXCLUDES1 superficial bite of eyelid and periocular area (S00.26, S00.27)

S01.151 Open bite of right eyelid and periocular area

S01.152 Open bite of left eyelid and periocular area

S01.159 Open bite of unspecified eyelid and periocular area

S01.2 Open wound of nose

S01.20 Unspecified open wound of nose

S01.21 Laceration without foreign body of nose

S01.22 Laceration with foreign body of nose

S01.23 Puncture wound without foreign body of nose

S01.24 Puncture wound with foreign body of nose

S01.25 Open bite of nose

Bite of nose NOS

EXCLUDES1 superficial bite of nose (S00.36, S00.37)

S01.3 Open wound of ear

S01.30 Unspecified open wound of ear

S01.301 Unspecified open wound of right ear

S01.302 Unspecified open wound of left ear

S01.309 Unspecified open wound of unspecified ear

S01.31 Laceration without foreign body of ear

S01.311 Laceration without foreign body of right ear

S01.312 Laceration without foreign body of left ear

S01.319 Laceration without foreign body of unspecified ear

S01.32 Laceration with foreign body of ear

S01.321 Laceration with foreign body of right ear

S01.322 Laceration with foreign body of left ear

S01.329 Laceration with foreign body of unspecified ear

S01.33 Puncture wound without foreign body of ear

S01.331 Puncture wound without foreign body of right ear

S01.332 Puncture wound without foreign body of left ear

S01.339 Puncture wound without foreign body of unspecified ear

S01.34 Puncture wound with foreign body of ear

S01.341 Puncture wound with foreign body of right ear

S01.342 Puncture wound with foreign body of left ear

S01.349 Puncture wound with foreign body of unspecified ear

S01.35 Open bite of ear

Bite of ear NOS

EXCLUDES1 superficial bite of ear (S00.46, S00.47)

S01.351 Open bite of right ear

S01.352 Open bite of left ear

S01.359 Open bite of unspecified ear

S01.4 Open wound of cheek and temporomandibular area

S01.40 Unspecified open wound of cheek and temporomandibular area

S01.401 Unspecified open wound of right cheek and temporomandibular area

S01.402 Unspecified open wound of left cheek and temporomandibular area

S01.409 Unspecified open wound of unspecified cheek and temporomandibular area

S01.41 Laceration without foreign body of cheek and temporomandibular area

S01.411 Laceration without foreign body of right cheek and temporomandibular area

S01.412 Laceration without foreign body of left cheek and temporomandibular area

S01.419 Laceration without foreign body of unspecified cheek and temporomandibular area

S01.42 Laceration with foreign body of cheek and temporomandibular area

S01.421 Laceration with foreign body of right cheek and temporomandibular area

S01.422 Laceration with foreign body of left cheek and temporomandibular area

S01.429 Laceration with foreign body of unspecified cheek and temporomandibular area

S01.43 Puncture wound without foreign body of cheek and temporomandibular area

S01.431 Puncture wound without foreign body of right cheek and temporomandibular area

S01.432 Puncture wound without foreign body of left cheek and temporomandibular area

S01.439 Puncture wound without foreign body of unspecified cheek and temporomandibular area

S01.44 Puncture wound with foreign body of cheek and temporomandibular area

S01.441 Puncture wound with foreign body of right cheek and temporomandibular area

S01.442 Puncture wound with foreign body of left cheek and temporomandibular area

Unspecified Code	Other Specified Code	N Newborn Age: 0	P Pediatric Age: 0-17	M Maternity Age: 12-55
A Adult Age: 15-124	♂ Male	♀ Female	● New Code	▲ Revised Code Title ►◄ Revised Text

[7th] **S01.449 Puncture wound with foreign body of unspecified cheek and temporomandibular area**

[6th] **S01.45 Open bite of cheek and temporomandibular area**
Bite of cheek and temporomandibular area NOS
[EXCLUDES2] *superficial bite of cheek and temporomandibular area (S00.86, S00.87)*

[7th] **S01.451 Open bite of right cheek and temporomandibular area**

[7th] **S01.452 Open bite of left cheek and temporomandibular area**

[7th] **S01.459 Open bite of unspecified cheek and temporomandibular area**

[5th] **S01.5 Open wound of lip and oral cavity**
[EXCLUDES2] *tooth dislocation (S03.2)*
tooth fracture (S02.5)

[6th] **S01.50 Unspecified open wound of lip and oral cavity**

[7th] **S01.501 Unspecified open wound of lip**

[7th] **S01.502 Unspecified open wound of oral cavity**

[6th] **S01.51 Laceration of lip and oral cavity without foreign body**

[7th] **S01.511 Laceration without foreign body of lip**

[7th] **S01.512 Laceration without foreign body of oral cavity**

[6th] **S01.52 Laceration of lip and oral cavity with foreign body**

[7th] **S01.521 Laceration with foreign body of lip**

[7th] **S01.522 Laceration with foreign body of oral cavity**

[6th] **S01.53 Puncture wound of lip and oral cavity without foreign body**

[7th] **S01.531 Puncture wound without foreign body of lip**

[7th] **S01.532 Puncture wound without foreign body of oral cavity**

[6th] **S01.54 Puncture wound of lip and oral cavity with foreign body**

[7th] **S01.541 Puncture wound with foreign body of lip**

[7th] **S01.542 Puncture wound with foreign body of oral cavity**

[6th] **S01.55 Open bite of lip and oral cavity**

[7th] **S01.551 Open bite of lip**
Bite of lip NOS
[EXCLUDES1] *superficial bite of lip (S00.571)*

[7th] **S01.552 Open bite of oral cavity**
Bite of oral cavity NOS
[EXCLUDES1] *superficial bite of oral cavity (S00.572)*

[5th] **S01.8 Open wound of other parts of head**

[7th] **S01.80 Unspecified open wound of other part of head**

[7th] **S01.81 Laceration without foreign body of other part of head**

[7th] **S01.82 Laceration with foreign body of other part of head**

[7th] **S01.83 Puncture wound without foreign body of other part of head**

[7th] **S01.84 Puncture wound with foreign body of other part of head**

[7th] **S01.85 Open bite of other part of head**
Bite of other part of head NOS
[EXCLUDES1] *superficial bite of other part of head (S00.85)*

[5th] **S01.9 Open wound of unspecified part of head**

[7th] **S01.90 Unspecified open wound of unspecified part of head**

[7th] **S01.91 Laceration without foreign body of unspecified part of head**

[7th] **S01.92 Laceration with foreign body of unspecified part of head**

[7th] **S01.93 Puncture wound without foreign body of unspecified part of head**

[7th] **S01.94 Puncture wound with foreign body of unspecified part of head**

[7th] **S01.95 Open bite of unspecified part of head**
Bite of head NOS
[EXCLUDES1] *superficial bite of head NOS (S00.97)*

[4th] **S02 Fracture of skull and facial bones**
[NOTES] A fracture not indicated as open or closed should be coded to closed
Code also any associated intracranial injury (S06.-)
The appropriate 7th character is to be added to each code from category S02
A = initial encounter for closed fracture
B = initial encounter for open fracture
D = subsequent encounter for fracture with routine healing
G = subsequent encounter for fracture with delayed healing
K = subsequent encounter for fracture with nonunion
S = sequela

[7th] **S02.0 Fracture of vault of skull**
Fracture of frontal bone
Fracture of parietal bone

[5th] **S02.1 Fracture of base of skull**
[EXCLUDES1] *orbit NOS (S02.8)*
[EXCLUDES2] *orbital floor (S02.3-)*

[7th] **S02.10 Unspecified fracture of base of skull**

[6th] **S02.11 Fracture of occiput**

[7th] **S02.110 Type I occipital condyle fracture**

[7th] **S02.111 Type II occipital condyle fracture**

[7th] **S02.112 Type III occipital condyle fracture**

[7th] **S02.113 Unspecified occipital condyle fracture**

[7th] **S02.118 Other fracture of occiput**

[7th] **S02.119 Unspecified fracture of occiput**

[7th] **S02.19 Other fracture of base of skull**
Fracture of anterior fossa of base of skull
Fracture of ethmoid sinus
Fracture of frontal sinus
Fracture of middle fossa of base of skull
Fracture of orbital roof
Fracture of posterior fossa of base of skull
Fracture of sphenoid
Fracture of temporal bone

[7th] **S02.2 Fracture of nasal bones**

[7th] **S02.3 Fracture of orbital floor**
[EXCLUDES1] *orbit NOS (S02.8)*
[EXCLUDES2] *orbital roof (S02.1-)*

[5th] **S02.4 Fracture of malar, maxillary and zygoma bones**
Fracture of superior maxilla
Fracture of upper jaw (bone)
Fracture of zygomatic process of temporal bone

[6th] **S02.40 Fracture of malar, maxillary and zygoma bones, unspecified**

[7th] **S02.400 Malar fracture unspecified**

[7th] **S02.401 Maxillary fracture, unspecified**

[7th] **S02.402 Zygomatic fracture, unspecified**

[6th] **S02.41 LeFort fracture**

[7th] **S02.411 LeFort I fracture**

[7th] **S02.412 LeFort II fracture**

[7th] **S02.413 LeFort III fracture**

[7th] **S02.42 Fracture of alveolus of maxilla**

[7th] **S02.5 Fracture of tooth (traumatic)**
Broken tooth
[EXCLUDES1] *cracked tooth (nontraumatic) (K03.81)*

[5th] **S02.6 Fracture of mandible**
Fracture of lower jaw (bone)

[6th] **S02.60 Fracture of mandible, unspecified**

[4th] 4th character required [5th] 5th character required [6th] 6th character required [7th] 7th character required [7th] Extension 'X' Alert
[EXCLUDES1] Not coded here [EXCLUDES2] Not included here [PDx] Primary Diagnosis Only Manifestation Code

🄬 S02.600 Fracture of unspecified part of body of mandible
🄬 S02.609 Fracture of mandible, unspecified
🄬 S02.61 Fracture of condylar process of mandible
🄬 S02.62 Fracture of subcondylar process of mandible
🄬 S02.63 Fracture of coronoid process of mandible
🄬 S02.64 Fracture of ramus of mandible
🄬 S02.65 Fracture of angle of mandible
🄬 S02.66 Fracture of symphysis of mandible
🄬 S02.67 Fracture of alveolus of mandible
🄬 S02.69 Fracture of mandible of other specified site
🄬 S02.8 Fractures of other specified skull and facial bones
Fracture of orbit NOS
Fracture of palate
EXCLUDES1 fracture of orbital floor (S02.3-)
fracture of orbital roof (S02.1-)
🄻 S02.9 Fracture of unspecified skull and facial bones
🄬 S02.91 Unspecified fracture of skull
🄬 S02.92 Unspecified fracture of facial bones
🄸 S03 Dislocation and sprain of joints and ligaments of head
INCLUDES avulsion of joint (capsule) or ligament of head
laceration of cartilage, joint (capsule) or ligament of head
sprain of cartilage, joint (capsule) or ligament of head
traumatic hemarthrosis of joint or ligament of head
traumatic rupture of joint or ligament of head
traumatic subluxation of joint or ligament of head
traumatic tear of joint or ligament of head
Code also any associated open wound
EXCLUDES2 Strain of muscle or tendon of head (S09.1)
The appropriate 7th character is to be added to each code from category S03
A = initial encounter
D = subsequent encounter
S = sequela
🄬 S03.0 Dislocation of jaw
Dislocation of jaw (cartilage) (meniscus)
Dislocation of mandible
Dislocation of temporomandibular (joint)
🄬 S03.1 Dislocation of septal cartilage of nose
🄬 S03.2 Dislocation of tooth
🄬 S03.4 Sprain of jaw
Sprain of temporomandibular (joint) (ligament)
🄬 S03.8 Sprain of joints and ligaments of other parts of head
🄬 S03.9 Sprain of joints and ligaments of unspecified parts of head

The Cranial Nerves

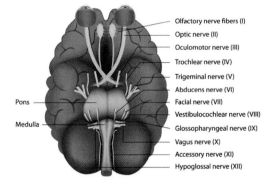

Olfactory nerve fibers (I)
Optic nerve (II)
Oculomotor nerve (III)
Trochlear nerve (IV)
Trigeminal nerve (V)
Abducens nerve (VI)
Facial nerve (VII)
Vestibulocochlear nerve (VIII)
Glossopharyngeal nerve (IX)
Vagus nerve (X)
Accessory nerve (XI)
Hypoglossal nerve (XII)
Pons
Medulla

Figure 15.1 The Cranial Nerves

🄸 S04 Injury of cranial nerve
The selection of side should be based on the side of the body being affected
Code first any associated intracranial injury (S06.-)
Code also any associated:
open wound of head (S01.-)
skull fracture (S02.-)
The appropriate 7th character is to be added to each code from category S04
A = initial encounter
D = subsequent encounter
S = sequela
🄻 S04.0 Injury of optic nerve and pathways
Use additional code to identify any visual field defect or blindness (H53.4-, H54)
🄼 S04.01 Injury of optic nerve
Injury of 2nd cranial nerve
🄬 S04.011 Injury of optic nerve, right eye
🄬 S04.012 Injury of optic nerve, left eye
🄬 S04.019 Injury of optic nerve, unspecified eye
Injury of optic nerve NOS
🄬 S04.02 Injury of optic chiasm
🄼 S04.03 Injury of optic tract and pathways
Injury of optic radiation
🄬 S04.031 Injury of optic tract and pathways, right eye
🄬 S04.032 Injury of optic tract and pathways, left eye
🄬 S04.039 Injury of optic tract and pathways, unspecified eye
Injury of optic tract and pathways NOS
🄼 S04.04 Injury of visual cortex
🄬 S04.041 Injury of visual cortex, right eye
🄬 S04.042 Injury of visual cortex, left eye
🄬 S04.049 Injury of visual cortex, unspecified eye
Injury of visual cortex NOS
🄻 S04.1 Injury of oculomotor nerve
Injury of 3rd cranial nerve
🄬 S04.10 Injury of oculomotor nerve, unspecified side
🄬 S04.11 Injury of oculomotor nerve, right side
🄬 S04.12 Injury of oculomotor nerve, left side
🄻 S04.2 Injury of trochlear nerve
Injury of 4th cranial nerve
🄬 S04.20 Injury of trochlear nerve, unspecified side
🄬 S04.21 Injury of trochlear nerve, right side
🄬 S04.22 Injury of trochlear nerve, left side
🄻 S04.3 Injury of trigeminal nerve
Injury of 5th cranial nerve
🄬 S04.30 Injury of trigeminal nerve, unspecified side
🄬 S04.31 Injury of trigeminal nerve, right side
🄬 S04.32 Injury of trigeminal nerve, left side
🄻 S04.4 Injury of abducent nerve
Injury of 6th cranial nerve
🄬 S04.40 Injury of abducent nerve, unspecified side
🄬 S04.41 Injury of abducent nerve, right side
🄬 S04.42 Injury of abducent nerve, left side
🄻 S04.5 Injury of facial nerve
Injury of 7th cranial nerve
🄬 S04.50 Injury of facial nerve, unspecified side
🄬 S04.51 Injury of facial nerve, right side
🄬 S04.52 Injury of facial nerve, left side
🄻 S04.6 Injury of acoustic nerve
Injury of auditory nerve
Injury of 8th cranial nerve
🄬 S04.60 Injury of acoustic nerve, unspecified side
🄬 S04.61 Injury of acoustic nerve, right side
🄬 S04.62 Injury of acoustic nerve, left side
🄻 S04.7 Injury of accessory nerve
Injury of 11th cranial nerve

Unspecified Code   Other Specified Code   Ⓝ Newborn Age: 0   Ⓟ Pediatric Age: 0-17   Ⓜ Maternity Age: 12-55
Ⓐ Adult Age: 15-124   ♂ Male   ♀ Female   ● New Code   ▲ Revised Code Title   ►◄ Revised Text

⑦ S04.70 Injury of accessory nerve, unspecified side
⑦ S04.71 Injury of accessory nerve, right side
⑦ S04.72 Injury of accessory nerve, left side
⑤ S04.8 Injury of other cranial nerves
⑥ S04.81 Injury of olfactory [1st] nerve
⑦ S04.811 Injury of olfactory [1st] nerve, right side
⑦ S04.812 Injury of olfactory [1st] nerve, left side
⑦ S04.819 Injury of olfactory [1st] nerve, unspecified side
⑥ S04.89 Injury of other cranial nerves
        Injury of vagus [10th] nerve
⑦ S04.891 Injury of other cranial nerves, right side
⑦ S04.892 Injury of other cranial nerves, left side
⑦ S04.899 Injury of other cranial nerves, unspecified side
④ S04.9 Injury of unspecified cranial nerve
④ S05 Injury of eye and orbit

> INCLUDES   open wound of eye and orbit
> EXCLUDES2   2nd cranial [optic] nerve injury (S04.0-)
>   3rd cranial [oculomotor] nerve injury (S04.1-)
>   open wound of eyelid and periocular area
>   (S01.1-)
>   orbital bone fracture (S02.1-, S02.3-, S02.8-)
>   superficial injury of eyelid (S00.1-S00.2)

The appropriate 7th character is to be added to each code from category S05
A = initial encounter
D = subsequent encounter
S = sequela

⑤ S05.0 Injury of conjunctiva and corneal abrasion without foreign body

> EXCLUDES1   foreign body in conjunctival sac (T15.1)
>   foreign body in cornea (T15.0)

⑦ S05.00 Injury of conjunctiva and corneal abrasion without foreign body, unspecified eye
⑦ S05.01 Injury of conjunctiva and corneal abrasion without foreign body, right eye
⑦ S05.02 Injury of conjunctiva and corneal abrasion without foreign body, left eye
⑤ S05.1 Contusion of eyeball and orbital tissues
        Traumatic hyphema

> EXCLUDES2   black eye NOS (S00.1)
>   contusion of eyelid and periocular area (S00.1)

⑦ S05.10 Contusion of eyeball and orbital tissues, unspecified eye
⑦ S05.11 Contusion of eyeball and orbital tissues, right eye
⑦ S05.12 Contusion of eyeball and orbital tissues, left eye
⑤ S05.2 Ocular laceration and rupture with prolapse or loss of intraocular tissue
⑦ S05.20 Ocular laceration and rupture with prolapse or loss of intraocular tissue, unspecified eye
⑦ S05.21 Ocular laceration and rupture with prolapse or loss of intraocular tissue, right eye
⑦ S05.22 Ocular laceration and rupture with prolapse or loss of intraocular tissue, left eye
⑤ S05.3 Ocular laceration without prolapse or loss of intraocular tissue
        Laceration of eye NOS
⑦ S05.30 Ocular laceration without prolapse or loss of intraocular tissue, unspecified eye
⑦ S05.31 Ocular laceration without prolapse or loss of intraocular tissue, right eye
⑦ S05.32 Ocular laceration without prolapse or loss of intraocular tissue, left eye
⑤ S05.4 Penetrating wound of orbit with or without foreign body

> EXCLUDES2   retained (old) foreign body following penetrating wound in orbit (H05.5-)

⑦ S05.40 Penetrating wound of orbit with or without foreign body, unspecified eye
⑦ S05.41 Penetrating wound of orbit with or without foreign body, right eye
⑦ S05.42 Penetrating wound of orbit with or without foreign body, left eye
⑤ S05.5 Penetrating wound with foreign body of eyeball

> EXCLUDES2   retained (old) intraocular foreign body (H44.6-, H44.7)

⑦ S05.50 Penetrating wound with foreign body of unspecified eyeball
⑦ S05.51 Penetrating wound with foreign body of right eyeball
⑦ S05.52 Penetrating wound with foreign body of left eyeball
⑤ S05.6 Penetrating wound without foreign body of eyeball
        Ocular penetration NOS
⑦ S05.60 Penetrating wound without foreign body of unspecified eyeball
⑦ S05.61 Penetrating wound without foreign body of right eyeball
⑦ S05.62 Penetrating wound without foreign body of left eyeball
⑤ S05.7 Avulsion of eye
        Traumatic enucleation
⑦ S05.70 Avulsion of unspecified eye
⑦ S05.71 Avulsion of right eye
⑦ S05.72 Avulsion of left eye
⑤ S05.8 Other injuries of eye and orbit
        Lacrimal duct injury
⑥ S05.8X Other injuries of eye and orbit
⑦ S05.8X1 Other injuries of right eye and orbit
⑦ S05.8X2 Other injuries of left eye and orbit
⑦ S05.8X9 Other injuries of unspecified eye and orbit
⑤ S05.9 Unspecified injury of eye and orbit
        Injury of eye NOS
⑦ S05.90 Unspecified injury of unspecified eye and orbit
⑦ S05.91 Unspecified injury of right eye and orbit
⑦ S05.92 Unspecified injury of left eye and orbit
④ S06 Intracranial injury

> INCLUDES   traumatic brain injury
> Code also any associated:
> open wound of head (S01.-)
> skull fracture (S02.-)
> EXCLUDES1   head injury NOS (S09.90)

The appropriate 7th character is to be added to each code from category S06
A = initial encounter
D = subsequent encounter
S = sequela

⑤ S06.0 Concussion
        Commotio cerebri

> EXCLUDES1   concussion with other intracranial injuries classified in category S06- code to specified intracranial injury

⑥ S06.0X Concussion
⑦ S06.0X0 Concussion without loss of consciousness
⑦ S06.0X1 Concussion with loss of consciousness of 30 minutes or less
⑦ S06.0X2 Concussion with loss of consciousness of 31 minutes to 59 minutes
⑦ S06.0X3 Concussion with loss of consciousness of 1 hour to 5 hours 59 minutes
⑦ S06.0X4 Concussion with loss of consciousness of 6 hours to 24 hours
⑦ S06.0X5 Concussion with loss of consciousness greater than 24 hours with return to pre-existing conscious level

---

④ 4th character required   ⑤ 5th character required   ⑥ 6th character required   ⑦ 7th character required   ⑦ Extension 'X' Alert
EXCLUDES 1 Not coded here   EXCLUDES 2 Not included here   PDx Primary Diagnosis Only   Manifestation Code

[7th] S06.0X6 Concussion with loss of consciousness greater than 24 hours without return to pre-existing conscious level with patient surviving
[7th] S06.0X7 Concussion with loss of consciousness of any duration with death due to brain injury prior to regaining consciousness
[7th] S06.0X8 Concussion with loss of consciousness of any duration with death due to other cause prior to regaining consciousness
[7th] S06.0X9 Concussion with loss of consciousness of unspecified duration
Concussion NOS

[5th] **S06.1 Traumatic cerebral edema**
Diffuse traumatic cerebral edema
Focal traumatic cerebral edema

[6th] **S06.1X Traumatic cerebral edema**
[7th] S06.1X0 Traumatic cerebral edema without loss of consciousness
[7th] S06.1X1 Traumatic cerebral edema with loss of consciousness of 30 minutes or less
[7th] S06.1X2 Traumatic cerebral edema with loss of consciousness of 31 minutes to 59 minutes
[7th] S06.1X3 Traumatic cerebral edema with loss of consciousness of 1 hour to 5 hours 59 minutes
[7th] S06.1X4 Traumatic cerebral edema with loss of consciousness of 6 hours to 24 hours
[7th] S06.1X5 Traumatic cerebral edema with loss of consciousness greater than 24 hours with return to pre-existing conscious level
[7th] S06.1X6 Traumatic cerebral edema with loss of consciousness greater than 24 hours without return to pre-existing conscious level with patient surviving
[7th] S06.1X7 Traumatic cerebral edema with loss of consciousness of any duration with death due to brain injury prior to regaining consciousness
[7th] S06.1X8 Traumatic cerebral edema with loss of consciousness of any duration with death due to other cause prior to regaining consciousness
[7th] S06.1X9 Traumatic cerebral edema with loss of consciousness of unspecified duration
Traumatic cerebral edema NOS

[5th] **S06.2 Diffuse traumatic brain injury**
Diffuse axonal brain injury
[EXCLUDES1] *traumatic diffuse cerebral edema (S06.1X-)*

[6th] **S06.2X Diffuse traumatic brain injury**
[7th] S06.2X0 Diffuse traumatic brain injury without loss of consciousness
[7th] S06.2X1 Diffuse traumatic brain injury with loss of consciousness of 30 minutes or less
[7th] S06.2X2 Diffuse traumatic brain injury with loss of consciousness of 31 minutes to 59 minutes
[7th] S06.2X3 Diffuse traumatic brain injury with loss of consciousness of 1 hour to 5 hours 59 minutes
[7th] S06.2X4 Diffuse traumatic brain injury with loss of consciousness of 6 hours to 24 hours
[7th] S06.2X5 Diffuse traumatic brain injury with loss of consciousness greater than 24 hours with return to pre-existing conscious levels
[7th] S06.2X6 Diffuse traumatic brain injury with loss of consciousness greater than 24 hours without return to pre-existing conscious level with patient surviving
[7th] S06.2X7 Diffuse traumatic brain injury with loss of consciousness of any duration with death due to brain injury prior to regaining consciousness
[7th] S06.2X8 Diffuse traumatic brain injury with loss of consciousness of any duration with death due to other cause prior to regaining consciousness
[7th] S06.2X9 Diffuse traumatic brain injury with loss of consciousness of unspecified duration
Diffuse traumatic brain injury NOS

[5th] **S06.3 Focal traumatic brain injury**
[EXCLUDES1] *any condition classifiable to S06.4-S06.6*
focal cerebral edema (S06.1)

[6th] **S06.30 Unspecified focal traumatic brain injury**
[7th] S06.300 Unspecified focal traumatic brain injury without loss of consciousness
[7th] S06.301 Unspecified focal traumatic brain injury with loss of consciousness of 30 minutes or less
[7th] S06.302 Unspecified focal traumatic brain injury with loss of consciousness of 31 minutes to 59 minutes
[7th] S06.303 Unspecified focal traumatic brain injury with loss of consciousness of 1 hour to 5 hours 59 minutes
[7th] S06.304 Unspecified focal traumatic brain injury with loss of consciousness of 6 hours to 24 hours
[7th] S06.305 Unspecified focal traumatic brain injury with loss of consciousness greater than 24 hours with return to pre-existing conscious level
[7th] S06.306 Unspecified focal traumatic brain injury with loss of consciousness greater than 24 hours without return to pre-existing conscious level with patient surviving
[7th] S06.307 Unspecified focal traumatic brain injury with loss of consciousness of any duration with death due to brain injury prior to regaining consciousness
[7th] S06.308 Unspecified focal traumatic brain injury with loss of consciousness of any duration with death due to other cause prior to regaining consciousness
[7th] S06.309 Unspecified focal traumatic brain injury with loss of consciousness of unspecified duration
Unspecified focal traumatic brain injury NOS

[6th] **S06.31 Contusion and laceration of right cerebrum**
[7th] S06.310 Contusion and laceration of right cerebrum without loss of consciousness
[7th] S06.311 Contusion and laceration of right cerebrum with loss of consciousness of 30 minutes or less
[7th] S06.312 Contusion and laceration of right cerebrum with loss of consciousness of 31 minutes to 59 minutes
[7th] S06.313 Contusion and laceration of right cerebrum with loss of consciousness of 1 hour to 5 hours 59 minutes
[7th] S06.314 Contusion and laceration of right cerebrum with loss of consciousness of 6 hours to 24 hours
[7th] S06.315 Contusion and laceration of right cerebrum with loss of consciousness greater than 24 hours with return to pre-existing conscious level

Unspecified Code | Other Specified Code | [N] Newborn Age: 0 | [P] Pediatric Age: 0-17 | [M] Maternity Age: 12-55
[A] Adult Age: 15-124 | ♂ Male | ♀ Female | ● New Code | ▲ Revised Code Title | ►◄ Revised Text

S06.316 Contusion and laceration of right cerebrum with loss of consciousness greater than 24 hours without return to pre-existing conscious level with patient surviving

S06.317 Contusion and laceration of right cerebrum with loss of consciousness of any duration with death due to brain injury prior to regaining consciousness

S06.318 Contusion and laceration of right cerebrum with loss of consciousness of any duration with death due to other cause prior to regaining consciousness

S06.319 Contusion and laceration of right cerebrum with loss of consciousness of unspecified duration
Contusion and laceration of right cerebrum NOS

S06.32 Contusion and laceration of left cerebrum

S06.320 Contusion and laceration of left cerebrum without loss of consciousness

S06.321 Contusion and laceration of left cerebrum with loss of consciousness of 30 minutes or less

S06.322 Contusion and laceration of left cerebrum with loss of consciousness of 31 minutes to 59 minutes

S06.323 Contusion and laceration of left cerebrum with loss of consciousness of 1 hour to 5 hours 59 minutes

S06.324 Contusion and laceration of left cerebrum with loss of consciousness of 6 hours to 24 hours

S06.325 Contusion and laceration of left cerebrum with loss of consciousness greater than 24 hours with return to pre-existing conscious level

S06.326 Contusion and laceration of left cerebrum with loss of consciousness greater than 24 hours without return to pre-existing conscious level with patient surviving

S06.327 Contusion and laceration of left cerebrum with loss of consciousness of any duration with death due to brain injury prior to regaining consciousness

S06.328 Contusion and laceration of left cerebrum with loss of consciousness of any duration with death due to other cause prior to regaining consciousness

S06.329 Contusion and laceration of left cerebrum with loss of consciousness of unspecified duration
Contusion and laceration of left cerebrum NOS

S06.33 Contusion and laceration of cerebrum, unspecified

S06.330 Contusion and laceration of cerebrum, unspecified, without loss of consciousness

S06.331 Contusion and laceration of cerebrum, unspecified, with loss of consciousness of 30 minutes or less

S06.332 Contusion and laceration of cerebrum, unspecified, with loss of consciousness of 31 minutes to 59 minutes

S06.333 Contusion and laceration of cerebrum, unspecified, with loss of consciousness of 1 hour to 5 hours 59 minutes

S06.334 Contusion and laceration of cerebrum, unspecified, with loss of consciousness of 6 hours to 24 hours

S06.335 Contusion and laceration of cerebrum, unspecified, with loss of consciousness greater than 24 hours with return to pre-existing conscious level

S06.336 Contusion and laceration of cerebrum, unspecified, with loss of consciousness greater than 24 hours without return to pre-existing conscious level with patient surviving

S06.337 Contusion and laceration of cerebrum, unspecified, with loss of consciousness of any duration with death due to brain injury prior to regaining consciousness

S06.338 Contusion and laceration of cerebrum, unspecified, with loss of consciousness of any duration with death due to other cause prior to regaining consciousness

S06.339 Contusion and laceration of cerebrum, unspecified, with loss of consciousness of unspecified duration
Contusion and laceration of cerebrum NOS

S06.34 Traumatic hemorrhage of right cerebrum
Traumatic intracerebral hemorrhage and hematoma of right cerebrum

S06.340 Traumatic hemorrhage of right cerebrum without loss of consciousness

S06.341 Traumatic hemorrhage of right cerebrum with loss of consciousness of 30 minutes or less

S06.342 Traumatic hemorrhage of right cerebrum with loss of consciousness of 31 minutes to 59 minutes

S06.343 Traumatic hemorrhage of right cerebrum with loss of consciousness of 1 hours to 5 hours 59 minutes

S06.344 Traumatic hemorrhage of right cerebrum with loss of consciousness of 6 hours to 24 hours

S06.345 Traumatic hemorrhage of right cerebrum with loss of consciousness greater than 24 hours with return to pre-existing conscious level

S06.346 Traumatic hemorrhage of right cerebrum with loss of consciousness greater than 24 hours without return to pre-existing conscious level with patient surviving

S06.347 Traumatic hemorrhage of right cerebrum with loss of consciousness of any duration with death due to brain injury prior to regaining consciousness

S06.348 Traumatic hemorrhage of right cerebrum with loss of consciousness of any duration with death due to other cause prior to regaining consciousness

S06.349 Traumatic hemorrhage of right cerebrum with loss of consciousness of unspecified duration
Traumatic hemorrhage of right cerebrum NOS

S06.35 Traumatic hemorrhage of left cerebrum
Traumatic intracerebral hemorrhage and hematoma of left cerebrum

S06.350 Traumatic hemorrhage of left cerebrum without loss of consciousness

S06.351 Traumatic hemorrhage of left cerebrum with loss of consciousness of 30 minutes or less

S06.352 Traumatic hemorrhage of left cerebrum with loss of consciousness of 31 minutes to 59 minutes

S06.353 Traumatic hemorrhage of left cerebrum with loss of consciousness of 1 hours to 5 hours 59 minutes

---

4️⃣ 4th character required   5️⃣ 5th character required   6️⃣ 6th character required   7️⃣ 7th character required   Ⓧ Extension 'X' Alert

EXCLUDES 1 Not coded here   **EXCLUDES 2** Not included here   PDx Primary Diagnosis Only   Manifestation Code

S06.354 Traumatic hemorrhage of left cerebrum with loss of consciousness of 6 hours to 24 hours

S06.355 Traumatic hemorrhage of left cerebrum with loss of consciousness greater than 24 hours with return to pre-existing conscious level

S06.356 Traumatic hemorrhage of left cerebrum with loss of consciousness greater than 24 hours without return to pre-existing conscious level with patient surviving

S06.357 Traumatic hemorrhage of left cerebrum with loss of consciousness of any duration with death due to brain injury prior to regaining consciousness

S06.358 Traumatic hemorrhage of left cerebrum with loss of consciousness of any duration with death due to other cause prior to regaining consciousness

S06.359 Traumatic hemorrhage of left cerebrum with loss of consciousness of unspecified duration

Traumatic hemorrhage of left cerebrum NOS

S06.36 Traumatic hemorrhage of cerebrum, unspecified

Traumatic intracerebral hemorrhage and hematoma, unspecified

S06.360 Traumatic hemorrhage of cerebrum, unspecified, without loss of consciousness

S06.361 Traumatic hemorrhage of cerebrum, unspecified, with loss of consciousness of 30 minutes or less

S06.362 Traumatic hemorrhage of cerebrum, unspecified, with loss of consciousness of 31 minutes to 59 minutes

S06.363 Traumatic hemorrhage of cerebrum, unspecified, with loss of consciousness of 1 hours to 5 hours 59 minutes

S06.364 Traumatic hemorrhage of cerebrum, unspecified, with loss of consciousness of 6 hours to 24 hours

S06.365 Traumatic hemorrhage of cerebrum, unspecified, with loss of consciousness greater than 24 hours with return to pre-existing conscious level

S06.366 Traumatic hemorrhage of cerebrum, unspecified, with loss of consciousness greater than 24 hours without return to pre-existing conscious level with patient surviving

S06.367 Traumatic hemorrhage of cerebrum, unspecified, with loss of consciousness of any duration with death due to brain injury prior to regaining consciousness

S06.368 Traumatic hemorrhage of cerebrum, unspecified, with loss of consciousness of any duration with death due to other cause prior to regaining consciousness

S06.369 Traumatic hemorrhage of cerebrum, unspecified, with loss of consciousness of unspecified duration

Traumatic hemorrhage of cerebrum NOS

S06.37 Contusion, laceration, and hemorrhage of cerebellum

S06.370 Contusion, laceration, and hemorrhage of cerebellum without loss of consciousness

S06.371 Contusion, laceration, and hemorrhage of cerebellum with loss of consciousness of 30 minutes or less

S06.372 Contusion, laceration, and hemorrhage of cerebellum with loss of consciousness of 31 minutes to 59 minutes

S06.373 Contusion, laceration, and hemorrhage of cerebellum with loss of consciousness of 1 hour to 5 hours 59 minutes

S06.374 Contusion, laceration, and hemorrhage of cerebellum with loss of consciousness of 6 hours to 24 hours

S06.375 Contusion, laceration, and hemorrhage of cerebellum with loss of consciousness greater than 24 hours with return to pre-existing conscious level

S06.376 Contusion, laceration, and hemorrhage of cerebellum with loss of consciousness greater than 24 hours without return to pre-existing conscious level with patient surviving

S06.377 Contusion, laceration, and hemorrhage of cerebellum with loss of consciousness of any duration with death due to brain injury prior to regaining consciousness

S06.378 Contusion, laceration, and hemorrhage of cerebellum with loss of consciousness of any duration with death due to other cause prior to regaining consciousness

S06.379 Contusion, laceration, and hemorrhage of cerebellum with loss of consciousness of unspecified duration

Contusion, laceration, and hemorrhage of cerebellum NOS

S06.38 Contusion, laceration, and hemorrhage of brainstem

S06.380 Contusion, laceration, and hemorrhage of brainstem without loss of consciousness

S06.381 Contusion, laceration, and hemorrhage of brainstem with loss of consciousness of 30 minutes or less

S06.382 Contusion, laceration, and hemorrhage of brainstem with loss of consciousness of 31 minutes to 59 minutes

S06.383 Contusion, laceration, and hemorrhage of brainstem with loss of consciousness of 1 hour to 5 hours 59 minutes

S06.384 Contusion, laceration, and hemorrhage of brainstem with loss of consciousness of 6 hours to 24 hours

S06.385 Contusion, laceration, and hemorrhage of brainstem with loss of consciousness greater than 24 hours with return to pre-existing conscious level

S06.386 Contusion, laceration, and hemorrhage of brainstem with loss of consciousness greater than 24 hours without return to pre-existing conscious level with patient surviving

S06.387 Contusion, laceration, and hemorrhage of brainstem with loss of consciousness of any duration with death due to brain injury prior to regaining consciousness

S06.388 Contusion, laceration, and hemorrhage of brainstem with loss of consciousness of any duration with death due to other cause prior to regaining consciousness

S06.389 Contusion, laceration, and hemorrhage of brainstem with loss of consciousness of unspecified duration

Contusion, laceration, and hemorrhage of brainstem NOS

| Unspecified Code | Other Specified Code | N Newborn Age: 0 | P Pediatric Age: 0-17 | M Maternity Age: 12-55 |
| A Adult Age: 15-124 | ♂ Male | ♀ Female | ● New Code | ▲ Revised Code Title | ►◄ Revised Text |

5ᵗʰ S06.4 Epidural hemorrhage
  Extradural hemorrhage NOS
  Extradural hemorrhage (traumatic)
  6ᵗʰ S06.4X Epidural hemorrhage
    7ᵗʰ S06.4X0 Epidural hemorrhage without loss of consciousness
    7ᵗʰ S06.4X1 Epidural hemorrhage with loss of consciousness of 30 minutes or less
    7ᵗʰ S06.4X2 Epidural hemorrhage with loss of consciousness of 31 minutes to 59 minutes
    7ᵗʰ S06.4X3 Epidural hemorrhage with loss of consciousness of 1 hour to 5 hours 59 minutes
    7ᵗʰ S06.4X4 Epidural hemorrhage with loss of consciousness of 6 hours to 24 hours
    7ᵗʰ S06.4X5 Epidural hemorrhage with loss of consciousness greater than 24 hours with return to pre-existing conscious level
    7ᵗʰ S06.4X6 Epidural hemorrhage with loss of consciousness greater than 24 hours without return to pre-existing conscious level with patient surviving
    7ᵗʰ S06.4X7 Epidural hemorrhage with loss of consciousness of any duration with death due to brain injury prior to regaining consciousness
    7ᵗʰ S06.4X8 Epidural hemorrhage with loss of consciousness of any duration with death due to other causes prior to regaining consciousness
    7ᵗʰ S06.4X9 Epidural hemorrhage with loss of consciousness of unspecified duration
      Epidural hemorrhage NOS
5ᵗʰ S06.5 Traumatic subdural hemorrhage
  6ᵗʰ S06.5X Traumatic subdural hemorrhage
    7ᵗʰ S06.5X0 Traumatic subdural hemorrhage without loss of consciousness
    7ᵗʰ S06.5X1 Traumatic subdural hemorrhage with loss of consciousness of 30 minutes or less
    7ᵗʰ S06.5X2 Traumatic subdural hemorrhage with loss of consciousness of 31 minutes to 59 minutes
    7ᵗʰ S06.5X3 Traumatic subdural hemorrhage with loss of consciousness of 1 hour to 5 hours 59 minutes
    7ᵗʰ S06.5X4 Traumatic subdural hemorrhage with loss of consciousness of 6 hours to 24 hours
    7ᵗʰ S06.5X5 Traumatic subdural hemorrhage with loss of consciousness greater than 24 hours with return to pre-existing conscious level
    7ᵗʰ S06.5X6 Traumatic subdural hemorrhage with loss of consciousness greater than 24 hours without return to pre-existing conscious level with patient surviving
    7ᵗʰ S06.5X7 Traumatic subdural hemorrhage with loss of consciousness of any duration with death due to brain injury before regaining consciousness
    7ᵗʰ S06.5X8 Traumatic subdural hemorrhage with loss of consciousness of any duration with death due to other cause before regaining consciousness
    7ᵗʰ S06.5X9 Traumatic subdural hemorrhage with loss of consciousness of unspecified duration
      Traumatic subdural hemorrhage NOS
5ᵗʰ S06.6 Traumatic subarachnoid hemorrhage
  6ᵗʰ S06.6X Traumatic subarachnoid hemorrhage
    7ᵗʰ S06.6X0 Traumatic subarachnoid hemorrhage without loss of consciousness
    7ᵗʰ S06.6X1 Traumatic subarachnoid hemorrhage with loss of consciousness of 30 minutes or less

7ᵗʰ S06.6X2 Traumatic subarachnoid hemorrhage with loss of consciousness of 31 minutes to 59 minutes
7ᵗʰ S06.6X3 Traumatic subarachnoid hemorrhage with loss of consciousness of 1 hour to 5 hours 59 minutes
7ᵗʰ S06.6X4 Traumatic subarachnoid hemorrhage with loss of consciousness of 6 hours to 24 hours
7ᵗʰ S06.6X5 Traumatic subarachnoid hemorrhage with loss of consciousness greater than 24 hours with return to pre-existing conscious level
7ᵗʰ S06.6X6 Traumatic subarachnoid hemorrhage with loss of consciousness greater than 24 hours without return to pre-existing conscious level with patient surviving
7ᵗʰ S06.6X7 Traumatic subarachnoid hemorrhage with loss of consciousness of any duration with death due to brain injury prior to regaining consciousness
7ᵗʰ S06.6X8 Traumatic subarachnoid hemorrhage with loss of consciousness of any duration with death due to other cause prior to regaining consciousness
7ᵗʰ S06.6X9 Traumatic subarachnoid hemorrhage with loss of consciousness of unspecified duration
  Traumatic subarachnoid hemorrhage NOS
5ᵗʰ S06.8 Other specified intracranial injuries
  6ᵗʰ S06.81 Injury of right internal carotid artery, intracranial portion, not elsewhere classified
    7ᵗʰ S06.810 Injury of right internal carotid artery, intracranial portion, not elsewhere classified without loss of consciousness
    7ᵗʰ S06.811 Injury of right internal carotid artery, intracranial portion, not elsewhere classified with loss of consciousness of 30 minutes or less
    7ᵗʰ S06.812 Injury of right internal carotid artery, intracranial portion, not elsewhere classified with loss of consciousness of 31 minutes to 59 minutes
    7ᵗʰ S06.813 Injury of right internal carotid artery, intracranial portion, not elsewhere classified with loss of consciousness of 1 hour to 5 hours 59 minutes
    7ᵗʰ S06.814 Injury of right internal carotid artery, intracranial portion, not elsewhere classified with loss of consciousness of 6 hours to 24 hours
    7ᵗʰ S06.815 Injury of right internal carotid artery, intracranial portion, not elsewhere classified with loss of consciousness greater than 24 hours with return to pre-existing conscious level
    7ᵗʰ S06.816 Injury of right internal carotid artery, intracranial portion, not elsewhere classified with loss of consciousness greater than 24 hours without return to pre-existing conscious level with patient surviving
    7ᵗʰ S06.817 Injury of right internal carotid artery, intracranial portion, not elsewhere classified with loss of consciousness of any duration with death due to brain injury prior to regaining consciousness
    7ᵗʰ S06.818 Injury of right internal carotid artery, intracranial portion, not elsewhere classified with loss of consciousness of any duration with death due to other cause prior to regaining consciousness

---

4️⃣ 4ᵗʰ character required   5️⃣ 5ᵗʰ character required   6️⃣ 6ᵗʰ character required   7️⃣ 7ᵗʰ character required   Ⓧ Extension 'X' Alert

EXCLUDES 1 Not coded here   **EXCLUDES 2** Not included here   ᴘᴅx Primary Diagnosis Only   Manifestation Code

[7th] S06.819 Injury of right internal carotid artery, intracranial portion, not elsewhere classified with loss of consciousness of unspecified duration
Injury of right internal carotid artery, intracranial portion, not elsewhere classified NOS

[6th] S06.82 Injury of left internal carotid artery, intracranial portion, not elsewhere classified
[7th] S06.820 Injury of left internal carotid artery, intracranial portion, not elsewhere classified without loss of consciousness
[7th] S06.821 Injury of left internal carotid artery, intracranial portion, not elsewhere classified with loss of consciousness of 30 minutes or less
[7th] S06.822 Injury of left internal carotid artery, intracranial portion, not elsewhere classified with loss of consciousness of 31 minutes to 59 minutes
[7th] S06.823 Injury of left internal carotid artery, intracranial portion, not elsewhere classified with loss of consciousness of 1 hour to 5 hours 59 minutes
[7th] S06.824 Injury of left internal carotid artery, intracranial portion, not elsewhere classified with loss of consciousness of 6 hours to 24 hours
[7th] S06.825 Injury of left internal carotid artery, intracranial portion, not elsewhere classified with loss of consciousness greater than 24 hours with return to pre-existing conscious level
[7th] S06.826 Injury of left internal carotid artery, intracranial portion, not elsewhere classified with loss of consciousness greater than 24 hours without return to pre-existing conscious level with patient surviving
[7th] S06.827 Injury of left internal carotid artery, intracranial portion, not elsewhere classified with loss of consciousness of any duration with death due to brain injury prior to regaining consciousness
[7th] S06.828 Injury of left internal carotid artery, intracranial portion, not elsewhere classified with loss of consciousness of any duration with death due to other cause prior to regaining consciousness
[7th] S06.829 Injury of left internal carotid artery, intracranial portion, not elsewhere classified with loss of consciousness of unspecified duration
Injury of left internal carotid artery, intracranial portion, not elsewhere classified NOS

[6th] S06.89 Other specified intracranial injury
[7th] S06.890 Other specified intracranial injury without loss of consciousness
[7th] S06.891 Other specified intracranial injury with loss of consciousness of 30 minutes or less
[7th] S06.892 Other specified intracranial injury with loss of consciousness of 31 minutes to 59 minutes
[7th] S06.893 Other specified intracranial injury with loss of consciousness of 1 hour to 5 hours 59 minutes
[7th] S06.894 Other specified intracranial injury with loss of consciousness of 6 hours to 24 hours
[7th] S06.895 Other specified intracranial injury with loss of consciousness greater than 24 hours with return to pre-existing conscious level
[7th] S06.896 Other specified intracranial injury with loss of consciousness greater than 24 hours without return to pre-existing conscious level with patient surviving
[7th] S06.897 Other specified intracranial injury with loss of consciousness of any duration with death due to brain injury prior to regaining consciousness
[7th] S06.898 Other specified intracranial injury with loss of consciousness of any duration with death due to other cause prior to regaining consciousness
[7th] S06.899 Other specified intracranial injury with loss of consciousness of unspecified duration

[5th] S06.9 Unspecified intracranial injury
Brain injury NOS
Head injury NOS with loss of consciousness
[EXCLUDES1] *head injury NOS (S09.90)*

[6th] S06.9X Unspecified intracranial injury
[7th] S06.9X0 Unspecified intracranial injury without loss of consciousness
[7th] S06.9X1 Unspecified intracranial injury with loss of consciousness of 30 minutes or less
[7th] S06.9X2 Unspecified intracranial injury with loss of consciousness of 31 minutes to 59 minutes
[7th] S06.9X3 Unspecified intracranial injury with loss of consciousness of 1 hour to 5 hours 59 minutes
[7th] S06.9X4 Unspecified intracranial injury with loss of consciousness of 6 hours to 24 hours
[7th] S06.9X5 Unspecified intracranial injury with loss of consciousness greater than 24 hours with return to pre-existing conscious level
[7th] S06.9X6 Unspecified intracranial injury with loss of consciousness greater than 24 hours without return to pre-existing conscious level with patient surviving
[7th] S06.9X7 Unspecified intracranial injury with loss of consciousness of any duration with death due to brain injury prior to regaining consciousness
[7th] S06.9X8 Unspecified intracranial injury with loss of consciousness of any duration with death due to other cause prior to regaining consciousness
[7th] S06.9X9 Unspecified intracranial injury with loss of consciousness of unspecified duration

[4th] S07 Crushing injury of head
Use additional code for all associated injuries, such as:
intracranial injuries (S06.-)
skull fractures (S02.-)

The appropriate 7th character is to be added to each code from category S07
A = initial encounter
D = subsequent encounter
S = sequela

[7th] S07.0 Crushing injury of face
[7th] S07.1 Crushing injury of skull
[7th] S07.8 Crushing injury of other parts of head
[7th] S07.9 Crushing injury of head, part unspecified

[4th] **S08 Avulsion and traumatic amputation of part of head**
An amputation not identified as partial or complete should be coded to complete
The appropriate 7th character is to be added to each code from category S08
A = initial encounter
D = subsequent encounter
S = sequela

[7th] **S08.0 Avulsion of scalp**
[5th] **S08.1 Traumatic amputation of ear**
[6th] **S08.11 Complete traumatic amputation of ear**
[7th] **S08.111 Complete traumatic amputation of right ear**
[7th] **S08.112 Complete traumatic amputation of left ear**
[7th] **S08.119 Complete traumatic amputation of unspecified ear**
[6th] **S08.12 Partial traumatic amputation of ear**
[7th] **S08.121 Partial traumatic amputation of right ear**
[7th] **S08.122 Partial traumatic amputation of left ear**
[7th] **S08.129 Partial traumatic amputation of unspecified ear**
[5th] **S08.8 Traumatic amputation of other parts of head**
[6th] **S08.81 Traumatic amputation of nose**
[7th] **S08.811 Complete traumatic amputation of nose**
[7th] **S08.812 Partial traumatic amputation of nose**
[7th] **S08.89 Traumatic amputation of other parts of head**

[4th] **S09 Other and unspecified injuries of head**
The appropriate 7th character is to be added to each code from category S09
A = initial encounter
D = subsequent encounter
S = sequela

[7th] **S09.0 Injury of blood vessels of head, not elsewhere classified**
[EXCLUDES1] *injury of cerebral blood vessels (S06.-)*
injury of precerebral blood vessels (S15.-)

[5th] **S09.1 Injury of muscle and tendon of head**
Code also any associated open wound (S01.-)
[EXCLUDES2] *sprain to joints and ligament of head (S03.9)*

[7th] **S09.10 Unspecified injury of muscle and tendon of head**
Injury of muscle and tendon of head NOS
[7th] **S09.11 Strain of muscle and tendon of head**
[7th] **S09.12 Laceration of muscle and tendon of head**
[7th] **S09.19 Other specified injury of muscle and tendon of head**
[5th] **S09.2 Traumatic rupture of ear drum**
[EXCLUDES1] *traumatic rupture of ear drum due to blast injury (S09.31-)*

[7th] **S09.20 Traumatic rupture of unspecified ear drum**
[7th] **S09.21 Traumatic rupture of right ear drum**
[7th] **S09.22 Traumatic rupture of left ear drum**

[5th] **S09.3 Other specified and unspecified injury of middle and inner ear**
[EXCLUDES1] *injury to ear NOS (S09.91-)*
[EXCLUDES2] *injury to external ear (S00.4-, S01.3-, S08.1-)*

[6th] **S09.30 Unspecified injury of middle and inner ear**
[7th] **S09.301 Unspecified injury of right middle and inner ear**
[7th] **S09.302 Unspecified injury of left middle and inner ear**
[7th] **S09.309 Unspecified injury of unspecified middle and inner ear**
[6th] **S09.31 Primary blast injury of ear**
Blast injury of ear NOS
[7th] **S09.311 Primary blast injury of right ear**
[7th] **S09.312 Primary blast injury of left ear**
[7th] **S09.313 Primary blast injury of ear, bilateral**
[7th] **S09.319 Primary blast injury of unspecified ear**
[6th] **S09.39 Other specified injury of middle and inner ear**
Secondary blast injury to ear
[7th] **S09.391 Other specified injury of right middle and inner ear**
[7th] **S09.392 Other specified injury of left middle and inner ear**
[7th] **S09.399 Other specified injury of unspecified middle and inner ear**
[7th] **S09.8 Other specified injuries of head**
[5th] **S09.9 Unspecified injury of face and head**
[7th] **S09.90 Unspecified injury of head**
Head injury NOS
[EXCLUDES1] *brain injury NOS (S06.9-)*
head injury NOS with loss of consciousness (S06.9-)
intracranial injury NOS (S06.9-)
[7th] **S09.91 Unspecified injury of ear**
Injury of ear NOS
[7th] **S09.92 Unspecified injury of nose**
Injury of nose NOS
[7th] **S09.93 Unspecified injury of face**
Injury of face NOS

Injuries to the neck (S10-S19)

[INCLUDES] *injuries of nape*
injuries of supraclavicular region
injuries of throat

[EXCLUDES2] *burns and corrosions (T20-T32)*
effects of foreign body in esophagus (T18.1)
effects of foreign body in larynx (T17.3)
effects of foreign body in pharynx (T17.2)
effects of foreign body in trachea (T17.4)
frostbite (T33-T34)
insect bite or sting, venomous (T63.4)

[4th] **S10 Superficial injury of neck**
The appropriate 7th character is to be added to each code from category S10
A = initial encounter
D = subsequent encounter
S = sequela

[7th] **S10.0 Contusion of throat**
Contusion of cervical esophagus
Contusion of larynx
Contusion of pharynx
Contusion of trachea
[5th] **S10.1 Other and unspecified superficial injuries of throat**
[7th] **S10.10 Unspecified superficial injuries of throat**
[7th] **S10.11 Abrasion of throat**
[7th] **S10.12 Blister (nonthermal) of throat**
[7th] **S10.14 External constriction of part of throat**
[7th] **S10.15 Superficial foreign body of throat**
Splinter in the throat
[7th] **S10.16 Insect bite (nonvenomous) of throat**
[7th] **S10.17 Other superficial bite of throat**
[EXCLUDES1] *open bite of throat (S11.85)*
[5th] **S10.8 Superficial injury of other specified parts of neck**
[7th] **S10.80 Unspecified superficial injury of other specified part of neck**
[7th] **S10.81 Abrasion of other specified part of neck**
[7th] **S10.82 Blister (nonthermal) of other specified part of neck**
[7th] **S10.83 Contusion of other specified part of neck**
[7th] **S10.84 External constriction of other specified part of neck**
[7th] **S10.85 Superficial foreign body of other specified part of neck**
Splinter in other specified part of neck

⑰ S10.86 Insect bite of other specified part of neck
⑰ S10.87 Other superficial bite of other specified part of neck

> EXCLUDES1 *open bite of other specified parts of neck (S11.85)*

5ᵗʰ S10.9 Superficial injury of unspecified part of neck
⑰ S10.90 Unspecified superficial injury of unspecified part of neck
⑰ S10.91 Abrasion of unspecified part of neck
⑰ S10.92 Blister (nonthermal) of unspecified part of neck
⑰ S10.93 Contusion of unspecified part of neck
⑰ S10.94 External constriction of unspecified part of neck
⑰ S10.95 Superficial foreign body of unspecified part of neck
⑰ S10.96 Insect bite of unspecified part of neck
⑰ S10.97 Other superficial bite of unspecified part of neck

④ S11 Open wound of neck

> Code also any associated:
> spinal cord injury (S14.0, S14.1-)
> wound infection
> EXCLUDES2 *open fracture of vertebra (S12.- with 7th character B)*

> **The appropriate 7th character is to be added to each code from category S11**
> **A = initial encounter**
> **D = subsequent encounter**
> **S = sequela**

5ᵗʰ S11.0 Open wound of larynx and trachea
6ᵗʰ S11.01 Open wound of larynx

> EXCLUDES2 *open wound of vocal cord (S11.03)*

⑰ S11.011 Laceration without foreign body of larynx
⑰ S11.012 Laceration with foreign body of larynx
⑰ S11.013 Puncture wound without foreign body of larynx
⑰ S11.014 Puncture wound with foreign body of larynx
⑰ S11.015 Open bite of larynx
> Bite of larynx NOS
⑰ S11.019 Unspecified open wound of larynx
6ᵗʰ S11.02 Open wound of trachea
> Open wound of cervical trachea
> Open wound of trachea NOS
> EXCLUDES2 *open wound of thoracic trachea (S27.5-)*
⑰ S11.021 Laceration without foreign body of trachea
⑰ S11.022 Laceration with foreign body of trachea
⑰ S11.023 Puncture wound without foreign body of trachea
⑰ S11.024 Puncture wound with foreign body of trachea
⑰ S11.025 Open bite of trachea
> Bite of trachea NOS
⑰ S11.029 Unspecified open wound of trachea
6ᵗʰ S11.03 Open wound of vocal cord
⑰ S11.031 Laceration without foreign body of vocal cord
⑰ S11.032 Laceration with foreign body of vocal cord
⑰ S11.033 Puncture wound without foreign body of vocal cord
⑰ S11.034 Puncture wound with foreign body of vocal cord
⑰ S11.035 Open bite of vocal cord
> Bite of vocal cord NOS
⑰ S11.039 Unspecified open wound of vocal cord
5ᵗʰ S11.1 Open wound of thyroid gland
⑰ S11.10 Unspecified open wound of thyroid gland
⑰ S11.11 Laceration without foreign body of thyroid gland
⑰ S11.12 Laceration with foreign body of thyroid gland
⑰ S11.13 Puncture wound without foreign body of thyroid gland
⑰ S11.14 Puncture wound with foreign body of thyroid gland

⑰ S11.15 Open bite of thyroid gland
> Bite of thyroid gland NOS
5ᵗʰ S11.2 Open wound of pharynx and cervical esophagus
> EXCLUDES1 *open wound of esophagus NOS (S27.8-)*
⑰ S11.20 Unspecified open wound of pharynx and cervical esophagus
⑰ S11.21 Laceration without foreign body of pharynx and cervical esophagus
⑰ S11.22 Laceration with foreign body of pharynx and cervical esophagus
⑰ S11.23 Puncture wound without foreign body of pharynx and cervical esophagus
⑰ S11.24 Puncture wound with foreign body of pharynx and cervical esophagus
⑰ S11.25 Open bite of pharynx and cervical esophagus
> Bite of pharynx and cervical esophagus NOS
5ᵗʰ S11.8 Open wound of other specified parts of neck
⑰ S11.80 Unspecified open wound of other specified part of neck
⑰ S11.81 Laceration without foreign body of other specified part of neck
⑰ S11.82 Laceration with foreign body of other specified part of neck
⑰ S11.83 Puncture wound without foreign body of other specified part of neck
⑰ S11.84 Puncture wound with foreign body of other specified part of neck
⑰ S11.85 Open bite of other specified part of neck
> Bite of other specified part of neck NOS
> EXCLUDES1 *superficial bite of other specified part of neck (S10.87)*
⑰ S11.89 Other open wound of other specified part of neck
5ᵗʰ S11.9 Open wound of unspecified part of neck
⑰ S11.90 Unspecified open wound of unspecified part of neck
⑰ S11.91 Laceration without foreign body of unspecified part of neck
⑰ S11.92 Laceration with foreign body of unspecified part of neck
⑰ S11.93 Puncture wound without foreign body of unspecified part of neck
⑰ S11.94 Puncture wound with foreign body of unspecified part of neck
⑰ S11.95 Open bite of unspecified part of neck
> Bite of neck NOS
> EXCLUDES1 *superficial bite of neck (S10.97)*

④ S12 Fracture of cervical vertebra and other parts of neck
> **NOTES** A fracture not indicated as displaced or nondisplaced should be coded to displaced
> A fracture not indicated as open or closed should be coded to closed

> INCLUDES *fracture of cervical neural arch*
> *fracture of cervical spine*
> *fracture of cervical spinous process*
> *fracture of cervical transverse process*
> *fracture of cervical vertebral arch*
> *fracture of neck*

> **The appropriate 7th character is to be added to all codes from subcategories S12.0-S12.6**
> **A = initial encounter for closed fracture**
> **B = initial encounter for open fracture**
> **D = subsequent encounter for fracture with routine healing**
> **G = subsequent encounter for fracture with delayed healing**
> **K = subsequent encounter for fracture with nonunion**
> **S = sequela**

> Code first any associated cervical spinal cord injury (S14.0, S14.1-)

Unspecified Code   Other Specified Code   Ⓝ Newborn Age: 0   Ⓟ Pediatric Age: 0-17   Ⓜ Maternity Age: 12-55
Ⓐ Adult Age: 15-124   ♂ Male   ♀ Female   ● New Code   ▲ Revised Code Title   ►◄ Revised Text

S10.86 - S12

CHAPTER 19: INJURY, POISONING, AND CERTAIN OTHER CONSEQUENCES OF EXTERNAL CAUSES (S00-T88)

S12.0 Fracture of first cervical vertebra
Atlas
- **S12.00** Unspecified fracture of first cervical vertebra
  - **S12.000** Unspecified displaced fracture of first cervical vertebra
  - **S12.001** Unspecified nondisplaced fracture of first cervical vertebra
- **S12.01** Stable burst fracture of first cervical vertebra
- **S12.02** Unstable burst fracture of first cervical vertebra
- **S12.03** Posterior arch fracture of first cervical vertebra
  - **S12.030** Displaced posterior arch fracture of first cervical vertebra
  - **S12.031** Nondisplaced posterior arch fracture of first cervical vertebra
- **S12.04** Lateral mass fracture of first cervical vertebra
  - **S12.040** Displaced lateral mass fracture of first cervical vertebra
  - **S12.041** Nondisplaced lateral mass fracture of first cervical vertebra
- **S12.09** Other fracture of first cervical vertebra
  - **S12.090** Other displaced fracture of first cervical vertebra
  - **S12.091** Other nondisplaced fracture of first cervical vertebra

S12.1 Fracture of second cervical vertebra
Axis
- **S12.10** Unspecified fracture of second cervical vertebra
  - **S12.100** Unspecified displaced fracture of second cervical vertebra
  - **S12.101** Unspecified nondisplaced fracture of second cervical vertebra
- **S12.11** Type II dens fracture
  - **S12.110** Anterior displaced Type II dens fracture
  - **S12.111** Posterior displaced Type II dens fracture
  - **S12.112** Nondisplaced Type II dens fracture
- **S12.12** Other dens fracture
  - **S12.120** Other displaced dens fracture
  - **S12.121** Other nondisplaced dens fracture
- **S12.13** Unspecified traumatic spondylolisthesis of second cervical vertebra
  - **S12.130** Unspecified traumatic displaced spondylolisthesis of second cervical vertebra
  - **S12.131** Unspecified traumatic nondisplaced spondylolisthesis of second cervical vertebra
- **S12.14** Type III traumatic spondylolisthesis of second cervical vertebra
- **S12.15** Other traumatic spondylolisthesis of second cervical vertebra
  - **S12.150** Other traumatic displaced spondylolisthesis of second cervical vertebra
  - **S12.151** Other traumatic nondisplaced spondylolisthesis of second cervical vertebra
- **S12.19** Other fracture of second cervical vertebra
  - **S12.190** Other displaced fracture of second cervical vertebra
  - **S12.191** Other nondisplaced fracture of second cervical vertebra

S12.2 Fracture of third cervical vertebra
- **S12.20** Unspecified fracture of third cervical vertebra
  - **S12.200** Unspecified displaced fracture of third cervical vertebra
  - **S12.201** Unspecified nondisplaced fracture of third cervical vertebra
- **S12.23** Unspecified traumatic spondylolisthesis of third cervical vertebra
  - **S12.230** Unspecified traumatic displaced spondylolisthesis of third cervical vertebra
  - **S12.231** Unspecified traumatic nondisplaced spondylolisthesis of third cervical vertebra
- **S12.24** Type III traumatic spondylolisthesis of third cervical vertebra
- **S12.25** Other traumatic spondylolisthesis of third cervical vertebra
  - **S12.250** Other traumatic displaced spondylolisthesis of third cervical vertebra
  - **S12.251** Other traumatic nondisplaced spondylolisthesis of third cervical vertebra
- **S12.29** Other fracture of third cervical vertebra
  - **S12.290** Other displaced fracture of third cervical vertebra
  - **S12.291** Other nondisplaced fracture of third cervical vertebra

S12.3 Fracture of fourth cervical vertebra
- **S12.30** Unspecified fracture of fourth cervical vertebra
  - **S12.300** Unspecified displaced fracture of fourth cervical vertebra
  - **S12.301** Unspecified nondisplaced fracture of fourth cervical vertebra
- **S12.33** Unspecified traumatic spondylolisthesis of fourth cervical vertebra
  - **S12.330** Unspecified traumatic displaced spondylolisthesis of fourth cervical vertebra
  - **S12.331** Unspecified traumatic nondisplaced spondylolisthesis of fourth cervical vertebra
- **S12.34** Type III traumatic spondylolisthesis of fourth cervical vertebra
- **S12.35** Other traumatic spondylolisthesis of fourth cervical vertebra
  - **S12.350** Other traumatic displaced spondylolisthesis of fourth cervical vertebra
  - **S12.351** Other traumatic nondisplaced spondylolisthesis of fourth cervical vertebra
- **S12.39** Other fracture of fourth cervical vertebra
  - **S12.390** Other displaced fracture of fourth cervical vertebra
  - **S12.391** Other nondisplaced fracture of fourth cervical vertebra

S12.4 Fracture of fifth cervical vertebra
- **S12.40** Unspecified fracture of fifth cervical vertebra
  - **S12.400** Unspecified displaced fracture of fifth cervical vertebra
  - **S12.401** Unspecified nondisplaced fracture of fifth cervical vertebra
- **S12.43** Unspecified traumatic spondylolisthesis of fifth cervical vertebra
  - **S12.430** Unspecified traumatic displaced spondylolisthesis of fifth cervical vertebra
  - **S12.431** Unspecified traumatic nondisplaced spondylolisthesis of fifth cervical vertebra
- **S12.44** Type III traumatic spondylolisthesis of fifth cervical vertebra
- **S12.45** Other traumatic spondylolisthesis of fifth cervical vertebra
  - **S12.450** Other traumatic displaced spondylolisthesis of fifth cervical vertebra
  - **S12.451** Other traumatic nondisplaced spondylolisthesis of fifth cervical vertebra
- **S12.49** Other fracture of fifth cervical vertebra
  - **S12.490** Other displaced fracture of fifth cervical vertebra
  - **S12.491** Other nondisplaced fracture of fifth cervical vertebra

S12.5 Fracture of sixth cervical vertebra
- **S12.50** Unspecified fracture of sixth cervical vertebra

4th character required 5th character required 6th character required 7th character required Extension 'X' Alert

EXCLUDES 1 Not coded here *EXCLUDES 2* Not included here PDx Primary Diagnosis Only Manifestation Code

S12.500 Unspecified displaced fracture of sixth cervical vertebra

S12.501 Unspecified nondisplaced fracture of sixth cervical vertebra

S12.53 Unspecified traumatic spondylolisthesis of sixth cervical vertebra

S12.530 Unspecified traumatic displaced spondylolisthesis of sixth cervical vertebra

S12.531 Unspecified traumatic nondisplaced spondylolisthesis of sixth cervical vertebra

S12.54 Type III traumatic spondylolisthesis of sixth cervical vertebra

S12.55 Other traumatic spondylolisthesis of sixth cervical vertebra

S12.550 Other traumatic displaced spondylolisthesis of sixth cervical vertebra

S12.551 Other traumatic nondisplaced spondylolisthesis of sixth cervical vertebra

S12.59 Other fracture of sixth cervical vertebra

S12.590 Other displaced fracture of sixth cervical vertebra

S12.591 Other nondisplaced fracture of sixth cervical vertebra

S12.6 Fracture of seventh cervical vertebra

S12.60 Unspecified fracture of seventh cervical vertebra

S12.600 Unspecified displaced fracture of seventh cervical vertebra

S12.601 Unspecified nondisplaced fracture of seventh cervical vertebra

S12.63 Unspecified traumatic spondylolisthesis of seventh cervical vertebra

S12.630 Unspecified traumatic displaced spondylolisthesis of seventh cervical vertebra

S12.631 Unspecified traumatic nondisplaced spondylolisthesis of seventh cervical vertebra

S12.64 Type III traumatic spondylolisthesis of seventh cervical vertebra

S12.65 Other traumatic spondylolisthesis of seventh cervical vertebra

S12.650 Other traumatic displaced spondylolisthesis of seventh cervical vertebra

S12.651 Other traumatic nondisplaced spondylolisthesis of seventh cervical vertebra

S12.69 Other fracture of seventh cervical vertebra

S12.690 Other displaced fracture of seventh cervical vertebra

S12.691 Other nondisplaced fracture of seventh cervical vertebra

S12.8 Fracture of other parts of neck
The appropriate 7th character is to be added to code S12.8
A = initial encounter
D = subsequent encounter
S = sequela
Hyoid bone
Larynx
Thyroid cartilage
Trachea

S12.9 Fracture of neck, unspecified
The appropriate 7th character is to be added to code S12.9
A = initial encounter
D = subsequent encounter
S = sequela
Fracture of neck NOS
Fracture of cervical spine NOS
Fracture of cervical vertebra NOS

S13 Dislocation and sprain of joints and ligaments at neck level

INCLUDES
avulsion of joint or ligament at neck level
laceration of cartilage, joint or ligament at neck level
sprain of cartilage, joint or ligament at neck level
traumatic hemarthrosis of joint or ligament at neck level
traumatic rupture of joint or ligament at neck level
traumatic subluxation of joint or ligament at neck level
traumatic tear of joint or ligament at neck level

Code also any associated open wound

EXCLUDES2 strain of muscle or tendon at neck level (S16.1)

The appropriate 7th character is to be added to each code from category S13
A = initial encounter
D = subsequent encounter
S = sequela

S13.0 Traumatic rupture of cervical intervertebral disc

EXCLUDES1 rupture or displacement (nontraumatic) of cervical intervertebral disc NOS (M50.-)

S13.1 Subluxation and dislocation of cervical vertebrae
Code also any associated:
open wound of neck (S11.-)
spinal cord injury (S14.1-)

EXCLUDES2 fracture of cervical vertebrae (S12.0-S12.3-)

S13.10 Subluxation and dislocation of unspecified cervical vertebrae

S13.100 Subluxation of unspecified cervical vertebrae

S13.101 Dislocation of unspecified cervical vertebrae

S13.11 Subluxation and dislocation of C0/C1 cervical vertebrae

Subluxation and dislocation of atlantooccipital joint
Subluxation and dislocation of atloidooccipital joint
Subluxation and dislocation of occipitoatloid joint

S13.110 Subluxation of C0/C1 cervical vertebrae

S13.111 Dislocation of C0/C1 cervical vertebrae

S13.12 Subluxation and dislocation of C1/C2 cervical vertebrae

Subluxation and dislocation of atlantoaxial joint

S13.120 Subluxation of C1/C2 cervical vertebrae

S13.121 Dislocation of C1/C2 cervical vertebrae

S13.13 Subluxation and dislocation of C2/C3 cervical vertebrae

S13.130 Subluxation of C2/C3 cervical vertebrae

S13.131 Dislocation of C2/C3 cervical vertebrae

S13.14 Subluxation and dislocation of C3/C4 cervical vertebrae

S13.140 Subluxation of C3/C4 cervical vertebrae

S13.141 Dislocation of C3/C4 cervical vertebrae

S13.15 Subluxation and dislocation of C4/C5 cervical vertebrae

S13.150 Subluxation of C4/C5 cervical vertebrae

S13.151 Dislocation of C4/C5 cervical vertebrae

S13.16 Subluxation and dislocation of C5/C6 cervical vertebrae

S13.160 Subluxation of C5/C6 cervical vertebrae

Unspecified Code	Other Specified Code	N Newborn Age: 0	P Pediatric Age: 0-17	M Maternity Age: 12-55	
A Adult Age: 15-124	♂ Male	♀ Female	● New Code	▲ Revised Code Title	►◄ Revised Text

7ᵗʰ S13.161 Dislocation of C5/C6 cervical vertebrae

6ᵗʰ S13.17 **Subluxation and dislocation of** C6/C7 **cervical vertebrae**

    7ᵗʰ S13.170 Subluxation of C6/C7 cervical vertebrae

    7ᵗʰ S13.171 Dislocation of C6/C7 cervical vertebrae

6ᵗʰ S13.18 **Subluxation and dislocation of** C7/T1 **cervical vertebrae**

    7ᵗʰ S13.180 Subluxation of C7/T1 cervical vertebrae

    7ᵗʰ S13.181 Dislocation of C7/T1 cervical vertebrae

5ᵗʰ S13.2 **Dislocation of other and unspecified parts of neck**

    6ᵗʰ S13.20 **Dislocation of unspecified parts of neck**

    6ᵗʰ S13.29 **Dislocation of other parts of neck**

5ᵗʰ S13.4 **Sprain of ligaments of cervical spine**

    Sprain of anterior longitudinal (ligament), cervical
    Sprain of atlanto-axial (joints)
    Sprain of atlanto-occipital (joints)
    Whiplash injury of cervical spine

5ᵗʰ S13.5 **Sprain of thyroid region**

    Sprain of cricoarytenoid (joint) (ligament)
    Sprain of cricothyroid (joint) (ligament)
    Sprain of thyroid cartilage

7ᵗʰ S13.8 **Sprain of joints and ligaments of other parts of neck**

7ᵗʰ S13.9 **Sprain of joints and ligaments of unspecified parts of neck**

4ᵗʰ S14 **Injury of nerves and spinal cord at neck level**

NOTES   Code to highest level of cervical cord injury
    Code also any associated:
    fracture of cervical vertebra (S12.0--S12.6.-)
    open wound of neck (S11.-)
    transient paralysis (R29.5)

    The appropriate 7th character is to be added to each code from category S14
    A = initial encounter
    D = subsequent encounter
    S = sequela

7ᵗʰ S14.0 **Concussion and edema of cervical spinal cord**

5ᵗʰ S14.1 **Other and unspecified injuries of cervical spinal cord**

    6ᵗʰ S14.10 Unspecified injury of cervical spinal cord

       7ᵗʰ S14.101 **Unspecified injury at** C1 **level of cervical spinal cord**

       7ᵗʰ S14.102 **Unspecified injury at** C2 **level of cervical spinal cord**

       7ᵗʰ S14.103 **Unspecified injury at** C3 **level of cervical spinal cord**

       7ᵗʰ S14.104 **Unspecified injury at** C4 **level of cervical spinal cord**

       7ᵗʰ S14.105 **Unspecified injury at** C5 **level of cervical spinal cord**

       7ᵗʰ S14.106 **Unspecified injury at** C6 **level of cervical spinal cord**

       7ᵗʰ S14.107 **Unspecified injury at** C7 **level of cervical spinal cord**

       7ᵗʰ S14.108 **Unspecified injury at** C8 **level of cervical spinal cord**

       7ᵗʰ S14.109 **Unspecified injury at** unspecified **level of cervical spinal cord**

          Injury of cervical spinal cord NOS

    6ᵗʰ S14.11 Complete lesion of cervical spinal cord

       7ᵗʰ S14.111 **Complete lesion at** C1 **level of cervical spinal cord**

       7ᵗʰ S14.112 **Complete lesion at** C2 **level of cervical spinal cord**

       7ᵗʰ S14.113 **Complete lesion at** C3 **level of cervical spinal cord**

       7ᵗʰ S14.114 **Complete lesion at** C4 **level of cervical spinal cord**

       7ᵗʰ S14.115 **Complete lesion at** C5 **level of cervical spinal cord**

7ᵗʰ S14.116 **Complete lesion at** C6 **level of cervical spinal cord**

7ᵗʰ S14.117 **Complete lesion at** C7 **level of cervical spinal cord**

7ᵗʰ S14.118 **Complete lesion at** C8 **level of cervical spinal cord**

7ᵗʰ S14.119 **Complete lesion at unspecified level of cervical spinal cord**

6ᵗʰ S14.12 Central cord syndrome of cervical spinal cord

    7ᵗʰ S14.121 **Central cord syndrome at** C1 **level of cervical spinal cord**

    7ᵗʰ S14.122 **Central cord syndrome at** C2 **level of cervical spinal cord**

    7ᵗʰ S14.123 **Central cord syndrome at** C3 **level of cervical spinal cord**

    7ᵗʰ S14.124 **Central cord syndrome at** C4 **level of cervical spinal cord**

    7ᵗʰ S14.125 **Central cord syndrome at** C5 **level of cervical spinal cord**

    7ᵗʰ S14.126 **Central cord syndrome at** C6 **level of cervical spinal cord**

    7ᵗʰ S14.127 **Central cord syndrome at** C7 **level of cervical spinal cord**

    7ᵗʰ S14.128 **Central cord syndrome at** C8 **level of cervical spinal cord**

    7ᵗʰ S14.129 **Central cord syndrome at unspecified level of cervical spinal cord**

6ᵗʰ S14.13 Anterior cord syndrome of cervical spinal cord

    7ᵗʰ S14.131 **Anterior cord syndrome at** C1 **level of cervical spinal cord**

    7ᵗʰ S14.132 **Anterior cord syndrome at** C2 **level of cervical spinal cord**

    7ᵗʰ S14.133 **Anterior cord syndrome at** C3 **level of cervical spinal cord**

    7ᵗʰ S14.134 **Anterior cord syndrome at** C4 **level of cervical spinal cord**

    7ᵗʰ S14.135 **Anterior cord syndrome at** C5 **level of cervical spinal cord**

    7ᵗʰ S14.136 **Anterior cord syndrome at** C6 **level of cervical spinal cord**

    7ᵗʰ S14.137 **Anterior cord syndrome at** C7 **level of cervical spinal cord**

    7ᵗʰ S14.138 **Anterior cord syndrome at** C8 **level of cervical spinal cord**

    7ᵗʰ S14.139 **Anterior cord syndrome at unspecified level of cervical spinal cord**

6ᵗʰ S14.14 Brown-Séquard syndrome of cervical spinal cord

    7ᵗʰ S14.141 **Brown-Séquard syndrome at** C1 **level of cervical spinal cord**

    7ᵗʰ S14.142 **Brown-Séquard syndrome at** C2 **level of cervical spinal cord**

    7ᵗʰ S14.143 **Brown-Séquard syndrome at** C3 **level of cervical spinal cord**

    7ᵗʰ S14.144 **Brown-Séquard syndrome at** C4 **level of cervical spinal cord**

    7ᵗʰ S14.145 **Brown-Séquard syndrome at** C5 **level of cervical spinal cord**

    7ᵗʰ S14.146 **Brown-Séquard syndrome at** C6 **level of cervical spinal cord**

    7ᵗʰ S14.147 **Brown-Séquard syndrome at** C7 **level of cervical spinal cord**

    7ᵗʰ S14.148 **Brown-Séquard syndrome at** C8 **level of cervical spinal cord**

    7ᵗʰ S14.149 **Brown-Séquard syndrome at unspecified level of cervical spinal cord**

6ᵗʰ S14.15 Other incomplete lesions of cervical spinal cord

    Incomplete lesion of cervical spinal cord NOS
    Posterior cord syndrome of cervical spinal cord

4ᵗʰ 4ᵗʰ character required   5ᵗʰ 5ᵗʰ character required   6ᵗʰ 6ᵗʰ character required   7ᵗʰ 7ᵗʰ character required   Extension 'X' Alert

EXCLUDES 1 Not coded here   **EXCLUDES 2** Not included here   PDx Primary Diagnosis Only   Manifestation Code

[7th] S14.151 Other incomplete lesion at C1 level of cervical spinal cord
[7th] S14.152 Other incomplete lesion at C2 level of cervical spinal cord
[7th] S14.153 Other incomplete lesion at C3 level of cervical spinal cord
[7th] S14.154 Other incomplete lesion at C4 level of cervical spinal cord
[7th] S14.155 Other incomplete lesion at C5 level of cervical spinal cord
[7th] S14.156 Other incomplete lesion at C6 level of cervical spinal cord
[7th] S14.157 Other incomplete lesion at C7 level of cervical spinal cord
[7th] S14.158 Other incomplete lesion at C8 level of cervical spinal cord
[7th] S14.159 Other incomplete lesion at unspecified level of cervical spinal cord

[7th] S14.2 Injury of nerve root of cervical spine
[7th] S14.3 Injury of brachial plexus
[7th] S14.4 Injury of peripheral nerves of neck
[7th] S14.5 Injury of cervical sympathetic nerves
[7th] S14.8 Injury of other specified nerves of neck
[7th] S14.9 Injury of unspecified nerves of neck

[4th] S15 Injury of blood vessels at neck level

Code also any associated open wound (S11.-)

The appropriate 7th character is to be added to each code from category S15
A = initial encounter
D = subsequent encounter
S = sequela

[5th] S15.0 Injury of carotid artery of neck

Injury of carotid artery (common) (external) (internal, extracranial portion)
Injury of carotid artery NOS

[EXCLUDES1] *injury of internal carotid artery, intracranial portion (S06.8)*

[6th] S15.00 Unspecified injury of carotid artery
[7th] S15.001 Unspecified injury of right carotid artery
[7th] S15.002 Unspecified injury of left carotid artery
[7th] S15.009 Unspecified injury of unspecified carotid artery

[6th] S15.01 Minor laceration of carotid artery

Incomplete transection of carotid artery
Laceration of carotid artery NOS
Superficial laceration of carotid artery

[7th] S15.011 Minor laceration of right carotid artery
[7th] S15.012 Minor laceration of left carotid artery
[7th] S15.019 Minor laceration of unspecified carotid artery

[6th] S15.02 Major laceration of carotid artery

Complete transection of carotid artery
Traumatic rupture of carotid artery

[7th] S15.021 Major laceration of right carotid artery
[7th] S15.022 Major laceration of left carotid artery
[7th] S15.029 Major laceration of unspecified carotid artery

[6th] S15.09 Other specified injury of carotid artery
[7th] S15.091 Other specified injury of right carotid artery
[7th] S15.092 Other specified injury of left carotid artery
[7th] S15.099 Other specified injury of unspecified carotid artery

[5th] S15.1 Injury of vertebral artery

[6th] S15.10 Unspecified injury of vertebral artery
[7th] S15.101 Unspecified injury of right vertebral artery
[7th] S15.102 Unspecified injury of left vertebral artery
[7th] S15.109 Unspecified injury of unspecified vertebral artery

[6th] S15.11 Minor laceration of vertebral artery

Incomplete transection of vertebral artery
Laceration of vertebral artery NOS
Superficial laceration of vertebral artery

[7th] S15.111 Minor laceration of right vertebral artery
[7th] S15.112 Minor laceration of left vertebral artery
[7th] S15.119 Minor laceration of unspecified vertebral artery

[6th] S15.12 Major laceration of vertebral artery

Complete transection of vertebral artery
Traumatic rupture of vertebral artery

[7th] S15.121 Major laceration of right vertebral artery
[7th] S15.122 Major laceration of left vertebral artery
[7th] S15.129 Major laceration of unspecified vertebral artery

[6th] S15.19 Other specified injury of vertebral artery
[7th] S15.191 Other specified injury of right vertebral artery
[7th] S15.192 Other specified injury of left vertebral artery
[7th] S15.199 Other specified injury of unspecified vertebral artery

[5th] S15.2 Injury of external jugular vein

[6th] S15.20 Unspecified injury of external jugular vein
[7th] S15.201 Unspecified injury of right external jugular vein
[7th] S15.202 Unspecified injury of left external jugular vein
[7th] S15.209 Unspecified injury of unspecified external jugular vein

[6th] S15.21 Minor laceration of external jugular vein

Incomplete transection of external jugular vein
Laceration of external jugular vein NOS
Superficial laceration of external jugular vein

[7th] S15.211 Minor laceration of right external jugular vein
[7th] S15.212 Minor laceration of left external jugular vein
[7th] S15.219 Minor laceration of unspecified external jugular vein

[6th] S15.22 Major laceration of external jugular vein

Complete transection of external jugular vein
Traumatic rupture of external jugular vein

[7th] S15.221 Major laceration of right external jugular vein
[7th] S15.222 Major laceration of left external jugular vein
[7th] S15.229 Major laceration of unspecified external jugular vein

[6th] S15.29 Other specified injury of external jugular vein
[7th] S15.291 Other specified injury of right external jugular vein
[7th] S15.292 Other specified injury of left external jugular vein
[7th] S15.299 Other specified injury of unspecified external jugular vein

[5th] S15.3 Injury of internal jugular vein

[6th] S15.30 Unspecified injury of internal jugular vein
[7th] S15.301 Unspecified injury of right internal jugular vein
[7th] S15.302 Unspecified injury of left internal jugular vein
[7th] S15.309 Unspecified injury of unspecified internal jugular vein

[6th] S15.31 Minor laceration of internal jugular vein

Incomplete transection of internal jugular vein
Laceration of internal jugular vein NOS
Superficial laceration of internal jugular vein

[7th] S15.311 Minor laceration of right internal jugular vein
[7th] S15.312 Minor laceration of left internal jugular vein

Unspecified Code | Other Specified Code | [N] Newborn Age: 0 | [P] Pediatric Age: 0-17 | [M] Maternity Age: 12-55
[A] Adult Age: 15-124 | ♂ Male | ♀ Female | ● New Code | ▲ Revised Code Title | ►◄ Revised Text

S15.319 **Minor laceration of unspecified internal jugular vein**

S15.32 **Major laceration of internal jugular vein**
    Complete transection of internal jugular vein
    Traumatic rupture of internal jugular vein

S15.321 **Major laceration of right internal jugular vein**

S15.322 **Major laceration of left internal jugular vein**

S15.329 **Major laceration of unspecified internal jugular vein**

S15.39 **Other specified injury of internal jugular vein**

S15.391 **Other specified injury of right internal jugular vein**

S15.392 **Other specified injury of left internal jugular vein**

S15.399 **Other specified injury of unspecified internal jugular vein**

S15.8 **Injury of other specified blood vessels at neck level**

S15.9 **Injury of unspecified blood vessel at neck level**

S16 **Injury of muscle, fascia and tendon at neck level**
    Code also any associated open wound (S11.-)
    EXCLUDES2 sprain of joint or ligament at neck level (S13.9)
    The appropriate 7th character is to be added to each code from category S16
    A = initial encounter
    D = subsequent encounter
    S = sequela

S16.1 **Strain of muscle, fascia and tendon at neck level**

S16.2 **Laceration of muscle, fascia and tendon at neck level**

S16.8 **Other specified injury of muscle, fascia and tendon at neck level**

S16.9 **Unspecified injury of muscle, fascia and tendon at neck level**

S17 **Crushing injury of neck**
    Use additional code for all associated injuries, such as:
    injury of blood vessels (S15.-)
    open wound of neck (S11.-)
    spinal cord injury (S14.0, S14.1-)
    vertebral fracture (S12.0--S12.3-)
    The appropriate 7th character is to be added to each code from category S17
    A = initial encounter
    D = subsequent encounter
    S = sequela

S17.0 **Crushing injury of larynx and trachea**

S17.8 **Crushing injury of other specified parts of neck**

S17.9 **Crushing injury of neck, part unspecified**

S19 **Other specified and unspecified injuries of neck**
    The appropriate 7th character is to be added to each code from category S19
    A = initial encounter
    D = subsequent encounter
    S = sequela

S19.8 **Other specified injuries of neck**

S19.80 **Other specified injuries of unspecified part of neck**

S19.81 **Other specified injuries of larynx**

S19.82 **Other specified injuries of cervical trachea**
    EXCLUDES2 other specified injury of thoracic trachea (S27.5-)

S19.83 **Other specified injuries of vocal cord**

S19.84 **Other specified injuries of thyroid gland**

S19.85 **Other specified injuries of pharynx and cervical esophagus**

S19.89 **Other specified injuries of other specified part of neck**

S19.9 **Unspecified injury of neck**

Injuries to the thorax (S20-S29)

    INCLUDES injuries of breast
    injuries of chest (wall)
    injuries of interscapular area
    EXCLUDES2 burns and corrosions (T20-T32)
    effects of foreign body in bronchus (T17.5)
    effects of foreign body in esophagus (T18.1)
    effects of foreign body in lung (T17.8)
    effects of foreign body in trachea (T17.4)
    frostbite (T33-T34)
    injuries of axilla
    injuries of clavicle
    injuries of scapular region
    injuries of shoulder
    insect bite or sting, venomous (T63.4)

S20 **Superficial injury of thorax**
    The appropriate 7th character is to be added to each code from category S20
    A = initial encounter
    D = subsequent encounter
    S = sequela

S20.0 **Contusion of breast**

S20.00 **Contusion of breast, unspecified breast**

S20.01 **Contusion of right breast**

S20.02 **Contusion of left breast**

S20.1 **Other and unspecified superficial injuries of breast**

S20.10 **Unspecified superficial injuries of breast**

S20.101 **Unspecified superficial injuries of breast, right breast**

S20.102 **Unspecified superficial injuries of breast, left breast**

S20.109 **Unspecified superficial injuries of breast, unspecified breast**

S20.11 **Abrasion of breast**

S20.111 **Abrasion of breast, right breast**

S20.112 **Abrasion of breast, left breast**

S20.119 **Abrasion of breast, unspecified breast**

S20.12 **Blister (nonthermal) of breast**

S20.121 **Blister (nonthermal) of breast, right breast**

S20.122 **Blister (nonthermal) of breast, left breast**

S20.129 **Blister (nonthermal) of breast, unspecified breast**

S20.14 **External constriction of part of breast**

S20.141 **External constriction of part of breast, right breast**

S20.142 **External constriction of part of breast, left breast**

S20.149 **External constriction of part of breast, unspecified breast**

S20.15 **Superficial foreign body of breast**
    Splinter in the breast

S20.151 **Superficial foreign body of breast, right breast**

S20.152 **Superficial foreign body of breast, left breast**

S20.159 **Superficial foreign body of breast, unspecified breast**

S20.16 **Insect bite (nonvenomous) of breast**

S20.161 **Insect bite (nonvenomous) of breast, right breast**

S20.162 **Insect bite (nonvenomous) of breast, left breast**

S20.169 **Insect bite (nonvenomous) of breast, unspecified breast**

S20.17 **Other superficial bite of breast**
    EXCLUDES1 open bite of breast (S21.05-)

S20.171 **Other superficial bite of breast, right breast**

- [7th] S20.172 Other superficial bite of breast, left breast
- [7th] S20.179 Other superficial bite of breast, unspecified breast

[5th] S20.2 Contusion of thorax
- [7th] S20.20 Contusion of thorax, unspecified
- [6th] S20.21 Contusion of front wall of thorax
  - [7th] S20.211 Contusion of right front wall of thorax
  - [7th] S20.212 Contusion of left front wall of thorax
  - [7th] S20.219 Contusion of unspecified front wall of thorax
- [6th] S20.22 Contusion of back wall of thorax
  - [7th] S20.221 Contusion of right back wall of thorax
  - [7th] S20.222 Contusion of left back wall of thorax
  - [7th] S20.229 Contusion of unspecified back wall of thorax

[5th] S20.3 Other and unspecified superficial injuries of front wall of thorax
- [6th] S20.30 Unspecified superficial injuries of front wall of thorax
  - [7th] S20.301 Unspecified superficial injuries of right front wall of thorax
  - [7th] S20.302 Unspecified superficial injuries of left front wall of thorax
  - [7th] S20.309 Unspecified superficial injuries of unspecified front wall of thorax
- [6th] S20.31 Abrasion of front wall of thorax
  - [7th] S20.311 Abrasion of right front wall of thorax
  - [7th] S20.312 Abrasion of left front wall of thorax
  - [7th] S20.319 Abrasion of unspecified front wall of thorax
- [6th] S20.32 Blister (nonthermal) of front wall of thorax
  - [7th] S20.321 Blister (nonthermal) of right front wall of thorax
  - [7th] S20.322 Blister (nonthermal) of left front wall of thorax
  - [7th] S20.329 Blister (nonthermal) of unspecified front wall of thorax
- [6th] S20.34 External constriction of front wall of thorax
  - [7th] S20.341 External constriction of right front wall of thorax
  - [7th] S20.342 External constriction of left front wall of thorax
  - [7th] S20.349 External constriction of unspecified front wall of thorax
- [6th] S20.35 Superficial foreign body of front wall of thorax

  Splinter in front wall of thorax
  - [7th] S20.351 Superficial foreign body of right front wall of thorax
  - [7th] S20.352 Superficial foreign body of left front wall of thorax
  - [7th] S20.359 Superficial foreign body of unspecified front wall of thorax
- [6th] S20.36 Insect bite (nonvenomous) of front wall of thorax
  - [7th] S20.361 Insect bite (nonvenomous) of right front wall of thorax
  - [7th] S20.362 Insect bite (nonvenomous) of left front wall of thorax
  - [7th] S20.369 Insect bite (nonvenomous) of unspecified front wall of thorax
- [6th] S20.37 Other superficial bite of front wall of thorax

  [EXCLUDES1] *open bite of front wall of thorax (S21.14)*
  - [7th] S20.371 Other superficial bite of right front wall of thorax
  - [7th] S20.372 Other superficial bite of left front wall of thorax
  - [7th] S20.379 Other superficial bite of unspecified front wall of thorax

[5th] S20.4 Other and unspecified superficial injuries of back wall of thorax
- [6th] S20.40 Unspecified superficial injuries of back wall of thorax
  - [7th] S20.401 Unspecified superficial injuries of right back wall of thorax
  - [7th] S20.402 Unspecified superficial injuries of left back wall of thorax
  - [7th] S20.409 Unspecified superficial injuries of unspecified back wall of thorax
- [6th] S20.41 Abrasion of back wall of thorax
  - [7th] S20.411 Abrasion of right back wall of thorax
  - [7th] S20.412 Abrasion of left back wall of thorax
  - [7th] S20.419 Abrasion of unspecified back wall of thorax
- [6th] S20.42 Blister (nonthermal) of back wall of thorax
  - [7th] S20.421 Blister (nonthermal) of right back wall of thorax
  - [7th] S20.422 Blister (nonthermal) of left back wall of thorax
  - [7th] S20.429 Blister (nonthermal) of unspecified back wall of thorax
- [6th] S20.44 External constriction of back wall of thorax
  - [7th] S20.441 External constriction of right back wall of thorax
  - [7th] S20.442 External constriction of left back wall of thorax
  - [7th] S20.449 External constriction of unspecified back wall of thorax
- [6th] S20.45 Superficial foreign body of back wall of thorax

  Splinter of back wall of thorax
  - [7th] S20.451 Superficial foreign body of right back wall of thorax
  - [7th] S20.452 Superficial foreign body of left back wall of thorax
  - [7th] S20.459 Superficial foreign body of unspecified back wall of thorax
- [6th] S20.46 Insect bite (nonvenomous) of back wall of thorax
  - [7th] S20.461 Insect bite (nonvenomous) of right back wall of thorax
  - [7th] S20.462 Insect bite (nonvenomous) of left back wall of thorax
  - [7th] S20.469 Insect bite (nonvenomous) of unspecified back wall of thorax
- [6th] S20.47 Other superficial bite of back wall of thorax

  [EXCLUDES1] *open bite of back wall of thorax (S21.24)*
  - [7th] S20.471 Other superficial bite of right back wall of thorax
  - [7th] S20.472 Other superficial bite of left back wall of thorax
  - [7th] S20.479 Other superficial bite of unspecified back wall of thorax

[5th] S20.9 Superficial injury of unspecified parts of thorax

[EXCLUDES1] *contusion of thorax NOS (S20.20)*
- [7th] S20.90 Unspecified superficial injury of unspecified parts of thorax

  Superficial injury of thoracic wall NOS
- [7th] S20.91 Abrasion of unspecified parts of thorax
- [7th] S20.92 Blister (nonthermal) of unspecified parts of thorax
- [7th] S20.94 External constriction of unspecified parts of thorax
- [7th] S20.95 Superficial foreign body of unspecified parts of thorax

  Splinter in thorax NOS
- [7th] S20.96 Insect bite (nonvenomous) of unspecified parts of thorax
- [7th] S20.97 Other superficial bite of unspecified parts of thorax

  [EXCLUDES1] *open bite of thorax NOS (S21.95)*

Unspecified Code | Other Specified Code | [N] Newborn Age: 0 | [P] Pediatric Age: 0-17 | [M] Maternity Age: 12-55
[A] Adult Age: 15-124 | ♂ Male | ♀ Female | ● New Code | ▲ Revised Code Title | ►◄ Revised Text

[4th] S21 Open wound of thorax
Code also any associated injury, such as: :
injury of heart (S26.-)
injury of intrathoracic organs (S27.-)
rib fracture (S22.3-, S22.4-)
spinal cord injury (S24.0-, S24.1-)
traumatic hemothorax (S27.1)
traumatic hemopneumothorax (S27.3)
traumatic pneumothorax (S27.0)
wound infection
EXCLUDES1 *traumatic amputation (partial) of thorax (S28.1)*
The appropriate 7th character is to be added to each code from category S21
A = initial encounter
D = subsequent encounter
S = sequela

[5th] S21.0 Open wound of breast
[6th] S21.00 Unspecified open wound of breast
[7th] S21.001 Unspecified open wound of right breast
[7th] S21.002 Unspecified open wound of left breast
[7th] S21.009 Unspecified open wound of unspecified breast
[6th] S21.01 Laceration without foreign body of breast
[7th] S21.011 Laceration without foreign body of right breast
[7th] S21.012 Laceration without foreign body of left breast
[7th] S21.019 Laceration without foreign body of unspecified breast
[6th] S21.02 Laceration with foreign body of breast
[7th] S21.021 Laceration with foreign body of right breast
[7th] S21.022 Laceration with foreign body of left breast
[7th] S21.029 Laceration with foreign body of unspecified breast
[6th] S21.03 Puncture wound without foreign body of breast
[7th] S21.031 Puncture wound without foreign body of right breast
[7th] S21.032 Puncture wound without foreign body of left breast
[7th] S21.039 Puncture wound without foreign body of unspecified breast
[6th] S21.04 Puncture wound with foreign body of breast
[7th] S21.041 Puncture wound with foreign body of right breast
[7th] S21.042 Puncture wound with foreign body of left breast
[7th] S21.049 Puncture wound with foreign body of unspecified breast
[6th] S21.05 Open bite of breast
Bite of breast NOS
EXCLUDES1 *superficial bite of breast (S20.17)*
[7th] S21.051 Open bite of right breast
[7th] S21.052 Open bite of left breast
[7th] S21.059 Open bite of unspecified breast

[5th] S21.1 Open wound of front wall of thorax without penetration into thoracic cavity
Open wound of chest without penetration into thoracic cavity
[6th] S21.10 Unspecified open wound of front wall of thorax without penetration into thoracic cavity
[7th] S21.101 Unspecified open wound of right front wall of thorax without penetration into thoracic cavity
[7th] S21.102 Unspecified open wound of left front wall of thorax without penetration into thoracic cavity
[7th] S21.109 Unspecified open wound of unspecified front wall of thorax without penetration into thoracic cavity
[6th] S21.11 Laceration without foreign body of front wall of thorax without penetration into thoracic cavity
[7th] S21.111 Laceration without foreign body of right front wall of thorax without penetration into thoracic cavity
[7th] S21.112 Laceration without foreign body of left front wall of thorax without penetration into thoracic cavity
[7th] S21.119 Laceration without foreign body of unspecified front wall of thorax without penetration into thoracic cavity
[6th] S21.12 Laceration with foreign body of front wall of thorax without penetration into thoracic cavity
[7th] S21.121 Laceration with foreign body of right front wall of thorax without penetration into thoracic cavity
[7th] S21.122 Laceration with foreign body of left front wall of thorax without penetration into thoracic cavity
[7th] S21.129 Laceration with foreign body of unspecified front wall of thorax without penetration into thoracic cavity
[6th] S21.13 Puncture wound without foreign body of front wall of thorax without penetration into thoracic cavity
[7th] S21.131 Puncture wound without foreign body of right front wall of thorax without penetration into thoracic cavity
[7th] S21.132 Puncture wound without foreign body of left front wall of thorax without penetration into thoracic cavity
[7th] S21.139 Puncture wound without foreign body of unspecified front wall of thorax without penetration into thoracic cavity
[6th] S21.14 Puncture wound with foreign body of front wall of thorax without penetration into thoracic cavity
[7th] S21.141 Puncture wound with foreign body of right front wall of thorax without penetration into thoracic cavity
[7th] S21.142 Puncture wound with foreign body of left front wall of thorax without penetration into thoracic cavity
[7th] S21.149 Puncture wound with foreign body of unspecified front wall of thorax without penetration into thoracic cavity
[6th] S21.15 Open bite of front wall of thorax without penetration into thoracic cavity
Bite of front wall of thorax NOS
EXCLUDES1 *superficial bite of front wall of thorax (S20.37)*
[7th] S21.151 Open bite of right front wall of thorax without penetration into thoracic cavity
[7th] S21.152 Open bite of left front wall of thorax without penetration into thoracic cavity
[7th] S21.159 Open bite of unspecified front wall of thorax without penetration into thoracic cavity

[5th] S21.2 Open wound of back wall of thorax without penetration into thoracic cavity
[6th] S21.20 Unspecified open wound of back wall of thorax without penetration into thoracic cavity
[7th] S21.201 Unspecified open wound of right back wall of thorax without penetration into thoracic cavity
[7th] S21.202 Unspecified open wound of left back wall of thorax without penetration into thoracic cavity
[7th] S21.209 Unspecified open wound of unspecified back wall of thorax without penetration into thoracic cavity

[4] 4th character required [5] 5th character required [6] 6th character required [7] 7th character required [7] Extension 'X' Alert
EXCLUDES 1 Not coded here EXCLUDES 2 Not included here PDx Primary Diagnosis Only Manifestation Code

S21.21 Laceration without foreign body of back wall of thorax without penetration into thoracic cavity

S21.211 Laceration without foreign body of right back wall of thorax without penetration into thoracic cavity

S21.212 Laceration without foreign body of left back wall of thorax without penetration into thoracic cavity

S21.219 Laceration without foreign body of unspecified back wall of thorax without penetration into thoracic cavity

S21.22 Laceration with foreign body of back wall of thorax without penetration into thoracic cavity

S21.221 Laceration with foreign body of right back wall of thorax without penetration into thoracic cavity

S21.222 Laceration with foreign body of left back wall of thorax without penetration into thoracic cavity

S21.229 Laceration with foreign body of unspecified back wall of thorax without penetration into thoracic cavity

S21.23 Puncture wound without foreign body of back wall of thorax without penetration into thoracic cavity

S21.231 Puncture wound without foreign body of right back wall of thorax without penetration into thoracic cavity

S21.232 Puncture wound without foreign body of left back wall of thorax without penetration into thoracic cavity

S21.239 Puncture wound without foreign body of unspecified back wall of thorax without penetration into thoracic cavity

S21.24 Puncture wound with foreign body of back wall of thorax without penetration into thoracic cavity

S21.241 Puncture wound with foreign body of right back wall of thorax without penetration into thoracic cavity

S21.242 Puncture wound with foreign body of left back wall of thorax without penetration into thoracic cavity

S21.249 Puncture wound with foreign body of unspecified back wall of thorax without penetration into thoracic cavity

S21.25 Open bite of back wall of thorax without penetration into thoracic cavity

Bite of back wall of thorax NOS

EXCLUDES1 superficial bite of back wall of thorax (S20.47)

S21.251 Open bite of right back wall of thorax without penetration into thoracic cavity

S21.252 Open bite of left back wall of thorax without penetration into thoracic cavity

S21.259 Open bite of unspecified back wall of thorax without penetration into thoracic cavity

S21.3 Open wound of front wall of thorax with penetration into thoracic cavity

Open wound of chest with penetration into thoracic cavity

S21.30 Unspecified open wound of front wall of thorax with penetration into thoracic cavity

S21.301 Unspecified open wound of right front wall of thorax with penetration into thoracic cavity

S21.302 Unspecified open wound of left front wall of thorax with penetration into thoracic cavity

S21.309 Unspecified open wound of unspecified front wall of thorax with penetration into thoracic cavity

S21.31 Laceration without foreign body of front wall of thorax with penetration into thoracic cavity

S21.311 Laceration without foreign body of right front wall of thorax with penetration into thoracic cavity

S21.312 Laceration without foreign body of left front wall of thorax with penetration into thoracic cavity

S21.319 Laceration without foreign body of unspecified front wall of thorax with penetration into thoracic cavity

S21.32 Laceration with foreign body of front wall of thorax with penetration into thoracic cavity

S21.321 Laceration with foreign body of right front wall of thorax with penetration into thoracic cavity

S21.322 Laceration with foreign body of left front wall of thorax with penetration into thoracic cavity

S21.329 Laceration with foreign body of unspecified front wall of thorax with penetration into thoracic cavity

S21.33 Puncture wound without foreign body of front wall of thorax with penetration into thoracic cavity

S21.331 Puncture wound without foreign body of right front wall of thorax with penetration into thoracic cavity

S21.332 Puncture wound without foreign body of left front wall of thorax with penetration into thoracic cavity

S21.339 Puncture wound without foreign body of unspecified front wall of thorax with penetration into thoracic cavity

S21.34 Puncture wound with foreign body of front wall of thorax with penetration into thoracic cavity

S21.341 Puncture wound with foreign body of right front wall of thorax with penetration into thoracic cavity

S21.342 Puncture wound with foreign body of left front wall of thorax with penetration into thoracic cavity

S21.349 Puncture wound with foreign body of unspecified front wall of thorax with penetration into thoracic cavity

S21.35 Open bite of front wall of thorax with penetration into thoracic cavity

EXCLUDES1 superficial bite of front wall of thorax (S20.37)

S21.351 Open bite of right front wall of thorax with penetration into thoracic cavity

S21.352 Open bite of left front wall of thorax with penetration into thoracic cavity

S21.359 Open bite of unspecified front wall of thorax with penetration into thoracic cavity

S21.4 Open wound of back wall of thorax with penetration into thoracic cavity

S21.40 Unspecified open wound of back wall of thorax with penetration into thoracic cavity

S21.401 Unspecified open wound of right back wall of thorax with penetration into thoracic cavity

S21.402 Unspecified open wound of left back wall of thorax with penetration into thoracic cavity

S21.409 Unspecified open wound of unspecified back wall of thorax with penetration into thoracic cavity

S21.41 Laceration without foreign body of back wall of thorax with penetration into thoracic cavity

---

Unspecified Code	Other Specified Code	N Newborn Age: 0	P Pediatric Age: 0-17	M Maternity Age: 12-55
A Adult Age: 15-124	♂ Male	♀ Female	● New Code	▲ Revised Code Title	►◄ Revised Text

[7th] S21.411 Laceration without foreign body of right back wall of thorax with penetration into thoracic cavity
[7th] S21.412 Laceration without foreign body of left back wall of thorax with penetration into thoracic cavity
[7th] S21.419 Laceration without foreign body of unspecified back wall of thorax with penetration into thoracic cavity
[6th] S21.42 Laceration with foreign body of back wall of thorax with penetration into thoracic cavity
[7th] S21.421 Laceration with foreign body of right back wall of thorax with penetration into thoracic cavity
[7th] S21.422 Laceration with foreign body of left back wall of thorax with penetration into thoracic cavity
[7th] S21.429 Laceration with foreign body of unspecified back wall of thorax with penetration into thoracic cavity
[6th] S21.43 Puncture wound without foreign body of back wall of thorax with penetration into thoracic cavity
[7th] S21.431 Puncture wound without foreign body of right back wall of thorax with penetration into thoracic cavity
[7th] S21.432 Puncture wound without foreign body of left back wall of thorax with penetration into thoracic cavity
[7th] S21.439 Puncture wound without foreign body of unspecified back wall of thorax with penetration into thoracic cavity
[6th] S21.44 Puncture wound with foreign body of back wall of thorax with penetration into thoracic cavity
[7th] S21.441 Puncture wound with foreign body of right back wall of thorax with penetration into thoracic cavity
[7th] S21.442 Puncture wound with foreign body of left back wall of thorax with penetration into thoracic cavity
[7th] S21.449 Puncture wound with foreign body of unspecified back wall of thorax with penetration into thoracic cavity
[6th] S21.45 Open bite of back wall of thorax with penetration into thoracic cavity
Bite of back wall of thorax NOS
[EXCLUDES1] *superficial bite of back wall of thorax (S20.47)*
[7th] S21.451 Open bite of right back wall of thorax with penetration into thoracic cavity
[7th] S21.452 Open bite of left back wall of thorax with penetration into thoracic cavity
[7th] S21.459 Open bite of unspecified back wall of thorax with penetration into thoracic cavity
[5th] S21.9 Open wound of unspecified part of thorax
Open wound of thoracic wall NOS
[x7th] S21.90 Unspecified open wound of unspecified part of thorax
[x7th] S21.91 Laceration without foreign body of unspecified part of thorax
[x7th] S21.92 Laceration with foreign body of unspecified part of thorax
[x7th] S21.93 Puncture wound without foreign body of unspecified part of thorax
[x7th] S21.94 Puncture wound with foreign body of unspecified part of thorax
[x7th] S21.95 Open bite of unspecified part of thorax
[EXCLUDES1] *superficial bite of thorax (S20.97)*

[4th] S22 Fracture of rib(s), sternum and thoracic spine
[NOTES] A fracture not indicated as displaced or nondisplaced should be coded to displaced
A fracture not indicated as open or closed should be coded to closed
[INCLUDES] *fracture of thoracic neural arch*
fracture of thoracic spinous process
fracture of thoracic transverse process
fracture of thoracic vertebra
fracture of thoracic vertebral arch
Code first any associated:
injury of intrathoracic organ (S27.-)
spinal cord injury (S24.0-, S24.1-)
[EXCLUDES1] *transection of thorax (S28.1)*
[EXCLUDES2] *fracture of clavicle (S42.0-)*
fracture of scapula (S42.1-)
The appropriate 7th character is to be added to each code from category S22
A = initial encounter for closed fracture
B = initial encounter for open fracture
D = subsequent encounter for fracture with routine healing
G = subsequent encounter for fracture with delayed healing
K = subsequent encounter for fracture with nonunion
S = sequela
[5th] S22.0 Fracture of thoracic vertebra
[6th] S22.00 Fracture of unspecified thoracic vertebra
[7th] S22.000 Wedge compression fracture of unspecified thoracic vertebra
[7th] S22.001 Stable burst fracture of unspecified thoracic vertebra
[7th] S22.002 Unstable burst fracture of unspecified thoracic vertebra
[7th] S22.008 Other fracture of unspecified thoracic vertebra
[7th] S22.009 Unspecified fracture of unspecified thoracic vertebra
[6th] S22.01 Fracture of first thoracic vertebra
[7th] S22.010 Wedge compression fracture of first thoracic vertebra
[7th] S22.011 Stable burst fracture of first thoracic vertebra
[7th] S22.012 Unstable burst fracture of first thoracic vertebra
[7th] S22.018 Other fracture of first thoracic vertebra
[7th] S22.019 Unspecified fracture of first thoracic vertebra
[6th] S22.02 Fracture of second thoracic vertebra
[7th] S22.020 Wedge compression fracture of second thoracic vertebra
[7th] S22.021 Stable burst fracture of second thoracic vertebra
[7th] S22.022 Unstable burst fracture of second thoracic vertebra
[7th] S22.028 Other fracture of second thoracic vertebra
[7th] S22.029 Unspecified fracture of second thoracic vertebra
[6th] S22.03 Fracture of third thoracic vertebra
[7th] S22.030 Wedge compression fracture of third thoracic vertebra
[7th] S22.031 Stable burst fracture of third thoracic vertebra
[7th] S22.032 Unstable burst fracture of third thoracic vertebra
[7th] S22.038 Other fracture of third thoracic vertebra
[7th] S22.039 Unspecified fracture of third thoracic vertebra
[6th] S22.04 Fracture of fourth thoracic vertebra

[4th] 4th character required [5th] 5th character required [6th] 6th character required [7th] 7th character required [x7th] Extension 'X' Alert
[EXCLUDES1] Not coded here [EXCLUDES2] Not included here [PDx] Primary Diagnosis Only Manifestation Code

7️⃣ **S22.040** Wedge compression fracture of fourth thoracic vertebra

7️⃣ **S22.041** Stable burst fracture of fourth thoracic vertebra

7️⃣ **S22.042** Unstable burst fracture of fourth thoracic vertebra

7️⃣ **S22.048** Other fracture of fourth thoracic vertebra

7️⃣ **S22.049** Unspecified fracture of fourth thoracic vertebra

6️⃣ **S22.05** Fracture of T5-T6 vertebra

7️⃣ **S22.050** Wedge compression fracture of T5-T6 vertebra

7️⃣ **S22.051** Stable burst fracture of T5-T6 vertebra

7️⃣ **S22.052** Unstable burst fracture of T5-T6 vertebra

7️⃣ **S22.058** Other fracture of T5-T6 vertebra

7️⃣ **S22.059** Unspecified fracture of T5-T6 vertebra

6️⃣ **S22.06** Fracture of T7-T8 vertebra

7️⃣ **S22.060** Wedge compression fracture of T7-T8 vertebra

7️⃣ **S22.061** Stable burst fracture of T7-T8 vertebra

7️⃣ **S22.062** Unstable burst fracture of T7-T8 vertebra

7️⃣ **S22.068** Other fracture of T7-T8 thoracic vertebra

7️⃣ **S22.069** Unspecified fracture of T7-T8 vertebra

6️⃣ **S22.07** Fracture of T9-T10 vertebra

7️⃣ **S22.070** Wedge compression fracture of T9-T10 vertebra

7️⃣ **S22.071** Stable burst fracture of T9-T10 vertebra

7️⃣ **S22.072** Unstable burst fracture of T9-T10 vertebra

7️⃣ **S22.078** Other fracture of T9-T10 vertebra

7️⃣ **S22.079** Unspecified fracture of T9-T10 vertebra

6️⃣ **S22.08** Fracture of T11-T12 vertebra

7️⃣ **S22.080** Wedge compression fracture of T11-T12 vertebra

7️⃣ **S22.081** Stable burst fracture of T11-T12 vertebra

7️⃣ **S22.082** Unstable burst fracture of T11-T12 vertebra

7️⃣ **S22.088** Other fracture of T11-T12 vertebra

7️⃣ **S22.089** Unspecified fracture of T11-T12 vertebra

5️⃣ **S22.2** Fracture of sternum

7️⃣ **S22.20** Unspecified fracture of sternum

7️⃣ **S22.21** Fracture of manubrium

7️⃣ **S22.22** Fracture of body of sternum

7️⃣ **S22.23** Sternal manubrial dissociation

7️⃣ **S22.24** Fracture of xiphoid process

5️⃣ **S22.3** Fracture of one rib

7️⃣ **S22.31** Fracture of one rib, right side

7️⃣ **S22.32** Fracture of one rib, left side

7️⃣ **S22.39** Fracture of one rib, unspecified side

5️⃣ **S22.4** Multiple fractures of ribs

Fractures of two or more ribs

EXCLUDES1 flail chest (S22.5-)

7️⃣ **S22.41** Multiple fractures of ribs, right side

7️⃣ **S22.42** Multiple fractures of ribs, left side

7️⃣ **S22.43** Multiple fractures of ribs, bilateral

7️⃣ **S22.49** Multiple fractures of ribs, unspecified side

7️⃣ **S22.5** Flail chest

7️⃣ **S22.9** Fracture of bony thorax, part unspecified

4️⃣ **S23** Dislocation and sprain of joints and ligaments of thorax

INCLUDES avulsion of joint or ligament of thorax
laceration of cartilage, joint or ligament of thorax
sprain of cartilage, joint or ligament of thorax
traumatic hemarthrosis of joint or ligament of thorax
traumatic rupture of joint or ligament of thorax
traumatic subluxation of joint or ligament of thorax
traumatic tear of joint or ligament of thorax

Code also any associated open wound

(handwritten annotations: S22.41XA, S22.41)

EXCLUDES2 dislocation, sprain of sternoclavicular joint (S43.2, S43.6)
strain of muscle or tendon of thorax (S29.01-)

The appropriate 7th character is to be added to each code from category S23
A = initial encounter
D = subsequent encounter
S = sequela

7️⃣ **S23.0** Traumatic rupture of thoracic intervertebral disc

EXCLUDES1 rupture or displacement (nontraumatic) of thoracic intervertebral disc NOS (M51.- with fifth character 4)

5️⃣ **S23.1** Subluxation and dislocation of thoracic vertebra

Code also any associated
open wound of thorax (S21.-)
spinal cord injury (S24.0-, S24.1-)

EXCLUDES2 fracture of thoracic vertebrae (S22.0-)

6️⃣ **S23.10** Subluxation and dislocation of unspecified thoracic vertebra

7️⃣ **S23.100** Subluxation of unspecified thoracic vertebra

7️⃣ **S23.101** Dislocation of unspecified thoracic vertebra

6️⃣ **S23.11** Subluxation and dislocation of T1/T2 thoracic vertebra

7️⃣ **S23.110** Subluxation of T1/T2 thoracic vertebra

7️⃣ **S23.111** Dislocation of T1/T2 thoracic vertebra

6️⃣ **S23.12** Subluxation and dislocation of T2/T3-T3/T4 thoracic vertebra

7️⃣ **S23.120** Subluxation of T2/T3 thoracic vertebra

7️⃣ **S23.121** Dislocation of T2/T3 thoracic vertebra

7️⃣ **S23.122** Subluxation of T3/T4 thoracic vertebra

7️⃣ **S23.123** Dislocation of T3/T4 thoracic vertebra

6️⃣ **S23.13** Subluxation and dislocation of T4/T5-T5/T6 thoracic vertebra

7️⃣ **S23.130** Subluxation of T4/T5 thoracic vertebra

7️⃣ **S23.131** Dislocation of T4/T5 thoracic vertebra

7️⃣ **S23.132** Subluxation of T5/T6 thoracic vertebra

7️⃣ **S23.133** Dislocation of T5/T6 thoracic vertebra

6️⃣ **S23.14** Subluxation and dislocation of T6/T7-T7/T8 thoracic vertebra

7️⃣ **S23.140** Subluxation of T6/T7 thoracic vertebra

7️⃣ **S23.141** Dislocation of T6/T7 thoracic vertebra

7️⃣ **S23.142** Subluxation of T7/T8 thoracic vertebra

7️⃣ **S23.143** Dislocation of T7/T8 thoracic vertebra

6️⃣ **S23.15** Subluxation and dislocation of T8/T9-T9/T10 thoracic vertebra

7️⃣ **S23.150** Subluxation of T8/T9 thoracic vertebra

7️⃣ **S23.151** Dislocation of T8/T9 thoracic vertebra

7️⃣ **S23.152** Subluxation of T9/T10 thoracic vertebra

7️⃣ **S23.153** Dislocation of T9/T10 thoracic vertebra

6️⃣ **S23.16** Subluxation and dislocation of T10/T11-T11/T12 thoracic vertebra

7️⃣ **S23.160** Subluxation of T10/T11 thoracic vertebra

7️⃣ **S23.161** Dislocation of T10/T11 thoracic vertebra

7️⃣ **S23.162** Subluxation of T11/T12 thoracic vertebra

7️⃣ **S23.163** Dislocation of T11/T12 thoracic vertebra

6️⃣ **S23.17** Subluxation and dislocation of T12/L1 thoracic vertebra

7️⃣ **S23.170** Subluxation of T12/L1 thoracic vertebra

7️⃣ **S23.171** Dislocation of T12/L1 thoracic vertebra

5️⃣ **S23.2** Dislocation of other and unspecified parts of thorax

7️⃣ **S23.20** Dislocation of unspecified part of thorax

7️⃣ **S23.29** Dislocation of other parts of thorax

7️⃣ **S23.3** Sprain of ligaments of thoracic spine

5️⃣ **S23.4** Sprain of ribs and sternum

7️⃣ **S23.41** Sprain of ribs

6️⃣ **S23.42** Sprain of sternum

7️⃣ **S23.420** Sprain of sternoclavicular (joint) (ligament)

7️⃣ **S23.421** Sprain of chondrosternal joint

7️⃣ **S23.428** Other sprain of sternum

Unspecified Code | Other Specified Code | N Newborn Age: 0 | P Pediatric Age: 0-17 | M Maternity Age: 12-55
A Adult Age: 15-124 | ♂ Male | ♀ Female | ● New Code | ▲ Revised Code Title | ►◄ Revised Text

[7th] S23.429 Unspecified sprain of sternum

[X] S23.8 Sprain of other specified parts of thorax

[X] S23.9 Sprain of unspecified parts of thorax

[4th] **S24 Injury of nerves and spinal cord at thorax level**

[NOTES] Code to highest level of thoracic spinal cord injury. Injuries to the spinal cord (S24.0 and S24.1) refer to the cord level and not bone level injury, and can affectnerve roots at and below the level given.

Code also any associated:
fracture of thoracic vertebra (S22.0-)
open wound of thorax (S21.-)
transient paralysis (R29.5)

[EXCLUDES2] *injury of brachial plexus (S14.3)*

The appropriate 7th character is to be added to each code from category S24
A = initial encounter
D = subsequent encounter
S = sequela

[X] S24.0 Concussion and edema of thoracic spinal cord

[5th] S24.1 Other and unspecified injuries of thoracic spinal cord

[6th] S24.10 Unspecified injury of thoracic spinal cord

[7th] S24.101 Unspecified injury at T1 level of thoracic spinal cord

[7th] S24.102 Unspecified injury at T2-T6 level of thoracic spinal cord

[7th] S24.103 Unspecified injury at T7-T10 level of thoracic spinal cord

[7th] S24.104 Unspecified injury at T11-T12 level of thoracic spinal cord

[7th] S24.109 Unspecified injury at unspecified level of thoracic spinal cord
Injury of thoracic spinal cord NOS

[6th] S24.11 Complete lesion of thoracic spinal cord

[7th] S24.111 Complete lesion at T1 level of thoracic spinal cord

[7th] S24.112 Complete lesion at T2-T6 level of thoracic spinal cord

[7th] S24.113 Complete lesion at T7-T10 level of thoracic spinal cord

[7th] S24.114 Complete lesion at T11-T12 level of thoracic spinal cord

[7th] S24.119 Complete lesion at unspecified level of thoracic spinal cord

[6th] S24.13 Anterior cord syndrome of thoracic spinal cord

[7th] S24.131 Anterior cord syndrome at T1 level of thoracic spinal cord

[7th] S24.132 Anterior cord syndrome at T2-T6 level of thoracic spinal cord

[7th] S24.133 Anterior cord syndrome at T7-T10 level of thoracic spinal cord

[7th] S24.134 Anterior cord syndrome at T11-T12 level of thoracic spinal cord

[7th] S24.139 Anterior cord syndrome at unspecified level of thoracic spinal cord

[6th] S24.14 Brown-Séquard syndrome of thoracic spinal cord

[7th] S24.141 Brown-Séquard syndrome at T1 level of thoracic spinal cord

[7th] S24.142 Brown-Séquard syndrome at T2-T6 level of thoracic spinal cord

[7th] S24.143 Brown-Séquard syndrome at T7-T10 level of thoracic spinal cord

[7th] S24.144 Brown-Séquard syndrome at T11-T12 level of thoracic spinal cord

[7th] S24.149 Brown-Séquard syndrome at unspecified level of thoracic spinal cord

[6th] S24.15 Other incomplete lesions of thoracic spinal cord
Incomplete lesion of thoracic spinal cord NOS
Posterior cord syndrome of thoracic spinal cord

[7th] S24.151 Other incomplete lesion at T1 level of thoracic spinal cord

[7th] S24.152 Other incomplete lesion at T2-T6 level of thoracic spinal cord

[7th] S24.153 Other incomplete lesion at T7-T10 level of thoracic spinal cord

[7th] S24.154 Other incomplete lesion at T11-T12 level of thoracic spinal cord

[7th] S24.159 Other incomplete lesion at unspecified level of thoracic spinal cord

[X] S24.2 Injury of nerve root of thoracic spine

[X] S24.3 Injury of peripheral nerves of thorax

[X] S24.4 Injury of thoracic sympathetic nervous system
Injury of cardiac plexus
Injury of esophageal plexus
Injury of pulmonary plexus
Injury of stellate ganglion
Injury of thoracic sympathetic ganglion

[X] S24.8 Injury of other specified nerves of thorax

[X] S24.9 Injury of unspecified nerve of thorax

[4th] **S25 Injury of blood vessels of thorax**

Code also any associated open wound (S21.-)

The appropriate 7th character is to be added to each code from category S25
A = initial encounter
D = subsequent encounter
S = sequela

[5th] S25.0 Injury of thoracic aorta
Injury of aorta NOS

[X] S25.00 Unspecified injury of thoracic aorta

[X] S25.01 Minor laceration of thoracic aorta
Incomplete transection of thoracic aorta
Laceration of thoracic aorta NOS
Superficial laceration of thoracic aorta

[X] S25.02 Major laceration of thoracic aorta
Complete transection of thoracic aorta
Traumatic rupture of thoracic aorta

[X] S25.09 Other specified injury of thoracic aorta

[5th] S25.1 Injury of innominate or subclavian artery

[6th] S25.10 Unspecified injury of innominate or subclavian artery

[7th] S25.101 Unspecified injury of right innominate or subclavian artery

[7th] S25.102 Unspecified injury of left innominate or subclavian artery

[7th] S25.109 Unspecified injury of unspecified innominate or subclavian artery

[6th] S25.11 Minor laceration of innominate or subclavian artery
Incomplete transection of innominate or subclavian artery
Laceration of innominate or subclavian artery NOS
Superficial laceration of innominate or subclavian artery

[7th] S25.111 Minor laceration of right innominate or subclavian artery

[7th] S25.112 Minor laceration of left innominate or subclavian artery

[7th] S25.119 Minor laceration of unspecified innominate or subclavian artery

[6th] S25.12 Major laceration of innominate or subclavian artery
Complete transection of innominate or subclavian artery
Traumatic rupture of innominate or subclavian artery

[7th] S25.121 Major laceration of right innominate or subclavian artery

[7th] S25.122 Major laceration of left innominate or subclavian artery

[4th] 4th character required [5th] 5th character required [6th] 6th character required [7th] 7th character required [X] Extension 'X' Alert
[EXCLUDES1] Not coded here [EXCLUDES2] Not included here [PDx] Primary Diagnosis Only Manifestation Code

[7th] S25.129 Major laceration of unspecified innominate or subclavian artery
[6th] S25.19 Other specified injury of innominate or subclavian artery
[7th] S25.191 Other specified injury of right innominate or subclavian artery
[7th] S25.192 Other specified injury of left innominate or subclavian artery
[7th] S25.199 Other specified injury of unspecified innominate or subclavian artery
[5th] S25.2 Injury of superior vena cava
Injury of vena cava NOS
[7th] S25.20 Unspecified injury of superior vena cava
[7th] S25.21 Minor laceration of superior vena cava
Incomplete transection of superior vena cava
Laceration of superior vena cava NOS
Superficial laceration of superior vena cava
[7th] S25.22 Major laceration of superior vena cava
Complete transection of superior vena cava
Traumatic rupture of superior vena cava
[7th] S25.29 Other specified injury of superior vena cava
[5th] S25.3 Injury of innominate or subclavian vein
[6th] S25.30 Unspecified injury of innominate or subclavian vein
[7th] S25.301 Unspecified injury of right innominate or subclavian vein
[7th] S25.302 Unspecified injury of left innominate or subclavian vein
[7th] S25.309 Unspecified injury of unspecified innominate or subclavian vein
[6th] S25.31 Minor laceration of innominate or subclavian vein
Incomplete transection of innominate or subclavian vein
Laceration of innominate or subclavian vein NOS
Superficial laceration of innominate or subclavian vein
[7th] S25.311 Minor laceration of right innominate or subclavian vein
[7th] S25.312 Minor laceration of left innominate or subclavian vein
[7th] S25.319 Minor laceration of unspecified innominate or subclavian vein
[6th] S25.32 Major laceration of innominate or subclavian vein
Complete transection of innominate or subclavian vein
Traumatic rupture of innominate or subclavian vein
[7th] S25.321 Major laceration of right innominate or subclavian vein
[7th] S25.322 Major laceration of left innominate or subclavian vein
[7th] S25.329 Major laceration of unspecified innominate or subclavian vein
[6th] S25.39 Other specified injury of innominate or subclavian vein
[7th] S25.391 Other specified injury of right innominate or subclavian vein
[7th] S25.392 Other specified injury of left innominate or subclavian vein
[7th] S25.399 Other specified injury of unspecified innominate or subclavian vein
[5th] S25.4 Injury of pulmonary blood vessels
[6th] S25.40 Unspecified injury of pulmonary blood vessels
[7th] S25.401 Unspecified injury of right pulmonary blood vessels
[7th] S25.402 Unspecified injury of left pulmonary blood vessels
[7th] S25.409 Unspecified injury of unspecified pulmonary blood vessels
[6th] S25.41 Minor laceration of pulmonary blood vessels
Incomplete transection of pulmonary blood vessels
Laceration of pulmonary blood vessels NOS
Superficial laceration of pulmonary blood vessels
[7th] S25.411 Minor laceration of right pulmonary blood vessels
[7th] S25.412 Minor laceration of left pulmonary blood vessels
[7th] S25.419 Minor laceration of unspecified pulmonary blood vessels
[6th] S25.42 Major laceration of pulmonary blood vessels
Complete transection of pulmonary blood vessels
Traumatic rupture of pulmonary blood vessels
[7th] S25.421 Major laceration of right pulmonary blood vessels
[7th] S25.422 Major laceration of left pulmonary blood vessels
[7th] S25.429 Major laceration of unspecified pulmonary blood vessels
[6th] S25.49 Other specified injury of pulmonary blood vessels
[7th] S25.491 Other specified injury of right pulmonary blood vessels
[7th] S25.492 Other specified injury of left pulmonary blood vessels
[7th] S25.499 Other specified injury of unspecified pulmonary blood vessels
[5th] S25.5 Injury of intercostal blood vessels
[6th] S25.50 Unspecified injury of intercostal blood vessels
[7th] S25.501 Unspecified injury of intercostal blood vessels, right side
[7th] S25.502 Unspecified injury of intercostal blood vessels, left side
[7th] S25.509 Unspecified injury of intercostal blood vessels, unspecified side
[6th] S25.51 Laceration of intercostal blood vessels
[7th] S25.511 Laceration of intercostal blood vessels, right side
[7th] S25.512 Laceration of intercostal blood vessels, left side
[7th] S25.519 Laceration of intercostal blood vessels, unspecified side
[6th] S25.59 Other specified injury of intercostal blood vessels
[7th] S25.591 Other specified injury of intercostal blood vessels, right side
[7th] S25.592 Other specified injury of intercostal blood vessels, left side
[7th] S25.599 Other specified injury of intercostal blood vessels, unspecified side
[5th] S25.8 Injury of other blood vessels of thorax
Injury of azygos vein
Injury of mammary artery or vein
[6th] S25.80 Unspecified injury of other blood vessels of thorax
[7th] S25.801 Unspecified injury of other blood vessels of thorax, right side
[7th] S25.802 Unspecified injury of other blood vessels of thorax, left side
[7th] S25.809 Unspecified injury of other blood vessels of thorax, unspecified side
[6th] S25.81 Laceration of other blood vessels of thorax
[7th] S25.811 Laceration of other blood vessels of thorax, right side

Unspecified Code | Other Specified Code | [N] Newborn Age: 0 | [P] Pediatric Age: 0-17 | [M] Maternity Age: 12-55
[A] Adult Age: 15-124 | ♂ Male | ♀ Female | ● New Code | ▲ Revised Code Title | ►◄ Revised Text

S25.812 Laceration of other blood vessels of thorax, left side

S25.819 Laceration of other blood vessels of thorax, unspecified side

S25.89 Other specified injury of other blood vessels of thorax

    S25.891 Other specified injury of other blood vessels of thorax, right side

    S25.892 Other specified injury of other blood vessels of thorax, left side

    S25.899 Other specified injury of other blood vessels of thorax, unspecified side

S25.9 Injury of unspecified blood vessel of thorax

    S25.90 Unspecified injury of unspecified blood vessel of thorax

    S25.91 Laceration of unspecified blood vessel of thorax

    S25.99 Other specified injury of unspecified blood vessel of thorax

S26 Injury of heart

Code also any associated:
open wound of thorax (S21.-)
traumatic hemopneumothorax (S27.2)
traumatic hemothorax (S27.1)
traumatic pneumothorax (S27.0)

The appropriate 7th character is to be added to each code from category S26
A = initial encounter
D = subsequent encounter
S = sequela

S26.0 Injury of heart with hemopericardium

    S26.00 Unspecified injury of heart with hemopericardium

    S26.01 Contusion of heart with hemopericardium

    S26.02 Laceration of heart with hemopericardium

        S26.020 Mild laceration of heart with hemopericardium

        Laceration of heart without penetration of heart chamber

        S26.021 Moderate laceration of heart with hemopericardium

        Laceration of heart with penetration of heart chamber

        S26.022 Major laceration of heart with hemopericardium

        Laceration of heart with penetration of multiple heart chambers

    S26.09 Other injury of heart with hemopericardium

S26.1 Injury of heart without hemopericardium

    S26.10 Unspecified injury of heart without hemopericardium

    S26.11 Contusion of heart without hemopericardium

    S26.12 Laceration of heart without hemopericardium

    S26.19 Other injury of heart without hemopericardium

S26.9 Injury of heart, unspecified with or without hemopericardium

    S26.90 Unspecified injury of heart, unspecified with or without hemopericardium

    S26.91 Contusion of heart, unspecified with or without hemopericardium

    S26.92 Laceration of heart, unspecified with or without hemopericardium

    Laceration of heart NOS

    S26.99 Other injury of heart, unspecified with or without hemopericardium

S27 Injury of other and unspecified intrathoracic organs

Code also any associated open wound of thorax (S21.-)

EXCLUDES2 injury of cervical esophagus (S10-S19)
                injury of trachea (cervical) (S10-S19)

The appropriate 7th character is to be added to each code from category S27
A = initial encounter
D = subsequent encounter
S = sequela

S27.0 Traumatic pneumothorax

    EXCLUDES1 spontaneous pneumothorax (J93.-)

S27.1 Traumatic hemothorax

S27.2 Traumatic hemopneumothorax

S27.3 Other and unspecified injuries of lung

    S27.30 Unspecified injury of lung

        S27.301 Unspecified injury of lung, unilateral

        S27.302 Unspecified injury of lung, bilateral

        S27.309 Unspecified injury of lung, unspecified

    S27.31 Primary blast injury of lung

        Blast injury of lung NOS

        S27.311 Primary blast injury of lung, unilateral

        S27.312 Primary blast injury of lung, bilateral

        S27.319 Primary blast injury of lung, unspecified

    S27.32 Contusion of lung

        S27.321 Contusion of lung, unilateral

        S27.322 Contusion of lung, bilateral

        S27.329 Contusion of lung, unspecified

    S27.33 Laceration of lung

        S27.331 Laceration of lung, unilateral

        S27.332 Laceration of lung, bilateral

        S27.339 Laceration of lung, unspecified

    S27.39 Other injuries of lung

        Secondary blast injury of lung

        S27.391 Other injuries of lung, unilateral

        S27.392 Other injuries of lung, bilateral

        S27.399 Other injuries of lung, unspecified

S27.4 Injury of bronchus

    S27.40 Unspecified injury of bronchus

        S27.401 Unspecified injury of bronchus, unilateral

        S27.402 Unspecified injury of bronchus, bilateral

        S27.409 Unspecified injury of bronchus, unspecified

    S27.41 Primary blast injury of bronchus

        Blast injury of bronchus NOS

        S27.411 Primary blast injury of bronchus, unilateral

        S27.412 Primary blast injury of bronchus, bilateral

        S27.419 Primary blast injury of bronchus, unspecified

    S27.42 Contusion of bronchus

        S27.421 Contusion of bronchus, unilateral

        S27.422 Contusion of bronchus, bilateral

        S27.429 Contusion of bronchus, unspecified

    S27.43 Laceration of bronchus

        S27.431 Laceration of bronchus, unilateral

        S27.432 Laceration of bronchus, bilateral

        S27.439 Laceration of bronchus, unspecified

    S27.49 Other injury of bronchus

        Secondary blast injury of bronchus

        S27.491 Other injury of bronchus, unilateral

        S27.492 Other injury of bronchus, bilateral

        S27.499 Other injury of bronchus, unspecified

S27.5 Injury of thoracic trachea

    S27.50 Unspecified injury of thoracic trachea

    S27.51 Primary blast injury of thoracic trachea

        Blast injury of thoracic trachea NOS

    S27.52 Contusion of thoracic trachea

    S27.53 Laceration of thoracic trachea

4️⃣ 4th character required   5️⃣ 5th character required   6️⃣ 6th character required   7️⃣ 7th character required   Extension 'X' Alert

EXCLUDES 1 Not coded here   EXCLUDES 2 Not included here   Pdx Primary Diagnosis Only   Manifestation Code

○7 S27.59 Other injury of thoracic trachea

　　Secondary blast injury of thoracic trachea

○5 S27.6 Injury of pleura

　○7 S27.60 Unspecified injury of pleura

　○7 S27.63 Laceration of pleura

　○7 S27.69 Other injury of pleura

○5 S27.8 Injury of other specified intrathoracic organs

　○6 S27.80 Injury of diaphragm

　　○7 S27.802 Contusion of diaphragm

　　○7 S27.803 Laceration of diaphragm

　　○7 S27.808 Other injury of diaphragm

　　○7 S27.809 Unspecified injury of diaphragm

　○6 S27.81 Injury of esophagus (thoracic part)

　　○7 S27.812 Contusion of esophagus (thoracic part)

　　○7 S27.813 Laceration of esophagus (thoracic part)

　　○7 S27.818 Other injury of esophagus (thoracic part)

　　○7 S27.819 Unspecified injury of esophagus (thoracic part)

　○6 S27.89 Injury of other specified intrathoracic organs

　　　Injury of lymphatic thoracic duct
　　　Injury of thymus gland

　　○7 S27.892 Contusion of other specified intrathoracic organs

　　○7 S27.893 Laceration of other specified intrathoracic organs

　　○7 S27.898 Other injury of other specified intrathoracic organs

　　○7 S27.899 Unspecified injury of other specified intrathoracic organs

○7 S27.9 Injury of unspecified intrathoracic organ

○4 S28 Crushing injury of thorax, and traumatic amputation of part of thorax

> The appropriate 7th character is to be added to each code from category S28
> A = initial encounter
> D = subsequent encounter
> S = sequela

○7 S28.0 Crushed chest

　　Use additional code for all associated injuries

　　EXCLUDES1 flail chest (S22.5)

○7 S28.1 Traumatic amputation (partial) of part of thorax, except breast

○5 S28.2 Traumatic amputation of breast

　○6 S28.21 Complete traumatic amputation of breast

　　Traumatic amputation of breast NOS

　　○7 S28.211 Complete traumatic amputation of right breast

　　○7 S28.212 Complete traumatic amputation of left breast

　　○7 S28.219 Complete traumatic amputation of unspecified breast

　○6 S28.22 Partial traumatic amputation of breast

　　○7 S28.221 Partial traumatic amputation of right breast

　　○7 S28.222 Partial traumatic amputation of left breast

　　○7 S28.229 Partial traumatic amputation of unspecified breast

○4 S29 Other and unspecified injuries of thorax

　　Code also any associated open wound (S21.-)

> The appropriate 7th character is to be added to each code from category S29
> A = initial encounter
> D = subsequent encounter
> S = sequela

○5 S29.0 Injury of muscle and tendon at thorax level

　○6 S29.00 Unspecified injury of muscle and tendon of thorax

　　○7 S29.001 Unspecified injury of muscle and tendon of front wall of thorax

　　○7 S29.002 Unspecified injury of muscle and tendon of back wall of thorax

　　○7 S29.009 Unspecified injury of muscle and tendon of unspecified wall of thorax

　○6 S29.01 Strain of muscle and tendon of thorax

　　○7 S29.011 Strain of muscle and tendon of front wall of thorax

　　○7 S29.012 Strain of muscle and tendon of back wall of thorax

　　○7 S29.019 Strain of muscle and tendon of unspecified wall of thorax

　○6 S29.02 Laceration of muscle and tendon of thorax

　　○7 S29.021 Laceration of muscle and tendon of front wall of thorax

　　○7 S29.022 Laceration of muscle and tendon of back wall of thorax

　　○7 S29.029 Laceration of muscle and tendon of unspecified wall of thorax

　○5 S29.09 Other injury of muscle and tendon of thorax

　　○7 S29.091 Other injury of muscle and tendon of front wall of thorax

　　○7 S29.092 Other injury of muscle and tendon of back wall of thorax

　　○7 S29.099 Other injury of muscle and tendon of unspecified wall of thorax

○7 S29.8 Other specified injuries of thorax

○7 S29.9 Unspecified injury of thorax

Injuries to the abdomen, lower back, lumbar spine, pelvis and external genitals (S30-S39)

INCLUDES　injuries to the abdominal wall
　　　　　injuries to the anus
　　　　　injuries to the buttock
　　　　　injuries to the external genitalia
　　　　　injuries to the flank
　　　　　injuries to the groin

EXCLUDES2　burns and corrosions (T20-T32)
　　　　　effects of foreign body in anus and rectum (T18.5)
　　　　　effects of foreign body in genitourinary tract (T19.-)
　　　　　effects of foreign body in stomach, small intestine and colon (T18.2-T18.4)
　　　　　frostbite (T33-T34)
　　　　　insect bite or sting, venomous (T63.4)

○4 S30 Superficial injury of abdomen, lower back, pelvis and external genitals

　　EXCLUDES2 superficial injury of hip (S70.-)

> The appropriate 7th character is to be added to each code from category S30
> A = initial encounter
> D = subsequent encounter
> S = sequela

○7 S30.0 Contusion of lower back and pelvis

　　Contusion of buttock

○7 S30.1 Contusion of abdominal wall

　　Contusion of flank
　　Contusion of groin

○5 S30.2 Contusion of external genital organs

　○6 S30.20 Contusion of unspecified external genital organ

　　○7 S30.201 Contusion of unspecified external genital organ, male

　　○7 S30.202 Contusion of unspecified external genital organ, female

　○7 S30.21 Contusion of penis

　○7 S30.22 Contusion of scrotum and testes

　○7 S30.23 Contusion of vagina and vulva

○7 S30.3 Contusion of anus

Unspecified Code	Other Specified Code	N Newborn Age: 0	P Pediatric Age: 0-17	M Maternity Age: 12-55	
A Adult Age: 15-124	♂ Male	♀ Female	● New Code	▲ Revised Code Title	►◄ Revised Text

[5th] S30.8 Other superficial injuries of abdomen, lower back, pelvis and external genitals
- [6th] S30.81 Abrasion of abdomen, lower back, pelvis and external genitals
  - [7th] S30.810 Abrasion of lower back and pelvis
  - [7th] S30.811 Abrasion of abdominal wall
  - [7th] S30.812 Abrasion of penis
  - [7th] S30.813 Abrasion of scrotum and testes
  - [7th] S30.814 Abrasion of vagina and vulva
  - [7th] S30.815 Abrasion of unspecified external genital organs, male
  - [7th] S30.816 Abrasion of unspecified external genital organs, female
  - [7th] S30.817 Abrasion of anus
- [6th] S30.82 Blister (nonthermal) of abdomen, lower back, pelvis and external genitals
  - [7th] S30.820 Blister (nonthermal) of lower back and pelvis
  - [7th] S30.821 Blister (nonthermal) of abdominal wall
  - [7th] S30.822 Blister (nonthermal) of penis
  - [7th] S30.823 Blister (nonthermal) of scrotum and testes
  - [7th] S30.824 Blister (nonthermal) of vagina and vulva
  - [7th] S30.825 Blister (nonthermal) of unspecified external genital organs, male
  - [7th] S30.826 Blister (nonthermal) of unspecified external genital organs, female
  - [7th] S30.827 Blister (nonthermal) of anus
- [6th] S30.84 External constriction of abdomen, lower back, pelvis and external genitals
  - [7th] S30.840 External constriction of lower back and pelvis
  - [7th] S30.841 External constriction of abdominal wall
  - [7th] S30.842 External constriction of penis

    Hair tourniquet syndrome of penis

    Use additional cause code to identify the constricting item (W49.0-)
  - [7th] S30.843 External constriction of scrotum and testes
  - [7th] S30.844 External constriction of vagina and vulva
  - [7th] S30.845 External constriction of unspecified external genital organs, male
  - [7th] S30.846 External constriction of unspecified external genital organs, female
- [6th] S30.85 Superficial foreign body of abdomen, lower back, pelvis and external genitals

  Splinter in the abdomen, lower back, pelvis and external genitals
  - [7th] S30.850 Superficial foreign body of lower back and pelvis
  - [7th] S30.851 Superficial foreign body of abdominal wall
  - [7th] S30.852 Superficial foreign body of penis
  - [7th] S30.853 Superficial foreign body of scrotum and testes
  - [7th] S30.854 Superficial foreign body of vagina and vulva
  - [7th] S30.855 Superficial foreign body of unspecified external genital organs, male
  - [7th] S30.856 Superficial foreign body of unspecified external genital organs, female
  - [7th] S30.857 Superficial foreign body of anus
- [6th] S30.86 Insect bite (nonvenomous) of abdomen, lower back, pelvis and external genitals
  - [7th] S30.860 Insect bite (nonvenomous) of lower back and pelvis
  - [7th] S30.861 Insect bite (nonvenomous) of abdominal wall
  - [7th] S30.862 Insect bite (nonvenomous) of penis
  - [7th] S30.863 Insect bite (nonvenomous) of scrotum and testes
  - [7th] S30.864 Insect bite (nonvenomous) of vagina and vulva
  - [7th] S30.865 Insect bite (nonvenomous) of unspecified external genital organs, male
  - [7th] S30.866 Insect bite (nonvenomous) of unspecified external genital organs, female
  - [7th] S30.867 Insect bite (nonvenomous) of anus
- [6th] S30.87 Other superficial bite of abdomen, lower back, pelvis and external genitals

  [EXCLUDES1] *open bite of abdomen, lower back, pelvis and external genitals (S31.05, S31.15, S31.25, S31.35, S31.45, S31.55)*
  - [7th] S30.870 Other superficial bite of lower back and pelvis
  - [7th] S30.871 Other superficial bite of abdominal wall
  - [7th] S30.872 Other superficial bite of penis
  - [7th] S30.873 Other superficial bite of scrotum and testes
  - [7th] S30.874 Other superficial bite of vagina and vulva
  - [7th] S30.875 Other superficial bite of unspecified external genital organs, male
  - [7th] S30.876 Other superficial bite of unspecified external genital organs, female
  - [7th] S30.877 Other superficial bite of anus

[5th] S30.9 Unspecified superficial injury of abdomen, lower back, pelvis and external genitals
- [7th] S30.91 Unspecified superficial injury of lower back and pelvis
- [7th] S30.92 Unspecified superficial injury of abdominal wall
- [7th] S30.93 Unspecified superficial injury of penis
- [7th] S30.94 Unspecified superficial injury of scrotum and testes
- [7th] S30.95 Unspecified superficial injury of vagina and vulva
- [7th] S30.96 Unspecified superficial injury of unspecified external genital organs, male
- [7th] S30.97 Unspecified superficial injury of unspecified external genital organs, female
- [7th] S30.98 Unspecified superficial injury of anus

[4th] S31 Open wound of abdomen, lower back, pelvis and external genitals

Code also any associated:
spinal cord injury (S24.0, S24.1-, S34.0-, S34.1-)
wound infection

[EXCLUDES1] *traumatic amputation of part of abdomen, lower back and pelvis (S38.2-, S38.3)*

[EXCLUDES2] *open wound of hip (S71.00-S71.02)*
open fracture of pelvis (S32.1--S32.9 with 7th character B)

The appropriate 7th character is to be added to each code from category S31
A = initial encounter
D = subsequent encounter
S = sequela

[5th] S31.0 Open wound of lower back and pelvis
- [6th] S31.00 Unspecified open wound of lower back and pelvis
  - [7th] S31.000 Unspecified open wound of lower back and pelvis without penetration into retroperitoneum

    Unspecified open wound of lower back and pelvis NOS
  - [7th] S31.001 Unspecified open wound of lower back and pelvis with penetration into retroperitoneum
- [6th] S31.01 Laceration without foreign body of lower back and pelvis
  - [7th] S31.010 Laceration without foreign body of lower back and pelvis without penetration into retroperitoneum

[4th] 4th character required [5th] 5th character required [6th] 6th character required [7th] 7th character required [7th] Extension 'X' Alert
[EXCLUDES1] Not coded here [EXCLUDES2] Not included here [PDx] Primary Diagnosis Only Manifestation Code

Laceration without foreign body of lower back and pelvis NOS

🟡 S31.011 Laceration without foreign body of lower back and pelvis with penetration into retroperitoneum

6️⃣ S31.02 Laceration with foreign body of lower back and pelvis

🟡 S31.020 Laceration with foreign body of lower back and pelvis without penetration into retroperitoneum

Laceration with foreign body of lower back and pelvis NOS

🟡 S31.021 Laceration with foreign body of lower back and pelvis with penetration into retroperitoneum

6️⃣ S31.03 Puncture wound without foreign body of lower back and pelvis

🟡 S31.030 Puncture wound without foreign body of lower back and pelvis without penetration into retroperitoneum

Puncture wound without foreign body of lower back and pelvis NOS

🟡 S31.031 Puncture wound without foreign body of lower back and pelvis with penetration into retroperitoneum

6️⃣ S31.04 Puncture wound with foreign body of lower back and pelvis

🟡 S31.040 Puncture wound with foreign body of lower back and pelvis without penetration into retroperitoneum

Puncture wound with foreign body of lower back and pelvis NOS

🟡 S31.041 Puncture wound with foreign body of lower back and pelvis with penetration into retroperitoneum

6️⃣ S31.05 Open bite of lower back and pelvis

Bite of lower back and pelvis NOS

EXCLUDES1 superficial bite of lower back and pelvis (S30.860, S30.870)

🟡 S31.050 Open bite of lower back and pelvis without penetration into retroperitoneum

Open bite of lower back and pelvis NOS

🟡 S31.051 Open bite of lower back and pelvis with penetration into retroperitoneum

5️⃣ S31.1 Open wound of abdominal wall without penetration into peritoneal cavity

Open wound of abdominal wall NOS

EXCLUDES2 open wound of abdominal wall with penetration into peritoneal cavity (S31.6-)

6️⃣ S31.10 Unspecified open wound of abdominal wall without penetration into peritoneal cavity

🟡 S31.100 Unspecified open wound of abdominal wall, right upper quadrant without penetration into peritoneal cavity

🟡 S31.101 Unspecified open wound of abdominal wall, left upper quadrant without penetration into peritoneal cavity

🟡 S31.102 Unspecified open wound of abdominal wall, epigastric region without penetration into peritoneal cavity

🟡 S31.103 Unspecified open wound of abdominal wall, right lower quadrant without penetration into peritoneal cavity

🟡 S31.104 Unspecified open wound of abdominal wall, left lower quadrant without penetration into peritoneal cavity

🟡 S31.105 Unspecified open wound of abdominal wall, periumbilic region without penetration into peritoneal cavity

🟡 S31.109 Unspecified open wound of abdominal wall, unspecified quadrant without penetration into peritoneal cavity

Unspecified open wound of abdominal wall NOS

6️⃣ S31.11 Laceration without foreign body of abdominal wall without penetration into peritoneal cavity

🟡 S31.110 Laceration without foreign body of abdominal wall, right upper quadrant without penetration into peritoneal cavity

🟡 S31.111 Laceration without foreign body of abdominal wall, left upper quadrant without penetration into peritoneal cavity

🟡 S31.112 Laceration without foreign body of abdominal wall, epigastric region without penetration into peritoneal cavity

🟡 S31.113 Laceration without foreign body of abdominal wall, right lower quadrant without penetration into peritoneal cavity

🟡 S31.114 Laceration without foreign body of abdominal wall, left lower quadrant without penetration into peritoneal cavity

🟡 S31.115 Laceration without foreign body of abdominal wall, periumbilic region without penetration into peritoneal cavity

🟡 S31.119 Laceration without foreign body of abdominal wall, unspecified quadrant without penetration into peritoneal cavity

6️⃣ S31.12 Laceration with foreign body of abdominal wall without penetration into peritoneal cavity

🟡 S31.120 Laceration of abdominal wall with foreign body, right upper quadrant without penetration into peritoneal cavity

🟡 S31.121 Laceration of abdominal wall with foreign body, left upper quadrant without penetration into peritoneal cavity

🟡 S31.122 Laceration of abdominal wall with foreign body, epigastric region without penetration into peritoneal cavity

🟡 S31.123 Laceration of abdominal wall with foreign body, right lower quadrant without penetration into peritoneal cavity

🟡 S31.124 Laceration of abdominal wall with foreign body, left lower quadrant without penetration into peritoneal cavity

🟡 S31.125 Laceration of abdominal wall with foreign body, periumbilic region without penetration into peritoneal cavity

🟡 S31.129 Laceration of abdominal wall with foreign body, unspecified quadrant without penetration into peritoneal cavity

6️⃣ S31.13 Puncture wound of abdominal wall without foreign body without penetration into peritoneal cavity

🟡 S31.130 Puncture wound of abdominal wall without foreign body, right upper quadrant without penetration into peritoneal cavity

🟡 S31.131 Puncture wound of abdominal wall without foreign body, left upper quadrant without penetration into peritoneal cavity

🟡 S31.132 Puncture wound of abdominal wall without foreign body, epigastric region without penetration into peritoneal cavity

🟡 S31.133 Puncture wound of abdominal wall without foreign body, right lower quadrant without penetration into peritoneal cavity

🟡 S31.134 Puncture wound of abdominal wall without foreign body, left lower quadrant without penetration into peritoneal cavity

🟡 S31.135 Puncture wound of abdominal wall without foreign body, periumbilic region without penetration into peritoneal cavity

Unspecified Code	Other Specified Code	Ⓝ Newborn Age: 0 Ⓟ Pediatric Age: 0-17 Ⓜ Maternity Age: 12-55
Ⓐ Adult Age: 15-124	♂ Male ♀ Female	● New Code ▲ Revised Code Title ►◄ Revised Text

7️⃣ **S31.139** Puncture wound of abdominal wall without foreign body, unspecified quadrant without penetration into peritoneal cavity

6️⃣ **S31.14** Puncture wound of abdominal wall with foreign body without penetration into peritoneal cavity

7️⃣ **S31.140** Puncture wound of abdominal wall with foreign body, right upper quadrant without penetration into peritoneal cavity

7️⃣ **S31.141** Puncture wound of abdominal wall with foreign body, left upper quadrant without penetration into peritoneal cavity

7️⃣ **S31.142** Puncture wound of abdominal wall with foreign body, epigastric region without penetration into peritoneal cavity

7️⃣ **S31.143** Puncture wound of abdominal wall with foreign body, right lower quadrant without penetration into peritoneal cavity

7️⃣ **S31.144** Puncture wound of abdominal wall with foreign body, left lower quadrant without penetration into peritoneal cavity

7️⃣ **S31.145** Puncture wound of abdominal wall with foreign body, periumbilic region without penetration into peritoneal cavity

7️⃣ **S31.149** Puncture wound of abdominal wall with foreign body, unspecified quadrant without penetration into peritoneal cavity

6️⃣ **S31.15** Open bite of abdominal wall without penetration into peritoneal cavity

Bite of abdominal wall NOS

EXCLUDES1 superficial bite of abdominal wall (S30.871)

7️⃣ **S31.150** Open bite of abdominal wall, right upper quadrant without penetration into peritoneal cavity

7️⃣ **S31.151** Open bite of abdominal wall, left upper quadrant without penetration into peritoneal cavity

7️⃣ **S31.152** Open bite of abdominal wall, epigastric region without penetration into peritoneal cavity

7️⃣ **S31.153** Open bite of abdominal wall, right lower quadrant without penetration into peritoneal cavity

7️⃣ **S31.154** Open bite of abdominal wall, left lower quadrant without penetration into peritoneal cavity

7️⃣ **S31.155** Open bite of abdominal wall, periumbilic region without penetration into peritoneal cavity

7️⃣ **S31.159** Open bite of abdominal wall, unspecified quadrant without penetration into peritoneal cavity

5️⃣ **S31.2** Open wound of penis

7️⃣ **S31.20** Unspecified open wound of penis

7️⃣ **S31.21** Laceration without foreign body of penis

7️⃣ **S31.22** Laceration with foreign body of penis

7️⃣ **S31.23** Puncture wound without foreign body of penis

7️⃣ **S31.24** Puncture wound with foreign body of penis

7️⃣ **S31.25** Open bite of penis

Bite of penis NOS

EXCLUDES1 superficial bite of penis (S30.862, S30.872)

5️⃣ **S31.3** Open wound of scrotum and testes

7️⃣ **S31.30** Unspecified open wound of scrotum and testes

7️⃣ **S31.31** Laceration without foreign body of scrotum and testes

7️⃣ **S31.32** Laceration with foreign body of scrotum and testes

7️⃣ **S31.33** Puncture wound without foreign body of scrotum and testes

7️⃣ **S31.34** Puncture wound with foreign body of scrotum and testes

7️⃣ **S31.35** Open bite of scrotum and testes

Bite of scrotum and testes NOS

EXCLUDES1 superficial bite of scrotum and testes (S30.863, S30.873)

5️⃣ **S31.4** Open wound of vagina and vulva

EXCLUDES1 injury to vagina and vulva during delivery (O70.-, O71.4)

7️⃣ **S31.40** Unspecified open wound of vagina and vulva

7️⃣ **S31.41** Laceration without foreign body of vagina and vulva

7️⃣ **S31.42** Laceration with foreign body of vagina and vulva

7️⃣ **S31.43** Puncture wound without foreign body of vagina and vulva

7️⃣ **S31.44** Puncture wound with foreign body of vagina and vulva

7️⃣ **S31.45** Open bite of vagina and vulva

Bite of vagina and vulva NOS

EXCLUDES1 superficial bite of vagina and vulva (S30.864, S30.874)

5️⃣ **S31.5** Open wound of unspecified external genital organs

EXCLUDES1 traumatic amputation of external genital organs (S38.21, S38.22)

6️⃣ **S31.50** Unspecified open wound of unspecified external genital organs

7️⃣ **S31.501** Unspecified open wound of unspecified external genital organs, male

7️⃣ **S31.502** Unspecified open wound of unspecified external genital organs, female

6️⃣ **S31.51** Laceration without foreign body of unspecified external genital organs

7️⃣ **S31.511** Laceration without foreign body of unspecified external genital organs, male

7️⃣ **S31.512** Laceration without foreign body of unspecified external genital organs, female

6️⃣ **S31.52** Laceration with foreign body of unspecified external genital organs

7️⃣ **S31.521** Laceration with foreign body of unspecified external genital organs, male

7️⃣ **S31.522** Laceration with foreign body of unspecified external genital organs, female

6️⃣ **S31.53** Puncture wound without foreign body of unspecified external genital organs

7️⃣ **S31.531** Puncture wound without foreign body of unspecified external genital organs, male

7️⃣ **S31.532** Puncture wound without foreign body of unspecified external genital organs, female

6️⃣ **S31.54** Puncture wound with foreign body of unspecified external genital organs

7️⃣ **S31.541** Puncture wound with foreign body of unspecified external genital organs, male

7️⃣ **S31.542** Puncture wound with foreign body of unspecified external genital organs, female

6️⃣ **S31.55** Open bite of unspecified external genital organs

Bite of unspecified external genital organs NOS

EXCLUDES1 superficial bite of unspecified external genital organs (S30.865, S30.866, S30.875, S30.876)

7️⃣ **S31.551** Open bite of unspecified external genital organs, male

7️⃣ **S31.552** Open bite of unspecified external genital organs, female

5️⃣ **S31.6** Open wound of abdominal wall with penetration into peritoneal cavity

6️⃣ **S31.60** Unspecified open wound of abdominal wall with penetration into peritoneal cavity

4️⃣ 4th character required   5️⃣ 5th character required   6️⃣ 6th character required   7️⃣ 7th character required   Ⓧ Extension 'X' Alert

EXCLUDES 1 Not coded here   *EXCLUDES 2* Not included here   Pᴅx Primary Diagnosis Only   Manifestation Code

566   ICD-10-CM 2015

- 7ᵈ **S31.600** Unspecified open wound of abdominal wall, right upper quadrant with penetration into peritoneal cavity
- 7ᵈ **S31.601** Unspecified open wound of abdominal wall, left upper quadrant with penetration into peritoneal cavity
- 7ᵈ **S31.602** Unspecified open wound of abdominal wall, epigastric region with penetration into peritoneal cavity
- 7ᵈ **S31.603** Unspecified open wound of abdominal wall, right lower quadrant with penetration into peritoneal cavity
- 7ᵈ **S31.604** Unspecified open wound of abdominal wall, left lower quadrant with penetration into peritoneal cavity
- 7ᵈ **S31.605** Unspecified open wound of abdominal wall, periumbilic region with penetration into peritoneal cavity
- 7ᵈ **S31.609** Unspecified open wound of abdominal wall, unspecified quadrant with penetration into peritoneal cavity
- 6ᵈ **S31.61** Laceration without foreign body of abdominal wall with penetration into peritoneal cavity
- 7ᵈ **S31.610** Laceration without foreign body of abdominal wall, right upper quadrant with penetration into peritoneal cavity
- 7ᵈ **S31.611** Laceration without foreign body of abdominal wall, left upper quadrant with penetration into peritoneal cavity
- 7ᵈ **S31.612** Laceration without foreign body of abdominal wall, epigastric region with penetration into peritoneal cavity
- 7ᵈ **S31.613** Laceration without foreign body of abdominal wall, right lower quadrant with penetration into peritoneal cavity
- 7ᵈ **S31.614** Laceration without foreign body of abdominal wall, left lower quadrant with penetration into peritoneal cavity
- 7ᵈ **S31.615** Laceration without foreign body of abdominal wall, periumbilic region with penetration into peritoneal cavity
- 7ᵈ **S31.619** Laceration without foreign body of abdominal wall, unspecified quadrant with penetration into peritoneal cavity
- 6ᵈ **S31.62** Laceration with foreign body of abdominal wall with penetration into peritoneal cavity
- 7ᵈ **S31.620** Laceration with foreign body of abdominal wall, right upper quadrant with penetration into peritoneal cavity
- 7ᵈ **S31.621** Laceration with foreign body of abdominal wall, left upper quadrant with penetration into peritoneal cavity
- 7ᵈ **S31.622** Laceration with foreign body of abdominal wall, epigastric region with penetration into peritoneal cavity
- 7ᵈ **S31.623** Laceration with foreign body of abdominal wall, right lower quadrant with penetration into peritoneal cavity
- 7ᵈ **S31.624** Laceration with foreign body of abdominal wall, left lower quadrant with penetration into peritoneal cavity
- 7ᵈ **S31.625** Laceration with foreign body of abdominal wall, periumbilic region with penetration into peritoneal cavity
- 7ᵈ **S31.629** Laceration with foreign body of abdominal wall, unspecified quadrant with penetration into peritoneal cavity
- 6ᵈ **S31.63** Puncture wound without foreign body of abdominal wall with penetration into peritoneal cavity

- 7ᵈ **S31.630** Puncture wound without foreign body of abdominal wall, right upper quadrant with penetration into peritoneal cavity
- 7ᵈ **S31.631** Puncture wound without foreign body of abdominal wall, left upper quadrant with penetration into peritoneal cavity
- 7ᵈ **S31.632** Puncture wound without foreign body of abdominal wall, epigastric region with penetration into peritoneal cavity
- 7ᵈ **S31.633** Puncture wound without foreign body of abdominal wall, right lower quadrant with penetration into peritoneal cavity
- 7ᵈ **S31.634** Puncture wound without foreign body of abdominal wall, left lower quadrant with penetration into peritoneal cavity
- 7ᵈ **S31.635** Puncture wound without foreign body of abdominal wall, periumbilic region with penetration into peritoneal cavity
- 7ᵈ **S31.639** Puncture wound without foreign body of abdominal wall, unspecified quadrant with penetration into peritoneal cavity
- 6ᵈ **S31.64** Puncture wound with foreign body of abdominal wall with penetration into peritoneal cavity
- 7ᵈ **S31.640** Puncture wound with foreign body of abdominal wall, right upper quadrant with penetration into peritoneal cavity
- 7ᵈ **S31.641** Puncture wound with foreign body of abdominal wall, left upper quadrant with penetration into peritoneal cavity
- 7ᵈ **S31.642** Puncture wound with foreign body of abdominal wall, epigastric region with penetration into peritoneal cavity
- 7ᵈ **S31.643** Puncture wound with foreign body of abdominal wall, right lower quadrant with penetration into peritoneal cavity
- 7ᵈ **S31.644** Puncture wound with foreign body of abdominal wall, left lower quadrant with penetration into peritoneal cavity
- 7ᵈ **S31.645** Puncture wound with foreign body of abdominal wall, periumbilic region with penetration into peritoneal cavity
- 7ᵈ **S31.649** Puncture wound with foreign body of abdominal wall, unspecified quadrant with penetration into peritoneal cavity
- 6ᵈ **S31.65** Open bite of abdominal wall with penetration into peritoneal cavity
  - EXCLUDES1 superficial bite of abdominal wall (S30.861, S30.871)
  - 7ᵈ **S31.650** Open bite of abdominal wall, right upper quadrant with penetration into peritoneal cavity
  - 7ᵈ **S31.651** Open bite of abdominal wall, left upper quadrant with penetration into peritoneal cavity
  - 7ᵈ **S31.652** Open bite of abdominal wall, epigastric region with penetration into peritoneal cavity
  - 7ᵈ **S31.653** Open bite of abdominal wall, right lower quadrant with penetration into peritoneal cavity
  - 7ᵈ **S31.654** Open bite of abdominal wall, left lower quadrant with penetration into peritoneal cavity
  - 7ᵈ **S31.655** Open bite of abdominal wall, periumbilic region with penetration into peritoneal cavity
  - 7ᵈ **S31.659** Open bite of abdominal wall, unspecified quadrant with penetration into peritoneal cavity

---

Unspecified Code Other Specified Code N Newborn Age: 0 P Pediatric Age: 0-17 M Maternity Age: 12-55
A Adult Age: 15-124 ♂ Male ♀ Female ● New Code ▲ Revised Code Title ►◄ Revised Text

[5th] S31.8 Open wound of other parts of abdomen, lower back and pelvis
- [6th] S31.80 Open wound of unspecified buttock
  - [7th] S31.801 Laceration without foreign body of unspecified buttock
  - [7th] S31.802 Laceration with foreign body of unspecified buttock
  - [7th] S31.803 Puncture wound without foreign body of unspecified buttock
  - [7th] S31.804 Puncture wound with foreign body of unspecified buttock
  - [7th] S31.805 Open bite of unspecified buttock
    Bite of buttock NOS
    EXCLUDES1 *superficial bite of buttock (S30.870)*
  - [7th] S31.809 Unspecified open wound of unspecified buttock
- [6th] S31.81 Open wound of right buttock
  - [7th] S31.811 Laceration without foreign body of right buttock
  - [7th] S31.812 Laceration with foreign body of right buttock
  - [7th] S31.813 Puncture wound without foreign body of right buttock
  - [7th] S31.814 Puncture wound with foreign body of right buttock
  - [7th] S31.815 Open bite of right buttock
    Bite of right buttock NOS
    EXCLUDES1 *superficial bite of buttock (S30.870)*
  - [7th] S31.819 Unspecified open wound of right buttock
- [6th] S31.82 Open wound of left buttock
  - [7th] S31.821 Laceration without foreign body of left buttock
  - [7th] S31.822 Laceration with foreign body of left buttock
  - [7th] S31.823 Puncture wound without foreign body of left buttock
  - [7th] S31.824 Puncture wound with foreign body of left buttock
  - [7th] S31.825 Open bite of left buttock
    Bite of left buttock NOS
    EXCLUDES1 *superficial bite of buttock (S30.870)*
  - [7th] S31.829 Unspecified open wound of left buttock
- [6th] S31.83 Open wound of anus
  - [7th] S31.831 Laceration without foreign body of anus
  - [7th] S31.832 Laceration with foreign body of anus
  - [7th] S31.833 Puncture wound without foreign body of anus
  - [7th] S31.834 Puncture wound with foreign body of anus
  - [7th] S31.835 Open bite of anus
    Bite of anus NOS
    EXCLUDES1 *superficial bite of anus (S30.877)*
  - [7th] S31.839 Unspecified open wound of anus

[4th] **S32 Fracture of lumbar spine and pelvis**

NOTES A fracture not indicated as displaced or nondisplaced should be coded to displaced
A fracture not indicated as opened or closed should be coded to closed

INCLUDES *fracture of lumbosacral neural arch*
fracture of lumbosacral spinous process
fracture of lumbosacral transverse process
fracture of lumbosacral vertebra
fracture of lumbosacral vertebral arch

Code first any associated spinal cord and spinal nerve injury (S34.-)

EXCLUDES1 *transection of abdomen (S38.3)*

EXCLUDES2 *fracture of hip NOS (S72.0-)*

The appropriate 7th character is to be added to each code from category S32
A = initial encounter for closed fracture
B = initial encounter for open fracture
D = subsequent encounter for fracture with routine healing
G = subsequent encounter for fracture with delayed healing
K = subsequent encounter for fracture with nonunion
S = sequela

[5th] S32.0 Fracture of lumbar vertebra
Fracture of lumbar spine NOS
- [6th] S32.00 Fracture of unspecified lumbar vertebra
  - [7th] S32.000 Wedge compression fracture of unspecified lumbar vertebra
  - [7th] S32.001 Stable burst fracture of unspecified lumbar vertebra
  - [7th] S32.002 Unstable burst fracture of unspecified lumbar vertebra
  - [7th] S32.008 Other fracture of unspecified lumbar vertebra
  - [7th] S32.009 Unspecified fracture of unspecified lumbar vertebra
- [6th] S32.01 Fracture of first lumbar vertebra
  - [7th] S32.010 Wedge compression fracture of first lumbar vertebra
  - [7th] S32.011 Stable burst fracture of first lumbar vertebra
  - [7th] S32.012 Unstable burst fracture of first lumbar vertebra
  - [7th] S32.018 Other fracture of first lumbar vertebra
  - [7th] S32.019 Unspecified fracture of first lumbar vertebra
- [6th] S32.02 Fracture of second lumbar vertebra
  - [7th] S32.020 Wedge compression fracture of second lumbar vertebra
  - [7th] S32.021 Stable burst fracture of second lumbar vertebra
  - [7th] S32.022 Unstable burst fracture of second lumbar vertebra
  - [7th] S32.028 Other fracture of second lumbar vertebra
  - [7th] S32.029 Unspecified fracture of second lumbar vertebra
- [6th] S32.03 Fracture of third lumbar vertebra
  - [7th] S32.030 Wedge compression fracture of third lumbar vertebra
  - [7th] S32.031 Stable burst fracture of third lumbar vertebra
  - [7th] S32.032 Unstable burst fracture of third lumbar vertebra
  - [7th] S32.038 Other fracture of third lumbar vertebra
  - [7th] S32.039 Unspecified fracture of third lumbar vertebra
- [6th] S32.04 Fracture of fourth lumbar vertebra
  - [7th] S32.040 Wedge compression fracture of fourth lumbar vertebra
  - [7th] S32.041 Stable burst fracture of fourth lumbar vertebra
  - [7th] S32.042 Unstable burst fracture of fourth lumbar vertebra
  - [7th] S32.048 Other fracture of fourth lumbar vertebra
  - [7th] S32.049 Unspecified fracture of fourth lumbar vertebra
- [6th] S32.05 Fracture of fifth lumbar vertebra
  - [7th] S32.050 Wedge compression fracture of fifth lumbar vertebra
  - [7th] S32.051 Stable burst fracture of fifth lumbar vertebra
  - [7th] S32.052 Unstable burst fracture of fifth lumbar vertebra

- [7th] S32.058 Other fracture of fifth lumbar vertebra
- [7th] S32.059 Unspecified fracture of fifth lumbar vertebra

[5th] S32.1 Fracture of sacrum
For vertical fractures, code to most medial fracture extension
Use two codes if both a vertical and transverse fracture are present
Code also any associated fracture of pelvic ring (S32.8-)

- [7th] S32.10 Unspecified fracture of sacrum
- [6th] S32.11 Zone I fracture of sacrum
  Vertical sacral ala fracture of sacrum
  - [7th] S32.110 Nondisplaced Zone I fracture of sacrum
  - [7th] S32.111 Minimally displaced Zone I fracture of sacrum
  - [7th] S32.112 Severely displaced Zone I fracture of sacrum
  - [7th] S32.119 Unspecified Zone I fracture of sacrum
- [6th] S32.12 Zone II fracture of sacrum
  Vertical foraminal region fracture of sacrum
  - [7th] S32.120 Nondisplaced Zone II fracture of sacrum
  - [7th] S32.121 Minimally displaced Zone II fracture of sacrum
  - [7th] S32.122 Severely displaced Zone II fracture of sacrum
  - [7th] S32.129 Unspecified Zone II fracture of sacrum
- [6th] S32.13 Zone III fracture of sacrum
  Vertical fracture into spinal canal region of sacrum
  - [7th] S32.130 Nondisplaced Zone III fracture of sacrum
  - [7th] S32.131 Minimally displaced Zone III fracture of sacrum
  - [7th] S32.132 Severely displaced Zone III fracture of sacrum
  - [7th] S32.139 Unspecified Zone III fracture of sacrum
- [7th] S32.14 Type 1 fracture of sacrum
  Transverse flexion fracture of sacrum without displacement
- [7th] S32.15 Type 2 fracture of sacrum
  Transverse flexion fracture of sacrum with posterior displacement
- [7th] S32.16 Type 3 fracture of sacrum
  Transverse extension fracture of sacrum with anterior displacement
- [7th] S32.17 Type 4 fracture of sacrum
  Transverse segmental comminution of upper sacrum
- [7th] S32.19 Other fracture of sacrum

[7th] S32.2 Fracture of coccyx

[5th] S32.3 Fracture of ilium
[EXCLUDES1] *fracture of ilium with associated disruption of pelvic ring (S32.8-)*

- [6th] S32.30 Unspecified fracture of ilium
  - [7th] S32.301 Unspecified fracture of right ilium
  - [7th] S32.302 Unspecified fracture of left ilium
  - [7th] S32.309 Unspecified fracture of unspecified ilium
- [6th] S32.31 Avulsion fracture of ilium
  - [7th] S32.311 Displaced avulsion fracture of right ilium
  - [7th] S32.312 Displaced avulsion fracture of left ilium
  - [7th] S32.313 Displaced avulsion fracture of unspecified ilium
  - [7th] S32.314 Nondisplaced avulsion fracture of right ilium
  - [7th] S32.315 Nondisplaced avulsion fracture of left ilium
  - [7th] S32.316 Nondisplaced avulsion fracture of unspecified ilium
- [6th] S32.39 Other fracture of ilium
  - [7th] S32.391 Other fracture of right ilium
  - [7th] S32.392 Other fracture of left ilium
  - [7th] S32.399 Other fracture of unspecified ilium

[5th] S32.4 Fracture of acetabulum
Code also any associated fracture of pelvic ring (S32.8-)

- [6th] S32.40 Unspecified fracture of acetabulum
  - [7th] S32.401 Unspecified fracture of right acetabulum
  - [7th] S32.402 Unspecified fracture of left acetabulum
  - [7th] S32.409 Unspecified fracture of unspecified acetabulum
- [6th] S32.41 Fracture of anterior wall of acetabulum
  - [7th] S32.411 Displaced fracture of anterior wall of right acetabulum
  - [7th] S32.412 Displaced fracture of anterior wall of left acetabulum
  - [7th] S32.413 Displaced fracture of anterior wall of unspecified acetabulum
  - [7th] S32.414 Nondisplaced fracture of anterior wall of right acetabulum
  - [7th] S32.415 Nondisplaced fracture of anterior wall of left acetabulum
  - [7th] S32.416 Nondisplaced fracture of anterior wall of unspecified acetabulum
- [6th] S32.42 Fracture of posterior wall of acetabulum
  - [7th] S32.421 Displaced fracture of posterior wall of right acetabulum
  - [7th] S32.422 Displaced fracture of posterior wall of left acetabulum
  - [7th] S32.423 Displaced fracture of posterior wall of unspecified acetabulum
  - [7th] S32.424 Nondisplaced fracture of posterior wall of right acetabulum
  - [7th] S32.425 Nondisplaced fracture of posterior wall of left acetabulum
  - [7th] S32.426 Nondisplaced fracture of posterior wall of unspecified acetabulum
- [6th] S32.43 Fracture of anterior column [iliopubic] of acetabulum
  - [7th] S32.431 Displaced fracture of anterior column [iliopubic] of right acetabulum
  - [7th] S32.432 Displaced fracture of anterior column [iliopubic] of left acetabulum
  - [7th] S32.433 Displaced fracture of anterior column [iliopubic] of unspecified acetabulum
  - [7th] S32.434 Nondisplaced fracture of anterior column [iliopubic] of right acetabulum
  - [7th] S32.435 Nondisplaced fracture of anterior column [iliopubic] of left acetabulum
  - [7th] S32.436 Nondisplaced fracture of anterior column [iliopubic] of unspecified acetabulum
- [6th] S32.44 Fracture of posterior column [ilioischial] of acetabulum
  - [7th] S32.441 Displaced fracture of posterior column [ilioischial] of right acetabulum
  - [7th] S32.442 Displaced fracture of posterior column [ilioischial] of left acetabulum
  - [7th] S32.443 Displaced fracture of posterior column [ilioischial] of unspecified acetabulum
  - [7th] S32.444 Nondisplaced fracture of posterior column [ilioischial] of right acetabulum
  - [7th] S32.445 Nondisplaced fracture of posterior column [ilioischial] of left acetabulum
  - [7th] S32.446 Nondisplaced fracture of posterior column [ilioischial] of unspecified acetabulum
- [6th] S32.45 Transverse fracture of acetabulum
  - [7th] S32.451 Displaced transverse fracture of right acetabulum
  - [7th] S32.452 Displaced transverse fracture of left acetabulum
  - [7th] S32.453 Displaced transverse fracture of unspecified acetabulum

S32.454 Nondisplaced transverse fracture of right acetabulum

S32.455 Nondisplaced transverse fracture of left acetabulum

S32.456 Nondisplaced transverse fracture of unspecified acetabulum

S32.46 Associated transverse-posterior fracture of acetabulum

S32.461 Displaced associated transverse-posterior fracture of right acetabulum

S32.462 Displaced associated transverse-posterior fracture of left acetabulum

S32.463 Displaced associated transverse-posterior fracture of unspecified acetabulum

S32.464 Nondisplaced associated transverse-posterior fracture of right acetabulum

S32.465 Nondisplaced associated transverse-posterior fracture of left acetabulum

S32.466 Nondisplaced associated transverse-posterior fracture of unspecified acetabulum

S32.47 Fracture of medial wall of acetabulum

S32.471 Displaced fracture of medial wall of right acetabulum

S32.472 Displaced fracture of medial wall of left acetabulum

S32.473 Displaced fracture of medial wall of unspecified acetabulum

S32.474 Nondisplaced fracture of medial wall of right acetabulum

S32.475 1 fracture of medial wall of left acetabulum

S32.476 Nondisplaced fracture of medial wall of unspecified acetabulum

S32.48 Dome fracture of acetabulum

S32.481 Displaced dome fracture of right acetabulum

S32.482 Displaced dome fracture of left acetabulum

S32.483 Displaced dome fracture of unspecified acetabulum

S32.484 Nondisplaced dome fracture of right acetabulum

S32.485 Nondisplaced dome fracture of left acetabulum

S32.486 Nondisplaced dome fracture of unspecified acetabulum

S32.49 Other specified fracture of acetabulum

S32.491 Other specified fracture of right acetabulum

S32.492 Other specified fracture of left acetabulum

S32.499 Other specified fracture of unspecified acetabulum

S32.5 Fracture of pubis

EXCLUDES1 fracture of pubis with associated disruption of pelvic ring (S32.8-)

S32.50 Unspecified fracture of pubis

S32.501 Unspecified fracture of right pubis

S32.502 Unspecified fracture of left pubis

S32.509 Unspecified fracture of unspecified pubis

S32.51 Fracture of superior rim of pubis

S32.511 Fracture of superior rim of right pubis

S32.512 Fracture of superior rim of left pubis

S32.519 Fracture of superior rim of unspecified pubis

S32.59 Other specified fracture of pubis

S32.591 Other specified fracture of right pubis

S32.592 Other specified fracture of left pubis

S32.599 Other specified fracture of unspecified pubis

S32.6 Fracture of ischium

EXCLUDES1 fracture of ischium with associated disruption of pelvic ring (S32.8-)

S32.60 Unspecified fracture of ischium

S32.601 Unspecified fracture of right ischium

S32.602 Unspecified fracture of left ischium

S32.609 Unspecified fracture of unspecified ischium

S32.61 Avulsion fracture of ischium

S32.611 Displaced avulsion fracture of right ischium

S32.612 Displaced avulsion fracture of left ischium

S32.613 Displaced avulsion fracture of unspecified ischium

S32.614 Nondisplaced avulsion fracture of right ischium

S32.615 Nondisplaced avulsion fracture of left ischium

S32.616 Nondisplaced avulsion fracture of unspecified ischium

S32.69 Other specified fracture of ischium

S32.691 Other specified fracture of right ischium

S32.692 Other specified fracture of left ischium

S32.699 Other specified fracture of unspecified ischium

S32.8 Fracture of other parts of pelvis

Code also any associated:
fracture of acetabulum (S32.4-)
sacral fracture (S32.1-)

S32.81 Multiple fractures of pelvis with disruption of pelvic ring

Multiple pelvic fractures with disruption of pelvic circle

S32.810 Multiple fractures of pelvis with stable disruption of pelvic ring

S32.811 Multiple fractures of pelvis with unstable disruption of pelvic ring

S32.82 Multiple fractures of pelvis without disruption of pelvic ring

Multiple pelvic fractures without disruption of pelvic circle

S32.89 Fracture of other parts of pelvis

S32.9 Fracture of unspecified parts of lumbosacral spine and pelvis

Fracture of lumbosacral spine NOS
Fracture of pelvis NOS

S33 Dislocation and sprain of joints and ligaments of lumbar spine and pelvis

INCLUDES avulsion of joint or ligament of lumbar spine and pelvis
laceration of cartilage, joint or ligament of lumbar spine and pelvis
sprain of cartilage, joint or ligament of lumbar spine and pelvis
traumatic hemarthrosis of joint or ligament of lumbar spine and pelvis
traumatic rupture of joint or ligament of lumbar spine and pelvis
traumatic subluxation of joint or ligament of lumbar spine and pelvis
traumatic tear of joint or ligament of lumbar spine and pelvis

Code also any associated open wound

EXCLUDES1 nontraumatic rupture or displacement of lumbar intervertebral disc NOS (M51.-)
obstetric damage to pelvic joints and ligaments (O71.6)

EXCLUDES2 dislocation and sprain of joints and ligaments of hip (S73.-)
strain of muscle of lower back and pelvis (S39.01-)

4th character required   5th character required   6th character required   7th character required   Extension 'X' Alert
EXCLUDES1 Not coded here   EXCLUDES2 Not included here   Primary Diagnosis Only   Manifestation Code

The appropriate 7th character is to be added to each code from category S33
A = initial encounter
D = subsequent encounter
S = sequela

S33.0 Traumatic rupture of lumbar intervertebral disc
> EXCLUDES1 rupture or displacement (nontraumatic) of lumbar intervertebral disc NOS (M51.- with fifth character 6)

S33.1 Subluxation and dislocation of lumbar vertebra
> Code also any associated:
> open wound of abdomen, lower back and pelvis (S31)
> spinal cord injury (S24.0, S24.1-, S34.0-, S34.1-)
> EXCLUDES2 fracture of lumbar vertebrae (S32.0-)

S33.10 Subluxation and dislocation of unspecified lumbar vertebra
> S33.100 Subluxation of unspecified lumbar vertebra
> S33.101 Dislocation of unspecified lumbar vertebra

S33.11 Subluxation and dislocation of L1/L2 lumbar vertebra
> S33.110 Subluxation of L1/L2 lumbar vertebra
> S33.111 Dislocation of L1/L2 lumbar vertebra

S33.12 Subluxation and dislocation of L2/L3 lumbar vertebra
> S33.120 Subluxation of L2/L3 lumbar vertebra
> S33.121 Dislocation of L2/L3 lumbar vertebra

S33.13 Subluxation and dislocation of L3/L4 lumbar vertebra
> S33.130 Subluxation of L3/L4 lumbar vertebra
> S33.131 Dislocation of L3/L4 lumbar vertebra

S33.14 Subluxation and dislocation of L4/L5 lumbar vertebra
> S33.140 Subluxation of L4/L5 lumbar vertebra
> S33.141 Dislocation of L4/L5 lumbar vertebra

S33.2 Dislocation of sacroiliac and sacrococcygeal joint

S33.3 Dislocation of other and unspecified parts of lumbar spine and pelvis
> S33.30 Dislocation of unspecified parts of lumbar spine and pelvis
> S33.39 Dislocation of other parts of lumbar spine and pelvis

S33.4 Traumatic rupture of symphysis pubis
S33.5 Sprain of ligaments of lumbar spine
S33.6 Sprain of sacroiliac joint
S33.8 Sprain of other parts of lumbar spine and pelvis
S33.9 Sprain of unspecified parts of lumbar spine and pelvis

S34 Injury of lumbar and sacral spinal cord and nerves at abdomen, lower back and pelvis level
> NOTES Code to highest level of lumbar cord injury.
> Injuries to the spinal cord (S34.0 and S34.1) refer to the cord level and not bone level injury, and can affect nerve roots at and below the level given.
> Code also any associated:
> fracture of vertebra (S22.0-, S32.0-)
> open wound of abdomen, lower back and pelvis (S31.-)
> transient paralysis (R29.5)
>
> The appropriate 7th character is to be added to each code from category S34
> A = initial encounter
> D = subsequent encounter
> S = sequela

S34.0 Concussion and edema of lumbar and sacral spinal cord
> S34.01 Concussion and edema of lumbar spinal cord
> S34.02 Concussion and edema of sacral spinal cord
> > Concussion and edema of conus medullaris

S34.1 Other and unspecified injury of lumbar and sacral spinal cord

S34.10 Unspecified injury to lumbar spinal cord
> S34.101 Unspecified injury to L1 level of lumbar spinal cord
> S34.102 Unspecified injury to L2 level of lumbar spinal cord
> S34.103 Unspecified injury to L3 level of lumbar spinal cord
> S34.104 Unspecified injury to L4 level of lumbar spinal cord
> S34.105 Unspecified injury to L5 level of lumbar spinal cord
> S34.109 Unspecified injury to unspecified level of lumbar spinal cord

S34.11 Complete lesion of lumbar spinal cord
> S34.111 Complete lesion of L1 level of lumbar spinal cord
> S34.112 Complete lesion of L2 level of lumbar spinal cord
> S34.113 Complete lesion of L3 level of lumbar spinal cord
> S34.114 Complete lesion of L4 level of lumbar spinal cord
> S34.115 Complete lesion of L5 level of lumbar spinal cord
> S34.119 Complete lesion of unspecified level of lumbar spinal cord

S34.12 Incomplete lesion of lumbar spinal cord
> S34.121 Incomplete lesion of L1 level of lumbar spinal cord
> S34.122 Incomplete lesion of L2 level of lumbar spinal cord
> S34.123 Incomplete lesion of L3 level of lumbar spinal cord
> S34.124 Incomplete lesion of L4 level of lumbar spinal cord
> S34.125 Incomplete lesion of L5 level of lumbar spinal cord
> S34.129 Incomplete lesion of unspecified level of lumbar spinal cord

S34.13 Other and unspecified injury to sacral spinal cord
> Other injury to conus medullaris
> S34.131 Complete lesion of sacral spinal cord
> > Complete lesion of conus medullaris
> S34.132 Incomplete lesion of sacral spinal cord
> > Incomplete lesion of conus medullaris
> S34.139 Unspecified injury to sacral spinal cord
> > Unspecified injury of conus medullaris

S34.2 Injury of nerve root of lumbar and sacral spine
> S34.21 Injury of nerve root of lumbar spine
> S34.22 Injury of nerve root of sacral spine

S34.3 Injury of cauda equina
S34.4 Injury of lumbosacral plexus
S34.5 Injury of lumbar, sacral and pelvic sympathetic nerves
> Injury of celiac ganglion or plexus
> Injury of hypogastric plexus
> Injury of mesenteric plexus (inferior) (superior)
> Injury of splanchnic nerve

S34.6 Injury of peripheral nerve(s) at abdomen, lower back and pelvis level
S34.8 Injury of other nerves at abdomen, lower back and pelvis level
S34.9 Injury of unspecified nerves at abdomen, lower back and pelvis level

---

Unspecified Code | Other Specified Code | N Newborn Age: 0 | P Pediatric Age: 0-17 | M Maternity Age: 12-55
A Adult Age: 15-124 | ♂ Male | ♀ Female | ● New Code | ▲ Revised Code Title | ►◄ Revised Text

S35   **Injury of blood vessels at abdomen, lower back and pelvis level**

Code also any associated open wound (S31.-)

The appropriate 7th character is to be added to each code from category S35
A = initial encounter
D = subsequent encounter
S = sequela

S35.0   **Injury of** abdominal aorta

    EXCLUDES1   injury of aorta NOS (S25.0)

S35.00   **Unspecified injury of abdominal aorta**

S35.01   Minor laceration **of abdominal aorta**

    Incomplete transection of abdominal aorta
    Laceration of abdominal aorta NOS
    Superficial laceration of abdominal aorta

S35.02   Major laceration **of abdominal aorta**

    Complete transection of abdominal aorta
    Traumatic rupture of abdominal aorta

S35.09   **Other injury of abdominal aorta**

S35.1   **Injury of inferior vena cava**

    Injury of hepatic vein

    EXCLUDES1   injury of vena cava NOS (S25.2)

S35.10   **Unspecified injury of inferior vena cava**

S35.11   Minor laceration **of inferior vena cava**

    Incomplete transection of inferior vena cava
    Laceration of inferior vena cava NOS
    Superficial laceration of inferior vena cava

S35.12   Major laceration **of inferior vena cava**

    Complete transection of inferior vena cava
    Traumatic rupture of inferior vena cava

S35.19   **Other injury of inferior vena cava**

S35.2   **Injury of** celiac or mesenteric artery **and branches**

S35.21   **Injury of celiac artery**

S35.211   Minor laceration **of celiac artery**

    Incomplete transection of celiac artery
    Laceration of celiac artery NOS
    Superficial laceration of celiac artery

S35.212   Major laceration **of celiac artery**

    Complete transection of celiac artery
    Traumatic rupture of celiac artery

S35.218   **Other injury of celiac artery**

S35.219   **Unspecified injury of celiac artery**

S35.22   **Injury of** superior mesenteric artery

S35.221   Minor laceration **of superior mesenteric artery**

    Incomplete transection of superior mesenteric artery
    Laceration of superior mesenteric artery NOS
    Superficial laceration of superior mesenteric artery

S35.222   Major laceration **of superior mesenteric artery**

    Complete transection of superior mesenteric artery
    Traumatic rupture of superior mesenteric artery

S35.228   **Other injury of superior mesenteric artery**

S35.229   **Unspecified injury of superior mesenteric artery**

S35.23   **Injury of** inferior mesenteric artery

S35.231   Minor laceration **of inferior mesenteric artery**

    Incomplete transection of inferior mesenteric artery
    Laceration of inferior mesenteric artery NOS
    Superficial laceration of inferior mesenteric artery

S35.232   Major laceration **of inferior mesenteric artery**

    Complete transection of inferior mesenteric artery
    Traumatic rupture of inferior mesenteric artery

S35.238   **Other injury of inferior mesenteric artery**

S35.239   **Unspecified injury of inferior mesenteric artery**

S35.29   **Injury of** branches of celiac and mesenteric artery

    Injury of gastric artery
    Injury of gastroduodenal artery
    Injury of hepatic artery
    Injury of splenic artery

S35.291   Minor laceration **of branches of celiac and mesenteric artery**

    Incomplete transection of branches of celiac and mesenteric artery
    Laceration of branches of celiac and mesenteric artery NOS
    Superficial laceration of branches of celiac and mesenteric artery

S35.292   Major laceration **of branches of celiac and mesenteric artery**

    Complete transection of branches of celiac and mesenteric artery
    Traumatic rupture of branches of celiac and mesenteric artery

S35.298   **Other injury of branches of celiac and mesenteric artery**

S35.299   **Unspecified injury of branches of celiac and mesenteric artery**

S35.3   **Injury of** portal or splenic **vein and branches**

S35.31   **Injury of** portal vein

S35.311   Laceration **of portal vein**

S35.318   **Other specified injury of portal vein**

S35.319   **Unspecified injury of portal vein**

S35.32   **Injury of** splenic vein

S35.321   Laceration **of splenic vein**

S35.328   **Other specified injury of splenic vein**

S35.329   **Unspecified injury of splenic vein**

S35.33   **Injury of** superior mesenteric vein

S35.331   Laceration **of superior mesenteric vein**

S35.338   **Other specified injury of superior mesenteric vein**

S35.339   **Unspecified injury of superior mesenteric vein**

S35.34   **Injury of** inferior mesenteric vein

S35.341   Laceration **of inferior mesenteric vein**

S35.348   **Other specified injury of inferior mesenteric vein**

S35.349   **Unspecified injury of inferior mesenteric vein**

S35.4   **Injury of** renal **blood vessels**

S35.40   Unspecified **injury of renal blood vessel**

S35.401   **Unspecified injury of** right **renal** artery

S35.402   **Unspecified injury of** left **renal** artery

S35.403   **Unspecified injury of unspecified renal** artery

S35.404   **Unspecified injury of** right **renal** vein

S35.405   **Unspecified injury of** left **renal** vein

S35.406   **Unspecified injury of unspecified renal** vein

S35.41   Laceration **of renal blood vessel**

S35.411   **Laceration of** right **renal** artery

S35.412   **Laceration of** left **renal** artery

S35.413   **Laceration of unspecified renal** artery

---

④ 4ᵗʰ character required   ⑤ 5ᵗʰ character required   ⑥ 6ᵗʰ character required   ⑦ 7ᵗʰ character required   ⑦ Extension 'X' Alert

EXCLUDES 1 Not coded here   *EXCLUDES 2* Not included here   PDx Primary Diagnosis Only   Manifestation Code

[7th] S35.414 Laceration of right renal vein
[7th] S35.415 Laceration of left renal vein
[7th] S35.416 Laceration of unspecified renal vein
[6th] S35.49 Other specified injury of renal blood vessel
[7th] S35.491 Other specified injury of right renal artery
[7th] S35.492 Other specified injury of left renal artery
[7th] S35.493 Other specified injury of unspecified renal artery
[7th] S35.494 Other specified injury of right renal vein
[7th] S35.495 Other specified injury of left renal vein
[7th] S35.496 Other specified injury of unspecified renal vein
[5th] S35.5 Injury of iliac blood vessels
[7th] S35.50 Injury of unspecified iliac blood vessel(s)
[6th] S35.51 Injury of iliac artery or vein
Injury of hypogastric artery or vein
[7th] S35.511 Injury of right iliac artery
[7th] S35.512 Injury of left iliac artery
[7th] S35.513 Injury of unspecified iliac artery
[7th] S35.514 Injury of right iliac vein
[7th] S35.515 Injury of left iliac vein
[7th] S35.516 Injury of unspecified iliac vein
[6th] S35.53 Injury of uterine artery or vein
[7th] S35.531 Injury of right uterine artery
[7th] S35.532 Injury of left uterine artery
[7th] S35.533 Injury of unspecified uterine artery
[7th] S35.534 Injury of right uterine vein
[7th] S35.535 Injury of left uterine vein
[7th] S35.536 Injury of unspecified uterine vein
[7th] S35.59 Injury of other iliac blood vessels
[5th] S35.8 Injury of other blood vessels at abdomen, lower back and pelvis level
Injury of ovarian artery or vein
[6th] S35.8X Injury of other blood vessels at abdomen, lower back and pelvis level
[7th] S35.8X1 Laceration of other blood vessels at abdomen, lower back and pelvis level
[7th] S35.8X8 Other specified injury of other blood vessels at abdomen, lower back and pelvis level
[7th] S35.8X9 Unspecified injury of other blood vessels at abdomen, lower back and pelvis level
[5th] S35.9 Injury of unspecified blood vessel at abdomen, lower back and pelvis level
[7th] S35.90 Unspecified injury of unspecified blood vessel at abdomen, lower back and pelvis level
[7th] S35.91 Laceration of unspecified blood vessel at abdomen, lower back and pelvis level
[7th] S35.99 Other specified injury of unspecified blood vessel at abdomen, lower back and pelvis level
[4th] S36 Injury of intra-abdominal organs
Code also any associated open wound (S31.-)
The appropriate 7th character is to be added to each code from category S36
A = initial encounter
D = subsequent encounter
S = sequela
[5th] S36.0 Injury of spleen
[7th] S36.00 Unspecified injury of spleen
[6th] S36.02 Contusion of spleen
[7th] S36.020 Minor contusion of spleen
Contusion of spleen less than 2 cm
[7th] S36.021 Major contusion of spleen
Contusion of spleen greater than 2 cm
[7th] S36.029 Unspecified contusion of spleen
[6th] S36.03 Laceration of spleen
[7th] S36.030 Superficial (capsular) laceration of spleen
Laceration of spleen less than 1 cm
Minor laceration of spleen
[7th] S36.031 Moderate laceration of spleen
Laceration of spleen 1 to 3 cm
[7th] S36.032 Major laceration of spleen
Avulsion of spleen
Laceration of spleen greater than 3 cm
Massive laceration of spleen
Multiple moderate lacerations of spleen
Stellate laceration of spleen
[7th] S36.039 Unspecified laceration of spleen
[7th] S36.09 Other injury of spleen
[5th] S36.1 Injury of liver and gallbladder and bile duct
[6th] S36.11 Injury of liver
[7th] S36.112 Contusion of liver
[7th] S36.113 Laceration of liver, unspecified degree
[7th] S36.114 Minor laceration of liver
Laceration involving capsule only, or, without significant involvement of hepatic parenchyma [i.e., less than 1 cm deep]
[7th] S36.115 Moderate laceration of liver
Laceration involving parenchyma but without major disruption of parenchyma [i.e., less than 10 cm long and less than 3 cm deep]
[7th] S36.116 Major laceration of liver
Laceration with significant disruption of hepatic parenchyma [i.e., greater than 10 cm long and 3 cm deep]
Multiple moderate lacerations, with or without hematoma
Stellate laceration of liver
[7th] S36.118 Other injury of liver
[7th] S36.119 Unspecified injury of liver
[6th] S36.12 Injury of gallbladder
[7th] S36.122 Contusion of gallbladder
[7th] S36.123 Laceration of gallbladder
[7th] S36.128 Other injury of gallbladder
[7th] S36.129 Unspecified injury of gallbladder
[7th] S36.13 Injury of bile duct
[5th] S36.2 Injury of pancreas
[6th] S36.20 Unspecified injury of pancreas
[7th] S36.200 Unspecified injury of head of pancreas
[7th] S36.201 Unspecified injury of body of pancreas
[7th] S36.202 Unspecified injury of tail of pancreas
[7th] S36.209 Unspecified injury of unspecified part of pancreas
[6th] S36.22 Contusion of pancreas
[7th] S36.220 Contusion of head of pancreas
[7th] S36.221 Contusion of body of pancreas
[7th] S36.222 Contusion of tail of pancreas
[7th] S36.229 Contusion of unspecified part of pancreas
[6th] S36.23 Laceration of pancreas, unspecified degree
[7th] S36.230 Laceration of head of pancreas, unspecified degree
[7th] S36.231 Laceration of body of pancreas, unspecified degree
[7th] S36.232 Laceration of tail of pancreas, unspecified degree
[7th] S36.239 Laceration of unspecified part of pancreas, unspecified degree
[6th] S36.24 Minor laceration of pancreas
[7th] S36.240 Minor laceration of head of pancreas
[7th] S36.241 Minor laceration of body of pancreas
[7th] S36.242 Minor laceration of tail of pancreas
[7th] S36.249 Minor laceration of unspecified part of pancreas
[6th] S36.25 Moderate laceration of pancreas

Unspecified Code | Other Specified Code | [N] Newborn Age: 0 | [P] Pediatric Age: 0-17 | [M] Maternity Age: 12-55
[A] Adult Age: 15-124 | ♂ Male | ♀ Female | ● New Code | ▲ Revised Code Title | ►◄ Revised Text

S36.250 Moderate laceration of head of pancreas
S36.251 Moderate laceration of body of pancreas
S36.252 Moderate laceration of tail of pancreas
S36.259 Moderate laceration of unspecified part of pancreas

S36.26 Major laceration of pancreas
S36.260 Major laceration of head of pancreas
S36.261 Major laceration of body of pancreas
S36.262 Major laceration of tail of pancreas
S36.269 Major laceration of unspecified part of pancreas

S36.29 Other injury of pancreas
S36.290 Other injury of head of pancreas
S36.291 Other injury of body of pancreas
S36.292 Other injury of tail of pancreas
S36.299 Other injury of unspecified part of pancreas

S36.3 Injury of stomach
S36.30 Unspecified injury of stomach
S36.32 Contusion of stomach
S36.33 Laceration of stomach
S36.39 Other injury of stomach

S36.4 Injury of small intestine
S36.40 Unspecified injury of small intestine
S36.400 Unspecified injury of duodenum
S36.408 Unspecified injury of other part of small intestine
S36.409 Unspecified injury of unspecified part of small intestine

S36.41 Primary blast injury of small intestine
Blast injury of small intestine NOS
S36.410 Primary blast injury of duodenum
S36.418 Primary blast injury of other part of small intestine
S36.419 Primary blast injury of unspecified part of small intestine

S36.42 Contusion of small intestine
S36.420 Contusion of duodenum
S36.428 Contusion of other part of small intestine
S36.429 Contusion of unspecified part of small intestine

S36.43 Laceration of small intestine
S36.430 Laceration of duodenum
S36.438 Laceration of other part of small intestine
S36.439 Laceration of unspecified part of small intestine

S36.49 Other injury of small intestine
S36.490 Other injury of duodenum
S36.498 Other injury of other part of small intestine
S36.499 Other injury of unspecified part of small intestine

S36.5 Injury of colon
EXCLUDES2 injury of rectum (S36.6-)
S36.50 Unspecified injury of colon
S36.500 Unspecified injury of ascending [right] colon
S36.501 Unspecified injury of transverse colon
S36.502 Unspecified injury of descending [left] colon
S36.503 Unspecified injury of sigmoid colon
S36.508 Unspecified injury of other part of colon
S36.509 Unspecified injury of unspecified part of colon

S36.51 Primary blast injury of colon
Blast injury of colon NOS
S36.510 Primary blast injury of ascending [right] colon
S36.511 Primary blast injury of transverse colon
S36.512 Primary blast injury of descending [left] colon

S36.513 Primary blast injury of sigmoid colon
S36.518 Primary blast injury of other part of colon
S36.519 Primary blast injury of unspecified part of colon

S36.52 Contusion of colon
S36.520 Contusion of ascending [right] colon
S36.521 Contusion of transverse colon
S36.522 Contusion of descending [left] colon
S36.523 Contusion of sigmoid colon
S36.528 Contusion of other part of colon
S36.529 Contusion of unspecified part of colon

S36.53 Laceration of colon
S36.530 Laceration of ascending [right] colon
S36.531 Laceration of transverse colon
S36.532 Laceration of descending [left] colon
S36.533 Laceration of sigmoid colon
S36.538 Laceration of other part of colon
S36.539 Laceration of unspecified part of colon

S36.59 Other injury of colon
Secondary blast injury of colon
S36.590 Other injury of ascending [right] colon
S36.591 Other injury of transverse colon
S36.592 Other injury of descending [left] colon
S36.593 Other injury of sigmoid colon
S36.598 Other injury of other part of colon
S36.599 Other injury of unspecified part of colon

S36.6 Injury of rectum
S36.60 Unspecified injury of rectum
S36.61 Primary blast injury of rectum
Blast injury of rectum NOS
S36.62 Contusion of rectum
S36.63 Laceration of rectum
S36.69 Other injury of rectum
Secondary blast injury of rectum

S36.8 Injury of other intra-abdominal organs
S36.81 Injury of peritoneum

S36.89 Injury of other intra-abdominal organs
Injury of retroperitoneum
S36.892 Contusion of other intra-abdominal organs
S36.893 Laceration of other intra-abdominal organs
S36.898 Other injury of other intra-abdominal organs
S36.899 Unspecified injury of other intra-abdominal organs

S36.9 Injury of unspecified intra-abdominal organ
S36.90 Unspecified injury of unspecified intra-abdominal organ
S36.92 Contusion of unspecified intra-abdominal organ
S36.93 Laceration of unspecified intra-abdominal organ
S36.99 Other injury of unspecified intra-abdominal organ

S37 Injury of urinary and pelvic organs
Code also any associated open wound (S31.-)
EXCLUDES1 obstetric trauma to pelvic organs (O71.-)
EXCLUDES2 injury of peritoneum (S36.81)
injury of retroperitoneum (S36.89-)
The appropriate 7th character is to be added to each code from category S37
A = initial encounter
D = subsequent encounter
S = sequela

S37.0 Injury of kidney
EXCLUDES2 acute kidney injury (nontraumatic) (N17.9)
S37.00 Unspecified injury of kidney
S37.001 Unspecified injury of right kidney
S37.002 Unspecified injury of left kidney

4️⃣ 4th character required   5️⃣ 5th character required   6️⃣ 6th character required   7️⃣ 7th character required   Extension 'X' Alert

EXCLUDES 1 Not coded here   EXCLUDES 2 Not included here   PDX Primary Diagnosis Only   Manifestation Code

S37.009 Unspecified injury of unspecified kidney
S37.01 Minor contusion of kidney
  Contusion of kidney less than 2 cm
  Contusion of kidney NOS
  S37.011 Minor contusion of right kidney
  S37.012 Minor contusion of left kidney
  S37.019 Minor contusion of unspecified kidney
S37.02 Major contusion of kidney
  Contusion of kidney greater than 2 cm
  S37.021 Major contusion of right kidney
  S37.022 Major contusion of left kidney
  S37.029 Major contusion of unspecified kidney
S37.03 Laceration of kidney, unspecified degree
  S37.031 Laceration of right kidney, unspecified degree
  S37.032 Laceration of left kidney, unspecified degree
  S37.039 Laceration of unspecified kidney, unspecified degree
S37.04 Minor laceration of kidney
  Laceration of kidney less than 1 cm
  S37.041 Minor laceration of right kidney
  S37.042 Minor laceration of left kidney
  S37.049 Minor laceration of unspecified kidney
S37.05 Moderate laceration of kidney
  Laceration of kidney 1 to 3 cm
  S37.051 Moderate laceration of right kidney
  S37.052 Moderate laceration of left kidney
  S37.059 Moderate laceration of unspecified kidney
S37.06 Major laceration of kidney
  Avulsion of kidney
  Laceration of kidney greater than 3 cm
  Massive laceration of kidney
  Multiple moderate lacerations of kidney
  Stellate laceration of kidney
  S37.061 Major laceration of right kidney
  S37.062 Major laceration of left kidney
  S37.069 Major laceration of unspecified kidney
S37.09 Other injury of kidney
  S37.091 Other injury of right kidney
  S37.092 Other injury of left kidney
  S37.099 Other injury of unspecified kidney
S37.1 Injury of ureter
  S37.10 Unspecified injury of ureter
  S37.12 Contusion of ureter
  S37.13 Laceration of ureter
  S37.19 Other injury of ureter
S37.2 Injury of bladder
  S37.20 Unspecified injury of bladder
  S37.22 Contusion of bladder
  S37.23 Laceration of bladder
  S37.29 Other injury of bladder
S37.3 Injury of urethra
  S37.30 Unspecified injury of urethra
  S37.32 Contusion of urethra
  S37.33 Laceration of urethra
  S37.39 Other injury of urethra
S37.4 Injury of ovary
  S37.40 Unspecified injury of ovary
    S37.401 Unspecified injury of ovary, unilateral
    S37.402 Unspecified injury of ovary, bilateral
    S37.409 Unspecified injury of ovary, unspecified
  S37.42 Contusion of ovary
    S37.421 Contusion of ovary, unilateral
    S37.422 Contusion of ovary, bilateral
    S37.429 Contusion of ovary, unspecified
  S37.43 Laceration of ovary

S37.431 Laceration of ovary, unilateral
S37.432 Laceration of ovary, bilateral
S37.439 Laceration of ovary, unspecified
S37.49 Other injury of ovary
  S37.491 Other injury of ovary, unilateral
  S37.492 Other injury of ovary, bilateral
  S37.499 Other injury of ovary, unspecified
S37.5 Injury of fallopian tube
  S37.50 Unspecified injury of fallopian tube
    S37.501 Unspecified injury of fallopian tube, unilateral
    S37.502 Unspecified injury of fallopian tube, bilateral
    S37.509 Unspecified injury of fallopian tube, unspecified
  S37.51 Primary blast injury of fallopian tube
    Blast injury of fallopian tube NOS
    S37.511 Primary blast injury of fallopian tube, unilateral
    S37.512 Primary blast injury of fallopian tube, bilateral
    S37.519 Primary blast injury of fallopian tube, unspecified
  S37.52 Contusion of fallopian tube
    S37.521 Contusion of fallopian tube, unilateral
    S37.522 Contusion of fallopian tube, bilateral
    S37.529 Contusion of fallopian tube, unspecified
  S37.53 Laceration of fallopian tube
    S37.531 Laceration of fallopian tube, unilateral
    S37.532 Laceration of fallopian tube, bilateral
    S37.539 Laceration of fallopian tube, unspecified
  S37.59 Other injury of fallopian tube
    Secondary blast injury fallopian tube
    S37.591 Other injury of fallopian tube, unilateral
    S37.592 Other injury of fallopian tube, bilateral
    S37.599 Other injury of fallopian tube, unspecified
S37.6 Injury of uterus
  EXCLUDES1 injury to gravid uterus (O9A.2-)
              injury to uterus during delivery (O71.-)
  S37.60 Unspecified injury of uterus
  S37.62 Contusion of uterus
  S37.63 Laceration of uterus
  S37.69 Other injury of uterus
S37.8 Injury of other urinary and pelvic organs
  S37.81 Injury of adrenal gland
    S37.812 Contusion of adrenal gland
    S37.813 Laceration of adrenal gland
    S37.818 Other injury of adrenal gland
    S37.819 Unspecified injury of adrenal gland
  S37.82 Injury of prostate
    S37.822 Contusion of prostate
    S37.823 Laceration of prostate
    S37.828 Other injury of prostate
    S37.829 Unspecified injury of prostate
  S37.89 Injury of other urinary and pelvic organ
    S37.892 Contusion of other urinary and pelvic organ
    S37.893 Laceration of other urinary and pelvic organ
    S37.898 Other injury of other urinary and pelvic organ
    S37.899 Unspecified injury of other urinary and pelvic organ
S37.9 Injury of unspecified urinary and pelvic organ
  S37.90 Unspecified injury of unspecified urinary and pelvic organ
  S37.92 Contusion of unspecified urinary and pelvic organ

Unspecified Code	Other Specified Code	N Newborn Age: 0	P Pediatric Age: 0-17	M Maternity Age: 12-55
A Adult Age: 15-124	♂ Male	♀ Female	● New Code	▲ Revised Code Title	►◄ Revised Text

S37.93 Laceration of unspecified urinary and pelvic organ

S37.99 Other injury of unspecified urinary and pelvic organ

S38 Crushing injury and traumatic amputation of abdomen, lower back, pelvis and external genitals

An amputation not identified as partial or complete should be coded to complete

The appropriate 7th character is to be added to each code from category S38
A = initial encounter
D = subsequent encounter
S = sequela

S38.0 Crushing injury of external genital organs
Use additional code for any associated injuries

S38.00 Crushing injury of unspecified external genital organs

S38.001 Crushing injury of unspecified external genital organs, male

S38.002 Crushing injury of unspecified external genital organs, female

S38.01 Crushing injury of penis

S38.02 Crushing injury of scrotum and testis

S38.03 Crushing injury of vulva

S38.1 Crushing injury of abdomen, lower back, and pelvis
Use additional code for all associated injuries, such as:
fracture of thoracic or lumbar spine and pelvis (S22.0-, S32.-)
injury to intra-abdominal organs (S36.-)
injury to urinary and pelvic organs (S37.-)
open wound of abdominal wall (S31.-)
spinal cord injury (S34.0, S34.1-)

EXCLUDES2 crushing injury of external genital organs (S38.0-)

S38.2 Traumatic amputation of external genital organs

S38.21 Traumatic amputation of female external genital organs

Traumatic amputation of clitoris
Traumatic amputation of labium (majus) (minus)
Traumatic amputation of vulva

S38.211 Complete traumatic amputation of female external genital organs

S38.212 Partial traumatic amputation of female external genital organs

S38.22 Traumatic amputation of penis

S38.221 Complete traumatic amputation of penis

S38.222 Partial traumatic amputation of penis

S38.23 Traumatic amputation of scrotum and testis

S38.231 Complete traumatic amputation of scrotum and testis

S38.232 Partial traumatic amputation of scrotum and testis

S38.3 Transection (partial) of abdomen

S39 Other and unspecified injuries of abdomen, lower back, pelvis and external genitals

Code also any associated open wound (S31.-)

EXCLUDES2 sprain of joints and ligaments of lumbar spine and pelvis (S33.-)

The appropriate 7th character is to be added to each code from category S39
A = initial encounter
D = subsequent encounter
S = sequela

S39.0 Injury of muscle, fascia and tendon of abdomen, lower back and pelvis

S39.00 Unspecified injury of muscle, fascia and tendon of abdomen, lower back and pelvis

S39.001 Unspecified injury of muscle, fascia and tendon of abdomen

S39.002 Unspecified injury of muscle, fascia and tendon of lower back

S39.003 Unspecified injury of muscle, fascia and tendon of pelvis

S39.01 Strain of muscle, fascia and tendon of abdomen, lower back and pelvis

S39.011 Strain of muscle, fascia and tendon of abdomen

S39.012 Strain of muscle, fascia and tendon of lower back

S39.013 Strain of muscle, fascia and tendon of pelvis

S39.02 Laceration of muscle, fascia and tendon of abdomen, lower back and pelvis

S39.021 Laceration of muscle, fascia and tendon of abdomen

S39.022 Laceration of muscle, fascia and tendon of lower back

S39.023 Laceration of muscle, fascia and tendon of pelvis

S39.09 Other injury of muscle, fascia and tendon of abdomen, lower back and pelvis

S39.091 Other injury of muscle, fascia and tendon of abdomen

S39.092 Other injury of muscle, fascia and tendon of lower back

S39.093 Other injury of muscle, fascia and tendon of pelvis

S39.8 Other specified injuries of abdomen, lower back, pelvis and external genitals

S39.81 Other specified injuries of abdomen

S39.82 Other specified injuries of lower back

S39.83 Other specified injuries of pelvis

S39.84 Other specified injuries of external genitals

S39.840 Fracture of corpus cavernosum penis

S39.848 Other specified injuries of external genitals

S39.9 Unspecified injury of abdomen, lower back, pelvis and external genitals

S39.91 Unspecified injury of abdomen

S39.92 Unspecified injury of lower back

S39.93 Unspecified injury of pelvis

S39.94 Unspecified injury of external genitals

Injuries to the shoulder and upper arm (S40-S49)

INCLUDES   injuries of axilla
injuries of scapular region

EXCLUDES2   burns and corrosions (T20-T32)
frostbite (T33-T34)
injuries of elbow (S50-S59)
insect bite or sting, venomous (T63.4)

S40 Superficial injury of shoulder and upper arm

The appropriate 7th character is to be added to each code from category S40
A = initial encounter
D = subsequent encounter
S = sequela

S40.0 Contusion of shoulder and upper arm

S40.01 Contusion of shoulder

S40.011 Contusion of right shoulder

S40.012 Contusion of left shoulder

S40.019 Contusion of unspecified shoulder

S40.02 Contusion of upper arm

S40.021 Contusion of right upper arm

S40.022 Contusion of left upper arm

S40.029 Contusion of unspecified upper arm

4th character required   5th character required   6th character required   7th character required   Extension 'X' Alert

EXCLUDES 1 Not coded here   EXCLUDES 2 Not included here   PDx Primary Diagnosis Only   Manifestation Code

S40.2 Other superficial injuries of shoulder
- S40.21 Abrasion of shoulder
  - S40.211 Abrasion of right shoulder
  - S40.212 Abrasion of left shoulder
  - S40.219 Abrasion of unspecified shoulder
- S40.22 Blister (nonthermal) of shoulder
  - S40.221 Blister (nonthermal) of right shoulder
  - S40.222 Blister (nonthermal) of left shoulder
  - S40.229 Blister (nonthermal) of unspecified shoulder
- S40.24 External constriction of shoulder
  - S40.241 External constriction of right shoulder
  - S40.242 External constriction of left shoulder
  - S40.249 External constriction of unspecified shoulder
- S40.25 Superficial foreign body of shoulder
  Splinter in the shoulder
  - S40.251 Superficial foreign body of right shoulder
  - S40.252 Superficial foreign body of left shoulder
  - S40.259 Superficial foreign body of unspecified shoulder
- S40.26 Insect bite (nonvenomous) of shoulder
  - S40.261 Insect bite (nonvenomous) of right shoulder
  - S40.262 Insect bite (nonvenomous) of left shoulder
  - S40.269 Insect bite (nonvenomous) of unspecified shoulder
- S40.27 Other superficial bite of shoulder
  EXCLUDES1 open bite of shoulder (S41.05)
  - S40.271 Other superficial bite of right shoulder
  - S40.272 Other superficial bite of left shoulder
  - S40.279 Other superficial bite of unspecified shoulder

S40.8 Other superficial injuries of upper arm
- S40.81 Abrasion of upper arm
  - S40.811 Abrasion of right upper arm
  - S40.812 Abrasion of left upper arm
  - S40.819 Abrasion of unspecified upper arm
- S40.82 Blister (nonthermal) of upper arm
  - S40.821 Blister (nonthermal) of right upper arm
  - S40.822 Blister (nonthermal) of left upper arm
  - S40.829 Blister (nonthermal) of unspecified upper arm
- S40.84 External constriction of upper arm
  - S40.841 External constriction of right upper arm
  - S40.842 External constriction of left upper arm
  - S40.849 External constriction of unspecified upper arm
- S40.85 Superficial foreign body of upper arm
  Splinter in the upper arm
  - S40.851 Superficial foreign body of right upper arm
  - S40.852 Superficial foreign body of left upper arm
  - S40.859 Superficial foreign body of unspecified upper arm
- S40.86 Insect bite (nonvenomous) of upper arm
  - S40.861 Insect bite (nonvenomous) of right upper arm
  - S40.862 Insect bite (nonvenomous) of left upper arm
  - S40.869 Insect bite (nonvenomous) of unspecified upper arm
- S40.87 Other superficial bite of upper arm
  EXCLUDES1 open bite of upper arm (S41.14)
  EXCLUDES2 other superficial bite of shoulder (S40.27-)
  - S40.871 Other superficial bite of right upper arm
  - S40.872 Other superficial bite of left upper arm
  - S40.879 Other superficial bite of unspecified upper arm

S40.9 Unspecified superficial injury of shoulder and upper arm

- S40.91 Unspecified superficial injury of shoulder
  - S40.911 Unspecified superficial injury of right shoulder
  - S40.912 Unspecified superficial injury of left shoulder
  - S40.919 Unspecified superficial injury of unspecified shoulder
- S40.92 Unspecified superficial injury of upper arm
  - S40.921 Unspecified superficial injury of right upper arm
  - S40.922 Unspecified superficial injury of left upper arm
  - S40.929 Unspecified superficial injury of unspecified upper arm

S41 Open wound of shoulder and upper arm
  Code also any associated wound infection
  EXCLUDES1 traumatic amputation of shoulder and upper arm (S48.-)
  EXCLUDES2 open fracture of shoulder and upper arm (S42.- with 7th character B or C)
  The appropriate 7th character is to be added to each code from category S41
  A = initial encounter
  D = subsequent encounter
  S = sequela

S41.0 Open wound of shoulder
- S41.00 Unspecified open wound of shoulder
  - S41.001 Unspecified open wound of right shoulder
  - S41.002 Unspecified open wound of left shoulder
  - S41.009 Unspecified open wound of unspecified shoulder
- S41.01 Laceration without foreign body of shoulder
  - S41.011 Laceration without foreign body of right shoulder
  - S41.012 Laceration without foreign body of left shoulder
  - S41.019 Laceration without foreign body of unspecified shoulder
- S41.02 Laceration with foreign body of shoulder
  - S41.021 Laceration with foreign body of right shoulder
  - S41.022 Laceration with foreign body of left shoulder
  - S41.029 Laceration with foreign body of unspecified shoulder
- S41.03 Puncture wound without foreign body of shoulder
  - S41.031 Puncture wound without foreign body of right shoulder
  - S41.032 Puncture wound without foreign body of left shoulder
  - S41.039 Puncture wound without foreign body of unspecified shoulder
- S41.04 Puncture wound with foreign body of shoulder
  - S41.041 Puncture wound with foreign body of right shoulder
  - S41.042 Puncture wound with foreign body of left shoulder
  - S41.049 Puncture wound with foreign body of unspecified shoulder
- S41.05 Open bite of shoulder
  Bite of shoulder NOS
  EXCLUDES1 superficial bite of shoulder (S40.27)
  - S41.051 Open bite of right shoulder
  - S41.052 Open bite of left shoulder
  - S41.059 Open bite of unspecified shoulder

S41.1 Open wound of upper arm
- S41.10 Unspecified open wound of upper arm

7️⃣ S41.101 Unspecified open wound of right upper arm
7️⃣ S41.102 Unspecified open wound of left upper arm
7️⃣ S41.109 Unspecified open wound of unspecified upper arm
6️⃣ S41.11 Laceration without foreign body of upper arm
7️⃣ S41.111 Laceration without foreign body of right upper arm
7️⃣ S41.112 Laceration without foreign body of left upper arm
7️⃣ S41.119 Laceration without foreign body of unspecified upper arm
6️⃣ S41.12 Laceration with foreign body of upper arm
7️⃣ S41.121 Laceration with foreign body of right upper arm
7️⃣ S41.122 Laceration with foreign body of left upper arm
7️⃣ S41.129 Laceration with foreign body of unspecified upper arm
6️⃣ S41.13 Puncture wound without foreign body of upper arm
7️⃣ S41.131 Puncture wound without foreign body of right upper arm
7️⃣ S41.132 Puncture wound without foreign body of left upper arm
7️⃣ S41.139 Puncture wound without foreign body of unspecified upper arm
6️⃣ S41.14 Puncture wound with foreign body of upper arm
7️⃣ S41.141 Puncture wound with foreign body of right upper arm
7️⃣ S41.142 Puncture wound with foreign body of left upper arm
7️⃣ S41.149 Puncture wound with foreign body of unspecified upper arm
5️⃣ S41.15 Open bite of upper arm
Bite of upper arm NOS
EXCLUDES1 superficial bite of upper arm (S40.87)
7️⃣ S41.151 Open bite of right upper arm
7️⃣ S41.152 Open bite of left upper arm
7️⃣ S41.159 Open bite of unspecified upper arm
4️⃣ S42 Fracture of shoulder and upper arm
NOTES A fracture not indicated as displaced or nondisplaced should be coded to displaced
A fracture not indicated as open or closed should be coded to closed
EXCLUDES1 traumatic amputation of shoulder and upper arm (S48.-)
The appropriate 7th character is to be added to all codes from category S42
A = initial encounter for closed fracture
B = initial encounter for open fracture
D = subsequent encounter for fracture with routine healing
G = subsequent encounter for fracture with delayed healing
K = subsequent encounter for fracture with nonunion
P = subsequent encounter for fracture with malunion
S = sequela
5️⃣ S42.0 Fracture of clavicle
6️⃣ S42.00 Fracture of unspecified part of clavicle
7️⃣ S42.001 Fracture of unspecified part of right clavicle
7️⃣ S42.002 Fracture of unspecified part of left clavicle
7️⃣ S42.009 Fracture of unspecified part of unspecified clavicle
6️⃣ S42.01 Fracture of sternal end of clavicle
7️⃣ S42.011 Anterior displaced fracture of sternal end of right clavicle
7️⃣ S42.012 Anterior displaced fracture of sternal end of left clavicle

7️⃣ S42.013 Anterior displaced fracture of sternal end of unspecified clavicle
Displaced fracture of sternal end of clavicle NOS
7️⃣ S42.014 Posterior displaced fracture of sternal end of right clavicle
7️⃣ S42.015 Posterior displaced fracture of sternal end of left clavicle
7️⃣ S42.016 Posterior displaced fracture of sternal end of unspecified clavicle
7️⃣ S42.017 Nondisplaced fracture of sternal end of right clavicle
7️⃣ S42.018 Nondisplaced fracture of sternal end of left clavicle
7️⃣ S42.019 Nondisplaced fracture of sternal end of unspecified clavicle
5️⃣ S42.02 Fracture of shaft of clavicle
7️⃣ S42.021 Displaced fracture of shaft of right clavicle
7️⃣ S42.022 Displaced fracture of shaft of left clavicle
7️⃣ S42.023 Displaced fracture of shaft of unspecified clavicle
7️⃣ S42.024 Nondisplaced fracture of shaft of right clavicle
7️⃣ S42.025 Nondisplaced fracture of shaft of left clavicle
7️⃣ S42.026 Nondisplaced fracture of shaft of unspecified clavicle
5️⃣ S42.03 Fracture of lateral end of clavicle
Fracture of acromial end of clavicle
7️⃣ S42.031 Displaced fracture of lateral end of right clavicle
7️⃣ S42.032 Displaced fracture of lateral end of left clavicle
7️⃣ S42.033 Displaced fracture of lateral end of unspecified clavicle
7️⃣ S42.034 Nondisplaced fracture of lateral end of right clavicle
7️⃣ S42.035 Nondisplaced fracture of lateral end of left clavicle
7️⃣ S42.036 Nondisplaced fracture of lateral end of unspecified clavicle
5️⃣ S42.1 Fracture of scapula
6️⃣ S42.10 Fracture of unspecified part of scapula
7️⃣ S42.101 Fracture of unspecified part of scapula, right shoulder
7️⃣ S42.102 Fracture of unspecified part of scapula, left shoulder
7️⃣ S42.109 Fracture of unspecified part of scapula, unspecified shoulder
6️⃣ S42.11 Fracture of body of scapula
7️⃣ S42.111 Displaced fracture of body of scapula, right shoulder
7️⃣ S42.112 Displaced fracture of body of scapula, left shoulder
7️⃣ S42.113 Displaced fracture of body of scapula, unspecified shoulder
7️⃣ S42.114 Nondisplaced fracture of body of scapula, right shoulder
7️⃣ S42.115 Nondisplaced fracture of body of scapula, left shoulder
7️⃣ S42.116 Nondisplaced fracture of body of scapula, unspecified shoulder
6️⃣ S42.12 Fracture of acromial process
7️⃣ S42.121 Displaced fracture of acromial process, right shoulder
7️⃣ S42.122 Displaced fracture of acromial process, left shoulder
7️⃣ S42.123 Displaced fracture of acromial process, unspecified shoulder
7️⃣ S42.124 1 fracture of acromial process, right shoulder

4️⃣ 4th character required   5️⃣ 5th character required   6️⃣ 6th character required   7️⃣ 7th character required   Extension 'X' Alert
EXCLUDES1 Not coded here   EXCLUDES2 Not included here   PDx Primary Diagnosis Only   Manifestation Code

578 **ICD-10-CM 2015**

(7ᵗʰ) **S42.125** Nondisplaced fracture of acromial process, left shoulder

(7ᵗʰ) **S42.126** Nondisplaced fracture of acromial process, unspecified shoulder

(6ᵗʰ) **S42.13** Fracture of coracoid process

(7ᵗʰ) **S42.131** Displaced fracture of coracoid process, right shoulder

(7ᵗʰ) **S42.132** Displaced fracture of coracoid process, left shoulder

(7ᵗʰ) **S42.133** Displaced fracture of coracoid process, unspecified shoulder

(7ᵗʰ) **S42.134** Nondisplaced fracture of coracoid process, right shoulder

(7ᵗʰ) **S42.135** Nondisplaced fracture of coracoid process, left shoulder

(7ᵗʰ) **S42.136** Nondisplaced fracture of coracoid process, unspecified shoulder

(6ᵗʰ) **S42.14** Fracture of glenoid cavity of scapula

(7ᵗʰ) **S42.141** Displaced fracture of glenoid cavity of scapula, right shoulder

(7ᵗʰ) **S42.142** Displaced fracture of glenoid cavity of scapula, left shoulder

(7ᵗʰ) **S42.143** Displaced fracture of glenoid cavity of scapula, unspecified shoulder

(7ᵗʰ) **S42.144** Nondisplaced fracture of glenoid cavity of scapula, right shoulder

(7ᵗʰ) **S42.145** Nondisplaced fracture of glenoid cavity of scapula, left shoulder

(7ᵗʰ) **S42.146** Nondisplaced fracture of glenoid cavity of scapula, unspecified shoulder

(6ᵗʰ) **S42.15** Fracture of neck of scapula

(7ᵗʰ) **S42.151** Displaced fracture of neck of scapula, right shoulder

(7ᵗʰ) **S42.152** Displaced fracture of neck of scapula, left shoulder

(7ᵗʰ) **S42.153** Displaced fracture of neck of scapula, unspecified shoulder

(7ᵗʰ) **S42.154** Nondisplaced fracture of neck of scapula, right shoulder

(7ᵗʰ) **S42.155** Nondisplaced fracture of neck of scapula, left shoulder

(7ᵗʰ) **S42.156** Nondisplaced fracture of neck of scapula, unspecified shoulder

(6ᵗʰ) **S42.19** Fracture of other part of scapula

(7ᵗʰ) **S42.191** Fracture of other part of scapula, right shoulder

(7ᵗʰ) **S42.192** Fracture of other part of scapula, left shoulder

(7ᵗʰ) **S42.199** Fracture of other part of scapula, unspecified shoulder

(5ᵗʰ) **S42.2** Fracture of upper end of humerus

Fracture of proximal end of humerus

EXCLUDES2   fracture of shaft of humerus (S42.3-)

physeal fracture of upper end of humerus (S49.0-)

(6ᵗʰ) **S42.20** Unspecified fracture of upper end of humerus

(7ᵗʰ) **S42.201** Unspecified fracture of upper end of right humerus

(7ᵗʰ) **S42.202** Unspecified fracture of upper end of left humerus

(7ᵗʰ) **S42.209** Unspecified fracture of upper end of unspecified humerus

(6ᵗʰ) **S42.21** Unspecified fracture of surgical neck of humerus

Fracture of neck of humerus NOS

(7ᵗʰ) **S42.211** Unspecified displaced fracture of surgical neck of right humerus

(7ᵗʰ) **S42.212** Unspecified displaced fracture of surgical neck of left humerus

(7ᵗʰ) **S42.213** Unspecified displaced fracture of surgical neck of unspecified humerus

(7ᵗʰ) **S42.214** Unspecified nondisplaced fracture of surgical neck of right humerus

(7ᵗʰ) **S42.215** Unspecified nondisplaced fracture of surgical neck of left humerus

(7ᵗʰ) **S42.216** Unspecified nondisplaced fracture of surgical neck of unspecified humerus

(6ᵗʰ) **S42.22** 2-part fracture of surgical neck of humerus

(7ᵗʰ) **S42.221** 2-part displaced fracture of surgical neck of right humerus

(7ᵗʰ) **S42.222** 2-part displaced fracture of surgical neck of left humerus

(7ᵗʰ) **S42.223** 2-part displaced fracture of surgical neck of unspecified humerus

(7ᵗʰ) **S42.224** 2-part nondisplaced fracture of surgical neck of right humerus

(7ᵗʰ) **S42.225** 2-part nondisplaced fracture of surgical neck of left humerus

(7ᵗʰ) **S42.226** 2-part nondisplaced fracture of surgical neck of unspecified humerus

(6ᵗʰ) **S42.23** 3-part fracture of surgical neck of humerus

(7ᵗʰ) **S42.231** 3-part fracture of surgical neck of right humerus

(7ᵗʰ) **S42.232** 3-part fracture of surgical neck of left humerus

(7ᵗʰ) **S42.239** 3-part fracture of surgical neck of unspecified humerus

(6ᵗʰ) **S42.24** 4-part fracture of surgical neck of humerus

(7ᵗʰ) **S42.241** 4-part fracture of surgical neck of right humerus

(7ᵗʰ) **S42.242** 4-part fracture of surgical neck of left humerus

(7ᵗʰ) **S42.249** 4-part fracture of surgical neck of unspecified humerus

(6ᵗʰ) **S42.25** Fracture of greater tuberosity of humerus

(7ᵗʰ) **S42.251** Displaced fracture of greater tuberosity of right humerus

(7ᵗʰ) **S42.252** Displaced fracture of greater tuberosity of left humerus

(7ᵗʰ) **S42.253** Displaced fracture of greater tuberosity of unspecified humerus

(7ᵗʰ) **S42.254** Nondisplaced fracture of greater tuberosity of right humerus

(7ᵗʰ) **S42.255** Nondisplaced fracture of greater tuberosity of left humerus

(7ᵗʰ) **S42.256** Nondisplaced fracture of greater tuberosity of unspecified humerus

(6ᵗʰ) **S42.26** Fracture of lesser tuberosity of humerus

(7ᵗʰ) **S42.261** Displaced fracture of lesser tuberosity of right humerus

(7ᵗʰ) **S42.262** Displaced fracture of lesser tuberosity of left humerus

(7ᵗʰ) **S42.263** Displaced fracture of lesser tuberosity of unspecified humerus

(7ᵗʰ) **S42.264** Nondisplaced fracture of lesser tuberosity of right humerus

(7ᵗʰ) **S42.265** Nondisplaced fracture of lesser tuberosity of left humerus

(7ᵗʰ) **S42.266** Nondisplaced fracture of lesser tuberosity of unspecified humerus

(6ᵗʰ) **S42.27** Torus fracture of upper end of humerus

The appropriate 7th character is to be added to all codes in subcategory S42.27

A = initial encounter for closed fracture

D = subsequent encounter for fracture with routine healing

G = subsequent encounter for fracture with delayed healing

K = subsequent encounter for fracture with nonunion

P = subsequent encounter for fracture with malunion

S = sequela

Unspecified Code   Other Specified Code   N Newborn Age: 0   P Pediatric Age: 0-17   M Maternity Age: 12-55

A Adult Age: 15-124   ♂ Male   ♀ Female   ● New Code   ▲ Revised Code Title   ►◄ Revised Text

⑦ S42.271 Torus fracture of upper end of right humerus

⑦ S42.272 Torus fracture of upper end of left humerus

⑦ S42.279 Torus fracture of upper end of unspecified humerus

⑥ S42.29 Other fracture of upper end of humerus

    Fracture of anatomical neck of humerus

    Fracture of articular head of humerus

⑦ S42.291 Other displaced fracture of upper end of right humerus

⑦ S42.292 Other displaced fracture of upper end of left humerus

⑦ S42.293 Other displaced fracture of upper end of unspecified humerus

⑦ S42.294 Other nondisplaced fracture of upper end of right humerus

⑦ S42.295 Other nondisplaced fracture of upper end of left humerus

⑦ S42.296 Other nondisplaced fracture of upper end of unspecified humerus

⑤ S42.3 Fracture of shaft of humerus

    Fracture of humerus NOS

    Fracture of upper arm NOS

    EXCLUDES2 *physeal fractures of upper end of humerus (S49.0-)*

    physeal fractures of lower end of humerus (S49.1-)

⑥ S42.30 Unspecified fracture of shaft of humerus

⑦ S42.301 Unspecified fracture of shaft of humerus, right arm

⑦ S42.302 Unspecified fracture of shaft of humerus, left arm

⑦ S42.309 Unspecified fracture of shaft of humerus, unspecified arm

⑥ S42.31 Greenstick fracture of shaft of humerus

    The appropriate 7th character is to be added to all codes in subcategory S42.31

    A = initial encounter for closed fracture

    D = subsequent encounter for fracture with routine healing

    G = subsequent encounter for fracture with delayed healing

    K = subsequent encounter for fracture with nonunion

    P = subsequent encounter for fracture with malunion

    S = sequela

⑦ S42.311 Greenstick fracture of shaft of humerus, right arm

⑦ S42.312 Greenstick fracture of shaft of humerus, left arm

⑦ S42.319 Greenstick fracture of shaft of humerus, unspecified arm

⑥ S42.32 Transverse fracture of shaft of humerus

⑦ S42.321 Displaced transverse fracture of shaft of humerus, right arm

⑦ S42.322 Displaced transverse fracture of shaft of humerus, left arm

⑦ S42.323 Displaced transverse fracture of shaft of humerus, unspecified arm

⑦ S42.324 Nondisplaced transverse fracture of shaft of humerus, right arm

⑦ S42.325 Nondisplaced transverse fracture of shaft of humerus, left arm

⑦ S42.326 Nondisplaced transverse fracture of shaft of humerus, unspecified arm

⑥ S42.33 Oblique fracture of shaft of humerus

⑦ S42.331 Displaced oblique fracture of shaft of humerus, right arm

⑦ S42.332 Displaced oblique fracture of shaft of humerus, left arm

⑦ S42.333 Displaced oblique fracture of shaft of humerus, unspecified arm

⑦ S42.334 Nondisplaced oblique fracture of shaft of humerus, right arm

⑦ S42.335 Nondisplaced oblique fracture of shaft of humerus, left arm

⑦ S42.336 Nondisplaced oblique fracture of shaft of humerus, unspecified arm

⑥ S42.34 Spiral fracture of shaft of humerus

⑦ S42.341 Displaced spiral fracture of shaft of humerus, right arm

⑦ S42.342 Displaced spiral fracture of shaft of humerus, left arm

⑦ S42.343 Displaced spiral fracture of shaft of humerus, unspecified arm

⑦ S42.344 Nondisplaced spiral fracture of shaft of humerus, right arm

⑦ S42.345 Nondisplaced spiral fracture of shaft of humerus, left arm

⑦ S42.346 Nondisplaced spiral fracture of shaft of humerus, unspecified arm

⑥ S42.35 Comminuted fracture of shaft of humerus

⑦ S42.351 Displaced comminuted fracture of shaft of humerus, right arm

⑦ S42.352 Displaced comminuted fracture of shaft of humerus, left arm

⑦ S42.353 Displaced comminuted fracture of shaft of humerus, unspecified arm

⑦ S42.354 Nondisplaced comminuted fracture of shaft of humerus, right arm

⑦ S42.355 Nondisplaced comminuted fracture of shaft of humerus, left arm

⑦ S42.356 Nondisplaced comminuted fracture of shaft of humerus, unspecified arm

⑥ S42.36 Segmental fracture of shaft of humerus

⑦ S42.361 Displaced segmental fracture of shaft of humerus, right arm

⑦ S42.362 Displaced segmental fracture of shaft of humerus, left arm

⑦ S42.363 Displaced segmental fracture of shaft of humerus, unspecified arm

⑦ S42.364 Nondisplaced segmental fracture of shaft of humerus, right arm

⑦ S42.365 Nondisplaced segmental fracture of shaft of humerus, left arm

⑦ S42.366 Nondisplaced segmental fracture of shaft of humerus, unspecified arm

⑥ S42.39 Other fracture of shaft of humerus

⑦ S42.391 Other fracture of shaft of right humerus

⑦ S42.392 Other fracture of shaft of left humerus

⑦ S42.399 Other fracture of shaft of unspecified humerus

⑤ S42.4 Fracture of lower end of humerus

    Fracture of distal end of humerus

    EXCLUDES2 *fracture of shaft of humerus (S42.3-)*

    physeal fracture of lower end of humerus (S49.1-)

⑥ S42.40 Unspecified fracture of lower end of humerus

    Fracture of elbow NOS

⑦ S42.401 Unspecified fracture of lower end of right humerus

⑦ S42.402 Unspecified fracture of lower end of left humerus

⑦ S42.409 Unspecified fracture of lower end of unspecified humerus

⑥ S42.41 Simple supracondylar fracture without intercondylar fracture of humerus

⑦ S42.411 Displaced simple supracondylar fracture without intercondylar fracture of right humerus

---

④ 4th character required   ⑤ 5th character required   ⑥ 6th character required   ⑦ 7th character required   ⑦ₓ Extension 'X' Alert

EXCLUDES1 Not coded here   EXCLUDES2 Not included here   PDx Primary Diagnosis Only   Manifestation Code

580   **ICD-10-CM 2015**

[7th] S42.412 Displaced simple supracondylar fracture without intercondylar fracture of left humerus
[7th] S42.413 Displaced simple supracondylar fracture without intercondylar fracture of unspecified humerus
[7th] S42.414 Nondisplaced simple supracondylar fracture without intercondylar fracture of right humerus
[7th] S42.415 Nondisplaced simple supracondylar fracture without intercondylar fracture of left humerus
[7th] S42.416 Nondisplaced simple supracondylar fracture without intercondylar fracture of unspecified humerus

[6th] S42.42 Comminuted supracondylar fracture without intercondylar fracture of humerus
[7th] S42.421 Displaced comminuted supracondylar fracture without intercondylar fracture of right humerus
[7th] S42.422 Displaced comminuted supracondylar fracture without intercondylar fracture of left humerus
[7th] S42.423 Displaced comminuted supracondylar fracture without intercondylar fracture of unspecified humerus
[7th] S42.424 Nondisplaced comminuted supracondylar fracture without intercondylar fracture of right humerus
[7th] S42.425 Nondisplaced comminuted supracondylar fracture without intercondylar fracture of left humerus
[7th] S42.426 Nondisplaced comminuted supracondylar fracture without intercondylar fracture of unspecified humerus

[6th] S42.43 Fracture (avulsion) of lateral epicondyle of humerus
[7th] S42.431 Displaced fracture (avulsion) of lateral epicondyle of right humerus
[7th] S42.432 Displaced fracture (avulsion) of lateral epicondyle of left humerus
[7th] S42.433 Displaced fracture (avulsion) of lateral epicondyle of unspecified humerus
[7th] S42.434 Nondisplaced fracture (avulsion) of lateral epicondyle of right humerus
[7th] S42.435 Nondisplaced fracture (avulsion) of lateral epicondyle of left humerus
[7th] S42.436 Nondisplaced fracture (avulsion) of lateral epicondyle of unspecified humerus

[6th] S42.44 Fracture (avulsion) of medial epicondyle of humerus
[7th] S42.441 Displaced fracture (avulsion) of medial epicondyle of right humerus
[7th] S42.442 Displaced fracture (avulsion) of medial epicondyle of left humerus
[7th] S42.443 Displaced fracture (avulsion) of medial epicondyle of unspecified humerus
[7th] S42.444 Nondisplaced fracture (avulsion) of medial epicondyle of right humerus
[7th] S42.445 Nondisplaced fracture (avulsion) of medial epicondyle of left humerus
[7th] S42.446 Nondisplaced fracture (avulsion) of medial epicondyle of unspecified humerus
[7th] S42.447 Incarcerated fracture (avulsion) of medial epicondyle of right humerus
[7th] S42.448 Incarcerated fracture (avulsion) of medial epicondyle of left humerus
[7th] S42.449 Incarcerated fracture (avulsion) of medial epicondyle of unspecified humerus

[6th] S42.45 Fracture of lateral condyle of humerus
Fracture of capitellum of humerus
[7th] S42.451 Displaced fracture of lateral condyle of right humerus
[7th] S42.452 Displaced fracture of lateral condyle of left humerus
[7th] S42.453 Displaced fracture of lateral condyle of unspecified humerus
[7th] S42.454 Nondisplaced fracture of lateral condyle of right humerus
[7th] S42.455 Nondisplaced fracture of lateral condyle of left humerus
[7th] S42.456 Nondisplaced fracture of lateral condyle of unspecified humerus

[6th] S42.46 Fracture of medial condyle of humerus
Trochlea fracture of humerus
[7th] S42.461 Displaced fracture of medial condyle of right humerus
[7th] S42.462 Displaced fracture of medial condyle of left humerus
[7th] S42.463 Displaced fracture of medial condyle of unspecified humerus
[7th] S42.464 Nondisplaced fracture of medial condyle of right humerus
[7th] S42.465 Nondisplaced fracture of medial condyle of left humerus
[7th] S42.466 Nondisplaced fracture of medial condyle of unspecified humerus

[6th] S42.47 Transcondylar fracture of humerus
[7th] S42.471 Displaced transcondylar fracture of right humerus
[7th] S42.472 Displaced transcondylar fracture of left humerus
[7th] S42.473 Displaced transcondylar fracture of unspecified humerus
[7th] S42.474 Nondisplaced transcondylar fracture of right humerus
[7th] S42.475 Nondisplaced transcondylar fracture of left humerus
[7th] S42.476 Nondisplaced transcondylar fracture of unspecified humerus

[6th] S42.48 Torus fracture of lower end of humerus
The appropriate 7th character is to be added to all codes in subcategory S42.48
A = initial encounter for closed fracture
D = subsequent encounter for fracture with routine healing
G = subsequent encounter for fracture with delayed healing
K = subsequent encounter for fracture with nonunion
P = subsequent encounter for fracture with malunion
S = sequela
[7th] S42.481 Torus fracture of lower end of right humerus
[7th] S42.482 Torus fracture of lower end of left humerus
[7th] S42.489 Torus fracture of lower end of unspecified humerus

[6th] S42.49 Other fracture of lower end of humerus
[7th] S42.491 Other displaced fracture of lower end of right humerus
[7th] S42.492 Other displaced fracture of lower end of left humerus
[7th] S42.493 Other displaced fracture of lower end of unspecified humerus
[7th] S42.494 Other nondisplaced fracture of lower end of right humerus
[7th] S42.495 Other nondisplaced fracture of lower end of left humerus
[7th] S42.496 Other nondisplaced fracture of lower end of unspecified humerus

[5th] S42.9 Fracture of shoulder girdle, part unspecified
Fracture of shoulder NOS

Unspecified Code | Other Specified Code | [N] Newborn Age: 0 | [P] Pediatric Age: 0-17 | [M] Maternity Age: 12-55
[A] Adult Age: 15-124 | ♂ Male | ♀ Female | ● New Code | ▲ Revised Code Title | ►◄ Revised Text

[7th] S42.90 Fracture of unspecified shoulder girdle, part unspecified
[7th] S42.91 Fracture of right shoulder girdle, part unspecified
[7th] S42.92 Fracture of left shoulder girdle, part unspecified

[4th] S43 Dislocation and sprain of joints and ligaments of shoulder girdle

INCLUDES *avulsion of joint or ligament of shoulder girdle*
laceration of cartilage, joint or ligament of shoulder girdle
sprain of cartilage, joint or ligament of shoulder girdle
traumatic hemarthrosis of joint or ligament of shoulder girdle
traumatic rupture of joint or ligament of shoulder girdle
traumatic subluxation of joint or ligament of shoulder girdle
traumatic tear of joint or ligament of shoulder girdle

Code also any associated open wound

EXCLUDES2 *strain of muscle, fascia and tendon of shoulder and upper arm (S46.-)*

The appropriate 7th character is to be added to each code from category S43
A = initial encounter
D = subsequent encounter
S = sequela

[5th] S43.0 Subluxation and dislocation of shoulder joint
Dislocation of glenohumeral joint
Subluxation of glenohumeral joint

[6th] S43.00 Unspecified subluxation and dislocation of shoulder joint
Dislocation of humerus NOS
Subluxation of humerus NOS
[7th] S43.001 Unspecified subluxation of right shoulder joint
[7th] S43.002 Unspecified subluxation of left shoulder joint
[7th] S43.003 Unspecified subluxation of unspecified shoulder joint
[7th] S43.004 Unspecified dislocation of right shoulder joint
[7th] S43.005 Unspecified dislocation of left shoulder joint
[7th] S43.006 Unspecified dislocation of unspecified shoulder joint

[6th] S43.01 Anterior subluxation and dislocation of humerus
[7th] S43.011 Anterior subluxation of right humerus
[7th] S43.012 Anterior subluxation of left humerus
[7th] S43.013 Anterior subluxation of unspecified humerus
[7th] S43.014 Anterior dislocation of right humerus
[7th] S43.015 Anterior dislocation of left humerus
[7th] S43.016 Anterior dislocation of unspecified humerus

[6th] S43.02 Posterior subluxation and dislocation of humerus
[7th] S43.021 Posterior subluxation of right humerus
[7th] S43.022 Posterior subluxation of left humerus
[7th] S43.023 Posterior subluxation of unspecified humerus
[7th] S43.024 Posterior dislocation of right humerus
[7th] S43.025 Posterior dislocation of left humerus
[7th] S43.026 Posterior dislocation of unspecified humerus

[6th] S43.03 Inferior subluxation and dislocation of humerus
[7th] S43.031 Inferior subluxation of right humerus
[7th] S43.032 Inferior subluxation of left humerus
[7th] S43.033 Inferior subluxation of unspecified humerus
[7th] S43.034 Inferior dislocation of right humerus
[7th] S43.035 Inferior dislocation of left humerus
[7th] S43.036 Inferior dislocation of unspecified humerus

[6th] S43.08 Other subluxation and dislocation of shoulder joint
[7th] S43.081 Other subluxation of right shoulder joint
[7th] S43.082 Other subluxation of left shoulder joint
[7th] S43.083 Other subluxation of unspecified shoulder joint
[7th] S43.084 Other dislocation of right shoulder joint
[7th] S43.085 Other dislocation of left shoulder joint
[7th] S43.086 Other dislocation of unspecified shoulder joint

[5th] S43.1 Subluxation and dislocation of acromioclavicular joint

[6th] S43.10 Unspecified dislocation of acromioclavicular joint
[7th] S43.101 Unspecified dislocation of right acromioclavicular joint
[7th] S43.102 Unspecified dislocation of left acromioclavicular joint
[7th] S43.109 Unspecified dislocation of unspecified acromioclavicular joint

[6th] S43.11 Subluxation of acromioclavicular joint
[7th] S43.111 Subluxation of right acromioclavicular joint
[7th] S43.112 Subluxation of left acromioclavicular joint
[7th] S43.119 Subluxation of unspecified acromioclavicular joint

[6th] S43.12 Dislocation of acromioclavicular joint, 100%-200% displacement
[7th] S43.121 Dislocation of right acromioclavicular joint, 100%-200% displacement
[7th] S43.122 Dislocation of left acromioclavicular joint, 100%-200% displacement
[7th] S43.129 Dislocation of unspecified acromioclavicular joint, 100%-200% displacement

[6th] S43.13 Dislocation of acromioclavicular joint, greater than 200% displacement
[7th] S43.131 Dislocation of right acromioclavicular joint, greater than 200% displacement
[7th] S43.132 Dislocation of left acromioclavicular joint, greater than 200% displacement
[7th] S43.139 Dislocation of unspecified acromioclavicular joint, greater than 200% displacement

[6th] S43.14 Inferior dislocation of acromioclavicular joint
[7th] S43.141 Inferior dislocation of right acromioclavicular joint
[7th] S43.142 Inferior dislocation of left acromioclavicular joint
[7th] S43.149 Inferior dislocation of unspecified acromioclavicular joint

[6th] S43.15 Posterior dislocation of acromioclavicular joint
[7th] S43.151 Posterior dislocation of right acromioclavicular joint
[7th] S43.152 Posterior dislocation of left acromioclavicular joint
[7th] S43.159 Posterior dislocation of unspecified acromioclavicular joint

[5th] S43.2 Subluxation and dislocation of sternoclavicular joint

[6th] S43.20 Unspecified subluxation and dislocation of sternoclavicular joint
[7th] S43.201 Unspecified subluxation of right sternoclavicular joint
[7th] S43.202 Unspecified subluxation of left sternoclavicular joint
[7th] S43.203 Unspecified subluxation of unspecified sternoclavicular joint

[4th] 4th character required [5th] 5th character required [6th] 6th character required [7th] 7th character required [7th] Extension 'X' Alert
EXCLUDES1 Not coded here EXCLUDES2 Not included here [PDx] Primary Diagnosis Only Manifestation Code

[7th] S43.204 Unspecified dislocation of right sternoclavicular joint
[7th] S43.205 Unspecified dislocation of left sternoclavicular joint
[7th] S43.206 Unspecified dislocation of unspecified sternoclavicular joint
[6th] S43.21 Anterior subluxation and dislocation of sternoclavicular joint
[7th] S43.211 Anterior subluxation of right sternoclavicular joint
[7th] S43.212 Anterior subluxation of left sternoclavicular joint
[7th] S43.213 Anterior subluxation of unspecified sternoclavicular joint
[7th] S43.214 Anterior dislocation of right sternoclavicular joint
[7th] S43.215 Anterior dislocation of left sternoclavicular joint
[7th] S43.216 Anterior dislocation of unspecified sternoclavicular joint
[6th] S43.22 Posterior subluxation and dislocation of sternoclavicular joint
[7th] S43.221 Posterior subluxation of right sternoclavicular joint
[7th] S43.222 Posterior subluxation of left sternoclavicular joint
[7th] S43.223 Posterior subluxation of unspecified sternoclavicular joint
[7th] S43.224 Posterior dislocation of right sternoclavicular joint
[7th] S43.225 Posterior dislocation of left sternoclavicular joint
[7th] S43.226 Posterior dislocation of unspecified sternoclavicular joint
[5th] S43.3 Subluxation and dislocation of other and unspecified parts of shoulder girdle
[6th] S43.30 Subluxation and dislocation of unspecified parts of shoulder girdle
Dislocation of shoulder girdle NOS
Subluxation of shoulder girdle NOS
[7th] S43.301 Subluxation of unspecified parts of right shoulder girdle
[7th] S43.302 Subluxation of unspecified parts of left shoulder girdle
[7th] S43.303 Subluxation of unspecified parts of unspecified shoulder girdle
[7th] S43.304 Dislocation of unspecified parts of right shoulder girdle
[7th] S43.305 Dislocation of unspecified parts of left shoulder girdle
[7th] S43.306 Dislocation of unspecified parts of unspecified shoulder girdle
[6th] S43.31 Subluxation and dislocation of scapula
[7th] S43.311 Subluxation of right scapula
[7th] S43.312 Subluxation of left scapula
[7th] S43.313 Subluxation of unspecified scapula
[7th] S43.314 Dislocation of right scapula
[7th] S43.315 Dislocation of left scapula
[7th] S43.316 Dislocation of unspecified scapula
[6th] S43.39 Subluxation and dislocation of other parts of shoulder girdle
[7th] S43.391 Subluxation of other parts of right shoulder girdle
[7th] S43.392 Subluxation of other parts of left shoulder girdle
[7th] S43.393 Subluxation of other parts of unspecified shoulder girdle
[7th] S43.394 Dislocation of other parts of right shoulder girdle
[7th] S43.395 Dislocation of other parts of left shoulder girdle
[7th] S43.396 Dislocation of other parts of unspecified shoulder girdle
[5th] S43.4 Sprain of shoulder joint
[6th] S43.40 Unspecified sprain of shoulder joint
[7th] S43.401 Unspecified sprain of right shoulder joint
[7th] S43.402 Unspecified sprain of left shoulder joint
[7th] S43.409 Unspecified sprain of unspecified shoulder joint
[6th] S43.41 Sprain of coracohumeral (ligament)
[7th] S43.411 Sprain of right coracohumeral (ligament)
[7th] S43.412 Sprain of left coracohumeral (ligament)
[7th] S43.419 Sprain of unspecified coracohumeral (ligament)
[6th] S43.42 Sprain of rotator cuff capsule
[EXCLUDES1] *rotator cuff syndrome (complete) (incomplete), not specified as traumatic (M75.1-)*
[EXCLUDES2] *injury of tendon of rotator cuff (S46.0-)*
[7th] S43.421 Sprain of right rotator cuff capsule
[7th] S43.422 Sprain of left rotator cuff capsule
[7th] S43.429 Sprain of unspecified rotator cuff capsule
[6th] S43.43 Superior glenoid labrum lesion
SLAP lesion
[7th] S43.431 Superior glenoid labrum lesion of right shoulder
[7th] S43.432 Superior glenoid labrum lesion of left shoulder
[7th] S43.439 Superior glenoid labrum lesion of unspecified shoulder
[6th] S43.49 Other sprain of shoulder joint
[7th] S43.491 Other sprain of right shoulder joint
[7th] S43.492 Other sprain of left shoulder joint
[7th] S43.499 Other sprain of unspecified shoulder joint
[5th] S43.5 Sprain of acromioclavicular joint
Sprain of acromioclavicular ligament
[7th] S43.50 Sprain of unspecified acromioclavicular joint
[7th] S43.51 Sprain of right acromioclavicular joint
[7th] S43.52 Sprain of left acromioclavicular joint
[5th] S43.6 Sprain of sternoclavicular joint
[7th] S43.60 Sprain of unspecified sternoclavicular joint
[7th] S43.61 Sprain of right sternoclavicular joint
[7th] S43.62 Sprain of left sternoclavicular joint
[5th] S43.8 Sprain of other specified parts of shoulder girdle
[7th] S43.80 Sprain of other specified parts of unspecified shoulder girdle
[7th] S43.81 Sprain of other specified parts of right shoulder girdle
[7th] S43.82 Sprain of other specified parts of left shoulder girdle
[5th] S43.9 Sprain of unspecified parts of shoulder girdle
[7th] S43.90 Sprain of unspecified parts of unspecified shoulder girdle
Sprain of shoulder girdle NOS
[7th] S43.91 Sprain of unspecified parts of right shoulder girdle
[7th] S43.92 Sprain of unspecified parts of left shoulder girdle
[4th] S44 Injury of nerves at shoulder and upper arm level
Code also any associated open wound (S41.-)
[EXCLUDES2] *injury of brachial plexus (S14.3-)*
The appropriate 7th character is to be added to each code from category S44
A = initial encounter
D = subsequent encounter
S = sequela
[5th] S44.0 Injury of ulnar nerve at upper arm level
[EXCLUDES1] *ulnar nerve NOS (S54.0)*

Unspecified Code | Other Specified Code | [N] Newborn Age: 0 | [P] Pediatric Age: 0-17 | [M] Maternity Age: 12-55
[A] Adult Age: 15-124 | ♂ Male | ♀ Female | ● New Code | ▲ Revised Code Title | ►◄ Revised Text

[7th] S44.00 Injury of ulnar nerve at upper arm level, unspecified arm
[7th] S44.01 Injury of ulnar nerve at upper arm level, right arm
[7th] S44.02 Injury of ulnar nerve at upper arm level, left arm
[5th] S44.1 Injury of median nerve at upper arm level
EXCLUDES1 *median nerve NOS (S54.1)*
[7th] S44.10 Injury of median nerve at upper arm level, unspecified arm
[7th] S44.11 Injury of median nerve at upper arm level, right arm
[7th] S44.12 Injury of median nerve at upper arm level, left arm
[5th] S44.2 Injury of radial nerve at upper arm level
EXCLUDES1 *radial nerve NOS (S54.2)*
[7th] S44.20 Injury of radial nerve at upper arm level, unspecified arm
[7th] S44.21 Injury of radial nerve at upper arm level, right arm
[7th] S44.22 Injury of radial nerve at upper arm level, left arm
[5th] S44.3 Injury of axillary nerve
[7th] S44.30 Injury of axillary nerve, unspecified arm
[7th] S44.31 Injury of axillary nerve, right arm
[7th] S44.32 Injury of axillary nerve, left arm
[5th] S44.4 Injury of musculocutaneous nerve
[7th] S44.40 Injury of musculocutaneous nerve, unspecified arm
[7th] S44.41 Injury of musculocutaneous nerve, right arm
[7th] S44.42 Injury of musculocutaneous nerve, left arm
[5th] S44.5 Injury of cutaneous sensory nerve at shoulder and upper arm level
[7th] S44.50 Injury of cutaneous sensory nerve at shoulder and upper arm level, unspecified arm
[7th] S44.51 Injury of cutaneous sensory nerve at shoulder and upper arm level, right arm
[7th] S44.52 Injury of cutaneous sensory nerve at shoulder and upper arm level, left arm
[5th] S44.8 Injury of other nerves at shoulder and upper arm level
[6th] S44.8X Injury of other nerves at shoulder and upper arm level
[7th] S44.8X1 Injury of other nerves at shoulder and upper arm level, right arm
[7th] S44.8X2 Injury of other nerves at shoulder and upper arm level, left arm
[7th] S44.8X9 Injury of other nerves at shoulder and upper arm level, unspecified arm
[5th] S44.9 Injury of unspecified nerve at shoulder and upper arm level
[7th] S44.90 Injury of unspecified nerve at shoulder and upper arm level, unspecified arm
[7th] S44.91 Injury of unspecified nerve at shoulder and upper arm level, right arm
[7th] S44.92 Injury of unspecified nerve at shoulder and upper arm level, left arm
[4th] S45 Injury of blood vessels at shoulder and upper arm level
Code also any associated open wound (S41.-)
EXCLUDES2 *injury of subclavian artery (S25.1)*
injury of subclavian vein (S25.3)
The appropriate 7th character is to be added to each code from category S45
A = initial encounter
D = subsequent encounter
S = sequela
[5th] S45.0 Injury of axillary artery
[6th] S45.00 Unspecified injury of axillary artery
[7th] S45.001 Unspecified injury of axillary artery, right side
[7th] S45.002 Unspecified injury of axillary artery, left side
[7th] S45.009 Unspecified injury of axillary artery, unspecified side
[6th] S45.01 Laceration of axillary artery
[7th] S45.011 Laceration of axillary artery, right side
[7th] S45.012 Laceration of axillary artery, left side
[7th] S45.019 Laceration of axillary artery, unspecified side
[6th] S45.09 Other specified injury of axillary artery
[7th] S45.091 Other specified injury of axillary artery, right side
[7th] S45.092 Other specified injury of axillary artery, left side
[7th] S45.099 Other specified injury of axillary artery, unspecified side
[5th] S45.1 Injury of brachial artery
[6th] S45.10 Unspecified injury of brachial artery
[7th] S45.101 Unspecified injury of brachial artery, right side
[7th] S45.102 Unspecified injury of brachial artery, left side
[7th] S45.109 Unspecified injury of brachial artery, unspecified side
[6th] S45.11 Laceration of brachial artery
[7th] S45.111 Laceration of brachial artery, right side
[7th] S45.112 Laceration of brachial artery, left side
[7th] S45.119 Laceration of brachial artery, unspecified side
[6th] S45.19 Other specified injury of brachial artery
[7th] S45.191 Other specified injury of brachial artery, right side
[7th] S45.192 Other specified injury of brachial artery, left side
[7th] S45.199 Other specified injury of brachial artery, unspecified side
[5th] S45.2 Injury of axillary or brachial vein
[6th] S45.20 Unspecified injury of axillary or brachial vein
[7th] S45.201 Unspecified injury of axillary or brachial vein, right side
[7th] S45.202 Unspecified injury of axillary or brachial vein, left side
[7th] S45.209 Unspecified injury of axillary or brachial vein, unspecified side
[6th] S45.21 Laceration of axillary or brachial vein
[7th] S45.211 Laceration of axillary or brachial vein, right side
[7th] S45.212 Laceration of axillary or brachial vein, left side
[7th] S45.219 Laceration of axillary or brachial vein, unspecified side
[6th] S45.29 Other specified injury of axillary or brachial vein
[7th] S45.291 Other specified injury of axillary or brachial vein, right side
[7th] S45.292 Other specified injury of axillary or brachial vein, left side
[7th] S45.299 Other specified injury of axillary or brachial vein, unspecified side
[5th] S45.3 Injury of superficial vein at shoulder and upper arm level
[6th] S45.30 Unspecified injury of superficial vein at shoulder and upper arm level
[7th] S45.301 Unspecified injury of superficial vein at shoulder and upper arm level, right arm
[7th] S45.302 Unspecified injury of superficial vein at shoulder and upper arm level, left arm
[7th] S45.309 Unspecified injury of superficial vein at shoulder and upper arm level, unspecified arm

[4th] 4th character required [5th] 5th character required [6th] 6th character required [7th] 7th character required [7th] Extension 'X' Alert
EXCLUDES1 Not coded here EXCLUDES2 Not included here PDx Primary Diagnosis Only Manifestation Code

6ᵗʰ S45.31 Laceration of superficial vein at shoulder and upper arm level
7ᵗʰ S45.311 Laceration of superficial vein at shoulder and upper arm level, right arm
7ᵗʰ S45.312 Laceration of superficial vein at shoulder and upper arm level, left arm
7ᵗʰ S45.319 Laceration of superficial vein at shoulder and upper arm level, unspecified arm
6ᵗʰ S45.39 Other specified injury of superficial vein at shoulder and upper arm level
7ᵗʰ S45.391 Other specified injury of superficial vein at shoulder and upper arm level, right arm
7ᵗʰ S45.392 Other specified injury of superficial vein at shoulder and upper arm level, left arm
7ᵗʰ S45.399 Other specified injury of superficial vein at shoulder and upper arm level, unspecified arm
5ᵗʰ S45.8 Injury of other specified blood vessels at shoulder and upper arm level
6ᵗʰ S45.80 Unspecified injury of other specified blood vessels at shoulder and upper arm level
7ᵗʰ S45.801 Unspecified injury of other specified blood vessels at shoulder and upper arm level, right arm
7ᵗʰ S45.802 Unspecified injury of other specified blood vessels at shoulder and upper arm level, left arm
7ᵗʰ S45.809 Unspecified injury of other specified blood vessels at shoulder and upper arm level, unspecified arm
6ᵗʰ S45.81 Laceration of other specified blood vessels at shoulder and upper arm level
7ᵗʰ S45.811 Laceration of other specified blood vessels at shoulder and upper arm level, right arm
7ᵗʰ S45.812 Laceration of other specified blood vessels at shoulder and upper arm level, left arm
7ᵗʰ S45.819 Laceration of other specified blood vessels at shoulder and upper arm level, unspecified arm
6ᵗʰ S45.89 Other specified injury of other specified blood vessels at shoulder and upper arm level
7ᵗʰ S45.891 Other specified injury of other specified blood vessels at shoulder and upper arm level, right arm
7ᵗʰ S45.892 Other specified injury of other specified blood vessels at shoulder and upper arm level, left arm
7ᵗʰ S45.899 Other specified injury of other specified blood vessels at shoulder and upper arm level, unspecified arm
5ᵗʰ S45.9 Injury of unspecified blood vessel at shoulder and upper arm level
6ᵗʰ S45.90 Unspecified injury of unspecified blood vessel at shoulder and upper arm level
7ᵗʰ S45.901 Unspecified injury of unspecified blood vessel at shoulder and upper arm level, right arm
7ᵗʰ S45.902 Unspecified injury of unspecified blood vessel at shoulder and upper arm level, left arm
7ᵗʰ S45.909 Unspecified injury of unspecified blood vessel at shoulder and upper arm level, unspecified arm
6ᵗʰ S45.91 Laceration of unspecified blood vessel at shoulder and upper arm level
7ᵗʰ S45.911 Laceration of unspecified blood vessel at shoulder and upper arm level, right arm
7ᵗʰ S45.912 Laceration of unspecified blood vessel at shoulder and upper arm level, left arm

7ᵗʰ S45.919 Laceration of unspecified blood vessel at shoulder and upper arm level, unspecified arm
6ᵗʰ S45.99 Other specified injury of unspecified blood vessel at shoulder and upper arm level
7ᵗʰ S45.991 Other specified injury of unspecified blood vessel at shoulder and upper arm level, right arm
7ᵗʰ S45.992 Other specified injury of unspecified blood vessel at shoulder and upper arm level, left arm
7ᵗʰ S45.999 Other specified injury of unspecified blood vessel at shoulder and upper arm level, unspecified arm
4ᵗʰ S46 Injury of muscle, fascia and tendon at shoulder and upper arm level

Code also any associated open wound (S41.-)

EXCLUDES2 injury of muscle, fascia and tendon at elbow (S56.-)
sprain of joints and ligaments of shoulder girdle (S43.9)

The appropriate 7th character is to be added to each code from category S46
A = initial encounter
D = subsequent encounter
S = sequela

5ᵗʰ S46.0 Injury of muscle(s) and tendon(s) of the rotator cuff of shoulder
6ᵗʰ S46.00 Unspecified injury of muscle(s) and tendon(s) of the rotator cuff of shoulder
7ᵗʰ S46.001 Unspecified injury of muscle(s) and tendon(s) of the rotator cuff of right shoulder
7ᵗʰ S46.002 Unspecified injury of muscle(s) and tendon(s) of the rotator cuff of left shoulder
7ᵗʰ S46.009 Unspecified injury of muscle(s) and tendon(s) of the rotator cuff of unspecified shoulder
6ᵗʰ S46.01 Strain of muscle(s) and tendon(s) of the rotator cuff of shoulder
7ᵗʰ S46.011 Strain of muscle(s) and tendon(s) of the rotator cuff of right shoulder
7ᵗʰ S46.012 Strain of muscle(s) and tendon(s) of the rotator cuff of left shoulder
7ᵗʰ S46.019 Strain of muscle(s) and tendon(s) of the rotator cuff of unspecified shoulder
6ᵗʰ S46.02 Laceration of muscle(s) and tendon(s) of the rotator cuff of shoulder
7ᵗʰ S46.021 Laceration of muscle(s) and tendon(s) of the rotator cuff of right shoulder
7ᵗʰ S46.022 Laceration of muscle(s) and tendon(s) of the rotator cuff of left shoulder
7ᵗʰ S46.029 Laceration of muscle(s) and tendon(s) of the rotator cuff of unspecified shoulder
6ᵗʰ S46.09 Other injury of muscle(s) and tendon(s) of the rotator cuff of shoulder
7ᵗʰ S46.091 Other injury of muscle(s) and tendon(s) of the rotator cuff of right shoulder
7ᵗʰ S46.092 Other injury of muscle(s) and tendon(s) of the rotator cuff of left shoulder
7ᵗʰ S46.099 Other injury of muscle(s) and tendon(s) of the rotator cuff of unspecified shoulder
5ᵗʰ S46.1 Injury of muscle, fascia and tendon of long head of biceps
6ᵗʰ S46.10 Unspecified injury of muscle, fascia and tendon of long head of biceps
7ᵗʰ S46.101 Unspecified injury of muscle, fascia and tendon of long head of biceps, right arm
7ᵗʰ S46.102 Unspecified injury of muscle, fascia and tendon of long head of biceps, left arm

Unspecified Code Other Specified Code N Newborn Age: 0 P Pediatric Age: 0-17 M Maternity Age: 12-55
A Adult Age: 15-124 ♂ Male ♀ Female ● New Code ▲ Revised Code Title ►◄ Revised Text

[7th] S46.109 Unspecified injury of muscle, fascia and tendon of long head of biceps, unspecified arm

[6th] S46.11 Strain of muscle, fascia and tendon of long head of biceps

[7th] S46.111 Strain of muscle, fascia and tendon of long head of biceps, right arm

[7th] S46.112 Strain of muscle, fascia and tendon of long head of biceps, left arm

[7th] S46.119 Strain of muscle, fascia and tendon of long head of biceps, unspecified arm

[6th] S46.12 Laceration of muscle, fascia and tendon of long head of biceps

[7th] S46.121 Laceration of muscle, fascia and tendon of long head of biceps, right arm

[7th] S46.122 Laceration of muscle, fascia and tendon of long head of biceps, left arm

[7th] S46.129 Laceration of muscle, fascia and tendon of long head of biceps, unspecified arm

[6th] S46.19 Other injury of muscle, fascia and tendon of long head of biceps

[7th] S46.191 Other injury of muscle, fascia and tendon of long head of biceps, right arm

[7th] S46.192 Other injury of muscle, fascia and tendon of long head of biceps, left arm

[7th] S46.199 Other injury of muscle, fascia and tendon of long head of biceps, unspecified arm

[5th] S46.2 Injury of muscle, fascia and tendon of other parts of biceps

[6th] S46.20 Unspecified injury of muscle, fascia and tendon of other parts of biceps

[7th] S46.201 Unspecified injury of muscle, fascia and tendon of other parts of biceps, right arm

[7th] S46.202 Unspecified injury of muscle, fascia and tendon of other parts of biceps, left arm

[7th] S46.209 Unspecified injury of muscle, fascia and tendon of other parts of biceps, unspecified arm

[6th] S46.21 Strain of muscle, fascia and tendon of other parts of biceps

[7th] S46.211 Strain of muscle, fascia and tendon of other parts of biceps, right arm

[7th] S46.212 Strain of muscle, fascia and tendon of other parts of biceps, left arm

[7th] S46.219 Strain of muscle, fascia and tendon of other parts of biceps, unspecified arm

[6th] S46.22 Laceration of muscle, fascia and tendon of other parts of biceps

[7th] S46.221 Laceration of muscle, fascia and tendon of other parts of biceps, right arm

[7th] S46.222 Laceration of muscle, fascia and tendon of other parts of biceps, left arm

[7th] S46.229 Laceration of muscle, fascia and tendon of other parts of biceps, unspecified arm

[6th] S46.29 Other injury of muscle, fascia and tendon of other parts of biceps

[7th] S46.291 Other injury of muscle, fascia and tendon of other parts of biceps, right arm

[7th] S46.292 Other injury of muscle, fascia and tendon of other parts of biceps, left arm

[7th] S46.299 Other injury of muscle, fascia and tendon of other parts of biceps, unspecified arm

[5th] S46.3 Injury of muscle, fascia and tendon of triceps

[6th] S46.30 Unspecified injury of muscle, fascia and tendon of triceps

[7th] S46.301 Unspecified injury of muscle, fascia and tendon of triceps, right arm

[7th] S46.302 Unspecified injury of muscle, fascia and tendon of triceps, left arm

[7th] S46.309 Unspecified injury of muscle, fascia and tendon of triceps, unspecified arm

[6th] S46.31 Strain of muscle, fascia and tendon of triceps

[7th] S46.311 Strain of muscle, fascia and tendon of triceps, right arm

[7th] S46.312 Strain of muscle, fascia and tendon of triceps, left arm

[7th] S46.319 Strain of muscle, fascia and tendon of triceps, unspecified arm

[6th] S46.32 Laceration of muscle, fascia and tendon of triceps

[7th] S46.321 Laceration of muscle, fascia and tendon of triceps, right arm

[7th] S46.322 Laceration of muscle, fascia and tendon of triceps, left arm

[7th] S46.329 Laceration of muscle, fascia and tendon of triceps, unspecified arm

[6th] S46.39 Other injury of muscle, fascia and tendon of triceps

[7th] S46.391 Other injury of muscle, fascia and tendon of triceps, right arm

[7th] S46.392 Other injury of muscle, fascia and tendon of triceps, left arm

[7th] S46.399 Other injury of muscle, fascia and tendon of triceps, unspecified arm

[5th] S46.8 Injury of other muscles, fascia and tendons at shoulder and upper arm level

[6th] S46.80 Unspecified injury of other muscles, fascia and tendons at shoulder and upper arm level

[7th] S46.801 Unspecified injury of other muscles, fascia and tendons at shoulder and upper arm level, right arm

[7th] S46.802 Unspecified injury of other muscles, fascia and tendons at shoulder and upper arm level, left arm

[7th] S46.809 Unspecified injury of other muscles, fascia and tendons at shoulder and upper arm level, unspecified arm

[6th] S46.81 Strain of other muscles, fascia and tendons at shoulder and upper arm level

[7th] S46.811 Strain of other muscles, fascia and tendons at shoulder and upper arm level, right arm

[7th] S46.812 Strain of other muscles, fascia and tendons at shoulder and upper arm level, left arm

[7th] S46.819 Strain of other muscles, fascia and tendons at shoulder and upper arm level, unspecified arm

[6th] S46.82 Laceration of other muscles, fascia and tendons at shoulder and upper arm level

[7th] S46.821 Laceration of other muscles, fascia and tendons at shoulder and upper arm level, right arm

[7th] S46.822 Laceration of other muscles, fascia and tendons at shoulder and upper arm level, left arm

[7th] S46.829 Laceration of other muscles, fascia and tendons at shoulder and upper arm level, unspecified arm

[6th] S46.89 Other injury of other muscles, fascia and tendons at shoulder and upper arm level

[7th] S46.891 Other injury of other muscles, fascia and tendons at shoulder and upper arm level, right arm

[7th] S46.892 Other injury of other muscles, fascia and tendons at shoulder and upper arm level, left arm

[7th] S46.899 Other injury of other muscles, fascia and tendons at shoulder and upper arm level, unspecified arm

[4th] 4th character required [5th] 5th character required [6th] 6th character required [7th] 7th character required [X] Extension 'X' Alert
[EXCLUDES1] Not coded here [EXCLUDES2] Not included here [PDx] Primary Diagnosis Only Manifestation Code

(6) **S46.9** Injury of unspecified muscle, fascia and tendon at shoulder and upper arm level

  (6) **S46.90** Unspecified injury of unspecified muscle, fascia and tendon at shoulder and upper arm level

    (7) **S46.901** Unspecified injury of unspecified muscle, fascia and tendon at shoulder and upper arm level, right arm

    (7) **S46.902** Unspecified injury of unspecified muscle, fascia and tendon at shoulder and upper arm level, left arm

    (7) **S46.909** Unspecified injury of unspecified muscle, fascia and tendon at shoulder and upper arm level, unspecified arm

  (6) **S46.91** Strain of unspecified muscle, fascia and tendon at shoulder and upper arm level

    (7) **S46.911** Strain of unspecified muscle, fascia and tendon at shoulder and upper arm level, right arm

    (7) **S46.912** Strain of unspecified muscle, fascia and tendon at shoulder and upper arm level, left arm

    (7) **S46.919** Strain of unspecified muscle, fascia and tendon at shoulder and upper arm level, unspecified arm

  (6) **S46.92** Laceration of unspecified muscle, fascia and tendon at shoulder and upper arm level

    (7) **S46.921** Laceration of unspecified muscle, fascia and tendon at shoulder and upper arm level, right arm

    (7) **S46.922** Laceration of unspecified muscle, fascia and tendon at shoulder and upper arm level, left arm

    (7) **S46.929** Laceration of unspecified muscle, fascia and tendon at shoulder and upper arm level, unspecified arm

  (6) **S46.99** Other injury of unspecified muscle, fascia and tendon at shoulder and upper arm level

    (7) **S46.991** Other injury of unspecified muscle, fascia and tendon at shoulder and upper arm level, right arm

    (7) **S46.992** Other injury of unspecified muscle, fascia and tendon at shoulder and upper arm level, left arm

    (7) **S46.999** Other injury of unspecified muscle, fascia and tendon at shoulder and upper arm level, unspecified arm

(4) **S47** Crushing injury of shoulder and upper arm

  Use additional code for all associated injuries

  EXCLUDES2 crushing injury of elbow (S57.0-)

  The appropriate 7th character is to be added to each code from category S47

  A = initial encounter
  D = subsequent encounter
  S = sequela

  (7) **S47.1** Crushing injury of right shoulder and upper arm

  (7) **S47.2** Crushing injury of left shoulder and upper arm

  (7) **S47.9** Crushing injury of shoulder and upper arm, unspecified arm

(4) **S48** Traumatic amputation of shoulder and upper arm

  An amputation not identified as partial or complete should be coded to complete

  EXCLUDES1 traumatic amputation at elbow level (S58.0)

  The appropriate 7th character is to be added to each code from category S48

  A = initial encounter
  D = subsequent encounter
  S = sequela

  (5) **S48.0** Traumatic amputation at shoulder joint

  (6) **S48.01** Complete traumatic amputation at shoulder joint

    (7) **S48.011** Complete traumatic amputation at right shoulder joint

    (7) **S48.012** Complete traumatic amputation at left shoulder joint

    (7) **S48.019** Complete traumatic amputation at unspecified shoulder joint

  (6) **S48.02** Partial traumatic amputation at shoulder joint

    (7) **S48.021** Partial traumatic amputation at right shoulder joint

    (7) **S48.022** Partial traumatic amputation at left shoulder joint

    (7) **S48.029** Partial traumatic amputation at unspecified shoulder joint

  (5) **S48.1** Traumatic amputation at level between shoulder and elbow

  (6) **S48.11** Complete traumatic amputation at level between shoulder and elbow

    (7) **S48.111** Complete traumatic amputation at level between right shoulder and elbow

    (7) **S48.112** Complete traumatic amputation at level between left shoulder and elbow

    (7) **S48.119** Complete traumatic amputation at level between unspecified shoulder and elbow

  (6) **S48.12** Partial traumatic amputation at level between shoulder and elbow

    (7) **S48.121** Partial traumatic amputation at level between right shoulder and elbow

    (7) **S48.122** Partial traumatic amputation at level between left shoulder and elbow

    (7) **S48.129** Partial traumatic amputation at level between unspecified shoulder and elbow

  (5) **S48.9** Traumatic amputation of shoulder and upper arm, level unspecified

  (6) **S48.91** Complete traumatic amputation of shoulder and upper arm, level unspecified

    (7) **S48.911** Complete traumatic amputation of right shoulder and upper arm, level unspecified

    (7) **S48.912** Complete traumatic amputation of left shoulder and upper arm, level unspecified

    (7) **S48.919** Complete traumatic amputation of unspecified shoulder and upper arm, level unspecified

  (6) **S48.92** Partial traumatic amputation of shoulder and upper arm, level unspecified

    (7) **S48.921** Partial traumatic amputation of right shoulder and upper arm, level unspecified

    (7) **S48.922** Partial traumatic amputation of left shoulder and upper arm, level unspecified

    (7) **S48.929** Partial traumatic amputation of unspecified shoulder and upper arm, level unspecified

(4) **S49** Other and unspecified injuries of shoulder and upper arm

  The appropriate 7th character is to be added to each code from subcategories S49.0 and S49.1

  A = initial encounter for closed fracture
  D = subsequent encounter for fracture with routine healing
  G = subsequent encounter for fracture with delayed healing
  K = subsequent encounter for fracture with nonunion
  P = subsequent encounter for fracture with malunion
  S = sequela

  (5) **S49.0** Physeal fracture of upper end of humerus

  (6) **S49.00** Unspecified physeal fracture of upper end of humerus

    (7) **S49.001** Unspecified physeal fracture of upper end of humerus, right arm

Unspecified Code   Other Specified Code   N Newborn Age: 0   P Pediatric Age: 0-17   M Maternity Age: 12-55
A Adult Age: 15-124   ♂ Male   ♀ Female   ● New Code   ▲ Revised Code Title   ►◄ Revised Text

ICD-10-CM 2015   **587**

S49.002 Unspecified physeal fracture of upper end of humerus, left arm

S49.009 Unspecified physeal fracture of upper end of humerus, unspecified arm

S49.01 Salter-Harris Type I physeal fracture of upper end of humerus

S49.011 Salter-Harris Type I physeal fracture of upper end of humerus, right arm

S49.012 Salter-Harris Type I physeal fracture of upper end of humerus, left arm

S49.019 Salter-Harris Type I physeal fracture of upper end of humerus, unspecified arm

S49.02 Salter-Harris Type II physeal fracture of upper end of humerus

S49.021 Salter-Harris Type II physeal fracture of upper end of humerus, right arm

S49.022 Salter-Harris Type II physeal fracture of upper end of humerus, left arm

S49.029 Salter-Harris Type II physeal fracture of upper end of humerus, unspecified arm

S49.03 Salter-Harris Type III physeal fracture of upper end of humerus

S49.031 Salter Harris Type III physeal fracture of upper end of humerus, right arm

S49.032 Salter Harris Type III physeal fracture of upper end of humerus, left arm

S49.039 Salter Harris Type III physeal fracture of upper end of humerus, unspecified arm

S49.04 Salter-Harris Type IV physeal fracture of upper end of humerus

S49.041 Salter-Harris Type IV physeal fracture of upper end of humerus, right arm

S49.042 Salter-Harris Type IV physeal fracture of upper end of humerus, left arm

S49.049 Salter-Harris Type IV physeal fracture of upper end of humerus, unspecified arm

S49.09 Other physeal fracture of upper end of humerus

S49.091 Other physeal fracture of upper end of humerus, right arm

S49.092 Other physeal fracture of upper end of humerus, left arm

S49.099 Other physeal fracture of upper end of humerus, unspecified arm

S49.1 Physeal fracture of lower end of humerus

S49.10 Unspecified physeal fracture of lower end of humerus

S49.101 Unspecified physeal fracture of lower end of humerus, right arm

S49.102 Unspecified physeal fracture of lower end of humerus, left arm

S49.109 Unspecified physeal fracture of lower end of humerus, unspecified arm

S49.11 Salter-Harris Type I physeal fracture of lower end of humerus

S49.111 Salter-Harris Type I physeal fracture of lower end of humerus, right arm

S49.112 Salter-Harris Type I physeal fracture of lower end of humerus, left arm

S49.119 Salter-Harris Type I physeal fracture of lower end of humerus, unspecified arm

S49.12 Salter-Harris Type II physeal fracture of lower end of humerus

S49.121 Salter-Harris Type II physeal fracture of lower end of humerus, right arm

S49.122 Salter-Harris Type II physeal fracture of lower end of humerus, left arm

S49.129 Salter-Harris Type II physeal fracture of lower end of humerus, unspecified arm

S49.13 Salter Harris Type III physeal fracture of lower end of humerus

S49.131 Salter Harris Type III physeal fracture of lower end of humerus, right arm

S49.132 Salter Harris Type III physeal fracture of lower end of humerus, left arm

S49.139 Salter Harris Type III physeal fracture of lower end of humerus, unspecified arm

S49.14 Salter-Harris Type IV physeal fracture of lower end of humerus

S49.141 Salter-Harris Type IV physeal fracture of lower end of humerus, right arm

S49.142 Salter-Harris Type IV physeal fracture of lower end of humerus, left arm

S49.149 Salter-Harris Type IV physeal fracture of lower end of humerus, unspecified arm

S49.19 Other physeal fracture of lower end of humerus

S49.191 Other physeal fracture of lower end of humerus, right arm

S49.192 Other physeal fracture of lower end of humerus, left arm

S49.199 Other physeal fracture of lower end of humerus, unspecified arm

S49.8 Other specified injuries of shoulder and upper arm

The appropriate 7th character is to be added to each code in subcategory S49.8

A = initial encounter
D = subsequent encounter
S = sequela

S49.80 Other specified injuries of shoulder and upper arm, unspecified arm

S49.81 Other specified injuries of right shoulder and upper arm

S49.82 Other specified injuries of left shoulder and upper arm

S49.9 Unspecified injury of shoulder and upper arm

The appropriate 7th character is to be added to each code in subcategory S49.9

A = initial encounter
D = subsequent encounter
S = sequela

S49.90 Unspecified injury of shoulder and upper arm, unspecified arm

S49.91 Unspecified injury of right shoulder and upper arm

S49.92 Unspecified injury of left shoulder and upper arm

Injuries to the elbow and forearm (S50-S59)

EXCLUDES2 burns and corrosions (T20-T32)
frostbite (T33-T34)
injuries of wrist and hand (S60-S69)
insect bite or sting, venomous (T63.4)

S50 Superficial injury of elbow and forearm

EXCLUDES2 superficial injury of wrist and hand (S60.-)

The appropriate 7th character is to be added to each code from category S50

A = initial encounter
D = subsequent encounter
S = sequela

S50.0 Contusion of elbow

S50.00 Contusion of unspecified elbow

S50.01 Contusion of right elbow

S50.02 Contusion of left elbow

S50.1 Contusion of forearm

S50.10 Contusion of unspecified forearm

S50.11 Contusion of right forearm

S50.12 Contusion of left forearm

4ᵗʰ 4ᵗʰ character required   5ᵗʰ 5ᵗʰ character required   6ᵗʰ 6ᵗʰ character required   7ᵗʰ 7ᵗʰ character required   7ᵗʰ Extension 'X' Alert

EXCLUDES 1 Not coded here   EXCLUDES 2 Not included here   PDX Primary Diagnosis Only   Manifestation Code

588

ICD-10-CM 2015

[5th] S50.3 Other superficial injuries of elbow
- [6th] S50.31 Abrasion of elbow
  - [7th] S50.311 Abrasion of right elbow
  - [7th] S50.312 Abrasion of left elbow
  - [7th] S50.319 Abrasion of unspecified elbow
- [6th] S50.32 Blister (nonthermal) of elbow
  - [7th] S50.321 Blister (nonthermal) of right elbow
  - [7th] S50.322 Blister (nonthermal) of left elbow
  - [7th] S50.329 Blister (nonthermal) of unspecified elbow
- [6th] S50.34 External constriction of elbow
  - [7th] S50.341 External constriction of right elbow
  - [7th] S50.342 External constriction of left elbow
  - [7th] S50.349 External constriction of unspecified elbow
- [6th] S50.35 Superficial foreign body of elbow

  Splinter in the elbow
  - [7th] S50.351 Superficial foreign body of right elbow
  - [7th] S50.352 Superficial foreign body of left elbow
  - [7th] S50.359 Superficial foreign body of unspecified elbow
- [6th] S50.36 Insect bite (nonvenomous) of elbow
  - [7th] S50.361 Insect bite (nonvenomous) of right elbow
  - [7th] S50.362 Insect bite (nonvenomous) of left elbow
  - [7th] S50.369 Insect bite (nonvenomous) of unspecified elbow
- [6th] S50.37 Other superficial bite of elbow

  EXCLUDES1 *open bite of elbow (S51.04)*
  - [7th] S50.371 Other superficial bite of right elbow
  - [7th] S50.372 Other superficial bite of left elbow
  - [7th] S50.379 Other superficial bite of unspecified elbow

[5th] S50.8 Other superficial injuries of forearm
- [6th] S50.81 Abrasion of forearm
  - [7th] S50.811 Abrasion of right forearm
  - [7th] S50.812 Abrasion of left forearm
  - [7th] S50.819 Abrasion of unspecified forearm
- [6th] S50.82 Blister (nonthermal) of forearm
  - [7th] S50.821 Blister (nonthermal) of right forearm
  - [7th] S50.822 Blister (nonthermal) of left forearm
  - [7th] S50.829 Blister (nonthermal) of unspecified forearm
- [6th] S50.84 External constriction of forearm
  - [7th] S50.841 External constriction of right forearm
  - [7th] S50.842 External constriction of left forearm
  - [7th] S50.849 External constriction of unspecified forearm
- [6th] S50.85 Superficial foreign body of forearm

  Splinter in the forearm
  - [7th] S50.851 Superficial foreign body of right forearm
  - [7th] S50.852 Superficial foreign body of left forearm
  - [7th] S50.859 Superficial foreign body of unspecified forearm
- [6th] S50.86 Insect bite (nonvenomous) of forearm
  - [7th] S50.861 Insect bite (nonvenomous) of right forearm
  - [7th] S50.862 Insect bite (nonvenomous) of left forearm
  - [7th] S50.869 Insect bite (nonvenomous) of unspecified forearm
- [6th] S50.87 Other superficial bite of forearm

  EXCLUDES1 *open bite of forearm (S51.84)*
  - [7th] S50.871 Other superficial bite of right forearm
  - [7th] S50.872 Other superficial bite of left forearm
  - [7th] S50.879 Other superficial bite of unspecified forearm

[5th] S50.9 Unspecified superficial injury of elbow and forearm
- [6th] S50.90 Unspecified superficial injury of elbow
  - [7th] S50.901 Unspecified superficial injury of right elbow
  - [7th] S50.902 Unspecified superficial injury of left elbow
  - [7th] S50.909 Unspecified superficial injury of unspecified elbow
- [6th] S50.91 Unspecified superficial injury of forearm
  - [7th] S50.911 Unspecified superficial injury of right forearm
  - [7th] S50.912 Unspecified superficial injury of left forearm
  - [7th] S50.919 Unspecified superficial injury of unspecified forearm

[4th] S51 Open wound of elbow and forearm

Code also any associated wound infection

EXCLUDES1 *open fracture of elbow and forearm (S52.- with open fracture 7th character)*
traumatic amputation of elbow and forearm (S58.-)

EXCLUDES2 *open wound of wrist and hand (S61.-)*

The appropriate 7th character is to be added to each code from category S51
A = initial encounter
D = subsequent encounter
S = sequela

[5th] S51.0 Open wound of elbow
- [6th] S51.00 Unspecified open wound of elbow
  - [7th] S51.001 Unspecified open wound of right elbow
  - [7th] S51.002 Unspecified open wound of left elbow
  - [7th] S51.009 Unspecified open wound of unspecified elbow

    Open wound of elbow NOS
- [6th] S51.01 Laceration without foreign body of elbow
  - [7th] S51.011 Laceration without foreign body of right elbow
  - [7th] S51.012 Laceration without foreign body of left elbow
  - [7th] S51.019 Laceration without foreign body of unspecified elbow
- [6th] S51.02 Laceration with foreign body of elbow
  - [7th] S51.021 Laceration with foreign body of right elbow
  - [7th] S51.022 Laceration with foreign body of left elbow
  - [7th] S51.029 Laceration with foreign body of unspecified elbow
- [6th] S51.03 Puncture wound without foreign body of elbow
  - [7th] S51.031 Puncture wound without foreign body of right elbow
  - [7th] S51.032 Puncture wound without foreign body of left elbow
  - [7th] S51.039 Puncture wound without foreign body of unspecified elbow
- [6th] S51.04 Puncture wound with foreign body of elbow
  - [7th] S51.041 Puncture wound with foreign body of right elbow
  - [7th] S51.042 Puncture wound with foreign body of left elbow
  - [7th] S51.049 Puncture wound with foreign body of unspecified elbow
- [6th] S51.05 Open bite of elbow

  Bite of elbow NOS

  EXCLUDES1 *superficial bite of elbow (S50.36, S50.37)*
  - [7th] S51.051 Open bite, right elbow
  - [7th] S51.052 Open bite, left elbow
  - [7th] S51.059 Open bite, unspecified elbow

[5th] S51.8 Open wound of forearm

EXCLUDES2 *open wound of elbow (S51.0-)*
- [6th] S51.80 Unspecified open wound of forearm
  - [7th] S51.801 Unspecified open wound of right forearm
  - [7th] S51.802 Unspecified open wound of left forearm
  - [7th] S51.809 Unspecified open wound of unspecified forearm

    Open wound of forearm NOS
- [6th] S51.81 Laceration without foreign body of forearm
  - [7th] S51.811 Laceration without foreign body of right forearm

Unspecified Code | Other Specified Code | [N] Newborn Age: 0 | [P] Pediatric Age: 0-17 | [M] Maternity Age: 12-55
[A] Adult Age: 15-124 | ♂ Male | ♀ Female | ● New Code | ▲ Revised Code Title | ►◄ Revised Text

[7th] S51.812 Laceration without foreign body of left forearm
[7th] S51.819 Laceration without foreign body of unspecified forearm

[6th] S51.82 Laceration with foreign body of forearm
[7th] S51.821 Laceration with foreign body of right forearm
[7th] S51.822 Laceration with foreign body of left forearm
[7th] S51.829 Laceration with foreign body of unspecified forearm

[6th] S51.83 Puncture wound without foreign body of forearm
[7th] S51.831 Puncture wound without foreign body of right forearm
[7th] S51.832 Puncture wound without foreign body of left forearm
[7th] S51.839 Puncture wound without foreign body of unspecified forearm

[6th] S51.84 Puncture wound with foreign body of forearm
[7th] S51.841 Puncture wound with foreign body of right forearm
[7th] S51.842 Puncture wound with foreign body of left forearm
[7th] S51.849 Puncture wound with foreign body of unspecified forearm

[6th] S51.85 Open bite of forearm
Bite of forearm NOS
[EXCLUDES1] *superficial bite of forearm (S50.86, S50.87)*
[7th] S51.851 Open bite of right forearm
[7th] S51.852 Open bite of left forearm
[7th] S51.859 Open bite of unspecified forearm

[4th] S52 Fracture of forearm
[NOTES] A fracture not indicated as displaced or nondisplaced should be coded to displaced
A fracture not indicated as open or closed should be coded to closed
The open fracture designations are based on the Gustilo open fracture classification
[EXCLUDES1] *traumatic amputation of forearm (S58.-)*
[EXCLUDES2] *fracture at wrist and hand level (S62.-)*
The appropriate 7th character is to be added to all codes from category S52
A = initial encounter for closed fracture
B = initial encounter for open fracture type I or II
C = initial encounter for open fracture type IIIA, IIIB, or IIIC
D = subsequent encounter for closed fracture with routine healing
E = subsequent encounter for open fracture type I or II with routine healing
F = subsequent encounter for open fracture type IIIA, IIIB, or IIIC with routine healing
G = subsequent encounter for closed fracture with delayed healing
H = subsequent encounter for open fracture type I or II with delayed healing
J = subsequent encounter for open fracture type IIIA, IIIB, or IIIC with delayed healing
K = subsequent encounter for closed fracture with nonunion
M = subsequent encounter for open fracture type I or II with nonunion
N = subsequent encounter for open fracture type IIIA, IIIB, or IIIC with nonunion
P = subsequent encounter for closed fracture with malunion
Q = subsequent encounter for open fracture type I or II with malunion
R = subsequent encounter for open fracture type IIIA, IIIB, or IIIC with malunion
S = sequela

[5th] S52.0 Fracture of upper end of ulna
Fracture of proximal end of ulna
[EXCLUDES2] *fracture of elbow NOS (S42.40-)*
fractures of shaft of ulna (S52.2-)

[6th] S52.00 Unspecified fracture of upper end of ulna
[7th] S52.001 Unspecified fracture of upper end of right ulna
[7th] S52.002 Unspecified fracture of upper end of left ulna
[7th] S52.009 Unspecified fracture of upper end of unspecified ulna

[6th] S52.01 Torus fracture of upper end of ulna
The appropriate 7th character is to be added to all codes in subcategory S52.01
A = initial encounter for closed fracture
D = subsequent encounter for fracture with routine healing
G = subsequent encounter for fracture with delayed healing
K = subsequent encounter for fracture with nonunion
P = subsequent encounter for fracture with malunion
S = sequela
[7th] S52.011 Torus fracture of upper end of right ulna
[7th] S52.012 Torus fracture of upper end of left ulna
[7th] S52.019 Torus fracture of upper end of unspecified ulna

[6th] S52.02 Fracture of olecranon process without intraarticular extension of ulna
[7th] S52.021 Displaced fracture of olecranon process without intraarticular extension of right ulna
[7th] S52.022 Displaced fracture of olecranon process without intraarticular extension of left ulna
[7th] S52.023 Displaced fracture of olecranon process without intraarticular extension of unspecified ulna
[7th] S52.024 Nondisplaced fracture of olecranon process without intraarticular extension of right ulna
[7th] S52.025 Nondisplaced fracture of olecranon process without intraarticular extension of left ulna
[7th] S52.026 Nondisplaced fracture of olecranon process without intraarticular extension of unspecified ulna

[6th] S52.03 Fracture of olecranon process with intraarticular extension of ulna
[7th] S52.031 Displaced fracture of olecranon process with intraarticular extension of right ulna
[7th] S52.032 Displaced fracture of olecranon process with intraarticular extension of left ulna
[7th] S52.033 Displaced fracture of olecranon process with intraarticular extension of unspecified ulna
[7th] S52.034 Nondisplaced fracture of olecranon process with intraarticular extension of right ulna
[7th] S52.035 Nondisplaced fracture of olecranon process with intraarticular extension of left ulna
[7th] S52.036 Nondisplaced fracture of olecranon process with intraarticular extension of unspecified ulna

[6th] S52.04 Fracture of coronoid process of ulna
[7th] S52.041 Displaced fracture of coronoid process of right ulna
[7th] S52.042 Displaced fracture of coronoid process of left ulna
[7th] S52.043 Displaced fracture of coronoid process of unspecified ulna
[7th] S52.044 Nondisplaced fracture of coronoid process of right ulna

[4th] 4th character required [5th] 5th character required [6th] 6th character required [7th] 7th character required [7th] Extension 'X' Alert
[EXCLUDES1] Not coded here [EXCLUDES2] Not included here [PDx] Primary Diagnosis Only Manifestation Code

7ᵗʰ S52.045 Nondisplaced fracture of coronoid process of left ulna

7ᵗʰ S52.046 Nondisplaced fracture of coronoid process of unspecified ulna

6ᵗʰ S52.09 Other fracture of upper end of ulna

7ᵗʰ S52.091 Other fracture of upper end of right ulna

7ᵗʰ S52.092 Other fracture of upper end of left ulna

7ᵗʰ S52.099 Other fracture of upper end of unspecified ulna

5ᵗʰ S52.1 Fracture of upper end of radius

Fracture of proximal end of radius

EXCLUDES2 physeal fractures of upper end of radius (S59.2-)
fracture of shaft of radius (S52.3-)

6ᵗʰ S52.10 Unspecified fracture of upper end of radius

7ᵗʰ S52.101 Unspecified fracture of upper end of right radius

7ᵗʰ S52.102 Unspecified fracture of upper end of left radius

7ᵗʰ S52.109 Unspecified fracture of upper end of unspecified radius

6ᵗʰ S52.11 Torus fracture of upper end of radius

The appropriate 7th character is to be added to all codes in subcategory S52.11

A = initial encounter for closed fracture

D = subsequent encounter for fracture with routine healing

G = subsequent encounter for fracture with delayed healing

K = subsequent encounter for fracture with nonunion

P = subsequent encounter for fracture with malunion

S = sequela

7ᵗʰ S52.111 Torus fracture of upper end of right radius

7ᵗʰ S52.112 Torus fracture of upper end of left radius

7ᵗʰ S52.119 Torus fracture of upper end of unspecified radius

6ᵗʰ S52.12 Fracture of head of radius

7ᵗʰ S52.121 Displaced fracture of head of right radius

7ᵗʰ S52.122 Displaced fracture of head of left radius

7ᵗʰ S52.123 Displaced fracture of head of unspecified radius

7ᵗʰ S52.124 Nondisplaced fracture of head of right radius

7ᵗʰ S52.125 Nondisplaced fracture of head of left radius

7ᵗʰ S52.126 Nondisplaced fracture of head of unspecified radius

6ᵗʰ S52.13 Fracture of neck of radius

7ᵗʰ S52.131 Displaced fracture of neck of right radius

7ᵗʰ S52.132 Displaced fracture of neck of left radius

7ᵗʰ S52.133 Displaced fracture of neck of unspecified radius

7ᵗʰ S52.134 Nondisplaced fracture of neck of right radius

7ᵗʰ S52.135 Nondisplaced fracture of neck of left radius

7ᵗʰ S52.136 Nondisplaced fracture of neck of unspecified radius

6ᵗʰ S52.18 Other fracture of upper end of radius

7ᵗʰ S52.181 Other fracture of upper end of right radius

7ᵗʰ S52.182 Other fracture of upper end of left radius

7ᵗʰ S52.189 Other fracture of upper end of unspecified radius

5ᵗʰ S52.2 Fracture of shaft of ulna

6ᵗʰ S52.20 Unspecified fracture of shaft of ulna

Fracture of ulna NOS

7ᵗʰ S52.201 Unspecified fracture of shaft of right ulna

7ᵗʰ S52.202 Unspecified fracture of shaft of left ulna

7ᵗʰ S52.209 Unspecified fracture of shaft of unspecified ulna

6ᵗʰ S52.21 Greenstick fracture of shaft of ulna

The appropriate 7th character is to be added to all codes in subcategory S52.21

A = initial encounter for closed fracture

D = subsequent encounter for fracture with routine healing

G = subsequent encounter for fracture with delayed healing

K = subsequent encounter for fracture with nonunion

P = subsequent encounter for fracture with malunion

S = sequela

7ᵗʰ S52.211 Greenstick fracture of shaft of right ulna

7ᵗʰ S52.212 Greenstick fracture of shaft of left ulna

7ᵗʰ S52.219 Greenstick fracture of shaft of unspecified ulna

6ᵗʰ S52.22 Transverse fracture of shaft of ulna

7ᵗʰ S52.221 Displaced transverse fracture of shaft of right ulna

7ᵗʰ S52.222 Displaced transverse fracture of shaft of left ulna

7ᵗʰ S52.223 Displaced transverse fracture of shaft of unspecified ulna

7ᵗʰ S52.224 Nondisplaced transverse fracture of shaft of right ulna

7ᵗʰ S52.225 Nondisplaced transverse fracture of shaft of left ulna

7ᵗʰ S52.226 Nondisplaced transverse fracture of shaft of unspecified ulna

6ᵗʰ S52.23 Oblique fracture of shaft of ulna

7ᵗʰ S52.231 Displaced oblique fracture of shaft of right ulna

7ᵗʰ S52.232 Displaced oblique fracture of shaft of left ulna

7ᵗʰ S52.233 Displaced oblique fracture of shaft of unspecified ulna

7ᵗʰ S52.234 Nondisplaced oblique fracture of shaft of right ulna

7ᵗʰ S52.235 Nondisplaced oblique fracture of shaft of left ulna

7ᵗʰ S52.236 Nondisplaced oblique fracture of shaft of unspecified ulna

6ᵗʰ S52.24 Spiral fracture of shaft of ulna

7ᵗʰ S52.241 Displaced spiral fracture of shaft of ulna, right arm

7ᵗʰ S52.242 Displaced spiral fracture of shaft of ulna, left arm

7ᵗʰ S52.243 Displaced spiral fracture of shaft of ulna, unspecified arm

7ᵗʰ S52.244 Nondisplaced spiral fracture of shaft of ulna, right arm

7ᵗʰ S52.245 Nondisplaced spiral fracture of shaft of ulna, left arm

7ᵗʰ S52.246 Nondisplaced spiral fracture of shaft of ulna, unspecified arm

6ᵗʰ S52.25 Comminuted fracture of shaft of ulna

7ᵗʰ S52.251 Displaced comminuted fracture of shaft of ulna, right arm

7ᵗʰ S52.252 Displaced comminuted fracture of shaft of ulna, left arm

7ᵗʰ S52.253 Displaced comminuted fracture of shaft of ulna, unspecified arm

7ᵗʰ S52.254 Nondisplaced comminuted fracture of shaft of ulna, right arm

7ᵗʰ S52.255 Nondisplaced comminuted fracture of shaft of ulna, left arm

7ᵗʰ S52.256 Nondisplaced comminuted fracture of shaft of ulna, unspecified arm

6ᵗʰ S52.26 Segmental fracture of shaft of ulna

7ᵗʰ S52.261 Displaced segmental fracture of shaft of ulna, right arm

[7th] S52.262 Displaced segmental fracture of shaft of ulna, left arm
[7th] S52.263 Displaced segmental fracture of shaft of ulna, unspecified arm
[7th] S52.264 Nondisplaced segmental fracture of shaft of ulna, right arm
[7th] S52.265 Nondisplaced segmental fracture of shaft of ulna, left arm
[7th] S52.266 Nondisplaced segmental fracture of shaft of ulna, unspecified arm
[6th] S52.27 Monteggia's fracture of ulna
Fracture of upper shaft of ulna with dislocation of radial head
[7th] S52.271 Monteggia's fracture of right ulna
[7th] S52.272 Monteggia's fracture of left ulna
[7th] S52.279 Monteggia's fracture of unspecified ulna
[6th] S52.28 Bent bone of ulna
[7th] S52.281 Bent bone of right ulna
[7th] S52.282 Bent bone of left ulna
[7th] S52.283 Bent bone of unspecified ulna
[6th] S52.29 Other fracture of shaft of ulna
[7th] S52.291 Other fracture of shaft of right ulna
[7th] S52.292 Other fracture of shaft of left ulna
[7th] S52.299 Other fracture of shaft of unspecified ulna
[5th] S52.3 Fracture of shaft of radius
[6th] S52.30 Unspecified fracture of shaft of radius
[7th] S52.301 Unspecified fracture of shaft of right radius
[7th] S52.302 Unspecified fracture of shaft of left radius
[7th] S52.309 Unspecified fracture of shaft of unspecified radius
[6th] S52.31 Greenstick fracture of shaft of radius
The appropriate 7th character is to be added to all codes in subcategory S52.31
A = initial encounter for closed fracture
D = subsequent encounter for fracture with routine healing
G = subsequent encounter for fracture with delayed healing
K = subsequent encounter for fracture with nonunion
P = subsequent encounter for fracture with malunion
S = sequela
[7th] S52.311 Greenstick fracture of shaft of radius, right arm
[7th] S52.312 Greenstick fracture of shaft of radius, left arm
[7th] S52.319 Greenstick fracture of shaft of radius, unspecified arm
[6th] S52.32 Transverse fracture of shaft of radius
[7th] S52.321 Displaced transverse fracture of shaft of right radius
[7th] S52.322 Displaced transverse fracture of shaft of left radius
[7th] S52.323 Displaced transverse fracture of shaft of unspecified radius
[7th] S52.324 Nondisplaced transverse fracture of shaft of right radius
[7th] S52.325 Nondisplaced transverse fracture of shaft of left radius
[7th] S52.326 Nondisplaced transverse fracture of shaft of unspecified radius
[6th] S52.33 Oblique fracture of shaft of radius
[7th] S52.331 Displaced oblique fracture of shaft of right radius
[7th] S52.332 Displaced oblique fracture of shaft of left radius
[7th] S52.333 Displaced oblique fracture of shaft of unspecified radius
[7th] S52.334 Nondisplaced oblique fracture of shaft of right radius
[7th] S52.335 Nondisplaced oblique fracture of shaft of left radius
[7th] S52.336 Nondisplaced oblique fracture of shaft of unspecified radius
[6th] S52.34 Spiral fracture of shaft of radius
[7th] S52.341 Displaced spiral fracture of shaft of radius, right arm
[7th] S52.342 Displaced spiral fracture of shaft of radius, left arm
[7th] S52.343 Displaced spiral fracture of shaft of radius, unspecified arm
[7th] S52.344 Nondisplaced spiral fracture of shaft of radius, right arm
[7th] S52.345 Nondisplaced spiral fracture of shaft of radius, left arm
[7th] S52.346 Nondisplaced spiral fracture of shaft of radius, unspecified arm
[6th] S52.35 Comminuted fracture of shaft of radius
[7th] S52.351 Displaced comminuted fracture of shaft of radius, right arm
[7th] S52.352 Displaced comminuted fracture of shaft of radius, left arm
[7th] S52.353 Displaced comminuted fracture of shaft of radius, unspecified arm
[7th] S52.354 Nondisplaced comminuted fracture of shaft of radius, right arm
[7th] S52.355 Nondisplaced comminuted fracture of shaft of radius, left arm
[7th] S52.356 Nondisplaced comminuted fracture of shaft of radius, unspecified arm
[6th] S52.36 Segmental fracture of shaft of radius
[7th] S52.361 Displaced segmental fracture of shaft of radius, right arm
[7th] S52.362 Displaced segmental fracture of shaft of radius, left arm
[7th] S52.363 Displaced segmental fracture of shaft of radius, unspecified arm
[7th] S52.364 Nondisplaced segmental fracture of shaft of radius, right arm
[7th] S52.365 Nondisplaced segmental fracture of shaft of radius, left arm
[7th] S52.366 Nondisplaced segmental fracture of shaft of radius, unspecified arm
[6th] S52.37 Galeazzi's fracture
Fracture of lower shaft of radius with radioulnar joint dislocation
[7th] S52.371 Galeazzi's fracture of right radius
[7th] S52.372 Galeazzi's fracture of left radius
[7th] S52.379 Galeazzi's fracture of unspecified radius
[6th] S52.38 Bent bone of radius
[7th] S52.381 Bent bone of right radius
[7th] S52.382 Bent bone of left radius
[7th] S52.389 Bent bone of unspecified radius
[6th] S52.39 Other fracture of shaft of radius
[7th] S52.391 Other fracture of shaft of radius, right arm
[7th] S52.392 Other fracture of shaft of radius, left arm
[7th] S52.399 Other fracture of shaft of radius, unspecified arm
[5th] S52.5 Fracture of lower end of radius
Fracture of distal end of radius
[EXCLUDES2] *physeal fractures of lower end of radius (S59.2-)*
[6th] S52.50 Unspecified fracture of the lower end of radius
[7th] S52.501 Unspecified fracture of the lower end of right radius
[7th] S52.502 Unspecified fracture of the lower end of left radius

[4th] 4th character required [5th] 5th character required [6th] 6th character required [7th] 7th character required [x7th] Extension 'X' Alert
[EXCLUDES1] Not coded here [EXCLUDES2] Not included here [PDx] Primary Diagnosis Only Manifestation Code

[7th] S52.509 Unspecified fracture of the lower end of unspecified radius

[6th] S52.51 Fracture of radial styloid process

[7th] S52.511 Displaced fracture of right radial styloid process

[7th] S52.512 Displaced fracture of left radial styloid process

[7th] S52.513 Displaced fracture of unspecified radial styloid process

[7th] S52.514 Nondisplaced fracture of right radial styloid process

[7th] S52.515 Nondisplaced fracture of left radial styloid process

[7th] S52.516 Nondisplaced fracture of unspecified radial styloid process

[6th] S52.52 Torus fracture of lower end of radius

The appropriate 7th character is to be added to all codes in subcategory S52.52
A = initial encounter for closed fracture
D = subsequent encounter for fracture with routine healing
G = subsequent encounter for fracture with delayed healing
K = subsequent encounter for fracture with nonunion
P = subsequent encounter for fracture with malunion
S = sequela

[7th] S52.521 Torus fracture of lower end of right radius

[7th] S52.522 Torus fracture of lower end of left radius

[7th] S52.529 Torus fracture of lower end of unspecified radius

[6th] S52.53 Colles' fracture

[7th] S52.531 Colles' fracture of right radius

[7th] S52.532 Colles' fracture of left radius

[7th] S52.539 Colles' fracture of unspecified radius

[6th] S52.54 Smith's fracture

[7th] S52.541 Smith's fracture of right radius

[7th] S52.542 Smith's fracture of left radius

[7th] S52.549 Smith's fracture of unspecified radius

[6th] S52.55 Other extraarticular fracture of lower end of radius

[7th] S52.551 Other extraarticular fracture of lower end of right radius

[7th] S52.552 Other extraarticular fracture of lower end of left radius

[7th] S52.559 Other extraarticular fracture of lower end of unspecified radius

[6th] S52.56 Barton's fracture

[7th] S52.561 Barton's fracture of right radius

[7th] S52.562 Barton's fracture of left radius

[7th] S52.569 Barton's fracture of unspecified radius

[6th] S52.57 Other intraarticular fracture of lower end of radius

[7th] S52.571 Other intraarticular fracture of lower end of right radius

[7th] S52.572 Other intraarticular fracture of lower end of left radius

[7th] S52.579 Other intraarticular fracture of lower end of unspecified radius

[6th] S52.59 Other fractures of lower end of radius

[7th] S52.591 Other fractures of lower end of right radius

[7th] S52.592 Other fractures of lower end of left radius

[7th] S52.599 Other fractures of lower end of unspecified radius

[5th] S52.6 Fracture of lower end of ulna

[6th] S52.60 Unspecified fracture of lower end of ulna

[7th] S52.601 Unspecified fracture of lower end of right ulna

[7th] S52.602 Unspecified fracture of lower end of left ulna

[7th] S52.609 Unspecified fracture of lower end of unspecified ulna

[6th] S52.61 Fracture of ulna styloid process

[7th] S52.611 Displaced fracture of right ulna styloid process

[7th] S52.612 Displaced fracture of left ulna styloid process

[7th] S52.613 Displaced fracture of unspecified ulna styloid process

[7th] S52.614 Nondisplaced fracture of right ulna styloid process

[7th] S52.615 Nondisplaced fracture of left ulna styloid process

[7th] S52.616 Nondisplaced fracture of unspecified ulna styloid process

[6th] S52.62 Torus fracture of lower end of ulna

The appropriate 7th character is to be added to all codes in subcategory S52.62
A = initial encounter for closed fracture
D = subsequent encounter for fracture with routine healing
G = subsequent encounter for fracture with delayed healing
K = subsequent encounter for fracture with nonunion
P = subsequent encounter for fracture with malunion
S = sequela

[7th] S52.621 Torus fracture of lower end of right ulna

[7th] S52.622 Torus fracture of lower end of left ulna

[7th] S52.629 Torus fracture of lower end of unspecified ulna

[6th] S52.69 Other fracture of lower end of ulna

[7th] S52.691 Other fracture of lower end of right ulna

[7th] S52.692 Other fracture of lower end of left ulna

[7th] S52.699 Other fracture of lower end of unspecified ulna

[5th] S52.9 Unspecified fracture of forearm

[7th] S52.90 Unspecified fracture of unspecified forearm

[7th] S52.91 Unspecified fracture of right forearm

[7th] S52.92 Unspecified fracture of left forearm

[4th] S53 Dislocation and sprain of joints and ligaments of elbow

[INCLUDES] *avulsion of joint or ligament of elbow*
laceration of cartilage, joint or ligament of elbow
sprain of cartilage, joint or ligament of elbow
traumatic hemarthrosis of joint or ligament of elbow
traumatic rupture of joint or ligament of elbow
traumatic subluxation of joint or ligament of elbow
traumatic tear of joint or ligament of elbow

Code also any associated open wound

[EXCLUDES2] *strain of muscle, fascia and tendon at forearm level (S56.-)*

The appropriate 7th character is to be added to each code from category S53
A = initial encounter
D = subsequent encounter
S = sequela

[5th] S53.0 Subluxation and dislocation of radial head

Dislocation of radiohumeral joint
Subluxation of radiohumeral joint

[EXCLUDES1] *Monteggia's fracture-dislocation (S52.27-)*

[6th] S53.00 Unspecified subluxation and dislocation of radial head

[7th] S53.001 Unspecified subluxation of right radial head

[7th] S53.002 Unspecified subluxation of left radial head

[7th] S53.003 Unspecified subluxation of unspecified radial head

Unspecified Code | Other Specified Code | [N] Newborn Age: 0 | [P] Pediatric Age: 0-17 | [M] Maternity Age: 12-55
[A] Adult Age: 15-124 | ♂ Male | ♀ Female | ● New Code | ▲ Revised Code Title | ►◄ Revised Text

7️⃣ S53.004 Unspecified dislocation of right radial head
7️⃣ S53.005 Unspecified dislocation of left radial head
7️⃣ S53.006 Unspecified dislocation of unspecified radial head

6️⃣ S53.01 Anterior subluxation and dislocation of radial head

　Anteriomedial subluxation and dislocation of radial head

7️⃣ S53.011 Anterior subluxation of right radial head
7️⃣ S53.012 Anterior subluxation of left radial head
7️⃣ S53.013 Anterior subluxation of unspecified radial head
7️⃣ S53.014 Anterior dislocation of right radial head
7️⃣ S53.015 Anterior dislocation of left radial head
7️⃣ S53.016 Anterior dislocation of unspecified radial head

6️⃣ S53.02 Posterior subluxation and dislocation of radial head

　Posteriolateral subluxation and dislocation of radial head

7️⃣ S53.021 Posterior subluxation of right radial head
7️⃣ S53.022 Posterior subluxation of left radial head
7️⃣ S53.023 Posterior subluxation of unspecified radial head
7️⃣ S53.024 Posterior dislocation of right radial head
7️⃣ S53.025 Posterior dislocation of left radial head
7️⃣ S53.026 Posterior dislocation of unspecified radial head

6️⃣ S53.03 Nursemaid's elbow

7️⃣ S53.031 Nursemaid's elbow, right elbow
7️⃣ S53.032 Nursemaid's elbow, left elbow
7️⃣ S53.033 Nursemaid's elbow, unspecified elbow

6️⃣ S53.09 Other subluxation and dislocation of radial head

7️⃣ S53.091 Other subluxation of right radial head
7️⃣ S53.092 Other subluxation of left radial head
7️⃣ S53.093 Other subluxation of unspecified radial head
7️⃣ S53.094 Other dislocation of right radial head
7️⃣ S53.095 Other dislocation of left radial head
7️⃣ S53.096 Other dislocation of unspecified radial head

5️⃣ S53.1 Subluxation and dislocation of ulnohumeral joint

　Subluxation and dislocation of elbow NOS
　EXCLUDES1 dislocation of radial head alone (S53.0-)

6️⃣ S53.10 Unspecified subluxation and dislocation of ulnohumeral joint

7️⃣ S53.101 Unspecified subluxation of right ulnohumeral joint
7️⃣ S53.102 Unspecified subluxation of left ulnohumeral joint
7️⃣ S53.103 Unspecified subluxation of unspecified ulnohumeral joint
7️⃣ S53.104 Unspecified dislocation of right ulnohumeral joint
7️⃣ S53.105 Unspecified dislocation of left ulnohumeral joint
7️⃣ S53.106 Unspecified dislocation of unspecified ulnohumeral joint

6️⃣ S53.11 Anterior subluxation and dislocation of ulnohumeral joint

7️⃣ S53.111 Anterior subluxation of right ulnohumeral joint
7️⃣ S53.112 Anterior subluxation of left ulnohumeral joint
7️⃣ S53.113 Anterior subluxation of unspecified ulnohumeral joint
7️⃣ S53.114 Anterior dislocation of right ulnohumeral joint
7️⃣ S53.115 Anterior dislocation of left ulnohumeral joint

7️⃣ S53.116 Anterior dislocation of unspecified ulnohumeral joint

6️⃣ S53.12 Posterior subluxation and dislocation of ulnohumeral joint

7️⃣ S53.121 Posterior subluxation of right ulnohumeral joint
7️⃣ S53.122 Posterior subluxation of left ulnohumeral joint
7️⃣ S53.123 Posterior subluxation of unspecified ulnohumeral joint
7️⃣ S53.124 Posterior dislocation of right ulnohumeral joint
7️⃣ S53.125 Posterior dislocation of left ulnohumeral joint
7️⃣ S53.126 Posterior dislocation of unspecified ulnohumeral joint

6️⃣ S53.13 Medial subluxation and dislocation of ulnohumeral joint

7️⃣ S53.131 Medial subluxation of right ulnohumeral joint
7️⃣ S53.132 Medial subluxation of left ulnohumeral joint
7️⃣ S53.133 Medial subluxation of unspecified ulnohumeral joint
7️⃣ S53.134 Medial dislocation of right ulnohumeral joint
7️⃣ S53.135 Medial dislocation of left ulnohumeral joint
7️⃣ S53.136 Medial dislocation of unspecified ulnohumeral joint

6️⃣ S53.14 Lateral subluxation and dislocation of ulnohumeral joint

7️⃣ S53.141 Lateral subluxation of right ulnohumeral joint
7️⃣ S53.142 Lateral subluxation of left ulnohumeral joint
7️⃣ S53.143 Lateral subluxation of unspecified ulnohumeral joint
7️⃣ S53.144 Lateral dislocation of right ulnohumeral joint
7️⃣ S53.145 Lateral dislocation of left ulnohumeral joint
7️⃣ S53.146 Lateral dislocation of unspecified ulnohumeral joint

6️⃣ S53.19 Other subluxation and dislocation of ulnohumeral joint

7️⃣ S53.191 Other subluxation of right ulnohumeral joint
7️⃣ S53.192 Other subluxation of left ulnohumeral joint
7️⃣ S53.193 Other subluxation of unspecified ulnohumeral joint
7️⃣ S53.194 Other dislocation of right ulnohumeral joint
7️⃣ S53.195 Other dislocation of left ulnohumeral joint
7️⃣ S53.196 Other dislocation of unspecified ulnohumeral joint

5️⃣ S53.2 Traumatic rupture of radial collateral ligament
　EXCLUDES1 sprain of radial collateral ligament NOS (S53.43-)

7️⃣ S53.20 Traumatic rupture of unspecified radial collateral ligament
7️⃣ S53.21 Traumatic rupture of right radial collateral ligament
7️⃣ S53.22 Traumatic rupture of left radial collateral ligament

5️⃣ S53.3 Traumatic rupture of ulnar collateral ligament
　EXCLUDES1 sprain of ulnar collateral ligament (S53.44-)

7️⃣ S53.30 Traumatic rupture of unspecified ulnar collateral ligament
7️⃣ S53.31 Traumatic rupture of right ulnar collateral ligament
7️⃣ S53.32 Traumatic rupture of left ulnar collateral ligament

5️⃣ S53.4 Sprain of elbow

4️⃣ 4th character required　　5️⃣ 5th character required　　6️⃣ 6th character required　　7️⃣ 7th character required　　🄰 Extension 'X' Alert

EXCLUDES1 Not coded here　　EXCLUDES2 Not included here　　PDx Primary Diagnosis Only　　Manifestation Code

EXCLUDES2 *traumatic rupture of radial collateral ligament (S53.2-)*
traumatic rupture of ulnar collateral ligament (S53.3-)

- S53.40 Unspecified sprain of elbow
  - S53.401 Unspecified sprain of right elbow
  - S53.402 Unspecified sprain of left elbow
  - S53.409 Unspecified sprain of unspecified elbow
    Sprain of elbow NOS
- S53.41 Radiohumeral (joint) sprain
  - S53.411 Radiohumeral (joint) sprain of right elbow
  - S53.412 Radiohumeral (joint) sprain of left elbow
  - S53.419 Radiohumeral (joint) sprain of unspecified elbow
- S53.42 Ulnohumeral (joint) sprain
  - S53.421 Ulnohumeral (joint) sprain of right elbow
  - S53.422 Ulnohumeral (joint) sprain of left elbow
  - S53.429 Ulnohumeral (joint) sprain of unspecified elbow
- S53.43 Radial collateral ligament sprain
  - S53.431 Radial collateral ligament sprain of right elbow
  - S53.432 Radial collateral ligament sprain of left elbow
  - S53.439 Radial collateral ligament sprain of unspecified elbow
- S53.44 Ulnar collateral ligament sprain
  - S53.441 Ulnar collateral ligament sprain of right elbow
  - S53.442 Ulnar collateral ligament sprain of left elbow
  - S53.449 Ulnar collateral ligament sprain of unspecified elbow
- S53.49 Other sprain of elbow
  - S53.491 Other sprain of right elbow
  - S53.492 Other sprain of left elbow
  - S53.499 Other sprain of unspecified elbow

- S54 Injury of nerves at forearm level
  Code also any associated open wound (S51.-)
  EXCLUDES2 *injury of nerves at wrist and hand level (S64.-)*
  The appropriate 7th character is to be added to each code from category S54
  A = initial encounter
  D = subsequent encounter
  S = sequela
  - S54.0 Injury of ulnar nerve at forearm level
    Injury of ulnar nerve NOS
    - S54.00 Injury of ulnar nerve at forearm level, unspecified arm
    - S54.01 Injury of ulnar nerve at forearm level, right arm
    - S54.02 Injury of ulnar nerve at forearm level, left arm
  - S54.1 Injury of median nerve at forearm level
    Injury of median nerve NOS
    - S54.10 Injury of median nerve at forearm level, unspecified arm
    - S54.11 Injury of median nerve at forearm level, right arm
    - S54.12 Injury of median nerve at forearm level, left arm
  - S54.2 Injury of radial nerve at forearm level
    Injury of radial nerve NOS
    - S54.20 Injury of radial nerve at forearm level, unspecified arm
    - S54.21 Injury of radial nerve at forearm level, right arm
    - S54.22 Injury of radial nerve at forearm level, left arm
  - S54.3 Injury of cutaneous sensory nerve at forearm level
    - S54.30 Injury of cutaneous sensory nerve at forearm level, unspecified arm
    - S54.31 Injury of cutaneous sensory nerve at forearm level, right arm
    - S54.32 Injury of cutaneous sensory nerve at forearm level, left arm
  - S54.8 Injury of other nerves at forearm level
    - S54.8X Unspecified injury of other nerves at forearm level
      - S54.8X1 Unspecified injury of other nerves at forearm level, right arm
      - S54.8X2 Unspecified injury of other nerves at forearm level, left arm
      - S54.8X9 Unspecified injury of other nerves at forearm level, unspecified arm
  - S54.9 Injury of unspecified nerve at forearm level
    - S54.90 Injury of unspecified nerve at forearm level, unspecified arm
    - S54.91 Injury of unspecified nerve at forearm level, right arm
    - S54.92 Injury of unspecified nerve at forearm level, left arm

- S55 Injury of blood vessels at forearm level
  Code also any associated open wound (S51.-)
  EXCLUDES2 *injury of blood vessels at wrist and hand level (S65.-)*
  injury of brachial vessels (S45.1-S45.2)
  The appropriate 7th character is to be added to each code from category S55
  A = initial encounter
  D = subsequent encounter
  S = sequela
  - S55.0 Injury of ulnar artery at forearm level
    - S55.00 Unspecified injury of ulnar artery at forearm level
      - S55.001 Unspecified injury of ulnar artery at forearm level, right arm
      - S55.002 Unspecified injury of ulnar artery at forearm level, left arm
      - S55.009 Unspecified injury of ulnar artery at forearm level, unspecified arm
    - S55.01 Laceration of ulnar artery at forearm level
      - S55.011 Laceration of ulnar artery at forearm level, right arm
      - S55.012 Laceration of ulnar artery at forearm level, left arm
      - S55.019 Laceration of ulnar artery at forearm level, unspecified arm
    - S55.09 Other specified injury of ulnar artery at forearm level
      - S55.091 Other specified injury of ulnar artery at forearm level, right arm
      - S55.092 Other specified injury of ulnar artery at forearm level, left arm
      - S55.099 Other specified injury of ulnar artery at forearm level, unspecified arm
  - S55.1 Injury of radial artery at forearm level
    - S55.10 Unspecified injury of radial artery at forearm level
      - S55.101 Unspecified injury of radial artery at forearm level, right arm
      - S55.102 Unspecified injury of radial artery at forearm level, left arm
      - S55.109 Unspecified injury of radial artery at forearm level, unspecified arm
    - S55.11 Laceration of radial artery at forearm level
      - S55.111 Laceration of radial artery at forearm level, right arm
      - S55.112 Laceration of radial artery at forearm level, left arm

Unspecified Code	Other Specified Code	N Newborn Age: 0	P Pediatric Age: 0-17	M Maternity Age: 12-55	
A Adult Age: 15-124	♂ Male	♀ Female	● New Code	▲ Revised Code Title	►◄ Revised Text

7️⃣ S55.119 Laceration of radial artery at forearm level, unspecified arm

6️⃣ S55.19 Other specified injury of radial artery at forearm level

7️⃣ S55.191 Other specified injury of radial artery at forearm level, right arm

7️⃣ S55.192 Other specified injury of radial artery at forearm level, left arm

7️⃣ S55.199 Other specified injury of radial artery at forearm level, unspecified arm

5️⃣ S55.2 Injury of vein at forearm level

6️⃣ S55.20 Unspecified injury of vein at forearm level

7️⃣ S55.201 Unspecified injury of vein at forearm level, right arm

7️⃣ S55.202 Unspecified injury of vein at forearm level, left arm

7️⃣ S55.209 Unspecified injury of vein at forearm level, unspecified arm

6️⃣ S55.21 Laceration of vein at forearm level

7️⃣ S55.211 Laceration of vein at forearm level, right arm

7️⃣ S55.212 Laceration of vein at forearm level, left arm

7️⃣ S55.219 Laceration of vein at forearm level, unspecified arm

6️⃣ S55.29 Other specified injury of vein at forearm level

7️⃣ S55.291 Other specified injury of vein at forearm level, right arm

7️⃣ S55.292 Other specified injury of vein at forearm level, left arm

7️⃣ S55.299 Other specified injury of vein at forearm level, unspecified arm

5️⃣ S55.8 Injury of other blood vessels at forearm level

6️⃣ S55.80 Unspecified injury of other blood vessels at forearm level

7️⃣ S55.801 Unspecified injury of other blood vessels at forearm level, right arm

7️⃣ S55.802 Unspecified injury of other blood vessels at forearm level, left arm

7️⃣ S55.809 Unspecified injury of other blood vessels at forearm level, unspecified arm

6️⃣ S55.81 Laceration of other blood vessels at forearm level

7️⃣ S55.811 Laceration of other blood vessels at forearm level, right arm

7️⃣ S55.812 Laceration of other blood vessels at forearm level, left arm

7️⃣ S55.819 Laceration of other blood vessels at forearm level, unspecified arm

6️⃣ S55.89 Other specified injury of other blood vessels at forearm level

7️⃣ S55.891 Other specified injury of other blood vessels at forearm level, right arm

7️⃣ S55.892 Other specified injury of other blood vessels at forearm level, left arm

7️⃣ S55.899 Other specified injury of other blood vessels at forearm level, unspecified arm

5️⃣ S55.9 Injury of unspecified blood vessel at forearm level

6️⃣ S55.90 Unspecified injury of unspecified blood vessel at forearm level

7️⃣ S55.901 Unspecified injury of unspecified blood vessel at forearm level, right arm

7️⃣ S55.902 Unspecified injury of unspecified blood vessel at forearm level, left arm

7️⃣ S55.909 Unspecified injury of unspecified blood vessel at forearm level, unspecified arm

6️⃣ S55.91 Laceration of unspecified blood vessel at forearm level

7️⃣ S55.911 Laceration of unspecified blood vessel at forearm level, right arm

7️⃣ S55.912 Laceration of unspecified blood vessel at forearm level, left arm

7️⃣ S55.919 Laceration of unspecified blood vessel at forearm level, unspecified arm

6️⃣ S55.99 Other specified injury of unspecified blood vessel at forearm level

7️⃣ S55.991 Other specified injury of unspecified blood vessel at forearm level, right arm

7️⃣ S55.992 Other specified injury of unspecified blood vessel at forearm level, left arm

7️⃣ S55.999 Other specified injury of unspecified blood vessel at forearm level, unspecified arm

4️⃣ S56 Injury of muscle, fascia and tendon at forearm level

Code also any associated open wound (S51.-)

EXCLUDES2 injury of muscle, fascia and tendon at or below wrist (S66.-)
sprain of joints and ligaments of elbow (S53.4-)

The appropriate 7th character is to be added to each code from category S56
A = initial encounter
D = subsequent encounter
S = sequela

5️⃣ S56.0 Injury of flexor muscle, fascia and tendon of thumb at forearm level

6️⃣ S56.00 Unspecified injury of flexor muscle, fascia and tendon of thumb at forearm level

7️⃣ S56.001 Unspecified injury of flexor muscle, fascia and tendon of right thumb at forearm level

7️⃣ S56.002 Unspecified injury of flexor muscle, fascia and tendon of left thumb at forearm level

7️⃣ S56.009 Unspecified injury of flexor muscle, fascia and tendon of unspecified thumb at forearm level

6️⃣ S56.01 Strain of flexor muscle, fascia and tendon of thumb at forearm level

7️⃣ S56.011 Strain of flexor muscle, fascia and tendon of right thumb at forearm level

7️⃣ S56.012 Strain of flexor muscle, fascia and tendon of left thumb at forearm level

7️⃣ S56.019 Strain of flexor muscle, fascia and tendon of unspecified thumb at forearm level

6️⃣ S56.02 Laceration of flexor muscle, fascia and tendon of thumb at forearm level

7️⃣ S56.021 Laceration of flexor muscle, fascia and tendon of right thumb at forearm level

7️⃣ S56.022 Laceration of flexor muscle, fascia and tendon of left thumb at forearm level

7️⃣ S56.029 Laceration of flexor muscle, fascia and tendon of unspecified thumb at forearm level

6️⃣ S56.09 Other injury of flexor muscle, fascia and tendon of thumb at forearm level

7️⃣ S56.091 Other injury of flexor muscle, fascia and tendon of right thumb at forearm level

7️⃣ S56.092 Other injury of flexor muscle, fascia and tendon of left thumb at forearm level

7️⃣ S56.099 Other injury of flexor muscle, fascia and tendon of unspecified thumb at forearm level

5️⃣ S56.1 Injury of flexor muscle, fascia and tendon of other and unspecified finger at forearm level

6️⃣ S56.10 Unspecified injury of flexor muscle, fascia and tendon of other and unspecified finger at forearm level

7️⃣ S56.101 Unspecified injury of flexor muscle, fascia and tendon of right index finger at forearm level

7️⃣ S56.102 Unspecified injury of flexor muscle, fascia and tendon of left index finger at forearm level

---

4️⃣ 4th character required   5️⃣ 5th character required   6️⃣ 6th character required   7️⃣ 7th character required   Ⓧ Extension 'X' Alert

EXCLUDES1 Not coded here   EXCLUDES2 Not included here   PDx Primary Diagnosis Only   Manifestation Code

[7th] S56.103 Unspecified injury of flexor muscle, fascia and tendon of right middle finger at forearm level
[7th] S56.104 Unspecified injury of flexor muscle, fascia and tendon of left middle finger at forearm level
[7th] S56.105 Unspecified injury of flexor muscle, fascia and tendon of right ring finger at forearm level
[7th] S56.106 Unspecified injury of flexor muscle, fascia and tendon of left ring finger at forearm level
[7th] S56.107 Unspecified injury of flexor muscle, fascia and tendon of right little finger at forearm level
[7th] S56.108 Unspecified injury of flexor muscle, fascia and tendon of left little finger at forearm level
[7th] S56.109 Unspecified injury of flexor muscle, fascia and tendon of unspecified finger at forearm level

[6th] S56.11 Strain of flexor muscle, fascia and tendon of other and unspecified finger at forearm level
[7th] S56.111 Strain of flexor muscle, fascia and tendon of right index finger at forearm level
[7th] S56.112 Strain of flexor muscle, fascia and tendon of left index finger at forearm level
[7th] S56.113 Strain of flexor muscle, fascia and tendon of right middle finger at forearm level
[7th] S56.114 Strain of flexor muscle, fascia and tendon of left middle finger at forearm level
[7th] S56.115 Strain of flexor muscle, fascia and tendon of right ring finger at forearm level
[7th] S56.116 Strain of flexor muscle, fascia and tendon of left ring finger at forearm level
[7th] S56.117 Strain of flexor muscle, fascia and tendon of right little finger at forearm level
[7th] S56.118 Strain of flexor muscle, fascia and tendon of left little finger at forearm level
[7th] S56.119 Strain of flexor muscle, fascia and tendon of finger of unspecified finger at forearm level

[6th] S56.12 Laceration of flexor muscle, fascia and tendon of other and unspecified finger at forearm level
[7th] S56.121 Laceration of flexor muscle, fascia and tendon of right index finger at forearm level
[7th] S56.122 Laceration of flexor muscle, fascia and tendon of left index finger at forearm level
[7th] S56.123 Laceration of flexor muscle, fascia and tendon of right middle finger at forearm level
[7th] S56.124 Laceration of flexor muscle, fascia and tendon of left middle finger at forearm level
[7th] S56.125 Laceration of flexor muscle, fascia and tendon of right ring finger at forearm level
[7th] S56.126 Laceration of flexor muscle, fascia and tendon of left ring finger at forearm level
[7th] S56.127 Laceration of flexor muscle, fascia and tendon of right little finger at forearm level
[7th] S56.128 Laceration of flexor muscle, fascia and tendon of left little finger at forearm level
[7th] S56.129 Laceration of flexor muscle, fascia and tendon of unspecified finger at forearm level

[6th] S56.19 Other injury of flexor muscle, fascia and tendon of other and unspecified finger at forearm level
[7th] S56.191 Other injury of flexor muscle, fascia and tendon of right index finger at forearm level
[7th] S56.192 Other injury of flexor muscle, fascia and tendon of left index finger at forearm level
[7th] S56.193 Other injury of flexor muscle, fascia and tendon of right middle finger at forearm level
[7th] S56.194 Other injury of flexor muscle, fascia and tendon of left middle finger at forearm level
[7th] S56.195 Other injury of flexor muscle, fascia and tendon of right ring finger at forearm level
[7th] S56.196 Other injury of flexor muscle, fascia and tendon of left ring finger at forearm level
[7th] S56.197 Other injury of flexor muscle, fascia and tendon of right little finger at forearm level
[7th] S56.198 Other injury of flexor muscle, fascia and tendon of left little finger at forearm level
[7th] S56.199 Other injury of flexor muscle, fascia and tendon of unspecified finger at forearm level

[5th] S56.2 Injury of other flexor muscle, fascia and tendon at forearm level
[6th] S56.20 Unspecified injury of other flexor muscle, fascia and tendon at forearm level
[7th] S56.201 Unspecified injury of other flexor muscle, fascia and tendon at forearm level, right arm
[7th] S56.202 Unspecified injury of other flexor muscle, fascia and tendon at forearm level, left arm
[7th] S56.209 Unspecified injury of other flexor muscle, fascia and tendon at forearm level, unspecified arm

[6th] S56.21 Strain of other flexor muscle, fascia and tendon at forearm level
[7th] S56.211 Strain of other flexor muscle, fascia and tendon at forearm level, right arm
[7th] S56.212 Strain of other flexor muscle, fascia and tendon at forearm level, left arm
[7th] S56.219 Strain of other flexor muscle, fascia and tendon at forearm level, unspecified arm

[6th] S56.22 Laceration of other flexor muscle, fascia and tendon at forearm level
[7th] S56.221 Laceration of other flexor muscle, fascia and tendon at forearm level, right arm
[7th] S56.222 Laceration of other flexor muscle, fascia and tendon at forearm level, left arm
[7th] S56.229 Laceration of other flexor muscle, fascia and tendon at forearm level, unspecified arm

[6th] S56.29 Other injury of other flexor muscle, fascia and tendon at forearm level
[7th] S56.291 Other injury of other flexor muscle, fascia and tendon at forearm level, right arm
[7th] S56.292 Other injury of other flexor muscle, fascia and tendon at forearm level, left arm
[7th] S56.299 Other injury of other flexor muscle, fascia and tendon at forearm level, unspecified arm

[5th] S56.3 Injury of extensor or abductor muscles, fascia and tendons of thumb at forearm level
[6th] S56.30 Unspecified injury of extensor or abductor muscles, fascia and tendons of thumb at forearm level
[7th] S56.301 Unspecified injury of extensor or abductor muscles, fascia and tendons of right thumb at forearm level
[7th] S56.302 Unspecified injury of extensor or abductor muscles, fascia and tendons of left thumb at forearm level
[7th] S56.309 Unspecified injury of extensor or abductor muscles, fascia and tendons of unspecified thumb at forearm level

[6th] S56.31 Strain of extensor or abductor muscles, fascia and tendons of thumb at forearm level

Unspecified Code | Other Specified Code | [N] Newborn Age: 0 | [P] Pediatric Age: 0-17 | [M] Maternity Age: 12-55
[A] Adult Age: 15-124 | ♂ Male | ♀ Female | ● New Code | ▲ Revised Code Title | ►◄ Revised Text

7️⃣ S56.311 Strain of extensor or abductor muscles, fascia and tendons of right thumb at forearm level

7️⃣ S56.312 Strain of extensor or abductor muscles, fascia and tendons of left thumb at forearm level

7️⃣ S56.319 Strain of extensor or abductor muscles, fascia and tendons of unspecified thumb at forearm level

6️⃣ S56.32 Laceration of extensor or abductor muscles, fascia and tendons of thumb at forearm level

7️⃣ S56.321 Laceration of extensor or abductor muscles, fascia and tendons of right thumb at forearm level

7️⃣ S56.322 Laceration of extensor or abductor muscles, fascia and tendons of left thumb at forearm level

7️⃣ S56.329 Laceration of extensor or abductor muscles, fascia and tendons of unspecified thumb at forearm level

6️⃣ S56.39 Other injury of extensor or abductor muscles, fascia and tendons of thumb at forearm level

7️⃣ S56.391 Other injury of extensor or abductor muscles, fascia and tendons of right thumb at forearm level

7️⃣ S56.392 Other injury of extensor or abductor muscles, fascia and tendons of left thumb at forearm level

7️⃣ S56.399 Other injury of extensor or abductor muscles, fascia and tendons of unspecified thumb at forearm level

5️⃣ S56.4 Injury of extensor muscle, fascia and tendon of other and unspecified finger at forearm level

6️⃣ S56.40 Unspecified injury of extensor muscle, fascia and tendon of other and unspecified finger at forearm level

7️⃣ S56.401 Unspecified injury of extensor muscle, fascia and tendon of right index finger at forearm level

7️⃣ S56.402 Unspecified injury of extensor muscle, fascia and tendon of left index finger at forearm level

7️⃣ S56.403 Unspecified injury of extensor muscle, fascia and tendon of right middle finger at forearm level

7️⃣ S56.404 Unspecified injury of extensor muscle, fascia and tendon of left middle finger at forearm level

7️⃣ S56.405 Unspecified injury of extensor muscle, fascia and tendon of right ring finger at forearm level

7️⃣ S56.406 Unspecified injury of extensor muscle, fascia and tendon of left ring finger at forearm level

7️⃣ S56.407 Unspecified injury of extensor muscle, fascia and tendon of right little finger at forearm level

7️⃣ S56.408 Unspecified injury of extensor muscle, fascia and tendon of left little finger at forearm level

7️⃣ S56.409 Unspecified injury of extensor muscle, fascia and tendon of unspecified finger at forearm level

6️⃣ S56.41 Strain of extensor muscle, fascia and tendon of other and unspecified finger at forearm level

7️⃣ S56.411 Strain of extensor muscle, fascia and tendon of right index finger at forearm level

7️⃣ S56.412 Strain of extensor muscle, fascia and tendon of left index finger at forearm level

7️⃣ S56.413 Strain of extensor muscle, fascia and tendon of right middle finger at forearm level

7️⃣ S56.414 Strain of extensor muscle, fascia and tendon of left middle finger at forearm level

7️⃣ S56.415 Strain of extensor muscle, fascia and tendon of right ring finger at forearm level

7️⃣ S56.416 Strain of extensor muscle, fascia and tendon of left ring finger at forearm level

7️⃣ S56.417 Strain of extensor muscle, fascia and tendon of right little finger at forearm level

7️⃣ S56.418 Strain of extensor muscle, fascia and tendon of left little finger at forearm level

7️⃣ S56.419 Strain of extensor muscle, fascia and tendon of finger, unspecified finger at forearm level

6️⃣ S56.42 Laceration of extensor muscle, fascia and tendon of other and unspecified finger at forearm level

7️⃣ S56.421 Laceration of extensor muscle, fascia and tendon of right index finger at forearm level

7️⃣ S56.422 Laceration of extensor muscle, fascia and tendon of left index finger at forearm level

7️⃣ S56.423 Laceration of extensor muscle, fascia and tendon of right middle finger at forearm level

7️⃣ S56.424 Laceration of extensor muscle, fascia and tendon of left middle finger at forearm level

7️⃣ S56.425 Laceration of extensor muscle, fascia and tendon of right ring finger at forearm level

7️⃣ S56.426 Laceration of extensor muscle, fascia and tendon of left ring finger at forearm level

7️⃣ S56.427 Laceration of extensor muscle, fascia and tendon of right little finger at forearm level

7️⃣ S56.428 Laceration of extensor muscle, fascia and tendon of left little finger at forearm level

7️⃣ S56.429 Laceration of extensor muscle, fascia and tendon of unspecified finger at forearm level

6️⃣ S56.49 Other injury of extensor muscle, fascia and tendon of other and unspecified finger at forearm level

7️⃣ S56.491 Other injury of extensor muscle, fascia and tendon of right index finger at forearm level

7️⃣ S56.492 Other injury of extensor muscle, fascia and tendon of left index finger at forearm level

7️⃣ S56.493 Other injury of extensor muscle, fascia and tendon of right middle finger at forearm level

7️⃣ S56.494 Other injury of extensor muscle, fascia and tendon of left middle finger at forearm level

7️⃣ S56.495 Other injury of extensor muscle, fascia and tendon of right ring finger at forearm level

7️⃣ S56.496 Other injury of extensor muscle, fascia and tendon of left ring finger at forearm level

7️⃣ S56.497 Other injury of extensor muscle, fascia and tendon of right little finger at forearm level

7️⃣ S56.498 Other injury of extensor muscle, fascia and tendon of left little finger at forearm level

7️⃣ S56.499 Other injury of extensor muscle, fascia and tendon of unspecified finger at forearm level

5️⃣ S56.5 Injury of other extensor muscle, fascia and tendon at forearm level

6️⃣ S56.50 Unspecified injury of other extensor muscle, fascia and tendon at forearm level

7️⃣ S56.501 Unspecified injury of other extensor muscle, fascia and tendon at forearm level, right arm

7️⃣ S56.502 Unspecified injury of other extensor muscle, fascia and tendon at forearm level, left arm

7️⃣ S56.509 Unspecified injury of other extensor muscle, fascia and tendon at forearm level, unspecified arm

---

4️⃣ 4th character required 5️⃣ 5th character required 6️⃣ 6th character required 7️⃣ 7th character required ⓧ Extension 'X' Alert

EXCLUDES 1 Not coded here EXCLUDES 2 Not included here PDx Primary Diagnosis Only Manifestation Code

[6th] S56.51 Strain of other extensor muscle, fascia and tendon at forearm level
- [7th] S56.511 Strain of other extensor muscle, fascia and tendon at forearm level, right arm
- [7th] S56.512 Strain of other extensor muscle, fascia and tendon at forearm level, left arm
- [7th] S56.519 Strain of other extensor muscle, fascia and tendon at forearm level, unspecified arm

[6th] S56.52 Laceration of other extensor muscle, fascia and tendon at forearm level
- [7th] S56.521 Laceration of other extensor muscle, fascia and tendon at forearm level, right arm
- [7th] S56.522 Laceration of other extensor muscle, fascia and tendon at forearm level, left arm
- [7th] S56.529 Laceration of other extensor muscle, fascia and tendon at forearm level, unspecified arm

[6th] S56.59 Other injury of other extensor muscle, fascia and tendon at forearm level
- [7th] S56.591 Other injury of other extensor muscle, fascia and tendon at forearm level, right arm
- [7th] S56.592 Other injury of other extensor muscle, fascia and tendon at forearm level, left arm
- [7th] S56.599 Other injury of other extensor muscle, fascia and tendon at forearm level, unspecified arm

[5th] S56.8 Injury of other muscles, fascia and tendons at forearm level

[6th] S56.80 Unspecified injury of other muscles, fascia and tendons at forearm level
- [7th] S56.801 Unspecified injury of other muscles, fascia and tendons at forearm level, right arm
- [7th] S56.802 Unspecified injury of other muscles, fascia and tendons at forearm level, left arm
- [7th] S56.809 Unspecified injury of other muscles, fascia and tendons at forearm level, unspecified arm

[6th] S56.81 Strain of other muscles, fascia and tendons at forearm level
- [7th] S56.811 Strain of other muscles, fascia and tendons at forearm level, right arm
- [7th] S56.812 Strain of other muscles, fascia and tendons at forearm level, left arm
- [7th] S56.819 Strain of other muscles, fascia and tendons at forearm level, unspecified arm

[6th] S56.82 Laceration of other muscles, fascia and tendons at forearm level
- [7th] S56.821 Laceration of other muscles, fascia and tendons at forearm level, right arm
- [7th] S56.822 Laceration of other muscles, fascia and tendons at forearm level, left arm
- [7th] S56.829 Laceration of other muscles, fascia and tendons at forearm level, unspecified arm

[6th] S56.89 Other injury of other muscles, fascia and tendons at forearm level
- [7th] S56.891 Other injury of other muscles, fascia and tendons at forearm level, right arm
- [7th] S56.892 Other injury of other muscles, fascia and tendons at forearm level, left arm
- [7th] S56.899 Other injury of other muscles, fascia and tendons at forearm level, unspecified arm

[5th] S56.9 Injury of unspecified muscles, fascia and tendons at forearm level

[6th] S56.90 Unspecified injury of unspecified muscles, fascia and tendons at forearm level
- [7th] S56.901 Unspecified injury of unspecified muscles, fascia and tendons at forearm level, right arm
- [7th] S56.902 Unspecified injury of unspecified muscles, fascia and tendons at forearm level, left arm
- [7th] S56.909 Unspecified injury of unspecified muscles, fascia and tendons at forearm level, unspecified arm

[6th] S56.91 Strain of unspecified muscles, fascia and tendons at forearm level
- [7th] S56.911 Strain of unspecified muscles, fascia and tendons at forearm level, right arm
- [7th] S56.912 Strain of unspecified muscles, fascia and tendons at forearm level, left arm
- [7th] S56.919 Strain of unspecified muscles, fascia and tendons at forearm level, unspecified arm

[6th] S56.92 Laceration of unspecified muscles, fascia and tendons at forearm level
- [7th] S56.921 Laceration of unspecified muscles, fascia and tendons at forearm level, right arm
- [7th] S56.922 Laceration of unspecified muscles, fascia and tendons at forearm level, left arm
- [7th] S56.929 Laceration of unspecified muscles, fascia and tendons at forearm level, unspecified arm

[6th] S56.99 Other injury of unspecified muscles, fascia and tendons at forearm level
- [7th] S56.991 Other injury of unspecified muscles, fascia and tendons at forearm level, right arm
- [7th] S56.992 Other injury of unspecified muscles, fascia and tendons at forearm level, left arm
- [7th] S56.999 Other injury of unspecified muscles, fascia and tendons at forearm level, unspecified arm

[4th] S57 Crushing injury of elbow and forearm

Use additional code(s) for all associated injuries

[EXCLUDES2] *crushing injury of wrist and hand (S67.-)*

The appropriate 7th character is to be added to each code from category S57
- A = initial encounter
- D = subsequent encounter
- S = sequela

[5th] S57.0 Crushing injury of elbow
- [7th] S57.00 Crushing injury of unspecified elbow
- [7th] S57.01 Crushing injury of right elbow
- [7th] S57.02 Crushing injury of left elbow

[5th] S57.8 Crushing injury of forearm
- [7th] S57.80 Crushing injury of unspecified forearm
- [7th] S57.81 Crushing injury of right forearm
- [7th] S57.82 Crushing injury of left forearm

[4th] S58 Traumatic amputation of elbow and forearm

An amputation not identified as partial or complete should be coded to complete

[EXCLUDES1] *traumatic amputation of wrist and hand (S68.-)*

The appropriate 7th character is to be added to each code from category S58
- A = initial encounter
- D = subsequent encounter
- S = sequela

[5th] S58.0 Traumatic amputation at elbow level

[6th] S58.01 Complete traumatic amputation at elbow level
- [7th] S58.011 Complete traumatic amputation at elbow level, right arm
- [7th] S58.012 Complete traumatic amputation at elbow level, left arm
- [7th] S58.019 Complete traumatic amputation at elbow level, unspecified arm

[6th] S58.02 Partial traumatic amputation at elbow level
- [7th] S58.021 Partial traumatic amputation at elbow level, right arm

[7th] S58.022 Partial traumatic amputation at elbow level, left arm

[7th] S58.029 Partial traumatic amputation at elbow level, unspecified arm

[5th] S58.1 Traumatic amputation at level between elbow and wrist

[6th] S58.11 Complete traumatic amputation at level between elbow and wrist

[7th] S58.111 Complete traumatic amputation at level between elbow and wrist, right arm

[7th] S58.112 Complete traumatic amputation at level between elbow and wrist, left arm

[7th] S58.119 Complete traumatic amputation at level between elbow and wrist, unspecified arm

[6th] S58.12 Partial traumatic amputation at level between elbow and wrist

[7th] S58.121 Partial traumatic amputation at level between elbow and wrist, right arm

[7th] S58.122 Partial traumatic amputation at level between elbow and wrist, left arm

[7th] S58.129 Partial traumatic amputation at level between elbow and wrist, unspecified arm

[5th] S58.9 Traumatic amputation of forearm, level unspecified

[EXCLUDES1] *traumatic amputation of wrist (S68.-)*

[6th] S58.91 Complete traumatic amputation of forearm, level unspecified

[7th] S58.911 Complete traumatic amputation of right forearm, level unspecified

[7th] S58.912 Complete traumatic amputation of left forearm, level unspecified

[7th] S58.919 Complete traumatic amputation of unspecified forearm, level unspecified

[6th] S58.92 Partial traumatic amputation of forearm, level unspecified

[7th] S58.921 Partial traumatic amputation of right forearm, level unspecified

[7th] S58.922 Partial traumatic amputation of left forearm, level unspecified

[7th] S58.929 Partial traumatic amputation of unspecified forearm, level unspecified

[4th] S59 Other and unspecified injuries of elbow and forearm

[EXCLUDES2] *other and unspecified injuries of wrist and hand (S69.-)*

The appropriate 7th character is to be added to each code from subcategories S59.0, S59.1, and S59.2

A = initial encounter for closed fracture

D = subsequent encounter for fracture with routine healing

G = subsequent encounter for fracture with delayed healing

K = subsequent encounter for fracture with nonunion

P = subsequent encounter for fracture with malunion

S = sequela

[5th] S59.0 Physeal fracture of lower end of ulna

[6th] S59.00 Unspecified physeal fracture of lower end of ulna

[7th] S59.001 Unspecified physeal fracture of lower end of ulna, right arm

[7th] S59.002 Unspecified physeal fracture of lower end of ulna, left arm

[7th] S59.009 Unspecified physeal fracture of lower end of ulna, unspecified arm

[6th] S59.01 Salter-Harris Type I physeal fracture of lower end of ulna

[7th] S59.011 Salter-Harris Type I physeal fracture of lower end of ulna, right arm

[7th] S59.012 Salter-Harris Type I physeal fracture of lower end of ulna, left arm

[7th] S59.019 Salter-Harris Type I physeal fracture of lower end of ulna, unspecified arm

[6th] S59.02 Salter-Harris Type II physeal fracture of lower end of ulna

[7th] S59.021 Salter-Harris Type II physeal fracture of lower end of ulna, right arm

[7th] S59.022 Salter-Harris Type II physeal fracture of lower end of ulna, left arm

[7th] S59.029 Salter-Harris Type II physeal fracture of lower end of ulna, unspecified arm

[6th] S59.03 Salter-Harris Type III physeal fracture of lower end of ulna

[7th] S59.031 Salter-Harris Type III physeal fracture of lower end of ulna, right arm

[7th] S59.032 Salter-Harris Type III physeal fracture of lower end of ulna, left arm

[7th] S59.039 Salter-Harris Type III physeal fracture of lower end of ulna, unspecified arm

[6th] S59.04 Salter-Harris Type IV physeal fracture of lower end of ulna

[7th] S59.041 Salter-Harris Type IV physeal fracture of lower end of ulna, right arm

[7th] S59.042 Salter-Harris Type IV physeal fracture of lower end of ulna, left arm

[7th] S59.049 Salter-Harris Type IV physeal fracture of lower end of ulna, unspecified arm

[6th] S59.09 Other physeal fracture of lower end of ulna

[7th] S59.091 Other physeal fracture of lower end of ulna, right arm

[7th] S59.092 Other physeal fracture of lower end of ulna, left arm

[7th] S59.099 Other physeal fracture of lower end of ulna, unspecified arm

[5th] S59.1 Physeal fracture of upper end of radius

[6th] S59.10 Unspecified physeal fracture of upper end of radius

[7th] S59.101 Unspecified physeal fracture of upper end of radius, right arm

[7th] S59.102 Unspecified physeal fracture of upper end of radius, left arm

[7th] S59.109 Unspecified physeal fracture of upper end of radius, unspecified arm

[6th] S59.11 Salter-Harris Type I physeal fracture of upper end of radius

[7th] S59.111 Salter-Harris Type I physeal fracture of upper end of radius, right arm

[7th] S59.112 Salter-Harris Type I physeal fracture of upper end of radius, left arm

[7th] S59.119 Salter-Harris Type I physeal fracture of upper end of radius, unspecified arm

[6th] S59.12 Salter-Harris Type II physeal fracture of upper end of radius

[7th] S59.121 Salter-Harris Type II physeal fracture of upper end of radius, right arm

[7th] S59.122 Salter-Harris Type II physeal fracture of upper end of radius, left arm

[7th] S59.129 Salter-Harris Type II physeal fracture of upper end of radius, unspecified arm

[6th] S59.13 Salter-Harris Type III physeal fracture of upper end of radius

[7th] S59.131 Salter-Harris Type III physeal fracture of upper end of radius, right arm

[7th] S59.132 Salter-Harris Type III physeal fracture of upper end of radius, left arm

[7th] S59.139 Salter-Harris Type III physeal fracture of upper end of radius, unspecified arm

[6th] S59.14 Salter-Harris Type IV physeal fracture of upper end of radius

[7th] S59.141 Salter-Harris Type IV physeal fracture of upper end of radius, right arm

[4th] 4th character required [5th] 5th character required [6th] 6th character required [7th] 7th character required [x] Extension 'X' Alert
[EXCLUDES1] Not coded here [EXCLUDES2] Not included here [PDx] Primary Diagnosis Only Manifestation Code

[7th] S59.142 Salter-Harris Type IV physeal fracture of upper end of radius, left arm
[7th] S59.149 Salter-Harris Type IV physeal fracture of upper end of radius, unspecified arm
[6th] S59.19 Other physeal fracture of upper end of radius
[7th] S59.191 Other physeal fracture of upper end of radius, right arm
[7th] S59.192 Other physeal fracture of upper end of radius, left arm
[7th] S59.199 Other physeal fracture of upper end of radius, unspecified arm
[5th] S59.2 Physeal fracture of lower end of radius
[6th] S59.20 Unspecified physeal fracture of lower end of radius
[7th] S59.201 Unspecified physeal fracture of lower end of radius, right arm
[7th] S59.202 Unspecified physeal fracture of lower end of radius, left arm
[7th] S59.209 Unspecified physeal fracture of lower end of radius, unspecified arm
[6th] S59.21 Salter-Harris Type I physeal fracture of lower end of radius
[7th] S59.211 Salter-Harris Type I physeal fracture of lower end of radius, right arm
[7th] S59.212 Salter-Harris Type I physeal fracture of lower end of radius, left arm
[7th] S59.219 Salter-Harris Type I physeal fracture of lower end of radius, unspecified arm
[6th] S59.22 Salter-Harris Type II physeal fracture of lower end of radius
[7th] S59.221 Salter-Harris Type II physeal fracture of lower end of radius, right arm
[7th] S59.222 Salter-Harris Type II physeal fracture of lower end of radius, left arm
[7th] S59.229 Salter-Harris Type II physeal fracture of lower end of radius, unspecified arm
[6th] S59.23 Salter-Harris Type III physeal fracture of lower end of radius
[7th] S59.231 Salter-Harris Type III physeal fracture of lower end of radius, right arm
[7th] S59.232 Salter-Harris Type III physeal fracture of lower end of radius, left arm
[7th] S59.239 Salter-Harris Type III physeal fracture of lower end of radius, unspecified arm
[6th] S59.24 Salter-Harris Type IV physeal fracture of lower end of radius
[7th] S59.241 Salter-Harris Type IV physeal fracture of lower end of radius, right arm
[7th] S59.242 Salter-Harris Type IV physeal fracture of lower end of radius, left arm
[7th] S59.249 Salter-Harris Type IV physeal fracture of lower end of radius, unspecified arm
[6th] S59.29 Other physeal fracture of lower end of radius
[7th] S59.291 Other physeal fracture of lower end of radius, right arm
[7th] S59.292 Other physeal fracture of lower end of radius, left arm
[7th] S59.299 Other physeal fracture of lower end of radius, unspecified arm
[5th] S59.8 Other specified injuries of elbow and forearm
The appropriate 7th character is to be added to each code in subcategory S59.8
A = initial encounter
D = subsequent encounter
S = sequela
[6th] S59.80 Other specified injuries of elbow
[7th] S59.801 Other specified injuries of right elbow
[7th] S59.802 Other specified injuries of left elbow
[7th] S59.809 Other specified injuries of unspecified elbow
[6th] S59.81 Other specified injuries of forearm
[7th] S59.811 Other specified injuries right forearm
[7th] S59.812 Other specified injuries left forearm
[7th] S59.819 Other specified injuries unspecified forearm
[5th] S59.9 Unspecified injury of elbow and forearm
The appropriate 7th character is to be added to each code in subcategory S59.9
A = initial encounter
D = subsequent encounter
S = sequela
[6th] S59.90 Unspecified injury of elbow
[7th] S59.901 Unspecified injury of right elbow
[7th] S59.902 Unspecified injury of left elbow
[7th] S59.909 Unspecified injury of unspecified elbow
[6th] S59.91 Unspecified injury of forearm
[7th] S59.911 Unspecified injury of right forearm
[7th] S59.912 Unspecified injury of left forearm
[7th] S59.919 Unspecified injury of unspecified forearm

Injuries to the wrist, hand and fingers (S60-S69)

[EXCLUDES2] *burns and corrosions (T20-T32)*
frostbite (T33-T34)
insect bite or sting, venomous (T63.4)

[4th] S60 Superficial injury of wrist, hand and fingers
The appropriate 7th character is to be added to each code from category S60
A = initial encounter
D = subsequent encounter
S = sequela
[5th] S60.0 Contusion of finger without damage to nail
[EXCLUDES1] *contusion involving nail (matrix) (S60.1)*
[7th] S60.00 Contusion of unspecified finger without damage to nail
Contusion of finger(s) NOS
[6th] S60.01 Contusion of thumb without damage to nail
[7th] S60.011 Contusion of right thumb without damage to nail
[7th] S60.012 Contusion of left thumb without damage to nail
[7th] S60.019 Contusion of unspecified thumb without damage to nail
[6th] S60.02 Contusion of index finger without damage to nail
[7th] S60.021 Contusion of right index finger without damage to nail
[7th] S60.022 Contusion of left index finger without damage to nail
[7th] S60.029 Contusion of unspecified index finger without damage to nail
[6th] S60.03 Contusion of middle finger without damage to nail
[7th] S60.031 Contusion of right middle finger without damage to nail
[7th] S60.032 Contusion of left middle finger without damage to nail
[7th] S60.039 Contusion of unspecified middle finger without damage to nail
[6th] S60.04 Contusion of ring finger without damage to nail
[7th] S60.041 Contusion of right ring finger without damage to nail
[7th] S60.042 Contusion of left ring finger without damage to nail
[7th] S60.049 Contusion of unspecified ring finger without damage to nail
[6th] S60.05 Contusion of little finger without damage to nail
[7th] S60.051 Contusion of right little finger without damage to nail
[7th] S60.052 Contusion of left little finger without damage to nail
[7th] S60.059 Contusion of unspecified little finger without damage to nail
[5th] S60.1 Contusion of finger with damage to nail
[7th] S60.10 Contusion of unspecified finger with damage to nail
[6th] S60.11 Contusion of thumb with damage to nail

Unspecified Code | Other Specified Code | [N] Newborn Age: 0 | [P] Pediatric Age: 0-17 | [M] Maternity Age: 12-55
[A] Adult Age: 15-124 | ♂ Male | ♀ Female | ● New Code | ▲ Revised Code Title | ►◄ Revised Text

S60.111 Contusion of right thumb with damage to nail

S60.112 Contusion of left thumb with damage to nail

S60.119 Contusion of unspecified thumb with damage to nail

S60.12 Contusion of index finger with damage to nail

S60.121 Contusion of right index finger with damage to nail

S60.122 Contusion of left index finger with damage to nail

S60.129 Contusion of unspecified index finger with damage to nail

S60.13 Contusion of middle finger with damage to nail

S60.131 Contusion of right middle finger with damage to nail

S60.132 Contusion of left middle finger with damage to nail

S60.139 Contusion of unspecified middle finger with damage to nail

S60.14 Contusion of ring finger with damage to nail

S60.141 Contusion of right ring finger with damage to nail

S60.142 Contusion of left ring finger with damage to nail

S60.149 Contusion of unspecified ring finger with damage to nail

S60.15 Contusion of little finger with damage to nail

S60.151 Contusion of right little finger with damage to nail

S60.152 Contusion of left little finger with damage to nail

S60.159 Contusion of unspecified little finger with damage to nail

S60.2 Contusion of wrist and hand

> EXCLUDES2 contusion of fingers (S60.0-, S60.1-)

S60.21 Contusion of wrist

S60.211 Contusion of right wrist

S60.212 Contusion of left wrist

S60.219 Contusion of unspecified wrist

S60.22 Contusion of hand

S60.221 Contusion of right hand

S60.222 Contusion of left hand

S60.229 Contusion of unspecified hand

S60.3 Other superficial injuries of thumb

S60.31 Abrasion of thumb

S60.311 Abrasion of right thumb

S60.312 Abrasion of left thumb

S60.319 Abrasion of unspecified thumb

S60.32 Blister (nonthermal) of thumb

S60.321 Blister (nonthermal) of right thumb

S60.322 Blister (nonthermal) of left thumb

S60.329 Blister (nonthermal) of unspecified thumb

S60.34 External constriction of thumb

> Hair tourniquet syndrome of thumb
> Use additional cause code to identify the constricting item (W49.0-)

S60.341 External constriction of right thumb

S60.342 External constriction of left thumb

S60.349 External constriction of unspecified thumb

S60.35 Superficial foreign body of thumb

> Splinter in the thumb

S60.351 Superficial foreign body of right thumb

S60.352 Superficial foreign body of left thumb

S60.359 Superficial foreign body of unspecified thumb

S60.36 Insect bite (nonvenomous) of thumb

S60.361 Insect bite (nonvenomous) of right thumb

S60.362 Insect bite (nonvenomous) of left thumb

S60.369 Insect bite (nonvenomous) of unspecified thumb

S60.37 Other superficial bite of thumb

> EXCLUDES1 open bite of thumb (S61.05-, S61.15-)

S60.371 Other superficial bite of right thumb

S60.372 Other superficial bite of left thumb

S60.379 Other superficial bite of unspecified thumb

S60.39 Other superficial injuries of thumb

S60.391 Other superficial injuries of right thumb

S60.392 Other superficial injuries of left thumb

S60.399 Other superficial injuries of unspecified thumb

S60.4 Other superficial injuries of other fingers

S60.41 Abrasion of fingers

S60.410 Abrasion of right index finger

S60.411 Abrasion of left index finger

S60.412 Abrasion of right middle finger

S60.413 Abrasion of left middle finger

S60.414 Abrasion of right ring finger

S60.415 Abrasion of left ring finger

S60.416 Abrasion of right little finger

S60.417 Abrasion of left little finger

S60.418 Abrasion of other finger

> Abrasion of specified finger with unspecified laterality

S60.419 Abrasion of unspecified finger

S60.42 Blister (nonthermal) of fingers

S60.420 Blister (nonthermal) of right index finger

S60.421 Blister (nonthermal) of left index finger

S60.422 Blister (nonthermal) of right middle finger

S60.423 Blister (nonthermal) of left middle finger

S60.424 Blister (nonthermal) of right ring finger

S60.425 Blister (nonthermal) of left ring finger

S60.426 Blister (nonthermal) of right little finger

S60.427 Blister (nonthermal) of left little finger

S60.428 Blister (nonthermal) of other finger

> Blister (nonthermal) of specified finger with unspecified laterality

S60.429 Blister (nonthermal) of unspecified finger

S60.44 External constriction of fingers

> Hair tourniquet syndrome of finger
> Use additional cause code to identify the constricting item (W49.0-)

S60.440 External constriction of right index finger

S60.441 External constriction of left index finger

S60.442 External constriction of right middle finger

S60.443 External constriction of left middle finger

S60.444 External constriction of right ring finger

S60.445 External constriction of left ring finger

S60.446 External constriction of right little finger

S60.447 External constriction of left little finger

S60.448 External constriction of other finger

> External constriction of specified finger with unspecified laterality

S60.449 External constriction of unspecified finger

S60.45 Superficial foreign body of fingers

> Splinter in the finger(s)

S60.450 Superficial foreign body of right index finger

S60.451 Superficial foreign body of left index finger

S60.452 Superficial foreign body of right middle finger

S60.453 Superficial foreign body of left middle finger

S60.454 Superficial foreign body of right ring finger

S60.455 Superficial foreign body of left ring finger

4th character required   5th character required   6th character required   7th character required   Extension 'X' Alert

EXCLUDES1 Not coded here   EXCLUDES2 Not included here   PDx Primary Diagnosis Only   Manifestation Code

[7th] S60.456 Superficial foreign body of right little finger
[7th] S60.457 Superficial foreign body of left little finger
[7th] S60.458 Superficial foreign body of other finger
Superficial foreign body of specified finger with unspecified laterality
[7th] S60.459 Superficial foreign body of unspecified finger

[6th] S60.46 Insect bite (nonvenomous) of fingers
[7th] S60.460 Insect bite (nonvenomous) of right index finger
[7th] S60.461 Insect bite (nonvenomous) of left index finger
[7th] S60.462 Insect bite (nonvenomous) of right middle finger
[7th] S60.463 Insect bite (nonvenomous) of left middle finger
[7th] S60.464 Insect bite (nonvenomous) of right ring finger
[7th] S60.465 Insect bite (nonvenomous) of left ring finger
[7th] S60.466 Insect bite (nonvenomous) of right little finger
[7th] S60.467 Insect bite (nonvenomous) of left little finger
[7th] S60.468 Insect bite (nonvenomous) of other finger
Insect bite (nonvenomous) of specified finger with unspecified laterality
[7th] S60.469 Insect bite (nonvenomous) of unspecified finger

[6th] S60.47 Other superficial bite of fingers
[EXCLUDES1] *open bite of fingers (S61.25-, S61.35-)*
[7th] S60.470 Other superficial bite of right index finger
[7th] S60.471 Other superficial bite of left index finger
[7th] S60.472 Other superficial bite of right middle finger
[7th] S60.473 Other superficial bite of left middle finger
[7th] S60.474 Other superficial bite of right ring finger
[7th] S60.475 Other superficial bite of left ring finger
[7th] S60.476 Other superficial bite of right little finger
[7th] S60.477 Other superficial bite of left little finger
[7th] S60.478 Other superficial bite of other finger
Other superficial bite of specified finger with unspecified laterality
[7th] S60.479 Other superficial bite of unspecified finger

[5th] S60.5 Other superficial injuries of hand
[EXCLUDES2] *superficial injuries of fingers (S60.3-, S60.4-)*

[6th] S60.51 Abrasion of hand
[7th] S60.511 Abrasion of right hand
[7th] S60.512 Abrasion of left hand
[7th] S60.519 Abrasion of unspecified hand

[6th] S60.52 Blister (nonthermal) of hand
[7th] S60.521 Blister (nonthermal) of right hand
[7th] S60.522 Blister (nonthermal) of left hand
[7th] S60.529 Blister (nonthermal) of unspecified hand

[6th] S60.54 External constriction of hand
[7th] S60.541 External constriction of right hand
[7th] S60.542 External constriction of left hand
[7th] S60.549 External constriction of unspecified hand

[6th] S60.55 Superficial foreign body of hand
Splinter in the hand
[7th] S60.551 Superficial foreign body of right hand
[7th] S60.552 Superficial foreign body of left hand
[7th] S60.559 Superficial foreign body of unspecified hand

[6th] S60.56 Insect bite (nonvenomous) of hand
[7th] S60.561 Insect bite (nonvenomous) of right hand
[7th] S60.562 Insect bite (nonvenomous) of left hand
[7th] S60.569 Insect bite (nonvenomous) of unspecified hand

[6th] S60.57 Other superficial bite of hand
[EXCLUDES1] *open bite of hand (S61.45-)*
[7th] S60.571 Other superficial bite of hand of right hand
[7th] S60.572 Other superficial bite of hand of left hand
[7th] S60.579 Other superficial bite of hand of unspecified hand

[5th] S60.8 Other superficial injuries of wrist

[6th] S60.81 Abrasion of wrist
[7th] S60.811 Abrasion of right wrist
[7th] S60.812 Abrasion of left wrist
[7th] S60.819 Abrasion of unspecified wrist

[6th] S60.82 Blister (nonthermal) of wrist
[7th] S60.821 Blister (nonthermal) of right wrist
[7th] S60.822 Blister (nonthermal) of left wrist
[7th] S60.829 Blister (nonthermal) of unspecified wrist

[6th] S60.84 External constriction of wrist
[7th] S60.841 External constriction of right wrist
[7th] S60.842 External constriction of left wrist
[7th] S60.849 External constriction of unspecified wrist

[6th] S60.85 Superficial foreign body of wrist
Splinter in the wrist
[7th] S60.851 Superficial foreign body of right wrist
[7th] S60.852 Superficial foreign body of left wrist
[7th] S60.859 Superficial foreign body of unspecified wrist

[6th] S60.86 Insect bite (nonvenomous) of wrist
[7th] S60.861 Insect bite (nonvenomous) of right wrist
[7th] S60.862 Insect bite (nonvenomous) of left wrist
[7th] S60.869 Insect bite (nonvenomous) of unspecified wrist

[6th] S60.87 Other superficial bite of wrist
[EXCLUDES1] *open bite of wrist (S61.55)*
[7th] S60.871 Other superficial bite of right wrist
[7th] S60.872 Other superficial bite of left wrist
[7th] S60.879 Other superficial bite of unspecified wrist

[5th] S60.9 Unspecified superficial injury of wrist, hand and fingers

[6th] S60.91 Unspecified superficial injury of wrist
[7th] S60.911 Unspecified superficial injury of right wrist
[7th] S60.912 Unspecified superficial injury of left wrist
[7th] S60.919 Unspecified superficial injury of unspecified wrist

[6th] S60.92 Unspecified superficial injury of hand
[7th] S60.921 Unspecified superficial injury of right hand
[7th] S60.922 Unspecified superficial injury of left hand
[7th] S60.929 Unspecified superficial injury of unspecified hand

[6th] S60.93 Unspecified superficial injury of thumb
[7th] S60.931 Unspecified superficial injury of right thumb
[7th] S60.932 Unspecified superficial injury of left thumb
[7th] S60.939 Unspecified superficial injury of unspecified thumb

[6th] S60.94 Unspecified superficial injury of other fingers
[7th] S60.940 Unspecified superficial injury of right index finger
[7th] S60.941 Unspecified superficial injury of left index finger
[7th] S60.942 Unspecified superficial injury of right middle finger
[7th] S60.943 Unspecified superficial injury of left middle finger
[7th] S60.944 Unspecified superficial injury of right ring finger
[7th] S60.945 Unspecified superficial injury of left ring finger
[7th] S60.946 Unspecified superficial injury of right little finger

Unspecified Code | Other Specified Code | [N] Newborn Age: 0 | [P] Pediatric Age: 0-17 | [M] Maternity Age: 12-55
[A] Adult Age: 15-124 | ♂ Male | ♀ Female | ● New Code | ▲ Revised Code Title | ►◄ Revised Text

[7th] S60.947 Unspecified superficial injury of left little finger
[7th] S60.948 Unspecified superficial injury of other finger
Unspecified superficial injury of specified finger with unspecified laterality
[7th] S60.949 Unspecified superficial injury of unspecified finger

[4th] S61 Open wound of wrist, hand and fingers
Code also any associated wound infection
EXCLUDES1 *open fracture of wrist, hand and finger (S62.- with 7th character B)*
traumatic amputation of wrist and hand (S68.-)
The appropriate 7th character is to be added to each code from category S61
A = initial encounter
D = subsequent encounter
S = sequela

[5th] S61.0 Open wound of thumb without damage to nail
EXCLUDES1 *open wound of thumb with damage to nail (S61.1-)*
[6th] S61.00 Unspecified open wound of thumb without damage to nail
[7th] S61.001 Unspecified open wound of right thumb without damage to nail
[7th] S61.002 Unspecified open wound of left thumb without damage to nail
[7th] S61.009 Unspecified open wound of unspecified thumb without damage to nail
[6th] S61.01 Laceration without foreign body of thumb without damage to nail
[7th] S61.011 Laceration without foreign body of right thumb without damage to nail
[7th] S61.012 Laceration without foreign body of left thumb without damage to nail
[7th] S61.019 Laceration without foreign body of unspecified thumb without damage to nail
[6th] S61.02 Laceration with foreign body of thumb without damage to nail
[7th] S61.021 Laceration with foreign body of right thumb without damage to nail
[7th] S61.022 Laceration with foreign body of left thumb without damage to nail
[7th] S61.029 Laceration with foreign body of unspecified thumb without damage to nail
[6th] S61.03 Puncture wound without foreign body of thumb without damage to nail
[7th] S61.031 Puncture wound without foreign body of right thumb without damage to nail
[7th] S61.032 Puncture wound without foreign body of left thumb without damage to nail
[7th] S61.039 Puncture wound without foreign body of unspecified thumb without damage to nail
[6th] S61.04 Puncture wound with foreign body of thumb without damage to nail
[7th] S61.041 Puncture wound with foreign body of right thumb without damage to nail
[7th] S61.042 Puncture wound with foreign body of left thumb without damage to nail
[7th] S61.049 Puncture wound with foreign body of unspecified thumb without damage to nail
[6th] S61.05 Open bite of thumb without damage to nail
Bite of thumb NOS
EXCLUDES1 *superficial bite of thumb (S60.36-, S60.37-)*
[7th] S61.051 Open bite of right thumb without damage to nail
[7th] S61.052 Open bite of left thumb without damage to nail
[7th] S61.059 Open bite of unspecified thumb without damage to nail

[5th] S61.1 Open wound of thumb with damage to nail
[6th] S61.10 Unspecified open wound of thumb with damage to nail
[7th] S61.101 Unspecified open wound of right thumb with damage to nail
[7th] S61.102 Unspecified open wound of left thumb with damage to nail
[7th] S61.109 Unspecified open wound of unspecified thumb with damage to nail
[6th] S61.11 Laceration without foreign body of thumb with damage to nail
[7th] S61.111 Laceration without foreign body of right thumb with damage to nail
[7th] S61.112 Laceration without foreign body of left thumb with damage to nail
[7th] S61.119 Laceration without foreign body of unspecified thumb with damage to nail
[6th] S61.12 Laceration with foreign body of thumb with damage to nail
[7th] S61.121 Laceration with foreign body of right thumb with damage to nail
[7th] S61.122 Laceration with foreign body of left thumb with damage to nail
[7th] S61.129 Laceration with foreign body of unspecified thumb with damage to nail
[6th] S61.13 Puncture wound without foreign body of thumb with damage to nail
[7th] S61.131 Puncture wound without foreign body of right thumb with damage to nail
[7th] S61.132 Puncture wound without foreign body of left thumb with damage to nail
[7th] S61.139 Puncture wound without foreign body of unspecified thumb with damage to nail
[6th] S61.14 Puncture wound with foreign body of thumb with damage to nail
[7th] S61.141 Puncture wound with foreign body of right thumb with damage to nail
[7th] S61.142 Puncture wound with foreign body of left thumb with damage to nail
[7th] S61.149 Puncture wound with foreign body of unspecified thumb with damage to nail
[6th] S61.15 Open bite of thumb with damage to nail
Bite of thumb with damage to nail NOS
EXCLUDES1 *superficial bite of thumb (S60.36-, S60.37-)*
[7th] S61.151 Open bite of right thumb with damage to nail
[7th] S61.152 Open bite of left thumb with damage to nail
[7th] S61.159 Open bite of unspecified thumb with damage to nail

[5th] S61.2 Open wound of other finger without damage to nail
EXCLUDES1 *open wound of finger involving nail (matrix) (S61.3-)*
EXCLUDES2 *open wound of thumb without damage to nail (S61.0-)*
[6th] S61.20 Unspecified open wound of other finger without damage to nail
[7th] S61.200 Unspecified open wound of right index finger without damage to nail
[7th] S61.201 Unspecified open wound of left index finger without damage to nail
[7th] S61.202 Unspecified open wound of right middle finger without damage to nail
[7th] S61.203 Unspecified open wound of left middle finger without damage to nail

[4th] 4th character required [5th] 5th character required [6th] 6th character required [7th] 7th character required [X7th] Extension 'X' Alert
EXCLUDES1 Not coded here EXCLUDES2 Not included here [PDx] Primary Diagnosis Only Manifestation Code

7ᵈ **S61.204** Unspecified open wound of right ring finger without damage to nail

7ᵈ **S61.205** Unspecified open wound of left ring finger without damage to nail

7ᵈ **S61.206** Unspecified open wound of right little finger without damage to nail

7ᵈ **S61.207** Unspecified open wound of left little finger without damage to nail

7ᵈ **S61.208** Unspecified open wound of other finger without damage to nail

Unspecified open wound of specified finger with unspecified laterality without damage to nail

7ᵈ **S61.209** Unspecified open wound of unspecified finger without damage to nail

6ᵈ **S61.21** Laceration without foreign body of finger without damage to nail

7ᵈ **S61.210** Laceration without foreign body of right index finger without damage to nail

7ᵈ **S61.211** Laceration without foreign body of left index finger without damage to nail

7ᵈ **S61.212** Laceration without foreign body of right middle finger without damage to nail

7ᵈ **S61.213** Laceration without foreign body of left middle finger without damage to nail

7ᵈ **S61.214** Laceration without foreign body of right ring finger without damage to nail

7ᵈ **S61.215** Laceration without foreign body of left ring finger without damage to nail

7ᵈ **S61.216** Laceration without foreign body of right little finger without damage to nail

7ᵈ **S61.217** Laceration without foreign body of left little finger without damage to nail

7ᵈ **S61.218** Laceration without foreign body of other finger without damage to nail

Laceration without foreign body of specified finger with unspecified laterality without damage to nail

7ᵈ **S61.219** Laceration without foreign body of unspecified finger without damage to nail

6ᵈ **S61.22** Laceration with foreign body of finger without damage to nail

7ᵈ **S61.220** Laceration with foreign body of right index finger without damage to nail

7ᵈ **S61.221** Laceration with foreign body of left index finger without damage to nail

7ᵈ **S61.222** Laceration with foreign body of right middle finger without damage to nail

7ᵈ **S61.223** Laceration with foreign body of left middle finger without damage to nail

7ᵈ **S61.224** Laceration with foreign body of right ring finger without damage to nail

7ᵈ **S61.225** Laceration with foreign body of left ring finger without damage to nail

7ᵈ **S61.226** Laceration with foreign body of right little finger without damage to nail

7ᵈ **S61.227** Laceration with foreign body of left little finger without damage to nail

7ᵈ **S61.228** Laceration with foreign body of other finger without damage to nail

Laceration with foreign body of specified finger with unspecified laterality without damage to nail

7ᵈ **S61.229** Laceration with foreign body of unspecified finger without damage to nail

6ᵈ **S61.23** Puncture wound without foreign body of finger without damage to nail

7ᵈ **S61.230** Puncture wound without foreign body of right index finger without damage to nail

7ᵈ **S61.231** Puncture wound without foreign body of left index finger without damage to nail

7ᵈ **S61.232** Puncture wound without foreign body of right middle finger without damage to nail

7ᵈ **S61.233** Puncture wound without foreign body of left middle finger without damage to nail

7ᵈ **S61.234** Puncture wound without foreign body of right ring finger without damage to nail

7ᵈ **S61.235** Puncture wound without foreign body of left ring finger without damage to nail

7ᵈ **S61.236** Puncture wound without foreign body of right little finger without damage to nail

7ᵈ **S61.237** Puncture wound without foreign body of left little finger without damage to nail

7ᵈ **S61.238** Puncture wound without foreign body of other finger without damage to nail

Puncture wound without foreign body of specified finger with unspecified laterality without damage to nail

7ᵈ **S61.239** Puncture wound without foreign body of unspecified finger without damage to nail

6ᵈ **S61.24** Puncture wound with foreign body of finger without damage to nail

7ᵈ **S61.240** Puncture wound with foreign body of right index finger without damage to nail

7ᵈ **S61.241** Puncture wound with foreign body of left index finger without damage to nail

7ᵈ **S61.242** Puncture wound with foreign body of right middle finger without damage to nail

7ᵈ **S61.243** Puncture wound with foreign body of left middle finger without damage to nail

7ᵈ **S61.244** Puncture wound with foreign body of right ring finger without damage to nail

7ᵈ **S61.245** Puncture wound with foreign body of left ring finger without damage to nail

7ᵈ **S61.246** Puncture wound with foreign body of right little finger without damage to nail

7ᵈ **S61.247** Puncture wound with foreign body of left little finger without damage to nail

7ᵈ **S61.248** Puncture wound with foreign body of other finger without damage to nail

Puncture wound with foreign body of specified finger with unspecified laterality without damage to nail

7ᵈ **S61.249** Puncture wound with foreign body of unspecified finger without damage to nail

6ᵈ **S61.25** Open bite of finger without damage to nail

Bite of finger without damage to nail NOS

EXCLUDES1 superficial bite of finger (S60.46-, S60.47-)

7ᵈ **S61.250** Open bite of right index finger without damage to nail

7ᵈ **S61.251** Open bite of left index finger without damage to nail

7ᵈ **S61.252** Open bite of right middle finger without damage to nail

7ᵈ **S61.253** Open bite of left middle finger without damage to nail

7ᵈ **S61.254** Open bite of right ring finger without damage to nail

7ᵈ **S61.255** Open bite of left ring finger without damage to nail

7ᵈ **S61.256** Open bite of right little finger without damage to nail

7ᵈ **S61.257** Open bite of left little finger without damage to nail

7ᵈ **S61.258** Open bite of other finger without damage to nail

Open bite of specified finger with unspecified laterality without damage to nail

7ᵈ **S61.259** Open bite of unspecified finger without damage to nail

5ᵈ **S61.3** Open wound of other finger with damage to nail

S61.30 Unspecified open wound of finger with damage to nail

- S61.300 Unspecified open wound of right index finger with damage to nail
- S61.301 Unspecified open wound of left index finger with damage to nail
- S61.302 Unspecified open wound of right middle finger with damage to nail
- S61.303 Unspecified open wound of left middle finger with damage to nail
- S61.304 Unspecified open wound of right ring finger with damage to nail
- S61.305 Unspecified open wound of left ring finger with damage to nail
- S61.306 Unspecified open wound of right little finger with damage to nail
- S61.307 Unspecified open wound of left little finger with damage to nail
- S61.308 Unspecified open wound of other finger with damage to nail

   Unspecified open wound of specified finger with unspecified laterality with damage to nail
- S61.309 Unspecified open wound of unspecified finger with damage to nail

S61.31 Laceration without foreign body of finger with damage to nail

- S61.310 Laceration without foreign body of right index finger with damage to nail
- S61.311 Laceration without foreign body of left index finger with damage to nail
- S61.312 Laceration without foreign body of right middle finger with damage to nail
- S61.313 Laceration without foreign body of left middle finger with damage to nail
- S61.314 Laceration without foreign body of right ring finger with damage to nail
- S61.315 Laceration without foreign body of left ring finger with damage to nail
- S61.316 Laceration without foreign body of right little finger with damage to nail
- S61.317 Laceration without foreign body of left little finger with damage to nail
- S61.318 Laceration without foreign body of other finger with damage to nail

   Laceration without foreign body of specified finger with unspecified laterality with damage to nail
- S61.319 Laceration without foreign body of unspecified finger with damage to nail

S61.32 Laceration with foreign body of finger with damage to nail

- S61.320 Laceration with foreign body of right index finger with damage to nail
- S61.321 Laceration with foreign body of left index finger with damage to nail
- S61.322 Laceration with foreign body of right middle finger with damage to nail
- S61.323 Laceration with foreign body of left middle finger with damage to nail
- S61.324 Laceration with foreign body of right ring finger with damage to nail
- S61.325 Laceration with foreign body of left ring finger with damage to nail
- S61.326 Laceration with foreign body of right little finger with damage to nail
- S61.327 Laceration with foreign body of left little finger with damage to nail
- S61.328 Laceration with foreign body of other finger with damage to nail

   Laceration with foreign body of specified finger with unspecified laterality with damage to nail
- S61.329 Laceration with foreign body of unspecified finger with damage to nail

S61.33 Puncture wound without foreign body of finger with damage to nail

- S61.330 Puncture wound without foreign body of right index finger with damage to nail
- S61.331 Puncture wound without foreign body of left index finger with damage to nail
- S61.332 Puncture wound without foreign body of right middle finger with damage to nail
- S61.333 Puncture wound without foreign body of left middle finger with damage to nail
- S61.334 Puncture wound without foreign body of right ring finger with damage to nail
- S61.335 Puncture wound without foreign body of left ring finger with damage to nail
- S61.336 Puncture wound without foreign body of right little finger with damage to nail
- S61.337 Puncture wound without foreign body of left little finger with damage to nail
- S61.338 Puncture wound without foreign body of other finger with damage to nail

   Puncture wound without foreign body of specified finger with unspecified laterality with damage to nail
- S61.339 Puncture wound without foreign body of unspecified finger with damage to nail

S61.34 Puncture wound with foreign body of finger with damage to nail

- S61.340 Puncture wound with foreign body of right index finger with damage to nail
- S61.341 Puncture wound with foreign body of left index finger with damage to nail
- S61.342 Puncture wound with foreign body of right middle finger with damage to nail
- S61.343 Puncture wound with foreign body of left middle finger with damage to nail
- S61.344 Puncture wound with foreign body of right ring finger with damage to nail
- S61.345 Puncture wound with foreign body of left ring finger with damage to nail
- S61.346 Puncture wound with foreign body of right little finger with damage to nail
- S61.347 Puncture wound with foreign body of left little finger with damage to nail
- S61.348 Puncture wound with foreign body of other finger with damage to nail

   Puncture wound with foreign body of specified finger with unspecified laterality with damage to nail
- S61.349 Puncture wound with foreign body of unspecified finger with damage to nail

S61.35 Open bite of finger with damage to nail

   Bite of finger with damage to nail NOS

   EXCLUDES1 superficial bite of finger (S60.46-, S60.47-)
- S61.350 Open bite of right index finger with damage to nail
- S61.351 Open bite of left index finger with damage to nail
- S61.352 Open bite of right middle finger with damage to nail
- S61.353 Open bite of left middle finger with damage to nail
- S61.354 Open bite of right ring finger with damage to nail
- S61.355 Open bite of left ring finger with damage to nail

4️⃣ 4th character required   5️⃣ 5th character required   6️⃣ 6th character required   7️⃣ 7th character required   Extension 'X' Alert

EXCLUDES 1 Not coded here   **EXCLUDES 2** Not included here   PDx Primary Diagnosis Only   Manifestation Code

[7th] S61.356 Open bite of right little finger with damage to nail
[7th] S61.357 Open bite of left little finger with damage to nail
[7th] S61.358 Open bite of other finger with damage to nail
Open bite of specified finger with unspecified laterality with damage to nail
[7th] S61.359 Open bite of unspecified finger with damage to nail
[5th] S61.4 Open wound of hand
[6th] S61.40 Unspecified open wound of hand
[7th] S61.401 Unspecified open wound of right hand
[7th] S61.402 Unspecified open wound of left hand
[7th] S61.409 Unspecified open wound of unspecified hand
[6th] S61.41 Laceration without foreign body of hand
[7th] S61.411 Laceration without foreign body of right hand
[7th] S61.412 Laceration without foreign body of left hand
[7th] S61.419 Laceration without foreign body of unspecified hand
[6th] S61.42 Laceration with foreign body of hand
[7th] S61.421 Laceration with foreign body of right hand
[7th] S61.422 Laceration with foreign body of left hand
[7th] S61.429 Laceration with foreign body of unspecified hand
[6th] S61.43 Puncture wound without foreign body of hand
[7th] S61.431 Puncture wound without foreign body of right hand
[7th] S61.432 Puncture wound without foreign body of left hand
[7th] S61.439 Puncture wound without foreign body of unspecified hand
[6th] S61.44 Puncture wound with foreign body of hand
[7th] S61.441 Puncture wound with foreign body of right hand
[7th] S61.442 Puncture wound with foreign body of left hand
[7th] S61.449 Puncture wound with foreign body of unspecified hand
[6th] S61.45 Open bite of hand
Bite of hand NOS
[EXCLUDES1] *superficial bite of hand (S60.56-, S60.57-)*
[7th] S61.451 Open bite of right hand
[7th] S61.452 Open bite of left hand
[7th] S61.459 Open bite of unspecified hand
[5th] S61.5 Open wound of wrist
[6th] S61.50 Unspecified open wound of wrist
[7th] S61.501 Unspecified open wound of right wrist
[7th] S61.502 Unspecified open wound of left wrist
[7th] S61.509 Unspecified open wound of unspecified wrist
[6th] S61.51 Laceration without foreign body of wrist
[7th] S61.511 Laceration without foreign body of right wrist
[7th] S61.512 Laceration without foreign body of left wrist
[7th] S61.519 Laceration without foreign body of unspecified wrist
[6th] S61.52 Laceration with foreign body of wrist
[7th] S61.521 Laceration with foreign body of right wrist
[7th] S61.522 Laceration with foreign body of left wrist
[7th] S61.529 Laceration with foreign body of unspecified wrist
[6th] S61.53 Puncture wound without foreign body of wrist
[7th] S61.531 Puncture wound without foreign body of right wrist
[7th] S61.532 Puncture wound without foreign body of left wrist
[7th] S61.539 Puncture wound without foreign body of unspecified wrist
[6th] S61.54 Puncture wound with foreign body of wrist
[7th] S61.541 Puncture wound with foreign body of right wrist
[7th] S61.542 Puncture wound with foreign body of left wrist
[7th] S61.549 Puncture wound with foreign body of unspecified wrist
[6th] S61.55 Open bite of wrist
Bite of wrist NOS
[EXCLUDES1] *superficial bite of wrist (S60.86-, S60.87-)*
[7th] S61.551 Open bite of right wrist
[7th] S61.552 Open bite of left wrist
[7th] S61.559 Open bite of unspecified wrist
[4th] S62 Fracture at wrist and hand level
[NOTES] A fracture not indicated as displaced or nondisplaced should be coded to displaced
A fracture not indicated as open or closed should be coded to closed
[EXCLUDES1] *traumatic amputation of wrist and hand (S68.-)*
[EXCLUDES2] *fracture of distal parts of ulna and radius (S52.-)*
The appropriate 7th character is to be added to each code from category S62
A = initial encounter for closed fracture
B = initial encounter for open fracture
D = subsequent encounter for fracture with routine healing
G = subsequent encounter for fracture with delayed healing
K = subsequent encounter for fracture with nonunion
P = subsequent encounter for fracture with malunion
S = sequela
[5th] S62.0 Fracture of navicular [scaphoid] bone of wrist
[6th] S62.00 Unspecified fracture of navicular [scaphoid] bone of wrist
[7th] S62.001 Unspecified fracture of navicular [scaphoid] bone of right wrist
[7th] S62.002 Unspecified fracture of navicular [scaphoid] bone of left wrist
[7th] S62.009 Unspecified fracture of navicular [scaphoid] bone of unspecified wrist
[6th] S62.01 Fracture of distal pole of navicular [scaphoid] bone of wrist
Fracture of volar tuberosity of navicular [scaphoid] bone of wrist
[7th] S62.011 Displaced fracture of distal pole of navicular [scaphoid] bone of right wrist
[7th] S62.012 Displaced fracture of distal pole of navicular [scaphoid] bone of left wrist
[7th] S62.013 Displaced fracture of distal pole of navicular [scaphoid] bone of unspecified wrist
[7th] S62.014 Nondisplaced fracture of distal pole of navicular [scaphoid] bone of right wrist
[7th] S62.015 Nondisplaced fracture of distal pole of navicular [scaphoid] bone of left wrist
[7th] S62.016 Nondisplaced fracture of distal pole of navicular [scaphoid] bone of unspecified wrist
[6th] S62.02 Fracture of middle third of navicular [scaphoid] bone of wrist
[7th] S62.021 Displaced fracture of middle third of navicular [scaphoid] bone of right wrist
[7th] S62.022 Displaced fracture of middle third of navicular [scaphoid] bone of left wrist
[7th] S62.023 Displaced fracture of middle third of navicular[scaphoid]boneofunspecifiedwrist
[7th] S62.024 Nondisplaced fracture of middle third of navicular [scaphoid] bone of right wrist

7️⃣ S62.025 Nondisplaced fracture of middle third of navicular [scaphoid] bone of left wrist

7️⃣ S62.026 Nondisplaced fracture of middle third of navicular [scaphoid] bone of unspecified wrist

6️⃣ S62.03 Fracture of proximal third of navicular [scaphoid] bone of wrist

7️⃣ S62.031 Displaced fracture of proximal third of navicular [scaphoid] bone of right wrist

7️⃣ S62.032 Displaced fracture of proximal third of navicular [scaphoid] bone of left wrist

7️⃣ S62.033 Displaced fracture of proximal third of navicular [scaphoid] bone of unspecified wrist

7️⃣ S62.034 Nondisplaced fracture of proximal third of navicular [scaphoid] bone of right wrist

7️⃣ S62.035 Nondisplaced fracture of proximal third of navicular [scaphoid] bone of left wrist

7️⃣ S62.036 Nondisplaced fracture of proximal third of navicular [scaphoid] bone of unspecified wrist

5️⃣ S62.1 Fracture of other and unspecified carpal bone(s)

EXCLUDES2 fracture of scaphoid of wrist (S62.0-)

6️⃣ S62.10 Fracture of unspecified carpal bone

Fracture of wrist NOS

7️⃣ S62.101 Fracture of unspecified carpal bone, right wrist

7️⃣ S62.102 Fracture of unspecified carpal bone, left wrist

7️⃣ S62.109 Fracture of unspecified carpal bone, unspecified wrist

6️⃣ S62.11 Fracture of triquetrum [cuneiform] bone of wrist

7️⃣ S62.111 Displaced fracture of triquetrum [cuneiform] bone, right wrist

7️⃣ S62.112 Displaced fracture of triquetrum [cuneiform] bone, left wrist

7️⃣ S62.113 Displaced fracture of triquetrum [cuneiform] bone, unspecified wrist

7️⃣ S62.114 Nondisplaced fracture of triquetrum [cuneiform] bone, right wrist

7️⃣ S62.115 Nondisplaced fracture of triquetrum [cuneiform] bone, left wrist

7️⃣ S62.116 Nondisplaced fracture of triquetrum [cuneiform] bone, unspecified wrist

6️⃣ S62.12 Fracture of lunate [semilunar]

7️⃣ S62.121 Displaced fracture of lunate [semilunar], right wrist

7️⃣ S62.122 Displaced fracture of lunate [semilunar], left wrist

7️⃣ S62.123 Displaced fracture of lunate [semilunar], unspecified wrist

7️⃣ S62.124 Nondisplaced fracture of lunate [semilunar], right wrist

7️⃣ S62.125 Nondisplaced fracture of lunate [semilunar], left wrist

7️⃣ S62.126 Nondisplaced fracture of lunate [semilunar], unspecified wrist

6️⃣ S62.13 Fracture of capitate [os magnum] bone

7️⃣ S62.131 Displaced fracture of capitate [os magnum] bone, right wrist

7️⃣ S62.132 Displaced fracture of capitate [os magnum] bone, left wrist

7️⃣ S62.133 Displaced fracture of capitate [os magnum] bone, unspecified wrist

7️⃣ S62.134 Nondisplaced fracture of capitate [os magnum] bone, right wrist

7️⃣ S62.135 Nondisplaced fracture of capitate [os magnum] bone, left wrist

7️⃣ S62.136 Nondisplaced fracture of capitate [os magnum] bone, unspecified wrist

6️⃣ S62.14 Fracture of body of hamate [unciform] bone

Fracture of hamate [unciform] bone NOS

7️⃣ S62.141 Displaced fracture of body of hamate [unciform] bone, right wrist

7️⃣ S62.142 Displaced fracture of body of hamate [unciform] bone, left wrist

7️⃣ S62.143 Displaced fracture of body of hamate [unciform] bone, unspecified wrist

7️⃣ S62.144 Nondisplaced fracture of body of hamate [unciform] bone, right wrist

7️⃣ S62.145 Nondisplaced fracture of body of hamate [unciform] bone, left wrist

7️⃣ S62.146 Nondisplaced fracture of body of hamate [unciform] bone, unspecified wrist

6️⃣ S62.15 Fracture of hook process of hamate [unciform] bone

Fracture of unciform process of hamate [unciform] bone

7️⃣ S62.151 Displaced fracture of hook process of hamate [unciform] bone, right wrist

7️⃣ S62.152 Displaced fracture of hook process of hamate [unciform] bone, left wrist

7️⃣ S62.153 Displaced fracture of hook process of hamate [unciform] bone, unspecified wrist

7️⃣ S62.154 Nondisplaced fracture of hook process of hamate [unciform] bone, right wrist

7️⃣ S62.155 Nondisplaced fracture of hook process of hamate [unciform] bone, left wrist

7️⃣ S62.156 Nondisplaced fracture of hook process of hamate [unciform] bone, unspecified wrist

6️⃣ S62.16 Fracture of pisiform

7️⃣ S62.161 Displaced fracture of pisiform, right wrist

7️⃣ S62.162 Displaced fracture of pisiform, left wrist

7️⃣ S62.163 Displaced fracture of pisiform, unspecified wrist

7️⃣ S62.164 Nondisplaced fracture of pisiform, right wrist

7️⃣ S62.165 Nondisplaced fracture of pisiform, left wrist

7️⃣ S62.166 Nondisplaced fracture of pisiform, unspecified wrist

6️⃣ S62.17 Fracture of trapezium [larger multangular]

7️⃣ S62.171 Displaced fracture of trapezium [larger multangular], right wrist

7️⃣ S62.172 Displaced fracture of trapezium [larger multangular], left wrist

7️⃣ S62.173 Displaced fracture of trapezium [larger multangular], unspecified wrist

7️⃣ S62.174 Nondisplaced fracture of trapezium [larger multangular], right wrist

7️⃣ S62.175 Nondisplaced fracture of trapezium [larger multangular], left wrist

7️⃣ S62.176 Nondisplaced fracture of trapezium [larger multangular], unspecified wrist

6️⃣ S62.18 Fracture of trapezoid [smaller multangular]

7️⃣ S62.181 Displaced fracture of trapezoid [smaller multangular], right wrist

7️⃣ S62.182 Displaced fracture of trapezoid [smaller multangular], left wrist

7️⃣ S62.183 Displaced fracture of trapezoid [smaller multangular], unspecified wrist

7️⃣ S62.184 Nondisplaced fracture of trapezoid [smaller multangular], right wrist

7️⃣ S62.185 Nondisplaced fracture of trapezoid [smaller multangular], left wrist

7️⃣ S62.186 Nondisplaced fracture of trapezoid [smaller multangular], unspecified wrist

5️⃣ S62.2 Fracture of first metacarpal bone

6️⃣ S62.20 Unspecified fracture of first metacarpal bone

4️⃣ 4th character required   5️⃣ 5th character required   6️⃣ 6th character required   7️⃣ 7th character required   Extension 'X' Alert

EXCLUDES1 Not coded here   EXCLUDES2 Not included here   PDx Primary Diagnosis Only   Manifestation Code

7ᵗʰ **S62.201** Unspecified fracture of first metacarpal bone, right hand

7ᵗʰ **S62.202** Unspecified fracture of first metacarpal bone, left hand

7ᵗʰ **S62.209** Unspecified fracture of first metacarpal bone, unspecified hand

6ᵗʰ **S62.21** Bennett's fracture

7ᵗʰ **S62.211** Bennett's fracture, right hand

7ᵗʰ **S62.212** Bennett's fracture, left hand

7ᵗʰ **S62.213** Bennett's fracture, unspecified hand

6ᵗʰ **S62.22** Rolando's fracture

7ᵗʰ **S62.221** Displaced Rolando's fracture, right hand

7ᵗʰ **S62.222** Displaced Rolando's fracture, left hand

7ᵗʰ **S62.223** Displaced Rolando's fracture, unspecified hand

7ᵗʰ **S62.224** Nondisplaced Rolando's fracture, right hand

7ᵗʰ **S62.225** Nondisplaced Rolando's fracture, left hand

7ᵗʰ **S62.226** Nondisplaced Rolando's fracture, unspecified hand

6ᵗʰ **S62.23** Other fracture of base of first metacarpal bone

7ᵗʰ **S62.231** Other displaced fracture of base of first metacarpal bone, right hand

7ᵗʰ **S62.232** Other displaced fracture of base of first metacarpal bone, left hand

7ᵗʰ **S62.233** Other displaced fracture of base of first metacarpal bone, unspecified hand

7ᵗʰ **S62.234** Other nondisplaced fracture of base of first metacarpal bone, right hand

7ᵗʰ **S62.235** Other nondisplaced fracture of base of first metacarpal bone, left hand

7ᵗʰ **S62.236** Other nondisplaced fracture of base of first metacarpal bone, unspecified hand

6ᵗʰ **S62.24** Fracture of shaft of first metacarpal bone

7ᵗʰ **S62.241** Displaced fracture of shaft of first metacarpal bone, right hand

7ᵗʰ **S62.242** Displaced fracture of shaft of first metacarpal bone, left hand

7ᵗʰ **S62.243** Displaced fracture of shaft of first metacarpal bone, unspecified hand

7ᵗʰ **S62.244** Nondisplaced fracture of shaft of first metacarpal bone, right hand

7ᵗʰ **S62.245** Nondisplaced fracture of shaft of first metacarpal bone, left hand

7ᵗʰ **S62.246** Nondisplaced fracture of shaft of first metacarpal bone, unspecified hand

6ᵗʰ **S62.25** Fracture of neck of first metacarpal bone

7ᵗʰ **S62.251** Displaced fracture of neck of first metacarpal bone, right hand

7ᵗʰ **S62.252** Displaced fracture of neck of first metacarpal bone, left hand

7ᵗʰ **S62.253** Displaced fracture of neck of first metacarpal bone, unspecified hand

7ᵗʰ **S62.254** Nondisplaced fracture of neck of first metacarpal bone, right hand

7ᵗʰ **S62.255** Nondisplaced fracture of neck of first metacarpal bone, left hand

7ᵗʰ **S62.256** Nondisplaced fracture of neck of first metacarpal bone, unspecified hand

6ᵗʰ **S62.29** Other fracture of first metacarpal bone

7ᵗʰ **S62.291** Other fracture of first metacarpal bone, right hand

7ᵗʰ **S62.292** Other fracture of first metacarpal bone, left hand

7ᵗʰ **S62.299** Other fracture of first metacarpal bone, unspecified hand

5ᵗʰ **S62.3** Fracture of other and unspecified metacarpal bone

EXCLUDES2 fracture of first metacarpal bone (S62.2-)

6ᵗʰ **S62.30** Unspecified fracture of other metacarpal bone

7ᵗʰ **S62.300** Unspecified fracture of second metacarpal bone, right hand

7ᵗʰ **S62.301** Unspecified fracture of second metacarpal bone, left hand

7ᵗʰ **S62.302** Unspecified fracture of third metacarpal bone, right hand

7ᵗʰ **S62.303** Unspecified fracture of third metacarpal bone, left hand

7ᵗʰ **S62.304** Unspecified fracture of fourth metacarpal bone, right hand

7ᵗʰ **S62.305** Unspecified fracture of fourth metacarpal bone, left hand

7ᵗʰ **S62.306** Unspecified fracture of fifth metacarpal bone, right hand

7ᵗʰ **S62.307** Unspecified fracture of fifth metacarpal bone, left hand

7ᵗʰ **S62.308** Unspecified fracture of other metacarpal bone

Unspecified fracture of specified metacarpal bone with unspecified laterality

7ᵗʰ **S62.309** Unspecified fracture of unspecified metacarpal bone

6ᵗʰ **S62.31** Displaced fracture of base of other metacarpal bone

7ᵗʰ **S62.310** Displaced fracture of base of second metacarpal bone, right hand

7ᵗʰ **S62.311** Displaced fracture of base of second metacarpal bone. left hand

7ᵗʰ **S62.312** Displaced fracture of base of third metacarpal bone, right hand

7ᵗʰ **S62.313** Displaced fracture of base of third metacarpal bone, left hand

7ᵗʰ **S62.314** Displaced fracture of base of fourth metacarpal bone, right hand

7ᵗʰ **S62.315** Displaced fracture of base of fourth metacarpal bone, left hand

7ᵗʰ **S62.316** Displaced fracture of base of fifth metacarpal bone, right hand

7ᵗʰ **S62.317** Displaced fracture of base of fifth metacarpal bone. left hand

7ᵗʰ **S62.318** Displaced fracture of base of other metacarpal bone

Displaced fracture of base of specified metacarpal bone with unspecified laterality

7ᵗʰ **S62.319** Displaced fracture of base of unspecified metacarpal bone

6ᵗʰ **S62.32** Displaced fracture of shaft of other metacarpal bone

7ᵗʰ **S62.320** Displaced fracture of shaft of second metacarpal bone, right hand

7ᵗʰ **S62.321** Displaced fracture of shaft of second metacarpal bone, left hand

7ᵗʰ **S62.322** Displaced fracture of shaft of third metacarpal bone, right hand

7ᵗʰ **S62.323** Displaced fracture of shaft of third metacarpal bone, left hand

7ᵗʰ **S62.324** Displaced fracture of shaft of fourth metacarpal bone, right hand

7ᵗʰ **S62.325** Displaced fracture of shaft of fourth metacarpal bone, left hand

7ᵗʰ **S62.326** Displaced fracture of shaft of fifth metacarpal bone, right hand

7ᵗʰ **S62.327** Displaced fracture of shaft of fifth metacarpal bone, left hand

7ᵗʰ **S62.328** Displaced fracture of shaft of other metacarpal bone

Displaced fracture of shaft of specified metacarpal bone with unspecified laterality

---

Unspecified Code   Other Specified Code   Ⓝ Newborn Age: 0   Ⓟ Pediatric Age: 0-17   Ⓜ Maternity Age: 12-55

Ⓐ Adult Age: 15-124   ♂ Male   ♀ Female   ● New Code   ▲ Revised Code Title   ►◄ Revised Text

[7th] S62.329 Displaced fracture of shaft of unspecified metacarpal bone

[6th] S62.33 Displaced fracture of neck of other metacarpal bone

[7th] S62.330 Displaced fracture of neck of second metacarpal bone, right hand

[7th] S62.331 Displaced fracture of neck of second metacarpal bone, left hand

[7th] S62.332 Displaced fracture of neck of third metacarpal bone, right hand

[7th] S62.333 Displaced fracture of neck of third metacarpal bone, left hand

[7th] S62.334 Displaced fracture of neck of fourth metacarpal bone, right hand

[7th] S62.335 Displaced fracture of neck of fourth metacarpal bone, left hand

[7th] S62.336 Displaced fracture of neck of fifth metacarpal bone, right hand

[7th] S62.337 Displaced fracture of neck of fifth metacarpal bone, left hand

[7th] S62.338 Displaced fracture of neck of other metacarpal bone

Displaced fracture of neck of specified metacarpal bone with unspecified laterality

[7th] S62.339 Displaced fracture of neck of unspecified metacarpal bone

[6th] S62.34 Nondisplaced fracture of base of other metacarpal bone

[7th] S62.340 Nondisplaced fracture of base of second metacarpal bone, right hand

[7th] S62.341 Nondisplaced fracture of base of second metacarpal bone. left hand

[7th] S62.342 Nondisplaced fracture of base of third metacarpal bone, right hand

[7th] S62.343 Nondisplaced fracture of base of third metacarpal bone, left hand

[7th] S62.344 Nondisplaced fracture of base of fourth metacarpal bone, right hand

[7th] S62.345 Nondisplaced fracture of base of fourth metacarpal bone, left hand

[7th] S62.346 Nondisplaced fracture of base of fifth metacarpal bone, right hand

[7th] S62.347 Nondisplaced fracture of base of fifth metacarpal bone. left hand

[7th] S62.348 Nondisplaced fracture of base of other metacarpal bone

Nondisplaced fracture of base of specified metacarpal bone with unspecified laterality

[7th] S62.349 Nondisplaced fracture of base of unspecified metacarpal bone

[6th] S62.35 Nondisplaced fracture of shaft of other metacarpal bone

[7th] S62.350 Nondisplaced fracture of shaft of second metacarpal bone, right hand

[7th] S62.351 Nondisplaced fracture of shaft of second metacarpal bone, left hand

[7th] S62.352 Nondisplaced fracture of shaft of third metacarpal bone, right hand

[7th] S62.353 Nondisplaced fracture of shaft of third metacarpal bone, left hand

[7th] S62.354 Nondisplaced fracture of shaft of fourth metacarpal bone, right hand

[7th] S62.355 Nondisplaced fracture of shaft of fourth metacarpal bone, left hand

[7th] S62.356 Nondisplaced fracture of shaft of fifth metacarpal bone, right hand

[7th] S62.357 Nondisplaced fracture of shaft of fifth metacarpal bone, left hand

[7th] S62.358 Nondisplaced fracture of shaft of other metacarpal bone

Nondisplaced fracture of shaft of specified metacarpal bone with unspecified laterality

[7th] S62.359 Nondisplaced fracture of shaft of unspecified metacarpal bone

[6th] S62.36 Nondisplaced fracture of neck of other metacarpal bone

[7th] S62.360 Nondisplaced fracture of neck of second metacarpal bone, right hand

[7th] S62.361 Nondisplaced fracture of neck of second metacarpal bone, left hand

[7th] S62.362 Nondisplaced fracture of neck of third metacarpal bone, right hand

[7th] S62.363 Nondisplaced fracture of neck of third metacarpal bone, left hand

[7th] S62.364 Nondisplaced fracture of neck of fourth metacarpal bone, right hand

[7th] S62.365 Nondisplaced fracture of neck of fourth metacarpal bone, left hand

[7th] S62.366 Nondisplaced fracture of neck of fifth metacarpal bone, right hand

[7th] S62.367 Nondisplaced fracture of neck of fifth metacarpal bone, left hand

[7th] S62.368 Nondisplaced fracture of neck of other metacarpal bone

Nondisplaced fracture of neck of specified metacarpal bone with unspecified laterality

[7th] S62.369 Nondisplaced fracture of neck of unspecified metacarpal bone

[6th] S62.39 Other fracture of other metacarpal bone

[7th] S62.390 Other fracture of second metacarpal bone, right hand

[7th] S62.391 Other fracture of second metacarpal bone, left hand

[7th] S62.392 Other fracture of third metacarpal bone, right hand

[7th] S62.393 Other fracture of third metacarpal bone, left hand

[7th] S62.394 Other fracture of fourth metacarpal bone, right hand

[7th] S62.395 Other fracture of fourth metacarpal bone, left hand

[7th] S62.396 Other fracture of fifth metacarpal bone, right hand

[7th] S62.397 Other fracture of fifth metacarpal bone, left hand

[7th] S62.398 Other fracture of other metacarpal bone

Other fracture of specified metacarpal bone with unspecified laterality

[7th] S62.399 Other fracture of unspecified metacarpal bone

[5th] S62.5 Fracture of thumb

[6th] S62.50 Fracture of unspecified phalanx of thumb

[7th] S62.501 Fracture of unspecified phalanx of right thumb

[7th] S62.502 Fracture of unspecified phalanx of left thumb

[7th] S62.509 Fracture of unspecified phalanx of unspecified thumb

[6th] S62.51 Fracture of proximal phalanx of thumb

[7th] S62.511 Displaced fracture of proximal phalanx of right thumb

[7th] S62.512 Displaced fracture of proximal phalanx of left thumb

[7th] S62.513 Displaced fracture of proximal phalanx of unspecified thumb

[7th] S62.514 Nondisplaced fracture of proximal phalanx of right thumb

[4th] 4th character required [5th] 5th character required [6th] 6th character required [7th] 7th character required [7th] Extension 'X' Alert
EXCLUDES 1 Not coded here EXCLUDES 2 Not included here PDx Primary Diagnosis Only Manifestation Code

[7th] S62.515 Nondisplaced fracture of proximal phalanx of left thumb
[7th] S62.516 Nondisplaced fracture of proximal phalanx of unspecified thumb
[6th] S62.52 Fracture of distal phalanx of thumb
[7th] S62.521 Displaced fracture of distal phalanx of right thumb
[7th] S62.522 Displaced fracture of distal phalanx of left thumb
[7th] S62.523 Displaced fracture of distal phalanx of unspecified thumb
[7th] S62.524 Nondisplaced fracture of distal phalanx of right thumb
[7th] S62.525 Nondisplaced fracture of distal phalanx of left thumb
[7th] S62.526 Nondisplaced fracture of distal phalanx of unspecified thumb
[5th] S62.6 Fracture of other and unspecified finger(s)
[EXCLUDES2] *fracture of thumb (S62.5-)*
[6th] S62.60 Fracture of unspecified phalanx of finger
[7th] S62.600 Fracture of unspecified phalanx of right index finger
[7th] S62.601 Fracture of unspecified phalanx of left index finger
[7th] S62.602 Fracture of unspecified phalanx of right middle finger
[7th] S62.603 Fracture of unspecified phalanx of left middle finger
[7th] S62.604 Fracture of unspecified phalanx of right ring finger
[7th] S62.605 Fracture of unspecified phalanx of left ring finger
[7th] S62.606 Fracture of unspecified phalanx of right little finger
[7th] S62.607 Fracture of unspecified phalanx of left little finger
[7th] S62.608 Fracture of unspecified phalanx of other finger
Fracture of unspecified phalanx of specified finger with unspecified laterality
[7th] S62.609 Fracture of unspecified phalanx of unspecified finger
[6th] S62.61 Displaced fracture of proximal phalanx of finger
[7th] S62.610 Displaced fracture of proximal phalanx of right index finger
[7th] S62.611 Displaced fracture of proximal phalanx of left index finger
[7th] S62.612 Displaced fracture of proximal phalanx of right middle finger
[7th] S62.613 Displaced fracture of proximal phalanx of left middle finger
[7th] S62.614 Displaced fracture of proximal phalanx of right ring finger
[7th] S62.615 Displaced fracture of proximal phalanx of left ring finger
[7th] S62.616 Displaced fracture of proximal phalanx of right little finger
[7th] S62.617 Displaced fracture of proximal phalanx of left little finger
[7th] S62.618 Displaced fracture of proximal phalanx of other finger
Displaced fracture of proximal phalanx of specified finger with unspecified laterality
[7th] S62.619 Displaced fracture of proximal phalanx of unspecified finger
[6th] S62.62 Displaced fracture of medial phalanx of finger
[7th] S62.620 Displaced fracture of medial phalanx of right index finger
[7th] S62.621 Displaced fracture of medial phalanx of left index finger
[7th] S62.622 Displaced fracture of medial phalanx of right middle finger
[7th] S62.623 Displaced fracture of medial phalanx of left middle finger
[7th] S62.624 Displaced fracture of medial phalanx of right ring finger
[7th] S62.625 Displaced fracture of medial phalanx of left ring finger
[7th] S62.626 Displaced fracture of medial phalanx of right little finger
[7th] S62.627 Displaced fracture of medial phalanx of left little finger
[7th] S62.628 Displaced fracture of medial phalanx of other finger
Displaced fracture of medial phalanx of specified finger with unspecified laterality
[7th] S62.629 Displaced fracture of medial phalanx of unspecified finger
[6th] S62.63 Displaced fracture of distal phalanx of finger
[7th] S62.630 Displaced fracture of distal phalanx of right index finger
[7th] S62.631 Displaced fracture of distal phalanx of left index finger
[7th] S62.632 Displaced fracture of distal phalanx of right middle finger
[7th] S62.633 Displaced fracture of distal phalanx of left middle finger
[7th] S62.634 Displaced fracture of distal phalanx of right ring finger
[7th] S62.635 Displaced fracture of distal phalanx of left ring finger
[7th] S62.636 Displaced fracture of distal phalanx of right little finger
[7th] S62.637 Displaced fracture of distal phalanx of left little finger
[7th] S62.638 Displaced fracture of distal phalanx of other finger
Displaced fracture of distal phalanx of specified finger with unspecified laterality
[7th] S62.639 Displaced fracture of distal phalanx of unspecified finger
[6th] S62.64 Nondisplaced fracture of proximal phalanx of finger
[7th] S62.640 Nondisplaced fracture of proximal phalanx of right index finger
[7th] S62.641 Nondisplaced fracture of proximal phalanx of left index finger
[7th] S62.642 Nondisplaced fracture of proximal phalanx of right middle finger
[7th] S62.643 Nondisplaced fracture of proximal phalanx of left middle finger
[7th] S62.644 Nondisplaced fracture of proximal phalanx of right ring finger
[7th] S62.645 Nondisplaced fracture of proximal phalanx of left ring finger
[7th] S62.646 Nondisplaced fracture of proximal phalanx of right little finger
[7th] S62.647 Nondisplaced fracture of proximal phalanx of left little finger
[7th] S62.648 Nondisplaced fracture of proximal phalanx of other finger
Nondisplaced fracture of proximal phalanx of specified finger with unspecified laterality
[7th] S62.649 Nondisplaced fracture of proximal phalanx of unspecified finger
[6th] S62.65 Nondisplaced fracture of medial phalanx of finger

Unspecified Code | Other Specified Code | [N] Newborn Age: 0 | [P] Pediatric Age: 0-17 | [M] Maternity Age: 12-55
[A] Adult Age: 15-124 | ♂ Male | ♀ Female | ● New Code | ▲ Revised Code Title | ►◄ Revised Text

S62.650 Nondisplaced fracture of medial phalanx of right index finger

S62.651 Nondisplaced fracture of medial phalanx of left index finger

S62.652 Nondisplaced fracture of medial phalanx of right middle finger

S62.653 Nondisplaced fracture of medial phalanx of left middle finger

S62.654 Nondisplaced fracture of medial phalanx of right ring finger

S62.655 Nondisplaced fracture of medial phalanx of left ring finger

S62.656 Nondisplaced fracture of medial phalanx of right little finger

S62.657 Nondisplaced fracture of medial phalanx of left little finger

S62.658 Nondisplaced fracture of medial phalanx of other finger

Nondisplaced fracture of medial phalanx of specified finger with unspecified laterality

S62.659 Nondisplaced fracture of medial phalanx of unspecified finger

S62.66 Nondisplaced fracture of distal phalanx of finger

S62.660 Nondisplaced fracture of distal phalanx of right index finger

S62.661 Nondisplaced fracture of distal phalanx of left index finger

S62.662 Nondisplaced fracture of distal phalanx of right middle finger

S62.663 Nondisplaced fracture of distal phalanx of left middle finger

S62.664 Nondisplaced fracture of distal phalanx of right ring finger

S62.665 Nondisplaced fracture of distal phalanx of left ring finger

S62.666 Nondisplaced fracture of distal phalanx of right little finger

S62.667 Nondisplaced fracture of distal phalanx of left little finger

S62.668 Nondisplaced fracture of distal phalanx of other finger

Nondisplaced fracture of distal phalanx of specified finger with unspecified laterality

S62.669 Nondisplaced fracture of distal phalanx of unspecified finger

S62.9 Unspecified fracture of wrist and hand

S62.90 Unspecified fracture of unspecified wrist and hand

S62.91 Unspecified fracture of right wrist and hand

S62.92 Unspecified fracture of left wrist and hand

S63 Dislocation and sprain of joints and ligaments at wrist and hand level

> INCLUDES   avulsion of joint or ligament at wrist and hand level
> laceration of cartilage, joint or ligament at wrist and hand level
> sprain of cartilage, joint or ligament at wrist and hand level
> traumatic hemarthrosis of joint or ligament at wrist and hand level
> traumatic rupture of joint or ligament at wrist and hand level
> traumatic subluxation of joint or ligament at wrist and hand level
> traumatic tear of joint or ligament at wrist and hand level

Code also any associated open wound

> EXCLUDES2   strain of muscle, fascia and tendon of wrist and hand (S66.-)

The appropriate 7th character is to be added to each code from category S63
A = initial encounter
D = subsequent encounter
S = sequela

S63.0 Subluxation and dislocation of wrist and hand joints

S63.00 Unspecified subluxation and dislocation of wrist and hand

Dislocation of carpal bone NOS
Dislocation of distal end of radius NOS
Subluxation of carpal bone NOS
Subluxation of distal end of radius NOS

S63.001 Unspecified subluxation of right wrist and hand

S63.002 Unspecified subluxation of left wrist and hand

S63.003 Unspecified subluxation of unspecified wrist and hand

S63.004 Unspecified dislocation of right wrist and hand

S63.005 Unspecified dislocation of left wrist and hand

S63.006 Unspecified dislocation of unspecified wrist and hand

S63.01 Subluxation and dislocation of distal radioulnar joint

S63.011 Subluxation of distal radioulnar joint of right wrist

S63.012 Subluxation of distal radioulnar joint of left wrist

S63.013 Subluxation of distal radioulnar joint of unspecified wrist

S63.014 Dislocation of distal radioulnar joint of right wrist

S63.015 Dislocation of distal radioulnar joint of left wrist

S63.016 Dislocation of distal radioulnar joint of unspecified wrist

S63.02 Subluxation and dislocation of radiocarpal joint

S63.021 Subluxation of radiocarpal joint of right wrist

S63.022 Subluxation of radiocarpal joint of left wrist

S63.023 Subluxation of radiocarpal joint of unspecified wrist

S63.024 Dislocation of radiocarpal joint of right wrist

S63.025 Dislocation of radiocarpal joint of left wrist

S63.026 Dislocation of radiocarpal joint of unspecified wrist

S63.03 Subluxation and dislocation of midcarpal joint

S63.031 Subluxation of midcarpal joint of right wrist

S63.032 Subluxation of midcarpal joint of left wrist

S63.033 Subluxation of midcarpal joint of unspecified wrist

S63.034 Dislocation of midcarpal joint of right wrist

S63.035 Dislocation of midcarpal joint of left wrist

S63.036 Dislocation of midcarpal joint of unspecified wrist

S63.04 Subluxation and dislocation of carpometacarpal joint of thumb

> EXCLUDES2   interphalangeal subluxation and dislocation of thumb (S63.1-)

S63.041 Subluxation of carpometacarpal joint of right thumb

S63.042 Subluxation of carpometacarpal joint of left thumb

S63.043 Subluxation of carpometacarpal joint of unspecified thumb

S63.044 Dislocation of carpometacarpal joint of right thumb

4th character required   5th character required   6th character required   7th character required   Extension 'X' Alert

EXCLUDES 1 Not coded here   EXCLUDES 2 Not included here   PDx Primary Diagnosis Only   Manifestation Code

- [7th] S63.045 Dislocation of carpometacarpal joint of left thumb
- [7th] S63.046 Dislocation of carpometacarpal joint of unspecified thumb

[6th] **S63.05 Subluxation and dislocation of other carpometacarpal joint**

[EXCLUDES2] *subluxation and dislocation of carpometacarpal joint of thumb (S63.04-)*

- [7th] S63.051 Subluxation of other carpometacarpal joint of right hand
- [7th] S63.052 Subluxation of other carpometacarpal joint of left hand
- [7th] S63.053 Subluxation of other carpometacarpal joint of unspecified hand
- [7th] S63.054 Dislocation of other carpometacarpal joint of right hand
- [7th] S63.055 Dislocation of other carpometacarpal joint of left hand
- [7th] S63.056 Dislocation of other carpometacarpal joint of unspecified hand

[6th] **S63.06 Subluxation and dislocation of metacarpal (bone), proximal end**

- [7th] S63.061 Subluxation of metacarpal (bone), proximal end of right hand
- [7th] S63.062 Subluxation of metacarpal (bone), proximal end of left hand
- [7th] S63.063 Subluxation of metacarpal (bone), proximal end of unspecified hand
- [7th] S63.064 Dislocation of metacarpal (bone), proximal end of right hand
- [7th] S63.065 Dislocation of metacarpal (bone), proximal end of left hand
- [7th] S63.066 Dislocation of metacarpal (bone), proximal end of unspecified hand

[6th] **S63.07 Subluxation and dislocation of distal end of ulna**

- [7th] S63.071 Subluxation of distal end of right ulna
- [7th] S63.072 Subluxation of distal end of left ulna
- [7th] S63.073 Subluxation of distal end of unspecified ulna
- [7th] S63.074 Dislocation of distal end of right ulna
- [7th] S63.075 Dislocation of distal end of left ulna
- [7th] S63.076 Dislocation of distal end of unspecified ulna

[6th] **S63.09 Other subluxation and dislocation of wrist and hand**

- [7th] S63.091 Other subluxation of right wrist and hand
- [7th] S63.092 Other subluxation of left wrist and hand
- [7th] S63.093 Other subluxation of unspecified wrist and hand
- [7th] S63.094 Other dislocation of right wrist and hand
- [7th] S63.095 Other dislocation of left wrist and hand
- [7th] S63.096 Other dislocation of unspecified wrist and hand

[5th] **S63.1 Subluxation and dislocation of thumb**

[6th] **S63.10 Unspecified subluxation and dislocation of thumb**

- [7th] S63.101 Unspecified subluxation of right thumb
- [7th] S63.102 Unspecified subluxation of left thumb
- [7th] S63.103 Unspecified subluxation of unspecified thumb
- [7th] S63.104 Unspecified dislocation of right thumb
- [7th] S63.105 Unspecified dislocation of left thumb
- [7th] S63.106 Unspecified dislocation of unspecified thumb

[6th] **S63.11 Subluxation and dislocation of metacarpophalangeal joint of thumb**

- [7th] S63.111 Subluxation of metacarpophalangeal joint of right thumb
- [7th] S63.112 Subluxation of metacarpophalangeal joint of left thumb
- [7th] S63.113 Subluxation of metacarpophalangeal joint of unspecified thumb
- [7th] S63.114 Dislocation of metacarpophalangeal joint of right thumb
- [7th] S63.115 Dislocation of metacarpophalangeal joint of left thumb
- [7th] S63.116 Dislocation of metacarpophalangeal joint of unspecified thumb

[6th] **S63.12 Subluxation and dislocation of unspecified interphalangeal joint of thumb**

- [7th] S63.121 Subluxation of unspecified interphalangeal joint of right thumb
- [7th] S63.122 Subluxation of unspecified interphalangeal joint of left thumb
- [7th] S63.123 Subluxation of unspecified interphalangeal joint of unspecified thumb
- [7th] S63.124 Dislocation of unspecified interphalangeal joint of right thumb
- [7th] S63.125 Dislocation of unspecified interphalangeal joint of left thumb
- [7th] S63.126 Dislocation of unspecified interphalangeal joint of unspecified thumb

[6th] **S63.13 Subluxation and dislocation of proximal interphalangeal joint of thumb**

- [7th] S63.131 Subluxation of proximal interphalangeal joint of right thumb
- [7th] S63.132 Subluxation of proximal interphalangeal joint of left thumb
- [7th] S63.133 Subluxation of proximal interphalangeal joint of unspecified thumb
- [7th] S63.134 Dislocation of proximal interphalangeal joint of right thumb
- [7th] S63.135 Dislocation of proximal interphalangeal joint of left thumb
- [7th] S63.136 Dislocation of proximal interphalangeal joint of unspecified thumb

[6th] **S63.14 Subluxation and dislocation of distal interphalangeal joint of thumb**

- [7th] S63.141 Subluxation of distal interphalangeal joint of right thumb
- [7th] S63.142 Subluxation of distal interphalangeal joint of left thumb
- [7th] S63.143 Subluxation of distal interphalangeal joint of unspecified thumb
- [7th] S63.144 Dislocation of distal interphalangeal joint of right thumb
- [7th] S63.145 Dislocation of distal interphalangeal joint of left thumb
- [7th] S63.146 Dislocation of distal interphalangeal joint of unspecified thumb

[5th] **S63.2 Subluxation and dislocation of other finger(s)**

[EXCLUDES2] *subluxation and dislocation of thumb (S63.1-)*

[6th] **S63.20 Unspecified subluxation of other finger**

- [7th] S63.200 Unspecified subluxation of right index finger
- [7th] S63.201 Unspecified subluxation of left index finger
- [7th] S63.202 Unspecified subluxation of right middle finger
- [7th] S63.203 Unspecified subluxation of left middle finger
- [7th] S63.204 Unspecified subluxation of right ring finger
- [7th] S63.205 Unspecified subluxation of left ring finger
- [7th] S63.206 Unspecified subluxation of right little finger
- [7th] S63.207 Unspecified subluxation of left little finger
- [7th] S63.208 Unspecified subluxation of other finger
  Unspecified subluxation of specified finger with unspecified laterality

Unspecified Code | Other Specified Code | [N] Newborn Age: 0 | [P] Pediatric Age: 0-17 | [M] Maternity Age: 12-55
[A] Adult Age: 15-124 | ♂ Male | ♀ Female | ● New Code | ▲ Revised Code Title | ►◄ Revised Text

7ᵗʰ **S63.209** Unspecified subluxation of unspecified finger

6ᵗʰ **S63.21** Subluxation of metacarpophalangeal joint of finger

7ᵗʰ **S63.210** Subluxation of metacarpophalangeal joint of right index finger

7ᵗʰ **S63.211** Subluxation of metacarpophalangeal joint of left index finger

7ᵗʰ **S63.212** Subluxation of metacarpophalangeal joint of right middle finger

7ᵗʰ **S63.213** Subluxation of metacarpophalangeal joint of left middle finger

7ᵗʰ **S63.214** Subluxation of metacarpophalangeal joint of right ring finger

7ᵗʰ **S63.215** Subluxation of metacarpophalangeal joint of left ring finger

7ᵗʰ **S63.216** Subluxation of metacarpophalangeal joint of right little finger

7ᵗʰ **S63.217** Subluxation of metacarpophalangeal joint of left little finger

7ᵗʰ **S63.218** Subluxation of metacarpophalangeal joint of other finger

Subluxation of metacarpophalangeal joint of specified finger with unspecified laterality

7ᵗʰ **S63.219** Subluxation of metacarpophalangeal joint of unspecified finger

6ᵗʰ **S63.22** Subluxation of unspecified interphalangeal joint of finger

7ᵗʰ **S63.220** Subluxation of unspecified interphalangeal joint of right index finger

7ᵗʰ **S63.221** Subluxation of unspecified interphalangeal joint of left index finger

7ᵗʰ **S63.222** Subluxation of unspecified interphalangeal joint of right middle finger

7ᵗʰ **S63.223** Subluxation of unspecified interphalangeal joint of left middle finger

7ᵗʰ **S63.224** Subluxation of unspecified interphalangeal joint of right ring finger

7ᵗʰ **S63.225** Subluxation of unspecified interphalangeal joint of left ring finger

7ᵗʰ **S63.226** Subluxation of unspecified interphalangeal joint of right little finger

7ᵗʰ **S63.227** Subluxation of unspecified interphalangeal joint of left little finger

7ᵗʰ **S63.228** Subluxation of unspecified interphalangeal joint of other finger

Subluxation of unspecified interphalangeal joint of specified finger with unspecified laterality

7ᵗʰ **S63.229** Subluxation of unspecified interphalangeal joint of unspecified finger

6ᵗʰ **S63.23** Subluxation of proximal interphalangeal joint of finger

7ᵗʰ **S63.230** Subluxation of proximal interphalangeal joint of right index finger

7ᵗʰ **S63.231** Subluxation of proximal interphalangeal joint of left index finger

7ᵗʰ **S63.232** Subluxation of proximal interphalangeal joint of right middle finger

7ᵗʰ **S63.233** Subluxation of proximal interphalangeal joint of left middle finger

7ᵗʰ **S63.234** Subluxation of proximal interphalangeal joint of right ring finger

7ᵗʰ **S63.235** Subluxation of proximal interphalangeal joint of left ring finger

7ᵗʰ **S63.236** Subluxation of proximal interphalangeal joint of right little finger

7ᵗʰ **S63.237** Subluxation of proximal interphalangeal joint of left little finger

7ᵗʰ **S63.238** Subluxation of proximal interphalangeal joint of other finger

Subluxation of proximal interphalangeal joint of specified finger with unspecified laterality

7ᵗʰ **S63.239** Subluxation of proximal interphalangeal joint of unspecified finger

6ᵗʰ **S63.24** Subluxation of distal interphalangeal joint of finger

7ᵗʰ **S63.240** Subluxation of distal interphalangeal joint of right index finger

7ᵗʰ **S63.241** Subluxation of distal interphalangeal joint of left index finger

7ᵗʰ **S63.242** Subluxation of distal interphalangeal joint of right middle finger

7ᵗʰ **S63.243** Subluxation of distal interphalangeal joint of left middle finger

7ᵗʰ **S63.244** Subluxation of distal interphalangeal joint of right ring finger

7ᵗʰ **S63.245** Subluxation of distal interphalangeal joint of left ring finger

7ᵗʰ **S63.246** Subluxation of distal interphalangeal joint of right little finger

7ᵗʰ **S63.247** Subluxation of distal interphalangeal joint of left little finger

7ᵗʰ **S63.248** Subluxation of distal interphalangeal joint of other finger

Subluxation of distal interphalangeal joint of specified finger with unspecified laterality

7ᵗʰ **S63.249** Subluxation of distal interphalangeal joint of unspecified finger

6ᵗʰ **S63.25** Unspecified dislocation of other finger

7ᵗʰ **S63.250** Unspecified dislocation of right index finger

7ᵗʰ **S63.251** Unspecified dislocation of left index finger

7ᵗʰ **S63.252** Unspecified dislocation of right middle finger

7ᵗʰ **S63.253** Unspecified dislocation of left middle finger

7ᵗʰ **S63.254** Unspecified dislocation of right ring finger

7ᵗʰ **S63.255** Unspecified dislocation of left ring finger

7ᵗʰ **S63.256** Unspecified dislocation of right little finger

7ᵗʰ **S63.257** Unspecified dislocation of left little finger

7ᵗʰ **S63.258** Unspecified dislocation of other finger

Unspecified dislocation of specified finger with unspecified laterality

7ᵗʰ **S63.259** Unspecified dislocation of unspecified finger

Unspecified dislocation of specified finger with unspecified laterality

6ᵗʰ **S63.26** Dislocation of metacarpophalangeal joint of finger

7ᵗʰ **S63.260** Dislocation of metacarpophalangeal joint of right index finger

7ᵗʰ **S63.261** Dislocation of metacarpophalangeal joint of left index finger

7ᵗʰ **S63.262** Dislocation of metacarpophalangeal joint of right middle finger

7ᵗʰ **S63.263** Dislocation of metacarpophalangeal joint of left middle finger

7ᵗʰ **S63.264** Dislocation of metacarpophalangeal joint of right ring finger

7ᵗʰ **S63.265** Dislocation of metacarpophalangeal joint of left ring finger

7ᵗʰ **S63.266** Dislocation of metacarpophalangeal joint of right little finger

7ᵗʰ **S63.267** Dislocation of metacarpophalangeal joint of left little finger

7ᵗʰ **S63.268** Dislocation of metacarpophalangeal joint of other finger

Dislocation of metacarpophalangeal joint of specified finger with unspecified laterality

---

4ᵗʰ 4ᵗʰ character required   5ᵗʰ 5ᵗʰ character required   6ᵗʰ 6ᵗʰ character required   7ᵗʰ 7ᵗʰ character required   7ˣ Extension 'X' Alert

EXCLUDES 1 Not coded here   **EXCLUDES 2** Not included here   PDx Primary Diagnosis Only   Manifestation Code

[7th] S63.045 Dislocation of carpometacarpal joint of left thumb
[7th] S63.046 Dislocation of carpometacarpal joint of unspecified thumb
[6th] S63.05 Subluxation and dislocation of other carpometacarpal joint
EXCLUDES2 *subluxation and dislocation of carpometacarpal joint of thumb (S63.04-)*
[7th] S63.051 Subluxation of other carpometacarpal joint of right hand
[7th] S63.052 Subluxation of other carpometacarpal joint of left hand
[7th] S63.053 Subluxation of other carpometacarpal joint of unspecified hand
[7th] S63.054 Dislocation of other carpometacarpal joint of right hand
[7th] S63.055 Dislocation of other carpometacarpal joint of left hand
[7th] S63.056 Dislocation of other carpometacarpal joint of unspecified hand
[6th] S63.06 Subluxation and dislocation of metacarpal (bone), proximal end
[7th] S63.061 Subluxation of metacarpal (bone), proximal end of right hand
[7th] S63.062 Subluxation of metacarpal (bone), proximal end of left hand
[7th] S63.063 Subluxation of metacarpal (bone), proximal end of unspecified hand
[7th] S63.064 Dislocation of metacarpal (bone), proximal end of right hand
[7th] S63.065 Dislocation of metacarpal (bone), proximal end of left hand
[7th] S63.066 Dislocation of metacarpal (bone), proximal end of unspecified hand
[6th] S63.07 Subluxation and dislocation of distal end of ulna
[7th] S63.071 Subluxation of distal end of right ulna
[7th] S63.072 Subluxation of distal end of left ulna
[7th] S63.073 Subluxation of distal end of unspecified ulna
[7th] S63.074 Dislocation of distal end of right ulna
[7th] S63.075 Dislocation of distal end of left ulna
[7th] S63.076 Dislocation of distal end of unspecified ulna
[6th] S63.09 Other subluxation and dislocation of wrist and hand
[7th] S63.091 Other subluxation of right wrist and hand
[7th] S63.092 Other subluxation of left wrist and hand
[7th] S63.093 Other subluxation of unspecified wrist and hand
[7th] S63.094 Other dislocation of right wrist and hand
[7th] S63.095 Other dislocation of left wrist and hand
[7th] S63.096 Other dislocation of unspecified wrist and hand
[5th] S63.1 Subluxation and dislocation of thumb
[6th] S63.10 Unspecified subluxation and dislocation of thumb
[7th] S63.101 Unspecified subluxation of right thumb
[7th] S63.102 Unspecified subluxation of left thumb
[7th] S63.103 Unspecified subluxation of unspecified thumb
[7th] S63.104 Unspecified dislocation of right thumb
[7th] S63.105 Unspecified dislocation of left thumb
[7th] S63.106 Unspecified dislocation of unspecified thumb
[6th] S63.11 Subluxation and dislocation of metacarpophalangeal joint of thumb
[7th] S63.111 Subluxation of metacarpophalangeal joint of right thumb
[7th] S63.112 Subluxation of metacarpophalangeal joint of left thumb
[7th] S63.113 Subluxation of metacarpophalangeal joint of unspecified thumb
[7th] S63.114 Dislocation of metacarpophalangeal joint of right thumb
[7th] S63.115 Dislocation of metacarpophalangeal joint of left thumb
[7th] S63.116 Dislocation of metacarpophalangeal joint of unspecified thumb
[6th] S63.12 Subluxation and dislocation of unspecified interphalangeal joint of thumb
[7th] S63.121 Subluxation of unspecified interphalangeal joint of right thumb
[7th] S63.122 Subluxation of unspecified interphalangeal joint of left thumb
[7th] S63.123 Subluxation of unspecified interphalangeal joint of unspecified thumb
[7th] S63.124 Dislocation of unspecified interphalangeal joint of right thumb
[7th] S63.125 Dislocation of unspecified interphalangeal joint of left thumb
[7th] S63.126 Dislocation of unspecified interphalangeal joint of unspecified thumb
[6th] S63.13 Subluxation and dislocation of proximal interphalangeal joint of thumb
[7th] S63.131 Subluxation of proximal interphalangeal joint of right thumb
[7th] S63.132 Subluxation of proximal interphalangeal joint of left thumb
[7th] S63.133 Subluxation of proximal interphalangeal joint of unspecified thumb
[7th] S63.134 Dislocation of proximal interphalangeal joint of right thumb
[7th] S63.135 Dislocation of proximal interphalangeal joint of left thumb
[7th] S63.136 Dislocation of proximal interphalangeal joint of unspecified thumb
[6th] S63.14 Subluxation and dislocation of distal interphalangeal joint of thumb
[7th] S63.141 Subluxation of distal interphalangeal joint of right thumb
[7th] S63.142 Subluxation of distal interphalangeal joint of left thumb
[7th] S63.143 Subluxation of distal interphalangeal joint of unspecified thumb
[7th] S63.144 Dislocation of distal interphalangeal joint of right thumb
[7th] S63.145 Dislocation of distal interphalangeal joint of left thumb
[7th] S63.146 Dislocation of distal interphalangeal joint of unspecified thumb
[5th] S63.2 Subluxation and dislocation of other finger(s)
EXCLUDES2 *subluxation and dislocation of thumb (S63.1-)*
[6th] S63.20 Unspecified subluxation of other finger
[7th] S63.200 Unspecified subluxation of right index finger
[7th] S63.201 Unspecified subluxation of left index finger
[7th] S63.202 Unspecified subluxation of right middle finger
[7th] S63.203 Unspecified subluxation of left middle finger
[7th] S63.204 Unspecified subluxation of right ring finger
[7th] S63.205 Unspecified subluxation of left ring finger
[7th] S63.206 Unspecified subluxation of right little finger
[7th] S63.207 Unspecified subluxation of left little finger
[7th] S63.208 Unspecified subluxation of other finger
Unspecified subluxation of specified finger with unspecified laterality

Unspecified Code | Other Specified Code | [N] Newborn Age: 0 | [P] Pediatric Age: 0-17 | [M] Maternity Age: 12-55
[A] Adult Age: 15-124 | ♂ Male | ♀ Female | ● New Code | ▲ Revised Code Title | ►◄ Revised Text

[7th] S63.209 **Unspecified subluxation of unspecified finger**

[6th] S63.21 **Subluxation of metacarpophalangeal joint of finger**

[7th] S63.210 **Subluxation of metacarpophalangeal joint of right index finger**

[7th] S63.211 **Subluxation of metacarpophalangeal joint of left index finger**

[7th] S63.212 **Subluxation of metacarpophalangeal joint of right middle finger**

[7th] S63.213 **Subluxation of metacarpophalangeal joint of left middle finger**

[7th] S63.214 **Subluxation of metacarpophalangeal joint of right ring finger**

[7th] S63.215 **Subluxation of metacarpophalangeal joint of left ring finger**

[7th] S63.216 **Subluxation of metacarpophalangeal joint of right little finger**

[7th] S63.217 **Subluxation of metacarpophalangeal joint of left little finger**

[7th] S63.218 **Subluxation of metacarpophalangeal joint of other finger**
Subluxation of metacarpophalangeal joint of specified finger with unspecified laterality

[7th] S63.219 **Subluxation of metacarpophalangeal joint of unspecified finger**

[6th] S63.22 **Subluxation of unspecified interphalangeal joint of finger**

[7th] S63.220 **Subluxation of unspecified interphalangeal joint of right index finger**

[7th] S63.221 **Subluxation of unspecified interphalangeal joint of left index finger**

[7th] S63.222 **Subluxation of unspecified interphalangeal joint of right middle finger**

[7th] S63.223 **Subluxation of unspecified interphalangeal joint of left middle finger**

[7th] S63.224 **Subluxation of unspecified interphalangeal joint of right ring finger**

[7th] S63.225 **Subluxation of unspecified interphalangeal joint of left ring finger**

[7th] S63.226 **Subluxation of unspecified interphalangeal joint of right little finger**

[7th] S63.227 **Subluxation of unspecified interphalangeal joint of left little finger**

[7th] S63.228 **Subluxation of unspecified interphalangeal joint of other finger**
Subluxation of unspecified interphalangeal joint of specified finger with unspecified laterality

[7th] S63.229 **Subluxation of unspecified interphalangeal joint of unspecified finger**

[6th] S63.23 **Subluxation of proximal interphalangeal joint of finger**

[7th] S63.230 **Subluxation of proximal interphalangeal joint of right index finger**

[7th] S63.231 **Subluxation of proximal interphalangeal joint of left index finger**

[7th] S63.232 **Subluxation of proximal interphalangeal joint of right middle finger**

[7th] S63.233 **Subluxation of proximal interphalangeal joint of left middle finger**

[7th] S63.234 **Subluxation of proximal interphalangeal joint of right ring finger**

[7th] S63.235 **Subluxation of proximal interphalangeal joint of left ring finger**

[7th] S63.236 **Subluxation of proximal interphalangeal joint of right little finger**

[7th] S63.237 **Subluxation of proximal interphalangeal joint of left little finger**

[7th] S63.238 **Subluxation of proximal interphalangeal joint of other finger**
Subluxation of proximal interphalangeal joint of specified finger with unspecified laterality

[7th] S63.239 **Subluxation of proximal interphalangeal joint of unspecified finger**

[6th] S63.24 **Subluxation of distal interphalangeal joint of finger**

[7th] S63.240 **Subluxation of distal interphalangeal joint of right index finger**

[7th] S63.241 **Subluxation of distal interphalangeal joint of left index finger**

[7th] S63.242 **Subluxation of distal interphalangeal joint of right middle finger**

[7th] S63.243 **Subluxation of distal interphalangeal joint of left middle finger**

[7th] S63.244 **Subluxation of distal interphalangeal joint of right ring finger**

[7th] S63.245 **Subluxation of distal interphalangeal joint of left ring finger**

[7th] S63.246 **Subluxation of distal interphalangeal joint of right little finger**

[7th] S63.247 **Subluxation of distal interphalangeal joint of left little finger**

[7th] S63.248 **Subluxation of distal interphalangeal joint of other finger**
Subluxation of distal interphalangeal joint of specified finger with unspecified laterality

[7th] S63.249 **Subluxation of distal interphalangeal joint of unspecified finger**

[6th] S63.25 **Unspecified dislocation of other finger**

[7th] S63.250 **Unspecified dislocation of right index finger**

[7th] S63.251 **Unspecified dislocation of left index finger**

[7th] S63.252 **Unspecified dislocation of right middle finger**

[7th] S63.253 **Unspecified dislocation of left middle finger**

[7th] S63.254 **Unspecified dislocation of right ring finger**

[7th] S63.255 **Unspecified dislocation of left ring finger**

[7th] S63.256 **Unspecified dislocation of right little finger**

[7th] S63.257 **Unspecified dislocation of left little finger**

[7th] S63.258 **Unspecified dislocation of other finger**
Unspecified dislocation of specified finger with unspecified laterality

[7th] S63.259 **Unspecified dislocation of unspecified finger**
Unspecified dislocation of specified finger with unspecified laterality

[6th] S63.26 **Dislocation of metacarpophalangeal joint of finger**

[7th] S63.260 **Dislocation of metacarpophalangeal joint of right index finger**

[7th] S63.261 **Dislocation of metacarpophalangeal joint of left index finger**

[7th] S63.262 **Dislocation of metacarpophalangeal joint of right middle finger**

[7th] S63.263 **Dislocation of metacarpophalangeal joint of left middle finger**

[7th] S63.264 **Dislocation of metacarpophalangeal joint of right ring finger**

[7th] S63.265 **Dislocation of metacarpophalangeal joint of left ring finger**

[7th] S63.266 **Dislocation of metacarpophalangeal joint of right little finger**

[7th] S63.267 **Dislocation of metacarpophalangeal joint of left little finger**

[7th] S63.268 **Dislocation of metacarpophalangeal joint of other finger**
Dislocation of metacarpophalangeal joint of specified finger with unspecified laterality

S63.269 Dislocation of metacarpophalangeal joint of unspecified finger

S63.27 Dislocation of unspecified interphalangeal joint of finger

S63.270 Dislocation of unspecified interphalangeal joint of right index finger

S63.271 Dislocation of unspecified interphalangeal joint of left index finger

S63.272 Dislocation of unspecified interphalangeal joint of right middle finger

S63.273 Dislocation of unspecified interphalangeal joint of left middle finger

S63.274 Dislocation of unspecified interphalangeal joint of right ring finger

S63.275 Dislocation of unspecified interphalangeal joint of left ring finger

S63.276 Dislocation of unspecified interphalangeal joint of right little finger

S63.277 Dislocation of unspecified interphalangeal joint of left little finger

S63.278 Dislocation of unspecified interphalangeal joint of other finger

Dislocation of unspecified interphalangeal joint of specified finger with unspecified laterality

S63.279 Dislocation of unspecified interphalangeal joint of unspecified finger

Dislocation of unspecified interphalangeal joint of specified finger without specified laterality

S63.28 Dislocation of proximal interphalangeal joint of finger

S63.280 Dislocation of proximal interphalangeal joint of right index finger

S63.281 Dislocation of proximal interphalangeal joint of left index finger

S63.282 Dislocation of proximal interphalangeal joint of right middle finger

S63.283 Dislocation of proximal interphalangeal joint of left middle finger

S63.284 Dislocation of proximal interphalangeal joint of right ring finger

S63.285 Dislocation of proximal interphalangeal joint of left ring finger

S63.286 Dislocation of proximal interphalangeal joint of right little finger

S63.287 Dislocation of proximal interphalangeal joint of left little finger

S63.288 Dislocation of proximal interphalangeal joint of other finger

Dislocation of proximal interphalangeal joint of specified finger with unspecified laterality

S63.289 Dislocation of proximal interphalangeal joint of unspecified finger

S63.29 Dislocation of distal interphalangeal joint of finger

S63.290 Dislocation of distal interphalangeal joint of right index finger

S63.291 Dislocation of distal interphalangeal joint of left index finger

S63.292 Dislocation of distal interphalangeal joint of right middle finger

S63.293 Dislocation of distal interphalangeal joint of left middle finger

S63.294 Dislocation of distal interphalangeal joint of right ring finger

S63.295 Dislocation of distal interphalangeal joint of left ring finger

S63.296 Dislocation of distal interphalangeal joint of right little finger

S63.297 Dislocation of distal interphalangeal joint of left little finger

S63.298 Dislocation of distal interphalangeal joint of other finger

Dislocation of distal interphalangeal joint of specified finger with unspecified laterality

S63.299 Dislocation of distal interphalangeal joint of unspecified finger

S63.3 Traumatic rupture of ligament of wrist

S63.30 Traumatic rupture of unspecified ligament of wrist

S63.301 Traumatic rupture of unspecified ligament of right wrist

S63.302 Traumatic rupture of unspecified ligament of left wrist

S63.309 Traumatic rupture of unspecified ligament of unspecified wrist

S63.31 Traumatic rupture of collateral ligament of wrist

S63.311 Traumatic rupture of collateral ligament of right wrist

S63.312 Traumatic rupture of collateral ligament of left wrist

S63.319 Traumatic rupture of collateral ligament of unspecified wrist

S63.32 Traumatic rupture of radiocarpal ligament

S63.321 Traumatic rupture of right radiocarpal ligament

S63.322 Traumatic rupture of left radiocarpal ligament

S63.329 Traumatic rupture of unspecified radiocarpal ligament

S63.33 Traumatic rupture of ulnocarpal (palmar) ligament

S63.331 Traumatic rupture of right ulnocarpal (palmar) ligament

S63.332 Traumatic rupture of left ulnocarpal (palmar) ligament

S63.339 Traumatic rupture of unspecified ulnocarpal (palmar) ligament

S63.39 Traumatic rupture of other ligament of wrist

S63.391 Traumatic rupture of other ligament of right wrist

S63.392 Traumatic rupture of other ligament of left wrist

S63.399 Traumatic rupture of other ligament of unspecified wrist

S63.4 Traumatic rupture of ligament of finger at metacarpophalangeal and interphalangeal joint(s)

S63.40 Traumatic rupture of unspecified ligament of finger at metacarpophalangeal and interphalangeal joint

S63.400 Traumatic rupture of unspecified ligament of right index finger at metacarpophalangeal and interphalangeal joint

S63.401 Traumatic rupture of unspecified ligament of left index finger at metacarpophalangeal and interphalangeal joint

S63.402 Traumatic rupture of unspecified ligament of right middle finger at metacarpophalangeal and interphalangeal joint

S63.403 Traumatic rupture of unspecified ligament of left middle finger at metacarpophalangeal and interphalangeal joint

7️⃣ **S63.404** Traumatic rupture of unspecified ligament of right ring finger at metacarpophalangeal and interphalangeal joint

7️⃣ **S63.405** Traumatic rupture of unspecified ligament of left ring finger at metacarpophalangeal and interphalangeal joint

7️⃣ **S63.406** Traumatic rupture of unspecified ligament of right little finger at metacarpophalangeal and interphalangeal joint

7️⃣ **S63.407** Traumatic rupture of unspecified ligament of left little finger at metacarpophalangeal and interphalangeal joint

7️⃣ **S63.408** Traumatic rupture of unspecified ligament of other finger at metacarpophalangeal and interphalangeal joint

Traumatic rupture of unspecified ligament of specified finger with unspecified laterality at metacarpophalangeal and interphalangeal joint

7️⃣ **S63.409** Traumatic rupture of unspecified ligament of unspecified finger at metacarpophalangeal and interphalangeal joint

6️⃣ **S63.41** Traumatic rupture of collateral ligament of finger at metacarpophalangeal and interphalangeal joint

7️⃣ **S63.410** Traumatic rupture of collateral ligament of right index finger at metacarpophalangeal and interphalangeal joint

7️⃣ **S63.411** Traumatic rupture of collateral ligament of left index finger at metacarpophalangeal and interphalangeal joint

7️⃣ **S63.412** Traumatic rupture of collateral ligament of right middle finger at metacarpophalangeal and interphalangeal joint

7️⃣ **S63.413** Traumatic rupture of collateral ligament of left middle finger at metacarpophalangeal and interphalangeal joint

7️⃣ **S63.414** Traumatic rupture of collateral ligament of right ring finger at metacarpophalangeal and interphalangeal joint

7️⃣ **S63.415** Traumatic rupture of collateral ligament of left ring finger at metacarpophalangeal and interphalangeal joint

7️⃣ **S63.416** Traumatic rupture of collateral ligament of right little finger at metacarpophalangeal and interphalangeal joint

7️⃣ **S63.417** Traumatic rupture of collateral ligament of left little finger at metacarpophalangeal and interphalangeal joint

7️⃣ **S63.418** Traumatic rupture of collateral ligament of other finger at metacarpophalangeal and interphalangeal joint

Traumatic rupture of collateral ligament of specified finger with unspecified laterality at metacarpophalangeal and interphalangeal joint

7️⃣ **S63.419** Traumatic rupture of collateral ligament of unspecified finger at metacarpophalangeal and interphalangeal joint

6️⃣ **S63.42** Traumatic rupture of palmar ligament of finger at metacarpophalangeal and interphalangeal joint

7️⃣ **S63.420** Traumatic rupture of palmar ligament of right index finger at metacarpophalangeal and interphalangeal joint

7️⃣ **S63.421** Traumatic rupture of palmar ligament of left index finger at metacarpophalangeal and interphalangeal joint

7️⃣ **S63.422** Traumatic rupture of palmar ligament of right middle finger at metacarpophalangeal and interphalangeal joint

7️⃣ **S63.423** Traumatic rupture of palmar ligament of left middle finger at metacarpophalangeal and interphalangeal joint

7️⃣ **S63.424** Traumatic rupture of palmar ligament of right ring finger at metacarpophalangeal and interphalangeal joint

7️⃣ **S63.425** Traumatic rupture of palmar ligament of left ring finger at metacarpophalangeal and interphalangeal joint

7️⃣ **S63.426** Traumatic rupture of palmar ligament of right little finger at metacarpophalangeal and interphalangeal joint

7️⃣ **S63.427** Traumatic rupture of palmar ligament of left little finger at metacarpophalangeal and interphalangeal joint

7️⃣ **S63.428** Traumatic rupture of palmar ligament of other finger at metacarpophalangeal and interphalangeal joint

Traumatic rupture of palmar ligament of specified finger with unspecified laterality at metacarpophalangeal and interphalangeal joint

7️⃣ **S63.429** Traumatic rupture of palmar ligament of unspecified finger at metacarpophalangeal and interphalangeal joint

6️⃣ **S63.43** Traumatic rupture of volar plate of finger at metacarpophalangeal and interphalangeal joint

7️⃣ **S63.430** Traumatic rupture of volar plate of right index finger at metacarpophalangeal and interphalangeal joint

7️⃣ **S63.431** Traumatic rupture of volar plate of left index finger at metacarpophalangeal and interphalangeal joint

7️⃣ **S63.432** Traumatic rupture of volar plate of right middle finger at metacarpophalangeal and interphalangeal joint

7️⃣ **S63.433** Traumatic rupture of volar plate of left middle finger at metacarpophalangeal and interphalangeal joint

7️⃣ **S63.434** Traumatic rupture of volar plate of right ring finger at metacarpophalangeal and interphalangeal joint

7️⃣ **S63.435** Traumatic rupture of volar plate of left ring finger at metacarpophalangeal and interphalangeal joint

7️⃣ **S63.436** Traumatic rupture of volar plate of right little finger at metacarpophalangeal and interphalangeal joint

7️⃣ **S63.437** Traumatic rupture of volar plate of left little finger at metacarpophalangeal and interphalangeal joint

7️⃣ **S63.438** Traumatic rupture of volar plate of other finger at metacarpophalangeal and interphalangeal joint

Traumatic rupture of volar plate of specified finger with unspecified laterality at metacarpophalangeal and interphalangeal joint

7️⃣ **S63.439** Traumatic rupture of volar plate of unspecified finger at metacarpophalangeal and interphalangeal joint

6️⃣ **S63.49** Traumatic rupture of other ligament of finger at metacarpophalangeal and interphalangeal joint

7️⃣ **S63.490** Traumatic rupture of other ligament of right index finger at metacarpophalangeal and interphalangeal joint

7️⃣ **S63.491** Traumatic rupture of other ligament of left index finger at metacarpophalangeal and interphalangeal joint

---

4️⃣ 4ᵗʰ character required 5️⃣ 5ᵗʰ character required 6️⃣ 6ᵗʰ character required 7️⃣ 7ᵗʰ character required Extension 'X' Alert

EXCLUDES 1 Not coded here EXCLUDES 2 Not included here PDx Primary Diagnosis Only Manifestation Code

[7th] S63.492 Traumatic rupture of other ligament of right middle finger at metacarpophalangeal and interphalangeal joint
[7th] S63.493 Traumatic rupture of other ligament of left middle finger at metacarpophalangeal and interphalangeal joint
[7th] S63.494 Traumatic rupture of other ligament of right ring finger at metacarpophalangeal and interphalangeal joint
[7th] S63.495 Traumatic rupture of other ligament of left ring finger at metacarpophalangeal and interphalangeal joint
[7th] S63.496 Traumatic rupture of other ligament of right little finger at metacarpophalangeal and interphalangeal joint
[7th] S63.497 Traumatic rupture of other ligament of left little finger at metacarpophalangeal and interphalangeal joint
[7th] S63.498 Traumatic rupture of other ligament of other finger at metacarpophalangeal and interphalangeal joint
Traumatic rupture of ligament of specified finger with unspecified laterality at metacarpophalangeal and interphalangeal joint
[7th] S63.499 Traumatic rupture of other ligament of unspecified finger at metacarpophalangeal and interphalangeal joint

[5th] S63.5 Other and unspecified sprain of wrist
[6th] S63.50 Unspecified sprain of wrist
[7th] S63.501 Unspecified sprain of right wrist
[7th] S63.502 Unspecified sprain of left wrist
[7th] S63.509 Unspecified sprain of unspecified wrist
[6th] S63.51 Sprain of carpal (joint)
[7th] S63.511 Sprain of carpal joint of right wrist
[7th] S63.512 Sprain of carpal joint of left wrist
[7th] S63.519 Sprain of carpal joint of unspecified wrist
[6th] S63.52 Sprain of radiocarpal joint
[EXCLUDES1] *traumatic rupture of radiocarpal ligament (S63.32-)*
[7th] S63.521 Sprain of radiocarpal joint of right wrist
[7th] S63.522 Sprain of radiocarpal joint of left wrist
[7th] S63.529 Sprain of radiocarpal joint of unspecified wrist
[6th] S63.59 Other specified sprain of wrist
[7th] S63.591 Other specified sprain of right wrist
[7th] S63.592 Other specified sprain of left wrist
[7th] S63.599 Other specified sprain of unspecified wrist

[5th] S63.6 Other and unspecified sprain of finger(s)
[EXCLUDES1] *traumatic rupture of ligament of finger at metacarpophalangeal and interphalangeal joint(s) (S63.4-)*
[6th] S63.60 Unspecified sprain of thumb
[7th] S63.601 Unspecified sprain of right thumb
[7th] S63.602 Unspecified sprain of left thumb
[7th] S63.609 Unspecified sprain of unspecified thumb
[6th] S63.61 Unspecified sprain of other and unspecified finger(s)
[7th] S63.610 Unspecified sprain of right index finger
[7th] S63.611 Unspecified sprain of left index finger
[7th] S63.612 Unspecified sprain of right middle finger
[7th] S63.613 Unspecified sprain of left middle finger
[7th] S63.614 Unspecified sprain of right ring finger
[7th] S63.615 Unspecified sprain of left ring finger
[7th] S63.616 Unspecified sprain of right little finger
[7th] S63.617 Unspecified sprain of left little finger
[7th] S63.618 Unspecified sprain of other finger
Unspecified sprain of specified finger with unspecified laterality
[7th] S63.619 Unspecified sprain of unspecified finger
[6th] S63.62 Sprain of interphalangeal joint of thumb
[7th] S63.621 Sprain of interphalangeal joint of right thumb
[7th] S63.622 Sprain of interphalangeal joint of left thumb
[7th] S63.629 Sprain of interphalangeal joint of unspecified thumb
[6th] S63.63 Sprain of interphalangeal joint of other and unspecified finger(s)
[7th] S63.630 Sprain of interphalangeal joint of right index finger
[7th] S63.631 Sprain of interphalangeal joint of left index finger
[7th] S63.632 Sprain of interphalangeal joint of right middle finger
[7th] S63.633 Sprain of interphalangeal joint of left middle finger
[7th] S63.634 Sprain of interphalangeal joint of right ring finger
[7th] S63.635 Sprain of interphalangeal joint of left ring finger
[7th] S63.636 Sprain of interphalangeal joint of right little finger
[7th] S63.637 Sprain of interphalangeal joint of left little finger
[7th] S63.638 Sprain of interphalangeal joint of other finger
[7th] S63.639 Sprain of interphalangeal joint of unspecified finger
[6th] S63.64 Sprain of metacarpophalangeal joint of thumb
[7th] S63.641 Sprain of metacarpophalangeal joint of right thumb
[7th] S63.642 Sprain of metacarpophalangeal joint of left thumb
[7th] S63.649 Sprain of metacarpophalangeal joint of unspecified thumb
[6th] S63.65 Sprain of metacarpophalangeal joint of other and unspecified finger(s)
[7th] S63.650 Sprain of metacarpophalangeal joint of right index finger
[7th] S63.651 Sprain of metacarpophalangeal joint of left index finger
[7th] S63.652 Sprain of metacarpophalangeal joint of right middle finger
[7th] S63.653 Sprain of metacarpophalangeal joint of left middle finger
[7th] S63.654 Sprain of metacarpophalangeal joint of right ring finger
[7th] S63.655 Sprain of metacarpophalangeal joint of left ring finger
[7th] S63.656 Sprain of metacarpophalangeal joint of right little finger
[7th] S63.657 Sprain of metacarpophalangeal joint of left little finger
[7th] S63.658 Sprain of metacarpophalangeal joint of other finger
Sprain of metacarpophalangeal joint of specified finger with unspecified laterality
[7th] S63.659 Sprain of metacarpophalangeal joint of unspecified finger
[6th] S63.68 Other sprain of thumb
[7th] S63.681 Other sprain of right thumb
[7th] S63.682 Other sprain of left thumb
[7th] S63.689 Other sprain of unspecified thumb
[6th] S63.69 Other sprain of other and unspecified finger(s)
[7th] S63.690 Other sprain of right index finger
[7th] S63.691 Other sprain of left index finger
[7th] S63.692 Other sprain of right middle finger
[7th] S63.693 Other sprain of left middle finger

Unspecified Code | Other Specified Code | [N] Newborn Age: 0 | [P] Pediatric Age: 0-17 | [M] Maternity Age: 12-55
[A] Adult Age: 15-124 | ♂ Male | ♀ Female | ● New Code | ▲ Revised Code Title | ►◄ Revised Text

S63.694 Other sprain of right ring finger
S63.695 Other sprain of left ring finger
S63.696 Other sprain of right little finger
S63.697 Other sprain of left little finger
S63.698 Other sprain of other finger
Other sprain of specified finger with unspecified laterality
S63.699 Other sprain of unspecified finger
S63.8 Sprain of other part of wrist and hand
S63.8X Sprain of other part of wrist and hand
S63.8X1 Sprain of other part of right wrist and hand
S63.8X2 Sprain of other part of left wrist and hand
S63.8X9 Sprain of other part of unspecified wrist and hand
S63.9 Sprain of unspecified part of wrist and hand
S63.90 Sprain of unspecified part of unspecified wrist and hand
S63.91 Sprain of unspecified part of right wrist and hand
S63.92 Sprain of unspecified part of left wrist and hand
S64 Injury of nerves at wrist and hand level
Code also any associated open wound (S61.-)
The appropriate 7th character is to be added to each code from category S64
A = initial encounter
D = subsequent encounter
S = sequela
S64.0 Injury of ulnar nerve at wrist and hand level
S64.00 Injury of ulnar nerve at wrist and hand level of unspecified arm
S64.01 Injury of ulnar nerve at wrist and hand level of right arm
S64.02 Injury of ulnar nerve at wrist and hand level of left arm
S64.1 Injury of median nerve at wrist and hand level
S64.10 Injury of median nerve at wrist and hand level of unspecified arm
S64.11 Injury of median nerve at wrist and hand level of right arm
S64.12 Injury of median nerve at wrist and hand level of left arm
S64.2 Injury of radial nerve at wrist and hand level
S64.20 Injury of radial nerve at wrist and hand level of unspecified arm
S64.21 Injury of radial nerve at wrist and hand level of right arm
S64.22 Injury of radial nerve at wrist and hand level of left arm
S64.3 Injury of digital nerve of thumb
S64.30 Injury of digital nerve of unspecified thumb
S64.31 Injury of digital nerve of right thumb
S64.32 Injury of digital nerve of left thumb
S64.4 Injury of digital nerve of other and unspecified finger
S64.40 Injury of digital nerve of unspecified finger
S64.49 Injury of digital nerve of other finger
S64.490 Injury of digital nerve of right index finger
S64.491 Injury of digital nerve of left index finger
S64.492 Injury of digital nerve of right middle finger
S64.493 Injury of digital nerve of left middle finger
S64.494 Injury of digital nerve of right ring finger
S64.495 Injury of digital nerve of left ring finger
S64.496 Injury of digital nerve of right little finger
S64.497 Injury of digital nerve of left little finger
S64.498 Injury of digital nerve of other finger
Injury of digital nerve of specified finger with unspecified laterality

S64.8 Injury of other nerves at wrist and hand level
S64.8X Injury of other nerves at wrist and hand level
S64.8X1 Injury of other nerves at wrist and hand level of right arm
S64.8X2 Injury of other nerves at wrist and hand level of left arm
S64.8X9 Injury of other nerves at wrist and hand level of unspecified arm
S64.9 Injury of unspecified nerve at wrist and hand level
S64.90 Injury of unspecified nerve at wrist and hand level of unspecified arm
S64.91 Injury of unspecified nerve at wrist and hand level of right arm
S64.92 Injury of unspecified nerve at wrist and hand level of left arm
S65 Injury of blood vessels at wrist and hand level
Code also any associated open wound (S61.-)
The appropriate 7th character is to be added to each code from category S65
A = initial encounter
D = subsequent encounter
S = sequela
S65.0 Injury of ulnar artery at wrist and hand level
S65.00 Unspecified injury of ulnar artery at wrist and hand level
S65.001 Unspecified injury of ulnar artery at wrist and hand level of right arm
S65.002 Unspecified injury of ulnar artery at wrist and hand level of left arm
S65.009 Unspecified injury of ulnar artery at wrist and hand level of unspecified arm
S65.01 Laceration of ulnar artery at wrist and hand level
S65.011 Laceration of ulnar artery at wrist and hand level of right arm
S65.012 Laceration of ulnar artery at wrist and hand level of left arm
S65.019 Laceration of ulnar artery at wrist and hand level of unspecified arm
S65.09 Other specified injury of ulnar artery at wrist and hand level
S65.091 Other specified injury of ulnar artery at wrist and hand level of right arm
S65.092 Other specified injury of ulnar artery at wrist and hand level of left arm
S65.099 Other specified injury of ulnar artery at wrist and hand level of unspecified arm
S65.1 Injury of radial artery at wrist and hand level
S65.10 Unspecified injury of radial artery at wrist and hand level
S65.101 Unspecified injury of radial artery at wrist and hand level of right arm
S65.102 Unspecified injury of radial artery at wrist and hand level of left arm
S65.109 Unspecified injury of radial artery at wrist and hand level of unspecified arm
S65.11 Laceration of radial artery at wrist and hand level
S65.111 Laceration of radial artery at wrist and hand level of right arm
S65.112 Laceration of radial artery at wrist and hand level of left arm
S65.119 Laceration of radial artery at wrist and hand level of unspecified arm
S65.19 Other specified injury of radial artery at wrist and hand level
S65.191 Other specified injury of radial artery at wrist and hand level of right arm
S65.192 Other specified injury of radial artery at wrist and hand level of left arm

④ 4th character required   ⑤ 5th character required   ⑥ 6th character required   ⑦ 7th character required   ⑦ˣ Extension 'X' Alert

EXCLUDES 1 Not coded here   EXCLUDES 2 Not included here   PDx Primary Diagnosis Only   Manifestation Code

618   ICD-10-CM 2015

7️⃣ S65.199 Other specified injury of radial artery at wrist and hand level of unspecified arm

5️⃣ S65.2 Injury of superficial palmar arch
 6️⃣ S65.20 Unspecified injury of superficial palmar arch
  7️⃣ S65.201 Unspecified injury of superficial palmar arch of right hand
  7️⃣ S65.202 Unspecified injury of superficial palmar arch of left hand
  7️⃣ S65.209 Unspecified injury of superficial palmar arch of unspecified hand
 6️⃣ S65.21 Laceration of superficial palmar arch
  7️⃣ S65.211 Laceration of superficial palmar arch of right hand
  7️⃣ S65.212 Laceration of superficial palmar arch of left hand
  7️⃣ S65.219 Laceration of superficial palmar arch of unspecified hand
 6️⃣ S65.29 Other specified injury of superficial palmar arch
  7️⃣ S65.291 Other specified injury of superficial palmar arch of right hand
  7️⃣ S65.292 Other specified injury of superficial palmar arch of left hand
  7️⃣ S65.299 Other specified injury of superficial palmar arch of unspecified hand

5️⃣ S65.3 Injury of deep palmar arch
 6️⃣ S65.30 Unspecified injury of deep palmar arch
  7️⃣ S65.301 Unspecified injury of deep palmar arch of right hand
  7️⃣ S65.302 Unspecified injury of deep palmar arch of left hand
  7️⃣ S65.309 Unspecified injury of deep palmar arch of unspecified hand
 6️⃣ S65.31 Laceration of deep palmar arch
  7️⃣ S65.311 Laceration of deep palmar arch of right hand
  7️⃣ S65.312 Laceration of deep palmar arch of left hand
  7️⃣ S65.319 Laceration of deep palmar arch of unspecified hand
 6️⃣ S65.39 Other specified injury of deep palmar arch
  7️⃣ S65.391 Other specified injury of deep palmar arch of right hand
  7️⃣ S65.392 Other specified injury of deep palmar arch of left hand
  7️⃣ S65.399 Other specified injury of deep palmar arch of unspecified hand

5️⃣ S65.4 Injury of blood vessel of thumb
 6️⃣ S65.40 Unspecified injury of blood vessel of thumb
  7️⃣ S65.401 Unspecified injury of blood vessel of right thumb
  7️⃣ S65.402 Unspecified injury of blood vessel of left thumb
  7️⃣ S65.409 Unspecified injury of blood vessel of unspecified thumb
 6️⃣ S65.41 Laceration of blood vessel of thumb
  7️⃣ S65.411 Laceration of blood vessel of right thumb
  7️⃣ S65.412 Laceration of blood vessel of left thumb
  7️⃣ S65.419 Laceration of blood vessel of unspecified thumb
 6️⃣ S65.49 Other specified injury of blood vessel of thumb
  7️⃣ S65.491 Other specified injury of blood vessel of right thumb
  7️⃣ S65.492 Other specified injury of blood vessel of left thumb
  7️⃣ S65.499 Other specified injury of blood vessel of unspecified thumb

5️⃣ S65.5 Injury of blood vessel of other and unspecified finger
 6️⃣ S65.50 Unspecified injury of blood vessel of other and unspecified finger

7️⃣ S65.500 Unspecified injury of blood vessel of right index finger
7️⃣ S65.501 Unspecified injury of blood vessel of left index finger
7️⃣ S65.502 Unspecified injury of blood vessel of right middle finger
7️⃣ S65.503 Unspecified injury of blood vessel of left middle finger
7️⃣ S65.504 Unspecified injury of blood vessel of right ring finger
7️⃣ S65.505 Unspecified injury of blood vessel of left ring finger
7️⃣ S65.506 Unspecified injury of blood vessel of right little finger
7️⃣ S65.507 Unspecified injury of blood vessel of left little finger
7️⃣ S65.508 Unspecified injury of blood vessel of other finger
    Unspecified injury of blood vessel of specified finger with unspecified laterality
7️⃣ S65.509 Unspecified injury of blood vessel of unspecified finger

6️⃣ S65.51 Laceration of blood vessel of other and unspecified finger
  7️⃣ S65.510 Laceration of blood vessel of right index finger
  7️⃣ S65.511 Laceration of blood vessel of left index finger
  7️⃣ S65.512 Laceration of blood vessel of right middle finger
  7️⃣ S65.513 Laceration of blood vessel of left middle finger
  7️⃣ S65.514 Laceration of blood vessel of right ring finger
  7️⃣ S65.515 Laceration of blood vessel of left ring finger
  7️⃣ S65.516 Laceration of blood vessel of right little finger
  7️⃣ S65.517 Laceration of blood vessel of left little finger
  7️⃣ S65.518 Laceration of blood vessel of other finger
    Laceration of blood vessel of specified finger with unspecified laterality
  7️⃣ S65.519 Laceration of blood vessel of unspecified finger

6️⃣ S65.59 Other specified injury of blood vessel of other and unspecified finger
  7️⃣ S65.590 Other specified injury of blood vessel of right index finger
  7️⃣ S65.591 Other specified injury of blood vessel of left index finger
  7️⃣ S65.592 Other specified injury of blood vessel of right middle finger
  7️⃣ S65.593 Other specified injury of blood vessel of left middle finger
  7️⃣ S65.594 Other specified injury of blood vessel of right ring finger
  7️⃣ S65.595 Other specified injury of blood vessel of left ring finger
  7️⃣ S65.596 Other specified injury of blood vessel of right little finger
  7️⃣ S65.597 Other specified injury of blood vessel of left little finger
  7️⃣ S65.598 Other specified injury of blood vessel of other finger
    Other specified injury of blood vessel of specified finger with unspecified laterality
  7️⃣ S65.599 Other specified injury of blood vessel of unspecified finger

5️⃣ S65.8 Injury of other blood vessels at wrist and hand level

| Unspecified Code | Other Specified Code | N Newborn Age: 0 | P Pediatric Age: 0-17 | W Maternity Age: 12-55 |
| A Adult Age: 15-124 | ♂ Male | ♀ Female | ● New Code | ▲ Revised Code Title | ►◄ Revised Text |

6ᵗʰ **S65.80** Unspecified injury of other blood vessels at wrist and hand level

    7ᵗʰ **S65.801** Unspecified injury of other blood vessels at wrist and hand level of right arm

    7ᵗʰ **S65.802** Unspecified injury of other blood vessels at wrist and hand level of left arm

    7ᵗʰ **S65.809** Unspecified injury of other blood vessels at wrist and hand level of unspecified arm

6ᵗʰ **S65.81** Laceration of other blood vessels at wrist and hand level

    7ᵗʰ **S65.811** Laceration of other blood vessels at wrist and hand level of right arm

    7ᵗʰ **S65.812** Laceration of other blood vessels at wrist and hand level of left arm

    7ᵗʰ **S65.819** Laceration of other blood vessels at wrist and hand level of unspecified arm

6ᵗʰ **S65.89** Other specified injury of other blood vessels at wrist and hand level

    7ᵗʰ **S65.891** Other specified injury of other blood vessels at wrist and hand level of right arm

    7ᵗʰ **S65.892** Other specified injury of other blood vessels at wrist and hand level of left arm

    7ᵗʰ **S65.899** Other specified injury of other blood vessels at wrist and hand level of unspecified arm

5ᵗʰ **S65.9** Injury of unspecified blood vessel at wrist and hand level

6ᵗʰ **S65.90** Unspecified injury of unspecified blood vessel at wrist and hand level

    7ᵗʰ **S65.901** Unspecified injury of unspecified blood vessel at wrist and hand level of right arm

    7ᵗʰ **S65.902** Unspecified injury of unspecified blood vessel at wrist and hand level of left arm

    7ᵗʰ **S65.909** Unspecified injury of unspecified blood vessel at wrist and hand level of unspecified arm

6ᵗʰ **S65.91** Laceration of unspecified blood vessel at wrist and hand level

    7ᵗʰ **S65.911** Laceration of unspecified blood vessel at wrist and hand level of right arm

    7ᵗʰ **S65.912** Laceration of unspecified blood vessel at wrist and hand level of left arm

    7ᵗʰ **S65.919** Laceration of unspecified blood vessel at wrist and hand level of unspecified arm

6ᵗʰ **S65.99** Other specified injury of unspecified blood vessel at wrist and hand level

    7ᵗʰ **S65.991** Other specified injury of unspecified blood vessel at wrist and hand of right arm

    7ᵗʰ **S65.992** Other specified injury of unspecified blood vessel at wrist and hand of left arm

    7ᵗʰ **S65.999** Other specified injury of unspecified blood vessel at wrist and hand of unspecified arm

4ᵗʰ **S66 Injury of muscle, fascia and tendon at wrist and hand level**

    Code also any associated open wound (S61.-)

    EXCLUDES2 sprain of joints and ligaments of wrist and hand (S63.-)

    The appropriate 7th character is to be added to each code from category S66
    A = initial encounter
    D = subsequent encounter
    S = sequela

5ᵗʰ **S66.0** Injury of long flexor muscle, fascia and tendon of thumb at wrist and hand level

6ᵗʰ **S66.00** Unspecified injury of long flexor muscle, fascia and tendon of thumb at wrist and hand level

    7ᵗʰ **S66.001** Unspecified injury of long flexor muscle, fascia and tendon of right thumb at wrist and hand level

    7ᵗʰ **S66.002** Unspecified injury of long flexor muscle, fascia and tendon of left thumb at wrist and hand level

    7ᵗʰ **S66.009** Unspecified injury of long flexor muscle, fascia and tendon of unspecified thumb at wrist and hand level

6ᵗʰ **S66.01** Strain of long flexor muscle, fascia and tendon of thumb at wrist and hand level

    7ᵗʰ **S66.011** Strain of long flexor muscle, fascia and tendon of right thumb at wrist and hand level

    7ᵗʰ **S66.012** Strain of long flexor muscle, fascia and tendon of left thumb at wrist and hand level

    7ᵗʰ **S66.019** Strain of long flexor muscle, fascia and tendon of unspecified thumb at wrist and hand level

6ᵗʰ **S66.02** Laceration of long flexor muscle, fascia and tendon of thumb at wrist and hand level

    7ᵗʰ **S66.021** Laceration of long flexor muscle, fascia and tendon of right thumb at wrist and hand level

    7ᵗʰ **S66.022** Laceration of long flexor muscle, fascia and tendon of left thumb at wrist and hand level

    7ᵗʰ **S66.029** Laceration of long flexor muscle, fascia and tendon of unspecified thumb at wrist and hand level

6ᵗʰ **S66.09** Other specified injury of long flexor muscle, fascia and tendon of thumb at wrist and hand level

    7ᵗʰ **S66.091** Other specified injury of long flexor muscle, fascia and tendon of right thumb at wrist and hand level

    7ᵗʰ **S66.092** Other specified injury of long flexor muscle, fascia and tendon of left thumb at wrist and hand level

    7ᵗʰ **S66.099** Other specified injury of long flexor muscle, fascia and tendon of unspecified thumb at wrist and hand level

5ᵗʰ **S66.1** Injury of flexor muscle, fascia and tendon of other and unspecified finger at wrist and hand level

    EXCLUDES2 Injury of long flexor muscle, fascia and tendon of thumb at wrist and hand level (S66.0-)

6ᵗʰ **S66.10** Unspecified injury of flexor muscle, fascia and tendon of other and unspecified finger at wrist and hand level

    7ᵗʰ **S66.100** Unspecified injury of flexor muscle, fascia and tendon of right index finger at wrist and hand level

    7ᵗʰ **S66.101** Unspecified injury of flexor muscle, fascia and tendon of left index finger at wrist and hand level

    7ᵗʰ **S66.102** Unspecified injury of flexor muscle, fascia and tendon of right middle finger at wrist and hand level

    7ᵗʰ **S66.103** Unspecified injury of flexor muscle, fascia and tendon of left middle finger at wrist and hand level

    7ᵗʰ **S66.104** Unspecified injury of flexor muscle, fascia and tendon of right ring finger at wrist and hand level

    7ᵗʰ **S66.105** Unspecified injury of flexor muscle, fascia and tendon of left ring finger at wrist and hand level

    7ᵗʰ **S66.106** Unspecified injury of flexor muscle, fascia and tendon of right little finger at wrist and hand level

    7ᵗʰ **S66.107** Unspecified injury of flexor muscle, fascia and tendon of left little finger at wrist and hand level

---

4ᵗʰ 4ᵗʰ character required   5ᵗʰ 5ᵗʰ character required   6ᵗʰ 6ᵗʰ character required   7ᵗʰ 7ᵗʰ character required   Extension 'X' Alert

EXCLUDES1 Not coded here   *EXCLUDES2* Not included here   PDx Primary Diagnosis Only   Manifestation Code

[7th] **S66.108 Unspecified injury of flexor muscle, fascia and tendon of other finger at wrist and hand level**

Unspecified injury of flexor muscle, fascia and tendon of specified finger with unspecified laterality at wrist and hand level

[7th] **S66.109 Unspecified injury of flexor muscle, fascia and tendon of unspecified finger at wrist and hand level**

[6th] **S66.11 Strain of flexor muscle, fascia and tendon of other and unspecified finger at wrist and hand level**

[7th] **S66.110 Strain of flexor muscle, fascia and tendon of right index finger at wrist and hand level**

[7th] **S66.111 Strain of flexor muscle, fascia and tendon of left index finger at wrist and hand level**

[7th] **S66.112 Strain of flexor muscle, fascia and tendon of right middle finger at wrist and hand level**

[7th] **S66.113 Strain of flexor muscle, fascia and tendon of left middle finger at wrist and hand level**

[7th] **S66.114 Strain of flexor muscle, fascia and tendon of right ring finger at wrist and hand level**

[7th] **S66.115 Strain of flexor muscle, fascia and tendon of left ring finger at wrist and hand level**

[7th] **S66.116 Strain of flexor muscle, fascia and tendon of right little finger at wrist and hand level**

[7th] **S66.117 Strain of flexor muscle, fascia and tendon of left little finger at wrist and hand level**

[7th] **S66.118 Strain of flexor muscle, fascia and tendon of other finger at wrist and hand level**

Strain of flexor muscle, fascia and tendon of specified finger with unspecified laterality at wrist and hand level

[7th] **S66.119 Strain of flexor muscle, fascia and tendon of unspecified finger at wrist and hand level**

[6th] **S66.12 Laceration of flexor muscle, fascia and tendon of other and unspecified finger at wrist and hand level**

[7th] **S66.120 Laceration of flexor muscle, fascia and tendon of right index finger at wrist and hand level**

[7th] **S66.121 Laceration of flexor muscle, fascia and tendon of left index finger at wrist and hand level**

[7th] **S66.122 Laceration of flexor muscle, fascia and tendon of right middle finger at wrist and hand level**

[7th] **S66.123 Laceration of flexor muscle, fascia and tendon of left middle finger at wrist and hand level**

[7th] **S66.124 Laceration of flexor muscle, fascia and tendon of right ring finger at wrist and hand level**

[7th] **S66.125 Laceration of flexor muscle, fascia and tendon of left ring finger at wrist and hand level**

[7th] **S66.126 Laceration of flexor muscle, fascia and tendon of right little finger at wrist and hand level**

[7th] **S66.127 Laceration of flexor muscle, fascia and tendon of left little finger at wrist and hand level**

[7th] **S66.128 Laceration of flexor muscle, fascia and tendon of other finger at wrist and hand level**

Laceration of flexor muscle, fascia and tendon of specified finger with unspecified laterality at wrist and hand level

[7th] **S66.129 Laceration of flexor muscle, fascia and tendon of unspecified finger at wrist and hand level**

[6th] **S66.19 Other injury of flexor muscle, fascia and tendon of other and unspecified finger at wrist and hand level**

[7th] **S66.190 Other injury of flexor muscle, fascia and tendon of right index finger at wrist and hand level**

[7th] **S66.191 Other injury of flexor muscle, fascia and tendon of left index finger at wrist and hand level**

[7th] **S66.192 Other injury of flexor muscle, fascia and tendon of right middle finger at wrist and hand level**

[7th] **S66.193 Other injury of flexor muscle, fascia and tendon of left middle finger at wrist and hand level**

[7th] **S66.194 Other injury of flexor muscle, fascia and tendon of right ring finger at wrist and hand level**

[7th] **S66.195 Other injury of flexor muscle, fascia and tendon of left ring finger at wrist and hand level**

[7th] **S66.196 Other injury of flexor muscle, fascia and tendon of right little finger at wrist and hand level**

[7th] **S66.197 Other injury of flexor muscle, fascia and tendon of left little finger at wrist and hand level**

[7th] **S66.198 Other injury of flexor muscle, fascia and tendon of other finger at wrist and hand level**

Other injury of flexor muscle, fascia and tendon of specified finger with unspecified laterality at wrist and hand level

[7th] **S66.199 Other injury of flexor muscle, fascia and tendon of unspecified finger at wrist and hand level**

[5th] **S66.2 Injury of extensor muscle, fascia and tendon of thumb at wrist and hand level**

[6th] **S66.20 Unspecified injury of extensor muscle, fascia and tendon of thumb at wrist and hand level**

[7th] **S66.201 Unspecified injury of extensor muscle, fascia and tendon of right thumb at wrist and hand level**

[7th] **S66.202 Unspecified injury of extensor muscle, fascia and tendon of left thumb at wrist and hand level**

[7th] **S66.209 Unspecified injury of extensor muscle, fascia and tendon of unspecified thumb at wrist and hand level**

[6th] **S66.21 Strain of extensor muscle, fascia and tendon of thumb at wrist and hand level**

[7th] **S66.211 Strain of extensor muscle, fascia and tendon of right thumb at wrist and hand level**

[7th] **S66.212 Strain of extensor muscle, fascia and tendon of left thumb at wrist and hand level**

[7th] **S66.219 Strain of extensor muscle, fascia and tendon of unspecified thumb at wrist and hand level**

[6th] **S66.22 Laceration of extensor muscle, fascia and tendon of thumb at wrist and hand level**

[7th] **S66.221 Laceration of extensor muscle, fascia and tendon of right thumb at wrist and hand level**

[7th] **S66.222 Laceration of extensor muscle, fascia and tendon of left thumb at wrist and hand level**

[7th] **S66.229 Laceration of extensor muscle, fascia and tendon of unspecified thumb at wrist and hand level**

[6th] **S66.29 Other specified injury of extensor muscle, fascia and tendon of thumb at wrist and hand level**

Unspecified Code | Other Specified Code | [N] Newborn Age: 0 | [P] Pediatric Age: 0-17 | [M] Maternity Age: 12-55
[A] Adult Age: 15-124 | ♂ Male | ♀ Female | ● New Code | ▲ Revised Code Title | ▶◀ Revised Text

7ᵗʰ S66.291 Other specified injury of extensor muscle, fascia and tendon of right thumb at wrist and hand level

7ᵗʰ S66.292 Other specified injury of extensor muscle, fascia and tendon of left thumb at wrist and hand level

7ᵗʰ S66.299 Other specified injury of extensor muscle, fascia and tendon of unspecified thumb at wrist and hand level

5ᵗʰ S66.3 Injury of extensor muscle, fascia and tendon of other and unspecified finger at wrist and hand level

> EXCLUDES2 Injury of extensor muscle, fascia and tendon of thumb at wrist and hand level (S66.2-)

6ᵗʰ S66.30 Unspecified injury of extensor muscle, fascia and tendon of other and unspecified finger at wrist and hand level

7ᵗʰ S66.300 Unspecified injury of extensor muscle, fascia and tendon of right index finger at wrist and hand level

7ᵗʰ S66.301 Unspecified injury of extensor muscle, fascia and tendon of left index finger at wrist and hand level

7ᵗʰ S66.302 Unspecified injury of extensor muscle, fascia and tendon of right middle finger at wrist and hand level

7ᵗʰ S66.303 Unspecified injury of extensor muscle, fascia and tendon of left middle finger at wrist and hand level

7ᵗʰ S66.304 Unspecified injury of extensor muscle, fascia and tendon of right ring finger at wrist and hand level

7ᵗʰ S66.305 Unspecified injury of extensor muscle, fascia and tendon of left ring finger at wrist and hand level

7ᵗʰ S66.306 Unspecified injury of extensor muscle, fascia and tendon of right little finger at wrist and hand level

7ᵗʰ S66.307 Unspecified injury of extensor muscle, fascia and tendon of left little finger at wrist and hand level

7ᵗʰ S66.308 Unspecified injury of extensor muscle, fascia and tendon of other finger at wrist and hand level

Unspecified injury of extensor muscle, fascia and tendon of specified finger with unspecified laterality at wrist and hand level

7ᵗʰ S66.309 Unspecified injury of extensor muscle, fascia and tendon of unspecified finger at wrist and hand level

5ᵗʰ S66.31 Strain of extensor muscle, fascia and tendon of other and unspecified finger at wrist and hand level

7ᵗʰ S66.310 Strain of extensor muscle, fascia and tendon of right index finger at wrist and hand level

7ᵗʰ S66.311 Strain of extensor muscle, fascia and tendon of left index finger at wrist and hand level

7ᵗʰ S66.312 Strain of extensor muscle, fascia and tendon of right middle finger at wrist and hand level

7ᵗʰ S66.313 Strain of extensor muscle, fascia and tendon of left middle finger at wrist and hand level

7ᵗʰ S66.314 Strain of extensor muscle, fascia and tendon of right ring finger at wrist and hand level

7ᵗʰ S66.315 Strain of extensor muscle, fascia and tendon of left ring finger at wrist and hand level

7ᵗʰ S66.316 Strain of extensor muscle, fascia and tendon of right little finger at wrist and hand level

7ᵗʰ S66.317 Strain of extensor muscle, fascia and tendon of left little finger at wrist and hand level

7ᵗʰ S66.318 Strain of extensor muscle, fascia and tendon of other finger at wrist and hand level

Strain of extensor muscle, fascia and tendon of specified finger with unspecified laterality at wrist and hand level

7ᵗʰ S66.319 Strain of extensor muscle, fascia and tendon of unspecified finger at wrist and hand level

6ᵗʰ S66.32 Laceration of extensor muscle, fascia and tendon of other and unspecified finger at wrist and hand level

7ᵗʰ S66.320 Laceration of extensor muscle, fascia and tendon of right index finger at wrist and hand level

7ᵗʰ S66.321 Laceration of extensor muscle, fascia and tendon of left index finger at wrist and hand level

7ᵗʰ S66.322 Laceration of extensor muscle, fascia and tendon of right middle finger at wrist and hand level

7ᵗʰ S66.323 Laceration of extensor muscle, fascia and tendon of left middle finger at wrist and hand level

7ᵗʰ S66.324 Laceration of extensor muscle, fascia and tendon of right ring finger at wrist and hand level

7ᵗʰ S66.325 Laceration of extensor muscle, fascia and tendon of left ring finger at wrist and hand level

7ᵗʰ S66.326 Laceration of extensor muscle, fascia and tendon of right little finger at wrist and hand level

7ᵗʰ S66.327 Laceration of extensor muscle, fascia and tendon of left little finger at wrist and hand level

7ᵗʰ S66.328 Laceration of extensor muscle, fascia and tendon of other finger at wrist and hand level

Laceration of extensor muscle, fascia and tendon of specified finger with unspecified laterality at wrist and hand level

7ᵗʰ S66.329 Laceration of extensor muscle, fascia and tendon of unspecified finger at wrist and hand level

6ᵗʰ S66.39 Other injury of extensor muscle, fascia and tendon of other and unspecified finger at wrist and hand level

7ᵗʰ S66.390 Other injury of extensor muscle, fascia and tendon of right index finger at wrist and hand level

7ᵗʰ S66.391 Other injury of extensor muscle, fascia and tendon of left index finger at wrist and hand level

7ᵗʰ S66.392 Other injury of extensor muscle, fascia and tendon of right middle finger at wrist and hand level

7ᵗʰ S66.393 Other injury of extensor muscle, fascia and tendon of left middle finger at wrist and hand level

7ᵗʰ S66.394 Other injury of extensor muscle, fascia and tendon of right ring finger at wrist and hand level

7ᵗʰ S66.395 Other injury of extensor muscle, fascia and tendon of left ring finger at wrist and hand level

7ᵗʰ S66.396 Other injury of extensor muscle, fascia and tendon of right little finger at wrist and hand level

---

4ᵗʰ 4ᵗʰ character required   5ᵗʰ 5ᵗʰ character required   6ᵗʰ 6ᵗʰ character required   7ᵗʰ 7ᵗʰ character required   7ᵗʰ Extension 'X' Alert

EXCLUDES 1 Not coded here   EXCLUDES 2 Not included here   PDX Primary Diagnosis Only   Manifestation Code

[7th] S66.397 Other injury of extensor muscle, fascia and tendon of left little finger at wrist and hand level

[7th] S66.398 Other injury of extensor muscle, fascia and tendon of other finger at wrist and hand level

Other injury of extensor muscle, fascia and tendon of specified finger with unspecified laterality at wrist and hand level

[7th] S66.399 Other injury of extensor muscle, fascia and tendon of unspecified finger at wrist and hand level

[5th] S66.4 Injury of intrinsic muscle, fascia and tendon of thumb at wrist and hand level

[6th] S66.40 Unspecified injury of intrinsic muscle, fascia and tendon of thumb at wrist and hand level

[7th] S66.401 Unspecified injury of intrinsic muscle, fascia and tendon of right thumb at wrist and hand level

[7th] S66.402 Unspecified injury of intrinsic muscle, fascia and tendon of left thumb at wrist and hand level

[7th] S66.409 Unspecified injury of intrinsic muscle, fascia and tendon of unspecified thumb at wrist and hand level

[6th] S66.41 Strain of intrinsic muscle, fascia and tendon of thumb at wrist and hand level

[7th] S66.411 Strain of intrinsic muscle, fascia and tendon of right thumb at wrist and hand level

[7th] S66.412 Strain of intrinsic muscle, fascia and tendon of left thumb at wrist and hand level

[7th] S66.419 Strain of intrinsic muscle, fascia and tendon of unspecified thumb at wrist and hand level

[6th] S66.42 Laceration of intrinsic muscle, fascia and tendon of thumb at wrist and hand level

[7th] S66.421 Laceration of intrinsic muscle, fascia and tendon of right thumb at wrist and hand level

[7th] S66.422 Laceration of intrinsic muscle, fascia and tendon of left thumb at wrist and hand level

[7th] S66.429 Laceration of intrinsic muscle, fascia and tendon of unspecified thumb at wrist and hand level

[6th] S66.49 Other specified injury of intrinsic muscle, fascia and tendon of thumb at wrist and hand level

[7th] S66.491 Other specified injury of intrinsic muscle, fascia and tendon of right thumb at wrist and hand level

[7th] S66.492 Other specified injury of intrinsic muscle, fascia and tendon of left thumb at wrist and hand level

[7th] S66.499 Other specified injury of intrinsic muscle, fascia and tendon of unspecified thumb at wrist and hand level

[5th] S66.5 Injury of intrinsic muscle, fascia and tendon of other and unspecified finger at wrist and hand level

[EXCLUDES2] *injury of intrinsic muscle, fascia and tendon of thumb at wrist and hand level (S66.4-)*

[6th] S66.50 Unspecified injury of intrinsic muscle, fascia and tendon of other and unspecified finger at wrist and hand level

[7th] S66.500 Unspecified injury of intrinsic muscle, fascia and tendon of right index finger at wrist and hand level

[7th] S66.501 Unspecified injury of intrinsic muscle, fascia and tendon of left index finger at wrist and hand level

[7th] S66.502 Unspecified injury of intrinsic muscle, fascia and tendon of right middle finger at wrist and hand level

[7th] S66.503 Unspecified injury of intrinsic muscle, fascia and tendon of left middle finger at wrist and hand level

[7th] S66.504 Unspecified injury of intrinsic muscle, fascia and tendon of right ring finger at wrist and hand level

[7th] S66.505 Unspecified injury of intrinsic muscle, fascia and tendon of left ring finger at wrist and hand level

[7th] S66.506 Unspecified injury of intrinsic muscle, fascia and tendon of right little finger at wrist and hand level

[7th] S66.507 Unspecified injury of intrinsic muscle, fascia and tendon of left little finger at wrist and hand level

[7th] S66.508 Unspecified injury of intrinsic muscle, fascia and tendon of other finger at wrist and hand level

Unspecified injury of intrinsic muscle, fascia and tendon of specified finger with unspecified laterality at wrist and hand level

[7th] S66.509 Unspecified injury of intrinsic muscle, fascia and tendon of unspecified finger at wrist and hand level

[6th] S66.51 Strain of intrinsic muscle, fascia and tendon of other and unspecified finger at wrist and hand level

[7th] S66.510 Strain of intrinsic muscle, fascia and tendon of right index finger at wrist and hand level

[7th] S66.511 Strain of intrinsic muscle, fascia and tendon of left index finger at wrist and hand level

[7th] S66.512 Strain of intrinsic muscle, fascia and tendon of right middle finger at wrist and hand level

[7th] S66.513 Strain of intrinsic muscle, fascia and tendon of left middle finger at wrist and hand level

[7th] S66.514 Strain of intrinsic muscle, fascia and tendon of right ring finger at wrist and hand level

[7th] S66.515 Strain of intrinsic muscle, fascia and tendon of left ring finger at wrist and hand level

[7th] S66.516 Strain of intrinsic muscle, fascia and tendon of right little finger at wrist and hand level

[7th] S66.517 Strain of intrinsic muscle, fascia and tendon of left little finger at wrist and hand level

[7th] S66.518 Strain of intrinsic muscle, fascia and tendon of other finger at wrist and hand level

Strain of intrinsic muscle, fascia and tendon of specified finger with unspecified laterality at wrist and hand level

[7th] S66.519 Strain of intrinsic muscle, fascia and tendon of unspecified finger at wrist and hand level

[6th] S66.52 Laceration of intrinsic muscle, fascia and tendon of other and unspecified finger at wrist and hand level

[7th] S66.520 Laceration of intrinsic muscle, fascia and tendon of right index finger at wrist and hand level

[7th] S66.521 Laceration of intrinsic muscle, fascia and tendon of left index finger at wrist and hand level

[7th] S66.522 Laceration of intrinsic muscle, fascia and tendon of right middle finger at wrist and hand level

[7th] S66.523 Laceration of intrinsic muscle, fascia and tendon of left middle finger at wrist and hand level

7ᵗʰ **S66.524** Laceration of intrinsic muscle, fascia and tendon of right ring finger at wrist and hand level

7ᵗʰ **S66.525** Laceration of intrinsic muscle, fascia and tendon of left ring finger at wrist and hand level

7ᵗʰ **S66.526** Laceration of intrinsic muscle, fascia and tendon of right little finger at wrist and hand level

7ᵗʰ **S66.527** Laceration of intrinsic muscle, fascia and tendon of left little finger at wrist and hand level

7ᵗʰ **S66.528** Laceration of intrinsic muscle, fascia and tendon of other finger at wrist and hand level

Laceration of intrinsic muscle, fascia and tendon of specified finger with unspecified laterality at wrist and hand level

7ᵗʰ **S66.529** Laceration of intrinsic muscle, fascia and tendon of unspecified finger at wrist and hand level

6ᵗʰ **S66.59** Other injury of intrinsic muscle, fascia and tendon of other and unspecified finger at wrist and hand level

7ᵗʰ **S66.590** Other injury of intrinsic muscle, fascia and tendon of right index finger at wrist and hand level

7ᵗʰ **S66.591** Other injury of intrinsic muscle, fascia and tendon of left index finger at wrist and hand level

7ᵗʰ **S66.592** Other injury of intrinsic muscle, fascia and tendon of right middle finger at wrist and hand level

7ᵗʰ **S66.593** Other injury of intrinsic muscle, fascia and tendon of left middle finger at wrist and hand level

7ᵗʰ **S66.594** Other injury of intrinsic muscle, fascia and tendon of right ring finger at wrist and hand level

7ᵗʰ **S66.595** Other injury of intrinsic muscle, fascia and tendon of left ring finger at wrist and hand level

7ᵗʰ **S66.596** Other injury of intrinsic muscle, fascia and tendon of right little finger at wrist and hand level

7ᵗʰ **S66.597** Other injury of intrinsic muscle, fascia and tendon of left little finger at wrist and hand level

7ᵗʰ **S66.598** Other injury of intrinsic muscle, fascia and tendon of other finger at wrist and hand level

Other injury of intrinsic muscle, fascia and tendon of specified finger with unspecified laterality at wrist and hand level

7ᵗʰ **S66.599** Other injury of intrinsic muscle, fascia and tendon of unspecified finger at wrist and hand level

5ᵗʰ **S66.8** Injury of other specified muscles, fascia and tendons at wrist and hand level

6ᵗʰ **S66.80** Unspecified injury of other specified muscles, fascia and tendons at wrist and hand level

7ᵗʰ **S66.801** Unspecified injury of other specified muscles, fascia and tendons at wrist and hand level, right hand

7ᵗʰ **S66.802** Unspecified injury of other specified muscles, fascia and tendons at wrist and hand level, left hand

7ᵗʰ **S66.809** Unspecified injury of other specified muscles, fascia and tendons at wrist and hand level, unspecified hand

6ᵗʰ **S66.81** Strain of other specified muscles, fascia and tendons at wrist and hand level

7ᵗʰ **S66.811** Strain of other specified muscles, fascia and tendons at wrist and hand level, right hand

7ᵗʰ **S66.812** Strain of other specified muscles, fascia and tendons at wrist and hand level, left hand

7ᵗʰ **S66.819** Strain of other specified muscles, fascia and tendons at wrist and hand level, unspecified hand

6ᵗʰ **S66.82** Laceration of other specified muscles, fascia and tendons at wrist and hand level

7ᵗʰ **S66.821** Laceration of other specified muscles, fascia and tendons at wrist and hand level, right hand

7ᵗʰ **S66.822** Laceration of other specified muscles, fascia and tendons at wrist and hand level, left hand

7ᵗʰ **S66.829** Laceration of other specified muscles, fascia and tendons at wrist and hand level, unspecified hand

6ᵗʰ **S66.89** Other injury of other specified muscles, fascia and tendons at wrist and hand level

7ᵗʰ **S66.891** Other injury of other specified muscles, fascia and tendons at wrist and hand level, right hand

7ᵗʰ **S66.892** Other injury of other specified muscles, fascia and tendons at wrist and hand level, left hand

7ᵗʰ **S66.899** Other injury of other specified muscles, fascia and tendons at wrist and hand level, unspecified hand

5ᵗʰ **S66.9** Injury of unspecified muscle, fascia and tendon at wrist and hand level

6ᵗʰ **S66.90** Unspecified injury of unspecified muscle, fascia and tendon at wrist and hand level

7ᵗʰ **S66.901** Unspecified injury of unspecified muscle, fascia and tendon at wrist and hand level, right hand

7ᵗʰ **S66.902** Unspecified injury of unspecified muscle, fascia and tendon at wrist and hand level, left hand

7ᵗʰ **S66.909** Unspecified injury of unspecified muscle, fascia and tendon at wrist and hand level, unspecified hand

6ᵗʰ **S66.91** Strain of unspecified muscle, fascia and tendon at wrist and hand level

7ᵗʰ **S66.911** Strain of unspecified muscle, fascia and tendon at wrist and hand level, right hand

7ᵗʰ **S66.912** Strain of unspecified muscle, fascia and tendon at wrist and hand level, left hand

7ᵗʰ **S66.919** Strain of unspecified muscle, fascia and tendon at wrist and hand level, unspecified hand

6ᵗʰ **S66.92** Laceration of unspecified muscle, fascia and tendon at wrist and hand level

7ᵗʰ **S66.921** Laceration of unspecified muscle, fascia and tendon at wrist and hand level, right hand

7ᵗʰ **S66.922** Laceration of unspecified muscle, fascia and tendon at wrist and hand level, left hand

7ᵗʰ **S66.929** Laceration of unspecified muscle, fascia and tendon at wrist and hand level, unspecified hand

6ᵗʰ **S66.99** Other injury of unspecified muscle, fascia and tendon at wrist and hand level

7ᵗʰ **S66.991** Other injury of unspecified muscle, fascia and tendon at wrist and hand level, right hand

7ᵗʰ **S66.992** Other injury of unspecified muscle, fascia and tendon at wrist and hand level, left hand

[7th] S66.999 Other injury of unspecified muscle, fascia and tendon at wrist and hand level, unspecified hand

[4th] S67 Crushing injury of wrist, hand and fingers
Use additional code for all associated injuries, such as:
fracture of wrist and hand (S62.-)
open wound of wrist and hand (S61.-)
The appropriate 7th character is to be added to each code from category S67
A = initial encounter
D = subsequent encounter
S = sequela

[5th] S67.0 Crushing injury of thumb
[7th] S67.00 Crushing injury of unspecified thumb
[7th] S67.01 Crushing injury of right thumb
[7th] S67.02 Crushing injury of left thumb

[5th] S67.1 Crushing injury of other and unspecified finger(s)
[EXCLUDES2] *crushing injury of thumb (S67.0-)*
[7th] S67.10 Crushing injury of unspecified finger(s)
[6th] S67.19 Crushing injury of other finger(s)
[7th] S67.190 Crushing injury of right index finger
[7th] S67.191 Crushing injury of left index finger
[7th] S67.192 Crushing injury of right middle finger
[7th] S67.193 Crushing injury of left middle finger
[7th] S67.194 Crushing injury of right ring finger
[7th] S67.195 Crushing injury of left ring finger
[7th] S67.196 Crushing injury of right little finger
[7th] S67.197 Crushing injury of left little finger
[7th] S67.198 Crushing injury of other finger
Crushing injury of specified finger with unspecified laterality

[5th] S67.2 Crushing injury of hand
[EXCLUDES2] *crushing injury of fingers (S67.1-)*
crushing injury of thumb (S67.0-)
[7th] S67.20 Crushing injury of unspecified hand
[7th] S67.21 Crushing injury of right hand
[7th] S67.22 Crushing injury of left hand

[5th] S67.3 Crushing injury of wrist
[7th] S67.30 Crushing injury of unspecified wrist
[7th] S67.31 Crushing injury of right wrist
[7th] S67.32 Crushing injury of left wrist

[5th] S67.4 Crushing injury of wrist and hand
[EXCLUDES1] *crushing injury of hand alone (S67.2-)*
crushing injury of wrist alone (S67.3-)
[EXCLUDES2] *crushing injury of fingers (S67.1-)*
crushing injury of thumb (S67.0-)
[7th] S67.40 Crushing injury of unspecified wrist and hand
[7th] S67.41 Crushing injury of right wrist and hand
[7th] S67.42 Crushing injury of left wrist and hand

[5th] S67.9 Crushing injury of unspecified part(s) of wrist, hand and fingers
[7th] S67.90 Crushing injury of unspecified part(s) of unspecified wrist, hand and fingers
[7th] S67.91 Crushing injury of unspecified part(s) of right wrist, hand and fingers
[7th] S67.92 Crushing injury of unspecified part(s) of left wrist, hand and fingers

[4th] S68 Traumatic amputation of wrist, hand and fingers
An amputation not identified as partial or complete should be coded to complete
The appropriate 7th character is to be added to each code from category S68
A = initial encounter
D = subsequent encounter
S = sequela

[5th] S68.0 Traumatic metacarpophalangeal amputation of thumb
Traumatic amputation of thumb NOS
[6th] S68.01 Complete traumatic metacarpophalangeal amputation of thumb
[7th] S68.011 Complete traumatic metacarpophalangeal amputation of right thumb
[7th] S68.012 Complete traumatic metacarpophalangeal amputation of left thumb
[7th] S68.019 Complete traumatic metacarpophalangeal amputation of unspecified thumb
[6th] S68.02 Partial traumatic metacarpophalangeal amputation of thumb
[7th] S68.021 Partial traumatic metacarpophalangeal amputation of right thumb
[7th] S68.022 Partial traumatic metacarpophalangeal amputation of left thumb
[7th] S68.029 Partial traumatic metacarpophalangeal amputation of unspecified thumb

[5th] S68.1 Traumatic metacarpophalangeal amputation of other and unspecified finger
Traumatic amputation of finger NOS
[EXCLUDES2] *traumatic metacarpophalangeal amputation of thumb (S68.0-)*
[6th] S68.11 Complete traumatic metacarpophalangeal amputation of other and unspecified finger
[7th] S68.110 Complete traumatic metacarpophalangeal amputation of right index finger
[7th] S68.111 Complete traumatic metacarpophalangeal amputation of left index finger
[7th] S68.112 Complete traumatic metacarpophalangeal amputation of right middle finger
[7th] S68.113 Complete traumatic metacarpophalangeal amputation of left middle finger
[7th] S68.114 Complete traumatic metacarpophalangeal amputation of right ring finger
[7th] S68.115 Complete traumatic metacarpophalangeal amputation of left ring finger
[7th] S68.116 Complete traumatic metacarpophalangeal amputation of right little finger
[7th] S68.117 Complete traumatic metacarpophalangeal amputation of left little finger
[7th] S68.118 Complete traumatic metacarpophalangeal amputation of other finger
Complete traumatic metacarpophalangeal amputation of specified finger with unspecified laterality
[7th] S68.119 Complete traumatic metacarpophalangeal amputation of unspecified finger
[6th] S68.12 Partial traumatic metacarpophalangeal amputation of other and unspecified finger
[7th] S68.120 Partial traumatic metacarpophalangeal amputation of right index finger
[7th] S68.121 Partial traumatic metacarpophalangeal amputation of left index finger
[7th] S68.122 Partial traumatic metacarpophalangeal amputation of right middle finger
[7th] S68.123 Partial traumatic metacarpophalangeal amputation of left middle finger
[7th] S68.124 Partial traumatic metacarpophalangeal amputation of right ring finger
[7th] S68.125 Partial traumatic metacarpophalangeal amputation of left ring finger
[7th] S68.126 Partial traumatic metacarpophalangeal amputation of right little finger
[7th] S68.127 Partial traumatic metacarpophalangeal amputation of left little finger

Unspecified Code | Other Specified Code | [N] Newborn Age: 0 | [P] Pediatric Age: 0-17 | [M] Maternity Age: 12-55
[A] Adult Age: 15-124 | ♂ Male | ♀ Female | ● New Code | ▲ Revised Code Title | ►◄ Revised Text

7ᵗʰ S68.128 Partial traumatic metacarpophalangeal amputation of other finger

> Partial traumatic metacarpophalangeal amputation of specified finger with unspecified laterality

7ᵗʰ S68.129 Partial traumatic metacarpophalangeal amputation of unspecified finger

5ᵗʰ S68.4 Traumatic amputation of hand at wrist level

> Traumatic amputation of hand NOS
> Traumatic amputation of wrist

6ᵗʰ S68.41 Complete traumatic amputation of hand at wrist level

7ᵗʰ S68.411 Complete traumatic amputation of right hand at wrist level

7ᵗʰ S68.412 Complete traumatic amputation of left hand at wrist level

7ᵗʰ S68.419 Complete traumatic amputation of unspecified hand at wrist level

6ᵗʰ S68.42 Partial traumatic amputation of hand at wrist level

7ᵗʰ S68.421 Partial traumatic amputation of right hand at wrist level

7ᵗʰ S68.422 Partial traumatic amputation of left hand at wrist level

7ᵗʰ S68.429 Partial traumatic amputation of unspecified hand at wrist level

5ᵗʰ S68.5 Traumatic transphalangeal amputation of thumb

> Traumatic interphalangeal joint amputation of thumb

6ᵗʰ S68.51 Complete traumatic transphalangeal amputation of thumb

7ᵗʰ S68.511 Complete traumatic transphalangeal amputation of right thumb

7ᵗʰ S68.512 Complete traumatic transphalangeal amputation of left thumb

7ᵗʰ S68.519 Complete traumatic transphalangeal amputation of unspecified thumb

6ᵗʰ S68.52 Partial traumatic transphalangeal amputation of thumb

7ᵗʰ S68.521 Partial traumatic transphalangeal amputation of right thumb

7ᵗʰ S68.522 Partial traumatic transphalangeal amputation of left thumb

7ᵗʰ S68.529 Partial traumatic transphalangeal amputation of unspecified thumb

5ᵗʰ S68.6 Traumatic transphalangeal amputation of other and unspecified finger

6ᵗʰ S68.61 Complete traumatic transphalangeal amputation of other and unspecified finger(s)

7ᵗʰ S68.610 Complete traumatic transphalangeal amputation of right index finger

7ᵗʰ S68.611 Complete traumatic transphalangeal amputation of left index finger

7ᵗʰ S68.612 Complete traumatic transphalangeal amputation of right middle finger

7ᵗʰ S68.613 Complete traumatic transphalangeal amputation of left middle finger

7ᵗʰ S68.614 Complete traumatic transphalangeal amputation of right ring finger

7ᵗʰ S68.615 Complete traumatic transphalangeal amputation of left ring finger

7ᵗʰ S68.616 Complete traumatic transphalangeal amputation of right little finger

7ᵗʰ S68.617 Complete traumatic transphalangeal amputation of left little finger

7ᵗʰ S68.618 Complete traumatic transphalangeal amputation of other finger

> Complete traumatic transphalangeal amputation of specified finger with unspecified laterality

7ᵗʰ S68.619 Complete traumatic transphalangeal amputation of unspecified finger

6ᵗʰ S68.62 Partial traumatic transphalangeal amputation of other and unspecified finger

7ᵗʰ S68.620 Partial traumatic transphalangeal amputation of right index finger

7ᵗʰ S68.621 Partial traumatic transphalangeal amputation of left index finger

7ᵗʰ S68.622 Partial traumatic transphalangeal amputation of right middle finger

7ᵗʰ S68.623 Partial traumatic transphalangeal amputation of left middle finger

7ᵗʰ S68.624 Partial traumatic transphalangeal amputation of right ring finger

7ᵗʰ S68.625 Partial traumatic transphalangeal amputation of left ring finger

7ᵗʰ S68.626 Partial traumatic transphalangeal amputation of right little finger

7ᵗʰ S68.627 Partial traumatic transphalangeal amputation of left little finger

7ᵗʰ S68.628 Partial traumatic transphalangeal amputation of other finger

> Partial traumatic transphalangeal amputation of specified finger with unspecified laterality

7ᵗʰ S68.629 Partial traumatic transphalangeal amputation of unspecified finger

5ᵗʰ S68.7 Traumatic transmetacarpal amputation of hand

6ᵗʰ S68.71 Complete traumatic transmetacarpal amputation of hand

7ᵗʰ S68.711 Complete traumatic transmetacarpal amputation of right hand

7ᵗʰ S68.712 Complete traumatic transmetacarpal amputation of left hand

7ᵗʰ S68.719 Complete traumatic transmetacarpal amputation of unspecified hand

6ᵗʰ S68.72 Partial traumatic transmetacarpal amputation of hand

7ᵗʰ S68.721 Partial traumatic transmetacarpal amputation of right hand

7ᵗʰ S68.722 Partial traumatic transmetacarpal amputation of left hand

7ᵗʰ S68.729 Partial traumatic transmetacarpal amputation of unspecified hand

4ᵗʰ S69 Other and unspecified injuries of wrist, hand and finger(s)

> The appropriate 7th character is to be added to each code from category S69
> A = initial encounter
> D = subsequent encounter
> S = sequela

5ᵗʰ S69.8 Other specified injuries of wrist, hand and finger(s)

7ᵗʰ S69.80 Other specified injuries of unspecified wrist, hand and finger(s)

7ᵗʰ S69.81 Other specified injuries of right wrist, hand and finger(s)

7ᵗʰ S69.82 Other specified injuries of left wrist, hand and finger(s)

5ᵗʰ S69.9 Unspecified injury of wrist, hand and finger(s)

7ᵗʰ S69.90 Unspecified injury of unspecified wrist, hand and finger(s)

7ᵗʰ S69.91 Unspecified injury of right wrist, hand and finger(s)

7ᵗʰ S69.92 Unspecified injury of left wrist, hand and finger(s)

Injuries to the hip and thigh (S70-S79)

> EXCLUDES2   burns and corrosions (T20-T32)
> frostbite (T33-T34)
> snake bite (T63.0-)
> venomous insect bite or sting (T63.4-)

4ᵗʰ 4ᵗʰ character required   5ᵗʰ 5ᵗʰ character required   6ᵗʰ 6ᵗʰ character required   7ᵗʰ 7ᵗʰ character required   Extension 'X' Alert

EXCLUDES 1 Not coded here   EXCLUDES 2 Not included here   PDx Primary Diagnosis Only   Manifestation Code

[4th] S70 Superficial injury of hip and thigh
The appropriate 7th character is to be added to each code from category S70
A = initial encounter
D = subsequent encounter
S = sequela
[5th] S70.0 Contusion of hip
[7th] S70.00 Contusion of unspecified hip
[7th] S70.01 Contusion of right hip
[7th] S70.02 Contusion of left hip
[5th] S70.1 Contusion of thigh
[7th] S70.10 Contusion of unspecified thigh
[7th] S70.11 Contusion of right thigh
[7th] S70.12 Contusion of left thigh
[5th] S70.2 Other superficial injuries of hip
[6th] S70.21 Abrasion of hip
[7th] S70.211 Abrasion, right hip
[7th] S70.212 Abrasion, left hip
[7th] S70.219 Abrasion, unspecified hip
[6th] S70.22 Blister (nonthermal) of hip
[7th] S70.221 Blister (nonthermal), right hip
[7th] S70.222 Blister (nonthermal), left hip
[7th] S70.229 Blister (nonthermal), unspecified hip
[6th] S70.24 External constriction of hip
[7th] S70.241 External constriction, right hip
[7th] S70.242 External constriction, left hip
[7th] S70.249 External constriction, unspecified hip
[6th] S70.25 Superficial foreign body of hip
Splinter in the hip
[7th] S70.251 Superficial foreign body, right hip
[7th] S70.252 Superficial foreign body, left hip
[7th] S70.259 Superficial foreign body, unspecified hip
[6th] S70.26 Insect bite (nonvenomous) of hip
[7th] S70.261 Insect bite (nonvenomous), right hip
[7th] S70.262 Insect bite (nonvenomous), left hip
[7th] S70.269 Insect bite (nonvenomous), unspecified hip
[6th] S70.27 Other superficial bite of hip
[EXCLUDES1] *open bite of hip (S71.05-)*
[7th] S70.271 Other superficial bite of hip, right hip
[7th] S70.272 Other superficial bite of hip, left hip
[7th] S70.279 Other superficial bite of hip, unspecified hip
[5th] S70.3 Other superficial injuries of thigh
[6th] S70.31 Abrasion of thigh
[7th] S70.311 Abrasion, right thigh
[7th] S70.312 Abrasion, left thigh
[7th] S70.319 Abrasion, unspecified thigh
[6th] S70.32 Blister (nonthermal) of thigh
[7th] S70.321 Blister (nonthermal), right thigh
[7th] S70.322 Blister (nonthermal), left thigh
[7th] S70.329 Blister (nonthermal), unspecified thigh
[6th] S70.34 External constriction of thigh
[7th] S70.341 External constriction, right thigh
[7th] S70.342 External constriction, left thigh
[7th] S70.349 External constriction, unspecified thigh
[6th] S70.35 Superficial foreign body of thigh
Splinter in the thigh
[7th] S70.351 Superficial foreign body, right thigh
[7th] S70.352 Superficial foreign body, left thigh
[7th] S70.359 Superficial foreign body, unspecified thigh
[6th] S70.36 Insect bite (nonvenomous) of thigh
[7th] S70.361 Insect bite (nonvenomous), right thigh
[7th] S70.362 Insect bite (nonvenomous), left thigh
[7th] S70.369 Insect bite (nonvenomous), unspecified thigh
[6th] S70.37 Other superficial bite of thigh
[EXCLUDES1] *open bite of thigh (S71.15)*
[7th] S70.371 Other superficial bite of right thigh
[7th] S70.372 Other superficial bite of left thigh
[7th] S70.379 Other superficial bite of unspecified thigh
[5th] S70.9 Unspecified superficial injury of hip and thigh
[6th] S70.91 Unspecified superficial injury of hip
[7th] S70.911 Unspecified superficial injury of right hip
[7th] S70.912 Unspecified superficial injury of left hip
[7th] S70.919 Unspecified superficial injury of unspecified hip
[6th] S70.92 Unspecified superficial injury of thigh
[7th] S70.921 Unspecified superficial injury of right thigh
[7th] S70.922 Unspecified superficial injury of left thigh
[7th] S70.929 Unspecified superficial injury of unspecified thigh

[4th] S71 Open wound of hip and thigh
Code also any associated wound infection
[EXCLUDES1] *open fracture of hip and thigh (S72.-)*
traumatic amputation of hip and thigh (S78.-)
[EXCLUDES2] *bite of venomous animal (T63.-)*
open wound of ankle, foot and toes (S91.-)
open wound of knee and lower leg (S81.-)
The appropriate 7th character is to be added to each code from category S71
A = initial encounter
D = subsequent encounter
S = sequela
[5th] S71.0 Open wound of hip
[6th] S71.00 Unspecified open wound of hip
[7th] S71.001 Unspecified open wound, right hip
[7th] S71.002 Unspecified open wound, left hip
[7th] S71.009 Unspecified open wound, unspecified hip
[6th] S71.01 Laceration without foreign body of hip
[7th] S71.011 Laceration without foreign body, right hip
[7th] S71.012 Laceration without foreign body, left hip
[7th] S71.019 Laceration without foreign body, unspecified hip
[6th] S71.02 Laceration with foreign body of hip
[7th] S71.021 Laceration with foreign body, right hip
[7th] S71.022 Laceration with foreign body, left hip
[7th] S71.029 Laceration with foreign body, unspecified hip
[6th] S71.03 Puncture wound without foreign body of hip
[7th] S71.031 Puncture wound without foreign body, right hip
[7th] S71.032 Puncture wound without foreign body, left hip
[7th] S71.039 Puncture wound without foreign body, unspecified hip
[6th] S71.04 Puncture wound with foreign body of hip
[7th] S71.041 Puncture wound with foreign body, right hip
[7th] S71.042 Puncture wound with foreign body, left hip
[7th] S71.049 Puncture wound with foreign body, unspecified hip
[6th] S71.05 Open bite of hip
Bite of hip NOS
[EXCLUDES1] *superficial bite of hip (S70.26, S70.27)*
[7th] S71.051 Open bite, right hip
[7th] S71.052 Open bite, left hip
[7th] S71.059 Open bite, unspecified hip
[5th] S71.1 Open wound of thigh
[6th] S71.10 Unspecified open wound of thigh
[7th] S71.101 Unspecified open wound, right thigh
[7th] S71.102 Unspecified open wound, left thigh
[7th] S71.109 Unspecified open wound, unspecified thigh
[6th] S71.11 Laceration without foreign body of thigh
[7th] S71.111 Laceration without foreign body, right thigh

Unspecified Code | Other Specified Code | [N] Newborn Age: 0 | [P] Pediatric Age: 0-17 | [M] Maternity Age: 12-55
[A] Adult Age: 15-124 | ♂ Male | ♀ Female | ● New Code | ▲ Revised Code Title | ►◄ Revised Text

[7th] S71.112 Laceration without foreign body, left thigh
[7th] S71.119 Laceration without foreign body, unspecified thigh
[6th] S71.12 Laceration with foreign body of thigh
[7th] S71.121 Laceration with foreign body, right thigh
[7th] S71.122 Laceration with foreign body, left thigh
[7th] S71.129 Laceration with foreign body, unspecified thigh
[6th] S71.13 Puncture wound without foreign body of thigh
[7th] S71.131 Puncture wound without foreign body, right thigh
[7th] S71.132 Puncture wound without foreign body, left thigh
[7th] S71.139 Puncture wound without foreign body, unspecified thigh
[6th] S71.14 Puncture wound with foreign body of thigh
[7th] S71.141 Puncture wound with foreign body, right thigh
[7th] S71.142 Puncture wound with foreign body, left thigh
[7th] S71.149 Puncture wound with foreign body, unspecified thigh
[6th] S71.15 Open bite of thigh
Bite of thigh NOS
[EXCLUDES1] *superficial bite of thigh (S70.37-)*
[7th] S71.151 Open bite, right thigh
[7th] S71.152 Open bite, left thigh
[7th] S71.159 Open bite, unspecified thigh

Types of Bone Fractures

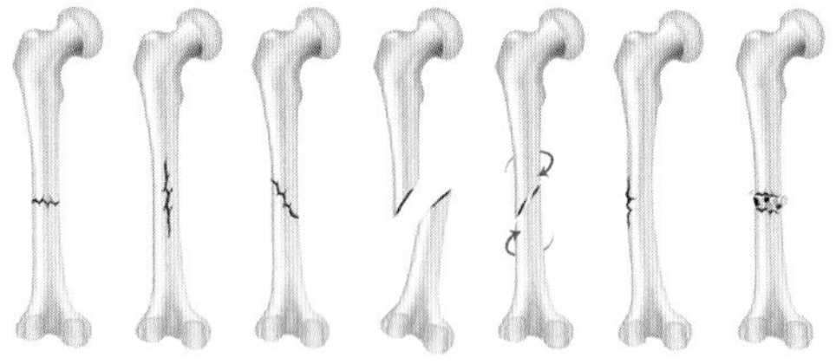

Transverse | Linear | Oblique, nondisplaced | Oblique, displaced | Spiral | Greenstick | Comminuted

Figure 16.1 Types of Bone fractures

[4th] S72 Fracture of femur
[NOTES] A fracture not indicated as displaced or nondisplaced should be coded to displaced
A fracture not indicated as open or closed should be coded to closed
The open fracture designations are based on the Gustilo open fracture classification
[EXCLUDES1] *traumatic amputation of hip and thigh (S78.-)*
[EXCLUDES2] *fracture of lower leg and ankle (S82.-)*
fracture of foot (S92.-)
periprosthetic fracture of prosthetic implant of hip (T84.040, T84.041)

The appropriate 7th character is to be added to all codes from category S72
A = initial encounter for closed fracture
B = initial encounter for open fracture type I or II
C = initial encounter for open fracture type IIIA, IIIB, or IIIC
D = subsequent encounter for closed fracture with routine healing
E = subsequent encounter for open fracture type I or II with routine healing
F = subsequent encounter for open fracture type IIIA, IIIB, or IIIC with routine healing
G = subsequent encounter for closed fracture with delayed healing
H = subsequent encounter for open fracture type I or II with delayed healing
J = subsequent encounter for open fracture type IIIA, IIIB, or IIIC with delayed healing
K = subsequent encounter for closed fracture with nonunion
M = subsequent encounter for open fracture type I or II with nonunion
N = subsequent encounter for open fracture type IIIA, IIIB, or IIIC with nonunion
P = subsequent encounter for closed fracture with malunion
Q = subsequent encounter for open fracture type I or II with malunion
R = subsequent encounter for open fracture type IIIA, IIIB, or IIIC with malunion
S = sequela

[5th] S72.0 Fracture of head and neck of femur
[EXCLUDES2] *physeal fracture of upper end of femur (S79.0-)*
[6th] S72.00 Fracture of unspecified part of neck of femur
Fracture of hip NOS
Fracture of neck of femur NOS
[7th] S72.001 Fracture of unspecified part of neck of right femur
[7th] S72.002 Fracture of unspecified part of neck of left femur
[7th] S72.009 Fracture of unspecified part of neck of unspecified femur
[6th] S72.01 Unspecified intracapsular fracture of femur
Subcapital fracture of femur
[7th] S72.011 Unspecified intracapsular fracture of right femur
[7th] S72.012 Unspecified intracapsular fracture of left femur
[7th] S72.019 Unspecified intracapsular fracture of unspecified femur
[6th] S72.02 Fracture of epiphysis (separation) (upper) of femur
Transepiphyseal fracture of femur
[EXCLUDES1] *capital femoral epiphyseal fracture (pediatric) of femur (S79.01-)*
Salter-Harris Type I physeal fracture of upper end of femur (S79.01-)
[7th] S72.021 Displaced fracture of epiphysis (separation) (upper) of right femur
[7th] S72.022 Displaced fracture of epiphysis (separation) (upper) of left femur
[7th] S72.023 Displaced fracture of epiphysis (separation) (upper) of unspecified femur
[7th] S72.024 Nondisplaced fracture of epiphysis (separation) (upper) of right femur
[7th] S72.025 Nondisplaced fracture of epiphysis (separation) (upper) of left femur
[7th] S72.026 Nondisplaced fracture of epiphysis (separation) (upper) of unspecified femur
[6th] S72.03 Midcervical fracture of femur
Transcervical fracture of femur NOS
[7th] S72.031 Displaced midcervical fracture of right femur
[7th] S72.032 Displaced midcervical fracture of left femur
[7th] S72.033 Displaced midcervical fracture of unspecified femur
[7th] S72.034 Nondisplaced midcervical fracture of right femur

[4th] 4th character required [5th] 5th character required [6th] 6th character required [7th] 7th character required [X] Extension 'X' Alert
[EXCLUDES 1] Not coded here [EXCLUDES 2] Not included here [PDx] Primary Diagnosis Only Manifestation Code

[7th] S72.035 Nondisplaced midcervical fracture of left femur
[7th] S72.036 Nondisplaced midcervical fracture of unspecified femur
[6th] S72.04 Fracture of base of neck of femur
Cervicotrochanteric fracture of femur
[7th] S72.041 Displaced fracture of base of neck of right femur
[7th] S72.042 Displaced fracture of base of neck of left femur
[7th] S72.043 Displaced fracture of base of neck of unspecified femur
[7th] S72.044 Nondisplaced fracture of base of neck of right femur
[7th] S72.045 Nondisplaced fracture of base of neck of left femur
[7th] S72.046 Nondisplaced fracture of base of neck of unspecified femur
[6th] S72.05 Unspecified fracture of head of femur
Fracture of head of femur NOS
[7th] S72.051 Unspecified fracture of head of right femur
[7th] S72.052 Unspecified fracture of head of left femur
[7th] S72.059 Unspecified fracture of head of unspecified femur
[6th] S72.06 Articular fracture of head of femur
[7th] S72.061 Displaced articular fracture of head of right femur
[7th] S72.062 Displaced articular fracture of head of left femur
[7th] S72.063 Displaced articular fracture of head of unspecified femur
[7th] S72.064 Nondisplaced articular fracture of head of right femur
[7th] S72.065 Nondisplaced articular fracture of head of left femur
[7th] S72.066 Nondisplaced articular fracture of head of unspecified femur
[6th] S72.09 Other fracture of head and neck of femur
[7th] S72.091 Other fracture of head and neck of right femur
[7th] S72.092 Other fracture of head and neck of left femur
[7th] S72.099 Other fracture of head and neck of unspecified femur
[5th] S72.1 Pertrochanteric fracture
[6th] S72.10 Unspecified trochanteric fracture of femur
Fracture of trochanter NOS
[7th] S72.101 Unspecified trochanteric fracture of right femur
[7th] S72.102 Unspecified trochanteric fracture of left femur
[7th] S72.109 Unspecified trochanteric fracture of unspecified femur
[6th] S72.11 Fracture of greater trochanter of femur
[7th] S72.111 Displaced fracture of greater trochanter of right femur
[7th] S72.112 Displaced fracture of greater trochanter of left femur
[7th] S72.113 Displaced fracture of greater trochanter of unspecified femur
[7th] S72.114 Nondisplaced fracture of greater trochanter of right femur
[7th] S72.115 Nondisplaced fracture of greater trochanter of left femur
[7th] S72.116 Nondisplaced fracture of greater trochanter of unspecified femur
[6th] S72.12 Fracture of lesser trochanter of femur
[7th] S72.121 Displaced fracture of lesser trochanter of right femur
[7th] S72.122 Displaced fracture of lesser trochanter of left femur
[7th] S72.123 Displaced fracture of lesser trochanter of unspecified femur
[7th] S72.124 Nondisplaced fracture of lesser trochanter of right femur
[7th] S72.125 Nondisplaced fracture of lesser trochanter of left femur
[7th] S72.126 Nondisplaced fracture of lesser trochanter of unspecified femur
[6th] S72.13 Apophyseal fracture of femur
[EXCLUDES1] *chronic (nontraumatic) slipped upper femoral epiphysis (M93.0-)*
[7th] S72.131 Displaced apophyseal fracture of right femur
[7th] S72.132 Displaced apophyseal fracture of left femur
[7th] S72.133 Displaced apophyseal fracture of unspecified femur
[7th] S72.134 Nondisplaced apophyseal fracture of right femur
[7th] S72.135 Nondisplaced apophyseal fracture of left femur
[7th] S72.136 Nondisplaced apophyseal fracture of unspecified femur
[6th] S72.14 Intertrochanteric fracture of femur
[7th] S72.141 Displaced intertrochanteric fracture of right femur
[7th] S72.142 Displaced intertrochanteric fracture of left femur
[7th] S72.143 Displaced intertrochanteric fracture of unspecified femur
[7th] S72.144 Nondisplaced intertrochanteric fracture of right femur
[7th] S72.145 Nondisplaced intertrochanteric fracture of left femur
[7th] S72.146 Nondisplaced intertrochanteric fracture of unspecified femur
[5th] S72.2 Subtrochanteric fracture of femur
[7th] S72.21 Displaced subtrochanteric fracture of right femur
[7th] S72.22 Displaced subtrochanteric fracture of left femur
[7th] S72.23 Displaced subtrochanteric fracture of unspecified femur
[7th] S72.24 Nondisplaced subtrochanteric fracture of right femur
[7th] S72.25 Nondisplaced subtrochanteric fracture of left femur
[7th] S72.26 Nondisplaced subtrochanteric fracture of unspecified femur
[5th] S72.3 Fracture of shaft of femur
[6th] S72.30 Unspecified fracture of shaft of femur
[7th] S72.301 Unspecified fracture of shaft of right femur
[7th] S72.302 Unspecified fracture of shaft of left femur
[7th] S72.309 Unspecified fracture of shaft of unspecified femur
[6th] S72.32 Transverse fracture of shaft of femur
[7th] S72.321 Displaced transverse fracture of shaft of right femur
[7th] S72.322 Displaced transverse fracture of shaft of left femur
[7th] S72.323 Displaced transverse fracture of shaft of unspecified femur
[7th] S72.324 Nondisplaced transverse fracture of shaft of right femur
[7th] S72.325 Nondisplaced transverse fracture of shaft of left femur
[7th] S72.326 Nondisplaced transverse fracture of shaft of unspecified femur
[6th] S72.33 Oblique fracture of shaft of femur

Unspecified Code | Other Specified Code | [N] Newborn Age: 0 | [P] Pediatric Age: 0-17 | [M] Maternity Age: 12-55 | [A] Adult Age: 15-124 | ♂ Male | ♀ Female | ● New Code | ▲ Revised Code Title | ►◄ Revised Text

[7th] S72.331 Displaced oblique fracture of shaft of right femur
[7th] S72.332 Displaced oblique fracture of shaft of left femur
[7th] S72.333 Displaced oblique fracture of shaft of unspecified femur
[7th] S72.334 Nondisplaced oblique fracture of shaft of right femur
[7th] S72.335 Nondisplaced oblique fracture of shaft of left femur
[7th] S72.336 Nondisplaced oblique fracture of shaft of unspecified femur

[6th] S72.34 Spiral fracture of shaft of femur
[7th] S72.341 Displaced spiral fracture of shaft of right femur
[7th] S72.342 Displaced spiral fracture of shaft of left femur
[7th] S72.343 Displaced spiral fracture of shaft of unspecified femur
[7th] S72.344 Nondisplaced spiral fracture of shaft of right femur
[7th] S72.345 Nondisplaced spiral fracture of shaft of left femur
[7th] S72.346 Nondisplaced spiral fracture of shaft of unspecified femur

[6th] S72.35 Comminuted fracture of shaft of femur
[7th] S72.351 Displaced comminuted fracture of shaft of right femur
[7th] S72.352 Displaced comminuted fracture of shaft of left femur
[7th] S72.353 Displaced comminuted fracture of shaft of unspecified femur
[7th] S72.354 Nondisplaced comminuted fracture of shaft of right femur
[7th] S72.355 Nondisplaced comminuted fracture of shaft of left femur
[7th] S72.356 Nondisplaced comminuted fracture of shaft of unspecified femur

[6th] S72.36 Segmental fracture of shaft of femur
[7th] S72.361 Displaced segmental fracture of shaft of right femur
[7th] S72.362 Displaced segmental fracture of shaft of left femur
[7th] S72.363 Displaced segmental fracture of shaft of unspecified femur
[7th] S72.364 Nondisplaced segmental fracture of shaft of right femur
[7th] S72.365 Nondisplaced segmental fracture of shaft of left femur
[7th] S72.366 Nondisplaced segmental fracture of shaft of unspecified femur

[6th] S72.39 Other fracture of shaft of femur
[7th] S72.391 Other fracture of shaft of right femur
[7th] S72.392 Other fracture of shaft of left femur
[7th] S72.399 Other fracture of shaft of unspecified femur

[5th] S72.4 Fracture of lower end of femur

Fracture of distal end of femur

[EXCLUDES2] *fracture of shaft of femur (S72.3-)*
physeal fracture of lower end of femur (S79.1-)

[6th] S72.40 Unspecified fracture of lower end of femur
[7th] S72.401 Unspecified fracture of lower end of right femur
[7th] S72.402 Unspecified fracture of lower end of left femur
[7th] S72.409 Unspecified fracture of lower end of unspecified femur

[6th] S72.41 Unspecified condyle fracture of lower end of femur

Condyle fracture of femur NOS

[7th] S72.411 Displaced unspecified condyle fracture of lower end of right femur
[7th] S72.412 Displaced unspecified condyle fracture of lower end of left femur
[7th] S72.413 Displaced unspecified condyle fracture of lower end of unspecified femur
[7th] S72.414 Nondisplaced unspecified condyle fracture of lower end of right femur
[7th] S72.415 Nondisplaced unspecified condyle fracture of lower end of left femur
[7th] S72.416 Nondisplaced unspecified condyle fracture of lower end of unspecified femur

[6th] S72.42 Fracture of lateral condyle of femur
[7th] S72.421 Displaced fracture of lateral condyle of right femur
[7th] S72.422 Displaced fracture of lateral condyle of left femur
[7th] S72.423 Displaced fracture of lateral condyle of unspecified femur
[7th] S72.424 Nondisplaced fracture of lateral condyle of right femur
[7th] S72.425 Nondisplaced fracture of lateral condyle of left femur
[7th] S72.426 Nondisplaced fracture of lateral condyle of unspecified femur

[6th] S72.43 Fracture of medial condyle of femur
[7th] S72.431 Displaced fracture of medial condyle of right femur
[7th] S72.432 Displaced fracture of medial condyle of left femur
[7th] S72.433 Displaced fracture of medial condyle of unspecified femur
[7th] S72.434 Nondisplaced fracture of medial condyle of right femur
[7th] S72.435 Nondisplaced fracture of medial condyle of left femur
[7th] S72.436 Nondisplaced fracture of medial condyle of unspecified femur

[6th] S72.44 Fracture of lower epiphysis (separation) of femur

[EXCLUDES1] *Salter-Harris Type I physeal fracture of lower end of femur (S79.11-)*

[7th] S72.441 Displaced fracture of lower epiphysis (separation) of right femur
[7th] S72.442 Displaced fracture of lower epiphysis (separation) of left femur
[7th] S72.443 Displaced fracture of lower epiphysis (separation) of unspecified femur
[7th] S72.444 Nondisplaced fracture of lower epiphysis (separation) of right femur
[7th] S72.445 Nondisplaced fracture of lower epiphysis (separation) of left femur
[7th] S72.446 Nondisplaced fracture of lower epiphysis (separation) of unspecified femur

[6th] S72.45 Supracondylar fracture without intracondylar extension of lower end of femur

Supracondylar fracture of lower end of femur NOS

[EXCLUDES1] *supracondylar fracture with intracondylar extension of lower end of femur (S72.46-)*

[7th] S72.451 Displaced supracondylar fracture without intracondylar extension of lower end of right femur
[7th] S72.452 Displaced supracondylar fracture without intracondylar extension of lower end of left femur
[7th] S72.453 Displaced supracondylar fracture without intracondylar extension of lower end of unspecified femur

[4th] 4th character required [5th] 5th character required [6th] 6th character required [7th] 7th character required [X] Extension 'X' Alert
[EXCLUDES1] Not coded here [EXCLUDES2] Not included here [PDx] Primary Diagnosis Only Manifestation Code

7️⃣ **S72.454** Nondisplaced **supracondylar fracture without intracondylar extension of lower end of** right **femur**

7️⃣ **S72.455** Nondisplaced **supracondylar fracture without intracondylar extension of lower end of** left **femur**

7️⃣ **S72.456** Nondisplaced **supracondylar fracture without intracondylar extension of lower end of unspecified femur**

6️⃣ **S72.46** Supracondylar **fracture with intracondylar extension of lower end of femur**

> EXCLUDES1 *supracondylar fracture without intracondylar extension of lower end of femur (S72.45-)*

7️⃣ **S72.461** Displaced **supracondylar fracture with intracondylar extension of lower end of** right **femur**

7️⃣ **S72.462** Displaced **supracondylar fracture with intracondylar extension of lower end of** left **femur**

7️⃣ **S72.463** Displaced **supracondylar fracture with intracondylar extension of lower end of unspecified femur**

7️⃣ **S72.464** Nondisplaced **supracondylar fracture with intracondylar extension of lower end of** right **femur**

7️⃣ **S72.465** Nondisplaced **supracondylar fracture with intracondylar extension of lower end of** left **femur**

7️⃣ **S72.466** Nondisplaced **supracondylar fracture with intracondylar extension of lower end of unspecified femur**

6️⃣ **S72.47** Torus **fracture of lower end of femur**

The appropriate 7th character is to be added to all codes in subcategory S72.47
A = initial encounter for closed fracture
D = subsequent encounter for fracture with routine healing
G = subsequent encounter for fracture with delayed healing
K = subsequent encounter for fracture with nonunion
P = subsequent encounter for fracture with malunion
S = sequela

7️⃣ **S72.471** Torus fracture of lower end of right **femur**
7️⃣ **S72.472** Torus fracture of lower end of left **femur**
7️⃣ **S72.479** Torus fracture of lower end of unspecified **femur**

6️⃣ **S72.49** Other **fracture of lower end of femur**
7️⃣ **S72.491** Other fracture of lower end of right **femur**
7️⃣ **S72.492** Other fracture of lower end of left **femur**
7️⃣ **S72.499** Other fracture of lower end of unspecified **femur**

5️⃣ **S72.8** Other fracture of femur
6️⃣ **S72.8X** Other fracture of femur
7️⃣ **S72.8X1** Other fracture of right **femur**
7️⃣ **S72.8X2** Other fracture of left **femur**
7️⃣ **S72.8X9** Other fracture of unspecified **femur**

5️⃣ **S72.9** Unspecified fracture of femur
Fracture of thigh NOS
Fracture of upper leg NOS

> EXCLUDES1 *fracture of hip NOS (S72.00-, S72.01-)*

7️⃣ **S72.90** Unspecified fracture of unspecified femur
7️⃣ **S72.91** Unspecified fracture of right **femur**
7️⃣ **S72.92** Unspecified fracture of left **femur**

4️⃣ **S73** Dislocation and sprain of joint and ligaments of hip

> INCLUDES *avulsion of joint or ligament of hip*
> *laceration of cartilage, joint or ligament of hip*
> *sprain of cartilage, joint or ligament of hip*
> *traumatic hemarthrosis of joint or ligament of*

hip
traumatic rupture of joint or ligament of hip
traumatic subluxation of joint or ligament of hip
traumatic tear of joint or ligament of hip

Code also any associated open wound

> EXCLUDES2 *strain of muscle, fascia and tendon of hip and thigh (S76.-)*

The appropriate 7th character is to be added to each code from category S73
A = initial encounter
D = subsequent encounter
S = sequela

5️⃣ **S73.0** Subluxation and dislocation of hip

> EXCLUDES2 *dislocation and subluxation of hip prosthesis (T84.020, T84.021)*

6️⃣ **S73.00** Unspecified **subluxation and dislocation of hip**
Dislocation of hip NOS
Subluxation of hip NOS
7️⃣ **S73.001** Unspecified subluxation of right **hip**
7️⃣ **S73.002** Unspecified subluxation of left **hip**
7️⃣ **S73.003** Unspecified subluxation of unspecified **hip**
7️⃣ **S73.004** Unspecified dislocation of right **hip**
7️⃣ **S73.005** Unspecified dislocation of left **hip**
7️⃣ **S73.006** Unspecified dislocation of unspecified **hip**

6️⃣ **S73.01** Posterior **subluxation and dislocation of hip**
7️⃣ **S73.011** Posterior subluxation of right **hip**
7️⃣ **S73.012** Posterior subluxation of left **hip**
7️⃣ **S73.013** Posterior subluxation of unspecified **hip**
7️⃣ **S73.014** Posterior dislocation of right **hip**
7️⃣ **S73.015** Posterior dislocation of left **hip**
7️⃣ **S73.016** Posterior dislocation of unspecified **hip**

6️⃣ **S73.02** Obturator **subluxation and dislocation of hip**
7️⃣ **S73.021** Obturator subluxation of right **hip**
7️⃣ **S73.022** Obturator subluxation of left **hip**
7️⃣ **S73.023** Obturator subluxation of unspecified **hip**
7️⃣ **S73.024** Obturator dislocation of right **hip**
7️⃣ **S73.025** Obturator dislocation of left **hip**
7️⃣ **S73.026** Obturator dislocation of unspecified **hip**

6️⃣ **S73.03** Other anterior **dislocation of hip**
7️⃣ **S73.031** Other anterior subluxation of right **hip**
7️⃣ **S73.032** Other anterior subluxation of left **hip**
7️⃣ **S73.033** Other anterior subluxation of unspecified **hip**
7️⃣ **S73.034** Other anterior dislocation of right **hip**
7️⃣ **S73.035** Other anterior dislocation of left **hip**
7️⃣ **S73.036** Other anterior dislocation of unspecified **hip**

6️⃣ **S73.04** Central **dislocation of hip**
7️⃣ **S73.041** Central subluxation of right **hip**
7️⃣ **S73.042** Central subluxation of left **hip**
7️⃣ **S73.043** Central subluxation of unspecified **hip**
7️⃣ **S73.044** Central dislocation of right **hip**
7️⃣ **S73.045** Central dislocation of left **hip**
7️⃣ **S73.046** Central dislocation of unspecified **hip**

5️⃣ **S73.1** Sprain of hip
6️⃣ **S73.10** Unspecified **sprain of hip**
7️⃣ **S73.101** Unspecified sprain of right **hip**
7️⃣ **S73.102** Unspecified sprain of left **hip**
7️⃣ **S73.109** Unspecified sprain of unspecified **hip**

6️⃣ **S73.11** Iliofemoral ligament **sprain of hip**
7️⃣ **S73.111** Iliofemoral ligament sprain of right **hip**
7️⃣ **S73.112** Iliofemoral ligament sprain of left **hip**
7️⃣ **S73.119** Iliofemoral ligament sprain of unspecified **hip**

6️⃣ **S73.12** Ischiocapsular **(ligament) sprain of hip**
7️⃣ **S73.121** Ischiocapsular ligament sprain of right **hip**
7️⃣ **S73.122** Ischiocapsular ligament sprain of left **hip**

Unspecified Code	Other Specified Code	N Newborn Age: 0	P Pediatric Age: 0-17	M Maternity Age: 12-55
A Adult Age: 15-124	♂ Male	♀ Female	● New Code	▲ Revised Code Title ▶◀ Revised Text

       7ᵗʰ **S73.129** **Ischiocapsular ligament sprain of unspecified hip**

     6ᵗʰ **S73.19** Other **sprain of hip**

       7ᵗʰ **S73.191** **Other sprain of** right **hip**

       7ᵗʰ **S73.192** **Other sprain of** left **hip**

       7ᵗʰ **S73.199** **Other sprain of unspecified hip**

4ᵗʰ **S74** **Injury of nerves at hip and thigh level**

     Code also any associated open wound (S71.-)

     EXCLUDES2 *injury of nerves at ankle and foot level (S94.-)*
              injury of nerves at lower leg level (S84.-)

     The appropriate 7th character is to be added to each code from category S74
     A = initial encounter
     D = subsequent encounter
     S = sequela

    5ᵗʰ **S74.0** **Injury of** sciatic nerve **at hip and thigh level**

     7ᵗʰ **S74.00** **Injury of sciatic nerve at hip and thigh level, unspecified leg**

     7ᵗʰ **S74.01** **Injury of sciatic nerve at hip and thigh level,** right **leg**

     7ᵗʰ **S74.02** **Injury of sciatic nerve at hip and thigh level,** left **leg**

    5ᵗʰ **S74.1** **Injury of** femoral nerve **at hip and thigh level**

     7ᵗʰ **S74.10** **Injury of femoral nerve at hip and thigh level, unspecified leg**

     7ᵗʰ **S74.11** **Injury of femoral nerve at hip and thigh level,** right **leg**

     7ᵗʰ **S74.12** **Injury of femoral nerve at hip and thigh level,** left **leg**

    5ᵗʰ **S74.2** **Injury of** cutaneous sensory nerve **at hip and thigh level**

     7ᵗʰ **S74.20** **Injury of cutaneous sensory nerve at hip and thigh level, unspecified leg**

     7ᵗʰ **S74.21** **Injury of cutaneous sensory nerve at hip and high level,** right **leg**

     7ᵗʰ **S74.22** **Injury of cutaneous sensory nerve at hip and thigh level,** left **leg**

    5ᵗʰ **S74.8** **Injury of** other nerves **at hip and thigh level**

     6ᵗʰ **S74.8X** **Injury of other nerves at hip and thigh level**

       7ᵗʰ **S74.8X1** **Injury of other nerves at hip and thigh level,** right **leg**

       7ᵗʰ **S74.8X2** **Injury of other nerves at hip and thigh level,** left **leg**

       7ᵗʰ **S74.8X9** **Injury of other nerves at hip and thigh level, unspecified leg**

    5ᵗʰ **S74.9** **Injury of** unspecified nerve **at hip and thigh level**

     7ᵗʰ **S74.90** **Injury of unspecified nerve at hip and thigh level, unspecified leg**

     7ᵗʰ **S74.91** **Injury of unspecified nerve at hip and thigh level,** right **leg**

     7ᵗʰ **S74.92** **Injury of unspecified nerve at hip and thigh level,** left **leg**

4ᵗʰ **S75** **Injury of blood vessels at hip and thigh level**

     Code also any associated open wound (S71.-)

     EXCLUDES2 *injury of blood vessels at lower leg level (S85.-)*
              injury of popliteal artery (S85.0)

     The appropriate 7th character is to be added to each code from category S75
     A = initial encounter
     D = subsequent encounter
     S = sequela

    5ᵗʰ **S75.0** **Injury of** femoral artery

     6ᵗʰ **S75.00** Unspecified **injury of femoral artery**

       7ᵗʰ **S75.001** **Unspecified injury of femoral artery,** right **leg**

       7ᵗʰ **S75.002** **Unspecified injury of femoral artery,** left **leg**

       7ᵗʰ **S75.009** **Unspecified injury of femoral artery, unspecified leg**

     6ᵗʰ **S75.01** Minor laceration **of femoral artery**

       Incomplete transection of femoral artery
       Laceration of femoral artery NOS
       Superficial laceration of femoral artery

       7ᵗʰ **S75.011** **Minor laceration of femoral artery,** right **leg**

       7ᵗʰ **S75.012** **Minor laceration of femoral artery,** left **leg**

       7ᵗʰ **S75.019** **Minor laceration of femoral artery, unspecified leg**

     6ᵗʰ **S75.02** Major laceration **of femoral artery**

       Complete transection of femoral artery
       Traumatic rupture of femoral artery

       7ᵗʰ **S75.021** **Major laceration of femoral artery,** right **leg**

       7ᵗʰ **S75.022** **Major laceration of femoral artery,** left **leg**

       7ᵗʰ **S75.029** **Major laceration of femoral artery, unspecified leg**

     6ᵗʰ **S75.09** Other **specified injury of femoral artery**

       7ᵗʰ **S75.091** **Other specified injury of femoral artery,** right **leg**

       7ᵗʰ **S75.092** **Other specified injury of femoral artery,** left **leg**

       7ᵗʰ **S75.099** **Other specified injury of femoral artery, unspecified leg**

    5ᵗʰ **S75.1** **Injury of** femoral vein **at hip and thigh level**

     6ᵗʰ **S75.10** Unspecified **injury of femoral vein at hip and thigh level**

       7ᵗʰ **S75.101** **Unspecified injury of femoral vein at hip and thigh level,** right **leg**

       7ᵗʰ **S75.102** **Unspecified injury of femoral vein at hip and thigh level,** left **leg**

       7ᵗʰ **S75.109** **Unspecified injury of femoral vein at hip and thigh level, unspecified leg**

     6ᵗʰ **S75.11** Minor laceration **of femoral vein at hip and thigh level**

       Incomplete transection of femoral vein at hip and thigh level
       Laceration of femoral vein at hip and thigh level NOS
       Superficial laceration of femoral vein at hip and thigh level

       7ᵗʰ **S75.111** **Minor laceration of femoral vein at hip and thigh level,** right **leg**

       7ᵗʰ **S75.112** **Minor laceration of femoral vein at hip and thigh level,** left **leg**

       7ᵗʰ **S75.119** **Minor laceration of femoral vein at hip and thigh level, unspecified leg**

     6ᵗʰ **S75.12** Major laceration **of femoral vein at hip and thigh level**

       Complete transection of femoral vein at hip and thigh level
       Traumatic rupture of femoral vein at hip and thigh level

       7ᵗʰ **S75.121** **Major laceration of femoral vein at hip and thigh level,** right **leg**

       7ᵗʰ **S75.122** **Major laceration of femoral vein at hip and thigh level,** left **leg**

       7ᵗʰ **S75.129** **Major laceration of femoral vein at hip and thigh level, unspecified leg**

     6ᵗʰ **S75.19** Other **specified injury of femoral vein at hip and thigh level**

       7ᵗʰ **S75.191** **Other specified injury of femoral vein at hip and thigh level,** right **leg**

       7ᵗʰ **S75.192** **Other specified injury of femoral vein at hip and thigh level,** left **leg**

       7ᵗʰ **S75.199** **Other specified injury of femoral vein at hip and thigh level, unspecified leg**

    5ᵗʰ **S75.2** **Injury of** greater saphenous vein **at hip and thigh level**

     EXCLUDES1 *greater saphenous vein NOS (S85.3)*

     6ᵗʰ **S75.20** Unspecified **injury of greater saphenous vein at hip and thigh level**

     4ᵗʰ 4ᵗʰ character required   5ᵗʰ 5ᵗʰ character required   6ᵗʰ 6ᵗʰ character required   7ᵗʰ 7ᵗʰ character required   7ᵗʰ Extension 'X' Alert

     EXCLUDES 1 Not coded here   EXCLUDES 2 Not included here   PDx Primary Diagnosis Only   Manifestation Code

7ᵗʰ **S75.201** Unspecified injury of greater saphenous vein at hip and thigh level, right leg

7ᵗʰ **S75.202** Unspecified injury of greater saphenous vein at hip and thigh level, left leg

7ᵗʰ **S75.209** Unspecified injury of greater saphenous vein at hip and thigh level, unspecified leg

6ᵗʰ **S75.21** Minor laceration of greater saphenous vein at hip and thigh level

Incomplete transection of greater saphenous vein at hip and thigh level

Laceration of greater saphenous vein at hip and thigh level NOS

Superficial laceration of greater saphenous vein at hip and thigh level

7ᵗʰ **S75.211** Minor laceration of greater saphenous vein at hip and thigh level, right leg

7ᵗʰ **S75.212** Minor laceration of greater saphenous vein at hip and thigh level, left leg

7ᵗʰ **S75.219** Minor laceration of greater saphenous vein at hip and thigh level, unspecified leg

6ᵗʰ **S75.22** Major laceration of greater saphenous vein at hip and thigh level

Complete transection of greater saphenous vein at hip and thigh level

Traumatic rupture of greater saphenous vein at hip and thigh level

7ᵗʰ **S75.221** Major laceration of greater saphenous vein at hip and thigh level, right leg

7ᵗʰ **S75.222** Major laceration of greater saphenous vein at hip and thigh level, left leg

7ᵗʰ **S75.229** Major laceration of greater saphenous vein at hip and thigh level, unspecified leg

6ᵗʰ **S75.29** Other specified injury of greater saphenous vein at hip and thigh level

7ᵗʰ **S75.291** Other specified injury of greater saphenous vein at hip and thigh level, right leg

7ᵗʰ **S75.292** Other specified injury of greater saphenous vein at hip and thigh level, left leg

7ᵗʰ **S75.299** Other specified injury of greater saphenous vein at hip and thigh level, unspecified leg

5ᵗʰ **S75.8** Injury of other blood vessels at hip and thigh level

6ᵗʰ **S75.80** Unspecified injury of other blood vessels at hip and thigh level

7ᵗʰ **S75.801** Unspecified injury of other blood vessels at hip and thigh level, right leg

7ᵗʰ **S75.802** Unspecified injury of other blood vessels at hip and thigh level, left leg

7ᵗʰ **S75.809** Unspecified injury of other blood vessels at hip and thigh level, unspecified leg

6ᵗʰ **S75.81** Laceration of other blood vessels at hip and thigh level

7ᵗʰ **S75.811** Laceration of other blood vessels at hip and thigh level, right leg

7ᵗʰ **S75.812** Laceration of other blood vessels at hip and thigh level, left leg

7ᵗʰ **S75.819** Laceration of other blood vessels at hip and thigh level, unspecified leg

6ᵗʰ **S75.89** Other specified injury of other blood vessels at hip and thigh level

7ᵗʰ **S75.891** Other specified injury of other blood vessels at hip and thigh level, right leg

7ᵗʰ **S75.892** Other specified injury of other blood vessels at hip and thigh level, left leg

7ᵗʰ **S75.899** Other specified injury of other blood vessels at hip and thigh level, unspecified leg

5ᵗʰ **S75.9** Injury of unspecified blood vessel at hip and thigh level

6ᵗʰ **S75.90** Unspecified injury of unspecified blood vessel at hip and thigh level

7ᵗʰ **S75.901** Unspecified injury of unspecified blood vessel at hip and thigh level, right leg

7ᵗʰ **S75.902** Unspecified injury of unspecified blood vessel at hip and thigh level, left leg

7ᵗʰ **S75.909** Unspecified injury of unspecified blood vessel at hip and thigh level, unspecified leg

6ᵗʰ **S75.91** Laceration of unspecified blood vessel at hip and thigh level

7ᵗʰ **S75.911** Laceration of unspecified blood vessel at hip and thigh level, right leg

7ᵗʰ **S75.912** Laceration of unspecified blood vessel at hip and thigh level, left leg

7ᵗʰ **S75.919** Laceration of unspecified blood vessel at hip and thigh level, unspecified leg

6ᵗʰ **S75.99** Other specified injury of unspecified blood vessel at hip and thigh level

7ᵗʰ **S75.991** Other specified injury of unspecified blood vessel at hip and thigh level, right leg

7ᵗʰ **S75.992** Other specified injury of unspecified blood vessel at hip and thigh level, left leg

7ᵗʰ **S75.999** Other specified injury of unspecified blood vessel at hip and thigh level, unspecified leg

4ᵗʰ **S76** Injury of muscle, fascia and tendon at hip and thigh level

Code also any associated open wound (S71.-)

EXCLUDES2 injury of muscle, fascia and tendon at lower leg level (S86)
sprain of joint and ligament of hip (S73.1)

The appropriate 7th character is to be added to each code from category S76
A = initial encounter
D = subsequent encounter
S = sequela

5ᵗʰ **S76.0** Injury of muscle, fascia and tendon of hip

6ᵗʰ **S76.00** Unspecified injury of muscle, fascia and tendon of hip

7ᵗʰ **S76.001** Unspecified injury of muscle, fascia and tendon of right hip

7ᵗʰ **S76.002** Unspecified injury of muscle, fascia and tendon of left hip

7ᵗʰ **S76.009** Unspecified injury of muscle, fascia and tendon of unspecified hip

6ᵗʰ **S76.01** Strain of muscle, fascia and tendon of hip

7ᵗʰ **S76.011** Strain of muscle, fascia and tendon of right hip

7ᵗʰ **S76.012** Strain of muscle, fascia and tendon of left hip

7ᵗʰ **S76.019** Strain of muscle, fascia and tendon of unspecified hip

6ᵗʰ **S76.02** Laceration of muscle, fascia and tendon of hip

7ᵗʰ **S76.021** Laceration of muscle, fascia and tendon of right hip

7ᵗʰ **S76.022** Laceration of muscle, fascia and tendon of left hip

7ᵗʰ **S76.029** Laceration of muscle, fascia and tendon of unspecified hip

6ᵗʰ **S76.09** Other specified injury of muscle, fascia and tendon of hip

7ᵗʰ **S76.091** Other specified injury of muscle, fascia and tendon of right hip

7ᵗʰ **S76.092** Other specified injury of muscle, fascia and tendon of left hip

7ᵗʰ **S76.099** Other specified injury of muscle, fascia and tendon of unspecified hip

5ᵗʰ **S76.1** Injury of quadriceps muscle, fascia and tendon

Injury of patellar ligament (tendon)

6ᵗʰ **S76.10** Unspecified injury of quadriceps muscle, fascia and tendon

7ᵗʰ **S76.101** Unspecified injury of right quadriceps muscle, fascia and tendon

Unspecified Code | Other Specified Code | N Newborn Age: 0 | P Pediatric Age: 0-17 | M Maternity Age: 12-55
A Adult Age: 15-124 | ♂ Male | ♀ Female | ● New Code | ▲ Revised Code Title | ►◄ Revised Text

[7th] S76.102 Unspecified injury of left quadriceps muscle, fascia and tendon
[7th] S76.109 Unspecified injury of unspecified quadriceps muscle, fascia and tendon
[6th] S76.11 Strain of quadriceps muscle, fascia and tendon
[7th] S76.111 Strain of right quadriceps muscle, fascia and tendon
[7th] S76.112 Strain of left quadriceps muscle, fascia and tendon
[7th] S76.119 Strain of unspecified quadriceps muscle, fascia and tendon
[6th] S76.12 Laceration of quadriceps muscle, fascia and tendon
[7th] S76.121 Laceration of right quadriceps muscle, fascia and tendon
[7th] S76.122 Laceration of left quadriceps muscle, fascia and tendon
[7th] S76.129 Laceration of unspecified quadriceps muscle, fascia and tendon
[6th] S76.19 Other specified injury of quadriceps muscle, fascia and tendon
[7th] S76.191 Other specified injury of right quadriceps muscle, fascia and tendon
[7th] S76.192 Other specified injury of left quadriceps muscle, fascia and tendon
[7th] S76.199 Other specified injury of unspecified quadriceps muscle, fascia and tendon
[5th] S76.2 Injury of adductor muscle, fascia and tendon of thigh
[6th] S76.20 Unspecified injury of adductor muscle, fascia and tendon of thigh
[7th] S76.201 Unspecified injury of adductor muscle, fascia and tendon of right thigh
[7th] S76.202 Unspecified injury of adductor muscle, fascia and tendon of left thigh
[7th] S76.209 Unspecified injury of adductor muscle, fascia and tendon of unspecified thigh
[6th] S76.21 Strain of adductor muscle, fascia and tendon of thigh
[7th] S76.211 Strain of adductor muscle, fascia and tendon of right thigh
[7th] S76.212 Strain of adductor muscle, fascia and tendon of left thigh
[7th] S76.219 Strain of adductor muscle, fascia and tendon of unspecified thigh
[6th] S76.22 Laceration of adductor muscle, fascia and tendon of thigh
[7th] S76.221 Laceration of adductor muscle, fascia and tendon of right thigh
[7th] S76.222 Laceration of adductor muscle, fascia and tendon of left thigh
[7th] S76.229 Laceration of adductor muscle, fascia and tendon of unspecified thigh
[6th] S76.29 Other injury of adductor muscle, fascia and tendon of thigh
[7th] S76.291 Other injury of adductor muscle, fascia and tendon of right thigh
[7th] S76.292 Other injury of adductor muscle, fascia and tendon of left thigh
[7th] S76.299 Other injury of adductor muscle, fascia and tendon of unspecified thigh
[5th] S76.3 Injury of muscle, fascia and tendon of the posterior muscle group at thigh level
[6th] S76.30 Unspecified injury of muscle, fascia and tendon of the posterior muscle group at thigh level
[7th] S76.301 Unspecified injury of muscle, fascia and tendon of the posterior muscle group at thigh level, right thigh
[7th] S76.302 Unspecified injury of muscle, fascia and tendon of the posterior muscle group at thigh level, left thigh
[7th] S76.309 Unspecified injury of muscle, fascia and tendon of the posterior muscle group at thigh level, unspecified thigh
[6th] S76.31 Strain of muscle, fascia and tendon of the posterior muscle group at thigh level
[7th] S76.311 Strain of muscle, fascia and tendon of the posterior muscle group at thigh level, right thigh
[7th] S76.312 Strain of muscle, fascia and tendon of the posterior muscle group at thigh level, left thigh
[7th] S76.319 Strain of muscle, fascia and tendon of the posterior muscle group at thigh level, unspecified thigh
[6th] S76.32 Laceration of muscle, fascia and tendon of the posterior muscle group at thigh level
[7th] S76.321 Laceration of muscle, fascia and tendon of the posterior muscle group at thigh level, right thigh
[7th] S76.322 Laceration of muscle, fascia and tendon of the posterior muscle group at thigh level, left thigh
[7th] S76.329 Laceration of muscle, fascia and tendon of the posterior muscle group at thigh level, unspecified thigh
[6th] S76.39 Other specified injury of muscle, fascia and tendon of the posterior muscle group at thigh level
[7th] S76.391 Other specified injury of muscle, fascia and tendon of the posterior muscle group at thigh level, right thigh
[7th] S76.392 Other specified injury of muscle, fascia and tendon of the posterior muscle group at thigh level, left thigh
[7th] S76.399 Other specified injury of muscle, fascia and tendon of the posterior muscle group at thigh level, unspecified thigh
[5th] S76.8 Injury of other specified muscles, fascia and tendons at thigh level
[6th] S76.80 Unspecified injury of other specified muscles, fascia and tendons at thigh level
[7th] S76.801 Unspecified injury of other specified muscles, fascia and tendons at thigh level, right thigh
[7th] S76.802 Unspecified injury of other specified muscles, fascia and tendons at thigh level, left thigh
[7th] S76.809 Unspecified injury of other specified muscles, fascia and tendons at thigh level, unspecified thigh
[6th] S76.81 Strain of other specified muscles, fascia and tendons at thigh level
[7th] S76.811 Strain of other specified muscles, fascia and tendons at thigh level, right thigh
[7th] S76.812 Strain of other specified muscles, fascia and tendons at thigh level, left thigh
[7th] S76.819 Strain of other specified muscles, fascia and tendons at thigh level, unspecified thigh
[6th] S76.82 Laceration of other specified muscles, fascia and tendons at thigh level
[7th] S76.821 Laceration of other specified muscles, fascia and tendons at thigh level, right thigh
[7th] S76.822 Laceration of other specified muscles, fascia and tendons at thigh level, left thigh
[7th] S76.829 Laceration of other specified muscles, fascia and tendons at thigh level, unspecified thigh

[4] 4th character required [5] 5th character required [6] 6th character required [7] 7th character required [7th] Extension 'X' Alert
EXCLUDES 1 Not coded here EXCLUDES 2 Not included here [PDx] Primary Diagnosis Only Manifestation Code

S76.89 Other injury of other specified muscles, fascia and tendons at thigh level

S76.891 Other injury of other specified muscles, fascia and tendons at thigh level, right thigh

S76.892 Other injury of other specified muscles, fascia and tendons at thigh level, left thigh

S76.899 Other injury of other specified muscles, fasciaandtendonsatthighlevel,unspecifiedthigh

S76.9 Injury of unspecified muscles, fascia and tendons at thigh level

S76.90 Unspecified injury of unspecified muscles, fascia and tendons at thigh level

S76.901 Unspecified injury of unspecified muscles, fascia and tendons at thigh level, right thigh

S76.902 Unspecified injury of unspecified muscles, fascia and tendons at thigh level, left thigh

S76.909 Unspecified injury of unspecified muscles, fascia and tendons at thigh level, unspecified thigh

S76.91 Strain of unspecified muscles, fascia and tendons at thigh level

S76.911 Strain of unspecified muscles, fascia and tendons at thigh level, right thigh

S76.912 Strain of unspecified muscles, fascia and tendons at thigh level, left thigh

S76.919 Strain of unspecified muscles, fascia and tendons at thigh level, unspecified thigh

S76.92 Laceration of unspecified muscles, fascia and tendons at thigh level

S76.921 Laceration of unspecified muscles, fascia and tendons at thigh level, right thigh

S76.922 Laceration of unspecified muscles, fascia and tendons at thigh level, left thigh

S76.929 Laceration of unspecified muscles, fascia and tendons at thigh level, unspecified thigh

S76.99 Other specified injury of unspecified muscles, fascia and tendons at thigh level

S76.991 Other specified injury of unspecified muscles, fascia and tendons at thigh level, right thigh

S76.992 Other specified injury of unspecified muscles, fascia and tendons at thigh level, left thigh

S76.999 Other specified injury of unspecified muscles, fascia and tendons at thigh level, unspecified thigh

S77 Crushing injury of hip and thigh

Use additional code(s) for all associated injuries

EXCLUDES2 crushing injury of ankle and foot (S97.-)
crushing injury of lower leg (S87.-)

The appropriate 7th character is to be added to each code from category S77

A = initial encounter
D = subsequent encounter
S = sequela

S77.0 Crushing injury of hip

S77.00 Crushing injury of unspecified hip

S77.01 Crushing injury of right hip

S77.02 Crushing injury of left hip

S77.1 Crushing injury of thigh

S77.10 Crushing injury of unspecified thigh

S77.11 Crushing injury of right thigh

S77.12 Crushing injury of left thigh

S77.2 Crushing injury of hip with thigh

S77.20 Crushing injury of unspecified hip with thigh

S77.21 Crushing injury of right hip with thigh

S77.22 Crushing injury of left hip with thigh

S78 Traumatic amputation of hip and thigh

An amputation not identified as partial or complete should be coded to complete

EXCLUDES1 traumatic amputation of knee (S88.0-)

The appropriate 7th character is to be added to each code from category S78

A = initial encounter
D = subsequent encounter
S = sequela

S78.0 Traumatic amputation at hip joint

S78.01 Complete traumatic amputation at hip joint

S78.011 Complete traumatic amputation at right hip joint

S78.012 Complete traumatic amputation at left hip joint

S78.019 Complete traumatic amputation at unspecified hip joint

S78.02 Partial traumatic amputation at hip joint

S78.021 Partial traumatic amputation at right hip joint

S78.022 Partial traumatic amputation at left hip joint

S78.029 Partial traumatic amputation at unspecified hip joint

S78.1 Traumatic amputation at level between hip and knee

EXCLUDES1 traumatic amputation of knee (S88.0-)

S78.11 Complete traumatic amputation at level between hip and knee

S78.111 Complete traumatic amputation at level between right hip and knee

S78.112 Complete traumatic amputation at level between left hip and knee

S78.119 Complete traumatic amputation at level between unspecified hip and knee

S78.12 Partial traumatic amputation at level between hip and knee

S78.121 Partial traumatic amputation at level between right hip and knee

S78.122 Partial traumatic amputation at level between left hip and knee

S78.129 Partial traumatic amputation at level between unspecified hip and knee

S78.9 Traumatic amputation of hip and thigh, level unspecified

S78.91 Complete traumatic amputation of hip and thigh, level unspecified

S78.911 Complete traumatic amputation of right hip and thigh, level unspecified

S78.912 Complete traumatic amputation of left hip and thigh, level unspecified

S78.919 Complete traumatic amputation of unspecified hip and thigh, level unspecified

S78.92 Partial traumatic amputation of hip and thigh, level unspecified

S78.921 Partial traumatic amputation of right hip and thigh, level unspecified

S78.922 Partial traumatic amputation of left hip and thigh, level unspecified

S78.929 Partial traumatic amputation of unspecified hip and thigh, level unspecified

S79 Other and unspecified injuries of hip and thigh

NOTES A fracture not indicated as open or closed should be coded to closed

The appropriate 7th character is to be added to each code from subcategories S79.0 and S79.1

A = initial encounter for closed fracture
D = subsequent encounter for fracture with routine healing
G = subsequent encounter for fracture with delayed healing
K = subsequent encounter for fracture with nonunion
P = subsequent encounter for fracture with malunion
S = sequela

S79.0 Physeal fracture of upper end of femur

Unspecified Code	Other Specified Code	N Newborn Age: 0	P Pediatric Age: 0-17	M Maternity Age: 12-55

A Adult Age: 15-124   ♂ Male   ♀ Female   ● New Code   ▲ Revised Code Title   ►◄ Revised Text

[EXCLUDES1] *apophyseal fracture of upper end of femur (S72.13-)*
nontraumatic slipped upper femoral epiphysis (M93.0-)

[6th] **S79.00 Unspecified physeal fracture of upper end of femur**
- [7th] **S79.001 Unspecified physeal fracture of upper end of right femur**
- [7th] **S79.002 Unspecified physeal fracture of upper end of left femur**
- [7th] **S79.009 Unspecified physeal fracture of upper end of unspecified femur**

[6th] **S79.01 Salter-Harris Type I physeal fracture of upper end of femur**

Acute on chronic slipped capital femoral epiphysis (traumatic)
Acute slipped capital femoral epiphysis (traumatic)
Capital femoral epiphyseal fracture

[EXCLUDES1] *chronic slipped upper femoral epiphysis (nontraumatic) (M93.02-)*

- [7th] **S79.011 Salter-Harris Type I physeal fracture of upper end of right femur**
- [7th] **S79.012 Salter-Harris Type I physeal fracture of upper end of left femur**
- [7th] **S79.019 Salter-Harris Type I physeal fracture of upper end of unspecified femur**

[6th] **S79.09 Other physeal fracture of upper end of femur**
- [7th] **S79.091 Other physeal fracture of upper end of right femur**
- [7th] **S79.092 Other physeal fracture of upper end of left femur**
- [7th] **S79.099 Other physeal fracture of upper end of unspecified femur**

[5th] **S79.1 Physeal fracture of lower end of femur**

[6th] **S79.10 Unspecified physeal fracture of lower end of femur**
- [7th] **S79.101 Unspecified physeal fracture of lower end of right femur**
- [7th] **S79.102 Unspecified physeal fracture of lower end of left femur**
- [7th] **S79.109 Unspecified physeal fracture of lower end of unspecified femur**

[6th] **S79.11 Salter-Harris Type I physeal fracture of lower end of femur**
- [7th] **S79.111 Salter-Harris Type I physeal fracture of lower end of right femur**
- [7th] **S79.112 Salter-Harris Type I physeal fracture of lower end of left femur**
- [7th] **S79.119 Salter-Harris Type I physeal fracture of lower end of unspecified femur**

[6th] **S79.12 Salter-Harris Type II physeal fracture of lower end of femur**
- [7th] **S79.121 Salter-Harris Type II physeal fracture of lower end of right femur**
- [7th] **S79.122 Salter-Harris Type II physeal fracture of lower end of left femur**
- [7th] **S79.129 Salter-Harris Type II physeal fracture of lower end of unspecified femur**

[6th] **S79.13 Salter-Harris Type III physeal fracture of lower end of femur**
- [7th] **S79.131 Salter-Harris Type III physeal fracture of lower end of right femur**
- [7th] **S79.132 Salter-Harris Type III physeal fracture of lower end of left femur**
- [7th] **S79.139 Salter-Harris Type III physeal fracture of lower end of unspecified femur**

[6th] **S79.14 Salter-Harris Type IV physeal fracture of lower end of femur**
- [7th] **S79.141 Salter-Harris Type IV physeal fracture of lower end of right femur**
- [7th] **S79.142 Salter-Harris Type IV physeal fracture of lower end of left femur**
- [7th] **S79.149 Salter-Harris Type IV physeal fracture of lower end of unspecified femur**

[6th] **S79.19 Other physeal fracture of lower end of femur**
- [7th] **S79.191 Other physeal fracture of lower end of right femur**
- [7th] **S79.192 Other physeal fracture of lower end of left femur**
- [7th] **S79.199 Other physeal fracture of lower end of unspecified femur**

[5th] **S79.8 Other specified injuries of hip and thigh**

The appropriate 7th character is to be added to each code in subcategory S79.8
A = initial encounter
D = subsequent encounter
S = sequela

[6th] **S79.81 Other specified injuries of hip**
- [7th] **S79.811 Other specified injuries of right hip**
- [7th] **S79.812 Other specified injuries of left hip**
- [7th] **S79.819 Other specified injuries of unspecified hip**

[6th] **S79.82 Other specified injuries of thigh**
- [7th] **S79.821 Other specified injuries of right thigh**
- [7th] **S79.822 Other specified injuries of left thigh**
- [7th] **S79.829 Other specified injuries of unspecified thigh**

[5th] **S79.9 Unspecified injury of hip and thigh**

The appropriate 7th character is to be added to each code in subcategory S79.9
A = initial encounter
D = subsequent encounter
S = sequela

[6th] **S79.91 Unspecified injury of hip**
- [7th] **S79.911 Unspecified injury of right hip**
- [7th] **S79.912 Unspecified injury of left hip**
- [7th] **S79.919 Unspecified injury of unspecified hip**

[6th] **S79.92 Unspecified injury of thigh**
- [7th] **S79.921 Unspecified injury of right thigh**
- [7th] **S79.922 Unspecified injury of left thigh**
- [7th] **S79.929 Unspecified injury of unspecified thigh**

Injuries to the knee and lower leg (S80-S89)

[EXCLUDES2] *burns and corrosions (T20-T32)*
frostbite (T33-T34)
injuries of ankle and foot, except fracture of ankle and malleolus (S90-S99)
insect bite or sting, venomous (T63.4)

[4th] **S80 Superficial injury of knee and lower leg**

[EXCLUDES2] *superficial injury of ankle and foot (S90.-)*

The appropriate 7th character is to be added to each code from category S80
A = initial encounter
D = subsequent encounter
S = sequela

[5th] **S80.0 Contusion of knee**
- [7th] **S80.00 Contusion of unspecified knee**
- [7th] **S80.01 Contusion of right knee**
- [7th] **S80.02 Contusion of left knee**

[5th] **S80.1 Contusion of lower leg**
- [7th] **S80.10 Contusion of unspecified lower leg**
- [7th] **S80.11 Contusion of right lower leg**
- [7th] **S80.12 Contusion of left lower leg**

[5th] **S80.2 Other superficial injuries of knee**

[6th] **S80.21 Abrasion of knee**
- [7th] **S80.211 Abrasion, right knee**
- [7th] **S80.212 Abrasion, left knee**
- [7th] **S80.219 Abrasion, unspecified knee**

[6th] **S80.22 Blister (nonthermal) of knee**

[4th] 4th character required [5th] 5th character required [6th] 6th character required [7th] 7th character required [7th] Extension 'X' Alert
[EXCLUDES1] Not coded here [EXCLUDES2] Not included here [PDx] Primary Diagnosis Only Manifestation Code

S80.221 Blister (nonthermal), right knee
S80.222 Blister (nonthermal), left knee
S80.229 Blister (nonthermal), unspecified knee
S80.24 External constriction of knee
S80.241 External constriction, right knee
S80.242 External constriction, left knee
S80.249 External constriction, unspecified knee
S80.25 Superficial foreign body of knee
Splinter in the knee
S80.251 Superficial foreign body, right knee
S80.252 Superficial foreign body, left knee
S80.259 Superficial foreign body, unspecified knee
S80.26 Insect bite (nonvenomous) of knee
S80.261 Insect bite (nonvenomous), right knee
S80.262 Insect bite (nonvenomous), left knee
S80.269 Insect bite (nonvenomous), unspecified knee
S80.27 Other superficial bite of knee
EXCLUDES1 open bite of knee (S81.05-)
S80.271 Other superficial bite of right knee
S80.272 Other superficial bite of left knee
S80.279 Other superficial bite of unspecified knee
S80.8 Other superficial injuries of lower leg
S80.81 Abrasion of lower leg
S80.811 Abrasion, right lower leg
S80.812 Abrasion, left lower leg
S80.819 Abrasion, unspecified lower leg
S80.82 Blister (nonthermal) of lower leg
S80.821 Blister (nonthermal), right lower leg
S80.822 Blister (nonthermal), left lower leg
S80.829 Blister (nonthermal), unspecified lower leg
S80.84 External constriction of lower leg
S80.841 External constriction, right lower leg
S80.842 External constriction, left lower leg
S80.849 External constriction, unspecified lower leg
S80.85 Superficial foreign body of lower leg
Splinter in the lower leg
S80.851 Superficial foreign body, right lower leg
S80.852 Superficial foreign body, left lower leg
S80.859 Superficial foreign body, unspecified lower leg
S80.86 Insect bite (nonvenomous) of lower leg
S80.861 Insect bite (nonvenomous), right lower leg
S80.862 Insect bite (nonvenomous), left lower leg
S80.869 Insect bite (nonvenomous), unspecified lower leg
S80.87 Other superficial bite of lower leg
EXCLUDES1 open bite of lower leg (S81.85-)
S80.871 Other superficial bite, right lower leg
S80.872 Other superficial bite, left lower leg
S80.879 Other superficial bite, unspecified lower leg
S80.9 Unspecified superficial injury of knee and lower leg
S80.91 Unspecified superficial injury of knee
S80.911 Unspecified superficial injury of right knee
S80.912 Unspecified superficial injury of left knee
S80.919 Unspecified superficial injury of unspecified knee
S80.92 Unspecified superficial injury of lower leg
S80.921 Unspecified superficial injury of right lower leg
S80.922 Unspecified superficial injury of left lower leg
S80.929 Unspecified superficial injury of unspecified lower leg
S81 Open wound of knee and lower leg

Code also any associated wound infection
EXCLUDES1 open fracture of knee and lower leg (S82.-)
traumatic amputation of lower leg (S88.-)
EXCLUDES2 open wound of ankle and foot (S91.-)
The appropriate 7th character is to be added to each code from category S81
A = initial encounter
D = subsequent encounter
S = sequela
S81.0 Open wound of knee
S81.00 Unspecified open wound of knee
S81.001 Unspecified open wound, right knee
S81.002 Unspecified open wound, left knee
S81.009 Unspecified open wound, unspecified knee
S81.01 Laceration without foreign body of knee
S81.011 Laceration without foreign body, right knee
S81.012 Laceration without foreign body, left knee
S81.019 Laceration without foreign body, unspecified knee
S81.02 Laceration with foreign body of knee
S81.021 Laceration with foreign body, right knee
S81.022 Laceration with foreign body, left knee
S81.029 Laceration with foreign body, unspecified knee
S81.03 Puncture wound without foreign body of knee
S81.031 Puncture wound without foreign body, right knee
S81.032 Puncture wound without foreign body, left knee
S81.039 Puncture wound without foreign body, unspecified knee
S81.04 Puncture wound with foreign body of knee
S81.041 Puncture wound with foreign body, right knee
S81.042 Puncture wound with foreign body, left knee
S81.049 Puncture wound with foreign body, unspecified knee
S81.05 Open bite of knee
Bite of knee NOS
EXCLUDES1 superficial bite of knee (S80.27-)
S81.051 Open bite, right knee
S81.052 Open bite, left knee
S81.059 Open bite, unspecified knee
S81.8 Open wound of lower leg
S81.80 Unspecified open wound of lower leg
S81.801 Unspecified open wound, right lower leg
S81.802 Unspecified open wound, left lower leg
S81.809 Unspecified open wound, unspecified lower leg
S81.81 Laceration without foreign body of lower leg
S81.811 Laceration without foreign body, right lower leg
S81.812 Laceration without foreign body, left lower leg
S81.819 Laceration without foreign body, unspecified lower leg
S81.82 Laceration with foreign body of lower leg
S81.821 Laceration with foreign body, right lower leg
S81.822 Laceration with foreign body, left lower leg
S81.829 Laceration with foreign body, unspecified lower leg
S81.83 Puncture wound without foreign body of lower leg
S81.831 Puncture wound without foreign body, right lower leg

⑦ **S81.832** Puncture wound without foreign body, left lower leg

⑦ **S81.839** Puncture wound without foreign body, unspecified lower leg

⑥ **S81.84** Puncture wound with foreign body of lower leg

⑦ **S81.841** Puncture wound with foreign body, right lower leg

⑦ **S81.842** Puncture wound with foreign body, left lower leg

⑦ **S81.849** Puncture wound with foreign body, unspecified lower leg

⑥ **S81.85** Open bite of lower leg

Bite of lower leg NOS

EXCLUDES1 superficial bite of lower leg (S80.86-, S80.87-)

⑦ **S81.851** Open bite, right lower leg

⑦ **S81.852** Open bite, left lower leg

⑦ **S81.859** Open bite, unspecified lower leg

④ **S82** Fracture of lower leg, including ankle

NOTES A fracture not indicated as displaced or nondisplaced should be coded to displaced

A fracture not indicated as open or closed should be coded to closed

The open fracture designations are based on the Gustilo open fracture classification

INCLUDES fracture of malleolus

EXCLUDES1 traumatic amputation of lower leg (S88.-)

EXCLUDES2 fracture of foot, except ankle (S92.-)
periprosthetic fracture of prosthetic implant of knee (T84.042, T84.043)

The appropriate 7th character is to be added to all codes from category S82

A = initial encounter for closed fracture

B = initial encounter for open fracture type I or II

C = initial encounter for open fracture type IIIA, IIIB, or IIIC

D = subsequent encounter for closed fracture with routine healing

E = subsequent encounter for open fracture type I or II with routine healing

F = subsequent encounter for open fracture type IIIA, IIIB, or IIIC with routine healing

G = subsequent encounter for closed fracture with delayed healing

H = subsequent encounter for open fracture type I or II with delayed healing

J = subsequent encounter for open fracture type IIIA, IIIB, or IIIC with delayed healing

K = subsequent encounter for closed fracture with nonunion

M = subsequent encounter for open fracture type I or II with nonunion

N = subsequent encounter for open fracture type IIIA, IIIB, or IIIC with nonunion

P = subsequent encounter for closed fracture with malunion

Q = subsequent encounter for open fracture type I or II with malunion

R = subsequent encounter for open fracture type IIIA, IIIB, or IIIC with malunion

S = sequela

⑤ **S82.0** Fracture of patella

Knee cap

⑥ **S82.00** Unspecified fracture of patella

⑦ **S82.001** Unspecified fracture of right patella

⑦ **S82.002** Unspecified fracture of left patella

⑦ **S82.009** Unspecified fracture of unspecified patella

⑥ **S82.01** Osteochondral fracture of patella

⑦ **S82.011** Displaced osteochondral fracture of right patella

⑦ **S82.012** Displaced osteochondral fracture of left patella

⑦ **S82.013** Displaced osteochondral fracture of unspecified patella

⑦ **S82.014** Nondisplaced osteochondral fracture of right patella

⑦ **S82.015** Nondisplaced osteochondral fracture of left patella

⑦ **S82.016** Nondisplaced osteochondral fracture of unspecified patella

⑥ **S82.02** Longitudinal fracture of patella

⑦ **S82.021** Displaced longitudinal fracture of right patella

⑦ **S82.022** Displaced longitudinal fracture of left patella

⑦ **S82.023** Displaced longitudinal fracture of unspecified patella

⑦ **S82.024** Nondisplaced longitudinal fracture of right patella

⑦ **S82.025** Nondisplaced longitudinal fracture of left patella

⑦ **S82.026** Nondisplaced longitudinal fracture of unspecified patella

⑥ **S82.03** Transverse fracture of patella

⑦ **S82.031** Displaced transverse fracture of right patella

⑦ **S82.032** Displaced transverse fracture of left patella

⑦ **S82.033** Displaced transverse fracture of unspecified patella

⑦ **S82.034** Nondisplaced transverse fracture of right patella

⑦ **S82.035** Nondisplaced transverse fracture of left patella

⑦ **S82.036** Nondisplaced transverse fracture of unspecified patella

⑥ **S82.04** Comminuted fracture of patella

⑦ **S82.041** Displaced comminuted fracture of right patella

⑦ **S82.042** Displaced comminuted fracture of left patella

⑦ **S82.043** Displaced comminuted fracture of unspecified patella

⑦ **S82.044** Nondisplaced comminuted fracture of right patella

⑦ **S82.045** Nondisplaced comminuted fracture of left patella

⑦ **S82.046** Nondisplaced comminuted fracture of unspecified patella

⑥ **S82.09** Other fracture of patella

⑦ **S82.091** Other fracture of right patella

⑦ **S82.092** Other fracture of left patella

⑦ **S82.099** Other fracture of unspecified patella

⑤ **S82.1** Fracture of upper end of tibia

Fracture of proximal end of tibia

EXCLUDES2 fracture of shaft of tibia (S82.2-)
physeal fracture of upper end of tibia (S89.0-)

⑥ **S82.10** Unspecified fracture of upper end of tibia

⑦ **S82.101** Unspecified fracture of upper end of right tibia

⑦ **S82.102** Unspecified fracture of upper end of left tibia

⑦ **S82.109** Unspecified fracture of upper end of unspecified tibia

⑥ **S82.11** Fracture of tibial spine

⑦ **S82.111** Displaced fracture of right tibial spine

---

④ 4th character required   ⑤ 5th character required   ⑥ 6th character required   ⑦ 7th character required   ⑦ᵡ Extension 'X' Alert

EXCLUDES1 Not coded here   EXCLUDES2 Not included here   ᴾᴰˣ Primary Diagnosis Only   Manifestation Code

638   **ICD-10-CM 2015**

- [7th] S82.112 Displaced fracture of left tibial spine
- [7th] S82.113 Displaced fracture of unspecified tibial spine
- [7th] S82.114 Nondisplaced fracture of right tibial spine
- [7th] S82.115 Nondisplaced fracture of left tibial spine
- [7th] S82.116 Nondisplaced fracture of unspecified tibial spine

[6th] S82.12 Fracture of lateral condyle of tibia

- [7th] S82.121 Displaced fracture of lateral condyle of right tibia
- [7th] S82.122 Displaced fracture of lateral condyle of left tibia
- [7th] S82.123 Displaced fracture of lateral condyle of unspecified tibia
- [7th] S82.124 Nondisplaced fracture of lateral condyle of right tibia
- [7th] S82.125 Nondisplaced fracture of lateral condyle of left tibia
- [7th] S82.126 Nondisplaced fracture of lateral condyle of unspecified tibia

[6th] S82.13 Fracture of medial condyle of tibia

- [7th] S82.131 Displaced fracture of medial condyle of right tibia
- [7th] S82.132 Displaced fracture of medial condyle of left tibia
- [7th] S82.133 Displaced fracture of medial condyle of unspecified tibia
- [7th] S82.134 Nondisplaced fracture of medial condyle of right tibia
- [7th] S82.135 Nondisplaced fracture of medial condyle of left tibia
- [7th] S82.136 Nondisplaced fracture of medial condyle of unspecified tibia

[6th] S82.14 Bicondylar fracture of tibia

Fracture of tibial plateau NOS

- [7th] S82.141 Displaced bicondylar fracture of right tibia
- [7th] S82.142 Displaced bicondylar fracture of left tibia
- [7th] S82.143 Displaced bicondylar fracture of unspecified tibia
- [7th] S82.144 Nondisplaced bicondylar fracture of right tibia
- [7th] S82.145 Nondisplaced bicondylar fracture of left tibia
- [7th] S82.146 Nondisplaced bicondylar fracture of unspecified tibia

[6th] S82.15 Fracture of tibial tuberosity

- [7th] S82.151 Displaced fracture of right tibial tuberosity
- [7th] S82.152 Displaced fracture of left tibial tuberosity
- [7th] S82.153 Displaced fracture of unspecified tibial tuberosity
- [7th] S82.154 Nondisplaced fracture of right tibial tuberosity
- [7th] S82.155 Nondisplaced fracture of left tibial tuberosity
- [7th] S82.156 Nondisplaced fracture of unspecified tibial tuberosity

[6th] S82.16 Torus fracture of upper end of tibia

The appropriate 7th character is to be added to all codes in subcategory S82.16
A = initial encounter for closed fracture
D = subsequent encounter for fracture with routine healing
G = subsequent encounter for fracture with delayed healing
K = subsequent encounter for fracture with nonunion
P = subsequent encounter for fracture with malunion
S = sequela

- [7th] S82.161 Torus fracture of upper end of right tibia
- [7th] S82.162 Torus fracture of upper end of left tibia
- [7th] S82.169 Torus fracture of upper end of unspecified tibia

[6th] S82.19 Other fracture of upper end of tibia

- [7th] S82.191 Other fracture of upper end of right tibia
- [7th] S82.192 Other fracture of upper end of left tibia
- [7th] S82.199 Other fracture of upper end of unspecified tibia

[5th] S82.2 Fracture of shaft of tibia

[6th] S82.20 Unspecified fracture of shaft of tibia

Fracture of tibia NOS

- [7th] S82.201 Unspecified fracture of shaft of right tibia
- [7th] S82.202 Unspecified fracture of shaft of left tibia
- [7th] S82.209 Unspecified fracture of shaft of unspecified tibia

[6th] S82.22 Transverse fracture of shaft of tibia

- [7th] S82.221 Displaced transverse fracture of shaft of right tibia
- [7th] S82.222 Displaced transverse fracture of shaft of left tibia
- [7th] S82.223 Displaced transverse fracture of shaft of unspecified tibia
- [7th] S82.224 Nondisplaced transverse fracture of shaft of right tibia
- [7th] S82.225 Nondisplaced transverse fracture of shaft of left tibia
- [7th] S82.226 Nondisplaced transverse fracture of shaft of unspecified tibia

[6th] S82.23 Oblique fracture of shaft of tibia

- [7th] S82.231 Displaced oblique fracture of shaft of right tibia
- [7th] S82.232 Displaced oblique fracture of shaft of left tibia
- [7th] S82.233 Displaced oblique fracture of shaft of unspecified tibia
- [7th] S82.234 Nondisplaced oblique fracture of shaft of right tibia
- [7th] S82.235 Nondisplaced oblique fracture of shaft of left tibia
- [7th] S82.236 Nondisplaced oblique fracture of shaft of unspecified tibia

[6th] S82.24 Spiral fracture of shaft of tibia

Toddler fracture

- [7th] S82.241 Displaced spiral fracture of shaft of right tibia
- [7th] S82.242 Displaced spiral fracture of shaft of left tibia
- [7th] S82.243 Displaced spiral fracture of shaft of unspecified tibia
- [7th] S82.244 Nondisplaced spiral fracture of shaft of right tibia
- [7th] S82.245 Nondisplaced spiral fracture of shaft of left tibia
- [7th] S82.246 Nondisplaced spiral fracture of shaft of unspecified tibia

[6th] S82.25 Comminuted fracture of shaft of tibia

- [7th] S82.251 Displaced comminuted fracture of shaft of right tibia
- [7th] S82.252 Displaced comminuted fracture of shaft of left tibia
- [7th] S82.253 Displaced comminuted fracture of shaft of unspecified tibia
- [7th] S82.254 Nondisplaced comminuted fracture of shaft of right tibia
- [7th] S82.255 Nondisplaced comminuted fracture of shaft of left tibia
- [7th] S82.256 Nondisplaced comminuted fracture of shaft of unspecified tibia

[6th] S82.26 Segmental fracture of shaft of tibia

- [7th] S82.261 Displaced segmental fracture of shaft of right tibia
- [7th] S82.262 Displaced segmental fracture of shaft of left tibia

- 7ᵗʰ S82.263 Displaced segmental fracture of shaft of unspecified tibia
- 7ᵗʰ S82.264 Nondisplaced segmental fracture of shaft of right tibia
- 7ᵗʰ S82.265 Nondisplaced segmental fracture of shaft of left tibia
- 7ᵗʰ S82.266 Nondisplaced segmental fracture of shaft of unspecified tibia
- 6ᵗʰ S82.29 Other fracture of shaft of tibia
  - 7ᵗʰ S82.291 Other fracture of shaft of right tibia
  - 7ᵗʰ S82.292 Other fracture of shaft of left tibia
  - 7ᵗʰ S82.299 Other fracture of shaft of unspecified tibia
- 5ᵗʰ S82.3 Fracture of lower end of tibia
  - EXCLUDES1 bimalleolar fracture of lower leg (S82.84-)
    fracture of medial malleolus alone (S82.5-)
    Maisonneuve's fracture (S82.86-)
    pilon fracture of distal tibia (S82.87-)
    trimalleolar fractures of lower leg (S82.85-)
  - 6ᵗʰ S82.30 Unspecified fracture of lower end of tibia
    - 7ᵗʰ S82.301 Unspecified fracture of lower end of right tibia
    - 7ᵗʰ S82.302 Unspecified fracture of lower end of left tibia
    - 7ᵗʰ S82.309 Unspecified fracture of lower end of unspecified tibia
  - 6ᵗʰ S82.31 Torus fracture of lower end of tibia
    The appropriate 7th character is to be added to all codes in subcategory S82.31
    A = initial encounter for closed fracture
    D = subsequent encounter for fracture with routine healing
    G = subsequent encounter for fracture with delayed healing
    K = subsequent encounter for fracture with nonunion
    P = subsequent encounter for fracture with malunion
    S = sequela
    - 7ᵗʰ S82.311 Torus fracture of lower end of right tibia
    - 7ᵗʰ S82.312 Torus fracture of lower end of left tibia
    - 7ᵗʰ S82.319 Torus fracture of lower end of unspecified tibia
  - 6ᵗʰ S82.39 Other fracture of lower end of tibia
    - 7ᵗʰ S82.391 Other fracture of lower end of right tibia
    - 7ᵗʰ S82.392 Other fracture of lower end of left tibia
    - 7ᵗʰ S82.399 Other fracture of lower end of unspecified tibia
- 5ᵗʰ S82.4 Fracture of shaft of fibula
  - EXCLUDES2 fracture of lateral malleolus alone (S82.6-)
  - 6ᵗʰ S82.40 Unspecified fracture of shaft of fibula
    - 7ᵗʰ S82.401 Unspecified fracture of shaft of right fibula
    - 7ᵗʰ S82.402 Unspecified fracture of shaft of left fibula
    - 7ᵗʰ S82.409 Unspecified fracture of shaft of unspecified fibula
  - 6ᵗʰ S82.42 Transverse fracture of shaft of fibula
    - 7ᵗʰ S82.421 Displaced transverse fracture of shaft of right fibula
    - 7ᵗʰ S82.422 Displaced transverse fracture of shaft of left fibula
    - 7ᵗʰ S82.423 Displaced transverse fracture of shaft of unspecified fibula
    - 7ᵗʰ S82.424 Nondisplaced transverse fracture of shaft of right fibula
    - 7ᵗʰ S82.425 Nondisplaced transverse fracture of shaft of left fibula
    - 7ᵗʰ S82.426 Nondisplaced transverse fracture of shaft of unspecified fibula
  - 6ᵗʰ S82.43 Oblique fracture of shaft of fibula
    - 7ᵗʰ S82.431 Displaced oblique fracture of shaft of right fibula

- 7ᵗʰ S82.432 Displaced oblique fracture of shaft of left fibula
- 7ᵗʰ S82.433 Displaced oblique fracture of shaft of unspecified fibula
- 7ᵗʰ S82.434 Nondisplaced oblique fracture of shaft of right fibula
- 7ᵗʰ S82.435 Nondisplaced oblique fracture of shaft of left fibula
- 7ᵗʰ S82.436 Nondisplaced oblique fracture of shaft of unspecified fibula
- 6ᵗʰ S82.44 Spiral fracture of shaft of fibula
  - 7ᵗʰ S82.441 Displaced spiral fracture of shaft of right fibula
  - 7ᵗʰ S82.442 Displaced spiral fracture of shaft of left fibula
  - 7ᵗʰ S82.443 Displaced spiral fracture of shaft of unspecified fibula
  - 7ᵗʰ S82.444 Nondisplaced spiral fracture of shaft of right fibula
  - 7ᵗʰ S82.445 Nondisplaced spiral fracture of shaft of left fibula
  - 7ᵗʰ S82.446 Nondisplaced spiral fracture of shaft of unspecified fibula
- 6ᵗʰ S82.45 Comminuted fracture of shaft of fibula
  - 7ᵗʰ S82.451 Displaced comminuted fracture of shaft of right fibula
  - 7ᵗʰ S82.452 Displaced comminuted fracture of shaft of left fibula
  - 7ᵗʰ S82.453 Displaced comminuted fracture of shaft of unspecified fibula
  - 7ᵗʰ S82.454 Nondisplaced comminuted fracture of shaft of right fibula
  - 7ᵗʰ S82.455 Nondisplaced comminuted fracture of shaft of left fibula
  - 7ᵗʰ S82.456 Nondisplaced comminuted fracture of shaft of unspecified fibula
- 6ᵗʰ S82.46 Segmental fracture of shaft of fibula
  - 7ᵗʰ S82.461 Displaced segmental fracture of shaft of right fibula
  - 7ᵗʰ S82.462 Displaced segmental fracture of shaft of left fibula
  - 7ᵗʰ S82.463 Displaced segmental fracture of shaft of unspecified fibula
  - 7ᵗʰ S82.464 Nondisplaced segmental fracture of shaft of right fibula
  - 7ᵗʰ S82.465 Nondisplaced segmental fracture of shaft of left fibula
  - 7ᵗʰ S82.466 Nondisplaced segmental fracture of shaft of unspecified fibula
- 6ᵗʰ S82.49 Other fracture of shaft of fibula
  - 7ᵗʰ S82.491 Other fracture of shaft of right fibula
  - 7ᵗʰ S82.492 Other fracture of shaft of left fibula
  - 7ᵗʰ S82.499 Other fracture of shaft of unspecified fibula
- 5ᵗʰ S82.5 Fracture of medial malleolus
  - EXCLUDES1 pilon fracture of distal tibia (S82.87-)
    Salter-Harris type III of lower end of tibia (S89.13-)
    Salter-Harris type IV of lower end of tibia (S89.14-)
  - 7ᵗʰ S82.51 Displaced fracture of medial malleolus of right tibia
  - 7ᵗʰ S82.52 Displaced fracture of medial malleolus of left tibia
  - 7ᵗʰ S82.53 Displaced fracture of medial malleolus of unspecified tibia
  - 7ᵗʰ S82.54 Nondisplaced fracture of medial malleolus of right tibia
  - 7ᵗʰ S82.55 Nondisplaced fracture of medial malleolus of left tibia

---

4ᵗʰ 4ᵗʰ character required   5ᵗʰ 5ᵗʰ character required   6ᵗʰ 6ᵗʰ character required   7ᵗʰ 7ᵗʰ character required   7ᵗʰ Extension 'X' Alert

EXCLUDES1 Not coded here   EXCLUDES2 Not included here   PDx Primary Diagnosis Only   Manifestation Code

[7th] S82.56 Nondisplaced fracture of medial malleolus of unspecified tibia

[5th] S82.6 Fracture of lateral malleolus

[EXCLUDES1] *pilon fracture of distal tibia (S82.87-)*

[7th] S82.61 Displaced fracture of lateral malleolus of right fibula

[7th] S82.62 Displaced fracture of lateral malleolus of left fibula

[7th] S82.63 Displaced fracture of lateral malleolus of unspecified fibula

[7th] S82.64 Nondisplaced fracture of lateral malleolus of right fibula

[7th] S82.65 Nondisplaced fracture of lateral malleolus of left fibula

[7th] S82.66 Nondisplaced fracture of lateral malleolus of unspecified fibula

[5th] S82.8 Other fractures of lower leg

[6th] S82.81 Torus fracture of upper end of fibula

The appropriate 7th character is to be added to all codes in subcategory S82.81
A = initial encounter for closed fracture
D = subsequent encounter for fracture with routine healing
G = subsequent encounter for fracture with delayed healing
K = subsequent encounter for fracture with nonunion
P = subsequent encounter for fracture with malunion
S = sequela

[7th] S82.811 Torus fracture of upper end of right fibula

[7th] S82.812 Torus fracture of upper end of left fibula

[7th] S82.819 Torus fracture of upper end of unspecified fibula

[6th] S82.82 Torus fracture of lower end of fibula

The appropriate 7th character is to be added to all codes in subcategory S82.82
A = initial encounter for closed fracture
D = subsequent encounter for fracture with routine healing
G = subsequent encounter for fracture with delayed healing
K = subsequent encounter for fracture with nonunion
P = subsequent encounter for fracture with malunion
S = sequela

[7th] S82.821 Torus fracture of lower end of right fibula

[7th] S82.822 Torus fracture of lower end of left fibula

[7th] S82.829 Torus fracture of lower end of unspecified fibula

[6th] S82.83 Other fracture of upper and lower end of fibula

[7th] S82.831 Other fracture of upper and lower end of right fibula

[7th] S82.832 Other fracture of upper and lower end of left fibula

[7th] S82.839 Other fracture of upper and lower end of unspecified fibula

[6th] S82.84 Bimalleolar fracture of lower leg

[7th] S82.841 Displaced bimalleolar fracture of right lower leg

[7th] S82.842 Displaced bimalleolar fracture of left lower leg

[7th] S82.843 Displaced bimalleolar fracture of unspecified lower leg

[7th] S82.844 Nondisplaced bimalleolar fracture of right lower leg

[7th] S82.845 Nondisplaced bimalleolar fracture of left lower leg

[7th] S82.846 Nondisplaced bimalleolar fracture of unspecified lower leg

[6th] S82.85 Trimalleolar fracture of lower leg

[7th] S82.851 Displaced trimalleolar fracture of right lower leg

[7th] S82.852 Displaced trimalleolar fracture of left lower leg

[7th] S82.853 Displaced trimalleolar fracture of unspecified lower leg

[7th] S82.854 Nondisplaced trimalleolar fracture of right lower leg

[7th] S82.855 Nondisplaced trimalleolar fracture of left lower leg

[7th] S82.856 Nondisplaced trimalleolar fracture of unspecified lower leg

[6th] S82.86 Maisonneuve's fracture

[7th] S82.861 Displaced Maisonneuve's fracture of right leg

[7th] S82.862 Displaced Maisonneuve's fracture of left leg

[7th] S82.863 Displaced Maisonneuve's fracture of unspecified leg

[7th] S82.864 Nondisplaced Maisonneuve's fracture of right leg

[7th] S82.865 Nondisplaced Maisonneuve's fracture of left leg

[7th] S82.866 Nondisplaced Maisonneuve's fracture of unspecified leg

[6th] S82.87 Pilon fracture of tibia

[7th] S82.871 Displaced pilon fracture of right tibia

[7th] S82.872 Displaced pilon fracture of left tibia

[7th] S82.873 Displaced pilon fracture of unspecified tibia

[7th] S82.874 Nondisplaced pilon fracture of right tibia

[7th] S82.875 Nondisplaced pilon fracture of left tibia

[7th] S82.876 Nondisplaced pilon fracture of unspecified tibia

[6th] S82.89 Other fractures of lower leg

Fracture of ankle NOS

[7th] S82.891 Other fracture of right lower leg

[7th] S82.892 Other fracture of left lower leg

[7th] S82.899 Other fracture of unspecified lower leg

[5th] S82.9 Unspecified fracture of lower leg

[7th] S82.90 Unspecified fracture of unspecified lower leg

[7th] S82.91 Unspecified fracture of right lower leg

[7th] S82.92 Unspecified fracture of left lower leg

[4th] S83 Dislocation and sprain of joints and ligaments of knee

[INCLUDES] *avulsion of joint or ligament of knee*
laceration of cartilage, joint or ligament of knee
sprain of cartilage, joint or ligament of knee
traumatic hemarthrosis of joint or ligament of knee
traumatic rupture of joint or ligament of knee
traumatic subluxation of joint or ligament of knee
traumatic tear of joint or ligament of knee

Code also any associated open wound

[EXCLUDES1] *derangement of patella (M22.0-M22.3)*
injury of patellar ligament (tendon) (S76.1-)
internal derangement of knee (M23.-)
old dislocation of knee (M24.36)
pathological dislocation of knee (M24.36)
recurrent dislocation of knee (M22.0)

[EXCLUDES2] *strain of muscle, fascia and tendon of lower leg (S86.-)*

The appropriate 7th character is to be added to each code from category S83
A = initial encounter
D = subsequent encounter
S = sequela

[5th] S83.0 Subluxation and dislocation of patella

[6th] S83.00 Unspecified subluxation and dislocation of patella

[7th] S83.001 Unspecified subluxation of right patella

🄬 S83.002 Unspecified subluxation of left patella
🄬 S83.003 Unspecified subluxation of unspecified patella
🄬 S83.004 Unspecified dislocation of right patella
🄬 S83.005 Unspecified dislocation of left patella
🄬 S83.006 Unspecified dislocation of unspecified patella
🄺 S83.01 Lateral subluxation and dislocation of patella
🄬 S83.011 Lateral subluxation of right patella
🄬 S83.012 Lateral subluxation of left patella
🄬 S83.013 Lateral subluxation of unspecified patella
🄬 S83.014 Lateral dislocation of right patella
🄬 S83.015 Lateral dislocation of left patella
🄬 S83.016 Lateral dislocation of unspecified patella
🄺 S83.09 Other subluxation and dislocation of patella
🄬 S83.091 Other subluxation of right patella
🄬 S83.092 Other subluxation of left patella
🄬 S83.093 Other subluxation of unspecified patella
🄬 S83.094 Other dislocation of right patella
🄬 S83.095 Other dislocation of left patella
🄬 S83.096 Other dislocation of unspecified patella
🄢 S83.1 Subluxation and dislocation of knee
  EXCLUDES2 instability of knee prosthesis (T84.022, T84.023)
🄺 S83.10 Unspecified subluxation and dislocation of knee
🄬 S83.101 Unspecified subluxation of right knee
🄬 S83.102 Unspecified subluxation of left knee
🄬 S83.103 Unspecified subluxation of unspecified knee
🄬 S83.104 Unspecified dislocation of right knee
🄬 S83.105 Unspecified dislocation of left knee
🄬 S83.106 Unspecified dislocation of unspecified knee
🄺 S83.11 Anterior subluxation and dislocation of proximal end of tibia
  Posterior subluxation and dislocation of distal end of femur
🄬 S83.111 Anterior subluxation of proximal end of tibia, right knee
🄬 S83.112 Anterior subluxation of proximal end of tibia, left knee
🄬 S83.113 Anterior subluxation of proximal end of tibia, unspecified knee
🄬 S83.114 Anterior dislocation of proximal end of tibia, right knee
🄬 S83.115 Anterior dislocation of proximal end of tibia, left knee
🄬 S83.116 Anterior dislocation of proximal end of tibia, unspecified knee
🄺 S83.12 Posterior subluxation and dislocation of proximal end of tibia
  Anterior dislocation of distal end of femur
🄬 S83.121 Posterior subluxation of proximal end of tibia, right knee
🄬 S83.122 Posterior subluxation of proximal end of tibia, left knee
🄬 S83.123 Posterior subluxation of proximal end of tibia, unspecified knee
🄬 S83.124 Posterior dislocation of proximal end of tibia, right knee
🄬 S83.125 Posterior dislocation of proximal end of tibia, left knee
🄬 S83.126 Posterior dislocation of proximal end of tibia, unspecified knee
🄺 S83.13 Medial subluxation and dislocation of proximal end of tibia
🄬 S83.131 Medial subluxation of proximal end of tibia, right knee
🄬 S83.132 Medial subluxation of proximal end of tibia, left knee

🄬 S83.133 Medial subluxation of proximal end of tibia, unspecified knee
🄬 S83.134 Medial dislocation of proximal end of tibia, right knee
🄬 S83.135 Medial dislocation of proximal end of tibia, left knee
🄬 S83.136 Medial dislocation of proximal end of tibia, unspecified knee
🄺 S83.14 Lateral subluxation and dislocation of proximal end of tibia
🄬 S83.141 Lateral subluxation of proximal end of tibia, right knee
🄬 S83.142 Lateral subluxation of proximal end of tibia, left knee
🄬 S83.143 Lateral subluxation of proximal end of tibia, unspecified knee
🄬 S83.144 Lateral dislocation of proximal end of tibia, right knee
🄬 S83.145 Lateral dislocation of proximal end of tibia, left knee
🄬 S83.146 Lateral dislocation of proximal end of tibia, unspecified knee
🄺 S83.19 Other subluxation and dislocation of knee
🄬 S83.191 Other subluxation of right knee
🄬 S83.192 Other subluxation of left knee
🄬 S83.193 Other subluxation of unspecified knee
🄬 S83.194 Other dislocation of right knee
🄬 S83.195 Other dislocation of left knee
🄬 S83.196 Other dislocation of unspecified knee
🄢 S83.2 Tear of meniscus, current injury
  EXCLUDES1 old bucket-handle tear (M23.2)
🄺 S83.20 Tear of unspecified meniscus, current injury
  Tear of meniscus of knee NOS
🄬 S83.200 Bucket-handle tear of unspecified meniscus, current injury, right knee
🄬 S83.201 Bucket-handle tear of unspecified meniscus, current injury, left knee
🄬 S83.202 Bucket-handle tear of unspecified meniscus, current injury, unspecified knee
🄬 S83.203 Other tear of unspecified meniscus, current injury, right knee
🄬 S83.204 Other tear of unspecified meniscus, current injury, left knee
🄬 S83.205 Other tear of unspecified meniscus, current injury, unspecified knee
🄬 S83.206 Unspecified tear of unspecified meniscus, current injury, right knee
🄬 S83.207 Unspecified tear of unspecified meniscus, current injury, left knee
🄬 S83.209 Unspecified tear of unspecified meniscus, current injury, unspecified knee
🄺 S83.21 Bucket-handle tear of medial meniscus, current injury
🄬 S83.211 Bucket-handle tear of medial meniscus, current injury, right knee
🄬 S83.212 Bucket-handle tear of medial meniscus, current injury, left knee
🄬 S83.219 Bucket-handle tear of medial meniscus, current injury, unspecified knee
🄺 S83.22 Peripheral tear of medial meniscus, current injury
🄬 S83.221 Peripheral tear of medial meniscus, current injury, right knee
🄬 S83.222 Peripheral tear of medial meniscus, current injury, left knee
🄬 S83.229 Peripheral tear of medial meniscus, current injury, unspecified knee
🄺 S83.23 Complex tear of medial meniscus, current injury

[7th] S83.231 Complex tear of medial meniscus, current injury, right knee
[7th] S83.232 Complex tear of medial meniscus, current injury, left knee
[7th] S83.239 Complex tear of medial meniscus, current injury, unspecified knee
[6th] S83.24 Other tear of medial meniscus, current injury
[7th] S83.241 Other tear of medial meniscus, current injury, right knee
[7th] S83.242 Other tear of medial meniscus, current injury, left knee
[7th] S83.249 Other tear of medial meniscus, current injury, unspecified knee
[6th] S83.25 Bucket-handle tear of lateral meniscus, current injury
[7th] S83.251 Bucket-handle tear of lateral meniscus, current injury, right knee
[7th] S83.252 Bucket-handle tear of lateral meniscus, current injury, left knee
[7th] S83.259 Bucket-handle tear of lateral meniscus, current injury, unspecified knee
[6th] S83.26 Peripheral tear of lateral meniscus, current injury
[7th] S83.261 Peripheral tear of lateral meniscus, current injury, right knee
[7th] S83.262 Peripheral tear of lateral meniscus, current injury, left knee
[7th] S83.269 Peripheral tear of lateral meniscus, current injury, unspecified knee
[6th] S83.27 Complex tear of lateral meniscus, current injury
[7th] S83.271 Complex tear of lateral meniscus, current injury, right knee
[7th] S83.272 Complex tear of lateral meniscus, current injury, left knee
[7th] S83.279 Complex tear of lateral meniscus, current injury, unspecified knee
[6th] S83.28 Other tear of lateral meniscus, current injury
[7th] S83.281 Other tear of lateral meniscus, current injury, right knee
[7th] S83.282 Other tear of lateral meniscus, current injury, left knee
[7th] S83.289 Other tear of lateral meniscus, current injury, unspecified knee
[5th] S83.3 Tear of articular cartilage of knee, current
[7th] S83.30 Tear of articular cartilage of unspecified knee, current
[7th] S83.31 Tear of articular cartilage of right knee, current
[7th] S83.32 Tear of articular cartilage of left knee, current
[5th] S83.4 Sprain of collateral ligament of knee
[6th] S83.40 Sprain of unspecified collateral ligament of knee
[7th] S83.401 Sprain of unspecified collateral ligament of right knee
[7th] S83.402 Sprain of unspecified collateral ligament of left knee
[7th] S83.409 Sprain of unspecified collateral ligament of unspecified knee
[6th] S83.41 Sprain of medial collateral ligament of knee
Sprain of tibial collateral ligament
[7th] S83.411 Sprain of medial collateral ligament of right knee
[7th] S83.412 Sprain of medial collateral ligament of left knee
[7th] S83.419 Sprain of medial collateral ligament of unspecified knee
[6th] S83.42 Sprain of lateral collateral ligament of knee
Sprain of fibular collateral ligament
[7th] S83.421 Sprain of lateral collateral ligament of right knee
[7th] S83.422 Sprain of lateral collateral ligament of left knee
[7th] S83.429 Sprain of lateral collateral ligament of unspecified knee
[5th] S83.5 Sprain of cruciate ligament of knee
[6th] S83.50 Sprain of unspecified cruciate ligament of knee
[7th] S83.501 Sprain of unspecified cruciate ligament of right knee
[7th] S83.502 Sprain of unspecified cruciate ligament of left knee
[7th] S83.509 Sprain of unspecified cruciate ligament of unspecified knee
[6th] S83.51 Sprain of anterior cruciate ligament of knee
[7th] S83.511 Sprain of anterior cruciate ligament of right knee
[7th] S83.512 Sprain of anterior cruciate ligament of left knee
[7th] S83.519 Sprain of anterior cruciate ligament of unspecified knee
[6th] S83.52 Sprain of posterior cruciate ligament of knee
[7th] S83.521 Sprain of posterior cruciate ligament of right knee
[7th] S83.522 Sprain of posterior cruciate ligament of left knee
[7th] S83.529 Sprain of posterior cruciate ligament of unspecified knee
[5th] S83.6 Sprain of the superior tibiofibular joint and ligament
[7th] S83.60 Sprain of the superior tibiofibular joint and ligament, unspecified knee
[7th] S83.61 Sprain of the superior tibiofibular joint and ligament, right knee
[7th] S83.62 Sprain of the superior tibiofibular joint and ligament, left knee
[5th] S83.8 Sprain of other specified parts of knee
[6th] S83.8X Sprain of other specified parts of knee
[7th] S83.8X1 Sprain of other specified parts of right knee
[7th] S83.8X2 Sprain of other specified parts of left knee
[7th] S83.8X9 Sprain of other specified parts of unspecified knee
[5th] S83.9 Sprain of unspecified site of knee
[7th] S83.90 Sprain of unspecified site of unspecified knee
[7th] S83.91 Sprain of unspecified site of right knee
[7th] S83.92 Sprain of unspecified site of left knee
[4th] S84 Injury of nerves at lower leg level
Code also any associated open wound (S81.-)
[EXCLUDES2] *injury of nerves at ankle and foot level (S94.-)*
The appropriate 7th character is to be added to each code from category S84
A = initial encounter
D = subsequent encounter
S = sequela
[5th] S84.0 Injury of tibial nerve at lower leg level
[7th] S84.00 Injury of tibial nerve at lower leg level, unspecified leg
[7th] S84.01 Injury of tibial nerve at lower leg level, right leg
[7th] S84.02 Injury of tibial nerve at lower leg level, left leg
[5th] S84.1 Injury of peroneal nerve at lower leg level
[7th] S84.10 Injury of peroneal nerve at lower leg level, unspecified leg
[7th] S84.11 Injury of peroneal nerve at lower leg level, right leg
[7th] S84.12 Injury of peroneal nerve at lower leg level, left leg
[5th] S84.2 Injury of cutaneous sensory nerve at lower leg level
[7th] S84.20 Injury of cutaneous sensory nerve at lower leg level, unspecified leg
[7th] S84.21 Injury of cutaneous sensory nerve at lower leg level, right leg
[7th] S84.22 Injury of cutaneous sensory nerve at lower leg level, left leg
[5th] S84.8 Injury of other nerves at lower leg level
[6th] S84.80 Injury of other nerves at lower leg level
[7th] S84.801 Injury of other nerves at lower leg level, right leg

Unspecified Code | Other Specified Code | [N] Newborn Age: 0 | [P] Pediatric Age: 0-17 | [M] Maternity Age: 12-55
[A] Adult Age: 15-124 | ♂ Male | ♀ Female | ● New Code | ▲ Revised Code Title | ►◄ Revised Text

S84.802 Injury of other nerves at lower leg level, left leg

S84.809 Injury of other nerves at lower leg level, unspecified leg

S84.9 Injury of unspecified nerve at lower leg level

S84.90 Injury of unspecified nerve at lower leg level, unspecified leg

S84.91 Injury of unspecified nerve at lower leg level, right leg

S84.92 Injury of unspecified nerve at lower leg level, left leg

S85 Injury of blood vessels at lower leg level

Code also any associated open wound (S81.-)

EXCLUDES2 injury of blood vessels at ankle and foot level (S95.-)

The appropriate 7th character is to be added to each code from category S85
A = initial encounter
D = subsequent encounter
S = sequela

S85.0 Injury of popliteal artery

S85.00 Unspecified injury of popliteal artery

S85.001 Unspecified injury of popliteal artery, right leg

S85.002 Unspecified injury of popliteal artery, left leg

S85.009 Unspecified injury of popliteal artery, unspecified leg

S85.01 Laceration of popliteal artery

S85.011 Laceration of popliteal artery, right leg

S85.012 Laceration of popliteal artery, left leg

S85.019 Laceration of popliteal artery, unspecified leg

S85.09 Other specified injury of popliteal artery

S85.091 Other specified injury of popliteal artery, right leg

S85.092 Other specified injury of popliteal artery, left leg

S85.099 Other specified injury of popliteal artery, unspecified leg

S85.1 Injury of tibial artery

S85.10 Unspecified injury of unspecified tibial artery

Injury of tibial artery NOS

S85.101 Unspecified injury of unspecified tibial artery, right leg

S85.102 Unspecified injury of unspecified tibial artery, left leg

S85.109 Unspecified injury of unspecified tibial artery, unspecified leg

S85.11 Laceration of unspecified tibial artery

S85.111 Laceration of unspecified tibial artery, right leg

S85.112 Laceration of unspecified tibial artery, left leg

S85.119 Laceration of unspecified tibial artery, unspecified leg

S85.12 Other specified injury of unspecified tibial artery

S85.121 Other specified injury of unspecified tibial artery, right leg

S85.122 Other specified injury of unspecified tibial artery, left leg

S85.129 Other specified injury of unspecified tibial artery, unspecified leg

S85.13 Unspecified injury of anterior tibial artery

S85.131 Unspecified injury of anterior tibial artery, right leg

S85.132 Unspecified injury of anterior tibial artery, left leg

S85.139 Unspecified injury of anterior tibial artery, unspecified leg

S85.14 Laceration of anterior tibial artery

S85.141 Laceration of anterior tibial artery, right leg

S85.142 Laceration of anterior tibial artery, left leg

S85.149 Laceration of anterior tibial artery, unspecified leg

S85.15 Other specified injury of anterior tibial artery

S85.151 Other specified injury of anterior tibial artery, right leg

S85.152 Other specified injury of anterior tibial artery, left leg

S85.159 Other specified injury of anterior tibial artery, unspecified leg

S85.16 Unspecified injury of posterior tibial artery

S85.161 Unspecified injury of posterior tibial artery, right leg

S85.162 Unspecified injury of posterior tibial artery, left leg

S85.169 Unspecified injury of posterior tibial artery, unspecified leg

S85.17 Laceration of posterior tibial artery

S85.171 Laceration of posterior tibial artery, right leg

S85.172 Laceration of posterior tibial artery, left leg

S85.179 Laceration of posterior tibial artery, unspecified leg

S85.18 Other specified injury of posterior tibial artery

S85.181 Other specified injury of posterior tibial artery, right leg

S85.182 Other specified injury of posterior tibial artery, left leg

S85.189 Other specified injury of posterior tibial artery, unspecified leg

S85.2 Injury of peroneal artery

S85.20 Unspecified injury of peroneal artery

S85.201 Unspecified injury of peroneal artery, right leg

S85.202 Unspecified injury of peroneal artery, left leg

S85.209 Unspecified injury of peroneal artery, unspecified leg

S85.21 Laceration of peroneal artery

S85.211 Laceration of peroneal artery, right leg

S85.212 Laceration of peroneal artery, left leg

S85.219 Laceration of peroneal artery, unspecified leg

S85.29 Other specified injury of peroneal artery

S85.291 Other specified injury of peroneal artery, right leg

S85.292 Other specified injury of peroneal artery, left leg

S85.299 Other specified injury of peroneal artery, unspecified leg

S85.3 Injury of greater saphenous vein at lower leg level

Injury of greater saphenous vein NOS
Injury of saphenous vein NOS

S85.30 Unspecified injury of greater saphenous vein at lower leg level

S85.301 Unspecified injury of greater saphenous vein at lower leg level, right leg

S85.302 Unspecified injury of greater saphenous vein at lower leg level, left leg

S85.309 Unspecified injury of greater saphenous vein at lower leg level, unspecified leg

S85.31 Laceration of greater saphenous vein at lower leg level

S85.311 Laceration of greater saphenous vein at lower leg level, right leg

4th character required   5th character required   6th character required   7th character required   Extension 'X' Alert
EXCLUDES 1 Not coded here   EXCLUDES 2 Not included here   PDx Primary Diagnosis Only   Manifestation Code

CHAPTER 19: INJURY, POISONING, AND CERTAIN OTHER CONSEQUENCES OF EXTERNAL CAUSES (S00-T88)

S84.802 - S85.311

[7th] S85.312 Laceration of greater saphenous vein at lower leg level, left leg
[7th] S85.319 Laceration of greater saphenous vein at lower leg level, unspecified leg
[6th] S85.39 Other specified injury of greater saphenous vein at lower leg level
[7th] S85.391 Other specified injury of greater saphenous vein at lower leg level, right leg
[7th] S85.392 Other specified injury of greater saphenous vein at lower leg level, left leg
[7th] S85.399 Other specified injury of greater saphenous vein at lower leg level, unspecified leg
[5th] S85.4 Injury of lesser saphenous vein at lower leg level
[6th] S85.40 Unspecified injury of lesser saphenous vein at lower leg level
[7th] S85.401 Unspecified injury of lesser saphenous vein at lower leg level, right leg
[7th] S85.402 Unspecified injury of lesser saphenous vein at lower leg level, left leg
[7th] S85.409 Unspecified injury of lesser saphenous vein at lower leg level, unspecified leg
[6th] S85.41 Laceration of lesser saphenous vein at lower leg level
[7th] S85.411 Laceration of lesser saphenous vein at lower leg level, right leg
[7th] S85.412 Laceration of lesser saphenous vein at lower leg level, left leg
[7th] S85.419 Laceration of lesser saphenous vein at lower leg level, unspecified leg
[6th] S85.49 Other specified injury of lesser saphenous vein at lower leg level
[7th] S85.491 Other specified injury of lesser saphenous vein at lower leg level, right leg
[7th] S85.492 Other specified injury of lesser saphenous vein at lower leg level, left leg
[7th] S85.499 Other specified injury of lesser saphenous vein at lower leg level, unspecified leg
[5th] S85.5 Injury of popliteal vein
[6th] S85.50 Unspecified injury of popliteal vein
[7th] S85.501 Unspecified injury of popliteal vein, right leg
[7th] S85.502 Unspecified injury of popliteal vein, left leg
[7th] S85.509 Unspecified injury of popliteal vein, unspecified leg
[6th] S85.51 Laceration of popliteal vein
[7th] S85.511 Laceration of popliteal vein, right leg
[7th] S85.512 Laceration of popliteal vein, left leg
[7th] S85.519 Laceration of popliteal vein, unspecified leg
[6th] S85.59 Other specified injury of popliteal vein
[7th] S85.591 Other specified injury of popliteal vein, right leg
[7th] S85.592 Other specified injury of popliteal vein, left leg
[7th] S85.599 Other specified injury of popliteal vein, unspecified leg
[5th] S85.8 Injury of other blood vessels at lower leg level
[6th] S85.80 Unspecified injury of other blood vessels at lower leg level
[7th] S85.801 Unspecified injury of other blood vessels at lower leg level, right leg
[7th] S85.802 Unspecified injury of other blood vessels at lower leg level, left leg
[7th] S85.809 Unspecified injury of other blood vessels at lower leg level, unspecified leg
[6th] S85.81 Laceration of other blood vessels at lower leg level
[7th] S85.811 Laceration of other blood vessels at lower leg level, right leg
[7th] S85.812 Laceration of other blood vessels at lower leg level, left leg
[7th] S85.819 Laceration of other blood vessels at lower leg level, unspecified leg
[6th] S85.89 Other specified injury of other blood vessels at lower leg level
[7th] S85.891 Other specified injury of other blood vessels at lower leg level, right leg
[7th] S85.892 Other specified injury of other blood vessels at lower leg level, left leg
[7th] S85.899 Other specified injury of other blood vessels at lower leg level, unspecified leg
[5th] S85.9 Injury of unspecified blood vessel at lower leg level
[6th] S85.90 Unspecified injury of unspecified blood vessel at lower leg level
[7th] S85.901 Unspecified injury of unspecified blood vessel at lower leg level, right leg
[7th] S85.902 Unspecified injury of unspecified blood vessel at lower leg level, left leg
[7th] S85.909 Unspecified injury of unspecified blood vessel at lower leg level, unspecified leg
[6th] S85.91 Laceration of unspecified blood vessel at lower leg level
[7th] S85.911 Laceration of unspecified blood vessel at lower leg level, right leg
[7th] S85.912 Laceration of unspecified blood vessel at lower leg level, left leg
[7th] S85.919 Laceration of unspecified blood vessel at lower leg level, unspecified leg
[6th] S85.99 Other specified injury of unspecified blood vessel at lower leg level
[7th] S85.991 Other specified injury of unspecified blood vessel at lower leg level, right leg
[7th] S85.992 Other specified injury of unspecified blood vessel at lower leg level, left leg
[7th] S85.999 Other specified injury of unspecified blood vessel at lower leg level, unspecified leg
[4th] S86 Injury of muscle, fascia and tendon at lower leg level
Code also any associated open wound (S81.-)
[EXCLUDES2] *injury of muscle, fascia and tendon at ankle (S96.-)*
injury of patellar ligament (tendon) (S76.1-)
sprain of joints and ligaments of knee (S83.-)
The appropriate 7th character is to be added to each code from category S86
A = initial encounter
D = subsequent encounter
S = sequela
[5th] S86.0 Injury of Achilles tendon
[6th] S86.00 Unspecified injury of Achilles tendon
[7th] S86.001 Unspecified injury of right Achilles tendon
[7th] S86.002 Unspecified injury of left Achilles tendon
[7th] S86.009 Unspecified injury of unspecified Achilles tendon
[6th] S86.01 Strain of Achilles tendon
[7th] S86.011 Strain of right Achilles tendon
[7th] S86.012 Strain of left Achilles tendon
[7th] S86.019 Strain of unspecified Achilles tendon
[6th] S86.02 Laceration of Achilles tendon
[7th] S86.021 Laceration of right Achilles tendon
[7th] S86.022 Laceration of left Achilles tendon
[7th] S86.029 Laceration of unspecified Achilles tendon
[6th] S86.09 Other specified injury of Achilles tendon
[7th] S86.091 Other specified injury of right Achilles tendon
[7th] S86.092 Other specified injury of left Achilles tendon
[7th] S86.099 Other specified injury of unspecified Achilles tendon

[5] S86.1 Injury of other muscle(s) and tendon(s) of posterior muscle group at lower leg level

[6] S86.10 Unspecified injury of other muscle(s) and tendon(s) of posterior muscle group at lower leg level

[7] S86.101 Unspecified injury of other muscle(s) and tendon(s) of posterior muscle group at lower leg level, right leg

[7] S86.102 Unspecified injury of other muscle(s) and tendon(s) of posterior muscle group at lower leg level, left leg

[7] S86.109 Unspecified injury of other muscle(s) and tendon(s) of posterior muscle group at lower leg level, unspecified leg

[6] S86.11 Strain of other muscle(s) and tendon(s) of posterior muscle group at lower leg level

[7] S86.111 Strain of other muscle(s) and tendon(s) of posterior muscle group at lower leg level, right leg

[7] S86.112 Strain of other muscle(s) and tendon(s) of posterior muscle group at lower leg level, left leg

[7] S86.119 Strain of other muscle(s) and tendon(s) of posterior muscle group at lower leg level, unspecified leg

[6] S86.12 Laceration of other muscle(s) and tendon(s) of posterior muscle group at lower leg level

[7] S86.121 Laceration of other muscle(s) and tendon(s) of posterior muscle group at lower leg level, right leg

[7] S86.122 Laceration of other muscle(s) and tendon(s) of posterior muscle group at lower leg level, left leg

[7] S86.129 Laceration of other muscle(s) and tendon(s) of posterior muscle group at lower leg level, unspecified leg

[6] S86.19 Other injury of other muscle(s) and tendon(s) of posterior muscle group at lower leg level

[7] S86.191 Other injury of other muscle(s) and tendon(s) of posterior muscle group at lower leg level, right leg

[7] S86.192 Other injury of other muscle(s) and tendon(s) of posterior muscle group at lower leg level, left leg

[7] S86.199 Other injury of other muscle(s) and tendon(s) of posterior muscle group at lower leg level, unspecified leg

[5] S86.2 Injury of muscle(s) and tendon(s) of anterior muscle group at lower leg level

[6] S86.20 Unspecified injury of muscle(s) and tendon(s) of anterior muscle group at lower leg level

[7] S86.201 Unspecified injury of muscle(s) and tendon(s) of anterior muscle group at lower leg level, right leg

[7] S86.202 Unspecified injury of muscle(s) and tendon(s) of anterior muscle group at lower leg level, left leg

[7] S86.209 Unspecified injury of muscle(s) and tendon(s) of anterior muscle group at lower leg level, unspecified leg

[6] S86.21 Strain of muscle(s) and tendon(s) of anterior muscle group at lower leg level

[7] S86.211 Strain of muscle(s) and tendon(s) of anterior muscle group at lower leg level, right leg

[7] S86.212 Strain of muscle(s) and tendon(s) of anterior muscle group at lower leg level, left leg

[7] S86.219 Strain of muscle(s) and tendon(s) of anterior muscle group at lower leg level, unspecified leg

[6] S86.22 Laceration of muscle(s) and tendon(s) of anterior muscle group at lower leg level

[7] S86.221 Laceration of muscle(s) and tendon(s) of anterior muscle group at lower leg level, right leg

[7] S86.222 Laceration of muscle(s) and tendon(s) of anterior muscle group at lower leg level, left leg

[7] S86.229 Laceration of muscle(s) and tendon(s) of anterior muscle group at lower leg level, unspecified leg

[6] S86.29 Other injury of muscle(s) and tendon(s) of anterior muscle group at lower leg level

[7] S86.291 Other injury of muscle(s) and tendon(s) of anterior muscle group at lower leg level, right leg

[7] S86.292 Other injury of muscle(s) and tendon(s) of anterior muscle group at lower leg level, left leg

[7] S86.299 Other injury of muscle(s) and tendon(s) of anterior muscle group at lower leg level, unspecified leg

[5] S86.3 Injury of muscle(s) and tendon(s) of peroneal muscle group at lower leg level

[6] S86.30 Unspecified injury of muscle(s) and tendon(s) of peroneal muscle group at lower leg level

[7] S86.301 Unspecified injury of muscle(s) and tendon(s) of peroneal muscle group at lower leg level, right leg

[7] S86.302 Unspecified injury of muscle(s) and tendon(s) of peroneal muscle group at lower leg level, left leg

[7] S86.309 Unspecified injury of muscle(s) and tendon(s) of peroneal muscle group at lower leg level, unspecified leg

[6] S86.31 Strain of muscle(s) and tendon(s) of peroneal muscle group at lower leg level

[7] S86.311 Strain of muscle(s) and tendon(s) of peroneal muscle group at lower leg level, right leg

[7] S86.312 Strain of muscle(s) and tendon(s) of peroneal muscle group at lower leg level, left leg

[7] S86.319 Strain of muscle(s) and tendon(s) of peroneal muscle group at lower leg level, unspecified leg

[6] S86.32 Laceration of muscle(s) and tendon(s) of peroneal muscle group at lower leg level

[7] S86.321 Laceration of muscle(s) and tendon(s) of peroneal muscle group at lower leg level, right leg

[7] S86.322 Laceration of muscle(s) and tendon(s) of peroneal muscle group at lower leg level, left leg

[7] S86.329 Laceration of muscle(s) and tendon(s) of peroneal muscle group at lower leg level, unspecified leg

[6] S86.39 Other injury of muscle(s) and tendon(s) of peroneal muscle group at lower leg level

[7] S86.391 Other injury of muscle(s) and tendon(s) of peroneal muscle group at lower leg level, right leg

[7] S86.392 Other injury of muscle(s) and tendon(s) of peroneal muscle group at lower leg level, left leg

[7] S86.399 Other injury of muscle(s) and tendon(s) of peroneal muscle group at lower leg level, unspecified leg

[5] S86.8 Injury of other muscles and tendons at lower leg level

[4] 4th character required [5] 5th character required [6] 6th character required [7] 7th character required [x7] Extension 'X' Alert
[EXCLUDES1] Not coded here [EXCLUDES2] Not included here [PDx] Primary Diagnosis Only Manifestation Code

S86.80 Unspecified injury of other muscles and tendons at lower leg level
- S86.801 Unspecified injury of other muscle(s) and tendon(s) at lower leg level, right leg
- S86.802 Unspecified injury of other muscle(s) and tendon(s) at lower leg level, left leg
- S86.809 Unspecified injury of other muscle(s) and tendon(s) at lower leg level, unspecified leg

S86.81 Strain of other muscles and tendons at lower leg level
- S86.811 Strain of other muscle(s) and tendon(s) at lower leg level, right leg
- S86.812 Strain of other muscle(s) and tendon(s) at lower leg level, left leg
- S86.819 Strain of other muscle(s) and tendon(s) at lower leg level, unspecified leg

S86.82 Laceration of other muscles and tendons at lower leg level
- S86.821 Laceration of other muscle(s) and tendon(s) at lower leg level, right leg
- S86.822 Laceration of other muscle(s) and tendon(s) at lower leg level, left leg
- S86.829 Laceration of other muscle(s) and tendon(s) at lower leg level, unspecified leg

S86.89 Other injury of other muscles and tendons at lower leg level
- S86.891 Other injury of other muscle(s) and tendon(s) at lower leg level, right leg
- S86.892 Other injury of other muscle(s) and tendon(s) at lower leg level, left leg
- S86.899 Other injury of other muscle(s) and tendon(s) at lower leg level, unspecified leg

S86.9 Injury of unspecified muscle and tendon at lower leg level
- S86.90 Unspecified injury of unspecified muscle and tendon at lower leg level
  - S86.901 Unspecified injury of unspecified muscle(s) and tendon(s) at lower leg level, right leg
  - S86.902 Unspecified injury of unspecified muscle(s) and tendon(s) at lower leg level, left leg
  - S86.909 Unspecified injury of unspecified muscle(s) and tendon(s) at lower leg level, unspecified leg
- S86.91 Strain of unspecified muscle and tendon at lower leg level
  - S86.911 Strain of unspecified muscle(s) and tendon(s) at lower leg level, right leg
  - S86.912 Strain of unspecified muscle(s) and tendon(s) at lower leg level, left leg
  - S86.919 Strain of unspecified muscle(s) and tendon(s) at lower leg level, unspecified leg
- S86.92 Laceration of unspecified muscle and tendon at lower leg level
  - S86.921 Laceration of unspecified muscle(s) and tendon(s) at lower leg level, right leg
  - S86.922 Laceration of unspecified muscle(s) and tendon(s) at lower leg level, left leg
  - S86.929 Laceration of unspecified muscle(s) and tendon(s) at lower leg level, unspecified leg
- S86.99 Other injury of unspecified muscle and tendon at lower leg level
  - S86.991 Other injury of unspecified muscle(s) and tendon(s) at lower leg level, right leg
  - S86.992 Other injury of unspecified muscle(s) and tendon(s) at lower leg level, left leg
  - S86.999 Other injury of unspecified muscle(s) and tendon(s) at lower leg level, unspecified leg

S87 Crushing injury of lower leg
Use additional code(s) for all associated injuries

EXCLUDES2 crushing injury of ankle and foot (S97.-)
The appropriate 7th character is to be added to each code from category S87
A = initial encounter
D = subsequent encounter
S = sequela

S87.0 Crushing injury of knee
- S87.00 Crushing injury of unspecified knee
- S87.01 Crushing injury of right knee
- S87.02 Crushing injury of left knee

S87.8 Crushing injury of lower leg
- S87.80 Crushing injury of unspecified lower leg
- S87.81 Crushing injury of right lower leg
- S87.82 Crushing injury of left lower leg

S88 Traumatic amputation of lower leg
An amputation not identified as partial or complete should be coded to complete
EXCLUDES1 traumatic amputation of ankle and foot (S98.-)
The appropriate 7th character is to be added to each code from category S88
A = initial encounter
D = subsequent encounter
S = sequela

S88.0 Traumatic amputation at knee level
- S88.01 Complete traumatic amputation at knee level
  - S88.011 Complete traumatic amputation at knee level, right lower leg
  - S88.012 Complete traumatic amputation at knee level, left lower leg
  - S88.019 Complete traumatic amputation at knee level, unspecified lower leg
- S88.02 Partial traumatic amputation at knee level
  - S88.021 Partial traumatic amputation at knee level, right lower leg
  - S88.022 Partial traumatic amputation at knee level, left lower leg
  - S88.029 Partial traumatic amputation at knee level, unspecified lower leg

S88.1 Traumatic amputation at level between knee and ankle
- S88.11 Complete traumatic amputation at level between knee and ankle
  - S88.111 Complete traumatic amputation at level between knee and ankle, right lower leg
  - S88.112 Complete traumatic amputation at level between knee and ankle, left lower leg
  - S88.119 Complete traumatic amputation at level between knee and ankle, unspecified lower leg
- S88.12 Partial traumatic amputation at level between knee and ankle
  - S88.121 Partial traumatic amputation at level between knee and ankle, right lower leg
  - S88.122 Partial traumatic amputation at level between knee and ankle, left lower leg
  - S88.129 Partial traumatic amputation at level between knee and ankle, unspecified lower leg

S88.9 Traumatic amputation of lower leg, level unspecified
- S88.91 Complete traumatic amputation of lower leg, level unspecified
  - S88.911 Complete traumatic amputation of right lower leg, level unspecified
  - S88.912 Complete traumatic amputation of left lower leg, level unspecified
  - S88.919 Complete traumatic amputation of unspecified lower leg, level unspecified
- S88.92 Partial traumatic amputation of lower leg, level unspecified

---

Unspecified Code   Other Specified Code   N Newborn Age: 0   P Pediatric Age: 0-17   M Maternity Age: 12-55
A Adult Age: 15-124   ♂ Male   ♀ Female   ● New Code   ▲ Revised Code Title   ►◄ Revised Text

[7th] S88.921 Partial traumatic amputation of right lower leg, level unspecified
[7th] S88.922 Partial traumatic amputation of left lower leg, level unspecified
[7th] S88.929 Partial traumatic amputation of unspecified lower leg, level unspecified

[4th] S89 Other and unspecified injuries of lower leg

[NOTES] A fracture not indicated as open or closed should be coded to closed

[EXCLUDES2] *other and unspecified injuries of ankle and foot (S99.-)*

The appropriate 7th character is to be added to each code from subcategories S89.0, S89.1, S89.2, and S89.3
A = initial encounter for closed fracture
D = subsequent encounter for fracture with routine healing
G = subsequent encounter for fracture with delayed healing
K = subsequent encounter for fracture with nonunion
P = subsequent encounter for fracture with malunion
S = sequela

[5th] S89.0 Physeal fracture of upper end of tibia
[6th] S89.00 Unspecified physeal fracture of upper end of tibia
[7th] S89.001 Unspecified physeal fracture of upper end of right tibia
[7th] S89.002 Unspecified physeal fracture of upper end of left tibia
[7th] S89.009 Unspecified physeal fracture of upper end of unspecified tibia
[6th] S89.01 Salter-Harris Type I physeal fracture of upper end of tibia
[7th] S89.011 Salter-Harris Type I physeal fracture of upper end of right tibia
[7th] S89.012 Salter-Harris Type I physeal fracture of upper end of left tibia
[7th] S89.019 Salter-Harris Type I physeal fracture of upper end of unspecified tibia
[6th] S89.02 Salter-Harris Type II physeal fracture of upper end of tibia
[7th] S89.021 Salter-Harris Type II physeal fracture of upper end of right tibia
[7th] S89.022 Salter-Harris Type II physeal fracture of upper end of left tibia
[7th] S89.029 Salter-Harris Type II physeal fracture of upper end of unspecified tibia
[6th] S89.03 Salter-Harris Type III physeal fracture of upper end of tibia
[7th] S89.031 Salter-Harris Type III physeal fracture of upper end of right tibia
[7th] S89.032 Salter-Harris Type III physeal fracture of upper end of left tibia
[7th] S89.039 Salter-Harris Type III physeal fracture of upper end of unspecified tibia
[6th] S89.04 Salter-Harris Type IV physeal fracture of upper end of tibia
[7th] S89.041 Salter-Harris Type IV physeal fracture of upper end of right tibia
[7th] S89.042 Salter-Harris Type IV physeal fracture of upper end of left tibia
[7th] S89.049 Salter-Harris Type IV physeal fracture of upper end of unspecified tibia
[6th] S89.09 Other physeal fracture of upper end of tibia
[7th] S89.091 Other physeal fracture of upper end of right tibia
[7th] S89.092 Other physeal fracture of upper end of left tibia
[7th] S89.099 Other physeal fracture of upper end of unspecified tibia

[5th] S89.1 Physeal fracture of lower end of tibia
[6th] S89.10 Unspecified physeal fracture of lower end of tibia
[7th] S89.101 Unspecified physeal fracture of lower end of right tibia
[7th] S89.102 Unspecified physeal fracture of lower end of left tibia
[7th] S89.109 Unspecified physeal fracture of lower end of unspecified tibia
[6th] S89.11 Salter-Harris Type I physeal fracture of lower end of tibia
[7th] S89.111 Salter-Harris Type I physeal fracture of lower end of right tibia
[7th] S89.112 Salter-Harris Type I physeal fracture of lower end of left tibia
[7th] S89.119 Salter-Harris Type I physeal fracture of lower end of unspecified tibia
[6th] S89.12 Salter-Harris Type II physeal fracture of lower end of tibia
[7th] S89.121 Salter-Harris Type II physeal fracture of lower end of right tibia
[7th] S89.122 Salter-Harris Type II physeal fracture of lower end of left tibia
[7th] S89.129 Salter-Harris Type II physeal fracture of lower end of unspecified tibia
[6th] S89.13 Salter-Harris Type III physeal fracture of lower end of tibia

[EXCLUDES1] *fracture of medial malleolus (adult) (S82.5-)*

[7th] S89.131 Salter-Harris Type III physeal fracture of lower end of right tibia
[7th] S89.132 Salter-Harris Type III physeal fracture of lower end of left tibia
[7th] S89.139 Salter-Harris Type III physeal fracture of lower end of unspecified tibia
[6th] S89.14 Salter-Harris Type IV physeal fracture of lower end of tibia

[EXCLUDES1] *fracture of medial malleolus (adult) (S82.5-)*

[7th] S89.141 Salter-Harris Type IV physeal fracture of lower end of right tibia
[7th] S89.142 Salter-Harris Type IV physeal fracture of lower end of left tibia
[7th] S89.149 Salter-Harris Type IV physeal fracture of lower end of unspecified tibia
[6th] S89.19 Other physeal fracture of lower end of tibia
[7th] S89.191 Other physeal fracture of lower end of right tibia
[7th] S89.192 Other physeal fracture of lower end of left tibia
[7th] S89.199 Other physeal fracture of lower end of unspecified tibia

[5th] S89.2 Physeal fracture of upper end of fibula
[6th] S89.20 Unspecified physeal fracture of upper end of fibula
[7th] S89.201 Unspecified physeal fracture of upper end of right fibula
[7th] S89.202 Unspecified physeal fracture of upper end of left fibula
[7th] S89.209 Unspecified physeal fracture of upper end of unspecified fibula
[6th] S89.21 Salter-Harris Type I physeal fracture of upper end of fibula
[7th] S89.211 Salter-Harris Type I physeal fracture of upper end of right fibula
[7th] S89.212 Salter-Harris Type I physeal fracture of upper end of left fibula
[7th] S89.219 Salter-Harris Type I physeal fracture of upper end of unspecified fibula
[6th] S89.22 Salter-Harris Type II physeal fracture of upper end of fibula

[4th] 4th character required [5th] 5th character required [6th] 6th character required [7th] 7th character required [X] Extension 'X' Alert
[EXCLUDES1] Not coded here [EXCLUDES2] Not included here [PDx] Primary Diagnosis Only Manifestation Code

[7th] S89.221 Salter-Harris Type II physeal fracture of upper end of right fibula
[7th] S89.222 Salter-Harris Type II physeal fracture of upper end of left fibula
[7th] S89.229 Salter-Harris Type II physeal fracture of upper end of unspecified fibula
[6th] S89.29 Other physeal fracture of upper end of fibula
[7th] S89.291 Other physeal fracture of upper end of right fibula
[7th] S89.292 Other physeal fracture of upper end of left fibula
[7th] S89.299 Other physeal fracture of upper end of unspecified fibula
[5th] S89.3 Physeal fracture of lower end of fibula
[6th] S89.30 Unspecified physeal fracture of lower end of fibula
[7th] S89.301 Unspecified physeal fracture of lower end of right fibula
[7th] S89.302 Unspecified physeal fracture of lower end of left fibula
[7th] S89.309 Unspecified physeal fracture of lower end of unspecified fibula
[6th] S89.31 Salter-Harris Type I physeal fracture of lower end of fibula
[7th] S89.311 Salter-Harris Type I physeal fracture of lower end of right fibula
[7th] S89.312 Salter-Harris Type I physeal fracture of lower end of left fibula
[7th] S89.319 Salter-Harris Type I physeal fracture of lower end of unspecified fibula
[6th] S89.32 Salter-Harris Type II physeal fracture of lower end of fibula
[7th] S89.321 Salter-Harris Type II physeal fracture of lower end of right fibula
[7th] S89.322 Salter-Harris Type II physeal fracture of lower end of left fibula
[7th] S89.329 Salter-Harris Type II physeal fracture of lower end of unspecified fibula
[6th] S89.39 Other physeal fracture of lower end of fibula
[7th] S89.391 Other physeal fracture of lower end of right fibula
[7th] S89.392 Other physeal fracture of lower end of left fibula
[7th] S89.399 Other physeal fracture of lower end of unspecified fibula
[5th] S89.8 Other specified injuries of lower leg

The appropriate 7th character is to be added to each code in subcategory S89.8
A = initial encounter
D = subsequent encounter
S = sequela

[7th] S89.80 Other specified injuries of unspecified lower leg
[7th] S89.81 Other specified injuries of right lower leg
[7th] S89.82 Other specified injuries of left lower leg
[5th] S89.9 Unspecified injury of lower leg

The appropriate 7th character is to be added to each code in subcategory S89.9
A = initial encounter
D = subsequent encounter
S = sequela

[7th] S89.90 Unspecified injury of unspecified lower leg
[7th] S89.91 Unspecified injury of right lower leg
[7th] S89.92 Unspecified injury of left lower leg

Injuries to the ankle and foot (S90-S99)

EXCLUDES2 *burns and corrosions (T20-T32)*
fracture of ankle and malleolus (S82.-)
frostbite (T33-T34)
insect bite or sting, venomous (T63.4)

[4th] S90 Superficial injury of ankle, foot and toes

The appropriate 7th character is to be added to each code from category S90
A = initial encounter
D = subsequent encounter
S = sequela

[5th] S90.0 Contusion of ankle
[7th] S90.00 Contusion of unspecified ankle
[7th] S90.01 Contusion of right ankle
[7th] S90.02 Contusion of left ankle
[5th] S90.1 Contusion of toe without damage to nail
[6th] S90.11 Contusion of great toe without damage to nail
[7th] S90.111 Contusion of right great toe without damage to nail
[7th] S90.112 Contusion of left great toe without damage to nail
[7th] S90.119 Contusion of unspecified great toe without damage to nail
[6th] S90.12 Contusion of lesser toe without damage to nail
[7th] S90.121 Contusion of right lesser toe(s) without damage to nail
[7th] S90.122 Contusion of left lesser toe(s) without damage to nail
[7th] S90.129 Contusion of unspecified lesser toe(s) without damage to nail
Contusion of toe NOS
[5th] S90.2 Contusion of toe with damage to nail
[6th] S90.21 Contusion of great toe with damage to nail
[7th] S90.211 Contusion of right great toe with damage to nail
[7th] S90.212 Contusion of left great toe with damage to nail
[7th] S90.219 Contusion of unspecified great toe with damage to nail
[6th] S90.22 Contusion of lesser toe with damage to nail
[7th] S90.221 Contusion of right lesser toe(s) with damage to nail
[7th] S90.222 Contusion of left lesser toe(s) with damage to nail
[7th] S90.229 Contusion of unspecified lesser toe(s) with damage to nail
[5th] S90.3 Contusion of foot
EXCLUDES2 *contusion of toes (S90.1-, S90.2-)*
[7th] S90.30 Contusion of unspecified foot
Contusion of foot NOS
[7th] S90.31 Contusion of right foot
[7th] S90.32 Contusion of left foot
[5th] S90.4 Other superficial injuries of toe
[6th] S90.41 Abrasion of toe
[7th] S90.411 Abrasion, right great toe
[7th] S90.412 Abrasion, left great toe
[7th] S90.413 Abrasion, unspecified great toe
[7th] S90.414 Abrasion, right lesser toe(s)
[7th] S90.415 Abrasion, left lesser toe(s)
[7th] S90.416 Abrasion, unspecified lesser toe(s)
[6th] S90.42 Blister (nonthermal) of toe
[7th] S90.421 Blister (nonthermal), right great toe
[7th] S90.422 Blister (nonthermal), left great toe
[7th] S90.423 Blister (nonthermal), unspecified great toe
[7th] S90.424 Blister (nonthermal), right lesser toe(s)
[7th] S90.425 Blister (nonthermal), left lesser toe(s)
[7th] S90.426 Blister (nonthermal), unspecified lesser toe(s)
[6th] S90.44 External constriction of toe
Hair tourniquet syndrome of toe
[7th] S90.441 External constriction, right great toe

Unspecified Code | Other Specified Code | [N] Newborn Age: 0 | [P] Pediatric Age: 0-17 | [M] Maternity Age: 12-55
[A] Adult Age: 15-124 | ♂ Male | ♀ Female | ● New Code | ▲ Revised Code Title | ►◄ Revised Text

7⃣ S90.442 External constriction, left great toe
7⃣ S90.443 External constriction, unspecified great toe
7⃣ S90.444 External constriction, right lesser toe(s)
7⃣ S90.445 External constriction, left lesser toe(s)
7⃣ S90.446 External constriction, unspecified lesser toe(s)
6⃣ S90.45 Superficial foreign body of toe
Splinter in the toe
7⃣ S90.451 Superficial foreign body, right great toe
7⃣ S90.452 Superficial foreign body, left great toe
7⃣ S90.453 Superficial foreign body, unspecified great toe
7⃣ S90.454 Superficial foreign body, right lesser toe(s)
7⃣ S90.455 Superficial foreign body, left lesser toe(s)
7⃣ S90.456 Superficial foreign body, unspecified lesser toe(s)
6⃣ S90.46 Insect bite (nonvenomous) of toe
7⃣ S90.461 Insect bite (nonvenomous), right great toe
7⃣ S90.462 Insect bite (nonvenomous), left great toe
7⃣ S90.463 Insect bite (nonvenomous), unspecified great toe
7⃣ S90.464 Insect bite (nonvenomous), right lesser toe(s)
7⃣ S90.465 Insect bite (nonvenomous), left lesser toe(s)
7⃣ S90.466 Insect bite (nonvenomous), unspecified lesser toe(s)
6⃣ S90.47 Other superficial bite of toe
EXCLUDES1 open bite of toe (S91.15-, S91.25-)
7⃣ S90.471 Other superficial bite of right great toe
7⃣ S90.472 Other superficial bite of left great toe
7⃣ S90.473 Other superficial bite of unspecified great toe
7⃣ S90.474 Other superficial bite of right lesser toe(s)
7⃣ S90.475 Other superficial bite of left lesser toe(s)
7⃣ S90.476 Other superficial bite of unspecified lesser toe(s)
5⃣ S90.5 Other superficial injuries of ankle
6⃣ S90.51 Abrasion of ankle
7⃣ S90.511 Abrasion, right ankle
7⃣ S90.512 Abrasion, left ankle
7⃣ S90.519 Abrasion, unspecified ankle
6⃣ S90.52 Blister (nonthermal) of ankle
7⃣ S90.521 Blister (nonthermal), right ankle
7⃣ S90.522 Blister (nonthermal), left ankle
7⃣ S90.529 Blister (nonthermal), unspecified ankle
6⃣ S90.54 External constriction of ankle
7⃣ S90.541 External constriction, right ankle
7⃣ S90.542 External constriction, left ankle
7⃣ S90.549 External constriction, unspecified ankle
6⃣ S90.55 Superficial foreign body of ankle
Splinter in the ankle
7⃣ S90.551 Superficial foreign body, right ankle
7⃣ S90.552 Superficial foreign body, left ankle
7⃣ S90.559 Superficial foreign body, unspecified ankle
6⃣ S90.56 Insect bite (nonvenomous) of ankle
7⃣ S90.561 Insect bite (nonvenomous), right ankle
7⃣ S90.562 Insect bite (nonvenomous), left ankle
7⃣ S90.569 Insect bite (nonvenomous), unspecified ankle
6⃣ S90.57 Other superficial bite of ankle
EXCLUDES1 open bite of ankle (S91.05-)
7⃣ S90.571 Other superficial bite of ankle, right ankle
7⃣ S90.572 Other superficial bite of ankle, left ankle
7⃣ S90.579 Other superficial bite of ankle, unspecified ankle
5⃣ S90.8 Other superficial injuries of foot
6⃣ S90.81 Abrasion of foot

7⃣ S90.811 Abrasion, right foot
7⃣ S90.812 Abrasion, left foot
7⃣ S90.819 Abrasion, unspecified foot
6⃣ S90.82 Blister (nonthermal) of foot
7⃣ S90.821 Blister (nonthermal), right foot
7⃣ S90.822 Blister (nonthermal), left foot
7⃣ S90.829 Blister (nonthermal), unspecified foot
6⃣ S90.84 External constriction of foot
7⃣ S90.841 External constriction, right foot
7⃣ S90.842 External constriction, left foot
7⃣ S90.849 External constriction, unspecified foot
6⃣ S90.85 Superficial foreign body of foot
Splinter in the foot
7⃣ S90.851 Superficial foreign body, right foot
7⃣ S90.852 Superficial foreign body, left foot
7⃣ S90.859 Superficial foreign body, unspecified foot
6⃣ S90.86 Insect bite (nonvenomous) of foot
7⃣ S90.861 Insect bite (nonvenomous), right foot
7⃣ S90.862 Insect bite (nonvenomous), left foot
7⃣ S90.869 Insect bite (nonvenomous), unspecified foot
6⃣ S90.87 Other superficial bite of foot
EXCLUDES1 open bite of foot (S91.35-)
7⃣ S90.871 Other superficial bite of right foot
7⃣ S90.872 Other superficial bite of left foot
7⃣ S90.879 Other superficial bite of unspecified foot
5⃣ S90.9 Unspecified superficial injury of ankle, foot and toe
6⃣ S90.91 Unspecified superficial injury of ankle
7⃣ S90.911 Unspecified superficial injury of right ankle
7⃣ S90.912 Unspecified superficial injury of left ankle
7⃣ S90.919 Unspecified superficial injury of unspecified ankle
6⃣ S90.92 Unspecified superficial injury of foot
7⃣ S90.921 Unspecified superficial injury of right foot
7⃣ S90.922 Unspecified superficial injury of left foot
7⃣ S90.929 Unspecified superficial injury of unspecified foot
6⃣ S90.93 Unspecified superficial injury of toes
7⃣ S90.931 Unspecified superficial injury of right great toe
7⃣ S90.932 Unspecified superficial injury of left great toe
7⃣ S90.933 Unspecified superficial injury of unspecified great toe
7⃣ S90.934 Unspecified superficial injury of right lesser toe(s)
7⃣ S90.935 Unspecified superficial injury of left lesser toe(s)
7⃣ S90.936 Unspecified superficial injury of unspecified lesser toe(s)
4⃣ S91 Open wound of ankle, foot and toes
Code also any associated wound infection
EXCLUDES1 open fracture of ankle, foot and toes (S92.-with 7th character B)
traumatic amputation of ankle and foot (S98.-)
The appropriate 7th character is to be added to each code from category S91
A = initial encounter
D = subsequent encounter
S = sequela
5⃣ S91.0 Open wound of ankle
6⃣ S91.00 Unspecified open wound of ankle
7⃣ S91.001 Unspecified open wound, right ankle
7⃣ S91.002 Unspecified open wound, left ankle
7⃣ S91.009 Unspecified open wound, unspecified ankle
6⃣ S91.01 Laceration without foreign body of ankle
7⃣ S91.011 Laceration without foreign body, right ankle
7⃣ S91.012 Laceration without foreign body, left ankle

4⃣ 4th character required   5⃣ 5th character required   6⃣ 6th character required   7⃣ 7th character required   ✖ Extension 'X' Alert
EXCLUDES 1 Not coded here   EXCLUDES 2 Not included here   PDx Primary Diagnosis Only   Manifestation Code

7️⃣ S91.019 Laceration without foreign body, unspecified ankle

6️⃣ S91.02 Laceration with foreign body of ankle
- 7️⃣ S91.021 Laceration with foreign body, right ankle
- 7️⃣ S91.022 Laceration with foreign body, left ankle
- 7️⃣ S91.029 Laceration with foreign body, unspecified ankle

6️⃣ S91.03 Puncture wound without foreign body of ankle
- 7️⃣ S91.031 Puncture wound without foreign body, right ankle
- 7️⃣ S91.032 Puncture wound without foreign body, left ankle
- 7️⃣ S91.039 Puncture wound without foreign body, unspecified ankle

6️⃣ S91.04 Puncture wound with foreign body of ankle
- 7️⃣ S91.041 Puncture wound with foreign body, right ankle
- 7️⃣ S91.042 Puncture wound with foreign body, left ankle
- 7️⃣ S91.049 Puncture wound with foreign body, unspecified ankle

6️⃣ S91.05 Open bite of ankle
> EXCLUDES1 superficial bite of ankle (S90.56-, S90.57-)
- 7️⃣ S91.051 Open bite, right ankle
- 7️⃣ S91.052 Open bite, left ankle
- 7️⃣ S91.059 Open bite, unspecified ankle

5️⃣ S91.1 Open wound of toe without damage to nail

6️⃣ S91.10 Unspecified open wound of toe without damage to nail
- 7️⃣ S91.101 Unspecified open wound of right great toe without damage to nail
- 7️⃣ S91.102 Unspecified open wound of left great toe without damage to nail
- 7️⃣ S91.103 Unspecified open wound of unspecified great toe without damage to nail
- 7️⃣ S91.104 Unspecified open wound of right lesser toe(s) without damage to nail
- 7️⃣ S91.105 Unspecified open wound of left lesser toe(s) without damage to nail
- 7️⃣ S91.106 Unspecified open wound of unspecified lesser toe(s) without damage to nail
- 7️⃣ S91.109 Unspecified open wound of unspecified toe(s) without damage to nail

6️⃣ S91.11 Laceration without foreign body of toe without damage to nail
- 7️⃣ S91.111 Laceration without foreign body of right great toe without damage to nail
- 7️⃣ S91.112 Laceration without foreign body of left great toe without damage to nail
- 7️⃣ S91.113 Laceration without foreign body of unspecified great toe without damage to nail
- 7️⃣ S91.114 Laceration without foreign body of right lesser toe(s) without damage to nail
- 7️⃣ S91.115 Laceration without foreign body of left lesser toe(s) without damage to nail
- 7️⃣ S91.116 Laceration without foreign body of unspecified lesser toe(s) without damage to nail
- 7️⃣ S91.119 Laceration without foreign body of unspecified toe without damage to nail

6️⃣ S91.12 Laceration with foreign body of toe without damage to nail
- 7️⃣ S91.121 Laceration with foreign body of right great toe without damage to nail
- 7️⃣ S91.122 Laceration with foreign body of left great toe without damage to nail
- 7️⃣ S91.123 Laceration with foreign body of unspecified great toe without damage to nail
- 7️⃣ S91.124 Laceration with foreign body of right lesser toe(s) without damage to nail
- 7️⃣ S91.125 Laceration with foreign body of left lesser toe(s) without damage to nail
- 7️⃣ S91.126 Laceration with foreign body of unspecified lesser toe(s) without damage to nail
- 7️⃣ S91.129 Laceration with foreign body of unspecified toe(s) without damage to nail

6️⃣ S91.13 Puncture wound without foreign body of toe without damage to nail
- 7️⃣ S91.131 Puncture wound without foreign body of right great toe without damage to nail
- 7️⃣ S91.132 Puncture wound without foreign body of left great toe without damage to nail
- 7️⃣ S91.133 Puncture wound without foreign body of unspecified great toe without damage to nail
- 7️⃣ S91.134 Puncture wound without foreign body of right lesser toe(s) without damage to nail
- 7️⃣ S91.135 Puncture wound without foreign body of left lesser toe(s) without damage to nail
- 7️⃣ S91.136 Puncture wound without foreign body of unspecified lesser toe(s) without damage to nail
- 7️⃣ S91.139 Puncture wound without foreign body of unspecified toe(s) without damage to nail

6️⃣ S91.14 Puncture wound with foreign body of toe without damage to nail
- 7️⃣ S91.141 Puncture wound with foreign body of right great toe without damage to nail
- 7️⃣ S91.142 Puncture wound with foreign body of left great toe without damage to nail
- 7️⃣ S91.143 Puncture wound with foreign body of unspecified great toe without damage to nail
- 7️⃣ S91.144 Puncture wound with foreign body of right lesser toe(s) without damage to nail
- 7️⃣ S91.145 Puncture wound with foreign body of left lesser toe(s) without damage to nail
- 7️⃣ S91.146 Puncture wound with foreign body of unspecified lesser toe(s) without damage to nail
- 7️⃣ S91.149 Puncture wound with foreign body of unspecified toe(s) without damage to nail

6️⃣ S91.15 Open bite of toe without damage to nail
Bite of toe NOS
> EXCLUDES1 superficial bite of toe (S90.46-, S90.47-)
- 7️⃣ S91.151 Open bite of right great toe without damage to nail
- 7️⃣ S91.152 Open bite of left great toe without damage to nail
- 7️⃣ S91.153 Open bite of unspecified great toe without damage to nail
- 7️⃣ S91.154 Open bite of right lesser toe(s) without damage to nail
- 7️⃣ S91.155 Open bite of left lesser toe(s) without damage to nail
- 7️⃣ S91.156 Open bite of unspecified lesser toe(s) without damage to nail
- 7️⃣ S91.159 Open bite of unspecified toe(s) without damage to nail

5️⃣ S91.2 Open wound of toe with damage to nail

6️⃣ S91.20 Unspecified open wound of toe with damage to nail
- 7️⃣ S91.201 Unspecified open wound of right great toe with damage to nail
- 7️⃣ S91.202 Unspecified open wound of left great toe with damage to nail

[7th] S91.203 Unspecified open wound of unspecified great toe with damage to nail
[7th] S91.204 Unspecified open wound of right lesser toe(s) with damage to nail
[7th] S91.205 Unspecified open wound of left lesser toe(s) with damage to nail
[7th] S91.206 Unspecified open wound of unspecified lesser toe(s) with damage to nail
[7th] S91.209 Unspecified open wound of unspecified toe(s) with damage to nail

[6th] S91.21 Laceration without foreign body of toe with damage to nail
[7th] S91.211 Laceration without foreign body of right great toe with damage to nail
[7th] S91.212 Laceration without foreign body of left great toe with damage to nail
[7th] S91.213 Laceration without foreign body of unspecified great toe with damage to nail
[7th] S91.214 Laceration without foreign body of right lesser toe(s) with damage to nail
[7th] S91.215 Laceration without foreign body of left lesser toe(s) with damage to nail
[7th] S91.216 Laceration without foreign body of unspecified lesser toe(s) with damage to nail
[7th] S91.219 Laceration without foreign body of unspecified toe(s) with damage to nail

[6th] S91.22 Laceration with foreign body of toe with damage to nail
[7th] S91.221 Laceration with foreign body of right great toe with damage to nail
[7th] S91.222 Laceration with foreign body of left great toe with damage to nail
[7th] S91.223 Laceration with foreign body of unspecified great toe with damage to nail
[7th] S91.224 Laceration with foreign body of right lesser toe(s) with damage to nail
[7th] S91.225 Laceration with foreign body of left lesser toe(s) with damage to nail
[7th] S91.226 Laceration with foreign body of unspecified lesser toe(s) with damage to nail
[7th] S91.229 Laceration with foreign body of unspecified toe(s) with damage to nail

[6th] S91.23 Puncture wound without foreign body of toe with damage to nail
[7th] S91.231 Puncture wound without foreign body of right great toe with damage to nail
[7th] S91.232 Puncture wound without foreign body of left great toe with damage to nail
[7th] S91.233 Puncture wound without foreign body of unspecified great toe with damage to nail
[7th] S91.234 Puncture wound without foreign body of right lesser toe(s) with damage to nail
[7th] S91.235 Puncture wound without foreign body of left lesser toe(s) with damage to nail
[7th] S91.236 Puncture wound without foreign body of unspecified lesser toe(s) with damage to nail
[7th] S91.239 Puncture wound without foreign body of unspecified toe(s) with damage to nail

[6th] S91.24 Puncture wound with foreign body of toe with damage to nail
[7th] S91.241 Puncture wound with foreign body of right great toe with damage to nail
[7th] S91.242 Puncture wound with foreign body of left great toe with damage to nail
[7th] S91.243 Puncture wound with foreign body of unspecified great toe with damage to nail
[7th] S91.244 Puncture wound with foreign body of right lesser toe(s) with damage to nail
[7th] S91.245 Puncture wound with foreign body of left lesser toe(s) with damage to nail
[7th] S91.246 Puncture wound with foreign body of unspecified lesser toe(s) with damage to nail
[7th] S91.249 Puncture wound with foreign body of unspecified toe(s) with damage to nail

[6th] S91.25 Open bite of toe with damage to nail
Bite of toe with damage to nail NOS
[EXCLUDES1] *superficial bite of toe (S90.46-, S90.47-)*
[7th] S91.251 Open bite of right great toe with damage to nail
[7th] S91.252 Open bite of left great toe with damage to nail
[7th] S91.253 Open bite of unspecified great toe with damage to nail
[7th] S91.254 Open bite of right lesser toe(s) with damage to nail
[7th] S91.255 Open bite of left lesser toe(s) with damage to nail
[7th] S91.256 Open bite of unspecified lesser toe(s) with damage to nail
[7th] S91.259 Open bite of unspecified toe(s) with damage to nail

[5th] S91.3 Open wound of foot
[6th] S91.30 Unspecified open wound of foot
[7th] S91.301 Unspecified open wound, right foot
[7th] S91.302 Unspecified open wound, left foot
[7th] S91.309 Unspecified open wound, unspecified foot
[6th] S91.31 Laceration without foreign body of foot
[7th] S91.311 Laceration without foreign body, right foot
[7th] S91.312 Laceration without foreign body, left foot
[7th] S91.319 Laceration without foreign body, unspecified foot
[6th] S91.32 Laceration with foreign body of foot
[7th] S91.321 Laceration with foreign body, right foot
[7th] S91.322 Laceration with foreign body, left foot
[7th] S91.329 Laceration with foreign body, unspecified foot
[6th] S91.33 Puncture wound without foreign body of foot
[7th] S91.331 Puncture wound without foreign body, right foot
[7th] S91.332 Puncture wound without foreign body, left foot
[7th] S91.339 Puncture wound without foreign body, unspecified foot
[6th] S91.34 Puncture wound with foreign body of foot
[7th] S91.341 Puncture wound with foreign body, right foot
[7th] S91.342 Puncture wound with foreign body, left foot
[7th] S91.349 Puncture wound with foreign body, unspecified foot
[6th] S91.35 Open bite of foot
[EXCLUDES1] *superficial bite of foot (S90.86-, S90.87-)*
[7th] S91.351 Open bite, right foot
[7th] S91.352 Open bite, left foot
[7th] S91.359 Open bite, unspecified foot

[4th] S92 Fracture of foot and toe, except ankle
[NOTES] A fracture not indicated as displaced or nondisplaced should be coded to displaced
A fracture not indicated as open or closed should be coded to closed
[EXCLUDES1] *traumatic amputation of ankle and foot (S98.-)*
[EXCLUDES2] *fracture of ankle (S82.-)*
fracture of malleolus (S82.-)

[4th] 4th character required [5th] 5th character required [6th] 6th character required [7th] 7th character required [X] Extension 'X' Alert
[EXCLUDES1] Not coded here [EXCLUDES2] Not included here [PDx] Primary Diagnosis Only Manifestation Code

The appropriate 7th character is to be added to each code from category S92
A = initial encounter for closed fracture
B = initial encounter for open fracture
D = subsequent encounter for fracture with routine healing
G = subsequent encounter for fracture with delayed healing
K = subsequent encounter for fracture with nonunion
P = subsequent encounter for fracture with malunion
S = sequela

S92.0 Fracture of calcaneus
Heel bone
Os calcis

S92.00 Unspecified fracture of calcaneus
- S92.001 Unspecified fracture of right calcaneus
- S92.002 Unspecified fracture of left calcaneus
- S92.009 Unspecified fracture of unspecified calcaneus

S92.01 Fracture of body of calcaneus
- S92.011 Displaced fracture of body of right calcaneus
- S92.012 Displaced fracture of body of left calcaneus
- S92.013 Displaced fracture of body of unspecified calcaneus
- S92.014 Nondisplaced fracture of body of right calcaneus
- S92.015 Nondisplaced fracture of body of left calcaneus
- S92.016 Nondisplaced fracture of body of unspecified calcaneus

S92.02 Fracture of anterior process of calcaneus
- S92.021 Displaced fracture of anterior process of right calcaneus
- S92.022 Displaced fracture of anterior process of left calcaneus
- S92.023 Displaced fracture of anterior process of unspecified calcaneus
- S92.024 Nondisplaced fracture of anterior process of right calcaneus
- S92.025 Nondisplaced fracture of anterior process of left calcaneus
- S92.026 Nondisplaced fracture of anterior process of unspecified calcaneus

S92.03 Avulsion fracture of tuberosity of calcaneus
- S92.031 Displaced avulsion fracture of tuberosity of right calcaneus
- S92.032 Displaced avulsion fracture of tuberosity of left calcaneus
- S92.033 Displaced avulsion fracture of tuberosity of unspecified calcaneus
- S92.034 Nondisplaced avulsion fracture of tuberosity of right calcaneus
- S92.035 Nondisplaced avulsion fracture of tuberosity of left calcaneus
- S92.036 Nondisplaced avulsion fracture of tuberosity of unspecified calcaneus

S92.04 Other fracture of tuberosity of calcaneus
- S92.041 Displaced other fracture of tuberosity of right calcaneus
- S92.042 Displaced other fracture of tuberosity of left calcaneus
- S92.043 Displaced other fracture of tuberosity of unspecified calcaneus
- S92.044 Nondisplaced other fracture of tuberosity of right calcaneus
- S92.045 Nondisplaced other fracture of tuberosity of left calcaneus
- S92.046 Nondisplaced other fracture of tuberosity of unspecified calcaneus

S92.05 Other extraarticular fracture of calcaneus
- S92.051 Displaced other extraarticular fracture of right calcaneus
- S92.052 Displaced other extraarticular fracture of left calcaneus
- S92.053 Displaced other extraarticular fracture of unspecified calcaneus
- S92.054 Nondisplaced other extraarticular fracture of right calcaneus
- S92.055 Nondisplaced other extraarticular fracture of left calcaneus
- S92.056 Nondisplaced other extraarticular fracture of unspecified calcaneus

S92.06 Intraarticular fracture of calcaneus
- S92.061 Displaced intraarticular fracture of right calcaneus
- S92.062 Displaced intraarticular fracture of left calcaneus
- S92.063 Displaced intraarticular fracture of unspecified calcaneus
- S92.064 Nondisplaced intraarticular fracture of right calcaneus
- S92.065 Nondisplaced intraarticular fracture of left calcaneus
- S92.066 Nondisplaced intraarticular fracture of unspecified calcaneus

S92.1 Fracture of talus
Astragalus

S92.10 Unspecified fracture of talus
- S92.101 Unspecified fracture of right talus
- S92.102 Unspecified fracture of left talus
- S92.109 Unspecified fracture of unspecified talus

S92.11 Fracture of neck of talus
- S92.111 Displaced fracture of neck of right talus
- S92.112 Displaced fracture of neck of left talus
- S92.113 Displaced fracture of neck of unspecified talus
- S92.114 Nondisplaced fracture of neck of right talus
- S92.115 Nondisplaced fracture of neck of left talus
- S92.116 Nondisplaced fracture of neck of unspecified talus

S92.12 Fracture of body of talus
- S92.121 Displaced fracture of body of right talus
- S92.122 Displaced fracture of body of left talus
- S92.123 Displaced fracture of body of unspecified talus
- S92.124 Nondisplaced fracture of body of right talus
- S92.125 Nondisplaced fracture of body of left talus
- S92.126 Nondisplaced fracture of body of unspecified talus

S92.13 Fracture of posterior process of talus
- S92.131 Displaced fracture of posterior process of right talus
- S92.132 Displaced fracture of posterior process of left talus
- S92.133 Displaced fracture of posterior process of unspecified talus
- S92.134 Nondisplaced fracture of posterior process of right talus
- S92.135 Nondisplaced fracture of posterior process of left talus
- S92.136 Nondisplaced fracture of posterior process of unspecified talus

S92.14 Dome fracture of talus
EXCLUDES1 osteochondritis dissecans (M93.2)
- S92.141 Displaced dome fracture of right talus

Unspecified Code   Other Specified Code   N Newborn Age: 0   P Pediatric Age: 0-17   M Maternity Age: 12-55
A Adult Age: 15-124   ♂ Male   ♀ Female   ● New Code   ▲ Revised Code Title   ►◄ Revised Text

- 7ᵗʰ S92.142 Displaced dome fracture of left talus
- 7ᵗʰ S92.143 Displaced dome fracture of unspecified talus
- 7ᵗʰ S92.144 Nondisplaced dome fracture of right talus
- 7ᵗʰ S92.145 Nondisplaced dome fracture of left talus
- 7ᵗʰ S92.146 Nondisplaced dome fracture of unspecified talus
- 6ᵗʰ S92.15 Avulsion fracture (chip fracture) of talus
  - 7ᵗʰ S92.151 Displaced avulsion fracture (chip fracture) of right talus
  - 7ᵗʰ S92.152 Displaced avulsion fracture (chip fracture) of left talus
  - 7ᵗʰ S92.153 Displaced avulsion fracture (chip fracture) of unspecified talus
  - 7ᵗʰ S92.154 Nondisplaced avulsion fracture (chip fracture) of right talus
  - 7ᵗʰ S92.155 Nondisplaced avulsion fracture (chip fracture) of left talus
  - 7ᵗʰ S92.156 Nondisplaced avulsion fracture (chip fracture) of unspecified talus
- 6ᵗʰ S92.19 Other fracture of talus
  - 7ᵗʰ S92.191 Other fracture of right talus
  - 7ᵗʰ S92.192 Other fracture of left talus
  - 7ᵗʰ S92.199 Other fracture of unspecified talus
- 5ᵗʰ S92.2 Fracture of other and unspecified tarsal bone(s)
  - 6ᵗʰ S92.20 Fracture of unspecified tarsal bone(s)
    - 7ᵗʰ S92.201 Fracture of unspecified tarsal bone(s) of right foot
    - 7ᵗʰ S92.202 Fracture of unspecified tarsal bone(s) of left foot
    - 7ᵗʰ S92.209 Fracture of unspecified tarsal bone(s) of unspecified foot
  - 6ᵗʰ S92.21 Fracture of cuboid bone
    - 7ᵗʰ S92.211 Displaced fracture of cuboid bone of right foot
    - 7ᵗʰ S92.212 Displaced fracture of cuboid bone of left foot
    - 7ᵗʰ S92.213 Displaced fracture of cuboid bone of unspecified foot
    - 7ᵗʰ S92.214 Nondisplaced fracture of cuboid bone of right foot
    - 7ᵗʰ S92.215 Nondisplaced fracture of cuboid bone of left foot
    - 7ᵗʰ S92.216 Nondisplaced fracture of cuboid bone of unspecified foot
  - 6ᵗʰ S92.22 Fracture of lateral cuneiform
    - 7ᵗʰ S92.221 Displaced fracture of lateral cuneiform of right foot
    - 7ᵗʰ S92.222 Displaced fracture of lateral cuneiform of left foot
    - 7ᵗʰ S92.223 Displaced fracture of lateral cuneiform of unspecified foot
    - 7ᵗʰ S92.224 Nondisplaced fracture of lateral cuneiform of right foot
    - 7ᵗʰ S92.225 Nondisplaced fracture of lateral cuneiform of left foot
    - 7ᵗʰ S92.226 Nondisplaced fracture of lateral cuneiform of unspecified foot
  - 6ᵗʰ S92.23 Fracture of intermediate cuneiform
    - 7ᵗʰ S92.231 Displaced fracture of intermediate cuneiform of right foot
    - 7ᵗʰ S92.232 Displaced fracture of intermediate cuneiform of left foot
    - 7ᵗʰ S92.233 Displaced fracture of intermediate cuneiform of unspecified foot
    - 7ᵗʰ S92.234 Nondisplaced fracture of intermediate cuneiform of right foot
    - 7ᵗʰ S92.235 Nondisplaced fracture of intermediate cuneiform of left foot

- 7ᵗʰ S92.236 Nondisplaced fracture of intermediate cuneiform of unspecified foot
- 6ᵗʰ S92.24 Fracture of medial cuneiform
  - 7ᵗʰ S92.241 Displaced fracture of medial cuneiform of right foot
  - 7ᵗʰ S92.242 Displaced fracture of medial cuneiform of left foot
  - 7ᵗʰ S92.243 Displaced fracture of medial cuneiform of unspecified foot
  - 7ᵗʰ S92.244 Nondisplaced fracture of medial cuneiform of right foot
  - 7ᵗʰ S92.245 Nondisplaced fracture of medial cuneiform of left foot
  - 7ᵗʰ S92.246 Nondisplaced fracture of medial cuneiform of unspecified foot
- 6ᵗʰ S92.25 Fracture of navicular [scaphoid] of foot
  - 7ᵗʰ S92.251 Displaced fracture of navicular [scaphoid] of right foot
  - 7ᵗʰ S92.252 Displaced fracture of navicular [scaphoid] of left foot
  - 7ᵗʰ S92.253 Displaced fracture of navicular [scaphoid] of unspecified foot
  - 7ᵗʰ S92.254 Nondisplaced fracture of navicular [scaphoid] of right foot
  - 7ᵗʰ S92.255 Nondisplaced fracture of navicular [scaphoid] of left foot
  - 7ᵗʰ S92.256 Nondisplaced fracture of navicular [scaphoid] of unspecified foot
- 5ᵗʰ S92.3 Fracture of metatarsal bone(s)
  - 6ᵗʰ S92.30 Fracture of unspecified metatarsal bone(s)
    - 7ᵗʰ S92.301 Fracture of unspecified metatarsal bone(s), right foot
    - 7ᵗʰ S92.302 Fracture of unspecified metatarsal bone(s), left foot
    - 7ᵗʰ S92.309 Fracture of unspecified metatarsal bone(s), unspecified foot
  - 6ᵗʰ S92.31 Fracture of first metatarsal bone
    - 7ᵗʰ S92.311 Displaced fracture of first metatarsal bone, right foot
    - 7ᵗʰ S92.312 Displaced fracture of first metatarsal bone, left foot
    - 7ᵗʰ S92.313 Displaced fracture of first metatarsal bone, unspecified foot
    - 7ᵗʰ S92.314 Nondisplaced fracture of first metatarsal bone, right foot
    - 7ᵗʰ S92.315 Nondisplaced fracture of first metatarsal bone, left foot
    - 7ᵗʰ S92.316 Nondisplaced fracture of first metatarsal bone, unspecified foot
  - 6ᵗʰ S92.32 Fracture of second metatarsal bone
    - 7ᵗʰ S92.321 Displaced fracture of second metatarsal bone, right foot
    - 7ᵗʰ S92.322 Displaced fracture of second metatarsal bone, left foot
    - 7ᵗʰ S92.323 Displaced fracture of second metatarsal bone, unspecified foot
    - 7ᵗʰ S92.324 Nondisplaced fracture of second metatarsal bone, right foot
    - 7ᵗʰ S92.325 Nondisplaced fracture of second metatarsal bone, left foot
    - 7ᵗʰ S92.326 Nondisplaced fracture of second metatarsal bone, unspecified foot
  - 6ᵗʰ S92.33 Fracture of third metatarsal bone
    - 7ᵗʰ S92.331 Displaced fracture of third metatarsal bone, right foot
    - 7ᵗʰ S92.332 Displaced fracture of third metatarsal bone, left foot
    - 7ᵗʰ S92.333 Displaced fracture of third metatarsal bone, unspecified foot
    - 7ᵗʰ S92.334 Nondisplaced fracture of third metatarsal bone, right foot

---

4ᵗʰ 4ᵗʰ character required   5ᵗʰ 5ᵗʰ character required   6ᵗʰ 6ᵗʰ character required   7ᵗʰ 7ᵗʰ character required   7ᵗʰˣ Extension 'X' Alert

EXCLUDES 1 Not coded here   EXCLUDES 2 Not included here   PDx Primary Diagnosis Only   Manifestation Code

7️⃣ S92.335 Nondisplaced fracture of third metatarsal bone, left foot
7️⃣ S92.336 Nondisplaced fracture of third metatarsal bone, unspecified foot
6️⃣ S92.34 Fracture of fourth metatarsal bone
7️⃣ S92.341 Displaced fracture of fourth metatarsal bone, right foot
7️⃣ S92.342 Displaced fracture of fourth metatarsal bone, left foot
7️⃣ S92.343 Displaced fracture of fourth metatarsal bone, unspecified foot
7️⃣ S92.344 Nondisplaced fracture of fourth metatarsal bone, right foot
7️⃣ S92.345 Nondisplaced fracture of fourth metatarsal bone, left foot
7️⃣ S92.346 Nondisplaced fracture of fourth metatarsal bone, unspecified foot
6️⃣ S92.35 Fracture of fifth metatarsal bone
7️⃣ S92.351 Displaced fracture of fifth metatarsal bone, right foot
7️⃣ S92.352 Displaced fracture of fifth metatarsal bone, left foot
7️⃣ S92.353 Displaced fracture of fifth metatarsal bone, unspecified foot
7️⃣ S92.354 Nondisplaced fracture of fifth metatarsal bone, right foot
7️⃣ S92.355 Nondisplaced fracture of fifth metatarsal bone, left foot
7️⃣ S92.356 Nondisplaced fracture of fifth metatarsal bone, unspecified foot
5️⃣ S92.4 Fracture of great toe
  6️⃣ S92.40 Unspecified fracture of great toe
7️⃣ S92.401 Displaced unspecified fracture of right great toe
7️⃣ S92.402 Displaced unspecified fracture of left great toe
7️⃣ S92.403 Displaced unspecified fracture of unspecified great toe
7️⃣ S92.404 Nondisplaced unspecified fracture of right great toe
7️⃣ S92.405 Nondisplaced unspecified fracture of left great toe
7️⃣ S92.406 Nondisplaced unspecified fracture of unspecified great toe
  6️⃣ S92.41 Fracture of proximal phalanx of great toe
7️⃣ S92.411 Displaced fracture of proximal phalanx of right great toe
7️⃣ S92.412 Displaced fracture of proximal phalanx of left great toe
7️⃣ S92.413 Displaced fracture of proximal phalanx of unspecified great toe
7️⃣ S92.414 Nondisplaced fracture of proximal phalanx of right great toe
7️⃣ S92.415 Nondisplaced fracture of proximal phalanx of left great toe
7️⃣ S92.416 Nondisplaced fracture of proximal phalanx of unspecified great toe
  6️⃣ S92.42 Fracture of distal phalanx of great toe
7️⃣ S92.421 Displaced fracture of distal phalanx of right great toe
7️⃣ S92.422 Displaced fracture of distal phalanx of left great toe
7️⃣ S92.423 Displaced fracture of distal phalanx of unspecified great toe
7️⃣ S92.424 Nondisplaced fracture of distal phalanx of right great toe
7️⃣ S92.425 Nondisplaced fracture of distal phalanx of left great toe
7️⃣ S92.426 Nondisplaced fracture of distal phalanx of unspecified great toe
  6️⃣ S92.49 Other fracture of great toe
7️⃣ S92.491 Other fracture of right great toe
7️⃣ S92.492 Other fracture of left great toe

7️⃣ S92.499 Other fracture of unspecified great toe
5️⃣ S92.5 Fracture of lesser toe(s)
  6️⃣ S92.50 Unspecified fracture of lesser toe(s)
7️⃣ S92.501 Displaced unspecified fracture of right lesser toe(s)
7️⃣ S92.502 Displaced unspecified fracture of left lesser toe(s)
7️⃣ S92.503 Displaced unspecified fracture of unspecified lesser toe(s)
7️⃣ S92.504 Nondisplaced unspecified fracture of right lesser toe(s)
7️⃣ S92.505 Nondisplaced unspecified fracture of left lesser toe(s)
7️⃣ S92.506 Nondisplaced unspecified fracture of unspecified lesser toe(s)
  6️⃣ S92.51 Fracture of proximal phalanx of lesser toe(s)
7️⃣ S92.511 Displaced fracture of proximal phalanx of right lesser toe(s)
7️⃣ S92.512 Displaced fracture of proximal phalanx of left lesser toe(s)
7️⃣ S92.513 Displaced fracture of proximal phalanx of unspecified lesser toe(s)
7️⃣ S92.514 Nondisplaced fracture of proximal phalanx of right lesser toe(s)
7️⃣ S92.515 Nondisplaced fracture of proximal phalanx of left lesser toe(s)
7️⃣ S92.516 Nondisplaced fracture of proximal phalanx of unspecified lesser toe(s)
  6️⃣ S92.52 Fracture of medial phalanx of lesser toe(s)
7️⃣ S92.521 Displaced fracture of medial phalanx of right lesser toe(s)
7️⃣ S92.522 Displaced fracture of medial phalanx of left lesser toe(s)
7️⃣ S92.523 Displaced fracture of medial phalanx of unspecified lesser toe(s)
7️⃣ S92.524 Nondisplaced fracture of medial phalanx of right lesser toe(s)
7️⃣ S92.525 Nondisplaced fracture of medial phalanx of left lesser toe(s)
7️⃣ S92.526 Nondisplaced fracture of medial phalanx of unspecified lesser toe(s)
  6️⃣ S92.53 Fracture of distal phalanx of lesser toe(s)
7️⃣ S92.531 Displaced fracture of distal phalanx of right lesser toe(s)
7️⃣ S92.532 Displaced fracture of distal phalanx of left lesser toe(s)
7️⃣ S92.533 Displaced fracture of distal phalanx of unspecified lesser toe(s)
7️⃣ S92.534 Nondisplaced fracture of distal phalanx of right lesser toe(s)
7️⃣ S92.535 Nondisplaced fracture of distal phalanx of left lesser toe(s)
7️⃣ S92.536 Nondisplaced fracture of distal phalanx of unspecified lesser toe(s)
  6️⃣ S92.59 Other fracture of lesser toe(s)
7️⃣ S92.591 Other fracture of right lesser toe(s)
7️⃣ S92.592 Other fracture of left lesser toe(s)
7️⃣ S92.599 Other fracture of unspecified lesser toe(s)
5️⃣ S92.9 Unspecified fracture of foot and toe
  6️⃣ S92.90 Unspecified fracture of foot
7️⃣ S92.901 Unspecified fracture of right foot
7️⃣ S92.902 Unspecified fracture of left foot
7️⃣ S92.909 Unspecified fracture of unspecified foot
  6️⃣ S92.91 Unspecified fracture of toe
7️⃣ S92.911 Unspecified fracture of right toe(s)
7️⃣ S92.912 Unspecified fracture of left toe(s)
7️⃣ S92.919 Unspecified fracture of unspecified toe(s)
4️⃣ S93 Dislocation and sprain of joints and ligaments at ankle, foot and toe level

Unspecified Code	Other Specified Code	N Newborn Age: 0	P Pediatric Age: 0-17	M Maternity Age: 12-55	
A Adult Age: 15-124	♂ Male	♀ Female	● New Code	▲ Revised Code Title	►◄ Revised Text

INCLUDES *avulsion of joint or ligament of ankle, foot and toe*
laceration of cartilage, joint or ligament of ankle, foot and toe
sprain of cartilage, joint or ligament of ankle, foot and toe
traumatic hemarthrosis of joint or ligament of ankle, foot and toe
traumatic rupture of joint or ligament of ankle, foot and toe
traumatic subluxation of joint or ligament of ankle, foot and toe
traumatic tear of joint or ligament of ankle, foot and toe

Code also any associated open wound

EXCLUDES2 strain of muscle and tendon of ankle and foot (S96.-)

The appropriate 7th character is to be added to each code from category S93
A = initial encounter
D = subsequent encounter
S = sequela

5️⃣ **S93.0 Subluxation and dislocation of** ankle joint
Subluxation and dislocation of astragalus
Subluxation and dislocation of fibula, lower end
Subluxation and dislocation of talus
Subluxation and dislocation of tibia, lower end
7️⃣ **S93.01** Subluxation of **right** ankle joint
7️⃣ **S93.02** Subluxation of **left** ankle joint
7️⃣ **S93.03** Subluxation of **unspecified** ankle joint
7️⃣ **S93.04** Dislocation of **right** ankle joint
7️⃣ **S93.05** Dislocation of **left** ankle joint
7️⃣ **S93.06** Dislocation of **unspecified** ankle joint

5️⃣ **S93.1 Subluxation and dislocation of** toe
6️⃣ **S93.10** Unspecified **subluxation and dislocation of toe**
Dislocation of toe NOS
Subluxation of toe NOS
7️⃣ **S93.101 Unspecified** subluxation of right **toe(s)**
7️⃣ **S93.102 Unspecified** subluxation of left **toe(s)**
7️⃣ **S93.103 Unspecified** subluxation of **unspecified toe(s)**
7️⃣ **S93.104 Unspecified** dislocation of right **toe(s)**
7️⃣ **S93.105 Unspecified** dislocation of left **toe(s)**
7️⃣ **S93.106 Unspecified** dislocation of **unspecified toe(s)**

6️⃣ **S93.11 Dislocation of** interphalangeal joint
7️⃣ **S93.111 Dislocation of interphalangeal joint of** right **great toe**
7️⃣ **S93.112 Dislocation of interphalangeal joint of** left **great toe**
7️⃣ **S93.113 Dislocation of interphalangeal joint of unspecified** great **toe**
7️⃣ **S93.114 Dislocation of interphalangeal joint of** right **lesser toe(s)**
7️⃣ **S93.115 Dislocation of interphalangeal joint of** left **lesser toe(s)**
7️⃣ **S93.116 Dislocation of interphalangeal joint of unspecified** lesser **toe(s)**
7️⃣ **S93.119 Dislocation of interphalangeal joint of unspecified toe(s)**

6️⃣ **S93.12 Dislocation of** metatarsophalangeal joint
7️⃣ **S93.121 Dislocation of metatarsophalangeal joint of** right great **toe**
7️⃣ **S93.122 Dislocation of metatarsophalangeal joint of** left great **toe**
7️⃣ **S93.123 Dislocation of metatarsophalangeal joint of unspecified** great **toe**
7️⃣ **S93.124 Dislocation of metatarsophalangeal joint of** right lesser **toe(s)**

7️⃣ **S93.125 Dislocation of metatarsophalangeal joint of** left lesser **toe(s)**
7️⃣ **S93.126 Dislocation of metatarsophalangeal joint of unspecified** lesser **toe(s)**
7️⃣ **S93.129 Dislocation of metatarsophalangeal joint of unspecified toe(s)**

6️⃣ **S93.13 Subluxation of** interphalangeal joint
7️⃣ **S93.131 Subluxation of interphalangeal joint of** right great **toe**
7️⃣ **S93.132 Subluxation of interphalangeal joint of** left great **toe**
7️⃣ **S93.133 Subluxation of interphalangeal joint of unspecified** great **toe**
7️⃣ **S93.134 Subluxation of interphalangeal joint of** right lesser **toe(s)**
7️⃣ **S93.135 Subluxation of interphalangeal joint of** left lesser **toe(s)**
7️⃣ **S93.136 Subluxation of interphalangeal joint of unspecified** lesser **toe(s)**
7️⃣ **S93.139 Subluxation of interphalangeal joint of unspecified toe(s)**

6️⃣ **S93.14 Subluxation of** metatarsophalangeal joint
7️⃣ **S93.141 Subluxation of metatarsophalangeal joint of** right great **toe**
7️⃣ **S93.142 Subluxation of metatarsophalangeal joint of** left great **toe**
7️⃣ **S93.143 Subluxation of metatarsophalangeal joint of unspecified** great **toe**
7️⃣ **S93.144 Subluxation of metatarsophalangeal joint of** right lesser **toe(s)**
7️⃣ **S93.145 Subluxation of metatarsophalangeal joint of** left lesser **toe(s)**
7️⃣ **S93.146 Subluxation of metatarsophalangeal joint of unspecified** lesser **toe(s)**
7️⃣ **S93.149 Subluxation of metatarsophalangeal joint of unspecified toe(s)**

5️⃣ **S93.3 Subluxation and dislocation of** foot
EXCLUDES2 dislocation of toe (S93.1-)
6️⃣ **S93.30** Unspecified **subluxation and dislocation of foot**
Dislocation of foot NOS
Subluxation of foot NOS
7️⃣ **S93.301 Unspecified** subluxation of right **foot**
7️⃣ **S93.302 Unspecified** subluxation of left **foot**
7️⃣ **S93.303 Unspecified** subluxation of unspecified **foot**
7️⃣ **S93.304 Unspecified** dislocation of right **foot**
7️⃣ **S93.305 Unspecified** dislocation of left **foot**
7️⃣ **S93.306 Unspecified** dislocation of unspecified **foot**

6️⃣ **S93.31 Subluxation and dislocation of** tarsal joint
7️⃣ **S93.311** Subluxation of tarsal joint of right **foot**
7️⃣ **S93.312** Subluxation of tarsal joint of left **foot**
7️⃣ **S93.313** Subluxation of tarsal joint of unspecified **foot**
7️⃣ **S93.314** Dislocation of tarsal joint of right **foot**
7️⃣ **S93.315** Dislocation of tarsal joint of left **foot**
7️⃣ **S93.316** Dislocation of tarsal joint of unspecified **foot**

6️⃣ **S93.32 Subluxation and dislocation of** tarsometatarsal joint
7️⃣ **S93.321** Subluxation of tarsometatarsal joint of right **foot**
7️⃣ **S93.322** Subluxation of tarsometatarsal joint of left **foot**
7️⃣ **S93.323** Subluxation of tarsometatarsal joint of unspecified **foot**
7️⃣ **S93.324** Dislocation of tarsometatarsal joint of right **foot**
7️⃣ **S93.325** Dislocation of tarsometatarsal joint of left **foot**

4️⃣ 4th character required   5️⃣ 5th character required   6️⃣ 6th character required   7️⃣ 7th character required   ⬤ Extension 'X' Alert
EXCLUDES1 Not coded here   EXCLUDES2 Not included here   PDx Primary Diagnosis Only   Manifestation Code

[7th] S93.326 Dislocation of tarsometatarsal joint of unspecified foot
[6th] S93.33 Other subluxation and dislocation of foot
[7th] S93.331 Other subluxation of right foot
[7th] S93.332 Other subluxation of left foot
[7th] S93.333 Other subluxation of unspecified foot
[7th] S93.334 Other dislocation of right foot
[7th] S93.335 Other dislocation of left foot
[7th] S93.336 Other dislocation of unspecified foot
[5th] S93.4 Sprain of ankle
[EXCLUDES2] *injury of Achilles tendon (S86.0-)*
[6th] S93.40 Sprain of unspecified ligament of ankle
Sprain of ankle NOS
Sprained ankle NOS
[7th] S93.401 Sprain of unspecified ligament of right ankle
[7th] S93.402 Sprain of unspecified ligament of left ankle
[7th] S93.409 Sprain of unspecified ligament of unspecified ankle
[6th] S93.41 Sprain of calcaneofibular ligament
[7th] S93.411 Sprain of calcaneofibular ligament of right ankle
[7th] S93.412 Sprain of calcaneofibular ligament of left ankle
[7th] S93.419 Sprain of calcaneofibular ligament of unspecified ankle
[6th] S93.42 Sprain of deltoid ligament
[7th] S93.421 Sprain of deltoid ligament of right ankle
[7th] S93.422 Sprain of deltoid ligament of left ankle
[7th] S93.429 Sprain of deltoid ligament of unspecified ankle
[6th] S93.43 Sprain of tibiofibular ligament
[7th] S93.431 Sprain of tibiofibular ligament of right ankle
[7th] S93.432 Sprain of tibiofibular ligament of left ankle
[7th] S93.439 Sprain of tibiofibular ligament of unspecified ankle
[6th] S93.49 Sprain of other ligament of ankle
Sprain of internal collateral ligament
Sprain of talofibular ligament
[7th] S93.491 Sprain of other ligament of right ankle
[7th] S93.492 Sprain of other ligament of left ankle
[7th] S93.499 Sprain of other ligament of unspecified ankle
[5th] S93.5 Sprain of toe
[6th] S93.50 Unspecified sprain of toe
[7th] S93.501 Unspecified sprain of right great toe
[7th] S93.502 Unspecified sprain of left great toe
[7th] S93.503 Unspecified sprain of unspecified great toe
[7th] S93.504 Unspecified sprain of right lesser toe(s)
[7th] S93.505 Unspecified sprain of left lesser toe(s)
[7th] S93.506 Unspecified sprain of unspecified lesser toe(s)
[7th] S93.509 Unspecified sprain of unspecified toe(s)
[6th] S93.51 Sprain of interphalangeal joint of toe
[7th] S93.511 Sprain of interphalangeal joint of right great toe
[7th] S93.512 Sprain of interphalangeal joint of left great toe
[7th] S93.513 Sprain of interphalangeal joint of unspecified great toe
[7th] S93.514 Sprain of interphalangeal joint of right lesser toe(s)
[7th] S93.515 Sprain of interphalangeal joint of left lesser toe(s)
[7th] S93.516 Sprain of interphalangeal joint of unspecified lesser toe(s)
[7th] S93.519 Sprain of interphalangeal joint of unspecified toe(s)
[6th] S93.52 Sprain of metatarsophalangeal joint of toe
[7th] S93.521 Sprain of metatarsophalangeal joint of right great toe
[7th] S93.522 Sprain of metatarsophalangeal joint of left great toe
[7th] S93.523 Sprain of metatarsophalangeal joint of unspecified great toe
[7th] S93.524 Sprain of metatarsophalangeal joint of right lesser toe(s)
[7th] S93.525 Sprain of metatarsophalangeal joint of left lesser toe(s)
[7th] S93.526 Sprain of metatarsophalangeal joint of unspecified lesser toe(s)
[7th] S93.529 Sprain of metatarsophalangeal joint of unspecified toe(s)
[5th] S93.6 Sprain of foot
[EXCLUDES2] *sprain of metatarsophalangeal joint of toe (S93.52-)*
sprain of toe (S93.5-)
[6th] S93.60 Unspecified sprain of foot
[7th] S93.601 Unspecified sprain of right foot
[7th] S93.602 Unspecified sprain of left foot
[7th] S93.609 Unspecified sprain of unspecified foot
[6th] S93.61 Sprain of tarsal ligament of foot
[7th] S93.611 Sprain of tarsal ligament of right foot
[7th] S93.612 Sprain of tarsal ligament of left foot
[7th] S93.619 Sprain of tarsal ligament of unspecified foot
[6th] S93.62 Sprain of tarsometatarsal ligament of foot
[7th] S93.621 Sprain of tarsometatarsal ligament of right foot
[7th] S93.622 Sprain of tarsometatarsal ligament of left foot
[7th] S93.629 Sprain of tarsometatarsal ligament of unspecified foot
[6th] S93.69 Other sprain of foot
[7th] S93.691 Other sprain of right foot
[7th] S93.692 Other sprain of left foot
[7th] S93.699 Other sprain of unspecified foot
[4th] S94 Injury of nerves at ankle and foot level
Code also any associated open wound (S91.-)
The appropriate 7th character is to be added to each code from category S94
A = initial encounter
D = subsequent encounter
S = sequela
[5th] S94.0 Injury of lateral plantar nerve
[7th] S94.00 Injury of lateral plantar nerve, unspecified leg
[7th] S94.01 Injury of lateral plantar nerve, right leg
[7th] S94.02 Injury of lateral plantar nerve, left leg
[5th] S94.1 Injury of medial plantar nerve
[7th] S94.10 Injury of medial plantar nerve, unspecified leg
[7th] S94.11 Injury of medial plantar nerve, right leg
[7th] S94.12 Injury of medial plantar nerve, left leg
[5th] S94.2 Injury of deep peroneal nerve at ankle and foot level
Injury of terminal, lateral branch of deep peroneal nerve
[7th] S94.20 Injury of deep peroneal nerve at ankle and foot level, unspecified leg
[7th] S94.21 Injury of deep peroneal nerve at ankle and foot level, right leg
[7th] S94.22 Injury of deep peroneal nerve at ankle and foot level, left leg
[5th] S94.3 Injury of cutaneous sensory nerve at ankle and foot level
[7th] S94.30 Injury of cutaneous sensory nerve at ankle and foot level, unspecified leg
[7th] S94.31 Injury of cutaneous sensory nerve at ankle and foot level, right leg
[7th] S94.32 Injury of cutaneous sensory nerve at ankle and foot level, left leg

Unspecified Code Other Specified Code [N] Newborn Age: 0 [P] Pediatric Age: 0-17 [M] Maternity Age: 12-55
[A] Adult Age: 15-124 ♂ Male ♀ Female ● New Code ▲ Revised Code Title ►◄ Revised Text

[5th] S94.8 Injury of other nerves at ankle and foot level
[6th] S94.8X Injury of other nerves at ankle and foot level
[7th] S94.8X1 Injury of other nerves at ankle and foot level, right leg
[7th] S94.8X2 Injury of other nerves at ankle and foot level, left leg
[7th] S94.8X9 Injury of other nerves at ankle and foot level, unspecified leg
[5th] S94.9 Injury of unspecified nerve at ankle and foot level
[7th] S94.90 Injury of unspecified nerve at ankle and foot level, unspecified leg
[7th] S94.91 Injury of unspecified nerve at ankle and foot level, right leg
[7th] S94.92 Injury of unspecified nerve at ankle and foot level, left leg

[4th] S95 Injury of blood vessels at ankle and foot level
Code also any associated open wound (S91.-)
EXCLUDES2 *injury of posterior tibial artery and vein (S85.1-, S85.8-)*
The appropriate 7th character is to be added to each code from category S95
A = initial encounter
D = subsequent encounter
S = sequela
[5th] S95.0 Injury of dorsal artery of foot
[6th] S95.00 Unspecified injury of dorsal artery of foot
[7th] S95.001 Unspecified injury of dorsal artery of right foot
[7th] S95.002 Unspecified injury of dorsal artery of left foot
[7th] S95.009 Unspecified injury of dorsal artery of unspecified foot
[6th] S95.01 Laceration of dorsal artery of foot
[7th] S95.011 Laceration of dorsal artery of right foot
[7th] S95.012 Laceration of dorsal artery of left foot
[7th] S95.019 Laceration of dorsal artery of unspecified foot
[6th] S95.09 Other specified injury of dorsal artery of foot
[7th] S95.091 Other specified injury of dorsal artery of right foot
[7th] S95.092 Other specified injury of dorsal artery of left foot
[7th] S95.099 Other specified injury of dorsal artery of unspecified foot
[5th] S95.1 Injury of plantar artery of foot
[6th] S95.10 Unspecified injury of plantar artery of foot
[7th] S95.101 Unspecified injury of plantar artery of right foot
[7th] S95.102 Unspecified injury of plantar artery of left foot
[7th] S95.109 Unspecified injury of plantar artery of unspecified foot
[6th] S95.11 Laceration of plantar artery of foot
[7th] S95.111 Laceration of plantar artery of right foot
[7th] S95.112 Laceration of plantar artery of left foot
[7th] S95.119 Laceration of plantar artery of unspecified foot
[6th] S95.19 Other specified injury of plantar artery of foot
[7th] S95.191 Other specified injury of plantar artery of right foot
[7th] S95.192 Other specified injury of plantar artery of left foot
[7th] S95.199 Other specified injury of plantar artery of unspecified foot
[5th] S95.2 Injury of dorsal vein of foot
[6th] S95.20 Unspecified injury of dorsal vein of foot
[7th] S95.201 Unspecified injury of dorsal vein of right foot
[7th] S95.202 Unspecified injury of dorsal vein of left foot
[7th] S95.209 Unspecified injury of dorsal vein of unspecified foot
[6th] S95.21 Laceration of dorsal vein of foot
[7th] S95.211 Laceration of dorsal vein of right foot
[7th] S95.212 Laceration of dorsal vein of left foot
[7th] S95.219 Laceration of dorsal vein of unspecified foot
[6th] S95.29 Other specified injury of dorsal vein of foot
[7th] S95.291 Other specified injury of dorsal vein of right foot
[7th] S95.292 Other specified injury of dorsal vein of left foot
[7th] S95.299 Other specified injury of dorsal vein of unspecified foot
[5th] S95.8 Injury of other blood vessels at ankle and foot level
[6th] S95.80 Unspecified injury of other blood vessels at ankle and foot level
[7th] S95.801 Unspecified injury of other blood vessels at ankle and foot level, right leg
[7th] S95.802 Unspecified injury of other blood vessels at ankle and foot level, left leg
[7th] S95.809 Unspecified injury of other blood vessels at ankle and foot level, unspecified leg
[6th] S95.81 Laceration of other blood vessels at ankle and foot level
[7th] S95.811 Laceration of other blood vessels at ankle and foot level, right leg
[7th] S95.812 Laceration of other blood vessels at ankle and foot level, left leg
[7th] S95.819 Laceration of other blood vessels at ankle and foot level, unspecified leg
[6th] S95.89 Other specified injury of other blood vessels at ankle and foot level
[7th] S95.891 Other specified injury of other blood vessels at ankle and foot level, right leg
[7th] S95.892 Other specified injury of other blood vessels at ankle and foot level, left leg
[7th] S95.899 Other specified injury of other blood vessels at ankle and foot level, unspecified leg
[5th] S95.9 Injury of unspecified blood vessel at ankle and foot level
[6th] S95.90 Unspecified injury of unspecified blood vessel at ankle and foot level
[7th] S95.901 Unspecified injury of unspecified blood vessel at ankle and foot level, right leg
[7th] S95.902 Unspecified injury of unspecified blood vessel at ankle and foot level, left leg
[7th] S95.909 Unspecified injury of unspecified blood vessel at ankle and foot level, unspecified leg
[6th] S95.91 Laceration of unspecified blood vessel at ankle and foot level
[7th] S95.911 Laceration of unspecified blood vessel at ankle and foot level, right leg
[7th] S95.912 Laceration of unspecified blood vessel at ankle and foot level, left leg
[7th] S95.919 Laceration of unspecified blood vessel at ankle and foot level, unspecified leg
[6th] S95.99 Other specified injury of unspecified blood vessel at ankle and foot level
[7th] S95.991 Other specified injury of unspecified blood vessel at ankle and foot level, right leg
[7th] S95.992 Other specified injury of unspecified blood vessel at ankle and foot level, left leg
[7th] S95.999 Other specified injury of unspecified blood vessel at ankle and foot level, unspecified leg

[4th] S96 Injury of muscle and tendon at ankle and foot level
Code also any associated open wound (S91.-)

[4] 4th character required [5] 5th character required [6] 6th character required [7] 7th character required [7] Extension 'X' Alert
EXCLUDES1 Not coded here EXCLUDES2 Not included here PDx Primary Diagnosis Only Manifestation Code

EXCLUDES2 *injury of Achilles tendon (S86.0-)*
sprain of joints and ligaments of ankle and foot (S93.-)

The appropriate 7th character is to be added to each code from category S96
A = initial encounter
D = subsequent encounter
S = sequela

5ᵗʰ **S96.0** Injury of muscle and tendon of long flexor muscle of toe at ankle and foot level

  6ᵗʰ **S96.00** Unspecified injury of muscle and tendon of long flexor muscle of toe at ankle and foot level

    7ᵗʰ **S96.001** Unspecified injury of muscle and tendon of long flexor muscle of toe at ankle and foot level, right foot

    7ᵗʰ **S96.002** Unspecified injury of muscle and tendon of long flexor muscle of toe at ankle and foot level, left foot

    7ᵗʰ **S96.009** Unspecified injury of muscle and tendon of long flexor muscle of toe at ankle and foot level, unspecified foot

  6ᵗʰ **S96.01** Strain of muscle and tendon of long flexor muscle of toe at ankle and foot level

    7ᵗʰ **S96.011** Strain of muscle and tendon of long flexor muscle of toe at ankle and foot level, right foot

    7ᵗʰ **S96.012** Strain of muscle and tendon of long flexor muscle of toe at ankle and foot level, left foot

    7ᵗʰ **S96.019** Strain of muscle and tendon of long flexor muscle of toe at ankle and foot level, unspecified foot

  6ᵗʰ **S96.02** Laceration of muscle and tendon of long flexor muscle of toe at ankle and foot level

    7ᵗʰ **S96.021** Laceration of muscle and tendon of long flexor muscle of toe at ankle and foot level, right foot

    7ᵗʰ **S96.022** Laceration of muscle and tendon of long flexor muscle of toe at ankle and foot level, left foot

    7ᵗʰ **S96.029** Laceration of muscle and tendon of long flexor muscle of toe at ankle and foot level, unspecified foot

  6ᵗʰ **S96.09** Other injury of muscle and tendon of long flexor muscle of toe at ankle and foot level

    7ᵗʰ **S96.091** Other injury of muscle and tendon of long flexor muscle of toe at ankle and foot level, right foot

    7ᵗʰ **S96.092** Other injury of muscle and tendon of long flexor muscle of toe at ankle and foot level, left foot

    7ᵗʰ **S96.099** Other injury of muscle and tendon of long flexor muscle of toe at ankle and foot level, unspecified foot

5ᵗʰ **S96.1** Injury of muscle and tendon of long extensor muscle of toe at ankle and foot level

  6ᵗʰ **S96.10** Unspecified injury of muscle and tendon of long extensor muscle of toe at ankle and foot level

    7ᵗʰ **S96.101** Unspecified injury of muscle and tendon of long extensor muscle of toe at ankle and foot level, right foot

    7ᵗʰ **S96.102** Unspecified injury of muscle and tendon of long extensor muscle of toe at ankle and foot level, left foot

    7ᵗʰ **S96.109** Unspecified injury of muscle and tendon of long extensor muscle of toe at ankle and foot level, unspecified foot

  6ᵗʰ **S96.11** Strain of muscle and tendon of long extensor muscle of toe at ankle and foot level

    7ᵗʰ **S96.111** Strain of muscle and tendon of long extensor muscle of toe at ankle and foot level, right foot

    7ᵗʰ **S96.112** Strain of muscle and tendon of long extensor muscle of toe at ankle and foot level, left foot

    7ᵗʰ **S96.119** Strain of muscle and tendon of long extensor muscle of toe at ankle and foot level, unspecified foot

  6ᵗʰ **S96.12** Laceration of muscle and tendon of long extensor muscle of toe at ankle and foot level

    7ᵗʰ **S96.121** Laceration of muscle and tendon of long extensor muscle of toe at ankle and foot level, right foot

    7ᵗʰ **S96.122** Laceration of muscle and tendon of long extensor muscle of toe at ankle and foot level, left foot

    7ᵗʰ **S96.129** Laceration of muscle and tendon of long extensor muscle of toe at ankle and foot level, unspecified foot

  6ᵗʰ **S96.19** Other specified injury of muscle and tendon of long extensor muscle of toe at ankle and foot level

    7ᵗʰ **S96.191** Other specified injury of muscle and tendon of long extensor muscle of toe at ankle and foot level, right foot

    7ᵗʰ **S96.192** Other specified injury of muscle and tendon of long extensor muscle of toe at ankle and foot level, left foot

    7ᵗʰ **S96.199** Other specified injury of muscle and tendon of long extensor muscle of toe at ankle and foot level, unspecified foot

5ᵗʰ **S96.2** Injury of intrinsic muscle and tendon at ankle and foot level

  6ᵗʰ **S96.20** Unspecified injury of intrinsic muscle and tendon at ankle and foot level

    7ᵗʰ **S96.201** Unspecified injury of intrinsic muscle and tendon at ankle and foot level, right foot

    7ᵗʰ **S96.202** Unspecified injury of intrinsic muscle and tendon at ankle and foot level, left foot

    7ᵗʰ **S96.209** Unspecified injury of intrinsic muscle and tendon at ankle and foot level, unspecified foot

  6ᵗʰ **S96.21** Strain of intrinsic muscle and tendon at ankle and foot level

    7ᵗʰ **S96.211** Strain of intrinsic muscle and tendon at ankle and foot level, right foot

    7ᵗʰ **S96.212** Strain of intrinsic muscle and tendon at ankle and foot level, left foot

    7ᵗʰ **S96.219** Strain of intrinsic muscle and tendon at ankle and foot level, unspecified foot

  6ᵗʰ **S96.22** Laceration of intrinsic muscle and tendon at ankle and foot level

    7ᵗʰ **S96.221** Laceration of intrinsic muscle and tendon at ankle and foot level, right foot

    7ᵗʰ **S96.222** Laceration of intrinsic muscle and tendon at ankle and foot level, left foot

    7ᵗʰ **S96.229** Laceration of intrinsic muscle and tendon at ankle and foot level, unspecified foot

  6ᵗʰ **S96.29** Other specified injury of intrinsic muscle and tendon at ankle and foot level

    7ᵗʰ **S96.291** Other specified injury of intrinsic muscle and tendon at ankle and foot level, right foot

    7ᵗʰ **S96.292** Other specified injury of intrinsic muscle and tendon at ankle and foot level, left foot

    7ᵗʰ **S96.299** Other specified injury of intrinsic muscle and tendon at ankle and foot level, unspecified foot

---

Unspecified Code   Other Specified Code   N Newborn Age: 0   P Pediatric Age: 0-17   M Maternity Age: 12-55
A Adult Age: 15-124   ♂ Male   ♀ Female   ● New Code   ▲ Revised Code Title   ►◄ Revised Text

⑤ᵗʰ S96.8 Injury of other specified muscles and tendons at ankle and foot level
⑥ᵗʰ S96.80 Unspecified injury of other specified muscles and tendons at ankle and foot level
⑦ᵗʰ S96.801 Unspecified injury of other specified muscles and tendons at ankle and foot level, right foot
⑦ᵗʰ S96.802 Unspecified injury of other specified muscles and tendons at ankle and foot level, left foot
⑦ᵗʰ S96.809 Unspecified injury of other specified muscles and tendons at ankle and foot level, unspecified foot
⑥ᵗʰ S96.81 Strain of other specified muscles and tendons at ankle and foot level
⑦ᵗʰ S96.811 Strain of other specified muscles and tendons at ankle and foot level, right foot
⑦ᵗʰ S96.812 Strain of other specified muscles and tendons at ankle and foot level, left foot
⑦ᵗʰ S96.819 Strain of other specified muscles and tendons at ankle and foot level, unspecified foot
⑥ᵗʰ S96.82 Laceration of other specified muscles and tendons at ankle and foot level
⑦ᵗʰ S96.821 Laceration of other specified muscles and tendons at ankle and foot level, right foot
⑦ᵗʰ S96.822 Laceration of other specified muscles and tendons at ankle and foot level, left foot
⑦ᵗʰ S96.829 Laceration of other specified muscles and tendons at ankle and foot level, unspecified foot
⑥ᵗʰ S96.89 Other specified injury of other specified muscles and tendons at ankle and foot level
⑦ᵗʰ S96.891 Other specified injury of other specified muscles and tendons at ankle and foot level, right foot
⑦ᵗʰ S96.892 Other specified injury of other specified muscles and tendons at ankle and foot level, left foot
⑦ᵗʰ S96.899 Other specified injury of other specified muscles and tendons at ankle and foot level, unspecified foot
⑤ᵗʰ S96.9 Injury of unspecified muscle and tendon at ankle and foot level
⑥ᵗʰ S96.90 Unspecified injury of unspecified muscle and tendon at ankle and foot level
⑦ᵗʰ S96.901 Unspecified injury of unspecified muscle and tendon at ankle and foot level, right foot
⑦ᵗʰ S96.902 Unspecified injury of unspecified muscle and tendon at ankle and foot level, left foot
⑦ᵗʰ S96.909 Unspecified injury of unspecified muscle and tendon at ankle and foot level, unspecified foot
⑥ᵗʰ S96.91 Strain of unspecified muscle and tendon at ankle and foot level
⑦ᵗʰ S96.911 Strain of unspecified muscle and tendon at ankle and foot level, right foot
⑦ᵗʰ S96.912 Strain of unspecified muscle and tendon at ankle and foot level, left foot
⑦ᵗʰ S96.919 Strain of unspecified muscle and tendon at ankle and foot level, unspecified foot
⑥ᵗʰ S96.92 Laceration of unspecified muscle and tendon at ankle and foot level
⑦ᵗʰ S96.921 Laceration of unspecified muscle and tendon at ankle and foot level, right foot
⑦ᵗʰ S96.922 Laceration of unspecified muscle and tendon at ankle and foot level, left foot

⑦ᵗʰ S96.929 Laceration of unspecified muscle and tendon at ankle and foot level, unspecified foot
⑥ᵗʰ S96.99 Other specified injury of unspecified muscle and tendon at ankle and foot level
⑦ᵗʰ S96.991 Other specified injury of unspecified muscle and tendon at ankle and foot level, right foot
⑦ᵗʰ S96.992 Other specified injury of unspecified muscle and tendon at ankle and foot level, left foot
⑦ᵗʰ S96.999 Other specified injury of unspecified muscle and tendon at ankle and foot level, unspecified foot
④ᵗʰ S97 Crushing injury of ankle and foot
Use additional code(s) for all associated injuries
The appropriate 7th character is to be added to each code from category S97
A = initial encounter
D = subsequent encounter
S = sequela
⑤ᵗʰ S97.0 Crushing injury of ankle
⑥ᵗʰ S97.00 Crushing injury of unspecified ankle
⑥ᵗʰ S97.01 Crushing injury of right ankle
⑥ᵗʰ S97.02 Crushing injury of left ankle
⑤ᵗʰ S97.1 Crushing injury of toe
⑥ᵗʰ S97.10 Crushing injury of unspecified toe(s)
⑦ᵗʰ S97.101 Crushing injury of unspecified right toe(s)
⑦ᵗʰ S97.102 Crushing injury of unspecified left toe(s)
⑦ᵗʰ S97.109 Crushing injury of unspecified toe(s)
Crushing injury of toe NOS
⑥ᵗʰ S97.11 Crushing injury of great toe
⑦ᵗʰ S97.111 Crushing injury of right great toe
⑦ᵗʰ S97.112 Crushing injury of left great toe
⑦ᵗʰ S97.119 Crushing injury of unspecified great toe
⑥ᵗʰ S97.12 Crushing injury of lesser toe(s)
⑦ᵗʰ S97.121 Crushing injury of right lesser toe(s)
⑦ᵗʰ S97.122 Crushing injury of left lesser toe(s)
⑦ᵗʰ S97.129 Crushing injury of unspecified lesser toe(s)
⑤ᵗʰ S97.8 Crushing injury of foot
⑥ᵗʰ S97.80 Crushing injury of unspecified foot
Crushing injury of foot NOS
⑥ᵗʰ S97.81 Crushing injury of right foot
⑥ᵗʰ S97.82 Crushing injury of left foot
④ᵗʰ S98 Traumatic amputation of ankle and foot
An amputation not identified as partial or complete should be coded to complete
The appropriate 7th character is to be added to each code from category S98
A = initial encounter
D = subsequent encounter
S = sequela
⑤ᵗʰ S98.0 Traumatic amputation of foot at ankle level
⑥ᵗʰ S98.01 Complete traumatic amputation of foot at ankle level
⑦ᵗʰ S98.011 Complete traumatic amputation of right foot at ankle level
⑦ᵗʰ S98.012 Complete traumatic amputation of left foot at ankle level
⑦ᵗʰ S98.019 Complete traumatic amputation of unspecified foot at ankle level
⑥ᵗʰ S98.02 Partial traumatic amputation of foot at ankle level
⑦ᵗʰ S98.021 Partial traumatic amputation of right foot at ankle level
⑦ᵗʰ S98.022 Partial traumatic amputation of left foot at ankle level
⑦ᵗʰ S98.029 Partial traumatic amputation of unspecified foot at ankle level

④ᵗʰ 4ᵗʰ character required ⑤ᵗʰ 5ᵗʰ character required ⑥ᵗʰ 6ᵗʰ character required ⑦ᵗʰ 7ᵗʰ character required ⓧ Extension 'X' Alert
EXCLUDES 1 Not coded here EXCLUDES 2 Not included here ᴾᴰˣ Primary Diagnosis Only Manifestation Code

[5th] S98.1 Traumatic amputation of one toe
[6th] S98.11 Complete traumatic amputation of great toe
[7th] S98.111 Complete traumatic amputation of right great toe
[7th] S98.112 Complete traumatic amputation of left great toe
[7th] S98.119 Complete traumatic amputation of unspecified great toe
[6th] S98.12 Partial traumatic amputation of great toe
[7th] S98.121 Partial traumatic amputation of right great toe
[7th] S98.122 Partial traumatic amputation of left great toe
[7th] S98.129 Partial traumatic amputation of unspecified great toe
[6th] S98.13 Complete traumatic amputation of one lesser toe
Traumatic amputation of toe NOS
[7th] S98.131 Complete traumatic amputation of one right lesser toe
[7th] S98.132 Complete traumatic amputation of one left lesser toe
[7th] S98.139 Complete traumatic amputation of one unspecified lesser toe
[6th] S98.14 Partial traumatic amputation of one lesser toe
[7th] S98.141 Partial traumatic amputation of one right lesser toe
[7th] S98.142 Partial traumatic amputation of one left lesser toe
[7th] S98.149 Partial traumatic amputation of one unspecified lesser toe
[5th] S98.2 Traumatic amputation of two or more lesser toes
[6th] S98.21 Complete traumatic amputation of two or more lesser toes
[7th] S98.211 Complete traumatic amputation of two or more right lesser toes
[7th] S98.212 Complete traumatic amputation of two or more left lesser toes
[7th] S98.219 Complete traumatic amputation of two or more unspecified lesser toes
[6th] S98.22 Partial traumatic amputation of two or more lesser toes
[7th] S98.221 Partial traumatic amputation of two or more right lesser toes
[7th] S98.222 Partial traumatic amputation of two or more left lesser toes
[7th] S98.229 Partial traumatic amputation of two or more unspecified lesser toes
[5th] S98.3 Traumatic amputation of midfoot
[6th] S98.31 Complete traumatic amputation of midfoot
[7th] S98.311 Complete traumatic amputation of right midfoot
[7th] S98.312 Complete traumatic amputation of left midfoot
[7th] S98.319 Complete traumatic amputation of unspecified midfoot
[6th] S98.32 Partial traumatic amputation of midfoot
[7th] S98.321 Partial traumatic amputation of right midfoot
[7th] S98.322 Partial traumatic amputation of left midfoot
[7th] S98.329 Partial traumatic amputation of unspecified midfoot
[5th] S98.9 Traumatic amputation of foot, level unspecified
[6th] S98.91 Complete traumatic amputation of foot, level unspecified
[7th] S98.911 Complete traumatic amputation of right foot, level unspecified
[7th] S98.912 Complete traumatic amputation of left foot, level unspecified
[7th] S98.919 Complete traumatic amputation of unspecified foot, level unspecified
[6th] S98.92 Partial traumatic amputation of foot, level unspecified
[7th] S98.921 Partial traumatic amputation of right foot, level unspecified
[7th] S98.922 Partial traumatic amputation of left foot, level unspecified
[7th] S98.929 Partial traumatic amputation of unspecified foot, level unspecified
[4th] S99 Other and unspecified injuries of ankle and foot
The appropriate 7th character is to be added to each code from category S99
A = initial encounter
D = subsequent encounter
S = sequela
[5th] S99.8 Other specified injuries of ankle and foot
[6th] S99.81 Other specified injuries of ankle
[7th] S99.811 Other specified injuries of right ankle
[7th] S99.812 Other specified injuries of left ankle
[7th] S99.819 Other specified injuries of unspecified ankle
[6th] S99.82 Other specified injuries of foot
[7th] S99.821 Other specified injuries of right foot
[7th] S99.822 Other specified injuries of left foot
[7th] S99.829 Other specified injuries of unspecified foot
[5th] S99.9 Unspecified injury of ankle and foot
[6th] S99.91 Unspecified injury of ankle
[7th] S99.911 Unspecified injury of right ankle
[7th] S99.912 Unspecified injury of left ankle
[7th] S99.919 Unspecified injury of unspecified ankle
[6th] S99.92 Unspecified injury of foot
[7th] S99.921 Unspecified injury of right foot
[7th] S99.922 Unspecified injury of left foot
[7th] S99.929 Unspecified injury of unspecified foot

Unspecified Code Other Specified Code [N] Newborn Age: 0 [P] Pediatric Age: 0-17 [M] Maternity Age: 12-55
[A] Adult Age: 15-124 ♂ Male ♀ Female ● New Code ▲ Revised Code Title ►◄ Revised Text

Injury, poisoning and certain other consequences of external causes (T07-T88)

Injuries involving multiple body regions (T07)

EXCLUDES1 *burns and corrosions (T20-T32)*
frostbite (T33-T34)
insect bite or sting, venomous (T63.4)
sunburn (L55.-)

T07 Unspecified multiple injuries
EXCLUDES1 *injury NOS (T14)*

Injury of unspecified body region (T14)

[4th] **T14 Injury of unspecified body region**
EXCLUDES1 *multiple unspecified injuries (T07)*
T14.8 Other injury of unspecified body region
Abrasion NOS
Contusion NOS
Crush injury NOS
Fracture NOS
Skin injury NOS
Vascular injury NOS
[5th] **T14.9 Unspecified injury**
T14.90 Injury, unspecified
Injury NOS
T14.91 Suicide attempt
Attempted suicide NOS

Effects of foreign body entering through natural orifice (T15-T19)

EXCLUDES2 *foreign body accidentally left in operation wound (T81.5-)*
foreign body in penetrating wound - See open wound by body region
residual foreign body in soft tissue (M79.5)
splinter, without open wound - See superficial injury by body region

[4th] **T15 Foreign body on external eye**
EXCLUDES2 *foreign body in penetrating wound of orbit and eye ball (S05.4-, S05.5-)*
open wound of eyelid and periocular area (S01.1-)
retained foreign body in eyelid (H02.8-)
retained (old) foreign body in penetrating wound of orbit and eye ball (H05.5-, H44.6-, H44.7-)
superficial foreign body of eyelid and periocular area (S00.25-)
The appropriate 7th character is to be added to each code from category T15
A = initial encounter
D = subsequent encounter
S = sequela
[5th] **T15.0 Foreign body in cornea**
[7th] **T15.00 Foreign body in cornea, unspecified eye**
[7th] **T15.01 Foreign body in cornea, right eye**
[7th] **T15.02 Foreign body in cornea, left eye**
[5th] **T15.1 Foreign body in conjunctival sac**
[7th] **T15.10 Foreign body in conjunctival sac, unspecified eye**
[7th] **T15.11 Foreign body in conjunctival sac, right eye**
[7th] **T15.12 Foreign body in conjunctival sac, left eye**
[5th] **T15.8 Foreign body in other and multiple parts of external eye**
Foreign body in lacrimal punctum
[7th] **T15.80 Foreign body in other and multiple parts of external eye, unspecified eye**
[7th] **T15.81 Foreign body in other and multiple parts of external eye, right eye**
[7th] **T15.82 Foreign body in other and multiple parts of external eye, left eye**
[5th] **T15.9 Foreign body on external eye, part unspecified**
[7th] **T15.90 Foreign body on external eye, part unspecified, unspecified eye**
[7th] **T15.91 Foreign body on external eye, part unspecified, right eye**
[7th] **T15.92 Foreign body on external eye, part unspecified, left eye**

[4th] **T16 Foreign body in ear**
INCLUDES *foreign body in auditory canal*
The appropriate 7th character is to be added to each code from category T16
A = initial encounter
D = subsequent encounter
S = sequela
[7th] **T16.1 Foreign body in right ear**
[7th] **T16.2 Foreign body in left ear**
[7th] **T16.9 Foreign body in ear, unspecified ear**

[4th] **T17 Foreign body in respiratory tract**
The appropriate 7th character is to be added to each code from category T17
A = initial encounter
D = subsequent encounter
S = sequela
[7th] **T17.0 Foreign body in nasal sinus**
[7th] **T17.1 Foreign body in nostril**
Foreign body in nose NOS
[5th] **T17.2 Foreign body in pharynx**
Foreign body in nasopharynx
Foreign body in throat NOS
[6th] **T17.20 Unspecified foreign body in pharynx**
[7th] **T17.200 Unspecified foreign body in pharynx causing asphyxiation**
[7th] **T17.208 Unspecified foreign body in pharynx causing other injury**
[6th] **T17.21 Gastric contents in pharynx**
Aspiration of gastric contents into pharynx
Vomitus in pharynx
[7th] **T17.210 Gastric contents in pharynx causing asphyxiation**
[7th] **T17.218 Gastric contents in pharynx causing other injury**
[6th] **T17.22 Food in pharynx**
Bones in pharynx
Seeds in pharynx
[7th] **T17.220 Food in pharynx causing asphyxiation**
[7th] **T17.228 Food in pharynx causing other injury**
[6th] **T17.29 Other foreign object in pharynx**
[7th] **T17.290 Other foreign object in pharynx causing asphyxiation**
[7th] **T17.298 Other foreign object in pharynx causing other injury**
[5th] **T17.3 Foreign body in larynx**
[6th] **T17.30 Unspecified foreign body in larynx**
[7th] **T17.300 Unspecified foreign body in larynx causing asphyxiation**
[7th] **T17.308 Unspecified foreign body in larynx causing other injury**
[6th] **T17.31 Gastric contents in larynx**
Aspiration of gastric contents into larynx
Vomitus in larynx
[7th] **T17.310 Gastric contents in larynx causing asphyxiation**
[7th] **T17.318 Gastric contents in larynx causing other injury**
[6th] **T17.32 Food in larynx**
ones in larynx
Seeds in larynx
[7th] **T17.320 Food in larynx causing asphyxiation**

[7th] T17.328 Food in larynx causing other injury

[6th] T17.39 Other foreign object in larynx

[7th] T17.390 Other foreign object in larynx causing asphyxiation

[7th] T17.398 Other foreign object in larynx causing other injury

[5th] T17.4 Foreign body in trachea

[6th] T17.40 Unspecified foreign body in trachea

[7th] T17.400 Unspecified foreign body in trachea causing asphyxiation

[7th] T17.408 Unspecified foreign body in trachea causing other injury

[6th] T17.41 Gastric contents in trachea

Aspiration of gastric contents into trachea
Vomitus in trachea

[7th] T17.410 Gastric contents in trachea causing asphyxiation

[7th] T17.418 Gastric contents in trachea causing other injury

[6th] T17.42 Food in trachea

Bones in trachea
Seeds in trachea

[7th] T17.420 Food in trachea causing asphyxiation

[7th] T17.428 Food in trachea causing other injury

[6th] T17.49 Other foreign object in trachea

[7th] T17.490 Other foreign object in trachea causing asphyxiation

[7th] T17.498 Other foreign object in trachea causing other injury

[5th] T17.5 Foreign body in bronchus

[6th] T17.50 Unspecified foreign body in bronchus

[7th] T17.500 Unspecified foreign body in bronchus causing asphyxiation

[7th] T17.508 Unspecified foreign body in bronchus causing other injury

[6th] T17.51 Gastric contents in bronchus

Aspiration of gastric contents into bronchus
Vomitus in bronchus

[7th] T17.510 Gastric contents in bronchus causing asphyxiation

[7th] T17.518 Gastric contents in bronchus causing other injury

[6th] T17.52 Food in bronchus

Bones in bronchus
Seeds in bronchus

[7th] T17.520 Food in bronchus causing asphyxiation

[7th] T17.528 Food in bronchus causing other injury

[6th] T17.59 Other foreign object in bronchus

[7th] T17.590 Other foreign object in bronchus causing asphyxiation

[7th] T17.598 Other foreign object in bronchus causing other injury

[5th] T17.8 Foreign body in other parts of respiratory tract

Foreign body in bronchioles
Foreign body in lung

[6th] T17.80 Unspecified foreign body in other parts of respiratory tract

[7th] T17.800 Unspecified foreign body in other parts of respiratory tract causing asphyxiation

[7th] T17.808 Unspecified foreign body in other parts of respiratory tract causing other injury

[6th] T17.81 Gastric contents in other parts of respiratory tract

Aspiration of gastric contents into other parts of respiratory tract
Vomitus in other parts of respiratory tract

[7th] T17.810 Gastric contents in other parts of respiratory tract causing asphyxiation

[7th] T17.818 Gastric contents in other parts of respiratory tract causing other injury

[6th] T17.82 Food in other parts of respiratory tract

Bones in other parts of respiratory tract
Seeds in other parts of respiratory tract

[7th] T17.820 Food in other parts of respiratory tract causing asphyxiation

[7th] T17.828 Food in other parts of respiratory tract causing other injury

[6th] T17.89 Other foreign object in other parts of respiratory tract

[7th] T17.890 Other foreign object in other parts of respiratory tract causing asphyxiation

[7th] T17.898 Other foreign object in other parts of respiratory tract causing other injury

[5th] T17.9 Foreign body in respiratory tract, part unspecified

[6th] T17.90 Unspecified foreign body in respiratory tract, part unspecified

[7th] T17.900 Unspecified foreign body in respiratory tract, part unspecified causing asphyxiation

[7th] T17.908 Unspecified foreign body in respiratory tract, part unspecified causing other injury

[6th] T17.91 Gastric contents in respiratory tract, part unspecified

Aspiration of gastric contents into respiratory tract, part unspecified
Vomitus in trachea respiratory tract, part unspecified

[7th] T17.910 Gastric contents in respiratory tract, part unspecified causing asphyxiation

[7th] T17.918 Gastric contents in respiratory tract, part unspecified causing other injury

[6th] T17.92 Food in respiratory tract, part unspecified

Bones in respiratory tract, part unspecified
Seeds in respiratory tract, part unspecified

[7th] T17.920 Food in respiratory tract, part unspecified causing asphyxiation

[7th] T17.928 Food in respiratory tract, part unspecified causing other injury

[6th] T17.99 Other foreign object in respiratory tract, part unspecified

[7th] T17.990 Other foreign object in respiratory tract, part unspecified in causing asphyxiation

[7th] T17.998 Other foreign object in respiratory tract, part unspecified causing other injury

[4th] T18 Foreign body in alimentary tract

[EXCLUDES2] *foreign body in pharynx (T17.2-)*

The appropriate 7th character is to be added to each code from category T18
A = initial encounter
D = subsequent encounter
S = sequela

[7th] T18.0 Foreign body in mouth

[5th] T18.1 Foreign body in esophagus

[EXCLUDES2] *foreign body in respiratory tract (T17.-)*

[6th] T18.10 Unspecified foreign body in esophagus

[7th] T18.100 Unspecified foreign body in esophagus causing compression of trachea

Unspecified foreign body in esophagus causing obstruction of respiration

[7th] T18.108 Unspecified foreign body in esophagus causing other injury

[6th] T18.11 Gastric contents in esophagus

Vomitus in esophagus

[7th] T18.110 Gastric contents in esophagus causing compression of trachea

Gastric contents in esophagus causing obstruction of respiration

[7th] **T18.118 Gastric contents in esophagus causing other injury**

[6th] **T18.12 Food in esophagus**

Bones in esophagus

Seeds in esophagus

[7th] **T18.120 Food in esophagus causing compression of trachea**

Food in esophagus causing obstruction of respiration

[7th] **T18.128 Food in esophagus causing other injury**

[6th] **T18.19 Other foreign object in esophagus**

[7th] **T18.190 Other foreign object in esophagus causing compression of trachea**

Other foreign body in esophagus causing obstruction of respiration

[7th] **T18.198 Other foreign object in esophagus causing other injury**

[x7th] **T18.2 Foreign body in stomach**

[x7th] **T18.3 Foreign body in small intestine**

[x7th] **T18.4 Foreign body in colon**

[x7th] **T18.5 Foreign body in anus and rectum**

Foreign body in rectosigmoid (junction)

[x7th] **T18.8 Foreign body in other parts of alimentary tract**

[x7th] **T18.9 Foreign body of alimentary tract, part unspecified**

Foreign body in digestive system NOS

Swallowed foreign body NOS

[4th] **T19 Foreign body in genitourinary tract**

[EXCLUDES2] *complications due to implanted mesh (T83.7-)*
mechanical complications of contraceptive device (intrauterine) (vaginal) (T83.3-)
presence of contraceptive device (intrauterine) (vaginal) (Z97.5)

The appropriate 7th character is to be added to each code from category T19
A = initial encounter
D = subsequent encounter
S = sequela

[x7th] **T19.0 Foreign body in urethra**

[x7th] **T19.1 Foreign body in bladder**

[x7th] **T19.2 Foreign body in vulva and vagina**

[x7th] **T19.3 Foreign body in uterus**

[x7th] **T19.4 Foreign body in penis**

[x7th] **T19.8 Foreign body in other parts of genitourinary tract**

[x7th] **T19.9 Foreign body in genitourinary tract, part unspecified**

Burns and corrosions (T20-T32)

INCLUDES *burns (thermal) from electrical heating appliances*
burns (thermal) from electricity
burns (thermal) from flame
burns (thermal) from friction
burns (thermal) from hot air and hot gases
burns (thermal) from hot objects
burns (thermal) from lightning
burns (thermal) from radiation
chemical burn [corrosion] (external) (internal)
scalds

[EXCLUDES2] *erythema [dermatitis] ab igne (L59.0)*
radiation-related disorders of the skin and subcutaneous tissue (L55-L59)
sunburn (L55.-)

Burns and corrosions of external body surface, specified by site (T20-T25)

Use additional code from category T31 or T32 to identify extent of body surface involved

INCLUDES *burns and corrosions of first degree [erythema]*
burns and corrosions of second degree [blisters][epidermal loss]
burns and corrosions of third degree [deep necrosis of underlying tissue] [full- thickness skin loss]

[4th] **T20 Burn and corrosion of head, face, and neck**

[EXCLUDES2] *burn and corrosion of ear drum (T28.41, T28.91)*
burn and corrosion of eye and adnexa (T26.-)
burn and corrosion of mouth and pharynx (T28.0)

The appropriate 7th character is to be added to each code from category T20
A = initial encounter
D = subsequent encounter
S = sequela

[5th] **T20.0 Burn of unspecified degree of head, face, and neck**

Use additional external cause code to identify the source, place and intent of the burn (X00-X19, X75-X77, X96-X98, Y92)

[x7th] **T20.00 Burn of unspecified degree of head, face, and neck, unspecified site**

[6th] **T20.01 Burn of unspecified degree of ear [any part, except ear drum]**

[EXCLUDES2] *burn of ear drum (T28.41-)*

[7th] **T20.011 Burn of unspecified degree of right ear [any part, except ear drum]**

[7th] **T20.012 Burn of unspecified degree of left ear [any part, except ear drum]**

[7th] **T20.019 Burn of unspecified degree of unspecified ear [any part, except ear drum]**

[x7th] **T20.02 Burn of unspecified degree of lip(s)**

[x7th] **T20.03 Burn of unspecified degree of chin**

[x7th] **T20.04 Burn of unspecified degree of nose (septum)**

[x7th] **T20.05 Burn of unspecified degree of scalp [any part]**

[x7th] **T20.06 Burn of unspecified degree of forehead and cheek**

[x7th] **T20.07 Burn of unspecified degree of neck**

[x7th] **T20.09 Burn of unspecified degree of multiple sites of head, face, and neck**

[5th] **T20.1 Burn of first degree of head, face, and neck**

Use additional external cause code to identify the source, place and intent of the burn (X00-X19, X75-X77, X96-X98, Y92)

[x7th] **T20.10 Burn of first degree of head, face, and neck, unspecified site**

[6th] **T20.11 Burn of first degree of ear [any part, except ear drum]**

[EXCLUDES2] *burn of ear drum (T28.41-)*

[7th] **T20.111 Burn of first degree of right ear [any part, except ear drum]**

[7th] **T20.112 Burn of first degree of left ear [any part, except ear drum]**

[7th] **T20.119 Burn of first degree of unspecified ear [any part, except ear drum]**

[x7th] **T20.12 Burn of first degree of lip(s)**

[x7th] **T20.13 Burn of first degree of chin**

[x7th] **T20.14 Burn of first degree of nose (septum)**

[x7th] **T20.15 Burn of first degree of scalp [any part]**

[x7th] **T20.16 Burn of first degree of forehead and cheek**

[x7th] **T20.17 Burn of first degree of neck**

[x7th] **T20.19 Burn of first degree of multiple sites of head, face, and neck**

[5th] **T20.2 Burn of second degree of head, face, and neck**

Use additional external cause code to identify the source, place and intent of the burn (X00-X19, X75-X77, X96-X98, Y92)

[4th] 4th character required [5th] 5th character required [6th] 6th character required [7th] 7th character required [x7th] Extension 'X' Alert
[EXCLUDES1] Not coded here [EXCLUDES2] Not included here [PDx] Primary Diagnosis Only Manifestation Code

- [7th] T20.20 Burn of second degree of head, face, and neck, unspecified site
- [6th] T20.21 Burn of second degree of ear [any part, except ear drum]
  - [EXCLUDES2] *burn of ear drum (T28.41-)*
  - [7th] T20.211 Burn of second degree of right ear [any part, except ear drum]
  - [7th] T20.212 Burn of second degree of left ear [any part, except ear drum]
  - [7th] T20.219 Burn of second degree of unspecified ear [any part, except ear drum]
- [7th] T20.22 Burn of second degree of lip(s)
- [7th] T20.23 Burn of second degree of chin
- [7th] T20.24 Burn of second degree of nose (septum)
- [7th] T20.25 Burn of second degree of scalp [any part]
- [7th] T20.26 Burn of second degree of forehead and cheek
- [7th] T20.27 Burn of second degree of neck
- [7th] T20.29 Burn of second degree of multiple sites of head, face, and neck

[5th] T20.3 Burn of third degree of head, face, and neck
Use additional external cause code to identify the source, place and intent of the burn (X00-X19, X75-X77, X96-X98, Y92)

- [7th] T20.30 Burn of third degree of head, face, and neck, unspecified site
- [6th] T20.31 Burn of third degree of ear [any part, except ear drum]
  - [EXCLUDES2] *burn of ear drum (T28.41-)*
  - [7th] T20.311 Burn of third degree of right ear [any part, except ear drum]
  - [7th] T20.312 Burn of third degree of left ear [any part, except ear drum]
  - [7th] T20.319 Burn of third degree of unspecified ear [any part, except ear drum]
- [7th] T20.32 Burn of third degree of lip(s)
- [7th] T20.33 Burn of third degree of chin
- [7th] T20.34 Burn of third degree of nose (septum)
- [7th] T20.35 Burn of third degree of scalp [any part]
- [7th] T20.36 Burn of third degree of forehead and cheek
- [7th] T20.37 Burn of third degree of neck
- [7th] T20.39 Burn of third degree of multiple sites of head, face, and neck

[5th] T20.4 Corrosion of unspecified degree of head, face, and neck
Code first (T51-T65) to identify chemical and intent
Use additional external cause code to identify place (Y92)

- [7th] T20.40 Corrosion of unspecified degree of head, face, and neck, unspecified site
- [6th] T20.41 Corrosion of unspecified degree of ear [any part, except ear drum]
  - [EXCLUDES2] *corrosion of ear drum (T28.91-)*
  - [7th] T20.411 Corrosion of unspecified degree of right ear [any part, except ear drum]
  - [7th] T20.412 Corrosion of unspecified degree of left ear [any part, except ear drum]
  - [7th] T20.419 Corrosion of unspecified degree of unspecified ear [any part, except ear drum]
- [7th] T20.42 Corrosion of unspecified degree of lip(s)
- [7th] T20.43 Corrosion of unspecified degree of chin
- [7th] T20.44 Corrosion of unspecified degree of nose (septum)
- [7th] T20.45 Corrosion of unspecified degree of scalp [any part]
- [7th] T20.46 Corrosion of unspecified degree of forehead and cheek
- [7th] T20.47 Corrosion of unspecified degree of neck
- [7th] T20.49 Corrosion of unspecified degree of multiple sites of head, face, and neck

[5th] T20.5 Corrosion of first degree of head, face, and neck
Code first (T51-T65) to identify chemical and intent
Use additional external cause code to identify place (Y92)

- [7th] T20.50 Corrosion of first degree of head, face, and neck, unspecified site
- [6th] T20.51 Corrosion of first degree of ear [any part, except ear drum]
  - [EXCLUDES2] *corrosion of ear drum (T28.91-)*
  - [7th] T20.511 Corrosion of first degree of right ear [any part, except ear drum]
  - [7th] T20.512 Corrosion of first degree of left ear [any part, except ear drum]
  - [7th] T20.519 Corrosion of first degree of unspecified ear [any part, except ear drum]
- [7th] T20.52 Corrosion of first degree of lip(s)
- [7th] T20.53 Corrosion of first degree of chin
- [7th] T20.54 Corrosion of first degree of nose (septum)
- [7th] T20.55 Corrosion of first degree of scalp [any part]
- [7th] T20.56 Corrosion of first degree of forehead and cheek ▲
- [7th] T20.57 Corrosion of first degree of neck
- [7th] T20.59 Corrosion of first degree of multiple sites of head, face, and neck

[5th] T20.6 Corrosion of second degree of head, face, and neck
Code first (T51-T65) to identify chemical and intent
Use additional external cause code to identify place (Y92)

- [7th] T20.60 Corrosion of second degree of head, face, and neck, unspecified site
- [6th] T20.61 Corrosion of second degree of ear [any part, except ear drum]
  - [EXCLUDES2] *corrosion of ear drum (T28.91-)*
  - [7th] T20.611 Corrosion of second degree of right ear [any part, except ear drum]
  - [7th] T20.612 Corrosion of second degree of left ear [any part, except ear drum]
  - [7th] T20.619 Corrosion of second degree of unspecified ear [any part, except ear drum]
- [7th] T20.62 Corrosion of second degree of lip(s)
- [7th] T20.63 Corrosion of second degree of chin
- [7th] T20.64 Corrosion of second degree of nose (septum)
- [7th] T20.65 Corrosion of second degree of scalp [any part]
- [7th] T20.66 Corrosion of second degree of forehead and cheek
- [7th] T20.67 Corrosion of second degree of neck
- [7th] T20.69 Corrosion of second degree of multiple sites of head, face, and neck

[5th] T20.7 Corrosion of third degree of head, face, and neck
Code first (T51-T65) to identify chemical and intent
Use additional external cause code to identify place (Y92)

- [7th] T20.70 Corrosion of third degree of head, face, and neck, unspecified site
- [6th] T20.71 Corrosion of third degree of ear [any part, except ear drum]
  - [EXCLUDES2] *corrosion of ear drum (T28.91-)*
  - [7th] T20.711 Corrosion of third degree of right ear [any part, except ear drum]
  - [7th] T20.712 Corrosion of third degree of left ear [any part, except ear drum]
  - [7th] T20.719 Corrosion of third degree of unspecified ear [any part, except ear drum]
- [7th] T20.72 Corrosion of third degree of lip(s)
- [7th] T20.73 Corrosion of third degree of chin
- [7th] T20.74 Corrosion of third degree of nose (septum)
- [7th] T20.75 Corrosion of third degree of scalp [any part]
- [7th] T20.76 Corrosion of third degree of forehead and cheek
- [7th] T20.77 Corrosion of third degree of neck

Unspecified Code | Other Specified Code | [N] Newborn Age: 0 | [P] Pediatric Age: 0-17 | [M] Maternity Age: 12-55
[A] Adult Age: 15-124 | ♂ Male | ♀ Female | ● New Code | ▲ Revised Code Title | ►◄ Revised Text

T20.79 **Corrosion of third degree of** multiple sites of head, face, and neck

T21 **Burn and corrosion of trunk**

INCLUDES   burns and corrosion of hip region

EXCLUDES2   burns and corrosion of axilla (T22.- with fifth character 4)
burns and corrosion of scapular region (T22.- with fifth character 6)
burns and corrosion of shoulder (T22.- with fifth character 5)

The appropriate 7th character is to be added to each code from category T21
A = initial encounter
D = subsequent encounter
S = sequela

T21.0 **Burn of** unspecified degree **of trunk**
Use additional external cause code to identify the source, place and intent of the burn (X00-X19, X75-X77, X96-X98, Y92)

T21.00 **Burn of unspecified degree of trunk, unspecified site**

T21.01 **Burn of unspecified degree of** chest wall
Burn of of unspecified degree of breast

T21.02 **Burn of unspecified degree of** abdominal wall
Burn of unspecified degree of flank
Burn of unspecified degree of groin

T21.03 **Burn of unspecified degree of** upper back
Burn of unspecified degree of interscapular region

T21.04 **Burn of unspecified degree of** lower back

T21.05 **Burn of unspecified degree of** buttock
Burn of unspecified degree of anus

T21.06 **Burn of unspecified degree of** male genital region
Burn of unspecified degree of penis
Burn of unspecified degree of scrotum
Burn of unspecified degree of testis

T21.07 **Burn of unspecified degree of** female genital region
Burn of unspecified degree of labium (majus) (minus)
Burn of unspecified degree of perineum
Burn of unspecified degree of vulva
EXCLUDES2 burn of vagina (T28.3)

T21.09 **Burn of unspecified degree of other site of trunk**

T21.1 **Burn of first degree of trunk**
Use additional external cause code to identify the source, place and intent of the burn (X00-X19, X75-X77, X96-X98, Y92)

T21.10 **Burn of first degree of trunk, unspecified site**

T21.11 **Burn of first degree of** chest wall
Burn of first degree of breast

T21.12 **Burn of first degree of** abdominal wall
Burn of first degree of flank
Burn of first degree of groin

T21.13 **Burn of first degree of** upper back
Burn of first degree of interscapular region

T21.14 **Burn of first degree of** lower back

T21.15 **Burn of first degree of** buttock
Burn of first degree of anus

T21.16 **Burn of first degree of** male genital region
Burn of first degree of penis
Burn of first degree of scrotum
Burn of first degree of testis

T21.17 **Burn of first degree of** female genital region
Burn of first degree of labium (majus) (minus)
Burn of first degree of perineum
Burn of first degree of vulva
EXCLUDES2 burn of vagina (T28.3)

T21.19 **Burn of first degree of other site of trunk**

T21.2 **Burn of** second degree **of trunk**
Use additional external cause code to identify the source, place and intent of the burn (X00-X19, X77, X96-X98, Y92)

T21.20 **Burn of second degree of trunk, unspecified site**

T21.21 **Burn of second degree of** chest wall
Burn of second degree of breast

T21.22 **Burn of second degree of** abdominal wall
Burn of second degree of flank
Burn of second degree of groin

T21.23 **Burn of second degree of** upper back
Burn of second degree of interscapular region

T21.24 **Burn of second degree of** lower back

T21.25 **Burn of second degree of** buttock
Burn of second degree of anus

T21.26 **Burn of second degree of** male genital region
Burn of second degree of penis
Burn of second degree of scrotum
Burn of second degree of testis

T21.27 **Burn of second degree of** female genital region
Burn of second degree of labium (majus) (minus)
Burn of second degree of perineum
Burn of second degree of vulva
EXCLUDES2 burn of vagina (T28.3)

T21.29 **Burn of second degree of other site of trunk**

T21.3 **Burn of** third degree **of trunk**
Use additional external cause code to identify the source, place and intent of the burn (X00-X19, X75-X77, X96-X98, Y92)

T21.30 **Burn of third degree of trunk, unspecified site**

T21.31 **Burn of third degree of** chest wall
Burn of third degree of breast

T21.32 **Burn of third degree of** abdominal wall
Burn of third degree of flank
Burn of third degree of groin

T21.33 **Burn of third degree of** upper back
Burn of third degree of interscapular region

T21.34 **Burn of third degree of** lower back

T21.35 **Burn of third degree of** buttock
Burn of third degree of anus

T21.36 **Burn of third degree of** male genital region
Burn of third degree of penis
Burn of third degree of scrotum
Burn of third degree of testis

T21.37 **Burn of third degree of** female genital region
Burn of third degree of labium (majus) (minus)
Burn of third degree of perineum
Burn of third degree of vulva
EXCLUDES2 burn of vagina (T28.3)

T21.39 **Burn of third degree of other site of trunk**

T21.4 **Corrosion of** unspecified degree **of trunk**
Code first (T51-T65) to identify chemical and intent
Use additional external cause code to identify place (Y92)

T21.40 **Corrosion of unspecified degree of trunk, unspecified site**

T21.41 **Corrosion of unspecified degree of** chest wall
Corrosion of unspecified degree of breast

T21.42 **Corrosion of unspecified degree of** abdominal wall
Corrosion of unspecified degree of flank
Corrosion of unspecified degree of groin

T21.43 **Corrosion of unspecified degree of** upper back
Corrosion of unspecified degree of interscapular region

4️⃣ 4ᵗʰ character required   5️⃣ 5ᵗʰ character required   6️⃣ 6ᵗʰ character required   7️⃣ 7ᵗʰ character required   Extension 'X' Alert

EXCLUDES1 Not coded here   EXCLUDES2 Not included here   PDX Primary Diagnosis Only   Manifestation Code

666   ICD-10-CM 2015

T21.44 **Corrosion of unspecified degree of** lower back

T21.45 **Corrosion of unspecified degree of** buttock

Corrosion of unspecified degree of anus

T21.46 **Corrosion of unspecified degree of** male genital region

Corrosion of unspecified degree of penis

Corrosion of unspecified degree of scrotum

Corrosion of unspecified degree of testis

T21.47 **Corrosion of unspecified degree of** female genital region

Corrosion of unspecified degree of labium (majus) (minus)

Corrosion of unspecified degree of perineum

Corrosion of unspecified degree of vulva

EXCLUDES2 corrosion of vagina (T28.8)

T21.49 **Corrosion of unspecified degree of other site of trunk**

T21.5 **Corrosion of** first degree **of trunk**

Code first (T51-T65) to identify chemical and intent

Use additional external cause code to identify place (Y92)

T21.50 **Corrosion of first degree of trunk, unspecified site**

T21.51 **Corrosion of first degree of** chest wall

Corrosion of first degree of breast

T21.52 **Corrosion of first degree of** abdominal wall

Corrosion of first degree of flank

Corrosion of first degree of groin

T21.53 **Corrosion of first degree of** upper back

Corrosion of first degree of interscapular region

T21.54 **Corrosion of first degree of** lower back

T21.55 **Corrosion of first degree of** buttock

Corrosion of first degree of anus

T21.56 **Corrosion of first degree of** male genital region

Corrosion of first degree of penis

Corrosion of first degree of scrotum

Corrosion of first degree of testis

T21.57 **Corrosion of first degree of** female genital region

Corrosion of first degree of labium (majus) (minus)

Corrosion of first degree of perineum

Corrosion of first degree of vulva

EXCLUDES2 corrosion of vagina (T28.8)

T21.59 **Corrosion of first degree of other site of trunk**

T21.6 **Corrosion of** second degree **of trunk**

Code first (T51-T65) to identify chemical and intent

Use additional external cause code to identify place (Y92)

T21.60 **Corrosion of second degree of trunk, unspecified site**

T21.61 **Corrosion of second degree of** chest wall

Corrosion of second degree of breast

T21.62 **Corrosion of second degree of** abdominal wall

Corrosion of second degree of flank

Corrosion of second degree of groin

T21.63 **Corrosion of second degree of** upper back

Corrosion of second degree of interscapular region

T21.64 **Corrosion of second degree of** lower back

T21.65 **Corrosion of second degree of** buttock

Corrosion of second degree of anus

T21.66 **Corrosion of second degree of** male genital region

Corrosion of second degree of penis

Corrosion of second degree of scrotum

Corrosion of second degree of testis

T21.67 **Corrosion of second degree of** female genital region

Corrosion of second degree of labium (majus) (minus)

Corrosion of second degree of perineum

Corrosion of second degree of vulva

EXCLUDES2 corrosion of vagina (T28.8)

T21.69 **Corrosion of second degree of other site of trunk**

T21.7 **Corrosion of** third degree **of trunk**

Code first (T51-T65) to identify chemical and intent

Use additional external cause code to identify place (Y92)

T21.70 **Corrosion of third degree of trunk, unspecified site**

T21.71 **Corrosion of third degree of** chest wall

Corrosion of third degree of breast

T21.72 **Corrosion of third degree of** abdominal wall

Corrosion of third degree of flank

Corrosion of third degree of groin

T21.73 **Corrosion of third degree of** upper back

Corrosion of third degree of interscapular region

T21.74 **Corrosion of third degree of** lower back

T21.75 **Corrosion of third degree of** buttock

Corrosion of third degree of anus

T21.76 **Corrosion of third degree of** male genital region

Corrosion of third degree of penis

Corrosion of third degree of scrotum

Corrosion of third degree of testis

T21.77 **Corrosion of third degree of** female genital region

Corrosion of third degree of labium (majus) (minus)

Corrosion of third degree of perineum

Corrosion of third degree of vulva

EXCLUDES2 corrosion of vagina (T28.8)

T21.79 **Corrosion of third degree of other site of trunk**

T22 **Burn and corrosion of shoulder and upper limb, except wrist and hand**

EXCLUDES2 burn and corrosion of interscapular region (T21.-)
burn and corrosion of wrist and hand (T23.-)

The appropriate 7th character is to be added to each code from category T22

A = initial encounter

D = subsequent encounter

S = sequela

T22.0 **Burn of** unspecified degree **of shoulder and upper limb, except wrist and hand**

Use additional external cause code to identify the source, place and intent of the burn (X00-X19, X75-X77, X96-X98, Y92)

T22.00 **Burn of unspecified degree of shoulder and upper limb, except wrist and hand, unspecified site**

T22.01 **Burn of unspecified degree of** forearm

T22.011 **Burn of unspecified degree of** right forearm

T22.012 **Burn of unspecified degree of** left forearm

T22.019 **Burn of unspecified degree of unspecified forearm**

T22.02 **Burn of unspecified degree of** elbow

T22.021 **Burn of unspecified degree of** right elbow

T22.022 **Burn of unspecified degree of** left elbow

T22.029 **Burn of unspecified degree of unspecified elbow**

T22.03 **Burn of unspecified degree of** upper arm

T22.031 **Burn of unspecified degree of** right upper arm

T22.032 **Burn of unspecified degree of** left upper arm

Unspecified Code	Other Specified Code	N Newborn Age: 0	P Pediatric Age: 0-17	M Maternity Age: 12-55	
A Adult Age: 15-124	♂ Male	♀ Female	● New Code	▲ Revised Code Title	►◄ Revised Text

⑦ T22.039 Burn of unspecified degree of unspecified upper arm
⑥ T22.04 Burn of unspecified degree of axilla
⑦ T22.041 Burn of unspecified degree of right axilla
⑦ T22.042 Burn of unspecified degree of left axilla
⑦ T22.049 Burn of unspecified degree of unspecified axilla
⑥ T22.05 Burn of unspecified degree of shoulder
⑦ T22.051 Burn of unspecified degree of right shoulder
⑦ T22.052 Burn of unspecified degree of left shoulder
⑦ T22.059 Burn of unspecified degree of unspecified shoulder
⑥ T22.06 Burn of unspecified degree of scapular region
⑦ T22.061 Burn of unspecified degree of right scapular region
⑦ T22.062 Burn of unspecified degree of left scapular region
⑦ T22.069 Burn of unspecified degree of unspecified scapular region
⑥ T22.09 Burn of unspecified degree of multiple sites of shoulder and upper limb, except wrist and hand
⑦ T22.091 Burn of unspecified degree of multiple sites of right shoulder and upper limb, except wrist and hand
⑦ T22.092 Burn of unspecified degree of multiple sites of left shoulder and upper limb, except wrist and hand
⑦ T22.099 Burn of unspecified degree of multiple sites of unspecified shoulder and upper limb, except wrist and hand
⑤ T22.1 Burn of first degree of shoulder and upper limb, except wrist and hand
Use additional external cause code to identify the source, place and intent of the burn (X00-X19, X75-X77, X96-X98, Y92)
⑦ T22.10 Burn of first degree of shoulder and upper limb, except wrist and hand, unspecified site
⑥ T22.11 Burn of first degree of forearm
⑦ T22.111 Burn of first degree of right forearm
⑦ T22.112 Burn of first degree of left forearm
⑦ T22.119 Burn of first degree of unspecified forearm
⑥ T22.12 Burn of first degree of elbow
⑦ T22.121 Burn of first degree of right elbow
⑦ T22.122 Burn of first degree of left elbow
⑦ T22.129 Burn of first degree of unspecified elbow
⑥ T22.13 Burn of first degree of upper arm
⑦ T22.131 Burn of first degree of right upper arm
⑦ T22.132 Burn of first degree of left upper arm
⑦ T22.139 Burn of first degree of unspecified upper arm
⑥ T22.14 Burn of first degree of axilla
⑦ T22.141 Burn of first degree of right axilla
⑦ T22.142 Burn of first degree of left axilla
⑦ T22.149 Burn of first degree of unspecified axilla
⑥ T22.15 Burn of first degree of shoulder
⑦ T22.151 Burn of first degree of right shoulder
⑦ T22.152 Burn of first degree of left shoulder
⑦ T22.159 Burn of first degree of unspecified shoulder
⑥ T22.16 Burn of first degree of scapular region
⑦ T22.161 Burn of first degree of right scapular region
⑦ T22.162 Burn of first degree of left scapular region
⑦ T22.169 Burn of first degree of unspecified scapular region
⑥ T22.19 Burn of first degree of multiple sites of shoulder and upper limb, except wrist and hand
⑦ T22.191 Burn of first degree of multiple sites of right shoulder and upper limb, except wrist and hand

⑦ T22.192 Burn of first degree of multiple sites of left shoulder and upper limb, except wrist and hand
⑦ T22.199 Burn of first degree of multiple sites of unspecified shoulder and upper limb, except wrist and hand
⑤ T22.2 Burn of second degree of shoulder and upper limb, except wrist and hand
Use additional external cause code to identify the source, place and intent of the burn (X00-X19, X75-X77, X96-X98, Y92)
⑦ T22.20 Burn of second degree of shoulder and upper limb, except wrist and hand, unspecified site
⑥ T22.21 Burn of second degree of forearm
⑦ T22.211 Burn of second degree of right forearm
⑦ T22.212 Burn of second degree of left forearm
⑦ T22.219 Burn of second degree of unspecified forearm
⑥ T22.22 Burn of second degree of elbow
⑦ T22.221 Burn of second degree of right elbow
⑦ T22.222 Burn of second degree of left elbow
⑦ T22.229 Burn of second degree of unspecified elbow
⑥ T22.23 Burn of second degree of upper arm
⑦ T22.231 Burn of second degree of right upper arm
⑦ T22.232 Burn of second degree of left upper arm
⑦ T22.239 Burn of second degree of unspecified upper arm
⑥ T22.24 Burn of second degree of axilla
⑦ T22.241 Burn of second degree of right axilla
⑦ T22.242 Burn of second degree of left axilla
⑦ T22.249 Burn of second degree of unspecified axilla
⑥ T22.25 Burn of second degree of shoulder
⑦ T22.251 Burn of second degree of right shoulder
⑦ T22.252 Burn of second degree of left shoulder
⑦ T22.259 Burn of second degree of unspecified shoulder
⑥ T22.26 Burn of second degree of scapular region
⑦ T22.261 Burn of second degree of right scapular region
⑦ T22.262 Burn of second degree of left scapular region
⑦ T22.269 Burn of second degree of unspecified scapular region
⑥ T22.29 Burn of second degree of multiple sites of shoulder and upper limb, except wrist and hand
⑦ T22.291 Burn of second degree of multiple sites of right shoulder and upper limb, except wrist and hand
⑦ T22.292 Burn of second degree of multiple sites of left shoulder and upper limb, except wrist and hand
⑦ T22.299 Burn of second degree of multiple sites of unspecified shoulder and upper limb, except wrist and hand
⑤ T22.3 Burn of third degree of shoulder and upper limb, except wrist and hand
Use additional external cause code to identify the source, place and intent of the burn (X00-X19, X75-X77, X96-X98, Y92)
⑦ T22.30 Burn of third degree of shoulder and upper limb, except wrist and hand, unspecified site
⑥ T22.31 Burn of third degree of forearm
⑦ T22.311 Burn of third degree of right forearm
⑦ T22.312 Burn of third degree of left forearm
⑦ T22.319 Burn of third degree of unspecified forearm
⑥ T22.32 Burn of third degree of elbow
⑦ T22.321 Burn of third degree of right elbow
⑦ T22.322 Burn of third degree of left elbow

④ 4th character required   ⑤ 5th character required   ⑥ 6th character required   ⑦ 7th character required   ⑩ Extension 'X' Alert

EXCLUDES 1 Not coded here   EXCLUDES 2 Not included here   PDx Primary Diagnosis Only   Manifestation Code

668   **ICD-10-CM 2015**

[7th] T22.329 Burn of third degree of unspecified elbow
[6th] T22.33 Burn of third degree of upper arm
[7th] T22.331 Burn of third degree of right upper arm
[7th] T22.332 Burn of third degree of left upper arm
[7th] T22.339 Burn of third degree of unspecified upper arm
[6th] T22.34 Burn of third degree of axilla
[7th] T22.341 Burn of third degree of right axilla
[7th] T22.342 Burn of third degree of left axilla
[7th] T22.349 Burn of third degree of unspecified axilla
[6th] T22.35 Burn of third degree of shoulder
[7th] T22.351 Burn of third degree of right shoulder
[7th] T22.352 Burn of third degree of left shoulder
[7th] T22.359 Burn of third degree of unspecified shoulder
[6th] T22.36 Burn of third degree of scapular region
[7th] T22.361 Burn of third degree of right scapular region
[7th] T22.362 Burn of third degree of left scapular region
[7th] T22.369 Burn of third degree of unspecified scapular region
[6th] T22.39 Burn of third degree of multiple sites of shoulder and upper limb, except wrist and hand
[7th] T22.391 Burn of third degree of multiple sites of right shoulder and upper limb, except wrist and hand
[7th] T22.392 Burn of third degree of multiple sites of left shoulder and upper limb, except wrist and hand
[7th] T22.399 Burn of third degree of multiple sites of unspecified shoulder and upper limb, except wrist and hand
[5th] T22.4 Corrosion of unspecified degree of shoulder and upper limb, except wrist and hand
Code first (T51-T65) to identify chemical and intent
Use additional external cause code to identify place (Y92)
[7th] T22.40 Corrosion of unspecified degree of shoulder and upper limb, except wrist and hand, unspecified site
[6th] T22.41 Corrosion of unspecified degree of forearm
[7th] T22.411 Corrosion of unspecified degree of right forearm
[7th] T22.412 Corrosion of unspecified degree of left forearm
[7th] T22.419 Corrosion of unspecified degree of unspecified forearm
[6th] T22.42 Corrosion of unspecified degree of elbow
[7th] T22.421 Corrosion of unspecified degree of right elbow
[7th] T22.422 Corrosion of unspecified degree of left elbow
[7th] T22.429 Corrosion of unspecified degree of unspecified elbow
[6th] T22.43 Corrosion of unspecified degree of upper arm
[7th] T22.431 Corrosion of unspecified degree of right upper arm
[7th] T22.432 Corrosion of unspecified degree of left upper arm
[7th] T22.439 Corrosion of unspecified degree of unspecified upper arm
[6th] T22.44 Corrosion of unspecified degree of axilla
[7th] T22.441 Corrosion of unspecified degree of right axilla
[7th] T22.442 Corrosion of unspecified degree of left axilla
[7th] T22.449 Corrosion of unspecified degree of unspecified axilla
[6th] T22.45 Corrosion of unspecified degree of shoulder
[7th] T22.451 Corrosion of unspecified degree of right shoulder
[7th] T22.452 Corrosion of unspecified degree of left shoulder
[7th] T22.459 Corrosion of unspecified degree of unspecified shoulder
[6th] T22.46 Corrosion of unspecified degree of scapular region
[7th] T22.461 Corrosion of unspecified degree of right scapular region
[7th] T22.462 Corrosion of unspecified degree of left scapular region
[7th] T22.469 Corrosion of unspecified degree of unspecified scapular region
[6th] T22.49 Corrosion of unspecified degree of multiple sites of shoulder and upper limb, except wrist and hand
[7th] T22.491 Corrosion of unspecified degree of multiple sites of right shoulder and upper limb, except wrist and hand
[7th] T22.492 Corrosion of unspecified degree of multiple sites of left shoulder and upper limb, except wrist and hand
[7th] T22.499 Corrosion of unspecified degree of multiple sites of unspecified shoulder and upper limb, except wrist and hand
[5th] T22.5 Corrosion of first degree of shoulder and upper limb, except wrist and hand
Code first (T51-T65) to identify chemical and intent
Use additional external cause code to identify place (Y92)
[7th] T22.50 Corrosion of first degree of shoulder and upper limb, except wrist and hand unspecified site
[6th] T22.51 Corrosion of first degree of forearm
[7th] T22.511 Corrosion of first degree of right forearm
[7th] T22.512 Corrosion of first degree of left forearm
[7th] T22.519 Corrosion of first degree of unspecified forearm
[6th] T22.52 Corrosion of first degree of elbow
[7th] T22.521 Corrosion of first degree of right elbow
[7th] T22.522 Corrosion of first degree of left elbow
[7th] T22.529 Corrosion of first degree of unspecified elbow
[6th] T22.53 Corrosion of first degree of upper arm
[7th] T22.531 Corrosion of first degree of right upper arm
[7th] T22.532 Corrosion of first degree of left upper arm
[7th] T22.539 Corrosion of first degree of unspecified upper arm
[6th] T22.54 Corrosion of first degree of axilla
[7th] T22.541 Corrosion of first degree of right axilla
[7th] T22.542 Corrosion of first degree of left axilla
[7th] T22.549 Corrosion of first degree of unspecified axilla
[6th] T22.55 Corrosion of first degree of shoulder
[7th] T22.551 Corrosion of first degree of right shoulder
[7th] T22.552 Corrosion of first degree of left shoulder
[7th] T22.559 Corrosion of first degree of unspecified shoulder
[6th] T22.56 Corrosion of first degree of scapular region
[7th] T22.561 Corrosion of first degree of right scapular region
[7th] T22.562 Corrosion of first degree of left scapular region
[7th] T22.569 Corrosion of first degree of unspecified scapular region
[6th] T22.59 Corrosion of first degree of multiple sites of shoulder and upper limb, except wrist and hand
[7th] T22.591 Corrosion of first degree of multiple sites of right shoulder and upper limb, except wrist and hand

Unspecified Code | Other Specified Code | [N] Newborn Age: 0 | [P] Pediatric Age: 0-17 | [M] Maternity Age: 12-55
[A] Adult Age: 15-124 | ♂ Male | ♀ Female | ● New Code | ▲ Revised Code Title | ►◄ Revised Text

7️⃣ T22.592 Corrosion of first degree of multiple sites of left shoulder and upper limb, except wrist and hand

7️⃣ T22.599 Corrosion of first degree of multiple sites of unspecified shoulder and upper limb, except wrist and hand

5️⃣ T22.6 Corrosion of second degree of shoulder and upper limb, except wrist and hand
Code first (T51-T65) to identify chemical and intent
Use additional external cause code to identify place (Y92)

6️⃣ T22.60 Corrosion of second degree of shoulder and upper limb, except wrist and hand, unspecified site

6️⃣ T22.61 Corrosion of second degree of forearm
7️⃣ T22.611 Corrosion of second degree of right forearm
7️⃣ T22.612 Corrosion of second degree of left forearm
7️⃣ T22.619 Corrosion of second degree of unspecified forearm

6️⃣ T22.62 Corrosion of second degree of elbow
7️⃣ T22.621 Corrosion of second degree of right elbow
7️⃣ T22.622 Corrosion of second degree of left elbow
7️⃣ T22.629 Corrosion of second degree of unspecified elbow

6️⃣ T22.63 Corrosion of second degree of upper arm
7️⃣ T22.631 Corrosion of second degree of right upper arm
7️⃣ T22.632 Corrosion of second degree of left upper arm
7️⃣ T22.639 Corrosion of second degree of unspecified upper arm

6️⃣ T22.64 Corrosion of second degree of axilla
7️⃣ T22.641 Corrosion of second degree of right axilla
7️⃣ T22.642 Corrosion of second degree of left axilla
7️⃣ T22.649 Corrosion of second degree of unspecified axilla

6️⃣ T22.65 Corrosion of second degree of shoulder
7️⃣ T22.651 Corrosion of second degree of right shoulder
7️⃣ T22.652 Corrosion of second degree of left shoulder
7️⃣ T22.659 Corrosion of second degree of unspecified shoulder

6️⃣ T22.66 Corrosion of second degree of scapular region
7️⃣ T22.661 Corrosion of second degree of right scapular region
7️⃣ T22.662 Corrosion of second degree of left scapular region
7️⃣ T22.669 Corrosion of second degree of unspecified scapular region

6️⃣ T22.69 Corrosion of second degree of multiple sites of shoulder and upper limb, except wrist and hand
7️⃣ T22.691 Corrosion of second degree of multiple sites of right shoulder and upper limb, except wrist and hand
7️⃣ T22.692 Corrosion of second degree of multiple sites of left shoulder and upper limb, except wrist and hand
7️⃣ T22.699 Corrosion of second degree of multiple sites of unspecified shoulder and upper limb, except wrist and hand

5️⃣ T22.7 Corrosion of third degree of shoulder and upper limb, except wrist and hand
Code first (T51-T65) to identify chemical and intent
Use additional external cause code to identify place (Y92)

6️⃣ T22.70 Corrosion of third degree of shoulder and upper limb, except wrist and hand, unspecified site

6️⃣ T22.71 Corrosion of third degree of forearm
7️⃣ T22.711 Corrosion of third degree of right forearm

7️⃣ T22.712 Corrosion of third degree of left forearm
7️⃣ T22.719 Corrosion of third degree of unspecified forearm

6️⃣ T22.72 Corrosion of third degree of elbow
7️⃣ T22.721 Corrosion of third degree of right elbow
7️⃣ T22.722 Corrosion of third degree of left elbow
7️⃣ T22.729 Corrosion of third degree of unspecified elbow

6️⃣ T22.73 Corrosion of third degree of upper arm
7️⃣ T22.731 Corrosion of third degree of right upper arm
7️⃣ T22.732 Corrosion of third degree of left upper arm
7️⃣ T22.739 Corrosion of third degree of unspecified upper arm

6️⃣ T22.74 Corrosion of third degree of axilla
7️⃣ T22.741 Corrosion of third degree of right axilla
7️⃣ T22.742 Corrosion of third degree of left axilla
7️⃣ T22.749 Corrosion of third degree of unspecified axilla

6️⃣ T22.75 Corrosion of third degree of shoulder
7️⃣ T22.751 Corrosion of third degree of right shoulder
7️⃣ T22.752 Corrosion of third degree of left shoulder
7️⃣ T22.759 Corrosion of third degree of unspecified shoulder

6️⃣ T22.76 Corrosion of third degree of scapular region
7️⃣ T22.761 Corrosion of third degree of right scapular region
7️⃣ T22.762 Corrosion of third degree of left scapular region
7️⃣ T22.769 Corrosion of third degree of unspecified scapular region

6️⃣ T22.79 Corrosion of third degree of multiple sites of shoulder and upper limb, except wrist and hand
7️⃣ T22.791 Corrosion of third degree of multiple sites of right shoulder and upper limb, except wrist and hand
7️⃣ T22.792 Corrosion of third degree of multiple sites of left shoulder and upper limb, except wrist and hand
7️⃣ T22.799 Corrosion of third degree of multiple sites of unspecified shoulder and upper limb, except wrist and hand

4️⃣ T23 Burn and corrosion of wrist and hand
The appropriate 7th character is to be added to each code from category T23
A = initial encounter
D = subsequent encounter
S = sequela

5️⃣ T23.0 Burn of unspecified degree of wrist and hand
Use additional external cause code to identify the source, place and intent of the burn (X00-X19, X75-X77, X96-X98, Y92)

6️⃣ T23.00 Burn of unspecified degree of hand, unspecified site
7️⃣ T23.001 Burn of unspecified degree of right hand, unspecified site
7️⃣ T23.002 Burn of unspecified degree of left hand, unspecified site
7️⃣ T23.009 Burn of unspecified degree of unspecified hand, unspecified site

6️⃣ T23.01 Burn of unspecified degree of thumb (nail)
7️⃣ T23.011 Burn of unspecified degree of right thumb (nail)
7️⃣ T23.012 Burn of unspecified degree of left thumb (nail)
7️⃣ T23.019 Burn of unspecified degree of unspecified thumb (nail)

6️⃣ T23.02 Burn of unspecified degree of single finger (nail) except thumb

---

4️⃣ 4th character required   5️⃣ 5th character required   6️⃣ 6th character required   7️⃣ 7th character required   7️⃣ Extension 'X' Alert

EXCLUDES 1 Not coded here   EXCLUDES 2 Not included here   PDx Primary Diagnosis Only   Manifestation Code

T23.021 Burn of unspecified degree of single right finger (nail) except thumb

T23.022 Burn of unspecified degree of single left finger (nail) except thumb

T23.029 Burn of unspecified degree of unspecified single finger (nail) except thumb

T23.03 Burn of unspecified degree of multiple fingers (nail), not including thumb

T23.031 Burn of unspecified degree of multiple right fingers (nail), not including thumb

T23.032 Burn of unspecified degree of multiple left fingers (nail), not including thumb

T23.039 Burn of unspecified degree of unspecified multiple fingers (nail), not including thumb

T23.04 Burn of unspecified degree of multiple fingers (nail), including thumb

T23.041 Burn of unspecified degree of multiple right fingers (nail), including thumb

T23.042 Burn of unspecified degree of multiple left fingers (nail), including thumb

T23.049 Burn of unspecified degree of unspecified multiple fingers (nail), including thumb

T23.05 Burn of unspecified degree of palm

T23.051 Burn of unspecified degree of right palm

T23.052 Burn of unspecified degree of left palm

T23.059 Burn of unspecified degree of unspecified palm

T23.06 Burn of unspecified degree of back of hand

T23.061 Burn of unspecified degree of back of right hand

T23.062 Burn of unspecified degree of back of left hand

T23.069 Burn of unspecified degree of back of unspecified hand

T23.07 Burn of unspecified degree of wrist

T23.071 Burn of unspecified degree of right wrist

T23.072 Burn of unspecified degree of left wrist

T23.079 Burn of unspecified degree of unspecified wrist

T23.09 Burn of unspecified degree of multiple sites of wrist and hand

T23.091 Burn of unspecified degree of multiple sites of right wrist and hand

T23.092 Burn of unspecified degree of multiple sites of left wrist and hand

T23.099 Burn of unspecified degree of multiple sites of unspecified wrist and hand

T23.1 Burn of first degree of wrist and hand
Use additional external cause code to identify the source, place and intent of the burn (X00-X19, X75-X77, X96-X98, Y92)

T23.10 Burn of first degree of hand, unspecified site

T23.101 Burn of first degree of right hand, unspecified site

T23.102 Burn of first degree of left hand, unspecified site

T23.109 Burn of first degree of unspecified hand, unspecified site

T23.11 Burn of first degree of thumb (nail)

T23.111 Burn of first degree of right thumb (nail)

T23.112 Burn of first degree of left thumb (nail)

T23.119 Burn of first degree of unspecified thumb (nail)

T23.12 Burn of first degree of single finger (nail) except thumb

T23.121 Burn of first degree of single right finger (nail) except thumb

T23.122 Burn of first degree of single left finger (nail) except thumb

T23.129 Burn of first degree of unspecified single finger (nail) except thumb

T23.13 Burn of first degree of multiple fingers (nail), not including thumb

T23.131 Burn of first degree of multiple right fingers (nail), not including thumb

T23.132 Burn of first degree of multiple left fingers (nail), not including thumb

T23.139 Burn of first degree of unspecified multiple fingers (nail), not including thumb

T23.14 Burn of first degree of multiple fingers (nail), including thumb

T23.141 Burn of first degree of multiple right fingers (nail), including thumb

T23.142 Burn of first degree of multiple left fingers (nail), including thumb

T23.149 Burn of first degree of unspecified multiple fingers (nail), including thumb

T23.15 Burn of first degree of palm

T23.151 Burn of first degree of right palm

T23.152 Burn of first degree of left palm

T23.159 Burn of first degree of unspecified palm

T23.16 Burn of first degree of back of hand

T23.161 Burn of first degree of back of right hand

T23.162 Burn of first degree of back of left hand

T23.169 Burn of first degree of back of unspecified hand

T23.17 Burn of first degree of wrist

T23.171 Burn of first degree of right wrist

T23.172 Burn of first degree of left wrist

T23.179 Burn of first degree of unspecified wrist

T23.19 Burn of first degree of multiple sites of wrist and hand

T23.191 Burn of first degree of multiple sites of right wrist and hand

T23.192 Burn of first degree of multiple sites of left wrist and hand

T23.199 Burn of first degree of multiple sites of unspecified wrist and hand

T23.2 Burn of second degree of wrist and hand
Use additional external cause code to identify the source, place and intent of the burn (X00-X19, X75-X77, X96-X98, Y92)

T23.20 Burn of second degree of hand, unspecified site

T23.201 Burn of second degree of right hand, unspecified site

T23.202 Burn of second degree of left hand, unspecified site

T23.209 Burn of second degree of unspecified hand, unspecified site

T23.21 Burn of second degree of thumb (nail)

T23.211 Burn of second degree of right thumb (nail)

T23.212 Burn of second degree of left thumb (nail)

T23.219 Burn of second degree of unspecified thumb (nail)

T23.22 Burn of second degree of single finger (nail) except thumb

T23.221 Burn of second degree of single right finger (nail) except thumb

T23.222 Burn of second degree of single left finger (nail) except thumb

T23.229 Burn of second degree of unspecified single finger (nail) except thumb

T23.23 Burn of second degree of multiple fingers (nail), not including thumb

T23.231 Burn of second degree of multiple right fingers (nail), not including thumb

T23.232 Burn of second degree of multiple left fingers (nail), not including thumb

Unspecified Code	Other Specified Code	N Newborn Age: 0	P Pediatric Age: 0-17	M Maternity Age: 12-55
A Adult Age: 15-124	♂ Male	♀ Female	● New Code	▲ Revised Code Title	►◄ Revised Text

[7th] T23.239 Burn of second degree of unspecified multiple fingers (nail), not including thumb

[6th] T23.24 Burn of second degree of multiple fingers (nail), including thumb

[7th] T23.241 Burn of second degree of multiple right fingers (nail), including thumb

[7th] T23.242 Burn of second degree of multiple left fingers (nail), including thumb

[7th] T23.249 Burn of second degree of unspecified multiple fingers (nail), including thumb

[6th] T23.25 Burn of second degree of palm

[7th] T23.251 Burn of second degree of right palm

[7th] T23.252 Burn of second degree of left palm

[7th] T23.259 Burn of second degree of unspecified palm

[6th] T23.26 Burn of second degree of back of hand

[7th] T23.261 Burn of second degree of back of right hand

[7th] T23.262 Burn of second degree of back of left hand

[7th] T23.269 Burn of second degree of back of unspecified hand

[6th] T23.27 Burn of second degree of wrist

[7th] T23.271 Burn of second degree of right wrist

[7th] T23.272 Burn of second degree of left wrist

[7th] T23.279 Burn of second degree of unspecified wrist

[6th] T23.29 Burn of second degree of multiple sites of wrist and hand

[7th] T23.291 Burn of second degree of multiple sites of right wrist and hand

[7th] T23.292 Burn of second degree of multiple sites of left wrist and hand

[7th] T23.299 Burn of second degree of multiple sites of unspecified wrist and hand

[5th] T23.3 Burn of third degree of wrist and hand

Use additional external cause code to identify the source, place and intent of the burn (X00-X19, X75-X77, X96-X98, Y92)

[6th] T23.30 Burn of third degree of hand, unspecified site

[7th] T23.301 Burn of third degree of right hand, unspecified site

[7th] T23.302 Burn of third degree of left hand, unspecified site

[7th] T23.309 Burn of third degree of unspecified hand, unspecified site

[6th] T23.31 Burn of third degree of thumb (nail)

[7th] T23.311 Burn of third degree of right thumb (nail)

[7th] T23.312 Burn of third degree of left thumb (nail)

[7th] T23.319 Burn of third degree of unspecified thumb (nail)

[6th] T23.32 Burn of third degree of single finger (nail) except thumb

[7th] T23.321 Burn of third degree of single right finger (nail) except thumb

[7th] T23.322 Burn of third degree of single left finger (nail) except thumb

[7th] T23.329 Burn of third degree of unspecified single finger (nail) except thumb

[6th] T23.33 Burn of third degree of multiple fingers (nail), not including thumb

[7th] T23.331 Burn of third degree of multiple right fingers (nail), not including thumb

[7th] T23.332 Burn of third degree of multiple left fingers (nail), not including thumb

[7th] T23.339 Burn of third degree of unspecified multiple fingers (nail), not including thumb

[6th] T23.34 Burn of third degree of multiple fingers (nail), including thumb

[7th] T23.341 Burn of third degree of multiple right fingers (nail), including thumb

[7th] T23.342 Burn of third degree of multiple left fingers (nail), including thumb

[7th] T23.349 Burn of third degree of unspecified multiple fingers (nail), including thumb

[6th] T23.35 Burn of third degree of palm

[7th] T23.351 Burn of third degree of right palm

[7th] T23.352 Burn of third degree of left palm

[7th] T23.359 Burn of third degree of unspecified palm

[6th] T23.36 Burn of third degree of back of hand

[7th] T23.361 Burn of third degree of back of right hand

[7th] T23.362 Burn of third degree of back of left hand

[7th] T23.369 Burn of third degree of back of unspecified hand

[6th] T23.37 Burn of third degree of wrist

[7th] T23.371 Burn of third degree of right wrist

[7th] T23.372 Burn of third degree of left wrist

[7th] T23.379 Burn of third degree of unspecified wrist

[6th] T23.39 Burn of third degree of multiple sites of wrist and hand

[7th] T23.391 Burn of third degree of multiple sites of right wrist and hand

[7th] T23.392 Burn of third degree of multiple sites of left wrist and hand

[7th] T23.399 Burn of third degree of multiple sites of unspecified wrist and hand

[5th] T23.4 Corrosion of unspecified degree of wrist and hand

Code first (T51-T65) to identify chemical and intent

Use additional external cause code to identify place (Y92)

[6th] T23.40 Corrosion of unspecified degree of hand, unspecified site

[7th] T23.401 Corrosion of unspecified degree of right hand, unspecified site

[7th] T23.402 Corrosion of unspecified degree of left hand, unspecified site

[7th] T23.409 Corrosion of unspecified degree of unspecified hand, unspecified site

[6th] T23.41 Corrosion of unspecified degree of thumb (nail)

[7th] T23.411 Corrosion of unspecified degree of right thumb (nail)

[7th] T23.412 Corrosion of unspecified degree of left thumb (nail)

[7th] T23.419 Corrosion of unspecified degree of unspecified thumb (nail)

[6th] T23.42 Corrosion of unspecified degree of single finger (nail) except thumb

[7th] T23.421 Corrosion of unspecified degree of single right finger (nail) except thumb

[7th] T23.422 Corrosion of unspecified degree of single left finger (nail) except thumb

[7th] T23.429 Corrosion of unspecified degree of unspecified single finger (nail) except thumb

[6th] T23.43 Corrosion of unspecified degree of multiple fingers (nail), not including thumb

[7th] T23.431 Corrosion of unspecified degree of multiple right fingers (nail), not including thumb

[7th] T23.432 Corrosion of unspecified degree of multiple left fingers (nail), not including thumb

[7th] T23.439 Corrosion of unspecified degree of unspecified multiple fingers (nail), not including thumb

[6th] T23.44 Corrosion of unspecified degree of multiple fingers (nail), including thumb

[7th] T23.441 Corrosion of unspecified degree of multiple right fingers (nail), including thumb

[7th] T23.442 Corrosion of unspecified degree of multiple left fingers (nail), including thumb

[7th] T23.449 Corrosion of unspecified degree of unspecified multiple fingers (nail), including thumb

[4th] 4th character required [5th] 5th character required [6th] 6th character required [7th] 7th character required [7th] Extension 'X' Alert
[EXCLUDES1] Not coded here [EXCLUDES2] Not included here [PDx] Primary Diagnosis Only Manifestation Code

6ᵗʰ T23.45 Corrosion of unspecified degree of palm
  7ᵗʰ T23.451 Corrosion of unspecified degree of right palm
  7ᵗʰ T23.452 Corrosion of unspecified degree of left palm
  7ᵗʰ T23.459 Corrosion of unspecified degree of unspecified palm
6ᵗʰ T23.46 Corrosion of unspecified degree of back of hand
  7ᵗʰ T23.461 Corrosion of unspecified degree of back of right hand
  7ᵗʰ T23.462 Corrosion of unspecified degree of back of left hand
  7ᵗʰ T23.469 Corrosion of unspecified degree of back of unspecified hand
6ᵗʰ T23.47 Corrosion of unspecified degree of wrist
  7ᵗʰ T23.471 Corrosion of unspecified degree of right wrist
  7ᵗʰ T23.472 Corrosion of unspecified degree of left wrist
  7ᵗʰ T23.479 Corrosion of unspecified degree of unspecified wrist
6ᵗʰ T23.49 Corrosion of unspecified degree of multiple sites of wrist and hand
  7ᵗʰ T23.491 Corrosion of unspecified degree of multiple sites of right wrist and hand
  7ᵗʰ T23.492 Corrosion of unspecified degree of multiple sites of left wrist and hand
  7ᵗʰ T23.499 Corrosion of unspecified degree of multiple sites of unspecified wrist and hand
5ᵗʰ T23.5 Corrosion of first degree of wrist and hand
    Code first (T51-T65) to identify chemical and intent
    Use additional external cause code to identify place (Y92)
6ᵗʰ T23.50 Corrosion of first degree of hand, unspecified site
  7ᵗʰ T23.501 Corrosion of first degree of right hand, unspecified site
  7ᵗʰ T23.502 Corrosion of first degree of left hand, unspecified site
  7ᵗʰ T23.509 Corrosion of first degree of unspecified hand, unspecified site
6ᵗʰ T23.51 Corrosion of first degree of thumb (nail)
  7ᵗʰ T23.511 Corrosion of first degree of right thumb (nail)
  7ᵗʰ T23.512 Corrosion of first degree of left thumb (nail)
  7ᵗʰ T23.519 Corrosion of first degree of unspecified thumb (nail)
6ᵗʰ T23.52 Corrosion of first degree of single finger (nail) except thumb
  7ᵗʰ T23.521 Corrosion of first degree of single right finger (nail) except thumb
  7ᵗʰ T23.522 Corrosion of first degree of single left finger (nail) except thumb
  7ᵗʰ T23.529 Corrosion of first degree of unspecified single finger (nail) except thumb
6ᵗʰ T23.53 Corrosion of first degree of multiple fingers (nail), not including thumb
  7ᵗʰ T23.531 Corrosion of first degree of multiple right fingers (nail), not including thumb
  7ᵗʰ T23.532 Corrosion of first degree of multiple left fingers (nail), not including thumb
  7ᵗʰ T23.539 Corrosion of first degree of unspecified multiple fingers (nail), not including thumb
6ᵗʰ T23.54 Corrosion of first degree of multiple fingers (nail), including thumb
  7ᵗʰ T23.541 Corrosion of first degree of multiple right fingers (nail), including thumb
  7ᵗʰ T23.542 Corrosion of first degree of multiple left fingers (nail), including thumb
  7ᵗʰ T23.549 Corrosion of first degree of unspecified multiple fingers (nail), including thumb
6ᵗʰ T23.55 Corrosion of first degree of palm

7ᵗʰ T23.551 Corrosion of first degree of right palm
7ᵗʰ T23.552 Corrosion of first degree of left palm
7ᵗʰ T23.559 Corrosion of first degree of unspecified palm
6ᵗʰ T23.56 Corrosion of first degree of back of hand
  7ᵗʰ T23.561 Corrosion of first degree of back of right hand
  7ᵗʰ T23.562 Corrosion of first degree of back of left hand
  7ᵗʰ T23.569 Corrosion of first degree of back of unspecified hand
6ᵗʰ T23.57 Corrosion of first degree of wrist
  7ᵗʰ T23.571 Corrosion of first degree of right wrist
  7ᵗʰ T23.572 Corrosion of first degree of left wrist
  7ᵗʰ T23.579 Corrosion of first degree of unspecified wrist
6ᵗʰ T23.59 Corrosion of first degree of multiple sites of wrist and hand
  7ᵗʰ T23.591 Corrosion of first degree of multiple sites of right wrist and hand
  7ᵗʰ T23.592 Corrosion of first degree of multiple sites of left wrist and hand
  7ᵗʰ T23.599 Corrosion of first degree of multiple sites of unspecified wrist and hand
5ᵗʰ T23.6 Corrosion of second degree of wrist and hand
    Code first (T51-T65) to identify chemical and intent
    Use additional external cause code to identify place (Y92)
6ᵗʰ T23.60 Corrosion of second degree of hand, unspecified site
  7ᵗʰ T23.601 Corrosion of second degree of right hand, unspecified site
  7ᵗʰ T23.602 Corrosion of second degree of left hand, unspecified site
  7ᵗʰ T23.609 Corrosion of second degree of unspecified hand, unspecified site
6ᵗʰ T23.61 Corrosion of second degree of thumb (nail)
  7ᵗʰ T23.611 Corrosion of second degree of right thumb (nail)
  7ᵗʰ T23.612 Corrosion of second degree of left thumb (nail)
  7ᵗʰ T23.619 Corrosion of second degree of unspecified thumb (nail)
6ᵗʰ T23.62 Corrosion of second degree of single finger (nail) except thumb
  7ᵗʰ T23.621 Corrosion of second degree of single right finger (nail) except thumb
  7ᵗʰ T23.622 Corrosion of second degree of single left finger (nail) except thumb
  7ᵗʰ T23.629 Corrosion of second degree of unspecified single finger (nail) except thumb
6ᵗʰ T23.63 Corrosion of second degree of multiple fingers (nail), not including thumb
  7ᵗʰ T23.631 Corrosion of second degree of multiple right fingers (nail), not including thumb
  7ᵗʰ T23.632 Corrosion of second degree of multiple left fingers (nail), not including thumb
  7ᵗʰ T23.639 Corrosion of second degree of unspecified multiple fingers (nail), not including thumb
6ᵗʰ T23.64 Corrosion of second degree of multiple fingers (nail), including thumb
  7ᵗʰ T23.641 Corrosion of second degree of multiple right fingers (nail), including thumb
  7ᵗʰ T23.642 Corrosion of second degree of multiple left fingers (nail), including thumb
  7ᵗʰ T23.649 Corrosion of second degree of unspecified multiple fingers (nail), including thumb
6ᵗʰ T23.65 Corrosion of second degree of palm
  7ᵗʰ T23.651 Corrosion of second degree of right palm
  7ᵗʰ T23.652 Corrosion of second degree of left palm

| Unspecified Code | Other Specified Code | Ⓝ Newborn Age: 0 | Ⓟ Pediatric Age: 0-17 | Ⓜ Maternity Age: 12-55 |
| Ⓐ Adult Age: 15-124 | ♂ Male | ♀ Female | ● New Code | ▲ Revised Code Title | ►◄ Revised Text |

7️⃣ T23.659 Corrosion of second degree of unspecified palm

6️⃣ T23.66 Corrosion of second degree of back of hand
   7️⃣ T23.661 Corrosion of second degree back of right hand
   7️⃣ T23.662 Corrosion of second degree back of left hand
   7️⃣ T23.669 Corrosion of second degree back of unspecified hand

6️⃣ T23.67 Corrosion of second degree of wrist
   7️⃣ T23.671 Corrosion of second degree of right wrist
   7️⃣ T23.672 Corrosion of second degree of left wrist
   7️⃣ T23.679 Corrosion of second degree of unspecified wrist

5️⃣ T23.69 Corrosion of second degree of multiple sites of wrist and hand
   7️⃣ T23.691 Corrosion of second degree of multiple sites of right wrist and hand
   7️⃣ T23.692 Corrosion of second degree of multiple sites of left wrist and hand
   7️⃣ T23.699 Corrosion of second degree of multiple sites of unspecified wrist and hand

5️⃣ T23.7 Corrosion of third degree of wrist and hand
   Code first (T51-T65) to identify chemical and intent
   Use additional external cause code to identify place (Y92)

6️⃣ T23.70 Corrosion of third degree of hand, unspecified site
   7️⃣ T23.701 Corrosion of third degree of right hand, unspecified site
   7️⃣ T23.702 Corrosion of third degree of left hand, unspecified site
   7️⃣ T23.709 Corrosion of third degree of unspecified hand, unspecified site

6️⃣ T23.71 Corrosion of third degree of thumb (nail)
   7️⃣ T23.711 Corrosion of third degree of right thumb (nail)
   7️⃣ T23.712 Corrosion of third degree of left thumb (nail)
   7️⃣ T23.719 Corrosion of third degree of unspecified thumb (nail)

6️⃣ T23.72 Corrosion of third degree of single finger (nail) except thumb
   7️⃣ T23.721 Corrosion of third degree of single right finger (nail) except thumb
   7️⃣ T23.722 Corrosion of third degree of single left finger (nail) except thumb
   7️⃣ T23.729 Corrosion of third degree of unspecified single finger (nail) except thumb

6️⃣ T23.73 Corrosion of third degree of multiple fingers (nail), not including thumb
   7️⃣ T23.731 Corrosion of third degree of multiple right fingers (nail), not including thumb
   7️⃣ T23.732 Corrosion of third degree of multiple left fingers (nail), not including thumb
   7️⃣ T23.739 Corrosion of third degree of unspecified multiple fingers (nail), not including thumb

6️⃣ T23.74 Corrosion of third degree of multiple fingers (nail), including thumb
   7️⃣ T23.741 Corrosion of third degree of multiple right fingers (nail), including thumb
   7️⃣ T23.742 Corrosion of third degree of multiple left fingers (nail), including thumb
   7️⃣ T23.749 Corrosion of third degree of unspecified multiple fingers (nail), including thumb

6️⃣ T23.75 Corrosion of third degree of palm
   7️⃣ T23.751 Corrosion of third degree of right palm
   7️⃣ T23.752 Corrosion of third degree of left palm
   7️⃣ T23.759 Corrosion of third degree of unspecified palm

6️⃣ T23.76 Corrosion of third degree of back of hand
   7️⃣ T23.761 Corrosion of third degree of back of right hand
   7️⃣ T23.762 Corrosion of third degree of back of left hand
   7️⃣ T23.769 Corrosion of third degree back of unspecified hand

6️⃣ T23.77 Corrosion of third degree of wrist
   7️⃣ T23.771 Corrosion of third degree of right wrist
   7️⃣ T23.772 Corrosion of third degree of left wrist
   7️⃣ T23.779 Corrosion of third degree of unspecified wrist

6️⃣ T23.79 Corrosion of third degree of multiple sites of wrist and hand
   7️⃣ T23.791 Corrosion of third degree of multiple sites of right wrist and hand
   7️⃣ T23.792 Corrosion of third degree of multiple sites of left wrist and hand
   7️⃣ T23.799 Corrosion of third degree of multiple sites of unspecified wrist and hand

4️⃣ T24 Burn and corrosion of lower limb, except ankle and foot
   EXCLUDES2 burn and corrosion of ankle and foot (T25.-)
             burn and corrosion of hip region (T21.-)
   The appropriate 7th character is to be added to each code from category T24
   A = initial encounter
   D = subsequent encounter
   S = sequela

5️⃣ T24.0 Burn of unspecified degree of lower limb, except ankle and foot
   Use additional external cause code to identify the source, place and intent of the burn (X00-X19, X75-X77, X96-X98, Y92)

6️⃣ T24.00 Burn of unspecified degree of unspecified site of lower limb, except ankle and foot
   7️⃣ T24.001 Burn of unspecified degree of unspecified site of right lower limb, except ankle and foot
   7️⃣ T24.002 Burn of unspecified degree of unspecified site of left lower limb, except ankle and foot
   7️⃣ T24.009 Burn of unspecified degree of unspecified site of unspecified lower limb, except ankle and foot

6️⃣ T24.01 Burn of unspecified degree of thigh
   7️⃣ T24.011 Burn of unspecified degree of right thigh
   7️⃣ T24.012 Burn of unspecified degree of left thigh
   7️⃣ T24.019 Burn of unspecified degree of unspecified thigh

6️⃣ T24.02 Burn of unspecified degree of knee
   7️⃣ T24.021 Burn of unspecified degree of right knee
   7️⃣ T24.022 Burn of unspecified degree of left knee
   7️⃣ T24.029 Burn of unspecified degree of unspecified knee

6️⃣ T24.03 Burn of unspecified degree of lower leg
   7️⃣ T24.031 Burn of unspecified degree of right lower leg
   7️⃣ T24.032 Burn of unspecified degree of left lower leg
   7️⃣ T24.039 Burn of unspecified degree of unspecified lower leg

6️⃣ T24.09 Burn of unspecified degree of multiple sites of lower limb, except ankle and foot
   7️⃣ T24.091 Burn of unspecified degree of multiple sites of right lower limb, except ankle and foot
   7️⃣ T24.092 Burn of unspecified degree of multiple sites of left lower limb, except ankle and foot
   7️⃣ T24.099 Burn of unspecified degree of multiple sites of unspecified lower limb, except ankle and foot

4️⃣ 4th character required   5️⃣ 5th character required   6️⃣ 6th character required   7️⃣ 7th character required   7️⃣ Extension 'X' Alert

EXCLUDES 1 Not coded here   EXCLUDES 2 Not included here   PDx Primary Diagnosis Only   Manifestation Code

674   **ICD-10-CM 2015**

5ᵗʰ T24.1 Burn of first degree of lower limb, except ankle and foot

Use additional external cause code to identify the source, place and intent of the burn (X00-X19, X75-X77, X96-X98, Y92)

6ᵗʰ T24.10 Burn of first degree of unspecified site of lower limb, except ankle and foot

7ᵗʰ T24.101 Burn of first degree of unspecified site of right lower limb, except ankle and foot

7ᵗʰ T24.102 Burn of first degree of unspecified site of left lower limb, except ankle and foot

7ᵗʰ T24.109 Burn of first degree of unspecified site of unspecified lower limb, except ankle and foot

6ᵗʰ T24.11 Burn of first degree of thigh

7ᵗʰ T24.111 Burn of first degree of right thigh

7ᵗʰ T24.112 Burn of first degree of left thigh

7ᵗʰ T24.119 Burn of first degree of unspecified thigh

6ᵗʰ T24.12 Burn of first degree of knee

7ᵗʰ T24.121 Burn of first degree of right knee

7ᵗʰ T24.122 Burn of first degree of left knee

7ᵗʰ T24.129 Burn of first degree of unspecified knee

6ᵗʰ T24.13 Burn of first degree of lower leg

7ᵗʰ T24.131 Burn of first degree of right lower leg

7ᵗʰ T24.132 Burn of first degree of left lower leg

7ᵗʰ T24.139 Burn of first degree of unspecified lower leg

6ᵗʰ T24.19 Burn of first degree of multiple sites of lower limb, except ankle and foot

7ᵗʰ T24.191 Burn of first degree of multiple sites of right lower limb, except ankle and foot

7ᵗʰ T24.192 Burn of first degree of multiple sites of left lower limb, except ankle and foot

7ᵗʰ T24.199 Burn of first degree of multiple sites of unspecified lower limb, except ankle and foot

5ᵗʰ T24.2 Burn of second degree of lower limb, except ankle and foot

Use additional external cause code to identify the source, place and intent of the burn (X00-X19, X75-X77, X96-X98, Y92)

6ᵗʰ T24.20 Burn of second degree of unspecified site of lower limb, except ankle and foot

7ᵗʰ T24.201 Burn of second degree of unspecified site of right lower limb, except ankle and foot

7ᵗʰ T24.202 Burn of second degree of unspecified site of left lower limb, except ankle and foot

7ᵗʰ T24.209 Burn of second degree of unspecified site of unspecified lower limb, except ankle and foot

6ᵗʰ T24.21 Burn of second degree of thigh

7ᵗʰ T24.211 Burn of second degree of right thigh

7ᵗʰ T24.212 Burn of second degree of left thigh

7ᵗʰ T24.219 Burn of second degree of unspecified thigh

6ᵗʰ T24.22 Burn of second degree of knee

7ᵗʰ T24.221 Burn of second degree of right knee

7ᵗʰ T24.222 Burn of second degree of left knee

7ᵗʰ T24.229 Burn of second degree of unspecified knee

6ᵗʰ T24.23 Burn of second degree of lower leg

7ᵗʰ T24.231 Burn of second degree of right lower leg

7ᵗʰ T24.232 Burn of second degree of left lower leg

7ᵗʰ T24.239 Burn of second degree of unspecified lower leg

6ᵗʰ T24.29 Burn of second degree of multiple sites of lower limb, except ankle and foot

7ᵗʰ T24.291 Burn of second degree of multiple sites of right lower limb, except ankle and foot

7ᵗʰ T24.292 Burn of second degree of multiple sites of left lower limb, except ankle and foot

7ᵗʰ T24.299 Burn of second degree of multiple sites of unspecified lower limb, except ankle and foot

5ᵗʰ T24.3 Burn of third degree of lower limb, except ankle and foot

Use additional external cause code to identify the source, place and intent of the burn (X00-X19, X75-X77, X96-X98, Y92)

6ᵗʰ T24.30 Burn of third degree of unspecified site of lower limb, except ankle and foot

7ᵗʰ T24.301 Burn of third degree of unspecified site of right lower limb, except ankle and foot

7ᵗʰ T24.302 Burn of third degree of unspecified site of left lower limb, except ankle and foot

7ᵗʰ T24.309 Burn of third degree of unspecified site of unspecified lower limb, except ankle and foot

6ᵗʰ T24.31 Burn of third degree of thigh

7ᵗʰ T24.311 Burn of third degree of right thigh

7ᵗʰ T24.312 Burn of third degree of left thigh

7ᵗʰ T24.319 Burn of third degree of unspecified thigh

6ᵗʰ T24.32 Burn of third degree of knee

7ᵗʰ T24.321 Burn of third degree of right knee

7ᵗʰ T24.322 Burn of third degree of left knee

7ᵗʰ T24.329 Burn of third degree of unspecified knee

6ᵗʰ T24.33 Burn of third degree of lower leg

7ᵗʰ T24.331 Burn of third degree of right lower leg

7ᵗʰ T24.332 Burn of third degree of left lower leg

7ᵗʰ T24.339 Burn of third degree of unspecified lower leg

6ᵗʰ T24.39 Burn of third degree of multiple sites of lower limb, except ankle and foot

7ᵗʰ T24.391 Burn of third degree of multiple sites of right lower limb, except ankle and foot

7ᵗʰ T24.392 Burn of third degree of multiple sites of left lower limb, except ankle and foot

7ᵗʰ T24.399 Burn of third degree of multiple sites of unspecified lower limb, except ankle and foot

5ᵗʰ T24.4 Corrosion of unspecified degree of lower limb, except ankle and foot

Code first (T51-T65) to identify chemical and intent

Use additional external cause code to identify place (Y92)

6ᵗʰ T24.40 Corrosion of unspecified degree of unspecified site of lower limb, except ankle and foot

7ᵗʰ T24.401 Corrosion of unspecified degree of unspecified site of right lower limb, except ankle and foot

7ᵗʰ T24.402 Corrosion of unspecified degree of unspecified site of left lower limb, except ankle and foot

7ᵗʰ T24.409 Corrosion of unspecified degree of unspecified site of unspecified lower limb, except ankle and foot

6ᵗʰ T24.41 Corrosion of unspecified degree of thigh

7ᵗʰ T24.411 Corrosion of unspecified degree of right thigh

7ᵗʰ T24.412 Corrosion of unspecified degree of left thigh

7ᵗʰ T24.419 Corrosion of unspecified degree of unspecified thigh

6ᵗʰ T24.42 Corrosion of unspecified degree of knee

7ᵗʰ T24.421 Corrosion of unspecified degree of right knee

7ᵗʰ T24.422 Corrosion of unspecified degree of left knee

7ᵗʰ T24.429 Corrosion of unspecified degree of unspecified knee

6ᵗʰ T24.43 Corrosion of unspecified degree of lower leg

Unspecified Code	Other Specified Code	N Newborn Age: 0	P Pediatric Age: 0-17	M Maternity Age: 12-55
A Adult Age: 15-124	♂ Male	♀ Female	● New Code	▲ Revised Code Title	►◄ Revised Text

[7th] T24.431 Corrosion of unspecified degree of right lower leg
[7th] T24.432 Corrosion of unspecified degree of left lower leg
[7th] T24.439 Corrosion of unspecified degree of unspecified lower leg
[6th] T24.49 Corrosion of unspecified degree of multiple sites of lower limb, except ankle and foot
[7th] T24.491 Corrosion of unspecified degree of multiple sites of right lower limb, except ankle and foot
[7th] T24.492 Corrosion of unspecified degree of multiple sites of left lower limb, except ankle and foot
[7th] T24.499 Corrosion of unspecified degree of multiple sites of unspecified lower limb, except ankle and foot
[5th] T24.5 Corrosion of first degree of lower limb, except ankle and foot
Code first (T51-T65) to identify chemical and intent
Use additional external cause code to identify place (Y92)
[6th] T24.50 Corrosion of first degree of unspecified site of lower limb, except ankle and foot
[7th] T24.501 Corrosion of first degree of unspecified site of right lower limb, except ankle and foot
[7th] T24.502 Corrosion of first degree of unspecified site of left lower limb, except ankle and foot
[7th] T24.509 Corrosion of first degree of unspecified site of unspecified lower limb, except ankle and foot
[6th] T24.51 Corrosion of first degree of thigh
[7th] T24.511 Corrosion of first degree of right thigh
[7th] T24.512 Corrosion of first degree of left thigh
[7th] T24.519 Corrosion of first degree of unspecified thigh
[6th] T24.52 Corrosion of first degree of knee
[7th] T24.521 Corrosion of first degree of right knee
[7th] T24.522 Corrosion of first degree of left knee
[7th] T24.529 Corrosion of first degree of unspecified knee
[6th] T24.53 Corrosion of first degree of lower leg
[7th] T24.531 Corrosion of first degree of right lower leg
[7th] T24.532 Corrosion of first degree of left lower leg
[7th] T24.539 Corrosion of first degree of unspecified lower leg
[6th] T24.59 Corrosion of first degree of multiple sites of lower limb, except ankle and foot
[7th] T24.591 Corrosion of first degree of multiple sites of right lower limb, except ankle and foot
[7th] T24.592 Corrosion of first degree of multiple sites of left lower limb, except ankle and foot
[7th] T24.599 Corrosion of first degree of multiple sites of unspecified lower limb, except ankle and foot
[5th] T24.6 Corrosion of second degree of lower limb, except ankle and foot
Code first (T51-T65) to identify chemical and intent
Use additional external cause code to identify place (Y92)
[6th] T24.60 Corrosion of second degree of unspecified site of lower limb, except ankle and foot
[7th] T24.601 Corrosion of second degree of unspecified site of right lower limb, except ankle and foot
[7th] T24.602 Corrosion of second degree of unspecified site of left lower limb, except ankle and foot
[7th] T24.609 Corrosion of second degree of unspecified site of unspecified lower limb, except ankle and foot
[6th] T24.61 Corrosion of second degree of thigh
[7th] T24.611 Corrosion of second degree of right thigh
[7th] T24.612 Corrosion of second degree of left thigh
[7th] T24.619 Corrosion of second degree of unspecified thigh
[6th] T24.62 Corrosion of second degree of knee
[7th] T24.621 Corrosion of second degree of right knee
[7th] T24.622 Corrosion of second degree of left knee
[7th] T24.629 Corrosion of second degree of unspecified knee
[6th] T24.63 Corrosion of second degree of lower leg
[7th] T24.631 Corrosion of second degree of right lower leg
[7th] T24.632 Corrosion of second degree of left lower leg
[7th] T24.639 Corrosion of second degree of unspecified lower leg
[6th] T24.69 Corrosion of second degree of multiple sites of lower limb, except ankle and foot
[7th] T24.691 Corrosion of second degree of multiple sites of right lower limb, except ankle and foot
[7th] T24.692 Corrosion of second degree of multiple sites of left lower limb, except ankle and foot
[7th] T24.699 Corrosion of second degree of multiple sites of unspecified lower limb, except ankle and foot
[5th] T24.7 Corrosion of third degree of lower limb, except ankle and foot
Code first (T51-T65) to identify chemical and intent
Use additional external cause code to identify place (Y92)
[6th] T24.70 Corrosion of third degree of unspecified site of lower limb, except ankle and foot
[7th] T24.701 Corrosion of third degree of unspecified site of right lower limb, except ankle and foot
[7th] T24.702 Corrosion of third degree of unspecified site of left lower limb, except ankle and foot
[7th] T24.709 Corrosion of third degree of unspecified site of unspecified lower limb, except ankle and foot
[6th] T24.71 Corrosion of third degree of thigh
[7th] T24.711 Corrosion of third degree of right thigh
[7th] T24.712 Corrosion of third degree of left thigh
[7th] T24.719 Corrosion of third degree of unspecified thigh
[6th] T24.72 Corrosion of third degree of knee
[7th] T24.721 Corrosion of third degree of right knee
[7th] T24.722 Corrosion of third degree of left knee
[7th] T24.729 Corrosion of third degree of unspecified knee
[6th] T24.73 Corrosion of third degree of lower leg
[7th] T24.731 Corrosion of third degree of right lower leg
[7th] T24.732 Corrosion of third degree of left lower leg
[7th] T24.739 Corrosion of third degree of unspecified lower leg
[6th] T24.79 Corrosion of third degree of multiple sites of lower limb, except ankle and foot
[7th] T24.791 Corrosion of third degree of multiple sites of right lower limb, except ankle and foot
[7th] T24.792 Corrosion of third degree of multiple sites of left lower limb, except ankle and foot
[7th] T24.799 Corrosion of third degree of multiple sites of unspecified lower limb, except ankle and foot
[4th] T25 Burn and corrosion of ankle and foot
The appropriate 7th character is to be added to each code from category T25
A = initial encounter
D = subsequent encounter
S = sequela

[4th] 4th character required [5th] 5th character required [6th] 6th character required [7th] 7th character required [X] Extension 'X' Alert
[EXCLUDES 1] Not coded here [EXCLUDES 2] Not included here [PDx] Primary Diagnosis Only Manifestation Code

T25.0 Burn of unspecified degree of ankle and foot
Use additional external cause code to identify the source, place and intent of the burn (X00-X19, X75-X77, X96-X98, Y92)

T25.01 Burn of unspecified degree of ankle
- T25.011 Burn of unspecified degree of right ankle
- T25.012 Burn of unspecified degree of left ankle
- T25.019 Burn of unspecified degree of unspecified ankle

T25.02 Burn of unspecified degree of foot
EXCLUDES2 burn of unspecified degree of toe(s) (nail) (T25.03-)
- T25.021 Burn of unspecified degree of right foot
- T25.022 Burn of unspecified degree of left foot
- T25.029 Burn of unspecified degree of unspecified foot

T25.03 Burn of unspecified degree of toe(s) (nail)
- T25.031 Burn of unspecified degree of right toe(s) (nail)
- T25.032 Burn of unspecified degree of left toe(s) (nail)
- T25.039 Burn of unspecified degree of unspecified toe(s) (nail)

T25.09 Burn of unspecified degree of multiple sites of ankle and foot
- T25.091 Burn of unspecified degree of multiple sites of right ankle and foot
- T25.092 Burn of unspecified degree of multiple sites of left ankle and foot
- T25.099 Burn of unspecified degree of multiple sites of unspecified ankle and foot

T25.1 Burn of first degree of ankle and foot
Use additional external cause code to identify the source, place and intent of the burn (X00-X19, X75-X77, X96-X98, Y92)

T25.11 Burn of first degree of ankle
- T25.111 Burn of first degree of right ankle
- T25.112 Burn of first degree of left ankle
- T25.119 Burn of first degree of unspecified ankle

T25.12 Burn of first degree of foot
EXCLUDES2 burn of first degree of toe(s) (nail) (T25.13-)
- T25.121 Burn of first degree of right foot
- T25.122 Burn of first degree of left foot
- T25.129 Burn of first degree of unspecified foot

T25.13 Burn of first degree of toe(s) (nail)
- T25.131 Burn of first degree of right toe(s) (nail)
- T25.132 Burn of first degree of left toe(s) (nail)
- T25.139 Burn of first degree of unspecified toe(s) (nail)

T25.19 Burn of first degree of multiple sites of ankle and foot
- T25.191 Burn of first degree of multiple sites of right ankle and foot
- T25.192 Burn of first degree of multiple sites of left ankle and foot
- T25.199 Burn of first degree of multiple sites of unspecified ankle and foot

T25.2 Burn of second degree of ankle and foot
Use additional external cause code to identify the source, place and intent of the burn (X00-X19, X75-X77, X96-X98, Y92)

T25.21 Burn of second degree of ankle
- T25.211 Burn of second degree of right ankle
- T25.212 Burn of second degree of left ankle
- T25.219 Burn of second degree of unspecified ankle

T25.22 Burn of second degree of foot
EXCLUDES2 burn of second degree of toe(s) (nail) (T25.23-)
- T25.221 Burn of second degree of right foot
- T25.222 Burn of second degree of left foot

- T25.229 Burn of second degree of unspecified foot

T25.23 Burn of second degree of toe(s) (nail)
- T25.231 Burn of second degree of right toe(s) (nail)
- T25.232 Burn of second degree of left toe(s) (nail)
- T25.239 Burn of second degree of unspecified toe(s) (nail)

T25.29 Burn of second degree of multiple sites of ankle and foot
- T25.291 Burn of second degree of multiple sites of right ankle and foot
- T25.292 Burn of second degree of multiple sites of left ankle and foot
- T25.299 Burn of second degree of multiple sites of unspecified ankle and foot

T25.3 Burn of third degree of ankle and foot
Use additional external cause code to identify the source, place and intent of the burn (X00-X19, X75-X77, X96-X98, Y92)

T25.31 Burn of third degree of ankle
- T25.311 Burn of third degree of right ankle
- T25.312 Burn of third degree of left ankle
- T25.319 Burn of third degree of unspecified ankle

T25.32 Burn of third degree of foot
EXCLUDES2 burn of third degree of toe(s) (nail) (T25.33-)
- T25.321 Burn of third degree of right foot
- T25.322 Burn of third degree of left foot
- T25.329 Burn of third degree of unspecified foot

T25.33 Burn of third degree of toe(s) (nail)
- T25.331 Burn of third degree of right toe(s) (nail)
- T25.332 Burn of third degree of left toe(s) (nail)
- T25.339 Burn of third degree of unspecified toe(s) (nail)

T25.39 Burn of third degree of multiple sites of ankle and foot
- T25.391 Burn of third degree of multiple sites of right ankle and foot
- T25.392 Burn of third degree of multiple sites of left ankle and foot
- T25.399 Burn of third degree of multiple sites of unspecified ankle and foot

T25.4 Corrosion of unspecified degree of ankle and foot
Code first (T51-T65) to identify chemical and intent
Use additional external cause code to identify place (Y92)

T25.41 Corrosion of unspecified degree of ankle
- T25.411 Corrosion of unspecified degree of right ankle
- T25.412 Corrosion of unspecified degree of left ankle
- T25.419 Corrosion of unspecified degree of unspecified ankle

T25.42 Corrosion of unspecified degree of foot
EXCLUDES2 corrosion of unspecified degree of toe(s) (nail) (T25.43-)
- T25.421 Corrosion of unspecified degree of right foot
- T25.422 Corrosion of unspecified degree of left foot
- T25.429 Corrosion of unspecified degree of unspecified foot

T25.43 Corrosion of unspecified degree of toe(s) (nail)
- T25.431 Corrosion of unspecified degree of right toe(s) (nail)
- T25.432 Corrosion of unspecified degree of left toe(s) (nail)
- T25.439 Corrosion of unspecified degree of unspecified toe(s) (nail)

T25.49 Corrosion of unspecified degree of multiple sites of ankle and foot

Unspecified Code	Other Specified Code	N Newborn Age: 0	P Pediatric Age: 0-17	M Maternity Age: 12-55
A Adult Age: 15-124	♂ Male	♀ Female	● New Code	▲ Revised Code Title	►◄ Revised Text

⑦ T25.491 Corrosion of unspecified degree of multiple sites of right ankle and foot
⑦ T25.492 Corrosion of unspecified degree of multiple sites of left ankle and foot
⑦ T25.499 Corrosion of unspecified degree of multiple sites of unspecified ankle and foot
⑤ T25.5 Corrosion of first degree of ankle and foot
　Code first (T51-T65) to identify chemical and intent
　Use additional external cause code to identify place (Y92)
⑥ T25.51 Corrosion of first degree of ankle
⑦ T25.511 Corrosion of first degree of right ankle
⑦ T25.512 Corrosion of first degree of left ankle
⑦ T25.519 Corrosion of first degree of unspecified ankle
⑥ T25.52 Corrosion of first degree of foot
　EXCLUDES2 corrosion of first degree of toe(s) (nail) (T25.53-)
⑦ T25.521 Corrosion of first degree of right foot
⑦ T25.522 Corrosion of first degree of left foot
⑦ T25.529 Corrosion of first degree of unspecified foot
⑥ T25.53 Corrosion of first degree of toe(s) (nail)
⑦ T25.531 Corrosion of first degree of right toe(s) (nail)
⑦ T25.532 Corrosion of first degree of left toe(s) (nail)
⑦ T25.539 Corrosion of first degree of unspecified toe(s) (nail)
⑥ T25.59 Corrosion of first degree of multiple sites of ankle and foot
⑦ T25.591 Corrosion of first degree of multiple sites of right ankle and foot
⑦ T25.592 Corrosion of first degree of multiple sites of left ankle and foot
⑦ T25.599 Corrosion of first degree of multiple sites of unspecified ankle and foot
⑤ T25.6 Corrosion of second degree of ankle and foot
　Code first (T51-T65) to identify chemical and intent
　Use additional external cause code to identify place (Y92)
⑥ T25.61 Corrosion of second degree of ankle
⑦ T25.611 Corrosion of second degree of right ankle
⑦ T25.612 Corrosion of second degree of left ankle
⑦ T25.619 Corrosion of second degree of unspecified ankle
⑥ T25.62 Corrosion of second degree of foot
　EXCLUDES2 corrosion of second degree of toe(s) (nail) (T25.63-)
⑦ T25.621 Corrosion of second degree of right foot
⑦ T25.622 Corrosion of second degree of left foot
⑦ T25.629 Corrosion of second degree of unspecified foot
⑥ T25.63 Corrosion of second degree of toe(s) (nail)
⑦ T25.631 Corrosion of second degree of right toe(s) (nail)
⑦ T25.632 Corrosion of second degree of left toe(s) (nail)
⑦ T25.639 Corrosion of second degree of unspecified toe(s) (nail)
⑥ T25.69 Corrosion of second degree of multiple sites of ankle and foot
⑦ T25.691 Corrosion of second degree of right ankle and foot
⑦ T25.692 Corrosion of second degree of left ankle and foot
⑦ T25.699 Corrosion of second degree of unspecified ankle and foot
⑤ T25.7 Corrosion of third degree of ankle and foot
　Code first (T51-T65) to identify chemical and intent
　Use additional external cause code to identify place (Y92)

⑥ T25.71 Corrosion of third degree of ankle
⑦ T25.711 Corrosion of third degree of right ankle
⑦ T25.712 Corrosion of third degree of left ankle
⑦ T25.719 Corrosion of third degree of unspecified ankle
⑥ T25.72 Corrosion of third degree of foot
　EXCLUDES2 corrosion of third degree of toe(s) (nail) (T25.73-)
⑦ T25.721 Corrosion of third degree of right foot
⑦ T25.722 Corrosion of third degree of left foot
⑦ T25.729 Corrosion of third degree of unspecified foot
⑥ T25.73 Corrosion of third degree of toe(s) (nail)
⑦ T25.731 Corrosion of third degree of right toe(s) (nail)
⑦ T25.732 Corrosion of third degree of left toe(s) (nail)
⑦ T25.739 Corrosion of third degree of unspecified toe(s) (nail)
⑥ T25.79 Corrosion of third degree of multiple sites of ankle and foot
⑦ T25.791 Corrosion of third degree of multiple sites of right ankle and foot
⑦ T25.792 Corrosion of third degree of multiple sites of left ankle and foot
⑦ T25.799 Corrosion of third degree of multiple sites of unspecified ankle and foot

Burns and corrosions confined to eye and internal organs (T26-T28)

④ T26 Burn and corrosion confined to eye and adnexa
　The appropriate 7th character is to be added to each code from category T26
　A = initial encounter
　D = subsequent encounter
　S = sequela
⑤ T26.0 Burn of eyelid and periocular area
　Use additional external cause code to identify the source, place and intent of the burn (X00-X19, X75-X77, X96-X98, Y92)
⑦ T26.00 Burn of unspecified eyelid and periocular area
⑦ T26.01 Burn of right eyelid and periocular area
⑦ T26.02 Burn of left eyelid and periocular area
⑤ T26.1 Burn of cornea and conjunctival sac
　Use additional external cause code to identify the source, place and intent of the burn (X00-X19, X75-X77, X96-X98, Y92)
⑦ T26.10 Burn of cornea and conjunctival sac, unspecified eye
⑦ T26.11 Burn of cornea and conjunctival sac, right eye
⑦ T26.12 Burn of cornea and conjunctival sac, left eye
⑤ T26.2 Burn with resulting rupture and destruction of eyeball
　Use additional external cause code to identify the source, place and intent of the burn (X00-X19, X75-X77, X96-X98, Y92)
⑦ T26.20 Burn with resulting rupture and destruction of unspecified eyeball
⑦ T26.21 Burn with resulting rupture and destruction of right eyeball
⑦ T26.22 Burn with resulting rupture and destruction of left eyeball
⑤ T26.3 Burns of other specified parts of eye and adnexa
　Use additional external cause code to identify the source, place and intent of the burn (X00-X19, X75-X77, X96-X98, Y92)
⑦ T26.30 Burns of other specified parts of unspecified eye and adnexa
⑦ T26.31 Burns of other specified parts of right eye and adnexa

⑰ T26.32 Burns of other specified parts of left eye and adnexa
⑤ T26.4 Burn of eye and adnexa, part unspecified
   Use additional external cause code to identify the source, place and intent of the burn (X00-X19, X75-X77, X96-X98, Y92)
   ⑰ T26.40 Burn of unspecified eye and adnexa, part unspecified
   ⑰ T26.41 Burn of right eye and adnexa, part unspecified
   ⑰ T26.42 Burn of left eye and adnexa, part unspecified
⑤ T26.5 Corrosion of eyelid and periocular area
   Code first (T51-T65) to identify chemical and intent
   Use additional external cause code to identify place (Y92)
   ⑰ T26.50 Corrosion of unspecified eyelid and periocular area
   ⑰ T26.51 Corrosion of right eyelid and periocular area
   ⑰ T26.52 Corrosion of left eyelid and periocular area
⑤ T26.6 Corrosion of cornea and conjunctival sac
   Code first (T51-T65) to identify chemical and intent
   Use additional external cause code to identify place (Y92)
   ⑰ T26.60 Corrosion of cornea and conjunctival sac, unspecified eye
   ⑰ T26.61 Corrosion of cornea and conjunctival sac, right eye
   ⑰ T26.62 Corrosion of cornea and conjunctival sac, left eye
⑤ T26.7 Corrosion with resulting rupture and destruction of eyeball
   Code first (T51-T65) to identify chemical and intent
   Use additional external cause code to identify place (Y92)
   ⑰ T26.70 Corrosion with resulting rupture and destruction of unspecified eyeball
   ⑰ T26.71 Corrosion with resulting rupture and destruction of right eyeball
   ⑰ T26.72 Corrosion with resulting rupture and destruction of left eyeball
⑤ T26.8 Corrosions of other specified parts of eye and adnexa
   Code first (T51-T65) to identify chemical and intent
   Use additional external cause code to identify place (Y92)
   ⑰ T26.80 Corrosions of other specified parts of unspecified eye and adnexa
   ⑰ T26.81 Corrosions of other specified parts of right eye and adnexa
   ⑰ T26.82 Corrosions of other specified parts of left eye and adnexa
⑤ T26.9 Corrosion of eye and adnexa, part unspecified
   Code first (T51-T65) to identify chemical and intent
   Use additional external cause code to identify place (Y92)
   ⑰ T26.90 Corrosion of unspecified eye and adnexa, part unspecified
   ⑰ T26.91 Corrosion of right eye and adnexa, part unspecified
   ⑰ T26.92 Corrosion of left eye and adnexa, part unspecified
④ T27 Burn and corrosion of respiratory tract
   Use additional external cause code to identify the source and intent of the burn (X00-X19, X75-X77, X96-X98)
   external cause code to identify place (Y92)
   The appropriate 7th character is to be added to each code from category T27
   A = initial encounter
   D = subsequent encounter
   S = sequela
   ⑰ T27.0 Burn of larynx and trachea
⑰ T27.1 Burn involving larynx and trachea with lung
⑰ T27.2 Burn of other parts of respiratory tract
   Burn of thoracic cavity
⑰ T27.3 Burn of respiratory tract, part unspecified
   Code first (T51-T65) to identify chemical and intent for codes T27.4-T27.7
⑰ T27.4 Corrosion of larynx and trachea
⑰ T27.5 Corrosion involving larynx and trachea with lung
⑰ T27.6 Corrosion of other parts of respiratory tract
⑰ T27.7 Corrosion of respiratory tract, part unspecified
④ T28 Burn and corrosion of other internal organs
   Use additional external cause code to identify the source and intent of the burn (X00-X19, X75-X77, X96-X98)
   external cause code to identify place (Y92)
   The appropriate 7th character is to be added to each code from category T28
   A = initial encounter
   D = subsequent encounter
   S = sequela
   ⑰ T28.0 Burn of mouth and pharynx
   ⑰ T28.1 Burn of esophagus
   ⑰ T28.2 Burn of other parts of alimentary tract
   ⑰ T28.3 Burn of internal genitourinary organs
   ⑤ T28.4 Burns of other and unspecified internal organs
      ⑰ T28.40 Burn of unspecified internal organ
      ⑤ T28.41 Burn of ear drum
         ⑰ T28.411 Burn of right ear drum
         ⑰ T28.412 Burn of left ear drum
         ⑰ T28.419 Burn of unspecified ear drum
      ⑰ T28.49 Burn of other internal organ
         Code first (T51-T65) to identify chemical and intent for T28.5-T28.9-
   ⑰ T28.5 Corrosion of mouth and pharynx
   ⑰ T28.6 Corrosion of esophagus
   ⑰ T28.7 Corrosion of other parts of alimentary tract
   ⑰ T28.8 Corrosion of internal genitourinary organs
   ⑤ T28.9 Corrosions of other and unspecified internal organs
      ⑰ T28.90 Corrosions of unspecified internal organs
      ⑤ T28.91 Corrosions of ear drum
         ⑰ T28.911 Corrosions of right ear drum
         ⑰ T28.912 Corrosions of left ear drum
         ⑰ T28.919 Corrosions of unspecified ear drum
      ⑰ T28.99 Corrosions of other internal organs

Burns and corrosions of multiple and unspecified body regions (T30-T32)

④ T30 Burn and corrosion, body region unspecified
   T30.0 Burn of unspecified body region, unspecified degree
      This code is not for inpatient use. Code to specified site and degree of burns
      Burn NOS
      Multiple burns NOS
   T30.4 Corrosion of unspecified body region, unspecified degree
      This code is not for inpatient use. Code to specified site and degree of corrosion
      Corrosion NOS
      Multiple corrosion NOS

Unspecified Code	Other Specified Code	N Newborn Age: 0 P Pediatric Age: 0-17 M Maternity Age: 12-55
A Adult Age: 15-124 ♂ Male ♀ Female ● New Code ▲ Revised Code Title ►◄ Revised Text		

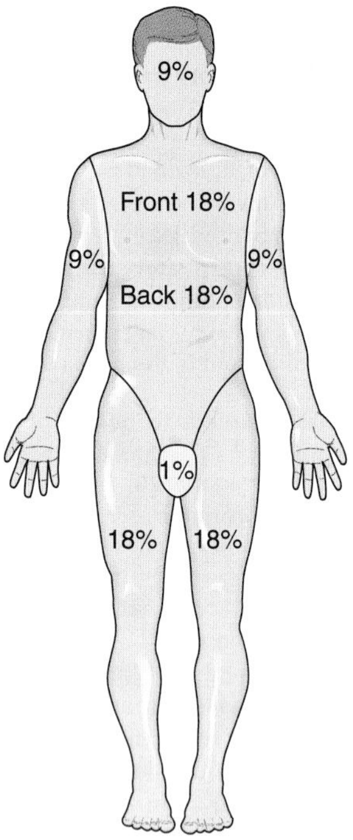

Figure 17.1 Rule of Nine: Percentage of burn areas

[4] **T31 Burns classified according to extent of body surface involved**

[NOTES] This category is to be used as the primary code only when the site of the burn is unspecified. It should be used as a supplementary code with categories T20-T25 when the site is specified.

T31.0 Burns involving less than 10% of body surface

[5] **T31.1 Burns involving 10-19% of body surface**

T31.10 Burns involving 10-19% of body surface with 0% to 9% third degree burns

Burns involving 10-19% of body surface NOS

T31.11 Burns involving 10-19% of body surface with 10-19% third degree burns

[5] **T31.2 Burns involving 20-29% of body surface**

T31.20 Burns involving 20-29% of body surface with 0% to 9% third degree burns

Burns involving 20-29% of body surface NOS

T31.21 Burns involving 20-29% of body surface with 10-19% third degree burns

T31.22 Burns involving 20-29% of body surface with 20-29% third degree burns

[5] **T31.3 Burns involving 30-39% of body surface**

T31.30 Burns involving 30-39% of body surface with 0% to 9% third degree burns

Burns involving 30-39% of body surface NOS

T31.31 Burns involving 30-39% of body surface with 10-19% third degree burns

T31.32 Burns involving 30-39% of body surface with 20-29% third degree burns

T31.33 Burns involving 30-39% of body surface with 30-39% third degree burns

[5] **T31.4 Burns involving 40-49% of body surface**

T31.40 Burns involving 40-49% of body surface with 0% to 9% third degree burns

Burns involving 40-49% of body surface NOS

T31.41 Burns involving 40-49% of body surface with 10-19% third degree burns

T31.42 Burns involving 40-49% of body surface with 20-29% third degree burns

T31.43 Burns involving 40-49% of body surface with 30-39% third degree burns

T31.44 Burns involving 40-49% of body surface with 40-49% third degree burns

[5] **T31.5 Burns involving 50-59% of body surface**

T31.50 Burns involving 50-59% of body surface with 0% to 9% third degree burns

Burns involving 50-59% of body surface NOS

T31.51 Burns involving 50-59% of body surface with 10-19% third degree burns

T31.52 Burns involving 50-59% of body surface with 20-29% third degree burns

T31.53 Burns involving 50-59% of body surface with 30-39% third degree burns

T31.54 Burns involving 50-59% of body surface with 40-49% third degree burns

T31.55 Burns involving 50-59% of body surface with 50-59% third degree burns

[5] **T31.6 Burns involving 60-69% of body surface**

T31.60 Burns involving 60-69% of body surface with 0% to 9% third degree burns

Burns involving 60-69% of body surface NOS

T31.61 Burns involving 60-69% of body surface with 10-19% third degree burns

T31.62 Burns involving 60-69% of body surface with 20-29% third degree burns

T31.63 Burns involving 60-69% of body surface with 30-39% third degree burns

T31.64 Burns involving 60-69% of body surface with 40-49% third degree burns

T31.65 Burns involving 60-69% of body surface with 50-59% third degree burns

T31.66 Burns involving 60-69% of body surface with 60-69% third degree burns

[5] **T31.7 Burns involving 70-79% of body surface**

T31.70 Burns involving 70-79% of body surface with 0% to 9% third degree burns

Burns involving 70-79% of body surface NOS

T31.71 Burns involving 70-79% of body surface with 10-19% third degree burns

T31.72 Burns involving 70-79% of body surface with 20-29% third degree burns

T31.73 Burns involving 70-79% of body surface with 30-39% third degree burns

T31.74 Burns involving 70-79% of body surface with 40-49% third degree burns

T31.75 Burns involving 70-79% of body surface with 50-59% third degree burns

T31.76 Burns involving 70-79% of body surface with 60-69% third degree burns

T31.77 Burns involving 70-79% of body surface with 70-79% third degree burns

[5] **T31.8 Burns involving 80-89% of body surface**

T31.80 Burns involving 80-89% of body surface with 0% to 9% third degree burns

Burns involving 80-89% of body surface NOS

T31.81 Burns involving 80-89% of body surface with 10-19% third degree burns

T31.82 Burns involving 80-89% of body surface with 20-29% third degree burns

T31.83 Burns involving 80-89% of body surface with 30-39% third degree burns

T31.84 Burns involving 80-89% of body surface with 40-49% third degree burns

T31.85 Burns involving 80-89% of body surface with 50-59% third degree burns

[4] 4th character required [5] 5th character required [6] 6th character required [7] 7th character required [7] Extension 'X' Alert
[EXCLUDES 1] Not coded here [EXCLUDES 2] Not included here [PDx] Primary Diagnosis Only Manifestation Code

T31.86 Burns involving 80-89% of body surface with 60-69% third degree **burns**

T31.87 Burns involving 80-89% of body surface with 70-79% third degree **burns**

T31.88 Burns involving 80-89% of body surface with 80-89% third degree **burns**

🔟 T31.9 Burns involving 90% or more of body surface

T31.90 Burns involving 90% or more of body surface with 0% to 9% third degree **burns**

Burns involving 90% or more of body surface NOS

T31.91 Burns involving 90% or more of body surface with 10-19% third degree **burns**

T31.92 Burns involving 90% or more of body surface with 20-29% third degree **burns**

T31.93 Burns involving 90% or more of body surface with 30-39% third degree **burns**

T31.94 Burns involving 90% or more of body surface with 40-49% third degree **burns**

T31.95 Burns involving 90% or more of body surface with 50-59% third degree **burns**

T31.96 Burns involving 90% or more of body surface with 60-69% third degree **burns**

T31.97 Burns involving 90% or more of body surface with 70-79% third degree **burns**

T31.98 Burns involving 90% or more of body surface with 80-89% third degree **burns**

T31.99 Burns involving 90% or more of body surface with 90% or more third degree burns

🔟 T32 Corrosions **classified** according to extent of body surface involved

NOTES This category is to be used as the primary code only when the site of the corrosion is unspecified. It may be used as a supplementary code with categories T20-T25 when the site is specified.

T32.0 Corrosions involving less than 10% of body surface

🔟 T32.1 Corrosions involving 10-19% of body surface

T32.10 Corrosions involving 10-19% of body surface with 0% to 9% third degree **corrosion**

Corrosions involving 10-19% of body surface NOS

T32.11 Corrosions involving 10-19% of body surface with 10-19% third degree **corrosion**

🔟 T32.2 Corrosions involving 20-29% of body surface

T32.20 Corrosions involving 20-29% of body surface with 0% to 9% third degree **corrosion**

T32.21 Corrosions involving 20-29% of body surface with 10-19% third degree **corrosion**

T32.22 Corrosions involving 20-29% of body surface with 20-29% third degree **corrosion**

🔟 T32.3 Corrosions involving 30-39% of body surface

T32.30 Corrosions involving 30-39% of body surface with 0% to 9% third degree **corrosion**

T32.31 Corrosions involving 30-39% of body surface with 10-19% third degree **corrosion**

T32.32 Corrosions involving 30-39% of body surface with 20-29% third degree **corrosion**

T32.33 Corrosions involving 30-39% of body surface with 30-39% third degree **corrosion**

🔟 T32.4 Corrosions involving 40-49% of body surface

T32.40 Corrosions involving 40-49% of body surface with 0% to 9% third degree **corrosion**

T32.41 Corrosions involving 40-49% of body surface with 10-19% third degree corrosion

T32.42 Corrosions involving 40-49% of body surface with 20-29% third degree **corrosion**

T32.43 Corrosions involving 40-49% of body surface with 30-39% third degree **corrosion**

T32.44 Corrosions involving 40-49% of body surface with 40-49% third degree **corrosion**

🔟 T32.5 Corrosions involving 50-59% of body surface

T32.50 Corrosions involving 50-59% of body surface with 0% to 9% third degree **corrosion**

T32.51 Corrosions involving 50-59% of body surface with 10-19% third degree **corrosion**

T32.52 Corrosions involving 50-59% of body surface with 20-29% third degree **corrosion**

T32.53 Corrosions involving 50-59% of body surface with 30-39% third degree **corrosion**

T32.54 Corrosions involving 50-59% of body surface with 40-49% third degree **corrosion**

T32.55 Corrosions involving 50-59% of body surface with 50-59% third degree **corrosion**

🔟 T32.6 Corrosions involving 60-69% of body surface

T32.60 Corrosions involving 60-69% of body surface with 0% to 9% third degree **corrosion**

T32.61 Corrosions involving 60-69% of body surface with 10-19% third degree **corrosion**

T32.62 Corrosions involving 60-69% of body surface with 20-29% third degree **corrosion**

T32.63 Corrosions involving 60-69% of body surface with 30-39% third degree **corrosion**

T32.64 Corrosions involving 60-69% of body surface with 40-49% third degree **corrosion**

T32.65 Corrosions involving 60-69% of body surface with 50-59% third degree **corrosion**

T32.66 Corrosions involving 60-69% of body surface with 60-69% third degree **corrosion**

🔟 T32.7 Corrosions involving 70-79% of body surface

T32.70 Corrosions involving 70-79% of body surface with 0% to 9% third degree **corrosion**

T32.71 Corrosions involving 70-79% of body surface with 10-19% third degree **corrosion**

T32.72 Corrosions involving 70-79% of body surface with 20-29% third degree **corrosion**

T32.73 Corrosions involving 70-79% of body surface with 30-39% third degree **corrosion**

T32.74 Corrosions involving 70-79% of body surface with 40-49% third degree **corrosion**

T32.75 Corrosions involving 70-79% of body surface with 50-59% third degree **corrosion**

T32.76 Corrosions involving 70-79% of body surface with 60-69% third degree **corrosion**

T32.77 Corrosions involving 70-79% of body surface with 70-79% third degree **corrosion**

🔟 T32.8 Corrosions involving 80-89% of body surface

T32.80 Corrosions involving 80-89% of body surface with 0% to 9% third degree **corrosion**

T32.81 Corrosions involving 80-89% of body surface with 10-19% third degree **corrosion**

T32.82 Corrosions involving 80-89% of body surface with 20-29% third degree **corrosion**

T32.83 Corrosions involving 80-89% of body surface with 30-39% third degree **corrosion**

T32.84 Corrosions involving 80-89% of body surface with 40-49% third degree **corrosion**

T32.85 Corrosions involving 80-89% of body surface with 50-59% third degree **corrosion**

T32.86 Corrosions involving 80-89% of body surface with 60-69% third degree **corrosion**

T32.87 Corrosions involving 80-89% of body surface with 70-79% third degree **corrosion**

T32.88 Corrosions involving 80-89% of body surface with 80-89% third degree **corrosion**

🔟 T32.9 Corrosions involving 90% or more of body surface

T32.90 Corrosions involving 90% or more of body surface with 0% to 9% third degree **corrosion**

T32.91 Corrosions involving 90% or more of body surface with 10-19% third degree **corrosion**

T32.92 Corrosions involving 90% or more of body surface with 20-29% third degree corrosion

T32.93 Corrosions involving 90% or more of body surface with 30-39% third degree corrosion

T32.94 Corrosions involving 90% or more of body surface with 40-49% third degree corrosion

T32.95 Corrosions involving 90% or more of body surface with 50-59% third degree corrosion

T32.96 Corrosions involving 90% or more of body surface with 60-69% third degree corrosion

T32.97 Corrosions involving 90% or more of body surface with 70-79% third degree corrosion

T32.98 Corrosions involving 90% or more of body surface with 80-89% third degree corrosion

T32.99 Corrosions involving 90% or more of body surface with 90% or more third degree corrosion

Frostbite (T33-T34)

 EXCLUDES2 *hypothermia and other effects of reduced temperature (T68, T69.-)*

T33 Superficial frostbite

 INCLUDES *frostbite with partial thickness skin loss*

 The appropriate 7th character is to be added to each code from category T33
 A = initial encounter
 D = subsequent encounter
 S = sequela

T33.0 Superficial frostbite of head

 T33.01 Superficial frostbite of ear

  T33.011 Superficial frostbite of right ear

  T33.012 Superficial frostbite of left ear

  T33.019 Superficial frostbite of unspecified ear

 T33.02 Superficial frostbite of nose

 T33.09 Superficial frostbite of other part of head

T33.1 Superficial frostbite of neck

T33.2 Superficial frostbite of thorax

T33.3 Superficial frostbite of abdominal wall, lower back and pelvis

T33.4 Superficial frostbite of arm

 EXCLUDES2 *superficial frostbite of wrist and hand (T33.5-)*

 T33.40 Superficial frostbite of unspecified arm

 T33.41 Superficial frostbite of right arm

 T33.42 Superficial frostbite of left arm

T33.5 Superficial frostbite of wrist, hand, and fingers

 T33.51 Superficial frostbite of wrist

  T33.511 Superficial frostbite of right wrist

  T33.512 Superficial frostbite of left wrist

  T33.519 Superficial frostbite of unspecified wrist

 T33.52 Superficial frostbite of hand

  EXCLUDES2 *superficial frostbite of fingers (T33.53-)*

  T33.521 Superficial frostbite of right hand

  T33.522 Superficial frostbite of left hand

  T33.529 Superficial frostbite of unspecified hand

 T33.53 Superficial frostbite of finger(s)

  T33.531 Superficial frostbite of right finger(s)

  T33.532 Superficial frostbite of left finger(s)

  T33.539 Superficial frostbite of unspecified finger(s)

T33.6 Superficial frostbite of hip and thigh

 T33.60 Superficial frostbite of unspecified hip and thigh

 T33.61 Superficial frostbite of right hip and thigh

 T33.62 Superficial frostbite of left hip and thigh

T33.7 Superficial frostbite of knee and lower leg

 EXCLUDES2 *superficial frostbite of ankle and foot (T33.8-)*

 T33.70 Superficial frostbite of unspecified knee and lower leg

 T33.71 Superficial frostbite of right knee and lower leg

 T33.72 Superficial frostbite of left knee and lower leg

T33.8 Superficial frostbite of ankle, foot, and toe(s)

 T33.81 Superficial frostbite of ankle

  T33.811 Superficial frostbite of right ankle

  T33.812 Superficial frostbite of left ankle

  T33.819 Superficial frostbite of unspecified ankle

 T33.82 Superficial frostbite of foot

  T33.821 Superficial frostbite of right foot

  T33.822 Superficial frostbite of left foot

  T33.829 Superficial frostbite of unspecified foot

 T33.83 Superficial frostbite of toe(s)

  T33.831 Superficial frostbite of right toe(s)

  T33.832 Superficial frostbite of left toe(s)

  T33.839 Superficial frostbite of unspecified toe(s)

T33.9 Superficial frostbite of other and unspecified sites

 T33.90 **Superficial frostbite of unspecified sites**

  Superficial frostbite NOS

 T33.99 **Superficial frostbite of other sites**

  Superficial frostbite of leg NOS
  Superficial frostbite of trunk NOS

T34 Frostbite with tissue necrosis

 The appropriate 7th character is to be added to each code from category T34
 A = initial encounter
 D = subsequent encounter
 S = sequela

T34.0 Frostbite with tissue necrosis of head

 T34.01 Frostbite with tissue necrosis of ear

  T34.011 Frostbite with tissue necrosis of right ear

  T34.012 Frostbite with tissue necrosis of left ear

  T34.019 **Frostbite with tissue necrosis of unspecified ear**

 T34.02 Frostbite with tissue necrosis of nose

 T34.09 **Frostbite with tissue necrosis of other part of head**

T34.1 Frostbite with tissue necrosis of neck

T34.2 Frostbite with tissue necrosis of thorax

T34.3 Frostbite with tissue necrosis of abdominal wall, lower back and pelvis

T34.4 Frostbite with tissue necrosis of arm

 EXCLUDES2 *frostbite with tissue necrosis of wrist and hand (T34.5-)*

 T34.40 Frostbite with tissue necrosis of unspecified arm

 T34.41 Frostbite with tissue necrosis of right arm

 T34.42 Frostbite with tissue necrosis of left arm

T34.5 Frostbite with tissue necrosis of wrist, hand, and finger(s)

 T34.51 Frostbite with tissue necrosis of wrist

  T34.511 Frostbite with tissue necrosis of right wrist

  T34.512 Frostbite with tissue necrosis of left wrist

  T34.519 **Frostbite with tissue necrosis of unspecified wrist**

 T34.52 Frostbite with tissue necrosis of hand

  EXCLUDES2 *frostbite with tissue necrosis of finger(s) (T34.53-)*

  T34.521 Frostbite with tissue necrosis of right hand

  T34.522 Frostbite with tissue necrosis of left hand

  T34.529 **Frostbite with tissue necrosis of unspecified hand**

 T34.53 Frostbite with tissue necrosis of finger(s)

  T34.531 Frostbite with tissue necrosis of right finger(s)

  T34.532 Frostbite with tissue necrosis of left finger(s)

  T34.539 **Frostbite with tissue necrosis of unspecified finger(s)**

T34.6 Frostbite with tissue necrosis of hip and thigh

 T34.60 **Frostbite with tissue necrosis of unspecified hip and thigh**

---

 4 4th character required **5** 5th character required **6** 6th character required **7** 7th character required **⑦** Extension 'X' Alert

 EXCLUDES 1 Not coded here **EXCLUDES 2** Not included here PDx Primary Diagnosis Only Manifestation Code

[7th] T34.61 Frostbite with tissue necrosis of right hip and thigh
[7th] T34.62 Frostbite with tissue necrosis of left hip and thigh
[5th] T34.7 Frostbite with tissue necrosis of knee and lower leg
EXCLUDES2 *frostbite with tissue necrosis of ankle and foot (T34.8-)*
[7th] T34.70 Frostbite with tissue necrosis of unspecified knee and lower leg
[7th] T34.71 Frostbite with tissue necrosis of right knee and lower leg
[7th] T34.72 Frostbite with tissue necrosis of left knee and lower leg
[5th] T34.8 Frostbite with tissue necrosis of ankle, foot, and toe(s)
[6th] T34.81 Frostbite with tissue necrosis of ankle
[7th] T34.811 Frostbite with tissue necrosis of right ankle
[7th] T34.812 Frostbite with tissue necrosis of left ankle
[7th] T34.819 Frostbite with tissue necrosis of unspecified ankle
[6th] T34.82 Frostbite with tissue necrosis of foot
[7th] T34.821 Frostbite with tissue necrosis of right foot
[7th] T34.822 Frostbite with tissue necrosis of left foot
[7th] T34.829 Frostbite with tissue necrosis of unspecified foot
[6th] T34.83 Frostbite with tissue necrosis of toe(s)
[7th] T34.831 Frostbite with tissue necrosis of right toe(s)
[7th] T34.832 Frostbite with tissue necrosis of left toe(s)
[7th] T34.839 Frostbite with tissue necrosis of unspecified toe(s)
[5th] T34.9 Frostbite with tissue necrosis of other and unspecified sites
[7th] T34.90 Frostbite with tissue necrosis of unspecified sites
Frostbite with tissue necrosis NOS
[7th] T34.99 Frostbite with tissue necrosis of other sites
Frostbite with tissue necrosis of leg NOS
Frostbite with tissue necrosis of trunk NOS

Poisoning by, adverse effects of and underdosing of drugs, medicaments and biological substances (T36-T50)

Code first, for adverse effects, the nature of the adverse effect, such as:
adverse effect NOS (T88.7)
aspirin gastritis (K29.-)
blood disorders (D56-D76)
contact dermatitis (L23-L25)
dermatitis due to substances taken internally (L27.-)
nephropathy (N14.0-N14.2)

INCLUDES *adverse effect of correct substance properly administered*
poisoning by overdose of substance
poisoning by wrong substance given or taken in error
underdosing by (inadvertently) (deliberately) taking less substance than prescribed or instructed

NOTES The drug giving rise to the adverse effect should be identified by use of codes from categories T36-T50 with fifth or sixth character 5.

Use additional code(s) to specify:
manifestations of poisoning
underdosing or failure in dosage during medical and surgical care (Y63.6, Y63.8-Y63.9)
underdosing of medication regimen (Z91.12-, Z91.13-)

EXCLUDES1 *toxic reaction to local anesthesia in pregnancy (O29.3-)*

EXCLUDES2 *abuse and dependence of psychoactive substances (F10-F19)*
abuse of non-dependence-producing substances (F55.-)
drug reaction and poisoning affecting newborn (P00-P96)
pathological drug intoxication (inebriation) (F10-F19)

[4th] T36 Poisoning by, adverse effect of and underdosing of systemic antibiotics
EXCLUDES1 *antineoplastic antibiotics (T45.1-)*
locally applied antibiotic NEC (T49.0)
topically used antibiotic for ear, nose and throat (T49.6)
topically used antibiotic for eye (T49.5)

The appropriate 7th character is to be added to each code from category T36
A = initial encounter
D = subsequent encounter
S = sequela

[5th] T36.0 Poisoning by, adverse effect of and underdosing of penicillins
[6th] T36.0X Poisoning by, adverse effect of and underdosing of penicillins
[7th] T36.0X1 Poisoning by penicillins, accidental (unintentional)
Poisoning by penicillins NOS
[7th] T36.0X2 Poisoning by penicillins, intentional self-harm
[7th] T36.0X3 Poisoning by penicillins, assault
[7th] T36.0X4 Poisoning by penicillins, undetermined
[7th] T36.0X5 Adverse effect of penicillins
[7th] T36.0X6 Underdosing of penicillins
[5th] T36.1 Poisoning by, adverse effect of and underdosing of cephalosporins and other beta-lactam antibiotics
[6th] T36.1X Poisoning by, adverse effect of and underdosing of cephalosporins and other beta-lactam antibiotics
[7th] T36.1X1 Poisoning by cephalosporins and other beta-lactam antibiotics, accidental (unintentional)
Poisoning by cephalosporins and other beta-lactam antibiotics NOS
[7th] T36.1X2 Poisoning by cephalosporins and other beta-lactam antibiotics, intentional self-harm
[7th] T36.1X3 Poisoning by cephalosporins and other beta-lactam antibiotics, assault
[7th] T36.1X4 Poisoning by cephalosporins and other beta-lactam antibiotics, undetermined
[7th] T36.1X5 Adverse effect of cephalosporins and other beta-lactam antibiotics
[7th] T36.1X6 Underdosing of cephalosporins and other beta-lactam antibiotics
[5th] T36.2 Poisoning by, adverse effect of and underdosing of chloramphenicol group
[6th] T36.2X Poisoning by, adverse effect of and underdosing of chloramphenicol group
[7th] T36.2X1 Poisoning by chloramphenicol group, accidental (unintentional)
Poisoning by chloramphenicol group NOS
[7th] T36.2X2 Poisoning by chloramphenicol group, intentional self-harm
[7th] T36.2X3 Poisoning by chloramphenicol group, assault
[7th] T36.2X4 Poisoning by chloramphenicol group, undetermined
[7th] T36.2X5 Adverse effect of chloramphenicol group
[7th] T36.2X6 Underdosing of chloramphenicol group
[5th] T36.3 Poisoning by, adverse effect of and underdosing of macrolides
[6th] T36.3X Poisoning by, adverse effect of and underdosing of macrolides
[7th] T36.3X1 Poisoning by macrolides, accidental (unintentional)
Poisoning by macrolides NOS

T36.3X2 Poisoning by macrolides, intentional self-harm

T36.3X3 Poisoning by macrolides, assault

T36.3X4 Poisoning by macrolides, undetermined

T36.3X5 Adverse effect of macrolides

T36.3X6 Underdosing of macrolides

T36.4 Poisoning by, adverse effect of and underdosing of tetracyclines

T36.4X Poisoning by, adverse effect of and underdosing of tetracyclines

T36.4X1 Poisoning by tetracyclines, accidental (unintentional)

Poisoning by tetracyclines NOS

T36.4X2 Poisoning by tetracyclines, intentional self-harm

T36.4X3 Poisoning by tetracyclines, assault

T36.4X4 Poisoning by tetracyclines, undetermined

T36.4X5 Adverse effect of tetracyclines

T36.4X6 Underdosing of tetracyclines

T36.5 Poisoning by, adverse effect of and underdosing of aminoglycosides

Poisoning by, adverse effect of and underdosing of streptomycin

T36.5X Poisoning by, adverse effect of and underdosing of aminoglycosides

T36.5X1 Poisoning by aminoglycosides, accidental (unintentional)

Poisoning by aminoglycosides NOS

T36.5X2 Poisoning by aminoglycosides, intentional self-harm

T36.5X3 Poisoning by aminoglycosides, assault

T36.5X4 Poisoning by aminoglycosides, undetermined

T36.5X5 Adverse effect of aminoglycosides

T36.5X6 Underdosing of aminoglycosides

T36.6 Poisoning by, adverse effect of and underdosing of rifampicins

T36.6X Poisoning by, adverse effect of and underdosing of rifampicins

T36.6X1 Poisoning by rifampicins, accidental (unintentional)

Poisoning by rifampicins NOS

T36.6X2 Poisoning by rifampicins, intentional self-harm

T36.6X3 Poisoning by rifampicins, assault

T36.6X4 Poisoning by rifampicins, undetermined

T36.6X5 Adverse effect of rifampicins

T36.6X6 Underdosing of rifampicins

T36.7 Poisoning by, adverse effect of and underdosing of antifungal antibiotics, systemically used

T36.7X Poisoning by, adverse effect of and underdosing of antifungal antibiotics, systemically used

T36.7X1 Poisoning by antifungal antibiotics, systemically used, accidental (unintentional)

Poisoning by antifungal antibiotics, systemically used NOS

T36.7X2 Poisoning by antifungal antibiotics, systemically used, intentional self-harm

T36.7X3 Poisoning by antifungal antibiotics, systemically used, assault

T36.7X4 Poisoning by antifungal antibiotics, systemically used, undetermined

T36.7X5 Adverse effect of antifungal antibiotics, systemically used

T36.7X6 Underdosing of antifungal antibiotics, systemically used

T36.8 Poisoning by, adverse effect of and underdosing of other systemic antibiotics

T36.8X Poisoning by, adverse effect of and underdosing of other systemic antibiotics

T36.8X1 Poisoning by other systemic antibiotics, accidental (unintentional)

Poisoning by other systemic antibiotics NOS

T36.8X2 Poisoning by other systemic antibiotics, intentional self-harm

T36.8X3 Poisoning by other systemic antibiotics, assault

T36.8X4 Poisoning by other systemic antibiotics, undetermined

T36.8X5 Adverse effect of other systemic antibiotics

T36.8X6 Underdosing of other systemic antibiotics

T36.9 Poisoning by, adverse effect of and underdosing of unspecified systemic antibiotic

T36.91 Poisoning by unspecified systemic antibiotic, accidental (unintentional)

Poisoning by systemic antibiotic NOS

T36.92 Poisoning by unspecified systemic antibiotic, intentional self-harm

T36.93 Poisoning by unspecified systemic antibiotic, assault

T36.94 Poisoning by unspecified systemic antibiotic, undetermined

T36.95 Adverse effect of unspecified systemic antibiotic

T36.96 Underdosing of unspecified systemic antibiotic

T37 Poisoning by, adverse effect of and underdosing of other systemic anti- infectives and antiparasitics

EXCLUDES1 anti-infectives topically used for ear, nose and throat (T49.6-)
anti-infectives topically used for eye (T49.5-)
locally applied anti-infectives NEC (T49.0-)

The appropriate 7th character is to be added to each code from category T37

A = initial encounter

D = subsequent encounter

S = sequela

T37.0 Poisoning by, adverse effect of and underdosing of sulfonamides

T37.0X Poisoning by, adverse effect of and underdosing of sulfonamides

T37.0X1 Poisoning by sulfonamides, accidental (unintentional)

Poisoning by sulfonamides NOS

T37.0X2 Poisoning by sulfonamides, intentional self-harm

T37.0X3 Poisoning by sulfonamides, assault

T37.0X4 Poisoning by sulfonamides, undetermined

T37.0X5 Adverse effect of sulfonamides

T37.0X6 Underdosing of sulfonamides

T37.1 Poisoning by, adverse effect of and underdosing of antimycobacterial drugs

EXCLUDES1 rifampicins (T36.6-)
streptomycin (T36.5-)

T37.1X Poisoning by, adverse effect of and underdosing of antimycobacterial drugs

T37.1X1 Poisoning by antimycobacterial drugs, accidental (unintentional)

Poisoning by antimycobacterial drugs NOS

T37.1X2 Poisoning by antimycobacterial drugs, intentional self-harm

T37.1X3 Poisoning by antimycobacterial drugs, assault

T37.1X4 Poisoning by antimycobacterial drugs, undetermined

T37.1X5 Adverse effect of antimycobacterial drugs

T37.1X6 Underdosing of antimycobacterial drugs

| 4th character required | 5th character required | 6th character required | 7th character required | Extension 'X' Alert |

EXCLUDES 1 Not coded here   EXCLUDES 2 Not included here   PDx Primary Diagnosis Only   Manifestation Code

Ⓢ T37.2 Poisoning by, adverse effect of and underdosing of antimalarials and drugs acting on other blood protozoa

EXCLUDES1 *hydroxyquinoline derivatives (T37.8-)*

Ⓖ T37.2X Poisoning by, adverse effect of and underdosing of antimalarials and drugs acting on other blood protozoa

Ⓣ T37.2X1 Poisoning by antimalarials and drugs acting on other blood protozoa, accidental (unintentional)

Poisoning by antimalarials and drugs acting on other blood protozoa NOS

Ⓣ T37.2X2 Poisoning by antimalarials and drugs acting on other blood protozoa, intentional self-harm

Ⓣ T37.2X3 Poisoning by antimalarials and drugs acting on other blood protozoa, assault

Ⓣ T37.2X4 Poisoning by antimalarials and drugs acting on other blood protozoa, undetermined

Ⓣ T37.2X5 Adverse effect of antimalarials and drugs acting on other blood protozoa

Ⓣ T37.2X6 Underdosing of antimalarials and drugs acting on other blood protozoa

Ⓢ T37.3 Poisoning by, adverse effect of and underdosing of other antiprotozoal drugs

Ⓖ T37.3X Poisoning by, adverse effect of and underdosing of other antiprotozoal drugs

Ⓣ T37.3X1 Poisoning by other antiprotozoal drugs, accidental (unintentional)

Poisoning by other antiprotozoal drugs NOS

Ⓣ T37.3X2 Poisoning by other antiprotozoal drugs, intentional self-harm

Ⓣ T37.3X3 Poisoning by other antiprotozoal drugs, assault

Ⓣ T37.3X4 Poisoning by other antiprotozoal drugs, undetermined

Ⓣ T37.3X5 Adverse effect of other antiprotozoal drugs

Ⓣ T37.3X6 Underdosing of other antiprotozoal drugs

Ⓢ T37.4 Poisoning by, adverse effect of and underdosing of anthelminthics

Ⓖ T37.4X Poisoning by, adverse effect of and underdosing of anthelminthics

Ⓣ T37.4X1 Poisoning by anthelminthics, accidental (unintentional)

Poisoning by anthelminthics NOS

Ⓣ T37.4X2 Poisoning by anthelminthics, intentional self-harm

Ⓣ T37.4X3 Poisoning by anthelminthics, assault

Ⓣ T37.4X4 Poisoning by anthelminthics, undetermined

Ⓣ T37.4X5 Adverse effect of anthelminthics

Ⓣ T37.4X6 Underdosing of anthelminthics

Ⓢ T37.5 Poisoning by, adverse effect of and underdosing of antiviral drugs

EXCLUDES1 *amantadine (T42.8-)*
cytarabine (T45.1-)

Ⓖ T37.5X Poisoning by, adverse effect of and underdosing of antiviral drugs

Ⓣ T37.5X1 Poisoning by antiviral drugs, accidental (unintentional)

Poisoning by antiviral drugs NOS

Ⓣ T37.5X2 Poisoning by antiviral drugs, intentional self-harm

Ⓣ T37.5X3 Poisoning by antiviral drugs, assault

Ⓣ T37.5X4 Poisoning by antiviral drugs, undetermined

Ⓣ T37.5X5 Adverse effect of antiviral drugs

Ⓣ T37.5X6 Underdosing of antiviral drugs

Ⓢ T37.8 Poisoning by, adverse effect of and underdosing of other specified systemic anti-infectives and antiparasitics

Poisoning by, adverse effect of and underdosing of hydroxyquinoline derivatives

EXCLUDES1 *antimalarial drugs (T37.2-)*

Ⓖ T37.8X Poisoning by, adverse effect of and underdosing of other specified systemic anti-infectives and antiparasitics

Ⓣ T37.8X1 Poisoning by other specified systemic anti-infectives and antiparasitics, accidental (unintentional)

Poisoning by other specified systemic anti-infectives and antiparasitics NOS

Ⓣ T37.8X2 Poisoning by other specified systemic anti-infectives and antiparasitics, intentional self-harm

Ⓣ T37.8X3 Poisoning by other specified systemic anti-infectives and antiparasitics, assault

Ⓣ T37.8X4 Poisoning by other specified systemic anti-infectives and antiparasitics, undetermined

Ⓣ T37.8X5 Adverse effect of other specified systemic anti-infectives and antiparasitics

Ⓣ T37.8X6 Underdosing of other specified systemic anti-infectives and antiparasitics

Ⓢ T37.9 Poisoning by, adverse effect of and underdosing of unspecified systemic anti-infective and antiparasitics

Ⓣ T37.91 Poisoning by unspecified systemic anti-infective and antiparasitics, accidental (unintentional)

Poisoning by, adverse effect of and underdosing of systemic anti-infective and antiparasitics NOS

Ⓣ T37.92 Poisoning by unspecified systemic anti-infective and antiparasitics, intentional self-harm

Ⓣ T37.93 Poisoning by unspecified systemic anti-infective and antiparasitics, assault

Ⓣ T37.94 Poisoning by unspecified systemic anti-infective and antiparasitics, undetermined

Ⓣ T37.95 Adverse effect of unspecified systemic anti-infective and antiparasitic

Ⓣ T37.96 Underdosing of unspecified systemic anti-infectives and antiparasitics

Ⓒ T38 Poisoning by, adverse effect of and underdosing of hormones and their synthetic substitutes and antagonists, not elsewhere classified

EXCLUDES1 *mineralocorticoids and their antagonists (T50.0-)*
oxytocic hormones (T48.0-)
parathyroid hormones and derivatives (T50.9-)

The appropriate 7th character is to be added to each code from category T38
A = initial encounter
D = subsequent encounter
S = sequela

Ⓢ T38.0 Poisoning by, adverse effect of and underdosing of glucocorticoids and synthetic analogues

EXCLUDES1 *glucocorticoids, topically used (T49.-)*

Ⓖ T38.0X Poisoning by, adverse effect of and underdosing of glucocorticoids and synthetic analogues

Ⓣ T38.0X1 Poisoning by glucocorticoids and synthetic analogues, accidental (unintentional)

Poisoning by glucocorticoids and synthetic analogues NOS

Ⓣ T38.0X2 Poisoning by glucocorticoids and synthetic analogues, intentional self-harm

Ⓣ T38.0X3 Poisoning by glucocorticoids and synthetic analogues, assault

Ⓣ T38.0X4 Poisoning by glucocorticoids and synthetic analogues, undetermined

Ⓣ T38.0X5 Adverse effect of glucocorticoids and synthetic analogues

Unspecified Code	Other Specified Code	Ⓝ Newborn Age: 0	Ⓟ Pediatric Age: 0-17	Ⓜ Maternity Age: 12-55
Ⓐ Adult Age: 15-124	♂ Male	♀ Female	● New Code	▲ Revised Code Title	►◄ Revised Text

CHAPTER 19: INJURY, POISONING, AND CERTAIN OTHER CONSEQUENCES OF EXTERNAL CAUSES (S00-T88)

T38.0X6 - T38.7X6

🗙 T38.0X6 Underdosing of glucocorticoids and synthetic analogues

5ᵗʰ T38.1 Poisoning by, adverse effect of and underdosing of thyroid hormones and substitutes

6ᵗʰ T38.1X Poisoning by, adverse effect of and underdosing of thyroid hormones and substitutes

🗙 T38.1X1 Poisoning by thyroid hormones and substitutes, accidental (unintentional)

Poisoning by thyroid hormones and substitutes NOS

🗙 T38.1X2 Poisoning by thyroid hormones and substitutes, intentional self-harm

🗙 T38.1X3 Poisoning by thyroid hormones and substitutes, assault

🗙 T38.1X4 Poisoning by thyroid hormones and substitutes, undetermined

🗙 T38.1X5 Adverse effect of thyroid hormones and substitutes

🗙 T38.1X6 Underdosing of thyroid hormones and substitutes

5ᵗʰ T38.2 Poisoning by, adverse effect of and underdosing of antithyroid drugs

6ᵗʰ T38.2X Poisoning by, adverse effect of and underdosing of antithyroid drugs

🗙 T38.2X1 Poisoning by antithyroid drugs, accidental (unintentional)

Poisoning by antithyroid drugs NOS

🗙 T38.2X2 Poisoning by antithyroid drugs, intentional self-harm

🗙 T38.2X3 Poisoning by antithyroid drugs, assault

🗙 T38.2X4 Poisoning by antithyroid drugs, undetermined

🗙 T38.2X5 Adverse effect of antithyroid drugs

🗙 T38.2X6 Underdosing of antithyroid drugs

5ᵗʰ T38.3 Poisoning by, adverse effect of and underdosing of insulin and oral hypoglycemic [antidiabetic] drugs

6ᵗʰ T38.3X Poisoning by, adverse effect of and underdosing of insulin and oral hypoglycemic [antidiabetic] drugs

🗙 T38.3X1 Poisoning by insulin and oral hypoglycemic [antidiabetic] drugs, accidental (unintentional)

Poisoning by insulin and oral hypoglycemic [antidiabetic] drugs NOS

🗙 T38.3X2 Poisoning by insulin and oral hypoglycemic [antidiabetic] drugs, intentional self-harm

🗙 T38.3X3 Poisoning by insulin and oral hypoglycemic [antidiabetic] drugs, assault

🗙 T38.3X4 Poisoning by insulin and oral hypoglycemic [antidiabetic] drugs, undetermined

🗙 T38.3X5 Adverse effect of insulin and oral hypoglycemic [antidiabetic] drugs

🗙 T38.3X6 Underdosing of insulin and oral hypoglycemic [antidiabetic] drugs

5ᵗʰ T38.4 Poisoning by, adverse effect of and underdosing of oral contraceptives

Poisoning by, adverse effect of and underdosing of multiple- and single-ingredient oral contraceptive preparations

6ᵗʰ T38.4X Poisoning by, adverse effect of and underdosing of oral contraceptives

🗙 T38.4X1 Poisoning by oral contraceptives, accidental (unintentional)

Poisoning by oral contraceptives NOS

🗙 T38.4X2 Poisoning by oral contraceptives, intentional self-harm

🗙 T38.4X3 Poisoning by oral contraceptives, assault

🗙 T38.4X4 Poisoning by oral contraceptives, undetermined

🗙 T38.4X5 Adverse effect of oral contraceptives

🗙 T38.4X6 Underdosing of oral contraceptives

5ᵗʰ T38.5 Poisoning by, adverse effect of and underdosing of other estrogens and progestogens

Poisoning by, adverse effect of and underdosing of estrogens and progestogens mixtures and substitutes

6ᵗʰ T38.5X Poisoning by, adverse effect of and underdosing of other estrogens and progestogens

🗙 T38.5X1 Poisoning by other estrogens and progestogens, accidental (unintentional)

Poisoning by other estrogens and progestogens NOS

🗙 T38.5X2 Poisoning by other estrogens and progestogens, intentional self-harm

🗙 T38.5X3 Poisoning by other estrogens and progestogens, assault

🗙 T38.5X4 Poisoning by other estrogens and progestogens, undetermined

🗙 T38.5X5 Adverse effect of other estrogens and progestogens

🗙 T38.5X6 Underdosing of other estrogens and progestogens

5ᵗʰ T38.6 Poisoning by, adverse effect of and underdosing of antigonadotrophins, antiestrogens, antiandrogens, not elsewhere classified

Poisoning by, adverse effect of and underdosing of tamoxifen

6ᵗʰ T38.6X Poisoning by, adverse effect of and underdosing of antigonadotrophins, antiestrogens, antiandrogens, not elsewhere classified

🗙 T38.6X1 Poisoning by antigonadotrophins, antiestrogens, antiandrogens, not elsewhere classified, accidental (unintentional)

Poisoning by antigonadotrophins, antiestrogens, antiandrogens, not elsewhere classified NOS

🗙 T38.6X2 Poisoning by antigonadotrophins, antiestrogens, antiandrogens, not elsewhere classified, intentional self-harm

🗙 T38.6X3 Poisoning by antigonadotrophins, antiestrogens, antiandrogens, not elsewhere classified, assault

🗙 T38.6X4 Poisoning by antigonadotrophins, antiestrogens, antiandrogens, not elsewhere classified, undetermined

🗙 T38.6X5 Adverse effect of antigonadotrophins, antiestrogens, antiandrogens, not elsewhere classified

🗙 T38.6X6 Underdosing of antigonadotrophins, antiestrogens, antiandrogens, not elsewhere classified

5ᵗʰ T38.7 Poisoning by, adverse effect of and underdosing of androgens and anabolic congeners

6ᵗʰ T38.7X Poisoning by, adverse effect of and underdosing of androgens and anabolic congeners

🗙 T38.7X1 Poisoning by androgens and anabolic congeners, accidental (unintentional)

Poisoning by androgens and anabolic congeners NOS

🗙 T38.7X2 Poisoning by androgens and anabolic congeners, intentional self-harm

🗙 T38.7X3 Poisoning by androgens and anabolic congeners, assault

🗙 T38.7X4 Poisoning by androgens and anabolic congeners, undetermined

🗙 T38.7X5 Adverse effect of androgens and anabolic congeners

🗙 T38.7X6 Underdosing of androgens and anabolic congeners

4ᵗʰ 4ᵗʰ character required	5ᵗʰ 5ᵗʰ character required	6ᵗʰ 6ᵗʰ character required	7ᵗʰ 7ᵗʰ character required	🗙 Extension 'X' Alert
EXCLUDES 1 Not coded here	**EXCLUDES 2** Not included here	PDx Primary Diagnosis Only	Manifestation Code	

[5th] T38.8 Poisoning by, adverse effect of and underdosing of other and unspecified hormones and synthetic substitutes
 [6th] T38.80 Poisoning by, adverse effect of and underdosing of unspecified hormones and synthetic substitutes
  [7th] T38.801 Poisoning by unspecified hormones and synthetic substitutes, accidental (unintentional)
   Poisoning by unspecified hormones and synthetic substitutes NOS
  [7th] T38.802 Poisoning by unspecified hormones and synthetic substitutes, intentional self-harm
  [7th] T38.803 Poisoning by unspecified hormones and synthetic substitutes, assault
  [7th] T38.804 Poisoning by unspecified hormones and synthetic substitutes, undetermined
  [7th] T38.805 Adverse effect of unspecified hormones and synthetic substitutes
  [7th] T38.806 Underdosing of unspecified hormones and synthetic substitutes
 [6th] T38.81 Poisoning by, adverse effect of and underdosing of anterior pituitary [adenohypophyseal] hormones
  [7th] T38.811 Poisoning by anterior pituitary [adenohypophyseal] hormones, accidental (unintentional)
   Poisoning by anterior pituitary [adenohypophyseal] hormones NOS
  [7th] T38.812 Poisoning by anterior pituitary [adenohypophyseal] hormones, intentional self-harm
  [7th] T38.813 Poisoning by anterior pituitary [adenohypophyseal] hormones, assault
  [7th] T38.814 Poisoning by anterior pituitary [adenohypophyseal] hormones, undetermined
  [7th] T38.815 Adverse effect of anterior pituitary [adenohypophyseal] hormones
  [7th] T38.816 Underdosing of anterior pituitary [adenohypophyseal] hormones
 [6th] T38.89 Poisoning by, adverse effect of and underdosing of other hormones and synthetic substitutes
  [7th] T38.891 Poisoning by other hormones and synthetic substitutes, accidental (unintentional)
   Poisoning by other hormones and synthetic substitutes NOS
  [7th] T38.892 Poisoning by other hormones and synthetic substitutes, intentional self-harm
  [7th] T38.893 Poisoning by other hormones and synthetic substitutes, assault
  [7th] T38.894 Poisoning by other hormones and synthetic substitutes, undetermined
  [7th] T38.895 Adverse effect of other hormones and synthetic substitutes
  [7th] T38.896 Underdosing of other hormones and synthetic substitutes
[5th] T38.9 Poisoning by, adverse effect of and underdosing of other and unspecified hormone antagonists
 [6th] T38.90 Poisoning by, adverse effect of and underdosing of unspecified hormone antagonists
  [7th] T38.901 Poisoning by unspecified hormone antagonists, accidental (unintentional)
   Poisoning by unspecified hormone antagonists NOS
  [7th] T38.902 Poisoning by unspecified hormone antagonists, intentional self-harm
  [7th] T38.903 Poisoning by unspecified hormone antagonists, assault
  [7th] T38.904 Poisoning by unspecified hormone antagonists, undetermined
  [7th] T38.905 Adverse effect of unspecified hormone antagonists
  [7th] T38.906 Underdosing of unspecified hormone antagonists
 [6th] T38.99 Poisoning by, adverse effect of and underdosing of other hormone antagonists
  [7th] T38.991 Poisoning by other hormone antagonists, accidental (unintentional)
   Poisoning by other hormone antagonists NOS
  [7th] T38.992 Poisoning by other hormone antagonists, intentional self-harm
  [7th] T38.993 Poisoning by other hormone antagonists, assault
  [7th] T38.994 Poisoning by other hormone antagonists, undetermined
  [7th] T38.995 Adverse effect of other hormone antagonists
  [7th] T38.996 Underdosing of other hormone antagonists

[4th] T39 Poisoning by, adverse effect of and underdosing of nonopioid analgesics, antipyretics and antirheumatics
 The appropriate 7th character is to be added to each code from category T39
 A = initial encounter
 D = subsequent encounter
 S = sequela
[5th] T39.0 Poisoning by, adverse effect of and underdosing of salicylates
 [6th] T39.01 Poisoning by, adverse effect of and underdosing of aspirin
  Poisoning by, adverse effect of and underdosing of acetylsalicylic acid
  [7th] T39.011 Poisoning by aspirin, accidental (unintentional)
  [7th] T39.012 Poisoning by aspirin, intentional self-harm
  [7th] T39.013 Poisoning by aspirin, assault
  [7th] T39.014 Poisoning by aspirin, undetermined
  [7th] T39.015 Adverse effect of aspirin
  [7th] T39.016 Underdosing of aspirin
 [6th] T39.09 Poisoning by, adverse effect of and underdosing of other salicylates
  [7th] T39.091 Poisoning by salicylates, accidental (unintentional)
   Poisoning by salicylates NOS
  [7th] T39.092 Poisoning by salicylates, intentional self-harm
  [7th] T39.093 Poisoning by salicylates, assault
  [7th] T39.094 Poisoning by salicylates, undetermined
  [7th] T39.095 Adverse effect of salicylates
  [7th] T39.096 Underdosing of salicylates
[5th] T39.1 Poisoning by, adverse effect of and underdosing of 4-Aminophenol derivatives
 [6th] T39.1X Poisoning by, adverse effect of and underdosing of 4-Aminophenol derivatives
  [7th] T39.1X1 Poisoning by 4-Aminophenol derivatives, accidental (unintentional)
   Poisoning by 4-Aminophenol derivatives NOS
  [7th] T39.1X2 Poisoning by 4-Aminophenol derivatives, intentional self-harm
  [7th] T39.1X3 Poisoning by 4-Aminophenol derivatives, assault
  [7th] T39.1X4 Poisoning by 4-Aminophenol derivatives, undetermined
  [7th] T39.1X5 Adverse effect of 4-Aminophenol derivatives
  [7th] T39.1X6 Underdosing of 4-Aminophenol derivatives
[5th] T39.2 Poisoning by, adverse effect of and underdosing of pyrazolone derivatives

Unspecified Code | Other Specified Code | [N] Newborn Age: 0 | [P] Pediatric Age: 0-17 | [M] Maternity Age: 12-55
[A] Adult Age: 15-124 | ♂ Male | ♀ Female | ● New Code | ▲ Revised Code Title | ►◄ Revised Text

[6th] T39.2X Poisoning by, adverse effect of and underdosing of pyrazolone derivatives

[7th] T39.2X1 Poisoning by pyrazolone derivatives, accidental (unintentional)

Poisoning by pyrazolone derivatives NOS

[7th] T39.2X2 Poisoning by pyrazolone derivatives, intentional self-harm

[7th] T39.2X3 Poisoning by pyrazolone derivatives, assault

[7th] T39.2X4 Poisoning by pyrazolone derivatives, undetermined

[7th] T39.2X5 Adverse effect of pyrazolone derivatives

[7th] T39.2X6 Underdosing of pyrazolone derivatives

[5th] T39.3 Poisoning by, adverse effect of and underdosing of other nonsteroidal anti-inflammatory drugs [NSAID]

[6th] T39.31 Poisoning by, adverse effect of and underdosing of propionic acid derivatives

Poisoning by, adverse effect of and underdosing of fenoprofen

Poisoning by, adverse effect of and underdosing of flurbiprofen

Poisoning by, adverse effect of and underdosing of ibuprofen

Poisoning by, adverse effect of and underdosing of ketoprofen

Poisoning by, adverse effect of and underdosing of naproxen

Poisoning by, adverse effect of and underdosing of oxaprozin

[7th] T39.311 Poisoning by propionic acid derivatives, accidental (unintentional)

[7th] T39.312 Poisoning by propionic acid derivatives, intentional self-harm

[7th] T39.313 Poisoning by propionic acid derivatives, assault

[7th] T39.314 Poisoning by propionic acid derivatives, undetermined

[7th] T39.315 Adverse effect of propionic acid derivatives

[7th] T39.316 Underdosing of propionic acid derivatives

[6th] T39.39 Poisoning by, adverse effect of and underdosing of other nonsteroidal anti-inflammatory drugs [NSAID]

[7th] T39.391 Poisoning by other nonsteroidal anti-inflammatory drugs [NSAID], accidental (unintentional)

Poisoning by other nonsteroidal anti-inflammatory drugs NOS

[7th] T39.392 Poisoning by other nonsteroidal anti-inflammatory drugs [NSAID], intentional self-harm

[7th] T39.393 Poisoning by other nonsteroidal anti-inflammatory drugs [NSAID], assault

[7th] T39.394 Poisoning by other nonsteroidal anti-inflammatory drugs [NSAID], undetermined

[7th] T39.395 Adverse effect of other nonsteroidal anti-inflammatory drugs [NSAID]

[7th] T39.396 Underdosing of other nonsteroidal anti-inflammatory drugs [NSAID]

[5th] T39.4 Poisoning by, adverse effect of and underdosing of antirheumatics, not elsewhere classified

[EXCLUDES1] *poisoning by, adverse effect of and underdosing of glucocorticoids (T38.0-)*
poisoning by, adverse effect of and underdosing of salicylates (T39.0-)

[6th] T39.4X Poisoning by, adverse effect of and underdosing of antirheumatics, not elsewhere classified

[7th] T39.4X1 Poisoning by antirheumatics, not elsewhere classified, accidental (unintentional)

Poisoning by antirheumatics, not elsewhere classified NOS

[7th] T39.4X2 Poisoning by antirheumatics, not elsewhere classified, intentional self-harm

[7th] T39.4X3 Poisoning by antirheumatics, not elsewhere classified, assault

[7th] T39.4X4 Poisoning by antirheumatics, not elsewhere classified, undetermined

[7th] T39.4X5 Adverse effect of antirheumatics, not elsewhere classified

[7th] T39.4X6 Underdosing of antirheumatics, not elsewhere classified

[5th] T39.8 Poisoning by, adverse effect of and underdosing of other nonopioid analgesics and antipyretics, not elsewhere classified

[6th] T39.8X Poisoning by, adverse effect of and underdosing of other nonopioid analgesics and antipyretics, not elsewhere classified

[7th] T39.8X1 Poisoning by other nonopioid analgesics and antipyretics, not elsewhere classified, accidental (unintentional)

Poisoning by other nonopioid analgesics and antipyretics, not elsewhere classified NOS

[7th] T39.8X2 Poisoning by other nonopioid analgesics and antipyretics, not elsewhere classified, intentional self-harm

[7th] T39.8X3 Poisoning by other nonopioid analgesics and antipyretics, not elsewhere classified, assault

[7th] T39.8X4 Poisoning by other nonopioid analgesics and antipyretics, not elsewhere classified, undetermined

[7th] T39.8X5 Adverse effect of other nonopioid analgesics and antipyretics, not elsewhere classified

[7th] T39.8X6 Underdosing of other nonopioid analgesics and antipyretics, not elsewhere classified

[5th] T39.9 Poisoning by, adverse effect of and underdosing of unspecified nonopioid analgesic, antipyretic and antirheumatic

[7th] T39.91 Poisoning by unspecified nonopioid analgesic, antipyretic and antirheumatic, accidental (unintentional)

Poisoning by nonopioid analgesic, antipyretic and antirheumatic NOS

[7th] T39.92 Poisoning by unspecified nonopioid analgesic, antipyretic and antirheumatic, intentional self-harm

[7th] T39.93 Poisoning by unspecified nonopioid analgesic, antipyretic and antirheumatic, assault

[7th] T39.94 Poisoning by unspecified nonopioid analgesic, antipyretic and antirheumatic, undetermined

[7th] T39.95 Adverse effect of unspecified nonopioid analgesic, antipyretic and antirheumatic

[7th] T39.96 Underdosing of unspecified nonopioid analgesic, antipyretic and antirheumatic

[4th] T40 Poisoning by, adverse effect of and underdosing of narcotics and psychodysleptics [hallucinogens]

[EXCLUDES2] *drug dependence and related mental and behavioral disorders due to psychoactive substance use (F10.-F19.-)*

The appropriate 7th character is to be added to each code from category T40

A = initial encounter

D = subsequent encounter

S = sequela

[5th] T40.0 Poisoning by, adverse effect of and underdosing of opium

[4th] 4th character required [5th] 5th character required [6th] 6th character required [7th] 7th character required [X] Extension 'X' Alert
[EXCLUDES1] Not coded here [EXCLUDES2] Not included here [PDx] Primary Diagnosis Only Manifestation Code

[6th] T40.0X Poisoning by, adverse effect of and underdosing of opium
- [7th] T40.0X1 Poisoning by opium, accidental (unintentional)
  Poisoning by opium NOS
- [7th] T40.0X2 Poisoning by opium, intentional self-harm
- [7th] T40.0X3 Poisoning by opium, assault
- [7th] T40.0X4 Poisoning by opium, undetermined
- [7th] T40.0X5 Adverse effect of opium
- [7th] T40.0X6 Underdosing of opium

[5th] T40.1 Poisoning by and adverse effect of heroin

[6th] T40.1X Poisoning by and adverse effect of heroin
- [7th] T40.1X1 Poisoning by heroin, accidental (unintentional)
  Poisoning by heroin NOS
- [7th] T40.1X2 Poisoning by heroin, intentional self-harm
- [7th] T40.1X3 Poisoning by heroin, assault
- [7th] T40.1X4 Poisoning by heroin, undetermined

[5th] T40.2 Poisoning by, adverse effect of and underdosing of other opioids

[6th] T40.2X Poisoning by, adverse effect of and underdosing of other opioids
- [7th] T40.2X1 Poisoning by other opioids, accidental (unintentional)
  Poisoning by other opioids NOS
- [7th] T40.2X2 Poisoning by other opioids, intentional self-harm
- [7th] T40.2X3 Poisoning by other opioids, assault
- [7th] T40.2X4 Poisoning by other opioids, undetermined
- [7th] T40.2X5 Adverse effect of other opioids
- [7th] T40.2X6 Underdosing of other opioids

[5th] T40.3 Poisoning by, adverse effect of and underdosing of methadone

[6th] T40.3X Poisoning by, adverse effect of and underdosing of methadone
- [7th] T40.3X1 Poisoning by methadone, accidental (unintentional)
  Poisoning by methadone NOS
- [7th] T40.3X2 Poisoning by methadone, intentional self-harm
- [7th] T40.3X3 Poisoning by methadone, assault
- [7th] T40.3X4 Poisoning by methadone, undetermined
- [7th] T40.3X5 Adverse effect of methadone
- [7th] T40.3X6 Underdosing of methadone

[5th] T40.4 Poisoning by, adverse effect of and underdosing of other synthetic narcotics

[6th] T40.4X Poisoning by, adverse effect of and underdosing of other synthetic narcotics
- [7th] T40.4X1 Poisoning by other synthetic narcotics, accidental (unintentional)
  Poisoning by other synthetic narcotics NOS
- [7th] T40.4X2 Poisoning by other synthetic narcotics, intentional self-harm
- [7th] T40.4X3 Poisoning by other synthetic narcotics, assault
- [7th] T40.4X4 Poisoning by other synthetic narcotics, undetermined
- [7th] T40.4X5 Adverse effect of other synthetic narcotics
- [7th] T40.4X6 Underdosing of other synthetic narcotics

[5th] T40.5 Poisoning by, adverse effect of and underdosing of cocaine

[6th] T40.5X Poisoning by, adverse effect of and underdosing of cocaine
- [7th] T40.5X1 Poisoning by cocaine, accidental (unintentional)
  Poisoning by cocaine NOS
- [7th] T40.5X2 Poisoning by cocaine, intentional self-harm
- [7th] T40.5X3 Poisoning by cocaine, assault
- [7th] T40.5X4 Poisoning by cocaine, undetermined
- [7th] T40.5X5 Adverse effect of cocaine
- [7th] T40.5X6 Underdosing of cocaine

[5th] T40.6 Poisoning by, adverse effect of and underdosing of other and unspecified narcotics

[6th] T40.60 Poisoning by, adverse effect of and underdosing of unspecified narcotics
- [7th] T40.601 Poisoning by unspecified narcotics, accidental (unintentional)
  Poisoning by narcotics NOS
- [7th] T40.602 Poisoning by unspecified narcotics, intentional self-harm
- [7th] T40.603 Poisoning by unspecified narcotics, assault
- [7th] T40.604 Poisoning by unspecified narcotics, undetermined
- [7th] T40.605 Adverse effect of unspecified narcotics
- [7th] T40.606 Underdosing of unspecified narcotics

[6th] T40.69 Poisoning by, adverse effect of and underdosing of other narcotics
- [7th] T40.691 Poisoning by other narcotics, accidental (unintentional)
  Poisoning by other narcotics NOS
- [7th] T40.692 Poisoning by other narcotics, intentional self-harm
- [7th] T40.693 Poisoning by other narcotics, assault
- [7th] T40.694 Poisoning by other narcotics, undetermined
- [7th] T40.695 Adverse effect of other narcotics
- [7th] T40.696 Underdosing of other narcotics

[5th] T40.7 Poisoning by, adverse effect of and underdosing of cannabis (derivatives)

[6th] T40.7X Poisoning by, adverse effect of and underdosing of cannabis (derivatives)
- [7th] T40.7X1 Poisoning by cannabis (derivatives), accidental (unintentional)
  Poisoning by cannabis NOS
- [7th] T40.7X2 Poisoning by cannabis (derivatives), intentional self-harm
- [7th] T40.7X3 Poisoning by cannabis (derivatives), assault
- [7th] T40.7X4 Poisoning by cannabis (derivatives), undetermined
- [7th] T40.7X5 Adverse effect of cannabis (derivatives)
- [7th] T40.7X6 Underdosing of cannabis (derivatives)

[5th] T40.8 Poisoning by and adverse effect of lysergide [LSD]

[6th] T40.8X Poisoning by and adverse effect of lysergide [LSD]
- [7th] T40.8X1 Poisoning by lysergide [LSD], accidental (unintentional)
  Poisoning by lysergide [LSD]NOS
- [7th] T40.8X2 Poisoning by lysergide [LSD], intentional self-harm
- [7th] T40.8X3 Poisoning by lysergide [LSD], assault
- [7th] T40.8X4 Poisoning by lysergide [LSD], undetermined

[5th] T40.9 Poisoning by, adverse effect of and underdosing of other and unspecified psychodysleptics [hallucinogens]

[6th] T40.90 Poisoning by, adverse effect of and underdosing of unspecified psychodysleptics [hallucinogens]
- [7th] T40.901 Poisoning by unspecified psychodysleptics [hallucinogens], accidental (unintentional)
- [7th] T40.902 Poisoning by unspecified psychodysleptics [hallucinogens], intentional self-harm
- [7th] T40.903 Poisoning by unspecified psychodysleptics [hallucinogens], assault
- [7th] T40.904 Poisoning by unspecified psychodysleptics [hallucinogens], undetermined
- [7th] T40.905 Adverse effect of unspecified psychodysleptics [hallucinogens]
- [7th] T40.906 Underdosing of unspecified psychodysleptics

Unspecified Code | Other Specified Code | [N] Newborn Age: 0 | [P] Pediatric Age: 0-17 | [M] Maternity Age: 12-55
[A] Adult Age: 15-124 | ♂ Male | ♀ Female | ● New Code | ▲ Revised Code Title | ►◄ Revised Text

[6th] **T40.99 Poisoning by, adverse effect of and underdosing of other psychodysleptics [hallucinogens]**

[7th] **T40.991 Poisoning by other psychodysleptics [hallucinogens], accidental (unintentional)**
Poisoning by other psychodysleptics [hallucinogens] NOS

[7th] **T40.992 Poisoning by other psychodysleptics [hallucinogens], intentional self-harm**

[7th] **T40.993 Poisoning by other psychodysleptics [hallucinogens], assault**

[7th] **T40.994 Poisoning by other psychodysleptics [hallucinogens], undetermined**

[7th] **T40.995 Adverse effect of other psychodysleptics [hallucinogens]**

[7th] **T40.996 Underdosing of other psychodysleptics**

[4th] **T41 Poisoning by, adverse effect of and underdosing of anesthetics and therapeutic gases**

EXCLUDES1 *benzodiazepines (T42.4-)*
cocaine (T40.5-)
complications of anesthesia during pregnancy (O29.-)
complications of anesthesia during labor and delivery (O74.-)
complications of anesthesia during the puerperium (O89.-)
opioids (T40.0-T40.2-)

The appropriate 7th character is to be added to each code from category T41
A = initial encounter
D = subsequent encounter
S = sequela

[5th] **T41.0 Poisoning by, adverse effect of and underdosing of inhaled anesthetics**

EXCLUDES1 *oxygen (T41.5-)*

[6th] **T41.0X Poisoning by, adverse effect of and underdosing of inhaled anesthetics**

[7th] **T41.0X1 Poisoning by inhaled anesthetics, accidental (unintentional)**
Poisoning by inhaled anesthetics NOS

[7th] **T41.0X2 Poisoning by inhaled anesthetics, intentional self-harm**

[7th] **T41.0X3 Poisoning by inhaled anesthetics, assault**

[7th] **T41.0X4 Poisoning by inhaled anesthetics, undetermined**

[7th] **T41.0X5 Adverse effect of inhaled anesthetics**

[7th] **T41.0X6 Underdosing of inhaled anesthetics**

[5th] **T41.1 Poisoning by, adverse effect of and underdosing of intravenous anesthetics**
Poisoning by, adverse effect of and underdosing of thiobarbiturates

[6th] **T41.1X Poisoning by, adverse effect of and underdosing of intravenous anesthetics**

[7th] **T41.1X1 Poisoning by intravenous anesthetics, accidental (unintentional)**
Poisoning by intravenous anesthetics NOS

[7th] **T41.1X2 Poisoning by intravenous anesthetics, intentional self-harm**

[7th] **T41.1X3 Poisoning by intravenous anesthetics, assault**

[7th] **T41.1X4 Poisoning by intravenous anesthetics, undetermined**

[7th] **T41.1X5 Adverse effect of intravenous anesthetics**

[7th] **T41.1X6 Underdosing of intravenous anesthetics**

[5th] **T41.2 Poisoning by, adverse effect of and underdosing of other and unspecified general anesthetics**

[6th] **T41.20 Poisoning by, adverse effect of and underdosing of unspecified general anesthetics**

[7th] **T41.201 Poisoning by unspecified general anesthetics, accidental (unintentional)**
Poisoning by general anesthetics NOS

[7th] **T41.202 Poisoning by unspecified general anesthetics, intentional self-harm**

[7th] **T41.203 Poisoning by unspecified general anesthetics, assault**

[7th] **T41.204 Poisoning by unspecified general anesthetics, undetermined**

[7th] **T41.205 Adverse effect of unspecified general anesthetics**

[7th] **T41.206 Underdosing of unspecified general anesthetics**

[6th] **T41.29 Poisoning by, adverse effect of and underdosing of other general anesthetics**

[7th] **T41.291 Poisoning by other general anesthetics, accidental (unintentional)**
Poisoning by other general anesthetics NOS

[7th] **T41.292 Poisoning by other general anesthetics, intentional self-harm**

[7th] **T41.293 Poisoning by other general anesthetics, assault**

[7th] **T41.294 Poisoning by other general anesthetics, undetermined**

[7th] **T41.295 Adverse effect of other general anesthetics**

[7th] **T41.296 Underdosing of other general anesthetics**

[5th] **T41.3 Poisoning by, adverse effect of and underdosing of local anesthetics**
Cocaine (topical)

EXCLUDES2 *poisoning by cocaine used as a central nervous system stimulant (T40.5X1-T40.5X4)*

[6th] **T41.3X Poisoning by, adverse effect of and underdosing of local anesthetics**

[7th] **T41.3X1 Poisoning by local anesthetics, accidental (unintentional)**
Poisoning by local anesthetics NOS

[7th] **T41.3X2 Poisoning by local anesthetics, intentional self-harm**

[7th] **T41.3X3 Poisoning by local anesthetics, assault**

[7th] **T41.3X4 Poisoning by local anesthetics, undetermined**

[7th] **T41.3X5 Adverse effect of local anesthetics**

[7th] **T41.3X6 Underdosing of local anesthetics**

[5th] **T41.4 Poisoning by, adverse effect of and underdosing of unspecified anesthetic**

[7th] **T41.41 Poisoning by unspecified anesthetic, accidental (unintentional)**
Poisoning by anesthetic NOS

[7th] **T41.42 Poisoning by unspecified anesthetic, intentional self-harm**

[7th] **T41.43 Poisoning by unspecified anesthetic, assault**

[7th] **T41.44 Poisoning by unspecified anesthetic, undetermined**

[7th] **T41.45 Adverse effect of unspecified anesthetic**

[7th] **T41.46 Underdosing of unspecified anesthetics**

[5th] **T41.5 Poisoning by, adverse effect of and underdosing of therapeutic gases**

[6th] **T41.5X Poisoning by, adverse effect of and underdosing of therapeutic gases**

[7th] **T41.5X1 Poisoning by therapeutic gases, accidental (unintentional)**
Poisoning by therapeutic gases NOS

[7th] **T41.5X2 Poisoning by therapeutic gases, intentional self-harm**

[7th] **T41.5X3 Poisoning by therapeutic gases, assault**

[7th] **T41.5X4 Poisoning by therapeutic gases, undetermined**

[7th] **T41.5X5 Adverse effect of therapeutic gases**

[7th] **T41.5X6 Underdosing of therapeutic gases**

[4th] 4th character required [5th] 5th character required [6th] 6th character required [7th] 7th character required [7th] Extension 'X' Alert
EXCLUDES1 Not coded here EXCLUDES2 Not included here [PDx] Primary Diagnosis Only Manifestation Code

🔵 T42 **Poisoning by, adverse effect of and underdosing of antiepileptic, sedative- hypnotic and antiparkinsonism drugs**

> *EXCLUDES2* *drug dependence and related mental and behavioral disorders due to psychoactive substance use (F10.--F19.-)*

The appropriate 7th character is to be added to each code from category T42
A = initial encounter
D = subsequent encounter
S = sequela

🔵 T42.0 **Poisoning by, adverse effect of and underdosing of hydantoin derivatives**

🔵 T42.0X **Poisoning by, adverse effect of and underdosing of** hydantoin derivatives

🔵 T42.0X1 **Poisoning by hydantoin derivatives,** accidental **(unintentional)**

Poisoning by hydantoin derivatives NOS

🔵 T42.0X2 **Poisoning by hydantoin derivatives,** intentional self-harm

🔵 T42.0X3 **Poisoning by hydantoin derivatives,** assault

🔵 T42.0X4 **Poisoning by hydantoin derivatives,** undetermined

🔵 T42.0X5 Adverse effect **of hydantoin derivatives**

🔵 T42.0X6 Underdosing **of hydantoin derivatives**

🔵 T42.1 **Poisoning by, adverse effect of and underdosing of iminostilbenes**

Poisoning by, adverse effect of and underdosing of carbamazepine

🔵 T42.1X **Poisoning by, adverse effect of and underdosing of** iminostilbenes

🔵 T42.1X1 **Poisoning by iminostilbenes,** accidental **(unintentional)**

Poisoning by iminostilbenes NOS

🔵 T42.1X2 **Poisoning by iminostilbenes,** intentional self-harm

🔵 T42.1X3 **Poisoning by iminostilbenes,** assault

🔵 T42.1X4 **Poisoning by iminostilbenes,** undetermined

🔵 T42.1X5 Adverse effect **of iminostilbenes**

🔵 T42.1X6 Underdosing **of iminostilbenes**

🔵 T42.2 **Poisoning by, adverse effect of and underdosing of succinimides and oxazolidinediones**

🔵 T42.2X **Poisoning by, adverse effect of and underdosing of** succinimides and oxazolidinediones

🔵 T42.2X1 **Poisoning by succinimides and oxazolidinediones,** accidental **(unintentional)**

Poisoning by succinimides and oxazolidinediones NOS

🔵 T42.2X2 **Poisoning by succinimides and oxazolidinediones,** intentional self-harm

🔵 T42.2X3 **Poisoning by succinimides and oxazolidinediones,** assault

🔵 T42.2X4 **Poisoning by succinimides and oxazolidinediones,** undetermined

🔵 T42.2X5 Adverse effect **of succinimides and oxazolidinediones**

🔵 T42.2X6 Underdosing **of succinimides and oxazolidinediones**

🔵 T42.3 **Poisoning by, adverse effect of and underdosing of barbiturates**

> *EXCLUDES1* *poisoning by, adverse effect of and underdosing of thiobarbiturates (T41.1-)*

🔵 T42.3X **Poisoning by, adverse effect of and underdosing of** barbiturates

🔵 T42.3X1 **Poisoning by barbiturates,** accidental **(unintentional)**

Poisoning by barbiturates NOS

🔵 T42.3X2 **Poisoning by barbiturates,** intentional self-harm

🔵 T42.3X3 **Poisoning by barbiturates,** assault

🔵 T42.3X4 **Poisoning by barbiturates,** undetermined

🔵 T42.3X5 Adverse effect **of barbiturates**

🔵 T42.3X6 Underdosing **of barbiturates**

🔵 T42.4 **Poisoning by, adverse effect of and underdosing of benzodiazepines**

🔵 T42.4X **Poisoning by, adverse effect of and underdosing of** benzodiazepines

🔵 T42.4X1 **Poisoning by benzodiazepines,** accidental **(unintentional)**

Poisoning by benzodiazepines NOS

🔵 T42.4X2 **Poisoning by benzodiazepines,** intentional self-harm

🔵 T42.4X3 **Poisoning by benzodiazepines,** assault

🔵 T42.4X4 **Poisoning by benzodiazepines,** undetermined

🔵 T42.4X5 Adverse effect **of benzodiazepines**

🔵 T42.4X6 Underdosing **of benzodiazepines**

🔵 T42.5 **Poisoning by, adverse effect of and underdosing of mixed antiepileptics**

🔵 T42.5X **Poisoning by, adverse effect of and underdosing of** antiepileptics

🔵 T42.5X1 **Poisoning by mixed antiepileptics,** accidental **(unintentional)**

Poisoning by mixed antiepileptics NOS

🔵 T42.5X2 **Poisoning by mixed antiepileptics,** intentional self-harm

🔵 T42.5X3 **Poisoning by mixed antiepileptics,** assault

🔵 T42.5X4 **Poisoning by mixed antiepileptics,** undetermined

🔵 T42.5X5 Adverse effect **of mixed antiepileptics**

🔵 T42.5X6 Underdosing **of mixed antiepileptics**

🔵 T42.6 **Poisoning by, adverse effect of and underdosing of other antiepileptic and sedative-hypnotic drugs**

Poisoning by, adverse effect of and underdosing of methaqualone

Poisoning by, adverse effect of and underdosing of valproic acid

> *EXCLUDES1* *poisoning by, adverse effect of and underdosing of carbamazepine (T42.1-)*

🔵 T42.6X **Poisoning by, adverse effect of and underdosing of** other antiepileptic and sedative-hypnotic drugs

🔵 T42.6X1 **Poisoning by other antiepileptic and sedative-hypnotic drugs,** accidental **(unintentional)**

Poisoning by other antiepileptic and sedative-hypnotic drugs NOS

🔵 T42.6X2 **Poisoning by other antiepileptic and sedative-hypnotic drugs,** intentional self-harm

🔵 T42.6X3 **Poisoning by other antiepileptic and sedative-hypnotic drugs,** assault

🔵 T42.6X4 **Poisoning by other antiepileptic and sedative-hypnotic drugs,** undetermined

🔵 T42.6X5 Adverse effect **of other antiepileptic and sedative-hypnotic drugs**

🔵 T42.6X6 Underdosing **of other antiepileptic and sedative-hypnotic drugs**

🔵 T42.7 **Poisoning by, adverse effect of and underdosing of** unspecified antiepileptic and sedative-hypnotic drugs

🔵 T42.71 **Poisoning by unspecified antiepileptic and sedative-hypnotic drugs,** accidental **(unintentional)**

Poisoning by antiepileptic and sedative-hypnotic drugs NOS

🔵 T42.72 **Poisoning by unspecified antiepileptic and sedative-hypnotic drugs,** intentional self-harm

Unspecified Code	Other Specified Code	N Newborn Age: 0	P Pediatric Age: 0 17	M Maternity Age: 12 55
A Adult Age: 15-124	♂ Male	♀ Female	● New Code	▲ Revised Code Title ►◄ Revised Text

⑦ **T42.73** **Poisoning by unspecified antiepileptic and sedative-hypnotic drugs,** assault

⑦ **T42.74** **Poisoning by unspecified antiepileptic and sedative-hypnotic drugs,** undetermined

⑦ **T42.75** Adverse effect **of unspecified antiepileptic and sedative-hypnotic drugs**

⑦ **T42.76** Underdosing **of unspecified antiepileptic and sedative-hypnotic drugs**

⑤ **T42.8** **Poisoning by, adverse effect of and underdosing of antiparkinsonism drugs and other central muscle-tone depressants**

Poisoning by, adverse effect of and underdosing of amantadine

⑥ **T42.8X** **Poisoning by, adverse effect of and underdosing of** antiparkinsonism drugs and other central muscle-tone depressants

⑦ **T42.8X1** **Poisoning by antiparkinsonism drugs and other central muscle-tone depressants,** accidental **(unintentional)**

Poisoning by antiparkinsonism drugs and other central muscle-tone depressants NOS

⑦ **T42.8X2** **Poisoning by antiparkinsonism drugs and other central muscle-tone depressants,** intentional self-harm

⑦ **T42.8X3** **Poisoning by antiparkinsonism drugs and other central muscle-tone depressants,** assault

⑦ **T42.8X4** **Poisoning by antiparkinsonism drugs and other central muscle-tone depressants,** undetermined

⑦ **T42.8X5** Adverse effect **of antiparkinsonism drugs and other central muscle-tone depressants**

⑦ **T42.8X6** Underdosing **of antiparkinsonism drugs and other central muscle-tone depressants**

④ **T43** **Poisoning by, adverse effect of and underdosing of psychotropic drugs, not elsewhere classified**

EXCLUDES1 *appetite depressants (T50.5-)*
barbiturates (T42.3-)
benzodiazepines (T42.4-)
methaqualone (T42.6-)
psychodysleptics [hallucinogens] (T40.7-T40.9-)

EXCLUDES2 *drug dependence and related mental and behavioral disorders due to psychoactive substance use (F10.- -F19.-)*

The appropriate 7th character is to be added to each code from category T43
A = initial encounter
D = subsequent encounter
S = sequela

⑤ **T43.0** **Poisoning by, adverse effect of and underdosing of tricyclic and tetracyclic antidepressants**

⑥ **T43.01** **Poisoning by, adverse effect of and underdosing of** tricyclic antidepressants

⑦ **T43.011** **Poisoning by tricyclic antidepressants,** accidental **(unintentional)**

Poisoning by tricyclic antidepressants NOS

⑦ **T43.012** **Poisoning by tricyclic antidepressants,** intentional self-harm

⑦ **T43.013** **Poisoning by tricyclic antidepressants,** assault

⑦ **T43.014** **Poisoning by tricyclic antidepressants,** undetermined

⑦ **T43.015** Adverse effect **of tricyclic antidepressants**

⑦ **T43.016** Underdosing **of tricyclic antidepressants**

⑥ **T43.02** **Poisoning by, adverse effect of and underdosing of** tetracyclic antidepressants

⑦ **T43.021** **Poisoning by tetracyclic antidepressants,** accidental **(unintentional)**

Poisoning by tetracyclic antidepressants NOS

⑦ **T43.022** **Poisoning by tetracyclic antidepressants,** intentional self-harm

⑦ **T43.023** **Poisoning by tetracyclic antidepressants,** assault

⑦ **T43.024** **Poisoning by tetracyclic antidepressants,** undetermined

⑦ **T43.025** Adverse effect **of tetracyclic antidepressants**

⑦ **T43.026** Underdosing **of tetracyclic antidepressants**

⑤ **T43.1** **Poisoning by, adverse effect of and underdosing of monoamine-oxidase-inhibitor antidepressants**

⑥ **T43.1X** **Poisoning by, adverse effect of and underdosing of** monoamine-oxidase-inhibitor antidepressants

⑦ **T43.1X1** **Poisoning by monoamine-oxidase-inhibitor antidepressants,** accidental **(unintentional)**

Poisoning by monoamine-oxidase-inhibitor antidepressants NOS

⑦ **T43.1X2** **Poisoning by monoamine-oxidase-inhibitor antidepressants,** intentional self-harm

⑦ **T43.1X3** **Poisoning by monoamine-oxidase-inhibitor antidepressants,** assault

⑦ **T43.1X4** **Poisoning by monoamine-oxidase-inhibitor antidepressants,** undetermined

⑦ **T43.1X5** Adverse effect **of monoamine-oxidase-inhibitor antidepressants**

⑦ **T43.1X6** Underdosing **of monoamine-oxidase-inhibitor antidepressants**

⑤ **T43.2** **Poisoning by, adverse effect of and underdosing of other and unspecified antidepressants**

⑥ **T43.20** **Poisoning by, adverse effect of and underdosing of** unspecified antidepressants

⑦ **T43.201** **Poisoning by unspecified antidepressants,** accidental **(unintentional)**

Poisoning by antidepressants NOS

⑦ **T43.202** **Poisoning by unspecified antidepressants,** intentional self-harm

⑦ **T43.203** **Poisoning by unspecified antidepressants,** assault

⑦ **T43.204** **Poisoning by unspecified antidepressants,** undetermined

⑦ **T43.205** Adverse effect **of unspecified antidepressants**

⑦ **T43.206** Underdosing **of unspecified antidepressants**

⑥ **T43.21** **Poisoning by, adverse effect of and underdosing of** selective serotonin and norepinephrine reuptake inhibitors

Poisoning by, adverse effect of and underdosing of SSNRI antidepressants

⑦ **T43.211** **Poisoning by selective serotonin and norepinephrine reuptake inhibitors,** accidental **(unintentional)**

⑦ **T43.212** **Poisoning by selective serotonin and norepinephrine reuptake inhibitors,** intentional self-harm

⑦ **T43.213** **Poisoning by selective serotonin and norepinephrine reuptake inhibitors,** assault

⑦ **T43.214** **Poisoning by selective serotonin and norepinephrine reuptake inhibitors,** undetermined

⑦ **T43.215** Adverse effect **of selective serotonin and norepinephrine reuptake inhibitors**

⑦ **T43.216** Underdosing **of selective serotonin and norepinephrine reuptake inhibitors**

⑥ **T43.22** **Poisoning by, adverse effect of and underdosing of** selective serotonin reuptake inhibitors

Poisoning by, adverse effect of and underdosing of SSRI antidepressants

⑦ **T43.221** **Poisoning by selective serotonin reuptake inhibitors,** accidental **(unintentional)**

---

④ 4th character required   ⑤ 5th character required   ⑥ 6th character required   ⑦ 7th character required   ⑦ₓ Extension 'X' Alert

EXCLUDES1 Not coded here   EXCLUDES2 Not included here   PDx Primary Diagnosis Only   Manifestation Code

[7th] T43.222 Poisoning by selective serotonin reuptake inhibitors, intentional self-harm
[7th] T43.223 Poisoning by selective serotonin reuptake inhibitors, assault
[7th] T43.224 Poisoning by selective serotonin reuptake inhibitors, undetermined
[7th] T43.225 Adverse effect of selective serotonin reuptake inhibitors
[7th] T43.226 Underdosing of selective serotonin reuptake inhibitors
[6th] T43.29 Poisoning by, adverse effect of and underdosing of other antidepressants
[7th] T43.291 Poisoning by other antidepressants, accidental (unintentional)
Poisoning by other antidepressants NOS
[7th] T43.292 Poisoning by other antidepressants, intentional self-harm
[7th] T43.293 Poisoning by other antidepressants, assault
[7th] T43.294 Poisoning by other antidepressants, undetermined
[7th] T43.295 Adverse effect of other antidepressants
[7th] T43.296 Underdosing of other antidepressants
[5th] T43.3 Poisoning by, adverse effect of and underdosing of phenothiazine antipsychotics and neuroleptics
[6th] T43.3X Poisoning by, adverse effect of and underdosing of phenothiazine antipsychotics and neuroleptics
[7th] T43.3X1 Poisoning by phenothiazine antipsychotics and neuroleptics, accidental (unintentional)
Poisoning by phenothiazine antipsychotics and neuroleptics NOS
[7th] T43.3X2 Poisoning by phenothiazine antipsychotics and neuroleptics, intentional self-harm
[7th] T43.3X3 Poisoning by phenothiazine antipsychotics and neuroleptics, assault
[7th] T43.3X4 Poisoning by phenothiazine antipsychotics and neuroleptics, undetermined
[7th] T43.3X5 Adverse effect of phenothiazine antipsychotics and neuroleptics
[7th] T43.3X6 Underdosing of phenothiazine antipsychotics and neuroleptics
[5th] T43.4 Poisoning by, adverse effect of and underdosing of butyrophenone and thiothixene neuroleptics
[6th] T43.4X Poisoning by, adverse effect of and underdosing of butyrophenone and thiothixene neuroleptics
[7th] T43.4X1 Poisoning by butyrophenone and thiothixene neuroleptics, accidental (unintentional)
Poisoning by butyrophenone and thiothixene neuroleptics NOS
[7th] T43.4X2 Poisoning by butyrophenone and thiothixene neuroleptics, intentional self-harm
[7th] T43.4X3 Poisoning by butyrophenone and thiothixene neuroleptics, assault
[7th] T43.4X4 Poisoning by butyrophenone and thiothixene neuroleptics, undetermined
[7th] T43.4X5 Adverse effect of butyrophenone and thiothixene neuroleptics
[7th] T43.4X6 Underdosing of butyrophenone and thiothixene neuroleptics
[5th] T43.5 Poisoning by, adverse effect of and underdosing of other and unspecified antipsychotics and neuroleptics
[EXCLUDES1] *poisoning by, adverse effect of and underdosing of rauwolfia (T46.5-)*
[6th] T43.50 Poisoning by, adverse effect of and underdosing of unspecified antipsychotics and neuroleptics
[7th] T43.501 Poisoning by unspecified antipsychotics and neuroleptics, accidental (unintentional)
Poisoning by antipsychotics and neuroleptics NOS
[7th] T43.502 Poisoning by unspecified antipsychotics and neuroleptics, intentional self-harm
[7th] T43.503 Poisoning by unspecified antipsychotics and neuroleptics, assault
[7th] T43.504 Poisoning by unspecified antipsychotics and neuroleptics, undetermined
[7th] T43.505 Adverse effect of unspecified antipsychotics and neuroleptics
[7th] T43.506 Underdosing of unspecified antipsychotics and neuroleptics
[6th] T43.59 Poisoning by, adverse effect of and underdosing of other antipsychotics and neuroleptics
[7th] T43.591 Poisoning by other antipsychotics and neuroleptics, accidental (unintentional)
Poisoning by other antipsychotics and neuroleptics NOS
[7th] T43.592 Poisoning by other antipsychotics and neuroleptics, intentional self-harm
[7th] T43.593 Poisoning by other antipsychotics and neuroleptics, assault
[7th] T43.594 Poisoning by other antipsychotics and neuroleptics, undetermined
[7th] T43.595 Adverse effect of other antipsychotics and neuroleptics
[7th] T43.596 Underdosing of other antipsychotics and neuroleptics
[5th] T43.6 Poisoning by, adverse effect of and underdosing of psychostimulants
[EXCLUDES1] *poisoning by, adverse effect of and underdosing of cocaine (T40.5-)*
[6th] T43.60 Poisoning by, adverse effect of and underdosing of unspecified psychostimulant
[7th] T43.601 Poisoning by unspecified psychostimulants, accidental (unintentional)
Poisoning by psychostimulants NOS
[7th] T43.602 Poisoning by unspecified psychostimulants, intentional self-harm
[7th] T43.603 Poisoning by unspecified psychostimulants, assault
[7th] T43.604 Poisoning by unspecified psychostimulants, undetermined
[7th] T43.605 Adverse effect of unspecified psychostimulants
[7th] T43.606 Underdosing of unspecified psychostimulants
[6th] T43.61 Poisoning by, adverse effect of and underdosing of caffeine
[7th] T43.611 Poisoning by caffeine, accidental (unintentional)
Poisoning by caffeine NOS
[7th] T43.612 Poisoning by caffeine, intentional self-harm
[7th] T43.613 Poisoning by caffeine, assault
[7th] T43.614 Poisoning by caffeine, undetermined
[7th] T43.615 Adverse effect of caffeine
[7th] T43.616 Underdosing of caffeine
[6th] T43.62 Poisoning by, adverse effect of and underdosing of amphetamines
Poisoning by, adverse effect of and underdosing of methamphetamines
[7th] T43.621 Poisoning by amphetamines, accidental (unintentional)
Poisoning by amphetamines NOS
[7th] T43.622 Poisoning by amphetamines, intentional self-harm

Unspecified Code | Other Specified Code | [N] Newborn Age: 0 | [P] Pediatric Age: 0-17 | [M] Maternity Age: 12-55
[A] Adult Age: 15-124 | ♂ Male | ♀ Female | ● New Code | ▲ Revised Code Title | ►◄ Revised Text

- T43.623 Poisoning by amphetamines, assault
- T43.624 Poisoning by amphetamines, undetermined
- T43.625 Adverse effect of amphetamines
- T43.626 Underdosing of amphetamines
- T43.63 Poisoning by, adverse effect of and underdosing of methylphenidate
  - T43.631 Poisoning by methylphenidate, accidental (unintentional)
    Poisoning by methylphenidate NOS
  - T43.632 Poisoning by methylphenidate, intentional self-harm
  - T43.633 Poisoning by methylphenidate, assault
  - T43.634 Poisoning by methylphenidate, undetermined
  - T43.635 Adverse effect of methylphenidate
  - T43.636 Underdosing of methylphenidate
- T43.69 Poisoning by, adverse effect of and underdosing of other psychostimulants
  - T43.691 Poisoning by other psychostimulants, accidental (unintentional)
    Poisoning by other psychostimulants NOS
  - T43.692 Poisoning by other psychostimulants, intentional self-harm
  - T43.693 Poisoning by other psychostimulants, assault
  - T43.694 Poisoning by other psychostimulants, undetermined
  - T43.695 Adverse effect of other psychostimulants
  - T43.696 Underdosing of other psychostimulants
- T43.8 Poisoning by, adverse effect of and underdosing of other psychotropic drugs
  - T43.8X Poisoning by, adverse effect of and underdosing of other psychotropic drugs
    - T43.8X1 Poisoning by other psychotropic drugs, accidental (unintentional)
      Poisoning by other psychotropic drugs NOS
    - T43.8X2 Poisoning by other psychotropic drugs, intentional self-harm
    - T43.8X3 Poisoning by other psychotropic drugs, assault
    - T43.8X4 Poisoning by other psychotropic drugs, undetermined
    - T43.8X5 Adverse effect of other psychotropic drugs
    - T43.8X6 Underdosing of other psychotropic drugs
- T43.9 Poisoning by, adverse effect of and underdosing of unspecified psychotropic drug
  - T43.91 Poisoning by unspecified psychotropic drug, accidental (unintentional)
    Poisoning by psychotropic drug NOS
  - T43.92 Poisoning by unspecified psychotropic drug, intentional self-harm
  - T43.93 Poisoning by unspecified psychotropic drug, assault
  - T43.94 Poisoning by unspecified psychotropic drug, undetermined
  - T43.95 Adverse effect of unspecified psychotropic drug
  - T43.96 Underdosing of unspecified psychotropic drug
- T44 Poisoning by, adverse effect of and underdosing of drugs primarily affecting the autonomic nervous system
  The appropriate 7th character is to be added to each code from category T44
  A = initial encounter
  D = subsequent encounter
  S = sequela
  - T44.0 Poisoning by, adverse effect of and underdosing of anticholinesterase agents
    - T44.0X Poisoning by, adverse effect of and underdosing of anticholinesterase agents
      - T44.0X1 Poisoning by anticholinesterase agents, accidental (unintentional)
        Poisoning by anticholinesterase agents NOS
      - T44.0X2 Poisoning by anticholinesterase agents, intentional self-harm
      - T44.0X3 Poisoning by anticholinesterase agents, assault
      - T44.0X4 Poisoning by anticholinesterase agents, undetermined
      - T44.0X5 Adverse effect of anticholinesterase agents
      - T44.0X6 Underdosing of anticholinesterase agents
  - T44.1 Poisoning by, adverse effect of and underdosing of other parasympathomimetics [cholinergics]
    - T44.1X Poisoning by, adverse effect of and underdosing of other parasympathomimetics [cholinergics]
      - T44.1X1 Poisoning by other parasympathomimetics [cholinergics], accidental (unintentional)
        Poisoning by other parasympathomimetics [cholinergics] NOS
      - T44.1X2 Poisoning by other parasympathomimetics [cholinergics], intentional self-harm
      - T44.1X3 Poisoning by other parasympathomimetics [cholinergics], assault
      - T44.1X4 Poisoning by other parasympathomimetics [cholinergics], undetermined
      - T44.1X5 Adverse effect of other parasympathomimetics [cholinergics]
      - T44.1X6 Underdosing of other parasympathomimetics
  - T44.2 Poisoning by, adverse effect of and underdosing of ganglionic blocking drugs
    - T44.2X Poisoning by, adverse effect of and underdosing of ganglionic blocking drugs
      - T44.2X1 Poisoning by ganglionic blocking drugs, accidental (unintentional)
        Poisoning by ganglionic blocking drugs NOS
      - T44.2X2 Poisoning by ganglionic blocking drugs, intentional self-harm
      - T44.2X3 Poisoning by ganglionic blocking drugs, assault
      - T44.2X4 Poisoning by ganglionic blocking drugs, undetermined
      - T44.2X5 Adverse effect of ganglionic blocking drugs
      - T44.2X6 Underdosing of ganglionic blocking drugs
  - T44.3 Poisoning by, adverse effect of and underdosing of other parasympatholytics [anticholinergics and antimuscarinics] and spasmolytics
    Poisoning by, adverse effect of and underdosing of papaverine
    - T44.3X Poisoning by, adverse effect of and underdosing of other parasympatholytics [anticholinergics and antimuscarinics] and spasmolytics
      - T44.3X1 Poisoning by other parasympatholytics [anticholinergics and antimuscarinics] and spasmolytics, accidental (unintentional)
        Poisoning by other parasympatholytics [anticholinergics and antimuscarinics] and spasmolytics NOS
      - T44.3X2 Poisoning by other parasympatholytics [anticholinergics and antimuscarinics] and spasmolytics, intentional self-harm
      - T44.3X3 Poisoning by other parasympatholytics [anticholinergics and antimuscarinics] and spasmolytics, assault
      - T44.3X4 Poisoning by other parasympatholytics [anticholinergics and antimuscarinics] and spasmolytics, undetermined
      - T44.3X5 Adverse effect of other parasympatholytics [anticholinergics and antimuscarinics] and spasmolytics
      - T44.3X6 Underdosing of other parasympatholytics [anticholinergics and antimuscarinics] and spasmolytics

4 4th character required   5 5th character required   6 6th character required   7 7th character required   Extension 'X' Alert

EXCLUDES 1 Not coded here   EXCLUDES 2 Not included here   PDx Primary Diagnosis Only   Manifestation Code

5ᵂ T44.4 **Poisoning by, adverse effect of and underdosing of predominantly alpha-adrenoreceptor agonists**
Poisoning by, adverse effect of and underdosing of metaraminol

6ᵂ T44.4X **Poisoning by, adverse effect of and underdosing of** predominantly alpha-adrenoreceptor agonists

7ᵂ T44.4X1 **Poisoning by predominantly alpha-adrenoreceptor agonists,** accidental **(unintentional)**
Poisoning by predominantly alpha-adrenoreceptor agonists NOS

7ᵂ T44.4X2 **Poisoning by predominantly alpha-adrenoreceptor agonists,** intentional self-harm

7ᵂ T44.4X3 **Poisoning by predominantly alpha-adrenoreceptor agonists,** assault

7ᵂ T44.4X4 **Poisoning by predominantly alpha-adrenoreceptor agonists,** undetermined

7ᵂ T44.4X5 Adverse effect **of predominantly alpha-adrenoreceptor agonists**

7ᵂ T44.4X6 Underdosing **of predominantly alpha-adrenoreceptor agonists**

5ᵂ T44.5 **Poisoning by, adverse effect of and underdosing of predominantly beta-adrenoreceptor agonists**
EXCLUDES1 *poisoning by, adverse effect of and underdosing of beta-adrenoreceptor agonists used in asthma therapy (T48.6-)*

6ᵂ T44.5X **Poisoning by, adverse effect of and underdosing of** predominantly beta-adrenoreceptor agonists

7ᵂ T44.5X1 **Poisoning by predominantly beta-adrenoreceptor agonists,** accidental **(unintentional)**
Poisoning by predominantly beta-adrenoreceptor agonists NOS

7ᵂ T44.5X2 **Poisoning by predominantly beta-adrenoreceptor agonists,** intentional self-harm

7ᵂ T44.5X3 **Poisoning by predominantly beta-adrenoreceptor agonists,** assault

7ᵂ T44.5X4 **Poisoning by predominantly beta-adrenoreceptor agonists,** undetermined

7ᵂ T44.5X5 Adverse effect **of predominantly beta-adrenoreceptor agonists**

7ᵂ T44.5X6 Underdosing **of predominantly beta-adrenoreceptor agonists**

5ᵂ T44.6 **Poisoning by, adverse effect of and underdosing of alpha-adrenoreceptor antagonists**
EXCLUDES1 *poisoning by, adverse effect of and underdosing of ergot alkaloids (T48.0)*

6ᵂ T44.6X **Poisoning by, adverse effect of and underdosing of** alpha-adrenoreceptor antagonists

7ᵂ T44.6X1 **Poisoning by alpha-adrenoreceptor antagonists,** accidental **(unintentional)**
Poisoning by alpha-adrenoreceptor antagonists NOS

7ᵂ T44.6X2 **Poisoning by alpha-adrenoreceptor antagonists,** intentional self-harm

7ᵂ T44.6X3 **Poisoning by alpha-adrenoreceptor antagonists,** assault

7ᵂ T44.6X4 **Poisoning by alpha-adrenoreceptor antagonists,** undetermined

7ᵂ T44.6X5 Adverse effect **of alpha-adrenoreceptor antagonists**

7ᵂ T44.6X6 Underdosing **of alpha-adrenoreceptor antagonists**

5ᵂ T44.7 **Poisoning by, adverse effect of and underdosing of beta-adrenoreceptor antagonists**

6ᵂ T44.7X **Poisoning by, adverse effect of and underdosing of** beta-adrenoreceptor antagonists

7ᵂ T44.7X1 **Poisoning by beta-adrenoreceptor antagonists,** accidental **(unintentional)**

Poisoning by beta-adrenoreceptor antagonists NOS

7ᵂ T44.7X2 **Poisoning by beta-adrenoreceptor antagonists,** intentional self-harm

7ᵂ T44.7X3 **Poisoning by beta-adrenoreceptor antagonists,** assault

7ᵂ T44.7X4 **Poisoning by beta-adrenoreceptor antagonists,** undetermined

7ᵂ T44.7X5 Adverse effect **of beta-adrenoreceptor antagonists**

7ᵂ T44.7X6 Underdosing **of beta-adrenoreceptor antagonists**

5ᵂ T44.8 **Poisoning by, adverse effect of and underdosing of centrally-acting and adrenergic-neuron- blocking agents**
EXCLUDES1 *poisoning by, adverse effect of and underdosing of clonidine (T46.5)*
poisoning by, adverse effect of and underdosing of guanethidine (T46.5)

6ᵂ T44.8X **Poisoning by, adverse effect of and underdosing of** centrally-acting and adrenergic- neuron-blocking agents

7ᵂ T44.8X1 **Poisoning by centrally-acting and adrenergic-neuron-blocking agents,** accidental **(unintentional)**

Poisoning by centrally-acting and adrenergic-neuron-blocking agents NOS

7ᵂ T44.8X2 **Poisoning by centrally-acting and adrenergic-neuron-blocking agents,** intentional self-harm

7ᵂ T44.8X3 **Poisoning by centrally-acting and adrenergic-neuron-blocking agents,** assault

7ᵂ T44.8X4 **Poisoning by centrally-acting and adrenergic-neuron-blocking agents,** undetermined

7ᵂ T44.8X5 Adverse effect **of centrally-acting and adrenergic-neuron-blocking agents**

7ᵂ T44.8X6 Underdosing **of centrally-acting and adrenergic-neuron-blocking agents**

5ᵂ T44.9 **Poisoning by, adverse effect of and underdosing of** other and unspecified drugs primarily affecting the autonomic nervous system
Poisoning by, adverse effect of and underdosing of drug stimulating both alpha and beta-adrenoreceptors

6ᵂ T44.90 **Poisoning by, adverse effect of and underdosing of** unspecified **drugs primarily affecting the autonomic nervous system**

7ᵂ T44.901 **Poisoning by unspecified drugs primarily affecting the autonomic nervous system,** accidental **(unintentional)**
Poisoning by unspecified drugs primarily affecting the autonomic nervous system NOS

7ᵂ T44.902 **Poisoning by unspecified drugs primarily affecting the autonomic nervous system,** intentional self-harm

7ᵂ T44.903 **Poisoning by unspecified drugs primarily affecting the autonomic nervous system,** assault

7ᵂ T44.904 **Poisoning by unspecified drugs primarily affecting the autonomic nervous system,** undetermined

7ᵂ T44.905 Adverse effect **of unspecified drugs primarily affecting the autonomic nervous system**

7ᵂ T44.906 Underdosing **of unspecified drugs primarily affecting the autonomic nervous system**

6ᵂ T44.99 **Poisoning by, adverse effect of and underdosing of** other **drugs primarily affecting the autonomic nervous system**

Unspecified Code	Other Specified Code	N Newborn Age: 0	P Pediatric Age: 0-17	M Maternity Age: 12-55	
A Adult Age: 15-124	♂ Male	♀ Female	● New Code	▲ Revised Code Title	►◄ Revised Text

⑦ **T44.991 Poisoning by other drug primarily affecting the autonomic nervous system, accidental (unintentional)**
Poisoning by other drugs primarily affecting the autonomic nervous system NOS

⑦ **T44.992 Poisoning by other drug primarily affecting the autonomic nervous system, intentional self-harm**

⑦ **T44.993 Poisoning by other drug primarily affecting the autonomic nervous system, assault**

⑦ **T44.994 Poisoning by other drug primarily affecting the autonomic nervous system, undetermined**

⑦ **T44.995 Adverse effect of other drug primarily affecting the autonomic nervous system**

⑦ **T44.996 Underdosing of other drug primarily affecting the autonomic nervous system**

④ **T45 Poisoning by, adverse effect of and underdosing of primarily systemic and hematological agents, not elsewhere classified**

The appropriate 7th character is to be added to each code from category T45
A = initial encounter
D = subsequent encounter
S = sequela

⑤ **T45.0 Poisoning by, adverse effect of and underdosing of antiallergic and antiemetic drugs**

> EXCLUDES1 *poisoning by, adverse effect of and underdosing of phenothiazine-based neuroleptics (T43.3)*

⑥ **T45.0X Poisoning by, adverse effect of and underdosing of antiallergic and antiemetic drugs**

⑦ **T45.0X1 Poisoning by antiallergic and antiemetic drugs, accidental (unintentional)**
Poisoning by antiallergic and antiemetic drugs NOS

⑦ **T45.0X2 Poisoning by antiallergic and antiemetic drugs, intentional self-harm**

⑦ **T45.0X3 Poisoning by antiallergic and antiemetic drugs, assault**

⑦ **T45.0X4 Poisoning by antiallergic and antiemetic drugs, undetermined**

⑦ **T45.0X5 Adverse effect of antiallergic and antiemetic drugs**

⑦ **T45.0X6 Underdosing of antiallergic and antiemetic drugs**

⑤ **T45.1 Poisoning by, adverse effect of and underdosing of antineoplastic and immunosuppressive drugs**

> EXCLUDES1 *poisoning by, adverse effect of and underdosing of tamoxifen (T38.6)*

⑥ **T45.1X Poisoning by, adverse effect of and underdosing of antineoplastic and immunosuppressive drugs**

⑦ **T45.1X1 Poisoning by antineoplastic and immunosuppressive drugs, accidental (unintentional)**
Poisoning by antineoplastic and immunosuppressive drugs NOS

⑦ **T45.1X2 Poisoning by antineoplastic and immunosuppressive drugs, intentional self-harm**

⑦ **T45.1X3 Poisoning by antineoplastic and immunosuppressive drugs, assault**

⑦ **T45.1X4 Poisoning by antineoplastic and immunosuppressive drugs, undetermined**

⑦ **T45.1X5 Adverse effect of antineoplastic and immunosuppressive drugs**

⑦ **T45.1X6 Underdosing of antineoplastic and immunosuppressive drugs**

⑤ **T45.2 Poisoning by, adverse effect of and underdosing of vitamins**

> EXCLUDES2 *poisoning by, adverse effect of and underdosing of nicotinic acid (derivatives) (T46.7)*

poisoning by, adverse effect of and underdosing of iron (T45.4)
poisoning by, adverse effect of and underdosing of vitamin K (T45.7)

⑥ **T45.2X Poisoning by, adverse effect of and underdosing of vitamins**

⑦ **T45.2X1 Poisoning by vitamins, accidental (unintentional)**
Poisoning by vitamins NOS

⑦ **T45.2X2 Poisoning by vitamins, intentional self-harm**

⑦ **T45.2X3 Poisoning by vitamins, assault**

⑦ **T45.2X4 Poisoning by vitamins, undetermined**

⑦ **T45.2X5 Adverse effect of vitamins**

⑦ **T45.2X6 Underdosing of vitamins**

> EXCLUDES1 *vitamin deficiencies (E50-E56)*

⑤ **T45.3 Poisoning by, adverse effect of and underdosing of enzymes**

⑥ **T45.3X Poisoning by, adverse effect of and underdosing of enzymes**

⑦ **T45.3X1 Poisoning by enzymes, accidental (unintentional)**
Poisoning by enzymes NOS

⑦ **T45.3X2 Poisoning by enzymes, intentional self-harm**

⑦ **T45.3X3 Poisoning by enzymes, assault**

⑦ **T45.3X4 Poisoning by enzymes, undetermined**

⑦ **T45.3X5 Adverse effect of enzymes**

⑦ **T45.3X6 Underdosing of enzymes**

⑤ **T45.4 Poisoning by, adverse effect of and underdosing of iron and its compounds**

⑥ **T45.4X Poisoning by, adverse effect of and underdosing of iron and its compounds**

⑦ **T45.4X1 Poisoning by iron and its compounds, accidental (unintentional)**
Poisoning by iron and its compounds NOS

⑦ **T45.4X2 Poisoning by iron and its compounds, intentional self-harm**

⑦ **T45.4X3 Poisoning by iron and its compounds, assault**

⑦ **T45.4X4 Poisoning by iron and its compounds, undetermined**

⑦ **T45.4X5 Adverse effect of iron and its compounds**

⑦ **T45.4X6 Underdosing of iron and its compounds**

> EXCLUDES1 *iron deficiency (E61.1)*

⑤ **T45.5 Poisoning by, adverse effect of and underdosing of anticoagulants and antithrombotic drugs**

⑥ **T45.51 Poisoning by, adverse effect of and underdosing of anticoagulants**

⑦ **T45.511 Poisoning by anticoagulants, accidental (unintentional)**
Poisoning by anticoagulants NOS

⑦ **T45.512 Poisoning by anticoagulants, intentional self-harm**

⑦ **T45.513 Poisoning by anticoagulants, assault**

⑦ **T45.514 Poisoning by anticoagulants, undetermined**

⑦ **T45.515 Adverse effect of anticoagulants**

⑦ **T45.516 Underdosing of anticoagulants**

⑥ **T45.52 Poisoning by, adverse effect of and underdosing of antithrombotic drugs**
Poisoning by, adverse effect of and underdosing of antiplatelet drugs

> EXCLUDES2 *poisoning by, adverse effect of and underdosing of aspirin (T39.01-)*
> *poisoning by, adverse effect of and underdosing of acetylsalicylic acid (T39.01-)*

⑦ **T45.521 Poisoning by antithrombotic drugs, accidental (unintentional)**
Poisoning by antithrombotic drug NOS

---

④ 4th character required   ⑤ 5th character required   ⑥ 6th character required   ⑦ 7th character required   ⓧ Extension 'X' Alert

EXCLUDES1 Not coded here   EXCLUDES2 Not included here   PDx Primary Diagnosis Only   Manifestation Code

7ᵈ T45.522 Poisoning by antithrombotic drugs, intentional self-harm

7ᵈ T45.523 Poisoning by antithrombotic drugs, assault

7ᵈ T45.524 Poisoning by antithrombotic drugs, undetermined

7ᵈ T45.525 Adverse effect of antithrombotic drugs

7ᵈ T45.526 Underdosing of antithrombotic drugs

5ᵈ T45.6 Poisoning by, adverse effect of and underdosing of fibrinolysis-affecting drugs

6ᵈ T45.60 Poisoning by, adverse effect of and underdosing of unspecified fibrinolysis-affecting drugs

7ᵈ T45.601 Poisoning by unspecified fibrinolysis-affecting drugs, accidental (unintentional)

Poisoning by fibrinolysis-affecting drug NOS

7ᵈ T45.602 Poisoning by unspecified fibrinolysis-affecting drugs, intentional self-harm

7ᵈ T45.603 Poisoning by unspecified fibrinolysis-affecting drugs, assault

7ᵈ T45.604 Poisoning by unspecified fibrinolysis-affecting drugs, undetermined

7ᵈ T45.605 Adverse effect of unspecified fibrinolysis-affecting drugs

7ᵈ T45.606 Underdosing of unspecified fibrinolysis-affecting drugs

6ᵈ T45.61 Poisoning by, adverse effect of and underdosing of thrombolytic drugs

7ᵈ T45.611 Poisoning by thrombolytic drug, accidental (unintentional)

Poisoning by thrombolytic drug NOS

7ᵈ T45.612 Poisoning by thrombolytic drug, intentional self-harm

7ᵈ T45.613 Poisoning by thrombolytic drug, assault

7ᵈ T45.614 Poisoning by thrombolytic drug, undetermined

7ᵈ T45.615 Adverse effect of thrombolytic drugs

7ᵈ T45.616 Underdosing of thrombolytic drugs

6ᵈ T45.62 Poisoning by, adverse effect of and underdosing of hemostatic drugs

7ᵈ T45.621 Poisoning by hemostatic drug, accidental (unintentional)

Poisoning by hemostatic drug NOS

7ᵈ T45.622 Poisoning by hemostatic drug, intentional self-harm

7ᵈ T45.623 Poisoning by hemostatic drug, assault

7ᵈ T45.624 Poisoning by hemostatic drug, undetermined

7ᵈ T45.625 Adverse effect of hemostatic drug

7ᵈ T45.626 Underdosing of hemostatic drugs

6ᵈ T45.69 Poisoning by, adverse effect of and underdosing of other fibrinolysis-affecting drugs

7ᵈ T45.691 Poisoning by other fibrinolysis-affecting drugs, accidental (unintentional)

Poisoning by other fibrinolysis-affecting drug NOS

7ᵈ T45.692 Poisoning by other fibrinolysis-affecting drugs, intentional self-harm

7ᵈ T45.693 Poisoning by other fibrinolysis-affecting drugs, assault

7ᵈ T45.694 Poisoning by other fibrinolysis-affecting drugs, undetermined

7ᵈ T45.695 Adverse effect of other fibrinolysis-affecting drugs

7ᵈ T45.696 Underdosing of other fibrinolysis-affecting drugs

5ᵈ T45.7 Poisoning by, adverse effect of and underdosing of anticoagulant antagonists, vitamin K and other coagulants

6ᵈ T45.7X Poisoning by, adverse effect of and underdosing of anticoagulant antagonists, vitamin K and other coagulants

7ᵈ T45.7X1 Poisoning by anticoagulant antagonists, vitamin K and other coagulants, accidental (unintentional)

Poisoning by anticoagulant antagonists, vitamin K and other coagulants NOS

7ᵈ T45.7X2 Poisoning by anticoagulant antagonists, vitamin K and other coagulants, intentional self-harm

7ᵈ T45.7X3 Poisoning by anticoagulant antagonists, vitamin K and other coagulants, assault

7ᵈ T45.7X4 Poisoning by anticoagulant antagonists, vitamin K and other coagulants, undetermined

7ᵈ T45.7X5 Adverse effect of anticoagulant antagonists, vitamin K and other coagulants

7ᵈ T45.7X6 Underdosing of anticoagulant antagonist, vitamin K and other coagulants

EXCLUDES1 vitamin K deficiency (E56.1)

5ᵈ T45.8 Poisoning by, adverse effect of and underdosing of other primarily systemic and hematological agents

Poisoning by, adverse effect of and underdosing of liver preparations and other antianemic agents

Poisoning by, adverse effect of and underdosing of natural blood and blood products

Poisoning by, adverse effect of and underdosing of plasma substitute

EXCLUDES2 poisoning by, adverse effect of and underdosing of immunoglobulin (T50.Z1)
poisoning by, adverse effect of and underdosing of iron (T45.4)
transfusion reactions (T80.-)

6ᵈ T45.8X Poisoning by, adverse effect of and underdosing of other primarily systemic and hematological agents

7ᵈ T45.8X1 Poisoning by other primarily systemic and hematological agents, accidental (unintentional)

Poisoning by other primarily systemic and hematological agents NOS

7ᵈ T45.8X2 Poisoning by other primarily systemic and hematological agents, intentional self-harm

7ᵈ T45.8X3 Poisoning by other primarily systemic and hematological agents, assault

7ᵈ T45.8X4 Poisoning by other primarily systemic and hematological agents, undetermined

7ᵈ T45.8X5 Adverse effect of other primarily systemic and hematological agents

7ᵈ T45.8X6 Underdosing of other primarily systemic and hematological agents

5ᵈ T45.9 Poisoning by, adverse effect of and underdosing of unspecified primarily systemic and hematological agent

7ᵈ T45.91 Poisoning by unspecified primarily systemic and hematological agent, accidental (unintentional)

Poisoning by primarily systemic and hematological agent NOS

7ᵈ T45.92 Poisoning by unspecified primarily systemic and hematological agent, intentional self-harm

7ᵈ T45.93 Poisoning by unspecified primarily systemic and hematological agent, assault

7ᵈ T45.94 Poisoning by unspecified primarily systemic and hematological agent, undetermined

7ᵈ T45.95 Adverse effect of unspecified primarily systemic and hematological agent

7ᵈ T45.96 Underdosing of unspecified primarily systemic and hematological agent

Unspecified Code	Other Specified Code	N Newborn Age: 0	P Pediatric Age: 0-17	M Maternity Age: 12-55
A Adult Age: 15-124	♂ Male	♀ Female	● New Code	▲ Revised Code Title	►◄ Revised Text

④ T46 **Poisoning by, adverse effect of and underdosing of agents primarily affecting the cardiovascular system**

> *EXCLUDES1* *poisoning by, adverse effect of and underdosing of metaraminol (T44.4)*

> **The appropriate 7th character is to be added to each code from category T46**
> **A = initial encounter**
> **D = subsequent encounter**
> **S = sequela**

⑤ T46.0 **Poisoning by, adverse effect of and underdosing of cardiac-stimulant glycosides and drugs of similar action**

⑥ T46.0X **Poisoning by, adverse effect of and underdosing of** cardiac-stimulant glycosides **and drugs of similar action**

⑦ T46.0X1 **Poisoning by cardiac-stimulant glycosides and drugs of similar action,** accidental **(unintentional)**

Poisoning by cardiac-stimulant glycosides and drugs of similar action NOS

⑦ T46.0X2 **Poisoning by cardiac-stimulant glycosides and drugs of similar action,** intentional self-harm

⑦ T46.0X3 **Poisoning by cardiac-stimulant glycosides and drugs of similar action,** assault

⑦ T46.0X4 **Poisoning by cardiac-stimulant glycosides and drugs of similar action,** undetermined

⑦ T46.0X5 Adverse effect **of cardiac-stimulant glycosides and drugs of similar action**

⑦ T46.0X6 Underdosing **of cardiac-stimulant glycosides and drugs of similar action**

⑤ T46.1 **Poisoning by, adverse effect of and underdosing of** calcium-channel blockers

⑥ T46.1X **Poisoning by, adverse effect of and underdosing of calcium-channel blockers**

⑦ T46.1X1 **Poisoning by calcium-channel blockers,** accidental **(unintentional)**

Poisoning by calcium-channel blockers NOS

⑦ T46.1X2 **Poisoning by calcium-channel blockers,** intentional self-harm

⑦ T46.1X3 **Poisoning by calcium-channel blockers,** assault

⑦ T46.1X4 **Poisoning by calcium-channel blockers,** undetermined

⑦ T46.1X5 Adverse effect **of calcium-channel blockers**

⑦ T46.1X6 Underdosing **of calcium-channel blockers**

⑤ T46.2 **Poisoning by, adverse effect of and underdosing of other antidysrhythmic drugs, not elsewhere classified**

> *EXCLUDES1* *poisoning by, adverse effect of and underdosing of beta-adrenoreceptor antagonists (T44.7-)*

⑥ T46.2X **Poisoning by, adverse effect of and underdosing of** other antidysrhythmic **drugs**

⑦ T46.2X1 **Poisoning by other antidysrhythmic drugs,** accidental **(unintentional)**

Poisoning by other antidysrhythmic drugs NOS

⑦ T46.2X2 **Poisoning by other antidysrhythmic drugs,** intentional self-harm

⑦ T46.2X3 **Poisoning by other antidysrhythmic drugs,** assault

⑦ T46.2X4 **Poisoning by other antidysrhythmic drugs,** undetermined

⑦ T46.2X5 Adverse effect **of other antidysrhythmic drugs**

⑦ T46.2X6 Underdosing **of other antidysrhythmic drugs**

⑤ T46.3 **Poisoning by, adverse effect of and underdosing of coronary vasodilators**

Poisoning by, adverse effect of and underdosing of dipyridamole

> *EXCLUDES1* *poisoning by, adverse effect of and underdosing of calcium-channel blockers (T46.1)*

⑥ T46.3X **Poisoning by, adverse effect of and underdosing of** coronary vasodilators

⑦ T46.3X1 **Poisoning by coronary vasodilators,** accidental **(unintentional)**

Poisoning by coronary vasodilators NOS

⑦ T46.3X2 **Poisoning by coronary vasodilators,** intentional self-harm

⑦ T46.3X3 **Poisoning by coronary vasodilators,** assault

⑦ T46.3X4 **Poisoning by coronary vasodilators,** undetermined

⑦ T46.3X5 Adverse effect **of coronary vasodilators**

⑦ T46.3X6 Underdosing **of coronary vasodilators**

⑤ T46.4 **Poisoning by, adverse effect of and underdosing of angiotensin-converting-enzyme inhibitors**

⑥ T46.4X **Poisoning by, adverse effect of and underdosing of** angiotensin-converting-enzyme inhibitors

⑦ T46.4X1 **Poisoning by angiotensin-converting-enzyme inhibitors,** accidental **(unintentional)**

Poisoning by angiotensin-converting-enzyme inhibitors NOS

⑦ T46.4X2 **Poisoning by angiotensin-converting-enzyme inhibitors,** intentional self-harm

⑦ T46.4X3 **Poisoning by angiotensin-converting-enzyme inhibitors,** assault

⑦ T46.4X4 **Poisoning by angiotensin-converting-enzyme inhibitors,** undetermined

⑦ T46.4X5 Adverse effect **of angiotensin-converting-enzyme inhibitors**

⑦ T46.4X6 Underdosing **of angiotensin-converting-enzyme inhibitors**

⑤ T46.5 **Poisoning by, adverse effect of and underdosing of other antihypertensive drugs**

> *EXCLUDES2* *poisoning by, adverse effect of and underdosing of beta-adrenoreceptor antagonists (T44.7)*
> *poisoning by, adverse effect of and underdosing of calcium-channel blockers (T46.1)*
> *poisoning by, adverse effect of and underdosing of diuretics (T50.0-T50.2)*

⑥ T46.5X **Poisoning by, adverse effect of and underdosing of** other antihypertensive **drugs**

⑦ T46.5X1 **Poisoning by other antihypertensive drugs, accidental (unintentional)**

Poisoning by other antihypertensive drugs NOS

⑦ T46.5X2 **Poisoning by other antihypertensive drugs,** intentional self-harm

⑦ T46.5X3 **Poisoning by other antihypertensive drugs,** assault

⑦ T46.5X4 **Poisoning by other antihypertensive drugs,** undetermined

⑦ T46.5X5 Adverse effect **of other antihypertensive drugs**

⑦ T46.5X6 Underdosing **of other antihypertensive drugs**

⑤ T46.6 **Poisoning by, adverse effect of and underdosing of antihyperlipidemic and antiarteriosclerotic drugs**

⑥ T46.6X **Poisoning by, adverse effect of and underdosing of** antihyperlipidemic and antiarteriosclerotic drugs

⑦ T46.6X1 **Poisoning by antihyperlipidemic and antiarteriosclerotic drugs,** accidental **(unintentional)**

Poisoning by antihyperlipidemic and antiarteriosclerotic drugs NOS

---

④ 4ᵗʰ character required   ⑤ 5ᵗʰ character required   ⑥ 6ᵗʰ character required   ⑦ 7ᵗʰ character required   ⓧ Extension 'X' Alert

EXCLUDES 1 Not coded here   *EXCLUDES 2* Not included here   PDx Primary Diagnosis Only   Manifestation Code

7️⃣ **T46.6X2** Poisoning by antihyperlipidemic and antiarteriosclerotic drugs, intentional self-harm

7️⃣ **T46.6X3** Poisoning by antihyperlipidemic and antiarteriosclerotic drugs, assault

7️⃣ **T46.6X4** Poisoning by antihyperlipidemic and antiarteriosclerotic drugs, undetermined

7️⃣ **T46.6X5** Adverse effect of antihyperlipidemic and antiarteriosclerotic drugs

7️⃣ **T46.6X6** Underdosing of antihyperlipidemic and antiarteriosclerotic drugs

5️⃣ **T46.7** Poisoning by, adverse effect of and underdosing of peripheral vasodilators

Poisoning by, adverse effect of and underdosing of nicotinic acid (derivatives)

EXCLUDES1 poisoning by, adverse effect of and underdosing of papaverine (T44.3)

6️⃣ **T46.7X** Poisoning by, adverse effect of and underdosing of peripheral vasodilators

7️⃣ **T46.7X1** Poisoning by peripheral vasodilators, accidental (unintentional)

Poisoning by peripheral vasodilators NOS

7️⃣ **T46.7X2** Poisoning by peripheral vasodilators, intentional self-harm

7️⃣ **T46.7X3** Poisoning by peripheral vasodilators, assault

7️⃣ **T46.7X4** Poisoning by peripheral vasodilators, undetermined

7️⃣ **T46.7X5** Adverse effect of peripheral vasodilators

7️⃣ **T46.7X6** Underdosing of peripheral vasodilators

5️⃣ **T46.8** Poisoning by, adverse effect of and underdosing of antivaricose drugs, including sclerosing agents

6️⃣ **T46.8X** Poisoning by, adverse effect of and underdosing of antivaricose drugs, including sclerosing agents

7️⃣ **T46.8X1** Poisoning by antivaricose drugs, including sclerosing agents, accidental (unintentional)

Poisoning by antivaricose drugs, including sclerosing agents NOS

7️⃣ **T46.8X2** Poisoning by antivaricose drugs, including sclerosing agents, intentional self-harm

7️⃣ **T46.8X3** Poisoning by antivaricose drugs, including sclerosing agents, assault

7️⃣ **T46.8X4** Poisoning by antivaricose drugs, including sclerosing agents, undetermined

7️⃣ **T46.8X5** Adverse effect of antivaricose drugs, including sclerosing agents

7️⃣ **T46.8X6** Underdosing of antivaricose drugs, including sclerosing agents

5️⃣ **T46.9** Poisoning by, adverse effect of and underdosing of other and unspecified agents primarily affecting the cardiovascular system

6️⃣ **T46.90** Poisoning by, adverse effect of and underdosing of unspecified agents primarily affecting the cardiovascular system

7️⃣ **T46.901** Poisoning by unspecified agents primarily affecting the cardiovascular system, accidental (unintentional)

7️⃣ **T46.902** Poisoning by unspecified agents primarily affecting the cardiovascular system, intentional self-harm

7️⃣ **T46.903** Poisoning by unspecified agents primarily affecting the cardiovascular system, assault

7️⃣ **T46.904** Poisoning by unspecified agents primarily affecting the cardiovascular system, undetermined

7️⃣ **T46.905** Adverse effect of unspecified agents primarily affecting the cardiovascular system

7️⃣ **T46.906** Underdosing of unspecified agents primarily affecting the cardiovascular system

6️⃣ **T46.99** Poisoning by, adverse effect of and underdosing of other agents primarily affecting the cardiovascular system

7️⃣ **T46.991** Poisoning by other agents primarily affecting the cardiovascular system, accidental (unintentional)

7️⃣ **T46.992** Poisoning by other agents primarily affecting the cardiovascular system, intentional self-harm

7️⃣ **T46.993** Poisoning by other agents primarily affecting the cardiovascular system, assault

7️⃣ **T46.994** Poisoning by other agents primarily affecting the cardiovascular system, undetermined

7️⃣ **T46.995** Adverse effect of other agents primarily affecting the cardiovascular system

7️⃣ **T46.996** Underdosing of other agents primarily affecting the cardiovascular system

4️⃣ **T47** Poisoning by, adverse effect of and underdosing of agents primarily affecting the gastrointestinal system

The appropriate 7th character is to be added to each code from category T47
A = initial encounter
D = subsequent encounter
S = sequela

5️⃣ **T47.0** Poisoning by, adverse effect of and underdosing of histamine H2-receptor blockers

6️⃣ **T47.0X** Poisoning by, adverse effect of and underdosing of histamine H2-receptor blockers

7️⃣ **T47.0X1** Poisoning by histamine H2-receptor blockers, accidental (unintentional)

Poisoning by histamine H2-receptor blockers NOS

7️⃣ **T47.0X2** Poisoning by histamine H2-receptor blockers, intentional self-harm

7️⃣ **T47.0X3** Poisoning by histamine H2-receptor blockers, assault

7️⃣ **T47.0X4** Poisoning by histamine H2-receptor blockers, undetermined

7️⃣ **T47.0X5** Adverse effect of histamine H2-receptor blockers

7️⃣ **T47.0X6** Underdosing of histamine H2-receptor blockers

5️⃣ **T47.1** Poisoning by, adverse effect of and underdosing of other antacids and anti-gastric-secretion drugs

6️⃣ **T47.1X** Poisoning by, adverse effect of and underdosing of other antacids and anti-gastric-secretion drugs

7️⃣ **T47.1X1** Poisoning by other antacids and anti-gastric-secretion drugs, accidental (unintentional)

Poisoning by other antacids and anti-gastric-secretion drugs NOS

7️⃣ **T47.1X2** Poisoning by other antacids and anti-gastric-secretion drugs, intentional self-harm

7️⃣ **T47.1X3** Poisoning by other antacids and anti-gastric-secretion drugs, assault

7️⃣ **T47.1X4** Poisoning by other antacids and anti-gastric-secretion drugs, undetermined

7️⃣ **T47.1X5** Adverse effect of other antacids and anti-gastric-secretion drugs

7️⃣ **T47.1X6** Underdosing of other antacids and anti-gastric-secretion drugs

5️⃣ **T47.2** Poisoning by, adverse effect of and underdosing of stimulant laxatives

T47.2X Poisoning by, adverse effect of and underdosing of stimulant laxatives
- T47.2X1 Poisoning by stimulant laxatives, accidental (unintentional)
  Poisoning by stimulant laxatives NOS
- T47.2X2 Poisoning by stimulant laxatives, intentional self-harm
- T47.2X3 Poisoning by stimulant laxatives, assault
- T47.2X4 Poisoning by stimulant laxatives, undetermined
- T47.2X5 Adverse effect of stimulant laxatives
- T47.2X6 Underdosing of stimulant laxatives

T47.3 Poisoning by, adverse effect of and underdosing of saline and osmotic laxatives
- T47.3X Poisoning by and adverse effect of saline and osmotic laxatives
  - T47.3X1 Poisoning by saline and osmotic laxatives, accidental (unintentional)
    Poisoning by saline and osmotic laxatives NOS
  - T47.3X2 Poisoning by saline and osmotic laxatives, intentional self-harm
  - T47.3X3 Poisoning by saline and osmotic laxatives, assault
  - T47.3X4 Poisoning by saline and osmotic laxatives, undetermined
  - T47.3X5 Adverse effect of saline and osmotic laxatives
  - T47.3X6 Underdosing of saline and osmotic laxatives

T47.4 Poisoning by, adverse effect of and underdosing of other laxatives
- T47.4X Poisoning by, adverse effect of and underdosing of other laxatives
  - T47.4X1 Poisoning by other laxatives, accidental (unintentional)
    Poisoning by other laxatives NOS
  - T47.4X2 Poisoning by other laxatives, intentional self-harm
  - T47.4X3 Poisoning by other laxatives, assault
  - T47.4X4 Poisoning by other laxatives, undetermined
  - T47.4X5 Adverse effect of other laxatives
  - T47.4X6 Underdosing of other laxatives

T47.5 Poisoning by, adverse effect of and underdosing of digestants
- T47.5X Poisoning by, adverse effect of and underdosing of digestants
  - T47.5X1 Poisoning by digestants, accidental (unintentional)
    Poisoning by digestants NOS
  - T47.5X2 Poisoning by digestants, intentional self-harm
  - T47.5X3 Poisoning by digestants, assault
  - T47.5X4 Poisoning by digestants, undetermined
  - T47.5X5 Adverse effect of digestants
  - T47.5X6 Underdosing of digestants

T47.6 Poisoning by, adverse effect of and underdosing of antidiarrheal drugs
  EXCLUDES2 poisoning by, adverse effect of and underdosing of systemic antibiotics and other anti-infectives (T36-T37)
- T47.6X Poisoning by, adverse effect of and underdosing of antidiarrheal drugs
  - T47.6X1 Poisoning by antidiarrheal drugs, accidental (unintentional)
    Poisoning by antidiarrheal drugs NOS
  - T47.6X2 Poisoning by antidiarrheal drugs, intentional self-harm
  - T47.6X3 Poisoning by antidiarrheal drugs, assault
  - T47.6X4 Poisoning by antidiarrheal drugs, undetermined
  - T47.6X5 Adverse effect of antidiarrheal drugs
  - T47.6X6 Underdosing of antidiarrheal drugs

T47.7 Poisoning by, adverse effect of and underdosing of emetics
- T47.7X Poisoning by, adverse effect of and underdosing of emetics
  - T47.7X1 Poisoning by emetics, accidental (unintentional)
    Poisoning by emetics NOS
  - T47.7X2 Poisoning by emetics, intentional self-harm
  - T47.7X3 Poisoning by emetics, assault
  - T47.7X4 Poisoning by emetics, undetermined
  - T47.7X5 Adverse effect of emetics
  - T47.7X6 Underdosing of emetics

T47.8 Poisoning by, adverse effect of and underdosing of other agents primarily affecting gastrointestinal system
- T47.8X Poisoning by, adverse effect of and underdosing of other agents primarily affecting gastrointestinal system
  - T47.8X1 Poisoning by other agents primarily affecting gastrointestinal system, accidental (unintentional)
    Poisoning by other agents primarily affecting gastrointestinal system NOS
  - T47.8X2 Poisoning by other agents primarily affecting gastrointestinal system, intentional self-harm
  - T47.8X3 Poisoning by other agents primarily affecting gastrointestinal system, assault
  - T47.8X4 Poisoning by other agents primarily affecting gastrointestinal system, undetermined
  - T47.8X5 Adverse effect of other agents primarily affecting gastrointestinal system
  - T47.8X6 Underdosing of other agents primarily affecting gastrointestinal system

T47.9 Poisoning by, adverse effect of and underdosing of unspecified agents primarily affecting the gastrointestinal system
- T47.91 Poisoning by unspecified agents primarily affecting the gastrointestinal system, accidental (unintentional)
  Poisoning by agents primarily affecting the gastrointestinal system NOS
- T47.92 Poisoning by unspecified agents primarily affecting the gastrointestinal system, intentional self-harm
- T47.93 Poisoning by unspecified agents primarily affecting the gastrointestinal system, assault
- T47.94 Poisoning by unspecified agents primarily affecting the gastrointestinal system, undetermined
- T47.95 Adverse effect of unspecified agents primarily affecting the gastrointestinal system
- T47.96 Underdosing of unspecified agents primarily affecting the gastrointestinal system

T48 Poisoning by, adverse effect of and underdosing of agents primarily acting on smooth and skeletal muscles and the respiratory system

The appropriate 7th character is to be added to each code from category T48
A = initial encounter
D = subsequent encounter
S = sequela

4th character required   5th character required   6th character required   7th character required   Extension 'X' Alert

EXCLUDES1 Not coded here   EXCLUDES2 Not included here   PDx Primary Diagnosis Only   Manifestation Code

T48.0 **Poisoning by, adverse effect of and underdosing of oxytocic drugs**

EXCLUDES1 *poisoning by, adverse effect of and underdosing of estrogens, progestogens and antagonists (T38.4-T38.6)*

T48.0X **Poisoning by, adverse effect of and underdosing of oxytocic drugs**

T48.0X1 **Poisoning by oxytocic drugs, accidental (unintentional)**

Poisoning by oxytocic drugs NOS

T48.0X2 **Poisoning by oxytocic drugs, intentional self-harm**

T48.0X3 **Poisoning by oxytocic drugs, assault**

T48.0X4 **Poisoning by oxytocic drugs, undetermined**

T48.0X5 Adverse effect of oxytocic drugs

T48.0X6 Underdosing of oxytocic drugs

T48.1 **Poisoning by, adverse effect of and underdosing of skeletal muscle relaxants [neuromuscular blocking agents]**

T48.1X **Poisoning by, adverse effect of and underdosing of skeletal muscle relaxants [neuromuscular blocking agents]**

T48.1X1 **Poisoning by skeletal muscle relaxants [neuromuscular blocking agents], accidental (unintentional)**

Poisoning by skeletal muscle relaxants [neuromuscular blocking agents] NOS

T48.1X2 **Poisoning by skeletal muscle relaxants [neuromuscular blocking agents], intentional self-harm**

T48.1X3 **Poisoning by skeletal muscle relaxants [neuromuscular blocking agents], assault**

T48.1X4 **Poisoning by skeletal muscle relaxants [neuromuscular blocking agents], undetermined**

T48.1X5 Adverse effect of skeletal muscle relaxants [neuromuscular blocking agents]

T48.1X6 Underdosing of skeletal muscle relaxants [neuromuscular blocking agents]

T48.2 **Poisoning by, adverse effect of and underdosing of other and unspecified drugs acting on muscles**

T48.20 **Poisoning by, adverse effect of and underdosing of unspecified drugs acting on muscles**

T48.201 **Poisoning by unspecified drugs acting on muscles, accidental (unintentional)**

Poisoning by unspecified drugs acting on muscles NOS

T48.202 **Poisoning by unspecified drugs acting on muscles, intentional self-harm**

T48.203 **Poisoning by unspecified drugs acting on muscles, assault**

T48.204 **Poisoning by unspecified drugs acting on muscles, undetermined**

T48.205 Adverse effect of unspecified drugs acting on muscles

T48.206 Underdosing of unspecified drugs acting on muscles

T48.29 **Poisoning by, adverse effect of and underdosing of other drugs acting on muscles**

T48.291 **Poisoning by other drugs acting on muscles, accidental (unintentional)**

Poisoning by other drugs acting on muscles NOS

T48.292 **Poisoning by other drugs acting on muscles, intentional self-harm**

T48.293 **Poisoning by other drugs acting on muscles, assault**

T48.294 **Poisoning by other drugs acting on muscles, undetermined**

T48.295 Adverse effect of other drugs acting on muscles

T48.296 Underdosing of other drugs acting on muscles

T48.3 **Poisoning by, adverse effect of and underdosing of antitussives**

T48.3X **Poisoning by, adverse effect of and underdosing of antitussives**

T48.3X1 **Poisoning by antitussives, accidental (unintentional)**

Poisoning by antitussives NOS

T48.3X2 **Poisoning by antitussives, intentional self-harm**

T48.3X3 **Poisoning by antitussives, assault**

T48.3X4 **Poisoning by antitussives, undetermined**

T48.3X5 Adverse effect of antitussives

T48.3X6 Underdosing of antitussives

T48.4 **Poisoning by, adverse effect of and underdosing of expectorants**

T48.4X **Poisoning by, adverse effect of and underdosing of expectorants**

T48.4X1 **Poisoning by expectorants, accidental (unintentional)**

Poisoning by expectorants NOS

T48.4X2 **Poisoning by expectorants, intentional self-harm**

T48.4X3 **Poisoning by expectorants, assault**

T48.4X4 **Poisoning by expectorants, undetermined**

T48.4X5 Adverse effect of expectorants

T48.4X6 Underdosing of expectorants

T48.5 **Poisoning by, adverse effect of and underdosing of other anti-common-cold drugs**

Poisoning by, adverse effect of and underdosing of decongestants

EXCLUDES2 *poisoning by, adverse effect of and underdosing of antipyretics, NEC (T39.9-)*
poisoning by, adverse effect of and underdosing of non-steroidal antiinflammatory drugs (T39.3-)
poisoning by, adverse effect of and underdosing of salicylates (T39.0-)

T48.5X **Poisoning by, adverse effect of and underdosing of other anti-common-cold drugs**

T48.5X1 **Poisoning by other anti-common-cold drugs, accidental (unintentional)**

Poisoning by other anti-common-cold drugs NOS

T48.5X2 **Poisoning by other anti-common-cold drugs, intentional self-harm**

T48.5X3 **Poisoning by other anti-common-cold drugs, assault**

T48.5X4 **Poisoning by other anti-common-cold drugs, undetermined**

T48.5X5 Adverse effect of other anti-common-cold drugs

T48.5X6 Underdosing of other anti-common-cold drugs

T48.6 **Poisoning by, adverse effect of and underdosing of antiasthmatics, not elsewhere classified**

Poisoning by, adverse effect of and underdosing of beta-adrenoreceptor agonists used in asthma therapy

EXCLUDES1 *poisoning by, adverse effect of and underdosing of beta-adrenoreceptor agonists not used in asthma therapy (T44.5)*
poisoning by, adverse effect of and underdosing of anterior pituitary [adenohypophyseal] hormones (T38.8)

T48.6X **Poisoning by, adverse effect of and underdosing of antiasthmatics**

Unspecified Code Other Specified Code N Newborn Age: 0 P Pediatric Age: 0-17 M Maternity Age: 12-55
A Adult Age: 15-124 ♂ Male ♀ Female ● New Code ▲ Revised Code Title ►◄ Revised Text

ICD-10-CM 2015 701

T48.6X1 Poisoning by antiasthmatics, accidental (unintentional)

Poisoning by antiasthmatics NOS

T48.6X2 Poisoning by antiasthmatics, intentional self-harm

T48.6X3 Poisoning by antiasthmatics, assault

T48.6X4 Poisoning by antiasthmatics, undetermined

T48.6X5 Adverse effect of antiasthmatics

T48.6X6 Underdosing of antiasthmatics

T48.9 Poisoning by, adverse effect of and underdosing of other and unspecified agents primarily acting on the respiratory system

T48.90 Poisoning by, adverse effect of and underdosing of unspecified agents primarily acting on the respiratory system

T48.901 Poisoning by unspecified agents primarily acting on the respiratory system, accidental (unintentional)

T48.902 Poisoning by unspecified agents primarily acting on the respiratory system, intentional self-harm

T48.903 Poisoning by unspecified agents primarily acting on the respiratory system, assault

T48.904 Poisoning by unspecified agents primarily acting on the respiratory system, undetermined

T48.905 Adverse effect of unspecified agents primarily acting on the respiratory system

T48.906 Underdosing of unspecified agents primarily acting on the respiratory system

T48.99 Poisoning by, adverse effect of and underdosing of other agents primarily acting on the respiratory system

T48.991 Poisoning by other agents primarily acting on the respiratory system, accidental (unintentional)

T48.992 Poisoning by other agents primarily acting on the respiratory system, intentional self-harm

T48.993 Poisoning by other agents primarily acting on the respiratory system, assault

T48.994 Poisoning by other agents primarily acting on the respiratory system, undetermined

T48.995 Adverse effect of other agents primarily acting on the respiratory system

T48.996 Underdosing of other agents primarily acting on the respiratory system

T49 Poisoning by, adverse effect of and underdosing of topical agents primarily affecting skin and mucous membrane and by ophthalmological, otorhinorlaryngological and dental drugs

INCLUDES   poisoning by, adverse effect of and underdosing of glucocorticoids, topically used

The appropriate 7th character is to be added to each code from category T49
A = initial encounter
D = subsequent encounter
S = sequela

T49.0 Poisoning by, adverse effect of and underdosing of local antifungal, anti-infective and anti-inflammatory drugs

T49.0X Poisoning by, adverse effect of and underdosing of local antifungal, anti-infective and anti-inflammatory drugs

T49.0X1 Poisoning by local antifungal, anti-infective and anti-inflammatory drugs, accidental (unintentional)

Poisoning by local antifungal, anti-infective and anti-inflammatory drugs NOS

T49.0X2 Poisoning by local antifungal, anti-infective and anti-inflammatory drugs, intentional self-harm

T49.0X3 Poisoning by local antifungal, anti-infective and anti-inflammatory drugs, assault

T49.0X4 Poisoning by local antifungal, anti-infective and anti-inflammatory drugs, undetermined

T49.0X5 Adverse effect of local antifungal, anti-infective and anti-inflammatory drugs

T49.0X6 Underdosing of local antifungal, anti-infective and anti-inflammatory drugs

T49.1 Poisoning by, adverse effect of and underdosing of antipruritics

T49.1X Poisoning by, adverse effect of and underdosing of antipruritics

T49.1X1 Poisoning by antipruritics, accidental (unintentional)

Poisoning by antipruritics NOS

T49.1X2 Poisoning by antipruritics, intentional self-harm

T49.1X3 Poisoning by antipruritics, assault

T49.1X4 Poisoning by antipruritics, undetermined

T49.1X5 Adverse effect of antipruritics

T49.1X6 Underdosing of antipruritics

T49.2 Poisoning by, adverse effect of and underdosing of local astringents and local detergents

T49.2X Poisoning by, adverse effect of and underdosing of local astringents and local detergents

T49.2X1 Poisoning by local astringents and local detergents, accidental (unintentional)

Poisoning by local astringents and local detergents NOS

T49.2X2 Poisoning by local astringents and local detergents, intentional self-harm

T49.2X3 Poisoning by local astringents and local detergents, assault

T49.2X4 Poisoning by local astringents and local detergents, undetermined

T49.2X5 Adverse effect of local astringents and local detergents

T49.2X6 Underdosing of local astringents and local detergents

T49.3 Poisoning by, adverse effect of and underdosing of emollients, demulcents and protectants

T49.3X Poisoning by, adverse effect of and underdosing of emollients, demulcents and protectants

T49.3X1 Poisoning by emollients, demulcents and protectants, accidental (unintentional)

Poisoning by emollients, demulcents and protectants NOS

T49.3X2 Poisoning by emollients, demulcents and protectants, intentional self-harm

T49.3X3 Poisoning by emollients, demulcents and protectants, assault

T49.3X4 Poisoning by emollients, demulcents and protectants, undetermined

T49.3X5 Adverse effect of emollients, demulcents and protectants

T49.3X6 Underdosing of emollients, demulcents and protectants

T49.4 Poisoning by, adverse effect of and underdosing of keratolytics, keratoplastics, and other hair treatment drugs and preparations

T49.4X Poisoning by, adverse effect of and underdosing of keratolytics, keratoplastics, and other hair treatment drugs and preparations

T49.4X1 Poisoning by keratolytics, keratoplastics, and other hair treatment drugs and preparations, accidental (unintentional)

Poisoning by keratolytics, keratoplastics, and other hair treatment drugs and preparations NOS

---

❹ 4ᵗʰ character required   ❺ 5ᵗʰ character required   ❻ 6ᵗʰ character required   ❼ 7ᵗʰ character required   ⓧ Extension 'X' Alert

EXCLUDES 1 Not coded here   **EXCLUDES 2** Not included here   ᴾᴰˣ Primary Diagnosis Only   Manifestation Code

702   **ICD-10-CM 2015**

7ᵗʰ T49.4X2 Poisoning by keratolytics, keratoplastics, and other hair treatment drugs and preparations, intentional self-harm
7ᵗʰ T49.4X3 Poisoning by keratolytics, keratoplastics, and other hair treatment drugs and preparations, assault
7ᵗʰ T49.4X4 Poisoning by keratolytics, keratoplastics, and other hair treatment drugs and preparations, undetermined
7ᵗʰ T49.4X5 Adverse effect of keratolytics, keratoplastics, and other hair treatment drugs and preparations
7ᵗʰ T49.4X6 Underdosing of keratolytics, keratoplastics, and other hair treatment drugs and preparations

5ᵗʰ T49.5 Poisoning by, adverse effect of and underdosing of ophthalmological drugs and preparations
6ᵗʰ T49.5X Poisoning by, adverse effect of and underdosing of ophthalmological drugs and preparations
7ᵗʰ T49.5X1 Poisoning by ophthalmological drugs and preparations, accidental (unintentional)
Poisoning by ophthalmological drugs and preparations NOS
7ᵗʰ T49.5X2 Poisoning by ophthalmological drugs and preparations, intentional self-harm
7ᵗʰ T49.5X3 Poisoning by ophthalmological drugs and preparations, assault
7ᵗʰ T49.5X4 Poisoning by ophthalmological drugs and preparations, undetermined
7ᵗʰ T49.5X5 Adverse effect of ophthalmological drugs and preparations
7ᵗʰ T49.5X6 Underdosing of ophthalmological drugs and preparations

5ᵗʰ T49.6 Poisoning by, adverse effect of and underdosing of otorhinolaryngological drugs and preparations
6ᵗʰ T49.6X Poisoning by, adverse effect of and underdosing of otorhinolaryngological drugs and preparations
7ᵗʰ T49.6X1 Poisoning by otorhinolaryngological drugs and preparations, accidental (unintentional)
Poisoning by otorhinolaryngological drugs and preparations NOS
7ᵗʰ T49.6X2 Poisoning by otorhinolaryngological drugs and preparations, intentional self-harm
7ᵗʰ T49.6X3 Poisoning by otorhinolaryngological drugs and preparations, assault
7ᵗʰ T49.6X4 Poisoning by otorhinolaryngological drugs and preparations, undetermined
7ᵗʰ T49.6X5 Adverse effect of otorhinolaryngological drugs and preparations
7ᵗʰ T49.6X6 Underdosing of otorhinolaryngological drugs and preparations

5ᵗʰ T49.7 Poisoning by, adverse effect of and underdosing of dental drugs, topically applied
6ᵗʰ T49.7X Poisoning by, adverse effect of and underdosing of dental drugs, topically applied
7ᵗʰ T49.7X1 Poisoning by dental drugs, topically applied, accidental (unintentional)
Poisoning by dental drugs, topically applied NOS
7ᵗʰ T49.7X2 Poisoning by dental drugs, topically applied, intentional self-harm
7ᵗʰ T49.7X3 Poisoning by dental drugs, topically applied, assault
7ᵗʰ T49.7X4 Poisoning by dental drugs, topically applied, undetermined
7ᵗʰ T49.7X5 Adverse effect of dental drugs, topically applied

7ᵗʰ T49.7X6 Underdosing of dental drugs, topically applied

5ᵗʰ T49.8 Poisoning by, adverse effect of and underdosing of other topical agents
Poisoning by, adverse effect of and underdosing of spermicides
6ᵗʰ T49.8X Poisoning by, adverse effect of and underdosing of other topical agents
7ᵗʰ T49.8X1 Poisoning by other topical agents, accidental (unintentional)
Poisoning by other topical agents NOS
7ᵗʰ T49.8X2 Poisoning by other topical agents, intentional self-harm
7ᵗʰ T49.8X3 Poisoning by other topical agents, assault
7ᵗʰ T49.8X4 Poisoning by other topical agents, undetermined
7ᵗʰ T49.8X5 Adverse effect of other topical agents
7ᵗʰ T49.8X6 Underdosing of other topical agents

5ᵗʰ T49.9 Poisoning by, adverse effect of and underdosing of unspecified topical agent
7ᵗʰ T49.91 Poisoning by unspecified topical agent, accidental (unintentional)
7ᵗʰ T49.92 Poisoning by unspecified topical agent, intentional self-harm
7ᵗʰ T49.93 Poisoning by unspecified topical agent, assault
7ᵗʰ T49.94 Poisoning by unspecified topical agent, undetermined
7ᵗʰ T49.95 Adverse effect of unspecified topical agent
7ᵗʰ T49.96 Underdosing of unspecified topical agent

4ᵗʰ T50 Poisoning by, adverse effect of and underdosing of diuretics and other and unspecified drugs, medicaments and biological substances

The appropriate 7th character is to be added to each code from category T50
A = initial encounter
D = subsequent encounter
S = sequela

5ᵗʰ T50.0 Poisoning by, adverse effect of and underdosing of mineralocorticoids and their antagonists
6ᵗʰ T50.0X Poisoning by, adverse effect of and underdosing of mineralocorticoids and their antagonists
7ᵗʰ T50.0X1 Poisoning by mineralocorticoids and their antagonists, accidental (unintentional)
Poisoning by mineralocorticoids and their antagonists NOS
7ᵗʰ T50.0X2 Poisoning by mineralocorticoids and their antagonists, intentional self-harm
7ᵗʰ T50.0X3 Poisoning by mineralocorticoids and their antagonists, assault
7ᵗʰ T50.0X4 Poisoning by mineralocorticoids and their antagonists, undetermined
7ᵗʰ T50.0X5 Adverse effect of mineralocorticoids and their antagonists
7ᵗʰ T50.0X6 Underdosing of mineralocorticoids and their antagonists

5ᵗʰ T50.1 Poisoning by, adverse effect of and underdosing of loop [high-ceiling] diuretics
6ᵗʰ T50.1X Poisoning by, adverse effect of and underdosing of loop [high-ceiling] diuretics
7ᵗʰ T50.1X1 Poisoning by loop [high-ceiling] diuretics, accidental (unintentional)
Poisoning by loop [high-ceiling] diuretics NOS
7ᵗʰ T50.1X2 Poisoning by loop [high-ceiling] diuretics, intentional self-harm
7ᵗʰ T50.1X3 Poisoning by loop [high-ceiling] diuretics, assault
7ᵗʰ T50.1X4 Poisoning by loop [high-ceiling] diuretics, undetermined

---

Unspecified Code   Other Specified Code   Ⓝ Newborn Age: 0   Ⓟ Pediatric Age: 0-17   Ⓜ Maternity Age: 12-55
Ⓐ Adult Age: 15-124   ♂ Male   ♀ Female   ● New Code   ▲ Revised Code Title   ►◄ Revised Text

T50.1X5 Adverse effect of loop [high-ceiling] diuretics

T50.1X6 Underdosing of loop [high-ceiling] diuretics

5ᵗʰ T50.2 Poisoning by, adverse effect of and underdosing of carbonic-anhydrase inhibitors, benzothiadiazides and other diuretics

Poisoning by, adverse effect of and underdosing of acetazolamide

6ᵗʰ T50.2X Poisoning by, adverse effect of and underdosing of carbonic-anhydrase inhibitors, benzothiadiazides and other diuretics

7ᵗʰ T50.2X1 Poisoning by carbonic-anhydrase inhibitors, benzothiadiazides and other diuretics, accidental (unintentional)

Poisoning by carbonic-anhydrase inhibitors, benzothiadiazides and other diuretics NOS

7ᵗʰ T50.2X2 Poisoning by carbonic-anhydrase inhibitors, benzothiadiazides and other diuretics, intentional self-harm

7ᵗʰ T50.2X3 Poisoning by carbonic-anhydrase inhibitors, benzothiadiazides and other diuretics, assault

7ᵗʰ T50.2X4 Poisoning by carbonic-anhydrase inhibitors, benzothiadiazides and other diuretics, undetermined

7ᵗʰ T50.2X5 Adverse effect of carbonic-anhydrase inhibitors, benzothiadiazides and other diuretics

7ᵗʰ T50.2X6 Underdosing of carbonic-anhydrase inhibitors, benzothiadiazides and other diuretics

5ᵗʰ T50.3 Poisoning by, adverse effect of and underdosing of electrolytic, caloric and water-balance agents

Poisoning by, adverse effect of and underdosing of oral rehydration salts

6ᵗʰ T50.3X Poisoning by, adverse effect of and underdosing of electrolytic, caloric and water-balance agents

7ᵗʰ T50.3X1 Poisoning by electrolytic, caloric and water-balance agents, accidental (unintentional)

Poisoning by electrolytic, caloric and water-balance agents NOS

7ᵗʰ T50.3X2 Poisoning by electrolytic, caloric and water-balance agents, intentional self-harm

7ᵗʰ T50.3X3 Poisoning by electrolytic, caloric and water-balance agents, assault

7ᵗʰ T50.3X4 Poisoning by electrolytic, caloric and water-balance agents, undetermined

7ᵗʰ T50.3X5 Adverse effect of electrolytic, caloric and water-balance agents

7ᵗʰ T50.3X6 Underdosing of electrolytic, caloric and water-balance agents

5ᵗʰ T50.4 Poisoning by, adverse effect of and underdosing of drugs affecting uric acid metabolism

6ᵗʰ T50.4X Poisoning by, adverse effect of and underdosing of drugs affecting uric acid metabolism

7ᵗʰ T50.4X1 Poisoning by drugs affecting uric acid metabolism, accidental (unintentional)

Poisoning by drugs affecting uric acid metabolism NOS

7ᵗʰ T50.4X2 Poisoning by drugs affecting uric acid metabolism, intentional self-harm

7ᵗʰ T50.4X3 Poisoning by drugs affecting uric acid metabolism, assault

7ᵗʰ T50.4X4 Poisoning by drugs affecting uric acid metabolism, undetermined

7ᵗʰ T50.4X5 Adverse effect of drugs affecting uric acid metabolism

7ᵗʰ T50.4X6 Underdosing of drugs affecting uric acid metabolism

5ᵗʰ T50.5 Poisoning by, adverse effect of and underdosing of appetite depressants

6ᵗʰ T50.5X Poisoning by, adverse effect of and underdosing of appetite depressants

7ᵗʰ T50.5X1 Poisoning by appetite depressants, accidental (unintentional)

Poisoning by appetite depressants NOS

7ᵗʰ T50.5X2 Poisoning by appetite depressants, intentional self-harm

7ᵗʰ T50.5X3 Poisoning by appetite depressants, assault

7ᵗʰ T50.5X4 Poisoning by appetite depressants, undetermined

7ᵗʰ T50.5X5 Adverse effect of appetite depressants

7ᵗʰ T50.5X6 Underdosing of appetite depressants

5ᵗʰ T50.6 Poisoning by, adverse effect of and underdosing of antidotes and chelating agents

Poisoning by, adverse effect of and underdosing of alcohol deterrents

6ᵗʰ T50.6X Poisoning by, adverse effect of and underdosing of antidotes and chelating agents

7ᵗʰ T50.6X1 Poisoning by antidotes and chelating agents, accidental (unintentional)

Poisoning by antidotes and chelating agents NOS

7ᵗʰ T50.6X2 Poisoning by antidotes and chelating agents, intentional self-harm

7ᵗʰ T50.6X3 Poisoning by antidotes and chelating agents, assault

7ᵗʰ T50.6X4 Poisoning by antidotes and chelating agents, undetermined

7ᵗʰ T50.6X5 Adverse effect of antidotes and chelating agents

7ᵗʰ T50.6X6 Underdosing of antidotes and chelating agents

5ᵗʰ T50.7 Poisoning by, adverse effect of and underdosing of analeptics and opioid receptor antagonists

6ᵗʰ T50.7X Poisoning by, adverse effect of and underdosing of analeptics and opioid receptor antagonists

7ᵗʰ T50.7X1 Poisoning by analeptics and opioid receptor antagonists, accidental (unintentional)

Poisoning by analeptics and opioid receptor antagonists NOS

7ᵗʰ T50.7X2 Poisoning by analeptics and opioid receptor antagonists, intentional self-harm

7ᵗʰ T50.7X3 Poisoning by analeptics and opioid receptor antagonists, assault

7ᵗʰ T50.7X4 Poisoning by analeptics and opioid receptor antagonists, undetermined

7ᵗʰ T50.7X5 Adverse effect of analeptics and opioid receptor antagonists

7ᵗʰ T50.7X6 Underdosing of analeptics and opioid receptor antagonists

5ᵗʰ T50.8 Poisoning by, adverse effect of and underdosing of diagnostic agents

6ᵗʰ T50.8X Poisoning by, adverse effect of and underdosing of diagnostic agents

7ᵗʰ T50.8X1 Poisoning by diagnostic agents, accidental (unintentional)

Poisoning by diagnostic agents NOS

7ᵗʰ T50.8X2 Poisoning by diagnostic agents, intentional self-harm

7ᵗʰ T50.8X3 Poisoning by diagnostic agents, assault

7ᵗʰ T50.8X4 Poisoning by diagnostic agents, undetermined

7ᵗʰ T50.8X5 Adverse effect of diagnostic agents

7ᵗʰ T50.8X6 Underdosing of diagnostic agents

5ᵗʰ T50.A Poisoning by, adverse effect of and underdosing of bacterial vaccines

④ 4ᵗʰ character required	⑤ 5ᵗʰ character required	⑥ 6ᵗʰ character required	⑦ 7ᵗʰ character required	Ⓧ Extension 'X' Alert
EXCLUDES 1 Not coded here	EXCLUDES 2 Not included here	PDx Primary Diagnosis Only	Manifestation Code	

- T50.A1 Poisoning by, adverse effect of and underdosing of pertussis vaccine, including combinations with a pertussis component
  - T50.A11 Poisoning by pertussis vaccine, including combinations with a pertussis component, accidental (unintentional)
  - T50.A12 Poisoning by pertussis vaccine, including combinations with a pertussis component, intentional self-harm
  - T50.A13 Poisoning by pertussis vaccine, including combinations with a pertussis component, assault
  - T50.A14 Poisoning by pertussis vaccine, including combinations with a pertussis component, undetermined
  - T50.A15 Adverse effect of pertussis vaccine, including combinations with a pertussis component
  - T50.A16 Underdosing of pertussis vaccine, including combinations with a pertussis component
- T50.A2 Poisoning by, adverse effect of and underdosing of mixed bacterial vaccines without a pertussis component
  - T50.A21 Poisoning by mixed bacterial vaccines without a pertussis component, accidental (unintentional)
  - T50.A22 Poisoning by mixed bacterial vaccines without a pertussis component, intentional self-harm
  - T50.A23 Poisoning by mixed bacterial vaccines without a pertussis component, assault
  - T50.A24 Poisoning by mixed bacterial vaccines without a pertussis component, undetermined
  - T50.A25 Adverse effect of mixed bacterial vaccines without a pertussis component
  - T50.A26 Underdosing of mixed bacterial vaccines without a pertussis component
- T50.A9 Poisoning by, adverse effect of and underdosing of other bacterial vaccines
  - T50.A91 Poisoning by other bacterial vaccines, accidental (unintentional)
  - T50.A92 Poisoning by other bacterial vaccines, intentional self-harm
  - T50.A93 Poisoning by other bacterial vaccines, assault
  - T50.A94 Poisoning by other bacterial vaccines, undetermined
  - T50.A95 Adverse effect of other bacterial vaccines
  - T50.A96 Underdosing of other bacterial vaccines
- T50.B Poisoning by, adverse effect of and underdosing of viral vaccines
  - T50.B1 Poisoning by, adverse effect of and underdosing of smallpox vaccines
    - T50.B11 Poisoning by smallpox vaccines, accidental (unintentional)
    - T50.B12 Poisoning by smallpox vaccines, intentional self-harm
    - T50.B13 Poisoning by smallpox vaccines, assault
    - T50.B14 Poisoning by smallpox vaccines, undetermined
    - T50.B15 Adverse effect of smallpox vaccines
    - T50.B16 Underdosing of smallpox vaccines
  - T50.B9 Poisoning by, adverse effect of and underdosing of other viral vaccines
    - T50.B91 Poisoning by other viral vaccines, accidental (unintentional)
    - T50.B92 Poisoning by other viral vaccines, intentional self-harm
    - T50.B93 Poisoning by other viral vaccines, assault

- T50.B94 Poisoning by other viral vaccines, undetermined
- T50.B95 Adverse effect of other viral vaccines
- T50.B96 Underdosing of other viral vaccines
- T50.Z Poisoning by, adverse effect of and underdosing of other vaccines and biological substances
  - T50.Z1 Poisoning by, adverse effect of and underdosing of immunoglobulin
    - T50.Z11 Poisoning by immunoglobulin, accidental (unintentional)
    - T50.Z12 Poisoning by immunoglobulin, intentional self-harm
    - T50.Z13 Poisoning by immunoglobulin, assault
    - T50.Z14 Poisoning by immunoglobulin, undetermined
    - T50.Z15 Adverse effect of immunoglobulin
    - T50.Z16 Underdosing of immunoglobulin
  - T50.Z9 Poisoning by, adverse effect of and underdosing of other vaccines and biological substances
    - T50.Z91 Poisoning by other vaccines and biological substances, accidental (unintentional)
    - T50.Z92 Poisoning by other vaccines and biological substances, intentional self-harm
    - T50.Z93 Poisoning by other vaccines and biological substances, assault
    - T50.Z94 Poisoning by other vaccines and biological substances, undetermined
    - T50.Z95 Adverse effect of other vaccines and biological substances
    - T50.Z96 Underdosing of other vaccines and biological substances
- T50.9 Poisoning by, adverse effect of and underdosing of other and unspecified drugs, medicaments and biological substances
  - T50.90 Poisoning by, adverse effect of and underdosing of unspecified drugs, medicaments and biological substances
    - T50.901 Poisoning by unspecified drugs, medicaments and biological substances, accidental (unintentional)
    - T50.902 Poisoning by unspecified drugs, medicaments and biological substances, intentional self-harm
    - T50.903 Poisoning by unspecified drugs, medicaments and biological substances, assault
    - T50.904 Poisoning by unspecified drugs, medicaments and biological substances, undetermined
    - T50.905 Adverse effect of unspecified drugs, medicaments and biological substances
    - T50.906 Underdosing of unspecified drugs, medicaments and biological substances
  - T50.99 Poisoning by, adverse effect of and underdosing of other drugs, medicaments and biological substances
    - T50.991 Poisoning by other drugs, medicaments and biological substances, accidental (unintentional)
    - T50.992 Poisoning by other drugs, medicaments and biological substances, intentional self-harm
    - T50.993 Poisoning by other drugs, medicaments and biological substances, assault
    - T50.994 Poisoning by other drugs, medicaments and biological substances, undetermined
    - T50.995 Adverse effect of other drugs, medicaments and biological substances
    - T50.996 Underdosing of other drugs, medicaments and biological substances

Unspecified Code	Other Specified Code	N Newborn Age: 0	P Pediatric Age: 0-17	M Maternity Age: 12-55	
A Adult Age: 15-124	♂ Male	♀ Female	● New Code	▲ Revised Code Title	►◄ Revised Text

Toxic effects of substances chiefly nonmedicinal as to source (T51-T65)

[NOTES] When no intent is indicated code to accidental. Undetermined intent is only for use when there is specific documentation in the record that the intent of the toxic effect cannot be determined.
Use additional code(s):
for all associated manifestations of toxic effect, such as: respiratory conditions due to external agents (J60-J70)
personal history of foreign body fully removed (Z87.821)
to identify any retained foreign body, if applicable (Z18.-)

[EXCLUDES1] *contact with and (suspected) exposure to toxic substances (Z77.-)*

④ **T51 Toxic effect of alcohol**

The appropriate 7th character is to be added to each code from category T51
A = initial encounter
D = subsequent encounter
S = sequela

⑤ **T51.0 Toxic effect of ethanol**
Toxic effect of ethyl alcohol
[EXCLUDES2] *acute alcohol intoxication or 'hangover' effects (F10.129, F10.229, F10.929)*
drunkenness (F10.129, F10.229, F10.929)
pathological alcohol intoxication (F10.129, F10.229, F10.929)

⑥ **T51.0X Toxic effect of ethanol**
⑦ **T51.0X1 Toxic effect of ethanol, accidental (unintentional)**
Toxic effect of ethanol NOS
⑦ **T51.0X2 Toxic effect of ethanol, intentional self-harm**
⑦ **T51.0X3 Toxic effect of ethanol, assault**
⑦ **T51.0X4 Toxic effect of ethanol, undetermined**

⑤ **T51.1 Toxic effect of methanol**
Toxic effect of methyl alcohol
⑥ **T51.1X Toxic effect of methanol**
⑦ **T51.1X1 Toxic effect of methanol, accidental (unintentional)**
Toxic effect of methanol NOS
⑦ **T51.1X2 Toxic effect of methanol, intentional self-harm**
⑦ **T51.1X3 Toxic effect of methanol, assault**
⑦ **T51.1X4 Toxic effect of methanol, undetermined**

⑤ **T51.2 Toxic effect of 2-Propanol**
Toxic effect of isopropyl alcohol
⑥ **T51.2X Toxic effect of 2-Propanol**
⑦ **T51.2X1 Toxic effect of 2-Propanol, accidental (unintentional)**
Toxic effect of 2-Propanol NOS
⑦ **T51.2X2 Toxic effect of 2-Propanol, intentional self-harm**
⑦ **T51.2X3 Toxic effect of 2-Propanol, assault**
⑦ **T51.2X4 Toxic effect of 2-Propanol, undetermined**

⑤ **T51.3 Toxic effect of fusel oil**
Toxic effect of amyl alcohol
Toxic effect of butyl [1-butanol] alcohol
Toxic effect of propyl [1-propanol] alcohol
⑥ **T51.3X Toxic effect of fusel oil**
⑦ **T51.3X1 Toxic effect of fusel oil, accidental (unintentional)**
Toxic effect of fusel oil NOS
⑦ **T51.3X2 Toxic effect of fusel oil, intentional self-harm**
⑦ **T51.3X3 Toxic effect of fusel oil, assault**
⑦ **T51.3X4 Toxic effect of fusel oil, undetermined**

⑤ **T51.8 Toxic effect of other alcohols**
⑥ **T51.8X Toxic effect of other alcohols**
⑦ **T51.8X1 Toxic effect of other alcohols, accidental (unintentional)**
Toxic effect of other alcohols NOS
⑦ **T51.8X2 Toxic effect of other alcohols, intentional self-harm**
⑦ **T51.8X3 Toxic effect of other alcohols, assault**
⑦ **T51.8X4 Toxic effect of other alcohols, undetermined**

⑤ **T51.9 Toxic effect of unspecified alcohol**
⑦ **T51.91 Toxic effect of unspecified alcohol, accidental (unintentional)**
⑦ **T51.92 Toxic effect of unspecified alcohol, intentional self-harm**
⑦ **T51.93 Toxic effect of unspecified alcohol, assault**
⑦ **T51.94 Toxic effect of unspecified alcohol, undetermined**

④ **T52 Toxic effect of organic solvents**
[EXCLUDES1] *halogen derivatives of aliphatic and aromatic hydrocarbons (T53.-)*

The appropriate 7th character is to be added to each code from category T52
A = initial encounter
D = subsequent encounter
S = sequela

⑤ **T52.0 Toxic effects of petroleum products**
Toxic effects of gasoline [petrol]
Toxic effects of kerosene [paraffin oil]
Toxic effects of paraffin wax
Toxic effects of ether petroleum
Toxic effects of naphtha petroleum
Toxic effects of spirit petroleum
⑥ **T52.0X Toxic effects of petroleum products**
⑦ **T52.0X1 Toxic effect of petroleum products, accidental (unintentional)**
Toxic effects of petroleum products NOS
⑦ **T52.0X2 Toxic effect of petroleum products, intentional self-harm**
⑦ **T52.0X3 Toxic effect of petroleum products, assault**
⑦ **T52.0X4 Toxic effect of petroleum products, undetermined**

⑤ **T52.1 Toxic effects of benzene**
[EXCLUDES1] *homologues of benzene (T52.2)*
nitroderivatives and aminoderivatives of benzene and its homologues (T65.3)
⑥ **T52.1X Toxic effects of benzene**
⑦ **T52.1X1 Toxic effect of benzene, accidental (unintentional)**
Toxic effects of benzene NOS
⑦ **T52.1X2 Toxic effect of benzene, intentional self-harm**
⑦ **T52.1X3 Toxic effect of benzene, assault**
⑦ **T52.1X4 Toxic effect of benzene, undetermined**

⑤ **T52.2 Toxic effects of homologues of benzene**
Toxic effects of toluene [methylbenzene]
Toxic effects of xylene [dimethylbenzene]
⑥ **T52.2X Toxic effects of homologues of benzene**
⑦ **T52.2X1 Toxic effect of homologues of benzene, accidental (unintentional)**
Toxic effects of homologues of benzene NOS
⑦ **T52.2X2 Toxic effect of homologues of benzene, intentional self-harm**
⑦ **T52.2X3 Toxic effect of homologues of benzene, assault**
⑦ **T52.2X4 Toxic effect of homologues of benzene, undetermined**

⑤ **T52.3 Toxic effects of glycols**
⑥ **T52.3X Toxic effects of glycols**
⑦ **T52.3X1 Toxic effect of glycols, accidental (unintentional)**
Toxic effects of glycols NOS

④ 4th character required ⑤ 5th character required ⑥ 6th character required ⑦ 7th character required ⑦ Extension 'X' Alert
[EXCLUDES1] Not coded here [EXCLUDES2] Not included here [PDx] Primary Diagnosis Only Manifestation Code

T52.3X2 Toxic effect of glycols, intentional self-harm
T52.3X3 Toxic effect of glycols, assault
T52.3X4 Toxic effect of glycols, undetermined
T52.4 Toxic effects of ketones
T52.4X Toxic effects of ketones
T52.4X1 Toxic effect of ketones, accidental (unintentional)
Toxic effects of ketones NOS
T52.4X2 Toxic effect of ketones, intentional self-harm
T52.4X3 Toxic effect of ketones, assault
T52.4X4 Toxic effect of ketones, undetermined
T52.8 Toxic effects of other organic solvents
T52.8X Toxic effects of other organic solvents
T52.8X1 Toxic effect of other organic solvents, accidental (unintentional)
Toxic effects of other organic solvents NOS
T52.8X2 Toxic effect of other organic solvents, intentional self-harm
T52.8X3 Toxic effect of other organic solvents, assault
T52.8X4 Toxic effect of other organic solvents, undetermined
T52.9 Toxic effects of unspecified organic solvent
T52.91 Toxic effect of unspecified organic solvent, accidental (unintentional)
T52.92 Toxic effect of unspecified organic solvent, intentional self-harm
T52.93 Toxic effect of unspecified organic solvent, assault
T52.94 Toxic effect of unspecified organic solvent, undetermined
T53 Toxic effect of halogen derivatives of aliphatic and aromatic hydrocarbons

The appropriate 7th character is to be added to each code from category T53
A = initial encounter
D = subsequent encounter
S = sequela

T53.0 Toxic effects of carbon tetrachloride
Toxic effects of tetrachloromethane
T53.0X Toxic effects of carbon tetrachloride
T53.0X1 Toxic effect of carbon tetrachloride, accidental (unintentional)
Toxic effects of carbon tetrachloride NOS
T53.0X2 Toxic effect of carbon tetrachloride, intentional self-harm
T53.0X3 Toxic effect of carbon tetrachloride, assault
T53.0X4 Toxic effect of carbon tetrachloride, undetermined
T53.1 Toxic effects of chloroform
Toxic effects of trichloromethane
T53.1X Toxic effects of chloroform
T53.1X1 Toxic effect of chloroform, accidental (unintentional)
Toxic effects of chloroform NOS
T53.1X2 Toxic effect of chloroform, intentional self-harm
T53.1X3 Toxic effect of chloroform, assault
T53.1X4 Toxic effect of chloroform, undetermined
T53.2 Toxic effects of trichloroethylene
Toxic effects of trichloroethene
T53.2X Toxic effects of trichloroethylene
T53.2X1 Toxic effect of trichloroethylene, accidental (unintentional)
Toxic effects of trichloroethylene NOS
T53.2X2 Toxic effect of trichloroethylene, intentional self-harm
T53.2X3 Toxic effect of trichloroethylene, assault

T53.2X4 Toxic effect of trichloroethylene, undetermined
T53.3 Toxic effects of tetrachloroethylene
Toxic effects of perchloroethylene
Toxic effect of tetrachloroethene
T53.3X Toxic effects of tetrachloroethylene
T53.3X1 Toxic effect of tetrachloroethylene, accidental (unintentional)
Toxic effects of tetrachloroethylene NOS
T53.3X2 Toxic effect of tetrachloroethylene, intentional self-harm
T53.3X3 Toxic effect of tetrachloroethylene, assault
T53.3X4 Toxic effect of tetrachloroethylene, undetermined
T53.4 Toxic effects of dichloromethane
Toxic effects of methylene chloride
T53.4X Toxic effects of dichloromethane
T53.4X1 Toxic effect of dichloromethane, accidental (unintentional)
Toxic effects of dichloromethane NOS
T53.4X2 Toxic effect of dichloromethane, intentional self-harm
T53.4X3 Toxic effect of dichloromethane, assault
T53.4X4 Toxic effect of dichloromethane, undetermined
T53.5 Toxic effects of chlorofluorocarbons
T53.5X Toxic effects of chlorofluorocarbons
T53.5X1 Toxic effect of chlorofluorocarbons, accidental (unintentional)
Toxic effects of chlorofluorocarbons NOS
T53.5X2 Toxic effect of chlorofluorocarbons, intentional self-harm
T53.5X3 Toxic effect of chlorofluorocarbons, assault
T53.5X4 Toxic effect of chlorofluorocarbons, undetermined
T53.6 Toxic effects of other halogen derivatives of aliphatic hydrocarbons
T53.6X Toxic effects of other halogen derivatives of aliphatic hydrocarbons
T53.6X1 Toxic effect of other halogen derivatives of aliphatic hydrocarbons, accidental (unintentional)
Toxic effects of other halogen derivatives of aliphatic hydrocarbons NOS
T53.6X2 Toxic effect of other halogen derivatives of aliphatic hydrocarbons, intentional self-harm
T53.6X3 Toxic effect of other halogen derivatives of aliphatic hydrocarbons, assault
T53.6X4 Toxic effect of other halogen derivatives of aliphatic hydrocarbons, undetermined
T53.7 Toxic effects of other halogen derivatives of aromatic hydrocarbons
T53.7X Toxic effects of other halogen derivatives of aromatic hydrocarbons
T53.7X1 Toxic effect of other halogen derivatives of aromatic hydrocarbons, accidental (unintentional)
Toxic effects of other halogen derivatives of aromatic hydrocarbons NOS
T53.7X2 Toxic effect of other halogen derivatives of aromatic hydrocarbons, intentional self-harm
T53.7X3 Toxic effect of other halogen derivatives of aromatic hydrocarbons, assault
T53.7X4 Toxic effect of other halogen derivatives of aromatic hydrocarbons, undetermined
T53.9 Toxic effects of unspecified halogen derivatives of aliphatic and aromatic hydrocarbons

Unspecified Code	Other Specified Code	N Newborn Age: 0	P Pediatric Age: 0-17	M Maternity Age: 12-55
A Adult Age: 15-124	♂ Male	♀ Female	● New Code	▲ Revised Code Title	►◄ Revised Text

T53.91 **Toxic effect of unspecified halogen derivatives of aliphatic and aromatic hydrocarbons,** accidental **(unintentional)**

T53.92 **Toxic effect of unspecified halogen derivatives of aliphatic and aromatic hydrocarbons,** intentional self-harm

T53.93 **Toxic effect of unspecified halogen derivatives of aliphatic and aromatic hydrocarbons,** assault

T53.94 **Toxic effect of unspecified halogen derivatives of aliphatic and aromatic hydrocarbons,** undetermined

T54 **Toxic effect of corrosive substances**

> **The appropriate 7th character is to be added to each code from category T54**
> **A = initial encounter**
> **D = subsequent encounter**
> **S = sequela**

T54.0 **Toxic effects of phenol and phenol homologues**

T54.0X **Toxic effects of** phenol and phenol homologues

T54.0X1 **Toxic effect of phenol and phenol homologues,** accidental **(unintentional)**

Toxic effects of phenol and phenol homologues NOS

T54.0X2 **Toxic effect of phenol and phenol homologues,** intentional self-harm

T54.0X3 **Toxic effect of phenol and phenol homologues,** assault

T54.0X4 **Toxic effect of phenol and phenol homologues,** undetermined

T54.1 **Toxic effects of other corrosive organic compounds**

T54.1X **Toxic effects of** other **corrosive** organic compounds

T54.1X1 **Toxic effect of other corrosive organic compounds,** accidental **(unintentional)**

Toxic effects of other corrosive organic compounds NOS

T54.1X2 **Toxic effect of other corrosive organic compounds,** intentional self-harm

T54.1X3 **Toxic effect of other corrosive organic compounds,** assault

T54.1X4 **Toxic effect of other corrosive organic compounds,** undetermined

T54.2 **Toxic effects of corrosive acids and acid-like substances**

Toxic effects of hydrochloric acid
Toxic effects of sulfuric acid

T54.2X **Toxic effects of corrosive** acids and acid-like substances

T54.2X1 **Toxic effect of corrosive acids and acid-like substances,** accidental **(unintentional)**

Toxic effects of corrosive acids and acid-like substances NOS

T54.2X2 **Toxic effect of corrosive acids and acid-like substances,** intentional self-harm

T54.2X3 **Toxic effect of corrosive acids and acid-like substances,** assault

T54.2X4 **Toxic effect of corrosive acids and acid-like substances,** undetermined

T54.3 **Toxic effects of corrosive alkalis and alkali-like substances**

Toxic effects of potassium hydroxide
Toxic effects of sodium hydroxide

T54.3X **Toxic effects of** corrosive alkalis and alkali-like substances

T54.3X1 **Toxic effect of corrosive alkalis and alkali-like substances,** accidental **(unintentional)**

Toxic effects of corrosive alkalis and alkali-like substances NOS

T54.3X2 **Toxic effect of corrosive alkalis and alkali-like substances,** intentional self-harm

T54.3X3 **Toxic effect of corrosive alkalis and alkali-like substances,** assault

T54.3X4 **Toxic effect of corrosive alkalis and alkali-like substances,** undetermined

T54.9 **Toxic effects of** unspecified **corrosive substance**

T54.91 **Toxic effect of unspecified corrosive substance,** accidental **(unintentional)**

T54.92 **Toxic effect of unspecified corrosive substance,** intentional self-harm

T54.93 **Toxic effect of unspecified corrosive substance,** assault

T54.94 **Toxic effect of unspecified corrosive substance,** undetermined

T55 **Toxic effect of soaps and detergents**

> **The appropriate 7th character is to be added to each code from category T55**
> **A = initial encounter**
> **D = subsequent encounter**
> **S = sequela**

T55.0 **Toxic effect of soaps**

T55.0X **Toxic effect of** soaps

T55.0X1 **Toxic effect of soaps,** accidental **(unintentional)**

Toxic effect of soaps NOS

T55.0X2 **Toxic effect of soaps,** intentional self-harm

T55.0X3 **Toxic effect of soaps,** assault

T55.0X4 **Toxic effect of soaps,** undetermined

T55.1 **Toxic effect of detergents**

T55.1X **Toxic effect of** detergents

T55.1X1 **Toxic effect of detergents,** accidental **(unintentional)**

Toxic effect of detergents NOS

T55.1X2 **Toxic effect of detergents,** intentional self-harm

T55.1X3 **Toxic effect of detergents,** assault

T55.1X4 **Toxic effect of detergents,** undetermined

T56 **Toxic effect of metals**

> INCLUDES   toxic effects of fumes and vapors of metals
> toxic effects of metals from all sources, except medicinal substances

> **Use additional code to identify any retained metal foreign body, if applicable (Z18.0-, T18.1-)**

> EXCLUDES1   arsenic and its compounds (T57.0)
> manganese and its compounds (T57.2)

> **The appropriate 7th character is to be added to each code from category T56**
> **A = initial encounter**
> **D = subsequent encounter**
> **S = sequela**

T56.0 **Toxic effects of lead and its compounds**

T56.0X **Toxic effects of** lead and its compounds

T56.0X1 **Toxic effect of lead and its compounds,** accidental **(unintentional)**

Toxic effects of lead and its compounds NOS

T56.0X2 **Toxic effect of lead and its compounds,** intentional self-harm

T56.0X3 **Toxic effect of lead and its compounds,** assault

T56.0X4 **Toxic effect of lead and its compounds,** undetermined

T56.1 **Toxic effects of mercury and its compounds**

T56.1X **Toxic effects of** mercury and its compounds

T56.1X1 **Toxic effect of mercury and its compounds,** accidental **(unintentional)**

Toxic effects of mercury and its compounds NOS

---

④ 4th character required   ⑤ 5th character required   ⑥ 6th character required   ⑦ 7th character required   ⑦ₓ Extension 'X' Alert

EXCLUDES 1 Not coded here   EXCLUDES 2 Not included here   PDx Primary Diagnosis Only   Manifestation Code

[7th] T56.1X2 Toxic effect of mercury and its compounds, intentional self-harm
[7th] T56.1X3 Toxic effect of mercury and its compounds, assault
[7th] T56.1X4 Toxic effect of mercury and its compounds, undetermined
[5th] T56.2 Toxic effects of chromium and its compounds
[6th] T56.2X Toxic effects of chromium and its compounds
[7th] T56.2X1 Toxic effect of chromium and its compounds, accidental (unintentional)
Toxic effects of chromium and its compounds NOS
[7th] T56.2X2 Toxic effect of chromium and its compounds, intentional self-harm
[7th] T56.2X3 Toxic effect of chromium and its compounds, assault
[7th] T56.2X4 Toxic effect of chromium and its compounds, undetermined
[5th] T56.3 Toxic effects of cadmium and its compounds
[6th] T56.3X Toxic effects of cadmium and its compounds
[7th] T56.3X1 Toxic effect of cadmium and its compounds, accidental (unintentional)
Toxic effects of cadmium and its compounds NOS
[7th] T56.3X2 Toxic effect of cadmium and its compounds, intentional self-harm
[7th] T56.3X3 Toxic effect of cadmium and its compounds, assault
[7th] T56.3X4 Toxic effect of cadmium and its compounds, undetermined
[5th] T56.4 Toxic effects of copper and its compounds
[6th] T56.4X Toxic effects of copper and its compounds
[7th] T56.4X1 Toxic effect of copper and its compounds, accidental (unintentional)
Toxic effects of copper and its compounds NOS
[7th] T56.4X2 Toxic effect of copper and its compounds, intentional self-harm
[7th] T56.4X3 Toxic effect of copper and its compounds, assault
[7th] T56.4X4 Toxic effect of copper and its compounds, undetermined
[5th] T56.5 Toxic effects of zinc and its compounds
[6th] T56.5X Toxic effects of zinc and its compounds
[7th] T56.5X1 Toxic effect of zinc and its compounds, accidental (unintentional)
Toxic effects of zinc and its compounds NOS
[7th] T56.5X2 Toxic effect of zinc and its compounds, intentional self-harm
[7th] T56.5X3 Toxic effect of zinc and its compounds, assault
[7th] T56.5X4 Toxic effect of zinc and its compounds, undetermined
[5th] T56.6 Toxic effects of tin and its compounds
[6th] T56.6X Toxic effects of tin and its compounds
[7th] T56.6X1 Toxic effect of tin and its compounds, accidental (unintentional)
Toxic effects of tin and its compounds NOS
[7th] T56.6X2 Toxic effect of tin and its compounds, intentional self-harm
[7th] T56.6X3 Toxic effect of tin and its compounds, assault
[7th] T56.6X4 Toxic effect of tin and its compounds, undetermined
[5th] T56.7 Toxic effects of beryllium and its compounds
[6th] T56.7X Toxic effects of beryllium and its compounds
[7th] T56.7X1 Toxic effect of beryllium and its compounds, accidental (unintentional)
Toxic effects of beryllium and its compounds NOS
[7th] T56.7X2 Toxic effect of beryllium and its compounds, intentional self-harm
[7th] T56.7X3 Toxic effect of beryllium and its compounds, assault
[7th] T56.7X4 Toxic effect of beryllium and its compounds, undetermined
[5th] T56.8 Toxic effects of other metals
[6th] T56.81 Toxic effect of thallium
[7th] T56.811 Toxic effect of thallium, accidental (unintentional)
Toxic effect of thallium NOS
[7th] T56.812 Toxic effect of thallium, intentional self-harm
[7th] T56.813 Toxic effect of thallium, assault
[7th] T56.814 Toxic effect of thallium, undetermined
[6th] T56.89 Toxic effects of other metals
[7th] T56.891 Toxic effect of other metals, accidental (unintentional)
Toxic effects of other metals NOS
[7th] T56.892 Toxic effect of other metals, intentional self-harm
[7th] T56.893 Toxic effect of other metals, assault
[7th] T56.894 Toxic effect of other metals, undetermined
[5th] T56.9 Toxic effects of unspecified metal
[7th] T56.91 Toxic effect of unspecified metal, accidental (unintentional)
[7th] T56.92 Toxic effect of unspecified metal, intentional self-harm
[7th] T56.93 Toxic effect of unspecified metal, assault
[7th] T56.94 Toxic effect of unspecified metal, undetermined
[4th] T57 Toxic effect of other inorganic substances
The appropriate 7th character is to be added to each code from category T57
A = initial encounter
D = subsequent encounter
S = sequela
[5th] T57.0 Toxic effect of arsenic and its compounds
[6th] T57.0X Toxic effect of arsenic and its compounds
[7th] T57.0X1 Toxic effect of arsenic and its compounds, accidental (unintentional)
Toxic effect of arsenic and its compounds NOS
[7th] T57.0X2 Toxic effect of arsenic and its compounds, intentional self-harm
[7th] T57.0X3 Toxic effect of arsenic and its compounds, assault
[7th] T57.0X4 Toxic effect of arsenic and its compounds, undetermined
[5th] T57.1 Toxic effect of phosphorus and its compounds
[EXCLUDES1] *organophosphate insecticides (T60.0)*
[6th] T57.1X Toxic effect of phosphorus and its compounds
[7th] T57.1X1 Toxic effect of phosphorus and its compounds, accidental (unintentional)
Toxic effect of phosphorus and its compounds NOS
[7th] T57.1X2 Toxic effect of phosphorus and its compounds, intentional self-harm
[7th] T57.1X3 Toxic effect of phosphorus and its compounds, assault
[7th] T57.1X4 Toxic effect of phosphorus and its compounds, undetermined
[5th] T57.2 Toxic effect of manganese and its compounds
[6th] T57.2X Toxic effect of manganese and its compounds
[7th] T57.2X1 Toxic effect of manganese and its compounds, accidental (unintentional)
Toxic effect of manganese and its compounds NOS

Unspecified Code | Other Specified Code | [N] Newborn Age: 0 | [P] Pediatric Age: 0-17 | [M] Maternity Age: 12-55
[A] Adult Age: 15-124 | ♂ Male | ♀ Female | ● New Code | ▲ Revised Code Title | ►◄ Revised Text

- 7️⃣ T57.2X2 Toxic effect of manganese and its compounds, intentional self-harm
- 7️⃣ T57.2X3 Toxic effect of manganese and its compounds, assault
- 7️⃣ T57.2X4 Toxic effect of manganese and its compounds, undetermined
- 5️⃣ T57.3 Toxic effect of hydrogen cyanide
  - 6️⃣ T57.3X Toxic effect of hydrogen cyanide
    - 7️⃣ T57.3X1 Toxic effect of hydrogen cyanide, accidental (unintentional)

      Toxic effect of hydrogen cyanide NOS
    - 7️⃣ T57.3X2 Toxic effect of hydrogen cyanide, intentional self-harm
    - 7️⃣ T57.3X3 Toxic effect of hydrogen cyanide, assault
    - 7️⃣ T57.3X4 Toxic effect of hydrogen cyanide, undetermined
- 5️⃣ T57.8 Toxic effect of other specified inorganic substances
  - 6️⃣ T57.8X Toxic effect of other specified inorganic substances
    - 7️⃣ T57.8X1 Toxic effect of other specified inorganic substances, accidental (unintentional)

      Toxic effect of other specified inorganic substances NOS
    - 7️⃣ T57.8X2 Toxic effect of other specified inorganic substances, intentional self-harm
    - 7️⃣ T57.8X3 Toxic effect of other specified inorganic substances, assault
    - 7️⃣ T57.8X4 Toxic effect of other specified inorganic substances, undetermined
- 5️⃣ T57.9 Toxic effect of unspecified inorganic substance
  - 7️⃣ T57.91 Toxic effect of unspecified inorganic substance, accidental (unintentional)
  - 7️⃣ T57.92 Toxic effect of unspecified inorganic substance, intentional self-harm
  - 7️⃣ T57.93 Toxic effect of unspecified inorganic substance, assault
  - 7️⃣ T57.94 Toxic effect of unspecified inorganic substance, undetermined
- 4️⃣ T58 Toxic effect of carbon monoxide

  INCLUDES   asphyxiation from carbon monoxide
              toxic effect of carbon monoxide from all sources

  The appropriate 7th character is to be added to each code from category T58
  A = initial encounter
  D = subsequent encounter
  S = sequela
  - 5️⃣ T58.0 Toxic effect of carbon monoxide from motor vehicle exhaust

    Toxic effect of exhaust gas from gas engine
    Toxic effect of exhaust gas from motor pump
    - 7️⃣ T58.01 Toxic effect of carbon monoxide from motor vehicle exhaust, accidental (unintentional)
    - 7️⃣ T58.02 Toxic effect of carbon monoxide from motor vehicle exhaust, intentional self-harm
    - 7️⃣ T58.03 Toxic effect of carbon monoxide from motor vehicle exhaust, assault
    - 7️⃣ T58.04 Toxic effect of carbon monoxide from motor vehicle exhaust, undetermined
  - 5️⃣ T58.1 Toxic effect of carbon monoxide from utility gas

    Toxic effect of acetylene
    Toxic effect of gas NOS used for lighting, heating, cooking
    Toxic effect of water gas
    - 7️⃣ T58.11 Toxic effect of carbon monoxide from utility gas, accidental (unintentional)
    - 7️⃣ T58.12 Toxic effect of carbon monoxide from utility gas, intentional self-harm

- 7️⃣ T58.13 Toxic effect of carbon monoxide from utility gas, assault
- 7️⃣ T58.14 Toxic effect of carbon monoxide from utility gas, undetermined
- 5️⃣ T58.2 Toxic effect of carbon monoxide from incomplete combustion of other domestic fuels

  Toxic effect of carbon monoxide from incomplete combustion of coal, coke, kerosene, wood
  - 6️⃣ T58.2X Toxic effect of carbon monoxide from incomplete combustion of other domestic fuels
    - 7️⃣ T58.2X1 Toxic effect of carbon monoxide from incomplete combustion of other domestic fuels, accidental (unintentional)
    - 7️⃣ T58.2X2 Toxic effect of carbon monoxide from incomplete combustion of other domestic fuels, intentional self-harm
    - 7️⃣ T58.2X3 Toxic effect of carbon monoxide from incomplete combustion of other domestic fuels, assault
    - 7️⃣ T58.2X4 Toxic effect of carbon monoxide from incomplete combustion of other domestic fuels, undetermined
- 5️⃣ T58.8 Toxic effect of carbon monoxide from other source

  Toxic effect of carbon monoxide from blast furnace gas
  Toxic effect of carbon monoxide from fuels in industrial use
  Toxic effect of carbon monoxide from kiln vapor
  - 6️⃣ T58.8X Toxic effect of carbon monoxide from other source
    - 7️⃣ T58.8X1 Toxic effect of carbon monoxide from other source, accidental (unintentional)
    - 7️⃣ T58.8X2 Toxic effect of carbon monoxide from other source, intentional self-harm
    - 7️⃣ T58.8X3 Toxic effect of carbon monoxide from other source, assault
    - 7️⃣ T58.8X4 Toxic effect of carbon monoxide from other source, undetermined
- 5️⃣ T58.9 Toxic effect of carbon monoxide from unspecified source
  - 7️⃣ T58.91 Toxic effect of carbon monoxide from unspecified source, accidental (unintentional)
  - 7️⃣ T58.92 Toxic effect of carbon monoxide from unspecified source, intentional self-harm
  - 7️⃣ T58.93 Toxic effect of carbon monoxide from unspecified source, assault
  - 7️⃣ T58.94 Toxic effect of carbon monoxide from unspecified source, undetermined
- 4️⃣ T59 Toxic effect of other gases, fumes and vapors

  INCLUDES   aerosol propellants
  EXCLUDES1   chlorofluorocarbons (T53.5)
  The appropriate 7th character is to be added to each code from category T59
  A = initial encounter
  D = subsequent encounter
  S = sequela
  - 5️⃣ T59.0 Toxic effect of nitrogen oxides
    - 6️⃣ T59.0X Toxic effect of nitrogen oxides
      - 7️⃣ T59.0X1 Toxic effect of nitrogen oxides, accidental (unintentional)

        Toxic effect of nitrogen oxides NOS
      - 7️⃣ T59.0X2 Toxic effect of nitrogen oxides, intentional self-harm
      - 7️⃣ T59.0X3 Toxic effect of nitrogen oxides, assault
      - 7️⃣ T59.0X4 Toxic effect of nitrogen oxides, undetermined
  - 5️⃣ T59.1 Toxic effect of sulfur dioxide
    - 6️⃣ T59.1X Toxic effect of sulfur dioxide
      - 7️⃣ T59.1X1 Toxic effect of sulfur dioxide, accidental (unintentional)

        Toxic effect of sulfur dioxide NOS

4️⃣ 4th character required   5️⃣ 5th character required   6️⃣ 6th character required   7️⃣ 7th character required   ⑦ Extension 'X' Alert

EXCLUDES 1 Not coded here   *EXCLUDES 2* Not included here   PDx Primary Diagnosis Only   Manifestation Code

🔟 T59.1X2 Toxic effect of sulfur dioxide, intentional self-harm
🔟 T59.1X3 Toxic effect of sulfur dioxide, assault
🔟 T59.1X4 Toxic effect of sulfur dioxide, undetermined
5️⃣ T59.2 Toxic effect of formaldehyde
6️⃣ T59.2X Toxic effect of formaldehyde
🔟 T59.2X1 Toxic effect of formaldehyde, accidental (unintentional)
Toxic effect of formaldehyde NOS
🔟 T59.2X2 Toxic effect of formaldehyde, intentional self-harm
🔟 T59.2X3 Toxic effect of formaldehyde, assault
🔟 T59.2X4 Toxic effect of formaldehyde, undetermined
5️⃣ T59.3 Toxic effect of lacrimogenic gas
Toxic effect of tear gas
6️⃣ T59.3X Toxic effect of lacrimogenic gas
🔟 T59.3X1 Toxic effect of lacrimogenic gas, accidental (unintentional)
Toxic effect of lacrimogenic gas NOS
🔟 T59.3X2 Toxic effect of lacrimogenic gas, intentional self-harm
🔟 T59.3X3 Toxic effect of lacrimogenic gas, assault
🔟 T59.3X4 Toxic effect of lacrimogenic gas, undetermined
5️⃣ T59.4 Toxic effect of chlorine gas
6️⃣ T59.4X Toxic effect of chlorine gas
🔟 T59.4X1 Toxic effect of chlorine gas, accidental (unintentional)
Toxic effect of chlorine gas NOS
🔟 T59.4X2 Toxic effect of chlorine gas, intentional self-harm
🔟 T59.4X3 Toxic effect of chlorine gas, assault
🔟 T59.4X4 Toxic effect of chlorine gas, undetermined
5️⃣ T59.5 Toxic effect of fluorine gas and hydrogen fluoride
6️⃣ T59.5X Toxic effect of fluorine gas and hydrogen fluoride
🔟 T59.5X1 Toxic effect of fluorine gas and hydrogen fluoride, accidental (unintentional)
Toxic effect of fluorine gas and hydrogen fluoride NOS
🔟 T59.5X2 Toxic effect of fluorine gas and hydrogen fluoride, intentional self-harm
🔟 T59.5X3 Toxic effect of fluorine gas and hydrogen fluoride, assault
🔟 T59.5X4 Toxic effect of fluorine gas and hydrogen fluoride, undetermined
5️⃣ T59.6 Toxic effect of hydrogen sulfide
6️⃣ T59.6X Toxic effect of hydrogen sulfide
🔟 T59.6X1 Toxic effect of hydrogen sulfide, accidental (unintentional)
Toxic effect of hydrogen sulfide NOS
🔟 T59.6X2 Toxic effect of hydrogen sulfide, intentional self-harm
🔟 T59.6X3 Toxic effect of hydrogen sulfide, assault
🔟 T59.6X4 Toxic effect of hydrogen sulfide, undetermined
5️⃣ T59.7 Toxic effect of carbon dioxide
6️⃣ T59.7X Toxic effect of carbon dioxide
🔟 T59.7X1 Toxic effect of carbon dioxide, accidental (unintentional)
Toxic effect of carbon dioxide NOS
🔟 T59.7X2 Toxic effect of carbon dioxide, intentional self-harm
🔟 T59.7X3 Toxic effect of carbon dioxide, assault
🔟 T59.7X4 Toxic effect of carbon dioxide, undetermined
5️⃣ T59.8 Toxic effect of other specified gases, fumes and vapors

6️⃣ T59.81 Toxic effect of smoke
Smoke inhalation
EXCLUDES2 toxic effect of cigarette (tobacco) smoke (T65.22-)
🔟 T59.811 Toxic effect of smoke, accidental (unintentional)
Toxic effect of smoke NOS
🔟 T59.812 Toxic effect of smoke, intentional self-harm
🔟 T59.813 Toxic effect of smoke, assault
🔟 T59.814 Toxic effect of smoke, undetermined
6️⃣ T59.89 Toxic effect of other specified gases, fumes and vapors
🔟 T59.891 Toxic effect of other specified gases, fumes and vapors, accidental (unintentional)
🔟 T59.892 Toxic effect of other specified gases, fumes and vapors, intentional self-harm
🔟 T59.893 Toxic effect of other specified gases, fumes and vapors, assault
🔟 T59.894 Toxic effect of other specified gases, fumes and vapors, undetermined
5️⃣ T59.9 Toxic effect of unspecified gases, fumes and vapors
🔟 T59.91 Toxic effect of unspecified gases, fumes and vapors, accidental (unintentional)
🔟 T59.92 Toxic effect of unspecified gases, fumes and vapors, intentional self-harm
🔟 T59.93 Toxic effect of unspecified gases, fumes and vapors, assault
🔟 T59.94 Toxic effect of unspecified gases, fumes and vapors, undetermined
4️⃣ T60 Toxic effect of pesticides
INCLUDES toxic effect of wood preservatives
The appropriate 7th character is to be added to each code from category T60
A = initial encounter
D = subsequent encounter
S = sequela
5️⃣ T60.0 Toxic effect of organophosphate and carbamate insecticides
6️⃣ T60.0X Toxic effect of organophosphate and carbamate insecticides
🔟 T60.0X1 Toxic effect of organophosphate and carbamate insecticides, accidental (unintentional)
Toxic effect of organophosphate and carbamate insecticides NOS
🔟 T60.0X2 Toxic effect of organophosphate and carbamate insecticides, intentional self-harm
🔟 T60.0X3 Toxic effect of organophosphate and carbamate insecticides, assault
🔟 T60.0X4 Toxic effect of organophosphate and carbamate insecticides, undetermined
5️⃣ T60.1 Toxic effect of halogenated insecticides
EXCLUDES1 chlorinated hydrocarbon (T53.-)
6️⃣ T60.1X Toxic effect of halogenated insecticides
🔟 T60.1X1 Toxic effect of halogenated insecticides, accidental (unintentional)
Toxic effect of halogenated insecticides NOS
🔟 T60.1X2 Toxic effect of halogenated insecticides, intentional self-harm
🔟 T60.1X3 Toxic effect of halogenated insecticides, assault
🔟 T60.1X4 Toxic effect of halogenated insecticides, undetermined
5️⃣ T60.2 Toxic effect of other insecticides
6️⃣ T60.2X Toxic effect of other insecticides
🔟 T60.2X1 Toxic effect of other insecticides, accidental (unintentional)
Toxic effect of other insecticides NOS

⑦ T60.2X2 Toxic effect of other insecticides, intentional self-harm
⑦ T60.2X3 Toxic effect of other insecticides, assault
⑦ T60.2X4 Toxic effect of other insecticides, undetermined
⑤ T60.3 Toxic effect of herbicides and fungicides
⑥ T60.3X Toxic effect of herbicides and fungicides
⑦ T60.3X1 Toxic effect of herbicides and fungicides, accidental (unintentional)
Toxic effect of herbicides and fungicides NOS
⑦ T60.3X2 Toxic effect of herbicides and fungicides, intentional self-harm
⑦ T60.3X3 Toxic effect of herbicides and fungicides, assault
⑦ T60.3X4 Toxic effect of herbicides and fungicides, undetermined
⑤ T60.4 Toxic effect of rodenticides
EXCLUDES1 strychnine and its salts (T65.1)
thallium (T56.81-)
⑥ T60.4X Toxic effect of rodenticides
⑦ T60.4X1 Toxic effect of rodenticides, accidental (unintentional)
Toxic effect of rodenticides NOS
⑦ T60.4X2 Toxic effect of rodenticides, intentional self-harm
⑦ T60.4X3 Toxic effect of rodenticides, assault
⑦ T60.4X4 Toxic effect of rodenticides, undetermined
⑤ T60.8 Toxic effect of other pesticides
⑥ T60.8X Toxic effect of other pesticides
⑦ T60.8X1 Toxic effect of other pesticides, accidental (unintentional)
Toxic effect of other pesticides NOS
⑦ T60.8X2 Toxic effect of other pesticides, intentional self-harm
⑦ T60.8X3 Toxic effect of other pesticides, assault
⑦ T60.8X4 Toxic effect of other pesticides, undetermined
⑤ T60.9 Toxic effect of unspecified pesticide
⑦ T60.91 Toxic effect of unspecified pesticide, accidental (unintentional)
⑦ T60.92 Toxic effect of unspecified pesticide, intentional self-harm
⑦ T60.93 Toxic effect of unspecified pesticide, assault
⑦ T60.94 Toxic effect of unspecified pesticide, undetermined
④ T61 Toxic effect of noxious substances eaten as seafood
EXCLUDES1 allergic reaction to food, such as:
anaphylactic reaction or shock due to adverse food reaction (T78.0-)
bacterial foodborne intoxications (A05.-)

dermatitis (L23.6, L25.4, L27.2)
gastroenteritis (noninfective) (K52.2)
toxic effect of aflatoxin and other mycotoxins (T64)
toxic effect of cyanides (T65.0-)
toxic effect of harmful algae bloom (T65.82-)
toxic effect of hydrogen cyanide (T57.3-)
toxic effect of mercury (T56.1-)
toxic effect of red tide (T65.82-)
The appropriate 7th character is to be added to each code from category T61
A = initial encounter
D = subsequent encounter
S = sequela
⑤ T61.0 Ciguatera fish poisoning
⑦ T61.01 Ciguatera fish poisoning, accidental (unintentional)
⑦ T61.02 Ciguatera fish poisoning, intentional self-harm
⑦ T61.03 Ciguatera fish poisoning, assault

⑦ T61.04 Ciguatera fish poisoning, undetermined
⑤ T61.1 Scombroid fish poisoning
Histamine-like syndrome
⑦ T61.11 Scombroid fish poisoning, accidental (unintentional)
⑦ T61.12 Scombroid fish poisoning, intentional self-harm
⑦ T61.13 Scombroid fish poisoning, assault
⑦ T61.14 Scombroid fish poisoning, undetermined
⑤ T61.7 Other fish and shellfish poisoning
⑥ T61.77 Other fish poisoning
⑦ T61.771 Other fish poisoning, accidental (unintentional)
⑦ T61.772 Other fish poisoning, intentional self-harm
⑦ T61.773 Other fish poisoning, assault
⑦ T61.774 Other fish poisoning, undetermined
⑥ T61.78 Other shellfish poisoning
⑦ T61.781 Other shellfish poisoning, accidental (unintentional)
⑦ T61.782 Other shellfish poisoning, intentional self-harm
⑦ T61.783 Other shellfish poisoning, assault
⑦ T61.784 Other shellfish poisoning, undetermined
⑤ T61.8 Toxic effect of other seafood
⑥ T61.8X Toxic effect of other seafood
⑦ T61.8X1 Toxic effect of other seafood, accidental (unintentional)
⑦ T61.8X2 Toxic effect of other seafood, intentional self-harm
⑦ T61.8X3 Toxic effect of other seafood, assault
⑦ T61.8X4 Toxic effect of other seafood, undetermined
⑤ T61.9 Toxic effect of unspecified seafood
⑦ T61.91 Toxic effect of unspecified seafood, accidental (unintentional)
⑦ T61.92 Toxic effect of unspecified seafood, intentional self-harm
⑦ T61.93 Toxic effect of unspecified seafood, assault
⑦ T61.94 Toxic effect of unspecified seafood, undetermined
④ T62 Toxic effect of other noxious substances eaten as food
EXCLUDES1 allergic reaction to food, such as:
anaphylactic shock (reaction) due to adverse food reaction (T78.0-)
bacterial food borne intoxications (A05.-)
dermatitis (L23.6, L25.4, L27.2)
gastroenteritis (noninfective) (K52.2)
toxic effect of aflatoxin and other mycotoxins (T64)
toxic effect of cyanides (T65.0-)
toxic effect of hydrogen cyanide (T57.3-)
toxic effect of mercury (T56.1-)
The appropriate 7th character is to be added to each code from category T62
A = initial encounter
D = subsequent encounter
S = sequela
⑤ T62.0 Toxic effect of ingested mushrooms
⑥ T62.0X Toxic effect of ingested mushrooms
⑦ T62.0X1 Toxic effect of ingested mushrooms, accidental (unintentional)
Toxic effect of ingested mushrooms NOS
⑦ T62.0X2 Toxic effect of ingested mushrooms, intentional self-harm
⑦ T62.0X3 Toxic effect of ingested mushrooms, assault
⑦ T62.0X4 Toxic effect of ingested mushrooms, undetermined
⑤ T62.1 Toxic effect of ingested berries
⑥ T62.1X Toxic effect of ingested berries

---

④ 4th character required   ⑤ 5th character required   ⑥ 6th character required   ⑦ 7th character required   ⑩ Extension 'X' Alert
EXCLUDES 1 Not coded here   EXCLUDES 2 Not included here   PDx Primary Diagnosis Only   Manifestation Code

[7th] T62.1X1 Toxic effect of ingested berries, accidental (unintentional)
Toxic effect of ingested berries NOS
[7th] T62.1X2 Toxic effect of ingested berries, intentional self-harm
[7th] T62.1X3 Toxic effect of ingested berries, assault
[7th] T62.1X4 Toxic effect of ingested berries, undetermined

[5th] T62.2 Toxic effect of other ingested (parts of) plant(s)
[6th] T62.2X Toxic effect of other ingested (parts of) plant(s)
[7th] T62.2X1 Toxic effect of other ingested (parts of) plant(s), accidental (unintentional)
Toxic effect of other ingested (parts of) plant(s) NOS
[7th] T62.2X2 Toxic effect of other ingested (parts of) plant(s), intentional self-harm
[7th] T62.2X3 Toxic effect of other ingested (parts of) plant(s), assault
[7th] T62.2X4 Toxic effect of other ingested (parts of) plant(s), undetermined

[5th] T62.8 Toxic effect of other specified noxious substances eaten as food
[6th] T62.8X Toxic effect of other specified noxious substances eaten as food
[7th] T62.8X1 Toxic effect of other specified noxious substances eaten as food, accidental (unintentional)
Toxic effect of other specified noxious substances eaten as food NOS
[7th] T62.8X2 Toxic effect of other specified noxious substances eaten as food, intentional self-harm
[7th] T62.8X3 Toxic effect of other specified noxious substances eaten as food, assault
[7th] T62.8X4 Toxic effect of other specified noxious substances eaten as food, undetermined

[5th] T62.9 Toxic effect of unspecified noxious substance eaten as food
[7th] T62.91 Toxic effect of unspecified noxious substance eaten as food, accidental (unintentional)
Toxic effect of unspecified noxious substance eaten as food NOS
[7th] T62.92 Toxic effect of unspecified noxious substance eaten as food, intentional self-harm
[7th] T62.93 Toxic effect of unspecified noxious substance eaten as food, assault
[7th] T62.94 Toxic effect of unspecified noxious substance eaten as food, undetermined

[4th] T63 Toxic effect of contact with venomous animals and plants
INCLUDES *bite or touch of venomous animal*
pricked or stuck by thorn or leaf
EXCLUDES2 *ingestion of toxic animal or plant (T61.-, T62.-)*

The appropriate 7th character is to be added to each code from category T63
A = initial encounter
D = subsequent encounter
S = sequela

[5th] T63.0 Toxic effect of snake venom
[6th] T63.00 Toxic effect of unspecified snake venom
[7th] T63.001 Toxic effect of unspecified snake venom, accidental (unintentional)
Toxic effect of unspecified snake venom NOS
[7th] T63.002 Toxic effect of unspecified snake venom, intentional self-harm
[7th] T63.003 Toxic effect of unspecified snake venom, assault
[7th] T63.004 Toxic effect of unspecified snake venom, undetermined

[6th] T63.01 Toxic effect of rattlesnake venom
[7th] T63.011 Toxic effect of rattlesnake venom, accidental (unintentional)
Toxic effect of rattlesnake venom NOS
[7th] T63.012 Toxic effect of rattlesnake venom, intentional self-harm
[7th] T63.013 Toxic effect of rattlesnake venom, assault
[7th] T63.014 Toxic effect of rattlesnake venom, undetermined

[6th] T63.02 Toxic effect of coral snake venom
[7th] T63.021 Toxic effect of coral snake venom, accidental (unintentional)
Toxic effect of coral snake venom NOS
[7th] T63.022 Toxic effect of coral snake venom, intentional self-harm
[7th] T63.023 Toxic effect of coral snake venom, assault
[7th] T63.024 Toxic effect of coral snake venom, undetermined

[6th] T63.03 Toxic effect of taipan venom
[7th] T63.031 Toxic effect of taipan venom, accidental (unintentional)
Toxic effect of taipan venom NOS
[7th] T63.032 Toxic effect of taipan venom, intentional self-harm
[7th] T63.033 Toxic effect of taipan venom, assault
[7th] T63.034 Toxic effect of taipan venom, undetermined

[6th] T63.04 Toxic effect of cobra venom
[7th] T63.041 Toxic effect of cobra venom, accidental (unintentional)
Toxic effect of cobra venom NOS
[7th] T63.042 Toxic effect of cobra venom, intentional self-harm
[7th] T63.043 Toxic effect of cobra venom, assault
[7th] T63.044 Toxic effect of cobra venom, undetermined

[6th] T63.06 Toxic effect of venom of other North and South American snake
[7th] T63.061 Toxic effect of venom of other North and South American snake, accidental (unintentional)
Toxic effect of venom of other North and South American snake NOS
[7th] T63.062 Toxic effect of venom of other North and South American snake, intentional self-harm
[7th] T63.063 Toxic effect of venom of other North and South American snake, assault
[7th] T63.064 Toxic effect of venom of other North and South American snake, undetermined

[6th] T63.07 Toxic effect of venom of other Australian snake
[7th] T63.071 Toxic effect of venom of other Australian snake, accidental (unintentional)
Toxic effect of venom of other Australian snake NOS
[7th] T63.072 Toxic effect of venom of other Australian snake, intentional self-harm
[7th] T63.073 Toxic effect of venom of other Australian snake, assault
[7th] T63.074 Toxic effect of venom of other Australian snake, undetermined

[6th] T63.08 Toxic effect of venom of other African and Asian snake
[7th] T63.081 Toxic effect of venom of other African and Asian snake, accidental (unintentional)
Toxic effect of venom of other African and Asian snake NOS
[7th] T63.082 Toxic effect of venom of other African and Asian snake, intentional self-harm
[7th] T63.083 Toxic effect of venom of other African and Asian snake, assault

Unspecified Code | Other Specified Code | [N] Newborn Age: 0 | [P] Pediatric Age: 0-17 | [M] Maternity Age: 12-55
[A] Adult Age: 15-124 | ♂ Male | ♀ Female | ● New Code | ▲ Revised Code Title | ►◄ Revised Text

[7th] T63.084 Toxic effect of venom of other African and Asian snake, undetermined

[6th] T63.09 Toxic effect of venom of other snake

[7th] T63.091 Toxic effect of venom of other snake, accidental (unintentional)

Toxic effect of venom of other snake NOS

[7th] T63.092 Toxic effect of venom of other snake, intentional self-harm

[7th] T63.093 Toxic effect of venom of other snake, assault

[7th] T63.094 Toxic effect of venom of other snake, undetermined

[5th] T63.1 Toxic effect of venom of other reptiles

[6th] T63.11 Toxic effect of venom of gila monster

[7th] T63.111 Toxic effect of venom of gila monster, accidental (unintentional)

Toxic effect of venom of gila monster NOS

[7th] T63.112 Toxic effect of venom of gila monster, intentional self-harm

[7th] T63.113 Toxic effect of venom of gila monster, assault

[7th] T63.114 Toxic effect of venom of gila monster, undetermined

[6th] T63.12 Toxic effect of venom of other venomous lizard

[7th] T63.121 Toxic effect of venom of other venomous lizard, accidental (unintentional)

Toxic effect of venom of other venomous lizard NOS

[7th] T63.122 Toxic effect of venom of other venomous lizard, intentional self-harm

[7th] T63.123 Toxic effect of venom of other venomous lizard, assault

[7th] T63.124 Toxic effect of venom of other venomous lizard, undetermined

[6th] T63.19 Toxic effect of venom of other reptiles

[7th] T63.191 Toxic effect of venom of other reptiles, accidental (unintentional)

Toxic effect of venom of other reptiles NOS

[7th] T63.192 Toxic effect of venom of other reptiles, intentional self-harm

[7th] T63.193 Toxic effect of venom of other reptiles, assault

[7th] T63.194 Toxic effect of venom of other reptiles, undetermined

[5th] T63.2 Toxic effect of venom of scorpion

[6th] T63.2X Toxic effect of venom of scorpion

[7th] T63.2X1 Toxic effect of venom of scorpion, accidental (unintentional)

Toxic effect of venom of scorpion NOS

[7th] T63.2X2 Toxic effect of venom of scorpion, intentional self-harm

[7th] T63.2X3 Toxic effect of venom of scorpion, assault

[7th] T63.2X4 Toxic effect of venom of scorpion, undetermined

[5th] T63.3 Toxic effect of venom of spider

[6th] T63.30 Toxic effect of unspecified spider venom

[7th] T63.301 Toxic effect of unspecified spider venom, accidental (unintentional)

[7th] T63.302 Toxic effect of unspecified spider venom, intentional self-harm

[7th] T63.303 Toxic effect of unspecified spider venom, assault

[7th] T63.304 Toxic effect of unspecified spider venom, undetermined

[6th] T63.31 Toxic effect of venom of black widow spider

[7th] T63.311 Toxic effect of venom of black widow spider, accidental (unintentional)

[7th] T63.312 Toxic effect of venom of black widow spider, intentional self-harm

[7th] T63.313 Toxic effect of venom of black widow spider, assault

[7th] T63.314 Toxic effect of venom of black widow spider, undetermined

[6th] T63.32 Toxic effect of venom of tarantula

[7th] T63.321 Toxic effect of venom of tarantula, accidental (unintentional)

[7th] T63.322 Toxic effect of venom of tarantula, intentional self-harm

[7th] T63.323 Toxic effect of venom of tarantula, assault

[7th] T63.324 Toxic effect of venom of tarantula, undetermined

[6th] T63.33 Toxic effect of venom of brown recluse spider

[7th] T63.331 Toxic effect of venom of brown recluse spider, accidental (unintentional)

[7th] T63.332 Toxic effect of venom of brown recluse spider, intentional self-harm

[7th] T63.333 Toxic effect of venom of brown recluse spider, assault

[7th] T63.334 Toxic effect of venom of brown recluse spider, undetermined

[6th] T63.39 Toxic effect of venom of other spider

[7th] T63.391 Toxic effect of venom of other spider, accidental (unintentional)

[7th] T63.392 Toxic effect of venom of other spider, intentional self-harm

[7th] T63.393 Toxic effect of venom of other spider, assault

[7th] T63.394 Toxic effect of venom of other spider, undetermined

[5th] T63.4 Toxic effect of venom of other arthropods

[6th] T63.41 Toxic effect of venom of centipedes and venomous millipedes

[7th] T63.411 Toxic effect of venom of centipedes and venomous millipedes, accidental (unintentional)

[7th] T63.412 Toxic effect of venom of centipedes and venomous millipedes, intentional self-harm

[7th] T63.413 Toxic effect of venom of centipedes and venomous millipedes, assault

[7th] T63.414 Toxic effect of venom of centipedes and venomous millipedes, undetermined

[6th] T63.42 Toxic effect of venom of ants

[7th] T63.421 Toxic effect of venom of ants, accidental (unintentional)

[7th] T63.422 Toxic effect of venom of ants, intentional self-harm

[7th] T63.423 Toxic effect of venom of ants, assault

[7th] T63.424 Toxic effect of venom of ants, undetermined

[6th] T63.43 Toxic effect of venom of caterpillars

[7th] T63.431 Toxic effect of venom of caterpillars, accidental (unintentional)

[7th] T63.432 Toxic effect of venom of caterpillars, intentional self-harm

[7th] T63.433 Toxic effect of venom of caterpillars, assault

[7th] T63.434 Toxic effect of venom of caterpillars, undetermined

[6th] T63.44 Toxic effect of venom of bees

[7th] T63.441 Toxic effect of venom of bees, accidental (unintentional)

[7th] T63.442 Toxic effect of venom of bees, intentional self-harm

[7th] T63.443 Toxic effect of venom of bees, assault

[7th] T63.444 Toxic effect of venom of bees, undetermined

[6th] T63.45 Toxic effect of venom of hornets

[7th] T63.451 Toxic effect of venom of hornets, accidental (unintentional)

[7th] T63.452 Toxic effect of venom of hornets, intentional self-harm

[7th] T63.453 Toxic effect of venom of hornets, assault

[4th] 4th character required [5th] 5th character required [6th] 6th character required [7th] 7th character required [X] Extension 'X' Alert
[EXCLUDES1] Not coded here [EXCLUDES2] Not included here [PDx] Primary Diagnosis Only Manifestation Code

[7th] T63.454 Toxic effect of venom of hornets, undetermined

[6th] T63.46 Toxic effect of venom of wasps
Toxic effect of yellow jacket

[7th] T63.461 Toxic effect of venom of wasps, accidental (unintentional)
[7th] T63.462 Toxic effect of venom of wasps, intentional self-harm
[7th] T63.463 Toxic effect of venom of wasps, assault
[7th] T63.464 Toxic effect of venom of wasps, undetermined

[6th] T63.48 Toxic effect of venom of other arthropod

[7th] T63.481 Toxic effect of venom of other arthropod, accidental (unintentional)
[7th] T63.482 Toxic effect of venom of other arthropod, intentional self-harm
[7th] T63.483 Toxic effect of venom of other arthropod, assault
[7th] T63.484 Toxic effect of venom of other arthropod, undetermined

[5th] T63.5 Toxic effect of contact with venomous fish
[EXCLUDES2] *poisoning by ingestion of fish (T61.-)*

[6th] T63.51 Toxic effect of contact with stingray

[7th] T63.511 Toxic effect of contact with stingray, accidental (unintentional)
[7th] T63.512 Toxic effect of contact with stingray, intentional self-harm
[7th] T63.513 Toxic effect of contact with stingray, assault
[7th] T63.514 Toxic effect of contact with stingray, undetermined

[6th] T63.59 Toxic effect of contact with other venomous fish

[7th] T63.591 Toxic effect of contact with other venomous fish, accidental (unintentional)
[7th] T63.592 Toxic effect of contact with other venomous fish, intentional self-harm
[7th] T63.593 Toxic effect of contact with other venomous fish, assault
[7th] T63.594 Toxic effect of contact with other venomous fish, undetermined

[5th] T63.6 Toxic effect of contact with other venomous marine animals
[EXCLUDES1] *sea-snake venom (T63.09)*
[EXCLUDES2] *poisoning by ingestion of shellfish (T61.78-)*

[6th] T63.61 Toxic effect of contact with Portugese Man-o-war
Toxic effect of contact with bluebottle

[7th] T63.611 Toxic effect of contact with Portugese Man-o-war, accidental (unintentional)
[7th] T63.612 Toxic effect of contact with Portugese Man-o-war, intentional self-harm
[7th] T63.613 Toxic effect of contact with Portugese Man-o-war, assault
[7th] T63.614 Toxic effect of contact with Portugese Man-o-war, undetermined

[6th] T63.62 Toxic effect of contact with other jellyfish

[7th] T63.621 Toxic effect of contact with other jellyfish, accidental (unintentional)
[7th] T63.622 Toxic effect of contact with other jellyfish, intentional self-harm
[7th] T63.623 Toxic effect of contact with other jellyfish, assault
[7th] T63.624 Toxic effect of contact with other jellyfish, undetermined

[6th] T63.63 Toxic effect of contact with sea anemone

[7th] T63.631 Toxic effect of contact with sea anemone, accidental (unintentional)
[7th] T63.632 Toxic effect of contact with sea anemone, intentional self-harm
[7th] T63.633 Toxic effect of contact with sea anemone, assault
[7th] T63.634 Toxic effect of contact with sea anemone, undetermined

[6th] T63.69 Toxic effect of contact with other venomous marine animals

[7th] T63.691 Toxic effect of contact with other venomous marine animals, accidental (unintentional)
[7th] T63.692 Toxic effect of contact with other venomous marine animals, intentional self-harm
[7th] T63.693 Toxic effect of contact with other venomous marine animals, assault
[7th] T63.694 Toxic effect of contact with other venomous marine animals, undetermined

[5th] T63.7 Toxic effect of contact with venomous plant

[6th] T63.71 Toxic effect of contact with venomous marine plant

[7th] T63.711 Toxic effect of contact with venomous marine plant, accidental (unintentional)
[7th] T63.712 Toxic effect of contact with venomous marine plant, intentional self-harm
[7th] T63.713 Toxic effect of contact with venomous marine plant, assault
[7th] T63.714 Toxic effect of contact with venomous marine plant, undetermined

[6th] T63.79 Toxic effect of contact with other venomous plant

[7th] T63.791 Toxic effect of contact with other venomous plant, accidental (unintentional)
[7th] T63.792 Toxic effect of contact with other venomous plant, intentional self-harm
[7th] T63.793 Toxic effect of contact with other venomous plant, assault
[7th] T63.794 Toxic effect of contact with other venomous plant, undetermined

[5th] T63.8 Toxic effect of contact with other venomous animals

[6th] T63.81 Toxic effect of contact with venomous frog
[EXCLUDES1] *contact with nonvenomous frog (W62.0)*

[7th] T63.811 Toxic effect of contact with venomous frog, accidental (unintentional)
[7th] T63.812 Toxic effect of contact with venomous frog, intentional self-harm
[7th] T63.813 Toxic effect of contact with venomous frog, assault
[7th] T63.814 Toxic effect of contact with venomous frog, undetermined

[6th] T63.82 Toxic effect of contact with venomous toad
[EXCLUDES1] *contact with nonvenomous toad (W62.1)*

[7th] T63.821 Toxic effect of contact with venomous toad, accidental (unintentional)
[7th] T63.822 Toxic effect of contact with venomous toad, intentional self-harm
[7th] T63.823 Toxic effect of contact with venomous toad, assault
[7th] T63.824 Toxic effect of contact with venomous toad, undetermined

[6th] T63.83 Toxic effect of contact with other venomous amphibian
[EXCLUDES1] *contact with nonvenomous amphibian (W62.9)*

[7th] T63.831 Toxic effect of contact with other venomous amphibian, accidental (unintentional)
[7th] T63.832 Toxic effect of contact with other venomous amphibian, intentional self-harm
[7th] T63.833 Toxic effect of contact with other venomous amphibian, assault
[7th] T63.834 Toxic effect of contact with other venomous amphibian, undetermined

[6th] T63.89 Toxic effect of contact with other venomous animals

Unspecified Code | Other Specified Code | [N] Newborn Age: 0 | [P] Pediatric Age: 0-17 | [M] Maternity Age: 12-55
[A] Adult Age: 15-124 | ♂ Male | ♀ Female | ● New Code | ▲ Revised Code Title | ►◄ Revised Text

CHAPTER 19: INJURY, POISONING, AND CERTAIN OTHER CONSEQUENCES OF EXTERNAL CAUSES (S00-T88)

T63.891 - T65.4X4

- T63.891 Toxic effect of contact with other venomous animals, accidental (unintentional)
- T63.892 Toxic effect of contact with other venomous animals, intentional self-harm
- T63.893 Toxic effect of contact with other venomous animals, assault
- T63.894 Toxic effect of contact with other venomous animals, undetermined
- T63.9 Toxic effect of contact with unspecified venomous animal
  - T63.91 Toxic effect of contact with unspecified venomous animal, accidental (unintentional)
  - T63.92 Toxic effect of contact with unspecified venomous animal, intentional self-harm
  - T63.93 Toxic effect of contact with unspecified venomous animal, assault
  - T63.94 Toxic effect of contact with unspecified venomous animal, undetermined
- T64 Toxic effect of aflatoxin and other mycotoxin food contaminants

  The appropriate 7th character is to be added to each code from category T64
  A = initial encounter
  D = subsequent encounter
  S = sequela
  - T64.0 Toxic effect of aflatoxin
    - T64.01 Toxic effect of aflatoxin, accidental (unintentional)
    - T64.02 Toxic effect of aflatoxin, intentional self-harm
    - T64.03 Toxic effect of aflatoxin, assault
    - T64.04 Toxic effect of aflatoxin, undetermined
  - T64.8 Toxic effect of other mycotoxin food contaminants
    - T64.81 Toxic effect of other mycotoxin food contaminants, accidental (unintentional)
    - T64.82 Toxic effect of other mycotoxin food contaminants, intentional self-harm
    - T64.83 Toxic effect of other mycotoxin food contaminants, assault
    - T64.84 Toxic effect of other mycotoxin food contaminants, undetermined
- T65 Toxic effect of other and unspecified substances

  The appropriate 7th character is to be added to each code from category T65
  A = initial encounter
  D = subsequent encounter
  S = sequela
  - T65.0 Toxic effect of cyanides

    EXCLUDES1 hydrogen cyanide (T57.3-)
    - T65.0X Toxic effect of cyanides
      - T65.0X1 Toxic effect of cyanides, accidental (unintentional)

        Toxic effect of cyanides NOS
      - T65.0X2 Toxic effect of cyanides, intentional self-harm
      - T65.0X3 Toxic effect of cyanides, assault
      - T65.0X4 Toxic effect of cyanides, undetermined
  - T65.1 Toxic effect of strychnine and its salts
    - T65.1X Toxic effect of strychnine and its salts
      - T65.1X1 Toxic effect of strychnine and its salts, accidental (unintentional)

        Toxic effect of strychnine and its salts NOS
      - T65.1X2 Toxic effect of strychnine and its salts, intentional self-harm
      - T65.1X3 Toxic effect of strychnine and its salts, assault
      - T65.1X4 Toxic effect of strychnine and its salts, undetermined

- T65.2 Toxic effect of tobacco and nicotine

  EXCLUDES2 nicotine dependence (F17.-)
  - T65.21 Toxic effect of chewing tobacco
    - T65.211 Toxic effect of chewing tobacco, accidental (unintentional)

      Toxic effect of chewing tobacco NOS
    - T65.212 Toxic effect of chewing tobacco, intentional self-harm
    - T65.213 Toxic effect of chewing tobacco, assault
    - T65.214 Toxic effect of chewing tobacco, undetermined
  - T65.22 Toxic effect of tobacco cigarettes

    Toxic effect of tobacco smoke
    Use additional code for exposure to second hand tobacco smoke (Z57.31, Z77.22)
    - T65.221 Toxic effect of tobacco cigarettes, accidental (unintentional)

      Toxic effect of tobacco cigarettes NOS
    - T65.222 Toxic effect of tobacco cigarettes, intentional self-harm
    - T65.223 Toxic effect of tobacco cigarettes, assault
    - T65.224 Toxic effect of tobacco cigarettes, undetermined
  - T65.29 Toxic effect of other tobacco and nicotine
    - T65.291 Toxic effect of other tobacco and nicotine, accidental (unintentional)

      Toxic effect of other tobacco and nicotine NOS
    - T65.292 Toxic effect of other tobacco and nicotine, intentional self-harm
    - T65.293 Toxic effect of other tobacco and nicotine, assault
    - T65.294 Toxic effect of other tobacco and nicotine, undetermined
  - T65.3 Toxic effect of nitroderivatives and aminoderivatives of benzene and its homologues

    Toxic effect of anilin [benzenamine]
    Toxic effect of nitrobenzene
    Toxic effect of trinitrotoluene
    - T65.3X Toxic effect of nitroderivatives and aminoderivatives of benzene and its homologues
      - T65.3X1 Toxic effect of nitroderivatives and aminoderivatives of benzene and its homologues, accidental (unintentional)

        Toxic effect of nitroderivatives and aminoderivatives of benzene and its homologues NOS
      - T65.3X2 Toxic effect of nitroderivatives and aminoderivatives of benzene and its homologues, intentional self-harm
      - T65.3X3 Toxic effect of nitroderivatives and aminoderivatives of benzene and its homologues, assault
      - T65.3X4 Toxic effect of nitroderivatives and aminoderivatives of benzene and its homologues, undetermined
  - T65.4 Toxic effect of carbon disulfide
    - T65.4X Toxic effect of carbon disulfide
      - T65.4X1 Toxic effect of carbon disulfide, accidental (unintentional)

        Toxic effect of carbon disulfide NOS
      - T65.4X2 Toxic effect of carbon disulfide, intentional self-harm
      - T65.4X3 Toxic effect of carbon disulfide, assault
      - T65.4X4 Toxic effect of carbon disulfide, undetermined

---

4ᵗʰ character required   5ᵗʰ character required   6ᵗʰ character required   7ᵗʰ character required   Extension 'X' Alert

EXCLUDES 1 Not coded here   EXCLUDES 2 Not included here   PDx Primary Diagnosis Only   Manifestation Code

[5th] T65.5 Toxic effect of nitroglycerin and other nitric acids and esters
Toxic effect of 1,2,3-Propanetriol trinitrate
[6th] T65.5X Toxic effect of nitroglycerin and other nitric acids and esters
[7th] T65.5X1 Toxic effect of nitroglycerin and other nitric acids and esters, accidental (unintentional)
Toxic effect of nitroglycerin and other nitric acids and esters NOS
[7th] T65.5X2 Toxic effect of nitroglycerin and other nitric acids and esters, intentional self-harm
[7th] T65.5X3 Toxic effect of nitroglycerin and other nitric acids and esters, assault
[7th] T65.5X4 Toxic effect of nitroglycerin and other nitric acids and esters, undetermined
[5th] T65.6 Toxic effect of paints and dyes, not elsewhere classified
[6th] T65.6X Toxic effect of paints and dyes, not elsewhere classified
[7th] T65.6X1 Toxic effect of paints and dyes, not elsewhere classified, accidental (unintentional)
Toxic effect of paints and dyes NOS
[7th] T65.6X2 Toxic effect of paints and dyes, not elsewhere classified, intentional self-harm
[7th] T65.6X3 Toxic effect of paints and dyes, not elsewhere classified, assault
[7th] T65.6X4 Toxic effect of paints and dyes, not elsewhere classified, undetermined
[5th] T65.8 Toxic effect of other specified substances
[6th] T65.81 Toxic effect of latex
[7th] T65.811 Toxic effect of latex, accidental (unintentional)
Toxic effect of latex NOS
[7th] T65.812 Toxic effect of latex, intentional self-harm
[7th] T65.813 Toxic effect of latex, assault
[7th] T65.814 Toxic effect of latex, undetermined
[6th] T65.82 Toxic effect of harmful algae and algae toxins
Toxic effect of (harmful) algae bloom NOS
Toxic effect of blue-green algae bloom
Toxic effect of brown tide
Toxic effect of cyanobacteria bloom
Toxic effect of Florida red tide
Toxic effect of pfiesteria piscicida
Toxic effect of red tide
[7th] T65.821 Toxic effect of harmful algae and algae toxins, accidental (unintentional)
Toxic effect of harmful algae and algae toxins NOS
[7th] T65.822 Toxic effect of harmful algae and algae toxins, intentional self-harm
[7th] T65.823 Toxic effect of harmful algae and algae toxins, assault
[7th] T65.824 Toxic effect of harmful algae and algae toxins, undetermined
[6th] T65.83 Toxic effect of fiberglass
[7th] T65.831 Toxic effect of fiberglass, accidental (unintentional)
Toxic effect of fiberglass NOS
[7th] T65.832 Toxic effect of fiberglass, intentional self-harm
[7th] T65.833 Toxic effect of fiberglass, assault
[7th] T65.834 Toxic effect of fiberglass, undetermined
[6th] T65.89 Toxic effect of other specified substances
[7th] T65.891 Toxic effect of other specified substances, accidental (unintentional)
Toxic effect of other specified substances NOS
[7th] T65.892 Toxic effect of other specified substances, intentional self-harm
[7th] T65.893 Toxic effect of other specified substances, assault
[7th] T65.894 Toxic effect of other specified substances, undetermined
[5th] T65.9 Toxic effect of unspecified substance
[7th] T65.91 Toxic effect of unspecified substance, accidental (unintentional)
Poisoning NOS
[7th] T65.92 Toxic effect of unspecified substance, intentional self-harm
[7th] T65.93 Toxic effect of unspecified substance, assault
[7th] T65.94 Toxic effect of unspecified substance, undetermined

Other and unspecified effects of external causes (T66-T78)

[7th] T66 Radiation sickness, unspecified
[EXCLUDES1] *specified adverse effects of radiation, such as:*
burns (T20-T31)
leukemia (C91-C95)
radiation gastroenteritis and colitis (K52.0)
radiation pneumonitis (J70.0)
radiation related disorders of the skin and subcutaneous tissue (L55-L59)
sunburn (L55.-)
The appropriate 7th character is to be added to code T66
A = initial encounter
D = subsequent encounter
S = sequela
[4th] T67 Effects of heat and light
[EXCLUDES1] *erythema [dermatitis] ab igne (L59.0)*
malignant hyperpyrexia due to anesthesia (T88.3)
radiation-related disorders of the skin and subcutaneous tissue (L55-L59)
[EXCLUDES2] *burns (T20-T31)*
sunburn (L55.-)
sweat disorder due to heat (L74-L75)
The appropriate 7th character is to be added to each code from category T67
A = initial encounter
D = subsequent encounter
S = sequela
[7th] T67.0 Heatstroke and sunstroke
Heat apoplexy
Heat pyrexia
Siriasis
Thermoplegia
Use additional code(s) to identify any associated complications of heatstroke, such as:
coma and stupor (R40.-)
systemic inflammatory response syndrome (R65.1-)
[7th] T67.1 Heat syncope
Heat collapse
[7th] T67.2 Heat cramp
[7th] T67.3 Heat exhaustion, anhydrotic
Heat prostration due to water depletion
[EXCLUDES1] *heat exhaustion due to salt depletion (T67.4)*
[7th] T67.4 Heat exhaustion due to salt depletion
Heat prostration due to salt (and water) depletion
[7th] T67.5 Heat exhaustion, unspecified
Heat prostration NOS
[7th] T67.6 Heat fatigue, transient
[7th] T67.7 Heat edema
[7th] T67.8 Other effects of heat and light
[7th] T67.9 Effect of heat and light, unspecified

Unspecified Code | Other Specified Code | [N] Newborn Age: 0 | [P] Pediatric Age: 0-17 | [M] Maternity Age: 12-55
[A] Adult Age: 15-124 | ♂ Male | ♀ Female | ● New Code | ▲ Revised Code Title | ►◄ Revised Text

[7th] **T68 Hypothermia**

Accidental hypothermia
Hypothermia NOS
Use additional code to identify source of exposure:
Exposure to excessive cold of man-made origin (W93)
Exposure to excessive cold of natural origin (X31)

[EXCLUDES1] *hypothermia following anesthesia (T88.51)*
hypothermia not associated with low environmental temperature (R68.0)
hypothermia of newborn (P80.-)

[EXCLUDES2] *frostbite (T33-T34)*

The appropriate 7th character is to be added to code T68
A = initial encounter
D = subsequent encounter
S = sequela

[4th] **T69 Other effects of reduced temperature**

Use additional code to identify source of exposure:
Exposure to excessive cold of man-made origin (W93)
Exposure to excessive cold of natural origin (X31)

[EXCLUDES2] *frostbite (T33-T34)*

The appropriate 7th character is to be added to each code from category T69
A = initial encounter
D = subsequent encounter
S = sequela

[5th] **T69.0 Immersion hand and foot**
[6th] **T69.01 Immersion hand**
[7th] **T69.011 Immersion hand, right hand**
[7th] **T69.012 Immersion hand, left hand**
[7th] **T69.019 Immersion hand, unspecified hand**
[6th] **T69.02 Immersion foot**
Trench foot
[7th] **T69.021 Immersion foot, right foot**
[7th] **T69.022 Immersion foot, left foot**
[7th] **T69.029 Immersion foot, unspecified foot**
[7th] **T69.1 Chilblains**
[7th] **T69.8 Other specified effects of reduced temperature**
[7th] **T69.9 Effect of reduced temperature, unspecified**

[4th] **T70 Effects of air pressure and water pressure**

The appropriate 7th character is to be added to each code from category T70
A = initial encounter
D = subsequent encounter
S = sequela

[7th] **T70.0 Otitic barotrauma**
Aero-otitis media
Effects of change in ambient atmospheric pressure or water pressure on ears
[7th] **T70.1 Sinus barotrauma**
Aerosinusitis
Effects of change in ambient atmospheric pressure on sinuses
[5th] **T70.2 Other and unspecified effects of high altitude**
[EXCLUDES2] *polycythemia due to high altitude (D75.1)*
[7th] **T70.20 Unspecified effects of high altitude**
[7th] **T70.29 Other effects of high altitude**
Alpine sickness
Anoxia due to high altitude
Barotrauma NOS
Hypobaropathy
Mountain sickness
[7th] **T70.3 Caisson disease [decompression sickness]**
Compressed-air disease
Diver's palsy or paralysis
[7th] **T70.4 Effects of high-pressure fluids**
Hydraulic jet injection (industrial)
Pneumatic jet injection (industrial)
Traumatic jet injection (industrial)
[7th] **T70.8 Other effects of air pressure and water pressure**
[7th] **T70.9 Effect of air pressure and water pressure, unspecified**

[4th] **T71 Asphyxiation**

Mechanical suffocation
Traumatic suffocation

[EXCLUDES1] *acute respiratory distress (syndrome) (J80)*
anoxia due to high altitude (T70.2)
asphyxia NOS (R09.01)
asphyxia from carbon monoxide (T58.-)
asphyxia from inhalation of food or foreign body (T17.-)
asphyxia from other gases, fumes and vapors (T59.-)
respiratory distress (syndrome) in newborn (P22.-)

The appropriate 7th character is to be added to each code from category T71
A = initial encounter
D = subsequent encounter
S = sequela

[5th] **T71.1 Asphyxiation due to mechanical threat to breathing**
Suffocation due to mechanical threat to breathing
[6th] **T71.11 Asphyxiation due to smothering under pillow**
[7th] **T71.111 Asphyxiation due to smothering under pillow, accidental**
Asphyxiation due to smothering under pillow NOS
[7th] **T71.112 Asphyxiation due to smothering under pillow, intentional self-harm**
[7th] **T71.113 Asphyxiation due to smothering under pillow, assault**
[7th] **T71.114 Asphyxiation due to smothering under pillow, undetermined**
[6th] **T71.12 Asphyxiation due to plastic bag**
[7th] **T71.121 Asphyxiation due to plastic bag, accidental**
Asphyxiation due to plastic bag NOS
[7th] **T71.122 Asphyxiation due to plastic bag, intentional self-harm**
[7th] **T71.123 Asphyxiation due to plastic bag, assault**
[7th] **T71.124 Asphyxiation due to plastic bag, undetermined**
[6th] **T71.13 Asphyxiation due to being trapped in bed linens**
[7th] **T71.131 Asphyxiation due to being trapped in bed linens, accidental**
Asphyxiation due to being trapped in bed linens NOS
[7th] **T71.132 Asphyxiation due to being trapped in bed linens, intentional self-harm**
[7th] **T71.133 Asphyxiation due to being trapped in bed linens, assault**
[7th] **T71.134 Asphyxiation due to being trapped in bed linens, undetermined**
[6th] **T71.14 Asphyxiation due to smothering under another person's body (in bed)**
[7th] **T71.141 Asphyxiation due to smothering under another person's body (in bed), accidental**
Asphyxiation due to smothering under another person's body (in bed) NOS
[7th] **T71.143 Asphyxiation due to smothering under another person's body (in bed), assault**
[7th] **T71.144 Asphyxiation due to smothering under another person's body (in bed), undetermined**

DRAFT

[4th] 4th character required [5th] 5th character required [6th] 6th character required [7th] 7th character required [7th] Extension 'X' Alert
[EXCLUDES1] Not coded here [EXCLUDES2] Not included here [PDx] Primary Diagnosis Only Manifestation Code

6ᵈ **T71.15 Asphyxiation due to** smothering in furniture

7ᵈ **T71.151 Asphyxiation due to smothering in furniture,** accidental

Asphyxiation due to smothering in furniture NOS

7ᵈ **T71.152 Asphyxiation due to smothering in furniture,** intentional self-harm

7ᵈ **T71.153 Asphyxiation due to smothering in furniture,** assault

7ᵈ **T71.154 Asphyxiation due to smothering in furniture,** undetermined

6ᵈ **T71.16 Asphyxiation due to** hanging

Hanging by window shade cord
Use additional code for any associated injuries, such as:
crushing injury of neck (S17.-)
fracture of cervical vertebrae (S12.0-S12.2-)
open wound of neck (S11.-)

7ᵈ **T71.161 Asphyxiation due to hanging,** accidental

Asphyxiation due to hanging NOS
Hanging NOS

7ᵈ **T71.162 Asphyxiation due to hanging,** intentional self-harm

7ᵈ **T71.163 Asphyxiation due to hanging,** assault

7ᵈ **T71.164 Asphyxiation due to hanging,** undetermined

6ᵈ **T71.19 Asphyxiation due to mechanical threat to breathing** due to other causes

7ᵈ **T71.191 Asphyxiation due to mechanical threat to breathing due to other causes,** accidental

Asphyxiation due to other causes NOS

7ᵈ **T71.192 Asphyxiation due to mechanical threat to breathing due to other causes,** intentional self-harm

7ᵈ **T71.193 Asphyxiation due to mechanical threat to breathing due to other causes,** assault

7ᵈ **T71.194 Asphyxiation due to mechanical threat to breathing due to other causes,** undetermined

5ᵈ **T71.2 Asphyxiation due to** systemic oxygen deficiency due to low oxygen content in ambient air

Suffocation due to systemic oxygen deficiency due to low oxygen content in ambient air

7ᵈ **T71.20 Asphyxiation due to systemic oxygen deficiency due to low oxygen content in ambient air due to unspecified cause**

7ᵈ **T71.21 Asphyxiation due to** cave-in or falling earth

Use additional code for any associated cataclysm (X34-X38)

6ᵈ **T71.22 Asphyxiation due to** being trapped in a car trunk

7ᵈ **T71.221 Asphyxiation due to being trapped in a car trunk,** accidental

7ᵈ **T71.222 Asphyxiation due to being trapped in a car trunk,** intentional self-harm

7ᵈ **T71.223 Asphyxiation due to being trapped in a car trunk,** assault

7ᵈ **T71.224 Asphyxiation due to being trapped in a car trunk,** undetermined

6ᵈ **T71.23 Asphyxiation due to being** trapped in a (discarded) refrigerator

7ᵈ **T71.231 Asphyxiation due to being trapped in a (discarded) refrigerator,** accidental

7ᵈ **T71.232 Asphyxiation due to being trapped in a (discarded) refrigerator,** intentional self-harm

7ᵈ **T71.233 Asphyxiation due to being trapped in a (discarded) refrigerator,** assault

7ᵈ **T71.234 Asphyxiation due to being trapped in a (discarded) refrigerator,** undetermined

7ᵈ **T71.29 Asphyxiation due to being trapped in other low oxygen environment**

7ᵈ **T71.9 Asphyxiation due to unspecified cause**

Suffocation (by strangulation) due to unspecified cause
Suffocation NOS
Systemic oxygen deficiency due to low oxygen content in ambient air due to unspecified cause
Systemic oxygen deficiency due to mechanical threat to breathing due to unspecified cause
Traumatic asphyxia NOS

4ᵈ **T73 Effects of other deprivation**

The appropriate 7th character is to be added to each code from category T73
A = initial encounter
D = subsequent encounter
S = sequela

7ᵈ **T73.0 Starvation**

Deprivation of food

7ᵈ **T73.1 Deprivation of water**

7ᵈ **T73.2 Exhaustion due to exposure**

7ᵈ **T73.3 Exhaustion due to excessive exertion**

Exhaustion due to overexertion

7ᵈ **T73.8 Other effects of deprivation**

7ᵈ **T73.9 Effect of deprivation, unspecified**

4ᵈ **T74 Adult and child abuse, neglect and other maltreatment, confirmed**

Use additional code, if applicable, to identify any associated current injury
external cause code to identify perpetrator, if known (Y07.-)

EXCLUDES1 abuse and maltreatment in pregnancy (O9A.3-, O9A.4-, O9A.5-)
adult and child maltreatment, suspected (T76.-)

The appropriate 7th character is to be added to each code from category T74
A = initial encounter
D = subsequent encounter
S = sequela

5ᵈ **T74.0 Neglect or abandonment, confirmed**

7ᵈ **T74.01 Adult neglect or abandonment, confirmed**

7ᵈ **T74.02 Child neglect or abandonment, confirmed**

5ᵈ **T74.1 Physical abuse, confirmed**

EXCLUDES2 sexual abuse (T74.2-)

7ᵈ **T74.11 Adult physical abuse, confirmed**

7ᵈ **T74.12 Child physical abuse, confirmed**

EXCLUDES2 shaken infant syndrome (T74.4)

5ᵈ **T74.2 Sexual abuse, confirmed**

Rape, confirmed
Sexual assault, confirmed

7ᵈ **T74.21 Adult sexual abuse, confirmed**

7ᵈ **T74.22 Child sexual abuse, confirmed**

5ᵈ **T74.3 Psychological abuse, confirmed**

7ᵈ **T74.31 Adult psychological abuse, confirmed**

7ᵈ **T74.32 Child psychological abuse, confirmed**

7ᵈ **T74.4 Shaken infant syndrome**

5ᵈ **T74.9 Unspecified maltreatment, confirmed**

7ᵈ **T74.91 Unspecified adult maltreatment, confirmed**

7ᵈ **T74.92 Unspecified child maltreatment, confirmed**

4ᵈ **T75 Other and unspecified effects of other external causes**

EXCLUDES1 adverse effects NEC (T78.-)
EXCLUDES2 burns (electric) (T20-T31)

The appropriate 7th character is to be added to each code from category T75
A = initial encounter
D = subsequent encounter
S = sequela

Unspecified Code   Other Specified Code   N Newborn Age: 0   P Pediatric Age: 0 17   M Maternity Age: 12-55
A Adult Age: 15-124   ♂ Male   ♀ Female   ● New Code   ▲ Revised Code Title   ►◄ Revised Text

[5th] **T75.0 Effects of lightning**
Struck by lightning
[7th] **T75.00 Unspecified effects of lightning**
Struck by lightning NOS
[7th] **T75.01 Shock due to being struck by lightning**
[7th] **T75.09 Other effects of lightning**
Use additional code for other effects of lightning
[7th] **T75.1 Unspecified effects of drowning and nonfatal submersion**
Immersion
EXCLUDES1 *specified effects of drowning- code to effects*
[5th] **T75.2 Effects of vibration**
[7th] **T75.20 Unspecified effects of vibration**
[7th] **T75.21 Pneumatic hammer syndrome**
[7th] **T75.22 Traumatic vasospastic syndrome**
[7th] **T75.23 Vertigo from infrasound**
EXCLUDES1 *vertigo NOS (R42)*
[7th] **T75.29 Other effects of vibration**
[7th] **T75.3 Motion sickness**
Airsickness
Seasickness
Travel sickness
Use additional external cause code to identify vehicle or type of motion (Y92.81-, Y93.5-)
[7th] **T75.4 Electrocution**
Shock from electric current
Shock from electroshock gun (taser)
[5th] **T75.8 Other specified effects of external causes**
[7th] **T75.81 Effects of abnormal gravitation [G] forces**
[7th] **T75.82 Effects of weightlessness**
[7th] **T75.89 Other specified effects of external causes**
[4th] **T76 Adult and child abuse, neglect and other maltreatment, suspected**
Use additional code, if applicable, to identify any associated current injury
EXCLUDES1 *adult and child maltreatment, confirmed (T74.-)*
suspected abuse and maltreatment in pregnancy (O9A.3-, O9A.4-, O9A.5-)
suspected adult physical abuse, ruled out (Z04.71)
suspected adult sexual abuse, ruled out (Z04.41)
suspected child physical abuse, ruled out (Z04.72)
suspected child sexual abuse, ruled out (Z04.42)
The appropriate 7th character is to be added to each code from category T76
A = initial encounter
D = subsequent encounter
S = sequela
[5th] **T76.0 Neglect or abandonment, suspected**
[7th] **T76.01 Adult neglect or abandonment, suspected**
[7th] **T76.02 Child neglect or abandonment, suspected**
[5th] **T76.1 Physical abuse, suspected**
[7th] **T76.11 Adult physical abuse, suspected**
[7th] **T76.12 Child physical abuse, suspected**
[5th] **T76.2 Sexual abuse, suspected**
Rape, suspected
Sexual abuse, suspected
EXCLUDES1 *alleged abuse, ruled out (Z04.7)*
[7th] **T76.21 Adult sexual abuse, suspected**
[7th] **T76.22 Child sexual abuse, suspected**
[5th] **T76.3 Psychological abuse, suspected**
[7th] **T76.31 Adult psychological abuse, suspected**
[7th] **T76.32 Child psychological abuse, suspected**
[5th] **T76.9 Unspecified maltreatment, suspected**
[7th] **T76.91 Unspecified adult maltreatment, suspected**
[7th] **T76.92 Unspecified child maltreatment, suspected**

[4th] **T78 Adverse effects, not elsewhere classified**
EXCLUDES2 *complications of surgical and medical care NEC (T80-T88)*
The appropriate 7th character is to be added to each code from category T78
A = initial encounter
D = subsequent encounter
S = sequela
[5th] **T78.0 Anaphylactic reaction due to food**
Anaphylactic reaction due to adverse food reaction
Anaphylactic shock or reaction due to nonpoisonous foods
Anaphylactoid reaction due to food
[7th] **T78.00 Anaphylactic reaction due to unspecified food**
[7th] **T78.01 Anaphylactic reaction due to peanuts**
[7th] **T78.02 Anaphylactic reaction due to shellfish (crustaceans)**
[7th] **T78.03 Anaphylactic reaction due to other fish**
[7th] **T78.04 Anaphylactic reaction due to fruits and vegetables**
[7th] **T78.05 Anaphylactic reaction due to tree nuts and seeds**
EXCLUDES1 *anaphylactic reaction due to peanuts (T78.01)*
[7th] **T78.06 Anaphylactic reaction due to food additives**
[7th] **T78.07 Anaphylactic reaction due to milk and dairy products**
[7th] **T78.08 Anaphylactic reaction due to eggs**
[7th] **T78.09 Anaphylactic reaction due to other food products**
[7th] **T78.1 Other adverse food reactions, not elsewhere classified**
Use additional code to identify the type of reaction
EXCLUDES1 *anaphylactic reaction or shock due to adverse food reaction (T78.0-)*
anaphylactic reaction due to food (T78.0-)
bacterial food borne intoxications (A05.-)
EXCLUDES2 *allergic and dietetic gastroenteritis and colitis (K52.2)*
allergic rhinitis due to food (J30.5)
dermatitis due to food in contact with skin (L23.6, L24.6, L25.4)
dermatitis due to ingested food (L27.2)
[7th] **T78.2 Anaphylactic shock, unspecified**
Allergic shock
Anaphylactic reaction
Anaphylaxis
EXCLUDES1 *anaphylactic reaction or shock due to adverse effect of correct medicinal substance properly administered (T88.6)*
anaphylactic reaction or shock due to adverse food reaction (T78.0-)
anaphylactic reaction or shock due to serum (T80.5-)
[7th] **T78.3 Angioneurotic edema**
Allergic angioedema
Giant urticaria
Quincke's edema
EXCLUDES1 *serum urticaria (T80.6-)*
urticaria (L50.-)
[5th] **T78.4 Other and unspecified allergy**
EXCLUDES1 *specified types of allergic reaction such as:*
allergic diarrhea (K52.2)
allergic gastroenteritis and colitis (K52.2)
dermatitis (L23-L25, L27.-)
hay fever (J30.1)
[7th] **T78.40 Allergy, unspecified**
Allergic reaction NOS
Hypersensitivity NOS
[7th] **T78.41 Arthus phenomenon**
Arthus reaction
[7th] **T78.49 Other allergy**
[7th] **T78.8 Other adverse effects, not elsewhere classified**

[4th] 4th character required [5th] 5th character required [6th] 6th character required [7th] 7th character required [7th] Extension 'X' Alert
EXCLUDES1 Not coded here EXCLUDES2 Not included here PDx Primary Diagnosis Only Manifestation Code

Certain early complications of trauma (T79)

Ⓛ **T79 Certain early complications of trauma, not elsewhere classified**

> EXCLUDES2 *acute respiratory distress syndrome (J80)*
> *complications occurring during or following medical procedures (T80-T88)*
> *complications of surgical and medical care NEC (T80-T88)*
> *newborn respiratory distress syndrome (P22.0)*

> **The appropriate 7th character is to be added to each code from category T79**
> **A = initial encounter**
> **D = subsequent encounter**
> **S = sequela**

Ⓣ **T79.0 Air embolism (traumatic)**

> EXCLUDES1 *air embolism complicating abortion or ectopic or molar pregnancy (O00-O07, O08.2)*
> *air embolism complicating pregnancy, childbirth and the puerperium (O88.0)*
> *air embolism following infusion, transfusion, and therapeutic injection (T80.0)*
> *air embolism following procedure NEC (T81.7-)*

Ⓣ **T79.1 Fat embolism (traumatic)**

> EXCLUDES1 *fat embolism complicating:*
> *abortion or ectopic or molar pregnancy (O00-O07, O08.2)*
> *pregnancy, childbirth and the puerperium (O88.8)*

Ⓣ **T79.2 Traumatic secondary and recurrent hemorrhage and seroma**

Ⓣ **T79.4 Traumatic shock**

> Shock (immediate) (delayed) following injury
> EXCLUDES1 *anaphylactic shock due to adverse food reaction (T78.0-)*
> *anaphylactic shock due to correct medicinal substance properly administered (T88.6)*
> *anaphylactic shock due to serum (T80.5-)*
> *anaphylactic shock NOS (T78.2)*
> *anesthetic shock (T88.2)*
> *electric shock (T75.4)*
> *nontraumatic shock NEC (R57.-)*
> *obstetric shock (O75.1)*
> *postprocedural shock (T81.1-)*
> *septic shock (R65.21)*
> *shock complicating abortion or ectopic or molar pregnancy (O00-O07, O08.3)*
> *shock due to lightning (T75.01)*
> *shock NOS (R57.9)*

Ⓣ **T79.5 Traumatic anuria**

> Crush syndrome
> Renal failure following crushing

Ⓣ **T79.6 Traumatic ischemia of muscle**

> Traumatic rhabdomyolysis
> Volkmann's ischemic contracture
> EXCLUDES2 *anterior tibial syndrome (M76.8)*
> *compartment syndrome (traumatic) (T79.A-)*
> *nontraumatic ischemia of muscle (M62.2-)*

Ⓣ **T79.7 Traumatic subcutaneous emphysema**

> EXCLUDES1 *emphysema NOS (J43)*
> *emphysema (subcutaneous) resulting from a procedure (T81.82)*

Ⓢ **T79.A Traumatic compartment syndrome**

> EXCLUDES1 *fibromyalgia (M79.7)*
> *nontraumatic compartment syndrome (M79.A-)*
> *traumatic ischemic infarction of muscle (T79.6)*

Ⓣ **T79.A0 Compartment syndrome, unspecified**

> Compartment syndrome NOS

Ⓢ **T79.A1 Traumatic compartment syndrome of** upper extremity

> Traumatic compartment syndrome of shoulder, arm, forearm, wrist, hand, and fingers

Ⓣ **T79.A11 Traumatic compartment syndrome of** right upper extremity

Ⓣ **T79.A12 Traumatic compartment syndrome of** left upper extremity

Ⓣ **T79.A19 Traumatic compartment syndrome of** unspecified upper extremity

Ⓢ **T79.A2 Traumatic compartment syndrome of** lower extremity

> Traumatic compartment syndrome of hip, buttock, thigh, leg, foot, and toes

Ⓣ **T79.A21 Traumatic compartment syndrome of** right lower extremity

Ⓣ **T79.A22 Traumatic compartment syndrome of** left lower extremity

Ⓣ **T79.A29 Traumatic compartment syndrome of** unspecified lower extremity

Ⓣ **T79.A3 Traumatic compartment syndrome of abdomen**

Ⓣ **T79.A9 Traumatic compartment syndrome of other sites**

Ⓣ **T79.8 Other early complications of trauma**

Ⓣ **T79.9 Unspecified early complication of trauma**

Complications of surgical and medical care, not elsewhere classified (T80-T88)

> Use additional code for adverse effect, if applicable, to identify drug (T36-T50 with fifth or sixth character 5)
> code(s) to identify the specified condition resulting from the complication
> code to identify devices involved and details of circumstances (Y62-Y82)

> EXCLUDES2 *any encounters with medical care for postprocedural conditions in which no complications are present, such as:*
> *artificial opening status (Z93.-)*
> *closure of external stoma (Z43.-)*
> *fitting and adjustment of external prosthetic device (Z44.-)*
> *burns and corrosions from local applications and irradiation (T20-T32)*
> *complications of surgical procedures during pregnancy, childbirth and the puerperium (O00-O9A)*
> *mechanical complication of respirator [ventilator] (J95.850)*
> *poisoning and toxic effects of drugs and chemicals (T36-T65 with fifth or sixth character 1-4 or 6)*
> *postprocedural fever (R50.82)*
> *specified complications classified elsewhere, such as:*
> *cerebrospinal fluid leak from spinal puncture (G97.0)*
> *colostomy malfunction (K94.0-)*
> *disorders of fluid and electrolyte imbalance (E86-E87)*
> *functional disturbances following cardiac surgery (I97.0-I97.1)*
> *intraoperative and postprocedural complications of specified body systems (D78.-, E36.-, E89.-, G97.3-, G97.4, H59.3-, H59.-, H95.2-, H95.3, I97.4-, I97.5, J95.6-, J95.7, K91.6-, L76.-, M96.-, N99.-)*
> *ostomy complications (J95.0-, K94.-, N99.5-)*
> *postgastric surgery syndromes (K91.1)*
> *postlaminectomy syndrome NEC (M96.1)*
> *postmastectomy lymphedema syndrome (I97.2)*
> *postsurgical blind-loop syndrome (K91.2)*
> *ventilator associated pneumonia (J95.851)*

Unspecified Code	Other Specified Code	Ⓝ Newborn Age: 0	Ⓟ Pediatric Age: 0-17	Ⓜ Maternity Age: 12-55
Ⓐ Adult Age: 15-124	♂ Male	♀ Female	● New Code	▲ Revised Code Title ▶◀ Revised Text

[4th] **T80 Complications following infusion, transfusion and therapeutic injection**

INCLUDES *complications following perfusion*

EXCLUDES2 *bone marrow transplant rejection (T86.01)*
febrile nonhemolytic transfusion reaction (R50.84)
fluid overload due to transfusion (E87.71)
posttransfusion purpura (D69.51)
transfusion associated circulatory overload (TACO) (E87.71)
transfusion (red blood cell) associated hemochromatosis (E83.111)
transfusion related acute lung injury (TRALI) (J95.84)

The appropriate 7th character is to be added to each code from category T80
A = initial encounter
D = subsequent encounter
S = sequela

[7th] **T80.0 Air embolism following infusion, transfusion and therapeutic injection**

[7th] **T80.1 Vascular complications following infusion, transfusion and therapeutic injection**
Use additional code to identify the vascular complication

EXCLUDES2 *extravasation of vesicant agent (T80.81-)*
infiltration of vesicant agent (T80.81-)
vascular complications specified as due to prosthetic devices, implants and grafts (T82.8-, T83.8, T84.8-, T85.8)
postprocedural vascular complications (T81.7-)

[5th] **T80.2 Infections following infusion, transfusion and therapeutic injection**
Use additional code to identify the specific infection, such as:
sepsis (A41.9)
code (R65.2-) to identify severe sepsis, if applicable

EXCLUDES2 *infections specified as due to prosthetic devices, implants and grafts (T82.6-T82.7, T83.5-T83.6, T84.5-T84.7, T85.7)*
postprocedural infections (T81.4)

[6th] **T80.21 Infection due to central venous catheter**

[7th] **T80.211 Bloodstream infection due to central venous catheter**
Catheter-related bloodstream infection (CRBSI) NOS
Central line-associated bloodstream infection (CLABSI)
Bloodstream infection due to Hickman catheter
Bloodstream infection due to peripherally inserted central catheter (PICC)
Bloodstream infection due to portacath (port-a-cath)
Bloodstream infection due to triple lumen catheter
Bloodstream infection due to umbilical venous catheter

[7th] **T80.212 Local infection due to central venous catheter**
Exit or insertion site infection
Local infection due to Hickman catheter
Local infection due to peripherally inserted central catheter (PICC)
Local infection due to portacath (port-a-cath)
Local infection due to triple lumen catheter
Local infection due to umbilical venous catheter
Port or reservoir infection
Tunnel infection

[7th] **T80.218 Other infection due to central venous catheter**
Other central line-associated infection
Other infection due to Hickman catheter
Other infection due to peripherally inserted central catheter (PICC)
Other infection due to portacath (port-a-cath)
Other infection due to triple lumen catheter
Other infection due to umbilical venous catheter

[7th] **T80.219 Unspecified infection due to central venous catheter**
Central line-associated infection NOS
Unspecified infection due to Hickman catheter
Unspecified infection due to peripherally inserted central catheter (PICC)
Unspecified infection due to portacath (port-a-cath)
Unspecified infection due to triple lumen catheter
Unspecified infection due to umbilical venous catheter

[7th] **T80.22 Acute infection following transfusion, infusion, or injection of blood and blood products**

[7th] **T80.29 Infection following other infusion, transfusion and therapeutic injection**

[5th] **T80.3 ABO incompatibility reaction due to transfusion of blood or blood products**

EXCLUDES1 *minor blood group antigens reactions (Duffy) (E) (K(ell)) (Kidd) (Lewis) (M) (N) (P) (S) (T80.A)*

[7th] **T80.30 ABO incompatibility reaction due to transfusion of blood or blood products, unspecified**
ABO incompatibility blood transfusion NOS
Reaction to ABO incompatibility from transfusion NOS

[6th] **T80.31 ABO incompatibility with hemolytic transfusion reaction**

[7th] **T80.310 ABO incompatibility with acute hemolytic transfusion reaction**
ABO incompatibility with hemolytic transfusion reaction less than 24 hours after transfusion
Acute hemolytic transfusion reaction (AHTR) due to ABO incompatibility

[7th] **T80.311 ABO incompatibility with delayed hemolytic transfusion reaction**
ABO incompatibility with hemolytic transfusion reaction 24 hours or more after transfusion
Delayed hemolytic transfusion reaction (DHTR) due to ABO incompatibility

[7th] **T80.319 ABO incompatibility with hemolytic transfusion reaction, unspecified**
ABO incompatibility with hemolytic transfusion reaction at unspecified time after transfusion
Hemolytic transfusion reaction (HTR) due to ABO incompatibility NOS

[7th] **T80.39 Other ABO incompatibility reaction due to transfusion of blood or blood products**
Delayed serologic transfusion reaction (DSTR) from ABO incompatibility
Other ABO incompatible blood transfusion
Other reaction to ABO incompatible blood transfusion

[4th] 4th character required [5th] 5th character required [6th] 6th character required [7th] 7th character required [X] Extension 'X' Alert
EXCLUDES1 Not coded here EXCLUDES2 Not included here [PDx] Primary Diagnosis Only Manifestation Code

5ᵗʰ **T80.4** Rh incompatibility **reaction due to transfusion of blood or blood products**

Reaction due to incompatibility of Rh antigens (C) (c) (D) (E) (e)

6ᵗʰ **T80.40 Rh incompatibility reaction due to transfusion of blood or blood products, unspecified**

Reaction due to Rh factor in transfusion NOS
Rh incompatible blood transfusion NOS

6ᵗʰ **T80.41 Rh incompatibility** with hemolytic transfusion reaction

7ᵗʰ **T80.410 Rh incompatibility with** acute **hemolytic transfusion reaction**

Acute hemolytic transfusion reaction (AHTR) due to Rh incompatibility
Rh incompatibility with hemolytic transfusion reaction less than 24 hours after transfusion

7ᵗʰ **T80.411 Rh incompatibility with** delayed **hemolytic transfusion reaction**

Delayed hemolytic transfusion reaction (DHTR) due to Rh incompatibility
Rh incompatibility with hemolytic transfusion reaction 24 hours or more after transfusion

7ᵗʰ **T80.419 Rh incompatibility with hemolytic transfusion reaction, unspecified**

Rh incompatibility with hemolytic transfusion reaction at unspecified time after transfusion
Hemolytic transfusion reaction (HTR) due to Rh incompatibility NOS

7ᵗʰ **T80.49 Other Rh incompatibility reaction due to transfusion of blood or blood products**

Delayed serologic transfusion reaction (DSTR) from Rh incompatibility
Other reaction to Rh incompatible blood transfusion

5ᵗʰ **T80.A** Non-ABO incompatibility **reaction due to transfusion of blood or blood products**

Reaction due to incompatibility of minor antigens (Duffy) (Kell) (Kidd) (Lewis) (M) (N) (P) (S)

6ᵗʰ **T80.A0 Non-ABO incompatibility reaction due to transfusion of blood or blood products, unspecified**

Non-ABO antigen incompatibility reaction from transfusion NOS

6ᵗʰ **T80.A1 Non-ABO incompatibility** with hemolytic transfusion reaction

7ᵗʰ **T80.A10 Non-ABO incompatibility with** acute **hemolytic transfusion reaction**

Acute hemolytic transfusion reaction (AHTR) due to non-ABO incompatibility
Non-ABO incompatibility with hemolytic transfusion reaction less than 24 hours after transfusion

7ᵗʰ **T80.A11 Non-ABO incompatibility with** delayed **hemolytic transfusion reaction**

Delayed hemolytic transfusion reaction (DHTR) due to non-ABO incompatibility
Non-ABO incompatibility with hemolytic transfusion reaction 24 or more hours after transfusion

7ᵗʰ **T80.A19 Non-ABO incompatibility with hemolytic transfusion reaction, unspecified**

Hemolytic transfusion reaction (HTR) due to non-ABO incompatibility NOS
Non-ABO incompatibility with hemolytic transfusion reaction at unspecified time after transfusion

7ᵗʰ **T80.A9 Other non-ABO incompatibility reaction due to transfusion of blood or blood products**

Delayed serologic transfusion reaction (DSTR) from non-ABO incompatibility
Other reaction to non-ABO incompatible blood transfusion

5ᵗʰ **T80.5 Anaphylactic reaction due to serum**

Allergic shock due to serum
Anaphylactic shock due to serum
Anaphylactoid reaction due to serum
Anaphylaxis due to serum

EXCLUDES1 *ABO incompatibility reaction due to transfusion of blood or blood products (T80.3-)*
allergic reaction or shock NOS (T78.2)
anaphylactic reaction or shock NOS (T78.2)
anaphylactic reaction or shock due to adverse effect of correct medicinal substance properly administered (T88.6)
other serum reaction (T80.6-)

6ᵗʰ **T80.51 Anaphylactic reaction due to** administration of blood and blood products

6ᵗʰ **T80.52 Anaphylactic reaction due to** vaccination

6ᵗʰ **T80.59 Anaphylactic reaction due to other serum**

5ᵗʰ **T80.6 Other serum reactions**

Intoxication by serum
Protein sickness
Serum rash
Serum sickness
Serum urticaria

EXCLUDES2 *serum hepatitis (B16.-)*

6ᵗʰ **T80.61 Other serum reaction** due to administration of blood and blood products

6ᵗʰ **T80.62 Other serum reaction** due to vaccination

6ᵗʰ **T80.69 Other serum reaction due to other** serum

5ᵗʰ **T80.8 Other complications following infusion, transfusion and therapeutic injection**

6ᵗʰ **T80.81 Extravasation of vesicant agent**

Infiltration of vesicant agent

7ᵗʰ **T80.810 Extravasation of vesicant antineoplastic chemotherapy**

Infiltration of vesicant antineoplastic chemotherapy

7ᵗʰ **T80.818 Extravasation of other vesicant agent**

Infiltration of other vesicant agent

6ᵗʰ **T80.89 Other complications following infusion, transfusion and therapeutic injection**

Delayed serologic transfusion reaction (DSTR), unspecified incompatibility
Use additional code to identify graft-versus-host reaction, if applicable, (D89.81-)

5ᵗʰ **T80.9 Unspecified complication following infusion, transfusion and therapeutic injection**

6ᵗʰ **T80.90 Unspecified complication** following infusion and therapeutic injection

6ᵗʰ **T80.91** Hemolytic transfusion reaction, **unspecified incompatibility**

EXCLUDES1 *ABO incompatibility with hemolytic transfusion reaction (T80.31-)*
Non-ABO incompatibility with hemolytic transfusion reaction (T80.A1-)
Rh incompatibility with hemolytic transfusion reaction (T80.41-)

7ᵗʰ **T80.910** Acute **hemolytic transfusion reaction, unspecified incompatibility**

7ᵗʰ **T80.911** Delayed **hemolytic transfusion reaction, unspecified incompatibility**

Unspecified Code	Other Specified Code	N Newborn Age: 0	P Pediatric Age: 0-17	M Maternity Age: 12-55
A Adult Age: 15-124	♂ Male	♀ Female	● New Code	▲ Revised Code Title	►◄ Revised Text

7️⃣ **T80.919 Hemolytic transfusion reaction, unspecified incompatibility, unspecified as acute or delayed**

Hemolytic transfusion reaction NOS

7️⃣ **T80.92 Unspecified transfusion reaction**

Transfusion reaction NOS

4️⃣ **T81 Complications of procedures, not elsewhere classified**

Use additional code for adverse effect, if applicable, to identify drug (T36-T50 with fifth or sixth character 5)

EXCLUDES2 *complications following immunization (T88.0-T88.1)*
complications following infusion, transfusion and therapeutic injection (T80.-)
complications of transplanted organs and tissue (T86.-)
specified complications classified elsewhere, such as:
complication of prosthetic devices, implants and grafts (T82-T85)
dermatitis due to drugs and medicaments (L23.3, L24.4, L25.1, L27.0-L27.1)
endosseous dental implant failure (M27.6-)
floppy iris syndrome (IFIS) (intraoperative) H21.81
intraoperative and postprocedural complications of specific body system (D78.-, E36.-, E89.-, G97.3-, G97.4, H59.3-, H59.-, H95.2-, H95.3, I97.4-, I97.5, J95, K91.-, L76.-, M96.-, N99.-)
ostomy complications (J95.0-, K94.-, N99.5-)
plateau iris syndrome (post-iridectomy) (postprocedural) H21.82
poisoning and toxic effects of drugs and chemicals (T36-T65 with fifth or sixth character 1-4 or 6)

The appropriate 7th character is to be added to each code from category T81
A = initial encounter
D = subsequent encounter
S = sequela

5️⃣ **T81.1 Postprocedural shock**

Shock during or resulting from a procedure, not elsewhere classified

EXCLUDES1 *anaphylactic shock NOS (T78.2)*
anaphylactic shock due to correct substance properly administered (T88.6)
anaphylactic shock due to serum (T80.5-)
anesthetic shock (T88.2)
electric shock (T75.4)
obstetric shock (O75.1)
septic shock (R65.21)
shock following abortion or ectopic or molar pregnancy (O00-O07, O08.3)
traumatic shock (T79.4)

7️⃣ **T81.10 Postprocedural shock unspecified**

Collapse NOS during or resulting from a procedure, not elsewhere classified
Postprocedural failure of peripheral circulation
Postprocedural shock NOS

7️⃣ **T81.11 Postprocedural cardiogenic shock**

7️⃣ **T81.12 Postprocedural septic shock**

Postprocedural endotoxic shock during or resulting from a procedure, not elsewhere classified
Postprocedural gram-negative shock during or resulting from a procedure, not elsewhere classified
Code first underlying infection
Use additional code, to identify any associated acute organ dysfunction, if applicable

7️⃣ **T81.19 Other postprocedural shock**

Postprocedural hypovolemic shock

5️⃣ **T81.3 Disruption of wound, not elsewhere classified**

Disruption of any suture materials or other closure methods

EXCLUDES1 *breakdown (mechanical) of permanent sutures (T85.612)*
displacement of permanent sutures (T85.622)
disruption of cesarean delivery wound (O90.0)
disruption of perineal obstetric wound (O90.1)
mechanical complication of permanent sutures NEC (T85.692)

7️⃣ **T81.30 Disruption of wound, unspecified**

Disruption of wound NOS

7️⃣ **T81.31 Disruption of external operation (surgical) wound, not elsewhere classified**

Dehiscence of operation wound NOS
Disruption of operation wound NOS
Disruption or dehiscence of closure of cornea
Disruption or dehiscence of closure of mucosa
Disruption or dehiscence of closure of skin and subcutaneous tissue
Full-thickness skin disruption or dehiscence
Superficial disruption or dehiscence of operation wound

EXCLUDES1 *dehiscence of amputation stump (T87.81)*

7️⃣ **T81.32 Disruption of internal operation (surgical) wound, not elsewhere classified**

Deep disruption or dehiscence of operation wound NOS
Disruption or dehiscence of closure of internal organ or other internal tissue
Disruption or dehiscence of closure of muscle or muscle flap
Disruption or dehiscence of closure of ribs or rib cage
Disruption or dehiscence of closure of skull or craniotomy
Disruption or dehiscence of closure of sternum or sternotomy
Disruption or dehiscence of closure of tendon or ligament
Disruption or dehiscence of closure of superficial or muscular fascia

7️⃣ **T81.33 Disruption of traumatic injury wound repair**

Disruption or dehiscence of closure of traumatic laceration (external) (internal)

7️⃣ **T81.4 Infection following a procedure**

Intra-abdominal abscess following a procedure
Postprocedural infection, not elsewhere classified
Sepsis following a procedure
Stitch abscess following a procedure
Subphrenic abscess following a procedure
Wound abscess following a procedure
Use additional code to identify infection
code (R65.2-) to identify severe sepsis, if applicable

EXCLUDES1 *obstetric surgical wound infection (O86.0)*
postprocedural fever NOS (R50.82)
postprocedural retroperitoneal abscess (K68.11)

EXCLUDES2 *bleb associated endophthalmitis (H59.4-)*
infection due to infusion, transfusion and therapeutic injection (T80.2-)
infection due to prosthetic devices, implants and grafts (T82.6-T82.7, T83.5-T83.6, T84.5-T84.7, T85.7)

5️⃣ **T81.5 Complications of foreign body accidentally left in body following procedure**

6️⃣ **T81.50 Unspecified complication of foreign body accidentally left in body following procedure**

4️⃣ 4th character required   5️⃣ 5th character required   6️⃣ 6th character required   7️⃣ 7th character required   Ⓧ Extension 'X' Alert

EXCLUDES 1 Not coded here   EXCLUDES 2 Not included here   Pdx Primary Diagnosis Only   Manifestation Code

T81.500 Unspecified complication of foreign body accidentally left in body following surgical operation

T81.501 Unspecified complication of foreign body accidentally left in body following infusion or transfusion

T81.502 Unspecified complication of foreign body accidentally left in body following kidney dialysis

T81.503 Unspecified complication of foreign body accidentally left in body following injection or immunization

T81.504 Unspecified complication of foreign body accidentally left in body following endoscopic examination

T81.505 Unspecified complication of foreign body accidentally left in body following heart catheterization

T81.506 Unspecified complication of foreign body accidentally left in body following aspiration, puncture or other catheterization

T81.507 Unspecified complication of foreign body accidentally left in body following removal of catheter or packing

T81.508 Unspecified complication of foreign body accidentally left in body following other procedure

T81.509 Unspecified complication of foreign body accidentally left in body following unspecified procedure

T81.51 Adhesions due to foreign body accidentally left in body following procedure

T81.510 Adhesions due to foreign body accidentally left in body following surgical operation

T81.511 Adhesions due to foreign body accidentally left in body following infusion or transfusion

T81.512 Adhesions due to foreign body accidentally left in body following kidney dialysis

T81.513 Adhesions due to foreign body accidentally left in body following injection or immunization

T81.514 Adhesions due to foreign body accidentally left in body following endoscopic examination

T81.515 Adhesions due to foreign body accidentally left in body following heart catheterization

T81.516 Adhesions due to foreign body accidentally left in body following aspiration, puncture or other catheterization

T81.517 Adhesions due to foreign body accidentally left in body following removal of catheter or packing

T81.518 Adhesions due to foreign body accidentally left in body following other procedure

T81.519 Adhesions due to foreign body accidentally left in body following unspecified procedure

T81.52 Obstruction due to foreign body accidentally left in body following procedure

T81.520 Obstruction due to foreign body accidentally left in body following surgical operation

T81.521 Obstruction due to foreign body accidentally left in body following infusion or transfusion

T81.522 Obstruction due to foreign body accidentally left in body following kidney dialysis

T81.523 Obstruction due to foreign body accidentally left in body following injection or immunization

T81.524 Obstruction due to foreign body accidentally left in body following endoscopic examination

T81.525 Obstruction due to foreign body accidentally left in body following heart catheterization

T81.526 Obstruction due to foreign body accidentally left in body following aspiration, puncture or other catheterization

T81.527 Obstruction due to foreign body accidentally left in body following removal of catheter or packing

T81.528 Obstruction due to foreign body accidentally left in body following other procedure

T81.529 Obstruction due to foreign body accidentally left in body following unspecified procedure

T81.53 Perforation due to foreign body accidentally left in body following procedure

T81.530 Perforation due to foreign body accidentally left in body following surgical operation

T81.531 Perforation due to foreign body accidentally left in body following infusion or transfusion

T81.532 Perforation due to foreign body accidentally left in body following kidney dialysis

T81.533 Perforation due to foreign body accidentally left in body following injection or immunization

T81.534 Perforation due to foreign body accidentally left in body following endoscopic examination

T81.535 Perforation due to foreign body accidentally left in body following heart catheterization

T81.536 Perforation due to foreign body accidentally left in body following aspiration, puncture or other catheterization

T81.537 Perforation due to foreign body accidentally left in body following removal of catheter or packing

T81.538 Perforation due to foreign body accidentally left in body following other procedure

T81.539 Perforation due to foreign body accidentally left in body following unspecified procedure

T81.59 Other complications of foreign body accidentally left in body following procedure

> EXCLUDES2 obstruction or perforation due to prosthetic devices and implants intentionally left in body (T82.0-T82.5, T83.0-T83.4, T83.7, T84.0-T84.4, T85.0-T85.6)

T81.590 Other complications of foreign body accidentally left in body following surgical operation

T81.591 Other complications of foreign body accidentally left in body following infusion or transfusion

T81.592 Other complications of foreign body accidentally left in body following kidney dialysis

T81.593 Other complications of foreign body accidentally left in body following injection or immunization

T81.594 Other complications of foreign body accidentally left in body following endoscopic examination

---

Unspecified Code	Other Specified Code	N Newborn Age: 0	P Pediatric Age: 0 17	M Maternity Age: 12-55
A Adult Age: 15-124	♂ Male	♀ Female	● New Code	▲ Revised Code Title	►◄ Revised Text

[7th] T81.595 Other complications of foreign body accidentally left in body following heart catheterization

[7th] T81.596 Other complications of foreign body accidentally left in body following aspiration, puncture or other catheterization

[7th] T81.597 Other complications of foreign body accidentally left in body following removal of catheter or packing

[7th] T81.598 Other complications of foreign body accidentally left in body following other procedure

[7th] T81.599 Other complications of foreign body accidentally left in body following unspecified procedure

[5th] T81.6 Acute reaction to foreign substance accidentally left during a procedure

EXCLUDES2 *complications of foreign body accidentally left in body cavity or operation wound following procedure (T81.5-)*

[7th] T81.60 Unspecified acute reaction to foreign substance accidentally left during a procedure

[7th] T81.61 Aseptic peritonitis due to foreign substance accidentally left during a procedure

Chemical peritonitis

[7th] T81.69 Other acute reaction to foreign substance accidentally left during a procedure

[5th] T81.7 Vascular complications following a procedure, not elsewhere classified

Air embolism following procedure NEC

Phlebitis or thrombophlebitis resulting from a procedure

EXCLUDES1 *embolism complicating abortion or ectopic or molar pregnancy (O00-O07, O08.2)*
embolism complicating pregnancy, childbirth and the puerperium (O88.-)
traumatic embolism (T79.0)

EXCLUDES2 *embolism due to prosthetic devices, implants and grafts (T82.8-, T83.8, T84.8-, T85.8)*
embolism following infusion, transfusion and therapeutic injection (T80.0)

[6th] T81.71 Complication of artery following a procedure, not elsewhere classified

[7th] T81.710 Complication of mesenteric artery following a procedure, not elsewhere classified

[7th] T81.711 Complication of renal artery following a procedure, not elsewhere classified

[7th] T81.718 Complication of other artery following a procedure, not elsewhere classified

[7th] T81.719 Complication of unspecified artery following a procedure, not elsewhere classified

[7th] T81.72 Complication of vein following a procedure, not elsewhere classified

[5th] T81.8 Other complications of procedures, not elsewhere classified

EXCLUDES2 *hypothermia following anesthesia (T88.51)*
malignant hyperpyrexia due to anesthesia (T88.3)

[7th] T81.81 Complication of inhalation therapy

[7th] T81.82 Emphysema (subcutaneous) resulting from a procedure

[7th] T81.83 Persistent postprocedural fistula

[7th] T81.89 Other complications of procedures, not elsewhere classified

Use additional code to specify complication, such as: postprocedural delirium (F05)

[7th] T81.9 Unspecified complication of procedure

[4th] T82 Complications of cardiac and vascular prosthetic devices, implants and grafts

EXCLUDES2 *failure and rejection of transplanted organs and tissue (T86.-)*

The appropriate 7th character is to be added to each code from category T82
A = initial encounter
D = subsequent encounter
S = sequela

[5th] T82.0 Mechanical complication of heart valve prosthesis

Mechanical complication of artificial heart valve

EXCLUDES1 *mechanical complication of biological heart valve graft (T82.22-)*

[7th] T82.01 Breakdown (mechanical) of heart valve prosthesis

[7th] T82.02 Displacement of heart valve prosthesis

Malposition of heart valve prosthesis

[7th] T82.03 Leakage of heart valve prosthesis

[7th] T82.09 Other mechanical complication of heart valve prosthesis

Obstruction (mechanical) of heart valve prosthesis
Perforation of heart valve prosthesis
Protrusion of heart valve prosthesis

[5th] T82.1 Mechanical complication of cardiac electronic device

[6th] T82.11 Breakdown (mechanical) of cardiac electronic device

[7th] T82.110 Breakdown (mechanical) of cardiac electrode

[7th] T82.111 Breakdown (mechanical) of cardiac pulse generator (battery)

[7th] T82.118 Breakdown (mechanical) of other cardiac electronic device

[7th] T82.119 Breakdown (mechanical) of unspecified cardiac electronic device

[6th] T82.12 Displacement of cardiac electronic device

Malposition of cardiac electronic device

[7th] T82.120 Displacement of cardiac electrode

[7th] T82.121 Displacement of cardiac pulse generator (battery)

[7th] T82.128 Displacement of other cardiac electronic device

[7th] T82.129 Displacement of unspecified cardiac electronic device

[6th] T82.19 Other mechanical complication of cardiac electronic device

Leakage of cardiac electronic device
Obstruction of cardiac electronic device
Perforation of cardiac electronic device
Protrusion of cardiac electronic device

[7th] T82.190 Other mechanical complication of cardiac electrode

[7th] T82.191 Other mechanical complication of cardiac pulse generator (battery)

[7th] T82.198 Other mechanical complication of other cardiac electronic device

[7th] T82.199 Other mechanical complication of unspecified cardiac device

[5th] T82.2 Mechanical complication of coronary artery bypass graft and biological heart valve graft

EXCLUDES1 *mechanical complication of artificial heart valve prosthesis (T82.0-)*

[6th] T82.21 Mechanical complication of coronary artery bypass graft

[7th] T82.211 Breakdown (mechanical) of coronary artery bypass graft

[7th] T82.212 Displacement of coronary artery bypass graft

Malposition of coronary artery bypass graft

[4th] 4th character required [5th] 5th character required [6th] 6th character required [7th] 7th character required [7th] Extension 'X' Alert
EXCLUDES1 Not coded here EXCLUDES2 Not included here PDx Primary Diagnosis Only Manifestation Code

- 7th T82.213 Leakage of coronary artery bypass graft
- 7th T82.218 Other mechanical complication of coronary artery bypass graft

    Obstruction, mechanical of coronary artery bypass graft

    Perforation of coronary artery bypass graft

    Protrusion of coronary artery bypass graft

- 6th T82.22 Mechanical complication of biological heart valve graft
- 7th T82.221 Breakdown (mechanical) of biological heart valve graft
- 7th T82.222 Displacement of biological heart valve graft

    Malposition of biological heart valve graft

- 7th T82.223 Leakage of biological heart valve graft
- 7th T82.228 Other mechanical complication of biological heart valve graft

    Obstruction of biological heart valve graft

    Perforation of biological heart valve graft

    Protrusion of biological heart valve graft

- 5th T82.3 Mechanical complication of other vascular grafts
- 6th T82.31 Breakdown (mechanical) of other vascular grafts
- 7th T82.310 Breakdown (mechanical) of aortic (bifurcation) graft (replacement)
- 7th T82.311 Breakdown (mechanical) of carotid arterial graft (bypass)
- 7th T82.312 Breakdown (mechanical) of femoral arterial graft (bypass)
- 7th T82.318 Breakdown (mechanical) of other vascular grafts
- 7th T82.319 Breakdown (mechanical) of unspecified vascular grafts
- 6th T82.32 Displacement of other vascular grafts

    Malposition of other vascular grafts

- 7th T82.320 Displacement of aortic (bifurcation) graft (replacement)
- 7th T82.321 Displacement of carotid arterial graft (bypass)
- 7th T82.322 Displacement of femoral arterial graft (bypass)
- 7th T82.328 Displacement of other vascular grafts
- 7th T82.329 Displacement of unspecified vascular grafts
- 6th T82.33 Leakage of other vascular grafts
- 7th T82.330 Leakage of aortic (bifurcation) graft (replacement)
- 7th T82.331 Leakage of carotid arterial graft (bypass)
- 7th T82.332 Leakage of femoral arterial graft (bypass)
- 7th T82.338 Leakage of other vascular grafts
- 7th T82.339 Leakage of unspecified vascular graft
- 6th T82.39 Other mechanical complication of other vascular grafts

    Obstruction (mechanical) of other vascular grafts

    Perforation of other vascular grafts

    Protrusion of other vascular grafts

- 7th T82.390 Other mechanical complication of aortic (bifurcation) graft (replacement)
- 7th T82.391 Other mechanical complication of carotid arterial graft (bypass)
- 7th T82.392 Other mechanical complication of femoral arterial graft (bypass)
- 7th T82.398 Other mechanical complication of other vascular grafts
- 7th T82.399 Other mechanical complication of unspecified vascular grafts
- 5th T82.4 Mechanical complication of vascular dialysis catheter

    Mechanical complication of hemodialysis catheter

    EXCLUDES1 mechanical complication of intraperitoneal dialysis catheter (T85.62)

- 7th T82.41 Breakdown (mechanical) of vascular dialysis catheter
- 7th T82.42 Displacement of vascular dialysis catheter

    Malposition of vascular dialysis catheter

- 7th T82.43 Leakage of vascular dialysis catheter
- 7th T82.49 Other complication of vascular dialysis catheter

    Obstruction (mechanical) of vascular dialysis catheter

    Perforation of vascular dialysis catheter

    Protrusion of vascular dialysis catheter

- 5th T82.5 Mechanical complication of other cardiac and vascular devices and implants

    EXCLUDES2 mechanical complication of epidural and subdural infusion catheter (T85.61)

- 6th T82.51 Breakdown (mechanical) of other cardiac and vascular devices and implants
- 7th T82.510 Breakdown (mechanical) of surgically created arteriovenous fistula
- 7th T82.511 Breakdown (mechanical) of surgically created arteriovenous shunt
- 7th T82.512 Breakdown (mechanical) of artificial heart
- 7th T82.513 Breakdown (mechanical) of balloon (counterpulsation) device
- 7th T82.514 Breakdown (mechanical) of infusion catheter
- 7th T82.515 Breakdown (mechanical) of umbrella device
- 7th T82.518 Breakdown (mechanical) of other cardiac and vascular devices and implants
- 7th T82.519 Breakdown (mechanical) of unspecified cardiac and vascular devices and implants
- 6th T82.52 Displacement of other cardiac and vascular devices and implants

    Malposition of other cardiac and vascular devices and implants

- 7th T82.520 Displacement of surgically created arteriovenous fistula
- 7th T82.521 Displacement of surgically created arteriovenous shunt
- 7th T82.522 Displacement of artificial heart
- 7th T82.523 Displacement of balloon (counterpulsation) device
- 7th T82.524 Displacement of infusion catheter
- 7th T82.525 Displacement of umbrella device
- 7th T82.528 Displacement of other cardiac and vascular devices and implants
- 7th T82.529 Displacement of unspecified cardiac and vascular devices and implants
- 6th T82.53 Leakage of other cardiac and vascular devices and implants
- 7th T82.530 Leakage of surgically created arteriovenous fistula
- 7th T82.531 Leakage of surgically created arteriovenous shunt
- 7th T82.532 Leakage of artificial heart
- 7th T82.533 Leakage of balloon (counterpulsation) device
- 7th T82.534 Leakage of infusion catheter
- 7th T82.535 Leakage of umbrella device
- 7th T82.538 Leakage of other cardiac and vascular devices and implants
- 7th T82.539 Leakage of unspecified cardiac and vascular devices and implants
- 6th T82.59 Other mechanical complication of other cardiac and vascular devices and implants

    Obstruction (mechanical) of other cardiac and vascular devices and implants

    Perforation of other cardiac and vascular devices and implants

    Protrusion of other cardiac and vascular devices and implants

7️⃣ T82.590 Other mechanical complication of surgically created arteriovenous fistula

7️⃣ T82.591 Other mechanical complication of surgically created arteriovenous shunt

7️⃣ T82.592 Other mechanical complication of artificial heart

7️⃣ T82.593 Other mechanical complication of balloon (counterpulsation) device

7️⃣ T82.594 Other mechanical complication of infusion catheter

7️⃣ T82.595 Other mechanical complication of umbrella device

7️⃣ T82.598 Other mechanical complication of other cardiac and vascular devices and implants

7️⃣ T82.599 Other mechanical complication of unspecified cardiac and vascular devices and implants

7️⃣ **T82.6** Infection and inflammatory reaction due to cardiac valve prosthesis

Use additional code to identify infection

7️⃣ **T82.7** Infection and inflammatory reaction due to other cardiac and vascular devices, implants and grafts

Use additional code to identify infection

5️⃣ **T82.8** Other specified complications of cardiac and vascular prosthetic devices, implants and grafts

6️⃣ T82.81 Embolism of cardiac and vascular prosthetic devices, implants and grafts

7️⃣ T82.817 Embolism of cardiac prosthetic devices, implants and grafts

7️⃣ T82.818 Embolism of vascular prosthetic devices, implants and grafts

6️⃣ T82.82 Fibrosis of cardiac and vascular prosthetic devices, implants and grafts

7️⃣ T82.827 Fibrosis of cardiac prosthetic devices, implants and grafts

7️⃣ T82.828 Fibrosis of vascular prosthetic devices, implants and grafts

6️⃣ T82.83 Hemorrhage of cardiac and vascular prosthetic devices, implants and grafts

7️⃣ T82.837 Hemorrhage of cardiac prosthetic devices, implants and grafts

7️⃣ T82.838 Hemorrhage of vascular prosthetic devices, implants and grafts

6️⃣ T82.84 Pain from cardiac and vascular prosthetic devices, implants and grafts

7️⃣ T82.847 Pain from cardiac prosthetic devices, implants and grafts

7️⃣ T82.848 Pain from vascular prosthetic devices, implants and grafts

6️⃣ T82.85 Stenosis of cardiac and vascular prosthetic devices, implants and grafts

7️⃣ T82.857 Stenosis of cardiac prosthetic devices, implants and grafts

7️⃣ T82.858 Stenosis of vascular prosthetic devices, implants and grafts

6️⃣ T82.86 Thrombosis of cardiac and vascular prosthetic devices, implants and grafts

7️⃣ T82.867 Thrombosis of cardiac prosthetic devices, implants and grafts

7️⃣ T82.868 Thrombosis of vascular prosthetic devices, implants and grafts

6️⃣ T82.89 Other specified complication of cardiac and vascular prosthetic devices, implants and grafts

7️⃣ T82.897 Other specified complication of cardiac prosthetic devices, implants and grafts

7️⃣ T82.898 Other specified complication of vascular prosthetic devices, implants and grafts

T82.9 Unspecified complication of cardiac and vascular prosthetic device, implant and graft

4️⃣ **T83** Complications of genitourinary prosthetic devices, implants and grafts

EXCLUDES2 *failure and rejection of transplanted organs and tissue (T86.-)*

The appropriate 7th character is to be added to each code from category T83
A = initial encounter
D = subsequent encounter
S = sequela

5️⃣ **T83.0** Mechanical complication of urinary (indwelling) catheter

EXCLUDES2 *complications of stoma of urinary tract (N99.5-)*

6️⃣ T83.01 Breakdown (mechanical) of urinary (indwelling) catheter

7️⃣ T83.010 Breakdown (mechanical) of cystostomy catheter

7️⃣ T83.018 Breakdown (mechanical) of other indwelling urethral catheter

6️⃣ T83.02 Displacement of urinary (indwelling) catheter

Malposition of urinary (indwelling) catheter

7️⃣ T83.020 Displacement of cystostomy catheter

7️⃣ T83.028 Displacement of other indwelling urethral catheter

6️⃣ T83.03 Leakage of urinary (indwelling) catheter

7️⃣ T83.030 Leakage of cystostomy catheter

7️⃣ T83.038 Leakage of other indwelling urethral catheter

6️⃣ T83.09 Other mechanical complication of urinary (indwelling) catheter

Obstruction (mechanical) of urinary (indwelling) catheter
Perforation of urinary (indwelling) catheter
Protrusion of urinary (indwelling) catheter

7️⃣ T83.090 Other mechanical complication of cystostomy catheter

7️⃣ T83.098 Other mechanical complication of other indwelling urethral catheter

5️⃣ **T83.1** Mechanical complication of other urinary devices and implants

6️⃣ T83.11 Breakdown (mechanical) of other urinary devices and implants

7️⃣ T83.110 Breakdown (mechanical) of urinary electronic stimulator device

7️⃣ T83.111 Breakdown (mechanical) of urinary sphincter implant

7️⃣ T83.112 Breakdown (mechanical) of urinary stent

7️⃣ T83.118 Breakdown (mechanical) of other urinary devices and implants

6️⃣ T83.12 Displacement of other urinary devices and implants

Malposition of other urinary devices and implants

7️⃣ T83.120 Displacement of urinary electronic stimulator device

7️⃣ T83.121 Displacement of urinary sphincter implant

7️⃣ T83.122 Displacement of urinary stent

7️⃣ T83.128 Displacement of other urinary devices and implants

6️⃣ T83.19 Other mechanical complication of other urinary devices and implants

Leakage of other urinary devices and implants
Obstruction (mechanical) of other urinary devices and implants
Perforation of other urinary devices and implants
Protrusion of other urinary devices and implants

7️⃣ T83.190 Other mechanical complication of urinary electronic stimulator device

7️⃣ T83.191 Other mechanical complication of urinary sphincter implant

---

4️⃣ 4th character required　　5️⃣ 5th character required　　6️⃣ 6th character required　　7️⃣ 7th character required　　🔟 Extension 'X' Alert

EXCLUDES1 Not coded here　　EXCLUDES2 Not included here　　Pdx Primary Diagnosis Only　　Manifestation Code

T83.192 Other mechanical complication of urinary stent

T83.198 Other mechanical complication of other urinary devices and implants

T83.2 Mechanical complication of graft of urinary organ

T83.21 Breakdown (mechanical) of graft of urinary organ

T83.22 Displacement of graft of urinary organ

Malposition of graft of urinary organ

T83.23 Leakage of graft of urinary organ

T83.29 Other mechanical complication of graft of urinary organ

Obstruction (mechanical) of graft of urinary organ
Perforation of graft of urinary organ
Protrusion of graft of urinary organ

T83.3 Mechanical complication of intrauterine contraceptive device

T83.31 Breakdown (mechanical) of intrauterine contraceptive device

T83.32 Displacement of intrauterine contraceptive device

Malposition of intrauterine contraceptive device

T83.39 Other mechanical complication of intrauterine contraceptive device

Leakage of intrauterine contraceptive device
Obstruction (mechanical) of intrauterine contraceptive device
Perforation of intrauterine contraceptive device
Protrusion of intrauterine contraceptive device

T83.4 Mechanical complication of other prosthetic devices, implants and grafts of genital tract

T83.41 Breakdown (mechanical) of other prosthetic devices, implants and grafts of genital tract

T83.410 Breakdown (mechanical) of penile (implanted) prosthesis

T83.418 Breakdown (mechanical) of other prosthetic devices, implants and grafts of genital tract

T83.42 Displacement of other prosthetic devices, implants and grafts of genital tract

Malposition of other prosthetic devices, implants and grafts of genital tract

T83.420 Displacement of penile (implanted) prosthesis

T83.428 Displacement of other prosthetic devices, implants and grafts of genital tract

T83.49 Other mechanical complication of other prosthetic devices, implants and grafts of genital tract

Leakage of other prosthetic devices, implants and grafts of genital tract
Obstruction, mechanical of other prosthetic devices, implants and grafts of genital tract
Perforation of other prosthetic devices, implants and grafts of genital tract
Protrusion of other prosthetic devices, implants and grafts of genital tract

T83.490 Other mechanical complication of penile (implanted) prosthesis

T83.498 Other mechanical complication of other prosthetic devices, implants and grafts of genital tract

T83.5 Infection and inflammatory reaction due to prosthetic device, implant and graft in urinary system

Use additional code to identify infection

T83.51 Infection and inflammatory reaction due to indwelling urinary catheter

EXCLUDES2 complications of stoma of urinary tract (N99.5-)

T83.59 Infection and inflammatory reaction due to prosthetic device, implant and graft in urinary system

T83.6 Infection and inflammatory reaction due to prosthetic device, implant and graft in genital tract

Use additional code to identify infection

T83.7 Complications due to implanted mesh and other prosthetic materials

T83.71 Erosion of implanted mesh and other prosthetic materials to surrounding organ or tissue

T83.711 Erosion of implanted vaginal mesh and other prosthetic materials to surrounding organ or tissue

Erosion of implanted vaginal mesh and other prosthetic materials into pelvic floor muscles

T83.718 Erosion of other implanted mesh and other prosthetic materials to surrounding organ or tissue

T83.72 Exposure of implanted mesh and other prosthetic materials into surrounding organ or tissue

T83.721 Exposure of implanted vaginal mesh and other prosthetic materials into vagina

Exposure of implanted vaginal mesh and other prosthetic materials through vaginal wall

T83.728 Exposure of other implanted mesh and other prosthetic materials to surrounding organ or tissue

T83.8 Other specified complications of genitourinary prosthetic devices, implants and grafts

T83.81 Embolism of genitourinary prosthetic devices, implants and grafts

T83.82 Fibrosis of genitourinary prosthetic devices, implants and grafts

T83.83 Hemorrhage of genitourinary prosthetic devices, implants and grafts

T83.84 Pain from genitourinary prosthetic devices, implants and grafts

T83.85 Stenosis of genitourinary prosthetic devices, implants and grafts

T83.86 Thrombosis of genitourinary prosthetic devices, implants and grafts

T83.89 Other specified complication of genitourinary prosthetic devices, implants and grafts

T83.9 Unspecified complication of genitourinary prosthetic device, implant and graft

T84 Complications of internal orthopedic prosthetic devices, implants and grafts

EXCLUDES2 failure and rejection of transplanted organs and tissues (T86.-)
fracture of bone following insertion of orthopedic implant, joint prosthesis or bone plate (M96.6)

The appropriate 7th character is to be added to each code from category T84
A = initial encounter
D = subsequent encounter
S = sequela

T84.0 Mechanical complication of internal joint prosthesis

T84.01 Broken internal joint prosthesis

Breakage (fracture) of prosthetic joint
Broken prosthetic joint implant

EXCLUDES1 periprosthetic joint implant fracture (T84.04)

T84.010 Broken internal right hip prosthesis

T84.011 Broken internal left hip prosthesis

T84.012 Broken internal right knee prosthesis

T84.013 Broken internal left knee prosthesis

T84.018 Broken internal joint prosthesis, other site

Use additional code to identify the joint (Z96.6-)

Unspecified Code | Other Specified Code | N Newborn Age: 0 | P Pediatric Age: 0-17 | M Maternity Age: 12-55
A Adult Age: 15-124 | ♂ Male | ♀ Female | ● New Code | ▲ Revised Code Title | ►◄ Revised Text

[7th] T84.019 Broken internal joint prosthesis, unspecified site

[6th] T84.02 Dislocation of internal joint prosthesis
Instability of internal joint prosthesis
Subluxation of internal joint prosthesis

[7th] T84.020 Dislocation of internal right hip prosthesis
[7th] T84.021 Dislocation of internal left hip prosthesis
[7th] T84.022 Instability of internal right knee prosthesis
[7th] T84.023 Instability of internal left knee prosthesis
[7th] T84.028 Dislocation of other internal joint prosthesis
Use additional code to identify the joint (Z96.6-)
[7th] T84.029 Dislocation of unspecified internal joint prosthesis

[6th] T84.03 Mechanical loosening of internal prosthetic joint
Aseptic loosening of prosthetic joint

[7th] T84.030 Mechanical loosening of internal right hip prosthetic joint
[7th] T84.031 Mechanical loosening of internal left hip prosthetic joint
[7th] T84.032 Mechanical loosening of internal right knee prosthetic joint
[7th] T84.033 Mechanical loosening of internal left knee prosthetic joint
[7th] T84.038 Mechanical loosening of other internal prosthetic joint
Use additional code to identify the joint (Z96.6-)
[7th] T84.039 Mechanical loosening of unspecified internal prosthetic joint

[6th] T84.04 Periprosthetic fracture around internal prosthetic joint
[EXCLUDES2] *breakage (fracture) of prosthetic joint (T84.01)*

[7th] T84.040 Periprosthetic fracture around internal prosthetic right hip joint
[7th] T84.041 Periprosthetic fracture around internal prosthetic left hip joint
[7th] T84.042 Periprosthetic fracture around internal prosthetic right knee joint
[7th] T84.043 Periprosthetic fracture around internal prosthetic left knee joint
[7th] T84.048 Periprosthetic fracture around other internal prosthetic joint
Use additional code to identify the joint (Z96.6-)
[7th] T84.049 Periprosthetic fracture around unspecified internal prosthetic joint

[6th] T84.05 Periprosthetic osteolysis of internal prosthetic joint
Use additional code to identify major osseous defect, if applicable (M89.7-)

[7th] T84.050 Periprosthetic osteolysis of internal prosthetic right hip joint
[7th] T84.051 Periprosthetic osteolysis of internal prosthetic left hip joint
[7th] T84.052 Periprosthetic osteolysis of internal prosthetic right knee joint
[7th] T84.053 Periprosthetic osteolysis of internal prosthetic left knee joint
[7th] T84.058 Periprosthetic osteolysis of other internal prosthetic joint
Use additional code to identify the joint (Z96.6-)
[7th] T84.059 Periprosthetic osteolysis of unspecified internal prosthetic joint

[6th] T84.06 Wear of articular bearing surface of internal prosthetic joint

[7th] T84.060 Wear of articular bearing surface of internal prosthetic right hip joint
[7th] T84.061 Wear of articular bearing surface of internal prosthetic left hip joint
[7th] T84.062 Wear of articular bearing surface of internal prosthetic right knee joint
[7th] T84.063 Wear of articular bearing surface of internal prosthetic left knee joint
[7th] T84.068 Wear of articular bearing surface of other internal prosthetic joint
Use additional code to identify the joint (Z96.6-)
[7th] T84.069 Wear of articular bearing surface of unspecified internal prosthetic joint

[6th] T84.09 Other mechanical complication of internal joint prosthesis
Prosthetic joint implant failure NOS

[7th] T84.090 Other mechanical complication of internal right hip prosthesis
[7th] T84.091 Other mechanical complication of internal left hip prosthesis
[7th] T84.092 Other mechanical complication of internal right knee prosthesis
[7th] T84.093 Other mechanical complication of internal left knee prosthesis
[7th] T84.098 Other mechanical complication of other internal joint prosthesis
Use additional code to identify the joint (Z96.6-)
[7th] T84.099 Other mechanical complication of unspecified internal joint prosthesis

[5th] T84.1 Mechanical complication of internal fixation device of bones of limb
[EXCLUDES2] *mechanical complication of internal fixation device of bones of feet (T84.2-)*
mechanical complication of internal fixation device of bones of fingers (T84.2-)
mechanical complication of internal fixation device of bones of hands (T84.2-)
mechanical complication of internal fixation device of bones of toes (T84.2-)

[6th] T84.11 Breakdown (mechanical) of internal fixation device of bones of limb

[7th] T84.110 Breakdown (mechanical) of internal fixation device of right humerus
[7th] T84.111 Breakdown (mechanical) of internal fixation device of left humerus
[7th] T84.112 Breakdown (mechanical) of internal fixation device of bone of right forearm
[7th] T84.113 Breakdown (mechanical) of internal fixation device of bone of left forearm
[7th] T84.114 Breakdown (mechanical) of internal fixation device of right femur
[7th] T84.115 Breakdown (mechanical) of internal fixation device of left femur
[7th] T84.116 Breakdown (mechanical) of internal fixation device of bone of right lower leg
[7th] T84.117 Breakdown (mechanical) of internal fixation device of bone of left lower leg
[7th] T84.119 Breakdown (mechanical) of internal fixation device of unspecified bone of limb

[6th] T84.12 Displacement of internal fixation device of bones of limb
Malposition of internal fixation device of bones of limb

[7th] T84.120 Displacement of internal fixation device of right humerus
[7th] T84.121 Displacement of internal fixation device of left humerus
[7th] T84.122 Displacement of internal fixation device of bone of right forearm
[7th] T84.123 Displacement of internal fixation device of bone of left forearm
[7th] T84.124 Displacement of internal fixation device of right femur

[4th] 4th character required [5th] 5th character required [6th] 6th character required [7th] 7th character required [x7th] Extension 'X' Alert
[EXCLUDES1] Not coded here [EXCLUDES2] Not included here [PDx] Primary Diagnosis Only Manifestation Code

[7th] T84.125 Displacement of internal fixation device of left femur
[7th] T84.126 Displacement of internal fixation device of bone of right lower leg
[7th] T84.127 Displacement of internal fixation device of bone of left lower leg
[7th] T84.129 Displacement of internal fixation device of unspecified bone of limb
[6th] T84.19 Other mechanical complication of internal fixation device of bones of limb
Obstruction (mechanical) of internal fixation device of bones of limb
Perforation of internal fixation device of bones of limb
Protrusion of internal fixation device of bones of limb
[7th] T84.190 Other mechanical complication of internal fixation device of right humerus
[7th] T84.191 Other mechanical complication of internal fixation device of left humerus
[7th] T84.192 Other mechanical complication of internal fixation device of bone of right forearm
[7th] T84.193 Other mechanical complication of internal fixation device of bone of left forearm
[7th] T84.194 Other mechanical complication of internal fixation device of right femur
[7th] T84.195 Other mechanical complication of internal fixation device of left femur
[7th] T84.196 Other mechanical complication of internal fixation device of bone of right lower leg
[7th] T84.197 Other mechanical complication of internal fixation device of bone of left lower leg
[7th] T84.199 Other mechanical complication of internal fixation device of unspecified bone of limb
[5th] T84.2 Mechanical complication of internal fixation device of other bones
[6th] T84.21 Breakdown (mechanical) of internal fixation device of other bones
[7th] T84.210 Breakdown (mechanical) of internal fixation device of bones of hand and fingers
[7th] T84.213 Breakdown (mechanical) of internal fixation device of bones of foot and toes
[7th] T84.216 Breakdown (mechanical) of internal fixation device of vertebrae
[7th] T84.218 Breakdown (mechanical) of internal fixation device of other bones
[6th] T84.22 Displacement of internal fixation device of other bones
Malposition of internal fixation device of other bones
[7th] T84.220 Displacement of internal fixation device of bones of hand and fingers
[7th] T84.223 Displacement of internal fixation device of bones of foot and toes
[7th] T84.226 Displacement of internal fixation device of vertebrae
[7th] T84.228 Displacement of internal fixation device of other bones
[6th] T84.29 Other mechanical complication of internal fixation device of other bones
Obstruction (mechanical) of internal fixation device of other bones
Perforation of internal fixation device of other bones
Protrusion of internal fixation device of other bones
[7th] T84.290 Other mechanical complication of internal fixation device of bones of hand and fingers
[7th] T84.293 Other mechanical complication of internal fixation device of bones of foot and toes
[7th] T84.296 Other mechanical complication of internal fixation device of vertebrae
[7th] T84.298 Other mechanical complication of internal fixation device of other bones
[5th] T84.3 Mechanical complication of other bone devices, implants and grafts
[EXCLUDES2] *other complications of bone graft (T86.83-)*
[6th] T84.31 Breakdown (mechanical) of other bone devices, implants and grafts
[7th] T84.310 Breakdown (mechanical) of electronic bone stimulator
[7th] T84.318 Breakdown (mechanical) of other bone devices, implants and grafts
[6th] T84.32 Displacement of other bone devices, implants and grafts
Malposition of other bone devices, implants and grafts
[7th] T84.320 Displacement of electronic bone stimulator
[7th] T84.328 Displacement of other bone devices, implants and grafts
[6th] T84.39 Other mechanical complication of other bone devices, implants and grafts
Obstruction (mechanical) of other bone devices, implants and grafts
Perforation of other bone devices, implants and grafts
Protrusion of other bone devices, implants and grafts
[7th] T84.390 Other mechanical complication of electronic bone stimulator
[7th] T84.398 Other mechanical complication of other bone devices, implants and grafts
[5th] T84.4 Mechanical complication of other internal orthopedic devices, implants and grafts
[6th] T84.41 Breakdown (mechanical) of other internal orthopedic devices, implants and grafts
[7th] T84.410 Breakdown (mechanical) of muscle and tendon graft
[7th] T84.418 Breakdown (mechanical) of other internal orthopedic devices, implants and grafts
[6th] T84.42 Displacement of other internal orthopedic devices, implants and grafts
Malposition of other internal orthopedic devices, implants and grafts
[7th] T84.420 Displacement of muscle and tendon graft
[7th] T84.428 Displacement of other internal orthopedic devices, implants and grafts
[6th] T84.49 Other mechanical complication of other internal orthopedic devices, implants and grafts
Mechanical complication of other internal orthopedic devices, implants and grafts NOS
Obstruction (mechanical) of other internal orthopedic devices, implants and grafts
Perforation of other internal orthopedic devices, implants and grafts
Protrusion of other internal orthopedic devices, implants and grafts
[7th] T84.490 Other mechanical complication of muscle and tendon graft
[7th] T84.498 Other mechanical complication of other internal orthopedic devices, implants and grafts
[5th] T84.5 Infection and inflammatory reaction due to internal joint prosthesis
Use additional code to identify infection
[7th] T84.50 Infection and inflammatory reaction due to unspecified internal joint prosthesis

Unspecified Code | Other Specified Code | [N] Newborn Age: 0 | [P] Pediatric Age: 0-17 | [M] Maternity Age: 12-55
[A] Adult Age: 15-124 | ♂ Male | ♀ Female | ● New Code | ▲ Revised Code Title | ▶◀ Revised Text

T84.51 Infection and inflammatory reaction due to internal right hip prosthesis

T84.52 Infection and inflammatory reaction due to internal left hip prosthesis

T84.53 Infection and inflammatory reaction due to internal right knee prosthesis

T84.54 Infection and inflammatory reaction due to internal left knee prosthesis

T84.59 Infection and inflammatory reaction due to other internal joint prosthesis

T84.6 Infection and inflammatory reaction due to internal fixation device
Use additional code to identify infection

T84.60 Infection and inflammatory reaction due to internal fixation device of unspecified site

T84.61 Infection and inflammatory reaction due to internal fixation device of arm

T84.610 Infection and inflammatory reaction due to internal fixation device of right humerus

T84.611 Infection and inflammatory reaction due to internal fixation device of left humerus

T84.612 Infection and inflammatory reaction due to internal fixation device of right radius

T84.613 Infection and inflammatory reaction due to internal fixation device of left radius

T84.614 Infection and inflammatory reaction due to internal fixation device of right ulna

T84.615 Infection and inflammatory reaction due to internal fixation device of left ulna

T84.619 Infection and inflammatory reaction due to internal fixation device of unspecified bone of arm

T84.62 Infection and inflammatory reaction due to internal fixation device of leg

T84.620 Infection and inflammatory reaction due to internal fixation device of right femur

T84.621 Infection and inflammatory reaction due to internal fixation device of left femur

T84.622 Infection and inflammatory reaction due to internal fixation device of right tibia

T84.623 Infection and inflammatory reaction due to internal fixation device of left tibia

T84.624 Infection and inflammatory reaction due to internal fixation device of right fibula

T84.625 Infection and inflammatory reaction due to internal fixation device of left fibula

T84.629 Infection and inflammatory reaction due to internal fixation device of unspecified bone of leg

T84.63 Infection and inflammatory reaction due to internal fixation device of spine

T84.69 Infection and inflammatory reaction due to internal fixation device of other site

T84.7 Infection and inflammatory reaction due to other internal orthopedic prosthetic devices, implants and grafts
Use additional code to identify infection

T84.8 Other specified complications of internal orthopedic prosthetic devices, implants and grafts

T84.81 Embolism due to internal orthopedic prosthetic devices, implants and grafts

T84.82 Fibrosis due to internal orthopedic prosthetic devices, implants and grafts

T84.83 Hemorrhage due to internal orthopedic prosthetic devices, implants and grafts

T84.84 Pain due to internal orthopedic prosthetic devices, implants and grafts

T84.85 Stenosis due to internal orthopedic prosthetic devices, implants and grafts

T84.86 Thrombosis due to internal orthopedic prosthetic devices, implants and grafts

T84.89 Other specified complication of internal orthopedic prosthetic devices, implants and grafts

T84.9 Unspecified complication of internal orthopedic prosthetic device, implant and graft

T85 Complications of other internal prosthetic devices, implants and grafts

EXCLUDES2 failure and rejection of transplanted organs and tissue (T86.-)

The appropriate 7th character is to be added to each code from category T85
A = initial encounter
D = subsequent encounter
S = sequela

T85.0 Mechanical complication of ventricular intracranial (communicating) shunt

T85.01 Breakdown (mechanical) of ventricular intracranial (communicating) shunt

T85.02 Displacement of ventricular intracranial (communicating) shunt
Malposition of ventricular intracranial (communicating) shunt

T85.03 Leakage of ventricular intracranial (communicating) shunt

T85.09 Other mechanical complication of ventricular intracranial (communicating) shunt
Obstruction (mechanical) of ventricular intracranial (communicating) shunt
Perforation of ventricular intracranial (communicating) shunt
Protrusion of ventricular intracranial (communicating) shunt

T85.1 Mechanical complication of implanted electronic stimulator of nervous system

T85.11 Breakdown (mechanical) of implanted electronic stimulator of nervous system

T85.110 Breakdown (mechanical) of implanted electronic neurostimulator (electrode) of brain

T85.111 Breakdown (mechanical) of implanted electronic neurostimulator (electrode) of peripheral nerve

T85.112 Breakdown (mechanical) of implanted electronic neurostimulator (electrode) of spinal cord

T85.118 Breakdown (mechanical) of other implanted electronic stimulator of nervous system

T85.12 Displacement of implanted electronic stimulator of nervous system
Malposition of implanted electronic stimulator of nervous system

T85.120 Displacement of implanted electronic neurostimulator (electrode) of brain

T85.121 Displacement of implanted electronic neurostimulator (electrode) of peripheral nerve

T85.122 Displacement of implanted electronic neurostimulator (electrode) of spinal cord

T85.128 Displacement of other implanted electronic stimulator of nervous system

T85.19 Other mechanical complication of implanted electronic stimulator of nervous system
Leakage of implanted electronic stimulator of nervous system
Obstruction (mechanical) of implanted electronic stimulator of nervous system
Perforation of implanted electronic stimulator of nervous system
Protrusion of implanted electronic stimulator of nervous system

---

4th character required   5th character required   6th character required   7th character required   Extension 'X' Alert

EXCLUDES 1 Not coded here   EXCLUDES 2 Not included here   PDx Primary Diagnosis Only   Manifestation Code

[7th] T85.190 Other mechanical complication of implanted electronic neurostimulator (electrode) of brain

[7th] T85.191 Other mechanical complication of implanted electronic neurostimulator (electrode) of peripheral nerve

[7th] T85.192 Other mechanical complication of implanted electronic neurostimulator (electrode) of spinal cord

[7th] T85.199 Other mechanical complication of other implanted electronic stimulator of nervous system

[5th] T85.2 Mechanical complication of intraocular lens

[7th] T85.21 Breakdown (mechanical) of intraocular lens

[7th] T85.22 Displacement of intraocular lens
Malposition of intraocular lens

[7th] T85.29 Other mechanical complication of intraocular lens
Obstruction (mechanical) of intraocular lens
Perforation of intraocular lens
Protrusion of intraocular lens

[5th] T85.3 Mechanical complication of other ocular prosthetic devices, implants and grafts
[EXCLUDES2] *other complications of corneal graft (T86.84-)*

[6th] T85.31 Breakdown (mechanical) of other ocular prosthetic devices, implants and grafts

[7th] T85.310 Breakdown (mechanical) of prosthetic orbit of right eye

[7th] T85.311 Breakdown (mechanical) of prosthetic orbit of left eye

[7th] T85.318 Breakdown (mechanical) of other ocular prosthetic devices, implants and grafts

[6th] T85.32 Displacement of other ocular prosthetic devices, implants and grafts
Malposition of other ocular prosthetic devices, implants and grafts

[7th] T85.320 Displacement of prosthetic orbit of right eye

[7th] T85.321 Displacement of prosthetic orbit of left eye

[7th] T85.328 Displacement of other ocular prosthetic devices, implants and grafts

[6th] T85.39 Other mechanical complication of other ocular prosthetic devices, implants and grafts
Obstruction (mechanical) of other ocular prosthetic devices, implants and grafts
Perforation of other ocular prosthetic devices, implants and grafts
Protrusion of other ocular prosthetic devices, implants and grafts

[7th] T85.390 Other mechanical complication of prosthetic orbit of right eye

[7th] T85.391 Other mechanical complication of prosthetic orbit of left eye

[7th] T85.398 Other mechanical complication of other ocular prosthetic devices, implants and grafts

[5th] T85.4 Mechanical complication of breast prosthesis and implant

[7th] T85.41 Breakdown (mechanical) of breast prosthesis and implant

[7th] T85.42 Displacement of breast prosthesis and implant
Malposition of breast prosthesis and implant

[7th] T85.43 Leakage of breast prosthesis and implant

[7th] T85.44 Capsular contracture of breast implant

[7th] T85.49 Other mechanical complication of breast prosthesis and implant
Obstruction (mechanical) of breast prosthesis and implant
Perforation of breast prosthesis and implant
Protrusion of breast prosthesis and implant

[5th] T85.5 Mechanical complication of gastrointestinal prosthetic devices, implants and grafts

[6th] T85.51 Breakdown (mechanical) of gastrointestinal prosthetic devices, implants and grafts

[7th] T85.510 Breakdown (mechanical) of bile duct prosthesis

[7th] T85.511 Breakdown (mechanical) of esophageal anti-reflux device

[7th] T85.518 Breakdown (mechanical) of other gastrointestinal prosthetic devices, implants and grafts

[6th] T85.52 Displacement of gastrointestinal prosthetic devices, implants and grafts
Malposition of gastrointestinal prosthetic devices, implants and grafts

[7th] T85.520 Displacement of bile duct prosthesis

[7th] T85.521 Displacement of esophageal anti-reflux device

[7th] T85.528 Displacement of other gastrointestinal prosthetic devices, implants and grafts

[6th] T85.59 Other mechanical complication of gastrointestinal prosthetic devices, implants and
Obstruction, mechanical of gastrointestinal prosthetic devices, implants and grafts
Perforation of gastrointestinal prosthetic devices, implants and grafts
Protrusion of gastrointestinal prosthetic devices, implants and grafts

[7th] T85.590 Other mechanical complication of bile duct prosthesis

[7th] T85.591 Other mechanical complication of esophageal anti-reflux device

[7th] T85.598 Other mechanical complication of other gastrointestinal prosthetic devices, implants and grafts

[5th] T85.6 Mechanical complication of other specified internal and external prosthetic devices, implants and grafts

[6th] T85.61 Breakdown (mechanical) of other specified internal prosthetic devices, implants and grafts

[7th] T85.610 Breakdown (mechanical) of epidural and subdural infusion catheter

[7th] T85.611 Breakdown (mechanical) of intraperitoneal dialysis catheter
[EXCLUDES1] *mechanical complication of vascular dialysis catheter (T82.4-)*

[7th] T85.612 Breakdown (mechanical) of permanent sutures
[EXCLUDES1] *mechanical complication of permanent (wire) suture used in bone repair (T84.1-T84.2)*

[7th] T85.613 Breakdown (mechanical) of artificial skin graft and decellularized allodermis
Failure of artificial skin graft and decellularized allodermis
Non-adherence of artificial skin graft and decellularized allodermis
Poor incorporation of artificial skin graft and decellularized allodermis
Shearing of artificial skin graft and decellularized allodermis

[7th] T85.614 Breakdown (mechanical) of insulin pump

T85.618 Breakdown (mechanical) of other specified internal prosthetic devices, implants and grafts

T85.62 Displacement of other specified internal prosthetic devices, implants and grafts

Malposition of other specified internal prosthetic devices, implants and grafts

T85.620 Displacement of epidural and subdural infusion catheter

T85.621 Displacement of intraperitoneal dialysis catheter

EXCLUDES1 mechanical complication of vascular dialysis catheter (T82.4-)

T85.622 Displacement of permanent sutures

EXCLUDES1 mechanical complication of permanent (wire) suture used in bone repair (T84.1-T84.2)

T85.623 Displacement of artificial skin graft and decellularized allodermis

Dislodgement of artificial skin graft and decellularized allodermis

Displacement of artificial skin graft and decellularized allodermis

T85.624 Displacement of insulin pump

T85.628 Displacement of other specified internal prosthetic devices, implants and grafts

T85.63 Leakage of other specified internal prosthetic devices, implants and grafts

T85.630 Leakage of epidural and subdural infusion catheter

T85.631 Leakage of intraperitoneal dialysis catheter

EXCLUDES1 mechanical complication of vascular dialysis catheter (T82.4)

T85.633 Leakage of insulin pump

T85.638 Leakage of other specified internal prosthetic devices, implants and grafts

T85.69 Other mechanical complication of other specified internal prosthetic devices, implants and grafts

Obstruction, mechanical of other specified internal prosthetic devices, implants and grafts

Perforation of other specified internal prosthetic devices, implants and grafts

Protrusion of other specified internal prosthetic devices, implants and grafts

T85.690 Other mechanical complication of epidural and subdural infusion catheter

T85.691 Other mechanical complication of intraperitoneal dialysis catheter

EXCLUDES1 mechanical complication of vascular dialysis catheter (T82.4)

T85.692 Other mechanical complication of permanent sutures

EXCLUDES1 mechanical complication of permanent (wire) suture used in bone repair (T84.1-T84.2)

T85.693 Other mechanical complication of artificial skin graft and decellularized allodermis

T85.694 Other mechanical complication of insulin pump

T85.698 Other mechanical complication of other specified internal prosthetic devices, implants and grafts

Mechanical complication of nonabsorbable surgical material NOS

T85.7 Infection and inflammatory reaction due to other internal prosthetic devices, implants and grafts

Use additional code to identify infection

T85.71 Infection and inflammatory reaction due to peritoneal dialysis catheter

T85.72 Infection and inflammatory reaction due to insulin pump

T85.79 Infection and inflammatory reaction due to other internal prosthetic devices, implants and grafts

T85.8 Other specified complications of internal prosthetic devices, implants and grafts, not elsewhere classified

T85.81 Embolism due to internal prosthetic devices, implants and grafts, not elsewhere classified

T85.82 Fibrosis due to internal prosthetic devices, implants and grafts, not elsewhere classified

T85.83 Hemorrhage due to internal prosthetic devices, implants and grafts, not elsewhere classified

T85.84 Pain due to internal prosthetic devices, implants and grafts, not elsewhere classified

T85.85 Stenosis due to internal prosthetic devices, implants and grafts, not elsewhere classified

T85.86 Thrombosis due to internal prosthetic devices, implants and grafts, not elsewhere classified

T85.89 Other specified complication of internal prosthetic devices, implants and grafts, not elsewhere classified

T85.9 Unspecified complication of internal prosthetic device, implant and graft

Complication of internal prosthetic device, implant and graft NOS

T86 Complications of transplanted organs and tissue

Use additional code to identify other transplant complications, such as:
graft-versus-host disease (D89.81-)
malignancy associated with organ transplant (C80.2)
post-transplant lymphoproliferative disorders (PTLD) (D47.Z1)

T86.0 Complications of bone marrow transplant

T86.00 Unspecified complication of bone marrow transplant

T86.01 Bone marrow transplant rejection

T86.02 Bone marrow transplant failure

T86.03 Bone marrow transplant infection

T86.09 Other complications of bone marrow transplant

T86.1 Complications of kidney transplant

T86.10 Unspecified complication of kidney transplant

T86.11 Kidney transplant rejection

T86.12 Kidney transplant failure

T86.13 Kidney transplant infection

Use additional code to specify infection

T86.19 Other complication of kidney transplant

T86.2 Complications of heart transplant

EXCLUDES1 complication of:
artificial heart device (T82.5)
heart-lung transplant (T86.3)

T86.20 Unspecified complication of heart transplant

T86.21 Heart transplant rejection

T86.22 Heart transplant failure

T86.23 Heart transplant infection

Use additional code to specify infection

T86.29 Other complications of heart transplant

T86.290 Cardiac allograft vasculopathy

EXCLUDES1 atherosclerosis of coronary arteries (I25.75-, I25.76-, I25.81-)

T86.298 Other complications of heart transplant

T86.3 Complications of heart-lung transplant

T86.30 Unspecified complication of heart-lung transplant

T86.31 Heart-lung transplant rejection

T86.32 Heart-lung transplant failure

T86.33 Heart-lung transplant infection

Use additional code to specify infection

T86.39 Other complications of heart-lung transplant

4th character required   5th character required   6th character required   7th character required   Extension 'X' Alert

EXCLUDES 1 Not coded here   EXCLUDES 2 Not included here   PDx Primary Diagnosis Only   Manifestation Code

T86.4 Complications of liver transplant
  T86.40 Unspecified complication of liver transplant
  T86.41 Liver transplant rejection
  T86.42 Liver transplant failure
  T86.43 Liver transplant infection
    Use additional code to identify infection, such as:
    Cytomegalovirus (CMV) infection (B25.-)
  T86.49 Other complications of liver transplant
T86.5 Complications of stem cell transplant
    Complications from stem cells from peripheral blood
    Complications from stem cells from umbilical cord
T86.8 Complications of other transplanted organs and tissues
  T86.81 Complications of lung transplant
    EXCLUDES1 complication of heart-lung transplant (T86.3-)
    T86.810 Lung transplant rejection
    T86.811 Lung transplant failure
    T86.812 Lung transplant infection
      Use additional code to specify infection
    T86.818 Other complications of lung transplant
    T86.819 Unspecified complication of lung transplant
  T86.82 Complications of skin graft (allograft) (autograft)
    EXCLUDES2 complication of artificial skin graft (T85.693)
    T86.820 Skin graft (allograft) rejection
    T86.821 Skin graft (allograft) (autograft) failure
    T86.822 Skin graft (allograft) (autograft) infection
      Use additional code to specify infection
    T86.828 Other complications of skin graft (allograft) (autograft)
    T86.829 Unspecified complication of skin graft (allograft) (autograft)
  T86.83 Complications of bone graft
    EXCLUDES2 mechanical complications of bone graft (T84.3-)
    T86.830 Bone graft rejection
    T86.831 Bone graft failure
    T86.832 Bone graft infection
      Use additional code to specify infection
    T86.838 Other complications of bone graft
    T86.839 Unspecified complication of bone graft
  T86.84 Complications of corneal transplant
    EXCLUDES2 mechanical complications of corneal graft (T85.3-)
    T86.840 Corneal transplant rejection
    T86.841 Corneal transplant failure
    T86.842 Corneal transplant infection
      Use additional code to specify infection
    T86.848 Other complications of corneal transplant
    T86.849 Unspecified complication of corneal transplant
  T86.85 Complication of intestine transplant
    T86.850 Intestine transplant rejection
    T86.851 Intestine transplant failure
    T86.852 Intestine transplant infection
      Use additional code to specify infection
    T86.858 Other complications of intestine transplant
    T86.859 Unspecified complication of intestine transplant
  T86.89 Complications of other transplanted tissue
    Transplant failure or rejection of pancreas
    T86.890 Other transplanted tissue rejection
    T86.891 Other transplanted tissue failure
    T86.892 Other transplanted tissue infection
      Use additional code to specify infection
    T86.898 Other complications of other transplanted tissue

    T86.899 Unspecified complication of other transplanted tissue
T86.9 Complication of unspecified transplanted organ and tissue
  T86.90 Unspecified complication of unspecified transplanted organ and tissue
  T86.91 Unspecified transplanted organ and tissue rejection
  T86.92 Unspecified transplanted organ and tissue failure
  T86.93 Unspecified transplanted organ and tissue infection
    Use additional code to specify infection
  T86.99 Other complications of unspecified transplanted organ and tissue
T87 Complications peculiar to reattachment and amputation
  T87.0 Complications of reattached (part of) upper extremity
    T87.0X Complications of reattached (part of) upper extremity
      T87.0X1 Complications of reattached (part of) right upper extremity
      T87.0X2 Complications of reattached (part of) left upper extremity
      T87.0X9 Complications of reattached (part of) unspecified upper extremity
  T87.1 Complications of reattached (part of) lower extremity
    T87.1X Complications of reattached (part of) lower extremity
      T87.1X1 Complications of reattached (part of) right lower extremity
      T87.1X2 Complications of reattached (part of) left lower extremity
      T87.1X9 Complications of reattached (part of) unspecified lower extremity
  T87.2 Complications of other reattached body part
  T87.3 Neuroma of amputation stump
    T87.30 Neuroma of amputation stump, unspecified extremity
    T87.31 Neuroma of amputation stump, right upper extremity
    T87.32 Neuroma of amputation stump, left upper extremity
    T87.33 Neuroma of amputation stump, right lower extremity
    T87.34 Neuroma of amputation stump, left lower extremity
  T87.4 Infection of amputation stump
    T87.40 Infection of amputation stump, unspecified extremity
    T87.41 Infection of amputation stump, right upper extremity
    T87.42 Infection of amputation stump, left upper extremity
    T87.43 Infection of amputation stump, right lower extremity
    T87.44 Infection of amputation stump, left lower extremity
  T87.5 Necrosis of amputation stump
    T87.50 Necrosis of amputation stump, unspecified extremity
    T87.51 Necrosis of amputation stump, right upper extremity
    T87.52 Necrosis of amputation stump, left upper extremity
    T87.53 Necrosis of amputation stump, right lower extremity
    T87.54 Necrosis of amputation stump, left lower extremity

| Unspecified Code | Other Specified Code | N Newborn Age: 0 | P Pediatric Age: 0-17 | M Maternity Age: 12-55 |
| A Adult Age: 15-124 | ♂ Male | ♀ Female | ● New Code | ▲ Revised Code Title | ►◄ Revised Text |

CHAPTER 19: INJURY, POISONING, AND CERTAIN OTHER CONSEQUENCES OF EXTERNAL CAUSES (S00-T88)

T87.8 - T88.8

5ᵗʰ **T87.8** Other complications of amputation stump

  T87.81 Dehiscence of amputation stump

  T87.89 Other complications of amputation stump
    Amputation stump contracture
    Amputation stump contracture of next proximal joint
    Amputation stump flexion
    Amputation stump edema
    Amputation stump hematoma
    EXCLUDES2 *phantom limb syndrome (G54.6-G54.7)*

  T87.9 Unspecified complications of amputation stump

4ᵗʰ **T88** Other complications of surgical and medical care, not elsewhere classified

    EXCLUDES2 *complication following infusion, transfusion and therapeutic injection (T80.-)*
      complication following procedure NEC (T81.-)
      complications of anesthesia in labor and delivery (O74.-)
      complications of anesthesia in pregnancy (O29.-)
      complications of anesthesia in puerperium (O89.-)
      complications of devices, implants and grafts (T82-T85)
      complications of obstetric surgery and procedure (O75.4)
      dermatitis due to drugs and medicaments (L23.3, L24.4, L25.1, L27.0-L27.1)
      poisoning and toxic effects of drugs and chemicals (T36-T65 with fifth or sixth character 1-4 or 6)
      specified complications classified elsewhere

    The appropriate 7th character is to be added to each code from category T88
    A = initial encounter
    D = subsequent encounter
    S = sequela

7ᵗʰ **T88.0** Infection following immunization
    Sepsis following immunization

7ᵗʰ **T88.1** Other complications following immunization, not elsewhere classified
    Generalized vaccinia
    Rash following immunization
    EXCLUDES1 *vaccinia not from vaccine (B08.011)*
    EXCLUDES2 *anaphylactic shock due to serum (T80.5-)*
      other serum reactions (T80.6-)
      postimmunization arthropathy (M02.2)
      postimmunization encephalitis (G04.02)
      postimmunization fever (R50.83)

7ᵗʰ **T88.2** Shock due to anesthesia
    Use additional code for adverse effect, if applicable, to identify drug (T41.- with fifth or sixth character 5)
    EXCLUDES1 *complications of anesthesia (in):*
      labor and delivery (O74.-)
      pregnancy (O29.-)
      puerperium (O89.-)
      postprocedural shock NOS (T81.1-)

7ᵗʰ **T88.3** Malignant hyperthermia due to anesthesia
    Use additional code for adverse effect, if applicable, to identify drug (T41.- with fifth or sixth character 5)

7ᵗʰ **T88.4** Failed or difficult intubation

5ᵗʰ **T88.5** Other complications of anesthesia
    Use additional code for adverse effect, if applicable, to identify drug (T41.- with fifth or sixth character 5)

  7ᵗʰ **T88.51** Hypothermia following anesthesia

  7ᵗʰ **T88.52** Failed moderate sedation during procedure
    Failed conscious sedation during procedure
    EXCLUDES2 *personal history of failed moderate sedation (Z92.83)*

  7ᵗʰ **T88.59** Other complications of anesthesia

7ᵗʰ **T88.6** Anaphylactic reaction due to adverse effect of correct drug or medicament properly administered
    Anaphylactic shock due to adverse effect of correct drug or medicament properly administered
    Anaphylactoid reaction NOS
    Use additional code for adverse effect, if applicable, to identify drug (T36-T50 with fifth or sixth character 5)
    EXCLUDES1 *anaphylactic reaction due to serum (T80.5-)*
      anaphylactic shock or reaction due to adverse food reaction (T78.0-)

7ᵗʰ **T88.7** Unspecified adverse effect of drug or medicament
    Drug hypersensitivity NOS
    Drug reaction NOS
    Use additional code for adverse effect, if applicable, to identify drug (T36-T50 with fifth or sixth character 5)
    EXCLUDES1 *specified adverse effects of drugs and medicaments (A00-R94 and T80-T88.6, T88.8)*

7ᵗʰ **T88.8** Other specified complications of surgical and medical care, not elsewhere classified
    Use additional code to identify the complication

  7ᵗʰ **T88.9** Complication of surgical and medical care, unspecified

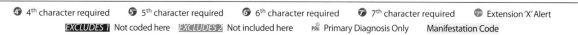

4 4ᵗʰ character required   **5** 5ᵗʰ character required   **6** 6ᵗʰ character required   **7** 7ᵗʰ character required   **7ˣ** Extension 'X' Alert

EXCLUDES 1 Not coded here   *EXCLUDES 2* Not included here   ᴾᴰˣ Primary Diagnosis Only   Manifestation Code

Chapter 20: External Causes of Morbidity (V00-Y99)

Chapter Specific Coding Guidelines

The external causes of morbidity codes should never be sequenced as the first-listed or principal diagnosis.

External cause codes are intended to provide data for injury research and evaluation of injury prevention strategies. These codes capture how the injury or health condition happened (cause), the intent (unintentional or accidental; or intentional, such as suicide or assault), the place where the event occurred the activity of the patient at the time of the event, and the person's status (e.g., civilian, military).

There is no national requirement for mandatory ICD-10-CM external cause code reporting. Unless a provider is subject to a state-based external cause code reporting mandate or these codes are required by a particular payer, reporting of ICD-10-CM codes in Chapter 20, External Causes of Morbidity, is not required. In the absence of a mandatory reporting requirement, providers are encouraged to voluntarily report external cause codes, as they provide valuable data for injury research and evaluation of injury prevention strategies.

a. General External Cause Coding Guidelines
   1) **Used with any code in the range of A00.0-T88.9, Z00-Z99**
   An external cause code may be used with any code in the range of A00.0-T88.9, Z00-Z99, classification that is a health condition due to an external cause. Though they are most applicable to injuries, they are also valid for use with such things as infections or diseases due to an external source, and other health conditions, such as a heart attack that occurs during strenuous physical activity.

   2) **External cause code used for length of treatment**
   Assign the external cause code, with the appropriate 7th character (initial encounter, subsequent encounter or sequela) for each encounter for which the injury or condition is being treated.

   3) **Use the full range of external cause codes**
   Use the full range of external cause codes to completely describe the cause, the intent, the place of occurrence, and if applicable, the activity of the patient at the time of the event, and the patient's status, for all injuries, and other health conditions due to an external cause.

   4) **Assign as many external cause codes as necessary**
   Assign as many external cause codes as necessary to fully explain each cause. If only one external code can be recorded, assign the code most related to the principal diagnosis.

   5) **The selection of the appropriate external cause code**
   The selection of the appropriate external cause code is guided by the Alphabetic Index of External Causes and by Inclusion and Exclusion notes in the Tabular List.

   6) **External cause code can never be a principal diagnosis**
   An external cause code can never be a principal (first-listed) diagnosis.

   7) **Combination external cause codes**
   Certain of the external cause codes are combination codes that identify sequential events that result in an injury, such as a fall which results in striking against an object. The injury may be due to either event or both. The combination external cause code used should correspond to the sequence of events regardless of which caused the most serious injury.

   8) **No external cause code needed in certain circumstances**
   No external cause code from Chapter 20 is needed if the external cause and intent are included in a code from another chapter (e.g. T36.0X1- Poisoning by penicillins, accidental (unintentional)).

b. **Place of Occurrence Guideline**

Codes from category Y92, Place of occurrence of the external cause, are secondary codes for use after other external cause codes to identify the location of the patient at the time of injury or other condition.

A place of occurrence code is used only once, at the initial encounter for treatment. No 7th characters are used for Y92. Only one code from Y92 should be recorded on a medical record.

Do not use place of occurrence code Y92.9 if the place is not stated or is not applicable.

c. **Activity Code**
Assign a code from category Y93, Activity code, to describe the activity of the patient at the time the injury or other health condition occurred.

An activity code is used only once, at the initial encounter for treatment. Only one code from Y93 should be recorded on a medical record.

The activity codes are not applicable to poisonings, adverse effects, misadventures or sequela .

Do not assign Y93.9, Unspecified activity, if the activity is not stated.

A code from category Y93 is appropriate for use with external cause and intent codes if identifying the activity provides additional information about the event.

d. **Place of Occurrence, Activity, and Status Codes Used with other External Cause Code**
When applicable, place of occurrence, activity, and external cause status codes are sequenced after the main external cause code(s). Regardless of the number of external cause codes assigned, there should be only one place of occurrence code, one activity code, and one external cause status code assigned to an encounter.

e. **If the Reporting Format Limits the Number of External Cause Codes**
If the reporting format limits the number of external cause codes that can be used in reporting clinical data, report the code for the cause/intent most related to the principal diagnosis. If the format permits capture of additional external cause codes, the cause/intent, including medical misadventures, of the additional events should be reported rather than the codes for place, activity, or external status.

f. **Multiple External Cause Coding Guidelines**
More than one external cause code is required to fully describe the external cause of an illness or injury. The assignment of external cause codes should be sequenced in the following priority:

If two or more events cause separate injuries, an external cause code should be assigned for each cause. The first-listed external cause code will be selected in the following order:

External codes for child and adult abuse take priority over all other external cause codes.

See Section I.C.19., Child and Adult abuse guidelines.

External cause codes for terrorism events take priority over all other external cause codes except child and adult abuse.

External cause codes for cataclysmic events take priority over all other external cause codes except child and adult abuse and terrorism.

External cause codes for transport accidents take priority over all other external cause codes except cataclysmic events, child and adult abuse and terrorism.

Activity and external cause status codes are assigned following all causal (intent) external cause codes.

The first-listed external cause code should correspond to the cause of the most serious diagnosis due to an assault, accident, or self-harm, following the order of hierarchy listed above.

g. **Child and Adult Abuse Guideline**

Adult and child abuse, neglect and maltreatment are classified as assault. Any of the assault codes may be used to indicate the external cause of any injury resulting from the confirmed abuse.

For confirmed cases of abuse, neglect and maltreatment, when the perpetrator is known, a code from Y07, Perpetrator of maltreatment and neglect, should accompany any other assault codes.

See Section I.C.19. Adult and child abuse, neglect and other maltreatment

h. **Unknown or Undetermined Intent Guideline**

If the intent (accident, self-harm, assault) of the cause of an injury or other condition is unknown or unspecified, code the intent as accidental intent. All transport accident categories assume accidental intent.

1) **Use of undetermined intent**

External cause codes for events of undetermined intent are only for use if the documentation in the record specifies that the intent cannot be determined.

i. **Sequelae (Late Effects) of External Cause Guidelines**

1) **Sequelae external cause codes**

Sequela are reported using the external cause code with the 7th character "S" for sequela. These codes should be used with any report of a late effect or sequela resulting from a previous injury.

2) **Sequela external cause code with a related current injury**

A sequela external cause code should never be used with a related current nature of injury code.

3) **Use of sequela external cause codes for subsequent visits**

Use a late effect external cause code for subsequent visits when a late effect of the initial injury is being treated. Do not use a late effect external cause code for subsequent visits for follow-up care (e.g., to assess healing, to receive rehabilitative therapy) of the injury when no late effect of the injury has been documented.

j. **Terrorism Guidelines**

1) **Cause of injury identified by the Federal Government (FBI) as terrorism**

When the cause of an injury is identified by the Federal Government (FBI) as terrorism, the first-listed external cause code should be a code from category Y38, Terrorism. The definition of terrorism employed by the FBI is found at the inclusion note at the beginning of category Y38. Use additional code for place of occurrence (Y92.-). More than one Y38 code may be assigned if the injury is the result of more than one mechanism of terrorism.

2) **Cause of an injury is suspected to be the result of terrorism**

When the cause of an injury is suspected to be the result of terrorism a code from category Y38 should not be assigned. Suspected cases should be classified as assault.

3) **Code Y38.9, Terrorism, secondary effects**

Assign code Y38.9, Terrorism, secondary effects, for conditions occurring subsequent to the terrorist event. This code should not be assigned for conditions that are due to the initial terrorist act.

It is acceptable to assign code Y38.9 with another code from Y38 if there is an injury due to the initial terrorist event and an injury that is a subsequent result of the terrorist event.

k. **External cause status**

A code from category Y99, External cause status, should be assigned whenever any other external cause code is assigned for an encounter, including an Activity code, except for the events noted below. Assign a code from category Y99, External cause status, to indicate the work status of the person at the time the event occurred. The status code indicates whether the event occurred during military activity, whether a non-military person was at work, whether an individual including a student or volunteer was involved in a non-work activity at the time of the causal event.

A code from Y99, External cause status, should be assigned, when applicable, with other external cause codes, such as transport accidents and falls. The external cause status codes are not applicable to poisonings, adverse effects, misadventures or late effects.

Do not assign a code from category Y99 if no other external cause codes (cause, activity) are applicable for the encounter.

An external cause status code is used only once, at the initial encounter for treatment. Only one code from Y99 should be recorded on a medical record.

Do not assign code Y99.9, Unspecified external cause status, if the status is not stated.

External causes of morbidity (V00-Y99)

NOTES This chapter permits the classification of environmental events and circumstances as the cause of injury, and other adverse effects. Where a code from this section is applicable, it is intended that it shall be used secondary to a code from another chapter of the Classification indicating the nature of the condition. Most often, the condition will be classifiable to Chapter 19, Injury, poisoning and certain other consequences of external causes (S00-T88). Other conditions that may be stated to be due to external causes are classified in Chapters I to XVIII. For these conditions, codes from Chapter 20 should be used to provide additional information as to the cause of the condition.

Accidents (V00-X58)

Transport accidents (V00-V99)

NOTES This section is structured in 12 groups. Those relating to land transport accidents (V01- V89) reflect the victim's mode of transport and are subdivided to identify the victim's 'counterpart' or the type of event. The vehicle of which the injured person is an occupant is identified in the first two characters since it is seen as the most important factor to identify for prevention purposes. A transport accident is one in which the vehicle involved must be moving or running or in use for transport purposes at the time of the accident.

NOTES Definitions of transport vehicles:
(a) A transport accident is any accident involving a device designed primarily for, or used at the time primarily for, conveying persons or good from one place to another.
(b) A public highway [trafficway] or street is the entire width between property lines (or other boundary lines) of land open to the public as a matter of right or custom for purposes of moving persons or property from one place to another. A roadway is that part of the public highway designed, improved and customarily used for vehicular traffic.
(c) A traffic accident is any vehicle accident occurring on the public highway [i.e. originating on, terminating on, or involving a vehicle partially on the highway]. A vehicle accident is assumed to have occurred on the public highway unless another place is specified, except in the case of accidents involving only off-road motor vehicles, which are classified as nontraffic accidents unless the contrary is stated.
(d) A nontraffic accident is any vehicle accident that occurs entirely in any place other than a public highway.
(e) A pedestrian is any person involved in an accident who was not at the time of the accident riding in or on a motor vehicle, railway train, streetcar or animal-drawn or other vehicle, or on a pedal cycle or animal. This includes, a person changing a tire or working on a parked car. It also includes the use of a pedestrian conveyance such as a baby carriage, ice-skates, roller skates, a skateboard, nonmotorized or motorized wheelchair, motorized mobility scooter, or nonmotorized scooter.
(f) A driver is an occupant of a transport vehicle who is operating or intending to operate it.
(g) A passenger is any occupant of a transport vehicle other than the driver, except a person traveling on the outside of the vehicle.
(h) A person on the outside of a vehicle is any person being transported by a vehicle but not occupying the space normally reserved for the driver or passengers, or the space intended for the transport of property. This includes the body, bumper, fender, roof, running board or step of a vehicle.
(i) A pedal cycle is any land transport vehicle operated solely by nonmotorized pedals including a bicycle or tricycle.
(j) A pedal cyclist is any person riding a pedal cycle or in a sidecar or trailer attached to a pedal cycle.
(k) A motorcycle is a two-wheeled motor vehicle with one or two riding saddles and sometimes with a third wheel for the support of a sidecar. The sidecar is considered part of the motorcycle.
(l) A motorcycle rider is any person riding a motorcycle or in a sidecar or trailer attached to the motorcycle.
(m) A three-wheeled motor vehicle is a motorized tricycle designed primarily for on-road use. This includes a motor-driven tricycle, a motorized rickshaw, or a three-wheeled motor car.
(n) A car [automobile] is a four-wheeled motor vehicle designed primarily for carrying up to 7 persons. A trailer being towed by the car is considered part of the car.
(o) A pick-up truck or van is a four or six-wheeled motor vehicle designed for carrying passengers as well as property or cargo weighing less than the local limit for classification as a heavy goods vehicle, and not requiring a special driver's license. This includes a minivan and a sport-utility vehicle (SUV).
(p) A heavy transport vehicle is a motor vehicle designed primarily for carrying property, meeting local criteria for classification as a heavy goods vehicle in terms of weight and requiring a special driver's license.
(q) A bus (coach) is a motor vehicle designed or adapted primarily for carrying more than 10 passengers, and requiring a special driver's license.
(r) A railway train or railway vehicle is any device, with or without freight or passenger cars couple to it, designed for traffic on a railway track. This includes subterranean (subways) or elevated trains.
(s) A streetcar, is a device designed and used primarily for transporting passengers within a municipality, running on rails, usually subject to normal traffic control signals, and operated principally on a right-of-way that forms part of the roadway. This includes a tram or trolley that runs on rails. A trailer being towed by a streetcar is considered part of the streetcar.
(t) A special vehicle mainly used on industrial premises is a motor vehicle designed primarily for use within the buildings and premises of industrial or commercial establishments. This includes battery-powered trucks, forklifts, coal-cars in a coal mine, logging cars and trucks used in mines or quarries.
(u) A special vehicle mainly used in agriculture is a motor vehicle designed specifically for use in farming and agriculture (horticulture), to work the land, tend and harvest crops and transport materials on the farm. This includes harvesters, farm machinery and tractor and trailers.
(v) A special construction vehicle is a motor vehicle designed specifically for use on construction and demolition sites. This includes bulldozers, diggers, earth levellers, dump trucks. backhoes, front-end loaders, pavers, and mechanical shovels.
(w) A special all-terrain vehicle is a motor vehicle of special design to enable it to negotiate over rough or soft terrain , snow or sand. This includes snow mobiles, All-terrain vehicles (ATV), and dune buggies. It does not include passenger vehicle designated as Sport Utility Vehicles. (SUV)
(x) A watercraft is any device designed for transporting passengers or goods on water. This includes motor or sail boats, ships, and hovercraft.
(y) An aircraft is any device for transporting passengers or goods in the air. This includes hot-air balloons, gliders, helicopters and airplanes.
(z) A military vehicle is any motorized vehicle operating on a public roadway owned by the military and being operated by a member of the military.
Use additional code to identify:
Airbag injury (W22.1)
Type of street or road (Y92.4-)
Use of cellular telephone and other electronic equipment at the time of the transport accident (Y93.C-)

[EXCLUDES1] *agricultural vehicles in stationary use or maintenance (W31.-)*
assault by crashing of motor vehicle (Y03.-)
automobile or motor cycle in stationary use or maintenance- code to type of accident
crashing of motor vehicle, undetermined intent (Y32)
intentional self-harm by crashing of motor vehicle (X82)

[EXCLUDES2] *transport accidents due to cataclysm (X34-X38)*

Pedestrian injured in transport accident (V00-V09)

[INCLUDES] *person changing tire on transport vehicle*
person examining engine of vehicle broken down in (on side of) road

[EXCLUDES1] *fall due to non-transport collision with other person (W03)*
pedestrian on foot falling (slipping) on ice and snow (W00.-)
struck or bumped by another person (W51)

[4] **V00 Pedestrian conveyance accident**

Use additional place of occurrence and activity external cause codes, if known (Y92.-, Y93.-)

[EXCLUDES1] *collision with another person without fall (W51)*
fall due to person on foot colliding with another person on foot (W03)
fall from non-moving wheelchair, nonmotorized scooter and motorized mobility scooter without collision (W05.-)
pedestrian (conveyance) collision with other land transport vehicle (V01-V09)
pedestrian on foot falling (slipping) on ice and snow (W00.-)

The appropriate 7th character is to be added to each code from category V00
A = initial encounter
D = subsequent encounter
S = sequela

[5] V00.0 Pedestrian on foot injured in collision with pedestrian conveyance
- [7th] V00.01 Pedestrian on foot injured in collision with roller-skater
- [7th] V00.02 Pedestrian on foot injured in collision with skateboarder
- [7th] V00.09 Pedestrian on foot injured in collision with other pedestrian conveyance

[5] V00.1 Rolling-type pedestrian conveyance accident

[EXCLUDES1] *accident with babystroller (V00.82-)*
accident with wheelchair (powered) (V00.81-)
accident with motorized mobility scooter (V00.83-)

[6] V00.11 In-line roller-skate accident
- [7] V00.111 Fall from in-line roller-skates
- [7] V00.112 In-line roller-skater colliding with stationary object
- [7] V00.118 Other in-line roller-skate accident

[EXCLUDES1] *roller-skater collision with other land transport vehicle (V01-V09 with 5th character 1)*

[6] V00.12 Non-in- line roller-skate accident
- [7] V00.121 Fall from non-in-line roller-skates
- [7] V00.122 Non-in-line roller-skater colliding with stationary object
- [7] V00.128 Other non-in-line roller-skating accident

[EXCLUDES1] *roller-skater collision with other land transport vehicle (V01-V09 with 5th character 1)*

[6] V00.13 Skateboard accident
- [7] V00.131 Fall from skateboard
- [7] V00.132 Skateboarder colliding with stationary object
- [7] V00.138 Other skateboard accident

[EXCLUDES1] *skateboarder collision with other land transport vehicle (V01-V09 with 5th character 2)*

[6] V00.14 Scooter (nonmotorized) accident

[EXCLUDES1] *motorscooter accident (V20-V29)*

- [7] V00.141 Fall from scooter (nonmotorized)
- [7] V00.142 Scooter (nonmotorized) colliding with stationary object
- [7] V00.148 Other scooter (nonmotorized) accident

[EXCLUDES1] *scooter (nonmotorized) collision with other land transport vehicle (V01-V09 with fifth character 9)*

[6] V00.15 Heelies accident
Rolling shoe
Wheeled shoe
Wheelies accident
- [7] V00.151 Fall from heelies
- [7] V00.152 Heelies colliding with stationary object
- [7] V00.158 Other heelies accident

[6] V00.18 Accident on other rolling-type pedestrian conveyance
- [7] V00.181 Fall from other rolling-type pedestrian conveyance
- [7] V00.182 Pedestrian on other rolling-type pedestrian conveyance colliding with stationary object
- [7] V00.188 Other accident on other rolling-type pedestrian conveyance

[5] V00.2 Gliding-type pedestrian conveyance accident

[6] V00.21 Ice-skates accident
- [7] V00.211 Fall from ice-skates
- [7] V00.212 Ice-skater colliding with stationary object
- [7] V00.218 Other ice-skates accident

[EXCLUDES1] *ice-skater collision with other land transport vehicle (V01-V09 with 5th digit 9)*

[6] V00.22 Sled accident
- [7] V00.221 Fall from sled
- [7] V00.222 Sledder colliding with stationary object
- [7] V00.228 Other sled accident

[EXCLUDES1] *sled collision with other land transport vehicle (V01-V09 with 5th digit 9)*

[6] V00.28 Other gliding-type pedestrian conveyance accident
- [7] V00.281 Fall from other gliding-type pedestrian conveyance
- [7] V00.282 Pedestrian on other gliding-type pedestrian conveyance colliding with stationary object
- [7] V00.288 Other accident on other gliding-type pedestrian conveyance

[EXCLUDES1] *gliding-type pedestrian conveyance collision with other land transport vehicle (V01-V09 with 5th digit 9)*

[5] V00.3 Flat-bottomed pedestrian conveyance accident

[6] V00.31 Snowboard accident
- [7] V00.311 Fall from snowboard
- [7] V00.312 Snowboarder colliding with stationary object
- [7] V00.318 Other snowboard accident

[EXCLUDES1] *snowboarder collision with other land transport vehicle (V01-V09 with 5th digit 9)*

[6] V00.32 Snow-ski accident
- [7] V00.321 Fall from snow-skis
- [7] V00.322 Snow-skier colliding with stationary object
- [7] V00.328 Other snow-ski accident

[EXCLUDES1] *snow-skier collision with other land transport vehicle (V01-V09 with 5th digit 9)*

[6] V00.38 Other flat-bottomed pedestrian conveyance accident
- [7] V00.381 Fall from other flat-bottomed pedestrian conveyance

[4] 4th character required [5] 5th character required [6] 6th character required [7] 7th character required [7th] Extension 'X' Alert
[EXCLUDES1] Not coded here [EXCLUDES2] Not included here [PDx] Primary Diagnosis Only Manifestation Code

⑦ **V00.382** Pedestrian on other flat-bottomed pedestrian conveyance colliding with stationary object

⑦ **V00.388** Other accident on other flat-bottomed pedestrian conveyance

⑤ **V00.8** Accident on other pedestrian conveyance

⑥ **V00.81** Accident with wheelchair (powered)

⑦ **V00.811** Fall from moving wheelchair (powered)

EXCLUDES1 fall from non-moving wheelchair (W05.0)

⑦ **V00.812** Wheelchair (powered) colliding with stationary object

⑦ **V00.818** Other accident with wheelchair (powered)

⑥ **V00.82** Accident with babystroller

⑦ **V00.821** Fall from babystroller

⑦ **V00.822** Babystroller colliding with stationary object

⑦ **V00.828** Other accident with babystroller

⑥ **V00.83** Accident with motorized mobility scooter

⑦ **V00.831** Fall from motorized mobility scooter

EXCLUDES1 fall from non-moving motorized mobility scooter (W05.2)

⑦ **V00.832** Motorized mobility scooter colliding with stationary object

⑦ **V00.838** Other accident with motorized mobility scooter

⑥ **V00.89** Accident on other pedestrian conveyance

⑦ **V00.891** Fall from other pedestrian conveyance

⑦ **V00.892** Pedestrian on other pedestrian conveyance colliding with stationary object

⑦ **V00.898** Other accident on other pedestrian conveyance

EXCLUDES1 other pedestrian (conveyance) collision with other land transport vehicle (V01-V09 with 5th digit 9)

④ **V01 Pedestrian injured in collision with pedal cycle**
The appropriate 7th character is to be added to each code from category V01
A = initial encounter
D = subsequent encounter
S = sequela

⑤ **V01.0** Pedestrian injured in collision with pedal cycle in nontraffic accident

⑦ **V01.00** Pedestrian on foot injured in collision with pedal cycle in nontraffic accident

Pedestrian NOS injured in collision with pedal cycle in nontraffic accident

⑦ **V01.01** Pedestrian on roller-skates injured in collision with pedal cycle in nontraffic accident

⑦ **V01.02** Pedestrian on skateboard injured in collision with pedal cycle in nontraffic accident

⑦ **V01.09** Pedestrian with other conveyance injured in collision with pedal cycle in nontraffic accident

Pedestrian with babystroller injured in collision with pedal cycle in nontraffic accident
Pedestrian on ice-skates injured in collision with pedal cycle in nontraffic accident
Pedestrian on nonmotorized scooter injured in collision with pedal cycle in nontraffic accident
Pedestrian on sled injured in collision with pedal cycle in nontraffic accident
Pedestrian on snowboard injured in collision with pedal cycle in nontraffic accident

Pedestrian on snow-skis injured in collision with pedal cycle in nontraffic accident
Pedestrian in wheelchair (powered) injured in collision with pedal cycle in nontraffic accident
Pedestrian in motorized mobility scooter injured in collision with pedal cycle in nontraffic accident

⑤ **V01.1** Pedestrian injured in collision with pedal cycle in traffic accident

⑦ **V01.10** Pedestrian on foot injured in collision with pedal cycle in traffic accident

Pedestrian NOS injured in collision with pedal cycle in traffic accident

⑦ **V01.11** Pedestrian on roller-skates injured in collision with pedal cycle in traffic accident

⑦ **V01.12** Pedestrian on skateboard injured in collision with pedal cycle in traffic accident

⑦ **V01.19** Pedestrian with other conveyance injured in collision with pedal cycle in traffic accident

Pedestrian with babystroller injured in collision with pedal cycle in traffic accident
Pedestrian on ice-skates injured in collision with pedal cycle in traffic accident
Pedestrian on nonmotorized scooter injured in collision with pedal cycle in traffic accident
Pedestrian on sled injured in collision with pedal cycle in traffic accident
Pedestrian on snowboard injured in collision with pedal cycle in traffic accident
Pedestrian on snow-skis injured in collision with pedal cycle in traffic accident
Pedestrian in wheelchair (powered) injured in collision with pedal cycle in traffic accident
Pedestrian in motorized mobility scooter injured in collision with pedal cycle in traffic accident

⑤ **V01.9** Pedestrian injured in collision with pedal cycle, unspecified whether traffic or nontraffic accident

⑦ **V01.90** Pedestrian on foot injured in collision with pedal cycle, unspecified whether traffic or nontraffic accident

Pedestrian NOS injured in collision with pedal cycle, unspecified whether traffic or nontraffic accident

⑦ **V01.91** Pedestrian on roller-skates injured in collision with pedal cycle, unspecified whether traffic or nontraffic accident

⑦ **V01.92** Pedestrian on skateboard injured in collision with pedal cycle, unspecified whether traffic or nontraffic accident

⑦ **V01.99** Pedestrian with other conveyance injured in collision with pedal cycle, unspecified whether traffic or nontraffic accident

Pedestrian with babystroller injured in collision with pedal cycle, unspecified whether traffic or nontraffic accident
Pedestrian on ice-skates injured in collision with pedal cycle unspecified, whether traffic or nontraffic accident
Pedestrian on nonmotorized scooter injured in collision with pedal cycle, unspecified whether traffic or nontraffic accident
Pedestrian on sled injured in collision with pedal cycle unspecified, whether traffic or nontraffic accident
Pedestrian on snowboard injured in collision with pedal cycle, unspecified whether traffic or nontraffic accident
Pedestrian on snow-skis injured in collision with pedal cycle, unspecified whether traffic or nontraffic accident
Pedestrian in wheelchair (powered) injured in collision with pedal cycle, unspecified whether traffic or nontraffic accident
Pedestrian in motorized mobility scooter injured in collision with pedal cycle, unspecified whether traffic or nontraffic accident

---

Unspecified Code	Other Specified Code	N Newborn Age: 0	P Pediatric Age: 0-17	M Maternity Age: 12-55
A Adult Age: 15-124	♂ Male	♀ Female	● New Code	▲ Revised Code Title ►◄ Revised Text

V02 - V02.99

CHAPTER 20: EXTERNAL CAUSES OF MORBIDITY (V00-Y99)

④ V02 Pedestrian injured in collision with two- or three-wheeled motor vehicle

The appropriate 7th character is to be added to each code from category V02

A = initial encounter
D = subsequent encounter
S = sequela

⑤ V02.0 Pedestrian injured in collision with two- or three-wheeled motor vehicle in nontraffic accident

⑦ V02.00 Pedestrian on foot injured in collision with two- or three-wheeled motor vehicle in nontraffic accident

Pedestrian NOS injured in collision with two- or three-wheeled motor vehicle in nontraffic accident

⑦ V02.01 Pedestrian on roller-skates injured in collision with two- or three-wheeled motor vehicle in nontraffic accident

⑦ V02.02 Pedestrian on skateboard injured in collision with two- or three-wheeled motor vehicle in nontraffic accident

⑦ V02.09 Pedestrian with other conveyance injured in collision with two- or three-wheeled motor vehicle in nontraffic accident

Pedestrian with babystroller injured in collision with two- or three-wheeled motor vehicle in nontraffic accident

Pedestrian on ice-skates injured in collision with two- or three-wheeled motor vehicle in nontraffic accident

Pedestrian on nonmotorized scooter injured in collision with two- or three-wheeled motor vehicle in nontraffic accident

Pedestrian on sled injured in collision with two- or three-wheeled motor vehicle in nontraffic accident

Pedestrian on snowboard injured in collision with two- or three-wheeled motor vehicle in nontraffic accident

Pedestrian on snow-skis injured in collision with two- or three-wheeled motor vehicle in nontraffic accident

Pedestrian in wheelchair (powered) injured in collision with two- or three-wheeled motor vehicle in nontraffic accident

Pedestrian in motorized mobility scooter injured in collision with two- or three-wheeled motor vehicle in nontraffic accident

⑤ V02.1 Pedestrian injured in collision with two- or three-wheeled motor vehicle in traffic accident

⑦ V02.10 Pedestrian on foot injured in collision with two- or three-wheeled motor vehicle in traffic accident

Pedestrian NOS injured in collision with two- or three-wheeled motor vehicle in traffic accident

⑦ V02.11 Pedestrian on roller-skates injured in collision with two- or three-wheeled motor vehicle in traffic accident

⑦ V02.12 Pedestrian on skateboard injured in collision with two- or three-wheeled motor vehicle in traffic accident

⑦ V02.19 Pedestrian with other conveyance injured in collision with two- or three-wheeled motor vehicle in traffic accident

Pedestrian with babystroller injured in collision with two- or three-wheeled motor vehicle in traffic accident

Pedestrian on ice-skates injured in collision with two- or three-wheeled motor vehicle in traffic accident

Pedestrian on nonmotorized scooter injured in collision with two- or three-wheeled motor vehicle in traffic accident

Pedestrian on sled injured in collision with two- or three-wheeled motor vehicle in traffic accident

Pedestrian on snowboard injured in collision with two- or three-wheeled motor vehicle in traffic accident

Pedestrian on snow-skis injured in collision with two- or three-wheeled motor vehicle in traffic accident

Pedestrian in wheelchair (powered) injured in collision with two- or three-wheeled motor vehicle in traffic accident

Pedestrian in motorized mobility scooter injured in collision with two- or three-wheeled motor vehicle in traffic accident

⑤ V02.9 Pedestrian injured in collision with two- or three-wheeled motor vehicle, unspecified whether traffic or nontraffic accident

⑦ V02.90 Pedestrian on foot injured in collision with two- or three-wheeled motor vehicle, unspecified whether traffic or nontraffic accident

Pedestrian NOS injured in collision with two- or three-wheeled motor vehicle, unspecified whether traffic or nontraffic accident

⑦ V02.91 Pedestrian on roller-skates injured in collision with two- or three-wheeled motor vehicle, unspecified whether traffic or nontraffic accident

⑦ V02.92 Pedestrian on skateboard injured in collision with two- or three-wheeled motor vehicle, unspecified whether traffic or nontraffic accident

⑦ V02.99 Pedestrian with other conveyance injured in collision with two- or three-wheeled motor vehicle, unspecified whether traffic or nontraffic accident

Pedestrian with babystroller injured in collision with two- or three-wheeled motor vehicle, unspecified whether traffic or nontraffic accident

Pedestrian on ice-skates injured in collision with two- or three-wheeled motor vehicle, unspecified whether traffic or nontraffic accident

Pedestrian on nonmotorized scooter injured in collision with two- or three-wheeled motor vehicle, unspecified whether traffic or nontraffic accident

Pedestrian on sled injured in collision with two- or three-wheeled motor vehicle, unspecified whether traffic or nontraffic accident

Pedestrian on snowboard injured in collision with two- or three-wheeled motor vehicle, unspecified whether traffic or nontraffic accident

Pedestrian on snow-skis injured in collision with two- or three-wheeled motor vehicle, unspecified whether traffic or nontraffic accident

Pedestrian in wheelchair (powered) injured in collision with two- or three-wheeled motor vehicle, unspecified whether traffic or nontraffic accident

Pedestrian in motorized mobility scooter injured in collision with two- or three-wheeled motor vehicle, unspecified whether traffic or nontraffic accident

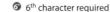

④ 4th character required   ⑤ 5th character required   ⑥ 6th character required   ⑦ 7th character required   Ⓧ Extension 'X' Alert

EXCLUDES 1 Not coded here   EXCLUDES 2 Not included here   PDx Primary Diagnosis Only   Manifestation Code

[4] **V03 Pedestrian injured in collision** with car, pick-up truck or van

The appropriate 7th character is to be added to each code from category V03
A = initial encounter
D = subsequent encounter
S = sequela

[5] **V03.0 Pedestrian injured in collision with car, pick-up truck or van** in nontraffic accident

[7th] **V03.00 Pedestrian** on foot **injured in collision with car, pick-up truck or van in nontraffic accident**
Pedestrian NOS injured in collision with car, pick-up truck or van in nontraffic accident

[7th] **V03.01 Pedestrian** on roller-skates **injured in collision with car, pick-up truck or van in nontraffic accident**

[7th] **V03.02 Pedestrian** on skateboard **injured in collision with car, pick-up truck or van in nontraffic accident**

[7th] **V03.09 Pedestrian with** other conveyance **injured in collision with car, pick-up truck or van in nontraffic accident**
Pedestrian with babystroller injured in collision with car, pick-up truck or van in nontraffic accident
Pedestrian on ice-skates injured in collision with car, pick-up truck or van in nontraffic accident
Pedestrian on nonmotorized scooter injured in collision with car, pick-up truck or van in nontraffic accident
Pedestrian on sled injured in collision with car, pick-up truck or van in nontraffic accident
Pedestrian on snowboard injured in collision with car, pick-up truck or van in nontraffic accident
Pedestrian on snow-skis injured in collision with car, pick-up truck or van in nontraffic accident
Pedestrian in wheelchair (powered) injured in collision with car, pick-up truck or van in nontraffic accident
Pedestrian in motorized mobility scooter injured in collision with car, pick-up truck or van in nontraffic accident

[5] **V03.1 Pedestrian injured in collision with car, pick-up truck or van** in traffic accident

[7th] **V03.10 Pedestrian** on foot **injured in collision with car, pick-up truck or van in traffic accident**
Pedestrian NOS injured in collision with car, pick-up truck or van in traffic accident

[7th] **V03.11 Pedestrian** on roller-skates **injured in collision with car, pick-up truck or van in traffic accident**

[7th] **V03.12 Pedestrian** on skateboard **injured in collision with car, pick-up truck or van in traffic accident**

[7th] **V03.19 Pedestrian with** other conveyance **injured in collision with car, pick-up truck or van in traffic accident**
Pedestrian with babystroller injured in collision with car, pick-up truck or van in traffic accident
Pedestrian on ice-skates injured in collision with car, pick-up truck or van in traffic accident
Pedestrian on nonmotorized scooter injured in collision with car, pick-up truck or van in traffic accident
Pedestrian on sled injured in collision with car, pick-up truck or van in traffic accident
Pedestrian on snowboard injured in collision with car, pick-up truck or van in traffic accident
Pedestrian on snow-skis injured in collision with car, pick-up truck or van in traffic accident
Pedestrian in wheelchair (powered) injured in collision with car, pick-up truck or van in traffic accident
Pedestrian in motorized mobility scooter injured in collision with car, pick-up truck or van in traffic accident

[5] **V03.9 Pedestrian injured in collision with car, pick-up truck or van,** unspecified whether traffic or nontraffic accident

[7th] **V03.90 Pedestrian** on foot **injured in collision with car, pick-up truck or van, unspecified whether traffic or nontraffic accident**
Pedestrian NOS injured in collision with car, pick-up truck or van, unspecified whether traffic or nontraffic accident

[7th] **V03.91 Pedestrian** on roller-skates **injured in collision with car, pick-up truck or van, unspecified whether traffic or nontraffic accident**

[7th] **V03.92 Pedestrian** on skateboard **injured in collision with car, pick-up truck or van, unspecified whether traffic or nontraffic accident**

[7th] **V03.99 Pedestrian with** other conveyance **injured in collision with car, pick-up truck or van, unspecified whether traffic or nontraffic accident**
Pedestrian with babystroller injured in collision with car, pick-up truck or van, unspecified whether traffic or nontraffic accident
Pedestrian on ice-skates injured in collision with car, pick-up truck or van, unspecified whether traffic or nontraffic accident
Pedestrian on nonmotorized scooter injured in collision with car, pick-up truck or van, unspecified whether traffic or nontraffic accident
Pedestrian on sled injured in collision with car, pick-up truck or van in nontraffic accident
Pedestrian on snowboard injured in collision with car, pick-up truck or van, unspecified whether traffic or nontraffic accident
Pedestrian on snow-skis injured in collision with car, pick-up truck or van, unspecified whether traffic or nontraffic accident
Pedestrian in wheelchair (powered) injured in collision with car, pick-up truck or van, unspecified whether traffic or nontraffic accident
Pedestrian in motorized mobility scooter injured in collision with car, pick-up truck or van, unspecified whether traffic or nontraffic accident

[4] **V04 Pedestrian injured in collision** with heavy transport vehicle or bus

[EXCLUDES1] *pedestrian injured in collision with military vehicle (V09.01, V09.21)*

The appropriate 7th character is to be added to each code from category V04
A = initial encounter
D = subsequent encounter
S = sequela

[5] **V04.0 Pedestrian injured in collision with heavy transport vehicle or bus** in nontraffic accident

[7th] **V04.00 Pedestrian** on foot **injured in collision with heavy transport vehicle or bus in nontraffic accident**
Pedestrian NOS injured in collision with heavy transport vehicle or bus in nontraffic accident

[7th] **V04.01 Pedestrian** on roller-skates **injured in collision with heavy transport vehicle or bus in nontraffic accident**

[7th] **V04.02 Pedestrian** on skateboard **injured in collision with heavy transport vehicle or bus in nontraffic accident**

[7th] **V04.09 Pedestrian with other conveyance injured in collision with heavy transport vehicle or bus in nontraffic accident**

Pedestrian with babystroller injured in collision with heavy transport vehicle or bus in nontraffic accident
Pedestrian on ice-skates injured in collision with heavy transport vehicle or bus in nontraffic accident
Pedestrian on nonmotorized scooter injured in collision with heavy transport vehicle or bus in nontraffic accident
Pedestrian on sled injured in collision with heavy transport vehicle or bus in nontraffic accident
Pedestrian on snowboard injured in collision with heavy transport vehicle or bus in nontraffic accident
Pedestrian on snow-skis injured in collision with heavy transport vehicle or bus in nontraffic accident
Pedestrian in wheelchair (powered) injured in collision with heavy transport vehicle or bus in nontraffic accident
Pedestrian in motorized mobility scooter injured in collision with heavy transport vehicle or bus in nontraffic accident

[5] **V04.1 Pedestrian injured in collision with heavy transport vehicle or bus in traffic accident**

[7th] **V04.10 Pedestrian on foot injured in collision with heavy transport vehicle or bus in traffic accident**

Pedestrian NOS injured in collision with heavy transport vehicle or bus in traffic accident

[7th] **V04.11 Pedestrian on roller-skates injured in collision with heavy transport vehicle or bus in traffic accident**

[7th] **V04.12 Pedestrian on skateboard injured in collision with heavy transport vehicle or bus in traffic accident**

[7th] **V04.19 Pedestrian with other conveyance injured in collision with heavy transport vehicle or bus in traffic accident**

Pedestrian with babystroller injured in collision with heavy transport vehicle or bus in traffic accident
Pedestrian on ice-skates injured in collision with heavy transport vehicle or bus in traffic accident
Pedestrian on nonmotorized scooter injured in collision with heavy transport vehicle or bus in traffic accident
Pedestrian on sled injured in collision with heavy transport vehicle or bus in traffic accident
Pedestrian on snowboard injured in collision with heavy transport vehicle or bus in traffic accident
Pedestrian on snow-skis injured in collision with heavy transport vehicle or bus in traffic accident
Pedestrian in wheelchair (powered) injured in collision with heavy transport vehicle or bus in traffic accident
Pedestrian in motorized mobility scooter injured in collision with heavy transport vehicle or bus in traffic accident

[5] **V04.9 Pedestrian injured in collision with heavy transport vehicle or bus, unspecified whether traffic or nontraffic accident**

[7th] **V04.90 Pedestrian on foot injured in collision with heavy transport vehicle or bus, unspecified whether traffic or nontraffic accident**

Pedestrian NOS injured in collision with heavy transport vehicle or bus, unspecified whether traffic or nontraffic accident

[7th] **V04.91 Pedestrian on roller-skates injured in collision with heavy transport vehicle or bus, unspecified whether traffic or nontraffic accident**

[7th] **V04.92 Pedestrian on skateboard injured in collision with heavy transport vehicle or bus, unspecified whether traffic or nontraffic accident**

[7th] **V04.99 Pedestrian with other conveyance injured in collision with heavy transport vehicle or bus, unspecified whether traffic or nontraffic accident**

Pedestrian with babystroller injured in collision with heavy transport vehicle or bus, unspecified whether traffic or nontraffic accident
Pedestrian on ice-skates injured in collision with heavy transport vehicle or bus, unspecified whether traffic or nontraffic accident
Pedestrian on nonmotorized scooter injured in collision with heavy transport vehicle or bus, unspecified whether traffic or nontraffic accident
Pedestrian on sled injured in collision with heavy transport vehicle or bus, unspecified whether traffic or nontraffic accident
Pedestrian on snowboard injured in collision with heavy transport vehicle or bus, unspecified whether traffic or nontraffic accident
Pedestrian on snow-skis injured in collision with heavy transport vehicle or bus, unspecified whether traffic or nontraffic accident
Pedestrian in wheelchair (powered) injured in collision with heavy transport vehicle or bus, unspecified whether traffic or nontraffic accident
Pedestrian in motorized mobility scooter injured in collision with heavy transport vehicle or bus, unspecified whether traffic or nontraffic accident

[4] **V05 Pedestrian injured in collision with railway train or railway vehicle**

The appropriate 7th character is to be added to each code from category V05
A = initial encounter
D = subsequent encounter
S = sequela

[5] **V05.0 Pedestrian injured in collision with railway train or railway vehicle in nontraffic accident**

[7th] **V05.00 Pedestrian on foot injured in collision with railway train or railway vehicle in nontraffic accident**

Pedestrian NOS injured in collision with railway train or railway vehicle in nontraffic accident

[7th] **V05.01 Pedestrian on roller-skates injured in collision with railway train or railway vehicle in nontraffic accident**

[7th] **V05.02 Pedestrian on skateboard injured in collision with railway train or railway vehicle in nontraffic accident**

[7th] **V05.09 Pedestrian with other conveyance injured in collision with railway train or railway vehicle in nontraffic accident**

Pedestrian with babystroller injured in collision with railway train or railway vehicle in nontraffic accident
Pedestrian on ice-skates injured in collision with railway train or railway vehicle in nontraffic accident
Pedestrian on nonmotorized scooter injured in collision with railway train or railway vehicle in nontraffic accident
Pedestrian on sled injured in collision with railway train or railway vehicle in nontraffic accident
Pedestrian on snowboard injured in collision with railway train or railway vehicle in nontraffic accident
Pedestrian on snow-skis injured in collision with railway train or railway vehicle in nontraffic accident
Pedestrian in wheelchair (powered) injured in collision with railway train or railway vehicle in nontraffic accident
Pedestrian in motorized mobility scooter injured in collision with railway train or railway vehicle in nontraffic accident

[5] **V05.1 Pedestrian injured in collision with railway train or railway vehicle in traffic accident**

[4] 4th character required [5] 5th character required [6] 6th character required [7] 7th character required [7th] Extension 'X' Alert
[EXCLUDES 1] Not coded here [EXCLUDES 2] Not included here [PDx] Primary Diagnosis Only Manifestation Code

🄥 **V05.10** Pedestrian on foot injured in collision with railway train or railway vehicle in traffic accident

Pedestrian NOS injured in collision with railway train or railway vehicle in traffic accident

🄥 **V05.11** Pedestrian on roller-skates injured in collision with railway train or railway vehicle in traffic accident

🄥 **V05.12** Pedestrian on skateboard injured in collision with railway train or railway vehicle in traffic accident

🄥 **V05.19** Pedestrian with other conveyance injured in collision with railway train or railway vehicle in traffic accident

Pedestrian with babystroller injured in collision with railway train or railway vehicle in traffic accident

Pedestrian on ice-skates injured in collision with railway train or railway vehicle in traffic accident

Pedestrian on nonmotorized scooter injured in collision with railway train or railway vehicle in traffic accident

Pedestrian on sled injured in collision with railway train or railway vehicle in traffic accident

Pedestrian on snowboard injured in collision with railway train or railway vehicle in traffic accident

Pedestrian on snow-skis injured in collision with railway train or railway vehicle in traffic accident

Pedestrian in wheelchair (powered) injured in collision with railway train or railway vehicle in traffic accident

Pedestrian in motorized mobility scooter injured in collision with railway train or railway vehicle in traffic accident

🄯 **V05.9** Pedestrian injured in collision with railway train or railway vehicle, unspecified whether traffic or nontraffic accident

🄥 **V05.90** Pedestrian on foot injured in collision with railway train or railway vehicle, unspecified whether traffic or nontraffic accident

Pedestrian NOS injured in collision with railway train or railway vehicle, unspecified whether traffic or nontraffic accident

🄥 **V05.91** Pedestrian on roller-skates injured in collision with railway train or railway vehicle, unspecified whether traffic or nontraffic accident

🄥 **V05.92** Pedestrian on skateboard injured in collision with railway train or railway vehicle, unspecified whether traffic or nontraffic accident

🄥 **V05.99** Pedestrian with other conveyance injured in collision with railway train or railway vehicle, unspecified whether traffic or nontraffic accident

Pedestrian with babystroller injured in collision with railway train or railway vehicle, unspecified whether traffic or nontraffic

Pedestrian on ice-skates injured in collision with railway train or railway vehicle, unspecified whether traffic or nontraffic

Pedestrian on nonmotorized scooter injured in collision with railway train or railway vehicle, unspecified whether traffic or nontraffic

Pedestrian on sled injured in collision with railway train or railway vehicle, unspecified whether traffic or nontraffic

Pedestrian on snowboard injured in collision with railway train or railway vehicle, unspecified whether traffic or nontraffic

Pedestrian on snow-skis injured in collision with railway train or railway vehicle, unspecified whether traffic or nontraffic

Pedestrian in wheelchair (powered) injured in collision with railway train or railway vehicle, unspecified whether traffic or nontraffic

Pedestrian in motorized mobility scooter injured in collision with railway train or railway vehicle, unspecified whether traffic or nontraffic

🄬 **V06** Pedestrian injured in collision with other nonmotor vehicle

> INCLUDES collision with animal-drawn vehicle, animal being ridden, nonpowered streetcar
>
> EXCLUDES1 pedestrian injured in collision with pedestrian conveyance (V00.0-)

The appropriate 7th character is to be added to each code from category V06
A = initial encounter
D = subsequent encounter
S = sequela

🄯 **V06.0** Pedestrian injured in collision with other nonmotor vehicle in nontraffic accident

🄥 **V06.00** Pedestrian on foot injured in collision with other nonmotor vehicle in nontraffic accident

Pedestrian NOS injured in collision with other nonmotor vehicle in nontraffic accident

🄥 **V06.01** Pedestrian on roller-skates injured in collision with other nonmotor vehicle in nontraffic accident

🄥 **V06.02** Pedestrian on skateboard injured in collision with other nonmotor vehicle in nontraffic accident

🄥 **V06.09** Pedestrian with other conveyance injured in collision with other nonmotor vehicle in nontraffic accident

Pedestrian with babystroller injured in collision with other nonmotor vehicle in nontraffic accident

Pedestrian on ice-skates injured in collision with other nonmotor vehicle in nontraffic accident

Pedestrian on nonmotorized scooter injured in collision with other nonmotor vehicle in nontraffic accident

Pedestrian on sled injured in collision with other nonmotor vehicle in nontraffic accident

Pedestrian on snowboard injured in collision with other nonmotor vehicle in nontraffic accident

Pedestrian on snow-skis injured in collision with other nonmotor vehicle in nontraffic accident

Pedestrian in wheelchair (powered) injured in collision with other nonmotor vehicle in nontraffic accident

Pedestrian in motorized mobility scooter injured in collision with other nonmotor vehicle in nontraffic accident

🄯 **V06.1** Pedestrian injured in collision with other nonmotor vehicle in traffic accident

🄥 **V06.10** Pedestrian on foot injured in collision with other nonmotor vehicle in traffic accident

Pedestrian NOS injured in collision with other nonmotor vehicle in traffic accident

🄥 **V06.11** Pedestrian on roller-skates injured in collision with other nonmotor vehicle in traffic accident

🄥 **V06.12** Pedestrian on skateboard injured in collision with other nonmotor vehicle in traffic accident

🄥 **V06.19** Pedestrian with other conveyance injured in collision with other nonmotor vehicle in traffic accident

Pedestrian with babystroller injured in collision with other nonmotor vehicle in nontraffic accident

Pedestrian on ice-skates injured in collision with other nonmotor vehicle in traffic accident

Pedestrian on nonmotorized scooter injured in collision with other nonmotor vehicle in traffic accident

Pedestrian on sled injured in collision with other nonmotor vehicle in traffic accident

Pedestrian on snowboard injured in collision with other nonmotor vehicle in traffic accident

Pedestrian on snow-skis injured in collision with

| Unspecified Code | Other Specified Code | N Newborn Age: 0 | P Pediatric Age: 0-17 | M Maternity Age: 12-55 |
| A Adult Age: 15-124 | ♂ Male | ♀ Female | ● New Code | ▲ Revised Code Title | ►◄ Revised Text |

ICD-10-CM 2015

745

other nonmotor vehicle in traffic accident

Pedestrian in wheelchair (powered) injured in collision with other nonmotor vehicle in traffic accident

Pedestrian in motorized mobility scooter injured in collision with other nonmotor vehicle in traffic accident

⑤ **V06.9** **Pedestrian injured in collision with other nonmotor vehicle,** unspecified whether traffic or nontraffic accident

⑦ **V06.90** **Pedestrian** on foot **injured in collision with other nonmotor vehicle, unspecified whether traffic or nontraffic accident**

Pedestrian NOS injured in collision with other nonmotor vehicle, unspecified whether traffic or nontraffic accident

⑦ **V06.91** **Pedestrian** on roller-skates **injured in collision with other nonmotor vehicle, unspecified whether traffic or nontraffic accident**

⑦ **V06.92** **Pedestrian** on skateboard **injured in collision with other nonmotor vehicle, unspecified whether traffic or nontraffic accident**

⑦ **V06.99** **Pedestrian with** other conveyance **injured in collision with other nonmotor vehicle, unspecified whether traffic or nontraffic accident**

Pedestrian with babystroller injured in collision with other nonmotor vehicle, unspecified whether traffic or nontraffic accident

Pedestrian on ice-skates injured in collision with other nonmotor vehicle, unspecified whether traffic or nontraffic accident

Pedestrian on nonmotorized scooter injured in collision with other nonmotor vehicle, unspecified whether traffic or nontraffic accident

Pedestrian on sled injured in collision with other nonmotor vehicle, unspecified whether traffic or nontraffic accident

Pedestrian on snowboard injured in collision with other nonmotor vehicle, unspecified whether traffic or nontraffic accident

Pedestrian on snow-skis injured in collision with other nonmotor vehicle, unspecified whether traffic or nontraffic accident

Pedestrian in wheelchair (powered) injured in collision with other nonmotor vehicle, unspecified whether traffic or nontraffic accident

Pedestrian in motorized mobility scooter injured in collision with other nonmotor vehicle, unspecified whether traffic or nontraffic accident

④ **V09** **Pedestrian injured in** other and unspecified transport accidents

The appropriate 7th character is to be added to each code from category V09

A = initial encounter
D = subsequent encounter
S = sequela

⑤ **V09.0** **Pedestrian injured** in nontraffic accident **involving other and unspecified motor vehicles**

⑦ **V09.00** **Pedestrian injured in nontraffic accident involving unspecified motor vehicles**

⑦ **V09.01** **Pedestrian injured in nontraffic accident involving** military **vehicle**

⑦ **V09.09** **Pedestrian injured in nontraffic accident involving other motor vehicles**

Pedestrian injured in nontraffic accident by special vehicle

⑤ **V09.1** **Pedestrian injured in unspecified** nontraffic **accident**

⑤ **V09.2** **Pedestrian injured** in traffic accident **involving other and unspecified motor vehicles**

⑦ **V09.20** **Pedestrian injured in traffic accident involving unspecified motor vehicles**

⑦ **V09.21** **Pedestrian injured in traffic accident involving** military **vehicle**

⑦ **V09.29** **Pedestrian injured in traffic accident involving other motor vehicles**

⑦ **V09.3** **Pedestrian injured in unspecified** traffic accident

⑦ **V09.9** **Pedestrian injured in unspecified** transport accident

Pedal cycle rider injured in transport accident (V10-V19)

INCLUDES   any non-motorized vehicle, excluding an animal-drawn vehicle, or a sidecar or trailer attached to the pedal cycle

EXCLUDES2   rupture of pedal cycle tire (W37.0)

④ **V10** **Pedal cycle rider injured in collision with pedestrian or animal**

EXCLUDES1   pedal cycle rider collision with animal-drawn vehicle or animal being ridden (V16.-)

The appropriate 7th character is to be added to each code from category V10

A = initial encounter
D = subsequent encounter
S = sequela

⑦ **V10.0** **Pedal cycle** driver **injured in collision with pedestrian or animal** in nontraffic accident

⑦ **V10.1** **Pedal cycle** passenger **injured in collision with pedestrian or animal** in nontraffic accident

⑦ **V10.2** Unspecified **pedal cyclist injured in collision with pedestrian or animal** in nontraffic accident

⑦ **V10.3** Person boarding or alighting **a pedal cycle injured in collision with pedestrian or animal**

⑦ **V10.4** **Pedal cycle** driver **injured in collision with pedestrian or animal** in traffic accident

⑦ **V10.5** **Pedal cycle** passenger **injured in collision with pedestrian or animal** in traffic accident

⑦ **V10.9** Unspecified **pedal cyclist injured in collision with pedestrian or animal** in traffic accident

④ **V11** **Pedal cycle rider injured in** collision with other pedal cycle

The appropriate 7th character is to be added to each code from category V11

A = initial encounter
D = subsequent encounter
S = sequela

⑦ **V11.0** **Pedal cycle** driver **injured in collision with other pedal cycle in** nontraffic accident

⑦ **V11.1** **Pedal cycle** passenger **injured in collision with other pedal cycle in** nontraffic accident

⑦ **V11.2** Unspecified **pedal cyclist injured in collision with other pedal cycle in** nontraffic accident

⑦ **V11.3** Person boarding or alighting **a pedal cycle injured in collision with other pedal cycle**

⑦ **V11.4** **Pedal cycle** driver **injured in collision with other pedal cycle in** traffic accident

⑦ **V11.5** **Pedal cycle** passenger **injured in collision with other pedal cycle in** traffic accident

⑦ **V11.9** Unspecified **pedal cyclist injured in collision with other pedal cycle in** traffic accident

④ **V12** **Pedal cycle rider injured in** collision with two- or three-wheeled motor vehicle

The appropriate 7th character is to be added to each code from category V12

A = initial encounter
D = subsequent encounter
S = sequela

⑦ **V12.0** **Pedal cycle** driver **injured in collision with two- or three-wheeled motor vehicle in** nontraffic accident

⑦ **V12.1** **Pedal cycle** passenger **injured in collision with two- or three-wheeled motor vehicle in** nontraffic accident

---

④ 4th character required   ⑤ 5th character required   ⑥ 6th character required   ⑦ 7th character required   ⑦ Extension 'X' Alert

EXCLUDES 1 Not coded here   EXCLUDES 2 Not included here   PDx Primary Diagnosis Only   Manifestation Code

ⓣ V12.2 Unspecified pedal cyclist injured in collision with two- or three-wheeled motor vehicle in nontraffic accident

ⓣ V12.3 Person boarding or alighting a pedal cycle injured in collision with two- or three-wheeled motor vehicle

ⓣ V12.4 Pedal cycle driver injured in collision with two- or three-wheeled motor vehicle in traffic accident

ⓣ V12.5 Pedal cycle passenger injured in collision with two- or three-wheeled motor vehicle in traffic accident

ⓣ V12.9 Unspecified pedal cyclist injured in collision with two- or three-wheeled motor vehicle in traffic accident

④ V13 Pedal cycle rider injured in collision with car, pick-up truck or van

The appropriate 7th character is to be added to each code from category V13
A = initial encounter
D = subsequent encounter
S = sequela

ⓣ V13.0 Pedal cycle driver injured in collision with car, pick-up truck or van in nontraffic accident

ⓣ V13.1 Pedal cycle passenger injured in collision with car, pick-up truck or van in nontraffic accident

ⓣ V13.2 Unspecified pedal cyclist injured in collision with car, pick-up truck or van in nontraffic accident

ⓣ V13.3 Person boarding or alighting a pedal cycle injured in collision with car, pick-up truck or van

ⓣ V13.4 Pedal cycle driver injured in collision with car, pick-up truck or van in traffic accident

ⓣ V13.5 Pedal cycle passenger injured in collision with car, pick-up truck or van in traffic accident

ⓣ V13.9 Unspecified pedal cyclist injured in collision with car, pick-up truck or van in traffic accident

④ V14 Pedal cycle rider injured in collision with heavy transport vehicle or bus

EXCLUDES1 *pedal cycle rider injured in collision with military vehicle (V19.81)*

The appropriate 7th character is to be added to each code from category V14
A = initial encounter
D = subsequent encounter
S = sequela

ⓣ V14.0 Pedal cycle driver injured in collision with heavy transport vehicle or bus in nontraffic accident

ⓣ V14.1 Pedal cycle passenger injured in collision with heavy transport vehicle or bus in nontraffic accident

ⓣ V14.2 Unspecified pedal cyclist injured in collision with heavy transport vehicle or bus in nontraffic accident

ⓣ V14.3 Person boarding or alighting a pedal cycle injured in collision with heavy transport vehicle or bus

ⓣ V14.4 Pedal cycle driver injured in collision with heavy transport vehicle or bus in traffic accident

ⓣ V14.5 Pedal cycle passenger injured in collision with heavy transport vehicle or bus in traffic accident

ⓣ V14.9 Unspecified pedal cyclist injured in collision with heavy transport vehicle or bus in traffic accident

④ V15 Pedal cycle rider injured in collision with railway train or railway vehicle

The appropriate 7th character is to be added to each code from category V15
A = initial encounter
D = subsequent encounter
S = sequela

ⓣ V15.0 Pedal cycle driver injured in collision with railway train or railway vehicle in nontraffic accident

ⓣ V15.1 Pedal cycle passenger injured in collision with railway train or railway vehicle in nontraffic accident

ⓣ V15.2 Unspecified pedal cyclist injured in collision with railway train or railway vehicle in nontraffic accident

ⓣ V15.3 Person boarding or alighting a pedal cycle injured in collision with railway train or railway vehicle

ⓣ V15.4 Pedal cycle driver injured in collision with railway train or railway vehicle in traffic accident

ⓣ V15.5 Pedal cycle passenger injured in collision with railway train or railway vehicle in traffic accident

ⓣ V15.9 Unspecified pedal cyclist injured in collision with railway train or railway vehicle in traffic accident

④ V16 Pedal cycle rider injured in collision with other nonmotor vehicle

INCLUDES *collision with animal-drawn vehicle, animal being ridden, streetcar*

The appropriate 7th character is to be added to each code from category V16
A = initial encounter
D = subsequent encounter
S = sequela

ⓣ V16.0 Pedal cycle driver injured in collision with other nonmotor vehicle in nontraffic accident

ⓣ V16.1 Pedal cycle passenger injured in collision with other nonmotor vehicle in nontraffic accident

ⓣ V16.2 Unspecified pedal cyclist injured in collision with other nonmotor vehicle in nontraffic accident

ⓣ V16.3 Person boarding or alighting a pedal cycle injured in collision with other nonmotor vehicle in nontraffic accident

ⓣ V16.4 Pedal cycle driver injured in collision with other nonmotor vehicle in traffic accident

ⓣ V16.5 Pedal cycle passenger injured in collision with other nonmotor vehicle in traffic accident

ⓣ V16.9 Unspecified pedal cyclist injured in collision with other nonmotor vehicle in traffic accident

④ V17 Pedal cycle rider injured in collision with fixed or stationary object

The appropriate 7th character is to be added to each code from category V17
A = initial encounter
D = subsequent encounter
S = sequela

ⓣ V17.0 Pedal cycle driver injured in collision with fixed or stationary object in nontraffic accident

ⓣ V17.1 Pedal cycle passenger injured in collision with fixed or stationary object in nontraffic accident

ⓣ V17.2 Unspecified pedal cyclist injured in collision with fixed or stationary object in nontraffic accident

ⓣ V17.3 Person boarding or alighting a pedal cycle injured in collision with fixed or stationary object

ⓣ V17.4 Pedal cycle driver injured in collision with fixed or stationary object in traffic accident

ⓣ V17.5 Pedal cycle passenger injured in collision with fixed or stationary object in traffic accident

ⓣ V17.9 Unspecified pedal cyclist injured in collision with fixed or stationary object in traffic accident

④ V18 Pedal cycle rider injured in noncollision transport accident

INCLUDES *fall or thrown from pedal cycle (without antecedent collision)*
overturning pedal cycle NOS
overturning pedal cycle without collision

The appropriate 7th character is to be added to each code from category V18
A = initial encounter
D = subsequent encounter
S = sequela

ⓣ V18.0 Pedal cycle driver injured in noncollision transport accident in nontraffic accident

ⓣ V18.1 Pedal cycle passenger injured in noncollision transport accident in nontraffic accident

ⓣ V18.2 Unspecified pedal cyclist injured in noncollision transport accident in nontraffic accident

ⓣ V18.3 Person boarding or alighting a pedal cycle injured in noncollision transport accident

Unspecified Code	Other Specified Code	Ⓝ Newborn Age: 0	Ⓟ Pediatric Age: 0-17	Ⓜ Maternity Age: 12-55
Ⓐ Adult Age: 15-124	♂ Male	♀ Female	● New Code	▲ Revised Code Title	►◄ Revised Text

[7th] V18.4 Pedal cycle driver injured in noncollision transport accident in traffic accident

[7th] V18.5 Pedal cycle passenger injured in noncollision transport accident in traffic accident

[7th] V18.9 Unspecified pedal cyclist injured in noncollision transport accident in traffic accident

[4th] V19 Pedal cycle rider injured in other and unspecified transport accidents

The appropriate 7th character is to be added to each code from category V19
A = initial encounter
D = subsequent encounter
S = sequela

[5th] V19.0 Pedal cycle driver injured in collision with other and unspecified motor vehicles in nontraffic accident

[7th] V19.00 Pedal cycle driver injured in collision with unspecified motor vehicles in nontraffic accident

[7th] V19.09 Pedal cycle driver injured in collision with other motor vehicles in nontraffic accident

[5th] V19.1 Pedal cycle passenger injured in collision with other and unspecified motor vehicles in nontraffic accident

[7th] V19.10 Pedal cycle passenger injured in collision with unspecified motor vehicles in nontraffic accident

[7th] V19.19 Pedal cycle passenger injured in collision with other motor vehicles in nontraffic accident

[5th] V19.2 Unspecified pedal cyclist injured in collision with other and unspecified motor vehicles in nontraffic accident

[7th] V19.20 Unspecified pedal cyclist injured in collision with unspecified motor vehicles in nontraffic accident

Pedal cycle collision NOS, nontraffic

[7th] V19.29 Unspecified pedal cyclist injured in collision with other motor vehicles in nontraffic accident

[7th] V19.3 Pedal cyclist (driver) (passenger) injured in unspecified nontraffic accident

Pedal cycle accident NOS, nontraffic
Pedal cyclist injured in nontraffic accident NOS

[5th] V19.4 Pedal cycle driver injured in collision with other and unspecified motor vehicles in traffic accident

[7th] V19.40 Pedal cycle driver injured in collision with unspecified motor vehicles in traffic accident

[7th] V19.49 Pedal cycle driver injured in collision with other motor vehicles in traffic accident

[5th] V19.5 Pedal cycle passenger injured in collision with other and unspecified motor vehicles in traffic accident

[7th] V19.50 Pedal cycle passenger injured in collision with unspecified motor vehicles in traffic accident

[7th] V19.59 Pedal cycle passenger injured in collision with other motor vehicles in traffic accident

[5th] V19.6 Unspecified pedal cyclist injured in collision with other and unspecified motor vehicles in traffic accident

[7th] V19.60 Unspecified pedal cyclist injured in collision with unspecified motor vehicles in traffic accident

Pedal cycle collision NOS (traffic)

[7th] V19.69 Unspecified pedal cyclist injured in collision with other motor vehicles in traffic accident

[5th] V19.8 Pedal cyclist (driver) (passenger) injured in other specified transport accidents

[7th] V19.81 Pedal cyclist (driver) (passenger) injured in transport accident with military vehicle

[7th] V19.88 Pedal cyclist (driver) (passenger) injured in other specified transport accidents

[7th] V19.9 Pedal cyclist (driver) (passenger) injured in unspecified traffic accident

Pedal cycle accident NOS

Motorcycle rider injured in transport accident (V20-V29)

INCLUDES *moped*
motorcycle with sidecar
motorized bicycle
motor scooter

EXCLUDES1 *three-wheeled motor vehicle (V30-V39)*

[4th] V20 Motorcycle rider injured in collision with pedestrian or animal

EXCLUDES1 *motorcycle rider collision with animal-drawn vehicle or animal being ridden (V26.-)*

The appropriate 7th character is to be added to each code from category V20
A = initial encounter
D = subsequent encounter
S = sequela

[7th] V20.0 Motorcycle driver injured in collision with pedestrian or animal in nontraffic accident

[7th] V20.1 Motorcycle passenger injured in collision with pedestrian or animal in nontraffic accident

[7th] V20.2 Unspecified motorcycle rider injured in collision with pedestrian or animal in nontraffic accident

[7th] V20.3 Person boarding or alighting a motorcycle injured in collision with pedestrian or animal

[7th] V20.4 Motorcycle driver injured in collision with pedestrian or animal in traffic accident

[7th] V20.5 Motorcycle passenger injured in collision with pedestrian or animal in traffic accident

[7th] V20.9 Unspecified motorcycle rider injured in collision with pedestrian or animal in traffic accident

[4th] V21 Motorcycle rider injured in collision with pedal cycle

The appropriate 7th character is to be added to each code from category V21
A = initial encounter
D = subsequent encounter
S = sequela

[7th] V21.0 Motorcycle driver injured in collision with pedal cycle in nontraffic accident

[7th] V21.1 Motorcycle passenger injured in collision with pedal cycle in nontraffic accident

[7th] V21.2 Unspecified motorcycle rider injured in collision with pedal cycle in nontraffic accident

[7th] V21.3 Person boarding or alighting a motorcycle injured in collision with pedal cycle

[7th] V21.4 Motorcycle driver injured in collision with pedal cycle in traffic accident

[7th] V21.5 Motorcycle passenger injured in collision with pedal cycle in traffic accident

[7th] V21.9 Unspecified motorcycle rider injured in collision with pedal cycle in traffic accident

[4th] V22 Motorcycle rider injured in collision with two- or three-wheeled motor vehicle

The appropriate 7th character is to be added to each code from category V22
A = initial encounter
D = subsequent encounter
S = sequela

[7th] V22.0 Motorcycle driver injured in collision with two- or three-wheeled motor vehicle in nontraffic accident

[7th] V22.1 Motorcycle passenger injured in collision with two- or three-wheeled motor vehicle in nontraffic accident

[7th] V22.2 Unspecified motorcycle rider injured in collision with two- or three-wheeled motor vehicle in nontraffic accident

[7th] V22.3 Person boarding or alighting a motorcycle injured in collision with two- or three-wheeled motor vehicle

[7th] V22.4 Motorcycle driver injured in collision with two- or three-wheeled motor vehicle in traffic accident

[7th] V22.5 Motorcycle passenger injured in collision with two- or three-wheeled motor vehicle in traffic accident

V22.9 Unspecified motorcycle rider injured in collision with two- or three-wheeled motor vehicle in traffic accident

V23 Motorcycle rider injured in collision with car, pick-up truck or van

The appropriate 7th character is to be added to each code from category V23
A = initial encounter
D = subsequent encounter
S = sequela

V23.0 Motorcycle driver injured in collision with car, pick-up truck or van in nontraffic accident

V23.1 Motorcycle passenger injured in collision with car, pick-up truck or van in nontraffic accident

V23.2 Unspecified motorcycle rider injured in collision with car, pick-up truck or van in nontraffic accident

V23.3 Person boarding or alighting a motorcycle injured in collision with car, pick-up truck or van

V23.4 Motorcycle driver injured in collision with car, pick-up truck or van in traffic accident

V23.5 Motorcycle passenger injured in collision with car, pick-up truck or van in traffic accident

V23.9 Unspecified motorcycle rider injured in collision with car, pick-up truck or van in traffic accident

V24 Motorcycle rider injured in collision with heavy transport vehicle or bus

EXCLUDES1 motorcycle rider injured in collision with military vehicle (V29.81)

The appropriate 7th character is to be added to each code from category V24
A = initial encounter
D = subsequent encounter
S = sequela

V24.0 Motorcycle driver injured in collision with heavy transport vehicle or bus in nontraffic accident

V24.1 Motorcycle passenger injured in collision with heavy transport vehicle or bus in nontraffic accident

V24.2 Unspecified motorcycle rider injured in collision with heavy transport vehicle or bus in nontraffic accident

V24.3 Person boarding or alighting a motorcycle injured in collision with heavy transport vehicle or bus

V24.4 Motorcycle driver injured in collision with heavy transport vehicle or bus in traffic accident

V24.5 Motorcycle passenger injured in collision with heavy transport vehicle or bus in traffic accident

V24.9 Unspecified motorcycle rider injured in collision with heavy transport vehicle or bus in traffic accident

V25 Motorcycle rider injured in collision with railway train or railway vehicle

The appropriate 7th character is to be added to each code from category V25
A = initial encounter
D = subsequent encounter
S = sequela

V25.0 Motorcycle driver injured in collision with railway train or railway vehicle in nontraffic accident

V25.1 Motorcycle passenger injured in collision with railway train or railway vehicle in nontraffic accident

V25.2 Unspecified motorcycle rider injured in collision with railway train or railway vehicle in nontraffic accident

V25.3 Person boarding or alighting a motorcycle injured in collision with railway train or railway vehicle

V25.4 Motorcycle driver injured in collision with railway train or railway vehicle in traffic accident

V25.5 Motorcycle passenger injured in collision with railway train or railway vehicle in traffic accident

V25.9 Unspecified motorcycle rider injured in collision with railway train or railway vehicle in traffic accident

V26 Motorcycle rider injured in collision with other nonmotor vehicle

INCLUDES collision with animal-drawn vehicle, animal being ridden, streetcar

The appropriate 7th character is to be added to each code from category V26
A = initial encounter
D = subsequent encounter
S = sequela

V26.0 Motorcycle driver injured in collision with other nonmotor vehicle in nontraffic accident

V26.1 Motorcycle passenger injured in collision with other nonmotor vehicle in nontraffic accident

V26.2 Unspecified motorcycle rider injured in collision with other nonmotor vehicle in nontraffic accident

V26.3 Person boarding or alighting a motorcycle injured in collision with other nonmotor vehicle

V26.4 Motorcycle driver injured in collision with other nonmotor vehicle in traffic accident

V26.5 Motorcycle passenger injured in collision with other nonmotor vehicle in traffic accident

V26.9 Unspecified motorcycle rider injured in collision with other nonmotor vehicle in traffic accident

V27 Motorcycle rider injured in collision with fixed or stationary object

The appropriate 7th character is to be added to each code from category V27
A = initial encounter
D = subsequent encounter
S = sequela

V27.0 Motorcycle driver injured in collision with fixed or stationary object in nontraffic accident

V27.1 Motorcycle passenger injured in collision with fixed or stationary object in nontraffic accident

V27.2 Unspecified motorcycle rider injured in collision with fixed or stationary object in nontraffic accident

V27.3 Person boarding or alighting a motorcycle injured in collision with fixed or stationary object

V27.4 Motorcycle driver injured in collision with fixed or stationary object in traffic accident

V27.5 Motorcycle passenger injured in collision with fixed or stationary object in traffic accident

V27.9 Unspecified motorcycle rider injured in collision with fixed or stationary object in traffic accident

V28 Motorcycle rider injured in noncollision transport accident

INCLUDES fall or thrown from motorcycle (without antecedent collision)
overturning motorcycle NOS
overturning motorcycle without collision

The appropriate 7th character is to be added to each code from category V28
A = initial encounter
D = subsequent encounter
S = sequela

V28.0 Motorcycle driver injured in noncollision transport accident in nontraffic accident

V28.1 Motorcycle passenger injured in noncollision transport accident in nontraffic accident

V28.2 Unspecified motorcycle rider injured in noncollision transport accident in nontraffic accident

V28.3 Person boarding or alighting a motorcycle injured in noncollision transport accident

V28.4 Motorcycle driver injured in noncollision transport accident in traffic accident

V28.5 Motorcycle passenger injured in noncollision transport accident in traffic accident

V28.9 Unspecified motorcycle rider injured in noncollision transport accident in traffic accident

Unspecified Code   Other Specified Code   N Newborn Age: 0   P Pediatric Age: 0-17   M Maternity Age: 12-55   A Adult Age: 15-124   ♂ Male   ♀ Female   ● New Code   ▲ Revised Code Title   ►◄ Revised Text

ICD-10-CM 2015   **749**

[4] V29 Motorcycle rider injured in other and unspecified transport accidents

The appropriate 7th character is to be added to each code from category V29
A = initial encounter
D = subsequent encounter
S = sequela

[5] V29.0 Motorcycle driver injured in collision with other and unspecified motor vehicles in nontraffic accident
[7] V29.00 Motorcycle driver injured in collision with unspecified motor vehicles in nontraffic accident
[7] V29.09 Motorcycle driver injured in collision with other motor vehicles in nontraffic accident
[5] V29.1 Motorcycle passenger injured in collision with other and unspecified motor vehicles in nontraffic accident
[7] V29.10 Motorcycle passenger injured in collision with unspecified motor vehicles in nontraffic accident
[7] V29.19 Motorcycle passenger injured in collision with other motor vehicles in nontraffic accident
[5] V29.2 Unspecified motorcycle rider injured in collision with other and unspecified motor vehicles in nontraffic accident
[7] V29.20 Unspecified motorcycle rider injured in collision with unspecified motor vehicles in nontraffic accident
Motorcycle collision NOS, nontraffic
[7] V29.29 Unspecified motorcycle rider injured in collision with other motor vehicles in nontraffic accident
[7] V29.3 Motorcycle rider (driver) (passenger) injured in unspecified nontraffic accident
Motorcycle accident NOS, nontraffic
Motorcycle rider injured in nontraffic accident NOS
[5] V29.4 Motorcycle driver injured in collision with other and unspecified motor vehicles in traffic accident
[7] V29.40 Motorcycle driver injured in collision with unspecified motor vehicles in traffic accident
[7] V29.49 Motorcycle driver injured in collision with other motor vehicles in traffic accident
[5] V29.5 Motorcycle passenger injured in collision with other and unspecified motor vehicles in traffic accident
[7] V29.50 Motorcycle passenger injured in collision with unspecified motor vehicles in traffic accident
[7] V29.59 Motorcycle passenger injured in collision with other motor vehicles in traffic accident
[5] V29.6 Unspecified motorcycle rider injured in collision with other and unspecified motor vehicles in traffic accident
[7] V29.60 Unspecified motorcycle rider injured in collision with unspecified motor vehicles in traffic accident
Motorcycle collision NOS (traffic)
[7] V29.69 Unspecified motorcycle rider injured in collision with other motor vehicles in traffic accident
[5] V29.8 Motorcycle rider (driver) (passenger) injured in other specified transport accidents
[7] V29.81 Motorcycle rider (driver) (passenger) injured in transport accident with military vehicle
[7] V29.88 Motorcycle rider (driver) (passenger) injured in other specified transport accidents
[7] V29.9 Motorcycle rider (driver) (passenger) injured in unspecified traffic accident
Motorcycle accident NOS

Occupant of three-wheeled motor vehicle injured in transport accident (V30-V39)

[INCLUDES] *motorized tricycle*
motorized rickshaw
three-wheeled motor car

[EXCLUDES1] *all-terrain vehicles (V86.-)*
motorcycle with sidecar (V20-V29)
vehicle designed primarily for off-road use (V86.-)

[4] V30 Occupant of three-wheeled motor vehicle injured in collision with pedestrian or animal

[EXCLUDES1] *three-wheeled motor vehicle collision with animal-drawn vehicle or animal being ridden (V36.-)*

The appropriate 7th character is to be added to each code from category V30
A = initial encounter
D = subsequent encounter
S = sequela

[7] V30.0 Driver of three-wheeled motor vehicle injured in collision with pedestrian or animal in nontraffic accident
[7] V30.1 Passenger in three-wheeled motor vehicle injured in collision with pedestrian or animal in nontraffic accident
[7] V30.2 Person on outside of three-wheeled motor vehicle injured in collision with pedestrian or animal in nontraffic accident
[7] V30.3 Unspecified occupant of three-wheeled motor vehicle injured in collision with pedestrian or animal in nontraffic accident
[7] V30.4 Person boarding or alighting a three-wheeled motor vehicle injured in collision with pedestrian or animal
[7] V30.5 Driver of three-wheeled motor vehicle injured in collision with pedestrian or animal in traffic accident
[7] V30.6 Passenger in three-wheeled motor vehicle injured in collision with pedestrian or animal in traffic accident
[7] V30.7 Person on outside of three-wheeled motor vehicle injured in collision with pedestrian or animal in traffic accident
[7] V30.9 Unspecified occupant of three-wheeled motor vehicle injured in collision with pedestrian or animal in traffic accident

[4] V31 Occupant of three-wheeled motor vehicle injured in collision with pedal cycle

The appropriate 7th character is to be added to each code from category V31
A = initial encounter
D = subsequent encounter
S = sequela

[7] V31.0 Driver of three-wheeled motor vehicle injured in collision with pedal cycle in nontraffic accident
[7] V31.1 Passenger in three-wheeled motor vehicle injured in collision with pedal cycle in nontraffic accident
[7] V31.2 Person on outside of three-wheeled motor vehicle injured in collision with pedal cycle in nontraffic accident
[7] V31.3 Unspecified occupant of three-wheeled motor vehicle injured in collision with pedal cycle in nontraffic accident
[7] V31.4 Person boarding or alighting a three-wheeled motor vehicle injured in collision with pedal cycle
[7] V31.5 Driver of three-wheeled motor vehicle injured in collision with pedal cycle in traffic accident
[7] V31.6 Passenger in three-wheeled motor vehicle injured in collision with pedal cycle in traffic accident
[7] V31.7 Person on outside of three-wheeled motor vehicle injured in collision with pedal cycle in traffic accident
[7] V31.9 Unspecified occupant of three-wheeled motor vehicle injured in collision with pedal cycle in traffic accident

[4] 4th character required [5] 5th character required [6] 6th character required [7] 7th character required [X] Extension 'X' Alert
[EXCLUDES1] Not coded here [EXCLUDES2] Not included here [PDx] Primary Diagnosis Only Manifestation Code

④ **V32** Occupant of three-wheeled motor vehicle injured in collision with two- or three-wheeled motor vehicle

The appropriate 7th character is to be added to each code from category V32
A = initial encounter
D = subsequent encounter
S = sequela

⑦ V32.0 Driver of three-wheeled motor vehicle injured in collision with two- or three-wheeled motor vehicle in nontraffic accident

⑦ V32.1 Passenger in three-wheeled motor vehicle injured in collision with two- or three-wheeled motor vehicle in nontraffic accident

⑦ V32.2 Person on outside of three-wheeled motor vehicle injured in collision with two- or three-wheeled motor vehicle in nontraffic accident

⑦ V32.3 Unspecified occupant of three-wheeled motor vehicle injured in collision with two- or three-wheeled motor vehicle in nontraffic accident

⑦ V32.4 Person boarding or alighting a three-wheeled motor vehicle injured in collision with two- or three-wheeled motor vehicle

⑦ V32.5 Driver of three-wheeled motor vehicle injured in collision with two- or three-wheeled motor vehicle in traffic accident

⑦ V32.6 Passenger in three-wheeled motor vehicle injured in collision with two- or three-wheeled motor vehicle in traffic accident

⑦ V32.7 Person on outside of three-wheeled motor vehicle injured in collision with two- or three-wheeled motor vehicle in traffic accident

⑦ V32.9 Unspecified occupant of three-wheeled motor vehicle injured in collision with two- or three-wheeled motor vehicle in traffic accident

④ **V33** Occupant of three-wheeled motor vehicle injured in collision with car, pick-up truck or van

The appropriate 7th character is to be added to each code from category V33
A = initial encounter
D = subsequent encounter
S = sequela

⑦ V33.0 Driver of three-wheeled motor vehicle injured in collision with car, pick-up truck or van in nontraffic accident

⑦ V33.1 Passenger in three-wheeled motor vehicle injured in collision with car, pick-up truck or van in nontraffic accident

⑦ V33.2 Person on outside of three-wheeled motor vehicle injured in collision with car, pick-up truck or van in nontraffic accident

⑦ V33.3 Unspecified occupant of three-wheeled motor vehicle injured in collision with car, pick-up truck or van in nontraffic accident

⑦ V33.4 Person boarding or alighting a three-wheeled motor vehicle injured in collision with car, pick-up truck or van

⑦ V33.5 Driver of three-wheeled motor vehicle injured in collision with car, pick-up truck or van in traffic accident

⑦ V33.6 Passenger in three-wheeled motor vehicle injured in collision with car, pick-up truck or van in traffic accident

⑦ V33.7 Person on outside of three-wheeled motor vehicle injured in collision with car, pick-up truck or van in traffic accident

⑦ V33.9 Unspecified occupant of three-wheeled motor vehicle injured in collision with car, pick-up truck or van in traffic accident

④ **V34** Occupant of three-wheeled motor vehicle injured in collision with heavy transport vehicle or bus

> EXCLUDES1 occupant of three-wheeled motor vehicle injured in collision with military vehicle (V39.81)

The appropriate 7th character is to be added to each code from category V34
A = initial encounter
D = subsequent encounter
S = sequela

⑦ V34.0 Driver of three-wheeled motor vehicle injured in collision with heavy transport vehicle or bus in nontraffic accident

⑦ V34.1 Passenger in three-wheeled motor vehicle injured in collision with heavy transport vehicle or bus in nontraffic accident

⑦ V34.2 Person on outside of three-wheeled motor vehicle injured in collision with heavy transport vehicle or bus in nontraffic accident

⑦ V34.3 Unspecified occupant of three-wheeled motor vehicle injured in collision with heavy transport vehicle or bus in nontraffic accident

⑦ V34.4 Person boarding or alighting a three-wheeled motor vehicle injured in collision with heavy transport vehicle or bus

⑦ V34.5 Driver of three-wheeled motor vehicle injured in collision with heavy transport vehicle or bus in traffic accident

⑦ V34.6 Passenger in three-wheeled motor vehicle injured in collision with heavy transport vehicle or bus in traffic accident

⑦ V34.7 Person on outside of three-wheeled motor vehicle injured in collision with heavy transport vehicle or bus in traffic accident

⑦ V34.9 Unspecified occupant of three-wheeled motor vehicle injured in collision with heavy transport vehicle or bus in traffic accident

④ **V35** Occupant of three-wheeled motor vehicle injured in collision with railway train or railway vehicle

The appropriate 7th character is to be added to each code from category V35
A = initial encounter
D = subsequent encounter
S = sequela

⑦ V35.0 Driver of three-wheeled motor vehicle injured in collision with railway train or railway vehicle in nontraffic accident

⑦ V35.1 Passenger in three-wheeled motor vehicle injured in collision with railway train or railway vehicle in nontraffic accident

⑦ V35.2 Person on outside of three-wheeled motor vehicle injured in collision with railway train or railway vehicle in nontraffic accident

⑦ V35.3 Unspecified occupant of three-wheeled motor vehicle injured in collision with railway train or railway vehicle in nontraffic accident

⑦ V35.4 Person boarding or alighting a three-wheeled motor vehicle injured in collision with railway train or railway vehicle

⑦ V35.5 Driver of three-wheeled motor vehicle injured in collision with railway train or railway vehicle in traffic accident

⑦ V35.6 Passenger in three-wheeled motor vehicle injured in collision with railway train or railway vehicle in traffic accident

⑦ V35.7 Person on outside of three-wheeled motor vehicle injured in collision with railway train or railway vehicle in traffic accident

⑦ V35.9 Unspecified occupant of three-wheeled motor vehicle injured in collision with railway train or railway vehicle in traffic accident

---

Unspecified Code   Other Specified Code   N Newborn Age: 0   P Pediatric Age: 0-17   M Maternity Age: 12-55
A Adult Age: 15-124   ♂ Male   ♀ Female   ● New Code   ▲ Revised Code Title   ►◄ Revised Text

[4th] **V36 Occupant of three-wheeled motor vehicle injured in collision with other nonmotor vehicle**

INCLUDES *collision with animal-drawn vehicle, animal being ridden, streetcar*

The appropriate 7th character is to be added to each code from category V36
A = initial encounter
D = subsequent encounter
S = sequela

[x7th] **V36.0 Driver of three-wheeled motor vehicle injured in collision with other nonmotor vehicle in nontraffic accident**

[x7th] **V36.1 Passenger in three-wheeled motor vehicle injured in collision with other nonmotor vehicle in nontraffic accident**

[x7th] **V36.2 Person on outside of three-wheeled motor vehicle injured in collision with other nonmotor vehicle in nontraffic accident**

[x7th] **V36.3 Unspecified occupant of three-wheeled motor vehicle injured in collision with other nonmotor vehicle in nontraffic accident**

[x7th] **V36.4 Person boarding or alighting a three-wheeled motor vehicle injured in collision with other nonmotor vehicle**

[x7th] **V36.5 Driver of three-wheeled motor vehicle injured in collision with other nonmotor vehicle in traffic accident**

[x7th] **V36.6 Passenger in three-wheeled motor vehicle injured in collision with other nonmotor vehicle in traffic accident**

[x7th] **V36.7 Person on outside of three-wheeled motor vehicle injured in collision with other nonmotor vehicle in traffic accident**

[x7th] **V36.9 Unspecified occupant of three-wheeled motor vehicle injured in collision with other nonmotor vehicle in traffic accident**

[4th] **V37 Occupant of three-wheeled motor vehicle injured in collision with fixed or stationary object**

The appropriate 7th character is to be added to each code from category V37
A = initial encounter
D = subsequent encounter
S = sequela

[x7th] **V37.0 Driver of three-wheeled motor vehicle injured in collision with fixed or stationary object in nontraffic accident**

[x7th] **V37.1 Passenger in three-wheeled motor vehicle injured in collision with fixed or stationary object in nontraffic accident**

[x7th] **V37.2 Person on outside of three-wheeled motor vehicle injured in collision with fixed or stationary object in nontraffic accident**

[x7th] **V37.3 Unspecified occupant of three-wheeled motor vehicle injured in collision with fixed or stationary object in nontraffic accident**

[x7th] **V37.4 Person boarding or alighting a three-wheeled motor vehicle injured in collision with fixed or stationary object**

[x7th] **V37.5 Driver of three-wheeled motor vehicle injured in collision with fixed or stationary object in traffic accident**

[x7th] **V37.6 Passenger in three-wheeled motor vehicle injured in collision with fixed or stationary object in traffic accident**

[x7th] **V37.7 Person on outside of three-wheeled motor vehicle injured in collision with fixed or stationary object in traffic accident**

[x7th] **V37.9 Unspecified occupant of three-wheeled motor vehicle injured in collision with fixed or stationary object in traffic accident**

[4th] **V38 Occupant of three-wheeled motor vehicle injured in noncollision transport accident**

INCLUDES *fall or thrown from three-wheeled motor vehicle*
overturning of three-wheeled motor vehicle NOS
overturning of three-wheeled motor vehicle without collision

The appropriate 7th character is to be added to each code from category V38
A = initial encounter
D = subsequent encounter
S = sequela

[x7th] **V38.0 Driver of three-wheeled motor vehicle injured in noncollision transport accident in nontraffic accident**

[x7th] **V38.1 Passenger in three-wheeled motor vehicle injured in noncollision transport accident in nontraffic accident**

[x7th] **V38.2 Person on outside of three-wheeled motor vehicle injured in noncollision transport accident in nontraffic accident**

[x7th] **V38.3 Unspecified occupant of three-wheeled motor vehicle injured in noncollision transport accident in nontraffic accident**

[x7th] **V38.4 Person boarding or alighting a three-wheeled motor vehicle injured in noncollision transport accident**

[x7th] **V38.5 Driver of three-wheeled motor vehicle injured in noncollision transport accident in traffic accident**

[x7th] **V38.6 Passenger in three-wheeled motor vehicle injured in noncollision transport accident in traffic accident**

[x7th] **V38.7 Person on outside of three-wheeled motor vehicle injured in noncollision transport accident in traffic accident**

[x7th] **V38.9 Unspecified occupant of three-wheeled motor vehicle injured in noncollision transport accident in traffic accident**

[4th] **V39 Occupant of three-wheeled motor vehicle injured in other and unspecified transport accidents**

The appropriate 7th character is to be added to each code from category V39
A = initial encounter
D = subsequent encounter
S = sequela

[5th] **V39.0 Driver of three-wheeled motor vehicle injured in collision with other and unspecified motor vehicles in nontraffic accident**

[x7th] **V39.00 Driver of three-wheeled motor vehicle injured in collision with unspecified motor vehicles in nontraffic accident**

[x7th] **V39.09 Driver of three-wheeled motor vehicle injured in collision with other motor vehicles in nontraffic accident**

[5th] **V39.1 Passenger in three-wheeled motor vehicle injured in collision with other and unspecified motor vehicles in nontraffic accident**

[x7th] **V39.10 Passenger in three-wheeled motor vehicle injured in collision with unspecified motor vehicles in nontraffic accident**

[x7th] **V39.19 Passenger in three-wheeled motor vehicle injured in collision with other motor vehicles in nontraffic accident**

[5th] **V39.2 Unspecified occupant of three-wheeled motor vehicle injured in collision with other and unspecified motor vehicles in nontraffic accident**

[x7th] **V39.20 Unspecified occupant of three-wheeled motor vehicle injured in collision with unspecified motor vehicles in nontraffic accident**

Collision NOS involving three-wheeled motor vehicle, nontraffic

[x7th] **V39.29 Unspecified occupant of three-wheeled motor vehicle injured in collision with other motor vehicles in nontraffic accident**

[4th] 4th character required [5th] 5th character required [6th] 6th character required [7th] 7th character required [x7th] Extension 'X' Alert
EXCLUDES1 Not coded here EXCLUDES2 Not included here PDx Primary Diagnosis Only Manifestation Code

🔟 **V39.3** Occupant (driver) (passenger) of three-wheeled motor vehicle injured in unspecified nontraffic accident

Accident NOS involving three-wheeled motor vehicle, nontraffic

Occupant of three-wheeled motor vehicle injured in nontraffic accident NOS

5️⃣ **V39.4** Driver of three-wheeled motor vehicle injured in collision with other and unspecified motor vehicles in traffic accident

🔟 **V39.40** Driver of three-wheeled motor vehicle injured in collision with unspecified motor vehicles in traffic accident

🔟 **V39.49** Driver of three-wheeled motor vehicle injured in collision with other motor vehicles in traffic accident

5️⃣ **V39.5** Passenger in three-wheeled motor vehicle injured in collision with other and unspecified motor vehicles in traffic accident

🔟 **V39.50** Passenger in three-wheeled motor vehicle injured in collision with unspecified motor vehicles in traffic accident

🔟 **V39.59** Passenger in three-wheeled motor vehicle injured in collision with other motor vehicles in traffic accident

5️⃣ **V39.6** Unspecified occupant of three-wheeled motor vehicle injured in collision with other and unspecified motor vehicles in traffic accident

🔟 **V39.60** Unspecified occupant of three-wheeled motor vehicle injured in collision with unspecified motor vehicles in traffic accident

Collision NOS involving three-wheeled motor vehicle (traffic)

🔟 **V39.69** Unspecified occupant of three-wheeled motor vehicle injured in collision with other motor vehicles in traffic accident

5️⃣ **V39.8** Occupant (driver) (passenger) of three-wheeled motor vehicle injured in other specified transport accidents

🔟 **V39.81** Occupant (driver) (passenger) of three-wheeled motor vehicle injured in transport accident with military vehicle

🔟 **V39.89** Occupant (driver) (passenger) of three-wheeled motor vehicle injured in other specified transport accidents

🔟 **V39.9** Occupant (driver) (passenger) of three-wheeled motor vehicle injured in unspecified traffic accident

Accident NOS involving three-wheeled motor vehicle

Car occupant injured in transport accident (V40-V49)

INCLUDES   a four-wheeled motor vehicle designed primarily for carrying passengers
automobile (pulling a trailer or camper)

EXCLUDES1   bus (V50-V59)
minibus (V50-V59)
minivan (V50-V59)
motorcoach (V70-V79)
pick-up truck (V50-V59)
sport utility vehicle (SUV) (V50-V59)

4️⃣ **V40** Car occupant injured in collision with pedestrian or animal

EXCLUDES1   car collision with animal-drawn vehicle or animal being ridden (V46.-)

The appropriate 7th character is to be added to each code from category V40
A = initial encounter
D = subsequent encounter
S = sequela

🔟 **V40.0** Car driver injured in collision with pedestrian or animal in nontraffic accident

🔟 **V40.1** Car passenger injured in collision with pedestrian or animal in nontraffic accident

🔟 **V40.2** Person on outside of car injured in collision with pedestrian or animal in nontraffic accident

🔟 **V40.3** Unspecified car occupant injured in collision with pedestrian or animal in nontraffic accident

🔟 **V40.4** Person boarding or alighting a car injured in collision with pedestrian or animal

🔟 **V40.5** Car driver injured in collision with pedestrian or animal in traffic accident

🔟 **V40.6** Car passenger injured in collision with pedestrian or animal in traffic accident

🔟 **V40.7** Person on outside of car injured in collision with pedestrian or animal in traffic accident

🔟 **V40.9** Unspecified car occupant injured in collision with pedestrian or animal in traffic accident

4️⃣ **V41** Car occupant injured in collision with pedal cycle

The appropriate 7th character is to be added to each code from category V41
A = initial encounter
D = subsequent encounter
S = sequela

🔟 **V41.0** Car driver injured in collision with pedal cycle in nontraffic accident

🔟 **V41.1** Car passenger injured in collision with pedal cycle in nontraffic accident

🔟 **V41.2** Person on outside of car injured in collision with pedal cycle in nontraffic accident

🔟 **V41.3** Unspecified car occupant injured in collision with pedal cycle in nontraffic accident

🔟 **V41.4** Person boarding or alighting a car injured in collision with pedal cycle

🔟 **V41.5** Car driver injured in collision with pedal cycle in traffic accident

🔟 **V41.6** Car passenger injured in collision with pedal cycle in traffic accident

🔟 **V41.7** Person on outside of car injured in collision with pedal cycle in traffic accident

🔟 **V41.9** Unspecified car occupant injured in collision with pedal cycle in traffic accident

4️⃣ **V42** Car occupant injured in collision with two- or three-wheeled motor vehicle

The appropriate 7th character is to be added to each code from category V42
A = initial encounter
D = subsequent encounter
S = sequela

🔟 **V42.0** Car driver injured in collision with two- or three-wheeled motor vehicle in nontraffic accident

🔟 **V42.1** Car passenger injured in collision with two- or three-wheeled motor vehicle in nontraffic accident

🔟 **V42.2** Person on outside of car injured in collision with two- or three-wheeled motor vehicle in nontraffic accident

🔟 **V42.3** Unspecified car occupant injured in collision with two- or three-wheeled motor vehicle in nontraffic accident

🔟 **V42.4** Person boarding or alighting a car injured in collision with two- or three-wheeled motor vehicle

🔟 **V42.5** Car driver injured in collision with two- or three-wheeled motor vehicle in traffic accident

🔟 **V42.6** Car passenger injured in collision with two- or three-wheeled motor vehicle in traffic accident

🔟 **V42.7** Person on outside of car injured in collision with two- or three-wheeled motor vehicle in traffic accident

🔟 **V42.9** Unspecified car occupant injured in collision with two- or three-wheeled motor vehicle in traffic accident

Unspecified Code	Other Specified Code	N Newborn Age: 0	P Pediatric Age: 0 17	M Maternity Age: 12-55
A Adult Age: 15-124	♂ Male	♀ Female	● New Code	▲ Revised Code Title	►◄ Revised Text

[4] **V43 Car occupant injured in collision with car, pick-up truck or van**

The appropriate 7th character is to be added to each code from category V43
A = initial encounter
D = subsequent encounter
S = sequela

- [5] **V43.0** Car driver injured in collision with car, pick-up truck or van in nontraffic accident
  - [7th] **V43.01** Car driver injured in collision with sport utility vehicle in nontraffic accident
  - [7th] **V43.02** Car driver injured in collision with other type car in nontraffic accident
  - [7th] **V43.03** Car driver injured in collision with pick-up truck in nontraffic accident
  - [7th] **V43.04** Car driver injured in collision with van in nontraffic accident
- [5] **V43.1** Car passenger injured in collision with car, pick-up truck or van in nontraffic accident
  - [7th] **V43.11** Car passenger injured in collision with sport utility vehicle in nontraffic accident
  - [7th] **V43.12** Car passenger injured in collision with other type car in nontraffic accident
  - [7th] **V43.13** Car passenger injured in collision with pick-up in nontraffic accident
  - [7th] **V43.14** Car passenger injured in collision with van in nontraffic accident
- [5] **V43.2** Person on outside of car injured in collision with car, pick-up truck or van in nontraffic accident
  - [7th] **V43.21** Person on outside of car injured in collision with sport utility vehicle in nontraffic accident
  - [7th] **V43.22** Person on outside of car injured in collision with other type car in nontraffic accident
  - [7th] **V43.23** Person on outside of car injured in collision with pick-up truck in nontraffic accident
  - [7th] **V43.24** Person on outside of car injured in collision with van in nontraffic accident
- [5] **V43.3** Unspecified car occupant injured in collision with car, pick-up truck or van in nontraffic accident
  - [7th] **V43.31** Unspecified car occupant injured in collision with sport utility vehicle in nontraffic accident
  - [7th] **V43.32** Unspecified car occupant injured in collision with other type car in nontraffic accident
  - [7th] **V43.33** Unspecified car occupant injured in collision with pick-up truck in nontraffic accident
  - [7th] **V43.34** Unspecified car occupant injured in collision with van in nontraffic accident
- [5] **V43.4** Person boarding or alighting a car injured in collision with car, pick-up truck or van
  - [7th] **V43.41** Person boarding or alighting a car injured in collision with sport utility vehicle
  - [7th] **V43.42** Person boarding or alighting a car injured in collision with other type car
  - [7th] **V43.43** Person boarding or alighting a car injured in collision with pick-up truck
  - [7th] **V43.44** Person boarding or alighting a car injured in collision with van
- [5] **V43.5** Car driver injured in collision with car, pick-up truck or van in traffic accident
  - [7th] **V43.51** Car driver injured in collision with sport utility vehicle in traffic accident
  - [7th] **V43.52** Car driver injured in collision with other type car in traffic accident
  - [7th] **V43.53** Car driver injured in collision with pick-up truck in traffic accident
  - [7th] **V43.54** Car driver injured in collision with van in traffic accident
- [5] **V43.6** Car passenger injured in collision with car, pick-up truck or van in traffic accident
  - [7th] **V43.61** Car passenger injured in collision with sport utility vehicle in traffic accident
  - [7th] **V43.62** Car passenger injured in collision with other type car in traffic accident
  - [7th] **V43.63** Car passenger injured in collision with pick-up truck in traffic accident
  - [7th] **V43.64** Car passenger injured in collision with van in traffic accident
- [5] **V43.7** Person on outside of car injured in collision with car, pick-up truck or van in traffic accident
  - [7th] **V43.71** Person on outside of car injured in collision with sport utility vehicle in traffic accident
  - [7th] **V43.72** Person on outside of car injured in collision with other type car in traffic accident
  - [7th] **V43.73** Person on outside of car injured in collision with pick-up truck in traffic accident
  - [7th] **V43.74** Person on outside of car injured in collision with van in traffic accident
- [5] **V43.9** Unspecified car occupant injured in collision with car, pick-up truck or van in traffic accident
  - [7th] **V43.91** Unspecified car occupant injured in collision with sport utility vehicle in traffic accident
  - [7th] **V43.92** Unspecified car occupant injured in collision with other type car in traffic accident
  - [7th] **V43.93** Unspecified car occupant injured in collision with pick-up truck in traffic accident
  - [7th] **V43.94** Unspecified car occupant injured in collision with van in traffic accident

[4] **V44 Car occupant injured in collision with heavy transport vehicle or bus**

[EXCLUDES1] *car occupant injured in collision with military vehicle (V49.81)*

The appropriate 7th character is to be added to each code from category V44
A = initial encounter
D = subsequent encounter
S = sequela

- [7th] **V44.0** Car driver injured in collision with heavy transport vehicle or bus in nontraffic accident
- [7th] **V44.1** Car passenger injured in collision with heavy transport vehicle or bus in nontraffic accident
- [7th] **V44.2** Person on outside of car injured in collision with heavy transport vehicle or bus in nontraffic accident
- [7th] **V44.3** Unspecified car occupant injured in collision with heavy transport vehicle or bus in nontraffic accident
- [7th] **V44.4** Person boarding or alighting a car injured in collision with heavy transport vehicle or bus
- [7th] **V44.5** Car driver injured in collision with heavy transport vehicle or bus in traffic accident
- [7th] **V44.6** Car passenger injured in collision with heavy transport vehicle or bus in traffic accident
- [7th] **V44.7** Person on outside of car injured in collision with heavy transport vehicle or bus in traffic accident
- [7th] **V44.9** Unspecified car occupant injured in collision with heavy transport vehicle or bus in traffic accident

[4] **V45 Car occupant injured in collision with railway train or railway vehicle**

The appropriate 7th character is to be added to each code from category V45
A = initial encounter
D = subsequent encounter
S = sequela

- [7th] **V45.0** Car driver injured in collision with railway train or railway vehicle in nontraffic accident
- [7th] **V45.1** Car passenger injured in collision with railway train or railway vehicle in nontraffic accident
- [7th] **V45.2** Person on outside of car injured in collision with railway train or railway vehicle in nontraffic accident

- V45.3 Unspecified car occupant injured in collision with railway train or railway vehicle in nontraffic accident
- V45.4 Person boarding or alighting a car injured in collision with railway train or railway vehicle
- V45.5 Car driver injured in collision with railway train or railway vehicle in traffic accident
- V45.6 Car passenger injured in collision with railway train or railway vehicle in traffic accident
- V45.7 Person on outside of car injured in collision with railway train or railway vehicle in traffic accident
- V45.9 Unspecified car occupant injured in collision with railway train or railway vehicle in traffic accident
- V46 Car occupant injured in collision with other nonmotor vehicle

  INCLUDES   collision with animal-drawn vehicle, animal being ridden, streetcar

The appropriate 7th character is to be added to each code from category V46
A = initial encounter
D = subsequent encounter
S = sequela

- V46.0 Car driver injured in collision with other nonmotor vehicle in nontraffic accident
- V46.1 Car passenger injured in collision with other nonmotor vehicle in nontraffic accident
- V46.2 Person on outside of car injured in collision with other nonmotor vehicle in nontraffic accident
- V46.3 Unspecified car occupant injured in collision with other nonmotor vehicle in nontraffic accident
- V46.4 Person boarding or alighting a car injured in collision with other nonmotor vehicle
- V46.5 Car driver injured in collision with other nonmotor vehicle in traffic accident
- V46.6 Car passenger injured in collision with other nonmotor vehicle in traffic accident
- V46.7 Person on outside of car injured in collision with other nonmotor vehicle in traffic accident
- V46.9 Unspecified car occupant injured in collision with other nonmotor vehicle in traffic accident
- V47 Car occupant injured in collision with fixed or stationary object

The appropriate 7th character is to be added to each code from category V47
A = initial encounter
D = subsequent encounter
S = sequela

- V47.0 Car driver injured in collision with fixed or stationary object in nontraffic accident
  - V47.01 Driver of sport utility vehicle injured in collision with fixed or stationary object in nontraffic accident
  - V47.02 Driver of other type car injured in collision with fixed or stationary object in nontraffic accident
- V47.1 Car passenger injured in collision with fixed or stationary object in nontraffic accident
  - V47.11 Passenger of sport utility vehicle injured in collision with fixed or stationary object in nontraffic accident
  - V47.12 Passenger of other type car injured in collision with fixed or stationary object in nontraffic accident
- V47.2 Person on outside of car injured in collision with fixed or stationary object in nontraffic accident
- V47.3 Unspecified car occupant injured in collision with fixed or stationary object in nontraffic accident
  - V47.31 Unspecified occupant of sport utility vehicle injured in collision with fixed or stationary object in nontraffic accident

- V47.32 Unspecified occupant of other type car injured in collision with fixed or stationary object in nontraffic accident
- V47.4 Person boarding or alighting a car injured in collision with fixed or stationary object
- V47.5 Car driver injured in collision with fixed or stationary object in traffic accident
  - V47.51 Driver of sport utility vehicle injured in collision with fixed or stationary object in traffic accident
  - V47.52 Driver of other type car injured in collision with fixed or stationary object in traffic accident
- V47.6 Car passenger injured in collision with fixed or stationary object in traffic accident
  - V47.61 Passenger of sport utility vehicle injured in collision with fixed or stationary object in traffic accident
  - V47.62 Passenger of other type car injured in collision with fixed or stationary object in traffic accident
- V47.7 Person on outside of car injured in collision with fixed or stationary object in traffic accident
- V47.9 Unspecified car occupant injured in collision with fixed or stationary object in traffic accident
  - V47.91 Unspecified occupant of sport utility vehicle injured in collision with fixed or stationary object in traffic accident
  - V47.92 Unspecified occupant of other type car injured in collision with fixed or stationary object in traffic accident
- V48 Car occupant injured in noncollision transport accident

  INCLUDES   overturning car NOS
             overturning car without collision

The appropriate 7th character is to be added to each code from category V48
A = initial encounter
D = subsequent encounter
S = sequela

- V48.0 Car driver injured in noncollision transport accident in nontraffic accident
- V48.1 Car passenger injured in noncollision transport accident in nontraffic accident
- V48.2 Person on outside of car injured in noncollision transport accident in nontraffic accident
- V48.3 Unspecified car occupant injured in noncollision transport accident in nontraffic accident
- V48.4 Person boarding or alighting a car injured in noncollision transport accident
- V48.5 Car driver injured in noncollision transport accident in traffic accident
- V48.6 Car passenger injured in noncollision transport accident in traffic accident
- V48.7 Person on outside of car injured in noncollision transport accident in traffic accident
- V48.9 Unspecified car occupant injured in noncollision transport accident in traffic accident
- V49 Car occupant injured in other and unspecified transport accidents

The appropriate 7th character is to be added to each code from category V49
A = initial encounter
D = subsequent encounter
S = sequela

- V49.0 Driver injured in collision with other and unspecified motor vehicles in nontraffic accident
  - V49.00 Driver injured in collision with unspecified motor vehicles in nontraffic accident
  - V49.09 Driver injured in collision with other motor vehicles in nontraffic accident
- V49.1 Passenger injured in collision with other and unspecified motor vehicles in nontraffic accident

[7th] V49.10 Passenger injured in collision with unspecified motor vehicles in nontraffic accident

[7th] V49.19 Passenger injured in collision with other motor vehicles in nontraffic accident

[5] V49.2 Unspecified car occupant injured in collision with other and unspecified motor vehicles in nontraffic accident

[7th] V49.20 Unspecified car occupant injured in collision with unspecified motor vehicles in nontraffic accident

Car collision NOS, nontraffic

[7th] V49.29 Unspecified car occupant injured in collision with other motor vehicles in nontraffic accident

[7th] V49.3 Car occupant (driver) (passenger) injured in unspecified nontraffic accident

Car accident NOS, nontraffic

Car occupant injured in nontraffic accident NOS

[5] V49.4 Driver injured in collision with other and unspecified motor vehicles in traffic accident

[7th] V49.40 Driver injured in collision with unspecified motor vehicles in traffic accident

[7th] V49.49 Driver injured in collision with other motor vehicles in traffic accident

[5] V49.5 Passenger injured in collision with other and unspecified motor vehicles in traffic accident

[7th] V49.50 Passenger injured in collision with unspecified motor vehicles in traffic accident

[7th] V49.59 Passenger injured in collision with other motor vehicles in traffic accident

[5] V49.6 Unspecified car occupant injured in collision with other and unspecified motor vehicles in traffic accident

[7th] V49.60 Unspecified car occupant injured in collision with unspecified motor vehicles in traffic accident

Car collision NOS (traffic)

[7th] V49.69 Unspecified car occupant injured in collision with other motor vehicles in traffic accident

[5] V49.8 Car occupant (driver) (passenger) injured in other specified transport accidents

[7th] V49.81 Car occupant (driver) (passenger) injured in transport accident with military vehicle

[7th] V49.88 Car occupant (driver) (passenger) injured in other specified transport accidents

[7th] V49.9 Car occupant (driver) (passenger) injured in unspecified traffic accident

Car accident NOS

Occupant of pick-up truck or van injured in transport accident (V50-V59)

INCLUDES *a four or six wheel motor vehicle designed primarily for carrying passengers and property but weighing less than the local limit for classification as a heavy goods vehicle*
minibus
minivan
sport utility vehicle (SUV)
truck
van

EXCLUDES1 *heavy transport vehicle (V60-V69)*

[4] V50 Occupant of pick-up truck or van injured in collision with pedestrian or animal

EXCLUDES1 *pick-up truck or van collision with animal-drawn vehicle or animal being ridden (V56.-)*

The appropriate 7th character is to be added to each code from category V50
A = initial encounter
D = subsequent encounter
S = sequela

[7th] V50.0 Driver of pick-up truck or van injured in collision with pedestrian or animal in nontraffic accident

[7th] V50.1 Passenger in pick-up truck or van injured in collision with pedestrian or animal in nontraffic accident

[7th] V50.2 Person on outside of pick-up truck or van injured in collision with pedestrian or animal in nontraffic accident

[7th] V50.3 Unspecified occupant of pick-up truck or van injured in collision with pedestrian or animal in nontraffic accident

[7th] V50.4 Person boarding or alighting a pick-up truck or van injured in collision with pedestrian or animal

[7th] V50.5 Driver of pick-up truck or van injured in collision with pedestrian or animal in traffic accident

[7th] V50.6 Passenger in pick-up truck or van injured in collision with pedestrian or animal in traffic accident

[7th] V50.7 Person on outside of pick-up truck or van injured in collision with pedestrian or animal in traffic accident

[7th] V50.9 Unspecified occupant of pick-up truck or van injured in collision with pedestrian or animal in traffic accident

[4] V51 Occupant of pick-up truck or van injured in collision with pedal cycle

The appropriate 7th character is to be added to each code from category V51
A = initial encounter
D = subsequent encounter
S = sequela

[7th] V51.0 Driver of pick-up truck or van injured in collision with pedal cycle in nontraffic accident

[7th] V51.1 Passenger in pick-up truck or van injured in collision with pedal cycle in nontraffic accident

[7th] V51.2 Person on outside of pick-up truck or van injured in collision with pedal cycle in nontraffic accident

[7th] V51.3 Unspecified occupant of pick-up truck or van injured in collision with pedal cycle in nontraffic accident

[7th] V51.4 Person boarding or alighting a pick-up truck or van injured in collision with pedal cycle

[7th] V51.5 Driver of pick-up truck or van injured in collision with pedal cycle in traffic accident

[7th] V51.6 Passenger in pick-up truck or van injured in collision with pedal cycle in traffic accident

[7th] V51.7 Person on outside of pick-up truck or van injured in collision with pedal cycle in traffic accident

[7th] V51.9 Unspecified occupant of pick-up truck or van injured in collision with pedal cycle in traffic accident

[4] V52 Occupant of pick-up truck or van injured in collision with two- or three-wheeled motor vehicle

The appropriate 7th character is to be added to each code from category V52
A = initial encounter
D = subsequent encounter
S = sequela

[7th] V52.0 Driver of pick-up truck or van injured in collision with two- or three-wheeled motor vehicle in nontraffic accident

[7th] V52.1 Passenger in pick-up truck or van injured in collision with two- or three-wheeled motor vehicle in nontraffic accident

[7th] V52.2 Person on outside of pick-up truck or van injured in collision with two- or three-wheeled motor vehicle in nontraffic accident

[7th] V52.3 Unspecified occupant of pick-up truck or van injured in collision with two- or three-wheeled motor vehicle in nontraffic accident

[7th] V52.4 Person boarding or alighting a pick-up truck or van injured in collision with two- or three-wheeled motor vehicle

[4] 4th character required [5] 5th character required [6] 6th character required [7] 7th character required [X] Extension 'X' Alert
EXCLUDES1 Not coded here EXCLUDES2 Not included here PDx Primary Diagnosis Only Manifestation Code

- V52.5 Driver of pick-up truck or van injured in collision with two- or three-wheeled motor vehicle in traffic accident
- V52.6 Passenger in pick-up truck or van injured in collision with two- or three-wheeled motor vehicle in traffic accident
- V52.7 Person on outside of pick-up truck or van injured in collision with two- or three-wheeled motor vehicle in traffic accident
- V52.9 Unspecified occupant of pick-up truck or van injured in collision with two- or three-wheeled motor vehicle in traffic accident

V53 Occupant of pick-up truck or van injured in collision with car, pick-up truck or van

The appropriate 7th character is to be added to each code from category V53
A = initial encounter
D = subsequent encounter
S = sequela

- V53.0 Driver of pick-up truck or van injured in collision with car, pick-up truck or van in nontraffic accident
- V53.1 Passenger in pick-up truck or van injured in collision with car, pick-up truck or van in nontraffic accident
- V53.2 Person on outside of pick-up truck or van injured in collision with car, pick-up truck or van in nontraffic accident
- V53.3 Unspecified occupant of pick-up truck or van injured in collision with car, pick-up truck or van in nontraffic accident
- V53.4 Person boarding or alighting a pick-up truck or van injured in collision with car, pick-up truck or van
- V53.5 Driver of pick-up truck or van injured in collision with car, pick-up truck or van in traffic accident
- V53.6 Passenger in pick-up truck or van injured in collision with car, pick-up truck or van in traffic accident
- V53.7 Person on outside of pick-up truck or van injured in collision with car, pick-up truck or van in traffic accident
- V53.9 Unspecified occupant of pick-up truck or van injured in collision with car, pick-up truck or van in traffic accident

V54 Occupant of pick-up truck or van injured in collision with heavy transport vehicle or bus

EXCLUDES1 occupant of pick-up truck or van injured in collision with military vehicle (V59.81)

The appropriate 7th character is to be added to each code from category V54
A = initial encounter
D = subsequent encounter
S = sequela

- V54.0 Driver of pick-up truck or van injured in collision with heavy transport vehicle or bus in nontraffic accident
- V54.1 Passenger in pick-up truck or van injured in collision with heavy transport vehicle or bus in nontraffic accident
- V54.2 Person on outside of pick-up truck or van injured in collision with heavy transport vehicle or bus in nontraffic accident
- V54.3 Unspecified occupant of pick-up truck or van injured in collision with heavy transport vehicle or bus in nontraffic accident
- V54.4 Person boarding or alighting a pick-up truck or van injured in collision with heavy transport vehicle or bus
- V54.5 Driver of pick-up truck or van injured in collision with heavy transport vehicle or bus in traffic accident
- V54.6 Passenger in pick-up truck or van injured in collision with heavy transport vehicle or bus in traffic accident

- V54.7 Person on outside of pick-up truck or van injured in collision with heavy transport vehicle or bus in traffic accident
- V54.9 Unspecified occupant of pick-up truck or van injured in collision with heavy transport vehicle or bus in traffic accident

V55 Occupant of pick-up truck or van injured in collision with railway train or railway vehicle

The appropriate 7th character is to be added to each code from category V55
A = initial encounter
D = subsequent encounter
S = sequela

- V55.0 Driver of pick-up truck or van injured in collision with railway train or railway vehicle in nontraffic accident
- V55.1 Passenger in pick-up truck or van injured in collision with railway train or railway vehicle in nontraffic accident
- V55.2 Person on outside of pick-up truck or van injured in collision with railway train or railway vehicle in nontraffic accident
- V55.3 Unspecified occupant of pick-up truck or van injured in collision with railway train or railway vehicle in nontraffic accident
- V55.4 Person boarding or alighting a pick-up truck or van injured in collision with railway train or railway vehicle
- V55.5 Driver of pick-up truck or van injured in collision with railway train or railway vehicle in traffic accident
- V55.6 Passenger in pick-up truck or van injured in collision with railway train or railway vehicle in traffic accident
- V55.7 Person on outside of pick-up truck or van injured in collision with railway train or railway vehicle in traffic accident
- V55.9 Unspecified occupant of pick-up truck or van injured in collision with railway train or railway vehicle in traffic accident

V56 Occupant of pick-up truck or van injured in collision with other nonmotor vehicle

INCLUDES collision with animal-drawn vehicle, animal being ridden, streetcar

The appropriate 7th character is to be added to each code from category V56
A = initial encounter
D = subsequent encounter
S = sequela

- V56.0 Driver of pick-up truck or van injured in collision with other nonmotor vehicle in nontraffic accident
- V56.1 Passenger in pick-up truck or van injured in collision with other nonmotor vehicle in nontraffic accident
- V56.2 Person on outside of pick-up truck or van injured in collision with other nonmotor vehicle in nontraffic accident
- V56.3 Unspecified occupant of pick-up truck or van injured in collision with other nonmotor vehicle in nontraffic accident
- V56.4 Person boarding or alighting a pick-up truck or van injured in collision with other nonmotor vehicle
- V56.5 Driver of pick-up truck or van injured in collision with other nonmotor vehicle in traffic accident
- V56.6 Passenger in pick-up truck or van injured in collision with other nonmotor vehicle in traffic accident
- V56.7 Person on outside of pick-up truck or van injured in collision with other nonmotor vehicle in traffic accident
- V56.9 Unspecified occupant of pick-up truck or van injured in collision with other nonmotor vehicle in traffic accident

V57 Occupant of pick-up truck or van injured in collision with fixed or stationary object

The appropriate 7th character is to be added to each code from category V57
A = initial encounter
D = subsequent encounter
S = sequela

V57.0 Driver of pick-up truck or van injured in collision with fixed or stationary object in nontraffic accident

V57.1 Passenger in pick-up truck or van injured in collision with fixed or stationary object in nontraffic accident

V57.2 Person on outside of pick-up truck or van injured in collision with fixed or stationary object in nontraffic accident

V57.3 Unspecified occupant of pick-up truck or van injured in collision with fixed or stationary object in nontraffic accident

V57.4 Person boarding or alighting a pick-up truck or van injured in collision with fixed or stationary object

V57.5 Driver of pick-up truck or van injured in collision with fixed or stationary object in traffic accident

V57.6 Passenger in pick-up truck or van injured in collision with fixed or stationary object in traffic accident

V57.7 Person on outside of pick-up truck or van injured in collision with fixed or stationary object in traffic accident

V57.9 Unspecified occupant of pick-up truck or van injured in collision with fixed or stationary object in traffic accident

V58 Occupant of pick-up truck or van injured in noncollision transport accident

INCLUDES   overturning pick-up truck or van NOS
overturning pick-up truck or van without collision

The appropriate 7th character is to be added to each code from category V58
A = initial encounter
D = subsequent encounter
S = sequela

V58.0 Driver of pick-up truck or van injured in noncollision transport accident in nontraffic accident

V58.1 Passenger in pick-up truck or van injured in noncollision transport accident in nontraffic accident

V58.2 Person on outside of pick-up truck or van injured in noncollision transport accident in nontraffic accident

V58.3 Unspecified occupant of pick-up truck or van injured in noncollision transport accident in nontraffic accident

V58.4 Person boarding or alighting a pick-up truck or van injured in noncollision transport accident

V58.5 Driver of pick-up truck or van injured in noncollision transport accident in traffic accident

V58.6 Passenger in pick-up truck or van injured in noncollision transport accident in traffic accident

V58.7 Person on outside of pick-up truck or van injured in noncollision transport accident in traffic accident

V58.9 Unspecified occupant of pick-up truck or van injured in noncollision transport accident in traffic accident

V59 Occupant of pick-up truck or van injured in other and unspecified transport accidents

The appropriate 7th character is to be added to each code from category V59
A = initial encounter
D = subsequent encounter
S = sequela

V59.0 Driver of pick-up truck or van injured in collision with other and unspecified motor vehicles in nontraffic accident

V59.00 Driver of pick-up truck or van injured in collision with unspecified motor vehicles in nontraffic accident

V59.09 Driver of pick-up truck or van injured in collision with other motor vehicles in nontraffic accident

V59.1 Passenger in pick-up truck or van injured in collision with other and unspecified motor vehicles in nontraffic accident

V59.10 Passenger in pick-up truck or van injured in collision with unspecified motor vehicles in nontraffic accident

V59.19 Passenger in pick-up truck or van injured in collision with other motor vehicles in nontraffic accident

V59.2 Unspecified occupant of pick-up truck or van injured in collision with other and unspecified motor vehicles in nontraffic accident

V59.20 Unspecified occupant of pick-up truck or van injured in collision with unspecified motor vehicles in nontraffic accident
Collision NOS involving pick-up truck or van, nontraffic

V59.29 Unspecified occupant of pick-up truck or van injured in collision with other motor vehicles in nontraffic accident

V59.3 Occupant (driver) (passenger) of pick-up truck or van injured in unspecified nontraffic accident
Accident NOS involving pick-up truck or van, nontraffic
Occupant of pick-up truck or van injured in nontraffic accident NOS

V59.4 Driver of pick-up truck or van injured in collision with other and unspecified motor vehicles in traffic accident

V59.40 Driver of pick-up truck or van injured in collision with unspecified motor vehicles in traffic accident

V59.49 Driver of pick-up truck or van injured in collision with other motor vehicles in traffic accident

V59.5 Passenger in pick-up truck or van injured in collision with other and unspecified motor vehicles in traffic accident

V59.50 Passenger in pick-up truck or van injured in collision with unspecified motor vehicles in traffic accident

V59.59 Passenger in pick-up truck or van injured in collision with other motor vehicles in traffic accident

V59.6 Unspecified occupant of pick-up truck or van injured in collision with other and unspecified motor vehicles in traffic accident

V59.60 Unspecified occupant of pick-up truck or van injured in collision with unspecified motor vehicles in traffic accident
Collision NOS involving pick-up truck or van (traffic)

V59.69 Unspecified occupant of pick-up truck or van injured in collision with other motor vehicles in traffic accident

V59.8 Occupant (driver) (passenger) of pick-up truck or van injured in other specified transport accidents

V59.81 Occupant (driver) (passenger) of pick-up truck or van injured in transport accident with military vehicle

V59.88 Occupant (driver) (passenger) of pick-up truck or van injured in other specified transport accidents

V59.9 Occupant (driver) (passenger) of pick-up truck or van injured in unspecified traffic accident
Accident NOS involving pick-up truck or van

---

❹ 4th character required   ❺ 5th character required   ❻ 6th character required   ❼ 7th character required   Extension 'X' Alert
EXCLUDES 1 Not coded here   EXCLUDES 2 Not included here   PDx Primary Diagnosis Only   Manifestation Code

Occupant of heavy transport vehicle injured in transport accident (V60-V69)

INCLUDES   18 wheeler
armored car
panel truck

EXCLUDES1   bus
motorcoach

⊙ **V60** Occupant of heavy transport vehicle injured in collision with pedestrian or animal

EXCLUDES1   heavy transport vehicle collision with animal-drawn vehicle or animal being ridden (V66.-)

The appropriate 7th character is to be added to each code from category V60
A = initial encounter
D = subsequent encounter
S = sequela

⊙ **V60.0** Driver of heavy transport vehicle injured in collision with pedestrian or animal in nontraffic accident

⊙ **V60.1** Passenger in heavy transport vehicle injured in collision with pedestrian or animal in nontraffic accident

⊙ **V60.2** Person on outside of heavy transport vehicle injured in collision with pedestrian or animal in nontraffic accident

⊙ **V60.3** Unspecified occupant of heavy transport vehicle injured in collision with pedestrian or animal in nontraffic accident

⊙ **V60.4** Person boarding or alighting a heavy transport vehicle injured in collision with pedestrian or animal

⊙ **V60.5** Driver of heavy transport vehicle injured in collision with pedestrian or animal in traffic accident

⊙ **V60.6** Passenger in heavy transport vehicle injured in collision with pedestrian or animal in traffic accident

⊙ **V60.7** Person on outside of heavy transport vehicle injured in collision with pedestrian or animal in traffic accident

⊙ **V60.9** Unspecified occupant of heavy transport vehicle injured in collision with pedestrian or animal in traffic accident

⊙ **V61** Occupant of heavy transport vehicle injured in collision with pedal cycle

The appropriate 7th character is to be added to each code from category V61
A = initial encounter
D = subsequent encounter
S = sequela

⊙ **V61.0** Driver of heavy transport vehicle injured in collision with pedal cycle in nontraffic accident

⊙ **V61.1** Passenger in heavy transport vehicle injured in collision with pedal cycle in nontraffic accident

⊙ **V61.2** Person on outside of heavy transport vehicle injured in collision with pedal cycle in nontraffic accident

⊙ **V61.3** Unspecified occupant of heavy transport vehicle injured in collision with pedal cycle in nontraffic accident

⊙ **V61.4** Person boarding or alighting a heavy transport vehicle injured in collision with pedal cycle while boarding or alighting

⊙ **V61.5** Driver of heavy transport vehicle injured in collision with pedal cycle in traffic accident

⊙ **V61.6** Passenger in heavy transport vehicle injured in collision with pedal cycle in traffic accident

⊙ **V61.7** Person on outside of heavy transport vehicle injured in collision with pedal cycle in traffic accident

⊙ **V61.9** Unspecified occupant of heavy transport vehicle injured in collision with pedal cycle in traffic accident

⊙ **V62** Occupant of heavy transport vehicle injured in collision with two- or three-wheeled motor vehicle

The appropriate 7th character is to be added to each code from category V62
A = initial encounter
D = subsequent encounter
S = sequela

⊙ **V62.0** Driver of heavy transport vehicle injured in collision with two- or three-wheeled motor vehicle in nontraffic accident

⊙ **V62.1** Passenger in heavy transport vehicle injured in collision with two- or three-wheeled motor vehicle in nontraffic accident

⊙ **V62.2** Person on outside of heavy transport vehicle injured in collision with two- or three-wheeled motor vehicle in nontraffic accident

⊙ **V62.3** Unspecified occupant of heavy transport vehicle injured in collision with two- or three-wheeled motor vehicle in nontraffic accident

⊙ **V62.4** Person boarding or alighting a heavy transport vehicle injured in collision with two- or three-wheeled motor vehicle

⊙ **V62.5** Driver of heavy transport vehicle injured in collision with two- or three-wheeled motor vehicle in traffic accident

⊙ **V62.6** Passenger in heavy transport vehicle injured in collision with two- or three-wheeled motor vehicle in traffic accident

⊙ **V62.7** Person on outside of heavy transport vehicle injured in collision with two- or three-wheeled motor vehicle in traffic accident

⊙ **V62.9** Unspecified occupant of heavy transport vehicle injured in collision with two- or three-wheeled motor vehicle in traffic accident

⊙ **V63** Occupant of heavy transport vehicle injured in collision with car, pick-up truck or van

The appropriate 7th character is to be added to each code from category V63
A = initial encounter
D = subsequent encounter
S = sequela

⊙ **V63.0** Driver of heavy transport vehicle injured in collision with car, pick-up truck or van in nontraffic accident

⊙ **V63.1** Passenger in heavy transport vehicle injured in collision with car, pick-up truck or van in nontraffic accident

⊙ **V63.2** Person on outside of heavy transport vehicle injured in collision with car, pick-up truck or van in nontraffic accident

⊙ **V63.3** Unspecified occupant of heavy transport vehicle injured in collision with car, pick-up truck or van in nontraffic accident

⊙ **V63.4** Person boarding or alighting a heavy transport vehicle injured in collision with car, pick-up truck or van

⊙ **V63.5** Driver of heavy transport vehicle injured in collision with car, pick-up truck or van in traffic accident

⊙ **V63.6** Passenger in heavy transport vehicle injured in collision with car, pick-up truck or van in traffic accident

⊙ **V63.7** Person on outside of heavy transport vehicle injured in collision with car, pick-up truck or van in traffic accident

⊙ **V63.9** Unspecified occupant of heavy transport vehicle injured in collision with car, pick-up truck or van in traffic accident

Unspecified Code   Other Specified Code   N Newborn Age: 0   P Pediatric Age: 0-17   M Maternity Age: 12-55
A Adult Age: 15-124   ♂ Male   ♀ Female   ● New Code   ▲ Revised Code Title   ►◄ Revised Text

[4th] **V64 Occupant of heavy transport vehicle injured in collision with heavy transport vehicle or bus**

[EXCLUDES1] *occupant of heavy transport vehicle injured in collision with military vehicle (V69.81)*

The appropriate 7th character is to be added to each code from category V64
A = initial encounter
D = subsequent encounter
S = sequela

- [7th] **V64.0** Driver of heavy transport vehicle injured in collision with heavy transport vehicle or bus in nontraffic accident
- [7th] **V64.1** Passenger in heavy transport vehicle injured in collision with heavy transport vehicle or bus in nontraffic accident
- [7th] **V64.2** Person on outside of heavy transport vehicle injured in collision with heavy transport vehicle or bus in nontraffic accident
- [7th] **V64.3** Unspecified occupant of heavy transport vehicle injured in collision with heavy transport vehicle or bus in nontraffic accident
- [7th] **V64.4** Person boarding or alighting a heavy transport vehicle injured in collision with heavy transport vehicle or bus while boarding or alighting
- [7th] **V64.5** Driver of heavy transport vehicle injured in collision with heavy transport vehicle or bus in traffic accident
- [7th] **V64.6** Passenger in heavy transport vehicle injured in collision with heavy transport vehicle or bus in traffic accident
- [7th] **V64.7** Person on outside of heavy transport vehicle injured in collision with heavy transport vehicle or bus in traffic accident
- [7th] **V64.9** Unspecified occupant of heavy transport vehicle injured in collision with heavy transport vehicle or bus in traffic accident

[4th] **V65 Occupant of heavy transport vehicle injured in collision with railway train or railway vehicle**

The appropriate 7th character is to be added to each code from category V65
A = initial encounter
D = subsequent encounter
S = sequela

- [7th] **V65.0** Driver of heavy transport vehicle injured in collision with railway train or railway vehicle in nontraffic accident
- [7th] **V65.1** Passenger in heavy transport vehicle injured in collision with railway train or railway vehicle in nontraffic accident
- [7th] **V65.2** Person on outside of heavy transport vehicle injured in collision with railway train or railway vehicle in nontraffic accident
- [7th] **V65.3** Unspecified occupant of heavy transport vehicle injured in collision with railway train or railway vehicle in nontraffic accident
- [7th] **V65.4** Person boarding or alighting a heavy transport vehicle injured in collision with railway train or railway vehicle
- [7th] **V65.5** Driver of heavy transport vehicle injured in collision with railway train or railway vehicle in traffic accident
- [7th] **V65.6** Passenger in heavy transport vehicle injured in collision with railway train or railway vehicle in traffic accident
- [7th] **V65.7** Person on outside of heavy transport vehicle injured in collision with railway train or railway vehicle in traffic accident
- [7th] **V65.9** Unspecified occupant of heavy transport vehicle injured in collision with railway train or railway vehicle in traffic accident

[4th] **V66 Occupant of heavy transport vehicle injured in collision with other nonmotor vehicle**

[INCLUDES] *collision with animal-drawn vehicle, animal being ridden, streetcar*

The appropriate 7th character is to be added to each code from category V66
A = initial encounter
D = subsequent encounter
S = sequela

- [7th] **V66.0** Driver of heavy transport vehicle injured in collision with other nonmotor vehicle in nontraffic accident
- [7th] **V66.1** Passenger in heavy transport vehicle injured in collision with other nonmotor vehicle in nontraffic accident
- [7th] **V66.2** Person on outside of heavy transport vehicle injured in collision with other nonmotor vehicle in nontraffic accident
- [7th] **V66.3** Unspecified occupant of heavy transport vehicle injured in collision with other nonmotor vehicle in nontraffic accident
- [7th] **V66.4** Person boarding or alighting a heavy transport vehicle injured in collision with other nonmotor vehicle
- [7th] **V66.5** Driver of heavy transport vehicle injured in collision with other nonmotor vehicle in traffic accident
- [7th] **V66.6** Passenger in heavy transport vehicle injured in collision with other nonmotor vehicle in traffic accident
- [7th] **V66.7** Person on outside of heavy transport vehicle injured in collision with other nonmotor vehicle in traffic accident
- [7th] **V66.9** Unspecified occupant of heavy transport vehicle injured in collision with other nonmotor vehicle in traffic accident

[4th] **V67 Occupant of heavy transport vehicle injured in collision with fixed or stationary object**

The appropriate 7th character is to be added to each code from category V67
A = initial encounter
D = subsequent encounter
S = sequela

- [7th] **V67.0** Driver of heavy transport vehicle injured in collision with fixed or stationary object in nontraffic accident
- [7th] **V67.1** Passenger in heavy transport vehicle injured in collision with fixed or stationary object in nontraffic accident
- [7th] **V67.2** Person on outside of heavy transport vehicle injured in collision with fixed or stationary object in nontraffic accident
- [7th] **V67.3** Unspecified occupant of heavy transport vehicle injured in collision with fixed or stationary object in nontraffic accident
- [7th] **V67.4** Person boarding or alighting a heavy transport vehicle injured in collision with fixed or stationary object
- [7th] **V67.5** Driver of heavy transport vehicle injured in collision with fixed or stationary object in traffic accident
- [7th] **V67.6** Passenger in heavy transport vehicle injured in collision with fixed or stationary object in traffic accident
- [7th] **V67.7** Person on outside of heavy transport vehicle injured in collision with fixed or stationary object in traffic accident
- [7th] **V67.9** Unspecified occupant of heavy transport vehicle injured in collision with fixed or stationary object in traffic accident

[4th] 4th character required [5th] 5th character required [6th] 6th character required [7th] 7th character required [X] Extension 'X' Alert
[EXCLUDES1] Not coded here [EXCLUDES2] Not included here [PDx] Primary Diagnosis Only Manifestation Code

④ **V68 Occupant of heavy transport vehicle injured in** noncollision transport accident

> INCLUDES   overturning heavy transport vehicle NOS
> overturning heavy transport vehicle without collision

The appropriate 7th character is to be added to each code from category V68
A = initial encounter
D = subsequent encounter
S = sequela

⑦ **V68.0** Driver **of heavy transport vehicle injured in noncollision transport accident in** nontraffic accident

⑦ **V68.1** Passenger **in heavy transport vehicle injured in noncollision transport accident in** nontraffic accident

⑦ **V68.2** Person on outside **of heavy transport vehicle injured in noncollision transport accident in** nontraffic accident

⑦ **V68.3** Unspecified **occupant of heavy transport vehicle injured in noncollision transport accident in** nontraffic accident

⑦ **V68.4** Person boarding or alighting **a heavy transport vehicle injured in noncollision transport accident**

⑦ **V68.5** Driver **of heavy transport vehicle injured in noncollision transport accident in** traffic accident

⑦ **V68.6** Passenger **in heavy transport vehicle injured in noncollision transport accident in** traffic accident

⑦ **V68.7** Person on outside **of heavy transport vehicle injured in noncollision transport accident in** traffic accident

⑦ **V68.9** Unspecified **occupant of heavy transport vehicle injured in noncollision transport accident in** traffic accident

④ **V69 Occupant of heavy transport vehicle injured in** other and unspecified **transport accidents**

The appropriate 7th character is to be added to each code from category V69
A = initial encounter
D = subsequent encounter
S = sequela

⑤ **V69.0** Driver **of heavy transport vehicle injured in collision with other and unspecified motor vehicles in** nontraffic accident

⑦ **V69.00 Driver of heavy transport vehicle injured in collision with unspecified motor vehicles in nontraffic accident**

⑦ **V69.09** Driver of heavy transport vehicle injured in collision with other motor vehicles in nontraffic accident

⑤ **V69.1** Passenger **in heavy transport vehicle injured in collision with other and unspecified motor vehicles in** nontraffic accident

⑦ **V69.10 Passenger in heavy transport vehicle injured in collision with unspecified motor vehicles in nontraffic accident**

⑦ **V69.19** Passenger in heavy transport vehicle injured in collision with other motor vehicles in nontraffic accident

⑤ **V69.2** Unspecified **occupant of heavy transport vehicle injured in collision with other and unspecified motor vehicles in** nontraffic accident

⑦ **V69.20 Unspecified occupant of heavy transport vehicle injured in collision with unspecified motor vehicles in nontraffic accident**

> Collision NOS involving heavy transport vehicle, nontraffic

⑦ **V69.29 Unspecified occupant of heavy transport vehicle injured in collision with other motor vehicles in nontraffic accident**

⑦ **V69.3** Occupant (driver) (passenger) **of heavy transport vehicle injured in unspecified** nontraffic accident

> Accident NOS involving heavy transport vehicle, nontraffic
> Occupant of heavy transport vehicle injured in nontraffic accident NOS

⑤ **V69.4** Driver **of heavy transport vehicle injured in collision with other and unspecified motor vehicles in** traffic accident

⑦ **V69.40 Driver of heavy transport vehicle injured in collision with unspecified motor vehicles in traffic accident**

⑦ **V69.49** Driver of heavy transport vehicle injured in collision with other motor vehicles in traffic accident

⑤ **V69.5** Passenger **in heavy transport vehicle injured in collision with other and unspecified motor vehicles in** traffic accident

⑦ **V69.50 Passenger in heavy transport vehicle injured in collision with unspecified motor vehicles in traffic accident**

⑦ **V69.59** Passenger in heavy transport vehicle injured in collision with other motor vehicles in traffic accident

⑤ **V69.6** Unspecified **occupant of heavy transport vehicle injured in collision with other and unspecified motor vehicles in** traffic accident

⑦ **V69.60 Unspecified occupant of heavy transport vehicle injured in collision with unspecified motor vehicles in traffic accident**

> Collision NOS involving heavy transport vehicle (traffic)

⑦ **V69.69 Unspecified occupant of heavy transport vehicle injured in collision with other motor vehicles in traffic accident**

⑤ **V69.8** Occupant (driver) (passenger) **of heavy transport vehicle injured in other specified transport accidents**

⑦ **V69.81 Occupant (driver) (passenger) of heavy transport vehicle injured in transport accidents with** military vehicle

⑦ **V69.88 Occupant (driver) (passenger) of heavy transport vehicle injured in other specified transport accidents**

⑦ **V69.9** Occupant (driver) (passenger) **of heavy transport vehicle injured in unspecified** traffic accident

> Accident NOS involving heavy transport vehicle

Bus occupant injured in transport accident (V70-V79)

> INCLUDES   motorcoach
> EXCLUDES1   minibus (V50-V59)

④ **V70 Bus occupant injured in collision** with pedestrian or animal
The appropriate 7th character is to be added to each code from category V70
A = initial encounter
D = subsequent encounter
S = sequela

> EXCLUDES1   bus collision with animal-drawn vehicle or animal being ridden (V76.-)

⑦ **V70.0** Driver **of bus injured in collision with pedestrian or animal in** nontraffic accident

⑦ **V70.1** Passenger **on bus injured in collision with pedestrian or animal in** nontraffic accident

⑦ **V70.2** Person on outside **of bus injured in collision with pedestrian or animal in** nontraffic accident

⑦ **V70.3** Unspecified **occupant of bus injured in collision with pedestrian or animal in** nontraffic accident

⑦ **V70.4** Person boarding or alighting **from bus injured in collision with pedestrian or animal**

⑦ **V70.5** Driver **of bus injured in collision with pedestrian or animal in** traffic accident

Unspecified Code	Other Specified Code	ℕ Newborn Age: 0	ℙ Pediatric Age: 0-17	𝕄 Maternity Age: 12-55
🅐 Adult Age: 15-124	♂ Male	♀ Female	● New Code	▲ Revised Code Title	►◄ Revised Text

[7th] V70.6 Passenger on bus injured in collision with pedestrian or animal in traffic accident
[7th] V70.7 Person on outside of bus injured in collision with pedestrian or animal in traffic accident
[7th] V70.9 Unspecified occupant of bus injured in collision with pedestrian or animal in traffic accident

[4th] V71 Bus occupant injured in collision with pedal cycle

The appropriate 7th character is to be added to each code from category V71
A = initial encounter
D = subsequent encounter
S = sequela

[7th] V71.0 Driver of bus injured in collision with pedal cycle in nontraffic accident
[7th] V71.1 Passenger on bus injured in collision with pedal cycle in nontraffic accident
[7th] V71.2 Person on outside of bus injured in collision with pedal cycle in nontraffic accident
[7th] V71.3 Unspecified occupant of bus injured in collision with pedal cycle in nontraffic accident
[7th] V71.4 Person boarding or alighting from bus injured in collision with pedal cycle
[7th] V71.5 Driver of bus injured in collision with pedal cycle in traffic accident
[7th] V71.6 Passenger on bus injured in collision with pedal cycle in traffic accident
[7th] V71.7 Person on outside of bus injured in collision with pedal cycle in traffic accident
[7th] V71.9 Unspecified occupant of bus injured in collision with pedal cycle in traffic accident

[4th] V72 Bus occupant injured in collision with two- or three-wheeled motor vehicle

The appropriate 7th character is to be added to each code from category V72
A = initial encounter
D = subsequent encounter
S = sequela

[7th] V72.0 Driver of bus injured in collision with two- or three-wheeled motor vehicle in nontraffic accident
[7th] V72.1 Passenger on bus injured in collision with two- or three-wheeled motor vehicle in nontraffic accident
[7th] V72.2 Person on outside of bus injured in collision with two- or three-wheeled motor vehicle in nontraffic accident
[7th] V72.3 Unspecified occupant of bus injured in collision with two- or three-wheeled motor vehicle in nontraffic accident
[7th] V72.4 Person boarding or alighting from bus injured in collision with two- or three-wheeled motor vehicle
[7th] V72.5 Driver of bus injured in collision with two- or three-wheeled motor vehicle in traffic accident
[7th] V72.6 Passenger on bus injured in collision with two- or three-wheeled motor vehicle in traffic accident
[7th] V72.7 Person on outside of bus injured in collision with two- or three-wheeled motor vehicle in traffic accident
[7th] V72.9 Unspecified occupant of bus injured in collision with two- or three-wheeled motor vehicle in traffic accident

[4th] V73 Bus occupant injured in collision with car, pick-up truck or van

The appropriate 7th character is to be added to each code from category V73
A = initial encounter
D = subsequent encounter
S = sequela

[7th] V73.0 Driver of bus injured in collision with car, pick-up truck or van in nontraffic accident
[7th] V73.1 Passenger on bus injured in collision with car, pick-up truck or van in nontraffic accident
[7th] V73.2 Person on outside of bus injured in collision with car, pick-up truck or van in nontraffic accident
[7th] V73.3 Unspecified occupant of bus injured in collision with car, pick-up truck or van in nontraffic accident
[7th] V73.4 Person boarding or alighting from bus injured in collision with car, pick-up truck or van
[7th] V73.5 Driver of bus injured in collision with car, pick-up truck or van in traffic accident
[7th] V73.6 Passenger on bus injured in collision with car, pick-up truck or van in traffic accident
[7th] V73.7 Person on outside of bus injured in collision with car, pick-up truck or van in traffic accident
[7th] V73.9 Unspecified occupant of bus injured in collision with car, pick-up truck or van in traffic accident

[4th] V74 Bus occupant injured in collision with heavy transport vehicle or bus

[EXCLUDES1] *bus occupant injured in collision with military vehicle (V79.81)*

The appropriate 7th character is to be added to each code from category V74
A = initial encounter
D = subsequent encounter
S = sequela

[7th] V74.0 Driver of bus injured in collision with heavy transport vehicle or bus in nontraffic accident
[7th] V74.1 Passenger on bus injured in collision with heavy transport vehicle or bus in nontraffic accident
[7th] V74.2 Person on outside of bus injured in collision with heavy transport vehicle or bus in nontraffic accident
[7th] V74.3 Unspecified occupant of bus injured in collision with heavy transport vehicle or bus in nontraffic accident
[7th] V74.4 Person boarding or alighting from bus injured in collision with heavy transport vehicle or bus
[7th] V74.5 Driver of bus injured in collision with heavy transport vehicle or bus in traffic accident
[7th] V74.6 Passenger on bus injured in collision with heavy transport vehicle or bus in traffic accident
[7th] V74.7 Person on outside of bus injured in collision with heavy transport vehicle or bus in traffic accident
[7th] V74.9 Unspecified occupant of bus injured in collision with heavy transport vehicle or bus in traffic accident

[4th] V75 Bus occupant injured in collision with railway train or railway vehicle

The appropriate 7th character is to be added to each code from category V75
A = initial encounter
D = subsequent encounter
S = sequela

[7th] V75.0 Driver of bus injured in collision with railway train or railway vehicle in nontraffic accident
[7th] V75.1 Passenger on bus injured in collision with railway train or railway vehicle in nontraffic accident
[7th] V75.2 Person on outside of bus injured in collision with railway train or railway vehicle in nontraffic accident
[7th] V75.3 Unspecified occupant of bus injured in collision with railway train or railway vehicle in nontraffic accident
[7th] V75.4 Person boarding or alighting from bus injured in collision with railway train or railway vehicle
[7th] V75.5 Driver of bus injured in collision with railway train or railway vehicle in traffic accident
[7th] V75.6 Passenger on bus injured in collision with railway train or railway vehicle in traffic accident
[7th] V75.7 Person on outside of bus injured in collision with railway train or railway vehicle in traffic accident
[7th] V75.9 Unspecified occupant of bus injured in collision with railway train or railway vehicle in traffic accident

[4th] **V76 Bus occupant injured in collision with other nonmotor vehicle**

INCLUDES *collision with animal-drawn vehicle, animal being ridden, streetcar*

The appropriate 7th character is to be added to each code from category V76
A = initial encounter
D = subsequent encounter
S = sequela

[7th] **V76.0 Driver of bus injured in collision with other nonmotor vehicle in nontraffic accident**
[7th] **V76.1 Passenger on bus injured in collision with other nonmotor vehicle in nontraffic accident**
[7th] **V76.2 Person on outside of bus injured in collision with other nonmotor vehicle in nontraffic accident**
[7th] **V76.3 Unspecified occupant of bus injured in collision with other nonmotor vehicle in nontraffic accident**
[7th] **V76.4 Person boarding or alighting from bus injured in collision with other nonmotor vehicle**
[7th] **V76.5 Driver of bus injured in collision with other nonmotor vehicle in traffic accident**
[7th] **V76.6 Passenger on bus injured in collision with other nonmotor vehicle in traffic accident**
[7th] **V76.7 Person on outside of bus injured in collision with other nonmotor vehicle in traffic accident**
[7th] **V76.9 Unspecified occupant of bus injured in collision with other nonmotor vehicle in traffic accident**

[4th] **V77 Bus occupant injured in collision with fixed or stationary object**

The appropriate 7th character is to be added to each code from category V77
A = initial encounter
D = subsequent encounter
S = sequela

[7th] **V77.0 Driver of bus injured in collision with fixed or stationary object in nontraffic accident**
[7th] **V77.1 Passenger on bus injured in collision with fixed or stationary object in nontraffic accident**
[7th] **V77.2 Person on outside of bus injured in collision with fixed or stationary object in nontraffic accident**
[7th] **V77.3 Unspecified occupant of bus injured in collision with fixed or stationary object in nontraffic accident**
[7th] **V77.4 Person boarding or alighting from bus injured in collision with fixed or stationary object**
[7th] **V77.5 Driver of bus injured in collision with fixed or stationary object in traffic accident**
[7th] **V77.6 Passenger on bus injured in collision with fixed or stationary object in traffic accident**
[7th] **V77.7 Person on outside of bus injured in collision with fixed or stationary object in traffic accident**
[7th] **V77.9 Unspecified occupant of bus injured in collision with fixed or stationary object in traffic accident**

[4th] **V78 Bus occupant injured in noncollision transport accident**

INCLUDES *overturning bus NOS*
overturning bus without collision

The appropriate 7th character is to be added to each code from category V78
A = initial encounter
D = subsequent encounter
S = sequela

[7th] **V78.0 Driver of bus injured in noncollision transport accident in nontraffic accident**
[7th] **V78.1 Passenger on bus injured in noncollision transport accident in nontraffic accident**
[7th] **V78.2 Person on outside of bus injured in noncollision transport accident in nontraffic accident**
[7th] **V78.3 Unspecified occupant of bus injured in noncollision transport accident in nontraffic accident**
[7th] **V78.4 Person boarding or alighting from bus injured in noncollision transport accident**
[7th] **V78.5 Driver of bus injured in noncollision transport accident in traffic accident**
[7th] **V78.6 Passenger on bus injured in noncollision transport accident in traffic accident**
[7th] **V78.7 Person on outside of bus injured in noncollision transport accident in traffic accident**
[7th] **V78.9 Unspecified occupant of bus injured in noncollision transport accident in traffic accident**

[4th] **V79 Bus occupant injured in other and unspecified transport accidents**

The appropriate 7th character is to be added to each code from category V79
A = initial encounter
D = subsequent encounter
S = sequela

[5th] **V79.0 Driver of bus injured in collision with other and unspecified motor vehicles in nontraffic accident**
[7th] **V79.00 Driver of bus injured in collision with unspecified motor vehicles in nontraffic accident**
[7th] **V79.09 Driver of bus injured in collision with other motor vehicles in nontraffic accident**
[5th] **V79.1 Passenger on bus injured in collision with other and unspecified motor vehicles in nontraffic accident**
[7th] **V79.10 Passenger on bus injured in collision with unspecified motor vehicles in nontraffic accident**
[7th] **V79.19 Passenger on bus injured in collision with other motor vehicles in nontraffic accident**
[5th] **V79.2 Unspecified bus occupant injured in collision with other and unspecified motor vehicles in nontraffic accident**
[7th] **V79.20 Unspecified bus occupant injured in collision with unspecified motor vehicles in nontraffic accident**
Bus collision NOS, nontraffic
[7th] **V79.29 Unspecified bus occupant injured in collision with other motor vehicles in nontraffic accident**
[7th] **V79.3 Bus occupant (driver) (passenger) injured in unspecified nontraffic accident**
Bus accident NOS, nontraffic
Bus occupant injured in nontraffic accident NOS
[5th] **V79.4 Driver of bus injured in collision with other and unspecified motor vehicles in traffic accident**
[7th] **V79.40 Driver of bus injured in collision with unspecified motor vehicles in traffic accident**
[7th] **V79.49 Driver of bus injured in collision with other motor vehicles in traffic accident**
[5th] **V79.5 Passenger on bus injured in collision with other and unspecified motor vehicles in traffic accident**
[7th] **V79.50 Passenger on bus injured in collision with unspecified motor vehicles in traffic accident**
[7th] **V79.59 Passenger on bus injured in collision with other motor vehicles in traffic accident**
[5th] **V79.6 Unspecified bus occupant injured in collision with other and unspecified motor vehicles in traffic accident**
[7th] **V79.60 Unspecified bus occupant injured in collision with unspecified motor vehicles in traffic accident**
Bus collision NOS (traffic)
[7th] **V79.69 Unspecified bus occupant injured in collision with other motor vehicles in traffic accident**
[5th] **V79.8 Bus occupant (driver) (passenger) injured in other specified transport accidents**
[7th] **V79.81 Bus occupant (driver) (passenger) injured in transport accidents with military vehicle**
[7th] **V79.88 Bus occupant (driver) (passenger) injured in other specified transport accidents**
[7th] **V79.9 Bus occupant (driver) (passenger) injured in unspecified traffic accident**
Bus accident NOS

Unspecified Code | Other Specified Code | [N] Newborn Age: 0 | [P] Pediatric Age: 0-17 | [M] Maternity Age: 12-55
[A] Adult Age: 15-124 | ♂ Male | ♀ Female | ● New Code | ▲ Revised Code Title | ►◄ Revised Text

Other land transport accidents (V80-V89)

④ **V80** Animal-rider or occupant of animal-drawn vehicle injured in transport accident

The appropriate 7th character is to be added to each code from category V80
A = initial encounter
D = subsequent encounter
S = sequela

⑤ **V80.0** Animal-rider or occupant of animal drawn vehicle injured by fall from or being thrown from animal or animal-drawn vehicle in noncollision accident

⑥ **V80.01** Animal-rider injured by fall from or being thrown from animal in noncollision accident

⑦ **V80.010** Animal-rider injured by fall from or being thrown from horse in noncollision accident

⑦ **V80.018** Animal-rider injured by fall from or being thrown from other animal in noncollision accident

⑦ **V80.02** Occupant of animal-drawn vehicle injured by fall from or being thrown from animal-drawn vehicle in noncollision accident

Overturning animal-drawn vehicle NOS
Overturning animal-drawn vehicle without collision

⑤ **V80.1** Animal-rider or occupant of animal-drawn vehicle injured in collision with pedestrian or animal

EXCLUDES1 animal-rider or animal-drawn vehicle collision with animal-drawn vehicle or animal being ridden (V80.7)

⑦ **V80.11** Animal-rider injured in collision with pedestrian or animal

⑦ **V80.12** Occupant of animal-drawn vehicle injured in collision with pedestrian or animal

⑤ **V80.2** Animal-rider or occupant of animal-drawn vehicle injured in collision with pedal cycle

⑦ **V80.21** Animal-rider injured in collision with pedal cycle

⑦ **V80.22** Occupant of animal-drawn vehicle injured in collision with pedal cycle

⑤ **V80.3** Animal-rider or occupant of animal-drawn vehicle injured in collision with two- or three-wheeled motor vehicle

⑦ **V80.31** Animal-rider injured in collision with two- or three-wheeled motor vehicle

⑦ **V80.32** Occupant of animal-drawn vehicle injured in collision with two- or three-wheeled motor vehicle

⑤ **V80.4** Animal-rider or occupant of animal-drawn vehicle injured in collision with car, pick-up truck, van, heavy transport vehicle or bus

EXCLUDES1 animal-rider injured in collision with military vehicle (V80.910)
occupant of animal-drawn vehicle injured in collision with military vehicle (V80.920)

⑦ **V80.41** Animal-rider injured in collision with car, pick-up truck, van, heavy transport vehicle or bus

⑦ **V80.42** Occupant of animal-drawn vehicle injured in collision with car, pick-up truck, van, heavy transport vehicle or bus

⑤ **V80.5** Animal-rider or occupant of animal-drawn vehicle injured in collision with other specified motor vehicle

⑦ **V80.51** Animal-rider injured in collision with other specified motor vehicle

⑦ **V80.52** Occupant of animal-drawn vehicle injured in collision with other specified motor vehicle

⑤ **V80.6** Animal-rider or occupant of animal-drawn vehicle injured in collision with railway train or railway vehicle

⑦ **V80.61** Animal-rider injured in collision with railway train or railway vehicle

⑦ **V80.62** Occupant of animal-drawn vehicle injured in collision with railway train or railway vehicle

⑤ **V80.7** Animal-rider or occupant of animal-drawn vehicle injured in collision with other nonmotor vehicles

⑥ **V80.71** Animal-rider or occupant of animal-drawn vehicle injured in collision with animal being ridden

⑦ **V80.710** Animal-rider injured in collision with other animal being ridden

⑦ **V80.711** Occupant of animal-drawn vehicle injured in collision with animal being ridden

⑥ **V80.72** Animal-rider or occupant of animal-drawn vehicle injured in collision with other animal-drawn vehicle

⑦ **V80.720** Animal-rider injured in collision with animal-drawn vehicle

⑦ **V80.721** Occupant of animal-drawn vehicle injured in collision with other animal-drawn vehicle

⑥ **V80.73** Animal-rider or occupant of animal-drawn vehicle injured in collision with streetcar

⑦ **V80.730** Animal-rider injured in collision with streetcar

⑦ **V80.731** Occupant of animal-drawn vehicle injured in collision with streetcar

⑥ **V80.79** Animal-rider or occupant of animal-drawn vehicle injured in collision with other nonmotor vehicles

⑦ **V80.790** Animal-rider injured in collision with other nonmotor vehicles

⑦ **V80.791** Occupant of animal-drawn vehicle injured in collision with other nonmotor vehicles

⑤ **V80.8** Animal-rider or occupant of animal-drawn vehicle injured in collision with fixed or stationary object

⑦ **V80.81** Animal-rider injured in collision with fixed or stationary object

⑦ **V80.82** Occupant of animal-drawn vehicle injured in collision with fixed or stationary object

⑤ **V80.9** Animal-rider or occupant of animal-drawn vehicle injured in other and unspecified transport accidents

⑥ **V80.91** Animal-rider injured in other and unspecified transport accidents

⑦ **V80.910** Animal-rider injured in transport accident with military vehicle

⑦ **V80.918** Animal-rider injured in other transport accident

⑦ **V80.919** Animal-rider injured in unspecified transport accident
Animal rider accident NOS

⑥ **V80.92** Occupant of animal-drawn vehicle injured in other and unspecified transport accidents

⑦ **V80.920** Occupant of animal-drawn vehicle injured in transport accident with military vehicle

⑦ **V80.928** Occupant of animal-drawn vehicle injured in other transport accident

⑦ **V80.929** Occupant of animal-drawn vehicle injured in unspecified transport accident
Animal-drawn vehicle accident NOS

④ **V81** Occupant of railway train or railway vehicle injured in transport accident

INCLUDES derailment of railway train or railway vehicle
person on outside of train

EXCLUDES1 streetcar (V82.-)

The appropriate 7th character is to be added to each code from category V81
A = initial encounter
D = subsequent encounter
S = sequela

⑦ **V81.0** Occupant of railway train or railway vehicle injured in collision with motor vehicle in nontraffic accident

EXCLUDES1 Occupant of railway train or railway vehicle injured due to collision with military vehicle (V81.83)

---

④ 4th character required   ⑤ 5th character required   ⑥ 6th character required   ⑦ 7th character required   ⑩ Extension 'X' Alert
EXCLUDES 1 Not coded here   EXCLUDES 2 Not included here   PDx Primary Diagnosis Only   Manifestation Code

[7th] V81.1 Occupant of railway train or railway vehicle injured in collision with motor vehicle in traffic accident
[EXCLUDES1] *Occupant of railway train or railway vehicle injured due to collision with military vehicle (V81.83)*

[7th] V81.2 Occupant of railway train or railway vehicle injured in collision with or hit by rolling stock

[7th] V81.3 Occupant of railway train or railway vehicle injured in collision with other object
Railway collision NOS

[7th] V81.4 Person injured while boarding or alighting from railway train or railway vehicle

[7th] V81.5 Occupant of railway train or railway vehicle injured by fall in railway train or railway vehicle

[7th] V81.6 Occupant of railway train or railway vehicle injured by fall from railway train or railway vehicle

[7th] V81.7 Occupant of railway train or railway vehicle injured in derailment without antecedent collision

[5th] V81.8 Occupant of railway train or railway vehicle injured in other specified railway accidents

[7th] V81.81 Occupant of railway train or railway vehicle injured due to explosion or fire on train

[7th] V81.82 Occupant of railway train or railway vehicle injured due to object falling onto train
Occupant of railway train or railway vehicle injured due to falling earth onto train
Occupant of railway train or railway vehicle injured due to falling rocks onto train
Occupant of railway train or railway vehicle injured due to falling snow onto train
Occupant of railway train or railway vehicle injured due to falling trees onto train

[7th] V81.83 Occupant of railway train or railway vehicle injured due to collision with military vehicle

[7th] V81.89 Occupant of railway train or railway vehicle injured due to other specified railway accident

[7th] V81.9 Occupant of railway train or railway vehicle injured in unspecified railway accident
Railway accident NOS

[4th] V82 Occupant of powered streetcar injured in transport accident
[INCLUDES] *interurban electric car*
person on outside of streetcar
tram (car)
trolley (car)
[EXCLUDES1] *bus (V70-V79)*
motorcoach (V70-V79)
nonpowered streetcar (V76.-)
train (V81.-)

The appropriate 7th character is to be added to each code from category V82
A = initial encounter
D = subsequent encounter
S = sequela

[7th] V82.0 Occupant of streetcar injured in collision with motor vehicle in nontraffic accident

[7th] V82.1 Occupant of streetcar injured in collision with motor vehicle in traffic accident

[7th] V82.2 Occupant of streetcar injured in collision with or hit by rolling stock

[7th] V82.3 Occupant of streetcar injured in collision with other object
[EXCLUDES1] *collision with animal-drawn vehicle or animal being ridden (V82.8)*

[7th] V82.4 Person injured while boarding or alighting from streetcar

[7th] V82.5 Occupant of streetcar injured by fall in streetcar
[EXCLUDES1] *fall in streetcar:*
while boarding or alighting (V82.4)
with antecedent collision (V82.0-V82.3)

[7th] V82.6 Occupant of streetcar injured by fall from streetcar
[EXCLUDES1] *fall from streetcar:*
while boarding or alighting (V82.4)
with antecedent collision (V82.0-V82.3)

[7th] V82.7 Occupant of streetcar injured in derailment without antecedent collision
[EXCLUDES1] *occupant of streetcar injured in derailment with antecedent collision (V82.0-V82.3)*

[7th] V82.8 Occupant of streetcar injured in other specified transport accidents
Streetcar collision with military vehicle
Streetcar collision with train or nonmotor vehicles

[7th] V82.9 Occupant of streetcar injured in unspecified traffic accident
Streetcar accident NOS

[4th] V83 Occupant of special vehicle mainly used on industrial premises injured in transport accident
[INCLUDES] *battery-powered airport passenger vehicle*
battery-powered truck (baggage) (mail)
coal-car in mine
forklift (truck)
logging car
self-propelled industrial truck
station baggage truck (powered)
tram, truck, or tub (powered) in mine or quarry
[EXCLUDES1] *special construction vehicles (V85.-)*
special industrial vehicle in stationary use or maintenance (W31.-)

The appropriate 7th character is to be added to each code from category V83
A = initial encounter
D = subsequent encounter
S = sequela

[7th] V83.0 Driver of special industrial vehicle injured in traffic accident

[7th] V83.1 Passenger of special industrial vehicle injured in traffic accident

[7th] V83.2 Person on outside of special industrial vehicle injured in traffic accident

[7th] V83.3 Unspecified occupant of special industrial vehicle injured in traffic accident

[7th] V83.4 Person injured while boarding or alighting from special industrial vehicle

[7th] V83.5 Driver of special industrial vehicle injured in nontraffic accident

[7th] V83.6 Passenger of special industrial vehicle injured in nontraffic accident

[7th] V83.7 Person on outside of special industrial vehicle injured in nontraffic accident

[7th] V83.9 Unspecified occupant of special industrial vehicle injured in nontraffic accident
Special-industrial-vehicle accident NOS

[4th] V84 Occupant of special vehicle mainly used in agriculture injured in transport accident
[INCLUDES] *self-propelled farm machinery*
tractor (and trailer)
[EXCLUDES1] *animal-powered farm machinery accident (W30.8-)*
contact with combine harvester (W30.0)
special agricultural vehicle in stationary use or maintenance (W30.-)

The appropriate 7th character is to be added to each code from category V84
A = initial encounter
D = subsequent encounter
S = sequela

[7th] V84.0 Driver of special agricultural vehicle injured in traffic accident

Unspecified Code | Other Specified Code | [N] Newborn Age: 0 | [P] Pediatric Age: 0-17 | [M] Maternity Age: 12-55
[A] Adult Age: 15-124 | ♂ Male | ♀ Female | ● New Code | ▲ Revised Code Title | ►◄ Revised Text

- V84.1 Passenger of special agricultural vehicle injured in traffic accident
- V84.2 Person on outside of special agricultural vehicle injured in traffic accident
- V84.3 Unspecified occupant of special agricultural vehicle injured in traffic accident
- V84.4 Person injured while boarding or alighting from special agricultural vehicle
- V84.5 Driver of special agricultural vehicle injured in nontraffic accident
- V84.6 Passenger of special agricultural vehicle injured in nontraffic accident
- V84.7 Person on outside of special agricultural vehicle injured in nontraffic accident
- V84.9 Unspecified occupant of special agricultural vehicle injured in nontraffic accident

Special-agricultural vehicle accident NOS

- V85 Occupant of special construction vehicle injured in transport accident

  INCLUDES bulldozer
            digger
            dump truck
            earth-leveller
            mechanical shovel
            road-roller

  EXCLUDES1 special industrial vehicle (V83.-)
             special construction vehicle in stationary use or maintenance (W31.-)

The appropriate 7th character is to be added to each code from category V85
A = initial encounter
D = subsequent encounter
S = sequela

- V85.0 Driver of special construction vehicle injured in traffic accident
- V85.1 Passenger of special construction vehicle injured in traffic accident
- V85.2 Person on outside of special construction vehicle injured in traffic accident
- V85.3 Unspecified occupant of special construction vehicle injured in traffic accident
- V85.4 Person injured while boarding or alighting from special construction vehicle
- V85.5 Driver of special construction vehicle injured in nontraffic accident
- V85.6 Passenger of special construction vehicle injured in nontraffic accident
- V85.7 Person on outside of special construction vehicle injured in nontraffic accident
- V85.9 Unspecified occupant of special construction vehicle injured in nontraffic accident

Special-construction-vehicle accident NOS

- V86 Occupant of special all-terrain or other off-road motor vehicle, injured in transport accident

  EXCLUDES1 special all-terrain vehicle in stationary use or maintenance (W31.-)
             sport-utility vehicle (V50-V59)
             three-wheeled motor vehicle designed for on-road use (V30-V39)

The appropriate 7th character is to be added to each code from category V86
A = initial encounter
D = subsequent encounter
S = sequela

- V86.0 Driver of special all-terrain or other off-road motor vehicle injured in traffic accident
  - V86.01 Driver of ambulance or fire engine injured in traffic accident
  - V86.02 Driver of snowmobile injured in traffic accident

- V86.03 Driver of dune buggy injured in traffic accident
- V86.04 Driver of military vehicle injured in traffic accident
- V86.09 Driver of other special all-terrain or other off-road motor vehicle injured in traffic accident

  Driver of dirt bike injured in traffic accident
  Driver of go cart injured in traffic accident
  Driver of golf cart injured in traffic accident
- V86.1 Passenger of special all-terrain or other off-road motor vehicle injured in traffic accident
  - V86.11 Passenger of ambulance or fire engine injured in traffic accident
  - V86.12 Passenger of snowmobile injured in traffic accident
  - V86.13 Passenger of dune buggy injured in traffic accident
  - V86.14 Passenger of military vehicle injured in traffic accident
  - V86.19 Passenger of other special all-terrain or other off-road motor vehicle injured in traffic accident

    Passenger of dirt bike injured in traffic accident
    Passenger of go cart injured in traffic accident
    Passenger of golf cart injured in traffic accident
- V86.2 Person on outside of special all-terrain or other off-road motor vehicle injured in traffic accident
  - V86.21 Person on outside of ambulance or fire engine injured in traffic accident
  - V86.22 Person on outside of snowmobile injured in traffic accident
  - V86.23 Person on outside of dune buggy injured in traffic accident
  - V86.24 Person on outside of military vehicle injured in traffic accident
  - V86.29 Person on outside of other special all-terrain or other off-road motor vehicle injured in traffic accident

    Person on outside of dirt bike injured in traffic accident
    Person on outside of go cart in traffic accident
    Person on outside of golf cart injured in traffic accident
- V86.3 Unspecified occupant of special all-terrain or other off-road motor vehicle injured in traffic accident
  - V86.31 Unspecified occupant of ambulance or fire engine injured in traffic accident
  - V86.32 Unspecified occupant of snowmobile injured in traffic accident
  - V86.33 Unspecified occupant of dune buggy injured in traffic accident
  - V86.34 Unspecified occupant of military vehicle injured in traffic accident
  - V86.39 Unspecified occupant of other special all-terrain or other off-road motor vehicle injured in traffic accident

    Unspecified occupant of dirt bike injured in traffic accident
    Unspecified occupant of go cart injured in traffic accident
    Unspecified occupant of golf cart injured in traffic accident
- V86.4 Person injured while boarding or alighting from special all-terrain or other off-road motor vehicle
  - V86.41 Person injured while boarding or alighting from ambulance or fire engine
  - V86.42 Person injured while boarding or alighting from snowmobile
  - V86.43 Person injured while boarding or alighting from dune buggy
  - V86.44 Person injured while boarding or alighting from military vehicle

---

4th character required   5th character required   6th character required   7th character required   Extension 'X' Alert
EXCLUDES1 Not coded here   EXCLUDES2 Not included here   PDx Primary Diagnosis Only   Manifestation Code

🔟 **V86.49** Person injured while boarding or alighting from other special all-terrain or other off-road motor vehicle

Person injured while boarding or alighting from dirt bike

Person injured while boarding or alighting from go cart

Person injured while boarding or alighting from golf cart

5️⃣ **V86.5** Driver of special all-terrain or other off-road motor vehicle injured in nontraffic accident

🔟 **V86.51** Driver of ambulance or fire engine injured in nontraffic accident

🔟 **V86.52** Driver of snowmobile injured in nontraffic accident

🔟 **V86.53** Driver of dune buggy injured in nontraffic accident

🔟 **V86.54** Driver of military vehicle injured in nontraffic accident

🔟 **V86.59** Driver of other special all-terrain or other off-road motor vehicle injured in nontraffic accident

Driver of dirt bike injured in nontraffic accident

Driver of go cart injured in nontraffic accident

Driver of golf cart injured in nontraffic accident

5️⃣ **V86.6** Passenger of special all-terrain or other off-road motor vehicle injured in nontraffic accident

🔟 **V86.61** Passenger of ambulance or fire engine injured in nontraffic accident

🔟 **V86.62** Passenger of snowmobile injured in nontraffic accident

🔟 **V86.63** Passenger of dune buggy injured in nontraffic accident

🔟 **V86.64** Passenger of military vehicle injured in nontraffic accident

🔟 **V86.69** Passenger of other special all-terrain or other off-road motor vehicle injured in nontraffic accident

Passenger of dirt bike injured in nontraffic accident

Passenger of go cart injured in nontraffic accident

Passenger of golf cart injured in nontraffic accident

5️⃣ **V86.7** Person on outside of special all-terrain or other off-road motor vehicle injured in nontraffic accident

🔟 **V86.71** Person on outside of ambulance or fire engine injured in nontraffic accident

🔟 **V86.72** Person on outside of snowmobile injured in nontraffic accident

🔟 **V86.73** Person on outside of dune buggy injured in nontraffic accident

🔟 **V86.74** Person on outside of military vehicle injured in nontraffic accident

🔟 **V86.79** Person on outside of other special all-terrain or other off-road motor vehicles injured in nontraffic accident

Person on outside of dirt bike injured in nontraffic accident

Person on outside of go cart injured in nontraffic accident

Person on outside of golf cart injured in nontraffic accident

5️⃣ **V86.9** Unspecified occupant of special all-terrain or other off-road motor vehicle injured in nontraffic accident

🔟 **V86.91** Unspecified occupant of ambulance or fire engine injured in nontraffic accident

🔟 **V86.92** Unspecified occupant of snowmobile injured in nontraffic accident

🔟 **V86.93** Unspecified occupant of dune buggy injured in nontraffic accident

🔟 **V86.94** Unspecified occupant of military vehicle injured in nontraffic accident

🔟 **V86.99** Unspecified occupant of other special all-terrain or other off-road motor vehicle injured in nontraffic accident

All-terrain motor-vehicle accident NOS

Off-road motor-vehicle accident NOS

Other motor-vehicle accident NOS

Unspecified occupant of dirt bike injured in nontraffic accident

Unspecified occupant of go cart injured in nontraffic accident

Unspecified occupant of golf cart injured in nontraffic accident

4️⃣ **V87** Traffic accident of specified type but victim's mode of transport unknown

> EXCLUDES1   collision involving:
> pedal cycle (V10-V19)
> pedestrian (V01-V09)

The appropriate 7th character is to be added to each code from category V87

A = initial encounter

D = subsequent encounter

S = sequela

🔟 **V87.0** Person injured in collision between car and two- or three-wheeled powered vehicle (traffic)

🔟 **V87.1** Person injured in collision between other motor vehicle and two- or three-wheeled motor vehicle (traffic)

🔟 **V87.2** Person injured in collision between car and pick-up truck or van (traffic)

🔟 **V87.3** Person injured in collision between car and bus (traffic)

🔟 **V87.4** Person injured in collision between car and heavy transport vehicle (traffic)

🔟 **V87.5** Person injured in collision between heavy transport vehicle and bus (traffic)

🔟 **V87.6** Person injured in collision between railway train or railway vehicle and car (traffic)

🔟 **V87.7** Person injured in collision between other specified motor vehicles (traffic)

🔟 **V87.8** Person injured in other specified noncollision transport accidents involving motor vehicle (traffic)

🔟 **V87.9** Person injured in other specified (collision)(noncollision) transport accidents involving nonmotor vehicle (traffic)

4️⃣ **V88** Nontraffic accident of specified type but victim's mode of transport unknown

> EXCLUDES1   collision involving:
> pedal cycle (V10-V19)
> pedestrian (V01-V09)

The appropriate 7th character is to be added to each code from category V88

A = initial encounter

D = subsequent encounter

S = sequela

🔟 **V88.0** Person injured in collision between car and two- or three-wheeled motor vehicle, nontraffic

🔟 **V88.1** Person injured in collision between other motor vehicle and two- or three-wheeled motor vehicle, nontraffic

🔟 **V88.2** Person injured in collision between car and pick-up truck or van, nontraffic

🔟 **V88.3** Person injured in collision between car and bus, nontraffic

🔟 **V88.4** Person injured in collision between car and heavy transport vehicle, nontraffic

🔟 **V88.5** Person injured in collision between heavy transport vehicle and bus, nontraffic

🔟 **V88.6** Person injured in collision between railway train or railway vehicle and car, nontraffic

---

Unspecified Code	Other Specified Code	🅽 Newborn Age: 0	🅿 Pediatric Age: 0-17	🅼 Maternity Age: 12-55
🅰 Adult Age: 15-124	♂ Male	♀ Female	● New Code	▲ Revised Code Title ▶◀ Revised Text

V88.7 **Person injured in collision between** other specified motor vehicle, **nontraffic**

V88.8 **Person injured in other** specified noncollision transport accidents involving motor vehicle, **nontraffic**

V88.9 **Person injured in** other specified (collision)(noncollision) transport accidents **involving** nonmotor vehicle, **nontraffic**

V89 **Motor- or nonmotor-vehicle accident, type of vehicle unspecified**

The appropriate 7th character is to be added to each code from category V89
A = initial encounter
D = subsequent encounter
S = sequela

V89.0 **Person injured in unspecified** motor-vehicle **accident,** nontraffic

Motor-vehicle accident NOS, nontraffic

V89.1 **Person injured in unspecified** nonmotor-vehicle **accident,** nontraffic

Nonmotor-vehicle accident NOS (nontraffic)

V89.2 **Person injured in unspecified** motor-vehicle **accident,** traffic

Motor-vehicle accident [MVA] NOS
Road (traffic) accident [RTA] NOS

V89.3 **Person injured in unspecified** nonmotor-vehicle **accident,** traffic

Nonmotor-vehicle traffic accident NOS

V89.9 **Person injured in** unspecified vehicle **accident**

Collision NOS

Water transport accidents (V90-V94)

V90 **Drowning and submersion due to accident to watercraft**

> EXCLUDES1 civilian water transport accident involving military watercraft (V94.81-)
> fall into water not from watercraft (W16.-)
> military watercraft accident in military or war operations (Y36.0-, Y37.0-)
> water-transport-related drowning or submersion without accident to watercraft (V92.-)

The appropriate 7th character is to be added to each code from category V90
A = initial encounter
D = subsequent encounter
S = sequela

V90.0 **Drowning and submersion due to** watercraft overturning

V90.00 **Drowning and submersion due to** merchant ship **overturning**

V90.01 **Drowning and submersion due to** passenger ship **overturning**

Drowning and submersion due to Ferry-boat overturning
Drowning and submersion due to Liner overturning

V90.02 **Drowning and submersion due to** fishing boat **overturning**

V90.03 **Drowning and submersion due to** other powered watercraft **overturning**

Drowning and submersion due to Hovercraft (on open water) overturning
Drowning and submersion due to Jet ski overturning

V90.04 **Drowning and submersion due to** sailboat **overturning**

V90.05 **Drowning and submersion due to** canoe or kayak **overturning**

V90.06 **Drowning and submersion due to** (nonpowered) inflatable craft **overturning**

V90.08 **Drowning and submersion due to** other unpowered watercraft **overturning**

Drowning and submersion due to windsurfer overturning

V90.09 **Drowning and submersion due to unspecified watercraft overturning**

Drowning and submersion due to boat NOS overturning
Drowning and submersion due to ship NOS overturning
Drowning and submersion due to watercraft NOS overturning

V90.1 **Drowning and submersion due to** watercraft sinking

V90.10 **Drowning and submersion due to** merchant ship **sinking**

V90.11 **Drowning and submersion due to** passenger ship **sinking**

Drowning and submersion due to Ferry-boat sinking
Drowning and submersion due to Liner sinking

V90.12 **Drowning and submersion due to** fishing boat **sinking**

V90.13 **Drowning and submersion due to** other powered watercraft **sinking**

Drowning and submersion due to Hovercraft (on open water) sinking
Drowning and submersion due to Jet ski sinking

V90.14 **Drowning and submersion due to** sailboat **sinking**

V90.15 **Drowning and submersion due to** canoe or kayak **sinking**

V90.16 **Drowning and submersion due to** (nonpowered) inflatable craft **sinking**

V90.18 **Drowning and submersion due to** other unpowered watercraft **sinking**

V90.19 **Drowning and submersion due to unspecified watercraft sinking**

Drowning and submersion due to boat NOS sinking
Drowning and submersion due to ship NOS sinking
Drowning and submersion due to watercraft NOS sinking

V90.2 **Drowning and submersion due to** falling or jumping from burning **watercraft**

V90.20 **Drowning and submersion due to falling or jumping from burning** merchant ship

V90.21 **Drowning and submersion due to falling or jumping from burning** passenger ship

Drowning and submersion due to falling or jumping from burning Ferry-boat
Drowning and submersion due to falling or jumping from burning Liner

V90.22 **Drowning and submersion due to falling or jumping from burning** fishing boat

V90.23 **Drowning and submersion due to falling or jumping from** other burning powered **watercraft**

Drowning and submersion due to falling and jumping from burning Hovercraft (on open water)
Drowning and submersion due to falling and jumping from burning Jet ski

V90.24 **Drowning and submersion due to falling or jumping from burning** sailboat

V90.25 **Drowning and submersion due to falling or jumping from burning** canoe or kayak

V90.26 **Drowning and submersion due to falling or jumping from burning** (nonpowered) inflatable craft

V90.27 **Drowning and submersion due to falling or jumping from burning** water-skis

V90.28 **Drowning and submersion due to falling or jumping from other burning** unpowered watercraft

---

④ 4th character required ⑤ 5th character required ⑥ 6th character required ⑦ 7th character required ⑩ Extension 'X' Alert

EXCLUDES 1 Not coded here   EXCLUDES 2 Not included here   PDx Primary Diagnosis Only   Manifestation Code

Drowning and submersion due to falling and jumping from burning surf-board

Drowning and submersion due to falling and jumping from burning windsurfer

🅐 **V90.29 Drowning and submersion due to falling or jumping from unspecified burning watercraft**

Drowning and submersion due to falling or jumping from burning boat NOS

Drowning and submersion due to falling or jumping from burning ship NOS

Drowning and submersion due to falling or jumping from burning watercraft NOS

🄯 **V90.3 Drowning and submersion due to falling or jumping from crushed watercraft**

🅐 **V90.30 Drowning and submersion due to falling or jumping from crushed merchant ship**

🅐 **V90.31 Drowning and submersion due to falling or jumping from crushed passenger ship**

Drowning and submersion due to falling and jumping from crushed Ferry boat

Drowning and submersion due to falling and jumping from crushed Liner

🅐 **V90.32 Drowning and submersion due to falling or jumping from crushed fishing boat**

🅐 **V90.33 Drowning and submersion due to falling or jumping from other crushed powered watercraft**

Drowning and submersion due to falling and jumping from crushed Hovercraft

Drowning and submersion due to falling and jumping from crushed Jet ski

🅐 **V90.34 Drowning and submersion due to falling or jumping from crushed sailboat**

🅐 **V90.35 Drowning and submersion due to falling or jumping from crushed canoe or kayak**

🅐 **V90.36 Drowning and submersion due to falling or jumping from crushed (nonpowered) inflatable craft**

🅐 **V90.37 Drowning and submersion due to falling or jumping from crushed water-skis**

🅐 **V90.38 Drowning and submersion due to falling or jumping from other crushed unpowered watercraft**

Drowning and submersion due to falling and jumping from crushed surf-board

Drowning and submersion due to falling and jumping from crushed windsurfer

🅐 **V90.39 Drowning and submersion due to falling or jumping from crushed unspecified watercraft**

Drowning and submersion due to falling and jumping from crushed boat NOS

Drowning and submersion due to falling and jumping from crushed ship NOS

Drowning and submersion due to falling and jumping from crushed watercraft NOS

🄯 **V90.8 Drowning and submersion due to other accident to watercraft**

🅐 **V90.80 Drowning and submersion due to other accident to merchant ship**

🅐 **V90.81 Drowning and submersion due to other accident to passenger ship**

Drowning and submersion due to other accident to Ferry-boat

Drowning and submersion due to other accident to Liner

🅐 **V90.82 Drowning and submersion due to other accident to fishing boat**

🅐 **V90.83 Drowning and submersion due to other accident to other powered watercraft**

Drowning and submersion due to other accident to Hovercraft (on open water)

Drowning and submersion due to other accident to Jet ski

🅐 **V90.84 Drowning and submersion due to other accident to sailboat**

🅐 **V90.85 Drowning and submersion due to other accident to canoe or kayak**

🅐 **V90.86 Drowning and submersion due to other accident to (nonpowered) inflatable craft**

🅐 **V90.87 Drowning and submersion due to other accident to water-skis**

🅐 **V90.88 Drowning and submersion due to other accident to other unpowered watercraft**

Drowning and submersion due to other accident to surf-board

Drowning and submersion due to other accident to windsurfer

🅐 **V90.89 Drowning and submersion due to other accident to unspecified watercraft**

Drowning and submersion due to other accident to boat NOS

Drowning and submersion due to other accident to ship NOS

Drowning and submersion due to other accident to watercraft NOS

🄯 **V91 Other injury due to accident to watercraft**

> *INCLUDES*   any injury except drowning and submersion as a result of an accident to watercraft

> *EXCLUDES1*   civilian water transport accident involving military watercraft (V94.81-)
> military watercraft accident in military or war operations (Y36, Y37.-)

> *EXCLUDES2*   drowning and submersion due to accident to watercraft (V90.-)

The appropriate 7th character is to be added to each code from category V91

A = initial encounter

D = subsequent encounter

S = sequela

🄯 **V91.0 Burn due to watercraft on fire**

> *EXCLUDES1*   burn from localized fire or explosion on board ship without accident to watercraft (V93.-)

🅐 **V91.00 Burn due to merchant ship on fire**

🅐 **V91.01 Burn due to passenger ship on fire**

Burn due to Ferry-boat on fire

Burn due to Liner on fire

🅐 **V91.02 Burn due to fishing boat on fire**

🅐 **V91.03 Burn due to other powered watercraft on fire**

Burn due to Hovercraft (on open water) on fire

Burn due to Jet ski on fire

🅐 **V91.04 Burn due to sailboat on fire**

🅐 **V91.05 Burn due to canoe or kayak on fire**

🅐 **V91.06 Burn due to (nonpowered) inflatable craft on fire**

🅐 **V91.07 Burn due to water-skis on fire**

🅐 **V91.08 Burn due to other unpowered watercraft on fire**

🅐 **V91.09 Burn due to unspecified watercraft on fire**

Burn due to boat NOS on fire

Burn due to ship NOS on fire

Burn due to watercraft NOS on fire

🄯 **V91.1 Crushed between watercraft and other watercraft or other object due to collision**

Crushed by lifeboat after abandoning ship in a collision

> *NOTES*   select the specified type of watercraft that the victim was on at the time of the collision

🅐 **V91.10 Crushed between merchant ship and other watercraft or other object due to collision**

Unspecified Code   Other Specified Code   Ⓝ Newborn Age: 0   Ⓟ Pediatric Age: 0-17   Ⓜ Maternity Age: 12-55

Ⓐ Adult Age: 15-124   ♂ Male   ♀ Female   ● New Code   ▲ Revised Code Title   ►◄ Revised Text

V91.11 Crushed between passenger ship and other watercraft or other object due to collision

Crushed between Ferry-boat and other watercraft or other object due to collision

Crushed between Liner and other watercraft or other object due to collision

V91.12 Crushed between fishing boat and other watercraft or other object due to collision

V91.13 Crushed between other powered watercraft and other watercraft or other object due to collision

Crushed between Hovercraft (on open water) and other watercraft or other object due to collision

Crushed between Jet ski and other watercraft or other object due to collision

V91.14 Crushed between sailboat and other watercraft or other object due to collision

V91.15 Crushed between canoe or kayak and other watercraft or other object due to collision

V91.16 Crushed between (nonpowered) inflatable craft and other watercraft or other object due to collision

V91.18 Crushed between other unpowered watercraft and other watercraft or other object due to collision

Crushed between surfboard and other watercraft or other object due to collision

Crushed between windsurfer and other watercraft or other object due to collision

V91.19 Crushed between unspecified watercraft and other watercraft or other object due to collision

Crushed between boat NOS and other watercraft or other object due to collision

Crushed between ship NOS and other watercraft or other object due to collision

Crushed between watercraft NOS and other watercraft or other object due to collision

V91.2 Fall due to collision between watercraft and other watercraft or other object

Fall while remaining on watercraft after collision

NOTES select the specified type of watercraft that the victim was on at the time of the collision

EXCLUDES1 crushed between watercraft and other watercraft and other object due to collision (V91.1-) drowning and submersion due to falling from crushed watercraft (V90.3-)

V91.20 Fall due to collision between merchant ship and other watercraft or other object

V91.21 Fall due to collision between passenger ship and other watercraft or other object

Fall due to collision between Ferry-boat and other watercraft or other object

Fall due to collision between Liner and other watercraft or other object

V91.22 Fall due to collision between fishing boat and other watercraft or other object

V91.23 Fall due to collision between other powered watercraft and other watercraft or other object

Fall due to collision between Hovercraft (on open water) and other watercraft or other object

Fall due to collision between Jet ski and other watercraft or other object

V91.24 Fall due to collision between sailboat and other watercraft or other object

V91.25 Fall due to collision between canoe or kayak and other watercraft or other object

V91.26 Fall due to collision between (nonpowered) inflatable craft and other watercraft or other object

V91.29 Fall due to collision between unspecified watercraft and other watercraft or other object

Fall due to collision between boat NOS and other watercraft or other object

Fall due to collision between ship NOS and other watercraft or other object

Fall due to collision between watercraft NOS and other watercraft or other object

V91.3 Hit or struck by falling object due to accident to watercraft

Hit or struck by falling object (part of damaged watercraft or other object) after falling or jumping from damaged watercraft

EXCLUDES2 drowning or submersion due to fall or jumping from damaged watercraft (V90.2-, V90.3-)

V91.30 Hit or struck by falling object due to accident to merchant ship

V91.31 Hit or struck by falling object due to accident to passenger ship

Hit or struck by falling object due to accident to Ferry-boat

Hit or struck by falling object due to accident to Liner

V91.32 Hit or struck by falling object due to accident to fishing boat

V91.33 Hit or struck by falling object due to accident to other powered watercraft

Hit or struck by falling object due to accident to Hovercraft (on open water)

Hit or struck by falling object due to accident to Jet ski

V91.34 Hit or struck by falling object due to accident to sailboat

V91.35 Hit or struck by falling object due to accident to canoe or kayak

V91.36 Hit or struck by falling object due to accident to (nonpowered) inflatable craft

V91.37 Hit or struck by falling object due to accident to water-skis

Hit by water-skis after jumping off of waterskis

V91.38 Hit or struck by falling object due to accident to other unpowered watercraft

Hit or struck by surf-board after falling off damaged surf-board

Hit or struck by object after falling off damaged windsurfer

V91.39 Hit or struck by falling object due to accident to unspecified watercraft

Hit or struck by falling object due to accident to boat NOS

Hit or struck by falling object due to accident to ship NOS

Hit or struck by falling object due to accident to watercraft NOS

V91.8 Other injury due to other accident to watercraft

V91.80 Other injury due to other accident to merchant ship

V91.81 Other injury due to other accident to passenger ship

Other injury due to other accident to Ferry-boat

Other injury due to other accident to Liner

V91.82 Other injury due to other accident to fishing boat

V91.83 Other injury due to other accident to other powered watercraft

Other injury due to other accident to Hovercraft (on open water)

Other injury due to other accident to Jet ski

V91.84 Other injury due to other accident to sailboat

V91.85 Other injury due to other accident to canoe or kayak

4ᵗʰ character required   5ᵗʰ character required   6ᵗʰ character required   7ᵗʰ character required   Extension 'X' Alert

EXCLUDES 1 Not coded here   *EXCLUDES 2* Not included here   PDx Primary Diagnosis Only   Manifestation Code

[7th] **V91.86 Other injury due to other accident to (nonpowered) inflatable craft**

[7th] **V91.87 Other injury due to other accident to water-skis**

[7th] **V91.88 Other injury due to other accident to other unpowered watercraft**

Other injury due to other accident to surf-board
Other injury due to other accident to windsurfer

[7th] **V91.89 Other injury due to other accident to unspecified watercraft**

Other injury due to other accident to boat NOS
Other injury due to other accident to ship NOS
Other injury due to other accident to watercraft NOS

[4] **V92 Drowning and submersion due to accident on board watercraft, without accident to watercraft**

[EXCLUDES1] *civilian water transport accident involving military watercraft (V94.81-)*
drowning or submersion due to accident to watercraft (V90-V91)
drowning or submersion of diver who voluntarily jumps from boat not involved in an accident (W16.711, W16.721)
fall into water without watercraft (W16.-)
military watercraft accident in military or war operations (Y36, Y37)

The appropriate 7th character is to be added to each code from category V92
A = initial encounter
D = subsequent encounter
S = sequela

[5] **V92.0 Drowning and submersion due to fall off watercraft**

Drowning and submersion due to fall from gangplank of watercraft
Drowning and submersion due to fall overboard watercraft

[EXCLUDES2] *hitting head on object or bottom of body of water due to fall from watercraft (V94.0-)*

[7th] **V92.00 Drowning and submersion due to fall off merchant ship**

[7th] **V92.01 Drowning and submersion due to fall off passenger ship**

Drowning and submersion due to fall off Ferry-boat
Drowning and submersion due to fall off Liner

[7th] **V92.02 Drowning and submersion due to fall off fishing boat**

[7th] **V92.03 Drowning and submersion due to fall off other powered watercraft**

Drowning and submersion due to fall off Hovercraft (on open water)
Drowning and submersion due to fall off Jet ski

[7th] **V92.04 Drowning and submersion due to fall off sailboat**

[7th] **V92.05 Drowning and submersion due to fall off canoe or kayak**

[7th] **V92.06 Drowning and submersion due to fall off (nonpowered) inflatable craft**

[7th] **V92.07 Drowning and submersion due to fall off water-skis**

[EXCLUDES1] *drowning and submersion due to falling off burning water-skis (V90.27)*
drowning and submersion due to falling off crushed water-skis (V90.37)
hit by boat while water-skiing NOS (V94.X)

[7th] **V92.08 Drowning and submersion due to fall off other unpowered watercraft**

Drowning and submersion due to fall off surf-board
Drowning and submersion due to fall off windsurfer

[EXCLUDES1] *drowning and submersion due to fall off burning unpowered watercraft (V90.28)*
drowning and submersion due to fall off crushed unpowered watercraft (V90.38)
drowning and submersion due to fall off damaged unpowered watercraft (V90.88)
drowning and submersion due to rider of nonpowered watercraft being hit by other watercraft (V94.-)
other injury due to rider of nonpowered watercraft being hit by other watercraft (V94.-)

[7th] **V92.09 Drowning and submersion due to fall off unspecified watercraft**

Drowning and submersion due to fall off boat NOS
Drowning and submersion due to fall off ship
Drowning and submersion due to fall off watercraft NOS

[5] **V92.1 Drowning and submersion due to being thrown overboard by motion of watercraft**

[EXCLUDES1] *drowning and submersion due to fall off surf-board (V92.08)*
drowning and submersion due to fall off water-skis (V92.07)
drowning and submersion due to fall off windsurfer (V92.08)

[7th] **V92.10 Drowning and submersion due to being thrown overboard by motion of merchant ship**

[7th] **V92.11 Drowning and submersion due to being thrown overboard by motion of passenger ship**

Drowning and submersion due to being thrown overboard by motion of Ferry-boat
Drowning and submersion due to being thrown overboard by motion of Liner

[7th] **V92.12 Drowning and submersion due to being thrown overboard by motion of fishing boat**

[7th] **V92.13 Drowning and submersion due to being thrown overboard by motion of other powered watercraft**

Drowning and submersion due to being thrown overboard by motion of Hovercraft

[7th] **V92.14 Drowning and submersion due to being thrown overboard by motion of sailboat**

[7th] **V92.15 Drowning and submersion due to being thrown overboard by motion of canoe or kayak**

[7th] **V92.16 Drowning and submersion due to being thrown overboard by motion of (nonpowered) inflatable craft**

[7th] **V92.19 Drowning and submersion due to being thrown overboard by motion of unspecified watercraft**

Drowning and submersion due to being thrown overboard by motion of boat NOS
Drowning and submersion due to being thrown overboard by motion of ship NOS
Drowning and submersion due to being thrown overboard by motion of watercraft NOS

[5] **V92.2 Drowning and submersion due to being washed overboard from watercraft**

Code first any associated cataclysm (X37.0-)

[7th] **V92.20 Drowning and submersion due to being washed overboard from merchant ship**

[7th] **V92.21 Drowning and submersion due to being washed overboard from passenger ship**

Drowning and submersion due to being washed overboard from Ferry-boat
Drowning and submersion due to being washed overboard from Liner

[7th] **V92.22 Drowning and submersion due to being washed overboard from fishing boat**

[7th] **V92.23 Drowning and submersion due to being washed overboard from other powered watercraft**

Drowning and submersion due to being washed overboard from Hovercraft (on open water)
Drowning and submersion due to being washed overboard from Jet ski

V92.24 Drowning and submersion due to being washed overboard from sailboat

V92.25 Drowning and submersion due to being washed overboard from canoe or kayak

V92.26 Drowning and submersion due to being washed overboard from (nonpowered) inflatable craft

V92.27 Drowning and submersion due to being washed overboard from water-skis

> EXCLUDES1 drowning and submersion due to fall off water-skis (V92.07)

V92.28 Drowning and submersion due to being washed overboard from other unpowered watercraft

Drowning and submersion due to being washed overboard from surf-board

Drowning and submersion due to being washed overboard from windsurfer

V92.29 Drowning and submersion due to being washed overboard from unspecified watercraft

Drowning and submersion due to being washed overboard from boat NOS

Drowning and submersion due to being washed overboard from ship NOS

Drowning and submersion due to being washed overboard from watercraft NOS

V93 Other injury due to accident on board watercraft, without accident to watercraft

> EXCLUDES1 civilian water transport accident involving military watercraft (V94.81-)
> other injury due to accident to watercraft (V91.-)
> military watercraft accident in military or war operations (Y36, Y37.-)
> EXCLUDES2 drowning and submersion due to accident on board watercraft, without accident to watercraft (V92.-)

The appropriate 7th character is to be added to each code from category V93

A = initial encounter
D = subsequent encounter
S = sequela

V93.0 Burn due to localized fire on board watercraft

> EXCLUDES1 burn due to watercraft on fire (V91.0-)

V93.00 Burn due to localized fire on board merchant vessel

V93.01 Burn due to localized fire on board passenger vessel

Burn due to localized fire on board Ferry-boat
Burn due to localized fire on board Liner

V93.02 Burn due to localized fire on board fishing boat

V93.03 Burn due to localized fire on board other powered watercraft

Burn due to localized fire on board Hovercraft
Burn due to localized fire on board Jet ski

V93.04 Burn due to localized fire on board sailboat

V93.09 Burn due to localized fire on board unspecified watercraft

Burn due to localized fire on board boat NOS
Burn due to localized fire on board ship NOS
Burn due to localized fire on board watercraft NOS

V93.1 Other burn on board watercraft

Burn due to source other than fire on board watercraft

> EXCLUDES1 burn due to watercraft on fire (V91.0-)

V93.10 Other burn on board merchant vessel

V93.11 Other burn on board passenger vessel

Other burn on board Ferry-boat
Other burn on board Liner

V93.12 Other burn on board fishing boat

V93.13 Other burn on board other powered watercraft

Other burn on board Hovercraft
Other burn on board Jet ski

V93.14 Other burn on board sailboat

V93.19 Other burn on board unspecified watercraft

Other burn on board boat NOS
Other burn on board ship NOS
Other burn on board watercraft NOS

V93.2 Heat exposure on board watercraft

> EXCLUDES1 exposure to man-made heat not aboard watercraft (W92)
> exposure to natural heat while on board watercraft (X30)
> exposure to sunlight while on board watercraft (X32)
> EXCLUDES2 burn due to fire on board watercraft (V93.0-)

V93.20 Heat exposure on board merchant ship

V93.21 Heat exposure on board passenger ship

Heat exposure on board Ferry-boat
Heat exposure on board Liner

V93.22 Heat exposure on board fishing boat

V93.23 Heat exposure on board other powered watercraft

Heat exposure on board hovercraft

V93.24 Heat exposure on board sailboat

V93.29 Heat exposure on board unspecified watercraft

Heat exposure on board boat NOS
Heat exposure on board ship NOS
Heat exposure on board watercraft NOS

V93.3 Fall on board watercraft

> EXCLUDES1 fall due to collision of watercraft (V91.2-)

V93.30 Fall on board merchant ship

V93.31 Fall on board passenger ship

Fall on board Ferry-boat
Fall on board Liner

V93.32 Fall on board fishing boat

V93.33 Fall on board other powered watercraft

Fall on board Hovercraft (on open water)
Fall on board Jet ski

V93.34 Fall on board sailboat

V93.35 Fall on board canoe or kayak

V93.36 Fall on board (nonpowered) inflatable craft

V93.38 Fall on board other unpowered watercraft

V93.39 Fall on board unspecified watercraft

Fall on board boat NOS
Fall on board ship NOS
Fall on board watercraft NOS

V93.4 Struck by falling object on board watercraft

Hit by falling object on board watercraft

> EXCLUDES1 struck by falling object due to accident to watercraft (V91.3)

V93.40 Struck by falling object on merchant ship

V93.41 Struck by falling object on passenger ship

Struck by falling object on Ferry-boat
Struck by falling object on Liner

V93.42 Struck by falling object on fishing boat

V93.43 Struck by falling object on other powered watercraft

Struck by falling object on Hovercraft

V93.44 Struck by falling object on sailboat

V93.48 Struck by falling object on other unpowered watercraft

V93.49 Struck by falling object on unspecified watercraft

4th character required 5th character required 6th character required 7th character required Extension 'X' Alert
EXCLUDES 1 Not coded here EXCLUDES 2 Not included here PDx Primary Diagnosis Only Manifestation Code

772 ICD-10-CM 2015

[5] **V93.5 Explosion on board watercraft**
Boiler explosion on steamship
[EXCLUDES2] *fire on board watercraft (V93.0-)*
[7th] **V93.50 Explosion on board merchant ship**
[7th] **V93.51 Explosion on board passenger ship**
Explosion on board Ferry-boat
Explosion on board Liner
[7th] **V93.52 Explosion on board fishing boat**
[7th] **V93.53 Explosion on board other powered watercraft**
Explosion on board Hovercraft
Explosion on board Jet ski
[7th] **V93.54 Explosion on board sailboat**
[7th] **V93.59 Explosion on board unspecified watercraft**
Explosion on board boat NOS
Explosion on board ship NOS
Explosion on board watercraft NOS
[5] **V93.6 Machinery accident on board watercraft**
[EXCLUDES1] *machinery explosion on board watercraft (V93.4-)*
machinery fire on board watercraft (V93.0-)
[7th] **V93.60 Machinery accident on board merchant ship**
[7th] **V93.61 Machinery accident on board passenger ship**
Machinery accident on board Ferry-boat
Machinery accident on board Liner
[7th] **V93.62 Machinery accident on board fishing boat**
[7th] **V93.63 Machinery accident on board other powered watercraft**
Machinery accident on board Hovercraft
[7th] **V93.64 Machinery accident on board sailboat**
[7th] **V93.69 Machinery accident on board unspecified watercraft**
Machinery accident on board boat NOS
Machinery accident on board ship NOS
Machinery accident on board watercraft NOS
[5] **V93.8 Other injury due to other accident on board watercraft**
Accidental poisoning by gases or fumes on watercraft
[7th] **V93.80 Other injury due to other accident on board merchant ship**
[7th] **V93.81 Other injury due to other accident on board passenger ship**
Other injury due to other accident on board Ferry-boat
Other injury due to other accident on board Liner
[7th] **V93.82 Other injury due to other accident on board fishing boat**
[7th] **V93.83 Other injury due to other accident on board other powered watercraft**
Other injury due to other accident on board Hovercraft
Other injury due to other accident on board Jet ski
[7th] **V93.84 Other injury due to other accident on board sailboat**
[7th] **V93.85 Other injury due to other accident on board canoe or kayak**
[7th] **V93.86 Other injury due to other accident on board (nonpowered) inflatable craft**
[7th] **V93.87 Other injury due to other accident on board water-skis**
Hit or struck by object while waterskiing
[7th] **V93.88 Other injury due to other accident on board other unpowered watercraft**
Hit or struck by object while surfing
Hit or struck by object while on board windsurfer
[7th] **V93.89 Other injury due to other accident on board unspecified watercraft**
Other injury due to other accident on board boat NOS
Other injury due to other accident on board ship NOS
Other injury due to other accident on board watercraft NOS

[4] **V94 Other and unspecified water transport accidents**
[EXCLUDES1] *military watercraft accidents in military or war operations (Y36, Y37)*

The appropriate 7th character is to be added to each code from category V94
A = initial encounter
D = subsequent encounter
S = sequela

[7th] **V94.0 Hitting object or bottom of body of water due to fall from watercraft**
[EXCLUDES2] *drowning and submersion due to fall from watercraft (V92.0-)*
[5] **V94.1 Bather struck by watercraft**
Swimmer hit by watercraft
[7th] **V94.11 Bather struck by powered watercraft**
[7th] **V94.12 Bather struck by nonpowered watercraft**
[5] **V94.2 Rider of nonpowered watercraft struck by other watercraft**
[7th] **V94.21 Rider of nonpowered watercraft struck by other nonpowered watercraft**
Canoer hit by other nonpowered watercraft
Surfer hit by other nonpowered watercraft
Windsurfer hit by other nonpowered watercraft
[7th] **V94.22 Rider of nonpowered watercraft struck by powered watercraft**
Canoer hit by motorboat
Surfer hit by motorboat
Windsurfer hit by motorboat
[5] **V94.3 Injury to rider of (inflatable) watercraft being pulled behind other watercraft**
[7th] **V94.31 Injury to rider of (inflatable) recreational watercraft being pulled behind other watercraft**
Injury to rider of inner-tube pulled behind motor boat
[7th] **V94.32 Injury to rider of non-recreational watercraft being pulled behind other watercraft**
Injury to occupant of dingy being pulled behind boat or ship
Injury to occupant of life-raft being pulled behind boat or ship
[7th] **V94.4 Injury to barefoot water-skier**
Injury to person being pulled behind boat or ship
[5] **V94.8 Other water transport accident**
[6] **V94.81 Water transport accident involving military watercraft**
[7] **V94.810 Civilian watercraft involved in water transport accident with military watercraft**
Passenger on civilian watercraft injured due to accident with military watercraft
[7] **V94.811 Civilian in water injured by military watercraft**
[7] **V94.818 Other water transport accident involving military watercraft**
[7th] **V94.89 Other water transport accident**
[7th] **V94.9 Unspecified water transport accident**
Water transport accident NOS

Unspecified Code | Other Specified Code | [N] Newborn Age: 0 | [P] Pediatric Age: 0-17 | [M] Maternity Age: 12-55
[A] Adult Age: 15-124 | ♂ Male | ♀ Female | ● New Code | ▲ Revised Code Title | ►◄ Revised Text

Air and space transport accidents (V95-V97)

EXCLUDES1 *military aircraft accidents in military or war operations (Y36, Y37)*

④ **V95** **Accident to** powered aircraft **causing injury to occupant**

The appropriate 7th character is to be added to each code from category V95

A = initial encounter
D = subsequent encounter
S = sequela

⑤ **V95.0** Helicopter **accident injuring occupant**
⑥ **V95.00** **Unspecified helicopter accident injuring occupant**
⑦ **V95.01** **Helicopter** crash **injuring occupant**
⑦ **V95.02** Forced landing **of helicopter injuring occupant**
⑦ **V95.03** **Helicopter** collision **injuring occupant**
   Helicopter collision with any object, fixed, movable or moving
⑦ **V95.04** **Helicopter** fire **injuring occupant**
⑦ **V95.05** **Helicopter** explosion **injuring occupant**
⑦ **V95.09** Other **helicopter accident injuring occupant**

⑤ **V95.1** Ultralight, microlight or powered-glider **accident injuring occupant**
⑥ **V95.10** **Unspecified ultralight, microlight or powered-glider accident injuring occupant**
⑦ **V95.11** **Ultralight, microlight or powered-glider** crash **injuring occupant**
⑦ **V95.12** Forced landing **of ultralight, microlight or powered-glider injuring occupant**
⑦ **V95.13** **Ultralight, microlight or powered-glider** collision **injuring occupant**
   Ultralight, microlight or powered-glider collision with any object, fixed, movable or moving
⑦ **V95.14** **Ultralight, microlight or powered-glider** fire **injuring occupant**
⑦ **V95.15** **Ultralight, microlight or powered-glider** explosion **injuring occupant**
⑦ **V95.19** Other **ultralight, microlight or powered-glider accident injuring occupant**

⑤ **V95.2** Other private fixed-wing aircraft **accident injuring occupant**
⑦ **V95.20** **Unspecified accident to other private fixed-wing aircraft, injuring occupant**
⑦ **V95.21** **Other private fixed-wing aircraft** crash **injuring occupant**
⑦ **V95.22** Forced landing **of other private fixed-wing aircraft injuring occupant**
⑦ **V95.23** **Other private fixed-wing aircraft** collision **injuring occupant**
   Other private fixed-wing aircraft collision with any object, fixed, movable or moving
⑦ **V95.24** **Other private fixed-wing aircraft** fire **injuring occupant**
⑦ **V95.25** **Other private fixed-wing aircraft** explosion **injuring occupant**
⑦ **V95.29** Other **accident to other private fixed-wing aircraft injuring occupant**

⑤ **V95.3** Commercial fixed-wing aircraft **accident injuring occupant**
⑦ **V95.30** **Unspecified accident to commercial fixed-wing aircraft injuring occupant**
⑦ **V95.31** **Commercial fixed-wing aircraft** crash **injuring occupant**
⑦ **V95.32** Forced landing **of commercial fixed-wing aircraft injuring occupant**
⑦ **V95.33** **Commercial fixed-wing aircraft** collision **injuring occupant**
   Commercial fixed-wing aircraft collision with any object, fixed, moving

⑦ **V95.34** **Commercial fixed-wing aircraft** fire **injuring occupant**
⑦ **V95.35** **Commercial fixed-wing aircraft** explosion **injuring occupant**
⑦ **V95.39** Other **accident to commercial fixed-wing aircraft injuring occupant**

⑤ **V95.4** Spacecraft **accident injuring occupant**
⑦ **V95.40** **Unspecified spacecraft accident injuring occupant**
⑦ **V95.41** **Spacecraft** crash **injuring occupant**
⑦ **V95.42** Forced landing **of spacecraft injuring occupant**
⑦ **V95.43** **Spacecraft** collision **injuring occupant**
   Spacecraft collision with any object, fixed, moveable or moving
⑦ **V95.44** **Spacecraft** fire **injuring occupant**
⑦ **V95.45** **Spacecraft** explosion **injuring occupant**
⑦ **V95.49** Other **spacecraft accident injuring occupant**
⑦ **V95.8** **Other powered aircraft accidents injuring occupant**
⑦ **V95.9** **Unspecified aircraft accident injuring occupant**
   Aircraft accident NOS
   Air transport accident NOS

④ **V96** **Accident to** nonpowered aircraft **causing injury to occupant**

The appropriate 7th character is to be added to each code from category V96

A = initial encounter
D = subsequent encounter
S = sequela

⑤ **V96.0** Balloon **accident injuring occupant**
⑦ **V96.00** **Unspecified balloon accident injuring occupant**
⑦ **V96.01** **Balloon** crash **injuring occupant**
⑦ **V96.02** Forced landing **of balloon injuring occupant**
⑦ **V96.03** **Balloon** collision **injuring occupant**
   Balloon collision with any object, fixed, moveable or moving
⑦ **V96.04** **Balloon** fire **injuring occupant**
⑦ **V96.05** **Balloon** explosion **injuring occupant**
⑦ **V96.09** **Other balloon accident injuring occupant**

⑤ **V96.1** Hang-glider **accident injuring occupant**
⑦ **V96.10** **Unspecified hang-glider accident injuring occupant**
⑦ **V96.11** **Hang-glider** crash **injuring occupant**
⑦ **V96.12** Forced landing **of hang-glider injuring occupant**
⑦ **V96.13** **Hang-glider** collision **injuring occupant**
   Hang-glider collision with any object, fixed, moveable or moving
⑦ **V96.14** **Hang-glider** fire **injuring occupant**
⑦ **V96.15** **Hang-glider** explosion **injuring occupant**
⑦ **V96.19** **Other hang-glider accident injuring occupant**

⑤ **V96.2** Glider (nonpowered) **accident injuring occupant**
⑦ **V96.20** **Unspecified glider (nonpowered) accident injuring occupant**
⑦ **V96.21** **Glider (nonpowered)** crash **injuring occupant**
⑦ **V96.22** Forced landing **of glider (nonpowered) injuring occupant**
⑦ **V96.23** **Glider (nonpowered)** collision **injuring occupant**
   Glider (nonpowered) collision with any object, fixed, moveable or moving
⑦ **V96.24** **Glider (nonpowered)** fire **injuring occupant**
⑦ **V96.25** **Glider (nonpowered)** explosion **injuring occupant**
⑦ **V96.29** **Other glider (nonpowered) accident injuring occupant**

⑦ **V96.8** **Other nonpowered-aircraft accidents injuring occupant**
   Kite carrying a person accident injuring occupant
⑦ **V96.9** **Unspecified nonpowered-aircraft accident injuring occupant**
   Nonpowered-aircraft accident NOS

---

④ 4th character required   ⑤ 5th character required   ⑥ 6th character required   ⑦ 7th character required   ⑦ Extension 'X' Alert

EXCLUDES 1 Not coded here   *EXCLUDES 2* Not included here   PDx Primary Diagnosis Only   Manifestation Code

🔵 **V97** Other specified air transport accidents
The appropriate 7th character is to be added to each code from category V97
A = initial encounter
D = subsequent encounter
S = sequela

V97.0 Occupant of aircraft injured in other specified air transport accidents

Fall in, on or from aircraft in air transport accident

EXCLUDES1 accident while boarding or alighting aircraft (V97.1)

V97.1 Person injured while boarding or alighting from aircraft

🔵 **V97.2** Parachutist accident

V97.21 Parachutist entangled in object
Parachutist landing in tree

V97.22 Parachutist injured on landing

V97.29 Other parachutist accident

🔵 **V97.3** Person on ground injured in air transport accident

V97.31 Hit by object falling from aircraft
Hit by crashing aircraft
Injured by aircraft hitting house
Injured by aircraft hitting car

V97.32 Injured by rotating propeller

V97.33 Sucked into jet engine

V97.39 Other injury to person on ground due to air transport accident

🔵 **V97.8** Other air transport accidents, not elsewhere classified

EXCLUDES1 aircraft accident NOS (V95.9)
exposure to changes in air pressure during ascent or descent (W94.-)

🔵 **V97.81** Air transport accident involving military aircraft

V97.810 Civilian aircraft involved in air transport accident with military aircraft
Passenger in civilian aircraft injured due to accident with military aircraft

V97.811 Civilian injured by military aircraft

V97.818 Other air transport accident involving military aircraft

V97.89 Other air transport accidents, not elsewhere classified
Injury from machinery on aircraft

Other and unspecified transport accidents (V98-V99)

EXCLUDES1 vehicle accident, type of vehicle unspecified (V89.-)

🔵 **V98** Other specified transport accidents
The appropriate 7th character is to be added to each code from category V98
A = initial encounter
D = subsequent encounter
S = sequela

V98.0 Accident to, on or involving cable-car, not on rails
Caught or dragged by cable-car, not on rails
Fall or jump from cable-car, not on rails
Object thrown from or in cable-car, not on rails

V98.1 Accident to, on or involving land-yacht

V98.2 Accident to, on or involving ice yacht

V98.3 Accident to, on or involving ski lift
Accident to, on or involving ski chair-lift
Accident to, on or involving ski-lift with gondola

V98.8 Other specified transport accidents

V99 Unspecified transport accident
The appropriate 7th character is to be added to code V99
A = initial encounter
D = subsequent encounter
S = sequela

Other external causes of accidental injury (W00-X58)

Slipping, tripping, stumbling and falls (W00-W19)

EXCLUDES1 assault involving a fall (Y01-Y02)
fall from animal (V80.-)
fall from machinery (in operation) (W28-W31)
fall from transport vehicle (V01-V99)
intentional self-harm involving a fall (X80-X81)

EXCLUDES2 at risk for fall (history of fall) Z91.81
fall (in) (from) burning building (X00.-)
fall into fire (X00-X04, X08-X09)

🔵 **W00** Fall due to ice and snow

INCLUDES pedestrian on foot falling (slipping) on ice and snow

EXCLUDES1 fall on (from) ice and snow involving pedestrian conveyance (V00.-)
fall from stairs and steps not due to ice and snow (W10.-)

The appropriate 7th character is to be added to each code from category W00
A = initial encounter
D = subsequent encounter
S = sequela

W00.0 Fall on same level due to ice and snow

W00.1 Fall from stairs and steps due to ice and snow

W00.2 Other fall from one level to another due to ice and snow

W00.9 Unspecified fall due to ice and snow

🔵 **W01** Fall on same level from slipping, tripping and stumbling

INCLUDES fall on moving sidewalk

EXCLUDES1 fall due to bumping (striking) against object (W18.0-)
fall in shower or bathtub (W18.2-)
fall on same level NOS (W18.30)
fall on same level from slipping, tripping and stumbling due to ice or snow (W00.0)
fall off or from toilet (W18.1-)
slipping, tripping and stumbling NOS (W18.40)
slipping, tripping and stumbling without falling (W18.4-)

The appropriate 7th character is to be added to each code from category W01
A = initial encounter
D = subsequent encounter
S = sequela

W01.0 Fall on same level from slipping, tripping and stumbling without subsequent striking against object
Falling over animal

🔵 **W01.1** Fall on same level from slipping, tripping and stumbling with subsequent striking against object

W01.10 Fall on same level from slipping, tripping and stumbling with subsequent striking against unspecified object

🔵 **W01.11** Fall on same level from slipping, tripping and stumbling with subsequent striking against sharp object

W01.110 Fall on same level from slipping, tripping and stumbling with subsequent striking against sharp glass

W01.111 Fall on same level from slipping, tripping and stumbling with subsequent striking against power tool or machine

W01.118 Fall on same level from slipping, tripping and stumbling with subsequent striking against other sharp object

---

| Unspecified Code | Other Specified Code | N Newborn Age: 0 | P Pediatric Age: 0-17 | M Maternity Age: 12-55 |
| A Adult Age: 15-124 | ♂ Male | ♀ Female | ● New Code | ▲ Revised Code Title | ►◄ Revised Text |

[7] W01.119 Fall on same level from slipping, tripping and stumbling with subsequent striking against unspecified sharp object

[6] W01.19 Fall on same level from slipping, tripping and stumbling with subsequent striking against other object

[7] W01.190 Fall on same level from slipping, tripping and stumbling with subsequent striking against furniture

[7] W01.198 Fall on same level from slipping, tripping and stumbling with subsequent striking against other object

[7] W03 Other fall on same level due to collision with another person

Fall due to non-transport collision with other person

EXCLUDES1 *collision with another person without fall (W51)*
crushed or pushed by a crowd or human stampede (W52)
fall involving pedestrian conveyance (V00-V09)
fall due to ice or snow (W00)
fall on same level NOS (W18.30)

The appropriate 7th character is to be added to code W03
A = initial encounter
D = subsequent encounter
S = sequela

[7] W04 Fall while being carried or supported by other persons

Accidentally dropped while being carried

The appropriate 7th character is to be added to code W04
A = initial encounter
D = subsequent encounter
S = sequela

[4] W05 Fall from non-moving wheelchair, nonmotorized scooter and motorized mobility scooter

EXCLUDES1 *fall from moving wheelchair (powered) (V00.811)*
fall from moving motorized mobility scooter (V00.831)
fall from nonmotorized scooter (V00.141)

The appropriate 7th character is to be added to each code from category W05
A = initial encounter
D = subsequent encounter
S = sequela

[7x] W05.0 Fall from non-moving wheelchair
[7x] W05.1 Fall from non-moving nonmotorized scooter
[7x] W05.2 Fall from non-moving motorized mobility scooter

[7] W06 Fall from bed

The appropriate 7th character is to be added to code W06
A = initial encounter
D = subsequent encounter
S = sequela

[7] W07 Fall from chair

The appropriate 7th character is to be added to code W07
A = initial encounter
D = subsequent encounter
S = sequela

[7] W08 Fall from other furniture

The appropriate 7th character is to be added to code W08
A = initial encounter
D = subsequent encounter
S = sequela

[4] W09 Fall on and from playground equipment

EXCLUDES1 *fall involving recreational machinery (W31)*

The appropriate 7th character is to be added to each code from category W09
A = initial encounter
D = subsequent encounter
S = sequela

[7x] W09.0 Fall on or from playground slide
[7x] W09.1 Fall from playground swing
[7x] W09.2 Fall on or from jungle gym
[7x] W09.8 Fall on or from other playground equipment

[4] W10 Fall on and from stairs and steps

EXCLUDES1 *Fall from stairs and steps due to ice and snow (W00.1)*

The appropriate 7th character is to be added to each code from category W10
A = initial encounter
D = subsequent encounter
S = sequela

[7x] W10.0 Fall (on)(from) escalator
[7x] W10.1 Fall (on)(from) sidewalk curb
[7x] W10.2 Fall (on)(from) incline

Fall (on) (from) ramp

[7x] W10.8 Fall (on) (from) other stairs and steps
[7x] W10.9 Fall (on) (from) unspecified stairs and steps

[7] W11 Fall on and from ladder

The appropriate 7th character is to be added to code W11
A = initial encounter
D = subsequent encounter
S = sequela

[7] W12 Fall on and from scaffolding

The appropriate 7th character is to be added to code W12
A = initial encounter
D = subsequent encounter
S = sequela

[4] W13 Fall from, out of or through building or structure

The appropriate 7th character is to be added to each code from category W13
A = initial encounter
D = subsequent encounter
S = sequela

[7x] W13.0 Fall from, out of or through balcony

Fall from, out of or through railing

[7x] W13.1 Fall from, out of or through bridge
[7x] W13.2 Fall from, out of or through roof
[7x] W13.3 Fall through floor
[7x] W13.4 Fall from, out of or through window

EXCLUDES2 *fall with subsequent striking against sharp glass (W01.110)*

[7x] W13.8 Fall from, out of or through other building or structure

Fall from, out of or through viaduct
Fall from, out of or through wall
Fall from, out of or through flag-pole

[7x] W13.9 Fall from, out of or through building, not otherwise specified

EXCLUDES1 *collapse of a building or structure (W20.-)*
fall or jump from burning building or structure (X00.-)

[7] W14 Fall from tree

The appropriate 7th character is to be added to code W14
A = initial encounter
D = subsequent encounter
S = sequela

[7] W15 Fall from cliff

The appropriate 7th character is to be added to code W15
A = initial encounter
D = subsequent encounter
S = sequela

[4] 4th character required [5] 5th character required [6] 6th character required [7] 7th character required [7x] Extension 'X' Alert
EXCLUDES1 Not coded here EXCLUDES2 Not included here [PDx] Primary Diagnosis Only Manifestation Code

[4] **W16 Fall, jump or diving into water**

[EXCLUDES1] *accidental non-watercraft drowning and submersion not involving fall (W65-W74)*
effects of air pressure from diving (W94.-)
fall into water from watercraft (V90-V94)
hitting an object or against bottom when falling from watercraft (V94.0)

[EXCLUDES2] *striking or hitting diving board (W21.4)*

The appropriate 7th character is to be added to each code from category W16
A = initial encounter
D = subsequent encounter
S = sequela

[5] **W16.0 Fall into swimming pool**
Fall into swimming pool NOS
[EXCLUDES1] *fall into empty swimming pool (W17.3)*

[6] **W16.01 Fall into swimming pool striking water surface**

[7] **W16.011 Fall into swimming pool striking water surface causing drowning and submersion**
[EXCLUDES1] *drowning and submersion while in swimming pool without fall (W67)*

[7] **W16.012 Fall into swimming pool striking water surface causing other injury**

[6] **W16.02 Fall into swimming pool striking bottom**

[7] **W16.021 Fall into swimming pool striking bottom causing drowning and submersion**
[EXCLUDES1] *drowning and submersion while in swimming pool without fall (W67)*

[7] **W16.022 Fall into swimming pool striking bottom causing other injury**

[6] **W16.03 Fall into swimming pool striking wall**

[7] **W16.031 Fall into swimming pool striking wall causing drowning and submersion**
[EXCLUDES1] *drowning and submersion while in swimming pool without fall (W67)*

[7] **W16.032 Fall into swimming pool striking wall causing other injury**

[5] **W16.1 Fall into natural body of water**
Fall into lake
Fall into open sea
Fall into river
Fall into stream

[6] **W16.11 Fall into natural body of water striking water surface**

[7] **W16.111 Fall into natural body of water striking water surface causing drowning and submersion**
[EXCLUDES1] *drowning and submersion while in natural body of water without fall (W69)*

[7] **W16.112 Fall into natural body of water striking water surface causing other injury**

[6] **W16.12 Fall into natural body of water striking bottom**

[7] **W16.121 Fall into natural body of water striking bottom causing drowning and submersion**
[EXCLUDES1] *drowning and submersion while in natural body of water without fall (W69)*

[7] **W16.122 Fall into natural body of water striking bottom causing other injury**

[6] **W16.13 Fall into natural body of water striking side**

[7] **W16.131 Fall into natural body of water striking side causing drowning and submersion**
[EXCLUDES1] *drowning and submersion while in natural body of water without fall (W69)*

[7] **W16.132 Fall into natural body of water striking side causing other injury**

[5] **W16.2 Fall in (into) filled bathtub or bucket of water**

[6] **W16.21 Fall in (into) filled bathtub**
[EXCLUDES1] *fall into empty bathtub (W18.2)*

[7] **W16.211 Fall in (into) filled bathtub causing drowning and submersion**
[EXCLUDES1] *drowning and submersion while in filled bathtub without fall (W65)*

[7] **W16.212 Fall in (into) filled bathtub causing other injury**

[6] **W16.22 Fall in (into) bucket of water**

[7] **W16.221 Fall in (into) bucket of water causing drowning and submersion**

[7] **W16.222 Fall in (into) bucket of water causing other injury**

[5] **W16.3 Fall into other water**
Fall into fountain
Fall into reservoir

[6] **W16.31 Fall into other water striking water surface**

[7] **W16.311 Fall into other water striking water surface causing drowning and submersion**
[EXCLUDES1] *drowning and submersion while in other water without fall (W73)*

[7] **W16.312 Fall into other water striking water surface causing other injury**

[6] **W16.32 Fall into other water striking bottom**

[7] **W16.321 Fall into other water striking bottom causing drowning and submersion**
[EXCLUDES1] *drowning and submersion while in other water without fall (W73)*

[7] **W16.322 Fall into other water striking bottom causing other injury**

[6] **W16.33 Fall into other water striking wall**

[7] **W16.331 Fall into other water striking wall causing drowning and submersion**
[EXCLUDES1] *drowning and submersion while in other water without fall (W73)*

[7] **W16.332 Fall into other water striking wall causing other injury**

[5] **W16.4 Fall into unspecified water**

[7th] **W16.41 Fall into unspecified water causing drowning and submersion**

[7th] **W16.42 Fall into unspecified water causing other injury**

[5] **W16.5 Jumping or diving into swimming pool**

[6] **W16.51 Jumping or diving into swimming pool striking water surface**

[7] **W16.511 Jumping or diving into swimming pool striking water surface causing drowning and submersion**
[EXCLUDES1] *drowning and submersion while in swimming pool without jumping or diving (W67)*

[7] **W16.512 Jumping or diving into swimming pool striking water surface causing other injury**

[6] **W16.52 Jumping or diving into swimming pool striking bottom**

[7] **W16.521 Jumping or diving into swimming pool striking bottom causing drowning and submersion**
[EXCLUDES1] *drowning and submersion while in swimming pool without jumping or diving (W67)*

[7] **W16.522 Jumping or diving into swimming pool striking bottom causing other injury**

[6] **W16.53 Jumping or diving into swimming pool striking wall**

[7] **W16.531 Jumping or diving into swimming pool striking wall causing drowning and submersion**
[EXCLUDES1] *drowning and submersion while in swimming pool without jumping or diving (W67)*

[7] **W16.532 Jumping or diving into swimming pool striking wall causing other injury**

Unspecified Code | Other Specified Code | [N] Newborn Age: 0 | [P] Pediatric Age: 0-17 | [M] Maternity Age: 12-55
[A] Adult Age: 15-124 | ♂ Male | ♀ Female | ● New Code | ▲ Revised Code Title | ►◄ Revised Text

[5] W16.6 Jumping or diving into natural body of water
Jumping or diving into lake
Jumping or diving into open sea
Jumping or diving into river
Jumping or diving into stream
[6] W16.61 Jumping or diving into natural body of water striking water surface
[7] W16.611 Jumping or diving into natural body of water striking water surface causing drowning and submersion
EXCLUDES1 *drowning and submersion while in natural body of water without jumping or diving (W69)*
[7] W16.612 Jumping or diving into natural body of water striking water surface causing other injury
[6] W16.62 Jumping or diving into natural body of water striking bottom
[7] W16.621 Jumping or diving into natural body of water striking bottom causing drowning and submersion
EXCLUDES1 *drowning and submersion while in natural body of water without jumping or diving (W69)*
[7] W16.622 Jumping or diving into natural body of water striking bottom causing other injury
[5] W16.7 Jumping or diving from boat
EXCLUDES1 *Fall from boat into water -see watercraft accident (V90-V94)*
[6] W16.71 Jumping or diving from boat striking water surface
[7] W16.711 Jumping or diving from boat striking water surface causing drowning and submersion
[7] W16.712 Jumping or diving from boat striking water surface causing other injury
[6] W16.72 Jumping or diving from boat striking bottom
[7] W16.721 Jumping or diving from boat striking bottom causing drowning and submersion
[7] W16.722 Jumping or diving from boat striking bottom causing other injury
[5] W16.8 Jumping or diving into other water
Jumping or diving into fountain
Jumping or diving into reservoir
[6] W16.81 Jumping or diving into other water striking water surface
[7] W16.811 Jumping or diving into other water striking water surface causing drowning and submersion
EXCLUDES1 *drowning and submersion while in other water without jumping or diving (W73)*
[7] W16.812 Jumping or diving into other water striking water surface causing other injury
[6] W16.82 Jumping or diving into other water striking bottom
[7] W16.821 Jumping or diving into other water striking bottom causing drowning and submersion
EXCLUDES1 *drowning and submersion while in other water without jumping or diving (W73)*
[7] W16.822 Jumping or diving into other water striking bottom causing other injury
[6] W16.83 Jumping or diving into other water striking wall
[7] W16.831 Jumping or diving into other water striking wall causing drowning and submersion
EXCLUDES1 *drowning and submersion while in other water without jumping or diving (W73)*
[7] W16.832 Jumping or diving into other water striking wall causing other injury
[5] W16.9 Jumping or diving into unspecified water
[7X] W16.91 Jumping or diving into unspecified water causing drowning and submersion
[7X] W16.92 Jumping or diving into unspecified water causing other injury
[4] W17 Other fall from one level to another
The appropriate 7th character is to be added to each code from category W17
A = initial encounter
D = subsequent encounter
S = sequela
[7X] W17.0 Fall into well
[7X] W17.1 Fall into storm drain or manhole
[7X] W17.2 Fall into hole
Fall into pit
[7X] W17.3 Fall into empty swimming pool
EXCLUDES1 *fall into filled swimming pool (W16.0-)*
[7X] W17.4 Fall from dock
[5] W17.8 Other fall from one level to another
[7X] W17.81 Fall down embankment (hill)
[7X] W17.82 Fall from (out of) grocery cart
Fall due to grocery cart tipping over
[7X] W17.89 Other fall from one level to another
Fall from cherry picker
Fall from lifting device
Fall from mobile elevated work platform [MEWP]
Fall from sky lift
[4] W18 Other slipping, tripping and stumbling and falls
The appropriate 7th character is to be added to each code from category W18
A = initial encounter
D = subsequent encounter
S = sequela
[5] W18.0 Fall due to bumping against object
Striking against object with subsequent fall
EXCLUDES1 *fall on same level due to slipping, tripping, or stumbling with subsequent striking against object (W01.1-)*
[7X] W18.00 Striking against unspecified object with subsequent fall
[7X] W18.01 Striking against sports equipment with subsequent fall
[7X] W18.02 Striking against glass with subsequent fall
[7X] W18.09 Striking against other object with subsequent fall
[5] W18.1 Fall from or off toilet
[7X] W18.11 Fall from or off toilet without subsequent striking against object
Fall from (off) toilet NOS
[7X] W18.12 Fall from or off toilet with subsequent striking against object
[7X] W18.2 Fall in (into) shower or empty bathtub
EXCLUDES1 *fall in full bathtub causing drowning or submersion (W16.21-)*
[5] W18.3 Other and unspecified fall on same level
[7X] W18.30 Fall on same level, unspecified
[7X] W18.31 Fall on same level due to stepping on an object
Fall on same level due to stepping on an animal
EXCLUDES1 *slipping, tripping and stumbling without fall due to stepping on animal (W18.41)*
[7X] W18.39 Other fall on same level
[5] W18.4 Slipping, tripping and stumbling without falling
EXCLUDES1 *collision with another person without fall (W51)*
[7X] W18.40 Slipping, tripping and stumbling without falling, unspecified
[7X] W18.41 Slipping, tripping and stumbling without falling due to stepping on object
Slipping, tripping and stumbling without falling due to stepping on animal
EXCLUDES1 *slipping, tripping and stumbling with fall due to stepping on animal (W18.31)*
[7X] W18.42 Slipping, tripping and stumbling without falling due to stepping into hole or opening

[4] 4th character required [5] 5th character required [6] 6th character required [7] 7th character required [7X] Extension 'X' Alert
EXCLUDES1 Not coded here EXCLUDES2 Not included here PDx Primary Diagnosis Only Manifestation Code

W18.43 Slipping, tripping and stumbling without falling due to stepping from one level to another

W18.49 Other slipping, tripping and stumbling without falling

W19 Unspecified fall

Accidental fall NOS

The appropriate 7th character is to be added to code W19

A = initial encounter
D = subsequent encounter
S = sequela

Exposure to inanimate mechanical forces (W20-W49)

EXCLUDES1 assault (X92-Y08)
contact or collision with animals or persons (W50-W64)
exposure to inanimate mechanical forces involving military or war operations (Y36.-, Y37.-)
intentional self-harm (X71-X83)

W20 Struck by thrown, projected or falling object

Code first any associated:
cataclysm (X34-X39)
lightning strike (T75.00)

EXCLUDES1 falling object in machinery accident (W24, W28-W31)
falling object in transport accident (V01-V99)
object set in motion by explosion (W35-W40)
object set in motion by firearm (W32-W34)
struck by thrown sports equipment (W21.-)

The appropriate 7th character is to be added to each code from category W20

A = initial encounter
D = subsequent encounter
S = sequela

W20.0 Struck by falling object in cave-in

EXCLUDES2 asphyxiation due to cave-in (T71.21)

W20.1 Struck by object due to collapse of building

EXCLUDES1 struck by object due to collapse of burning building (X00.2, X02.2)

W20.8 Other cause of strike by thrown, projected or falling object

EXCLUDES1 struck by thrown sports equipment (W21.-)

W21 Striking against or struck by sports equipment

EXCLUDES1 assault with sports equipment (Y08.0-)
striking against or struck by sports equipment with subsequent fall (W18.01)

The appropriate 7th character is to be added to each code from category W21

A = initial encounter
D = subsequent encounter
S = sequela

W21.0 Struck by hit or thrown ball

W21.00 Struck by hit or thrown ball, unspecified type

W21.01 Struck by football

W21.02 Struck by soccer ball

W21.03 Struck by baseball

W21.04 Struck by golf ball

W21.05 Struck by basketball

W21.06 Struck by volleyball

W21.07 Struck by softball

W21.09 Struck by other hit or thrown ball

W21.1 Struck by bat, racquet or club

W21.11 Struck by baseball bat

W21.12 Struck by tennis racquet

W21.13 Struck by golf club

W21.19 Struck by other bat, racquet or club

W21.2 Struck by hockey stick or puck

W21.21 Struck by hockey stick

W21.210 Struck by ice hockey stick

W21.211 Struck by field hockey stick

W21.22 Struck by hockey puck

W21.220 Struck by ice hockey puck

W21.221 Struck by field hockey puck

W21.3 Struck by sports foot wear

W21.31 Struck by shoe cleats

Stepped on by shoe cleats

W21.32 Struck by skate blades

Skated over by skate blades

W21.39 Struck by other sports foot wear

W21.4 Striking against diving board

Use additional code for subsequent falling into water, if applicable (W16.-)

W21.8 Striking against or struck by other sports equipment

W21.81 Striking against or struck by football helmet

W21.89 Striking against or struck by other sports equipment

W21.9 Striking against or struck by unspecified sports equipment

W22 Striking against or struck by other objects

EXCLUDES1 striking against or struck by object with subsequent fall (W18.09)

The appropriate 7th character is to be added to each code from category W22

A = initial encounter
D = subsequent encounter
S = sequela

W22.0 Striking against stationary object

EXCLUDES1 striking against stationary sports equipment (W21.8)

W22.01 Walked into wall

W22.02 Walked into lamppost

W22.03 Walked into furniture

W22.04 Striking against wall of swimming pool

W22.041 Striking against wall of swimming pool causing drowning and submersion

EXCLUDES1 drowning and submersion while swimming without striking against wall (W67)

W22.042 Striking against wall of swimming pool causing other injury

W22.09 Striking against other stationary object

W22.1 Striking against or struck by automobile airbag

W22.10 Striking against or struck by unspecified automobile airbag

W22.11 Striking against or struck by driver side automobile airbag

W22.12 Striking against or struck by front passenger side automobile airbag

W22.19 Striking against or struck by other automobile airbag

W22.8 Striking against or struck by other objects

Striking against or struck by object NOS

EXCLUDES1 struck by thrown, projected or falling object (W20.-)

Unspecified Code | Other Specified Code | N Newborn Age: 0 | P Pediatric Age: 0-17 | M Maternity Age: 12-55 | A Adult Age: 15-124 | ♂ Male | ♀ Female | ● New Code | ▲ Revised Code Title | ►◄ Revised Text

[4] **W23 Caught, crushed, jammed or pinched in or between objects**
[EXCLUDES1] *injury caused by cutting or piercing instruments (W25-W27)*
injury caused by firearms malfunction (W32.1, W33.1-, W34.1-)
injury caused by lifting and transmission devices (W24.-)
injury caused by machinery (W28-W31)
injury caused by nonpowered hand tools (W27.-)
injury caused by transport vehicle being used as a means of transportation (V01-V99)
injury caused by struck by thrown, projected or falling object (W20.-)
The appropriate 7th character is to be added to each code from category W23
A = initial encounter
D = subsequent encounter
S = sequela
[7th] **W23.0 Caught, crushed, jammed, or pinched between moving objects**
[7th] **W23.1 Caught, crushed, jammed, or pinched between stationary objects**

[4] **W24 Contact with lifting and transmission devices, not elsewhere classified**
[EXCLUDES1] *transport accidents (V01-V99)*
The appropriate 7th character is to be added to each code from category W24
A = initial encounter
D = subsequent encounter
S = sequela
[7th] **W24.0 Contact with lifting devices, not elsewhere classified**
Contact with chain hoist
Contact with drive belt
Contact with pulley (block)
[7th] **W24.1 Contact with transmission devices, not elsewhere classified**
Contact with transmission belt or cable

[7] **W25 Contact with sharp glass**
Code first any associated:
injury due to flying glass from explosion or firearm discharge (W32-W40)
transport accident (V00-V99)
[EXCLUDES1] *fall on same level due to slipping, tripping and stumbling with subsequent striking against sharp glass (W01.10)*
striking against sharp glass with subsequent fall (W18.02)
The appropriate 7th character is to be added to code W25
A = initial encounter
D = subsequent encounter
S = sequela

[4] **W26 Contact with knife, sword or dagger**
The appropriate 7th character is to be added to each code from category W26
A = initial encounter
D = subsequent encounter
S = sequela
[7th] **W26.0 Contact with knife**
[EXCLUDES1] *contact with electric knife (W29.1)*
[7th] **W26.1 Contact with sword or dagger**

[4] **W27 Contact with nonpowered hand tool**
The appropriate 7th character is to be added to each code from category W27
A = initial encounter
D = subsequent encounter
S = sequela
[7th] **W27.0 Contact with workbench tool**
Contact with auger
Contact with axe
Contact with chisel
Contact with handsaw
Contact with screwdriver
[7th] **W27.1 Contact with garden tool**
Contact with hoe
Contact with nonpowered lawn mower
Contact with pitchfork
Contact with rake
[7th] **W27.2 Contact with scissors**
[7th] **W27.3 Contact with needle (sewing)**
[EXCLUDES1] *contact with hypodermic needle (W46.-)*
[7th] **W27.4 Contact with kitchen utensil**
Contact with fork
Contact with ice-pick
Contact with can-opener NOS
[7th] **W27.5 Contact with paper-cutter**
[7th] **W27.8 Contact with other nonpowered hand tool**
Contact with nonpowered sewing machine
Contact with shovel

[7] **W28 Contact with powered lawn mower**
Powered lawn mower (commercial) (residential)
[EXCLUDES1] *contact with nonpowered lawn mower (W27.1)*
[EXCLUDES2] *exposure to electric current (W86.-)*
The appropriate 7th character is to be added to code W28
A = initial encounter
D = subsequent encounter
S = sequela

[4] **W29 Contact with other powered hand tools and household machinery**
[EXCLUDES1] *contact with commercial machinery (W31.82)*
contact with hot household appliance (X15)
contact with nonpowered hand tool (W27.-)
exposure to electric current (W86)
The appropriate 7th character is to be added to each code from category W29
A = initial encounter
D = subsequent encounter
S = sequela
[7th] **W29.0 Contact with powered kitchen appliance**
Contact with blender
Contact with can-opener
Contact with garbage disposal
Contact with mixer
[7th] **W29.1 Contact with electric knife**
[7th] **W29.2 Contact with other powered household machinery**
Contact with electric fan
Contact with powered dryer (clothes) (powered) (spin)
Contact with washing-machine
Contact with sewing machine
[7th] **W29.3 Contact with powered garden and outdoor hand tools and machinery**
Contact with chainsaw
Contact with edger
Contact with garden cultivator (tiller)
Contact with hedge trimmer
Contact with other powered garden tool
[EXCLUDES1] *contact with powered lawn mower (W28)*
[7th] **W29.4 Contact with nail gun**
[7th] **W29.8 Contact with other powered powered hand tools and household machinery**
Contact with do-it-yourself tool NOS

[4] **W30 Contact with agricultural machinery**
[INCLUDES] *animal-powered farm machine*
[EXCLUDES1] *agricultural transport vehicle accident (V01-V99)*
explosion of grain store (W40.8)
exposure to electric current (W86.-)
The appropriate 7th character is to be added to each code from category W30
A = initial encounter
D = subsequent encounter
S = sequela

[4] 4th character required [5] 5th character required [6] 6th character required [7] 7th character required [7th] Extension 'X' Alert
[EXCLUDES1] Not coded here [EXCLUDES2] Not included here [PDx] Primary Diagnosis Only Manifestation Code

W30.0 **Contact with** combine harvester
Contact with reaper
Contact with thresher
W30.1 **Contact with** power take-off devices (PTO)
W30.2 **Contact with** hay derrick
W30.3 **Contact with** grain storage elevator
EXCLUDES1 explosion of grain store (W40.8)
W30.8 **Contact with** other specified **agricultural machinery**
W30.81 **Contact with agricultural transport vehicle in stationary use**
Contact with agricultural transport vehicle under repair, not on public roadway
EXCLUDES1 agricultural transport vehicle accident (V01-V99)
W30.89 **Contact with other specified agricultural machinery**
W30.9 **Contact with** unspecified **agricultural machinery**
Contact with farm machinery NOS
W31 **Contact with** other and unspecified **machinery**
EXCLUDES1 contact with agricultural machinery (W30.-)
contact with machinery in transport under own power or being towed by a vehicle (V01-V99)
exposure to electric current (W86)

The appropriate 7th character is to be added to each code from category W31
A = initial encounter
D = subsequent encounter
S = sequela

W31.0 **Contact with** mining and earth-drilling **machinery**
Contact with bore or drill (land) (seabed)
Contact with shaft hoist
Contact with shaft lift
Contact with undercutter
W31.1 **Contact with** metalworking **machines**
Contact with abrasive wheel
Contact with forging machine
Contact with lathe
Contact with mechanical shears
Contact with metal drilling machine
Contact with milling machine
Contact with power press
Contact with rolling-mill
Contact with metal sawing machine
W31.2 **Contact with** powered woodworking and forming **machines**
Contact with band saw
Contact with bench saw
Contact with circular saw
Contact with molding machine
Contact with overhead plane
Contact with powered saw
Contact with radial saw
Contact with sander
EXCLUDES1 nonpowered woodworking tools (W27.0)
W31.3 **Contact with** prime movers
Contact with gas turbine
Contact with internal combustion engine
Contact with steam engine
Contact with water driven turbine
W31.8 **Contact with** other specified **machinery**
W31.81 **Contact with** recreational **machinery**
Contact with roller coaster
W31.82 **Contact with** other commercial **machinery**
Contact with commercial electric fan
Contact with commercial kitchen appliances
Contact with commercial powered dryer (clothes) (powered) (spin)

Contact with commercial washing-machine
Contact with commercial sewing machine
EXCLUDES1 contact with household machinery (W29.-)
contact with powered lawn mower (W28)
W31.83 **Contact with** special construction vehicle in stationary use
Contact with special construction vehicle under repair, not on public roadway
EXCLUDES1 special construction vehicle accident (V01-V99)
W31.89 **Contact with other specified machinery**
W31.9 **Contact with** unspecified **machinery**
Contact with machinery NOS
W32 **Accidental** handgun **discharge and malfunction**
INCLUDES accidental discharge and malfunction of gun for single hand use
accidental discharge and malfunction of pistol
accidental discharge and malfunction of revolver
Handgun discharge and malfunction NOS
EXCLUDES1 accidental airgun discharge and malfunction (W34.010, W34.110)
accidental BB gun discharge and malfunction (W34.010, W34.110)
accidental pellet gun discharge and malfunction (W34.010, W34.110)
accidental shotgun discharge and malfunction (W33.01, W33.11)
assault by handgun discharge (X93)
handgun discharge involving legal intervention (Y35.0-)
handgun discharge involving military or war operations (Y36.4-)
intentional self-harm by handgun discharge (X72)
Very pistol discharge and malfunction (W34.09, W34.19)

The appropriate 7th character is to be added to each code from category W32
A = initial encounter
D = subsequent encounter
S = sequela
W32.0 **Accidental handgun** discharge
W32.1 **Accidental handgun** malfunction
Injury due to explosion of handgun (parts)
Injury due to malfunction of mechanism or component of handgun
Injury due to recoil of handgun
Powder burn from handgun
W33 **Accidental** rifle, shotgun and larger firearm **discharge and malfunction**
INCLUDES rifle, shotgun and larger firearm discharge and malfunction NOS
EXCLUDES1 accidental airgun discharge and malfunction (W34.010, W34.110)
accidental BB gun discharge and malfunction (W34.010, W34.110)
accidental handgun discharge and malfunction (W32.-)
accidental pellet gun discharge and malfunction (W34.010, W34.110)
assault by rifle, shotgun and larger firearm discharge (X94)
firearm discharge involving legal intervention (Y35.0-)
firearm discharge involving military or war operations (Y36.4-)
intentional self-harm by rifle, shotgun and larger firearm discharge (X73)

The appropriate 7th character is to be added to each code from category W33
A = initial encounter
D = subsequent encounter
S = sequela

Unspecified Code   Other Specified Code   **N** Newborn Age: 0   **P** Pediatric Age: 0-17   **M** Maternity Age: 12-55
A Adult Age: 15-124   ♂ Male   ♀ Female   ● New Code   ▲ Revised Code Title   ►◄ Revised Text

[5] W33.0 Accidental rifle, shotgun and larger firearm discharge
[7th] W33.00 Accidental discharge of unspecified larger firearm
Discharge of unspecified larger firearm NOS
[7th] W33.01 Accidental discharge of shotgun
Discharge of shotgun NOS
[7th] W33.02 Accidental discharge of hunting rifle
Discharge of hunting rifle NOS
[7th] W33.03 Accidental discharge of machine gun
Discharge of machine gun NOS
[7th] W33.09 Accidental discharge of other larger firearm
Discharge of other larger firearm NOS
[5] W33.1 Accidental rifle, shotgun and larger firearm malfunction
Injury due to explosion of rifle, shotgun and larger firearm (parts)
Injury due to malfunction of mechanism or component of rifle, shotgun and larger firearm
Injury due to piercing, cutting, crushing or pinching due to (by) slide trigger mechanism, scope or other gun part
Injury due to recoil of rifle, shotgun and larger firearm
Powder burn from rifle, shotgun and larger firearm
[7th] W33.10 Accidental malfunction of unspecified larger firearm
Malfunction of unspecified larger firearm NOS
[7th] W33.11 Accidental malfunction of shotgun
Malfunction of shotgun NOS
[7th] W33.12 Accidental malfunction of hunting rifle
Malfunction of hunting rifle NOS
[7th] W33.13 Accidental malfunction of machine gun
Malfunction of machine gun NOS
[7th] W33.19 Accidental malfunction of other larger firearm
Malfunction of other larger firearm NOS
[4] W34 Accidental discharge and malfunction from other and unspecified firearms and guns
The appropriate 7th character is to be added to each code from category W34
A = initial encounter
D = subsequent encounter
S = sequela
[5] W34.0 Accidental discharge from other and unspecified firearms and guns
[7th] W34.00 Accidental discharge from unspecified firearms or gun
Discharge from firearm NOS
Gunshot wound NOS
Shot NOS
[6] W34.01 Accidental discharge of gas, air or spring-operated guns
[7] W34.010 Accidental discharge of airgun
Accidental discharge of BB gun
Accidental discharge of pellet gun
[7] W34.011 Accidental discharge of paintball gun
Accidental injury due to paintball discharge
[7] W34.018 Accidental discharge of other gas, air or spring-operated gun
[7th] W34.09 Accidental discharge from other specified firearms
Accidental discharge from Very pistol [flare]
[5] W34.1 Accidental malfunction from other and unspecified firearms and guns
[7th] W34.10 Accidental malfunction from unspecified firearms or gun
Firearm malfunction NOS
[6] W34.11 Accidental malfunction of gas, air or spring-operated guns
[7] W34.110 Accidental malfunction of airgun
Accidental malfunction of BB gun
Accidental malfunction of pellet gun
[7] W34.111 Accidental malfunction of paintball gun
Accidental injury due to paintball gun malfunction
[7] W34.118 Accidental malfunction of other gas, air or spring-operated gun
[7th] W34.19 Accidental malfunction from other specified firearms
Accidental malfunction from Very pistol [flare]
[7] W35 Explosion and rupture of boiler
[EXCLUDES1] *explosion and rupture of boiler on watercraft (V93.4)*
The appropriate 7th character is to be added to code W35
A = initial encounter
D = subsequent encounter
S = sequela
[4] W36 Explosion and rupture of gas cylinder
The appropriate 7th character is to be added to each code from category W36
A = initial encounter
D = subsequent encounter
S = sequela
[7th] W36.1 Explosion and rupture of aerosol can
[7th] W36.2 Explosion and rupture of air tank
[7th] W36.3 Explosion and rupture of pressurized-gas tank
[7th] W36.8 Explosion and rupture of other gas cylinder
[7th] W36.9 Explosion and rupture of unspecified gas cylinder
[4] W37 Explosion and rupture of pressurized tire, pipe or hose
The appropriate 7th character is to be added to each code from category W37
A = initial encounter
D = subsequent encounter
S = sequela
[7th] W37.0 Explosion of bicycle tire
[7th] W37.8 Explosion and rupture of other pressurized tire, pipe or hose
[7] W38 Explosion and rupture of other specified pressurized devices
The appropriate 7th character is to be added to code W38
A = initial encounter
D = subsequent encounter
S = sequela
[7] W39 Discharge of firework
The appropriate 7th character is to be added to code W39
A = initial encounter
D = subsequent encounter
S = sequela
[4] W40 Explosion of other materials
[EXCLUDES1] *assault by explosive material (X96)*
explosion involving legal intervention (Y35.1-)
explosion involving military or war operations (Y36.0-, Y36.2-)
intentional self-harm by explosive material (X75)
The appropriate 7th character is to be added to each code from category W40
A = initial encounter
D = subsequent encounter
S = sequela
[7th] W40.0 Explosion of blasting material
Explosion of blasting cap
Explosion of detonator
Explosion of dynamite
Explosion of explosive (any) used in blasting operations
[7th] W40.1 Explosion of explosive gases
Explosion of acetylene
Explosion of butane
Explosion of coal gas

[4] 4th character required [5] 5th character required [6] 6th character required [7] 7th character required [7th] Extension 'X' Alert
[EXCLUDES1] Not coded here [EXCLUDES2] Not included here [PDx] Primary Diagnosis Only Manifestation Code

Explosion in mine NOS
Explosion of explosive gas
Explosion of fire damp
Explosion of gasoline fumes
Explosion of methane
Explosion of propane

[7th] W40.8 Explosion of other specified explosive materials
Explosion in dump NOS
Explosion in factory NOS
Explosion in grain store
Explosion in munitions
EXCLUDES1 *explosion involving legal intervention (Y35.1-)*
explosion involving military or war operations (Y36.0-, Y36.2-)

[7th] W40.9 Explosion of unspecified explosive materials
Explosion NOS

[4th] W42 Exposure to noise
The appropriate 7th character is to be added to each code from category W42
A = initial encounter
D = subsequent encounter
S = sequela

[7th] W42.0 Exposure to supersonic waves
[7th] W42.9 Exposure to other noise
Exposure to sound waves NOS

[4th] W45 Foreign body or object entering through skin
EXCLUDES2 *contact with hand tools (nonpowered) (powered) (W27-W29)*
contact with knife, sword or dagger (W26.-)
contact with sharp glass (W25.-)
struck by objects (W20-W22)
The appropriate 7th character is to be added to each code from category W45
A = initial encounter
D = subsequent encounter
S = sequela

[7th] W45.0 Nail entering through skin
[7th] W45.1 Paper entering through skin
Paper cut
[7th] W45.2 Lid of can entering through skin
[7th] W45.8 Other foreign body or object entering through skin
Splinter in skin NOS

[4th] W46 Contact with hypodermic needle
The appropriate 7th character is to be added to each code from category W46
A = initial encounter
D = subsequent encounter
S = sequela

[7th] W46.0 Contact with hypodermic needle
Hypodermic needle stick NOS
[7th] W46.1 Contact with contaminated hypodermic needle

[4th] W49 Exposure to other inanimate mechanical forces
INCLUDES *exposure to abnormal gravitational [G] forces*
exposure to inanimate mechanical forces NEC
EXCLUDES1 *exposure to inanimate mechanical forces involving military or war operations (Y36.-, Y37.-)*
The appropriate 7th character is to be added to each code from category W49
A = initial encounter
D = subsequent encounter
S = sequela

[5th] W49.0 Item causing external constriction
[7th] W49.01 Hair causing external constriction
[7th] W49.02 String or thread causing external constriction
[7th] W49.03 Rubber band causing external constriction
[7th] W49.04 Ring or other jewelry causing external constriction
[7th] W49.09 Other specified item causing external constriction
[7th] W49.9 Exposure to other inanimate mechanical forces

Exposure to animate mechanical forces (W50-W64)

EXCLUDES1 *Toxic effect of contact with venomous animals and plants (T63.-)*

[4th] W50 Accidental hit, strike, kick, twist, bite or scratch by another person
INCLUDES *hit, strike, kick, twist, bite, or scratch by another person NOS*
EXCLUDES1 *assault by bodily force (Y04)*
struck by objects (W20-W22)
The appropriate 7th character is to be added to each code from category W50
A = initial encounter
D = subsequent encounter
S = sequela

[7th] W50.0 Accidental hit or strike by another person
Hit or strike by another person NOS
[7th] W50.1 Accidental kick by another person
Kick by another person NOS
[7th] W50.2 Accidental twist by another person
Twist by another person NOS
[7th] W50.3 Accidental bite by another person
Human bite
Bite by another person NOS
[7th] W50.4 Accidental scratch by another person
Scratch by another person NOS

[7th] W51 Accidental striking against or bumped into by another person
EXCLUDES1 *assault by striking against or bumping into by another person (Y04.2)*
fall due to collision with another person (W03)
The appropriate 7th character is to be added to code W51
A = initial encounter
D = subsequent encounter
S = sequela

[7th] W52 Crushed, pushed or stepped on by crowd or human stampede
Crushed, pushed or stepped on by crowd or human stampede with or without fall
The appropriate 7th character is to be added to code W52
A = initial encounter
D = subsequent encounter
S = sequela

[4th] W53 Contact with rodent
INCLUDES *contact with saliva, feces or urine of rodent*
The appropriate 7th character is to be added to each code from category W53
A = initial encounter
D = subsequent encounter
S = sequela

[5th] W53.0 Contact with mouse
[7th] W53.01 Bitten by mouse
[7th] W53.09 Other contact with mouse
[5th] W53.1 Contact with rat
[7th] W53.11 Bitten by rat
[7th] W53.19 Other contact with rat
[5th] W53.2 Contact with squirrel
[7th] W53.21 Bitten by squirrel
[7th] W53.29 Other contact with squirrel
[5th] W53.8 Contact with other rodent
[7th] W53.81 Bitten by other rodent
[7th] W53.89 Other contact with other rodent

Unspecified Code | Other Specified Code | [N] Newborn Age: 0 | [P] Pediatric Age: 0-17 | [M] Maternity Age: 12-55
[A] Adult Age: 15-124 | ♂ Male | ♀ Female | ● New Code | ▲ Revised Code Title | ►◄ Revised Text

④ **W54 Contact with** dog

> INCLUDES   *contact with saliva, feces or urine of dog*

The appropriate 7th character is to be added to each code from category W54
A = initial encounter
D = subsequent encounter
S = sequela

⑥ **W54.0** Bitten **by dog**

⑥ **W54.1** Struck **by dog**
> Knocked over by dog

⑥ **W54.8 Other contact with dog**

④ **W55 Contact with** other mammals

> INCLUDES   *contact with saliva, feces or urine of mammal*
> EXCLUDES1 *animal being ridden- see transport accidents*
> *bitten or struck by dog (W54)*
> *bitten or struck by rodent (W53.-)*
> *contact with marine mammals (W56.X-)*

The appropriate 7th character is to be added to each code from category W55
A = initial encounter
D = subsequent encounter
S = sequela

⑤ **W55.0 Contact with** cat
⑥ **W55.01** Bitten **by cat**
⑥ **W55.03** Scratched **by cat**
⑥ **W55.09 Other contact with cat**

⑤ **W55.1 Contact with** horse
⑥ **W55.11** Bitten **by horse**
⑥ **W55.12** Struck **by horse**
⑥ **W55.19 Other contact with horse**

⑤ **W55.2 Contact with** cow
> Contact with bull
⑥ **W55.21** Bitten **by cow**
⑥ **W55.22** Struck **by cow**
> Gored by bull
⑥ **W55.29 Other contact with cow**

⑤ **W55.3 Contact with** other hoof stock
> Contact with goats
> Contact with sheep
⑥ **W55.31** Bitten **by other hoof stock**
⑥ **W55.32** Struck **by other hoof stock**
> Gored by goat
> Gored by ram
⑥ **W55.39 Other contact with other hoof stock**

⑤ **W55.4 Contact with** pig
⑥ **W55.41** Bitten **by pig**
⑥ **W55.42** Struck **by pig**
⑥ **W55.49 Other contact with pig**

⑤ **W55.5 Contact with** raccoon
⑥ **W55.51** Bitten **by raccoon**
⑥ **W55.52** Struck **by raccoon**
⑥ **W55.59 Other contact with raccoon**

⑤ **W55.8 Contact with** other mammals
⑥ **W55.81 Bitten by other mammals**
⑥ **W55.82 Struck by other mammals**
⑥ **W55.89 Other contact with other mammals**

④ **W56 Contact with** nonvenomous marine animal
> EXCLUDES1 *contact with venomous marine animal (T63.-)*

The appropriate 7th character is to be added to each code from category W56
A = initial encounter
D = subsequent encounter
S = sequela

⑤ **W56.0 Contact with** dolphin
⑥ **W56.01** Bitten **by dolphin**
⑥ **W56.02** Struck **by dolphin**
⑥ **W56.09 Other contact with dolphin**

⑤ **W56.1 Contact with** sea lion
⑥ **W56.11** Bitten **by sea lion**
⑥ **W56.12** Struck **by sea lion**
⑥ **W56.19 Other contact with sea lion**

⑤ **W56.2 Contact with** orca
> Contact with killer whale
⑥ **W56.21** Bitten **by orca**
⑥ **W56.22** Struck **by orca**
⑥ **W56.29 Other contact with orca**

⑤ **W56.3 Contact with** other marine mammals
⑥ **W56.31** Bitten **by other marine mammals**
⑥ **W56.32** Struck **by other marine mammals**
⑥ **W56.39 Other contact with other marine mammals**

⑤ **W56.4 Contact with** shark
⑥ **W56.41** Bitten **by shark**
⑥ **W56.42** Struck **by shark**
⑥ **W56.49 Other contact with shark**

⑤ **W56.5 Contact with** other fish
⑥ **W56.51** Bitten **by other fish**
⑥ **W56.52** Struck **by other fish**
⑥ **W56.59 Other contact with other fish**

⑤ **W56.8 Contact with** other nonvenomous marine animals
⑥ **W56.81** Bitten **by other nonvenomous marine animals**
⑥ **W56.82** Struck **by other nonvenomous marine animals**
⑥ **W56.89 Other contact with other nonvenomous marine animals**

⑦ **W57 Bitten or stung by nonvenomous** insect and other nonvenomous arthropods
> EXCLUDES1 *contact with venomous insects and arthropods (T63.2-, T63.3-, T63.4-)*

The appropriate 7th character is to be added to code W57
A = initial encounter
D = subsequent encounter
S = sequela

④ **W58 Contact with** crocodile or alligator

The appropriate 7th character is to be added to each code from category W58
A = initial encounter
D = subsequent encounter
S = sequela

⑤ **W58.0 Contact with** alligator
⑥ **W58.01** Bitten **by alligator**
⑥ **W58.02** Struck **by alligator**
⑥ **W58.03** Crushed **by alligator**
⑥ **W58.09 Other contact with alligator**

⑤ **W58.1 Contact with** crocodile
⑥ **W58.11** Bitten **by crocodile**
⑥ **W58.12** Struck **by crocodile**
⑥ **W58.13** Crushed **by crocodile**
⑥ **W58.19 Other contact with crocodile**

④ **W59 Contact with** other nonvenomous reptiles
> EXCLUDES1 *contact with venomous reptile (T63.0-, T63.1-)*

The appropriate 7th character is to be added to each code from category W59
A = initial encounter
D = subsequent encounter
S = sequela

⑤ **W59.0 Contact with nonvenomous** lizards
⑥ **W59.01** Bitten **by nonvenomous lizards**
⑥ **W59.02** Struck **by nonvenomous lizards**
⑥ **W59.09 Other contact with nonvenomous lizards**
> Exposure to nonvenomous lizards

⑤ **W59.1 Contact with nonvenomous** snakes
⑥ **W59.11** Bitten **by nonvenomous snake**
⑥ **W59.12** Struck **by nonvenomous snake**
⑥ **W59.13** Crushed **by nonvenomous snake**
⑥ **W59.19 Other contact with nonvenomous snake**

---

④ 4th character required   ⑤ 5th character required   ⑥ 6th character required   ⑦ 7th character required   ⑩ Extension 'X' Alert
EXCLUDES1 Not coded here   EXCLUDES2 Not included here   📕 Primary Diagnosis Only   Manifestation Code

[5th] W59.2 Contact with turtles
[EXCLUDES1] *contact with tortoises (W59.8-)*
[7th] W59.21 Bitten by turtle
[7th] W59.22 Struck by turtle
[7th] W59.29 Other contact with turtle
Exposure to turtles
[5th] W59.8 Contact with other nonvenomous reptiles
[7th] W59.81 Bitten by other nonvenomous reptiles
[7th] W59.82 Struck by other nonvenomous reptiles
[7th] W59.83 Crushed by other nonvenomous reptiles
[7th] W59.89 Other contact with other nonvenomous reptiles

[7th] W60 Contact with nonvenomous plant thorns and spines and sharp leaves
[EXCLUDES1] *Contact with venomous plants (T63.7-)*
The appropriate 7th character is to be added to code W60
A = initial encounter
D = subsequent encounter
S = sequela

[4th] W61 Contact with birds (domestic) (wild)
[INCLUDES] *contact with excreta of birds*
The appropriate 7th character is to be added to each code from category W61
A = initial encounter
D = subsequent encounter
S = sequela
[5th] W61.0 Contact with parrot
[7th] W61.01 Bitten by parrot
[7th] W61.02 Struck by parrot
[7th] W61.09 Other contact with parrot
Exposure to parrots
[5th] W61.1 Contact with macaw
[7th] W61.11 Bitten by macaw
[7th] W61.12 Struck by macaw
[7th] W61.19 Other contact with macaw
Exposure to macaws
[5th] W61.2 Contact with other psittacines
[7th] W61.21 Bitten by other psittacines
[7th] W61.22 Struck by other psittacines
[7th] W61.29 Other contact with other psittacines
Exposure to other psittacines
[5th] W61.3 Contact with chicken
[7th] W61.32 Struck by chicken
[7th] W61.33 Pecked by chicken
[7th] W61.39 Other contact with chicken
Exposure to chickens
[5th] W61.4 Contact with turkey
[7th] W61.42 Struck by turkey
[7th] W61.43 Pecked by turkey
[7th] W61.49 Other contact with turkey
[5th] W61.5 Contact with goose
[7th] W61.51 Bitten by goose
[7th] W61.52 Struck by goose
[7th] W61.59 Other contact with goose
[5th] W61.6 Contact with duck
[7th] W61.61 Bitten by duck
[7th] W61.62 Struck by duck
[7th] W61.69 Other contact with duck
[5th] W61.9 Contact with other birds
[7th] W61.91 Bitten by other birds
[7th] W61.92 Struck by other birds
[7th] W61.99 Other contact with other birds
Contact with bird NOS

[4th] W62 Contact with nonvenomous amphibians
[EXCLUDES1] *contact with venomous amphibians (T63.81-R63.83)*
The appropriate 7th character is to be added to each code from category W62
A = initial encounter
D = subsequent encounter
S = sequela
[7th] W62.0 Contact with nonvenomous frogs
[7th] W62.1 Contact with nonvenomous toads
[7th] W62.9 Contact with other nonvenomous amphibians

[7th] W64 Exposure to other animate mechanical forces
[INCLUDES] *exposure to nonvenomous animal NOS*
[EXCLUDES1] *contact with venomous animal (T63.-)*
The appropriate 7th character is to be added to code W64
A = initial encounter
D = subsequent encounter
S = sequela

Accidental non-transport drowning and submersion (W65-W74)

[EXCLUDES1] *accidental drowning and submersion due to fall into water (W16.-)*
accidental drowning and submersion due to water transport accident (V90.-, V92.-)
[EXCLUDES2] *accidental drowning and submersion due to cataclysm (X34-X39)*

[7th] W65 Accidental drowning and submersion while in bath-tub
[EXCLUDES1] *accidental drowning and submersion due to fall in (into) bathtub (W16.211)*
The appropriate 7th character is to be added to code W65
A = initial encounter
D = subsequent encounter
S = sequela

[7th] W67 Accidental drowning and submersion while in swimming-pool
[EXCLUDES1] *accidental drowning and submersion due to fall into swimming pool (W16.011, W16.021, W16.031)*
accidental drowning and submersion due to striking into wall of swimming pool (W22.041)
The appropriate 7th character is to be added to code W67
A = initial encounter
D = subsequent encounter
S = sequela

[7th] W69 Accidental drowning and submersion while in natural water
Accidental drowning and submersion while in lake
Accidental drowning and submersion while in open sea
Accidental drowning and submersion while in river
Accidental drowning and submersion while in stream
[EXCLUDES1] *accidental drowning and submersion due to fall into natural body of water (W16.111, W16.121, W16.131)*
The appropriate 7th character is to be added to code W69
A = initial encounter
D = subsequent encounter
S = sequela

[7th] W73 Other specified cause of accidental non-transport drowning and submersion
Accidental drowning and submersion while in quenching tank
Accidental drowning and submersion while in reservoir
[EXCLUDES1] *accidental drowning and submersion due to fall into other water (W16.311, W16.321, W16.331)*
The appropriate 7th character is to be added to code W73
A = initial encounter
D = subsequent encounter
S = sequela

Unspecified Code | Other Specified Code | [N] Newborn Age: 0 | [P] Pediatric Age: 0-17 | [M] Maternity Age: 12-55
[A] Adult Age: 15-124 | ♂ Male | ♀ Female | ● New Code | ▲ Revised Code Title | ►◄ Revised Text

[7] W74 Unspecified cause of accidental drowning and submersion
Drowning NOS
The appropriate 7th character is to be added to code W74
A = initial encounter
D = subsequent encounter
S = sequela

Exposure to electric current, radiation and extreme ambient air temperature and pressure (W85-W99)

[EXCLUDES1] *exposure to:*
failure in dosage of radiation or temperature during surgical and medical care (Y63.2-Y63.5)
lightning (T75.0-)
natural cold (X31)
natural heat (X30)
natural radiation NOS (X39)
radiological procedure and radiotherapy (Y84.2)
sunlight (X32)

[7] W85 Exposure to electric transmission lines
Broken power line
The appropriate 7th character is to be added to code W85
A = initial encounter
D = subsequent encounter
S = sequela

[4] W86 Exposure to other specified electric current
The appropriate 7th character is to be added to each code from category W86
A = initial encounter
D = subsequent encounter
S = sequela
[7th] W86.0 Exposure to domestic wiring and appliances
[7th] W86.1 Exposure to industrial wiring, appliances and electrical machinery
Exposure to conductors
Exposure to control apparatus
Exposure to electrical equipment and machinery
Exposure to transformers
[7th] W86.8 Exposure to other electric current
Exposure to wiring and appliances in or on farm (not farmhouse)
Exposure to wiring and appliances outdoors
Exposure to wiring and appliances in or on public building
Exposure to wiring and appliances in or on residential institutions
Exposure to wiring and appliances in or on schools

[4] W88 Exposure to ionizing radiation
[EXCLUDES1] *exposure to sunlight (X32)*
The appropriate 7th character is to be added to each code from category W88
A = initial encounter
D = subsequent encounter
S = sequela
[7th] W88.0 Exposure to X-rays
[7th] W88.1 Exposure to radioactive isotopes
[7th] W88.8 Exposure to other ionizing radiation

[4] W89 Exposure to man-made visible and ultraviolet light
[INCLUDES] *exposure to welding light (arc)*
[EXCLUDES2] *exposure to sunlight (X32)*
The appropriate 7th character is to be added to each code from category W89
A = initial encounter
D = subsequent encounter
S = sequela
[7th] W89.0 Exposure to welding light (arc)
[7th] W89.1 Exposure to tanning bed
[7th] W89.8 Exposure to other man-made visible and ultraviolet light
[7th] W89.9 Exposure to unspecified man-made visible and ultraviolet light

[4] W90 Exposure to other nonionizing radiation
[EXCLUDES1] *exposure to sunlight (X32)*
The appropriate 7th character is to be added to each code from category W90
A = initial encounter
D = subsequent encounter
S = sequela
[7th] W90.0 Exposure to radiofrequency
[7th] W90.1 Exposure to infrared radiation
[7th] W90.2 Exposure to laser radiation
[7th] W90.8 Exposure to other nonionizing radiation

[7] W92 Exposure to excessive heat of man-made origin
The appropriate 7th character is to be added to code W92
A = initial encounter
D = subsequent encounter
S = sequela

[4] W93 Exposure to excessive cold of man-made origin
The appropriate 7th character is to be added to each code from category W93
A = initial encounter
D = subsequent encounter
S = sequela
[5] W93.0 Contact with or inhalation of dry ice
[7th] W93.01 Contact with dry ice
[7th] W93.02 Inhalation of dry ice
[5] W93.1 Contact with or inhalation of liquid air
[7th] W93.11 Contact with liquid air
Contact with liquid hydrogen
Contact with liquid nitrogen
[7th] W93.12 Inhalation of liquid air
Inhalation of liquid hydrogen
Inhalation of liquid nitrogen
[7th] W93.2 Prolonged exposure in deep freeze unit or refrigerator
[7th] W93.8 Exposure to other excessive cold of man-made origin

[4] W94 Exposure to high and low air pressure and changes in air pressure
The appropriate 7th character is to be added to each code from category W94
A = initial encounter
D = subsequent encounter
S = sequela
[7th] W94.0 Exposure to prolonged high air pressure
[5] W94.1 Exposure to prolonged low air pressure
[7th] W94.11 Exposure to residence or prolonged visit at high altitude
[7th] W94.12 Exposure to other prolonged low air pressure
[5] W94.2 Exposure to rapid changes in air pressure during ascent
[7th] W94.21 Exposure to reduction in atmospheric pressure while surfacing from deep-water diving
[7th] W94.22 Exposure to reduction in atmospheric pressure while surfacing from underground
[7th] W94.23 Exposure to sudden change in air pressure in aircraft during ascent
[7th] W94.29 Exposure to other rapid changes in air pressure during ascent
[5] W94.3 Exposure to rapid changes in air pressure during descent
[7th] W94.31 Exposure to sudden change in air pressure in aircraft during descent ▲
[7th] W94.32 Exposure to high air pressure from rapid descent in water

🌐 W94.39 **Exposure to other rapid changes in air pressure during descent**

❼ W99 **Exposure to** other man-made **environmental factors**
The appropriate 7th character is to be added to code W99
A = initial encounter
D = subsequent encounter
S = sequela

Exposure to smoke, fire and flames (X00-X08)

> EXCLUDES1 arson (X97)
> EXCLUDES2 explosions (W35-W40)
>   lightning (T75.0-)
>   transport accident (V01-V99)

❹ X00 **Exposure to** uncontrolled fire **in building or structure**

> INCLUDES conflagration in building or structure
> Code first any associated cataclysm
> EXCLUDES2 Exposure to ignition or melting of nightwear (X05)
>   Exposure to ignition or melting of other clothing and apparel (X06.-)
>   Exposure to other specified smoke, fire and flames (X08.-)

The appropriate 7th character is to be added to each code from category X00
A = initial encounter
D = subsequent encounter
S = sequela

🌐 X00.0 **Exposure to** flames **in uncontrolled fire in building or structure**

🌐 X00.1 **Exposure to** smoke **in uncontrolled fire in building or structure**

🌐 X00.2 Injury due to collapse **of burning building or structure in uncontrolled fire**

> EXCLUDES1 injury due to collapse of building not on fire (W20.1)

🌐 X00.3 Fall from **burning building or structure in uncontrolled fire**

🌐 X00.4 Hit by object **from burning building or structure in uncontrolled fire**

🌐 X00.5 Jump from **burning building or structure in uncontrolled fire**

🌐 X00.8 **Other exposure to uncontrolled fire in building or structure**

❹ X01 **Exposure to uncontrolled fire,** not in building or structure

> INCLUDES exposure to forest fire

The appropriate 7th character is to be added to each code from category X01
A = initial encounter
D = subsequent encounter
S = sequela

🌐 X01.0 **Exposure to** flames **in uncontrolled fire, not in building or structure**

🌐 X01.1 **Exposure to** smoke **in uncontrolled fire, not in building or structure**

🌐 X01.3 Fall due to **uncontrolled fire, not in building or structure**

🌐 X01.4 Hit by object **due to uncontrolled fire, not in building or structure**

🌐 X01.8 **Other exposure to uncontrolled fire, not in building or structure**

❹ X02 **Exposure to** controlled fire **in building or structure**

> INCLUDES exposure to fire in fireplace
>   exposure to fire in stove

The appropriate 7th character is to be added to each code from category X02
A = initial encounter
D = subsequent encounter
S = sequela

🌐 X02.0 **Exposure to** flames **in controlled fire in building or structure**

🌐 X02.1 **Exposure to** smoke **in controlled fire in building or structure**

🌐 X02.2 Injury due to collapse **of burning building or structure in controlled fire**

> EXCLUDES1 injury due to collapse of building not on fire (W20.1)

🌐 X02.3 Fall from **burning building or structure in controlled fire**

🌐 X02.4 Hit by object **from burning building or structure in controlled fire**

🌐 X02.5 Jump from **burning building or structure in controlled fire**

🌐 X02.8 **Other exposure to controlled fire in building or structure**

❹ X03 **Exposure to controlled fire,** not in building or structure

> INCLUDES exposure to bon fire
>   exposure to camp-fire
>   exposure to trash fire

The appropriate 7th character is to be added to each code from category X03
A = initial encounter
D = subsequent encounter
S = sequela

🌐 X03.0 **Exposure to** flames **in controlled fire, not in building or structure**

🌐 X03.1 **Exposure to** smoke **in controlled fire, not in building or structure**

🌐 X03.3 Fall due to **controlled fire, not in building or structure**

🌐 X03.4 Hit by object **due to controlled fire, not in building or structure**

🌐 X03.8 **Other exposure to controlled fire, not in building or structure**

❼ X04 **Exposure to ignition of highly flammable material**

Exposure to ignition of gasoline
Exposure to ignition of kerosene
Exposure to ignition of petrol

> EXCLUDES2 exposure to ignition or melting of nightwear (X05)
>   exposure to ignition or melting of other clothing and apparel (X06)

The appropriate 7th character is to be added to code X04
A = initial encounter
D = subsequent encounter
S = sequela

❼ X05 **Exposure to ignition or melting of nightwear**

> EXCLUDES2 exposure to uncontrolled fire in building or structure (X00.-)
>   exposure to uncontrolled fire, not in building or structure (X01.-)
>   exposure to controlled fire in building or structure (X02.-)
>   exposure to controlled fire, not in building or structure (X03.-)
>   exposure to ignition of highly flammable materials (X04.-)

The appropriate 7th character is to be added to code X05
A = initial encounter
D = subsequent encounter
S = sequela

Unspecified Code Other Specified Code 🅝 Newborn Age: 0 🅟 Pediatric Age: 0-17 🅜 Maternity Age: 12-55
🅐 Adult Age: 15-124 ♂ Male ♀ Female ● New Code ▲ Revised Code Title ►◄ Revised Text

⚂ X06 **Exposure to ignition or melting of** other clothing and apparel

> EXCLUDES2 *exposure to uncontrolled fire in building or structure (X00.-)*
> *exposure to uncontrolled fire, not in building or structure (X01.-)*
> *exposure to controlled fire in building or structure (X02.-)*
> *exposure to controlled fire, not in building or structure (X03.-)*
> *exposure to ignition of highly flammable materials (X04.-)*

The appropriate 7th character is to be added to each code from category X06
A = initial encounter
D = subsequent encounter
S = sequela

⚃ X06.0 Exposure to ignition of plastic jewelry
⚃ X06.1 Exposure to melting of plastic jewelry
⚃ X06.2 Exposure to ignition of other clothing and apparel
⚃ X06.3 Exposure to melting of other clothing and apparel

⚂ X08 **Exposure to** other specified **smoke, fire and flames**

The appropriate 7th character is to be added to each code from category X08
A = initial encounter
D = subsequent encounter
S = sequela

⚃ X08.0 **Exposure to** bed fire

Exposure to mattress fire

⚄ X08.00 Exposure to bed fire due to unspecified burning material
⚄ X08.01 Exposure to bed fire due to burning cigarette
⚄ X08.09 Exposure to bed fire due to other burning material

⚃ X08.1 **Exposure to** sofa fire

⚄ X08.10 Exposure to sofa fire due to unspecified burning material
⚄ X08.11 Exposure to sofa fire due to burning cigarette
⚄ X08.19 Exposure to sofa fire due to other burning material

⚃ X08.2 **Exposure to** other furniture fire

⚄ X08.20 Exposure to other furniture fire due to unspecified burning material
⚄ X08.21 Exposure to other furniture fire due to burning cigarette
⚄ X08.29 Exposure to other furniture fire due to other burning material

⚄ X08.8 **Exposure to** other specified **smoke, fire and flames**

Contact with heat and hot substances (X10-X19)

> EXCLUDES1 *exposure to excessive natural heat (X30)*
> *exposure to fire and flames (X00-X09)*

⚁ X10 **Contact with hot drinks, food, fats and cooking oils**

The appropriate 7th character is to be added to each code from category X10
A = initial encounter
D = subsequent encounter
S = sequela

⚄ X10.0 **Contact with** hot drinks
⚄ X10.1 **Contact with** hot food
⚄ X10.2 **Contact with** fats and cooking oils

⚁ X11 **Contact with** hot tap-water

> INCLUDES *contact with boiling tap-water*
> *contact with boiling water NOS*
> EXCLUDES1 *contact with water heated on stove (X12)*

The appropriate 7th character is to be added to each code from category X11
A = initial encounter
D = subsequent encounter
S = sequela

⚄ X11.0 **Contact with hot water in** bath or tub

> EXCLUDES1 *contact with running hot water in bath or tub (X11.1)*

⚄ X11.1 **Contact with** running hot water

Contact with hot water running out of hose
Contact with hot water running out of tap

⚄ X11.8 **Contact with** other **hot tap-water**

Contact with hot water in bucket
Contact with hot tap-water NOS

⚆ X12 **Contact with** other hot fluids

Contact with water heated on stove

> EXCLUDES1 *hot (liquid) metals (X18)*

The appropriate 7th character is to be added to code X12
A = initial encounter
D = subsequent encounter
S = sequela

⚁ X13 **Contact with** steam and other hot vapors

The appropriate 7th character is to be added to each code from category X13
A = initial encounter
D = subsequent encounter
S = sequela

⚄ X13.0 Inhalation of steam and other hot vapors
⚄ X13.1 Other contact with steam and other hot vapors

⚁ X14 **Contact with** hot air and other hot gases

The appropriate 7th character is to be added to each code from category X14
A = initial encounter
D = subsequent encounter
S = sequela

⚄ X14.0 Inhalation of hot air and gases
⚄ X14.1 Other contact with hot air and other hot gases

⚁ X15 **Contact with** hot household appliances

> EXCLUDES1 *contact with heating appliances (X16)*
> *contact with powered household appliances (W29.-)*
> *exposure to controlled fire in building or structure due to household appliance (X02.8)*
> *exposure to household appliances electrical current (W86.0)*

The appropriate 7th character is to be added to each code from category X15
A = initial encounter
D = subsequent encounter
S = sequela

⚄ X15.0 **Contact with hot** stove (kitchen)
⚄ X15.1 **Contact with hot** toaster
⚄ X15.2 **Contact with** hotplate
⚄ X15.3 **Contact with hot** saucepan or skillet
⚄ X15.8 **Contact with** other **hot household appliances**

Contact with cooker
Contact with kettle
Contact with light bulbs

⚆ X16 **Contact with** hot heating appliances, radiators and pipes

> EXCLUDES1 *contact with powered appliances (W29.-)*
> *exposure to controlled fire in building or structure due to appliance (X02.8)*
> *exposure to industrial appliances electrical current (W86.1)*

The appropriate 7th character is to be added to code X16
A = initial encounter
D = subsequent encounter
S = sequela

⚁ 4th character required   ⚃ 5th character required   ⚄ 6th character required   ⚆ 7th character required   ⚇ Extension 'X' Alert

EXCLUDES 1 Not coded here   EXCLUDES 2 Not included here   PDx Primary Diagnosis Only   Manifestation Code

788

ICD-10-CM 2015

[7] **X17 Contact with hot engines, machinery and tools**
[EXCLUDES1] *contact with hot heating appliances, radiators and pipes (X16)*
contact with hot household appliances (X15)
The appropriate 7th character is to be added to code X17
A = initial encounter
D = subsequent encounter
S = sequela

[7] **X18 Contact with other hot metals**
Contact with liquid metal
The appropriate 7th character is to be added to code X18
A = initial encounter
D = subsequent encounter
S = sequela

[7] **X19 Contact with other heat and hot substances**
[EXCLUDES1] *objects that are not normally hot, e.g., an object made hot by a house fire (X00-X09)*
The appropriate 7th character is to be added to code X19
A = initial encounter
D = subsequent encounter
S = sequela

Exposure to forces of nature (X30-X39)

[7] **X30 Exposure to excessive natural heat**
Exposure to excessive heat as the cause of sunstroke
Exposure to heat NOS
[EXCLUDES1] *excessive heat of man-made origin (W92)*
exposure to man-made radiation (W89)
exposure to sunlight (X32)
exposure to tanning bed (W89)
The appropriate 7th character is to be added to code X30
A = initial encounter
D = subsequent encounter
S = sequela

[7] **X31 Exposure to excessive natural cold**
Excessive cold as the cause of chilblains NOS
Excessive cold as the cause of immersion foot or hand
Exposure to cold NOS
Exposure to weather conditions
[EXCLUDES1] *cold of man-made origin (W93.-)*
contact with or inhalation of dry ice (W93.-)
contact with or inhalation of liquefied gas (W93.-)
The appropriate 7th character is to be added to code X31
A = initial encounter
D = subsequent encounter
S = sequela

[7] **X32 Exposure to sunlight**
[EXCLUDES1] *radiation-related disorders of the skin and subcutaneous tissue (L55-L59)*
man-made radiation (tanning bed) (W89)
The appropriate 7th character is to be added to code X32
A = initial encounter
D = subsequent encounter
S = sequela

[7] **X34 Earthquake**
[EXCLUDES2] *tidal wave (tsunami) due to earthquake (X37.41)*
The appropriate 7th character is to be added to code X34
A = initial encounter
D = subsequent encounter
S = sequela

[7] **X35 Volcanic eruption**
[EXCLUDES2] *tidal wave (tsunami) due to volcanic eruption (X37.41)*
The appropriate 7th character is to be added to code X35
A = initial encounter
D = subsequent encounter
S = sequela

[4] **X36 Avalanche, landslide and other earth movements**
[INCLUDES] *victim of mudslide of cataclysmic nature*
[EXCLUDES1] *earthquake (X34)*
[EXCLUDES2] *transport accident involving collision with avalanche or landslide not in motion (V01-V99)*
The appropriate 7th character is to be added to each code from category X36
A = initial encounter
D = subsequent encounter
S = sequela

[7th] **X36.0 Collapse of dam or man-made structure causing earth movement**
[7th] **X36.1 Avalanche, landslide, or mudslide**

[4] **X37 Cataclysmic storm**
The appropriate 7th character is to be added to each code from category X37
A = initial encounter
D = subsequent encounter
S = sequela

[7th] **X37.0 Hurricane**
Storm surge
Typhoon
[7th] **X37.1 Tornado**
Cyclone
Twister
[7th] **X37.2 Blizzard (snow)(ice)**
[7th] **X37.3 Dust storm**
[5] **X37.4 Tidalwave**
[7th] **X37.41 Tidal wave due to earthquake or volcanic eruption**
Tidal wave NOS
Tsunami
[7th] **X37.42 Tidal wave due to storm**
[7th] **X37.43 Tidal wave due to landslide**
[7th] **X37.8 Other cataclysmic storms**
Cloudburst
Torrential rain
[EXCLUDES2] *flood (X38)*
[7th] **X37.9 Unspecified cataclysmic storm**
Storm NOS
[EXCLUDES1] *collapse of dam or man-made structure causing earth movement (X39.0)*

[7] **X38 Flood**
Flood arising from remote storm
Flood of cataclysmic nature arising from melting snow
Flood resulting directly from storm
[EXCLUDES1] *collapse of dam or man-made structure causing earth movement (X39.0)*
tidal wave NOS (X37.41)
tidal wave caused by storm (X37.2)
The appropriate 7th character is to be added to code X38
A = initial encounter
D = subsequent encounter
S = sequela

[4] **X39 Exposure to other forces of nature**
The appropriate 7th character is to be added to each code from category X39
A = initial encounter
D = subsequent encounter
S = sequela

[5] **X39.0 Exposure to natural radiation**
[EXCLUDES1] *contact with and (suspected) exposure to radon and other naturally occuring radiation (Z77.122)*
exposure to man-made radiation (W88-W90)
exposure to sunlight (X32)
[7th] **X39.01 Exposure to radon**
[7th] **X39.08 Exposure to other natural radiation**
[7th] **X39.8 Other exposure to forces of nature**

Unspecified Code | Other Specified Code | [N] Newborn Age: 0 | [P] Pediatric Age: 0-17 | [M] Maternity Age: 12-55
[A] Adult Age: 15-124 | ♂ Male | ♀ Female | ● New Code | ▲ Revised Code Title | ▶◀ Revised Text

Accidental exposure to other specified factors (X52, X58)

[7] X52 Prolonged stay in weightless environment
Weightlessness in spacecraft (simulator)
The appropriate 7th character is to be added to code X52
A = initial encounter
D = subsequent encounter
S = sequela

[7] X58 Exposure to other specified factors
Accident NOS
Exposure NOS
The appropriate 7th character is to be added to code X58
A = initial encounter
D = subsequent encounter
S = sequela

Intentional self-harm (X71-X83)

Purposely self-inflicted injury
Suicide (attempted)

[4] X71 Intentional self-harm by drowning and submersion
The appropriate 7th character is to be added to each code from category X71
A = initial encounter
D = subsequent encounter
S = sequela
- [X] X71.0 Intentional self-harm by drowning and submersion while in bathtub
- [X] X71.1 Intentional self-harm by drowning and submersion while in swimming pool
- [X] X71.2 Intentional self-harm by drowning and submersion after jump into swimming pool
- [X] X71.3 Intentional self-harm by drowning and submersion in natural water
- [X] X71.8 Other intentional self-harm by drowning and submersion
- [X] X71.9 Intentional self-harm by drowning and submersion, unspecified

[7] X72 Intentional self-harm by handgun discharge
Intentional self-harm by gun for single hand use
Intentional self-harm by pistol
Intentional self-harm by revolver
[EXCLUDES1] *Very pistol (X74.8)*
The appropriate 7th character is to be added to code X72
A = initial encounter
D = subsequent encounter
S = sequela

[4] X73 Intentional self-harm by rifle, shotgun and larger firearm discharge
[EXCLUDES1] *airgun (X74.01)*
The appropriate 7th character is to be added to each code from category X73
A = initial encounter
D = subsequent encounter
S = sequela
- [X] X73.0 Intentional self-harm by shotgun discharge
- [X] X73.1 Intentional self-harm by hunting rifle discharge
- [X] X73.2 Intentional self-harm by machine gun discharge
- [X] X73.8 Intentional self-harm by other larger firearm discharge
- [X] X73.9 Intentional self-harm by unspecified larger firearm discharge

[4] X74 Intentional self-harm by other and unspecified firearm and gun discharge
The appropriate 7th character is to be added to each code from category X74
A = initial encounter
D = subsequent encounter
S = sequela
- [5] X74.0 Intentional self-harm by gas, air or spring-operated guns
  - [X] X74.01 Intentional self-harm by airgun
    Intentional self-harm by BB gun discharge
    Intentional self-harm by pellet gun discharge
  - [X] X74.02 Intentional self-harm by paintball gun
  - [X] X74.09 Intentional self-harm by other gas, air or spring-operated gun
- [X] X74.8 Intentional self-harm by other firearm discharge
  Intentional self-harm by Very pistol [flare] discharge
- [X] X74.9 Intentional self-harm by unspecified firearm discharge

[7] X75 Intentional self-harm by explosive material
The appropriate 7th character is to be added to code X75
A = initial encounter
D = subsequent encounter
S = sequela

[7] X76 Intentional self-harm by smoke, fire and flames
The appropriate 7th character is to be added to code X76
A = initial encounter
D = subsequent encounter
S = sequela

[4] X77 Intentional self-harm by steam, hot vapors and hot objects
The appropriate 7th character is to be added to each code from category X77
A = initial encounter
D = subsequent encounter
S = sequela
- [X] X77.0 Intentional self-harm by steam or hot vapors
- [X] X77.1 Intentional self-harm by hot tap water
- [X] X77.2 Intentional self-harm by other hot fluids
- [X] X77.3 Intentional self-harm by hot household appliances
- [X] X77.8 Intentional self-harm by other hot objects
- [X] X77.9 Intentional self-harm by unspecified hot objects

[4] X78 Intentional self-harm by sharp object
The appropriate 7th character is to be added to each code from category X78
A = initial encounter
D = subsequent encounter
S = sequela
- [X] X78.0 Intentional self-harm by sharp glass
- [X] X78.1 Intentional self-harm by knife
- [X] X78.2 Intentional self-harm by sword or dagger
- [X] X78.8 Intentional self-harm by other sharp object
- [X] X78.9 Intentional self-harm by unspecified sharp object

[7] X79 Intentional self-harm by blunt object
The appropriate 7th character is to be added to code X79
A = initial encounter
D = subsequent encounter
S = sequela

[7] X80 Intentional self-harm by jumping from a high place
Intentional fall from one level to another
The appropriate 7th character is to be added to code X80
A = initial encounter
D = subsequent encounter
S = sequela

[4] X81 Intentional self-harm by jumping or lying in front of moving object
The appropriate 7th character is to be added to each code from category X81
A = initial encounter
D = subsequent encounter
S = sequela
- [X] X81.0 Intentional self-harm by jumping or lying in front of motor vehicle
- [X] X81.1 Intentional self-harm by jumping or lying in front of (subway) train

[4] 4th character required [5] 5th character required [6] 6th character required [7] 7th character required [X] Extension 'X' Alert
[EXCLUDES1] Not coded here [EXCLUDES2] Not included here [PDx] Primary Diagnosis Only Manifestation Code

X81.8 Intentional self-harm by jumping or lying in front of other moving object

X82 Intentional self-harm by crashing of motor vehicle

The appropriate 7th character is to be added to each code from category X82
A = initial encounter
D = subsequent encounter
S = sequela

X82.0 Intentional collision of motor vehicle with other motor vehicle

X82.1 Intentional collision of motor vehicle with train

X82.2 Intentional collision of motor vehicle with tree

X82.8 Other intentional self-harm by crashing of motor vehicle

X83 Intentional self-harm by other specified means

EXCLUDES1 intentional self-harm by poisoning or contact with toxic substance- See Table of Drugs and Chemicals

The appropriate 7th character is to be added to each code from category X83
A = initial encounter
D = subsequent encounter
S = sequela

X83.0 Intentional self-harm by crashing of aircraft

X83.1 Intentional self-harm by electrocution

X83.2 Intentional self-harm by exposure to extremes of cold

X83.8 Intentional self-harm by other specified means

Assault (X92-Y08)

INCLUDES homicide
injuries inflicted by another person with intent to injure or kill, by any means

EXCLUDES1 injuries due to legal intervention (Y35.-)
injuries due to operations of war (Y36.-)
injuries due to terrorism (Y38.-)

X92 Assault by drowning and submersion

The appropriate 7th character is to be added to each code from category X92
A = initial encounter
D = subsequent encounter
S = sequela

X92.0 Assault by drowning and submersion while in bathtub

X92.1 Assault by drowning and submersion while in swimming pool

X92.2 Assault by drowning and submersion after push into swimming pool

X92.3 Assault by drowning and submersion in natural water

X92.8 Other assault by drowning and submersion

X92.9 Assault by drowning and submersion, unspecified

X93 Assault by handgun discharge

Assault by discharge of gun for single hand use
Assault by discharge of pistol
Assault by discharge of revolver

EXCLUDES1 Very pistol (X95.8)

The appropriate 7th character is to be added to code X93
A = initial encounter
D = subsequent encounter
S = sequela

X94 Assault by rifle, shotgun and larger firearm discharge

EXCLUDES1 airgun (X95.01)

The appropriate 7th character is to be added to each code from category X94
A = initial encounter
D = subsequent encounter
S = sequela

X94.0 Assault by shotgun

X94.1 Assault by hunting rifle

X94.2 Assault by machine gun

X94.8 Assault by other larger firearm discharge

X94.9 Assault by unspecified larger firearm discharge

X95 Assault by other and unspecified firearm and gun discharge

The appropriate 7th character is to be added to each code from category X95
A = initial encounter
D = subsequent encounter
S = sequela

X95.0 Assault by gas, air or spring-operated guns

X95.01 Assault by airgun discharge
Assault by BB gun discharge
Assault by pellet gun discharge

X95.02 Assault by paintball gun discharge

X95.09 Assault by other gas, air or spring-operated gun

X95.8 Assault by other firearm discharge
Assault by very pistol [flare] discharge

X95.9 Assault by unspecified firearm discharge

X96 Assault by explosive material

EXCLUDES1 incendiary device (X97)
terrorism involving explosive material (Y38.2-)

The appropriate 7th character is to be added to each code from category X96
A = initial encounter
D = subsequent encounter
S = sequela

X96.0 Assault by antipersonnel bomb

EXCLUDES1 antipersonnel bomb use in military or war (Y36.2-)

X96.1 Assault by gasoline bomb

X96.2 Assault by letter bomb

X96.3 Assault by fertilizer bomb

X96.4 Assault by pipe bomb

X96.8 Assault by other specified explosive

X96.9 Assault by unspecified explosive

X97 Assault by smoke, fire and flames

Assault by arson
Assault by cigarettes
Assault by incendiary device

The appropriate 7th character is to be added to code X97
A = initial encounter
D = subsequent encounter
S = sequela

X98 Assault by steam, hot vapors and hot objects

The appropriate 7th character is to be added to each code from category X98
A = initial encounter
D = subsequent encounter
S = sequela

X98.0 Assault by steam or hot vapors

X98.1 Assault by hot tap water

X98.2 Assault by hot fluids

X98.3 Assault by hot household appliances

X98.8 Assault by other hot objects

X98.9 Assault by unspecified hot objects

X99 Assault by sharp object

EXCLUDES1 assault by strike by sports equipment (Y08.0-)

The appropriate 7th character is to be added to each code from category X99
A = initial encounter
D = subsequent encounter
S = sequela

X99.0 Assault by sharp glass

X99.1 Assault by knife

X99.2 Assault by sword or dagger

X99.8 Assault by other sharp object

X99.9 Assault by unspecified sharp object
Assault by stabbing NOS

Unspecified Code   Other Specified Code   N Newborn Age: 0   P Pediatric Age: 0-17   M Maternity Age: 12-55

A Adult Age: 15-124   ♂ Male   ♀ Female   ● New Code   ▲ Revised Code Title   ►◄ Revised Text

[7] **Y00 Assault by blunt object**

[EXCLUDES1] *assault by strike by sports equipment (Y08.0-)*

The appropriate 7th character is to be added to code Y00
A = initial encounter
D = subsequent encounter
S = sequela

[7] **Y01 Assault by pushing from high place**

The appropriate 7th character is to be added to code Y01
A = initial encounter
D = subsequent encounter
S = sequela

[4] **Y02 Assault by pushing or placing victim in front of moving object**

The appropriate 7th character is to be added to each code from category Y02
A = initial encounter
D = subsequent encounter
S = sequela

[X] **Y02.0 Assault by pushing or placing victim in front of motor vehicle**
[X] **Y02.1 Assault by pushing or placing victim in front of (subway) train**
[X] **Y02.8 Assault by pushing or placing victim in front of other moving object**

[4] **Y03 Assault by crashing of motor vehicle**

The appropriate 7th character is to be added to each code from category Y03
A = initial encounter
D = subsequent encounter
S = sequela

[X] **Y03.0 Assault by being hit or run over by motor vehicle**
[X] **Y03.8 Other assault by crashing of motor vehicle**

[4] **Y04 Assault by bodily force**

[EXCLUDES1] *assault by:*
submersion (X92.-)
use of weapon (X93-X95, X99, Y00)

The appropriate 7th character is to be added to each code from category Y04
A = initial encounter
D = subsequent encounter
S = sequela

[X] **Y04.0 Assault by unarmed brawl or fight**
[X] **Y04.1 Assault by human bite**
[X] **Y04.2 Assault by strike against or bumped into by another person**
[X] **Y04.8 Assault by other bodily force**
Assault by bodily force NOS

[4] **Y07 Perpetrator of assault, maltreatment and neglect**

[NOTES] Codes from this category are for use only in cases of confirmed abuse (T74.-)
Selection of the correct perpetrator code is based on the relationship between the perpetrator and the victim

[INCLUDES] *perpetrator of abandonment*
perpetrator of emotional neglect
perpetrator of mental cruelty
perpetrator of physical abuse
perpetrator of physical neglect
perpetrator of sexual abuse
perpetrator of torture

[5] **Y07.0 Spouse or partner, perpetrator of maltreatment and neglect**
Spouse or partner, perpetrator of maltreatment and neglect against spouse or partner

Y07.01 Husband, perpetrator of maltreatment and neglect
Y07.02 Wife, perpetrator of maltreatment and neglect
Y07.03 Male partner, perpetrator of maltreatment and neglect
Y07.04 Female partner, perpetrator of maltreatment and neglect

[5] **Y07.1 Parent (adoptive) (biological), perpetrator of maltreatment and neglect**

Y07.11 Biological father, perpetrator of maltreatment and neglect
Y07.12 Biological mother, perpetrator of maltreatment and neglect
Y07.13 Adoptive father, perpetrator of maltreatment and neglect
Y07.14 Adoptive mother, perpetrator of maltreatment and neglect

[5] **Y07.4 Other family member, perpetrator of maltreatment and neglect**

[6] **Y07.41 Sibling, perpetrator of maltreatment and neglect**

[EXCLUDES1] *stepsibling, perpetrator of maltreatment and neglect (Y07.435, Y07.436)*

Y07.410 Brother, perpetrator of maltreatment and neglect
Y07.411 Sister, perpetrator of maltreatment and neglect

[6] **Y07.42 Foster parent, perpetrator of maltreatment and neglect**

Y07.420 Foster father, perpetrator of maltreatment and neglect
Y07.421 Foster mother, perpetrator of maltreatment and neglect

[6] **Y07.43 Stepparent or stepsibling, perpetrator of maltreatment and neglect**

Y07.430 Stepfather, perpetrator of maltreatment and neglect
Y07.432 Male friend of parent (co-residing in household), perpetrator of maltreatment and neglect
Y07.433 Stepmother, perpetrator of maltreatment and neglect
Y07.434 Female friend of parent (co-residing in household), perpetrator of maltreatment and neglect
Y07.435 Stepbrother, perpetrator or maltreatment and neglect
Y07.436 Stepsister, perpetrator of maltreatment and neglect

[6] **Y07.49 Other family member, perpetrator of maltreatment and neglect**

Y07.490 Male cousin, perpetrator of maltreatment and neglect
Y07.491 Female cousin, perpetrator of maltreatment and neglect
Y07.499 Other family member, perpetrator of maltreatment and neglect

[5] **Y07.5 Non-family member, perpetrator of maltreatment and neglect**

Y07.50 Unspecified non-family member, perpetrator of maltreatment and neglect

[6] **Y07.51 Daycare provider, perpetrator of maltreatment and neglect**

Y07.510 At-home childcare provider, perpetrator of maltreatment and neglect
Y07.511 Daycare center childcare provider, perpetrator of maltreatment and neglect
Y07.512 At-home adultcare provider, perpetrator of maltreatment and neglect
Y07.513 Adultcare center provider, perpetrator of maltreatment and neglect
Y07.519 Unspecified daycare provider, perpetrator of maltreatment and neglect

[6] **Y07.52 Healthcare provider, perpetrator of maltreatment and neglect**

Y07.521 Mental health provider, **perpetrator of maltreatment and neglect**

Y07.528 Other therapist or healthcare provider, **perpetrator of maltreatment and neglect**

Nurse perpetrator of maltreatment and neglect
Occupational therapist perpetrator of maltreatment and neglect
Physical therapist perpetrator of maltreatment and neglect
Speech therapist perpetrator of maltreatment and neglect

Y07.529 Unspecified healthcare provider, **perpetrator of maltreatment and neglect**

Y07.53 Teacher or instructor, **perpetrator of maltreatment and neglect**

Coach, perpetrator of maltreatment and neglect

Y07.59 Other **non-family member, perpetrator of maltreatment and neglect**

Y07.9 Unspecified **perpetrator of maltreatment and neglect**

Y08 Assault by other specified **means**

The appropriate 7th character is to be added to each code from category Y08
A = initial encounter
D = subsequent encounter
S = sequela

Y08.0 **Assault by** strike by sport equipment
Y08.01 **Assault by strike by** hockey stick
Y08.02 **Assault by strike by** baseball bat
Y08.09 **Assault by strike by other specified type of sport equipment**

Y08.8 **Assault by** other specified **means**
Y08.81 **Assault by** crashing of aircraft
Y08.89 **Assault by other specified means**

Y09 **Assault by unspecified means**

Assassination (attempted) NOS
Homicide (attempted) NOS
Manslaughter (attempted) NOS
Murder (attempted) NOS

Event of undetermined intent (Y21-Y33)

Undetermined intent is only for use when there is specific documentation in the record that the intent of the injury cannot bedetermined. If no such documentation is present, code to accidental (unintentional)

Y21 **Drowning and submersion, undetermined intent**

The appropriate 7th character is to be added to each code from category Y21
A = initial encounter
D = subsequent encounter
S = sequela

Y21.0 **Drowning and submersion** while in bathtub, **undetermined intent**
Y21.1 **Drowning and submersion** after fall into bathtub, **undetermined intent**
Y21.2 **Drowning and submersion** while in swimming pool, **undetermined intent**
Y21.3 **Drowning and submersion** after fall into swimming pool, **undetermined intent**
Y21.4 **Drowning and submersion** in natural water, **undetermined intent**
Y21.8 Other **drowning and submersion, undetermined intent**
Y21.9 Unspecified **drowning and submersion, undetermined intent**

Y22 Handgun **discharge, undetermined intent**

Discharge of gun for single hand use, undetermined intent

Discharge of pistol, undetermined intent
Discharge of revolver, undetermined intent

EXCLUDES2 *very pistol (Y24.8)*

The appropriate 7th character is to be added to code Y22
A = initial encounter
D = subsequent encounter
S = sequela

Y23 Rifle, shotgun and larger firearm **discharge, undetermined intent**

EXCLUDES2 *airgun (Y24.0)*

The appropriate 7th character is to be added to each code from category Y23
A = initial encounter
D = subsequent encounter
S = sequela

Y23.0 Shotgun **discharge, undetermined intent**
Y23.1 Hunting rifle **discharge, undetermined intent**
Y23.2 Military firearm **discharge, undetermined intent**
Y23.3 Machine gun **discharge, undetermined intent**
Y23.8 Other **larger firearm discharge, undetermined intent**
Y23.9 Unspecified **larger firearm discharge, undetermined intent**

Y24 Other and unspecified **firearm discharge, undetermined intent**

The appropriate 7th character is to be added to each code from category Y24
A = initial encounter
D = subsequent encounter
S = sequela

Y24.0 Airgun **discharge, undetermined intent**
BB gun discharge, undetermined intent
Pellet gun discharge, undetermined intent
Y24.8 Other **firearm discharge, undetermined intent**
Paintball gun discharge, undetermined intent
Very pistol [flare] discharge, undetermined intent
Y24.9 Unspecified **firearm discharge, undetermined intent**

Y25 **Contact with explosive material, undetermined intent**
The appropriate 7th character is to be added to code Y25
A = initial encounter
D = subsequent encounter
S = sequela

Y26 **Exposure to smoke, fire and flames, undetermined intent**
The appropriate 7th character is to be added to code Y26
A = initial encounter
D = subsequent encounter
S = sequela

Y27 **Contact with steam, hot vapors and hot objects, undetermined intent**
The appropriate 7th character is to be added to each code from category Y27
A = initial encounter
D = subsequent encounter
S = sequela

Y27.0 **Contact with** steam and hot vapors, **undetermined intent**
Y27.1 **Contact with** hot tap water, **undetermined intent**
Y27.2 **Contact with** hot fluids, **undetermined intent**
Y27.3 **Contact with** hot household appliance, **undetermined intent**
Y27.8 **Contact with** other hot objects, **undetermined intent**
Y27.9 **Contact with unspecified hot objects, undetermined intent**

Unspecified Code   Other Specified Code   N Newborn Age: 0   P Pediatric Age: 0-17   M Maternity Age: 12-55
A Adult Age: 15-124   ♂ Male   ♀ Female   ● New Code   ▲ Revised Code Title   ►◄ Revised Text

ICD-10-CM 2015

793

④ Y28 Contact with sharp object, undetermined intent

The appropriate 7th character is to be added to each code from category Y28

A = initial encounter
D = subsequent encounter
S = sequela

⑦ Y28.0 Contact with sharp glass, undetermined intent
⑦ Y28.1 Contact with knife, undetermined intent
⑦ Y28.2 Contact with sword or dagger, undetermined intent
⑦ Y28.8 Contact with other sharp object, undetermined intent
⑦ Y28.9 Contact with unspecified sharp object, undetermined intent

⑦ Y29 Contact with blunt object, undetermined intent

The appropriate 7th character is to be added to code Y29

A = initial encounter
D = subsequent encounter
S = sequela

⑦ Y30 Falling, jumping or pushed from a high place, undetermined intent

Victim falling from one level to another, undetermined intent

The appropriate 7th character is to be added to code Y30

A = initial encounter
D = subsequent encounter
S = sequela

⑦ Y31 Falling, lying or running before or into moving object, undetermined intent

The appropriate 7th character is to be added to code Y31

A = initial encounter
D = subsequent encounter
S = sequela

⑦ Y32 Crashing of motor vehicle, undetermined intent

The appropriate 7th character is to be added to code Y32

A = initial encounter
D = subsequent encounter
S = sequela

⑦ Y33 Other specified events, undetermined intent

The appropriate 7th character is to be added to code Y33

A = initial encounter
D = subsequent encounter
S = sequela

Legal intervention, operations of war, military operations, and terrorism (Y35-Y38)

④ Y35 Legal intervention

INCLUDES   any injury sustained as a result of an encounter with any law enforcement official, serving in any capacity at the time of the encounter, whether on-duty or off-duty. Includes: injury to law enforcement official, suspect and bystander

The appropriate 7th character is to be added to each code from category Y35

A = initial encounter
D = subsequent encounter
S = sequela

⑤ Y35.0 Legal intervention involving firearm discharge
⑥ Y35.00 Legal intervention involving unspecified firearm discharge

Legal intervention involving gunshot wound
Legal intervention involving shot NOS

⑦ Y35.001 Legal intervention involving unspecified firearm discharge, law enforcement official injured
⑦ Y35.002 Legal intervention involving unspecified firearm discharge, bystander injured
⑦ Y35.003 Legal intervention involving unspecified firearm discharge, suspect injured

⑥ Y35.01 Legal intervention involving injury by machine gun
⑦ Y35.011 Legal intervention involving injury by machine gun, law enforcement official injured
⑦ Y35.012 Legal intervention involving injury by machine gun, bystander injured
⑦ Y35.013 Legal intervention involving injury by machine gun, suspect injured

⑥ Y35.02 Legal intervention involving injury by handgun
⑦ Y35.021 Legal intervention involving injury by handgun, law enforcement official injured
⑦ Y35.022 Legal intervention involving injury by handgun, bystander injured
⑦ Y35.023 Legal intervention involving injury by handgun, suspect injured

⑥ Y35.03 Legal intervention involving injury by rifle pellet
⑦ Y35.031 Legal intervention involving injury by rifle pellet, law enforcement official injured
⑦ Y35.032 Legal intervention involving injury by rifle pellet, bystander injured
⑦ Y35.033 Legal intervention involving injury by rifle pellet, suspect injured

⑥ Y35.04 Legal intervention involving injury by rubber bullet
⑦ Y35.041 Legal intervention involving injury by rubber bullet, law enforcement official injured
⑦ Y35.042 Legal intervention involving injury by rubber bullet, bystander injured
⑦ Y35.043 Legal intervention involving injury by rubber bullet, suspect injured

⑥ Y35.09 Legal intervention involving other firearm discharge
⑦ Y35.091 Legal intervention involving other firearm discharge, law enforcement official injured
⑦ Y35.092 Legal intervention involving other firearm discharge, bystander injured
⑦ Y35.093 Legal intervention involving other firearm discharge, suspect injured

⑤ Y35.1 Legal intervention involving explosives
⑥ Y35.10 Legal intervention involving unspecified explosives
⑦ Y35.101 Legal intervention involving unspecified explosives, law enforcement official injured
⑦ Y35.102 Legal intervention involving unspecified explosives, bystander injured
⑦ Y35.103 Legal intervention involving unspecified explosives, suspect injured

⑥ Y35.11 Legal intervention involving injury by dynamite
⑦ Y35.111 Legal intervention involving injury by dynamite, law enforcement official injured
⑦ Y35.112 Legal intervention involving injury by dynamite, bystander injured
⑦ Y35.113 Legal intervention involving injury by dynamite, suspect injured

⑥ Y35.12 Legal intervention involving injury by explosive shell
⑦ Y35.121 Legal intervention involving injury by explosive shell, law enforcement official injured
⑦ Y35.122 Legal intervention involving injury by explosive shell, bystander injured
⑦ Y35.123 Legal intervention involving injury by explosive shell, suspect injured

⑥ Y35.19 Legal intervention involving other explosives

Legal intervention involving injury by grenade
Legal intervention involving injury by mortar bomb

---

④ 4th character required   ⑤ 5th character required   ⑥ 6th character required   ⑦ 7th character required   ⑩ Extension 'X' Alert

EXCLUDES 1 Not coded here   *EXCLUDES 2* Not included here   PDx Primary Diagnosis Only   Manifestation Code

⑦ Y35.191 **Legal intervention involving other explosives,** law enforcement official injured

⑦ Y35.192 **Legal intervention involving other explosives,** bystander injured

⑦ Y35.193 **Legal intervention involving other explosives,** suspect injured

⑤ Y35.2 **Legal intervention involving** gas

Legal intervention involving asphyxiation by gas

Legal intervention involving poisoning by gas

⑥ Y35.20 **Legal intervention involving** unspecified gas

⑦ Y35.201 **Legal intervention involving unspecified gas,** law enforcement official injured

⑦ Y35.202 **Legal intervention involving unspecified gas,** bystander injured

⑦ Y35.203 **Legal intervention involving unspecified gas,** suspect injured

⑥ Y35.21 **Legal intervention involving injury by** tear gas

⑦ Y35.211 **Legal intervention involving injury by tear gas,** law enforcement official injured

⑦ Y35.212 **Legal intervention involving injury by tear gas,** bystander injured

⑦ Y35.213 **Legal intervention involving injury by tear gas,** suspect injured

⑥ Y35.29 **Legal intervention involving** other gas

⑦ Y35.291 **Legal intervention involving other gas,** law enforcement official injured

⑦ Y35.292 **Legal intervention involving other gas,** bystander injured

⑦ Y35.293 **Legal intervention involving other gas,** suspect injured

⑤ Y35.3 **Legal intervention involving** blunt objects

Legal intervention involving being hit or struck by blunt object

⑥ Y35.30 **Legal intervention involving** unspecified **blunt objects**

⑦ Y35.301 **Legal intervention involving unspecified blunt objects,** law enforcement official injured

⑦ Y35.302 **Legal intervention involving unspecified blunt objects,** bystander injured

⑦ Y35.303 **Legal intervention involving unspecified blunt objects,** suspect injured

⑥ Y35.31 **Legal intervention involving** baton

⑦ Y35.311 **Legal intervention involving baton,** law enforcement official injured

⑦ Y35.312 **Legal intervention involving baton,** bystander injured

⑦ Y35.313 **Legal intervention involving baton,** suspect injured

⑥ Y35.39 **Legal intervention involving** other blunt objects

⑦ Y35.391 **Legal intervention involving other blunt objects,** law enforcement official injured

⑦ Y35.392 **Legal intervention involving other blunt objects,** bystander injured

⑦ Y35.393 **Legal intervention involving other blunt objects,** suspect injured

⑤ Y35.4 **Legal intervention involving** sharp objects

Legal intervention involving being cut by sharp objects

Legal intervention involving being stabbed by sharp objects

⑥ Y35.40 **Legal intervention involving** unspecified **sharp objects**

⑦ Y35.401 **Legal intervention involving unspecified sharp objects,** law enforcement official injured

⑦ Y35.402 **Legal intervention involving unspecified sharp objects,** bystander injured

⑦ Y35.403 **Legal intervention involving unspecified sharp objects,** suspect injured

⑥ Y35.41 **Legal intervention involving** bayonet

⑦ Y35.411 **Legal intervention involving bayonet,** law enforcement official injured

⑦ Y35.412 **Legal intervention involving bayonet,** bystander injured

⑦ Y35.413 **Legal intervention involving bayonet,** suspect injured

⑥ Y35.49 **Legal intervention involving** other sharp objects

⑦ Y35.491 **Legal intervention involving other sharp objects,** law enforcement official injured

⑦ Y35.492 **Legal intervention involving other sharp objects,** bystander injured

⑦ Y35.493 **Legal intervention involving other sharp objects,** suspect injured

⑤ Y35.8 **Legal intervention involving** other specified means

⑥ Y35.81 **Legal intervention involving** manhandling

⑦ Y35.811 **Legal intervention involving manhandling,** law enforcement official injured

⑦ Y35.812 **Legal intervention involving manhandling,** bystander injured

⑦ Y35.813 **Legal intervention involving manhandling,** suspect injured

⑥ Y35.89 **Legal intervention involving** other specified means

⑦ Y35.891 **Legal intervention involving other specified means,** law enforcement official injured

⑦ Y35.892 **Legal intervention involving other specified means,** bystander injured

⑦ Y35.893 **Legal intervention involving other specified means,** suspect injured

⑤ Y35.9 **Legal intervention, means** unspecified

⑦ Y35.91 **Legal intervention, means unspecified,** law enforcement official injured

⑦ Y35.92 **Legal intervention, means unspecified,** bystander injured

⑦ Y35.93 **Legal intervention, means unspecified,** suspect injured

④ Y36 **Operations of war**

> *INCLUDES*   *injuries to military personnel and civilians caused by war, civil insurrection, and peacekeeping missions*
>
> *EXCLUDES1*   *injury to military personnel occurring during peacetime military operations (Y37.-)*
> *military vehicles involved in transport accidents with non-military vehicle during peacetime (V09.01, V09.21, V19.81, V29.81, V39.81, V49.81, V59.81, V69.81, V79.81)*

The appropriate 7th character is to be added to each code from category Y36

A = initial encounter

D = subsequent encounter

S = sequela

⑤ Y36.0 **War operations involving** explosion of marine weapons

⑥ Y36.00 **War operations involving explosion of** unspecified **marine weapon**

War operations involving underwater blast NOS

⑦ Y36.000 **War operations involving explosion of unspecified marine weapon,** military personnel

⑦ Y36.001 **War operations involving explosion of unspecified marine weapon,** civilian

⑥ Y36.01 **War operations involving explosion of** depth-charge

⑦ Y36.010 **War operations involving explosion of depth-charge,** military personnel

⑦ Y36.011 **War operations involving explosion of depth-charge,** civilian

---

⑥ Y36.02 War operations involving explosion of marine mine

War operations involving explosion of marine mine, at sea or in harbor

　⑦ Y36.020 War operations involving explosion of marine mine, military personnel

　⑦ Y36.021 War operations involving explosion of marine mine, civilian

⑥ Y36.03 War operations involving explosion of sea-based artillery shell

　⑦ Y36.030 War operations involving explosion of sea-based artillery shell, military personnel

　⑦ Y36.031 War operations involving explosion of sea-based artillery shell, civilian

⑥ Y36.04 War operations involving explosion of torpedo

　⑦ Y36.040 War operations involving explosion of torpedo, military personnel

　⑦ Y36.041 War operations involving explosion of torpedo, civilian

⑥ Y36.05 War operations involving accidental detonation of onboard marine weapons

　⑦ Y36.050 War operations involving accidental detonation of onboard marine weapons, military personnel

　⑦ Y36.051 War operations involving accidental detonation of onboard marine weapons, civilian

⑥ Y36.09 War operations involving explosion of other marine weapons

　⑦ Y36.090 War operations involving explosion of other marine weapons, military personnel

　⑦ Y36.091 War operations involving explosion of other marine weapons, civilian

⑤ Y36.1 War operations involving destruction of aircraft

⑥ Y36.10 War operations involving unspecified destruction of aircraft

　⑦ Y36.100 War operations involving unspecified destruction of aircraft, military personnel

　⑦ Y36.101 War operations involving unspecified destruction of aircraft, civilian

⑥ Y36.11 War operations involving destruction of aircraft due to enemy fire or explosives

War operations involving destruction of aircraft due to air to air missile

War operations involving destruction of aircraft due to explosive placed on aircraft

War operations involving destruction of aircraft due to rocket propelled grenade [RPG]

War operations involving destruction of aircraft due to small arms fire

War operations involving destruction of aircraft due to surface to air missile

　⑦ Y36.110 War operations involving destruction of aircraft due to enemy fire or explosives, military personnel

　⑦ Y36.111 War operations involving destruction of aircraft due to enemy fire or explosives, civilian

⑥ Y36.12 War operations involving destruction of aircraft due to collision with other aircraft

　⑦ Y36.120 War operations involving destruction of aircraft due to collision with other aircraft, military personnel

　⑦ Y36.121 War operations involving destruction of aircraft due to collision with other aircraft, civilian

⑥ Y36.13 War operations involving destruction of aircraft due to onboard fire

　⑦ Y36.130 War operations involving destruction of aircraft due to onboard fire, military personnel

　⑦ Y36.131 War operations involving destruction of aircraft due to onboard fire, civilian

⑥ Y36.14 War operations involving destruction of aircraft due to accidental detonation of onboard munitions and explosives

　⑦ Y36.140 War operations involving destruction of aircraft due to accidental detonation of onboard munitions and explosives, military personnel

　⑦ Y36.141 War operations involving destruction of aircraft due to accidental detonation of onboard munitions and explosives, civilian

⑥ Y36.19 War operations involving other destruction of aircraft

　⑦ Y36.190 War operations involving other destruction of aircraft, military personnel

　⑦ Y36.191 War operations involving other destruction of aircraft, civilian

⑤ Y36.2 War operations involving other explosions and fragments

　EXCLUDES1 war operations involving explosion of aircraft (Y36.1-)

war operations involving explosion of marine weapons (Y36.0-)

war operations involving explosion of nuclear weapons (Y36.5-)

war operations involving explosion occurring after cessation of hostilities (Y36.8-)

⑥ Y36.20 War operations involving unspecified explosion and fragments

War operations involving air blast NOS

War operations involving blast NOS

War operations involving blast fragments NOS

War operations involving blast wave NOS

War operations involving blast wind NOS

War operations involving explosion NOS

War operations involving explosion of bomb NOS

　⑦ Y36.200 War operations involving unspecified explosion and fragments, military personnel

　⑦ Y36.201 War operations involving unspecified explosion and fragments, civilian

⑥ Y36.21 War operations involving explosion of aerial bomb

　⑦ Y36.210 War operations involving explosion of aerial bomb, military personnel

　⑦ Y36.211 War operations involving explosion of aerial bomb, civilian

⑥ Y36.22 War operations involving explosion of guided missile

　⑦ Y36.220 War operations involving explosion of guided missile, military personnel

　⑦ Y36.221 War operations involving explosion of guided missile, civilian

⑥ Y36.23 War operations involving explosion of improvised explosive device [IED]

War operations involving explosion of person-borne improvised explosive device [IED]

War operations involving explosion of vehicle-borne improvised explosive device [IED]

War operations involving explosion of roadside improvised explosive device [IED]

　⑦ Y36.230 War operations involving explosion of improvised explosive device [IED], military personnel

　⑦ Y36.231 War operations involving explosion of improvised explosive device [IED], civilian

---

④ 4th character required　　⑤ 5th character required　　⑥ 6th character required　　⑦ 7th character required　　ⓧ Extension 'X' Alert

EXCLUDES1 Not coded here　　EXCLUDES2 Not included here　　PDx Primary Diagnosis Only　　Manifestation Code

[6] Y36.24 War operations involving explosion due to accidental detonation and discharge of own munitions or munitions launch device

[7] Y36.240 War operations involving explosion due to accidental detonation and discharge of own munitions or munitions launch device, military personnel

[7] Y36.241 War operations involving explosion due to accidental detonation and discharge of own munitions or munitions launch device, civilian

[6] Y36.25 War operations involving fragments from munitions

[7] Y36.250 War operations involving fragments from munitions, military personnel

[7] Y36.251 War operations involving fragments from munitions, civilian

[6] Y36.26 War operations involving fragments of improvised explosive device [IED]

War operations involving fragments of person-borne improvised explosive device [IED]
War operations involving fragments of vehicle-borne improvised explosive device [IED]
War operations involving fragments of roadside improvised explosive device [IED]

[7] Y36.260 War operations involving fragments of improvised explosive device [IED], military personnel

[7] Y36.261 War operations involving fragments of improvised explosive device [IED], civilian

[6] Y36.27 War operations involving fragments from weapons

[7] Y36.270 War operations involving fragments from weapons, military personnel

[7] Y36.271 War operations involving fragments from weapons, civilian

[6] Y36.29 War operations involving other explosions and fragments

War operations involving explosion of grenade
War operations involving explosions of land mine
War operations involving shrapnel NOS

[7] Y36.290 War operations involving other explosions and fragments, military personnel

[7] Y36.291 War operations involving other explosions and fragments, civilian

[5] Y36.3 War operations involving fires, conflagrations and hot substances

War operations involving smoke, fumes, and heat from fires, conflagrations and hot substances

[EXCLUDES1] *war operations involving fires and conflagrations aboard military aircraft (Y36.1-)*
war operations involving fires and conflagrations aboard military watercraft (Y36.0-)
war operations involving fires and conflagrations caused indirectly by conventional weapons (Y36.2-)
war operations involving fires and thermal effects of nuclear weapons (Y36.53-)

[6] Y36.30 War operations involving unspecified fire, conflagration and hot substance

[7] Y36.300 War operations involving unspecified fire, conflagration and hot substance, military personnel

[7] Y36.301 War operations involving unspecified fire, conflagration and hot substance, civilian

[6] Y36.31 War operations involving gasoline bomb

War operations involving incendiary bomb
War operations involving petrol bomb

[7] Y36.310 War operations involving gasoline bomb, military personnel

[7] Y36.311 War operations involving gasoline bomb, civilian

[6] Y36.32 War operations involving incendiary bullet

[7] Y36.320 War operations involving incendiary bullet, military personnel

[7] Y36.321 War operations involving incendiary bullet, civilian

[6] Y36.33 War operations involving flamethrower

[7] Y36.330 War operations involving flamethrower, military personnel

[7] Y36.331 War operations involving flamethrower, civilian

[6] Y36.39 War operations involving other fires, conflagrations and hot substances

[7] Y36.390 War operations involving other fires, conflagrations and hot substances, military personnel

[7] Y36.391 War operations involving other fires, conflagrations and hot substances, civilian

[5] Y36.4 War operations involving firearm discharge and other forms of conventional warfare

[6] Y36.41 War operations involving rubber bullets

[7] Y36.410 War operations involving rubber bullets, military personnel

[7] Y36.411 War operations involving rubber bullets, civilian

[6] Y36.42 War operations involving firearms pellets

[7] Y36.420 War operations involving firearms pellets, military personnel

[7] Y36.421 War operations involving firearms pellets, civilian

[6] Y36.43 War operations involving other firearms discharge

War operations involving bullets NOS

[EXCLUDES1] *war operations involving munitions fragments (Y36.25-)*
war operations involving incendiary bullets (Y36.32-)

[7] Y36.430 War operations involving other firearms discharge, military personnel

[7] Y36.431 War operations involving other firearms discharge, civilian

[6] Y36.44 War operations involving unarmed hand to hand combat

[EXCLUDES1] *war operations involving combat using blunt or piercing object (Y36.45-)*
war operations involving intentional restriction of air and airway (Y36.46-)
war operations involving unintentional restriction of air and airway (Y36.47-)

[7] Y36.440 War operations involving unarmed hand to hand combat, military personnel

[7] Y36.441 War operations involving unarmed hand to hand combat, civilian

[6] Y36.45 War operations involving combat using blunt or piercing object

[7] Y36.450 War operations involving combat using blunt or piercing object, military personnel

[7] Y36.451 War operations involving combat using blunt or piercing object, civilian

[6] Y36.46 War operations involving intentional restriction of air and airway

[7] Y36.460 War operations involving intentional restriction of air and airway, military personnel

[7] Y36.461 War operations involving intentional restriction of air and airway, civilian

Unspecified Code | Other Specified Code | [N] Newborn Age: 0 | [P] Pediatric Age: 0-17 | [M] Maternity Age: 12-55
[A] Adult Age: 15-124 | ♂ Male | ♀ Female | ● New Code | ▲ Revised Code Title | ►◄ Revised Text

[6] Y36.47 War operations involving unintentional restriction of air and airway
[7] Y36.470 War operations involving unintentional restriction of air and airway, military personnel
[7] Y36.471 War operations involving unintentional restriction of air and airway, civilian
[6] Y36.49 War operations involving other forms of conventional warfare
[7] Y36.490 War operations involving other forms of conventional warfare, military personnel
[7] Y36.491 War operations involving other forms of conventional warfare, civilian
[5] Y36.5 War operations involving nuclear weapons
War operations involving dirty bomb NOS
[6] Y36.50 War operations involving unspecified effect of nuclear weapon
[7] Y36.500 War operations involving unspecified effect of nuclear weapon, military personnel
[7] Y36.501 War operations involving unspecified effect of nuclear weapon, civilian
[6] Y36.51 War operations involving direct blast effect of nuclear weapon
War operations involving blast pressure of nuclear weapon
[7] Y36.510 War operations involving direct blast effect of nuclear weapon, military personnel
[7] Y36.511 War operations involving direct blast effect of nuclear weapon, civilian
[6] Y36.52 War operations involving indirect blast effect of nuclear weapon
War operations involving being thrown by blast of nuclear weapon
War operations involving being struck or crushed by blast debris of nuclear weapon
[7] Y36.520 War operations involving indirect blast effect of nuclear weapon, military personnel
[7] Y36.521 War operations involving indirect blast effect of nuclear weapon, civilian
[6] Y36.53 War operations involving thermal radiation effect of nuclear weapon
War operations involving direct heat from nuclear weapon
War operation involving fireball effects from nuclear weapon
[7] Y36.530 War operations involving thermal radiation effect of nuclear weapon, military personnel
[7] Y36.531 War operations involving thermal radiation effect of nuclear weapon, civilian
[6] Y36.54 War operation involving nuclear radiation effects of nuclear weapon
War operation involving acute radiation exposure from nuclear weapon
War operation involving exposure to immediate ionizing radiation from nuclear weapon
War operation involving fallout exposure from nuclear weapon
War operation involving secondary effects of nuclear weapons
[7] Y36.540 War operation involving nuclear radiation effects of nuclear weapon, military personnel
[7] Y36.541 War operation involving nuclear radiation effects of nuclear weapon, civilian
[6] Y36.59 War operation involving other effects of nuclear weapons
[7] Y36.590 War operation involving other effects of nuclear weapons, military personnel
[7] Y36.591 War operation involving other effects of nuclear weapons, civilian
[5] Y36.6 War operations involving biological weapons
[6] Y36.6X War operations involving biological weapons
[7] Y36.6X0 War operations involving biological weapons, military personnel
[7] Y36.6X1 War operations involving biological weapons, civilian
[5] Y36.7 War operations involving chemical weapons and other forms of unconventional warfare
[EXCLUDES1] *war operations involving incendiary devices (Y36.3-, Y36.5-)*
[6] Y36.7X War operations involving chemical weapons and other forms of unconventional warfare
[7] Y36.7X0 War operations involving chemical weapons and other forms of unconventional warfare, military personnel
[7] Y36.7X1 War operations involving chemical weapons and other forms of unconventional warfare, civilian
[5] Y36.8 War operations occurring after cessation of hostilities
War operations classifiable to categories Y36.0-Y36.8 but occurring after cessation of hostilities
[6] Y36.81 Explosion of mine placed during war operations but exploding after cessation of hostilities
[7] Y36.810 Explosion of mine placed during war operations but exploding after cessation of hostilities, military personnel
[7] Y36.811 Explosion of mine placed during war operations but exploding after cessation of hostilities, civilian
[6] Y36.82 Explosion of bomb placed during war operations but exploding after cessation of hostilities
[7] Y36.820 Explosion of bomb placed during war operations but exploding after cessation of hostilities, military personnel
[7] Y36.821 Explosion of bomb placed during war operations but exploding after cessation of hostilities, civilian
[6] Y36.88 Other war operations occurring after cessation of hostilities
[7] Y36.880 Other war operations occurring after cessation of hostilities, military personnel
[7] Y36.881 Other war operations occurring after cessation of hostilities, civilian
[6] Y36.89 Unspecified war operations occurring after cessation of hostilities
[7] Y36.890 Unspecified war operations occurring after cessation of hostilities, military personnel
[7] Y36.891 Unspecified war operations occurring after cessation of hostilities, civilian
[5] Y36.9 Other and unspecified war operations
[7th] Y36.90 War operations, unspecified
[7th] Y36.91 War operations involving unspecified weapon of mass destruction [WMD]
[7th] Y36.92 War operations involving friendly fire

[4] 4th character required [5] 5th character required [6] 6th character required [7] 7th character required [7th] Extension 'X' Alert
[EXCLUDES1] Not coded here [EXCLUDES2] Not included here [PDx] Primary Diagnosis Only Manifestation Code

[4] Y37 Military operations

[INCLUDES] *injuries to military personnel and civilians occurring during peacetime on military property and during routine military exercises and operations*

[EXCLUDES1] *military aircraft involved in aircraft accident with civilian aircraft (V97.81-)*
military vehicles involved in transport accident with civilian vehicle (V09.01, V09.21, V19.81, V29.81, V39.81, V49.81, V59.81, V69.81, V79.81)
military watercraft involved in water transport accident with civilian watercraft (V94.81-)
war operations (Y36.-)

The appropriate 7th character is to be added to each code from category Y37
A = initial encounter
D = subsequent encounter
S = sequela

[5] Y37.0 Military operations involving explosion of marine weapons

[6] Y37.00 Military operations involving explosion of unspecified marine weapon
Military operations involving underwater blast NOS

[7] Y37.000 Military operations involving explosion of unspecified marine weapon, military personnel

[7] Y37.001 Military operations involving explosion of unspecified marine weapon, civilian

[6] Y37.01 Military operations involving explosion of depth-charge

[7] Y37.010 Military operations involving explosion of depth-charge, military personnel

[7] Y37.011 Military operations involving explosion of depth-charge, civilian

[6] Y37.02 Military operations involving explosion of marine mine
Military operations involving explosion of marine mine, at sea or in harbor

[7] Y37.020 Military operations involving explosion of marine mine, military personnel

[7] Y37.021 Military operations involving explosion of marine mine, civilian

[6] Y37.03 Military operations involving explosion of sea-based artillery shell

[7] Y37.030 Military operations involving explosion of sea-based artillery shell, military personnel

[7] Y37.031 Military operations involving explosion of sea-based artillery shell, civilian

[6] Y37.04 Military operations involving explosion of torpedo

[7] Y37.040 Military operations involving explosion of torpedo, military personnel

[7] Y37.041 Military operations involving explosion of torpedo, civilian

[6] Y37.05 Military operations involving accidental detonation of onboard marine weapons

[7] Y37.050 Military operations involving accidental detonation of onboard marine weapons, military personnel

[7] Y37.051 Military operations involving accidental detonation of onboard marine weapons, civilian

[6] Y37.09 Military operations involving explosion of other marine weapons

[7] Y37.090 Military operations involving explosion of other marine weapons, military personnel

[7] Y37.091 Military operations involving explosion of other marine weapons, civilian

[5] Y37.1 Military operations involving destruction of aircraft

[6] Y37.10 Military operations involving unspecified destruction of aircraft

[7] Y37.100 Military operations involving unspecified destruction of aircraft, military personnel

[7] Y37.101 Military operations involving unspecified destruction of aircraft, civilian

[6] Y37.11 Military operations involving destruction of aircraft due to enemy fire or explosives
Military operations involving destruction of aircraft due to air to air missile
Military operations involving destruction of aircraft due to explosive placed on aircraft
Military operations involving destruction of aircraft due to rocket propelled grenade [RPG]
Military operations involving destruction of aircraft due to small arms fire
Military operations involving destruction of aircraft due to surface to air missile

[7] Y37.110 Military operations involving destruction of aircraft due to enemy fire or explosives, military personnel

[7] Y37.111 Military operations involving destruction of aircraft due to enemy fire or explosives, civilian

[6] Y37.12 Military operations involving destruction of aircraft due to collision with other aircraft

[7] Y37.120 Military operations involving destruction of aircraft due to collision with other aircraft, military personnel

[7] Y37.121 Military operations involving destruction of aircraft due to collision with other aircraft, civilian

[6] Y37.13 Military operations involving destruction of aircraft due to onboard fire

[7] Y37.130 Military operations involving destruction of aircraft due to onboard fire, military personnel

[7] Y37.131 Military operations involving destruction of aircraft due to onboard fire, civilian

[6] Y37.14 Military operations involving destruction of aircraft due to accidental detonation of onboard munitions and explosives

[7] Y37.140 Military operations involving destruction of aircraft due to accidental detonation of onboard munitions and explosives, military personnel

[7] Y37.141 Military operations involving destruction of aircraft due to accidental detonation of onboard munitions and explosives, civilian

[6] Y37.19 Military operations involving other destruction of aircraft

[7] Y37.190 Military operations involving other destruction of aircraft, military personnel

[7] Y37.191 Military operations involving other destruction of aircraft, civilian

[5] Y37.2 Military operations involving other explosions and fragments

[EXCLUDES1] *military operations involving explosion of aircraft (Y37.1-)*
military operations involving explosion of marine weapons (Y37.0-)
military operations involving explosion of nuclear weapons (Y37.5-)

[6] Y37.20 Military operations involving unspecified explosion and fragments
Military operations involving air blast NOS
Military operations involving blast NOS
Military operations involving blast fragments NOS
Military operations involving blast wave NOS
Military operations involving blast wind NOS
Military operations involving explosion NOS
Military operations involving explosion of bomb NOS

Unspecified Code | Other Specified Code | [N] Newborn Age: 0 | [P] Pediatric Age: 0-17 | [M] Maternity Age: 12-55
[A] Adult Age: 15-124 | ♂ Male | ♀ Female | ● New Code | ▲ Revised Code Title | ►◄ Revised Text

[7] Y37.200 **Military operations involving unspecified explosion and fragments,** military personnel

[7] Y37.201 **Military operations involving unspecified explosion and fragments,** civilian

[6] Y37.21 **Military operations involving explosion of** aerial bomb

[7] Y37.210 **Military operations involving explosion of aerial bomb,** military personnel

[7] Y37.211 **Military operations involving explosion of aerial bomb,** civilian

[6] Y37.22 **Military operations involving** explosion of guided missile

[7] Y37.220 **Military operations involving explosion of guided missile,** military personnel

[7] Y37.221 **Military operations involving explosion of guided missile,** civilian

[6] Y37.23 **Military operations involving** explosion of improvised explosive device [IED]

Military operations involving explosion of person-borne improvised explosive device [IED]
Military operations involving explosion of vehicle-borne improvised explosive device [IED]
Military operations involving explosion of roadside improvised explosive device [IED]

[7] Y37.230 **Military operations involving explosion of improvised explosive device [IED],** military personnel

[7] Y37.231 **Military operations involving explosion of improvised explosive device [IED],** civilian

[6] Y37.24 **Military operations involving explosion** due to accidental detonation and discharge of own munitions or munitions launch device

[7] Y37.240 **Military operations involving explosion due to accidental detonation and discharge of own munitions or munitions launch device,** military personnel

[7] Y37.241 **Military operations involving explosion due to accidental detonation and discharge of own munitions or munitions launch device,** civilian

[6] Y37.25 **Military operations involving** fragments from munitions

[7] Y37.250 **Military operations involving fragments from munitions,** military personnel

[7] Y37.251 **Military operations involving fragments from munitions,** civilian

[6] Y37.26 **Military operations involving fragments of** improvised explosive device [IED]

Military operations involving fragments of person-borne improvised explosive device [IED]
Military operations involving fragments of vehicle-borne improvised explosive device [IED]
Military operations involving fragments of roadside improvised explosive device [IED]

[7] Y37.260 **Military operations involving fragments of improvised explosive device [IED],** military personnel

[7] Y37.261 **Military operations involving fragments of improvised explosive device [IED],** civilian

[6] Y37.27 **Military operations involving fragments from** weapons

[7] Y37.270 **Military operations involving fragments from weapons,** military personnel

[7] Y37.271 **Military operations involving fragments from weapons,** civilian

[6] Y37.29 **Military operations involving** other **explosions and fragments**

Military operations involving explosion of grenade
Military operations involving explosions of land mine
Military operations involving shrapnel NOS

[7] Y37.290 **Military operations involving other explosions and fragments,** military personnel

[7] Y37.291 **Military operations involving other explosions and fragments,** civilian

[5] Y37.3 **Military operations involving** fires, conflagrations and hot substances

Military operations involving smoke, fumes, and heat from fires, conflagrations and hot substances

EXCLUDES1 *military operations involving fires and conflagrations aboard military aircraft (Y37.1-)*
military operations involving fires and conflagrations aboard military watercraft (Y37.0-)
military operations involving fires and conflagrations caused indirectly by conventional weapons (Y37.2-)
military operations involving fires and thermal effects of nuclear weapons (Y36.53-)

[6] Y37.30 **Military operations involving** unspecified **fire, conflagration and hot substance**

[7] Y37.300 **Military operations involving unspecified fire, conflagration and hot substance,** military personnel

[7] Y37.301 **Military operations involving unspecified fire, conflagration and hot substance,** civilian

[6] Y37.31 **Military operations involving** gasoline bomb

Military operations involving incendiary bomb
Military operations involving petrol bomb

[7] Y37.310 **Military operations involving gasoline bomb,** military personnel

[7] Y37.311 **Military operations involving gasoline bomb,** civilian

[6] Y37.32 **Military operations involving** incendiary bullet

[7] Y37.320 **Military operations involving incendiary bullet,** military personnel

[7] Y37.321 **Military operations involving incendiary bullet,** civilian

[6] Y37.33 **Military operations involving** flamethrower

[7] Y37.330 **Military operations involving flamethrower,** military personnel

[7] Y37.331 **Military operations involving flamethrower,** civilian

[6] Y37.39 **Military operations involving** other **fires, conflagrations and hot substances**

[7] Y37.390 **Military operations involving other fires, conflagrations and hot substances,** military personnel

[7] Y37.391 **Military operations involving other fires, conflagrations and hot substances,** civilian

[5] Y37.4 **Military operations involving firearm discharge and other forms of conventional warfare**

[6] Y37.41 **Military operations involving** rubber bullets

[7] Y37.410 **Military operations involving rubber bullets,** military personnel

[7] Y37.411 **Military operations involving rubber bullets,** civilian

[6] Y37.42 **Military operations involving** firearms pellets

[7] Y37.420 **Military operations involving firearms pellets,** military personnel

[7] Y37.421 **Military operations involving firearms pellets,** civilian

[6] Y37.43 **Military operations involving** other firearms discharge

Military operations involving bullets NOS

EXCLUDES1 *military operations involving munitions fragments (Y37.25-)*
military operations involving incendiary bullets (Y37.32-)

[7] Y37.430 **Military operations involving other firearms discharge,** military personnel

[4] 4th character required [5] 5th character required [6] 6th character required [7] 7th character required [X] Extension 'X' Alert
EXCLUDES 1 Not coded here EXCLUDES 2 Not included here [PDx] Primary Diagnosis Only Manifestation Code

[7] **Y37.431 Military operations involving other firearms discharge, civilian**

[6] **Y37.44 Military operations involving unarmed hand to hand combat**

[EXCLUDES1] *military operations involving combat using blunt or piercing object (Y37.45-)*
military operations involving intentional restriction of air and airway (Y37.46-)
military operations involving unintentional restriction of air and airway (Y37.47-)

[7] **Y37.440 Military operations involving unarmed hand to hand combat, military personnel**

[7] **Y37.441 Military operations involving unarmed hand to hand combat, civilian**

[6] **Y37.45 Military operations involving combat using blunt or piercing object**

[7] **Y37.450 Military operations involving combat using blunt or piercing object, military personnel**

[7] **Y37.451 Military operations involving combat using blunt or piercing object, civilian**

[6] **Y37.46 Military operations involving intentional restriction of air and airway**

[7] **Y37.460 Military operations involving intentional restriction of air and airway, military personnel**

[7] **Y37.461 Military operations involving intentional restriction of air and airway, civilian**

[6] **Y37.47 Military operations involving unintentional restriction of air and airway**

[7] **Y37.470 Military operations involving unintentional restriction of air and airway, military personnel**

[7] **Y37.471 Military operations involving unintentional restriction of air and airway, civilian**

[6] **Y37.49 Military operations involving other forms of conventional warfare**

[7] **Y37.490 Military operations involving other forms of conventional warfare, military personnel**

[7] **Y37.491 Military operations involving other forms of conventional warfare, civilian**

[5] **Y37.5 Military operations involving nuclear weapons**

Military operation involving dirty bomb NOS

[6] **Y37.50 Military operations involving unspecified effect of nuclear weapon**

[7] **Y37.500 Military operations involving unspecified effect of nuclear weapon, military personnel**

[7] **Y37.501 Military operations involving unspecified effect of nuclear weapon, civilian**

[6] **Y37.51 Military operations involving direct blast effect of nuclear weapon**

Military operations involving blast pressure of nuclear weapon

[7] **Y37.510 Military operations involving direct blast effect of nuclear weapon, military personnel**

[7] **Y37.511 Military operations involving direct blast effect of nuclear weapon, civilian**

[6] **Y37.52 Military operations involving indirect blast effect of nuclear weapon**

Military operations involving being thrown by blast of nuclear weapon
Military operations involving being struck or crushed by blast debris of nuclear weapon

[7] **Y37.520 Military operations involving indirect blast effect of nuclear weapon, military personnel**

[7] **Y37.521 Military operations involving indirect blast effect of nuclear weapon, civilian**

[6] **Y37.53 Military operations involving thermal radiation effect of nuclear weapon**

Military operations involving direct heat from nuclear weapon
Military operation involving fireball effects from nuclear weapon

[7] **Y37.530 Military operations involving thermal radiation effect of nuclear weapon, military personnel**

[7] **Y37.531 Military operations involving thermal radiation effect of nuclear weapon, civilian**

[6] **Y37.54 Military operation involving nuclear radiation effects of nuclear weapon**

Military operation involving acute radiation exposure from nuclear weapon
Military operation involving exposure to immediate ionizing radiation from nuclear weapon
Military operation involving fallout exposure from nuclear weapon
Military operation involving secondary effects of nuclear weapons

[7] **Y37.540 Military operation involving nuclear radiation effects of nuclear weapon, military personnel**

[7] **Y37.541 Military operation involving nuclear radiation effects of nuclear weapon, civilian**

[6] **Y37.59 Military operation involving other effects of nuclear weapons**

[7] **Y37.590 Military operation involving other effects of nuclear weapons, military personnel**

[7] **Y37.591 Military operation involving other effects of nuclear weapons, civilian**

[5] **Y37.6 Military operations involving biological weapons**

[6] **Y37.6X Military operations involving biological weapons**

[7] **Y37.6X0 Military operations involving biological weapons, military personnel**

[7] **Y37.6X1 Military operations involving biological weapons, civilian**

[5] **Y37.7 Military operations involving chemical weapons and other forms of unconventional warfare**

[EXCLUDES1] *military operations involving incendiary devices (Y36.3-, Y36.5-)*

[6] **Y37.7X Military operations involving chemical weapons and other forms of unconventional warfare**

[7] **Y37.7X0 Military operations involving chemical weapons and other forms of unconventional warfare, military personnel**

[7] **Y37.7X1 Military operations involving chemical weapons and other forms of unconventional warfare, civilian**

[5] **Y37.9 Other and unspecified military operations**

[7] **Y37.90 Military operations, unspecified**

[7] **Y37.91 Military operations involving unspecified weapon of mass destruction [WMD]**

[7] **Y37.92 Military operations involving friendly fire**

[4] **Y38 Terrorism**

These codes are for use to identify injuries resulting from the unlawful use of force or violence against persons or property to intimidate or coerce a Government, the civilian population, or any segment thereof, in furtherance of political or social objective

Use additional code for place of occurrence (Y92.-)

The appropriate 7th character is to be added to each code from category Y38
A = initial encounter
D = subsequent encounter
S = sequela

[5] **Y38.0 Terrorism involving explosion of marine weapons**

Terrorism involving depth-charge
Terrorism involving marine mine
Terrorism involving mine NOS, at sea or in harbor
Terrorism involving sea-based artillery shell
Terrorism involving torpedo
Terrorism involving underwater blast

Unspecified Code | Other Specified Code | [N] Newborn Age: 0 | [P] Pediatric Age: 0-17 | [M] Maternity Age: 12-55
[A] Adult Age: 15-124 | ♂ Male | ♀ Female | ● New Code | ▲ Revised Code Title | ►◄ Revised Text

[6] **Y38.0X Terrorism involving explosion of marine weapons**
[7] **Y38.0X1 Terrorism involving explosion of marine weapons, public safety official injured**
[7] **Y38.0X2 Terrorism involving explosion of marine weapons, civilian injured**
[7] **Y38.0X3 Terrorism involving explosion of marine weapons, terrorist injured**

[5] **Y38.1 Terrorism involving destruction of aircraft**
Terrorism involving aircraft burned
Terrorism involving aircraft exploded
Terrorism involving aircraft being shot down
Terrorism involving aircraft used as a weapon
[6] **Y38.1X Terrorism involving destruction of aircraft**
[7] **Y38.1X1 Terrorism involving destruction of aircraft, public safety official injured**
[7] **Y38.1X2 Terrorism involving destruction of aircraft, civilian injured**
[7] **Y38.1X3 Terrorism involving destruction of aircraft, terrorist injured**

[5] **Y38.2 Terrorism involving other explosions and fragments**
Terrorism involving antipersonnel (fragments) bomb
Terrorism involving blast NOS
Terrorism involving explosion NOS
Terrorism involving explosion of breech block
Terrorism involving explosion of cannon block
Terrorism involving explosion (fragments) of artillery shell
Terrorism involving explosion (fragments) of bomb
Terrorism involving explosion (fragments) of grenade
Terrorism involving explosion (fragments) of guided missile
Terrorism involving explosion (fragments) of land mine
Terrorism involving explosion of mortar bomb
Terrorism involving explosion of munitions
Terrorism involving explosion (fragments) of rocket
Terrorism involving explosion (fragments) of shell
Terrorism involving shrapnel
Terrorism involving mine NOS, on land
[EXCLUDES1] *terrorism involving explosion of nuclear weapon (Y38.5)*
terrorism involving suicide bomber (Y38.81)
[6] **Y38.2X Terrorism involving other explosions and fragments**
[7] **Y38.2X1 Terrorism involving other explosions and fragments, public safety official injured**
[7] **Y38.2X2 Terrorism involving other explosions and fragments, civilian injured**
[7] **Y38.2X3 Terrorism involving other explosions and fragments, terrorist injured**

[5] **Y38.3 Terrorism involving fires, conflagration and hot substances**
Terrorism involving conflagration NOS
Terrorism involving fire NOS
Terrorism involving petrol bomb
[EXCLUDES1] *terrorism involving fire or heat of nuclear weapon (Y38.5)*
[6] **Y38.3X Terrorism involving fires, conflagration and hot substances**
[7] **Y38.3X1 Terrorism involving fires, conflagration and hot substances, public safety official injured**
[7] **Y38.3X2 Terrorism involving fires, conflagration and hot substances, civilian injured**
[7] **Y38.3X3 Terrorism involving fires, conflagration and hot substances, terrorist injured**

[5] **Y38.4 Terrorism involving firearms**
Terrorism involving carbine bullet
Terrorism involving machine gun bullet
Terrorism involving pellets (shotgun)
Terrorism involving pistol bullet
Terrorism involving rifle bullet
Terrorism involving rubber (rifle) bullet
[6] **Y38.4X Terrorism involving firearms**
[7] **Y38.4X1 Terrorism involving firearms, public safety official injured**
[7] **Y38.4X2 Terrorism involving firearms, civilian injured**
[7] **Y38.4X3 Terrorism involving firearms, terrorist injured**

[5] **Y38.5 Terrorism involving nuclear weapons**
Terrorism involving blast effects of nuclear weapon
Terrorism involving exposure to ionizing radiation from nuclear weapon
Terrorism involving fireball effect of nuclear weapon
Terrorism involving heat from nuclear weapon
[6] **Y38.5X Terrorism involving nuclear weapons**
[7] **Y38.5X1 Terrorism involving nuclear weapons, public safety official injured**
[7] **Y38.5X2 Terrorism involving nuclear weapons, civilian injured**
[7] **Y38.5X3 Terrorism involving nuclear weapons, terrorist injured**

[5] **Y38.6 Terrorism involving biological weapons**
Terrorism involving anthrax
Terrorism involving cholera
Terrorism involving smallpox
[6] **Y38.6X Terrorism involving biological weapons**
[7] **Y38.6X1 Terrorism involving biological weapons, public safety official injured**
[7] **Y38.6X2 Terrorism involving biological weapons, civilian injured**
[7] **Y38.6X3 Terrorism involving biological weapons, terrorist injured**

[5] **Y38.7 Terrorism involving chemical weapons**
Terrorism involving gases, fumes, chemicals
Terrorism involving hydrogen cyanide
Terrorism involving phosgene
Terrorism involving sarin
[6] **Y38.7X Terrorism involving chemical weapons**
[7] **Y38.7X1 Terrorism involving chemical weapons, public safety official injured**
[7] **Y38.7X2 Terrorism involving chemical weapons, civilian injured**
[7] **Y38.7X3 Terrorism involving chemical weapons, terrorist injured**

[5] **Y38.8 Terrorism involving other and unspecified means**
[7X] **Y38.80 Terrorism involving unspecified means**
Terrorism NOS
[6] **Y38.81 Terrorism involving suicide bomber**
[7] **Y38.811 Terrorism involving suicide bomber, public safety official injured**
[7] **Y38.812 Terrorism involving suicide bomber, civilian injured**
[6] **Y38.89 Terrorism involving other means**
Terrorism involving drowning and submersion
Terrorism involving lasers
Terrorism involving piercing or stabbing instruments
[7] **Y38.891 Terrorism involving other means, public safety official injured**
[7] **Y38.892 Terrorism involving other means, civilian injured**
[7] **Y38.893 Terrorism involving other means, terrorist injured**

[5] **Y38.9 Terrorism, secondary effects**
[NOTES] This code is for use to identify conditions occurring subsequent to a terrorist attack not those that are due to the initial terrorist attack

[4] 4th character required [5] 5th character required [6] 6th character required [7] 7th character required [7X] Extension 'X' Alert
[EXCLUDES1] Not coded here [EXCLUDES2] Not included here [PDx] Primary Diagnosis Only Manifestation Code

[6] Y38.9X Terrorism, secondary effects
[7] Y38.9X1 Terrorism, secondary effects, public safety official injured
[7] Y38.9X2 Terrorism, secondary effects, civilian injured

Complications of medical and surgical care (Y62-Y84)

INCLUDES *complications of medical devices*
surgical and medical procedures as the cause of abnormal reaction of the patient, or of later complication, without mention of misadventure at the time of the procedure

Misadventures to patients during surgical and medical care (Y62-Y69)

EXCLUDES2 *breakdown or malfunctioning of medical device (during procedure) (after implantation) (ongoing use) (Y70-Y82)*
surgical and medical procedures as the cause of abnormal reaction of the patient, without mention of misadventure at the time of the procedure (Y83-Y84)

[4] **Y62 Failure of sterile precautions during surgical and medical care**
Y62.0 Failure of sterile precautions during surgical operation
Y62.1 Failure of sterile precautions during infusion or transfusion
Y62.2 Failure of sterile precautions during kidney dialysis and other perfusion
Y62.3 Failure of sterile precautions during injection or immunization
Y62.4 Failure of sterile precautions during endoscopic examination
Y62.5 Failure of sterile precautions during heart catheterization
Y62.6 Failure of sterile precautions during aspiration, puncture and other catheterization
Y62.8 Failure of sterile precautions during other surgical and medical care
Y62.9 Failure of sterile precautions during unspecified surgical and medical care

[4] **Y63 Failure in dosage during surgical and medical care**
EXCLUDES2 *accidental overdose of drug or wrong drug given in error (T36-T50)*
Y63.0 Excessive amount of blood or other fluid given during transfusion or infusion
Y63.1 Incorrect dilution of fluid used during infusion
Y63.2 Overdose of radiation given during therapy
Y63.3 Inadvertent exposure of patient to radiation during medical care
Y63.4 Failure in dosage in electroshock or insulin-shock therapy
Y63.5 Inappropriate temperature in local application and packing
Y63.6 Underdosing and nonadministration of necessary drug, medicament or biological substance
Y63.8 Failure in dosage during other surgical and medical care
Y63.9 Failure in dosage during unspecified surgical and medical care

[4] **Y64 Contaminated medical or biological substances**
Y64.0 Contaminated medical or biological substance, transfused or infused
Y64.1 Contaminated medical or biological substance, injected or used for immunization
Y64.8 Contaminated medical or biological substance administered by other means
Y64.9 Contaminated medical or biological substance administered by unspecified means
Administered contaminated medical or biological substance NOS

[4] **Y65 Other misadventures during surgical and medical care**
Y65.0 Mismatched blood in transfusion
Y65.1 Wrong fluid used in infusion
Y65.2 Failure in suture or ligature during surgical operation
Y65.3 Endotracheal tube wrongly placed during anesthetic procedure
Y65.4 Failure to introduce or to remove other tube or instrument
[5] Y65.5 Performance of wrong procedure (operation)
Y65.51 Performance of wrong procedure (operation) on correct patient
Wrong device implanted into correct surgical site
EXCLUDES1 *performance of correct procedure (operation) on wrong side or body part (Y65.53)*
Y65.52 Performance of procedure (operation) on patient not scheduled for surgery
Performance of procedure (operation) intended for another patient
Performance of procedure (operation) on wrong patient
Y65.53 Performance of correct procedure (operation) on wrong side or body part
Performance of correct procedure (operation) on wrong side
Performance of correct procedure (operation) on wrong site
Y65.8 Other specified misadventures during surgical and medical care

Y66 Nonadministration of surgical and medical care
Premature cessation of surgical and medical care
EXCLUDES1 *DNR status (Z66)*
palliative care (Z51.5)

Y69 Unspecified misadventure during surgical and medical care

Medical devices associated with adverse incidents in diagnostic and therapeutic use (Y70-Y82)

INCLUDES *breakdown or malfunction of medical devices (during use) (after implantation) (ongoing use)*
EXCLUDES1 *misadventure to patients during surgical and medical care, classifiable to (Y62-Y69)*
later complications following use of medical devices without breakdown or malfunctioning of device (Y83-Y84)

[4] **Y70 Anesthesiology devices associated with adverse incidents**
Y70.0 Diagnostic and monitoring anesthesiology devices associated with adverse incidents
Y70.1 Therapeutic (nonsurgical) and rehabilitative anesthesiology devices associated with adverse incidents
Y70.2 Prosthetic and other implants, materials and accessory anesthesiology devices associated with adverse incidents
Y70.3 Surgical instruments, materials and anesthesiology devices (including sutures) associated with adverse incidents
Y70.8 Miscellaneous anesthesiology devices associated with adverse incidents, not elsewhere classified

[4] **Y71 Cardiovascular devices associated with adverse incidents**
Y71.0 Diagnostic and monitoring cardiovascular devices associated with adverse incidents
Y71.1 Therapeutic (nonsurgical) and rehabilitative cardiovascular devices associated with adverse incidents

Unspecified Code   Other Specified Code   [N] Newborn Age: 0   [P] Pediatric Age: 0-17   [M] Maternity Age: 12-55
[A] Adult Age: 15-124   ♂ Male   ♀ Female   ● New Code   ▲ Revised Code Title   ►◄ Revised Text

Y71.2 Prosthetic and other implants, materials and accessory cardiovascular devices associated with adverse incidents
Y71.3 Surgical instruments, materials and cardiovascular devices (including sutures) associated with adverse incidents
Y71.8 Miscellaneous cardiovascular devices associated with adverse incidents, not elsewhere classified

[4] Y72 Otorhinolaryngological devices associated with adverse incidents
Y72.0 Diagnostic and monitoring otorhinolaryngological devices associated with adverse incidents
Y72.1 Therapeutic (nonsurgical) and rehabilitative otorhinolaryngological devices associated with adverse incidents
Y72.2 Prosthetic and other implants, materials and accessory otorhinolaryngological devices associated with adverse incidents
Y72.3 Surgical instruments, materials and otorhinolaryngological devices (including sutures) associated with adverse incidents
Y72.8 Miscellaneous otorhinolaryngological devices associated with adverse incidents, not elsewhere classified

[4] Y73 Gastroenterology and urology devices associated with adverse incidents
Y73.0 Diagnostic and monitoring gastroenterology and urology devices associated with adverse incidents
Y73.1 Therapeutic (nonsurgical) and rehabilitative gastroenterology and urology devices associated with adverse incidents
Y73.2 Prosthetic and other implants, materials and accessory gastroenterology and urology devices associated with adverse incidents
Y73.3 Surgical instruments, materials and gastroenterology and urology devices (including sutures) associated with adverse incidents
Y73.8 Miscellaneous gastroenterology and urology devices associated with adverse incidents, not elsewhere classified

[4] Y74 General hospital and personal-use devices associated with adverse incidents
Y74.0 Diagnostic and monitoring general hospital and personal-use devices associated with adverse incidents
Y74.1 Therapeutic (nonsurgical) and rehabilitative general hospital and personal-use devices associated with adverse incidents
Y74.2 Prosthetic and other implants, materials and accessory general hospital and personal-use devices associated with adverse incidents
Y74.3 Surgical instruments, materials and general hospital and personal-use devices (including sutures) associated with adverse incidents
Y74.8 Miscellaneous general hospital and personal-use devices associated with adverse incidents, not elsewhere classified

[4] Y75 Neurological devices associated with adverse incidents
Y75.0 Diagnostic and monitoring neurological devices associated with adverse incidents
Y75.1 Therapeutic (nonsurgical) and rehabilitative neurological devices associated with adverse incidents
Y75.2 Prosthetic and other implants, materials and neurological devices associated with adverse incidents
Y75.3 Surgical instruments, materials and neurological devices (including sutures) associated with adverse incidents
Y75.8 Miscellaneous neurological devices associated with adverse incidents, not elsewhere classified

[4] Y76 Obstetric and gynecological devices associated with adverse incidents
Y76.0 Diagnostic and monitoring obstetric and gynecological devices associated with adverse incidents ♀
Y76.1 Therapeutic (nonsurgical) and rehabilitative obstetric and gynecological devices associated with adverse incidents ♀
Y76.2 Prosthetic and other implants, materials and accessory obstetric and gynecological devices associated with adverse incidents ♀
Y76.3 Surgical instruments, materials and obstetric and gynecological devices (including sutures) associated with adverse incidents ♀
Y76.8 Miscellaneous obstetric and gynecological devices associated with adverse incidents, not elsewhere classified ♀

[4] Y77 Ophthalmic devices associated with adverse incidents
Y77.0 Diagnostic and monitoring ophthalmic devices associated with adverse incidents
Y77.1 Therapeutic (nonsurgical) and rehabilitative ophthalmic devices associated with adverse incidents
Y77.2 Prosthetic and other implants, materials and accessory ophthalmic devices associated with adverse incidents
Y77.3 Surgical instruments, materials and ophthalmic devices (including sutures) associated with adverse incidents
Y77.8 Miscellaneous ophthalmic devices associated with adverse incidents, not elsewhere classified

[4] Y78 Radiological devices associated with adverse incidents
Y78.0 Diagnostic and monitoring radiological devices associated with adverse incidents
Y78.1 Therapeutic (nonsurgical) and rehabilitative radiological devices associated with adverse incidents
Y78.2 Prosthetic and other implants, materials and accessory radiological devices associated with adverse incidents
Y78.3 Surgical instruments, materials and radiological devices (including sutures) associated with adverse incidents
Y78.8 Miscellaneous radiological devices associated with adverse incidents, not elsewhere classified

[4] Y79 Orthopedic devices associated with adverse incidents
Y79.0 Diagnostic and monitoring orthopedic devices associated with adverse incidents
Y79.1 Therapeutic (nonsurgical) and rehabilitative orthopedic devices associated with adverse incidents
Y79.2 Prosthetic and other implants, materials and accessory orthopedic devices associated with adverse incidents
Y79.3 Surgical instruments, materials and orthopedic devices (including sutures) associated with adverse incidents
Y79.8 Miscellaneous orthopedic devices associated with adverse incidents, not elsewhere classified

[4] Y80 Physical medicine devices associated with adverse incidents
Y80.0 Diagnostic and monitoring physical medicine devices associated with adverse incidents
Y80.1 Therapeutic (nonsurgical) and rehabilitative physical medicine devices associated with adverse incidents
Y80.2 Prosthetic and other implants, materials and accessory physical medicine devices associated with adverse incidents

[4] 4th character required [5] 5th character required [6] 6th character required [7] 7th character required [7x] Extension 'X' Alert
[EXCLUDES 1] Not coded here [EXCLUDES 2] Not included here [PDx] Primary Diagnosis Only Manifestation Code

Y80.3 **Surgical instruments**, materials and physical medicine devices (including sutures) associated with adverse incidents

Y80.8 **Miscellaneous** physical medicine devices associated with adverse incidents, not elsewhere classified

④ Y81 General- and plastic-surgery devices associated with adverse incidents

Y81.0 Diagnostic and monitoring **general- and plastic-surgery** devices associated with adverse incidents

Y81.1 Therapeutic (nonsurgical) and rehabilitative **general- and plastic-surgery** devices associated with adverse incidents

Y81.2 Prosthetic and other implants, **materials and accessory general- and plastic-surgery devices associated with adverse incidents**

Y81.3 Surgical instruments, **materials and general- and plastic-surgery devices (including sutures) associated with adverse incidents**

Y81.8 Miscellaneous **general- and plastic-surgery devices associated with adverse incidents, not elsewhere classified**

④ Y82 Other and unspecified **medical devices associated with adverse incidents**

Y82.8 Other medical devices associated with adverse incidents

Y82.9 Unspecified medical devices associated with adverse incidents

Surgical and other medical procedures as the cause of abnormal reaction of the patient, or of later complication, without mention of misadventure at the time of the procedure (Y83-Y84)

> EXCLUDES1 *misadventures to patients during surgical and medical care, classifiable to (Y62-Y69)*

④ Y83 Surgical operation and other surgical procedures **as the cause of abnormal reaction of the patient, or of later complication, without mention of misadventure at the time of the procedure**

Y83.0 **Surgical operation** with transplant of whole organ **as the cause of abnormal reaction of the patient, or of later complication, without mention of misadventure at the time of the procedure**

Y83.1 **Surgical operation** with implant of artificial internal device **as the cause of abnormal reaction of the patient, or of later complication, without mention of misadventure at the time of the procedure**

Y83.2 **Surgical operation** with anastomosis, bypass or graft **as the cause of abnormal reaction of the patient, or of later complication, without mention of misadventure at the time of the procedure**

Y83.3 **Surgical operation** with formation of external stoma **as the cause of abnormal reaction of the patient, or of later complication, without mention of misadventure at the time of the procedure**

Y83.4 Other reconstructive surgery **as the cause of abnormal reaction of the patient, or of later complication, without mention of misadventure at the time of the procedure**

Y83.5 Amputation of limb(s) **as the cause of abnormal reaction of the patient, or of later complication, without mention of misadventure at the time of the procedure**

Y83.6 Removal of other organ (partial) (total) **as the cause of abnormal reaction of the patient, or of later complication, without mention of misadventure at the time of the procedure**

Y83.8 Other surgical procedures as the cause of abnormal reaction of the patient, or of later complication, without mention of misadventure at the time of the procedure

Y83.9 **Surgical procedure, unspecified as the cause of abnormal reaction of the patient, or of later complication, without mention of misadventure at the time of the procedure**

④ Y84 Other medical procedures **as the cause of abnormal reaction of the patient, or of later complication, without mention of misadventure at the time of the procedure**

Y84.0 Cardiac catheterization **as the cause of abnormal reaction of the patient, or of later complication, without mention of misadventure at the time of the procedure**

Y84.1 Kidney dialysis **as the cause of abnormal reaction of the patient, or of later complication, without mention of misadventure at the time of the procedure**

Y84.2 Radiological procedure and radiotherapy **as the cause of abnormal reaction of the patient, or of later complication, without mention of misadventure at the time of the procedure**

Y84.3 Shock therapy **as the cause of abnormal reaction of the patient, or of later complication, without mention of misadventure at the time of the procedure**

Y84.4 Aspiration of fluid **as the cause of abnormal reaction of the patient, or of later complication, without mention of misadventure at the time of the procedure**

Y84.5 Insertion of gastric or duodenal sound **as the cause of abnormal reaction of the patient, or of later complication, without mention of misadventure at the time of the procedure**

Y84.6 Urinary catheterization **as the cause of abnormal reaction of the patient, or of later complication, without mention of misadventure at the time of the procedure**

Y84.7 Blood-sampling **as the cause of abnormal reaction of the patient, or of later complication, without mention of misadventure at the time of the procedure**

Y84.8 Other medical procedures as the cause of abnormal reaction of the patient, or of later complication, without mention of misadventure at the time of the procedure

Y84.9 **Medical procedure, unspecified as the cause of abnormal reaction of the patient, or of later complication, without mention of misadventure at the time of the procedure**

Supplementary factors related to causes of morbidity classified elsewhere (Y90-Y99)

> NOTES These categories may be used to provide supplementary information concerning causes of morbidity. They are not to be used for single-condition coding.

④ Y90 **Evidence of alcohol involvement determined by blood alcohol level**

> Code first any associated alcohol related disorders (F10)

Y90.0 **Blood alcohol level of** less than 20 mg/100 ml

Y90.1 **Blood alcohol level of** 20-39 mg/100 ml

Y90.2 **Blood alcohol level of** 40-59 mg/100 ml

Y90.3 **Blood alcohol level of** 60-79 mg/100 ml

Y90.4 **Blood alcohol level of** 80-99 mg/100 ml

Y90.5 **Blood alcohol level of** 100-119 mg/100 ml

Y90.6 **Blood alcohol level of** 120-199 mg/100 ml

Y90.7 **Blood alcohol level of** 200-239 mg/100 ml

Y90.8 **Blood alcohol level of** 240 mg/100 ml or more

Y90.9 **Presence of alcohol in blood, level not specified**

④ Y92 **Place of occurrence of the external cause**

> The following category is for use, when relevant, to identify the place of occurrence of the external cause.
> Use in conjunction with an activity code.
> Place of occurrence should be recorded only at the initial encounter for treatment

---

Unspecified Code	Other Specified Code	Ⓝ Newborn Age: 0	Ⓟ Pediatric Age: 0-17	Ⓜ Maternity Age: 12-55
Ⓐ Adult Age: 15-124	♂ Male	♀ Female	● New Code	▲ Revised Code Title	►◄ Revised Text

[5] **Y92.0 Non-institutional (private) residence as the place of occurrence of the external cause**

EXCLUDES1 *abandoned or derelict house (Y92.89)*
home under construction but not yet occupied (Y92.6-)
institutional place of residence (Y92.1-)

[6] **Y92.00 Unspecified non-institutional (private) residence as the place of occurrence of the external cause**

Y92.000 Kitchen of unspecified non-institutional (private) residence as the place of occurrence of the external cause

Y92.001 Dining room of unspecified non-institutional (private) residence as the place of occurrence of the external cause

Y92.002 Bathroom of unspecified non-institutional (private) residence single-family (private) house as the place of occurrence of the external cause ▲

Y92.003 Bedroom of unspecified non-institutional (private) residence as the place of occurrence of the external cause

Y92.007 Garden or yard of unspecified non-institutional (private) residence as the place of occurrence of the external cause

Y92.008 Other place in unspecified non-institutional (private) residence as the place of occurrence of the external cause

Y92.009 Unspecified place in unspecified non-institutional (private) residence as the place of occurrence of the external cause

Home (NOS) as the place of occurrence of the external cause

[6] **Y92.01 Single-family non-institutional (private) house as the place of occurrence of the external cause**

Farmhouse as the place of occurrence of the external cause

EXCLUDES1 *barn (Y92.71)*
chicken coop or hen house (Y92.72)
farm field (Y92.73)
orchard (Y92.74)
single family mobile home or trailer (Y92.02-)
slaughter house (Y92.86)

Y92.010 Kitchen of single-family (private) house as the place of occurrence of the external cause

Y92.011 Dining room of single-family (private) house as the place of occurrence of the external cause

Y92.012 Bathroom of single-family (private) house as the place of occurrence of the external cause

Y92.013 Bedroom of single-family (private) house as the place of occurrence of the external cause

Y92.014 Private driveway to single-family (private) house as the place of occurrence of the external cause

Y92.015 Private garage of single-family (private) house as the place of occurrence of the external cause

Y92.016 Swimming-pool in single-family (private) house or garden as the place of occurrence of the external cause

Y92.017 Garden or yard in single-family (private) house as the place of occurrence of the external cause

Y92.018 Other place in single-family (private) house as the place of occurrence of the external cause

Y92.019 Unspecified place in single-family (private) house as the place of occurrence of the external cause

[6] **Y92.02 Mobile home as the place of occurrence of the external cause**

Y92.020 Kitchen in mobile home as the place of occurrence of the external cause

Y92.021 Dining room in mobile home as the place of occurrence of the external cause

Y92.022 Bathroom in mobile home as the place of occurrence of the external cause

Y92.023 Bedroom in mobile home as the place of occurrence of the external cause

Y92.024 Driveway of mobile home as the place of occurrence of the external cause

Y92.025 Garage of mobile home as the place of occurrence of the external cause

Y92.026 Swimming-pool of mobile home as the place of occurrence of the external cause

Y92.027 Garden or yard of mobile home as the place of occurrence of the external cause

Y92.028 Other place in mobile home as the place of occurrence of the external cause

Y92.029 Unspecified place in mobile home as the place of occurrence of the external cause

[6] **Y92.03 Apartment as the place of occurrence of the external cause**

Condominium as the place of occurrence of the external cause
Co-op apartment as the place of occurrence of the external cause

Y92.030 Kitchen in apartment as the place of occurrence of the external cause

Y92.031 Bathroom in apartment as the place of occurrence of the external cause

Y92.032 Bedroom in apartment as the place of occurrence of the external cause

Y92.038 Other place in apartment as the place of occurrence of the external cause

Y92.039 Unspecified place in apartment as the place of occurrence of the external cause

[6] **Y92.04 Boarding-house as the place of occurrence of the external cause**

Y92.040 Kitchen in boarding-house as the place of occurrence of the external cause

Y92.041 Bathroom in boarding-house as the place of occurrence of the external cause

Y92.042 Bedroom in boarding-house as the place of occurrence of the external cause

Y92.043 Driveway of boarding-house as the place of occurrence of the external cause

Y92.044 Garage of boarding-house as the place of occurrence of the external cause

Y92.045 Swimming-pool of boarding-house as the place of occurrence of the external cause

Y92.046 Garden or yard of boarding-house as the place of occurrence of the external cause

Y92.048 Other place in boarding-house as the place of occurrence of the external cause

Y92.049 Unspecified place in boarding-house as the place of occurrence of the external cause

[6] **Y92.09 Other non-institutional residence as the place of occurrence of the external cause**

Y92.090 Kitchen in other non-institutional residence as the place of occurrence of the external cause

Y92.091 Bathroom in other non-institutional residence as the place of occurrence of the external cause

[4] 4th character required [5] 5th character required [6] 6th character required [7] 7th character required [X] Extension 'X' Alert
EXCLUDES 1 Not coded here EXCLUDES 2 Not included here PDx Primary Diagnosis Only Manifestation Code

Y92.092 Bedroom in other non-institutional residence as the place of occurrence of the external cause

Y92.093 Driveway of other non-institutional residence as the place of occurrence of the external cause

Y92.094 Garage of other non-institutional residence as the place of occurrence of the external cause

Y92.095 Swimming-pool of other non-institutional residence as the place of occurrence of the external cause

Y92.096 Garden or yard of other non-institutional residence as the place of occurrence of the external cause

Y92.098 Other place in other non-institutional residence as the place of occurrence of the external cause

Y92.099 Unspecified place in other non-institutional residence as the place of occurrence of the external cause

Y92.1 Institutional (nonprivate) residence as the place of occurrence of the external cause

Y92.10 Unspecified residential institution as the place of occurrence of the external cause

Y92.11 Children's home and orphanage as the place of occurrence of the external cause

Y92.110 Kitchen in children's home and orphanage as the place of occurrence of the external cause

Y92.111 Bathroom in children's home and orphanage as the place of occurrence of the external cause

Y92.112 Bedroom in children's home and orphanage as the place of occurrence of the external cause

Y92.113 Driveway of children's home and orphanage as the place of occurrence of the external cause

Y92.114 Garage of children's home and orphanage as the place of occurrence of the external cause

Y92.115 Swimming-pool of children's home and orphanage as the place of occurrence of the external cause

Y92.116 Garden or yard of children's home and orphanage as the place of occurrence of the external cause

Y92.118 Other place in children's home and orphanage as the place of occurrence of the external cause

Y92.119 Unspecified place in children's home and orphanage as the place of occurrence of the external cause

Y92.12 Nursing home as the place of occurrence of the external cause

Home for the sick as the place of occurrence of the external cause

Hospice as the place of occurrence of the external cause

Y92.120 Kitchen in nursing home as the place of occurrence of the external cause

Y92.121 Bathroom in nursing home as the place of occurrence of the external cause

Y92.122 Bedroom in nursing home as the place of occurrence of the external cause

Y92.123 Driveway of nursing home as the place of occurrence of the external cause

Y92.124 Garage of nursing home as the place of occurrence of the external cause

Y92.125 Swimming-pool of nursing home as the place of occurrence of the external cause

Y92.126 Garden or yard of nursing home as the place of occurrence of the external cause

Y92.128 Other place in nursing home as the place of occurrence of the external cause

Y92.129 Unspecified place in nursing home as the place of occurrence of the external cause

Y92.13 Military base as the place of occurrence of the external cause

EXCLUDES1 military training grounds (Y92.83)

Y92.130 Kitchen on military base as the place of occurrence of the external cause

Y92.131 Mess hall on military base as the place of occurrence of the external cause

Y92.133 Barracks on military base as the place of occurrence of the external cause

Y92.135 Garage on military base as the place of occurrence of the external cause

Y92.136 Swimming-pool on military base as the place of occurrence of the external cause

Y92.137 Garden or yard on military base as the place of occurrence of the external cause

Y92.138 Other place on military base as the place of occurrence of the external cause

Y92.139 Unspecified place military base as the place of occurrence of the external cause

Y92.14 Prison as the place of occurrence of the external cause

Y92.140 Kitchen in prison as the place of occurrence of the external cause

Y92.141 Dining room in prison as the place of occurrence of the external cause

Y92.142 Bathroom in prison as the place of occurrence of the external cause

Y92.143 Cell of prison as the place of occurrence of the external cause

Y92.146 Swimming-pool of prison as the place of occurrence of the external cause

Y92.147 Courtyard of prison as the place of occurrence of the external cause

Y92.148 Other place in prison as the place of occurrence of the external cause

Y92.149 Unspecified place in prison as the place of occurrence of the external cause

Y92.15 Reform school as the place of occurrence of the external cause

Y92.150 Kitchen in reform school as the place of occurrence of the external cause

Y92.151 Dining room in reform school as the place of occurrence of the external cause

Y92.152 Bathroom in reform school as the place of occurrence of the external cause

Y92.153 Bedroom in reform school as the place of occurrence of the external cause

Y92.154 Driveway of reform school as the place of occurrence of the external cause

Y92.155 Garage of reform school as the place of occurrence of the external cause

Y92.156 Swimming-pool of reform school as the place of occurrence of the external cause

Y92.157 Garden or yard of reform school as the place of occurrence of the external cause

Y92.158 Other place in reform school as the place of occurrence of the external cause

Y92.159 Unspecified place in reform school as the place of occurrence of the external cause

Unspecified Code	Other Specified Code	N Newborn Age: 0	P Pediatric Age: 0-17	M Maternity Age: 12-55
A Adult Age: 15-124	♂ Male	♀ Female	● New Code	▲ Revised Code Title	►◄ Revised Text

[6] Y92.16 School dormitory as the place of occurrence of the external cause

EXCLUDES1 *reform school as the place of occurrence of the external cause (Y92.15-)*
school buildings and grounds as the place of occurrence of the external cause (Y92.2-)
school sports and athletic areas as the place of occurrence of the external cause (Y92.3-)

Y92.160 Kitchen in school dormitory as the place of occurrence of the external cause
Y92.161 Dining room in school dormitory as the place of occurrence of the external cause
Y92.162 Bathroom in school dormitory as the place of occurrence of the external cause
Y92.163 Bedroom in school dormitory as the place of occurrence of the external cause
Y92.168 Other place in school dormitory as the place of occurrence of the external cause
Y92.169 Unspecified place in school dormitory as the place of occurrence of the external cause

[6] Y92.19 Other specified residential institution as the place of occurrence of the external cause

Y92.190 Kitchen in other specified residential institution as the place of occurrence of the external cause
Y92.191 Dining room in other specified residential institution as the place of occurrence of the external cause
Y92.192 Bathroom in other specified residential institution as the place of occurrence of the external cause
Y92.193 Bedroom in other specified residential institution as the place of occurrence of the external cause
Y92.194 Driveway of other specified residential institution as the place of occurrence of the external cause
Y92.195 Garage of other specified residential institution as the place of occurrence of the external cause
Y92.196 Pool of other specified residential institution as the place of occurrence of the external cause
Y92.197 Garden or yard of other specified residential institution as the place of occurrence of the external cause
Y92.198 Other place in other specified residential institution as the place of occurrence of the external cause
Y92.199 Unspecified place in other specified residential institution as the place of occurrence of the external cause

[5] Y92.2 School, other institution and public administrative area as the place of occurrence of the external cause

Building and adjacent grounds used by the general public or by a particular group of the public

EXCLUDES1 *building under construction as the place of occurrence of the external cause (Y92.6)*
residential institution as the place of occurrence of the external cause (Y92.1)
school dormitory as the place of occurrence of the external cause (Y92.16-)
sports and athletics area of schools as the place of occurrence of the external cause (Y92.3-)

[6] Y92.21 School (private) (public) (state) as the place of occurrence of the external cause

Y92.210 Daycare center as the place of occurrence of the external cause
Y92.211 Elementary school as the place of occurrence of the external cause
Kindergarten as the place of occurrence of the external cause
Y92.212 Middle school as the place of occurrence of the external cause
Y92.213 High school as the place of occurrence of the external cause
Y92.214 College as the place of occurrence of the external cause
University as the place of occurrence of the external cause
Y92.215 Trade school as the place of occurrence of the external cause
Y92.218 Other school as the place of occurrence of the external cause
Y92.219 Unspecified school as the place of occurrence of the external cause

Y92.22 Religious institution as the place of occurrence of the external cause

Church as the place of occurrence of the external cause
Mosque as the place of occurrence of the external cause
Synagogue as the place of occurrence of the external cause

[6] Y92.23 Hospital as the place of occurrence of the external cause

EXCLUDES1 *ambulatory (outpatient) health services establishments (Y92.53-)*
home for the sick as the place of occurrence of the external cause (Y92.12-)
hospice as the place of occurrence of the external cause (Y92.12-)
nursing home as the place of occurrence of the external cause (Y92.12-)

Y92.230 Patient room in hospital as the place of occurrence of the external cause
Y92.231 Patient bathroom in hospital as the place of occurrence of the external cause
Y92.232 Corridor of hospital as the place of occurrence of the external cause
Y92.233 Cafeteria of hospital as the place of occurrence of the external cause
Y92.234 Operating room of hospital as the place of occurrence of the external cause
Y92.238 Other place in hospital as the place of occurrence of the external cause
Y92.239 Unspecified place in hospital as the place of occurrence of the external cause

[6] Y92.24 Public administrative building as the place of occurrence of the external cause

Y92.240 Courthouse as the place of occurrence of the external cause
Y92.241 Library as the place of occurrence of the external cause
Y92.242 Post office as the place of occurrence of the external cause
Y92.243 City hall as the place of occurrence of the external cause
Y92.248 Other public administrative building as the place of occurrence of the external cause

[6] Y92.25 Cultural building as the place of occurrence of the external cause

Y92.250 Art Gallery as the place of occurrence of the external cause
Y92.251 Museum as the place of occurrence of the external cause
Y92.252 Music hall as the place of occurrence of the external cause

[4] 4th character required [5] 5th character required [6] 6th character required [7] 7th character required [7x] Extension 'X' Alert
EXCLUDES1 Not coded here EXCLUDES2 Not included here [PDx] Primary Diagnosis Only Manifestation Code

Y92.253 Opera house **as the place of occurrence of the external cause**

Y92.254 Theater (live) **as the place of occurrence of the external cause**

Y92.258 **Other cultural public building as the place of occurrence of the external cause**

Y92.26 Movie house or cinema **as the place of occurrence of the external cause**

Y92.29 **Other specified public building as the place of occurrence of the external cause**

Assembly hall as the place of occurrence of the external cause

Clubhouse as the place of occurrence of the external cause

⑤ Y92.3 Sports and athletics area **as the place of occurrence of the external cause**

⑥ Y92.31 Athletic court **as the place of occurrence of the external cause**

EXCLUDES1 *tennis court in private home or garden (Y92.09)*

Y92.310 Basketball court **as the place of occurrence of the external cause**

Y92.311 Squash court **as the place of occurrence of the external cause**

Y92.312 Tennis court **as the place of occurrence of the external cause**

Y92.318 **Other athletic court as the place of occurrence of the external cause**

⑥ Y92.32 Athletic field **as the place of occurrence of the external cause**

Y92.320 Baseball field **as the place of occurrence of the external cause**

Y92.321 Football field **as the place of occurrence of the external cause**

Y92.322 Soccer field **as the place of occurrence of the external cause**

Y92.328 **Other athletic field as the place of occurrence of the external cause**

Cricket field as the place of occurrence of the external cause

Hockey field as the place of occurrence of the external cause

⑥ Y92.33 Skating rink **as the place of occurrence of the external cause**

Y92.330 Ice skating **rink (indoor) (outdoor) as the place of occurrence of the external cause**

Y92.331 Roller skating **rink as the place of occurrence of the external cause**

Y92.34 Swimming pool (public) **as the place of occurrence of the external cause**

EXCLUDES1 *swimming pool in private home or garden (Y92.016)*

Y92.39 **Other specified sports and athletic area as the place of occurrence of the external cause**

Golf-course as the place of occurrence of the external cause

Gymnasium as the place of occurrence of the external cause

Riding-school as the place of occurrence of the external cause

Stadium as the place of occurrence of the external cause

⑤ Y92.4 **Street , highway and other paved roadways as the place of occurrence of the external cause**

EXCLUDES1 *private driveway of residence (Y92.014, Y92.024, Y92.043, Y92.093, Y92.113, Y92.123, Y92.154,Y92.194)*

⑥ Y92.41 Street and highway **as the place of occurrence of the external cause**

Y92.410 **Unspecified street and highway as the place of occurrence of the external cause**

Road NOS as the place of occurrence of the external cause

Y92.411 Interstate highway **as the place of occurrence of the external cause**

Freeway as the place of occurrence of the external cause

Motorway as the place of occurrence of the external cause

Y92.412 Parkway **as the place of occurrence of the external cause**

Y92.413 State road **as the place of occurrence of the external cause**

Y92.414 Local residential or business street **as the place of occurrence of the external cause**

Y92.415 Exit ramp or entrance ramp **of street or highway as the place of occurrence of the external cause**

⑥ Y92.48 Other paved roadways **as the place of occurrence of the external cause**

Y92.480 Sidewalk **as the place of occurrence of the external cause**

Y92.481 Parking lot **as the place of occurrence of the external cause**

Y92.482 Bike path **as the place of occurrence of the external cause**

Y92.488 **Other paved roadways as the place of occurrence of the external cause**

⑤ Y92.5 Trade and service area **as the place of occurrence of the external cause**

EXCLUDES1 *garage in private home (Y92.015) schools and other public administration buildings (Y92.2-)*

⑥ Y92.51 Private commercial establishments **as the place of occurrence of the external cause**

Y92.510 Bank **as the place of occurrence of the external cause**

Y92.511 Restaurant or café **as the place of occurrence of the external cause**

Y92.512 Supermarket, store or market **as the place of occurrence of the external cause**

Y92.513 Shop (commercial) **as the place of occurrence of the external cause**

⑥ Y92.52 Service areas **as the place of occurrence of the external cause**

Y92.520 Airport **as the place of occurrence of the external cause**

Y92.521 Bus station **as the place of occurrence of the external cause**

Y92.522 Railway station **as the place of occurrence of the external cause**

Y92.523 Highway rest stop **as the place of occurrence of the external cause**

Y92.524 Gas station **as the place of occurrence of the external cause**

Petroleum station as the place of occurrence of the external cause

Service station as the place of occurrence of the external cause

⑥ Y92.53 Ambulatory health services establishments **as the place of occurrence of the external cause**

Y92.530 Ambulatory surgery center **as the place of occurrence of the external cause**

Outpatient surgery center, including that connected with a hospital as the place of occurrence of the external cause

Same day surgery center, including that connected with a hospital as the place of occurrence of the external cause

Unspecified Code	Other Specified Code	N Newborn Age: 0	P Pediatric Age: 0-17	M Maternity Age: 12-55
A Adult Age: 15-124	♂ Male	♀ Female	● New Code	▲ Revised Code Title	►◄ Revised Text

Y92.531 Health care provider office **as the place of occurrence of the external cause**
Physician office as the place of occurrence of the external cause
Y92.532 Urgent care center **as the place of occurrence of the external cause**
Y92.538 **Other ambulatory health services establishments as the place of occurrence of the external cause**
Y92.59 **Other** trade areas **as the place of occurrence of the external cause**
Office building as the place of occurrence of the external cause
Casino as the place of occurrence of the external cause
Garage (commercial) as the place of occurrence of the external cause
Hotel as the place of occurrence of the external cause
Radio or television station as the place of occurrence of the external cause
Shopping mall as the place of occurrence of the external cause
Warehouse as the place of occurrence of the external cause
[5] Y92.6 Industrial and construction area **as the place of occurrence of the external cause**
Y92.61 Building [any] under construction **as the place of occurrence of the external cause**
Y92.62 Dock or shipyard **as the place of occurrence of the external cause**
Dockyard as the place of occurrence of the external cause
Dry dock as the place of occurrence of the external cause
Shipyard as the place of occurrence of the external cause
Y92.63 Factory **as the place of occurrence of the external cause**
Factory building as the place of occurrence of the external cause
Factory premises as the place of occurrence of the external cause
Industrial yard as the place of occurrence of the external cause
Y92.64 Mine or pit **as the place of occurrence of the external cause**
Mine as the place of occurrence of the external cause
Y92.65 Oil rig **as the place of occurrence of the external cause**
Pit (coal) (gravel) (sand) as the place of occurrence of the external cause
Y92.69 **Other specified industrial and construction area as the place of occurrence of the external cause**
Gasworks as the place of occurrence of the external cause
Power-station (coal) (nuclear) (oil) as the place of occurrence of the external cause
Tunnel under construction as the place of occurrence of the external cause
Workshop as the place of occurrence of the external cause
[5] Y92.7 Farm **as the place of occurrence of the external cause**
Ranch as the place of occurrence of the external cause
EXCLUDES1 *farmhouse and home premises of farm (Y92.01-)*
Y92.71 Barn **as the place of occurrence of the external cause**
Y92.72 Chicken coop **as the place of occurrence of the external cause**
Hen house as the place of occurrence of the external cause
Y92.73 Farm field **as the place of occurrence of the external cause**
Y92.74 Orchard **as the place of occurrence of the external cause**
Y92.79 **Other farm location as the place of occurrence of the external cause**
[5] Y92.8 Other places **as the place of occurrence of the external cause**
[6] Y92.81 Transport vehicle **as the place of occurrence of the external cause**
EXCLUDES1 *transport accidents (V00-V99)*
Y92.810 Car **as the place of occurrence of the external cause**
Y92.811 Bus **as the place of occurrence of the external cause**
Y92.812 Truck **as the place of occurrence of the external cause**
Y92.813 Airplane **as the place of occurrence of the external cause**
Y92.814 Boat **as the place of occurrence of the external cause**
Y92.815 Train **as the place of occurrence of the external cause**
Y92.816 Subway car **as the place of occurrence of the external cause**
Y92.818 **Other transport vehicle as the place of occurrence of the external cause**
[6] Y92.82 Wilderness area
Y92.820 Desert **as the place of occurrence of the external cause**
Y92.821 Forest **as the place of occurrence of the external cause**
Y92.828 **Other wilderness area as the place of occurrence of the external cause**
Swamp as the place of occurrence of the external cause
Mountain as the place of occurrence of the external cause
Marsh as the place of occurrence of the external cause
Prairie as the place of occurrence of the external cause
[6] Y92.83 Recreation area **as the place of occurrence of the external cause**
Y92.830 Public park **as the place of occurrence of the external cause**
Y92.831 Amusement park **as the place of occurrence of the external cause**
Y92.832 Beach **as the place of occurrence of the external cause**
Seashore as the place of occurrence of the external cause
Y92.833 Campsite **as the place of occurrence of the external cause**
Y92.834 Zoological garden (Zoo) **as the place of occurrence of the external cause**
Y92.838 **Other recreation area as the place of occurrence of the external cause**
Y92.84 Military training ground **as the place of occurrence of the external cause**
Y92.85 Railroad track **as the place of occurrence of the external cause**
Y92.86 Slaughter house **as the place of occurrence of the external cause**
Y92.89 **Other specified places as the place of occurrence of the external cause**
Derelict house as the place of occurrence of the external cause
Y92.9 **Unspecified place or not applicable**

[4] 4th character required [5] 5th character required [6] 6th character required [7] 7th character required [X] Extension 'X' Alert
EXCLUDES1 Not coded here EXCLUDES2 Not included here PDx Primary Diagnosis Only Manifestation Code

[4] **Y93 Activity codes**

[NOTES] Category Y93 is provided for use to indicate the activity of the person seeking healthcare for an injury or health condition, such as a heart attack while shoveling snow, which resulted from, or was contributed to, by the activity. These codes are appropriate for use for both acute injuries, such as those from chapter 19, and conditions that are due to the long-term, cumulative effects of an activity, such as those from chapter 13. They are also appropriate for use with external cause codes for cause and intent if identifying the activity provides additional information on the event. These codes should be used in conjunction with codes for external cause status (Y99) and place of occurrence (Y92).

This section contains the following broad activity categories:

Y93.0 Activities involving walking and running
Y93.1 Activities involving water and water craft
Y93.2 Activities involving ice and snow
Y93.3 Activities involving climbing, rappelling, and jumping off
Y93.4 Activities involving dancing and other rhythmic movement
Y93.5 Activities involving other sports and athletics played individually
Y93.6 Activities involving other sports and athletics played as a team or group
Y93.7 Activities involving other specified sports and athletics
Y93.A Activities involving other cardiorespiratory exercise
Y93.B Activities involving other muscle strengthening exercises
Y93.C Activities involving computer technology and electronic devices
Y93.D Activities involving arts and handcrafts
Y93.E Activities involving personal hygiene and interior property and clothing maintenance
Y93.F Activities involving caregiving
Y93.G Activities involving food preparation, cooking and grilling
Y93.H Activities involving exterior property and land maintenance, building and construction
Y93.I Activities involving roller coasters and other types of external motion
Y93.J Activities involving playing musical instrument
Y93.K Activities involving animal care
Y93.8 Activities, other specified
Y93.9 Activity, unspecified

[5] **Y93.0 Activities involving walking and running**

[EXCLUDES1] *activity, walking an animal (Y93.K1)*
activity, walking or running on a treadmill (Y93.A1)

Y93.01 Activity, walking, marching and hiking
Activity, walking, marching and hiking on level or elevated terrain
[EXCLUDES1] *activity, mountain climbing (Y93.31)*

Y93.02 Activity, running

[5] **Y93.1 Activities involving water and water craft**

[EXCLUDES1] *activities involving ice (Y93.2-)*

Y93.11 Activity, swimming
Y93.12 Activity, springboard and platform diving
Y93.13 Activity, water polo
Y93.14 Activity, water aerobics and water exercise
Y93.15 Activity, underwater diving and snorkeling
Activity, SCUBA diving
Y93.16 Activity, rowing, canoeing, kayaking, rafting and tubing
Activity, canoeing, kayaking, rafting and tubing in calm and turbulent water
Y93.17 Activity, water skiing and wake boarding
Y93.18 Activity, surfing, windsurfing and boogie boarding
Activity, water sliding
Y93.19 Activity, other involving water and watercraft
Activity involving water NOS
Activity, parasailing
Activity, water survival training and testing

[5] **Y93.2 Activities involving ice and snow**

[EXCLUDES1] *activity, shoveling ice and snow (Y93.H1)*

Y93.21 Activity, ice skating
Activity, figure skating (singles) (pairs)
Activity, ice dancing
[EXCLUDES1] *activity, ice hockey (Y93.22)*
Y93.22 Activity, ice hockey
Y93.23 Activity, snow (alpine) (downhill) skiing, snow boarding, sledding, tobogganing and snow tubing
[EXCLUDES1] *activity, cross country skiing (Y93.24)*
Y93.24 Activity, cross country skiing
Activity, nordic skiing
Y93.29 Activity, other involving ice and snow
Activity involving ice and snow NOS

[5] **Y93.3 Activities involving climbing, rappelling and jumping off**

[EXCLUDES1] *activity, hiking on level or elevated terrain (Y93.01)*
activity, jumping rope (Y93.56)
activity, trampoline jumping (Y93.44)

Y93.31 Activity, mountain climbing, rock climbing and wall climbing
Y93.32 Activity, rappelling
Y93.33 Activity, BASE jumping
Activity, Building, Antenna, Span, Earth jumping
Y93.34 Activity, bungee jumping
Y93.35 Activity, hang gliding
Y93.39 Activity, other involving climbing, rappelling and jumping off

[5] **Y93.4 Activities involving dancing and other rhythmic movement**

[EXCLUDES1] *activity, martial arts (Y93.75)*

Y93.41 Activity, dancing
Y93.42 Activity, yoga
Y93.43 Activity, gymnastics
Activity, rhythmic gymnastics
[EXCLUDES1] *activity, trampolining (Y93.44)*
Y93.44 Activity, trampolining
Y93.45 Activity, cheerleading
Y93.49 Activity, other involving dancing and other rhythmic movements

[5] **Y93.5 Activities involving other sports and athletics played individually**

[EXCLUDES1] *activity, dancing (Y93.41)*
activity, gymnastic (Y93.43)
activity, trampolining (Y93.44)
activity, yoga (Y93.42)

Y93.51 Activity, roller skating (inline) and skateboarding
Y93.52 Activity, horseback riding
Y93.53 Activity, golf
Y93.54 Activity, bowling
Y93.55 Activity, bike riding
Y93.56 Activity, jumping rope
Y93.57 Activity, non-running track and field events
[EXCLUDES1] *activity, running (any form) (Y93.02)*
Y93.59 Activity, other involving other sports and athletics played individually
[EXCLUDES1] *activities involving climbing, rappelling, and jumping (Y93.3-)*
activities involving ice and snow (Y93.2-)
activities involving walking and running (Y93.0-)
activities involving water and watercraft (Y93.1-)

Unspecified Code | Other Specified Code | [N] Newborn Age: 0 | [P] Pediatric Age: 0-17 | [M] Maternity Age: 12-55
[A] Adult Age: 15-124 | ♂ Male | ♀ Female | ● New Code | ▲ Revised Code Title | ►◄ Revised Text

⑤ **Y93.6** Activities involving other sports and athletics played as a team or group

> EXCLUDES1 activity, ice hockey (Y93.22)
> activity, water polo (Y93.13)

Y93.61 Activity, american tackle football

Activity, football NOS

Y93.62 Activity, american flag or touch football

Y93.63 Activity, rugby

Y93.64 Activity, baseball

Activity, softball

Y93.65 Activity, lacrosse and field hockey

Y93.66 Activity, soccer

Y93.67 Activity, basketball

Y93.68 Activity, volleyball (beach) (court)

Y93.6A Activity, physical games generally associated with school recess, summer camp and children

Activity, capture the flag

Activity, dodge ball

Activity, four square

Activity, kickball ⓟ

Y93.69 Activity, other involving other sports and athletics played as a team or group

Activity, cricket

⑤ **Y93.7** Activities involving other specified sports and athletics

Y93.71 Activity, boxing

Y93.72 Activity, wrestling

Y93.73 Activity, racquet and hand sports

Activity, handball

Activity, racquetball

Activity, squash

Activity, tennis

Y93.74 Activity, frisbee

Activity, ultimate frisbee

Y93.75 Activity, martial arts

Activity, combatives

Y93.79 Activity, other specified sports and athletics

> EXCLUDES1 sports and athletics activities specified in categories Y93.0-Y93.6

⑤ **Y93.A** Activities involving other cardiorespiratory exercise

Activities involving physical training

Y93.A1 Activity, exercise machines **primarily for cardiorespiratory conditioning**

Activity, elliptical and stepper machines

Activity, stationary bike

Activity, treadmill

Y93.A2 Activity, calisthenics

Activity, jumping jacks

Activity, warm up and cool down

Y93.A3 Activity, aerobic and step exercise

Y93.A4 Activity, circuit training

Y93.A5 Activity, obstacle course

Activity, challenge course

Activity, confidence course

Y93.A6 Activity, grass drills

Activity, guerilla drills

Y93.A9 Activity, other involving cardiorespiratory exercise

> EXCLUDES1 activities involving cardiorespiratory exercise specified in categories Y93.0-Y93.7

⑤ **Y93.B** Activities involving other muscle strengthening exercises

Y93.B1 Activity, exercise machines **primarily for muscle strengthening**

Y93.B2 Activity, push-ups, pull-ups, sit-ups

Y93.B3 Activity, free weights

Activity, barbells

Activity, dumbbells

Y93.B4 Activity, pilates

Y93.B9 Activity, other involving muscle strengthening exercises

> EXCLUDES1 activities involving muscle strengthening specified in categories Y93.0-Y93.A

⑤ **Y93.C** Activities involving computer technology and electronic devices

> EXCLUDES1 activity, electronic musical keyboard or instruments (Y93.J-)

Y93.C1 Activity, computer keyboarding

Activity, electronic game playing using keyboard or other stationary device

Y93.C2 Activity, hand held interactive electronic device

Activity, cellular telephone and communication device

Activity, electronic game playing using interactive device

> EXCLUDES1 activity, electronic game playing using keyboard or other stationary device (Y93.C1)

Y93.C9 Activity, other involving computer technology and electronic devices

⑤ **Y93.D** Activities involving arts and handcrafts

> EXCLUDES1 activities involving playing musical instrument (Y93.J-)

Y93.D1 Activity, knitting and crocheting

Y93.D2 Activity, sewing

Y93.D3 Activity, furniture building and finishing

Activity, furniture repair

Y93.D9 Activity, other involving arts and handcrafts

⑤ **Y93.E** Activities involving personal hygiene and interior property and clothing maintenance

> EXCLUDES1 activities involving cooking and grilling (Y93.G-)
> activities involving exterior property and land maintenance, building and construction (Y93.H-)
> activities involving caregiving (Y93.F-)
> activity, dishwashing (Y93.G1)
> activity, food preparation (Y93.G1)
> activity, gardening (Y93.H2)

Y93.E1 Activity, personal bathing and showering

Y93.E2 Activity, laundry

Y93.E3 Activity, vacuuming

Y93.E4 Activity, ironing

Y93.E5 Activity, floor mopping and cleaning

Y93.E6 Activity, residential relocation

Activity, packing up and unpacking involved in moving to a new residence

Y93.E8 Activity, other personal hygiene

Y93.E9 Activity, other interior property and clothing maintenance

⑤ **Y93.F** Activities involving caregiving

Activity involving the provider of caregiving

Y93.F1 Activity, caregiving, bathing

Y93.F2 Activity, caregiving, lifting

Y93.F9 Activity, other **caregiving**

⑤ **Y93.G** Activities involving food preparation, cooking and grilling

Y93.G1 Activity, food preparation and clean up

Activity, dishwashing

Y93.G2 Activity, grilling and smoking food

Y93.G3 Activity, cooking and baking

Activity, use of stove, oven and microwave oven

Y93.G9 Activity, other involving cooking and grilling

---

④ 4th character required   ⑤ 5th character required   ⑥ 6th character required   ⑦ 7th character required   ⓧ Extension 'X' Alert

EXCLUDES1 Not coded here   EXCLUDES2 Not included here   ⓟⓓⓧ Primary Diagnosis Only   Manifestation Code

812

ICD-10-CM 2015

[5] Y93.H Activities involving exterior property and land maintenance, building and construction

Y93.H1 Activity, digging, shoveling and raking
Activity, dirt digging
Activity, raking leaves
Activity, snow shoveling

Y93.H2 Activity, gardening and landscaping
Activity, pruning, trimming shrubs, weeding

Y93.H3 Activity, building and construction

Y93.H9 Activity, other involving exterior property and land maintenance, building and construction

[5] Y93.I Activities involving roller coasters and other types of external motion

Y93.I1 Activity, roller coaster riding

Y93.I9 Activity, other involving external motion

[5] Y93.J Activities involving playing musical instrument
Activity involving playing electric musical instrument

Y93.J1 Activity, piano playing
Activity, musical keyboard (electronic) playing

Y93.J2 Activity, drum and other percussion instrument playing

Y93.J3 Activity, string instrument playing

Y93.J4 Activity, winds and brass instrument playing

[5] Y93.K Activities involving animal care
[EXCLUDES1] *activity, horseback riding (Y93.52)*

Y93.K1 Activity, walking an animal

Y93.K2 Activity, milking an animal

Y93.K3 Activity, grooming and shearing an animal

Y93.K9 Activity, other involving animal care

[5] Y93.8 Activities, other specified

Y93.81 Activity, refereeing a sports activity

Y93.82 Activity, spectator at an event

Y93.83 Activity, rough housing and horseplay

Y93.84 Activity, sleeping

Y93.89 Activity, other specified

Y93.9 Activity, unspecified

Y95 Nosocomial condition

[4] Y99 External cause status
[NOTES] A single code from category Y99 should be used in conjunction with the external cause code(s) assigned to a record to indicate the status of the person at the time the event occurred.

Y99.0 Civilian activity done for income or pay
Civilian activity done for financial or other compensation
[EXCLUDES1] *military activity (Y99.1)*
volunteer activity (Y99.2)

Y99.1 Military activity
[EXCLUDES1] *activity of off duty military personnel (Y99.8)*

Y99.2 Volunteer activity
[EXCLUDES1] *activity of child or other family member assisting in compensated work of other family member (Y99.8)*

Y99.8 Other external cause status
Activity NEC
Activity of child or other family member assisting in compensated work of other family member
Hobby not done for income
Leisure activity
Off-duty activity of military personnel
Recreation or sport not for income or while a student
Student activity
[EXCLUDES1] *civilian activity done for income or compensation (Y99.0)*
military activity (Y99.1)

Y99.9 Unspecified external cause status

Unspecified Code | Other Specified Code | [N] Newborn Age: 0 | [P] Pediatric Age: 0-17 | [M] Maternity Age: 12-55
[A] Adult Age: 15-124 | ♂ Male | ♀ Female | ● New Code | ▲ Revised Code Title | ►◄ Revised Text

This page intentionally left blank

Chapter 21: Factors Influencing Health Status and Contact with Health Services (Z00-Z99)

Chapter Specific Coding Guidelines

Note: The chapter specific guidelines provide additional information about the use of Z codes for specified encounters.

a. Use of Z codes in any healthcare setting
Z codes are for use in any healthcare setting. Z codes may be used as either a first-listed (principal diagnosis code in the inpatient setting) or secondary code, depending on the circumstances of the encounter. Certain Z codes may only be used as first-listed or principal diagnosis.

b. Z Codes indicate a reason for an encounter
Z codes are not procedure codes. A corresponding procedure code must accompany a Z code to describe any procedure performed.

c. Categories of Z Codes
1) Contact/Exposure
Category Z20 indicates contact with, and suspected exposure to, communicable diseases. These codes are for patients who do not show any sign or symptom of a disease but are suspected to have been exposed to it by close personal contact with an infected individual or are in an area where a disease is epidemic.

Category Z77, indicates contact with and suspected exposures hazardous to health.

Contact/exposure codes may be used as a first-listed code to explain an encounter for testing, or, more commonly, as a secondary code to identify a potential risk.

2) Inoculations and vaccinations
Code Z23 is for encounters for inoculations and vaccinations. It indicates that a patient is being seen to receive a prophylactic inoculation against a disease. Procedure codes are required to identify the actual administration of the injection and the type(s) of immunizations given. Code Z23 may be used as a secondary code if the inoculation is given as a routine part of preventive health care, such as a well-baby visit.

3) Status
Status codes indicate that a patient is either a carrier of a disease or has the sequelae or residual of a past disease or condition. This includes such things as the presence of prosthetic or mechanical devices resulting from past treatment. A status code is informative, because the status may affect the course of treatment and its outcome. A status code is distinct from a history code. The history code indicates that the patient no longer has the condition.

A status code should not be used with a diagnosis code from one of the body system chapters, if the diagnosis code includes the information provided by the status code. For example, code Z94.1, Heart transplant status, should not be used with a code from subcategory T86.2, Complications of heart transplant. The status code does not provide additional information. The complication code indicates that the patient is a heart transplant patient.

For encounters for weaning from a mechanical ventilator, assign a code from subcategory J96.1, Chronic respiratory failure, followed by code Z99.11, Dependence on respirator [ventilator] status.

The status Z codes/categories are:

Z14   Genetic carrier

Genetic carrier status indicates that a person carries a gene, associated with a particular disease, which may be passed to offspring who may develop that disease. The person does not have the disease and is not at risk of developing the disease.

Z15   Genetic susceptibility to disease

Genetic susceptibility indicates that a person has a gene that increases the risk of that person developing the disease.

Codes from category Z15 should not be used as principal or first-listed codes. If the patient has the condition to which he/she is susceptible, and that condition is the reason for the encounter, the code for the current condition should be sequenced first. If the patient is being seen for follow-up after completed treatment for this condition, and the condition no longer exists, a follow-up code should be sequenced first, followed by the appropriate personal history and genetic susceptibility codes. If the purpose of the encounter is genetic counseling associated with procreative management, code Z31.5, Encounter for genetic counseling, should be assigned as the first-listed code, followed by a code from category Z15. Additional codes should be assigned for any applicable family or personal history.

Z16   Resistance to antimicrobial drugs

This code indicates that a patient has a condition that is resistant to antimicrobial drug treatment. Sequence the infection code first.

Z17   Estrogen receptor status

Z18   Retained foreign body fragments

Z21   Asymptomatic HIV infection status

This code indicates that a patient has tested positive for HIV but has manifested no signs or symptoms of the disease.

Z22   Carrier of infectious disease

Carrier status indicates that a person harbors the specific organisms of a disease without manifest symptoms and is capable of transmitting the infection.

Z28.3 Underimmunization status

Z33.1 Pregnant state, incidental

This code is a secondary code only for use when the pregnancy is in no way complicating the reason for visit. Otherwise, a code from the obstetric chapter is required.

Z66   Do not resuscitate

This code may be used when it is documented by the provider that a patient is on do not resuscitate status at any time during the stay.

Z67   Blood type

Z68   Body mass index (BMI)

Z74.01 Bed confinement status

Z76.82 Awaiting organ transplant status

Z78   Other specified health status

Code Z78.1, Physical restraint status, may be used when it is documented by the provider that a patient has been put in restraints during the current encounter. Please note that this code should not be reported when it is documented by the provider that a patient is temporarily restrained during a procedure.

Z79   Long-term (current) drug therapy

Codes from this category indicate a patient's continuous use of a prescribed drug (including such things as aspirin therapy) for the long-term treatment of a condition or for prophylactic use. It is not for use for patients who have addictions to drugs. This subcategory is not for use of medications for detoxification or maintenance programs to prevent withdrawal symptoms in patients with drug dependence (e.g., methadone maintenance for opiate dependence). Assign the appropriate code for the drug dependence instead.

Assign a code from Z79 if the patient is receiving a medication for an extended period as a prophylactic measure (such as for the prevention of deep vein thrombosis) or as treatment of a chronic condition (such as arthritis) or a disease requiring a lengthy course of treatment (such as cancer). Do not assign a code from category Z79 for medication being administered for a brief period of time to treat an acute illness or injury (such as a course of antibiotics to treat acute bronchitis).

Z88 Allergy status to drugs, medicaments and biological substances

Except: Z88.9, Allergy status to unspecified drugs, medicaments and biological substances status

Z89 Acquired absence of limb

Z90 Acquired absence of organs, not elsewhere classified

Z91.0- Allergy status, other than to drugs and biological substances

Z92.82 Status post administration of tPA (rtPA) in a different facility within the last 24 hours prior to admission to a current facility

Assign code Z92.82, Status post administration of tPA (rtPA) in a different facility within the last 24 hours prior to admission to current facility, as a secondary diagnosis when a patient is received by transfer into a facility and documentation indicates they were administered tissue plasminogen activator (tPA) within the last 24 hours prior to admission to the current facility.

This guideline applies even if the patient is still receiving the tPA at the time they are received into the current facility.

The appropriate code for the condition for which the tPA was administered (such as cerebrovascular disease or myocardial infarction) should be assigned first.

Code Z92.82 is only applicable to the receiving facility record and not to the transferring facility record.

Z93 Artificial opening status

Z94 Transplanted organ and tissue status

Z95 Presence of cardiac and vascular implants and grafts

Z96 Presence of other functional implants

Z97 Presence of other devices

Z98 Other postprocedural states

Assign code Z98.85, Transplanted organ removal status, to indicate that a transplanted organ has been previously removed. This code should not be assigned for the encounter in which the transplanted organ is removed. The complication necessitating removal of the transplant organ should be assigned for that encounter.

See section I.C19. for information on the coding of organ transplant complications.

Z99 Dependence on enabling machines and devices, not elsewhere classified

Note: Categories Z89-Z90 and Z93-Z99 are for use only if there are no complications or malfunctions of the organ or tissue replaced, the amputation site or the equipment on which the patient is dependent.

4) **History (of)**

There are two types of history Z codes, personal and family. Personal history codes explain a patient's past medical condition that no longer exists and is not receiving any treatment, but that has the potential for recurrence, and therefore may require continued monitoring.

Family history codes are for use when a patient has a family member(s) who has had a particular disease that causes the patient to be at higher risk of also contracting the disease.

Personal history codes may be used in conjunction with follow-up codes and family history codes may be used in conjunction with screening codes to explain the need for a test or procedure. History codes are also acceptable on any medical record regardless of the reason for visit. A history of an illness, even if no longer present, is important information that may alter the type of treatment ordered.

The history Z code categories are:

Z80 Family history of primary malignant neoplasm

Z81 Family history of mental and behavioral disorders

Z82 Family history of certain disabilities and chronic diseases (leading to disablement)

Z83 Family history of other specific disorders

Z84 Family history of other conditions

Z85 Personal history of malignant neoplasm

Z86 Personal history of certain other diseases

Z87 Personal history of other diseases and conditions

Z91.4- Personal history of psychological trauma, not elsewhere classified

Z91.5 Personal history of self-harm

Z91.8- Other specified personal risk factors, not elsewhere classified

Exception: Z91.83, Wandering in diseases classified elsewhere

Z92 Personal history of medical treatment

Except: Z92.0, Personal history of contraception

Except: Z92.82, Status post administration of tPA (rtPA) in a different facility within the last 24 hours prior to admission to a current facility

5) **Screening**

Screening is the testing for disease or disease precursors in seemingly well individuals so that early detection and treatment can be provided for those who test positive for the disease (e.g., screening mammogram).

The testing of a person to rule out or confirm a suspected diagnosis because the patient has some sign or symptom is a diagnostic examination, not a screening. In these cases, the sign or symptom is used to explain the reason for the test.

A screening code may be a first-listed code if the reason for the visit is specifically the screening exam. It may also be used as an additional code if the screening is done during an office visit for other health problems. A screening code is not necessary if the screening is inherent to a routine examination, such as a pap smear done during a routine pelvic examination.

Should a condition be discovered during the screening then the code for the condition may be assigned as an additional diagnosis.

The Z code indicates that a screening exam is planned. A procedure code is required to confirm that the screening was performed.

The screening Z codes/categories:

Z11   Encounter for screening for infectious and parasitic diseases

Z12   Encounter for screening for malignant neoplasms

Z13   Encounter for screening for other diseases and disorders

Except: Z13.9, Encounter for screening, unspecified

Z36   Encounter for antenatal screening for mother

6) **Observation**

There are two observation Z code categories. They are for use in very limited circumstances when a person is being observed for a suspected condition that is ruled out. The observation codes are not for use if an injury or illness or any signs or symptoms related to the suspected condition are present. In such cases the diagnosis/symptom code is used with the corresponding external cause code.

The observation codes are to be used as principal diagnosis only. Additional codes may be used in addition to the observation code but only if they are unrelated to the suspected condition being observed.

Codes from subcategory Z03.7, Encounter for suspected maternal and fetal conditions ruled out, may either be used as a first-listed or as an additional code assignment depending on the case. They are for use in very limited circumstances on a maternal record when an encounter is for a suspected maternal or fetal condition that is ruled out during that encounter (for example, a maternal or fetal condition may be suspected due to an abnormal test result). These codes should not be used when the condition is confirmed. In those cases, the confirmed condition should be coded. In addition, these codes are not for use if an illness or any signs or symptoms related to the suspected condition or problem are present. In such cases the diagnosis/symptom code is used.

Additional codes may be used in addition to the code from subcategory Z03.7, but only if they are unrelated to the suspected condition being evaluated.

Codes from subcategory Z03.7 may not be used for encounters for antenatal screening of mother. *See Section I.C.21. Screening.*

For encounters for suspected fetal condition that are inconclusive following testing and evaluation, assign the appropriate code from category O35, O36, O40 or O41.

The observation Z code categories:

Z03   Encounter for medical observation for suspected diseases and conditions ruled out

Z04   Encounter for examination and observation for other reasons

Except: Z04.9, Encounter for examination and observation for unspecified reason

7) **Aftercare**

Aftercare visit codes cover situations when the initial treatment of a disease has been performed and the patient requires continued care during the healing or recovery phase, or for the long-term consequences of the disease. The aftercare Z code should not be used if treatment is directed at a current, acute disease. The diagnosis code is to be used in these cases. Exceptions to this rule are codes Z51.0, Encounter for antineoplastic radiation therapy, and codes from subcategory Z51.1, Encounter for antineoplastic chemotherapy and immunotherapy. These codes are to be first-listed, followed by the diagnosis code when a patient's encounter is solely to receive radiation therapy, chemotherapy, or immunotherapy for the treatment of a neoplasm. If the reason for the encounter is more than one type of antineoplastic therapy, code Z51.0 and a code from subcategory Z51.1 may be assigned together, in which

case one of these codes would be reported as a secondary diagnosis.

The aftercare Z codes should also not be used for aftercare for injuries. For aftercare of an injury, assign the acute injury code with the appropriate 7th character (for subsequent encounter).

The aftercare codes are generally first-listed to explain the specific reason for the encounter. An aftercare code may be used as an additional code when some type of aftercare is provided in addition to the reason for admission and no diagnosis code is applicable. An example of this would be the closure of a colostomy during an encounter for treatment of another condition.

Aftercare codes should be used in conjunction with other aftercare codes or diagnosis codes to provide better detail on the specifics of an aftercare encounter visit, unless otherwise directed by the classification. Should a patient receive multiple types of antineoplastic therapy during the same encounter, code Z51.0, Encounter for antineoplastic radiation therapy, and codes from subcategory Z51.1, Encounter for antineoplastic chemotherapy and immunotherapy, may be used together on a record. The sequencing of multiple aftercare codes depends on the circumstances of the encounter.

Certain aftercare Z code categories need a secondary diagnosis code to describe the resolving condition or sequelae. For others, the condition is included in the code title.

Additional Z code aftercare category terms include fitting and adjustment, and attention to artificial openings.

Status Z codes may be used with aftercare Z codes to indicate the nature of the aftercare. For example code Z95.1, Presence of aortocoronary bypass graft, may be used with code Z48.812,

Encounter for surgical aftercare following surgery on the circulatory system, to indicate the surgery for which the aftercare is being performed. A status code should not be used when the aftercare code indicates the type of status, such as using Z43.0, Encounter for attention to tracheostomy, with Z93.0, Tracheostomy status.

The aftercare Z category/codes:

Z42   Encounter for plastic and reconstructive surgery following medical procedure or healed injury

Z43   Encounter for attention to artificial openings

Z44   Encounter for fitting and adjustment of external prosthetic device

Z45   Encounter for adjustment and management of implanted device

Z46   Encounter for fitting and adjustment of other devices

Z47   Orthopedic aftercare

Z48   Encounter for other postprocedural aftercare

Z49   Encounter for care involving renal dialysis

Z51   Encounter for other aftercare

8) **Follow-up**

The follow-up codes are used to explain continuing surveillance following completed treatment of a disease, condition, or injury. They imply that the condition has been fully treated and no longer exists. They should not be confused with aftercare codes, or injury codes with a 7th character for subsequent encounter, that explain ongoing care of a healing condition or its sequelae. Follow-up codes may be used in conjunction with history codes to provide the full picture of the healed condition and its treatment. The follow-up code is sequenced first, followed by the history code.

A follow-up code may be used to explain multiple visits. Should a condition be found to have recurred on the follow-up visit, then the diagnosis code for the condition should be assigned in place of the follow-up code.

The follow-up Z code categories:

Z08 Encounter for follow-up examination after completed treatment for malignant neoplasm

Z09 Encounter for follow-up examination after completed treatment for conditions other than malignant neoplasm

Z39 Encounter for maternal postpartum care and examination

9) Donor
Codes in category Z52, Donors of organs and tissues, are used for living individuals who are donating blood or other body tissue. These codes are only for individuals donating for others, not for self-donations. They are not used to identify cadaveric donations.

10) Counseling
Counseling Z codes are used when a patient or family member receives assistance in the aftermath of an illness or injury, or when support is required in coping with family or social problems. They are not used in conjunction with a diagnosis code when the counseling component of care is considered integral to standard treatment.

The counseling Z codes/categories:

Z30.0- Encounter for general counseling and advice on contraception

Z31.5 Encounter for genetic counseling

Z31.6- Encounter for general counseling and advice on procreation

Z32.2 Encounter for childbirth instruction

Z32.3 Encounter for childcare instruction

Z69 Encounter for mental health services for victim and perpetrator of abuse

Z70 Counseling related to sexual attitude, behavior and orientation

Z71 Persons encountering health services for other counseling and medical advice, not elsewhere classified

Z76.81 Expectant mother prebirth pediatrician visit

11) Encounters for Obstetrical and Reproductive Services
See Section I.C.15. Pregnancy, Childbirth, and the Puerperium, for further instruction on the use of these codes.

Z codes for pregnancy are for use in those circumstances when none of the problems or complications included in the codes from the Obstetrics chapter exist (a routine prenatal visit or postpartum care). Codes in category Z34, Encounter for supervision of normal pregnancy, are always first-listed and are not to be used with any other code from the OB chapter.

Codes in category Z3A, Weeks of gestation, may be assigned to provide additional information about the pregnancy. **The date of the admission should be used to determine weeks of gestation for inpatient admissions that encompass more than one gestational week.**

The outcome of delivery, category Z37, should be included on all maternal delivery records. It is always a secondary code. Codes in category Z37 should not be used on the newborn record.

Z codes for family planning (contraceptive) or procreative management and counseling should be included on an obstetric record either during the pregnancy or the postpartum stage, if applicable.

Z codes/categories for obstetrical and reproductive services:

Z30 Encounter for contraceptive management

Z31 Encounter for procreative management

Z32.2 Encounter for childbirth instruction

Z32.3 Encounter for childcare instruction

Z33 Pregnant state

Z34 Encounter for supervision of normal pregnancy

Z36 Encounter for antenatal screening of mother

Z3A Weeks of gestation

Z37 Outcome of delivery

Z39 Encounter for maternal postpartum care and examination

Z76.81 Expectant mother prebirth pediatrician visit

12) Newborns and Infants
See Section I.C.16. Newborn (Perinatal) Guidelines, for further instruction on the use of these codes.

Newborn Z codes/categories:

Z76.1 Encounter for health supervision and care of foundling

Z00.1- Encounter for routine child health examination

Z38 Liveborn infants according to place of birth and type of delivery

13) Routine and Administrative Examinations
The Z codes allow for the description of encounters for routine examinations, such as, a general check-up, or, examinations for administrative purposes, such as, a pre-employment physical. The codes are not to be used if the examination is for diagnosis of a suspected condition or for treatment purposes. In such cases the diagnosis code is used. During a routine exam, should a diagnosis or condition be discovered, it should be coded as an additional code. Pre-existing and chronic conditions and history codes may also be included as additional codes as long as the examination is for administrative purposes and not focused on any particular condition.

Some of the codes for routine health examinations distinguish between "with" and "without" abnormal findings. Code assignment depends on the information that is known at the time the encounter is being coded. For example, if no abnormal findings were found during the examination, but the encounter is being coded before test results are back, it is acceptable to assign the code for "without abnormal findings." When assigning a code for "with abnormal findings," additional code(s) should be assigned to identify the specific abnormal finding(s).

Pre-operative examination and pre-procedural laboratory examination Z codes are for use only in those situations when a patient is being cleared for a procedure or surgery and no treatment is given.

The Z codes/categories for routine and administrative examinations:

Z00 Encounter for general examination without complaint, suspected or reported diagnosis

Z01 Encounter for other special examination without complaint, suspected or reported diagnosis

Z02 Encounter for administrative examination

Except: Z02.9, Encounter for administrative examinations, unspecified

Z32.0- Encounter for pregnancy test

14) Miscellaneous Z Codes
The miscellaneous Z codes capture a number of other health care encounters that do not fall into one of the other categories. Certain of these codes identify the reason for the encounter; others are for use as additional codes that provide useful information on circumstances that may affect a patient's care and treatment.

Prophylactic Organ Removal

For encounters specifically for prophylactic removal of an organ (such as prophylactic removal of breasts due to a genetic susceptibility to cancer or a family history of cancer), the principal or first-listed code should be a code from category Z40, Encounter for prophylactic surgery, followed by the appropriate codes to identify the associated risk factor (such as genetic susceptibility or family history).

If the patient has a malignancy of one site and is having prophylactic removal at another site to prevent either a new primary malignancy or metastatic disease, a code for the malignancy should also be assigned in addition to a code from subcategory Z40.0, Encounter for prophylactic surgery for risk factors related to malignant neoplasms. A Z40.0 code should not be assigned if the patient is having organ removal for treatment of a malignancy, such as the removal of the testes for the treatment of prostate cancer.

Miscellaneous Z codes/categories:

Z28	Immunization not carried out
	Except: Z28.3, Underimmunization status
Z40	Encounter for prophylactic surgery
Z41	Encounter for procedures for purposes other than remedying health state
	Except: Z41.9, Encounter for procedure for purposes other than remedying health state, unspecified
Z53	Persons encountering health services for specific procedures and treatment, not carried out
Z55	Problems related to education and literacy
Z56	Problems related to employment and unemployment
Z57	Occupational exposure to risk factors
Z58	Problems related to physical environment
Z59	Problems related to housing and economic circumstances
Z60	Problems related to social environment
Z62	Problems related to upbringing
Z63	Other problems related to primary support group, including family circumstances
Z64	Problems related to certain psychosocial circumstances
Z65	Problems related to other psychosocial circumstances
Z72	Problems related to lifestyle
Z73	Problems related to life management difficulty
Z74	Problems related to care provider dependency
	Except: Z74.01, Bed confinement status
Z75	Problems related to medical facilities and other health care
Z76.0	Encounter for issue of repeat prescription
Z76.3	Healthy person accompanying sick person
Z76.4	Other boarder to healthcare facility
Z76.5	Malingerer [conscious simulation]
Z91.1-	Patient's noncompliance with medical treatment and regimen
Z91.83	Wandering in diseases classified elsewhere
Z91.89	Other specified personal risk factors, not elsewhere classified

15) **Nonspecific Z codes**
Certain Z codes are so non-specific, or potentially redundant with other codes in the classification, that there can be little

justification for their use in the inpatient setting. Their use in the outpatient setting should be limited to those instances when there is no further documentation to permit more precise coding. Otherwise, any sign or symptom or any other reason for visit that is captured in another code should be used.

Nonspecific Z codes/categories:

Z02.9	Encounter for administrative examinations, unspecified
Z04.9	Encounter for examination and observation for unspecified reason
Z13.9	Encounter for screening, unspecified
Z41.9	Encounter for procedure for purposes other than remedying health state, unspecified
Z52.9	Donor of unspecified organ or tissue
Z86.59	Personal history of other mental and behavioral disorders
Z88.9	Allergy status to unspecified drugs, medicaments and biological substances status
Z92.0	Personal history of contraception

16) **Z Codes That May Only be Principal/First-Listed Diagnosis**
The following Z codes/categories may only be reported as the principal/first-listed diagnosis, except when there are multiple encounters on the same day and the medical records for the encounters are combined:

Z00	Encounter for general examination without complaint, suspected or reported diagnosis
Z01	Encounter for other special examination without complaint, suspected or reported diagnosis
Z02	Encounter for administrative examination
Z03	Encounter for medical observation for suspected diseases and conditions ruled out
Z04	Encounter for examination and observation for other reasons
Z33.2	Encounter for elective termination of pregnancy
Z31.81	Encounter for male factor infertility in female patient
Z31.82	Encounter for Rh incompatibility status
Z31.83	Encounter for assisted reproductive fertility procedure cycle
Z31.84	Encounter for fertility preservation procedure
Z34	Encounter for supervision of normal pregnancy
Z39	Encounter for maternal postpartum care and examination
Z38	Liveborn infants according to place of birth and type of delivery
Z42	Encounter for plastic and reconstructive surgery following medical procedure or healed injury
Z51.0	Encounter for antineoplastic radiation therapy
Z51.1-	Encounter for antineoplastic chemotherapy and immunotherapy
Z52	Donors of organs and tissues
	Except: Z52.9, Donor of unspecified organ or tissue
Z76.1	Encounter for health supervision and care of foundling
Z76.2	Encounter for health supervision and care of other healthy infant and child
Z99.12	Encounter for respirator [ventilator] dependence during power failure

This page intentionally left blank

Factors influencing health status and contact with health services (Z00-Z99)

NOTES   Z codes represent reasons for encounters. A corresponding procedure code must accompany a Z code if a procedure is performed. Categories Z00-Z99 are provided for occasions when circumstances other than a disease, injury or external cause classifiable to categories A00-Y89 are recorded as 'diagnoses' or 'problems'. This can arise in two main ways:
(a)   When a person who may or may not be sick encounters the health services for some specific purpose, such as to receive limited care or service for a current condition, to donate an organ or tissue, to receive prophylactic vaccination (immunization), or to discuss a problem which is in itself not a disease or injury.
(b)   When some circumstance or problem is present which influences the person's health status but is not in itself a current illness or injury.

Persons encountering health services for examinations (Z00-Z13)

NOTES   Nonspecific abnormal findings disclosed at the time of these examinations are classified to categories R70-R94.
   EXCLUDES1 *examinations related to pregnancy and reproduction (Z30-Z36, Z39.-)*

Z00 **Encounter for general examination without complaint, suspected or reported diagnosis**
   EXCLUDES1 *encounter for examination for administrative purposes (Z02.-)*
   EXCLUDES2 *encounter for pre-procedural examinations (Z01.81-)*
   special screening examinations (Z11-Z13)

Z00.0 **Encounter for general** adult medical **examination**
Encounter for adult periodic examination (annual) (physical) and any associated laboratory and radiologic examinations
   EXCLUDES1 *encounter for examination of sign or symptom-code to sign or symptom*
   general health check-up of infant or child (Z00.12.-)

Z00.00 **Encounter for general adult medical examination** without abnormal findings
Encounter for adult health check-up NOS

Z00.01 **Encounter for general adult medical examination** with abnormal findings
Use additional code to identify abnormal findings

Z00.1 **Encounter for** newborn, infant and child health **examinations**

Z00.11 Newborn **health examination**
Health check for child under 29 days old
Use additional code to identify any abnormal findings
   EXCLUDES1 *health check for child over 28 days old (Z00.12-)*

Z00.110 **Health examination for newborn** under 8 days old
Health check for newborn under 8 days old

Z00.111 **Health examination for newborn** 8 to 28 days old
Health check for newborn 8 to 28 days old
Newborn weight check

Z00.12 **Encounter for** routine child **health examination**
Encounter for development testing of infant or child
Health check (routine) for child over 28 days old
   EXCLUDES1 *health check for child under 29 days old (Z00.11-)*
   health supervision of foundling or other healthy infant or child (Z76.1-Z76.2)
   newborn health examination (Z00.11-)

Z00.121 **Encounter for routine child health examination** with abnormal findings
Use additional code to identify abnormal findings

Z00.129 **Encounter for routine child health examination** without abnormal findings
Encounter for routine child health examination NOS

Z00.2 **Encounter for examination for** period of rapid growth in childhood

Z00.3 **Encounter for examination for** adolescent development **state**
Encounter for puberty development state

Z00.5 **Encounter for examination of** potential donor of organ and tissue

Z00.6 **Encounter for examination for** normal comparison and control in clinical research program
Examination of participant or control in clinical research program

Z00.7 **Encounter for examination for period of** delayed growth in childhood

Z00.70 **Encounter for examination for period of delayed growth in childhood** without abnormal findings

Z00.71 **Encounter for examination for period of delayed growth in childhood** with abnormal findings
Use additional code to identify abnormal findings

Z00.8 **Encounter for other general examination**
Encounter for health examination in population surveys

Z01 **Encounter for other** special examination **without complaint, suspected or reported diagnosis**
   INCLUDES *routine examination of specific system*

NOTES   Codes from category Z01 represent the reason for the encounter. A separate procedure code is required to identify any examinations or procedures performed
   EXCLUDES1 *encounter for examination for administrative purposes (Z02.-)*
   encounter for examination for suspected conditions, proven not to exist (Z03.-)
   encounter for laboratory and radiologic examinations as a component of general medical examinations (Z00.0-)
   encounter for laboratory, radiologic and imaging examinations for sign(s) and symptom(s) - code to the sign(s) or symptom(s)
   EXCLUDES2 *screening examinations (Z11-Z13)*

Z01.0 **Encounter for examination of** eyes and vision
   EXCLUDES1 *examination for driving license (Z02.4)*

Z01.00 **Encounter for examination of eyes and vision** without abnormal findings
Encounter for examination of eyes and vision NOS

Z01.01 **Encounter for examination of eyes and vision** with abnormal findings
Use additional code to identify abnormal findings

Z01.1 **Encounter for examination of** ears and hearing

Z01.10 **Encounter for examination of ears and hearing** without abnormal findings
Encounter for examination of ears and hearing NOS

Z01.11 **Encounter for examination of ears and hearing** with abnormal findings

Z01.110 **Encounter for hearing examination following** failed hearing screening

Z01.118 **Encounter for examination of ears and hearing with other abnormal findings**
Use additional code to identify abnormal findings

Z01.12 **Encounter for** hearing conservation and treatment

Z01.2 **Encounter for** dental examination and cleaning

Z01.20 **Encounter for dental examination and cleaning** without abnormal findings
Encounter for dental examination and cleaning NOS

Z01.21 **Encounter for dental examination and cleaning** with abnormal findings
Use additional code to identify abnormal findings

Unspecified Code	Other Specified Code	N Newborn Age: 0	P Pediatric Age: 0-17	M Maternity Age: 12-55
A Adult Age: 15-124	♂ Male	♀ Female	● New Code	▲ Revised Code Title	►◄ Revised Text

[5] **Z01.3 Encounter for examination of** blood pressure

Z01.30 Encounter for examination of blood pressure without abnormal findings

Encounter for examination of blood pressure NOS

Z01.31 Encounter for examination of blood pressure with abnormal findings

Use additional code to identify abnormal findings

[5] **Z01.4 Encounter for** gynecological **examination**

EXCLUDES2 *pregnancy examination or test (Z32.0-)*
routine examination for contraceptive maintenance (Z30.4-)

[6] **Z01.41 Encounter for** routine **gynecological examination**

Encounter for general gynecological examination with or without cervical smear

Encounter for gynecological examination (general) (routine) NOS

Encounter for pelvic examination (annual) (periodic)

Use additional code:
for screening for human papillomavirus, if applicable, (Z11.51)
for screening vaginal pap smear, if applicable (Z12.72)
to identify acquired absence of uterus, if applicable (Z90.71-)

EXCLUDES1 *gynecologic examination status-post hysterectomy for malignant condition (Z08)*
screening cervical pap smear not a part of a routine gynecological examination (Z12.4)

Z01.411 Encounter for gynecological examination (general) (routine) with abnormal findings ♀ [PDx]

Z01.419 Encounter for gynecological examination (general) (routine) without abnormal findings

Use additional code to identify abnormal findings ♀ [PDx]

Z01.42 Encounter for cervical smear to confirm findings **of recent normal smear following initial abnormal smear** ♀ [PDx]

[5] **Z01.8 Encounter for** other **specified** special **examinations**

[6] **Z01.81 Encounter for** preprocedural **examinations**

Encounter for preoperative examinations

Encounter for radiological and imaging examinations as part of preprocedural examination

Z01.810 Encounter for preprocedural cardiovascular **examination**

Z01.811 Encounter for preprocedural respiratory **examination**

Z01.812 Encounter for preprocedural laboratory **examination**

Blood and urine tests prior to treatment or procedure

Z01.818 Encounter for other preprocedural examination

Encounter for preprocedural examination NOS

Encounter for examinations prior to antineoplastic chemotherapy

Z01.82 Encounter for allergy testing

EXCLUDES1 *encounter for antibody response examination (Z01.84)*

Z01.83 Encounter for blood typing

Encounter for Rh typing

Z01.84 Encounter for antibody response examination

Encounter for immunity status testing

EXCLUDES1 *encounter for allergy testing (Z01.82)*

Z01.89 Encounter for other specified special examinations

[4] **Z02 Encounter for** administrative **examination** [PDx]

Z02.0 Encounter for examination for admission to educational institution

Encounter for examination for admission to preschool (education)

Encounter for examination for re-admission to school following illness or medical treatment

Z02.1 Encounter for pre-employment **examination**

Z02.2 Encounter for examination for admission to residential institution

EXCLUDES1 *examination for admission to prison (Z02.89)*

Z02.3 Encounter for examination for recruitment to armed forces

Z02.4 Encounter for examination for driving license

Z02.5 Encounter for examination for participation in sport

EXCLUDES1 *blood-alcohol and blood-drug test (Z02.83)*

Z02.6 Encounter for examination for insurance purposes

[5] **Z02.7 Encounter for** issue of medical certificate

EXCLUDES1 *encounter for general medical examination (Z00-Z01, Z02.0-Z02.6, Z02.8-Z02.9,)*

Z02.71 Encounter for disability determination

Encounter for issue of medical certificate of incapacity

Encounter for issue of medical certificate of invalidity

Z02.79 Encounter for issue of other medical certificate

[5] **Z02.8 Encounter for** other **administrative examinations**

Z02.81 Encounter for paternity testing

Z02.82 Encounter for adoption services

Z02.83 Encounter for blood-alcohol and blood-drug test

Use additional code for findings of alcohol or drugs in blood (R78.-)

Z02.89 Encounter for other administrative examinations

Encounter for examination for admission to prison

Encounter for examination for admission to summer camp

Encounter for immigration examination

Encounter for naturalization examination

Encounter for premarital examination

EXCLUDES1 *health supervision of foundling or other healthy infant or child (Z76.1-Z76.2)*

Z02.9 Encounter for administrative examinations, unspecified

[4] **Z03 Encounter for** medical observation **for suspected diseases and conditions ruled out**

This category is to be used when a person without a diagnosis is suspected of having an abnormal condition, without signs or symptoms, which requires study, but after examination and observation, is ruled out. This category is also for use for administrative and legal observation status.

EXCLUDES1 *contact with and (suspected) exposures hazardous to health (Z77.-)*
newborn observation for suspected condition, ruled out (P00-P04)
person with feared complaint in whom no diagnosis is made (Z71.1)
signs or symptoms under study- code to signs or symptoms [PDx]

Z03.6 Encounter for observation for suspected toxic effect from ingested substance **ruled out**

Encounter for observation for suspected adverse effect from drug

Encounter for observation for suspected poisoning

[4] 4th character required [5] 5th character required [6] 6th character required [7] 7th character required [X] Extension 'X' Alert
EXCLUDES1 Not coded here EXCLUDES2 Not included here [PDx] Primary Diagnosis Only Manifestation Code

[5] **Z03.7 Encounter for suspected maternal and fetal conditions ruled out**
Encounter for suspected maternal and fetal conditions not found
[EXCLUDES1] *known or suspected fetal anomalies affecting management of mother, not ruled out (O26.-, O35.-, O36.-, O40.-, O41.-)*

Z03.71 Encounter for suspected problem with amniotic cavity and membrane ruled out
Encounter for suspected oligohydramnios ruled out
Encounter for suspected polyhydramnios ruled out [M] ♀ [PDx]

Z03.72 Encounter for suspected placental problem ruled out [M] ♀ [PDx]

Z03.73 Encounter for suspected fetal anomaly ruled out [M] ♀ [PDx]

Z03.74 Encounter for suspected problem with fetal growth ruled out [M] ♀ [PDx]

Z03.75 Encounter for suspected cervical shortening ruled out [M] ♀ [PDx]

Z03.79 Encounter for other suspected maternal and fetal conditions ruled out [M] ♀ [PDx]

[5] **Z03.8 Encounter for observation for other suspected diseases and conditions ruled out**

[6] **Z03.81 Encounter for observation for suspected exposure to biological agents ruled out**

Z03.810 Encounter for observation for suspected exposure to anthrax ruled out

Z03.818 Encounter for observation for suspected exposure to other biological agents ruled out

Z03.89 Encounter for observation for other suspected diseases and conditions ruled out

[4] **Z04 Encounter for examination and observation for other reasons**
[INCLUDES] *encounter for examination for medicolegal reasons*
This category is to be used when a person without a diagnosis is suspected of having an abnormal condition, without signs or symptoms, which requires study, but after examination and observation, is ruled-out. This category is also for use for administrative and legal observation status. [PDx]

Z04.1 Encounter for examination and observation following transport accident
[EXCLUDES1] *encounter for examination and observation following work accident (Z04.2)*

Z04.2 Encounter for examination and observation following work accident

Z04.3 Encounter for examination and observation following other accident

[5] **Z04.4 Encounter for examination and observation following alleged rape**
Encounter for examination and observation of victim following alleged rape
Encounter for examination and observation of victim following alleged sexual abuse

Z04.41 Encounter for examination and observation following alleged adult rape
Suspected adult rape, ruled out
Suspected adult sexual abuse, ruled out [A] [PDx]

Z04.42 Encounter for examination and observation following alleged child rape
Suspected child rape, ruled out
Suspected child sexual abuse, ruled out [P] [PDx]

Z04.6 Encounter for general psychiatric examination, requested by authority

[5] **Z04.7 Encounter for examination and observation following alleged physical abuse**

Z04.71 Encounter for examination and observation following alleged adult physical abuse
Suspected adult physical abuse, ruled out
[EXCLUDES1] *confirmed case of adult physical abuse (T74.-)*
encounter for examination and observation following alleged adult sexual abuse (Z04.41)
suspected case of adult physical abuse, not ruled out (T76.-) [A] [PDx]

Z04.72 Encounter for examination and observation following alleged child physical abuse
Suspected child physical abuse, ruled out
[EXCLUDES1] *confirmed case of child physical abuse (T74.-)*
encounter for examination and observation following alleged child sexual abuse (Z04.42)
suspected case of child physical abuse, not ruled out (T76.-) [P] [PDx]

Z04.8 Encounter for examination and observation for other specified reasons
Encounter for examination and observation for request for expert evidence

Z04.9 Encounter for examination and observation for unspecified reason
Encounter for observation NOS

Z08 Encounter for follow-up examination after completed treatment for malignant neoplasm
Medical surveillance following completed treatment
Use additional code to identify any acquired absence of organs (Z90.-)
code to identify the personal history of malignant neoplasm (Z85.-)
[EXCLUDES1] *aftercare following medical care (Z43-Z49, Z51)*

Z09 Encounter for follow-up examination after completed treatment for conditions other than malignant neoplasm
Medical surveillance following completed treatment
Use additional code to identify any applicable history of disease code (Z86.-. Z87.-)
[EXCLUDES1] *aftercare following medical care (Z43-Z49, Z51)*
surveillance of contraception (Z30.4-)
surveillance of prosthetic and other medical devices (Z44-Z46)

[4] **Z11 Encounter for screening for infectious and parasitic diseases**
Screening is the testing for disease or disease precursors in asymptomatic individuals so that early detection and treatment can be provided for those who test positive for the disease.
[EXCLUDES1] *encounter for diagnostic examination-code to sign or symptom*

Z11.0 Encounter for screening for intestinal infectious diseases

Z11.1 Encounter for screening for respiratory tuberculosis

Z11.2 Encounter for screening for other bacterial diseases

Z11.3 Encounter for screening for infections with a predominantly sexual mode of transmission
[EXCLUDES2] *encounter for screening for human immunodeficiency virus [HIV] (Z11.4)*
encounter for screening for human papillomavirus (Z11.51)

Z11.4 Encounter for screening for human immunodeficiency virus [HIV]

[5] **Z11.5 Encounter for screening for other viral diseases**
[EXCLUDES2] *encounter for screening for viral intestinal disease (Z11.0)*

Z11.51 Encounter for screening for human papillomavirus (HPV)

Unspecified Code | Other Specified Code | [N] Newborn Age: 0 | [P] Pediatric Age: 0-17 | [M] Maternity Age: 12-55 | [A] Adult Age: 15-124 | ♂ Male | ♀ Female | ● New Code | ▲ Revised Code Title | ►◄ Revised Text

Z11.59 **Encounter for screening for other viral diseases**

Z11.6 **Encounter for screening for other protozoal diseases and helminthiases**

[EXCLUDES2] *encounter for screening for protozoal intestinal disease (Z11.0)*

Z11.8 **Encounter for screening for other infectious and parasitic diseases**

Encounter for screening for chlamydia
Encounter for screening for rickettsial
Encounter for screening for spirochetal
Encounter for screening for mycoses

Z11.9 **Encounter for screening for infectious and parasitic diseases, unspecified**

[4] Z12 **Encounter for screening for malignant neoplasms**

Screening is the testing for disease or disease precursors in asymptomatic individuals so that early detection and treatment can be provided for those who test positive for the disease.

Use additional code to identify any family history of malignant neoplasm (Z80.-)

[EXCLUDES1] *encounter for diagnostic examination-code to sign or symptom*

Z12.0 **Encounter for screening for malignant neoplasm of stomach**

[5] Z12.1 **Encounter for screening for malignant neoplasm of intestinal tract**

Z12.10 **Encounter for screening for malignant neoplasm of intestinal tract, unspecified**

Z12.11 **Encounter for screening for malignant neoplasm of colon**

Encounter for screening colonoscopy NOS

Z12.12 **Encounter for screening for malignant neoplasm of rectum**

Z12.13 **Encounter for screening for malignant neoplasm of small intestine**

Z12.2 **Encounter for screening for malignant neoplasm of respiratory organs**

[5] Z12.3 **Encounter for screening for malignant neoplasm of breast**

Z12.31 **Encounter for screening mammogram for malignant neoplasm of breast**

[EXCLUDES1] *inconclusive mammogram (R92.2)*

Z12.39 **Encounter for other screening for malignant neoplasm of breast**

Z12.4 **Encounter for screening for malignant neoplasm of cervix**

Encounter for screening pap smear for malignant neoplasm of cervix

[EXCLUDES1] *encounter for screening for human papillomavirus (Z11.51)*
when screening is part of general gynecological examination (Z01.4-) ♀

Z12.5 **Encounter for screening for malignant neoplasm of prostate** ♂

Z12.6 **Encounter for screening for malignant neoplasm of bladder**

[5] Z12.7 **Encounter for screening for malignant neoplasm of other genitourinary organs**

Z12.71 **Encounter for screening for malignant neoplasm of testis** ♂

Z12.72 **Encounter for screening for malignant neoplasm of vagina**

Vaginal pap smear status-post hysterectomy for non-malignant condition

Use additional code to identify acquired absence of uterus (Z90.71-)

[EXCLUDES1] *vaginal pap smear status-post hysterectomy for malignant conditions (Z08)* ♀

Z12.73 **Encounter for screening for malignant neoplasm of ovary** ♀

Z12.79 **Encounter for screening for malignant neoplasm of other genitourinary organs**

[5] Z12.8 **Encounter for screening for malignant neoplasm of other sites**

Z12.81 **Encounter for screening for malignant neoplasm of oral cavity**

Z12.82 **Encounter for screening for malignant neoplasm of nervous system**

Z12.83 **Encounter for screening for malignant neoplasm of skin**

Z12.89 **Encounter for screening for malignant neoplasm of other sites**

Z12.9 **Encounter for screening for malignant neoplasm, site unspecified**

[4] Z13 **Encounter for screening for other diseases and disorders**

Screening is the testing for disease or disease precursors in asymptomatic individuals so that early detection and treatment can be provided for those who test positive for the disease.

[EXCLUDES1] *encounter for diagnostic examination-code to sign or symptom*

Z13.0 **Encounter for screening for diseases of the blood and blood-forming organs and certain disorders involving the immune mechanism**

Z13.1 **Encounter for screening for diabetes mellitus**

[5] Z13.2 **Encounter for screening for nutritional, metabolic and other endocrine disorders**

Z13.21 **Encounter for screening for nutritional disorder**

[6] Z13.22 **Encounter for screening for metabolic disorder**

Z13.220 **Encounter for screening for lipoid disorders**

Encounter for screening for cholesterol level
Encounter for screening for hypercholesterolemia
Encounter for screening for hyperlipidemia

Z13.228 **Encounter for screening for other metabolic disorders**

Z13.29 **Encounter for screening for other suspected endocrine disorder**

[EXCLUDES1] *encounter for screening for diabetes mellitus (Z13.1)*

Z13.4 **Encounter for screening for certain developmental disorders in childhood**

Encounter for screening for developmental handicaps in early childhood

[EXCLUDES1] *routine development testing of infant or child (Z00.1-)* [P]

Z13.5 **Encounter for screening for eye and ear disorders**

[EXCLUDES2] *encounter for general hearing examination (Z01.1-)*
encounter for general vision examination (Z01.0-)

Z13.6 **Encounter for screening for cardiovascular disorders**

[5] Z13.7 **Encounter for screening for genetic and chromosomal anomalies**

[EXCLUDES1] *genetic testing for procreative management (Z31.4-)*

Z13.71 **Encounter for nonprocreative screening for genetic disease carrier status**

Z13.79 **Encounter for other screening for genetic and chromosomal anomalies**

[5] Z13.8 **Encounter for screening for other specified diseases and disorders**

[EXCLUDES2] *screening for malignant neoplasms (Z12.-)*

[6] Z13.81 **Encounter for screening for digestive system disorders**

Z13.810 **Encounter for screening for upper gastrointestinal disorder**

Z13.811 **Encounter for screening for lower gastrointestinal disorder**

[4] 4th character required [5] 5th character required [6] 6th character required [7] 7th character required [X] Extension 'X' Alert
[EXCLUDES1] Not coded here [EXCLUDES2] Not included here [PDX] Primary Diagnosis Only Manifestation Code

[EXCLUDES1] *encounter for screening for intestinal infectious disease (Z11.0)*

Z13.818 Encounter for screening for other digestive system disorders

[6] Z13.82 Encounter for screening for musculoskeletal disorder

Z13.820 Encounter for screening for osteoporosis

Z13.828 Encounter for screening for other musculoskeletal disorder

Z13.83 Encounter for screening for respiratory disorder NEC

[EXCLUDES1] *encounter for screening for respiratory tuberculosis (Z11.1)*

Z13.84 Encounter for screening for dental disorders

[6] Z13.85 Encounter for screening for nervous system disorders

Z13.850 Encounter for screening for traumatic brain injury

Z13.858 Encounter for screening for other nervous system disorders

Z13.88 Encounter for screening for disorder due to exposure to contaminants

[EXCLUDES1] *those exposed to contaminants without suspected disorders (Z57.-, Z77.-)*

Z13.89 Encounter for screening for other disorder

Encounter for screening for genitourinary disorders

Z13.9 Encounter for screening, unspecified

Genetic carrier and genetic susceptibility to disease (Z14-Z15)

[4] Z14 Genetic carrier

[5] Z14.0 Hemophilia A carrier

Z14.01 Asymptomatic hemophilia A carrier

Z14.02 Symptomatic hemophilia A carrier

Z14.1 Cystic fibrosis carrier

Z14.8 Genetic carrier of other disease

[4] Z15 Genetic susceptibility to disease

[INCLUDES] *confirmed abnormal gene*

Use additional code, if applicable, for any associated family history of the disease (Z80-Z84)

[EXCLUDES1] *chromosomal anomalies (Q90-Q99)*

[5] Z15.0 Genetic susceptibility to malignant neoplasm

Code first , if applicable, any current malignant neoplasm (C00-C75, C81-C96)

Use additional code, if applicable, for any personal history of malignant neoplasm (Z85.-)

Z15.01 Genetic susceptibility to malignant neoplasm of breast

Z15.02 Genetic susceptibility to malignant neoplasm of ovary ♀

Z15.03 Genetic susceptibility to malignant neoplasm of prostate ♂

Z15.04 Genetic susceptibility to malignant neoplasm of endometrium ♀

Z15.09 Genetic susceptibility to other malignant neoplasm

[5] Z15.8 Genetic susceptibility to other disease

Z15.81 Genetic susceptibility to multiple endocrine neoplasia [MEN]

[EXCLUDES1] *multiple endocrine neoplasia [MEN] syndromes (E31.2-)*

Z15.89 Genetic susceptibility to other disease

Resistance to antimicrobial drugs (Z16)

[4] Z16 Resistance to antimicrobial drugs

[NOTES] The codes in this category are provided for use as additional codes to identify the resistance and non-responsiveness of a condition to antimicrobial drugs.

Code first the infection

[EXCLUDES1] *Methicillin resistant Staphylococcus aureus infection (A49.02)*
Methicillin resistant Staphylococcus aureus infection in diseases classified elsewhere (B95.62)
Methicillin resistant Staphylococcus aureus pneumonia (J15.212)
Sepsis due to Methicillin resistant Staphylococcus aureus (A41.02)

[5] Z16.1 Resistance to beta lactam antibiotics

Z16.10 Resistance to unspecified beta lactam antibiotics

Z16.11 Resistance to penicillins

Resistance to amoxicillin

Resistance to ampicillin

Z16.12 Extended spectrum beta lactamase (ESBL) resistance

Z16.19 Resistance to other specified beta lactam antibiotics

Resistance to cephalosporins

[5] Z16.2 Resistance to other antibiotics

Z16.20 Resistance to unspecified antibiotic

Resistance to antibiotics NOS

Z16.21 Resistance to vancomycin

Z16.22 Resistance to vancomycin related antibiotics

Z16.23 Resistance to quinolones and fluoroquinolones

Z16.24 Resistance to multiple antibiotics

Z16.29 Resistance to other single specified antibiotic

Resistance to aminoglycosides

Resistance to macrolides

Resistance to sulfonamides

Resistance to tetracyclines

[5] Z16.3 Resistance to other antimicrobial drugs

[EXCLUDES1] *resistance to antibiotics (Z16.1-, Z16.2-)*

Z16.30 Resistance to unspecified antimicrobial drugs

Drug resistance NOS

Z16.31 Resistance to antiparasitic drug(s)

Resistance to quinine and related compounds

Z16.32 Resistance to antifungal drug(s)

Z16.33 Resistance to antiviral drug(s)

[6] Z16.34 Resistance to antimycobacterial drug(s)

Resistance to tuberculostatics

Z16.341 Resistance to single antimycobacterial drug

Resistance to antimycobacterial drug NOS

Z16.342 Resistance to multiple antimycobacterial drugs

Z16.35 Resistance to multiple antimicrobial drugs

[EXCLUDES1] *Resistance to multiple antibiotics only (Z16.24)*

Z16.39 Resistance to other specified antimicrobial drug

Estrogen receptor status (Z17)

[4] Z17 Estrogen receptor status

Code first malignant neoplasm of breast (C50.-)

Z17.0 Estrogen receptor positive status [ER+]

Z17.1 Estrogen receptor negative status [ER-]

Retained foreign body fragments (Z18)

[4] Z18 Retained foreign body fragments

[INCLUDES] *embedded fragment (status)*
embedded splinter (status)
retained foreign body status

[EXCLUDES1] *artificial joint prosthesis status (Z96.6-)*
foreign body accidentally left during a procedure (T81.5-)
foreign body entering through orifice (T15-T19)
in situ cardiac device (Z95.-)
organ or tissue replaced by means other than transplant (Z96.-, Z97.-)
organ or tissue replaced by transplant (Z94.-)
personal history of retained foreign body fully removed Z87.821
superficial foreign body (non-embedded splinter) - code to superficial foreign body, by site

Unspecified Code | Other Specified Code | [N] Newborn Age: 0 | [P] Pediatric Age: 0-17 | [M] Maternity Age: 12-55 | [A] Adult Age: 15-124 | ♂ Male | ♀ Female | ● New Code | ▲ Revised Code Title | ►◄ Revised Text

⑤ **Z18.0** **Retained** radioactive **fragments**

    Z18.01 **Retained** depleted uranium **fragments**

    Z18.09 **Other retained radioactive fragments**

        Other retained depleted isotope fragments

        Retained nontherapeutic radioactive fragments

⑤ **Z18.1** **Retained** metal **fragments**

    EXCLUDES1 *retained radioactive metal fragments (Z18.01-Z18.09)*

    Z18.10 **Retained metal fragments, unspecified**

        Retained metal fragment NOS

    Z18.11 **Retained** magnetic **metal fragments**

    Z18.12 **Retained** nonmagnetic **metal fragments**

Z18.2 **Retained** plastic **fragments**

    Acrylics fragments

    Diethylhexylphthalates fragments

    Isocyanate fragments

⑤ **Z18.3** **Retained** organic **fragments**

    Z18.31 **Retained** animal quills or spines

    Z18.32 **Retained** tooth

    Z18.33 **Retained** wood **fragments**

    Z18.39 **Other retained organic fragments**

⑤ **Z18.8** Other **specified retained foreign body**

    Z18.81 **Retained** glass **fragments**

    Z18.83 **Retained** stone or crystalline **fragments**

        Retained concrete or cement fragments

    Z18.89 **Other specified retained foreign body fragments**

Z18.9 **Retained foreign body fragments, unspecified material**

Persons with potential health hazards related to communicable diseases (Z20-Z28)

④ **Z20** **Contact with and (suspected) exposure to communicable diseases**

    EXCLUDES1 *carrier of infectious disease (Z22.-)*
               diagnosed current infectious or parasitic disease -see Alphabetic Index

    EXCLUDES2 *personal history of infectious and parasitic diseases (Z86.1-)*

⑤ **Z20.0** **Contact with and (suspected) exposure to** intestinal infectious diseases

    Z20.01 **Contact with and (suspected) exposure to intestinal infectious diseases due to** Escherichia coli (E. coli)

    Z20.09 **Contact with and (suspected) exposure to other intestinal infectious diseases**

Z20.1 **Contact with and (suspected) exposure to** tuberculosis

Z20.2 **Contact with and (suspected) exposure to infections with a** predominantly sexual mode of transmission

Z20.3 **Contact with and (suspected) exposure to** rabies

Z20.4 **Contact with and (suspected) exposure to** rubella

Z20.5 **Contact with and (suspected) exposure to** viral hepatitis

Z20.6 **Contact with and (suspected) exposure to** human immunodeficiency virus **[HIV]**

    EXCLUDES1 *asymptomatic human immunodeficiency virus [HIV]*
               HIV infection status (Z21)

Z20.7 **Contact with and (suspected) exposure to** pediculosis, acariasis and other **infestations**

⑤ **Z20.8** **Contact with and (suspected) exposure to** other communicable **diseases**

  ⑥ **Z20.81** **Contact with and (suspected) exposure to other** bacterial **communicable diseases**

    Z20.810 **Contact with and (suspected) exposure to** anthrax

    Z20.811 **Contact with and (suspected) exposure to** meningococcus

    Z20.818 **Contact with and (suspected) exposure to other bacterial communicable diseases**

  ⑥ **Z20.82** **Contact with and (suspected) exposure to other** viral **communicable diseases**

    Z20.820 **Contact with and (suspected) exposure to** varicella

    Z20.828 **Contact with and (suspected) exposure to other viral communicable diseases**

  Z20.89 **Contact with and (suspected) exposure to other communicable diseases**

Z20.9 **Contact with and (suspected) exposure to unspecified communicable disease**

Z21 **Asymptomatic human immunodeficiency virus [HIV] infection status**

    HIV positive NOS

    Code first Human immunodeficiency virus [HIV] disease complicating pregnancy, childbirth and the puerperium, if applicable (O98.7-)

    EXCLUDES1 *acquired immunodeficiency syndrome (B20)*
               contact with human immunodeficiency virus [HIV] (Z20.6)
               exposure to human immunodeficiency virus [HIV] (Z20.6)
               human immunodeficiency virus [HIV] disease (B20)
               inconclusive laboratory evidence of human immunodeficiency virus [HIV] (R75)

④ **Z22** **Carrier of infectious disease**

    INCLUDES *colonization status*
           suspected carrier

Z22.0 **Carrier of** typhoid

Z22.1 **Carrier of other** intestinal **infectious diseases**

Z22.2 **Carrier of** diphtheria

⑤ **Z22.3** **Carrier of** other **specified bacterial diseases**

    Z22.31 **Carrier of bacterial disease due to** meningococci

  ⑤ **Z22.32** **Carrier of bacterial disease due to** staphylococci

    Z22.321 **Carrier or suspected carrier of** Methicillin susceptible **Staphylococcus aureus**

        MSSA colonization

    Z22.322 **Carrier or suspected carrier of** Methicillin resistant **Staphylococcus aureus**

        MRSA colonization

  ⑥ **Z22.33** **Carrier of bacterial disease due to** streptococci

    Z22.330 **Carrier of** Group B **streptococcus**

    Z22.338 **Carrier of other streptococcus**

    Z22.39 **Carrier of other specified bacterial diseases**

Z22.4 **Carrier of infections with a predominantly sexual mode of transmission**

⑤ **Z22.5** **Carrier of** viral hepatitis

    Z22.50 **Carrier of unspecified viral hepatitis**

    Z22.51 **Carrier of viral hepatitis** B

        Hepatitis B surface antigen [HBsAg] carrier

    Z22.52 **Carrier of viral hepatitis** C

    Z22.59 **Carrier of other viral hepatitis**

Z22.6 **Carrier of** human T-lymphotropic virus type-1 **[HTLV-1] infection**

Z22.8 **Carrier of other infectious diseases**

Z22.9 **Carrier of infectious disease, unspecified**

Z23 **Encounter for immunization**

    Code first any routine childhood examination

    NOTES procedure codes are required to identify the types of immunizations given

④ **Z28** **Immunization not carried out and underimmunization status**

    INCLUDES *vaccination not carried out*

---

    ④ 4th character required   ⑤ 5th character required   ⑥ 6th character required   ⑦ 7th character required   ⑩ Extension 'X' Alert

          EXCLUDES1 Not coded here   EXCLUDES2 Not included here   PDx Primary Diagnosis Only   Manifestation Code

[5] **Z28.0 Immunization not carried out because of contraindication**

Z28.01 Immunization not carried out because of acute illness of patient

Z28.02 Immunization not carried out because of chronic illness or condition of patient

Z28.03 Immunization not carried out because of immune compromised state of patient

Z28.04 Immunization not carried out because of patient allergy to vaccine or component

Z28.09 Immunization not carried out because of other contraindication

Z28.1 Immunization not carried out because of patient decision for reasons of belief or group pressure

Immunization not carried out because of religious belief

[5] **Z28.2 Immunization not carried out because of patient decision for other and unspecified reason**

Z28.20 Immunization not carried out because of patient decision for unspecified reason

Z28.21 Immunization not carried out because of patient refusal

Z28.29 Immunization not carried out because of patient decision for other reason

Z28.3 Underimmunization status

Delinquent immunization status

Lapsed immunization schedule status

[5] **Z28.8 Immunization not carried out for other reason**

Z28.81 Immunization not carried out due to patient having had the disease

Z28.82 Immunization not carried out because of caregiver refusal

Immunization not carried out because of guardian refusal

Immunization not carried out because of parent refusal

[EXCLUDES1] *immunization not carried out because of caregiver refusal because of religious belief (Z28.1)*

Z28.89 Immunization not carried out for other reason

Z28.9 Immunization not carried out for unspecified reason

Persons encountering health services in circumstances related to reproduction (Z30-Z39)

[4] **Z30 Encounter for contraceptive management**

[5] **Z30.0 Encounter for general counseling and advice on contraception**

[6] **Z30.01 Encounter for initial prescription of contraceptives**

[EXCLUDES1] *encounter for surveillance of contraceptives (Z30.4-)*

Z30.011 Encounter for initial prescription of contraceptive pills ♀

Z30.012 Encounter for prescription of emergency contraception

Encounter for postcoital contraception ♀

Z30.013 Encounter for initial prescription of injectable contraceptive ♀

Z30.014 Encounter for initial prescription of intrauterine contraceptive device

[EXCLUDES1] *encounter for insertion of intrauterine contraceptive device (Z30.430, Z30.432)* ♀

Z30.018 Encounter for initial prescription of other contraceptives ♀

Z30.019 Encounter for initial prescription of contraceptives, unspecified ♀

Z30.02 Counseling and instruction in natural family planning to avoid pregnancy

Z30.09 Encounter for other general counseling and advice on contraception

Encounter for family planning advice NOS

Z30.2 Encounter for sterilization

[5] **Z30.4 Encounter for surveillance of contraceptives**

Z30.40 Encounter for surveillance of contraceptives, unspecified

Z30.41 Encounter for surveillance of contraceptive pills

Encounter for repeat prescription for contraceptive pill ♀

Z30.42 Encounter for surveillance of injectable contraceptive ♀

[6] **Z30.43 Encounter for surveillance of intrauterine contraceptive device**

Z30.430 Encounter for insertion of intrauterine contraceptive device ♀

Z30.431 Encounter for routine checking of intrauterine contraceptive device ♀

Z30.432 Encounter for removal of intrauterine contraceptive device ♀

Z30.433 Encounter for removal and reinsertion of intrauterine contraceptive device

Encounter for replacement of intrauterine contraceptive device ♀

Z30.49 Encounter for surveillance of other contraceptives ♀

Z30.8 Encounter for other contraceptive management

Encounter for postvasectomy sperm count

Encounter for routine examination for contraceptive maintenance

[EXCLUDES1] *sperm count following sterilization reversal (Z31.42)*
sperm count for fertility testing (Z31.41)

Z30.9 Encounter for contraceptive management, unspecified

[4] **Z31 Encounter for procreative management**

[EXCLUDES1] *complications associated with artificial fertilization (N98.-)*
female infertility (N97.-)
male infertility (N46.-)

Z31.0 Encounter for reversal of previous sterilization

[5] **Z31.4 Encounter for procreative investigation and testing**

[EXCLUDES1] *postvasectomy sperm count (Z30.8)*

Z31.41 Encounter for fertility testing

Encounter for fallopian tube patency testing

Encounter for sperm count for fertility testing

Z31.42 Aftercare following sterilization reversal

Sperm count following sterilization reversal

[6] **Z31.43 Encounter for genetic testing of female for procreative management**

Use additional code for recurrent pregnancy loss, if applicable (N96, O26.2-)

[EXCLUDES1] *nonprocreative genetic testing (Z13.7-)*

Z31.430 Encounter of female for testing for genetic disease carrier status for procreative management ♀

Z31.438 Encounter for other genetic testing of female for procreative management ♀

[6] **Z31.44 Encounter for genetic testing of male for procreative management**

[EXCLUDES1] *nonprocreative genetic testing (Z13.7-)*

Z31.440 Encounter of male for testing for genetic disease carrier status for procreative management ♂

Z31.441 Encounter for testing of male partner of patient with recurrent pregnancy loss [A] ♂

Unspecified Code | Other Specified Code | [N] Newborn Age: 0 | [P] Pediatric Age: 0-17 | [M] Maternity Age: 12-55
[A] Adult Age: 15-124 | ♂ Male | ♀ Female | ● New Code | ▲ Revised Code Title | ►◄ Revised Text

Z31.448 Encounter for other genetic testing of male for procreative management [A] ♂

Z31.49 Encounter for other procreative investigation and testing

Z31.5 Encounter for genetic counseling

[5] Z31.6 Encounter for general counseling and advice on procreation

Z31.61 Procreative counseling and advice using natural family planning

Z31.62 Encounter for fertility preservation counseling
Encounter for fertility preservation counseling prior to cancer therapy
Encounter for fertility preservation counseling prior to surgical removal of gonads

Z31.69 Encounter for other general counseling and advice on procreation

[5] Z31.8 Encounter for other procreative management

Z31.81 Encounter for male factor infertility in female patient ♀ [PDx]

Z31.82 Encounter for Rh incompatibility status ♀ [PDx]

Z31.83 Encounter for assisted reproductive fertility procedure cycle
Patient undergoing in vitro fertilization cycle
Use additional code to identify the type of infertility
[EXCLUDES1] *pre-cycle diagnosis and testing - code to reason for encounter* ♀ [PDx]

Z31.84 Encounter for fertility preservation procedure
Encounter for fertility preservation procedure prior to cancer therapy
Encounter for fertility preservation procedure prior to surgical removal of gonads [PDx]

Z31.89 Encounter for other procreative management

Z31.9 Encounter for procreative management, unspecified

[4] Z32 Encounter for pregnancy test and childbirth and childcare instruction

[5] Z32.0 Encounter for pregnancy test

Z32.00 Encounter for pregnancy test, result unknown
Encounter for pregnancy test NOS ♀

Z32.01 Encounter for pregnancy test, result positive [M] ♀

Z32.02 Encounter for pregnancy test, result negative ♀

Z32.2 Encounter for childbirth instruction

Z32.3 Encounter for childcare instruction
Encounter for prenatal or postpartum childcare instruction

[4] Z33 Pregnant state

Z33.1 Pregnant state, incidental
Pregnant state NOS
[EXCLUDES1] *complications of pregnancy (O00-O9A)* [M] ♀

Z33.2 Encounter for elective termination of pregnancy
[EXCLUDES1] *early fetal death with retention of dead fetus (O02.1)*
late fetal death (O36.4)
spontaneous abortion (O03) [M] ♀ [PDx]

[4] Z34 Encounter for supervision of normal pregnancy
[EXCLUDES1] *any complication of pregnancy (O00-O9A)*
encounter for pregnancy test (Z32.0-)
encounter for supervision of high risk pregnancy (O09.-) [PDx]

[5] Z34.0 Encounter for supervision of normal first pregnancy

Z34.00 Encounter for supervision of normal first pregnancy, unspecified trimester [M] ♀ [PDx]

Z34.01 Encounter for supervision of normal first pregnancy, first trimester [M] ♀ [PDx]

Z34.02 Encounter for supervision of normal first pregnancy, second trimester [M] ♀ [PDx]

Z34.03 Encounter for supervision of normal first pregnancy, third trimester [M] ♀ [PDx]

[5] Z34.8 Encounter for supervision of other normal pregnancy

Z34.80 Encounter for supervision of other normal pregnancy, unspecified trimester [M] ♀ [PDx]

Z34.81 Encounter for supervision of other normal pregnancy, first trimester [M] ♀ [PDx]

Z34.82 Encounter for supervision of other normal pregnancy, second trimester [M] ♀ [PDx]

Z34.83 Encounter for supervision of other normal pregnancy, third trimester [M] ♀ [PDx]

[5] Z34.9 Encounter for supervision of normal pregnancy, unspecified

Z34.90 Encounter for supervision of normal pregnancy, unspecified, unspecified trimester [M] ♀ [PDx]

Z34.91 Encounter for supervision of normal pregnancy, unspecified, first trimester [M] ♀ [PDx]

Z34.92 Encounter for supervision of normal pregnancy, unspecified, second trimester [M] ♀ [PDx]

Z34.93 Encounter for supervision of normal pregnancy, unspecified, third trimester [M] ♀ [PDx]

Z36 Encounter for antenatal screening of mother
[EXCLUDES1] *abnormal findings on antenatal screening of mother (O28.-)*
diagnostic examination- code to sign or symptom
encounter for suspected maternal and fetal conditions ruled out (Z03.7-)
suspected fetal condition affecting management of pregnancy - code to condition in Chapter 15
[EXCLUDES2] *genetic counseling and testing (Z31.43-, Z31.5)*
routine prenatal care (Z34) ♀

[4] Z3A Weeks of gestation
[NOTES] Codes from category Z3A are for use, only on the maternal record, to indicate the weeks of gestation of the pregnancy.
Code first complications of pregnancy, childbirth and the puerperium (O00-O9A)

[5] Z3A.0 Weeks of gestation of pregnancy, unspecified or less than 10 weeks

Z3A.00 Weeks of gestation of pregnancy not specified [M] ♀

Z3A.01 Less than 8 weeks gestation of pregnancy [M] ♀

Z3A.08 8 weeks gestation of pregnancy [M] ♀

Z3A.09 9 weeks gestation of pregnancy [M] ♀

[5] Z3A.1 Weeks of gestation of pregnancy, weeks 10-19

Z3A.10 10 weeks gestation of pregnancy [M] ♀

Z3A.11 11 weeks gestation of pregnancy [M] ♀

Z3A.12 12 weeks gestation of pregnancy [M] ♀

Z3A.13 13 weeks gestation of pregnancy [M] ♀

Z3A.14 14 weeks gestation of pregnancy [M] ♀

Z3A.15 15 weeks gestation of pregnancy [M] ♀

Z3A.16 16 weeks gestation of pregnancy [M] ♀

Z3A.17 17 weeks gestation of pregnancy [M] ♀

Z3A.18 18 weeks gestation of pregnancy [M] ♀

Z3A.19 19 weeks gestation of pregnancy [M] ♀

[5] Z3A.2 Weeks of gestation of pregnancy, weeks 20-29

Z3A.20 20 weeks gestation of pregnancy [M] ♀

Z3A.21 21 weeks gestation of pregnancy [M] ♀

Z3A.22 22 weeks gestation of pregnancy [M] ♀

Z3A.23 23 weeks gestation of pregnancy [M] ♀

Z3A.24 24 weeks gestation of pregnancy [M] ♀

Z3A.25 25 weeks gestation of pregnancy [M] ♀

Z3A.26 26 weeks gestation of pregnancy [M] ♀

Z3A.27 27 weeks gestation of pregnancy [M] ♀

Z3A.28 28 weeks gestation of pregnancy [M] ♀

[4] 4th character required [5] 5th character required [6] 6th character required [7] 7th character required [X] Extension 'X' Alert
[EXCLUDES1] Not coded here [EXCLUDES2] Not included here [PDx] Primary Diagnosis Only Manifestation Code

Z3A.29 29 weeks **gestation of pregnancy** M ♀
⑤ **Z3A.3 Weeks of gestation of pregnancy, weeks** 30-39
Z3A.30 30 weeks **gestation of pregnancy** M ♀
Z3A.31 31 weeks **gestation of pregnancy** M ♀
Z3A.32 32 weeks **gestation of pregnancy** M ♀
Z3A.33 33 weeks **gestation of pregnancy** M ♀
Z3A.34 34 weeks **gestation of pregnancy** M ♀
Z3A.35 35 weeks **gestation of pregnancy** M ♀
Z3A.36 36 weeks **gestation of pregnancy** M ♀
Z3A.37 37 weeks **gestation of pregnancy** M ♀
Z3A.38 38 weeks **gestation of pregnancy** M ♀
Z3A.39 39 weeks **gestation of pregnancy** M ♀
⑤ **Z3A.4 Weeks of gestation of pregnancy, weeks** 40 or greater
Z3A.40 40 weeks **gestation of pregnancy** M ♀
Z3A.41 41 weeks **gestation of pregnancy** M ♀
Z3A.42 42 weeks **gestation of pregnancy** M ♀
Z3A.49 Greater than 42 weeks **gestation of pregnancy** M ♀
④ **Z37 Outcome of delivery**

This category is intended for use as an additional code to identify the outcome of delivery on the mother's record. It is not for use on the newborn record.

EXCLUDES1 stillbirth (P95)

Z37.0 Single live birth M ♀
Z37.1 Single stillbirth M ♀
Z37.2 Twins, both liveborn M ♀
Z37.3 Twins, one liveborn and one stillborn M ♀
Z37.4 Twins, both stillborn M ♀
⑤ **Z37.5 Other multiple births, all liveborn**
Z37.50 Multiple births, unspecified, all liveborn M ♀
Z37.51 Triplets, all liveborn M ♀
Z37.52 Quadruplets, all liveborn M ♀
Z37.53 Quintuplets, all liveborn M ♀
Z37.54 Sextuplets, all liveborn M ♀
Z37.59 Other multiple births, all liveborn M ♀
⑤ **Z37.6 Other multiple births, some liveborn**
Z37.60 Multiple births, unspecified, some liveborn M ♀
Z37.61 Triplets, some liveborn M ♀
Z37.62 Quadruplets, some liveborn M ♀
Z37.63 Quintuplets, some liveborn M ♀
Z37.64 Sextuplets, some liveborn M ♀
Z37.69 Other multiple births, some liveborn M ♀
Z37.7 Other multiple births, all stillborn M ♀
Z37.9 Outcome of delivery, unspecified
Multiple birth NOS
Single birth NOS M ♀
④ **Z38 Liveborn infants according to place of birth and type of delivery**

This category is for use as the principal code on the initial record of a newborn baby. It is to be used for the initial birth record only. It is not to be used on the mother's record. Pdx

⑤ **Z38.0 Single liveborn infant,** born in hospital
Single liveborn infant, born in birthing center or other health care facility
Z38.00 Single liveborn infant, delivered vaginally N Pdx
Z38.01 Single liveborn infant, delivered by cesarean N Pdx
Z38.1 Single liveborn infant, born outside hospital N Pdx
Z38.2 Single liveborn infant, unspecified as to place of birth
Single liveborn infant NOS N Pdx
⑤ **Z38.3 Twin liveborn infant,** born in hospital
Z38.30 Twin liveborn infant, delivered vaginally N Pdx
Z38.31 Twin liveborn infant, delivered by cesarean N Pdx
Z38.4 Twin liveborn infant, born outside hospital N Pdx

Z38.5 Twin liveborn infant, unspecified as to place of birth N Pdx
⑤ **Z38.6 Other multiple liveborn infant,** born in hospital
Z38.61 Triplet liveborn infant, delivered vaginally N Pdx
Z38.62 Triplet liveborn infant, delivered by cesarean N Pdx
Z38.63 Quadruplet liveborn infant, delivered vaginally N Pdx
Z38.64 Quadruplet liveborn infant, delivered by cesarean N Pdx
Z38.65 Quintuplet liveborn infant, delivered vaginally N Pdx
Z38.66 Quintuplet liveborn infant, delivered by cesarean N Pdx
Z38.68 Other multiple liveborn infant, delivered vaginally N Pdx
Z38.69 Other multiple liveborn infant, delivered by cesarean N Pdx
Z38.7 Other multiple liveborn infant, born outside hospital N Pdx
Z38.8 Other multiple liveborn infant, unspecified as to place of birth N Pdx
④ **Z39 Encounter for maternal postpartum care and examination** Pdx
Z39.0 Encounter for care and examination of mother immediately after delivery
Care and observation in uncomplicated cases when the delivery occurs outside a healthcare facility
EXCLUDES1 care for postpartum complication- see Alphabetic index M ♀ Pdx
Z39.1 Encounter for care and examination of lactating mother
Encounter for supervision of lactation
EXCLUDES1 disorders of lactation (O92.-) M ♀ Pdx
Z39.2 Encounter for routine postpartum **follow-up** M ♀ Pdx

Encounters for other specific health care (Z40-Z53)

NOTES Categories Z40-Z53 are intended for use to indicate a reason for care. They may be used for patients who have already been treated for a disease or injury, but who are receiving aftercare or prophylactic care, or care to consolidate the treatment, or to deal with a residual state
EXCLUDES2 follow-up examination for medical surveillance after treatment (Z08-Z09)

④ **Z40 Encounter for prophylactic surgery**
EXCLUDES1 organ donations (Z52.-)
therapeutic organ removal-code to condition
⑤ **Z40.0 Encounter for prophylactic surgery for** risk factors related to malignant neoplasms
Admission for prophylactic organ removal
Use additional code to identify risk factor
Z40.00 Encounter for prophylactic removal of unspecified organ
Z40.01 Encounter for prophylactic removal of breast
Z40.02 Encounter for prophylactic removal of ovary ♀
Z40.09 Encounter for prophylactic removal of other organ
Z40.8 Encounter for other prophylactic **surgery**
Z40.9 Encounter for prophylactic surgery, unspecified
④ **Z41 Encounter for procedures for purposes other than remedying health state**
Z41.1 Encounter for cosmetic surgery
Encounter for cosmetic breast implant
Encounter for cosmetic procedure
EXCLUDES1 encounter for plastic and reconstructive surgery following medical procedure or healed injury (Z42.-)
encounter for post-mastectomy breast implantation (Z42.1)
Z41.2 Encounter for routine and ritual male circumcision ♂

Unspecified Code	Other Specified Code	N Newborn Age: 0	P Pediatric Age: 0-17	M Maternity Age: 12-55
A Adult Age: 15-124	♂ Male	♀ Female	● New Code	▲ Revised Code Title	►◄ Revised Text

Z41.3 Encounter for ear piercing

Z41.8 Encounter for other procedures for purposes other than remedying health state

Z41.9 Encounter for procedure for purposes other than remedying health state, unspecified

④ **Z42** Encounter for plastic and reconstructive surgery following medical procedure or healed injury

    EXCLUDES1   *encounter for cosmetic plastic surgery (Z41.1)*
                  encounter for plastic surgery for treatment of current injury - code to relevent injury   PDx

Z42.1 Encounter for breast reconstruction following mastectomy

    EXCLUDES1   *deformity and disproportion of reconstructed breast (N65.1-)*   A   PDx

Z42.8 Encounter for other plastic and reconstructive surgery following medical procedure or healed injury

④ **Z43** Encounter for attention to artificial openings

    INCLUDES   *closure of artificial openings*
                passage of sounds or bougies through artificial openings
                reforming artificial openings
                removal of catheter from artificial openings
                toilet or cleansing of artificial openings

    EXCLUDES1   *artificial opening status only, without need for care (Z93.-)*
                  complications of external stoma (J95.0-, K94.-, N99.5-)

    EXCLUDES2   *fitting and adjustment of prosthetic and other devices (Z44-Z46)*

Z43.0 Encounter for attention to tracheostomy

Z43.1 Encounter for attention to gastrostomy

Z43.2 Encounter for attention to ileostomy

Z43.3 Encounter for attention to colostomy

Z43.4 Encounter for attention to other artificial openings of digestive tract

Z43.5 Encounter for attention to cystostomy

Z43.6 Encounter for attention to other artificial openings of urinary tract

    Encounter for attention to nephrostomy
    Encounter for attention to ureterostomy
    Encounter for attention to urethrostomy

Z43.7 Encounter for attention to artificial vagina

Z43.8 Encounter for attention to other artificial openings

Z43.9 Encounter for attention to unspecified artificial opening

④ **Z44** Encounter for fitting and adjustment of external prosthetic device

    INCLUDES   *removal or replacement of external prosthetic device*

    EXCLUDES1   *malfunction or other complications of device - see Alphabetical Index*
                  presence of prosthetic device (Z97.-)

⑤ **Z44.0** Encounter for fitting and adjustment of artificial arm

   ⑥ **Z44.00** Encounter for fitting and adjustment of unspecified artificial arm

      Z44.001 Encounter for fitting and adjustment of unspecified right artificial arm

      Z44.002 Encounter for fitting and adjustment of unspecified left artificial arm

      Z44.009 Encounter for fitting and adjustment of unspecified artificial arm, unspecified arm

   ⑥ **Z44.01** Encounter for fitting and adjustment of complete artificial arm

      Z44.011 Encounter for fitting and adjustment of complete right artificial arm

      Z44.012 Encounter for fitting and adjustment of complete left artificial arm

      Z44.019 Encounter for fitting and adjustment of complete artificial arm, unspecified arm

   ⑥ **Z44.02** Encounter for fitting and adjustment of partial artificial arm

      Z44.021 Encounter for fitting and adjustment of partial artificial right arm

      Z44.022 Encounter for fitting and adjustment of partial artificial left arm

      Z44.029 Encounter for fitting and adjustment of partial artificial arm, unspecified arm

⑤ **Z44.1** Encounter for fitting and adjustment of artificial leg

   ⑥ **Z44.10** Encounter for fitting and adjustment of unspecified artificial leg

      Z44.101 Encounter for fitting and adjustment of unspecified right artificial leg

      Z44.102 Encounter for fitting and adjustment of unspecified left artificial leg

      Z44.109 Encounter for fitting and adjustment of unspecified artificial leg, unspecified leg

   ⑥ **Z44.11** Encounter for fitting and adjustment of complete artificial leg

      Z44.111 Encounter for fitting and adjustment of complete right artificial leg

      Z44.112 Encounter for fitting and adjustment of complete left artificial leg

      Z44.119 Encounter for fitting and adjustment of complete artificial leg, unspecified leg

   ⑥ **Z44.12** Encounter for fitting and adjustment of partial artificial leg

      Z44.121 Encounter for fitting and adjustment of partial artificial right leg

      Z44.122 Encounter for fitting and adjustment of partial artificial left leg

      Z44.129 Encounter for fitting and adjustment of partial artificial leg, unspecified leg

⑤ **Z44.2** Encounter for fitting and adjustment of artificial eye

    EXCLUDES1   *mechanical complication of ocular prosthesis (T85.3)*

   Z44.20 Encounter for fitting and adjustment of artificial eye, unspecified

   Z44.21 Encounter for fitting and adjustment of artificial right eye

   Z44.22 Encounter for fitting and adjustment of artificial left eye

⑤ **Z44.3** Encounter for fitting and adjustment of external breast prosthesis

    EXCLUDES1   *complications of breast implant (T85.4-)*
                  encounter for adjustment or removal of breast implant (Z45.81-)
                  encounter for initial breast implant insertion for cosmetic breast augmentation (Z41.1)
                  encounter for breast reconstruction following mastectomy (Z42.1)

   Z44.30 Encounter for fitting and adjustment of external breast prosthesis, unspecified breast   ♀

   Z44.31 Encounter for fitting and adjustment of external right breast prosthesis   ♀

   Z44.32 Encounter for fitting and adjustment of external left breast prosthesis   ♀

Z44.8 Encounter for fitting and adjustment of other external prosthetic devices

Z44.9 Encounter for fitting and adjustment of unspecified external prosthetic device

④ **Z45** Encounter for adjustment and management of implanted device

    INCLUDES   *removal or replacement of implanted device*

    EXCLUDES1   *malfunction or other complications of device - see Alphabetical Index*
                  presence of prosthetic and other devices (Z95-Z97)

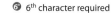

④ 4ᵗʰ character required   ⑤ 5ᵗʰ character required   ⑥ 6ᵗʰ character required   ⑦ 7ᵗʰ character required   ⑦ˣ Extension 'X' Alert

EXCLUDES 1 Not coded here   *EXCLUDES 2* Not included here   PDx Primary Diagnosis Only   Manifestation Code

EXCLUDES2 encounter for fitting and adjustment of non-implanted device (Z46.-)

Z45.0 Encounter for adjustment and management of cardiac device

Z45.01 Encounter for adjustment and management of cardiac pacemaker

EXCLUDES1 encounter for adjustment and management of automatic implantable cardiac defibrillator with synchronous cardiac pacemaker (Z45.02)

Z45.010 Encounter for checking and testing of cardiac pacemaker pulse generator [battery]

Encounter for replacing cardiac pacemaker pulse generator [battery]

Z45.018 Encounter for adjustment and management of other part of cardiac pacemaker

Z45.02 Encounter for adjustment and management of automatic implantable cardiac defibrillator

Encounter for adjustment and management of automatic implantable cardiac defibrillator with synchronous cardiac pacemaker

Z45.09 Encounter for adjustment and management of other cardiac device

Z45.1 Encounter for adjustment and management of infusion pump

Z45.2 Encounter for adjustment and management of vascular access device

Encounter for adjustment and management of vascular catheters

EXCLUDES1 encounter for adjustment and management of renal dialysis catheter (Z49.01)

Z45.3 Encounter for adjustment and management of implanted devices of the special senses

Z45.31 Encounter for adjustment and management of implanted visual substitution device

Z45.32 Encounter for adjustment and management of implanted hearing device

EXCLUDES1 Encounter for fitting and adjustment of hearing aide (Z46.1)

Z45.320 Encounter for adjustment and management of bone conduction device

Z45.321 Encounter for adjustment and management of cochlear device

Z45.328 Encounter for adjustment and management of other implanted hearing device

Z45.4 Encounter for adjustment and management of implanted nervous system device

Z45.41 Encounter for adjustment and management of cerebrospinal fluid drainage device

Encounter for adjustment and management of cerebral ventricular (communicating) shunt

Z45.42 Encounter for adjustment and management of neuropacemaker (brain) (peripheral nerve) (spinal cord)

Z45.49 Encounter for adjustment and management of other implanted nervous system device

Z45.8 Encounter for adjustment and management of other implanted devices

Z45.81 Encounter for adjustment or removal of breast implant

Encounter for elective implant exchange (different material) (different size)

Encounter removal of tissue expander without synchronous insertion of permanent implant

EXCLUDES1 complications of breast implant (T85.4-)
encounter for initial breast implant insertion for cosmetic breast augmentation (Z41.1)
encounter for breast reconstruction following mastectomy (Z42.1)

Z45.811 Encounter for adjustment or removal of right breast implant ♀

Z45.812 Encounter for adjustment or removal of left breast implant ♀

Z45.819 Encounter for adjustment or removal of unspecified breast implant ♀

Z45.82 Encounter for adjustment or removal of myringotomy device (stent) (tube)

Z45.89 Encounter for adjustment and management of other implanted devices

Z45.9 Encounter for adjustment and management of unspecified implanted device

Z46 Encounter for fitting and adjustment of other devices

INCLUDES removal or replacement of other device

EXCLUDES1 malfunction or other complications of device - see Alphabetical Index

EXCLUDES2 encounter for fitting and management of implanted devices (Z45.-)
issue of repeat prescription only (Z76.0)
presence of prosthetic and other devices (Z95-Z97)

Z46.0 Encounter for fitting and adjustment of spectacles and contact lenses

Z46.1 Encounter for fitting and adjustment of hearing aid

EXCLUDES1 encounter for adjustment and management of implanted hearing device (Z45.32-)

Z46.2 Encounter for fitting and adjustment of other devices related to nervous system and special senses

EXCLUDES2 encounter for adjustment and management of implanted nervous system device (Z45.4-)
encounter for adjustment and management of implanted visual substitution device (Z45.31)

Z46.3 Encounter for fitting and adjustment of dental prosthetic device

Encounter for fitting and adjustment of dentures

Z46.4 Encounter for fitting and adjustment of orthodontic device

Z46.5 Encounter for fitting and adjustment of other gastrointestinal appliance and device

EXCLUDES1 encounter for attention to artificial openings of digestive tract (Z43.1-Z43.4)

Z46.51 Encounter for fitting and adjustment of gastric lap band

Z46.59 Encounter for fitting and adjustment of other gastrointestinal appliance and device

Z46.6 Encounter for fitting and adjustment of urinary device

EXCLUDES2 attention to artificial openings of urinary tract (Z43.5, Z43.6)

Z46.8 Encounter for fitting and adjustment of other specified devices

Z46.81 Encounter for fitting and adjustment of insulin pump

Encounter for insulin pump titration

Encounter for insulin pump instruction and training

Z46.82 Encounter for fitting and adjustment of non-vascular catheter

Z46.89 Encounter for fitting and adjustment of other specified devices

Encounter for fitting and adjustment of wheelchair

Z46.9 Encounter for fitting and adjustment of unspecified device

Z47 Orthopedic aftercare

EXCLUDES1 aftercare for healing fracture-code to fracture with 7th character D

Z47.1 Aftercare following joint replacement surgery

Use additional code to identify the joint (Z96.6-)

Unspecified Code   Other Specified Code   N Newborn Age: 0   P Pediatric Age: 0-17   M Maternity Age: 12-55
A Adult Age: 15-124   ♂ Male   ♀ Female   ● New Code   ▲ Revised Code Title   ►◄ Revised Text

ICD-10-CM 2015

831

Z47.2 Encounter for removal of internal fixation device

[EXCLUDES1] *encounter for adjustment of internal fixation device for fracture treatment- code to fracture with appropriate 7th character*
encounter for removal of external fixation device- code to fracture with 7th character D
infection or inflammatory reaction to internal fixation device (T84.6-)
mechanical complication of internal fixation device (T84.1-)

[5] **Z47.3 Aftercare following explantation of joint prosthesis**
Aftercare following explantation of joint prosthesis, staged procedure
Encounter for joint prosthesis insertion following prior explantation of joint prosthesis

Z47.31 Aftercare following explantation of shoulder joint prosthesis

[EXCLUDES1] *acquired absence of shoulder joint following prior explantation of shoulder joint prosthesis (Z89.23-)*
shoulder joint prosthesis explantation status (Z89.23-)

Z47.32 Aftercare following explantation of hip joint prosthesis

[EXCLUDES1] *acquired absence of hip joint following prior explantation of hip joint prosthesis (Z89.62-)*
hip joint prosthesis explantation status (Z89.62-)

Z47.33 Aftercare following explantation of knee joint prosthesis

[EXCLUDES1] *acquired absence of knee joint following prior explantation of knee prosthesis (Z89.52-*
knee joint prosthesis explantation status (Z89.52-)

[5] **Z47.8 Encounter for other orthopedic aftercare**

Z47.81 Encounter for orthopedic aftercare following surgical amputation
Use additional code to identify the limb amputated (Z89.-)

Z47.82 Encounter for orthopedic aftercare following scoliosis surgery

Z47.89 Encounter for other orthopedic aftercare

[4] **Z48 Encounter for other postprocedural aftercare**

[EXCLUDES1] *encounter for follow-up examination after completed treatment (Z08-Z09)*

[EXCLUDES2] *encounter for attention to artificial openings (Z43.-)*
encounter for fitting and adjustment of prosthetic and other devices (Z44-Z46)

[5] **Z48.0 Encounter for attention to dressings, sutures and drains**

[EXCLUDES1] *encounter for planned postprocedural wound closure (Z48.1)*

Z48.00 Encounter for change or removal of nonsurgical wound dressing
Encounter for change or removal of wound dressing NOS

Z48.01 Encounter for change or removal of surgical wound dressing

Z48.02 Encounter for removal of sutures
Encounter for removal of staples

Z48.03 Encounter for change or removal of drains

Z48.1 Encounter for planned postprocedural wound closure

[EXCLUDES1] *encounter for attention to dressings and sutures (Z48.0-)*

[5] **Z48.2 Encounter for aftercare following organ transplant**

Z48.21 Encounter for aftercare following heart transplant

Z48.22 Encounter for aftercare following kidney transplant

Z48.23 Encounter for aftercare following liver transplant

Z48.24 Encounter for aftercare following lung transplant

[6] **Z48.28 Encounter for aftercare following multiple organ transplant**

Z48.280 Encounter for aftercare following heart-lung transplant

Z48.288 Encounter for aftercare following multiple organ transplant

[6] **Z48.29 Encounter for aftercare following other organ transplant**

Z48.290 Encounter for aftercare following bone marrow transplant

Z48.298 Encounter for aftercare following other organ transplant

Z48.3 Aftercare following surgery for neoplasm
Use additional code to identify the neoplasm

[5] **Z48.8 Encounter for other specified postprocedural aftercare**

[6] **Z48.81 Encounter for surgical aftercare following surgery on specified body systems**
These codes identify the body system requiring aftercare. They are for use in conjunction with other aftercare codes to fully explain the aftercare encounter. The condition treated should also be coded if still present.

[EXCLUDES1] *aftercare for injury- code the injury with 7th character D*
aftercare following surgery for neoplasm (Z48.3)

[EXCLUDES2] *aftercare following organ transplant (Z48.2-)*
orthopedic aftercare (Z47.-)

Z48.810 Encounter for surgical aftercare following surgery on the sense organs

Z48.811 Encounter for surgical aftercare following surgery on the nervous system

[EXCLUDES2] *encounter for surgical aftercare following surgery on the sense organs (Z48.810)*

Z48.812 Encounter for surgical aftercare following surgery on the circulatory system

Z48.813 Encounter for surgical aftercare following surgery on the respiratory system

Z48.814 Encounter for surgical aftercare following surgery on the teeth or oral cavity

Z48.815 Encounter for surgical aftercare following surgery on the digestive system

Z48.816 Encounter for surgical aftercare following surgery on the genitourinary system

[EXCLUDES1] *encounter for aftercare following sterilization reversal (Z31.42)*

Z48.817 Encounter for surgical aftercare following surgery on the skin and subcutaneous tissue

Z48.89 Encounter for other specified surgical aftercare

[4] **Z49 Encounter for care involving renal dialysis**
Code also associated end stage renal disease (N18.6)

[5] **Z49.0 Preparatory care for renal dialysis**
Encounter for dialysis instruction and training

Z49.01 Encounter for fitting and adjustment of extracorporeal dialysis catheter
Removal or replacement of renal dialysis catheter
Toilet or cleansing of renal dialysis catheter

Z49.02 Encounter for fitting and adjustment of peritoneal dialysis catheter

[5] **Z49.3 Encounter for adequacy testing for dialysis**

Z49.31 Encounter for adequacy testing for hemodialysis

Z49.32 Encounter for adequacy testing for peritoneal dialysis
Encounter for peritoneal equilibration test

[4] 4th character required [5] 5th character required [6] 6th character required [7] 7th character required [7th] Extension 'X' Alert
[EXCLUDES1] Not coded here [EXCLUDES2] Not included here [PDx] Primary Diagnosis Only Manifestation Code

[4] **Z51 Encounter for other aftercare**
Code also condition requiring care
[EXCLUDES1] *follow-up examination after treatment (Z08-Z09)*
Z51.0 Encounter for antineoplastic radiation therapy [PDx]
[5] **Z51.1 Encounter for antineoplastic chemotherapy and immunotherapy**
[EXCLUDES2] *encounter for chemotherapy and immunotherapy for nonneoplastic condition - code to condition* [PDx]
Z51.11 Encounter for antineoplastic chemotherapy
Z51.12 Encounter for antineoplastic immunotherapy
Z51.5 Encounter for palliative care
[5] **Z51.8 Encounter for other specified aftercare**
[EXCLUDES1] *holiday relief care (Z75.5)*
Z51.81 Encounter for therapeutic drug level monitoring
Code also any long-term (current) drug therapy (Z79.-)
[EXCLUDES1] *encounter for blood-drug test for administrative or medicolegal reasons (Z02.83)*
Z51.89 Encounter for other specified aftercare

[4] **Z52 Donors of organs and tissues**
[INCLUDES] *autologous and other living donors*
[EXCLUDES1] *cadaveric donor - omit code*
examination of potential donor (Z00.5) [PDx]
[5] **Z52.0 Blood donor** [PDx]
[6] **Z52.00 Unspecified blood donor** [PDx]
Z52.000 Unspecified donor, whole blood [PDx]
Z52.001 Unspecified donor, stem cells [PDx]
Z52.008 Unspecified donor, other blood [PDx]
[6] **Z52.01 Autologous blood donor** [PDx]
Z52.010 Autologous donor, whole blood [PDx]
Z52.011 Autologous donor, stem cells [PDx]
Z52.018 Autologous donor, other blood [PDx]
[6] **Z52.09 Other blood donor**
Volunteer donor [PDx]
Z52.090 Other blood donor, whole blood [PDx]
Z52.091 Other blood donor, stem cells [PDx]
Z52.098 Other blood donor, other blood [PDx]
[5] **Z52.1 Skin donor** [PDx]
Z52.10 Skin donor, unspecified [PDx]
Z52.11 Skin donor, autologous [PDx]
Z52.19 Skin donor, other [PDx]
[5] **Z52.2 Bone donor** [PDx]
Z52.20 Bone donor, unspecified [PDx]
Z52.21 Bone donor, autologous [PDx]
Z52.29 Bone donor, other [PDx]
Z52.3 Bone marrow donor [PDx]
Z52.4 Kidney donor [PDx]
Z52.5 Cornea donor [PDx]
Z52.6 Liver donor [PDx]
[5] **Z52.8 Donor of other specified organs or tissues** [PDx]
[6] **Z52.81 Egg (Oocyte) donor** [PDx]
Z52.810 Egg (Oocyte) donor under age 35, anonymous recipient
Egg donor under age 35 NOS ♀ [PDx]
Z52.811 Egg (Oocyte) donor under age 35, designated recipient ♀ [PDx]
Z52.812 Egg (Oocyte) donor age 35 and over, anonymous recipient
Egg donor age 35 and over NOS ♀ [PDx]
Z52.813 Egg (Oocyte) donor age 35 and over, designated recipient ♀ [PDx]
Z52.819 Egg (Oocyte) donor, unspecified ♀ [PDx]
Z52.89 Donor of other specified organs or tissues [PDx]
Z52.9 Donor of unspecified organ or tissue
Donor NOS

[4] **Z53 Persons encountering health services for specific procedures and treatment, not carried out**
[5] **Z53.0 Procedure and treatment not carried out because of contraindication**
Z53.01 Procedure and treatment not carried out due to patient smoking
Z53.09 Procedure and treatment not carried out because of other contraindication
Z53.1 Procedure and treatment not carried out because of patient's decision for reasons of belief and group pressure
[5] **Z53.2 Procedure and treatment not carried out because of patient's decision for other and unspecified reasons**
Z53.20 Procedure and treatment not carried out because of patient's decision for unspecified reasons
Z53.21 Procedure and treatment not carried out due to patient leaving prior to being seen by health care provider
Z53.29 Procedure and treatment not carried out because of patient's decision for other reasons
Z53.8 Procedure and treatment not carried out for other reasons
Z53.9 Procedure and treatment not carried out, unspecified reason

Persons with potential health hazards related to socioeconomic and psychosocial circumstances (Z55-Z65)

[4] **Z55 Problems related to education and literacy**
[EXCLUDES1] *disorders of psychological development (F80-F89)*
Z55.0 Illiteracy and low-level literacy
Z55.1 Schooling unavailable and unattainable
Z55.2 Failed school examinations
Z55.3 Underachievement in school
Z55.4 Educational maladjustment and discord with teachers and classmates
Z55.8 Other problems related to education and literacy
Problems related to inadequate teaching
Z55.9 Problems related to education and literacy, unspecified
Academic problems NOS

[4] **Z56 Problems related to employment and unemployment**
[EXCLUDES2] *occupational exposure to risk factors (Z57.-)*
problems related to housing and economic circumstances (Z59.-)
Z56.0 Unemployment, unspecified
Z56.1 Change of job [A]
Z56.2 Threat of job loss
Z56.3 Stressful work schedule
Z56.4 Discord with boss and workmates
Z56.5 Uncongenial work environment
Difficult conditions at work
Z56.6 Other physical and mental strain related to work
[5] **Z56.8 Other problems related to employment**
Z56.81 Sexual harassment on the job
Z56.82 Military deployment status
Individual (civilian or military) currently deployed in theater or in support of military war, peacekeeping and humanitarian operations
Z56.89 Other problems related to employment
Z56.9 Unspecified problems related to employment
Occupational problems NOS

[4] **Z57 Occupational exposure to risk factors**
Z57.0 Occupational exposure to noise
Z57.1 Occupational exposure to radiation
Z57.2 Occupational exposure to dust

Unspecified Code | Other Specified Code | [N] Newborn Age: 0 | [P] Pediatric Age: 0-17 | [M] Maternity Age: 12-55
[A] Adult Age: 15-124 | ♂ Male | ♀ Female | ● New Code | ▲ Revised Code Title | ►◄ Revised Text

[5] Z57.3 Occupational exposure to other air contaminants
Z57.31 Occupational exposure to environmental tobacco smoke
[EXCLUDES2] *exposure to environmental tobacco smoke (Z77.22)*
Z57.39 Occupational exposure to other air contaminants

Z57.4 Occupational exposure to toxic agents in agriculture
Occupational exposure to solids, liquids, gases or vapors in agriculture
Z57.5 Occupational exposure to toxic agents in other industries
Occupational exposure to solids, liquids, gases or vapors in other industries
Z57.6 Occupational exposure to extreme temperature
Z57.7 Occupational exposure to vibration
Z57.8 Occupational exposure to other risk factors
Z57.9 Occupational exposure to unspecified risk factor
[4] Z59 Problems related to housing and economic circumstances
[EXCLUDES2] *problems related to upbringing (Z62.-)*
Z59.0 Homelessness
Z59.1 Inadequate housing
Lack of heating
Restriction of space
Technical defects in home preventing adequate care
Unsatisfactory surroundings
[EXCLUDES1] *problems related to the natural and physical environment (Z77.1-)*
Z59.2 Discord with neighbors, lodgers and landlord
Z59.3 Problems related to living in residential institution
Boarding-school resident
[EXCLUDES1] *institutional upbringing (Z62.2)*
Z59.4 Lack of adequate food and safe drinking water
Inadequate drinking water supply
[EXCLUDES1] *effects of hunger (T73.0)*
inappropriate diet or eating habits (Z72.4)
malnutrition (E40-E46)
Z59.5 Extreme poverty
Z59.6 Low income
Z59.7 Insufficient social insurance and welfare support
Z59.8 Other problems related to housing and economic circumstances
Foreclosure on loan
Isolated dwelling
Problems with creditors
Z59.9 Problem related to housing and economic circumstances, unspecified
[4] Z60 Problems related to social environment
Z60.0 Problems of adjustment to life-cycle transitions
Empty nest syndrome
Phase of life problem
Problem with adjustment to retirement [pension]
Z60.2 Problems related to living alone
Z60.3 Acculturation difficulty
Problem with migration
Problem with social transplantation
Z60.4 Social exclusion and rejection
Exclusion and rejection on the basis of personal characteristics, such as unusual physical appearance, illness or behavior.
[EXCLUDES1] *target of adverse discrimination such as for racial or religious reasons (Z60.5)*
Z60.5 Target of (perceived) adverse discrimination and persecution
[EXCLUDES1] *social exclusion and rejection (Z60.4)*
Z60.8 Other problems related to social environment
Z60.9 Problem related to social environment, unspecified
[4] Z62 Problems related to upbringing
[INCLUDES] *current and past negative life events in childhood*
current and past problems of a child related to upbringing
[EXCLUDES2] *maltreatment syndrome (T74.-)*
problems related to housing and economic circumstances (Z59.-)
Z62.0 Inadequate parental supervision and control
Z62.1 Parental overprotection
[5] Z62.2 Upbringing away from parents
[EXCLUDES1] *problems with boarding school (Z59.3)*
Z62.21 Child in welfare custody
Child in care of non-parental family member
Child in foster care
[EXCLUDES2] *problem for parent due to child in welfare custody (Z63.5)* [P]
Z62.22 Institutional upbringing
Child living in orphanage or group home
Z62.29 Other upbringing away from parents
Z62.3 Hostility towards and scapegoating of child [P]
Z62.6 Inappropriate (excessive) parental pressure
[5] Z62.8 Other specified problems related to upbringing
[6] Z62.81 Personal history of abuse in childhood
Z62.810 Personal history of physical and sexual abuse in childhood
[EXCLUDES1] *current child physical abuse (T74.12, T76.12)*
current child sexual abuse (T74.22, T76.22)
Z62.811 Personal history of psychological abuse in childhood
[EXCLUDES1] *current child psychological abuse (T74.32, T76.32)*
Z62.812 Personal history of neglect in childhood
[EXCLUDES1] *current child neglect (T74.02, T76.02)*
Z62.819 Personal history of unspecified abuse in childhood
[EXCLUDES1] *current child abuse NOS (T74.92, T76.92)*
[6] Z62.82 Parent-child conflict
Z62.820 Parent-biological child conflict
Parent-child problem NOS
Z62.821 Parent-adopted child conflict
Z62.822 Parent-foster child conflict
[6] Z62.89 Other specified problems related to upbringing
Z62.890 Parent-child estrangement NEC
Z62.891 Sibling rivalry
Z62.898 Other specified problems related to upbringing
Z62.9 Problem related to upbringing, unspecified
[4] Z63 Other problems related to primary support group, including family circumstances
[EXCLUDES2] *maltreatment syndrome (T74.-, T76)*
parent-child problems (Z62.-)
problems related to negative life events in childhood (Z62.-)
problems related to upbringing (Z62.-)
Z63.0 Problems in relationship with spouse or partner
[EXCLUDES1] *counseling for spousal or partner abuse problems (Z69.1)*
counseling related to sexual attitude, behavior, and orientation (Z70.-)
Z63.1 Problems in relationship with in-laws

[5] Z63.3 Absence of family member
[EXCLUDES1] *absence of family member due to disappearance and death (Z63.4)*

[4] 4th character required [5] 5th character required [6] 6th character required [7] 7th character required [X] Extension 'X' Alert
[EXCLUDES1] Not coded here [EXCLUDES2] Not included here [PDx] Primary Diagnosis Only Manifestation Code

absence of family member due to separation and divorce (Z63.5)

Z63.31 **Absence of family member due to military deployment**

Individual or family affected by other family member being on military deployment

EXCLUDES1 *family disruption due to return of family member from military deployment (Z63.71)*

Z63.32 Other absence of family member

Z63.4 **Disappearance and death of family member**

Assumed death of family member
Bereavement

Z63.5 **Disruption of family by separation and divorce**

Marital estrangement

Z63.6 **Dependent relative needing care at home**

Z63.7 Other stressful life events affecting family and household

Z63.71 **Stress on family due to return of family member from military deployment**

Individual or family affected by family member having returned from military deployment (current or past conflict)

Z63.72 **Alcoholism and drug addiction in family**

Z63.79 Other stressful life events affecting family and household

Anxiety (normal) about sick person in family
Health problems within family
Ill or disturbed family member
Isolated family

Z63.8 Other specified problems related to primary support group

Family discord NOS
Family estrangement NOS
High expressed emotional level within family
Inadequate family support NOS
Inadequate or distorted communication within family

Z63.9 **Problem related to primary support group, unspecified**

Relationship disorder NOS

Z64 Problems related to certain psychosocial circumstances

Z64.0 **Problems related to unwanted pregnancy** Ⓜ ♀

Z64.1 **Problems related to multiparity** ♀

Z64.4 **Discord with counselors**

Discord with probation officer
Discord with social worker

Z65 Problems related to other psychosocial circumstances

Z65.0 **Conviction in civil and criminal proceedings without imprisonment**

Z65.1 **Imprisonment and other incarceration**

Z65.2 **Problems related to release from prison**

Z65.3 **Problems related to other legal circumstances**

Arrest
Child custody or support proceedings
Litigation
Prosecution

Z65.4 **Victim of crime and terrorism**

Victim of torture

Z65.5 **Exposure to disaster, war and other hostilities**

EXCLUDES1 *target of perceived discrimination or persecution (Z60.5)*

Z65.8 Other specified problems related to psychosocial circumstances

Z65.9 **Problem related to unspecified psychosocial circumstances**

Do not resuscitate status (Z66)

Z66 **Do not resuscitate**

DNR status

Blood type (Z67)

Z67 **Blood type**

Z67.1 Type A blood

Z67.10 **Type A blood,** Rh positive

Z67.11 **Type A blood,** Rh negative

Z67.2 Type B blood

Z67.20 **Type B blood,** Rh positive

Z67.21 **Type B blood,** Rh negative

Z67.3 Type AB blood

Z67.30 **Type AB blood,** Rh positive

Z67.31 **Type AB blood,** Rh negative

Z67.4 Type O blood

Z67.40 **Type O blood,** Rh positive

Z67.41 **Type O blood,** Rh negative

Z67.9 Unspecified blood type

Z67.90 **Unspecified blood type,** Rh positive

Z67.91 **Unspecified blood type,** Rh negative

Body mass index [BMI] (Z68)

Z68 **Body mass index [BMI]**

Kilograms per meters squared

NOTES BMI adult codes are for use for persons 21 years of age or older
BMI pediatric codes are for use for persons 2-20 years of age. These percentiles are based on the growth charts published by the Centers for Disease Control and Prevention (CDC)

Z68.1 **Body mass index (BMI)** 19 or less, **adult** Ⓐ

Z68.2 **Body mass index (BMI)** 20-29, adult

Z68.20 **Body mass index (BMI)** 20.0-20.9, **adult** Ⓐ
Z68.21 **Body mass index (BMI)** 21.0-21.9, **adult** Ⓐ
Z68.22 **Body mass index (BMI)** 22.0-22.9, **adult** Ⓐ
Z68.23 **Body mass index (BMI)** 23.0-23.9, **adult** Ⓐ
Z68.24 **Body mass index (BMI)** 24.0-24.9, **adult** Ⓐ
Z68.25 **Body mass index (BMI)** 25.0-25.9, **adult** Ⓐ
Z68.26 **Body mass index (BMI)** 26.0-26.9, **adult** Ⓐ
Z68.27 **Body mass index (BMI)** 27.0-27.9, **adult** Ⓐ
Z68.28 **Body mass index (BMI)** 28.0-28.9, **adult** Ⓐ
Z68.29 **Body mass index (BMI)** 29.0-29.9, **adult** Ⓐ

Z68.3 **Body mass index (BMI)** 30-39, adult

Z68.30 **Body mass index (BMI)** 30.0-30.9, **adult** Ⓐ
Z68.31 **Body mass index (BMI)** 31.0-31.9, **adult** Ⓐ
Z68.32 **Body mass index (BMI)** 32.0-32.9, **adult** Ⓐ
Z68.33 **Body mass index (BMI)** 33.0-33.9, **adult** Ⓐ
Z68.34 **Body mass index (BMI)** 34.0-34.9, **adult** Ⓐ
Z68.35 **Body mass index (BMI)** 35.0-35.9, **adult** Ⓐ
Z68.36 **Body mass index (BMI)** 36.0-36.9, **adult** Ⓐ
Z68.37 **Body mass index (BMI)** 37.0-37.9, **adult** Ⓐ
Z68.38 **Body mass index (BMI)** 38.0-38.9, **adult** Ⓐ
Z68.39 **Body mass index (BMI)** 39.0-39.9, **adult** Ⓐ

Z68.4 **Body mass index (BMI)** 40 or greater, **adult**

Z68.41 **Body mass index (BMI)** 40.0-44.9, **adult** Ⓐ
Z68.42 **Body mass index (BMI)** 45.0-49.9, **adult** Ⓐ
Z68.43 **Body mass index (BMI)** 50-59.9 , **adult** Ⓐ
Z68.44 **Body mass index (BMI)** 60.0-69.9, **adult** Ⓐ
Z68.45 **Body mass index (BMI)** 70 or greater, **adult** Ⓐ

Z68.5 **Body mass index (BMI)** pediatric

Z68.51 **Body mass index (BMI) pediatric,** less than 5th percentile for age Ⓟ
Z68.52 **Body mass index (BMI) pediatric,** 5th percentile to less than 85th percentile for age Ⓟ

Unspecified Code	Other Specified Code	Ⓝ Newborn Age: 0	Ⓟ Pediatric Age: 0-17	Ⓜ Maternity Age: 12-55
Ⓐ Adult Age: 15-124	♂ Male	♀ Female	● New Code	▲ Revised Code Title	►◄ Revised Text

Z68.53 Body mass index (BMI) pediatric, 85th percentile to less than 95th percentile for age [P]
Z68.54 Body mass index (BMI) pediatric, greater than or equal to 95th percentile for age [P]

Persons encountering health services in other circumstances (Z69-Z76)

[4] **Z69 Encounter for mental health services for victim and perpetrator of abuse**
INCLUDES *counseling for victims and perpetrators of abuse*
[5] **Z69.0 Encounter for mental health services for child abuse problems**
[6] **Z69.01 Encounter for mental health services for parental child abuse**
Z69.010 Encounter for mental health services for victim of parental child abuse [P]
Z69.011 Encounter for mental health services for perpetrator of parental child abuse
EXCLUDES1 *encounter for mental health services for non-parental child abuse (Z69.02-)*
[6] **Z69.02 Encounter for mental health services for non-parental child abuse**
Z69.020 Encounter for mental health services for victim of non-parental child abuse [P]
Z69.021 Encounter for mental health services for perpetrator of non-parental child abuse
[5] **Z69.1 Encounter for mental health services for spousal or partner abuse problems**
Z69.11 Encounter for mental health services for victim of spousal or partner abuse
Z69.12 Encounter for mental health services for perpetrator of spousal or partner abuse
[5] **Z69.8 Encounter for mental health services for victim or perpetrator of other abuse**
Z69.81 Encounter for mental health services for victim of other abuse
Encounter for rape victim counseling
Z69.82 Encounter for mental health services for perpetrator of other abuse

[4] **Z70 Counseling related to sexual attitude, behavior and orientation**
INCLUDES *encounter for mental health services for sexual attitude, behavior and orientation*
EXCLUDES2 *contraceptive or procreative counseling (Z30-Z31)*
Z70.0 Counseling related to sexual attitude
Z70.1 Counseling related to patient's sexual behavior and orientation
Patient concerned regarding impotence
Patient concerned regarding non-responsiveness
Patient concerned regarding promiscuity
Patient concerned regarding sexual orientation
Z70.2 Counseling related to sexual behavior and orientation of third party
Advice sought regarding sexual behavior and orientation of child
Advice sought regarding sexual behavior and orientation of partner
Advice sought regarding sexual behavior and orientation of spouse
Z70.3 Counseling related to combined concerns regarding sexual attitude, behavior and orientation
Z70.8 Other sex counseling
Encounter for sex education
Z70.9 Sex counseling, unspecified

[4] **Z71 Persons encountering health services for other counseling and medical advice, not elsewhere classified**
EXCLUDES2 *contraceptive or procreation counseling (Z30-Z31)*
sex counseling (Z70.-)
Z71.0 Person encountering health services to consult on behalf of another person
Person encountering health services to seek advice or treatment for non-attending third party
EXCLUDES2 *anxiety (normal) about sick person in family (Z63.7)*
expectant (adoptive) parent(s) pre-birth pediatrician visit (Z76.81)
Z71.1 Person with feared health complaint in whom no diagnosis is made
Person encountering health services with feared condition which was not demonstrated
Person encountering health services in which problem was normal state
'Worried well'
EXCLUDES1 *medical observation for suspected diseases and conditions proven not to exist (Z03.-)*
Z71.2 Person consulting for explanation of examination or test findings
Z71.3 Dietary counseling and surveillance
Use additional code for any associated underlying medical condition
code to identify body mass index (BMI), if known (Z68.-)
[5] **Z71.4 Alcohol abuse counseling and surveillance**
Use additional code for alcohol abuse or dependence (F10.-)
Z71.41 Alcohol abuse counseling and surveillance of alcoholic
Z71.42 Counseling for family member of alcoholic
Counseling for significant other, partner, or friend of alcoholic
[5] **Z71.5 Drug abuse counseling and surveillance**
Use additional code for drug abuse or dependence (F11-F16, F18-F19)
Z71.51 Drug abuse counseling and surveillance of drug abuser
Z71.52 Counseling for family member of drug abuser
Counseling for significant other, partner, or friend of drug abuser
Z71.6 Tobacco abuse counseling
Use additional code for nicotine dependence (F17.-)
Z71.7 Human immunodeficiency virus [HIV] counseling
[5] **Z71.8 Other specified counseling**
EXCLUDES2 *counseling for contraception (Z30.0-)*
counseling for genetics (Z31.5)
counseling for procreative management (Z31.6-)
Z71.81 Spiritual or religious counseling
Z71.89 Other specified counseling
Z71.9 Counseling, unspecified
Encounter for medical advice NOS

[4] **Z72 Problems related to lifestyle**
EXCLUDES2 *problems related to life-management difficulty (Z73.-)*
problems related to socioeconomic and psychosocial circumstances (Z55-Z65)
Z72.0 Tobacco use
Tobacco use NOS
EXCLUDES1 *history of tobacco dependence (Z87.891)*
nicotine dependence (F17.2-)
tobacco dependence (F17.2-)
tobacco use during pregnancy (O99.33-)
Z72.3 Lack of physical exercise
Z72.4 Inappropriate diet and eating habits
EXCLUDES1 *behavioral eating disorders of infancy or childhood (F98.2.-F98.3)*
eating disorders (F50.-)
lack of adequate food (Z59.4)

[4] 4th character required [5] 5th character required [6] 6th character required [7] 7th character required [X] Extension 'X' Alert
EXCLUDES1 Not coded here EXCLUDES2 Not included here [PDx] Primary Diagnosis Only Manifestation Code

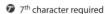

malnutrition and other nutritional deficiencies (E40-E64)

[5] **Z72.5 High risk sexual behavior**
Promiscuity
[EXCLUDES1] *paraphilias (F65)*
Z72.51 High risk heterosexual behavior
Z72.52 High risk homosexual behavior
Z72.53 High risk bisexual behavior
Z72.6 Gambling and betting
[EXCLUDES1] *compulsive or pathological gambling (F63.0)*

[5] **Z72.8 Other problems related to lifestyle**
[6] **Z72.81 Antisocial behavior**
[EXCLUDES1] *conduct disorders (F91.-)*
Z72.810 Child and adolescent antisocial behavior
Antisocial behavior (child) (adolescent) without manifest psychiatric disorder
Delinquency NOS
Group delinquency
Offenses in the context of gang membership
Stealing in company with others
Truancy from school [P]
Z72.811 Adult antisocial behavior
Adult antisocial behavior without manifest psychiatric disorder [A]
[6] **Z72.82 Problems related to sleep**
Z72.820 Sleep deprivation
Lack of adequate sleep
[EXCLUDES1] *insomnia (G47.0-)*
Z72.821 Inadequate sleep hygiene
Bad sleep habits
Irregular sleep habits
Unhealthy sleep wake schedule
[EXCLUDES1] *insomnia (F51.0-, G47.0-)*
Z72.89 Other problems related to lifestyle
Self-damaging behavior
Z72.9 Problem related to lifestyle, unspecified

[4] **Z73 Problems related to life management difficulty**
[EXCLUDES2] *problems related to socioeconomic and psychosocial circumstances (Z55-Z65)*
Z73.0 Burn-out
Z73.1 Type A behavior pattern
Z73.2 Lack of relaxation and leisure
Z73.3 Stress, not elsewhere classified
Physical and mental strain NOS
[EXCLUDES1] *stress related to employment or unemployment (Z56.-)*
Z73.4 Inadequate social skills, not elsewhere classified
Z73.5 Social role conflict, not elsewhere classified
Z73.6 Limitation of activities due to disability
[EXCLUDES1] *care-provider dependency (Z74.-)*
[5] **Z73.8 Other problems related to life management difficulty**
[6] **Z73.81 Behavioral insomnia of childhood**
Z73.810 Behavioral insomnia of childhood, sleep-onset association type [P]
Z73.811 Behavioral insomnia of childhood, limit setting type [P]
Z73.812 Behavioral insomnia of childhood, combined type [P]
Z73.819 Behavioral insomnia of childhood, unspecified type [P]
Z73.82 Dual sensory impairment
Z73.89 Other problems related to life management difficulty
Z73.9 Problem related to life management difficulty, unspecified

[4] **Z74 Problems related to care provider dependency**
[EXCLUDES2] *dependence on enabling machines or devices NEC (Z99.-)*
[5] **Z74.0 Reduced mobility**
Z74.01 Bed confinement status
Bedridden
Z74.09 Other reduced mobility
Chairridden
Reduced mobility NOS
[EXCLUDES2] *wheelchair dependence (Z99.3)*
Z74.1 Need for assistance with personal care
Z74.2 Need for assistance at home and no other household member able to render care
Z74.3 Need for continuous supervision
Z74.8 Other problems related to care provider dependency
Z74.9 Problem related to care provider dependency, unspecified

[4] **Z75 Problems related to medical facilities and other health care**
Z75.0 Medical services not available in home
[EXCLUDES1] *no other household member able to render care (Z74.2)*
Z75.1 Person awaiting admission to adequate facility elsewhere
Z75.2 Other waiting period for investigation and treatment
Z75.3 Unavailability and inaccessibility of health-care facilities
[EXCLUDES1] *bed unavailable (Z75.1)*
Z75.4 Unavailability and inaccessibility of other helping agencies
Z75.5 Holiday relief care
Z75.8 Other problems related to medical facilities and other health care
Z75.9 Unspecified problem related to medical facilities and other health care

[4] **Z76 Persons encountering health services in other circumstances**
Z76.0 Encounter for issue of repeat prescription
Encounter for issue of repeat prescription for appliance
Encounter for issue of repeat prescription for medicaments
Encounter for issue of repeat prescription for spectacles
[EXCLUDES2] *issue of medical certificate (Z02.7)*
repeat prescription for contraceptive (Z30.4-)
Z76.1 Encounter for health supervision and care of foundling [PDx]
Z76.2 Encounter for health supervision and care of other healthy infant and child
Encounter for medical or nursing care or supervision of healthy infant under circumstances such as adverse socioeconomic conditions at home
Encounter for medical or nursing care or supervision of healthy infant under circumstances such as awaiting foster or adoptive placement
Encounter for medical or nursing care or supervision of healthy infant under circumstances such as maternal illness
Encounter for medical or nursing care or supervision of healthy infant under circumstances such as number of children at home preventing or interfering with normal care [P] [PDx]
Z76.3 Healthy person accompanying sick person
Z76.4 Other boarder to healthcare facility
[EXCLUDES1] *homelessness (Z59.0)*
Z76.5 Malingerer [conscious simulation]
Person feigning illness (with obvious motivation)
[EXCLUDES1] *factitious disorder (F68.1-)*
peregrinating patient (F68.1-)
[5] **Z76.8 Persons encountering health services in other specified circumstances**
Z76.81 Expectant parent(s) prebirth pediatrician visit
Pre-adoption pediatrician visit for adoptive parent(s)
Z76.82 Awaiting organ transplant status
Patient waiting for organ availability
Z76.89 Persons encountering health services in other specified circumstances
Persons encountering health services NOS

Unspecified Code | Other Specified Code | [N] Newborn Age: 0 | [P] Pediatric Age: 0-17 | [M] Maternity Age: 12-55
[A] Adult Age: 15-124 | ♂ Male | ♀ Female | ● New Code | ▲ Revised Code Title | ►◄ Revised Text

Persons with potential health hazards related to family and personal history and certain conditions influencing health status (Z77-Z99)

Code also any follow-up examination (Z08-Z09)

[4] **Z77 Other contact with and (suspected) exposures hazardous to health**

[INCLUDES] *contact with and (suspected) exposures to potential hazards to health*

[EXCLUDES2] *contact with and (suspected) exposure to communicable diseases (Z20.-)*
exposure to (parental) (environmental) tobacco smoke in the perinatal period (P96.81)
newborn (suspected to be) affected by noxious substances transmitted via placenta or breast milk (P04.-)
occupational exposure to risk factors (Z57.-)
retained foreign body (Z18.-)
retained foreign body fully removed (Z87.821)
toxic effects of substances chiefly nonmedicinal as to source (T51-T65)

[5] **Z77.0 Contact with and (suspected) exposure to** hazardous, chiefly nonmedicinal, chemicals

[6] **Z77.01 Contact with and (suspected) exposure to hazardous** metals

Z77.010 Contact with and (suspected) exposure to arsenic

Z77.011 Contact with and (suspected) exposure to lead

Z77.012 Contact with and (suspected) exposure to uranium

[EXCLUDES1] *retained depleted uranium fragments (Z18.01)*

Z77.018 Contact with and (suspected) exposure to other hazardous metals

Contact with and (suspected) exposure to chromium compounds

Contact with and (suspected) exposure to nickel dust

[6] **Z77.02 Contact with and (suspected) exposure to hazardous** aromatic compounds

Z77.020 Contact with and (suspected) exposure to aromatic amines

Z77.021 Contact with and (suspected) exposure to benzene

Z77.028 Contact with and (suspected) exposure to other hazardous aromatic compounds

Aromatic dyes NOS

Polycyclic aromatic hydrocarbons

[6] **Z77.09 Contact with and (suspected) exposure to other hazardous, chiefly** nonmedicinal, chemicals

Z77.090 Contact with and (suspected) exposure to asbestos

Z77.098 Contact with and (suspected) exposure to other hazardous, chiefly nonmedicinal, chemicals

Dyes NOS

[5] **Z77.1 Contact with and (suspected) exposure to environmental pollution and** hazards in the physical environment

[6] **Z77.11 Contact with and (suspected) exposure to** environmental pollution

Z77.110 Contact with and (suspected) exposure to air **pollution**

Z77.111 Contact with and (suspected) exposure to water **pollution**

Z77.112 Contact with and (suspected) exposure to soil **pollution**

Z77.118 Contact with and (suspected) exposure to other environmental pollution

[6] **Z77.12 Contact with and (suspected) exposure to hazards in the physical environment**

Z77.120 Contact with and (suspected) exposure to mold **(toxic)**

Z77.121 Contact with and (suspected) exposure to harmful algae and algae toxins

Contact with and (suspected) exposure to (harmful) algae bloom NOS

Contact with and (suspected) exposure to blue-green algae bloom

Contact with and (suspected) exposure to brown tide

Contact with and (suspected) exposure to cyanobacteria bloom

Contact with and (suspected) exposure to Florida red tide

Contact with and (suspected) exposure to pfiesteria piscicida

Contact with and (suspected) exposure to red tide

Z77.122 Contact with and (suspected) exposure to noise

Z77.123 Contact with and (suspected) exposure to radon and other naturally occuring radiation

[EXCLUDES2] *radiation exposure as the cause of a confirmed condition (W88-W90, X39.0-)*
radiation sickness NOS (T66)

Z77.128 Contact with and (suspected) exposure to other hazards in the physical environment

[5] **Z77.2 Contact with and (suspected) exposure to** other **hazardous substances**

Z77.21 Contact with and (suspected) exposure to potentially hazardous body fluids

Z77.22 Contact with and (suspected) exposure to environmental tobacco smoke **(acute) (chronic)**

Exposure to second hand tobacco smoke (acute) (chronic)

Passive smoking (acute) (chronic)

[EXCLUDES1] *nicotine dependence (F17.-)*
tobacco use (Z72.0)

[EXCLUDES2] *occupational exposure to environmental tobacco smoke (Z57.31)*

Z77.29 Contact with and (suspected) exposure to other hazardous substances

Z77.9 Other contact with and (suspected) exposures hazardous to health

[4] **Z78 Other specified health status**

[EXCLUDES2] *asymptomatic human immunodeficiency virus [HIV] infection status (Z21)*
postprocedural status (Z93-Z99)
sex reassignment status (Z87.890)

Z78.0 Asymptomatic menopausal state

Menopausal state NOS

Postmenopausal status NOS

[EXCLUDES2] *symptomatic menopausal state (N95.1)* [A] ♀

Z78.1 Physical restraint status

[EXCLUDES1] *physical restraint due to a procedure - omit code*

Z78.9 Other specified health status

[4] **Z79 Long term (current) drug therapy**

[INCLUDES] *long term (current) drug use for prophylactic purposes*

Code also any therapeutic drug level monitoring (Z51.81)

[EXCLUDES2] *drug abuse and dependence (F11-F19)*
drug use complicating pregnancy, childbirth, and the puerperium (O99.32-)

[4] 4th character required [5] 5th character required [6] 6th character required [7] 7th character required [X] Extension 'X' Alert
[EXCLUDES 1] Not coded here [EXCLUDES 2] Not included here [PDx] Primary Diagnosis Only Manifestation Code

[5] Z79.0 Long term (current) use of anticoagulants and antithrombotics/antiplatelets

EXCLUDES2 *long term (current) use of aspirin (Z79.82)*

Z79.01 Long term (current) use of anticoagulants
Z79.02 Long term (current) use of antithrombotics/antiplatelets

Z79.1 Long term (current) use of non-steroidal anti-inflammatories (NSAID)

EXCLUDES2 *long term (current) use of aspirin (Z79.82)*

Z79.2 Long term (current) use of antibiotics
Z79.3 Long term (current) use of hormonal contraceptives

Long term (current) use of birth control pill or patch

Z79.4 Long term (current) use of insulin

[5] Z79.5 Long term (current) use of steroids

Z79.51 Long term (current) use of inhaled steroids
Z79.52 Long term (current) use of systemic steroids

[5] Z79.8 Other long term (current) drug therapy

[6] Z79.81 Long term (current) use of agents affecting estrogen receptors and estrogen levels

Code first , if applicable:
malignant neoplasm of breast (C50.-)
malignant neoplasm of prostate (C61)

Use additional code, if applicable, to identify:
estrogen receptor positive status (Z17.0)
family history of breast cancer (Z80.3)
genetic susceptibility to malignant neoplasm (cancer) (Z15.0-)
personal history of breast cancer (Z85.3)
personal history of prostate cancer (Z85.46)
postmenopausal status (Z78.0)

EXCLUDES1 *hormone replacement therapy (postmenopausal) (Z79.890)*

Z79.810 Long term (current) use of selective estrogen receptor modulators (SERMs)

Long term (current) use of raloxifene (Evista)
Long term (current) use of tamoxifen (Nolvadex)
Long term (current) use of toremifene (Fareston)

Z79.811 Long term (current) use of aromatase inhibitors

Long term (current) use of anastrozole (Arimidex)
Long term (current) use of exemestane (Aromasin)
Long term (current) use of letrozole (Femara)

Z79.818 Long term (current) use of other agents affecting estrogen receptors and estrogen levels

Long term (current) use of estrogen receptor downregulators
Long term (current) use of fulvestrant (Faslodex)
Long term (current) use of gonadotropin-releasing hormone (GnRH) agonist
Long term (current) use of goserelin acetate (Zoladex)
Long term (current) use of leuprolide acetate (leuprorelin) (Lupron)
Long term (current) use of megestrol acetate (Megace)

Z79.82 Long term (current) use of aspirin
Z79.83 Long term (current) use of bisphosphonates

[6] Z79.89 Other long term (current) drug therapy

Z79.890 Hormone replacement therapy (postmenopausal) ♀
Z79.891 Long term (current) use of opiate analgesic

Long term (current) use of methadone for pain management

EXCLUDES1 *methodone use NOS (F11.2-)*
use of methodone for treatment of heroin addiction (F11.2-)

Z79.899 Other long term (current) drug therapy

[4] Z80 Family history of primary malignant neoplasm

Z80.0 Family history of malignant neoplasm of digestive organs

Conditions classifiable to C15-C26

Z80.1 Family history of malignant neoplasm of trachea, bronchus and lung

Conditions classifiable to C33-C34

Z80.2 Family history of malignant neoplasm of other respiratory and intrathoracic organs

Conditions classifiable to C30-C32, C37-C39

Z80.3 Family history of malignant neoplasm of breast

Conditions classifiable to C50.-

[5] Z80.4 Family history of malignant neoplasm of genital organs

Conditions classifiable to C51-C63

Z80.41 Family history of malignant neoplasm of ovary ♀
Z80.42 Family history of malignant neoplasm of prostate ♂
Z80.43 Family history of malignant neoplasm of testis ♂
Z80.49 Family history of malignant neoplasm of other genital organs

[5] Z80.5 Family history of malignant neoplasm of urinary tract

Conditions classifiable to C64-C68

Z80.51 Family history of malignant neoplasm of kidney
Z80.52 Family history of malignant neoplasm of bladder
Z80.59 Family history of malignant neoplasm of other urinary tract organ

Z80.6 Family history of leukemia

Conditions classifiable to C91-C95

Z80.7 Family history of other malignant neoplasms of lymphoid, hematopoietic and related tissues

Conditions classifiable to C81-C90, C96.-

Z80.8 Family history of malignant neoplasm of other organs or systems

Conditions classifiable to C00-C14, C40-C49, C69-C79

Z80.9 Family history of malignant neoplasm, unspecified

Conditions classifiable to C80.1

[4] Z81 Family history of mental and behavioral disorders

Z81.0 Family history of intellectual disabilities

Conditions classifiable to F70-F79

Z81.1 Family history of alcohol abuse and dependence

Conditions classifiable to F10.-

Z81.2 Family history of tobacco abuse and dependence

Conditions classifiable to F17.-

Z81.3 Family history of other psychoactive substance abuse and dependence

Conditions classifiable to F11-F16, F18-F19

Z81.4 Family history of other substance abuse and dependence

Conditions classifiable to F55

Z81.8 Family history of other mental and behavioral disorders

Conditions classifiable elsewhere in F01-F99

[4] Z82 Family history of certain disabilities and chronic diseases (leading to disablement)

Z82.0 Family history of epilepsy and other diseases of the nervous system

Conditions classifiable to G00-G99

Z82.1 Family history of blindness and visual loss

Conditions classifiable to H54.-

Z82.2 Family history of deafness and hearing loss

Conditions classifiable to H90-H91

Unspecified Code | Other Specified Code | [N] Newborn Age: 0 | [P] Pediatric Age: 0-17 | [M] Maternity Age: 12-55
[A] Adult Age: 15-124 | ♂ Male | ♀ Female | ● New Code | ▲ Revised Code Title | ►◄ Revised Text

Z82.3 Family history of stroke
Conditions classifiable to I60-I64

[5] Z82.4 Family history of ischemic heart disease and other diseases of the circulatory system
Conditions classifiable to I00-I52, I65-I99

Z82.41 Family history of sudden cardiac death

Z82.49 Family history of ischemic heart disease and other diseases of the circulatory system

Z82.5 Family history of asthma and other chronic lower respiratory diseases
Conditions classifiable to J40-J47
EXCLUDES2 *family history of other diseases of the respiratory system (Z83.6)*

[5] Z82.6 Family history of arthritis and other diseases of the musculoskeletal system and connective tissue
Conditions classifiable to M00-M99

Z82.61 Family history of arthritis

Z82.62 Family history of osteoporosis

Z82.69 Family history of other diseases of the musculoskeletal system and connective tissue

[5] Z82.7 Family history of congenital malformations, deformations and chromosomal abnormalities
Conditions classifiable to Q00-Q99

Z82.71 Family history of polycystic kidney

Z82.79 Family history of other congenital malformations, deformations and chromosomal abnormalities

Z82.8 Family history of other disabilities and chronic diseases leading to disablement, not elsewhere classified

[4] Z83 Family history of other specific disorders
EXCLUDES2 *contact with and (suspected) exposure to communicable disease in the family (Z20.-)*

Z83.0 Family history of human immunodeficiency virus [HIV] disease
Conditions classifiable to B20

Z83.1 Family history of other infectious and parasitic diseases
Conditions classifiable to A00-B19, B25-B94, B99

Z83.2 Family history of diseases of the blood and blood-forming organs and certain disorders involving the immune mechanism
Conditions classifiable to D50-D89

Z83.3 Family history of diabetes mellitus
Conditions classifiable to E08-E13

[5] Z83.4 Family history of other endocrine, nutritional and metabolic diseases
Conditions classifiable to E00-E07, E15-E88

Z83.41 Family history of multiple endocrine neoplasia [MEN] syndrome

Z83.49 Family history of other endocrine, nutritional and metabolic diseases

[5] Z83.5 Family history of eye and ear disorders

[6] Z83.51 Family history of eye disorders
Conditions classifiable to H00-H53, H55-H59
EXCLUDES2 *family history of blindness and visual loss (Z82.1)*

Z83.511 Family history of glaucoma

Z83.518 Family history of other specified eye disorder

Z83.52 Family history of ear disorders
Conditions classifiable to H60-H83, H92-H95
EXCLUDES2 *family history of deafness and hearing loss (Z82.2)*

Z83.6 Family history of other diseases of the respiratory system
Conditions classifiable to J00-J39, J60-J99
EXCLUDES2 *family history of asthma and other chronic lower respiratory diseases (Z82.5)*

[5] Z83.7 Family history of diseases of the digestive system
Conditions classifiable to K00-K93

Z83.71 Family history of colonic polyps
EXCLUDES1 *family history of malignant neoplasm of digestive organs (Z80.0)*

Z83.79 Family history of other diseases of the digestive system

[4] Z84 Family history of other conditions

Z84.0 Family history of diseases of the skin and subcutaneous tissue
Conditions classifiable to L00-L99

Z84.1 Family history of disorders of kidney and ureter
Conditions classifiable to N00-N29

Z84.2 Family history of other diseases of the genitourinary system
Conditions classifiable to N30-N99

Z84.3 Family history of consanguinity

[5] Z84.8 Family history of other specified conditions

Z84.81 Family history of carrier of genetic disease

Z84.89 Family history of other specified conditions

[4] Z85 Personal history of malignant neoplasm
Code first any follow-up examination after treatment of malignant neoplasm (Z08)
Use additional code to identify:
alcohol use and dependence (F10.-)
exposure to environmental tobacco smoke (Z77.22)
history of tobacco use (Z87.891)
occupational exposure to environmental tobacco smoke (Z57.31)
tobacco dependence (F17.-)
tobacco use (Z72.0)
EXCLUDES2 *personal history of benign neoplasm (Z86.01-)*
personal history of carcinoma-in-situ (Z86.00-)

[5] Z85.0 Personal history of malignant neoplasm of digestive organs

Z85.00 Personal history of malignant neoplasm of unspecified digestive organ

Z85.01 Personal history of malignant neoplasm of esophagus
Conditions classifiable to C15

[6] Z85.02 Personal history of malignant neoplasm of stomach

Z85.020 Personal history of malignant carcinoid tumor of stomach
Conditions classifiable to C7A.092

Z85.028 Personal history of other malignant neoplasm of stomach
Conditions classifiable to C16

[6] Z85.03 Personal history of malignant neoplasm of large intestine

Z85.030 Personal history of malignant carcinoid tumor of large intestine
Conditions classifiable to C7A.022-C7A.025, C7A.029

Z85.038 Personal history of other malignant neoplasm of large intestine
Conditions classifiable to C18

[6] Z85.04 Personal history of malignant neoplasm of rectum, rectosigmoid junction, and anus

Z85.040 Personal history of malignant carcinoid tumor of rectum
Conditions classifiable to C7A.026

Z85.048 Personal history of other malignant neoplasm of rectum, rectosigmoid junction, and anus
Conditions classifiable to C19-C21

[4] 4th character required [5] 5th character required [6] 6th character required [7] 7th character required [7th] Extension 'X' Alert
EXCLUDES1 Not coded here EXCLUDES2 Not included here [PDx] Primary Diagnosis Only Manifestation Code

Z85.05 Personal history of malignant neoplasm of liver
Conditions classifiable to C22
[6] Z85.06 Personal history of malignant neoplasm of small intestine
Z85.060 Personal history of malignant carcinoid tumor of small intestine
Conditions classifiable to C7A.01-
Z85.068 Personal history of other malignant neoplasm of small intestine
Conditions classifiable to C17
Z85.07 Personal history of malignant neoplasm of pancreas
Conditions classifiable to C25
Z85.09 Personal history of malignant neoplasm of other digestive organs
[5] Z85.1 Personal history of malignant neoplasm of trachea, bronchus and lung
[6] Z85.11 Personal history of malignant neoplasm of bronchus and lung
Z85.110 Personal history of malignant carcinoid tumor of bronchus and lung
Conditions classifiable to C7A.090
Z85.118 Personal history of other malignant neoplasm of bronchus and lung
Conditions classifiable to C34
Z85.12 Personal history of malignant neoplasm of trachea
Conditions classifiable to C33
[5] Z85.2 Personal history of malignant neoplasm of other respiratory and intrathoracic organs
Z85.20 Personal history of malignant neoplasm of unspecified respiratory organ
Z85.21 Personal history of malignant neoplasm of larynx
Conditions classifiable to C32
Z85.22 Personal history of malignant neoplasm of nasal cavities, middle ear, and accessory sinuses
Conditions classifiable to C30-C31
[6] Z85.23 Personal history of malignant neoplasm of thymus
Z85.230 Personal history of malignant carcinoid tumor of thymus
Conditions classifiable to C7A.091
Z85.238 Personal history of other malignant neoplasm of thymus
Conditions classifiable to C37
Z85.29 Personal history of malignant neoplasm of other respiratory and intrathoracic organs
Z85.3 Personal history of malignant neoplasm of breast
Conditions classifiable to C50.-
[5] Z85.4 Personal history of malignant neoplasm of genital organs
Conditions classifiable to C51-C63
Z85.40 Personal history of malignant neoplasm of unspecified female genital organ ♀
Z85.41 Personal history of malignant neoplasm of cervix uteri ♀
Z85.42 Personal history of malignant neoplasm of other parts of uterus ♀
Z85.43 Personal history of malignant neoplasm of ovary ♀
Z85.44 Personal history of malignant neoplasm of other female genital organs ♀
Z85.45 Personal history of malignant neoplasm of unspecified male genital organ ♂
Z85.46 Personal history of malignant neoplasm of prostate ♂
Z85.47 Personal history of malignant neoplasm of testis ♂
Z85.48 Personal history of malignant neoplasm of epididymis ♂
Z85.49 Personal history of malignant neoplasm of other male genital organs ♂
[5] Z85.5 Personal history of malignant neoplasm of urinary tract
Conditions classifiable to C64-C68
Z85.50 Personal history of malignant neoplasm of unspecified urinary tract organ
Z85.51 Personal history of malignant neoplasm of bladder
[6] Z85.52 Personal history of malignant neoplasm of kidney
[EXCLUDES1] *personal history of malignant neoplasm of renal pelvis (Z85.53)*
Z85.520 Personal history of malignant carcinoid tumor of kidney
Conditions classifiable to C7A.093
Z85.528 Personal history of other malignant neoplasm of kidney
Conditions classifiable to C64
Z85.53 Personal history of malignant neoplasm of renal pelvis
Z85.54 Personal history of malignant neoplasm of ureter
Z85.59 Personal history of malignant neoplasm of other urinary tract organ
Z85.6 Personal history of leukemia
Conditions classifiable to C91-C95
[EXCLUDES1] *leukemia in remission C91.0-C95.9 with 5th character 1*
[5] Z85.7 Personal history of other malignant neoplasms of lymphoid, hematopoietic and related tissues
Z85.71 Personal history of Hodgkin lymphoma
Conditions classifiable to C81
Z85.72 Personal history of non-Hodgkin lymphomas
Conditions classifiable to C82-C85
Z85.79 Personal history of other malignant neoplasms of lymphoid, hematopoietic and related tissues
Conditions classifiable to C88-C90, C96
[EXCLUDES1] *multiple myeloma in remission (C90.01)*
plasma cell leukemia in remission (C90.11)
plasmacytoma in remission (C90.21)
[5] Z85.8 Personal history of malignant neoplasms of other organs and systems
Conditions classifiable to C00-C14, C40-C49, C69-C79, C7A.098
[6] Z85.81 Personal history of malignant neoplasm of lip, oral cavity, and pharynx
Z85.810 Personal history of malignant neoplasm of tongue
Z85.818 Personal history of malignant neoplasm of other sites of lip, oral cavity, and pharynx
Z85.819 Personal history of malignant neoplasm of unspecified site of lip, oral cavity, and pharynx
[6] Z85.82 Personal history of malignant neoplasm of skin
Z85.820 Personal history of malignant melanoma of skin
Conditions classifiable to C43
Z85.821 Personal history of Merkel cell carcinoma
Conditions classifiable to C4A
Z85.828 Personal history of other malignant neoplasm of skin
Conditions classifiable to C44
[6] Z85.83 Personal history of malignant neoplasm of bone and soft tissue

Unspecified Code | Other Specified Code | [N] Newborn Age: 0 | [P] Pediatric Age: 0-17 | [M] Maternity Age: 12-55
[A] Adult Age: 15-124 | ♂ Male | ♀ Female | ● New Code | ▲ Revised Code Title | ►◄ Revised Text

Z85.830 Personal history of malignant neoplasm of bone

Z85.831 Personal history of malignant neoplasm of soft tissue

[EXCLUDES2] personal history of malignant neoplasm of skin (Z85.82-)

[6] Z85.84 Personal history of malignant neoplasm of eye and nervous tissue

Z85.840 Personal history of malignant neoplasm of eye

Z85.841 Personal history of malignant neoplasm of brain

Z85.848 Personal history of malignant neoplasm of other parts of nervous tissue

[6] Z85.85 Personal history of malignant neoplasm of endocrine glands

Z85.850 Personal history of malignant neoplasm of thyroid

Z85.858 Personal history of malignant neoplasm of other endocrine glands

Z85.89 Personal history of malignant neoplasm of other organs and systems

Z85.9 Personal history of malignant neoplasm, unspecified

Conditions classifiable to C7A.00, C80.1

[4] Z86 Personal history of certain other diseases

Code first any follow-up examination after treatment (Z09)

[5] Z86.0 Personal history of in-situ and benign neoplasms and neoplasms of uncertain behavior

[EXCLUDES2] personal history of malignant neoplasms (Z85.-)

[6] Z86.00 Personal history of in-situ neoplasm

Z86.000 Personal history of in-situ neoplasm of breast

Z86.001 Personal history of in-situ neoplasm of cervix uteri ♀

Z86.008 Personal history of in-situ neoplasm of other site

[6] Z86.01 Personal history of benign neoplasm

Z86.010 Personal history of colonic polyps

Z86.011 Personal history of benign neoplasm of the brain

Z86.012 Personal history of benign carcinoid tumor

Z86.018 Personal history of other benign neoplasm

Z86.03 Personal history of neoplasm of uncertain behavior

[5] Z86.1 Personal history of infectious and parasitic diseases

Conditions classifiable to A00-B89, B99

[EXCLUDES1] personal history of infectious diseases specific to a body system
sequelae of infectious and parasitic diseases (B90-B94)

Z86.11 Personal history of tuberculosis

Z86.12 Personal history of poliomyelitis

Z86.13 Personal history of malaria

Z86.14 Personal history of Methicillin resistant Staphylococcus aureus infection

Personal history of MRSA infection

Z86.19 Personal history of other infectious and parasitic diseases

Z86.2 Personal history of diseases of the blood and blood-forming organs and certain disorders involving the immune mechanism

Conditions classifiable to D50-D89

[5] Z86.3 Personal history of endocrine, nutritional and metabolic diseases

Conditions classifiable to E00-E88

Z86.31 Personal history of diabetic foot ulcer

[EXCLUDES2] current diabetic foot ulcer (E08.621, E09.621, E10.621, E11.621, E13.621)

Z86.32 Personal history of gestational diabetes

Personal history of conditions classifiable to O24.4-

[EXCLUDES1] gestational diabetes mellitus in current pregnancy (O24.4-) ♀

Z86.39 Personal history of other endocrine, nutritional and metabolic disease

[5] Z86.5 Personal history of mental and behavioral disorders

Conditions classifiable to F40-F59

Z86.51 Personal history of combat and operational stress reaction [A]

Z86.59 Personal history of other mental and behavioral disorders

[5] Z86.6 Personal history of diseases of the nervous system and sense organs

Conditions classifiable to G00-G99, H00-H95

Z86.61 Personal history of infections of the central nervous system

Personal history of encephalitis
Personal history of meningitis

Z86.69 Personal history of other diseases of the nervous system and sense organs

[5] Z86.7 Personal history of diseases of the circulatory system

Conditions classifiable to I00-I99

[EXCLUDES2] old myocardial infarction (I25.2)
personal history of anaphylactic shock (Z87.892)
postmyocardial infarction syndrome (I24.1)

[6] Z86.71 Personal history of venous thrombosis and embolism

Z86.711 Personal history of pulmonary embolism

Z86.718 Personal history of other venous thrombosis and embolism

Z86.72 Personal history of thrombophlebitis

Z86.73 Personal history of transient ischemic attack (TIA), and cerebral infarction without residual deficits

Personal history of prolonged reversible ischemic neurological deficit (PRIND)
Personal history of stroke NOS without residual deficits

[EXCLUDES1] personal history of traumatic brain injury (Z87.820)
sequelae of cerebrovascular disease (I69.-)

Z86.74 Personal history of sudden cardiac arrest

Personal history of sudden cardiac death successfully resuscitated

Z86.79 Personal history of other diseases of the circulatory system

[4] Z87 Personal history of other diseases and conditions

Code first any follow-up examination after treatment (Z09)

[5] Z87.0 Personal history of diseases of the respiratory system

Conditions classifiable to J00-J99

Z87.01 Personal history of pneumonia (recurrent)

Z87.09 Personal history of other diseases of the respiratory system

[5] Z87.1 Personal history of diseases of the digestive system

Conditions classifiable to K00-K93

Z87.11 Personal history of peptic ulcer disease

Z87.19 Personal history of other diseases of the digestive system

Z87.2 Personal history of diseases of the skin and subcutaneous tissue

Conditions classifiable to L00-L99

[EXCLUDES2] personal history of diabetic foot ulcer (Z86.31)

[5] Z87.3 Personal history of diseases of the musculoskeletal system and connective tissue

Conditions classifiable to M00-M99

[4] 4th character required [5] 5th character required [6] 6th character required [7] 7th character required [X] Extension 'X' Alert
[EXCLUDES1] Not coded here [EXCLUDES2] Not included here [PDx] Primary Diagnosis Only Manifestation Code

EXCLUDES2 *personal history of (healed) traumatic fracture (Z87.81)*

Z87.31 **Personal history of (healed)** nontraumatic fracture

 Z87.310 **Personal history of (healed)** osteoporosis fracture

  Personal history of (healed) fragility fracture

  Personal history of (healed) collapsed vertebra due to osteoporosis

 Z87.311 **Personal history of (healed) other pathological fracture**

  Personal history of (healed) collapsed vertebra NOS

  EXCLUDES2 *personal history of osteoporosis fracture (Z87.310)*

 Z87.312 **Personal history of (healed)** stress fracture

  Personal history of (healed) fatigue fracture

Z87.39 **Personal history of other diseases of the musculoskeletal system and connective tissue**

Z87.4 **Personal history of diseases of** genitourinary system

 Conditions classifiable to N00-N99

Z87.41 **Personal history of** dysplasia of the female genital tract

 EXCLUDES1 *personal history of malignant neoplasm of female genital tract (Z85.40-Z85.44)*

 Z87.410 **Personal history of** cervical dysplasia ♀

 Z87.411 **Personal history of** vaginal dysplasia ♀

 Z87.412 **Personal history of** vulvar dysplasia ♀

Z87.42 **Personal history of other diseases of the** female genital tract ♀

Z87.43 **Personal history of diseases of** male genital organs

 Z87.430 **Personal history of** prostatic dysplasia

 EXCLUDES1 *personal history of malignant neoplasm of prostate (Z85.46)*

 Z87.438 **Personal history of other diseases of** male genital organs

Z87.44 **Personal history of diseases of** urinary system

 EXCLUDES1 *personal history of malignant neoplasm of cervix uteri (Z85.41)*

 Z87.440 **Personal history of** urinary (tract) infections

 Z87.441 **Personal history of** nephrotic syndrome

 Z87.442 **Personal history of** urinary calculi

  Personal history of kidney stones

 Z87.448 **Personal history of other diseases of urinary system**

Z87.5 **Personal history of complications of** pregnancy, childbirth and the puerperium

 Conditions classifiable to O00-O9A

 EXCLUDES2 *recurrent pregnancy loss (N96)*

Z87.51 **Personal history of** pre-term labor

 EXCLUDES1 *current pregnancy with history of pre-term labor (O09.21-)* ♀

Z87.59 **Personal history of other** complications of **pregnancy, childbirth and the puerperium**

 Personal history of trophoblastic disease ♀

Z87.7 **Personal history of (corrected)** congenital malformations

 Conditions classifiable to Q00-Q89 that have been repaired or corrected

 EXCLUDES1 *congenital malformations that have been partially corrected or repair but which still require medical treatment - code to condition*

 EXCLUDES2 *other postprocedural states (Z98.-)*
personal history of medical treatment (Z92.-)
presence of cardiac and vascular implants and grafts (Z95.-)
presence of other devices (Z97.-)

presence of other functional implants (Z96.-)
transplanted organ and tissue status (Z94.-)

Z87.71 **Personal history of (corrected) congenital malformations of** genitourinary system

 Z87.710 **Personal history of (corrected)** hypospadias ♂

 Z87.718 **Personal history of other specified (corrected) congenital malformations of genitourinary system**

Z87.72 **Personal history of (corrected) congenital malformations of** nervous system and sense organs

 Z87.720 **Personal history of (corrected) congenital malformations of** eye

 Z87.721 **Personal history of (corrected) congenital malformations of** ear

 Z87.728 **Personal history of other specified (corrected) congenital malformations of nervous system and sense organs**

Z87.73 **Personal history of (corrected) congenital malformations of** digestive system

 Z87.730 **Personal history of (corrected)** cleft lip and palate

 Z87.738 **Personal history of other specified (corrected) congenital malformations of digestive system**

Z87.74 **Personal history of (corrected) congenital malformations of** heart and circulatory system

Z87.75 **Personal history of (corrected) congenital malformations of** respiratory system

Z87.76 **Personal history of (corrected) congenital malformations of** integument, limbs and musculoskeletal system

Z87.79 **Personal history of** other **(corrected) congenital malformations**

 Z87.790 **Personal history of (corrected) congenital malformations of** face and neck

 Z87.798 **Personal history of other (corrected) congenital malformations**

Z87.8 **Personal history of other specified conditions**

 EXCLUDES2 *personal history of self harm (Z91.5)*

Z87.81 **Personal history of (healed)** traumatic fracture

 EXCLUDES2 *personal history of (healed) nontraumatic fracture (Z87.31-)*

Z87.82 **Personal history of other (healed)** physical injury and trauma

 Conditions classifiable to S00-T88, except traumatic fractures

 Z87.820 **Personal history of traumatic** brain injury

 EXCLUDES1 *personal history of transient ischemic attack (TIA), and cerebral infarction without residual deficits (Z86.73)*

 Z87.821 **Personal history of** retained foreign body fully removed

 Z87.828 **Personal history of other (healed) physical injury and trauma**

Z87.89 **Personal history of** other specified **conditions**

 Z87.890 **Personal history of** sex reassignment

 Z87.891 **Personal history of** nicotine dependence

 EXCLUDES1 *current nicotine dependence (F17.2-)*

 Z87.892 **Personal history of** anaphylaxis

  Code also allergy status such as:
  allergy status to drugs, medicaments and biological substances (Z88.-)
  allergy status, other than to drugs and biological substances (Z91.0-)

 Z87.898 **Personal history of other specified conditions**

[4th] **Z88 Allergy status to drugs, medicaments and biological substances**

EXCLUDES2 *Allergy status, other than to drugs and biological substances (Z91.0-)*

Z88.0 Allergy status to penicillin
Z88.1 Allergy status to other antibiotic agents status
Z88.2 Allergy status to sulfonamides status
Z88.3 Allergy status to other anti-infective agents status
Z88.4 Allergy status to anesthetic agent status
Z88.5 Allergy status to narcotic agent status
Z88.6 Allergy status to analgesic agent status
Z88.7 Allergy status to serum and vaccine status
Z88.8 Allergy status to other drugs, medicaments and biological substances status
Z88.9 Allergy status to unspecified drugs, medicaments and biological substances status

[4th] **Z89 Acquired absence of limb**

INCLUDES *amputation status*
postprocedural loss of limb
post-traumatic loss of limb

EXCLUDES1 *acquired deformities of limbs (M20-M21)*
congenital absence of limbs (Q71-Q73)

[5th] Z89.0 Acquired absence of thumb and other finger(s)
[6th] Z89.01 Acquired absence of thumb
Z89.011 Acquired absence of right thumb
Z89.012 Acquired absence of left thumb
Z89.019 Acquired absence of unspecified thumb
[6th] Z89.02 Acquired absence of other finger(s)
EXCLUDES2 *acquired absence of thumb (Z89.01-)*
Z89.021 Acquired absence of right finger(s)
Z89.022 Acquired absence of left finger(s)
Z89.029 Acquired absence of unspecified finger(s)
[5th] Z89.1 Acquired absence of hand and wrist
[6th] Z89.11 Acquired absence of hand
Z89.111 Acquired absence of right hand
Z89.112 Acquired absence of left hand
Z89.119 Acquired absence of unspecified hand
[6th] Z89.12 Acquired absence of wrist
Disarticulation at wrist
Z89.121 Acquired absence of right wrist
Z89.122 Acquired absence of left wrist
Z89.129 Acquired absence of unspecified wrist
[5th] Z89.2 Acquired absence of upper limb above wrist
[6th] Z89.20 Acquired absence of upper limb, unspecified level
Z89.201 Acquired absence of right upper limb, unspecified level
Z89.202 Acquired absence of left upper limb, unspecified level
Z89.209 Acquired absence of unspecified upper limb, unspecified level
Acquired absence of arm NOS
[6th] Z89.21 Acquired absence of upper limb below elbow
Z89.211 Acquired absence of right upper limb below elbow
Z89.212 Acquired absence of left upper limb below elbow
Z89.219 Acquired absence of unspecified upper limb below elbow
[6th] Z89.22 Acquired absence of upper limb above elbow
Disarticulation at elbow
Z89.221 Acquired absence of right upper limb above elbow
Z89.222 Acquired absence of left upper limb above elbow
Z89.229 Acquired absence of unspecified upper limb above elbow
[6th] Z89.23 Acquired absence of shoulder
Acquired absence of shoulder joint following explantation of shoulder joint prosthesis, with or without presence of antibiotic-impregnated cement spacer
Z89.231 Acquired absence of right shoulder
Z89.232 Acquired absence of left shoulder
Z89.239 Acquired absence of unspecified shoulder
[5th] Z89.4 Acquired absence of toe(s), foot, and ankle
[6th] Z89.41 Acquired absence of great toe
Z89.411 Acquired absence of right great toe
Z89.412 Acquired absence of left great toe
Z89.419 Acquired absence of unspecified great toe
[6th] Z89.42 Acquired absence of other toe(s)
EXCLUDES2 *acquired absence of great toe (Z89.41-)*
Z89.421 Acquired absence of other right toe(s)
Z89.422 Acquired absence of other left toe(s)
Z89.429 Acquired absence of other toe(s), unspecified side
[6th] Z89.43 Acquired absence of foot
Z89.431 Acquired absence of right foot
Z89.432 Acquired absence of left foot
Z89.439 Acquired absence of unspecified foot
[6th] Z89.44 Acquired absence of ankle
Disarticulation of ankle
Z89.441 Acquired absence of right ankle
Z89.442 Acquired absence of left ankle
Z89.449 Acquired absence of unspecified ankle
[5th] Z89.5 Acquired absence of leg below knee
[6th] Z89.51 Acquired absence of leg below knee
Z89.511 Acquired absence of right leg below knee
Z89.512 Acquired absence of left leg below knee
Z89.519 Acquired absence of unspecified leg below knee
[6th] Z89.52 Acquired absence of knee
Acquired absence of knee joint following explantation of knee joint prosthesis, with or without presence of antibiotic-impregnated cement spacer
Z89.521 Acquired absence of right knee
Z89.522 Acquired absence of left knee
Z89.529 Acquired absence of unspecified knee
[5th] Z89.6 Acquired absence of leg above knee
[6th] Z89.61 Acquired absence of leg above knee
Acquired absence of leg NOS
Disarticulation at knee
Z89.611 Acquired absence of right leg above knee
Z89.612 Acquired absence of left leg above knee
Z89.619 Acquired absence of unspecified leg above knee
[6th] Z89.62 Acquired absence of hip
Acquired absence of hip joint following explantation of hip joint prosthesis, with or without presence of antibiotic-impregnated cement spacer
Disarticulation at hip
Z89.621 Acquired absence of right hip joint
Z89.622 Acquired absence of left hip joint
Z89.629 Acquired absence of unspecified hip joint
Z89.9 Acquired absence of limb, unspecified

[4th] **Z90 Acquired absence of organs, not elsewhere classified**

INCLUDES *postprocedural or post-traumatic loss of body part NEC*

EXCLUDES1 *congenital absence - see Alphabetical Index*

EXCLUDES2 *postprocedural absence of endocrine glands (E89.-)*

[5th] Z90.0 Acquired absence of part of head and neck
Z90.01 Acquired absence of eye
Z90.02 Acquired absence of larynx
Z90.09 Acquired absence of other part of head and neck
Acquired absence of nose
EXCLUDES2 *teeth (K08.1)*
[5th] Z90.1 Acquired absence of breast and nipple

[4th] 4th character required [5th] 5th character required [6th] 6th character required [7th] 7th character required [7th] Extension 'X' Alert
EXCLUDES1 Not coded here EXCLUDES2 Not included here [PDx] Primary Diagnosis Only Manifestation Code

Z90.10 Acquired absence of unspecified breast and nipple
Z90.11 Acquired absence of right breast and nipple
Z90.12 Acquired absence of left breast and nipple
Z90.13 Acquired absence of bilateral breasts and nipples
Z90.2 Acquired absence of lung [part of]
Z90.3 Acquired absence of stomach [part of]
[5] Z90.4 Acquired absence of other specified parts of digestive tract
[6] Z90.41 Acquired absence of pancreas
Use additional code to identify any associated:
insulin use (Z79.4)
diabetes mellitus, postpancreatectomy (E13.-)
Z90.410 Acquired total absence of pancreas
Acquired absence of pancreas NOS
Z90.411 Acquired partial absence of pancreas
Z90.49 Acquired absence of other specified parts of digestive tract
Z90.5 Acquired absence of kidney
Z90.6 Acquired absence of other parts of urinary tract
Acquired absence of bladder
[5] Z90.7 Acquired absence of genital organ(s)
[EXCLUDES1] *personal history of sex reassignment (Z87.890)*
[EXCLUDES2] *female genital mutilation status (N90.81-)*
[6] Z90.71 Acquired absence of cervix and uterus
Z90.710 Acquired absence of both cervix and uterus
Acquired absence of uterus NOS
Status post total hysterectomy ♀
Z90.711 Acquired absence of uterus with remaining cervical stump
Status post partial hysterectomy with remaining cervical stump ♀
Z90.712 Acquired absence of cervix with remaining uterus ♀
[6] Z90.72 Acquired absence of ovaries
Z90.721 Acquired absence of ovaries, unilateral ♀
Z90.722 Acquired absence of ovaries, bilateral ♀
Z90.79 Acquired absence of other genital organ(s)
[5] Z90.8 Acquired absence of other organs
Z90.81 Acquired absence of spleen
Z90.89 Acquired absence of other organs
[4] Z91 Personal risk factors, not elsewhere classified
[EXCLUDES2] *contact with and (suspected) exposures hazardous to health (Z77.-)*
exposure to pollution and other problems related to physical environment (Z77.1-)
personal history of physical injury and trauma (Z87.81, Z87.82-)
occupational exposure to risk factors (Z57.-)
[5] Z91.0 Allergy status, other than to drugs and biological substances
[EXCLUDES2] *Allergy status to drugs, medicaments, and biological substances (Z88.-)*
[6] Z91.01 Food allergy status
[EXCLUDES2] *food additives allergy status (Z91.02)*
Z91.010 Allergy to peanuts
Z91.011 Allergy to milk products
[EXCLUDES1] *lactose intolerance (E73.-)*
Z91.012 Allergy to eggs
Z91.013 Allergy to seafood
Allergy to shellfish
Allergy to octopus or squid ink
Z91.018 Allergy to other foods
Allergy to nuts other than peanuts
Z91.02 Food additives allergy status
[6] Z91.03 Insect allergy status
Z91.030 Bee allergy status
Z91.038 Other insect allergy status
[6] Z91.04 Nonmedicinal substance allergy status
Z91.040 Latex allergy status
Latex sensitivity status
Z91.041 Radiographic dye allergy status
Allergy status to contrast media used for diagnostic X-ray procedure
Z91.048 Other nonmedicinal substance allergy status
Z91.09 Other allergy status, other than to drugs and biological substances
[5] Z91.1 Patient's noncompliance with medical treatment and regimen
Z91.11 Patient's noncompliance with dietary regimen
[6] Z91.12 Patient's intentional underdosing of medication regimen
Code first underdosing of medication (T36-T50) with fifth or sixth character 6
[EXCLUDES1] *adverse effect of prescribed drug taken as directed- code to adverse effect*
poisoning (overdose) -code to poisoning
Z91.120 Patient's intentional underdosing of medication regimen due to financial hardship
Z91.128 Patient's intentional underdosing of medication regimen for other reason
[6] Z91.13 Patient's unintentional underdosing of medication regimen
Code first underdosing of medication (T36-T50) with fifth or sixth character 6
[EXCLUDES1] *adverse effect of prescribed drug taken as directed- code to adverse effect*
poisoning (overdose) -code to poisoning
Z91.130 Patient's unintentional underdosing of medication regimen due to age-related debility
Z91.138 Patient's unintentional underdosing of medication regimen for other reason
Z91.14 Patient's other noncompliance with medication regimen
Patient's underdosing of medication NOS
Z91.15 Patient's noncompliance with renal dialysis
Z91.19 Patient's noncompliance with other medical treatment and regimen
[5] Z91.4 Personal history of psychological trauma, not elsewhere classified
[6] Z91.41 Personal history of adult abuse
[EXCLUDES2] *personal history of abuse in childhood (Z62.81-)*
Z91.410 Personal history of adult physical and sexual abuse
[EXCLUDES1] *current adult physical abuse (T74.11, T76.11)*
current adult sexual abuse (T74.21, T76.11) [A]
Z91.411 Personal history of adult psychological abuse [A]
Z91.412 Personal history of adult neglect
[EXCLUDES1] *current adult neglect (T74.01, T76.01)* [A]
Z91.419 Personal history of unspecified adult abuse [A]
Z91.49 Other personal history of psychological trauma, not elsewhere classified
Z91.5 Personal history of self-harm
Personal history of parasuicide
Personal history of self-poisoning
Personal history of suicide attempt
[5] Z91.8 Other specified personal risk factors, not elsewhere classified
Z91.81 History of falling
At risk for falling

Unspecified Code | Other Specified Code | [N] Newborn Age: 0 | [P] Pediatric Age: 0-17 | [M] Maternity Age: 12-55
[A] Adult Age: 15-124 | ♂ Male | ♀ Female | ● New Code | ▲ Revised Code Title | ▶◀ Revised Text

Z91.82 Personal history of military deployment
Individual (civilian or military) with past history of military war, peacekeeping and humanitarian deployment (current or past conflict)
Returned from military deployment [A]

Z91.83 Wandering in diseases classified elsewhere
Code first underlying disorder such as:
Alzheimer's disease (G30.-)
autism or pervasive developmental disorder (F84.-)
intellectual disabilities (F70-F79)
unspecified dementia with behavioral disturbance (F03.9-)

Z91.89 Other specified personal risk factors, not elsewhere classified

[4] Z92 Personal history of medical treatment
EXCLUDES2 *postprocedural states (Z98.-)*

Z92.0 Personal history of contraception
EXCLUDES1 *counseling or management of current contraceptive practices (Z30.-)*
long term (current) use of contraception (Z79.3)
presence of (intrauterine) contraceptive device (Z97.5)

[5] Z92.2 Personal history of drug therapy
EXCLUDES2 *long term (current) drug therapy (Z79.-)*

Z92.21 Personal history of antineoplastic chemotherapy
Z92.22 Personal history of monoclonal drug therapy
Z92.23 Personal history of estrogen therapy
[6] Z92.24 Personal history of steroid therapy
Z92.240 Personal history of inhaled steroid therapy
Z92.241 Personal history of systemic steroid therapy
Personal history of steroid therapy NOS
Z92.25 Personal history of immunosupression therapy
EXCLUDES2 *personal history of steroid therapy (Z92.24)*
Z92.29 Personal history of other drug therapy

Z92.3 Personal history of irradiation
Personal history of exposure to therapeutic radiation
EXCLUDES1 *exposure to radiation in the physical environment (Z77.12)*
occupational exposure to radiation (Z57.1)

[5] Z92.8 Personal history of other medical treatment
Z92.81 Personal history of extracorporeal membrane oxygenation (ECMO)
Z92.82 Status post administration of tPA (rtPA) in a different facility within the last 24 hours prior to admission to current facility
Code first condition requiring tPA administration, such as:
acute cerebral infarction (I63.-)
acute myocardial infarction (I21.-, I22.-)
Z92.83 Personal history of failed moderate sedation
Personal history of failed conscious sedation
EXCLUDES2 *failed moderate sedation during procedure (T88.52)*
Z92.89 Personal history of other medical treatment

[4] Z93 Artificial opening status
EXCLUDES1 *artificial openings requiring attention or management (Z43.-)*
complications of external stoma (J95.0-, K94.-, N99.5-)

Z93.0 Tracheostomy status
Z93.1 Gastrostomy status
Z93.2 Ileostomy status
Z93.3 Colostomy status
Z93.4 Other artificial openings of gastrointestinal tract status
[5] Z93.5 Cystostomy status
Z93.50 Unspecified cystostomy status
Z93.51 Cutaneous-vesicostomy status
Z93.52 Appendico-vesicostomy status
Z93.59 Other cystostomy status
Z93.6 Other artificial openings of urinary tract status
Nephrostomy status
Ureterostomy status
Urethrostomy status
Z93.8 Other artificial opening status
Z93.9 Artificial opening status, unspecified

[4] Z94 Transplanted organ and tissue status
INCLUDES *organ or tissue replaced by heterogenous or homogenous transplant*
EXCLUDES1 *complications of transplanted organ or tissue - see Alphabetical Index*
EXCLUDES2 *presence of vascular grafts (Z95.-)*

Z94.0 Kidney transplant status
Z94.1 Heart transplant status
EXCLUDES1 *artificial heart status (Z95.812)*
heart-valve replacement status (Z95.2-Z95.4)
Z94.2 Lung transplant status
Z94.3 Heart and lungs transplant status
Z94.4 Liver transplant status
Z94.5 Skin transplant status
Autogenous skin transplant status
Z94.6 Bone transplant status
Z94.7 Corneal transplant status
[5] Z94.8 Other transplanted organ and tissue status
Z94.81 Bone marrow transplant status
Z94.82 Intestine transplant status
Z94.83 Pancreas transplant status
Z94.84 Stem cells transplant status
Z94.89 Other transplanted organ and tissue status
Z94.9 Transplanted organ and tissue status, unspecified

[4] Z95 Presence of cardiac and vascular implants and grafts
EXCLUDES1 *complications of cardiac and vascular devices, implants and grafts (T82.-)*

Z95.0 Presence of cardiac pacemaker
EXCLUDES1 *adjustment or management of cardiac pacemaker (Z45.0)*
presence of automatic (implantable) cardiac defibrillator with synchronous cardiac pacemaker (Z95.810)
Z95.1 Presence of aortocoronary bypass graft
Z95.2 Presence of prosthetic heart valve
Presence of heart valve NOS
Z95.3 Presence of xenogenic heart valve
Z95.4 Presence of other heart-valve replacement
Z95.5 Presence of coronary angioplasty implant and graft
EXCLUDES1 *coronary angioplasty status without implant and graft (Z98.61)*
[5] Z95.8 Presence of other cardiac and vascular implants and grafts
[6] Z95.81 Presence of other cardiac implants and grafts
Z95.810 Presence of automatic (implantable) cardiac defibrillator
Presence of automatic (implantable) cardiac defibrillator with synchronous cardiac pacemaker
Z95.811 Presence of heart assist device
Z95.812 Presence of fully implantable artificial heart
Z95.818 Presence of other cardiac implants and grafts
[6] Z95.82 Presence of other vascular implants and grafts
Z95.820 Peripheral vascular angioplasty status with implants and grafts
EXCLUDES1 *peripheral vascular angioplasty without implant and graft (Z98.62)*
Z95.828 Presence of other vascular implants and grafts
Presence of intravascular prosthesis NEC

[4] 4th character required [5] 5th character required [6] 6th character required [7] 7th character required [7] Extension 'X' Alert
EXCLUDES1 Not coded here EXCLUDES2 Not included here [PDx] Primary Diagnosis Only Manifestation Code

Z95.9 Presence of cardiac and vascular implant and graft, unspecified

[4] Z96 Presence of other functional implants

[EXCLUDES2] *complications of internal prosthetic devices, implants and grafts (T82-T85)*
fitting and adjustment of prosthetic and other devices (Z44-Z46)

Z96.0 Presence of urogenital implants

Z96.1 Presence of intraocular lens

Presence of pseudophakia

[5] Z96.2 Presence of otological and audiological implants

Z96.20 Presence of otological and audiological implant, unspecified

Z96.21 Cochlear implant status

Z96.22 Myringotomy tube(s) status

Z96.29 Presence of other otological and audiological implants

Presence of bone-conduction hearing device
Presence of eustachian tube stent
Stapes replacement

Z96.3 Presence of artificial larynx

[5] Z96.4 Presence of endocrine implants

Z96.41 Presence of insulin pump (external) (internal)

Z96.49 Presence of other endocrine implants

Z96.5 Presence of tooth-root and mandibular implants

[5] Z96.6 Presence of orthopedic joint implants

Z96.60 Presence of unspecified orthopedic joint implant

[6] Z96.61 Presence of artificial shoulder joint

Z96.611 Presence of right artificial shoulder joint

Z96.612 Presence of left artificial shoulder joint

Z96.619 Presence of unspecified artificial shoulder joint

[6] Z96.62 Presence of artificial elbow joint

Z96.621 Presence of right artificial elbow joint

Z96.622 Presence of left artificial elbow joint

Z96.629 Presence of unspecified artificial elbow joint

[6] Z96.63 Presence of artificial wrist joint

Z96.631 Presence of right artificial wrist joint

Z96.632 Presence of left artificial wrist joint

Z96.639 Presence of unspecified artificial wrist joint

[6] Z96.64 Presence of artificial hip joint

Hip-joint replacement (partial) (total)

Z96.641 Presence of right artificial hip joint

Z96.642 Presence of left artificial hip joint

Z96.643 Presence of artificial hip joint, bilateral

Z96.649 Presence of unspecified artificial hip joint

[6] Z96.65 Presence of artificial knee joint

Z96.651 Presence of right artificial knee joint

Z96.652 Presence of left artificial knee joint

Z96.653 Presence of artificial knee joint, bilateral

Z96.659 Presence of unspecified artificial knee joint

[6] Z96.66 Presence of artificial ankle joint

Z96.661 Presence of right artificial ankle joint

Z96.662 Presence of left artificial ankle joint

Z96.669 Presence of unspecified artificial ankle joint

[6] Z96.69 Presence of other orthopedic joint implants

Z96.691 Finger-joint replacement of right hand

Z96.692 Finger-joint replacement of left hand

Z96.693 Finger-joint replacement, bilateral

Z96.698 Presence of other orthopedic joint implants

Z96.7 Presence of other bone and tendon implants

Presence of skull plate

[5] Z96.8 Presence of other specified functional implants

Z96.81 Presence of artificial skin

Z96.89 Presence of other specified functional implants

Z96.9 Presence of functional implant, unspecified

[4] Z97 Presence of other devices

[EXCLUDES1] *complications of internal prosthetic devices, implants and grafts (T82-T85)*
fitting and adjustment of prosthetic and other devices (Z44-Z46)

[EXCLUDES2] *presence of cerebrospinal fluid drainage device (Z98.2)*

Z97.0 Presence of artificial eye

[5] Z97.1 Presence of artificial limb (complete) (partial)

Z97.10 Presence of artificial limb (complete) (partial), unspecified

Z97.11 Presence of artificial right arm (complete) (partial)

Z97.12 Presence of artificial left arm (complete) (partial)

Z97.13 Presence of artificial right leg (complete) (partial)

Z97.14 Presence of artificial left leg (complete) (partial)

Z97.15 Presence of artificial arms, bilateral (complete) (partial)

Z97.16 Presence of artificial legs, bilateral (complete) (partial)

Z97.2 Presence of dental prosthetic device (complete) (partial)

Presence of dentures (complete) (partial)

Z97.3 Presence of spectacles and contact lenses

Z97.4 Presence of external hearing-aid

Z97.5 Presence of (intrauterine) contraceptive device

[EXCLUDES1] *checking, reinsertion or removal of contraceptive device (Z30.43)* ♀

Z97.8 Presence of other specified devices

[4] Z98 Other postprocedural states

[EXCLUDES2] *aftercare (Z43-Z49, Z51)*
follow-up medical care (Z08-Z09)
postprocedural complication - see Alphabetical Index

Z98.0 Intestinal bypass and anastomosis status

[EXCLUDES2] *bariatric surgery status (Z98.84)*
gastric bypass status (Z98.84)
obesity surgery status (Z98.84)

Z98.1 Arthrodesis status

Z98.2 Presence of cerebrospinal fluid drainage device

Presence of CSF shunt

Z98.3 Post therapeutic collapse of lung status

Code first underlying disease

[5] Z98.4 Cataract extraction status

Use additional code to identify intraocular lens implant status (Z96.1)

[EXCLUDES1] *aphakia (H27.0)*

Z98.41 Cataract extraction status, right eye

Z98.42 Cataract extraction status, left eye

Z98.49 Cataract extraction status, unspecified eye

[5] Z98.5 Sterilization status

[EXCLUDES1] *female infertility (N97.-)*
male infertility (N46.-)

Z98.51 Tubal ligation status ♀

Z98.52 Vasectomy status [A] ♂

[5] Z98.6 Angioplasty status

Z98.61 Coronary angioplasty status

[EXCLUDES1] *coronary angioplasty status with implant and graft (Z95.5)*

Z98.62 Peripheral vascular angioplasty status

[EXCLUDES1] *peripheral vascular angioplasty status with implant and graft (Z95.820)*

Unspecified Code | Other Specified Code | [N] Newborn Age: 0 | [P] Pediatric Age: 0-17 | [M] Maternity Age: 12-55
[A] Adult Age: 15-124 | ♂ Male | ♀ Female | ● New Code | ▲ Revised Code Title | ►◄ Revised Text

⑤ **Z98.8** Other specified postprocedural states
　　⑥ **Z98.81** Dental procedure status
　　　　Z98.810 Dental sealant status
　　　　Z98.811 Dental restoration status
　　　　　Dental crown status
　　　　　Dental fillings status
　　　　Z98.818 Other dental procedure status
　　Z98.82 Breast implant status
　　　EXCLUDES1 breast implant removal status (Z98.86)
　　Z98.83 Filtering (vitreous) bleb after glaucoma surgery status
　　　EXCLUDES1 Inflammation (infection) of postprocedural bleb (H59.4-)
　　Z98.84 Bariatric surgery status
　　　Gastric banding status
　　　Gastric bypass status for obesity
　　　Obesity surgery status
　　　EXCLUDES1 bariatric surgery status complicating pregnancy, childbirth, or the puerperium (O99.84)
　　　EXCLUDES2 intestinal bypass and anastomosis status (Z98.0)
　　Z98.85 Transplanted organ removal status
　　　Transplanted organ previously removed due to complication, failure, rejection or infection
　　　EXCLUDES1 encounter for removal of transplanted organ -code to complication of transplanted organ (T86.-)
　　Z98.86 Personal history of breast implant removal
　　⑥ **Z98.87** Personal history of in utero procedure
　　　　Z98.870 Personal history of in utero procedure during pregnancy
　　　　EXCLUDES2 complications from in utero procedure for current pregnancy (O35.7)
　　　　　supervision of current pregnancy with history of in utero procedure during previous pregnancy (O09.82-) ♀
　　　　Z98.871 Personal history of in utero procedure while a fetus
　　Z98.89 Other specified postprocedural states
　　　Personal history of surgery, not elsewhere classified

④ **Z99** Dependence on enabling machines and devices, not elsewhere classified
　　　EXCLUDES1 cardiac pacemaker status (Z95.0)
　　Z99.0 Dependence on aspirator
　⑤ **Z99.1** Dependence on respirator
　　　Dependence on ventilator
　　　Z99.11 Dependence on respirator [ventilator] status
　　　Z99.12 Encounter for respirator [ventilator] dependence during power failure
　　　　EXCLUDES1 mechanical complication of respirator [ventilator] (J95.850) 🄿🄳🅇
　　Z99.2 Dependence on renal dialysis
　　　Hemodialysis status
　　　Peritoneal dialysis status
　　　Presence of arteriovenous shunt for dialysis
　　　Renal dialysis status NOS
　　　EXCLUDES1 encounter for fitting and adjustment of dialysis catheter (Z49.0-)
　　　　noncompliance with renal dialysis (Z91.15)

　　Z99.3 Dependence on wheelchair
　　　Wheelchair confinement status
　　　Code first cause of dependence, such as:
　　　muscular dystrophy (G71.0)
　　　obesity (E66.-)

⑤ **Z99.8** Dependence on other enabling machines and devices
　　Z99.81 Dependence on supplemental oxygen
　　　Dependence on long-term oxygen
　　Z99.89 Dependence on other enabling machines and devices
　　　Dependence on machine or device NOS

---

④ 4ᵗʰ character required　　⑤ 5ᵗʰ character required　　⑥ 6ᵗʰ character required　　⑦ 7ᵗʰ character required　　⑦ˣ Extension 'X' Alert

EXCLUDES 1 Not coded here　　*EXCLUDES 2* Not included here　　🄿🄳🅇 Primary Diagnosis Only　　Manifestation Code

ICD-10-CM 2015